1972

AVMA votes to accredit training programs for animal technicians. The AVMA Committee on Accreditation of Training for Animal Technicians (CATAT) is formed.

The first national continuing education meeting for animal technicians and assistants in the United States is held at the Western States Veterinary Conference in Las Vegas, Nevada.

1973

MSU and Nebraska College of Technical Agriculture are the first programs accredited by the AVMA.

The Association of Animal Technician Educators (AATE) is formed at the Third Symposium on Animal Technician Training.

AVMA House of Delegates passes a resolution proposing "registration" but not "licensing" of animal technicians. The Committee on Accreditation for Training of Animal Technicians changes its name to the Committee on Animal Technician Activities and Training.

1975

Washington State Association of Veterinary Technicians (WSAVT) is established. The AATE constitution is adopted and the first officers are elected. The name of the organization is later changed to the Association of Veterinary Technician Educators (AVTE).

1976

CATAT is recognized by the U.S. Office of Education as the accrediting body for animal technician training programs.

The first professional journal for veterinary technicians is published in the US and is titled: *Methods: The Journal for Animal Health Technicians.*

The Veterinary Technicians and Assistants Association of Pennsylvania (VTAAP) is created.

1977

New York offers the first written state examination for animal health technicians.

1978

The Virginia Association of Licensed Veterinary Technicians is established.

AVMA's annual conference includes continuing education classes for animal health technicians for the first time.

The Alberta Association of Animal Health Technologists is formed.

1980

At the AVMA's annual conference in Washington, an ad hoc committee of Canadian and U.S. veterinary technicians and members of the AATE agree to develop an international veterinary technician's association. Plans are made to continue the discussion at the 1981 Western States Veterinary Conference and 1981 AATE Symposium (JAVMA Vol 177 #7 p 596).

The Compendium on Continuing Education for the Animal Health Technician (later called Veterinary Technician) is first published.

Association Technician Sante Animal du Quebec (ATSAQ) begins, with 25 members.

1981

At the AATE Symposium at Michigan State University, groundwork for the establishment of the North American Veterinary Technician Association (NAVTA) occurs. A name for the new organization, a constitution and pro-tem officers are established this year. The Association of Zoo Veterinary Technicians is formed.

1982

NAVTA publishes *The Compendium on Continuing Education for the Animal Health Technician.* The title of this publication is changed in 1984 to include the term "veterinary technician."

NAVTA proposes a professional oath.

1984

NAVTA adopts a national code of ethics for veterinary technicians. First student chapter of NAVTA is formed at Michigan State University.

1985

The AVMA Executive Board establishes the Animal Technician Testing Committee, which generates the Animal Technician National Examination (ATNE) in conjunction with Professional Education Services (PES).

The Association of Animal Technician Educators (AATE) changes its name to the Association of Veterinary Technician Educators (AVTE).

1986

The first ATNE is given in Maine. The NAVTA Newsletter is developed and distributed.

1988

In Canada, the Eastern Veterinary Technician Association (EVTA) is established. The AVMA votes no to a resolution that would change terminology from "animal technician" to "veterinary technician."

WESTERN
WVC

McCURNIN'S

Clinical Textbook for Veterinary Technicians

Eighth Edition

Joanna M. Bassert, VMD

Professor and Director
Program of Veterinary Technology
Manor College
Jenkintown, Pennsylvania

John A. Thomas, DVM

Assistant Professor
Program of Veterinary Technology
Cuyahoga Community College
Cleveland, Ohio

With 1639 illustrations

ELSEVIER

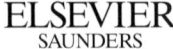

SAUNDERS

3251 Riverport Lane
St. Louis, Missouri 63043

MCCURNIN'S CLINICAL TEXTBOOK FOR VETERINARY TECHNICIANS   ISBN: 978-1-4377-2680-0

Notices

Knowledge and best practice in this field are constantly changing. As new research and experience broaden
our understanding, changes in research methods, professional practices, or medical treatment may become
necessary.

Practitioners and researchers must always rely on their own experience and knowledge in evaluating and
using any information, methods, compounds, or experiments described herein. In using such information
or methods, they should be mindful of their own safety and the safety of others, including parties for
whom they have a professional responsibility.

With respect to any drug or pharmaceutical products identified, readers are advised to check the most
current information provided (i) on procedures featured or (ii) by the manufacturer of each product to be
administered, to verify the recommended dose or formula, the method and duration of administration,
and contraindications. It is the responsibility of practitioners, relying on their own experience and
knowledge of their patients, to make diagnoses, to determine dosages and the best treatment for each
individual patient, and to take all appropriate safety precautions.

To the fullest extent of the law, neither the Publisher nor the authors, contributors, or editors assume any
liability for any injury and/or damage to persons or property as a matter of product liability, negligence, or
otherwise, or from any use or operation of any methods, products, instructions, or ideas contained in the
material herein.

Library of Congress Cataloging-in-Publication Data or Control Number

McCurnin's clinical textbook for veterinary technicians / [edited by] Joanna M. Bassert, John A. Thomas.
—8th ed.
    p. ; cm.
   Clinical textbook for veterinary technicians
   Includes bibliographical references and index.
   ISBN 978-1-4377-2680-0 (hardcover : alk. paper)
   I. Bassert, Joanna M.   II. Thomas, John A. (John Alfred), 1956-   III. McCurnin, Dennis M. McCurnin's
clinical textbook for veterinary technicians.   IV. Title: Clinical textbook for veterinary technicians.
   [DNLM: 1. Veterinary Medicine.   2. Animal Diseases—nursing.   3. Animal Technicians. SF 745]
   636.089—dc23

                2012043121

Vice President and Publisher: Linda Duncan
Content Strategy Director: Penny Rudolph
Content Manager: Shelly Stringer
Publishing Services Manager: Catherine Jackson
Senior Project Manager: Rachel E. McMullen
Design Direction: Amy Buxton

**Working together to grow
libraries in developing countries**

www.elsevier.com | www.bookaid.org | www.sabre.org

ELSEVIER   BOOK AID International   Sabre Foundation

Printed in China

Last digit is the print number: 9   8   7   6   5   4   3   2   1

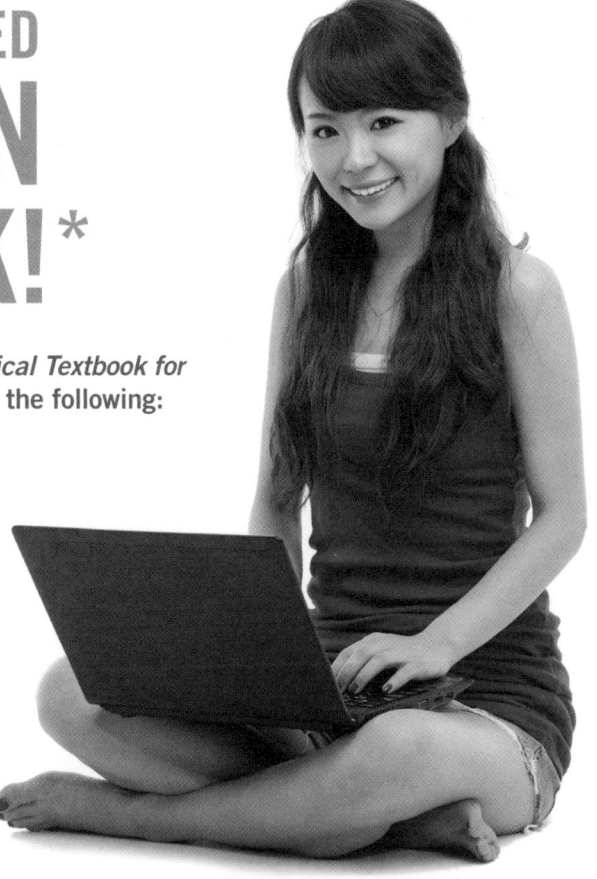
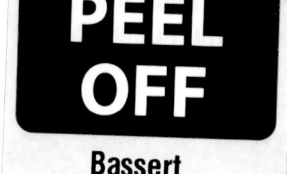

To our students …

who are the fuel that feeds our passion for teaching, and who make every day in the classroom a new and enjoyable adventure.

And

To Teri Merchant …

Rarely does one find packed into a single person the exceptional levels of creativity, intelligence, and wisdom that constitute Teri Merchant, Managing Editor at Elsevier. Certainly, among our greatest professional experiences has been the opportunity to work with her and to learn from her example. Although short in stature, Teri is a force of determination to see a project through … a skilled defender of the deadline, yet, at the same time, an understanding supporter of harried professors who necessarily must take on too much in their professional lives. In the face of this stress, Teri seems to keep the more important truths in view, and this is well exemplified in her delivery of an occasional and brilliantly timed wise-crack. One must fully understand the state of affairs to see the humor in it. In this way, Teri is both clear-sighted in her vision and compassionate in her lightness of heart. She reminds us that we are not writing and editing machines, but human beings … and that there is indeed a life to be lived beyond our laptops.

Teri will be sorely missed by all who had the good fortune to work with her during her remarkable and lengthy tenure at Elsevier.

JMB and JAT

Contributors

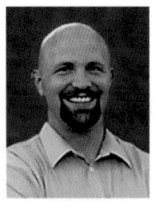

Shawn L. Archibeque, BS, MS, PhD, PAS
Associate Professor
Department of Animal Sciences
Colorado State University
Fort Collins, Colorado

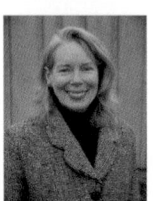

Joanna M. Bassert, VMD
Program Director and Professor
Program of Veterinary Technology
Manor College
Jenkintown, Pennsylvania

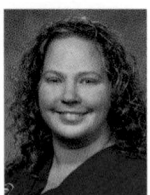

Courtney Beiter, RVT, VTS (Anesthesia)
Service Coordinator SAFR
Small Animal ECC
The Ohio State University Veterinary
    Medical Center
Columbus, Ohio

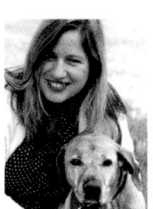

Amy I. Bentz, VMD, Dipl ACVIM
Course Instructor
Program of Veterinary Technology
Manor College
Jenkintown, Pennsylvania
Co-founder
EquineVeterinarian.com
Academic Veterinary Solutions LLC
Chadds Ford, Pennsylvania

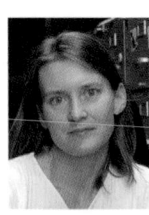

Loretta J. Bubenik-Angapen, DVM, MS, Dipl ACVS
Diplomate American College of
    Veterinary Surgeons
Surgery
Sugar Land Veterinary Specialists
Sugar Land, Texas

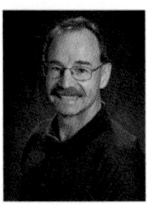

Daniel J. Burba, DVM, Dipl ACVS
Professor, Equine Surgery
Veterinary Clinical Sciences
Louisiana State University
Baton Rouge, Louisiana

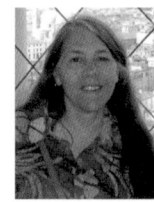

Margret L. Casal, Dr med vet, PhD, Dipl ECAR
Associate Professor of Medical Genetics,
    Pediatrics, and Reproduction
School of Veterinary Medicine
University of Pennsylvania
Philadelphia, Pennsylvania

Richard E. Cober, DV, MS
Clinical Instructor
Cardiology and Interventional Medicine
Veterinary Clinical Sciences
The Ohio State University Veterinary
    Medical Center
Columbus, Ohio

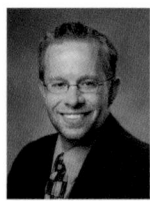

Edward Cooper, VMD, MS, Dipl ACVECC
Assistant Professor
Clinical, Small Animal Emergency and
    Critical Care
Veterinary Clinical Sciences
The Ohio State University
Columbus, Ohio
Head of Service
Small Animal Emergency and Critical Care
Veterinary Medical Center
The Ohio State University
Columbus, Ohio

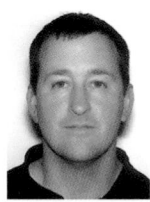

William T.N. Culp, VMD, Dipl ACVS
Assistant Professor
Department of Surgical and Radiological
    Sciences
University of California–Davis
Davis, California

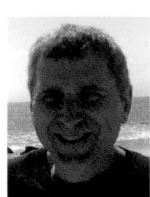

Craig Datz, DVM, MS, Dipl ABVP, Dipl ACVN
Assistant Professor
Veterinary Medicine and Surgery
College of Veterinary Medicine
University of Missouri
Columbia, Missouri

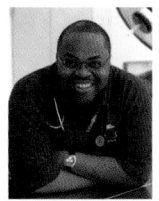

Harold Davis, RVT, VTS (ECC) (Anesth)
Manager
Small Animal Veterinary Emergency and
 Critical Care Service
University of California–Davis
Davis, California

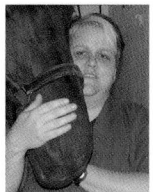

Barbara Dugan, AS Veterinary Technology, CVT
Adjunct Instructor
Program of Veterinary Technology
Manor College
Jenkintown, Pennsylvania
Certified Veterinary Technician
Nursing
University of Pennsylvania
New Bolton Center
Kennett Square, Pennsylvania

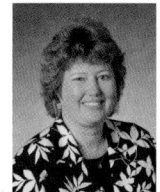

Karen E. Felsted, CPA, MS, DVM, CVPM
President
Felsted Veterinary Consultants, Inc.
Dallas, Texas

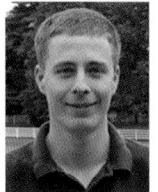

Jonathan R.O. Garber, VMD
Lecturer in Field Service
Clinical Studies
New Bolton Center
University of Pennsylvania
School of Veterinary Medicine
Kennett Square, Pennsylvania

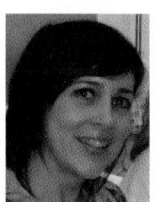

Lorrie Gaschen, PhD, DVM, Dr med vet, Dipl ECVDI
Professor
Veterinary Clinical Sciences
Louisiana State University
Baton Rouge, Louisiana

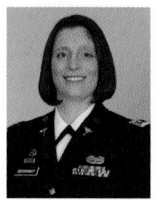

Michelle E. Goodnight, MA, MS, DVM, DACVEEC
Resident
Small Animal Emergency and Critical Care
The Ohio State University
Veterinary Medical Center
Columbus, Ohio
Chief of Clinical Services
Fort Bragg Veterinary Center
Fort Bragg, North Carolina
Major
United Sates Army Veterinary Corps

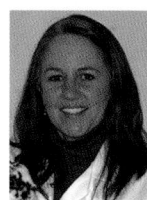

Tamara Grubb, DVM, MS, Dipl ACVA
Assistant Clinical Professor
Anesthesia and Analgesia
Veterinary Clinical Sciences
College of Veterinary Medicine
Washington State University
Pullman, Washington

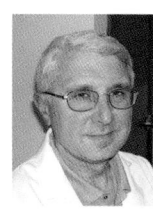

Perry L. Habecker, VMD, Dipl ACVP
Chief
Large Animal Pathology Service
Department of Pathobiology
School of Veterinary Medicine
University of Pennsylvania
Philadelphia, Pennsylvania

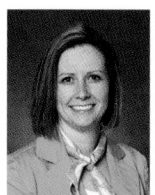

Carolyn J. Hammer, DVM, PhD
Director
Equine Science
Department of Animal Sciences
North Dakota State University
Fargo, North Dakota

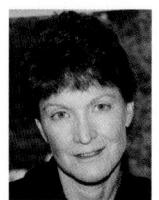

Elizabeth A. Hanie, DVM, MS
Honors College
University of North Carolina at Charlotte
Charlotte, North Carolina

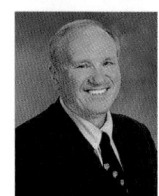

Charles M. Hendrix, DVM, PhD
Professor
Department of Pathobiology
College of Veterinary Medicine
Auburn University
Auburn, Alabama

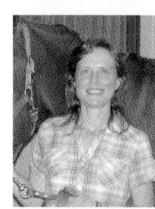

Tanja M. Hess, MV, MSc, PhD
Assistant Professor
Equine Science/Animal Science
Colorado State University
Fort Collins, Colorado

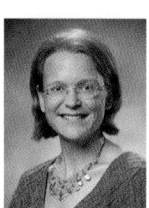

Bianca F. Hettlich, Dr med vet, Dipl ACVS (Small Animal)
Assistant Professor
Small Animal Orthopedics
Department of Veterinary Clinical Sciences
The Ohio State University
Columbus, Ohio

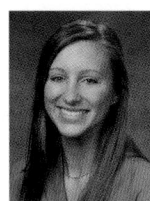

Olivia M. Holt Williams, RVT
Equine ICU
The Ohio State University
Columbus, Ohio

**Laura H. Javsicas, VMD,
    Dipl ACVIM**
Internal Medicine Specialist
Upstate Equine Medical Center
Schuylerville, New York

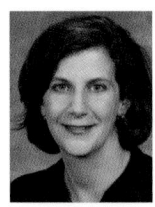

Stephanie W. Johnson, LCSW
Instructor
Veterinary Clinical Science
Louisiana State University
School of Veterinary Medicine
Baton Rouge, Louisiana

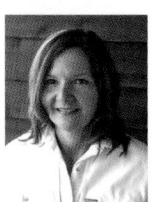

Christine Jurek, DVM
Associate Veterinarian
TOPS Veterinary Rehabilitation
Grayslake, Illinois

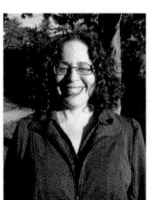

Kathianne Komurek, DVM, MA
Program Coordinator
Veterinary Technology
Manor College
Jenkintown, Pennsylvania

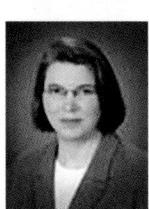

**Sara D. Lawhon, DVM, PhD,
    Dipl ACVM**
Assistant Professor
Veterinary Pathobiology
Texas A&M University
College Station, Texas
Associate Director
Clinical Microbiology
Veterinary Medical Teaching Hospital
College Station, Texas

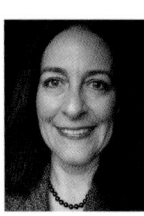

Teresa Lazo, Esquire
Assistant Counsel
Governor's Office of General Counsel
Harrisburg, Pennsylvania;
Adjunct Professor, Animal Law
Penn State University Dickinson
    School of Law
Carlisle, Pennsylvania

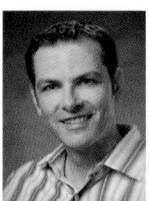

Phillip Lerche, BVSc, PhD, DipACVA
Assistant Professor–Clinical
Veterinary Clinical Sciences
The Ohio State University
Columbus, Ohio

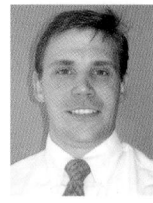

**John R. Lewis, VMD, FAVD,
    Dipl AVDC**
Assistant Professor of Dentistry and Oral
    Surgery
Department of Clinical Studies
School of Veterinary Medicine
University of Pennsylvania
Philadelphia, Pennsylvania

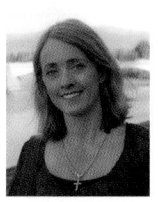

Laurie McCauley, DVM
Medical Director
TOPS Veterinary Rehabilitation
Grayslake, Illinois
Faculty
Canine Rehabilitation Institute
Wellington, Florida

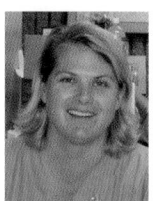

Kristin Miguel, BS, RVT, VTS (LAIM)
Supervisor
Large Animal Critical Care
University of California–Davis
William R. Pritchard Veterinary Medical
    Teaching Hospital
Davis, California

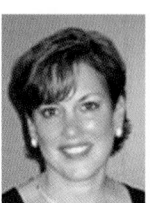

Bonnie R. Miller, RDH, BS
Registered Dental Hygienist
Dentistry and Oral Surgery Service
Matthew J. Ryan Veterinary Hospital
University of Pennsylvania
Philadelphia, Pennsylvania

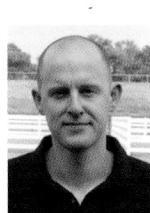

**Colin F. Mitchell, BVM&S, MS,
    Dipl ACVS**
Associate Professor
Equine Surgery
Veterinary Clinical Sciences
Louisiana State University
Baton Rouge, Louisiana

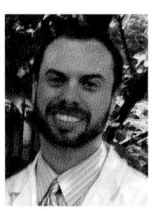

Chris Montgomery, DVM
Relief Veterinarian
Avian, Zoo, and Exotic Animal Medicine
    and Surgery
Lafayette, Louisiana

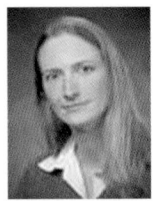

Margaret Mudge, VMD, Dipl ACVS, Dipl ACVECC
The Ohio State University
Veterinary Medical Center
Columbus, Ohio

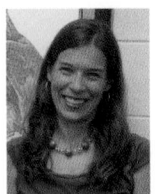

Sara-Louise Roberts Newcomer, DVM
Clinical Instructor
Department of Clinical Sciences
Auburn University
College of Veterinary Medicine
Auburn, Alabama

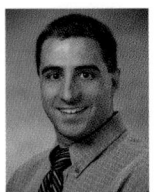

Andrew J. Niehaus, DVM, MS, Dipl ACVS
Assistant Professor
Veterinary Clinical Sciences
The Ohio State University
Columbus, Ohio

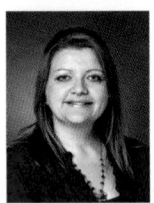

Stacey M. Ostby, BS, LVT
Veterinary Technologist
Animal Science
North Dakota State University
Fargo, North Dakota

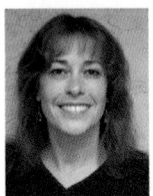

Marika Pappagianis, BS, RVT, VTS (LAIM)
Large Animal Clinic Nursing Manger
Large Animal Clinic
William R. Pritchard Veterinary Medical
    Teaching Hospital
Davis, California

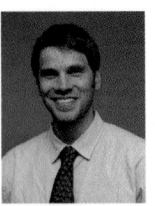

James A. Perry, DVM, PhD, Dipl ACVIM
Oncology and Surgery
Aspen Meadow Veterinary Specialists
Longmont, Colorado

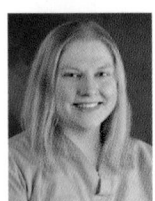

Ann M. Peruski, DVM, MS, Dipl ACVECC
Small Animal Criticalist
Cincinnati Animal Referral and Emergency
    Center
Cincinnati, Ohio

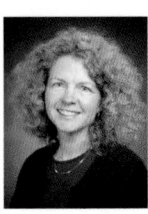

M. Judith Radin, DVM, PhD, Dipl ACVP
Professor
Department of Veterinary Biosciences
The Ohio State University
College of Veterinary Medicine
Columbus, Ohio

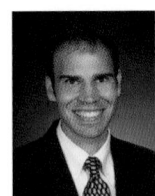

Christopher T. Reetz, DVM
Adjunct Professor
Program of Veterinary Technology
Manor College
Jenkintown, Pennsylvania

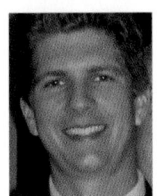

Darren W. Remsburg, DVM
Black Horse Animal Hospital
Kinzers, Pennsylvania

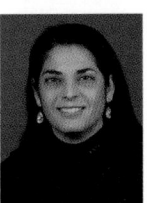

Darlene L. Riel, RVT, VTS (SAIM)
Manager
Gourley Clinical Teaching Center
School of Veterinary Medicine
University of California–Davis
Davis, California

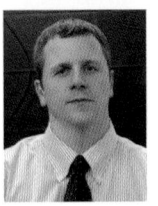

Mark Rondeau, DMV, Dipl ACVIM (SAIM)
Department of Clinical
    Studies–Philadelphia
University of Pennsylvania
School of Veterinary Medicine
Philadelphia, Pennsylvania

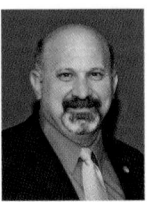

Philip J. Seibert, Jr., CVT
SafetyVet
Calhoun, Tennessee

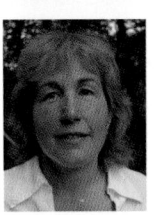

Nancy Shaffran, CVT, VTS (ECC)
Private Lecturer/Consultant
Erwinna, Pennsylvania

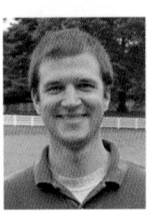

Matthew L. Stock, VMD
Department of Biomedical Sciences
Iowa State University
Ames, Iowa

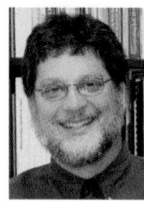

Joseph Taboada, DVM, Dipl ACVIM
Associate Dean
Office of Student and Academic Affairs
School of Veterinary Medicine
Louisiana State University
Baton Rouge, Louisiana
Professor
Small Animal Internal Medicine
Department of Veterinary Clinical Sciences
School of Veterinary Medicine
Louisiana State University
Baton Rouge, Louisiana

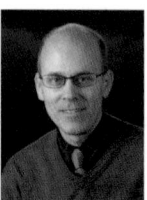

John A. Thomas, DVM
Assistant Professor
Veterinary Technology
Cuyahoga Community College
Cleveland, Ohio

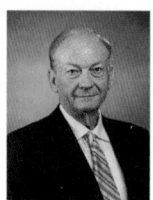

**Walter R. Threlfall, DVM, MS, PhD,
   DACT**
Professor Emeritus
Department of Veterinary Clinical Sciences
College of Veterinary Medicine
The Ohio State University
Columbus, Ohio
Theriogenology Consultant
Powell, Ohio

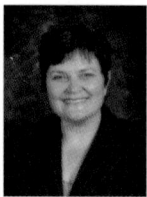

Monica M. Tighe, RVT, BA, MEd
Coordinator
St Clair College
Veterinary Technician Program
Windsor, Ontario
Canada

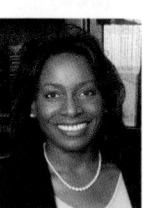

Karen Todd-Jenkins, VMD
Owner
Independent Veterinary Relief Services
Ewing, New Jersey

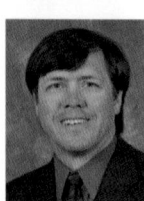

**Thomas N. Tully, Jr., DVM, MS,
   Dipl ABVP (Avian), ECZM (Avian)**
Professor
Zoological Medicine
Veterinary Clinical Sciences
Louisiana State University
School of Veterinary Medicine
Baton Rouge, Louisiana

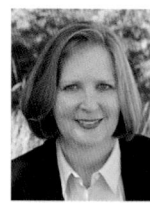

Valarie V. Tynes, DVM, Dipl ACVB
Owner
Premier Veterinary Behavior Consulting
Sweetwater, Texas

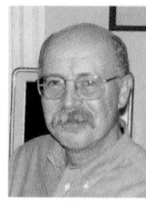

**Thomas J. Van Winkle, VMD,
   Dipl ACVP**
Professor
Department of Pathobiology
School of Veterinary Medicine
University of Pennsylvania
Philadelphia, Pennsylvania

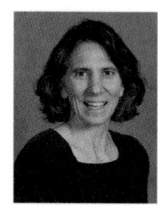

**Katrina R. Viviano, DVM, PhD,
   Dipl ACVIM, Dipl ACVCP**
Clinical Assistant Professor
Department of Medical Sciences
University of Wisconsin
School of Veterinary Medicine
Madison, Wisconsin

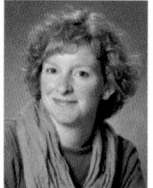

**Sarah A. Wagner, DVM, PhD,
   Dipl ACVCP**
Associate Professor of Veterinary
   Technology
Department of Animal Sciences
North Dakota State University
Fargo, North Dakota

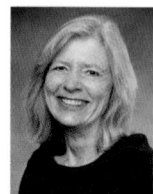

**Maxey L. Wellman, DVM, MS, PhD,
   Dipl ACVP (Clinical Pathology)**
Professor
Department of Veterinary Biosciences
The Ohio State University
Columbus, Ohio

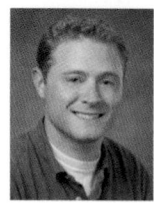

**Jarred Matthew Williams, MS,
   DVM, Dipl ACVS-LA**
Equine Emergency and Critical Care
   Fellow
Ohio State University
Columbus, Ohio

Preface

It gives me great satisfaction to present to you the Eighth Edition of *McCurnin's Clinical Textbook for Veterinary Technicians*. Like previous editions, this text reflects some of the important changes in the profession since the release of the last edition 4 years ago. Among them is the unprecedented rise in the number of accredited programs of veterinary technology in the United States and Canada, including more than 25 accredited distance learning programs. Never before has education in veterinary technology been as accessible as it is today. Employment opportunities, particularly in emergency, critical care, and specialty practices, have also expanded. Once limited to emergency, critical care, and university veterinary teaching hospitals, veterinary specialty practice is now widely available in cities throughout the United States and Canada, giving veterinary technicians greater opportunity to pursue one of the many specialties approved by the National Association of Veterinary Technicians in America (NAVTA). As of this printing, NAVTA has approved 11 specialties in veterinary technology range from emergency and critical care nursing to veterinary clinical pathology. Although many general veterinary practices continue to function with the exclusive aid of veterinary assistants, emergency, critical care, and specialty practices require veterinary technicians and veterinary technician specialists. Therefore, never before have veterinary technicians been in such demand, and never before has the profession asked so much of them.

Among the most important and challenging skills for veterinary technicians to master is the art of independent, critical thinking and decision making. As veterinary technicians are given greater levels of responsibility for patient care, they are expected to accurately assess the patient, collect and evaluate data, and independently develop a list of technician evaluations and interventions. Whereas the veterinarian is charged with diagnosing and curing the patient, the veterinary technician assesses the patient's responses to disease and formulates methods to ameliorate those responses as well as carries out the orders of the veterinarian. The disciplined, cyclic, step-by-step approach of the veterinary technician practice model ensures that excellent nursing care is consistently provided to each and every patient. Because of its importance, the technician practice model is introduced in Chapter 1 and is further developed in subsequent chapters. In addition, clinical applications that exemplify use of the veterinary technician practice model have been placed throughout the Textbook. In this way, it is hoped that the 8th edition of *McCurnin's Clinical Textbook for Veterinary Technicians* will help prepare veterinary technician students to perform the independent critical thinking and decision making required in today's state of the art veterinary practices.

Sensitive to the growing size of the textbook, this edition has been thoughtfully revised to maximize content and value without extending its length. This is a particular challenge for any editing team and could not have been possible without the talent of my new co-editor, Dr. John Thomas, whom I am delighted to welcome to our team.

KEY FEATURES

This edition continues to be heavily illustrated with hundreds of photographs and line drawings in full color, and it includes numerous tables and boxes. Each chapter begins with a list of **key terms** and a series of **learning objectives**. **Technician notes** continue to be a helpful study tool for students. A comprehensive **glossary** that has been assembled from the key terms appears at the end of the text.

NEW FEATURES

A major goal of this edition is to introduce the concept of the Veterinary Technician Practice Model, a list of Technician Evaluations (analogous to the Nursing Diagnosis), and the importance of critical thinking in clinical practice. These themes have been threaded throughout the textbook in the form of expanded numbers of case presentations, but also directly in Chapters 1, 2, and 3 (Introduction, Laws and Ethics, and Medical Record Keeping), and in Chapters 19 and 20 (Small and Large Animal Medicine). Chapter 24, "Fluid Therapy and Transfusion Medicine," is a brand new chapter. As in former editions, one-third of the textbook has been completely rewritten, with new authors, ideas, and approaches. We have taken on the challenge of generating a fresh, new textbook without expanding its length and weight. Therefore, we have selected its content carefully. In addition, chapter outlines have been expanded to facilitate navigation through each chapter. Finally, each of the 29 new contributors to this edition is an expert in his or her respective field.

ORGANIZATION

The book is divided into eight sections that are delineated by different colored pages:
- Part One is an introduction to the profession; it focuses on practice management, computer applications, medical records, and health and safety.
- Part Two transitions into basic nursing topics such as restraint, handling, physical examination, and preventive health medicine.

- Part Three covers clinical sciences, including diagnostic imaging.
- Part Four, Medical Nursing, includes diagnostic sampling and therapeutic techniques as well as a chapter that presents large animal procedures and sequential illustrations of techniques, which emphasize the role of the vet tech in collecting specimens. This part also provides information on small animal medical nursing and alternative medicine. The "Large Animal Medical Nursing" and "Physical Therapy, Rehabilitation, and Alternative Medical Nursing" chapters enable students to integrate the basics of physical rehabilitation into patient care.

THE LEARNING PACKAGE

The Eighth Edition of *McCurnin's Clinical Textbook for Veterinary Technicians* is designed as a comprehensive learning package.

The student package includes:
- The textbook
- Student Workbook
- Evolve website

The faculty package includes:
- The textbook
- TEACH Instructor Resources
- Student Workbook
- Evolve website

The entire package has been designed with the student and the educator in mind. The ease of reading each comprehensive chapter along with the additional materials provides students with the maximum opportunity to learn. The driving force in the development of this package was the creation of a proficient veterinary technician.

STUDENT WORKBOOK

The Student Workbook is designed to be a supplement to the learning process. The content of the Workbook matches the book chapter by chapter to help students master and apply key concepts and procedures in a clinical situation. Included are multiple choice questions, matching exercises, photo quizzes, labeling exercises, crossword puzzles, and other activities to guide the studying process.

TEACH INSTRUCTOR RESOURCES

Available on Evolve, TEACH Instructor Resources are designed to save the instructor time and to take the guesswork out of classroom planning and preparation. They include Chapter Focus, Teaching Tips, completely updated Lesson Plans, an updated Test Bank, and answers to the Workbook Exercises.

EVOLVE WEBSITE

Elsevier has created a website that is dedicated solely to support this learning package: http://evolve.elsevier.com/Bassert/McCurnin/. The website includes both a Student site and an Instructor site.

Student site resources include:
- Medical Record Forms: 25 medical records that correlate directly with the medical records chapter in the book. These full-size forms can be printed and used. They are listed alphabetically.
- Student Activities:
  - Crossword Puzzles: created for each chapter using the key words from the text
  - Picture-It Exercises: drag-and-drop activities that help to identify labels on critical illustrations
  - Hangman: word-building activity
  - Quiz Shows: may be played as a group activity or individually

Faculty site resources include:
- TEACH Instructor Resources
  - Lesson Plans
  - PowerPoint Lecture Presentations
  - Test Bank in Examview consisting of 2000 questions
  - Answer Key: contains answers to the questions included in the Workbook
- Image collection: contains all of the images from within the book, plus some additional images
- Access to all student resources

SUPPORT

If you have questions or need assistance with ordering or adopting the learning package for *McCurnin's Textbook for Veterinary Technicians,* contact Faculty Support at 1-800-222-9570, or via e-mail at sales.inquiry@elsevier.com.

Joanna M. Bassert
John A. Thomas

Acknowledgments

This textbook would not be possible without the help of many energetic souls. The development and production teams at Elsevier, including Teri Merchant, Jaime Pendill, Shelly Stringer, Rachel E. McMullen, and Kristen Mandava, were especially instrumental in transforming 36 chapters of manuscript into a cohesive and graphically beautiful textbook. We are grateful to Dr. Rustin Moore for his invaluable assistance in recruiting authors for several chapters, and to the many veterinary practices in the Greater Philadelphia area that opened their doors to Dr. Bassert, so she could take photos of technicians in action. These include Eva Rager and Vickie Byard at Rau Animal Hospital; Dr. Robert Orsher, Deb Blades, and Rebecca Orsher at the Veterinary Specialty and Emergency Center (VSEC); Ania Wozniak at the Center for Animal Referral and Emergency Services (CARES); and Daryl Wampler and Mandy Fellouzis Hilbert at Fox Chase Farm. Photographs for the historical time line were provided by Patrick Navarre and the National Association of Veterinary Technicians in America (NAVTA). The introduction of the veterinary technician practice model in this edition was the result of many animated discussions with Drs. Jody Rockett and Kathianne Komurek based on the book *Patient Assessment, Intervention, and Documentation for the Veterinary Technician*, by Jody Rockett, Cynthia Lattanzio, and Katie Anderson. Finally, we are grateful to Sandy Sponaugle, Dan Walsh, Amanda Hadley, and Rachel Bedard for their support.

Joanna M. Bassert
John A. Thomas

Contents

Part One: Veterinary Technology: An Overview

1. **Introduction to Veterinary Technology: Its Laws and Ethics,** *1*
   Joanna M. Bassert, Teresa Lazo, and Monica M. Tighe

2. **Veterinary Practice Management,** *37*
   Karen E. Felsted

3. **Veterinary Medical Records,** *80*
   Joanna M. Bassert

4. **Occupational Health and Safety in Veterinary Hospitals,** *114*
   Philip J. Seibert, Jr.

Part Two: Patient Management and Nutrition

5. **Animal Behavior,** *133*
   Valarie V. Tynes

6. **Restraint and Handling of Animals,** *176*
   Karen Todd-Jenkins, Barbara Dugan, Darren W. Remsburg, and Chris Montgomery

7. **History and Physical Examination,** *221*
   Mark Rondeau and Elizabeth A. Hanie

8. **Preventive Health Programs,** *258*
   Carolyn J. Hammer, Stacey M. Ostby, Christopher T. Reetz, and Sarah A. Wagner

9. **Small Animal Nutrition,** *291*
   Craig Datz

10. **Large Animal Nutrition,** *337*
    Tanja M. Hess and Shawn L. Archibeque

11. **Animal Reproduction (Theriogenology),** *366*
    Walter R. Threlfall

Part Three: Clinical Sciences

12. **Hematology and Cytology,** *397*
    Maxey L. Wellman and M. Judith Radin

13. **Clinical Chemistry, Serology, and Urinalysis,** *423*
    M. Judith Radin and Maxey L. Wellman

14. **Parasitology,** *438*
    Sara-Louise Roberts Newcomer and Charles M. Hendrix

15. **Clinical Microbiology,** *482*
    Sara D. Lawhon

16. **Diagnostic Imaging,** *516*
    Lorrie Gaschen

17. **Basic Necropsy Procedures,** *561*
    Thomas J. Van Winkle and Perry L. Habecker

Part Four: Medical Nursing

18. **Diagnostic Sampling and Therapeutic Techniques,** *583*
    Harold Davis, Darlene L. Riel, Marika Pappagianis, and Kristin Miguel

19. **Small Animal Medical Nursing,** *672*
    Kathianne Komurek

20. **Large Animal Medical Nursing,** *720*
    Amy I. Bentz, Laura H. Javsicas, Jonathan R.O. Garber, and Matthew L. Stock

21. **Neonatal Care of the Puppy, Kitten, and Foal,** *787*
    Margret L. Casal and Amy I. Bentz

22. **Care of Birds, Reptiles, and Small Mammals,** *810*
    Thomas N. Tully, Jr.

23. **Physical Therapy, Rehabilitation, and Alternative Medical Nursing,** *845*
    Laurie McCauley and Christine Jurek

Part Five: Emergency and Critical Care

24. Fluid Therapy and Transfusion Medicine, *881*

Courtney Beiter, Edward Cooper, Olivia M. Holt Williams, and Margaret Mudge

25. Emergency and Critical Care Nursing, *905*

Ann M. Peruski, Michelle E. Goodnight, Richard E. Cober, Jarred Matthew Williams, and Andrew J. Niehaus

26. Wound Management and Bandaging, *971*

Bianca F. Hettlich and Daniel J. Burba

Part Six: Pharmacology, Analgesia, and Anesthesia

27. Pharmacology and Pharmacy, *1009*

Katrina R. Viviano

28. Pain Management, *1045*

Nancy Shaffran and Tamara Grubb

29. Veterinary Anesthesia, *1075*

John A. Thomas and Phillip Lerche

Part Seven: Surgical Nursing

30. Surgical Instruments and Aseptic Technique, *1129*

James A. Perry, William T.N. Culp, and Daniel J. Burba

31. Surgical Assistance and Suture Material, *1186*

William T.N. Culp and Daniel J. Burba

32. Small Animal Surgical Nursing, *1212*

Loretta J. Bubenik-Angapen

33. Large Animal Surgical Nursing, *1259*

Colin F. Mitchell

34. Veterinary Dentistry, *1297*

John R. Lewis and Bonnie R. Miller

Part Eight: End of Life

35. Geriatric and Hospice Care: Supporting the Aged and Dying Patient, *1355*

Karen Todd-Jenkins and Amy I. Bentz

36. The Human-Animal Bond, Bereavement, and Euthanasia, *1377*

Joseph Taboada and Stephanie W. Johnson

Glossary, *1399*

How to Use This Learning Package

McCurnin's Clinical Textbook for Veterinary Technicians is the ultimate learning package for preparing students to become veterinary technicians. It provides a solid foundation for the basic and advanced clinical skills that students must master to achieve competence, and its student-friendly style clarifies even the most complex concepts and procedures to help prepare for the VTNE and certification.

TEXTBOOK FEATURES

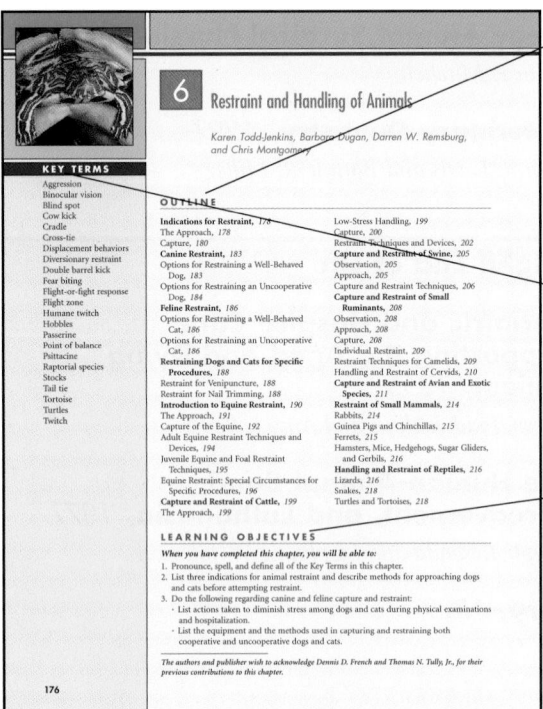

A simple Chapter Outline introduces you to the chapter material as a whole, allowing you to see at a glance how the subject material is organized. It also helps you focus on one topic at a time by showing you relationships to other topics in the chapter.

Key Terms listed on the chapter opening page reinforce new terminology.

Learning Objectives help you focus on key concepts and procedures for mastery on completion of the chapter.

Introduction gives an overview of the chapter that distills the key points and focuses your study.

- List the advantages and disadvantages of chemical restraint in dogs and cats.
- Describe various positions for restraining cats and dogs specifically for nail trimming and venipuncture of the cephalic vein.
4. Do the following regarding equine capture and restraint:
  - Explain the principles that affect equine perception and behavior.
  - Describe the physical abilities of horses and how these affect the ways in which horses are handled.
  - Describe methods for approaching and capturing adult and juvenile equine patients, including using restraint equipment, diversions, and pharmaceutical products, and identify special restraint techniques for horses and the circumstances in which they are used.
5. Do the following regarding capture and restraint of cattle:
  - Describe the principles that affect cattle behavior and list principles used to move cattle and individuals in an effective and low-stress manner.
  - Explain the differences in housing between dairy and beef cattle and describe how these differences affect methods to handle and restrain them.
  - List the type of bulls known to be particularly dangerous to handle.
  - List the equipment used to restrain cattle in general and specific parts of their bodies. Also, describe the circumstances of their use.
6. Describe methods for observing and approaching swine of each gender and age group, and discuss methods used to capture and restrain adult and young pigs.
7. Do the following regarding small ruminant capture and restraint:
  - Describe the behavioral tendencies of small ruminants and explain how these influence the approach and capture of herds.
  - List factors that affect levels of aggression in camelids and describe how aggression presents in these species.
  - Describe the approach, capture, and restraint of individual sheep, goats, and camelids.
  - List additional restraint techniques used in camelids, but not in sheep or goats.
  - Define cervids and explain methods for their restraint and handling.
8. Describe restraint and handling techniques used with birds, small mammals, and reptiles.

INTRODUCTION

Most people entering the field of veterinary technology have had experience with animals, but few have had the experience necessary to deal with all the species that might be encountered. To assume that all animals respond to a particular situation in the same manner is incorrect and can be a dangerous assumption to make. Restraint techniques differ markedly among species, and even among conspecies, the responses of individuals can be highly variable. People can protect themselves by understanding the body language of animals and by anticipating a particular array of responses. In this way, appropriate actions can be taken in advance to manage the animal.

This chapter is intended to be a guide to the handling and restraint of animals commonly encountered in veterinary practice. It is intended not to be an exhaustive text, but rather to provide a range of techniques to build confidence and competence in the veterinary technician.

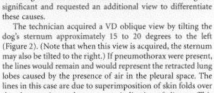

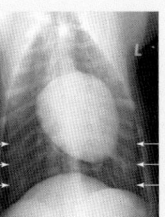

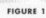

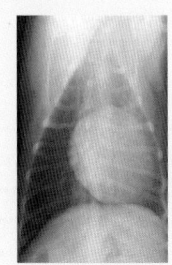

Case Presentations challenge you to apply your knowledge of chapter content to realistic clinical scenarios to solve problems and make appropriate decisions.

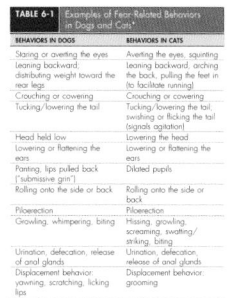

Technician Notes are interspersed throughout each chapter to help you retain key information related to the technician's role.

Procedure boxes present clear, step-by-step guidelines for performing important tasks.

Glossary with definitions of Key Terms from each chapter reinforces new terminology and helps you comprehend the reading material.

STUDENT WORKBOOK

The Workbook, sold separately, includes review exercises for all chapters, including definitions of Key Terms; matching, fill-in-the-blank, short answer, true-false, and review questions; and Photo Quizzes, Word Searches, and Crossword Puzzles.

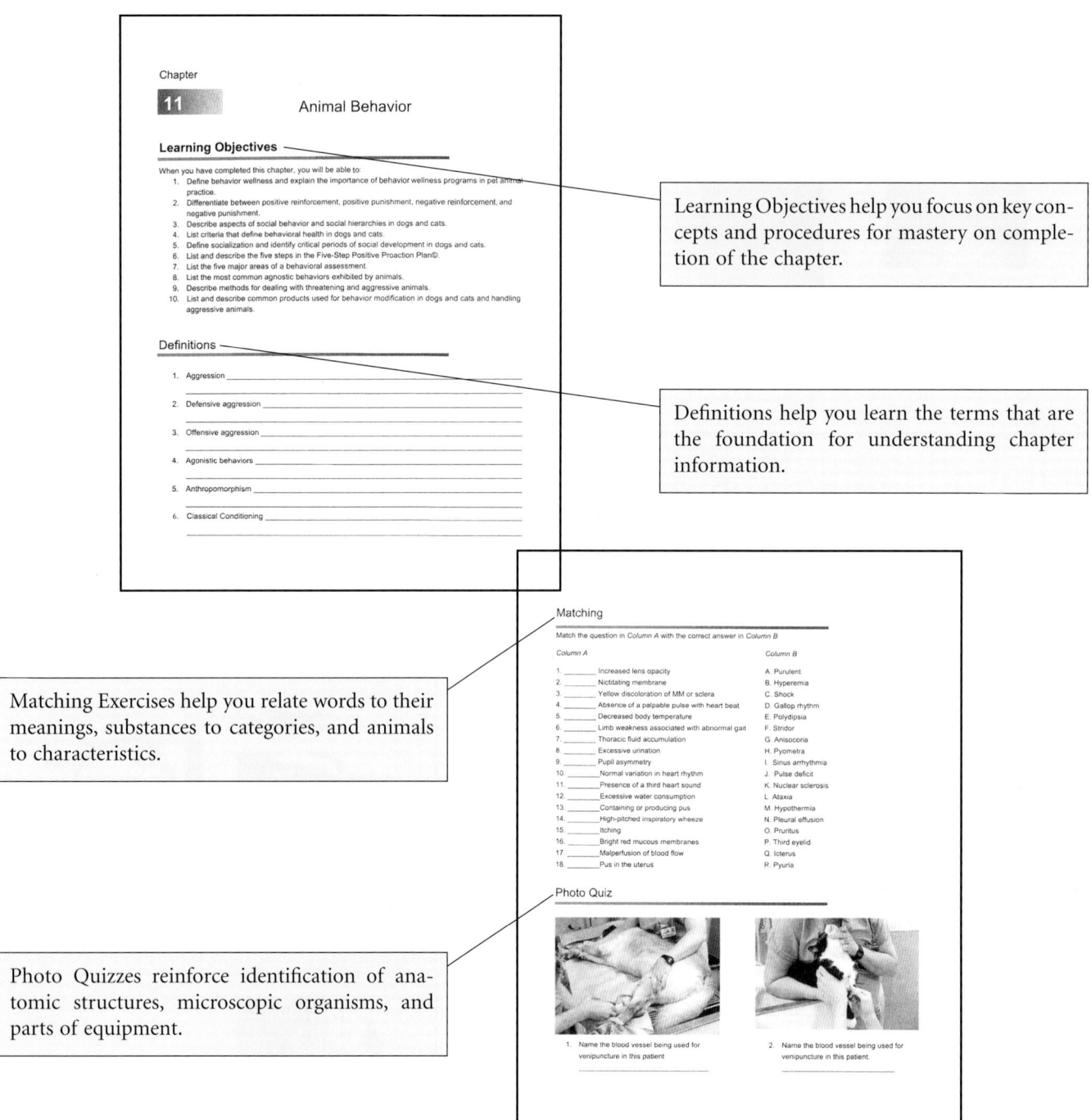

Learning Objectives help you focus on key concepts and procedures for mastery on completion of the chapter.

Definitions help you learn the terms that are the foundation for understanding chapter information.

Matching Exercises help you relate words to their meanings, substances to categories, and animals to characteristics.

Photo Quizzes reinforce identification of anatomic structures, microscopic organisms, and parts of equipment.

EVOLVE WEBSITE

The Evolve website includes learning resources available to instructors and students using *McCurnin's Clinical Textbook for Veterinary Technicians*. At the front of this textbook is a page introducing the Evolve site. All you need to get started is a computer with an Internet connection. To register as a Student or Instructor, enter the following URL: http://evolve.elsevier.com/Bassert/McCurnin/. Follow the directions for "Instructors" or "Students" to create an Evolve account. You will have to do this only one time.

Student resources include the following:

- Medical Record Forms: 25 medical records that correlate directly with the medical records chapter in the book. These are full-size forms that can be printed and used. They are listed alphabetically.
- Student Activities:
  - Crossword Puzzles: created for each chapter using Key Words from the text
  - Picture-It Exercises: drag-and-drop activities that help identify labels on critical illustrations
  - Hangman: word-building activity
  - Quiz Shows: may be played as a group activity or individually

Faculty resources include the following:

- TEACH Instructor Resources
  - Lesson Plans
  - PowerPoint Lecture Presentations
  - Test Bank in Examview, including 1120 questions
  - Answer Key: contains answers to the questions provided in the Workbook
- Image Collection: contains all of the images from within the book, plus some additional images
- Access to all student resources

ADDITIONAL RESOURCES

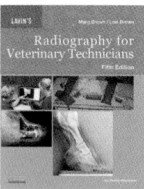

Brown & Brown
Lavin's Radiography for Veterinary Technicians, 5e
This concise, step-by-step text gives students the knowledge and skills they need to produce excellent radiographic images. It covers the physics of radiography, the origin of film artifacts, and positioning and restraint of small, large, avian, and exotic animals.

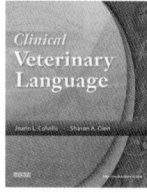

Colville & Oien
Clinical Veterinary Language
Clinically-focused, this all new terminology book is filled with innovative activities that teach students how to build and deconstruct medical terms and to use their new vocabulary by interpreting case studies and medical reports.

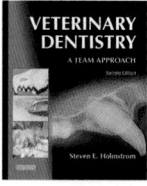

Holmstrom
Veterinary Dentistry: A Team Approach, 2e
From radiology to anesthesia to patient needs and client education, this handy full-color guide covers everything students need to know about veterinary dentistry!

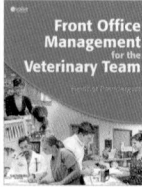

Prendergast
Front Office Management for the Veterinary Team
Focusing on the day-to-day duties of the veterinary team, this book offers a complete guide to scheduling appointments, billing and accounting, communicating effectively and compassionately with clients, managing medical records, budgeting, marketing your practice, managing inventory, and using outside diagnostic laboratory services.

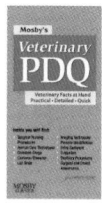

Sirois
Mosby's Veterinary PDQ
This full-color, pocket-sized reference offers instant access to hundreds of veterinary medicine facts, formulas, drug calculations, lab values, procedures, and photographs of parasites, laboratory diagnostic samples, and instruments for easy identification.

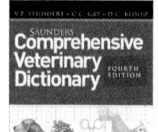

Studdert, Gay, & Blood
Saunders Comprehensive Veterinary Dictionary, 4e
This is the most comprehensive dictionary in the field, offering a wide range of full-color illustrations and over 60,000 main entries and subentries including large animals, small animals and exotics, in an all new user-friendly format.

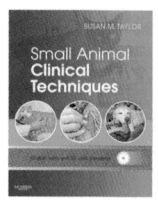

Taylor
Small Animal Clinical Techniques
With step-by-step instructions for 53 procedures, this must-have text includes everything you need to learn the techniques you need for everyday practice.

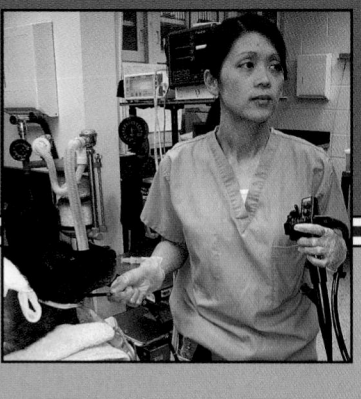

1 Introduction to Veterinary Technology: Its Laws and Ethics

Joanna M. Bassert, Teresa Lazo, and Monica M. Tighe

OUTLINE

History of Veterinary Technology, *3*
The Veterinary Technician Today, *3*
Employment Prospects, Salaries, and
   Attrition, *5*
Education, *6*
Programs of Veterinary Technology, *6*
Continuing Education, *7*
**The Veterinary Technician National
   Examination (VTNE),** *7*
**The Profession of Veterinary
   Technology,** *8*
The Veterinary Technician Practice
   Model, *8*
Scope of Practice, *9*
Responsibilities of the Veterinary
   Technician in Practice, *9*
**Terminology and the Veterinary Health
   Care Team,** *14*
Veterinarian, *14*
Veterinary Technician Specialist, *15*
Veterinary Technologist, *15*
Veterinary Technician, *15*
Veterinary Assistant, *16*
Laboratory Animal Technicians and
   Technologists, *17*
Professionalism, *17*
Professional Appearance, *18*

Professional Conduct, *20*
Professional Communication, *20*
**Professional Organizations and
   Acronyms,** *21*
National Association of Veterinary
   Technicians in America (NAVTA), *21*
Canadian Association of Animal Health
   Technologists and Technicians/
   l'Association Canadienne des Techniciens
   et Technologistes en Santé Animale
   (CAAHTT), *23*
Professional Ethics, *23*
**Profession-Related Laws and
   Regulations,** *24*
Laws (Statutes), *24*
Rules and Regulations, *25*
Entry Into Practice, *26*
Grounds for Disciplinary Action, *29*
Process of Disciplinary Action, *32*
**Additional Laws Governing Veterinary
   Practice,** *34*
Labor Laws, *34*
Medical Waste Management Laws, *34*
Controlled Substances, *34*
Animal-Related Laws, *35*
Laws Specific to Canada, *36*

KEY TERMS

CAAHTT
NAVTA
Practice acts
Rules and regulations
Technician evaluation
Technician intervention
Veterinary technician
Veterinary technician
   practice model
Veterinarian
Veterinary assistant
Veterinary technician
   specialist
Veterinary technologist
Veterinary technology
VTNE
Walter E. Collins, DVM

LEARNING OBJECTIVES

When you have completed this chapter, you will be able to:

1. Pronounce, define, and spell all of the Key Terms in this chapter.
2. Describe the events from 1963 to 1990 that led to the development of modern
   veterinary technology in the United States and Canada.
3. Describe the educational and credentialing requirements established in most states for
   entry into the profession of veterinary technology.
4. Explain the structure, format, and scheduling of the VTNE.
5. List the six features that characterize a profession.
6. Describe the five steps of the veterinary technician practice model.

7. Describe the scope of practice for veterinary technicians and list five duties performed only by veterinarians.
8. Describe areas of responsibility for veterinary technicians in clinical practice.
9. List the members of the veterinary health care team and describe their respective roles. In your description of veterinary technician specialists include a list of the veterinary technician academies recognized by NAVTA.
10. Describe professional appearance, conduct, and communication.
11. Name the organizations represented by the acronyms AVMA, CVMA, CVTEA, NAVTA, and AAVSB, and describe their roles in the education and credentialing of veterinary technicians.
12. Describe professional ethics.
13. Differentiate between statutes (laws) and regulations.
14. Describe the role of state boards in the credentialing of veterinary professionals.
15. List possible grounds for disciplinary action by state or provincial boards, list three levels of supervision defined in the NAVTA Model Rules and Regulations, and describe how these levels affect the veterinary technician's scope of practice.
16. Describe steps and possible sanctions carried out during disciplinary action against a licensee.
17. Describe how laws related to labor, medical waste, controlled substances, and animals relate to the profession of veterinary technology.
18. Name and describe laws that are specific to Canada regarding animals.

INTRODUCTION

The veterinary technician has emerged as a critical component of the veterinary health care team. Like the registered nurse in the human health care field, the veterinary technician gathers clinical information about each patient, analyzes the data, and generates a plan for nursing care. As part of the veterinary health care team, the veterinary technician carries out the orders of the **veterinarian** and is aided by veterinary assistants. However, unlike registered nurses, veterinary technicians are expected to perform the duties of radiology and laboratory technicians and those of medical, surgical, and anesthesia nurses (Figure 1-1). In addition, veterinary technicians must be prepared to work with multiple species rather than just one. For these reasons, the veterinary technician has a surprisingly broad range of clinical responsibilities. Over the past 50 years, veterinary medicine has become highly sophisticated. Many veterinarians find that they can no longer meet their practice goals in terms of both providing a high level of medical care and attaining acceptable profit margins, without the assistance of veterinary technicians. The veterinary technician has become a skilled practitioner of patient assessment and critical thinking, independently generating and enacting plans for patient care.

In addition, the development of veterinary-centered television programs has heightened awareness of **veterinary technology** and has led to an increased expectation, for both the practitioner and the pet owner, that animal patients will receive excellent veterinary nursing care.

This chapter presents an overview of the profession of veterinary technology along with the profession's history, educational requirements, range of duties, salaries, specialties, professional organizations, and expectations for professional conduct. It provides an introduction to the **veterinary technician practice model** and the steps that define the nursing process. In addition, the laws and ethics that define the profession of veterinary technology and that govern the credentialing process and those that support animal welfare are discussed.

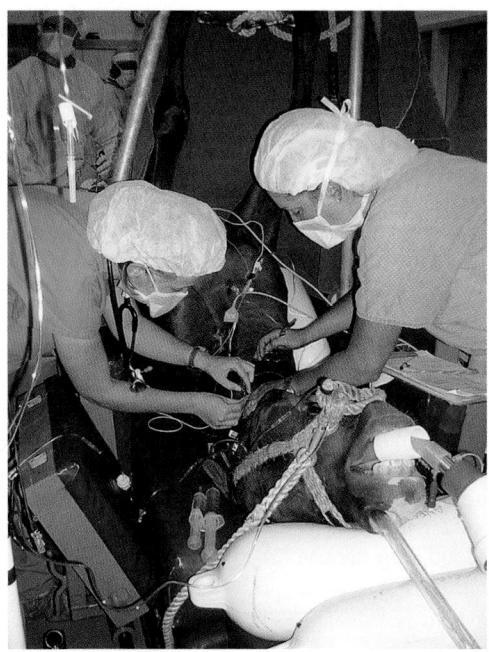

FIGURE 1-1 The veterinary technician has emerged as a critical component of the veterinary health care team. These veterinary technicians work at the New Bolton Center, University of Pennsylvania School of Veterinary Medicine. (Courtesy Dr. Joanna Bassert.)

I solemnly dedicate myself to aiding animals and society by providing excellent care and services for animals, by alleviating animal suffering, and by promoting public health.

I accept my obligations to practice my profession conscientiously and with sensitivity, adhering to the profession's Code of Ethics and furthering my knowledge and competence through a commitment to lifelong learning.
Veterinary Technician Oath

HISTORY OF VETERINARY TECHNOLOGY

Historically, many veterinarians practiced independently and performed many of the laboratory and nursing duties themselves. Often spouses and other laypersons served as veterinary assistants, receptionists, and office managers. Today, many practices employ multiple veterinarians and require a staff of veterinary technicians, assistants, receptionists, and kennel workers to carry out the many duties required in running a successful practice. This team approach is a fundamental part of veterinary practice management today, and the veterinary technician often serves as an important link between the veterinarian and support personnel.

The profession of veterinary technology began to take form in the early 1960s with establishment of the first formal university level program for the education of animal health technicians. The period following 1960 is rich with the accomplishments of dedicated veterinarians and veterinary technicians (see the Timeline in the front of this textbook).

Of particular importance are the accomplishments of **Walter E. Collins, DVM** (Box 1-1), who is considered the

father of veterinary technology in North America. Veterinary technicians were first called *animal health technicians*. The adjective "veterinary" referred exclusively to veterinarians until 1989, when the term *veterinary technician* was approved for use by the House of Delegates of the American Veterinary Medical Association (AVMA). Now, hundreds of accredited programs of veterinary technology are available in Canada and in the United States, and this number is steadily increasing. Current listings of these programs can be found at www.avma.org for programs accredited by the AVMA, and at www.caahtt-acttsa.ca for programs accredited by the Canadian Veterinary Medical Association (CVMA). Thousands of individuals have graduated from these programs, and the number of veterinary technology programs continues to grow as the demand for educated, skilled personnel increases.

THE VETERINARY TECHNICIAN TODAY

Veterinary technicians work in a wide range of facilities, perform many different kinds of tasks, and may encounter all types of animal species. Veterinary technicians may work in private veterinary practices, such as companion animal, large animal, or mixed practices. (A mixed practice is one that treats both farm and companion animals.) Veterinary technicians also may work in zoos, aquariums, wildlife rehabilitation centers, and research facilities, and in industry as sales representatives of veterinary products. They may become entrepreneurs by establishing their own kennel facility or pet-sitting business. Qualified veterinary technicians may also become instructors in veterinary technology programs or other academic programs. The range of job opportunities for the veterinary technician today is broader than ever before.

Within this diverse array of opportunities, veterinary technicians may narrow their field of work and concentrate on specific areas. For example, a technician working in a practice that treats exotic species, such as birds and reptiles, will develop skills and knowledge particular to that aspect of veterinary medicine. In addition, some veterinary practices are called *specialty* or *referral* practices because they employ veterinarians who have completed special training in a particular aspect of veterinary medicine, such as dermatology, surgery, internal medicine, radiology, or ophthalmology.

Veterinarians who are general practitioners may refer particularly challenging or difficult cases to specialty practices. Specialized veterinary technicians who work in specialty practices see unusual cases and become skilled in addressing the particular needs of these critically ill patients. It is not uncommon for specialty practices to share their facility with an emergency and trauma practice. Some veterinary technicians prefer the challenge and excitement of emergency practice and have dedicated their careers to this aspect of veterinary technology.

After a growing number of veterinary technicians expressed an interest in furthering their education

BOX 1-1   Walter Emmett Collins, DVM, Father of Veterinary Technology

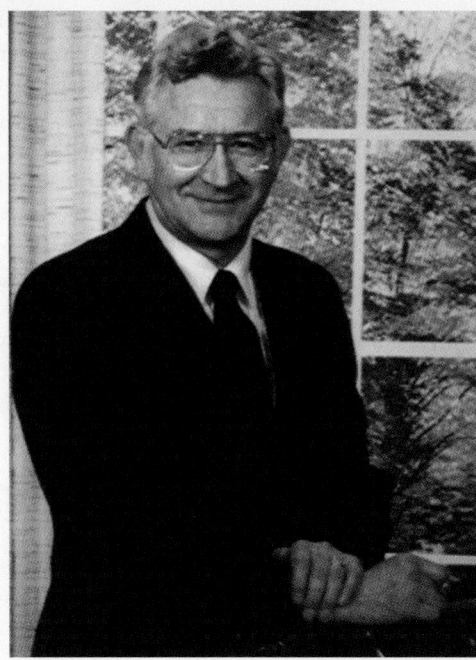

On November 19, 1930, Dr. Walter Collins was born on a small farm in Milford, New York. Like many children reared in a bucolic setting, Dr. Collins grew to love the expansive fields of crops and the many farm animals that were part of his young life. In 1948, after graduation from high school, his interest in agriculture led him to the State University of New York (SUNY) at Delhi, where he studied general agriculture for 2 years. Afterward, he served as a dairy herd improvement supervisor for 2 years before entering the U.S. Air Force. Dr. Collins believed that he was fortunate to be assigned to the Veterinary Department at Webb Air Force Base in Big Spring, Texas, where he worked under the direction of three "understanding and stimulating" veterinarian commanding officers, who encouraged him to pursue a career in veterinary medicine. When his tour ended in the spring of 1956, Dr. Collins moved to Ithaca, New York, where he studied pre-veterinary science and subsequently attended New York State College of Veterinary Medicine at Cornell University. He graduated and received a doctor of veterinary medicine (DVM) degree in June 1961 and later returned to Delhi, where he joined a large animal practice. After 1 year, he opted to establish his own private veterinary practice in Delhi.

In the fall of 1964, while still practicing part time in Delhi, Dr. Collins became a teacher for the first time by joining the faculty of the Animal Science Technology Program. He was hired by Dr. Winfield Stone, the director of the program, who

soon became an important mentor and friend. Several years later, in 1967, after Dr. Stone accepted another position on campus, Dr. Collins became the new program director at Delhi. During his tenure as director, Dr. Collins, as administrator, was awarded a grant from the U.S. Department of Health, Education, and Welfare to develop a model curriculum guide for training animal health technicians. From 1969 to 1975, Dr. Collins authored or coauthored several significant publications and the model curriculum.

In the early 1970s, Delhi's faculty was anxious to prove that the program was meeting real needs of New York practitioners. Dr. Collins decided to survey veterinarians and presented his findings at the 62nd New York State Conference for Veterinarians. Dr. Collins wrote, "For myself, I had felt the veterinary practitioner employer could use his/her new technician employee to relieve them of many non-professional duties, as was already being accomplished similarly in human medicine. Both my staff and I were gratified at the time by this small sampling survey, which certainly hinted that we were on the right track!"

After leaving Delhi, Dr. Collins served as program director for 1 year at Mountain View College in Dallas. He subsequently became an associate professor and coordinator of the Veterinary Technology Program at Michigan State University, where he stayed from 1977 until his retirement in 1990. In Michigan, he served on the Michigan Veterinary Medical Association (MVMA) Veterinary Technician Committee, which assisted in the development of legislation that defined veterinary technology for Michigan.

When asked about important events occurring in his professional life, Dr. Collins readily recalled his involvement in the formation of the Association of Animal Technician Educators (now the Association of Veterinary Technician Educators [AVTE]). In addition, he remembered well his service during the formative years on the American Veterinary Medical Association Committee on Animal Technician Activities and Training (now called the Committee on Veterinary Technician Education and Activities) and on the National Veterinary Technician Testing Committee, which was charged with developing the Veterinary Technician National Examination. Finally, Dr. Collins was proud to host the 1981 AVTE Symposium at Michigan State University, which gave rise to the first professional organization for veterinary technicians, the North American Veterinary Technician Association (now known as the National Association of Veterinary Technicians in America).

For these efforts and a lifetime of commitment to development of the profession, Dr. Collins is considered to be the "father of veterinary technology in the United States."

---

and credentials, the **National Association of Veterinary Technicians of America (NAVTA)** developed the **Committee on Veterinary Technician Specialties (CVTS)**. The CVTS provides a standardized list of criteria and assistance for societies interested in attaining academy status. Academies initiate and set the rigorous standards that veterinary technicians must meet and maintain to be awarded the

designation of **VTS (Veterinary Technician Specialist)** in their specific discipline. A veterinary technician awarded a VTS has completed a formal process of education, training, experience, and testing to qualify in a specific specialty. Societies have been formed for veterinary technicians with an interest in a specific discipline of veterinary medicine.

EMPLOYMENT PROSPECTS, SALARIES, AND ATTRITION

Presently, widespread shortages of veterinary technicians have been reported nationwide, and graduates of veterinary technology programs are finding ample job opportunities. Although job opportunities are plenty, salaries vary depending on the field of interest and the level of experience (Table 1-1). For example, in 2011, the U.S Bureau of Labor Statistics reported that the average salary for veterinary technicians nationwide was $31,570 per year. However, level of experience, location of work, and field of interest have an impact on income potential. The location of an employment position determines salaries. Technicians working in metropolitan areas earn more, on average, than those working in rural areas. Similarly, technicians working in industry and sales earn more than technicians working in companion animal practices. An experienced graduate veterinary technician, particularly one with management and technical responsibilities, working in a metropolitan setting, may earn from $43,000 to $65,000 per year. Income for an experienced veterinary technician specialist, the highest paid cohort working in clinical practice, may range from $45,000 to $90,000 for those working in large specialty practices.

In addition to salary compensation, many employers offer a range of benefits, including health care coverage, retirement plans, and payment for continuing education (CE) and professional membership fees. Large companies or practices are generally better equipped to provide more complete benefits packages than small private businesses. Some pharmaceutical companies offer educational packages that finance continued education in a related field. In this way, bachelor's and master's degrees have been financed by some corporate employers.

The profession of veterinary technology has a high rate of attrition. Graduate technicians report leaving the profession because of lack of appreciation, underutilization, low pay, and lack of advancement opportunities. Attrition from the profession is a critical part of the current shortage problem. Many states have shortages of veterinarians and veterinary assistants, as well as of veterinary technicians.

The National Commission on Veterinary Economic Issues (NCVEI) has established a website to help guide practice owners, practice managers, and staff toward more efficient

TABLE 1-1	National Estimate and Mean Wage Estimate for Veterinary Technologists and Technicians

EMPLOYMENT NO.	MEAN HOURLY WAGE	MEAN ANNUAL WAGE
78,800	$15.18	$31,570

Percentile Wage Estimates for This Occupation

PERCENTILE	10%	25%	50% (MEDIAN)	75%	90%
Hourly Wage	$10.04	$12.02	$14.49	$17.62	$21.51
Annual Wage	$20,880	$25,010	$30,140	$36,660	$44,740

Top Paying States for This Occupation

STATE	EMPLOYMENT	HOURLY MEAN WAGE	ANNUAL MEAN WAGE
Connecticut	1130	$17.62	$36,640
New York	3,930	$18.01	$37,460
Alaska	200	$18.36	$38,190
California	8,560	$17.07	$35,500
Massachusetts	2,880	$17.49	$36,380

Top Paying Metropolitan Areas for This Occupation

	EMPLOYMENT	HOURLY MEAN WAGE	ANNUAL MEAN WAGE
Sacramento–Arden-Arcade–Roseville, CA	620	$23.07	$47,990
Madison, WI	420	$22.39	$46,570
San Jose-Sunnyvale-Santa Clara, CA	360	$20.56	$42,770
Poughkeepsie-Newburgh-Middletown, NY	200	$20.53	$42,690
Reno-Sparks, NV	60	$20.06	$41,720
Newark-Union, NJ-PA Metropolitan Division	250	$19.68	$40,930
Hartford–West Hartford–East Hartford, CT	330	$19.50	$41,550
Athens-Clarke County, GA	40	$19.37	$40,290
New York-White Plains-Wayne, NY-NJ Metropolitan Division	1,420	$19.24	$40,010
Anchorage, AK	130	$19.17	$39,870

U.S. Bureau of Labor Statistics, May 2011.

management protocols (refer to www.ncvei.org). Because employee attrition is costly, both fiscally and in terms of the morale and efficiency of the veterinary health care team, improved staff management is particularly critical to the health of the practice. With improved understanding of the abilities of credentialed veterinary technicians, it is hoped that practices will allow them to apply their skills more fully. Statistics gathered by NCVEI indicate that the most financially sound practices are those that make full use of their staff. Veterinarians in these well-run practices complete only those tasks that by law they alone are permitted to do. All other animal care tasks are completed by veterinary technicians and veterinary assistants.

EDUCATION

PROGRAMS OF VETERINARY TECHNOLOGY

Like nursing schools in the human health care field, programs of veterinary technology may include 2, 3, or 4 years of undergraduate study and may bestow an associate's degree (2 or 3 years) or a baccalaureate degree (4 years). Programs in the United States are accredited by the Committee on Veterinary Technician Education and Activities (CVTEA), which is under the auspices of the AVMA. Programs in Canada are accredited by the Animal Health Technology/Veterinary Technician Program Accreditation Committee (AHT/VTPAC), which is under the auspices of the CVMA. When a program is accredited by the CVTEA, it must meet 11 essential criteria for curricula, faculty, facility, and admissions requirements. Each program must submit reports to the accrediting body for review semiannually, annually, or biannually, depending on the age and stability of the program. In addition, the accrediting body carries out on-site visits of each program. Based on on-site evaluation and preassessment documentation, recommendations by the accrediting body are classified into three categories: critical, major, and minor recommendations. Programs must report to the accrediting body any progress made in addressing the deficits cited by the on-site review committee. In June 2006, the CVTEA recognized the accreditation of the CVMA AHT/VTPAC as being equivalent to the CVTEA process. Shortly after, the CVMA followed suit. This allows graduates of AVMA-accredited programs to be eligible for licensure in Canadian provinces, and graduates of CVMA-accredited programs are eligible for recognition in the United States.

Two- and Four-Year Programs

The curriculum of veterinary technology programs includes general college level courses, such as biology and chemistry, and courses specific to clinical practice, such as veterinary parasitology, medicine, and clinical chemistry. More than 350 "essential" and "recommended" tasks are listed in the *Accreditation Policies and Procedures Handbook* of the CVTEA, which constitutes the foundation of the hands-on curriculum for laboratory and practical training (Figure 1-2). Many 4-year programs include the same veterinary

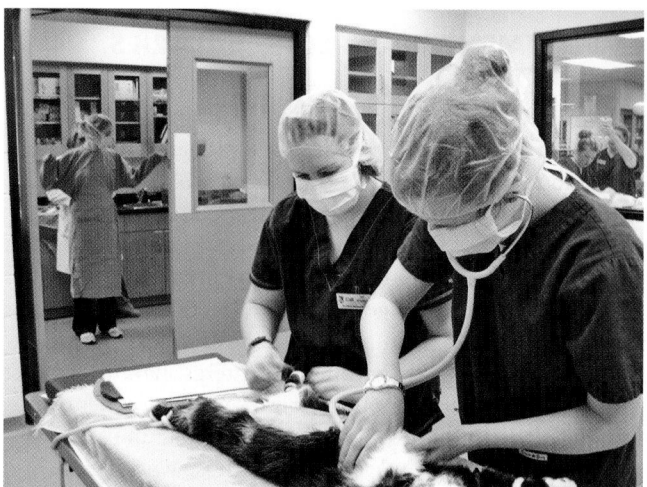

FIGURE 1-2 Students in a Canadian Veterinary Medical Association (CVMA)-accredited veterinary technician program at St. Clair College, Windsor, Ontario. (Courtesy Penny Rivait.)

BOX 1-2	Types of Courses Required in Veterinary Technology Programs

Basic Math and Science Courses
Technical Math
Biology
Chemistry
Microbiology
Comparative Mammalian Anatomy and Physiology
Medical Terminology
Computer Science

Veterinary Technology Courses
Introduction to Veterinary Technology
Veterinary Practice Management
Animal Management and Nutrition
Farm Animal Clinical Procedures
Companion Animal Clinical Procedures
Laboratory Animal Science
Animal Medicine
Veterinary Radiology
Animal Parasitology
Veterinary Hematology
Veterinary Clinical Chemistry and Urinalysis
Veterinary Surgical Assisting
Veterinary Pharmacology and Anesthesiology

---

technology curriculum as 2-year programs, along with greater numbers of liberal arts courses. Some 4-year programs include advanced veterinary technology courses in the junior and senior years, in addition to the standard curriculum required by the CVTEA. As the profession continues to grow, greater numbers of 4-year programs are expected to be established, and a few of these programs will offer increasing numbers of advanced veterinary technology courses. Refer to Box 1-2 for a list of courses typically offered in veterinary technology programs.

Standard Criteria

Through the development of standard criteria for each required task, programs ensure consistency of standards among various faculty members and classroom sections, and in distance education versus traditional courses. In addition, programs are required to document that every student successfully completes each of the required tasks before graduation.

Distance Education

Although most veterinary technology programs are offered to students in the traditional on-campus fashion, some programs are available via distance education using the Internet and teleconferencing. Distance education programs offered via the Internet provide educational opportunities to students around the world. The courses are rigorous and require a high degree of self-discipline from students, who often must work independently, although communication with teachers and classmates is encouraged via threaded discussions and e-mail listservs. The flexibility of distance education programs makes them particularly well suited for mature students who are already working in veterinary practices, and who may not live near a college or university with a traditional program.

Many distance education programs require that students work in veterinary practices while completing online course work. This enables students to be supervised by an employer or another mentor while developing required hands-on skills. In addition, it offers ready access to many of the materials and animals needed to complete required clinical tasks. As documentation, distant students are often asked to videotape themselves successfully completing tasks in keeping with the program's standard criteria and AVMA requirements. They may be asked to turn in the results of projects such as blood films and radiographs, as well as lab results, in addition to completing the usual written assignments and examinations that traditional students complete.

CONTINUING EDUCATION

Most states and provinces require veterinary technicians to attend continuing education (CE) lectures and workshops to maintain licensure, certification, or registration. These lectures are available at various national, regional, and local professional conferences and workshops throughout the United States and Canada, and through AVMA- and CVMA-accredited programs of veterinary technology. CE is also available online, via webinars or web-based lectures and through the websites of many professional associations and veterinary information centers. See Table 1-4 for a list of professional associations and veterinary information links. As veterinary medicine rapidly progresses and changes, it is particularly important for veterinary technicians to commit themselves to a career of lifelong learning.

THE VETERINARY TECHNICIAN NATIONAL EXAMINATION (VTNE)

After completing the requirements to graduate from a program of veterinary technology, students prepare to take the Veterinary Technician National Examination (**VTNE**), which is required in most states and provinces. The VTNE is developed under a contractual agreement between the American Association of Veterinary State Boards (AAVSB) and the Professional Examination Service (PES). The AAVSB is represented by the Veterinary Technician National Exam Committee (VTNEC), which is composed of veterinarians and veterinary technicians who are engaged in clinical practice, national professional associations, AVMA-affiliated specialty boards, and academia. Members of the committee are recommended by the executive boards of AVMA, NAVTA, the Association of Veterinary Technician Educators (AVTE), the Canadian Association of Animal Health Technologists and Technicians (CAAHTT), and the AAVSB, and then are appointed by the Board of Directors of the AAVSB.

The examination is computer based and consists of 150 multiple choice questions. PES provides the committee with three draft examinations for their review and validation. These drafts are developed from a computerized bank of questions, originally written by veterinarians and veterinary technicians from all aspects of the veterinary medical profession. The questions are reviewed independently for accuracy, relevance to the field of veterinary technology, and level of difficulty. In addition, the questions are screened for grammar, style, and conformity to psychometric principles.

Candidates are given 4 hours to complete the examination, which is offered at Prometric Centers throughout North America. Three 30-day windows are available for candidates to complete the VTNE: March 1 to 31, November 15 to December 15, and July 15 to August 15.

Applicants may apply to take the VTNE online at the AAVSB website at www.aavsb.org and can list their preferences for testing center location and date and time when they would like to take the examination. In addition, candidates must send proof to the AAVSB of having completed the following requirement:

1. Graduated from an AVMA- or CVMA-accredited veterinary technician program OR
2. Is within 6 months of graduation from an accredited program.

Candidates wanting to take the VTNE in Arizona, Delaware, Georgia, Illinois, Tennessee, or Washington must apply via these state boards to obtain information about additional requirements specific to the state **and must apply** through the AAVSB.

Immediately after the candidate completes the examination, a provisional pass or fail is given. Scaled scores are subsequently tallied by PES, and AAVSB distributes these scores electronically to both the candidate and the school from which the candidate graduated.

The examination is composed of 150 multiple choice questions that cover the following nine primary areas or domains within the profession of veterinary technology:

1. Pharmacy and Pharmacology 12%
2. Surgical Nursing 11%
3. Dentistry 7%
4. Laboratory Procedures 12%
5. Animal Care and Nursing 22%
6. Diagnostic Imaging 7%
7. Anesthesia 16%
8. Emergency Medicine/Critical Care 6%
9. Pain Management/Analgesia 7%

Twenty-five new questions are added to each examination. These additional questions do not count toward the final score of the candidate but are inserted to determine how well the candidates answer, and if they qualify as repeatable questions. Candidates are not aware of which questions are confirmed and which are untested.

Candidates who would like to have their VTNE scores sent to multiple state boards must register with the Veterinary Information Verifying Agency (VIVA) through AAVSB. A fee is required for registration with VIVA, along with a second fee for each transfer. It is important to note that requirements for credentialing veterinary technicians vary among states and provinces. Therefore, veterinary technicians who relocate to other states or provinces are encouraged to consult the AAVSB and the state or provincial board of the jurisdiction to which they are moving, to obtain information regarding credentialing requirements specific to the new jurisdiction.

THE PROFESSION OF VETERINARY TECHNOLOGY

Veterinary technicians administer nursing care to animals in a conscientious and knowledgeable manner. They assess each patient's health and subsequently develop and enact their own nursing plan to address the patient's reaction to illness, the patient's risk for future problems and the owner's knowledge-deficits and limitations in coping at home with pet care.

Professions such as veterinary technology are characterized by six features:

1. The profession comprises individuals who have completed specific undergraduate or graduate education programs within the framework of a liberal arts institution, and who have successfully passed national and/or state qualifying examinations.
2. The profession is based on a specific body of knowledge that leads to defined skills, abilities, and conduct.
3. The profession provides a specific service.
4. The profession comprises individuals who act independently and make decisions based on observation, knowledge, critical thinking, and independent analysis.
5. The profession has a code of ethics and conduct.
6. The profession is structured by **practice acts** and corresponding **rules and regulations** in each state or province.

These laws and regulations are enforced and upheld by an overseeing committee, which is typically the state licensing board or the state board of governors.

THE VETERINARY TECHNICIAN PRACTICE MODEL

The veterinary technician practice model provides a structured approach to patient assessment, critical thinking and analysis of patient data, and the development of individual patient care plans that are uniquely tailored to each patient. This structure provides a method for ensuring consistently excellent patient care and a mechanism for reevaluation and adjustment of nursing plans based on observation, analysis, and reason. For the veterinary technician student, it offers a systematic approach to critical thinking and problem solving.

The veterinary technician practice model consists of five steps. These steps are performed cyclically throughout a patient's hospitalization period:

1. Gather data about the patient.
2. Identify and prioritize patient evaluations.
3. Develop and implement a plan for patient care by establishing a series of technician interventions.
4. Evaluate the patient's response to the plan of care.
5. Gather additional data (go back to Step 1 and reevaluate the patient).

Step 1: Gather Data

When patients are admitted for hospitalization, veterinary technicians assist veterinarians in gathering an initial database. The database is composed of subjective and objective information. The subjective information includes observable information such as the patient's history and nonmeasurable physical examination findings. Examples of subjective data include observations about the patient's mentation, degree of edema, estimated levels of dehydration, and degree of appetite level.

Objective data include vital signs such as heart rate, respiratory rate, blood pressure, and body temperature, as well as laboratory results such as complete blood count (CBC) results and serum chemistry analysis.

Step 2: Identify and Prioritize Patient Evaluations

Once the database is collected, the veterinary technician uses reasoning to develop a list of patient evaluations. These evaluations reflect the animal's response to physiologic and psychological changes due to a particular disease process. Evaluations fall into one of three categories:

1. Evaluations that relate to actual physical and psychological problems of the patient, such as "hypovolemia," "abnormal eating behavior," and "fear."
2. Evaluations that relate to the risk of or potential for problems in the future, such as "risk for infection" and "risk of aspiration."
3. Evaluations that relate to the owner (also called the client), such as "client knowledge deficit" and "noncompliant owner."

Next, the veterinary technician prioritizes the evaluations so that the most life-threatening problems are addressed first (Table 1-2). The most critical problems are considered foundation issues because if they are not addressed first, the animal may not live. For this reason, the foundation evaluations are listed at the bottom of Table 1-2 in the same way that the foundation of a house, which is closest to the ground, is the most important component of a healthy, well-built building. Evaluations are divided into nine categories; the <u>most important</u> issues at the bottom relate to oxygenation, and the least important issue at the top pertains to utility. All evaluations that are related to oxygenation, such as "obstructed airway," "altered ventilation," and "altered gas diffusion," would be addressed early in the technician's plan of care.

Step 3: Develop Plan of Care and Implement Interventions

After the evaluations have been prioritized, the veterinary technician develops a written plan of care. The veterinary technician uses critical thinking and creativity to develop a unique series of technician interventions for the patient. These interventions are crafted to address the technician evaluations of the patient listed in Step 2. For example, if a **technician evaluation** indicates that the patient has hypothermia, the veterinary technician can include the intervention, "Give the patient hot water bottles or circulating heating pads and blankets," as part of the technician plan of care. Similarly, if the patient is experiencing pain, the technician can list the intervention, "Notify the veterinarian of pain," as part of the technician nursing plan, so that pain medication is ordered.

Step 4: Evaluate Patient Response

Reevaluation of the patient and of the technician plan of care ensures that the patient's condition is monitored as it improves or worsens with treatment. Evaluations and interventions can subsequently be adjusted to address changes in patient status. The technician may examine and reevaluate the patient several times throughout the day.

Step 5: Add Data

As the patient's condition changes with treatment and hospitalization, additional tests, laboratory studies, and physical examinations may be needed. These processes yield additional data for the technician to analyze and evaluate. In this way, this step is similar to Step 1, because it includes the continued collection of new or additional data that could influence the patient's recovery.

SCOPE OF PRACTICE

As the sophistication of veterinary medicine has increased, the responsibilities of the veterinary technician in clinical practice have broadened. However, much variability has been noted among veterinary practices in the ways in which veterinary technicians are employed. In a well-managed practice, veterinary technicians perform all duties associated with the care and treatment of animal patients except those tasks that by law can be performed only by the veterinarian. In addition, they are empowered to delegate appropriate tasks to veterinary assistants. Although state laws differ, it is widely accepted and has been proposed by both the American Veterinary Medical Association (AVMA) and the American Association of Veterinary State Boards (AAVSB) that *only* veterinarians may do the following:
1. Prescribe.
2. Diagnose.
3. Prognose.
4. Perform surgery.
5. Attest to health status.

In other words, veterinary technicians cannot diagnose or prognose; prescribe any treatments, drugs, medications, or appliances; [nor] perform surgery or attest to the health status of an animal, but they are at liberty to carry out all other patient care duties, including placement of catheters by all routes. Therefore, it is important that the veterinary technician, when completing veterinary medical records, enter the notation, "as per order," for each treatment, drug, medication, or appliance ordered by the veterinarian.

In addition to patient care and client education, the veterinary technician may be involved in nonclinical tasks, such as personnel management, management of facilities and equipment, and inventory control. Modern veterinary practices are organized into distinct working areas. A veterinary technician, depending on his or her job description and the size of the practice, may work in all, a few, or only one of the areas discussed in the following sections.

RESPONSIBILITIES OF THE VETERINARY TECHNICIAN IN PRACTICE
Reception Area

Although many practices hire receptionists, not veterinary technicians, to work in the reception area, it is important for the clinical staff to be cross-trained in this aspect of the practice, so that important information can be accessed easily when the receptionist is not available. The veterinary technician should be familiar with the computer network system and the practice management software used by the practice. This will facilitate obtaining existing records, creating new patient records, and accessing medical histories and billing information during emergencies that may occur after hours.

Examination Rooms and Outpatients

The veterinary technician helps to ensure that office visits are handled in an efficient and professional manner. This involves directing clients to the appropriate examination room or treatment area, obtaining a brief history, weighing the patient, and acquiring the vaccines, instruments, and materials needed for the visit. The veterinary technician may also collect blood at this time and may obtain skin scrapings and fecal, urine, and cytology samples for laboratory testing. In addition, the veterinary technician provides to clients important information regarding preventive care,

TABLE 1-2	Identification and Prioritization of Patient Evaluations in the Veterinary Technician Practice Model	
PRIORITY	**CATEGORY**	**EVALUATIONS**
9 Lowest Priority Address these evaluations last.	Utility	Aggression Anxiety Client Coping Deficit Client Knowledge Deficit Fear Inappropriate Elimination Reproductive Dysfunction
8	Activity	Exercise Intolerance Reduced Mobility Sleep Disturbance
7	Chronic Pain/Acute Pain (Mild to Moderate)	Mild-Moderate Acute Pain Chronic Pain
6	Noncritical Safety	Altered Mentation Altered Sensory Perception Noncompliant Owner Hyperthermia Hypothermia Impaired Tissue Integrity Owner Knowledge Deficit Risk of Infection Risk of Infection Transmission Self-Inflicted Injury Status Within Appropriate Limits
5 Middle	Nutrition	Altered Oral Health Abnormal Eating Behavior Ineffective Nursing Overweight Self-Care Deficit Underweight Vomiting/Diarrhea
4	Elimination	Altered Urinary Production Bowel Incontinence Constipation Diarrhea Inappropriate Elimination Self-Care Ceficit Urinary Incontinence
3	Hydration	Hypervolemia Hypovolemia
2	Critical Safety/Acute Pain (Severe)	Acute Pain Electrolyte Imbalance Hyperthermia (Severe) Hypothermia (Severe) Postoperative Compliance Preoperative Compliance
1 Highest Priority Address these evaluations first!	Oxygenation	Altered Gas Diffusion Altered Ventilation Cardiac Insufficiency Decreased Perfusion Obstructed Airway Risk of Aspiration

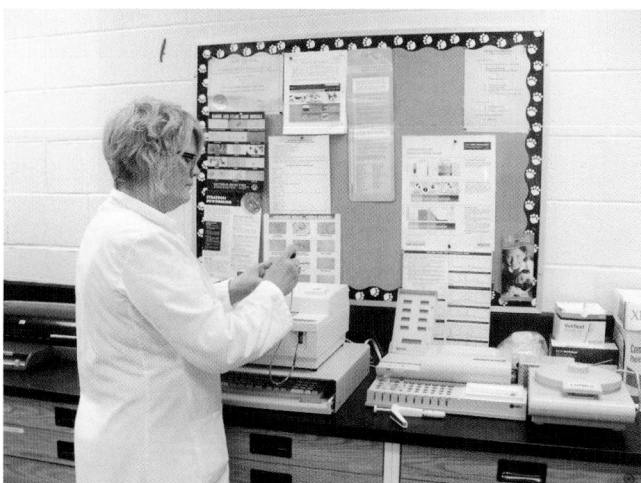

FIGURE 1-3 A registered veterinary technician completes laboratory tests using automated analyzers. (Courtesy Monica Tighe.)

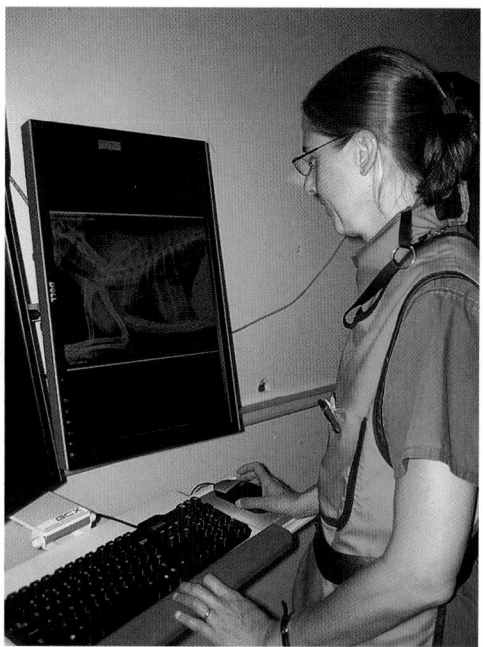

FIGURE 1-4 Veterinary technicians are skilled in the use of radiographic equipment. Today, digital radiographs, as shown, have proved quick to generate and easy to store. (Courtesy Dr. Joanna Bassert.)

diet, behavior modification, medication, discharge instructions, and spay and neutering procedures for their animals.

Because pet owners often feel more at ease talking to the veterinary technician than to the veterinarian, the technician can be a valuable support person for bereaved or worried pet owners. In addition, the veterinary technician answers clients' questions both in person and over the telephone and occasionally must address difficult or angry pet owners.

Laboratory and Pharmacy

The veterinary technician has the skills to perform laboratory tests used in practice (Figure 1-3). The number of laboratory tests actually performed on-site varies. In veterinary hospitals that make full use of these skills, veterinary technicians perform CBCs, differential counts, and morphologic examinations of blood. They perform urinalysis, including examination of urine sediment, and fecal analysis for evidence of parasites. Veterinary technicians are skilled in the use of enzyme-linked immunosorbent assay (ELISA) test kits, dextrometers, refractometers, and dry chemistry analyzers. In addition, veterinary technicians are familiar with interpreting common cytologic preparations, such as ear swabs and vaginal smears.

Once a diagnosis is made, the veterinarian prescribes, in writing or orally, a treatment for the animal patient. The veterinary technician interprets the prescription language, then fills and dispenses the medication to the pet owner, along with instructions for its use. In addition, veterinary technicians are often responsible for ensuring that the pharmacy is well stocked, that expired drugs are discarded, and that controlled substances are handled appropriately.

Radiology and Special Imaging

The x-ray (also known as a *radiograph*) is an important diagnostic tool in veterinary medicine. Veterinary technicians are skilled in radiographic techniques, including positioning the patient, selecting the proper settings, and taking exposures at appropriate times. In addition, technicians ensure that hospital staff members protect themselves from harmful radiation by wearing appropriate protective clothing, such as lead aprons, gloves, and thyroid shields, and that dosimeters are used routinely to monitor x-ray exposure. Technicians may be responsible for managing the ordering and mailing of dosimeters as well.

Many veterinary technology programs teach students to use digital radiographic equipment and to employ the corresponding software that allows for adjustment of the image to maximize accurate interpretation by the veterinarian (Figure 1-4). Digital imaging offers many advantages over standard radiographic techniques. It is faster to produce, easier to adjust, and convenient to store. In addition, images can be sent electronically via e-mail to specialists for a second opinion or to referring veterinary hospitals. Similarly, special imaging techniques, such as computed tomography (CT) and magnetic resonance imaging (MRI), are being used with increasing frequency in veterinary medicine (Figure 1-5), particularly in specialty practices and veterinary teaching hospitals. In addition, veterinary technicians are playing a greater role in collecting images using ultrasound and endoscopy (Figure 1-6) that are subsequently interpreted by a radiologist.

Treatment Room

Most veterinary hospitals have a treatment room to which patients are brought for various procedures and where animals are prepped for surgery. Often the treatment area is a large central room that may include a bank of cages for postoperative and critical care patients. This arrangement facilitates monitoring of hospitalized patients and enables the technical staff to be efficient in completing important

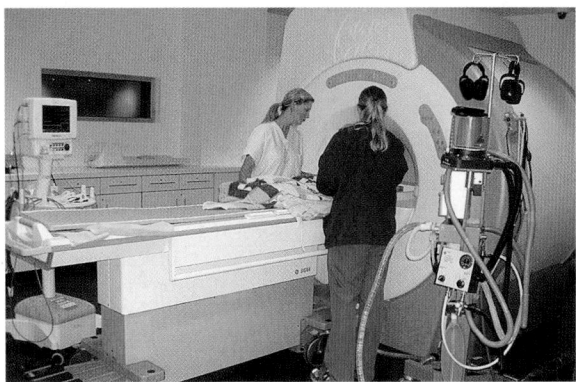

FIGURE 1-5 Advanced imaging techniques, such as the use of magnetic resonance imaging (MRI), as shown, are becoming an important diagnostic tool in veterinary medicine today. (Courtesy Dr. Joanna Bassert.)

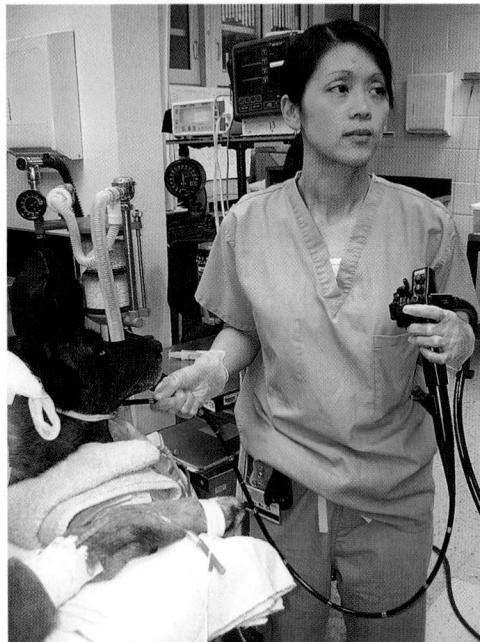

FIGURE 1-6 This veterinary technician works at the Mathew Ryan Veterinary Hospital of the University of Pennsylvania, where she has become proficient in using fiberoptic endoscopes. (Courtesy Dr. Joanna Bassert.)

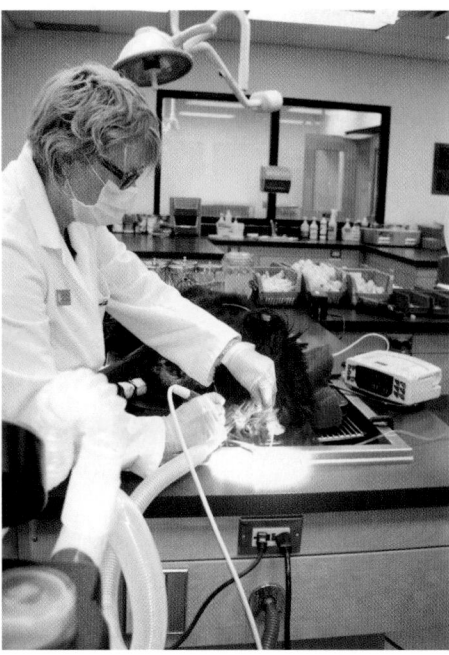

FIGURE 1-7 Performing oral examinations, dental charting, and prophylactic teeth cleaning are important aspects of veterinary technology. (Courtesy Monica Tighe.)

treatment duties. Dental units and procedure sinks may be used in the main treatment room, where dentistry and minor surgical procedures are completed.

Veterinary technicians are responsible for carrying out medication administration orders given by the veterinarian. This involves giving medications by all routes (i.e., orally, intramuscularly, and intravenously). It may also involve placing catheters and setting up and monitoring intravenous fluid administration. Small amounts of blood may be collected every few hours, and the animal may be routinely checked for alertness, temperature, pulse, respiration, urination, and defecation. For critical cases, treatment may include changing bandages, lavaging open wounds, placing and monitoring nasal oxygen, and maintaining chest, tracheal,

urethral, or abdominal tubes. Veterinary technicians are responsible for documenting in the patient's record all treatments, data, and physical findings. The patient record is an important legal document and serves as a means of ensuring that errors in treatment are not made.

The veterinary technician prepares the patient before entry into the operating room. This involves ensuring that the animal has not had anything to eat or drink, and that the animal urinates before surgery. The technician is responsible for weighing the animal and for calculating and administering preoperative anesthetic agents. In many veterinary practices, the veterinary technician is responsible for induction and maintenance of anesthesia. Although an animal can be anesthetized in many ways, this procedure usually involves placing an intravenous catheter, setting up fluids, placing an endotracheal tube, and administering intravenous and/or gas anesthetic agents. Monitoring equipment, such as a pulse oximeter, capnography, an esophageal stethoscope, a Dinamap monitor, a Doppler ultrasonography machine, or a blood pressure monitor, may be used by the technician in monitoring the anesthetized patient. Before moving the patient to the operating room, the technician clips hair from the region of the animal that will undergo surgery and performs an initial skin preparation of the area.

Often a technician is responsible for performing routine dental procedures that must be performed while the animal is anesthetized (Figure 1-7). In this situation, the technician must perform two important jobs at once: namely, monitor the patient under anesthesia, and complete oral examinations and dental health procedures, such as scaling and polishing the patient's teeth. The veterinary technician must be prepared for anesthetic emergencies and should be familiar

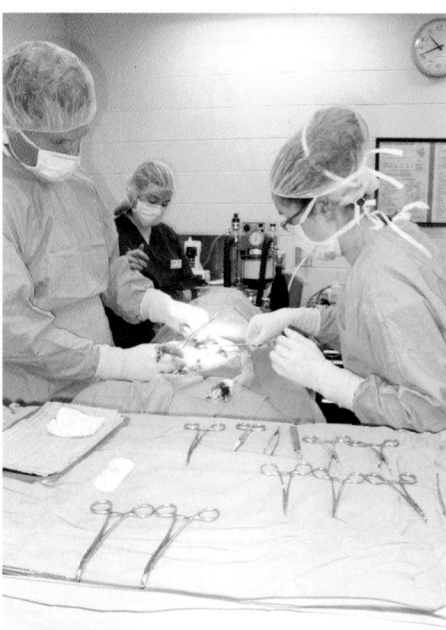

FIGURE 1-8 A veterinary technician student assists in surgery. (Courtesy Penny Rivait.)

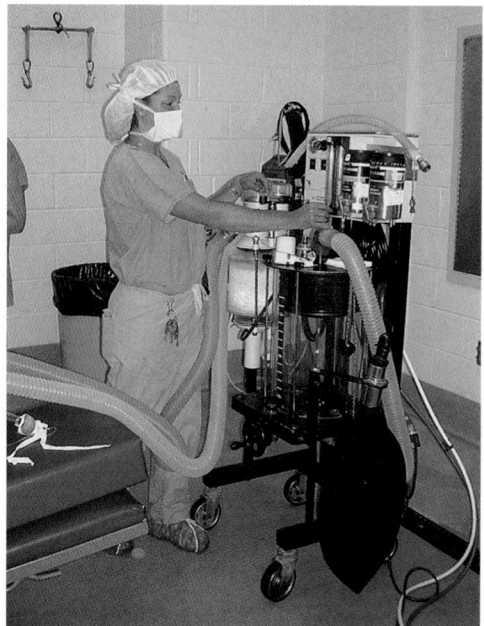

FIGURE 1-9 Administering anesthetics and monitoring anesthetized patients constitute one of the most challenging aspects of veterinary technology and are associated with a high level of responsibility for the life of the patient. (Courtesy Dr. Joanna Bassert.)

with emergency drugs and procedures needed to resuscitate animals in crisis.

Operating Room

The operating room (OR) technician, or the circulating nurse, positions the animal patient on the operating table and completes the final surgical scrub. Instruments, equipment, and materials needed by the surgeon are made available. The technician retrieves any additional materials requested during the procedure, adjusts surgery lights, tilts the surgery table, and, in general, does whatever is necessary to support the comfort of the surgeon (Figure 1-8). In some practices, the technician acts simultaneously as anesthetist and circulating nurse. Occasionally, technicians are asked to assist during a particularly challenging operation and must be skilled in proper sterile techniques, including gloving and gowning. After the procedure has been performed, the technician washes and dries the surgical instruments and reorganizes them into surgical packs for sterilization. The technician may also perform the duties of the postoperative care nurse for the recovering patient.

Being an anesthetist is one of the most important duties of the veterinary technician. In some practices, veterinary technicians are responsible for completing the dosage calculations for preoperative, postoperative, and intraoperative drugs. The technician is also responsible for induction and intubation of the patient and for intraoperative monitoring of blood pressure and heart and respiratory rates. A negative change in vital signs might require the veterinary technician to give compensational and resuscitative drugs. Although modern anesthetic agents are considered safe to use, risk continues to be present whenever an anesthetic is administered. Unexpected reactions to anesthetic agents, surgical

complications, and human error can be fatal to a patient. Anesthesia technicians must be meticulous about checking and rechecking the functionality of the anesthesia machine. Valves, tubing, vaporizer, oxygen levels, and rebreathing bags must be in impeccable condition and working order. The technician is responsible for checking and rechecking the equipment before commencing to anesthetize a patient (Figure 1-9).

Wards

Veterinary technicians play an important role on the wards, not only in ensuring that treatments are given correctly and in a timely manner, but also in providing animals with compassion and a gentle touch. Nurturing animals when they are sick is an important part of their recovery. Even healthy animals that are being boarded benefit from special care and reassurance from technical staff members.

The veterinary technician is often the first to observe changes in a patient's status (Figure 1-10). Difficulties with intravenous lines, infusion pumps, or monitoring equipment also are first noticed by the veterinary technician. Immediate patient assessment and interventions are carried out by the technician, documented in the medical record, and communicated to the veterinarian. Throughout the patient's hospitalization, the veterinary technician assesses and reassesses patient status, develops new evaluations, and adjusts the technician nursing plan. During these periodic patient assessments, the veterinary technician is keenly aware of pain levels experienced by the patient and ensures that appropriate pain management is provided as per order from the veterinarian.

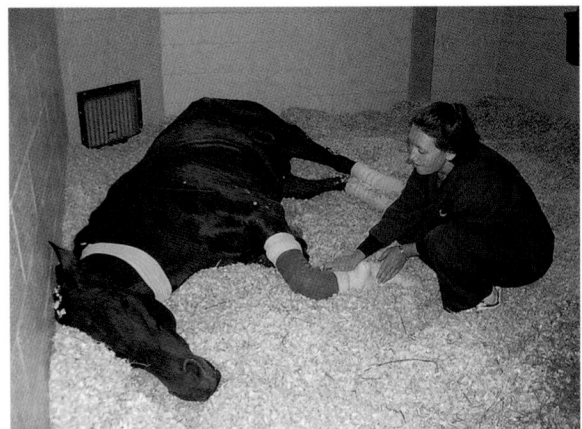

FIGURE 1-10 Veterinary technicians monitor hospitalized patients and are often the first to notice an animal in pain or distress. Technicians are responsible for alerting the attending veterinarian and ensuring that patients receive effective pain management and treatment. (Courtesy Dr. Joanna Bassert.)

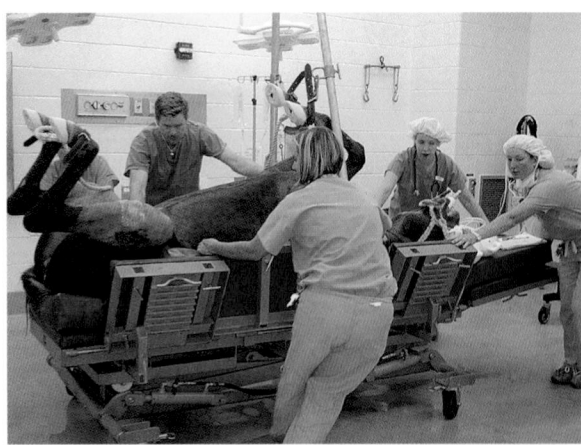

FIGURE 1-11 The veterinary health care team must work collaboratively to provide the best possible veterinary medical care. Here, a veterinary team rushes an anesthetized horse to recovery. (Courtesy Dr. Joanna Bassert.)

Hospital Management and Communications

Veterinary technicians, particularly those with an interest in business, may pursue additional training in hospital management and become employed as hospital managers. They may oversee the veterinary staff and assist with scheduling, hiring, personnel and client management, bookkeeping, and inventory control. Increasingly, veterinary technicians, particularly those in large practices, are drawn into management duties, such as management of technical staff and ordering of supplies. In states where it is legal for nonveterinarians to own veterinary practices, veterinary technicians have become practice owners and managers.

TERMINOLOGY AND THE VETERINARY HEALTH CARE TEAM

A productive and efficiently managed veterinary practice depends on the dedication of a team of veterinary professionals and support personnel (Table 1-3). As described in the following sections, each member of the team plays a collaborative role in helping to provide quality health care for the animal patient (Figure 1-11).

VETERINARIAN

A veterinarian typically completes 4 years of study at an AVMA- or CVMA-accredited school of veterinary medicine after completing 4 years of undergraduate study. Graduates of veterinary medical schools are distinguished by the initials DVM after their names, unless they have graduated from the University of Pennsylvania, in which case they will have the initials VMD after their names. To practice, veterinarians must be licensed by the state or province in which they work. Typically, this requires successful completion of national and state/provincial examinations and payment of a licensing fee. About 28 American and 5 Canadian colleges of veterinary medicine have been established, and this number is increasing. For a current listing of accredited colleges of veterinary

TABLE 1-3	Common Professional Terminology
ACRONYM	**NAME**
Veterinary Health Care Team	
ACT	Animal Care Technician
AHT	Animal Health Technician
CVPM	Certified Veterinary Practice Manager
CVT	Certified Veterinary Technician
DVM	Doctor of Veterinary Medicine
LVT	Licensed Veterinary Technician
OJT	On-the-Job–Trained (veterinary assistant)
RAHT	Registered Animal Health Technician
RVT	Registered Veterinary Technician
VA	Veterinary Assistant
VHM	Veterinary Hospital Manager
VMD	Veterinary Medical Doctor (University of Pennsylvania)
American Laboratory Animal Technology	
AALAS	American Association of Laboratory Animal Science
• ALAT	Assistant Laboratory Animal Technician
• LAT	Laboratory Animal Technician
• LATG	Laboratory Animal Technologist
Canadian Laboratory Animal Technology	
CALAS	Canadian Association of Laboratory Animal Science
• RLAT	Registered Laboratory Animal Technician
• RLAT (Res)	Registered Laboratory Animal Technician in Research
• RMLAT	Registered Master Laboratory Animal Technician
• RMLAT (Res)	Registered Master Laboratory Animal Technician in Research

medicine in the United States and Canada, go to www.avma.org and www.cvma.org, respectively.

In some states, exceptions for licensure are made for veterinarians who are employed in university veterinary teaching hospitals.

Veterinarians who have completed an educational program and examination in a particular medical or veterinary medical specialty are "board certified." In veterinary medicine, the specialty boards are associated with the AVMA. For example, a veterinarian may become board certified in surgery by the specialty organization known as the American College of Veterinary Surgeons (ACVS). A board certified veterinarian is permitted to use the initials "ACVS" behind her name and to advertise as a "specialist" in surgery. To maintain the specialty certification, the veterinarian must complete continuing education in her specialty as mandated by the specialty board. Board certified veterinarians often practice in groups in referral hospitals. Here they primarily see patients referred by other practicing veterinarians for a second opinion, or for performance of complex diagnostic, surgical, and therapeutic procedures.

VETERINARY TECHNICIAN SPECIALIST

In February 1994, NAVTA formed the Committee on Veterinary Technician Specialties (CVTS) to address growing interest among veterinary technicians who wanted to attain higher levels of skill and knowledge in a particular aspect of veterinary technology. For this reason, CVTS established a process and a list of criteria for the formation of academies in specialized fields of veterinary technology.

The first step in the process of forming a specialty is for a group of veterinary technicians who share an interest in a particular field of veterinary technology to establish a professional society. After the society has grown in size, it may then petition CVTS for recognition as an academy. The organizing committee of the proposed academy together with CVTS establishes the advanced requirements and the examination process for becoming a VTS in the field of interest. As of this printing, NAVTA (www.navta.net) has recognized eleven areas of specialty in veterinary technology (Box 1-3). NAVTA also recognizes the following societies: Society of Veterinary Behavior Technicians, American Association of Equine Veterinary Technicians, Association of Zoo Veterinary Technicians, and Veterinary Emergency and Critical Care Society.

Thus the VTS is a veterinary technician who has reached a higher level of skill and understanding in a particular field of veterinary technology (Box 1-4). The VTS must meet the following criteria:
- Must be a graduate of an AVMA-accredited program of veterinary technology and/or be legally credentialed to practice veterinary technology in his or her respective state, province, or country
- Must have successfully completed the education, training, and experience requirements established by the respective academy of specialists
- Must be reviewed and approved for specialist status by the academy

---

BOX 1-3	NAVTA Recognized Areas of Specialty for Veterinary Technicians

Veterinary Dental Technicians
Veterinary Technician Anesthetists
Internal Medicine for Veterinary Technicians
Veterinary Emergency and Critical Care Technicians
Veterinary Behavior Technicians
Veterinary Zoological Medicine Technicians
Equine Veterinary Nursing Technicians
Veterinary Surgical Technicians
Veterinary Technicians in Clinical Practice
Veterinary Nutrition Technicians
Veterinary Clinical Pathology Technicians

NAVTA, National Association of Veterinary Technicians in America.

In addition, it is strongly recommended that the applicant must be a member of national, state/province, and local veterinary technician associations and a member of the specialty society.

Veterinary technicians who have achieved specialty status are signified by the initials VTS (with their field of specialty in parentheses) after their names. For example, the technician Mary Jones, CVT, VTS (dentistry), is a specialist in veterinary dentistry.

The VTS often works in specialty and referral veterinary hospitals and in teaching hospitals associated with universities. In these environments, the VTS can concentrate on his or her field of interest and can share knowledge with veterinary medical and veterinary technology students.

VETERINARY TECHNOLOGIST

In the United States, the **veterinary technologist** holds a Bachelor of Science (BS) degree in veterinary technology from a 4-year, AVMA-accredited program. The veterinary technologist works in positions that may require a greater level of education than is required for the veterinary technician, such as project leader, practice supervisor, or teacher in a veterinary technology program. Some veterinary technologists, particularly those employed in teaching hospitals of veterinary medical schools, become highly skilled in a particular aspect of veterinary technology. Some institutions and practices use the term *veterinary technologist* to refer to a veterinary technician who holds a BS degree in any field.

In Canada, the term *veterinary technologist* is synonymous with the term *veterinary technician*, or a graduate of a 3-year college program in Ontario.

VETERINARY TECHNICIAN

A veterinary technician is a person who has earned an associate of science (AS) degree in veterinary technology from a 2- or 3-year, AVMA/CVMA-accredited program of veterinary technology. After graduating, veterinary technicians are required to complete national and state examinations before

---

BOX 1-4 | What Does It Take to Become a Specialist?

Each veterinary technician academy has its own requirements for becoming a technician specialist. Specific requirements can be found on each of the academy websites. The Academy of Emergency and Critical Care Technicians (AVECCT) is the first technician academy to be recognized by the National Association of Veterinary Technicians in America (NAVTA).

Following are the requirements for sitting for the AVECCT examination*:

Section 1. Credential requirements dictate that each applicant, before he or she is declared eligible for examination, must:

A. Be a graduate of an American Veterinary Medical Association (AVMA)-approved veterinary technician school and/or legally credentialed to practice as a veterinary technician in some state or province of the United States, Canada, or another country.

B. It is strongly encouraged that the candidate be a member of a local, state, provincial, or North American veterinary technician association, and a member of the Veterinary Emergency Critical Care Society.

C. After graduating from a recognized school of veterinary technology and/or becoming credentialed to practice as a veterinary technician and meet training requirements, as specified:

1. Three years' full-time work experience or its equivalent (5760 hour) in the field of veterinary emergency and critical care medicine. All experience must be completed within 5 years before the application.

   a) For the purpose of this eligibility requirement, the definitions of emergency care and critical care as established by the Veterinary Emergency Critical Care Society will be used.

   (1) Emergency care: action taken in response to an emergency. The term implies emergency action directed toward assessment, treatment, and stabilization of a patient with an urgent medical problem.

   (2) Critical care: care taken or required in response to a crisis; in medicine, treatment of a patient with a life-threatening or a potentially life-threatening illness or injury, whose condition is likely to change on a moment-to-moment or hour-to-hour basis. Such patients require intense and often constant monitoring, reassessment, and treatment.

2. A minimum of 25 hours' continuing education related to veterinary emergency and critical care.

a) Continuing education must be completed within the last 5 years before the application is submitted.

b) Continuing education must be received from a nationally recognized program. Proof of attendance is required.

D. Provide documentary evidence of advanced competency in veterinary emergency and critical care nursing through clinical experience.

1. Completion of the Advanced Veterinary Emergency Critical Care Nursing Skills Form. The skills form documents those nursing skills that have been mastered by the candidate and are necessary to practice veterinary emergency critical care nursing at an advanced level. The list will be provided by the Credentials Approval Committee. The skills form is subject to change based upon the current state of the art in veterinary emergency critical care nursing.

2. A case record log is maintained from January 1 to December 31 of the year immediately preceding submission of the application. A minimum of 50 cases should be recorded. These cases should reflect management of the emergent or critically ill patient and mastery of advanced nursing skills. The log should include the following: date, patient identification (name or number), species/breed, age, sex, weight, diagnosis, length of care, final outcome, and summary of nursing care techniques and procedures performed by the applicant on the patient.

3. Four case reports of no more than 5 pages each, double spaced. Case reports must demonstrate expertise in the nursing management of a variety of veterinary patients requiring emergency and critical care. Case reports should be selected from the case record log. Case reports must be the original work of the applicant.

4. Two letters of recommendation from an AVECCT member—a Veterinary Emergency Critical Care Society (VECCS) veterinarian or a Diplomate of the American College of Veterinary Emergency and Critical Care.

   a) Until sufficient numbers of the aforementioned are provided, letters of recommendations will be accepted from the following: non-VECCS emergency clinic veterinarians and Board certified specialists in anesthesia, internal medicine, and surgery.

Modified from the AVECCT website. Additional information can be found at www.avecct.org.
More information on specialties can be found at to https://www.navta.net/specialties/specialties.
*Requirements are subject to change.

---

they can be licensed, registered, or certified. Frequently, veterinary technicians are required to pay a fee to the state veterinary association to receive a license, certification, or registration. The term *veterinary nurse* rather than *veterinary technician* is used in European countries.

VETERINARY ASSISTANT

The term **veterinary assistant** is used to describe an individual who is involved in the care of animals who is not a veterinary technician, laboratory animal technician, or veterinarian. Typically, veterinary assistants are responsible for assisting the veterinary technician and the veterinarian by restraining animals, setting up equipment and supplies, cleaning and maintaining practice and laboratory facilities, and feeding and exercising patients. Most veterinary assistants are trained on the job by a supervising veterinary technician or veterinarian, but some assistants complete 4 to 6 months of training in a formal course of study.

The profession of veterinary technology started to take form in the early 1960s. Before this time, veterinary technicians, as defined today, did not exist, and veterinary practices depended exclusively on the skill of on-the-job–trained veterinary assistants. Today, veterinary assistants continue to constitute a large and important portion of the work force in veterinary practices nationwide. Veterinary technicians and veterinary assistants work together in many veterinary practices, and although AVMA and NAVTA make clear distinctions between the two groups, some states have confused these distinctions.

As the number of traditional and distance AVMA- and CVMA-accredited programs grows, education in the field of veterinary technology becomes increasingly accessible to veterinary support staff members who wish to become veterinary technicians.

LABORATORY ANIMAL TECHNICIANS AND TECHNOLOGISTS

The American Association for Laboratory Animal Science (AALAS) and the Canadian Association of Laboratory Animal Science (CALAS) have established a certification program that certifies the following three to four levels of animal technicians:

- Assistant Laboratory Animal Technician (ALAT)
- Laboratory Animal Technician (LAT)
- Laboratory Animal Technologist (LATG)
- Master Laboratory Animal Technologist (MLAT)— *Canada only*

AALAS- and CALAS-certified animal technicians care for the laboratory animals used in research facilities and teaching institutions. These facilities are registered by the U.S. Department of Agriculture (USDA) and may be located in pharmaceutical companies, universities, and colleges. A technician does not need to be a graduate of an AVMA- or CVMA-accredited program of veterinary technology to be eligible for AALAS or CALAS certification. Graduates of AVMA- and CVMA-accredited programs must complete 6 months of additional training in a registered facility before they are eligible for the Level 1 ALAT examination.

Like the VTNE, AALAS/CALAS certification examinations are developed and administered by the PES, but they fall under the auspices of AALAS rather than the AAVSB. All three levels of examinations consist of multiple choice questions, but each successive level becomes more rigorous and asks more questions. For example, the ALAT examination is composed of 120 questions; the LAT examination, 155 questions; and the LATG examination, 180 questions. After passing the examination, the candidate may use the designation of registered laboratory animal technician (RLAT), for

example. Candidates must complete a specified length of on-the-job experience to qualify for the next level of AALAS or CALAS certification (see Box 1-3).

CASE PRESENTATION 1-1

Two weeks ago Technician Larry learned that he had passed the VTNE and yesterday he received his state credentials. Today, Larry received a call from the Pleasant Valley Veterinary Practice where he had interviewed last week. They congratulate Larry and tell him that they decided to hire him as a "tech" beginning tomorrow. On his first day, Larry is prohibited from drawing blood from a patient by the "head tech" because he has not yet been authorized to do so. He is told that he must "work his way up the ladder" before he is allowed to perform that level of task. Larry recalls learning to draw blood during the first semester of his freshman year, and he is now proficient in performing phlebotomy as well as a wide range of other tasks such as inducing and monitoring anesthesia. Larry learns that there is a three-tier hierarchy of "techs" at the Practice and that he must advance through all three tiers before he can draw blood. It will take about a year to advance to the top level.

Larry also learns that the "head tech" has been employed at the practice for many years but is not credentialed in the state and did not graduate from an accredited Program of Veterinary Technology. As the day goes on, Larry finds himself prevented from performing many technician duties and is merely asked to hold and restrain animals. He also learns that half of the "techs" on staff are veterinary assistants, not veterinary technicians. On his second day, Larry notices that the veterinarians place catheters, intubate, and administer anesthesia themselves. He also notices that one of the senior "techs," who is a veterinary assistant, extracted two premolars using a root elevator while performing a dental prophy.

List concerns that you may have about the Pleasant Valley Veterinary Practice. What roles in the veterinary health care team are being confused, if any? It turns out that there is a high level of turnover among the credentialed veterinary technicians. How would you account for this? List changes you would make in staff management if you were the practice manager.

PROFESSIONALISM

As with all professions, veterinary technology is best represented by the excellent skill, ethical conduct, and passion of its members. Veterinary technicians are bound by a code of ethics and ideals established by NAVTA (Box 1-5) and by our societal expectations of what constitutes professionalism. Although the ethics and ideals of veterinary technology may be clearly defined in writing, the nuances of professional conduct may be less clear, much like the subtleties of social interpersonal conduct. Therefore, programs of veterinary technology are challenged to instill in their diverse student body a common understanding of professional manners. To this end, programs may have mandatory dress codes and

BOX 1-5 | NAVTA Veterinary Technician Code of Ethics

Introduction

Every veterinary technician has the obligation to uphold the trust invested in the profession by adhering to the profession's code of ethics.

A code of ethics is an essential characteristic of a profession and serves three main functions:

1. A code communicates to the public and to members of the profession the ideals of the profession.
2. A code is a general guide for professional ethical conduct.
3. A code of ethics provides standards of acceptable conduct that allow the profession to implement disciplinary procedures against those who fall below the standards.

No code can provide the answer to every ethical question faced by members of the profession. They shall continue to bear responsibility for reasoned and conscientious interpretation and application of the basic ethical principles embodied in the Code to individual cases.

Ethical standards are never less than those required by law; frequently they are more stringent.

Preamble

The code of ethics is based on the supposition that the honor and dignity of the profession of veterinary technology lie in a just and reasonable code of ethics. Veterinary technicians promote and maintain good health in animals; care for diseased and injured animals; and assist in the control of diseases transmissible from animals to human. The purpose of this code of ethics is to provide guidance to the veterinary technician for carrying out professional responsibilities, so as to meet the ethical obligations of the profession.

Code of Ethics

1. Veterinary technicians shall aid society and animals by providing excellent care and services for animals.
2. Veterinary technicians shall prevent and relieve the suffering of animals with competence and compassion.
3. Veterinary technicians shall remain competent through commitment to lifelong learning.

4. Veterinary technicians promote public health by assisting with control of zoonotic diseases and educating the public about these diseases.
5. Veterinary technicians shall collaborate with other members of the veterinary medical profession in efforts to ensure quality health care services for all animals.
6. Veterinary technicians shall protect confidential information provided by clients, unless required by law or to protect public health.
7. Veterinary technicians shall assume accountability for individual professional actions and judgments.
8. Veterinary technicians shall safeguard the public and the profession against individuals deficient in professional competence or ethics.
9. Veterinary technicians shall assist with efforts to ensure conditions of employment consistent with excellent care for animals.
10. Veterinary technicians shall uphold laws/regulations that apply to the technician's responsibilities as a member of the animal health care team.
11. Veterinary technicians shall represent their credentials or identify themselves with specialty organizations only if the designation has been awarded or earned.

Professional Ideals

In addition to adhering to the standards listed in the code of ethics, veterinary technicians must strive to attain a number of ideals. Some of these include the following:

- Veterinary technicians shall strive to participate in defining, upholding, and improving standards of professional practice, legislation, and education.
- Veterinary technicians shall strive to contribute to the profession's body of knowledge.
- Veterinary technicians shall strive to understand, support, and promote the human-animal bond.

This code has been developed by the NAVTA Ethics Committee. No part of it may be reproduced without the written permission of NAVTA. Copyright © 2007 NAVTA, Inc. All rights reserved. www.navta.net.

NAVTA, National Association of Veterinary Technicians in America.

rules about comportment on campus, particularly in the classroom. A portion of a laboratory grade, for example, may assess the professional conduct of the student. Did the student come to class on time, in uniform, and with a positive attitude? Did the student work well with classmates and teachers? These assessments help guide and prepare the student for work in a clinical environment in which they will be judged by pet owners and the employer.

The following guidelines outline the principal aspects of professionalism in veterinary technology.

PROFESSIONAL APPEARANCE

The first impression a veterinary technician makes is usually based simply on how he or she looks. Neat, clean, well-fitted, and ironed uniforms are essential. Long hair should be pulled back and fingernails kept short; little to no jewelry,

makeup, or perfume should be worn. Tattoos should be covered, if possible, and facial body piercings (such as those in the tongue, nose, and eyebrow) should be devoid of studs or rings.

Uniform

Veterinary technicians wear a variety of "uniforms" depending upon the field in which they work. In an equine practice, for example, many technicians wear collared shirts, khaki pants, and solid protective footwear, which have proved to be durable, warm, and practical in the rugged and often unheated setting of hospital barns (Figure 1-12, *A*). Sturdy leather boots, in particular, are important, to protect the feet from fracturing under the weight of a shod hoof. Clearly, sneakers, sandals, and other open-toed shoes would be inappropriate in a barn. Technicians who work in

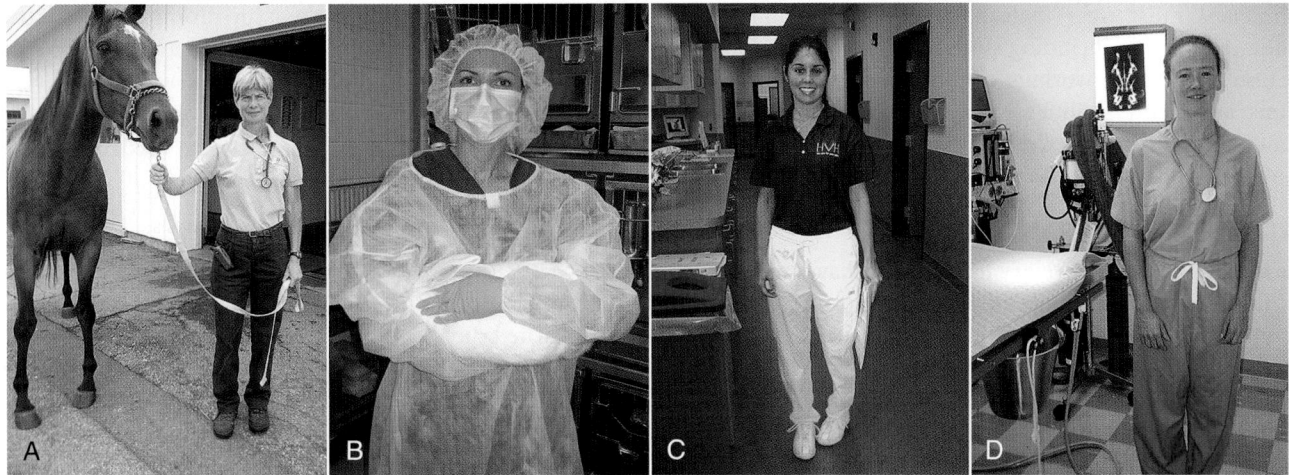

FIGURE 1-12 **A,** Many veterinary technicians who work in equine practice wear collared shirts, pants, and solid protective boots, which have proved to be practical in the rugged setting of hospital barns. **B,** A technician who works in a laboratory animal facility must wear gloves and protective gowns to ensure that contagions are not transmitted to the animals in the vivarium. **C,** Some veterinary technicians working in companion animal practice wear collared shirts that carry the practice name and logo. **D,** An operating room nurse wears clean scrubs and is equipped with a watch and a stethoscope to evaluate the status of anesthetized and recovering patients. (Courtesy Dr. Joanna Bassert.)

bovine practices are likely to wear insulated coveralls and weatherproof boots to stay warm while working in muddy cattle pens.

Veterinary technicians who work indoors as in laboratory animal facilities (Figure 1-12, *B*) and in companion animal practices often wear scrubs and clean white sneakers or orthopedic clogs. Some companion animal or mixed practices prefer that the staff wear collared shirts (or scrub shirts) with the practice name and khaki pants (Figure 1-12, *C*).

In a working environment in which one can become quickly covered by animal hair, saliva, blood, and other bodily fluids, a clean, neat uniform may be challenging to maintain. It is helpful to have garment brushes and adhesive rollers on hand to remove hair from one's uniform, particularly before entering an examination room with a client. Having an extra uniform available is essential when handling animals with suspected contagious disorders, such as parvoviral enteritis and panleukopenia, because the pathogens can be transmitted to other animals by contaminated clothing.

Uniforms must be clean and ironed; they must also fit well. In other words, bending over should not reveal cleavage or a backside. To instill this message in its students, one veterinary technology program uses the slogan, "Say no to crack, front and back." Thus, maintaining a professional appearance for many technicians includes wearing white crew-neck T-shirts under a V-neck scrub shirt, for example, and scrub pants with elastic waistbands rather than drawstrings. The pants should be hemmed to an appropriate length to avoid risk of tripping (Figure 1-12, *D*).

Veterinary technicians are encouraged to wear professional pins on their shirts and the name tag or practice logo required by the practice. Many programs of veterinary technology award college or university pins to graduating students. These pins bear the veterinary caduceus and the name of the college or university. In addition, NAVTA awards pins to its longtime members, as do several state veterinary technician associations. Although college rings are not acceptable, because they are prohibited in the operating room, wearing of pins as symbols of the profession is encouraged.

Finally, the uniform of all veterinary technicians, regardless of field of interest, must include a watch with a second hand. Taking vital signs and conducting appropriate patient assessments, which are important parts of veterinary nursing, cannot be completed without a suitable watch. Other items, such as a functional pen and a stethoscope, are also critical tools for the veterinary technician to have readily available at all times.

Hands and Nails

It is well known in the health industry that contagions can be spread from one patient to another on the hands, especially under the nails, of health care workers. For this reason, it is important to make a habit of washing hands several times a day, particularly between contacts with different animals. In addition, fingernails should be kept as short as possible and free of nail lacquer, which can chip off into sterile surgical fields. Not only can long nails harbor infectious agents, they also interfere with daily nursing tasks, such as scruffing cats, putting on surgical gloves, and placing IV catheters.

Jewelry, Face, and Hair

Veterinary technicians must be proficient in restraining animals and must be prepared to do so. Risk of injury to the technician and other staff members is increased if jewelry and long hair can be caught up in the fury of claws and flailing limbs. Necklaces, dangling earrings, and loose bracelets are particularly dangerous for technicians to wear. In addition, small items, such as studs, earrings, earring backs, and individual hairs, can accidentally fall into sterile surgical fields or, worse, into open surgical incisions. Veterinary technicians must wear their hair pulled back and must remove all jewelry, including studs, before working. Finally, because of the close working conditions of most operating rooms and ward facilities, veterinary technicians should avoid chewing gum and wearing strong cologne, which may be offensive to coworkers and to pet owners.

PROFESSIONAL CONDUCT

The way in which a veterinary technician behaves represents the most important aspect of his or her professionalism. Technicians, like many health care professionals, are held to a high standard of conduct. For this reason, NAVTA developed the list of professional ideals listed in Box 1-6. Below are specific guidelines for professional conduct both in and outside the workplace.

In the Workplace

1. Be honest and forthright in communications with coworkers and clients. Take responsibility for making a mistake and, if possible, take immediate action to correct the error.
2. Maintain a positive attitude and an even, controlled disposition. Be respectful of coworkers and pet owners at all times. Avoid expressing anger, sarcasm, and cynicism because this has a de-motivating effect on the veterinary health care team and often worsens the situation.
3. Be tactful and careful in both verbal and written communications. Avoid saying all that is thought and felt. Be considerate of the time, place, and quality of a query when asking questions.
4. Be a collaborative team player. Provide the ideas and positive energy needed to help improve the efficiency of the health care team and the quality of the medical services it provides.
5. Be attentive to the concerns and needs of both coworkers and pet owners. Avoid mentally tuning out. Take initiative to pitch in and help where needed.
6. Respect the veterinarian-client-patient relationship. Keep in mind that some communications are most appropriately delivered to clients by the veterinarian.
7. Be aware of the clinical and professional competence of others. When concerned about incompetence in

the workplace, address the issue promptly and tactfully to protect the integrity of the practice. Do not turn a blind eye.

8. When a conflict arises, address it promptly, privately, and calmly with those directly involved. Avoid drawing in those who are not directly involved in the conflict. Doing this undermines trust and is a poor substitute for direct communication.
9. Maintain the confidentiality of professional and personal information about clients and coworkers that was learned directly or indirectly. Do not gossip.
10. Be committed to being competent and skilled. Be receptive to new ideas and suggestions for improvement. Be enthusiastic about teaching others.
11. Be aware of and abide by the laws and regulations that define the scope of practice in your state.

Outside the Workplace

1. Join and participate in national, state, and local professional organizations.
2. Participate in high school career days, and give presentations about the profession when the opportunity arises.
3. Attend national, state, and local veterinary conferences. Stay current on issues affecting the profession.
4. Support legislation in your state that better defines and strengthens veterinary technology.
5. Maintain state licensure, certification, or registration.
6. Seek healthy ways to manage stress, such as exercise, meditation. and taking time for personal interests. Refer to Chapter 2 for additional information about managing stress.

PROFESSIONAL COMMUNICATION
Verbal Communication

Clear and frequent communication with coworkers and clients is an important part of an efficient health care team. Veterinary technicians should be sure to use correct grammar and articulated speech, and should avoid using words that might offend. For some who are accustomed to speaking in an informal manner, cleaning up one's language can be a challenge. To expedite the cleanup process, some veterinary technology programs penalize the professionalism portion of a student's grade for using inappropriate words and expletives in class. Cursing is universally considered to be unprofessional communication.

Written Communication
Medical Records

The medical record is a legal document owned by the veterinary practice or supervising institution. It can be subpoenaed by a court of law and subjected to detailed scrutiny. Errors in the document can render the medical record invalid; this could have adverse legal ramifications for the practice. In addition, medical records of animals used for teaching in veterinary technology programs and in schools of veterinary medicine are examined by the USDA inspector, who could cite deficiencies during an inspection if the

BOX 1-6	Questions to Help Determine a Good Course of Conduct

1. Do the practice act and the regulations of the state board require that the technician act in a certain manner or prohibit the technician from acting in a certain manner?
2. Do the ethics of the profession of veterinary medicine or veterinary technology require that the technician act in a certain manner or prohibit the technician from acting in a certain manner?
3. Do the individual technician's personal ethics require that the technician act in a certain manner or prohibit the technician from acting in a certain manner?

written record contains errors. Using correct spelling and grammar in these legal documents is important. Refer to Chapter 3 for additional information about addressing errors in medical records.

E-mail

E-mail is a common form of written communication today, and although e-mails are often considered less formal than letters, use of correct spelling and grammar in e-mails to clients and colleagues is important. It is helpful to get into the habit of doing the following when sending e-mails to professional contacts:

1. Begin with a salutation that includes the person's name to whom you are writing (e.g., "Hi, Mary," or "Good evening, Dr. Brown"). E-mail accounts can be shared, and it is important to be clear when identifying the intended recipient of the e-mail. Salutations may not be necessary during frequent exchanges but should be included when first making contact.
2. Write a concise e-mail that is grammatically correct. Use a spell-checker.
3. Keep in mind that e-mail can be forwarded, and that the tone can be misinterpreted. *Never* write an angry e-mail or one that is critical of a colleague or coworker. Be careful with the use of humor lest it be misinterpreted.
4. Always end with a closing and your name. Many professionals program their computers to automatically end each e-mail with a prewritten closing. Typically, this includes the person's full name, title, address, and telephone number.
5. Maintain an e-mail address that does not leave a bad impression. Silly, cute, and animal-related e-mail addresses, such as bunnyluvr@comcast.net or pintaday@msn.com, are not helpful toward the development of a professional image. A simple e-mail that includes your first initial and last name works well. Similarly, make sure that recorded answering machine greetings are appropriate for professional colleagues, particularly if you are actively searching for a new position and expect potential employers to call.

> **TECHNICIAN NOTE** Keep in mind that e-mail and text messages can be forwarded, and that the tone can be misinterpreted. NEVER write an angry e-mail (or text message) or one that is critical of a colleague or coworker.

Text Messaging

In some practices, text messaging or texting is now used for reminders or to let a pet owner know that a pet has come out of surgery. Accurate and professional communication is more difficult with texting than with e-mail or written letters. Text messages should be sent only to clients who wish to receive information that way and should be used only to send information that can be accurately and professionally conveyed in a few words. Tips for texting include the following:

- Do not use acronyms or emoticons that you are not sure the recipient will understand—the message needs to be unambiguous and crystal clear.
- Communicate briefly and succinctly.
- Do not use texting for serious topics or to send bad news.

PROFESSIONAL ORGANIZATIONS AND ACRONYMS

As the profession of veterinary technology matures, increasing numbers of professional organizations are being formed at national, state, and provincial or local levels. These organizations support the education, professional interests, and activities of the veterinary technician. NAVTA and CAAHTT, for example, represent the professional foundation of veterinary technology in the United States and Canada, respectively. However, numerous national organizations now forming are based on the special interests of their members. Examples include Association of Zoo Veterinary Technicians, Society of Veterinary Behavior Technicians, and American Association of Equine Veterinary Technicians. Continued growth of veterinary technology depends heavily on the efforts of individuals within these and other professionally related organizations (Tables 1-4 and 1-5). Graduate veterinary technicians can assist in advancing their profession by joining and participating as active members.

NATIONAL ASSOCIATION OF VETERINARY TECHNICIANS IN AMERICA (NAVTA)

NAVTA has been the leader in shaping and supporting the profession of veterinary technology in the United States. It has written the code of ethics, the veterinary technician oath, and the veterinary technician portion of the model practice act, and has brought about important changes in the terminology of the profession. In addition, NAVTA is an important source of support and information for veterinary technicians. Therefore, it is not surprising that the NAVTA mission statement reads as follows: "To represent and promote the profession of veterinary technology. NAVTA provides direction, education, support, and coordination for its members and works with other allied professional organizations for the competent care and humane treatment of animals." In addition, the goals of NAVTA are to help its members do the following:

1. Influence the future of veterinary technology.
2. Be part of the decision-making process that affects veterinary technology.
3. Foster high standards of veterinary care.
4. Promote the veterinary health care team.

To be an active member of NAVTA, you must live in the United States, must be a graduate of an AVMA-accredited program of veterinary technology, or must be licensed, certified, or registered as a veterinary technician. Associate members include veterinarians, veterinary technicians who live outside the United States, and veterinary assistants. Associate members may serve on committees but may not vote or hold an elected office.

TABLE 1-4	Professional Associations		
ORGANIZATION		**ACRONYM**	**WEBSITE**
American Association of Equine Practitioners		AAEP	www.aaep.org
American Association of Feline Practitioners		AAFP	www.aafponline.org
American Animal Hospital Association		AAHA	www.aahanet.org or www.healthypet.com
American Association for Laboratory Animal Science		AALAS	www.aalas.org
American Association of Veterinary Laboratory Diagnosticians		AAVLD	www.aavld.org
American Association of Veterinary Medical Colleges		AAVMC	www.aavmc.org
American Association of Veterinary State Boards		AAVSB	www.aavsb.org
American College of Laboratory Animal Medicine		ACLAM	www.aclam.org
American College of Veterinary Emergency and Critical Care		ACVECC	www.acvecc.org
American College of Veterinary Internal Medicine		ACVIM	www.acvim.org
American College of Veterinary Surgeons		ACVS	www.acvs.org
Animal Medical Center of New York		AMCNY	www.amcny.org
American Society of Laboratory Animal Practitioners		ASLAP	www.aslap.org
American Society for Veterinary Clinical Pathology		ASVCP	www.asvcp.org
American Veterinary Dental Society		AVDS	www.avds-online.org
American Veterinary Medical Association		AVMA	www.avma.org
Association of Veterinary Technician Educators		AVTE	www.avte.net
British Small Animal Veterinary Association		BSAVA	www.bsava.com
British Veterinary Nurses Association		BVNA	www.bvna.org.uk
Canadian Association for Laboratory Animal Medicine		CALAM	www.calam-acmal.org
Canadian Association of Animal Health Technologists and Technicians		CAAHTT	www.caahtt-acttsa.ca
Canadian Association for Laboratory Animal Science		CALAS	www.calas-acsal.org
Canadian Council on Animal Care		CCAC	www.ccac.ca
Centers for Disease Control		CDC	www.cdc.gov
Canadian Food Inspection Agency		CFIA	www.inspection.gc.ca
Canadian Veterinary Medical Association		CVMA	www.canadianveterinarians.net
Committee on Veterinary Technician Education and Activities		CVTEA	www.avma.org
Food and Drug Administration		FDA	www.fda.gov
Federation of European Companion Animal Veterinary Association		FECAVA	www.fecava.org
International Veterinary Emergency and Critical Care Symposium		IVECCS	www.veccs.org
International Veterinary Nurses and Technicians Association		IVNTA	www.ivnta.org
National Animal Health Laboratory Network		NAHLN	www.aphis.usda.gov
National Association for Veterinary Technicians in America		NAVTA	www.navta.net
National Board of Veterinary Medical Examiners		NBVME	www.nbvme.org
National Commission on Veterinary Economic Issues		NCVEI	www.ncvei.org
Occupational Safety and Health Administration		OSHA	www.osha.gov
Professional Examination Service		PES	www.proexam.org
Veterinary Emergency and Critical Care Society		VECCS	www.veccs.org
Veterinary European Transnational Network for Nursing Education and Training		VETNNET	www.vetnnet.com
Veterinary Hospital Managers Association, Inc.		VHMA	www.vhma.org
Veterinary Ophthalmic Technician Society		VOTS	www.votsweb.com
Veterinary Information Network		VIN	www.vin.org
Veterinary Support Personnel Network		VSPN	www.vspn.org
Work Hazard Material Information System		WHMIS	www.labour.gov.on.ca
World Small Animal Veterinary Association		WSAVA	www.wsava.org

TABLE 1-5	International Veterinary Nurses and Technician Associations	
COUNTRY	**ORGANIZATION**	**WEBSITE**
International Veterinary Nurses and Technicians Association	The IVNTA is an association of member countries that seeks to foster and promote links with veterinary nursing/veterinary technician staff worldwide by communication and cooperation.	www.ivnta.org
Australia	Veterinary Nurses Council of Australia	www.vnca.asn.au
Canada	Canadian Association of Animal Health Technologists and Technicians	www.caahtt-acttsa.ca
Finland	Klinikkaeläinhoitajat ry	www.klinikkaelainhoitajat.fi
Ireland	Irish Veterinary Nursing Association	www.ivna.ie
Japan	Japan Veterinary Nurses & Technicians Association	www5.plala.or.jp/VTNAHP
New Zealand	New Zealand Veterinary Nursing Association	www.nzvna.org.nz
Norway	Norsk Dyrepleier og Assistent Forening	www.dyrepleier.com
South Africa	Veterinary Nurses Association of South Africa	www.vnasa.co.za
Turkey	Veteriner SaĐlık Teknisyenleri DerneĐi (Association of Veterinary Technicians in Turkey)	www.vested.org.tr
United Kingdom	British Veterinary Nurses Association	www.bvna.org.uk
United States	National Association of Veterinary Technicians of America	www.navta.net

CANADIAN ASSOCIATION OF ANIMAL HEALTH TECHNOLOGISTS AND TECHNICIANS/L'ASSOCIATION CANADIENNE DES TECHNICIENS ET TECHNOLOGISTS EN SANTÉ ANIMALE (CAAHTT)

CAAHTT was founded in 1989 and represents the joining together of seven provincial associations. Each association maintains its own membership base and submits funding (proportionate to the size of its membership) to the CAAHTT. In this way, individuals who are members of a provincial association are automatically given membership in the CAAHTT.

Objectives of CAAHTT include the following:

1. Establish and maintain a national standard of membership.
2. Promote and assist in providing continuing education to animal health technologists and veterinary technicians.
3. Promote greater communication among various aspects of the profession, both nationally and internationally.
4. Promote the profession of animal health technology and veterinary technology within the animal health community and to the general public.
5. Be a resource to members of the profession and to the public regarding national and international issues.

> **TECHNICIAN NOTE**   NAVTA and CAAHTT have designated the third week in October as National Veterinary Technician Week! Mark your calendars! For more information, check www.navta.net or www.caahtt-acttsa.ca.

PROFESSIONAL ETHICS

"Rules or principles that govern right conduct. Each practitioner, upon entering a profession, is invested with the responsibility to adhere to the standards of ethical practice and conduct set by the profession."

Saunders Comprehensive Veterinary Dictionary, ed 3, St Louis, 2007, Saunders

How does one determine what is good and what is bad and what is right and what is wrong? Is the technician's primary concern the animal, the client, or the employer? In the practice of the healing arts, practitioners are frequently faced with situations where the right course of conduct is not immediately apparent. To some extent, this is magnified in veterinary medicine because not only are veterinarians and technicians responsible for the care of a patient, they also have responsibilities to the animal's owner and, in some cases, to the general public. For this reason, when considering the question of "right conduct," one first must ask, "Right for whom?"

Ethical questions are often complicated in veterinary medicine because veterinarians and technicians serve not only the patient, but also the client. Conflicts may arise when the recommendations of the veterinary medical team are not adopted by the client. The veterinary medical team must work within the limits set by the client, who often is balancing the desire to provide the best care for the animal with the constraints of financial, work, and familial commitments, which may or may not be known by the veterinary medical team. It is important in such situations to remember that, in most situations, the client is the owner of the animal and as such has the ultimate decision-making authority over the care provided to the animal.

To provide guidance to veterinary technicians, NAVTA has generated a code of professional ethics (see Box 1-5) and a curriculum of ethical queries to help veterinary technicians make professionally appropriate choices in practice. Finally, the technician will need to determine whether acting or not acting in a certain manner will conflict with his or her own personal ethics.

Meaningful discussions regarding professional ethics can arise when examples of situations frequently encountered by technicians in practice are considered, and when ethical queries are applied to help resolve dilemmas (see Box 1-6). The following two scenarios depict various legal and ethical issues. Use the reference material available in this chapter to assist you during your discussion of these scenarios.

CASE PRESENTATION 1-2

You have an employment interview scheduled with a veterinarian who has been in practice for 30 years. The veterinarian had told you that he has no other employees and is looking for someone to be his "right hand." Upon entering the practice, you notice a strong odor of urine, and your feet even stick to the floor as you walk through the facility. The veterinarian does not have equipment that you have been trained on (e.g., the facility has no oxygen and no gas anesthesia machine).

When you ask about the old equipment, Dr. Smith tells you that he has been using them for 30 years and they work just fine. You also notice that films at the practice do not have any identification on them. What should you do?

PROFESSION-RELATED LAWS AND REGULATIONS

The practices of professions and occupations, such as dentistry, engineering, and veterinary technology, are considered matters to be governed by each state. Therefore, most laws and regulations that govern the practice of veterinary technology are state based. A veterinary technician does not need to be an expert in all of the laws and regulations that affect the profession; however, a technician should have a strong grasp of the state law that provides for the licensing, professional conduct, and discipline of veterinary technicians and veterinarians. In addition, a veterinary technician should be familiar with some of the areas governed by federal law, so that if a question arises, the technician will know where to look for further information.

> **TECHNICIAN NOTE**   Most laws and regulations that govern the practice of veterinary technology are state based.

LAWS (STATUTES)

Each state or province has a practice act. The practice act is considered the primary law that governs the practice of veterinary medicine and veterinary technology. The practice act and any changes to the practice act must be "enacted" by the state legislature. In other words, the original act and any amendments to the act must be approved by both the state house of representatives and the state senate and signed into law by the governor. A proposed amendment or change to the practice act is called a *bill*.

The practice act is enacted to promote public health, safety, and welfare by ensuring the delivery of competent veterinary medical care. A practice act mandates that only licensed veterinarians or those who possess the personal and professional qualifications specified in the act can practice veterinary medicine in that specific jurisdiction (state or province). It may also include the function and outline the powers of the state board of veterinary medicine, licensing requirements, examinations, and possible disciplinary actions. Some veterinary practice acts of some states or provinces include jurisdiction over veterinary technicians; in other states there are separate veterinarian and veterinary technician practice acts.

It is important to keep in mind that if a veterinary technician violates the state's practice act, the penalty can include loss of licensure as well as fines or other disciplinary action. Some state practice acts include a provision that would allow criminal prosecution of individuals who violate the practice act or board regulations; however, criminal prosecution under these provisions virtually never occurs and must be investigated and charged by criminal authorities rather than by the licensing board. In these states, if a criminal violation of the practice act or board regulations is proven, penalties may include fines and imprisonment. Because practice acts vary from one jurisdiction to another, every veterinary technician must be sure to understand the laws that govern the practice of veterinary technology in the state or province in which the technician plans to practice.

AVMA, AAVSB, and NAVTA have proposed model practice acts as templates for states and provinces that are preparing to revise their practice acts. Refer to Box 1-7 for the model practice act for veterinary technicians developed by NAVTA, and to Box 1-8 for the AAVSB model practice act. Refer to the Evolve site for the complete AVMA model practice act.

The practice act usually defines the practice of veterinary medicine and veterinary technology, although in some states, the board has been left to define the practice of veterinary technology. Some states do not license veterinary technicians nor regulate the practice of veterinary technology. The definition of the practice is important not only because it informs veterinarians and technicians of the practices in which they may engage, but because when the practice is defined, persons who are not veterinarians or veterinary technicians are prohibited from practicing veterinary medicine or veterinary technology as it is defined.

BOX 1-7	NAVTA Model Practice Act for Veterinary Technicians

Section I. Title

This act shall be known and may be cited as the "Model Practice Act."

Section II. Legislative Intent and Purpose

The practice of veterinary technology is a privilege granted by legislative authority to maintain public health, safety, and welfare and to protect the public from being misled by unauthorized individuals.

Section III. Definitions

When used in the text that follows, except where otherwise indicated by context, the words and phrases below shall have the following meanings:

1. Animal: Any mammalian animal other than man, and any avian, amphibian, fish, or reptile, wild or domestic.
2. Board: The _____ State Board of Veterinary Medical Examiners or Board of Governors.
3. Veterinary technology: The science and art of providing all aspects of professional medical care and treatment for animals, with the exceptions of diagnosis, prognosis, surgery, and prescription.
4. Emergency: When an animal has been placed in a life-threatening condition and immediate treatment is necessary to sustain life; or when death is imminent and action is necessary to relieve pain or suffering.
5. Licensed veterinarian: An individual who is validly and currently licensed by the Board to practice veterinary medicine in _____.
6. Veterinary technician (licensed, registered, or certified): An individual who has graduated from a veterinary technology program that is accredited according to the standards adopted by the American Veterinary Medical Association Committee on Veterinary Technician Education and Activities, and who has passed the examination requirements as prescribed by the Board in _____, shall be known as a licensed, registered, or certified veterinary technician.

Section IV. Tasks

Certain tasks may be performed ONLY by a licensed veterinarian OR by a licensed, registered, or certified veterinary technician under the direction, supervision, and control of a veterinarian licensed to practice in the state of _____.

See the Rules and Regulations Document for a list of tasks.

Section V. Examination for Licensure, Registration, or Certification

Veterinary technicians applying for licensure, registration, or certification shall be required to pass the Veterinary Technician National Examination, with scores as set by the Board before licensure, registration, or certification.

See the Rules and Regulations section for specifics.

Section VI. Continuing Education

All licensed, registered, or certified veterinary technicians shall be required to continue their professional education as a condition of maintenance of their status in the state of _____.

See the Rules and Regulations section for specifics.

Section VII. Denial, Suspension, or Revocation of Veterinary Technician Licenses, Registrations, or Certifications

The Board may suspend, revoke, or deny the issuance or renewal of license, registration, or certification of any veterinary technician if, after a hearing by his or her peers, he or she has been found guilty of any of the following:

1. Fraud or misrepresentation in applying for license, registration, or certification.
2. Criminal offense related to veterinary medicine.
3. Any violation of the Uniform Controlled Substances Act or the Legend Drug Act.
4. Convicted of cruelty to animals.
5. Violation of any of the rules or regulations stated in the Rules and Regulations Document.

Modified from navta.net/files/Model_Practice_Act_-_Rev_2009.pdf.

The unlicensed practice of veterinary medicine or veterinary technology will subject the unlicensed individual to sanction (discipline) by the board; in most states, it is also a crime and may subject an unlicensed individual to criminal penalties, including imprisonment. Criminal violations must be investigated and charged by criminal authorities. It is more likely that an unlicensed individual purporting to practice veterinary medicine would be criminally charged with animal cruelty than with violating the veterinary or veterinary technology practice act. The practice act may set general or specific parameters for entry into practice and grounds for disciplining veterinarians and technicians. The practice act creates the board and authorizes it to oversee and regulate the professions.

> **TECHNICIAN NOTE** Violation of the state practice act or a board's regulations may subject the violator to loss of licensure or practice restrictions, if applicable, and to monetary penalties, and possibly even imprisonment.

RULES AND REGULATIONS

Rules and regulations are [often] written by each state's board of veterinary medicine, which is known simply as "the board." The review process of regulations varies from state to state, but in general, regulations do not have to be approved by the legislature or the governor. They are therefore usually easier and less costly to change and update than the practice act [amendments]. The [rules and] regulations, together

<table>
<tr><td>

BOX 1-8	American Association of Veterinary State Boards (AAVSB) Veterinary Technology State Practice Act Model

Veterinary technician means:

A person who is duly licensed to practice veterinary technology under the provisions of this Act.

The practice of veterinary technology means:

Any person practices veterinary technology with respect to animals when such person performs any one or more of the following:

1. Provides professional medical care and monitors and treats animals under supervision of a licensed veterinarian.
2. Represents oneself directly or indirectly as engaging in the practice of veterinary technology.
3. Uses any words, letters, or titles under such circumstance to induce the belief that the person using them is qualified to engage in the practice of veterinary technology, as defined. Such use shall be prima facie evidence of the intention to represent oneself as engaged in the practice of veterinary technology.

Nothing in this section shall be construed to permit a veterinary technician to do the following:

1. Surgery.
2. Diagnosis and prognosis of animal diseases.
3. Prescribing of drugs, medicine, and appliances.

Regulations Defining Tasks of Veterinary Technicians
The Board shall adopt regulations establishing animal health care tasks and the appropriate degree of supervision required for those tasks that may be performed only by a veterinary technician or a veterinarian.

</td></tr>
</table>

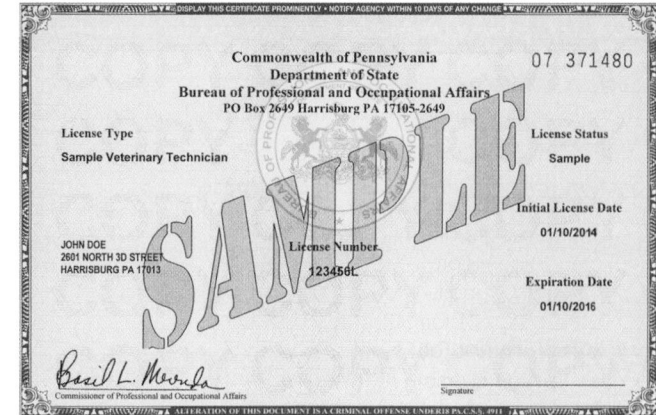

FIGURE 1-13 Sample of a license to practice veterinary technology from the state of Pennsylvania.

with the state practice act, are posted on the state board's website. It is important for veterinary technicians to be familiar with these documents and to understand that both the practice act and [rules and] regulations must be followed. Refer to Box 1-9 for the NAVTA model rules and regulations for veterinary technicians.

The overriding purpose of the board is to protect the public by enforcing the practice act[, as well as rules] and regulations. To do this, it ensures that those seeking professional licensure have completed all of the requirements set forth in the law to be licensed, and that the requirements for maintaining a license, such as completion of continuing education and payment of a renewal fee, are completed.

Regulations are said to have the "force and effect" of law because they must be followed, or the violator will be subject to sanction by the board. Because regulations have the force and effect of law, violating a regulation written by an agency, such as the board, will subject the violator to the possibility of the same sanctions as are available for violating the practice act itself. These sanctions include the imposition of a reprimand or a monetary penalty, restrictions placed on a license, suspension of a license, or revocation of a license. In other words, the license that the board giveth, the board can taketh away. Most state boards also have the authority to impose sanctions designed to remediate the conduct of the

violator. Remedial sanctions may include requiring that an individual practice with monitoring, or complete additional continuing education.

The public may have input into both the practice act and regulations. The public may influence laws by providing information and opinions to legislators. The public may affect regulations by providing information and opinions to the state board that is rewriting the regulation. You may influence regulations that affect your practice by providing information and your opinion to your state board of veterinary medicine.

Sometimes, the practice act and regulations do not address questions facing technicians. Technicians may write to their state board to ask for clarification and guidance; however, some state boards are prohibited from providing such guidance. In this case, a technician seeking advice may wish to contact the state veterinary technician society or a former professor in the technician's education program for guidance. The board may be able to inform the technician if other laws or regulations (e.g., regulations of the state department of agriculture related to rabies disclosure) affect the particular question facing the technician. The technician may consult model acts and regulations of organizations for additional guidance, while keeping in mind that model acts and regulations are not mandatory. In addition, the technician may consult codes of professional ethics set forth by NAVTA and the AVMA for guidance.

ENTRY INTO PRACTICE
Licenses, Certificates, and Registrations
Because the practice of veterinary technology is regulated by each state or province, some variety is noted in the terminology used to designate an individual whom the board has authorized to practice. This variety can be confusing because one state may issue a license, whereas another may issue a certificate. Granting of a license by a state board implies that the board has reviewed and approved the qualifications of the individual to practice (Figure 1-13). Granting of a certificate implies that some other entity has reviewed and approved the qualifications of the individual to practice, and

BOX 1-9 | NAVTA Model Rules and Regulations for Veterinary Technicians

I. Licensed, Registered, or Certified Veterinary Technician Activities

Tasks

Levels of supervision defined:

1. Immediate supervision—A licensed veterinarian is within direct eyesight and hearing range.
2. Direct supervision—A licensed veterinarian is on the premises and is readily available.
3. Indirect supervision—A licensed veterinarian is not on the premises but is able to perform the duties of a licensed veterinarian by maintaining direct communication.

The following tasks may be performed ONLY by a licensed, registered, or certified veterinary technician (or licensed veterinarian) under the direction, supervision, and control of a veterinarian licensed to practice in _____, provided said veterinarian makes a daily physical examination of the patient treated.

Immediate Supervision

- Induction of anesthesia
- Dental extraction not requiring sectioning of the tooth or resectioning of bone
- Surgical assistant to a licensed veterinarian within the rules and regulations issued by the Board of Veterinary Medical Examiners and the laws of the state of _____

Direct Supervision

- Euthanasia
- Blood or blood component collection, preparation, and administration
- Application of splints and slings
- Dental procedures including, but not limited to, removal of calculus, soft deposits, plaque, and stains; smoothing, filing, and polishing of teeth; or flotation or dressing of equine teeth

Indirect Supervision

- Administration and application of treatments, drugs, medications, and immunologic agents by parenteral and injectable routes (subcutaneous, intramuscular, intraperitoneal, and intravenous), except when in conflict with government regulations
  - Initiation of parenteral fluid administration
  - Intravenous catheterizations
  - Radiography, including settings, positioning, processing, and safety procedures
  - Collection of blood; collection of urine by expression, cystocentesis, or catheterization; collection and preparation of tissue, cellular, or microbiological samples by skin scrapings, impressions, or other nonsurgical methods, except when in conflict with government regulations
  - Routine laboratory test procedures
  - Supervision of handling of biohazardous waste materials
- Other services that a licensed, registered, or certified veterinary technician is competent to perform under the appropriate degree of supervision
  - Under conditions of emergency, a licensed, registered, or certified veterinary technician may render the following lifesaving aid and treatment:
    - Application of tourniquets and/or pressure bandages to control hemorrhage

- Pharmacologic agents and parenteral fluids shall be administered only after direct communication with a veterinarian authorized to practice in _____, and when such veterinarian is present or en route to the location of the distressed animals.
- Resuscitative procedures
- Application of temporary splints or bandages to prevent further injury to bones or soft tissue
- Application of appropriate wound dressings and external supportive treatment in severe wound and burn cases
- External supportive treatment in heat prostration cases

HOWEVER, nothing shall be construed to permit a licensed, registered, or certified veterinary technician to do the following:

- Make any diagnosis or prognosis
- Prescribe any treatments, drugs, medications, or appliances
- Perform surgery

II. Examinations

Examinations of applicants for licensure, registration, or certification as a veterinary technician in _____ shall be held at least annually at a time, place, and date set by the Board, no later than ninety (90) days before the scheduled examination.

An applicant shall be required to pass the veterinary technician national examination (VTNE) with scores as set by the Board before licensure, registration, or certification.

III. Continuing Education Requirements for Licensed, Registered, or Certified Veterinary Technicians

All licensed, registered, or certified veterinary technicians shall be required to continue their professional education as a condition of maintaining their license of veterinary technology in the state of _____ with hours of continuing education required annually.

IV. Removal of Veterinary Technician Licenses, Registrations, or Certifications

All licenses, registrations, or certifications issued to veterinary technicians in the state of _____ shall expire on _____ of every year unless renewed.

All license, registration, or certification holders shall submit renewal fees and a current mailing address by the dates determined by the Board on a renewal form that shall be provided by the Board and mailed to all license, registration, or certification holders.

All license, registration, or certification holders will be required to submit to the Board evidence of the necessary amount of continuing education in the fields of veterinary medicine, as required by the Board for license, registration, or certification renewal.

Failure to submit the appropriate license, registration, or certification renewal fee by the dates determined by the Board shall result in forfeiture of all privileges and rights extended by the license, registration, or certification, and the license, registration, or certification holder must immediately cease and desist in engaging further in performance of veterinary technician activities under the veterinary practice act until payment of a delinquency fee, in addition to the license, registration, or certification renewal fee, has been received by the Board.

has certified that the person is competent to practice. Some states issue a license but call a technician certified (e.g., in Pennsylvania, technicians' qualifications are reviewed by the board, and the board issues a license bestowing the title *Certified Veterinary Technician*). Some jurisdictions "register" rather than license technicians. The term *registered* implies that neither the board nor an independent entity has reviewed and approved the qualifications of the technician to practice; however, to lawfully practice veterinary technology, the individual must register and provide information to the board. Some boards that refer to registration actually do review and approve the qualifications of technicians. A technician should check with the state's board before beginning practice to ensure that he or she has obtained the proper authorization to practice.

The terminology used in the state or province in which you plan to practice is not as important as the distinction made between a person who has been authorized to practice and one who has <u>not</u> been authorized to practice. In most states, only a person who has been issued some credential by a state may perform the functions that the state defines as the practice of veterinary technology.

Demonstrating Good Moral Character

State and provincial laws vary widely in how the board determines whether an applicant possesses the good moral character required for licensure. In some jurisdictions, the applicant merely verifies (signs a statement under legal penalty of prosecution for perjury, or making a false statement) that he has good moral character. Other requirements can include submitting letters of recommendation attesting to the applicant's good moral character, a criminal history record check from the jurisdiction where the applicant has lived for the past 5 years, a federal criminal history record check, or a signed document verifying that the applicant has never been convicted of a crime.

Background Checks

The nationwide trend across all professions is to require applicants for licensure to submit criminal history record checks. Citations for "underage drinking," "disorderly conduct," "driving while under the influence of alcohol," and "driving while intoxicated" (DUI or DWI) are crimes that must be reported on your application for licensure. Generally, traffic offenses, such as "speeding" or "failure to yield," do not need to be reported. <u>Read the application carefully</u>, and err on the side of reporting any criminal convictions you believe you may have. If the board does not have the authority to refuse to issue a license based on the crime you have committed, the board will disregard the information.

How does a board view an applicant with a criminal record? To some extent, the answer to this question varies from state to state. Some states have absolute bars to licensure, meaning that if a person has been convicted of certain crimes, he or she may not be issued a license. It is rare to find a state that has an absolute lifetime bar to licensure regardless of the crime that the applicant has committed; to do so

would be contrary to the theory that a person who has committed a crime can be rehabilitated. It is not unusual, however, to see 5- and 10-year bars to licensure. For example, in some states, a person who has been convicted of a felony level criminal offense involving drugs may be barred from licensure for 10 years. In other states, a person who has been convicted of any violent crime may be barred from licensure for 5 years.

Refusal of Licensure

State boards may use an applicant's criminal convictions to support the board's finding that the applicant does not have good moral character and may then refuse to bestow licensure. The most common criminal convictions that lead boards to refuse to license an applicant are convictions involving **crimes of moral turpitude**. A crime of moral turpitude is a crime that involves dishonesty or deception, immorality or depravity, or interference with justice. All theft offenses, such as shoplifting, theft by unlawful taking, theft by deception, embezzlement, false swearing, forgery, and writing bad checks, are considered crimes of moral turpitude because they involve dishonesty. **Crimes of depravity** include murder, rape, and distribution of drugs, but also include misdemeanor offenses, such as stalking, harassment, and assault. Crimes that involve **interference with justice** include eluding a police officer and interfering with the conduct of a criminal investigation.

> **TECHNICIAN NOTE** The most common criminal convictions that lead boards to refuse to license an applicant are convictions involving crimes of moral turpitude.

If you have a criminal conviction in your background, you should review the practice act and regulations of the board in the jurisdiction in which you plan to practice to determine whether the conviction will bar you from being licensed in that jurisdiction. When a licensing board is faced with a decision on whether or not to license a person who has a background that includes a criminal conviction, it will seek to determine whether the person is rehabilitated (unlikely to commit further criminal offenses). Positive indications of rehabilitation include no additional criminal convictions, a steady work history, admission of responsibility for the crime, and a positive outlook toward the future.

Other information commonly required on an application for licensure includes whether the applicant has held any other professional license in any state, whether the applicant has ever had a license disciplined by a state, and whether the applicant is now or has ever been addicted to alcohol or drugs. In most states, the simple fact that a person has held a professional license that has been subject to discipline is a legal ground to deny the application for licensure. A veterinary technician in one state who has had his or her license revoked for stealing drugs from the practice will not likely be granted a veterinary technician license in another state.

> **TECHNICIAN NOTE** Report any criminal convictions to the board when you apply for a license, even if you do not think it is a reason for the board to refuse licensure. The board will determine whether the conviction prohibits you from licensure.

License Renewal and Continuing Education

Every state that issues a license to practice veterinary technology requires that the license be renewed. The length of time that a license is valid varies from state to state. In most states, you will be able to renew your license online.

To renew your license, you will be required to fill out a renewal application and pay a renewal fee. Although renewal applications vary from state to state, the common theme of renewal applications is to determine whether the licensee remains fit to hold the license. Some states (e.g., New Mexico) require veterinary technicians to annually register with the state board and inform the board of their employment. In addition, a technician may be required to inform the board whenever the technician changes employment.

Most jurisdictions require professional licensees, including veterinary technicians, to complete continuing education to renew their licenses. The number of hours and the types of continuing education required for licensure renewal vary from state to state. Be sure to check with the board in the jurisdiction in which you intend to practice for detailed information about the state's continuing education requirements.

A common scheme used by many states is to have a list of approved continuing education providers. For example, many states accept continuing education credits offered by the state's schools of veterinary technology, AVMA or the state veterinary medical association, NAVTA or the state technician association, programs approved by the Registry of Continuing Education (RACE) of the AAVSB, and most of the large national veterinary medical conferences. Some states limit the number of continuing education hours that may be earned from "distance learning" sources, which usually include Internet-based courses, teleconferences, and journal articles with test questions that are mailed to the journal's publisher.

Many states permit technicians to obtain continuing education credits for other educational activities, but technicians must seek board approval in advance for a nontraditional educational activity. A state board will approve an educational program for credit when it appears that the program will enhance the technician's knowledge and skills and will advance the practice of veterinary technology.

GROUNDS FOR DISCIPLINARY ACTION
Technical Violations

The grounds for which a board may discipline a licensee (or refuse to grant an application to an applicant for licensure) are set forth in the state practice act. Additional grounds for discipline may be set forth in the state board's regulations. Some violations of the practice act are spoken of as *technical violations*. These so-called technical violations include practicing on a lapsed license, failing to complete mandatory continuing education, having a record of a criminal conviction that is not related to the practice of the profession, and being disciplined by another state's licensing board. These violations are considered technical violations because there is no direct link between the licensee's misconduct and harm to an animal. It is important to note that in virtually every state, a licensee may be prosecuted and disciplined for misconduct, even if the licensee's misconduct did not cause any harm to an animal.

Substantive Violations

The so-called substantive violations of the practice act and regulations are violations that bear directly on the licensee's conduct in practicing the profession. Common grounds for discipline include unprofessional conduct, malpractice, incompetence, deviation from the standards of acceptable and prevailing practice, practicing beyond the scope of practice authorized in the state, violating any rules of the board or any rules set forth in the practice act, engaging in acts of moral turpitude, fraud, or deceit in the practice of the profession or during entry into the practice of the profession, misrepresentation, animal abuse, animal neglect or animal cruelty, engaging in any act that is illegal and is related to the profession, aiding another person to violate the practice act, impairment by reason of addiction to drugs or alcohol or by mental disease that prevents safe practice, and a criminal conviction.

Fraud and Deceit

A licensee may be prosecuted and disciplined for violating any rule of the board or any rule set forth in the practice act, even if it is not specifically mentioned as grounds for discipline. A licensee may be prosecuted and disciplined, or an applicant may be prevented entry into the practice of the profession, for committing fraud or deceit in the practice of the profession. This includes falsifying information submitted on an application for licensure, omitting requested information on an application, and cheating on the licensure examination. It also includes conduct such as falsifying a health certificate or other document and signing a form for the veterinarian that the veterinarian is required to sign. Finally, violations under this section may include fraudulent or deceitful conduct related to the client, such as charging for services not performed, and may include fraudulent or deceitful conduct related to the technician's employer, such as stealing from the practice.

> **TECHNICIAN NOTE** A licensee may be prosecuted and disciplined or an applicant may be prevented entry into the practice of the profession for committing fraud or deceit in the practice of the profession. This includes falsifying information submitted on an application for licensure, omitting requested information on an application, and cheating on the licensure examination.

Crimes of Moral Turpitude

In some states, a licensee may be prosecuted and disciplined for engaging in acts of moral turpitude and engaging in immoral conduct. Because *moral turpitude* is a well-defined term in criminal law, a licensing board will usually look to the criminal law in its state to determine what conduct by a licensee involves moral turpitude. (Refer to the earlier discussion regarding disclosing your criminal history on the application for licensure for additional information on crimes involving moral turpitude.) In addition to being authorized to discipline a licensee who has been convicted of a crime of moral turpitude, a licensing board may have the authority to discipline a licensee for engaging in acts of moral turpitude, even if the licensee was not convicted of a crime related to the conduct. Some state practice acts include a definition of immoral conduct, some reference criminal statutes for the definition of immoral conduct, and some do not specify what kind of conduct is considered immoral conduct.

Misrepresentation

A licensee may be prosecuted and disciplined for misrepresentation. Misrepresentation is saying something that is not accurate. Telling a client that a certain treatment will cure a patient is misrepresentation because virtually nothing in medicine is an absolute certainty and a technician may not give a prognosis. However, it is not a violation to say, "Your pet is in good hands. We are doing everything we can for your pet."

Animal Abuse

A licensee may be prosecuted and disciplined for animal abuse, animal neglect, or animal cruelty. States and provinces vary on whether the abuse, neglect, or cruelty applies to any animal or only to animals that are under the care of the technician. In some states, the board considers abuse, neglect, or cruelty to be a deviation from the standards of acceptable and prevailing practice, rather than a separate offense.

Committing or Aiding Illegal Professional Acts

A licensee may be prosecuted and disciplined for engaging in an illegal act that is related to the profession. For example, a licensee who provides a performance-enhancing drug to the owner of a competition animal could be prosecuted for engaging in an illegal act related to the profession.

A licensee may be prosecuted and disciplined for aiding another person to violate the practice act. If you were to give unauthorized assistance to another person in taking the licensing examination, you would be guilty of aiding another person to violate the practice act. The most common example of this misconduct occurs when an unlicensed person is working in a veterinary practice and the licensed persons in the practice know, or even instruct, the unlicensed person to perform acts that only licensed persons are allowed to perform. This situation occurs fairly often when veterinarians who are licensed to practice in another country come to the United States and become employed as noncredentialed veterinary assistants. It may take a year or longer for them to become licensed veterinarians in the United States. However, because they may have been practicing veterinary medicine outside the United States for a number of years, they may appear to be competent to perform a wide variety of tasks within a hospital. It is important to remember that unlicensed, noncredentialed individuals are limited to performing only those tasks that the statute and board regulations authorize, regardless of the knowledge or skill level of the individual. Any licensed person who assists an unlicensed person in performing tasks that the statute includes as the practice of the profession may be aiding unlicensed practice.

> **TECHNICIAN NOTE** The most common example of misconduct occurs when an unlicensed person is working in a veterinary practice, and licensed persons in the practice know, or even instruct, the unlicensed person to perform acts that only licensed persons are allowed to perform.

Working Impaired

Licensees may be prosecuted and disciplined for working while impaired by addiction to drugs or alcohol or by an untreated mental disease. Disciplinary action may require that the licensee practice only under supervision, and that the licensee must actively participate in a treatment program. In addition, the licensee must submit random observed urine samples that are tested for drugs of abuse, including alcohol.

> **TECHNICIAN NOTE** The most common reason why a technician is disciplined by a licensing board is that the technician has exceeded the scope of practice authorized by law.

CASE PRESENTATION 1-3

Technician Tina has a long history working with animal rights groups. She helped start the first no-kill shelter in her community. In order to further her knowledge and be able to better help animals, Tina became a veterinary technician. Tina now works for Dr. Jones. George has just become a client of the practice and brings his new puppy in for examination. The puppy is sickly; Dr. Jones diagnoses Parvo. George does not want to pay for the treatment, even though Dr. Jones advises George that the puppy should make a full recovery. George instructs Dr. Jones to put the puppy to sleep and pays for the procedure and cremation. After George leaves, Tina tells Dr. Jones that she is involved in the local shelter and that the shelter will pay for the puppy's treatment and then place the puppy for adoption. Can Dr. Jones begin the treatment and let Tina take the puppy? What should Dr. Jones do? What should Tina do?

A few weeks have passed at Dr. Jones' hospital. Barbara comes in for an appointment with her elderly cat. The cat has terminal cancer and has been crying the past 5 hours. Barbara elects euthanasia and then leaves the hospital. Dr. Jones directs Tina to administer the euthanasia solution. Tina is vehemently opposed to euthanasia and believes that animals should be permitted to die naturally when it is their time. Can Tina refuse Dr. Jones' instructions?

Practicing Beyond the Scope of Practice

A licensee may be prosecuted and disciplined for practicing beyond the scope of practice authorized in the state. This violation is considered among the most serious examples of misconduct that may be committed by a licensee because it demonstrates a fundamental misunderstanding of the role of the licensee or deliberate disregard for the role of the licensee.

Most states prohibit veterinary technicians from performing surgery, diagnosing an animal's ailment, attesting to an animal's health status, offering a prognosis for the animal, and prescribing treatments or drugs. In addition, states often require a level of supervision by a veterinarian for a veterinary technician to perform any particular task such as administration of an anesthetic. These items usually are set forth in the regulations of the state board.

NAVTA model rules and regulations for veterinary technicians (see Box 1-9) include three levels of supervision defined as follows:

1. Immediate supervision—A licensed veterinarian is within direct eyesight and hearing range.
2. Direct supervision—A licensed veterinarian is on the premises and is readily available.
3. Indirect supervision—A licensed veterinarian is not on the premises but is able to perform the duties of a licensed veterinarian by maintaining direct communication.

A wide variety of state regulations have addressed the authorized scope of practice of veterinary technicians, especially in particular areas. One such area that has recently undergone intense scrutiny by licensing boards nationwide is the appropriate scope of practice for technicians performing dental procedures. States range from permitting technicians to perform only cleaning and polishing without subgingival scaling to permitting technicians to perform certain types of extractions. Massachusetts permits a veterinary technician to clean and polish teeth under direct veterinary supervision. Georgia permits a veterinary technician who is under the direct supervision of a veterinarian to remove calculus, soft deposits, polish stains, and smooth and file teeth, and to perform dental extractions that do not require sectioning of the tooth or resectioning of bone.

At a hearing before a licensing board at which the allegation against the licensee is that the licensee practiced beyond the authorized scope of practice, the board will attempt to discern whether the licensee committed the violation because the licensee did not understand the proper role of a technician, or because the licensee disregarded the proper role. If the latter is found, the board will further attempt to discern the licensee's rationale for the misconduct. The board's findings on these key issues will determine the degree of culpability (guilt) of the licensee, which, in turn, will influence the disciplinary sanction imposed by the board.

If the technician is found to have deliberately practiced beyond the scope of practice authorized by the state, it is likely that the sanction imposed will be severe. The theory behind imposing a severe sanction, such as revocation or suspension of a license, is that the public can be protected only by prohibiting the individual from practicing. If, on the other hand, the board determines that the technician did not understand his role in the delivery of veterinary health care, the board is more likely to impose a sanction that seeks to educate the technician about the proper role of a technician, and to impose a probationary period during which the technician must practice under more intense monitoring and supervision to ensure that the technician does not err again.

TECHNICIAN NOTE If a veterinary technician is found to have deliberately practiced beyond the scope of practice authorized by the state, it is likely that the sanction imposed will be severe.

Unprofessional Conduct

A licensee may be prosecuted and disciplined for unprofessional conduct. Unprofessional conduct usually refers to conduct that disparages the profession in the eyes of the public.

Malpractice (Negligence)

A licensee may be prosecuted and disciplined for malpractice (also called *negligence*). *Malpractice* refers to deviation from or failure to conform to acceptable standards of practice. Licensing law borrows the concept of a "tort" from civil law; in civil law, a tort is a wrong or injury for which a court will provide a remedy. The usual remedy in a tort action is the award of monetary damages. For a person to recover damages for infliction of a negligent tort, the person must prove the existence of a legal duty owed to the person by another, the other's breach of the duty, a causal relationship between the breach and the person's injury, and damages suffered by the person. However, in laws governing professionals (unlike in civil lawsuits), the state's prosecuting attorney need only establish a duty to the patient and a breach of that duty by the licensed practitioner. The patient does not have to suffer any injury for the professional to be disciplined for malpractice. An additional difference is that a state board does not award monetary damages to the animal's owner; the state board's authority is limited to imposing disciplinary sanctions on the professional. Veterinarians can carry veterinarians' professional liability insurance, which is similar to malpractice insurance. The veterinarian's professional liability insurance covers acts, errors, and omissions performed while legally responsible to render professional services as a veterinarian or a veterinary technician.

Veterinarians can also be found negligent or guilty of malpractice owing to the actions of a staff member. Some veterinary technicians purchase errors and omissions insurance as part of the yearly state or provincial membership dues and licensing requirements.

The ultimate safeguard to ensure that there is proof of standard veterinary practice is a complete and thorough patient record that accurately documents all therapies conducted. Communications and discussions with clients regarding the patient should be documented by staff members who speak with the client. Refer to Chapter 3 for more information about documentation and completion of veterinary medical records.

> **TECHNICIAN NOTE**   In the laws governing professionals (unlike in civil lawsuits), the state's prosecuting attorney need only establish a duty to the patient and a breach of that duty by the licensed practitioner. The patient <u>DOES NOT</u> have to suffer any injury for the professional to be disciplined for malpractice.

Incompetence

Finally, a licensee may be prosecuted and disciplined for incompetence. Incompetence is conduct that increases the risk that negligence will occur, even if negligence has not yet actually occurred. For example, sloppy laboratory practices, incomplete record keeping, and improper sanitation may demonstrate incompetence because they increase the risk that something could go wrong. Sloppy laboratory practices increase the risk of tainted samples and misdiagnoses; incomplete record keeping increases the risk for an animal to be given the wrong medication; and improper sanitation increases the risk that animals (or humans) may be inflicted with a virus or infection.

Responsibility for Actions

As a credentialed professional, a veterinary technician is responsible for his or her conduct. Because a technician is employed by and acts under the supervision and direction of a veterinarian, the veterinarian is also responsible for the conduct of the technician. For this reason, as a general rule, whenever a veterinary technician is disciplined by a licensing board for exceeding the technician's authorized scope of practice, incompetence, or negligence or malpractice, the veterinarian responsible for supervising the technician may also be disciplined by the board.

PROCESS OF DISCIPLINARY ACTION

Notice

The board must notify the licensee in writing of the specific allegations that are initiating disciplinary action. For example, a state may allege that a technician is subject to

---

CASE PRESENTATION 1-5

Two weeks ago Technician Tom learned that he had passed the VTNE and yesterday he received your state credentials. Today Tom received a call from a busy four-veterinarian practice where he had interviewed last week. They congratulate Tom and tell him that they have decided to hire him as a technician beginning tomorrow. On his first day at work, Tom is assigned to shadow Annette. Annette is introduced to you as the "head technician" and he is told that she has been working at the practice for nine years and that she will show him how things are done in the "real world." Annette's nametag identifies her as "technician" and "behavior specialist." Tom notices that Annette does not have a technician license displayed in the facility where the other licenses are displayed.

Annette takes Tom to the back and introduces him to Bassie, a young Basset Hound that was dropped off that morning to be spayed. Annette takes the dog's vitals and listens to her heart. Annette tells Tom that everything is normal and that there is no need to do pre-operative blood work, which will make the owner happy when she gets her bill. Annette directs Tom to administer pre-anesthetic medications to Bassie and then carry the dog into the surgical room. Annette then administers IV medication to Beatrice, scrubs, clips and drapes her, and tells Tom to call Dr. White on his cell phone and let him know that Bassie is ready for surgery. Dr. White is just pulling up to the hospital when he takes Tom's call and tells you he will be right in. When Dr. White arrives, he asks Annette how everything is; Annette says everything is okay. Dr. White begins the surgery, but Bassie loses her heartbeat and cannot be revived. A necropsy reveals that Bassie had a serious heart condition that should have been audible on auscultation. Does Tom have any legal or ethical responsibilities in this situation?

---

discipline under the practice act because the technician has been convicted of a crime, and a particular section of the practice act gives the board the authority to take disciplinary action against licensees who have been convicted of certain crimes. The notice is usually sent by certified mail, return receipt requested, but may also be sent by first class mail. In some cases, a board will have the notice delivered to the accused licensee by personal service (i.e., hand delivery). If the board cannot locate the licensee because the licensee has moved and has not notified the board of the licensee's forwarding address, notice may be accomplished by publishing an announcement in a publication of legal record within the state. This publication is generally the same publication in which a board publishes notice of new regulations governing the practice of the profession.

Right to a Hearing

In addition to setting forth the factual allegations that give rise to the action against the licensee, the notice will inform the licensee that he or she has a right to a hearing to defend against the allegations and tell his or her side of the story. The hearing may be held before an administrative law judge or hearing officer or may be held before one or more members of the licensing board.

The licensee is not required to be represented by an attorney at a disciplinary hearing before a licensing authority. There is no "right" to an attorney in disciplinary matters, as there is in criminal matters; therefore, the state will not appoint (and pay for) an attorney to represent you if you cannot afford legal representation—a concept you are likely familiar with from television shows depicting the criminal legal process. However, an attorney is likely to tell you that you should have an attorney to represent you because the disciplinary action before the board is a legal proceeding, and attorneys have expertise in the law. The administrative law judge or hearing officer will often assist an unrepresented licensee in the technical aspects of presenting the evidence. Although it is not necessary to retain legal counsel, it is advisable.

Hearings Procedures

The opportunity to be heard requires that a licensing authority hold a hearing, so that the licensee can present evidence and provide responses to the allegations. Hearings are matters of public record, which means that the public may come to a hearing or may obtain a transcript of the hearing. In lieu of a hearing on alleged violations of the practice act, the state's attorney may offer the licensee a settlement (or consent) agreement. Settlement agreements are documents wherein the licensee admits that he or she violated the practice act and agrees to a sanction set forth in the agreement. In some cases, more lenient sanctions are offered if the licensee will agree to settle the matter through agreement because this resolution of a case saves the state time and money by not requiring the formal presentation of evidence at a hearing. The state board must approve the agreement before it is considered final.

A hearing generally begins with an announcement of the time and location that the hearing is being held and an introduction of the officials present. Generally, a presiding officer, usually an administrative law judge or hearing officer, will be present. A prosecuting attorney who works for the state will represent the state (the state's attorney). The licensee may have legal counsel or may proceed without legal counsel. The state's attorney will proceed first because the state bears the responsibility for demonstrating that the licensee has committed a violation of the law or regulations. The state's attorney may call witnesses, including the licensee, and may present documents. The licensee, in turn, may question the state's witnesses. Following the presentation of the state's case, the licensee will have an opportunity to call witnesses and produce documents. The state's attorney may question the licensee's witnesses. The hearing officer or any board member may also question any witness. The hearing usually concludes with closing arguments. Each side makes a statement about what it believes the evidence introduced at the hearing has shown, and whether or not it believes the licensee has violated the licensing law or regulations. The state's attorney and the licensee may also make

recommendations regarding the disciplinary sanction, if any, that they believe should be imposed. Following the hearing, the parties are generally given an opportunity to file a written argument regarding what they believe the evidence has shown. The board will issue a written opinion at a later date, generally anywhere from 2 months to a year after the hearing. The written opinion issued by the board will set forth what the board believes happened, and whether the licensee is subject to discipline. If the board finds that the licensee is subject to discipline, the written opinion will include an order setting forth the disciplinary sanction imposed by the board.

In some states, a licensing board may offer to resolve a matter through an "informal conference" rather than a formal hearing. Whether you are in a state that uses formal hearings or informal conferences to resolve disciplinary matters against licensees, you should learn as much as you can about the process that is followed and how you can dispute the outcome if it is not favorable to you.

Disciplinary Sanctions
Revocation of a License

Revocation of a license is considered the most severe sanction that a board may impose. In some states, revocation is the permanent preclusion of an individual from the practice of a profession. In other states, an individual may apply for re-licensure after 5 or 10 years. To be re-licensed, the individual must demonstrate all qualifications for licensure, including good moral character, and/or must retake the licensure examination.

Suspension of a License

Suspension is considered a severe sanction that may be imposed by a board because a suspension prohibits the sanctioned individual from practicing the profession. A suspension may be imposed for either a set period of time, or for an indefinite period of time, where the suspension is lifted after the licensee has completed specific tasks assigned by the board. For example, in a disciplinary case where the board found that the technician exceeded the scope of practice of the profession, the board might require the technician to cease practice until the technician has completed continuing education in the role of a veterinary technician and a continuing education course in the state's law governing veterinary technicians. When the sanctioned technician is permitted to return to practice, the board may further limit the technician by means of the terms of probation.

> **TECHNICIAN NOTE** Suspension of a license is considered a severe sanction because a suspension prohibits the sanctioned individual from practicing the profession.

Probation of Licensee

A licensing board may place a licensee on probation. A licensee who is on probationary status with the board is permitted to practice the profession; however, boards generally place limits on the practice of an individual who is on probation. Limits may include ongoing continuing education, practicing under a higher level of supervision, or restriction from performing specific tasks. For example, a technician who made an error in administering an anesthetic may be required to observe the administration of an anesthetic during 10 surgical procedures and then may be directly monitored by another technician for 10 surgical procedures before being able to resume normal practice.

Reprimand

A reprimand is a public censure of a licensee without suspension or probation. This sanction is generally reserved for violations or repeat violations that warrant more than a civil penalty.

Civil Penalty

A civil penalty is a fine paid to the licensing board. Virtually every state has statutory limits on the amount of the civil penalty that may be imposed for a violation of the state's licensing laws. Although this varies from state to state, caps are commonly set at $1000 (Pennsylvania, Tennessee), $5000 dollars (Illinois), and $10,000 (Connecticut) per violation. Some boards permit licensees who have been sanctioned with a civil penalty to make installment payments on the penalty.

> **TECHNICIAN NOTE**   A civil penalty is a fine paid to the licensing board. Virtually every state has statutory limits on the amount of the civil penalty that may be imposed for a violation of the state's licensing laws.

ADDITIONAL LAWS GOVERNING VETERINARY PRACTICE

LABOR LAWS

Labor laws define the rights and obligations of both employees and employers. They specify requirements for employment standards such as annual vacation pay, minimum wage, layoff procedures, and severance pay. Every jurisdiction has some type of labor law. Employees and employers should be aware of the labor legislation that governs employment in their state or province and should be familiar with the governmental agency that regulates these types of laws.

Hostile Work Environment

A hostile work environment can be defined as any workplace where:

1. The actions of workers or employers, including remarks, are overtly discriminatory with regard to age, race, gender, sexual orientation, sexual harassment, or disability.
2. An employee cannot reasonably perform his work owing to certain behaviors by management or coworkers.
3. A manager engages in behavior designed to make a worker quit in retaliation for previous actions.

4. A worker feels physically threatened. Violence is criminal in nature and should be reported to police. A police report will document the actions of the hostile person.

Many jurisdictions have few, if any, laws prohibiting hostile work environments. However, civil rights acts, discrimination in employment acts, and disabilities acts play a role in how a complaint is addressed, prosecuted, and resolved.

Safety in the Workplace

The Occupational Safety and Health Administration (OSHA), which resides in the Department of Labor, was created by Congress to enforce federal employment laws that help to ensure safe working environments for American workers. The primary goal of the Occupational Safety and Health Act is to prevent employment-related accidents and illnesses. It confirms that all workers have a fundamental right to a safe workplace. Safety is also supported by working with stakeholders to establish, promote, and enforce safe work practices, standards, and procedures. Stiff penalties or fines may be imposed on businesses that are noncompliant.

Most jurisdictions also have a Radiation Health and Safety Act that imposes minimum conditions for the protection of persons exposed to radiation and engaged in the operation and use of radiation equipment. Refer to Chapter 4 for additional information about OSHA compliance and safety in veterinary practices.

MEDICAL WASTE MANAGEMENT LAWS

Health care facilities, such as hospitals, physicians' offices, dental practices, and veterinary hospitals, generate a plethora of medical waste. Disposal of this waste is regulated by municipalities, states and provinces, and the federal government. Although states impose regulations for office, municipal, and medical waste, including potentially infectious waste, the federal government imposes regulations for hazardous waste, such as mercury and radioactive wastes. Medical waste includes cultures and stocks of infectious agents, body tissues, blood wastes and blood byproducts, sharps, contaminated carcasses and stall/cage beddings, surgery or autopsy waste that was once in contact with infectious agents, laboratory waste, medical equipment that has come in contact with infectious agents, and other contaminated biological materials.

In the United States, the Environmental Protection Agency (EPA) enforces the Medical Waste Tracking Act. This act defines medical waste, regulates its management and transport, and outlines enforcement processes. Most jurisdictions have a governmental agency that regulates the disposal of medical waste.

CONTROLLED SUBSTANCES

A *controlled substance* is a drug or chemical whose manufacture, possession, or use is regulated by government. In veterinary medicine, controlled substances are used on a daily basis. Federal and state laws legislation, such as the Federal and state Ccontrolled Ssubstance Aacts, establish[es] limitations and guidelines for possession, use, storage, exportation, and production of specific drugs. Controlled drugs are categorized into specific classes or schedules based on the drugs' capacity for addiction. In the United States, the Drug Enforcement Agency (DEA) has been empowered by Congress to enforce federal regulation of controlled substances. Controlled substance log books, used in many veterinary practices, are required by governmental regulatory agencies and legislation to document the distribution and use of controlled substances. State controlled substance acts frequently apply to all drugs and devices, not just those drugs that are on the state or Federal Controlled Substances lists. For example, in Pennsylvania, the state's controlled substance act prohibits a veterinarian from prescribing any drug for an animal unless the veterinarian has an established a veterinarian-client-patient relationship.

ANIMAL-RELATED LAWS

Animals Used in Research and Education

In the United States, the Animal Welfare Act (AWA) requires that minimum standards of care and treatment be provided for [most] some warm-blooded animals bred for commercial sale, used in research and higher education, transported commercially, and exhibited to the public. The AWA does not apply to mice, rats or birds, which represent approximately 90% of animals used in research and higher education. Animals regulated under this law include those exhibited in zoos, circuses, and marine mammal facilities, and pets transported on commercial airlines, as well as those used in research and for teaching purposes. The AWA prohibits staged dogfights, as well as bear and raccoon baiting.

The AWA was passed in 1966 and was amended in 1970, 1976, 1985, and 1990. Inspectors from Animal Care (a subsidiary of the USDA) conduct randomly scheduled, unannounced inspections to ensure that all regulated facilities are compliant. If an inspection reveals deficiencies in meeting AWA standards and regulations, the inspector instructs the facility to correct the problems within a specific time frame. If follow-up inspections show that the deficiencies are not corrected, the inspector documents repeat violations and may pursue more forceful legal action.

USDA-registered research facilities are required to have Institutional Animal Care and Use Committees (IACUCs) that help to enforce the AWA through the actions of employees within and near the institution. This form of self-assessment helps the institution stay on course with AWA compliance. Enforcing standards regarding animal housing, feeding, handling, and veterinary care and review of animal use protocols are included among the responsibilities of the IACUC. In Canada, the Animals in Research Act governs the use of animals in research and education. This act is enforced by the Canadian Council on Animal Care (CCAC), and registered research and educational institutions in Canada are required to have Animal Care Committees (ACCs) to help institutions oversee the care of institution-owned animals. Both IACUCs and ACCs are composed of at least one

veterinarian, an institutional member who is not a researcher, and a community or public member who is not affiliated with the institution and is not engaged in any aspect of laboratory animal science. The number of members on IACUCs and ACCs varies depending upon the size of the institution and the number of protocols reviewed annually.

AVMA-accredited programs of veterinary technology are required to have IACUC or ACC committees if the school owns regulated species. Each program must create protocols for clinical procedures conducted using animals. These protocols are subsequently reviewed by the IACUC or ACC for discussion, amendment, and approval.

Horse Protection Act

The U.S. Horse Protection Act (HPA) is a Federal law enacted in 1970 (P.L. 91-540, as amended, 15 U.S.C. § 1821 et seq.) to prohibit horses subjected to practices known as *soring* from participating in shows, sales, exhibitions, or auctions. Soring has been a widespread problem in the Tennessee Walking Horse show community and includes such horrific practices as the external application of caustic chemicals to the pasterns of horses coupled with exercising the horse with heavy chains fastened around its pasterns to create pain and various methods of "pressure shoeing" to cause pain to the horse every time the horse places its front feet on the ground. The law is enforced by USDA-APHIS, but the enforcement program has been underfunded for years and only a very small number of violators have been criminally prosecuted. In early 2011, the USDA announced new minimum civil penalties for violations of the act and regulations. The HPA also prohibits drivers from transporting sored horses to or from any of these events. Several states have specifically addressed soring as part of the state's criminal statutes related to prosecutions for animal cruelty. On June 14, 2012, the AVMA and AAEP (American Association of Equine Professionals) called for the USDA to ban all action devices and "performance packages" (a type of elevated shoeing) in both the training and showing of Tennessee Walking Horses.

Endangered Species Act

The primary goals of the Endangered Species Act are to prevent the extinction of imperiled plant and animal life, and to recover and maintain those populations by removing or lessening threats to their survival. This act is administered by two federal agencies—the U.S. Fish and Wildlife Service (FWS) and the National Oceanic and Atmospheric Administration (NOAA).

Animal Cruelty Prevention

In the United States, each state's criminal code prohibits animal cruelty. Variation is seen from state to state in the laws prohibiting animal cruelty both in the animals that are protected under the laws and the specific acts that are prohibited. Every state prohibits dog and cock fighting and intentional acts that injure or kill certain animals in a cruel manner. In addition, state anti-cruelty laws almost always exempt farmed animals from the protections provided by the laws. Most states also prohibit neglecting animals In Canada, regional ordinances often include cruelty laws. Humane investigators and police officers may investigate complaints of animal cruelty. At the Federal level in the United States, certain statutes intend to protect certain animals at very specific times. For example, the Humane Methods of Slaughter Act seeks to ensure that farmed animals are treated humanely on the property of a slaughterhouse.

LAWS SPECIFIC TO CANADA
Canadian Food Inspection Agency (CFIA)
The Canadian Food Inspection Agency enforces the criminal code through routine inspections, unannounced site inspections, and response to reports of noncompliance.

Provincial Legislation on Animal Welfare
Each province has legislation concerning animal welfare. Provincial legislation and regulations tend to be general in scope, covering a wide range of animal welfare interests. Some provinces have regulations pertaining to specific species.

Nongovernment Animal Welfare Organizations
A number of Canadian nongovernment organizations have animal welfare mandates and assume responsibility for various aspects of animal welfare. The National Farm Animal Care Council (NFACC), for example, facilitates collaboration among all of its members with respect to the care and management of farm animals. The NFACC also facilitates sharing of information and monitors trends and initiatives in domestic and international marketplaces.

Humane Transportation of Animals
The Canadian Food Inspection Agency ensures the humane transport of food animal species. Regulations prohibit overcrowding, transport of incompatible animals in the same stall, and transport of animals unfit for travel. These regulations specify appropriate conditions for loading and unloading animals, adequate feeding and watering regimes, maximum transit times, minimum rest periods, and bedding requirements. Regulations also require animal handlers to take animals to the nearest veterinary medical facility for care if they are compromised in transit.

Canadian Meat Inspection Act
The *Meat Inspection Act* established standards for the humane handling and slaughter of food animals in federally inspected slaughter facilities. The Canadian Food Inspection Agency places inspectors at federally registered slaughter establishments to monitor the handling and slaughter of food animals.

RECOMMENDED READINGS

Bassert JM, McCurnin DM: McCurnin's clinical textbook for veterinary technicians, ed 7, St Louis, 2010, Saunders Elsevier, pp 1–53.

Canadian Vet Tech (a newsmagazine for veterinary technologists and technicians). Features in-depth articles and continuing education specifically for veterinary technicians. This magazine is included for provincial Association members who belong to CAAHTT.

International Institute for Animal Law: Available at: www.animallaw.com (accessed June 27, 2011).

NAVTA Journal is the official publication of the National Association of Veterinary Technicians in America (NAVTA) and is exclusive to NAVTA members (www.navta.net).

Rockett J, Lattanzio C, Anderson K: Patient assessment, intervention and documentation for the veterinary technician: a guide to developing care plans and SOAP's, Florence, KY, 2008, Delmar Cengage Learning.

Rollin, Bernard E: The Well-Being of Farm Animals: Challenges and Solutions, ed 1, 2004, Wiley-Blackwell, ISBN 0-8138-0473-6.

Rollin, Bernard E: Animal Rights & Human Morality, ed 3, 2006, Prometheus Books, ISBN 1-59102-421-8.

Shapiro LS: Applied animal ethics, Albany, NY, 2000, Delmar Thomson Learning.

Technews, a journal for Canadian veterinary technicians (www.oavt.org).

U.S. Department of Agriculture, National Agriculture Library: Animal Welfare Act. Available at: http://awic.nal.usda.gov/nal_display/index.php? (accessed June 27, 2011).

Veterinary Technician Journal features in-depth articles and continuing education specifically for veterinary technicians (www.vetlearn.com).

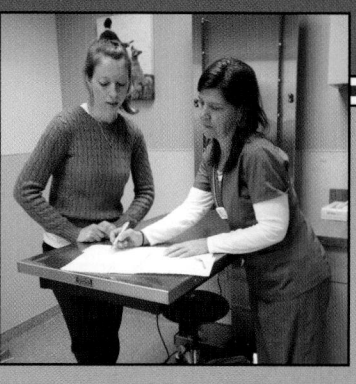

2

Veterinary Practice Management

Karen E. Felsted

OUTLINE

Types of Veterinary Practices, *39*
Typical Employee Positions, *39*
Management Personnel, *40*
Veterinarians, *42*
Veterinary Technicians and
    Technologists, *42*
Veterinary Assistants, *43*
Receptionists, *43*
Kennel, Ward, and Barn Attendants, *43*
Practice Facilities and Workflow, *44*
Small Animal General Practices, *45*
Small Animal House Call Practices, *51*
Specialty and Emergency Practices, *51*
Large Animal Mobile Units, *52*

Large Animal Haul-In Facilities, *52*
Clients and Client Services, *54*
Importance of Client Communication, *55*
Dealing With Difficult Clients, *57*
**Management of the Veterinary
    Practice,** *57*
Planning, *58*
Human Resources, *59*
Marketing, *62*
Financial, *68*
Operations, *71*
Computerization of the Veterinary
    Practice, *75*
Summary, *78*

LEARNING OBJECTIVES

When you have completed this chapter, you will be able to:

1. Pronounce, spell, and define each of the Key Terms in this chapter.
2. List the terms used to describe various types of veterinary facilities.
3. List the roles and responsibilities of each member of the veterinary health care team.
4. Describe the basic flow of clients, patients, and employees through a typical veterinary hospital.
5. Outline the key elements of effectively working with clients, including the importance of communication skills, myths about communication skills, and how to diffuse the anger of difficult clients.
6. Describe the major job management functions needed to effectively run a veterinary hospital.
7. Describe the components of a comprehensive business model.
8. Describe the primary components of excellent practice management.
9. List examples of stressors in the veterinary workplace, and describe ways to ameliorate the effects of those stressors on personnel.
10. Describe the major areas in which veterinary practices employ internal and external marketing techniques.
11. List some of the major tasks associated with good financial management.
12. List reasons why management and financial analysis are important to the business of veterinary medicine.
13. Discuss the importance of efficient operations for practice revenue.
14. Discuss key areas in which computerization adds to the efficiency and productivity of a veterinary practice.

*The authors and publisher wish to acknowledge Dennis M. McCurnin and Roger L. Lukens, for their
previous contributions to this chapter.*

KEY TERMS

Accounts receivable
Appointment system
Cash flow
Clinic
Consultation
Emergency facility
Gross revenue total
Haul-in facility
Hospital
Mobile facility
National Commission on
    Veterinary Economic
    Issues (NCVEI)
Net income
Office
On-call emergency
    service
Outpatient
Petty cash
Profits
Referral facility
Specialty facility
Strategic planning
Traffic flow
Veterinary teaching
    hospital
Walk-in system

INTRODUCTION

Veterinary technicians today have diverse employment opportunities available to them. Some of these include working in laboratory animal medicine and in the pharmaceutical industry. However, most veterinary technicians work in clinical practice. A vast majority of veterinary practices are operated as privately owned, for-profit businesses, and most offer a full complement of veterinary services, including care for sick and injured animals, as well as preventive and wellness care. A few practices, such as SPCA (Society for the Prevention of Cruelty to Animals) shelters, are operated by animal welfare organizations as nonprofit organizations; these practices commonly offer more limited services than those offered by for-profit practices.

The revenue and **profits** generated by a practice make it possible for veterinary health care team members to provide good quality medical care to patients. In the long run, it is not possible for a practice to offer excellent veterinary care if the practice is not economically successful. The revenue and profits earned by practices are reinvested in obtaining equipment, drugs, and supplies; in hiring staff; and in updating and maintaining the **hospital** building. In addition, revenue is used to pay all employees of the practice, including the practice owner. Only if the practice does well economically can the people who work in the practice thrive economically.

It is not easy to operate a veterinary practice successfully from a medical or a business standpoint. Much time and money must be invested in the activities necessary to make the practice a success. Effective management of a veterinary practice as a business has become complicated because of increased competition, growing malpractice threats, new technology, the availability of the Internet, shifting client expectations, and continued inflation of the costs of medical equipment, supplies, and personnel.

Not all practices are structured in the same way; some are focused solely on companion animals, and others treat horses exclusively; still others offer veterinary care for a variety of species, large and small. Some practices are located in their own facility; others offer only ambulatory care, and some provide both ambulatory and nonambulatory services. Most practices focus on general medicine, but a growing number offer emergency or specialty care. No matter the type of practice, most team members will have some role in management activities that allow the practice to thrive. Therefore, students need to develop a working knowledge of the principles of practice management to be effective technicians, to contribute to the financial success of the practice, and to prepare for future advancement in the veterinary technology profession. This understanding is critical for assessing practice differences when searching for the best employment opportunity.

TECHNICIAN NOTE In the long run, it is not possible for a practice to offer excellent veterinary care if the practice is not economically successful. Only if the practice does well financially can the people who work in the practice thrive financially.

TECHNICIAN NOTE Most team members will have some role in management activities that allow the practice to thrive. Management responsibilities are commonly divided into the following areas: planning, human resources, marketing, financial, operations, facility, and equipment.

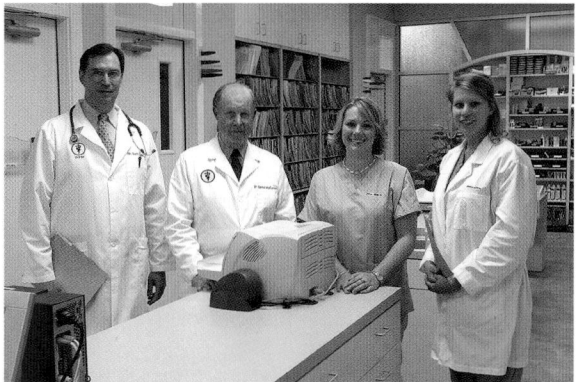

FIGURE 2-1 Members of the veterinary health care team.

TYPES OF VETERINARY PRACTICES

About two-thirds[1] of veterinarians in the United States work in private clinical practice, taking care of animals owned as pets or for production purposes. Most practices have between two and three full-time–equivalent veterinarians working in them, although they range in size from 1 veterinarian to 20 or more. Most practices are owned by veterinarians who also work in the practice. A small percentage of practices, perhaps 5% to 10%, are owned by corporate groups such as VCA Antech or National Veterinary Associates (NVA), which own large numbers of practices.

Most practices limit the types of animals they treat, for example, they may offer care only to a single species such as cats or horses, only to companion animals (dogs, cats, exotic pets), or only to large animals (livestock, horses). If the livestock population in an area is high, a group practice may have several large animal veterinarians, each focusing on a specific species. Some practices, called *mixed animal practices*, see a variety of species, including companion animals, livestock, and horses. A few practices are limited to exotic animals such as reptiles, birds, and small mammals. About 77% of veterinarians practice small animal medicine, 8% work in food animal practices, 6% in equine practices, and about 7% in mixed animal practices.[1]

Most practicing veterinarians are general practitioners who offer a primary care level of service. Complicated cases are often referred to veterinarians who are specialists working in **referral facilities** (secondary care providers) or veterinary schools (tertiary care providers). These veterinary specialists are board certified in surgery, internal medicine, dermatology, ophthalmology, or other areas. Veterinary technician specialists also work in referral practices and in hospitals affiliated with veterinary medical schools. Veterinary **emergency facilities** can be found in all major cities and in many smaller communities as well. Sometimes they are part of a referral and **specialty facility** or a veterinary teaching hospital, but often they are stand-alone businesses. These facilities are usually open when general practices are not, such as at night and on weekends and holidays. This network of referring practitioners not only provides access to the best quality of care possible, it also serves as the foundation of clinical research at tertiary care centers in veterinary medical schools. Ongoing clinical and basic science research is absolutely necessary to improve our understanding of the pathogenesis of diseases, new and effective diagnostics, and effective treatments.

Most general practices open between 7 AM and 8 AM, close around 6 PM during the week, and have some Saturday hours as well. Some practices are open in the evening on one or more days and some have Sunday hours. Specialty hospitals generally open around 8 AM and close between 5 PM and 6 PM. They usually do not offer Saturday or Sunday hours. Emergency practices are generally open nights, weekends, and holidays—all the times general practices are closed. Teaching hospitals at veterinary colleges tend to have similar hours for their general and specialty practices and accept emergencies 24 hours a day, 365 days per year.

Veterinary practices can be described in various ways such as a **clinic**, an **office**, or a **veterinary teaching hospital**. The American Veterinary Medical Association (AVMA) has developed guidelines (Box 2-1) for consistency in naming veterinary facilities to prevent confusion by the general public.[1]

TYPICAL EMPLOYEE POSITIONS

Regardless of the size and type of the practice, overall types of staff positions tend to be similar. Most practices have the following types of employees: management personnel, veterinarians, veterinary technicians and technologists, veterinary assistants, receptionists, and kennel, ward, or barn attendants (Figure 2-1). Veterinary technicians are graduates of an AVMA-accredited program of veterinary technology; veterinary technologists are those who have graduated from an accredited 4-year program. In large practices, the roles may be further subdivided, for example, the practice may have **outpatient** technicians and surgery technicians, or the management staff may consist of a hospital administrator, a practice manager, and an accounting staff. In smaller practices, staff members may have dual roles. For example, a veterinary technician may also handle some management duties, or a veterinary assistant may also work in the kennel. In these practices, staff members are often cross-trained in

BOX 2-1	Guidelines for Naming Veterinary Facilities

Veterinary teaching hospital: A veterinary teaching hospital is a facility in which consultative, clinical, and hospital services are rendered, and in which a large staff of basic and applied veterinary scientists perform significant research and teaching of professional veterinary students (DVM or equivalent degree) and house officers.

Hospital: A veterinary or animal hospital is a facility in which the practice conducted typically includes inpatient and outpatient diagnostics and treatment.

Clinic: A veterinary or animal clinic is a facility in which the practice conducted may include inpatient and outpatient diagnosis and treatment.

Outpatient clinic: A veterinary or animal outpatient clinic is a facility in which the practice conducted may include short-term admission of patients, but where all patients are discharged at the end of the workday.

Office: A veterinary office is a veterinary practice where a limited or consultative practice is conducted; it typically provides no facilities for housing or inpatient diagnostics or treatment.

Mobile facility: A mobile practice is a veterinary practice conducted from a vehicle with special medical or surgical facilities, or from a vehicle suitable for making house or farm calls. Regardless of mode of transportation, such practice shall have a permanent base of operations with a published address and telecommunication capabilities for making appointments or responding to emergency situations.

Emergency facility: A veterinary emergency facility is one with the primary function of receiving, treating, and monitoring emergency patients during its specified hours of operation. A veterinarian is in attendance at all hours of operation, and sufficient staff is available to provide timely and appropriate care. Veterinarians, support staff, instrumentation, medications, and supplies must be sufficient to provide an appropriate level of emergency care. A veterinary emergency service may be an independent, after-hours service; an independent 24-hour service; or part of a full-service hospital.

On-call emergency service: An **on-call emergency service** is a veterinary medical service where veterinarians and staff are not necessarily on the premises during all hours of operation, or one where, after initial triage and treatment are provided, veterinarians leave orders for continued patient care by staff and remain available on-call.

Specialty facility: A specialty facility is a veterinary/animal facility that provides services by board-certified veterinarian(s)/specialists.

Referral facility: A referral facility provides services by those veterinarians with a special interest in certain species or a particular area of veterinary medicine.

Center: The word "Center" in the name of a veterinary/animal facility strongly implies a unique depth or scope of practice (e.g., Animal Medical Center, Veterinary Imaging Center, Canine Sports Medicine Center).

several positions, so that the practice can continue to function when sickness, vacation, or emergencies arise and a key individual is out for the day. In most practices, everyone is expected to do some activities, for example, it may be the receptionist's job to answer the telephone, but if the receptionist is busy and the phone keeps ringing, everyone should be willing to answer it. Entering charges into a client's invoice may be the primary responsibility of the technician, but veterinarian, receptionist, and kennel workers sometimes will need to do this as well. In all practices, everyone is expected to communicate well and contribute to outstanding client service.

To be effective, the veterinarian-owner must act as the overall hospital chief executive officer (CEO) and must delegate appropriate areas of responsibility to veterinary technicians and other members of the team. In the best run practices, job duties are pushed down to the lowest-level person who can do the job well within the legal scope of practice.

> **TECHNICIAN NOTE** In the best run practices, job duties are delegated to the lowest-level person who can do the job well within the legal scope of practice. This is why successful practices delegate all clinical care duties to veterinary technicians and other members of the veterinary health care team, except those tasks that, by law, must be performed exclusively by veterinarians.

This kind of delegation is a key component of good management. In "real life," it is not uncommon to see veterinarians doing tasks that a well-trained technician is legally allowed to do and can do better. Many also hire veterinary technicians but have them perform the duties of veterinary assistants and caretakers. Consequently, the practice spends more money than necessary on personnel, causing frustration among veterinarians and veterinary technicians who are not given the opportunity to fully exercise the skills they were educated to perform. It is important to remember, however, that most veterinary practices are small and have a limited number of employees; except in the largest practices, it is difficult to fully limit duties to just one individual or staff position.

Regardless of position in the hospital setting, all personnel should have a detailed job description. A job description will allow both the employee and management to maintain a clear understanding of areas of responsibility. Job descriptions are also useful when new employees are hired or employees are replaced. Common duties of each employee are discussed in the following paragraphs; remember, however, that some variation may occur, depending on the way in which an individual practice is structured.

MANAGEMENT PERSONNEL

Veterinary practices are small businesses that must be efficiently operated and financially successful if they are to offer quality patient care. To survive as a veterinary hospital, the practice must survive as a <u>business</u>. Ensuring survival is the job of practice owners and management staff.

Historically, veterinarians who owned a veterinary practice often performed the management tasks necessary to keep the practice economically viable and running smoothly. As practices have gotten bigger and the challenges of management have become greater, increasing numbers of veterinarians are delegating business management responsibilities to trained managers. Unfortunately, the quality of management among veterinary practices varies widely; some practices are managed well and others poorly.

The organization of management staff varies according to practice size and management philosophy. Three commonly seen management positions are office manager, practice manager, and hospital administrator. No commonly accepted job descriptions are available for these positions, and the duties assigned to each position and the quality of work performed can vary widely. However, a typical division of labor is provided below:

- *Office manager*—Office managers generally report to the practice owner or the practice manager (if one has been hired). Their duties include hiring and training office and reception staff, scheduling shifts and supervising receptionists, acting as a client liaison when problems or complaints arise, preparing bank deposits, collecting **accounts receivable**, and performing clerical work.
- *Practice manager*—Practice managers generally report to the practice owner or to the hospital administrator (if there is one). They often have more extensive management training and experience than do office managers, and they have a wider range of management responsibilities. Typically, their duties include hiring, training, scheduling, and supervising all nondoctor staff, carrying out marketing activities, and preparing or supervising the preparation of accounting and financial documents such as accounts receivable, accounts payable, budgets, and financial analyses. Establishing budgets and fees, purchasing supplies and equipment including maintaining inventory control, serving as a client liaison, managing the computer network, and supervising and organizing workflow are additional responsibilities of the practice manager. Practice managers generally are not involved in medical management duties, although they may be in charge of the nonmedical aspects of veterinarians' work.
- *Hospital administrators*—These individuals are generally responsible for all activities of the hospital, both medical and administrative, and run the hospital in conjunction with practice owners. Hospital administrators are also responsible for the tasks commonly performed by office managers and practice managers, in addition to hiring and supervising veterinarians and veterinary technicians.

In some hospitals, head receptionists and head technicians may perform some management duties in their area, in addition to their regular responsibilities. Large hospitals may have management personnel solely responsible for human resources, finance, or marketing.

The size of the practice generally influences the management structure. In small practices, management tasks may be shared among several individuals. Practice owners, for example, may delegate some tasks to receptionists, technicians, or office managers, such as inventory control and staff scheduling, but may do planning-, finance-, and employee-related work themselves. Team members handling management tasks may report directly to the practice owner or to the office manager. Office managers report to practice owners.

Medium-sized practices often have a full-time practice manager whose responsibility is to handle the vast majority of management duties. Some duties may still be delegated to other team members, and the practice may also have employees in head technician and head receptionist positions. Practice owners generally remain involved in some high-level tasks such as hiring veterinarians, generating **strategic planning**, and managing financial issues. Most often, the head technician, the head receptionist, and others doing management tasks report to the practice manager, and the practice manager in turn reports to the practice owner.

Large to very large practices often have both a practice manager and a hospital administrator on staff and, in addition, may have a human resources (HR) manager, a finance manager, a bookkeeper or accounting department, and clerical staff. Usually, the HR manager, the finance manager, the accounting staff, and other low-level management personnel report to the practice manager. The practice manager reports to the hospital administrator, and the administrator to the practice owner.

Practices owned by large corporate groups generally have a hospital administrator and a practice manager, who are responsible for day-to-day management of the practice with support from the corporate group.

Many nonowner veterinarians working in clinical practice do not have formal management duties assigned to them. It would be expected, however, that they would demonstrate the traits of good managers and leaders in client service, communication, teamwork, and other areas.

It is not uncommon to see veterinary technicians who have an interest in management moving into the role of practice manager. The obvious advantage to this is that the technician generally has worked at the practice for a long time and knows how the practice operates. The disadvantage is that the technician may not have the management skills necessary to run the practice well and may have too many friendships among the staff to be able to effectively deal with personnel issues. Not all practice owners, many of whom are veterinarians, offer the training and support necessary for veterinary technicians to be successful in new management roles. Technicians who are interested in management can learn more about what management work entails by attending management-related continuing education classes before moving into these new roles.

TECHNICIAN NOTE   It is not uncommon to see veterinary technicians who have an interest in management moving into the role of practice manager.

The Veterinary Hospital Managers Association is the only organization that can certify veterinary practice managers. Managers who complete the program become certified veterinary practice managers (CVPMs). Candidates must document veterinary management work experience and completion of continuing education in management, must submit letters of recommendation, and must pass an examination administered by the CVPM board. The CVPM program is accredited by the Institute for Credentialing Excellence.

TECHNICIAN NOTE   The Veterinary Hospital Managers Association is the only organization that can certify veterinary practice managers. Managers who complete the program become certified veterinary practice managers (CVPMs).

VETERINARIANS

The primary activities of veterinarians in clinical practice include diagnosing and treating ill or injured animals and providing preventive or wellness care to animals to reduce the likelihood of disease or accident in the future. Generally, a full physical examination is performed on each animal presented for care, or an assessment of herd health is completed, and findings from these assessments, along with results from various laboratories and imaging and other diagnostic tests, are used to diagnose what is wrong with the animal. Treatment can consist of a broad range of activities, including surgery, dental cleaning and extractions, oral or parenteral medication, hospitalization, acupuncture, and many others.

Preventive or "wellness care" activities for companion animals include an annual physical examination, vaccinations, and administration and/or prescription of parasiticides. Pet owners, even those who have owned pets before, often do not understand what care is needed for their pets or why it is important. A critical component of veterinary care is communication about these issues with pet owners.

Large animal practitioners and those who work in shelter medicine focus on the care of the animal group as a whole, as well as on individual animals.

Ideally, the veterinarian delegates most animal care tasks (as allowed by the state practice act) to veterinary technicians and technologists; examples of these tasks include providing anesthesia, dental prophylaxes, imaging, laboratory procedures, and client communications. Delegation of these duties to the veterinary technician allows the veterinarian to increase his or her own efficiency and allows the veterinary technician to carry out the job that he or she was educated to do and in this way to have a meaningful role in the hospital.

VETERINARY TECHNICIANS AND TECHNOLOGISTS

As discussed in Chapter 1, a veterinary technician is a graduate of a 2- or 3-year AVMA-accredited program in veterinary technology, and a veterinary technologist is a graduate of a 4-year, AVMA-accredited program. Unlike the veterinarian, who is responsible for making a diagnosis and curing the patient, the veterinary technician and technologist evaluate and ameliorate the patient's reactions to disease. Assessing and reassessing the patient, making technician evaluations, and using independent critical thinking to develop and implement a nursing plan of care are the primary steps in the veterinary technician practice model. Veterinary technicians and technologists are responsible for carrying out the medical treatment plans of the veterinarian, alerting the veterinarian to changes in patient status, educating the client about disease processes and home treatment protocols, and completing medical record entries (Figure 2-2). Recognizing and addressing patient discomfort and anticipating potential complications are additional important responsibilities of the veterinary technician.

TECHNICIAN NOTE   Assessing and reassessing the patient, making technician evaluations, and using independent critical thinking to develop and implement a nursing plan of care are the primary steps in the veterinary technician practice model.

The role of veterinary technicians and assistants can vary greatly among veterinary hospitals, depending on the size of the hospital and the organization of workflow. Many hospitals do not have credentialed veterinary technicians;

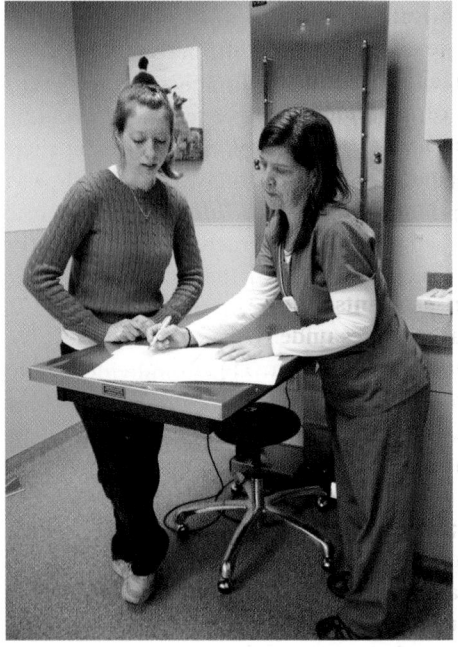

FIGURE 2-2 Technician explaining a diagnosis to a client using a visual aid. (Courtesy Dr. Joanna Bassert.)

therefore, veterinarians and veterinary assistants perform all animal care duties. Other hospitals have a mixture of technicians and assistants.

The term *technician* or *tech* is too often used erroneously in veterinary practices to describe many or all animal care personnel regardless of educational background, credential status, or skill set of the individual. It is important for veterinary practices to use proper terminology, so that clients are clear about the qualifications of each member of the veterinary health care team. Staff members who wear name tags that use unapproved terminology, such as *veterinary nurse*, and practices that make no distinction between veterinary assistants and veterinary technicians or technologists may confuse pet owners and are doing a disservice to their employees in not recognizing those with true credentials. Indeed, the Internet-educated client of today may construe these practices as an intentional effort, on the part of the practice, to deceive the client by inflating the image of noncredentialed personnel. The development of National Association of Veterinary Technicians in America (NAVTA)- and AVMA-approved terminology decades ago, together with official terminology as outlined in state practice acts, offers the pet owner and the veterinary practice owner clear terminology to distinguish credentialed from noncredentialed staff.[2]

> **TECHNICIAN NOTE** The development of NAVTA- and AVMA-approved terminology decades ago, together with official terminology outlined in state practice acts, offers the pet owner and the veterinary practice owner clear terminology to distinguish credentialed from noncredentialed veterinary staff.

Large private practices such as specialty and referral practices and veterinary teaching hospitals often have large caseloads that allow veterinary technicians to work exclusively in one area of a hospital, such as in the operating room, the intensive care unit, and the departments of anesthesiology, cardiology, internal medicine, ophthalmology, dermatology, radiology, and clinical pathology.

VETERINARY ASSISTANTS

Veterinary assistants generally perform animal care and ward maintenance duties under the supervision of a veterinarian or a veterinary technician. These duties may include using animal restraint; performing laboratory work; filling prescriptions; preparing patients for surgery; administering and monitoring treatments; bathing animals; cleaning cages; feeding, watering, and walking hospitalized patients and boarders; and performing other duties as needed to create a smooth patient flow in the hospital.

Assistants may be responsible for cleaning and maintaining the building, wards, and barn (in large animal practices). In some practices, some of these tasks may be performed by kennel or barn attendants instead of by veterinary assistants.

The role of the assistant is generally determined by the size and type of practice and the number of staff members.

RECEPTIONISTS

Receptionist is a key position in any hospital operation. Receptionists are the first and last person a client sees and are often instrumental in leaving the pet owner with a good impression. Typical receptionist duties include making appointments, answering questions in-person or on the phone, handling emergencies, greeting clients, updating client and patient information, setting up the medical record for the current visit, checking clients in and out, quoting fees, maintaining appointment schedules for veterinarians and veterinary technicians, handling money and bank deposits, and managing accounts receivable.

Movement of patients and their medical records from the receptionist in the front to the veterinary technician in the back is critical for an efficiently functioning hospital. Both receptionists and technicians should have some understanding of the other's duties and how their tasks affect others. They should regularly work together to resolve issues that are impeding the ability of each group to do its job well.

> **TECHNICIAN NOTE** Movement of patients and their medical records from the receptionist in the front to the veterinary technician in the back is critical for an efficiently functioning hospital. Both receptionists and technicians should have some understanding of each other's duties and how their tasks affect others.

KENNEL, WARD, AND BARN ATTENDANTS

Attendants perform the basic husbandry required to keep patients clean, groomed, fed, watered, and exercised, with the safety and comfort of each patient taken into consideration. Ward staff must observe and record the patient's appetites, attitudes, bowel movements, and urinary output and must alert the staff about observed abnormal behavior. They also move patients from wards to the treatment area, to the reception area for discharge, or to surgery. Ward staff can double as veterinary assistants through cross-training.

Attendants are usually responsible for ongoing cleaning and maintenance of all areas of the hospital. Cleaning and sanitation are critical in a hospital environment to prevent nosocomial infections—those inadvertently acquired by patients from the hospital environment (Box 2-2). Nosocomial infections in human hospitals are well known as *super bacteria* because they have developed resistance to commonly used antibiotics.

General maintenance within the building is an ongoing challenge. Floors, flat surfaces, walls, cages, runs, and stalls must be kept clean and odor free. Counters, magazine racks, and pictures need to be organized and dusted frequently. The reception room, examination rooms, and public bathrooms must be inspected and cleaned regularly throughout each day. Everyone in the practice must assume some of the

---

BOX 2-2 | Nosocomial Infections

Nosocomial infections are new infections acquired by patients while in the veterinary facility.

Examples of Nosocomial Infection Sources
- Staff: unwashed hands; contaminated equipment, including dirty needles, clothing, and boots; inadequate cleaning and disinfecting protocols; breaks in aseptic technique
- Other patients: direct contact, airborne droplets, hair, excrement, blood
- Environment: cages, drains, floors, walls, feed or water pans, dust, bedding

Preventing Nosocomial Infections
- Always wash hands between patients.
- Always wear clean clothing and boots.
- Always follow established cleaning, disinfecting, sterilizing, and aseptic protocols.
- Conduct ongoing training in these areas.

---

cleaning responsibility. One of the reasons why cleanup in a veterinary practice is so challenging is the larger quantity of hair shed by animals than humans. Hair is such a major problem that a vacuum system needs to be available and used before general mopping; otherwise, a buildup of hair is simply moved around the facility. Some practices have been built with a central vacuum system to improve the efficiency of hair reduction from the floors. Removal of hair from the environment is also extremely important for the proper care of electronic equipment and computers.

Clients notice hospital cleanliness. When one client actually complains, many other clients probably are quietly forming a negative impression of the practice. If the veterinary hospital is to be considered a modern and progressive medical facility, all personnel must rigidly monitor odors and sanitation. Whenever a pet soils an area or cage, it must be cleaned thoroughly as soon as possible. Appropriate disinfectants must be used to prevent odor buildup. Deodorizers may be of benefit to help clean the area but should not be used to cover up a sanitation problem. Appropriate ventilation systems should be in place throughout the building.

Equipment cleaning must be an ongoing activity. Each major piece of equipment should be assigned to a specified member of the hospital team to keep it well maintained. It is recommended that the person most familiar with each piece of equipment be assigned to maintain it. If this is done, all equipment will last longer and will always be ready for use when needed for quality patient care. Nonmedical equipment, such as typewriters, calculators, computers, air conditioning and heating units, lawn mowers, and related equipment, should also have regular maintenance. The responsibility to maintain this equipment is most commonly assigned to those who use it most often.

Important medical equipment, such as anesthesia machines, endoscopes, and ultrasound machines, should have a documented, regular maintenance schedule to ensure proper servicing and consistent functioning of the equipment.

Although each position in the hospital has its own specific responsibilities, it is essential that all employees work together as a team to maximize the veterinarians' effectiveness and productivity, as well as the pet owners' service experiences. Team members must be selected on the basis of their ability to work together efficiently as an effective team rather than their ability to perform isolated duties.

> **TECHNICIAN NOTE**   Although each position in the hospital has its own specific responsibilities, it is essential that all employees work together as a team to maximize the veterinarians' effectiveness and productivity, as well as the pet owners' service experiences.

PRACTICE FACILITIES AND WORKFLOW

The facilities of veterinary practices vary greatly based on the needs of clients and the species of animals seen by the practice. Facility design must accommodate the needs of patients, the number of clients served, the interests of the veterinarians, the level of care to be provided, and the level of financing available for investing in the facility.

As discussed previously, the practice may limit veterinary service to a single species (feline, equine, swine, cattle), to small animals (dogs, cats, exotic pets), to large animals (livestock and horses), or to exotic animals, or it may serve as a mixed practice (many species). Each type of practice has unique requirements for facility design and construction. Large animal and mixed practices may provide all veterinary services on the animal owner's premises, may have **haul-in facilities** for these species, or may provide both options as a convenience to the client. Some companion animal practices provide house calls, in addition to work done at the practice facility, and a few veterinarians operate house call–only practices.

Many state practice acts and other regulations that apply to veterinary practices not only have been updated to specify standards of practice and professional competency for both veterinarians and technicians, they also have adopted facility and equipment requirements. Some states require facility registration and have hired inspectors to ensure that standards established by the state are being met.

The American Animal Hospital Association (AAHA) offers voluntary accreditation programs for veterinary hospitals. The process generally takes 3 to 9 months to complete and is designed to help practices refine and improve their services in five areas:
1. Quality of care
2. Diagnostics and pharmacy
3. Management
4. Medical records
5. Facility

The most common type of veterinary facility is a small animal practice devoted to general care that employs two to three veterinarians; this will be used as the model for discussing facility design and client, patient, and employee workflow. Issues unique to larger general practices, referral hospitals, emergency clinics, veterinary teaching hospitals, large animal or mixed animal practices, and ambulatory practices will be discussed at the end of this section.

Hospital facilities are generally designed to provide overnight hospitalization, complete surgical facilities, and sufficient examination rooms to allow outpatient services. They must have ancillary support areas such as a reception room, a laboratory, a pharmacy, imaging, diagnostic procedures, treatment, and an inpatient ward space. Some hospitals also offer boarding and grooming services. The appropriate size and location of each area in the hospital are related to the types of services offered by the hospital, the numbers of veterinarians and support staff in the practice, and the numbers of clients and patients served.

SMALL ANIMAL GENERAL PRACTICES
Facility Exterior
Pet owners generally choose a practice that is convenient to their homes; therefore, most companion animal practices are located near populous residential areas. The practice facility, both inside and out, should convey an attractive and professional image and should meet the needs of patients, clients, and employees (Figure 2-3). In most communities, pet owners have many choices when it comes to selecting a veterinary practice. Practices that will be most successful are those that best meet the needs and expectations of the pet owner. Ideally, veterinary practices are located in areas of high visibility and easy access. Not only is well-placed, well-lit professional signage a marketing tool, it also allows clients to find the practice easily at night and during an emergency.

A client's initial impression of a practice is based on the appearance of the building and grounds. Regular maintenance, including painting and repair, is therefore very important. Landscaping should be regularly attended to as dead plants and weeds do not send the right message. The parking lot should be clean, neat, and well lighted and should offer easy access to the hospital entrance (Figure 2-4). The parking lot entrance and exit should be clearly marked by signs. Parking spaces should be reserved for clients only, with employee parking behind the building or in a remote area away from the building entrance.

The entrance to the veterinary facility should be in full view and should be well marked to allow easy access. If more than one entrance is available, as is occasionally done to separate small and large animals or canines and felines, each entrance should be well marked. To prevent client congestion, the entrance and the exit should be separate. Practice employees should not use the public entrance of the building. Further, those providing routine deliveries and service activities should enter and exit the building away from client contact when possible.

Professional activities within a veterinary hospital can be grouped into four areas: outpatient, inpatient, surgical, and support.

Outpatient Areas
Most patients visit a veterinary hospital as an outpatient. This means that the pet will not be admitted to the hospital and will not be staying overnight. Outpatient areas are composed primarily of the reception area and the examination rooms, but the laboratory and pharmacy areas are used for outpatients, as well as for hospitalized patients. Clients generally cannot judge the quality of medicine in a veterinary practice; much of their evaluation of the quality of the practice is based on their impressions of the facility and the level of client service. A disorganized, dirty, smelly, noisy hospital will not inspire confidence in clients about the level of patient care, nor will it convey value for the fees charged. It is important for employees to impress clients by wearing clean, neat uniforms and by maintaining a well-groomed appearance.

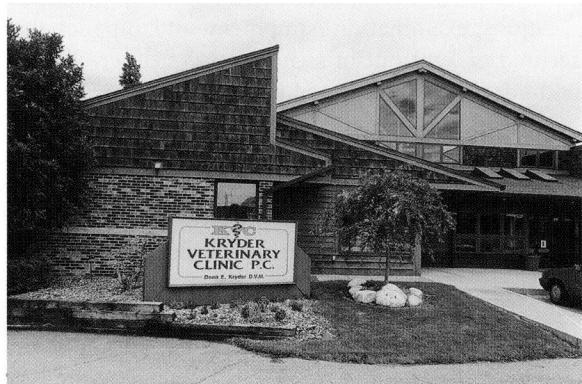

FIGURE 2-3 Exterior appearance of the hospital should provide a positive image.

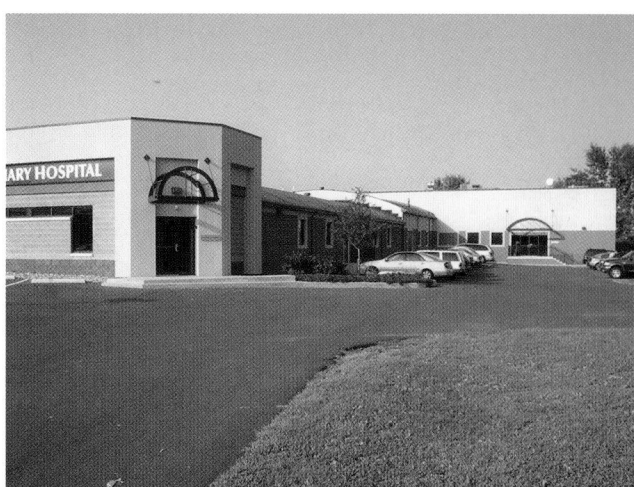

FIGURE 2-4 Client parking lot should be clearly designated and clean.

Clients and their pets typically first enter the reception area, where the admission process begins. Most reception rooms have a large counter behind which the receptionist sits. If the practice uses hard copy medical records, an area for filing them often adjoins the receptionist's work area. The receptionist checks the client in, locates the client record, and initiates the business and medical records needed for the visit. Some practices have a separate telephone area where additional receptionists take telephone calls and schedule appointments.

The waiting area for clients and their pets often dominates the reception space, but space is often devoted to the sale of pet food and other products as well. Clients often spend time waiting in the reception area, so it is important that this area be neatly organized, attractive, and clean. A bright reception area with attractive wall hangings and plants and warm colors may help clients to relax (Figure 2-5).

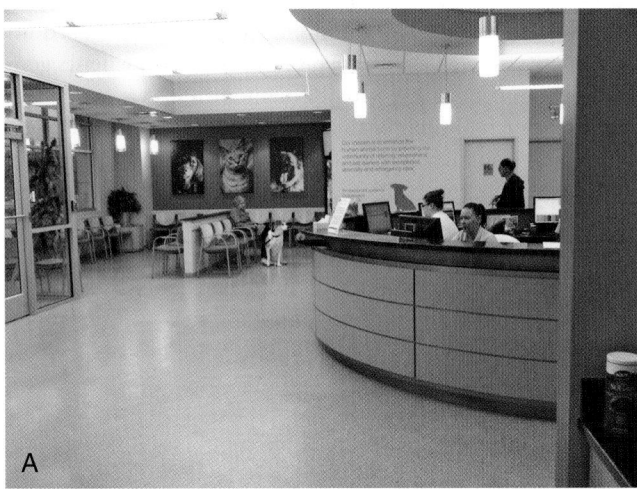

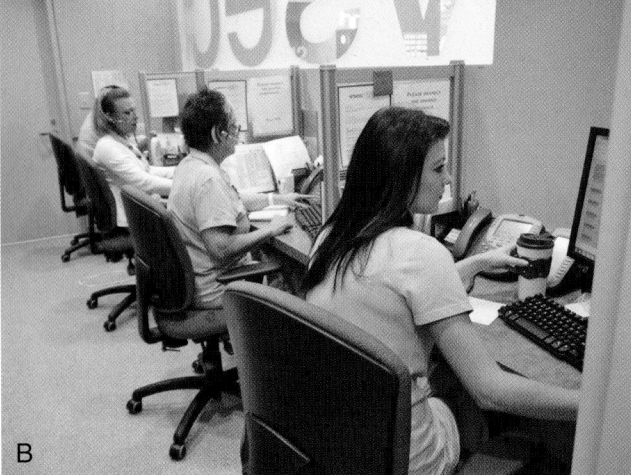

FIGURE 2-5 A and B, Reception area should give a warm, comfortable feeling to clients and staff. (B, Courtesy Dr. Joanna Bassert.)

However, dead or dying plants in the reception area, hairballs, and dirty floors will not send a positive message to the client. Seating should be comfortable, and tables or other raised areas on which pet owners can set carriers should be available. The waiting area should be scrupulously clean and should not smell of animal excretions. This is a hospital, and it should convey that image. Ideally, separate areas will be available in which dog owners and cat owners can sit; cats are very sensitive to the presence of dogs. The reception area should be reasonably quiet; interesting magazines and pet information should be available, as should a client restroom. Reading material should be complete and should not have torn or missing pages; pictures should be neatly framed and matted. Coffee or soft drinks are a welcome touch.

Receptionists should be mindful of how their conversations and actions are viewed by clients. Personal phone conversations, arguments among staff members in view of clients, and staff members who do not appear to be working while clients are waiting to be served do not give a good impression.

Clients do not want to wait. They should spend only a short period of time in the reception room before they are escorted to one of the examination rooms. This requires effective appointment scheduling and dedication to timely service. As a general rule, two examination rooms should be available in the outpatient area for each veterinarian working on a given day. Therefore, in the typical two-veterinarian practice, four examination rooms should be available.

A patient presented as an emergency always receives priority. If any question exists as to whether the case is truly an emergency, the pet should be placed in an examination room or taken back to the treatment room for immediate examination by a veterinarian. If the case is not an emergency, it can be worked back into the normal scheduling.

Examination rooms generally include an examination table, seating for the client, and a counter and cabinets to hold equipment and supplies needed by the veterinarian and other staff members. Computers and monitors are often present in each room. Examination areas should be clean, well organized, and attractive; the same guidelines described for reception areas apply to examination rooms as well (Figure 2-6). A soiled floor or wall covering, a dirty sink, or a marred door will be noted and remembered by the client. Medications, examination equipment, and supplies should be secured or kept out of sight, so that neither clients nor their children will be tempted to look at or play with them.

After the client is escorted into one of the examination rooms, a veterinary technician will often enter to obtain the pet's weight, temperature, pulse, and respiration (TPR) along with a brief history, and to prepare all materials needed for the visit. Sometimes a veterinarian does these tasks, but it is more efficient to have them delegated to a veterinary technician. Veterinarians typically perform a thorough physical examination on the pet and further discuss the pet's history with the client. A veterinary assistant should assist the veterinarian during the physical examination by restraining the patient as necessary. If blood, urine, or skin

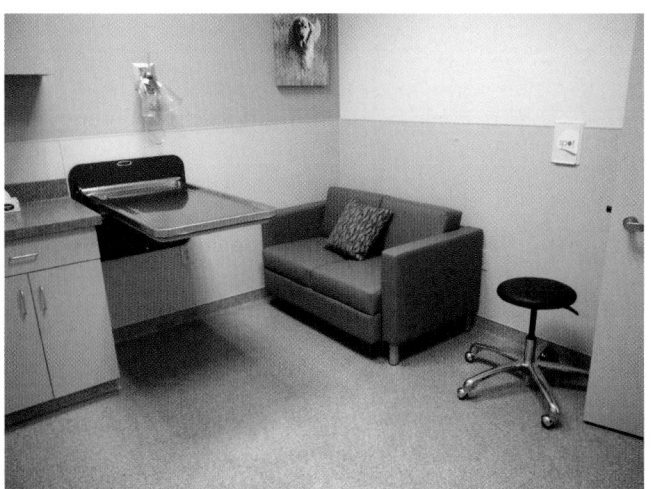

FIGURE 2-6 Examination rooms should be warmly decorated, clean, and in excellent condition.

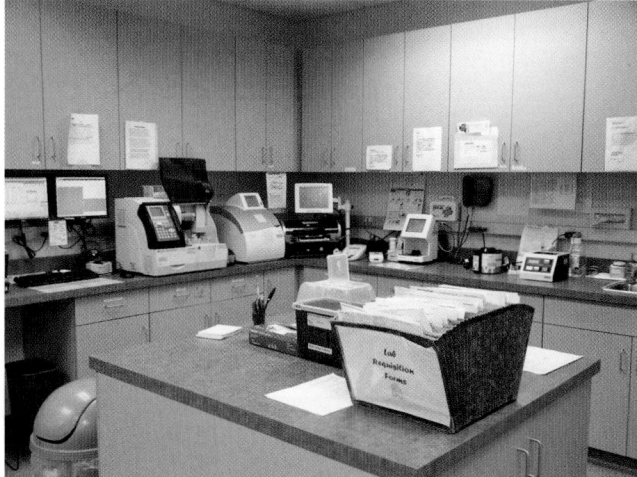

FIGURE 2-7 The laboratory is located just beyond the examination rooms.

specimens are needed, a technician will usually take the patient to the treatment room and will conduct these procedures away from the client with the help of an assistant while the veterinarian sees other patients. Clients should not be allowed to restrain their own pets because of the risk of being bitten.

After the examination and **consultation** are completed, results of the examination and of diagnostic procedures will be discussed with the client. Recommendations for additional diagnostics and for treatment or preventive care are made, if necessary. The veterinary technician will often administer treatments such as immunizations and will fill prescriptions as per order by the veterinarian. In addition, the veterinary technician will educate the owner regarding administration of home medications and treatments.

After the initial consultation with the veterinarian, some patients will be admitted to the hospital for further diagnostics and treatment. In this case, the patient will be taken to the wards or treatment areas, and the client will be escorted to the reception area to leave contact information for further follow-up with the veterinarian and staff. If the patient is going home, both client and patient will be escorted back to the reception area to settle the account and to schedule any necessary future appointments.

The laboratory and pharmacy areas are usually located near the examination rooms. They often separate the "front" of the hospital, which includes the reception area and examination rooms, from the "back," which includes the treatment area, the surgical area, hospital runs, wards, and the boarding area. This central location is important because the laboratory and the pharmacy are used by veterinarians when examining and treating both outpatients and those admitted to the hospital (Figures 2-7 and 2-8). Both of these areas should be well organized and clean. Clients occasionally will visit these areas and should always be accompanied by a hospital employee. In some practices, the laboratory and the pharmacy will be combined for more efficient use of floor space. The pharmacy may also house the material safety data sheets

(MSDS) required by the Occupational Safety and Health Administration (OSHA). Refer to Chapter 4 for more information about safety in a veterinary practice.

Inpatient Areas
Inpatients are those pets that have been admitted to the hospital for various kinds of diagnostics or treatments, including laboratory work, radiographs, dental care, and surgery. The pet may be admitted for an hour or two or for many days. The second work area in the hospital is devoted to these types of procedures and generally consists of a treatment area; special procedure rooms for x-ray, ultrasound, and endoscopy; patient wards; an isolation ward; an exercise area; a kitchen; boarding cages and runs; and a bathing and grooming area.

The treatment area is the central hub of the hospital (Figure 2-9). Patients from the wards (inpatients) and from examination rooms (outpatients) will be moved to this area for diagnostic procedures, medication administration, and recheck procedures such as cast, bandage, or splint changes. Veterinary technicians perform various prescribed medical treatments and nursing procedures while veterinarians perform surgery or see outpatients. The treatment room many also be used for the preparation of surgical patients.

> **TECHNICIAN NOTE** The treatment area is the central hub of the hospital. Patients from the wards (inpatients) and from examination rooms (outpatients) will be moved to this area for diagnostic procedures, medication administration, and recheck procedures such as cast, bandage, or splint changes.

In most hospitals, the radiology suite is near or connected to the treatment room and provides easy access to the surgery area as well (Figure 2-10). The radiology suite includes areas for taking, processing, and storing radiographs (film or digital), and for viewing, enhancing, and interpreting them.

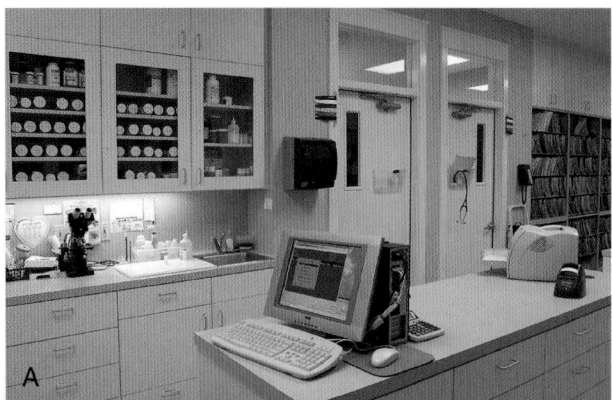

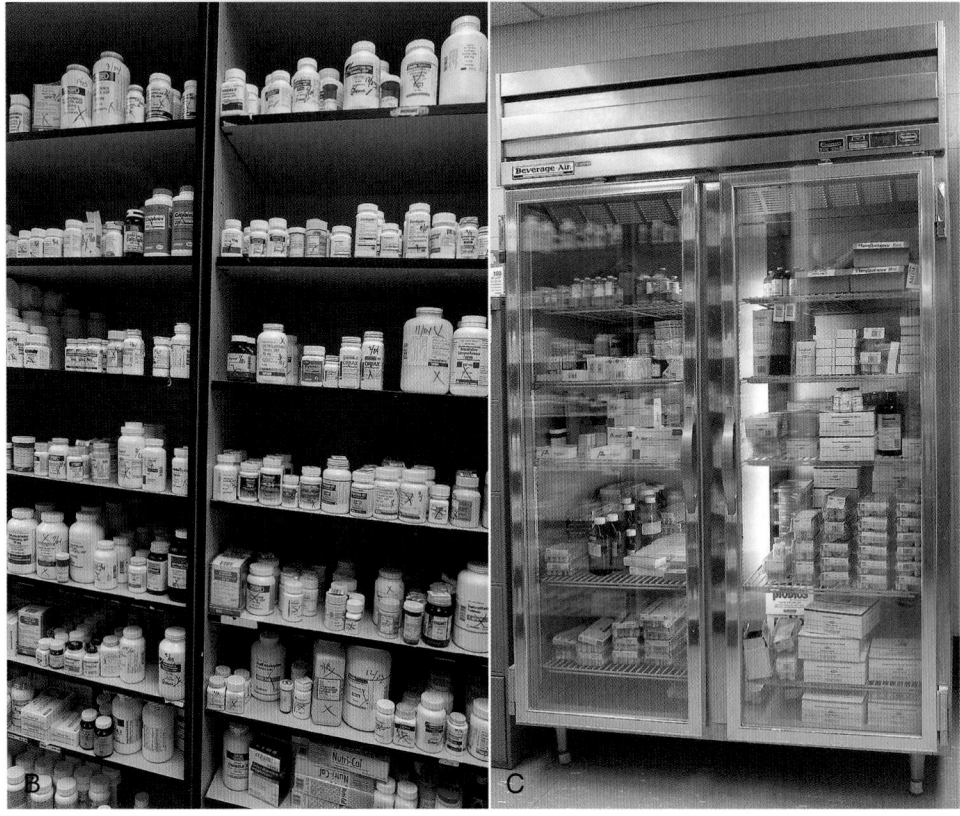

FIGURE 2-8 A, Pharmacy is located near examination rooms and inpatient treatment area. B, Drug shelf storage in pharmacy. C, Glass door refrigerator for storage of vaccines and biologicals.

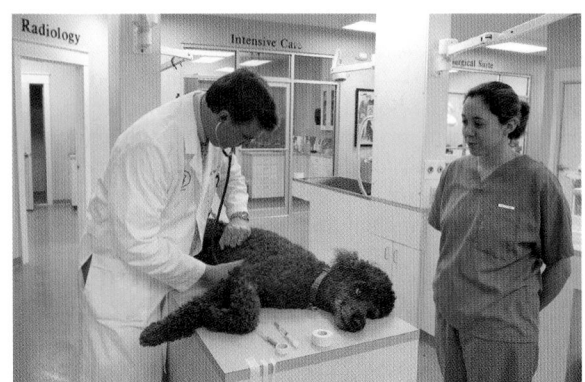

FIGURE 2-9 Centralized treatment area accommodates both outpatient and inpatient treatment.

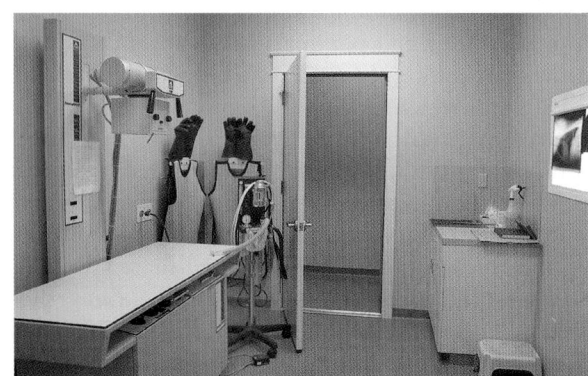

FIGURE 2-10 Radiology room with x-ray machine and protection equipment hanging on the wall. The automatic film processor is not visible through the open door.

Clients should not visit the radiology section when the x-ray machine is in use because of risk of exposure to radiation. All personnel in radiology should wear protective aprons, gloves, and film exposure badges. Thyroid shields and lead goggles are also helpful safety equipment. Some hospitals have other small rooms off the treatment area for ultrasound, dental, or other procedures.

Cages and runs for hospitalized patients are generally included in the treatment area, although some hospitals have small rooms off the treatment area for less seriously ill hospitalized patients. Critical patients are generally kept directly in the treatment area, where they can be easily monitored. Increasingly, cats are kept in quiet areas away from dogs to reduce their anxiety.

The veterinarian will establish the treatment regimen for each hospitalized patient. The veterinary technician assesses the hospitalized patient frequently and generates a list of nursing evaluations relevant to the patient. These evaluations are subsequently prioritized, and a technician plan of care is developed; specific interventions are developed and implemented. The veterinarian writes SOAP (subjective, objective, assessment, and plan) notes to assist in the diagnostic process; the veterinary technician prepares SOAP notes to support the nursing process and to ensure that all technician evaluations are addressed. Many practices, particularly those that employ electronic medical record keeping systems, employ a truncated method of making medical notations in the patient record. For purposes of instruction and for teaching critical thinking skills, veterinary medical schools and veterinary technology programs instruct students in the formal method of writing SOAP notes. This approach represents best practices but is time-consuming and is not always carried out in general practice. Refer to Chapters 1 and 3 for additional discussion about completing patient assessments and medical record keeping respectively.

During hospitalization, the veterinary technician carries out medical treatments and diagnostic tests ordered by the veterinarian and delegates exercising, feeding, restraining, and grooming of the patient to veterinary assistants and animal caretakers. Often daily communication with the client is carried out by the veterinary technician. A whiteboard in the treatment room may be used to summarize the diagnostic, treatment, and surgery schedules for hospitalized patients. Computerized schedules may be generated with the same information. All patients should be assessed several times each day by the attending veterinarian and veterinary technician, and these assessments should be documented with appropriate entries into the medical record. Daily ward rounds can be helpful in keeping each member of the veterinary health care team up-to-date on the status of hospitalized patients.

Constant attention must be given to these areas to maintain a clean, odor-free environment for the comfort of staff and pets, as well as to prevent nosocomial infections among patients. Cages and runs must be cleaned several times during the day. Hospitalized patients may require more frequent cleaning of their cages and runs than animals that are boarding because sick animals often cannot control urination and defecation. Patient wards must be well insulated to reduce noise both in the wards and in public areas of the hospital.

When animals with infectious and contagious diseases are hospitalized, they are placed in an isolation ward. The isolation area should have one entrance and exit preferably with access to the outside, so that infectious patients do not walk through the common areas of the hospital. Isolation areas are designed to restrict the shedding of infectious microbes to a single region that can be easily sanitized. Therefore, disinfectants and protective disposable gloves, booties, and gowns should be available at the entrance to the isolation ward. The air-handling system for the isolation area must be separate from that used in other parts of the building to prevent the aerosol transmission of contagions. In the event that adequate isolation facilities are not available on the premises, the case should be referred to a veterinarian who has the proper facility. All treatment and handling of the infectious patient should be done by just one or two persons. The patient should be treated and housed in the isolation facility and should never be taken to any other part of the hospital, including the main treatment room. Staff must be trained to follow stringent isolation protocols to prevent the transmission of nosocomial infections to other patients.

When hospitalized pets are ready for discharge, the client is given written instructions for home care. These instructions together with discharge forms are reviewed and discussed with the owner. The client may have a brief consultation with the veterinarian before the patient is discharged. Surgical incisions, bandages, splints, and casts must be clean and dry before the patient is discharged. The client may make a judgment about the surgeon's skill based on the size of the incision and the neatness of hair removal at the surgical site. Clients are often asked to settle their account before their pet is brought to them.

> **TECHNICIAN NOTE** When hospitalized pets are ready for discharge, the client is given written instructions for home care. These instructions together with discharge forms are reviewed and discussed with the owner.

Clients often wish to visit their pets when they are hospitalized. In this event, the client usually makes an appointment with the receptionist to visit the animal at a specific time that is convenient for both the client and the hospital operation. During the owner's visit with the pet, a technician or veterinarian should be present to answer questions concerning the status of the patient. Client visits are generally beneficial for both the hospitalized patient and the client. The mental attitudes of client and patient can be strengthened, and communication between veterinarian and client can be improved. Unfortunately, some practices discourage or limit client visits because they can disrupt normal operations.

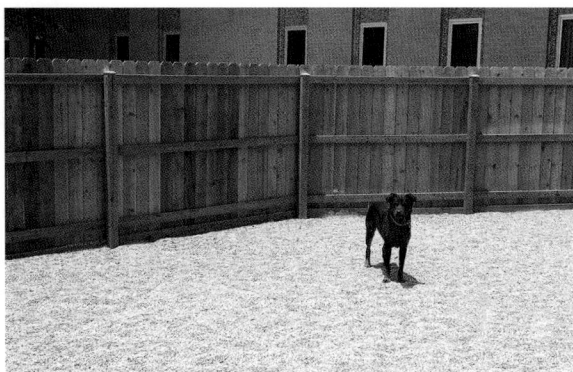

FIGURE 2-11 For security, fenced enclosures should always be used for outside exercise.

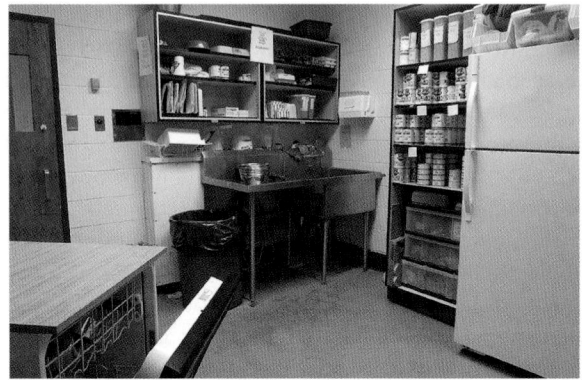

FIGURE 2-12 Hospital kitchen should contain diet materials, dishwasher, counter space, and refrigerator.

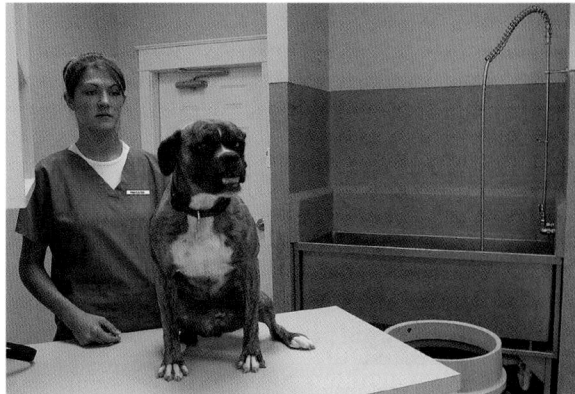

FIGURE 2-13 Custom pet-bathing tub in background designed to aid in controlling animal during bath.

Most hospitals have an inside or outside exercise area for dogs. Outside areas are enclosed in escape-proof fencing or walls and generally are positioned next to boarding kennels to decrease the likelihood that a kenneled animal may escape (Figure 2-11). The hospital and practice owners assume legal responsibility when hospitalized or boarded animals escape.

The food storage room is sometimes referred to as the *kitchen* (Figure 2-12). This room is used to store a variety of canned and dry foods kept in dry, rodent-proof containers. Automatic dishwashers are frequently used to sanitize food and water bowls. It is helpful to acquire quiet dishwashers if they are in close proximity to the wards and ones that heat water to high temperatures. A sink with hot and cold running water, plenty of countertop space, and a refrigerator should be available in the kitchen. OSHA regulations dictate that human food and drink must not be stored in the same refrigerator as pet food, biological samples, and pharmaceuticals.

With the exception of hospitalized patients, regional zoning laws may preclude practices from boarding animals. Most hospitals, however, do include kennels if zoning permits. Boarding facilities are typically located in the back of the hospital and often include separate areas for dogs and cats. If the hospital offers grooming services, they are often located in this area as well. Although some veterinary hospitals board only pets who are regular clients of the practice,

others offer boarding services for both clients and nonclients. Some practices have extensive and elaborate boarding, grooming, and pet spa areas; others offer a simpler array of services.

Not all practice owners find boarding and grooming to be profitable services. These services are often more labor intensive (and thus more expensive) than others offered by practices. In some regions, the clientele cannot support the increased costs associated with maintaining a kennel, so the hospital does not offer boarding.

However, many practices have found that, if done well, boarding kennels complement the medical side of the business and are profitable. Practices that offer luxury boarding with attractive dog suites and cat condos, extra playtimes, swimming, and socialization with other pets or people can charge more for these services and make this a very profitable enterprise. The second way of capitalizing on boarding and grooming is by generating as many spin-off medical services as possible. In hospitals that do this, technicians or doctors will give each boarding or grooming pet a mini-exam to identify obvious eye, ear, nose, teeth, skin, and other easily recognizable problems. Groomers and all those involved in working with the boarders will be trained to identify these issues and report them to a doctor for follow-up.

Even if a hospital does not offer grooming services, most practices have a small area for bathing pets (Figure 2-13). This usually consists of a raised bathroom tub, a combing table, and a dryer cage. It is important that all patients be clean and dry before they are discharged.

Some hospitals have a separate entrance and reception area for pets that are visiting solely for boarding or grooming; others check in and discharge animals to be groomed via the main hospital entrance and exit.

Surgical Area

The third work area in the hospital, the surgical area, consists of the surgical preparation room, operating rooms (ORs), and a recovery room. All three areas in the surgical section are typically in close proximity to one another.

As stated earlier, surgical prep may be done in the treatment room in some hospitals. All presurgical preparation of

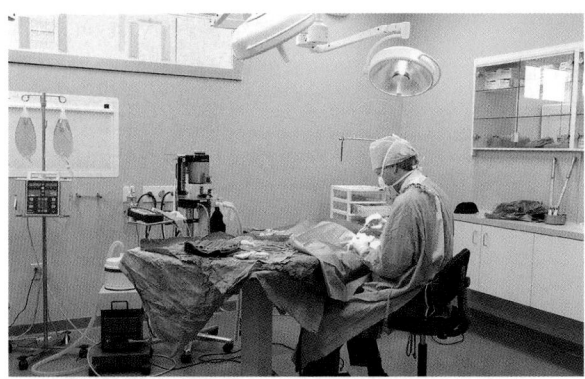

FIGURE 2-14 Surgical room with one door for entrance and exit, ceiling-mounted lights, and minimal countertops.

patient, surgeon, and technician should take place outside the OR to keep the OR as clean as possible. These presurgical activities include instrument preparation and sterilization, clipping and scrubbing of the patient, and hand scrubbing, gowning, and gloving of the surgical team.

The OR itself should be a "dead-end" room with only one entrance and exit (Figure 2-14). Dust-carrying bacteria are easily stirred into the air when people walk through the room and will settle into an open surgical incision. No one should enter the OR without proper clothing, shoes, cap, and mask. Clients will not be permitted in this area, except in unusual circumstances.

> **TECHNICIAN NOTE** Dust-carrying bacteria are easily stirred into the air when people walk through the room and will settle into an open surgical incision. No one should enter the OR without proper clothing, shoes, cap, and mask.

The OR should be used only for surgical procedures and must not double as a treatment or examination room. Storage cabinets should be kept to a minimum and should contain only items that are used in surgery. Items used elsewhere in the hospital should not be stored in the OR. Countertops should be kept to a minimum because flat surfaces collect dust and must be wiped down daily. Surgery lights, oxygen outlets, and patient monitors should be ceiling or wall mounted when possible. Floors, walls, and ceiling should be washable, smooth, and seam free to allow complete and easy cleaning. Cleaning under the surgery table base and on the top of surgical lights, as well as cleaning of the floor and flat surfaces (window ledges, countertop, etc.), should be performed daily. The air-handling system for the OR should be separate and should create slight positive pressure to prevent dust and other debris from entering the room from other rooms when the door is opened. All cleaning materials and utensils used in the OR should be restricted to use in this room. Mops and sponges that are used elsewhere in the building and then are used in the OR will bring additional contamination into the room. The cleanliness of the OR should be everyone's concern to prevent nosocomial infection of the surgical patient.

Some practices have a separate surgical recovery room; others place recovering pets in areas of the hospital ward where they can be carefully monitored. Whenever surgical recovery occurs, the patient should be closely monitored by the technical staff. Under no circumstances should any patient recovering from anesthesia be left unattended in the ward, in a stall, or elsewhere with an endotracheal tube in place.

Support Area
The fourth work area of the hospital is the hospital support area. This area contains, somewhat by default, the "leftover spaces," but it also contains the critical planning and management areas of the hospital. The support area includes the doctors' offices, the business management office, the library, the employee lounge, and storage areas. In smaller practices, the professional office, the business management office, and the library may be found in one room.

From a management viewpoint, hospital storage space is the most expensive floor space in the building because this space produces the least income. Therefore, storage areas must be given close attention, so that this valuable space will function as efficiently as possible. Supplies and equipment that are no longer used or usable should be removed to make room for essential items. Inventory control (avoiding overstocking or understocking) and space organization will ensure maximal use. Items that can be hung on the wall or ceiling should be removed from the floor. Metal or wooden shelving will organize space for bulk drugs, food, and cleaning supplies. Flammable or toxic materials should be safely marked and stored away from food or drugs (refer to Chapter 4 for additional information about safety).

The smaller the practice, the less distinct these four areas (outpatient, inpatient, surgery, and support) will be. Further, the smaller the practice, the fewer technical staff members and assistants will be needed, resulting in less opportunity for the veterinary technician to focus on one work area. This is not to imply that the smaller practice is less desirable. Sometimes the small practice can provide greater personal satisfaction because of closer contact with the entire operation and increased diversification of job roles.

SMALL ANIMAL HOUSE CALL PRACTICES
A few small animal practices do not have a permanent hospital facility but instead offer house call services and operate from a mobile veterinary vehicle that is especially equipped for treating pets at home. Veterinarians can perform basic surgical and diagnostic procedures in a **mobile facility**. In addition, ambulatory veterinarians frequently establish a relationship with a nearby veterinary hospital that allows use of the facility for treatment of more complicated house call cases.

SPECIALTY AND EMERGENCY PRACTICES
These practices are usually larger and offer more advanced care than most general practices. Although their facilities

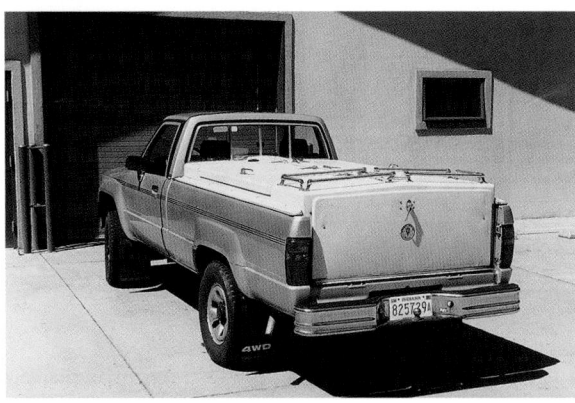

FIGURE 2-15 A veterinary mobile unit is equipped with hot water, a refrigerator, and many compartments for equipment and supplies.

include the same types of areas as are found in a general practice (reception area, examination rooms, surgical area, etc.), more space is allocated to each area, and the hospital may be divided by department. For example, internal medicine has its own examination rooms, treatment area, and hospitalization ward, as do the other services (surgery, dermatology, ophthalmology, etc.). Services often share an intensive care unit (ICU), some hospitalization space, and pharmacy and laboratory areas.

LARGE ANIMAL MOBILE UNITS

Many large animal veterinarians operate mobile units only. Some practice out of permanent facilities to which clients must bring their animals (haul-in practices), and some large animal practices offer both types of services.

Veterinary diagnostic and preventive medicine services for a herd of animals require the veterinarian to visit the owner's farm or stable. The large animal practice often makes use of a specially designed mobile vehicle for conducting farm visits (Figure 2-15). These visits require stringent sanitary precautions to prevent transmission of disease from one client facility to another. Washing hands, changing to clean coveralls, chemically disinfecting boots, and cleaning equipment between farm calls are paramount to prevent disease transmission among farms, and to gain and keep the confidence of the livestock or equine owner.

> **TECHNICIAN NOTE** Mobile large animal practices employ stringent sanitary precautions to prevent transmission of disease from one farm to another. Washing hands, changing to clean coveralls, chemically disinfecting boots, and cleaning equipment between farm calls are paramount to prevent disease transmission among farms.

Mobile facilities used to serve large animal patients and clients may vary from a car with a few portable "grips" in the trunk, to a van with a set of drawers and containers, to a specially designed mobile truck unit. Truck units usually are fully equipped with refrigeration for biologicals plus hot water and a supply of disinfectants, drugs, vaccines, medical

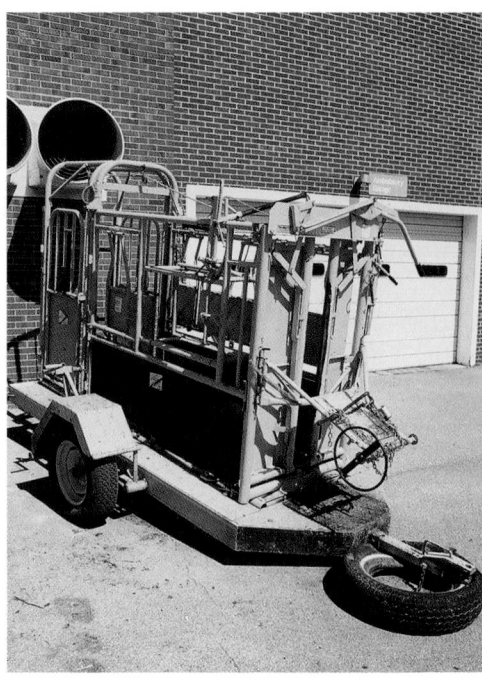

FIGURE 2-16 A portable cattle chute on wheels is pulled behind the ambulatory truck to the farm.

supplies, restraints, diagnostic and treatment equipment, and sometimes even mobile x-ray units. Everything needed for a series of planned visits plus unexpected emergencies must be on board. The water supply and disinfectants are used to clean and disinfect hands, boots, and equipment after every farm call. A portable cattle chute may be pulled behind the mobile unit to the farm to process herds of cattle (Figure 2-16).

A veterinary technician or assistant may be responsible for stocking, organizing, and maintaining the large animal mobile unit. The mobile unit inventory will vary depending on the nature of the practice, the preferences of the veterinarian, and the species served. Preparing inventory lists and organizational charts for this daily activity ensures that the veterinarian will have what is needed on every call. Obviously, a wide range of specific supplies is necessary for the routine practice of large animal veterinary medicine. This inventory must be replenished frequently, organized for easy and quick access, and cleaned and disinfected on a daily basis and after every farm call. Technicians often assist veterinarians on farm calls and become efficient at maintaining and organizing the mobile unit.

LARGE ANIMAL HAUL-IN FACILITIES

Some veterinarians with mixed and large animal practices provide haul-in facilities for individual patients to be trucked or brought by trailer into the practice (Figure 2-17). Unloading chutes and gates for cattle trucks and stock trailers are provided at the large animal outpatient entrance. A few even provide holding corrals and squeeze chutes for processing a truckload of cattle or sheep. Unloading chutes for cattle, sheep, and swine must adjust to different heights to

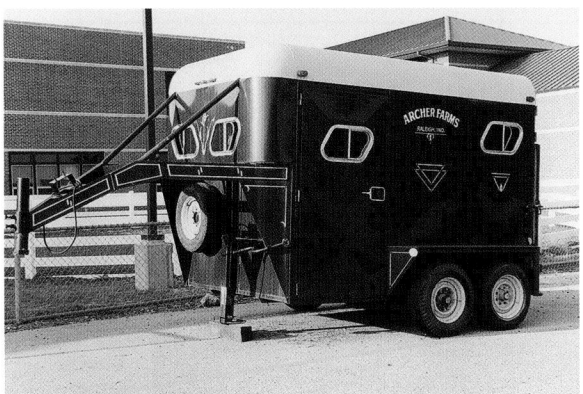

FIGURE 2-17 A stock trailer is used by animal owners to transport farm animals to the large animal hospital for treatment.

accommodate the trucks, pickups, and trailers used for transporting animals. It is paramount that fencing and panel arrangements be constructed to prevent escape from the premises if the animal escapes from the head-catch or alleyway, or when unloading.

When haul-in facilities for large animals are provided, each of the areas previously discussed for a small animal facility will be present for serving large animal patients. Frequently, some areas (e.g., reception area, laboratory, conference rooms, pharmacy) will be used for both small animal and large animal services. Large mixed animal hospitals may have a separate pharmacy for large animal supplies, separate public restrooms, and possibly a separate reception area. The nature of the large animal facilities of each practice is variable depending on the needs of the livestock and equine population and owners served by the practice.

The large animal inpatient treatment area may be the same as the outpatient examination area for large animal patients. An alleyway with a head-catch or a squeeze chute is used for bovine patients, a stock is used for equine patients, and pigs or sheep may be treated in their stalls. When haul-in facilities are available for large animals, patient wards with a few stalls are usually provided (Figure 2-18). These will often be provided indoors to protect patients from bad weather, although outdoor pens may be used in good weather. Isolation areas in a different barn are sometimes necessary to prevent the spread of infectious disease.

Examination rooms for large animals and small animals are always separate because large animal examinations require stocks for horses (Figure 2-19), a squeeze chute and head-catch for cattle, and large special examination tables for restraining cattle on their sides for hoof work or minor surgery. Because of the size of these species, the staff should be well trained in restraint and safety procedures; this ensures protection for large animal patients, owners, and staff. A variety of restraint procedures may be followed (see Chapter 6).

Most large animal practices also use the treatment area as a minor, nonsterile surgical room. Because of the large size of patients and the extensive amount of hair and excrement brought to these areas by large animals, high-pressure hoses

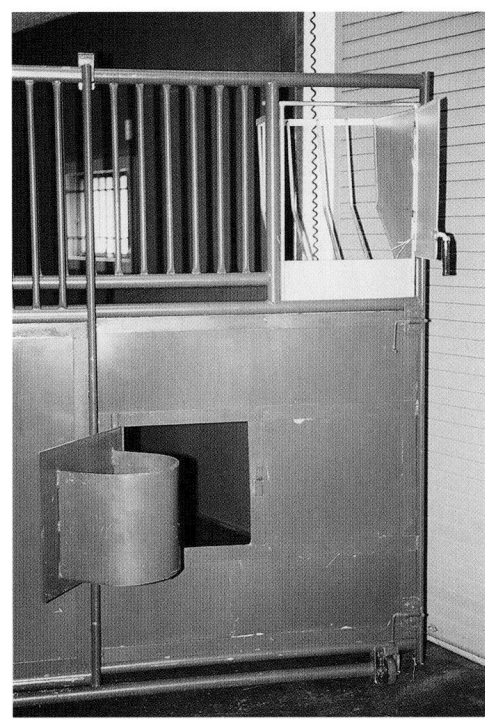

FIGURE 2-18 Large animal stall door has mini-doors to feed and water large animal patients without the need to enter the stall.

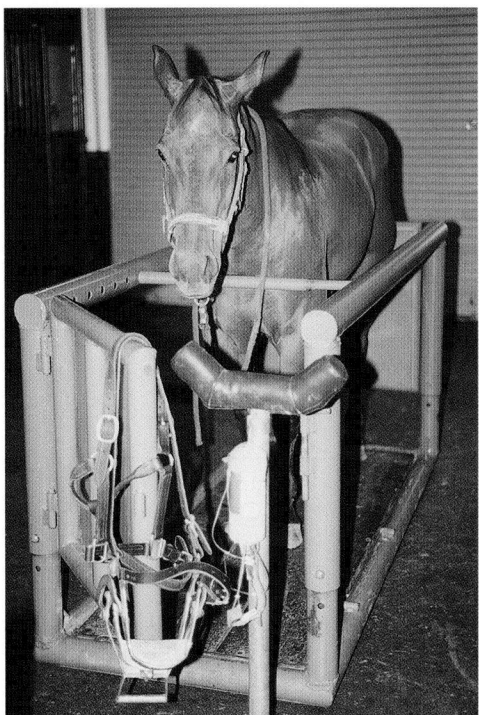

FIGURE 2-19 Horse in stocks with bar in front of chest to keep horse back against rear door. Mouth speculum is used to perform equine dental procedures.

and disinfectant systems are necessary, along with removable floor drain traps. Most mixed practices use the same support areas for small and large animal clients and patients, with the exception of areas used for storage of cleaning equipment, lawn mowers, large animal hoof equipment, general supplies, and bulk pharmacy items.

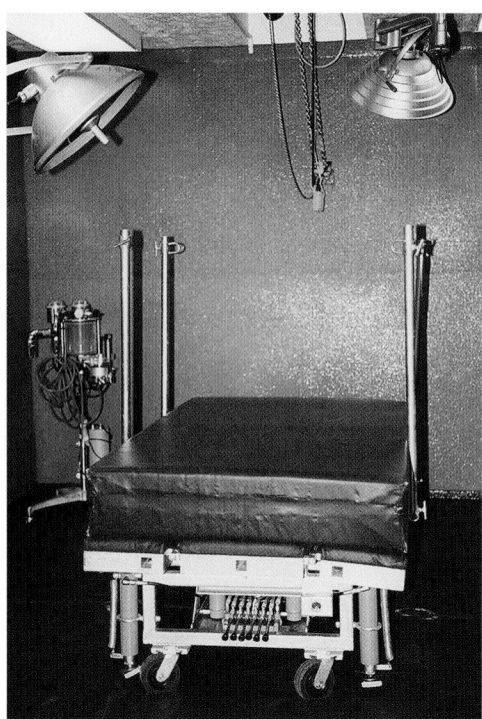

FIGURE 2-20 Large animal surgery table with anesthesia machine and padded walls of recovery room for recovering anesthetized horses.

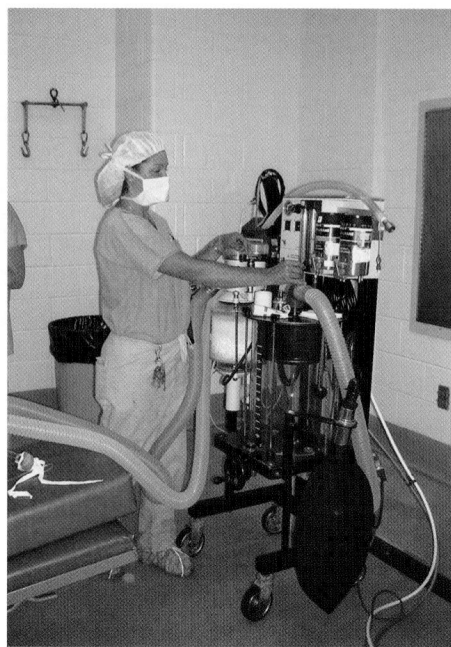

FIGURE 2-21 Large animal endotracheal tubes, rebreathing bags, and related anesthesia equipment stored on a rack for quick access.

The surgical room in the equine practice facility is organized to provide the same stringent asepsis as is provided in a small animal surgical area. However, because the patient is much larger, mechanical or hydraulic equipment designed to lift the horse is provided. Larger equine practices have an induction room (which may also serve as a treatment or minor surgery area), an OR with a large animal radiology machine, and a padded recovery room. The surgical area is equipped with a surgical table on which the horse is placed after induction of general anesthetic (Figures 2-20 and 2-21). Anesthesia is maintained with an equine gas anesthesia machine.

> **TECHNICIAN NOTE**   Larger equine practices have an induction room and an OR with a large animal radiology machine, along with a padded recovery room.

An area where a necropsy can be appropriately performed must be available (see Chapter 17). Necropsies are performed more frequently when a large animal dies than for a small animal. Because of the economic value of large herds or flocks, necropsies of dead animals are often done to determine whether the rest of the herd or flock is threatened. Confirmation of the diagnosis will often require the submission of specimens to a state or university diagnostic laboratory for testing and review by a board certified pathologist. Sometimes necropsy of several animals may be done (more common in sheep, pigs, and poultry) to determine which of several concurrent diseases is the probable cause of death. Necropsies are valuable as a preventive measure to stop the

spread of a disease and to prevent it in the future. They also serve as a great learning tool for use by the veterinary staff in becoming better prepared to recognize similar cases in the future.

Traffic flow patterns in large animal and mixed practices vary greatly. Facilities that primarily serve small animal patients but have a moderately used large animal facility attached have some mixing of traffic from the two groups. In some facilities, a practice that has many large animal patients may be organized with greater separation to reduce crossover of traffic patterns of small and large animal clients. Obviously, in an exclusive large animal facility (e.g., an equine practice), these areas are similar to those in a small animal practice in name, but the arrangement and size will depend on the types of horses routinely presented for treatment.

CLIENTS AND CLIENT SERVICES

The most important person in any practice is the client; no animal visits a veterinary practice without a human attached. The practice of veterinary medicine is truly a people business. Veterinarians and technicians who do not like working with clients should not be employed in practice because they will be ineffective in client communication and in serving the client's needs. Many other professional careers are now available for individuals who desire less public contact.

> **TECHNICIAN NOTE**   The most important person in any practice is the client; no animal visits a veterinary practice without a human attached. The practice of veterinary medicine is truly a people business.

Clients generally judge a practice based on client service, not on the quality of medicine. Although the availability of the Internet allows clients to be more educated about medical matters, it is still difficult for most clients to know whether or not they received good care unless an obvious mistake is made, such as amputation of the wrong leg. Clients tend to assume that all practices offer a similar level of medical care. Therefore, they use nonmedical factors to evaluate the quality of care. For example, to a client, dog urine in the reception room indicates a dirty hospital and thus poor care, because everyone knows that sanitation and sterility are required as part of good medicine.

It is important to realize that clients often judge a practice on the basis of <u>perception</u> of value rather than <u>true</u> value, regardless of whether they are looking at medical or surgical aspects. And unfortunately, it is easier for a practice with only average medical care to persuade its clients that the care is outstanding than for a practice with only average service to persuade a client that it provides outstanding care. Again, this comes back to the fact that clients understand service issues better than medical issues; good or bad service is more easily recognizable to them. For example, if the receptionist tells the client that Fluffy will be ready at 3 PM and the client stands around the reception area until 3:25 PM, the client KNOWS that a client service error has occurred. If the veterinarian does not remove all stones from the bladder during a cystotomy, the owner probably will never know.

Availability of veterinary services in the United States appears to be at an all-time high. New schools of veterinary medicine and expanded enrollment at existing schools have resulted in increased availability of graduate veterinarians. In addition, more than 200 AVMA-accredited programs of veterinary technology have been established in the United States. The net result of the increasing supply of veterinary personnel is increased competition for clients among established and new practices. Practices that will financially survive must offer an outstanding client service experience, in addition to outstanding care. The practice will collapse unless old clients are retained and new clients are continually entering the hospital. Clients are the lifeblood of the practice, and everyone in the practice works for the client. Loyalty is won with hard work and dedicated caring service to each client. If the staff attitude becomes one of negative feelings toward clients ("not another one of these!"), the practice clientele will dwindle. A practice's facilities, equipment, and techniques may be the finest available, but they will remain unused until enough clients willingly authorize or request that practice's services.

How does a client select a veterinary practice? Historically, most clients will select the practice with the most convenient location or one that is recommended by friends and colleagues. With increasing use of social media, pet owners also make use of online reviews.

Once a practice has been selected, it is judged on the following client service attributes:

- Professional, friendly, and caring personnel
- Attention to the client's needs and desires
- Consistency in care and service
- Availability of a wide range of services
- Convenience—hours, location, respect for clients' time
- Reliability
- Clean, attractive, and updated facility
- Clear and understandable communication of recommendations and benefits to client and pet

In large animal practices, retention and satisfaction issues are the same for clients as those encountered by small animal owners, with the addition of economic return. In food animal practices, the veterinarian must become an economic asset to overall farm profitability, or the client cannot afford to seek veterinary services. The sentimental and emotional attachment (human–animal bond) of the client to the animal extends that economic limit in companion animal and some equine practices but is not a factor in food animal practices.

IMPORTANCE OF CLIENT COMMUNICATION

In study after study, the importance of good communication skills in well-run veterinary practices has been demonstrated. Clear communication must occur not only among members of the veterinary staff, but also between staff members and clients.

> **TECHNICIAN NOTE** Most complaints against veterinary practices are the result of ineffective communication between the practice and the pet owner.

Communication Myths

Myths regarding communication skills abound. The first is that communication is a personality trait, and either you have it or you don't. In reality, communication consists of a series of learned skills, and anyone who wants to <u>can</u> learn them. Another myth is that experience is a good teacher of communication skills. In reality, experience alone tends to be a poor teacher of communication skills, because experience tends to reinforce habits, regardless of whether the habits are good or bad. Still another common myth is that it takes too long for veterinary health care team members to communicate well with clients. Practices are busy, and good communication is not feasibly done when the veterinary health care team is under pressure. In reality, good communication is more efficient in the long run because it results in fewer errors, greater client satisfaction, and better medical care for patients.

Six Aspects of Excellent Communication

Clear and frequent verbal communication with coworkers and clients is an important part of effective veterinary health care. Components of what makes good communication are listed and discussed here.

1. *Clarity*: Be clear in speech by using correct grammar and articulation.

2. *Courtesy*: Be courteous and respectful at all times. Avoid using words that might offend, such as curse words and unprofessional slang.
3. *Positive nonverbal communication*: Be aware of your own nonverbal communication, and use open body postures and direct eye contact to build trust.
4. *Open-ended inquiry*: Obtain important information from the client using open-ended inquiries.
5. *Reflective listening*: Employ active and reflective listening to let clients know that you understand what they are saying.
6. *Empathy*: Show sincere empathy by putting yourself in the position of others. Let them know that you understand how they must be feeling.

Clarity

Clarity is particularly important in medical communication. Only 57% of veterinary clients surveyed in the 2011 Bayer Veterinary Care Usage Study[3] fully agreed with the following statement: "My veterinarian communicates with me using language I understand." Only 44% agreed with the statement, "My veterinarian clearly explains when I need to bring my pet in for various procedures or tests." It is clear from this study that improvement is needed in the communication that veterinarians and other staff members have with clients.

It is easy for veterinarians and veterinary technicians to use medically precise words that mean nothing to a pet owner. Use terminology that the client will understand, and don't overwhelm the client with too much information. Make it clear exactly what needs to be done, why, and when. Simply *saying* this to a client is often not enough. Verbal communication needs to be followed up by written take-home information and a later reminder phone call or other communication.

Courtesy

Common courtesy, genuine concern, and respect are important parts of communication in all professions and businesses and in personal relationships. When a veterinary practice loses sight of the individual client, the personal service feeling is lost for both client and patient. Courtesy begins with acknowledging clients as soon as they enter the reception room, calling clients by name, asking about clients' families, and, in short, treating clients as important guests in the practice. Courtesy also extends to telephone manners. All calls should be answered promptly; the caller should be welcomed with a greeting such as, "Good morning, this is ABC Animal Hospital; this is Kathy speaking. How may I help you?" In this way, the caller immediately knows that he or she has reached the correct hospital, and that someone is there to help. Telephone courtesy is just as important as face-to-face courtesy because most clients have their first contact with the hospital by telephone.

Nothing is more important for the veterinary professional to do than talk to a client; one should not rush through information just because one is feeling hurried, or because the information asked for appears to be "common knowledge." Remember that what is common knowledge to a veterinarian or veterinary technician or other practice staff person is very likely new information to the client; do not assume a superior manner or tone to the extent that the client feels "put down."

Positive Nonverbal Communication

A large portion of communication is nonverbal. Nonverbal communication includes all the behavioral signals that pass between interacting individuals, exclusive of verbal content. For example, a client, when asked if all medication was given to the dog, may say "Yes" but with a tentativeness that indicates either "No" or "Not sure." Practicing open, nonverbal communication (uncrossing legs and arms, and maintaining good eye contact) builds greater levels of trust. Nonverbal signals are generally involuntary and are construed to more accurately reflect a person's true feelings. When mixed messages are sent, the nonverbal message is instinctively perceived as more accurate than the verbal message.

Open-Ended Inquiry

Open-ended questions are particularly important when a history is taken; they encourage the client to elaborate or to tell a story with no shaping or focusing of content by the recipient. The goal is to find the meaning of the communication, not just the facts. Simple examples include questions that start with "Tell me…" or "Describe for me…" "What" and "How" questions are also effective. "Why" questions are less effective; they tend to provoke defensiveness. Open-ended questions are part of a funnel approach to gathering information—start with the broad questions and end with more specific ones. For example, the first broad, open-ended question might be, "How does Fluffy behave in the morning when you see him acting strangely?" After the story comes out, the time is right to focus on specifics. Use closed-ended questions to clarify details, such as "Which leg do you think he is favoring?"

Reflective Listening

Listening is extremely important because it represents half of the communication process. The skill of active and reflective listening must be practiced on a regular basis. Many people prefer to talk rather than listen; when other individuals are speaking, they may be formulating their response rather than truly listening to what is being said. Clients have much to contribute to the diagnostic process by providing important clues in the patient history.

Active and reflective listening first involves offering encouragement to the speaker by nodding and making direct eye contact. After the speaker has finished talking, the listener reflects back to the speaker what was said and asks the speaker if the reflection is correct. This helps ensure that the listener has an accurate understanding of the information communicated and helps the speaker feel heard and understood. One example of reflective listening is verifying the facts: "So Fluffy threw up twice last night. Is that correct, Mrs. Jones?"

Empathy

Empathy is the ability to understand the position of another person and to communicate that understanding to the person. Examples include the following: "I can see how hard it is to make this decision about Fluffy," or "It sounds like you did all that you could for Fluffy."

DEALING WITH DIFFICULT CLIENTS

Dealing with an angry client is not easy and requires skill. There should be a clear understanding within the practice about how difficult clients are to be dealt with and whose role this is. Although there is no way to completely prepare for a client outburst, it does help to role-play such situations during staff training.

These guidelines may help to diffuse the situation:

- An angry client should immediately be "invited" to a private area such as an examination room or an office away from other clients, or to a place without distraction or interruption.
- A friendlier environment is created when people sit down side by side without a desk or an examination table between them.
- The staff member should immediately start the conversation by thanking the client, in a friendly fashion, for allowing the practice to find out what is wrong.
- Sometimes the client will burst out with everything that is wrong, in great detail. Although this may be unpleasant, it is essential for eventual resolution. If the client does not initiate a discussion, the staff member must speak first: "Could you explain to me what is wrong?"
- Active and reflective types of listening are employed. Being empathic helps staff members understand the client's point of view.
- Try to find points of agreement. At any part of the client's experience during which the pet owner confirms that something went well, or that he or she is satisfied, is beneficial for the process of resolving problems.
- Be careful not to justify a clinical action that the client is criticizing. If the client is correct that a mistake has been made, or that poor service has been delivered, this should be admitted and the situation corrected immediately.
- When it does become appropriate to explain hospital procedures, try to put them in a positive light, for example, clients hate to hear that their pet needs a rabies vaccination because it is your "policy." Talk to clients in terms of what constitutes the best health care for their pet: "Did you know that Texas has the highest incidence of rabies in the nation?"
- Try to find a solution, to create a "win-win" situation. It can help to ask the client what he or she would recommend to resolve the problem.
- Let the client save face whenever possible.
- Do not take problems and problem people personally—be professional, and see this as part of the job.

Even if it is the role of the practice manager to ultimately deal with an angry client, some of the tips already presented can be used by all staff members to help control the situation while the veterinarian or the practice manager is being located. It is always important to review the client's complaint after the situation has been resolved, to see if the practice should do some things differently in the future to avoid a repeat situation.

The most difficult people to reason with are those who have been drinking or are on drugs. Be careful how you handle these people. Do not argue or confront them because they could become violent and uncontrollable. In situations in which drugs or alcohol has been consumed to excess, law enforcement officials should be contacted to handle the situation.

MANAGEMENT OF THE VETERINARY PRACTICE

Effective management of the people, facilities, and processes in a veterinary hospital makes it possible for veterinarians, technicians, and other staff members to practice good quality medicine and to serve clients in a way that makes them want to return to the hospital. What would happen if no one was available to order drugs and medical supplies; to hire competent veterinarians, technicians, and receptionists; to make the sure the facility was clean and the equipment in good working order; and to promote the hospital while making sure the workflow was efficient? First of all, no clients would be present; second, even if clients did show up, no appropriately trained people or drugs and supplies would allow for the practice of good quality medicine. Management is not a side role in a veterinary hospital; it is essential for a quality operation. Management roles are commonly divided into the following categories:

- *Planning*—strategic and operational
- *Human resources*—hiring, managing, and training employees who work in the practice and fulfilling related legal and regulatory requirements
- *Marketing*—all activities necessary to obtain and retain clients and to enhance awareness and standing of the hospital in the community
- *Financial*—accounting, bookkeeping, financial analysis, capital acquisition, budgeting, pricing strategies, risk management, and related compliance with legal and regulatory requirements
- *Operations*—broad category that has to do with all systems, policies, and procedures that make the hospital operate smoothly on a day-to-day basis, including inventory control, patient and staff scheduling, purchasing, patient flow, management of the front desk, and many other activities
- *Facility and equipment*—acquisition and maintenance

Technicians have an ever-increasing role in practice management. In most practice situations, technicians are involved in management of patients, clients, equipment, and inventory. They may also be involved in hiring and supervising employees and in conducting training and marketing activities. To develop management skills, one must be willing to assume increasing levels of responsibility. As the practice changes in terms of staffing, numbers of cases, the facility, types of clients, new technologies, and so forth, the veterinary technician must adapt his or her management skills to these changes.

The role of the veterinary technician in management will vary depending on the type of practice and the previous experiences of the technician and the veterinarian. The technician who can (1) conceptualize the vision and goals set by the veterinarian for the practice, (2) efficiently organize each area in which he or she is given responsibility, (3) become a productive team player and a good communicator, and (4) develop the ability to solve problems constructively to enhance patient care and the veterinary team usually will be given a greater role in practice management, as well as greater responsibility overall and greater financial rewards.

It is not possible to cover in detail all of the management areas mentioned here; topics discussed in this section are considered to be particularly critical and include areas in which technicians are commonly involved.

PLANNING

Businesses that are most successful in the long run are those that can grow and adapt to changing circumstances. Medical and surgical standards necessary to provide quality care, expectations of clients and employees, and the business skills necessary to run a financially successful practice are not the same now as they were 10 years ago and will not be the same when 10 more years have passed. Practices that do not engage in formal planning activities will ultimately deteriorate and die. Some changes are forced upon a practice; examples include the following:

- Drug or vaccine recalls
- Changes in medical standards
- New and revised laws and regulations
- Changes in the economy and in discretionary spending by clients
- Availability of trained staff

TECHNICIAN NOTE Businesses that are most successful in the long run are those that can grow and adapt to changing circumstances.

Other changes occur internally and are obvious to an owner or manager as something that must be dealt with. Examples include deterioration of facility or equipment quality and hiring of poorly trained staff.

Other changes may not be as visible to a hospital owner or manager as those already mentioned, but they are identified through ongoing monitoring of practice metrics. Examples include lack of transaction growth and decline in profitability.

In addition to reacting to types of negative change discussed here, practices often wish to be proactive and engage in activities that will make the hospital a better one, such as those listed here:

- Adding new services
- Expanding staff training
- Adopting new forms of marketing
- Remodeling the current facility or building a new one

All practices need to have systems in place to identify problems and plan for the future. Some of these activities will be performed monthly or quarterly; others may be done annually or on an as needed basis.

One of the most important times for business planning is before a practice is started or purchased, or when a significant change is being made to the practice, for example, the addition of specialty services to a general practice, or the opening of a satellite clinic. The document prepared most frequently during this planning process is known as a *business plan*.

A business plan is a written document that describes the current nature of the business and plans for the future, both short-term and long-term. The business plan should cover all key areas of the business; sections commonly seen in a veterinary practice business plan include the following:

- Services offered or to be offered by the practice
- Description of the facility and equipment (both existing and desired)
- Veterinarians and support staff: numbers of and types of personnel; compensation and benefits
- Management personnel, activities, and key systems
- Current and projected financial statements
- Marketing and promotion strategies
- Competitor analyses
- Market analyses
- Operations plans
- Anticipated sources of capital to fund the acquisition, formation, or expansion of the business

TECHNICIAN NOTE One of the most important times for business planning is before a practice is started or purchased, or when a significant change is being made to the practice, for example, the addition of specialty services to a general practice, or the opening of a satellite clinic.

Preparing a business plan forces the practice owner to think through exactly how the practice will operate; this process is very useful for identifying potential problems and for setting up systems and processes before the business opens or goes through its expansion. The more detailed the plan, the more likely it is that the practice will run smoothly once open. Business plans are often required to obtain financing.

As noted previously, planning activities should be engaged in monthly, quarterly, and annually once the practice is operating. Common planning and monitoring activities include those listed here:

- Preparation of a monthly and annual budget with regular comparisons of budget versus actual figures

- Monthly tracking of revenue, expenses, and key performance indicators
- Compliance measurement
- Medical record audits

One of the things successful practices do is allot time in each year for formal planning. Ideally, this will involve a strategic retreat away from the practice and moderated by an outside party. The retreat will last 2 or 3 days and will include all key employees of the practice. Some of the areas covered in the retreat will include changes imposed upon or desired by the practice, evaluation of strengths and weakness of the practice, analysis of market threats and opportunities the practice could take advantage of, and the beginnings of the budget process. All areas of the practice should be analyzed, including medical and surgical services, client services, staffing, marketing, finance, operations, facilities, and general management. Practices that do the most effective job at planning will ask technicians and other staff members to contribute their thoughts about how the practice could function better, the kind of feedback they receive from clients, and other matters related to management of the hospital.

HUMAN RESOURCES

The term *human resources* is used to describe the department or activities related to hiring, training, managing, and terminating (if necessary) the people who work in a business. Finding and keeping good employees is arguably one of the most difficult tasks facing the veterinary profession today. Without these employees, veterinarians will not be able to offer the high levels of medical and surgical care that they wish to, nor will they be able to provide the type of client service that keeps clients returning to a practice, allowing the business to prosper financially.

Hiring

Hiring duties are handled differently in different practices depending on practice size, the presence of management personnel, and the management philosophy of the individuals involved. If the hospital has a practice manager, this person generally will be in charge of hiring lower-level management personnel, technicians, receptionists, veterinary assistants, and kennel/ward/barn personnel. Practice owners usually will be significantly involved in the hiring of doctors and upper-level management personnel. Other staff members may also participate in the process as part of formal and/or working interviews.

Before effective hiring can take place, the practice must understand the position it wishes to fill. Preparation or updating of two key documents will help with this task: the organizational chart and the job description.

An organizational chart (aka "org chart") is a visual representation of how departments and employee positions in a business are aligned. It shows how authority and responsibility flow between departments and individuals. All key individuals in the practice should be included in the org chart, along with indications of who reports to whom. Both direct and indirect reporting relationships may be noted. For

example, technicians may formally report to the practice manager but on a day-to-day basis may work regularly for and informally report to the veterinarians in the practice.

> **TECHNICIAN NOTE**   Before effective hiring can take place, the practice must understand the position it wishes to fill. Preparation or updating of two key documents will help with this task: the organizational chart and the job description.

A job description outlines the duties and other attributes of someone who fills a particular position. Job descriptions should be prepared for all positions in the practice and should be updated regularly. A job description will allow both employee and management to maintain a clear understanding of current and new areas of responsibility. Job descriptions are also useful when new employees are hired and when employees are replaced. Technicians are often involved in updating these descriptions for their particular positions. Components of a well-written job description include the following:

- Position title
- Reporting relationship
- Basic purpose or mission of the job
- Principal job duties and responsibilities (both technical and interpersonal)
- Minimum education, experience, and skill and personal characteristic requirements
- ADA requirements

Once the practice has a clear idea of the technical and interpersonal skills needed for the job, along with education and experience requirements, the next step of the hiring process can begin. Applicants can be attracted to the practice in a number of ways. Although some advertising is still done in newspapers and print publications, much of it has moved to the Internet. Practices sometimes use placement services to hire doctors and management personnel. Listings can also be sent to technician or veterinary schools for those particular positions. Suitable candidates are sometimes identified through personal contacts, vendor representatives, or current employees.

Once suitable applicants have been identified, the practice must obtain more detailed information about their skills and experience. This is usually done through the job application, resume, interview, and references. All applicants should fill out a job application (even if they submit a resume) because it contains information not usually seen in resumes, and it supports the practice's efforts at nondiscrimination.

The best way to gather this information and determine whether a candidate is a good fit for the practice is by conducting an interview. Current interviewing theory states that past behavior is the best predictor of future behavior. Therefore, the hiring manager's goal is to identify situations in candidates' past that are similar to circumstances that they will encounter in this job position, and to see how they reacted to them. Questions will also be asked that clarify or expand on information provided in the candidate's application and resume. Once all candidates have been interviewed and their references checked, a decision will be made about which to hire. Attitude and interpersonal skills are generally considered to be as important as, if not more important than, technical skills. All candidates should be notified of the practice's decision.

It is not uncommon for practices to have candidates participate in several interviews and to include technicians and other staff in these sessions. Some interview questions are unlawful or discriminatory and must not be asked (e.g., questions on race, religion, national origin, gender, handicaps, marital status); it is important that they not be asked by anyone in the practice. One of the most important techniques anyone involved in an interview should remember is to listen. It is more important to find out all you can about someone who may be coming to work in the practice than to talk about yourself or the hospital. Ask a lot of questions, and listen to the answers.

Compensation

Another key task performed by the HR department is determination of compensation for veterinarians, technicians, and other staff members. Total compensation is composed of both salaries/wages and benefits.

Objectives of a compensation system include the following:

- Attract, retain, and motivate high performers.
- Maintain internal consistency and external competitiveness.
- Recognize and reward performance.

The first step in creating an equitable and effective wage and compensation system is to develop a consistent procedure for setting pay levels for each position. It is essential to know not only the pay ranges for veterinary practices in the area, but also the going rates for positions in other businesses where current staff members or job candidates might apply for equivalent positions. To find and keep better-than-average people, it is necessary to pay better-than-average salaries.

Pay should be based on performance. A good correlation is generally found between the productivity of employees and their level of education, skill sets, and work experiences, although more experience and more education do not always translate into better work. In salary determination, the key is to make sure that the education, skills, and experiences being rewarded are specific requirements of the position that will contribute to better job performance. Seniority by itself is not a reason for higher pay. Those who do not perform should not be paid in the same manner as those who do.

> **TECHNICIAN NOTE** Good correlation is generally noted between the productivity of employees and their education level, skill set, and work experience.

Benefits vary among staff positions and between full-time and part-time employees. However, those often seen in veterinary practices include health insurance, vacation pay, sick pay, paid holidays, and reimbursement for dues, licenses, continuing education, and retirement plan contributions.

Training and Orientation

In an ideal world, all employees would come to the practice knowing everything they need to know to be a productive employee. Unfortunately, this is not the case. Even if a doctor, a technician, or a receptionist has worked in another practice, they will not know the policies and procedures in their new hospital. The quality of training programs can vary greatly among practices; the most successful hospitals are those with good quality, formalized training programs.

Employee orientation is usually the first training experience a new employee encounters. The goal of the orientation is to introduce the employee to colleagues, give the employee an overview of how the practice operates, instruct the employee in the policies and procedures necessary for efficient operation of the practice, provide OSHA training, and give the employee the basic, practical information needed for a successful start—work hours, pay dates, and so on.

Employees should then receive a longer, more detailed training program dedicated to their role in the hospital. Some components of the training will be the same across positions, for example, everyone needs to know how to use the practice information management system (PIMS). Other components of training will be specific to the position.

The best hospitals offer ongoing training in both medical and client service matters. Technology and medical standards change rapidly, and ongoing training of all employees is essential if good quality medicine and client services are to be offered. Ongoing training leads to improved efficiency, better work quality, and improved client service, and makes the job more interesting for employees.

Some ongoing training will be done internally, often as a part of staff meetings held weekly, monthly, or at other intervals. Another important aspect of ongoing training is the opportunity to attend outside veterinary meetings or veterinary conferences. In addition to attending sessions given by recognized experts in their field, these meetings give all staff members a chance to meet and talk with people from other hospitals. Information learned in these conversations can be as helpful as that learned in formal sessions.

Employee Management and Retention

Another formal task of the HR department is ongoing management of employees in the practice. In reality, however, some employee management falls to almost everyone in the practice.

The management process is a two-way street between the employer/manager and the employee. The employer/manager needs to communicate expectations to the employee and to work with the employee to set mutually agreed upon performance goals and contributions needed from the employee for clinic success. The employer/manager also needs to provide guidance and feedback to the employee as needed, as well as tools and resources needed by the employee to be successful. The employee has a role in this as well. The employee needs to work with the employer/manager in setting goals and expectations and must communicate any concerns about these during this planning process. The employee also needs to seek out training opportunities, guidance, and direction as needed, and to communicate to the manager in a professional manner problems and issues in the practice.

An important management task that is generally performed or coordinated by the HR staff is that of performance appraisals. One of the most common mistakes in personnel management is putting off regular employee evaluations. Personnel problems resulting from poor work performance do not just go away; they only become worse. Employees cannot improve their performance unless they are given an opportunity to identify shortcomings. Employers also need to identify and reward employees for work they do well.

Good managers do not wait for the annual performance review to let their employees know which areas they excel in and where they need help and guidance. However, it is important that this feedback be formally conveyed and documented at least annually. Written performance appraisals are a formalization of the day-to-day appraisal process. They often help to reduce misunderstandings, can be more convincing than words, and create a permanent record. However, nothing in the formal evaluation should be a surprise to the employee unless it has to do with an incident that occurred 5 minutes before the performance appraisal meeting with the person involved. All positive and negative feedback should have been communicated to the employee at the time the behavior occurred. Ideally, the performance review process is a positive one wherein management and employees work together to help the employee perform better and reach personal work goals as well.

> **TECHNICIAN NOTE** Good managers do not wait for the annual performance review to let their employees know which areas they excel in and where they need help and guidance. However, it is important that this feedback be formally conveyed and documented at least annually.

Formal reviews are typically given after 3 months for a new employee, and after that once a year. The appraisal should cover technical skills (e.g., Is the employee able/not able to do specific tasks?) as well as the employee's willingness, motivation, and general attitude toward his or her work.

Sometimes employees are asked to complete self-appraisal forms before the time of the review. Employees frequently know more about their performance than any other single person, and they often require higher standards of their own performance than do others. A self-appraisal form includes questions about the following:

- Accomplishments
- Areas where goals were not accomplished and why
- Assessment of strengths and weaknesses
- Factors impeding accomplishment of the job
- What the employee wants to accomplish in the next year in the form of skills, abilities, and goals

Even if the person performing the review has not asked the employee to do a self-assessment, this is a good exercise for the employee to go through in preparation for the meeting.

Addressing Employee Stress

Veterinary medicine, like other health care professions, includes a fair amount of stress. Veterinary personnel who work in clinical practices are on their feet for the vast majority of the day. Many technicians feel that they have little time for lunch or other breaks and are challenged to keep up with the pace of a busy practice. Animals can be uncooperative, and owners, who may be stressed themselves (particularly if their pet is ill), can be difficult at times. In addition, the closely knit staff that constitutes many veterinary health care teams can be particularly vulnerable to stress if conflict arises within the team. Finally, pet loss from euthanasia and illness, and particularly unexpected death, can bring sadness and lower morale, which in turn exacerbates an already stressful working environment. With time, experienced technicians learn to pace themselves and to recognize and address potentially stressful situations as they arise. Nevertheless, stress is an all too common aspect of working in veterinary technology.

Physical signs of stress include gastric reflux, ulcers, nausea, and muscle tension leading to muscular aches and pains. As stress gets worse or goes on for a longer period of time, anxiety, depression, anger, and a reduced ability to cope are commonly seen.

People will not experience stress in the same way. Whether or not a person can adapt to stress depends upon the situation, the level and duration of the stress, and the personality of the individual. Some personality types are susceptible to stress; others are stress resistant. People who have a tendency to be competitive, perfectionistic, and often angry are more vulnerable to stress. They are called type A personalities. In contrast, type B personalities are more stress resilient. They tend to have realistic expectations of what they can accomplish and are less worried about failure.

Stressors

The extent to which a person is self-confident and possesses self-esteem is important in the level of stress experienced by the person. For example, an individual who is confident in her abilities, intelligence, and organizational skills may be relatively calm while planning a wedding, working full-time, and volunteering to run the community fundraiser. On the other hand, a less confident individual might feel tremendously stressed when performing the simplest tasks.

Previous experiences, personal backgrounds, and the circumstances of one's living situation can make an individual more or less resilient to the stress of clinical practice. Life events play a key role in the performance of workers and in the level of stress they experience. A person who feels supported by family and friends, for example, is more stress resilient in the workplace than someone who does not have support. Stress can come both from positive events such as getting married and from negative events such as experiencing the death of a loved one. Both events are stressful. Employees who have overextended themselves in their activities outside of the workplace may feel tired and short tempered, even though the activities are designed to be fun. Thus, moderation is an important part of a balanced and happy life.

Reducing Stress in the Workplace

Veterinary technicians who are leaders within the veterinary health care team can help to create a positive working environment for the team by minimizing stress and by building a culture of collaboration (Box 2-3). Insisting on no gossip, for example, and removing staff members who incite conflict can alleviate a huge source of stress for the veterinary health care team. Technicians can help to create an environment in which staff members feel free to admit mistakes, and where individuals are not singled out and shamed. Finally, veterinary technician leaders can decrease stress by arranging regular meetings in which open and clear communication with team members can take place.

BOX 2-3 | Five Steps for Reducing Stress

1. Plan for the unexpected.
   - Keep time slots free for emergencies and delays.
   - Arrange for emergency backup personnel in the event that a team member unexpectedly cannot work, and when more emergencies than expected arrive for treatment.
   - Cross-train staff.
   - Have backup generators that keep the practice (and the computer system) functional during power failures.
   - Prepare written standard operating procedures, and review them with staff.
2. Create reasonable work schedules.
   - Avoid scheduling excessively long hours.
   - Insist that each member of the health care team take at least one break per 8-hour period.
   - Schedule and take vacation time.
3. Create a culture of collaboration, trust, and mutual support (rather than of gossip, blame, and fingerpointing).
   - Model professional behavior and respect for coworkers.
   - Never reprimand a staff member in front of others.
   - Keep emotions under control at all times.
4. Recognize and counsel staff members who are particularly stressed.
5. Provide clear communication with staff members.
   - Have regular staff meetings.
   - Support open communication, but at the same time, limit complaining.

Employee Substance Abuse and Stress

The combination of a stressful workplace and the availability of various drugs in veterinary practice puts veterinary personnel at risk of engaging in illegal drug use. The nervous system, brain, and emotions are dependent on the normal action of neurotransmitters; therefore, some individuals suffering from stress may turn to drugs and alcohol almost as a form of self-medication. Alcohol and drugs can enhance, distort, or even eliminate information normally exchanged by nerve cells. Evidence seems to indicate that a genetic vulnerability to substance abuse may be present as well. Some cultural groups have established patterns of use, and some age groups seem to be more vulnerable. In studies comparing occupations, physicians and health care professionals have been found to be more vulnerable than those in other occupations. When the individual has knowledge about drugs and has access to drugs, that individual is at risk. In general, a veterinarian or a veterinary staff member with a substance abuse problem will exhibit a change in behavior. Their behavior in the clinic may change, so that they neglect duties, appear disorganized, or exhibit poor judgment in the practice of veterinary medicine. Other signs may include prescriptions written for themselves, friends, or family, or drugs may go missing from the clinic during the hours in which they were on duty. Financial or legal problems may arise. Unexplained absences, conflicts with others, and career instability may result.

Some type of intervention and action is needed any time that substance abuse interferes with work activities. Client, patient, and coworker safety is of primary importance. The entire practice may be at risk of malpractice because of the substance abuser. In every state, a Board of Veterinary Medicine awards, reviews, and can suspend licenses of veterinarians (and veterinary technicians if licensed) in that state. Most governing boards for health care professionals have stipulations by which impairment of the professional prevents renewal. Generally speaking, the impaired professional should be confronted, preferably by a peer or a superior, and should be asked to seek treatment.

All 50 states offer resources and guidance for impaired veterinarians, through the governing board or through the state professional association. Because many states do not license veterinary technicians, fewer rehabilitation opportunities are available for them via state licensing boards or state technician associations. Most states have a list of qualified counselors and treatment centers that work with impaired doctors, dentists, and veterinarians. For these medical professionals, counselors will do an evaluation to determine what type of treatment is recommended.

MARKETING

The term *marketing* often gets confused with advertising; however, marketing is composed of much more than this. Marketing includes all activities necessary to obtain and retain clients and enhance awareness and standing of the hospital in the community. To obtain and retain clients, the practice must offer services/products that are of value to the pet owner, at a price consistent with that value and in a way that is appealing to the client. Marketing therefore is not only about the service/product itself, it is also about client service. And of course, part of marketing involves communicating the offerings of the hospital to clients and potential clients. Some professionals feel uncomfortable with the idea of marketing because the concept gets confused with the idea of sales or trying to get pet owners to buy something they don't really need. This is not what marketing is about. Another way to think of marketing is as client education, that is, helping pet owners understand the care needed for their pets to live a long and healthy life. The veterinary technician must understand marketing principles to be an effective communicator of professional services and goods offered by the practice.

> **TECHNICIAN NOTE** Marketing includes all activities necessary to obtain and retain clients and enhance awareness and standing of the hospital in the community.

Animals are totally dependent on the owner's awareness of their health care needs and the willingness of the owner to provide for those needs. Some practitioners believe that as long as high-quality medical and surgical skills are delivered, the client will continue to use their services based on this alone. However, the average client lacks the professional background to accurately judge the quality of medical or surgical services performed. Instead, clients judge the quality of services and caring communication that they receive, which influences their perception of the value of medical and surgical services received. Clients' perceived value of services is their reality of the quality of the practice.

Veterinary medicine is a people-service business. Veterinary professionals care for animals but ultimately provide services and products to their owners. As discussed in an earlier section, patients cannot come to the practice without owners. This is a key concept that should infuse everything a practice does. When clients call on the telephone, for example, this should not be regarded as an interruption of the veterinarian's or technician's time; those clients are the only reason the practice continues to exist. Only satisfied clients return and refer others.

Almost every activity the hospital engages in is a part of marketing. The professional appearance of the hospital, clinic, or ambulatory vehicle is suggestive of the quality of care it provides. Verbal and nonverbal communication between doctors or technicians and pet owners does not just convey factual information; it also conveys interest in the pet and the pet owner, warmth and concern, and a desire to help the pet owner. Technicians are actively involved in marketing the practice with everything they do.

Marketing activities are often broken into two types: internal and external. Internal marketing is generally aimed at the existing client base, and much of this is focused on

day-to-day client service and communication, and other activities that occur within each practice. External marketing is focused more outwardly, but current clients are also reached by external marketing. Much of the goal of these activities is to attract new clients. The line between the two is fuzzy; however, the purpose of both internal and external techniques is to increase the number of clients served by the practice and the frequency with which they visit.

Internal Marketing

Internal marketing is aimed primarily at the existing client base. Internal marketing techniques attempt to educate current clients about the health needs of their pets and the various veterinary services and service programs available to meet those needs. Much of the internal marketing carried on within a practice will be handled by veterinary team members, including technicians.

> **TECHNICIAN NOTE** Internal marketing is aimed primarily at the existing client base. Internal marketing techniques attempt to educate current clients about the health needs of their pets and about various veterinary services and service programs that are available to meet those needs.

The veterinarian and the support staff must work together as a service team, all delivering the same high-quality educational messages, care, and service.

Client Relationships

The most important technique that can be used in any marketing program is personalized, sincere care of the client. Most clients require as much attention and care as the patient. Personalized service that emphasizes each individual client is critical. This concern and caring cannot be faked; people who work in veterinary practices need to be genuinely concerned about the clients they serve.

Practice Appearance

The importance of the visual appearance of the clinic, hospital, or ambulatory vehicle was discussed previously. A practice facility does not have to be new or have the latest equipment to project a positive professional image, but it must be attractive and clean, and it must be given proper care and maintenance to send the desired marketing messages of warmth, caring, and professional competence.

Full-Service Care

Part of the marketing process involves identifying what clients want and providing it to them. In general, pet owners, like all other consumers in today's busy world, want convenience. One-stop shopping is the goal, particularly for single-parent families and families in which both husband and wife work. In a small animal practice, full-service care includes pet prepurchase counseling, human–animal bond and behavioral problem counseling, pediatric care, preventive medicine, nutritional counseling, nutritional management, veterinary-supervised boarding, geriatric care, dentistry, in-house emergency care, bereavement counseling, and cremation services, in addition to full routine veterinary care. Many clients also want their veterinary practice to offer online product purchase or delivery of medications and food purchases, nonmedical boarding, grooming, and puppy day care. Anything that makes it simpler and faster for pet owners to take care of their pets is important to them. Full-service care sends a strong marketing message regarding convenience and respect for the client's time and needs.

Particular concern among veterinarians about the lack of care provided to cats has been noted. Practice owners and managers are increasingly focusing on making cats and cat owners feel welcome and comfortable in their practice. Providing information to cat owners about acclimating cats to carriers and transporting them to the clinic can make it easier for cats to get the care they need. A separate reception area for cats combined with the practice of keeping cats in a separate ward eases both cat and cat owner anxiety.

Client Reminders

Most practices have a system in place in which reminders are sent to clients when it is time for various services to be performed, such as annual examinations, vaccinations, and medication refills. As noted previously, clients are increasingly busy and want to be reminded when care is due. All the most commonly used practice management computer software packages have the capability of capturing reminder information.

The most successful reminder protocols in practices have the following characteristics:

- Multiple reminders (usually up to three) will be sent if the client does not respond to the first or second one.
- Multiple reminders are sent in various formats; for example, the first reminder may be sent by direct mail, the second by e-mail, and the third by telephone.
- Reminders are sent not just for vaccinations but for a wide variety of services, including dental care, follow-up laboratory testing, food refills, ovariohysterectomy or castration, heartworm, and flea and tick or other medication refills.
- The language used in the reminder does not just name the recommended service; "FVRCP" means nothing to a client. Instead, the reminder should briefly describe the service offered and should emphasize the benefits for both pet and client.

In some practices, clients have the opportunity to choose the way they would like to receive reminders (i.e., by mail, by text, or by e-mail).

Personal Appearance

The personal appearance and hygiene of each staff member reflect the quality of the practice. Many clients relate personal appearance to sanitation and the level of medicine practiced. If someone does not care enough to change a dirty smock, coveralls, or boots, why should he or she care enough to provide the highest-quality medical care? Personal appearance marketing works the way building appearance marketing works—it serves as an outward signal of internal quality.

Handout Materials

Client handouts can range from a practice brochure (Figure 2-22) outlining hours and services to educational materials

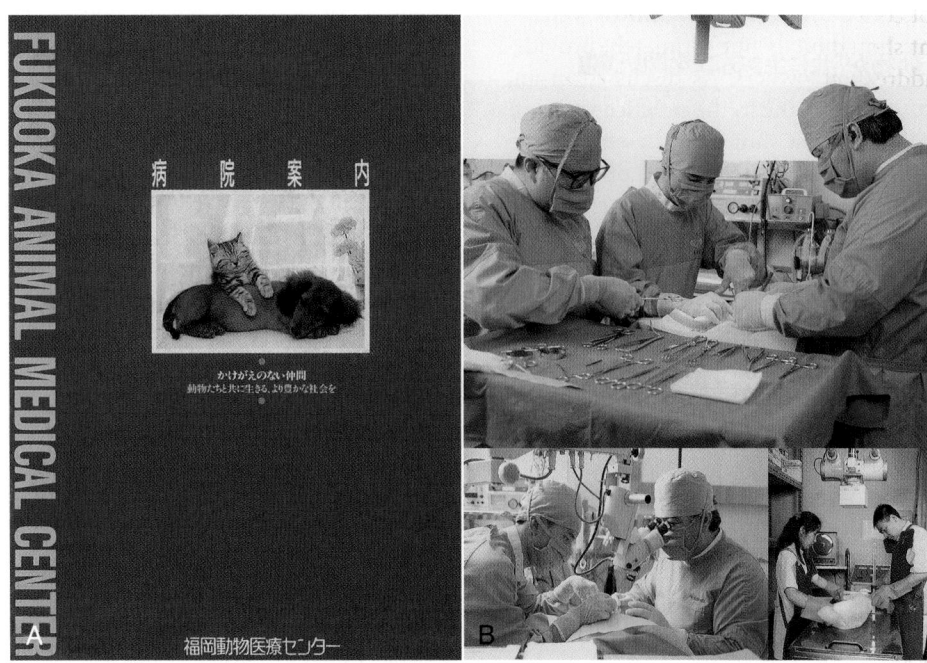

FIGURE 2-22 Practice information pamphlet. **A,** Cover. **B,** Inner page. (Courtesy Fukuoka Animal Medical Center, Fukuoka, Japan.)

discussing preventive care and specific diseases. Use of handouts is important for several reasons. Not only do they reinforce information that was provided at the practice, they also make it possible for others involved in the pet's care to understand the medical condition of the pet and the recommendations made by the practice.

Not everyone learns best by listening; some take in information better when reading, and others when seeing pictures, models, or the problem with the pet itself. Handouts are particularly useful for those who learn best by reading or through other visual means.

Some practices will create their own handouts; others use commercially available versions. The quantity and quality of handouts received from veterinary professional organizations such as AVMA, AAHA, or the American Association of Equine Practitioners (AAEP), or from companies in the animal health industry, are often excellent; however, these pieces should be carefully reviewed by the practice to make sure they conform to the philosophy and recommendations of the practice. A professional rubber stamp or printed stick-on labels that have the practice name, location, and telephone number on them can be purchased and used to personalize all commercial handout materials.

An important role of the veterinary technician in practice is client education. Veterinary technicians should be familiar with preprinted information brochures distributed by the practice and should have them available at each appointment. The client is most likely to read the information and benefit from it if the material is handed to them with an explanation provided by the veterinary technician (Figure 2-23).

Other examples of handout materials include a payment policy, invoices received at the end of a visit, discharge instructions, business cards, and letterhead stationery. All materials should have a consistent look and feel (logo, font, colors) and should not contain spelling or grammatical mistakes. Every document should contain the practice's contact information: name, address, phone, fax, e-mail address, and website.

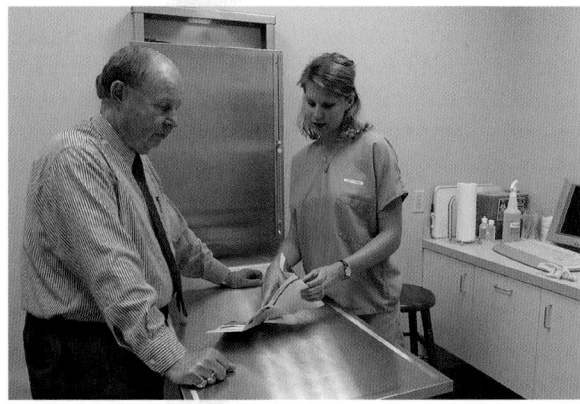

FIGURE 2-23 Technician explaining and providing a handout to client.

Sympathy and Thank You Communications

A sympathy card or a personal note sent to a client when a pet dies demonstrates concern for the feelings of the client during a time of bereavement. This expression helps the client deal with the loss and allows the client to understand the "I care" attitude of the practice for both client and pet.

Thank you notes to clients for referring another client, to new clients, or to those who bring cookies or other gifts to the practice are not only a common courtesy but reflect good marketing. The practice may choose to use commercially prepared cards or may develop a letter format on the computer that can be personalized. Regardless of the format used, the sentiments expressed should be sincere and professional.

Newsletters

Many practices reach out to their clients via a newsletter, usually sent either by regular mail or by e-mail. Newsletters help educate clients about husbandry items related to their animals, things the owner can do to keep them healthy, and necessary veterinary services. Practices often include human interest stories, as well as news about the practice. Photos, graphics, and an easy-to-read style all increase the likelihood that the newsletter will be read. Topics included can range from information about seasonal illnesses/accidents to signs and symptoms noticed by an owner that should be discussed with a veterinarian to the benefits of having a healthy pet. The newsletter should also refer the reader to the practice's website for further information on a specific subject found in the electronic library of the website.

Most veterinarians do not have the experience or the time to compose a complete newsletter 3 or 4 times per year. The practice manager, veterinary technicians, and receptionists may develop articles for a practice newsletter, or consideration can be given to purchasing a professionally edited newsletter service. A number of good quality options are available commercially and may be edited to include information specified by the practice.

As with handout materials, newsletters should have a consistent look and feel (logo, font, colors) and should not contain spelling or grammatical mistakes. Every document should contain the practice's contact information: name, address, phone, fax, e-mail address, and website.

Targeted Mail

Another way of educating clients is through targeted letters sent by regular mail or by e-mail. These are generally shorter than newsletters and focus on just one topic, for example, the importance of heartworm prevention. These mailings can be sent to specific segments of clients or to all clients, depending on the applicability of the information. The letters should talk about what the practice recommends, but also why it is important, and should identify the benefits provided to the client and the animal. In companion animal practices, these ideally are personalized with the pet's name and sex and should be easy to understand and read.

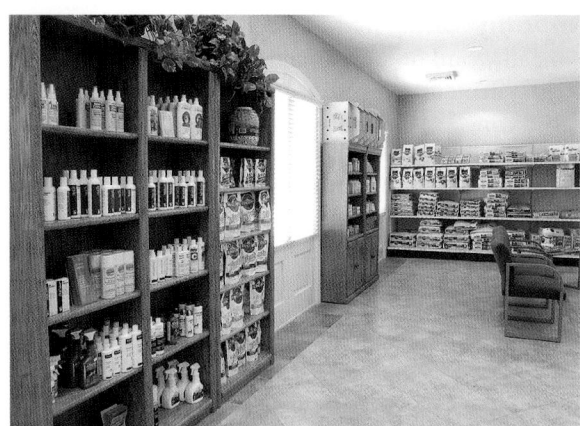

FIGURE 2-24 Professional display in reception area.

A few practices have the e-mail addresses of all of their clients, but most practices are still in their infancy in this regard. Receptionists should regularly ask all clients for this information, but follow-up by technicians will help keep the practice's database up-to-date.

Point-of-Sale Displays

Point-of-sale displays can be useful in educating clients about pet health products and offer a convenient way to purchase the products (Figure 2-24). When displays are being considered as an internal marketing technique, several important points must be contemplated if they are to be successful. First, the practice must define client needs. The specific products must be carefully selected and priced. An appropriate location or locations must be established in the clinic or hospital. The products must be attractively arranged and kept neat and clean. Prices must be clearly marked on all products. To add value above that offered at feed stores, pet stores, grocery stores, or other outlets, practice staff members should be readily available to answer questions and educate clients. The technician staff will play a key role in providing this information to the client.

Animal Care Talks

Results from the Bayer Veterinary Care Usage Study[3] indicate that a large number of pet owners do not have a good understanding of the care their pet needs to live a long and healthy life. Practice owners have a large opportunity to increase traffic at their practice and help pets get better care by educating pet owners about these matters. One way of doing this is to offer seminars about pet/animal care matters at the practice or in the community. Examples include kitten kindergarten classes offered at the practice, talks given to grade school or high school students, and seminars provided to members of community organizations.

> **TECHNICIAN NOTE** Results from the Bayer Veterinary Care Usage Study[3] indicate that a large number of pet owners do not have a good understanding of the care their pet needs to live a long and healthy life.

Veterinary technicians and veterinarians are often best suited to present these seminars because of their technical training. However, presentations should be interesting and entertaining, as well as educational, so it is important to select someone who has good public speaking skills. These presentations can provide information on routine animal health care, first aid activities, signs to look for when an animal is ill, and general information on the veterinary profession and the practice of veterinary medicine. Attendees should be provided with handout material to take home for future reference. When the education program is held at the practice, a complete tour of the facilities should be planned. Clients are interested in seeing hospital equipment and in understanding more about hospital care. A behind-the-scenes tour is something that most clients have not had an opportunity to experience. Many will be amazed to see x-ray, anesthesia, surgery, and laboratory equipment, "just like in a human hospital." Children are especially impressed with show-and-tell demonstrations using live animals.

External Marketing

As noted previously, the line between internal and external marketing is not a clear one; however, external marketing is focused more outwardly. Some of these marketing efforts will reach current clients as well, but much of the goal is to attract new clients.

External marketing activities are implemented by individual practices, veterinary professional organizations, and commercial companies in the animal health arena. Marketing done by professional organizations and the animal health industry focuses on general messages such as "Visit your veterinarian twice a year" or on specific product-related messages. External marketing efforts initiated by the practice generally include educational content but also focus on the benefits of visiting that particular practice.

Discussed in the following paragraphs are commonly seen types of external marketing efforts used by veterinary practices.

Advertising

The term *advertising* is generally used to refer to paid announcements in print, broadcast, or electronic media. Advertising most commonly done by veterinary hospitals includes telephone book listings, newspapers, magazines, radio, and direct mail. A great majority of professionals (physicians, dentists, attorneys, veterinarians) do not like advertising for a variety of reasons: It seems to be unprofessional and unethical, and it lowers status, credibility, and the sense of dignity. Therefore, many kinds of true advertising are not used in veterinary marketing as much as they are used in other fields.

All practices should have clear signage. This is important as a marketing tool to help clients locate the practice (Figure 2-25). Signs should be large and well lighted and should be placed in a highly visible area. They should be professionally created with messaging that can be changed or that will

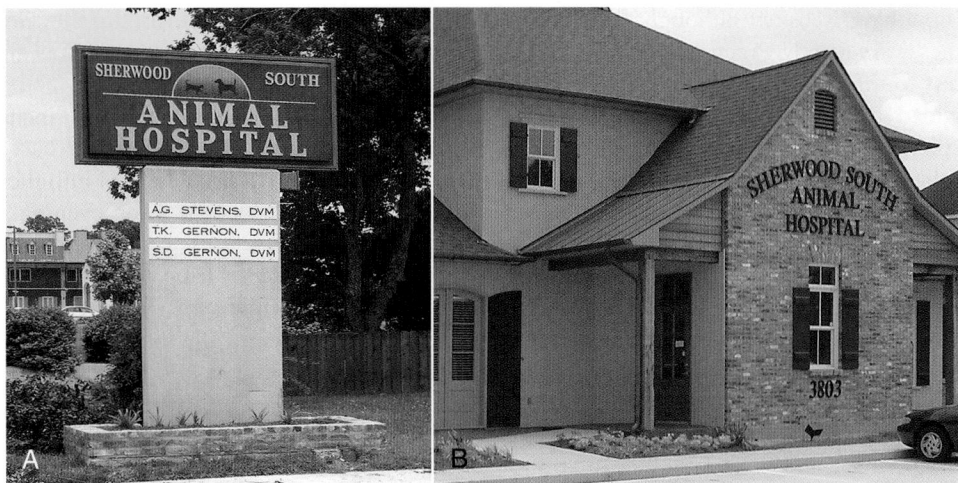

FIGURE 2-25 A, Hospital signs should be professional and clearly visible from the street. B, Signs directly on the building may also be used.

stand the test of time. Signage should be well maintained, along with the rest of the building exterior.

Telephone yellow page advertising has been a staple of veterinary marketing for many years but has been falling out of favor for some time. The proliferation of books within a community has increased the cost to the point where the cost/benefit analysis does not make sense. In addition, the advent of the Internet has shifted many consumers' business research habits. Consumers who used to use the yellow pages to locate businesses now go online. Most practices still have a listing or an ad in the yellow pages but have reduced the size of the ad and the number of books in which the ad appears.

Newspapers

Newspaper advertising is not used as frequently as yellow page advertising by most practices because of both cost and readership. Ongoing newspaper advertising is most effective in smaller community papers, where the readership is likely to comprise pet owners who live near enough to the practice to consider it as a viable option. Pet owners generally visit a practice that is within 3 to 5 miles of where they live, so many of the readers of a newspaper in a major metropolitan area would never cross town to visit a practice advertised in that paper. Practices that do successfully include newspaper advertising in their marketing program most often do so via the writing of an animal care information column. These weekly or monthly columns are often of interest to readers and serve as a good source of publicity for the practice.

Some practices will have a newspaper listing when opening a new practice, when relocating an existing practice, or when adding new associates to an existing practice.

Some veterinarians have a relationship with local newspapers and are called to comment on animal-related matters affecting the community.

Radio and Television

Occasionally, you will see a veterinary practice advertise on TV or radio, but this is very uncommon. Public service announcements and paid advertising by veterinary organizations sometimes occur. The most common use of radio and television advertising by practices is seen when the practice's veterinarians participate in talk shows devoted to animal care.

Not only does this participation market the services of a particular practice, it educates pet owners about the need for care and is good for the profession as a whole. As with newspapers, some veterinarians have a relationship with local radio and TV stations and are called to comment on animal-related matters affecting the community.

Popular television programs such as *Animal Planet* have had a large impact on marketing of the veterinary profession as a whole. Likewise, the earlier James Herriot books and televised Public Broadcasting System (PBS) series attracted many animal lovers to the profession. All these media events help increase public awareness of the need for veterinary care and the high level of care provided by the veterinary profession.

Community Activities

Veterinary practices that engage in community activities have found these activities to be personally rewarding, as well as a way to increase their client base. Many opportunities arise for veterinarians and technicians to become involved in community service through Girl Scouts, Boy Scouts, 4-H programs, school boards, humane societies, country clubs, Rotary clubs, Lions clubs, and church activities. Potential contacts with clients are made in the course of being involved with and contributing to these organizations. Practices will often sponsor local activities such as sports teams or animal fairs; this is another good way to get the practice's name out.

Web-Based Marketing

Web-based marketing represents the newest form of marketing for veterinary practices and organizations. It is evolving at lightning speed, and many practices are still trying to decide how to use these new forms of media.

Most practices now have websites, although the quality and usefulness of these vary greatly. Practices use websites to provide public access to information about the practice, its staff, services provided by the practice, and pet care in general. Graphics, pictures, and videos are commonly used and may include a virtual tour of the medical facility. A Web page may provide practice clientele with the ability to make an appointment online and to access their pets' health records. The practice Web page should be updated frequently and must be attractive and easy to use.

Facebook, Twitter, and blogs are being used more commonly by practices, although many are still struggling with how to use these tools effectively.

Many, many websites other than those created by veterinary practices offer veterinary and pet-related information. Some of these provide accurate information, but many do not. Clients are going to use the Internet, so practices should educate clients about how to tell whether or not a site has good information. Providing a list of recommended sites and keeping the practice's own website up-to-date and well stocked are critical components of this education.

Pet Portals

A number of companies are offering pet portal services to veterinary practices that combine with other options some of the internal and external marketing activities already discussed. These services vary in what they offer, but it is often a combination of client communication materials and home delivery for medications and pet food. Specific offerings may include a website, e-mail or mail reminders, pet birthday cards, targeted marketing, online shopping, pet medical record access, online appointment scheduling, a pet health library, pet ID cards, and more. Standardized and customized options are available. Practices are using these tools to improve client education and convenience.

FINANCIAL

Managing the finances of a practice well is critical. If the practice is not financially successful, it will not be able to offer good quality medicine and surgery, invest in its employees, nor, ultimately, survive. Some of the tasks associated with good financial management include the following:
- Bookkeeping and accounting, including payment of bills and collection of fees
- Management analysis
- Budgeting
- Price setting
- Capital acquisition
- Risk management
- Compliance with legal and regulatory requirements

Bookkeeping and Accounting

All small businesses, including veterinary practices, must perform the following bookkeeping tasks: collect payments for services performed or products sold; make payments for products purchased and services received; and run payroll and prepare financial statements. Most practices do not prepare their own tax returns, but they must keep the financial records in such a way as to allow their accountant to easily do so.

All client financial information, including invoices for services performed or products purchased, returns, credits, and payments, is initially entered into the practice information management system. Each evening, the daily transactions entered into this system are reconciled with the payments collected during the day, and a bank deposit is made. This information is then entered into the practice's accounting software. The most commonly used software in small businesses is QuickBooks. Bills are generally paid on a regular schedule, often weekly, and this information is also captured in the accounting software. Payroll is most often handled by an outside payroll service with the information entered into the practice accounting software.

The practice accounting software is used to generate regular reports for use in preparing the tax return and managing the practice's finances and operations. The most commonly used reports are the balance sheet, the income statement, and the statement of **cash flows**. A brief description of each of these reports is given here.

Balance Sheet

The balance sheet is one of the financial statements commonly prepared for a business internally or by the practice's outside accountant. This statement summarizes the financial position of the practice at a point in time, and shows all assets of the practice and all of its liabilities. Assets are the economic resources controlled by an entity and used to carry out its mission. Most assets are tangible in nature (cash, **petty cash**, equipment, buildings, drug and supplies inventory); however, some intangible assets such as goodwill are also recorded in the financial statements. Liabilities are obligations of the practice, generally payable in cash at some future date; examples include credit card payables, accounts payable, and loans. This report is particularly useful to practice owners/managers in terms of enhancing their understanding of inventory levels, debt levels, and the proportion of debt that must be paid off within the next year compared with the cash needed to do so.

Income Statement

The income statement is the second of the financial statements commonly prepared for a business; it reflects the financial performance of a business between two points in time. It includes the **gross revenue total** generated by the practice for a specified period of time (typically a month or a year) and expenses incurred to generate that revenue during the same time period. In a veterinary practice, a vast amount of revenue is derived from providing medical/surgical services to pet owners as well as from product sales. Typical expenses include compensation, benefits, drugs and medical supplies, laboratory expenses, pet food expenses, facility rental, utilities, advertising, accounting, and others. The income statement is often called by other names, including *profit and loss statement (P&L)*, *statement of operations*, and *statement of revenue and expenses*. The amount left over after the expenses are subtracted from the revenue is *net income*, which is hoped to be a positive number. This report helps practice owners/managers understand revenue growth or decline and whether expenses are within reasonable limits.

> **TECHNICIAN NOTE** The income statement is the second of the financial statements commonly prepared for a business; it reflects the financial performance of a business between two points in time and includes the gross revenue generated by the practice over a specified period of time (typically a month or a year) and expenses incurred to generate that revenue during the same time period.

Statement of Cash Flows

The statement of cash flows is another financial statement that is always prepared for big businesses and less commonly for small businesses. This is a mistake because the main reason why businesses fail is that they run out of cash, and this report helps a business understand what its cash position is. This statement reflects the sources and uses of cash during a particular period of time (again, typically a month or a year).

The accounting system must be set up to capture all financial data simply and accurately. Various checks and balances must be included in the system to identify inadvertent mistakes or deliberate fraud or theft. The people involved in all aspects of the accounting process must have the proper training to do this job properly; these are not generally tasks that employees can pick up intuitively. Technicians are not usually involved in the actual preparation of the accounting reports unless they have moved into a management role; however, they are often involved in some of the activities that feed into the accounting system, such as preparation of client invoices and inventory control. Performing these tasks properly is very important to the accuracy of financial reports.

Management Analysis

The accounting system is also used to generate information for management analysis (i.e., to gain a better understanding of how well the practice is doing operationally and financially and which areas could be improved). The financial statements discussed previously are used in this type of analysis; however, it is also important to review the other data described in the following paragraphs.

Profitability Calculation

Understanding the profitability of a practice is one of the most important concepts needed to manage a veterinary hospital well. Profitability is the one single number that shows whether or not a practice is financially successful. Calculating the true operating profits of a practice is not a simple task. None of the standard financial or management reports a practice usually gets shows this figure. This does not mean that those reports are improperly prepared; it simply means that the reports required by the IRS and

accounting standards for small businesses were not designed to determine profitability. Because practice owners and managers are not used to getting this kind of information, they generally do not know what the true profitability of their practice is.

Operating profit is the difference between operating revenues and expenses of a practice. Operating revenue and expenses include only items normally and necessarily seen in the day-to-day operations of the practice, such as fees for professional services and expenses for drugs and medical supplies. These items should be stated at fair market value rates. For ease of comparison with other practices, the profit margin is generally stated as a percentage—calculated as practice profits divided by gross revenue.

Net income per financial statements or the tax return is the starting point for the profitability figure. Various adjustments are made from there; the easiest way to get this figure is to use the National Commission on Veterinary Economic Issues (NCVEI)/VetPartners Profitability Estimator available on the NCVEI website (www.ncvei.org). The NCVEI is a nonprofit organization devoted to keeping veterinary medicine economically strong.

Key Performance Indicators

Key performance indicators (KPIs) are metrics used by the practice to evaluate performance. The term is used loosely and can include a wide range of figures, many of which come from the practice information management system. In addition to the items already discussed, some of the most commonly used include the following:

- Revenue and transactions per full-time-equivalent (FTE) doctor—an FTE doctor is usually considered to be one who works 40 hours/week, 52 weeks/year. FTE doctor figures are used instead of absolute numbers of doctors because doctors do not always work the same number of hours per week. Transactions are equivalent to client invoices; invoices are generated for all services provided and may range from a small dollar amount for a bag of food or a prescription refill to a much greater amount for a complicated surgical or medical case. These metrics are used to measure the productivity of doctors. Technicians are instrumental in helping doctors to be productive.
- Patient visits—patient visits are different from transactions. Transactions (invoices) include all services/products purchased by a client, whereas patient visit figures include only times that a patient actually visited the hospital and had some kind of procedure performed such as an examination, surgery, or dental work.
- Average transaction charge—this figure is calculated by dividing the total revenue of a practice by the total number of transactions; it represents the average amount a client spends during a visit to the practice.
- Revenue by category (dentistry, surgery, product sales, etc.)—these metrics are used to analyze the types of services clients are electing to receive.
- Numbers of new clients and active clients—a new client is considered to be one who has never visited the practice

before; an active client is one who has visited the practice within the last 12 months.

- Accounts receivable aging—accounts receivable represent amounts owed to the practice by clients who are allowed to charge at the practice (i.e., they do not pay for their services at the time of purchase but are billed later). The aging report shows the dollar amount owed by these clients and how long the money has been owed.
- Overtime hours—it is often difficult to schedule employee hours to exactly meet the needs of the practice because of emergencies and last minute additions to the appointment schedule; therefore, overtime is sometimes incurred by staff members. Overtime pay is more expensive than regular time pay, so practice owners and managers strive to keep it to a minimum.
- Number of staff calculated on an FTE basis and compared with the number of FTE doctors—both FTE doctors and staff members are considered to be those who work 40 hours/week, 52 weeks/year. This calculation helps a practice understand whether it has too many or too few staff people to help the doctors be most productive.
- Works hours per transaction—this metric is calculated by dividing the total number of hours worked by doctors and staff by the total number of transactions. The resulting figure serves as a measure of staff and doctor efficiency.

> **TECHNICIAN NOTE** Key performance indicators (KPIs) are metrics used by the practice to evaluate practice performance.

Clinical signs of poor business management that can be identified through the types of review described previously include increasing accounts receivable, reduced amounts of cash, increased debt, decline in gross revenue and/or profitability, increasing personnel costs, declining productivity, declining client numbers, and a declining average transaction charge. These are all fixable problems, but they must first be identified.

In general, the process for analyzing metrics is as follows:
- Identify areas the owner/manager wants to review or improve—these can be selected on the basis of their knowledge of the practice and what areas need help, or by looking at some of the areas commonly analyzed by other practices.
- Collect data from the practice and compare with industry studies with similar data or with trends within the practice.
- Determine whether improvement is necessary in one or more areas.
- Identify relevant strategies needed to effect change.
- Implement new systems and processes.
- Measure results and modify systems and processes if needed.

In addition to these metrics, practices will track metrics specific to programs they are instigating or areas in which

they are trying to improve. For example, if a practice is trying to increase the number of cats that receive care, it may monitor metrics such as the number of cats that have received care in the practice before, the number that have received an annual examination in the past 12 months, and the number that have received certain kinds of care (vaccinations, heartworm tests, etc.).

Technicians often are not involved in the management analysis itself, but they are instrumental in improving the operational and financial success of the practice through their client service, communication, and medical roles.

Budgeting

Budgeting, however dull or intimidating, is an essential tool for managing the finances of a veterinary hospital. A budget is generally prepared at the end of one fiscal year for the following year; it includes estimated amounts for revenue and expenses.

Besides providing very specific financial data, a budget forces planning, which helps in identifying problems early, in determining why circumstances might be expected to change in the future, and in deciding what can be done about this.

Budgeting is also an excellent way to communicate goals to the entire hospital staff, to ensure that these goals are coordinated, and to monitor actual performance against expectations.

Price Setting

Standard prices are not applied by all practices for certain services or products. (This type of price setting among competing practices would, in fact, be illegal.) Each practice determines its own fees based on what has been charged in the past, how much it costs to provide the service, what others in the community charge, and what value the practice believes the service brings to the client. Setting fees is as much of an art as a science.

For a long time, the cost of veterinary medicine was very low. Over the past 10 years or so, it has risen significantly, and client resistance to the cost of veterinary care has been observed. This increase in cost is not due just to increases in prices charged to clients; it has also occurred because of the expanded range of care now available for pets, and because pets live longer than they used to.

Practices will have to use more sophisticated fee strategies in the future and will strive to increase profitability through ways other than fee increases. Owners and managers need to understand the drivers of profitability. In addition to the fees charged to clients, key drivers include the number of clients in the practice, the frequency with which they visit the practice, the quantity of services they choose to accept each time they visit, the amounts of discounts or missed charges, and whether or not the amounts charged to clients are actually collected. All else being equal, fee increases will increase profitability, but those same fee increases may also cause declines in some of the other profitability drivers (e.g., number of new clients, the frequency with which pet owners visit the

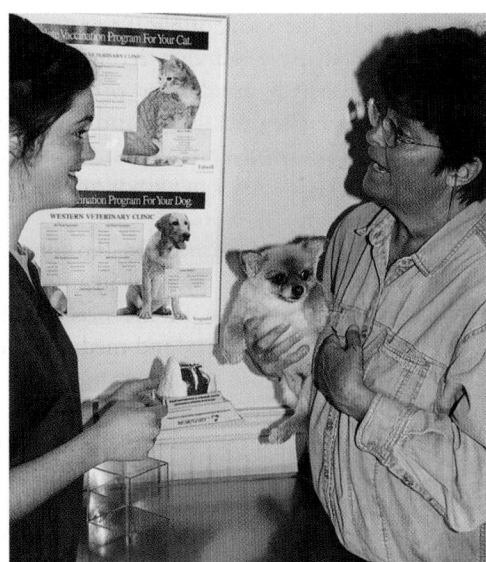

FIGURE 2-26 Veterinary technician uses a heartworm model to enhance client understanding of the impact of heartworm disease.

practice). The expected impact of all changes must be understood before the level of fee increases that are truly beneficial to the practice can be determined.

Whether or not a pet owner is willing to pay for a service or a product is not always about the absolute price charged for the item. Willingness to pay also has to do with whether or not an owner finds value in the item and thinks it is important to the pet's health. Findings from the Bayer Veterinary Care Usage Study[3] indicate that many pet owners do not understand the need for veterinary care. Technicians play a vital role in educating pet owners about veterinary care and in explaining why it can help their pets live happier, healthier lives (Figure 2-26).

Even if the price and the value are acceptable to the client, if they do not have the money in their checking account, they are not going to be able to afford the services. Therefore, the availability of payment options is critical. Even clients who are fully committed to providing quality care are looking at payment alternatives. Payment options for clients generally fall into four categories: in-house delayed billing of various types, third-party payment plans, pay by the month preventive care plans, and pet insurance. This is another area in which technicians have a critical role; they need to understand the various payment options offered by the practice and must be able to communicate this well to clients.

> **TECHNICIAN NOTE** Even if the price and the value of pet services are acceptable to clients, if they do not have the money in their checking account, they are not going to be able to afford the services. Therefore, the availability of payment options is critical.

It is also critical that everyone in the practice actually charge the stated fee for services and products sold. All charges related to the pet's care should be included on the invoice. Many practices offer reduced cost care to some deserving clients; any discounts included on an invoice by technicians should be approved by the practice owner/manager in advance.

The goal of the practice is to charge fair and equitable fees to cover the practice's cost of providing good quality care and service to clients. The fees should support investment in equipment, competitive salaries and benefits for doctors and staff, and a fair return on the investment to practice owners for the business risks involved.

> **TECHNICIAN NOTE** It is also critical that everyone in the practice charge the stated fee for services and products sold. All charges related to the pet's care should be included on the invoice.

OPERATIONS

As discussed earlier in the chapter, this is a broad category that has to do with all the systems, policies, and procedures that make the hospital operate smoothly on a day-to-day basis, including patient scheduling, client check-in and checkout, inventory control, patient flow, and many other activities. Activities related to client and patient flow have been discussed previously. Additional activities in which technicians are most likely to be involved or by which they may be affected are discussed in greater detail here.

Front Desk Management
Appointment Scheduling
Companion animal practices can operate through the use of an **appointment system** or a **walk-in system**. Each system has advantages and disadvantages, but most veterinarians prefer the appointment system. Appointments allow the practice to channel the flow of clients and patients into specific time periods that will improve the efficiency of the work schedule. When more clients are scheduled, more staff can be made available during the busier periods; on the other hand, when no appointments are scheduled, staff numbers can be reduced.

Practices using the appointment system generally schedule client/patient visits in 15, 20, or 30-minute blocks. When 15-minute blocks are used, four appointments per hour can be scheduled. Some practices book all appointments for the same length of time; others adjust appointment length depending on why the animal is visiting the practice. Companion animal practices often schedule 3 or 4 hours of appointment times in the morning and again in the afternoon. A typical appointment schedule might be from 8 AM to 12 PM and from 3 PM to 6 PM. Between noon and 3 PM, case workups, treatments, and surgery are performed.

Because of clients' work schedules, practices are now scheduling appointments in the evening as well, to help meet the needs of working animal owners. Saturdays are also very popular for the same reason; in many practices, Saturday is the busiest day of the week. Some practices are open on Sunday as well.

Practices that do not schedule appointments simply let clients "walk in," and they are seen on a first come, first served basis, except of course for emergencies. Advantages for the client include not having to make an appointment and having the ability to drop in at the practice whenever it is convenient. Disadvantages include the length of wait time and the congestion that may occur when several clients come in at the same time. For the practice, the major disadvantage is not having the ability to plan appropriate staffing and control the workload.

Many practices also take "drop-offs" (i.e., the client brings the pet and leaves it to be seen when a doctor is available). Examination of these pets is worked into the schedule when doctors become free. Some clients will just show up in practices that generally operate by appointment, and most practices try to accommodate them.

The receptionist generally makes appointments. The technician's role is to help ensure that clients and patients are seen at their scheduled time, and that all the various activities that need to occur during the appointment (physical examination, diagnostics, client communication) happen in a timely fashion. Doctors, technicians, receptionists, and other staff members must work as a team to make this happen. It is very frustrating for both clients and practice staff members when appointments run late.

Estimates and Client Payments

Once the pet has been examined and the veterinarian has discussed his or her recommendations with the pet owner, a written treatment plan/estimate should be prepared and agreed to by the client before care is provided. One clear exception to this is true life-threatening emergencies. However, once the pet has been stabilized, the treatment plan/estimate should be prepared.

The treatment plan estimate should be reviewed with the client after it is prepared. In some practices, this is done by the veterinarian, in others by a technician or another staff person. It is important that the person talking to the client can answer questions not only about the proposed charges but also about the need for care and why the recommended services are important. Client concerns about money more often reflect lack of understanding of the need for care than concern about the absolute cost. At this time, the practice's payment options can also be discussed.

Most practices require clients to pay in full at the time the service is provided. Traditionally, practices have accepted the same payment options seen at most retail businesses—cash, checks, and bank credit cards (MasterCard, Visa, Discover, American Express, etc.). Many practices also used in-house delayed billing plans to help clients who could not pay for their pet's care at the time of service. These generally took the form of held checks or statements sent post treatment with the idea that clients would pay when they received the statement, either in full or in installments.

The desire for payment options continues to rise as clients are dealing with the increasing costs of veterinary care resulting from the availability of more sophisticated medical options, the extended life span of pets, and fee increases. Because some hospitals have found it challenging to collect fees through the use of in-house delayed billing options, the preferred trend has been toward using third-party payment plans and pet insurance. Large animal ambulatory practices are an exception because livestock owners often are not available during farm calls and therefore are billed later. However, many ambulatory practitioners are now requiring credit cards for payment.

These payment options make a difference in the care that clients provide. A sophisticated study[4] conducted by one of the largest pet health insurance companies showed that the company's clients with pet health insurance on average had 41% higher stop-treatment levels, scheduled 40% more veterinary visits, and spent twice as much on veterinary care over the life of their pet. A cardholder survey by one of the leading third-party medical financing companies revealed that 71% of cardholders said that having this financing option affected their decision as to the level of treatment they could provide for their pet.[5]

Third-party medical payment plans are not all the same, but in general, their financing arrangements function like a credit card that can be used for multiple types of medical services such as veterinary care, dentistry, and optometry. Clients can apply for the cards while at the veterinary practice and receive immediate approval. The practice receives its money soon after it provides the care and is not responsible for collecting from the client.

As with regular credit cards, the practice pays a fee to the financing company. Sometimes these fees are higher than those charged with regular credit cards; however, advantages are associated with these dedicated medical credit cards. First, the ability to be approved for credit while at the practice means that pet owners can make an immediate decision to accept or not accept the practice's recommendations for pet care. Second, the higher fee allows the financing company to offer attractive interest-free plans that encourage client spending.

Another financial option for clients is pet health insurance. As with all insurance, this is a form of risk management. The transaction involves the pet owner (the insured) assuming a guaranteed and known relatively small loss in the form of a premium payment to the insurer in exchange for the insurer's promise to compensate the insured in case of a large, possibly devastating loss. Pet insurance is classified as indemnity insurance and is similar to other forms of indemnity insurance such as automobile insurance. Pet health insurance is very different from human health insurance.

As with third-party payment plans, an understanding of plan options and the companies providing them will help practice team members make intelligent and useful recommendations to clients. When veterinarians, their staff, or their clients become unhappy with pet insurance, this generally arises from lack of understanding of what is reasonable to expect from pet insurance. Points that will help both practice employees and clients understand their options include the following:

- Pet insurance is not right for all pet owners. Several factors for clients to consider in making the decision to insure their pet include their bond with the pet, their philosophical position about how much they would be willing to pay for a pet's care, the number of pets they want/need to insure, their level of risk tolerance, and the nature of their financial situation. Pet owners need to think about their ability to cover not only basic wellness care (annual examinations, vaccines, heartworm tests and preventive care, etc.) but also nonroutine accidents and illnesses. Some clients can cover the costs of this kind of care with some planning, a savings account, a credit card, and access to medical financing, as already discussed. But what happens if their pet needs care that is really complicated and expensive, or even catastrophic? These are the kinds of events that even the most financially responsible pet owner may have trouble finding the cash for. Pet insurance offers not just claims reimbursement but also peace of mind that when something of an expensive and catastrophic nature happens, care can be provided.

- All companies limit coverage in some way; if they didn't, they would pay out more in claims than they took in from premiums and would be bankrupt in months. These limitations come in several forms, including deductibles, co-pay percentages, annual or lifetime limits, the use of benefits schedules, and coverage exclusions. Practice team members and clients need to understand the coverage of the policy as a whole. Pet owners need to be aware of any breed-specific conditions that apply to their pets or to any particular types of procedures that they might want covered (e.g., dentistry, acupuncture), and to see whether their policy includes those items.

- For pet owners or veterinarians to expect that all owners will receive claims payments that equal or exceed what they pay in premiums is not even a realistic expectation. That does not happen with any kind of insurance. Some percentage of pet owners will pay more in premiums than they receive back in benefits; you could say they were unlucky with their pet insurance, or you could say they were lucky with their animal's health. Another group will pay much less in premiums than they get in benefits— these individuals own pets that were unlucky health-wise, but they were fortunate enough to have insured their pets. And most pet owners (or owners of any insurance) are going to be somewhere in the middle.

Once pet owners decide that pet insurance is for them, they need to pick a company and a plan. Many options are available out there, and it can be a bit daunting to sort through them all. Practices can help their clients by spending some time understanding the policies and recommending a couple of companies that they are comfortable with.

Technicians can play a large role in helping clients understand not only why the recommended care is so important, but also what their financial options are. Effective communication related to the cost of care begins with confident receptionists, technicians, and veterinarians who understand how the fee is computed and are confident that it is deserved

and fair and truly represents the quality of service provided. Clients will be more willing to accept the fees charged if they perceive value not only in the care recommendations but in the client service experience as well. Technicians can contribute significantly to increasing the value that clients receive.

Inventory Management

One of the most significant expense categories in veterinary practices is the one that includes inventory items such as pharmaceuticals, vaccines, pet food, surgical supplies, laboratory reagents and test kits, x-ray film, and other drugs and supplies necessary to provide medical and surgical care. Effective inventory management is important for keeping these costs under control and making sure that necessary items are on hand when needed. Inventory control is sometimes seen as a boring and tedious task, but it can have a huge impact on practice efficiency and profitability and is actually one of the easier things to do well in a practice.

Much money can be lost through inadequate inventory control procedures. This loss may occur because the business was billed for materials that were never shipped or never received at the practice or was double-billed for a single shipment, billed for damaged goods, or billed for more or different items than were received. Back orders that are not canceled when the product is reordered elsewhere double the inventory. Losses also occur when products expire and are no longer effective or legally safe to use. Oversupply also crowds the shelf and storage space, leading to misplacement and over-ordering.

Technicians are very frequently involved in inventory management and can do much to keep this part of the hospital running smoothly.

> **TECHNICIAN NOTE** Much money can be lost through inadequate inventory control procedures. This loss may occur because the business was billed for materials that were never shipped or never received at the practice or was double-billed for a single shipment, billed for damaged goods, or billed for more or different items than were received.

Goals of an effective inventory system include the following:
- The smallest quantities of drugs and supplies needed by the practice are maintained, procured at the lowest overall cost while providing the practice with everything needed to provide the highest quality care and without incurring stock-outs.
- Systems and controls are in place to keep theft and other shrinkage to a minimum, to insure accurate records are kept and that drugs and supplies are available when needed.
- Accurate records are readily available to evaluate the efficiency of the system and to improve upon it.
- The system is simple for all to use.
- Inventory is well organized within the facility and is easy to locate and is not vulnerable to theft or misplacement.

- Vendor numbers are kept to a minimum.
- Vendors selected are reputable, are interested in the success of the practice and of the profession, and provide products necessary within the practice, as well as good service and fair prices.
- All medications and products sold to clients are included on the invoice and are charged appropriately.
- Inventory is sold to clients before payment to the vendor has to be made (there will be some exceptions to this when good deals present themselves); generally, this means that inventory needs to turn over once a month.
- A reasonable profit is realized on sales.

Generally, one person should be put in charge of the inventory system, although in some hospitals, one person will be in charge of the drugs and supplies inventory, and another in charge of food inventory. This person may perform all or most of the tasks related to inventory or may delegate some activities while supervising the overall system. All tasks should be assigned to specific individuals to maintain accountability.

The inventory should be ordered on a regular basis, often weekly. The practice must have a system in place for determining what items need to be ordered. This can be done in many ways; sometimes a list is maintained, at other times reorder reports from the practice information management system are used, and in other hospitals the person doing the ordering goes through each cabinet to see what needs to be replenished.

Practices generally have a group of distributors and manufacturers from which they order; ideally, this list is kept relatively small. Item prices should be checked regularly, although not obsessively. Many practices have found that picking one distributor from whom they order most of their items works best; they get good service, and average prices tend to be reasonable and competitive.

A list of items ordered or actual purchase orders should be maintained for the items ordered. When the order is received, the list of items ordered should be compared with the items received, and the order list initialed by the person doing the comparison. Procedures should be in place to follow up on discrepancies and track back orders.

When supplies are delivered to the practice, the packing slip or invoice included in the box should be checked against the items actually received and discrepancies investigated. Quantities received and item prices should be entered into the computer after the order is received. The packing slip and invoices should then be given to the accounting department. If the practice receives both an invoice and a packing slip, items should be compared from one to the other and missing items investigated.

Procedures should be in place to identify, use, and/or return short-dated and out-of-date products.

One of the most important inventory management procedures involves regular counting of products on the shelves. Most practices do not count their inventory on a regular basis. At best, they do it once a year for tax purposes. The count done for tax purposes is not sufficient to make sure

that an inventory system is working effectively. All items need to be counted on a more regular basis.

Items most susceptible to theft include food, heartworm preventive, and flea/tick products; these should be counted monthly to make sure they are not being given to clients without charge or stolen. In the beginning, these items may need to be counted more frequently if the practice is having problems keeping track of inventory. Make a list of all of these items (list each size individually) and then divide it by four, so that each item is counted once a month. Count the product on hand and immediately check the balance indicated in the computer for this product. It is critical to do these two steps right after each other so that comparisons are between "apples and apples." If the product is counted at one time and the computer balance is checked later, the product could be sold or received and added or deducted from the computer balance, which then would not agree with the quantity counted. If discrepancies in the counts are noted, follow-up will be necessary:

- Are there any product purchase invoices that have not been entered into the inventory module?
- Was any product used in-house that has not been recorded in the inventory module (e.g., through a dummy client account)?
- Was any product sent home with clients or with employees that has not yet been recorded on an invoice? This is more often a problem with hospitalized or boarding patients than with outpatients.
- Was any product returned to the manufacturer that has not been deleted from the inventory module?
- Was product used for any other reason and not deleted from the inventory module?
- Is product stored in some other location that may not have been counted?
- Do staff members have any other ideas as to why the discrepancies exist?

> **TECHNICIAN NOTE** Items most susceptible to theft include food, heartworm preventive, and flea/tick products; these should be counted monthly to make sure they are not being given to clients without charge or stolen.

Depending on the extent of the discrepancies and whether or not reasonable explanations can be found for them, it may be necessary to institute more stringent inventory control procedures until the problem can be identified.

Unless the practice is experiencing a problem, counts on the other products usually do not need to be done as frequently. Frequency will be determined by the dollar value of the item, its likelihood of being stolen or given away, and experience with this product in the clinic. Do not forget that the records for controlled substance must be maintained exactly at all times.

Good physical control of the inventory is important for several reasons:

- Good physical control helps ensure that inventory is properly stored based on its physical requirements (e.g., temperature, light).
- Inventory that is well organized and easy to find makes it easier to assess how much is on hand, facilitates keeping track of short-dated product, and allows for quicker and more accurate physical counts.
- Proper organization and storage serves as a deterrent against theft and makes it easier to keep track of in-house usage.
- Sensible organization facilitates good record keeping.

In general, good physical control of the inventory requires the following:

- A locked central storage area with limited access—even here, only small quantities of product should be kept
- Small quantities of products kept in examination rooms, pharmacy and laboratory areas, and other areas easily accessible to employees
- Empty boxes displayed in public areas

Ideally, drugs would be used and replaced every 30 days (i.e., a turnover rate of 12 times per year). Unfortunately, the turnover rate is much lower in many practices.

It is also important to set up an inventory master list of all items stocked in the hospital; keep a pharmacy library of all company product inserts, catalogs, and ordering procedures; and keep a file of MSDSs for all products, as required by OSHA.

All practice information management systems have inventory modules, although practices frequently do not use them to their full capacity. It is almost impossible to have accurate inventory information without a computerized system.

COMPUTERIZATION OF THE VETERINARY PRACTICE

Today, the vast majority of veterinary practices use computers to perform practice management duties, including maintaining patient medical records, invoicing, and performing inventory and operational analyses. The wide range of management options available in software products has provided practices with an indispensable tool for increasing efficiency and productivity.

A commonly used acronym for these systems is PIMS (practice information management system). Currently, at least 25 systems are available for veterinary practices. A wide range of available features is seen in these systems, and although some activities are common to almost all systems (e.g., invoicing and inventory modules), other features such as the ability to interface with diagnostic equipment or the ability to enter all medical information about a pet may be available only on more sophisticated systems. The most commonly used systems are IDEXX Cornerstone, AVImark, ImproMed Infinity, IntraVet, and DVMax. Given the wide range of products that are now available, researching and selecting a particular software system can be a daunting but very important task for veterinary hospitals.

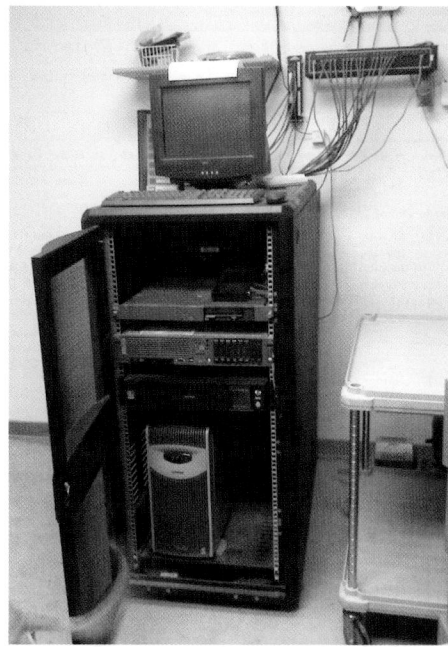

FIGURE 2-27 Practice management software and associated clinical data are housed on a server, the central computer hub that services a set of satellite computers.

Once the software and the hardware have been selected, an electronic network is established in a practice; this forms the platform for generating medical records and other information databases. Practice management software and associated clinical data are housed on a server, the central computer hub that services a set of satellite computers (Figure 2-27). Satellite computers are often called *workstations*. All practices have workstations located at the reception desk and often in other hospital locations as well. A common secondary location is the laboratory/pharmacy area, which is often adjacent to examination rooms; this allows for easy entry of patient information as the appointment progresses. Workstations may also be located in examination rooms or in doctors' offices. Some practices have the capability of using portable stations via laptops or tablet computers. All workstations are controlled by a central server, which backs up data entered into the workstation. In addition, many practices have an additional backup server. PIMS companies can upgrade and service their software remotely via the Internet. Updates to practice management software are often made automatically when the PIMS connects to the Internet.

Each client and pet combination has a central electronic patient record established during the first visit to the practice. Information is added with each client or patient visit or during communication between the pet owner and the veterinary health care team. During a visit, veterinary personnel enter information as procedures are performed on a particular patient. The receptionist, for example, collects and enters new or updated client and pet information. As the client moves from the waiting room to the examination room, the weight of the patient is obtained and is entered into the

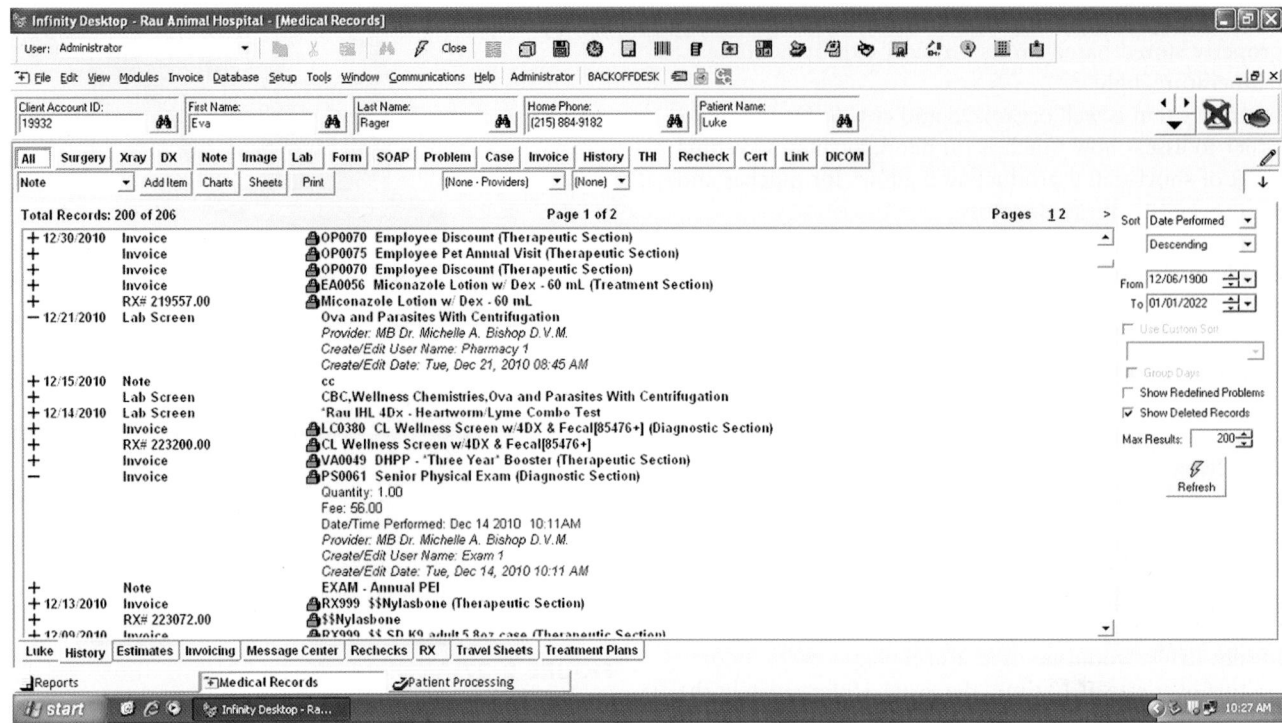

FIGURE 2-28 Screen showing a patient's medical record.

patient record by veterinary health care staff. The dates of previous inoculations and any existing medical problems are keyed into the computer. Findings from the physical examination and from diagnostics can also be entered. All of these data are stored in a database and become part of the patient's electronic medical record (Figure 2-28). At the conclusion of an office visit or hospitalization, the receptionist prints out an invoice that itemizes procedures performed on the pet. The PIMS is also used to record payments made by the client to the hospital.

Electronic Medical Records

Historically, a paper medical record would be generated for each patient in a veterinary practice. This record would include the history, physical examination and diagnostic testing results, and SOAP assessments. The patient's computerized record would include a list of all procedures done for the patient and amounts charged. Some practices have moved toward a complete electronic medical record for each pet, in which the information traditionally kept on paper is kept as part of the electronic medical record. Not all PIMSs provide this capability. Use of electronic medical records improves communication and efficiency within the veterinary health care team.

Patient Scheduling

An important feature in a PIMS is the appointment scheduler (Figure 2-29). When the appointment book is not computerized, only one staff member at a time can record or change appointments. Computers make it possible for multiple staff members to be able to add or delete appointments

concurrently. The veterinarian can schedule an appointment while speaking to the client, and the technician can schedule a recheck appointment while discharging the patient from surgery. Ideally, the appointment schedule should be available at a variety of workstations. This feature alone decreases the chaos at the front desk that is created when all client contact requires a receptionist.

Different software systems have different capabilities in the scheduling module; one example is the "Find next appointment" feature. If a client has forgotten when his or her next appointment is scheduled, the receptionist may enter the patient record, use a drop-down menu to gain access to the appointment scheduler, and select "Find next appointment." The computer will then search and display the appointment. This would be a tedious task without the help of a computer. A very important feature of some appointment schedulers is appointment time customization. Different types of appointments can be assigned specific lengths of time. Instead of a standard 15- or 30-minute appointment scheduled for all clients, appointment length can be customized to an appropriate length for the service to be provided. For example, suture removal may be set up as a 5-minute appointment, but a new client examination may require a 30-minute appointment.

Another related feature is the ability of the PIMS to show where patients physically are within the hospital. For example, all pets visiting the hospital for grooming are shown in the grooming section, all surgery patients are shown in surgery, and so on. This facilitates locating the patient if questions arise, or if the client calls for a progress update (Figure 2-30).

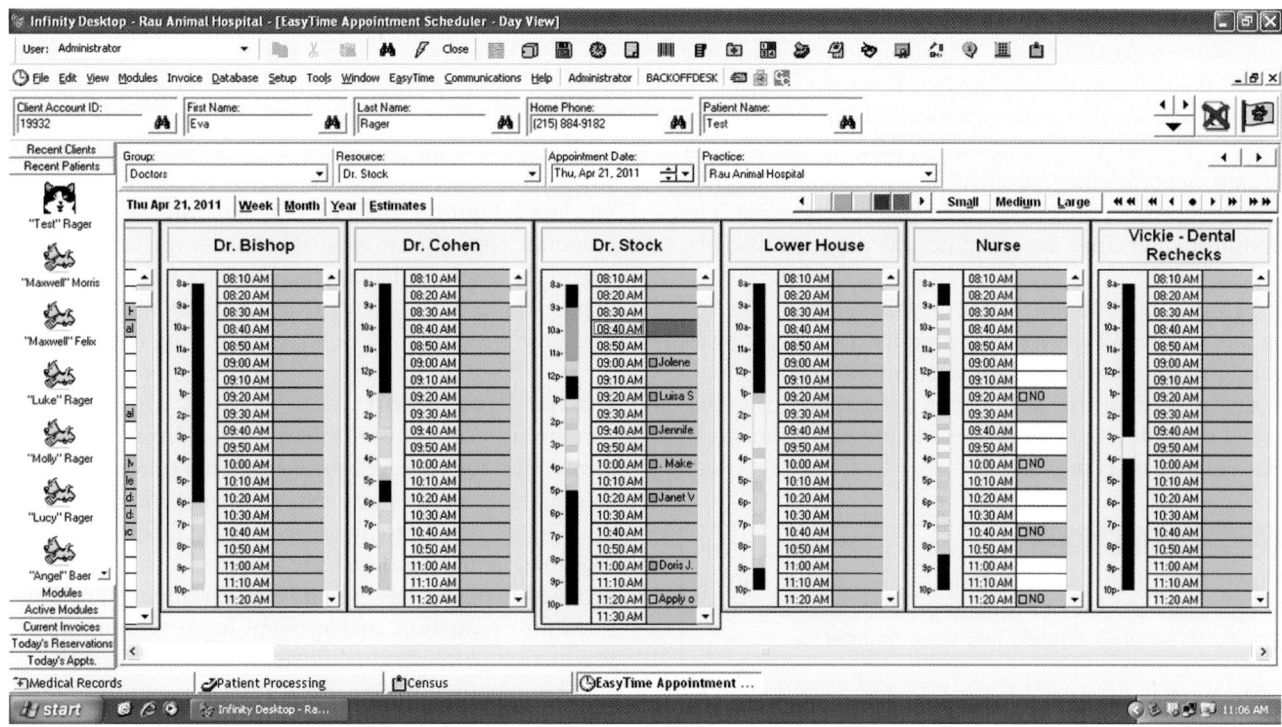

FIGURE 2-29 Screen showing the schedule of the health care team.

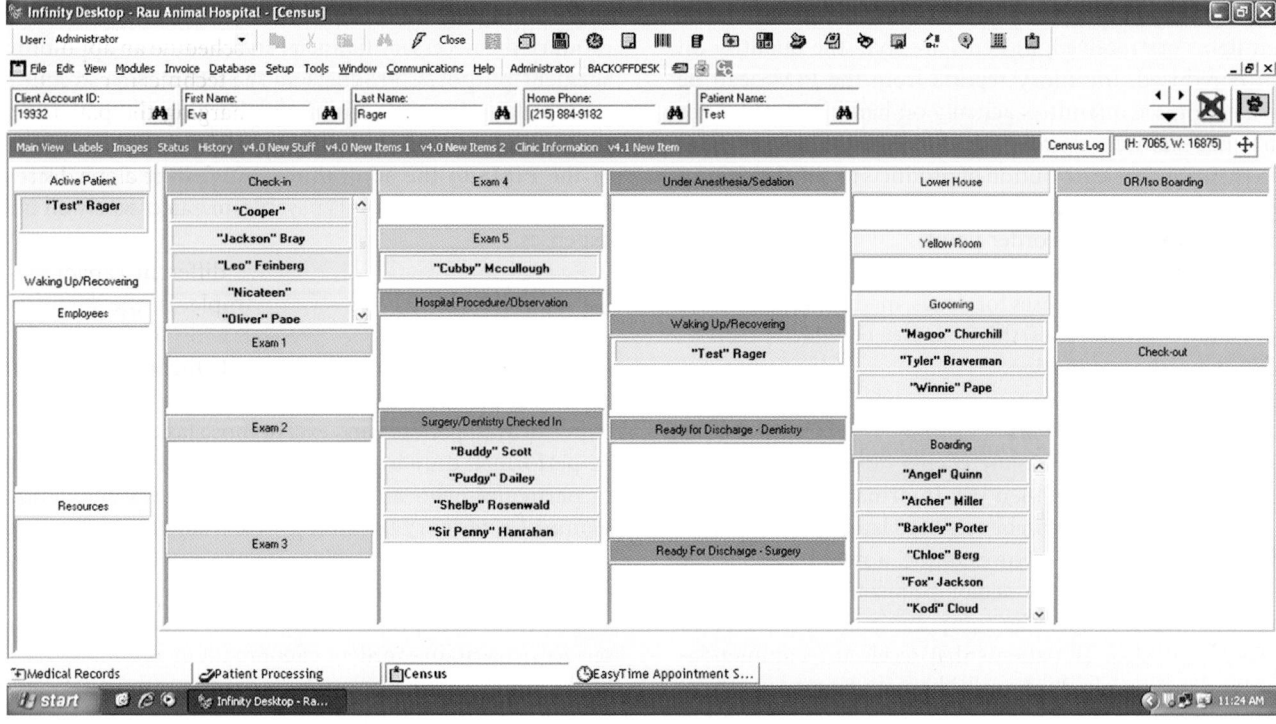

FIGURE 2-30 Screen showing locations of patients within the hospital.

Reminders

The reminder module includes information about services that each pet needs in the future and provides the practice with periodic information about upcoming care needed by particular pets. For example, at the time that vaccinations are provided, the pet's record will be updated with the date the next vaccinations are due. The reminder module can also be used for heartworm preventive and other medications, blood work related to drug monitoring, therapeutic diets, and other needed services or product refills. The PIMS can often be used to print reminder cards or labels, to generate e-mail reminders, or to provide a list for contact by other means.

Billing

An invoice is created for each patient upon entry into the practice. As staff members perform medical tasks or dispense products to clients, they enter those services directly into the computer. The veterinary software updates the invoice for each item entered. When the client is ready to check out, the receptionist prints a fully itemized invoice for the client. The receptionist enters into the computer the payment made by the client.

When the software system was installed, one of the first tasks was to enter all services and products sold by the practice and the amount charged to the client for each. Not only does automation of this task reduce the number of billing errors, it also allows practices to easily provide estimates to clients before care is provided.

> **TECHNICIAN NOTE**   An invoice is created for each patient upon entry into the practice. As staff members perform medical tasks or dispense products to clients, they enter those services directly into the computer.

Inventory

Inventory management is a critical module included in most PIMSs. Inventory items are entered into the system, along with information about the price to be charged to clients when items are received; as items are sold, the quantity on hand is reduced. Inventory reports from the PIMS can be used to compare quantities actually on hand in the practice with what should be on hand, thus identifying potential theft, shrinkage, or distribution of products to clients without charge. Other reports can be used to analyze the usage of particular products or reorder points.

Many practices do not use the PIMS inventory to its full advantage. Because expenses for drugs, medical supplies, and food are big in all practices, this is an area on which practices should focus more attention.

Client Communication

As discussed previously, many clients do not fully understand the care needed by their pet. Information entered into the pet's medical record can be retrieved later for educational and marketing purposes. For example, a mailing about the benefits of blood work for senior pets could be sent to all pets over 7 years of age. The computer could also be asked to produce a list of all patients that received recommendations for dental work. Phone calls then can be made to those clients who have not yet booked appointments. Many other similar educational and marketing activities can now be done much more easily with the advent of computerization in veterinary practice.

Accounts Receivable

As noted previously, when medical services are added to the medical record, charges are added to the invoice. When the receptionist cashiers out the client, the payment is recorded on the invoicing/payment screen. Most clients pay the full balance at the time of service, but some are allowed to pay off their invoices over time. The veterinary software keeps track of these accounts receivable—amounts owed to the practice.

The practice administrator sets a time within the system when accounts are considered overdue (30 days, 60 days, and 90 days). Monthly bills can be sent out to all past due accounts. The software is capable of adding a late fee depending on the length of delinquency. Today's software also makes it possible to block clients from charging fees in the event that they are habitually negligent in paying their bills.

Doctor Production

Another aspect of most PIMSs is their ability to track income production for each veterinarian. Some practices pay their veterinarians a base salary plus compensation based on production. As entries are made within the medical record, the veterinarian who ordered the service is credited with the production of that fee. Even if veterinarians are not compensated for production, management needs to understand the productivity of individual doctors.

Although the PIMS is an essential part of most practices, other software is needed for a few activities. None of the currently available PIMSs have a good quality accounting or general ledger program integrated within their software. Practices therefore need separate accounting software to produce the necessary financial statements for tax and management purposes. Products such as Peachtree Accounting or QuickBooks are commonly used. Bookkeepers input revenue information from the billing and invoicing features of the PIMS to the accounting software, and this financial software manages accounts payable, prints checks, and tracks expenses.

SUMMARY

Practices that flourish now and will continue to thrive into the future are those that leverage veterinary health care staff to perform all patient care, except those tasks that by law may be performed only by veterinarians. Veterinary technicians, in particular, who are educated in AVMA-accredited programs of veterinary technology, are trained to deliver excellent nursing care by carrying out the veterinary technician practice model. This input affects all areas of practice and helps practices to provide high-quality medical and surgical services, maintain excellent client–patient and internal communications, maintain thorough written and digital medical records, and assist in the management of attractive, efficient veterinary facilities. These flourishing practices will be exciting and rewarding enterprises for all who are affiliated with them, including the client and pet and the entire veterinary health care team.

REFERENCES

1. AVMA.org (accessed June 2, 2011).
2. AVMA report on veterinary practice business measures, 2011 edition.

3. Bayer veterinary care usage study, 2011.
4. VPI pet owner and client survey, veterinary pet insurance, California, 2006.
5. CareCredit cardholder survey (641 cardholders), CareCredit, California, August 2010.

RECOMMENDED READINGS

Ackerman L: Business basics for veterinarians, Lincoln, NE, 2002, ASJA Press.

Ackerman L: Management basics for veterinarians, Lincoln, NE, 2003, Universe.

Boss N: Educating your clients from A to Z: What to say and how to say it, Lakewood, CO, 2011, AAHA Press.

Compensation and benefits, ed 6, Lakewood, CO, 2010, AAHA Press.

Dobbs K: 101 veterinary technician questions answered, Lakewood, CO, 2009, AAHA Press.

Durrance D, Lagoni L: Connecting with clients: Practical communication for 10 common situations, Lakewood, CO, 2010, AAHA Press.

Guenther J: 101 veterinary inventory questions answered, Lakewood, CO, 2010, AAHA Press.

Heinke ML, McCarthy JB: Practice made perfect: A guide to veterinary practice management, Lakewood, CO, 2001, AAHA Press.

Smith C: Client satisfaction pays: Quality service for practice success, Lakewood, CO, 2009, AAHA Press.

Smith C, Rose R: Career choices for veterinary technicians, Lakewood, CO, 2009, AAHA Press.

Journals

DVM Newsmagazine, Cleveland, OH, Advanstar Communications, monthly.

Exceptional Veterinary Team, Tulsa, OK, Educational Concepts, LLC, bimonthly.

Trends, Denver, CO, American Animal Hospital Association, monthly.

Veterinary Economics, Lenexa, KS, Advanstar Communications, monthly.

Firstline, Lenexa, KS, Advanstar Communications, monthly.

Veterinary Practice News, BowTie, Mission Viejo, CA, monthly.

Veterinary Technician NAVTA Journal, NAVTA, Washington, DC, quarterly.

Management Short Courses

Veterinary Management Institute at Purdue University. Contact AAHA for details.

Internet Sites

www.avma.org (information on veterinary medicine and links to pet care sites)

www.avma.org/navta/ (veterinary technology profession information)

www.ncvei.org (financial information for the veterinary profession)

www.vhma.org

www.dvm360.com (information on veterinary practice management and news topics)

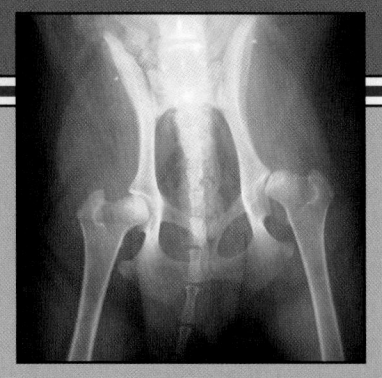

3

Veterinary Medical Records

Joanna M. Bassert

KEY TERMS

Master problem list
MAOR
Previous history
Problem-oriented
   veterinary medical
   record (POVMR)
Progress notes
Recent history
Signalment
SOAP
Source-oriented
   veterinary medical
   record (SOVMR)
Technician assessment
Veterinary medical
   database
Working problem list

OUTLINE

Functions of the Medical Record, *82*
Primary Purposes, *82*
Secondary Purposes, *82*
Medical and Legal Requirements, *82*
Veterinarian–Client–Patient Relationship
   (VCPR), *82*
Importance of Informed Consent, *83*
Documentation: Protection Against
   Complaints and Litigation, *84*
Ownership and Release of Medical
   Information, *85*
**Format of Veterinary Medical
   Records,** *86*
Source-Oriented Veterinary Medical Record
   (SOVMR), *86*
Problem-Oriented Veterinary Medical
   Record (POVMR), *86*
Components of the POVMR, *86*
The Database, *86*

Master Problem List and Working Problem
   List, *92*
Hospitalized Patient Records, *94*
**Management of Paper Medical
   Records,** *105*
Organization and Filing, *105*
File Purging, *107*
Lost Records, *107*
Logs, *107*
**Management of Electronic Medical
   Records,** *109*
Overview, *109*
Validating the Electronic Record, *110*
Risk of Loss, *111*
Advantages of Electronic Medical
   Records, *111*
**Management of Ambulatory Practice
   Records,** *111*
Veterinary Medical Database, *112*

LEARNING OBJECTIVES

When you have completed this chapter, you will be able to:

1. Pronounce, define, and spell all Key Terms within this chapter.
2. List and describe the primary and secondary purposes of the medical record.
3. Explain the legal issues related to ownership of medical records, release of medical information, and maintenance of medical records.
4. Describe methods for formatting medical records and explain their respective advantages and disadvantages.
5. List and describe each component of the problem-oriented veterinary medical record (POVMR).
6. Explain each portion of the technician SOAP note, the types of information included in each portion, and describe how each portion correlates to the steps in the veterinary technician practice model (presented in Chapter 1).
7. Describe the importance of cage cards, discharge instructions, and summary and MAOR forms and why they are valuable in organizing the care of hospitalized veterinary patients.
8. Compare and contrast the types of filing systems commonly used for paper medical records.
9. List and describe the types of paper-based forms and logs commonly used in veterinary practice.

Many thanks to Eva Rager and Vickie Byard, CVT, VTS (Dentistry), from the Rau Animal Hospital, for their provision of computer screen shots and valuable support during the development of this chapter.

10. Explain the advantages and disadvantages of electronic medical record keeping.
11. Describe methods for collecting and storing medical information in ambulatory veterinary medical practices.
12. Explain how veterinary medical databases support the advancement of research in veterinary medicine.

INTRODUCTION

Veterinary medical information includes a wide range of data that document the treatment and care of animal patients. Results of history taking, physical examination and patient assessment, laboratory tests, and diagnostic procedures such as radiographic imaging, ultrasound, electrocardiograms, and endoscopy are examples of information that is recorded and maintained for each patient. Treatments such as administration of medication and intravenous fluids, surgery, and wound care are also recorded, along with patient progress and daily observations. Finally, medical records document euthanasia and post-mortem examinations, communications with clients, and important authorization and consent agreements.

The term *medical record* refers to both the physical folder for each patient and the total body of information that constitutes each animal's health history. However, many practices use computers to store and organize all patient health information, so there is no physical folder in these practices. The medical record is the full body of patient information held within the computer system.

Given the plethora of information that is gathered for each patient and the thousands of patients that each practice might treat, it is not surprising that computers have become an essential tool for storing some, if not all, of this information. Although some practices continue to use written medical records, a vast majority of practices use computers to support some aspect of practice management and medical record keeping. Indeed, client and staff scheduling, billing, inventory management, payroll, marketing, data collection, accounting, and client communications and mailings all can be managed using computers.

This chapter offers an overview of the organization, components, and functions of the veterinary patient record using illustrations from both paper-based and electronic platforms. In addition, it discusses the ethical and legal issues that accompany the record keeping process and introduces the importance of consistently maintaining neat, thorough accounts of patient care. It also introduces the reader to technician **SOAP** (subjective, objective, assessment, planning) notes and to the veterinary technician patient nursing care plan and describes their importance in helping to support excellent patient care. Refer to Chapter 1 for a description of the veterinary technician practice model, and to Chapter 7 for information about patient assessment. Entire books have been written on the subject of medical information documentation both in North America and in Europe. Please refer to the "Recommended Readings" section at the end of this chapter for sources on these topics.

FUNCTIONS OF THE MEDICAL RECORD

The Institute of Medicine has organized the functions of the medical record into two broad categories: primary purposes and secondary purposes. Primary purposes support the patient's medical care and include documentation of diagnostic procedures, diagnoses, prognoses, and treatment. Secondary purposes are not clinically based; they include evaluations of medical information for business, legal, and research purposes.

PRIMARY PURPOSES

Supports Excellent Medical Care

The medical record is a critical tool that enables and supports in many ways the effective treatment and care of animals. First, it assists the veterinary health care team in correctly identifying the patient and the owner. After all, many black Labrador Retrievers look alike, and many owners may have the same last name. The medical record helps to prevent confusion among the identities of patients and their owners. Second, it helps in the generation of effective diagnostic and treatment plans. It documents physical examination findings of the veterinarian and the veterinary technician, lists diagnostic procedures and tests to be performed, and records the veterinarian's ideas regarding differential diagnoses. The medical record also enables the veterinary health care team to document the patient's responses to treatment, so that plans may be adjusted as needed. As time passes and members of the health care team change, the medical record supports continuity of care. It helps those who are not familiar with the patient to understand the medical history and conditions of the animal. In this way, it provides an avenue for communication between all members of the veterinary health care team, so that treatment can be accurately and effectively administered.

Documents Communications

The medical record also documents communications with the client; this is particularly important when many members of the veterinary health care team are assisting the same client. A copy of take-home instructions, for example, will be included in the medical record, so any confusion about home care provided by the client (owner) can be quickly clarified. In addition, the medical record assists in the generation of reminder cards that help pet owners stay current with their pet's preventive medical plan. In these ways, good communication is critical for providing a logical, continued plan of patient care for both health care providers and pet owners.

Interactions with clients and their pets are also aided by the use of medical records. Financial limitations, for example, and the behavioral idiosyncrasies of the pet may be recorded. In addition, the veterinarian–client relationship can be further enhanced when the names of other family members and important family activities are noted in the record as reminders for future topics of informal discussion.

SECONDARY PURPOSES

Supports Business and Legal Activities

The medical record lists all services rendered to the pet owner, whether they involve boarding a dog or spaying a cat. This documentation verifies billing and serves as legal evidence of services received by the owner. It can be used to assess the workloads of staff members, formulate income analyses, make budgetary plans, perform actuarial calculations, maintain inventory, and generate a marketing strategy. In addition, it plays an important role during hospital accreditations and helps assess compliance with standards of care.

The medical record is used as a legal document in a court of law and is valuable during litigation. It serves as evidence of procedures performed and treatments administered, and it provides specific dates and times of events. In this way, the medical record is critical in defending against malpractice suits. Special care must be taken to ensure that the record is complete and accurate. Keep in mind that in a court of law, the prevailing view is "not recorded, not done." In addition, insurance companies may require the medical record to assess whether a claim is to be paid.

Supports Research

The medical record is a key element in the preparation of case studies and presentations for conferences. Information from medical records is collected to develop registries and databases, which assist in the conduction of retrospective studies and in predicting clinical outcomes. It is used to teach veterinary medical and veterinary technician students. To maintain confidentiality, all patient markers are removed from the record before they are used for any purpose other than patient care (Box 3-1).

> **TECHNICIAN NOTE**   A comprehensive medical record supports excellent medical care, communication, and research and good business practices. It helps to protect practices during malpractice litigation, or when complaints are filed against a practice with the Board of Veterinary Medicine.

MEDICAL AND LEGAL REQUIREMENTS

VETERINARY–CLIENT–PATIENT RELATIONSHIP (VCPR)

The VCPR serves as the foundation of the interaction among veterinarians, their clients, and their patients. Medical records must be maintained for all patients with whom a veterinary-client-patient relationship exists (Box 3-2). According to the American Veterinary Medical Association, a VCPR occurs when all of the following conditions have been met:

- The veterinarian has assumed responsibility for making clinical judgments regarding the health of the animal(s)

BOX 3-1 | Summary Chart: *Functions of the Medical Record*

I. Primary Purposes
Supports Excellent Medical Care
A. Identifies correct patient and owner
B. Supports generation of diagnostic and treatment plans
C. Supports continuity of care
D. Supports communication
 1. Among health care team members
 2. With the owner
 3. Personalizes veterinarian–client relationship

II. Secondary Purposes
Supports Business and Legal Activities
A. Verifies billing
B. Supports actuarial calculations
 1. Income analysis
 2. Budgetary plans
 3. Staff workloads
C. Supports inventory maintenance
D. Supports formulation of marketing strategy
E. Supports hospital accreditation
F. Acts as a legal document

Supports Research
A. Case studies and presentations
B. Registries and databases
C. Education of veterinarians and veterinary technicians

BOX 3-2 | AVMA Ethics and Medical Records

A. Veterinary medical records are an integral part of veterinary care. These records must comply with standards established by state and federal law.
B. Medical records are the property of the practice and the practice owner. The original records must be retained by the practice for the period required by statute.
C. Ethically, the information within veterinary medical records is considered privileged and confidential. It must not be released except by court order or with consent of the owner of the patient.
D. Veterinarians are obligated to provide copies or summaries of medical records when requested by the client. Veterinarians should secure a written release to document that request.
E. Without the express permission of the practice owner, it is unethical for a veterinarian (or a veterinary technician) to remove, copy, or use medical records or any part of any record.

Source: The principles of veterinary medical ethics. www.AVMA.org.

---

and the need for medical treatment, and the client has agreed to follow the veterinarian's instructions.
- The veterinarian has sufficient knowledge of the animal(s) to initiate at least a general or preliminary diagnosis of the medical condition of the animal(s). This means that the veterinarian has recently seen and is personally acquainted with keeping and care of the animal(s) by virtue of an examination of the animal(s), or through medically appropriate and timely visits to the premises where the animal(s) are kept.
- The veterinarian is readily available or has arranged for emergency coverage for follow-up evaluation in the event of adverse reactions or failure of the treatment regimen.

IMPORTANCE OF INFORMED CONSENT

A common complaint of pet owners is that veterinary services were delivered that were not authorized, or were authorized but were not properly understood by the client. Euthanasia, expensive diagnostics, and high-risk procedures are particularly likely to be disputed by a client at a later date. Therefore, it is important for veterinary practices to demonstrate not only client consent, but *informed* client consent. In other words, the client or representative must be educated with regard to the pet's malady, diagnosis, prognosis, and treatment options, and with regard to justification for the cost of treatment. In addition, in-clinic and home care, monitoring procedures, follow-up and emergency procedures, and preventive health care plans should be discussed.

In documenting informed consent, communications with clients should be recorded in the medical record, including the content of face-to-face consultations, e-mail communications, and conversations on the phone. If an animal is co-owned, it may be helpful to note the specific party involved in the conversation because clients don't always communicate effectively with each other. Written communication with clients via e-mail should be maintained as it offers a dated and timed record. When consent is offered over the phone, it is preferable for the conversation to be witnessed by another staff member on speaker phone or on another line. This discussion should later be summarized in the medical record and signed by both the veterinarian and the staff/witness.

Consent and Authorization Forms
Consent and authorization forms document in writing an understanding between the veterinary practice and the pet owner. Forms outline specific conditions, risks of procedures, and responsibilities of both parties. In keeping with the doctrine of informed consent, completed authorization forms provide veterinary practices with legal evidence that the owner was informed of important information, and that the owner agreed to pursue a particular course of action based on the circumstances and information given to him or her. Be aware that consent must be given by legal adults 18 years of age or older. Consent by a juvenile is not consent.

From avma.org/animal_health/vcpr_poster.pdf.

In many practices, consent forms are generated in those areas where potential is greatest for bad feelings as a result of poor communication. Surgery, necropsy, and euthanasia are a few examples of situations where written owner permission and verbal communication are critical. During emergencies, for example, owners can be particularly emotional and may have difficulty making clear decisions. Owners who decide to euthanize their seriously injured pet may regret their decision later. They may blame the veterinary staff for feeling "pressured into it" or may believe that they were not given all information needed to make a sound choice. Authorization forms such as the one posted on the Evolve site at http://evolve.elsevier.com/McCurnin/vettech/ verify the identity of the owner and free the practice of liability in performing euthanasia. Because complications and complaints can arise months later, it is important to make consent forms a permanent part of the medical record.

A common source of consternation in veterinary practices is miscommunication regarding the cost of services. Many veterinary hospitals have developed forms for fee estimation and for treatment consent (see the Evolve site at http://evolve.elsevier.com/McCurnin/vettech/). These forms give owners a written estimate of the costs of procedures, verify ownership, and establish an agreement in the event that the animal is abandoned by the owner. This empowers the practice to take action in the event that the owner cannot meet his responsibility to pay for services and/or retrieve the pet.

Obtaining consent from the owner is recommended whenever indications suggest that a client might end up causing a problem. Often legal difficulties can be prevented by identifying potentially difficult clients in advance. Having the owner's written consent to restrain his or her own pet during an examination, for example, may protect the practice later if the client is bitten. Sometimes an owner who normally insists on holding the pet during an office visit may decide not to do so after reading and signing a consent form that lists the risks of restraining an animal.

DOCUMENTATION: PROTECTION AGAINST COMPLAINTS AND LITIGATION

When a lawsuit or a complaint is filed against a veterinarian, a veterinary technician, or a practice, a complete, accurate, and legible medical record is one of the most convincing pieces of evidence used to refute allegations. An inaccurate, illegible, or incomplete record may be construed as evidence of professional incompetence and substandard care, which may lead to stiff fines or worse imposed by the state board of veterinary medicine.

Disgruntled pet owners are often prepared at hearings with a plethora of evidence against the practice, including transcripts of phone conversations and office visits, retrieved foreign objects, copies of medical records, itemized receipts, pill vials, sworn witness testimony, and before and after photographs of their pet. Maintaining a discipline of generating consistently complete and accurate medical records is essential to ensure protection from legal action.

Keep in mind the following rules of thumb:
1. If it was not written down, it did not happen,
2. If the writing is illegible, it was not written down.
3. If one part of the medical record shows signs of tampering or is inaccurate, the integrity of the *entire* medical record is questionable.

Below are some guidelines for generating clear, complete, and accurate records:
1. Entries should be typed or written neatly in black ink. This improves clarity of images during copying or faxing.
2. In a court of law, handwriting alone is not an adequate way to identify the author of a notation. Therefore, all written entries should be signed by the author, and the author's credentials (e.g., CVT, DVM) and the date and time should be entered. Entries into electronic patient records similarly must verify the person making the entry and the date and time the entry is made.
3. Errors in written records should NOT be scratched out, erased, or blotted out with marker or correction fluid. Instead, a single line should be drawn through the mistake and the word "error" should be written in the margin along with the corrected information. This change should be signed and dated by the person who made the error, and a brief explanation for the correction should be entered. Any erasure or blotting out may suggest tampering with the record and could render the document inadmissible in a court of law. Computerized medical records must be able to track input, changes, and deletions. If the history of electronic entries, deletions, and changes cannot be tracked, the medical record is not credible as evidence.
4. Entries to written records may be initialed rather than signed if the form includes a signature box in which an individual's signature is listed with his or her initials.
5. Only approved, standard abbreviations should be used. Refer to the inside cover of this text for a list of commonly used abbreviations.

The medical record is considered legal evidence of services and procedures performed by the veterinary health care team. In the event of litigation, as during a malpractice or insurance suit, the record is often subpoenaed and admitted as evidence.

Legal guidelines for medical records vary from state to state and may dictate the type of information that should be included, how long the record should be kept, and restrictions on the release of medical information. It is recommended that all members of the veterinary health care team be familiar with the laws of the state in which they work.

TECHNICIAN NOTE Errors should not be scratched out, erased, or blotted out. Instead, a single line should be drawn through the mistake and the word "error" should be written in the margin, along with the corrected information. This change should be signed and dated by the person who made the error. Any erasure or blotting out may suggest tampering with the record and could render the document inadmissible in a court of law.

Progress Notes

Date/Time	Initials	Progress Notes	
7/7/13	JS	Notation: "Fluffy" exhibits moderate pain in the	
6 pm		cranioventral abdomen. ~~Small~~ Firm oval mass palpable	Error, Jane Smith 7/7/13 6:03pm
		approx. 2 cm x 2.5 cm.	

OWNERSHIP AND RELEASE OF MEDICAL INFORMATION

In general, veterinary medical records are the property of the veterinary practice and its owners. Although the client purchased the veterinary services that generated the medical information, the client is not, by law, the owner of the medical record. However, the client may make a written request at any time for a copy of a pet's medical record. It is customary for clients to request copies of their pet's medical record when they are moving and changing veterinary practices. This facilitates continued care of the patient and prevents repetition of immunizations or diagnostic tests. It is recommended that copies of medical records be mailed or e-mailed to the successive veterinarian and not hand delivered by the owner, who may be apt to misinterpret entries in the medical record. A cover letter should be included with the copy of the record, so that the original veterinary hospital and veterinarian can be easily contacted, if necessary. A fee may be charged for sending a copy of the record.

A signed authorization form (see the Evolve site at http://evolve.elsevier.com/McCurnin/vettech/) or a written letter of request for record copies should be obtained from the animal's owner before any information is released to the owner, another veterinarian, or another third party. The practice owner should be the only person to authorize the release of information contained in the record. Keep in mind that the patient record is confidential, and that its confidentiality must be guarded. Therefore, in most states, the patient record may be released to a third party only with permission from the client. The following circumstances are exceptions to this rule. In these instances, information in the medical record must be given to the appropriate authority without client permission.

- The veterinarian has diagnosed a reportable disease and must alert local, state, and federal agencies as required by law. *Reportable diseases* may be dangerous for the public or for the widespread health of animals and include a wide variety of diseases such as rabies, brucellosis, and equine encephalitis. Additional regulations regarding reportable diseases can be found in the *Animal Movement Quarantine Regulations Manual,* which is published by the U.S. Department of Agriculture (USDA).
- A court of law subpoenas the medical record.

Clients give permission for their pet's medical record to be copied and sent to a third party for a variety of reasons. Below are some examples.

- The patient is moving to another veterinary practice, and the client would like the new practice to have a copy of the medical record.
- The pet has bitten a person, and the client would like to give proof of the animal's immunization against rabies.
- The animal's health, life, or ability to perform is insured. The client cannot collect from an insurance company until official proof indicates that the animal did indeed die or become injured.
- Scientists studying epidemiology, zoonoses, and medical trends examine patient records for data that are relevant to their research. The client agrees to release patient information as long as the confidentiality of the owner is maintained.

FORMAT OF VETERINARY MEDICAL RECORDS

However important the medical record is in securing a strong legal defense, the most important reason for excelling at medical record keeping is to provide optimum patient care. Incomplete or lost medical information leads to incomplete and suboptimal patient care. Because it is impossible to remember all of the clinical details associated with each case, a thorough, well-written medical record can be extensive. The medical information therefore must be organized in such a way that veterinary personnel can locate pertinent details quickly and easily. Medical record information can be organized in several ways. Most methods fall into one of three categories:

1. Source-oriented veterinary medical record (SOVMR)
2. Problem-oriented veterinary medical record (POVMR)
3. Combination of source- and problem-oriented veterinary medical records

SOURCE-ORIENTED VETERINARY MEDICAL RECORD (SOVMR)

In an SOVMR, patient information is kept together by subject matter. Laboratory reports, for example, may be kept in one particular section of the record, while **progress notes** may be clipped together in the front of the record. The progress notes are written in chronological order using a paragraph format. Clinical observations are entered as they become evident. In this way, the most recent information is located last and the oldest information is found first.

The source-oriented method is easy to learn and takes little time to complete; however, it can lack detailed documentation, which may prove vital during litigation. Remember, if it is not written down, it didn't happen. In addition, and perhaps most important, individual medical problems may be difficult to monitor. A veterinary technician, for example, may have to leaf through several different sections of an SOVMR to follow the progress of a diabetic cat because blood work, physical examination findings, and diagnostic imaging details may be located in three different areas of the medical record. The organization of medical information in a SOVMR format may be further complicated in practices that include different departments and specialty groups.

PROBLEM-ORIENTED VETERINARY MEDICAL RECORD (POVMR)

The problem-oriented veterinary medical record provides an organized approach to clinical veterinary care in that information in the medical record is grouped by problem, and each problem is assigned a number and is addressed separately. Notes are written on progress forms using the SOAP format. SOAP stands for Subjective, Objective, Assessment, and Plan. A SOAP note is written for each problem. Both veterinarians and veterinary technicians may write SOAP notes in the POVMR, although their focus is different. The veterinarian focuses on identifying the cause of illness and subsequently a cure, and the veterinary technician focuses

on the patient's psychological and physiologic reactions to the malady. The POVMR fosters excellent communication and team-oriented medical care and encourages ongoing assessment and revision of the health care plan by all members of the health care team. The American Animal Hospital Association (AAHA) endorses the use of problem-oriented veterinary medical record keeping and insists upon its use in practices seeking AAHA certification.

COMPONENTS OF THE POVMR

Although POVMR medical records vary somewhat, they most commonly include the following:

1. Database
   a. Client and patient information
   b. History (current history, chief presenting complaint, and **previous history**)
   c. Physical examination findings
   d. Pertinent test results (radiography, special imaging, and laboratory reports)
2. **Master problem list** and working problem lists
3. Initial plan and progress notes
   a. Progress forms that include SOAP notes for each problem
   b. Treatment-related forms, medication administration/order record (**MAOR**) forms, surgical reports, and anesthesia forms
4. Case summary and discharge instructions

These components can be further subdivided into more specific units of information (Box 3-3).

THE DATABASE

A database is a collection of all available information that would contribute to the diagnostic process of a patient when originally seen for a particular problem. Initial data may include the following: client and patient information, details gleaned through interview with the owner regarding the pet's recent and prior histories, findings of health assessment or physical examination of the animal, and results of various laboratory and radiologic tests.

It is recommended that the database be as complete as possible, restricted only by potential risk to the patient including pain and by limitations of the owner's financial resources.

Client and Patient Information

Typically, the receptionist takes the name and contact information of the client (and/or agent of the client) when the first appointment is made. Contact information includes the client's mailing address; home, cell, and office phone numbers; fax number; and e-mail addresses. This information is confirmed later when the owner arrives for the appointment. It is particularly important to record the correct spelling of the owner's first and last names. Even seemingly simple names such as Megan Brown may be spelled Meaghan Brown or Meghan Browne. Do not presume to know the correct spelling of the client's name; always

| BOX 3-3 | Standard Information for Veterinary Medical Records |

Client Information
1. Name of owner
2. Address
3. Home, cell, work, and fax phone numbers
4. Additional information if co-owned:
   a. Other adult family members
   b. Alternate emergency contact information
5. If applicable, referring person

Patient Information
1. Name of animal
2. Signalment: species, breed, age, sex, and spayed or neutered
3. Color and markings
4. Tattoo, microchip number, and identification (ID) number

Pertinent History
1. Presenting complaint
2. Last normal
3. Frequency of episodes
4. Client observations and/or concerns
5. Current medications
6. Allergies
7. Current diet
8. Transfusion history
9. Recent travel history

Previous History
1. Previous problems
2. Previous treatments and responses
3. Previous surgeries
4. Previous medications
5. Previous diagnostic tests
6. Immunization history
7. Patient's weight history
8. Previous diet
9. Geographic region of origin/birth and travel history
10. Previous reactions to drugs, anesthesia, and transfusions

Physical Examination
1. Initial physical examination findings
2. Progress notes and SOAPs
3. Master problem list
4. Working problem list

Diagnosis
1. Tentative diagnoses
2. Definitive diagnoses

Prognoses

Diagnostic Results
1. Laboratory reports
2. Reports and assessments of diagnostic procedures (endoscopy, radiography, ultrasound, and special imaging)
3. Description of surgical and dental procedures, including duration of procedure and name of surgeon
4. Anesthesia record
5. Consultation reports with specialists or other referring veterinarians (dermatology, oncology, cardiology, ophthalmology, surgery, internal medicine, dentistry, and neurology)
6. Necropsy report

Therapeutic Plans
1. Changes in therapy
2. Medication administration and order record (MAOR)
   a. Name of medication
   b. Time
   c. Date
   d. Dosage and directions
   e. Fluid rate
   f. Route of administration
   g. Frequency
   h. Duration of treatment
   i. Identification of individuals

Cautionary Notes
1. Slaughter withdrawal and/or milk withholding dates (food animal)
2. Client communications
3. Signed consent forms
4. Client waivers or deferrals of recommendations
5. Client phone log
6. Discharge instructions

Financial Records

Derived from Peden AH: Comparative records for health information management, ed 2, Florence, KY, 2004, Delmar; and AVMA guidelines for basic information for records, and the American Animal Hospital Association standards of accreditation.

confirm it. This will prevent subsequent confusion and the risk of client or patient identity error.

In addition, the receptionist may want to have a general idea of the client's schedule for the day and where he or she can be reached and at what times. This is particularly critical if the pet is undergoing surgery or a procedure that requires anesthesia. Unexpected events or findings can occur during clinical procedures, and the veterinarian may need to consult the owner immediately. Sometimes the owner must make important decisions over the telephone, such as the extent of treatment to be performed, while the animal is on the surgery table and/or under an anesthetic. In this situation,

good communication and care provided for the patient are maximized if the client can be contacted immediately. In addition to client information, the receptionist records co-owner information and the name of the referring individual.

Patient identification is also recorded at the time of admission and includes the name of the animal, any electronic identification such as a microchip or tattoo number, species, breed, gender, reproductive status (e.g., intact, spayed, neutered, pregnant), age, color and any distinctive markings such as ear notches or cropping, scars, and tail docking. Collectively, this information identifies the individual patient and is known as the **signalment**. In some veterinary practices that use hard copy medical records, the patient's signalment is imprinted, together with the client information, on the top of each medical record form. Hospitals that employ computer-based patient records include this information automatically in each electronic view of the patient record. Many practices that use handwritten medical records employ a wide range of forms for various diagnostic tests and for different departments. In these hospitals, it is important to stamp each and every form with the client information and the patient's signalment, including the back of the form if it is two-sided. Refer to Figure 3-1, *A* and *B* for examples of hard copy and electronic client–patient information forms. Notice that computer-based records separate data into windows that can be opened separately and edited. In the patient information window, many practice management software programs issue alerts to veterinary personnel regarding special handling of the patient, drug allergies, and other important reminders (Figure 3-2, *A* and *B*).

Before the patient is examined, veterinary technicians and veterinarians obtain valuable information about the patient from the patient's signalment. Physiologic changes related to age, breed, and gender, for example, can influence a patient's rate of healing, as well as its resolve when stressed and its behavior toward other animals, respectively. In this way, signalment assists the veterinary technician to more accurately assess the patient and to anticipate potential risks during hospitalization.

History

A comprehensive history includes both previous and recent historical information. Previous historical information is typically taken during each new-patient visit. Some practices have two history forms: one on which the previous history information is recorded, and the other for **recent history** information. Refer to Figure 3-3 for an example of a form that includes both recent and previous historical information. Also, refer to Chapter 7 for an example of a completed form and instruction in documentation of patient histories.

Previous history information may include the following:

1. Origin: animal's birthplace and date
2. Preventive medicine program: immunizations, parasite control, dental care program, ear care program, spay/neutering, and exercise program
3. Behavior: usual disposition and temperament, unusual behavioral events
4. Environment: kept indoors or outdoors, presence of other pets and humans in the home, level of exposure to non–family-owned pets, travel history
5. Nutritional history: current weight, daily diet, and weight changes
6. Known allergies and reactions: atopy, food, contact with substances, medications, blood transfusions
7. Reproduction: neutered, estrus cycles; when bred, number of litters

8. Previous conditions: medical illness, trauma, or surgical operations
9. Medications, treatments, and responses
10. Prior referral history

Recent history information may include these items:

1. Presenting complaint and circumstances
2. Last normal
3. Location and character of problem such as quality, severity, onset, duration, time of day, frequency, triggers, associated problems, and progression
4. Current medications
5. Treatment efforts (if any)
6. Comments and concerns of the owner
7. Current diet
8. Recent changes in environment, household schedule, or pets/humans in household
9. Information from previous or referring veterinarian

Physical Examination

The physical examination (PE) is one of the most important diagnostic procedures. Although the physical examination of the veterinarian and that of the veterinary technician differ in their focus, both are important components of the patient's database. If performed carefully and systematically, the physical examination can provide veterinary technicians with valuable information to accurately assess hospitalized patients under their care. Typically, data entry is organized by anatomic system, and prompts to the examiner help support a thorough examination (Figure 3-4). Notes are made directly on the PE form or are entered into the computer at the time of the examination. In some veterinary hospitals, voice recognition software allows members of the veterinary health care team to dictate findings while completing the examination. Refer to Chapter 7 for an example of a completed physical examination form and instructions for performing a thorough examination.

Each anatomic system is examined, and abnormalities are typically recorded in detail; normal systems are noted with the notation "WNL" (within normal limits). This confirms that the system was indeed examined and was found to be normal. Electronic forms include a "short-hand" box to click if the system is within normal limits. Absence of "WNL" would imply that the system was not examined. Another common short-hand notation is "BAR" (bright, alert, and responsive). Use of standard abbreviations supports efficient and accurate medical record keeping and creates a common language for all referring and collaborating health care providers.

Laboratory, Diagnostic Imaging, and Other Pertinent Forms

Animals may have a variety of diagnostic tests performed such as complete blood count (CBC), chemistry profile, urine and fecal analysis, radiologic and ultrasonic studies, electrocardiographic (ECG) and electroencephalographic (EEG) studies, endoscopic examinations, scintigraphy, computed tomography (CT), and magnetic resonance

COMPANION ANIMAL CLIENT/PATIENT INFORMATION FORM

DATE_____ CASE NUMBER_____

Please provide the following information for our records: **PLEASE PRINT!**

OWNER INFORMATION

OWNER'S NAME

SOCIAL SECURITY NUMBER

STREET ADDRESS

CITY/STATE

ZIP CODE

PARISH OR COUNTY

TELEPHONE NUMBER(S) (Area Code, if long distance) → HOME   BUSINESS

DRIVER'S LICENSE NUMBER   PLACE OF EMPLOYMENT   HOW LONG?

ANIMAL INFORMATION

ANIMAL SPECIES (Dog, Cat, Other)   BREED

ANIMAL'S NAME   SEX   HAS ANIMAL BEEN SEXUALLY ALTERED? ☐ Yes ☐ No

COLOR   BIRTHDATE (Month/year, or approximate)   The undersigned owner or agent certifies that the herein described animal has a maximum value of approximately **$**

REFERRAL INFORMATION

WERE YOU REFERRED BY A VETERINARIAN? ☐ Yes ☐ No   IF YOU WERE REFERRED BY A VETERINARIAN, PLEASE COMPLETE THE FOLLOWING:

VETERINARIAN'S NAME   PHONE

STREET ADDRESS

CITY/STATE   ZIP CODE

You will be advised of estimated cost and anticipated procedures. Please feel free to discuss the proposed treatment and its cost with the veterinarian. A minimum deposit of 50% of the initial estimated charges will be required for hospitalization of an animal patient.

STATEMENT OF OWNERSHIP AND CONSENT: I am the owner of the above described animal, or have authorization from the owner to consent to its treatment.

I hereby authorize the performance of professionally accepted diagnostic, therapeutic, anesthetic, and surgical procedures necessary for its treatment.

I accept financial responsibility for these services.

I have read the above consent and understand why the above procedures may be necessary. I also have been told of the possible complications and alternatives to the listed procedures.

PAYMENT CHOICE: ☐ Cash ☐ Check ☐ Bank Card

SIGNATURE (Owner/Agent)   DATE

A

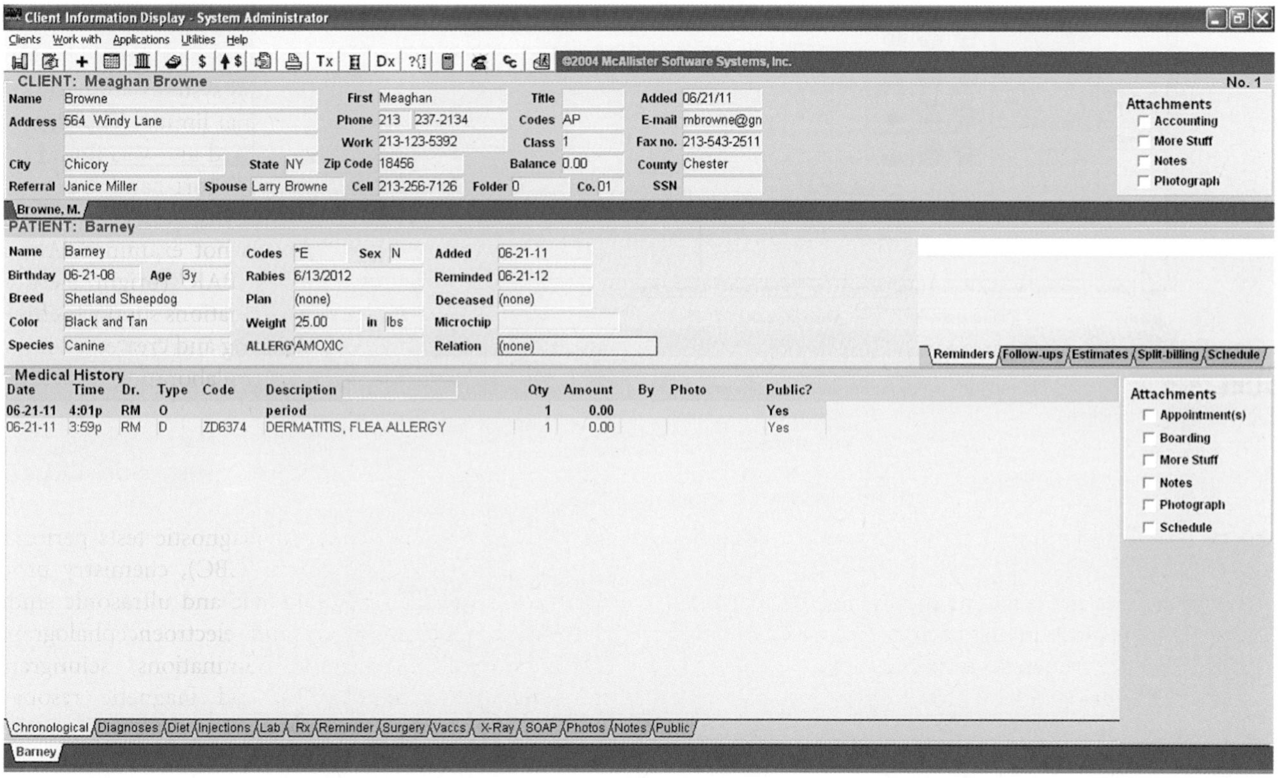

B

FIGURE 3-1 A, An example of a client and patient information form. **B,** Within practice management software, client and patient information is stored in specified windows. AVImark software (McAllister Software Systems, Inc., Piedmont, MO) combines client and patient information windows on the same screen.

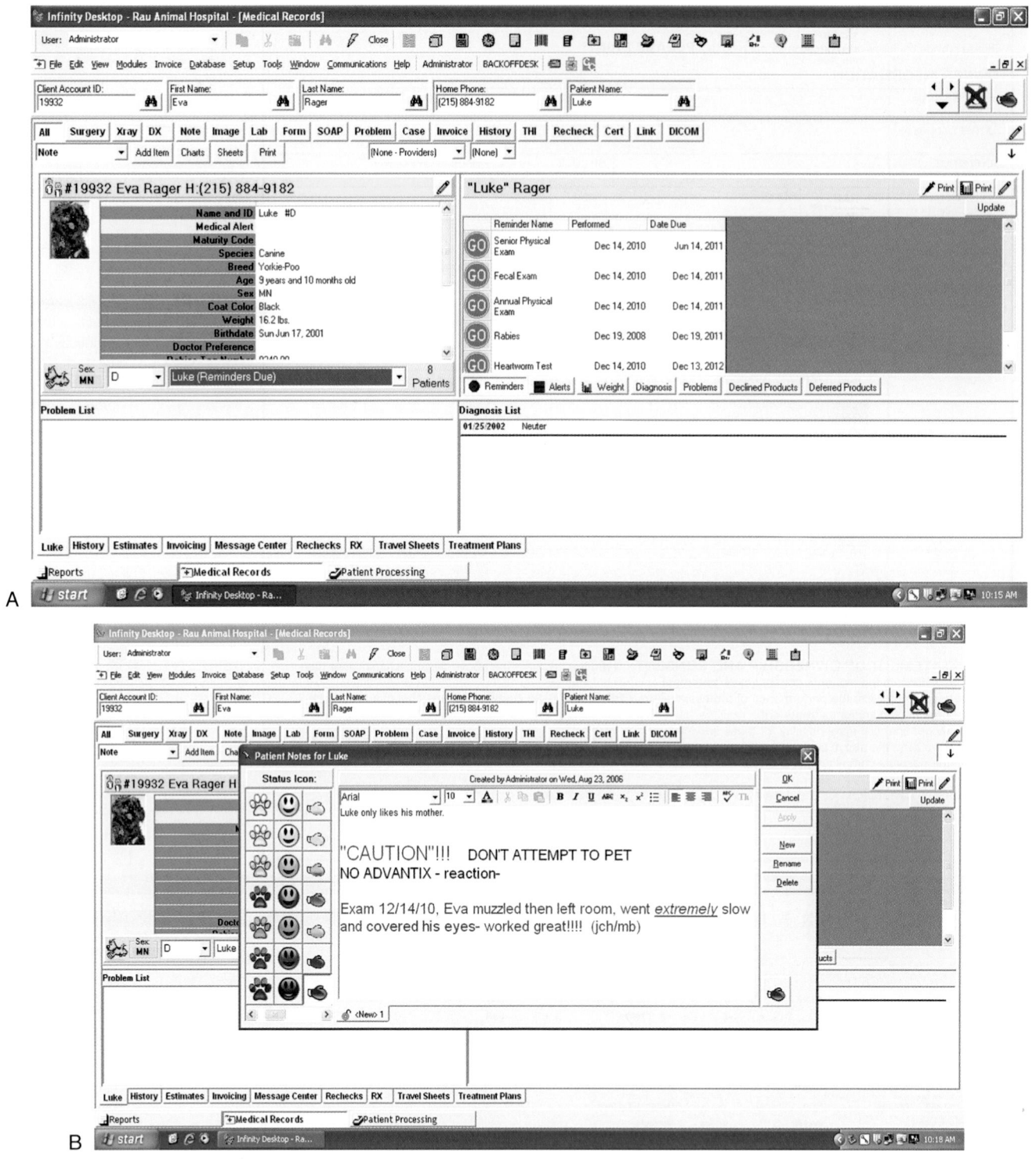

FIGURE 3-2 **A,** Patient information window for Infinity software (Infinity Software Development, Inc., Tallahassee, FL). **B,** Patient alert regarding special handling instructions.

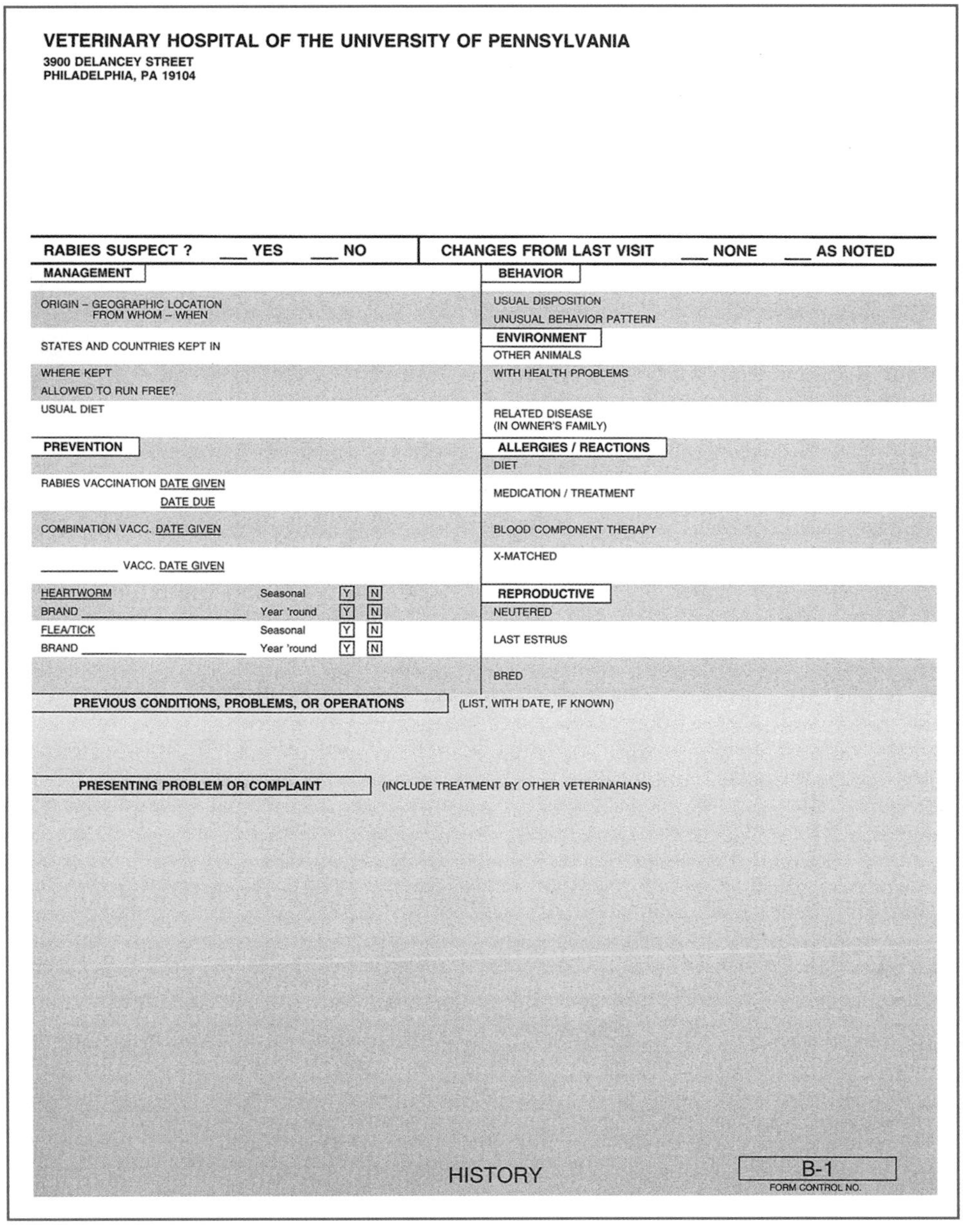

VETERINARY HOSPITAL OF THE UNIVERSITY OF PENNSYLVANIA
3900 DELANCEY STREET
PHILADELPHIA, PA 19104

RABIES SUSPECT ? ___ YES ___ NO	CHANGES FROM LAST VISIT ___ NONE ___ AS NOTED
MANAGEMENT	**BEHAVIOR**
ORIGIN – GEOGRAPHIC LOCATION FROM WHOM – WHEN	USUAL DISPOSITION
	UNUSUAL BEHAVIOR PATTERN
STATES AND COUNTRIES KEPT IN	**ENVIRONMENT**
	OTHER ANIMALS
WHERE KEPT	WITH HEALTH PROBLEMS
ALLOWED TO RUN FREE?	
USUAL DIET	RELATED DISEASE (IN OWNER'S FAMILY)
PREVENTION	**ALLERGIES / REACTIONS**
	DIET
RABIES VACCINATION _DATE GIVEN_	
DATE DUE	MEDICATION / TREATMENT
COMBINATION VACC. _DATE GIVEN_	BLOOD COMPONENT THERAPY
_____ VACC. _DATE GIVEN_	X-MATCHED
HEARTWORM Seasonal Y N	**REPRODUCTIVE**
BRAND _____ Year 'round Y N	NEUTERED
FLEA/TICK Seasonal Y N	
BRAND _____ Year 'round Y N	LAST ESTRUS
	BRED
PREVIOUS CONDITIONS, PROBLEMS, OR OPERATIONS (LIST, WITH DATE, IF KNOWN)	
PRESENTING PROBLEM OR COMPLAINT (INCLUDE TREATMENT BY OTHER VETERINARIANS)	

HISTORY | B-1 |
FORM CONTROL NO.

FIGURE 3-3 An example of a history form that includes both current and prior historical information. Refer to Chapter 7 for instructions on completing this form.

imaging (MRI). This part of the database can vary depending on the needs of the patient and the specific orders of the veterinarian. Depending on the size and caseload of the veterinary practice, separate forms may be used for different diagnostic procedures. For example, results of diagnostic procedures, such as radiography and endoscopy, and of laboratory tests may all be found in the medical record of an animal that had an esophageal foreign body (see the Evolve site at http://evolve.elsevier.com/McCurnin/vettech/).

Anesthesia, surgery, recovery, and pain management forms may also be pertinent to a patient that has undergone a surgical procedure (see the Evolve site at http://evolve.elsevier.com/McCurnin/vettech/).

Laboratory Diagnostic Summary and Flow Sheet

The laboratory diagnostic flow sheet is a compilation of laboratory data collected from an individual animal. It can be used for outpatients or inpatients. It shows at a glance the different laboratory values for tests that have been performed on the patient. Specific values on different dates can be compared for blood counts, chemistry panels, blood gases, urinalyses, and coagulation rates (see the Evolve site at http://evolve.elsevier.com/McCurnin/vettech/). This sheet is of particular value when internal medicine cases are evaluated, such as animals with diabetes or any of the following disorders: anemia, chronic renal failure, hepatic failure, Addison's disease, and Cushing's disease.

PHYSICAL EXAMINATION

Temp.	Pulse/min.	Resp./min.

Attitude at time of Exam (Circle one)
(Vicious, excited, alert, depressed, comatose, other_____)
Nutritional state (Circle one)
(Obese, overweight, normal, underweight, cachectic)

State of Hydration: good, fair, poor (Circle one)   Weight (from scale)   kg.

SYSTEMATIC EXAMINATION (Use space below as needed)

Oro-Pharyngeal

Eyes

Ears

Respiratory

Cardiovascular

Gastrointestinal and Anus

Rectal

Uro-Genital

Integument

Lymph Nodes

Musculo-Skeletal

Nervous

Physical Exam Performed By:

_____
(Student's signature)

PROBLEMS:
1.
2.
3.
4.

FIGURE 3-4 An example of a physical examination form. Refer to Chapter 7 for instructions on completing this form.

Consultants

Specialties such as behavior, dermatology, medicine, neurology, nutrition, oncology, ophthalmology, orthopedics, and surgery are examples of the departments that can make up referral and specialty hospitals. As cases are worked up, specialists may be consulted to address specific problems that the patient is experiencing. A consultation form would be completed, and the consulting veterinarian's findings, diagnosis, and recommendations would be recorded. These findings, together with results of special imaging or other diagnostic tests, would be e-mailed to the referring practice or practitioner. Refer to the Evolve site at http://evolve.elsevier.com/McCurnin/vettech/.

MASTER PROBLEM LIST AND WORKING PROBLEM LIST

A defining part of the POVMR is the master problem list. The master problem list includes the major medical disorders experienced by a patient during its lifetime. Each problem represents a conclusion or a decision resulting from examination, investigation, and analysis of the database. The master problem list is typically arranged in five columns: a chronological list of each problem, the date of onset, the action taken, the outcome or resolution, and the date of the outcome or resolution. In this way, the master problem list serves as an index to the patient's medical history. Problems may be added, and intervention or plans for intervention

```
JONATHAN HART DVM
2441 TREASURE HILL BLVD
HOUSTON, TEXAS  78550


210  389  4726
```

```
BERNARD DAVIS                    66444
1087 TARA BLVD
BATON ROUGE, LA  70825

CAN LAB F/S
BO BLK 11/30/96
```

IMMUNIZATION PREVENTATIVE RECORD

DATE	5/10/03	6/14/04								
RABIES	X	X								
DA2PL	X	X								
PARVO	X	X								
FVRCP										
FELV VACC.										
FELV/FIV										
FECAL	neg.	neg.								
HEARTWORM	neg.	neg.								

	PROBLEM LIST	DATE ENTERED	DATE RESOLVED
1.	Elective Ovariohysterectomy	8/10/95	8/10/95
2.	Malassezia-otitis externa	8/10/95	8/17/95
3.	Dental prophylaxis	11/3/98	11/3/98
4.	Gastroenteritis — small bowel diarrhea	3/15/99	3/18/99
5.	Uncomplicated UTI	2/3/05	2/16/05
6.	Recurrent UTI — E. Coli	3/14/05	3/28/05
7.	Recurrent UTI	6/10/05	6/20/05
8.	Right Renomegaly; Cystic kidney mass	6/20/05	
9.	Right unilateral nephrectomy	6/23/05	6/23/05
10.	Renal carcinoma	6/24/05	
11.	Lethary, anorexia	7/2/05	7/5/05
12.			
13.			

BREED=   SEX=

FIGURE 3-5 Immunization history record and master problem list.

may be changed. At a glance, the veterinary technician can determine what happened, when, and how long it lasted (Figure 3-5). A summary of the preventive medical history may accompany the master problem list, which includes the dates when immunizations were administered and the results of fecal analysis and routine screenings for heartworm and contagious viral diseases.

The **working problem list** (Figure 3-6) is often used in veterinary practices to assist the veterinary health care team in working through current problems. For example, if the patient is hospitalized and is subsequently diagnosed with autoimmune hemolytic anemia, the initial working problem list may include symptomatic and reactive problems until the final diagnosis is made by the veterinarian.

Whereas the master problem list is essentially a list of final diagnoses generated by the veterinarian, the working problem list is a dynamic tabulation of clinical problems and symptoms generated by the veterinary technician and the veterinarian. The technician may list exercise intolerance and the veterinarian might list nonregenerative anemia. In this way, the working problem list helps the veterinary health care team prioritize problems, think critically, and formulate interventions as problems become apparent without offering a specific diagnosis. When a final diagnosis such as autoimmune hemolytic anemia is reached by the veterinarian, it is added to the master problem list.

TECHNICIAN NOTE The working problem list helps the veterinarian and the veterinary technician identify and prioritize problems, think critically, and formulate an understanding of the patient's reactions to an illness.

Pamela Davis 1085 Tabia Road Melvorn, PA 19756 Fred Can Lab M/N BIK 3/14/xx	Melvorn Veterinary Hospital 76 Springhouse Drive Melvorn, PA 19756 **Working Problem List**		
Problem number	Active date	Problem	Date resolved
1	7/14/xx	Depression/lethargy	8/15/xx
2	7/14/xx	Pale, yellow mucus membranes	
3	7/14xx	Mild Tachycardia	7/20/xx
4	7/20/xx	Anemia	
5	7/20/xx	Icterus	
6	7/24/xx	Autoimmune hemolytic anemia	

FIGURE 3-6 Working problem list.

HOSPITALIZED PATIENT RECORDS

Overview

Each separate problem is named and described in the initial plan in progress notes using the SOAP format (Figure 3-7). If an animal is hospitalized, ongoing daily management of the patient is also documented in the progress notes. Therapeutic interventions and plans are evaluated and adjusted according to the progress of the patient, evaluations are made, and the working problem list is modified as needed. If diagnostic procedures are performed, findings relevant to the current problem may be entered in the SOAP or added later as a notation independent of the SOAP. Test results printed on separate laboratory forms included elsewhere in the medical record can be referenced in the SOAP or notation without the need to restate the results. If laboratory test results such as the results of an in-house CBC are printed on a small slip of paper, the slip can be taped directly to the progress sheet in the medical record. Placing a signature and a date across both the progress sheet and the piece of paper helps to authenticate the information. If a definitive diagnosis is made by the veterinarian, it is added to the medical record together with the patient's prognosis and therapeutic plans. Communications with the client and any changes in therapy are also noted on the progress sheets.

When the patient is ready to be discharged, a summary is written that relates the overall assessment of the animal and its progress during treatment with plans for follow-up or referral. The summary includes a review of all problems initially identified and encourages continuity of care for the patient at home and via subsequent follow-up visits or referral appointments. Medications and take-home instructions are dispensed and reviewed with the owner. Each subsequent time a patient visits the veterinary hospital, SOAP notes and notations are made to summarize the visit and address new problems.

Technician SOAP Notes

Patient evaluation and assessment are documented in the progress notes using a structured format called the SOAP.

Although SOAP notes may be written by both veterinarians and veterinary technicians, their notes have different focus. The veterinarian seeks to find a primary cause and a cure for illness, whereas the veterinary technician assesses the patient's physiologic and psychosocial responses to illness and strives to ameliorate those responses. In this way, the technician's evaluation of the patient is distinctly different from that of the veterinarian. The motivation of the veterinary nurse is to put the patient's comfort first. In addition to assessing the patient, the veterinary technician anticipates future changes, complications, and sequelae to current problems. This forward thinking is noted in the SOAP as risks, such as "risk for infection" or "risk for transmission of infection." Because veterinary technicians may not prescribe, dispensation and administration of medication are noted in the patient record by the veterinary technician "as per order." This verifies the role the veterinarian plays in prescribing medical treatment.

Subjective/Objective

Although it is widely agreed that information from the database constitutes the "S" and "O" portions of the SOAP note, differences of opinion have been put forth on what constitutes subjective and objective information. Different schools teach different approaches. In this chapter, all *nonmeasurable* information will be categorized as "subjective" and all *measurable* information as "objective." Relevant historical information, such as the presenting complaint, and most of the physical examination findings would therefore be entered in the subjective section. Observations of the patient's posture, attitude, and appetite may also be included, such as "standing, panting, and wagging tail," or "awake, in left lateral recumbency." Measurable data such as laboratory results, temperature, heart and respiratory rates, weight, skin retraction time, capillary refill time, numbers of bowel movements, and measured urine output would be noted in the objective section.

Assessment

Completion of the *assessment* portion of the SOAP requires analysis of all subjective and objective data that have been

Anatomy of In-Patient Progress Notes

(1) Patient Information

This includes the patient's signalment and the owner's name and mailing address, which together help confirm the correct identity of the patient. The signalment guides veterinary personnel towards a list of possible diagnoses relevant to the sex, age and breed of the patient.

(2) Signature and Credentials Verification

Veterinary personnel complete this section to correlate staff signatures with their respective initials. The "title" column identifies the role on the veterinary health care team member as either a veterinarian or veterinary technician.

(3) Date, Time, and Author of Entry

Because the medical record is a legal document, every entry must be dated and timed. In addition, the signature or initials of the author should be noted to indicate who made the entry and when.

(4) Subjective Patient Information

Assessment of the patient begins from a distance before the cage or stall door is opened and may include:
a. A brief summary of presenting complaint and recent historical information from the owner.
b. Subjective observations such as the patient's posture, behavior, mentation, and the appearance and frequency of defecation, urination and vomition.
c. Observations about food and water consumption are also noted.
A physical examination of the patient follows and all relevant, non-quantifiable findings are recorded.

IN-PATIENT PROGRESS NOTES

Patient ID	Allergies	Initials	Signature	Title
"Freddy" Henderson 3/18/XX Chow Mix, FS 14 Briar Cliff Road Misty, KY 23564	Clavamox	SP	Sarah Pace	CVT
	Weight: 54 lb			

Date	Time, Signature	SOAP	Progress Notes
9/3/XX	4:45 PM Sarah Pace, CVT	S	Owner reports patient is lethargic with poor appetite and licking flanks. PE: geriatric patient, slow stiff gate, multi-focal, ulcerative skin lesions with sl. serous exudate on R and L flanks, dull brittle coat, matting in perianal region and flanks. Flea dirt evident. PE othrwise WNL
		O	T=103.5F, P=80, RR=panting, MMC=blue (chow), MMM=tacky, BCS: 2/5, CRT=2.5 sec, Skin turgor= 2 sec., PCV=49%, TP=7.9 g/dl
		A	Hypovolemia, hyperthermia, impaired tissue integrity, risk of infection, pain/pruritis, self-inflicted injury, altered appetite, underweight, self-care deficit, client knowledge deficit, decreased mobility.
		P	1. Place IV catheter and administer 0.9% NaCl IV as per order of Dr. Fox. 2. Collect culture and sensitivity of affected dermal areas as per order. 3. Clip and lavage affected regions, remove mats. 4. Administer trimethoprim sulfa, Rymadil, Frontline as per order. 5. Install cage mat and soft bedding in cage. 6. Apply E-collar. 7. Client education re: flea control, import. of regular grooming and mod. exercise in geriatric animals. 8. Dispense prescription diet as per order

(5) Objective Patient Information

All quantifiable information such as vital signs, test results, capillary refill time, and dehydration indicators are recorded.

(6) Assessment

The veterinary technician identifies pertinent patient evaluations and prioritizes them in order of importance according to the physical and psychological needs of the patient. Risks for complications and client knowledge deficits are also noted and prioritized.

(7) Plan

Using logic and independent critical thinking, a technician intervention is formulated to address each of the technician evaluations listed in the Assessment section. In this way, a nursing care plan is formulated. The interventions are carried out in order of importance.

FIGURE 3-7 Anatomy of the veterinary technician's SOAP (subjective, objective, assessment, and planning).

BOX 3-4	Examples of Patient Evaluations Listed Alphabetically

Abnormal Eating Behavior	Decreased Perfusion	Overweight
Acute Pain	Dehydration	Postoperative Compliance
Aggression	Diarrhea	Preoperative Compliance
Altered Ambulation	Electrolyte Imbalance	Pruritus
Altered Gas Diffusion	Exercise Intolerance	Reduced Mobility
Altered Mentation	Fear	Reproductive Dysfunction
Altered Oral Health	Hypertension	Risk of Aspiration
Altered Sensory Perception	Hyperthermia	Risk of Dehydration
Altered Urinary Production	Hypervolemia	Risk of Infection
Altered Ventilation	Hypotension	Risk of Infection Transmission
Anxiety	Hypothermia	Self-Care Deficit
Bleeding/Blood Loss	Hypovolemia	Self-Inflicted Injury
Bowel Incontinence	Impaired Tissue Integrity	Sleep Disturbance
Bradycardia	Inappropriate Elimination	Status Within Appropriate Limits
Cardiac Insufficiency	Ineffective Nursing	Tachycardia
Chronic Pain	Infection	Underweight
Client Coping Deficit	Irregular Cardiac Rhythm	Urinary Incontinence
Client Knowledge Deficit	Noncompliant Owner	Vomiting/Nausea
Constipation	Obstructed Airway	

Modified from Figure 3-3, p. 57; Rockett J, Lattnzio C, Anderson K: Patient assessment and interventions and documentation for the veterinary technician, Clifton Park, NY, 2009, Delmar Cengage Learning.

gathered thus far. Based on these data, the veterinary technician uses critical thinking to generate a list of **patient evaluations** that reflect the animal's physical, psychological, social, and environmental conditions. In this way, the veterinary technician's assessment of the patient is holistic, taking into account all aspects of the individual's experience and generating a custom-tailored nursing plan to address each of the patient's needs. Refer to Box 3-4 for examples of patient evaluations.

In 1943, the famous psychiatrist Abraham Maslow developed a hierarchal pyramid of needs to account for motivating forces observed in the human psyche. This concept was later applied to the nursing profession to help guide the prioritization of clinical problems and to improve understanding in addressing the needs of patients. Veterinary technicians similarly can make use of Maslow's concept by prioritizing patient evaluations to generate an effective nursing plan that addresses the most important issues first. Table 3-1 illustrates a hierarchy of animal health needs and offers examples of corresponding **technician evaluations**. Notice that the most important needs of the patient are listed first and the less critical ones are listed below in decreasing order of importance. In SOAP notes, each patient evaluation is assigned a number such that the most important evaluation in the hierarchy of physiologic needs is number one. This organization supports the veterinary technician's practice model of addressing the most important health problems first. Refer to Chapter 1 for a discussion of the veterinary technician practice model. Examples of technician evaluations include hypothermia, altered mentation, inappropriate elimination, and risk of infection. Evaluations that require

urgent attention, such as those related to inappropriate oxygenation, are first in the hierarchy of patient needs. As part of the veterinary technician practice model, technicians reevaluate their patients and reassess and adjust the plan. Patient progress and adjustments to the list of evaluations are noted in the assessment portion of the technician SOAP notes.

Plan

In the last portion of the SOAP, the veterinary technician methodically develops an intervention for each of the evaluations listed in the assessment portion of the SOAP note. The compilation of these interventions constitutes *the plan* for patient care, and it is hoped that carrying out the plan will restore patient comfort and well-being. Plans may include, for example, client education, medications, moderate daily exercise, daily cold compresses, and follow-up appointments. Perhaps the patient will be discharged from the veterinary hospital, or perhaps the patient will require additional diagnostic testing and evaluation. As the patient is evaluated and reevaluated, the veterinary technician plan of care is adjusted to address any new developments and changes in status or prognosis.

Notations

Any incoming information that is entered in the progress notes but is independent of the SOAP is entered as a *notation*. Additional information from a referring veterinarian, for example, or communication with an animal's owner in person or by telephone may be recorded in the progress notes as a notation.

Progress Notes

Date/Time	Initials	Progress Notes
3/15/XX 5PM	RB, CVT	Notation: Canine SNAP test negative for Lyme Disease. Notified Dr. Wilcox.

TABLE 3-1	Prioritization of Technician Evaluations
	Based on Hierarchy of Patient's Physiologic Needs

PRIORITY	PHYSIOLOGIC NEED	TECHNICIAN EVALUATION	PRIORITY	PHYSIOLOGIC NEED	TECHNICIAN EVALUATION
1	Oxygenation	Altered Gas Diffusion Altered Ventilation Cardiac Insufficiency Decreased Perfusion Obstructed Airway Risk of Aspiration	6	Noncritical Safety	Altered Mentation Altered Sensory Perception Noncompliant Owner Hyperthermia Hypothermia Impaired Tissue Integrity Owner Knowledge Deficit Risk of Infection Risk of Infection Transmission Self-Inflicted Injury Status Within Appropriate Limits
2	Critical Safety and/or Severe Pain	Acute Pain Electrolyte Imbalance Hyperthermia (Severe) Hypothermia (Severe) Postoperative Compliance Preoperative Compliance	7	Chronic Pain or Mild-Moderate Acute Pain	Acute Pain Chronic Pain
3	Hydration	Hypervolemia Hypovolemia	8	Activity	Exercise Intolerance Reduced Mobility Sleep Disturbance
4	Elimination	Altered Urinary Production Bowel Incontinence Constipation Diarrhea Inappropriate Elimination Self-Care Deficit Urinary Incontinence	9	Utility	Aggression Anxiety Client Coping Deficit Client Knowledge Deficit Fear Inappropriate Elimination Reproductive Dysfunction
5	Nutrition	Altered Oral Health Abnormal Eating Behavior Ineffective Nursing Overweight Self-Care Deficit Underweight Vomiting and/or Diarrhea			

Modified from Figure 3-1; Rockett J, Lattnzio C, Anderson K: Patient assessment and interventions and documentation for the veterinary technician, Clifton Park, NY, 2009, Delmar Cengage Learning.

Small sheets of paper with laboratory results or physiologic test results may be taped directly onto the progress sheet near to the notation that references the test result. To further verify the authenticity of the addition, the veterinary technician should sign across the junction of the progress sheet and attached piece of paper. The entry should be dated and timed, and the date on the laboratory paper should be circled or underlined.

> **TECHNICIAN NOTE** To assist the veterinary health care team in carrying out treatment orders efficiently, MAOR sheets are used to record which treatments were delivered, when, and by whom. In addition, the MAOR offers an at-a-glance summary of the patient's management during hospitalization.

Medication Administration/Order Record (MAOR)

The MAOR, also known as a *ward treatment sheet*, is used to ensure that hospitalized patients are given treatments, diagnostic tests, and diet as requested by the attending veterinarian. Management of hospitalized patients can be complicated, particularly in busy practices with heavy caseloads and in those that treat emergency and critical care patients. To assist the veterinary health care team in carrying out treatment orders efficiently, grids are used to record which treatments were delivered, when, and by whom. In addition, the MAOR offers an at-a-glance summary of the patient's management during hospitalization (Figure 3-8). Treatments to be given and dates and specific times throughout the day when each of the treatments should be completed are listed on the MAOR. Doses, methods of administration, and cautionary notes should be written for each medication. In addition, MAORs should always include the patient's full name, patient ID number, and/or signalment, and any known allergies that the patient may have. MAORs should also include a signature chart that lists the full name of each member of the health care team with corresponding initials. This allows team members to use the short-hand approach of initialing boxes in the chart without having to sign their full name. Although MAORs are often used in hard copy, they can be generated and used electronically as well. Examples of specialized MAORs for equine patients with (A) colic or (B) diarrhea and (C) for foals housed in the intensive care unit can be found on the Evolve site at http://evolve.elsevier.com/McCurnin/vettech/.

When paper MAORs are completed, the following guidelines apply:

1. Each order entered in the MAOR should be written exactly as the veterinarian wrote it. The full name of the medication and its dose and route of administration should be listed. It is important for the veterinary technician to ask for clarification if instructions are not clear. Medications given during surgery or anesthesia are entered onto surgical or anesthesia forms and are *not* entered on the MAOR.

2. When a treatment is given, the person giving the treatment writes his or her initials in the column that indicates the time of administration. A treatment that is given 1 hour before or after the ordered time is typically considered "on time." However, when the time of administration is significantly different from the requested time, the veterinary technician enters the actual time that the treatment was administered.

3. When a treatment is not given, the initials "NG" should be entered into the appropriate column and box. In addition, the veterinary technician must notify the attending veterinarian if a treatment was not administered.

4. When a dose is ordered for a specific period of time, an "X" should be place in the boxes representing the dates when the medication is <u>not</u> to be given.

5. When a medication is discontinued, the veterinary technician should enter the word "discontinued." Erasure and crossing out or blotting out the record of a discontinued medication should never be done.

6. If the full recommended duration of medication was not given by hospital personnel because the patient was discharged, the remaining boxes of dates and times should be left blank.

In most practices, medications and supplies needed to complete treatments are kept near the patient for convenience. Some practices store a patient's medications and treatment supplies in bins on a table or shelf, along with the patient's medical record (Figure 3-9, *A*). Other practices prefer to use baskets that can be suspended from the patient's cage together with the MAOR (Figure 3-9, *B*). Hospitals for equine and food animal patients often maintain medications and supplies in treatment carts that can be wheeled easily in barn aisles from stall to stall. Regardless of the approach used, it is important to clearly label medications and supplies with the patient's name, signalment, and owner information.

Cage Cards and Patient Identification

Cage and stall cards are used to identify the patient and the reason for the hospitalization. The owner's and patient's information is stamped on the card. Many practices apply identifying collars to each patient so the cage card can be matched to the identification on the patient. In equine practices, the identification strip is applied to the horse's halter. In some practices that do not use separate ward treatment sheets or MAORs, the treatment grid is also stamped on the cage and stall card and lists the procedures to be performed. In some specialty and referral practices, the color of the cage card may be used to indicate the hospital division that is treating the patient. A red card, for example, might indicate surgery, whereas a blue card might indicate internal medicine or cardiology.

> **TECHNICIAN NOTE** Veterinary technicians need to be sure that owners have the necessary information and resources to continue any prescribed home care and home monitoring of their pet.

Discharge and Summary Forms

It is important to discharge patients in a fashion that ensures a desirable outcome for patient and owner. To this end, veterinary technicians need to ensure that owners have the necessary information and resources to continue any prescribed home care and home monitoring of their pet. A clear, concise summary of the pet's illness, prognosis, and treatment during hospitalization and specific discharge instructions are written in simple language that is understandable to the client. A printed copy of the form is given to the owner, and the veterinary technician reviews it with the owner before the animal leaves the hospital. In this way, the veterinary technician directly educates the pet owner about the pet's disease process and the clinical signs and symptoms of potential complications. Take-home instructions regarding

Medication Administration/Order Record
MAOR

Patient ID	Allergies	Initials	Signature	Title
"Freddy" Henderson 3/18/XX Chow, FS 14 Briar Cliff Road Misty, KY 23564	Clavamox	BJ	Beth Johnson	CVT
		MF	Mathew Fox	DVM
	Weight: 54 lb	CM	Cindy Miller	VTS (ECC)
		SP	Sarah Pace	CVT

Medication Administration

Date of Order	Medication	Time	9/3	9/4	9/5	9/6	9/7	9/8	9/9
9/3/XX	SS Trimethoprim sulfa One tablet PO BID for 10 days	7am	✕	CM	CM	CM			
		7pm	BJ	CM	MF	BJ			
9/3/XX	Frontline tube, apply topically at discharge	8pm	✕	✕	✕	BJ			
9/3/XX	Rymadil caplets PO BID 1mg/lb Pending lab results	7AM	✕	CM	CM	CM			
		7PM	✕	CM	MF	BJ			

Fluids and IV Drips

Date of Order	Medication	Time	9/3	9/4	9/5	9/6	9/7	9/8	9/9
9/3/XX	0.9% NaCl at 3cc/lb/hr for 6hrs	AM	✕	Stop 1:30am SP	✕	✕			
		PM	Start 7:30pm BJ	✕	✕	✕			
9/3/XX	Then 1.5cc/lb/hr for 12 hours	AM	✕	Start 1:30am SP	✕	✕			
		PM	✕	Stop 1:30pm CM	✕	✕			

FIGURE 3-8 An example of a medication administration/order record (MAOR) sheet.

Medication Administration/Order Record
MAOR-continued

Patient ID	Allergies	Initials	Signature	Title
"Freddy" Henderson 3/18/XX Chow, FS 14 Briar Cliff Road Misty, KY 23564	Clavamox	BJ	Beth Johnson	CVT
		MF	Mathew Fox	DVM
	Weight: 54 lb	CM	Cindy Miller	VTS (ECC)
		SP	Sarah Pace	CVT

Order Record

Treatments

Date of Order	Treatment	Time	9/3	9/4	9/5	9/6	9/7	9/8	9/9
9/3/XX	Clip fur in all affected areas, lavage with dilute nolvasan solution, dry well	7:30pm	SP						
9/3/XX	Heparinize catheter BID while on fluids	AM		CM	Discontinued				
		PM	SP	SP	Discontinued				

Tests

Date	Test	Time	9/3	9/4	9/5	9/6	9/7	9/8	9/9
9/3/XX	Dermal culture and sensitivity of affected areas	8pm	BJ						
9/3/XX	PCV/TS q 12hrs while on fluids		7:30pm SP	7:30am CM	Discontinued				
			7:30pm SP						

Diet

Date	Diet	Time	9/3	9/4	9/5	9/6	9/7	9/8	9/9
9/3/XX	Provide H2O and Hills G/D diet, encourage eating	AM		7A CM	7A CM	7:30A CM			
		PM	7pm BJ	6:30p CM	7pm CM	7pm BJ			

FIGURE 3-8, cont'd.

administration of medications and use of Elizabethan collars, for example, are also discussed directly with the client. Pre-printed instructional brochures may be attached to the instructions for further edification of the client. This one-on-one communication offers an opportunity for the pet owner to ask questions and allows the technician to ensure that appropriate care of the pet will be continued at home. Often the veterinary technician's name and contact information are included on the form, so the owner can call if questions or problems arise. Refer to Case Presentation 3-1 for an example of case summary and discharge instructions.

Through discharge information and procedures, the veterinary technician does the following:

- Provides a concise, written summary of the patient's malady and treatment followed by clear step-by-step instructions on how to care for the animal at home
- Verbally reviews instructions with the pet owner using language that is appropriate for the client; reviews

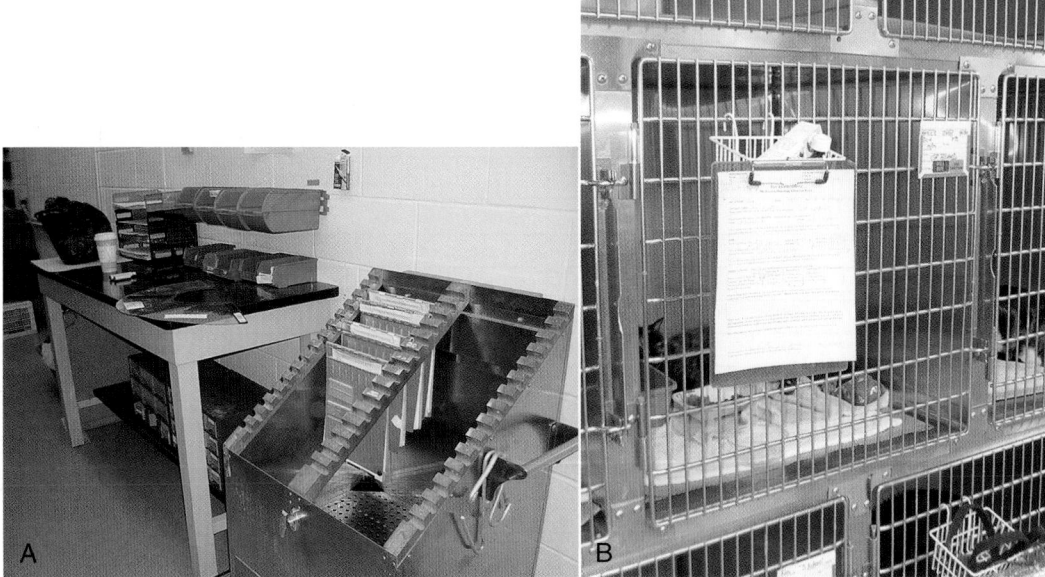

FIGURE 3-9 A, Some practices use individual bins to store the medications and supplies of each patient. These are kept near the medical record and are labeled with the patient's name. Notice that records kept on the wards are stored in protective metal holders. The record is removed from the holder before it is filed. B, Some practices store patient medications in wire baskets that can be attached directly to the door of the patient's cage. Medical records can also be attached to the cage. Both the record and the medications must be labeled clearly.

CASE PRESENTATION 3-1

A 12-year-old, female, spayed, black and tan Border collie mix named "Muffy" presented for halitosis and multiple dermal masses. No problems with mastication have been reported, but the dog occasionally paws at her mouth. The patient's immunizations are current and she receives monthly Heartgard Plus and Frontline. A recent SNAP 4 test indicated that the patient is positive for *Borrelia burdorferi* but negative for anaplasmosis, *Escherichia canis,* and heartworm.

Physical examination revealed extensive periodontal disease, particularly in the upper arcade, and eight subcutaneous soft masses ranging in size from 1 to 6 cm. Most of the masses were located on the lateral chest wall and the ventral chest and abdomen. A small meibomian cyst was present on the upper eyelid OS (of the left eye), where mild blepharospasm, increased tearing, and moderate scleral injection were noted. All other findings are WNL.

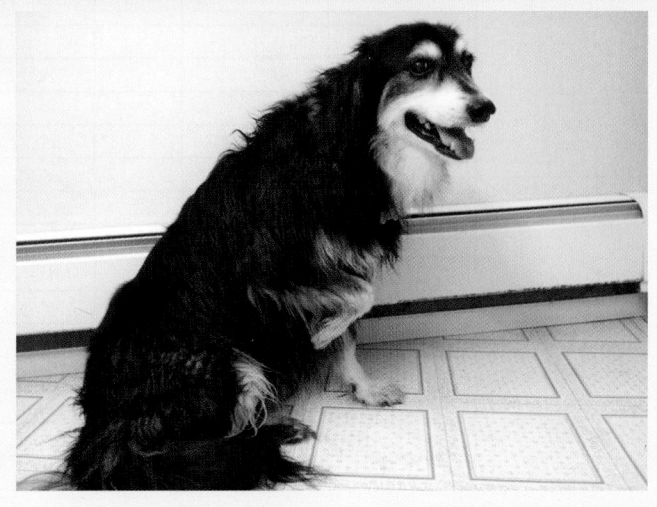

Continued

CASE PRESENTATION 3-1—cont'd

Surgery was scheduled in 1 week for a dental cleaning and oral examination, and for lumpectomies. Blood and urine samples were collected for presurgical analysis. The client was provided consent forms and a cost estimate. The owner was contacted before the date of surgery, was reminded of NPO instructions, and was informed that blood work results are normal.

On the day of surgery, NPO status and contact information were confirmed with the client. A presurgical physical examination was performed. Other than presenting complaints, PE was within normal limits. The dog was premedicated with hydromorphone, midazolam, and Dexdomitor IM and was placed in the surgical ward preoperatively. Induction occurred with intravenous (IV)

Progress Notes

Patient ID	Allergies	Initials	Signature	Title
"Muffy" Bennington 9/6/XX FS, Shetl. mix, Bk & Tan 65 Pine Road Kellersville, WI 43802	None	SP	Sarah Pace	CVT
		MF	Mike Feather	VMD
	Weight: 42 lb			

Date/Time	Initials	SOAP	Progress Notes
8/1/XX 8:30 AM	MF, VMD	S	BAR, small eyelid mass OS, sl. sclera injection, blepharospasm and epiphora, strong halitosis. Multiple soft, well circumscribed, SQ masses. Fine needle aspirate of masses consistent with Lipoma, mild DJD in coxofemeral joint, PE otherwise WNL
		O	T=100.8 F, P=80, RR=panting, MMC=pink, MMM=moist, CRT<2 sec, skin turgor <1 sec, BCS: 3.5/5, masses ranging from 1-6 cm.,
		A	Meibomian cyst OS, secondary conjunctivitis, advanced periodontal disease in upper arcade, multiple benign lipomas, oral pain
		P	1. Schedule oral examination, cleaning, root planning with likely extractions 2. Schedule same day lumpectomies 3. Collect blood for pre-surgical screening: CBC, CS, UA 4. Administer 250mg Clavamox PO for 7 days pre-op 5. Prescribe Rimadyl 75mg SID for oral and hip pain
8/2/xx 9:45 AM	SP, CVT		CBC, CS and UA results WNL
8/1/XX 8:30 AM	MF, VMD	S	Heart/lungs WNL, no murmurs or arrhythmias, pulses SnS. abdomen soft and non-painful, oral cavity and masses unchanged since 8/1.
		O	TPR=100.3F, 85bpm, 14bpm. MMM=moist, MM=pink, CRT<2 sec
		A	OK surg candidate
		P	lumpectomies and oral examination, cleaning and extractions

CASE PRESENTATION 3-1—cont'd

propofol, and inhalant isoflurane was administered throughout surgery.

Postoperatively, 4 mL of cefazolin was given slowly IV. Hydromorphone and Dexdomitor were administered intramuscularly. The dog recovered uneventfully. Orders for medication were placed by the attending veterinarian. A follow-up appointment for suture removal was scheduled at the time of discharge.

Progress Notes

See chart for detailed progress notes.

Postoperative Documentation

See the discharge instructions for postoperative documentation.

Progress Notes

Schools of thought vary regarding the way in which a database is divided into subjective and objective information.

Date/Time	Initials	SOAP	Progress Notes
8/7/xx	SP, CVT	S	Patient transferred to wards from OR recovery,
1:30 PM			patient AR, able to ambulate, mild ataxia, urination
			WNL, offered water-drank sm. amt, sutures intact,
			incision weeping small amt. serosanguinous fluid
			on caudal flank.
		O	T=99F, P=80, RR=15, MMC=pink, MMM=wet CRT<2
			sec, Skin turgor <1 sec., pulses strong/synch
		A	Post-operative compliance, impaired tissue integrity,
			acute pain, risk of infection, client knowledge deficit
		P	1. Prepare client discharge instructions
			2. Dispense medications as per order
			a. Triple antibiotic ophthalmic
			ointment OS BID
			b. Clavamox 250 mg 1 tab BID for
			7 days postop
			c. Tramadol 50mg 1/2 tablet BID
			3. Client education:
			a. Explain purpose and administration
			of medications.
			b. Check incision sites daily
			c. Applying E-collar when unsupervised
			d. Feed soft canned food X 7-10 days
			e. Instruction in teeth brushing/oral
			hygiene
			4. Schedule follow up appointment and suture
			removal in 10 days
			5. Call in 24 hours for progress report

Continued

Banner Animal Hospital
76 Meadow Lane
Unionville, WI 43802
(342) 567-1237

Date: 8/7/XX   Owner: Charlotte Bennington
Time of Discharge: 4:30pm   Route Home: On leash, CB drove
Patient: "Muffy"

Discharge Instructions

Case Summary:
Muffy was anesthetized and her teeth were examined, scaled, and polished. X-rays were taken of Muffy's teeth and several teeth were extracted. Multiple soft masses, located under the skin on her chest and abdomen, were removed. A small cyst on her left eyelid was also removed. Sutures have been placed where the cyst, and each of the masses, were located. Absorbable sutures were also placed inside her mouth where some of her teeth were pulled.

Home Care:
  A. Sedation or Anesthesia Aftercare:
    1. You can anticipate that Muffy may act quieter and sluggish when you first bring her home. She may be wobbly on her feet and should be kept away from stairs, slippery floors, or regions of the house where she may fall. Because sedation and anesthesia can interfere with temperature regulation, please keep Muffy indoors where the temperature is comfortable.
    2. Avoid giving large amounts of water initially. However, you may offer her small amounts of water, and if she keeps this down, you can offer more. You may also offer small amounts of food later today. Please read Dietary Restrictions section below before offering food.
    3. If Muffy vomits or has diarrhea, please call the office.
    4. Muffy should be brighter in 12 hours. If not, please call the office.

  B. Medications:
    Before giving medication, please read the attached handouts regarding medication side effects and cautions. If you believe that Muffy is having a reaction to the medication, please call right away.

    Please be sure that Muffy receives all of the medication as prescribed below. These medications do not require a refill.

    1. Triple antibiotic ophthalmic ointment:
       This is an antibiotic for the eyes to prevent infection.
        Apply a ribbon of gel to the inside lower lid of each eye twice daily (am and pm) until your next appointment.

    2. Clavamox 250mg 1 tablet BID for 7 days
       This is an antibiotic to prevent infection.
       Give one tablet by mouth twice a day (am and pm) for the next 7 days

    3. Tramadol 50mg ½ tablet BID
       This is a medication for pain.
       Give one half tablet by mouth twice a day (am and pm) until gone.

  C. Elizabethan Collar
    We are dispensing to you an E-collar for Muffy to wear when she is unattended. This is to prevent her from licking the surgical sites/wounds and sutures. Please be sure that Muffy wears it when you are not in her immediate presence. Please remove the E-collar when she is fed so that she can access food and water.

  D. Wound Monitoring:
    Please monitor Muffy's incision sites and sutures. You should expect the sites to have modest redness and swelling. However, if you observe any of the following, please contact us: increased swelling, increased redness, heat (to the touch), pain, discharge and/or gaping of the wound, suture loss.

  E. Dietary Restrictions:
    Muffy should be fed only soft canned dog food for the next 7-10 days.

Follow-up Appointment:
Muffy is due to have her sutures removed in 10-14 days. Please make an appointment for Muffy during this time period. Our receptionist can be reached at: (342) 567-1238.

Contacting Us:
If you have any questions or concerns, please call us at: (342) 567-1237.
Ask for Cindy Miller, CVT.

Community Resources:
Non-applicable

rehabilitation techniques and the family's responsibility for patient care

- Gives instruction regarding medications:
  - *When* to take each medication
  - *Why* the medication is prescribed
  - *What* the precautions and possible adverse reactions may be
  - *How* to get prescriptions refilled and how to contact the practice with any questions or concerns
- If possible, demonstrates and models the technique to be used, such as how to administer oral medication. Makes sure to give instructions regarding potential food–drug interactions and nutritional interventions via modified diets
- Reviews signs and symptoms of complications that should be reported, such as signs of infection
- Provides the name and contact information of the veterinary health care team member who should be contacted by the client in the event of complications
- Informs the client know of any unresolved problems and discusses a plan for continued care and follow-up appointments
- Gives the client information regarding community resources if pertinent
- Lists actual time of discharge and the name of the family member who transported the animal patient; lists the method used to transport the animal

Several days after a patient is discharged, the veterinary technician often completes a follow-up call to the owner. This enables the veterinary technician to assess the patient's progress at home and gives the owner an opportunity to ask questions. Pet owners are often grateful for and appreciative of the special care that a follow-up call represents.

MANAGEMENT OF PAPER MEDICAL RECORDS

ORGANIZATION AND FILING

The American Animal Hospital Association requires that each patient should have its own medical record, and that paper records should be stored in standard 8 × 10-inch folders (Figure 3-10). Tabs are located at the edge of one end of the folder to facilitate the placement of color-coded decals. Some folders have grids printed on the outside of the cover on which critical information, such as the animal's immunization history, can be written. In this way, the staff can quickly visualize key pieces of information. More commonly, however, veterinary practices use folders with a plain manila cover.

The folders are stored vertically on shelves, which are kept behind or near the receptionist's desk for easy retrieval. Some practices may have record rooms in which a mobile shelving system may be employed. In these systems, large shelves are mounted on tracks so that they can be moved easily from one location to another when pushed. Mobile shelving systems save space because shelves may be positioned up

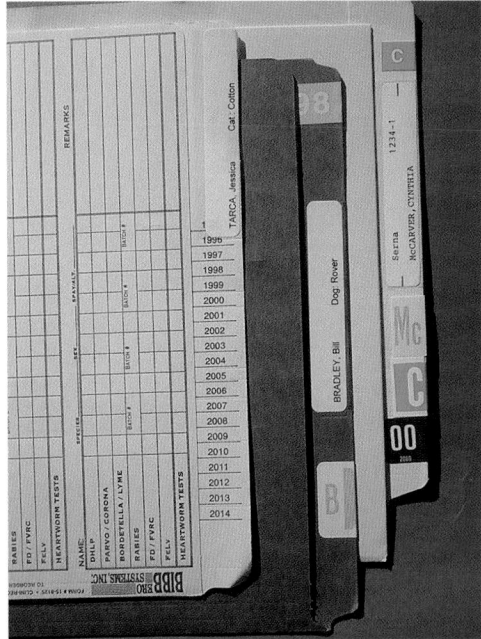

FIGURE 3-10 Shown are a variety of letter-size folders. The color and the style of the folders can vary, as can whether charting is stamped on the cover. Color-coded decals are placed on the edges of the folders to facilitate filing.

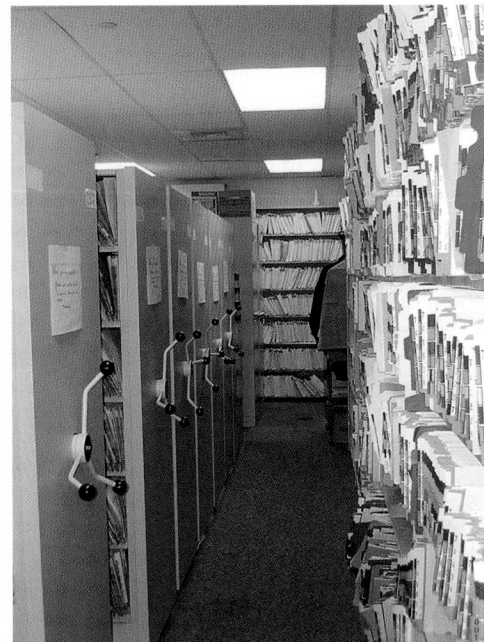

FIGURE 3-11 Mobile shelving creates more storage space for medical records. These shelves move on tracks that are fixed to the floor. Each shelf is moved by turning the wheel crank located on the side of the shelf.

against one another when access to the records is not needed (Figure 3-11).

Many veterinary hospitals use a folder system that is developed specifically for veterinary medicine. Several companies make a variety of systems, so they are easy to acquire (you can order them from a catalog); a wide selection of styles, sizes, and colors is available (see Figure 3-10). Most folders include internal flexible clips that hold forms in their

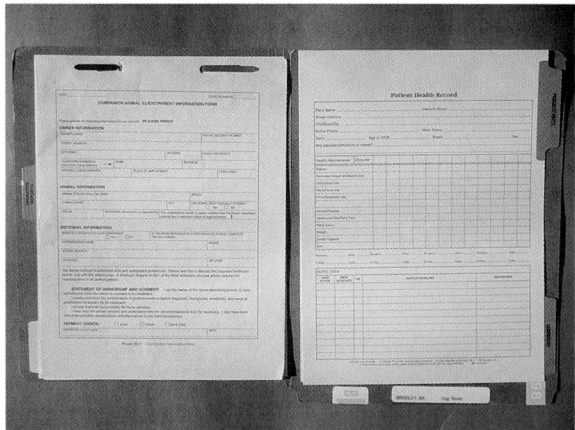

FIGURE 3-12 Letter-size folders contain flexible metal clips that hold forms in their correct order. Dividers allow for rapid retrieval of laboratory reports, operative notes, and progress notes.

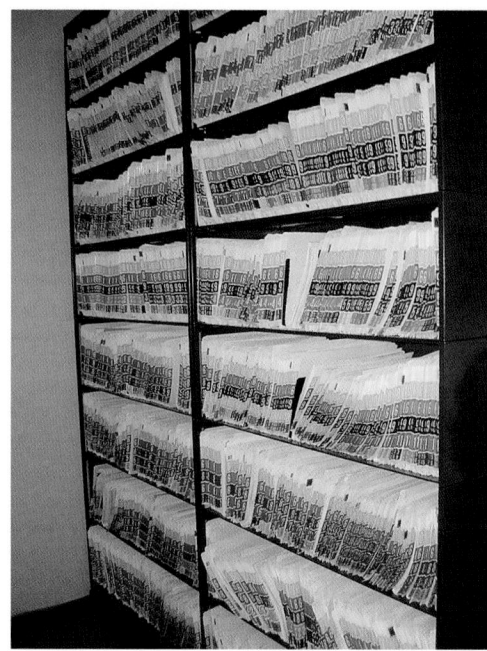

FIGURE 3-13 Numeric color-coding systems allow for rapid retrieval and filing.

FIGURE 3-14 Can you spot the filing error in these color-coded files?

correct order (Figure 3-12). In addition, the folders are designed to accommodate color-coded tabs or stickers (known as *signaling devices*) that are applied to the outer edge of the folder, making filing more efficient and filing errors easier to identify.

Alphabetic Filing

Colored stickers are sold separately, which allows the practice to choose the organizational scheme of the color-coding system. For example, it can be alphabetic, numeric, or a combination of the two. In the alphabetic system, a different color is given to each letter of the alphabet. The system is easy to learn and does not require cross-referencing with a master list of clients. The primary challenge of using the alphabetic system, however, is that the employee doing the filing must be careful to correctly apply the alphabetic order and spell clients' names correctly without exception. Unfortunately, errors in spelling and filing do occur from time to time, so misfiled records tend to be more common with the alphabetic system than with numeric systems.

> **TECHNICIAN NOTE**   The American Animal Hospital Association requires that each patient have its own medical record, and that paper records should be stored in standard 8 × 10-inch folders.

Numeric Filing

In the numeric system, each client is assigned a number. The number assigned to the file may be a hospital-generated number. Each digit in the number has a different color, and files are shelved numerically from lowest to highest (Figure 3-13). In this way, it is easy to correctly sequence the files, and any misfiled records are easily identified because the file color sequence does not match that of surrounding files. Can you see the misfiled record in Figure 3-14? To retrieve a particular file, the receptionist first must check a cross-reference that lists the client's name and the corresponding file number.

One of the advantages of the numeric filing system is that fewer filing errors occur because numbers are easier to read and interpret than letters, and spelling is not a factor. In addition, numeric filing systems are practical for large-volume practices because no file duplication occurs, whereas in the alphabetic system, many clients may have the same surname. The disadvantage of the numeric system, however, is that a cross-reference list must be generated and maintained.

Additional colored tabs can be applied to files to alert the receptionist to specific client–patient issues. For example, the records of animals that need immunizations and worming can be flagged to indicate that reminders should be mailed out. Colored flags may indicate those clients that have an outstanding bill, or that have not returned to the practice in a long time. In this way, colored signaling devices can be added to identify groups of files that need attention.

FILE PURGING

Periodically, the collection of medical records should be reviewed and purged of files that are not in current use. Each veterinary hospital has its own review and purging schedule; however, the following rules can serve as a helpful starting point:

1. The collection of medical records is reviewed at least once per year.
2. Active records covering a 3-year period are maintained in the primary medical records collection.
3. Records that have been inactive for 4 years or longer are moved to storage. Storage should be easily accessible.
4. Records 8 years old or older may be removed from storage and shredded.

Use of color-coded tabs with the year can be of particular value when the annual review of medical records is completed. They enable the receptionist to quickly identify 4-year-old and 8-year-old records by their specific colors.

LOST RECORDS

The risk of losing records in a small hospital and in a large hospital is problematic. They can be lost through misfiling, incorrect spelling of names, or misplacement. At times even after an exhaustive search, the record continues to be missing. Sometimes the loss is not discovered until the animal comes back to the practice for a return visit.

It is best, in this case, to explain to the client that the record has been misplaced. A new record should be started and information requested from the client and veterinarian. In addition, copies of laboratory data, pathology reports, and radiologic information should be obtained and added to reestablish the file.

Although the problem of lost records is embarrassing for the practice and inconvenient for the client, it will happen even with the most elaborate record keeping system; however, every effort should be made to quickly and accurately file each record after each visit. Clients feel more at ease and welcomed if the record is complete and is easily accessible.

LOGS

In addition to documents contained within the patient record, medical information is maintained continuously in logs that are located throughout the veterinary hospital. Many practices have logs for radiology and special imaging, surgery, anesthesia, controlled substances, ultrasound, clinical laboratory, and euthanasia. In addition, some practices have unexpected death, drug reaction, and medical waste logs. Any division of the veterinary hospital or any specific activity could conceivably have a log that records daily activity in that particular aspect of the hospital. Some large practices may have 8 to 12 different types of logs, whereas smaller practices may have 2 to 4 logs.

Logs serve two purposes:
1. They provide additional documentation for legal support.
2. They provide data for quick analysis and retrospective studies.

A practice that is interested in examining the average length of surgery, for example, can quickly calculate that figure based on data in the surgery log. In radiology, techniques could be evaluated by examining the recorded settings in the x-ray log. Typically, logs are kept in binders or in bound composition books so that pages cannot be lost or discarded accidentally.

Radiology Log

The radiology log records the technique used for every x-ray taken. This log might include some or all of the following:
- Patient's name and identification (ID) number
- Client's name
- Date
- Study type
- Measurement of body thickness
- Technique used: milliamperes (mA), time, kilovolts peak (kVp)
- Radiographic findings or diagnosis

The radiology log is typically completed by the veterinary technician (Figure 3-15) and is particularly helpful when improved exposure technique is desired and repeat films are requested.

> **TECHNICIAN NOTE** The radiology log is especially helpful for technicians who wish to review and improve previous exposure techniques.

Surgery Log

Although much variation is noted from practice to practice regarding the content and structure of the surgery log, most contain the following information:
- Date
- Animal's and owner's names
- Case number
- Patient's weight
- Name of surgeon
- Surgical procedure
- Duration of surgery
- Complications

Surgery and anesthesia logs are particularly helpful during completion of retrospective studies regarding the cost of performing each surgical procedure and regarding surgical complications (see the Evolve site at http://evolve.elsevier.com/McCurnin/vettech/). Some practices have separate surgery and anesthesia logs, whereas other practices combine the information to prevent redundancy.

Melvorn Veterinary Hospital
76 Springhouse Drive
Melvorn, PA 19756

Radiology Log

Date	Case No.	Owner	Patient	Species	Study	Grid	Thickness (cm)	KVP	MA	Time Sec.	MAs	Initials
5/10/05	3246	Marshall	"Ed"	K-9	Abd.	Yes	21	90	300	1/30	10	bh
5/10/05	2671	Edward	"Wayne"	K-9	FR ext	No	6	60	100	1/20	5	DF
5/10/05	6342	Kahn	"Nathanial"	Iguana	LF ext	No	1	50	100	1/20	5	CM
5/11/05	4563	Marshall	"Will"	Feline	Thorax	yes	8	60	75	1/10	7.5	JU
5/12/05	4532	Pattison	"Hatchie"	Feline	Abd	yes	10	60	100	1/10	10	GT
5/12/05	6543	Bassert	"Serena"	K-9	LH ext	No	6	60	100	1/20	5.0	GT
5/12/05	8964	Rose	"Suzie"	Feline	Thorax	yes	8	60	75	1/10	7.5	DF
5/12/05	8964	Rose	"Suzie"	Feline	Abd.	yes	5	50	100	1/10	10	CM
5/14/05	6751	Stern	"Gadget"	Snake	Skull	No	1	50	100	1/20	5.0	CM
5/14/05	7602	Berson	"Pete"	K-9	Abd	yes	14	76	300	1/40	7.5	MN
5/14/05	4398	Yates	"Mila"	K-9	Abd	yes	23	94	300	1/30	10	LK
5/10/05	3246	Marshall	"Ed"	K-9	Abd	Yes	21	90	300	1/30	10	LK

FIGURE 3-15 Example of a radiology log. Radiology logs are helpful to the veterinary health care team when radiographs need to be repeated and the initial technique must be adjusted.

Anesthesia Log

The anesthesia log documents the anesthetic protocol used in surgical and nonsurgical procedures. Dental procedures, thorough ear examinations, and bone marrow aspirates are examples of procedures that would require anesthesia but that might not be entered into the surgery log. Information contained in the anesthesia log might include the following:

- Patient's and owner's names
- Patient's weight
- Relative risk category or results of physical examination
- Anesthetic protocol, including type and dosage of each anesthetic agent
- Anesthesia start and end times
- Number of intubation attempts
- Surgical procedure and name of surgeon
- Anesthetist's name
- Complications

The anesthesia log complements the information entered on the anesthesia form (see the Evolve site at http://evolve.elsevier.com/McCurnin/vettech/). Some of the information is repeated and is found in both the log and the form. However, the advantage of the log is that it is easily accessible (the notebook often sits out) and represents a summary of all anesthesia cases. The anesthesia form, on the other hand, although it contains more detailed information, is not as accessible and contains information about only one anesthesia case.

Necropsy Log

The necropsy log is a compilation of data regarding the death of animals. It includes the date and cause of death and the type of necropsy performed (see the Evolve site at http://evolve.elsevier.com/McCurnin/vettech/). It also contains the owner's name, case number, species, name of the veterinarian performing the evaluation, histopathologic and gross findings, and special tissues submitted. The log is typically kept in the necropsy area.

Controlled Substances Log

The Comprehensive Drug Abuse and Control Act (the Act), a federal law that was passed by Congress in 1970, regulates the possession of drugs that have the potential to be abused. These drugs are called *controlled substances*. In the Act, drugs are categorized according to their potential for addiction. Categories range from Schedule I drugs, which are the most addictive, to Schedule V drugs, which are the least addictive. Schedule I drugs include lysergic acid diethylamide (LSD), heroin, crack cocaine, and peyote and have no accepted medical use. All other scheduled drugs (Schedules II, III, IV, and V) must be securely stored in a locked cabinet and inventoried separately from noncontrolled drugs. An inventory of all controlled substances must be taken every 2 years, although most practices do this annually. The inventory should include the following:

1. Name, address, and Drug Enforcement Agency (DEA) registration number
2. Date and time the inventory is performed
3. Contents of the inventory
4. Signature of the person taking the inventory

A separate inventory record must be kept for each Schedule II drug. Records for Schedule III, IV, and V drugs may be combined into one log, but must be kept separate from the other practice records. In addition, all drug-log information must be kept in a bound composition book or a book from which the pages cannot be torn out without notice. Although specific requirements vary from state to state, a typical controlled substances log includes the following:

1. Date
2. Owner's and patient's names
3. Starting volume
4. Ending volume
5. Amount used
6. Initials of the person who used the drug

All inventory records must be kept for 2 years.

MANAGEMENT OF ELECTRONIC MEDICAL RECORDS

OVERVIEW

A patient's medical record folder can be found in a variety of places—in the file cabinet, in a stack of records on the bookkeeper's desk, in a pile waiting to be re-filed, and even in a box in the attic as a result of inactivity. However, electronic medical records are easily retrievable and can be viewed by multiple people at the same time from different workstations. This convenience with greater accessibility allows practices to run more efficiently, faster, and with fewer errors caused by misplaced documents. Greater efficiency lends itself to better patient care and a better business model (Figure 3-16).

Computerization has also improved the quality of patient information. Entries into electronic medical records are consistently legible and organized. When notable findings are made, veterinarian personnel can type in the information or can select a finding from a menu.

With the use of templates for physical examinations that list all anatomic systems, the veterinarian and the veterinary technician are prompted to assess each aspect of the patient. In many of the software systems, the examiner may click on "within normal limits" to verify that a system was examined and was found to be normal.

To expedite the process of data entry, voice recognition software is sometimes employed in the operating room or in examination rooms that are wired for sound and recording. In these "smart" rooms, veterinary personnel can dictate physical examination findings or can describe the appearance of organs during an exploratory laparotomy, for example. Voice recognition software transcribes the spoken word into text that is subsequently cut and pasted into the patient's medical record.

Veterinary practice management software permits documents such as referral reports, electrocardiogram strips,

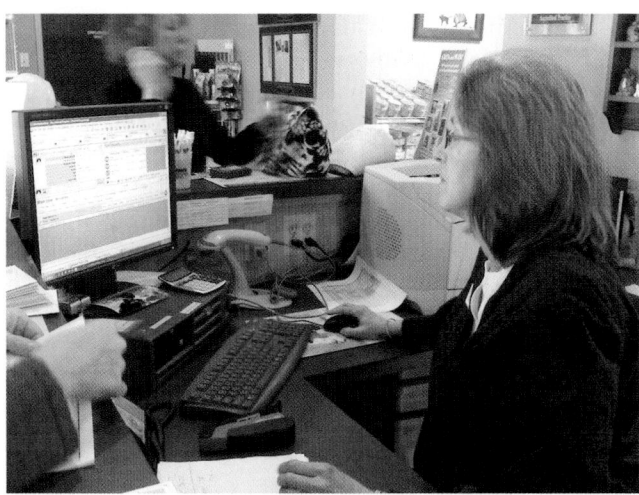

FIGURE 3-16 Electronic medical records are easily retrievable and can be viewed by multiple people at the same time from different workstations. This creates greater efficiency and improved organization and communication, which can lead to improved patient care.

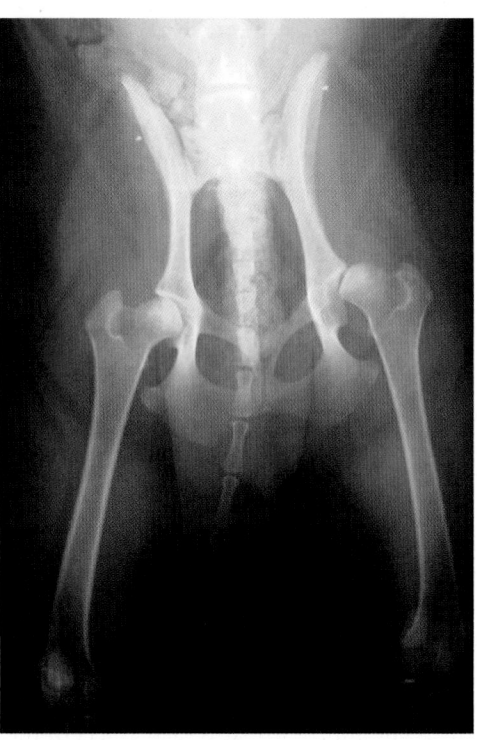

FIGURE 3-17 An example of a digital abdominal radiograph of a cat with a needle caught in the intestine. The photo is stored on the veterinary practice's server as a permanent part of the patient's electronic medical record.

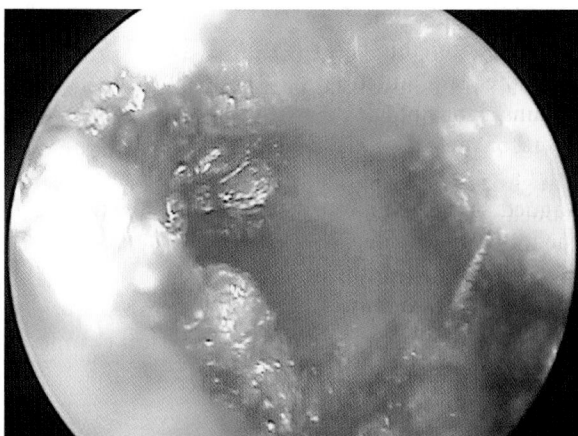

FIGURE 3-18 This digital image of an ear canal was taken using a video otoscope before the patient's ear was flushed. It was shown to the owner during the patient's discharge as part of the case summary and was used to help explain to the owner why home care of the external ear canal is important for this patient.

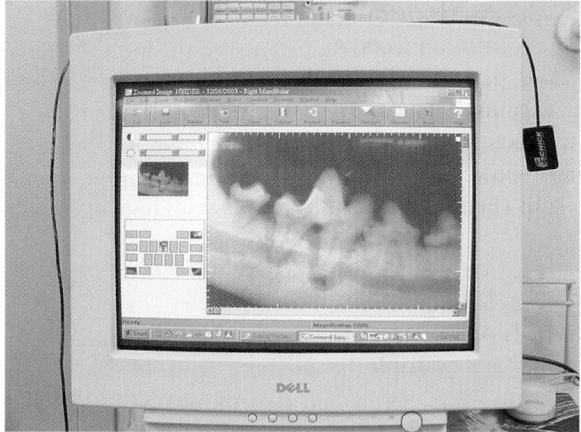

FIGURE 3-19 This photograph shows a screen shot of an intraoral radiograph taken with a digital sensor and a dental x-ray unit. The digital sensor is inserted into the patient's mouth instead of film. The probe is visible in this photo hanging to the right of the computer monitor.

radiographs, photos from endoscopic examinations (Figure 3-17), photos (Figure 3-18), microscopic images, and more to be scanned or imported directly into the patient's medical record. This reduces staff time spent searching for reports, pulling radiographs, and doing subsequent re-filing.

Most programs are capable of maintaining a digital photo of the client and the pet on the record. Digital photography can be used to take images of lesions or teeth (Figure 3-19), or a camera can be attached to a microscope to obtain images of cytologic or hematologic findings. These images can be imported into the patient's electronic medical record for future use or can be e-mailed to a referral specialist for a second opinion.

VALIDATING THE ELECTRONIC RECORD

As with all veterinary hospitals, it is important for paper-less practices to be able to show an accurate, neat, and complete medical record. The practice must also be able to demonstrate that the record is void of tampering, and that it gives an accurate representation of patient care administered. Because digital records are easy to change, it is important that a historical account of the electronic medical record be automatically collected and stored in the data management system. For example, some practice management software programs will allow the veterinary health care team to make entries into a patient record and to make changes to those entries within the first 24 to 48 hours of patient care. Entries made within this time frame are regarded as the primary document. After this period of time, however, the system records the date and time of all subsequent changes and maintains a copy of the primary document. For this reason, it is best for veterinarians and veterinary technicians to make prompt accurate entries. In a court of law or a hearing, it can be argued that information entered after the fact is more prone to inaccuracy owing to lapses in memory of the caregiver. Some practices make use of off-site services that store their electronic information in heavily secured servers. Companies that specialize in housing medical databases can also act as third-party agents to verify the originality of the records and the absence of tampering.

RISK OF LOSS

Risk of loss of digital information is a concern during lightning storms and unexpected power surges that can destroy hard drives in servers, as well as "take out" printers, monitors, TVs, and most electrical instrumentation and monitoring devices. Using surge suppressors and unplugging computers during storms is important to do and can save practices from unnecessary loss of equipment, as well as of valuable patient information. In addition, practices can guard against data loss by incorporating backup servers into their practice network and by using backup generators or battery power in the event of a regional brownout or blackout (Figure 3-20).

ADVANTAGES OF ELECTRONIC MEDICAL RECORDS

Hundreds of veterinary practice management software products are available today. Each program uses its own approach to management and organization of patient medical records. However, most if not all offer improved legibility, increased speed of access to data, and ease of use by multiple users at the same time. In addition, if appropriate precautions are employed, digital medical record keeping decreases the risk of loss. Finally, electronic medical records can include all patient information, including digital radiographs, laboratory results, endoscopic examination findings, surgical images, and ECG tracings. In these ways, electronic medical record keeping offers numerous advantages over standard paper-based patient records. Refer to Chapter 2 for more information about the use of computers in veterinary practice management.

MANAGEMENT OF AMBULATORY PRACTICE RECORDS

Ambulatory food animal and equine practitioners work long hours and put many miles on their trucks as they travel from farm to farm (Figure 3-21). Transporting lengthy medical record files is impractical in a situation where there is little storage space (in the truck), and where paper might blow out the window. Many ambulatory practitioners therefore make handwritten notes on carbonized invoice sheets that are loaded into a sturdy metal dispenser (Figure 3-22). Once procedures are performed, diagnostic, treatment, and billing information may be included on the invoice pages. A copy is given to the owner. Information from these sheets is later typed into the computerized record keeping system by administrative staff at the home office of the practice.

Many ambulatory practitioners have begun to use laptop computers in their trucks to assist with record keeping. The practitioner enters diagnostic, treatment, and billing information into a portable laptop computer that can be plugged into the cigarette lighter or can run on batteries. Data can be transmitted wirelessly if a signal is available or can be synchronized later with the practice's networked computer system when the veterinarian returns to the office to restock

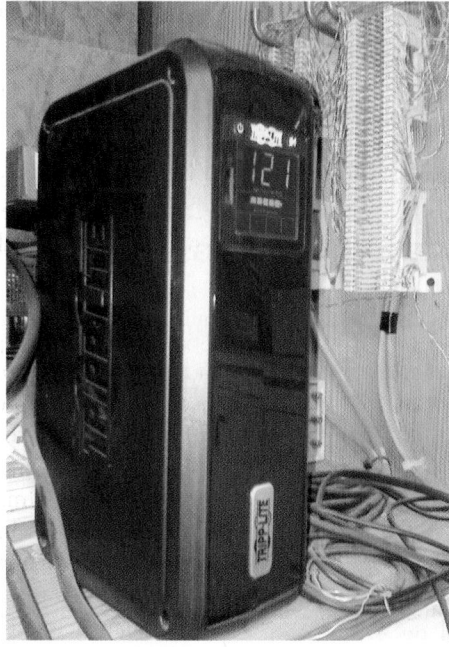

FIGURE 3-20 Battery power backup, such as the unit pictured above, can allow continued use of the practice's computer network and access to patient information during power failures.

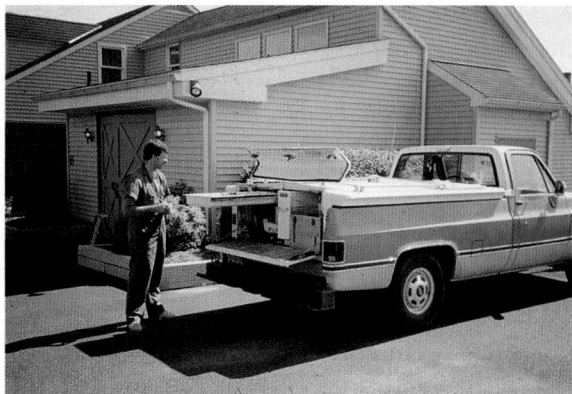

FIGURE 3-21 An ambulatory large animal veterinarian has little room in his truck for cumbersome medical records. Many practitioners now travel with laptop computers that run on batteries and can be kept recharged by adaptors that plug into the truck's cigarette lighter. Digital entries are subsequently transferred to the practice's main server.

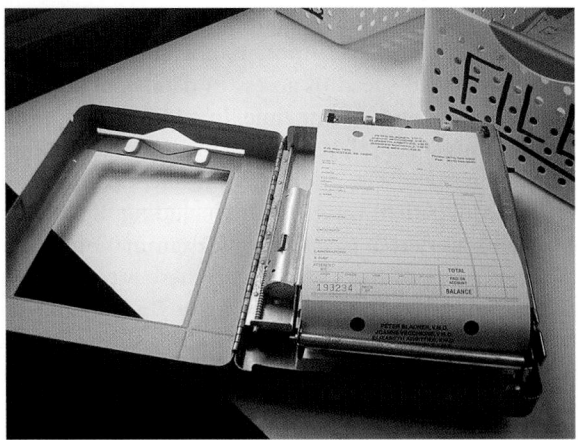

FIGURE 3-22 The resiliency, small size, and light weight of metal canisters that house carbonized billing sheets, such as the one pictured above, make them convenient when farm calls are performed. The carbonized sheets are returned to support staff at the home office, where medical and billing information is typed into the patient's electronic medical record.

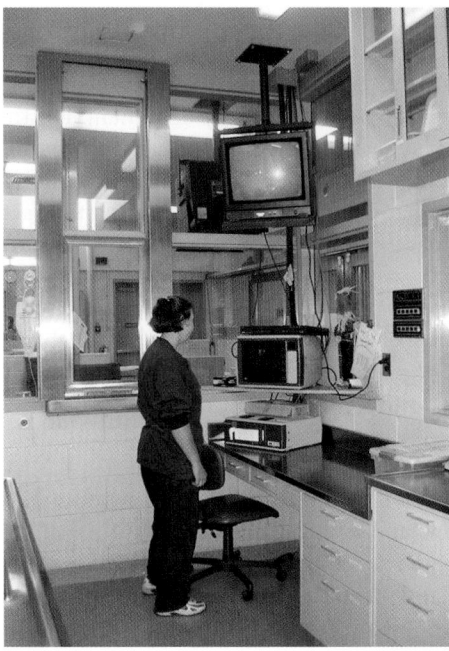

FIGURE 3-23 Computers and telemetry monitoring equipment can be housed in glass-enclosed nursing stations, such as the one shown above, to protect the delicate circuitry from exposure to dust and water. (Courtesy Joanna Bassert.)

the truck. Some ambulatory practitioners use an index of bar codes, each one representing a different diagnosis, procedure, or medication. The veterinarian scans the appropriate bar codes to create an invoice and to document the diagnosis and treatments rendered. Instructions to the owner might also be generated. A small portable printer carried in the truck would enable the document to be printed on-site and subsequently given to the owner.

It is impractical for food animal veterinarians who are responsible for the health of entire herds of livestock to maintain an individual record for every animal treated. In this situation, records are kept on the herd as a whole. Immunizations and reproductive histories are maintained for the group, although individual records may be generated for animals that have undergone special surgical or treatment procedures.

Large animal teaching hospitals and full-service large animal private practices commonly have hospitalized surgery, medicine, and neonatal patients. In this context, each large animal patient has its own medical record. In-house treatments and procedures are recorded in the medical record by hospital staff members on hard copy or electronically. Computer terminals and keyboards, although vulnerable to the dust commonly found in barns, work well in enclosed nurses' stations or treatment closets, which are commonly constructed in a central area of the wards (Figure 3-23). Dust covers help to protect computer hardware in particularly dusty areas when they are not in use. Computer terminals are also found in large animal treatment, radiologic, and surgical facilities for easy entry and retrieval of veterinary medical information.

VETERINARY MEDICAL DATABASE

The **Veterinary Medical Database (VMDB)** is a national data bank that contains computerized veterinary medical data supplied by 24 veterinary schools in the United States and Canada. Each institution submits data for the VMDB on a quarterly basis to a central processing center. Data consist of abstracted data from each clinical case seen at each teaching hospital. The national database allows studies of national trends in various animal diseases. It provides patient chart number, institution code, date of visit, length of stay, clinician code, gender, species, breed, discharge status, age, weight, diagnosis, and procedures for each animal. The VMDB is available for use in retrospective studies and in the evaluation of national and regional disease patterns.

RECOMMENDED READINGS

AAHA: Standard abbreviations for veterinary medical records, ed 3, Lakewood, CO, 2010, American Animal Hospital Association.

AAHA: Standards of accreditation CD-ROM, Lakewood, CO, 2003, American Animal Hospital Association.

Allen DG: The problem-oriented approach in Small Animal Medicine, Philadelphia, 1991, Lippincott.

Heinke ML, McCarthy JB: Practice made perfect: a guide to veterinary practice management, Lakewood, CO, 2001, American Animal Hospital Association.

Johns ML: Health information management technology: an applied approach, Chicago, 2007, American Health Information Management Association.

Johns ML: Information management for health professions, ed 2, Florence, KY, 2002, Delmar.

Rockett J, Christianson C: Case studies in veterinary technology: a scenario-based critical thinking approach, Heyburn, ID, 2010, Rockett House Publishing, LLC.

Rockett J, Lattnzio C, Anderson K: Patient assessment and interventions and documentation for the veterinary technician, Clifton Park, NY, 2009, Delmar Cengage Learning.

Peden AH: Veterinary settings. In Comparative records for health information management, Florence, KY, 1998, Delmar.

Potter PA, Perry AG: Fundamentals of nursing, ed 7, St Louis, 2009, Mosby.

For access to all of the medical record forms discussed in this chapter, see the Evolve site at http://evolve.elsevier.com/McCurnin/vettech/.

RELATED ASSOCIATIONS

American Animal Hospital Association, 12575 West Bayaud Ave., Lakewood, CO 80228

American Health Information Management Association, North Michigan Avenue, Suite 2150, Chicago, IL 60601-65800, www.ahima.org

American Veterinary Health Information Management Association, c/o Flo Nelson, University of Missouri, Veterinary Medical Teaching Hospital, 379 E. Campus Drive, Columbia, MO 65211

American Veterinary Medical Association, 1931 N. Meacham Road, Suite 100, Schaumburg, IL 60173-64360

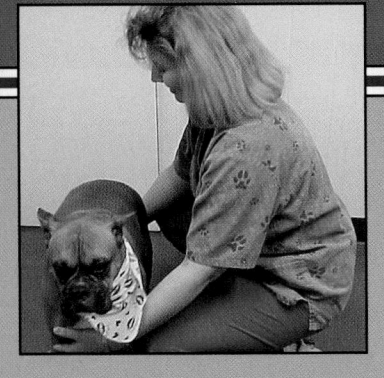

KEY TERMS

Carpal tunnel syndrome
Coccidia
Cutaneous larval
  migrans
Ergonomic injury
Giardia
Hazardous chemical
  (also known as
  hazardous material or
  hazmat)
Hazardous materials
  plan
Hospital safety manual
Lyme disease
Material safety data sheet
  (MSDS)
Occupational safety and
  health act
Occupational safety and
  health administration
  (OSHA)
Panleukopenia
Parvoviral enteritis
Personal protective
  equipment (PPE)
Rabies
Right to know law
Ringworm
Sarcoptic mange
Toxoplasmosis
Visceral larval migrans
Waste anesthetic gas
Zoonotic disease

4 Occupational Health and Safety in Veterinary Hospitals

Philip J. Seibert, Jr.

OUTLINE

Safety, *116*
Objectives of a Safety Program, *116*
Your Safety Rights, *116*
Your Safety Responsibilities, *116*
The Leadership's Rights, *116*
The Leadership's Responsibilities, *117*
General Workplace Hazards, *117*
Dressing Appropriately for the Job, *117*
Save Your Back!, *117*
Clean Up After Yourself, *118*
Everything in Its Place, *118*
Beware of Break Times, *118*
Machinery and Equipment, *119*
Electrical, *119*
Fire and Evacuation, *119*
Do Not Become a Victim of Violence, *120*

Hazardous Chemicals: Right to Know, *121*
Special Chemicals, *122*
Medical and Animal-Related Hazards, *123*
Noise, *123*
Bathing, Dipping, and Spraying Areas, *124*
Zoonotic Diseases, *124*
Nonzoonotic Diseases, *125*
**A Dirty Mouth? Precautions for Dentistry
  Operations,** *126*
Radiology, *126*
Anesthesia, *127*
Compressed Gases, *129*
Sharps and Medical Waste, *129*
**Hazardous Drugs and Pharmacy
  Operations,** *130*
Summary, *132*

LEARNING OBJECTIVES

When you have completed this chapter, you will be able to:

1. Pronounce, spell, and define all Key Terms in the chapter.
2. Do the following regarding safety in the veterinary hospital:
   - Explain the acronym OSHA and describe the role it plays in the development of safety programs in veterinary practices.
   - List the safety rights and responsibilities of employees in the workplace.
   - List the safety rights and responsibilities of workplace leaders.
3. List common workplace hazards in a veterinary facility and describe precautions that can be taken to reduce the risk of these hazards. Also do the following:
   - Explain proper methods for lifting objects and animals.
   - List hazards associated with the use of ethylene oxide, formalin, glutaraldehyde, anesthetic gases, and compressed gases.
   - Describe the requirements of the OSHA "right to know" law.
   - Explain the acronym MSDS and describe the components of an MSDS.
4. Do the following regarding medical and animal-related hazards:
   - List hazards related to the capture and restraint of small and large animals.
   - Explain risks associated with excessive noise and methods taken to minimize these risks.
   - Describe hazards related to bathing and dipping animals and explain methods to minimize these risks.
   - Define the term *zoonotic disease* and list zoonotic and nonzoonotic diseases commonly encountered in veterinary practices.
5. Explain the importance of wearing goggles, gloves, and a surgical mask when performing dental procedures on animals.

6. List methods to minimize the risks associated with exposure to radiation, anesthetic gases, and medical waste.
7. List the equipment and supplies needed to protect veterinary personnel when handling hazardous pharmaceuticals such as chemotherapeutic drugs and describe methods for safely handling contaminated bedding and waste from oncology patients.

INTRODUCTION

Most people who work in the veterinary health care professions do so because of a love for animals and a desire to help them. Working as a veterinary technician and as a part of the veterinary health care team can be deeply rewarding. However, with every reward comes responsibility. One of the responsibilities of a veterinary technician is to help ensure the safety of coworkers, patients, and clients and one's own safety. If you are hurt on the job, the injury incurred extends beyond the physical pain and disability you suffer. The hospital is also affected, both financially and operationally, because the veterinary health care team loses an important member—you. Other employees of the practice have to work harder to cover the personnel shortage. In addition, the quality of health care delivered to the animals may be adversely affected by having less than a full team of caregivers.

As a staff member in a veterinary hospital, you are exposed to hazards in the day-to-day routine of clinical practice. These hazards include exposure to infectious diseases, harmful chemicals, and radiation, and the risks of being scratched, bitten, shoved, stepped on, and kicked. That is the bad news. The good news is that these hazards, when properly identified, can be managed and the risk of injury minimized or even eliminated.

By reading this chapter and educating yourself about hazards in the veterinary health care field, you are taking the first step toward minimizing your risk of injury and of contracting a contagious disease. Some of the topics discussed will be familiar to you, whereas others will be new. The important point to remember is that all of the topics presented in this chapter are true health risks for the veterinary technician in clinical practice.

The second step toward minimizing health risks in the workplace is to integrate the safety procedures you learn in this chapter into the everyday habits of your job. You are the most important person in ensuring your safety on the job. As human beings, we operate from a set of habits for most of life's activities. Your safety should not be something you have to stop to think about—it should be automatic. The only way it becomes automatic is by developing and practicing good work habits.

SAFETY

OBJECTIVES OF A SAFETY PROGRAM

The purpose of any safety program is to reduce or eliminate the possibility of injury or illness for employees. The **Occupational Safety and Health Administration (OSHA)** enforces federal laws that help to ensure a safe workplace for American workers. These laws require employers to have a safety program, which includes educating employees about inherent risks of their jobs, providing them with appropriate safety equipment, and training them in safety procedures and the proper use of safety equipment. If you are receiving this training from your employer, she or he is fulfilling important OSHA requirements. If you are learning this material as a self-study program, you can take pride in the knowledge that you are becoming a "self-taught expert" in the field of occupational safety. Your knowledge and initiative will be welcomed by your veterinary health care team.

YOUR SAFETY RIGHTS

One can never eliminate every hazard completely, but each of us can minimize our exposure to hazards in most cases.

> **TECHNICIAN NOTE**   You have the right to expect your workplace to be reasonably free from unnecessary hazards.

The ability to participate in a safety program at work is an important part of your rights. It is often assumed that the owner or manager of a business knows all there is to know about the business. But too often, it is the employee who first becomes aware of potential safety problems. As an employee, you have the right and a responsibility to bring those concerns to the attention of the employer without fear of reprisal. In most instances, the complaint is first presented to the immediate supervisor, but be aware that not all complaints will bring about changes to the operation of the practice. Some complaints stem from lack of familiarity with standard safety procedures on the part of the employee, and in these cases, instruction by the employer is all that is needed to resolve the issue. However, if a complaint is not taken seriously by the employer, or if a dangerous situation is not adequately addressed, the employee has the right to bring the issue to the attention of the regional OSHA office.

When records such as medical evaluations or radiation exposure reports are collected by the veterinary hospital, these records must be made available to the employee for review. This does not mean that you are entitled to see private or sensitive information about other staff members, but it does mean that you are entitled to see data that are relevant to your safety. You are also entitled to know about the nature and type of accidents that have occurred in your hospital. If your practice employs more than 10 employees, you have the right to view the summary of work-related injuries and illnesses (OSHA Form 300A), which should be posted on the employee bulletin board at certain times of the year.

YOUR SAFETY RESPONSIBILITIES

It is your responsibility to learn and follow the safety rules and practices that have been established for your position in the veterinary hospital. Even though OSHA will not cite or fine the employee directly for violations of these responsibilities, he or she is required under the **Occupational Safety and Health Act** (the Act) to "comply with all occupational safety and health standards and all rules, regulations, and orders issued under the Act." Not only does this include specific OSHA standards, it also applies to workplace-specific rules established by the leadership at your hospital.

> **TECHNICIAN NOTE**   It is your responsibility to learn and follow the safety rules and practices that have been established for your position in the veterinary hospital.

Although you cannot be disciplined by your employer for exercising your rights under the act, you can be disciplined by your employer for willful violations of any safety rule or standard. In some cases, this discipline can be as simple as a verbal reprimand, but in severe or chronic situations, it can include termination. In most states, if you are terminated for the willful violation of safety rules, you will likely be denied unemployment benefits.

In addition to the responsibility to follow the rules, the Act requires you to do the following:
- Read the OSHA poster (Figure 4-1).
- Comply with all applicable standards.
- Wear or use prescribed **personal protective equipment (PPE)** while working.
- Report hazardous conditions to your supervisor.
- Report any job-related injury or illness to the proper person and seek treatment promptly.

THE LEADERSHIP'S RIGHTS

Although the act and OSHA require the leadership of a business to maintain safety standards, this is not meant to restrict the right of the business to set rules of conduct or operation for its staff. The practice owner, for example, has the right to set and enforce rules for his or her own practice as long as those rules are consistent with federal and state safety laws.

Practice owners must have ample time to correct any safety-related problems. In other words, the employee should not rush off to file a grievance with the regional OSHA office without first giving the employer ample time to correct the deficiency.

In the event that a practice is inspected, the practice owner has the right to be present because the practice is considered his or her personal property. An employee is not authorized to admit an OSHA inspector to the practice in the absence of the employer (unless, of course, the employer specifically gives the employee the authority to act on his or

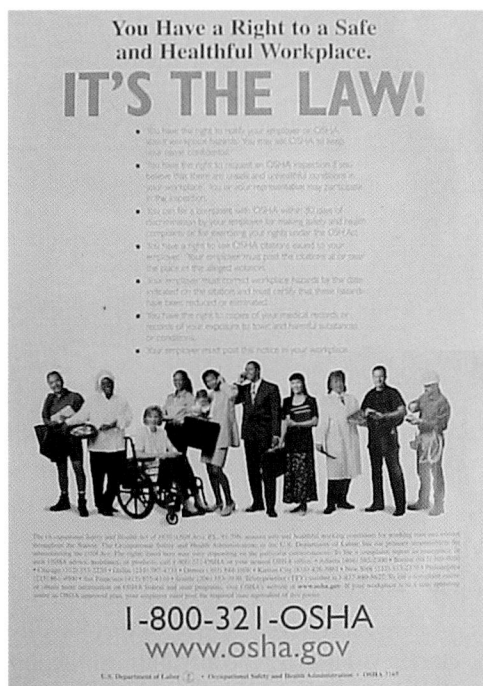

FIGURE 4-1 Locate and read all safety notices where you work.

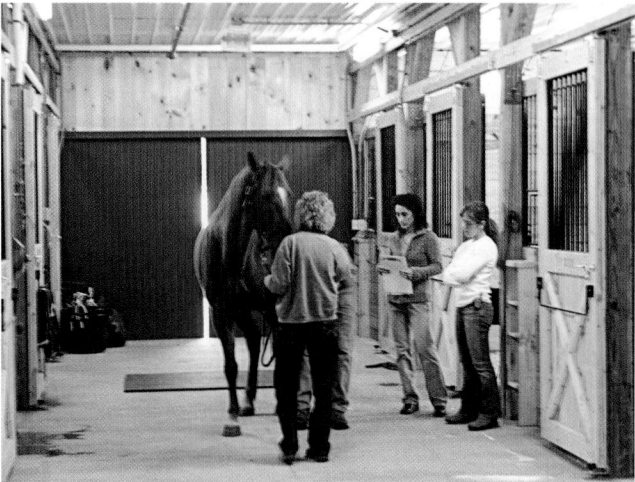

FIGURE 4-2 Safety training can be conducted in a formal session or it can be more "hands-on," but it needs to be practice specific.

her behalf). However, OSHA inspectors may enter a practice without the presence of the owner and without permission by the employee if the inspectors have a court order to do so.

THE LEADERSHIP'S RESPONSIBILITIES

The leadership of a veterinary practice is responsible for providing a safe work environment for employees. This does not mean providing a facility with no hazards—that would be impossible. It means that the leadership must make a reasonable effort to identify the hazards present, correct those that can be eliminated, and control the hazards that cannot be eliminated.

The practice must comply with laws and regulations pertaining to safety and health by establishing safety procedures for the hospital, including emergency procedures for addressing employee's accidents. The leadership must enforce these rules as diligently as it would be expected to enforce any other rule in the practice.

The employer is also responsible for providing practice-specific safety training to employees (Figure 4-2). Even if a veterinary technician has years of prior experience, the practice is required to make sure that the technician is capable of doing her or his job safely. This training can be provided in a formal setting, as in staff meetings or a continuing education course, or it can be given within the practice. A great deal of learning takes place in many practices every day. On-the-job training can be an effective way to obtain knowledge about safety, but be sure you know your limits and abilities. Ultimately, you are the best person to determine whether you are competent to do a job safely. If you think you need extra safety training in a particular area, do not hesitate to ask for

it. Tell your supervisor immediately, so that arrangements can be made for proper instruction.

GENERAL WORKPLACE HAZARDS

Every practice should have a collection of written safety-related policies known as the ***Hospital Safety Manual***. You should know where the *Hospital Safety Manual* is located in your practice and should take time to become familiar with it. Memorize the "do's and don'ts" for your particular veterinary hospital, and always follow the safety rules. No one can protect you from an injury or illness better than you can.

> **TECHNICIAN NOTE** Every practice should have a collection of written safety-related policies known as the *Hospital Safety Manual.*

DRESSING APPROPRIATELY FOR THE JOB

One of the first rules of safety is to dress appropriately for the job at hand. In the veterinary profession, this includes protective footwear and minimal, if any, jewelry. You can reduce the chances of getting injured by wearing sturdy shoes that cover your whole foot (not sandals or slip-on or open-toed shoes) and that have nonslip soles. Be especially cautious when walking on uneven or wet floors. Never run inside the hospital or on uneven footing. Excessive jewelry can present a hazard in many clinical situations, but particularly when an animal struggles during restraint and can inadvertently link an earring or necklace with a claw. This is definitely one of those circumstances when less is more.

SAVE YOUR BACK!

According to insurance statistics, back injuries account for one in every five workplace injuries among American workers. To minimize your chances of suffering one of these painful injuries, remember the rules for lifting: Keep your back straight and lift with your legs (Figure 4-3). Never bend

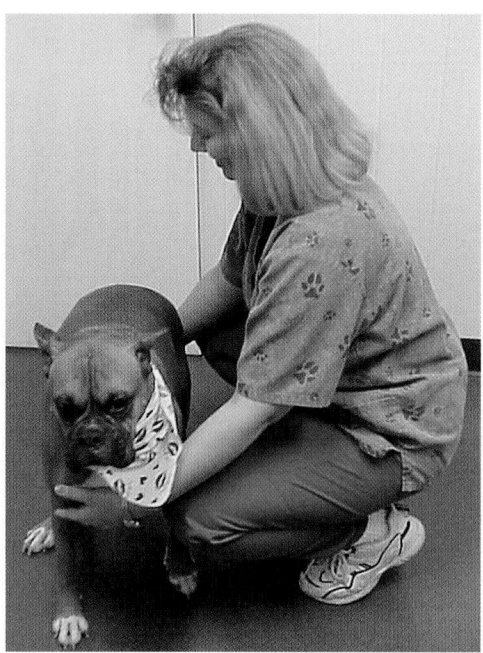

FIGURE 4-3 Remember to keep your back straight and to lift with your legs.

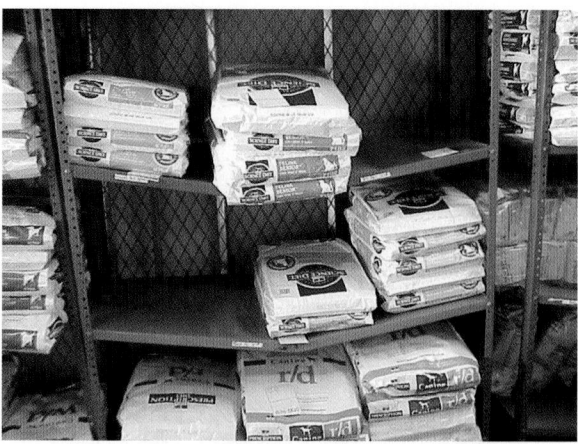

FIGURE 4-4 Improper storage of materials can lead to serious injury.

over at the waist to lift an object. This rule applies when lifting patients and inanimate objects, such as boxes or supplies. If your practice does not have a motorized lift table, get help when lifting patients weighing more than about 40 lb. Remember to follow sound ergonomic principles when positioning or restraining patients, especially when working with horses or food animals.

CASE PRESENTATION 4-1

A 22-year-old man has been a veterinary technician for 2 years. He worked at a companion animal practice in the past but has recently started working in an equine-only hospital. During his first week on the job, he suffered a debilitating back injury while trying to capture and restrain a fractious patient.

Because he has a background in companion animals, the technician viewed restraint as primarily a physical overpowering of the patient. Had he received proper training when he first started the job, he would have known that tranquilization and sedation are the primary methods of restraint used for horses that become fractious when physical restraint (such as placement in a stock) is not practical.

The technician was confined to bed for 3 days by the physician and was restricted in his physical activities for 2 weeks to overcome the muscle strain.

Because veterinary technicians perform such a variety of jobs in any given hour, it is rare for us to acquire the types of ergonomic injuries commonly seen in other industries (such as **carpal tunnel syndrome**). However, it is important to note that the best defense against almost all **ergonomic injuries** is to change your posture and routine frequently.

CLEAN UP AFTER YOURSELF

Some injuries are caused by cluttered or dirty work areas. In addition, clutter is known to contribute to the severity of accidents that otherwise would be minor. Cleanliness and organization are good business standards, especially in a health care facility. Always clean up spills as soon as they happen. You should always clean and return equipment to the proper storage place immediately after use. At least daily, remove all trash from your work area. Organize drawers, cabinets, and counters so that items can be found easily and clutter is reduced.

EVERYTHING IN ITS PLACE

Supplies and equipment should always be stored properly. Heavy supplies or equipment, for example, should be kept on lower shelves to prevent unnecessary strain in trying to lift them overhead and to reduce the risk of material falling on your head. Never use stairways or exit hallways as storage areas. Do not overload shelves or cabinets (Figure 4-4). Store liquids in containers with tight-fitting lids, and always replace the lids when finished using the product. Whenever possible, store chemicals on shelves at or below eye level; this will minimize the possibility of accidental spilling of the chemical on you when you are getting or replacing a container. Never climb into or on cabinets, shelves, chairs, buckets, or similar items. Use an appropriate ladder or step to reach high locations.

BEWARE OF BREAK TIMES

Ingestion of pathogenic organisms or harmful chemicals while eating on the job is a possibility in veterinary hospitals. This is why it is important to eat and drink only in areas designated for staff breaks that are free of toxic and biologically harmful substances. This also applies to the preparation of food and beverages. Make sure that coffeepots and utensils are well away from sources that could contaminate food, such as laboratories and treatment and bathing areas. Check the cabinets or shelves above food preparation areas to ensure that no hazards could spill onto the area. Always store food, drinks, condiments, and snacks in a separate refrigerator from the one used to store biological or chemical hazards such as vaccines, drugs, and laboratory samples.

> **TECHNICIAN NOTE** Always store food, drinks, condiments, and snacks in a separate refrigerator from the one used to store biological or chemical hazards such as vaccines, drugs, and laboratory samples.

MACHINERY AND EQUIPMENT

Never operate machinery or equipment without all proper guards in place. Items of equipment such as fans and cage dryers have moving parts that can severely hurt or even sever a finger. Long hair should be tied back or pinned up to prevent it from getting caught in fans or other moving parts. Avoid wearing excessively loose clothing or jewelry when working around machinery with moving parts.

When using equipment such as autoclaves, microwave ovens, cautery irons, or other heating devices, be sure to understand the proper rules for safe operation. Burns, especially from steam, are painful and serious and almost always can be prevented. Autoclaves also present a danger from the pressure that is used for proper sterilization. Before opening an autoclave, be sure to first release the pressure by activating the vent device, and at the same time keep your hands and face away from the steam. Let the steam dissipate completely before opening the door fully, and be careful when removing the packs because they may still be hot. Always assume that cautery devices and branding irons are hot, and use the insulated handle whenever you touch them. Never place heated irons on any surface where they could overheat and start a fire, or where someone might accidentally touch them.

ELECTRICAL

Many procedures performed on a daily basis require the use of electricity. Although new equipment and buildings have many safety features built into the design, you must be conscious of preventing a situation that could cause a fire or physical harm to yourself, another person, or a patient.

Do not remove light switch or electrical outlet covers. Always keep circuit-breaker boxes closed, and never block access by stacking supplies or equipment in front of them. Only persons trained to perform maintenance duties should repair electrical appliances, outlets, switches, fixtures, or breakers.

If you must use a portable dryer or other electrical equipment in a wet area, make sure it is properly grounded and is plugged into only a ground-fault circuit interruption (GFCI) type of outlet. Extension cords should be used only for temporary applications and should always be of the three-conductor, grounded type. Never run extension cords through windows or doors that may close and damage the wires, or across aisles or floors where a tripping hazard may be created.

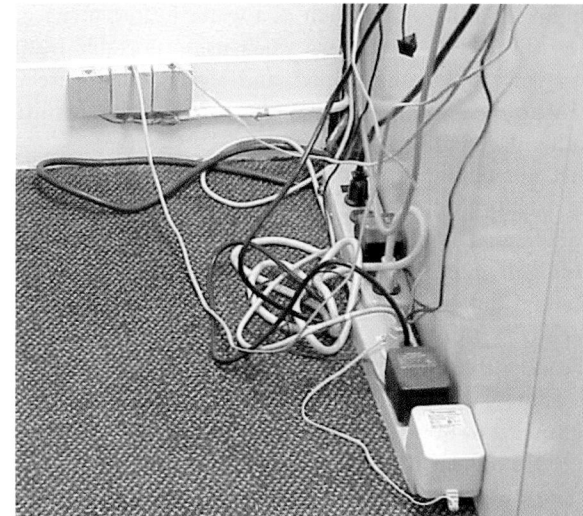

FIGURE 4-5 Overloaded surge suppressors or extension cords can start a fire.

Surge suppressors should be used to protect only sensitive electronic equipment and should never be overloaded (Figure 4-5). Surge suppressors should never be used with portable heaters, autoclaves, or coffeepots because they may overheat and cause a fire.

Equipment with grounded plugs must never be used with adaptors or with nongrounded extension cords. Never alter or remove the ground terminals on plugs. Appliances or equipment with defective ground terminals or plugs should not be used until repaired.

When changing a light bulb (especially a fluorescent bulb), be careful to remove and replace the bulb without breaking it. Inoperable bulbs should be disposed of directly into the outside dumpster or inside of a container to keep the bulb from breaking.

FIRE AND EVACUATION

The potential for dramatic loss of life (both human and animal) and destruction of property makes a hospital fire one of the most feared accidents imaginable. Fortunately, the danger of such an event can be significantly reduced with a few simple precautions.

Never use power adaptors or surge suppressors as a substitute for permanent wiring. Overloaded or faulty electrical cords can overheat or short out and start a fire, even when the equipment is turned off.

Always store flammable liquids properly; many fluids, such as gasoline, paint thinner, and ether, should never be stored inside the hospital except in an approved flammable storage cabinet. Some components of specialty dental and large animal acrylic repair kits are also flammable. Very small amounts of these components usually are not a problem, but always ensure that they are stored and used in an area with good ventilation, and that the containers have tight-fitting lids that are replaced immediately after use.

Flammable materials such as newspapers, boxes, and cleaning chemicals must always be stored at least 3 feet away from an ignition source such as a water heater, furnace, or stove. Always take extra care when using portable heaters. Never leave them unattended, and always make sure that they are placed no closer than 3 feet from any wall, furniture, or other flammable material.

Become familiar with the locations of emergency exits in your facility. Make sure that emergency exits are always unlocked and free from obstruction when you are in the building. If you must work in a building when security warrants that the doors be locked, make sure you have at least two clear exits from the building.

Learn the emergency warning system in your hospital. If the facility is equipped with an electronic alarm system, be sure you know how to activate it manually. In the absence of an electronic alarm system, a verbal alarm is effective. You can use the telephone intercom feature to alert everyone that there is a fire in the building (in small buildings, simply yell in a loud clear voice to get the message out).

Know your duties in the event of a fire. Remember that your first responsibility is to notify others about the fire and then to get out of the building safely if an evacuation is ordered. Leave the rescue duties to professionals who are trained and equipped to handle this dangerous task. If you do evacuate the building, immediately report to the designated assembly area for accountability and assignments. This is important because others will assume that you are trapped in the building if you are not present at the assembly area.

Know where the fire extinguishers are located and how to use them (Procedure 4-1). Most veterinary hospitals are equipped with dry chemical types of fire extinguishers. Before you decide to use a fire extinguisher, make sure the alarm has been sounded, everyone has left the building (or is in the process of leaving), and the fire department has been called.

> **TECHNICIAN NOTE** Become familiar with the locations of emergency exits in your facility. Make sure that emergency exits are always unlocked and free from obstruction when you are in the building.

PROCEDURE 4-1 | Using a Fire Extinguisher

- If you must use a portable fire extinguisher, remember the word PASS:
  - **P**ull the pin: Some extinguishers require releasing a lock latch, pressing a puncture lever, or another motion. (Check your extinguishers to be sure.)
  - **A**im low: Point the extinguisher (or its horn or hose) at the base of the fire.
  - **S**queeze the handle: This releases the extinguishing agent.
  - **S**weep from side to side at the base of the fire until it appears to be out.
- Watch the fire area. If a fire breaks out again, repeat use of the extinguisher.
- Most portable extinguishers work according to these directions, but read and follow the directions on your specific extinguisher.

The National Fire Protection Association recommends that you never attempt to fight a fire if any of these conditions are true:
- The fire is spreading beyond the immediate area where it started or involves any part of the building or structure.
- The fire could block your escape route.
- You are unsure of the proper operation of the extinguisher.
- You are in doubt that the extinguisher you are holding is designed for the type of fire at hand or is large enough to suppress the fire.

DO NOT BECOME A VICTIM OF VIOLENCE

Just as in any occupation, you are at risk of injury from accidents not directly related to your job. Vehicle accidents, personal assault, robbery, and even natural disasters have resulted in injury to veterinary technicians while on duty. Although no one can prevent every possible scenario, preparation can certainly help and sometimes will minimize injury. When outside the hospital building, be aware of your environment, and do your best to avoid placing yourself in a situation that could go bad.

Always keep "nonclient" doors locked from the outside to prevent anyone from gaining unauthorized or undetected entry into the building (Figure 4-6).

If you work in a critical care or 24-hour practice, you should use the "barriers" that are usually available. Things such as buzzers to control access through the front door and one-way locks on remaining doors (to let you out in case of an emergency, while keeping the door locked from the outside) are essential in these environments, so do not prop doors open, disassemble the locking system, or turn the

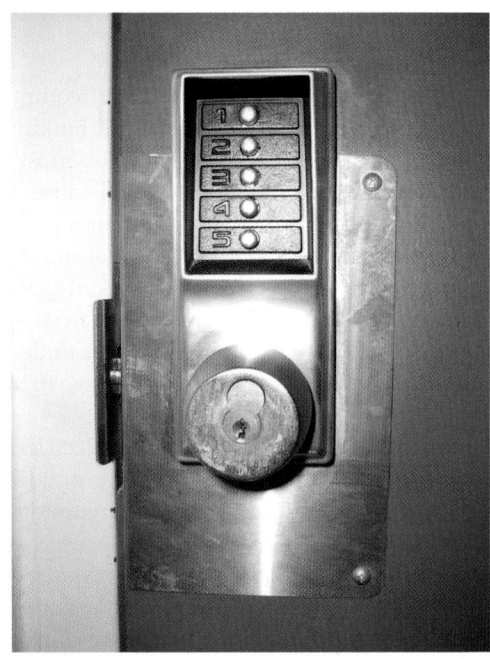

FIGURE 4-6 Personal safety includes the diligent use of locks and barriers to deter unauthorized persons from entering the facility.

system off. In any business that keeps money or that stores valuable items, there is a potential for robbery. If you ever find yourself in a situation where someone demands money, drugs, or other material items while threatening your personal safety—do not withhold the things they demand. As soon as safely is possible, let everyone else know of the situation. You should attempt to contact the police if this can be safely done without the person's knowledge; otherwise, do it immediately after the person has left.

Cooperate with the person's demands and give him what he wants, but do not go with the person. Resist physical assault or battery to the best of your abilities and preferably go outside the building, so that passersby can see what is happening and can render assistance or call the police.

HAZARDOUS CHEMICALS: RIGHT TO KNOW

You may not think about it, but many products that you use every day can be **hazardous chemicals**. Every chemical, even common ones, such as cleaning supplies, has the potential to cause you harm. Some chemicals contribute to health problems, whereas others may be flammable and pose a fire threat. The most common chemicals in use in the veterinary practice include the following:

- Cleaning and disinfecting agents
- Insecticides and pesticides
- Drugs and medications (including anesthetic gases)
- Sterilization agents
- Radiology processing fluids

Planning and training are the keys to safe handling of any chemical. Every business, including your practice, must follow the requirements of OSHA's **"right to know" law**. This law requires that you be informed of all chemicals you may be exposed to while doing your job. The right to know law also requires that you wear all safety equipment prescribed by the manufacturer and the practice when using any product containing a hazardous chemical. Safety equipment must be provided to you at no cost, but it is not optional—you must wear what is prescribed.

A key component of the right to know law is the **hazardous materials plan**. The hazardous materials plan includes instructions for organizing and maintaining the practice's "right to know" documents. When a product is used in a business such as your veterinary practice, you may be exposed to that product to a greater extent than the average consumer, so your risk may be different. Chemicals such as alcohol may be shipped in a large container by the manufacturer and may be subsequently transferred to smaller containers or spray bottles by hospital personnel to facilitate their use in the practice. It is important to remember to apply a secondary container hazard warning label (Figure 4-7) to the second container to ensure that the chemical is used safely. In addition, the manufacturer of a product that contains a hazardous chemical will prepare a **material safety data sheet (MSDS)** for that product. The MSDS will give you additional precautions, instructions, and advice for handling that product in the workplace (Figure 4-8). Your practice is required to keep an MSDS library for the chemicals that you

		Isopropyl Alcohol (70%)			
H	2				
F	3	Avoid contact with eyes. Do not inhale fumes. Avoid prolonged contact with skin. Do not ingest.			
R	0				
P	A				

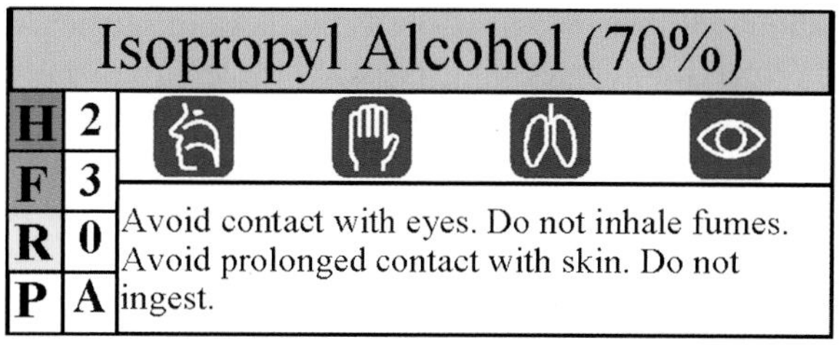

FIGURE 4-7 Example of a secondary container hazard warning label.

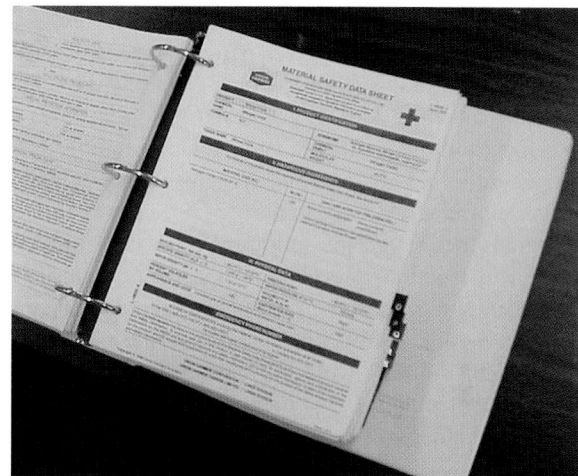

FIGURE 4-8 Material safety data sheets (MSDSs) contain safety information that may not be indicated on the product label.

use. Ask your supervisor where your hospital's MSDS library is located. Take the time to review the MSDSs for the products you use frequently. Although MSDSs may look complicated at first glance, the information that is important to you is easy to find: Review the health, protective equipment, and disposal sections to gain a better understanding of risks and precautions that you should know.

> **TECHNICIAN NOTE** Your practice is required to keep an MSDS library for the chemicals that you use. Ask your supervisor where your hospital's MSDS library is located.

Working bottles of hazardous products should always have tight-fitting, screw-on lids. Always remember to place the cap back on the bottle after using any chemical product. You should endeavor to store chemical bottles in a closed cabinet; this will help prevent animals from injury in the event that they escape. Ideally, the cabinet or shelf should be at or below eye level. This will minimize the chance of spilling the product in your face if the cap is not secure. Never store or use hazardous products near food, beverages, or food preparation areas.

Be cautious when mixing or diluting any chemical product. Try to keep the material from splashing on your hands, clothes, or face. If it is likely that the product will splash on you, wear a pair of protective latex or nitrile gloves and protective goggles or glasses. When making solutions from a concentrate, you should always start with the correct quantity of water, then add the concentrate. Never add water to the concentrate because the chemical may splash or react differently.

When two chemicals are mixed together, the result is seldom a simple mixture. It is often a new, sometimes different, and possibly dangerous chemical. Never mix any chemicals unless you are directed to do so by the label or an MSDS.

Minor spills of most chemicals can be cleaned up with paper towels or absorbent material (e.g., kitty litter) and disposed of in the trash; however, dangerous chemicals such as mercury require special procedures. Before you use a new chemical, review the MSDS, and learn the procedures you must follow for cleaning up a spill. When cleaning up any spill, remember to wear protective gloves and any other special equipment required on the MSDS. Keep other people and animals away from the spill until it is safe. Unless prohibited by instructions on the MSDS, wash the spill site and any contaminated equipment with a detergent soap and water—not with a disinfecting soap (Procedure 4-2).

Familiarize yourself with the locations of the eyewash stations in your practice. Test them regularly and know how to use them before you are in a position to need them.

PROCEDURE 4-2 | Chemical Spill Cleanup

Step 1. Keep unnecessary people and pets out of the area to prevent spreading of spilled material.

Step 2. If the area is small or if the fumes are extremely strong, increase ventilation by opening a window or turning on an exhaust fan. Do not use an electrical exhaust fan or electrical equipment, and avoid turning switches on or off when cleaning up spilled flammable materials.

Step 3. Put on a pair of protective latex or nitrile gloves. If it is likely that your clothing will become contaminated during the cleanup, put on a protective apron and protective eyewear.

Step 4. As soon as possible, cover the spill with absorbent materials such as paper towels or cat litter. Allow the absorbent material to fully collect the liquid.

Step 5. Using a broom, gently sweep the saturated absorbent into a dustpan, and deposit it into a plastic trash bag.

Step 6. When all material has been picked up, seal the trash bag and dispose of it as regular waste, unless your institution, city, or county requires you to do otherwise.

Step 7. Wash the contaminated area thoroughly with plain water or detergent soap (not with a disinfectant) if permissible by instructions in the material safety data sheet (MSDS). Allow the area to air-dry.

Step 8. Remove any protective equipment used during the cleanup. Dispose of single-use items as regular trash unless your institution, city, or county requires you to do otherwise.

Step 9. Wash your hands thoroughly and change any clothing that has become contaminated during the cleanup process.

Step 10. Replace used materials in the spill kit.

SPECIAL CHEMICALS
Ethylene Oxide

Many hospitals use gas sterilization for items that would be damaged by other procedures. Electrical drills, rubber products, and sharps are commonly exposed to ethylene oxide (EtO) as a sterilization agent in human and veterinary medicine. This method has distinct advantages, but because EtO is thought to be a human carcinogen, special precautions must be maintained:

- Read the MSDS carefully and follow all instructions.
- Store the ampules in a closed cabinet away from sources of heat.
- Use only approved devices for the procedure.
- Read, understand, and follow all written procedures and safety precautions relevant to your practice.
- Know the emergency procedures that should be performed in case of accidental release of EtO.

Formalin

Historically, formalin has been used in the veterinary profession for tissue preservation, diagnostic tests, and even sterilization. Because formaldehyde is also a suspected human carcinogen, OSHA takes its use seriously. Standards for the use of formaldehyde are similar to those put forth for the use of EtO:

- Read the MSDS carefully and follow all instructions.
- Store supplies safely (include museum jars).
- Use only with good ventilation in the room, and avoid breathing vapors.
- Wear gloves and goggles to prevent skin and eye contact.

Whenever possible, you should obtain formalin in small, premeasured containers (also called *biopsy jars*) so that serious risk is minimized (Figure 4-9). Often the diagnostic laboratory will supply prefilled biopsy jars at no charge, so be sure to ask.

Glutaraldehyde

Glutaraldehyde is a potent chemical used in the veterinary practice to sterilize hard instruments without the use of an autoclave. Because it is so effective at killing germs,

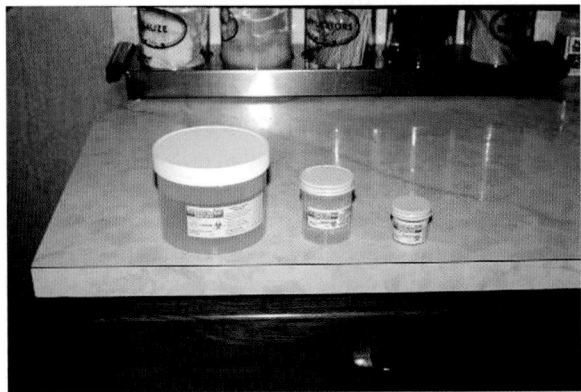

FIGURE 4-9 When possible, use only biopsy jars prefilled with formalin to prevent excessive exposure.

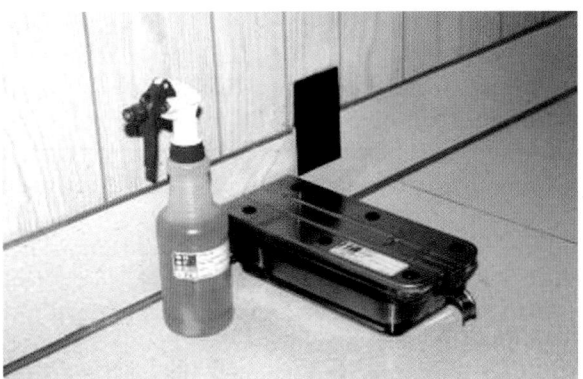

FIGURE 4-10 Disinfectants are designed to kill living organisms, so they must be handled safely.

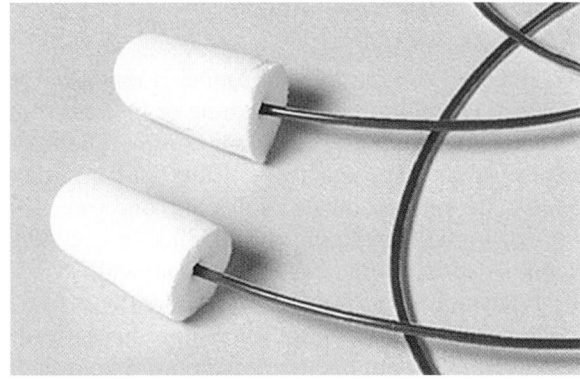

FIGURE 4-11 Hearing protectors should always be used in noisy kennels.

glutaraldehyde can be harmful to other living organisms, including you (Figure 4-10). When using this "cold-sterilization" solution, be sure to follow all safe handling rules put forth by the manufacturer, including washing your hands after handling instruments exposed to the solution and keeping trays covered to minimize evaporation.

MEDICAL AND ANIMAL-RELATED HAZARDS

We cannot forget that the overriding purpose of a veterinary practice is the care and treatment of animals. But sometimes handling our patients can be a hazard in itself. Anyone who has worked with animals under stress or in pain will relate personal accounts of injuries caused by patients. Insurance statistics show that animal-related accidents are the most common type of injury among workers in veterinary-related jobs, including veterinary technicians.

> **TECHNICIAN NOTE** Insurance statistics show that animal-related accidents are the most common type of injury among workers in veterinary-related jobs, including veterinary technicians.

Unfortunately, this hazard cannot be eliminated, so we have to do the next best thing—minimize it. The best way to protect oneself from this hazard is to obtain training and practice in animal restraint. The first safety rule when working around animals is to stay alert. Animals sometimes react to situations unexpectedly. Sudden noises, movements, or even light can be the stimulus that would cause an animal to react, so if you are the person responsible for restraining the animal, keep your attention focused on the animal's reactions, not on the procedure. You must learn the proper restraint positions for each of the species of animals with which you work. Refer to Chapter 6 for additional information about the restraint and handling of animals.

Remember that capture-restraint equipment is available if the animal is fractious or is not cooperating; sometimes just a piece of rope to hobble a leg or a piece of gauze for a hasty muzzle will make all the difference. Do not forget that

chemical restraint, rather than physical restraint, is often better for both you and the animal, but be sure to ask the veterinarian for approval before administering any medication to a patient.

Large animals such as horses and cattle are particularly dangerous and may severely injure or even kill a person when trying to escape restraint. Never put your hand or leg or any other part of your body between the animal and the side of the enclosure or chute; use a hook or a pole to pass ropes or belts through the chute. If you have to enter a stall, paddock, or trailer with a large animal, stay on the side of the animal nearest the door so that you can escape if the situation becomes hazardous. If you must capture a fractious animal from a cage or a pen, make sure that another person is present who can assist you if you get into trouble.

If your job entails handling exotic or nondomestic animals, remember that they all have their own unique methods of defense. You should know and understand their possible reactions before you attempt to restrain or treat them.

NOISE

Dogs in cages will inevitably bark, and barking dogs can adversely affect your hearing, especially if you work in an indoor kennel. Noise levels in dog wards can reach as high as 110 dB. Although relatively short-duration exposure to these noise levels such as going into the kennel just to retrieve a patient poses no serious damage to your hearing, chronic or long-term exposure can contribute to hearing loss. When working in noisy areas for extended periods of time (e.g., while cleaning cages), you must wear personal hearing protectors (Figure 4-11). It does not matter what style or type of hearing protector you use (earplugs or muffs), as long as it is rated to filter the noise by at least 20 dB (the package will indicate the rating).

> **TECHNICIAN NOTE** Dogs in cages will inevitably bark, and barking dogs can adversely affect your hearing, especially if you work in an indoor kennel. Noise levels in dog wards can reach as high as 110 dB.

BATHING, DIPPING, AND SPRAYING AREAS

Probably no area of an animal hospital is associated with greater risk for injury than the bathing or insecticide application area. Although newer parasite control products significantly reduce exposure to pesticides and insecticides, shampoos and medical dips are still a big concern.

Products used for bathing and dipping animals can be harmful to your health and the environment. Even "all natural" shampoos can cause eye irritation, and you can develop sensitivities to even the mildest products if you are exposed often enough. Because it is impossible to prevent splashing and shaking, it is important to always wear protective glasses or goggles when bathing or dipping animals. In most cases, it is also important to wear gloves and a protective apron to prevent the product from getting on your skin or clothing; this minimizes the amount absorbed through the skin.

Bottles of dips, shampoos, and insecticides should be stored in a cabinet at or below eye level. Bottles should be properly labeled with the contents and any hazard warning that is appropriate (refer to the discussion on chemicals in this chapter for additional details). Always replace the cap or lid on the container when you are finished using it, to prevent accidental spillage. Plastic containers recycled from other areas can be used for diluted shampoos and dips; however, use only the ones that have a screw-on cap or lid.

Always use a ventilation fan to keep the fumes from shampoos and dips at a safe level. When exhaust fans are too large, they waste heating or air conditioning, so you may be hesitant to use them in some situations. Ideally, a smaller fan installed directly over the tub will exhaust fumes without sacrificing comfort in the room.

Make sure you know where the eyewash station for this area is located. Learn how to properly use the eyewash device before it is needed. If you ever splash a chemical in your eyes, do not rub your eyes with your hands. Immediately call out for help; someone is usually nearby. With a coworker's assistance, go to the eyewash station and flush both eyes (even if only one eye is affected). Avoid using spray attachments for tubs and sinks because the water pressure is unregulated and streams of water from these devices can be fine enough to lacerate your cornea.

ZOONOTIC DISEASES

Infectious diseases that can be passed from animals to humans are known as **zoonotic diseases**. Some zoonotic diseases are not easily transmitted from animals to humans, whereas others are easily spread. You can be exposed to the organisms that cause disease by several means: inhalation, contact with broken skin, ingestion, contact with eyes and mucous membranes, and via accidental inoculation by a needle. A veterinary technician may be exposed to a wide variety of zoonotic agents—certainly more than can be discussed in this chapter. However, some important ones are discussed in the following sections.

Viral Infections

Rabies is a serious (almost always fatal) viral disease that can affect any warm-blooded animal (including humans). The virus is spread by contact with an infected animal's saliva. Usually the virus is transmitted through a bite, but it has also been transmitted when open wounds or mucous membranes come in contact with virus-rich saliva.

Although the disease is ever present in wild animal populations (primarily bats, raccoons, and skunks in the United States), in recent years many states have confirmed record high numbers of rabies cases in domestic species such as cats, dogs, horses, and cattle. Several university veterinary hospitals have recorded cases of rabies in horses, cattle, and companion animals. Some of those animals were even adopted from pet shops. Although rare, it is possible that you will encounter a rabid pet at the veterinary hospital where you work.

It is important that you are aware of the prevalence of rabies and its incidence among wild species in your area because it varies in each region of the country. If you work in a high-risk environment, such as with unvaccinated, stray, and homeless animals in a shelter or with wild animals at a rehabilitation center, you should be immunized with preexposure prophylaxis. Ask your hospital administrator about the availability of these vaccines. They are often available through the occupational health divisions of regional human hospitals. When you must handle an unvaccinated, wild, or stray animal, wear protective (rubber or latex) gloves; wear protective gowns and goggles in cases where the procedure may be "messy."

Bacterial Infections

You may be exposed to a wide variety of pathogenic and nonpathogenic bacteria during your professional life. Examples of pathogenic bacteria include *Salmonella* spp., *Pasteurella* spp., *Escherichia coli*, and *Pseudomonas* spp. Bacteria can be transferred by direct contact with animals and their exudates. This is particularly likely if you have any cuts or open sores. Some bacteria may be aerosolized and inhaled or absorbed through mucous membranes. The best protection against exposure to bacteria is simply good personal hygiene. Always follow the personal hygiene rules discussed later in this chapter.

Lyme Disease

Recently, **Lyme disease** has become a more serious concern for animals and people. When an infected deer tick bites a host (an animal or person) to feed, the bacterium *Borrelia burgdorferi* is transferred to the host. Lyme disease in humans is characterized by aches in the joints, fever, and a host of other flu-like symptoms. The best defense against this disease is to check oneself daily for ticks and remove them promptly. If you work in a food animal or mixed animal practice, it is a good idea to use an insect repellent when you go out into fields or woods to work.

Fungal Infections

Contrary to its name, **ringworm** is not a parasite or a worm. It is an infection of the skin caused by a fungus known as *Microsporum*. Ringworm is passed between animals and humans. Cats and horses are particularly susceptible to ringworm infection. The most effective protection from ringworm infection is to wear gloves when handling or treating animals diagnosed with the condition and to practice good personal hygiene. Be especially careful about preventing contamination of your clothing when treating patients with *Microsporum* spp. because it is believed that fungal spores can be carried to other locations (such as your home) on clothing and can infect other animals or other people.

Internal Parasites

Larval Migrans

When the eggs of common internal parasites such as roundworms infect humans, they usually do not mature into adult parasites, but they do cause other problems. Roundworm larvae can migrate to virtually any organ in the body and develop into a cyst-like growth known as **visceral larval migrans**. These "cysts" usually are not clinically noticeable unless they develop in a vital organ such as the eye, where they can do permanent damage to the retina and may cause blindness. Puppies almost always have some level of roundworm infestation because passage of worms from the bitch to the fetus occurs through the placenta and via lactation. When the infected puppy defecates in soil, roundworm eggs can survive for long periods of time until they are picked up and ingested by another mammal.

Another common internal parasite, hookworms, can also cause problems in humans by a condition known as **cutaneous larval migrans**. This condition is particularly prevalent in southern areas of the United States, where winters are warm and humid. Children who play barefoot where pets defecate frequently may be affected, as well as people who lie on the ground where dogs have defecated. Unlike the visceral cysts from roundworms, cutaneous larval migrans are relatively easy to spot and appear as small, red lines in the regions where the parasite has burrowed into the skin from the soil. Often these marks are itchy and lengthen as the parasite moves from one part of the body to another, subcutaneously.

Protozoal Infections

Infestation with a protozoan known as *Toxoplasma gondii* is called **toxoplasmosis**. Although it is usually not harmful to most adults, this event can have devastating effects on the development of a human fetus by causing hydrocephalus and mental retardation. Nonsporulated *Toxoplasma* eggs are shed in the feces of infected cats. These eggs sporulate approximately 2 to 4 days later. Three-day-old sporulated oocysts—if ingested by some pregnant women—are particularly dangerous to the fetus. Pregnant women can avoid potential exposure to *Toxoplasma* by taking the following steps:

1. Avoid cleaning cat litter pans when possible, particularly those that contain feces older than 2 days. If cleaning is unavoidable, be sure to wear gloves when handling the litter box, and wash your hands when you are finished.
2. Wash raw vegetables thoroughly (dirt on vegetables may contain oocysts).
3. Do not eat raw or uncooked meat, particularly lamb and pork, which can carry the encysted protozoan in the muscle tissue. Cook all meat thoroughly.
4. When gardening, wear gloves that can be removed easily. Under no circumstances should dirt accidentally enter your mouth (e.g., when removing a hair from your mouth).
5. Women in the veterinary profession are encouraged to have *Toxoplasma* titers evaluated before becoming pregnant, if at all possible. Your physician can give you more specific advice about *Toxoplasma* titers during your pregnancy.

Other zoonotic protozoal agents, such as ***Giardia*** and **coccidia,** may cause diarrhea and gastrointestinal cramping in humans. They are typically spread to people through contact with infected animals (particularly puppies and kittens), but they can be acquired by drinking contaminated water.

Because you will probably come in contact with some of these diseases in your job, particular attention to personal hygiene and sanitary work practices is essential. Good personal hygiene includes making sure your clothes do not become soiled by chemicals or biological material and, of course, performing regular hand washing. In general, you should wash your hands at the following times:

1. After handling medications or laboratory samples
2. After treating patients or cleaning cages
3. Before and after you use the restroom
4. Before lunch or meal breaks and before you leave work at the end of your shift

External Parasites

The irritating and itchy mite that causes **sarcoptic mange** can spread easily to humans from animals. Typically, this occurs in regions where clothing may be tight, such as along bra lines and waistbands. When treating animal patients for mange, always wear gloves and a protective gown, and wash your hands thoroughly with disinfecting soap immediately after the procedure.

NONZOONOTIC DISEASES

Some infectious agents such as **parvoviral enteritis** in dogs and **panleukopenia** in cats are not a serious concern for human health, but they are so highly contagious that you can carry the live virus home to your pets on your clothes and shoes. For this reason, some technicians when working with parvoviral cases at work leave their shoes outside the front door and change their clothes immediately upon entering the home; some even change clothes before they leave the hospital. In addition, technicians who work with cats that have certain viral upper respiratory conditions and chlamydia can themselves contract pinkeye or conjunctivitis. Therefore, when treating cases with contagious diseases, be sure to wear a protective apron, a surgical mask, examination gloves, and, when appropriate, eye protection. Thoroughly wash your hands with a disinfecting agent such as chlorhexidine or povidone-iodine scrub at the completion of treatment, and change your clothes before handling your own animals.

A DIRTY MOUTH? PRECAUTIONS FOR DENTISTRY OPERATIONS

Dental procedures that include use of a high-speed and ultrasonic scaler aerosolize oral microbes, making personal protection a necessity. One of the most common pathogens in the mouths of animals is *Pasteurella multocida,* an organism that has been linked to cardiac and pulmonary problems in humans and animals alike. Therefore, when performing dental procedures, be sure to wear goggles, gloves, and a surgical mask (Figure 4-12).

RADIOLOGY

The ability to "see inside the body" is a great tool in medicine. In most cases, the method of choice is diagnostic radiography (x-rays). Short-duration, infrequent exposure to radiation, as occurs when radiographs are taken of yourself, is considered an acceptable level of exposure (the benefits outweigh the risks). However, long-term exposure to low doses of radiation has been linked to many medical disorders. High-dose exposure can cause skin changes, cell damage, and gastrointestinal and bone marrow disorders that can be fatal. Fortunately, much is known about the properties of x-rays, and we are clear about the ways in which we need to protect ourselves. By following some simple safety precautions, you can safely use radiography in your practice.

Although modern radiographic machines have many safeguards integrated into their design, injury may occur if these tools are used incorrectly. When you are taking x-rays, always wear a lead apron and lead gloves. Lead thyroid collars and lead glasses are also recommended, particularly during extensive studies such as those performed with fluoroscopy. Although restraint of animals during radiographic studies can be challenging, never place any part of your body, even a gloved hand, in the primary beam (Figure 4-13).

Before you use an x-ray machine, make sure you know the purpose of every knob and button. Always use the collimator to restrict the primary beam to a size smaller than the size of the cassette—in other words, "cone down" to the area to be radiographed so that scatter radiation is

CASE PRESENTATION 4-2

A 40-year-old veterinary technician noticed dark-colored spots on her hands that are not typical aging spots. A visit to her dermatologist led to a diagnosis of skin cancer. It was later determined that the cancer was a type that is typically associated with exposure to radiation.

An investigation into the case revealed that the technician has worked at various veterinary hospitals and even in a research facility throughout her career. In most of these positions, her duties included exposure and processing of radiographs. Because the technician was "small in size," she found the protective gloves used for the procedure bulky and cumbersome. Therefore, she most often chose to restrain patients without the gloves. At one job in a mixed animal hospital, she even held the cassette for lameness evaluations with her bare hand. Her desire to help patients without regard for her own safety was compounded by the perpetual "hurry up and get it done" attitude that sometimes prevails in practice.

In this case, the damage was not evident and no physical pain occurred when the exposure happened, so the technician falsely assumed that the practice of taking radiographs without gloves was safe. Her failure to follow the instructions given when she was a technician student and the safety training that was continual throughout her career is the primary cause of her incurable condition.

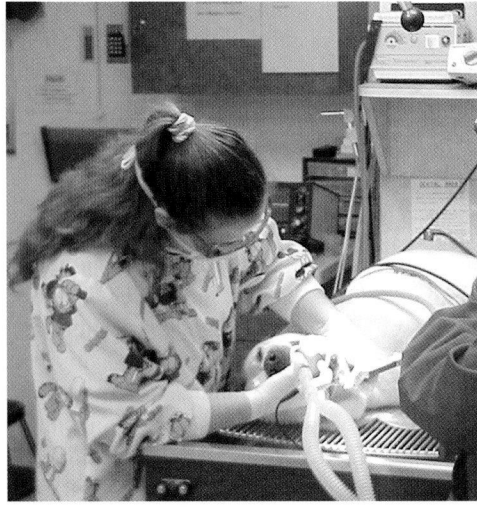

FIGURE 4-12 Always wear eye protection, a mask, and gloves when performing dental prophylactic procedures.

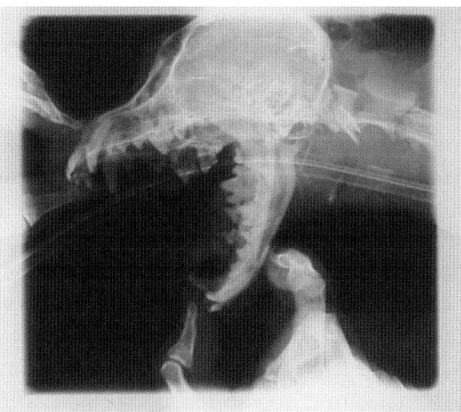

FIGURE 4-13 Never place your hand or any other part of your body in the primary beam when taking radiographs.

minimized. A properly collimated radiograph will have a small clear border around the entire film once developed.

Always follow the written operational and safety procedures provided by the hospital or the machine manufacturer. If you have not already done so, make an exposure chart specific to your machine so that you can replicate the best techniques for various studies. By following a proven technique chart and positioning the patient correctly the first time, you will have fewer "retakes" and will reduce unnecessary exposure.

Portable machines such as those used in large animal and mobile practices can be particularly dangerous because of their multipurpose abilities. These machines can be aimed in any direction, and because of their limited power, they must use longer exposure times to produce diagnostic images. When using a portable machine, always make sure no one is in the path of the primary beam (even at a distance). Always use a cassette-holding pole, and never hold a cassette with your hands while the exposure is made—even with gloves. Remember to wear a lead apron and gloves when near the machine during exposure.

If you are involved in the exposure portion of radiography, you must have and use an individual dosimetry badge. This badge is worn on your collar outside your protective apron during radiographic procedures, not as protection, but as a way to measure any incidental radiation you may receive during the procedure. It is important to return the badge to the designated storage location (outside the x-ray area) when not in use. Unless you are taking radiographs, do not wear your badge outside because exposure to sunlight will result in false readings. As a result of the relatively low numbers of radiographs taken in most practices, the availability of safer machines, and the use of good protective equipment, most technicians receive little, if any, occupational exposure to radiation.

Radiographic processing chemicals (the developer and fixer) can be corrosive to materials and organic tissues, so use protective gloves and goggles when mixing and pouring the chemicals. When using manual processing tanks, stir the chemicals with care and avoid splashing. After handling radiographic developing chemicals, always wash your hands. It is important to avoid breathing the fumes of processing chemicals, so make sure that ventilation in the darkroom is adequate; an exhaust fan is usually necessary.

Radiographic developing solutions can react dangerously with other chemicals. For this reason, never pour chemicals down the drain with developing solutions. Some liquid drain openers, when mixed with developer and fixer solutions, can produce toxic gases. Others can produce an exothermic reaction (can generate high temperatures) that can damage pipes.

ANESTHESIA

Anesthesia is as common to veterinary medicine as antiseptic wound care. The National Institute of Occupational Safety

and Health (NIOSH) estimates that more than 250,000 U.S. workers may be at risk from exposure to waste gases not metabolized by the patient. Long-term exposure to **waste anesthetic gases** (WAGs) has been linked to congenital abnormalities in children, spontaneous abortions, and even liver and kidney damage.

Although recent development and use of improved WAGs have lowered risk for patients and health care workers, no chemical is entirely without risk. Therefore, we must continue to take precautions to protect ourselves, even when using isoflurane and sevoflurane. OSHA has established a safe exposure limit for all halogenated anesthetic agents that is not to exceed 2 parts per million (ppm).

Using a proper scavenging system is the single most effective means of reducing exposure to WAGs. Three general types of scavenging systems are available: active scavenging, passive exhaust, and absorption. Each has a place, but rarely does one method fit all circumstances. Regardless of the system chosen, make sure it is fully operational and is in use before turning on the anesthesia machine. If you use absorption canisters, be sure to check them (by weighing with a gram scale) regularly and replace them as needed. Once the canister becomes saturated with gas, it is ineffective.

According to some research findings, as much as 90% of the anesthetic gas levels found in the room during a procedure can be attributed to leaks in the anesthesia machine, so be sure to perform a leak check before use (Procedure 4-3). Also make sure that correct sizes of hoses and rebreathing bags are used. Intubation tubes should be placed and the cuff inflated before the animal is connected to the anesthesia machine. Start the flow of anesthetic gases only after the patient is connected to the machine. When the surgical procedure is finished, turn off the vaporizer and increase the flow of oxygen to the patient. Be sure to use the "flush" feature to purge the circuit before disconnecting the patient.

Before filling the vaporizer, move the anesthesia machine to a well-ventilated area. Use a pouring funnel, and be careful to avoid overfilling the vaporizer or spilling the liquid anesthetic. If you accidentally break a bottle of anesthetic, immediately evacuate all nonessential people from the area. Any windows in the area should be opened, and all exhaust fans should be turned on. Quickly control the liquid with a generous amount of kitty litter, and place a plastic bag over the spill to reduce evaporation. Pick up the absorbed liquid and kitty litter with a dust pan, and place it inside a plastic garbage bag. Seal the bag tightly and dispose of it in an outside trash can. Leave the exhaust fans on and the windows open until you are sure the gas level has been reduced to a safe level.

Anesthetic protocols that involve masking the patient or using a tank for induction are more likely to generate a larger quantity of WAGs. When using these protocols, be sure to use an appropriate flow rate and a proper reservoir bag for the size of the patient—do not turn up the oxygen flowmeter to maximum when masking a patient. Induction chambers should always be connected to the scavenging system or absorption canisters to reduce the levels of escaping gases.

PROCEDURE 4-3 | Leak Check Your Anesthesia Machine Before Each Use

1. Assemble all hoses, canisters, valves, and tubes according to the manufacturer's instructions.
2. Turn on the oxygen supply to the machine.
3. Close the pressure relief (pop-off) valve.

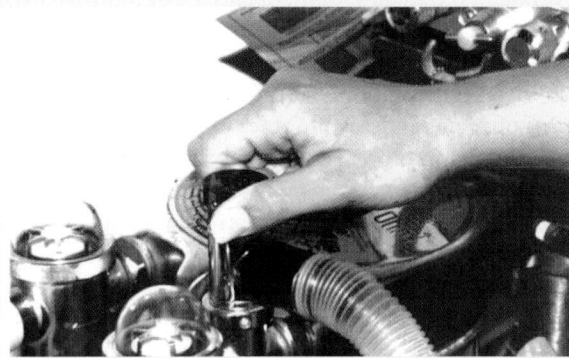

4. Use your thumb or palm to form a tight seal on the Y-piece (the part of the hose that attaches to the patient's endotracheal tube).

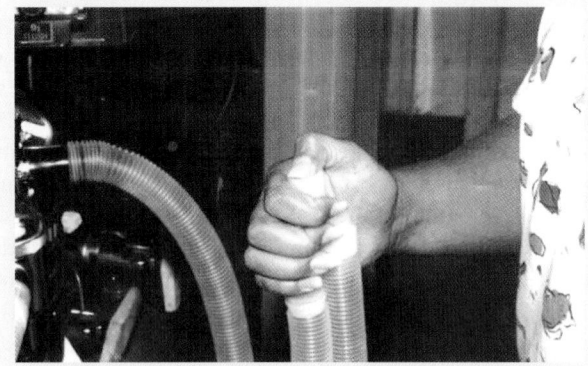

5. Turn on the oxygen until the bag is slightly overinflated (or when the pressure on the manometer reaches the 20 mark), then close the valve.

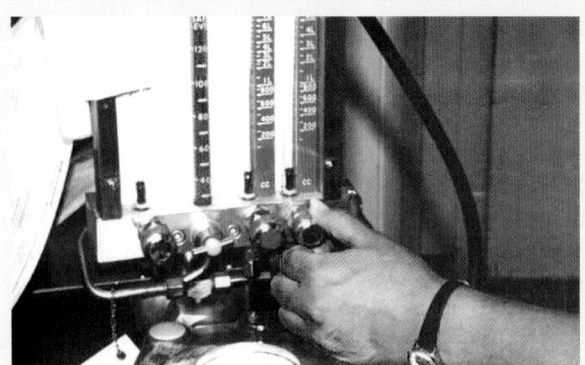

6. Observe the pressure in the system on the manometer, and watch closely for any decrease. (If your machine is not equipped with a manometer, observe the size of the bag closely.) If the pressure remains constant, the machine is leak free. If the pressure drops, a leak (or leaks) is present in the system. The faster the pressure drops, the larger the leak(s).

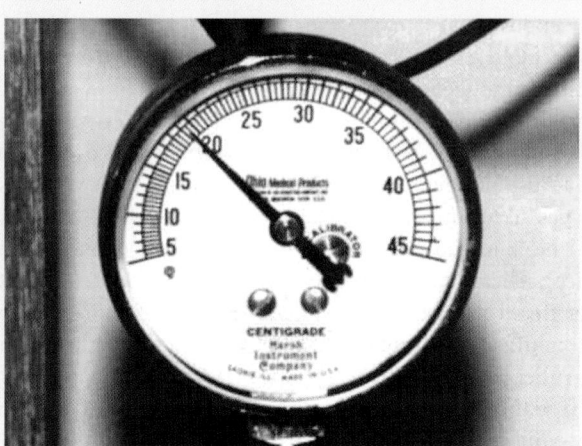

7. If a leak is detected, check the bag, hoses, and other rubber (plastic) parts for evidence of cracks or deterioration. Replace any parts that are damaged. Check all connections, especially the seals at the top and bottom of the soda lime canister and on the one-way valves (clear plastic domes). Tighten any loose connections that you find.
8. After checking all connections and hoses, if a leak is still noted, have the machine serviced by a qualified technician before use.
9. When the machine is leak free, reset the pressure relief (pop-off) valve to the proper position for normal use of the machine.

Make sure that ventilation in the room is good, and use local exhaust fans when available.

Anesthetized animals do not metabolize all of the anesthetic gas that they have inhaled. They exhale some of it into the room after they have been extubated and while they are recovering. When monitoring patients during their recovery, you should avoid putting your face close to the animal's face. In addition, keep the number of recovering patients to an acceptable number based on the size of the area and the capability of the ventilation system (Figure 4-14). As much as possible, delay extubation and allow the patient to recover while still connected to the anesthetic machine (oxygen only) and scavenging system.

When changing the soda lime (carbon dioxide absorbent) in anesthetic machines, wear rubber or latex gloves. When the soda lime is wet, as is often the case from humidity in the system, it can be caustic to tissues and some metals. Dispose of used soda lime granules in a plastic trash bag as regular trash.

Pregnant women should discuss with their physician the risks of exposure to anesthetic gases from unscavenged procedures. They should inform their supervisor of their condition as soon as possible so that safety procedures can be reviewed and adjusted, if necessary.

📎 *TECHNICIAN NOTE* Anesthetized animals do not metabolize all of the anesthetic gas that they have inhaled. They exhale some of it into the room after they have been extubated and while they are recovering.

COMPRESSED GASES

Every year, hundreds of workers are injured while working with compressed gas cylinders, usually because of improper storage or handling of these cylinders. Regardless of the size of the cylinder or whether the cylinder is empty, full, or in use, store cylinders in a dry, cool place, away from potential heat sources such as furnaces, water heaters, and direct sunlight. Always secure the tanks, even small ones, in an upright position by means of a chain or strap (Figure 4-15). Cylinders that are stored inside a closet should also be secured because they can fall against the door, causing injury when you open the door. If cylinders are equipped with a protective cap, this cap must be firmly screwed in place when the cylinder is not in use. If you have to move a large cylinder, do not roll or drag it; always use a hand truck or a handcart, and remember to strap the tank in.

SHARPS AND MEDICAL WASTE

The most serious hazard from needles or sharp objects in a veterinary medical environment involves the physical trauma (and possible bacterial infection) caused by a puncture or laceration. To prevent these types of accidents, always keep sharps, needles, scalpel blades, and other sharp instruments capped or sheathed until ready for use. Do not attempt to recap the needle after use unless the physical danger from sticks or lacerations cannot be prevented by any other means. When it is necessary to recap a needle, you should use the "one-handed" method (Procedure 4-4). Although some practice is needed before the one-handed method becomes second nature, it is the safest and most practical approach for most veterinary situations.

Do not remove the needle from the syringe for disposal because this unnecessary handling often results in injury. Whenever possible, the entire needle and syringe should be disposed of in the designated sharps containers immediately

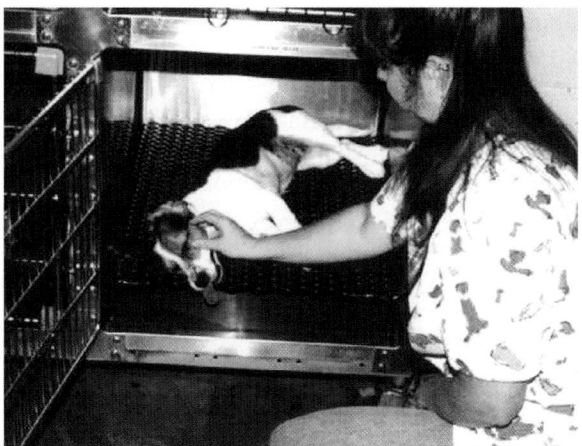

FIGURE 4-14 Monitor recovering anesthesia patients "at arm's length" to minimize exposure to gases emitted during respiration.

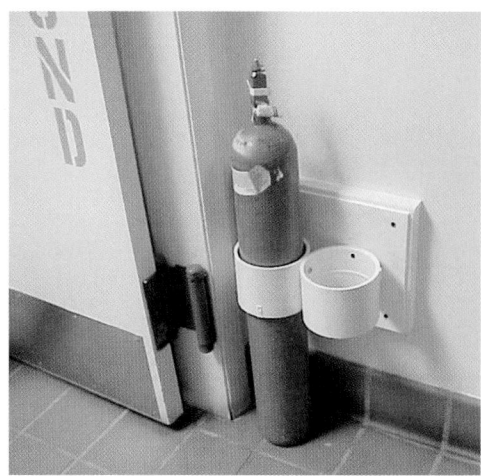

FIGURE 4-15 Small compressed-gas cylinders must be secured to prevent them from falling over.

PROCEDURE 4-4 | One-Handed Needle Recapping

Step 1. Place the cap on a flat surface such as the countertop or even the floor.

Step 2. Using only one hand, hold the syringe between the tips of your fingers with the needle pointing away from your body.

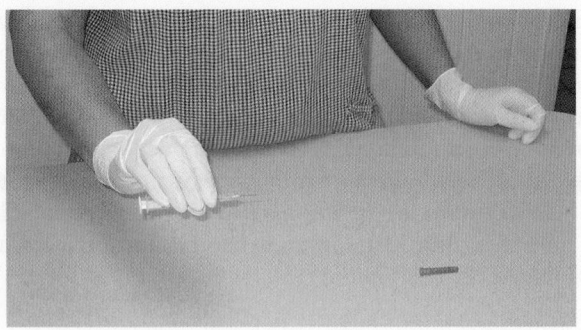

Step 3. Place your fingertips on the flat surface so that the needle and the syringe are parallel to and in line with the cap. Move your hand forward until the needle is inside the cap.

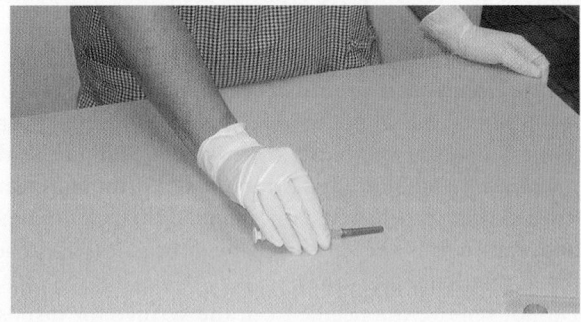

Step 4. You may then use your other hand to "seat" the cap firmly.

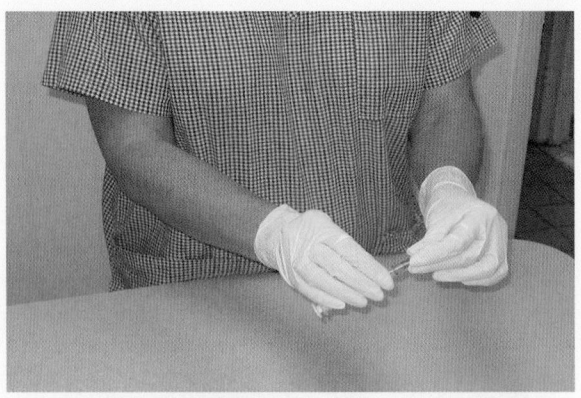

after use. Do not try to overfill a sharps container—when it is full, it is full! When the sharps container is full, seal it and replace it with a new one. Never open a sharps container that has already been sealed or stick your fingers into one for any reason.

Destroying the needle before disposal is not recommended because this may aerosolize the contents of the needle, increasing your exposure. Likewise, you should not collect sharps in a smaller container and transfer them to a larger container for disposal. Of course, never throw needles or sharps directly into regular trash containers, regardless of whether or not they are capped.

Table 4-1 explains which materials are usually considered hazardous and which are not. Although this chart is essentially accurate, some states have special rules for discarding medical waste, so be sure to follow the rules prescribed by your state.

HAZARDOUS DRUGS AND PHARMACY OPERATIONS

Medicines are designed to cure diseases and make patients better, but it is important to remember that all medicines are chemicals, and chemicals can be dangerous. In the veterinary pharmacy, you can be exposed to all kinds of drugs just by handling them. Liquids can splash in your eyes when you pour them, or they can release vapors that you may inhale. Handling, crushing, or breaking tablets can leave powder residue on your hands that will be ingested next time you put your hands near your mouth or mucous membranes.

Some drugs, such as cytotoxic drugs (CDs) used to treat patients with cancer, are so potent that even minute exposures can cause harm. When preparing CDs, always wear powder-free chemotherapy gloves and a disposable gown that is not used for any other purpose. Chemotherapy drugs should always be prepared inside of a biological safety cabinet (Figure 4-16). Be sure to follow all instructions on the MSDS, on the package insert, and in your practice's chemotherapy safety plan.

During administration of CDs, expect the unexpected. Keep unnecessary people out of the area, and wear protective equipment such as gloves, disposable aprons, surgical masks, and eyeglasses. You should avoid wearing contact lenses when preparing or administering CDs.

When handling patients that have received chemotherapeutic treatments, remember that some drugs are excreted in bodily fluids, so proper precautions are necessary when cleaning up their urine, feces, and other bodily excretions. Always wear powder-free chemotherapy gloves and avoid contaminating your clothes when cleaning cages or picking up waste from chemotherapy patients. Make sure you dispose of all soiled materials from these patients as medical waste and launder nondisposable items separately from general laundry.

The most important rule to remember when handling any medication is to practice good personal hygiene, especially by performing thorough handwashing.

TABLE 4-1	Typical Medical Waste Definitions	
MATERIAL	**MEDICAL WASTE**	**NORMAL TRASH**
Sharps (any device with characteristics that make it possible to puncture, lacerate, or penetrate the skin)	Any used needles and scalpel blades Glass or hard plastic that is contaminated with a *human disease*–causing agent	Glass or hard plastic that is not contaminated with *human disease*–causing agents can be disposed of as normal waste
Medical devices such as blood tubes, vials, catheters, IV tubes, etc.	Considered biomedical waste only when they contain *human* pathogens or they have been used for chemotherapy	Devices that simply contain or are contaminated with animal blood (except from primates) are normally not considered biomedical waste.
Animal blood or tissues	Only dead animals or animal parts that are infected with zoonotic diseases; these include but are not limited to rabies, brucellosis, systemic fungal diseases, tuberculosis, and atypical mycobacteriosis.	Tissues from routine surgical procedures (castration, ovariohysterectomy, etc.) should be considered regular waste.
Laboratory cultures	Microbiological cultures (bacterial, fungal, or viral) of *human* pathogens are considered biomedical waste.	In some cases, culture media from negative tests may be considered regular trash, but it is probably wise to just classify all laboratory cultures as biomedical waste for simplicity.
Bandages/sponges	Used absorbent materials such as bandages, gauze, or sponges that are saturated with blood or body fluids that contain *human* pathogens that may splash or drip	Sponges or bandages used on animals not infected with a disease transmissible to humans
Primate materials		Normally, waste generated from work on primates is considered regular waste *unless it fits into another category* (such as from research studies using human pathogens).
Animal waste	Waste from animals infected with a disease contagious to *humans* that can be transmitted by means of the waste. Waste from chemotherapy patients for up to 48 hours after the last treatment	Normally, waste from animals not infected with human disease–causing agents should be disposed of as regular trash.

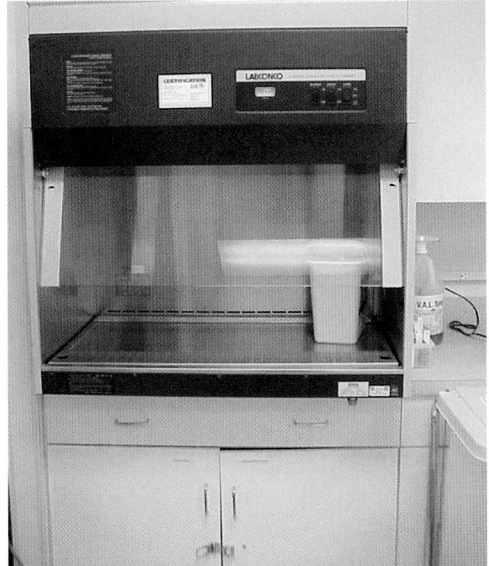

FIGURE 4-16 A biological safety cabinet (BSC) is required when cytotoxic drugs are prepared.

CASE PRESENTATION 4-3

A 25-year-old veterinary technician is working in private mixed animal hospital. She and her husband have been trying to conceive a child for several years without success. Her obstetrician has suggested that her exposure to hazards at work may be contributing to her inability to conceive. After a thorough analysis of the chemicals, pathogens, and physical hazards she is exposed to at work, it was determined that her failure to use proper precautions when handling patient medications, in particular chemotherapy drugs, contributed to unviable egg production.

After undergoing retraining and by practicing better personal hygiene when handling patients and medications, she became pregnant within a year.

SUMMARY

We all face dangers in life every day, but that does not mean we have to intentionally place ourselves in danger to get our job done. The successful person makes sure that the reward for an action far outweighs the risk.

In this chapter, we discussed your rights and responsibilities in a safety program, the hazards associated with your job from a general and a medical perspective, and the actions you should take to protect yourself. Employing good safety practices should not be the cause for additional work. If a job is safely completed and the correct protocol is followed, then it is done properly. Occupational risks should not keep you from doing your job; they should motivate you to do your job better, to pay attention to what you are doing, and to comply with the standard operating procedures established in your practice. Employing good safety practices will enable you to remain healthy and will therefore allow you to continue to practice your career for a long time.

Have fun and be safe!

INTERNET RESOURCES/RECOMMENDED READING

Canadian Centre for Occupational Health & Safety: www.ccohs.ca
Canadian OSHA: www.canoshweb.org
Centers for Disease Control and Prevention: www.cdc.gov
Department of Labor: www.dol.gov
Environmental Protection Agency: www.epa.gov
Infection Control Today: www.infectioncontroltoday.com
Lab Safety Supply: www.labsafety.com
National Institute of Occupational Safety and Health (NIOSH): www.cdc.gov/niosh
OSHA: www.osha.gov
SafetyVet: www.safetyvet.com
The Veterinary Information Network (VIN): www.vin.com
The Veterinary Support Personnel Network (VSPN): www.vspn.org
The Virtual Anesthesia Machine: http://vam.anest.ufl.edu/

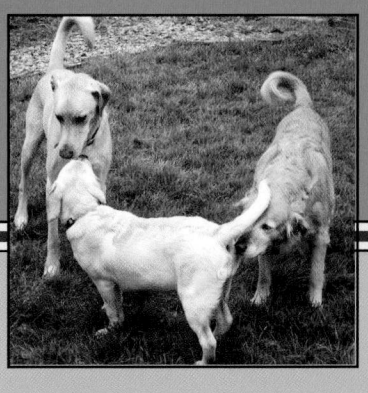

5 Animal Behavior

Valarie V. Tynes

OUTLINE

The Technician's Role in Behavior Counseling, *135*
Technician Specialists in Behavior, *135*
Taking a Behavior-Specific History, *135*
Learning and Animal Behavior Modification, *136*
Preventing Behavior Problems, *139*
Step 1: Elicit and Reinforce Appropriate Behavior, *140*
Step 2: Prevent or Minimize Inappropriate Behavior, *140*
Step 3: Meet the Pet's Behavioral and Developmental Needs, *141*
Step 4: Use the "Take Away" Method (Negative Punishment) to Discourage Inappropriate Behavior, *142*
Step 5: Minimize Discipline (Positive Punishment) and Use It Correctly When Necessary, *142*
Habituation to Handling, *143*
Choosing a Pet, *143*
Medications and Treating Behavior Problems, *144*
Canine, *146*
Development, *146*
Social Behavior, *147*

Reading Canine Body Language, *148*
Coping With Behavior in the Clinic, *149*
Introducing a New Dog, *150*
Common Behavior Problems, *150*
Feline, *155*
Development, *155*
Social Behavior, *156*
Reading Feline Body Language, *156*
Coping With Feline Behavior in the Clinic, *157*
Introducing a New Cat, *157*
Common Behavior Problems, *158*
Equine, *164*
Communication and the Senses, *164*
Social Behavior, *168*
Prey Behavior, *168*
Sexual Behavior of the Mare, *169*
Sexual Behavior of the Stallion, *169*
Maternal Behavior, *170*
Common Behavior Problems, *171*
Cattle and Small Ruminants, *172*
Species-Typical Behaviors, *172*
Sexual Behavior, *174*
Maternal Behavior, *174*
Common Behavior Problems, *174*

LEARNING OBJECTIVES

When you have completed this chapter, you will be able to:

1. Pronounce, spell, and define all Key Terms in the chapter.
2. Explain why behavior problems can be life threatening to pets.
3. Summarize the veterinary technician's role in supporting behavioral health.
4. List steps taken when gathering information for a behavioral history.
5. Do the following regarding learning and animal behavior modification:
   • Explain how animals learn and whether or not their behavior, like that of humans, is based on a moral code of conduct.

Dr. Tynes gratefully acknowledges the assistance of Drs. Jeannine Berger and Amanda Florsheim in the preparation of this chapter.

KEY TERMS

Affiliative behaviors
Allogrooming
Anxiety
Classical conditioning
Conflict-related aggression
Conspecific
Dominance aggression
Dominant role
Fear
Fear-related aggression
Food-related aggression
Frustration
Idiopathic aggression
Interdog (male/male)
Irritable aggression
Maternal aggression
Multiparous
Negative punishment
Negative reinforcement
Operant conditioning
Pain-related aggression
Phobia
Play-related aggression
Positive punishment
Positive reinforcement
Possessive aggression
Predatory aggression
Primiparous
Redirected aggression
Redirected behaviors
Social hierarchies
Social status/dominance aggression
Socialization
Stress
Submissive behaviors
Subordinate role
Territorial aggression

- Differentiate between positive reinforcement, positive punishment, negative reinforcement, and negative punishment.
- Explain the relationship between operant behaviors and continuous and intermittent reinforcement.
- Describe why extinction of a behavior is difficult to achieve.
- Differentiate between the following: desensitization, counter-conditioning, counter-commanding, and flooding.

6. Do the following regarding preventing behavior problems:
   - Describe each step in the Five-Step Positive Proaction Plan. List the criteria required for effective discipline.
   - Explain the importance of habituating young animals to handling.
   - Explain some of the challenges in habituating older animals to handling.
   - Describe ways in which a veterinary technician can assist a client in selecting a pet.
   - Describe the role medication plays in treating behavior problems.

7. Do the following regarding canine and feline development and behavior:
   - Describe the four stages of canine and feline development.
   - List important canine and feline behaviors that owners should be able to interpret correctly.
   - Explain how a veterinary technician's understanding of animal behavior can create a safer environment for workers, pet owners, and pets.
   - Describe methods for introducing a new dog or cat to existing pets.
   - List common behavior problems in dogs and cats and describe methods for addressing them.
   - Describe common circumstances in the dog and cat in which aggression can be problematic for the pet owner.

8. Do the following regarding equine behavior:
   - Explain how being a prey species influences the behavior of horses and their desire to be in a herd.
   - Describe how hierarchy affects the behavior of individual animals within a herd of horses.
   - Describe normal sexual behavior in mares and stallions.
   - Describe the behavior of mares with foal and explain why foal rejection is a behavior emergency.
   - List three common stable vices in horses.

9. Do the following regarding cattle and small ruminant behavior:
   - Describe how hierarchy affects the behavior of individual animals within a herd of cattle, sheep, or goats.
   - Describe how aggression commonly manifests in cattle, sheep, and goats.
   - Describe normal sexual and maternal behaviors in farm animals.
   - Describe common behavior problems in domestic livestock.

INTRODUCTION—WHY BEHAVIOR?

Multiple studies have shown that behavior problems are likely the leading cause of death in pets in the United States, in part because problem behavior is the most common reason for dogs and cats to be surrendered to animal shelters. Relinquishment often occurs because owners have unrealistic expectations of their pet, they do not recognize or understand normal behaviors or visual cues, and they often do not know that behavioral problems can be corrected. Pet owners may express concerns about their pet's behavior to their veterinarian, but if they are given inadequate guidance, clients are more likely to relinquish or euthanize their pet than to treat the behavior problem. Knowledge of both normal and abnormal animal behavior is therefore very important and may save lives. In addition, it can help to keep clients and veterinary personnel safe while handling animals and carrying out animal care duties. Finally, the correlation between **stress** and illness is well known and underscores the importance of providing animals with a psychologically safe environment in which they are free to carry out innate, species-appropriate behavior. Because an animal's behavior is a direct result of physiologic activity in the brain, behavior is an inextricable part of physiology. Knowledge of normal animal behavior is critical for the accurate assessment, and ultimately the successful treatment, of both medical and behavioral problems.

THE TECHNICIAN'S ROLE IN BEHAVIOR COUNSELING

Because veterinary technicians frequently are the first to interact with clients and their pets in the examination room, they are often the first to become aware of problem behaviors or the potential for problem behaviors. Many clients are embarrassed to admit their pet has a behavior problem; some feel that they must be at fault and will be blamed. Many owners are unaware that veterinary technicians and veterinarians are trained to assist with behavior problems, so it is important that technicians begin a dialogue with clients in a nonthreatening and empathetic manner. In the case of a new puppy, you might jokingly ask, "What product do you find is best for cleaning up those puppy accidents?" Or, "You haven't lost any good shoes yet, have you?" This light-hearted approach is more likely to elicit actual conversation than a simple yes or no question such as, "How is the housetraining going?" You can then proceed to helping educate the client about how to prevent behavior problems from forming and how to raise a dog that will be a pleasure to keep in the home.

Initiating dialogue when presented with older pets for the first time can be a little more challenging but can be made somewhat easier if the practice uses a new patient questionnaire containing questions about the pet's behavior. This questionnaire can include questions such as the following:

1. How many times has your pet eliminated in the home since 6 months of age?
2. Does your pet vocalize more than you would like it to?
3. Is there anything about your pet's behavior that you would like to change?

Although some of these may be yes or no questions, they demonstrate to the pet owner that the practice cares about the pet's behavior and wants to help. The technician can then use these responses to ask more questions and attempt to collect information that can be used to make an accurate assessment of the pet's behavior.

When pets are presented for certain problems, such as wounds encountered in a dog fight or potentially self-inflicted wounds, such as those incurred when an animal is attempting to escape from a crate, home, or yard (e.g., broken teeth or nails, lacerated paws), questions should be asked as to how the injuries came about. The technician may need to be particularly alert and prepared to ask questions about wounds or injuries because many pet owners will not mention how the injury was acquired. Some clients believe that the role of a veterinarian is merely to treat physical problems; the technician can explain that treating the pet's underlying behavioral problem is equally important. Simply treating wounds and sending the patient home is the equivalent of treating a symptom but not the disease. Demonstrating a desire to understand the cause of the problem shows the pet owner that you care about the animal's psychological and physical well-being.

In addition to collecting a behavioral history, veterinary technicians educate pet owners about behavioral problem prevention and early intervention. This can be done by distributing and discussing prepared handouts with the client about good training practices. At home, these documents serve as important reminders and references for the owner. Numerous good behavior-related handouts are commercially available and can be found in the references listed at the end of this chapter under "Recommended Readings."

> **TECHNICIAN NOTE** Veterinary technicians play a vital role in educating owners about their pet's normal behavior and appropriate responses to problem behaviors.

TECHNICIAN SPECIALISTS IN BEHAVIOR

The veterinary technician's role has become even more exciting in recent years with recognition of a specialty in veterinary behavior. In 2008, the National Association of Veterinary Technicians in America (NAVTA) recognized the Academy of Veterinary Behavior Technicians (AVBT), making veterinary behavior one of ten technician specialties recognized by NAVTA. The AVBT allows for certification of technicians with an interest in behavior medicine who demonstrate increased knowledge of "scientifically—and humanely—based techniques of behavior health, problem prevention, training, management, and behavior modification." Interested technicians must complete a formal training program and pass a test to be credentialed as a technician specialist. The American College of Veterinary Behaviorists (ACVB) eagerly supported the development of the behavior technician specialty and appreciates the role that veterinary technician specialists play as part of the veterinary health care team to provide the best possible physical and psychological health care for animals. Veterinary technician specialists provide behavior-specific education and patient assessment in general practice. In addition, their knowledge of behavior modification techniques makes them particularly well suited to work with Board-certified veterinary behaviorists. To learn more about the requirements for becoming a veterinary technician specialist in behavior, refer to the websites for the Society of Veterinary Behavior Technicians and AVBT (Box 5-1).

TAKING A BEHAVIOR-SPECIFIC HISTORY

Taking a behavior-specific history can be challenging because many owners describe their pet's behavior in terms of what *the owner* thinks the pet is experiencing (e.g., "Fluffy is mad at me for leaving him home alone," "Spot does not like my new boyfriend"). The owner is projecting his human perspective onto the animal to justify the troublesome actions of the pet. This is called *anthropomorphizing*, and it is commonly done by most pet owners. The veterinary technician must encourage owners to describe only the actions of the animal, not what they believe the pet was feeling or thinking. Examples of actions can be described as follows: "When I came home from work, I found that my shoes had been

---

BOX 5-1   Helpful Behavior-Related Resources

Academy of Veterinary Behavior Technicians—certifies technicians in the specialty of behavior: www.avbt.net

American College of Veterinary Behaviorists: www.dacvb.org

American Veterinary Society of Animal Behavior—position statements on punishment, puppy socialization, and guidelines for choosing trainers: www.avsabonline

Animal Behavior Society (ABS)—organization that certifies Applied Animal Behaviorists: www.animalbehaviorsociety.org

Association of Pet Dog Trainers: www.apdt.com (will also take you to the CCPDT site)

Certification Council for Professional Dog Trainers (CCPDT): www.ccpdt.org

Certified Applied Animal Behaviorists (with links to the ABS website): www.certfiedanimalbehaviorist.com

Delta Society from which the document Professional Standards for Dog Trainers: Effective, Humane Principles can be obtained: www.deltasociety.org

Society of Veterinary Behavior Technicians—for technicians interested in learning more about behavior: www.svbt.org

BOX 5-2   Questions for Collecting an Initial Behavioral History

- Describe the problem behavior (including any facial cues, body postures, and vocal cues).
- What was happening before it occurred and what happened afterward?
- What was your immediate response and how did the pet respond to that?
- When was this behavior first noted?
- How often does the behavior occur?
- What triggers appear to elicit the behavior?
- Where does the behavior occur? (Where does it never occur?)
- Does the behavior appear to be increasing in frequency? Worsening in severity?
- Who lives in the home with the pet, including all people and pets that interact with the pet on a regular basis?
- Who is the primary caretaker of the pet?
- What treatment(s) have been tried? What has worked and what has not worked?

If the problem behavior is aggression:

- Describe the behavior in detail (i.e., visual cues, growling, snapping, or biting). If biting, does the animal bite once and retreat, bite repeatedly, or cause minor lacerations or deep puncture wounds?
- Who is the target?
- Has medical care been required for the victim of any incident?

---

chewed up," and "Spot growled at my new boyfriend." Box 5-2 lists some of the questions that are included in a behavioral history. The history may be more or less detailed depending upon the role the veterinarians in the practice choose to take. If they have an interest in diagnosing and treating behavior problems, then the history will need to be more detailed and may be best collected by sending the client home with a questionnaire to fill out before returning for a behavioral appointment. If the veterinarian is more likely to choose to refer the owner to a specialist, the technician will collect only the historical information needed to assess the risk that the animal may pose to others, along with the extent of current or future damage to the human–animal bond. The history should also help the veterinarian to determine what diagnostic tests may be needed before a referral can be made.

> **TECHNICIAN NOTE**   While collecting a behavior-specific history, ask clients to describe the pet's *actions*, NOT what they believe the animal was *thinking* or *feeling*.

LEARNING AND ANIMAL BEHAVIOR MODIFICATION

How organisms learn has been the subject of scientific study for well over a hundred years. Yet most of what clients know is based on conventional wisdom that persists because it is often repeated, in many cases by celebrity figures or others who are able to reach millions with their message. Continued use of outdated methods of training or treating problem behaviors creates more problems, not fewer, and leads to needless suffering for animals and caregivers. A technician armed with an understanding of the science of learning has

the potential to save lives, simply by educating pet owners about appropriate training methods. In addition, because most animal species learn in the same way, this same knowledge can be applied to the wide variety of animals encountered by veterinary technicians in practice.

One of the most important messages that veterinary technicians can share with pet owners is that animals are unlikely to possess a sense of morality and most likely do not take actions or make decisions based upon a sense of "right" or "wrong." The impetus for an animal's behavior is most likely based on whether a previous action made the animal feel good or bad. Behaviors that made them feel good are repeated, and actions that gave rise to negativity are avoided. Most animals (with primates being the possible exception) do not perform behaviors out of spite or anger. Helping pet owners to understand this is an important first step in helping to resolve a pet's problem behavior because it moves the owner from feeling anger to feeling empathy. For example, an owner may be initially upset because the cat urinates on the living room wall. The owner may believe that the cat does this out of spite because it is left alone all day. However, questioning the owner reveals that a neighbor's cat loiters outside the front door, and that this is most likely very stressful for the territorially sensitive pet. When the owner is made to understand that the cat is defensively marking its territory by spraying, the owner may feel more empathy than anger and is more likely to seek out a solution to the behavioral problem, because the problem is understood and a resolution can be envisioned.

> **TECHNICIAN NOTE** Pets repeat behaviors that make them feel good and avoid those that do not.

One of the more common ways in which animals learn is referred to as *associative learning*. As the name suggests, associative learning occurs when an animal forms a learned association between two features or events. The development of these associations is dependent upon two factors: contiguity and contingency. Contiguity describes a relationship between two events in both time and place. Contingency describes the predictability of the association. For example, if a loud pan drops in the kitchen and scares a cat, it may or may not form an association between the **fear** it experiences and the place in which it is experienced. If it does, a consequence could be that the cat becomes fearful of entering the kitchen in the future owing to the contiguity of these events. Alternatively, it could associate the fear with the person who dropped the pan and become fearful of that person. What association the animal makes is dependent upon a variety of individual factors, including individual temperament and prior experiences. If *every* time the cat happens to be walking by the kitchen, a loud noise is made, the association between the kitchen and the fear may be reinforced owing to the contingency of the two events. Associations that are highly predictable will be learned most readily.

When describing how associations relate to the development of learned behaviors, behaviors are usually divided into two types: respondent and **operant conditioning**. Respondent behaviors are learned through a process referred to as *classical* or *Pavlovian conditioning*. Respondent behaviors should be considered relatively involuntary or reflexive types of behaviors such as salivation in response to food. Respondent behaviors depend on events that occur immediately before them. **Classical conditioning** occurs when a neutral stimulus comes to elicit a reflexive response when paired with a stimulus that normally elicits that response. For example, if a dog fears strangers simply because he did not meet many strangers during the first several weeks of life, his heart rate may go up (a normal physiologic response to fear) every time he sees a stranger. In this case, increased heart rate is the unconditioned response (UCR) and the stranger is the unconditioned stimulus (UCS). Through continued association with the appearance of a stranger, ringing of the doorbell may come to increase the dog's heart rate because it signals that a stranger will appear. The doorbell becomes the conditioned stimulus (CS) and the increased heart rate is now a conditioned response (CR). As mentioned earlier, this association is more readily made because the doorbell always signals the appearance of a stranger (contingency) and the stranger always appears within a few seconds of the doorbell being rung (contiguity). Owing to the way these associations develop, respondent behaviors are often referred to as

---

BOX 5-3	An Example of Classical Conditioning

Being milked (UCS) → Oxytocin release and milk letdown (UCR)

After repeated associations between entering the milking parlor and being milked:

Approaching milking parlor (sights and sounds associated with the parlor) (CS) → Oxytocin release and milk letdown (CR)

CR, Conditioned response; *CS*, conditioned stimulus; *UCR*, unconditioned response; *UCS*, unconditioned stimulus.

BOX 5-4	Important Definitions for Understanding How Animals Learn

Reinforcement is any stimulus that *increases* the chance of a behavior being repeated.

Positive reinforcement involves the *presentation* of something *pleasant* (such as food) that is likely to strengthen a behavior response. (It increases the likelihood that the behavior will be repeated.)

Negative reinforcement involves the *removal* of something *unpleasant* (such as escape from a fearful stimulus) that strengthens the behavior response.

Punishment is any stimulus that *decreases* the chance of a behavior being repeated.

Positive punishment involves the *application* of something *unpleasant or aversive*, such as a shock, verbal reprimand, squirting with water, threatening with a newspaper, etc.

Negative punishment involves the *removal* of something *pleasant*, such as play or social interaction.

---

stimulus-response (S-R) relationships. Refer to Box 5-3 for an example of classical conditioning.

> **TECHNICIAN NOTE** Respondent behaviors (those acquired by classical conditioning) are involuntary or reflexive types of behaviors.

Operant behaviors are learned through a process referred to as *operant, Skinnerian,* or *instrumental conditioning,* or "trial and error" learning. Operant behaviors depend on consequences. The animal performs a behavior and the likelihood that the behavior will increase or decrease in frequency depends on the consequence that occurs immediately after performance of the behavior. For this reason, operant behaviors are described as response-stimulus (R-S) relationships, where the stimulus that follows the response increases or decreases future responses. Terms used in the description of operant learning can be confusing and are commonly misused. *Punishment* and *negative reinforcement* are not the same things. Refer to Box 5-4 for definitions of these terms. Please be sure to note that, although frequently misinterpreted by many, the terms *positive* and *negative* are used like

TABLE 5-1	Consequences and Functions Involved in Operant Learning		
		FUNCTION	
		INCREASE THE BEHAVIOR	**DECREASE THE BEHAVIOR**
Operation	Addition +	Positive reinforcement (rewards)	Positive punishment (discipline)
	Subtraction −	Negative reinforcement (escape from something unpleasant)	Negative punishment (loss of something desirable)

mathematical operations. They do not imply any type of value judgment; they simply refer to the giving or taking away of something (Table 5-1).

> **TECHNICIAN NOTE** Punishment and negative reinforcement are not the same things.

One of the most important things to remember about reinforcement and punishment is that they must be defined by their effects, not by intended function. In other words, just because you think using a squirt bottle to squirt a dog is aversive, this does not necessarily mean that it is aversive to the dog. If the dog likes water, it may interpret this as play. It is the continual search, by the person training the animal, for an effective punisher that can lead to inhumane treatment of the animal. Often, the punishment necessary to stop a highly motivated or internally rewarding behavior must be very harsh and can lead to additional and often worse behavior problems. Similarly, reinforcement must be something that is considered by the animal to be very pleasant and worth working for. For some animals, this may be play or verbal reassurance; other animals may be best reinforced by food.

Two types of reinforcement are used: continuous and intermittent. It is important for veterinary technicians to explain to pet owners the differences between these types of reinforcement, because they can aid in training the pet *and* can contribute to problem behaviors without the owner's realization.

Continuous reinforcement, as the name suggests, means that you provide a reinforcement every single time the animal does something you want repeated. Continuous reinforcement is the best way to teach an animal a new behavior. It leads to a very rapid learned response.

Intermittent reinforcement, on the other hand, is given only periodically when the animal performs the desired behavior. Intermittent reinforcement is most useful for maintaining an already established behavior. In fact, it is the form of reinforcement that makes a behavior most resistant to extinction.

> **TECHNICIAN NOTE** Punishment and reinforcement are defined by their *actual* effect on animal behavior, not by their *intended* effect.

Extinction is the process by which an association between two events is broken. This is usually done by removing reinforcement for the behavior. If a normally reinforced behavior ceases to be reinforced, then the behavior should disappear. For example, if a dog has learned to bark to get attention from its owners, then ignoring the dog completely every time it barks will eventually stop the dog from barking for attention. Extinction can be challenging to achieve for many reasons. First, sudden withdrawal of reinforcement, especially of a behavior that has been reinforced for a long time, leads to a certain amount of **frustration** in the animal. The animal does not understand why this behavior that previously "worked" so well no longer "works" to achieve its desires. Most of the time, this leads to greatly increased frequency of the behavior initially, before a decrease is ever seen. This is called the *extinction burst* and can prove very difficult for pet owners, especially if they are not warned beforehand of the likelihood of this occurrence. Extinction can be difficult to achieve for other reasons:
1. The reinforcement has not been accurately identified.
2. The reinforcement is coming from more than one source.
3. The behavior is internally rewarding and thus is self-reinforcing.

One way to increase the efficacy of extinction is to positively reinforce an alternative behavior. For example, a dog likes to jump on people as they enter the house. If everyone who enters the house ignores the dog completely by turning away when it is jumping, not speaking to the dog or making eye contact with the dog, then the behavior may eventually be extinguished. However, if they wait a few minutes until the dog has calmed down (all the while ignoring it) and then ask it to sit, and give it a lot of attention for sitting, then the dog should very quickly learn to forego the jumping because sitting is what earns it attention.

> **TECHNICIAN NOTE** When attempting to use extinction to stop a problem behavior, owners must be warned about the likelihood of the *extinction burst*.

Operant learning is most useful for teaching pets appropriate or acceptable behaviors and for decreasing unwanted or unacceptable behaviors. However, many pet behavior problems are rooted in **anxiety** or fear. These behaviors are often exhibited through the effects of respondent learning. For example, the animal with separation anxiety learns through classical conditioning that when it is left alone, it feels fear or anxiety. After a time, the physiologic response of increased heart rate, panting, and trembling occurs every time the animal thinks its owners are preparing to leave. Its fear or anxiety becomes the CR to the owners' cues that they are departing, the CS. Three methods are well documented for treating respondent fear. These include systematic desensitization, counter-conditioning or counter-commanding, and response blocking or flooding.

Systematic desensitization is a procedure by which we change a dog's emotional response to a stimulus. This is done by gradually increasing exposure to the stimulus, starting at a level that does not cause an emotional response. Over a period of several sessions, exposure to the stimulus is gradually increased until the animal no longer responds to it at any level. During a successful desensitization process, the animal never experiences a fear response. This is critical for a positive outcome. When people increase the stimulus level faster than the animal can tolerate, a fear response will occur.

To use systematic desensitization appropriately, it helps to develop a hierarchy of stimuli from least to most stimulating. This can be a simple matter when desensitizing a dog to something like fireworks, for example, where there is a primary single stimulus—noise. Recordings of fireworks are commercially available and can be played at very low levels so that they do not elicit a fear response from the dog. Over time, the sound level is slowly increased until the dog no longer responds to the noise, even when played at a volume similar to real fireworks. Desensitization can take many weeks with multiple sessions per day, depending upon the individual.

Developing the hierarchy of stimuli can be more challenging when the fearful stimulus is something like the approach of strange dogs or people. In this case, several stimulus features have to be managed. For example, the dog's proximity to a strange individual, the size of the individual, how long the individual is in view, and the number of individuals approaching may all be variables to be addressed during the desensitization process. When multiple variables are involved, it is most effective to desensitize the animal to one at a time before moving to another. For example, begin by desensitizing an animal to the approach of a small dog, and once the animal remains calm in the presence of a small dog, move on to desensitizing the same animal to the approach of a large dog. Place the larger dog as far away as necessary, so as not to elicit any fear. Once the animal shows no fear of the larger dog, add more than one dog and so on. The efficacy of desensitization may be improved by combining it with counter-conditioning or counter-commanding.

Counter-conditioning is the process used to substitute an alternative emotional response or behavior that is incompatible with the problem behavior or emotional response you are trying to eliminate. This usually is performed most easily by using food rewards during systematic desensitization. If you are desensitizing a dog to a loud noise by using a recording, for example, you would simply sit with the dog and, as long as it remained calm, provide a continual stream of very small, special food treats. The pleasant emotional response triggered by eating is incompatible with the emotional response of fear or anxiety. This can be made easier to perform because most dogs will not eat when very anxious or fearful. If the dog stops accepting food during the desensitization process, this tells you that you have increased the stimulus too much, too fast.

Counter-commanding is similar to counter-conditioning because while exposing the animal to low levels of the stimulus that it fears, you simultaneously ask the animal to respond to a command such as "sit" and reward the animal (usually with food) for complying. When the animal responds to requests and accepts a food reward as the stimulus is gradually increased, the animal is learning a new behavior. Learning to sit calmly next to the owner rather than barking and lunging at a strange dog or person is an example of learned behavior using counter-commanding or response substitution. Although the techniques of desensitization can be effective tools for changing behavior, they require a great deal of patience, the ability to read subtle cues of fear in the animal, and "props" such as people and dogs to act as the fearful stimulus. When these techniques fail, it is usually because people increased the stimulus too soon, before the animal has had a chance to become fully desensitized to the stimulus at a lower level.

Flooding, also known as *response blocking*, is a technique that exposes an animal to a fearful stimulus at full intensity and prevents the animal from escaping until it ceases to be fearful. This technique can require very long sessions and, if a session ends before the animal stops responding, the animal's fear may intensify rather than diminish. This technique can be traumatic for both the pet and the owner. In addition, when the animal's ability to escape from something it fears is removed, an additional problem, called *learned helplessness* may develop. In cases of learned helplessness, animals learn that they have no control over events, and that how they respond cannot make a difference in their situation. Subsequently, these animals may cease to respond to any stimulus, and owners may find that their pet has new problem behaviors that did not exist before treatment.

> **TECHNICIAN NOTE**   Flooding is a training technique that should be avoided as a treatment for most problem behaviors in pets.

PREVENTING BEHAVIOR PROBLEMS

Many "problem behaviors" are normal, albeit unacceptable, behaviors for the species. Common complaints, such as jumping up on people, pulling on the leash, play biting, house soiling, and excessive vocalizations, often cause owners to relinquish their pet to an animal shelter. As is the case with most behavior problems, they are more easily prevented than cured. Pet owners need to understand that it is simpler to teach an animal acceptable behavior than to stop unacceptable behavior with punishment. When owners realize that inappropriate pet behaviors, such as aggression and house soiling, too often lead to euthanasia of animals in shelters, they may recognize the critical importance of effective training. Many problem behaviors can be approached by adhering to the following five-step plan[1] (Box 5-5).

BOX 5-5	Five-Step Positive Proaction Plan

1. Elicit and reinforce appropriate behavior.
2. Prevent or minimize inappropriate behavior.
3. Meet your pet's behavioral and developmental needs.
4. Use the "take away" method (negative punishment) to discourage inappropriate behavior.
5. Minimize discipline (positive punishment) and use it correctly when necessary.

From Hetts S, Heinke ML, Estep DQ: Behavior wellness concepts for general veterinary practice, J Am Vet Med Assoc 4:506–513, 2004.

BOX 5-6	Proper Use of Food Rewards

- Must be highly favored by animals; they should not get it any other time except when responding to commands
  - Examples for dogs: soft, chewy liver treats; small pieces of cut-up turkey franks or cheese, etc.
  - Examples for cats: whipping cream, cream cheese, tuna, etc.
- Must be very small pieces (about the size of a green pea)
- Once an animal has learned a command, food rewards should stay hidden until the animal responds appropriately; it is a *reward* not a *bribe*.
- When teaching a new behavior, give food every single time (continuous reinforcement) that the animal responds appropriately.
- Once the behavior is established, rewards should be given occasionally (intermittent reinforcement).

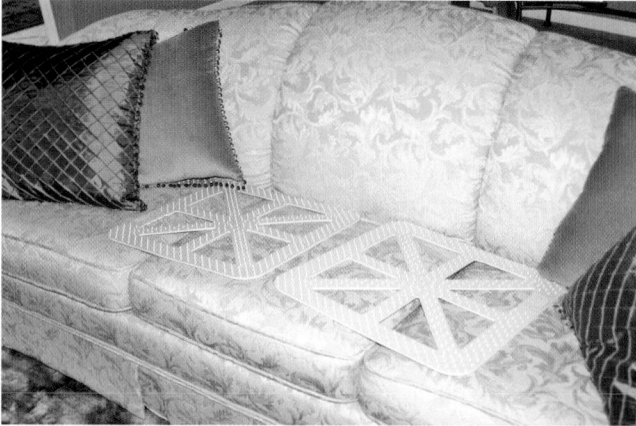

FIGURE 5-1 An example of commercially available products that can discourage a pet from using a particular area of the home.

STEP 1: ELICIT AND REINFORCE APPROPRIATE BEHAVIOR

Most owners are more reactive to their pet than proactive in preventing inappropriate behavior. The result is that pets are frequently scolded or disciplined for unwanted behaviors and are ignored when they behave in an acceptable manner. Veterinary technicians can instruct pet owners to reward their dog when they see it lying quietly and chewing on its own toys, for example, or when it goes to its crate and rests, or when it eliminates outside. In addition, the veterinary technician can assist the owner in determining ways to elicit appropriate behaviors at home. For example, teaching owners to keep food treats readily available when visitors arrive is one way to be proactive when training a dog not to jump up on guests. The dog should be asked to sit when people arrive and should be rewarded when it sits rather than scolded for jumping on people.

Veterinary technicians should also teach owners how to use food rewards appropriately (Box 5-6). Food rewards are often the best way to teach animals new behaviors. Once food rewards have been paired repeatedly with verbal praise, play, or attention, food rewards will not always be needed for the pet to behave appropriately. Initially, food can be used to lure a dog into the appropriate response. For example, using a food treat and passing it slowly over the dog's head toward

the tail will cause most dogs to sit as they follow the lure with their eyes. Once the dog sits, it is immediately given the food reward. The dog's sitting can then be paired with the word "sit," and eventually the treat will no longer have to be visible for the dog to respond to the request "sit." Many pet owners mistakenly believe that if they use food rewards, food will always be needed to get their dog to obey. This occurs only when people do not use food rewards correctly; it is not an inherent problem with using food.

> **TECHNICIAN NOTE**   Food rewards are the best way to teach most pets new behaviors.

The veterinary technician should also be able to direct the owner to websites and other resources to obtain additional information about training and to find an appropriate trainer for their pet (see Box 5-1).

STEP 2: PREVENT OR MINIMIZE INAPPROPRIATE BEHAVIOR

Pet owners should be taught to manage the pet's environment to minimize the unwanted behavior. Remind owners of the old adage "practice makes perfect." The more times an animal is able to practice an inappropriate behavior, such as chewing on furniture or eliminating in the house, the more established those behaviors will be. In the case of young animals, or animals that are in a new or unfamiliar environment, constant supervision is necessary for them to be prevented from making "mistakes." This can be done in many ways, including using crates, baby gates to limit the pet's access to non–pet-proofed rooms, and even tethering the pet to the owner or near the owner (Figure 5-1). Sometimes simply closing the doors to other rooms so that the pet cannot get out of the owners' view is effective.

Crate Training

Crates are one of the most useful tools that pet owners have for preventing unwanted behaviors, yet they are often misused by some clients and are avoided altogether by others, who have never been taught how to use them appropriately. It is true that the crate should not be a place that an adult dog spends most of its life, but it can be a useful training aid for most dogs. Much misinformation exists about crating dogs, such as the fact that the crate mimics a den—something the dog should be automatically comfortable with and even seek out. This is not entirely accurate because in the wild, dogs would never be left alone in a den; other puppies would be there even when the dam leaves. In addition, wild canids become acclimated to the den when they are puppies, but many domestic dogs are expected to adjust to crates as adults. Wild canids use a den only occasionally once they reach adulthood; many dogs are left in crates for several hours a day.

The crate must be appropriate for the size of the dog, and it may take some time to acclimate an adult dog to a crate. The crate must be large enough for the dog to stand at its full height, turn around, and lie down with its legs outstretched. If the dog soils its crate, the first instruction should not be to use a smaller crate. Possible causes for the "accident" should be investigated. For example, was the dog left confined for too long? Did the dog become anxious or frightened while in the crate, or does the dog have a medical condition leading to urgency or incontinence? A dog might soil its crate for many reasons. In these cases, a complete behavioral consult should be recommended. A smaller crate is rarely the answer. Refer to Box 5-7 on teaching a pet to be comfortable in a crate.

> **TECHNICIAN NOTE** When used appropriately, crates are an excellent tool for preventing many problem behaviors in pets.

Remind clients that just because a dog enters a crate willingly does not mean that it is entirely comfortable there alone. Clients should be instructed to watch for signs that the dog is not comfortable in the crate. Reluctance to enter the crate, trembling, and salivating can all be signs that the dog really is not comfortable with being confined to the crate. The best way to confirm this is to collect videotape of the dog while confined in the crate when the owner is gone. If the dog vocalizes, salivates heavily, eliminates in the crate, or attempts to get out of the crate, the dog is not comfortable there. Sometimes pet owners will note that when they come home, the crate has been moved. This usually occurs as the dog is trying frantically to escape from the crate. Injuries to the dog's mouth, feet, or pads are also strong indicators that the dog is not comfortable in the crate. If it is determined that the dog is not comfortable in the crate, the owners should stop confining it there, and other options should be considered. If the behavior is suggestive of separation anxiety, a behavior consultation is recommended.

> **TECHNICIAN NOTE** A dog that is showing fear of a crate should never be forced into the crate.

BOX 5-7 | Teaching a Pet to Be Comfortable in a Crate

- Begin with the crate in a quiet area of the house but not too far away from family activities.
- Leave the door propped open. Wire it open if necessary, so that it cannot close accidentally and frighten the pet.
- Make the crate a pleasant place by putting a comfortable bed or bedding inside.
- If the pet already seems afraid of the crate, begin by feeding it every meal next to the crate.
- After several days, begin moving the bowl closer to the crate, eventually placing it just inside the door of the crate.
- Once the pet eagerly eats out of the bowl, place it in the back of the crate and feed every meal there. Do not attempt to close the door at this point!
- Once the pet is comfortable eating in the crate, begin tossing treats into the crate occasionally, eventually leaving a larger, longer-lasting treat (stuffed Kongs, rawhides, etc.) inside the crate.
- Once the pet goes into the crate eagerly for the treat, spends time in there, and occasionally sleeps in there, you are ready to close the door.
- The first time you close the door, do so only for a few seconds, without leaving the room.
- Slowly increase the length of time that the pet is left in the closed crate, by just a few minutes at a time.
- Once the pet can stay in the crate for about 15 minutes, it can be left alone in the room.
- Initially, these periods should be kept short and increased very slowly.
- Once the pet is comfortable alone in the crate without the owner in the room, the owner can begin to leave the pet alone while leaving the home, again starting at a few minutes and increasing slowly.
- The owner should be advised to always try to avoid letting the pet out of the crate if it is whining or barking. This teaches the pet that it can get out by performing these behaviors. Waiting a few seconds for the pet to stop may be sufficient, but if the pet is vocalizing because it was left in the crate longer than it was comfortable, the owner needs to go back to the last length of time the dog was comfortable (e.g., if the dog begins to vocalize at 15 minutes, go back to 10 minutes at next session; if vocalizing at 10 minutes, go back to 5 minutes).

STEP 3: MEET THE PET'S BEHAVIORAL AND DEVELOPMENTAL NEEDS

Many problem behaviors arise simply because the pet's needs have not been considered and addressed. Veterinary technicians should begin educating pet owners about their pet's behavioral needs from the very first appointment. These discussions are no different from those aimed at teaching appropriate preventive health care. Too many pets are euthanized because they were acquired by someone who had no knowledge of the animal's needs and no ability to meet them. Therefore, it is better that these discussions begin right away. The cat owner who has just adopted a new kitten when he already had one or two cats at home needs to be informed right away of the need for additional litter boxes, because failing to meet this need may lead to house soiling problems.

Chewing is an important behavioral need for puppies, at least during their first 6 months of life. Owners should be instructed to provide the puppy with multiple appropriate objects to chew on, confining them so that they do not have access to inappropriate items and praising them for chewing on their own toys or chews. You should not simply punish the puppy for chewing on inappropriate items because he has a strong behavioral need to chew at this stage of development.

Another important requirement for most pets is physical and mental stimulation. The amount required depends on breed and age. This stimulation, sometimes referred to as *environmental enrichment,* can be provided via toys, exercise, and play. Many unwanted canine behaviors are a result of not having adequate play time or exercise. These can include, but are not limited to, hyperactivity; pushy, annoying, or pestering behavior; excessive vocalization; destructive behavior; and self-injury. Pets need time for social play with people or other animals and for play with toys. A variety of toys support the expression of different behaviors, such as chewing, chasing, stalking, and retrieving. Also, having an adequate number of toys that can be rotated helps hold the pet's interest.

> **TECHNICIAN NOTE** Most pets do not get enough physical exercise or mental stimulation; this often results in problem behaviors.

STEP 4: USE THE "TAKE AWAY" METHOD (NEGATIVE PUNISHMENT) TO DISCOURAGE INAPPROPRIATE BEHAVIOR

The "take away" method is a useful and relatively safe way to make behavioral changes. This is particularly true when training young animals that need to learn which behaviors are acceptable and which are not. The "take away" method, as described in the learning section (see Box 5-4 and Table 5-1), involves removing a valued object from the animal when its behavior becomes inappropriate. For example, if a puppy begins biting or playing too roughly, the owner should be instructed to immediately get up and walk away rather than pushing the puppy away or yelling at it. Responding consistently this way teaches the puppy that these types of behaviors make the fun stop. Cats meowing and dogs barking in an attempt to get attention are also best responded to in this manner. The horse that likes to approach and nibble on clothing can learn that this makes you leave. When animals learn that these behaviors cause people to leave the area and ignore them, they will quickly learn to try a different method for getting attention.

Clients should be instructed that not all behaviors can be changed with this method. Behaviors that are internally motivated will not be responsive to this method because they are not reliant upon any external reinforcement, and negative punishment is not powerful enough to affect these behaviors. For example, barking and meowing may serve to release tension due to feelings of anxiety so are unlikely to be affected by this method. If the horse is biting you because it wants you to leave, then withdrawing only reinforces the behavior rather than extinguishing it. This demonstrates why it is so important to always try to determine the underlying cause of a behavior. Different methods of treatment will be effective depending upon the motivation for the behavior.

STEP 5: MINIMIZE DISCIPLINE (POSITIVE PUNISHMENT) AND USE IT CORRECTLY WHEN NECESSARY

If the previous four steps are followed, discipline becomes unnecessary.

Using punishment appropriately and effectively can be very challenging. For punishment to be effective, it must meet the following criteria:

- *It must occur immediately after the unwanted behavior.* Unless punishment is administered within a couple of seconds of the behavior, the animal is unable to make the association between the punishment and the unwanted behavior. Within a few seconds of the unwanted behavior, the animal has likely performed another behavior, so the animal may even associate the punishment with that behavior rather than with the behavior the owner is trying to stop.

  Many owners mistakenly believe that their pet "knows what it did wrong" because it looks "guilty." The behavior that is interpreted as guilt is often the dog showing **submissive behaviors** when the owner is angry. Dogs are much better at interpreting body language than most people and are particularly aware of nonverbal communication from the owner. Dogs often learn to associate a mess on the floor and the owner's arrival with bad things happening. They therefore demonstrate submissive behaviors when the owner arrives and there is a mess on the floor, but not when the owner arrives and there is no mess on the floor. Dogs do not necessarily make an association between the act of making the mess and bad things happening, so they continue to perform unwanted behaviors and look "guilty" when the owner arrives.

- *It must follow the unwanted behavior every time it occurs.* Most owners are unable to be present every single time a pet performs an unwanted behavior. Because this is the case, many pets are able to perform the behavior some of the time without an unpleasant consequence. Because many unwanted behaviors are inherently rewarding to the pet, the behavior is being intermittently reinforced and made stronger. Punishment is even less likely to be effective. The absolute necessity of imposing punishment immediately after every performance of an unwanted behavior is so difficult that it is an inappropriate choice for managing most problem behaviors.

- *It must be of appropriate intensity to stop the behavior from occurring without causing fear, harm, or anxiety for the pet.* To make these criteria even more difficult to meet, animals learn to tolerate higher levels of aversive stimuli if they are increased gradually rather than being presented at a moderately high intensity immediately. For example, an owner may initially respond to a pet's unwanted behavior by saying "no" quietly. When the pet ignores it, she may say "no" a little louder. The pet may continue to ignore the "no" until the owner has to scream at the dog or even pick up a newspaper and slap the dog to get it to stop. If the owner had simply begun by saying "no" in a firm, authoritative voice, this might have stopped the behavior the first time. Unfortunately, in many cases, the stimulus that is aversive enough to stop an unwanted behavior may also cause fear or anxiety in the pet. Too often, this results in a pet that develops an actual fear of the owner and may be hesitant or nervous around her. The bond between pet and owner can be damaged beyond repair.
- *Remote punishment should be considered.* Remote punishment is one form of punishment that can be useful mostly because it prevents the pet from associating the punishment with the owner. When owners administer punishment, not only can animals learn to fear them, as described earlier, they may also learn simply to avoid the behavior in the owner's presence. For this reason, house soiling pets often learn to just wait until the owners leave the house or the room before eliminating. Administering remote punishment can be as simple as the pet owner hiding around a corner and quietly squirting water at the pet using a water bottle or water gun as the pet begins to perform an unwanted behavior. Because the owner may not always be able to be present to provide the remote punishment, a variety of devices that are commercially available can be effective in the owner's absence. These include motion-activated devices that shoot a blast of air, mats that emit a slight electrical shock when stepped on, and citronella anti-bark collars, to name a few. If remote punishment can be used so that it meets all of these criteria, it can be useful for solving some behavior problems. In addition, it is necessary for the owner to apply all of the first four steps.

> **TECHNICIAN NOTE** **Positive punishment** should be avoided as a response to most pet behavior problems because most pet owners cannot use it effectively.

HABITUATION TO HANDLING

A part of every new puppy and kitten visit should involve educating pet owners about how to raise a puppy or kitten that will be physically and behaviorally healthy. One aspect of this is teaching them how to habituate the pet to circumstances that it is likely to encounter during its lifetime.

All dogs and cats, regardless of their age, can be habituated to handling procedures. This is most easily performed when animals are still young; it can be accomplished in older animals as well, but this takes longer. In addition, some older animals that have developed fear of certain procedures will require desensitization and counter-conditioning. *Habituation* means that an animal should be exposed frequently, and in a nonthreatening manner, to gentle handling that mimics commonly performed procedures such as nail trimming, teeth brushing, taking rectal temperatures, examining and treating mouth and ears, and brushing. For example, in starting to habituate a pet to nail trims, the feet should be picked up and stroked then released several times a day. Every time this is done, the pet should immediately be given a very small food reward. After the pet seems used to having its feet handled gently, the next step might be to pick up the feet and extend the nail as if it were going to be cut. Again, every repetition should be followed by a food treat. Once the pet seems accustomed to this handling, feet can be picked up, and nail trimmers may be used to mimic cutting a nail, the pet is given a treat. After several repetitions, a nail might be cut; this is followed by a food treat. In the beginning, cutting just one nail at a time will ensure that the pet remains relaxed, unafraid, and focused on the treat that it now knows it will receive. After a period of a few weeks, most pets will be willing to have their nails trimmed because they have associated the procedure with receiving a treat.

> **TECHNICIAN NOTE** All animals can be habituated to restraint and common handling procedures, but beginning when they are young may make the task easier.

CHOOSING A PET

Although many behavior problems can be prevented with good **socialization**, this may not be enough to offset the plethora of problems associated with an owner's poor choice of pet. The species, breed, and gender of an animal should be thoughtfully considered by the owner before a selection is made. Potential owners should be encouraged to discuss possibilities with veterinary personnel before making an acquisition. With some knowledge of the owner's lifestyle, a veterinary technician may determine that the potential new pet owner does not have adequate time or living space to accommodate a dog, and that a cat may be a better choice.

Veterinary technicians may help pet owners select appropriate breeds by discussing with the owner the work the dog was bred to carry out. For example, a Border Collie that was bred to herd sheep all day may be a poor choice for a working couple living in a high rise in the city, unless they have a few hours every day to devote to exercising the dog in an appropriate manner. The Akita, which was bred as a hunting and guard dog in Japan, may not be the best choice for a family with small children. A variety of excellent texts are available to assist pet owners in learning more about dog breeds. One of these books, *The Perfect Puppy*, is included in the "Recommended Readings" list at the end of the chapter.

Potential dog owners should be encouraged to avoid choosing a breed because they met one dog of that breed. A single dog may not necessarily be representative of the breed. People should be encouraged to meet several dogs of the breed they are interested in, talk to several different people owning or breeding that breed, and review more than one book on the breed. Once a particular breed has been decided upon, owners should be educated on how to locate a responsible breeder. High-quality, responsible breeders should not sell puppies younger than 8 weeks of age and should be willing to provide some type of written guarantee as to the health and temperament of the dog. They should be willing to take the dog back if for some reason it proves to be a poor match for the family. When visiting the breeder, it should be possible to meet at least one, if not both, of the parents of the litter. The parents should exhibit behavior that you would find acceptable in your own home. If they are barking at or hiding from the visitors, that is a very good indication of the behavior that the chosen pup may display.

Choosing a puppy from the litter should be done with care. Although the idea of temperament testing puppies in an attempt to determine suitability to different homes has become popular in recent years, no test has yet been validated. In addition, the temperament of a puppy younger than 8 weeks of age is unlikely to be representative of its temperament or behavior as an adult. However, some common sense should be applied to choosing the puppy. A puppy that cowers away from visitors could grow into a fearful puppy, so very shy or fearful puppies should be avoided. Generally speaking, however, the behavior of the parents is the best guide as to the future behavior of the pups.

These same guidelines for choosing a puppy can be applied to choosing from a mixed breed litter. When a parent is not available, for example when choosing a shelter pup, one simply has to rely on the behavior of the pup and choose one that is not extremely fearful. Choosing older mixed breed dogs from a shelter can be a little bit more challenging but should not be avoided if one is not interested in purchasing a pure bred. The pet owner should be encouraged to choose a pet from a shelter that collects a behavioral history on dogs that are owner surrendered, performs some behavioral evaluation on all pets that it puts up for adoption, shares all of this information with the potential adopter, counsels with potential adopters at the time of adoption, and offers follow-up counseling should the owner have difficulty with the pet after they take it home. Breed-specific rescues can be a good choice for acquiring a new dog if someone is interested in a particular breed but for whatever reason would rather acquire an adult. Many breed rescues have individuals who foster the dogs in their home, so they can

tell you more about the temperament of the dog in their environment. It should be emphasized that following all of these suggestions does not guarantee a result. It simply increases the chance of success at choosing a pet that has the potential for developing into a well-behaved, normal animal.

MEDICATIONS AND TREATING BEHAVIOR PROBLEMS

Psychotropic drugs can be excellent tools for treating behavior problems. The main reason for using these medications to treat behavior problems is twofold: to prevent suffering, as in many cases of separation anxiety or severe **phobias**, and to assist with behavior modification. Used alone, medications rarely solve behavior problems. They may initially help enough to give the owners the impression that the problem is solved, but they do not usually lead to dramatic, lasting behavior changes. An active program of behavior modification is usually necessary to achieve that.

One common scenario in which medication alone may lead to a satisfactory outcome is the pet with thunderstorm or fireworks phobias. In the case of fireworks phobias, if the likelihood of fireworks is occasional and predictable, a medication such as a benzodiazepine may be all that is needed to keep the pet safe and comfortable and the owner satisfied. In cases of thunderstorm phobias, where the pet lives in an area where storms are mostly limited to a few months of the year and are somewhat predictable, medications alone may be adequate. Owners should be informed that desensitization to loud noises (see the section on learning) is highly effective and could be used to eliminate or at least decrease the need for medication.

When medications do appear to be working without behavior modification, clients should be aware that if they only give medication, the pet may require it for the rest of its life, and with some, tolerance may develop and their efficacy may decrease over time. When used in conjunction with behavior modification, the goal is often to eventually stop using medication, or at least to decrease the dosage to the lowest possible amount that will help with control of the problem behavior. However, there will always be some animals that will require medication for the remainder of their life.

At the time of this writing, only three psychotropic medications have been Food and Drug Administration (FDA) approved for use in animals with behavior problems: Clomicalm (clomipramine), Reconcile (fluoxetine), and Anipryl (selegiline). All other psychotropics, although used frequently in veterinary behavioral medicine, are being used in an off-label manner, and the practice should have an informed consent statement signed by the owner. See Table 5-2 for a list of some of these medications, dosages, common uses, side effects, and contraindications.

TABLE 5-2	Some of the Psychotropic Drugs More Commonly Used in Veterinary Behavior Medicine				
DRUG BY CLASS GENERIC (BRAND)	**DOG DOSE**	**CAT DOSE**	**POSSIBLE SIDE EFFECTS**	**CONTRAINDICATIONS**	**COMMONLY USED FOR**
Antipsychotics Acepromazine	0.5-2.0 mg/kg q 8 h or PRN	1.0-2.0 mg/kg PRN	Bradycardia, hypotension, seizures; with chronic use, tardive dyskinesia	Not safe for long-term use. Rarely an appropriate choice for problem behavior	Only for severe occasional anxiety where likelihood of injury is high; use to sedate
Azapirones Buspirone	0.5-2.0 mg/kg q 8-24 h	0.5-1.0 mg/kg q 12 h	Sedation; increased friendliness in cats	Use w/caution in patients on monoamine oxidase inhibitors (MAOIs), erythromycin, or itraconazole	Anxiety; inter-cat aggression; historically used for feline urine marking—less effective than selective serotonin reuptake inhibitors (SSRIs) or tricyclic antidepressants (TCAs)
Benzodiazepines Diazepam	0.5-2.0 mg/kg q 4 h	0.1-1.0 mg/kg q 4 h	Ataxia, sedation, increased appetite, hepatic necrosis, anxiety, hallucinations, insomnia, paradoxical excitation. Addictive! Withdraw slowly.	Use w/caution in patients w/kidney or liver damage or glaucoma and in pregnant or lactating females	Ideal for predictable, situational anxiety or for fear-related problems without aggression. Fast acting; not long acting. Historically useful for feline urine marking, but less effective than SSRIs or TCAs
Alprazolam	0.02-0.1 mg/kg q 4 h	0.0125-0.25 mg/kg q 8 h			
Hormones Progestins	Varies by product	Varies by product	Polyphagia, polydipsia, sedation; with long-term treatment, numerous irreversible effects possible	Many; should be a treatment of last resort after all other medications have been tried	Likely useful only to suppress behaviors influenced by androgens
MAOIs Selegiline	0.5-1 mg/kg q 24 h	0.5-1.0 mg/kg q 24 h	Restlessness, agitation, disorientation, vomiting, diarrhea	DO not give in conjunction with TCAs, SSRIs, or other MAOIs; use with caution in patients on metronidazole, prednisone, or trimethoprim-sulfamethoxazole; do not administer until 5 weeks after discontinuation of fluoxetine	Approved only for canine cognitive dysfunction; has been used in cats for cognitive dysfunction. In Europe has been used to treat a variety of disorders, including fears, phobias, anxiety, and aggression

Continued

TABLE 5-2	Some of the Psychotropic Drugs More Commonly Used in Veterinary Behavior Medicine—cont'd				
DRUG BY CLASS GENERIC (BRAND)	**DOG DOSE**	**CAT DOSE**	**POSSIBLE SIDE EFFECTS**	**CONTRAINDICATIONS**	**COMMONLY USED FOR**
Opioid Antagonists					
Naltrexone	1-2.2 mg/kg q 12-24 h	25-50 mg/cat q 24 h	Gastrointestinal effects, mainly diarrhea	Do not use in patients with severe liver, kidney, or heart disease	For treatment of stereotypic behaviors; may be most effective in very early stages of development of the behavior
SSRIs					
Fluoxetine	1.0-2.0 mg/ kg q 24 h	0.5-1.5 mg/kg q 24 h	*Uncommon but may include sedation, anorexia, nausea, constipation, tremors, irritability, agitation, aggression, mania, decreased libido, seizures	Use w/caution in patients w/diabetes. Do not use in patients w/glaucoma or liver or kidney dysfunction or in pregnant or lactating animals. Use w/caution in patients on TCAs, tramadol, chlorpheniramine, trazadone, buspirone, or any serotonergic compound (e.g., tryptophan)	Most any anxiety-related condition; feline urine marking, separation anxiety, generalized anxiety, fears, phobias, and compulsive disorders
Paroxetine	1.0-1.5 mg/ kg q 24 h	0.5-1.5 mg/kg q 24 h			
TCAs					
Amitriptyline	1-6 mg/kg q 12 h	0.5-2.0 mg/kg q 12 -24 h	Sedation, constipation, diarrhea, urinary retention, appetite changes, ataxia, decreased tear production, dry mouth, arrhythmias, tachycardia, mydriasis, and blood pressure alterations. All may be more likely with amitriptyline	Do not give in conjunction with MAOIs, antipsychotics, anticholinergics, antidepressants, antithyroid agents, or barbiturates. Avoid in breeding, pregnant, or lactating animals and in animals w/ liver disease, glaucoma, heart disease, or history of seizures. Clomipramine may decrease thyroxine levels	Most any anxiety-related condition; feline urine marking, separation anxiety, compulsive disorders. Some may be useful for neuropathic pain and pruritus
Clomipramine	1-3 mg/kg q 12 h	0.25-1.3 mg/ kg q 24 h			

Note: All doses are given orally.

*Most common side effects are sedation and anorexia.

CANINE

DEVELOPMENT

The behavior of every organism is a result of complex interactions between genetics, early developmental experiences, learning, and the environment in which the animal lives. Experiences that occur in utero have even been found to have varying effects on the behavior of the animal later in life. For example, it has been postulated that the female pup developing in a uterine horn surrounded by male pups and thus exposed to large quantities of androgens may ultimately display more behaviors typical of a male dog.

The early development of the dog has been studied extensively and has been divided into four stages or periods:
1. The neonatal period.
2. The transition period.
3. The socialization period.
4. The juvenile period.

During the neonatal period (approximately the first 2 weeks of life), puppies are completely helpless and reliant upon the dam for their survival. Their neurosensory systems are immature and motor skills are limited. The eyes and ears are completely closed, so they cannot see or hear. They cannot lift their body with their legs, so they move forward by paddling with their forelimbs. Neonatal puppies are very sensitive to tactile stimuli and olfactory cues, which allow them to search for and locate the nipple, and they spend most of their time sleeping and eating. During this period, the anogenital region must be stimulated for the puppy to eliminate. The dam usually does this by licking the area. Studies have shown that short periods of daily handling during this stage of development can have positive long-term effects such as increased confidence and exploratory behavior.

The transition period is marked by a rapid rate of sensory and motor development. The eyes open during this period (10 to 16 days) and the puppy begins to eliminate on its own, outside of the nest if possible. The puppy will begin walking and play fighting with littermates and can growl and wag its tail. It begins to show an interest in solid food at this time, and when the ear canals open at about 14 to 20 days, it begins to demonstrate the "startle" response to loud noises. By 3 to 4 weeks of age, the transition period ends and the socialization period begins. Although the socialization period is considered to last from about 4 to 14 weeks, it is important to understand that none of these periods is completely distinct, and much overlap occurs.

The socialization period is, as the name implies, the period of time in which the puppy learns about its environment and how to interact with its mother, its siblings, and humans. During this period, puppies are highly motivated to explore, but at the same time, they are somewhat fearful of novel stimuli. Puppies begin to demonstrate fearful postures at this time, such as tail tucking, and if separated from their dam or siblings during this period, they vocalize loudly. Puppies not exposed to a variety of stimuli during this period, including other dogs, people, sights, sounds, and substrates, are more likely to be fearful of novel stimuli as adults. Puppies not well socialized to a variety of dogs and people are likely to show fearful responses and even aggression toward strangers and strange dogs as adults.

> **TECHNICIAN NOTE** Proper socialization is critical if a puppy is to develop into a good pet.

Socialization during this period may be made more difficult if the puppy has a shy or fearful nature. Studies have demonstrated that fearfulness or shyness is a highly heritable trait in dogs, so socialization, although not impossible for these dogs, must be handled carefully. For socialization to be successful, experiences with novel stimuli must be positive ones. Ideally, all puppies should be exposed to a large variety of the environmental features that they are likely to encounter as an adult. However, these experiences must not be frightening. In some cases, as when meeting new people, it may be beneficial to have a stranger offer the puppy small, tasty treats, so that the puppy learns to associate strangers

with good things happening. Puppies that have good positive experiences with novelty during the socialization period are more likely to make good pets as adults. They will be less fearful, more confident, and more capable of dealing with novel stimuli later in life.

> **TECHNICIAN NOTE** Fearfulness and shyness are highly heritable traits in dogs.

During the socialization period, the dog develops its substrate preference for elimination. This is why some dogs acquired from kennels or pet stories after about 14 weeks of age may be difficult to housetrain. They may be used to eliminating on hard surfaces rather than grass, so they are more likely to be comfortable eliminating on the floor. Owners desiring a puppy that will ultimately eliminate outside should be taught the importance of helping the dog develop a substrate preference outdoors from a very early age. Although it is not impossible to change a dog's substrate preference once it is mature, it can be much more difficult than teaching it the desired substrate from a very early age.

The juvenile period could be considered simply an extension of the socialization period. This period, lasting up to 6 months, is the time at which most dogs reach puberty and may begin to show adult sexual behaviors. During this time, the dog should continue to be exposed to new people, places, and dogs in a positive and unthreatening way. Although sexually mature at 6 months of age, dogs are not considered socially mature until 18 months of age or later.

SOCIAL BEHAVIOR

The dog was the first species to be domesticated by man, several thousand years ago. Although domesticated from the wolf, domestication has made numerous critical changes in the dog's behavior, so any comparison must be made with caution. Unlike wolf packs, dog social groups are small and open to outsiders and are not typically made up of related individuals. Wolf packs form relatively stable social hierarchies; however, evidence suggests that groups of free-ranging dogs do not do this. Other misconceptions about dominance in the dog abound, including the idea that dominance is somehow a personality trait. In fact, dominance describes the role taken in a relationship between two individuals. It is common among dogs to see one take the **dominant role** in a relationship with one dog and a **subordinate role** with a different dog. These roles may even change between individuals depending on the context in which the interaction takes place. Many dogs are mistakenly labeled by their owner as "dominant," when in fact they are fearful. The misconception that dog behavior problems are caused by dominance has led to the application of a variety of cruel, unnecessary forms of dog training. Dog owners need to be warned against the mistaken belief that they must somehow physically dominate their dogs. Scruff shakes, alpha rolls, and other forms of physical intimidation are to be avoided at all costs. In some cases, they may result in the owner being bitten, and they are likely to make the fearful dog's behavior problems worse.

> ⓘ **TECHNICIAN NOTE** Dog owners should be instructed to avoid the use of physical intimidation with their dog; techniques such as scruff shakes and alpha rolls are likely to cause more problems than they solve.

Dogs use a variety of visual and olfactory cues when beginning, forming, and maintaining social relationships. When unfamiliar dogs meet, they usually begin by sniffing each other. Generally speaking, sniffing begins at the head and then moves toward the tail. Typically, the dog that approaches and begins to sniff first may resist being sniffed himself. Although the dog that is being sniffed is most likely to try to terminate the interaction, it is unlikely to attempt to sniff the other dog. A dog attempting to take the dominant role will usually approach the other dog in a "T-position" in relation to the other dog's shoulder and begin sniffing (Figure 5-2). The other dog, if accepting a subordinate role, will turn its head away from the approaching dog. If it does not want to accept the subordinate role, it may resist being sniffed and may attempt to sniff the other dog. Another way in which a dog may signal submission is by rolling over on it back and exposing the inguinal region. This area is then sniffed by the dominant dog. If a dog is being solicitous and not aggressive, it is likely to raise a paw loosely at the same time that it demonstrates a loosely wagging tail and play face (Figure 5-3). The play bow is the classic sign that often follows; it is used by the dog to indicate that what follows is play (Figure 5-4).

READING CANINE BODY LANGUAGE

The veterinary technician who is aware of the visual cues used by the dog will be able to interact with dogs more safely and to teach dog owners how to accurately interpret their dog's behavior, thus often keeping the dog owner safe as well. Fear, a common cause for many behavior problems, produces certain physiologic signs such as tachycardia, tachypnea, elevated blood pressure, and dilated pupils. In addition, fearful dogs may pant, salivate, and tremble. Dogs that are fearful or anxious will also display body postures consistent with these emotions. The fearful dog will lower the ears, head, and neck. The tail will be lowered and possibly even tucked between the rear legs and up against the abdomen. The fearful dog probably will avoid eye contact. The eyes will be wide open and the whites of the eyes may be showing. They may turn their entire body sideways to you and roll over in a posture of complete submission or may simply try

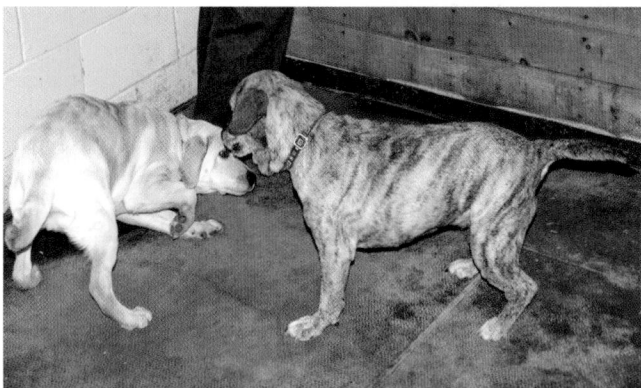

FIGURE 5-3 The pup (on the left) meets a dog that is behaving a little bit too aggressively. She is demonstrating a very submissive, somewhat fearful posture, along with the appeasement gesture of the raised forepaw.

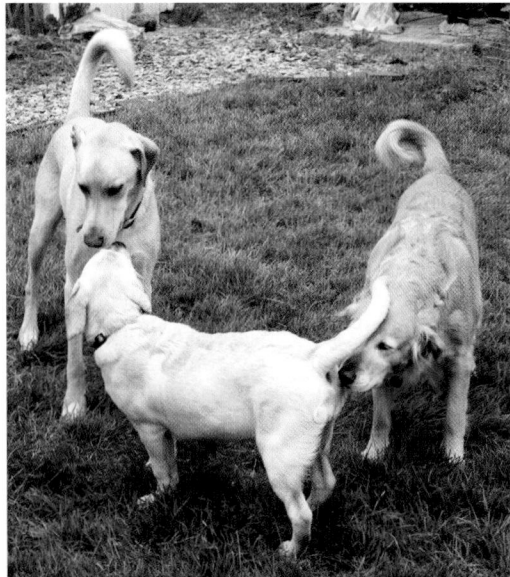

FIGURE 5-2 Two resident dogs greet a 5-month-old puppy. Note the "T" postures taken by the resident dogs and the upright forward manner of the dog on the left. The puppy is behaving confidently by greeting nose to nose but remains slightly submissive in her posture.

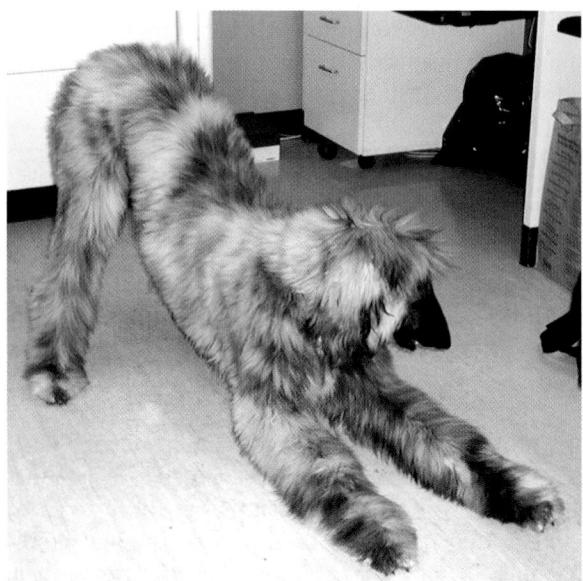

FIGURE 5-4 The typical "play bow" of the dog attempting to solicit play.

to escape the situation completely. The message being sent by the animal demonstrating these postures is "Don't come any closer!" If you continue to approach the dog displaying these signs, you should be prepared for it to bare teeth, snap, growl, or bite in a further attempt to stop the approach. The likelihood that the dog will progress quickly to biting, as opposed to just snarling or snapping, depends on many factors, including learning and experience. Many dogs that are punished for showing their teeth, snarling, or snapping will learn quickly to forego those gestures and bite first, so although not all dogs showing fearful signs will bite, they should be approached with caution, as if they may.

In addition to these more obvious visual signals, one should be aware that dogs show some very subtle signs of being anxious or uncomfortable, often in combination with the signs already discussed—sometimes before they even show those more obvious visual cues. Most commonly, anxious, fearful dogs will lick their lips repeatedly, yawn, look away, or suddenly sit and scratch or lick. These behaviors can be recognized as fear or anxiety reflected in the dog's overall appearance. The anxious dog will appear stiffer and not relaxed or loose as a comfortable dog will.

> **TECHNICIAN NOTE** Fearful dogs can show several subtle visual cues such as yawning, lip licking, or scratching, in addition to the more obvious cues such as shaking, panting, and salivating.

Most human directed aggression in dogs is **fear-related aggression** and does not indicate that the dog is trying to be "dominant," as many try to suggest. The dog's visual cues will clearly demonstrate this if one is observant and knows what to look for. The fearfully aggressive dog, as previously described, will probably have its ears and tail tucked. These dogs are likely to be backing away; although some dogs may lunge forward initially, most will then try to escape the situation. This directly contrasts with the offensively aggressive dog (one that may be trying to take the dominant role), whose body will be stiff, with weight on the forelegs and with the tail, ears, and head held upward and stiff. Even the bared teeth of an offensively aggressive dog differ from those of a fearful dog. The offensively aggressive dog will retract the lips around the most rostral part of the mouth, showing mostly canines and incisors (Figure 5-5). The fearful dog will be more likely to open its mouth wide and retract its lips in such a way as to show most or all of its teeth (Figure 5-6).

> **TECHNICIAN NOTE** Most problem behaviors occur as a result of fear or anxiety—not because the dog is trying to be dominant.

COPING WITH BEHAVIOR IN THE CLINIC

Most problem behaviors seen within the veterinary clinical setting occur as a result of fear. Because of the hectic schedule in most animal hospitals, little attention is usually paid

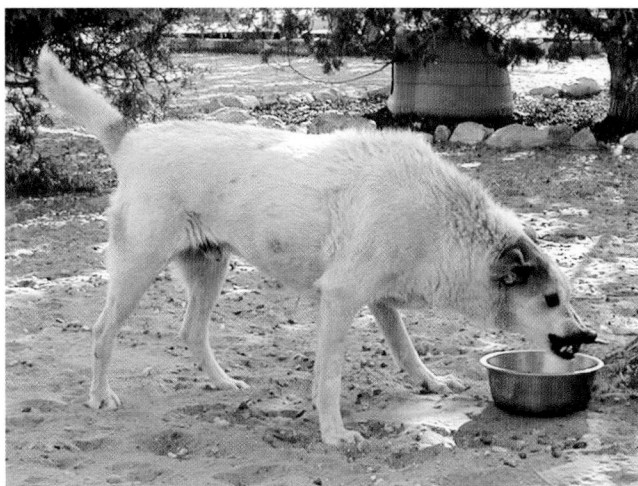

FIGURE 5-5 A dog demonstrating relatively offensive body postures over food. Note the lips retracted just over the rostral-most part of the mouth, the piloerection, the upright stiff tail, and the weight on the fore end.

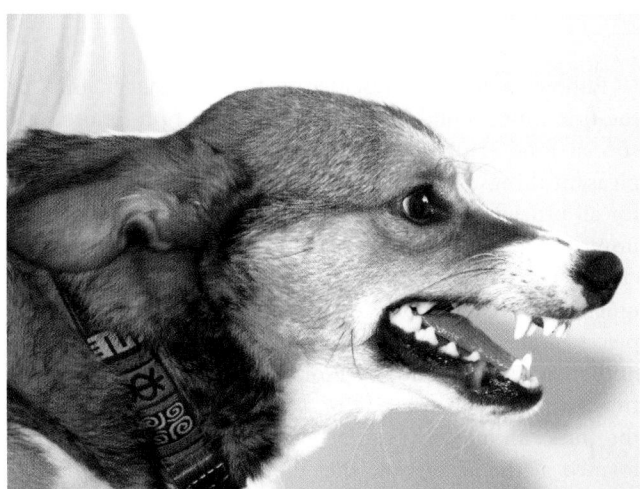

FIGURE 5-6 The face of a fearfully aggressive dog. Note the laid back ears, the dilated pupils, and the lips retracted to show all of the teeth and the open mouth. (Photo courtesy Heather Mohan-Gibbons.)

to what the dog is experiencing during the visit. If the dog is struggling, additional people may be called in to assist with restraint. By forcing the fearful dog to submit to frightening manipulation, it is essentially "taught" that going to the veterinary clinic is an experience to be afraid of, and the dog's future behavior is likely to be even worse. This problem develops as a result of classical conditioning (see the section on learning). The dog associates a fearful emotional state with the experience in the veterinary clinic. When these associations occur repeatedly, the dog soon begins to experience fear simply when approaching the veterinary clinic or walking in the front door. Dogs that travel in the car only to be taken to the veterinary clinic may eventually begin to display signs of fear as soon as they are placed in the car; some will soon begin to resist getting into the car.

The veterinary technician who has an understanding of these naturally occurring events can change the way he or she works with the animal and can prevent the dog from making these associations in the first place, for example, when presented with puppies for their first visits, or at least can work to decrease the fearful association in older dogs. How a person approaches a fearful dog is very important. The technician should avoid staring at and reaching over or bending over toward a fearful dog. The dog should be approached by turning sideways so as not to present the largest most fearful image. In addition, standing several feet from the dog, squatting down, looking at the dog with a sideways glance, and offering a slightly outstretched hand gives the dog the opportunity to make the first approach. This helps the technician to evaluate just how fearful the dog is. If it shrinks away, rather than approaching, or if it lifts its lips or growls, you have been warned that there is a greater likelihood that it will use aggression to protect itself.

> **TECHNICIAN NOTE**　One should avoid staring at and reaching or bending over a fearful animal.

Puppies and dogs presented to the veterinary clinic for the first time should be given lots of attention, praise, and special food treats, so that they associate the clinic with pleasant things. The least restraint possible should be used for all procedures, and every procedure should be followed immediately by a treat. These food rewards should be soft, chewy, very small pieces of food that the dog consumes quickly, so that it looks to the handler for another. Small pieces of cheese or turkey hot dogs, soft liver treats, peanut butter, and canned spray cheese are excellent for this purpose. In many cases when a dog or a puppy is not yet fearful of the clinic, an injection can be given or an examination performed at the same time that the puppy is eating. Peanut butter can be smeared on the examination table in front of the dog, or someone can stand in front of the dog, offering treats by hand.

One should be aware that a very frightened dog will not eat, so if the patient refuses the food, this is a signal that it is already afraid and should be handled in a special way. In these cases, only the necessary restraint should be used, and the dog should be removed from the examination table as soon as possible and provided with a food reward. Sometimes having the pet owner offer the food reward will increase the chance that the dog will take it. In cases where dogs are extremely fearful, sedation or even anesthesia (if the owner will allow it) will prevent the dog's association between its fearful emotional state and the clinic from being further reinforced. Desensitization of these dogs can then be recommended.

> **TECHNICIAN NOTE**　When a healthy dog refuses a highly palatable food treat, this is usually a sign that it is very afraid.

Owners of fearful dogs should be encouraged to bring their dogs to the clinic frequently only to be walked through the door, petted, and fed a few treats. If the dog has frequent regular exposure to the clinic with no frightening experiences, it can lose its fear of the clinic. Once this is accomplished, occasional visits should also include being placed on the examination table, given a treat, and allowed to back down. With time, treats should be associated with all procedures such as performing physical examinations, taking the temperature, trimming nails, and so forth.

INTRODUCING A NEW DOG

Many new pet introductions fail because pet owners are unaware of things they can do to make introductions less stressful and more likely to succeed. Dog introductions ideally should be made in a neutral area, rather than bringing a new dog into the home and immediately turning it loose in the territory of the existing pet. These introductions should be performed in any open area away from the house, even a neighbor's yard, as long as the existing dog does not spend much time there. Both dogs should be on a leash at this time and should be allowed to meet and interact while the owners observe for normal greeting behaviors and ideally some play solicitation. If both dogs take an offensive or aggressive stance, then the two should be separated for a while and reintroduced again the next day for a few minutes. These reintroductions should be repeated until the dogs appear more relaxed with each other, and at least one dog shows a willingness to display subordinate behaviors. Once both dogs seem comfortable and willing to interact in a relatively nonaggressive manner, they can be introduced in the owner's home or fenced-in yard. The dogs should simply have plenty of space for interacting and for withdrawing from the interaction if they desire. Once the dogs are behaving well with each other in this context, they may be ready to interact on a regular basis. However, keeping them separated except for times when the owner can supervise would be best for the first few days or weeks, depending on the degree of friendliness demonstrated by the dogs toward each other.

COMMON BEHAVIOR PROBLEMS
Unruly Behaviors

Unruly behaviors such as jumping on people, mouthing or playing too roughly, pulling on the leash, or barking excessively, although normal behaviors for the most part, can be very frustrating for dog owners. The veterinary technician can educate people about these behaviors and instruct them how to use the Five-Step Positive Proaction Plan to deal with them. For example, all dogs should be taught to sit for attention rather than jumping up to greet people face to face. The dog should be ignored completely when it is excited and jumping. This includes instructing people not to push it away or yell at it or even make eye contact. As soon as the dog has relaxed enough to respond to a command, it can be asked to sit and is given lots of attention as long as it remains sitting.

Mouthing and rough play (**play-related aggression**) can be approached in a similar way. When playing with a dog, the second it begins to play too roughly (or teeth make contact with skin), the owner must be prepared to get up and walk away. Once the dog learns that using its teeth on humans stops the play entirely, it will be less likely to repeat that behavior.

> **TECHNICIAN NOTE** Almost all unruly behaviors can be corrected by applying the Five-Step Positive Proaction Plan.

Leash walking can be very problematic, especially for owners of large dogs, and can severely detract from the pleasure people get from their pet. Head halters, such as the Gentle Leader, Snoot Loop, or Halti, and no-pull harnesses should be recommended rather than choke collars. Head halters give the owner more humane control because they are controlling the dog's head. Imagine trying to control a horse with a collar around its neck! Owners may need help in choosing the proper head collar for their pet; ideally, such collars should be fit by the technician because proper fit is critical to their efficacy. Selling head collars and charging for this service could serve as an excellent profit center for the clinic, in addition to aiding the client with control of their pet. Dogs wearing head halters can also be much easier to control in the clinic during examination and other minor procedures. The technician can teach dog owners one very helpful tip for walking their dog: When the leash is loose, keep walking. The minute the leash becomes tight around the dog's neck, for example, when the dog starts to forge ahead, stop walking. As soon as the dog stops, begin to walk again. Most dogs quickly learn that a loose leash means "go" and a tight leash means "stop." This simple lesson can greatly increase the pleasure owners get from walking their dog and can make the dog easier to bring to the clinic. Pets that are easy for the owner to bring to the clinic are much more likely to get appropriate preventive health care.

> **TECHNICIAN NOTE** Veterinary technicians should be knowledgeable about canine head halters. They should be prepared to recommend specific types of halters, to properly size them for the owner, and to provide instruction in how to put them on and use them for training.

Excessive barking can be an extremely challenging problem because if you cannot determine why the dog is barking, you cannot begin to control the problem. Dogs bark for many reasons: in play, in greeting, as a warning, to make contact, or to gain attention. Problem barking can thus develop when dogs learn to use it to get attention from their owner or secondarily as a result of fear, anxiety, territorial behaviors, or other aggressive threats. In some cases, barking can become repetitive and ritualized, sometimes in association with other repetitive behaviors, and can have a pathophysiologic basis. These cases are likely to require consultation with a specialist. Owners can be taught to prevent attention-seeking barking by never responding to a barking dog. Waiting several seconds after the dog has stopped barking before giving it attention will help to prevent it from learning that barking gets it what it wants.

Fear, Phobias, and Anxiety

One of the most common underlying causes for canine problem behaviors is fear or anxiety. No one understands fully why some dogs exhibit extreme fear, anxiety, or phobias, but this behavior is likely due to a combination of factors, including inherited temperament, early experiences, and/or lack of appropriate socialization. In some cases, a single traumatic incident can cause a dog to develop fear of a stimulus, and it may then generalize this fear to other similar stimuli. Evidence is increasing that many of these problems are a result of abnormalities at the neurophysiologic level within the brain.

Body language and some of the physiologic signs of fear and anxiety in dogs have already been reviewed. A fearful or anxious animal may demonstrate hypervigilance, avoidance behaviors, aberrant appetite, vomiting or diarrhea, and vocalization, ranging from whining to barking. Growling is likely with fearfully aggressive dogs. Animals under chronic stress will begin to show signs consistent with constant stimulation of the hypothalamic-pituitary-adrenal axis (HPA) and frequent release of glucocorticoids and glucose into the bloodstream. These can include weight loss, the presence of a stress leukogram, and decreased immunity to disease. Some pets under chronic stress demonstrate increased motor activity and repetitive activity that can lead to self-injury, such as lick granulomas. Injured pads and toenails as well as damage to teeth and gums, along with other abrasions or lacerations, are common in dogs that are attempting escape owing to severe fear or anxiety. The technician should be able to recognize these signs and teach pet owners how to recognize them.

> **TECHNICIAN NOTE** Chronic fear or anxiety can lead to stress and subsequently to illness.

Unless the fear or anxiety develops as the result of an extremely traumatic event, most cases will develop in adolescence or around the time of social maturity (18 to 36 months). Aged animals that are presented for sudden onset of fear- or anxiety-related problems should be assessed for other signs of canine cognitive dysfunction because fear and anxiety appear to occur commonly in association with canine cognitive dysfunction.

Technicians should also be aware that one of the most important things that they can do for owners of fearful or anxious dogs is to help them recognize the problem right away and understand how they can at least prevent fear or anxiety from worsening. As has already been described regarding fear of the veterinary clinic, fears and anxieties worsen with repeated experience. Unfortunately, many pet owners mistakenly believe that they can cure their pet's fear or anxiety by providing repeated exposure to the stimuli that they fear. They believe that they are "socializing" their dog. The technician can instruct owners that socialization is what you are doing when you expose a young animal to stimuli *that the dog does not already fear*. Once fear or anxiety is associated with a particular event or place (via classical conditioning), gradual desensitization is needed to decrease the dog's fear. Therefore, the best response initially to a dog with fear or anxiety is to prevent, to the greatest extent possible, its exposure to any of the things that cause it fear or anxiety. This may involve decreasing walks for dogs that display fear of strange people or dogs or other stimuli while walking. For owners living in apartments or condominiums, who must walk their dog for elimination, determining when the best time is and where the best places are for avoiding those stimuli may be the best that they can do. It is critical that you stress to pet owners that these avoidance tactics are not treatment for the problem. They are temporary interventions that will prevent the problem from worsening until a complete assessment, diagnosis, and treatment plan have been developed by a veterinarian or a qualified behaviorist.

> **TECHNICIAN NOTE** One of the first and most important steps in treating most behavior problems is avoidance of the stimulus that leads to the behaviors.

Separation anxiety is a very serious and common form of anxiety in dogs, so it is deserving of additional comment. Separation anxiety at its worst can lead to severe injury and even death to dogs that, in their panic to escape confinement, tear out nails, break teeth, or, upon escaping, are hit by a car. Even more tragic may be the dog that experiences great distress but only vocalizes, salivates, pants, or paces, because in this case, the owner may never be aware of how much the dog is suffering. Many people remain unaware of their dog's separation anxiety until it does some damage to the home that causes the owner distress. For this reason alone, the most valuable thing the technician can do when confronted with a dog that may have separation anxiety is to educate the owner about this condition.

Separation anxiety is a form of distress, anxiety, and often even panic that occurs in the absence (or in the perceived absence) of the owner or another attachment figure. The severity of separation anxiety varies, with some pets being relaxed as long as some person is present. Other dogs become distressed if they are separated from one particular person to whom they are attached, and the presence of other dogs or people does nothing to decrease the anxiety. Some dogs can demonstrate the same level of destruction, house soiling, and vocalization because they become aroused about other events that occur when their owner is gone. These can include thunderstorms, other loud noises or frightening events, the presence of other animals outside of the home,

and even the presence of small mammals under the home or in the walls. A young dog that is showing these same signs may simply be finding ways to entertain itself or may not yet be fully housetrained. The only way to differentiate separation anxiety from other forms of anxiety or arousal that may occur when the dog is alone is to collect video of the dog when left alone. In cases where the owner is afraid to leave the dog alone because it may harm itself or do more damage to the home, remind him that as little as 5 to 15 minutes of video can confirm the diagnosis.

Separation anxiety has achieved much attention in recent years because it is one of the first behavioral conditions in dogs for which a drug has received FDA approval. Both Clomicalm and Reconcile have been approved for the treatment of canine separation anxiety. It is critical that when a dog is diagnosed with separation anxiety and is prescribed one of these medications, the client should be informed that behavior modification must be combined with the medication to have the best chance for treatment success. Good behavior modification protocols have been developed for use with each of these medications (available from the manufacturer); the technician should take some time to review them with the pet owner at the time the medication is dispensed.

> **TECHNICIAN NOTE** Successful, lasting treatment for separation anxiety requires behavior modification in addition to antianxiety medications.

Destructive Behavior

Destructive behavior may be associated with separation anxiety, escape attempts, panic, and normal exploratory behavior. The Five-Step Positive Proaction Plan described previously can be used to prevent the development of problem destructive behaviors associated with young dogs. When an older dog begins to demonstrate destructive behaviors, the underlying motivation needs to be determined through collection of a through history. The history should include exactly when the dog is destructive, if destruction is limited to certain portions of the home or certain items, and what other events could be congruent with the destruction. For example, until the technician asks, "Do you know if there were thunderstorms on the day your dog was destructive?" it will not occur to many owners that their thunderstorm-phobic dog was panicking or attempting escape. When the areas targeted for destruction are windows, doors, gates, or other barriers, then separation anxiety, panic due to loud noises outside, and the presence of outdoor stimuli such as other dogs, cats, squirrels, etc., should be considered. It is ironic that dogs that panic over a thunderstorm or other loud noise will injure themselves in their attempts to get outside, where the loud noise is occurring. It is likely that in its panic, the dog simply does not realize that it will be more exposed to the fear-inducing stimuli once it gets outdoors. Dogs that are destructive of household items may behave this way for a variety of reasons. They may simply be dogs that have not been taught what is appropriate and what is not appropriate to chew on. Be aware that many dogs with separation anxiety seek out things that their owners have handled or worn. Although no one can know exactly what drives them to do this, it is likely that they chew on these items to interact with the familiar scent of their owner (this may be soothing) rather than out of spite or anger directed at the owner.

Canine Aggression

Aggression can be defined as any threat or harmful action directed toward another. Generally speaking, aggression can be divided into two categories: offensive aggression and defensive aggression. Offensive aggression is usually an attempt to gain a resource at the expense of another individual. Defensive aggression is usually performed by a victim and directed toward a perceived threat. A variety of different labels have been applied to the different forms of aggression (Box 5-8). The technician should keep in mind that these are descriptive labels. They do not reveal anything about the neurophysiologic basis for the behaviors. Labels are assigned to aggression based on the underlying motivation of the behavior. Understanding what motivates a behavior is the first step in the development of a treatment program; this requires very careful and thorough history taking.

It is also important to be aware that aggression is a normal form of communication among dogs, as it is with many social animals. However, the subtle visual cues and threats associated with aggression are often used in a highly ritualized manner between dogs, so that no injury is inflicted. Often, the extent of threats can be used to determine whether the behavior is "normal" or "abnormal." For example, a pair of household dogs that growl at each other over a toy, resulting in one animal taking the toy and the other deferring and walking away, could be considered normal. On the other hand, when one dog attacks another and the victim rolls over and demonstrates submission via its body postures and by not fighting back, but the aggressor continues attacking, this most likely could be considered abnormal aggression. When assessing any behavior problem, you should always start by trying to determine whether the behavior appears to be an acceptable response in the context of the given situation, and if the degree of response is modified for the degree of threat. A normal dog should be able to modify and appropriately inhibit its aggressive response to a perceived threat versus a true and serious threat.

BOX 5-8 | Some Labels Commonly Applied to Different Forms of Aggression

Conflict-related—Aggression toward people, often over resources and in similar contexts as **dominance aggression**, but with the dog showing ambivalent visual cues. These dogs are often submissive or fearful in other contexts and are likely to act submissive or fearful immediately after an attack. Many clients will say the dog acted like it "was sorry for what it did."

Fear-related (defensive)—Aggression displayed when the dog perceives a threat. Most dogs demonstrate fearful body postures and possibly physiologic signs. Over time, as the dog learns that these behaviors are effective, it may begin to demonstrate more offensive body postures.

Food-related—Aggression demonstrated only in the presence of food, bones, rawhides, human food, or other high-value food items used to prevent real or perceived attempts by others to access the food.

Idiopathic—Aggression that is unpredictable and severe and occurs in the absence of stimuli that would allow the aggression to be categorized otherwise. The form of aggression commonly referred to as *Springer rage* is likely a form of aggression that could be called *idiopathic*.

Inter-dog (male/male)—As the term implies, may occur as the result of fear of strange dogs, or may be related to hormonal influences when it occurs between two intact male dogs. Inter-dog aggression within a household may develop owing to a changing hierarchy between the dogs.

Irritable—Aggression that can be similar to pain-related but that may occur simply because a dog is tired or is just not desiring interaction. May be more common in older dogs and/ or dogs living with small children. May be difficult to differentiate from pain- or fear-related.

Maternal—Aggression typical of a female attempting to prevent access to her offspring (usually neonates). May also occur during pseudopregnancy (pseudocyesis) when females nest and guard items as if they are neonates, in the absence of actual pregnancy.

Pain-related—Aggression similar to fear-related, in that the dog may be aggressing because of discomfort, pain, or fear of pain (e.g., a dog with a history of painful ears may display aggression when the owner approaches with the ear medication).

Play-related—Behavior typical of play, usually nonaffective, and often simply referred to as *inappropriate play behavior* when directed toward humans.

Possessive—Aggression demonstrated in the presence of any high-value resource; used to prevent real or perceived attempts by others to access the resource.

Predatory—Aggression, consistent hunting; usually quiet, staring, and stalking with tail twitching and body lowered. When directed at small children or infant humans, should be considered an emergency situation in need of immediate assessment and management.

Redirected—Aggression toward a nearby individual that occurs when an animal is highly emotionally aroused, usually owing to some other stimulus (e.g., the dog that bites its owner when he or she tries to intervene in a dog fight).

Social status/dominance—Aggression toward people in an attempt to acquire or maintain resources. Dogs displaying this form of aggression should be demonstrating offensive rather than defensive or fear-related visual cues.

Territorial—Aggression demonstrated only in a particular, circumscribed area when approached by a perceived threat.

Aggression can be a problem in dogs of any gender, although it appears that male dogs are overrepresented in certain types of aggression. Recommending neutering is not an inappropriate response to any form of aggression because ideally, one would not want to propagate unwanted behaviors. However, the technician should inform pet owners as to what they can realistically expect to occur after neutering. Neutering is likely to affect only hormonally influenced behavior such as roaming, marking, and mounting behavior in male dogs. It is less likely to have an effect on aggression, unless the problem aggression is occurring between two male dogs. Many pet owners mistakenly believe that no benefit is gained by neutering the adult dog after it has been displaying problem behaviors for some time. Studies have shown, however, that this is not the case, and that even later neutering can have a very useful effect on hormonally influenced behaviors.

> **TECHNICIAN NOTE**   Neutering has minimal effect on most forms of aggression, but it is highly effective in decreasing marking, mounting, and roaming behaviors in male dogs.

Aggression problems can appear in very young animals but are most likely to occur at sexual maturity (5 to 9 months of age) or social maturity (12 to 36 months of age). When aggression appears later, in a middle-aged or geriatric animal, it is far more likely to be the result of an underlying medical condition causing pain, discomfort, or dementia. Although aggression could potentially be the result of an organic condition in the brain, such as brain tumors and/or seizure disorders, these conditions are not common in any age of dog.

The purposes for which certain breeds have been developed may make them more likely to exhibit certain types of aggression. For example, dogs bred for guarding might be predisposed to territorial aggression, and foxhounds (bred for hunting and chasing) may be predisposed to **predatory aggression**. However, any dog of any breed may develop aggression. Not all breed-specific characterizations are entirely accurate. The size and strength of the dog will ultimately be more important than the breed, especially when the potential threat posed by the dog is assessed.

When presented with a dog for aggression, the technician should collect enough history so as to determine the extent of the danger posed by the dog (Box 5-9). After educating the pet owner about normal social behavior in dogs, normal visual cues, and the important role that fear and anxiety play in aggression, the technician can instruct the pet owner as to the importance of avoiding triggers for aggression. As with fear- and anxiety-related issues, the first and most important thing that the pet owner can do is to avoid putting the dog in situations where it is likely to show aggression. For example, the dog that has shown **food-related aggression** should be fed while confined to another room or a crate. The dog that has demonstrated aggression when being reached

---

BOX 5-9	Risk Factors to Consider With Aggressive Dogs

- Size of the dog
- Number of bites that have occurred
- Severity of bites—degree of inhibition or lack thereof
- Owner is able to recognize and avoid triggers of aggression.
- Aggression is seen in response to very benign challenges.

for should not be reached for; it should be called to the owner and rewarded for coming. Again, the owner will need to be reminded that these interventions are not treatment for the problem; they are intended to keep everyone safe and to prevent the dog from practicing the unwanted behavior.

House Soiling

Canine house soiling can occur as a result of urine marking, separation anxiety (and possibly other fears and phobias), lack of complete housetraining, or any medical condition that may lead to urgency or incontinence. When a house soiling dog is presented, after the history has been collected, the most important steps will be physical examination and urinalysis. In some cases, even after a medical condition has been diagnosed and treated, the dog will have to be completely re-housetrained, as described in Box 5-10.

> **TECHNICIAN NOTE**   Successful housetraining of any dog requires very close supervision and an understanding of normal canine elimination behaviors.

Urine marking can be challenging to confirm because both male and female dogs may normally urinate with a lifted leg, so the presence or absence of leg lifting does not necessarily differentiate urine marking from elimination. The sudden development of urine marking in a neutered animal may suggest some degree of anxiety or stress, such as the presence of a new animal or person in the house or other changes in the living condition. Identifying these stressors is an important part of the assessment. The technician can then educate the owner as to how to remove the stressors or attempt to desensitize the dog to them.

Cognitive Dysfunction

Cognitive dysfunction is a syndrome that develops as a result of brain aging. Multiple neurologic changes occur in the aging brain and can result in deficits in learning and memory, as well as impaired awareness and decreased responsiveness to stimuli. Clinical signs associated with cognitive dysfunction can be remembered using the acronym DISHA (Box 5-11).

Subtle signs seen in very early stages of aging are often referred to as *cognitive decline*. Not all animals will suffer from cognitive decline as they age, and there appears to be

BOX 5-10	A Guide to Housetraining the Dog

- **Prevent** elimination in unacceptable places by constant supervision or confinement to a relatively small area.
- Supervision can be provided by tethering the dog to yourself or to a nearby piece of furniture, or by confining the dog to the room you are in, using child gates or closed doors. In these cases, the dog must be observed closely.
  - If while supervised the puppy is seen to begin sniffing the ground and/or circling, it should be quickly but calmly taken to the area preferred by the owner and rewarded if it finishes eliminating.
  - If constant supervision is not possible, confining the dog to a crate is ideal.
- The dog should be fed a measured amount of food at the same time every day. When the dog walks away, or after about 10 to 15 minutes, the food should be removed.
- The dog should be taken outside or to the desired elimination place on a **regular schedule** every day. For puppies about 8 weeks of age, this can be done every 1 to 2 hours, depending on their size. As the puppy matures, every 3 to 4 hours may be adequate. However, if a puppy eliminates in its crate, the first response should be to take it outside more frequently.
- Outside, the dog should be taken to the same place each time and allowed to sniff the area. Getting the puppy interested in the chosen area can be more easily accomplished by cleaning an "accident" in the house with a paper towel, and then bringing the urine-soaked towel to the area in which the owner would like the puppy to eliminate. If the puppy eliminates in the chosen area, it should be quietly **praised** immediately. After finishing, it can be praised more enthusiastically and given a small food reward and/or can be taken to another area and rewarded with some play before returning inside.
- If the puppy does not eliminate, it should be taken inside and placed in the crate or observed very carefully and taken back outside again in about 15 minutes to be given another opportunity.
- Be aware that puppies instinctively desire to eliminate after the following activities: after being confined, after eating and drinking, after playing, and after resting or sleeping. These rules apply to most adult dogs as well. About 15 minutes after any of these activities, the dog should be taken to the place for elimination.
- If the dog happens to have an accident in the house, **DO NOT SCOLD**! Simply clean up the mess and deodorize the area, and try to determine where you erred in preventing the mistake.
- Upon careful examination, you can see that the instructions given here closely follow the Five-Step Positive Proaction Plan.

BOX 5-11	Clinical Signs Commonly Associated With Cognitive Dysfunction in Dogs and Cats (DISHA)

D—Disorientation
- Dogs may act lost in familiar environments or may have trouble navigating them. Example: Dog goes to the wrong side of the door.

I—Interactions
- Decreased interaction with people and other pets may be observed. Example: Dog may play less; may seem irritable or uninterested in affection.

S—Sleep/wake cycle changes
- Dogs may sleep more during the day and less at night. Nighttime waking may occur and may include vocalizing, panting, and/or pacing.

H—House training
- Previously learned behaviors may be "forgotten." A general disinhibition of previously learned behaviors may occur. Example: Dog may begin house soiling, ignoring previously learned commands, and getting on furniture when it had been previously trained not to.

A—Activity alterations
- Changes in activity may mean that the dog is less active or interested in exploring the environment. Alternatively, it may become more restless or anxious. Some dogs may begin to perform repetitive behaviors.

this condition. Clients should be urged to give the medication a 1- to 2-month trial before deciding whether or not it is helping.

Regardless of whether clients choose to medicate or give supplements, they should be encouraged to modify the environment as needed for the aging pet. Aging dogs may not be able to wait as long between walks or being allowed outside. Some may even need to be managed as if they were a puppy being housetrained. Enriching the environment with regular play, walks, and social interaction should be encouraged, so as to keep the dog active and alert. Pet owners should be reminded to reinforce calm, quiet behaviors and to ignore anxiety-related behaviors such as pacing or whining.

FELINE

DEVELOPMENT

Kittens go through developmental periods similar to the dog, but they may be shorter and even less discrete. Similar to dogs, kittens are born with eyes and ears closed. For the first 2 weeks, they are capable only of dragging themselves about with their forelimbs and suckling when the queen initiates nursing. The kitten also requires stimulation from the queen for the first 2 weeks of life to eliminate. The kitten's eyes open at about 7 to 10 days, but full visual acuity develops slowly and is not present until 3 to 4 months of age. The kitten's ears open as early as 5 days but kittens do not begin to orient to sound until about 2 weeks of age.

no breed or gender predilection. Once decline begins, however, it is irreversible; the condition may be slowed but not necessarily halted. A variety of supplements with neuroprotective effects are available and may be more affective if started early on in the development of the condition. In addition, selegiline (Anipryl) is approved for treatment of

Studies have demonstrated that the sensitive period for socialization in the kitten occurs at about 2 to 7 weeks of age. Handling kittens as little as 15 minutes per day from 2 to 6 weeks will result in kittens that are friendlier. Friendliness in cats has also been shown to have a heritable component. Kittens of friendly fathers are more likely to be friendly than kittens whose fathers are unfriendly. This is not to suggest that maternal genetics do not also play a role, only that their contribution has not yet been elucidated as clearly as that of the father. It is more difficult to differentiate the role of maternal genetics from the role of the environment when kittens typically spend their first several weeks of life with their mother. It is likely that a kitten whose mother demonstrates a fear of humans will learn to act fearful of humans as well.

> **TECHNICIAN NOTE**   Temperament in kittens is highly heritable.

Kittens begin to play at 3 weeks of age, and their play consists mostly of pawing at each other. This social play increases from 4 to 11 weeks and eventually involves more biting, chasing, and rolling instead of pawing. Solitary play develops during the same period, and kittens will chase, pounce on, or bat at small moving objects. Social play decreases rapidly after 11 weeks, but solitary play does not begin to decline until after 4 months of age.

Kittens learn to hunt, kill, and eat prey by watching their mother. When kittens are between 4 and 8 weeks of age, the queen begins to bring live prey back to the nest. She attracts the kittens to the activity by vocalizing and then allowing the kittens to interact with the prey, so that they learn to kill and eat it. By 8 weeks of age, kittens can kill and eat mice.

SOCIAL BEHAVIOR

The ancestor of the domestic cat is believed to be the African Wild Cat *(Felis silvestris lybica),* a solitary, desert-dwelling animal. Domestic cats are often considered to be asocial animals, but this is not entirely correct. Domestication of the cat has led to a highly adaptable animal that can modify its social organization according to available resources. Free-ranging cats can live in large groups when living near a concentrated food source such as a dump, a fishing village, or a farm. However, these groups are almost always composed of related females that form a dominance hierarchy. A certain amount of aggression persists, and the more closely related the animals, the less aggression is demonstrated between those individuals. A dominant male's territory will encompass the territory of these females, and they will allow his presence when a female is in estrus. All other strange cats will be chased away from the territory.

Territoriality is particularly problematic in the intact male cat, which will naturally roam, urine mark, and fight when given the opportunity. This can result in injury caused by other cats, the spread of contagious disease, and high risk of being hit by cars. Castration is highly effective at limiting these behaviors, no matter the age at which the cat is castrated.

Domestic cats that live together may show a variety of **affiliative behaviors** such as cheek and tail rubbing. Nevertheless, aggression between cats in a household is a common problem, especially because most cat owners are unfamiliar with the visual signals used by cats. Cat signals can be very subtle, and differentiating play from true aggression can be challenging. Refer to the section in this chapter, "Reading Feline Body Language."

> **TECHNICIAN NOTE**   Cats are not asocial animals; however, their tolerance of other cats can be limited and is based on familiarity and individual temperament.

Introducing a new cat almost always results in aggression initially and should be done in a gradual systematic way, rather than by simply releasing a new cat into the home (see "Introducing the New Cat"). Whenever possible, the technician can educate clients about risks and challenges associated with adding cats to a household. The tendency to be aggressive toward other cats appears to be another heritable trait in cats, and clients should be warned that some cats simply do not seem to like living with other cats. When a new cat is added, even if this is done properly, there is no guarantee that the cats will eventually be friendly toward one another. Tolerance of each other may be more likely in a large home, where cats are given many resources (litter boxes, food and water dishes, resting places, etc.) and are not forced to interact with each other because of close confinement. Clients expecting to want more than two cats will find it easier to acquire two kittens and raise them together. Studies have shown that aggression is less likely in pairs of cats, the longer they have lived together. Clients that add new cats to their home regularly and/or maintain more than two or three cats at a time are more likely to have aggression and house soiling problems within the household.

READING FELINE BODY LANGUAGE

When feline visual cues are observed, body postures, as well as the face, head, ears, and tail, contribute to the message being sent. The cat's tail is high when it is greeting, investigating, or frustrated. A relaxed cat usually stands with its tail hanging and its ears pointed forward (Figure 5-7). The aggressive cat appears to be walking on tiptoe with its head down so that its rear end seems higher than its fore end. The tail is down but the tip is held away from the hocks, and the hair on the rump and tail may be piloerected. Its ears are erect but swiveled in such a way as to point the openings to the side (Figure 5-8). A frightened cat will crouch down with ears flattened back on the head and tail tucked under its body. The eyes of the frightened cat are likely to be dilated, and it is likely to hiss or spit. A fearfully aggressive cat looks like the typical "Halloween cat" with body arched, tail erect, and ears flattened to the head. This is the equivalent of the fear aggressive dog.

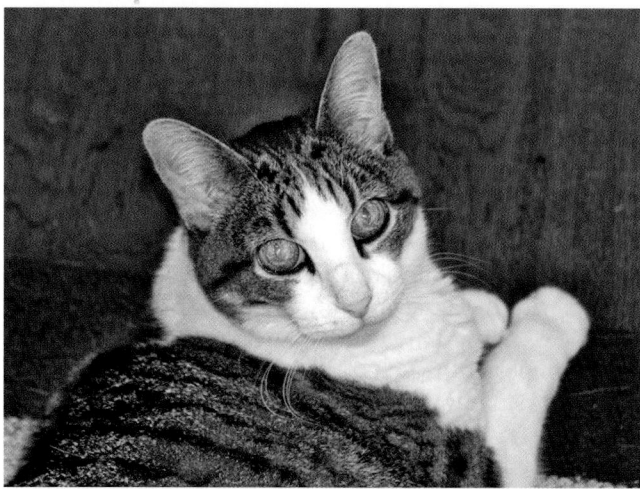

FIGURE 5-7 The face of a relaxed, alert cat.

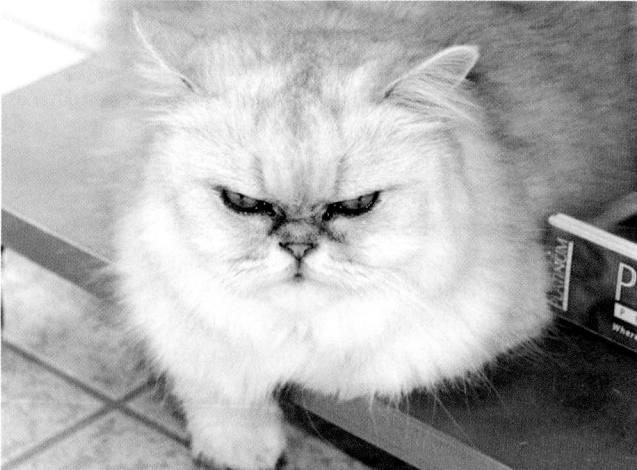

FIGURE 5-8 The cat demonstrating the outwardly directed ears typical of offensive aggression.

Cats that display predatory aggression exhibit unique visual cues. They carry their body as low to the ground as possible and move slowly forward without making a sound. They may pause momentarily, with just the end of the tail moving slightly, before pouncing on their prey.

COPING WITH FELINE BEHAVIOR IN THE CLINIC

Most domestic cats appear to dislike major changes in their environment, and they seem less likely to enjoy going places as many dogs do. To make matters worse, most cats are placed in their carrier and taken somewhere only once or twice a year, and that trip is usually to the veterinary clinic, where something at least mildly unpleasant takes place. As with other animals, the sights and smells of the veterinary clinic become associated with their feelings of fear or anxiety, and through classical conditioning, their fear and thus their behavior may become worse with each subsequent visit. It can be difficult to change this association once it is firmly established, but doing everything possible to decrease stimuli that contribute to fear is a good first step. For example, in

clinics that do not have separate dog and cat waiting areas, moving the cat owner into an examination room as quickly as possible can be helpful. Instructing owners to bring a towel or blanket with them so that the carrier can be covered may be similarly helpful. The cat that has to sit even in a crate, where dogs can see it, walk around it, and step up and sniff it, can be quite traumatized. If the cat is already fearfully aroused by this experience when it is taken to the examination room, removing it from the carrier and examining it will be even more difficult.

Cats are often even more difficult than fearful dogs to interest in food while in the clinic; however, food rewards can be helpful with many cats and should always be tried before the possibility is discarded. Meat-flavored baby food, dairy products such as whipped cream or cream cheese, and fish-flavored canned cat foods may be especially appealing to a cat. One of these products can be smeared on the examination table for the kitten or cat to lick while it is being examined and after any procedures have been completed. Some cats will lick these "treats" off of a tongue depressor while other, more invasive procedures, such as taking the rectal temperature, are being performed. If this use of food is initiated on the cat's first visit, before it has developed a fear of the clinic, it can be very helpful at preventing the development of fear, because the cat's last memory of the experience will be that of licking up a delicious treat.

Cat owners should be instructed on how to habituate their cat to a carrier as soon as it is acquired, but this can be done with the adult cat that is already fearful of a carrier as well. It simply takes a little longer. The technique is similar to acclimating a dog to a crate, as described in Box 5-7). The crate, with comfortable bedding inside, should always be left available to the cat somewhere in the home that is quiet. The cat then will never learn to associate the crate only with trips to the veterinary clinic.

> **TECHNICIAN NOTE** Cats whose carriers are used only for trips to the veterinarian are highly likely to fear the crate and be more difficult to place inside.

INTRODUCING A NEW CAT

Cat owners should be instructed to prepare their home for a new cat by first preparing a separate room in which it can be confined during its first few days in the home. The room should have a solid door that can be closed, a litter box, food and water, and ideally several vertical resting spaces for the cat. If the existing household cat and the new cat show an interest in interacting with each other beneath the door, that is fine. Occasionally, after the new cat has been allowed to settle in, the cats' places in the home should be exchanged, so that the existing household cat is confined and the new cat is allowed to explore the new home. In addition, a towel can be used to rub the new cat over its face and tail and then to rub the other cat on a daily basis. If the smell of the towel appears to alarm the cats, do not force them to accept rubbing; simply lay the towel in the environment so that they can investigate it whenever they wish. After a few days of this, as long as both cats are calm and relaxed about the situation, each of the cats can be confined to a crate for every mealtime. The first time this is done, the carriers should be separated by several feet or however much is necessary for the cats to ignore each other and eat their food. This should be repeated at every feeding and, ideally, the cats could be fed as many as three times per day so as to speed up the process. In this way, the cats learn to associate the pleasure of eating with the presence of the other cat. As long as no hissing, staring, or other signs of fear are demonstrated, the carriers can gradually be moved closer to each other over a period of several days. Once the cats can eat calmly side by side, the crates can be opened and the cats allowed to interact freely. As long as there is no staring or hissing or one cat chasing another, they can be allowed to roam the house freely together. However, confining them separately when they cannot be closely supervised, for an additional week or so, may be helpful. Their tolerance of each other should continue to improve with time as long as they are not forced into close association with each other.

> **TECHNICIAN NOTE** New cats should never be released into the home with an existing cat without first taking the time to familiarize the cats with each other in a very systematic way.

COMMON BEHAVIOR PROBLEMS
Unruly Behaviors

As with dogs, cats can exhibit a variety of behaviors that, although normal, may be unwanted by the owner. One of the behaviors most commonly reported to veterinarians is excessive vocalization and nocturnal activity. This problem may be more likely to occur in young animals or geriatric animals. Vocalization and activity may be a sign of underlying discomfort due to a medical problem, so possible medical causes should be explored. Nevertheless, the technician can inform owners that the ancestor of the cat is a nocturnal animal, and many domestic cats will revert to this pattern of behavior, especially if they are left alone all day to do as they please. Most cats spend most of the day sleeping and are then energetic and ready to interact with their owners when night falls. This problem can be dealt with by following the Five-Step Positive Proaction Plan described earlier. Owners will need to be sure to provide a highly enriched environment while they are gone, to increase the chance that the cat will play instead of sleep. In some cases, another cat may help. Owners should also schedule time before bed to interact with and exercise the cat in an attempt to tire it out. After this, the most important thing they can do is to completely ignore inappropriate behavior. This may make it necessary to close their bedroom door and prevent the cat's entry or confine the cat to another room. With excessively vocal cats, owners may wish to wear earplugs at night.

Destructive Behavior

Cats, like dogs, can be very destructive; they simply use their claws more often than their teeth. Some kittens and young cats will chew up items as a puppy will, and in these situations should be treated like puppies, where they are confined to a pet-proof room and are provided with items for chewing. When allowed complete access to the home, items that they are likely to chew should be removed.

Cats are far more likely to present a problem to their owners with their clawing and scratching behavior when it is directed toward household furnishings. Cats claw for several important reasons: to remove the dead outer layers of the claw, to leave a visual mark, and to make an olfactory mark (cats have sebaceous glands on their feet). Cats appear to be stretching and flexing their shoulders, feet, and legs when they scratch, so this may also be a form of exercise or body maintenance similar to grooming.

Teaching cats to scratch on appropriate objects rather than furniture, drapery, or carpet is similar to teaching a puppy what is appropriate to chew on and what is not. Again, the Five-Step Positive Proaction Plan lays the ground rules. Appropriate scratching areas must be provided and inappropriate places must be made inaccessible. Individual cats can be very choosy about what they prefer to scratch on, so a variety of different devices of different sizes, shapes, and textures should be provided until the owner can identify which the cat prefers (Figure 5-9). Not all cats want to stand up and scratch on a vertical scratching post. Many seem to prefer scratching devices that lie horizontally or slightly angled off the ground. In addition to texture, stability may be one of the most important features. If the device is not heavy enough for the cat to scratch on without it moving about, they are less likely to use it. If the cat is already scratching on particular surfaces in the home, the owner should be attentive to those choices and try to provide the cat with similar textures. Once owners have identified scratching devices that the cat prefers, they may wish to put one of those devices near each of the other inappropriate locations that the cat has chosen. The owner can then praise the cat every time it makes the right choice. Surfaces that the cat has chosen or is likely to choose can be changed by covering them with plastic or double-sided tape. Additionally, if preventing access to all of the inappropriate places that the cat may scratch is very difficult, owners may wish to confine the cat to an area with its food, water, litter pan, and scratching posts when the owner cannot supervise. When available to supervise, the owner can quietly squirt the cat with water when it makes an inappropriate choice. Remote punishing devices such as Scat Mats may be very useful for keeping cats from scratching on inappropriate surfaces.

> **TECHNICIAN NOTE** Cats can be taught which surfaces are appropriate to scratch on and which are not.

If all efforts at controlling a cat's scratching behavior fail, and the cat is in danger of euthanasia or relinquishment,

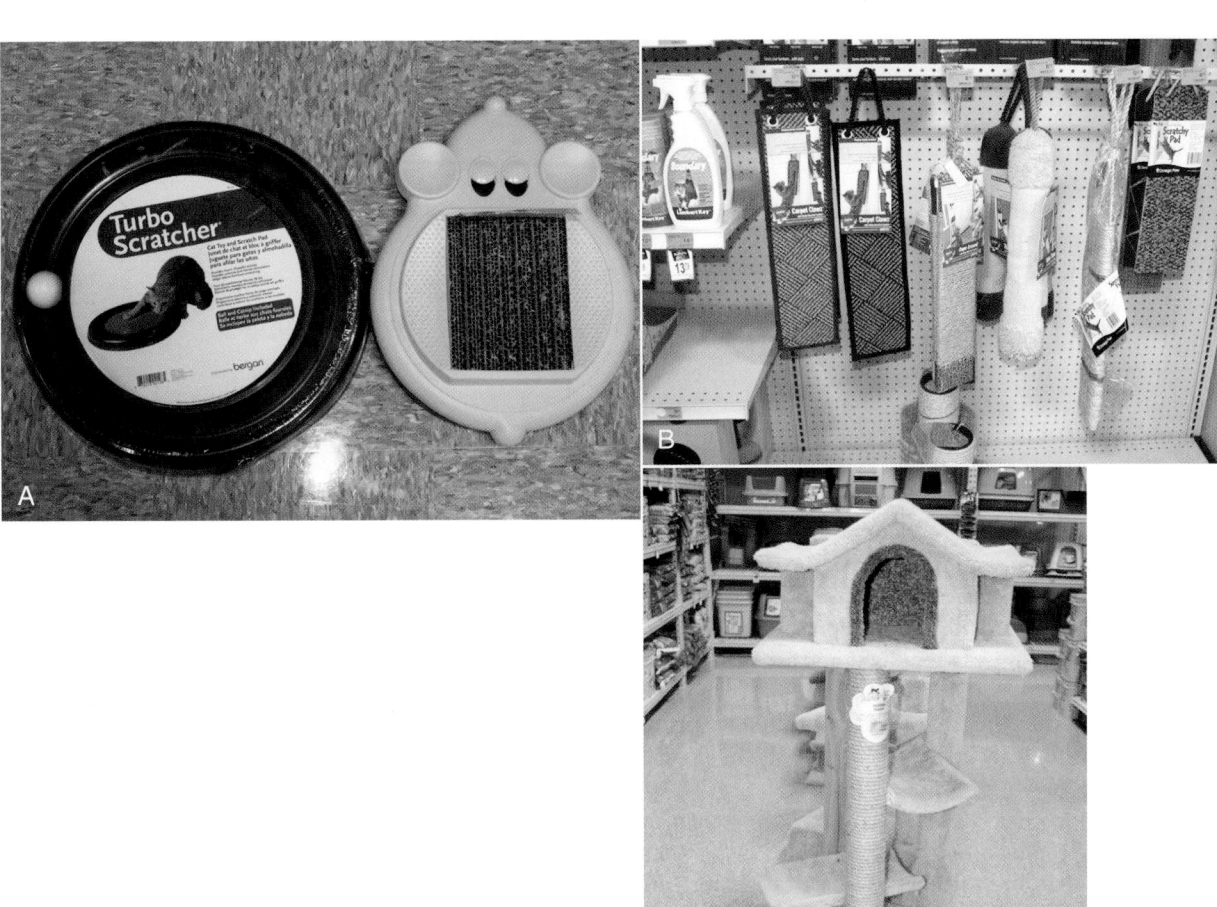

FIGURE 5-9 A through C, Examples of the variety of scratching "posts" commercially available for cats.

declawing is a reasonable consideration. Analgesic options for cats have been much improved over the past few decades, so the procedure can be performed humanely and without undue pain. In addition, no good evidence suggests that declawing leads to any other unwanted problem behaviors.

Feline Aggression
Inter-Cat Aggression
As was mentioned previously, multiple cats in the same household can present a problem, and often cat owners are unaware that there is a problem until one or both of the cats begins house soiling. Assessing the problem requires a detailed history that includes details about the visual and vocal cues being used by the cats involved (Figure 5-10). Offensively aggressive cats may simply stare at the other cat. A submissive cat may hiss and flatten its ears while standing its ground, or it may run or slink away. When two cats approach each other aggressively, they will do so as described previously—on tiptoe with their tail lashing. If one of the cats does not run away, they will eventually jump at each

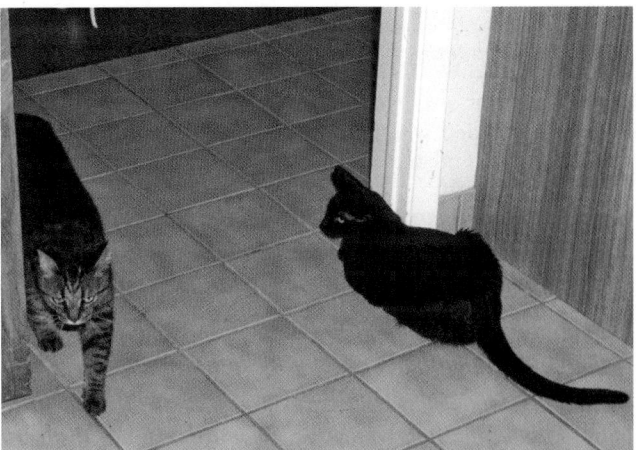

FIGURE 5-10 An easily overlooked agonistic encounter between two cats. The cat on the right is staring and his ears are directed outward. The cat on the left is making an effort to not get too close or look at the other cat, but its posture is relatively confident.

other with each cat attempting to bite the nape of the other cat. In an attempt to avoid being bitten on the neck, the cats will roll over and may end up belly to belly as they claw, vocalize, and attempt to bite each other. If one cat decides to flee, the victor is likely to pursue it.

Some owners have difficulty recognizing when two cats are playing and when they are being truly aggressive. This can be challenging because cat play and aggression can share many of the same components. In addition, some cats will begin by playing, and as the play progresses, they can become increasingly aroused until the play changes to an aggressive encounter. In these cases, usually one or more of the cats will hiss and run away. Pet owners can be taught to look for the staring that may precede an attack. They should be made aware that the cat that hisses is usually expressing fear of the other cat. This may provoke another cat to attack, but the hissing cat is usually the victim. If one cat in a household begins to spend most of its time hiding from the other cat(s), this is a sign that the cats are not getting along. When owners feel that they do not see any of these signs and are still unsure of whether or not the cats are having a problem, the technician should ask whether the cats spend any time grooming one another or sleeping together. If they do, this is a very good sign that they are comfortable with each other.

Households that contain multiple cats may be even more difficult to assess. Technicians can make owners aware that forcing multiple cats to live together in a crowded home can lead to a great deal of anxiety and stress, which can result in illness as well as problem behaviors such as house soiling. For all individuals in a multi-cat household to stay physically and behaviorally healthy, they need to be provided with abundant resources. This includes litter boxes, food and water stations, scratching posts, toys, and vertical resting areas. If cats that are not closely bonded are forced to encounter each other frequently while going about their day-to-day lives, anxiety and subsequent stress can pose severe problems.

> **TECHNICIAN NOTE**   Multi-cat households are prone to a variety of anxiety- and stress-related problems if cats are not provided with abundant resources and space for avoiding each other.

Aggression Toward People

Human directed aggression in the cat can take several forms. A common form of aggression occurs most often in young male cats; this is often referred to as *play aggression* or *inappropriate play,* and sometimes it may have some predatory components as well. These cats often stalk and pounce on people's feet or hands. If their bites are uninhibited, they can cause severe injury and be a serious problem, especially for elderly clients or those with children in the household. Oftentimes, these are cats that simply have more energy than the owner was prepared for and need increased exercise and in some cases another cat to play with. Sometimes these cats play inappropriately because they have never been taught

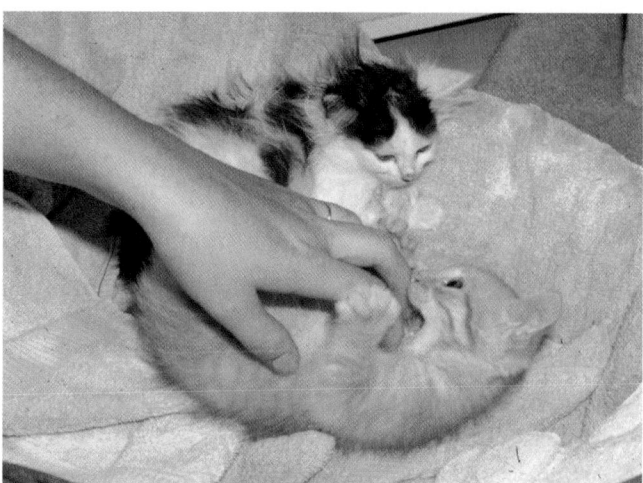

FIGURE 5-11 A good example of how NOT to play with a kitten.

acceptable play by their owners and have been rewarded for playing with hands or feet. Preventing this form of aggression is certainly easier than treating it, so all new kitten owners should be given some advice about appropriate play with their kitten (Figure 5-11). Hands and feet should never be used as toys. Ideal cat toys are those that involve stalking, pouncing, or chasing at a distance from the owner's hands. These can include the "fishing pole"–type toys that are commercially available under a variety of names. Catnip-stuffed balls and mice (anything that can be chased and grabbed) are also appropriate.

Another form of aggression, petting-related aggression, has also been referred to as *dominance-* or *status-related* or **irritable aggression;** it occurs when the cat is being stroked. The cat often chooses to sit in the owner's lap or near him and appears to enjoy the petting for a period of time (often purring while being petted) until it suddenly stops and turns and bites. In many cases, the cat continues to lie there, and in other cases it may run off. No one quite understands why cats do this, although several theories have been proposed. The best advice that the technician can give the owner is to help him understand that this may in fact be normal behavior for the cat. The cat may simply tire of this type of stroking and yet want to remain in the company of the owner, so it uses the only method it has to say "Stop that." Keeping the owner safe is paramount, so in a situation like this, where the cat's aggression is somewhat predictable, avoidance is the best advice. The owner can be instructed to not pet the cat but one or two strokes and then stop before the cat can become agitated. The client can also be instructed in how to watch for early warning signs that the cat is becoming uncomfortable, such as twitching tail, stiffening body, and dilated eyes. These signs may be subtle and easy to miss so should not be relied upon for safety. Many owners, once they understand the problem, live with it by limiting their petting of the cat. Others may desire treatment for the problem, in which case desensitization and counter-conditioning to petting can be practiced.

Redirected aggression is a potentially serious form of aggression in the cat. Similar to redirected aggression in the dog, cats usually display this behavior when they are aroused or frightened by another stimulus—often the presence of another cat. The cat turns and redirects its aggression toward the nearest person. In some cases, cats will redirect to their feline housemate, contributing to the development of a potentially serious inter-cat aggression problem. One aspect of this problem unique to cats is that once frightened or aroused, they tend to stay that way for several hours, sometimes days. In this state of heightened arousal, they can be very dangerous, and veterinarians may get calls from cat owners who have had to confine themselves to one room of the home to get away from the cat. Waiting for the cat to calm down is not always an option because it can take quite a while. Owners must be instructed to attempt to lure the cat into a separate room using food, so that they can close the door on it and leave it there as long as necessary for the cat to calm down. Litter pans and food and water bowls can be slipped through a partially open door and then the door closed and the cat ignored for 24 hours or longer as needed.

> **TECHNICIAN NOTE** Cats experiencing a traumatic event and redirected aggression can stay fearfully and aggressively aroused for several hours and even days.

Redirected aggression can also occur when a cat is startled by a loud noise or other surprising stimulus. Owners of a cat that have handled another cat may be targets of aggression by their cat when they arrive home; this may be another form of redirected aggression. Sometimes these cases are more accurately defined as fear related, but the response of the cat and the severity of the response are often very similar. In addition to remaining aroused for some time after these episodes, some cats appear to associate the event with a particular person or cat in the home, and they continue to demonstrate aggression toward that individual long after they have calmed down from the initial arousal. Desensitization and counter-conditioning to one of the family members may be necessary. If they have associated the frightening event with the presence of one of their feline housemates, procedures similar to those used for introducing new cats to the home may be needed.

Sudden development of an aggression problem in an older cat with no apparent frightening event can be due to a variety of medical conditions, including but not limited to hyperthyroidism, feline ischemic encephalopathy, and neoplasia.

House Soiling

House soiling is one of the most common presenting complaints for cats seen by veterinary behaviorists and is a likely reason for many cats being relinquished to animal shelters. House soiling can be a relatively straightforward problem to treat, with a high success rate, if you get a good detailed history and you have a solid understanding of normal feline

CASE PRESENTATION 5-1

Mrs. Appleford presents her cat, Fluffy, with the complaint that Fluffy is "peeing all over the house." Fluffy is a 5-year-old spayed female Maine Coon that Mrs. A purchased from a breeder when she was 8 weeks of age. Upon collecting the history, it is discovered that Mrs. A. just moved in with her daughter and her family a few weeks ago. There are no other pets within the household, but the home is large compared with the condominium in which she previously lived. Children are in the household so she has changed to a covered litter box for Fluffy and has changed the litter because the brand that she was familiar with was not available at the nearby store. Fluffy is still using her litter box for urine and feces, and Mrs. A. reports that she has always and still does cover her waste thoroughly. The litter box is now in her room in a large walk-in closet. When asked to describe the behavior, Mrs. A. says that she has never seen Fluffy urinate outside of her box; it appears that she may eliminate in the house mostly during the night. When asked to describe the mess, Mrs. A. says that it is often on the walls and baseboards around the backyard, but she has also found it on the curtains that hang on windows in the family room and one of the bedrooms. Both of these rooms face the backyard. Fluffy has also urinated against the stereo speakers in the family room.

The history is suggestive of urine marking, and when Mrs. A. talks to her daughter, she learns that there is a stray cat that hangs around the backyard, and the daughter has been leaving food on the back porch for the cat.

After a complete physical examination and urinalysis are determined to be within normal limits, Fluffy is started on fluoxetine once daily at 1 mg/kg. Mrs. A. is instructed to suggest that the stray cat no longer be fed, and that an attempt be made to keep the stray cat out of the yard. In addition, Mrs. A. says that temporarily she can confine Fluffy to the front part of the house by closing doors to the family room and the back bedroom. She is reminded to continue cleaning the litter box regularly and to try taking the top off of it for a while. She is instructed to clean all marked areas thoroughly with an enzymatic cleaner.

Four weeks later, a call to Mrs. A. reveals that Fluffy stopped urine marking within a week. The stray cat was caught in a live trap and was taken to a nearby animal shelter. Mrs. A. is instructed to keep Fluffy on medication and to begin to allow Fluffy supervised access to the family room.

A second call made to Mrs. A. 4 weeks later reveals that Fluffy still is not urine marking and is roaming the house again unsupervised. Mrs. A. is instructed to begin decreasing the dose of fluoxetine by half daily for 2 weeks, and then to give every other day for 2 weeks.

When Fluffy is seen a year later for an annual physical, she reports that Fluffy has not ever urine marked again.

elimination behavior. Unrealistic owner expectations and their unwillingness to make changes in their cat's environment are common causes of treatment failure. The technician with this knowledge not only can help cat owners prevent house soiling problems by educating cat owners about normal feline elimination behavior and the behavioral needs of the cat but will be in a better position to assist with early intervention in cases where a client complains about a house soiling cat.

House soiling usually occurs as a result of one of two different behaviors: marking or elimination. One would be wise to remember, however, that some cats will perform both in the same environment. Marking is usually but not always performed with the cat standing, backing up to a wall or other vertical surface, and squirting out a variable quantity of urine. The cat's tail may twitch, and it may perform a treading motion with some or all of its paws while depositing urine. This behavior in most cases is a result of the cat's desire to leave an olfactory message. Studies have suggested that the message is a result of anxiety associated with major changes in the environment, the presence of outdoor cats, and/or **conflict** with other household cats. In the author's experience, this is rare, but some cats will use feces to mark (also called *middening*). However, depositing of feces outside the litter box is most often a sign of a problem associated with the gastrointestinal tract, so medical problems should be ruled out first in these cases.

> **TECHNICIAN NOTE** When assessing the house soiling cat, the technician needs to collect the history that will allow for differentiation between marking and elimination.

Elimination, as opposed to urine marking, is usually performed with the cat in a squatting position and with the waste deposited on a horizontal surface. A rare cat will actually urinate on a regular basis from a standing position. A detailed history will help to determine the difference between this and marking behavior (Table 5-3). Elimination is simply a result of the cat needing to empty its bowels and/or bladder and usually is not associated with any kind of "message." Most cats that eliminate outside of their litter box do so because they dislike the box, litter, or location for some reason. A box that is not kept clean by the cat owner is one very common reason why a cat may try out a new toileting area. Clients should be taught that what seems clean to them may not be clean enough for the cat. In addition, human perception differs greatly from that of cats, and what we find pleasant smelling may be offensive to the cat. Sometimes we can never be sure of what initially triggered a cat to use an alternate toileting location, but with repeated use of the new location, many cats then develop a preference for the new location.

Urinary tract disorders, any condition causing polyuria and polydipsia, and conditions causing pain or discomfort when attempting to access the litter box have all been associated with a cat choosing an alternative location for elimination. Even after these conditions have been diagnosed and treated, a program of environmental and behavioral modification may be necessary in cases where the cat has developed an aversion to the litter box or a preference for another

TABLE 5-3	Criteria for Assessing House Soiling Problems	
SURFACE TARGETED POSTURE	**URINE MARKING VERTICAL STANDING**	**ELIMINATION HORIZONTAL SQUATTING**
Amount	May be a smaller amount	Large amount—complete voiding of the bladder or evacuation of the bowels
Behavior	No digging—will simply walk away	May dig or scratch at surface before or afterward
Location	Socially significant locations—doors, windows, new objects, furniture legs, objects that smell of the owner or other animals, high traffic areas	Locations not socially significant, likely to be in quiet, undisturbed or out-of-the-way places in the home
Unusual locations	Appliances, stereo speakers	Sinks, bath tubs—it is theorized that cats with lower urinary tract disease may be more likely to target these locations
Substrates	A variety of surfaces targeted	Usually consistent—for example, soft absorbent surfaces such as clothing, upholstery, carpeting, bedding, etc.

location or substrate. Every cat presented for eliminating outside the box should have a urinalysis, urine culture and sensitivity, complete blood count, and serum chemistry profile. Radiographs and/or ultrasound may be necessary in some cases. If evidence that the cat is strictly urine marking is particularly strong, these tests are less critical. Appropriate treatment for urine marking can be initiated, and if the problem does not improve dramatically within 1 to 2 weeks, additional diagnostics are recommended.

The most critical aspect of successful treatment for house soiling, after treatment of any underlying medical conditions, is that while inappropriately targeted sites are made less acceptable and/or inaccessible to the cat, the litter box is made more accessible and ideal for that individual cat. This requires that owners must be willing to make certain temporary changes in the environment. Rooms can be closed off so the cat cannot access them, or plastic drop cloths can be placed over targeted areas. In addition, a variety of commercially available products can be used to "booby trap" an area that the cat has been soiling. These include mats that shock, mats that have small upward pointing projections on them, and motion-sensing devices that spray a burst of air at the cat. It is critical that soiled areas be cleaned thoroughly so as to remove the odor of the waste, which also acts to draw the cat back to the area. A variety of cleansers are

BOX 5-12	Common Reasons for Cats to Choose an Alternate Toileting Location

- Type of box
  - Too small
  - Covered, may be problematic in a household with other cats or dogs
  - Too high for a geriatric or arthritic cat to get into comfortably
  - Box is dirty. Covered boxes may make it easier for the owner to go longer between cleaning.
  - Box is cleaned with strong smelling detergents and/or deodorizers
- Number
  - Not enough for the number of cats; may need a box for each cat plus one
- Type of litter
  - "Crystals," "pearls," rough clay litters, shredded paper, corn cob litter
- Location
  - Too busy
  - Too far away from the area where cat spends most of its time
  - Only one entry and exit point
  - In a place that the cat finds difficult or unpleasant to get to (e.g., basement)
- Traumatic events
  - Pain associated with a medical condition
  - Loud noises (on top of an appliance)
  - Startled or attacked by another animal
  - Caught by owner for medicating
- Medical conditions causing polyuria, polydipsia, pain, or discomfort associated with elimination, pain, or discomfort when getting to or into the box

BOX 5-13	Providing the Cat With a Toilet That Meets Its Behavioral Needs

- Large enough for the cat to walk around in—larger seems to be preferred
- Litter type—the finer the better, unscented, about 1½ to 2 inches deep
- Uncovered seems to be preferred.
- Liners may be unpleasant to some cats.
- Clean—sift daily, empty completely, and wash weekly with unscented mild detergents
- Cats appear to avoid citrus and floral scents, so these should be avoided in and around the box.
- Number of boxes—should be appropriate for the number of cats; boxes should not be placed adjacent to each other
- Location of boxes—easily accessible, someplace safe and quiet (not next to noisy appliances) with more than one escape route; not too close to food, water, or resting place

The geriatric cat may have additional requirements:
- Very shallow boxes (may use shallow baking pans)
- May need to have additional boxes, so the box is very easily accessible (e.g., the cat should not have to maneuver a flight of stairs to get to the box)

commercially available, but enzymatic cleansers may be most effective. In some cases, carpets and carpet pads may have to be removed completely.

> **TECHNICIAN NOTE** Some cats will use litter or a box that they do not like for years before one day, for reasons not always clear, they try another location and find it preferable.

Making the litter box more acceptable to the cat may require some understanding of what the cat dislikes about the box. Box 5-12 covers many of the reasons that cats will stop using their litter box. For example if the cat experienced pain or discomfort in the box, the entire box may need to be moved to an alternate location, or the box may even need to be changed to something that looks and seems completely different. Sometimes using large, shallow baking tins and placing litter in them may appeal to the cat. These can be especially helpful for cats with osteoarthritis that may make it difficult for them to step into a box with higher sides. See Box 5-13 for features to consider when providing a box that the cat will be most likely to use. In some cases, litter box

trials may be necessary where two to four different styles of litter box, all containing the same type of litter, are offered in an attempt to determine which box the cat finds acceptable. After a couple of weeks, a preference should emerge, and that box style should be used in the future.

Oftentimes, cats simply appear to dislike their litter. These cats may shake their paws after exiting the box, fail to dig or cover, or even stand on the edges of the box as if they do not want to touch the litter. When cats eliminate beside the box but not in it, this can be a clue that they do not like the litter. If this is suspected, litter trials should be initiated. This requires that the owner prepare two to four identical boxes and fill each of them with a different litter. The boxes should then be left down for at least 2 weeks, and the litter chosen most frequently should be noted. That litter should then be provided to the cat. In multi-cat households where some of the cats appear to like the current litter, it may be necessary to keep some boxes the same but provide the new litter in other boxes.

It is a common albeit puzzling fact that cats that dislike their litter may defecate in their box but not urinate there and, less commonly, may urinate in the box and defecate elsewhere. Nevertheless, these cats may not like their litter or litter box and should be given choices to test as already described. Many cats will use a litter for years, even though they clearly dislike it, and then one day, for reasons not always clear, they will discover another spot that they like better.

Owners must be encouraged to be patient while living with all of these recommended changes. They should be reassured that most are temporary. For example, even if the box must be placed in a completely different location to get the cat to use it again, once the cat begins using it reliably, the owner can begin to move the box, just a few inches every day, to the location that the owner prefers, assuming that that location can be made satisfactory to the cat. We simply cannot expect the 15-year-old cat to climb two flights of stairs to use the toilet, and we cannot expect a cat to use a litter box that is next to a washer and dryer, or the dog's food bowl, if that is what the cat finds frightening.

> **TECHNICIAN NOTE** Cat owners must keep the cat's needs in mind when providing the litter box, if they expect the cat to use it regularly.

The importance of differentiating urine marking from elimination is demonstrated by the treatments recommended. Urine marking has been shown to respond very well to antianxiety medications such as fluoxetine and clomipramine. Elimination outside of the box is not likely to be treated successfully with medication unless it is associated with anxiety due to conflict among cats in the household. If medication is to be used to treat either of these conditions, environmental modification and sometimes behavior modification will be necessary as well, if the client wishes to ever discontinue medication. In the case of the marking cats, triggers need to be identified and avoided or desensitization used to change the cat's response to them. Covering windows or moving favorite perching sites can be helpful if the cat is being stressed by cats hanging around outside. Treating any inter-cat aggression issues within the home or other fear- or anxiety-related problems may also be necessary to ensure long-term success.

Cognitive Dysfunction

Cats can suffer from cognitive decline, just as dogs do, although their decline often begins later. Clinical signs are similar to those seen in the dog and can similarly be evaluated using the DISHA acronym (see Box 5-11). In addition, cats with cognitive dysfunction are likely to vocalize in a random and apparently purposeless way. Because a variety of medical conditions can cause pain, discomfort, and anxiety in the cat, these will need to be ruled out before it can be assumed that a behavior change is due to cognitive dysfunction.

EQUINE

COMMUNICATION AND THE SENSES

Horses are highly social, grazing prey animals, so their sensory and communication systems have evolved for that lifestyle. Typical of most prey animals, horses' eyes are set laterally, allowing them to have a wide field of monocular vision to either side of their body, and a narrow binocular field of view directly in front of their noses. This leaves the horse with two blind spots: one directly behind the animal and one directly below the nose. It is necessary for the horse to raise and lower its head to change its field of vision and

its depth perception. Horses can see color, but their vision, similar to most mammals, is dichromatic, rather than trichromatic. This means that they mostly see shades of pale blue, green, gray, and yellow.

> **TECHNICIAN NOTE** Horses have a blind spot directly behind them and directly below their nose.

The herd behavior that the horse relies on for safety also requires excellent communication between herd members. Horses communicate a great deal by using visual cues. Horses' ears serve as one very important feature in nonvocal communication. When attending to something in front of it, the horse will rotate its ears forward. When attending to something behind, the ears will rotate backward. When frightened or aggressing, the ears will be pinned back. Generally speaking, when alarmed, the horse will lower its ears, but the opening to the aural canal will be directed outward. The aggressive horse will lower its ears in such a way as to turn the opening backward. Swiveling of the ears may be seen when a horse is in pain or is being irritated by flies. Figures 5-12 through 5-15 demonstrate the large array of messages that can be conveyed by horses' head and ear postures. Posture of the head, ear position, body posture, tail position, and appearance of the nostrils all combine to provide greater detail about what the horse is communicating at the time. The position of the tail should always be observed in combination with the other visual cues. Generally speaking, a lowered, relaxed tail is seen when the horse is standing and relaxed. A frightened horse or one attempting to escape from an alarming stimulus will hold its tail tightly against its hindquarters and between its rear legs. Figure 5-16 demonstrates tail postures seen during different displays by the horse.

> **TECHNICIAN NOTE** Close attention must be paid to the visual cues sent by the horse so as to work with and around the horse safely.

Horses also use foot-stomping and pawing as auditory signals. Foot-stomping can be a mild threat or a sign of discomfort; pawing often signals frustration.

Snapping (also called *champing* and *teeth clapping*) is a behavior peculiar to foals that is characterized by varying degrees of extension of the head, retraction of the lips with partial exposure of the teeth, and rapid snapping of the teeth with the ears turned so that the openings are pointed laterally. Sometimes the behavior is accompanied by sucking and tongue clicking sounds. It has been seen in a number of different contexts: during approach by other adult horses, with aggression directed toward the foal by an adult, during the courtship and copulatory behavior of the foal's dam and the stallion, and sometimes with no apparent trigger. Foals have been seen to direct this behavior toward cattle, people, and horse-rider pairs. The exact meaning of the behavior is still under debate.

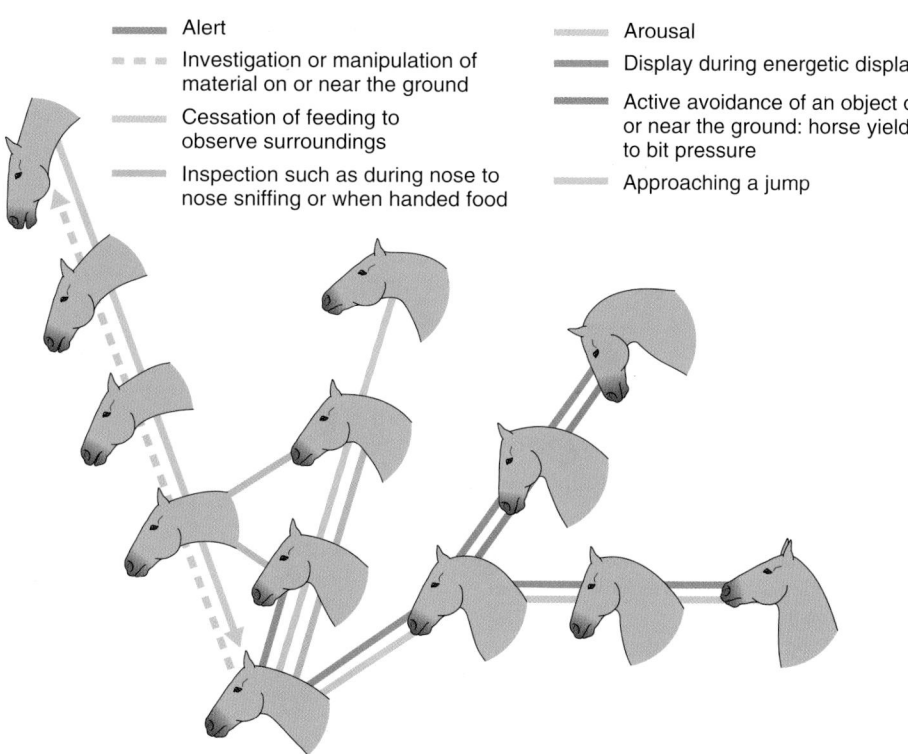

Legend:
- Alert
- Investigation or manipulation of material on or near the ground
- Cessation of feeding to observe surroundings
- Inspection such as during nose to nose sniffing or when handed food
- Arousal
- Display during energetic display
- Active avoidance of an object on or near the ground: horse yielding to bit pressure
- Approaching a jump

FIGURE 5-12 Expression of forward attention in the horse. (From McGreevy P: Equine behavior: a guide for veterinarians and equine scientists, St Louis, 2005, Saunders.)

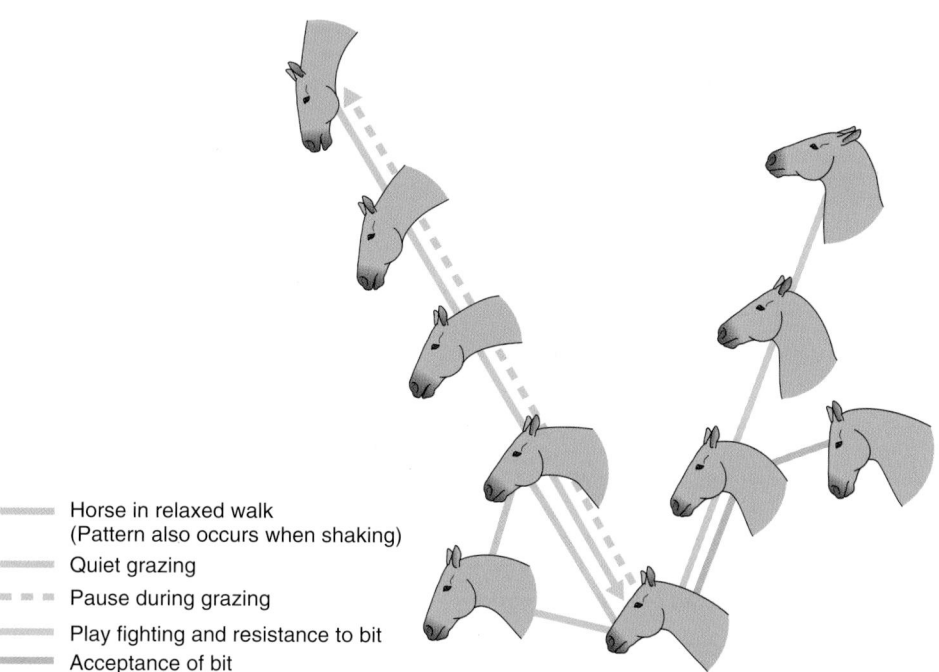

Legend:
- Horse in relaxed walk (Pattern also occurs when shaking)
- Quiet grazing
- Pause during grazing
- Play fighting and resistance to bit
- Acceptance of bit

FIGURE 5-13 Expressions of lateral attention. (From McGreevy P: Equine behavior: a guide for veterinarians and equine scientists, St Louis, 2005, Saunders.)

Vocalizations also play an important role in communication among horses, and they have a well-developed sense of hearing. The whinny or neigh is a greeting or separation call, usually used by the horse to help maintain contact between **conspecifics** (members of the same species). It is the vocalization most often produced by mares and foals when they are separated. Some horses will whinny when they see their owners.

The nicker is the care-giving or care-soliciting call of the horse. The mare will usually nicker to her foal when it returns

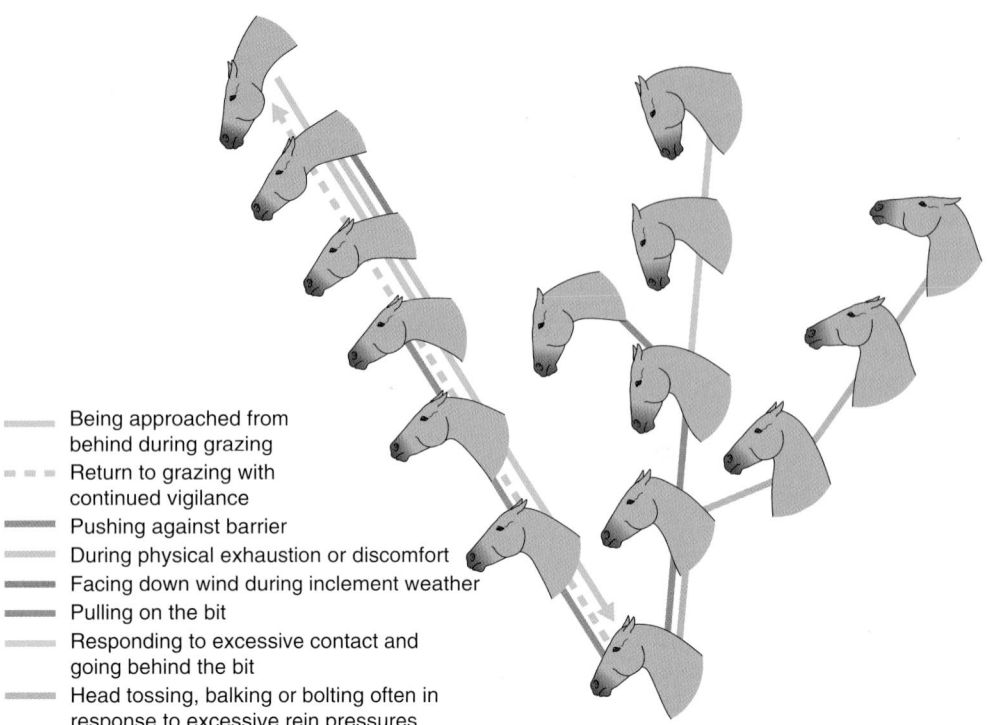

Being approached from behind during grazing

Return to grazing with continued vigilance

Pushing against barrier

During physical exhaustion or discomfort

Facing down wind during inclement weather

Pulling on the bit

Responding to excessive contact and going behind the bit

Head tossing, balking or bolting often in response to excessive rein pressures

FIGURE 5-14 Expressions of backward attention in the horse. (From McGreevy P: Equine behavior: a guide for veterinarians and equine scientists, St Louis, 2005, Saunders.)

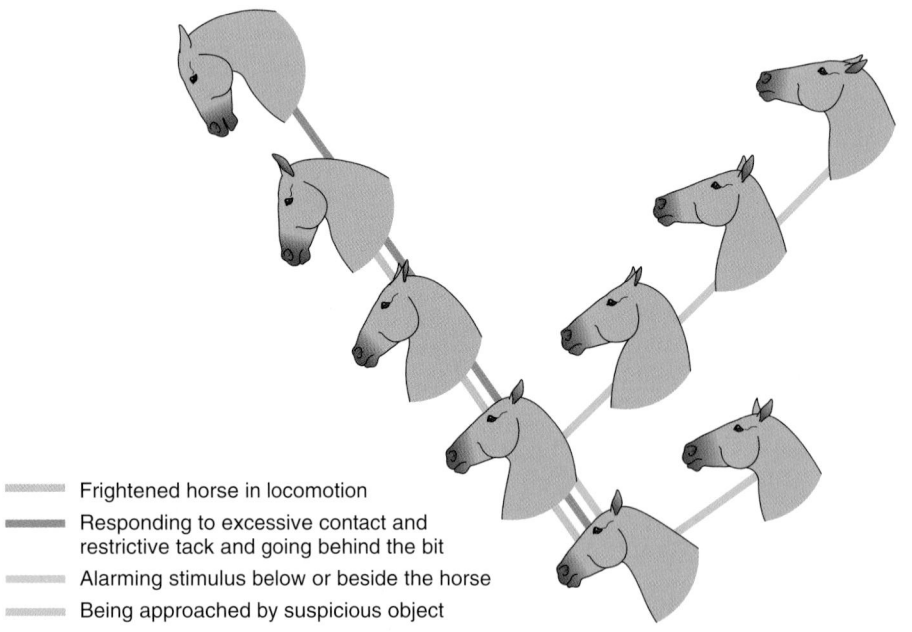

Frightened horse in locomotion

Responding to excessive contact and restrictive tack and going behind the bit

Alarming stimulus below or beside the horse

Being approached by suspicious object

FIGURE 5-15 Expressions of alarm. (From McGreevy P: Equine behavior: a guide for veterinarians and equine scientists, St Louis, 2005, Saunders.)

to her side. Horses will also nicker in greeting and when food is being delivered. Stallions often nicker as a part of their courtship behavior. Both nickers and whinnys are likely to elicit a reply.

The squeal is a close-mouthed vocalization associated with defense and/or aggression. Mares that are not in estrus may squeal when approached by the stallion. Horses may squeal when they are in pain, and if the squeal is particularly long and loud, it may be referred to as a scream. The snort may be produced in alarm and when a horse is frustrated or in conflict, as when being restrained. It may be heard when the horse is investigating an olfactory stimulus and is often associated with pain or fear. Horses may produce a soft groan usually when tired or uncomfortable.

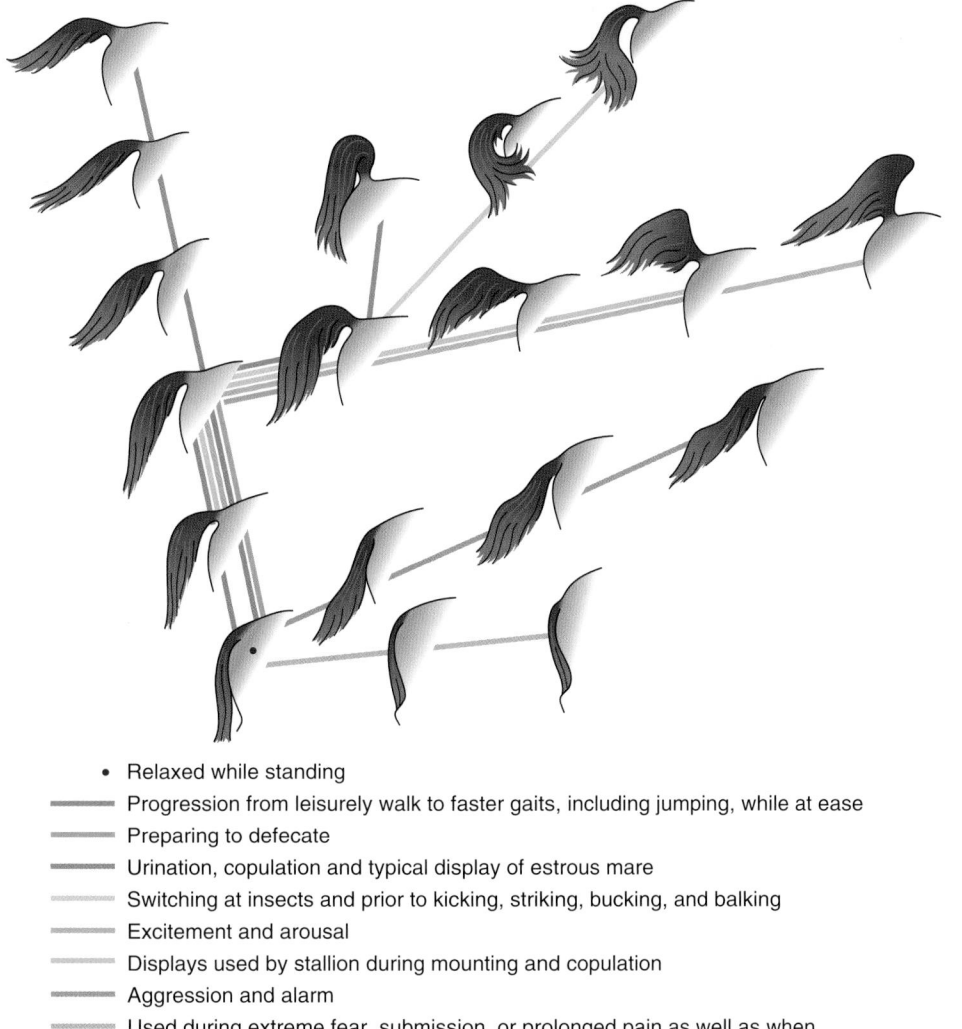

- • Relaxed while standing
- —— Progression from leisurely walk to faster gaits, including jumping, while at ease
- —— Preparing to defecate
- —— Urination, copulation and typical display of estrous mare
- —— Switching at insects and prior to kicking, striking, bucking, and balking
- —— Excitement and arousal
- —— Displays used by stallion during mounting and copulation
- —— Aggression and alarm
- —— Used during extreme fear, submission, or prolonged pain as well as when facing downwind during inclement weather

FIGURE 5-16 Tail positions associated with different displays. (From McGreevy P: Equine behavior: a guide for veterinarians and equine scientists, St Louis, 2005, Saunders.)

Olfaction is another important means of communication between horses. In addition to the conventional olfactory system, horses have a well-developed accessory olfactory system, the vomeronasal organ, or VNO (also referred to as *Jacobson's organ*). The vomeronasal organ is a paired tubular structure within the horse's hard palate that opens into the nasal cavity. When investigating other horses' urine or feces, and sometimes in response to novel smells or flavors, the horse may exhibit the flehmen response. Flehmen involves the horse extending its head, rotating its ears to the side, and everting its upper lip. This behavior forces air through slits in the nasal cavity and into the VNO, allowing the horse to detect and process pheromones and other volatile substances.

Horses recognize foods by their odor and investigate most foreign objects by smelling them. They also greet conspecifics nose to nose, smelling the "breath" from their nostrils. One method by which horses recognize individuals is by their odor, and odor plays an important role in a mare's recognition of her own foal. Stallions use odor cues as well as a variety of other cues to determine when a mare is in estrus.

Our frequent bathing, changing clothes, and using soaps, deodorants, and perfumes cause our odors to change and can interfere with the horse's ability to use olfactory cues alone to recognize us. Unlike our visual and olfactory features, our voice remains unique to us, so speaking to the horse provides it with a reliable means of recognizing us and a good way for us to begin to establish a bond with the horse.

The sensitivity of the horse's skin varies with location, and tactile communication is important between horses, as well as between horse and rider. The density of the skin receptors, as well as the thickness of the skin, contributes to differences in sensitivity. The buccal mucosa of the horse is as sensitive as skin to tactile stimuli, giving the horse the ability to "sift" through its feed and refuse inedible materials by dropping them out of the mouth. The vibrissae around the eye and muzzle are well innervated and help the horse to determine

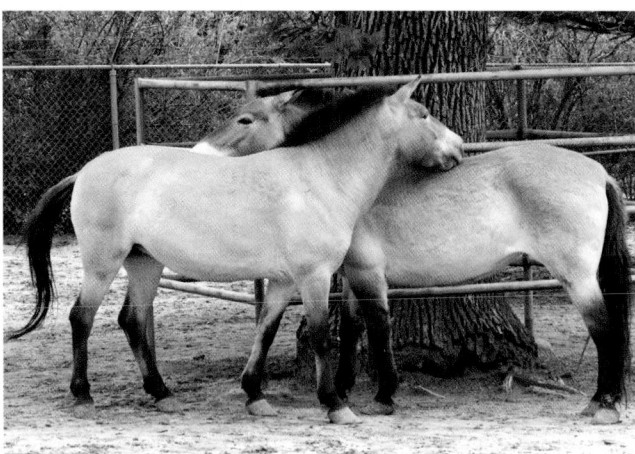

FIGURE 5-17 Two Przewalski horses demonstrating the typical allogrooming behavior of the horse.

the distance from its muzzle to a surface. The withers and flank and elbow regions are other sensitive areas. Some horses may be sensitive to having their ears, groin, area under the tail, or bulbs of the heels touched. When horses allogroom, they tend to stand shoulder to shoulder and nibble at the areas over each other's withers, neck, and back (Figure 5-17). The withers are a good place to begin stroking a horse after you have greeted it because grooming of this area has been shown to reduce heart rate in the horse.[2]

SOCIAL BEHAVIOR

Under free-ranging conditions, the horse is virtually never alone. Horses live in small groups called *bands*, consisting of several mares, their offspring under 3 years of age, and, in most cases, a single stallion. When young horses reach sexual maturity, they leave their natal band but quickly join up with other bands of horses. The mares in the herd form a relatively stable dominance hierarchy among themselves, and the oldest mare in the band is likely to be the highest ranking mare. The dominant mare in the group is usually responsible for leading the herd in flight and to resting areas, watering holes, and feeding areas. The stallion is not necessarily dominant to his mares and must spend most of his time attempting to keep his harem together and prevent their being lured away by other stallions. The dominance hierarchy is important to ensure the availability of resources such as food and water, but it may also ensure reproductive success. Free-ranging horses spend most of their day grazing.

> **TECHNICIAN NOTE** Free-ranging horses are never alone. This has many implications for how we house and manage the domestic horse because these management practices result in many of the problem behaviors seen in the horse.

When domestic horses are kept in groups, they will form similar hierarchies that can remain stable if the group membership remains unchanged. However, the hierarchy seems less determined by age or size; the dominant status is more reliant upon the individual horse's temperament and the position of its mother in the group. Mares are not necessarily dominant over their daughters, and, as is the case in free-ranging horses, daughters eventually achieve the same rank as their dam.

Within any group, horses usually have preferred associates. These individuals often will be related and similar in social rank. Possibly because of their similarity in rank, preferred associates receive more aggression than other members of the group, but it usually is seen in the form of mild threats. Preferred associates will allogroom and conduct most of their daily activities in close proximity. If they are at some distance from each other when a threat is perceived, they will often move closer together. When bonded pairs are separated, for whatever reason, varying degrees of distress may be seen among both parties.

Establishment and maintenance of a hierarchy is important for social animals because it decreases the amount of actual aggression that must occur. In other words, a threat to kick becomes as effective as actually kicking the conspecifc. Without a stable hierarchy, aggression would be necessary every time there was conflict over a resource. This takes time away from eating and other maintenance behaviors, increases the chance of injury, and may have reproductive costs (i.e., decreased conception rates and increased fetal and foal mortality). Once established, the dominance hierarchy is maintained by appeasement gestures and avoidance more than by threats of aggression. The submitting horse often will simply move away from the threatening dominant animal, lower the head, and avert its gaze.

The manner in which we keep horses today—frequently moving them from place to place for training, for competition, or because they are purchased by new owners, and often housing them singly—prevents them from establishing stable **social hierarchies** or forming normal relationships with conspecifics. The general lack of stable social relationships may serve as one of several predisposing factors to the variety of behavior problems that afflict the domestic horse.

PREY BEHAVIOR

One of the advantages of social living is the improved ability, due to mere numbers, to recognize danger more efficiently. Numbers provide each individual with a statistically better chance of not being the one caught by the predator. When a group of horses is alarmed, the response of those first seeing the alarming stimulus will be to raise their head and neck and focus all of their attention on the possible threat. After the initial alert response, the horse may investigate or take flight. Investigation of the stimulus is usually slow and cautious, with the horse making several circuitous approaches from different angles to investigate. Once the horse confirms a potential predator, it will take flight.

A solitary horse will be even more cautious, and one should be prepared for it to take flight more quickly, without taking time to investigate a perceived threat. Generally speaking, the behavior of a startled or frightened horse may be difficult to predict and may be one reason why those not accustomed to horses may think of them as flighty and dangerous animals. When handling unfamiliar horses, one must remember that temperaments and therefore responses to stimuli differ. In addition, the genetics, socialization, training, and other experiences the horse has had will influence its responses in startling or frightening situations. A good handler must remain calm and confident while constantly being alert to anything in the environment that may startle or frighten the horse, as well as always being prepared for a horse to startle or panic when no apparent stimuli can be seen by the handler. A frightened horse may attempt escape regardless of the harm it may cause itself or nearby individuals. Many horses are consistently calm and gentle; however, becoming complacent around horses can lead to serious and sometimes fatal injuries.

> **TECHNICIAN NOTE** A frightened horse can be a danger to its handler.

SEXUAL BEHAVIOR OF THE MARE

The mare in estrus (heat) will stand still and allow the stallion to investigate her by nibbling and smelling. When receptive, the mare will spread her rear legs and squat slightly while urinating frequently and will rhythmically evert the clitoris using her labial muscles. This behavior is known as *winking*. Mares rarely mount each other when in heat, as cows will, and the winking behavior is considered a fairly reliable sign of estrus or impending estrus. However, the most accurate way of determining estrus in most mares is observing her willingness to stand still and allow the stallion to mount. Once the stallion mounts, the mare is likely to exhibit a characteristic expression with her ears turned back, but not flattened, and her lips drooping slightly. Mares that are not receptive will not stand for mounting and will squeal and strike at the stallion if he persists in his attentions.

Today's common management practices of manipulating the estrous cycle using artificial lighting while transporting mares to a strange place to be bred by a strange stallion are likely responsible for many of the abnormal estrous behaviors seen in mares. Anestrus is one of the more common reproductive problems in mares. Although this may be due to physiologic abnormalities, mares may also fail to demonstrate behavioral signs of estrus. This problem is referred to as *silent heat*. It is known that mares demonstrate preferences for particular stallions, so when teasing mares to determine receptivity, several different stallions may have to be used. Other environmental factors such as being in a strange place and being handled by strange people may affect mares' estrous behaviors. Mares are often restrained and forcibly mated by the stallion (or artificially inseminated); in these cases, they may still conceive if they are actually in estrus and ovulation takes place normally.

SEXUAL BEHAVIOR OF THE STALLION

Seasonality affects stallions' reproductive behavior much less than that of mares. Although their peak sexual behavior occurs in the spring, stallions demonstrate a willingness to breed throughout the year. However, several environmental and social factors can affect the stallion's libido. It has been noted that stallions with a harem have higher levels of testosterone than those in a bachelor herd, and those in a bachelor herd have higher levels than stalled stallions.

When a mare and a stallion are allowed free access to each other, the stallion will begin by nipping and nuzzling at the mare's head and will gradually extend this exploration down her neck and back to the perineal area. During this time, he may also exhibit flehmen. Vocalizations in the form of nickers, neighs, and roars (the roar is a high-amplitude vocalization unique to the stallion) are also likely to occur. If the female continues to stand, the stallion becomes increasingly aroused and may lick and nibble her back and rear legs. Several minutes of this courtship behavior may be required for the stallion to become fully erect, and full erection is necessary for intromission to occur. However, the stallion might first attempt to mount a few times without an erection to test the mare's willingness to breed. Thus the stallion must be given adequate time to exhibit these behaviors leading to sexual arousal. Once full erection is achieved, the stallion may make several attempts to mount and intromit. When intromission is finally achieved, the stallion may rest his sternum on the mare's croup and sometimes will reach forward to bite her neck. After several thrusts, ejaculation occurs. Flagging of the stallion's tail usually indicates that ejaculation is complete. The stallion may also rest his head against the mare's neck. After ejaculation, the mare steps forward, allowing the stallion to dismount. Copulation is usually completed in less than a minute. Postcopulatory behavior of the stallion may include some genital sniffing, which typically prompts the flehmen response.

Sexual behavior problems are not uncommon in stallions and range from those showing relatively no libido to those in which the stallion shows an interest in the mare but will not mount, or if he mounts will not intromit or ejaculate. Other problems include injuring or "savaging" the mare or handlers, or being willing to mount a mare only in the presence of another particular horse. Young stallions that have been overused as breeders may suffer from low libido. Young, novice stallions may be hesitant to breed if confronted with a more dominant or aggressive mare. Stallions that have been overused as a stud may behave aggressively during attempted hand breeding, posing harm to both the mare and the handlers. This is more common in stallions that are used for breeding outside of the normal breeding season.

> **TECHNICIAN NOTE** Stallions should never be punished for normal sexual behaviors because this may result in problem behaviors when it is time to use the horse for breeding.

Punishing a stallion for sexual behavior may certainly lead to loss of libido, so proper handling of the stallion is critical. Handlers must be calm and confident, as well as knowledgeable about the breeding procedure, when handling any stallion. Attempting to breed a stallion in an area with slippery flooring may cause him to avoid mounting. Low roofs or overhangs can also pose a danger as the horse rears up to mount the mare. If he strikes his head, he can be injured, but he may also be inhibited about mounting a mare in the future for fear of hurting himself again.

Similar to many male animals, stallions may be stimulated by the presence of another stallion that may be perceived as a competitor. In some cases of low libido, simply bringing another stallion into the area may effectively increase the sexual behavior of an inhibited stallion.

Physical injuries that cause pain upon mounting or intromission should be considered possible causes for a stallion to be hesitant to breed. Genital injuries and limb or back pain can be a problem even after they are successfully treated, if the stallion has learned from prior experience that mounting or intromission might be painful.

Masturbation is a normal behavior of stallions and is accomplished by the stallion flipping the erect penis against the ventral side of his abdomen. Ejaculation is rare and masturbation is unlikely to contribute to breeding problems such as decreased libido or fertility. On the other hand, punishment for masturbation or the use of devices, such as stallion rings or brushes, to decrease masturbation may lead to a decrease in libido.

> **TECHNICIAN NOTE** Masturbation is a normal behavior of stallions and does not negatively affect their breeding potential.

Self-mutilation is a behavior problem that occurs most commonly in stallions. The behavior consists of biting at, or biting, the flanks and occasionally the chest. The horse may squeal and/or kick at the same time. The exact cause of the problem is unknown but is suspected to be related to sociosexual deprivation. It has never been documented in free-ranging stallions. Providing a stall companion or allowing the stallion to live with a mare is curative in many cases. Castration will sometimes but not always stop the behavior. It is critical that any medical condition that could cause pain or discomfort be ruled out before self-mutilation is treated strictly as a behavior problem.

Stallions not intended for breeding are often castrated in an attempt to stop unwanted sexual behaviors, such as aggression. However, castration should not be expected to be 100% effective at decreasing stallion-like behaviors. A variety of factors contribute to sexual behaviors in male animals, including learning and experience, as well as exposure to masculinizing hormones during development in utero. No evidence supports the commonly held misconception that a gelding showing stallion-like behavior has not been properly or completely castrated. In fact, horses of all sexes and ages can show some aspects of the behavior associated with breeding, and it is considered normal for some geldings to show stallion-like behavior.

MATERNAL BEHAVIOR

The mare begins licking and nuzzling her foal soon after birth. She may also investigate and lick any surface containing amniotic fluid. This behavior generally persists for 30 minutes to 1 hour and is likely critical to mare recognition of her foal and development of the mare–foal bond. Foals initially will follow any large moving object and may take as long as a week to selectively recognize their dam. This is just one reason why interruption of the mare and foal during this postparturient period may be detrimental and should be avoided when possible. Most foals will stand and begin nursing within 2 to 3 hours at most. Foals that have not found the udder by this time may need assistance.

Olfaction is the primary means by which mare and foal recognize each other, with visual cues and vocalizations playing a more minor role. The foal is responsible for maintaining contact with the mare except when sleeping; when the foal is recumbent, the mare will stay very close, often just standing and resting. At other times, she may circle the foal, grazing. Mares are very protective of their foals; some will display aggression toward people and other horses that approach too closely during this time.

> **TECHNICIAN NOTE** Interrupting normal mare and foal bonding during the first few hours after birth should be avoided whenever possible.

Free-ranging mares do not wean their foals until 5 to 15 weeks before the birth of their next foal. Before this time, as the foal begins to graze more, the mare's aggression toward the foal will peak in an attempt to prevent nursing. Today's management practices usually result in weaning when the foal is 4 to 6 months of age. Studies have shown that abrupt weaning is very stressful on the foal and may be a contributing cause to several different behavior problems. Gradual weaning, as occurs when the foal has partial contact with the mare through a fence for a period of time before complete separation, has been shown to be much less stressful. Group weaning, where mares and foals are together at pasture for a period of time before the mares are removed, also appears to be less stressful because the foals are left with other foals for companionship, and they remain in a familiar location.

A technique for improving adult equine behavior through early handling of foals, often called *imprint training*, has received much attention in recent years. This technique suggests a series of handling exercises that begin within 48 hours of birth. Studies looking to confirm the efficacy of this technique have been equivocal, and much concern has been expressed about interfering with mare–foal bonding, as well as with the foal's early nursing attempts (potentially preventing timely transfer of immunoglobulins), with this approach. Some studies have looked at the effects of similar habituation and desensitization techniques on older foals and have found them to be similarly effective without the potential negative side effects. Much remains to be learned about the sensitive period of the foal and the ideal time at which early handling and socialization will be most beneficial. Nevertheless, foals learn faster than adults, and early habituation to people can be achieved without interfering with the mare–foal bond. One should make an effort to ensure that all interactions with foals are positive ones, so as not to create a learned fear of human approach or handling. Gentle, regular handling of the mare in the foal's presence may be equally important.

Foal Rejection

Foal rejection is one of the few recognized behavior emergencies. It is critical to the foal's survival that it receives colostrum within several hours of birth. After 36 hours, the foal's digestive tract is incapable of absorbing the important macromolecules contained within the colostrum. Many mares, particularly primiparous mares, resent manipulation of the inguinal fold and the udder. These mares may avoid the foal's approach and may kick, squeal, and even bite when the foal attempts to nurse. Pain associated with mastitis, passage of the placenta, or uterine contractions that occur because of oxytocin released when the foal suckles may contribute to this problem.

A more serious form of foal rejection occurs when the mare acts as if she is afraid of the foal itself and actively attacks it. In these situations, the mare may attempt to escape the foal and may injure it in the process and/or kick the foal whenever it approaches. Other mares may attack the foal by biting it and throwing it across the stall. These mares often have a history of not having licked the fetal membranes or the foal in the minutes after birth and generally behave in a less protective manner toward the foal. These mares have been shown to have lower concentrations of serum progesterone than normal mares. Arabian mares appear to be more predisposed to foal rejection, and the behavior likely has a heritable component. Therefore, caution should be recommended when owners consider rebreeding mares that reject their foals. However, the likelihood of foal rejection does appear to decrease with parity.

A variety of methods have been used to manage and treat foal rejection. A combination of tranquilization and restraint can be used to allow the foal to nurse and to teach the mare that suckling relieves tension on the udder. A combination of gradual desensitization of the flank/udder region and counter-conditioning to change the mare's emotional response to the foal has also been used successfully to treat this problem.

> **TECHNICIAN NOTE** Foal rejection is an emergency behavior problem that can be successfully treated if addressed right away.

COMMON PROBLEM BEHAVIORS
Repetitive Behaviors (Stable Vices)

Horses may perform a number of different unwanted repetitive behaviors often referred to as *stable vices*. These include cribbing, wind-sucking, wood chewing, stall walking and weaving, stall kicking, and repetitive pawing to name a few. Some of these behaviors may accurately be considered displacement or **redirected behaviors**, some represent true stereotypies, and others may simply be reinforced, learned responses. They do not represent any sort of malicious intent or moral failing on the horse's part, so the term *stable vice* is inappropriate and should be removed from the vernacular.

Wood eating or chewing is essentially a normal behavior, equivalent to bark eating and chewing, that is seen in free-ranging horses. Wood eating or chewing may also represent a redirected ingestive behavior. Horses require high fiber content in their diet, and if it is not provided to them, they will eat wood, often doing great damage to the walls of a stall or paddock rails. Providing them with a diet higher in fiber usually significantly reduces the behavior. Wood chewing should not be confused with cribbing, a distinctly different behavior.

Pawing is a normal motor behavior for horses, which is often performed as they attempt to find food under snow or to break the ice over water. Repetitive pawing is often seen as a displacement activity in a stalled horse, especially around feeding time. Repetitive stall kicking can be a form of redirected aggression seen in the horse that cannot directly interact with other nearby horses and form a hierarchy.

Stereotypies have been described as repetitive, relatively invariant behaviors that are believed to serve no function. Cribbing, weaving, and stall walking are some of the most common stereotypies. These behaviors are not seen in free-ranging horses, yet they have been seen in captive wild equids, suggesting that they represent a response to captivity. Free-ranging equids spend most of their day walking and feeding. They rarely stand in one place longer than required to take a few mouthfuls of grass before moving a few steps. If allowed, the horse would eat many small meals throughout a 24 hour period. Yet in captivity, the average horse is not allowed to do any of these things. His locomotion is frequently limited to a stall or paddock, and meals are provided at the convenience of the owner or caretaker.

Cribbing, or crib-biting, is a behavior in which a horse grasps a fixed object with its incisor teeth, arches its neck, and leans backwards, while sometimes, but not always, gulping air and making a distinctive grunting noise. Cribbing has been linked to management factors such as diets that are low in forage and housing that limits normal social behavior between horses. However, many horses are kept stalled, with limited access to forage, and are fed concentrates twice daily, and they do not all become cribbers. This fact suggests that the origin of cribbing is complex and multifactorial, and research continues to provide fascinating information about this problem. Cribbing may be associated with the stress of coping with an abnormal environment in the adult horse, as well as the stress of weaning in foals. The likelihood of cribbing is greater in weanling foals given concentrate feeds. A high incidence of gastric ulcer has been recognized in horses on restricted diets, and it has been postulated that cribbing increases the flow of alkaline saliva, thus helping to decrease the gastric acidity associated with concentrates. Thus cribbing may serve as a partial substitute for eating.

Equine Aggression
Inter-Horse

Aggressive threats are common among groups of horses and, as mentioned earlier, are intended to decrease actual physical conflict. Generally speaking, offensive aggression arises from the fore end and includes the more common head threats, in addition to bite threats, bites, threats to strike, and actual strikes. Kicking and kick threats are believed by some to be limited to defensive behavior but may in fact be used whenever the danger or the opponent is closer to the hindquarters than the forequarters. When a head threat does not result in the offending party moving or otherwise deferring, teeth may be bared in a threat, or the aggressor may actually bite. Horses may also threaten to strike with their foreleg by simply moving one foreleg forward and pinning their ears. A kick threat may involve simply shifting weight or cocking a leg, but a thrashing tail may also be seen. Sometimes a slight hop on the hindquarters is performed before the horse kicks out with one or both legs. Horses can be very accurate in the placement of their strikes or kicks, so it should always be assumed that when they do not make contact, the intent was to only threaten. The subordinate horse will lower its head and look away. If still pursued, it may tuck its tail, drop its croup, and move away with head lowered. When a submitting horse is unable to move away from the aggressor, it may swing its head and roll its eyes, showing the sclera. When the subordinate horse does not perform deferential behaviors acceptable to the aggressor, the aggressor may actually chase the subordinate away.

Horses can cause serious injury to conspecifics in the process of forming a hierarchy. Injuries may be more likely if horses have been confined by themselves for a period of time, and if they are introduced in confined quarters. In preparing to house two horses together, they should first be allowed time to become acquainted while separated but able to have olfactory, visual, and limited tactile contact, without being able to harm each other. Aggression between horses already confined together may be decreased by spacing food buckets as far from each other as possible because much aggression occurs over competition for resources. In addition, the area holding multiple horses must be large enough that horses can use their normal visual cues for deference or appeasement, as well as have room to escape aggressors.

Aggression Toward Humans

Equine aggression directed toward humans is unfortunately common and is often seen in the stalled horse. In some instances, it may be a result of dominance directed toward the person, but in most cases, it is simply a learned response. Horses learn quickly that aggressive threats work to keep people away, so fear is often at the root of a horse's aggression. For example, the veterinarian who has caused some discomfort in the past may be feared. Farriers and handling of the feet can similarly elicit fear. Horses can develop a fear of being caught, clipped, saddled, or ridden. In many cases, chronic pain as well as the fear of pain may be the cause of the fear and the subsequent aggression. If a horse has subclinical orthopedic pain, it can learn quickly to use aggression to keep people from approaching if it expects the approaching person to catch, saddle, or ride it. Underlying pain or discomfort must always be ruled out as a contributing cause of aggression, irritability, and reluctance to work. Once pain has been ruled out or treated, the behavior modification techniques described earlier in the chapter can all be used to treat aggression in the horse. For example, horses can be desensitized to saddling, clipping, shoeing, injections, and so forth.

CATTLE AND SMALL RUMINANTS

SPECIES-TYPICAL BEHAVIORS

The most commonly kept domestic livestock are the hoofed ruminants: cattle, goats, and sheep. These three species are all highly social, herd-dwelling, grazing, and browsing (in the case of goats) prey animals. Their olfactory capabilities are excellent, and olfaction is one of their more critical senses for social behavior. Olfaction plays an important role in recognition of conspecifics, male ruminants use olfaction to assist in determining the stage of estrus of females, and olfaction aids in the mutual recognition of dam and offspring. All domestic male ruminants will display flehman in response to female urine.

Vocalizations are also important, although they have been less well studied than the vocalizations of many other species. Vocalizations in ruminants appear to be limited to distress calls and contact calls. Distress calls of sheep, goats, and cattle are all easily recognizable and tend to be drawn out, repeated calls that are higher pitched than most contact calls. Contact calls, as the name implies, are used by the ruminant to locate others when separated from the herd. Not unlike horses, these species are rarely alone of their own volition and when separated will work hard to regain contact with their herd mates. Distress calls are likely to be heard when separated, as well as when they are hungry or injured. Most ruminants will be less stressed in a frightening situation if they are with familiar animals.

> **TECHNICIAN NOTE** When ruminants are handled, most will be less distressed and thus easier to handle if they are with familiar conspecifics.

Cattle, sheep, and goats have visual capabilities that allow them to recognize different individuals, including humans. In addition to olfactory cues, visual cues play a role in recognizing behaviors associated with courtship and breeding, as well as with postures associated with dominance and submission. Sheep in particular watch their flock mates very closely. If one sheep raises it head to look at a stimulus, other nearby sheep will also raise their head and look. If one sheep flees, all of the others will flee with it.

Generally speaking, social facilitation plays a large role in the behavior of herding ruminants. They tend to eat at the same time, move at the same time, and rest at the same time. They are all likely to be more difficult to handle when completely separated from conspecifics and should be maintained in small groups whenever possible.

As is usually the case with social animals, ruminants will form social hierarchies within their herds. Development of the hierarchy may require some degree of aggression initially, but once established, the hierarchy is maintained mostly with visual threats and with avoidance behavior by subordinates.

Cattle in particular take about 24 to 48 hours to form the hierarchy, but it can be a full month before actual physical aggression is replaced by visual threats. Generally speaking, the hierarchy of the sheep is less well defined. A newcomer introduced to the herd may simply not be allowed to join the flock right away and may be forced to use less productive parts of the pasture. Goats display more overt aggressive behavior when establishing a hierarchy than sheep and tend to be more exploratory. Goats are likely to be most aggressive when food is present, and introduction of a novel food will lead to increased aggression.

Dominant/Aggressive Behaviors

Cattle threatening aggression will stand sideways (the broadside threat) with their head held low and perpendicular to the ground as if displaying horns. Their feet will be drawn well under their body. A bull may paw the ground and also drop to the ground on his forelegs, while making slashing movements in the dirt with his horns. When fighting, cattle will butt heads and shoulders and then struggle to reach the flank of the opponent. Once one individual reaches the flank of the other, it places its head between the legs and the udder, which is referred to as the *clinch*, where it has a decided advantage over the opponent. The individual held in the "clinch" is helpless and can run or can continue to attempt to get loose and take the flank advantage itself.

Sheep that demonstrate aggression may stamp their feet and strike with their forelimbs; when fighting, the dominant animal will hold its head low with its nose pointed up.

Goats demonstrate aggression by raring up on their hindlimbs and then charging and butting heads or horns with their opponent. Once the hierarchy is established, head/horn threats and rushes are common.

Submissive Behaviors

Cattle demonstrate submission by holding their head low but parallel to the ground with their ears turned outward.

Sheep demonstrating submission may shake their head and lower it while looking away and then moving away.

Goats will look away from the dominant animal and may move away to avoid conflict.

> **TECHNICIAN NOTE** If a bovid presents its side to you with its head held low and perpendicular to the ground, it is demonstrating an offensive aggressive threat.

When observing a herd of cattle, the technician should be aware that sick cows and cows with advanced pregnancies will withdraw from the herd and lose status temporarily. Upon returning to the herd, they assume their previous rank. When grazing, animals close in rank will be closer to one another; the lower the rank, the larger the inter-animal distance. In other words, if you are higher in rank, you do not have to be cautious about approaching another animal too closely. When cattle are driven, the least dominant animals will be first and the most dominant animals will remain in the middle of the group. This should be kept in mind when animals are moved into a crush; if subordinate animals and dominant animals are forced into each other, aggression is likely.

> **TECHNICIAN NOTE** Sick cattle and cows with advanced pregnancies will usually withdraw from the herd.

If aggression is going to occur in a herd of cattle with a stable hierarchy, it will usually occur when feeding at a trough. The animal that can supplant all others most likely will be the dominant animal. The farther apart cattle stand from each other at the trough, the greater the difference in their rank. If food is limited, the lowest ranking cow may not get to eat or may be forced to eat the less palatable choices. To minimize problems when cattle are mixed, they should never be mixed when they are hungry.

Allogrooming may assist in the maintenance of bonds between individual cattle. Cattle groom each other by licking the head and neck of the other individual. Grooming is more likely to involve kin, animals of the same age, or simply the nearest animal. Sheep and goats perform some muzzle-to-muzzle affiliative behaviors but minimal allogrooming.

When sheep are approached in a pen, the sheep the farthest away from the approaching person will be the most dominant. When working with sheep, especially if attempting to move them, the technician should be aware that when fewer than three sheep are in the group, they do not readily flock together. More sheep are needed if one hopes to get them to move from one place to another as a group.

SEXUAL BEHAVIOR

Male farm animals are usually selected for breeding and often are separately reared. This can have a large impact on their ability to exhibit normal sexual behaviors. In addition, because they are not forced to compete for females, as they do in the wild, and are not usually selected for sexual performance, breeding problems are not uncommon. For example, rams reared in all-male groups, fail to develop an interest in females and direct sexual behaviors only toward males. In some cases, this can be reversed by confinement for a period of time in an all-ewe group. The rearing environment does not appear to be as critical in cattle in that bulls raised in isolation still direct sexual behavior toward females, although they make more disoriented mounting attempts (at the side or the head) before learning to mount from the rear.

Maintaining libido in male animals that are frequently used for "hand breeding" can be challenging. Studies have shown that bulls allowed to watch other bulls while breeding show increased sexual performance. This is also effective in improving male dairy goat sexual performance, but not that of rams.

MATERNAL BEHAVIOR

Most breeds of domestic livestock, with dairy cows being the exception, are selected for good maternal behavior. Obvious problems arise when a dam does not care for her offspring. Ruminants in particular exhibit strong maternal behavior, especially in the minutes to hours after parturition when they lick, nuzzle, and smell their newborn. A sensitive period exists for responding to any neonate, and in some species it may be as short as a few minutes. During this period, they bond with their offspring. If their offspring is taken away before bonding develops, they may refuse it when presented again at a later time. Before the end of this sensitive period, they can also have other offspring presented and they are likely to accept them. Maternal experience plays an important role, with **primiparous** females more likely to reject a neonate that is separated from them within a few minutes of birth than **multiparous** females.

Fostering an orphaned or rejected neonate on another female is often necessary when raising livestock. It can be very challenging to do this if a dam has already bonded with her own offspring. Because olfactory cues play such an important role in recognition of a neonate by its dam, transferring odors from the real offspring to the fostered offspring can be effective. This has been attempted using a variety of different methods, many of which are effective much of the time. If the need occurs soon after parturition of the foster mom, the placenta and amniotic fluids from her own offspring can be rubbed on the neonate needing to be fostered. Another technique involves using orthopedic stockinette to make jackets for lambs. The jacket first is worn for a few

minutes by the dam's own offspring and then is placed on the animal that needs fostering. This results in immediate acceptance a large percentage of the time. This technique has also been found effective with cattle.

> **TECHNICIAN NOTE** Fostering calves and lambs can usually be achieved by making the fostered offspring smell like the actual offspring of the dam.

Different strategies for offspring care are apparent among different ruminant species. Lambs are referred to as *followers*, and calves and kids are *hiders*. This refers to the fact that lambs are very precocious and begin following their dam within minutes to hours of birth and subsequently stay near her wherever she goes until the time of maturity. Hider species are left alone while their dams go off to feed. The dam periodically returns to the area where she left her offspring and vocalizes. The young then stand and approach the dam and suckle. After a few days (cattle) or weeks (goats), the hider offspring begin to follow their dam and to socialize with other offspring. It is common to see these "nursery groups" of calves together in a field playing or resting.

COMMON BEHAVIOR PROBLEMS
Buller Steer Syndrome

Buller steer syndrome develops when one steer repeatedly stands and tolerates mounting by other steers. This problem has a large economic impact on feedlots, where it occurs most commonly, and may lead to loss second only to respiratory disease. No one understands fully why any particular steer develops this problem. A normal steer would not submit to mounting but should exhibit avoidance behaviors or turn and threaten the animal attempting to mount. Instead "buller" steers allow it and may be injured by the persistent mounting, often becoming debilitated and having to be removed from the pen. The only way known to stop the behavior is to remove the "buller" steer from the group.

Aggression to Humans

Most of the domestic livestock species have been selected for a certain amount of tolerance of human proximity and handling. Nevertheless, some individuals may display aggression toward humans. This may be more common among hand-raised individuals that direct their normal species-typical behaviors toward humans as if they are conspecifics. Whenever possible, orphaned animals should be raised with conspecifics or fostered so as to prevent these problems.

Cattle that spend much of their life on open range may also be more difficult to handle and more aggressive than other cattle. This is mostly a result of lack of habituation to human handling. Habituation can make a lot of difference in the ease with which cattle can be worked. Whenever possible, simply moving cattle through a chute without performing any procedures can be worth the time invested in the time saved when the cattle are actually worked.

Sometimes, this may need to be done only two or three times to make a difference in the cattle's behavior in the chute.

Dairy cows in particular are selected for ease of handling, but dairy bulls are notoriously aggressive and must be handled with a great degree of caution. The technician should remain aware that all livestock species can recognize people by their appearance and remember them. They have shown the ability to remember people who have treated them gently, as well as those who have not. Raised voices as well as slapping and hitting have been shown to be aversive to cattle. Patience and tolerance will pay off if the animals do not learn to associate your approach with fearful stimuli.

REFERENCES

1. Hetts S, Heinke ML, Estep DQ: Behavior wellness concepts for general veterinary practice, J Am Vet Med Assoc 4:506–513, 2004.
2. Feh C, De Mazières J: Grooming at preferred sites reduces heart rate in horses, Anim Behav 46:1191–1194, 1993.

RECOMMENDED READINGS

Bradshaw WS: The behaviour of the domestic cat, New York, 1992, CABI Publishing.

Hart BL, Hart LA: The perfect puppy: how to choose your dog by its behavior, New York, 1988, W.H. Freeman and Company.

Horwitz DF, Neilson JC: Blackwell's five minute veterinary consult clinical companion: canine and feline behavior, Ames, IA, 2007, Wiley-Blackwell.

Houpt KA: Domestic animal behavior for veterinarians and animal scientists, Ames, IA, 2011, Wiley-Blackwell.

Landsberg G, Hunthausen W, Ackerman L: Handbook of behavior problems of the dog and cat, London, 2003, Saunders.

McGreevy P: Equine behavior: a guide for veterinarians and equine scientists, London, 2005, Saunders.

Price EO: Principles and applications of domestic animal behavior, Oxfordshire, UK, 2008, CABI Publishing.

Serpell J: The domestic dog: its evolution, behaviour and interactions with people, Cambridge, 1995, Cambridge University Press.

The Behavior Perspective, newsletter of the Society of Veterinary Behavior Technicians.

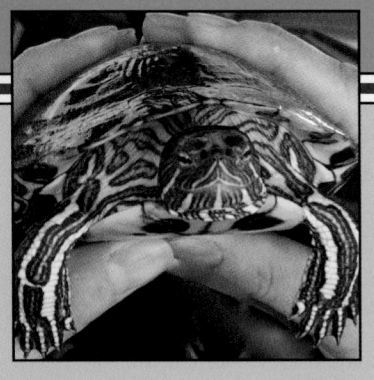

6 Restraint and Handling of Animals

Karen Todd-Jenkins, Barbara Dugan, Darren W. Remsburg, and Chris Montgomery

KEY TERMS

Aggression
Binocular vision
Blind spot
Cow kick
Cradle
Cross-tie
Displacement behaviors
Diversionary restraint
Double barrel kick
Fear biting
Flight-or-fight response
Flight zone
Humane twitch
Hobbles
Passerine
Point of balance
Psittacine
Raptorial species
Stocks
Tail tie
Tortoise
Turtles
Twitch

OUTLINE

Indications for Restraint, *178*
The Approach, *178*
Capture, *180*
Canine Restraint, *183*
Options for Restraining a Well-Behaved Dog, *183*
Options for Restraining an Uncooperative Dog, *184*
Feline Restraint, *186*
Options for Restraining a Well-Behaved Cat, *186*
Options for Restraining an Uncooperative Cat, *186*
Restraining Dogs and Cats for Specific Procedures, *188*
Restraint for Venipuncture, *188*
Restraint for Nail Trimming, *188*
Introduction to Equine Restraint, *190*
The Approach, *191*
Capture of the Equine, *192*
Adult Equine Restraint Techniques and Devices, *194*
Juvenile Equine and Foal Restraint Techniques, *195*
Equine Restraint: Special Circumstances for Specific Procedures, *196*
Capture and Restraint of Cattle, *199*
The Approach, *199*

Low-Stress Handling, *199*
Capture, *200*
Restraint Techniques and Devices, *202*
Capture and Restraint of Swine, *205*
Observation, *205*
Approach, *205*
Capture and Restraint Techniques, *206*
Capture and Restraint of Small Ruminants, *208*
Observation, *208*
Approach, *208*
Capture, *208*
Individual Restraint, *209*
Restraint Techniques for Camelids, *209*
Handling and Restraint of Cervids, *210*
Capture and Restraint of Avian and Exotic Species, *211*
Restraint of Small Mammals, *214*
Rabbits, *214*
Guinea Pigs and Chinchillas, *215*
Ferrets, *215*
Hamsters, Mice, Hedgehogs, Sugar Gliders, and Gerbils, *216*
Handling and Restraint of Reptiles, *216*
Lizards, *216*
Snakes, *218*
Turtles and Tortoises, *218*

LEARNING OBJECTIVES

When you have completed this chapter, you will be able to:

1. Pronounce, spell, and define all of the Key Terms in this chapter.
2. List three indications for animal restraint and describe methods for approaching dogs and cats before attempting restraint.
3. Do the following regarding canine and feline capture and restraint:
   - List actions taken to diminish stress among dogs and cats during physical examinations and hospitalization.
   - List the equipment and the methods used in capturing and restraining both cooperative and uncooperative dogs and cats.

- List the advantages and disadvantages of chemical restraint in dogs and cats.
- Describe various positions for restraining cats and dogs specifically for nail trimming and venipuncture of the cephalic vein.
4. Do the following regarding equine capture and restraint:
   - Explain the principles that affect equine perception and behavior.
   - Describe the physical abilities of horses and how these affect the ways in which horses are handled.
   - Describe methods for approaching and capturing adult and juvenile equine patients, including using restraint equipment, diversions, and pharmaceutical products, and identify special restraint techniques for horses and the circumstances in which they are used.
5. Do the following regarding capture and restraint of cattle:
   - Describe the principles that affect cattle behavior and list principles used to move cattle and individuals in an effective and low-stress manner.
   - Explain the differences in housing between dairy and beef cattle and describe how these differences affect methods to handle and restrain them.
   - List the type of bulls known to be particularly dangerous to handle.
   - List the equipment used to restrain cattle in general and specific parts of their bodies. Also, describe the circumstances of their use.
6. Describe methods for observing and approaching swine of each gender and age group, and discuss methods used to capture and restrain adult and young pigs.
7. Do the following regarding small ruminant capture and restraint:
   - Describe the behavioral tendencies of small ruminants and explain how these influence the approach and capture of herds.
   - List factors that affect levels of aggression in camelids and describe how aggression presents in these species.
   - Describe the approach, capture, and restraint of individual sheep, goats, and camelids.
   - List additional restraint techniques used in camelids, but not in sheep or goats.
   - Define cervids and explain methods for their restraint and handling.
8. Describe restraint and handling techniques used with birds, small mammals, and reptiles.

INTRODUCTION

Most people entering the field of veterinary technology have had experience with animals, but few have had the experience necessary to deal with all the species that might be encountered. To assume that all animals respond to a particular situation in the same manner is incorrect and can be a dangerous assumption to make. Restraint techniques differ markedly among species, and even among conspecies, the responses of individuals can be highly variable. People can protect themselves by understanding the body language of animals and by anticipating a particular array of responses. In this way, appropriate actions can be taken in advance to manage the animal.

This chapter is intended to be a guide to the handling and restraint of animals commonly encountered in veterinary practice. It is intended not to be an exhaustive text, but rather to provide a range of techniques to build confidence and competence in the veterinary technician.

INDICATIONS FOR RESTRAINT

Competent restraint of animals is critical in veterinary practice for the following reasons:

1. **To control an animal so that it can receive medical care.** Most animals resist physical examination and the administration of diagnostic and therapeutic procedures. Proper restraint of a sick animal may allow humans to save its life.

2. **To prevent the animal from harming itself while it is receiving medical care.** Animals must be restrained when panicked or when trying to flee from what they perceive as a dangerous situation. Jumping off an examination table, attempting to crash through a fence, and chewing the bars of confinement are examples of fleeing behavior that can have disastrous results. Maintaining a safe environment, including well-constructed stalls, cages, and fencing, is a critical part of protecting the animal from injury.

3. **To protect personnel.** The safety of veterinary personnel, clients, and handlers is of the utmost importance. Injury and even death of individuals can devastate families and veterinary practices. These events can lead to loss of wages, expensive litigation, anxiety, decreased morale, and loss of livelihood. Practice owners are responsible for any injuries incurred by veterinary personnel and clients during the performance of veterinary procedures. This liability begins when the client enters the practice, or when the truck stops in the driveway. For this reason, many practitioners believe that the ability to perform excellent animal restraint is the most important skill for a veterinary technician to master.

> **TECHNICIAN NOTE** Excellent skill in restraint is critical to ensure that the animal receives medical care without injury to patient or care-givers.

THE APPROACH

The interaction between a veterinary health care professional and a patient begins long before the pet is approached or touched. Many dogs and cats know "where they are going" as soon as they are placed into a pet carrier or loaded into a car. Other pets remember past experiences and react accordingly as soon as they see the parking lot or enter the door of the practice. Once inside, animals are continually observing everything around them. Sounds (including human voices and the voices of other pets in the area), smells, movements, and postures all are evaluated and interpreted. Pets' reactions to direct contact are modified by how they have interpreted the situation up to that point. That said, the manner in which patients are approached by veterinary personnel deserves significant consideration.

Observing the Pet Before Approaching

In a clinic setting, most aggressive behaviors in dogs and cats are based on fear or the perception of a threat. Although different types of **aggression** can play a role, such as a dominant personality, the primary motivation is generally fear and avoidance of injury. This distinction is important because corrective training methods that can improve the behavior of a pet with a dominance aggression problem can make the behavior of a pet worse if it has fear-related aggression. The reader is referred to Chapter 5 for specific information on animal behavior and how to interpret different types of aggression. For the purpose of facilitating safe and effective animal handling, this chapter will focus primarily on dealing with fearful pets.

A veterinary technician's ability to interpret nonverbal communication in patients is critical for safe and efficient patient handling and for providing medical care. Table 6-1 lists some behaviors and postural changes that can be observed in fearful pets. Certain behaviors, including vocalization and hissing, are warnings. When a fearful pet displays warnings, the situation can usually be improved by backing

TABLE 6-1	Examples of Fear-Related Behaviors in Dogs and Cats*
BEHAVIORS IN DOGS	**BEHAVIORS IN CATS**
Staring or averting the eyes	Averting the eyes, squinting
Leaning backward; distributing weight toward the rear legs	Leaning backward, arching the back, pulling the feet in (to facilitate running)
Crouching or cowering	Crouching or cowering
Tucking/lowering the tail	Tucking/lowering the tail; swishing or flicking the tail (signals agitation)
Head held low	Lowering the head
Lowering or flattening the ears	Lowering or flattening the ears
Panting, lips pulled back ("submissive grin")	Dilated pupils
Rolling onto the side or back	Rolling onto the side or back
Piloerection	Piloerection
Growling, whimpering, biting	Hissing, growling, screaming, swatting/striking, biting
Urination, defecation, release of anal glands	Urination, defecation, release of anal glands
Displacement behavior: yawning, scratching, licking lips	Displacement behavior: grooming

*This table lists some common demonstrations of fear and anxiety in dogs and cats. Not every pet will display all of these behaviors, and some of the changes can be very subtle (especially in cats). Pets demonstrating these behaviors may bite when handlers approach, reach into their space, lean over them, or proceed with any behaviors that make the pet feel threatened. In many cases, backing away slightly, using verbal reassurance, adopting a nonthreatening body posture, and taking other steps to reduce the pet's anxiety level can reverse the progression to increasingly demonstrative behaviors and eventual attack.

up and reducing the pet's perceived threat level. Continuing to engage the pet may result in aggression. It is worth noting that some pets may display "mixed signals" if they are uncertain of how to interpret the current threat level. Also, it is advisable to evaluate the entire animal instead of looking to tail movement, ear position, or any other single indicator of an animal's emotional state; a wagging tail does not necessarily mean a happy dog. Finally, veterinary care providers should be aware of **displacement behaviors** in fearful pets. These behaviors are a coping mechanism intended to help the pet reduce its anxiety level. Displacement behaviors such as grooming in cats, and yawning, scratching, and licking lips in dogs, may seem out of character in a fearful pet in that they seem to imply relaxation. However, displacement behaviors should not be misinterpreted as indicating that the pet is relaxed and is no longer fearful.

> **TECHNICIAN NOTE** No single behavior can indicate an animal's state of mind in all situations. Ear position, vocalization, tail movement, and other behaviors are open to interpretation and must be evaluated collectively to determine whether a patient is exhibiting threatening behavior.

If possible, pets should be observed from a distance while in the waiting room because their behavior in this setting can reveal valuable information about their emotional state. A dog that is happily engaging every person and pet in the waiting area is probably less anxious than a dog that is hiding under the owner's chair or aggressively lunging at anyone passing by. Also, observe how well the pet obeys the owner's commands in an unfamiliar setting like the waiting room. If the pet ignores commands while in the waiting area, it will likely continue to do so in the examination room.

Observation from a distance is more limited in cats because they are generally in a pet carrier, but nervous cats may crouch against the back wall of a pet carrier, growl when the carrier is approached, or show other evidence of anxiety. A cat that is head-butting the front of the carrier or reaching out to gently touch a nearby hand or finger is probably comfortable with the current situation. Placing a finger against the cage for the cat to sniff can facilitate an introduction, but avoid sticking fingers into the cage. Some veterinary professionals spray feline facial pheromone spray (Feliway, Ceva Animal Health, Inc., Saint Louis, MO) on their hands a few minutes before a feline appointment; this can have a calming effect on some cats. The spray can also be applied to any towels that will be used while handling the cat or (at home) to the towel inside the pet carrier. Ideally, the spray should be applied 30 minutes ahead of time to allow the alcohol-based solution to dry. If possible, the practice's waiting area can be modified to reduce the stress level for cats. This can include having a separate area (or a separate waiting room) for cats; providing space for benches or

shelves, so carriers don't have to be placed on the floor (where a dog can approach and sniff); and using plug-in feline pheromone in the feline waiting area.

> **TECHNICIAN NOTE** Cat owners should be advised to acclimate their cat to the carrier before veterinary office visits. Leaving the carrier open on the floor at home and placing catnip or treats inside can make the carrier more pleasant for the cat. Cat owners can also place catnip, treats, and a familiar towel in the carrier to help reduce the cat's anxiety during transportation.

Pets that are hospitalized should be observed momentarily before an attempt is made to approach them or enter a cage. If a hospitalized pet is sleeping, suddenly opening the cage may startle the patient and incite a fearful reaction. Consider gently speaking to the pet or softly calling it by name to wake it up before getting closer or opening the cage. If the pet is awake in the cage, observe its posture and activities and its reaction to people and other animals that pass by.

Approaching the Pet

Pets are observing their surroundings just as surely as veterinary care providers are observing their patients. Pets rely heavily on scents to interpret their environment, so the lingering aroma of anal gland secretions, urine, or feces can affect the behavior of the next pet that enters the area. It is recommended to wash hands in between each pet, and to keep the examination room, table, and waiting area as clean as possible in between appointments. Feline facial pheromone spray is helpful for improving the perception of aromas for cats. A dog-appeasing pheromone spray (D.A.P., Ceva Animal Health, Inc.) can be sprayed on towels, muzzles, or other equipment for use in dogs. Both pheromone products are available as plug-in atomizers that can be used in strategic areas around the practice.

When approaching a patient, note that certain behaviors and postures can be perceived as threatening. For example, staring directly at a dog or cat and approaching from the front can be perceived as hostile. Approaching on an angle from the side and in a nonthreatening manner is preferable. Avoid placing hands on hips or appearing tall; instead, try to appear smaller and nonthreatening. Making excessive or large arm movements, clapping hands, and making loud noises should be avoided. Speaking gently in a soft tone while saying the pet's name is helpful. Approaching too quickly (which can be interpreted as pursuit) should also be avoided. Instead, keep all movements purposeful and deliberate, and try to move at a moderately steady and consistent pace. Standing between a dog and its owners should be avoided if possible, especially if children are present. Dogs that are being protective or fearful may react negatively to this positioning. Once the pet and the owner are within reasonable range, greetings and introductions should be conducted using a pleasant, even tone. While speaking with the owner, any touching (including shaking hands) should be done very cautiously or avoided because some dogs can perceive a handshake as a lunge or another type of threat directed toward the owner. When the dog is close enough to reach, avoid leaning over the dog or reaching over its head. It is better to bend at the knees or squat. Offering a small treat may be appropriate, as long as this does not interfere with the reason for the veterinary visit. Place the treat on the floor near the dog or offer it in an outstretched palm if the dog seems trustworthy. When in doubt, placing the treat on the floor is safer than offering it by hand.

These precautions are recommended when encountering a new or unknown pet, but even dogs that have been to the practice many times and are familiar to staff members can experience behavior changes, especially if they are ill or in pain. Even a dog that seems engaging and is not exhibiting any signs of fear or aggression should be approached with some caution and briefly evaluated before further interaction takes place.

Pet owners can sometimes help determine how much caution should be exercised when dealing with their pet. Owners are sometimes willing to report whether their pet has needed "special handling" during previous veterinary visits, so questioning them can be helpful. However, ask the owner directly if the pet is "good at the vet's office." Simply asking if the pet is "nice" is inadequate, as the pet may be perfectly well behaved at the park or around friends and family but may display a completely different personality at the veterinarian's office.

Once the dog and the owner are close enough, the dog may approach a new person on its own and try to sniff a shoe, leg, or hand (held in a relaxed position close to the body). This is perfectly fine and can be rewarded by gently scratching the pet's chin or petting the head. However, reaching from above the dog's head can still be perceived as threatening and should be avoided. If appropriate, a small treat may be offered at this time.

If the dog does not approach willingly, some veterinary professionals offer the back of the hand (while approaching on an angle from the side, avoiding direct eye contact, and speaking the pet's name using a soothing voice), but this should be done very cautiously or avoided if the pet backs away or displays other signs of hostility or fear. Within reason, a fearful pet should be allowed to back away temporarily and should not be pursued or cornered; this may lead to more fear and potentially aggressive action. Some dogs can be coaxed forward by speaking gentle words of encouragement, using hand gestures to beckon them forward, assuming a less-threatening posture, and backing away so they feel less pursued. Speaking in a soft, confident voice can encourage the pet to become more comfortable. Offering a small treat (by placing it on the floor near the dog) may be worth a try, but a dog that is extremely stressed will likely not accept a treat from a stranger. If the dog has backed itself into a corner, under a chair, or into another inconvenient location, the owner may be able to coax the pet out,

after which the introduction can be repeated with the dog on a closer leash. If the dog still refuses to leave the corner, back away completely and allow the owner and the dog to enter the examination room together. Different strategies can be attempted within the closed area of an examination room.

CAPTURE

In many cases, attempting to capture a pet represents the first point during an interaction between a patient and a veterinary technician in which the pet is close enough to do significant harm. Attempts to pick up a small dog, remove a cat from a carrier, or touch a large dog should be made using caution—even if the pet seems fine and has been handled before. The **"fight or flight"** response occurs whenever an animal enters a state of alert—certainly when a threat is perceived. Stimulation of the sympathetic nervous system increases heart rate and blood pressure, increases blood flow to the skeletal muscles, lungs, and brain, and causes other changes in the body that prepare the animal to avoid a threat by escaping ("flight") or to resolve the threat by attacking ("fight"). When interaction with a patient progresses from observation and approach to capture, veterinary professionals are advised that the patient is likely in a state of physiologic excitement. If a pet is not permitted to escape (flee) and the stress level continues to escalate, the next logical step is to attack (fight). Fortunately, most pets would rather run than fight, so as long as the stress level can be controlled or reduced, most pets do not progress to a level where attack is their only perceived option. Some behaviorists have included a third term—"freeze"—along with "fight" and "flight." Many pets (especially cats) simply become very still when they are nervous. This allows easier handling but does not necessarily mean that the pet's stress level is under control, so continued caution is still warranted.

Because most unacceptable behavior exhibited at the veterinary office results from stress or fear, veterinary professionals should make every attempt to minimize anxiety for patients. If possible, equipment that will be needed during the appointment should be set up ahead of time to reduce the amount of time the pet spends on the examination table and to minimize excess noise and activity during the visit. Movements during the examination should be efficient and deliberate, and sudden movements or loud noises should be avoided. Fumbling and being indecisive can add to the pet's anxiety. Cats should be left in the carrier until handling and other examination procedures are ready to begin. Cats tend to be more stressed on the examination table than in the carrier, so the amount of time spent on the table should be minimized. Some cats are punished at home for being on tables and countertops, so they may be very nervous about being on a metal examination table. Placing a towel or mat on the table can help reduce this anxiety. If possible, dedicate an exam room to be used only for cats; leftover smells from dogs will be less prominent. Other touches like a Feliway outlet diffuser can be added, and feline-specific health literature can be provided for owners.

Capturing a Dog

Capturing a dog should be relatively straightforward if the dog is already on a leash. This is just one of many reasons why every dog in the practice should be on a leash. Owners of small dogs sometimes prefer to hold the dog on their shoulder or on their lap without a leash. This can be politely discouraged by offering a complimentary leash for use until the dog is ready to leave the office. Larger dogs are generally leashed, but owners using retractable leashes may have to be gently reminded to keep their dogs within a reasonable distance to help avoid mishaps in the reception area. With a leash in place, a well-behaved dog generally can be led up onto a platform scale or a lift table with very little effort. A dog that is fearful or that needs to be picked up requires more immediate control. Most dogs respond favorably to vocal reassurance, so this should be incorporated as often as possible during interactions with patients. Before picking up any dog, ask the owner if the dog seems painful anywhere; any painful areas should be avoided if possible. A small dog that is being held by the owner should be accepted in such a way that the face and the teeth are directed away from the face of the receiver. In picking up a small dog, one hand can be placed under the chest (between the front legs) while the other hand is placed behind or just in front of the rear legs to support the hind quarters. Medium-sized dogs can be picked up using a similar technique, but the arms can be used (one under the chest and the other just in front of or behind the rear legs) while the dog's trunk is cradled against the chest of the holder. Two or more people may be needed to lift large dogs safely, with a focus on adequately supporting the dog's front, spine, and rear. When possible, lift tables should be used for large dogs (Figure 6-1).

If a dog escapes, resist the natural inclination to pursue it. Chasing a dog will simply make it run faster, and cornering a dog can potentially cause it to fight. This is an example of **fear biting.** Instead, follow the dog from a safe distance and give it a few minutes to calm down (if this can be done safely). Continue to use vocal reassurance to encourage the dog to stop running. If the dog slows down or hesitates, it may be possible to approach, calmly slip a leash over its head, and regain control. Continue vocal reassurance; if the dog seems willing to accept petting, this can be offered as well. If the dog will not allow anyone to approach close enough to slip a leash over its head, using techniques described earlier (creating a small posture, speaking the dog's name using a gentle voice, offering treats) may encourage the dog to allow closer approach and recapture. Handlers are advised to watch the dog carefully for postural changes or any other signs of increasing anxiety. If necessary, the dog's owner may be able to coax the pet closer, but this must be done from a reasonable distance and without endangering the owner in

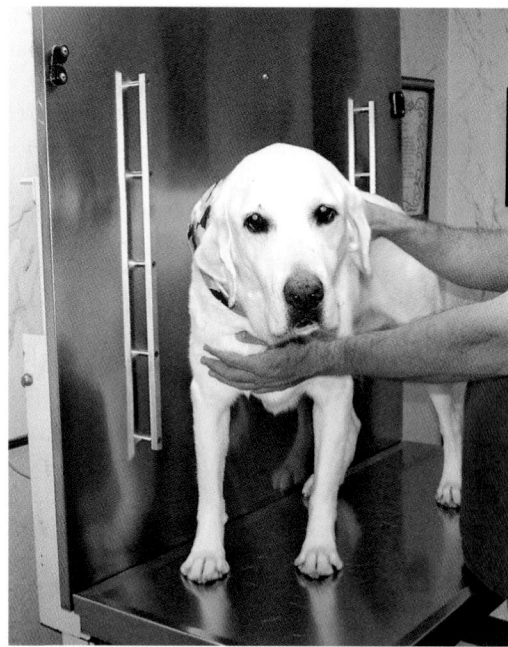

FIGURE 6-1 A lift table is helpful for examining large dogs. The table's platform lowers to within a few inches of the floor, allowing the dog to walk up onto the surface. The table can then be raised to the desired height. Dogs should never be left unattended on a lift table.

any way. As an absolute last resort, a long-distance restraint device (such as a rabies pole) can be used, but this should be done only by an experienced handler because the dog can easily be injured by such a device.

TECHNICIAN NOTE Even the most experienced technician may need help when handling a patient. It is better to ask for help than to risk injury (or harm to a patient).

Capturing a Cat

Before removing a cat from a pet carrier, close accessible doors and windows, and secure the examination room in case the cat escapes. Many cats willingly come out of a carrier on their own, given a little time or some gentle coaxing. If the cat is unwilling to come out but is lying on a towel or a rug inside the carrier, it may be possible to slowly pull the towel through the front door of the carrier and let the cat slide out on the towel. A variation on this idea involves slowly, gently lifting the rear of the carrier and allowing the cat to slide and/or walk toward the front door. If a towel is on the floor of the carrier, slowly pulling the towel can help the cat slide forward and through the open door.

Carriers that open from the front and top, or that disassemble so the top can be removed, facilitate removal of the pet. The cat can simply be lifted out and placed on the examination table. If the cat is nervous or fractious, place a towel over the cat before removing the pet from the open carrier. If necessary, the examination can be conducted with the cat sitting in the bottom of the opened carrier. However, a towel or other restraint device should be nearby in case additional control is needed. With traditional cardboard carriers or other carriers that open only from the top, a calm cat can simply be picked up, but be sure to support under the chest and hind quarters. A cat that is nervous should be draped in a towel before it is picked up.

If it is necessary to reach into a carrier to remove a cat, do so with extreme caution. If the cat is growling, hissing, or refusing to make eye contact, or has the ears pulled back, use another technique. If the cat seems calm but simply does not want to come out, stroke the cheek and chin for a few moments. If the cat is still calm, reach underneath the chest/body and remove the cat from the carrier. Another technique is to gently grasp the scruff with one hand and support the rest of the body with the other hand to help pull the cat forward through the front door (or top) of the carrier. Scruffing, however, is controversial; it will be discussed more thoroughly in the section on feline restraint techniques.

> **TECHNICIAN NOTE**   Most cats prefer to be stroked around the head, neck, and chin, but avoid this if the cat is trying to strike with the front claws, or if it is trying to bite.

By the time a cat reaches the examination table, it is likely to be more stressed than a dog in the same position. Capture at home, placement into a pet carrier, a car ride to the veterinary practice, and experience in the waiting room all culminate with the pet being extracted from its carrier and subsequently surrounded by unusual sounds, people, and aromas. A cat that is crouched in the rear of a pet carrier may have already gone through the "flight" stage and be ready to fight if not handled appropriately, so caution and care are warranted. Feline behavior signals tend to be more subtle than signals from dogs. Cats also tend to be faster than dogs and are capable of scratching very effectively with all four feet, in addition to being able to bite. Kittens have better flexibility than adult cats, so even though they are smaller, they can still cause significant injury. Consider these factors while observing, approaching, and capturing feline patients.

If a cat escapes in the examination room, recheck all windows and doors immediately. Cats tend to look for places to hide, so cabinets should be blocked off, as well as any small spaces that may be accessible. Cats have been known to climb upper cabinets and to jump into dropped-ceiling panels. It is important to remain as calm as possible, but try to recapture the cat before it can escape to an inaccessible location. Quickly covering the cat with a towel can facilitate recapture. However, make sure the cat is on a stable surface (on the floor or on a secure counter top) before trying to catch it. If the cat rolls onto its back and pushes the towel away, using a pair of clean gauntlets (Figure 6-2) may be an option. If the cat will not permit approach, it may be willing to run back into the open carrier. Place the open carrier on the floor near the cat and slowly slide the open door toward the cat.

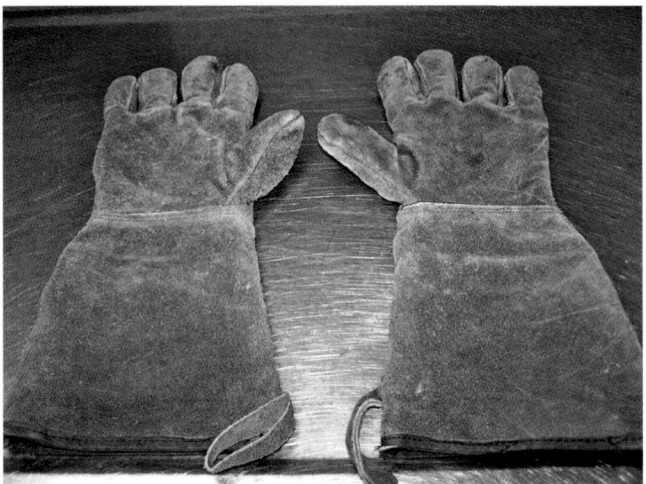

FIGURE 6-2 Long, heavy, leather gloves, known as *gauntlets*, can be helpful when restraining cats and small dogs. The gloves cover most of the forearms and reduce the risk of being scratched. However, pets can still bite through the gloves, so caution is warranted.

Once the cat is back inside the carrier, capture and handling can be renegotiated. As a last resort, a slip leash or snare can be used, but these tools must be used with extreme caution to avoid strangling or otherwise injuring the cat.

Removing a Pet From a Hospital Cage

When removing pets from cages or runs, the procedures described previously (observation, approach, and capture) can be used. For example, when removing a dog from a run or a large cage, try to approach from an angle, maintain a nonthreatening posture, and use verbal reassurance to get the dog to approach. Try to avoid blocking the entire doorway, which can make the dog feel cornered. Standing to the side of the entrance is better, but avoid leaving a large enough gap for the dog to escape. Once the dog approaches, a leash can be slipped over the head. If the dog refuses to approach, try to avoid entering the cage any farther than the very front. Use verbal reassurance and other techniques as previously described to encourage the dog to come forward.

When removing a small dog from a cage, stand slightly to the side and encourage the pet to come forward; avoid leaving a large enough space for the pet to escape. Once the pet approaches, a leash can be slipped over the head and/or a towel can be gently wrapped around the pet as it is picked up and transported. A similar approach can be used for cats. Allow the cat to come forward and sniff the handler. If the cat seems calm enough to be picked up, scoop up the body, taking care to support the rear legs. Wrapping the cat in a towel (sprayed with pheromone spray) for transportation is a good idea if practical.

Once the pet is removed from the cage, adequate control must be maintained to reduce the likelihood of escape or injury. Cats should be transported in a pet carrier or wrapped in a towel, with care taken to support the body securely. Small dogs can be carried in a similar way or walked on a leash. Large dogs should be leashed.

CANINE RESTRAINT

OPTIONS FOR RESTRAINING A WELL-BEHAVED DOG

Once a cooperative canine patient has been captured successfully, it can be helped onto the examination table. Small and medium-sized dogs can be picked up and placed onto the table.

When lifting pets, use the techniques previously described in this section. If the pet is injured, take this into consideration when lifting and otherwise restraining the patient.

Large dogs should be examined on a table. If a large dog is very fearful of the table, examination can be conducted on the floor; however, this situation is not ideal. The dog has greater mobility on the floor than on the table, so escape is easier. When restraining a dog on the floor, it is important to avoid leaning over the dog. This positioning can make a fearful or aggressive dog feel threatened. One option is to squat or kneel beside the dog (with one arm under the chest and the other arm under the midsection) or to stand next to the dog with a hand controlling the head and neck. Unfortunately, the mobility, balance, and reaction time of the holder are impaired when kneeling or squatting, and only very limited control of the patient is possible when only the head is restrained. Ideally, a large dog should be examined on a lift table. A cooperative patient will often walk onto a lift table with minimal coaxing. Placing a skid-proof mat on the table can help a dog feel more secure during examination. Once on the table, adequate restraint should continue until the examination is over and the pet is back on the floor. The front end and rear of the body should be supported to help prevent the dog from jumping or falling from the table. Most commonly, the handler can place one arm just in front of the rear legs and the other arm in front of the chest while cradling the head. Pulling the dog's body toward the handler's body helps provide additional support. As a general rule, use the least amount of restraint necessary (Figure 6-3). Dogs should never be left alone on an examination table; severe injury is possible if they fall or jump off. The vertical wall of some lift tables have hooks that are intended for securing a leash. These must be used with extreme caution, however, to reduce the risk of strangulation if the dog struggles, falls, or jumps off the table.

During examination, many dogs behave better if they can see their owners. If possible, position the dog so it is facing the owner. However, owners should not be permitted to hold or restrain their own pets, and during any potentially objectionable procedures (e.g., rectal temperature, nail trimming) the owner should be advised to stay away from the dog's face and mouth, in case the pet becomes startled and snaps. Many dogs do better with minimal restraint (Figure 6-4). Even a well-behaved dog may become tense and nervous if extreme restraint is suddenly applied. Similarly, a dog that is already nervous may become more nervous and uncooperative if

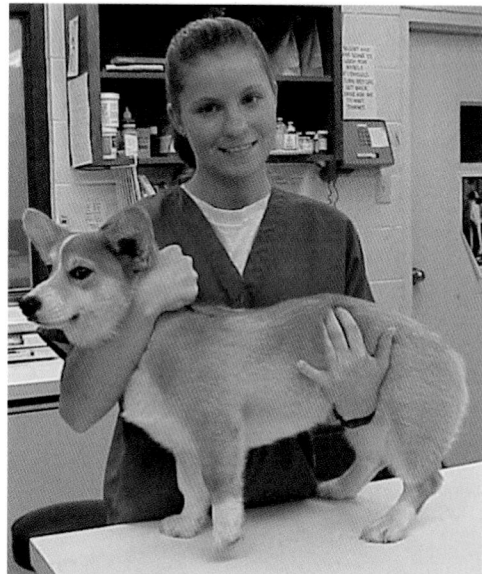

FIGURE 6-3 This handler is providing support for the dog and restraint for examination at the same time. If the dog tries to escape, the handler can pull the body closer to attain additional control. The arm that is in front of the chest hinders the dog's forward movement, and the arm that is under the abdomen helps keep the dog on its feet.

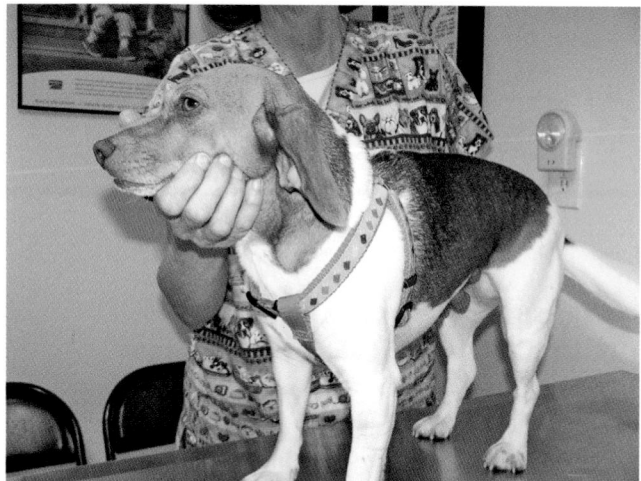

FIGURE 6-4 If minimal restraint is adequate for a well-behaved patient, simply controlling the head can be effective.

subjected to heavy restraint. In some cases, it is possible to accomplish more with a gentle hand, a soft voice, and distraction with a toy or with food than with heavier restraint. Also, if a dog seems to object strenuously to restraint, it is best to avoid wrestling with the dog. Instead, take a break and consider using less restraint or a different restraint technique (Box 6-1).

> **TECHNICIAN NOTE** When restraining a dog or cat, use the minimal amount of restraint necessary to prevent injury and facilitate examination. Many pets do much better with minimal restraint.

BOX 6-1 | Restraint Tips

Safely and effectively restraining a patient may be as much an art as it is a science. No single procedure or "trick" will work for every pet, so if one thing doesn't work, be prepared to try something else. Here are some general restraint tips to consider:

- **Never wrestle with a pet:** If it takes three or more people to restrain a pet, a different strategy is necessary. Wrestling with a patient creates a negative experience for the pet (one it will remember during future visits); a potentially dangerous situation for the pet, technician, and veterinarian; and an unnecessarily stressful episode for the pet owner. Clients expect better, gentler care of their pets, and veterinary patients deserve better care than being "manhandled."

- **Effective documentation can help improve future visits:** If a particular procedure worked well (e.g., pet is better away from the owner), or a certain size and type of muzzle fit particularly well, make a note in the record, so future visits can go more smoothly.

- **Don't rush:** Although movements during a patient examination should be purposeful and efficient, rushing is not advised. Sudden movements can be perceived by the patient as threatening.

- **Know when to take a break:** If a situation seems to be escalating out of control, tempers are flaring, or veterinary staffers are becoming impatient, it may be time to take a break and spend a few minutes thinking of a new strategy.

- **Check the patient periodically:** If a patient is struggling or seems particularly stressed or resentful of handling, check tongue color and respiratory rate/effort. If the pet experiences any bluish discoloration of the tongue or seems to have abnormal respiration, stop immediately and let the pet relax. If the pet does not return to normal within a few seconds, alert the veterinarian.

- **Communicate with colleagues:** If a pet is wriggling loose or if control is otherwise being lost, anyone working on the pet needs to know immediately. It takes only a second to say, "I'm losing him," "Wait," or "Stop." It also takes only a second for someone to be scratched or bitten because he or she didn't know that the pet was no longer being restrained. If possible, try to avoid letting go without first giving warning.

- **Prevent pet owners from restraining their own pets:** Pet owners know their pets better than anyone else, and some of them may feel that their pet will behave better if it is being restrained by someone familiar. Whether this is accurate or not, the legal implications associated with owners being injured outweigh arguments in favor of letting them restrain their pet. Instead, offer to have the owner stand close by (preferably in a location where the pet can still see him or her), and encourage the owner to talk to the pet if that helps keep the pet calm. However, owners should be advised to keep away from the pet's face and nails, particularly when something potentially uncomfortable is occurring (such as administration of an injection).

- **If necessary, get help:** Even the most experienced technician can encounter a situation that requires help or a second opinion on how to best proceed. If a pet is showing signs of aggression and previously successful techniques aren't working, it is prudent to ask for help.

OPTIONS FOR RESTRAINING AN UNCOOPERATIVE DOG

Muzzle

Muzzles offer a safe and effective first choice restraint device for uncooperative dogs. Most owners accept their dog being muzzled, particularly if they are witnessing their dog's unacceptable behavior and they are made to understand that the device is not painful or harmful to the dog. Despite this, veterinary professionals are sometimes reluctant to use muzzles. In a 2003 study conducted at a veterinary teaching hospital, less than 50% of dogs and cats considered likely to bite were muzzled.

Muzzles are available in several sizes and in a variety of styles, including cloth, leather, and basket-style. When choosing the right fit for a traditional cloth or leather muzzle, the muzzle should be snug enough that it cannot be pushed off, and the cone portion over the dog's nose should be tight enough to prevent biting. However, it is helpful if the dog has enough room to pant, as many stressed dogs need to do. The muzzle should also be loose enough for the dog's tongue color to be observed during examination. Basket muzzles can be a better option for dogs that are panting heavily; the "bird cage" around the dog's muzzle hinders biting, but the basket design facilitates panting. Brachycephalic dogs can be difficult to muzzle because their noses are too short to allow most muzzle styles to be secured. An Air Muzzle (Smart Practice, Phoenix, AZ) can be a good choice for brachycephalic dogs, as well as for small dogs and cats. The Air Muzzle is designed as a clear, hollow, plastic ball that fits over the dog's head (Figure 6-5). It allows panting and keeps the dog's entire face away from handlers. Gauze muzzles (Figure 6-6) offer an option for dogs that are difficult to approach and safely muzzle. However, dogs can easily remove gauze muzzles using their front paws, so the muzzle must be tied relatively tightly to be effective. This limits panting and observation of tongue color. Therefore, gauze muzzles can be useful but are not an ideal first choice. Creating a gauze muzzle is relatively simple (Procedure 6-1).

Towel

A towel can be an effective restraint device for a small dog. The towel can be draped over the entire dog, making it easier to pick the dog up without being bitten or scratched. A thick towel is best, in case the dog tries to bite through the towel. A towel can also be rolled lengthwise and wrapped around the back of the head just behind the ears, like a thick collar.

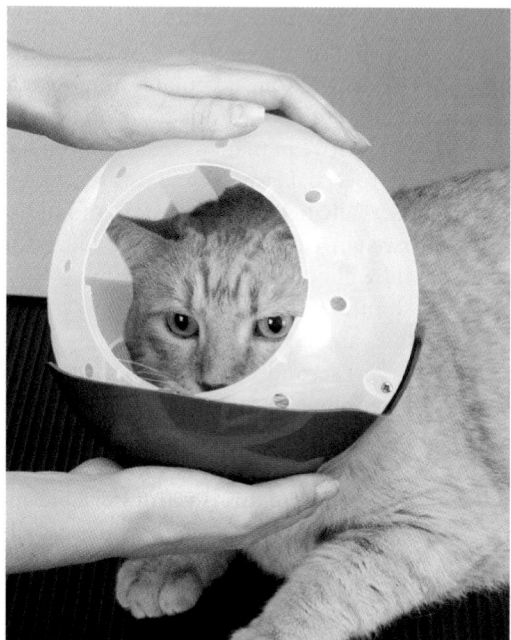

FIGURE 6-5 The Air Muzzle can work well for small dogs, brachycephalic dogs, and cats. The handler's hands are well protected during and after placement of the device. (Photo provided courtesy Smart Practice, Phoenix, AZ.)

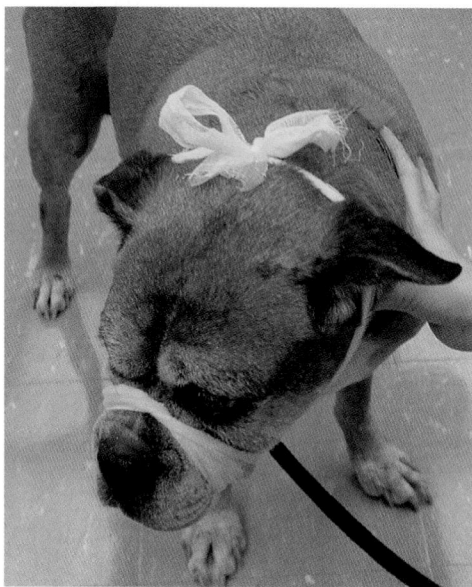

FIGURE 6-6 A makeshift gauze muzzle.

The thickness of the towel hinders head movement while the handler's hands are safely behind the dog's head. Use care to make sure the towel is not too tight, and monitor tongue color and breathing at all times.

Chemical Restraint

A variety of safe, effective agents are available for chemical restraint in dogs. However, this should be considered a last resort for several reasons. Even the safest sedative is associated with a minimal amount of risk, so administration can

PROCEDURE 6-1 | Gauze Muzzle Technique

A makeshift gauze muzzle can work well if no other muzzles are available, or if a dog will not permit anyone to get close enough to the face to properly apply a muzzle:

1. Start with a relatively long piece of gauze (4 to 5 feet may be reasonable for a medium-sized dog). A gauze strip that is too short requires that the restrainer be too close to the dog's teeth.
2. Tie a small knot in the center of the strip. This creates a tiny "weight" to facilitate slipping the light material over the dog's nose.
3. Make a loose loop in the center of the gauze with the "weight" at the bottom. Make sure the loop is large enough to fit over the dog's face. Tie a slip knot at the top (this will be tightened down once the loop is over the dog's nose).
4. Keeping fingers away from the dog's teeth, slip the loop over the dog's muzzle. If the dog is lunging or snapping at the loop, several attempts may be necessary.
5. Once the loop is over the muzzle, tighten it down with the "weight" on the bottom and the slip knot on the top.
6. While continuing to keep hands away from the dog's face, loop each end of the gauze strip under the dog's chin once. If possible, twist the ends once, so there is a makeshift "knot" under the bottom of the jaw. If the dog will permit, this looping can be repeated to give the muzzle a little more strength.
7. Bring each strip of gauze to the back of the head (under the dog's ears) and tie a bow behind the head (see Figure 6-6).
8. When the pet is ready to be released, undo the bow at the back of the head and pull both gauze strips forward. The muzzle should slide off quickly and easily.

have health consequences in some patients. Also, sedatives hinder physical assessment of a patient; physical parameters like heart rate, blood pressure, and respiratory rate can be altered by sedatives. Sedation also makes it nearly impossible to assess a pet's mental state, perform a neurologic examination, or localize pain. Finally, depending on which agent is used, some dogs can become so stressed and excited that they "override" the effect of the drug, dramatically limiting the expected response to the agent. Chemical restraint is very useful if a painful procedure is anticipated, or if the dog cannot be safely restrained using other techniques, so technicians are advised to become familiar with the modes of action and expected effects of sedatives (refer to Chapter 29, "Veterinary Anesthesia"). However, if sedation is not required, other restraint techniques should be employed if possible and practical.

TECHNICIAN NOTE Adopting safe, effective handling procedures protects everyone—the technician, the veterinarian, the pet, and the owner. It also strengthens the bond between the client and the practice.

FELINE RESTRAINT

OPTIONS FOR RESTRAINING A WELL-BEHAVED CAT

Once the cat is secured on the examination table, begin by using minimal restraint. Increase control only if the cat's behavior dictates more assertive handling. Cats should be allowed to move or change their position when it is not required for them to be still. For example, if the cat's head and ears are being examined, the cat should be free to rest on its side, stand, sit, or lie sternally until other areas of the body need to be maintained in a certain position. In most cases, a well-behaved cat can be examined relatively thoroughly with very little restraint. It may be prudent to keep one hand resting lightly near the back of the neck; this keeps the scruff within easy reach in case the cat tries to run away. This positioning also allows easy stroking of the head, cheek, chin, and neck, which can help calm a nervous cat. During the examination, move slowly and deliberately, maintain a pleasant voice, and remain calm; a cat may become anxious if surrounded by unpleasant movements and noises. A nervous cat that "freezes" can still be considered well-behaved and can be handled using minimal restraint. However, if the same cat becomes fidgety, tries to escape, or starts hissing or growling, more assertive restraint will be required.

OPTIONS FOR RESTRAINING AN UNCOOPERATIVE CAT

Towel

Whenever a feline patient is being handled, it is recommended to keep a thick towel nearby. The cat can be completely wrapped in the towel; keep one hand just behind the head and the other hand along the body to maintain control (Figure 6-7). The towel can be flipped back to expose the face and head when needed. The towel can also be manipulated to expose other parts of the body only when needed.

Scruffing and Alternate Holds

Traditionally, scruffing (grasping the cat by the scruff of the neck) has been considered an acceptable way to maintain control of a cat because it does not harm the cat if done properly, and it is effective in many cases. However, scruffing has become a controversial issue. Some cats react negatively to scruffing and actually fight harder instead of holding still. Also, some overweight cats have very little loose tissue to scruff, so the hold will be less effective.

In general, scruffing should be used only if minimal restraint techniques are not working. If scruffing seems necessary, try it for a few seconds. It the cat gets worse, discontinue and try something else. When scruffing a cat, use the minimum amount of force necessary and take care to avoid injuring the cat's neck. A cat should not be lifted or suspended by the scruff because this is uncomfortable and may make the cat's behavior worse. If scruffing does not discourage the cat from striking with the rear claws, the rear legs can also be restrained as shown in Figures 6-8 and 6-9.

Muzzle

Muzzles can be effective restraint devices for cats. The Air Muzzle works well because the entire head is kept away from the handler. Cloth feline muzzles are effective, but the feet must also be controlled to avoid scratching of the handler. When attempting to place a muzzle on a cat, wrapping the body and legs in a towel "burrito style" can help stop the cat from batting the muzzle away or striking out at the handler placing the muzzle (Figure 6-10). Once the muzzle is in place, make sure that the cat's nose is clearly through the opening, and that the cat can breathe normally (Figure 6-11).

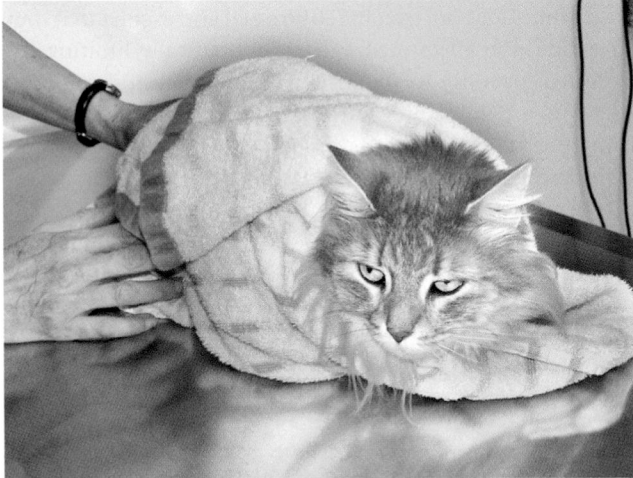

FIGURE 6-7 This cat is loosely wrapped in a towel. If necessary, the edge of the towel can be flipped over the head to hinder biting.

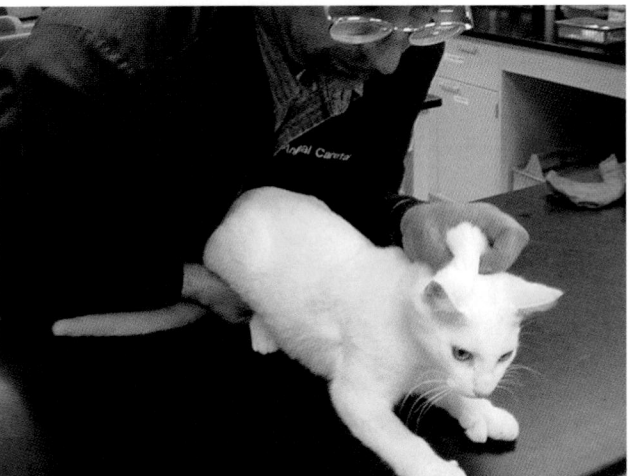

FIGURE 6-8 This cat can remain sternal while being scruffed. Controlling the rear legs reduces the likelihood of scratching or using the rear legs to propel the cat off the table. (From Sheldon CC, Sonshagen T, Topel JA: Animal restraint for veterinary professionals, St Louis, 2006, Mosby.)

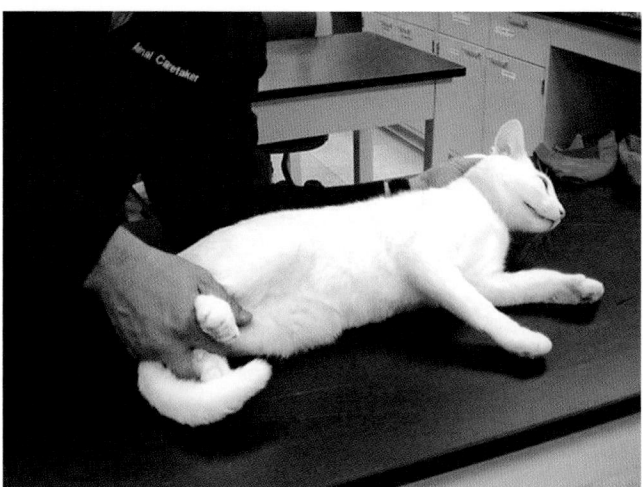

FIGURE 6-9 If more control is required while the cat's scruff is being secured, the rear legs can be stretched back slightly. (From Sheldon CC, Sonshagen T, Topel JA: Animal restraint for veterinary professionals, St Louis, 2006, Mosby.)

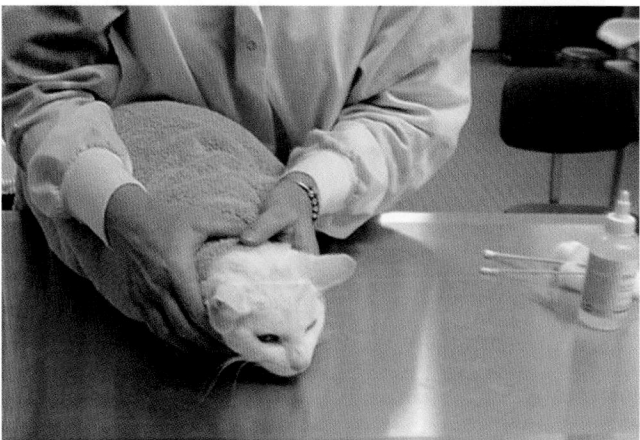

FIGURE 6-10 Wrapping the cat's entire body in a towel "burrito-style" secures all four feet, while leaving the face and head accessible for placement of a muzzle. (From Sheldon CC, Sonshagen T, Topel JA: Animal restraint for veterinary professionals, St Louis, 2006, Mosby.)

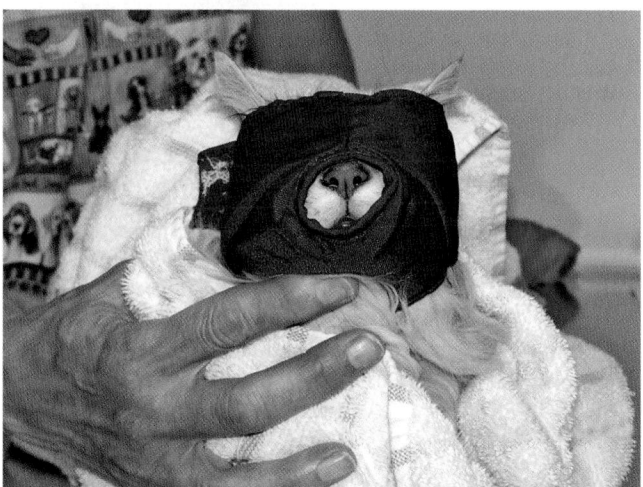

FIGURE 6-11 Cloth feline muzzle. Make sure the cat's nose is clearly uncovered. Otherwise, breathing is inhibited.

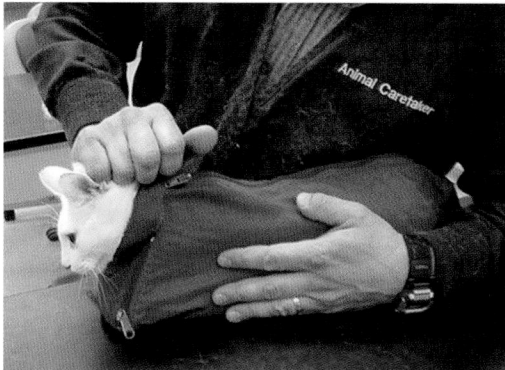

FIGURE 6-12 This cat has been secured using a cat bag. Zippers allow exposure of the legs when needed. (From Sheldon CC, Sonshagen T, Topel JA: Animal restraint for veterinary professionals, St Louis, 2006, Mosby.)

Gloves, Cat Bag, and Other Devices

Elbow-length leather gloves, known as *gauntlets*, can be used to help restrain an aggressive cat. However, the handler wearing these gloves has limited feeling and digital dexterity, so isolating individual feet, legs, etc., can be more difficult. Cats have also been known to bite through a leather glove, so the protection that gauntlets provide is not without limits. It is also acceptable to use some of these devices in combination, such as using a towel with gauntlets. Gloves, towels, and muzzles should be washed in between patients because cats can detect and react negatively to residual odors from a previous patient.

Some practitioners use cloth cat bags (Figure 6-12) to restrain the cat's legs and feet. This reduces the likelihood of being scratched but makes performing a physical examination difficult. Also, getting a fractious cat into the cat bag can be a challenge, and some cats struggle against the tight confines of a bag more than they might if wrapped in a towel. Nets and similar devices, such as the EZ-Nabber (Campbell Pet Company, Brush Prairie, WA), can be useful but must be used with caution to avoid catching a foot or a toe in the net. Physical examination is limited once the cat is restrained within the device. However, net-type devices can immobilize a fractious cat for an injection to be administered, facilitate extracting a fractious cat from a cage, or help catch a cat that has escaped. Slip leashes, snares, and similar devices that loop around the neck should be used only with extreme caution by experienced handlers. Inappropriate use of such devices can result in strangulation or other injury.

Chemical Restraint

As with dogs, safe, effective agents are available for chemical restraint in cats. The limitations and precautions associated with chemical restraint in cats are the same as those in dogs and include altering physiologic parameters and mental status. Technicians are advised to become familiar with drugs available for sedation in cats because chemical restraint is sometimes necessary, particularly if a painful procedure is anticipated. Most injectable sedatives for chemical restraint are administered subcutaneously or intramuscularly. If a cat is already in an EZ-Nabber or another restrictive type of restraint device, giving such an injection is much easier than if the cat is in a carrier or a cage and is difficult to approach. If the cat is truly unapproachable, some injectable sedatives can be given orally: after loading the syringe, remove the needle and connect an open-ended tomcat catheter to the end of the syringe. The agent can be squirted through the cage bars into the cat's mouth. However, be careful to avoid accidentally squirting the drug into the eyes.

> **TECHNICIAN NOTE** Pet owners expect their pet to be handled in a respectful, compassionate manner. Wrestling with a pet or using what may be perceived as excessive force can damage a client's perception of the practice and its staff.

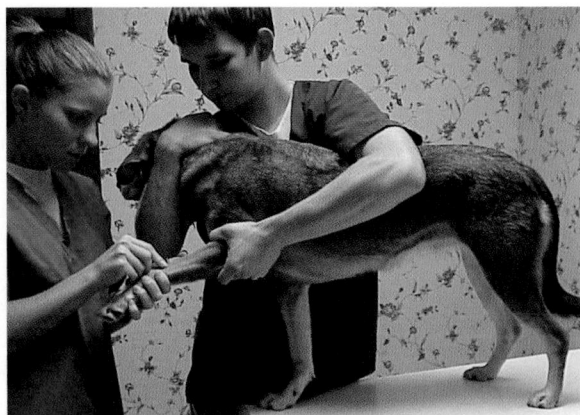

FIGURE 6-13 When a dog is restrained for cephalic venipuncture, the dog can stand (as shown) or sit. The vein is on the dorsal aspect of the leg, but rolling the vein slightly laterally improves visualization and access.

RESTRAINING DOGS AND CATS FOR SPECIFIC PROCEDURES

RESTRAINT FOR VENIPUNCTURE

When attempting to draw blood, continue to use the minimum level of restraint necessary, but try to keep the patient as still as possible. Movement can result in perivascular placement of the needle, or self-injury. The primary reason for struggling and movement during venipuncture is anxiety. Calm, affectionate handling with petting and soothing words can help alleviate anxiety. The most painful portion of the venipuncture is the piercing of skin and vessel; this is the point when the restraint must be most secure.

Positioning is the most critical part of a venipuncture because it allows accurate location of the vessel and successful drawing of blood. Fortunately, a variety of positions can be used to gain access to acceptable veins for venipuncture. Positioning options for jugular, medial saphenous, and lateral saphenous venipuncture in dogs and cats are described in Chapter 18, "Diagnostic Sampling and Treatment Techniques," along with a technique for accessing the marginal ear vein in a cat. Positioning for accessing the cephalic vein is very similar in dogs and cats. Dogs can stand or sit for this procedure; large dogs can remain on the floor if adequate control can be maintained. Cats should be sitting or lying in sternal recumbency. For very nervous or aggressive pets, a towel, a muzzle, or another restraint device may be helpful. Cats may try to swat the hands away or bite, whereas dogs are more likely to try to bite.

When positioning a dog for cephalic venipuncture, the handler stands (or kneels) beside the dog facing the venipuncturist (who is in front of the dog) and places one arm under the dog's neck, using the hand of that arm to hold the dog's head against the anterior shoulder. At the same time, the handler wraps the other arm over the back of the dog and uses the hand of that arm to encircle the dog's forearm just below the elbow. The thumb is used to cover the cephalic vein on the medial side, and gentle downward pressure is

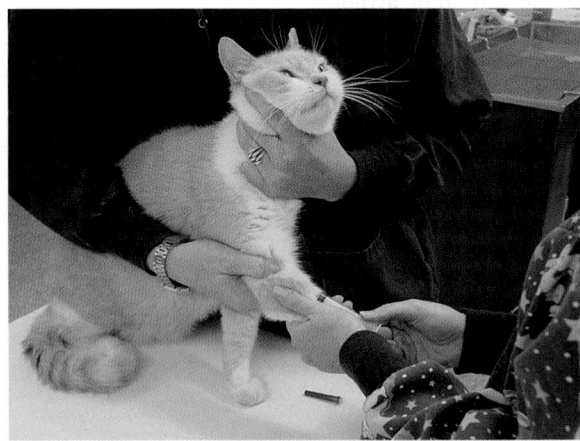

FIGURE 6-14 In a well-behaved cat, the holder can use the forearm and the body to control the cat's body and rear legs.

applied with the thumb to help raise the vein. The hand is then rotated laterally, pulling the skin and vessel as far to the outside as possible. Concurrently, the dog's elbow is pushed forward to extend and stabilize the leg (Figure 6-13).

Restraint and positioning for cats is very similar (Figure 6-14). If necessary, a towel can be used to wrap the body and rear claws while the handler controls the head and front legs, as described previously. Use of a muzzle may be advised because both of the handler's hands are close to the cat's teeth during this procedure. For a truly aggressive cat, medial saphenous venipuncture may be the safest approach because the entire body (including the head) can be wrapped in a towel while the rear leg is isolated for venipuncture. Cat bags are made with zippers so that a single limb may be withdrawn and used for cephalic or medial saphenous venipuncture.

RESTRAINT FOR NAIL TRIMMING

Although a well-behaved pet may need only one person to trim its nails, it is always prudent to have two people available. One person can restrain the pet while the other performs the nail trimming. It is important to use vocal reassurance and other calming techniques to reduce the patient's stress level during this procedure. It is also critically important to consider the pet's physical comfort. When lifting the feet and manipulating the limbs, remember the normal anatomic positions of the limbs, and consider the normal range of motion for the joints involved. Under ideal conditions, the front legs have a reasonable range of forward and backward motion but limited ability to extend laterally. The coxofemoral joint (hip) is technically a "ball-and-socket" joint, which means that it should be capable of a relatively circular range of motion. However, the knees do not have a comparable range of motion. Also, a surprisingly large number of veterinary patients (including young dogs with hip dysplasia or elbow dysplasia) may not have full range of motion in many of their joints. Pulling on the feet; squeezing the paws too firmly; pulling a leg too far laterally, forward, or backward; or lifting a limb unnaturally high can cause pain and should be avoided.

For a well-behaved dog, nail trimming can be performed with the pet standing. Using minimal restraint, the holder can simply control the dog's head while the person trimming isolates each paw as needed and trims the nails. For a medium-sized or large dog, the holder can gently **cradle** the dog's head against the chest as if holding for cephalic venipuncture (see Figure 6-13). However, slightly less control is needed because the dog does not have to be completely still during a nail trim. For smaller dogs, the holder can cup the dog's chin in the hand to gently control the head. A nervous dog may benefit from being muzzled. For a dog that is very fidgety, holding up contralateral legs at the same time can encourage the dog to stand still. For example, if the person trimming is working on (and therefore lifting) the right front paw, the holder can hold the left rear paw slightly off the ground. This encourages the dog to stand still because only the left front and right rear legs are available for balance (Figure 6-15). The dog may lean against the holder for additional support, but the technique is frequently effective. As the person trimming moves from paw to paw, the holder can adjust accordingly, lifting contralateral paws as needed. Sometimes, a fidgety dog can be encouraged to sit down; the front paws are easy to trim from this position, and the dog can stand momentarily while the rear claws are trimmed.

For additional control of an unruly dog, placing the dog in lateral recumbency can be effective. The holder should try to hold the legs by placing one arm just in front of the dog's shoulder and the other arm just in front of the rear legs, and reaching through the legs to grasp the front and rear paws (Figure 6-16). A muzzle is recommended if the dog tries to bite because controlling the head is more difficult when this hold is used.

Most well-behaved cats are willing to sit or stand for a nail trimming. For an uncooperative cat, lateral recumbency works well, as does wrapping the cat in a towel and exposing each paw only as it is being trimmed. "Stretching a cat out" can work for a nail trimming, but the holder must maintain control of the cat's scruff (Figure 6-17). Placing a folded

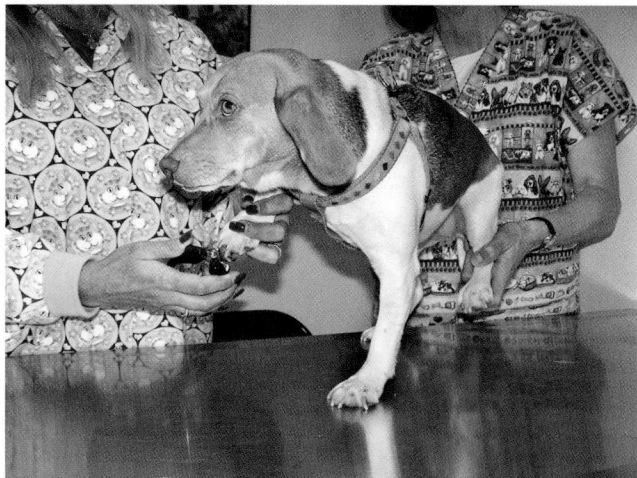

FIGURE 6-15 By holding up the contralateral leg slightly, this wriggly dog is encouraged to stand still. When trimming nails, be sure that joints are not positioned uncomfortably.

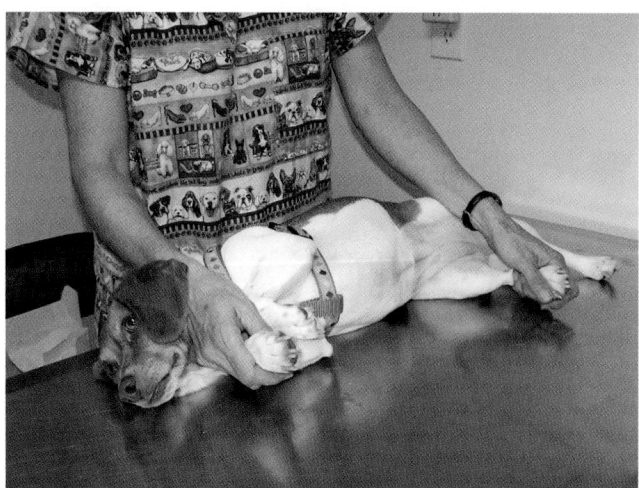

FIGURE 6-16 This dog is being held in lateral recumbency for a nail trimming. Controlling the dependent (downside) legs hinders the dog's ability to stand back up.

towel over the cat's head can help protect the person trimming (especially when the front claws are being trimmed). A cat bag can also work for an unruly cat because each leg can be isolated as it is needed.

With few exceptions, nail trimming is a cosmetic procedure. Wrestling with a pet to complete a nail trimming is ill advised and can lead to injury to veterinary personnel or to the pet. If three or more people are required to trim a pet's nails, it is best to consider other options such as postponing the procedure or (as a last resort) using chemical restraint. Some pet owners can be taught to trim their pets' nails at home, but this should not be advised if the pet is truly aggressive and the owner could be injured. Referring the owner for professional training sessions or behavior counseling is advised if the pet's aggression poses a risk to the owner.

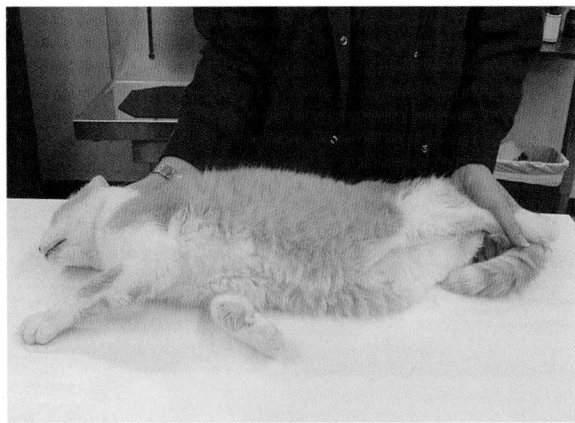

FIGURE 6-17 "Stretching" a cat for nail trimming can be effective, but other techniques (such as wrapping the cat in a towel) are preferable.

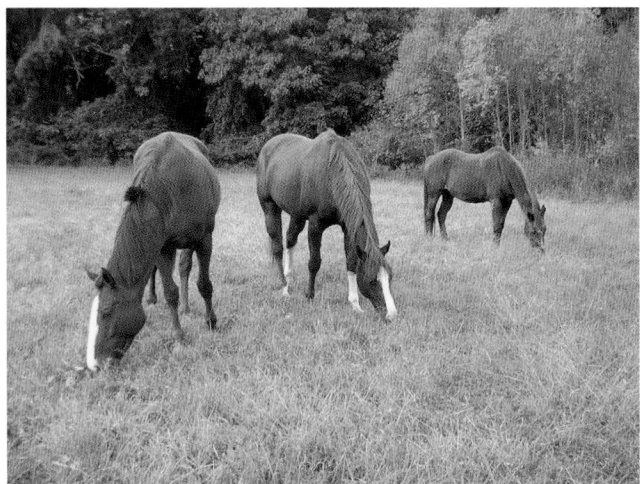

FIGURE 6-18 Typical behavior of a small herd of horses.

INTRODUCTION TO EQUINE RESTRAINT

Horses are herd animals, and within the herd there is a hierarchy. Horses may fight to establish their place in the herd; however, horses are not typically aggressive (Figure 6-18). Certain factors can make horses aggressive. The most antagonistic horses seem to be protecting something; mares with foals can become unpredictable as they defend their foals, stallions will guard their herd of mares, and even racehorses can become extremely protective of the stall. These horses can be very quick to bite strike or wheel around and kick at a perceived threat. More commonly, what veterinary professionals encounter when dealing with horses is fear or anxiety. Horses that are isolated from the herd owing to illness or injury can become anxious; being transported to a new environment full of strange people only increases equine stress levels. Remember that horses are prey animals and humans can be perceived (by the horse) as predators. The horse's instinct in this situation is to evade human contact and capture; this is similar to the flight-or-fight response seen in

nature. Fearful horses will try anything to escape capture; this can result in human or animal injury. Both aggressive and fearful horses can quickly turn away from the person attempting to restrain, leaving the handler in a potentially dangerous situation.

> **TECHNICIAN NOTE**   Horses are not typically aggressive.

The equine field of vision is almost 360 degrees. Horses have 60 to 70 degrees **binocular vision,** that is, vision in which both eyes are used synchronously to produce a single image. This makes judging distances directly in front of them difficult, without moving their head. Horses have three areas where their vision is extremely limited: directly behind them, directly in front of their nose, and between their eyes on the forehead. These locations are known as **blind spots;** to compensate for blind spots, horses will turn the head quickly toward objects in these areas to determine whether they are a threat. Blind spots are one reason why people should not approach if a horse that is not aware of their presence or the hind end is facing them.

Veterinary personnel need to be cautious when moving into and around equine blind spots, where they are more vulnerable to being injured by a kick. Horses generally give warning before kicking. Typical warnings of an impending kick include but are not limited to lifting the limb quickly, stomping a foot, and pawing. However, a frightened horse can be unpredictable and can kick without warning. Horses can kick with both front and hind legs. When horses use their front legs, this is known as *striking*. A single leg strike is the most common way to get injured when in front of the horse if the horse is prone to this behavior or is agitated. A single front leg strike usually is not fatal but can cause bruising, hematoma, or even a fractured limb. However, some horses, especially young horses, will rear up and strike out with both front feet, usually causing damage to the upper body or head. This reaction has the potential to cause serious if not fatal injury to the handler. The handler should position himself closer to the shoulder of the horse, keeping the body from being directly in front of the horse. Horses can kick in several ways, some of which can be fatal to humans and other animals. Horses can kick straight back with one or both hind legs ("**double barrel kick**"), to the side ("**cow kick**"), and as far forward as their ears. Fatal kicks usually occur with a straight back kick or a "double barrel" kick, when the limb/limbs are at full extension. These kicks can reach the chest and head of a person easily and have the most power behind them. It is important when working around horses' hind end to keep in close proximity to their body and to keep a firm hand on them to let them know where the handler is at all times. Staying close to the horse does not mean that it cannot or will not try to kick, strike, or step on the handler; however, this will reduce the chance that the injury will be fatal (Figure 6-19).

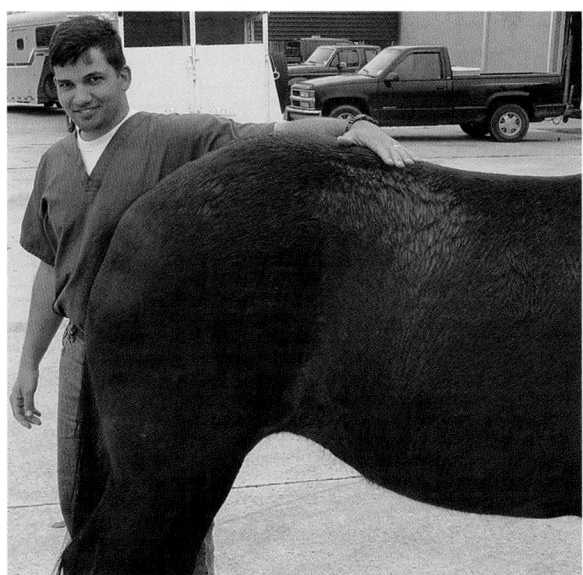

FIGURE 6-19 Maneuvering safely and properly when working around the hind end of a horse.

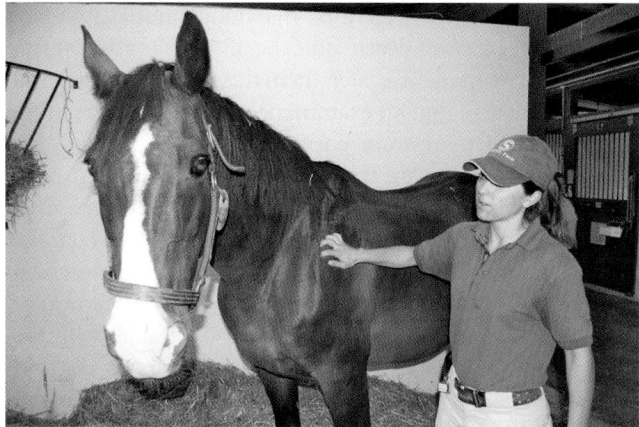

FIGURE 6-20 Safely approaching a horse for capture. This method simulates the way horses interact in nature.

> **TECHNICIAN NOTE** Whether working at the front or hind end of the horse, it is important to stay close to the horse with a hand on it at all times. Staying close to the horse does not mean that it cannot or will not try to kick, strike, or step on the handler; however, this will reduce the chance that the injury will be fatal.

Restraint is defined as control of an animal for the purpose of examination or treatment; with regard to equine restraint, this can be divided into three subcategories: physical restraint, **diversionary restraint,** and chemical restraint.
1. Physical restraint includes the use of halters and lead ropes.
2. Diversionary restraint uses varying techniques or devices to distract the horse. Diversionary restraint can be manual (tapping lightly on the horses head) or mechanical (use of a **twitch**).
3. Chemical restraint is the use of specific drugs to achieve the appropriate level of restraint for the protection of all involved.

In veterinary medicine, it is often the duty of technicians to restrain these animals for the safety of both the animal and the veterinarian who is performing the procedure. Veterinary technicians need to have a keen understanding of the restraint techniques used in multiple species.

Proper and safe restraint of the equine patient starts with observation of the horse's behavior and subtle cues as to how it will react to further encroachment into its territory. Horses are individuals; they have their own unique idiosyncrasies and personalities. Approaching the horse for restraint is best achieved with calm confidence, a gentle hand on the withers, and a soft voice. This method can go a long way toward easing a nervous horse (Figure 6-20). Certain breeds, for example, Arabians, Thoroughbreds, and

American Saddlebreds, can be more nervous ("high strung") than others. Finally, capturing the horse can be accomplished with low, slow movements and with patience. Once captured, the decision can be made whether further restraint is necessary; sometimes with equine restraint, less really is more.

> **TECHNICIAN NOTE** Proper and safe restraint of the equine patient starts with observation of the horse's behavior.

THE APPROACH

Equine restraint can be intimidating, even for those with horse experience. A horse's stature alone can be menacing, making restraint seem like a daunting task. Learning proper and safe techniques can ease any personal fears and can help achieve respect for the horse. Observe and assess the horse before entering any enclosure. Watch closely for signs of fear or aggression; a handler can observe subtle cues before approach and capture that can help suggest how the horse is going to react. Signs of aggression in horses include but are not limited to pinning ears, pawing at the ground, snorting, lunging forward, and turning the head quickly and biting. Signs of fear are much more subtle and include tension; tightening of muscles around the mouth, eyes, and neck; eyes wide with sclera (the whites of the eyes) obvious; and an increased respiratory rate. Nostrils will be flared and the horse will be taking deep breaths. Although the ears are forward and alert, the head is high, and awareness of everything around the horse is heightened. (For further information on equine behavior, refer to Chapter 5.)

Before physical contact with the horse, the veterinary team should develop a plan. This plan should include how to approach the horse, how much restraint will be required, and what escape route should be used if things should go wrong. The veterinary technician should have all necessary supplies prepared ahead of time. The key to successful restraint is to reduce the animal's stress. Always have a backup plan to allow for a horse that dodges initial approach and capture. Horses learn quickly; if they evade capture once, it will be harder to catch them the second time around. The plan ensures that an examination will follow even if the initial attempt to restrain goes awry. Horses generally are housed on farms or are transported by hauling companies. Oftentimes, an owner is not present during veterinary visits, but a farm manager may be. If an owner or a farm manager is present, question him about the horse. His input can sometimes be invaluable. Ask the about the horse's normal behavior and attitude. Ask about previous contact with veterinary personnel and procedures. Inquire about restraint techniques used by the owner/farm manager and by veterinary personnel during previous veterinary care visits. Listen to the owner, but ultimately the veterinary personnel should decide the best course of action with regard to restraint; even the best behaved horses can be unpredictable when sick or injured.

> **TECHNICIAN NOTE** The key to successful restraint is reducing the animal's stress.

When entering the horse's stall or field, personal safety comes first. A person capturing a horse should never enter an area if the horse is not aware of the person's presence. As a general rule, a stall should not be entered if the horse has its hind end facing you. A clicking noise made with the tongue or talking to the horse is usually enough to get its attention. The handler should not enter a stall without having the horse's attention. This can startle ("spook") the horse. A startled horse can wheel around quickly, pinning the handler into a corner or pressing him against the wall. A handler trapped in a stall with a nervous, stressed, and startled horse is a recipe for disaster. Make sure to leave room for escape if necessary. Once the horse is aware of the presence of the person, it is safe to approach and capture. Once the horse is restrained, the handler should always work on the same side of the horse as the examiner. Patience is imperative when working with horses; it will go a long way toward easing the horse's fears and keeping everyone safe.

> **TECHNICIAN NOTE** Patience is imperative when working with horses; it will go a long way toward easing the horse's fears and keeping everyone safe.

CAPTURE OF THE EQUINE

Adult equine patients who have been properly handled and trained seem relatively familiar with common restraint techniques. Horses typically and traditionally are handled on the left side, probably because people lead horses with their right hand. The left side of the horse is known as the *near side.* Horses handled this way tend to be more accepting of capture; this does not mean that they cannot and will not

lash out. Any horse that has teeth or feet can bite, strike, or kick. Try to remain calm when working around a horse; horses can sense when a person is nervous. Move gradually, keep hands low, talk in a light calm tone, and avoid quick jerking motions or loud noises. Patience is key; let the horse get used to the handler's presence in the stall. Reach out slowly and attempt to touch the horse near its withers. Rub the horse in this area and along the neck. These techniques are similar to the bonding and grooming rituals of horses in a herd. Once bonding and acceptance have occurred, a lead rope can be placed around the neck (Figure 6-21). The lead rope around the neck provides very minimal restraint but usually enough that a halter can be placed if it is not already on the horse. Once the halter is placed, the lead rope can be attached to the tie ring on the halter, and head control can be obtained. Keep in mind that slow, gentle movement and talking are still necessary so as not to "spook" the horse. Working this way around horses will minimize stress and unacceptable behaviors.

Hospitalized horses in a stall are somewhat more agreeable to being captured compared with horses in the field. Field service personnel can be faced with a bigger challenge when attempting to capture a horse for examination. Horses in an open field typically have a large **flight zone.** The normal flight distance of most horses is between approximately 10 and 30 feet; once inside this area, it is most important to remain calm and to never move quickly. Startling a horse or a herd of horses in the flight zone will cause the herd to run and can create a dangerous situation for all involved. Horses that evade capture may be enticed with some grain; often food is all that is needed to catch the horse. Veterinary personnel can ask the owner or farm manager to have the horse who needs examination caught or placed in a stall before their arrival. Sometimes utilizing the buddy system works well too. If personnel are able to capture a herd mate, this will often make capturing the patient easier. Difficult situations will occur and need to be addressed appropriately for the safety of all.

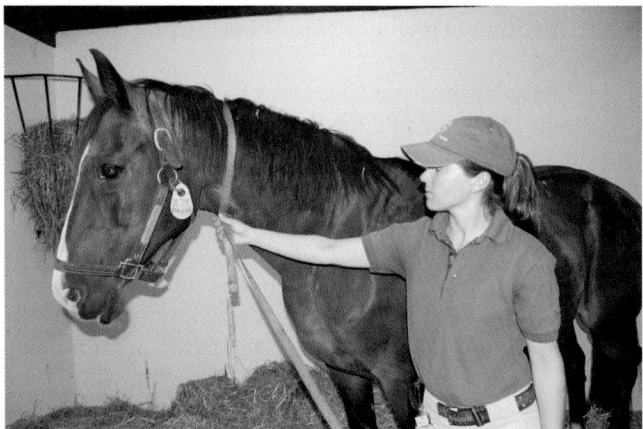

FIGURE 6-21 Use of the lead rope around the neck to aid in capture. A lead rope provides minimal restraint, but usually enough for application of the halter.

Juvenile horses (weanlings and yearlings), that is, horses between the ages of approximately 6 months and 2 years, present a unique challenge for veterinary personnel. Certain breeds will be introduced to handling only when veterinary care is needed, and these young horses often are just being introduced to halters and restraint. Young horses typically are more anxious than their adult counterparts; however, they often are more curious. The curiosity of the young horse can be used to your advantage. Squatting down, avoiding eye contact, and making the handler appear small will often make a nervous but inquisitive young horse come close enough to touch on the shoulder and scratch. Try scratching the withers at the caudal aspect of the neck, and work cranially without touching the halter. Grabbing the horse by the halter at this point or at any time is ill advised and dangerous. Juvenile horses most likely will pull back hard to escape, and when they realize that this maneuver is not working, they may try to rear up or flip over backward. To avoid injury, it is advised to use slow movements and a soothing voice. Handlers also can attempt to apply the lead rope to the tie ring under the chin without touching the young horse; as they are scratching with one hand, they can reach under with the other and clip the lead to the halter (Figure 6-22). Never put a chain over a juvenile horse's nose; the horse does not know what it is and will not react favorably to the application; this could make future attempts to handle the young horse very difficult. Sometimes it is necessary to use enticements like grass or grain to gain the juvenile horse's trust.

Foals require a lot of patience and understanding. Ideally, three people should be charged with capturing a foal: one to restrain the mare and two to catch the foal. However, this is not always the reality. The key to capturing a foal is using the mare. A foal that feels threatened will run behind the mare. The foal's head will be directly behind the mare. The foal's hind end will be facing the person who is attempting to capture; be careful to try to avoid being kicked. The handler needs to approach from the side of the foal farthest from the mare (Figure 6-23). Moving in between the mare and the foal can be detrimental to capturing the foal; instead, this could stress the mare out, especially if she cannot see the foal. She will most likely move, allowing the foal to escape. Foals, just like adult horses, will be more difficult to catch the second time around. The same techniques apply for the foal: slow steady movement and a calm relaxed tone. Scratch or rub the foal's neck or withers when first contact is made; then use only the arms and body to restrain (Figure 6-24).

Whether an adult, juvenile, or foal, once captured, it is important to allow the horse time to adjust before starting any examination or procedure. Rewarding the horse with a neck scratch and soothing words will help it to relax. Do not make the assumption that high levels of restraint are

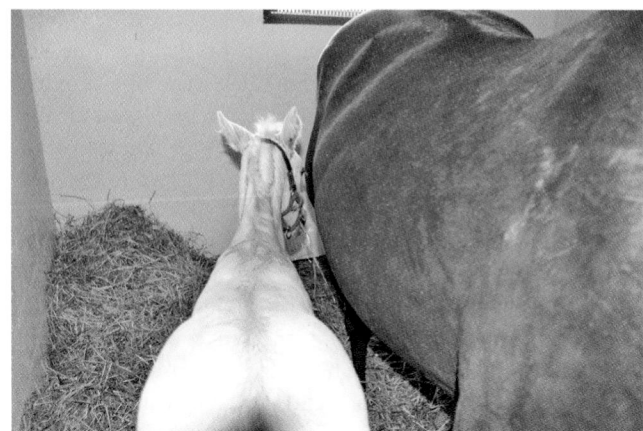

FIGURE 6-23 Normal foal behavior, running behind the mare for protection.

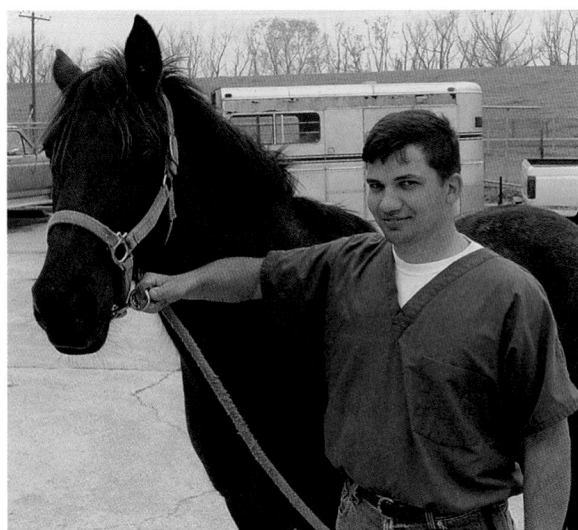

FIGURE 6-22 Proper restraint of the juvenile horse using only the halter and the lead rope.

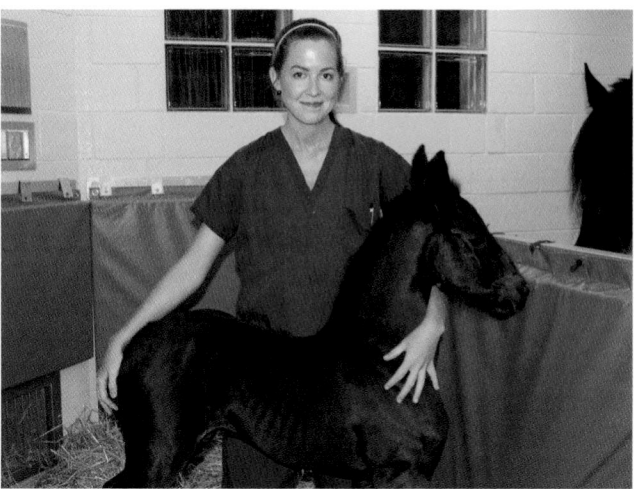

FIGURE 6-24 Proper restraint of the foal.

necessary. Begin with calm, pleasant interactions. If greater levels of restraint are needed, the horse will give behavioral signals. Wait until the animal gives these signals before increasing levels of restraint. Too much restraint can make some patients uncooperative.

ADULT EQUINE RESTRAINT TECHNIQUES AND DEVICES

Physical restraint of the adult equine begins with the halter. A halter is placed around the horse's head. Halters can be made of leather, nylon, or rope. The halter consists of the noseband (which consists of the nose piece and the chin piece), the connecting strap, the throat latch piece, a cheek piece that runs up either side of the face, the crown piece, a buckle, and/or a snap. Other pieces on the halter include the metal tie ring, the square metal nose pieces, and the metal cheek rings (Figure 6-25). Specialty halters are used for medical procedures such as anesthesia or laryngotomy. These halters usually are composed of burlap or nylon; they lack the connecting strap and the throat latch piece and are temporary. Anesthesia and laryngotomy halters provide little restraint. Veterinary technicians should know the different types of halters and should be able to list their parts in order for proper use and application.

Lead ropes can have a single snap or chain at one end and are made from rope or nylon. The lead rope provides some head control, and the rope end can be placed around the horse's neck for control while haltering. The lead rope, once attached to the halter, should be held close to the snap end with the right hand, and the extra length should be folded and grasped in the left hand. The lead rope, although similar to a dog leash, is not a dog leash and should never be wrapped around hands or arms. Mistaking a lead rope for a leash and wrapping it around an arm could lead to the handler getting dragged by a horse that "spooks" and decides to take off running. The rope end of the lead should not be allowed to drag on the ground; the person handling or the horse could step on the end. Stepping on the end of a lead

rope by horse or person can cause a horse to panic and potentially get injured.

> **TECHNICIAN NOTE**   A lead rope, although similar to a dog leash, is not a dog leash and should never be wrapped around hands or arms.

Chain shanks have a chain and a single snap on one end and can be made of rope, nylon, or leather. Chains can provide greater restraint than lead alone. A chain can be placed through the square metal nose pieces and over or under the nose or under the chin (Figure 6-26). This chain often is used to distract the horse and usually provides adequate restraint; however, for a fractious horse, the chain can be placed on the gums. This is known as a *gum* or *lip chain* and is a fairly severe form of restraint. The chain needs to be tight over the gums but should never be pulled across the gums or yanked on, once applied. Handlers using this technique should be skilled in this practice to avoid damage to the gums and additional stress to the horse (Figure 6-27).

> **TECHNICIAN NOTE**   A gum or lip chain is a fairly severe form of restraint. Handlers using this technique should be skilled in this practice to avoid damage to the gums and additional stress to the horse.

Diversionary restraint techniques are used to distract horses from unwanted behaviors during examination or procedures. Manual diversionary techniques use the handler's own hand to assist in providing restraint; this can be

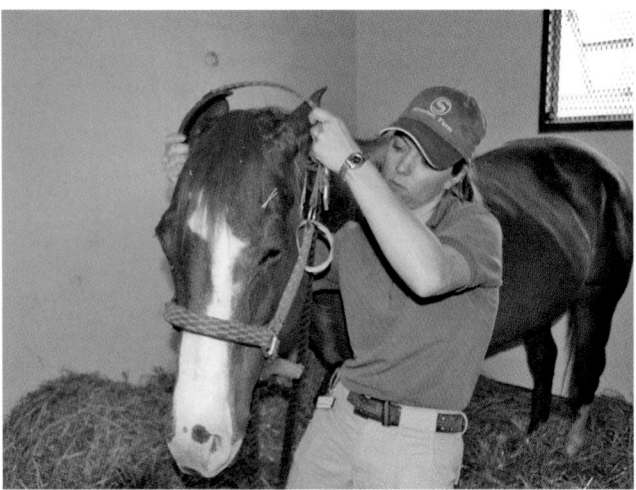

FIGURE 6-25 Proper application of a halter.

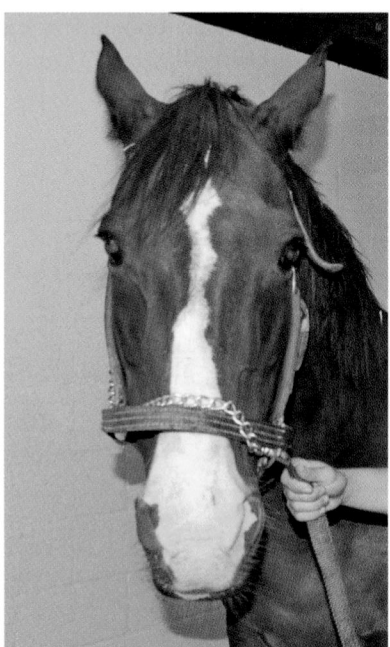

FIGURE 6-26 Proper placement of the chain over the nose. Use the nose band of the halter to prevent the chain from slipping or digging into the skin.

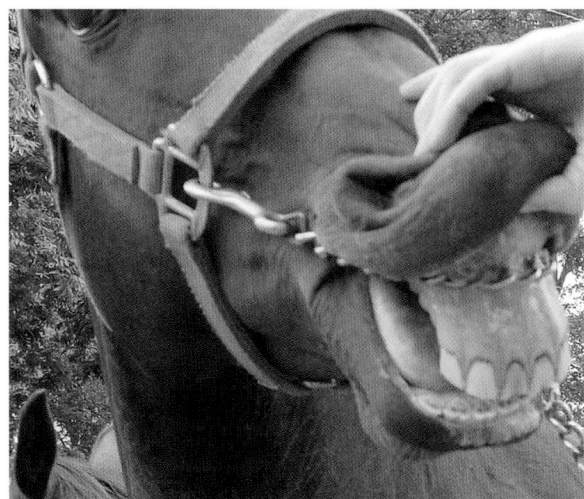

FIGURE 6-27 Proper placement of a lip/gum chain. Handlers should be skilled in this technique to avoid damage to the gums.

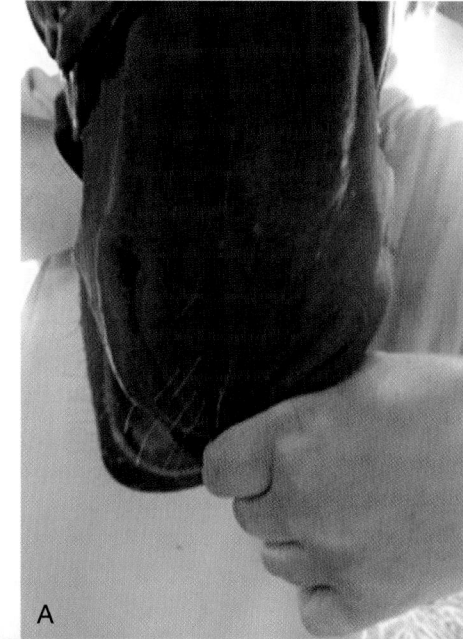

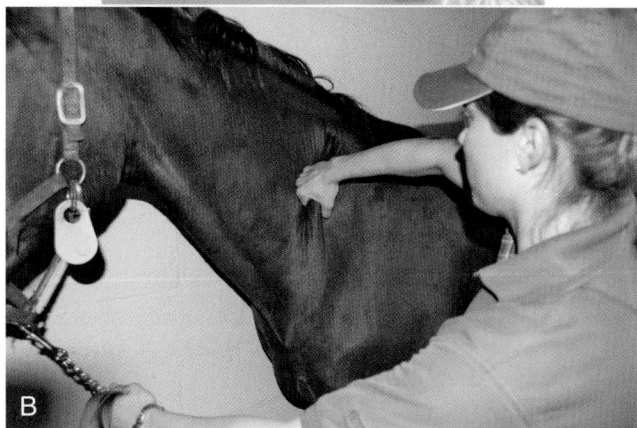

FIGURE 6-28 A, Proper application of a manual nose twitch. B, Proper application of a skin/neck twitch.

as simple as tapping on the forehead or under the eye to hold a horse's attention during simple procedures such as blood withdrawal. Other manual diversionary restraint techniques that utilize the hand are manual twitches. With a manual twitch, the handler can squeeze the horse's nose, pinch the skin along the lateral aspect of the neck, or squeeze an ear (Figure 6-28, A and B). All these forms of restraint can lose effectiveness and should be used for only a few minutes (Figure 6-29, A and B). Mechanical diversionary technique uses mechanical twitches for the purpose of restraint to achieve desired behaviors during examination or procedures. A mechanical twitch is a device used in restraining horses; it consists of a wooden handle and a chain loop or a rope loop that gets twisted around the horse's nose. It is believed that the nose is a pressure point, and once squeezed by the twitch, endorphins are released, relaxing the horse. This endorphin release is not immediate. Similar to chemicals used for sedation, it takes about 3 minutes for the release of endorphins, and they last only about 15 to 20 minutes. It is counterproductive to attempt any procedures when the twitch is initially applied. The use of a rope or a chain twitch requires two people: generally, the restrainer and the examiner. Several different types of twitches are available, but the most commonly used have a wooden handle and a rope loop (Figure 6-30). The **humane twitch** is a mechanical restraint device composed of a metal hinge, which is placed over the upper lip of the horse, squeezed, and clipped to the halter; it is designed for the person who has to perform procedures or examinations alone (Figure 6-31).

Chemical restraint is the use of tranquilizers, sedatives, and anesthetics to achieve a desired behavior. Chemical restraint is often used for horses that are violently painful, as can be the case with certain types of colic. It can also be used in horses that are generally uncooperative and resistant to certain procedures such as nasogastric intubation. Drugs commonly used for chemical restraint include acepromazine, butorphanol, detomidine, and xylazine. For further

information on pharmacology and equine pain management, refer to Chapters 27 and 28.

JUVENILE EQUINE AND FOAL RESTRAINT TECHNIQUES

Juvenile horses—weanlings and yearlings—generally are just being introduced to haltering and leading. They tend to be more nervous, especially away from familiar surroundings. For these young horses, a catch rope can sometimes be placed on the tie ring of the halter. Similar to the halter, it is unadvisable to grab the catch rope. Young, unbroken horses have a tendency to resist the halter being grabbed and can rear up, flip over, or, in trying to escape, slip on a stall floor and fall over. The best advice for catching a juvenile horse is to use a calm, quiet approach. Use treats as enticement, and once the handler is close enough, quietly clip the lead rope to the halter or stroke the horse's neck and withers, wait to gain its trust, and then attach the lead rope. Once the weanling or yearling is on the lead rope, go with it as it moves,

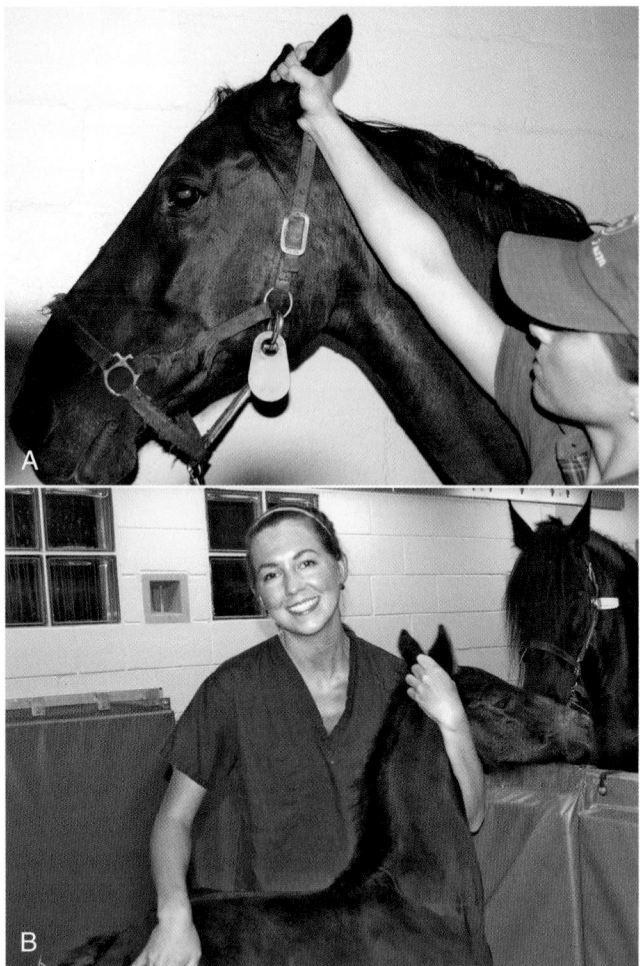

FIGURE 6-29 A, Use of a manual ear twitch in an adult equine. B, Use of a manual ear twitch in a foal.

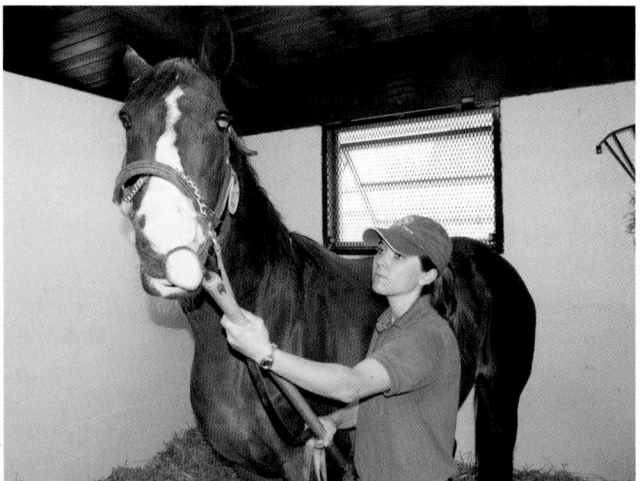

FIGURE 6-30 Proper application of a mechanical rope twitch.

and do not pull on the lead rope because this could cause the horse to pull back and rear up. Understand that a weanling or a yearling may panic and try to rear up or escape; this is when sticking with the horse, keeping calm, and having patience are most important. For the safety of the animal

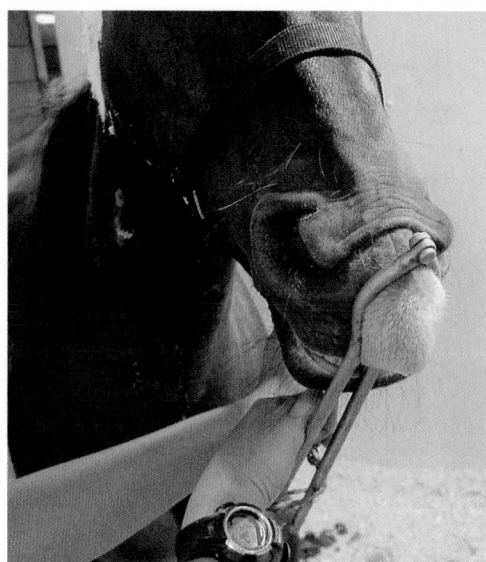

FIGURE 6-31 Use of a humane twitch.

and the handler, never use a chain over the nose of a juvenile horse for restraint.

> **TECHNICIAN NOTE** For the safety of the animal and the handler, never use a chain over the nose of a juvenile horse for restraint.

Foal restraint requires a lot of patience. Once caught and restrained, the foal will still fight and try to get away. Following easy guidelines for proper foal restraint will make restraint less stressful on the foal, the mare, and the handler. First, approach very gradually, so the foal does not startle and run. Remain calm, and once the foal is within reach, place an arm around the foal's chest and hind end. The foal will struggle to escape; just hold on until it settles down. During invasive procedures, it may be necessary to lay the foal down and sit on its front and hind legs, or to press the foal against a wall with the hind end firmly in a corner. Smaller foals can be laid down; larger foals need to be pressed against a wall, but be careful not to lift the foal off its feet. Any horse that cannot touch the ground with its feet can become frantic, causing injury to the animal or to personnel. If moving the foal is necessary, a lead rope without a chain can be wrapped around the chest and hind end in a figure eight (Figure 6-32). With foals, diversionary restraint is vital because mechanical restraint cannot be used; lifting the tail up, using a skin twitch, or squeezing an ear can help veterinary personnel perform examinations and procedures (Figure 6-33).

EQUINE RESTRAINT: SPECIAL CIRCUMSTANCES FOR SPECIFIC PROCEDURES

Tying a horse is generally done for noninvasive procedures such as grooming. Horses can be trained to ground tie,

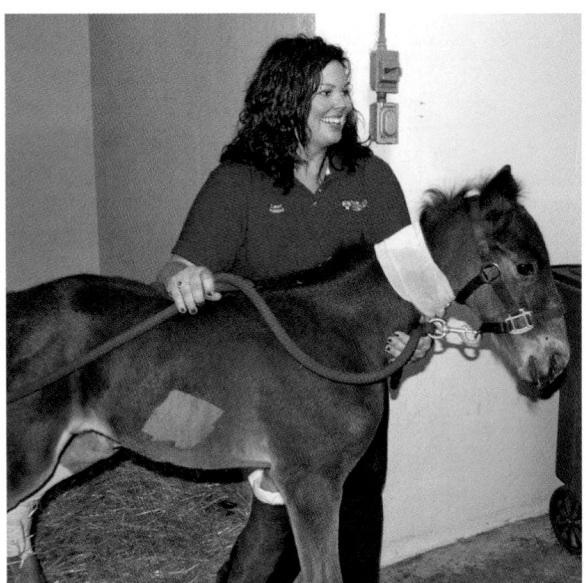

FIGURE 6-32 Application of a lead rope around the foal's body when moving from one location to another.

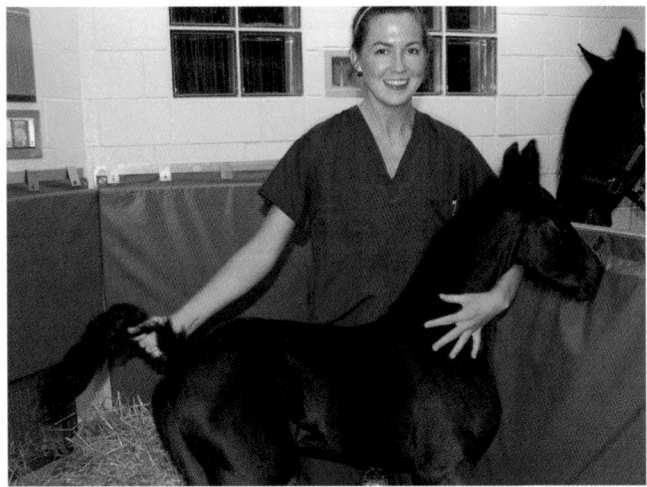

FIGURE 6-33 Holding the tail up is a diversionary restraint in foals.

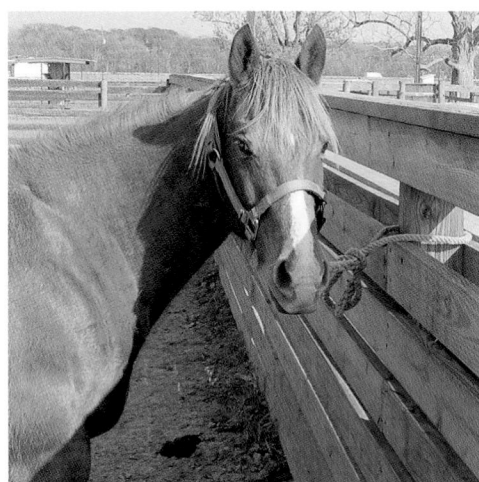

FIGURE 6-34 Tying a horse to a fence post for a noninvasive procedure.

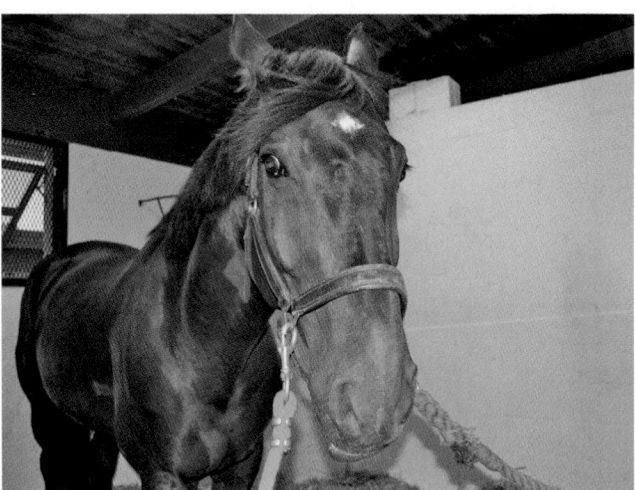

FIGURE 6-35 A horse that is cross-tied in the stall.

> **TECHNICIAN NOTE** Tying a horse is generally done for noninvasive procedures such as grooming. Any horse that is tied needs to be monitored closely and ideally not left alone.

cross-tie, or be tied to a ring in the stall, or to some other sturdy structure such as a fence post (Figure 6-34). Another reason to tie a horse is to prevent further injury, for example, in a horse that has had a severely fractured limb repaired; preventing this horse from lying down could be crucial for recovery, and the veterinarian may decide that this particular horse should be cross-tied (Figure 6-35). Any horse that is tied needs to be monitored closely and ideally not left alone. A horse should never be tied with the chain over the nose or under the chin because if the horse becomes anxious or tries to escape, it will be injured. A quick release knot or break-away snaps should always be used to set the horse free if it panics. Tying a horse should be done only when absolutely necessary, and invasive procedures should not be completed while the horse is tied.

Lifting a front or hind leg is done to keep other limbs on the ground. The thought process behind this type of restraint is that if you lift a front foot, the horse is less likely to kick with a hind foot. Lifting a limb is easy, but keeping the leg up can be difficult for the handler; horses sometimes will lean all their weight on the handler or will still try to kick (Figure 6-36). Examples of when lifting a leg could be a beneficial restraint technique include assisting with limb examinations and examining the prepuce, penis, or udder. **Hobbles** can also be used to keep horses from kicking; several versions of hobbles are available, although they are rarely used anymore. The general purpose of hobbles is to connect two limbs together, such as the hind legs. Breeding hobbles can be used to prevent a mare from kicking the

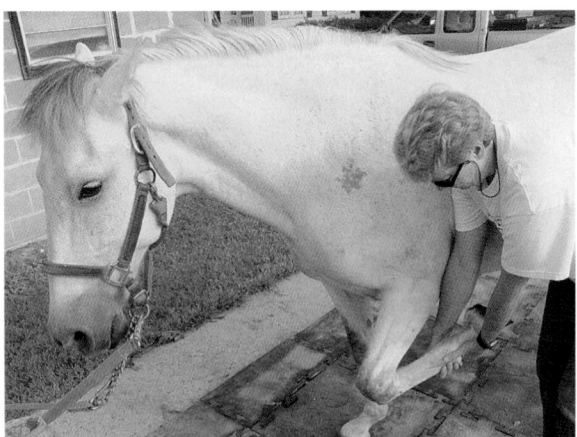

FIGURE 6-36 Lifting a front leg to aid in examination of limbs, prepuce, or udder.

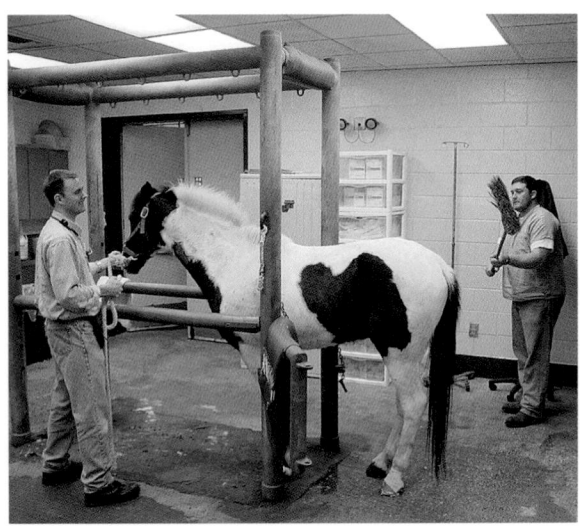

FIGURE 6-37 A horse being placed in stocks.

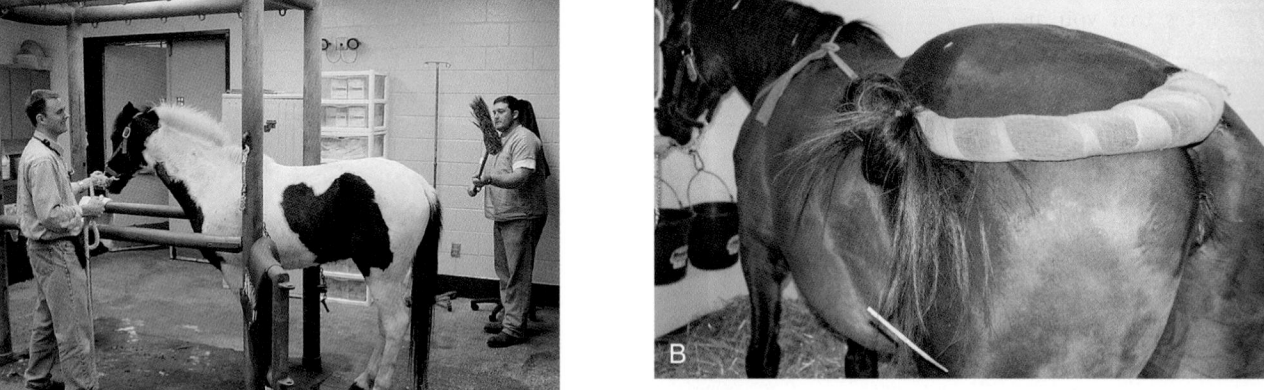

FIGURE 6-38 A, A horse wearing a cradle. B, Horse with brown gauze tail tie.

stallion during live cover. Nurse mares—mares used to provide rejected or orphaned foals nutrients—typically are hobbled on the hind limbs to prevent them from kicking the new foal during introduction and until bonding has occurred.

Stocks are vertical metal or wooden pillars, arranged in a rectangular shape and connected by horizontal bars and designed to restrain horses or cattle standing within. Stocks are commonly found in most large animal hospitals. They can be used during many procedures but commonly are used for rectal or vaginal examinations or procedures. Stocks serve as a safe alternative to handler restraint for these procedures; however, it must be noted that horses have been known to freak out and jump over or out of stocks, causing serious injury. Also, horses can still "cow kick" and strike out when in stocks. The handler should always be present when a horse is in stocks to ensure the safety of the animal and other barn personnel (Figure 6-37).

Other forms of restraint in horses are those that restrict movement in a specific area, such as the neck or the tail. The cradle is a barred restraint device. The bars are tied together

like a nonridged fence. The cradle is tied around the neck of a horse like a loose splint; it prevents the horse from biting or licking itself. A cradle can be used to prevent damage to bandages or to temporarily stop undesirable stall behaviors such as cribbing (Figure 6-38, *A*). A **tail tie** can be applied with rope or brown gauze and tied around the horse's neck and chest to prevent movement of the tail during rectal or vaginal examination. A brown gauze tail tie is more commonly used; it is applied at the base of the tail and is wrapped around the tail to the end of the tail bone. The hairs that hang from the end of the tail are then folded over and the brown gauze is wrapped around, creating a loop in the tail. The brown gauze is put through this loop and is stretched over the back and around the neck; it is then secured with a quick release knot (Figure 6-38, *B*). The purpose of the brown gauze wrap is to cover the bulk of the small hairs at the base of the tail and prevent them from getting into a clean field. A tail tie is applied to the hairs at the end of the tail and is secured in a similar fashion; however, small hair coverage will not be attained.

Many methods of restraint are known; however, no one way is the correct way. Every horse is different and should be treated as an individual. The entire situation should be assessed before restraint, and with regard to equine restraint, the safety of personnel should always be a priority. Learning and understanding proper and safe restraint techniques will minimize stress on the animal and will keep all those working with the animal safe.

CAPTURE AND RESTRAINT OF CATTLE

THE APPROACH

The fundamental difference between working with live-stock species and working with companion animals is the predator–prey interaction that serves as the foundation of human–livestock interactions. This relationship causes cattle to alter their behavior when they observe a predator, to avoid being chosen as prey. Therefore, it is important to complete as much of the physical examination as possible before the cow notices that you are evaluating it or are moving to restrain it. General conditions such as attitude, lameness, rumination/cud chewing, appetite, and respiratory rate can be included in an initial observation. The reaction of the cow or the herd when they do observe you can provide information about how to proceed. Cattle that startle at your presence and begin to flee need to be handled more carefully and quietly than cattle that approach you with curiosity. These initial observations are very helpful as you determine the best way to work with and restrain herds and individual cattle for medical interventions. Be particularly cautious when separating sick or injured animals from the larger herd. Elevated anxiety levels caused by separation can lead both the patient and members of the herd to be defensive and aggressive.

LOW-STRESS HANDLING

The predator–prey relationship already mentioned can be dangerous if cattle are stressed and feel threatened; however, it also serves as the basis of the way we work with cattle. Cows have an inherent fear of humans and will try to maintain a distance at which they feel safe. This distance is termed the *flight zone* and varies from zero to 25 feet, depending on the tameness of the animal (Figure 6-39). Adult dairy cattle tend to have smaller flight zones (5 to 10 ft) because of the daily contact that they have with farmers; beef cattle on range have a larger personal space (15 to 25 ft).

> **TECHNICIAN NOTE** Pet cattle will have no flight zone; the best method of moving these animals usually involves a rope halter.

When humans or other predators enter the flight zone of typical cattle, cows tend to bunch together and move away from the perceived threat. As they move to a more comfortable distance, they turn back and look at the

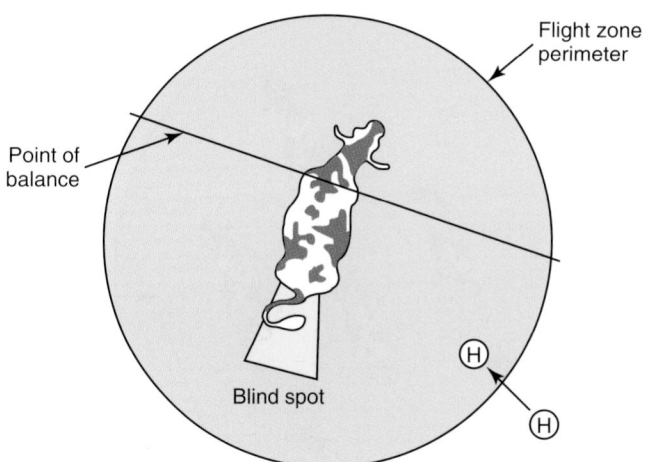

FIGURE 6-39 A graphic illustration of the cattle flight zone. As the handler (H) moves into the flight zone from behind the point of balance, this cow will move forward and to the left. (Redrawn from Jason C. Fisher, IAN Image Library, ian.umces.edu/imagelibrary.)

perceived threat. This is an indication that the flight zone has been reestablished.

These behavioral cues are important in that appropriate handling of cattle is based on a pressure and release system. Handlers move cattle by invading the flight zone by a couple of feet (pressure) and then allowing the animal to reestablish it (release). Repetition of this pressure and release system uses a cow's natural behavioral instincts to move her in the desired direction. It is critical that the "release" portion of the handling last as long as the cattle are moving in the desired direction. Only when they stop or need redirection should a new, corrective pressure be added. Questions concerning the welfare of cattle worked in this manner often arise (e.g., Is it humane to scare cattle into moving?) Current understanding of this behavior indicates that a properly implemented pressure and release system causes anxiety, not fear. Indeed, anxiety can be a positive motivating factor, such as the anxiety you feel about an upcoming examination that (hopefully) motivates you to study for it.

However, if the handler invades the flight zone of the cattle too aggressively, a fear response can be generated, and the cow will panic and flee. A frightened animal is a dangerous one; this is especially true of cattle because they are large and strong and can push through or jump over fences, potentially injuring themselves and their handlers (i.e., you) and certainly changing (and thus confusing) physical examination findings, such as heart rate and respiration rate.

The method in which people work with cattle also can affect the flight zone of cows. Cows should be worked calmly and quietly with deliberate movements. Quick or sudden movement or loud noises such as yelling can cause cattle to panic and attempt to flee. Also, remember that cows do not understand vocal commands, but they do understand body language. Calm and quiet handlers can often shrink the flight zone of cattle (i.e., get closer to the animal); aggressive, frustrated, and loud handlers can cause the flight zone to expand, causing cattle to flee greater distances.

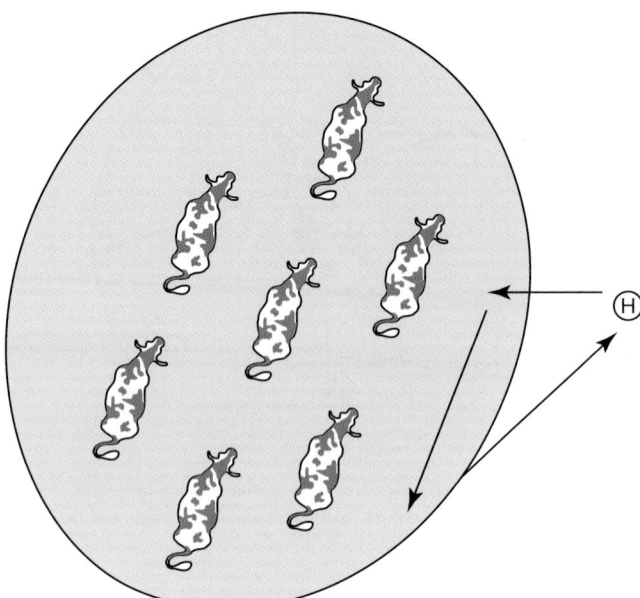

FIGURE 6-40 Moving groups. When moving a group of cattle, the initial movement should move the leading animals forward by directing movement behind the shoulder. As the handler (H) passes the second animal, it moves forward, and the handler exits the flight zone. (Redrawn from Jason C. Fisher, IAN Image Library, ian.umces.edu/imagelibrary.)

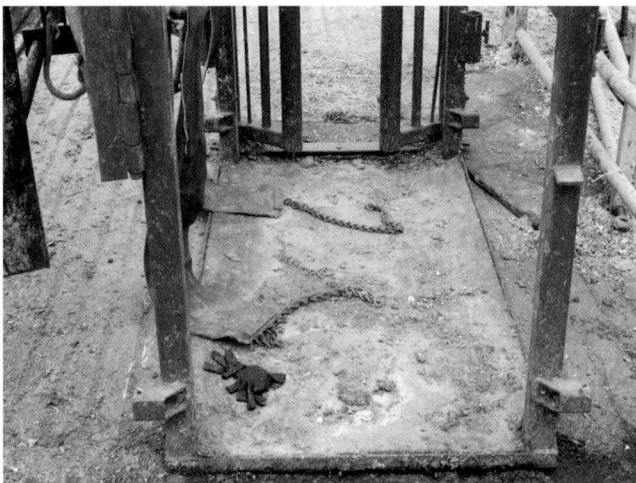

FIGURE 6-41 Common distractions in a cattle chute. A pair of black latex gloves (foreground) have been left from the previous treatment, and the chains used to support the cow during treatment should be removed to allow smoother entry into the chute.

An understanding of the flight zone of cattle and of the predator–prey relationship serves as a good foundation for working cattle. The next fundamental is to understand the **point of balance.** Simply, the point of balance is the part of the animal that if you took a step in either direction, the animal would move in the opposite direction. The shoulder is the point of balance of the cow. To move a single cow forward, approach the cow from the side, enter the flight zone from behind the shoulder, and wait for the cow to reestablish its comfort level. Remember, as long as the cow continues to move in the direction you want, no further pressure is needed. When it stops or begins to move in an undesired direction, corrective pressure can be added by reentering the cow's flight zone. Cattle prefer to stay in a group and will follow the leader. When groups of cattle are moved in a working chute system or in a pasture, pressure is placed on the point of balance of the leader or on the middle of the leading group to move the entire herd. Figure 6-40 shows the handler entering the flight zone near the front of the group, walking toward the rear of the group, and then exiting the flight zone. This triangular movement pattern moves the herd forward as the point of balance is crossed, then releases pressure as the flight zone is exited. The pattern can be repeated as necessary.

As cattle approach a holding area, handlers should initially move outside the flight zone, releasing pressure. If cattle balk at the entrance and turn back, a small amount of pressure should be added. However, continuous pressure can make a cow feel trapped and can make it begin to panic. This is especially dangerous if the handler is between the animal and the exit. Cattle will run over and through obstacles (such

as handlers) if they are pressured to the point of panic. Cows have very poor vertical vision and cannot focus at close distances. These traits result in cows balking at things that do not cause much concern for humans (Figure 6-41). Such traits may include shadows, changes in floor or wall color, flapping clothes or bags, extension cords, discarded cups or cans, and changes in flooring. Removal of the offending item is the easiest solution, although some items require more long-term planning. The use of electric prods to push cattle into or through a poorly designed system is unacceptable and in this author's opinion is inhumane. Electric prods should be used in less than 5% of cattle working through a chute system.

CAPTURE

Handling facilities differ significantly for beef and dairy cows. In the United States, most dairy cows are housed in a barn for some portion of the day, so the need to group and bring animals to a common handling facility is largely eliminated. Further, a restraint system for common management practices such as artificial insemination, vaccination, examination, and treatment often provides the veterinarian and/or veterinary technician easy access to animals. If better control is necessary, especially of the head, a rope halter can be placed on the cow's head (Figure 6-42). A cow halter is often made of braided rope and has two loops and a tail. The loop that is reduced in size when you pull on the tail goes over the nose and under the jaw. The other loop is changed in size by adjusting a portion of the nose loop; it is placed over the poll and around the ears. This author finds it easier to adjust the poll and ear loop and place it first, then place the nose and jaw loop, but either order is acceptable. The halter is secured by pulling on the tail of the halter after both loops are placed. Technically, the tail of the halter should exit from the left side of the cow's mandible, but head restraint will be more secure if the tail exits to the side of the cow

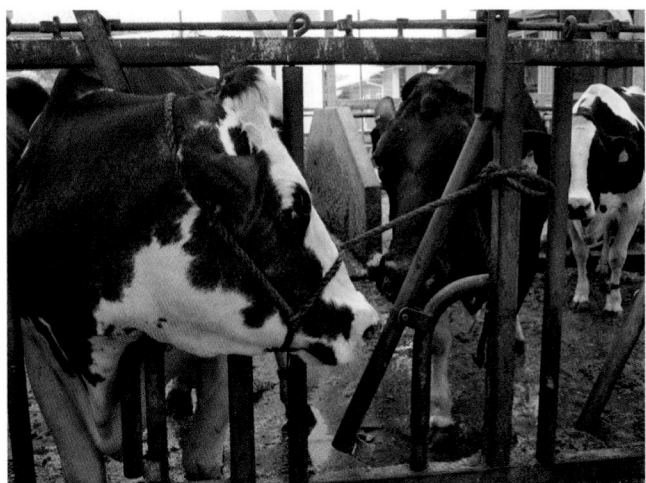

FIGURE 6-42 After the halter is placed, the cow's head is pulled through the stanchion and turned to the side. The halter is tied using a quick release knot. This position allows access to the jugular vein.

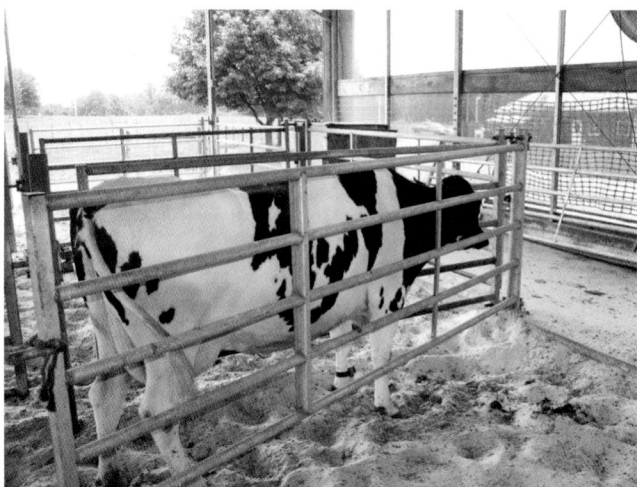

FIGURE 6-43 To restrain a cow in a pen, move the cow to a corner and swing the gate to squeeze the cow. This restraint may be sufficient for rapid procedures such as pregnancy examination by rectal palpation, or a halter can be placed if needed.

where it will be tied. If a cow has horns, they should be included in the loop that encompasses the poll and the ears.

> **TECHNICIAN NOTE** Placement of the halter upside down on a cow so that the part that tightens when the tail is pulled around the ears provides additional head control while maintaining the ability to open the cow's mouth.

When placing a halter over the poll, be very careful to keep your head from being directly over the cow's head. Cattle occasionally will lift their heads straight up, colliding with the restrainer's head, chin, and/or nose. To avoid this injury, ensure that your head does not occupy the space directly over the cow's head by keeping the cow at arm's length or approaching from the side instead of directly from the front. Sometimes cows will be in individual "box stalls" for additional treatment and care. In these situations, the cow often may be more nervous because it is separated from the herd. Successful placement of a halter in this situation may be aided by trapping the cow between two gates to limit movement (see Figure 6-43).

A smaller halter of identical design is used for calves. Adult halters may work but often have a nose piece that is too large. On dairy farms, calves typically are individually raised in their own hutch (Figure 6-44), and a halter provides sufficient restraint for most procedures. However, extreme caution should be exercised if you are attempting to restrain a calf in the same pen as the calf's dam. The predator–prey interaction is more intense in confined settings and is further exacerbated by maternal instincts of protection. Try to work with calves close to an exit, or separate the calf from the cow before conducting any procedures.

The halter should be tied with a quick release knot that maintains the desired length of lead and allows the handler to release the cow with one pull of the rope. This is critically important because some cows will react negatively to being

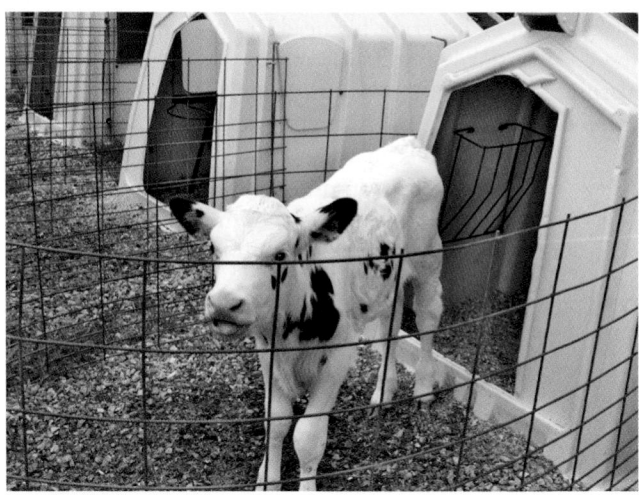

FIGURE 6-44 Dairy calf in an individual hutch. Calves are usually curious and easy to catch, and they are usually eager to see people because they associate humans with feeding time.

handled or treated and will lie down while tied. Depending on the type of restraint used, this can be potentially harmful to the cow, and a rapid release knot allows the animal to be quickly freed.

Beef cattle are typically handled less often than dairy cattle; additional handling facilities are required for working with them. In a commercial operation, a chute system is often used. This may be composed of a holding pen, a crowding pen, an alley, and a chute. Cattle are moved into the holding pen and the crowding pen using principles of pressure and release. Sometimes catwalks are built onto the side of the pens and the alley to allow handlers to treat animals before they enter the chute and to assist in moving the animals through the system. Movement into the holding pen can be safely and effectively conducted by using a simple flag attached to a stick. The same principles of pressure release and point of balance apply, but in this case, the stick serves as an extension, allowing the handler to work from the outside of the pen. The crowding pen often is round, allowing a large swinging gate to follow the cows into the alley. Cows enter the alley single file and follow the cow ahead. Alleys should have solid sides to avoid distractions, should be slightly wider than the cow without allowing it to turn around, and may be curved to take advantage of the cow's preference to return to where it came from. Handlers should avoid entering the alley without identified methods of escape. A frightened or injured cow is most dangerous and will seek an exit by moving forward or backward and through you if needed.

Extreme caution should be used when working with bulls. Beef and dairy bulls may be co-mingled with female cattle and can easily be overlooked; when handling cattle, always ask whether a bull is present. Beef bulls tend to be less aggressive toward humans than their dairy counterparts, but both can be deadly to handlers. If a bull is present, watch for signs that the bull is showcasing his size and is becoming aggressive. Such signs include the bull showing you his side, pawing the ground, or lowering his head. If you see a bull exhibit these signs, slowly back away out of the bull's flight zone. Turning and running away may invite being chased and injured by the bull. Exit the pen or pasture as soon as possible. Individual bulls may have nose rings as additional means of handling and restraint. The nose of a cow or a bull is very sensitive, and a ring placed in the nasal septum provides additional but not total control of the bull.

RESTRAINT TECHNIQUES AND DEVICES

When working animals through handling facilities, a chute with a head-gate or a head-catch is the final destination (Figure 6-45). This piece of equipment has two doors with a vertical opening in between. The doors are opened to allow the animal to see a path for escape. When the animal's head enters the opening, the gate is quickly closed and tightened around the neck. This restrains the cow and limits forward movement to the length between head and shoulder. The head-gate can also be self-locking, but this type is less common in a chute system because of the need to adjust the size for animals of different sizes and to prevent more frequent escapes. If a cow gets part of its shoulder through, it will escape and should be released before it or one of the handlers gets injured. On some chutes, additional restraint is provided by adding a collapsing side that squeezes the cow and prevents additional movement. These chutes can be manually run or operated hydraulically. Numerous commercial chute manufacturers and some home-made systems are available. Each chute operates slightly differently with multiple handles and moving parts; a little time should be taken to become familiar with the handling equipment to avoid injury. For dairy cattle, a simpler, automatic head-catch system may be used at the feed bunk and in a box stall. This head restraint system is called a *head-lock* (Figure 6-46). This system automatically secures a cow's head between two vertical bars when the cow puts her head down to eat. A head-lock system provides an opportunity to restrain an entire pen of cows for routine management practices while ensuring that they stay with the herd and have access to feed. However, care should be taken to prevent having cows locked up for longer than an hour because this impinges on a cow's time budget and prevents lying down and rumination.

A physical examination can often be completed with simple head restraint. In dairy cattle, head-locks are commonly used for routine postpartum health monitoring. In beef cattle, many chutes provide drop-down sides or windows in the side of the chute for access to the bovine. An oral examination can often be accomplished without further restraint, and the use of a halter is contraindicated because the halter tightens over the nose and under the jaw, effectively closing the mouth. A towel can be used to grasp and move the tongue to allow examination of the oral cavity and detection of the tongue paresis common in cases of botulism.

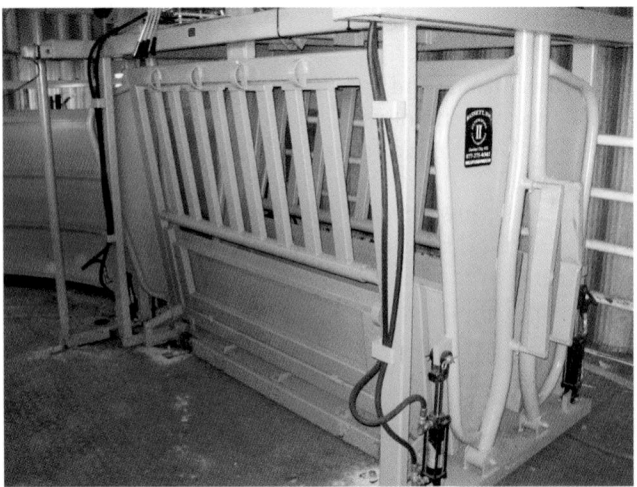

FIGURE 6-45 A hydraulic squeeze chute used for beef cattle. The head protrudes through the vertical doors, which open to release the cow when treatment is completed.

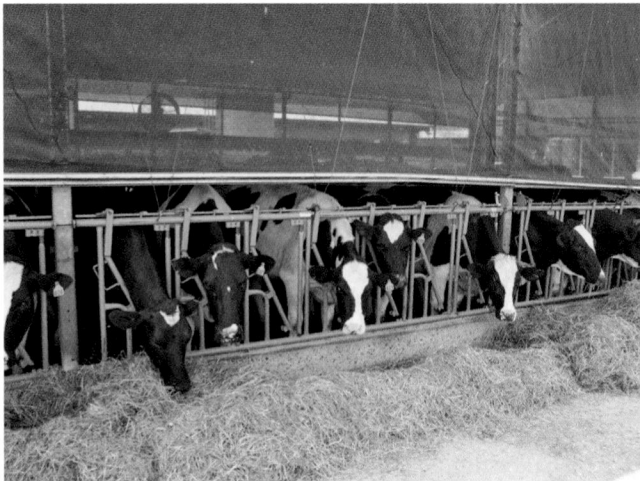

FIGURE 6-46 Dairy cows in a feed line head-lock system. Head-locks are "set" to restrain animals when needed. Otherwise, they serve to prevent dominant animals from clearing the bunk of competition.

Many cows can be administered oral medication or fluids using only a head-lock or a head-gate. Oral administration of boluses, a magnet, or fluids is often easier without a halter. To administer a bolus using a pill gun or a balling gun, stand on the cow's left side facing the same direction the cow is facing (i.e., with your back to the cow). Reach over the nose with your right hand, and brace the cow's head against your hip. Maintaining the cow's head and neck as straight as possible will facilitate administration of oral medications. Next, place your first two fingers into the mouth at the oral commissure. Recall that cows do not have upper incisors, so the risk of being bitten is very low, especially if you keep your fingers in the space between the lower incisors and the molars, termed the *dental pad*. Once your fingers are in the cow's mouth, the cow will open it slightly; move your fingers to the hard palate, and the cow will further open its mouth (Figure 6-47). Now insert the pill gun into the cow's mouth with your free hand. Placement of the pill gun is important: too rostral, and the bolus will easily be spit out, and too caudal can cause damage to the oropharynx. The pill gun should be directed medially over the torus linguae (the large bump on the back of the tongue) and the plunger depressed to administer the medication.

A similar approach can be used when administering oral fluids. For pumps that have soft rubber hosing, a speculum is required to prevent damage to the tubing caused by

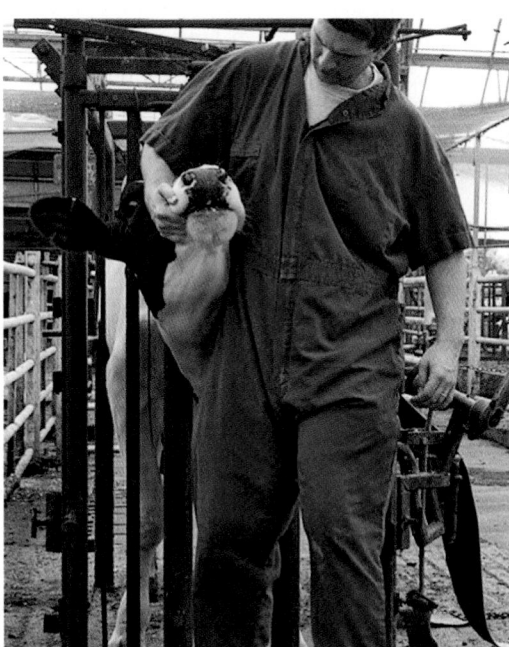

FIGURE 6-47 The technique used to open a cow's mouth for oral administration of fluids or boluses.

chewing and a potential rumen foreign body if the cow chews through the hose and swallows the distal portion. A Frick speculum can be placed in a similar manner to the pill gun and held in place by hand. Often a Frick speculum comes with a set of nose tongs attached that maintain placement of the speculum when an orogastric tube is placed and fluids are administered. Some pumps are made with protective metal encircling the esophageal tube, allowing the tube to be passed directly into the mouth without the need for a speculum. When passing an esophageal tube, care should be taken to keep the head level such that the nose stays below the poll. An inclined head (nose above poll) makes it easier to pass an orogastric tube into the trachea instead of into the esophagus.

Additional Head Restraint

To access the jugular vein or for more advanced or invasive procedures of the head, a halter must be utilized in combination with a head-lock or a head-gate to restrain the bovine patient. The cow should be pulled straight ahead to get the shoulder as close to the head-lock as possible before turning the cow's head and tying the halter. This procedure minimizes the ability of the cow to move in a cranial-caudal direction and exposes the maximum length of the jugular vein for venipuncture or catheter placement. In fractious bovine patients, applying pressure to the nasal septum can result in better control over the head.

Pressure can be applied by inserting metal nose tongs that squeeze the nasal septum. The tongs are connected to a rope, which can be tied off and allows the examiner to maintain use of both hands for procedures. Although useful when necessary, nose tongs occasionally elicit an escalation of fractious behavior, and some behavior experts have indicated that nose tongs may cause increased adverse reactions with repeated use.

Tail Restraint

During obstetric procedures such as dystocia correction or Caslick's surgery, the cow's tail can be restrained with a simple tail tie. A rope is tied into the hair at the end of the tail (the cow's switch) by folding the hair upward after the rope is laid horizontally across the switch. The rope is then tied into a quick release knot with the short end of the rope providing the release. The remainder of the rope should be tied to the cow, not to a surrounding structure. If the cow were to escape from its restraint, lie down unexpectedly, or move in an unexpected manner, injury to the tail could result. The preferred anchor for the tail tie is a quick release knot encircling the neck. A cow's collar or halter has also been used but still presents a potential risk if the cow escapes.

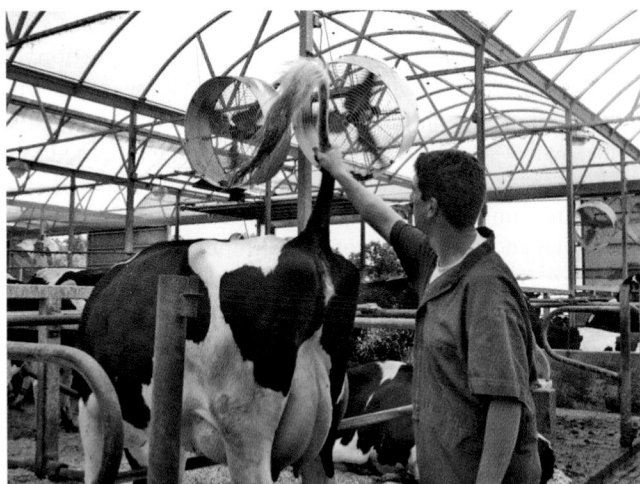

FIGURE 6-48 The tail jack technique. This is especially helpful if cows have to be examined or sampled in free stalls with no head restraint.

Another tail restraint method is the tail jack. This simple method of restraint is thought to provide nerve stimulation similar to that of the twitch in horses. It is a useful method of restraint for nervous patients when a minor procedure is being conducted such as the administration of local analgesia, infusion of intramammary mastitis treatment, and rectal palpation. The tail jack is accomplished by grasping the tail 6 to 10 inches from the tail head and pushing straight up and over the midline of the cow until it forms a 60-degree angle with the spine of the cow (Figure 6-48). This method of restraint is also useful for venipuncture because it provides access to the coccygeal vein and artery of the cow. For small quantities of blood (<20 mL), the author has found coccygeal venipuncture using a Vacutainer (BD, Franklin Lakes, NJ) and collection tube to be the easiest, safest, and most efficient method.

Foot Control and Restraint

Lameness is a common disease of dairy cows often requiring corrective trimming as treatment. Cattle are much more reluctant than horses to raise their feet for examination and treatment. Professional hoof trimmers will often use a tilt table to access all four feet simultaneously. This method secures the cow to a vertical wall with a large abdominal band and then lifts the cow, turning it 90 degrees to rest in lateral recumbency. Standing chutes are also available in which each individual foot, one at a time, is attached to a rope and is lifted by manual crank or hydraulic pressure to allow examination and treatment. When these restraint systems are not available, a pulley system can be constructed using a rope alone or a rope with block and tackle.

Lifting and restraining a cow's front foot is typically the most difficult step, perhaps because cows bear most of their weight on their forelimbs. The best approach for this author is to place a slip knot or use a rope with a quick release Honda to encircle the forelimb to examine, as close to the pastern as possible. Take the rope over a bar or beam and

come back to the foot. Loop back around the foot and over the same bar or beam. You've now constructed a double pulley system that will allow you to lift the foot with relative ease. Once the forelimb is lifted, secure it to an adjacent bar or pole for further restraint if needed. Always be cautious when lifting a cow's foot because this requires a shift in balance that may cause the cow to fall over, occasionally onto the person lifting the foot. This can also be caused by the cow's attempts to kick the examiner with the rear leg of the same side. Fortunately, approximately 90% of lameness occurs in the back feet, and they are relatively easier to handle.

In practice, this author has successfully used a 2-inch-wide leather strap fitted with a belt buckle and a semicircular metal fitting. This strap is applied tightly, proximal to the hock, to apply pressure to the calcaneus tendon and limit movement. A block and tackle is attached to the metal fitting and to a bar or beam above the cow, and the cow's foot is raised to the desired level. Alternatively, a rope can be tied with a slip knot or by using a Honda proximal to the hock. The rope is passed over a bar or beam, and the cow's rear leg is raised for examination. With both methods, the cow retains some ability to extend her leg, so the examiner must be cautious when trimming or applying treatment. Hoof knives and other lameness equipment can be dangerous to examiners when it is not under their control.

For lameness procedures causing moderate pain and distress, or for cattle unwilling to submit to the restraint required to deliver an appropriate treatment, regional analgesia is often very effective. In this case, a rubber IV hose is applied as a tourniquet just distal to the hock. The lateral branch of the saphenous vein is located, and 20 to 30 mL of 2% lidocaine is infused using a butterfly catheter. Analgesia develops in 10 to 15 minutes and persists for as long as the tourniquet remains in place. This author used this technique with increasing frequency when lame cows were presented that had hoof pathology extending to the soft tissue. It provided a safer working environment for the veterinarian and the cow and allowed the veterinarian to complete treatment in a more efficient manner.

Casting Cows

Occasionally, it becomes necessary to place a cow in lateral or dorsal recumbency for a treatment procedure. This straight forward procedure can usually be accomplished by one or two individuals without the need for great strength. First, the cow must be haltered and tied to a post or a bar that will withstand some force. The length of the rope should be such that the cow is able to lie down comfortably with her head and neck extended in a normal position. Second, one of two rope patterns is applied to the cow. The author's preference is the half-hitch pattern. This method uses a noose with a slip knot or Honda around the neck, followed by two half-hitch knots. After the noose is tied around the neck, the free end is dropped on the opposite side of the cow and is brought up and under the section originating from the noose, forming a half hitch. The free end is then run to just cranial to the hip, where the end is dropped underneath the cow and is picked up on the other side and run under the length of rope originating from the first half-hitch. This requires a bit of extra work, but after the restraint is complete and the noose is released, the rope can be easily removed from the recumbent cow without entangling the rope under the patient's abdomen. This can potentially cause damage to recent surgical sites and is often very difficult to retrieve. The udder or prepuce should not be included in the knot because pressure can cause inflammation and injury. The tail of the rope comes off the cow's spine with all three knots positioned dorsally. A strong pull of the free end should result in the cow's lying down.

> **TECHNICIAN NOTE** When the half-hitch method is used to cast a cow, a large loop can be made on one side to facilitate removal of the rope after the procedure is completed.

The other method is the Burley or "Running W" method. Again, after the patient is securely tied with a halter of sufficient length, the rope is placed over her back with its center at the point of the shoulder. The ends are carried between the forelegs and are crossed at the sternum. One end is carried up each side of the animal's body, and the two are crossed again over the back. Each end passes downward between the rear legs, going between the inner surface of the legs and under the udder or scrotum. Pulling on both ends of the rope applies pressure to the cow, causing it to lie down, with the cow favoring the side on which the greatest pressure is applied. With both methods, application of hobbles to the front and rear legs at the level of the pastern limits the bovine patient's ability to balance, resulting in quicker and easier progression to recumbency.

After the cow has been cast, kneeling on the head at the angle of the mandible or just caudal to the head on the neck of the cow maintains lateral recumbency, while additional positioning is completed. This procedure can also be used to maintain lateral recumbency after the casting rope has been removed. If hobbles were placed, they can be used to place the cow in dorsal recumbency. A small square bale of hay or straw can further aid in positioning and support of the cow. When cows are cast, the rumen should be carefully observed. Ruminants that are cast can suffer from bloat or regurgitation and from aspiration of rumen contents, especially if sedatives are used concurrently. The use of xylazine, an alpha-2 agonist often used for sedation of cattle, may exacerbate these issues.

Cows that are already in recumbency and are unable to rise owing to hypocalcemia, endotoxemia, or other disease causes can be tied to maintain recumbency during treatment. The bovine patient should be placed in sternal recumbency and can be braced with a straw bale if necessary. After a halter is placed on the cow's head, the cow's head is turned back to the side where her feet are visible. The free end of

end of the halter is then tied to the most lateral leg, above the hock, bringing the cow's nose as close as possible to the hock. A quick release knot is used to secure the halter. This enables exposure of the jugular vein for IV fluid administration while effectively restraining the cow.

CAPTURE AND RESTRAINT OF SWINE

OBSERVATION

Observation of pigs before handling and restraint is a critical part of the physical examination. This is especially true when the examiner is evaluating the herd, not just an individual pig. When and where pigs are lying, their interactions with each other, and their gait and dunging patterns are important parts of a thorough barn evaluation.

APPROACH

When the examiner enters the pen, adult pigs are often curious and may seek out the examiner using their excellent sense of smell to investigate. Adult pigs may also attempt to chew on the examiner's boots, coveralls, or legs, if given the opportunity. This is normal behavior and does not necessarily indicate that pigs are not being fed appropriately. When an examiner enters a farrowing room or nursery, nursing and weaned piglets may demonstrate additional avoidance behaviors. Often they will startle when the examiner is first observed and may run into a corner in an effort to escape (Figure 6-49). As with other livestock species, the lactating female with offspring, an injured animal, and an adult male should be considered dangerous and handled with extreme caution. Lactating sows may be confined in a crate during some or all of lactation to prevent crushing of their offspring (Figure 6-50). However, sows can reach through bars to bite handlers in some cases. Boars are kept on farms to elicit estrus behavior from gilts and sows during artificial insemination. When boars are exposed to a female in standing heat,

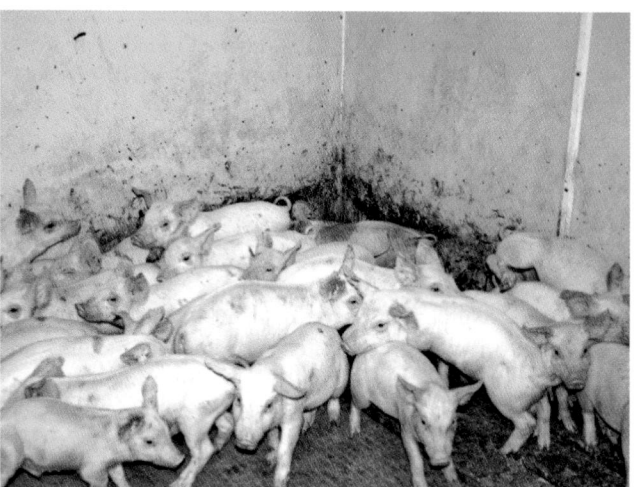

FIGURE 6-49 Piglets crowding into a corner when a handler approaches. As the handler gets closer, the piglets turn away, allowing the handler to quickly grasp a rear leg and lift the piglet for restraint.

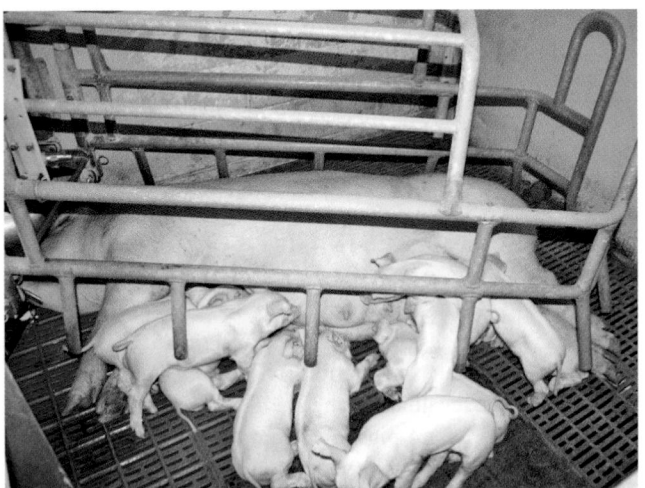

FIGURE 6-50 A farrowing crate with nursing piglets. Aggressive sows can injure handlers that attempt to catch and restrain piglets.

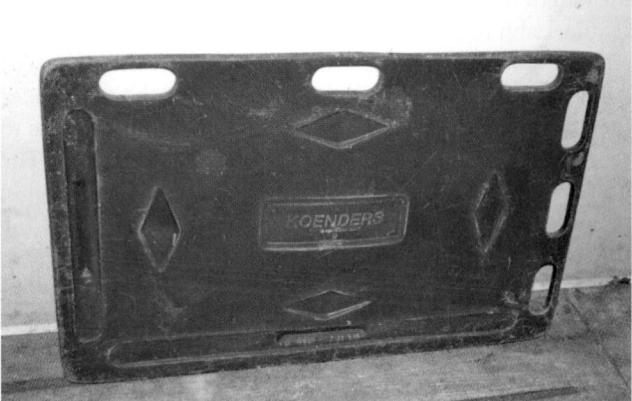

FIGURE 6-51 A pig board used as a barrier to guide and direct pigs for movement and restraint. Always make sure the board is flush to the floor to prevent pigs from rooting underneath it and escaping.

they often become aggressive and present a danger to the handler. Boars are strong and grow tusks that can impale and injure handlers. A solid board should always be used when handling boars and should be kept in between the handler and the boar.

Pigs have the least herding instinct of the food animal species, although they do become nervous when separated from herdmates. Swine have a flight zone similar to that of ruminants with a blind spot directly behind them. Compared with other livestock species, pigs can be more stubborn and difficult to move, perhaps because of their poor eyesight or their reliance on scent to investigate new environments. When pigs are moved within a barn or are loaded onto a ramp, the same principles of minimizing stress among livestock should be followed. The path should be cleared of obstacles or distractions to facilitate pig flow. Moving pigs in small groups of five or six allows them to remain in a group without the group becoming too large and uncontrollable.

> **TECHNICIAN NOTE** If you attempt to move a large group of pigs, the leaders often will turn back before entering the desired pen, making the remainder of the pen difficult to move successfully.

A pig board can be utilized to apply gentle movement pressure to the back of the group as they explore their new surroundings (Figure 6-51). Exertion of extra pressure, loud noises, and rough or aggressive treatment can cause the pigs to panic and makes any directed movement difficult. Handling equipment for pigs should adhere to the same principles that are followed for other livestock: solid walls of a bright and similar color and a well-lighted area facilitate pig flow. If a pig does turn to face you and the board, be sure the board is flush with the floor. Pigs have a natural rooting instinct and will pick the board up with their nose if given the opportunity. The board can be angled such that the end

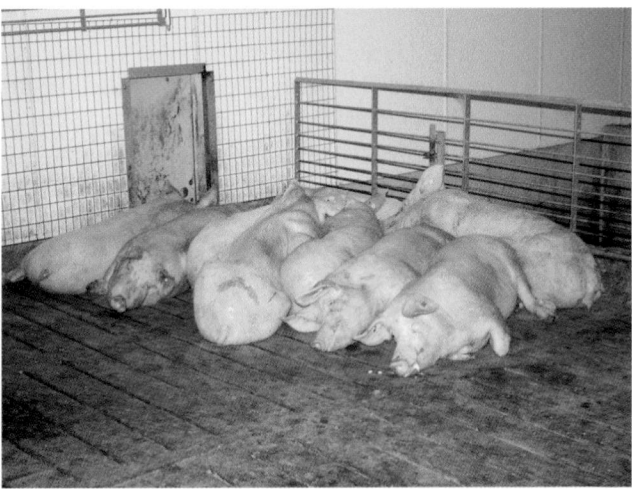

FIGURE 6-52 Sows resting in an open pen system. An experienced technician can deliver injections to sows in this group without the need for restraint.

closest to the pig is ahead of the other end. This provides leverage for the handler and prevents the pig from pushing through the board and past the handler.

When in open pens, adult pigs often can be approached while resting and given an injection with little need for capture or restraint (Figure 6-52). If this approach is not successful, they can be captured individually or worked in small groups. Pigs communicate through a complex series of grunts and squeals. When a pig is in distress, the squeals can become loud to the point of damaging the examiner's hearing. Always wear ear protection to protect your hearing when working with pigs.

CAPTURE AND RESTRAINT TECHNIQUES

In commercial operations, adult pigs are often housed in stalls or crates, reducing the need for capture. In open pen

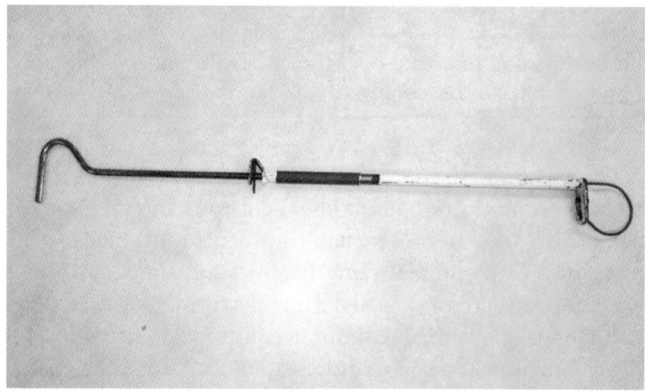

FIGURE 6-53 A hog snare. The loop on the left is placed in the hog's mouth and over the snout. The handle on the left is pulled to tighten the loop and restrain the pig.

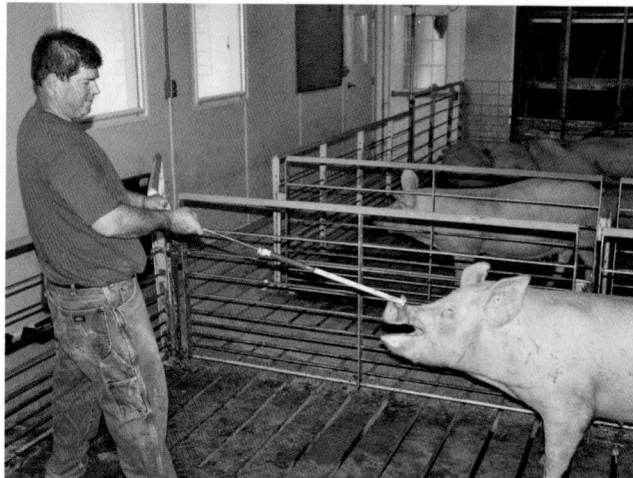

FIGURE 6-54 Restraint of a sow using a hog snare. A second person can now perform the procedure required. Always wear ear protection when snaring pigs.

systems or when new gilts are introduced into a barn, pigs can be crowded into a small stall to facilitate vaccination, ear tag placement/removal, or other necessary procedures. Handlers quickly discover the need to bring as many pigs into the pen as will fit to limit movement and minimize the length of time restraint is needed. Pigs are quickly agitated and can become hyperthermic during this procedure if they are restrained for an excessive period of time. A genetic predisposition to hyperthermia (porcine stress syndrome gene) has been largely eliminated in commercial hogs but still remains in the show pig industry. This author has had little problem with groups of 10 to 12 commercial pigs restrained in a 10′ × 10′ ft pen. To capture individual pigs, a pig board can be used as a third wall to trap the pig. The handler should move the pig into a corner using the solid board and the pig's point of balance. When the pig is facing the corner, the board is placed parallel with the pig and pressure is applied to the board, squeezing the pig between the wall and the board. As soon as treatment is completed, the pig should be released.

If greater control of the pig is needed, as in venipuncture, or if a more invasive procedure is required, a snare can be used (Figure 6-53). The loop of the snare is adjusted for the size of the pig and is placed into the mouth of the pig. Pigs are curious and like to chew; many will readily accept the wire loop into their mouth and over their snout and maxilla. The snare handle is held vertically while the loop is positioned as caudally as possible and then is tightened. The handler then secures the pig by keeping pressure on the handle while the procedure is completed by a second person (Figure 6-54). Two people are required to treat a pig using this technique. Do not tie the snare or otherwise try to secure it. The share should not be used to move the pig because this can cause injury to the palate and the oral cavity. As soon as the procedure is completed, the snare is released and the pig is returned to its pen. Both people should always wear ear protection when using a pig snare, to mitigate hearing loss. A pig's squeal can be as loud as 130 decibels, placing it on the scale between a jet engine

and a chainsaw and well above the 85 decibels needed for hearing loss.

For smaller pigs, lifting and manual restraining are preferred. Piglets are often weighed and vaccinated or administered iron, and boars are castrated in the first few days of life. As with other species, care should be taken when capturing piglets in a pen with a nursing dam. Piglets younger than a week old often weigh 3 to 5 lbs and can be grasped by the thorax from above and then retrained. For larger piglets, grasping a back leg provides an initial hold. Then slip your other hand under the chest to provide support while lifting the piglet in a horizontal position. The piglet can be held in a football-type hold with the piglet resting on the forearm with the rump toward the elbow and the head in the hand. The opposite hand is free to conduct an examination or administer treatment. Restraint for castration of male piglets can be done in a similar manner. The head is restrained between the handler's elbow and chest, while the hand of the same arm grasps the back feet. For larger nursery pigs, or as an alternative for small pigs, the piglet can be held upside down by the rear legs, which are held between the feet and the hock with the spine closest to the handler. The abdomen faces a second person, who can perform the castration or another procedure (Figure 6-55).

Pet Pigs
Pet pigs, whether pot-bellied or otherwise, are raised more as companion animals and should be handled and restrained accordingly when possible. These pigs are often trained to walk on a leash with a harness similar to that of a dog. Restraint of these pet pigs can be similar to that for a dog. These pigs can also be suspended in a mesh or canvas that allows all four legs to protrude through the ventral aspect of the sling. More invasive procedures may best be accomplished under sedation or general anesthesia for the benefit of the animal and the owner.

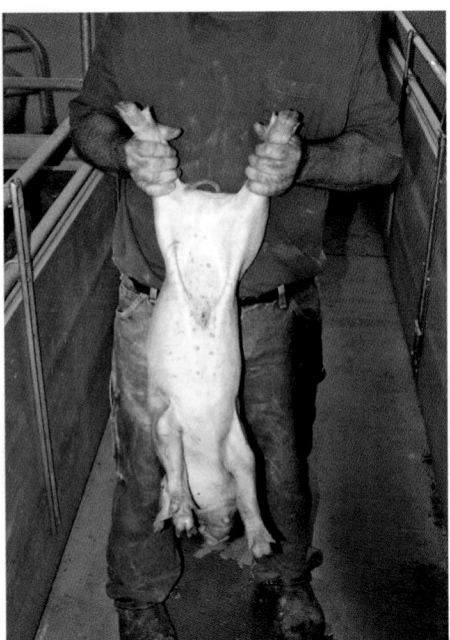

FIGURE 6-55 Restraint of a nursery pig by holding the rear legs. Pigs relax in this position and offer very little resistance. Male piglets can be castrated in this position by a second person.

> **TECHNICIAN NOTE** Pet pigs are pets first and pigs second. Treat them (and their owners) as if they were companion animals.

CAPTURE AND RESTRAINT OF SMALL RUMINANTS

OBSERVATION

Shifting population demographics and growing interest in alternative livestock enterprises have resulted in increasing numbers of small ruminant producers in the United States. Sheep, goats, and camelids, primarily llamas and alpacas, are discussed in this section. These species have similar predator–prey interactions as cattle when confronted with humans. Observation of these animals from a distance beyond their flight zone is therefore an important step in identifying animals in need of medical intervention.

APPROACH

Small ruminants flock together when confronted with a threat. This behavior can be used to the handler's advantage by first bunching the herd tightly and then moving them as a group. Sheep flocks demonstrate this behavioral trait most consistently. Some flock owners will employ dogs to bring flocks into holding facilities, although the owner should have complete control over the dog to avoid over-agitation of the flock or injury due to dog attack. Dogs are less commonly used in handling goat herds because some goats will challenge the dogs or become agitated and act unpredictably.

> **TECHNICIAN NOTE** Guardian dogs are sometimes used in small ruminant flocks to protect against predators and should not be confused with herding dogs.

Small ruminants have flight zones inversely proportional to their domestication level. The flight zone and the point of balance are used to move small ruminants into smaller pens to allow treatment. Handling facilities are similar to those used for cattle: solid walls with alleyways that are wide enough for one animal without permitting it to turn around. If an individual animal requires attention, it can be examined as part of a smaller group or separated from the flock or herd within the handling facilities.

Small ruminants are the safest of the livestock species to work with. Sheep and goats rarely kick or bite, and only aggressive males will challenge handlers. Working around camelids requires greater caution because they are known to spit fermented stomach contents up to 6 feet when agitated. A gurgling sound emits from a llama or an alpaca before expulsion of stomach contents. Camelids may also kick and bite when very agitated. The ear and tail positions of the camelid can provide information regarding the animal's attitude. Ears that are flattened caudally against the head and a vertical tail indicate a high level of aggression in the camelid patient. Conversely, a lowered head and a tail that is curled forward demonstrate submissive behavior, as is most commonly seen in imprinted camelids. Imprinted llamas and alpacas can also be dangerous, especially males. As they reach sexual maturity, they view humans as competitors instead of predators and will attack to defend their territory.

CAPTURE

When possible, small ruminants should be worked in small groups (three to four animals) to mitigate the panic associated with being separated from their peers. Sheep and goats can be confined in alleyways and small pens that allow handlers to deliver injections, place and remove ear tags, administer oral medications, perform FAMACHA scoring, and conduct a variety of other procedures. Caution should be taken when crowding or working heavily fleeced sheep during hot weather because they can develop hyperthermia.

> **TECHNICIAN NOTE** The normal temperature of sheep (101°F to 103°F) makes development of hyperthermia a greater risk. Be careful when working heavily fleeced sheep in hot weather.

Goats can also be crowded into small pens but may exhibit greater numbers of adverse reactions such as jumping over gates, pushing through weak spots in a fence, or lying down. Camelids can be crowded together into a corner or pen by stretching a rope of approximately 35 feet between two handlers, 3 to 4 feet off the ground. If the camelid challenges the rope, it may be worked through individual squeeze chutes similar to those used for cattle.

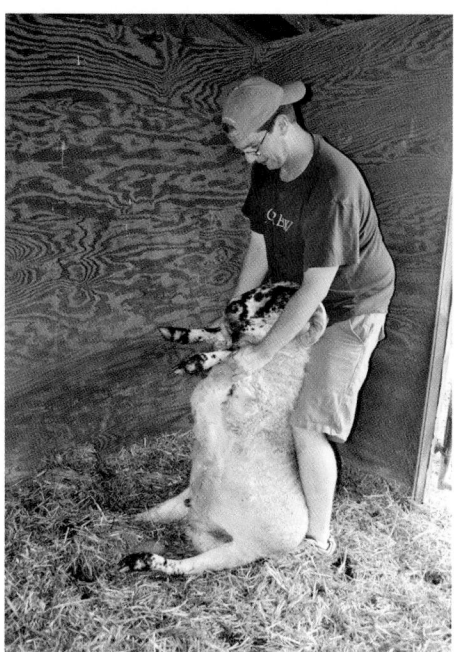

FIGURE 6-56 Restraint of the sheep after sitting it on its rump. Called *setting up* or *flipping*, this procedure allows a skilled handler to now treat, examine, or shear this sheep.

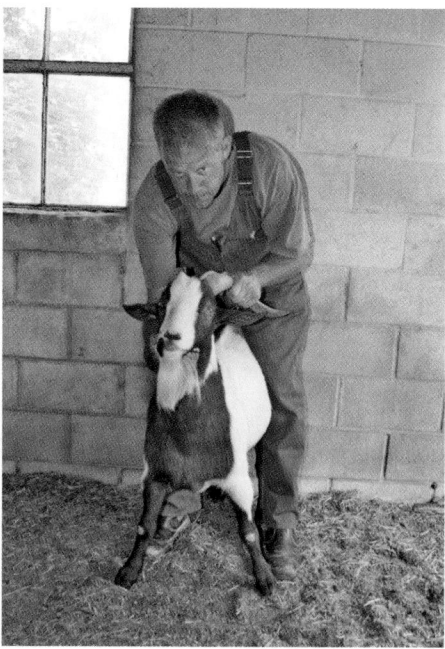

FIGURE 6-57 Restraint of an adult male goat. Note that the handler has backed the goat against a wall using one hand under the jaw. The other hand is grasping the horn for additional restraint.

INDIVIDUAL RESTRAINT

After the animal has been moved into a smaller pen, the first step of restraint for all small ruminant species is to control the head. This can be accomplished by grasping the neck just under the jaw. This is the first step in flipping a sheep into a sitting position. After the neck and head are controlled with the left hand, move the right hand to the sheep's right rear leg. By turning the sheep's nose back and toward the handler, and by lifting the right rear leg, the handler can push the sheep into a sitting position. A second method of setting sheep up is to use the right hand to apply firm pressure over the pelvis; the left hand can turn the sheep's nose back and away from the handler. The sheep's weight is shifted onto the handler's legs; take a step back with the right leg, and the sheep's right leg will begin to buckle. Continued flexion of the sheep's head will cause the sheep to sit down with its back leaning against the handler's legs. With both methods, once the sheep is sitting up, grasp the left forelimb with the left hand and the right forelimb with the right hand, and rest the weight of the sheep against your legs (Figure 6-56). With this position, the sheep can be administered medication, held for hoof trimming, or, in the case of lambs, castrated and docked.

Goats can be initially restrained by a hand under the jaw. However, they are more athletic than sheep and resist being tipped onto their rump like sheep. Instead, a goat can be held by placing the neck in the crook of the elbow and squeezing it to the restrainers chest while using the other hand to grab the tail. Caution should be employed, however, because goats that have horns may be able to injure the handler by head butting in this position. A safer alternative for restraining a goat is to back it into a corner with your hand on its jaw, then straddle the goat with its rump against the wall and

squeeze with your knees. Handlers can use the horns of mature goats as an additional method of restraint in this position (Figure 6-57). Immature goats should not be restrained by their horns because horns can fracture and break off. Dairy goats and goats accustomed to routine handling may be restrained using a halter, by their neck collar (if present), or on a milking or trimming stand.

> **TECHNICIAN NOTE** Never grab the wool or hair of a small ruminant as restraint. In addition to being painful, this can cause damage to the fiber and underlying meat, decreasing the value of both.

Camelids can also be restrained by initially placing a hand under the jaw, followed by squeezing the neck in a flexed elbow against your chest. The other hand can be used to grasp the tail or press down at the shoulders.

RESTRAINT TECHNIQUES FOR CAMELIDS

Additional restraint techniques can be used in camelids that are not useful in sheep or goats. If additional restraint is needed, pressure can be applied at the base of the ear. Similar to "earing" in the horse, the right hand is moved up the neck to the base of the ear, and pressure is applied. Twisting or other manipulation is not necessary and does not increase the restraint available to the handler. When pressure is initially applied, the llama or alpaca will retreat from the hold, so a firm grip should be employed and caution should be exercised to avoid sudden jerks of the animal's head, which may collide with the handler's face. Also similar to horses, halters and lead ropes can be applied to camelids as a method

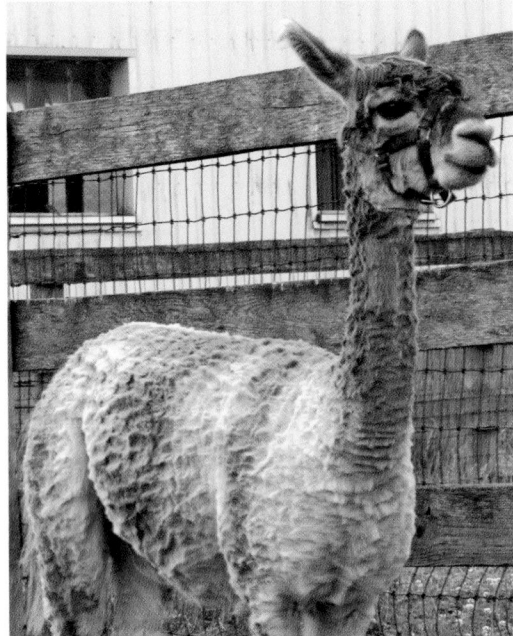

FIGURE 6-58 Alpacas and llamas can be captured and restrained using a miniature pony halter. Care should be taken to ensure that the nose piece of the halter is placed just rostral to the eyes to avoid its compression of soft nasal passages, causing the animal to panic.

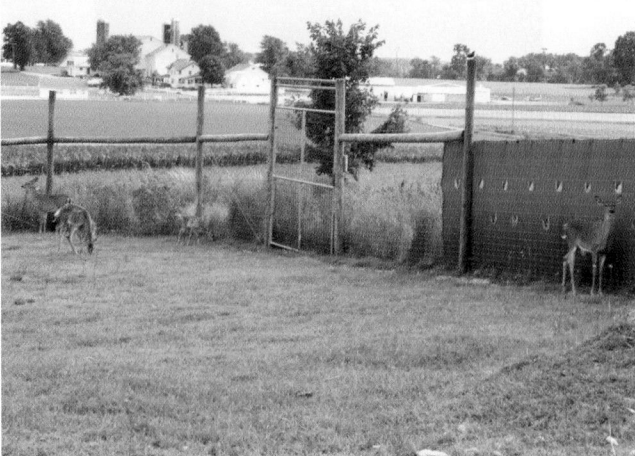

FIGURE 6-59 White-tailed deer farms require fences at least 10 feet tall with an additional visual barrier to mitigate stress. Note the alert posture and distance from the photographer demonstrating the extreme flight zone of cervids.

of control and restraint. The miniature pony halter is often used effectively to ensure that the nose strap does not pinch the soft tissue of the nasal passages (Figure 6-58). The nose strap should be just rostral to the eye to avoid this complication, which may lead to agitation and panic in the animal. Camelids that are accustomed to halters can also be cross-tied like a horse for examination and for minor procedures. When working with and restraining camelids, they may "kush," or lie down. Maintaining pressure over the back and shoulders with your hands can keep them in this position, enabling completion of treatment, examinations, and minor procedures.

HANDLING AND RESTRAINT OF CERVIDS

A small but growing population of farmers and ranchers are raising white-tailed deer, red deer, and reindeer for meat, and to stock commercial hunting operations (Figure 6-59). When handling or restraining these species, remember that they are only a few generations removed from wild cervids. Their flight zone is extremely large compared with livestock species previously discussed, and special holding and restraining facilities are required to examine or treat these animals. Female deer may be bottle-fed as fawns to acclimate them to human contact, but they become more wary as they age. White-tailed deer enclosures are regulated by the state where they are located but often are at least 10 feet tall and have fabric attached to the outside to block the deer's view of human traffic, vehicular traffic, and other distractions.

The two main methods of cervid restraint are chemical immobilization and restraint in a chute system. Female deer can be worked through a specialized chute system that

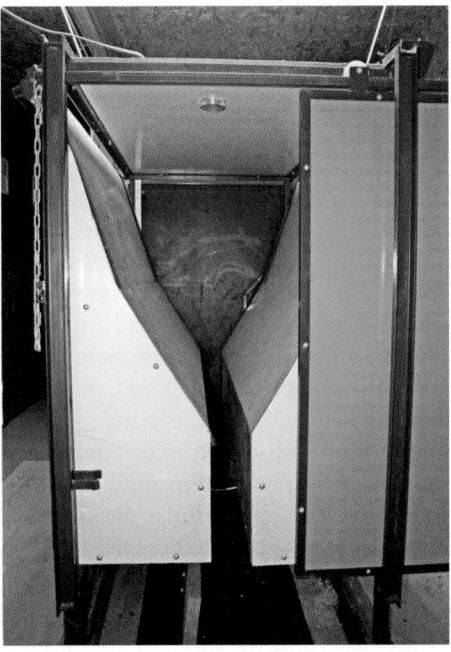

FIGURE 6-60 A specially designed chute for white-tailed deer. This picture is taken from the front of the chute, looking back toward the alleyway. The yellow door is closed when the deer enters the chute and the floor is removed. Note the two angled walls that provide a squeeze restraint.

employs the same principles as cattle handling facilities. Deer are brought into a holding pen using pressure and release handling. They then enter an enclosed alleyway single file, and this connects to a special squeeze chute. Installing on-demand lighting by the section in the alleyway and in the chute facilitates movement toward the end of the alleyway. The chute has two wedge-shaped walls and a floor that falls away (Figure 6-60). After the deer enters the chute, the floor is removed, causing the cervid to drop into the wedge. The animal then can be examined, treated, or inseminated. An alternative to the chute is separation of sick or injured deer into a dark room. These small rooms have no light, may have dirt or rubber mat flooring, and provide a place to treat deer that cannot or will not go through the chute. After treatment in the dark room, cervids are released. If a chute system is unavailable, or if the deer have antlers, chemical immobilization through darting is preferred. The stress of being handled has potent and long-lasting immune suppressive effects in deer. Often these animals are administered prophylactic antimicrobials at the time of handling to decrease the likelihood of infectious disease.

CAPTURE AND RESTRAINT OF AVIAN AND EXOTIC SPECIES

As the popularity of avian and exotic species increases, so too will the presence of these species in veterinary hospitals. Veterinary medical care is as important for birds and exotic animals as it is for domestic species. Veterinary technicians who work with exotic species therefore must have a solid understanding of the natural history, husbandry needs, and safe restraint techniques needed to provide competent medical care to these species. Typically, exotic pet practices see a variety of avian and exotic animals that can be categorized as predators or prey species. As with all animals, the hospital visit should be as stress free as possible because it is well known that convalescence is hindered by stress. One simple rule of thumb for reducing stress in hospitalized animals is to house predator and prey species separately.

RESTRAINT OF AVIAN SPECIES
Psittacines

The initial reaction of most avian species to an unfamiliar environment is fear; this may lead to a flight-or-fight response. As you can imagine, prey species such as **psittacines** (parrots, macaws, and parakeets) become guarded when sensing a predator species, such as cat, dog, or ferret, nearby. Fleeing birds tend to head for windows and can crash into glass panes or walls when panicked.

> **TECHNICIAN NOTE** Make sure all windows in examination and treatment rooms are closed and shaded with curtains or blinds. Fleeing birds will go straight for a clear glass pane during an escape and can critically injure themselves.

In addition, a psittacine can smell the scent of a predator on the hands of veterinary personnel during an examination and while being restrained. This can cause the animal to startle and try to flee without warning. Care must be taken to wash hands between appointments and after handling animals in the wards. Practicing good hygiene not only reduces the risk of spreading communicable diseases, it also decreases the possibility of the handler being bitten and of the patient being injured when attempting to flee what is perceived to be a dangerous environment.

Observation and Approach

Psittacines should be observed and evaluated from a distance before being handled. Subtle behaviors may provide information about the pet's stress level, attitude, and overall health. Psittacines that are stressed may emit an alarm call during most of the visit while a comfortable parrot might readily step out of its carrier and onto the owner's hand. Transferring a calm bird to a veterinary technician to restrain during the visit goes more smoothly if the animal is calm.

> **TECHNICIAN NOTE** To ensure the safety of all animals visiting a veterinary practice, exotic animals should be transported in enclosed carriers or cages.

Even when a bird is comfortable on the hand of its owner, the pet may not be willing to go to a new person. Parrots that lean backward when approached by a veterinary handler are expressing their resistance to being handled by a stranger. In addition, parrots will contract and dilate their pupils in rapid succession when they are focusing to strike at an object. This behavior is called *pinning* and is another warning sign to handlers. Ideally, stressed parrots are given time to acclimate to the new environment of the examination room before any attempt is made to handle. Offering parrots a favorite snack can also help diminish anxiety in the patient before the animal is restrained. As with any veterinary visit, all supplies needed to carry out the examination and veterinary care should be gathered and made available before the patient is restrained.

Restraint Techniques

A calm bird can be examined using hand restraint, but a stressed bird that makes repeated alarm calls and displays defensive body posture will have to be captured and restrained using a towel. With crushing beaks, sharp penetrating nails, and strong wings, psittacine birds, particularly large parrots, can injure veterinary personnel if not restrained properly and safely. Handling parrot species with leather gloves is fruitless because the traumatic power of their beaks is crushing, not tearing, as it is in raptors. An average Macaw can crack a Brazilian nut with minimal effort, making leather gloves a useless defense from its powerful bill. In addition, when working with multiple larger parrot species in a short period of time, ear protection should be worn by veterinary personnel. The alarm cry of the Hyacinth Macaw, for example, rivals in decibels the screams of swine.

> **TECHNICIAN NOTE** A Macaw can crack a Brazilian nut with minimal effort, making leather gloves a useless defense against its powerful bill.

Most parrot species, regardless of size, can be trained to accept hand restraint for grooming and medical examinations. To restrain small birds with one hand, gently control the head at the base of the mandible with the thumb and

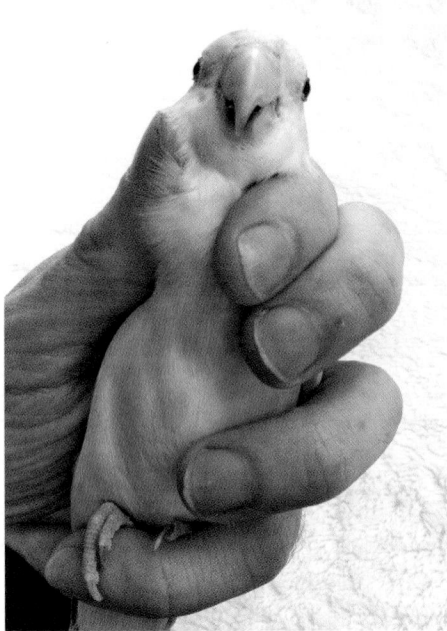

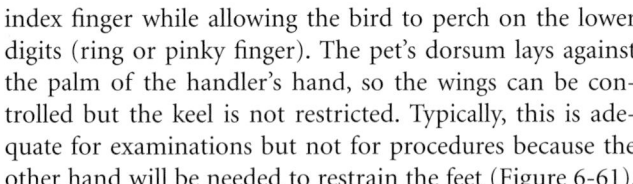

FIGURE 6-61 Single-handed restraint of a lovebird. With this method, the nonrestraining hand can deliver injections or oral medications.

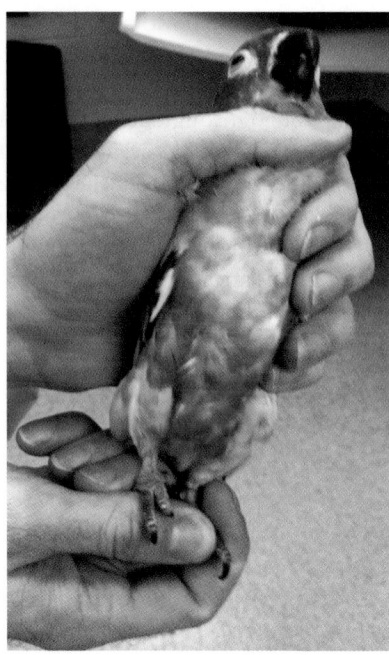

FIGURE 6-62 Two-handed restraint of a Sun Conure.

index finger while allowing the bird to perch on the lower digits (ring or pinky finger). The pet's dorsum lays against the palm of the handler's hand, so the wings can be controlled but the keel is not restricted. Typically, this is adequate for examinations but not for procedures because the other hand will be needed to restrain the feet (Figure 6-61).

To restrain small to medium-sized parrots with two hands, the head and wings are restrained as described earlier, but the opposite hand is used to restrain the legs. The legs are restrained at the level of the tibiotarsus, with the thumb and index finger holding one leg and the index finger and the middle finger holding the other leg (Figure 6-62). This technique has a few benefits. First, movement of the keel is not restricted, so the risk of compromising the bird's ability to breathe is reduced; second, the position of the bird affords both the handler and the veterinarian excellent visualization of the pet's respiratory effort and rate (Figure 6-63). Last, with this technique, the patient is less likely to overheat as it sometimes does with prolonged use of towels. The owner is the best person to train the pet to voluntarily accept gentle restraint for nail and feather trims and physical examinations (Figure 6-64). During training, owners should be sure to desensitize the pet to every aspect of the physical examination process. If any question about the temperament of a bird arises, always err on the side of caution during office visits, and use the restraint technique that is safest for both patient and veterinary personnel.

Many avian patients may be too big or too resistant to be restrained with hands alone. For these patients, making use of a towel is necessary. When wings and torso are wrapped in a towel, the handler can concentrate on restraining the head and feet. For small to medium-sized patients, the

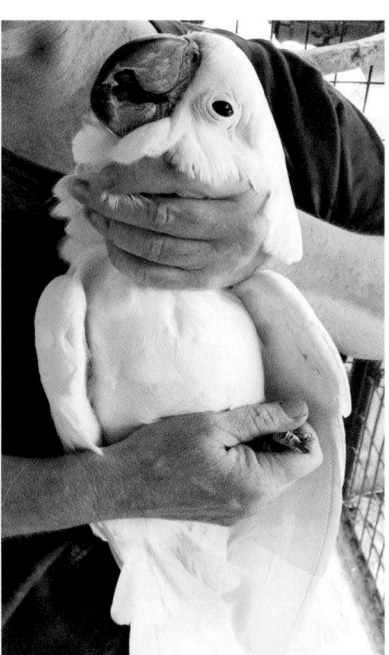

FIGURE 6-63 No towel restraint of a Cockatoo. The handler and the veterinarian can easily monitor respirations, and the animal is less likely to overheat.

capture technique is typically performed while the bird is perched on the handler's hand. While the owner grips the toes of the bird, a towel is slowly raised in front of the bird and is draped over it. The back of the head is then restrained, and the remainder of the bird is wrapped in the towel, being careful not to cover the face. This enables the bird to breathe without obstruction.

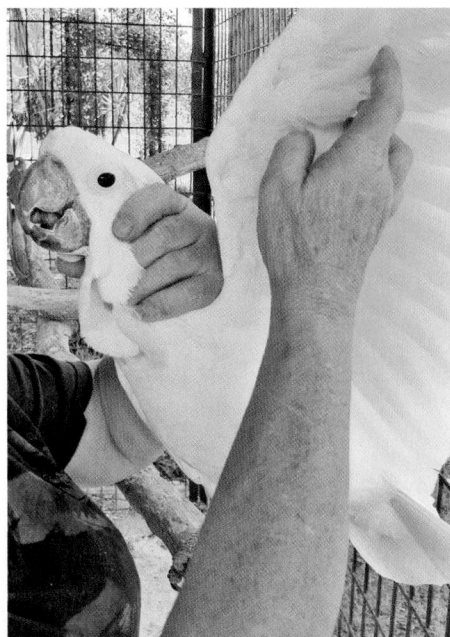

FIGURE 6-64 With training, this Cockatoo will voluntarily allow a physical examination and routine grooming with very minimal restraint of the head.

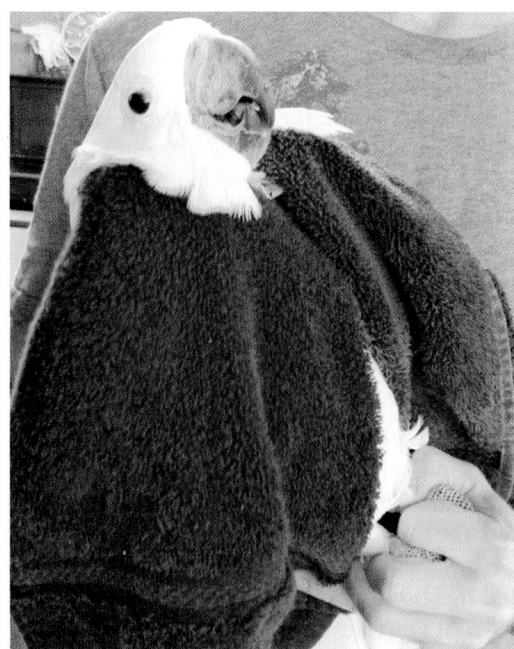

FIGURE 6-65 When a towel is used for restraint, make sure the keel is unrestricted but the wings are well restrained.

For particularly resistant birds, capture should be done with a towel while the patient is still in the carrier. The towel is used to gently cover the patient from the back and simultaneously restrain the bird's head and bill. Once the head and the beak are adequately restrained, the towel can be wrapped around the patient with the opening along the keel. This opening enables direct observation of the keel and associated respirations. It also provides easy access to the wings and feet but at the same time restricts wing motion until the wings are needed and are gently pulled from underneath the towel. Once the towel is in place and the head and bill are restrained, the feet are secured with the remaining hand (Figure 6-65). With towel restraint, one must pay special attention to respiratory rate and effort and to body temperature to ensure that the animal does not inadvertently suffocate or overheat. Because birds do not have diaphragms, respiration is dependent upon expansion of the thoracic wall. Holding a bird too tightly across the chest can therefore prohibit respiration.

TECHNICIAN NOTE When wrapping a bird in a towel, care must be taken not to restrict normal movement of the thoracic wall and cause inadvertent suffocation.

If the animal appears to be overheating, the physical examination should stop and the patient should be allowed to recover. With repeated towel restraint sessions for grooming or clinical procedures, the bird will grow to become fearful of towels and will react violently at even the sight of them. Desensitization techniques can be employed by owners to prevent the bird from developing a fear of towels.

Chemical Restraint

For those avian patients that are too anxious or are in need of prolonged restraint for clinical procedures, a dose of an anxiolytic medication such as midazolam given intramuscularly can aid in decreasing anxiety. If the animal is so stressed that it is refractory to the administration of medication, a brief "chill period" may be necessary. This should be followed by use of the inhalant isoflurane delivered via face mask to the point of twilight anesthesia or immobilization. Once immobilized, a physical examination and any nonpainful clinical procedures, such as grooming, blood sampling, and positioning for radiographs, can be performed with relative ease. If the animal is in need of a procedure that includes noxious stimuli, injectable analgesics and greater depths of inhalant anesthesia are needed for pain management.

Passerines

Small **passerines** such as finches and canaries are restrained very gently, as described in the section on small psittacines, using the single-handed method.

Birds of Prey

Because most birds of prey (**raptorial species**), such as falcons, vultures, hawks, owls, and eagles, have dangerously sharp beaks and talons, leather gloves must be worn by handlers when restraining these species. Once the animal has been captured, a gloved hand restraint technique is used. The aid of a towel may be helpful, depending upon the demeanor and size of the animal and the procedure to be performed. Because wild raptors are not accustomed to being handled by people, restraining them for physical examination typically requires use of a towel and gloves. However, raptors used as falconry animals and those that reside in wildlife sanctuaries or zoos are handled by people and are often calmed by applying a leather hood over the head and eyes. In addition, leather jesses are applied around the lower legs, enabling control of the legs via a string while the animal is perched on the handler's gloved hand.

RESTRAINT OF SMALL MAMMALS

RABBITS

The rabbit can be a highly stressed patient, especially when placed in an environment where predators may be detected. However, some rabbits are raised in households with many other species, such as dogs and cats, which desensitizes the rabbit to the presence of these predators. Rabbits raised without the constant presence of predators are not desensitized and therefore are more likely to be stressed in a veterinary hospital where cats and dogs share the same waiting and examination rooms. Questioning the client about the home environment and the presence or absence of other pets in the home can be helpful in predicting the level of stress experienced by a particular patient when it is removed from its carrier.

The posture and respiratory rate of rabbits may offer clues about stress levels and the type of restraint that would be appropriate for the patient. For example, if the animal is at the front of the carrier sniffing and trying to explore the world outside the carrier, it is likely that the rabbit is comfortable in the presence of humans and will require minimal restraint. A fearful rabbit, on the other hand, often hides in the back of the carrier, grunts, and has rapid breathing with flared nares. Some rabbits slap a hind paw onto the carrier floor, known as *thumping*, as an offensive warning. When threatened, they can charge veterinary personnel with forelimbs outstretched in a lurching motion.

Restraint

Removal of the animal from the carrier or hospital cage is accomplished by using a football hold. The handler places one arm under the ventrum, supporting both the chest and the hind quarters from underneath. While the supporting hand controls the hind legs, the rabbit's face is buried into the crux of the handler's forearm, and the opposite hand is placed on the dorsum of the animal. In essence, the rabbit is carried like a football, such that the handler has complete control of the head and back legs (Figure 6-66). Never carry a rabbit by the scruff alone.

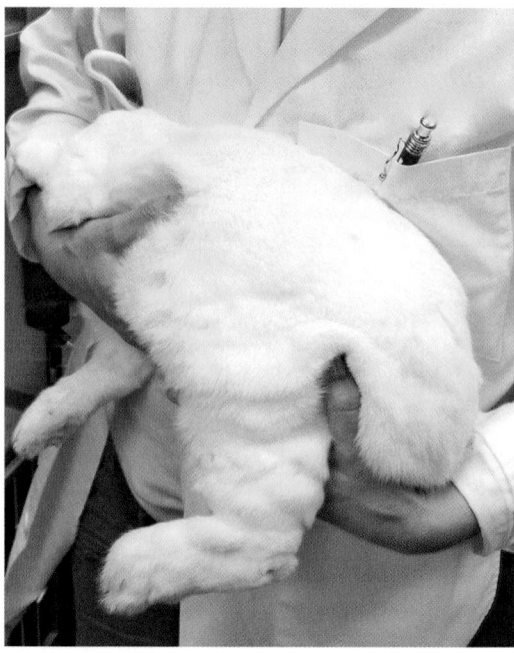

FIGURE 6-66 Rabbits are often comfortable when carried football style. This style also is very useful for blood sampling from the rear lateral saphenous vein. Note the handler supporting under the sternum and holding off the leg and supporting the back end at the same time.

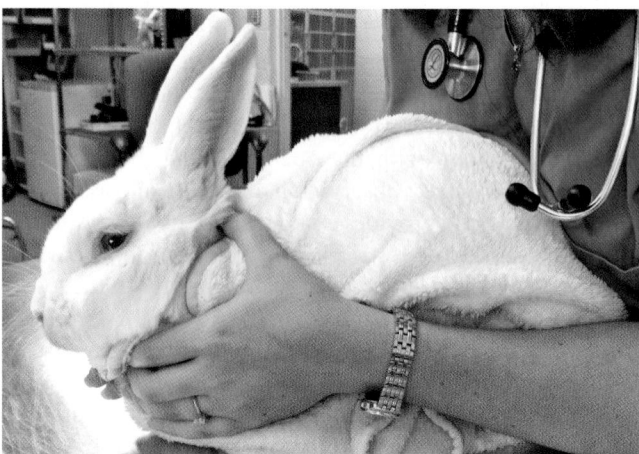

FIGURE 6-67 Rabbit wrapped in a towel for examination. Care must be taken to not allow the animal to overheat.

Using a towel is the safest way to restrain an uncooperative rabbit for nail trims, examinations, and nonpainful clinical procedures. The rabbit is placed on a towel, and both sides of the towel are lifted and wrapped around the patient, leaving the head exposed for examination and subsequent procedures (Figure 6-67).

TECHNICIAN NOTE An improperly restrained rabbit can kick forcefully with its hind legs and can subluxate or fracture thoracolumbar vertebrae, resulting in paralysis. Therefore, it is important that the hind legs be under the control of the handler.

TECHNICIAN NOTE Rabbits are obligate nasal breathers, meaning that they do not breathe through their oral cavity, only through their nose. Therefore, care must be taken to ensure that the nares are not obstructed during restraint.

To examine the perianal area, the rabbit can be rotated into a dorsal position (either toweled or untoweled) with the hind legs restrained by the handler. For those patients that are calm and acclimated to human handling, a towel may not be needed during most of the examination. However, most rabbits object to manual manipulation of the oral cavity, making toweling a common requirement for this portion of the examination.

Chemical Restraint

Anxiolytic medications, such as midazolam, can be beneficial during short, nonpainful clinical procedures on most rabbits such as blood sampling or positioning for radiographs. If further sedation is needed, a premedication cocktail that consists of midazolam and other analgesics, tranquilizers, and dissociative drugs can be given. Care must be taken when giving rabbits drug combinations that could potentially cause respiratory depression because rabbits can be *extremely difficult* to intubate without a great deal of practice. However, experienced veterinarians and veterinary technicians have become skilled in the procedure and can intubate rabbits without the use of a laryngoscope.

GUINEA PIGS AND CHINCHILLAS

As prey species, guinea pigs and chinchillas may be on high alert if not well socialized to the presence of and handling by humans. Guinea pigs tend to emit high-pitched alarm calls and can defend themselves by biting using their sharp incisors. Chinchillas often struggle and thrash during restraint in an attempt to flee.

Well-socialized guinea pigs typically need little restraint for grooming and examinations, whereas the best-behaved chinchilla is still a bit too restless for minimal restraint to be effective. Towel restraint as previously described for rabbits is ideal for both the uncooperative guinea pig and the squirmy chinchilla (Figure 6-68).

> **TECHNICIAN NOTE** Handling guinea pigs with intensely pruritic (itchy) dermatologic disorders, such as sarcoptic mange, can elicit a grand mal seizure of short duration. Always forewarn the owner of this potential complication before handling an extremely itchy guinea pig.

FERRETS

Ferrets are generally mild-tempered predators that eat and play for most of their waking hours. Be cautious in approaching ferrets because they can nip, particularly females, which tend to be more independent and aggressive than males. Ferrets explore the world by their exquisite sense of smell, making distraction with the use of treats and pheromones (Hills A/D Recovery Diet for Cats [Hill's Pet Nutrition Co.] and Ferre Tone Skin & Coat Daily Moist Treat [8 in 1 Co.]) an effective form of light restraint during physical examinations, minor clinical procedures, and grooming. Ferrets may react strongly to noxious smells such as isopropyl alcohol, which is used during venipuncture and ultrasound. Using a skin sanitation substance such as chlorhexidine surgical scrub instead of alcohol is helpful in reducing stress when ferret skin is prepared for IV catheter placement or phlebotomy. Warmed, unscented ultrasound gel used judiciously for ultrasound procedures is acceptable; however, some ferrets will groom the affected area for hours if it is not completely washed off at the end of the procedure.

Restraint

A gentle scruffing technique is effective in restraining ferrets. The handler scruffs the dorsum of the neck and holds the animal in vertical position with one hand while the other hand is used to stabilize the hind limbs (Figure 6-69). Ferrets

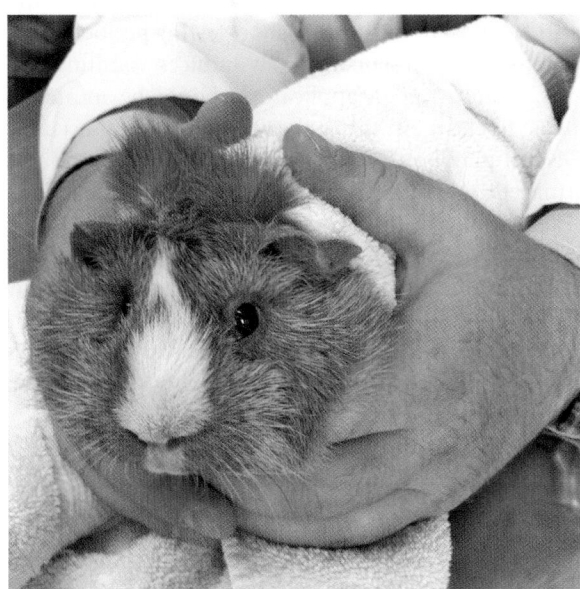

FIGURE 6-68 Guinea pig restrained in a towel, facilitating physical and dental examinations.

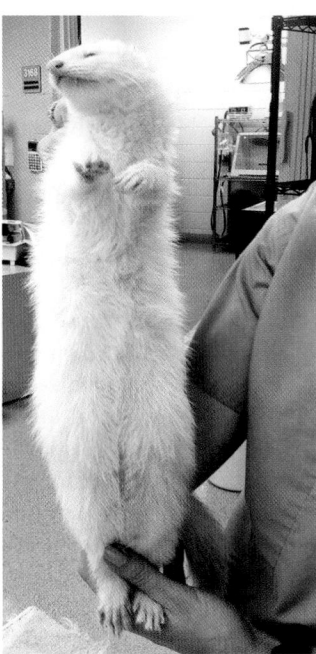

FIGURE 6-69 Ferret restraint. Scruffing a ferret induces a relaxed state that can be noticed when the patient yawns during scruffing.

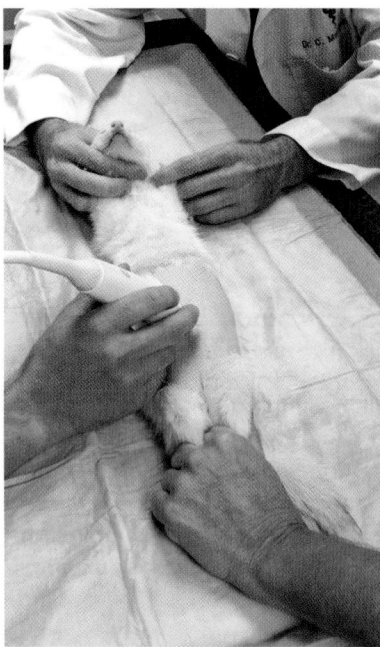

FIGURE 6-70 With low-dose butorphanol, this ferret is much more amendable to restraint and an ultrasound examination.

held in this position often make a yawn reflex, which facilitates an examination of the oral cavity. If the patient is uncooperative despite treat distractions and scruffing, the ferret can be scruffed and positioned in lateral recumbency in the same way that aggressive cats are restrained.

Chemical Restraint

Chemical restraint can be an effective form of restraint and is used as a last resort. In this author's experience, low-dose butorphanol adequately tranquilizes most ferrets for noninvasive diagnostic procedures such as blood collection and radiograph and ultrasound positioning (Figure 6-70).

HAMSTERS, MICE, HEDGEHOGS, SUGAR GLIDERS, AND GERBILS

Caution should be taken when capturing and handling hamsters. Most hamsters are aggressive and will bite aggressively when threatened. Scruffing is one option for restraint, but there is risk that the eyes will proptose bilaterally if the scruffing is too taught around the eyes and face. On the other hand, if the animal is scruffed along the neck to avoid the face, the animal can readily turn and bite the handler. A small hand towel is often successful in the safe restraint of hamsters. Inhalant isoflurane for immobilization is sometimes warranted after a small fasting period until the animal has emptied out its cheek pouches of foodstuffs. If seeds or food is present in the cheek pouches during gas sedation, the patient is at high risk of aspiration causing tracheal obstruction and suffocation.

Mice are more easily handled than hamsters, but their small size makes them difficult to control during clinical procedures. Mice can be gently restrained by scruffing the available skin along the neck and dorsum with the thumb and index finger while restraining the tail with the pinky finger. Chemical or gas immobilization may be needed for certain clinical procedures such as blood collection and radiography.

The quills of hedgehogs are a defensive feature worth respecting. The quills are modified hairs and are very stiff and sharp—similar to those found on porcupines. When threatened, hedgehogs quickly curl up, protecting their vulnerable abdomen. Contrary to common belief, hedgehogs cannot actively shoot their quills; rather, when threatened, the quills become easily epilated, allowing them to stay in the predator's mouth, tongue, and face, for example, when attacked. In addition, hedgehogs generate frothy sputum, which they apply to the tips of their own dorsal spines. No one knows the precise reason for this behavior, but it is thought to help conceal the scent of the hedgehog as the sticky froth readily absorbs odors from the surrounding environment. When handling hedgehogs, be sure to use leather gloves to prevent accidental injury from the quills. Use of inhalant anesthesia may be needed for completion of a thorough physical examination and any clinical procedures because the hedgehog will most likely curl up. Because they can vomit, a short fasting period and cotton-tipped applicators kept on hand to clean out the oral cavity when needed are advisable. Visual inspection of the patient from outside the carrier before the pet is removed for further study can be informative.

Sugar gliders are challenging to handle during a physical examination. They are agile animals and are excellent at jumping out of hand and gliding a good distance through the air. Sugar gliders have sharp nails used for climbing and have sharp incisors designed to extract gum from trees in their native habitat. These characteristics make sugar gliders extremely challenging to restrain. Control of the head is carried out with the thumb and index finger, with care taken not to damage the very large eyes, which are designed for seeing at night. Most clinicians elect to use isoflurane immobilization to facilitate completion of the physical examination and clinical procedures. A short fasting period is needed because gas anesthesia commonly induces vomiting in this species. Cotton-tipped applicators should be immediately available to clean out the oral cavity if vomiting occurs.

Gerbils may be restrained manually or with the use of pharmaceuticals, as described in the previous section on hamsters. When using manual restraint, be sure <u>not</u> to grab gerbils by their tails because the connective tissue under the skin loosens during stressful events, causing the skin and the fur of the tail to deglove. This is a defense mechanism called *fur slip*. Needless to say, witnessing fur slip is upsetting to gerbil owners because only the raw, exposed flesh of their pet's tail is left behind.

HANDLING AND RESTRAINT OF REPTILES

LIZARDS

Knowing the species of lizard and its temperament enables the handler to quickly select a safe form of restraint for each patient. The Green Iguana is probably the most challenging species of lizard to restrain because it is territorial and naturally aggressive, particularly during breeding season. These large lizards can reach 5 feet in length in captivity. They have remarkably sharp teeth and nails and a muscular tail, which the animal uses to defend itself by whipping it back and forth. These are the weapons that the handler must guard against when planning to restrain these large individuals. Some Green Iguanas that have been well socialized to humans may be complacent during an examination, but be careful not to confuse a well-behaved animal with an ill one. Indeed, most lizards and reptiles that present to veterinary hospitals are ill.

Care should be taken when approaching a patient for the first time to read its body language. A defensive lizard has a hunched back, and its tail may be whipped back and forth. In addition, some iguanas bob their heads up and down in a threatening gesture. The easiest and safest capture technique for most medium to large Green Iguanas and Chinese Crested Water Dragons and for most Monitor lizards is the towel restraint method. Capture should be attempted while the animal is still in its transport carrier. When attempting to capture a small lizard, keep in mind that these animals are particularly quick movers, making their escape relatively easy when the carrier door is opened or the top of the carrier is removed.

Towel restraint is usually the preferred method for medium-sized to large lizards; however, be careful to watch for signs of overstressing the patient or worse—inadvertently restricting respiration. Keep in mind that reptiles, like birds, lack diaphragms and therefore rely on movement of the thoracic wall to draw air into and out of the lungs. Restricting the movement of the thorax will suffocate a lizard. The towel must not be wrapped too tightly around the animal. Slipping a towel over the animal as the top of the carrier is being removed usually works well. However, carrying this approach out successfully requires at least two people. The person performing the restraint should be prepared with a towel and possibly leather gloves, depending on the skill and comfort level of the handler, and on the size and temperament of the patient (Figure 6-71). The towel should be slipped over the patient's head and back. The handler should quickly gain control of the head at the base of the neck while, at the same time, wrapping the animal's trunk with a towel that also restrains the legs and feet. When picking the animal up, one hand should maintain control of the head at all times. The opposite hand and forearm are slipped under the animal's trunk to support the body, and the tail is restrained between the handler's arm and the body wall (Figure 6-72).

> ⓘ **TECHNICIAN NOTE** As much as possible, use gentle restraint when capturing and examining reptiles. Many reptiles present to veterinary hospitals with calcium and vitamin D deficiencies—two of the many causes of metabolic bone disease, making them prone to iatrogenic bone fracture with rough handling.

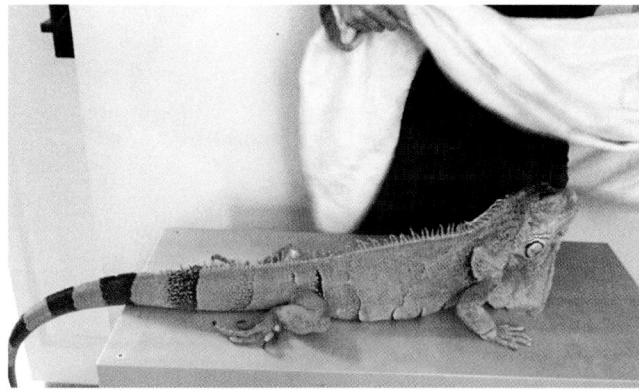

FIGURE 6-71 This Green Iguana is very comfortable with handling, as is shown by the relaxed posture of the animal. Note the relaxed abdomen and back with the head alert and curious, even with the handler approaching with a towel. This relaxation shows that reptile training and desensitization are very beneficial for decreasing stress levels during the examination.

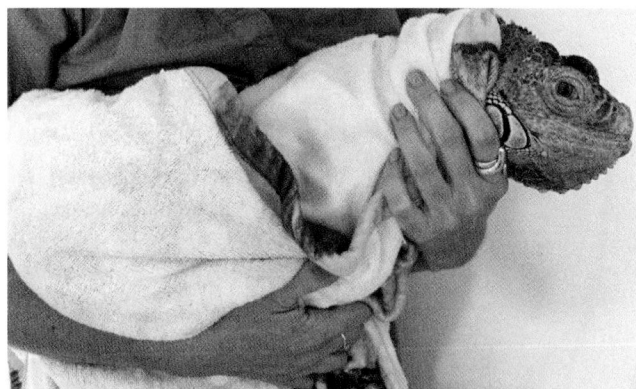

FIGURE 6-72 Properly towel restrained large Green Iguana.

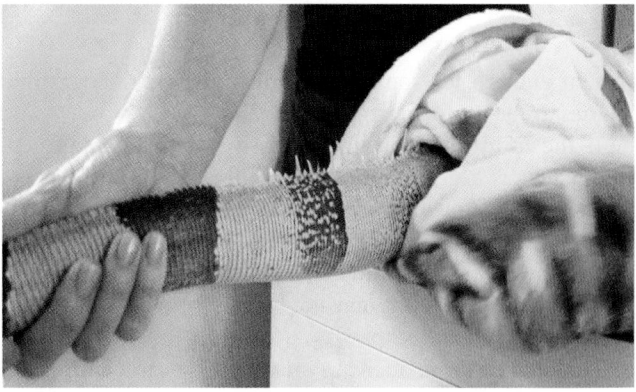

FIGURE 6-73 Easy access to the tail for blood sampling is accomplished as shown in this photograph.

For blood collection, once the animal is properly restrained using the towel method, the tail can be exposed to allow access to venipuncture of the tail veins. This can be accomplished with the patient in a dorsal or ventral position (Figures 6-73 and 6-74). In some cases with very calm or ill lizards, wrapping the head and covering the eyes with gauze while being careful not to obstruct the nose will relax the

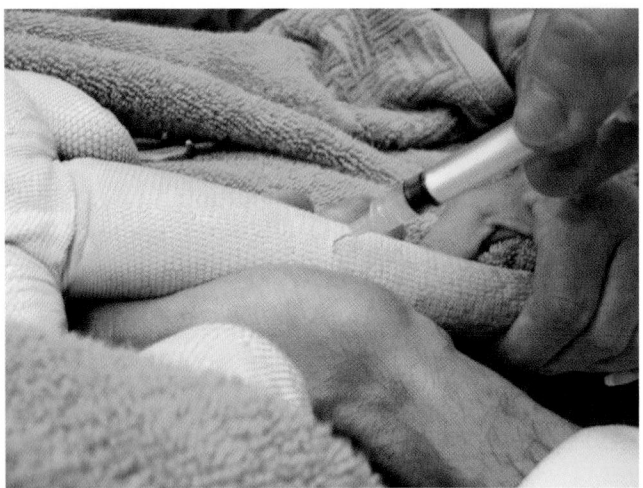

FIGURE 6-74 Green Iguana restraint for tail blood sampling while in dorsal recumbency.

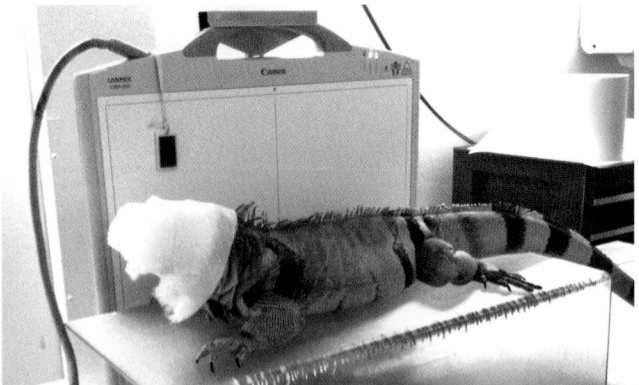

FIGURE 6-75 Green Iguana with bandage material hood to cover the eyes for short clinical procedures. Mild pressure of the hood over the eyes relaxes the animal, presumably through increased vagal tone.

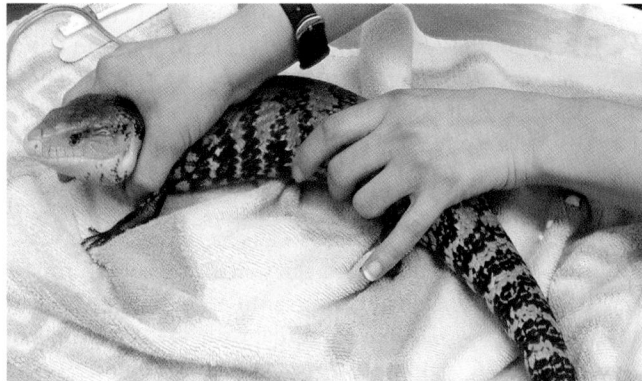

FIGURE 6-76 Restraint of small to medium-sized lizards, such as this blue-tongued skink, typically requires minimal restraint while controlling the head at all times.

patient enough for some procedures, such as radiographic studies, to be performed (Figure 6-75).

If the lizard is displaying defensive or threatening gestures, such as head bobbing and tail flicking, dim the overhead lights to allow the patient to calm down. Then, with the aid of another staff member, slowly cover and wrap the pet with a towel. Keep in mind that this technique works well with diurnal species but may not be as effective with nocturnal species such as geckos.

For smaller, more docile lizards, such as bearded dragons, uromastyx, and geckos, minimal hand restraint is typically all that is needed. However, these smaller creatures may inflict bite wounds, especially during minor procedures such as blood sampling, so be sure to have control of the head at all times (Figure 6-76).

SNAKES

Because both venomous and nonvenomous snakes can be purchased by pet owners, be sure to know the species of snake that is being presented for examination. Even if a quick Internet search is required to be sure of the species, it is

better to know in advance for the protection of all veterinary personnel. Never reach into a transport device without visually identifying the species beforehand because several venomous species are available on the market, and clients may not be forthcoming.

> **TECHNICIAN NOTE**   Never handle a venomous snake or lizard without proper training from an experienced herpetologist, such as a veterinarian, zoo keeper, or scientist. Handling venomous snakes requires special equipment such as Plexiglas restraint tubes and long-handled graspers. Emergency backup procedures should be in place in advance. Check with the local emergency response team to ensure that antivenin serum is immediately available in the event of accidental exposure.

Smaller species such as corn snakes, king snakes, and legless lizards (discussed here because the restraint is the same as for snakes) are docile and are easily handled. Large constrictors such as pythons and boas may not be complacent, and large snakes such as Burmese pythons may require multiple handlers—one to control the head, and several others to control and support the immense body. The safest way to restrain any nonvenomous snake is to control the head with thumb and middle finger just behind the animal's mandible, and with an index finger on top of the animal's head. The rest of the hand gently encompasses the neck. The opposite hand is then available to support the remainder of the snake's body (Figure 6-77).

Snakes may show defensive and threatening behavior by raising their heads and hissing. This behavior should not to be confused with signs that a snake is ill with a respiratory infection. Snakes in respiratory distress will extend their head and neck to facilitate breathing. They may also hiss and make gurgling sounds as they blow bubbles from the nares and mouth.

TURTLES AND TORTOISES

Turtles and **tortoises** are easily captured and held. During restraint, use caution around the head because the beak of

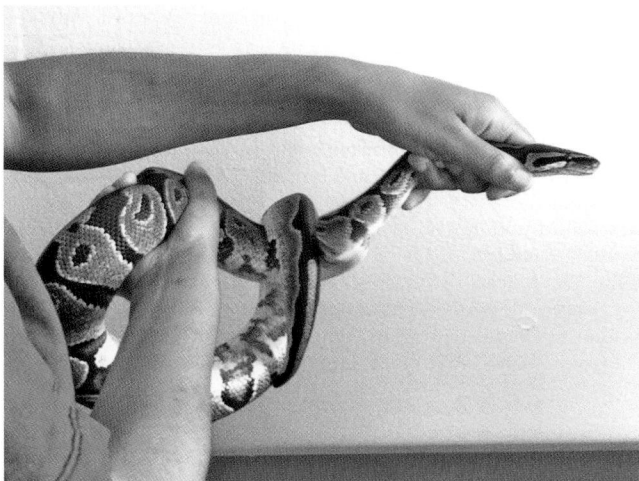

FIGURE 6-77 This photo demonstrates the proper way to maintain control of the head of a snake while supporting the body. (Photo Courtesy Dr. La'Toya Latney, 2011.)

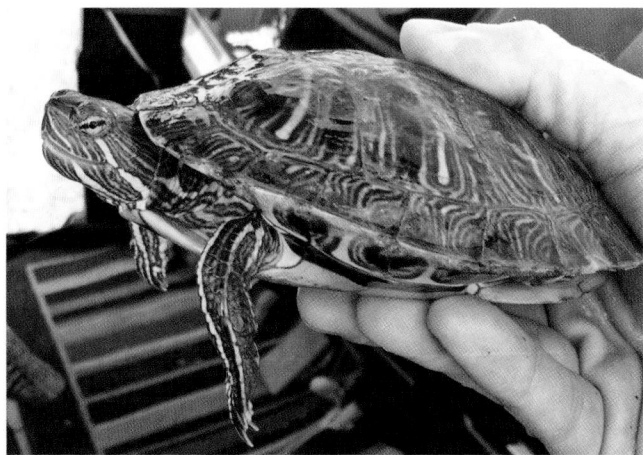

FIGURE 6-78 One-handed turtle restraint. Hand placement is intended to prevent the head from reaching the handler, and the legs are less likely to scratch the handler. However, one must expect some degree of voiding into the hand, perfect for fresh fecal sample collection.

these animals can inflict a serious wound, especially by snapping turtles. The nails of turtles, especially those on the forelimbs, can inflict deep scratch wounds if the animal is improperly restrained. Restraint can be accomplished in small to medium-sized animals by grasping behind the plastron (bottom shell) and carapace (top shell) with a one-handed "sandwich"-type grip. The other hand is then free to grasp the head just behind the mandibles when and if the animal relaxes and extrudes its head (Figure 6-78). This technique may be advantageous in restraining small snapping turtles because snapping turtles have remarkably long necks and can bite a hand that is not well out of the way. Box turtles have hinged plastrons and are able to close the cranial and caudal hinged portions over the front and back openings, respectively, creating a kind of box. Be careful that fingers are not injured by being closed into the "box." Medium-sized

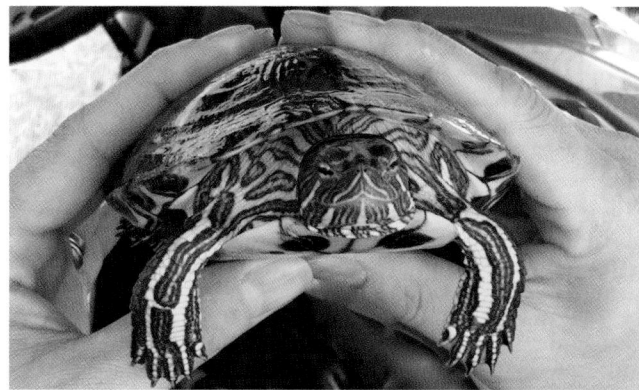

FIGURE 6-79 Two-handed technique for turtle or tortoise restraint.

turtles can be restrained using a two-handed sandwich method by grasping both sides of the shell (top and bottom) at the same time (Figure 6-79). A veterinary technician or a veterinarian will subsequently need to control the head.

> **TECHNICIAN NOTE**   Tongue depressors can be used as a protective barrier against a potential bite from a small to medium-sized turtle. This is particularly helpful when drawing blood from a forelimb. The tongue depressor can be placed between the head and the forelimb so that the turtle, despite its long neck, cannot bite the hand of the phlebotomist.

RECOMMENDED READINGS

Canine and Feline Restraint and Handling

Drobatz KJ, Smith G: Evaluation of risk factors for bite wounds inflicted on caregivers by dogs and cats in a veterinary teaching hospital. J Am Vet Med Assoc 223:312, 2003.

Moffat K: Addressing canine and feline aggression in the veterinary clinic. Vet Clin North Am Small Anim Pract 38:983, 2008.

Rodan I: Understanding feline behavior and application for appropriate handling and management. Topics Comp Anim Med 25:178, 2010.

Rodan I, Sundahl E, Carney H, et al: AAFP and ISFM feline-friendly handling guidelines. J Fel Med Surg 13:364, 2011. Also available at: http://catvets.com/uploads/PDF/2011FelineFriendlyHandling Guidelines.pdf (accessed on May 2011).

Equine Restraint and Handling

Hanie EA: Physical restraint of horses. In: Large animal clinical procedures for veterinary technicians, St Louis, 2006, Elsevier Mosby, p 47.

Higgins AJ, Snyder JR: The equine manual, ed 2, Edinburgh, 2005, Elsevier Saunders.

Marlborough LC, Knottenbelt DC: Basic management. In: Coumbe K, editor: Equine veterinary nursing manual, London, 2001, Blackwell Science Ltd, p 1.

Reeder D, Miller S, Wilfong DA, et al: AAEVT's equine manual for veterinary technicians, Ames, IA, 2009, Wiley-Blackwell.

Equine-Related Websites

http://research.vet.upenn.edu/Equine/Restraint
http://www.thehorse.com: Restraint Techniques
http://loudoun.nvcc.edu/vetonline/vet105/restraint_and_handling.htm

Cattle, Swine, Small Ruminants, Camelids, and Cervids

Fowler M: Medicine and surgery of South American camelids: llama, alpaca, vicuña, guanaco, ed 2, Ames, IA, 1998, Blackwell Publishing Professional.

Fowler M: Restraint and handling of wild and domestic animals, ed 3, Ames, IA, 2008, Wiley-Blackwell.

Hall LW, Clarke KW, Trim CM: Veterinary anesthesia, ed 10, Philadelphia, 2000, WB Saunders.

Grandin T: Behavioral principles of livestock handling, Professional Animal Scientist. American Registry of Professional Animal Scientists 5:1, 1989.

Grandin T: Teaching principles of behavior and equipment design for handling livestock, J Anim Sci 71:1065, 1993.

Miller L, Zeimet D, Schwab CV: Lend an ear to hearing protection, Iowa State Extension Fact Sheet, 1993. Available at: http://nasdonline.org/static_content/documents/1270/d001068.pdf. Accessed July 12, 2012.

Restraint and Handling of Exotic Species

Fowler M: Restraint and handling of wild and domestic animals, ed 3, Ames, IA, 2008, Wiley-Blackwell.

Mader D: Reptile medicine and surgery, ed 2, Philadelphia, 2006, Saunders.

Mitchell MA, Tully TN: Manual of exotic pet practice, Philadelphia, 2009, Saunders.

Tully TN, Mitchell MA: A technician guide to exotic animal care, Denver, 2001, American Animal Hospital Association.

Wilson L: Considerations on companion parrot behavior and avian veterinarians, J Avian Med Surg 14:273, 2000.

7 History and Physical Examination

Mark Rondeau and Elizabeth A. Hanie

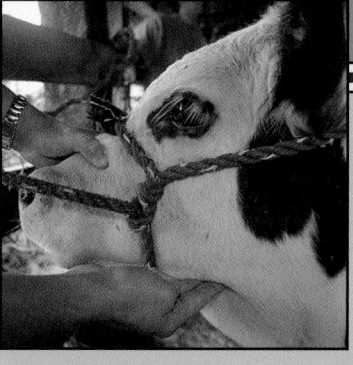

OUTLINE

HISTORY AND PHYSICAL EXAMINATION OF SMALL ANIMALS, *223*
History, *223*
The Role of the Veterinary Technician, *223*
The Information, *224*
Physical Examination, *226*
Documenting the Information, *228*
Surroundings, *228*
Temperature, Pulse, and Respiration, *228*
Systems Review, *230*

HISTORY AND PHYSICAL EXAMINATION OF LARGE ANIMALS, *243*

History, *244*
Owner/Agent Information, *244*
Signalment of the Animal, *244*
Individual History and Chief Complaint, *245*
Medical and Treatment History, *245*
Herd Health History, *245*
Physical Examination of Large Animals, *246*
Physical Examination of the Equine, *246*
Physical Examination of Ruminants, *254*

LEARNING OBJECTIVES

When you have completed this chapter, you will be able to:

1. Pronounce, spell, and define all of the Key Terms in this chapter.
2. Obtain an accurate and complete medical history by:
   - Explaining the role of the veterinary technician in obtaining the patient's medical history.
   - Listing questions commonly used to obtain a dog's or a cat's medical history.
   - Describing what a leading question is, and explaining why asking the owner leading questions can lead to inaccurate historical information.
   - Describing the type of information contained in each section of the patient's medical history for dogs and cats.
   - Explaining what a patient's signalment is and how it relates to patient assessment.
   - Listing six aspects of an animal's origin, background, and past medical history that may be relevant to a presenting complaint.
3. Describe the general procedures used to perform a physical examination in dogs and cats.
4. Discuss methods for performing a comprehensive evaluation of each of the body systems in large animal species.
5. Describe why the process of gathering historical information on herd health differs from taking an individual patient's history.
6. List and describe unique procedures used in the examination of horses and ruminants.

KEY TERMS

Abdominal pinging
Alopecia
Aortic stenosis
Ataxia
Aural
Axillary
Barbering
Body condition score
Borborygmus
Colitis
Excoriation
Fever
Glucosuria
Halitosis
Hyperthermia
Hypothermia
Hypovolemia
Icterus
Ileus
Mentation
Nares
Patent ductus arteriosus
Perineal hernia
Petechiation
Pleural effusion
Pneumothorax
Polydipsic
Pruritic
Pulmonary edema
Pulse deficit
Pulse pressure
Pyometra
Renomegaly
Shock
Signalment
Stertor
Stridor

The author and publisher wish to acknowledge Rebecca Marquardt for her previous contributions to this chapter.

INTRODUCTION

History and physical examination are the first steps in the technician's observation of any patient or group of patients. Information obtained from these processes serves as the basis for all subsequent assessment and intervention. It is essential that veterinary technicians are able to obtain complete and accurate historical information in both individual patient and herd assessments. Similarly, good physical examination skills allow rapid identification of significant problems followed by appropriate therapeutic measures. This can be lifesaving in emergency situations. The following chapter will stress the importance of a systematic approach to both obtaining historical information and performing a physical examination. The veterinary technician is often the first to observe changes in patient status, and the level to which she observes and correctly interprets physical examination findings may have a significant impact on the outcome for a patient. Significant differences have been noted between small animals and large animals in terms of how a patient's history and physical examination are performed. However, the basic premise that this information is an imperative part of the initial database in veterinary medicine holds true for all species.

History and Physical Examination of Small Animals

HISTORY

Obtaining a complete history is the first step toward creating a diagnostic and therapeutic plan for most veterinary patients. Pertinent historical information is an important part of a complete and accurate technician's observation and assessment of the patient. The veterinary technician should be sure to ask questions that clarify the nature of current and previous clinical problems and that confirm the accuracy of the information. This may require asking the same question more than once and repeating responses back to the owner, asking, "Do I have this correct?" Despite its importance, obtaining a thorough history is often overlooked by both veterinarians and veterinary technicians.

Obtaining a thorough history in a clear and organized manner is the foundation of a comprehensive patient's evaluation, but this can be challenging to do. For example, it is difficult to extract information from some owners because they may say too little or may talk incessantly about unrelated issues. When faced with the former, the veterinary technician must stress the importance of the information and explain to the owner that the more information he is able to provide, the more likely it is that the professional team will be able to help his pet. In the latter situation, the veterinary technician must constantly focus the owner on the problem she is trying to obtain information about. This may require interrupting the owner and suggesting, "Let's talk about that later, but let's focus now on this problem." In some cases, the person presenting the patient to the practice may not be the patient's owner and may not know the answers to the questions you are asking. Finally, certain problems or disease states may require specifically tailored questions. The goal of this discussion is to present an organized approach to obtaining a complete and accurate history for each and every patient. This method serves as a foundation upon which questions, based on the owner's knowledge and the patient's specific complaints and preexisting diseases, can be added.

> *TECHNICIAN NOTE* Using a consistent, organized system for obtaining historical information about each and every patient is important, to ensure that nothing is overlooked.

THE ROLE OF THE VETERINARY TECHNICIAN

The veterinary technician who is capable of obtaining a complete and accurate history can play a critical role in a busy veterinary practice. Obtaining information from clients is often time-consuming, and veterinary technicians who can do this well free veterinarians to complete other work. Using historical information, as well as other parts of the database, the veterinary technician should be able to generate technician evaluations and to formulate appropriate technician interventions to support the patient. The historical information obtained, however, is useful only if it is complete and accurate. Acquiring inaccurate information could be worse than obtaining no historical information at all. Faulty information might result in unnecessary diagnostic tests and treatments and lost client trust. To optimize the likelihood that the information obtained is complete and accurate, technicians must have excellent interpersonal skills and must gain the trust and confidence of the pet owner.

Developing Rapport With the Client

When obtaining a medical history, the first step is to introduce yourself to the client and explain what you are doing, so the client feels comfortable and is willing to share information with you. Always be certain to know the client's name and the pet's name and sex to prevent embarrassing mistakes when referring to the client or patient. In situations where the pet has been taken away from the client before the history is obtained (e.g., taken to the treatment area for cardiovascular stabilization following trauma), it is essential that you reassure the owner about the pet's status before asking questions. If the client is worried that his pet is in danger, he will not be able to focus on you and give you the information you need. Once you have established a rapport with the client, obtaining complete and accurate information will be easier. The next challenge is to ask questions in an effective manner.

Asking the Questions

The most important aspect of taking a history is understanding and respecting the pet owner. Some owners have medical training and can be spoken to using medical jargon; however, most owners do not understand medical terminology, and the veterinary technician must be careful to use simple language without belittling the client. For example, if the technician is doing a follow-up examination of a diabetic cat whose owner is checking the urine daily for glucose, it would be inappropriate to ask, "Have you noted **glucosuria** since your previous visit?" It would be equally inappropriate to ask, "Is the little square pad on your dipstick changing color when you dip it in Fluffy's pee pee?" Finding words that are appropriate for the client is important, so that he feels neither confused nor insulted. Technicians are safest when asking, "Has the urine strip been positive for sugar since your previous visit?" It is important to strike an appropriate balance and tailor your questions to the individual client to avoid losing trust.

It is also important to ask open-ended questions, rather than leading questions. An open-ended question is one that requires clients to fill in the information themselves, whereas a leading question is one that potentially guides them to an answer. For example, if you are trying to determine whether a pet is **polydipsic,** it is best to ask the open-ended question, "Have you noticed any changes in his water intake during this illness?" rather than "Has he been drinking more water than usual?" When leading questions are asked, clients sense which response the interviewer prefers and are likely to give it; pet owners are anxious to help resolve their animal's problems. Needless to say, asking leading questions can generate inaccurate historical information.

When questioning clients, try to avoid being judgmental of their care and management of their pet because this may make them feel uncomfortable about giving truthful answers. The questions you ask should not show your biases or personal beliefs. For example, when questioning an owner about his dog that has acute vomiting and diarrhea, it would be unhelpful to ask, "You don't feed her table scraps, do you?" Faced with that question, an owner is likely to say, "No, of course not," even if she really does feed her pet table scraps. It would be better to ask, "What is her normal diet?" or "Did she eat anything outside of her normal diet recently?" or "What human food does she typically eat?" Making clients feel comfortable with their decisions will improve the chances that you will receive accurate information.

> **TECHNICIAN NOTE** Explaining your position and role to clients and tailoring your questions to their level of understanding will allow you to gain the client's trust and obtain more detailed information.

Documenting the Information

Historical information is useless unless it is written carefully, neatly, and accurately in a structured medical record form. All veterinary hospitals should have a standardized history form as part of the medical record; this allows efficient recording of the information presented (Figure 7-1). The form provides prompts to remind you to obtain certain pieces of information. Information should be recorded in the medical record as it is obtained to prevent any subsequent misunderstanding. Practices that use medical practice management software enter historical data digitally into prescribed fields. If using a hard copy form, remember that entries must be written legibly or typed using appropriate medical terminology. Keep in mind that the medical record is a legal document and, as such, should be written with the utmost care and precision. The medical history will provide a reference for the veterinary health care team as it implements and revises treatment plans for the patient.

THE INFORMATION

The following sections provide a general listing of important information that should be obtained in most medical histories. Some additions or deletions may be appropriate in specific cases. This is meant to serve as a guideline to ensure that complete and accurate historical information is obtained in an efficient manner.

> **TECHNICIAN NOTE** The major focus of any medical history is the presenting complaint; however, it is equally important to obtain general background information.

Signalment

Every patient record should contain the pet's **signalment,** which includes age, breed (or dominant breed if mixed), sex, and reproductive status (spayed or neutered). It is important to confirm the signalment during the first meeting with the client because this information often provides important clues about the case. Certain diseases appear more commonly in animals of certain signalments. For example, congenital diseases are more likely to be diagnosed in very young patients than in very old patients.

Background Information
General Management

Background information should begin with a discussion of how long the pet has been owned and where and when it was obtained. Any previous medical problems should be recorded. If it was obtained from a breeder, it may be useful to note whether the client still has contact with the breeder, and if she knows of any diseases diagnosed in related dogs. When discussing the pet's origins, ask whether there has been any recent travel away from the pet's normal living areas. This information is most important when there is suspicion of a disease that is endemic to a region where the pet has visited within the past 6 months.

This is also a good time to find out where the pet is kept during the day and what its normal routine is. If it is kept indoors, is it in a crate or is it restricted to a certain part of the home? If it is kept outdoors, is it in a fenced yard or is it allowed to run free? You should always get a thorough diet history at this time. This should include the type of food eaten, the amount, and the frequency. It is also important to note whether any recent changes have been made to the diet, or if the animal was fed anything unusual (or if it got into something it should not have) just before the onset of illness.

Preventive Medicine

Complete information regarding vaccination history should be obtained if the pet is not a previous patient. Note which vaccines were given, when they were given, and the expiration date of the vaccine. This is also the time to ask about other preventive medications, such as heartworm and flea and tick prevention. Information regarding the consistency with which these medications are given is important, as is whether they are given year round or only during warmer months. When discussing flea and tick medication, it is a good idea to ask whether the owner has seen fleas or ticks on the pet.

Behavioral Information

Ascertain what the pet's normal behavior is on a day-to-day basis and, more important, note any changes in behavior relative to the illness. This is helpful in several ways. First, it lets you know if the pet is aggressive toward people or other animals, which may affect how you handle the animal when it comes time for a physical examination or hospitalization. Second, it allows you to determine whether any behavior changes may explain the underlying illness, such as increased

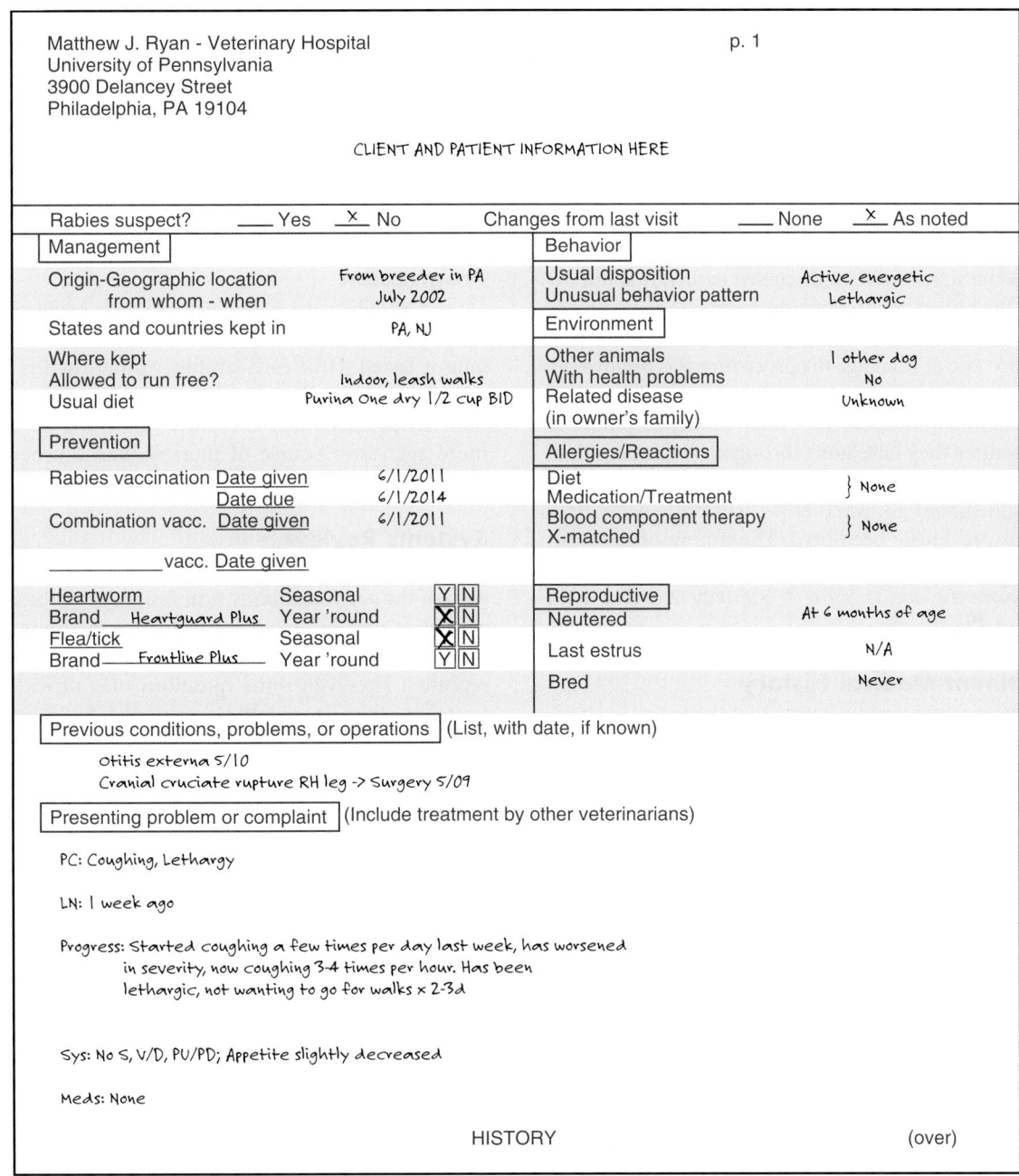

Matthew J. Ryan - Veterinary Hospital   p. 1
University of Pennsylvania
3900 Delancey Street
Philadelphia, PA 19104

CLIENT AND PATIENT INFORMATION HERE

Rabies suspect?   ____ Yes   _X_ No   Changes from last visit   ____ None   _X_ As noted

Management

Origin-Geographic location	From breeder in PA
from whom - when	July 2002
States and countries kept in	PA, NJ
Where kept	Indoor, leash walks
Allowed to run free?	
Usual diet	Purina One dry 1/2 cup BID

Prevention

Rabies vaccination Date given	6/1/2011
Date due	6/1/2014
Combination vacc. Date given	6/1/2011
_____ vacc. Date given	

Heartworm	Seasonal	Y [N]
Brand _Heartguard Plus_	Year 'round	[X] [N]
Flea/tick	Seasonal	[X] [N]
Brand _Frontline Plus_	Year 'round	Y [N]

Behavior

Usual disposition	Active, energetic
Unusual behavior pattern	Lethargic

Environment

Other animals	1 other dog
With health problems	No
Related disease	Unknown
(in owner's family)	

Allergies/Reactions

Diet	} None
Medication/Treatment	
Blood component therapy	} None
X-matched	

Reproductive

Neutered	At 6 months of age
Last estrus	N/A
Bred	Never

Previous conditions, problems, or operations (List, with date, if known)

    Otitis externa 5/10
    Cranial cruciate rupture RH leg -> Surgery 5/09

Presenting problem or complaint (Include treatment by other veterinarians)

PC: Coughing, Lethargy

LN: 1 week ago

Progress: Started coughing a few times per day last week, has worsened
         in severity, now coughing 3-4 times per hour. Has been
         lethargic, not wanting to go for walks x 2-3d

Sys: No S, V/D, PU/PD; Appetite slightly decreased

Meds: None

HISTORY   (over)

FIGURE 7-1 Sample of a completed history form.

aggression, disorientation, unusual elimination habits, and so on.

Household Information

The health status of other members of the patient's household can be important in determining the cause of the pet's illness, especially in cases of infectious disease. Determine to what extent the pet is exposed to other animals: what species, how many, and for what duration. You should also determine whether any of these animals are ill, regardless of whether symptoms are similar to those of the presenting patient. Remember to ask questions about illnesses among humans in the family. This is especially important in some

cases of infectious dermatologic disease, such as sarcoptic mange, and may provide information regarding the patient's exposure to toxins, such as medication belonging to family members.

Allergy History

Before instituting any medical therapy, it is important to note any known allergies or other adverse reactions to medications or food that the pet may have experienced. Even if these reactions have not been confirmed to be related to the exposure in question, they are important to note. Avoidance of medications to which there is even a suspicion of an allergy is sensible. At this time, also inquire about prior blood product transfusions and reactions. You should ask whether the pet has ever received a blood product transfusion. If it has, attempt to determine what product, when it was administered, whether any adverse reaction occurred, and if the pet's blood type is known. This information will help guide any subsequent blood product therapy.

Reproductive History

Although the current reproductive status of the patient will be noted in the signalment, as discussed earlier, it is important to ask for historical information regarding the patient's prior reproductive history. If an animal is neutered, it is important to note at what age the procedure was performed. This information may pertain to disease prevalence. For example, mammary tumors are much more common in female dogs after they have gone through a single heat than if they are spayed before their first heat. If an animal is not neutered, you should ask whether it is currently being bred and if it has previously been bred. The timing of the most recent heat cycle should be noted for all intact female dogs because **pyometra** occurs most commonly 2 weeks to 2 months after a heat cycle.

Past Pertinent Medical History

Identify any prior medical problems that the pet has experienced. Recurrent bouts of similar problems may represent a serious chronic disease. Some previous historical problems may be of no significance to the current presentation. These problems can be ignored. However, if a problem sounds as though it may be relevant to the current complaint, you will have the opportunity to question the owner more thoroughly about it.

Presenting Complaint

The presenting or chief complaint is the most important information to be addressed in the medical history. Every patient will have a presenting complaint, and owners are often anxious to discuss this. During emergencies, it is important to quickly obtain information regarding the presenting complaint before obtaining any background information because time is of the essence in treating life-threatening problems. The presenting complaint can be obtained simply by asking, "What brings you to the practice today?" A patient may have more than one presenting complaint. In this case, it is best to record and discuss each complaint separately. Do not assume that all symptoms can be tied to a single medical disorder.

> **TECHNICIAN NOTE**   In emergency situations where rapid patient stabilization is necessary, information regarding the presenting complaint should always be obtained first to assist in generating an immediate treatment plan for the patient.

Last Normal

A good way to get a sense of the duration of a problem is to ask the client, "When would you say your pet was last normal?" This often helps the client recall a pleasant time when the pet was acting normally, which is easier than trying to remember how long the pet has been sick. The duration of each presenting complaint varies. A clear timeline of clinical events offers diagnostic clues to the veterinarian and assists the veterinary technician in formulating technician evaluations and interventions in the event the patient is hospitalized.

Progression

Once a problem list is established, each problem is prioritized according to the order in which it appeared and how long it lasted. How each problem progressed is also ascertained. In other words, are the problems better, worse, or the same? A problem that is rapidly worsening may warrant a more aggressive course of therapy than a problem that is stable or improving.

Systems Review

The client should be asked a series of questions that review each of the pet's basic body systems. Some of these questions may have already been answered when the presenting complaint was discussed, in which case they should not be repeated. However, some questions may provide information that otherwise would be overlooked by owners because they are so focused on the presenting complaint. All clients should be asked about the presence of coughing, sneezing, vomiting, diarrhea, polyuria, and polydipsia. Current appetite and energy level should be addressed. Any perceived weight loss or weight gain should be noted.

Medications

All clients must be asked what medications, if any, they are currently giving their pet. This information should be as complete as possible. The goal should be to find out the following: type of medication, dose and frequency of medication, duration for which it has been given, reason it has being given, and whether it has provided benefit to the pet. When not all of this information is known by the owner, you should obtain as much of the information as possible. In addition to conventional medication, you must always ask about any vitamins or dietary supplements that are given to the pet. Ask specifically about the use of topical eye and ear preparations and medicated shampoos; some owners do not think of these as medications. Finally, be sure to review any preventive medications that are being given, such as heartworm and flea and tick products.

PHYSICAL EXAMINATION

A thorough physical examination is often the first and most important diagnostic test performed on a patient. Because we must rely on an owner's interpretation of the pet's illness, and because the symptoms that pets show are often vague, the physical examination may be more important than the medical history in determining the source of illness. The physical examination is the main component of the

Signalment: 6-year-old intact male Boston Terrier

Past pertinent history: None

Presenting complaint: Vomiting

Last normal: 3 days prior

Progression: The dog was normal when the owners left for work 3 days ago but was vomiting when they returned home. They took him to another veterinary hospital, where abdominal radiographs were taken. Based on normal radiographs and lack of abdominal pain, the dog was given subcutaneous fluids and was discharged with instructions to withhold food and water for 24 hours and then introduce a bland diet. Since discharge, he has continued to vomit and has become progressively more lethargic.

Systems: No coughing, sneezing, diarrhea, polyuria, or polydipsia noted. No recent weight loss

As the admitting technician, you are responsible for obtaining the patient's history. As you discuss the case with the owners, they recall that the dog was chewing a "cow trachea" when they left for work the day he was last normal. As you question them more carefully, it becomes clear that the dog is bringing up white foamy material in the absence of abdominal retching. You ask specific questions with the goal of determining whether the dog is truly vomiting or is actually displaying regurgitation (Table 1). You suspect that regurgitation is the actual presenting complaint.

Agreeing with your assessment that regurgitation may be the problem in this patient, the veterinarian orders cervical and thoracic radiographs (Figure 1). These reveal a radiopaque foreign body in the cervical esophagus with esophageal dilation proximal to the foreign body. An emergency endoscopy is performed and the presence of the foreign body is confirmed (Figure 2). The foreign body (a "cow trachea") is removed with endoscopic guidance (Figure 3), and the dog goes on to make a full recovery.

The owners are grateful that you took the time to obtain an accurate and complete history.

Summary: This is an example of how important good history-taking skills are. At the dog's initial visit, the individual obtaining the history was not able to discern that the dog was regurgitating. The erroneous historical diagnosis of vomiting resulted in the ordering of abdominal radiographs. This resulted in a missed diagnosis followed by inappropriate treatment. By taking the time to obtain a complete and accurate history, you will optimize the chances that diagnostic and therapeutic plans will be appropriate.

Table 1	Historical Differentiation Between Regurgitation and Vomiting	
	REGURGITATION	**VOMITING**
Bile	Rarely to never	Often
Digested food	Sometimes	Often
Active abdominal retch	Rarely to never	Always
Hypersalivation	Sometimes	Sometimes
Gagging	Sometimes	Rarely
Odynophagia	Often	Never

The most useful pieces of information are the presence or absence of bile in the expelled material and the presence or absence of active abdominal retching during expulsion.

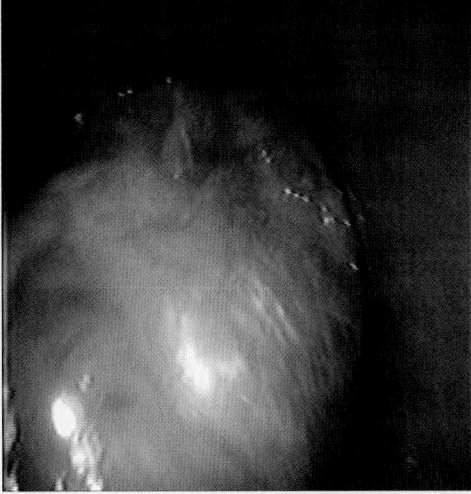

FIGURE 2 Endoscopic image of cervical esophagus obstructed with foreign body.

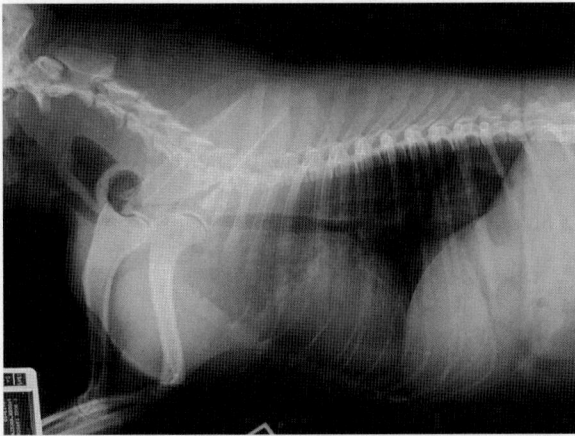

FIGURE 1 Lateral cervical and thoracic radiograph showing circular radiopaque foreign body in cervical esophagus with dilated esophagus proximal to it.

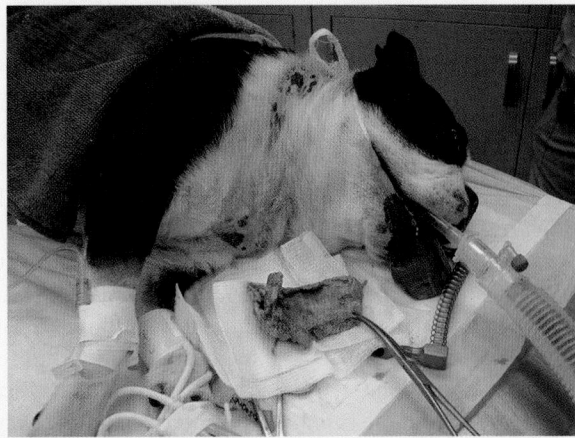

FIGURE 3 Cow trachea foreign body immediately after endoscopic removal from the patient.

technician's observation of a patient, both during the initial presentation and when monitoring changes in a hospitalized patient. As such, a good physical examination and recognition of changes in the physical examination will help guide the veterinary nursing process and will help the technician identify pertinent evaluations and subsequently formulate a list of technician interventions. Keep in mind that it is important for veterinary technicians to examine the patient frequently throughout the period of hospitalization and to maintain a dynamic nursing plan that effectively addresses changes in patient status. The key to a good physical examination is careful completion of all parts of the examination every time it is performed. You should perform all aspects of the physical examination in the same order in every patient. Developing this sort of routine will prevent you from forgetting to evaluate one area because you are overly focused on another. The routine you develop may have to vary slightly from patient to patient. You will find that certain areas of the examination will be covered more carefully in some patients than in others. For example, a complete neurologic examination may be unnecessary on a patient that is seen for coughing and is ambulating normally with no historical complaints about the nervous system. Similarly, in a patient that has hindlimb paralysis, you may limit your respiratory examination to a brief auscultation and spend more time performing a complete neurologic examination, including reflex testing. The key is to perform some evaluation of every system during every examination. The guidelines in the following paragraphs provide one example of the method by which a physical examination could be performed, but you can develop your own routine as you become more experienced. As long as you follow the same routine every time you perform a physical examination, you can be sure that your examination will be thorough.

> **TECHNICIAN NOTE**   As with the patient's history, following a consistent routine for every physical examination will prevent you from overlooking an important finding.

DOCUMENTING THE INFORMATION

As discussed for the medical history, the physical examination must be documented appropriately. All veterinary hospitals should have a standardized physical examination form as part of the medical record (Figure 7-2). This form should include areas for recording body weight, temperature, pulse rate, and respiratory rate. It should also provide prompts to remind you to examine each of the body systems discussed later as well as specified areas in which to record that information. As with any part of a medical record, recorded information should be typed or legibly written, medical terminology should be used, and content should always remain professional. Information should be documented in as much detail as possible so that findings can be compared with those of future physical examinations.

> **TECHNICIAN NOTE**   Historical and physical examination findings should be recorded thoroughly, professionally, and legibly in every patient's medical record.

SURROUNDINGS

Every physical examination should begin with a subjective assessment of the patient in its surroundings. Several pieces of useful information can be obtained with just a quick visual inspection of the animal from a distance as it behaves in the waiting room, the examination room, or the kennel. You can obtain a general sense for the animal's **mentation.** Is the patient bright, alert, and responsive? Is the patient quiet but alert and responsive? These states may suggest a less emergent condition. Is the patient dull, depressed, or even unresponsive? These states could indicate more serious disease or neurologic dysfunction. In addition to mentation, you can visually inspect the animal as it rests for increases in respiratory rate or effort. While the animal walks, quickly look for evidence of lameness, **ataxia,** or visual deficits. You may be able to identify asymmetry or swelling of the patient. This is a good time to evaluate the body condition of the patient and to assign a **body condition score.** The list of things that you can identify by careful visual inspection is extensive. All of this information is important to determine before you move forward with the remainder of your physical examination.

> **TECHNICIAN NOTE**   Taking a brief minute to observe the patient in its surroundings before performing a physical examination can provide important information.

TEMPERATURE, PULSE, AND RESPIRATION

Measurement of body temperature, pulse rate, and respiratory rate will be a part of every physical examination. Even if the veterinary technician will not be performing a complete physical examination, he or she will often be asked to obtain this information before the veterinarian's examination is performed. For the veterinarian and the veterinary technician, these values provide a quick reference to a substantial amount of information regarding the status of the patient. As mentioned previously, these values should be recorded in a dedicated area on the standard physical examination form or in designated fields in digital records.

The body temperature is optimally measured rectally by using a rectal probe thermometer. Most rectal thermometers in current use report the temperature through a digital display window (Figure 7-3). These thermometers work quickly and are safe and accurate. Still available but less commonly used are liquid capillary thermometers, which rely on a column of liquid (usually alcohol or mercury) rising inside the thermometer and being compared with a scale on the thermometer for temperature determination. Always use a protective cover with the thermometer to minimize disease transmission. Lubricating the probe will make insertion

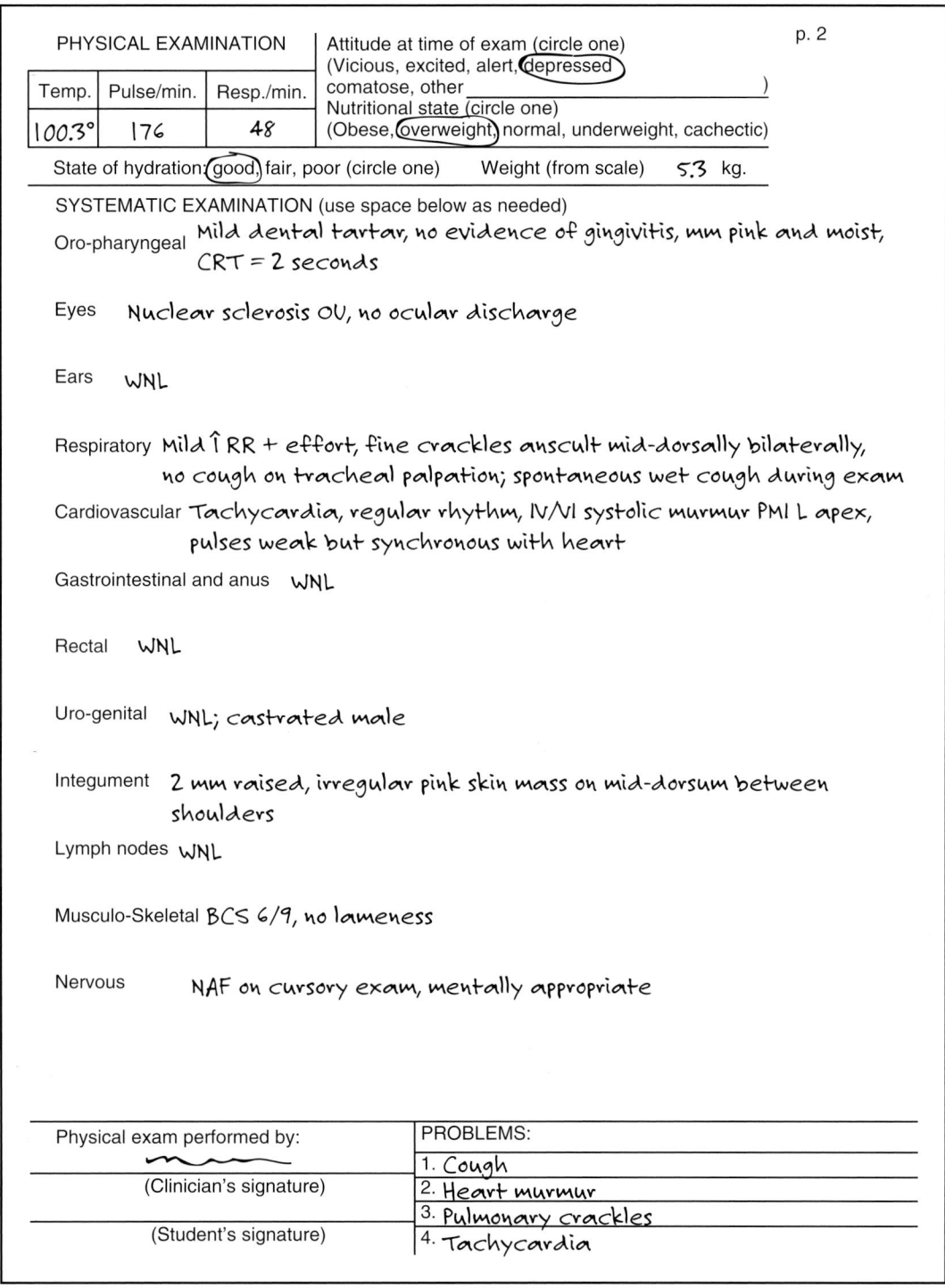

p. 2

PHYSICAL EXAMINATION

Attitude at time of exam (circle one)
(Vicious, excited, alert, ⟨depressed⟩, comatose, other _____)

Nutritional state (circle one)
(Obese, ⟨overweight⟩, normal, underweight, cachectic)

Temp.	Pulse/min.	Resp./min.
100.3°	176	48

State of hydration: ⟨good⟩, fair, poor (circle one)   Weight (from scale)   5.3 kg.

SYSTEMATIC EXAMINATION (use space below as needed)

Oro-pharyngeal   Mild dental tartar, no evidence of gingivitis, mm pink and moist, CRT = 2 seconds

Eyes   Nuclear sclerosis OU, no ocular discharge

Ears   WNL

Respiratory   Mild ↑ RR + effort, fine crackles anscult mid-dorsally bilaterally, no cough on tracheal palpation; spontaneous wet cough during exam

Cardiovascular   Tachycardia, regular rhythm, IV/VI systolic murmur PMI L apex, pulses weak but synchronous with heart

Gastrointestinal and anus   WNL

Rectal   WNL

Uro-genital   WNL; castrated male

Integument   2 mm raised, irregular pink skin mass on mid-dorsum between shoulders

Lymph nodes   WNL

Musculo-Skeletal   BCS 6/9, no lameness

Nervous   NAF on cursory exam, mentally appropriate

Physical exam performed by:
_____
(Clinician's signature)

_____
(Student's signature)

PROBLEMS:
1. Cough
2. Heart murmur
3. Pulmonary crackles
4. Tachycardia

FIGURE 7-2 Sample of a completed physical examination form.

much easier. When using the liquid capillary type of thermometer, remember to shake the thermometer with the insertion tip down so that the liquid level falls from where it was left after its most recent use. Forgetting this step could result in an inaccurate measurement. Whereas a rectal temperature measurement is optimal, an **axillary** or **aural** temperature measurement may be used in cases where the rectum or nearby anatomy is swollen or painful, as in severe **colitis** or with a **perineal hernia.** These methods are less accurate than a rectal measurement and should be used only when necessary.

Variations from normal body temperature can be useful in determining the nature or severity of a patient's illness. An elevated body temperature (**fever** or **hyperthermia**) usually signifies the presence of infection, inflammation, or neoplasia. However, mild elevations may be noted secondary to the stress or anxiety associated with a visit to the practice. Significant true hyperthermia may be present when

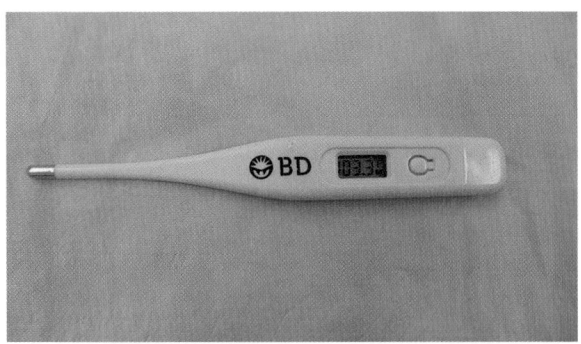

FIGURE 7-3 Digital rectal thermometer.

TABLE 7-1	Normal TPR Values for Adult Small Animals		
	RECTAL TEMPERATURE, °F	HEART RATE	RESPIRATORY RATE
Dog	100.0-102.2	60-160/minute (smaller breeds may have higher rates; puppies can have rates up to 200)	16-32/minute
Cat	100.0-102.2	140-220/minute	20-42/minute

heat-dissipating mechanisms cannot overcome excessive ambient temperatures (heatstroke) or secondary to certain drugs. Severe elevations (>107° F) can lead to organ dysfunction and can warrant initiation of gradual cooling mechanisms. Decreased body temperature (**hypothermia**) is seen less commonly and usually results from impaired thermoregulation in any sick animal, especially cats. Inability to maintain body temperature is more common in patients that are young, old, or thin. Conditions that commonly result in impaired thermoregulation include chronic renal failure, hypothyroidism, and central nervous system (CNS) disease. Severe hypothermia (<90° F) can be life threatening and requires immediate attention. Normal body temperature ranges for dogs and cats are noted in Table 7-1.

Peripheral arterial pulses should be palpated to determine pulse rate and pulse quality in every patient. Pulses generally are palpated by way of the femoral artery, which is located high on the medial thigh of the animal. Digital pressure should be applied over the femoral artery by using the tips of the fingers. Some degree of pressure will be required to feel the pulse, but excessive pressure could compress the vessel, making the pulse difficult to feel. The degree of pressure needed will vary from patient to patient. The pulse rate (per minute) is calculated by counting the number of pulses palpated for 15 seconds and multiplying by 4. Normal pulse rates for the dog and cat are listed in Table 7-1. It is essential to auscult the heart while palpating pulses. Heart rate and pulse rate should be identical, and a pulse of approximately

equal quality should be produced by each heartbeat. Absence of a palpable pulse (or a significant change in pulse quality) with an audible heartbeat is called a **pulse deficit.** Pulse deficits usually indicate an abnormal heart rhythm and warrant further evaluation, such as electrocardiography.

It is important to determine the pulse quality when palpating peripheral arterial pulses. The pressure you feel when palpating a pulse is called the **pulse pressure.** Pulse pressure represents the difference between systolic and diastolic arterial pressures. The intensity of the palpated pulse will vary depending on the body condition of the animal, appearing stronger in thin animals and weaker in obese or heavily muscled animals. Pulse quality is a subjective measurement that is likely to vary from technician to technician, according to the level of experience and comfort attained in palpating peripheral pulses. An attempt should be made to describe the intensity of the pulse using terms such as *weak, moderate,* or *strong.* In general, a weak peripheral pulse is indicative of poor perfusion and may be caused by decreased cardiac output (as in congestive heart failure or **hypovolemia**) or increased peripheral resistance (as in **shock**). Pulses may be described as slow to rise if the peak of intensity comes late in the pulse wave. This can be seen with obstruction to cardiac output, as occurs with **aortic stenosis.** A pulse that feels stronger than normal may also indicate a problem. Such pulses may be described as *bounding, tall,* or *hyperkinetic.* Bounding pulses may be palpated in hyperdynamic states (early septic shock, anemia) or when a rapid drop-off in diastolic pressure occurs (**patent ductus arteriosus**). Whenever pulse quality is abnormal, evaluation of blood pressure using direct or indirect means is warranted.

Respiratory rate and effort should be noted in all patients. An initial notation of respiratory rate and effort should be made before any stressful manipulation of the patient is performed because stress will commonly cause an increase in those parameters. Respiratory rates are generally obtained visually first and then by auscultation to actually hear lung sounds. To calculate the respiratory rate (per minute), count the number of breaths for 15 seconds and multiply by 4. Normal respiration rates for the dog and cat are listed in Table 7-1. Determination of respiratory effort is more subjective. Animals respiring with normal effort should appear comfortable and lack any abdominal effort. If abnormal effort is detected, you should attempt to determine the phase of respiration during which effort is increased. Increased inspiratory effort may indicate an upper airway problem, especially if an associated noise is noted, as with laryngeal paralysis. Increased expiratory effort may indicate small airway obstructive disease, such as asthma. However, many patients will display an increased effort throughout respiration; this is less useful in determining the source of the problem and will be discussed in greater detail later in the chapter.

SYSTEMS REVIEW

After visual inspection of the animal in its surroundings and notation of temperature, pulse, and respiration, a more thorough examination of individual body systems is in order. As discussed earlier, the body systems examinations should be done in the same order in every patient to prevent overlooking any aspect of the physical examination. A consistent routine will ensure thorough physical examinations. However, the degree of detail with which you examine each system will vary from patient to patient based on the presenting complaint.

> **TECHNICIAN NOTE** Every major body system should be examined briefly in every patient. Special attention may be paid to specific systems depending on the individual patient.

Oropharyngeal System

Diseases of the oral cavity may cause loss of appetite, difficulty chewing, or **halitosis.** Dental disease (such as periodontal disease) is common in small animal patients. As such, a good oropharyngeal examination is an important part of the physical examination. An oral examination can be easily performed in most patients by lifting the lips with the mouth closed and by opening the mouth. However, caution should be taken during an oral examination, especially in uncooperative patients. Teeth should be examined visually for any evidence of discoloration, fracture, or excessive tartar formation. Abnormal teeth should be gently palpated to assess for pain and to determine whether the tooth is loose (suggesting periodontal disease). Any missing teeth should be noted and recorded in the medical record. The gums should be examined for redness, which could indicate gingivitis, the precursor to periodontal disease. Any gingival swelling should be noted. Focal swellings could represent neoplastic masses or tooth root abscesses. More diffuse swelling can be seen with gingival hyperplasia. Gingival ulcers may be seen with renal disease, feline viral upper respiratory disease (herpesvirus, calicivirus), or ingestion of caustic substances. Examination with the mouth open will allow inspection of the lingual surfaces of teeth and gums. It also allows examination of the tongue for swelling, discoloration, or ulceration. You should always look under the tongue by pushing upward from under the jaw between the two rami of the mandible. Inspection under the tongue may reveal abnormalities such as masses (sublingual squamous cell carcinoma [Figure 7-4]), swelling (a ranula or a salivary mucocele), or foreign material (string around the base of a cat's tongue with a linear foreign body). An open-mouth examination also allows inspection of the roof of the oral cavity (soft and hard palate) and the back of the oral cavity (pharynx, larynx). These areas should similarly be visually inspected for any swelling or mass, discoloration, or foreign material. Some pharyngeal masses may be large enough that they can be palpated externally by feeling the area just caudal to the mandible and cranial to the tracheal cartilage. Greater detail regarding an oropharyngeal examination and dental disease can be found in Chapter 34.

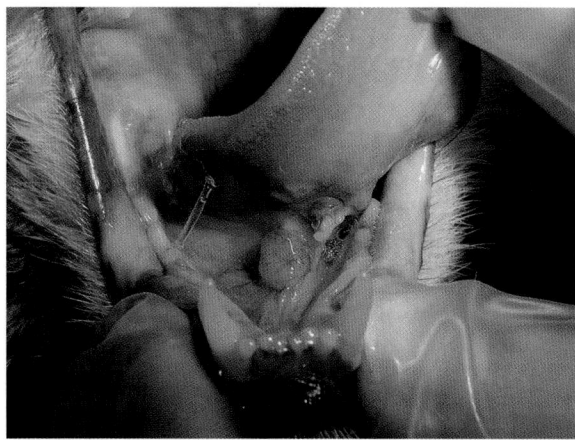

FIGURE 7-4 Sublingual squamous cell carcinoma visualized during an examination under the tongue of a cat.

> **TECHNICIAN NOTE** A thorough oropharyngeal examination should include both open- and closed-mouthed examinations.

Eyes

A good initial ocular examination can be performed with no specialized equipment and should include examination of the eyelids and of the external and internal structures of the eyes. It should also include an assessment of the patient's visual status. An examination of the eyelids should strive to identify any redness or swelling. Eyelid margins should be evaluated for evidence of masses or abnormal hairs (especially if they appear to be growing in toward the eye and causing irritation of the eye). Finally, the position of the lower eyelid should be examined to see whether the lower lid is rolling in toward the eye (entropion) or out away from the eye (ectropion) because both of these conditions can lead to ocular problems. Any ocular discharge should be noted and described with regard to symmetry (unilateral, bilateral) and character (serous, mucoid, purulent, hemorrhagic). Excessive tearing or squinting of the eye may indicate irritation and should be noted. A general visual inspection of the globes should be performed to determine whether they are symmetric, and whether they are enlarged and/or protruding (as can be seen with glaucoma or lesions behind the eye) or sunken. The globes can be gently pressed with the thumbs over the eyelids. They may feel extremely firm when intraocular pressure is high (as with glaucoma) or soft when intraocular pressure is low (as with uveitis). If the eyes cannot be pushed backward (retropulsed) slightly, a lesion (such as a mass) may be present behind one or both eyes.

> **TECHNICIAN NOTE** Although a complete ocular examination requires specialized ophthalmologic equipment, a significant amount of information can be obtained with no equipment.

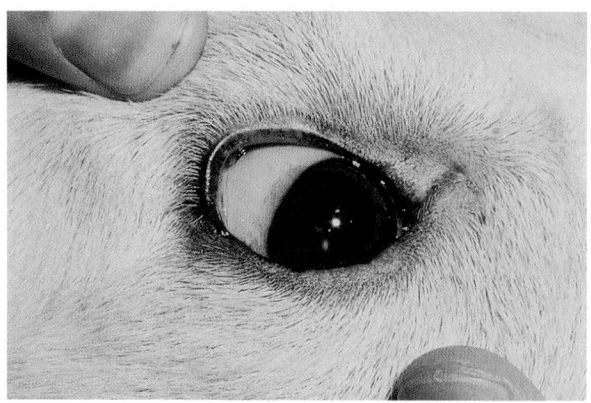

FIGURE 7-5 Yellow discoloration of the sclera seen with icterus.

The external parts of the eye that can be evaluated include the conjunctiva, sclera, nictitating membrane, and cornea. The conjunctiva is the pink membrane that can be seen by pulling back the upper or lower eyelids; it covers the outer part of the eye up to where the cornea begins. Redness of the conjunctiva (conjunctival hyperemia) is seen with many diseases of the external part of the eye, such as conjunctivitis. The sclera is the normally white part of the eye. It is an easy place to examine for the yellow discoloration seen with **icterus** (Figure 7-5). Redness noted in the sclera may be caused by conjunctival hyperemia (usually diffuse with small, movable blood vessels), episcleral injection (large, straight blood vessels, often indicative of internal ocular disease), or subconjunctival hemorrhage (usually large, round to irregular blotches). Any eye redness should be recorded and reported to the veterinarian for further evaluation. The nictitating membrane (third eyelid) usually is not visible or is only partially visible; it rests beneath the lower eyelid on the medial aspect of the orbit. If the nictitating membranes are visible, this is abnormal and should be noted. If not, they can be briefly examined by pressing inward on the eye, causing the nictitating membrane to rise. They should be evaluated for swelling, redness, masses, or foreign material. The cornea is the transparent covering of the front of the eye; it should be clear. It should be examined for cloudiness or other precipitates (such as pigment). Corneal ulcers are fairly common, and although fluorescein staining is usually required for recognition of a corneal ulcer, deeper ulcers may be identifiable with only visual inspection. A diseased cornea may have blood vessels growing into it (especially toward an area of ulceration to help with healing), and these should be noted.

The internal structures of the eye that can be evaluated without specialized equipment include the iris, lens, and anterior chamber. The iris is the colored part of the eye. It should be evaluated for swelling, discoloration, irregularity, or masses. The pupil is the opening of the iris. Pupils should always be evaluated for degree of constriction or dilation and for symmetry of size. If pupils are of differing sizes, this is referred to as *anisocoria*. The pupillary light response should be examined in all patients. When a light of sufficient strength is shined into one pupil, both that pupil and the opposite pupil should constrict. Anisocoria and abnormal pupillary light responses can indicate various ocular and neurologic diseases. The lens is the part of the eye responsible for focusing images onto the retina; it is located inside the pupillary opening. In a normal patient, the lens is not visible without specialized equipment. However, increased lens opacity may be seen with nuclear sclerosis (a normal aging change seen commonly in dogs) or cataract formation. The anterior chamber is the part of the eye behind the cornea but in front of the iris. This area should normally be clear, and you should have no difficulty seeing the structures behind it. Cloudiness, pus, or blood may be present in the anterior chamber in association with severe ocular inflammation. Rarely, masses may be seen in the anterior chamber.

A simple evaluation of the patient's visual ability can be made as it is walking into or around the examination room. Most blind patients have difficulty getting around in the unfamiliar setting of the veterinary hospital, even if they have accommodated for their blindness well at home. Another way to assess a patient's ability to see is to test its menace reflex by covering one eye (so you are testing only one eye at a time) and making a menacing gesture toward the other eye with your hand (making sure not to touch the patient or create excessive air movement that it could feel). A visual patient will close the eye in response to this gesture (assuming it is old enough to recognize that your gesture is menacing, and that it has an intact facial nerve and is capable of blinking). You may also assess vision by dropping cotton balls in front of the patient from above its head and noting whether it visually follows the cotton balls as they pass by.

Ears

Examination of the ears should begin with visualization and palpation of the pinnae. During visualization, the pinnae should be evaluated for symmetry (although in some patients asymmetry may be normal) and inspected inside and outside for swelling, redness, **alopecia,** crusting, or evidence of **excoriation.** Inside the pinnae is a common place to recognize **petechiation,** which is indicative of a primary hemostatic defect (such as thrombocytopenia) (Figure 7-6). Palpation of the pinnae will allow for recognition of focal swelling (as seen with aural hematoma) or diffuse thickening (as might be seen with chronic otitis). Lifting and/or pulling back the pinnae will allow visual inspection of the external ear canal. Canine and feline ear canals consist of a vertical canal that opens to the external environment and runs inward parallel to the skull, as well as a horizontal canal that is a short section between the vertical canal and the eardrum, which runs more perpendicular to the skull. Only the vertical canal may be visualized without specialized equipment. This area should be evaluated for discharge, thickening and/or swelling, or masses. Aural discharge should be described in terms of amount (mild, moderate, severe) and appearance (waxy, black, hemorrhagic, purulent). Evaluation of the horizontal canal and eardrum requires the use of an otoscope.

Most otoscopes found in veterinary practice are wall mounted or portable. They typically consist of a handle, which allows the examiner to hold the instrument, and a head, through which the examiner visualizes the structures. For otoscopy, a cone is attached to the head. The cone is a gradually tapering tube that fits nicely into the ear canal, through which the otoscope light shines to allow visualization. Most otoscopes can also be used as ophthalmoscopes by changing the head. Wall-mounted otoscopes usually have a base that plugs into an electrical outlet and hangs on the wall. The handle is attached to the base via a cord that supplies the power to light the otoscope. The handle is permanently attached to the base. The only assembly that is needed for use is changing the cone to match the size of the patient undergoing an examination. The cone should be large enough to allow clear visualization of structures inside the ear canal, but small enough so as not to cause the patient discomfort. Wall-mounted otoscopes offer the advantage of always being ready for use and requiring little assembly, but they lack the flexibility of the portable units in terms of where the patient is positioned.

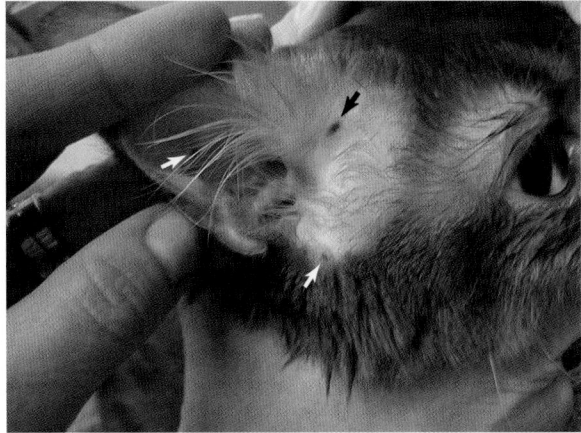

FIGURE 7-6 Petechiae (arrows) inside and in front of the pinna in a cat.

> **TECHNICIAN NOTE** An otoscopic examination must consist of a thorough ear examination performed by visualizing the vertical and horizontal canals.

With wall-mounted units, the patient must be fairly close to the wall-mounted base, but with portable units, the patient can be anywhere. The portable unit consists of a handle that contains a rechargeable battery to power the light source, a connecting piece that attaches the handle to the head, and the head (Figure 7-7). As with the wall-mounted unit, a cone must be attached to the head for an examination. Disadvantages of the portable otoscope are that the battery requires recharging and may not always be ready when needed, and that the otoscope needs to be assembled before use.

To examine the horizontal canal and eardrum using an otoscope, the pinnae are first gently pulled upward (opposite the direction of the patient's legs) to lessen the angle between vertical and horizontal canals. At this point, the otoscope cone is gently passed into the vertical canal while the examiner is looking through the head. The cone is gently advanced into the horizontal canal until the eardrum is visualized, or until the patient shows evidence of discomfort (Figure 7-8). During passage of the otoscope through the vertical and horizontal canals, those areas should be examined for evidence of redness, swelling, masses, discharge, excess hair, or foreign material. The eardrum should appear as a gray to white, slightly transparent, round membrane separating the inner ear from the external ear canal. Abnormalities of the eardrum that should be noted include tears or perforation of the eardrum, increased thickness (or decreased transparency), and evidence of discharge behind the eardrum. It should be noted that an otoscopic examination is technically challenging and is resisted by many patients. Visualization of the eardrum may be difficult for the novice technician; only through frequent practice will the technique of otoscopy become comfortable.

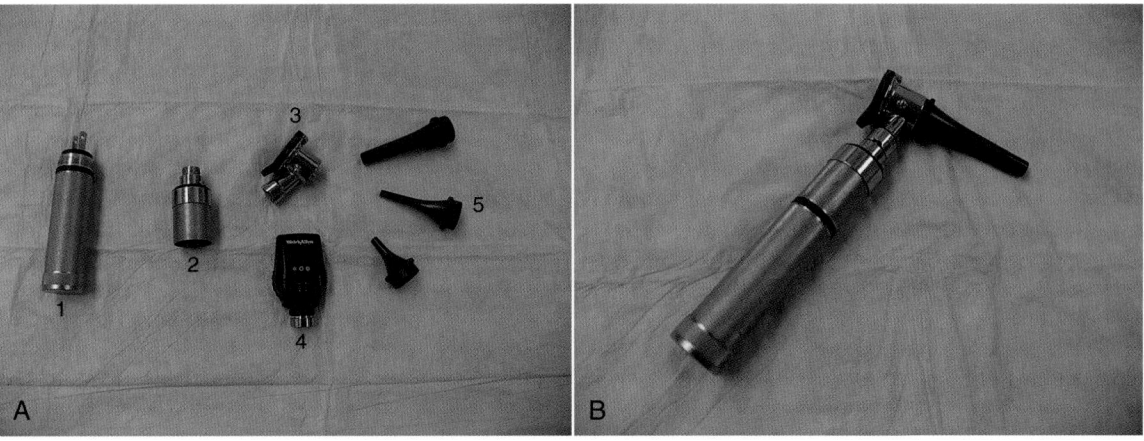

FIGURE 7-7 **A,** Components of a portable otoscope/ophthalmoscope. *1,* Handle. *2,* Connecting piece. *3,* Otoscope head. *4,* Ophthalmoscope head. *5,* Otoscope cones of varying size. **B,** Assembled portable otoscope.

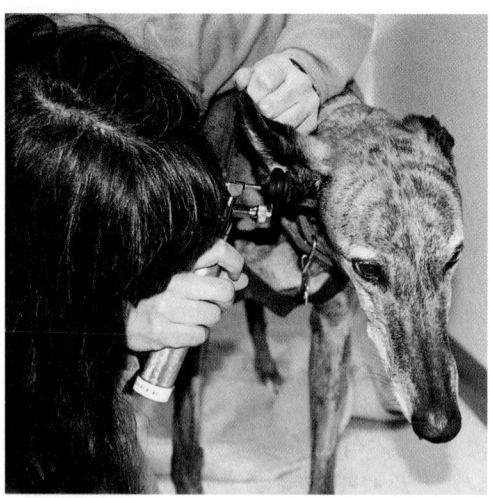

FIGURE 7-8 Technique for otoscopic examination.

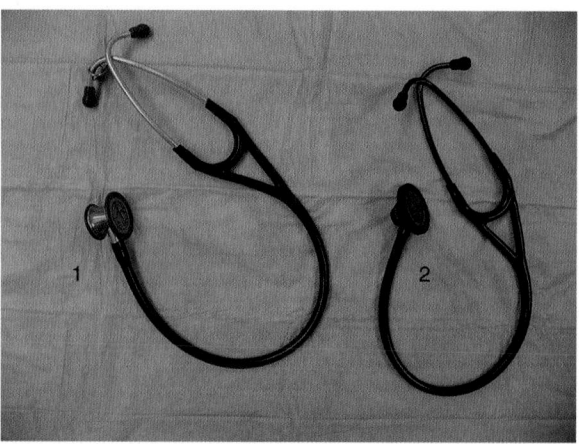

FIGURE 7-9 Stethoscopes. *1,* Chest piece with separate bell and diaphragm *2,* Chest piece with integrated bell and diaphragm.

Respiratory System

The initial examination of a patient's respiratory status involves visual determination of respiratory rate and effort as discussed previously. Patients in significant respiratory distress should be provided with supplemental oxygen and should be minimally stressed. The remainder of the physical examination should be brief or may be postponed until the patient is more stable.

> **TECHNICIAN NOTE** Patients in significant respiratory distress should be placed on oxygen and stabilized before a complete respiratory examination is performed.

In a stable patient, examination of the respiratory system should begin with an evaluation of the upper respiratory tract. The **nares** should be visually inspected to ensure symmetry and patency. Patency can be evaluated by holding a glass slide in front of the nares and looking for condensation to form from each nostril as the animal exhales. The nares should also be evaluated for normal opening size, especially in brachycephalic breeds of dogs, in which stenotic nares are common. Nasal discharge should be described in terms of symmetry (unilateral, bilateral), severity (mild, moderate, severe), and character (serous, mucoid, purulent, hemorrhagic). Opening the mouth and briefly visualizing the hard and soft palate at the roof of the mouth will allow a crude inspection of the nasopharynx for masses, which may appear as a bulging downward of the palate. Any clinical signs of upper airway disease noted during an examination should be recorded, such as sneezing, **stertor,** or **stridor.**

Auscultation using a stethoscope makes up the remainder of the respiratory examination. Most stethoscopes used in veterinary medicine are acoustic stethoscopes, which consist of a chest piece that contacts the patient and transmits sounds via hollow tubes to the examiner's ears (Figure 7-9).

Electronic stethoscopes are less common. A stethoscope should be used such that the earpieces are pointing toward the examiner's nose when they are placed into the ears. The

chest piece on most stethoscopes consists of two sides: a flat side called the *diaphragm* and a cup-shaped side called the *bell.* The diaphragm, which transmits high-frequency sounds, is used most commonly and is appropriate for lung auscultation. The bell, which transmits low-frequency sounds, is used less frequently and may enhance the ability to hear certain cardiac sounds, such as those associated with a gallop rhythm. Twisting the chest piece 180 degrees within the tubing will change whether the bell or the diaphragm is active. Some stethoscopes do not have a separate bell and diaphragm but can function as both if the pressure with which the chest piece is applied to the patient is varied.

When respiratory auscultation is performed, the patient should be in a quiet room. Many things can hamper your ability to effectively auscultate a patient, including ambient noise, patient movement (causing hair rubbing to be heard through the ear pieces), panting, and purring. The mouth should be held gently closed in a panting dog to improve auscultation. Attempts should be made to quiet a cat's purring, such as temporarily covering the nares, running water near the cat, or holding alcohol-soaked cotton to the nares. Once conditions are optimal, respiratory auscultation should begin with the chest piece over the trachea. Normal tracheal airflow is turbulent, and respiratory sounds should be loud and harsh. Abnormal sounds heard over the trachea suggest a problem in the upper airway (trachea or more cranial). For example, a high-pitched inspiratory sound may indicate partial upper airway obstruction, as can be seen with laryngeal paralysis. Although these abnormal upper airway sounds will likely be transmitted to the lungs and audible during lung auscultation, they do not indicate lung disease. The lungs should be auscultated on both sides of the patient, generally dividing the lung fields into nine quadrants on each side (Figure 7-10). Each quadrant should be auscultated through at least two to three respiratory cycles of inspiration and expiration. In a normal patient, air movement will be audible during both inspiration and expiration but should be of minimal intensity. The intensity of normal lung sounds will vary with the body condition of the patient;

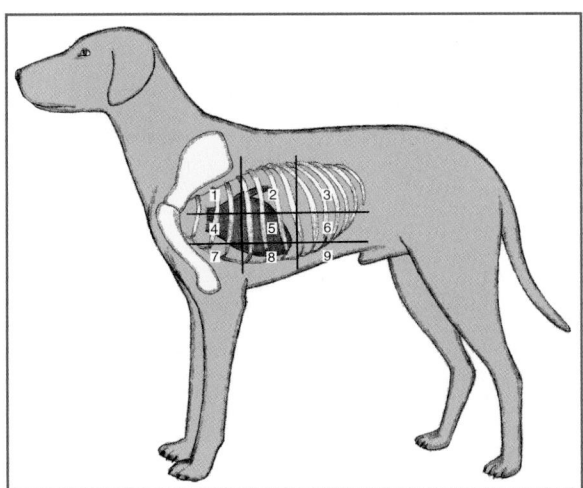

FIGURE 7-10 Division of the lungs into nine quadrants for auscultation and description of location of abnormal lung sounds. (From McCurnin DM, Poffenbarger EM: Small animal physical diagnosis and clinical procedures, St Louis, 1991, Saunders.)

sounds are more intense in thin patients and less intense in obese or well-muscled patients. The most commonly identified abnormal lung sounds are crackles and wheezes. Inspiratory crackles usually indicate the presence of fluid within alveoli, as can be seen with **pulmonary edema.** Wheezes may occur during inspiration and/or expiration when air is moving through a narrowed airway, as can be seen with feline asthma. Failure to hear any air movement is another sign of a problem. Lack of lung sounds in the ventral lung fields in the standing animal usually indicates **pleural effusion** because fluid tends to settle in the ventral areas. Conversely, a lack of sounds in the dorsal lung fields often indicates a **pneumothorax** because air will rise to the dorsal areas. Space-occupying masses and lung consolidation can also result in the absence of lung sounds. When abnormal lung sounds are auscultated (or lung sounds are absent), the technician should note whether they are occurring during inspiration or expiration, and in which lung fields they were identified.

Cardiovascular System

Examination of the cardiovascular system begins with a look into the mouth. Rather than looking for specific oral pathologic conditions, we are looking at the gingival mucous membranes to gain an assessment of perfusion status. The gingival mucous membranes should be pink and moist, although some animals will have normally pigmented gingivae. Pallor of the mucous membranes usually indicates anemia or poor perfusion. Hyperemia of the mucous membranes can occur in stressed animals or can be seen in hyperdynamic states, such as the early phase of septic shock. If the mucous membranes are not moist but are dry or tacky, this is usually an early sign of dehydration. However, in a patient that is panting excessively, the mucous membranes will be dried by air movement associated with panting, and mucous membranes will not be a good indicator of hydration status.

The gingival mucous membranes are also used for measuring capillary refill time, which serves as another indicator of perfusion. With the lip raised, the gingival surface is gently pressed with a finger to occlude blood flow until the color fades from the mucous membrane beneath the finger. The finger is removed, and the time it takes for the mucous membrane color to return to normal is measured (Figure 7-11). In a normal animal, this capillary refill time will be less than 2 seconds. Refill times longer than 2 seconds are indicative of poor perfusion, as can be seen in hypotensive states. Extremely rapid refill (<1 second) may be seen in stressed patients or in hyperdynamic states, such as the early phase of septic shock. Peripheral arterial pulse quality will also provide information regarding perfusion, as was discussed previously.

> **TECHNICIAN NOTE** A complete cardiac examination includes assessment of perfusion status, heart rate, heart rhythm, and heart sounds.

Cardiac auscultation will allow evaluation for abnormal heart rate, rhythm, and sounds. In dogs, the heart should be auscultated on each side of the chest around the level of the costochondral junction (just behind the level of the elbow when the patient is standing). By moving the chest piece around slightly, you will be able to auscultate in the vicinity of each heart valve. The pulmonic, aortic, and mitral valves can be auscultated best on the left side, whereas the tricuspid valve is auscultated best on the right side (Figure 7-12). Normal heart rates have been discussed previously. In cats, it is best to auscultate directly over the sternum initially and to move the chest piece gradually up to the left side and back over to the right side. Valve positions are similar to those in the dog, but in cats, abnormal heart sounds are more commonly auscultated in the sternal area. The heart rhythm should be regular, meaning that each heartbeat is separated from the following one by an identical time interval. Dogs may normally have a slight variation in heart rhythm, such that the heart rate increases slightly during inspiration and decreases slightly during expiration. This is called *respiratory sinus arrhythmia*, and it is a sign that a dog has normal cardiac function. To best evaluate cardiac rhythm, the pulses must be palpated during auscultation. As discussed previously, a pulse of approximately equal intensity should be generated with each heartbeat. In a patient with an abnormal heart rhythm or with pulse deficits, electrocardiography should be performed to determine the exact nature of the abnormality.

The heart sounds typically audible during auscultation in a normal patient are S_1 (the first heart sound), which is created by closure of the mitral and tricuspid valves at the start of systole, and S_2 (the second heart sound), which is created by closure of the aortic and pulmonic valves at the end of systole. These two short heart sounds result in the typical "lub-dub" sound of the normal heartbeat. The presence of a third heart sound is termed a *gallop rhythm* because

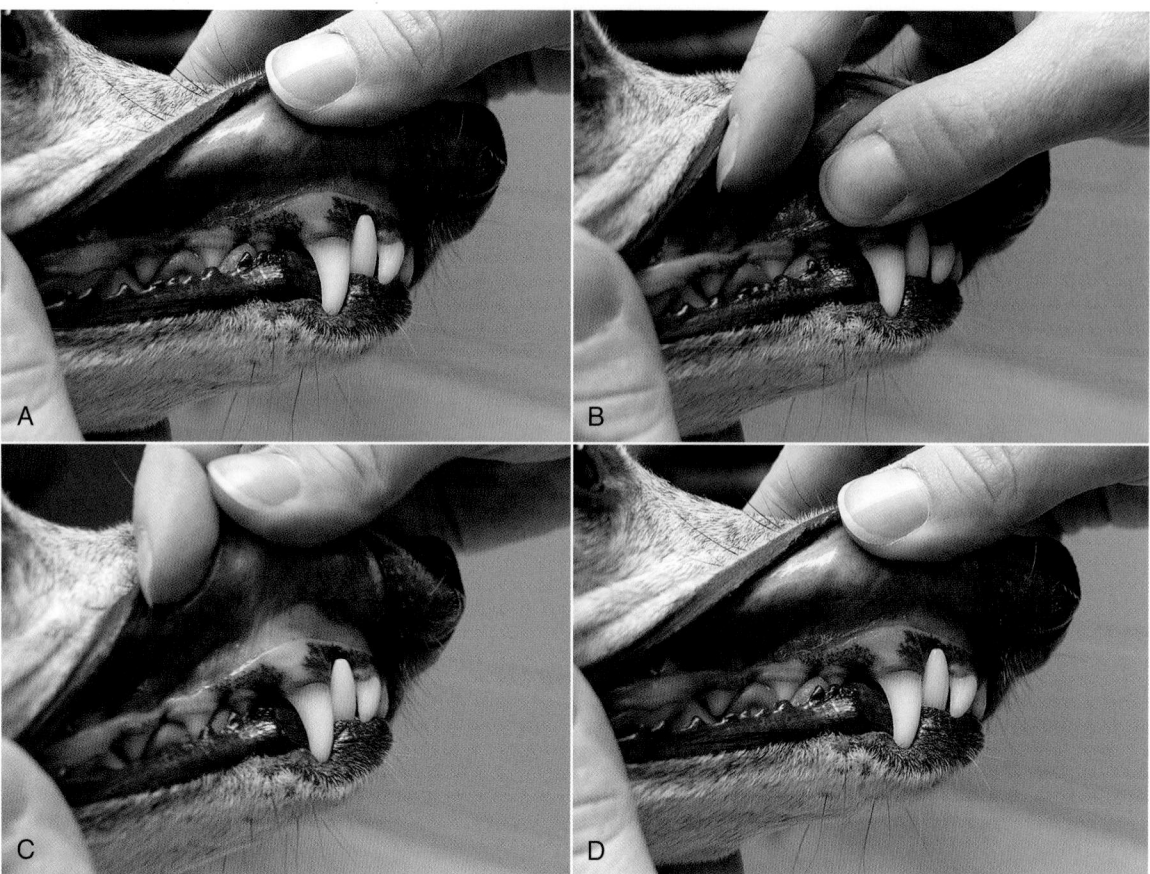

FIGURE 7-11 Assessing capillary refill time. **A,** Visualize the gingival mucous membranes by lifting the lip. **B,** Apply gentle pressure with the thumb onto the mucous membranes. **C,** Resultant area of pallor when the thumb is removed. **D,** Note time to return of normal mucous membrane color.

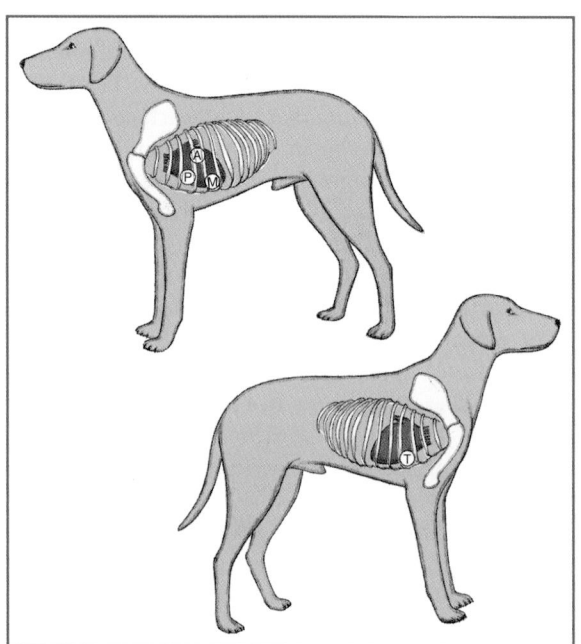

FIGURE 7-12 Location of heart valves as an aid in determination of the origin of a heart murmur. *A,* Aortic; *M,* mitral; *P,* pulmonic; *T,* tricuspid. (From McCurnin DM, Poffenbarger EM: *Small animal physical diagnosis and clinical procedures,* St Louis, 1991, Saunders.)

the resulting heart rhythm sounds like the galloping of a horse. A gallop rhythm is not actually an abnormal rhythm in the sense of electrical activity but is caused by an extra heart sound termed S_3 or S_4. S_3 is usually associated with ventricular dilation, as with dilated cardiomyopathy, whereas S_4 is usually associated with decreased ventricular compliance and hypertrophy, as with hypertrophic cardiomyopathy. S_3 and S_4 cannot be differentiated via auscultation. Rarely the second heart sound (S_2) may be split and may sound like a third heart sound. This phenomenon is uncommon.

A heart murmur is an abnormal sound caused by turbulent blood flow, which typically sounds like a "swishing" noise. Identification of heart murmurs can indicate cardiac disease, although they can occur with noncardiac disease (such as with anemia) or can be normal in some young animals. Heart murmurs should be described by their intensity, when they occur in the cardiac cycle, and where they are heard loudest. The intensity of a heart murmur is typically graded on a scale from I to VI, as shown in Table 7-2. Systolic murmurs occur between S_1 and S_2 (i.e., during systole) or may mask those two sounds. Diastolic murmurs occur after S_2 and before the next S_1 (i.e., during diastole). A continuous murmur occurs throughout the cardiac cycle. The area on the chest where a murmur is loudest is termed the *point of*

TABLE 7-2	Grading of Heart Murmurs in Small Animals
GRADE	DESCRIPTION
I	Very low intensity murmur that can be heard only in a quiet area
II	Murmur of soft intensity that can be heard immediately
III	Murmur of moderate intensity
IV	Loud murmur
V	Loud murmur with a palpable thrill on the body wall
VI	Loud murmur that can be heard with the stethoscope held some distance from the thoracic wall

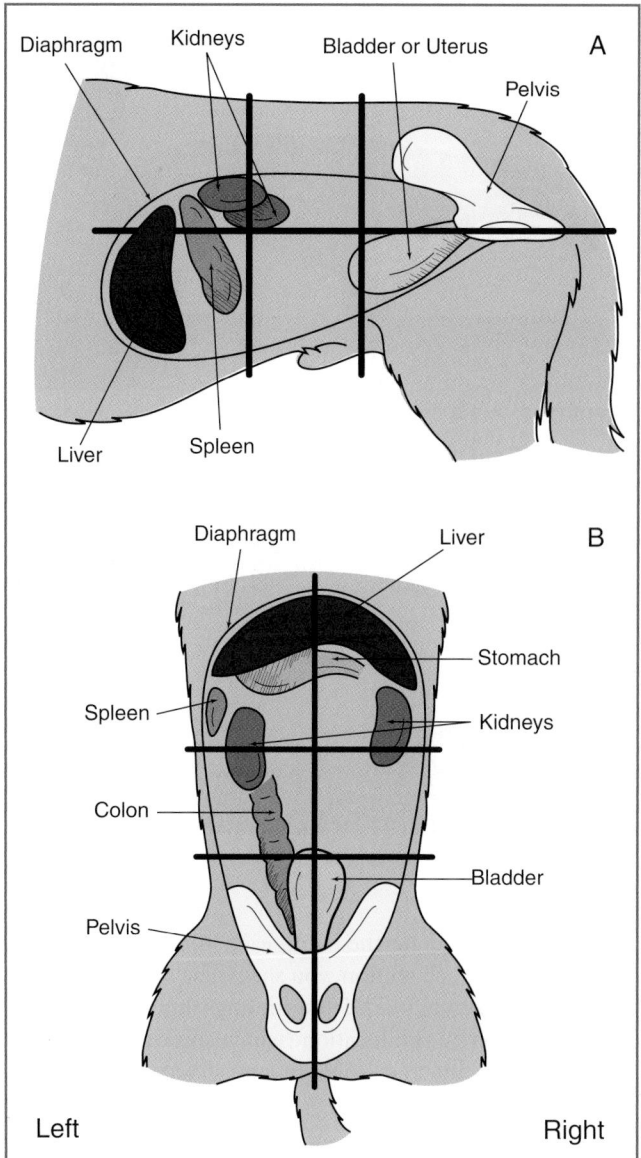

FIGURE 7-13 Location of internal organs within the abdominal quadrants. **A**, Lateral projection. **B**, Dorsoventral projection.

maximal intensity. For dogs, this point is usually identified in relation to the location of heart valves, as shown in Figure 7-12. For cats, this point may more easily be described in relation to the sternum (such as midsternum or left parasternum) because many feline murmurs are best auscultated in this area.

The final part of a thorough cardiovascular examination consists of evaluation of jugular veins. In a short-haired patient, the jugular veins can be visualized on either side of the trachea with the patient's muzzle lifted dorsally in a standing or sitting position. In animals with thicker or longer coats, the hair may need to be clipped or wet down to allow evaluation. Normal patients should have jugular pulsations that do not extend more than one-third up the neck. The jugular veins drain blood into the right atrium, and their pulsations and distention give a direct indication of right atrial pressure. Distended jugular veins extending farther up the neck can be seen in any disease causing elevated central venous pressure, especially those causing increased right atrial pressure, such as pericardial effusion or pulmonic stenosis.

Gastrointestinal System

This section of the physical examination would more appropriately be called *abdominal palpation* because it actually involves assessment of more than just the gastrointestinal (GI) tract. During abdominal palpation, other abdominal organs will be examined, including liver, spleen, kidneys, and urinary bladder. The technique of abdominal palpation can be difficult for the novice technician, but with practice, one can become proficient. As with the physical examination as a whole, following a consistent routine every time abdominal palpation is performed will ensure that nothing is missed. A thorough understanding of the anatomic location of abdominal organs within the abdominal cavity is essential for effective palpation. Figure 7-13 shows the location of abdominal organs within the abdomen. For the purposes of description, the abdomen can be divided into six sections (cranial-dorsal, cranial-ventral, mid-dorsal, mid-ventral, caudal-dorsal,

caudal-ventral). For most dogs, the two-handed technique is the best method (Figure 7-14). For small dogs and cats, a one-handed technique (Figure 7-15) may be easier, using the general principles discussed later for the two-handed technique. With the patient in the standing position, the examiner should stand just behind the patient or should stand straddling the caudal end of the patient. This will allow the placement of one hand on either side of the abdomen. The hands should be in a flat, relaxed position. Palpation should begin in one section (such as cranial-dorsal). The hands should be moved gently toward each other in a smooth, fluid motion. The hands and fingers should remain relaxed, and excessive pressure should not be exerted so the patient does not tense its abdominal muscles (as this makes delineation of organs difficult). The palpation should move slowly and methodically through all other sections of the abdomen. The

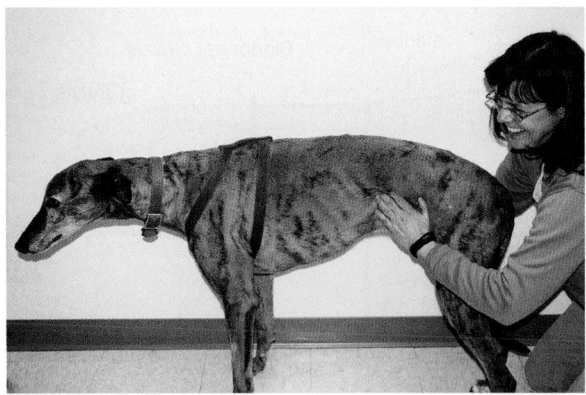

FIGURE 7-14 Two-handed abdominal palpation in the dog.

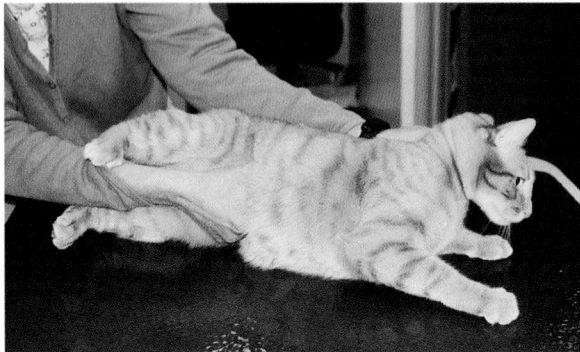

FIGURE 7-15 One-handed abdominal palpation in the cat.

progression should be the same each time you palpate a patient. Within each section, you should be noting any pain, swelling, firmness, or fluid. These findings should be recorded as to their severity and location (which section, left or right side). Be as specific as possible in your descriptions.

> **TECHNICIAN NOTE** Abdominal palpation should be performed using a consistent routine in every patient to avoid failure to evaluate any area.

Specific organs should be palpated in their respective regions. The liver should not be palpable in the normal animal, but if it is enlarged or contains a mass, it may be palpated in the cranial-ventral abdomen just caudal to the rib margin. The spleen is usually palpable in the cranial-ventral or midventral abdomen more on the left side. It should be gently palpated for enlargement or masses. The kidneys reside in the cranial-dorsal or middorsal abdomen and cannot be palpated in most dogs because they are encased in quite a bit of fat and are not movable. However, they may be palpated in thin dogs or when **renomegaly** is present. Pain in those sections of the abdomen may represent renal pain. In cats, the kidneys are much more movable and much more easily palpable. They usually are just caudal to the ribs in the dorsal abdomen and can be freely moved in most cats. They should be palpated for irregularities in size

or shape and for evidence of pain. The urinary bladder can be easily palpated in the caudal-ventral abdomen, assuming it is not empty and that the patient is cooperative. Identification of the urinary bladder makes cystocentesis possible. The urinary bladder should also be palpated for distention or thickness. On rare occasions, bladder stones may be palpable on physical examination. In male dogs, the prostate gland may be palpable in the caudal-dorsal abdomen, especially if it is significantly enlarged. However, the prostate usually is best examined via a rectal examination.

The GI tract can be examined to some extent during abdominal palpation. The stomach usually is not palpable if it is empty, but if gastric distention or a mass is present, it may be palpable in the cranial-dorsal abdomen (or farther caudal with severe distention). The small intestines are generally palpable as loops passing through your fingers in much of the midabdomen. It is not possible to delineate the different sections of small intestine by palpation. Small intestinal masses should be easily palpable, but other intestinal changes, such as wall thickening, are usually subtle and difficult to appreciate. The large intestine usually can be palpated in the middorsal and caudal-dorsal abdomen as it courses toward the rectum, assuming that it contains formed feces. If it is empty, it may not be as easily palpable. Good palpation may allow for identification of large intestinal masses or of constipation or obstipation. Remember that a complete GI examination includes an examination of the oral cavity, pharynx, rectum, and anus. Examination of these areas is discussed in other sections.

Rectal Examination

A rectal examination should be performed in almost every canine patient. In cats and small dogs, a rectal examination may be prohibitively painful and should be performed only in patients with a presenting complaint that may be referable to that area. A thorough rectal examination can be quick and can provide a significant amount of useful information. The examination is typically performed using a well-lubricated, gloved index finger (although the pinkie finger can be used in smaller patients). Before examining the rectum, the perineal area and anus should be examined for redness, swelling, masses, discharge, or other abnormalities. The finger is passed gently through the anal sphincter with the knuckles aimed dorsally. The finger is placed in as far as is comfortable for the patient, and structures are examined moving caudally. In the male dog, the prostate gland may be palpated ventral to the rectum cranial to the pelvic brim. It should be palpable in most intact dogs and in any dog with prostatomegaly. The normal gland is bilobed with a median raphe and should be smooth, symmetric, and nonpainful. Enlargement or pain on palpation may be indicative of prostatic infection or neoplasia. Moving caudally, the urethra can be palpated ventral to the rectum as it courses caudally from the urinary bladder. Feel carefully for any irregularities (such as stones or masses). Dorsal to the rectum, the medial iliac lymph nodes are present to either side of the midline and may be palpated if they are enlarged. The inner mucosa of

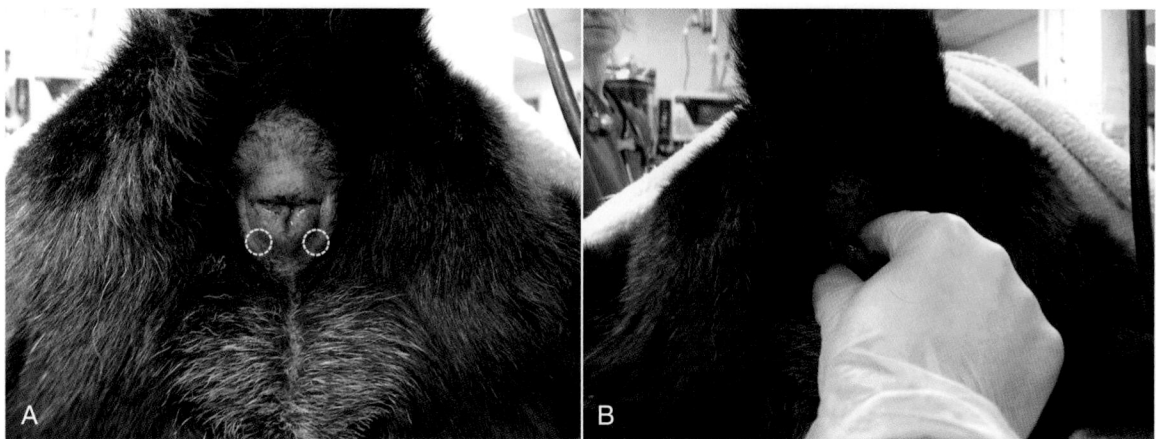

FIGURE 7-16 A, Approximate location of the anal sacs in a dog (dotted circles). B, Technique for expression of the left anal sac in a dog.

the rectum should be palpated during the examination by running the finger 360 degrees around the wall at various levels. The rectal wall should be evaluated for irregularity, thickness, or masses. The character of the stool within the rectum (if present) should be noted. If possible, a sample of stool should be removed with the gloved finger and examined. Finally, the anal sacs can be palpated. The anal sacs lie just behind the anal mucosa with one on either side, located at approximately 5 and 7 o'clock (Figure 7-16, A). The anal sacs can be palpated by moving the finger within the rectum laterally and caudally while gently pressing with the thumb on the outside of the anus. Normal anal sacs should be small (<1 cm) and firm but slightly fluctuant. Distended anal sacs likely contain normal anal sac fluid but could contain a mass. Both sacs must be fully expressed to confirm whether or not a mass is present. This should be done in any patient with a palpably distended anal sac. Each sac opens at the rectal-anal junction adjacent to the location of the sac. The anal sacs are expressed by gently applying pressure with the thumb and finger during palpation (Figure 7-16, B). Anal sac fluid can vary in appearance from whitish to dark brown and can vary in consistency from watery to fairly thick. Evidence of blood or pus may indicate anal sac infection. Thick material can result in an anal sac impaction, which can be uncomfortable for the patient and can lead to scooting of the rear end. Anal sac expression can be difficult in patients with an impaction and may require sedation.

> **TECHNICIAN NOTE** The rectal examination provides an impressive amount of useful information and should be performed on every patient except those that will experience significant discomfort from the examination.

Urogenital

Much of the urinary system is evaluated during abdominal palpation and a rectal examination, as discussed previously. The kidneys, urinary bladder, and proximal urethra have already been examined. The only part of the urinary system

left to be evaluated is the distal urethra, which opens at the tip of the penis in the male and into the vestibule in the female. In male dogs, the penis should be gently extruded by pulling back the skin of the prepuce. Any discharge within the prepuce should be noted. The penis should be evaluated to ensure that the urethral opening is normal and appears patent. Any masses or wounds on the penis should be noted. Penile examination is not typically performed in the male cat, except when the patient is sedated, such as would occur during urethral obstruction. Examination of the vagina and vestibule is not routinely performed in dogs and cats. In cases with a presenting complaint referable to the lower urinary tract, a vaginal examination may be indicated. A digital vaginal examination may be performed in the awake dog, but often sedation will be necessary. Sedation will always be required in the cat. In either case, the examiner should wear sterile gloves and should use copious lubrication to prevent trauma and discomfort for the patient.

In the United States, a vast majority of dogs and cats are neutered. Therefore, an examination of reproductive organs is not commonly performed. In the intact male dog or cat, the testicles should be examined. The scrotum should be gently palpated to ensure that both testicles are present. Testicles should descend into the scrotum by 8 weeks of age in most patients and by 6 months in all patients. The testicles should be gently palpated to assess for any asymmetry in size, masses, heat, or pain. The penis should be extruded and examined as described earlier. In the intact female dog or cat, the reproductive organs are not as easily examined. A vaginal examination may be performed as described previously but is not part of a routine examination. The uterus cannot be palpated during abdominal palpation unless it is enlarged, as with pregnancy or **pyometra.** The ovaries cannot be palpated. It is good practice to palpate the mammary chains in all female dogs and cats, but it is especially important in sexually intact patients because they have a much higher risk of mammary cancer. Most dogs and cats will have five mammary glands on each side of the ventral abdomen. They should be gently palpated for heat, swelling, masses, or discharge. In lactating animals, milk should be expressed and examined.

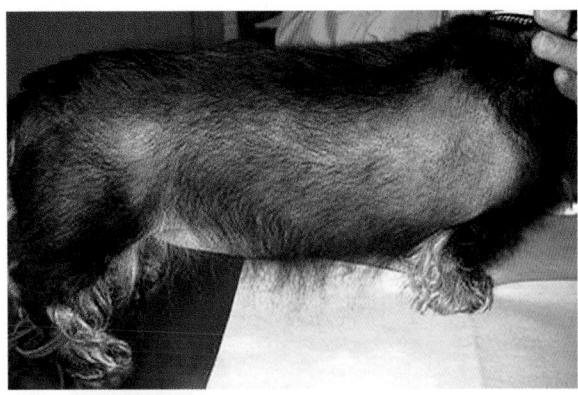

FIGURE 7-17 Bilaterally symmetric truncal alopecia in a dog with hyperadrenocorticism.

> **TECHNICIAN NOTE** A urogenital examination is most important in patients who are sexually intact.

Integument

A complete evaluation of the integumentary system will include an examination of the hair, skin (including footpads and nails), and subcutaneous tissues. The character of the normal hair coat can vary greatly between breeds and between individual patients, but in general, it should be thick and shiny. Abnormal hair coats may be dull or greasy. They may contain scale (flakes of shed epidermis). The coat should be visually evaluated for areas of thinning or alopecia (Figure 7-17). If alopecia is noted, it should be described in terms of location (focal vs. diffuse vs. patchy, unilateral vs. bilateral, symmetric vs. asymmetric) and degree (partial vs. complete). The coat should be inspected closely in alopecic areas. The examiner should look for evidence of broken hairs, which may indicate that the alopecia is caused by scratching or **barbering.** The skin should also be examined in the alopecic area for evidence of excoriation or underlying disease. The hair should be gently parted in several areas to look for evidence of ectoparasites, such as fleas. In highly suspicious cases, such as in extremely **pruritic** animals, a flea comb can be used to improve the chances of identifying live fleas or their excrement.

> **TECHNICIAN NOTE** Dermatologic diseases are common in small animal patients. Familiarity with the skin examination and with terminology of skin lesions will be useful.

The extent to which the skin is directly examined will depend on the presenting complaint of the patient. A patient with no complaints referable to the skin (such as pruritus, flaking, or odor) need only have a cursory skin examination. Patients with complaints referable to the skin warrant a more thorough evaluation. In any patient lacking alopecia, the hair must be parted to allow an evaluation of the skin. The ventral-caudal abdomen has a light covering of hair in many patients and is a good place to visualize the skin. Common abnormalities that can be identified on the skin include papules and pustules, which are seen commonly with bacterial skin infection. A papule is a pink or red elevated skin lesion smaller than 0.5 cm in diameter. A pustule is similar in size to a papule but is a raised area containing pus; it usually has a pink or red base with a white tip. Scales and crusts are caused by any inflammatory process affecting the outer layers of skin. Both appear as flakes and contain shed epidermal cells, but crusts also contain inflammatory cells. They can be difficult to differentiate based on visual inspection alone. Excoriations are areas of self-trauma caused by scratching in a pruritic animal. The skin is a good area in which to see petechiae and ecchymoses, which usually indicate a primary hemostatic defect. Erythema (redness) of the skin may be noted focally or diffusely. Nail beds and footpads should be examined, especially in patients with diseased skin, to evaluate for redness, discharge, or ulceration.

Masses are commonly found on the skin and within the subcutaneous tissues in veterinary patients. Most masses will be caused by benign neoplastic processes, although palpable masses may represent malignancy, vaccine reactions, abscesses, or swelling caused by trauma. It is important that any masses be noted in the medical record in great detail, so that any changes in their size or appearance can be noted. Masses should be described on the basis of their location, including whether they are on the surface of the skin (cutaneous) or under the skin (subcutaneous). Their exact location can be recorded in the medical record by using a body map. Such a map will allow the precise marking of the location of the mass and is much more effective than written descriptions for comparison in future examinations. The size and shape of the mass should be noted. The size is most precisely recorded using measuring calipers, although it can be estimated if calipers are not available. The mass should be described as soft, fluctuant, or firm. Its adherence to underlying structures should be noted by recording whether it is movable or fixed. Careful monitoring of cutaneous and subcutaneous masses is important in determining a diagnostic and therapeutic plan.

Lymph Nodes

In the normal patient, peripheral lymph nodes that can be palpated are mandibular, prescapular, and popliteal lymph nodes. Axillary and inguinal lymph nodes typically are palpable only when they are significantly enlarged. Similarly, enlarged medial iliac lymph nodes may be palpable via a rectal examination, as discussed earlier. The mandibular lymph nodes are located on either side of the neck just caudal-dorsal to the ramus of the mandible and cranial-ventral to the mandibular salivary glands. They can be differentiated from the salivary gland because they tend to be more movable, slightly firmer, and smaller (in the normal patient). The prescapular lymph nodes are located in the subcutaneous tissue just medial to the scapular-humeral joint on either side of the patient. These nodes often are encased in fat and may feel slightly softer than other normal

lymph nodes may be enlarged, firm, warm, or painful. The most common abnormality palpated is an enlarged lymph node. It should be noted that lymph nodes in young animals (younger than 6 months of age) are normally mildly enlarged as compared with the size they will be during adulthood. Lymph node enlargement may indicate that the node is infected, is reacting to local inflammation, or is neoplastic. Enlargement should be noted as focal (single node or single region) or generalized (all palpable nodes enlarged). The specific nodes that are enlarged should be noted and their size measured with calipers or estimated.

> **TECHNICIAN NOTE** The peripheral lymph nodes that should be palpable in every patient are the mandibular, prescapular, and popliteal lymph nodes.

Musculoskeletal System

Examination of the musculoskeletal system will vary greatly depending on the patient's presenting complaint. In a patient without symptoms referable to the musculoskeletal system (such as lameness, swelling, difficulty rising, or pain), the examination will be fairly cursory. All patients should be observed as they walk around the examination room or waiting area for signs of lameness that the owner may not have perceived. In patients lacking lameness, the musculoskeletal examination should include a visual inspection of the standing animal for asymmetry of the limbs. This is followed by gentle palpation of each limb and the vertebral column over the neck and back. Initial palpation of limbs should be performed such that opposite sides (i.e., left and right forelimbs, left and right hindlimbs) are examined simultaneously. This will allow for comparison with the opposite leg when swelling or pain is evaluated.

In a patient that is seen with a complaint referable to the musculoskeletal system, such as lameness, or in one in which the cursory musculoskeletal examination revealed an abnormality, a more thorough examination is indicated. This should start with observation of the animal walking or jogging on a lead for identification of lameness. Animals will put less weight on a painful limb when walking, shifting the weight to the good limb. This results in the patient putting the head down when stepping on the good limb and pulling the head up when stepping on the painful limb. Once the affected limb has been identified, the patient should be placed in lateral recumbency and each limb thoroughly examined one at a time. The soft tissues and long bones of the limb should be palpated with gradually increasing levels of pressure to identify swelling or pain. Then, starting at the toes, every joint should be put through a range of flexion and extension in an attempt to isolate the examined joint and not move any other joints. It is important to examine all limbs so that perceived discomfort in one limb can be compared with the opposite limb. If you identify pain in one limb and the patient does not show a similar response in the other limbs, you have likely identified a problem. The bones

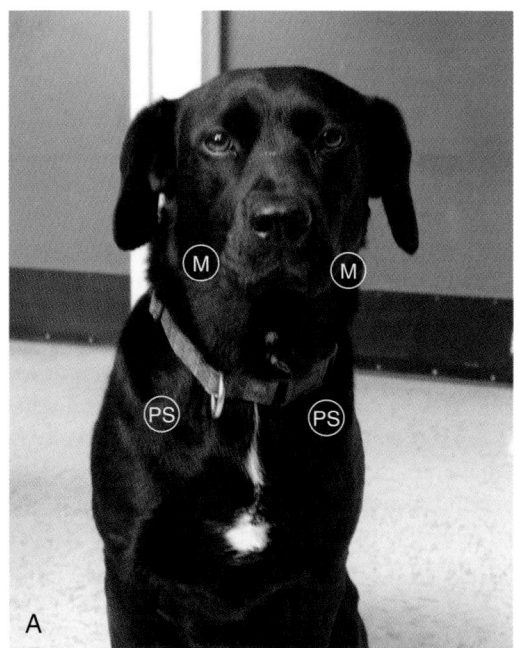
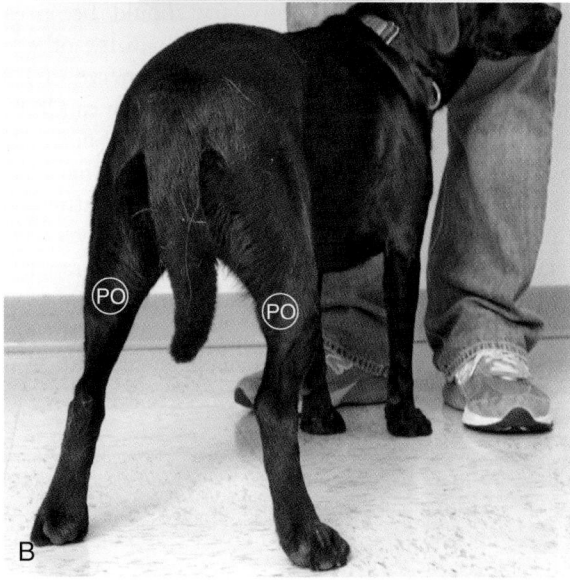

FIGURE 7-18 A, Dog showing the location of mandibular lymph nodes. B, Dog showing the location of popliteal lymph nodes.

nodes (Figure 7-18, *A*). The popliteal lymph nodes are located on the caudal aspect of each hindlimb at the level of the stifle joint (Figure 7-18, *B*). The axillary lymph nodes, if palpable, will be located in the subcutaneous space on the lateral aspect of the ventral thorax under the arm. The inguinal lymph nodes are located in the most caudal part of the ventral abdomen, just medial to the thighs, on either side of the midline.

Lymph nodes should be palpated by gently isolating them between thumb and index finger. Ideally, the left and right lymph nodes are palpated simultaneously at each location to determine whether they are identical in size and shape. Normal lymph nodes are round to oval in shape, slightly movable, and firm, but slightly compressible. Abnormal

of the vertebral column should be palpated one at a time by pressing down on their dorsal surface on the animal's back. The neck should be put through a full range of motion and any pain noted.

> **TECHNICIAN NOTE** In a patient with lameness, all limbs should be thoroughly examined to allow comparisons to be made and to isolate the affected area.

Nervous System

Similar to the musculoskeletal examination, the time allotted to the neurologic examination will vary greatly depending on the patient. The examination of every patient will include a subjective visual evaluation of mentation, visual acuity, and gait as it enters the examination room, as described in the section on observing patients in their surroundings. Most patients will have menace and pupillary light reflex testing performed as part of the eye examination. If these parameters are considered normal and the patient does not have any complaints that could be referable to the nervous system, the neurologic examination need not be any more extensive.

A patient with an abnormality noted on the cursory examination or one with a complaint that could be referable to the nervous system should have a more complete neurologic examination. Presenting complaints that could be referable to the nervous system include, but are not limited to, behavior changes, depression, lethargy, blindness, head tilt, circling, lameness, weakness, or paralysis. A complete neurologic examination includes an evaluation of mentation, gait and posture, muscle tone, cranial nerves, postural reactions, and reflexes. Mentation is assessed subjectively during visual observation of the patient and may be described as bright and alert, quiet, dull or obtunded (not interested in surroundings), stuporous (responsive only to noxious stimuli), or comatose (unresponsive to stimuli). Gait and posture are also observed. The patient should be walked or jogged on a lead and made to turn when gait is assessed. Although animals with neurologic disease can have normal gait and posture, ataxia is a common gait abnormality in these patients. *Ataxia* is a term used to describe uncoordinated muscle movements when walking. When a patient's gait is evaluated, ataxia is identified when you are unable to predict where the foot will fall on the patient's next step. Ataxia can vary in type and severity, and it is often confused with lameness by owners. Muscle tone is subjectively assessed by visual inspection and palpation. The evaluation of muscle tone should include determination of anal sphincter tone. During a rectal examination, the anal sphincter muscles should tighten around your finger. Muscle atrophy or decreased tone may be noted in denervated muscle.

A cranial nerve examination is an essential part of every complete neurologic examination. Cranial nerve reflex tests are summarized in Table 7-3. The olfactory nerve (cranial nerve I) is not routinely tested because a patient's response to scent is difficult to evaluate. The spinal accessory nerve

(cranial nerve XI) is not evaluated. Lesions in this nerve cause atrophy of the trapezius muscle, which can be difficult to identify. As discussed in the section on the eye examination, the pupils should be evaluated for size and symmetry, and menace and pupillary light reflex tests should be performed. These will evaluate the optic (cranial nerve II) and oculomotor nerves (cranial nerve III). The position of the eyes at rest and the doll's eye reflex (physiologic nystagmus) will evaluate oculomotor, trochlear (cranial nerve IV), and abducens nerves (cranial nerve VI). The doll's eye reflex is performed by turning the patient's muzzle and head from left to right. As the head moves in one direction, the eyes should initially move to the opposite direction and then snap back to the center. The palpebral reflex is tested by tapping the medial and lateral canthus of the eye to induce a blink. The corneal reflex is tested by holding the eyelids open and gently touching the cornea with a wet cotton swab. Gently pinching the lips with a hemostat or placing the hemostat inside either nostril should cause the patient to move away and will evaluate the sensory portion of the trigeminal nerve (cranial nerve V). Facial symmetry should be assessed because a droop to one side compared with the other can indicate a lesion of the facial nerve (cranial nerve VII). The eyes should be examined for nystagmus, which can indicate a lesion in the vestibulocochlear nerve (cranial nerve VIII). The gag reflex is performed by pressing with a finger on the back of the patient's tongue; this should elicit contraction of the pharyngeal muscles, which can be used to evaluate the glossopharyngeal nerve (cranial nerve IX) and branches of the vagus nerve (cranial nerve X). A visual examination of the tongue for determination of deviation to one side or another can identify lesions of the hypoglossal nerve (cranial nerve XII).

> **TECHNICIAN NOTE** A complete neurologic examination should include evaluation of mentation, gait and posture, muscle tone, cranial nerves, postural reactions, and reflexes.

A neurologic examination of the limbs involves assessment of postural reactions, reflexes, and sensation. Conscious proprioception is tested in the standing patient by picking up one paw and placing its dorsal surface onto the floor. The normal patient will quickly lift and turn the foot so that the palmar or plantar surface is touching the floor. This test should be performed on each leg. Note that patients with significant muscle weakness may not have the strength to lift the limb to turn it, so you should help to support the patient's weight. Limb strength can be assessed by forcing the patient to hop on one limb at a time and comparing their strength to do so between limbs. In small patients, this can be done easily by supporting the weight of the other three limbs while the patient is moved from side to side on one limb. In larger dogs, it may be necessary to hold up only one forelimb and move the patient from side to side on the opposite forelimb while keeping the hindlimbs fairly still. A

TABLE 7-3 | Examination of the Cranial Nerves

NERVE	TEST	TEST RESPONSE NORMAL	ABNORMAL
I. Olfactory	Volatile substance	Sniff, recoil, nose lick Blink	No response No blink
II. Optic	Menace Pupillary light reflex	Direct, consensual responses present	No direct or consensual responses
III. Oculomotor	Pupillary light reflex Observe eye following an object	Direct, consensual responses present Normal eye movement	No direct response, consensual intact Impaired ocular movement in ventral, dorsal, and medial directions Dorsomedial strabismus
IV. Trochlear	Observe Palpate temporalis Corneal reflex Palpebral reflex	Normal eye position Normal muscle tone Eye blink Eye blink	Muscle atrophy No blink No blink
V. Trigeminal	Observe ability to chew Palpate masseter muscle Pupillary light reflex	Normal jaw movement Normal muscle tone Direct, consensual responses present	Inability to chew Muscle atrophy No direct or consensual response present
VI. Abducens	Observe	Normal eye position	Medial strabismus
VII. Facial	Observe Corneal reflex Palpebral reflex Menace	Facial symmetry Eye blink Eye blink Eye blink	Lip droop No blink No blink No blink
VIII. Acoustic	Hand clap Move head horizontally, vertically	Startle response Normal nystagmus	No response No response, resting or positional nystagmus
IX. Glossopharyngeal	Gag reflex	Swallow	No response
X. Vagus	Gag reflex Oculocardiac reflex Laryngeal reflex	Swallow Bradycardia Cough	No response No response No response
XI. Accessory	Palpate neck muscles	Normal muscle tone	Muscle atrophy
XII. Hypoglossal	Tongue stretch	Retraction of tongue	No response

From McCurnin DM, Poffenbarger EM: Small animal and physical diagnosis and clinical procedures, Philadelphia, 1991, Saunders.

similar technique can be used to evaluate the hindlimbs. Reflex testing should be performed with the patient in lateral recumbency and relaxed. Forelimb reflexes to be tested include the withdrawal reflex, the biceps reflex, and the triceps reflex. Forelimb reflexes can be difficult to obtain, and the withdrawal reflex is the most reliable. It is performed by pinching the patient's toe, which should result in strong flexion of the limb. Hindlimb reflexes are more reliable and include the withdrawal reflex, the patellar reflex, and the cranial tibial reflex. Reflex responses should be scored from 0 to 4, as described in Table 7-4. Although not a limb reflex, the cutaneous trunci reflex can provide information regarding the integrity of spinal segments. It is performed by gently pinching the skin on either side of the lateral thorax, which should cause twitching of superficial muscles. Pinching the anal mucosa should result in a reflex contraction of the anal sphincter muscles (the perineal reflex). Sensation should be tested in paralyzed limbs by aggressively pinching the bones of the toes with a hemostat. The animal with intact sensation will vocalize or will try to bite. Note that pulling the leg back into flexion does not indicate normal sensation, but rather

TABLE 7-4 | Grading of Reflex Responses

GRADE	DESCRIPTION
0	No response
1	Hyporeflexia (less than normal response)
2	Normal response
3	Hyperreflexia (greater than normal response)
4	Clonus (repetitive response)

indicates an intact withdrawal reflex. Absence of sensation suggests a more severe lesion. Results of the complete neurologic examination should allow for anatomic localization of the source of neurologic symptoms.

History and Physical Examination of Large Animals

When a large animal patient is presented for an evaluation, a database that will become part of the medical record is generated. The history and physical examination are the most important parts of the database and serve as the starting point for identifying the patient's problems. After this initial information is collected, the database may be expanded to include laboratory tests, diagnostic imaging, and special examinations of body systems, depending on the purpose of the examination and the condition of the patient.

HISTORY

Husbandry practices, animal environments, and economic factors affecting large animals differ significantly from those of small animals; however, the basic approach to effective history taking is the same for both large and small animal patients. Experienced clients can provide an excellent history with little coaching, but most clients do not know how to give a concise, useful summary of their animal's condition. The technician will need to ask specific questions to obtain relevant information and will keep the information on an organized timeline. Once the history is obtained, the accuracy of the information must be evaluated because owners may unknowingly give inaccurate information, believing it to be true. Occasionally, owners provide false information to avoid embarrassment, not wanting to appear ignorant or to admit that they may have made a mistake in management of their animal.

Even though the history will focus on the chief clinical problem of an animal or group of animals, it is essential for the technician to keep the bigger picture of herd health and husbandry in mind when taking a history of large animal patients.

> **TECHNICIAN NOTE** The history of an individual animal is not complete without herd health information.

OWNER/AGENT INFORMATION

It is common for large animals to be attended by a person (or persons) other than the owner, such as a trainer, groomer, farmhand, stable owner, or lessee (animal lease agreements are not uncommon). It is important to determine the identity of the person presenting the animal and to establish his or her relationship to the animal. If the owner is not present, it is necessary to obtain appropriate contact information so that the veterinarian can communicate with the owner. It is also important to determine who has the decision-making responsibility for the animal because owners may entrust the trainer or agent to make decisions about the animal's treatment and care.

The insurance status of the animal should be determined. The economic value of certain large animals created a need many years ago for an insurance industry to protect owners' investments. In particular, equine insurance coverage is common in the United States, and valuable ruminant breeding animals also are often insured. *Mortality insurance* covers the value of the animal in case of death. *Surgical insurance* covers specific costs of surgery and hospitalization with some limitations—similar to human health insurance policies. *Loss of use insurance* states specifically the intended use of the animal (breeding, racing, etc.), and if the animal cannot perform its intended use because of illness or injury, the owner may be reimbursed for lost potential income. The insurance company's and insurance agent's contact numbers should be noted in the medical record because they may be involved in the decision-making process for the affected animal. The type of insurance policy and the estimated economic value of the animal should also be recorded because these factors often play an important role in the diagnostic and treatment options provided for the animal.

SIGNALMENT OF THE ANIMAL

The signalment of the animal typically includes age, sex, breed, color, and reproductive status. This information helps in formulating the patient's rule-out list of potential diagnoses because certain disease conditions have known predilections for subsets of the population according to signalment. For example, gray coat color in horses is associated with a higher incidence of melanoma than other coat colors; obstructive urolithiasis in ruminants is almost always associated with males; and β-mannosidase deficiency has been reported only in the Nubian breed of goats.

Another important part of large animal signalment is the intended use of the animal; most large animals are kept for specific purposes, such as breeding, athletic performance, and commercial production of meat, milk, hair, or other products. The animal's occupation may predispose it to certain diseases or injuries, such as the increased occurrence of osteochondral "chip" fractures in race horses versus pleasure horses, and the higher incidence of mastitis in dairy cattle than in beef cattle.

The terminology used by clients with large animals to describe their animals is species specific, and the technician should be familiar with commonly used terms for the sex, age, and reproductive status of large animal species (Tables 7-5 and 7-6).

TABLE 7-5	Age/Sex Terminology for the Horse
TERM	**DESCRIPTION**
Foal	Young horse, from birth to weaning (weaning usually at 4-7 months old)
Weanling	Young horse, from weaning to first birthday
Yearling	1 year-1½ years
Long yearling	1½ year to second birthday
Colt	Intact male from 2-3 years old
Filly	Female from 2-3 years old
Stallion	Intact male after third birthday
Mare	Female after third birthday
Gelding	Castrated male, of any age

TABLE 7-6	Age/Sex Terminology for Ruminants		
AGE	**CATTLE**	**SHEEP**	**GOAT**
Parturition (freshening)	Calving	Lambing	Kidding
Neonate	Calf	Lamb	Kid
Male (<1 year)	Bull calf	Ram lamb	Buck kid
Female (<1 year)	Heifer calf	Ewe lamb	Doe kid
Immature female (has not given birth)	Heifer	Yearling ewe	Yearling doe
Mature female	Cow	Ewe	Doe (nanny)
Mature male	Bull	Ram	Buck (billy)
Castrated male	Steer	Wether	Wether

INDIVIDUAL HISTORY AND CHIEF COMPLAINT

The history is usually obtained before the physical examination is begun because it may contain helpful information for the examiner. However, in emergency situations, it may be necessary to evaluate and stabilize the animal before proceeding with obtaining details about the animal's history. For example, an animal's vaccination and deworming history has little immediate value for an animal in need of treatment for severe shock.

> **TECHNICIAN NOTE** In an emergency situation, it may be necessary to perform the physical examination before taking a detailed history.

The individual history includes two major components: history of the current problem and the general history of the animal. The history of the current problem is usually taken first and includes the client's chief complaint. The chief complaint is the primary reason for requesting an examination, although it is not always the animal's primary problem. It is important to listen to the client and to avoid any perception of discounting or disregarding their concerns. Once the chief complaint has been determined, the technician can begin a more directed line of questioning to accurately characterize the problem in terms of duration, progression, severity, frequency, and response to therapy (if treatment has been attempted). Further questioning will focus on specific body systems affected by the current problem; in an animal with respiratory disease, the presence and character of a cough, nasal discharge, or respiratory noise are important to determine. Information on appetite, dental care, abdominal pain, and fecal volume and consistency is important in assessing an animal with GI disease.

The general history includes information on the animal before the current problem developed. Typically, this includes information on diet, exercise, preventive health maintenance, reproductive status, and previous medical problems and surgical procedures. Large animal clients are more likely than small animal owners to purchase and administer vaccines and deworming medications. Food animal producers commonly perform minor surgical procedures on their animals, such as dehorning, tail docking, and castration.

MEDICATION AND TREATMENT HISTORY

Most large animal facilities keep first aid kits and pharmaceuticals on the premises, and animals are often treated before the veterinarian is called. This situation is fairly common in large animal practices, especially with production animals, where economics often dictates whether the owner calls the vet immediately or attempts to solve the problem himself. Owners may be reluctant to admit this information and may need to be asked specifically whether they have treated the animal and what they have attempted to do for treatment.

HERD HEALTH HISTORY

Large animals are seldom kept as isolated individuals and therefore commonly share resources with other large animals. Similarly, animals often receive preventive health maintenance such as vaccination, deworming, and external parasite control as a group. After the individual history is obtained, it may be important to gather information on the size and nature of the group or herd and the resources that they share. Resources include not only food and water, but also shelter facilities and common land areas such as pastures and pens. Animals may be grouped randomly, but more commonly, large animals are grouped by age, sex, reproductive status, and other common attributes. If other animals are affected, the signalment of those animals can hold vital clues to the nature of the problem. Shared food, water, and grazing sources allow ready transmission of infectious agents and widespread distribution of parasites and toxins. Even horses that are housed in individual stalls are usually placed in common turnout areas for daily exercise, where they may contact other animals and/or their fecal material. Herd conditions may also create competition for food and water that prevents some individuals from getting adequate nutrition.

> **TECHNICIAN NOTE** Large animals often share resources, such as food, water, shelter, and turnout areas, with other animals.

The source of feed, hay, bedding, and water may not always be the farm on which the animals are kept. Under pasture conditions, stream, creek, or pond water may provide water for the animals' use. The purity of such water sources may be affected by "upstream" agricultural activities and runoff. Commonly, feed, hay, and bedding are purchased and are shipped to the farm by outside vendors; their quality and content may not be guaranteed. For example, poisonous plants may be inadvertently harvested when hay is cut and

BOX 7-1	Large Animal History

The following information should be obtained and recorded in the medical record:

Person Providing Information
Owner, agent, trainer, or farm employee

Insurance Information
Company name, contact information
Policy number
Type of insurance

Patient Signalment
Age, sex, breed, color, and identifying markings

Diet
Feed schedule
Forage/hay
    Type
    Source
Grain
    Type
    Source
Supplements
Dietary changes
    Intake: increased or decreased
    Change in appetite for certain foodstuffs
    Change in source of foodstuffs

Water
Sources
Availability

Housing Type

Reproductive Status

Vaccination History

Deworming History

Production History: Any Increase or Decrease in Production

Previous Illnesses/Surgical Procedures

Presenting (Chief) Complaint
Time of onset
Speed of onset: peracute, acute, or chronic
Duration
Progression of severity: improving, worsening, or static
Previous treatments/medications

Herd Information
Number of animals in herd
Number affected
Number of deaths

baled, producing toxicity when animals consume it. In certain areas of the country, black walnut trees may be included in the production of wood shavings, but no labeling requirements for packaging have been put forth; black walnut shavings may cause severe laminitis in horses when it is used for bedding.

A summary of basic large animal history information is presented in Box 7-1.

PHYSICAL EXAMINATION OF LARGE ANIMALS

Combined with a thorough history, the physical examination forms the basis for identifying a patient's true problems.

Most clinicians use a problem-oriented approach to diagnosis and treatment; this provides a logical method by which to work from the simplest to the most complicated medical and surgical cases. The history and physical examination also serve as the basis for the technician evaluation, which can be prioritized according to the urgency of the patient's physiologic needs.

Regardless of the size or species of animal, a consistent and systematic approach to the physical examination will increase the proficiency of the examiner and will decrease the likelihood of overlooking important findings.

PHYSICAL EXAMINATION OF THE EQUINE

When an animal is presented with medical or surgical problems, a physical examination is performed by the veterinarian for diagnostic purposes. The diagnostic physical examination may range from a basic temperature, pulse, and respiration (TPR) examination to a thorough multisystem or system-specific evaluation, depending on the patient's problems. In addition to the diagnostic type of physical examination, horse owners may request other types of "routine" physical examinations for their horses. The *insurance examination* is required by the insurance company before a horse can receive insurance coverage. It may range from a basic physical examination to a thorough, in-depth examination of all body systems; the type of insurance and the value of the animal will dictate the depth of examination required by the insurance company. The *prepurchase examination* is conducted before the sale of an animal is completed and is a common procedure in equine practice. A seller and a buyer are identified, and the veterinarian performing the examination is presumed to be working in the buyer's best interest (the veterinarian is paid by the buyer). Like the insurance examination, the scope of the prepurchase examination is dictated by the intended use of the horse and its estimated value; it may be a simple physical examination or an in-depth examination, including biopsies, blood samples, endoscopy, electrocardiogram (ECG) and/or echocardiogram, and diagnostic imaging. Prepurchase examinations are a potential source of lawsuits against the veterinarian; therefore, veterinarians go to great lengths to document the findings of prepurchase examinations and not to overstate their findings as predictions or guarantees of future performance.

The technician should understand the potentially sensitive nature of insurance and prepurchase examinations and should help ensure the accuracy and privacy of the results.

> **TECHNICIAN NOTE** Prepurchase examinations are a potential source of lawsuits, and examination results must be kept strictly confidential.

Getting Started

The basic physical examination always begins with observation of the animal from a distance. Good examiners will take advantage of this opportunity to observe the animal before applying restraint and will consider the total picture of the horse and its environment. The attitude, alertness, and general body condition of the horse are noted. Movements of the horse provide an opportunity to observe lameness. If food and water are available, appetite, mastication, and swallowing reflexes can be observed. Interactions with other animals can also provide useful information.

After the horse is observed and its temperament, presence or absence of pain, and possible body systems that will need to be evaluated are gauged, the most appropriate method of physical restraint can be selected. All physical examinations begin with appropriate physical restraint. Physical restraint is necessary for the safety of personnel and of the horse; it facilitates physical examination procedures. Depending on the body system (or systems) to be evaluated, the method of physical restraint may need to be changed during the examination. Chemical restraint may need to be applied to supplement physical restraint of painful or uncooperative patients (refer to Chapter 6 for more information about restraint and handling of animals).

After proper restraint has been applied, the hands-on physical examination can begin. A basic physical examination typically includes temperature, pulse, and respiration (TPR); heart and lung auscultation; abdominal auscultation; hydration status; examination of mucous membranes; and height and weight measurement.

Body Temperature

Temperature is almost always taken rectally, using a standard mercury or digital thermometer. Rarely, a vaginal temperature may be used.

Although any thermometer may be used on large animals, thermometers designed strictly for large animals are commercially available. Large animal thermometers are typically 5 inches long and have a thicker glass casing than regular thermometers. They often include a "ring top," which allows the user to attach a short (<12 inches) string. Strings are helpful for managing two commonly encountered situations: aspiration of the thermometer into the rectum and pushing the thermometer out of the rectum. Some horses may pull the anus inward while the thermometer is in place; occasionally, this results in aspiration of the entire thermometer into the rectum. This is potentially serious if the thermometer breaks inside the rectum, or if the horse strains to defecate; perforation of the rectum with the thermometer may occur and can be life threatening. The presence of the thermometer in the anus may also stimulate defecation; if this occurs, the thermometer will be passed out of the rectum, fall to the ground, and break. Broken thermometer glass can puncture hooves or skin or may be eaten as the horse browses for food. Because of these complications, it is necessary to maintain a firm grip on the thermometer for the entire procedure or to tie a string to the ring top and secure the string to the horse's tail hairs or hair coat (not the skin) with a clothespin or a small alligator clamp. If the horse aspirates the thermometer, the string can be used to gently

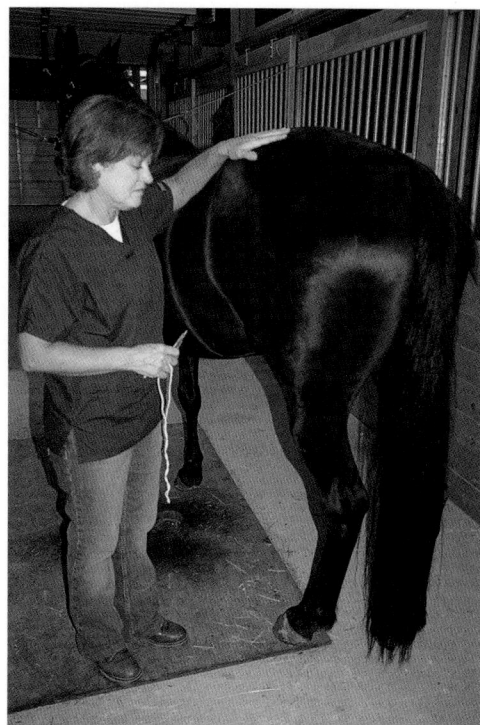

FIGURE 7-19 When taking rectal temperature, stand facing caudally and maintain contact with the horse.

retrieve it or to follow the string manually into the rectum to retrieve it. If the horse pushes the thermometer out of the rectum, the secured string should prevent it from falling on the ground. Strings longer than 12 inches should be avoided; long strings allow the thermometer to dangle against the legs, which causes some horses to kick.

Inserting the rectal thermometer requires some tact. The thermometer should be lubricated with petroleum jelly, mineral oil, or water, but dipping the thermometer in the horse's water bucket should be avoided; this practice gives the impression of disregard for sanitary procedure. Even if the thermometer has been properly disinfected, it is viewed by owners as a piece of equipment that has been in other horses' rectums and has no place in their horse's water bucket.

To insert the thermometer, stand next to the horse's hindquarters, facing caudally (Figure 7-19). Never stand directly behind the horse. If the horse resists by kicking or appears agitated by manipulations of the tail and hindquarters, the technician can stand behind a stall door or a stack of hay bales for protection. Grasp the tail near the base and elevate it or push it to the opposite side of the horse; it is not necessary to force the tail into an extreme position, which will only be met with resistance by the horse. Move the tail only enough to get clear entrance to the anus (Figure 7-20). Some horses respond best to gentle rubbing of the perianal area before the anus is touched with the thermometer, rather than thrusting the thermometer into the anus with no warning. The anal opening may be identified visually or by feel, and the thermometer gently inserted with a twisting motion.

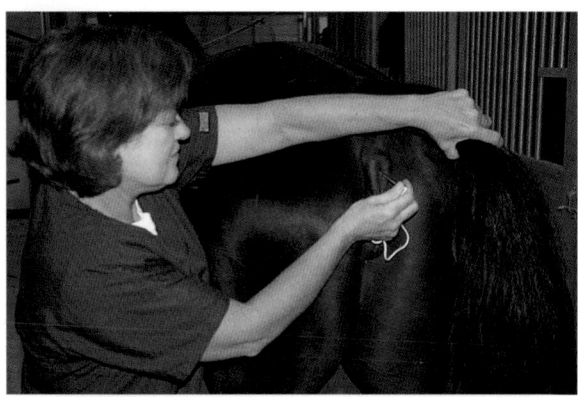

FIGURE 7-20 Grasp the tail at the base and move it gently to the side; the thermometer can then be inserted through the anus into the rectum.

If the thermometer does not easily advance, never force it; the rectal wall may be perforated with little effort. If the horse strains in resistance, try distracting it by offering feed or having someone tap on the horse's forehead while the thermometer is being inserted. The thermometer usually enters horizontally, but some horses require tipping of the thermometer slightly upward (dorsally) to enter the rectum.

> **TECHNICIAN NOTE**   Rectal thermometers should be inserted and advanced into the rectum without use of force.

The thermometer should be advanced several inches into the rectum, then either handheld or clipped to the tail hairs or coat hairs. It should be left in place for at least 60 seconds (mercury type) or until the audible or visual signal is heard or seen (digital type).

Normal rectal temperature varies by the age, breed, and environment of the animal. Body temperature is typically lowest in the morning. Normal rectal temperature of the adult horse at rest is 99.0°F to 101.5°F. From 101.5°F to 102.0°F is a "gray zone" that may be normal for some individuals, especially in hot weather. A temperature above 102.0°F is always suspicious, except following physical exercise, which can readily temporarily elevate temperature to this level and above. Normal values for TPR are given in Table 7-7.

Other factors may influence temperature. Large breeds and draft horses tend to have rectal temperatures at the lower end of the temperature range. Neonatal foals may lack the ability to generate body heat and often have low body temperatures immediately after birth. As heat-generating mechanisms develop, older foals may average approximately 1° higher than adults for the first few days to weeks after birth. Rectal procedures, such as a manual or endoscopic rectal examination, may allow air to enter the rectum, falsely lowering the rectal temperature; the temperature should be taken before any rectal procedure is performed.

If the rectum contains feces, the thermometer tip sometimes may be inadvertently inserted into a fecal ball. This is

TABLE 7-7	Normal TPR Values for Adult Large Animals		
	RECTAL TEMPERATURE, °F	**HEART RATE**	**RESPIRATORY RATE**
Horse	99.0-101.5	28-44/minute	6-16/minute
Cattle	101.5 (range, 100.4-103.1)	40-80/minute	10-30/minute
Sheep	102.5 (range, 102.0-104.0)	70-90/minute	12-25/minute
Goat	102.0 (range, 101.5-104.0)	70-90/minute	15-30/minute

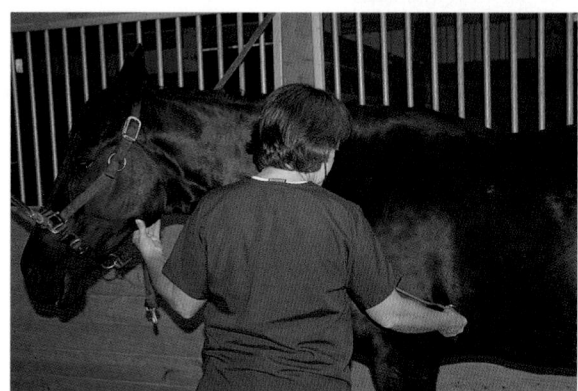

FIGURE 7-21 Simultaneous palpation of arterial pulse on the facial artery and auscultation of the heart for possible pulse deficit.

the most common cause of unusually low readings. If this occurs, the procedure should be repeated.

Pulse Rate/Heart Rate

Strictly speaking, heart rate and pulse rate are not the same; heart rate refers to the number of heartbeats/minute (beats/minute [bpm]); pulse rate refers to the number of palpable arterial pulse waves/minute. In normal animals, the heart rate and the pulse rate are equal.

The pulse rate is taken by palpation of arteries. As blood passes from arteries through capillary beds, a dampening effect on arterial blood pressure fluctuations (waves) is noted; therefore, veins do not have palpable pulses.

Auscultation of the heart is properly used for taking heart rate, not pulse rate. This is done because some heart abnormalities may produce audible heart sounds that are not necessarily accompanied by an arterial pulse. For accuracy, when the heart is auscultated, the arterial pulse should be simultaneously palpated to ensure that every audible heartbeat is accompanied by a palpable pulse wave (Figure 7-21). If each audible heartbeat is not accompanied by a pulse wave—a condition called *pulse deficit*—the clinician should be notified.

Arterial pulses may be palpated at several locations. The most convenient location is over the facial artery, where it crosses the ventral aspect of the mandible, rostral to the origin of the masseter muscle (Figure 7-22). Two or three

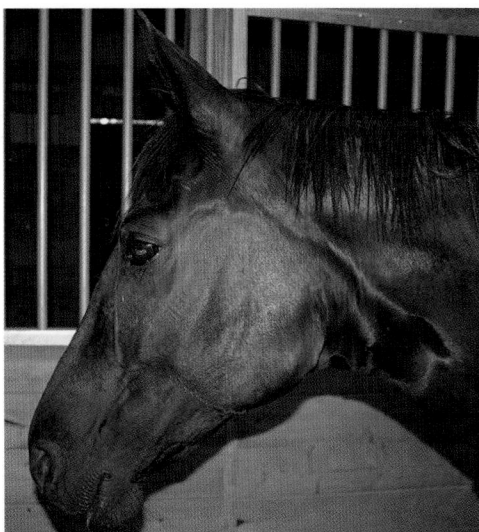

FIGURE 7-22 The facial artery courses along the rostral aspect of the masseter muscle and crosses the ventromedial aspect of the mandible.

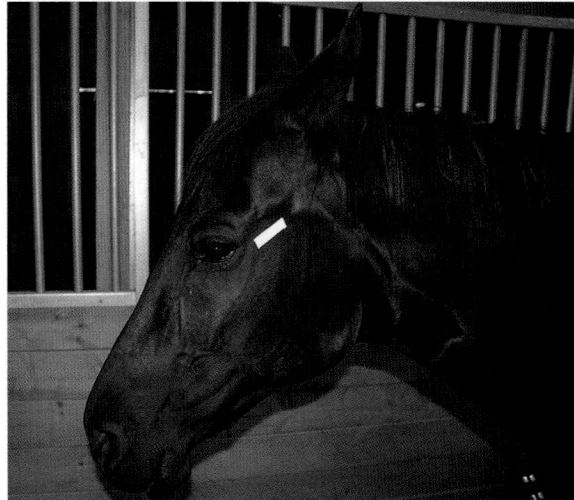

FIGURE 7-24 Location of the transverse facial artery.

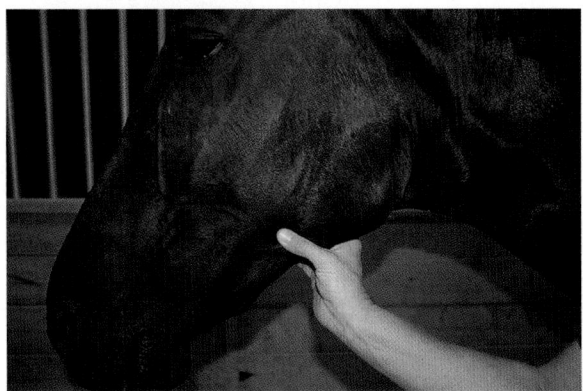

FIGURE 7-23 Press the vascular bundle firmly against the medial aspect of the mandible.

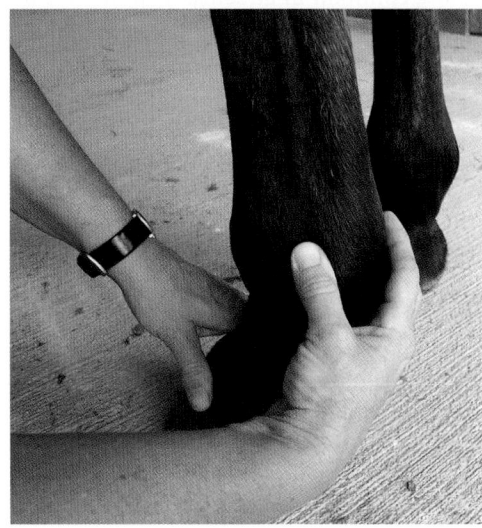

FIGURE 7-25 Palpation of the digital arteries over the proximal sesamoid bones.

fingers are lightly rolled back and forth across the ventromedial aspect of the mandible just rostral to the masseter muscle to identify the facial artery and facial vein; these vessels lie side by side and form a tubular, compressible type of structure. Once identified, the vascular bundle is firmly pressed against the mandible to feel the arterial pulse (Figure 7-23). If the bundle is pressed too tightly, the artery may be occluded and the pulse not easily felt. Large animal heart rates are much lower than their small animal counterparts, often requiring more patience to identify a palpable pulse.

> **TECHNICIAN NOTE** The facial artery where it crosses the ventromedial aspect of the mandible is the most convenient location for obtaining the pulse rate.

Other arteries are available for obtaining pulse rates. The transverse facial artery is located in a horizontal depression about 1 inch caudal to the lateral canthus of the eye, just below the zygomatic arch (Figure 7-24). The coccygeal artery supplies the tail and is located along the ventral midline of the tail. The dorsal metatarsal artery is located between metatarsals 3 and 4 (cannon bone and lateral splint bone) on the hindlimbs. The lateral and medial digital arteries can be palpated where they course over the abaxial aspect of the proximal sesamoid bones of each leg or just proximal to the collateral cartilages of each hoof (Figure 7-25). The carotid artery has a pulse wave, but it is difficult to accurately palpate in large animals because of its deep position and is seldom useful for palpation.

The main features of the pulse are rate and rhythm. The rate is recorded as the number of beats/minute (bpm). The pulse rate is normally 28 to 48 bpm in adult horses at rest. Foals have a rate of 60 to 80 bpm immediately after birth; this climbs to 75 to 100 bpm for the first week or 2 of life; it then gradually declines toward the adult rate over the next several weeks to months. Athletically fit horses may normally have rates less than 28 bpm; 24 bpm is not uncommon in fit race horses.

The pulse rhythm is recorded as regular or irregular. Irregular rhythm likely indicates an arrhythmia of the heart. The most common cause of pulse irregularity in horses is second-degree atrioventricular (AV) block, a heart arrhythmia caused by failure of the electric current generated by the atria to reach the ventricles. Intermittent blockage of current occurs at the AV node, resulting in "dropped" pulse beats. The dropped beats usually occur in *a regular pattern;* typically the dropped beat occurs every third or fourth heartbeat. Second-degree AV block is readily identified by palpating the pulse. The regular rhythm is interrupted by a single "lost" (dropped) beat, with "lost" beats occurring at regular intervals (beat-beat-beat-no beat-beat-beat-beat-no beat, etc.). Even though second-degree AV block is usually considered to be a normal finding in horses, its presence should be noted in the medical record. Horses with this arrhythmia may have low resting heart rates—less than 28 bpm. Second-degree AV block is more common in athletically fit horses and should disappear in any horse when the horse is exercised. It is believed to be caused by increased tone from the vagus nerve, which is part of the parasympathetic nervous system.

Pulse quality is often described as strong, bounding, weak, or thready, or in other nonspecific terms. The pulse quality is subjective; its usefulness depends on the experience of the person assessing the pulse and should not be overinterpreted.

Respiratory Rate

The number of respirations per minute can be counted in several ways: (1) A stethoscope can be used to listen to air movements into and out of the trachea or chest; (2) a hand can be used to feel the movement of air into and out of a nostril; and (3) most commonly, chest excursions (rise and fall of the thoracic wall) per minute can be visually counted.

Respirations should be characterized by their effort and depth. Respirations may be described as shallow, deep, labored, or gasping, and in other nonspecific terms. Horses normally use a combination of thoracic and abdominal muscles to breathe; this is called *costoabdominal breathing.* Some painful conditions of the chest may lead to increased use of abdominal muscles to breathe; this is referred to as an *increased abdominal effort* in the respiratory pattern.

Normal horses cannot breathe through the mouth. If mouth breathing is observed, it should be noted and brought to the attention of the clinician.

Respiratory noises are not uncommon in horses and are often significant findings. Noises may be characterized as wheezing, whistling, honking, snoring, fluttering, etc. Noises may be heard only at rest or only during exercise. It is important to note the horse's activity at the time the noise is heard. Equally important is to note whether the noise occurs during inspiration, expiration, or both.

The normal respiratory rate of an adult horse at rest is 6 to 16 breaths per minute. The rate is higher during hot weather and after physical activity. Foals have a high respiratory rate at birth as a result of residual fluid in the lower airways. Newborn foals may have a respiratory rate from 80 to 90; this will slow to 60 to 80 in the first 5 to 10 minutes after birth and will gradually decrease to 20 to 40 for the first week or two of life.

> **TECHNICIAN NOTE**   Respiratory noises should be characterized as inspiratory, expiratory, or both.

Heart Auscultation

Auscultation may be done on the left or right side of the chest, although most of the heart valves and sounds are heard best from the left side. However, the right side should not be overlooked; some murmurs are audible only on the right side and will be missed if the horse is auscultated only from the left.

Horses are athletes; the heart of the average horse may be as large as a basketball. The landmarks for basic auscultation of the heart are the same on either side of the chest. Landmarks for the dorsoventral position of the heart are the level of the shoulder joint for the heart base and the point of the elbow (olecranon) for the heart apex (Figure 7-26). The craniocaudal position is defined by the caudal border of the triceps muscle, which roughly divides the heart into cranial and caudal halves. Using these landmarks, the position of the heart can be estimated.

Usually, heart sounds are easier to hear when auscultation is performed cranial to the caudal border of the triceps muscle. However, the triceps muscle is too thick to allow any heart sounds to be heard through it; the head of the stethoscope must be placed directly against the chest wall. To expose the chest wall at this location, the triceps muscle can be gently elevated away from the chest wall before the stethoscope is positioned (Figure 7-27). Another approach is to advance the forelimb to a more forward position, as if the horse were taking a step forward, which moves the triceps cranially. However, many horses are reluctant to hold this position for any length of time.

The heart rate is counted as beats per minute. The cardiac sounds S_1 (lub) and S_2 (dub) are components of one heartbeat. A common error, especially for those accustomed to

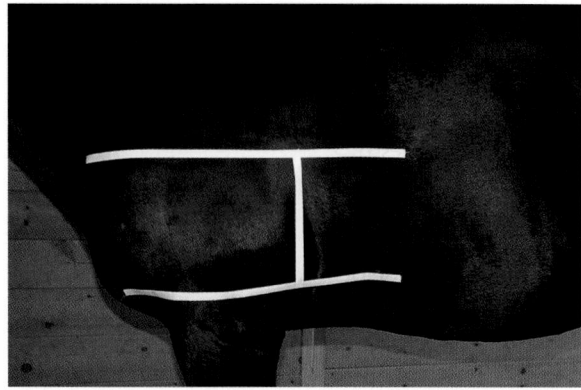

FIGURE 7-26 Landmarks for the heart: The horizontal marks indicate the level of the shoulder and elbow joints; the vertical mark indicates the caudal border of the triceps muscle.

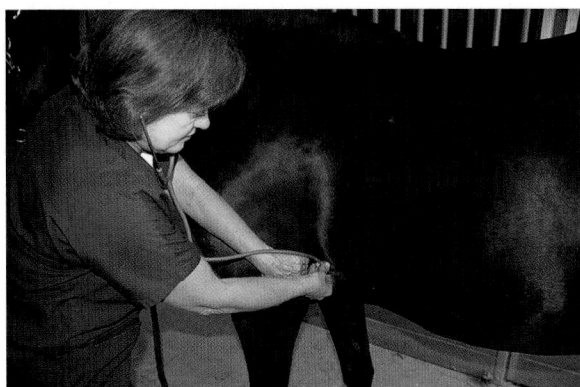

FIGURE 7-27 The triceps muscle is gently lifted away from the chest wall to provide access for the stethoscope.

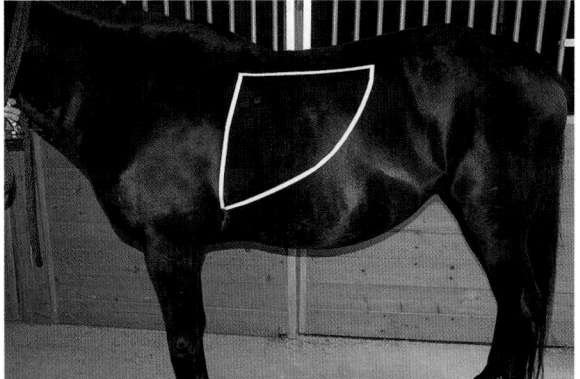

FIGURE 7-28 Borders of the left lung field for lung auscultation.

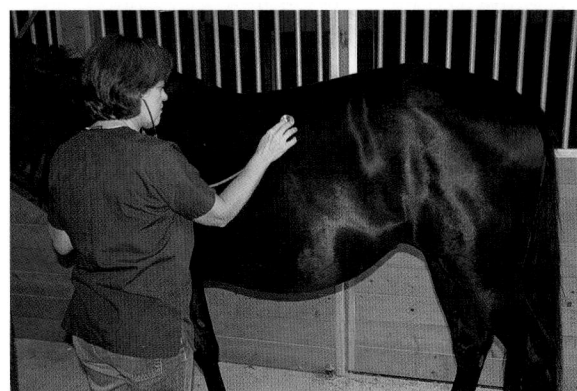

FIGURE 7-29 Auscultation of the left caudodorsal lung field.

small animal auscultation, is to count S_1 and S_2 as separate beats, essentially doubling the actual heart rate. The heart rate in large animals is slow, and heart sounds are usually loud and distinct, leading to possible confusion.

Auscultation is also used to detect abnormal heart sounds. Murmurs are not uncommon in horses, although most murmurs in the horse are actually normal heart sounds and are simply the result of large volumes of blood moving at high speeds through the heart valves. Because of the large heart size, these sounds are amplified and are referred to as *ejection murmurs*. Ejection murmurs are commonly heard in horses and should disappear when the horse is exercised. True cardiac disease is unusual in horses but usually will be accompanied by murmurs or other abnormal sounds.

Heart murmurs are assessed for loudness, character, and the timing of the murmur in the cardiac cycle (systolic, diastolic, or continuous). The horse may be exercised to see if the abnormal sound disappears, stays the same, or gets louder with exercise. Using these initial criteria, the veterinarian decides whether further evaluation of the cardiovascular system is warranted.

> **TECHNICIAN NOTE** Ejection murmurs are commonly auscultated in the horse and usually are normal findings.

Lung Auscultation

Despite the large size of equine lungs, breath sounds may be difficult to hear. A quiet environment is important for an accurate evaluation. Lung auscultation should *always* be performed on *both* sides of the chest. Respiratory diseases do not necessarily affect both lungs and pleural cavities equally and can result in markedly different auscultation findings over the right and left lung fields of a single individual. Because of the large size of the lungs and possible uneven distribution of disease, auscultation findings may vary even over different areas of the same lung.

The borders of the lung fields are the same for the right and left sides of the chest and are outlined in Figure 7-28. The lung field basically consists of a cranioventral area and a caudodorsal area; a part of the cranioventral field is

obscured by the shoulder musculature and cannot be heard. The stethoscope is placed in several locations within the lung field, and several breaths are listened to at each location (Figure 7-29). Normally, air movement into and out of the airways should be heard with each chest excursion; sounds may be amplified in foals, in thin animals, and in any animal after exercise. Occasionally, it is desirable to induce deep breathing to accentuate lung sounds; this is easily accomplished by occluding the nostrils temporarily until the horse begins to object to the lack of air; at the first sign of discomfort, the examiner releases the nostrils and immediately moves to auscultate the chest. Abnormal respiratory sounds include wheezes, crackles, and gurgling, moist sounds; the absence of breath sounds may also be significant. The veterinarian should be alerted when abnormal sounds are detected.

Abdominal Auscultation

A stethoscope is used to listen to abdominal sounds, which are created by movements of the intestines. This is commonly referred to as *gastrointestinal motility* or *GI motility*. In reality, this term is a misnomer because some sounds are generated by the passive movement of gas and liquids within the intestines without actually being propelled by the intestinal musculature. It is not completely accurate to assume that all intestinal sounds are due to functional intestines. This becomes important in the patient with GI disease; diseased portions of intestine may have little or no purposeful motility, yet passive fluid and gas sounds may be heard.

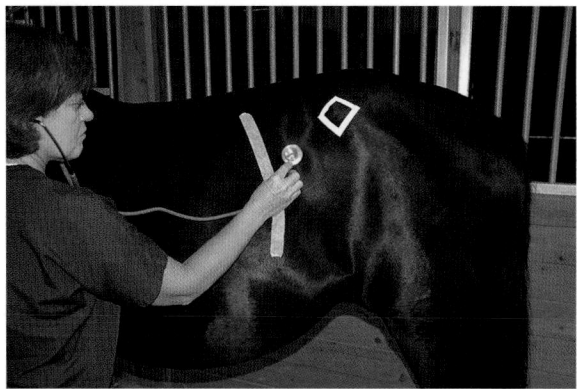

FIGURE 7-30 Landmarks for abdominal auscultation in the flank area are the point of the hip (tuber coxae) and the last rib.

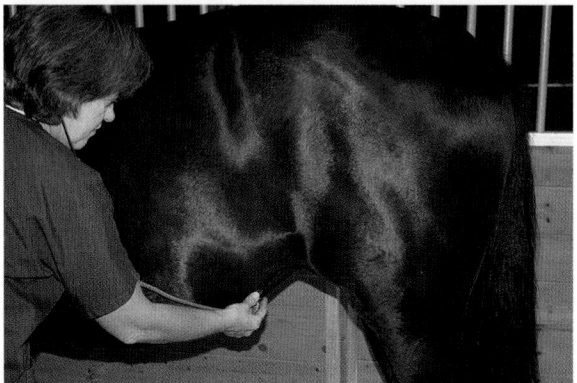

FIGURE 7-31 Auscultation of the lower left abdominal quadrant.

Experience is required to distinguish active motility from passive sounds.

Abdominal auscultation should be performed on both sides of the horse. Although auscultation can be performed at any location on the abdominal wall, common sites for auscultation are in the areas known as the right and left *flanks*. The flank is the slightly depressed area between the pelvis and the caudal margin of the rib cage. The point of the hip (tuber coxae) identifies the dorsal extent of the flank area (Figure 7-30). Horses may be sensitive in the flank and abdominal regions, so these areas should be approached slowly and gently. A good approach is to place the hand with the stethoscope on the horse's back and slowly slide it to the flank or lower abdominal area.

A standard four-point auscultation is sufficient for most patients. A stethoscope is used to auscultate the upper flank and the lower flank on both sides of the abdomen. The four points of auscultation are referred to as *upper left*, *upper right*, *lower left*, and *lower right abdominal quadrants* (Figure 7-31). Intestinal motility sounds, also called *borborygmi*, have been described as sounding like thunder rumbling or an approaching freight train. These sounds usually are associated with coordinated, normal patterns of large intestinal motility. The number of borborygmi per minute is counted in each abdominal quadrant; the stethoscope should be left in place for *at least 1 minute* at *each* of the four auscultation points to get an accurate count. "Normal" motility is considered to be one to three borborygmi per minute in each abdominal quadrant. More than this is

Findings from the four-point auscultation are recorded in the medical record using a grid that identifies each abdominal quadrant.

Upper Left Quadrant	Upper Right Quadrant
Lower Left Quadrant	Lower Right Quadrant

Results of auscultation at each location are recorded as follows:

0 = no motility heard
+1 = hypomotility (<1 borborygmus/minute)
+2 = normal motility (1-3 borborygmi/minute)
+3 = hypermotility (>3 borborygmi/minute)

For example, a horse with hypomotility in the lower right quadrant and a normal number of borborygmi in all other quadrants would be recorded as follows.

+2	+2
+2	+1

considered to be hypermotility, and less than this rate is considered to be hypomotility. The complete absence of **borborygmus** is equated with "intestinal standstill," properly termed ***ileus***. Ileus often indicates serious intestinal disease and is associated with increased morbidity and mortality in horses with colic. Auscultation in colic patients may be confusing because gas and fluid "tinkling" sounds may still be heard in horses with complete ileus. These are passive sounds and should not be confused with the motility of normally functioning intestines.

Findings of four-point abdominal auscultation are recorded in the medical record using the grid system in Box 7-2.

> **TECHNICIAN NOTE** The presence of intestinal sounds does not always indicate the presence of intestinal motility.

Mucous Membranes

Mucous membranes are tissues that have the ability to produce and secrete mucus. The mucous membrane color is helpful for disease diagnosis. Several mucous membranes are readily visible to the examiner: the gums (gingiva), conjunctiva of the eye, lining of the nostrils, and inner surfaces of the vulva in females (Figures 7-32 and 7-33). The inner surface of the ear pinna is not a mucous membrane, although it may be useful for detecting icterus and clotting disorders.

Mucous membrane color is usually light to dark pink. The color may change with abnormalities of blood perfusion and with oxygen content of the blood and other diseases. Cyanosis is a bluish tint that usually indicates extremely low oxygen

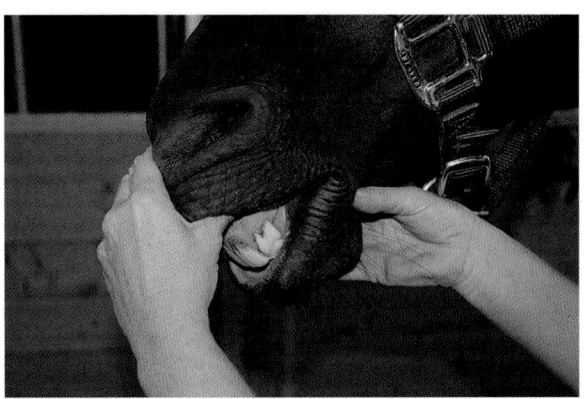

FIGURE 7-32 Examination of the gums. The upper lip is gently elevated to the extent necessary for the gum tissue to be seen.

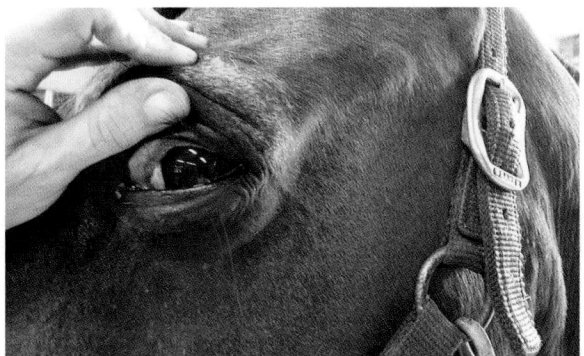

FIGURE 7-33 Examination of the conjunctiva. The upper lid is gently elevated upward, without pinching or pressing.

content in the tissue. Brick red coloration indicates bacterial septicemia and/or septic shock. Endotoxemia in the horse has the unique characteristic of producing a purple gum color that appears along the margin of the teeth and gums; this is commonly referred to as a *toxic line*. Yellowish coloring of the gums indicates icterus, usually resulting from liver dysfunction or abnormal hemolysis of red blood cells. Pale mucous membranes may indicate anemia or poor perfusion, although many normal horses have naturally pale pink gum color. Clotting disorders may produce visible hemorrhage in mucous membranes. Small pinpoint hemorrhages less than 1 mm in diameter are called *petechial hemorrhages* or *petechiae*; *ecchymotic hemorrhage* produces slightly larger hemorrhages 1 mm to 1 cm in diameter.

Mucous membranes are often assessed for moisture and are commonly described as moist, dry, or tacky, or in other subjective terms. This information is less useful than the membrane color.

Hydration Status

The hydration status of an animal is important information. It may be measured with laboratory tests or estimated from the physical examination. Two common methods of assessing the hydration of an animal on a physical examination are the skin turgor test and the capillary refill time.

Skin turgor is assessed by the *skin pinch* or *skin snap* test. Loose skin over the lateral aspect of the neck is briefly and firmly pinched with the fingers and is allowed to retract back

to its original position. In normally hydrated animals, the skin should return ("snap") promptly back to its original position in approximately 1 second or less. Dehydration (>5% dehydration) prolongs the response to greater than 1 second. Severely dehydrated animals may take 8 seconds or longer for the skin to retract. Skin turgor is less reliable in obese animals; fat in the cervical area may falsely improve the skin snap. Conversely, thin horses and horses older than 15 years may have delayed skin snap response, regardless of hydration status.

Capillary refill time (CRT) is a reflection of cardiac output, which is directly affected by hydration status. Prolonged CRT is usually associated with low cardiac output, which is most commonly caused by inadequate hydration of the animal. Low cardiac output can also result from decreased heart function. CRT is assessed by pressing briefly but firmly on the gums with a fingertip to produce a "blanched" white spot. The time for the original gum color to return to the blanched spot is counted in seconds. The original color should return in less than 2.5 seconds. A CRT greater than 2.5 seconds is considered abnormally delayed. Dehydration and shock are the most common causes of a prolonged CRT in the horse. Severe dehydration and severe shock may produce a greatly prolonged CRT—from 5 to 8 seconds.

> **TECHNICIAN NOTE** CRT is more accurate than skin turgor in assessing an animal's hydration status.

Height/Weight Measurement

Height and weight measurements are needed for a variety of purposes. A height measurement may be required as part of an insurance or prepurchase examination, for breed registration, or for entry into certain horse show classes. The weight measurement is usually obtained for calculating the proper dose of drugs and therapeutic substances and for formulating the diet of the animal.

Height may be estimated or measured precisely. Rough estimates may be made with a height-weight tape. This instrument is essentially a tape measure, marked on one side for height measurement in hands (1 hand = 4 inches) and on the other side for weight measurement. Ideally, the horse should stand on a firm, level surface with its weight distributed evenly on all four legs. The horse's head should not be elevated or lowered but should be in a horizontal position with the neck parallel to the ground. One end of the measuring tape is held on the ground just behind the horse's forelimb. The tape is then stretched vertically to the withers and the height read at the level of the highest point of the withers. The tape gives an approximation of the animal's height.

For precise determination of height, commercially made rigid measuring rulers are available. These rulers are made of metal and include bubble-style levels to ensure that the ruler is not tilted when the measurement is taken. The animal should stand squarely on a firm, level surface with the head and neck held parallel to the ground. The measurement is taken at the last mane hair or the highest point of the withers, depending on the breed registry or rules of competition.

Weight may be roughly estimated with the height-weight tape or taken more precisely with a livestock scale. The height-weight tape has one side that is calibrated for weight measurement; weight tick marks are based on measurements around the girth of the horse. The tape is applied to encircle the horse at its girth, which is the area caudal to the withers and just behind the forelimb (Figure 7-34). The weight tape is formulated from logarithms of "normal" animals and may be inaccurate for excessively thin or obese animals. The build of an animal may also affect the results. Height-weight tapes designed for cattle are not accurate for horses.

Precise weights for large animals may be obtained with livestock scales. Digital livestock scales have a walk-over design and are popular at many hospitals and practices. Traditional livestock scales are somewhat cumbersome to use and have largely been replaced by digital walk-over scales.

PHYSICAL EXAMINATION OF RUMINANTS

The physical examination begins with an initial visual observation of the animal from a distance. The animal's posture, behavior, body condition, and alertness are easily observed. More specific signs, such as breathing pattern, respiratory noise, lameness, skin wounds, and muscle atrophy, may also be noted. When working with any species, some understanding of basic instincts and typical behaviors is essential for interpreting what is seen through observation. Although ruminants share many physiologic traits, they do not share a common "mentality," and behavioral differences among various ruminant species must be appreciated. This is especially important when observing an individual's interactions with the herd.

> **TECHNICIAN NOTE** Valuable information can be obtained by observing an animal from a distance before the physical examination is performed.

CASE PRESENTATION 7-2

Signalment: 9-year-old, Standardbred gelding
Presenting complaint: Colic
History: A 9-year-old Standardbred gelding was admitted to the equine hospital with a history of abdominal pain of 3 days' duration. The referring veterinarian treated this horse on the farm with mineral oil and water administered via nasogastric intubation, and provided medication as needed for pain control. All grain and hay have been withheld since treatment began, but free access to water has been allowed. The horse has not been observed to pass manure in 3 days, and its discomfort is increasing. The horse was referred to the hospital for further assessment and treatment, including surgery if necessary.

Subjective:
Mentation: Alert but slightly depressed
Behavior: Paws occasionally; frequently assumes urination stance but does not urinate
Mucous membrane color: Pale pink with mild yellowish discoloration
Eyes: Mild yellowish discoloration of sclerae
GI motility: Hypomotility, all abdominal quadrants

Objective:
T 100.8; P 52; R 12
CRT= 3 seconds
Lays down and rolls 2-3×/hour
Defecated 3 hard, dry fecal balls during examination

Assessment (prioritized technician evaluations, with rationale):
1. Abdominal pain (patient displays clinical signs consistent with abdominal pain: pawing, stretching as if to urinate, rolling, elevated pulse rate).
2. Dehydration (increased CRT, increased pulse rate).
3. Icterus (yellowish cast to mucous membranes and sclerae).

Plan (prioritized technician evaluations, with interventions):
1. Abdominal pain: closely monitor for signs of increasing pain and notify veterinarian immediately if pain increases. Risk for self-trauma and injury to veterinary staff.
2. Dehydration: anticipate need for IV catheterization and IV fluid therapy. Monitor vital signs.
3. Icterus: anticipate need for blood work (CBC and chemistry panel).

Technician Case Notes
- The most accurate indicator of the need for exploratory abdominal surgery in a colic case is the horse's level of pain. Pain is more accurate than any other physical examination finding or laboratory result. Close monitoring of the patient's pain level is crucial in case management; signs of increasing pain constitute a true emergency.
- Although passing 3 fecal balls may seem insignificant compared with the normal volume of a typical defecation, when observing a colic patient this finding can be highly significant to the clinician. Not only should small fecal volumes be noted on the patient's chart, but also the character of the feces. If mineral oil has been administered via nasogastric intubation, its appearance on feces or around the anal/perineal area is highly significant and should be noted.
- Horses may develop icterus when food is withheld for 24 hours or longer. This type of icterus is properly referred to as *fasting hyperbilirubinemia* and usually occurs with no clinical signs of liver dysfunction. Serum chemistry will show an increase in total bilirubin (unconjugated), but all other liver parameters are typically normal. The icterus requires no special treatment and will resolve rapidly when the patient is allowed to eat.

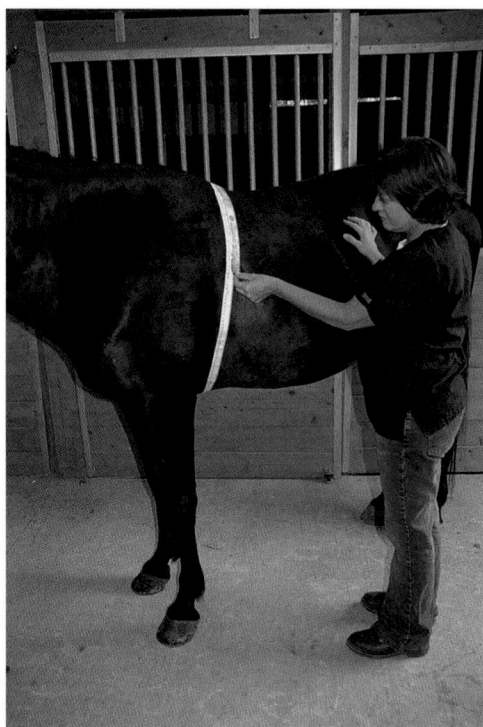

FIGURE 7-34 The weight tape is positioned around the thorax at the girth, just caudal to the withers.

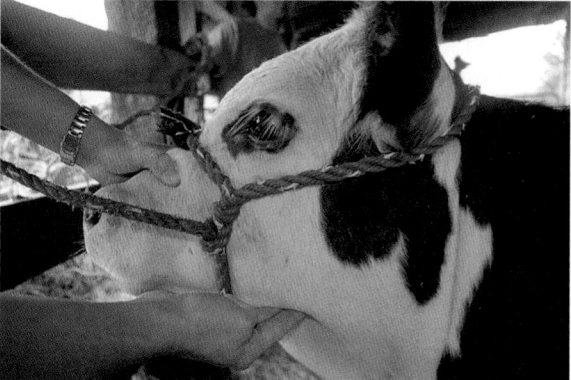

FIGURE 7-35 Palpation of the arterial pulse at the facial artery, where it crosses the ventromedial aspect of the mandible.

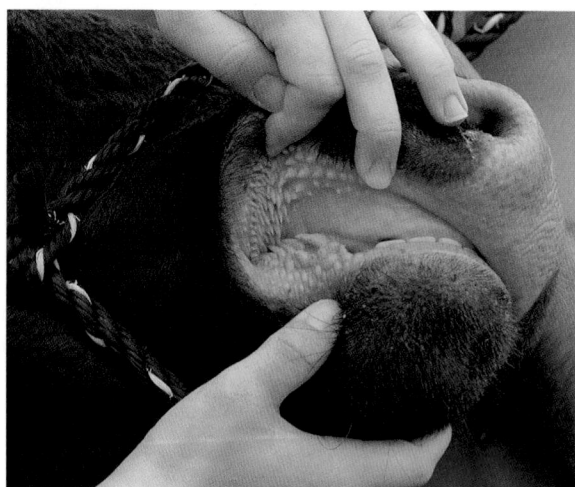

FIGURE 7-36 Normal mucous membranes in ruminants are pink and moist.

Direct "hands-on" physical examination typically includes the TPR, heart and lung auscultation, abdominal auscultation and assessment of rumen function, hydration status, and examination of mucous membranes. Animals must be adequately restrained for this portion of the physical examination, and methods of restraint used for cattle, sheep, and goats are quite different. Cattle are typically restrained in a chute, whereas sheep and goats are usually restrained manually (see Chapter 6 for additional information on restraint of large animals).

A temperature is taken rectally, similar to the procedure in horses. When the rectal temperature of the goat is taken, a dark brown, waxy material may be seen near the anus; this is a normal secretion produced by sebaceous glands under the tail head. The pulse can be palpated readily at the facial artery; the coccygeal, median (forelimb), and great metatarsal (hindlimb) arteries are also available (Figure 7-35). The femoral artery is useful in sheep and goats. The respiratory rate is best taken by counting chest excursions from a distance before herding or handling; the excitement and fear of herding and restraint can cause dramatic increases in respiratory rate, especially in hot environmental temperatures, which will not reflect the true respiratory rate of the animal at rest. Ruminants, unlike horses, are capable of open-mouth breathing; when observed, it is usually considered to be a sign of distress or heat stress (usually when environmental temperature exceeds 85° F). Abdominal breathing is normal in ruminants. Normal values for TPR are given in Table 7-7.

Heart auscultation is performed using the same anatomic landmarks as in the horse. The shoulder joint and the olecranon indicate the dorsal-ventral position of the heart. The caudal border of the triceps muscle indicates the cranial-caudal position, generally corresponding to the fourth to fifth intercostal space. Auscultated cardiac sounds are normally only S_1 and S_2 in cattle (unlike the horse, where any combination of S_3 and S_4 may accompany S_1 and S_2). Borders for lung auscultation in the ruminant are between the fifth rib cranially and the eleventh rib caudally. If it is necessary to induce deep breathing for lung auscultation, the nostrils and the mouth (because ruminants can mouth breathe) can be held closed for about a minute to stimulate deeper breathing and a higher respiratory rate.

The mucous membranes should be pink and moist, with a CRT of 1 to 2 seconds (Figure 7-36). If it is necessary to fully open the mouth for an examination, placing the fingers into the interdental space and pressing on the hard palate encourages opening of the mouth; the tongue can be quickly grasped and brought to the side at the commissure of the lips, where it encourages the animal to keep the mouth open. Alternatively, a mouth speculum may be used. The tongue of cattle has a single deep transverse groove across its dorsal surface; this groove is often mistaken for a laceration. The molars of ruminants may be sharp and jagged, and caution must be used whenever the hands are placed into the mouth. When examining the head and mouth area, be aware of the possibility of being struck with the animal's head if it is not properly restrained. Adult cattle especially can cause serious injury by striking with the head.

When standing near a ruminant or when auscultating the thorax or trachea, occasional low-pitched fluttering sounds may be heard; this is eructation (burping), which is normal in ruminants. Eructation rates are approximately 18/hour in cattle, and 10/hour in sheep and goats.

Evaluation of the ruminant abdomen includes an assessment of rumen contractions. The rumen occupies most of the left side of the abdominal cavity. The number of rumen contractions per minute may be counted by auscultation directly over the caudolateral rib cage or the paralumbar fossa on the left side. Rumen contractions sound like a deep-pitched rumbling or "thunderstorm" noise, which gets gradually louder as the contraction wave approaches the stethoscope. Rumen contractions can also be counted by ballottement (palpation) by pressing both fists firmly into the left paralumbar fossa (use one fist in the sheep and the goat). The fists are allowed to remain against the body wall for 1 minute. Each rumen contraction will be felt as a wave passing under the hands, pushing the hands slightly outward. The normal animal will have 1 to 2 contractions/minute. Hypomotility and absence of motility (ileus) are abnormal findings; hypermotility of the rumen is uncommon. Auscultation of the right side of the abdomen usually reveals few sounds; this is normal in ruminants.

The shape of the abdomen is observed by standing behind the animal, facing the head, and comparing the right and left abdominal outlines or "silhouettes." The overall shape of the right and left abdominal outlines should be similar, with the overall outline of the cow resembling a pear (wider at the lower flanks than at the paralumbar fossae) (Figure 7-37). The paralumbar fossae normally should be flat or slightly sunken. Accumulation of gas within certain portions of the GI tract (tympany or *"bloat"*) can produce asymmetry and enlargement of the abdominal wall. The most common location for bloat, the rumen, appears as an enlargement of the left paralumbar fossa; this has been referred to as a *papple*-shaped abdomen, where the left side resembles an apple and the right side a pear. Severe abdominal gas accumulation can cause protrusion of the paralumbar fossa on both sides of the animal, changing the normal pear shape to one that resembles an apple.

> **TECHNICIAN NOTE** The abdominal "silhouette," viewed from behind the animal, provides useful diagnostic information for possible GI diseases.

Gas accumulations can also be detected by simultaneous percussion and auscultation, a technique commonly known as **abdominal pinging.** The stethoscope is held in place with one hand, while the other hand is used to snap a finger

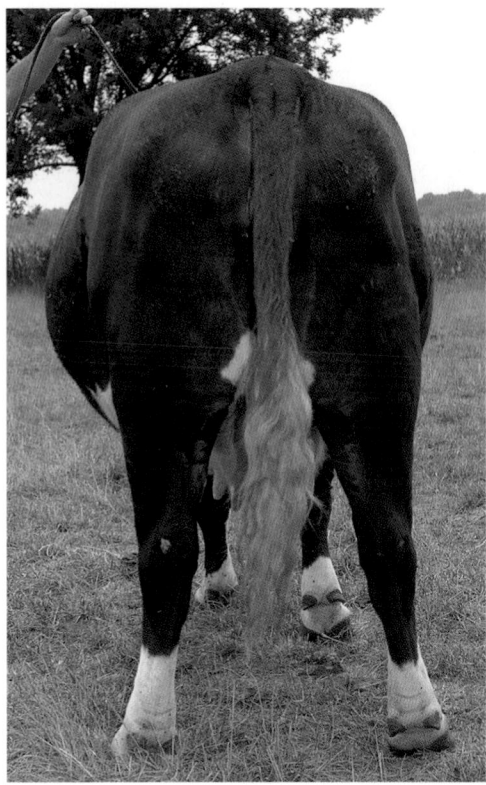

FIGURE 7-37 Normal "pear" abdominal shape of the cow as viewed from behind. As a result of the anatomic location of the rumen, the left side may appear slightly fuller than the right.

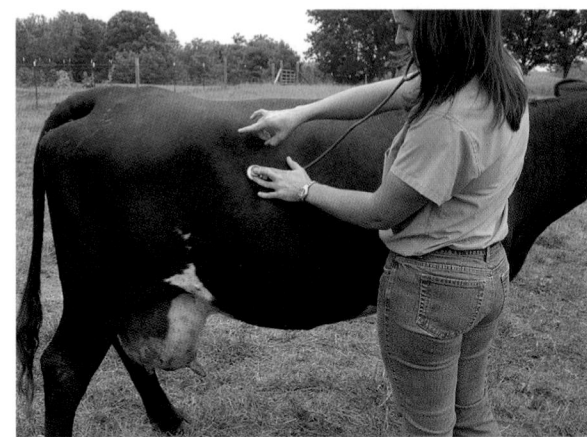

FIGURE 7-38 Proper technique for abdominal "pinging." The stethoscope is held in place while snapping a finger sharply against the abdominal wall in the vicinity of the stethoscope head.

against the abdominal wall at several locations around the stethoscope head (Figure 7-38). Gas accumulations make a resonant tympanic "ping" sound, like a high-pitched drum. Pings are significant findings and generally indicate abnormal position or contents of one or more GI tract organs. Note that solid organs and non-GI organs cannot accumulate gas (with the exception of the uterus, which is extremely rare) and do not create pings. Pinging should be performed on both sides of the abdomen and may detect abnormalities before they are visible as external enlargement of the abdomen.

The character of feces and urine, if available for observation, should be evaluated. Fecal character varies among ruminants. Cattle defecate 12 to 18 times/day; the feces have a semisolid "cow-plop" or "cow-pie" consistency, without distinct form. Goats produce well-formed feces in the shape of small, solid pellets. Sheep feces are also pelleted. The color of the feces depends on the diet, ranging from green to dark brown. Undigested roughage fibers in the fecal material are an abnormal finding that may indicate dysfunction of the rumen and/or reticulum.

RECOMMENDED READINGS

Fubini SL, Ducharme NG: Farm animal surgery, St Louis, 2004, Saunders.

Hanie EA: Large animal clinical procedures for veterinary technicians, St Louis, 2006, Mosby.

McCurnin DM, Poffenbarger EM: Small animal physical diagnosis and clinical procedures, Philadelphia, 1991, Saunders.

Pugh DG: Sheep and goat medicine, ed 2, St Louis, 2012, Saunders.

Smith MC, Sherman DM: Goat medicine, ed 2, Hoboken, 2009, Wiley-Blackwell.

Speirs VC: Clinical examination of horses, Philadelphia, 1997, Saunders.

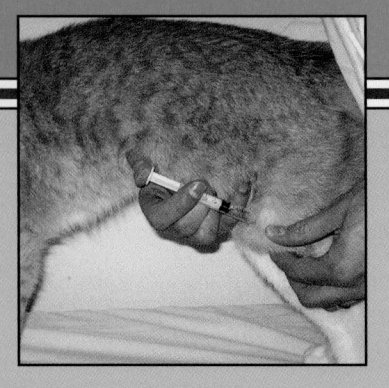

Preventive Health Programs

Carolyn J. Hammer, Stacey M. Ostby, Christopher T. Reetz, and Sarah A. Wagner

KEY TERMS

Active immunity
Adjuvant
Anaphylaxis
Antitoxin
Biosecurity
Colostrum
Congenital
Fomite
Needle teeth
Passive immunity
Toxoid

OUTLINE

Preventive Health Programs for Dogs and Cats, 260
Lifelong Wellness, 260
Grooming, 262
Immunity, 262
Parasite Prevention, 274
Preventive Health Program for Horses, 275
Physical Examination, 275
Vaccinations, 275

Parasites, 284
Dental Care, 284
Hoof Care, 285
Nutrition, 285
Preventive Health Program for Livestock Species, 285
Swine, 285
Cattle, 286
Small Ruminants: Sheep and Goats, 288

LEARNING OBJECTIVES

When you have completed this chapter, you will be able to:

1. Define, pronounce and spell all of the Key Terms.
2. Compare and contrast the issues and information discussed during wellness visits at various life stages of a dog or cat (puppy/kitten, adult, senior/geriatric).
3. Do the following regarding immunity in cats and dogs:
   - Differentiate between active and passive immunity, and discuss why it is necessary to administer a series of vaccinations to young puppies and kittens.
   - Differentiate between noninfectious and infectious types of vaccines, and explain the purpose of adjuvants.
   - Describe the storage, handling, reconstitution, and dosing of animal vaccines.
   - List the recommended administration locations for various canine and feline vaccinations.
   - Distinguish between core and noncore vaccines, and explain what is meant by duration of immunity.
   - Identify core and noncore vaccines for dogs and cats.
   - Describe potential adverse vaccine events and how to deal with various adverse events should they occur.
4. Explain the importance of discussing potential canine and feline parasitic infections with owners, and describe general preventive measures that can be taken.
5. Describe a routine preventive health program for horses including physical examination, vaccinations, prevention of parasitic infections, dental and hoof care, and nutrition.
6. Describe vaccines and other preventive measures that can be used during various life stages of pigs, cattle, sheep, and goats.

INTRODUCTION

Preventive health programs are an important part of veterinary practice and encompass a wide range of issues. Through these programs, veterinary health care team members have the opportunity to anticipate the risks of disease for each individual patient and to tailor recommendations to the owner based on information specific to the animal, such as its age and the environment in which it lives. In this way, many diseases and disorders that once were common can be entirely avoided or detected early on, when treating the condition successfully is more likely.

Preventive health programs are important for all stages of an animal's life. Although the focus may change depending on the age of the patient, underlying concepts remain the same. Routine examinations, screening tests, and client education are key components of responsible health care. Preventive health programs are especially important in situations where animals are housed in group situations, as in nonprofit animal shelters or animal-centered farming enterprises. In these situations, preventive health care can help to decrease the likelihood that large populations of animals may contract contagious diseases, which could have catastrophic consequences both for the health of the animals and for the economic viability of the business.

This chapter offers a general overview of preventive health measures for dogs, cats, horses, and common livestock species. For information about preventive health care specific to the neonate, refer to Chapter 21. Preventive health care information for geriatric patients can be found in Chapter 35. Finally, information about training young animals can be found in Chapter 5.

PREVENTIVE HEALTH PROGRAMS FOR DOGS AND CATS

LIFELONG WELLNESS

Regular wellness visits are important for maintaining health in dogs and cats throughout their life. The American Association of Feline Practitioners (AAFP) has identified six life stages in cats: Kitten (0 to 6 months), Junior (7 months to 2 years), Adult (3 to 6 years), Mature (7 to 10 years), Senior (11 to 14 years), and Geriatric. Refer to the AAFP's online Feline Life Stages Guidelines for specific recommendations regarding preventive health care in cats (http://www.catvets.com/uploads/PDF/Feline%20Life%20Stage%20Guidelines%20Final.pdf).

In the past, regular visits to a veterinary practice were predominantly driven by the need for pets to receive their annual immunizations. As vaccination recommendations have changed in more recent years, other important themes that were addressed during these visits are being emphasized more. A thorough physical examination should be performed during each appointment. Routine examinations establish what is normal for healthy patients and help detect abnormalities of which the owner may not be aware. When a problem is detected early in the disease process, a favorable outcome of treatment for the condition becomes more likely. Routine wellness visits also give the veterinary health care team an opportunity to update subjective patient data, such as changes in the animal's life, and to make recommendations accordingly. They provide an important opportunity to educate the client on various physical and psychological needs of the patient as the animal matures and to ensure client compliance when the pet becomes ill.

Wellness in Puppies and Kittens

The initial visit to a veterinary practice for a healthy puppy or kitten typically occurs at 6 to 8 weeks of age. A lot of information is discussed with the owner during this appointment; in many practices, extra time is designated for a pet's first visit. The pet is examined with emphasis on identifying any **congenital** defects that may be present. Depending on the contractual agreement of sale and on the laws of the state where the animal was purchased, the first appointment may identify a serious condition deemed unfit for purchase, and the owner may be entitled to reimbursement or may be allowed to exchange or return the animal to the dealer. For kittens, the initial visit often involves performing a blood test to check for feline leukemia virus (FeLV) and feline immunodeficiency virus (FIV). Other blood tests that address specific genetic diseases are available and may be discussed with and offered to owners of breeds predisposed to these problems. Parasite control is also addressed, and owners may be instructed to bring with them a fecal specimen from their pet for early detection and treatment of parasitism. This is an important opportunity to educate clients about the need for routine parasite control and the potential risks of certain parasites to humans, particularly of ocular larval migrans

in young children who are exposed to roundworm eggs. Depending on results of the fecal flotation test and any previous history of deworming, antiparasitic medications may be dispensed. Clients are educated about the risks of heartworm disease and flea infestation in both cats and dogs. Free samples of heartworm medication and flea control products may be dispensed to owners at this time, along with informational brochures about these samples.

The initial visit is also a good time for the veterinary health care team to educate the client on basic husbandry practices and the normal progression of a pet's development. This is especially important for new pet owners, who may not be aware of what is involved in properly caring for a pet. Topics that are typically addressed include the following:

1. Instruction on house-breaking puppies and litter box–training kittens.
2. Nutritional information, including appropriate pet food, amounts to feed, and frequency of feeding.
3. Basic socialization and animal training techniques.
4. Housing requirements for the pet, including appropriate outdoor shelters.
5. Tooth development, eruption times, and the importance of dental care throughout the animal's life.
6. Techniques on animal-proofing the house, including recognizing and removing potential foreign bodies from the pet's environment and informing owners about foods and common household products that are toxic to animals.
7. Exercise requirements.
8. Grooming requirements.
9. The importance of spaying and neutering and ideal ages when these procedures should be performed on pets.

Details about spaying or neutering should be discussed with owners if their pet is not to be bred. The client must be informed about both the medical benefits and the surgical and anesthetic risks of spaying and neutering. Spaying eliminates unwanted pregnancies, heat-related behaviors, ovarian cancer, and pyometra. It also decreases the likelihood of mammary carcinoma if performed before the second heat. Neutering may eliminate roaming, inter-male aggression, enlargement of the prostate, and testicular cancer. Surgical risk to the animal has been minimized with that use of state-of-the-art anesthetics and sterile techniques, but nevertheless, risks of adverse reactions to medications, unexpected hemorrhage, and postoperative complications are present. Informed consent forms should be signed by the owner before all surgical procedures are performed.

After the initial visit, puppies and kittens are examined 1 or 2 more times at 3- to 4-week intervals. During these visits, the pet is reexamined and receives booster vaccinations. At this time, the veterinary staff can get updates on how the pet is doing at home and can answer any questions that the owner may have.

Initial puppy and kitten wellness visits are extremely important in setting a client on a path toward responsible and reliable pet ownership. In addition, these initial appointments give the veterinary health care team an opportunity to provide excellent service and to create a positive experience for first-time clients in the hope that it will give rise to a lasting relationship for the life of the pet.

> **TECHNICIAN NOTE** Initial wellness visits for puppies and kittens typically occur every 3 to 4 weeks until the animal is approximately 16 weeks of age, and usually coincide with the animal's vaccination schedule.

Wellness in Adult Dogs and in Adult and Mature Cats

As young dogs and cats mature into adults, their physical and psychological needs change. New recommendations regarding the pet's nutrition must be made as the animal transitions from food required for growth to maintenance diets. Immunization protocols also change. After 1-year boosters have been administered, many of the core vaccines are recommended to be administered every 3 years. This does not mean, however, that adult dogs and cats do not need to continue to visit the veterinary practice regularly. According to current American Animal Hospital Association (AAHA)–American Veterinary Medical Association (AVMA) Canine and Feline Preventive Health Guidelines, dogs and cats should be examined annually, with some animals requiring more frequent examinations, based on the needs of each individual patient. Physical examination remains one of the most important aspects of these visits; it allows the veterinarian to detect potential changes that may have gone unnoticed by the owner and to address any current problems that the animal may be experiencing.

Dental health is assessed. As dogs and cats age, the amount of dental disease and tartar tends to increase, and by examining them regularly, the veterinary health care team can make recommendations on dental care. Testing for various regional infectious diseases, such as heartworm disease in dogs and cats, and Lyme disease in dogs, is also commonly performed during these visits. At this time, owners acquire medications for parasite control, such as heartworm prevention and flea and tick control. As the pet ages, routine blood and urine tests (complete blood count [CBC], chemistry panel, and urinalysis) are recommended to establish baseline levels and to screen for underlying disease.

Finally, these visits offer veterinary technicians important opportunities to educate clients about the changing requirements of their pet as it ages and to make recommendations based on risks and needs of the individual patient. It is especially important to impress upon clients the importance of regular preventive health care to ensure the long-term health of their pet.

> **TECHNICIAN NOTE** AAHA-AVMA Canine and Feline Preventive Health Guidelines recommend that adult dogs and cats be examined annually, with some animals requiring more frequent visits.

CASE PRESENTATION 8-1

Bailey, a gray and white, 4-year-old, spayed female, domestic shorthair cat, presents for her annual preventive health appointment. As the veterinary technician, you escort the client and the patient back to an examination room and obtain the following information about Bailey:
- Weight: 17 lbs
- Heart rate: 170 bpm
- Respiratory rate: 24 bpm
- Temperature: 101.5° F
- Information from owner: Bailey's appetite is good, and she has no problems that the owner has noticed. The cat is not on any medications. Bailey is indoor-only, but occasionally goes out onto a patio area that is enclosed by a fence. Bailey is the only pet in the house.

Physical Examination Findings

A moderate amount of tartar is present on the cat's teeth. When the cat is combed, a few small black flecks of material are visible in the comb mixed in with the hair. All other examination findings are unremarkable. You ask the client if she has noticed the cat scratching herself lately, and the client verifies that Bailey has been scratching herself occasionally, but by no means regularly.

You prepare vaccines and other materials for the veterinarian and enter the following information into the medical record using the SOAP format:

Date: 8/18/XX, Barb Smith, CVT

S: Good appetite; not on any medications; owner reports "indoor-only" but cat has access to enclosed patio; sole pet in household; no problems according to owner; moderate tartar on teeth, evidence of flea dirt; occasionally scratches; all other physical examination findings WNL

O: 17 lbs, HR = 170 bpm, RR = 24 bpm, T = 101.5° F

A: 1. Altered oral health
   2. Overweight
   3. Flea infestation and risk of transmission
   4. Client knowledge deficit

P: 1. If ordered, dispense:
- Dental and oral care products
- House treatment products and flea medications
- Prescription weight reduction diet

   2. Educate client:
- Treatment for fleas in home, in yard, and on pet
- Home dental health care
- Importance of regular professional dental cleaning
- Weight loss program

Senior and Geriatric Animal Wellness

According to the American Association of Feline Practitioners Senior Care Guidelines, cats are classified as "senior" when they are between the ages of 11 and 14 years. At 15 years and beyond, cats are considered geriatric. For dogs, exact age ranges are not as well defined because wide variations have been noted in the life span of large breed dogs versus small breed dogs. The American Animal Hospital Association Senior Care Guidelines for Dogs and Cats define seniors as those animals in the last 25% of their predicted life span. As animals reach this stage of their life, it becomes more likely that some sort of illness will develop. Because one of the goals of preventive health programs is to detect disease early in its onset, it is recommended that animals in this age group visit the veterinary practice every 6 months. Specific attention is paid to weight, mobility, dental health, and psychological needs. A thorough history is necessary to determine how the owner feels the pet is doing. Older animals may experience vision and hearing loss; it is important to establish whether this is occurring by asking pointed questions directed at these areas. It is also common for small animals to develop joint problems as they age, and nutraceuticals that promote joint health, regular moderate exercise, and use of nonsteroidal anti-inflammatory drugs (NSAIDs) may be beneficial in controlling pain caused by osteoarthritis (OA). Changes in weight must also be addressed because weight gain may occur in aging animals that are less active. This may add stress to arthritic joints, further decreasing their mobility. Unexpected weight loss is a common initial sign of illness that may be detected before the owner notices overt signs of clinical disease. Laboratory tests such as CBC, blood chemistry, and urinalysis are recommended to establish a minimum database for senior and geriatric pets. For cats, thyroxine (T_4) levels are often recommended because hyperthyroidism is common among elderly cats. In dogs, hypothyroidism can be problematic, particularly in large breed dogs, and obtaining T_4 levels in these animals can be beneficial. These tests help to detect disease in its early stages. Immunizations and parasite control continue to be addressed during elderly care appointments; as with all wellness visits, client education is paramount.

> **TECHNICIAN NOTE** It is recommended that wellness visits be scheduled every 6 months for senior and geriatric dogs and cats.

GROOMING

Proper grooming is an important exercise that can contribute to an animal's overall general health. Bathing, nail trimming, ear cleaning, brushing, and in some cases hair trimming are procedures that can help prevent dermatologic disease and can contribute to the pet's overall comfort. Regular ear cleaning, for example, may help prevent ear infection in dogs that routinely swim or in breeds predisposed to ear problems. Many grooming issues are initially addressed during a pet's first appointment. Information on techniques and the frequency of performing these tasks should be provided by veterinary health care team members. It is also important to make sure that owners of long-haired pets understand that many of these breeds require regular visits to a groomer for hair trimming. For new pet owners, it may be helpful to offer recommendations on local groomers that can offer these services. As animals age, their grooming needs may change. Older dogs, for example, that no longer go for long walks on the pavement because of degenerative joint disease and decreased mobility may require more frequent nail trims.

IMMUNITY

Active Immunity versus Passive Immunity

Immunity against disease can be acquired actively or passively. **Active immunity** occurs in the body when the immune system develops antibodies to antigens such as viruses, yeast, or bacteria. The animal can be exposed to the antigen via natural exposure from the environment or by injection with a noninfectious form of the antigen in a vaccine. When an animal is exposed to a pathogen in the environment, it may contract the illness and mount an active immune response subsequent to being ill.

Passive immunity can occur in the following three ways:
1. In utero when antibodies pass through the placenta from the dam to the fetus.
2. In newborns from the consumption of antibody-rich colostrum.
3. By intravenous infusion of antibody-rich plasma (usually given to foals that failed to gain adequate levels of antibodies in steps 1 and 2 above).

In dogs and cats, antibodies are transferred almost entirely via the consumption of **colostrum**, which the neonate must ingest within the first 24 hours after birth. Unfortunately, passive immunity lasts for a relatively short time, and the neonate eventually becomes susceptible to the diseases it was once protected against. Vaccinations therefore are administered to puppies and kittens to stimulate an active immune response in the animal, which protects it from disease for a longer time.

A protective level of passive immunity is determined by several factors, including the amount of colostrum ingested and absorbed, the concentrations of maternal antibodies in the colostrum, and the rate at which maternal antibodies are degraded in the puppy or the kitten. High levels of passively acquired antibodies in neonates render immunizations ineffective because maternal antibodies limit the neonate's ability to mount an active immune response. It is generally accepted that puppies and kittens are able to mount an active immune response (immune competence) sometime between 6 and 12 weeks of age. Because multiple factors contribute to the timing of when passive immunity is lost and when the animal is immunocompetent, it is difficult to know the precise times when the animal is immunologically vulnerable to disease, and when its immune system is mature enough to mount an active immune response to immunization. This is why certain vaccines are administered to puppies and kittens every 3 to 4 weeks until they are 16 weeks of age, the goal being to vaccinate the animal at the earliest possible opportunity to stimulate active immunity. On the other hand, only one or two vaccinations (depending on the vaccine) are necessary to stimulate an immune response in older animals because passive immunity can no longer interfere with the animal's own active immune response to the vaccine.

For certain diseases, young puppies and kittens require a series of vaccinations to ensure that an adequate active immune response to the antigen occurs at the earliest possible time, once passive immunity is lost.

Vaccine Types

Many different types of vaccines have been developed over the years, and each type works in a slightly different way. The ultimate goal of all vaccines, however, is the same. Vaccines are used to stimulate an active immune response, so that an animal (or human) develops immunity against a disease. At the same time, the vaccine must not cause the host to develop the disease itself, so the contents of the vaccine must be altered. In the 2011 American Animal Hospital Association Canine Vaccination Guidelines, vaccine types are classified into two major categories. Noninfectious vaccines include whole pathogens, which are killed, and subunits, which are parts of pathogens. As the name of the category implies, the contents of the vaccine are unable to infect the animal. Rabies vaccine is an example of a noninfectious vaccine. A limitation of using noninfectious contents in a vaccine is that the amount of antigen associated with pathogens in the vaccine may not be adequate to stimulate a strong enough immune response to produce protective immunity for the animal. Remember that the ultimate goal of the vaccine is for the animal to develop adequate levels of immunity to protect itself from actual natural exposure to the disease. To ensure that an adequate immune response occurs, **adjuvants** are typically added to the contents of the vaccine. Adjuvants are substances that help stimulate a stronger immune response to antigens contained within a vaccine. An example of an adjuvant is aluminum hydroxide. One way that a vaccine adjuvant may work is by prolonging the release of antigen into the body over an extended time. Advantages of noninfectious types of vaccines include that they are unable to cause the disease they are attempting to protect the animal against, and they are more stable than infectious types of vaccines. A disadvantage of noninfectious types of vaccines is that although hypersensitivity reactions to vaccines are rare, they are more likely to occur with noninfectious than infectious types of vaccines.

Infectious vaccines contain pathogens that are altered so that they are unable to cause the disease but are still able to infect cells within the host to stimulate immunity. Examples of infectious types of vaccines include modified live, attenuated, and recombinant. Canine distemper virus vaccine is an example of an infectious type of vaccine. An advantage of infectious types of vaccines is that they stimulate immunity in a way that would be similar to what would happen if the animal was naturally exposed to the disease. As a result, the immunity produced is more efficacious and lasts for a longer duration than that produced by noninfectious vaccines. A potential disadvantage is that certain types of infectious vaccines, such as modified live vaccines, could potentially cause disease if the pathogen was not altered in a successful manner.

New technology, however, has decreased the likelihood of this phenomenon occurring. An example of this is recombinant vaccine technology, which inserts DNA from a particular pathogen into a carrier (e.g., virus) that would be nonpathogenic to the animal receiving the vaccine, thereby eliminating any possibility that the host may contract the disease.

Adjuvants are substances that, when added to a noninfectious vaccine, stimulate a stronger immune response in the animal, with the adjuvant having no immunologic effect of its own.

Storage, Reconstitution, and Dosing

All vaccines should be stored per the manufacturer's direction; this involves refrigeration. Infectious vaccines tend to lack stability and are lyophilized (freeze-dried) to support vaccine efficacy and to extend the stability of the vaccine. Along with the lyophilized portion of the vaccine, a diluent will be provided by the manufacturer to reconstitute the product. It is important to use the diluent provided by the manufacturer because it is specially formulated with appropriate pH and preservatives (Figure 8-1). Vaccines are susceptible to inactivation if mixed with inappropriate substances, which then would render them ineffective. To reconstitute a vaccine, the diluent is drawn up into a syringe and is mixed into the vial containing the lyophilized product. The contents should be gently mixed before the vaccine product is drawn back up into the syringe. Once a vaccine is reconstituted, it is no longer stable. It is therefore recommended that the vaccine be administered within 1 hour of being reconstituted.

Noninfectious vaccines are more stable than infectious vaccines, and thus can be sold and stored in liquid form. It is important to gently mix the vial before drawing the vaccine up into the syringe, especially if multidose vials are being

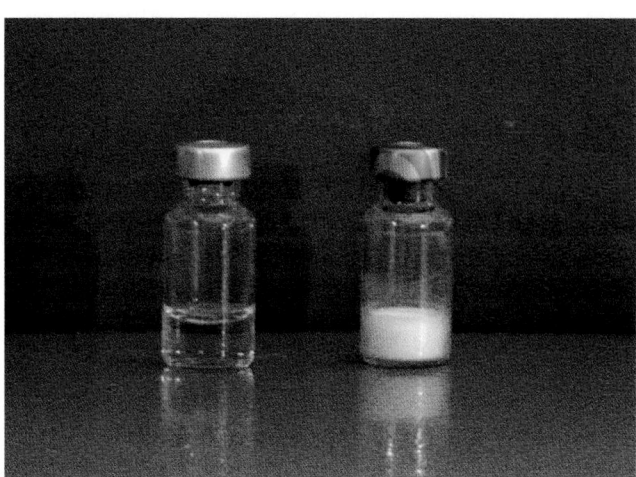

FIGURE 8-1 Examples of lyophilized vaccine *(right)* and diluent *(left)*. The vaccine must be reconstituted by mixing the diluent with the lyophilized product before administering it to the patient.

used. A disadvantage of using multidose vials is the issue of sterility. Because syringes must be introduced into the vial multiple times, contamination of the contents can occur; for this reason, sterile technique must be maintained.

Vaccination doses should be based on manufacturer recommendations and are typically 1 mL. It is important to remember that the quantity administered does not change according to the size or age of the animal. Different vaccinations should never be mixed into a single syringe, unless this is indicated by the manufacturer. All vaccines should be administered before their expiration date, which is located on the label.

> **TECHNICIAN NOTE** All dogs and cats should receive the same designated vaccine dose, per manufacturer recommendations, regardless of the age or size of the animal.

Routes of Administration

It is always important to follow manufacturer recommendations regarding routes of administration for various vaccines. Most immunizations are administered subcutaneously (SQ) or, less commonly, intramuscularly (IM). In the case of rabies vaccination, local laws may be more specific about the required route of administration. Certain infectious vaccines, such as kennel cough vaccines, are formulated to be administered intranasally to stimulate local immunity. The purpose of these vaccines is to improve immune defenses in the region of the body where the disease is typically contracted. Intranasal vaccines should never be administered subcutaneously or intramuscularly because infection or more serious side effects may result. Transdermal vaccine administration is an uncommon route of administration that requires special equipment to deliver and does not involve the use of needles. The canine oral melanoma vaccine is an example of an immunization delivered transdermally.

The site of vaccine administration should always be recorded in the medical record. Administering multiple vaccines in the same area should be avoided. Although rare, adverse vaccine events, including vaccine-induced sarcomas, are possible side effects of vaccine administration. To aid in documenting where a vaccine was administered, to help manage local vaccine reactions, and to avoid administration of multiple vaccines in the same area, the American Association of Feline Practitioners vaccine advisory panel has made recommendations regarding where particular vaccines should be administered (Table 8-1 and Figures 8-2 and 8-3). Although similar recommendations regarding locations for vaccine administration have not been established by the American Animal Hospital Association Canine Vaccination Guidelines, it is not uncommon for veterinary health care teams to follow a similar protocol, with rabies vaccines administered subcutaneously into the right hindlimb, DA₂PP (distemper, adenovirus 2, parainfluenza, parvovirus) vaccines administered subcutaneously into the right front limb (Figure 8-4), and noncore vaccines, such as leptospirosis or

TABLE 8-1	Recommended Sites of Administration of Feline Vaccines		
VACCINATION	**ROUTE**	**BODY REGION**	**LOCATION ON LIMB**
FVRCP	SQ	Right front leg	Lateral side, distal to elbow
FeLV or FIV	SQ	Left hind leg	Lateral side, distal to stifle
Rabies	SQ	Right hind leg	Lateral side, distal to stifle
Giardia	SQ	Left front leg	Lateral side, distal to elbow

FeLV, Feline leukemia virus; *FIV,* feline immunodeficiency virus; *FVRCP,* feline viral rhinotracheitis (herpesvirus), calicivirus, and panleukopenia virus; *SQ,* subcutaneous.
Based on recommendations made in the 2006 American Association of Feline Practitioners Feline Vaccine Advisory Panel Report.

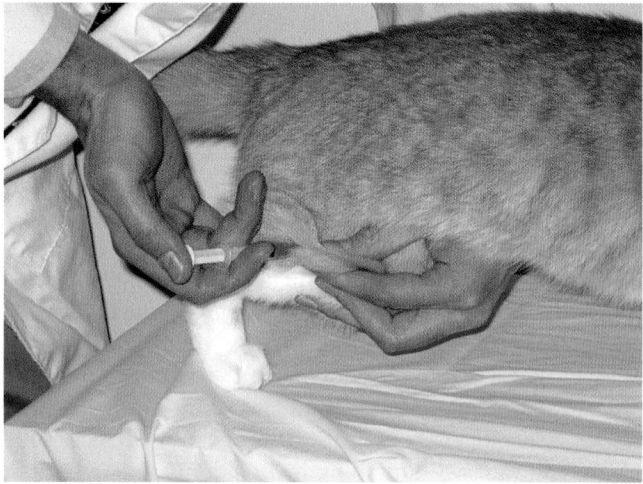

FIGURE 8-2 The American Association of Feline Practitioners recommends that the feline rabies vaccine be administered subcutaneously in the right hind leg, distal to the stifle.

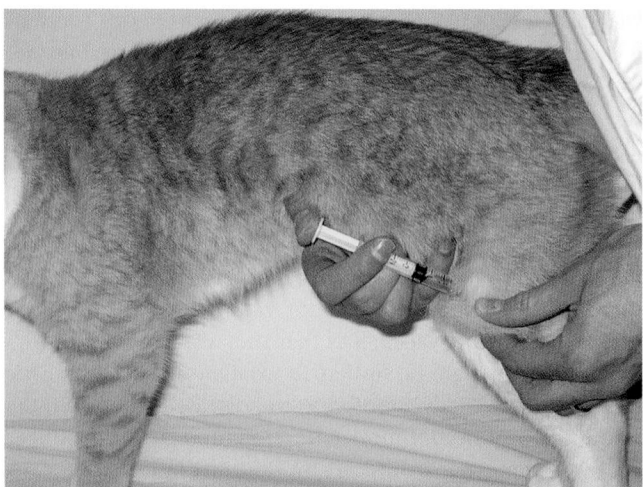

FIGURE 8-3 The American Association of Feline Practitioners recommends that the feline leukemia virus (FeLV) vaccine be administered subcutaneously in the left hind leg, distal to the stifle.

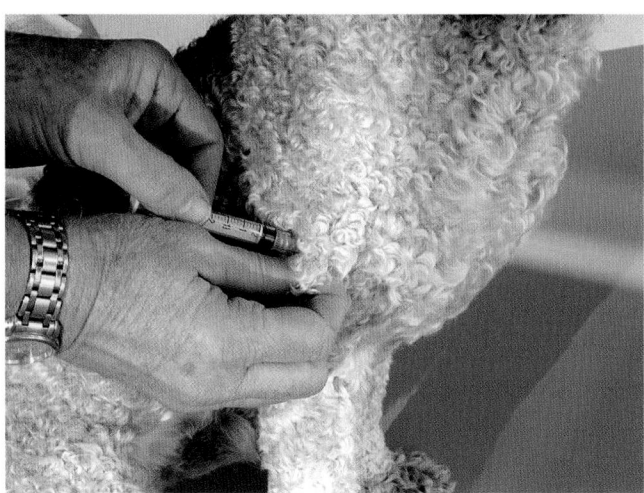

FIGURE 8-4 The right front limb is a common site of administration of the DA₂PP (distemper, adenovirus 2, parainfluenza, parvovirus) vaccine in dogs.

Borrelia burgdorferi (Lyme), administered subcutaneously into the left hindlimb. These administration sites may vary by veterinary practice and by veterinarian. Traditionally, many vaccines were administered subcutaneously between the shoulder blades; however, because of the invasive nature of vaccine-induced sarcomas, it is very difficult to surgically remove all tumor cells in this region. For this reason, immunizations are now recommended to be administered on the distal limb because in the event of a local vaccine-induced sarcoma, the leg could be amputated, if necessary, to completely remove the mass.

> **TECHNICIAN NOTE** Always be aware of the appropriate route of administration of a vaccine. Intranasal vaccines should never be administered subcutaneously or intramuscularly.

Core versus Noncore Vaccines

Vaccines have had a profound effect on preventing disease in both humans and animals. Despite all the good that has come from immunization, some risk is associated with vaccines. For this reason, it is not necessarily advisable to immunize every animal with every vaccine that exists for that species. Both the American Association of Feline Practitioners and the American Animal Hospital Association have published guidelines for vaccines that they consider core and those that they consider noncore (Tables 8-2 and 8-3). Core vaccines are those that are recommended for all animals of that species. These vaccinations stimulate immunity against diseases that are highly contagious and prevalent in the environment. In most cases, all animals, regardless of their lifestyle, have at least the potential to be exposed to these diseases. According to the 2011 American Animal Hospital Association Canine Vaccination Guidelines, core vaccines for dogs include rabies, distemper, hepatitis (adenovirus-2), and canine parvovirus. According to the American Association

of Feline Practitioners feline vaccine advisory panel, core vaccines for cats include rabies and the combination vaccine FVRCP, which protects against feline viral rhinotracheitis (herpesvirus), calicivirus, and panleukopenia.

Noncore vaccines, on the other hand, are not recommended for every animal. They are vaccinations that are specifically recommended for animals at risk for contracting the disease. Therefore, veterinary health care team members must discuss with the owner the lifestyle of the animal and must weigh the risks of the animal contracting the disease versus the risks of potential adverse effects of the vaccine. An example of a feline noncore vaccine is FeLV, which can be used to illustrate whether a noncore vaccine should be administered to an animal. Because FeLV is spread through saliva and nasal secretions of infected cats, an FeLV-negative cat must come in contact with an infected cat or its secretions to become infected. An adult cat that is indoor only and never has access to other cats is not at risk for contracting this disease; thus the vaccine would not typically be recommended because the risk of adverse reactions outweighs the benefits of protecting against a disease that the cat is unlikely to contract. On the other hand, the vaccine would be recommended for a cat that primarily lives outside and would come into contact with other cats because the risk that the outdoor cat may contract the disease is much greater than for the indoor-only cat.

Both the American Association of Feline Practitioners and the American Animal Hospital Association have classified a few vaccines as not recommended. In these cases, it is the opinion of the advisory committee that the vaccines have little to no indication for use because the vaccine has been associated with adverse events, or because it has failed to induce adequate protection against the disease.

> **TECHNICIAN NOTE** Core vaccinations are recommended for all animals of a particular species because they provide protection against highly contagious common pathogens.

Onset and Duration of Immunity

The onset of immunity varies between infectious and noninfectious vaccines; it generally takes longer for immunity to develop after administration of a noninfectious vaccination than after administration of an infectious vaccination.

Duration of immunity is the length of time that an animal retains an adequate level of immunity to protect itself from disease or infection if it were naturally exposed to the pathogenic organism. In many cases, infectious vaccines provide a longer duration of immunity than noninfectious vaccines. However, this is not an absolute rule because certain rabies vaccines (noninfectious) can provide immunity for 3 years in animals that have received two vaccines 1 year apart, but annual boosters are recommended for intranasal *Bordetella bronchiseptica* vaccines (infectious). After the initial puppy or kitten series and a 1-year booster, 3-year revaccinations intervals are recommended for both the canine combination

TABLE 8-2	Recommended Feline Vaccination Protocol

VACCINE TYPE	CATEGORY	ROUTE	INITIAL VACCINATION AGE (≥6 WK AND ≤16 WK) PROTOCOL	INITIAL VACCINATION AGE (>16 WK) PROTOCOL	BOOSTER INTERVAL FOLLOWING INITIAL VACCINATION SERIES	SUBSEQUENT REVACCINATION INTERVAL	COMMENTS
Rabies							
Canarypox virus–vectored recombinant, nonadjuvanted	Core	Injection	1 dose when ≥8 wk of age	Same as (≥6 wk and ≤16 wk) protocol	1 yr later	Every year	Must follow state/local regulations regarding interval, route, initial age, etc.
1-Year killed virus, adjuvanted	Core	Injection	1 dose when ≥12 wk of age	Same as (≥6 wk and ≤16 wk) protocol	1 yr later	Every year	Must follow state/local regulations regarding interval, route, initial age, etc.
3-Year killed virus, adjuvanted	Core	Injection	1 dose when ≥12 wk of age	Same as (≥6 wk and ≤16 wk) protocol	1 yr later	Every 3 yr	Must follow state/local regulations regarding interval, route, initial age, etc.
Feline Herpesvirus-1 and Feline Calicivirus							
MLV, nonadjuvanted	Core	Injection	Every 3-4 wk until 16 wk of age	2 doses 3-4 wk apart	1 yr later	Every 3 yr	
Killed virus, adjuvanted	Core	Injection	Every 3-4 wk until 16 wk of age	2 doses 3-4 wk apart	1 yr later	Every 3 yr	
MLV, nonadjuvanted	Core	Intranasal	Every 3-4 wk until 16 wk of age	2 doses 3-4 wk apart	1 yr later	Every 3 yr	
Feline Panleukopenia Virus							
MLV, nonadjuvanted	Core	Injection	Every 3-4 wk until 16 wk of age	2 doses 3-4 wk apart	1 yr later	≥Every 3 yr	
Killed virus, adjuvanted or nonadjuvanted	Core	Injection	Every 3-4 wk until 16 wk of age	2 doses 3-4 wk apart	1 yr later	≥Every 3 yr	
MLV, nonadjuvanted	Core	Intranasal	Every 3-4 wk until 16 wk of age	2 doses 3-4 wk apart	1 yr later	≥Every 3 yr	
Feline Leukemia Virus							
Canarypox virus–vectored recombinant, nonadjuvanted	Noncore	Transdermal	2 doses 3-4 wk apart when ≥8 wk of age	Same as (≥6 wk and ≤16 wk) protocol	1 yr later	Every year	AAFP highly recommends for all kittens
Killed virus, adjuvanted	Noncore	Injection	2 doses 3-4 wk apart when ≥8 wk of age	Same as (≥6 wk and ≤16 wk) protocol	1 yr later	Every year	AAFP highly recommends for all kittens

TABLE 8-2	Recommended Feline Vaccination Protocol—cont'd						
VACCINE TYPE	CATEGORY	ROUTE	INITIAL VACCINATION AGE (≥6 WK AND ≤16 WK) PROTOCOL	INITIAL VACCINATION AGE (>16 WK) PROTOCOL	BOOSTER INTERVAL FOLLOWING INITIAL VACCINATION SERIES	SUBSEQUENT REVACCINATION INTERVAL	COMMENTS
Feline Immunodeficiency Virus (FIV)							
Killed virus, adjuvanted	Noncore	Injection	3 doses 2-3 wk apart when ≥8 wk of age	Same as (≥6 wk and ≤16 wk) protocol	1 yr later	Every year	Vaccinates will test positive with antibody-based FIV test
Chlamydophila felis							
Avirulent live organism, nonadjuvanted	Noncore	Injection	2 doses 3-4 wk apart when ≥9 wk of age	Same as (≥6 wk and ≤16 wk) protocol	1 yr later	Every year	
Killed organism, adjuvanted	Noncore	Injection	2 doses 3-4 wk apart when ≥9 wk of age	Same as (≥6 wk and ≤16 wk) protocol	1 yr later	Every year	
Bordetella bronchiseptica							
Avirulent live organism, nonadjuvanted	Noncore	Intranasal	1 dose when ≥8 wk of age	Same as (≥6 wk and ≤16 wk) protocol	1 yr later	Every year	
Feline Coronavirus							
MLV, nonadjuvanted	Noncore	Intranasal	2 doses 3-4 wk apart when 16 wk of age	Same as (≥6 wk and ≤16 wk) protocol	1 yr later	Every year	AAFP generally does not recommend
Giardia lamblia							
Killed organism, adjuvanted	Noncore	Injection	2 doses 2-4 wk apart when ≥8 wk of age	Same as (≥6 wk and ≤16 wk) protocol	1 yr later	Every year	AAFP generally does not recommend

Based on recommendations made in the 2006 American Association of Feline Practitioners Feline Vaccine Advisory Panel Report.
AAFP, American Association of Feline Practitioners; *MLV,* modified live virus.

(DA₂PP) and the feline combination (FVRCP) core vaccines.

Feline Immunizations
The following recommendations are based on the 2006 American Association of Feline Practitioners Feline Advisory Panel Report. A summary of these recommendations can be found in Table 8-2.

Rabies (Core Vaccine)
Rabies is a zoonotic disease caused by a rhabdovirus, which affects the nervous system. It is spread through saliva and central nervous system (CNS) tissue and is most commonly transmitted through bite wounds. Rabies is an endemic disease in the United States, where skunks, bats, foxes, raccoons, and coyotes act as natural reservoirs of the disease. Clinical signs in animals vary widely but typically involve

neurologic signs, such as increased aggression, agitation, solitude seeking, incoordination, and/or paralysis. No treatment is available for the disease, and it is almost always fatal, following the onset of clinical signs. Rabies is a reportable disease. Injectable, adjuvanted, killed virus vaccines and nonadjuvanted, recombinant virus, canarypox-vectored vaccines are available. In many regions, pets are required by law to receive rabies vaccination, and the law may even dictate the route of administration (intramuscular vs. subcutaneous) and/or the frequency of administration (annually vs. triennially).

TECHNICIAN NOTE Veterinary health care team members must be aware of local or regional rabies immunization laws before administering the vaccination.

| TABLE 8-3 | Recommended Canine Vaccination Protocol |

VACCINE TYPE	CATEGORY	ROUTE	INITIAL VACCINATION AGE (≤16 WK) PROTOCOL	INITIAL VACCINATION AGE (>16 WK) PROTOCOL	BOOSTER INTERVAL FOLLOWING INITIAL VACCINATION SERIES	SUBSEQUENT REVACCINATION INTERVAL	COMMENTS
Rabies							
1-Year killed virus	Core	Injection	1 dose when ≥12 wk of age	Same as (≤16 wk) protocol	1 yr later	Every year	Must follow state/local regulations regarding interval, route, initial age, etc.
3-Year killed virus	Core	Injection	1 dose when ≥12 wk of age	Same as (≤16 wk) protocol	1 yr later	Every 3 yr	Must follow state/local regulations regarding interval, route, initial age, etc.
Canine Distemper Virus							
MLV or recombinant	Core	Injection	Every 3-4 wk when ≥6 wk until 14-16 wk of age	1 dose	1 yr later for (≤16 wk) protocol	≥Every 3 yr	
					≥3 yr later for (>16 wk) protocol	≥Every 3 yr	
Measles Virus							
MLV	Noncore	Injection (IM only)	1 dose when >6 wk and <12 wk of age	Not recommended	Not recommended	Not recommended	
Canine Adenovirus, Type 2							
MLV	Core	Injection	Every 3-4 wk when ≥6 wk until 14-16 wk of age	1 dose	1 yr later for (≤16 wk) protocol	≥Every 3 yr	
					≥3 yr later for (>16 wk) protocol	≥Every 3 yr	
MLV	Noncore	Intranasal	1 dose when ≥3-4 wk of age	Same as (≤16 wk) protocol	≤1 yr later	≤Every year	May not provide protection against CAV-1, and should not replace MLV injectable vaccine. Recommended for dogs at risk for infectious tracheobronchitis. Available only as a combination vaccine
Canine Parvovirus							
MLV	Core	Injection	Every 3-4 wk when ≥6 wk until 14-16 wk of age	1 dose	1 yr later for (≤16 wk) protocol	≥Every 3 yr	

TABLE 8-3 | Recommended Canine Vaccination Protocol—cont'd

VACCINE TYPE	CATEGORY	ROUTE	INITIAL VACCINATION AGE (≤16 WK) PROTOCOL	INITIAL VACCINATION AGE (>16 WK) PROTOCOL	BOOSTER INTERVAL FOLLOWING INITIAL VACCINATION SERIES	SUBSEQUENT REVACCINATION INTERVAL	COMMENTS
					≥3 yr later for (>16 wk) protocol	≥Every 3 yr	
Canine Parainfluenza Virus							
MLV	Noncore	Injection	Every 3-4 wk when ≥6 wk until 14-16 wk of age	1 dose	1 yr later for (≤16 wk) protocol ≥3 yr later for (>16 wk) protocol	≥Every 3 yr	Available only in combination with canine distemper virus, canine adenovirus type 2, and canine parvovirus
MLV	Noncore	Intranasal	1 dose when ≥3-4 wk of age	Same as (≤16 wk) protocol	≤1 yr later	≤Every yr	May be administered more often than annually for high-risk animals. Available only as a combination vaccine
Leptospira interrogans							
4-Way killed whole cell or subunit bacterin	Noncore	Injection	2 doses 2-4 wk apart when ≥12 wk of age	Same as (≤16 wk) protocol	1 yr later	Every year	
2-Way killed bacterin	Noncore	Injection					AAHA does not recommend
Bordetella bronchiseptica							
Inactivated cellular antigen extract	Noncore	Injection	Doses administered at 8 and 12 wk of age	2 doses 2-4 wk apart	1 yr later	Every year	2nd dose in initial vaccine series should be given ≥1 wk before exposure
Bordetella bronchiseptica							
Live avirulent bacteria	Noncore	Intranasal	1 dose when ≥3-4 wk of age	Same as (≤16 wk) protocol	≤1 yr later	≤Every year	May be administered more often than annually for high-risk animals
Borrelia burgdorferi							
Killed whole cell bacterin or recombinant subunit OspA	Noncore	Injection	2 doses 2-4 wk apart when ≥12 wk of age	Same as (≤16 wk) protocol	1 yr later	Every year	
Canine Influenza							
Killed virus	Noncore	Injection	2 doses 2-4 wk apart when ≥6 wk of age	Same as (≤16 wk) protocol	1 yr later	Every year	

Based on recommendations made in the 2011 American Animal Hospital Association Canine Vaccination Guidelines.
AAHA, American Animal Hospital Association; *CAV,* canine adenovirus; *IM,* intramuscular; *MLV,* modified live virus.

Feline Viral Rhinotracheitis (FHV-1) and Calicivirus (FCV) (Core Vaccine)

Feline rhinotracheitis virus is a herpesvirus that is a frequent cause of upper respiratory disease in cats. Common clinical signs include sneezing, ocular and nasal discharge, and fever. Feline calicivirus, of which there are many strains, is also a frequent cause of upper respiratory disease in cats. Calicivirus causes similar signs as feline rhinotracheitis virus but also may cause oral ulceration. In both cases, viruses are shed via oropharyngeal, conjunctival, and nasal secretions for up to 3 weeks. In addition, calicivirus can be shed in urine and feces. Calicivirus is able to survive in the environment for a longer period of time (up to a week); herpesvirus can survive in the environment for only 24 hours. Direct contact between cats is the most common means of viral spread, although indirect contact with infective secretions is also possible. Latent infections are normal with feline herpesvirus infection and involve the virus lying dormant within the cat for a period of time. After stressful episodes for the cat, clinical signs of upper respiratory disease and/or viral shedding typically recur. A carrier state is also possible in cats infected with feline calicivirus; however, these cats tend to shed virus continuously.

Both of these pathogens are commonly found in cat populations, making exposure to these organisms likely. Cats of any age are susceptible to upper respiratory disease, although kittens tend to be most severely affected. Both modified live and inactivated vaccines are available, and both types have relatively good efficacy in protecting against disease. These vaccines do not, however, protect against infection or carrier state. In the case of calicivirus, the vaccine does not cover against all strains. Vaccines are available in an injectable form, which is administered subcutaneously, as well as in an intranasal form. It is possible for vaccinates to develop mild signs of upper respiratory disease, especially following the intranasal vaccine, and lameness may develop secondary to the calicivirus component of the vaccine. FHV-1 and FCV vaccines are commonly combined with feline panleukopenia to form the combination vaccine FVRCP.

> **TECHNICIAN NOTE** Feline rhinotracheitis virus and calicivirus are common causes of upper respiratory disease in cats.

Feline Panleukopenia (FPV) (Core Vaccine)

Feline panleukopenia is caused by a parvovirus. It is highly contagious and is commonly found in the environment; cats of all ages are susceptible. Clinical signs include fever, lethargy, anorexia, dehydration, vomiting, and diarrhea. Sudden death is also possible, especially in younger cats. As the name implies, a low white blood cell count (leukopenia) is typical. Neurologic signs are possible because infection during late gestation or the first few weeks of life can lead to cerebellar hypoplasia. The virus is shed in all body secretions but is most commonly found in feces and urine, and the virus can survive in the environment for up to a year. Direct contact with an infected cat or with infectious secretions is the most common means of viral spread. Both modified live and inactivated vaccines are available in injectable forms and provide excellent immunity. An intranasal modified live vaccine is also available. It is possible for modified live vaccines to cause cerebellar disease in fetuses and neonates, so this vaccine type should not be administered to kittens younger than 4 weeks of age or to pregnant queens. FPV is commonly combined with feline rhinotracheitis and feline calicivirus to create the combination vaccine FVRCP.

Feline Leukemia Virus (FeLV) (Noncore Vaccine)

Feline leukemia virus is a retrovirus of the subfamily Oncornavirus. It is shed in saliva and nasal secretions and typically is spread through mutual grooming, sharing of food and water dishes, and biting. The disease can also be spread in utero, through nursing, and via blood transfusions. The virus can survive in the environment for up to 48 hours. Cats of all ages can be infected; however, kittens and young cats seem to be most susceptible. Cats infected with FeLV experience clinical signs secondary to immunosuppression, anemia, and/or lymphoma. Inactivated injectable, nonadjuvanted recombinant injectable, and nonadjuvanted recombinant transdermal vaccines are available. This immunization is recommended for cats that are at risk of contracting the disease, such as cats that have access to the outdoors or cats that have contact with cats of unknown FeLV status. It is also recommended that cats test negative for FeLV before vaccination. The American Association of Feline Practitioners Feline Vaccine Advisory Panel highly recommends vaccination of all kittens because of the potential for their risk status to change.

Feline Immunodeficiency Virus (FIV) (Noncore Vaccine)

Feline immunodeficiency virus is a lentivirus that causes immunosuppression in cats. It is spread primarily through saliva and blood via bites, wounds, and other fighting injuries. Adult male cats that have access to the outdoors are considered most susceptible owing to their predisposition for fighting. An inactivated injectable vaccine is available. Cats receiving the vaccine should test negative for FIV before their first injection. After vaccination, cats will test positive on the antibody-based FIV screening test. This is because the screening test is unable to differentiate between antibodies formed secondary to the vaccine and antibodies formed secondary to the actual disease. Therefore, it is important to educate owners on the implications associated with a cat with these test results. It is recommended that cats receiving this vaccine also receive a microchip identification to increase the likelihood that the cat will be returned to the owner and will not be euthanized because of its false-positive FIV test result, if it were ever to go missing. The FIV vaccine is recommended for cats at risk of contracting the disease, such as cats that have access to the outdoors and a predisposition to fighting and FIV-negative cats that live in a household with an FIV-positive cat.

Chlamydophila felis (Noncore Vaccine)

Chlamydophila felis is a bacterial disease that infects the conjunctiva and respiratory tract of cats. It primarily causes signs of conjunctivitis, including unilateral or bilateral serous ocular discharge, which may progress to mucopurulent discharge. Signs of upper respiratory tract disease, such as mild nasal discharge and sneezing, occur less commonly. The pathogen is spread by direct contact between cats and may be shed for months beyond clinical resolution of the disease. Infections are treatable. Some evidence suggests that zoonotic transmission of this organism is possible. Injectable inactivated adjuvanted and modified live vaccines are available and stimulate some protection against the disease. Similar to other vaccines that protect against feline upper respiratory disease, this immunization does not prevent infection or shedding. The vaccine is recommended for cats that live in multi-cat environments that have a previous history of *Chlamydophila felis* infection.

Bordetella bronchiseptica (Noncore Vaccine)

Bordetella bronchiseptica is a bacterial infection that is most commonly associated with infectious tracheobronchitis (kennel cough) in dogs. Clinical signs of upper respiratory disease occur less frequently in cats and include sneezing, submandibular lymphadenopathy, oculonasal discharge, and sometimes coughing. Cases most frequently occur in animal shelters and multi-cat households. The disease often is most severe in young kittens, but cats of all ages may be affected. *B. bronchiseptica* is shed in oropharyngeal and nasal secretions, and transmission occurs via direct contact with other cats or with secretions. The bacteria can be shed for up to 19 weeks post infection. It is possible for this organism to be transmitted between cats and dogs. A modified live intranasal vaccine is available and is recommended for cats at risk for contracting the disease, such as those entering boarding facilities, animal shelters, or catteries that have had confirmed cases of the disease. The vaccine should be administered at least 72 hours before the cat enters the facility.

Feline Coronavirus (FCoV) (Noncore Vaccine)

Feline coronavirus is the causative agent of feline infectious peritonitis (FIP); however, only certain strains of the virus actually cause the disease. It is not uncommon for cats to be exposed to feline coronavirus, but only a small percentage of cats actually develop FIP. Two forms of the disease have been identified. Clinical signs of the "dry" form include fever, decreased appetite, and weight loss. The main clinical sign of the "wet" form is effusion, which occurs in the abdomen and/or the thoracic cavity. Feline coronavirus is shed in feces, respiratory secretions, saliva, and urine. Transmission of the virus occurs through direct contact with secretions or excretions or via mutual grooming. Cats of all ages are susceptible, although kittens seem to be most at risk of developing the disease. An intranasal modified live vaccine is available, but its efficacy is controversial in that studies have shown varying results. It may be helpful in preventing the disease in cats that have never been exposed to feline coronavirus. Thus, testing for FCoV is recommended before vaccination. According to the American Association of Feline Practitioners Feline Vaccine Advisory report, this vaccine generally is not recommended.

Giardia lamblia (Noncore Vaccine)

Giardia lamblia is a protozoan parasite that causes gastrointestinal disease in many animals, including cats. If clinical signs occur, the most common sign is diarrhea. Weight loss is also reported. The organism is transmitted via the fecal-oral route, and infection commonly occurs secondary to ingestion of contaminated water or infected prey, sharing of litter boxes with an infected animal, and mutual grooming. The organism can survive in wet, cold environments for several months. An injectable adjuvanted inactivated vaccine is available. Owing to insufficient numbers of research studies, its efficacy is controversial. Therefore, it is not generally recommended by the American Association of Feline Practitioners Feline Vaccine Advisory Panel.

Canine Immunizations

The following recommendations are based on the 2011 American Animal Hospital Association Canine Vaccination Guidelines. A summary of these recommendations can be found in Table 8-3.

Rabies (Core Vaccine)

Rabies vaccination is required by law in many regions. State, local, and/or provincial laws may dictate the frequency of administration of the vaccine—either annually or triennially. The route of administration, which may be subcutaneous or intramuscular, is also specified by some laws. Injectable killed virus vaccines are available for use in dogs. For further information on the disease, please refer to the rabies paragraph found in the feline immunization section.

Canine Distemper Virus (CDV) (Core Vaccine)

Canine distemper is caused by a paramyxovirus. Many different clinical signs can be associated with the disease, including decreased appetite, fever, lethargy, and signs of respiratory disease. In more severe cases, vomiting, diarrhea, anorexia, and dehydration may occur. The disease has been associated with neurologic signs, such as seizures, ataxia, paresis, and/or hyperesthesia. Hyperkeratosis of the planum nasale and foot pads may also be observed later in the disease process. Dogs of any age may be affected; however, young dogs are most at risk. This disease can also affect many other species, including foxes, raccoons, skunks, wolves, and ferrets. The virus is shed in all secretions but is most commonly transmitted through respiratory exudates. The virus does not survive in the environment very long, under normal conditions. Injectable recombinant and modified live vaccines are available and are considered core vaccines. CDV is often combined with vaccines for other canine diseases to create the DA$_2$PP or DHPP (distemper, hepatitis, parainfluenza, parvovirus) vaccine. In addition, a measles virus vaccine is available for use in puppies younger than 16 weeks. The use of measles vaccine in young puppies can provide some temporary protection against canine distemper disease because the measles virus shares some similarities to distemper virus. It is also able to stimulate an immune response in the presence of lower levels of acquired maternal antibodies. Thus, the advantage of using this vaccine is that it is able to cross-protect young dogs against canine distemper at a potentially earlier age than distemper vaccine alone. Measles vaccine must be administered intramuscularly and is considered a noncore vaccine by the American Animal Hospital Association Canine Vaccination Task Force.

> **TECHNICIAN NOTE** Measles vaccine can provide some temporary cross-protection against canine distemper virus in young puppies.

Canine Adenovirus Type 2 (CAV-2) (Core Vaccine)

Canine adenovirus type 2 is one of the causes of canine infectious tracheobronchitis (kennel cough). Canine adenovirus type 1, on the other hand, causes infectious canine hepatitis. Signs of this disease include vomiting, diarrhea, abdominal pain, clotting disorders, and fever. Ocular signs, such as anterior uveitis and corneal edema, may occur as the dog recovers from the infection. Acute death may also occur, especially in young puppies. Dogs of all ages may be infected, although young dogs are most commonly affected. CAV-1–modified live vaccines were found to cause renal and ocular disease in some animals. The injectable modified live vaccine using CAV-2, however, rarely cause any side effects and induces protection against CAV-1 and CAV-2. This core vaccine is often combined with canine distemper, canine parvovirus, and canine parainfluenza to create the DA$_2$PP or DHPP vaccine. The "A$_2$" and "H" in these vaccine names are used interchangeably, depending on the brand, and stand for adenovirus type 2 and hepatitis, respectively. An intranasal vaccine for CAV-2 is also available and is used in combination with *B. bronchiseptica* and canine parainfluenza to provide protection against canine infectious tracheobronchitis. This form does not protect against CAV-1 and should not be used as a substitution for the injectable vaccine. The intranasal CAV-2 combination vaccine is classified as a noncore vaccine by the American Animal Hospital Association Canine Vaccination Task Force.

Canine Parvovirus (CPV-2) (Core Vaccine)

Canine parvoviral enteritis is a serious, highly contagious disease. Canine parvovirus is shed in the feces, and the disease is spread by fecal-oral transmission. The virus is resistant to many disinfectants and is able to survive in the environment for weeks to months. Parvocidal disinfectants and 1:30 solutions of dilute bleach are effective in killing the pathogen. Clinical signs of the disease include diarrhea, vomiting, dehydration, leukopenia, and fever. Dogs of all ages are susceptible to illness, but young dogs are at highest risk. Certain breeds, such as Doberman Pinschers and Rottweilers, have an increased incidence of the disease. Injectable modified live vaccines are available and are often combined with canine distemper, canine adenovirus type 2, and canine parainfluenza virus to create the DA$_2$PP combination vaccine. Modified live vaccines are expected to provide immunity to all variants of canine parvovirus.

> **TECHNICIAN NOTE** Canine parvoviral enteritis is a highly contagious disease; infected patients must be housed in designated isolation areas during hospitalization.

Canine Parainfluenza Virus (CPiV) (Noncore Vaccine)

Canine parainfluenza virus is a paramyxovirus that is one of the causes of canine infectious tracheobronchitis (kennel cough). The main clinical sign of the disease is a self-limiting cough, which is typically nonproductive. Both injectable and intranasal modified live vaccines are available. The injectable canine parainfluenza virus vaccine is available only in combination with canine distemper, canine parvovirus, and canine adenovirus type 2 vaccines (DA$_2$PP). The injectable form only protects against clinical signs and does not prevent infection or viral shedding. The intranasal canine parainfluenza virus vaccine is available only in combination with *B. bronchiseptica* and canine adenovirus type 2 vaccines. The intranasal form is considered superior in protection against parainfluenza virus because in addition to protecting against clinical signs, it prevents infection and viral shedding.

Leptospirosis (Noncore Vaccine)

Leptospirosis is caused by the bacteria *Leptospira*, of which there are many serovars. Leptospirosis is transmitted through exposure to contaminated water, food, soil, or bedding, as well as through bite wounds, by placental and venereal transfer, and through direct contact with infected urine. The bacterium can survive for weeks in warm moist environments. It is uncommon in dry, arid regions. Clinical signs in infected dogs are dependent in part on the infecting serovar and may include fever, anorexia, polyuria, polydipsia, vomiting, and diarrhea. Renal failure and/or liver disease is possible. Some of the most commonly implicated serovars in canine leptospirosis infection include *L. icterohemorrhagiae, L. grippotyphosa, L. pomona,* and *L. canicola*. Leptospirosis is a zoonotic disease, and precautions must be taken when treating animals that have or are suspected of having this disease. *Leptospira interrogans* 4-way injectable killed whole cell and subunit vaccines are available. Each type provides protection against *L. canicola, L. pomona, L. grippotyphosa,* and *L. icterohemorrhagiae*. The leptospirosis vaccine is considered a noncore vaccine and is recommended for animals at risk for contracting the disease based on prevalence of the disease in the area in which the animal lives and the risk that the animal has of being exposed to the pathogen. It should be kept in mind that several other serovars can cause leptospirosis, and existing vaccines do not protect against these other serovars. An older 2-way injectable killed bacterin vaccine, which contains serovars for *L. icterohemorrhagiae* and *L. canicola,* currently is not recommended by the American Animal Hospital Association Canine Vaccination Task Force. The 4-way *Leptospira interrogans* vaccine can be administered as an individual immunization or sometimes is combined with canine distemper, canine adenovirus type 2, canine parainfluenza, and canine parvovirus combination vaccine (DA$_2$PPL).

> **TECHNICIAN NOTE** Many serovars can cause leptospirosis. The vaccine provides protection against four of the most common ones.

Bordetella bronchiseptica (Noncore Vaccine)

Bordetella bronchiseptica is one of the primary causes of canine infectious tracheobronchitis (kennel cough). Clinical signs include a dry, honking cough and possible nasal discharge. Bacteria are shed in respiratory secretions and are transmitted via airborne contact with secretions or through direct dog-to-dog contact. The infection is easily spread in highly populated closed environments such as boarding kennels, animal shelters, and pet shops. An injectable inactivated-cellular antigen extract, as well as an intranasal live avirulent bacterial vaccine, are available. These vaccines are considered noncore and should be administered to animals at risk for contracting infectious tracheobronchitis. It is not uncommon for boarding facilities to require this immunization before admission. *B. bronchiseptica* vaccines may be administered individually or may be combined with canine parainfluenza and canine adenovirus type 2 vaccines.

> **TECHNICIAN NOTE** Intranasal *Bordetella bronchiseptica* vaccines are often preferred over injectable forms of the vaccine because they stimulate both local and systemic immunity.

Borrelia burgdorferi (Noncore Vaccine)

Canine Lyme disease is caused by the bacterium *Borrelia burgdorferi*. The disease is spread by ticks (*Ixodes* species). Although only a small percentage of infected dogs show evidence of clinical disease, signs may include fever and polyarthritis. A small portion of infected dogs may also develop a protein-losing glomerulopathy and experience signs associated with renal failure. Injectable killed whole cell bacterin and recombinant subunit OspA vaccines are available. OspA is an outer surface lipoprotein of *Borrelia burgdorferi*. The vaccine is recommended for use in dogs with increased risk of exposure, such as those living in or visiting areas where the risk of *Ixodes* tick exposure is high, or where the disease is endemic. Tick control plays an important role in prevention of Lyme disease.

Canine Influenza (Noncore Vaccine)

Canine influenza virus causes upper respiratory disease in dogs. Clinical signs include cough, fever, and possible nasal discharge. A small percentage of dogs may develop pneumonia, secondary to the infection. Currently, an injectable killed virus vaccine is available. It is listed as a noncore vaccine, according to the American Animal Hospital Association Canine Vaccination Task Force. Although the group does not make any specific recommendations regarding the vaccine, principles similar to those for other noncore upper respiratory disease vaccines would apply. Specifically, dogs that are at risk of contracting the disease, such as those animals that live in or are traveling to endemic areas or that will come in contact with dogs from regions where the disease is endemic, may benefit from immunization.

Canine Coronavirus (CCoV) (Noncore Vaccine)

Canine coronavirus causes an infectious form of enteritis that infrequently affects dogs. It is a highly contagious disease that spreads rapidly via fecal-oral transmission. Clinical signs include malodorous diarrhea, decreased appetite, lethargy, and possibly vomiting. Young animals tend to be most severely affected by the disease. Injectable killed virus and modified live virus vaccines are available. The vaccine provides incomplete protection by decreasing, but not entirely eliminating, canine coronavirus replication. This vaccine is not recommended by the American Animal Hospital Association Canine Vaccination Task Force.

Adverse Vaccine Events

Adverse vaccine events are side effects that may occur secondary to administration of a vaccine. Most of these events are transient, typically lasting a few days, and are not life threatening. Examples of side effects that typically do not require treatment include lethargy, mild fever, soreness at the injection site, and/or decreased appetite. Before their pet receives a vaccination, owners should be warned that these side effects may occur and should be instructed to contact a veterinary health care team member if signs last longer than 2 or 3 days or are otherwise progressive. With many intranasal vaccines, it is not uncommon for a small percentage of animals to develop mild signs of transient upper respiratory disease, such as sneezing, nasal discharge, and coughing. With any immunization, the client must also be instructed to monitor the pet for any signs of an allergic reaction. A veterinary health care team member should be contacted immediately if the client observes the pet displaying signs such as facial swelling, difficulty breathing, vomiting, diarrhea, urticaria (hives), and/or seizures. In the most severe cases, systemic **anaphylaxis** can occur; this is a severe allergic or hypersensitivity response to a foreign substance. In these cases, cardiovascular collapse, respiratory arrest, and death may result if treatment is not immediately instituted. Treatment for allergic reactions may involve administration of an injectable antihistamine and/or administration of an injectable steroid. For more severe cases, the animal may also require administration of epinephrine and intravenous fluids.

Many other types of adverse events have been implicated as potentially being secondary to vaccination, but it should be noted that direct causality has not necessarily been documented in each of these cases. In many instances, these events occur days to weeks (or more) after vaccination, and additional factors could play a role. Examples include immune-mediated hemolytic anemia, immune-mediated thrombocytopenia, immunosuppression, hypertrophic osteodystrophy, and thyroiditis.

Another potential adverse vaccine event is the development of a mass at the injection site, which has especially been an issue with cats. Although this is considered rare, it is possible for a sarcoma to develop in the location at which vaccines are administered. This is why it is recommended that immunizations be given over a limb instead of in the shoulder blade region, where tumor removal would be more difficult. Not all masses that develop in the region of a vaccine injection are cancerous, however. Sometimes benign inflammatory masses (granulomas) may develop in the region; these typically resolve within several weeks of vaccine administration. According to the Vaccine-Associated Feline Sarcoma Task Force, any mass that appears at an injection site should be documented. It is important to note the size, shape, and location of the mass, as well as when it was first observed. Initially, the owner should be instructed to monitor the mass for any changes. It is recommended by the task force that any mass that is greater than 2 cm in diameter, is still present 3 months after vaccination, and/or continues to enlarge beyond 1 month post injection should be biopsied to determine whether the mass is cancerous.

All adverse vaccine events should be reported to the manufacturer of the vaccine. If multiple vaccines were administered to an animal during the same appointment, all vaccine manufacturers involved should be contacted. In addition, adverse vaccine events should be reported to the USDA-APHIS (U.S. Department of Agriculture Animal and Plant Health Inspection Service) Center for Veterinary Biologics (CVB). Reports may be submitted online, via telephone (800) 752-6255, or by fax or mail. Links to online submission forms and a printable pdf file report form that can be used to submit the report by mail or fax can be found at the USDA-APHIS CVB website (http://www.aphis.usda.gov/animal_health/vet_biologics/vb_adverse_event.shtml).

It must be kept in mind that in general, adverse vaccine events are considered rare, and in most cases the protection afforded by immunization outweighs the small potential risk of an adverse event occurring in a naïve animal. For animals with suspected or known reactions to vaccines, the veterinary health care team must discuss with the owner the risks and benefits of administering the vaccine. Depending on the previous reaction, an antihistamine injection may be

recommended up to 30 minutes before vaccine administration. Another option may be to administer a different brand of vaccine. In other cases, the owner and the veterinarian may elect to forgo vaccinating the pet given demonstrated adequate antibody titer levels, which can be measured to determine whether protective immunity against the disease is present. Other potential actions that can be taken to decrease the likelihood of an adverse event occurring include selecting vaccine types that are less likely to cause local inflammation (nonadjuvanted) and/or spreading out the immunization process by placing priority on administering core vaccinations first and administering noncore vaccinations, if necessary, at a later time, when they can be given separately.

> **TECHNICIAN NOTE**   The "1-2-3" recommendations for biopsy or removal of a postvaccinal mass are as follows:
> 1. The mass is still growing after 1 month.
> 2. The mass is greater than 2 cm in diameter.
> 3. The mass persists for longer than 3 months.

PARASITE PREVENTION

Parasite control is an important aspect of preventive health programs. This is true not only because parasites can cause disease in their own right, but also because many parasites are carriers of other diseases that they transmit to pets. Fleas, for example, can cause flea allergy dermatitis, but if they are ingested by a cat or a dog, they can also transmit tapeworms. A primary concern of ticks is the transmission of tick-borne diseases, which include ehrlichiosis, Rocky Mountain spotted fever, and Lyme disease. Fortunately, many safe and effective products are currently available to treat and prevent fleas and ticks. These include oral medications that sterilize flea eggs or kill fleas in contact with the animal, as well as monthly topical spot-on treatments that kill and/or repel fleas and ticks. It is important to note that some tick products that are safe and effective for use in dogs are not safe for use in cats. It is especially important that owners are aware of this information if they have both dogs and cats in their household. The veterinary health care team should make recommendations to clients regarding which products are best indicated for their pets' needs, based on the animals' risk of infection and the animals' lifestyle.

Internal parasites also pose a risk for dogs and cats. Roundworms commonly infect many puppies and kittens and are a common cause of diarrhea. All puppies and kittens therefore should receive deworming medication. Annual fecal examinations to check for intestinal parasites are a regular occurrence at many practices and are useful for animals of all ages. In regions of the country where it is prevalent, many animals receive annual heartworm tests. A monthly heartworm preventive agent is recommended in areas where heartworm disease is endemic; an added advantage of this medication is that it also treats for common intestinal parasites (Table 8-4).

| TABLE 8-4 | Examples of Commonly Used Heartworm Preventive Products that Also Aid in the Treatment and Control of Other Parasites |

PRODUCT	HEARTWORMS	HOOKWORMS	ROUNDWORMS	WHIPWORMS	FLEAS	EAR MITES	SARCOPTIC MANGE	TICKS
Heartgard Plus Chewables (Ivermectin & pyrantel pamoate)								
Canine	+	+	+	–	–	–	–	–
Heartgard Chewables (Ivermectin)								
Feline	+	+	–	–	–	–	–	–
Revolution (Selamectin)								
Canine	+	–	–	–	Adults & eggs	+	+	Dermacentor variabilis
Feline	+	+	+	–	Adults & eggs	+	–	–
Interceptor (Milbemycin oxime)								
Canine	+	+	+	+	–	–	–	–
Feline	+	+	+	–	–	–	–	–
Sentinel (Milbemycin oxime & lufenuron)								
Canine	+	+	+	+	Eggs & larvae	–	–	–
Trifexis (Spinosad &milbemycin oxime)								
Canine	+	+	+	+	Adults	–	–	–

Wellness examinations are a good time to educate owners on the dangers that parasites pose to their pets, the benefits of these preventive products, and ease of applying or administering these products. For further information regarding diagnosis and treatment of parasites, please refer to Chapter 14, "Parasitology," and Chapter 27, "Pharmacology and Pharmacy."

PREVENTIVE HEALTH PROGRAM FOR HORSES

A preventive health program for horses should be designed to meet the specific needs of the individual animal or herd. Such programs generally vary from one stable to another and from one veterinary practice to another, depending on expected exposures, management styles, and personal preferences of attending veterinarians and horse owners. An example of one preventive health program for horses is outlined in Box 8-1.

PHYSICAL EXAMINATION

All new additions to a stable or an established herd should have a negative Coggins test result for equine infectious anemia before arrival. Ideally upon arrival, the horse(s) should immediately be placed in quarantine for 1 month before entering the general population. During this time, the first physical examination of the preventive health program can be performed (refer to Chapter 7, "History and Physical Examination," and Chapter 20, "Large Animal Medical Nursing"). If quarantine facilities are not available, at the very least a thorough physical examination should be performed before the horse is allowed contact with any animals from the resident population. Any signs of illness or of a parasite infection should be addressed before the new horse is turned in with resident horses.

VACCINATIONS

Vaccination schedules are based on the age of the horse, anticipated exposure to infectious organisms, and the

| BOX 8-1 | General Outline of a Preventive Health Program for Horses |

Spring
- Perform annual physical examination.
- Vaccinate all horses; vaccinate broadmares approximately 30 days before foaling.
- Obtain fecal egg count; deworm those with egg counts greater than 150 eggs/g.
- Perform annual dentistry examination; remove wolf teeth in 2-year-olds.
- Trim feet every 6 to 8 weeks.

Summer
- Give booster vaccinations for herpesvirus and influenza in high-risk animals.
- Vaccinate foals beginning at 3 to 4 months of age (can delay until 6 months of age for foals born to vaccinated dams)
- Trim feet every 6 to 8 weeks.
- Obtain fecal egg count; deworm those with egg counts greater than 150 eggs/g.

Fall
- Give booster vaccinations for herpesvirus and influenza in high-risk animals.
- Give booster vaccinations for equine encephalitis viruses (WEE, EEE, VEE) and WNV in endemic areas.
- Trim feet every 6 to 8 weeks.
- Obtain fecal egg count; deworm those with egg counts greater than 150 eggs/g.
- Perform dentistry examination on horses younger than 5 years and on horses with known dental problems.

Winter
- Trim feet every 6 to 8 weeks.
- Deworm all horses with ivermectin-praziquantel or moxidectin-praziquantel to treat tapeworms and bots acquired over the summer and fall.

EEE, Eastern equine encephalitis; *VEE*, Venezuelan equine encephalitis; *WEE*, Western equine encephalitis; *WNV*, West Nile virus.

duration of immunity provided by the vaccine. Tables 8-5 and 8-6 list the vaccination guidelines provided by the American Association of Equine Practitioners. A variety of commercially available vaccines are approved for use in healthy horses, and the choice of product often depends on geographic location and personal experience and familiarity.

Young horses that are immunologically naïve or any horse that has an unknown immunization history should receive an initial immunization followed by a second booster immunization. The time between initial and booster vaccinations can vary based on the type of vaccine and the manufacturer but is generally 4 weeks.

> **TECHNICIAN NOTE** Young horses and those with an unknown vaccination history should receive an initial immunization followed by a booster in 4 weeks.

In rare instances, anaphylactoid reactions can occur with the use of any vaccine. These life-threatening crises must be handled quickly. Accordingly, it is essential that epinephrine be available for the treatment of anaphylactoid reactions. Other complications, such as fever, lameness, and swelling or abscess formation at the injection site, may occur with routine use of the vaccines. The horse owner should always be informed of these possibilities before any vaccine is administered.

Common diseases and vaccines used as an aid in disease prevention are discussed in the following sections.

Tetanus Vaccines

Tetanus, or lockjaw, is a disease characterized by muscular rigidity that may culminate in death from respiratory arrest or convulsions. Tetanus is caused by toxins produced by the anaerobic bacterium *Clostridium tetani*. Active immunity to tetanus is produced by administration of a tetanus **toxoid**, which is a purified, inactivated toxin of *C. tetani*.

C. tetani is routinely found in the environment, and yearly vaccinations are recommended for all horses. Tetanus toxoid booster vaccinations are routinely given by many veterinarians when treating horses with penetrating injuries or at surgery.

Tetanus **antitoxin** is produced by hyperimmunization of donor horses with tetanus toxoid. Tetanus antitoxin provides protection by binding to the *C. tetani* toxin and can be used locally at the site of infection or given parenterally. Administration of tetanus antitoxin to unvaccinated horses induces immediate protection, which lasts approximately 2 weeks, but its use should be restricted to high-risk cases because it can cause acute hepatitis.

Tetanus antitoxin and tetanus toxoid should never be mixed in the same syringe and should be injected at distant sites if administered at the same time.

> **TECHNICIAN NOTE** Tetanus antitoxin and tetanus toxoid should never be mixed in the same syringe.

Western, Eastern, and Venezuelan Encephalitis Vaccines

Equine encephalomyelitis is a viral neurologic disease of horses caused by Eastern, Western, and Venezuelan viruses. These viruses are maintained in nature by bird and animal reservoirs and are transmitted to horses by biting insects. Venezuelan equine encephalomyelitis occurs primarily in South and Central America and has not been diagnosed in the United States for many years. The trivalent vaccine is commonly used for horses in states bordering Mexico to create a buffer zone, which may prevent the spread of Venezuelan equine encephalomyelitis into the United States.

The equine encephalomyelitis vaccines currently used for active immunization are inactivated-virus vaccines. They should be administered annually before the biting-insect

TABLE 8-5	Vaccinations for Foals*†		
DISEASE	**FOALS AND WEANLINGS (<12 MO OF AGE) OF MARES VACCINATED IN THE PREPARTUM PERIOD FOR THE DISEASE**	**FOALS AND WEANLINGS (<12 MO OF AGE) OF UNVACCINATED MARES**	**COMMENTS**
<u>*CORE VACCINATIONS*</u> Protect Against Diseases That Are Endemic to a Region, Those With Potential Health Significance, Required by Law, Virulent/Highly Infectious, and/or Those Posing a Risk of Severe Disease. Core Vaccines Have Clearly Demonstrated Efficacy and Safety, and Thus Exhibit a High Energy Level of Patient Benefit and Low Enough Level Risk to Justify Their Use in All Equids.			
Tetanus	3-Dose series: 1st dose at 4-6 mo of age 2nd dose 4-6 wk after first dose 3rd dose at 10-12 mo of age	3-Dose series: 1st dose at 1-4 mo of age 2nd dose 4 wk after 1st dose 3rd dose 4 wk after 2nd dose	
Eastern/Western equine encephalomyelitis (EEE/WEE)	3-Dose series: 1st dose at 4-6 mo of age‡ 2nd dose 4-6 wk after first dose 3rd dose at 10-12 mo of age, before onset of next vector season	3-Dose series: 1st dose at 3-4 mo of age§ 2nd dose 4 wk after first dose 3rd dose at 10-12 mo of age, before onset of next vector season	*Note:* Primary vaccination series scheduling may be amended with vaccinations administered earlier to younger foals that are at increased disease risk owing to the presence of vectors. A foal born during the vector season may warrant beginning vaccination at an earlier age than a foal born before the vector season.
Rabies	3-Dose series: 1st dose at 6 mo of age 2nd dose 4-6 wk after first dose 3rd dose at 10-12 mo of age	3-Dose series: 1st dose at 3-4 mo of age 2nd dose 4 wk after first dose 3rd dose at 10-12 mo of age	
West Nile virus (WNV)	*Inactivated vaccine*¶ 3-Dose series: 1st dose at 4-6 mo of age 2nd dose 4-6 wk after the first dose 3rd dose at 10-12 mo of age, before onset of next vector season	*Inactivated vaccine*¶ 3-Dose series: 1st dose at 3-4 mo of age 2nd dose 4 wk after first dose 3rd dose at 10-12 mo of age, before onset of next vector season	*Note:* Primary vaccination series scheduling may be amended with vaccinations administered earlier to younger foals that are at increased disease risk owing to the presence of vectors. A foal born during the vector season may warrant beginning vaccination at an earlier age than a foal born before the vector season.
	Recombinant canarypox vaccine 3-Dose series: 1st dose at 5-6 mo of age 2nd dose 4 wk after 1st dose 3rd dose at 10-12 mo of age, before onset of next vector season	*Recombinant canarypox vaccine* 3-Dose series: 1st dose at 5-6 mo of age 2nd dose 4 wk after 1st dose 3rd dose at 10-12 mo of age, before onset of next vector season	No data are available for use of the recombinant or chimera product in foals <5 mo of age. If either product is administered to foals at <5 mo of age, the recommended primary schedule should still be completed.
	Flavivirus chimera vaccine 2-Dose series: 1st dose at 5-6 mo of age 2nd dose at 10-12 mo of age, before onset of next vector season	*Flavivirus chimera vaccine* 2-Dose series: 1st dose at 5-6 mo of age 2nd dose at 10-12 mo of age, before onset of next vector season	

TABLE 8-5	Vaccinations for Foals*†—cont'd		
DISEASE	**FOALS AND WEANLINGS (<12 MO OF AGE) OF MARES VACCINATED IN THE PREPARTUM PERIOD FOR THE DISEASE**	**FOALS AND WEANLINGS (<12 MO OF AGE) OF UNVACCINATED MARES**	**COMMENTS**
RISK-BASED VACCINATIONS Are Those Having Applications That May Vary Between Individuals, Populations, and Geographic Regions. Risk Assessment Should Be Performed by, or in Consultation With, a Licensed Veterinarian to Identify Which Vaccines Are Appropriate for a Given Horse or Population of Horses. The Listing of a Vaccine Here is NOT a Recommendation for Its Inclusion in a Vaccination Program. Vaccine Scheduling Is Provided for Use After It Has Been Determined Which, if Any, Risk-Based Vaccines Are Indicated. _Note:_ Vaccines Are Listed in This Table in Alphabetical Order, Not in Order of Priority for Use.			
Anthrax	Not applicable. Because it is not recommended to vaccinate mares during pregnancy, no foals of mares will be vaccinated prepartum.	No age-specific guidelines are available for this vaccine. Manufacturer's recommendation is for primary series of 2 doses administered subcutaneously at 2-3 wk intervals.	Antimicrobial drugs must **not** be given concurrently with this vaccine. Caution should be used during storage, handling, and administration of this live bacterial product. Consult a physician immediately should accidental human exposure (via mucous membranes, conjunctiva, or broken skin) occur.
Botulism	3-Dose series: 1st dose 2-3 mo of age 2nd dose 4 wk after 1st dose 3rd dose 4 wk after 2nd dose	3-Dose series: 1st dose 1-3 mo of age 2nd dose 4 wk after 1st dose 3rd dose 4 wk after 2nd dose	Maternal antibody does not interfere with vaccination; foals at high risk may be vaccinated as early as 2 wk of age.
Equine herpes virus (EHV)	_Inactivated or modified live vaccine_ 3-Dose series: 1st dose 4-6 mo of age 2nd dose 4-6 wk after 1st dose 3rd dose at 10-12 mo of age Revaccinate at 6-mo intervals	_Inactivated or modified live vaccine_ 3-Dose series: 1st dose 4-6 mo of age 2nd dose 4-6 wk after 1st dose 3rd dose at 10-12 mo of age Revaccinate at 6-mo intervals	
Equine viral arteritis (EVA)	Colt (male) foals Single dose at 6-12 mo of age (see comments)	Colt (male) foals Single dose at 6-12 mo of age (see comments)	Before initial vaccination, colt (male) foals should undergo serologic testing and be confirmed negative for antibodies to EVA. Testing should be performed shortly before, or preferably at, the time of vaccination. Because foals can carry colostrum-derived antibodies to EVA for up to 6 mo, testing and vaccination should NOT be performed before 6 mo of age.
Equine influenza	_Inactivated vaccine_ 3-Dose series: 1st dose at 6 mo of age 2nd dose 3-4 wk after 1st dose 3rd dose at 10-12 mo of age	_Inactivated vaccine_ 3-Dose series: 1st dose at 6 mo of age 2nd dose 3-4 wk after 1st dose 3rd dose at 10-12 mo of age	Increased risk of disease may warrant vaccinations of younger foals. Because some maternal anti-influenza antibody is likely to be present, a complete series of primary vaccinations should still be given after 6 mo of age.
	Modified live vaccine 2-Dose series, administered intranasally: 1st dose at 6-7 mo of age 2nd dose at 11-12 mo of age Revaccinate at 6-mo intervals	_Modified live vaccine_ 2-Dose series, administered intranasally: 1st dose at 6-7 mo of age 2nd dose at 11-12 mo of age Revaccinate at 6-mo intervals	

TABLE 8-5	Vaccinations for Foals*†—cont'd		
DISEASE	**FOALS AND WEANLINGS (<12 MO OF AGE) OF MARES VACCINATED IN THE PREPARTUM PERIOD FOR THE DISEASE**	**FOALS AND WEANLINGS (<12 MO OF AGE) OF UNVACCINATED MARES**	**COMMENTS**
Potomac horse fever (PHF)	2-Dose series: 1st dose at 5 mo of age 2nd dose 3-4 wk after 1st dose	2-Dose series: 1st dose at 5 mo of age 2nd dose 3-4 wk after 1st dose	If risk warrants, vaccine may be administered to younger foals. Subsequent doses are to be administered at 4-wk intervals until 6 mo of age.
Rotavirus	Not recommended in foals	Not recommended in foals	
Strangles (*Streptococcus equi*)	*Killed vaccine* 3-Dose series: 1st dose at 4-6 mo of age 2nd dose 4-6 wk after 1st dose 3rd dose 4-6 wk after 2nd dose	*Killed vaccine* 3-Dose series: 1st dose at 4-6 mo of age 2nd dose 4-6 wk after 1st dose 3rd dose 4-6 wk after 2nd dose	Vaccination is NOT recommended as a strategy in outbreak mitigation. If risk warrants, the MLV may be safely administered to foals as young as 6 wk of age. However, vaccine efficacy in this age group has not been adequately studied. If MLV is administered to younger foals, a 3rd dose of vaccine should then be administered 2-4 wk before weaning.
	Modified live vaccine 3-Dose series, administered intranasally: 1st dose at 6-9 mo of age 2nd dose 3-4 wk after 1st dose 3rd dose at 11-12 mo of age	*Modified live vaccine* 3-Dose series, administered intranasally: 1st dose at 6-9 mo of age 2nd dose 3-4 wk after 1st dose 3rd dose at 11-12 mo of age	

MLV, Modified live virus.

*ALL vaccination programs should be developed in consultation with a licensed veterinarian.

†The two categories (core and risk-based vaccinations) reflect differences in the foal's susceptibility to disease and ability to mount an appropriate immune response to vaccination based on the presence (or absence) of maternal antibodies derived from colostrums. The phenomenon of maternal antibody interference is discussed in the text portion of these guidelines.

‡*Foals in the Southeastern U.S.*: The primary vaccination series should be initiated with an additional dose at 3 mo of age because of early seasonal vector presence.

§*Foals in the Southeastern U.S.*: The primary vaccination series should be initiated at 3 mo of age because of early seasonal vector presence.

¶*Foals in the Southeastern U.S.*: Owing to early seasonal vector presence, the primary vaccination series should be initiated earlier with the addition of a dose at 3 mo of age.

¶*Foals in the Southeastern U.S.*: The primary vaccination series should be initiated at 3 mo of age because of early seasonal vector presence.

season. Vaccine protection lasts approximately 6 to 8 months, and in areas where winter freezes are uncommon or in endemic areas, semiannual vaccinations are advisable.

Equine Herpesvirus Vaccines

Equine herpesvirus (EHV), also known as *rhinopneumonitis*, frequently causes respiratory disease, but can also cause abortion, neurologic disease, and neonatal illness. Although multiple herpesviruses have been identified, current vaccines offer protection against EHV-1 and EHV-4. These viruses cause respiratory disease; however, EHV-1 is also associated with infections of the central nervous system and the reproductive tract. EHV-4 is most frequently associated with upper respiratory tract disease in young horses and is rarely a cause of abortion.

Both inactivated and modified live virus (MLV) vaccines are available for protection against the respiratory form of EHV; no currently available vaccines are licensed for protection against neurologic disease. Because immunity is short-lived, high-risk animals should be vaccinated every 6 months. Pregnant mares should be vaccinated during the fifth, seventh, and ninth months of gestation with an approved vaccine to aid in control of abortion.

Equine Influenza Vaccines

Equine influenza is a highly contagious viral disease with worldwide distribution. Influenza is contracted through inhalation and infects the upper and lower airways. Influenza is frequently seen in mobile populations of horses, and disease outbreaks usually occur in horses 1 to 3 years of age after mixing with infected horses at racetracks, training barns, or show grounds.

Both inactivated and MLV vaccines are available. MLV vaccines for influenza are administered intranasally and provide a greater duration of immunity. Booster vaccines are recommended every 6 months in high-risk animals.

TABLE 8-6 | Vaccinations for Adult Horses*

CORE VACCINATIONS Protect Against Diseases That Are Endemic to a Region, Are Virulent/Highly Contagious, Pose a Risk of Severe Disease, Those Having Potential Public Health Significance, and/or Are Required by Law. Core Vaccines Have Clearly Demonstrable Efficacy and Safety, With a High Enough Level of Patient Benefit and Low Enough Level of Risk to Justify Their Use in All Equids.

DISEASE	BROODMARES	OTHER ADULT HORSES (>1 YR OF AGE) PREVIOUSLY VACCINATED FOR THE DISEASE	OTHER ADULT HORSES (>1 YR OF AGE) UNVACCINATED OR LACKING VACCINATION HISTORY	COMMENTS
Tetanus	_Previously vaccinated_ Annual, 4-6 wk prepartum _Previously unvaccinated or having unknown vaccination history_ 2-Dose series: 2nd dose 4-6 wk after 1st dose Revaccinate 4-6 wk prepartum	Annual	2-Dose series: 2nd dose 4-6 wk after 1st dose Annual revaccination	Booster at time of penetrating injury or before surgery if last dose was administered more than 6 mo previously
Eastern/Western equine encephalomyelitis (EEE/WEE)	_Previously vaccinated_ Annual, 4-6 wk prepartum _Previously unvaccinated or having unknown vaccination history_ 2-Dose series: 2nd dose 4 wk after 1st dose Revaccinate 4-6 wk prepartum	Annual: spring, before onset of vector season	2-Dose series: 2nd dose 4-6 wk after 1st dose Revaccinate before onset of next vector season	_Consider 6-mo revaccination interval for_ 1. Horses residing in endemic areas 2. Immunocompromised horses
Rabies	Annual: 4-6 wk prepartum or before breeding (see comments)	Annual	Single dose: annual revaccination	NOTE on before breeding: Owing to the relatively long duration of immunity, this vaccine may be given post foaling but before breeding and thus may reduce the number of vaccines given to a mare prepartum.
West Nile virus (WNV)	_Previously vaccinated_ Annual: 4-6 wk prepartum	Annual: spring, before onset of vector season	_Inactivated vaccine_ 2-Dose series: 2nd dose 4-6 wk after 1st dose Revaccinate before onset of next vector season	When using inactivated or recombinant product, consider 6-mo revaccination interval for: 1. Horses residing in endemic areas 2. Juvenile (<5 yr of age) 3. Geriatric horses (>15 yr of age) 4. Immunocompromised horses
	Unvaccinated or lacking vaccination history • It is preferable to vaccinate naïve mares when open • In areas of high risk, initiate primary series as described for unvaccinated adult horses		_Recombinant canarypox vaccine_ 2-Dose series: 2nd dose 4-6 wk after 1st dose Revaccinate before onset of next vector season	

TABLE 8-6	Vaccinations for Adult Horses*—cont'd

RISK-BASED VACCINES Are Selected for Use Based on Risk Assessment Performed by, or in Consultation With, a Licensed Veterinarian. Use of These Vaccines May Vary Between Individuals, Populations, and/or Geographic Regions. _Note:_ Vaccines Are Listed in This Table in Alphabetical Order, Not in Order of Priority of Use.

DISEASE	BROODMARES	OTHER ADULT HORSES (>1 YR OF AGE) PREVIOUSLY VACCINATED FOR THE DISEASE	OTHER ADULT HORSES (>1 YR OF AGE)UNVACCINATED OR LACKING VACCINATION HISTORY	COMMENTS
West Nile virus (WNV)—cont'd			_Flavivirus chimera vaccine_ Single dose Revaccinate before onset of next vector season	
Anthrax	Not recommended during gestation	Annual	2-Dose series: 2nd dose 3-4 wk after 1st dose Annual revaccination	Do not administer concurrently with antibiotics. Use caution during storage, handling, and administration. Consult a physician immediately if exposure occurs by accidental injection, ingestion, or otherwise through the conjunctiva or broken skin.
Botulism	_Previously vaccinated_ Annual: 4-6 wk prepartum _Previously unvaccinated or having unknown vaccination history_ 3-Dose series: 1st dose at 8 mo gestation 2nd dose 4 wk after 1st dose 3rd dose 4 wk after 2nd dose	Annual	3-Dose series: 2nd dose 4 wk after 1st dose 3rd dose 4 wk after 2nd dose Annual revaccination	
Equine herpes virus (EHV)	3-Dose series with product labeled for protection against EHV abortion: Give at 5, 7, 9 mo of gestation	Annual (see comments)	3-Dose series: 2nd dose 4-6 wk after 1st dose 3rd dose 4-6 wk after 2nd dose	Consider 6-mo revaccination interval for: • Horses younger than 5 yr of age • Horses on breeding farms or in contact with pregnant mares • Performance or show horses at high risk

TABLE 8-6 | Vaccinations for Adult Horses*—cont'd

DISEASE	BROODMARES	OTHER ADULT HORSES (>1 YR OF AGE) PREVIOUSLY VACCINATED FOR THE DISEASE	OTHER ADULT HORSES (>1 YR OF AGE) UNVACCINATED OR LACKING VACCINATION HISTORY	COMMENTS
Equine viral arteritis (EVA)	Not recommended unless high risk	Annual: Stallions, teasers: vaccinate 2-4 wk before breeding season Mares: vaccinate when open	Single dose (see comments)	Before initial vaccination, intact males and any horses potentially intended for export should undergo serologic testing and be confirmed negative for antibodies to EVA. Testing should be performed shortly before, or preferably at, the time of vaccination.
Influenza	*Previously vaccinated* *Inactivated vaccine* Semiannual with one dose administered 4-6 wk prepartum *Canarypox vector vaccine* Semiannual with one dose administered 4-6 wk prepartum *Previously unvaccinated or having unknown vaccination history* *Inactivated vaccine* 3-Dose series: 2nd dose 4-6 wk after 1st dose 3rd dose 4-6 wk prepartum *Canarypox vector vaccine* 2-Dose series: 2nd dose 4-6 wk after 1st dose but no later than 4 wk prepartum	*Horses with ongoing risk of exposure* Semiannual *Horses at low risk of exposure* Annual	*Modified live vaccine* Single dose administered intranasally Revaccinate semiannually to annually *Inactivated vaccine* 3-Dose series: 2nd dose 4-6 wk after 1st dose 3rd dose 3-6 mo after 2nd dose Revaccinate semiannually to annually *Canarypox vector vaccine* 2-Dose series: 2nd dose 4-6 wk after 1st dose Revaccinate semiannually	
Potomac horse fever (PHF)	*Previously vaccinated* Semiannual, with one dose given 4-6 wk prepartum *Previously unvaccinated or having unknown vaccination history* 2-Dose series: 1st dose 7-9 wk prepartum 2nd dose 4-6 wk prepartum	Semiannual to annual	2-Dose series: 2nd dose 3-4 wk after 1st dose Semiannual or annual booster	A revaccination interval of 3-4 mo may be considered in endemic areas when disease risk is high.
Rotavirus	3-Dose series: 1st dose at 8 mo gestation 2nd and 3rd doses at 4-wk intervals thereafter	Not applicable	Not applicable	

		TABLE 8-6 Vaccinations for Adult Horses*—cont'd		
DISEASE	BROODMARES	OTHER ADULT HORSES (>1 YR OF AGE) PREVIOUSLY VACCINATED FOR THE DISEASE	OTHER ADULT HORSES (>1 YR OF AGE)UNVACCINATED OR LACKING VACCINATION HISTORY	COMMENTS
Strangles (Streptococcus equi)	Previously vaccinated Killed vaccine containing M-protein Semiannual with one dose given 4-6 wk prepartum Previously unvaccinated or having unknown vaccination history Killed vaccine containing M-protein 3-Dose series: 2nd dose 2-4 wk after 1st dose 3rd dose 4-6 wk prepartum	Semiannual to annual	Killed vaccine containing M-protein 2-3–Dose series: 2nd dose 2-4 wk after 1st dose 3rd dose (where recommended by manufacturer) 2-4 wk after 2nd dose Revaccinate semiannually Modified live vaccine 2-Dose series: Administered intranasally 2nd dose 3 wk after 1st dose Revaccinate semiannually to annually	Vaccination is not recommended as a strategy in outbreak mitigation.

*ALL vaccination programs should be developed in consultation with a licensed veterinarian.

Strangles Vaccines

Strangles is a respiratory disease caused by infection with the bacterium *Streptococcus equi*. Strangles is easily transmitted through direct contact with mucopurulent discharge from infected horses or from contaminated **fomites**, such as feeding utensils, buckets, or other equipment. Strangles is characterized by sudden onset of fever and nasal discharge followed by acute swelling and abscess formation in submaxillary, submandibular, and retropharyngeal lymph nodes.

Several inactivated injectable vaccines and one low-virulence live strain IN vaccines are available to aid in control and prevention of strangles. IM strangles vaccinations may cause postinjection reactions or abscesses at the site of administration. Because of these adverse effects, vaccination against strangles is recommended only for horses with a high likelihood of exposure. Vaccination is not 100% effective for preventing disease but does often reduce the severity and incidence of disease. Purpura hemorrhagica (immune-mediated vasculitis) is a possible adverse effect of all strangles vaccines.

> **TECHNICIAN NOTE** Administration of IN vaccines often results in MLV contamination of hands and clothing. Therefore IN vaccines should be given last if a series of injections is being given, and hands should be washed thoroughly after administration.

Equine Viral Arteritis Vaccine

Equine viral arteritis (EVA) is a contagious viral disease. Although infection is rarely serious in healthy adult horses, it is a matter of concern to horse breeders because it can lead to abortion or neonatal death, and it can render stallions as permanent carriers of the virus.

Only one commercially available MLV vaccine is available against EVA. Vaccination is recommended for colts intended to be breeding stallions and for broodmares with no evidence of previous exposure to the virus before being bred to carrier stallions. Vaccination is tightly controlled in some states, and seropositive horses may have problems with import or export to certain countries.

Potomac Horse Fever Vaccines

Potomac horse fever (PHF) is caused by *Neorickettsia risticii* (formerly known as *Ehrlichia risticii*). It is most prevalent in the eastern United States, particularly near large waterways, but has been identified throughout the United States and in other countries.

Approved vaccines are available for use in the control and prevention of PHF, and their use should be considered in areas where the disease is known to occur. The antibody response to vaccination is reportedly poor; however, vaccinated animals may exhibit reduced severity of clinical signs.

Botulism Vaccine

Botulism is caused by toxins produced by the bacterium *Clostridium botulinum* and results in gradual progressive muscular weakness. Multiple types of *C. botulinum* exist, although type B is most common in horses and is associated with the consumption of decaying forage.

The currently available equine botulism vaccine is a *C. botulinum* type B toxoid and is recommended for use in endemic areas. This vaccine requires an initial three-dose series followed by annual vaccination. Foals from unvaccinated mares may benefit from vaccination beginning as early as 2 weeks of age.

Anthrax Vaccine

Anthrax is caused by the bacterium *Bacillus anthracis*. Infection results from ingestion of soil, forage, or water contaminated with spores.

The currently available vaccine is an avirulent live-spore vaccine. Because swelling and abscesses have been associated with vaccination, its use is generally limited to high-risk areas.

Rabies Vaccines

Rabies is a viral disease affecting the nervous system and resulting in death. Approved killed-virus vaccines are available for use in horses and should be used annually. Rabies vaccines induce a strong immunologic response; therefore, only a single dose is required annually in adult horses.

West Nile Virus Vaccines

West Nile virus (WNV) was a foreign animal disease before 1999, when the disease was detected in humans and horses on the East Coast of the United States; however, WNV is currently prevalent throughout the United States. The disease is caused by a flavivirus that infects numerous species of birds and mosquitoes; humans and horses are dead-end hosts.

Several vaccines are available for protection against WNV. They should be administered annually before the biting-insect season. Vaccine protection lasts approximately 6 months; in areas where winter freezes are uncommon, semi-annual vaccinations are advisable.

PARASITES

A good preventive health program should account for control of internal and external parasites. Heavy parasite burdens decrease athletic and reproductive performance and can cause weight loss and colic. A good deworming program should target ascarids, small and large strongyles, bots, and tapeworms (see Chapter 14, "Parasitology").

It is important that all horses maintained at a facility be on an effective deworming program. If all horses pastured together are not properly dewormed, the parasite control program for all horses will be ineffective. No standard program delineates the frequency of administration or the anthelmintic of choice; therefore, it is important to discuss available options with owners.

Although the standard has been to recommend deworming of all horses every 8 to 12 weeks, studies have demonstrated that a small number of horses on each farm are usually responsible for carrying the majority of all worms. Why some horses carry high worm burdens and some do not is still unknown. Although treating all horses similarly is easiest, it is not ideal. If possible, fecal flotations should be evaluated on 10% of the herd immediately before and 7 days after dewormer administration. Egg counts greater than 150 eggs/g before deworming indicate that the interval between treatments is too long. The presence of ova after treatment indicates resistance to the anthelmintic used.

> **TECHNICIAN NOTE** Developing deworming protocols based on fecal egg counts is generally more cost-effective than "blanket deworming" all horses at set time periods.

A variety of anthelmintics are available; benzimidazoles (fenbendazole, oxfendazole, and oxibendazole), pyrantel salts, ivermectin, and moxidectin are the most common. No anthelmintic is effective against all internal parasites, and a few differences should be pointed out:

1. Moxidectin and ivermectin are the only approved boticides.
2. Praziquantel is the only Food and Drug Administration (FDA)-approved product for tapeworms and is available in combination with moxidectin and ivermectin.
3. Moxidectin and fenbendazole (fenbendazole given for 5 days at double dose) are approved for removal of encysted small strongyles.

Daily deworming products are available that can be added to a horse's grain and fed each day. Products currently available are ineffective in controlling all species of internal parasites. Many horse owners incorrectly assume that because their horses are on daily dewormer, internal parasites are not a problem.

Feed additives are also available that are lethal to developing housefly and stable fly larvae in treated horse feces (but are not effective against existing adult flies). These types of feed additives should be used with caution because they are organophosphate larvicides with possible adverse effects if used concomitantly with other pharmaceutical products.

DENTAL CARE

Routine examination and care of the teeth is an important part of any horse's preventive health program. It is estimated that as many as 80% of horses have dental problems. Signs of a dental problem can range from obvious to subtle and include weight loss, bad breath, excessive drooling, swelling of the face or jaw, dropping feed while eating, head tossing, excessive chewing of the bit, and problems while being ridden (bucking, tail ringing, fighting against the bit). Proper and thorough examination of the oral cavity usually requires sedation, a light source (such as a headlamp or a flashlight), and a mouth speculum.

In the horse, the teeth are continually erupting, and the lower jaw is narrower than the upper jaw. As the horse grinds its food from side to side, the teeth are worn down unevenly. The inside (near the tongue) of the upper teeth is worn, as is the outside (near the cheek) of the lower teeth. Thus sharp points develop on the outside of the upper teeth and the inside of the lower teeth. These sharp enamel points can become severe, resulting in lacerations of the tongue and cheek. Most enamel points can be removed by floating (rasping). The cheek teeth of the upper jaw are often positioned slightly forward of the teeth in the lower jaw, and because of the offset positioning, hooks and ramps can form. Hooks are sharp points found on the first upper cheek teeth. Ramps are sharp points found on the last lower cheek teeth.

Wolf teeth are the small, pointed, rudimentary first premolars located just in front of the first cheek teeth. Wolf teeth do not appear in all horses, are more common in the upper jaw than in the lower jaw, and vary in size. In some horses, the position of these teeth causes interference with the position and function of the bit. For this reason, wolf teeth are often removed before a horse enters training (around 12 to 18 months of age). Wolf teeth are generally removed while the horse is standing and sedated.

Normally, the deciduous premolars are replaced by the permanent premolars without a problem between the ages of 2 and 4 years. Occasionally a deciduous premolar fails to fall out—a condition known as a *retained cap*. This can result in discomfort leading to decreased feed consumption and lowered performance. Caps are easily removed in standing, sedated horses.

Feed that becomes trapped around a tooth can lead to bacterial growth, resulting in infection. Other causes of infection include a fractured jaw and inflammation of the periodontal ligament (ligament that holds a tooth to the bone). An infected tooth usually leads to the more obvious clinical signs of dental disease, such as a swollen face or jaw, a draining abscess, trouble eating, and foul breath. Because the upper teeth are closely associated with the nasal sinuses, nasal discharge and sinusitis can also be signs of infection. Depending on the site of the infection and the length of the tooth root, the infected tooth may be pulled from the oral cavity or removed by accessing the roots via the maxillary sinus or mandible and driving the tooth forward into the oral cavity.

Routine dental maintenance can prevent or minimize many of the dental problems observed in horses. Yearly examinations are recommended for mature horses. Young horses (2 to 5 years) are losing deciduous teeth and gaining their permanent teeth. During this time, 24 teeth are lost and replaced, providing ample opportunity for dental problems to occur. Young horses should undergo a thorough dental examination before starting training and then twice yearly until all permanent teeth are in. Finally, horses with a history of dental problems should have their teeth examined biannually or even more frequently if required.

> **TECHNICIAN NOTE** Young horses (younger than 5 years) and those with a history of dental problems should have their teeth examined biannually.

HOOF CARE

The roles of the veterinarian and the veterinary technician in hoof care are largely advisory because most routine hoof care is provided by farriers. However, education of the client on the importance of proper and frequent hoof care for the prevention of lameness is important.

Horse hooves grow an average of one-quarter inch per month depending on ground surface, exercise frequency, nutrition, and individual growth rates. Based on the average growth rate, hooves should be trimmed every 6 to 8 weeks to maintain proper shape, balance, and movement. Keeping the hooves trimmed short and maintaining the correct hoof-pastern axis helps prevent excess stress on tendons and ligaments of the limb. In foals, some minor conformation problems, such as splayfoot or pigeon toe, can be corrected or minimized with frequent hoof trimming.

Cleaning out the bottom of the foot is also important. Hoof cleaning not only removes rocks and debris from the foot, it also helps in the prevention of thrush. Thrush is caused by anaerobic bacteria that grow in moist and dark conditions, such as in the sulci of the frog and under dirt that has accumulated and packed into the sole. Thrush appears as a moist, malodorous accumulation in the sulci of the frog and sometimes over the sole. Frequent cleaning removes dirt and exposes these bacteria to drying, aerobic conditions. Copper- or iodine-based solutions can be applied to the sulci and the frog to treat thrush.

NUTRITION

Proper nutrition is the foundation for any preventive health program. Many health issues, such as laminitis, colic, and ulcers, can be directly related to nutritional problems. Owners should be encouraged to feed a balanced diet and to work closely with their veterinarian or equine nutritionist to develop proper diets for their horse(s). Equine nutrition is discussed in greater detail in Chapter 10, Large Animal Nutrition.

PREVENTIVE HEALTH PROGRAMS FOR LIVESTOCK SPECIES

Preventive medicine is especially important in livestock species to maintain the productivity of the herd. Management, nutrition, and vaccination all play a role in minimizing the incidence of disease in livestock species. This section is not intended to provide a comprehensive review of all of the vaccines available for livestock; the goal is to describe typical preventive management procedures and commonly used vaccination programs.

SWINE
Birth to Weaning
Preventive medicine in swine herds begins with piglets, which must be kept in a warm, draft-free environment. When young pigs are are cold, they lie on top of each other, increas the risk of rectal prolapse. Within the first week of life, piglets have their **needle (canine) teeth** trimmed and tails docked to decrease chewing on each other. Baby pigs are commonly given a shot of iron within the first few days of life to prevent anemia, and male piglets that will not be used for breeding are castrated.

Growing Pigs

Pigs are vaccinated against erysipelas at weaning, when they are removed from the sow and placed into groups of growing pigs. Erysipelas, which is caused by the bacteria *Erysipelothrix rhusiopathiae,* is characterized by fever, skin lesions, and sudden death in infected pigs. Animals that survive the acute infection may develop chronic arthritis or endocarditis and consequently grow poorly. Pens into which weaned pigs are moved must be cleaned and disinfected, and they must be well ventilated without being cold or drafty. Newly grouped weaned pigs should not be mixed in pens or buildings with older pigs because this would increase stress and competition for food for the younger pigs and may expose them to diseases carried by the older pigs. Overcrowding must also be avoided. Because weaning is a stressful time for pigs, some farms will add antibiotics to the feed for a few weeks after weaning to help counteract the increased risk of infectious disease due to stress-induced suppression of the immune system during the post-weaning period. Pigs may be dewormed at weaning, if necessary, and some farms will vaccinate pigs at weaning against pathogens that may cause pneumonia, such as *Mycoplasma* bacteria.

Biosecurity (a protocol to prevent the introduction of disease organisms onto the farm) is practiced commonly and strictly in swine production. On some farms, all visitors, including veterinarians and their staff, are asked to shower and change into clothing provided by the farm before coming into contact with any animals. The risk of spreading disease may also be minimized by working with the youngest pigs first, then proceeding through progressively older groups of pigs.

Breeding Animals

Pigs are commonly vaccinated for leptospirosis, parvovirus, and again for erysipelas before entering the breeding herd. Leptospirosis, an infection with *L. pomona, L. bratislava,* or other members of the genus *Leptospira,* may cause infertility, abortion, stillbirth, or the birth of weak piglets. Animals purchased for breeding should be tested for brucellosis, and for pseudorabies if the animals are not from a pseudorabies-free area (commercial pigs in the United States are considered pseudorabies-free, but feral pigs in some southern states and California may still carry the disease). Brucellosis may cause abortion or infertility and it is zoonotic. Pseudorabies causes infertility, death in young pigs, and respiratory disease with the possibility of chronic infection in older animals. Animals entering a herd free of porcine reproductive and respiratory syndrome (PRRS) should also be tested for the PRRS virus, which causes reproductive failure, respiratory disease, and chronic infections. Depending on their origin, animals may need to be treated for internal and external parasites. New additions to the herd should always be quarantined away from the herd for 30 days or longer before they are introduced to the rest of the herd. Quarantine prevents new animals from spreading diseases that they may have been carrying asymptomatically when they were purchased

or diseases such as pneumonia that they may have developed during transport to the farm.

Sows in the breeding herd should have booster vaccinations against erysipelas and leptospirosis when their litters are weaned; boars may be given the same vaccines every 6 months. Sows and gilts (young sows) may also be vaccinated against *Escherichia coli* bacteria to diminish the occurrence of diarrhea in their offspring, and against parvovirus, which may cause infertility and abortion.

> **TECHNICIAN NOTE**   Because swine in modern production systems may never be outdoors, many pigs do not require deworming at any time.

CATTLE

Although beef and dairy production systems have many differences, they are discussed together here because many of the principles of disease control and diseases of concern are the same in both systems.

Birth to Weaning

In cattle, preventive medicine often starts before birth because many pregnant cows are vaccinated against *Escherichia coli,* rotavirus, and coronavirus to protect their calves from developing diarrhea. Colostrum from vaccinated cows provides extra protection to calves against diseases for which the cow has been vaccinated. Calves should be born into a dry, draft-free environment. It is essential that calves receive an adequate amount of good quality colostrum soon after birth. In beef herds, this is ensured by frequent monitoring of cows during calving season, whereas dairy herds typically hand-feed colostrum to newborn calves. Dairy farms will keep frozen colostrum or colostrum replacer on hand to feed orphan calves or calves from dams that fail to produce adequate colostrum or leak colostrum before calving.

> **TECHNICIAN NOTE**   The first step in keeping calves healthy is ensuring that they receive an adequate amount of good quality colostrum shortly after birth.

In calves, weaning is the discontinuation of milk consumption by the calf. Dairy calves are raised away from their dams, so weaning is primarily a dietary adjustment, although calves are often housed in larger groups after weaning than during the milk-feeding period. In beef calves, weaning is usually achieved by separating the calf from its dam. Vaccination in beef calves should begin before weaning because weaning is a stressful time, and stress may suppress the immune system, increasing the risk of developing infectious disease. Refer to Table 8-7 for a list of vaccines used in cattle. Weaning in dairy calves is done at a younger age than in beef calves (younger than 2 months of age vs. about 6 months), so vaccination is commonly delayed until after weaning in dairy calves. For any young cattle, vaccination at younger than 3 months of age is likely to be incompletely effective as

TABLE 8-7	Vaccines Used in Cattle	
DISEASE	**TYPICAL SCHEDULE**	**COMMENTS**
*Viral diseases (IBR-BVD-PI3-BRSV)	Two doses in calfhood, annually thereafter	IBR, BVD, PI3, and BRSV are respiratory pathogens. BVD can cause a variety of disease syndromes and depressed immune function.
*Leptospirosis	Two doses in calfhood, every 3-12 months in adulthood	Leptospirosis is commonly included in viral combination vaccines. Leptospirosis decreases reproductive performance.
*Brucellosis	One dose in calfhood, females only	Commonly called "Bangs" vaccine. Vaccination of heifers makes interstate shipment and sale easier. Brucellosis decreases reproductive performance.
*Clostridial diseases	Two doses in calfhood, optional in adults	Most vaccines include several clostridial components, often referred to as *7-way* or *Blackleg* vaccine.
Campylobacteriosis	Annually before breeding season in beef herds	Also called vibriosis or "vibrio"; decreases reproductive performance.
Bacterial respiratory diseases	Before weaning or upon entrance to the feedlot	These vaccines are often multivalent, including antigens from *Pasteurella, Mannheimia,* and *Haemophilus* bacteria.
Gram-negative mastitis	Follow label directions	Commonly used in dairy cows.
Rotavirus and coronavirus	Administered to pregnant cows	Designed to protect calves from diarrhea via antibodies in the cow's colostrum.

Vaccines may be used in other situations such as anaplasmosis, anthrax, Johne's disease, pinkeye *(Moraxella bovis)*, footrot, and trichomoniasis.

*Core vaccines.
This table is not intended to be comprehensive.
BRSV, Bovine respiratory syncytial virus; *BVD,* bovine diarrhea virus; *IBR,* infectious bovine rhinotracheitis; *PI3,* parainfluenza 3.

a result of interference from maternal antibodies obtained in colostrum; maternal antibodies against the antigen in a vaccine may bind the antigen and prevent it from stimulating a good response from the calf's own immune system. Calfhood vaccination programs usually include a clostridial vaccine, a viral respiratory and reproductive pathogen vaccine, and brucellosis vaccination (often called "Bangs" vaccination). Clostridial diseases, such as tetanus, blackleg, and malignant edema, are caused by bacteria from the genus *Clostridium,* occur primarily in young animals, and often are rapidly fatal. Viral respiratory and reproductive diseases are commonly included in one "5-way" or "6-way" product, usually with a brand name connoting strength rather than what the vaccine is designed to protect against. The viral reproductive and respiratory pathogens commonly included in combination vaccines are bovine diarrhea virus (BVD), which may cause diarrhea, mucosal ulcers, abortion, and immunosuppression, plus infectious bovine rhinotracheitis (IBR), parainfluenza 3 (PI3), and bovine respiratory syncytial virus (BRSV), which are primarily respiratory pathogens. These combination vaccines also frequently include the bacterial pathogens *Histophilus somnus,* which may cause sudden death or fever and depression, and/or *Leptospira* species, which cause infertility and abortion. Bangs vaccination protects against brucellosis, an infection with *Brucella abortus* that is associated with abortion and infertility. Brucellosis vaccination is reported to the USDA, and vaccinates are marked with an orange ear tag and a tattoo in the right

ear. Only heifers younger than 1 year may be legally vaccinated against brucellosis, and in some states, the maximum age for vaccination is less than 1 year. Vaccination against brucellosis is especially important for animals that may be sold as breeding stock. Special care is taken in the handling and administration of RB51, the brucellosis vaccine, because the vaccine contains live organisms and the disease is zoonotic. Unlike the clostridial and viral vaccines, the brucellosis vaccine is given only one time; there is no "booster" vaccination.

Beef and dairy cattle that naturally have horns are commonly dehorned to protect other animals from injury. In dairy calves, this is usually done within the first few weeks of life, whereas in beef animals, dehorning may be done at the time of weaning.

> **TECHNICIAN NOTE** Cattle vaccines should be administered as labeled (IM or SQ) only in the neck region to maintain meat quality. In addition, most vaccines for food animals have withdrawal or withholding periods wherein the animal and its products (such as milk) may not be sold for human consumption.

Growing Cattle

Disease in growing cattle is best prevented by appropriate nutrition and clean, well-ventilated housing (or good pasture), in addition to vaccination. Growing cattle that are at risk will need to be treated for external and internal parasites as necessary. Adequate fly control will help prevent infectious bovine keratoconjunctivitis (pinkeye), an infection of the eye caused by *Branhamella ovis* and/or *Moraxella bovis* bacteria, which are carried between animals on flies. Heifers commonly receive another dose of viral respiratory and reproductive vaccine before being bred for the first time. Beef cattle are typically given a repeat vaccination against viral respiratory pathogens upon entering the feedlot; in addition, such animals are commonly vaccinated against the bacterial respiratory pathogens *Histophilus somnus, Mannheimia hemolytica,* and *Pasteurella multocida.*

Breeding Animals

To protect the health of the herd, care must be taken when breeding bulls are obtained. Beef herds are more likely to purchase bulls because they generally employ natural breeding throughout the herd, whereas dairy herds use artificial insemination extensively. In addition to a breeding soundness examination for fertility, purchased bulls should at least have a negative test result for BVD, which may cause infertility, abortion, diarrhea, death, or a chronic poor condition. It is also advisable to test bulls for the venereal disease trichomoniasis, which is passed to cows during breeding and causes fertility problems. It is preferable to purchase the bull from a herd that is free of Johne's disease, which is caused by *Mycobacterium paratuberculosis* bacteria and is manifested by chronic diarrhea and weight loss, and bovine leukosis virus (BLV), which may cause cancer. Bulls should be vaccinated before the breeding season against the viral respiratory and reproductive pathogens; campylobacteriosis, which is caused by *Campylobacter fetus* bacteria and may be passed to cows when breeding and cause infertility; and leptospirosis. Cows also should be revaccinated against these diseases before the breeding season.

> **TECHNICIAN NOTE**   Nearly all adult cattle receive vaccinations against viral respiratory and reproductive pathogens (IBR, BVD, PI3, and BRSV), frequently combined with antigens for one or more bacterial pathogens, at least once per year.

In dairy cows, mastitis (an infection of the mammary gland) is an important disease and a key focus of preventive efforts. Dairy cows are commonly vaccinated against mastitis caused by *Escherichia coli,* which can be severe and life threatening. The vaccine does not prevent *E. coli* mastitis, but it does reduce the frequency and severity of the disease on the farm. Most cases of mastitis cannot be prevented by vaccination; prevention also relies on management steps. These include keeping cow housing and milking areas clean, cleaning the teats well before milking, dipping the teats into disinfectant before and after milking (called predipping and postdipping), and providing proper nutrition.

Only the most commonly used vaccines were mentioned previously, but many more are available. Not all available vaccines are considered effective. Vaccine protocols should be tailored to each herd specifically based on needs and risks in the herd. It must also be kept in mind that even an excellent vaccination protocol cannot overcome poor management and nutrition. Additional information about common infectious diseases in cattle may be found in Chapter 20 Large Animal Medical Nursing. Hoof trimming is especially important in dairy animals. They may not wear their hooves down as quickly as they grow, and animals that have suffered an episode of lameness may not wear their hooves evenly. Dairy cows should have their feet trimmed at least once a year; more often if problems develop. Because they walk more, beef animals do not usually need routine trimming, but this practice may be necessary for animals with abnormal hoof growth patterns, such as "corkscrew claws," in which the wall of the hoof spirals under the sole. This is thought to be a hereditary problem, so cows who display corkscrew claws probably should be removed from a breeding program.

As with bulls, purchased cows should be tested and quarantined before joining a herd. It is preferable to buy cows from a herd that is free of Johne's disease and BLV, and all animals should have a negative test result for BVD virus. In addition, the milk of purchased dairy cows should have a negative test result for the presence of mastitis infection.

SMALL RUMINANTS: SHEEP AND GOATS
Newborn and Growing Animals

As with cattle, preventive health programs for sheep and goats begin before birth, when pregnant ewes and does are vaccinated against *Clostridium perfringens* types C and D and *Clostridium tetani* bacteria, which cause the usually fatal diseases lamb dysentery, overeating disease, and tetanus. Protection for lambs and kids is provided through the colostrum of their vaccinated dams. Previously vaccinated ewes and does should be vaccinated against these clostridial diseases again at least 4 weeks before their due date; if they have not previously been vaccinated, they should be vaccinated twice during pregnancy. Refer to Table 8-8 for a list of vaccines used in sheep and goats. The offspring of vaccinated dams should be vaccinated twice between 6 and 10 weeks of age. If ewes and does do not get vaccinated during pregnancy, kids or lambs should be vaccinated just after birth and again at 2 to 3 weeks of age. In selenium-deficient areas, ewes should be supplemented with selenium orally or by injection to prevent weakness caused by selenium deficiency (white muscle disease) in their lambs.

During the first 2 weeks of life, most sheep in the United States have their tails "docked" or shortened. This is believed to decrease the accumulation of feces on the tail and the risk of infestation of the tail with fly larvae (maggots). In addition, sheep with docked tails may be easier to shear and fetch a higher price when sold for meat. Tail docking is usually performed using a hot metal instrument that cuts off the tail and cauterizes blood vessels at the same time, or by applying a very tight elastic band to the tail, which causes it to undergo necrosis (death) and to fall off after a few weeks. It is

TABLE 8-8	Vaccines Used in Sheep and Goats	
DISEASE	**TYPICAL SCHEDULE**	**COMMENTS**
*Clostridial diseases	Two doses while growing, periodically thereafter	Commonly called "CD-T"; includes protection against *Clostridium perfringens* types C and D (bloody scours and pulpy kidney disease) and *Clostridium tetani* (tetanus).
Sore mouth	Annually	Also called *contagious ecthyma* or *orf*. Caused by a poxvirus. Vaccine is live and should not be used on farms that do not already have sore mouth on the premises.
Rabies	Annually	Not practical or necessary in commercial flocks, but recommended for pets.

Vaccines may be used in other situations such as footrot, chlamydia, vibriosis, and caseous lymphadenitis.

*Core vaccine.
This table is not intended to be comprehensive.

recommended to leave the tail long enough to cover the animal's anus; too short docking of the tail may damage local nerves and increase the risk of rectal prolapse. Male animals that will not be sold young or used for breeding are usually castrated, either by surgically removing the testicles or by applying a tight elastic band to the scrotum, as may be done to remove tails.

Most goats will grow horns if they do not have their horn buds removed; this removal is best done in the first week of life and is usually performed using a hot iron instrument that destroys the horn-growing cells of the horn bud. If the horn bud is not removed when the goat is small, and an animal without horns is desired, the goat will have to be de-horned, which is a more complex procedure than disbudding a kid. Horns are moved to protect people and other animals from damage that may be caused by the horns.

At the time of castration, horn bud removal, dehorning, and/or tail docking, tetanus antitoxin should be administered to the offspring of ewes and does that were not vaccinated against clostridial diseases during pregnancy.

> **TECHNICIAN NOTE** Diseases caused by bacteria of the genus *Clostridium* are especially dangerous in sheep and goats. Pregnant ewes and does should be vaccinated against clostridial diseases to protect their offspring.

Small ruminants may also be vaccinated against contagious ecthyma, also called *orf* or *sore mouth*. It is a viral disease that causes painful lesions of the skin on the mouth of young animals and the mouth and teats of ewes and does, resulting in decreased nursing by young animals. Sore mouth vaccination is performed by scratching the skin in an area

without wool (inner ear or under the tail in older animals, inner thigh in young animals) and introducing a live virus into the scratch. This must be done well before lambing or kidding, so that newborn animals will not be affected. In addition, great care must be taken by the person administering the vaccine because it contains a live virus and the disease is zoonotic. The vaccine should not be used in herds that have not had problems with the disease.

Coccidia are present in all sheep and goats and may cause diarrhea, weight loss, and illness in young animals under stress. Coccidia are controlled by management steps such as preventing overcrowding, providing good sanitation, and not placing feed on the ground. A coccidiostatic drug, such as lasalocid or decoquinate, may be added to the feed to help prevent outbreaks of coccidiosis at times of stress.

The Breeding Herd

For small ruminants kept as pets, rabies vaccination is probably worthwhile, although it is not used in commercial flocks. As in other species, many other vaccines are available for use in sheep and goats; decisions about whether to use them in particular animals or herds should be made in consultation with a veterinarian and in consideration of specific needs and risks.

> **TECHNICIAN NOTE** Rabies vaccination is not practiced for all animals in commercial sheep and goat flocks, but it is a good idea for pet sheep and goats.

Parasitism is a serious problem in sheep and goats, particularly infestations with *Haemonchus contortus*, also called the *barber pole worm*. *H. contortus* attaches to the wall of the abomasum and consumes the animal's blood. If left untreated, infestation may lead to severe anemia and death. No strategy completely eliminates internal parasites in sheep and goats, but the burden can be reduced in several ways. One approach is good nutrition; well-nourished animals are less susceptible to parasitic illness. Feed should be elevated from the ground in a trough into which young animals cannot climb, to reduce contamination of feed with feces. Goats that are able to browse plants above the ground, instead of just grazing as sheep do, will have reduced parasite burdens. Parasitism in sheep may be reduced by rotating them through pastures that have been kept empty or have been used by cattle or horses (not goats) or crops for the previous 3 to 6 months. Culling of animals with chronic severe parasitism is recommended because such animals have low parasite resistance—a trait that may be passed on to offspring. Oral dewormers of the benzimidazole (e.g., thiabendazole) and avermectin (e.g., ivermectin) families are used in small ruminants, but these drugs must be used strategically because overuse promotes resistance. Some experts have recommended deworming only animals that show signs of disease. Sheep may develop external parasites, such as ticks and lice, which should be treated as necessary with sprays, dips, or ivermectin-type drugs.

> **TECHNICIAN NOTE** Sheep may be evaluated for anemia caused by parasitism with *Haemonchus contortus* by examining the conjunctiva of the eyes. If it is white, not pink, the animal is likely to be anemic and heavily parasitized.

SUMMARY

Many aspects of preventive medicine must be applied in livestock species. Vaccination is important, but it is not a substitute for proper management. In addition to vaccination, disease is prevented through proper nutrition, good hygiene, appropriate housing, and parasite control. New animals must be tested for disease and quarantined before they are mixed in with the herd, to prevent the introduction of disease into the herd.

RECOMMENDED READINGS

Dogs and Cats

Boss N, Holmstrom S, Vogt AH, et al: Development of new canine and feline preventive healthcare guidelines designed to improve pet health, J Am Anim Hosp Assoc 47:306, 2011. Available at: https://www.aahanet.org/Library/PreventiveHealthcare.aspx (accessed on December 30, 2011).

Day MJ: Immune system development in the dog and cat, J Comp Path 137:S10, 2007.

Epstein M, Kuehn NF, Landsberg G, et al: AAHA senior care guidelines for dogs and cats, J Am Anim Hosp Assoc 41:81, 2005. Available at: https://www.aahanet.org/Library/SeniorCare.aspx (accessed on December 30, 2011).

Greene CE: Infectious diseases of the dog and cat, ed 4, St Louis, 2012, Saunders.

Pittari J, Rodan I, Beekman G, et al: American Association of Feline Practitioners senior care guidelines, J Fel Med Surg 11:763, 2009. Available at: http://www.catvets.com/professionals/guidelines/publications/?Id=398 (accessed on December 30, 2011).

Richards JR, Elston TH, Ford RB, et al: The 2006 American Association of Feline Practitioners feline vaccine advisory panel report, J Am Vet Med Assoc 229:1405, 2006. Available at: http://www.catvets.com/professionals/guidelines/publications/?Id=176 (accessed on December 30, 2011).

United State Department of Agriculture, Animal and Plant Health Inspection Service. Adverse event reporting, 2010. Available at: http://www.aphis.usda.gov/animal_health/vet_biologics/vb_adverse_event.shtml (accessed on December 30, 2011).

Vaccine-Associated Feline Sarcoma Task Force: Vaccine-Associated Feline Sarcoma Task Force guidelines: diagnosis and management of suspected sarcomas, American Veterinary Medical Association website. Available at: http://www.avma.org/vafstf/tfguidelines99.asp (accessed on December 30, 2011).

Vogt AH, Rodan I, Brown M, et al: AAFP-AAHA feline life stage guidelines, J Am Anim Hosp Assoc 46:70, 2010. Available at: https://www.aahanet.org/library/felinelife.aspx (accessed on December 30, 2011).

Welborn LV, DeVries JG, Ford R, et al: 2011 AAHA canine vaccination guidelines, J Am Anim Hosp Assoc 47:1, 2011. Available at: https://www.aahanet.org/library/caninevaccine.aspx (accessed on December 30, 2011).

Horses

Ensminger ME, Hammer CJ: Ensminger's equine science, ed 8, Upper Saddle River, NJ, 2004, Pearson Prentice Hall.

Love S: Treatment and prevention of intestinal parasite-associated disease, Vet Clin North Am Equine Pract 3:791, 2003.

Smith BP: Large animal internal medicine, ed 4, St Louis, 2009, Mosby.

Livestock

Bagley CV: Vaccination program for beef calves. Available at: http://extension.usu.edu/files/publications/factsheet/ah_beef__40.pdf.

Bagley CV: Vaccination program for dairy young stock. Available at: http://extension.usu.edu/files/publications/factsheet/AH_Dairy_06.pdf.

Maryland small ruminant page: Available at: www.sheepandgoat.com.

Tubbs RC: Herd health programs for swine seedstock production. Available at: http://extension.missouri.edu/explore/agguides/ansci/g02508.htm (accessed on October 4, 2008).

Tubbs RC, Floss JL: Herd management for disease prevention. Available at: http://extension.missouri.edu/explore/agguides/ansci/g02507.htm (accessed on October 4, 2008).

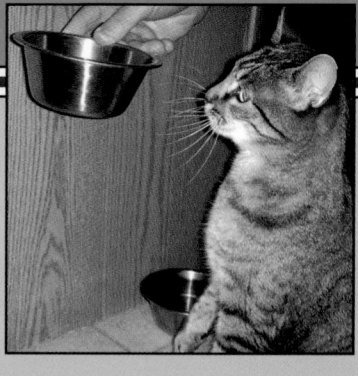

9

Small Animal Nutrition

Craig Datz

OUTLINE

Nutrients, *293*
Water, *293*
Protein, *293*
Fat, *293*
Carbohydrate, *294*
Vitamins, *294*
Minerals, *294*
Fiber, *295*
Supplements, *295*
Energy, *295*
Food Intake and Regulation, *295*
Energy Units, *295*
Energy Partitioning, *295*
Metabolizable Energy Measurement, *296*
Atwater Factors, *296*
Energy Density, *296*
Measurements of Energy Expenditure, *296*
Protein, *297*
Dietary Requirements, *297*
Protein Quality, *298*
Fat, *298*
Structure, *298*
Dietary Requirements, *299*
Carbohydrate, *300*
Dietary Requirements, *300*
Fiber, *300*
Dietary Requirements, *300*
Vitamins, *300*
Dietary Requirements, *300*
Minerals, *302*
Dietary Requirements, *302*
Commercial Pet Food, *304*
History, *304*
Types, *305*
Marketing, *305*
Veterinary Therapeutic Diets, *308*
Pet Food Regulation, *309*
Pet Food Labels, *310*
Home-Prepared Pet Food, *313*
Including or Avoiding Specific
   Ingredients, *313*

Chemicals, *313*
Preservatives, *313*
Additives, *314*
By-products, *314*
Perceived Low Quality of Pet Foods, *314*
Avoiding Contaminants and Toxins, *314*
Perceived Health Benefits, *315*
Food Allergy or Intolerance, *315*
Palatability, *315*
Cost, *315*
Human-Animal Bond, *315*
Recipes and Sources, *315*
Home Recipe Formulation, *317*

FEEDING HEALTHY DOGS AND
   CATS, *317*
Dogs, *317*
Neonatal Period, *317*
Weaning, *318*
Growth, *318*
Feeding Plan for Growth, *319*
Adult Maintenance, *320*
Feeding Plan for Adult Maintenance, *322*
Gestation, *323*
Parturition, *323*
Lactation, *323*
Working and Performance, *324*
Seniors, *324*
Feeding Plan for Seniors, *325*
Cats, *325*
Neonatal Period, *325*
Weaning, *325*
Growth, *325*
Feeding Plan for Growth, *327*
Adult Maintenance, *327*
Feeding Plan for Adult Maintenance, *328*
Reproduction, *328*
Seniors, *329*
Clinical Nutrition, *329*
Assisted Feeding, *329*
Nutritional Strategies for Obesity, *335*

KEY TERMS

Amino acid
Assisted feeding
Atwater factors
Body condition score
Calorie
Energy density
Esophagostomy tubes
Fatty acid
Kilojoule
Lipid
Metabolizable energy
Metabolizable
   (maintenance) energy
   requirement
Nutrient
Palatability

*The authors and the publisher wish to acknowledge Mary Tefend Campbell for her previous
contributions to this chapter.*

When you have completed this chapter, you will be able to:

1. Define, pronounce, and spell all of the Key Terms.
2. List the macronutrients and micronutrients found in pet food. Explain what building-block molecules compose these nutrients, if any.
3. Compare and contrast the concepts of energy units, energy partitioning, metabolizable energy measurement, Atwater factors, energy density, and measurements of energy expenditure.
4. Discuss the requirements for protein, fat, carbohydrates, fiber, vitamins, and minerals in the diet of dogs and cats.
5. Explain various aspects regarding commercial pet food, including the following:
   - Describe how commercial pet food manufacturing has developed since the late 19th century and compare the different types of pet food available today.
   - Describe which marketing language bears little nutritional significance and explain how veterinary therapeutic diets may be used appropriately and inappropriately.
   - Explain how pet food manufacturing is regulated in the United States and identify the government agencies and organizations involved in the regulation of pet food.
   - List the components of pet food labels and explain how the information provided in each component should be interpreted.
6. Compare and contrast the reasons why clients might feed home-cooked diets to their pets.
7. Describe feeding protocols for healthy dogs and cats at each stage of life, including pregnant and lactating bitches.
8. Explain the principles of clinical nutrition.
9. Describe methods of providing therapeutic enteral and parenteral nutrition.
10. Describe a safe and effective weight-loss program for dogs and cats.

INTRODUCTION

Nutrition is the story of **nutrients,** especially how they are obtained and how they are used in the bodies of all living organisms. With well over 100 years of research behind us, we have an advanced understanding of nutrition that allows us to feed animals for good health and long lives. There is still much to learn, however, about the differences between basic and optimal nutrition, the challenges of feeding during illness instead of health, and the interactions of both known and unknown nutrients and other substances in foods. This chapter emphasizes a nutrient-oriented approach to feeding dogs and cats. Basic information about nutrients found in foods and supplements is presented first. Practical information about diets and real-world feeding follows, including evaluation of commercial products and nutritional strategies for different life stages of both dogs and cats.

NUTRIENTS

A nutrient is usually defined as a substance that provides nourishment to an organism. A better definition is something essential that a plant or animal obtains from the environment for growth and maintenance of life. Nutrients are chemicals, but because the term "chemical" implies something artificial that is produced in a laboratory, we rarely use it. Nutrients usually are grouped into categories that help us understand their importance and function (Box 9-1). However, there is some overlap among these categories, and some nutrient-like substances are not easily categorized. Three types of nutrients, often referred to as *macronutrients,* can be used by the body for energy production: protein, fat, and carbohydrate. Other nutrients, called *micronutrients,* have many functions but do not provide energy. These include vitamins and minerals, along with certain supplements found in pet foods (Figure 9-1).

> **TECHNICIAN NOTE** Protein, fat, and carbohydrate are nutrients that supply energy.

BOX 9-1	Classification of Nutrients

1. Water
2. Macronutrients
   a. Protein
      i. Essential amino acids
      ii. Nonessential amino acids
   b. Fat
      i. Essential fatty acids
      ii. Nonessential fatty acids
   c. Carbohydrate
3. Micronutrients
   a. Vitamins
   b. Minerals
      i. Macrominerals
      ii. Microminerals

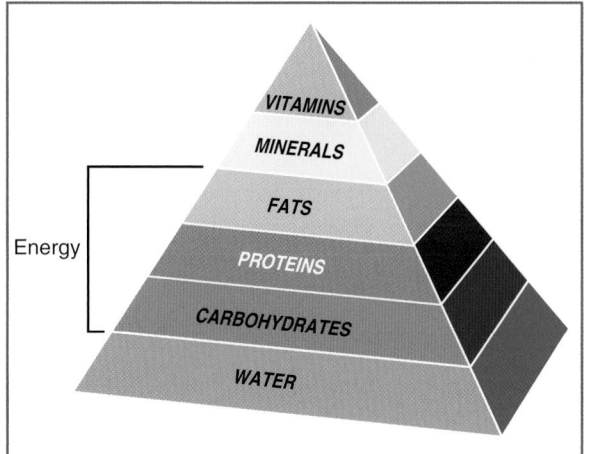

FIGURE 9-1 Six basic classes of nutrients are important for life sustenance. Among these six, carbohydrates, proteins, and fats provide energy and serve as structural components in the body.

WATER

Water is the most important nutrient, but it is often overlooked in discussions of nutrition. Approximately 50% to 70% of human or animal body weight is water. Without an adequate supply of water, other nutrients cannot be carried throughout the body via blood or used in chemical reactions. Water is necessary for temperature regulation, and it provides shape and structure to organs. A decrease in the amount of water present in the body is called *dehydration.*

Dogs and cats obtain water daily through drinking and from eating food. Typical dry pet foods contain approximately 10% water, and canned foods contain about 75% water. Therefore, animals tend to drink more water when fed dry compared with wet (canned) diets. All dogs and cats require constant access to fresh, clean water. Although daily minimum water requirements vary in dogs and cats, a rule of thumb is that milliliters (ml) of water per day is equivalent to kilocalories (kcal) per day. Many animals consume more water than is minimally required, and the excess water is excreted by the kidneys as urine.

PROTEIN

Proteins are large molecules made up of chains of smaller compounds called **amino acids**. Proteins come in many shapes and sizes, as do amino acids, and proteins sometimes are bound to other substances to form even more complex molecules. For example, proteins conjugated with carbohydrates are called *glycoproteins,* and those conjugated with **lipids** (fats) are called *lipoproteins.* In the body, proteins are used as structural components of organs and tissues. They also function as enzymes, hormones, and carriers of other molecules (e.g., hemoglobin is a protein that transports oxygen to tissues) and can be a source of energy.

Animals obtain protein and amino acids from many types of food. Dietary protein is digested in the stomach and intestines to smaller compounds such as amino acids and peptides, which are then absorbed from the intestines into the bloodstream. Some dietary protein and amino acids are excreted in feces rather than being absorbed in the intestine. Certain food sources of protein are said to be highly digestible if most of the amino acids are absorbed. Low digestibility means that a larger proportion of dietary protein is excreted. Proteins can be synthesized in the body from amino acids and other compounds, but protein is not stored. Every day, protein is lost from the body through breakdown (catabolism), metabolic processes, and skin and hair loss, as well as in waste products. Animals therefore need to consume dietary protein regularly to make up for normal losses.

> **TECHNICIAN NOTE** Protein is not stored in the body and is an important part of the daily diet.

FAT

Lipids, which consist of fats and oils, are simple to complex molecules with many functions, including providing and storing energy, making up cell membrane structure, acting as signaling agents and hormones, and forming other important compounds such as cholesterol. A basic neutral fat consists of a chain of glycerol with three **fatty acids** attached (a triglyceride). Fatty acids are classified in several ways, such as short-, medium-, and long-chain, or saturated, monounsaturated, and polyunsaturated. Many fats and fatty acids can be synthesized in the body from building blocks, but several must be supplied in the diet. These are called *essential fatty acids;* linoleic acid and alpha-linolenic acid are required for both dogs and cats, and arachidonic acid is required for cats.

> **TECHNICIAN NOTE**   Essential dietary fatty acids include linoleic acid and alpha-linolenic acid. Cats also need arachidonic acid from the diet, but dogs can synthesize it from other fatty acids.

Fats and oils are found in most types of food, including animal tissue (meat and fish) and plants (vegetable oils). Although dietary fat has a bad reputation in human nutrition, it is absolutely necessary to be supplied in animal diets. Fat, like protein, is digested in the stomach and intestines to smaller compounds, including individual fatty acids and monoglycerides. These compounds are then absorbed into intestinal cells and are repackaged into structures called *chylomicrons,* which contain triglycerides, lipoproteins, cholesterol, and other compounds. Chylomicrons are transported in the lymphatic system to the bloodstream, where they are later broken down by the liver and other tissues. All cells in the body use some of the fatty acids, and excessive amounts are stored as fat (adipose tissue). During times when the animal is not eating, stored fat can be broken down for daily needs.

CARBOHYDRATE

Sugars and starches are examples of dietary carbohydrates, which are used mainly for energy. They are a source of glucose and can be used as building blocks for other nutrients. Simple carbohydrates include glucose, sucrose (ordinary table sugar), and fructose (sugar found in fruit); complex carbohydrates include starches, glycogen (stored in the body), and certain fibers. Dietary carbohydrate is digested to glucose and other simple molecules and is absorbed mainly in the intestinal tract. Insulin and glucagons from the pancreas help to regulate blood glucose levels to keep them in a normal range. Excess glucose is stored in the liver and muscle tissue as glycogen, which can be converted to fat for long-term storage.

FIBER

Although fiber is often classified as a complex carbohydrate, it is not broken down into sugars. Technically it is not a nutrient, but is present in variable amounts in foods and has positive effects on health. Fiber resists digestion by enzymes in the stomach and the small intestine. Some types of fiber

are fermented by bacteria in the large intestine (often called *soluble* fiber), and other types pass into feces unchanged (*insoluble* fiber). Fiber is found in plant sources of food rather than animal tissue.

> **TECHNICIAN NOTE**   Many types of dietary fiber are known to have different characteristics and functions.

VITAMINS

A number of different compounds are classified as vitamins, which are used in many metabolic processes and are necessary in the diet to prevent deficiency syndromes. Vitamins are distinct from protein, fat, and carbohydrate; they are organic molecules found in animal and plant tissues, and some can be synthesized in the body (or produced in laboratories). Species differences in vitamin requirements have been noted—for example, humans and guinea pigs need vitamin C in the diet, but dogs and cats synthesize it on their own.

> **TECHNICIAN NOTE**   Vitamin requirements differ between humans, dogs, and cats.

Many vitamins have been discovered over the past 100 years and have been given both letter and chemical names (Table 9-1). They are classified into two groups: fat-soluble (A, D, E, and K) and water-soluble (B and C). Fat-soluble vitamins can be stored in the body and may accumulate to toxic levels. Water-soluble vitamins have limited storage and are excreted rapidly, making toxicity much less likely. An

TABLE 9-1	Vitamins
COMMON NAME	**CHEMICAL NAME(S)**
Fat-Soluble	
Vitamin A	Retinol, retinal, retinaldehyde, retinoic acid, carotenoid
Vitamin D	Cholecalciferol (D_3), ergocalciferol (D_2)
Vitamin E	α-, β-, γ-, δ-Tocopherol or tocotrienol
Vitamin K	Phylloquinone (K_1), menaquinone (K_2), menadione (K_3)
Water-Soluble	
Vitamin B_1	Thiamin, thiamine
Vitamin B_2	Riboflavin
Vitamin B_3	Niacin, nicotinic acid, nicotinamide, niacinamide
Vitamin B_6	Pyridoxine, pyridoxal, pyridoxamine
Vitamin B_{12}	Cobalamin
Pantothenic acid	Same
Folic acid	Folate, folinic acid
Vitamin C	Ascorbic acid, ascorbate
Biotin	Same
Choline	Same

animal that stops eating will become deficient in water-soluble vitamins much sooner than fat-soluble vitamins.

MINERALS

Minerals are necessary in the diet for metabolic processes and to provide structure (such as calcium making up bone). They are inorganic elements that make up "ash," a term found on pet food labels that refers to everything left over in a diet after combustion (heating at high temperatures). Minerals have many different functions in the body, and this makes them difficult to classify. Some are required in the diet in larger amounts (macrominerals) than others (microminerals). Both deficiencies and excesses of minerals can be harmful to health.

> **TECHNICIAN NOTE** The term "ash" may be found on a pet food label, but it does not indicate the quality of the diet. It refers to the inorganic material that is left over after food has been heated to high temperatures and has undergone combustion.

SUPPLEMENTS

In addition to the main categories of nutrients, several other compounds can be found in foods that may play a role in nutrition. Antioxidants are substances that delay or prevent oxidation (breakdown) of other compounds or structures such as cell membranes. Although certain vitamins and minerals serve as antioxidants (e.g., vitamin E, selenium), nonnutrients such as flavonoids and polyphenols can be found in certain plants used in pet food or may be added separately. Carotenoids are found in colorful vegetables and act both as provitamins (partially converted to vitamin A in the body) and as antioxidants. Choline is a compound that acts like a B-vitamin but usually is synthesized in the liver rather than being required in the diet. However, in some situations, choline can be an essential nutrient. Another vitamin-like compound is L-carnitine, which can be found in animal tissue (meat) and synthesized in the body. However, it is sometimes added to pet food for effects on health. Other examples of nutrient-like substances are included naturally in foods or may be added to pet foods; with continued research, some may eventually be considered essential.

> **TECHNICIAN NOTE** Antioxidants are added to pet foods for possible health benefits.

ENERGY

FOOD INTAKE AND REGULATION

The main reason to eat food is to obtain energy. Energy is not a nutrient by itself, but it is needed to fuel all body functions. When chemical bonds in foods are broken down, energy that can be used in various metabolic processes is released. The amount of food an animal eats in a day is regulated by energy needs in a complex system of feedback mechanisms. In simple terms, animals eat when they are hungry and stop eating when they are full. It is rare to observe obesity in stray or feral dogs and cats. However, in household pets, many factors interfere with normal food intake, leading to excess energy and weight gain. Highly palatable (tasty) foods, free-choice feeding, snacks and treats, and less opportunity for exercise are among the reasons why dogs and cats tend to become overweight.

> **TECHNICIAN NOTE** Animals eat mainly to satisfy energy requirements, not for specific nutrients.

ENERGY UNITS

In the United States, the usual measure of energy is the kilocalorie (abbreviated kcal); in other countries, **kilojoule** (kJ) is used. One **calorie** is defined as the energy needed to increase the temperature of 1 gram (g) of water from 14.5°C to 15.5°C. Because a calorie is too small a unit to be practical, the term *kilocalorie* is used instead (1 kcal = 1000 calories) in discussions of nutrition and energy. A kilojoule is the energy needed to move a 1 kilogram weight 1 meter by 1 newton (which is a measure of work instead of heat). To convert kJ to kcal, multiply by 4.184. To convert kcal to kJ, divide by 0.239. When speaking with pet owners, it is better to use the term "calories" to mean the same thing as kcal. When the word calorie is used to mean kilocalorie, it is capitalized. "Calorie" means kilocalorie or large calorie, and "calorie" means calorie or small calorie. However, most nutritionists and textbooks use kcal to be scientifically clear and accurate.

> **TECHNICIAN NOTE** Kilocalorie (kcal) is the standard measurement for energy. A calorie is $\frac{1}{1000}$ of a kcal and is not practical to use. Most nutritionists and dietitians use kcal and calories to mean the same thing.

ENERGY PARTITIONING

Some of the energy contained in food is not used by the body. To keep track of where energy goes, a series of measurements can be made. Gross energy (GE) is all of the potential energy available in a food or diet; it is measured by bomb calorimetry (burning the food to see how much heat is produced). Some energy is lost in feces, and subtracting fecal energy from GE results in digestible energy (DE). More energy is lost in urine and gases produced by the body, and subtracting that from DE results in **metabolizable energy** (ME). This is the most common estimate of the amount of energy available from pet foods, so ME is a good measure of what is available to the animal for body functions. One more term, net energy (NE), results from the measurement of how much energy is used for digesting, absorbing, and using food. Because the act of eating and digesting uses energy, subtracting this amount from ME provides an estimate of how much is left over for metabolism. To summarize the concepts of energy partitioning:

GE → DE + Energy in feces → ME + Energy in urine and gas → NE + Energy used for digestion

METABOLIZABLE ENERGY MEASUREMENT

Because ME is the term most commonly used in nutrition, it is helpful to understand how this value is measured or calculated. Most pet foods use estimates rather than direct measurements because of the complexity and expense of feeding experiments. The method used for directly measuring ME is to start with a group of 6 adult animals, feed the test diet for 5 days while collecting all feces and urine produced, then calculate the GE of the diet consumed and the GE of the feces and urine using bomb calorimetry. The average difference is the ME for that diet.

TECHNICIAN NOTE Metabolizable energy (ME) is the most common estimate of how much energy (kcal) is supplied by pet food.

ATWATER FACTORS

A vast majority of commercial pet foods use an estimate of energy content rather than a direct measurement. The typical method is to use modified Atwater factors, which assign energy (caloric) content to the three macronutrients (protein, fat, carbohydrate). For human foods that are highly digestible, the Atwater factors are as follows: protein 4 kcal/g, fat 9 kcal/g, and carbohydrate 4 kcal/g. Because commercial pet food is considered less digestible than foods sold for human consumption, modified Atwater factors are used instead: protein 3.5 kcal/g, fat 8.5 kcal/g, carbohydrate 3.5 kcal/g. These multipliers represent averages and are not exact for any given food or diet. To confirm how to use modified Atwater factors to estimate the energy content of a pet food and the contribution of each macronutrient to the total, consider the calculations (based on a popular dry diet for dogs) listed in Table 9-2.

Nutrients are most commonly listed on pet food labels as percentages. A percentage is the same as g/100 g. In other words, if protein is 20%, that is equivalent to 20 g/100 g, meaning that for every 100 g of pet food, 20 g of protein is included. Percentages are directly converted to g/100 g. It does not matter whether the % is "as fed" or "dry matter"—

either way will work when caloric content and the % each nutrient contributes are estimated on an ME basis.

TECHNICIAN NOTE Modified Atwater factors can be used to estimate the energy density (caloric content) of pet food and to determine how much energy is provided by protein, fat, and carbohydrate by percentage.

ENERGY DENSITY

The term **energy density** refers to the kcal per unit of a food ingredient or pet food. On pet food labels, this is commonly expressed as kcal/kg, meaning that for every 1 kg of pet food, a specific number of calories can be used by the animal (ME). On average, dry dog foods contain 3500 kcal/kg, and dry cat foods contain 4000 kcal/kg. The energy density of canned foods is much less than this because of increased water content (water does not supply any energy and dilutes out the calories present in food). A high–energy density pet food can be fed during life stages that require greater kcal intake, such as growth, reproduction, or performance. A low–energy density pet food should be fed to overweight or obese animals.

MEASUREMENTS OF ENERGY EXPENDITURE

In thinking about how much energy (how many kcal) we should feed animals, it is important to consider how much energy is being used or burned. This is called *energy expenditure (EE)*, which refers to the need to use or spend energy to maintain normal body processes and to supply extra energy for increased demands such as exercise or maintaining body heat in cold weather. Different methods may be used to measure or estimate EE, just as various methods are available to measure or estimate the energy content of foods. Direct measurement is difficult because it involves isolating an animal in an air-tight chamber and measuring oxygen and carbon dioxide levels.

Because it is not practical to measure EE, equations have been formulated for obtaining an estimate. One widely used estimate that works for many species of animals is called the Kleiber-Brody equation for **resting energy requirement** (RER). The RER is used for a normal animal at rest in a thermoneutral environment with no additional activity or exercise.

$$RER = 70 \times BW_{kg}^{0.75} \text{ kcal/day}$$

TABLE 9-2	Estimated Energy Content of a Pet Food Using Modified Atwater Factors			
NUTRIENT	% AS LISTED ON LABEL	MODIFIED ATWATER FACTOR	TOTAL KCAL	% OF TOTAL ENERGY (KCAL)
Protein	21	3.5 kcal/g	73.5	22.6
Fat	10	8.5 kcal/g	85	26.2
Carbohydrate	47.5	3.5 kcal/g	166.25	51.2
Total	78.5 (remainder is moisture, ash, fiber)		324.75	Calculated by dividing kcal of each by total

TABLE 9-3	Resting Energy Requirements (RER) for Common Body Weights (BW)				
	BW, KG LB	RER, KCAL/DAY		BW, KG LB	RER, KCAL/DAY
1	2.2	70	15	33	534
2	4.4	118	20	44	662
3	6.6	160	30	66	897
4	8.8	198	40	88	1113
5	11	234	50	110	1316
10	22	394	60	132	1509

TABLE 9-4	Classification of Amino Acids	
ESSENTIAL	**NONESSENTIAL**	**CONDITIONALLY ESSENTIAL**
Arginine	Alanine	Glutamine
Histidine	Asparagine	Taurine (dogs)
Isoleucine	Aspartate	
Leucine	Cystine, cysteine	
Lysine	Glutamate	
Methionine	Glycine	
Phenylalanine	Proline	
Taurine (cats)	Serine	
Threonine	Tyrosine	
Tryptophan		
Valine		

where BW_{kg} is body weight measured in kilograms and 0.75 is a constant exponent. Refer to Table 9-3 to see RER calculated for common body weights of dogs and cats. The RER kcal/day is often used for estimating how much to feed a hospitalized patient. Overweight or sedentary dogs or cats rarely require any more than RER, and sometimes need to be fed less for effective weight loss.

Once the RER for an individual animal is calculated, multipliers can be used to estimate the EE, or the daily amount to feed to maintain a healthy body weight. A healthy animal with normal daily activity and exercise is estimated to need a maintenance energy requirement (MER), which is also called the **metabolizable energy requirement** or the daily energy requirement (DER). The MER for a neutered adult dog is approximately 1.4 to 1.6 × RER, and the MER for a neutered adult cat is 1.2 to 1.4 × RER. An active adult animal may need 1.6 to 2.0 × RER to account for exercise or light work. A performance or working dog may need 2.0 to 6.0 × RER. Dogs and cats that are growing or reproducing also require higher amounts than RER—a fact that is discussed later. Because of differences in breeds, ages, metabolic rates, and so forth, the actual energy requirements for dogs and cats tend to vary by ±50% from the calculated MER. For example, the MER for a dog at a certain body weight may be estimated at 400 kcal/day, but the true amount can be as low as 200 kcal/day or as high as 600 kcal/day and still be normal.

> **TECHNICIAN NOTE** It is useful to be able to calculate RER for any dog or cat and then estimate MER using multiplication factors.

PROTEIN

DIETARY REQUIREMENTS

Protein is necessary in the diet because it supplies nitrogen and amino acids. Nitrogen is required to replace losses in urine, feces, sloughing of epithelial cells, sweat, hair, and other secretions. The daily maintenance protein requirement is based on the amount of nitrogen lost per day.

Amino acids are used to synthesize new protein in the body and have many other functions. They are divided into two groups: essential (indispensable) and nonessential (dispensable). Essential amino acids cannot be synthesized in the body and must come from the diet; nonessential amino acids can be formed in the body if dietary intake is not adequate. A third group, conditionally essential amino acids, includes those that may be required in the diet during certain disease states or life stages. A list of the common amino acids is presented in Table 9-4. Taurine is unique in that it is required in the diet for cats but not for dogs, because healthy dogs are able to synthesize taurine from other amino acids.

> **TECHNICIAN NOTE** Taurine is an essential amino acid for cats and is added to most cat foods. It is considered nonessential or conditionally essential for dogs.

To understand dietary protein and amino acid needs, it is important to first consider units of measurement and how requirements are expressed. A nutrient is measured in units of mass such as grams (g), milligrams (mg), or micrograms (μg or mcg). As part of a food or diet, nutrients can be expressed as a percentage (%) instead of mass. For example, if the protein requirement for an adult dog is said to be 18%, that means for every 100 g of pet food (dry-matter basis), at least 18 g of protein should be included (18/100 = 18%). However, it is usually more accurate to consider nutrient requirements based on the size of the animal (body weight). In this case, the recommended protein intake for an adult dog may be expressed as approximately 2 g per kg body weight. Therefore, a dog weighing 10 kg should be offered at least 20 g protein per day. Cats generally require at least 3 to 4 g protein per kg body weight.

The percentage method can be used in three different ways: as-fed basis, dry-matter (DM) basis, and metabolizable energy (ME) basis. "As fed" refers to pet food directly from a bag, can, or package. "Dry matter" refers to pet food without the water content, and can be estimated by subtracting the moisture content as listed on the label. For example, if a dry pet food contained 10% moisture, then 100 g of the diet "as fed" would consist of only 90 g "dry matter"

(100 − 10 = 90). The third method, the ME basis, refers only to the three nutrients that supply energy (kcal)—protein, fat, and carbohydrate. The % ME is a proportion of energy rather than weight. For example, a pet food that supplies 20% ME protein would provide 20 kcal of protein for every 100 kcal of total diet (20/100 = 20%).

> **TECHNICIAN NOTE**   Percentages of protein, fat, carbohydrate, and other nutrients may be expressed on an "as-fed," "dry matter," or "metabolizable energy" basis. These values are not interchangeable.

The daily protein requirement ranges on a DM or ME basis are listed in Table 9-5. Cats need more protein than dogs, and both dogs and cats that are growing or reproducing need more than adult animals at maintenance.

To be strictly accurate, animals do not have a true protein requirement, but they do need the amino acids and nitrogen supplied by dietary protein. A deficiency of protein can lead to detrimental effects on health. In dogs and cats, a diet deficient in protein will lead to poor growth and reproduction, reduced appetite, anemia, and poor hair coat. Over time, muscle and other tissues will be broken down, leading to muscle atrophy and decreased quantities of internal proteins such as albumin. Specific amino acid deficiencies also lead to diseases. For example, arginine deficiency causes a buildup of ammonia in the bloodstream, leading to vomiting in dogs and even death in cats. Methionine and cysteine deficiencies cause weight loss and skin disorders. In cats, taurine deficiency leads to blindness and heart failure.

Excessive dietary protein is usually tolerated by dogs and cats as the amino acids are broken down and converted to energy, and nitrogen waste is excreted. In disease conditions such as kidney failure or some types of liver disease, excess protein can lead to worsening of the disease. Whenever excess protein over requirements is fed to dogs and cats, it is not stored for later use and does not seem to have a health benefit. Instead, it is simply used to provide energy. Because protein is an expensive component of pet food, this leads to higher costs for pet owners, and very-high-protein products are usually not as palatable. As a general rule, pet foods for adult dogs should contain less than 40% and for adult cats less than 50% crude protein on a dry-matter basis.

> **TECHNICIAN NOTE**   Excessively high-protein pet foods are expensive and are not healthier than moderate-protein foods.

PROTEIN QUALITY

The quality of a commercial pet food or an individual ingredient is not well defined and is a topic of much controversy. In terms of protein quality, specific measurements help determine how well the protein is used in the animal's body. A simple definition of protein quality is whether the amino acid components of the protein are suitable for the animal and in a form that is digestible and available for use. A high-quality protein supplies all of the essential amino acids in correct proportions as needed by the animal. A low-quality protein may lack sufficient quantities of one or more amino acids, or it may have excesses that interfere with absorption. Digestibility affects protein quality, and cooking times or temperatures may increase or decrease availability (raw or overcooked). The fiber content of a diet can affect protein quality in that plant-based protein generally is less digestible than animal-based protein (meat, poultry, fish). Measures of protein quality are listed in Table 9-6.

FAT

STRUCTURE

As described earlier, fats are composed of triglycerides, which include three fatty acids attached to a glycerol chain. Different types of fatty acids are found in dietary sources and in the body based on chain length, location and number of double bonds, and function. The first variable to consider is how many carbon molecules the fatty acid contains. These are divided into short-chain (2 to 6), medium-chain (8 to 12), and long-chain (14 to 24) varieties. Short-chain fatty acids are building blocks and are not an important part of diet or function in dogs and cats. Medium-chain triglycerides (MCT) are found in mothers' milk and in certain foods such as coconuts. Coconut oil is rich in MCT and is the basis for commercial supplements (MCT oil) and certain pet foods that are intended to be easily digestible. Although only limited research has examined the effects and benefits of MCT compared with other triglycerides, it is thought to be more easily broken down and absorbed in the intestinal tract. MCT oil is less palatable than long-chain triglycerides

---

TABLE 9-5   Protein Requirements of Dogs and Cats

A. Dry-Matter Basis, %

LIFE STAGE	DOG		CAT	
	AAFCO*	NRC†	AAFCO	NRC
Growth	22	17.5	30	22.5
Maintenance	18	10	26	20

B. Metabolizable Energy Basis, g Protein per 1000 kcal

LIFE STAGE	DOG		CAT	
	AAFCO	NRC	AAFCO	NRC
Growth	62.9	43.8	75	56.3
Maintenance	51.4	25	65	50

AAFCO, Association of American Feed Control Officials; *NRC,* National Research Council.
*Minimum requirement.
†Recommended allowance.

TABLE 9-6	Measures of Protein Quality of Foods
MEASURE	**EQUATION**
Protein-efficiency ratio (PER) =	$\dfrac{\text{Weight gain of animal}}{\text{Protein intake of animal}}$
Biological value (BV) =	$\dfrac{(\text{Food nitrogen} - [\text{Fecal nitrogen} + \text{Urinary nitrogen}])}{(\text{Food nitrogen} + \text{Fecal nitrogen})}$
Net protein utilization (NPU) =	$\text{BV} \times \text{digestibility}$
Amino acid score (AAS) =	$\dfrac{\text{Amino acid, mg/Test protein, g}}{\text{Amino acid, mg/Reference protein, g}}$

Crude protein digestibility (CPD): measured in ileal-cannulated dogs.
Whole body nitrogen flux: stable isotopes.

so cannot be used as the only dietary source of fat. Long-chain fatty acids are the most common type found in foods and include linoleic and alpha-linolenic acids (essential for dogs and cats) and arachidonic acid (essential for cats).

The degree of saturation for each fatty acid is important in human nutrition but less so for dogs and cats. Saturated fats do not contain double bonds. These fatty acids are common in animal fat but less common in vegetable oil. Monounsaturated fats have one double bond, and polyunsaturated fats have two or more double bonds. As saturation increases, the fats become less solid and more liquid at room temperature. People should avoid excessive dietary saturated fat because it increases the risk of cardiovascular disease and stroke. Dogs and cats do not have the same fat metabolism or tendency to get atherosclerosis, so no risk is associated with feeding saturated (animal origin) fats.

Polyunsaturated fatty acids are further divided into three groups or series based on the location of the first double bond in the structure: omega-3, omega-6, and omega-9 (also called n-3, n-6, and n-9). These differences in structure result in different effects in the body.

> **TECHNICIAN NOTE** Dietary fatty acids can be classified in several ways, including carbon chain length, degree of saturation, and location of the first double bond in the chemical structure (omega- or n-nomenclature).

The first fatty acid found to be essential in human and animal diets was linoleic acid (LA), which has 18 carbons and 2 double bonds, and is in the omega-6 series. Vegetable oil is rich in LA and often is used as a dietary source. Deficiency of LA leads to poor hair coat, skin infection, weight loss, decreased immunity, and other problems in dogs and cats. Another important fatty acid in the omega-6 series is arachidonic acid (AA), which has 20 carbons and 4 double bonds. Dogs can convert LA to AA by adding a carbon group and 2 double bonds, but cats have limited ability to do this because of a lack of enzyme activity of Δ6 desaturase. Therefore, for optimal health, especially for reproductive capacity, cats require AA in the diet; it is found in animal but not plant sources of fat. This is one reason why cats should not be fed

vegetarian diets; AA deficiency may lead to impaired reproduction and growth.

> **TECHNICIAN NOTE** Arachidonic acid, which is essential for cats, is found only in animal-origin foods.

Omega-3 fatty acids have been widely studied for a number of effects on human and animal health. The three common ones found in foods are alpha-linolenic acid (ALA; 18 carbons, 3 double bonds), eicosapentaenoic acid (EPA; 20 carbons, 5 double bonds), and docosahexaenoic acid (DHA; 22 carbons, 6 double bonds). In humans, ALA can be converted to EPA and DHA, but in dogs and cats this pathway is not efficient. Therefore, EPA and DHA are typically provided in pet food in the form of fish or fish oil. Cold-water fish are rich in EPA and DHA mainly because of their diet of algae. In contrast, farmed fish have lower levels of EPA and DHA because they are often fed corn or other plant-based foods. Fish oil is extracted from various types of fish, most commonly menhaden, but also salmon, sardines, tuna, and anchovies, and can be incorporated into pet food or added as a separate supplement. EPA and DHA are important for retinal and nervous system development in young animals, and can compete with AA incorporation in cell membranes, where they are involved in the production of anti-inflammatory immunoregulatory compounds known as *resolvins* and *protectins*.

> **TECHNICIAN NOTE** Fish oil can be a beneficial supplement or additive to pet food through its anti-inflammatory effects.

DIETARY REQUIREMENTS

Dogs and cats require both fat and essential fatty acids in their diets. Daily ranges are listed in Table 9-7 on a DM and ME basis. Dogs and cats that are growing or reproducing need more fat than adult animals at maintenance. As with protein, the fat or fatty acid content of a pet food can be expressed on an as-fed, dry matter, or metabolizable energy basis. Excessive fat intake often leads to an overweight or

TABLE 9-7 | Fat Requirements of Dogs and Cats

A. Dry-Matter Basis, %

	DOG		CAT	
LIFE STAGE	AAFCO*	NRC†	AAFCO	NRC
Growth	8	8.5	9	9
Maintenance	5	5.5	9	9

B. Metabolizable Energy Basis, g Fat per 1000 kcal

	DOG		CAT	
LIFE STAGE	AAFCO	NRC	AAFCO	NRC
Growth	22.9	21.3	22.5	22.5
Maintenance	14.3	13.8	22.5	22.5

*Minimum requirement.
†Recommended allowance.
AAFCO, Association of American Feed Control Officials; *NRC*, National Research Council.

obese state, because fat supplies 2.25 times more kcal than an equivalent amount of protein or carbohydrate. High-fat diets are necessary for some working or performance dogs because of their increased energy expenditure. These diets require additional preservatives or antioxidants because dietary fat, especially polyunsaturated, is susceptible to per-oxidation (rancidity) over time. A condition called *pansteatitis* ("yellow fat disease") in animals results from excess dietary fat and deficient antioxidants. Clinical signs include anorexia, depression, fever, and inflammation of subcutaneous fat; treatment consists of dietary correction and supplemental vitamin E.

CARBOHYDRATE

DIETARY REQUIREMENTS

Simple and complex carbohydrates are present in foods of plant origin. Animals have limited storage as glycogen (present in liver and muscle tissues), so meat, poultry, and fish supply little or no carbohydrates. In dogs and cats, there is no minimum daily requirement. Their main function is to supply energy because they are easily converted to glucose, and can also supply body heat and serve as structures for other nutrients. Excess carbohydrate is converted to fat for long-term storage. During growth, gestation, and lactation, carbohydrates are used to supply the extra energy required and are usually considered conditionally essential nutrients during these phases. Starch consists of straight glucose chains, and most types of starch are more digestible if cooked.

> **TECHNICIAN NOTE** Dietary carbohydrate is conditionally essential and is used mainly for energy. Both dogs and cats can digest and absorb most types of carbohydrates.

TABLE 9-8 | Characteristics of Fiber Sources Used in Pet Food

FIBER TYPE	SOLUBLE	INSOLUBLE	VISCOUS
Psyllium	Yes	Yes	Yes
Guar gum	Yes	No	Yes
Pectin	Yes	No	Yes
Beet pulp	Yes	Yes	No
Wheat bran	No	Yes	No
Cellulose	No	Yes	No

FIBER

DIETARY REQUIREMENTS

Many types of complex carbohydrates found in plant food sources are not readily digestible or used for energy and are classified as fiber. Fibers differ from starches in that they are not digested in the stomach or the small intestine. Fiber may be subdivided into soluble or insoluble (based on ability to absorb water) or fermentable or nonfermentable (based on whether microbes in the lower intestinal tract can convert the compounds into gases and short-chain fatty acids). A characteristic of fiber is that it passes through the stomach and small intestine of dogs and cats mostly unchanged. After entering the large intestine, fiber is excreted in the feces and, depending on the type, is partially fermented to carbon dioxide, hydrogen, and methane, along with fatty acids such as acetate, propionate, and butyrate.

The purposes of dietary fiber are to increase water and fecal bulk and to help regulate normal bowel transit time and function. Various types of fiber are added to pet foods for beneficial effects on stool quality, for slower intestinal transit time, and to aid in satiety and weight loss, among other functions. Some fiber compounds such as oligosaccharides act as prebiotics in the diet, which means they stimulate the growth and activity of beneficial bacteria in the large intestine. A list of common types of dietary fiber along with classifications is found in Table 9-8.

No minimum daily requirement for fiber has been put forth, but most pet foods include one or more types of fiber as part of plant-based ingredients or as a separate additive. The guaranteed analysis found on pet food labels does not reflect total dietary fiber content because the assays used are not accurate for detecting all types.

VITAMINS

DIETARY REQUIREMENTS
Vitamin A

Vitamin A is necessary in the diet of all animals for formation and maintenance of the epithelium (skin, mucous membranes). It is also important for vision, growth, reproduction, and immunity. Animal products supply vitamin A and plant sources have carotenoids, which are found in

| TABLE 9-9 | Vitamins A and D and E Recommended Allowance (RA) and Safe Upper Limit (SUL), ME Basis, IU/1000 kcal, NRC |

Vitamin A

LIFE STAGE	DOG RA	DOG SUL	CAT RA	CAT SUL
Growth	1263	12,500	833	66,667
Maintenance	1263	53,333	833	83,333

Vitamin D

LIFE STAGE	DOG RA	DOG SUL	CAT RA	CAT SUL
Growth	136	800	56	7520
Maintenance	136	800	70	7520

Vitamin E

LIFE STAGE	DOG RA	CAT RA
Growth	7.5	9.4
Maintenance	7.5	10

ME, Metabolizable energy; NRC, National Research Council.

colorful vegetables. Carotenoids are also called *provitamin A*, in that they have to be converted in the body to the active form. Dogs can metabolize about half of dietary carotenoids to vitamin A. Cats, on the other hand, are inefficient at converting carotenoids to vitamin A, because they lack many of the necessary enzymes. Therefore, cats are inefficient at converting carotenoids to vitamin A; this is one example of why cats cannot eat a vegetarian diet alone (unless supplemented). Vitamin A deficiency is uncommon in animals because it is stored in the liver and other tissues. Clinical signs include night blindness, dry skin and mucous membranes, and poor growth, reproduction, and immunity. Excess vitamin A can be toxic; this problem is seen when an improper diet is fed to animals or high doses of supplements are given. Cats fed an all-liver diet often have hypervitaminosis A with skeletal malformations and bony hyperplasia of the cervical vertebrae. Vitamin A in the diet can be measured in international units (IU) or retinol equivalents (RE). One IU equals 0.3 μg of RE. The recommended allowance and safe upper limits are listed in Table 9-9.

Vitamin D

Vitamin D is a necessary vitamin in the diet of dogs and cats because they cannot use sunlight to convert provitamin D (7-dehydrocholesterol) found in the skin to the active form (unlike humans and many other mammals). The major function of vitamin D is to regulate absorption and mobilization of calcium in the body. The active form of vitamin D—1,25-dihydroxycholecalciferol (also called *calcitriol*)—is a hormone that works with parathyroid hormone, calcitonin, and circulating calcium and phosphorus in a tightly controlled feedback system. Animal products supply cholecalciferol and plant products supply ergocalciferol. Cholecalciferol has more activity and is more likely to lead to toxicity.

A deficiency of vitamin D can lead to rickets or osteoporosis (thin, brittle bones) and neurologic disorders. Because it is a fat-soluble vitamin, toxic levels can occur; this leads to increased circulating calcium (hypercalcemia) that in turn results in soft tissue mineralization, bony remodeling, and organ failure. Cod liver oil is rich in vitamins A and D and can cause toxicity in animals, so it is important to distinguish between "fish oil" (with no vitamins) and cod liver oil when recommending supplements. Dietary vitamin D is measured in IU or μg as cholecalciferol. One IU equals 0.025 μg of cholecalciferol. The recommended allowance and safe upper limits are listed in Table 9-9.

Vitamin E

Vitamin E is the general name for a group of compounds called *tocol* and *tocotrienol derivatives,* with α-tocopherol being the most active form. The main function is antioxidant activity, meaning that it helps protect against cell damage by reactive oxygen and other free radicals. This property of vitamin E makes it useful as a preservative in pet foods. A deficiency of dietary vitamin E leads to muscle disease, poor reproduction, and retinal degeneration. In cats, a condition called *steatitis* (yellow fat disease) can occur when oily fish is fed exclusively. The higher the fat content of the diet, the more vitamin E is required. Toxicity is rare but possible with excessive supplementation. Vitamin E may be measured in IU or in mg, which are approximately equivalent (1 IU equals 1 mg of α-tocopherol). Recommended amounts are listed in Table 9-9.

> **TECHNICIAN NOTE** Two of the fat-soluble vitamins, A and D, can cause toxicity with inappropriate diets or if supplemented.

Vitamin K

Vitamin K is a unique fat-soluble vitamin in that it can be absorbed from dietary sources or synthesized by microbes in the large intestine of dogs and cats. Both animal and plant sources can supply vitamin K, which functions mainly in the blood clotting system. It is also used in the production of osteocalcin, which helps to regulate bony growth. Naturally occurring deficiencies are rare but can be induced with anticoagulant rodenticides (rat poisons). The main clinical sign of a deficiency is spontaneous bleeding. Toxicities are rare, but excessive supplementation should be avoided. Daily requirements are not clear because it is naturally synthesized, but in some situations, vitamin K may be conditionally essential.

Thiamin

Thiamin, also called vitamin B$_1$, was the first water-soluble vitamin to be discovered. Only a few food sources are rich in thiamin, and this vitamin is labile (easily lost) during pet food processing. Certain raw fish contain thiaminases, which are compounds that destroy thiamin. Sulfites used as

TABLE 9-10	Vitamin B-Complex Recommended Allowance (RA), ME Basis, mg/1000 kcal, NRC		
NUTRIENT	DOG GROWTH	DOG MAINTENANCE	CAT GROWTH AND MAINTENANCE
Thiamin	0.34	0.56	1.4
Riboflavin	1.32	1.3	1.0
Pyridoxine	0.375	0.375	0.625
Niacin	4.25	4.25	10
Pantothenic acid	3.75	3.75	1.43
Cobalamin, μg	8.75	8.75	5.6
Folic acid, μg	68	67.5	188
Choline	425	425	637

ME, Metabolizable energy; *NRC,* National Research Council.

preservatives in food can also lead to thiamin loss. This vitamin is necessary for many metabolic reactions and is not stored in the body. Deficiencies lead to neurologic and cardiac disease in dogs. Cats are more susceptible to thiamin deficiency because they require approximately 4 times as much as dogs. They may display a characteristic ventroflexion of the head that may progress to seizures and death. Daily requirements for thiamin and other B-vitamins are listed in Table 9-10.

Riboflavin

Riboflavin (vitamin B_2) is involved in many biochemical reactions and is needed for energy metabolism. Deficiencies are not common because riboflavin is found in many foods, but excessive ultraviolet light can lead to losses.

Niacin

Niacin (vitamin B_3) was historically studied in relationship to pellagra, or "black tongue" disease. A dietary deficiency of niacin, or lack of bioavailability from certain foods such as corn, was found to cause pellagra in both humans and dogs. Dogs are able to synthesize niacin from tryptophan, an amino acid, but cats lack the necessary enzyme pathways. Niacin functions in metabolic processes, and although dietary deficiencies are rare, they can lead to reddening and ulceration of the tongue and mucous membranes, diarrhea, and neurologic disease.

Pyridoxine

Pyridoxine (vitamin B_6) is needed as a coenzyme for many enzymatic reactions. A deficiency may lead to anemia, kidney disease, and neurologic disorders.

Cobalamin

Cobalamin (vitamin B_{12}) is unique among the vitamins in that it is synthesized only by microorganisms. It is found in animal products, not in plant food sources, and functions in metabolic reactions. Deficiencies lead to weakness, poor growth, anemia, and bone marrow disease. Vegetarian diets need to be supplemented.

Pantothenic Acid

Pantothenic acid is found in most food sources and functions as a component of coenzyme A in energy metabolism. True deficiencies are very rare.

Folic Acid

Folic acid or folate is used as a cofactor in many metabolic reactions. Deficiencies are rare and cause anemia and poor growth.

Biotin

Biotin is not a true vitamin in that it is synthesized in the intestinal tract by microorganisms and is also found in many food sources. It serves as a cofactor in reactions. A glycoprotein called *avidin,* which is found in raw egg whites, can bind biotin, making it unavailable.

Choline

Choline is synthesized in the liver but sometimes is included among the B-vitamins. It is a component of phospholipids and is involved in several metabolic reactions.

Ascorbic Acid

Ascorbic acid, or vitamin C, is an important water-soluble nutrient but is not necessary in the diet of dogs and cats. Metabolism of glucose produces adequate amounts of vitamin C, which is a part of many reactions, including the synthesis of collagen and elastin. It also serves as an antioxidant.

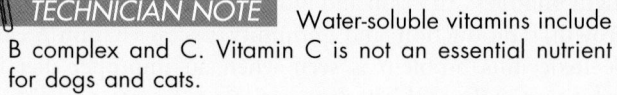

TECHNICIAN NOTE Water-soluble vitamins include B complex and C. Vitamin C is not an essential nutrient for dogs and cats.

MINERALS

DIETARY REQUIREMENTS

Twelve minerals are essential for dogs and cats, although continued research may prove that several others are necessary in the diet as well. Essential minerals are often divided into two groups: macrominerals (calcium, phosphorus, magnesium, sodium, potassium, chloride) and microminerals, also called *trace minerals* (iron, copper, zinc, manganese, selenium, iodine). The basic difference is that macrominerals are measured in gram amounts and microminerals are measured in milligram amounts in formulating pet diets.

Calcium

Calcium (Ca) is the most abundant mineral in the body, making up much of the skeleton and teeth. It is also needed for muscles, nerves, and blood clotting, and acts as a cellular

TABLE 9-11	Mineral Recommended Allowance (RA), ME Basis, mg/1000 kcal, NRC			
NUTRIENT	DOG GROWTH	DOG MAINTENANCE	CAT GROWTH	CAT MAINTENANCE
Calcium	3000	1000	2000	720
Phosphorus	2500	750	1800	640
Magnesium	100	150	100	100
Sodium	550	200	350	170
Potassium	1100	1000	1000	1300
Chloride	720	300	225	240
Iron	22	7.5	20	20
Copper	2.7	1.5	2.1	1.2
Zinc	25	15	18.5	18.5
Manganese	1.4	1.2	1.2	1.2
Selenium	0.0875	0.0875	0.075	0.075
Iodine	0.22	0.22	0.45	0.35

ME, Metabolizable energy; *NRC*, National Research Council.

messenger. Dietary sources often include supplements such as Ca phosphate or carbonate instead of foods (because Ca-rich dairy products are not commonly used as major ingredients of pet food). A deficiency of Ca causes nutritional secondary hyperparathyroidism, which leads to loss of bone structure (rickets) and pathologic fractures. Excessive Ca intake, especially during the growth phase, leads to osteochondrosis and other skeletal abnormalities. Dietary requirements are increased during growth, gestation, and lactation. Recommended allowances for Ca and other minerals are listed in Table 9-11.

> **TECHNICIAN NOTE** Calcium will be deficient in all-meat diets. Excesses can result from inappropriate supplementation.

Phosphorus
Phosphorus (P) is the second most abundant mineral. Most of the P in the body is found in bone, but muscle and other tissues have P as a structural component. In addition to providing structure, P is part of the high-energy phosphate compounds used in energy metabolism. Most food sources supply P, but if phytate is present, P is less bioavailable. Deficiencies and excesses of P alone are rare in animals and are noted with clinical signs of poor appetite and poor growth along with bony abnormalities.

Magnesium
Magnesium (Mg) serves as a cofactor in many enzyme systems and is used in metabolic reactions; it is also a part of bone and tooth structure. Animal and plant food sources supply Mg, but it can be supplemented in pet food as well. Deficiencies can cause musculoskeletal and neurologic problems; excesses have been linked to urinary stone formation in cats (although urine pH has greater influence).

Sodium
Sodium (Na) is found in bone, body fluids, and tissues. The major function of Na is to regulate body water and acid-base balance. It also helps maintain electrical potential in muscle, nerve, and other tissues. Unprocessed foods are generally low in Na, so salt (sodium chloride) is often added to pet foods. A dietary deficiency can cause loss of water, dehydration, and acid-base disruption. Excess Na is well tolerated in healthy dogs and cats but can be harmful in certain medical conditions such as heart failure and kidney disease.

Potassium
Potassium (K) is found mainly in intracellular fluid, with small amounts in bone, connective tissues, and plasma. It is involved in acid-base regulation, nerve transmission, and enzymatic and metabolic reactions. Many foods supply K, and supplements may be used as well. Dietary deficiencies of K lead to neurologic disease, especially ventroflexion of the head (similar to thiamin deficiency), along with weakness, poor growth, and cardiac abnormalities.

Chloride
Chloride (Cl) helps maintain osmolality of extracellular fluids and is involved in acid-base regulation. It is added to foods in combination with sodium (table salt) or other minerals such as potassium and calcium. Deficiencies are rare and result in fluid balance and acid-base alterations.

Iron
Iron (Fe) is a component of hemoglobin and therefore is found mostly in red blood cells. Muscle tissue (myoglobin) and other body cells also contain Fe. The main function of Fe is to bind and transport oxygen, and it plays a role in enzymatic reactions. Animal and plant food sources supply Fe, which can be added as a separate supplement to pet food. Fe oxide and Fe carbonate are not bioavailable

and should not be used. Deficiency results in anemia (microcytic hypochromic), weakness, and poor growth; excess amounts can be toxic and may cause gastrointestinal signs and death.

Copper

Copper (Cu) functions in many metabolic reactions and enzyme systems. It is stored in the liver and released into blood circulation bound to a protein called *ceruloplasmin*. For pet foods, Cu is added as a supplement as sulfate, chloride, or other salts, but Cu oxide should be avoided because that compound is not bioavailable in feed. Growth rates and hair pigmentation are reduced with dietary deficiency, and toxicity is possible with excess consumption or in dogs with a hereditary defect (copper storage disease).

Zinc

Zinc (Zn) is a cofactor in many enzymes and is widespread in the body in small amounts. It may be supplemented in pet foods because food sources have varied contents. Deficiency leads to skin lesions such as hair loss and crusting, especially around the head and foot pads. Excess dietary Zn is usually well tolerated, but toxicity occurs with ingestion of zinc-containing objects such as coins, leading to hemolytic anemia and gastroenteritis.

Manganese

Manganese (Mn) is another component of enzymes and is necessary for bone development and neurologic function. It is found in animal and plant foods and is often supplemented in the diet. Deficiencies and excesses are rare but result in poor growth and reproduction.

Selenium

Selenium (Se) is found in small amounts in most tissues and functions mainly as an antioxidant through its role in the enzyme glutathione peroxidase. Both animal and plant sources contain Se with varying bioavailability. Deficiencies may cause muscle disease, along with neurologic and other signs; excesses may result in anemia and liver disease.

Iodine

Iodine (I) is required in small amounts as a component of thyroid hormones. Dietary sources vary, so it is often added to pet food. A deficiency can lead to goiter (thyroid gland enlargement), poor hair coat, and weight gain secondary to low thyroid hormone concentrations. Excess dietary I leads to skin and hair coat problems and changes in thyroid gland function.

Other Minerals

Other minerals play a role in animal nutrition, but dietary requirements have not been established. These include molybdenum, boron, chromium, silicon, nickel, vanadium, and arsenic. Because these other minerals are naturally occurring, they are not added to pet foods or supplements.

TECHNICIAN NOTE   Minerals must be carefully balanced in pet foods to avoid deficiencies, excesses, and interactions.

COMMERCIAL PET FOOD

HISTORY

Dogs have been living with people for thousands of years, and for most of that time, dogs have eaten leftovers, table scraps, and even garbage discarded in and around human settlements. As omnivores, dogs survived on anything they could find to eat; therefore they tended not to be selective or finicky. The first commercial product intended as dog food was Spratt's dog biscuits, which were modeled after hardtack biscuits eaten by sailors on sea voyages. They were first sold in 1860 in England, but most dog owners did not see the need to purchase special food, and some stores refused to stock dog food on the same shelves as human food. It was almost 50 years before a commercial dog food was introduced in the United States—Milk-Bone biscuits. A canned dog food was first sold by Ken-L Ration in 1922, and then in 1925, Gaines dog meal was introduced. Canned dog foods made up most of the market until World War II, when tin and other metals were scarce and were no longer available for pet foods.

The first successful, widely sold dry dog food was Purina Dog Chow (introduced in 1957), which was manufactured using extrusion technology—similar to how breakfast cereals were made. Canned, soft-moist, and meal dog foods continued to be produced, but extruded kibble became the most popular type of product. In the late 1960s, the dog food market started to become differentiated, with premium and specialty products marketed toward veterinarians, breeders, and other professionals, and general products advertised to the general public.

It is believed that cats were first domesticated by humans who needed them for rodent control where grains and other foods were stored. Throughout most of history, cats have been free-roaming and were often found outdoors in barns, garages, and other structures. More recently, cats have become the most popular type of pet, especially in the United States, where they are routinely kept indoors as part of the household. Cats are carnivores and are more selective about their diet than dogs. Studies of stray and feral cats have shown that although rodents (mice, rats, small rabbits) are a large component of the diet, they also eat birds, amphibians, beetles, spiders, and insects. Cats are able to digest the stomach and intestinal contents of the prey, which are vegetarian (grains, seeds, etc.) in origin. They tend to avoid plant-based sources of food, but many cats nibble on green grasses and other vegetation. Spratt's company introduced a commercial cat food in 1876. A market for cat foods along with dog foods developed over time. Today, dry kibble is the most popular cat food, and canned varieties are also widely sold.

> **TECHNICIAN NOTE** Dogs are omnivores and tend to do well on animal-based or plant-based foods. Cats are carnivores, meaning that a large portion of their diet must consist of animal-based foods. However, cats can also digest and utilize plant products such as grains and starches.

TYPES

Most dog and cat foods are complete and balanced and are available in dry and wet (canned) varieties. A few products are semi-moist alone or mixed with dry kibble. Refrigerated and frozen pet foods are also available in many areas. Dry food is manufactured through an extrusion process. First, bulk ingredients are ground to small particles that resemble coarse flour and are mixed together. Next, liquids such as fats, oils, and other soft or moist ingredients are added, along with water and steam. An extruder, which looks like a large screw, propels, mixes, and cooks the combined ingredients into a consistent dough-like product. The dough is pushed through small openings in a die, which can have different shapes and sizes of cutouts. High temperature and pressure during this whole process cook the food and destroy microorganisms.

A knife cuts the rope-like extruded dough into small kibbles, which are then cooled and dried. A last step in manufacturing is applying liquid or dry coatings to the kibble (enrobing), usually fats and flavor enhancers. Filling machines are used to package the end product into bags or other containers.

Canning as a way to preserve food was invented in 1810, and is an important method to destroy bacteria and extend the shelf life of human and pet foods. As with dry foods, the ingredients are first ground, then are mixed with water and steam to a consistent moisture content. At this point, instead of entering an extruder, they are processed in a cooker/mixer. A filler/seamer machine is used to fill cans and seal the lids. Cans are placed in a machine called a *retort* because the process of retorting canned food is necessary to achieve sterilization. This heating and cooling step is sufficient to kill *Clostridium botulinum*, a bacterial pathogen that causes botulism.

Semi-moist pet foods have higher moisture levels than dry foods, so mold and bacteria inhibitors must be added to avoid spoilage and contamination. Humectants, which bind free water, are also necessary. These products must be packaged in moisture-proof bags or containers and kept sealed after opening, because otherwise the product will dry out.

Some pet owners express concern that commercial pet food is overly "processed" and therefore is not healthy or nutritionally complete. One way to explain how extruded pet food is made is to compare the process to making bread. Ingredients are ground (like flour), mixed with liquids, kneaded into dough, allowed to rise and be shaped, and finally cooked and sliced. Even people who try to avoid processed foods in their own diets often eat bread. Another concern is that nutritional value is destroyed during cooking because high temperatures and storage can affect certain nutrients, especially vitamins. This is true for both fat-soluble and water-soluble vitamins, so pet food companies routinely add more nutrients than the minimum requirement to allow for a percentage loss. Also, some nutrients are added after cooking during the enrobing process. Reputable companies that practice good quality control analyze the finished product for vitamin and other nutrient levels to ensure that recommended allowances are met. Ideally, products should be analyzed for nutrients after storage, up until the expiration date, so that animals receive the same nutritional value whether the food is fresh or is obtained from storage.

> **TECHNICIAN NOTE** Processed pet food from reputable companies contains adequate quantities of nutrients, although manufacturing procedures account for some loss during cooking and storage. There is no need to add vitamins or other nutrients to commercial pet food to make up for losses during processing.

MARKETING

Much of the commercial pet food market in the United States is made up of brands and products from four large companies: Mars, Nestlé Purina, Hill's, and Iams. Hundreds of smaller pet food companies sell thousands of varieties nationally, regionally, and locally. Even small independent mills that produce feed for cattle, swine, and poultry can easily mix batches of pet food and sell them locally. One general characteristic of large companies is that they do research, conduct feeding trials, and have extensive quality control measures throughout the manufacturing and distribution processes. Smaller companies typically do not have the resources, experience, and expertise to carry out similar procedures.

Pet foods are advertised and sold with a number of similar, different, and overlapping marketing claims. Both professionals and consumers should be aware that pet food companies often emphasize factors other than nutritional value to sell their products. The best pet foods may not be the ones heavily marketed. Although it is impossible to identify every type of marketing claim, the following are commonly used.

All-Purpose

All-purpose pet foods are intended for feeding healthy animals of any age or life stage. They are complete and balanced, meaning that they contain all known nutrients in adequate amounts, and that the nutrients are bioavailable. Ideally, these products have undergone feeding trials for growth of puppies or kittens, as well as reproduction (gestation and lactation), to ensure that they meet the increased nutritional demands (Figure 9-2).

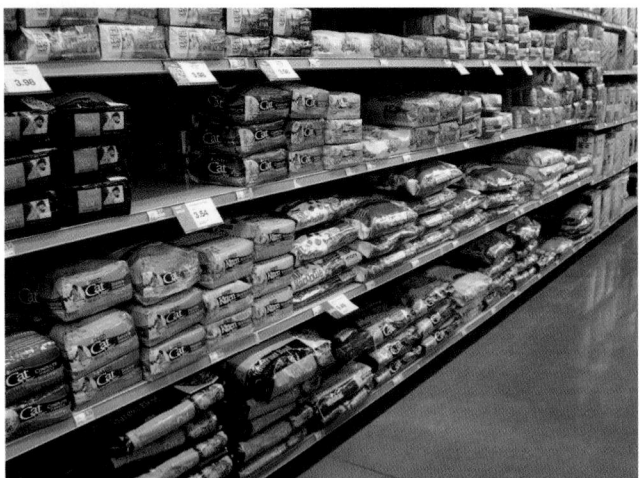

FIGURE 9-2 All-purpose pet foods are intended for feeding healthy animals of any age or life stage. All-purpose diets are complete and balanced.

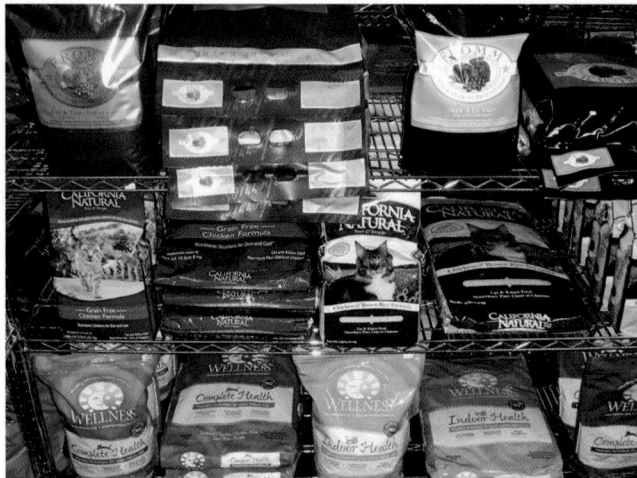

FIGURE 9-3 Premium pet foods, such as California Natural, Wellness, and FROMM brands *(pictured)*, may include more expensive ingredients and may cater to selective pet owners.

Specific-Purpose

Specific-purpose products are intended for certain life stages, such as growth, or for certain medical conditions such as obesity, kidney disease, hairballs, etc. Most veterinary therapeutic diets fall into this category, which should be prescribed and monitored by animal health professionals.

Value

Value or low-priced products are aimed at consumers looking for bargains or who are feeding multiple animals. Many store brands, private labels, and generic pet foods are positioned as low-cost, high-value. These are often sold at discount and grocery stores, feed stores, and warehouse clubs, and sometimes at pet retailers, as an alternative to higher-priced products. Value-oriented pet foods are typically complete and balanced and are acceptable for feeding healthy dogs and cats.

Premium

Premium products are sold on the basis that more expensive ingredients and foods are healthier than low-priced value products. Some companies market certain pet foods as "super-premium." Although no standard definition has been established, in general premium products are sold at specialty retailers such as pet stores, kennels, and veterinary clinics. By making some products exclusive to certain retailers, pet food companies hope to attract more demanding owners, or those consumers who equate high price with high quality. Some overlap in categories occurs because some pet foods once considered to be premium are sold in grocery stores and discount retailers. These products may have added **palatability** enhancers and often contain added ingredients not found in value- or all-purpose pet foods (Figure 9-3).

People Food

People food products are those in which the pet food is designed or marketed to look like recognizable human foods. For example, there may be chunks of "meat" or vegetables in a "stew." Shapes, textures, aromas, and even colors can be manipulated to make pet food resemble human food. It is difficult to maintain foods in their original state after they have been extruded or canned, but some frozen and refrigerated products attempt to preserve or re-create human-appearing foods. Owners should be advised that human-appearing foods are not necessarily any healthier or nutritionally complete than other pet foods. In fact, sometimes chunks of "meat" are actually composed of texturized vegetable protein with artificial colors such as red dye to mislead consumers into thinking they are serving real "meat."

Flavors and Varieties

Flavors and varieties are major factors in how pet foods are formulated and marketed. Dogs and cats often have distinct flavor preferences, which are typically measured in two-bowl feeding tests. Different products can be placed in separate bowls before a hungry dog or cat, and the one that is eaten first or the fastest is assumed to be preferred because of flavor, aroma, texture, etc. Consumers for the most part want their pets to "enjoy" their food, so they will experiment with different flavors and varieties to find those products that their pets consume willingly. In general, there are no significant nutritional differences in products that for example are beef-flavored instead of chicken-flavored, or those that contain fish, lamb, or other ingredients. A nearly infinite variety of ingredients and combinations can be used in pet foods, and the listing of ingredients on labels may not tell you the actual flavor characteristics, or whether an individual animal will "enjoy" the different foods.

Ingredients

Ingredients are also highly marketed characteristics of pet foods and are usually prominently displayed on package labels. Some products are sold because of the presence of ingredients (e.g., "with real chicken," "ocean fish"); others are sold because of the absence of ingredients (e.g., "contains no soy," "grain-free"). Unusual foods such as venison, rabbit, pheasant, barley, and so forth, may appeal to certain consumers, especially those who believe their animals are allergic or sensitive to more common ingredients.

> **TECHNICIAN NOTE** When evaluating pet foods, the ingredient list is the most accurate information about what is in the product. The name of the product or the advertising on the front of the label may not exactly match the ingredients.

Nutrients

Nutrients are similar to ingredients in that they may be featured on product labels. Consumers often think that "more is better" when it comes to nutrients in pet foods. The main example is protein, because many varieties of dog and cat foods have the claim of "high-protein." Owners willingly pay more for these products, thinking that extra protein is somehow better or healthier than "ordinary" pet foods. However, as noted earlier, protein is not stored in the body, and when fed in excessive amounts, it is used or stored as energy. Although protein requirements vary depending on life stage, medical conditions, age, and other factors, in general there is no reason to choose a "high-protein" pet food only for that characteristic. Other claims include "extra calcium," "high-fiber," or the addition of non-nutrients such as glucosamine. In other cases, "less is better" marketing claims are used to market products. For example, "low-fat" or "reduced-fat" claims often appear on products designed for overweight dogs and cats. "Low-carbohydrate" products are marketed for animals, often with no rationale.

Natural

Natural pet foods claim to avoid any chemically synthesized ingredients. This term most often applies to preservatives used in dry products (moist foods usually do not need added preservatives because the sealed cans prevent spoilage). Some consumers wish to avoid chemical preservatives but find natural preservatives such as vitamin E to be acceptable. At the present time, many pet foods that claim to be "all-natural" actually contain added vitamins, minerals, and trace nutrients that are chemically synthesized. As described earlier, many nutrients must be added to pet foods to meet minimum requirements because animal and plant food sources alone may not supply the correct amounts. Also, raw ingredients may have been preserved with "artificial chemicals" before arriving at the pet food processing plant. One example is fish, which always has to be preserved between the time it is caught and when it is made into pet food. The claim of natural should therefore be regarded with some skepticism, and in fact, most pet food companies have substituted "natural" preservatives for "artificial" chemicals to meet perceived consumer demand.

> **TECHNICIAN NOTE** "All-natural" pet foods almost always contain chemically synthesized ingredients such as vitamin supplements. There is no known health advantage to selecting "natural" dog or cat food.

Organic

Organic pet foods generally refer to those that use food ingredients that are not exposed to insecticides, pesticides, or, in the case of animals, medications such as antibiotics or growth promotants. At present, no complete and balanced pet food can be considered 100% organic because of the need to add inorganic vitamins, minerals, and trace nutrients. Although organic products appeal to consumers who try to avoid artificial chemicals, no evidence currently suggests that organic foods are by definition healthier or more nutritious.

Holistic

Holistic is a more recent product claim seen on certain pet food labels. There is no official definition or general agreement on what the term "holistic" means. In medical practice, holistic often implies considering the health of the whole person or animal instead of just treating a single symptom. Some health care professionals claim to practice "holistic medicine," and pet foods marketed as holistic may appeal to those professionals and the pet owners they serve.

> **TECHNICIAN NOTE** "Holistic" has no meaning and should be ignored in pet food marketing.

Raw

Raw pet foods and ingredients are marketed to those consumers who believe that food in its natural, uncooked state is healthier than cooked, or to those who think that nutrients are destroyed during processing, leading to unhealthy products. Some people attempt to eat only raw foods themselves for the same reasons. Proponents of raw feeding claim that dogs and cats in the wild eat uncooked food sources, and therefore pets should do the same. The main problem with offering raw foods to pets is that most of the meats and even some of the plant food sources sold in stores are contaminated with pathogenic bacteria. Raw or undercooked meat is a frequent cause of food poisoning, and outbreaks of foodborne illness in humans are common. Dogs and cats are likewise susceptible to illness from bacterial contamination of raw food. Animals can also acquire harmful bacteria from raw food and can spread disease to humans even if they remain apparently healthy. Another issue with raw foods is that overall diets are often incomplete and unbalanced unless they come from reputable companies that ensure the nutritional value of their products. Feeding of bones is

CASE PRESENTATION 9-1 EFFECTS OF RAW FOOD DIET ON GROWING PUPPY

A 10-week-old male German Shepherd puppy was presented for lethargy, weight loss, ataxia (stumbling while walking), and whimpering as if in pain. The owner had purchased the puppy from a breeder 2 weeks earlier. He had been active and in good health when first brought home, but progressively had become weaker and less responsive (Figure 1). A diet history was obtained. According to records from the breeder, this puppy and others in the litter were originally fed a complete and balanced commercial dry diet (Purina Pro Plan Large Breed Formula for Puppies). The new owner had researched on the Internet what to feed and had found many websites that recommended a raw meat diet. The owner decided to feed only raw chicken necks and backs to the puppy. On physical examination, the puppy showed signs of pain when the abdomen and bones and joints were palpated. Evidence of diarrhea was found, and fecal analysis revealed roundworm ova *(Toxacara canis)*. Abdominal radiographs showed evidence of bones in the stomach and intestines. A tentative diagnosis of enteritis

was made, likely caused by feeding bones and possibly bacterially-contaminated raw meat. Developmental orthopedic disease was also suspected because of the unbalanced diet deficient in calcium and other minerals. The puppy was treated with an antibiotic and dewormer, and the diet was switched to a canned commercial product (Hill's Science Diet Puppy). Over the next 2 weeks, the puppy gradually improved and began to gain weight (Figure 2). Ataxia and signs of pain resolved. The most likely cause of the puppy's illness was the switch from a complete and balanced diet to raw chicken, which is incomplete, unbalanced, and most likely contaminated with pathogenic bacteria. Switching back to a commercial diet formulated for puppy growth was essential in resolving the illness.

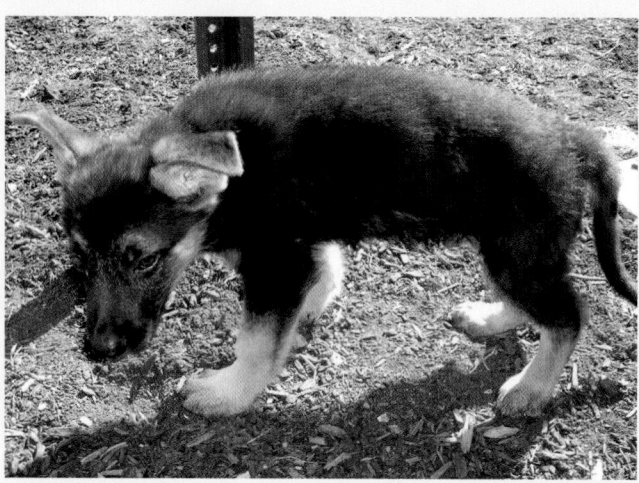

FIGURE 1 A puppy after 2 weeks of being fed an incomplete and unbalanced raw diet.

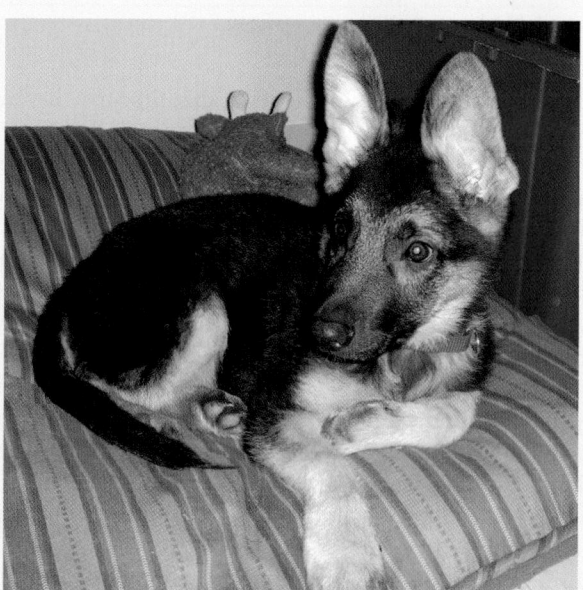

FIGURE 2 The same puppy after 4 weeks of being fed a complete and balanced commercial diet for growing dogs.

recommended by many raw feeders, but depending on the size and type, bones can cause gastrointestinal upset, obstruction, and even perforation and death. Frozen and refrigerated raw diets for pets are available, but owners should be advised to take as much care in preparing and handling these products as they would raw hamburger or raw chicken in their kitchen (Figure 9-4).

VETERINARY THERAPEUTIC DIETS

In the 1930s, a veterinarian named Mark Morris developed a recipe for a dog food to help treat a service dog that had kidney disease. The dog did well and lived longer than expected, and this experience led to an association between Dr. Morris and Hill's Packing Company in 1948. Since then, Hill's Pet Nutrition has introduced many pet foods that are formulated to help prevent, manage, and even cure various disease processes in dogs and cats. Other companies have

developed lines of veterinary diets, and today many choices are available.

The distinction between therapeutic diets and those sold over-the-counter (OTC) is not always clear. Veterinary therapeutic diets are intended to be dispensed under the supervision of veterinarians in the context of a valid veterinarian-client-patient relationship (VCPR). Although they are not strictly "prescription" items, such as pharmaceuticals, in most areas these products may be sold (dispensed) only at the veterinary clinic where the patient is seen. Often the label will have a phrase such as "Use under the direction of a veterinarian." To purchase therapeutic diets from other clinics, online pharmacies, or other suppliers, a veterinarian must prescribe or request the order. This is done to prevent dispensing or recommending an inappropriate product. Most of these diets are not harmful if fed to healthy animals, but serious consequences could result if different diseases are

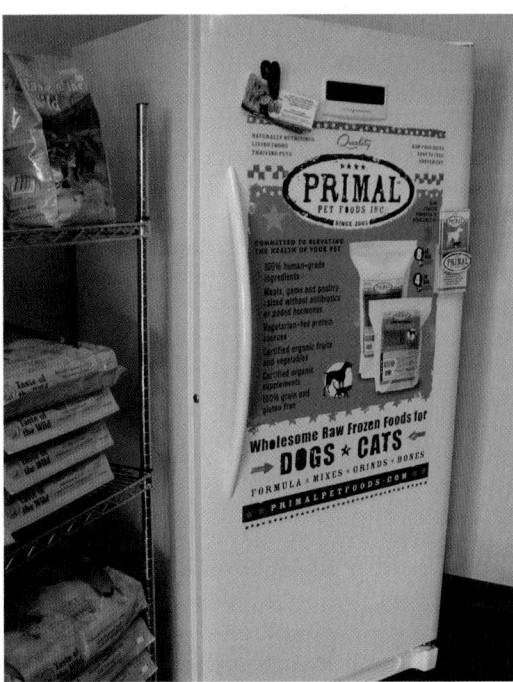

FIGURE 9-4 Frozen and refrigerated raw diets require care when storing, preparing, and handling them.

present. For example, feeding a kidney diet that is high in fat to an animal suffering from pancreatitis could lead to worsening of the illness or even death. Other examples that may be harmful include feeding a high-fiber diet formulated for weight loss to a very thin patient, or a restricted-protein diet to a young, growing animal. Therefore, veterinary diets are not sold OTC, and animal health professionals should be cautious about recommending and dispensing these products without a current VPCR.

Medicated pet food is not currently legal in the United States. Therefore, no pharmaceutical drugs may be added to products, and supplements that claim to have an effect on diseases or the structure/function of the animal are not permitted. Because it is impossible to have all animals receive an appropriate "dose" of an added drug or supplement, such pet foods are illegal. No pet food should claim the same effects as legally approved drugs and products. Many veterinary therapeutic diets contain unique combinations of foods and ingredients and may contain supplements or additives not found in OTC diets, such as urinary acidifiers in diets formulated to manage bladder stones or fiber mixtures in diets for weight loss. These are permitted to some extent, but all additives must be approved as safe and edible.

> **TECHNICIAN NOTE** Pet foods that claim to cure diseases—either on the labels or through advertising—are technically illegal and are best avoided.

PET FOOD REGULATION

In the United States, a number of different government agencies and organizations are involved in oversight of the pet food industry. Veterinary professionals should be familiar with these various groups and should have an understanding of the procedures and protocols in place to ensure a safe, nutritious pet food supply.

Food and Drug Administration–Center for Veterinary Medicine

The Food and Drug Administration (FDA) and its division, the Center for Veterinary Medicine (CVM), are the main regulators of the safety of pet foods. The FDA-CVM has authority over much of the information on pet food labels, including health and nutrition claims. As with human foods, all pet foods, treats, and snacks must be safe to eat, must be produced under sanitary conditions, must contain no harmful substances, and must be truthfully labeled. Any claims found on labels or in advertising and marketing literature from pet food companies are subject to oversight, especially those that state or imply that a food, ingredient, or supplement will prevent, treat, or affect a disease or any medical condition. Regulations involving control of microbial and chemical contamination of pet foods, along with additives such as supplements, are developed and enforced by FDA-CVM. Pet food recalls in the case of contamination (such as *Salmonella*, mycotoxins, or unapproved ingredients) are requested or mandated by the FDA and are subsequently monitored. The FDA-CVM has the power to shut down manufacturing facilities or distribution centers if unsafe or contaminated pet food is being produced or sold. Any questions or concerns about the safety of pet food should be reported to the FDA using an online Safety Reporting Portal, phone calls, faxes, or other means.

U.S. Department of Agriculture

The U.S. Department of Agriculture (USDA) is broadly responsible for agricultural products, including ingredients used in pet foods. The USDA conducts inspections of farms and pet food manufacturers to ensure safety and proper handling. Some labeling requirements fall under USDA jurisdiction, so that animal food is not mistaken for human food. Pet food companies that maintain research facilities with animals are subject to USDA inspection for proper care of animals, housing, record keeping, sanitation, etc.

Association of American Feed Control Officials

The Association of American Feed Control Officials (AAFCO) is a private, nongovernmental organization that does not have regulatory or enforcement power. However, many members of AAFCO are employed by federal and state governments as feed control officials. The organization develops definitions of feed ingredients, wording that is used on pet food labels, protocols for feeding studies, and other guidelines and standards that often become laws or official regulations after adoption by governmental agencies. Each year, AAFCO distributes an official publication (currently over 500 pages long) that contains model bills and regulations, model guidance documents, definitions of feed terms and ingredients, and reports from committees on future activities. Contrary to popular belief, AAFCO does not regulate, test, approve, or certify pet foods in any way. It is the pet food company's responsibility to formulate products according to the appropriate AAFCO standard. Actual regulatory authority lies with state feed control officials.

> **TECHNICIAN NOTE** Pet foods that claim to be "AAFCO-approved" are misleading, because AAFCO does not approve products.

Some of the most important AAFCO documents are the AAFCO Dog (and Cat) Food Nutrient Profiles based on dry matter and calorie content. These documents list all known essential nutrients, along with minimum values for "growth and reproduction" and "adult maintenance" (see Tables 9-5 and 9-7). For some nutrients, maximum values are listed. The profiles are used by nearly all pet food manufacturers to ensure that their products contain a complete spectrum of all nutrients that meet or exceed the minimum amounts. Other important guidelines are the AAFCO Dog and Cat Feeding Protocols, which describe in detail the minimum feeding protocols for proving that a dog or cat food supports adult maintenance, growth, gestation/lactation (reproduction), or "all life stages," which is a sequential combination of the reproduction and growth protocols.

National Research Council

The National Research Council (NRC) is a private, nonprofit organization that works under the guidance of the National Academy of Sciences. From time to time, the NRC develops a set of nutrient requirements for various animal species. The current volume of the *Nutrient Requirements of Dogs and Cats* was published by the National Academies Press in 2006 and contains a great deal of useful information about nutrients, physiology, feeding behavior, diet formulation and feed processing, and even physical activity and environment. The actual nutrient requirements are variably listed as minimal requirements, adequate intakes, recommended allowances, and safe upper limits. After each chapter, an extensive list of scientific references enables animal health professionals to consider and evaluate the scientific basis of the nutritional information. The AAFCO nutrient profiles are based on the NRC guidelines.

> **TECHNICIAN NOTE** The nutrient requirements for dogs and cats are based on AAFCO and NRC publications. These are updated periodically to incorporate new research findings.

The Federal Trade Commission

The Federal Trade Commission (FTC) regulates business practices in the United States. False, misleading, or deceptive marketing practices in the manufacture, distribution, and sale of pet food may be subject to FTC enforcement.

PET FOOD LABELS

Animal health professionals and consumers can obtain much information from product labels that helps in evaluating the suitability of the diet for an animal and in knowing how to use it (e.g., feeding guides). An important point is that it is difficult to judge the quality of any pet food based on its label. Some information is legally required to appear on labels, but other information is optional (Figure 9-5).

Principal Display Panel

The principal display panel of a pet food label refers to the front or main part of the product, and serves as identification (dog food, cat food) and to attract consumers with colors, illustrations, advertising, etc. The exact brand and product name must appear here (e.g., Purina Dog Chow, Hill's Science Diet Adult, Iams Chunks), along with the species of animal. The quantity of food contained in the package (by weight or liquid measure) is required. The principal display panel cannot be hidden by an outer container or wrapper. Any photos or illustrations of the product must be accurate and must not misrepresent the contents.

Information Panel

The information panel is the second required part of a pet food label. Among the requirements are a guaranteed analysis, an ingredient statement, a statement of nutritional adequacy or purpose, feeding directions, and the name and address of the manufacturer or distributor. A universal product code often appears, along with a company telephone number and a freshness date ("best before …").

Pet food regulations in other countries may differ from those in the United States. The following details further explain current U.S. rules and guidelines.

Product Identity

The product identity usually contains both a brand name and a product name, but the manufacturer's name can appear elsewhere on the label. The terms "all" or "100%" cannot be used in the product name if the pet food contains more than one ingredient (apart from water or trace amounts of preservatives or additives). Likewise, if the name of a food or ingredient is part of the product name, it must make up at least 70% of the product by weight (or 95% if water is excluded from the weight). For example, "Acme Beef Chunks for dogs" must contain at least 70% beef by weight. Products with less than 70% of a food ingredient are permitted as part of the product name, as long as a descriptor is used, such as "dinner," "platter," "entrée," "formula," or "recipe." In these cases, the food must make up at least 10% of the product weight (25% if water is excluded). So "Acme Beef Recipe for dogs" must have 10% or more beef by weight. A final descriptor is the word "with," which refers to a food that makes up at least 3% of the product excluding water. "Acme Dog Food with Chicken" must have at least 3% chicken. If more than one ingredient is in the product name, then ingredients must be listed in order of weight, and each must make up at least 3% excluding water. For example, "Acme Dog Food with

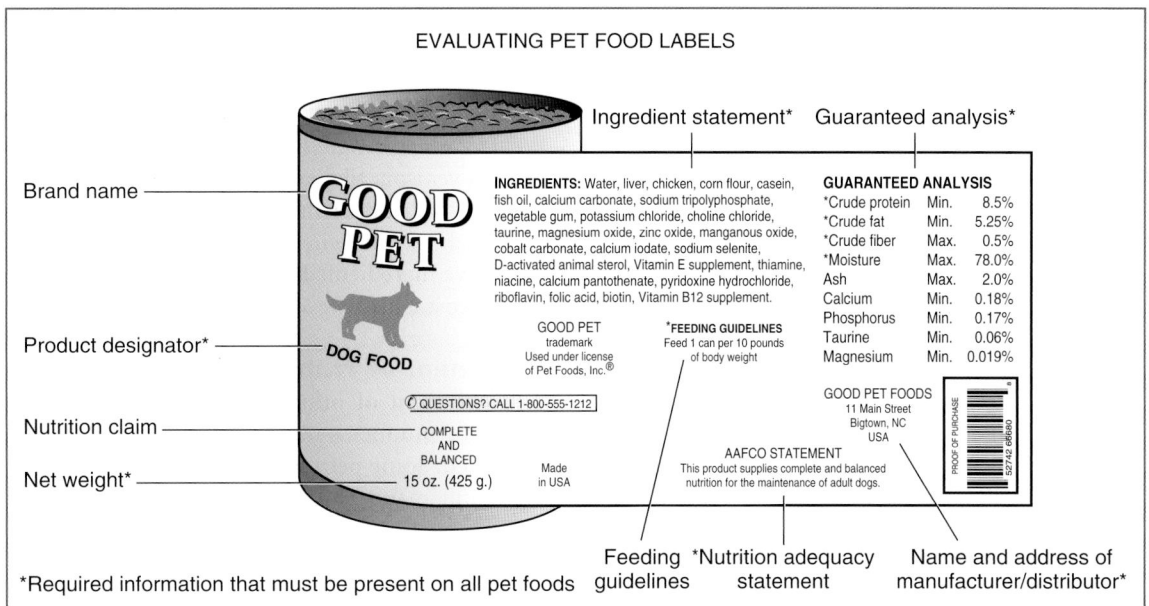

EVALUATING PET FOOD LABELS

Ingredient statement*   Guaranteed analysis*

Brand name

INGREDIENTS: Water, liver, chicken, corn flour, casein, fish oil, calcium carbonate, sodium tripolyphosphate, vegetable gum, potassium chloride, choline chloride, taurine, magnesium oxide, zinc oxide, manganous oxide, cobalt carbonate, calcium iodate, sodium selenite, D-activated animal sterol, Vitamin E supplement, thiamine, niacine, calcium pantothenate, pyridoxine hydrochloride, riboflavin, folic acid, biotin, Vitamin B12 supplement.

GUARANTEED ANALYSIS
*Crude protein   Min.   8.5%
*Crude fat   Min.   5.25%
*Crude fiber   Max.   0.5%
*Moisture   Max.   78.0%
Ash   Max.   2.0%
Calcium   Min.   0.18%
Phosphorus   Min.   0.17%
Taurine   Min.   0.06%
Magnesium   Min.   0.019%

GOOD PET
trademark
Used under license
of Pet Foods, Inc.®

Product designator*

*FEEDING GUIDELINES
Feed 1 can per 10 pounds
of body weight

GOOD PET FOODS
11 Main Street
Bigtown, NC
USA

© QUESTIONS? CALL 1-800-555-1212

Nutrition claim

COMPLETE
AND
BALANCED

Net weight*

15 oz. (425 g.)

Made
in USA

AAFCO STATEMENT
This product supplies complete and balanced
nutrition for the maintenance of adult dogs.

PROOF OF PURCHASE

Feeding   *Nutrition adequacy   Name and address of
guidelines   statement   manufacturer/distributor*

*Required information that must be present on all pet foods

FIGURE 9-5 A pet food label is a contract between the manufacturer and the consumer. A label provides information required by law and may include optional information, such as a statement of calorie content, the Universal Product Code, batch information, or a freshness date.

Lamb and Rice" must have 3% or more lamb and 3% or more rice, and the weight of the lamb must be higher than that of the rice. Flavor designations as part of the product identity (e.g., "beef-flavored," "with real fish flavor") must conform to the ingredient statement and must impart a distinctive characteristic to the product. Some pet food labels contain a highlighted "burst" or "flag," which draws attention to statements that might include "Improved" or "New." These are permitted only for 6 months of product production, then the burst or flag must be removed. Comparison or preference statements (e.g., "preferred 3 to 1 over the leading brand") are permitted for 1 year but must be substantiated by evidence. The claim may be resubstantiated after 1 year if the statement is to remain on the label.

> **TECHNICIAN NOTE** Consumers are easily misled by labels. It is helpful for animal health professionals to assist pet owners in understanding the advertising and marketing techniques commonly used by pet food companies.

Net Weight

The net weight of a product must adhere to the Fair Packaging and Label Act. In the United States, pounds and ounces must be used along with SI (metric) units such as grams and kilograms. For liquid products, the largest whole unit (quart, pint, cup) followed by smaller units (such as ounces) must appear along with SI units (liters, milliliters). If the product is divided into smaller packages, then the weight or measure of the smaller units is required as well.

Guaranteed Analysis

The guaranteed analysis (GA) is an important part of the information panel. It is also one of the most confusing

TABLE 9-12	Guaranteed Analysis Required on All Pet Food Labels (AAFCO)
NUTRIENT	**PERCENTAGE**
Crude protein	Minimum percentage
Crude fat	Minimum percentage
Crude fiber	Maximum percentage
Moisture	Maximum percentage
Optional	
Crude fat	Maximum percentage, required if pet food is labeled "lean," "low fat," "less fat," "reduced fat," or similar wording
Calcium	Minimum percentage
Phosphorus	Minimum percentage
Ash	Maximum percentage

AAFCO, Association of American Feed Control Officials.

statements found on pet food labels, so an understanding of its uses and limitations is important. A GA consists of four required diet components and amounts, along with several others that are optional but are found on many pet foods (Table 9-12). Only the minimum crude protein and crude fat amounts are required, along with the maximum fiber and moisture amounts. The actual contents of the diet may be more or less. For example, a GA that states "crude protein 18% min" can legally contain 18%, 20%, or any higher level. It cannot contain less than 18%. Most pet food companies automatically include higher amounts than the label minimums to account for losses during processing and for variations in foods and ingredients. Ash is sometimes listed in a GA as a maximum, and this contains the mineral portion of the food, but is not a measure of quality or exact amounts of calcium, phosphorus, etc. Moisture levels cannot exceed

78% of the diet by weight unless labeled as gravy, sauce, stew, broth, etc. The GA is often used to compare one diet with another, but usually incorrectly. As a hypothetical example, Diet A is a dry kibble and has 25% protein, and Diet B is canned and has 8% protein. A consumer might conclude that Diet A is "better" than Diet B because it has more protein. But because Diet B has more moisture, by calculating on a dry-matter basis (using an average 10% moisture in dry products and 75% moisture in canned), Diet B is actually higher in protein (8%/.25 = 32% compared with 25%/.90 = 28%). But in both cases, the true protein content may be higher and the moisture content lower than those listed in the GA. Also, the digestibility and bioavailability of the protein is not stated. Therefore, an accurate comparison cannot be made. Based on the GA alone, it is very difficult to evaluate the quality of a pet food.

Ingredient Statement

The ingredient statement, a key portion of a pet food label, should be reviewed whenever a product is purchased or recommended. Ingredients must be listed in order by weight, with the heaviest first and the lightest last. Units cannot be used (e.g., it is illegal to state "chicken 40%, rice 20%" or "beef 90 grams"). Each ingredient must use a standardized name as found in the feed definitions established by AAFCO, and no brand or trade names may be used. The ingredient statement is important for several reasons, but it also has shortcomings. One advantage is that a consumer can see what types of foods have been used in the product, which is helpful if an animal is allergic or sensitive to certain foods. Also, information can be compared with that on the principal display panel because many pet foods have one claim in their product name (e.g., a cat food may feature "real salmon and tuna"), but the actual list may not be consistent (e.g., chicken may be included as a main ingredient). Listing in order of weight is somewhat helpful but can be misleading. Water makes up a large percentage of meat (approximately 50% to 75%) by weight but does not have any nutritional value. If a company used, for example, 2 kg of chicken and 1 kg of corn meal in a product, a consumer would think that the nutrients mostly come from chicken. However, because chicken may be 70% moisture and corn meal is 10% moisture, the actual amounts are closer to 0.6 kg chicken and 0.9 kg corn. A similarly misleading feature of the ingredient statement is that similar products may have different names and may be listed separately. An example is wheat, wheat flour, and wheat germ meal, all of which come from the same grain and may make up a large portion of the diet, even if "meat" is the first ingredient. As a rule of thumb, the first few ingredients listed supply mostly protein and energy (carbohydrate), then fats and oils are listed, then supplements such as calcium and other minerals along with vitamins, with preservatives and additives appearing near the middle or end of the list. Consumers are often confused by chemical-sounding names that appear on the ingredient statement, but most of these are simply scientific names for vitamins, minerals, and preservatives. Many consumers and even health professionals do not understand terms such as "by-products" or "meal," or even what species "meat" represents. These definitions are hard to find but appear on some pet food company websites and in the AAFCO official publication. Finally, ingredients that sound expensive or unique, such as venison, tilapia, pheasant, barley, etc., do not necessarily provide better nutrition than more common ingredients such as chicken and rice. Products that incorporate expensive ingredients have a higher cost for consumers, but higher cost is not the same as higher quality.

Statement of Nutritional Adequacy

The statement of nutritional adequacy indicates what life stages the product is intended for and how the claim is substantiated. Some pet foods are for "all life stages," others are for "adult maintenance" or "growth" (or both), and a few claim "gestation/lactation." There is no life stage of "senior" or "mature" in the AAFCO definitions, so products intended and labeled for older animals do not have to follow any particular nutrient profiles. To show that their products support the life stage claim, companies can use one of three methods. The first is to compare the nutrients in their finished product versus the AAFCO nutrient profiles, and if all nutrients meet or exceed 100%, then the claim is "(Name of product) is formulated to meet the nutritional levels established by the AAFCO Dog (or Cat) Food Nutrient Profiles for (life stage)." The second method is to conduct a feeding test with AAFCO-approved protocols, and the claim would be "Animal feeding tests using AAFCO procedures substantiate that (name of product) provides complete and balanced nutrition for (life stage)." The third method is to use a product family, where a lead product is identified by feeding tests, and all other very similar products (recipes and formulations are very similar but may differ in flavor, texture, additives, etc.) may carry the claim, "(Name of product) is comparable in nutritional adequacy to a product that has been substantiated using AAFCO feeding tests." Consumers and professionals should determine whether a pet food has been through feeding tests or has simply been formulated to compare with nutrient profiles. Feeding tests are preferable in that they evaluate digestibility, bioavailability, and actual performance in animals; products justified by formulation alone do not guarantee results when fed.

> **TECHNICIAN NOTE** AAFCO does not do any testing of pet foods, but it publishes protocols that support statements of nutritional adequacy. Pet food companies or independent research facilities do the actual feed testing.

Feeding Directions

Feeding directions are included to help pet owners determine how much product is intended to be fed; they must be provided in common terms. At a minimum, the directions are required to state "feed (weight/unit) per (body weight) of dog (or cat)." Many pet foods include weight ranges, such as "10-20 lb, feed ½ to 1 cup; 20-40 lb, feed 1 to 2 cups"; etc.

For therapeutic diets, the statement "Use only as directed by your veterinarian" may be substituted for feeding directions. Because of the sedentary lifestyle of many pets and the tendency for people to feed human foods and treats, feeding guidelines should be used only as a starting point. If animals gain weight while eating the recommended amounts, gradual reductions should be made. However, the treatment of obesity is more complicated than simply feeding less; this topic is discussed later.

Descriptive terms such as "light," "less," "reduced calories," "lean," and "low fat" have special AAFCO definitions and cannot be used on pet food labels unless exact requirements are met. Comparative claims such as "less than" another product must include information on the comparison product and the percentage of reduction. The calorie content is not required to be listed on labels unless there is a "light" or similar claim. This regulation is scheduled to be changed in the near future, and all pet food products may be required to list caloric content as measured by bomb calorimetry or as estimated with modified Atwater factors.

> **TECHNICIAN NOTE** Feeding directions as found on pet food labels are only a starting point, and may be more or less than an individual animal requires to achieve and maintain a healthy body weight.

HOME-PREPARED PET FOOD

Many pet owners feed "human" foods in addition to or instead of commercial dog and cat diets. In a telephone survey of pet owners in the United States and Australia, owners reported they fed table scraps, leftovers, or homemade foods to 30% of dogs and 13% of cats in the study (635 dogs and 469 cats were reported). However, more than 93% of dogs and cats received at least half their diet as commercial pet food. Pet owners feed human foods for a variety of reasons.

INCLUDING OR AVOIDING SPECIFIC INGREDIENTS

Some owners believe that their pets need a certain food or type of food. Various meat and dairy products, eggs, grains, vegetables, fruits, or supplements are added to commercial foods or are substituted for part of the diet. If there is an inexpensive convenient source of food such as venison after deer season, owners may want to feed that instead of commercial pet food. Another motivation is that some owners perceive "organic" or "natural" foods to be better, so they seek out special types of foods to feed their pets. In contrast to wanting to include certain foods, owners may wish to avoid other foods or additives because of the perception that they are harmful or are not nutritionally beneficial.

CHEMICALS

Pet food labels often contain unusual or unfamiliar ingredients, which may be mistaken for "chemicals" and may be thought to be harmful. Most of these are vitamins and minerals; others may be preservatives. For example, one brand of "natural, organic" dog food contains chemical-sounding ingredients such as pyridoxine hydrochloride (a B-vitamin), cobalt proteinate (a mineral that does not have a dietary requirement), dicalcium pantothenate (a mineral combined with a B-vitamin), DL-methionine (an amino acid), and sodium ascorbate (vitamin C, which is not required by dogs and cats). A small number of pet owners may not want to feed commercial products if they do not recognize or understand the names or the purposes of the ingredients.

> **TECHNICIAN NOTE** Health professionals should become familiar with names of vitamins and other additives commonly used in pet food to help owners understand the "chemical"-sounding names.

PRESERVATIVES

Many consumers define natural foods as being free of preservatives. A basic definition of a preservative is a substance that inhibits or slows the growth of microorganisms or reduces the rate of decomposition or deterioration. Commercial dry and semi-moist pet food must contain some kind of preservative. Otherwise, the shelf life would be only a few days before spoilage would start to occur (similar to a loaf of bread left out on a kitchen counter with no preservatives). To enable production of dry pet foods economically and to ensure a reasonable shelf life of 1 or 2 years, preservatives are included in virtually all products. Canned pet foods do not always require preservatives because high-heat processing and the sealed containers prevent bacteria and mold from multiplying. The shelf life of canned food is longer than that of dry food but is not indefinite. For many years, the pet food industry used chemically synthesized preservatives such as ethoxyquin, butylated hydroxyanisole (BHA), and butylated hydroxytoluene (BHT), which act as antioxidants to prevent rancidity (oxidation of fats). Because of concerns about these types of preservatives causing cancer or adverse effects on human health and despite the lack of scientific data demonstrating these effects in pets, many companies no longer use these in pet food. Instead, commonly used "natural" preservatives include vitamin E (mixed tocopherols), vitamin C (ascorbic acid or ascorbate), and rosemary extract. The shelf life of "naturally" preserved products is shorter than that of products with "chemical" preservatives, so consumers should use pet foods within their "best before" dating period. Products should be stored in their original packaging, closed tightly, and protected from excessive heat or humidity. The practice of dumping a bag of dry pet food into another container and storing it in a garage or shed should be discouraged because this shortens the shelf-life considerably.

> **TECHNICIAN NOTE** Pet foods are best stored in their original containers at room temperature.

ADDITIVES

Some but not all pet foods include flavors, colors, binders, emulsifiers, and other ingredients that consumers may or may not recognize as nonfood additives. Anything added to a commercial pet food must be "generally recognized as safe" (GRAS), which is a classification regulated by the FDA. These additives may be subject to premarket review and approval or, if generally recognized by qualified experts, may be added without separate approval. Premarket approval takes the form of lengthy feeding studies (2 years or longer) in more than one species of animal to reveal short- and long-term effects on health. Benefits of additives include improved structure, texture, and color, along with improved binding and gelling of the finished product. Also, vitamins, antioxidants, glucosamine, and other substances may be considered additives for nutritional or health purposes. Pet owners may be concerned that artificial colors or flavors are harmful; in these cases, they can be assured that many pet foods do not contain these types of additives.

BY-PRODUCTS

These widely misunderstood ingredients are found in many pet foods. Many people assume that they are of poor quality, are not fit for consumption, do not qualify as human foods, or even consist of scraps swept off the floor. None of these beliefs is true. The basic definition of a *by-product* is that portion of a meat product that is not packaged and sold separately to consumers in typical grocery stores. Because these terms appear on pet food labels, "meat" refers to mostly skeletal (striate) muscle, and "meat by-products" include other parts of the animal (whether beef, pork, lamb, poultry). For example, in the case of pork, the carcass is first divided into the shoulder, loin, ham, and belly. These may be subdivided into pork chops, ribs, bacon, and other recognizable products. The remaining part of the pork carcass is considered a by-product, and includes organs such as lungs, spleen, kidneys, and liver. Although these sound unappetizing to consumers, they are in fact nutritious sources of highly digestible animal protein, vitamins, minerals, and fatty acids. By-products such as these are commonly found in processed meat products such as hot dogs, sausage, and deli meats, including bologna and salami. Pet owners who consider by-products harmful or of poor quality should be informed of what the term actually means. Contrary to popular belief, by-products cannot legally contain intestinal contents, hair, horns, teeth, hooves, or feathers (if poultry). The reasons why pet food companies use by-products in pet food are both nutritional and economic. Because by-products provide many essential nutrients at a lower cost than muscle meat (such as sirloin steak, chicken breast, pork loin, etc.), they are very suitable for animal feeding. Another fact to consider is that although U.S. consumers prefer muscle meat, people in other countries may consider by-products as delicacies. For example, beef tongue is widely used in Mexican, German, English, and Japanese cuisine. Kidneys are part of steak and kidney pie in Britain. Scottish haggish consists of sheep stomach stuffed with liver, heart, lungs, and other

ingredients. Pet owners can be assured that the same by-products that cause them concern are safely eaten by humans all over the world.

> **TECHNICIAN NOTE** By-products are safe and nutritious, and are not indicators of poor-quality pet foods.

PERCEIVED LOW QUALITY OF PET FOODS

Another concern that some owners express is that they want their pets to eat the same high-quality foods that they eat themselves. They may have heard that only poor-quality foods are found in pet food compared with better foods sold for humans. No scientific evidence indicates that foods combined in pet food formulations are of poor quality, at least those used by large, reputable companies. Digestibility of pet food in general may be somewhat less than human foods, but this depends on the overall diet and ingredients. It is possible that an inexpensive pet food produced by a local feed mill that mainly formulates diets for cattle and hogs could be of low quality. Often these pet foods can be easily identified by their price, their packaging, and the obscure names of their manufacturers and distributors. When poor-quality pet foods are fed to pets, observable health problems such as poor hair coat, skin problems (dry or oily), increased fecal material, weight loss, lethargy, etc., may be noted. If the suspect diet is replaced by a more reputable pet food and the problems are resolved, this would indicate that the diet is poorly balanced or incomplete, and/or that the ingredients are of poor quality or are not bioavailable.

AVOIDING CONTAMINANTS AND TOXINS

A final concern expressed by some pet owners is that pet foods may accidentally or purposefully contain substances that are harmful or toxic to dogs and cats. This concern is valid. In 2007, a number of commercial products were associated with dogs and cats becoming ill and dying of kidney failure. A rapid investigation found that vegetable proteins imported from China were purposefully contaminated with melamine, an unapproved product normally used to create plastics, cleaning products, glues, inks, and fertilizers. The pet food companies that had used the contaminated ingredients (wheat and rice gluten) recalled their products and stopped importing pet food ingredients from China. A criminal investigation led to indictments and penalties. This incident was tragic but was an intentional criminal act; it was not a result of pet food companies purposefully using poor-quality ingredients. Since then, reputable companies screen food products for melamine and other toxins. Another pet food recall in 2005 was a result of aflatoxin contamination of a single brand of dry food. The problem was traced to corn from a supplier that had not followed proper procedures to avoid aflatoxin, as well as improper screening at the pet food company. Bacterial contamination with organisms such as *Salmonella* also occurs in the pet (and human) food industry. Because food production, whether for humans or animals, has inherent risks, consumers should be comfortable with the reputation of companies for excellent quality control and its financial and personnel resources and expertise to identify hazards and minimize if not eliminate the risks. As discussed earlier, many smaller pet food (and human food) companies do not have the same resources or ability to screen ingredients and finished products for contamination, whether naturally occurring toxins such as aflatoxin, illegal additives such as melamine, or bacteria such as *Salmonella*, *Listeria*, *Escherichia coli*, and other common foodborne pathogens.

PERCEIVED HEALTH BENEFITS

Consumers may believe that there are properties of home-prepared human foods that are not found in commercial pet foods. They may assume that foods intended for human consumption are automatically healthier, or have special properties. There may be some truth in this, in that fresh vegetables, grains, fruits, etc., contain phytonutrients, antioxidants, and many compounds that may or may not be beneficial for health. It is difficult to research the effects of fresh foods on animal health because they can make up only a portion of the overall diet. In some cases, special foods, if needed, should be included in home-prepared diets rather than added to commercial products.

FOOD ALLERGY OR INTOLERANCE

Dogs and cats that develop skin problems such as itching or ear infection, or gastrointestinal problems such as vomiting and diarrhea, may have an underlying food allergy. This refers to a rare condition wherein some type of protein found in the diet stimulates a hypersensitivity (allergic) reaction. In cases where food allergy is suspected, an animal may be switched to a commercial diet that contains different ingredients. But a reasonable alternative is to offer the pet a home-prepared diet using a limited number of ingredients that have not been previously fed. If the clinical signs (itching, diarrhea) go away, there's a reasonable chance that food allergy or intolerance is present. At that point, a home diet can be continued, or commercial diets can be reintroduced to see if the pet reacts again.

> **TECHNICIAN NOTE** Food allergy can be a significant medical problem and requires a careful elimination food trial for diagnosis.

PALATABILITY

A common reason for owners to feed human foods or table scraps is that their pets refuse to eat commercial diets. If dogs or cats walk away from their bowls of pet food without eating, the owners begin to worry that the food does not taste good, and that their pets will starve if not fed something else. In general, modern pet foods have added palatability enhancers (flavors and textures) that ensure most pets will find them tasty and acceptable. Pets that develop a preference for human foods are often "spoiled," in that they simply beg and are rewarded for their behavior with table scraps, treats, or

complete diets made from human foods. Most pets who find success in avoiding the food in their bowls and instead beg for table scraps will continue that behavior long-term. The key is educating pet owners that most commercial diets are in fact palatable and acceptable to the vast majority of animals. In some cases, different flavors (meat, fish, poultry), types (dry, semi-moist, canned), or textures (small or large kibble, minced or ground or chunky canned foods) need to be offered before the pet will accept one. But continual switching of diets to encourage the pet to eat can lead to behavioral problems as well, in that they may eat new diets for a short period of time but then will refuse them and "beg" for something else. Owners often do not realize that animals express behaviors that result in rewards. One solution is to refuse to acknowledge the begging behavior and simply keep offering the diet until the animal starts to eat again. Overweight animals often are not hungry even if the owners perceive that they should be eating more at each meal. This "tough love" approach can extend to about 3 days, at which point another flavor or type of food should be offered if nothing has been eaten. However, during times of illness or old age, the only way to get a sick animal to eat is with highly palatable human foods.

COST

Owners may be concerned about the price of commercial pet foods, especially premium diets sold in specialty stores. They may believe that table scraps are sufficient for the nutrition of dogs and cats, or that they can duplicate a commercial product by preparing food at home. In reality, complete and balanced home diets are significantly more expensive than most commercial pet foods. Purchasing consumer quantities of meats and other ingredients at grocery stores is always much more expensive than the situation where pet food companies purchase ingredients by the ton. Supplemental minerals and vitamins are much more expensive than pre-mixes used by companies. Also, much time is involved in shopping for ingredients and preparing recipes, which makes home feeding not only more expensive but much less convenient.

HUMAN-ANIMAL BOND

Many owners have special relationships with their pets, and a part of expressing their bond may involve preparing and serving home-cooked foods. Just as a person may enjoy preparing food for family and friends, pet owners may prefer the ritual of cooking and feeding.

RECIPES AND SOURCES

For these and other reasons, pet owners may ask animal health professionals for advice on how to feed a home diet. They may find guidelines or recipes in books, in magazines, or on the Internet, or they may not follow a recipe and may simply offer human foods to their pets. In some cases, owners may present a recipe to a veterinarian or technician and ask if it is okay to feed. In evaluating home-prepared recipes for dogs and cats, a few basic principles apply. The recipe should provide for all of the 40+ nutrients that dogs and cats require with no deficiencies or excesses. It should be consistent rather than variable from day to day. The ingredients in the recipe should be recognizable and well defined, so that the different foods and supplements along with their amounts can be evaluated. Finally, the recipe should be safe and non-toxic and should include appropriate cooking directions to destroy bacterial pathogens associated with raw or under-cooked foods. More specific problems are described in the following paragraphs.

Not Complete and Balanced

Recipes found in books and on the Internet are almost always incomplete and unbalanced. Several studies have attempted to evaluate the nutrient content of these "generic" diet recipes and have found missing or deficient nutrients in the vast majority of cases. Some people claim that home recipes will be "balanced over time," meaning that nutrients not provided one day will be made up in the future. However, this concept is difficult to understand because a nutrient deficiency in the recipe cannot necessarily be corrected by an excessive amount at a different time. Although some proponents believe that human diets are not complete each day but over time balance out, this is a false assumption. Most Americans and most likely people in other countries do not eat complete, balanced diets daily or over time, which leads to many adverse effects later in life. On the other hand, pets that are provided at least 100% of their nutrient requirements daily are much more likely to live long, healthy lives than those with daily deficiencies.

TECHNICIAN NOTE   Almost all home-prepared pet food recipes found in books, in magazines, or on the Internet are not complete and balanced for long-term feeding.

Not Appropriate for Life Stage or Health

Generic recipes cannot account for the unique needs of individual pets. For example, a home recipe may not supply adequate nutrition for growth of puppies and kittens and may lead to musculoskeletal malformations and diseases. A "standard" recipe for all dogs may contain too much fat for a dog that cannot tolerate high levels. Medical conditions such as kidney disease, diabetes, or liver failure require specific nutrient profiles in individual animals. Or a standard recipe may contain ingredients not palatable to all dogs or cats.

Safety Concerns

Some recipes call for raw meat; as discussed previously, raw foods are commonly contaminated with bacterial pathogens and can cause foodborne illness in pets and in people who handle the foods and feeding bowls. Other recipes insist on bones, which are well known to cause gastrointestinal upset,

obstruction, or perforation. Claims that uncooked bones are safe should be ignored. Many veterinarians have had the experience of performing emergency surgery to remove bones stuck in the intestinal tract. Some foods such as garlic, onions, grapes, and raisins may be toxic. If the person formulating the recipe is not aware of medical concerns about potentially toxic foods, the pet could inadvertently be poisoned by a well-meaning owner.

Vague Recipes

Almost all recipes found in books, in magazines, and on the Internet do not define the ingredients or preparation instructions carefully enough that pet owners can follow them. The exact foods are often not defined. For example, a recipe may call for "chicken" but not the specific part of the chicken. Or if it says "chicken breast," it may not say whether skin is included or should be removed. In either case, the protein/fat/nutrient profile would be different depending on the chicken part (breast, thigh, leg, wing, giblet, back, neck, etc.). "Hamburger" or "ground beef" is often included in recipes, but a visit to the grocery store reveals that this product is sold as 70% lean/30% fat all the way up to 96% lean/4% fat and many varieties in between. The caloric content and the nutritional content of these types of ground beef are significantly different. Another common problem is that quantities and amounts are not accurately specified. Vague instructions may be provided, such as "1 part meat, 3 parts vegetables," which does not say whether that is measured by weight or volume. Ingredients have different measures depending on whether they are raw or cooked. For example, 2 cups of rice is a very different quantity if measured dry before cooking or wet after cooking. One key to evaluating a recipe is to predict that if different people followed the same recipe, they would all end up with the same finished product with the same nutritional value. Obviously, with vague ingredients and directions, this is very unlikely. Cooking instructions may not be specific as well. Undercooked meat can pose a health hazard because of bacterial contamination. Because vitamins and other nutrients can be lost during cooking, it is important that supplements are added after rather than before, but recipes may not state that. Unusual or expensive ingredients may be difficult to obtain or may not be available consistently at grocery stores, so owners turn to substituting or leaving ingredients out. Supplemental vitamins and minerals are required in home-prepared pet foods, but rarely do exact product names and amounts appear in generic recipes. Sometimes, the only instruction is a "pet vitamin" or a "good human vitamin-mineral supplement," which is vague, in that there are hundreds if not thousands of possible supplements—all with different quantities and mixtures of nutrients. A final concern with generic recipes is "diet drift," whereby owners start out preparing the food as instructed, but over time they start to change the types and quantities of the ingredients. Often this is a reaction to the animal's not wanting to eat the recipe, or to its picking out the tasty parts and leaving the rest uneaten.

Home Recipe Formulation

Home recipes can be formulated appropriately as long as potential problems are identified and managed. The first step in preparing a home diet is to evaluate the animal and determine the reason why a home diet is requested or necessary. A complete medical and diet history should be reviewed, so that previous commercial or home foods can be evaluated and medical problems can be identified. A diet for a 2-year-old healthy, large breed dog will be very different from a diet for a 15-year-old sick toy breed dog. Age, breed, activity level, food preferences, and owner commitment to the process should be assessed before the process of formulating a home diet is begun. The basic reasons why home diets are considered are that commercial diets are not palatable or acceptable, health or medical issues preclude regular diets, and/or owners prefer home diets. The second step in formulating a home diet is to establish nutrient ranges appropriate for the animal. For this step, daily minimum or recommended allowances according to AAFCO and NRC should be consulted. Any special needs, such as lower fat, increased potassium, decreased sodium, higher fiber, etc., should be determined. The third step is to choose ingredients that are acceptable to the owner and palatable to the pet. In general, inexpensive, easily obtained, consistent products are recommended (e.g., chicken, beef, or pork instead of duck, bison, or lamb, all of which are more expensive and are not as widely sold). Any food allergies or intolerances are noted and avoided in choosing ingredients. Supplemental vitamins and minerals are provided with pre-mixes or separate tablets and capsules. The fourth step is to enter the chosen foods and supplements into computer diet balancing software that will analyze the ingredients for nutrient content and compare the results with AAFCO or NRC guidelines to ensure that at least 100% of the requirements are met.

After the recipe is balanced for energy (caloric) content and appropriate levels of protein, fat, carbohydrate, vitamins, minerals, fiber, and water, specific cooking instructions should be included. Use of proper cooking temperatures of meats, grains, and vegetables to ensure safety and digestibility is important, as is stating whether supplements are added before or after cooking and cooling ("after" is preferred). The final step is to list feeding instructions, which include the quantity and frequency of the diet, along with guidelines for storage in the refrigerator or freezer. The owner should be educated on what to monitor in pets eating home diets, including acceptance, coat and skin quality, fecal quality and quantity, and improvement in medical conditions (if indicated). Because of the complexity of accurately formulating home diets, trained veterinary nutritionists should be consulted whenever possible. Veterinarians who have advanced training in nutrition and experience with home diets often offer consulting services to other veterinarians and owners, so that appropriate recipes can be formulated. Although the Internet is full of people claiming to be able to prepare home diets, it is best to check their credentials before requesting a consultation. Some are not veterinarians, others have no training or education in nutrition, and still others claim to have dubious degrees and certifications. The only current certification for veterinarians in the United States is Diplomate status conferred by the American College of Veterinary Nutrition (ACVN); this establishes advanced training and knowledge.

Feeding Healthy Dogs and Cats

After acquiring basic knowledge of nutrition, including an understanding of nutrients, foods, ingredients, and the pet food industry, animal health professionals can help pet owners select nutritional plans. The following sections contain information on feeding puppies and dogs, starting from birth throughout the life stages; then similar information is provided for kittens and cats.

DOGS

NEONATAL PERIOD

Puppies begin to nurse within a few hours after birth. The first secretions from the mammary glands of the bitch are called *colostrum*. Colostrum is rich in protein and contains immunoglobulins to transfer immunity from mother to puppies. Minerals such as Ca, P, Mg, Fe, Cu, and Zn are higher in colostrum, but lactose (milk sugar) is lower compared with milk. At 24 hours after whelping (postpartum), the colostrum gradually changes over to milk. The protein content drops by about half, and lactose increases for the first week, after which the milk is "mature" and is stable throughout lactation. Milk from healthy bitches is assumed to be a complete and balanced food for neonatal puppies. On an as-fed basis, the composition is approximately 77% moisture with at least 7.5% protein, 9.5% fat, and 3.3% lactose. Vitamins and minerals make up the rest. The osmolality is approximately 570 mOsm/kg and digestibility is high (>95%), leading to soft stools. Puppies generally nurse for 6 to 8 weeks, or until the bitch stops allowing by moving away and not lying still.

Neonatal puppies may need nutritional support if they are orphaned or are not able to nurse naturally. Signs of inadequate intake include failure to grow, weakness, lethargy, enlarged abdomen, restlessness, and frequent vocalization.

The most straightforward way to assess success of nursing is to weigh puppies daily on an accurate gram scale. It is also possible to weigh them before and after nursing if there are any concerns. Puppies should always maintain or gain weight on a gram basis each day, typically 10% to 15% of birth weight daily. If at any time body weight decreases, there is a problem with nutrition or illness. Supporting neonatal puppies involves choosing an appropriate milk replacer and a feeding method. A medical investigation may be necessary as well.

Commercial milk replacers that attempt to duplicate the nutrients and amounts found in bitches' milk are available for puppies. Both ready-to-feed liquids and powders are sold; the powders are generally less expensive. One widely sold liquid product contains 85% moisture, 4.5% protein, and 6.5% fat, with an energy content of 0.8 kcal/ml. Ingredients include condensed milk and cream (from cows), soybean oil, casein (milk protein), egg yolks, and supplemental minerals and vitamins. Another liquid product contains 78% moisture, 6.5% protein, and 6.5% fat, and the ingredients include corn oil, cows' milk, casein, corn syrup, soy protein, flavors, and vitamins and minerals. The suggested feeding amount for orphan puppies (complete replacement for nursing) is 30 ml (1 ounce) for every 115 g (4 ounces) body weight divided into frequent feedings. Actual requirements vary; therefore, daily or twice-daily weighing on a gram scale is helpful.

> **TECHNICIAN NOTE** Commercial milk replacers are superior to cow's milk or home recipes for feeding orphan puppies or for supplementing mother's milk.

Hand-feeding neonatal puppies can be done with eyedroppers, syringes, nursing bottles, and feeding tubes. The preferred method is bottle-feeding, although tube-feeding is faster and more efficient. For bottles, select a commercial plastic bottle and nipple appropriate for puppies, and make sure the opening is large but not too large. Milk should drip slowly but not flow out when the bottle is inverted. During feeding, the bottle should never be squeezed because a rapid flow rate could lead to aspiration of milk, pneumonia, and death. Puppies may be held in dorsal or sternal recumbency while bottle-feeding. When full, most puppies will voluntarily stop suckling at the bottle. The procedure for tube feeding is slightly more complicated but once mastered is much easier. A puppy infant feeding tube (5-French size for very small neonates, 8-French for older or larger puppies) and syringe is needed, along with a sterile lubricating jelly. The first step is to measure the length of insertion of the tube by holding the puppy horizontally and measuring from the tip of the nose to the last rib. Mark the tube with tape or indelible pen. Warm milk replacer can be given at body temperature (95°F), but be careful of microwaving because hot and cold spots may be found in the mixture. Shake well, then draw up an appropriate amount of milk into a syringe. Hold the puppy on its side, and slowly and gently insert the lubricated tip of the feeding tube into the mouth and down the esophagus. It is possible to accidentally insert the tube into the airway (trachea), so observe for easy, smooth passage with no distress or obstruction. After the tube is comfortably in place (tip at level of last rib), attach the syringe and slowly deliver the milk replacer. The stomach area can be palpated to see if filling; feeding should stop if it feels distended. Remove the syringe and pull the feeding tube out. Clean and rinse the outside and the inside of the tube, and allow to dry. Orphan puppies need stimulation to urinate and defecate. A moist cotton ball or a tip of a soft washcloth is rubbed on the ventral abdominal area, and any urine and feces are cleaned up. For additional information about caring for neonatal puppies and kittens, refer to Chapter 21.

> **TECHNICIAN NOTE** Tube feeding is quick and easy once the technique is learned, and it can be taught to owners.

WEANING

Beginning around 3 to 4 weeks of age, puppies are ready to be introduced to solid food. Their baby teeth erupt at this time, and they spend time exploring their environment away from their mothers. Puppies learn to wag their tails and playfight with littermates by 3 weeks of age. There is less crying behavior when separated from their mother or littermates. To start the weaning process, simply offer soft food (gruel consistency) appropriate for growth in a shallow or flat dish, and allow puppies to explore the food by smelling, tasting, and even walking in it. Canned food should be mixed with water in a 1:1 ratio; dry food should be mixed with water in a 3:1 or 4:1 ratio. If puppies show no interest in food, commercial milk replacer can be mixed in. Commercial weaning products (liquids and powders) are available but are rarely necessary with healthy litters. Added water can be gradually decreased over the next week until the puppies are eating an undiluted canned or dry diet. When puppies are eating adequate amounts of solid food and the mother's milk production starts to decline, usually at 5 to 6 weeks of age, complete separation will hasten the weaning process. The puppies can be removed and offered solid food or a gruel while the mother is fed ⅓ to ½ of what she was previously eating for 2 to 3 days; she can then be returned to the food and feeding schedule she was on before gestation.

GROWTH

From weaning until adulthood, which is reached at 10 to 18 months of age in most breeds of dogs, puppies should be fed an appropriate diet and amount to meet the needs of growth, maintenance, and activity. Compared with adult dogs at the same weight, puppies require approximately 2 to 3 times as much energy until 50% of adult weight is reached; they then require approximately 1.5 times adult energy until 80% to 100% of adult weight. Important considerations for feeding puppies include energy, protein, fat, calcium, and phosphorus. All nutrients are required in somewhat higher amounts for puppies compared with adults, but these have special significance.

Energy

As mentioned, puppies need energy for growth and for normal maintenance, including activities such as play and exercise. However, because the main nutritional problem in adult dogs is obesity, it is important to prevent puppies from overeating and gaining too much weight. Just as in adults, overfed puppies have excessive body fat and are at increased risk for musculoskeletal diseases such as hip dysplasia. It is difficult to put overweight puppies on a "diet" to induce weight loss without risking malnutrition, so prevention of an overweight or obese body condition is important.

> **TECHNICIAN NOTE** The most common error in feeding growing puppies is giving too much food.

Protein

The requirements for protein and amino acids are highest at weaning and gradually decrease throughout the growth period. The digestibility of the dietary protein source affects the requirement. Foods with lower digestibility and availability of amino acids are needed in higher amounts, but puppies may not be able to tolerate large quantities of food without experiencing vomiting and diarrhea. Therefore, the best diets for the growth stage include high-quality, highly digestible animal and plant sources of protein. On a dry-matter basis, puppy diets should include a minimum of 17.5% (NRC) to 22% (AAFCO) crude protein. On a metabolizable energy (ME) basis, the minimum is 44 g (NRC) to 63 g (AAFCO) crude protein per 1000 kcal. These differences can be explained by protein quality and digestibility. AAFCO nutrient profiles include a safety margin to account for variations in pet foods, and NRC-recommended allowances assume a high-quality diet. Most commercial puppy diets contain more protein than required, which is not dangerous, but if levels are excessive (e.g., over 40% dry matter base [DMB]), the diet may not be as palatable, and nutrients other than amino acids may be deficient.

Fat

The total fat content of a diet for puppies should be a minimum 8% (AAFCO) to 8.5% (NRC) on a DMB. On an ME basis, the amounts are 21 to 23 g/1000 kcal. Puppies require linoleic acid (LA), which is an essential fatty acid, at 1% to 1.3% DMB or 2.9 to 3.3 g/1000 kcal. Another essential fatty acid, alpha-linolenic (ALA), is required at lower amounts (approximately 10% of the LA requirement). Some studies have shown that puppies benefit from arachidonic acid (AA), eicosapentaenoic acid (EPA), and docosahexaenoic acid (DHA), which are longer-chain fatty acids. Dogs can synthesize AA from LA and EPA from ALA, but these conversions may not be sufficient. Therefore, some pet foods formulated for puppy growth are supplemented with these additional fatty acids. Excessive fat in puppy diets should be avoided because this increases energy density and can lead to an overweight or obese body condition. Overweight puppies are at greater risk of developing orthopedic diseases and other health problems. No more than 33% (NRC) total fat on a DMB should be fed to growing puppies.

Calcium and Phosphorus

Puppies require more Ca and P than adult dogs for development of bones and teeth. However, there is a common misconception that growing dogs need supplemental Ca and P because commercial diets are inadequate. Minimum amounts for Ca in growth diets are 1% (AAFCO) to 1.2% (NRC), and for P are 0.8% (AAFCO) to 1% (NRC) on a DMB. In addition, AAFCO recommends a Ca:P ratio of 1:1 to 2:1 for both puppies and adult dogs. Ratios are simply mathematical expressions and can be confusing and unreliable because inadequate or excessive Ca and P can still have appropriate ratios. Instead, growth diets should include correct levels of Ca, P, and other minerals because deficiencies or excesses can result in musculoskeletal disorders. Growth diets should not contain more than 1.8% to 2.5% Ca DMB or more than 1.6% P DMB. Supplementation with additional Ca or P is inappropriate. This is especially true in large breed and rapidly growing puppies. Adult dogs can regulate Ca absorption from the small intestine and are better able to tolerate excessive amounts. Puppies are less able to regulate Ca and are more susceptible to overdose.

> **TECHNICIAN NOTE** Calcium supplements should be avoided unless there is a specific medical indication.

FEEDING PLAN FOR GROWTH

Using knowledge of pet food regulation and key nutrients for the growth stage, it is possible to recommend appropriate types and amounts of food for puppies. A first consideration is whether the manufacturer is a large, reputable company that conducts research and feeding trials. Most manufacturers produce life stage diets, with separate product lines for puppies and adults. There are also all-purpose dog foods that can be used for all life stages. After selecting a reputable company, the puppy foods should be evaluated to see if they have been through AAFCO feeding protocols for growth. This test starts with at least 8-week-old puppies and lasts for a minimum of 10 weeks. The tested puppy food needs to support growth, overall health, and various lab work results to pass. Of course, 10 weeks is not long enough to evaluate all possible problems with diets, including musculoskeletal disorders that may take months or a year to develop. Therefore, reputable manufacturers often conduct longer feeding trials that are not specifically AAFCO protocols but help ensure that the pet food safely supports normal growth and development. This information can be obtained directly from companies.

For large breed puppies, many companies produce specialized diets that differ in composition and nutrients from regular puppy or small breed diets. However, no official

AAFCO or NRC guidelines are available for nutrient levels in large breed diets. Therefore, companies are free to formulate a wide range of products as long as they follow the basic growth diet minimum and maximum requirements. In general, large breed puppy diets are lower in energy density, which means that there are fewer kcal per cup or can compared with other growth diets. This helps owners avoid overfeeding of large breed puppies. Ca and P levels of large breed diets are controlled to avoid excessive amounts even if owners overfeed. The crude protein and fat content may be similar or somewhat different. Kibble shape, size, and texture may be modified for large breed compared with small breed puppies. In general, it is safe and appropriate to feed any high-quality growth diet from a reputable company to large breed puppies.

> **TECHNICIAN NOTE** The choice of a growth diet depends on factors such as reputation of the company, appropriate formulation (e.g., large breed diets when needed), availability, cost, palatability, and how the puppy responds.

Owners often ask how much to feed a growing puppy. As was previously discussed, in the growth stage, energy is required for maintenance, activity (play and exercise), and growth and development of body tissues. Some puppies will regulate their food intake and will not overeat, even if presented with large amounts. Other puppies will eat to excess. Free-choice (ad libitum) feeding is not recommended for puppies because of the health risks of obesity. Instead, controlled meal feeding is suitable for almost all puppies. Estimated daily energy needs should be offered in two or three meals per day (morning and evening for most puppies, but a third meal can be offered for small breeds or picky eaters that may not consume adequate amounts with two meals per day). Feeding guides on product labels can be used as starting points, but they often indicate ranges rather than exact amounts. Breed, age, body condition, activity level, predicted adult size, and other factors all help determine how much an individual puppy should eat. Animal health professionals should be able to calculate resting energy requirements (RER) for current body weight, then multiply by 2 or 3 to account for growth. Time-restricted meal feeding has been recommended, but studies have shown that this can lead to excessive energy intake and health problems. It is no longer appropriate to allow puppies to eat all they want within a time interval, such as 10 or 15 minutes. Instead, a premeasured amount of puppy food should be offered. If not completely eaten after 30 to 60 minutes, owners should remove the bowl and offer the next pre-measured meal at the next feeding time. Again, smaller breeds and very young puppies often require 3 instead of 2 meals per day because of stomach volume limitations and picky appetites.

To monitor whether food intake is meeting but not exceeding daily energy expenditure, owners should be taught to perform body condition assessments and scoring on a regular basis, such as weekly. Several **body condition score** (BCS) charts are available, and copies can be distributed to owners. Figure 9-6 provides one example. If puppies are gaining excessive weight beyond normal growth, visual and palpable evidence of increased body fat will be seen. Meal size should be decreased by approximately 10% if BCS is increasing, or increased if BCS is decreasing to below ideal. As puppies grow, their food intake should gradually increase as well. Special attention should be paid to treats, especially when used for training. The daily allotment of treats can be calculated, and the energy content (kcal) should be less than 10% of total daily intake. For example, if a puppy is eating 300 kcal/day, all treats and snacks combined should not exceed 30 kcal.

At 6 to 9 months of age, the growth rate slows, although most puppies maintain high activity levels. Food intake should continue to be increased, along with increased body weight, but regular BCS checks will help determine whether puppies are being overfed or underfed. Many puppies are spayed and neutered by this age, and daily energy needs decrease after this surgical procedure. To avoid overfeeding neutered pets, a general rule is to decrease the amount of food by 25% to 33% ($\frac{1}{4}$ to $\frac{1}{3}$ less food) immediately after surgery. The same puppy diet can be fed, and there is no reason to switch foods or to put the pet on a "diet." For example, if the puppy is eating 3 cups of food per day, the daily amount should be decreased after spaying or neutering to 2 to 2.5 cups/day. Depending on breed, size, growth rate, etc., this lower amount can still be gradually increased over time as the pup continues to grow. When the puppy has attained adult size, which occurs at 10 to 12 months of age for small and medium breeds, and at up to 18 to 24 months of age for large and giant breeds, the food can gradually be transitioned to an adult maintenance diet. In some cases, if the puppy food is an all-life-stage product, the same food can be continued into the adult stage with the daily amount controlled to avoid weight gain after growth is completed.

> **TECHNICIAN NOTE** Timed feeding or following label instructions exactly can lead to overfeeding. It is better to monitor a growing puppy's body condition and adjust food intake to support gradual, steady growth without excessive fat deposits.

ADULT MAINTENANCE

Normal, healthy young to middle-aged dogs tend to do well on a variety of commercial dog foods. The most common nutritional problem seen by animal health professionals is overfeeding, which results in overweight to obese dogs. Many dogs are relatively sedentary, in that they are confined to houses or crates for much of the day and night and are taken out for "walks" instead of runs or vigorous physical activity. An appropriate diet and feeding plan for adult dogs is one that meets all nutritional requirements while avoiding excessive energy intake. Nutrient deficiencies are rare, but excesses are possible, especially when commercial diets are supplemented. Adult diets can be evaluated for energy, protein, fat, and fiber content, but all of the 40+ required nutrients must be present at appropriate levels as well.

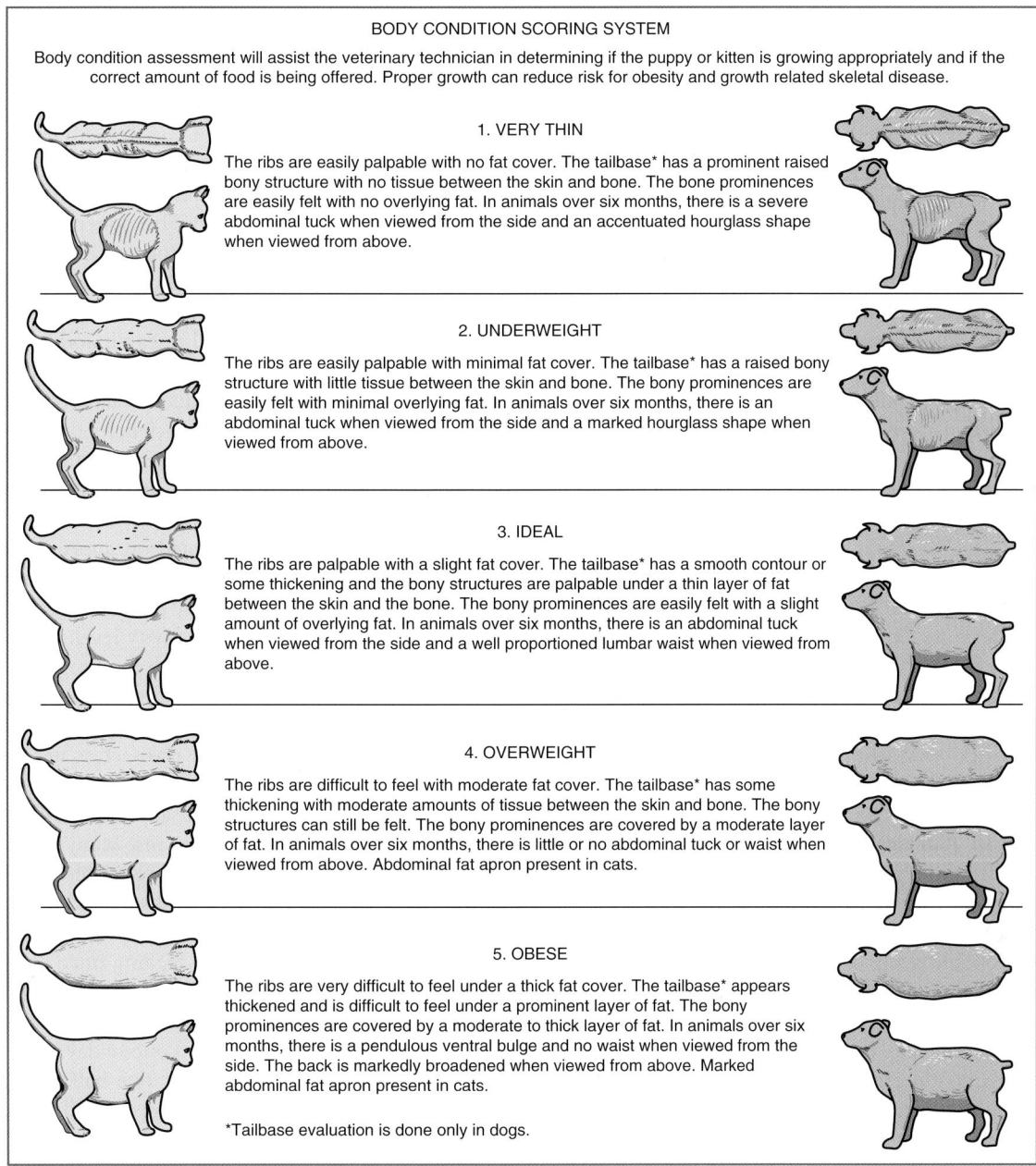

BODY CONDITION SCORING SYSTEM

Body condition assessment will assist the veterinary technician in determining if the puppy or kitten is growing appropriately and if the correct amount of food is being offered. Proper growth can reduce risk for obesity and growth related skeletal disease.

1. VERY THIN

The ribs are easily palpable with no fat cover. The tailbase* has a prominent raised bony structure with no tissue between the skin and bone. The bone prominences are easily felt with no overlying fat. In animals over six months, there is a severe abdominal tuck when viewed from the side and an accentuated hourglass shape when viewed from above.

2. UNDERWEIGHT

The ribs are easily palpable with minimal fat cover. The tailbase* has a raised bony structure with little tissue between the skin and bone. The bony prominences are easily felt with minimal overlying fat. In animals over six months, there is an abdominal tuck when viewed from the side and a marked hourglass shape when viewed from above.

3. IDEAL

The ribs are palpable with a slight fat cover. The tailbase* has a smooth contour or some thickening and the bony structures are palpable under a thin layer of fat between the skin and the bone. The bony prominences are easily felt with a slight amount of overlying fat. In animals over six months, there is an abdominal tuck when viewed from the side and a well proportioned lumbar waist when viewed from above.

4. OVERWEIGHT

The ribs are difficult to feel with moderate fat cover. The tailbase* has some thickening with moderate amounts of tissue between the skin and bone. The bony structures can still be felt. The bony prominences are covered by a moderate layer of fat. In animals over six months, there is little or no abdominal tuck or waist when viewed from above. Abdominal fat apron present in cats.

5. OBESE

The ribs are very difficult to feel under a thick fat cover. The tailbase* appears thickened and is difficult to feel under a prominent layer of fat. The bony prominences are covered by a moderate to thick layer of fat. In animals over six months, there is a pendulous ventral bulge and no waist when viewed from the side. The back is markedly broadened when viewed from above. Marked abdominal fat apron present in cats.

*Tailbase evaluation is done only in dogs.

FIGURE 9-6 A 5-point body condition scoring guide for dogs and cats. A 9-point system is also used in which 1-3 is below ideal weight, 4-5 is ideal, and 6-9 is above ideal weight.

Energy

Adult dogs need energy for normal maintenance, which includes basic physiologic requirements for rest and activities such as play and exercise. As discussed earlier in the section on energy expenditure, a starting point for estimating how much food an adult dog needs is to calculate RER $(70 \times BW_{kg}^{0.75}$ kcal/day), and then multiply the result by various factors to account for breed, age, and lifestyle. Sedentary dogs that are predisposed to being overweight often require 1.0 to 1.2 × RER, and active dogs at an ideal BCS may do well with 1.8 to 2.0 RER. Certain breeds such as Great Danes and terriers tend to require more energy, but Newfoundlands require less energy than typical dogs. Neutered dogs need less energy than intact dogs. Dogs used for hunting, sporting, and work require more energy. Older dogs are often less active, and so energy requirements may decrease with increasing age. As with puppies, the best way to monitor adult dogs for proper food intake is to measure BCS at regular intervals such as monthly. If BCS is increasing and excessive body fat is visualized or palpated, approximately 10% less food should be offered until a more ideal BCS is achieved. Overweight to obese dogs need more specific treatment, as discussed later.

Protein

It may be surprising to owners that adult dogs require relatively little protein for good health. Most commercial dog foods contain more protein than average dogs need, and the excess is converted to energy and is stored as fat rather than "building muscle" or other such advertising claims. The recommended allowances are outlined in Table 9-5. The overall quality of a pet food has very little to do with the amount of protein.

> **TECHNICIAN NOTE** The amount of protein in an adult maintenance pet food is not the most important factor and does not indicate quality.

Fat

Adult dogs require a small amount of fat and essential fatty acids daily, and most dogs tolerate higher amounts. However, high-fat diets predispose dogs to obesity and may be a factor in diseases such as arthritis, pancreatitis, and other inflammatory conditions. Fat lends flavor to pet foods and is necessary for absorption of fat-soluble vitamins. The recommended allowances are outlined in Table 9-7.

Fiber

Healthy dogs do well on low- or moderate-fiber diets. The amounts and types of fiber found in maintenance diets vary; higher-fiber diets are typically recommended for weight management, and lower-fiber diets are formulated for better digestibility. Dietary fiber becomes more of a concern when dogs have intestinal disorders. For most pet foods, the fiber content is higher than the guaranteed analysis percent because assays do not detect all types.

Vitamins and Minerals

Maintenance diets from reputable companies include appropriate amounts of micronutrients, typically with 20% or more than recommended allowances as a safety factor. Deficiencies are possible with commercial pet foods but are usually the result of errors in formulation or processing. Vitamins and minerals are supplied as a powdered or granulated pre-mix, which may come from a different manufacturer. Therefore, it is important that batches of pet food are frequently analyzed to ensure that all nutrients are present in adequate amounts. Smaller pet food companies that do not perform their own nutritional evaluations or quality control are at higher risk for errors.

FEEDING PLAN FOR ADULT MAINTENANCE

Pet owners are presented with hundreds of different diets that are marketed for adult dogs by many different companies. To narrow down the choices and make suitable recommendations, the first step is to look for a large, reputable company that performs research and feeding trials. Some but not all adult diets are tested with an AAFCO feeding protocol for maintenance. This test uses dogs older than 1 year of age and runs for at least 26 weeks. A minimum of eight dogs are used, along with observations and measurements of health and lab work. Products that pass the AAFCO protocol include a statement on their labels such as "Animal feeding tests using AAFCO procedures ..." Some companies perform additional or more stringent testing of their pet foods. Most adult dog foods are not fed in 26-week AAFCO studies, but instead are "formulated to meet the nutritional levels ...," which means that at least on paper, the diet contains all required nutrients at appropriate levels. However, even if a diet formulation looks correct on paper or by computer analysis, this method does not test digestibility or bioavailability. In general, AAFCO feeding tests are preferred for recommending adult diets, but because of time and expense, many products are never tested. This does not mean the diets are of low quality or are not appropriate. Large manufacturers usually perform AAFCO feeding trials on their popular, widely sold diets but not on their lesser-selling products. However, the same nutritional research and manufacturing procedures are used, so with reputable companies, pet owners can be assured that products will perform as expected and will not have nutritional deficiencies or excesses.

As previously discussed, the most common nutritional problem in adult dogs consists of overfeeding and overweight body conditions. Therefore, owners of adult dogs first and foremost should be educated on appropriate amounts to feed. As with puppies, a starting point is calculation of RER, which is then multiplied by factors ranging from 1.0 to 2.0 depending on breed, size, activity level, etc. A sedentary adult dog may require only enough food to meet daily RER, but an active dog at the same weight may eat twice as much. Dogs should be assessed for BCS regularly and weighed several times a year. One of the risk factors in weight gain is free-choice feeding. Owners that keep bowls full of dry dog food and allow their pets free access are contributing to obesity and related health problems. Many dogs, especially those that are spayed or neutered, are unable to regulate their food intake and tend to eat whenever food is available, not just when hungry. Although free-choice feeding is convenient, a better method is meal feeding once or twice a day. For a starting point, the feeding guidelines on the pet food label can be used, or a multiple of RER can be calculated. The total daily amount is offered once a day in the morning, or one-half in the morning and one-half in the evening. Because dogs vary widely in energy expenditure, the actual amounts fed to keep dogs at a healthy weight (not gaining or losing) may be more or less than recommended or calculated.

> **TECHNICIAN NOTE** Animal health professionals can calculate RER in kcal/day and can inform pet owners that many dogs need only that amount of food or slightly more (1.1 or 1.2 × RER) per day.

Owners may wonder whether they should feed the same product long-term or switch among varieties or brands. In general, a high-quality pet food can be fed to adult dogs for many years. As long as all required nutrients are present in adequate amounts, there is no nutritional or medical reason to switch to different diets. Although no simple or inexpensive tests for nutritional adequacy are available, owners and animal health professionals can monitor for changes in a dog's skin and hair coat (dry, oily, flaky skin or dull coat), stool quality (soft or excessively hard stools, gas or unusual odors), and for changes in body weight and condition (gain or loss of fat or lean body mass). If there is any concern that the pet is not doing well on the current diet, it is fairly straightforward to transition to a different dog food and monitor for improvement. Some dogs will eat a certain product well and then will seemingly tire of it. If the owner offers different foods every time this happens, the dog may learn that food refusal leads to more attention from the owner and tastier dog food. To avoid creating behavioral problems, owners should be willing to keep offering the same product for 1 to 2 days before offering something different.

Another concern is that commercial pet foods do not supply the nutrients and compounds found in fresh foods. One example is phytochemicals, which generally act as anti-oxidants and are found in colorful fruits and vegetables. Owners who wish to add human foods to commercial dog foods should be encouraged to keep the amounts less than 10% of the daily energy intake. If the dog is eating 400 kcal/day, for example, no more than 40 kcal of fruits, vegetables, or other foods should be offered. Higher amounts can lead to dilution of nutrients such as protein and over time can cause deficiencies. Dogs can be fed vegetables such as carrots, celery, green beans, broccoli, tomatoes, etc., and fruits such as apples and bananas. Grapes and raisins are potentially toxic and should never be fed. Onions, garlic, and chocolate are harmful in large amounts.

> **TECHNICIAN NOTE** A rule of thumb for treat or snack allowance is 10% of the daily energy (kcal) intake.

GESTATION

Breeding adult dogs to produce puppies is not recommended for average pet owners, but animal health professionals may be consulted by breeders for nutritional advice. Only healthy dogs in good body condition should be bred. Neither overweight nor underweight female dogs are good candidates for gestation or lactation. Ovulation, litter size, and milk production can be affected by poor body condition before breeding. There are no special considerations for male dogs, except that some dogs have poor appetites during mating season and may lose weight if continuously exposed to females in heat.

Similar to growing puppies, pregnant dogs have an increased need for energy and other nutrients. However, for the first 5 to 6 weeks of gestation, fetal growth is minimal, and so the nutritional requirements are the same as for adult maintenance. Beginning in week 5, a pregnant dog's energy intake should increase by approximately 30% to 60% depending on breed, size, number of puppies, and stage of gestation. However, the enlarging uterus limits the extent of stomach distention. Pregnant dogs may not be able to eat sufficient food to meet energy requirements if fed once or twice a day. An extra meal per day will help distribute the day's food into manageable portions. For example, if a dog is accustomed to eating 2 cups at one meal once a day, it may be difficult to increase to 3 cups at one time, and so she may do better with 1.5 cups twice a day. One recommendation

(NRC) for increased energy intake during pregnancy is to add 26 kcal/kg body weight. A 10-kg dog that normally eats 400 kcal/day may need an extra 260 kcal/day, or 660 kcal/day, during the last 4 to 5 weeks of pregnancy. Overfeeding should be avoided because obese dogs can have trouble with the reproductive process.

Protein and fat requirements also increase during the last 4 to 5 weeks of gestation. To meet these additional needs, pregnant dogs should be offered more food per day, as has been described. Recommendations range from 20% to 100% more dietary protein and from 20% to 60% more dietary fat. During the final weeks of gestation, it is reasonable to gradually switch from a maintenance diet to one formulated for growth (puppy food) or reproduction (gestation and lactation). An all-life-stage diet is also appropriate for late gestation. These diets, if high-quality products from reputable companies, will help support the additional nutrient requirements. Dietary minerals need to be increased as well, and these higher amounts are already included in reputable growth products. There is no need to give supplemental vitamins and minerals (especially calcium and phosphorus) to pregnant dogs. In fact, excessive amounts can be harmful and can interfere with healthy reproduction.

> **TECHNICIAN NOTE** Pregnant dogs should not be overfed or allowed to eat free-choice because obesity contributes to reproductive problems.

PARTURITION

Most dogs stop eating or reduce their intake approximately 24 hours before whelping. They usually do not start eating again until all puppies have been delivered and cleaned, and are settled down and nursing. This is an important reason to make sure that food intake is appropriate during late gestation, because dogs will be using stored energy for the whelping process and initial lactation.

LACTATION

The nutritional requirements for lactating dogs depend on the age of the puppies and the size of the litter. For adequate milk production, an increase in dietary energy, protein, fat, and minerals is necessary (similar to late gestation and growth). However, nursing a large litter causes extreme physiologic stress, and large quantities of energy-dense diets are appropriate. Although carbohydrate deficiency in general has not been reported in canine diets, during reproduction and lactation, carbohydrates are considered conditionally essential. Dry or canned diets formulated for growth or reproduction (or for all life stages) may be offered. To ensure adequate intake, free-choice feeding is best in most cases, or a minimum of 3 meals per day. Nursing mothers can be nervous, especially if this is the first litter, and may refuse to eat if stress, noise, or human activities surround the puppies.

During the first week postpartum, daily energy intake should be 25% to 50% higher than maintenance, and by week 4 or 5 of lactation, energy needs may be 100% to 200% higher. For example, a dog that typically eats 2 cups of dry food per day should be offered 3 cups in late gestation, then 4 cups per day after whelping, and up to 5 or 6 cups at week 4 or 5 postpartum. This is assuming a medium-size litter of 4 or 5 puppies. If the litter size is larger, more food is needed. Estimating meal size and appropriate daily amounts is difficult, which is why free-choice (ad libitum) feeding is ideal. Weight loss is common in lactating dogs, especially those with large litters. To prevent adverse health effects of loss of weight and lean body mass during lactation, recommendations should be given to owners concerning types of foods and the need to increase intake as puppies gain weight. As discussed previously, weaning should begin when puppies are 3 to 4 weeks of age. Offering solid food to puppies at an early age provides the benefit of reducing stress on the mother by reducing milk demand.

> **TECHNICIAN NOTE** Lactation is the most energy-demanding, stressful stage in a typical female dog's life.

WORKING AND PERFORMANCE

Heavy work and exercise are stressful to dogs and result in increased nutritional requirements, similar to lactation. Examples include hunting, racing, sledding, agility, and sporting competitions. Exercise may be short and high-intensity (racing), intermediate (hunting), or endurance (sledding). Temperature, humidity, and other environmental factors influence nutritional needs. Water is a key nutrient and is vital for exercising dogs. The energy density of diets should be high because stomach volume is a limiting factor in some types of exercise. For example, dogs involved in long-distance sled pulling may need 6000 to 10,000 kcal/day, which must be supplied by very energy-dense diets. If food is high in protein, carbohydrate, or fiber, the dog may not be able to consume that much energy per day. Because dietary fat supplies the greatest quantity of kcal/g, diets for sled dogs are formulated to be 60% to 80% fat. In contrast, the diet for a racing Greyhound dog may contain higher carbohydrate and lower fat levels to supply rapidly metabolized energy for sprinting. Protein requirements may be mildly higher for exercise than for maintenance to supply amino acids for muscle maintenance and repair. Vitamins and minerals should meet adult requirements, but no evidence suggests that greater amounts or supplementation of commercial diets is necessary.

SENIORS

Various commercial diets are formulated for older dogs. There is no clear definition of when a dog moves from the adult stage to the senior or geriatric stage, but estimates range from 10 to 12 years in small dogs, from 8 to 10 years in larger dogs, and from 6 to 8 years in giant breeds. Neither the NRC nor AAFCO has published nutrient profiles or recommended allowances for older dogs. They are assumed to be the same as for adult maintenance. However, this does not discourage pet food companies from formulating special diets and making health claims for older dogs.

> **TECHNICIAN NOTE** There are no regulations for or definitions of senior, mature, and geriatric pet foods.

Energy

Older dogs may need less energy than younger adults because they exercise less and may have more sedentary lifestyles. Senior diets often have lower energy density than maintenance diets or fewer kcal per cup or can. On the other hand, older dogs may have decreased appetites and may not be interested in eating. Restricting dietary energy in dogs with poor appetites is not recommended. Therefore, just as with puppies and adult dogs, seniors should have their body weight and BCS checked regularly and the amount of food adjusted to maintain a healthy weight and size.

Protein

A degree of controversy surrounds whether older dogs need less, more, or the same amount of protein as younger adults. One theory is that low-protein diets reduce the workload on the kidneys, and this can help prevent chronic kidney disease. This theory has never been proven. Another theory states that older dogs lose lean body tissue or muscle mass, and that high-protein diets are needed to prevent this loss. This condition is sometimes called *sarcopenia* (reduced muscle), and adequate dietary protein should be supplied as compensation. However, the appropriate amount of protein to prevent or reverse sarcopenia has not been determined. Highly digestible protein sources may be preferable because seniors may lose some ability to fully digest all food sources. From a medical point of view, older dogs should be evaluated through lab work and other diagnostic tests to look for evidence of kidney disease, protein loss in the GI or urinary tract, or other conditions in which dietary protein may need to be adjusted. Otherwise, healthy older dogs can continue on the same level of protein as younger adults.

Fat

Fat is required in the diets of older dogs and can be important when appetite is poor or food intake is decreased. Fat supplies more energy than protein and carbohydrate and enhances palatability and absorption of fat-soluble vitamins. Unless the older dog is overweight, dietary fat does not need to be restricted. Fatty acids such as EPA and DHA found in fish oil may be helpful as supplements or included in senior diets, and are commonly used to help with arthritis and inflammation.

Fiber

Senior diets can be low, high, or moderate in fiber content. The type of fiber (fermentable, nonfermentable) also varies depending on the diet. Older dogs sometimes have soft stools that can improve with fiber supplementation or a higher-fiber diet. Other dogs have harder stools or constipation, which also may respond to dietary fiber (different type or less). If the senior dog is gradually losing weight or has a poor appetite, high-fiber diets should be avoided because they are less digestible and have lower energy density.

Vitamins and Minerals

Although older dogs may require higher levels of these nutrients than young adults, this has not been proven in research studies. Deficiencies are possible but usually are related to overall lower food intake. Unless a clear medical indication is identified, there is no need to supplement vitamins and minerals.

FEEDING PLAN FOR SENIORS

Older dogs may be less active and less likely to beg for food or eat all that is offered. An extra meal per day can be helpful (2 or 3 feedings daily instead of 1 or 2). Moving food and water dishes closer to the dog's favorite spots may encourage better intake. The texture of the diet may influence food intake, and canned or moistened dry diets may be easier to eat. Warming diets may help with aromas and may stimulate appetite. As previously discussed, the same nutrient guidelines for adults are used for older dogs. However, seniors are more likely to develop diseases such as kidney, liver, heart, musculoskeletal, and even neurologic disorders that may respond to nutritional therapy. Regular veterinary examinations and diagnostic testing are important in older dogs, and results should be carefully interpreted in the context of diseases and typical old-age changes. If a dietary modification is needed, it should generally be done slowly over 1 to 4 weeks to allow for adaptation. Abrupt changes in types, amounts, flavors, or brands of diets can cause GI upset and other adverse reactions.

> **TECHNICIAN NOTE** Healthy older animals can continue to eat the same diet unless certain medical conditions develop.

CATS

NEONATAL PERIOD

Kittens are born at an average body weight of 100 g, with a typical range of 80 to 120 g. They begin to suckle within a few hours after birth, similar to puppies. Queens (mother cats) produce colostrum for the first 24 hours postpartum, and colostrum gradually changes over to milk by 72 hours. The function of colostrum is to provide immunoglobulins, growth factors, and enzymes, in addition to nutrients. Milk from healthy queens is assumed to be a complete and balanced food for neonatal kittens. On an as-fed basis, the composition is approximately 79% moisture with at least 7.5% protein, 8.5% fat, and 4.0% lactose. Vitamins and minerals make up the rest. Osmolality is approximately

329 mOsm/kg, and digestibility is high (>95%), leading to soft stools. Kittens generally nurse for 6 to 8 weeks, or until the queen stops allowing by moving away and not lying still.

Kittens can have problems with nursing and may require supplemental feeding. Commercial milk replacers are available for kittens in liquid and powder form. One widely sold liquid product contains 82% moisture, 7.5% protein, and 4.5% fat with an energy content of 0.8 kcal/ml. Ingredients include condensed skimmed milk, cream, and milk protein (cows' milk), soybean oil, egg yolks, and supplemental minerals and vitamins. Another liquid product contains 83% moisture, 7.0% protein, and 3.8% fat, and ingredients include nonfat dry milk (cows' milk), corn oil, soy protein, corn syrup, flavors, and vitamins and minerals. The suggested feeding amount for orphan kittens (complete replacement for nursing) is 15 ml ($\frac{1}{2}$ ounce) for every 55 g (2 oz) body weight divided into frequent feedings. The protocol for bottle- or tube-feeding is similar to that described for puppies (Figures 9-7 and 9-8).

WEANING

This process can begin as early as 3 to 4 weeks of age and is complete by 6 to 9 weeks of age. Kittens can be introduced to solid food in canned or moistened dry forms, with water added to make gruel (oatmeal-type consistency). Commercial diets formulated for kittens or all-life-stages foods can be offered for weaning.

GROWTH

Adulthood in cats is reached by 10 to 12 months of age. During the post-weaning period, kittens are usually active and playful. Energy requirements are 2 to 3 times that of adult cats on a body weight basis.

Energy

Just as with growing puppies, it is important to prevent kittens from overeating and gaining too much weight. Obese kittens are rare but are sometimes seen if they are overfed highly palatable diets and are not allowed to exercise. The energy density of diets formulated for kittens should be high to allow for sufficient nutrition if small amounts are eaten. Highly digestible products are also helpful in providing nutrients for growth.

Protein

Similar to kittens, the requirements for protein and amino acids are highest at weaning and gradually decrease until adulthood. The digestibility of the dietary protein source affects the requirement. On a dry-matter basis, puppy diets should include a minimum of 22.5% (NRC) to 30% (AAFCO) crude protein. On a metabolizable energy (ME) basis, the minimum is 56.3 g (NRC) to 75 g (AAFCO) crude protein per 1000 kcal. Most commercial kitten diets contain more protein than is required, which is not dangerous, but if levels are excessive (e.g., over 50% DMB), the diet may not be as palatable, and nutrients other than amino acids may be deficient.

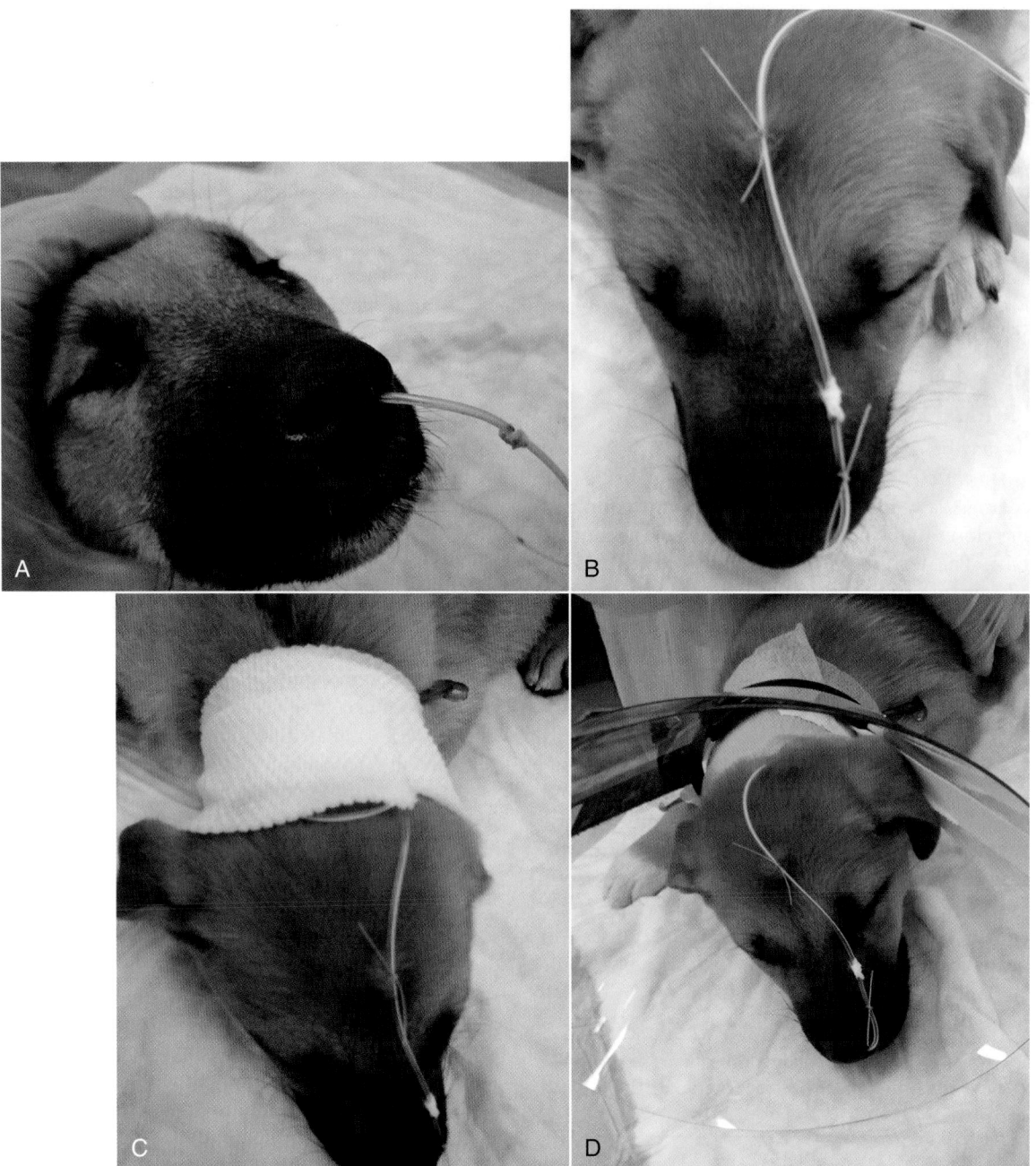

FIGURE 9-7 Placement of a nasogastric (NG) or nasoesophogeal (NE) tube in a puppy. **A,** One drop of local anesthetic may be placed in the nasal passage before insertion of the NG or NE tube. The tube is inserted in the ventromedial direction to avoid the ethmoid turbinates. **B,** After it is determined that the tube has been placed in the desired location, the tube is sutured in place on the rostrum and across the central forehead. **C,** A soft wrap is placed around the distal end of the feeding tube and where it secures the tube to the dorsal aspect of the neck. **D,** Bandage material is placed over the soft wrap, and an E-collar is placed on the patient, to prevent displacement of the tube.

> **TECHNICIAN NOTE** Cats require more protein than dogs, but very high-protein diets confer no added benefit.

Fat

The total fat content of a diet for kittens should be a minimum of 9% (AAFCO and NRC) on a DMB. On an ME basis, the amount is 22.5 g/1000 kcal. Kittens require linoleic acid (LA), which is an essential fatty acid, at 0.5% DMB or 1.4 g/1000 kcal. Other essential fatty acids—alpha-linolenic

(ALA) and arachidonic (AA) acids—are required at lesser amounts (each at approximately 5% of the LA requirement). Kittens also benefit from eicosapentaenoic acid (EPA) and docosahexaenoic acid (DHA), which are longer-chain fatty acids, at approximately half the LA or AA requirement.

Calcium and Phosphorus

Although growing kittens should be fed appropriate levels of minerals such as Ca and P, they are less sensitive than puppies to mild deficiencies or excesses. Developmental

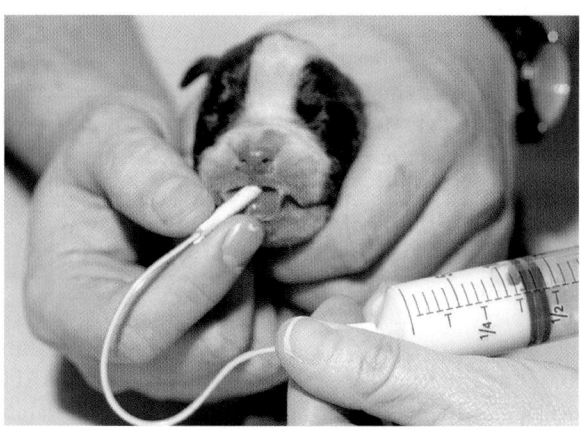

FIGURE 9-8 Tube feeding milk replacer fluid given to an orphaned neonate.

orthopedic diseases are much less common in kittens than in puppies.

FEEDING PLAN FOR GROWTH

The preceding discussion on how to choose commercial products suitable for growth in puppies is also valid for kittens. Diets formulated for growth or all life stages by reputable manufacturers are preferred for feeding kittens. Dry or canned products may be offered. Several advantages are associated with feeding moist (canned) foods as part or all of the diet. They contain more water and help prevent dehydration, which can occur if cats do not voluntarily drink water. Kittens may be better able to regulate food intake with canned food because the energy density is less, and may avoid overeating. Some disease conditions seen in older cats respond to wet diets, so making sure a growing kitten is accustomed to that form of food is helpful if a switch from dry to wet should be needed in the future.

Free-choice dry feeding with supplemental meals of canned food is a preferred method. For example, each morning, kittens can be offered a small amount of wet food for a meal, and dry food may be available for nibbling the rest of the day. An evening meal of wet food can also be given. Estimation of energy intake in terms of kcal/day usually is not necessary for kittens, but as with puppies, owners should be shown how to do body condition scoring and to adjust the diet more or less if kittens are lighter or heavier than expected for their age and body size. Spaying and neutering often are performed at or before 6 months of age in kittens. Food intake tends to increase after surgery, so to avoid overfeeding of neutered kittens, a general rule is to decrease the amount of food by 25% to 33% ($\frac{1}{4}$ to $\frac{1}{3}$ less food) immediately after surgery. There is no reason to use a weight-loss food or to place growing kittens on a "diet," but the quantity of kitten food offered should be carefully monitored after neutering. When kittens have reached an adult size and body weight, at approximately 10 to 12 months of age, a gradual transition to a maintenance diet is appropriate. However, if the cat is doing well on an all-life-stage diet, that product can be continued into adulthood as long as the amount is controlled to avoid overfeeding.

ADULT MAINTENANCE

Healthy cats in the age range of 1 to 10 years that are healthy can be fed maintenance diets. A wide variety of commercial dry, wet, and semi-moist diets are appropriate for adults, and some are used for both growth and maintenance (all life stages). Cats as well as dogs require 40+ nutrients for optimal health, and these need to be provided in a relatively small amount of food.

Energy

Cats that are intact (not spayed or neutered) tend to regulate their food intake and maintain a lean body condition. Almost all household pet cats are neutered, and numerous studies have shown that cats act hungrier and eat more food if available after surgical sterilization. Feline diets are generally more energy-dense than canine diets, which means that there are more calories per gram, ounce, or cup of food. On a dry-matter basis, many cat foods contain greater than 4000 kcal/kg diet. Daily metabolizable energy (ME) requirements for adult cats vary depending on the body condition score. Based on NRC guidelines, for a 10-lb (4.54-kg) cat, an estimated starting point is 275 kcal/day, assuming normal activity. For a 13-lb (6.2-kg) overweight cat, the starting point is 270 kcal/day. These calculations indicate that overweight cats need less energy on a weight basis to maintain (not lose). The same formula for RER works for dogs and cats ($70 \times BW_{kg}^{0.75}$ kcal/day), and multipliers of 1.0 to 1.4 are commonly used to account for exercise, play, and activity. Many cats have become habituated to a sedentary lifestyle. Cats kept indoors have limited opportunity to express normal behaviors such as stalking, hunting, chasing prey, and being chased. Their energy expenditure often is no higher than RER.

> **TECHNICIAN NOTE** Indoor, sedentary cats often do not exercise and usually do not need more food than daily RER.

Protein

It is well known that cats require more protein than dogs or humans. As a species, cats are carnivorous and have adapted to a diet of rodents, birds, and other prey. There is no need to choose cat foods that are excessively high in protein, however. Moderate levels of 25% to 30% DMB are adequate. Requirements are listed in Table 9-5.

Fat

As with dogs, cats require fat and essential fatty acids, but high-fat diets are a risk factor for obesity. A low- to moderate-fat diet (10% to 15% DMB) is adequate. Actual requirements are listed in Table 9-7.

Fiber

There is no absolute requirement for fiber in cat diets, but small amounts can help with normal gastrointestinal function, stool quality, prevention of hairballs, and weight control.

Vitamins and Minerals

Commercial products generally contain at least 120% of the daily recommended allowances for these nutrients. However, on occasion, cat foods have been found to be deficient in thiamin, which is a B-vitamin especially susceptible to loss during processing. Much attention has been given to mineral levels in cat foods because of the theory that excessive minerals (or high ash content) in commercial products can lead to urinary tract disease, bladder stones, and urethral obstruction. Neither excesses nor deficiencies of minerals are appropriate, and reputable pet food manufacturers formulate their diets to reduce the risk of urinary stones and diseases wherever possible. Recent research has identified a number of other causes of feline lower urinary tract disease that are not related to diet. Therefore, there is no reason to look for "low-ash" or "low-magnesium" products for healthy cats.

FEEDING PLAN FOR ADULT MAINTENANCE

A common way of feeding cats in the past was to place dry food in a bowl and simply refill the bowl whenever empty. Cats would self-regulate their food intake and eat multiple small meals throughout the day and night. Because of the high prevalence of overweight and obese cats, this practice is no longer recommended. The current theory is that spayed and neutered cats lose some of their appetite inhibition. When presented with free-choice food, cats cannot stop themselves from eating more than their energy expenditure. The result is excess body weight, especially fat mass. To reduce this risk, cats that act hungry and tend to overeat should be meal-fed twice a day (Figure 9-9). For active cats,

RER can be calculated on the basis of current body weight and then multiplied by 1.2 to 1.4 for an estimation of kcal/day. Sedentary cats need less food, or approximately 1.0 to 1.2 times RER. Portion control is very important because the actual amount of food placed into a measuring cup may exceed what is expected because of rounded scoops. As mentioned, cat foods are energy-dense, so a few extra kibbles beyond daily needs can lead to slowly progressive weight gain.

The preceding discussion on commercial products for adult dogs is also valid for cats. The choice of a diet should be based on the reputation of the manufacturer, AAFCO feeding statements, availability, cost, and palatability/acceptability to the cat. Dry cat foods are the most popular, but canned (wet) products are available in many different varieties and flavors. Cats respond to the texture and flavor of food, which helps explain why manufacturers offer different shapes of dry kibble and different types of canned food (chunky, sliced, minced, etc.). Unlike dogs, cats sometimes are reluctant to drink water from bowls, and they may become subclinically dehydrated from eating dry foods and taking no additional water. In these situations, owners can be informed about other ways of offering water, including using drinking fountains, leaving a faucet dripping, adding water to dry food, or using canned products for part or all of the daily feeding. Healthy adult cats rarely have problems with reduced water consumption, but it can become a significant problem for older cats or in certain disease states.

Cats are noted for being finicky, which means they may eat only certain types, textures, or flavors of cat food. Ideally, cats should be exposed to more than one type of food to avoid "addiction" to one brand or flavor. Manufacturers sometimes change recipes or discontinue certain products, or stores may stop carrying favored cat foods. If this happens, it is easier to transition a cat that is accustomed to eating more than one product. If canned products are needed in the future, such as in older age for medical conditions, it is helpful for the younger adult to be used to wet food. Owners often give cats human foods as treats, especially if cats display begging behavior. High-calorie treats and snacks such as meat, cheese, dairy, etc., should be limited to 20 to 25 kcal/day (no more than 10% of normal daily food intake should be treats).

> **TECHNICIAN NOTE**   Free-choice feeding for sedentary adult cats often leads to excessive intake. Dry and canned foods are ideally offered as meals once or twice a day.

REPRODUCTION

Cats are well suited to reproduction, and female cats are able to produce more than one litter per year. Because of the pet overpopulation problem, breeding of cats is highly discouraged. However, questions about nutrition during gestation, parturition, and lactation may be asked by breeders or owners. During estrus (heat cycles), female cats and males

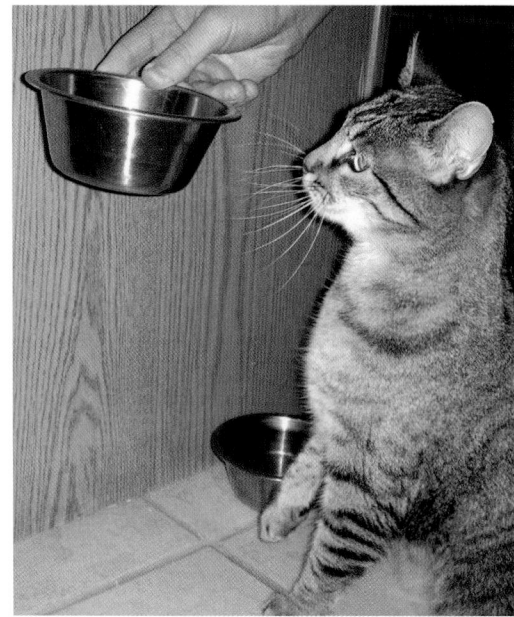

FIGURE 9-9 Cats that show high levels of hunger by begging for food frequently benefit from having the daily ration divided and fed 2 times each day rather than ad lib.

in the area often eat less and may lose weight. Highly palatable, energy-dense foods should be offered to both male and female cats intended for breeding. Food intake often increases naturally in the sixth to seventh week of pregnancy. A gradual increase to 25% to 50% higher energy is recommended in the last 3 weeks of gestation, and free-choice feeding typically supplies adequate energy and nutrients. Lactation is the most demanding physiologic stage in cats, and nutritional requirements are at their highest level. Milk production increases in the postpartum period until kittens are 3 to 4 weeks of age; then a gradual weaning process leads to a mild reduction if other sources of food are available (such as the queen's normal diet). Peak energy needs are seen at 6 to 7 weeks postpartum, and free-choice feeding of an appropriate diet generally meets these requirements. Less stress is placed on the queen if canned or moistened dry food is offered to kittens at 3 to 4 weeks of age to encourage early weaning.

Diets formulated for kitten growth are suitable for reproduction. Products intended for all life stages are also appropriate. Some adult maintenance diets, especially those formulated for weight control or "indoor cats," may be relatively deficient in energy and nutrients and not appropriate for reproduction. Therapeutic diets should be avoided unless a significant medical condition is present that requires nutritional intervention. For example, diets for urinary tract disease may be harmful for both queens and kittens during gestation and lactation.

> **TECHNICIAN NOTE** Pregnant and lactating cats require diets formulated for growth or all life stages.

SENIORS

Pet food manufacturers market products for older cats, but as with dogs, there are no AAFCO or NRC nutrient guidelines. Therefore, "mature" or "senior" cat foods may contain higher or lower levels of energy and nutrients compared with adult maintenance products. On average, cats live longer than dogs and are not considered geriatric until at least 10 years of age. The common nutritional problem of obesity continues from middle to old age, but many cats begin to gradually lose weight as they get older. Food intake may naturally decline, or health problems may lead to decreased appetite or increased energy expenditure. Offering both dry and wet foods may help encourage adequate intake. No consensus has been reached on whether older cats need more, less, or the same amounts of protein, fat, carbohydrate, fiber, vitamins, and minerals compared with younger adults. Feeding should be convenient for older cats that may lack the mobility to climb stairs. The texture and temperature of the food may need to be adjusted. The previous discussion about senior dog foods is also relevant to older cats.

CLINICAL NUTRITION

Animal health professionals are directly involved with nutritional planning and implementation for dogs and cats that do not fall into "healthy" categories such as growth, maintenance, and reproduction. Pets are often identified as having medical conditions or health issues in which nutrition is important as a cause, a direct treatment, or a means of supportive care. The following section presents an overview of clinical nutrition; additional details can be found in the recommended reading list.

ASSISTED FEEDING

Various types of malnutrition are seen in animals that are injured, sick, or hospitalized. The most common is lack of energy and protein intake because of reluctance or inability to eat voluntarily. Some pets are fed improperly, such as table scraps or raw meat only, and have deficiencies of vitamins and minerals. Cachexia refers to loss of lean body mass (muscle) and is seen with conditions such as cancer and congestive heart failure. Nutrition is necessary in sick patients for immune system function, tissue synthesis for healing, proper GI function, and regulation of many physiologic processes. Historically, in both human and veterinary medicine, sick patients often were not fed or were allowed to remain anorectic (poor to no appetite) in the belief that "resting" the GI and other systems from eating and digesting would be beneficial. However, research and clinical experience have shown that withholding food often leads to worsening of diseases and higher morbidity and mortality. Intentional starvation of patients during illness or hospitalization should no longer be practiced by conscientious health care providers.

A nutritional assessment should be performed on all sick, injured, and hospitalized dogs and cats. A medical and dietary history can be obtained from owners to gain information about the illness, as well as about current and previous diets and feeding plans. A complete physical examination of the patient is necessary to determine the extent of the medical problem, and an initial body weight and body condition score should be noted. For hospitalized patients, daily examinations and body weights help guide nutritional therapy. Problems such as vomiting, diarrhea, oral disease, etc., can complicate efforts to feed sick animals. Medical therapy is always indicated first to correct fluid and electrolyte imbalances, decreased perfusion (shock), infection, pain, and other significant problems. Assisted feeding is generally delayed until the patient has been stabilized. Indications for assisted feeding include 72 hours of hospitalization without eating, 10% or greater weight loss (or 5% in young animals), and presentation of the animal in a debilitated condition. These are only guidelines, and each case should be assessed individually.

> **TECHNICIAN NOTE** Sick, injured, and hospitalized pets should undergo nutritional assessment daily. Assisted feeding should be started by day 3 of anorexia at the latest.

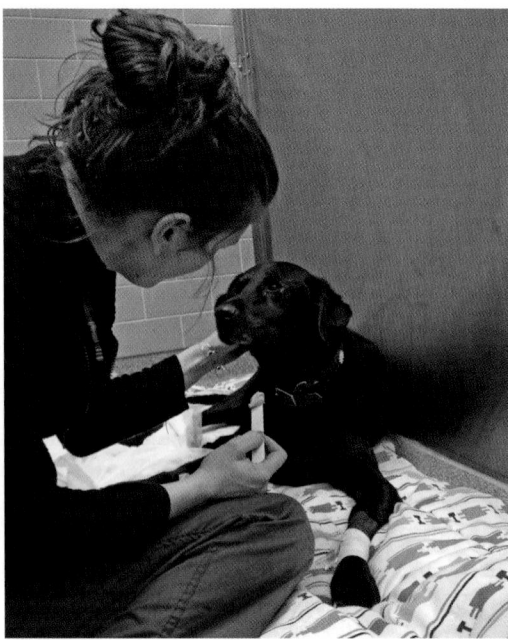

FIGURE 9-10 An encouraging veterinary technician gently offers food to an anorexic patient. (Courtesy Dr. Joanna Bassert.)

Enteral Assisted Feeding

When the veterinarian or the veterinary technician determines that a patient can be fed, the two main considerations are choice of diet and route of feeding. In some cases, the animal's regular diet may be adequate and eaten voluntarily. Oral feeding is the most physiologic and often the safest route. However, force-feeding is contraindicated in that it may cause food aversion and even aspiration pneumonia if the animal struggles. An appropriate diet is offered in a quiet, unstressed environment (Figure 9-10). Hand-feeding may be more effective than simply leaving food in a cage. If an animal refuses to eat voluntarily, food should be removed after 15 to 30 minutes and reintroduced at a later time.

> **TECHNICIAN NOTE**   Force-feeding and syringe-feeding are rarely tolerated by sick animals. Quietly offering food by hand in a low-stress environment may be more effective.

Nasoesophageal or Nasogastric Tubes

Nasoesophageal or nasogastric tubes (NE or NG tubes) are inexpensive, easy to place, and useful for short-term feeding support. The typical length of time that an NE or NG tube remains in place is 1 week or less, but in some cases, animals will tolerate nasal feeding tubes for up to 3 weeks if functioning well. NE tubes are better for preventing gastric reflux and are more physiologic. NG tubes are better for aspirating residual stomach contents. A 5-French polyurethane or silicone feeding tube is used for cats and small to medium-size dogs; an 8-French feeding tube is used for medium-size to large dogs. Red rubber catheters can be used if feeding tubes are not available. Other materials needed include local

anesthetic, tape, suture, suture or hypodermic needle, and an Elizabethan collar. The placement technique is as follows (see Figure 9-7):

1. Place a few drops up to 1 ml of local anesthetic solution (ophthalmic proparacaine 0.5% or lidocaine 2%) into one of the nostrils. Elevate the head to allow anesthetic to coat the nasal mucosa.
2. Extend the head and neck, and measure the length of the tube from the nose to the 8th to 10th rib (nasoesophageal) or the last rib (nasogastric). Mark the proximal tube with indelible ink or a piece of tape.
3. Lubricate the distal end of the tube with sterile gel (or 4% to 5% lidocaine gel). A stylet or a guide wire may be placed inside the tube to help with placement, but this is rarely necessary.
4. Insert the tube slowly in a ventromedial direction into the nostril. After 1 to 2 cm of the tube has been inserted, push the nose and nostrils in and up (to resemble a "pig snout"). Continue sliding the tube 2 to 4 cm, then relax pressure on the nose.
5. The animal may swallow as the tube passes the oropharynx. Continue inserting the tube to the predetermined length.
6. Attach a 6- to 12-ml syringe and aspirate. Negative pressure indicates proper placement. If air is easily aspirated, the tip of the tube may be in the airways. A radiograph should be taken to confirm that the tube is in the esophagus or the stomach and is not coiled or misplaced.
7. Slowly inject 3 to 5 ml of sterile saline into the tube, and observe for coughing.
8. After confirming successful placement, suture the tube into place. The proximal end of the tube can be tacked along the dorsal muzzle, between the eyes, and secured near the top of the head. Alternatively, the tube can run along the lateral muzzle ventral to the eye.
9. A 20- or 22-gauge hypodermic needle may be used to puncture a skin fold, then suture material is threaded from the point to the hub. A 10- to 15-cm length of suture is sufficient to place the first throw directly onto the skin; the tube is placed on top, then several throws are placed on top of the tube. Butterfly tape can also be used. Tissue glue is possible but is less secure and can be difficult to remove. Place an E-collar to reduce the risk of scratching and tugging at the tube.
10. Place a column of water into the tube, then cap when not being used. Only liquid diets can be used in 5- to 8-French tubes because blenderized slurries are too thick and will clog.
11. For NG tubes, an empty syringe is attached and stomach contents aspirated before each feeding. If significant fluid or liquid food is still in the stomach, the next feeding should be postponed. Aspiration is not possible with NE tubes, so the animal should be observed for signs of nausea or discomfort while feeding (Figure 9-11).
12. After feeding, flush the tube with 3 to 5 ml of water, and recap the proximal end.

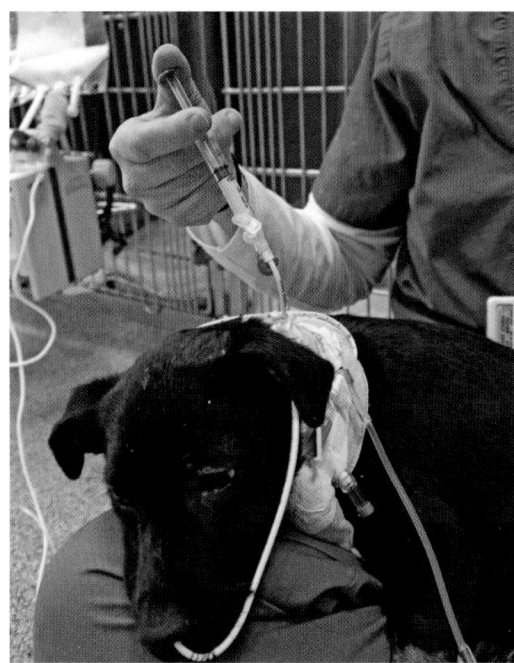

FIGURE 9-11 A puppy recovering from parvoviral enteritis is fed a liquid diet via nasoesophageal tube. (Courtesy Dr. Joanna Bassert.)

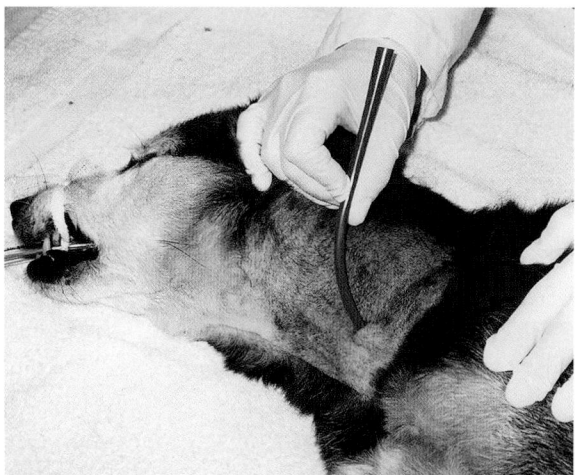

FIGURE 9-12 Esophagostomy tube for enteral feeding is placed into the midcervical esophagus on the left side of the neck.

Nasally-placed feeding tubes should not be used in animals with severe vomiting or with loss of a gag reflex and high risk of aspiration. Animals with upper airway disease, epistaxis, or nasal disease or irritation should be fed by other methods. Complications of these tubes include epistaxis, facial irritation, and premature dislodgment or removal.

13. Animals can eat and drink voluntarily while the tube is in place. When no longer needed, the tube is easily removed by clipping the suture knots and gently pulling the tube straight out.

Esophagostomy Tubes

Esophagostomy tubes (E-tubes) are indicated for longer-term support (weeks to months) and allow a variety of diets to be fed (Figure 9-12). Sizes range from 12- to 16-French for cats and small dogs, and from 12- to 24-French for larger dogs, and a variety of types are available, including silicone and red rubber. A short-acting general anesthetic or heavy sedation is required because the procedure involves minor surgery (incision into the skin and the esophagus). As with nasally placed feeding tubes, proper placement and location should be confirmed by taking a lateral radiograph. After placement, the tube is sutured using a finger-trap pattern or multiple encircling suture knots. A light wrap with roll gauze and bandage material around the neck helps secure the tube and keeps it clean. A column of water is used after each feeding to clear the tube. The skin around the tube is monitored daily for signs of redness, discharge, swelling, or abscess formation. The area can be cleaned and rewrapped daily or as needed. Larger-diameter tubes allow blenderized slurries (canned diets mixed with water or other liquids), so that appropriate nutritional strategies can be used.

Complications of these tubes include vomiting, skin infection, premature dislodgment or removal, coughing, and, rarely, esophageal stricture formation. Animals can eat and drink voluntarily while the tube is in place. When no longer needed, the tube is easily removed by clipping the suture knots and gently pulling the tube straight out. The opening in the skin heals quickly by second intention, and there is no need to suture. A light wrap or bandage can be used for 24 hours to keep the area clean.

Gastrostomy Tubes

Gastrostomy tubes (G-tubes) may be placed surgically or endoscopically (or sometimes blindly with a special applicator). They can be used for months or even a year or longer and allow feeding directly into the stomach, bypassing the oral cavity and the esophagus (Figure 9-13, *A* and *B*). Several types and sizes of tubes are available, most with a mushroom-shaped tip to prevent dislodgment (Figure 9-14). Blenderized slurries can be fed through these tubes. As with E-tubes, water should be flushed before and after each feeding and the tube capped when not in use. Do not feed for at least 12 hours after placement.

Proper placement and securing of the G-tube are essential, because if the tube is inadvertently placed or slips outside the stomach into the peritoneal cavity, peritonitis will result, leading to severe complications, including death. Other complications include gastric outflow obstruction, vomiting, tube clogging, skin irritation or infection, and premature dislodgment or removal. Unlike other types of feeding tubes, G-tubes must be left in place at least 1 week, so that adhesions will form. When the tube is no longer needed, removal can be scheduled. Food and water are withheld at least 6 hours before removal. Clip any sutures, then apply firm and steady traction and pull the tube straight out. The opening is left to heal by second intention, and a light wrap or bandage can be used to keep the area clean. It is best to leave G-tubes in place for 3 to 4 days after the animal has resumed normal daily water and food intake.

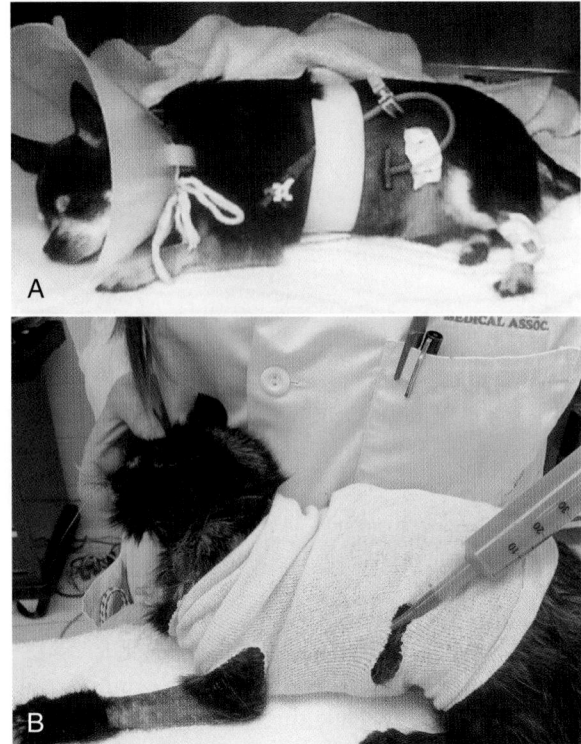

FIGURE 9-13 A, Gastrostomy tube is placed to feed a dog that has undergone esophageal surgery. The Elizabethan collar prevents chewing on the tube and on the catheter placed in the lateral saphenous vein. **B,** Gastrostomy tube feeding of an anorexic cat. A large range of diet formulations can be used because of ease of administration, facilitated by large tube diameter.

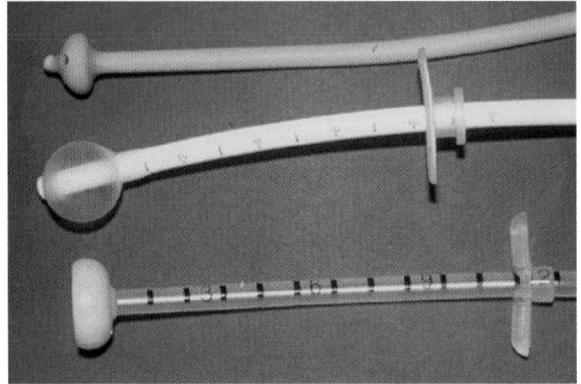

FIGURE 9-14 Examples of gastrostomy tubes. *From top to bottom:* Pezzer or mushroom tip; Foley balloon; and bumper or disc style.

Jejunostomy Tubes

Jejunostomy tubes (J-tubes) can be placed surgically during an abdominal exploratory operation or laparoscopically. Small-diameter (5- to 8-French) tubes are used; this limits the diet to liquids only. This technique bypasses the upper GI tract in cases of stomach or esophageal disease. Care of J-tubes is similar to that of G-tubes. Complications include intestinal perforation leading to peritonitis, subcutaneous leakage leading to cellulitis, skin irritation or infection, and premature dislodgment or removal. The tube must be left in place at least 5 days before removal so that adhesions will

TABLE 9-13	Liquid Diets for Dogs and Cats		
PRODUCT	**CLINICARE***	**CLINICARE* RF**	**ENTERALCARE† MLP**
Nutrient, g/100 kcal			
Protein	8.20	6.34	7.53
Fat	5.10	6.76	5.66
Carbohydrate	6.78	6.26	5.77
Energy Density, kcal/ml	1.05	1.04	1.20

*CliniCare, Abbott Animal Health, Abbott Park, IL.
†EnteralCare, PetAg, Hampshire, IL.

form. It should not be removed until the animal has resumed normal voluntary feeding. Removal is similar to that of other tubes in that the sutures are clipped and the tube pulled straight out. Healing is by second intention.

Enteral feeding has proved to be an excellent method for supporting nutritional status when oral intake is not possible. If the gastrointestinal tract is capable of digestion and absorption, food slurries, fluid, or medication can be administered through tubes placed directly into the esophagus, stomach, duodenum, or jejunum. The technician needs to be familiar with the technique that the veterinarian uses to place feeding tubes and must be knowledgeable about tube maintenance. Selection of the feeding tube is dependent upon several issues, including the expected duration of enteral support, aspiration risk, and the animal's temperament.

Nasoesophageal and nasogastric tubes are used for short-term feeding and for administration of medications. If a patient requires nutritional support beyond 10 days, placement of an esophagostomy or gastrostomy tube is preferred. Esophagostomy and gastrostomy tubes can remain long-term (weeks to months), although occasional replacement may be necessary depending on the construction and wear of the tube. If the stomach must be bypassed completely, a duodenostomy or jejunostomy tube is surgically placed.

Enteral feeding tubes of all types should be flushed before and after use. A small volume of warm water is administered to help prevent lumen obstructions. Fluids should always be injected slowly. Before injection of fluid into a gastrostomy tube, the tube is aspirated with a syringe to make certain the stomach contents have emptied from the previous feeding. If the stomach is still full, the veterinarian should be consulted; the full volume of the next meal should not be instilled into the gastrostomy tube until the previous meal has passed from the stomach. The tube insertion site and tube position are inspected daily to make certain that the tube has not shifted and that the skin is free from inflammation, redness, tenderness, and discharge.

Once a feeding tube has been properly placed, the type and amount of diet are selected. Complete and balanced liquid diets are available for dogs and cats (Table 9-13). They are used for NE, NG, and jejunostomy feeding. To calculate how much and how often to feed, the animal's current body weight is used to estimate the resting energy requirement (RER), which is $70 \times BW_{kg}^{0.75}$ kcal/day. Then the kcal/day is divided by kcal/ml of the product to calculate the daily volume to feed. On the first day, 50% RER can be fed while monitoring for tolerance. On the second day of assisted feeding, 100% RER is fed, and, if tolerated, 100% RER is continued on day 3 and subsequently until the animal is voluntarily eating. At that time, the tube may be removed. In some cases, a slower introduction is used, with 33% RER on day 1, 66% RER on day 2, and 100% RER on day 3. The number of ml/day to offer is divided by the number of feedings, for example, if 6 feedings per day are used (1 every 4 hours), ml/day is divided by 6, and that amount is fed each time. If an infusion pump is available, the liquid diet can be fed continuously, with kcal/day divided by 24 (hours per day) and the pump set to ml/hour. Most veterinary liquid diets are formulated to supply 1 to 1.2 kcal/ml metabolizable energy (ME), which makes calculations easy. Examples can be found in Box 9-2.

For esophagostomy and gastrostomy tubes, liquid diets can be fed but typically are much more expensive and not necessary. Instead, an appropriate canned diet is selected that meets the individual needs of the patient. The can is mixed with a certain amount of water in a blender and then is thoroughly mixed to form a slurry that easily passes through the size of tube used without risking a clog. After blenderizing, the slurry should be poured through a fine strainer to filter out any chunks or hard pieces of food that may obstruct the tube. In some cases, dry pet foods can be ground to fine particles in a food processor or blender and then diluted with water to form a slurry. For large tubes (at least 14-French), several products have a smooth, thin consistency and may be used undiluted (Table 9-14). These are often called *critical care* or *recovery diets*. The energy density (kcal/ml) of the slurry varies depending on the kcal/can of the product and on how much water is used.

TECHNICIAN NOTE It is important to be able to calculate RER for the patient and kcal/ml of liquid and blenderized diets so that appropriate amounts are fed.

In caring for feeding tubes, proper suturing and bandaging is important to secure the tube in place. The opening in the skin should be kept clean and antiseptic ointment applied around the edges. Elizabethan collars or other restraint devices help keep the animal from chewing on or dislodging the tube. All types should be flushed with warm water before and after feeding to clear any residual food material from the inside. Otherwise the remaining slurry may harden and cause narrowing or obstruction.

Complications of feeding tubes include clogging, aspiration, dislodgment, erosions, and dehiscence of sutures. Clogged tubes may be cleared by flushing with warm carbonated water or soda, or with a mixture of pancreatic enzymes, sodium bicarbonate, and water. Aspiration is best prevented by confirming that feeding tubes are marked at

---

BOX 9-2 | **Examples of Liquid Diet Feeding Plan for Nasal or Enterostomy Feeding Tubes**

1. A 5-French nasoesophageal feeding tube is placed in a 5-kg (11-lb) cat that has been anorectic for 3 days. Resting energy requirement (RER) at current body weight is 234 kcal/day (see Table 9-3), and the plan is to feed 50% RER on day 1 and 100% RER on day 2 and subsequently. Feedings are scheduled for 6 times a day (every 4 hours). The diet choice is EnteralCare MLP (see Table 9-13), which has an energy density of 1.2 kcal/ml. The calculations are as follows:

   Day 1: 50% RER = 234/2 = 117 kcal/day.
   117 kcal/1.2 kcal/ml = 98 ml/day
   98 ml/6 = 16 ml per feeding (every 4 hours)

   Day 2: 100% RER = 234 kcal/day.
   234 kcal/1.2 kcal/ml = 195 ml/day
   195 ml/6 = 32 ml per feeding (every 4 hours)

2. An 8-French jejunostomy feeding tube is placed in a 20-kg (44-lb) dog that has undergone intestinal surgery for removal of a foreign body. RER is 662 kcal/day, and the plan is to feed 33% RER on day 1, 66% on day 2, and 100% RER on day 3 and subsequently. A feeding pump is available, so the liquid diet will be administered continuously. The diet choice is CliniCare, which has an energy density of 1.05 kcal/ml.

   Day 1: 33% RER = 662 × 0.33 = 218 kcal/day.
   218 kcal/1.05 kcal/ml = 208 ml/day.
   208 ml/24 = 9 ml/hour. The pump is set at 9 ml/hour.

   Day 2: 66% RER = 662 × 0.66 = 437 kcal/day.
   437 kcal/1.05 kcal/ml = 416 ml/day.
   416 ml/24 = 17 ml/hour. The pump is set at 17 ml/hour.

   Day 3: 100% RER = 662 kcal/day.
   662 kcal/1.05 kcal/ml = 630 ml/day.
   630 ml/24 = 26 ml/hour. The pump is set at 26 ml/hour.

TABLE 9-14 | **Critical Care/Recovery Diets for Dogs and Cats**

PRODUCT	a/d*	MAXIMUM CALORIE†	RECOVERY RS‡
Nutrient g/100 kcal			
Protein	9.2	7.2	9.9
Fat	6.3	6.4	6.5
Carbohydrate	3.2	2.1	1.7
Energy Density, kcal/ml	1.2	2.1	1.1

*Hill's Pet Nutrition, Topeka, KS.
†Iams Company, Mason, OH
‡Royal Canin USA, St Charles, MO.

the exit point to make sure that they have not migrated in or out. Radiographs are helpful in determining feeding tube placement and for checking later regarding any questions of migration. Dislodgment can be avoided with E-collars, bandages, and sutures, along with close monitoring. Premature removal can lead to leakage, especially with gastrostomy tubes, with severe complications. Typically, 10 to 14 days is needed to form adhesions and a fistula before stomach tubes can be safely removed. Erosions can occur if tubes are left in place too long, or if red rubber catheters are used instead of appropriate feeding tube materials. Suturing the tube into place should be done carefully, avoiding pressure from tight knots and suturing too close to the incision line.

Metabolic complications of enteral nutrition include hyperglycemia and hyperlipidemia caused by introducing food too rapidly or by overfeeding. If parenteral fluid therapy is being used, the water used in the feeding plan must be accounted for because fluid overload is possible in some patients. Refeeding syndrome refers to a condition of decreased serum phosphorus, potassium, and magnesium that results from intracellular shift when food is introduced too quickly after a period of starvation. Nausea and vomiting occur when patients have preexisting GI or metabolic diseases, or when there is irritation from the feeding tube (improper placement or materials). If gastric emptying is delayed, food can build up in the stomach with frequent or continuous feedings. Before a stomach tube is used, aspiration of residual contents will help determine whether feeding amount and frequency are excessive.

> **TECHNICIAN NOTE** Refeeding syndrome is rare, but caution should be used when initiating feeding of starved patients.

Parenteral Assisted Feeding

When dogs or cats are not eating voluntarily and cannot be fed using the enteral route, parenteral nutrition (PN) is available, which is defined as providing nutrients intravenously (Figure 9-15). Patients that may benefit from PN include those with diffuse intestinal disease, at risk for aspiration if fed, or unable to be sedated or anesthetized for placement of a feeding tube. Before PN is considered, the animal should be stable, should not have fluid or electrolyte imbalances, and should be able to tolerate intravenous fluids. At least 3 days is the minimum recommended time for PN, so if the patient is expected to return to eating or can tolerate enteral nutrition within 3 days, PN is not needed. The clinic needs to have qualified personnel around the clock to monitor patients receiving PN and must have the ability to run in-house lab work. Patients must have a dedicated central IV catheter (usually jugular) for PN because of the high osmolality, although a peripheral vein can be used for partial PN. Therefore, PN is often limited to 24-hour emergency and specialty clinics. In some cases, PN can be administered during the day and stopped overnight, but this method is riskier.

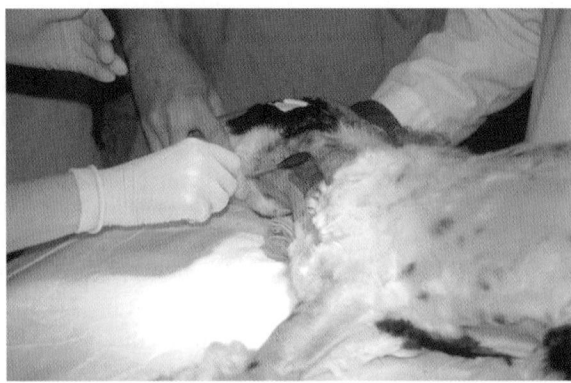

FIGURE 9-15 Dog being prepped for placement of a central venous catheter. Parenteral nutrition (PN) is typically administered through a central venous catheter, which can remain in place for a prolonged time.

The goal of total parenteral nutrition (TPN) is to supply enough energy to meet RER, amino acids to achieve a nitrogen balance, and essential fatty acids and vitamins, as well as some minerals. The most common form of TPN is a sterile admixture of an amino acid solution, a lipid solution, a dextrose solution, a vitamin B complex injection, and sometimes other minerals such as potassium, magnesium, and trace elements. Compounding a sterile mixture requires special equipment not found in most veterinary hospitals. In some situations, human PN services associated with hospitals or home services can formulate sterile admixtures if provided with an appropriate formulation ("recipe") for dogs and cats. Some veterinary nutrition specialists will compound and deliver solutions for other veterinarians to use.

After a sterile central IV catheter is placed, the TPN is infused slowly with a pump. As with enteral feeding, the RER is calculated, and on day 1, 50% RER is administered, followed by 100% RER on day 2 and on subsequent days. In some cases, a slower administration rate is used, with 33% RER on day 1, 66% RER on day 2, and 100% RER on day 3 and subsequently. All patients receiving TPN must be carefully monitored. While the infusion rate is started and increased, blood glucose should be checked every 4 to 6 hours, and then daily after rate is stabilized. Serum or plasma should be checked daily for lipemia or high triglycerides. The catheter, extension tubing, bandaging, etc., all need to be checked every 4 to 6 hours. Additionally, the patient's vital signs are recorded every 12 hours and body weight every 24 hours. Small blood samples are obtained daily to check packed cell volume/total protein, blood urea nitrogen (BUN), albumin, and electrolytes K, P, and Mg. Complications of TPN include metabolic (detected by physical examination observations and lab work), septic (infection at the catheter site), and mechanical events (catheter dysfunction or dislodgment, pinched or twisted lines, equipment failure). The entire veterinary staff should be aware of how to monitor animals receiving PN so that complications can be avoided if possible, or corrected early before more serious problems occur.

If a central line is not available, a peripheral vein (cephalic, saphenous) can be used to administer PN. This is called *partial (or peripheral) parenteral nutrition (PPN),* and the formulation must be more dilute to lower the osmolality. Otherwise, thrombophlebitis will occur at the catheter site. In general, only 50% to 70% of daily energy needs (RER) can be met with PPN unless a large volume of fluids is used at a high infusion rate. Potential complications and monitoring procedures are the same for PPN as for TPN. When the animal is ready to transition to voluntary oral or enteral assisted feeding, the PN rate is gradually reduced over 8 to 12 hours instead of being stopped abruptly.

> **TECHNICIAN NOTE** Intravenous feeding can be life-saving and cost-effective if 24-hour nursing care is provided and if experienced personnel are involved in the feeding protocols.

NUTRITIONAL STRATEGIES FOR OBESITY

As was previously discussed, the most common form of malnutrition in dogs and cats is overfeeding with resulting overweight and obese body conditions (Figure 9-16). There are no shortcuts or reliably consistent methods of treating obesity, and a team approach involving veterinarians and animal health professionals is necessary. The following is an example of a logical plan; it should be kept in mind that other techniques and approaches may work as well.

The first step is to recognize the problem. Dogs and cats should be weighed on accurate scales and scored for body condition at every veterinary visit and follow-up (see Figure 9-6). Owners can be taught to estimate BCS by feeling along the rib cage and checking for a waist and abdominal tuck. There are two systems commonly used to determine body condition in dogs and cats, a 5-point scale and a 9-point scale. A BCS of 5 on the 5-point scale or 9 on the 9-point scale indicates that the animal is obese. A score of one on both scales indicates that the animal is emaciated. Ideal weights are represented by scores of 3/5 or 4-5/9. Each point above or below 3 for the 5-point system is 20% overweight or underweight. Animals with a BCS of 6 on a 9-point scale

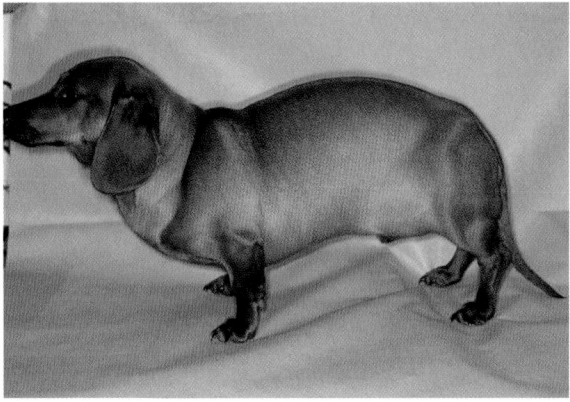

FIGURE 9-16 An obese dog. Once formed, fat cells are present for life, although they can shrink. Animals that eat too much as juveniles experience fat-cell division and are subsequently predisposed to excessive weight gain throughout their lives.

are approximately 10% to 15% overweight; 7/9 indicates 20% to 30%, 8/9 indicates 30% to 45%, and 9/9 over 45%. These rough estimates give guidelines as to how much weight should be lost while following a treatment plan. For example, a 15-lb cat with a BCS of 7/9 should lose 20% to 30% of body weight, or 3 to 4.5 lb, to attain a lean body weight.

> **TECHNICIAN NOTE** Animals with a BCS of 5 or higher on a 9-point body condition scale and a 3 or higher on a 5-point scale, benefit from a weight loss program.

The second step is to take a thorough diet history and ask about activity level, exercise, play behavior, indoor/outdoor status, and all other factors that influence energy intake and expenditure. It is common for owners to be unable to report exact brands or varieties or diets fed, and the total daily amount fed is often a guess rather than an exact measurement. Snacks, treats, table scraps, and other sources of food may be overlooked. The feeding method is important as well, such as free-choice (ad libitum), meal feeding, timed feeding, etc. The presence of other pets in the household will influence the diet history because animals may share a single large bowl or get into food intended for others.

After a diet history is collected, an attempt should be made to estimate daily energy intake. This can be done if owners supply name brands of pet foods and treats and report actual amounts fed (such as 2 measuring cups per day, or 1 can per day). The current daily amount may be leading to progressive weight gain or maintaining a stable (but excess) body weight. Therefore, the new feeding plan must supply fewer calories than the current amount. A mildly overweight animal (BCS 6/9) can be energy-restricted by 10%, or 90% of current intake. For example, if a dog is estimated to be eating 300 kcal/day, the new feeding plan should be 10% less (30 kcal), or 270 kcal/day. Moderately overweight animals (BCS 7/9 or 8/9) should be restricted by 20%. Extremely obese animals (BCS 9/9) can be restricted by 30% to 33%. When owners cannot provide an accurate diet history and when current energy intake is unknown, the resting energy requirement (RER) can be used as a substitute. The RER is calculated using current (not ideal) body weight, and then is reduced by 10% to 33% depending on BCS.

> **TECHNICIAN NOTE** When the current food and energy intake is known, a weight-loss plan is started by reducing this amount by 20%.

The fourth step is to select an appropriate diet to supply nutrients within the context of energy restriction. This is often the most misunderstood aspect of a weight-loss program. Many owners simply try to reduce the amount fed of the current diet, and animal health professionals may encourage this by recommending "feed less." However, this practice is no longer recommended for several reasons. Maintenance diets often have moderate to high levels of fat, and this leads to high energy density (because fat supplies at least twice as much energy as is supplied by protein and carbohydrate). A high level of fat is a risk factor for obesity and rarely is a successful strategy for weight loss. Most maintenance products meet or slightly exceed daily recommended allowances when fed at low amounts, but when energy is restricted enough to cause weight loss (10% to 30%), protein and other nutrients often fall below minimal requirements. This can be dangerous if continued long-term. For example, if a dog is eating 3 cups of dry food a day but is overweight, if intake if reduced to 2 cups per day, there is 33% less energy, but also 33% less protein, essential amino acids, fatty acids, vitamins, and minerals. Unless the product supplies at least 150% of all nutrients, it will be deficient if fed at 33% less than label recommendations. Also, maintenance diets often do not have formulations that help with satiety (feeling of being full) such as increased protein or fiber. For these and other reasons, it is not appropriate to continue the same diet at reduced amounts when the goal is weight loss.

Because maintenance diets are not optimal for weight loss, several pet food manufacturers have developed formulas that meet the needs of overweight pets without risking nutrient deficiencies. Although all products are different, common characteristics include decreased energy density, reduced fat, increased fiber, increased protein, and increased complex carbohydrates. Some products include supplements such as L-carnitine, which helps with energy metabolism, antioxidants, and other substances. One of the main features is the lower energy density, which leads to fewer kcal per cup or can of food. Because owners may feed with visual cues, such as how much food is in the bowl, reducing the kcal can be helpful in reducing energy intake. A low energy–density product allows owners to continue feeding reasonable amounts of food. Lower-fat diets help keep the energy density low and reduce the risk of adding more body fat. An increase in fiber can help with satiety because fiber provides bulk and dietary satisfaction without adding energy (no additional kcal when fiber is added). Higher-protein diets help with satiety and involve increased metabolic energy to digest and metabolize. Nutraceuticals and supplements may or may not help with weight loss but are often found in specialized diets.

Because weight-loss diets are designed to be fed at reduced amounts of energy, they include higher amounts of crude protein and amino acids, essential fatty acids, vitamins, and minerals than are typically found in maintenance diets. To use the previous example, instead of reducing a dog's food intake from 3 cups to 2 cups of a maintenance diet, the better strategy is to switch to a weight-loss diet and calculate the amount to feed from current intake or RER, as mentioned previously. A reasonable weight-loss goal is 1% to 2% of body weight per week, for example, a 50-lb dog that should weigh 40 lb needs to lose 20% of total body weight. At 1% weight loss per week, this will take 20 weeks (5 months), or at 2% per week, this will take 10 weeks (2.5 months). If weight loss is much slower than this, owners may become discouraged when results are not obvious. If weight loss is faster, this indicates that insufficient amounts of food are being offered, and the animal is at higher risk for rapidly regaining weight when the "diet" is over.

> **TECHNICIAN NOTE** A safe rate of body weight loss is 1% to 2% per week. Most pets require 3 to 6 months to lose significant weight.

After successful weight loss, most dogs should be gradually transitioned to a maintenance diet that is formulated for weight management instead of an all-purpose diet. A number of "light" and "reduced calorie" products can help maintain the animal at a healthy weight. Simply returning the pet to the previous diet and feeding plan inevitably results in weight gain. Another option is to continue feeding the weight-loss diet long-term because products are complete and balanced and their use should not result in nutrient deficiencies or excesses.

RECOMMENDED READINGS

Fascetti AJ, Delaney SJ: Applied veterinary clinical nutrition, Ames, IA, 2012, Wiley-Blackwell.

Association of American Feed Control Officials Incorporated: AAFCO 2012 official publication, Champaign, IL, 2012, AAFCO.

Canine and feline nutrition: a resource for companion animal professionals, ed 3, Maryland Heights, MO, 2011, Mosby Elsevier.

Companion animal nutrition: a manual for veterinary nurses and technicians, Philadelphia, 2008, Butterworth Heinemann Elsevier.

Encyclopedia of canine clinical nutrition, Paris, 2006, Aniwa SAS.

Encyclopedia of feline clinical nutrition, Paris, 2008, Aniwa SAS.

Nutrient requirements of dogs and cats, Washington, DC, 2006, The National Academies Press.

Nutrition for veterinary technicians and nurses, Ames, IA, 2007, Blackwell Publishing.

Small animal clinical nutrition, ed 5, Topeka, KS, 2010, Mark Morris Institute.

10 Large Animal Nutrition

Tanja M. Hess and Shawn L. Archibeque

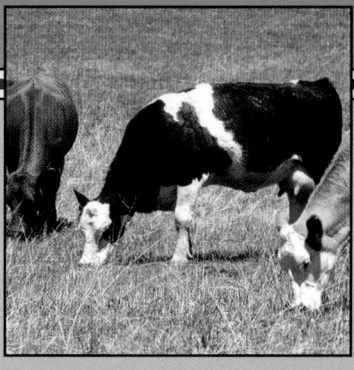

OUTLINE

Nutrients, *340*
Protein, *341*
Fats, *342*
Carbohydrates, *342*
Minerals and Vitamins, *343*
Water, *343*
Dairy Cattle, *343*
Energy, *346*
Protein, *348*
Minerals and Vitamins, *348*
Dairy Calves, *348*
Beef Cattle, *349*
Cow-Calf Production, *349*
Calves, *352*

Finishing Cattle, *352*
Sheep, *353*
Breeding Flock, *353*
Lambs, *356*
Swine, *356*
Breeding Herd, *356*
Starter Pigs, *358*
Growing/Finishing Pigs, *358*
Horses, *359*
Maintenance Horses, *359*
Gestation and Lactation, *361*
Foals, *362*
Working Horses, *363*
Feeding Sick Horses, *365*

KEY TERMS

Amino acids
Biological value
Concentrates
Digestible energy (DE)
Digestion
Forage
Gross energy (GE)
Maintenance nutrient requirements (MNRs)
Metabolizable energy (ME)
Net energy (NE)
Protein efficiency ratio
Reduced gastrointestinal monitoring
Total digestible nutrients (TDNs)

LEARNING OBJECTIVES

When you have completed this chapter, you will be able to:

1. Pronounce, spell, and define each of the Key Terms in the chapter.
2. Do the following regarding nutrients:
   - Explain the relationship between nutrition, productivity and profitability in livestock production.
   - List the building block molecules that makeup proteins, fats and carbohydrates.
   - List two ways in which carbohydrates are digested in horses.
   - List the energy-producing and non–energy-producing components of food.
   - List the variables affecting energy requirements of livestock.
   - Differentiate between microminerals and macrominerals and give examples of each.
   - Explain the importance of water in metabolic reactions.
3. Describe the two commonly used feeding systems for dairy cattle.
4. Compare and contrast the special considerations and protocols employed when feeding dairy cattle, beef cattle, sheep, and swine. Also do the following:
   - State the importance of water and list the factors affecting water intake of livestock.
   - Describe how the nutritional requirements of each of these species are affected by the animal's stage of life and by its energy expenditure (maintenance, growth, finishing, lactation, work, or wool).
   - List advantages and disadvantages of pasture feeding of livestock.
5. Do the following regarding nutrition in horses:
   - Explain the importance of grass and hays in the equine diet.
   - Describe how pregnancy and lactation alter a mare's nutritional requirements.
   - List steps taken to provide appropriate nutrition to foals and young, growing horses.
   - Describe how work-levels are classified in working horses and how these levels affect water, energy and mineral requirements.
   - Describe general guidelines for feeding sick and post-operative horses.

The authors and publisher wish to acknowledge the contributions of William D. Scoenherr, whose original work served as the foundation for this chapter.

INTRODUCTION

Optimal nutrition has often been identified as the most expensive element in achieving full productivity and profitability in livestock.[1] Veterinary technicians must have a strong fundamental knowledge of nutrient needs and must be able to identify risks for potential nutritional problems. Veterinary technicians must also feel comfortable educating clients about nutrition and giving specific instructions for feeding. The client who has the greatest need for this type of information is not the large, intensive livestock farmer who normally has feed professionally formulated for optimum production. Most often, questions will be asked by clients who run small operations, have family members raising livestock for 4-H or children's clubs' (e.g., Future Farmers of America) projects, or possess a "hobby farm." With these client needs in mind, this chapter focuses on common nutritional problems and sound principles to help the veterinary technician provide meaningful, relevant information about livestock and horses.

Nutritional disorders can be similar to an array of diseases and may not be identified easily by the livestock producer or the horse owner until problems become chronic and additional assistance is sought. It is essential to get a complete history, including a detailed feeding regimen, on any livestock or equine patient that is exhibiting signs of illness.

Dramatic advancements have been made in large animal nutrition, including studies that have increased our understanding of the specific nutrient needs of livestock. Being able to provide optimal nutrition will help clients maximize production, successful breeding, and the generation of high-quality, lean meat. Future research will continue to improve our understanding of animal physiology, and this will lead to improvements in livestock production and equine nutrition. (Table 10-1).

TABLE 10-1	Feeding Problems in Ruminants			
SYMPTOMS	**CAUSES**	**PREVENTION**	**COMMENTS**
Bloat			
Distention of the left flank and then the right flank Hypersalivation Profuse burning Froth or gas accumulation in the rumen Respiratory distress Cyanosis Death	Change in pasture with heavy fertilizer Genetics Bacterial overgrowth Excessive concentrate consumption	Feed coarse grasses or dry forage before turnout to quick-growing pastures. Allow continuous feed consumption. Avoid straight pastures. Avoid large consumption of concentrates. Avoid rapid diet changes. Keep stock on pasture continuously rather than sporadically. Allow full access to water and salt.	Watch legume exposure for all ruminants.
Enterotoxemia (Overeating Disease)			
Death is often the first symptom. Circling Progressive weakness Head butting Convulsions	Often occurs in faster-growing juveniles *Clostridium perfringens* Excess consumption of high-energy feed or lush pasture or heavy milk supply	Vaccinate with *Clostridium perfringens* type D for lambs and types C and D for breeding ewes. Avoid access to large meals of concentrates.	Applies primarily in sheep and goats; sometimes cattle If outbreak occurs, consider enterotoxemia antiserum for 21-day protection in lambs.
Fescue Toxicosis			
±Lameness Necrosis of tail end Milk production Abortion	Change in parasitized animal In malnourished animal Endophyte fungus *Acremonium coenophialum*	Avoid heavy parasitism and malnutrition. Use fungus-free fescue seed for planting.	Applies mostly for cattle and sheep (fescue foot) Highest occurrence is in fall and winter in all fescue pasture.
Grass Tetany (Hypomagnesemia)			
Disorientation Paddling Convulsions Muscle twitching	Most common in cows 4 years and older Occurrence during early lactation in heavy milking cows Pastures with $\downarrow Mg^{2+}$ and $\uparrow K^+$ and $\downarrow Ca^+$ availability	Start providing Mg^{2+} 30 days before high-risk times. $\uparrow Mg^{2+}$ in lactating and older cows and ewes Highest risk is during spring and early summer; lush, rapidly growing pastures Molasses supplement with Mg^{2+} may be required.	Stress from weather, movement, or environment increases risk. Mg^{2+} supplements have low palatability; make sure animals consume feed.
Milk Fever (Parturition, Paresis, or Hypocalcemia)			
Appetite Nervous behavior Collapse Wrenching of head toward back	Postcalving in high-producing cows $\downarrow$ Blood Ca^{2+}	Feed anionic salts 2-3 weeks before parturition. Feed balanced Ca^{2+}/P rations. Vitamin D intake provided 1 week before parturition. Avoid obesity.	Watch Ca^{2+} and P levels in dry periods. Choose feeds low in Na^+ and K^+.
Displaced Abomasum			
$\downarrow$ Appetite $\downarrow$ Milk production Diarrhea, discolored feces	Pregnancy Lack of bulk in diet Sudden jarring of fresh cows Poor muscle tone Mycotoxin exposure	Avoid acidosis or alkalosis. Adapt cattle to high-concentrate rations before parturition.	Occurs most frequently in high-producing, heavily fed dairy cattle near parturition

Continued

TABLE 10-1	Feeding Problems in Ruminants—cont'd		
SYMPTOMS	**CAUSES**	**PREVENTION**	**COMMENTS**
Ketosis Occurs: • 14-50 days after parturition in cattle • 2 weeks before parturition in sheep ↓ Milk production ↓ Appetite Sugary-acid breath ↓ Body weight Frequent urination Trembling Collapse	↑ Chances in multiple births with ewes and does Rapid loss of body fat and low availability of carbohydrates in diet	Maintain lean body condition and prevent excess fat. ↑ Energy intake before parturition in sheep Avoid sudden changes in the physical nature of the feed.	Ewes are at risk before lambing. Cows are typically at risk after calving. Animals that rapidly stop eating owing to disease or changes in diet are at risk.
Thiamin Deficiency Polio Decreased vision Incoordination Acute death Excitable	Excess S intake	Limit high-S feeds such as distiller's grains.	Occur primarily in feedlot and young cattle younger than 2 years old Goats may be affected while nursing young.
Rickets In young animals, enlarged joints Painful gait Leg bowing	Incorrect Ca^{2+}, P, vitamin intake	Provide balanced Ca^{2+}, P, and vitamin D diets.	
Urinary Calculi Difficult urination Bloody urine	↑ Increase in feedlots ↑ P, ↓ Ca^{2+}	Provide readily available water. Keep Ca/P ratio between 1.5:1 and 7:1.	Males have ↑ risk.
Urolithiasis Bloody urine	High K^+ consumption, ↑ P, ↓ Ca^{2+}	Balance P/Ca^{2+} ratio.	
Water Belly Kicking at abdomen Rupture of bladder	Excess silicate intake Urinary calculi	Avoid excess silicate intake. Balance Ca/P ratios to avoid urinary calculi.	
White Muscle Disease Irregular gait Hunched-back appearance Heart irregularities Death	Se and vitamin E deficiency Geographic distribution: ↓ Se in many areas of United States and Canada	↑ Se in dietary intake in known deficient areas ↑ Vitamin E provision to at risk animals	Most commonly occurs in most rapidly growing individuals in flock or herd

Data from Naylor JM, et al: Large animal clinical nutrition, St Louis, 1991, Mosby; McDonald P, et al: Animal nutrition, New York, 1995, Longman Scientific and Technical; Maynard LA, et al: Animal nutrition, ed 7, New York, 1979, McGraw-Hill; Ensminger ME, et al: Feeds and nutrition, Clovis, CA, 1990, Ensminger Publishing.

NUTRIENTS

Nutrients are ingested to support life. Livestock producers and horse owners want to obtain the most desirable results from the nutrients their animals consume at an economical rate and with an advantageous financial return. Ingested nutrients may be retained by the animal or excreted in the urine and feces. Retained nutrients are used for a wide array of body functions, such as homeostasis, replenishment and development of tissues, reproduction, and milk, wool, and meat production.

Maintenance nutrient requirements (MNRs) are the levels of nutrients needed to sustain body weight without gain or loss (Box 10-1). The MNR is the minimum level of dietary need; usually a vast percentage of published requirements are higher than this standard. As a general rule, one-half or more of consumed and absorbed nutrients are used to fulfill MNRs. Individual variation results in fluctuation

- Body size
- Health status
- Stress
- Environment
- Exercise
- Behavior
- Genetics
- Reproductive status
- Gender
- Breed

- Pasture and grasslands, 40.0%*
- Corn, 23.3%
- Hay, 12.2%
- Grains and high-protein feed, 16.9%
- Silage and miscellaneous, 7.6%

From the U.S. Department of Agriculture (USDA) Economic Research Service, 1983-1984.
*Varies significantly by season and pasture quality.

TECHNICIAN NOTE Protein is a common component of plants, and the highest concentration is found in the seed and leafy portions.

from this standard; be sure to evaluate need against all information to achieve the most accurate results.

Feeding standards are available listing the quantities of nutrients required by different species for specific productive purposes, such as maintenance, growth, finishing, lactation, work, wool, or eggs. The most widely used feeding standards in the United States are those published by the National Research Council (NRC), and they are established for beef cattle, dairy cattle, sheep, goats, swine, poultry, and horses (see "Recommended Readings"). Periodically, feeding standards are updated and published by a committee appointed by the NRC.

TECHNICIAN NOTE MNRs are the levels of nutrients needed to sustain body weight without gain or loss.

Digestion (the process of protein, carbohydrate, and fat breakdown into absorbable nutrients) is accomplished by chemical, enzymatic, microbial, and physical methods. It is essential to remember that it is not the alfalfa, hay, corn, or oats that are used by cells, but rather the digested and absorbed nutrients, such as **amino acids,** simple sugars, fatty acids, minerals, and vitamins that present at the cellular level. The quality, quantity, and cost of nutrients that can be provided by the feedstuff are of primary importance when ingredients are chosen for feeding farm animals.

PROTEIN

Protein is the principal constituent of organs and soft tissues. It is constructed of building blocks called *amino acids* that are linked together in a chain. The arrangement of amino acids in the chain and the length of the chain are two factors that help to determine the composition and functionality of the protein. A total of 10 essential and 12 nonessential amino acids have been identified. Essential amino acids must be supplied in the diet because the body of the animal cannot synthesize them fast enough to meet its requirement. Amino acids consist of nitrogen, carbon, oxygen, and sulfur. The deconstruction or deamination process releases these elements into the body's system, resulting in their elimination from the body or their use as energy.

Animal feed (Box 10-2) is identified often by crude protein content, but the measurement rarely illustrates the quality or use potential of the protein. Feed can possess high protein content, yet the *biological value* of that protein is low. Protein biological value is the percentage of true absorbed protein that is available for productive body functions. Conceptually, it is the "amino acid grade card" because it defines the available amino acids. In general, proteins of animal origin have greater **biological value** than do proteins of plant origin. The higher the biological value, the better the protein used for productive purposes. Protein quality is also measured as the **protein efficiency ratio,** which is the number of grams of body weight gained per unit of protein consumed.[2]

Animal and plant proteins vary greatly in their distribution of amino acids and their biological value. When combined in correct proportions with other protein (e.g., animal protein), protein that individually has very poor biological value (e.g., corn) may yield a biological value similar to that of a single high-quality protein. The quality of protein depends on disallowing overprocessing of feed and overheating in storage, and on the form of the feed (Figure 10-1).[3]

Use by Ruminants

Rumen digestion facilitated by microbes has the ability to convert most consumed proteins to peptides and amino acids, many of which are further degraded into ammonia, organic acids, and carbon dioxide. Ammonia released on microbial degradation of feed protein will be removed from the rumen by absorption through the rumen wall or used by microorganisms for synthesis of microbial protein. Microbial protein synthesis by the microorganisms results in a fairly constant supply of protein quality to the lower digestive tract. The protein quality from moderate to poor feed will usually be improved by rumen metabolism, whereas the opposite may occur with high-quality protein feed. Rumen microbes also have the ability to convert nonprotein nitrogen sources into microbial protein. Typical nonprotein nitrogen sources include urea, ammonium salts,

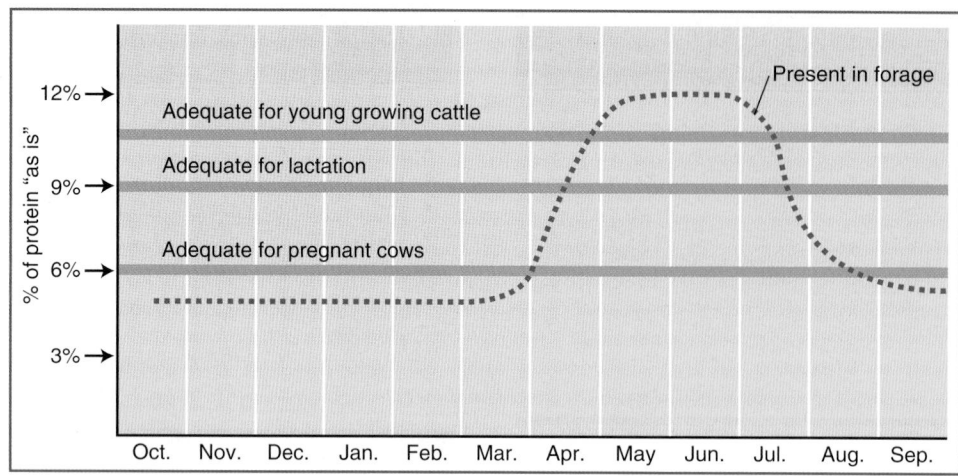

FIGURE 10-1 Nutrient content of forage varies with pasture quality and season.

ammoniated by-products, and free amino acids and are best used judiciously because excessive or unbalanced intake can be toxic.[4] Use of animal protein sources derived from ruminant species is not allowed in ruminant (i.e., cattle and sheep) rations to prevent the possible transmission of bovine spongiform encephalopathy (BSE).

FATS

Fats provide dietary energy and essential fatty acids and serve as sources of heat, insulation, and protection for vital organs. Fat has 2.25 times more energy per gram than protein or carbohydrate. Fats aids in the absorption of fat-soluble vitamins such as linoleic and alpha-linolenic acids. Linoleic acid is capable of being converted to arachidonic acid, which is important during the inflammatory process. Alpha-linolenic acid is converted to eicosapentaenoic and docosahexaenoic acids, which are important in mediating inflammation and in the formation of nerves.

> **TECHNICIAN NOTE**   Fat has more energy per gram than all other nutrients.

CARBOHYDRATES

Carbohydrates are the primary energy source in livestock rations. They are less expensive and more readily available than protein or fat. Most feedstuffs of plant origin are high in carbohydrates, especially cereal grains. Carbohydrates must be broken down into simple sugars such as glucose before they can be absorbed in the intestine. Carbohydrate catabolism requires digestive enzymes that are generated by the host or by microflora that live in the animal's digestive system. These carbohydrate-splitting enzymes are effective in splitting most complex carbohydrates into simple sugars but are less successful in splitting apart structural polysaccharides such as cellulose (fiber). Fortunately, microbes in the rumen and in the cecum of some nonruminants, such as horses and rabbits, produce an enzyme that breaks down fiber. Carbohydrates can be classified into three groups:

simple sugars, storage molecules such as starch and fructans, and structural polysaccharides such as hemicellulose and cellulose. In horses, complex carbohydrates can be broken down into simple sugars by hydrolytic enzymes in the stomach and small intestine. These are said to be hydrolyzable carbohydrates. The horse can gain nutritional value from nonhydrolyzable carbohydrates such as cellulose because microbes that live in the equine cecum consume fiber and subsequently release volatile fatty acids that are absorbed through the cecal wall. Because this process is microbial fermentation, structural carbohydrates like fiber are called *fermentable carbohydrates.*

Hydrolyzable carbohydrates include disaccharides, some oligosaccharides (e.g., maltotriose), and starch. Fermentable carbohydrates include hemicellulose, cellulose, legnocellulose, soluble fibers, and oligosaccharides (fructans, galactans), as well as starches resistant to hydrolysis. Carbohydrates in animal feed are commonly categorized as **concentrates,** such as grains, and as high-starch compounds or **forage,** such as grass, hays, and legumes. No minimum or maximum requirements have been put forth for carbohydrates because intake is related to activity levels and energy needs.

> **TECHNICIAN NOTE**   Carbohydrates are the primary energy source in livestock rations.

Feedstuff Energy

The largest function of feed is to provide energy for body processes. **Total digestible nutrients (TDNs), gross energy (GE), digestible energy (DE), metabolizable energy (ME),** and **net energy (NE)** are all different measures of feed energy value.

TDN (total digestible nutrients) is a general measure of the nutritive value of a feed. Digestibility coefficients are used to compute the content of TDN. The usefulness of TDN as a measure of feed energy is limited in that it does not take into account energy losses in urine, combustible

BOX 10-3	Variables Affecting Energy Requirements

- Activity
- Environment
- Body size
- Life stage
- Reproductive status

gases, and heat. Discrepancies can be large for forage-based feed because of the tendency to overestimate the energy available for productive purposes. TDN is expressed as a percentage of the ration or in units of weight, not as an actual caloric number.

Gross energy (GE) is the total energy (Box 10-3) potentially available in a feed consumed by an animal. All energy values used in the following scheme are expressed in kilocalories (kcal) or megacalories (Mcal) per unit of weight. During digestion and absorption, a portion of the GE escapes the body in the form of undigested food residue in the feces. Subtraction of energy lost in the feces from consumed GE reveals energy that was digested and absorbed, or digestible energy (DE). Measurement of DE uses the same elements as TDN and assigns similar energy values to feed. DE values and TDN are used extensively in horse feed. Energy that is digested and absorbed by the body is not used with 100% efficiency; a portion of the absorbed energy is lost in the urine and as combustible gases. Accounting for these energy losses leads to a step beyond DE or TDN—metabolizable energy (ME). Energy values for ME are used widely in the formulation of swine and poultry feed. One further refinement of this energy scheme involves accounting for heat lost from the body during metabolism of nutrients. Net energy (NE) represents the actual portion of energy available to the animal for use in maintaining body tissues or during pregnancy or lactation. NE values are used extensively in the beef, dairy, and sheep industry.

MINERALS AND VITAMINS

Minerals and vitamins are needed in small amounts compared with other nutrients, but they play integral roles in many metabolic processes. Minerals are divided into two categories: microminerals and macrominerals (Box 10-4). Lists of minerals and vitamins and their functions are given in Tables 10-2, 10-3, and 10-4.

WATER

Water is the cheapest and most abundant nutrient. It accounts for 65% to 85% of an animal's body weight at birth and 45% to 60% of body weight at maturity. Water is derived metabolically from the breakdown of organic nutrients in animal tissues or drinking water or is derived from foodstuffs. Because water is the largest constituent of the animal, deprivation of water of only a few percentages of body weight is life threatening. Clean, fresh water should be readily available to maintain a zero water balance (Table 10-5).

BOX 10-4	Mineral Categories

Macrominerals*
Salt (sodium chloride; NaCl)
Potassium (K)
Phosphorus (P)
Magnesium (Mg)
Calcium (Ca)
Sulfur (S)

Microminerals[†]
Zinc (Zn)
Selenium (Se)
Manganese (Mn)
Iodine (I)
Fluorine (F)
Chromium (Cr)
Copper (Cu)
Iron (Fe)
Silicon (Si)
Molybdenum (Mo)
Cobalt (Co)

*Measured in kg.
[†]Measured in ppm or mg/kg.

> **TECHNICIAN NOTE** Water is the cheapest and most abundant nutrient.

DAIRY CATTLE

The dairy industry is successfully using many different production systems. Systems are based on geographic area and feedstuff availability. The traditional pasture system continues to be used in areas with readily available land, whereas dry-lot systems are more popular in urban and suburban areas (Figure 10-2). Regardless of the dairy production system, two feeding programs are most frequently employed. Total mixed ration (TMR) is the practice of weighing and blending all feedstuffs into a complete ration. Each bite consumed by the cow contains all of the required levels of nutrients. The other program is a forage and grain diet fed separately. Animals are provided hay free-choice at all times, silage is offered once or twice per day, and feed concentrates are fed twice daily.

Feeding, more than any other single factor, determines the productivity of lactating dairy cows. Feed represents about 50% of the total cost of milk production. Therefore, a good feeding program is necessary for profitable milk production. Nutrient requirements for lactation are large and are often several times the MNR (Figure 10-3 and Tables 10-6, 10-7, and 10-8). Water is also important for dairy cows (Boxes 10-5 and 10-6).

> **TECHNICIAN NOTE** Feed represents 50% of the total costs of milk production.

TABLE 10-2	Macrominerals for Livestock		
USE	**TOXICITY**	**DEFICIENCY**	**SOURCES**
Calcium			
Nerve transmission	Calcium kidney stones	↓ Quality of bone and teeth	Alfalfa
Clotting cascade	↑ Calcium deposition into soft	↓ Milk production	Milk
Cardiac function	tissue	Fish by-products	Soybean meal
Muscle contraction	Osteomalacia	Osteoporosis	Bone meal
Milk production	↑ Blood calcium level	Hypocalcemia (tetany)	Dicalcium phosphate
	↓ Absorption of Zn, Mg, Fe, Cu	Rickets (young)	supplement
Phosphorus			
Milk secretion	↓ Absorption of Ca	Similar to Ca	Meat meals
Building muscle	Urinary stones if Ca low	Osteomalacia	Soybean oil meal
Teeth and bone development	Water belly	Rickets (young)	Wheat bran
Acid-base balance		Hematuria	Bone meal
Protein metabolism		Pica	Monosodium phosphate
		↓ Breeding capability	supplement
Sodium			
Muscle contraction	↑ Toxicity with ↓ H$_2$O intake	↓ Breeding capability	Molasses
Absorption of carbohydrates	Staggering	Cravings: urine drinking	Meat by-products
Part of sweat and bile	Blindness	↓ Growth rate	Salt and mineral blocks
Acid-base balance	Hypertension	↓ Milk production	Monosodium glutamate
Water balance	Neurologic disorders	Weight loss	Osmotic pressure supplement
		↓ Appetite	
Potassium			
Heart function	↓ Heart rate	↓ Growth	Molasses
Insulin secretion	↓ Mg use	Excess NaCl depletes K.	Forage
Acid-base balance	Exaggerated when ↓ Mg and	Irregular gait	Soy by-products
Muscle development	H$_2$O restricted	Pica	Carrots
		↓ Weight	Potassium gluconate supplement
Chlorine			
Water balance	Bone loss	↓ Appetite	Meat meals
Osmotic pressure	Metabolic acidosis	↓ Growth	Molasses
Acid-base balance	Rare	Alkalosis	Salt blocks (NaCl)
HCl production in stomach		↓ Respiratory rate	Potassium chloride supplement
		Muscle cramps	
		Convulsions	
		Alfalfa	
Magnesium			
Cellular energy metabolism	Rare	↑ Grass tetany	Meat and bone meal
Alkalinizer		↑ Body temperature	Molasses
Nerve impulse relaxant		Respiratory rate	Wheat bran
Bone and teeth		Hypersalivation	Alfalfa supplements
		Death	
Sulfur			
Carbohydrate metabolism	Hydrogen sulfide gas production	↓ Growth	Meat meal
Insulin production	Polioencephalomalacia	↓ Hair and wool production	Yeast
Hair and wool production			Whey
			Supplements

TABLE 10-3	Microminerals for Livestock		
USE	**TOXICITY**	**DEFICIENCY**	**SOURCES**
Zinc			
Skin	↓ Growth	↓ Growth	Meat meal
Hair	Anemia	↓ Appetite	Corn gluten or germ meal
Bone maintenance	Bone changes	Bone irregularities	Wheat by-product supplements
Synthesis of protein	↑ Appetite	↓ Wound healing	
Development of reproductive organs	Stiff gait	Wool and hair loss Parakeratosis	
Selenium			
Vitamin and sparing tissue damage	Weight loss	White muscle disease (sheep)	Poultry and fish meals
Fatty acid oxidation	Blind staggers	Liver necrosis (pigs)	Wheat by-products
	Lameness		Cereals
	Anemia		Oil-seed meals
	Paralysis		
Manganese			
Bone and cartilage growth	Rare	↓ Growth	Wheat
Clotting cascade	Iron deficiency	Lameness	Grass, alfalfa, hay
Metabolism of nutrients		Reproductive disorders	Corn
			Sorghum supplements
Iodine			
Hormone production	Hyperparathyroidism	↓ Hair quality	Molasses
Influence growth	Goiter	↓ Growth	Meat and bone meal
Muscle tissue development	↓ Use of iodine	Reproductive problems	Oats
Milk production		Abortion	Wheat
Nutrient metabolism			Iodized salt
			Soybean meal
Fluorine			
Bone	↓ Feed use	Rare	Fish meals
Teeth	↓ Hair and wool quality		Present in most foods
	Deformed teeth and bone		
Chromium			
Synthesis of some fatty acids	Rare	Hyperglycemia glucosuria	Wheat
↑ Insulin use		↓ Fat metabolism	Potatoes
Stabilizes DNA and RNA			Corn
			Vegetable oil
			Supplements
Copper			
Pigment of hair and wool	Although rare, sometimes	Swayback (lambs)	Safflower oil
Reproduction	seen in sheep ingestion	↓ Wool quality	Molasses
Skeletal structure	of copper foot bath	Lameness	Grass hays
Hemoglobin construction	Gastroenteritis	Anemia	Cotton seeds
Absorption of iron	Hypersalivation	Diarrhea	Mineral mix
	↓ Appetite		
	Thirst		
Iron			
Hemoglobin production	Irregularity in red blood	Anemia	Fish and meat meals
Muscle oxygenation	cell production	Pica	Safflower
Enzyme activation	Reproductive disorders	Diarrhea	Alfalfa
		↓ Hair coat quality	Corn gluten meal
		↓ Iron in milk	Supplements
Silicon			
Skeletal development	Calculi formation	Skeletal abnormalities	Meat by-products
			Grains

TABLE 10-3	Microminerals for Livestock—cont'd			
USE	**TOXICITY**	**DEFICIENCY**	**SOURCES**
Molybdenum			
Metabolism of fats, carbohydrates, proteins	Diarrhea	Rare	Grass, alfalfa, hay
	Weight		Meat meal
Growth promotion	↓ Hair quality		Corn
Enamel production	↓ Reproduction		Oats
			Wheat
Cobalt			
Formation of vitamin B_{12}	Low toxicity	↓ Skin and hair coat quality	Soybean meal
	May impair iron absorption	Abortion	Meat and poultry meal
		↓ Milk	Corn
		↓ Appetite	Wheat
			Molasses

BOX 10-5	Factors Affecting Water Intake

- Dry-matter intake
- Reproductive status
- Activity
- Type of feeding regimen
- Environment
- Weight
- Age
- Rate of gain

BOX 10-6	Importance of Water

- For digestion, absorption, and use of nutrients
- For production requirements
- Watering methods
- Free water always available
- Twice-daily watering
- Cleanliness
- Water heaters in winter to prevent freezing
- Troughs kept clean

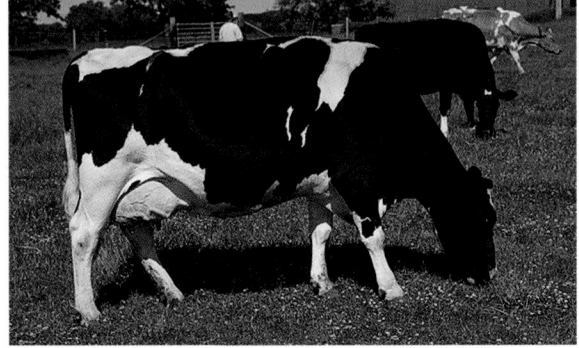

FIGURE 10-2 Holsteins are the predominant breed in the dairy industry.

BOX 10-7	Factors Affecting Dry-Matter Intake

- Stage of lactation
- Body condition
- Quality of feed
- Environment
- Size of cow
- Milk production
- Feeding regimen
- Age

ENERGY

Carbohydrates constitute 50% to 80% of energy on a dry-matter basis of much of the forage and of many grains. Forage possesses a significant fiber content that is broken down by the microbial population in the rumen and used as energy. This unique feature allows ruminants to use feeds that most other animals cannot.

Although the rumen capacity of the dairy cow is considerable, she cannot eat sufficient forage to meet her extensive nutrient needs during lactation. The estimated daily intake for forage is based on body weight and forage quality. A guide for estimating the consumption of forage (dry-matter basis) fed on a free-choice basis is provided in Box 10-7 and Table 10-8.

If cows are allowed to consume all the forage they want, they will not have sufficient rumen capacity to consume enough concentrate to meet the energy requirements for lactation. In general, most dairy farmers try to feed forage at a rate of 1.75% of body weight. The concentrate fed with the forage will vary with the kind of forage offered (a high-protein concentrate will be needed with a low-protein forage) and the availability and cost of the feedstuffs (Table 10-9). The concentrate provides more energy and usually is higher in protein than the forage. Fat use varies with age, environment, and reproductive status. Fat intake during lactation can be 5% to 6% of the total energy intake. Excessive

TABLE 10-4	Water-Soluble Vitamins for Livestock		
FUNCTION	**TOXICITY**	**DEFICIENCY**	**SOURCES**
B Complex			
Biotin			
Metabolism of carbohydrates, fats, proteins Enzyme activities	No known toxicity	↓ Growth ↓ Hair quality Lameness ↓ Reproduction	Young grasses Safflower meal Soybean meal supplements
Thiamin (Vitamin B₁) Coenzyme of energy metabolism Peripheral nerve function Maintenance and assistance of appetite	No known toxicity	Heart irregularities ↓ Body temperature	Wheat Millet Oil-seed meals Oats Supplements
Pyridoxine (Vitamin B₆) Nitrogen metabolism Fat and carbohydrate metabolism	Nontoxic	Anorexia ↓ Growth Eye discharge Anemia	Green pastures Meat and fish meals Corn gluten meal Safflower meal Alfalfa
Cobalamin (Vitamin B₁₂) Red blood cell formation Maintenance of nerve tissue DNA synthesis	Nontoxic	↓ Coordination (blackleg: pigs) ↓ Reproduction	Fish and meat meals Whey Brewer's yeast supplements
Niacin Growth ↓ Cholesterol levels Release of energy from fats, proteins, carbohydrates	Nontoxic	↓ Growth ↓ Appetite Diarrhea Unthriftiness	Wheat barley Yeast supplements
Folic Acid Construction of hemoglobin Manipulation of protein Choline synthesis	Nontoxic	Anemia Diarrhea ↓ Growth	Soybean meal Alfalfa Wheat Meat and fish meal Supplement
Pantothenic Acid Metabolism of fats, proteins, carbohydrates Hemoglobin production Maintenance of normal blood levels	Nontoxic	Neurologic disorder Goose stepping (swine) ↓ Hair quality Enteritis	Wheat bran Alfalfa Safflower meal Supplements
Riboflavin (Vitamin B₂) Metabolism of amino acids and fatty acids Retinal pigment Adrenal function	Nontoxic	↓ Growth Moon blindness (horses) Anemia Unthriftiness ↓ Reproduction (swine)	Alfalfa Green pastures Sweet and white clover Supplements
Vitamin C Absorption of iron Metabolism of folic acid Antioxidant Teeth and bone integrity	Rare in food animals	Rare in food animals	Green pastures Hay Synthesized by the animal

TABLE 10-5	Water Consumption Guidelines	
SPECIES	**WEIGHT, LB**	**CONSUMPTION, GAL/DAY**
Swine		
Pigs	30-125	0.3-2.0
Feeder pigs	126-200	2.0-3.2
Finisher pigs	201-250	3.2-4.0
Sow and boar	150-400	1.3-3.5
maintenance	401-600	3.5-5.2
Sow: late gestation	250-400	4.5-5.0
	401-600	5.0-7.5
Sow: lactation	250-400	5.5-6.5
	401-600	6.5-9.8
Sheep		
Lambs	20-50	0.4-0.6
Feeder lambs	50-110	0.5-1.4
Finisher lambs	111-125	1.4-1.8
Ewes: grain and hay intake*		
Maintenance	150-300	0.3-1.2
Lactation	150-300	0.5-2.4
Rams: grain and hay intake	150-300	0.3-2.0
Cattle		
Calves	100-200	1.2-2.5
	201-400	2.5-4.9
Developing steers and	401-600	4.5-6.2
heifers	601-800	6.0-8.2
	801-1000	8.0-9.8
Finishing Steers		
Pasture	1001-1200	8.5-10.2
Maintenance	800-1000	3.6-4.6
	1001-1200	4.4-7.2
	1201-1400	5.0-7.2
	1401-1600	6.0-9.0
Cows: late gestation	800-1000	4.4-5.5
	1001-1200	5.3-6.6
	1201-1400	6.4-7.9
	1401-1600	7.7-9.5
Beef cows: heifer lactation	800-1000	6.7-15.6
	1001-1200	8.3-18.8
	1201-1400	10.0-21.8
	1401-1600	11.7-25.0
Dairy cows: heifer peak	800-1000	14.8-20.6
lactation†	1001-1201	18.5-24.3
	1201-1400	22.5-28.8
	1401-1600	28.0-32.2
	1601-1800	30.5-36.0

*Intake is influenced dramatically by factors found in Box 14-6. Table is intended as a guideline.
†Dairy cattle intake varies on milk production more than beef cattle.

dietary fat intake can negatively affect rumen microbial activity, depressing fiber use.[5]

PROTEIN

Restriction of protein or energy during lactation can lead to reduced milk production and increased reproductive problems. Protein is supplied by the forage or by the concentrate and should be added at levels to ensure that minimum protein requirements are met (see Tables 10-6 to 10-8). Protein intake that exceeds the requirement is used as energy at a premium value. Protein is an expensive nutrient and is not an economic source of energy. Most cows are fed high-protein legume hay, such as alfalfa, which should supply most or all protein needs during lactation. Nonprotein nitrogen supplied as urea can be an effective feedstuff to supply protein equivalents in dairy rations.

MINERALS AND VITAMINS

Milk is composed of 0.7% minerals on a dry-weight basis. The average cow will lactate 140 lb of mineral as a portion of the milk produced per year. A balanced mineral intake is essential; mineral requirements for lactation are given in Tables 10-6 to 10-8.

Rumen microorganisms can synthesize water-soluble vitamins, whereas vitamin K is the only fat-soluble vitamin readily synthesized by microorganisms. Supplementation of water-soluble vitamins or vitamin K normally is not necessary in rations for ruminants.

Forage of good quality that is properly harvested normally contains adequate levels of vitamin E and the precursor of vitamin A, carotene. Vitamin A is stored for extended periods in the body. Vitamin D is synthesized through ultraviolet radiation by the skin or is added to a dairy ration as sun-cured forage or a vitamin supplement.

DAIRY CALVES

Newborn calves require the mother's colostrum within the first 72 hours of life to acquire energy and maternal immunity from disease. Peak benefits of colostrum intake are realized within the first 24 hours postpartum. Optimally, the first milking colostrum should be given to the calf at 10% to 12% of the calf's weight, with at least one-half administered within 4 to 6 hours after birth. Colostrum can be successfully frozen and used at a later date and diluted equally with water should diarrhea occur because of the richness of the colostrum. Initial sucking of the calf will create a bypass of the rumen, allowing the milk to go directly into the abomasum. This ability will decrease as the calf ages and the rumen becomes functional. Calves normally start on milk replacers and then are offered calf starters within the first week of life. Calf-starter rations are commonly fed until about 3 months of age at a rate of 5 to 7 lb of calf starter per day. During the first week of life, a forage source should be added to the diet selection along with free-choice water. Calves are typically weaned at 4 to 8 weeks of age and are accustomed to solid food.

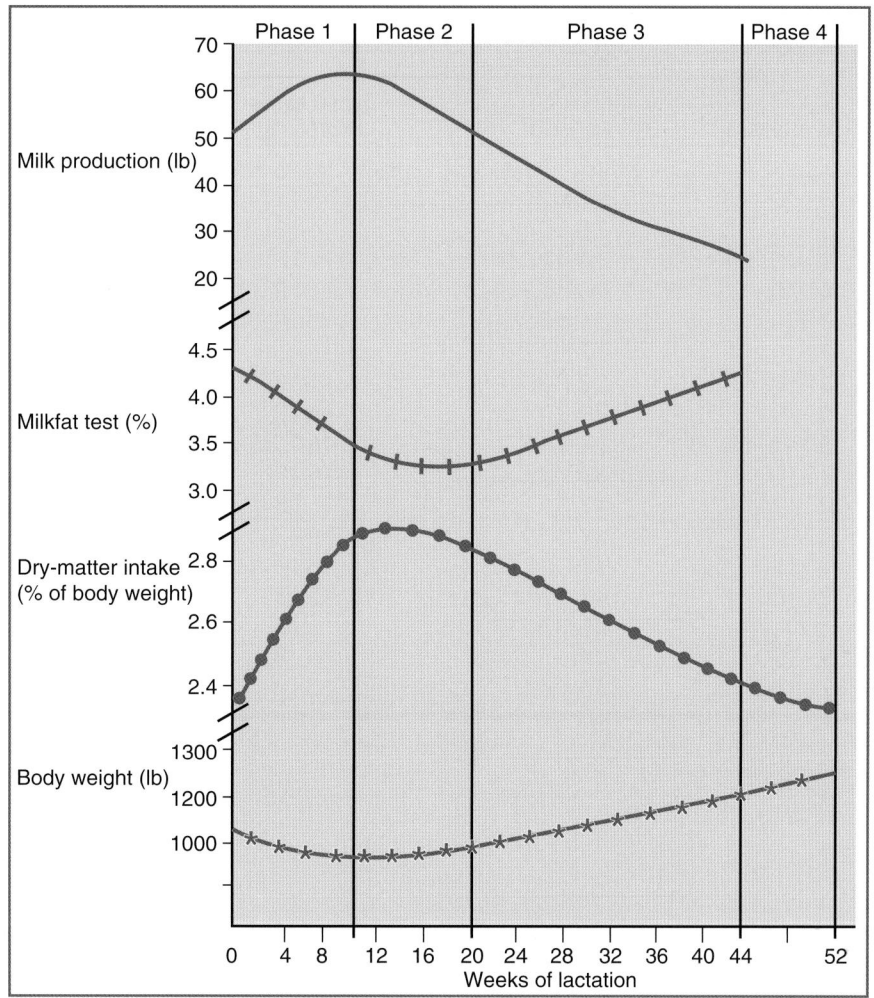

FIGURE 10-3 Milk production varies during a typical 52-week production phase. Disparity is also observed in milk fat content, dry-matter intake requirements, and body weight.

| TABLE 10-6 | Daily Feeding Considerations in Developing Female Dairy Cattle* |

WEIGHT, LB	NE, MCAL†	TOTAL CRUDE PROTEIN, %	MINERALS‡	
			CA²⁺	P
200-399	6.4-11.5	16-18	15-18	9-15
400-599	11.5-15.4	12-16	18-23	13-15
600-799	15.4-19.5	12-14	23-24	15-17
800-999	19.5-23.9	12-14	24-26	17-18
1000-1199	23.9-28.4	12-14	26-28	18-19
1200-1399	28.4-33.8	12-14	28-30	19-21

*Ranges shown in table are to be used as guidelines, with recognition that variations can occur as a result of breed, milk production levels, butter fat content, rate of gain, and lactation cycle.
†Net energy (NE) expressed in megacalories (Mcal).
‡Ca²⁺/phosphorus ratio needs to be maintained from 0.43% to 0.66%; levels above 0.95% to 100% can result in decreased performance and metabolic abnormalities.

BEEF CATTLE

Feeding represents almost three-fourths of the cost of production of beef cattle.[6] Beef producers control their profitability by attaining optimal nutrient intake with the least-cost feed formulation. Profitability hinges on their ability to balance the use of resources, such as pasture and feedlot, with the production of high-quality finishing animals generated by the breeding herd. Beef production usually is divided into two primary areas: cow-calf production and finishing cattle.

> *TECHNICIAN NOTE*   Feeding represents 75% of the cost of beef cattle production.

COW-CALF PRODUCTION

A live calf from each cow each year should be the goal of the profitable cow-calf producer. Nutrition has a large impact on

TABLE 10-7　Daily Guidelines for Lactating Dairy Cows*

WEIGHT, LB	MILK YIELD, LB	NE, MCAL†	TOTAL CRUDE PROTEIN, %	MINERALS† CA²⁺	MINERALS† P
800	15-45	13.1-21.6	12-16	40-77	25-49
	45-60	21.6-25.8	16-17	77-96	49-61
	61-75	25.8-34.0	16-18	96-115	61-78
1000	20-40	14.9-20.3	12-16	44-70	29-44
	41-70	20.3-25.6	16-18	70-114	44-73
	71-90	25.6-36.3	16-18	114-146	73-86
1200	20-40	17.0-23.7	12-16	50-81	33-52
	41-60	23.7-30.3	16-18	81-110	52-70
	61-80	30.3-37.0	16-18	110-139	70-87
1400	50-75	27.7-35.7	15-17	95-131	62-83
	76-100	35.7-43.7	16-18	131-165	83-104
	101-125	43.7-51.7	16-18	165-200	104-126
1600	60-90	31.0-40.0	15-17	108-146	69-92
	91-120	40.0-48.3	16-18	146-184	92-116
	121-150	48.3-57.0	16-18	184-221	116-137
1800	60-90	40.9-44.6	16-18	121-164	78-104
	91-120	44.6-54.4	16-18	164-207	104-131
	121-150	54.4-64.1	16-18	207-249	131-157

*This table is designed to be used only as a guideline. Feed to maintain body condition. Table assumes a 4% milk fat content of lactation.
†Net energy (NE) measured in megacalories (Mcal).
‡Mineral values assume that balance has been established. Variations occur with breed, lactation phase, milk yield, and age.

TABLE 10-8　Daily Nutrient Considerations for Dairy Cattle*

WEIGHT, LB	ME, MCAL†	TOTAL CRUDE PROTEIN, G	MINERALS, G‡ CA²⁺	MINERALS, G‡ P	VITAMINS, 1000 IU A	VITAMINS, 1000 IU D
Females: 60 Days Before Gestation						
800-1000	13.8-16.4	850-925	24-30	16-18	30-35	12-14
1000-1200	16.4-19.2	925-1000	30-35	18-22	35-42	14-17
1200-1400	19.2-21.5	1000-1100	35-42	22-26	42-48	17-19
1400-1600	21.5-23.6	1100-1200	42-45	26-30	48-56	19-22
Dairy Bulls						
1000-1300	14.3-17.8	775-900	16-20	10-12	17.00-21.00	2.7-3.3
1301-1500	17.8-19.7	900-1000	20-24	12-15	21.00-25.25	3.3-3.9
1501-1700	19.7-21.6	1000-1125	24-28	15-18	25.25-29.50	3.9-4.6
1701-1900	21.6-23.5	1125-1225	28-32	18-20	29.50-33.75	4.6-5.3
1901-2100	23.5-25.3	1225-1325	32-36	20-22	33.75-38.00	5.3-5.9
2101-2300	25.3-27.0	1325-1425	36-40	22-25	38.00-42.50	5.9-6.6
2301-2500	27.0-28.8	1425-1520	40-44	25-28	42.50-46.60	6.6-7.3
2501-2700	28.0-30.4	1520-1610	44-48	28-30	46.60-50.90	7.3-7.9
2701-2900	30.4-32.1	1610-1700	48-52	30-32	50.90-55.10	7.9-8.6

*Ranges shown in table are to be used as guidelines, with recognition that variations can occur because of milk production levels, butter fat content, rate of gain, and lactation cycle.
†Metabolizable energy (ME) measured in megacalories (Mcal).
‡Ca²⁺/phosphorus ratio needs to be maintained from 0.43% to 0.66%; levels above 0.95% to 100% can result in decreased performance and metabolic abnormalities.

TABLE 10-9	Forage Quality
FORAGE QUALITY	**DAILY INTAKE, % BODY WEIGHT**
Excellent	3.0
Good	2.5
Average	2.0
Fair	1.5
Poor	1.0

BOX 10-8 | Typical Grain: Nutritional Overview

- 20% (or less) protein
- 18% (or less) crude fiber
- Variable moisture
- 85% (or less) carbohydrate
- 6% (or less) fat
- 75% to 80% total digestible nutrients (TDNs)

BOX 10-9 | Signs of Undernutrition

- ↓ Growth
- ↓ Hair and/or skin quality
- Skeletal irregularities
- ↓ Reproductive capabilities
- ↓ Immune function
- Death

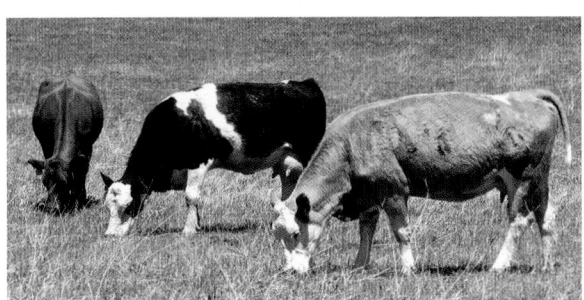

FIGURE 10-4 Beef cows constitute the majority of animals used in pasture production systems. Good pasture rotation management ensures optimal nutrition for grazing animals.

BOX 10-10 | Protein Deficiency and Toxicity in Cattle

- Deficiency
- ↓ Appetite
- Weight loss
- ↓ Growth
- ↓ Reproductive capability
- ↓ Milk production
- Toxicity
- Ammonia: avoid >40% excess protein or nonprotein nitrogen (NPN) intake

the beef-breeding herd. Cows gaining weight just before and during the breeding season have a shorter period between calving and the first estrus period and typically have higher conception rates.

Energy

Carbohydrates are the major energy source for beef cows, followed by proteins and fat. Forage commonly fed to beef cows possesses a significant fiber content that is broken down by the microbial population in the rumen and used as energy.

> **TECHNICIAN NOTE** Carbohydrates are the major energy source for beef cows.

Feeding of beef cows can be very economical because high-quality forage or pasture can supply all energy needs with no need for energy supplementation from grains or fats (Figure 10-4). In the summer, pasture normally will supply adequate energy for the cow. If pasture is inadequate, supplemental energy should be provided in the form of silage or hay. In the winter, pregnant cows are fed wintering rations (a combination of forage, grain, and a protein source supplemented with vitamins and minerals) to meet energy needs with minimal weight gain (Box 10-8). Cows in good condition are more tolerant to the stresses of winter and require less maintenance energy per unit of weight than do cows in poor condition.

Protein

Most pasture, silage, and forage contain adequate levels of protein to meet the needs of the breeding cow. If low-grade

roughage (e.g., cobs, straw, stalks) is fed over extended periods of time, the ration must be supplemented daily with 1 to 1.5 lb of a 35% to 45% crude protein supplement. A review of deficiency and toxicity signs can be found in Boxes 10-9 and 10-10. Use of animal protein sources derived from ruminant species *is not allowed* in beef-breeding–herd rations. This is done to prevent the possible transmission of BSE.

Minerals and Vitamins

Mineral supplementation will be necessary and usually is offered on a free-choice basis when animals are on pasture (Figure 10-5). Trace-mineral salt blocks and granular salt are popular methods of offering minerals and salt to animals on pasture. Good-quality pasture and roughage are adequate in vitamins A and E, with ample levels to meet the needs of breeding cows. Supplemental vitamin A should be provided when low-grade roughage or long-stored hays are used as a major source of energy in wintering rations. Some mineral mixes contain a stabilized form of vitamin A.

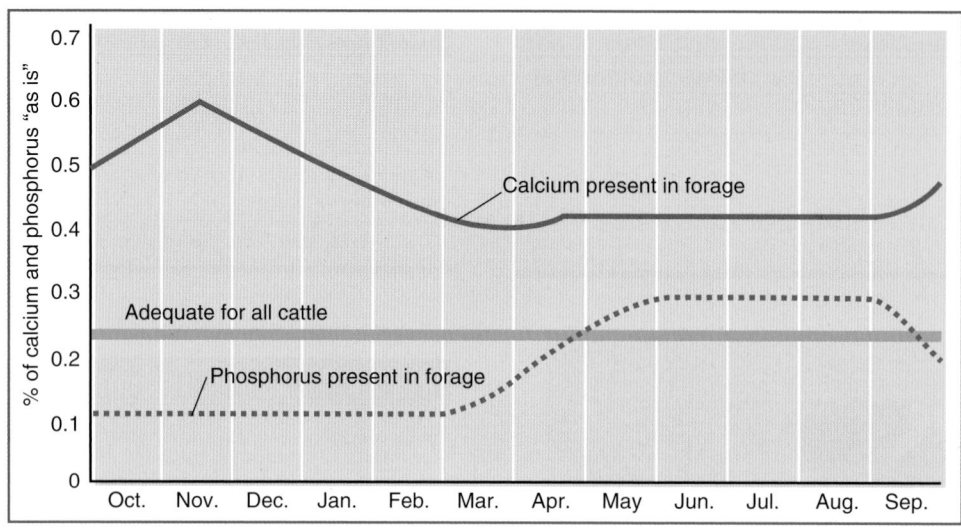

FIGURE 10-5 Availability of calcium and phosphorus varies greatly during the seasons of the year, and intake should be supplemented if inadequate amounts are present in livestock forage sources.

BOX 10-11	Feeding Considerations for Calves

Dairy Calves

Days 1 to 3: obtain colostrum from dam

Days 4 to 7: transition to milk replacer or other liquid feed; begin offering starter and free-choice water

Days 5 to 84: starter and free-choice water through weaning; begin to offer forage

Beef Calves

Ensure that calf nurses within 2 hours of birth to obtain vital colostrum.

Ensure that calf continues to thrive and that cow does not show signs of mastitis or decreased milk production.

Orphans

Can sometimes be grafted to another cow

Ensure that colostrum has been administered.

Feed like dairy calves

CALVES

Basic food for calves consists of mother's milk (Box 10-11) plus access to pasture or forage fed to the cows. Many cow-calf producers offer calves a highly palatable creep feed to supply additional nutrients, leading to improved weaning weight and decreased weight loss by nursing cows. Creep-fed calves will weigh an extra 30 to 50 lb by weaning time. The greatest response to creep feeding is seen when pasture is inadequate or the quality is poor. Beef calves generally are weaned at 7 to 8 months of age.

> **TECHNICIAN NOTE** Creep-fed calves can weigh 30 to 50 lb more by weaning time.

FINISHING CATTLE

The *finishing* of cattle refers to the time in the growth phase of growing cattle when they are fed to produce beef that is desirable to the food consumer. Most finished cattle are between 1 and 2 years of age and weigh more than 1000 lb. The goal of the finishing feeding program is to maintain a maximum feed intake and weight gain without causing digestive upsets (Table 10-10).

Energy

High-energy diets are used to increase weight gain, improve carcass characteristics, and decrease the cost of energy compared with diets high in fiber. Total dry-feed intake commonly will be 2% to 3% of the animal's body weight. The feed contains high levels of grains to supply readily available energy (Figure 10-6). Cattle fed these rations are prone to develop digestive upset (rumen acidosis), founder, or liver abscesses and require greater attention and management to prevent these problems.

Protein

Protein requirements (9% to 14%) are greatly affected by age, size of the animal, and growth rate. Young cattle require more protein (as a percentage of the diet) than do older cattle. Protein sources cost more than feed grains, but experienced finishing cattle producers know that a protein deficiency is more expensive than a slight protein excess in the ration. When protein is deficient, energy is not well used, and performance suffers.

Supplemental protein for finishing cattle can be provided by natural protein sources or nonprotein nitrogen (e.g., urea). Nonprotein nitrogen sources are used most efficiently by cattle consuming relatively high levels of grain. A normal range of urea intake for many finishing rations is 0.10 to 0.15 lb per animal per day.

Minerals and Vitamins

Calcium is often added to the high-grain diets fed to finishing cattle. Generally, when forage (especially legumes) constitutes more than 25% of a finishing ration, additional

TABLE 10-10	Daily Nutrient Considerations for Beef Cattle*			
			MINERALS, G	
WEIGHT, LB	**NE, MCAL†**	**TOTAL PROTEIN, LB**	**CA²⁺**	**P**
Growing/Finishing‡				
300-400	3.0-3.6	0.75-1.5	10-42	6-8
401-500	3.7-4.4	0.90-1.9	11-40	8-18
501-600	4.4-5.0	1.0-2.0	12-38	9-19
601-700	5.0-5.6	1.1-2.1	13-36	11-19
701-800	5.6-6.2	1.3-2.1	14-34	12-20
801-900	6.2-6.8	1.4-2.2	15-33	14-20
901-1000	6.8-7.3	1.5-2.3	16-37	16-22
1001-1100	7.3-7.5	1.6-2.3	19-35	18-23
1101-1200	7.5-7.8	1.7-2.4	20-34	20-24
1201-1300	7.8-8.4	1.8-2.4	20-32	20-24
Yearling Heifers, Early to Late Gestation				
700-800	8.0-8.6	1.3-1.6	19-28	19-22
801-900	8.6-9.1	1.4-1.7	21-28	15-19
901-1000	9.1-9.8	1.5-1.7	20-23	14-20
1001-1100	9.8-10.3	1.5-1.7	23-25	18-20
1101-1200	10.3-10.8	1.6-1.8	25-27	20-21
1201-1300	10.8-11.4	1.6-1.8	26-28	21-23
1301-1400	11.4-12.0	1.8-2.0	26-28	23-24
Lactating Cow/Heifer				
800-900	10.0-14.0	2.0-2.4	23-35	19-20
901-1000	10.4-14.5	1.9-2.5	24-36	19-20
1001-1100	11.0-15.0	2.0-2.6	25-38	20-22
1101-1200	11.5-15.5	2.0-2.7	27-39	22-23
1201-1300	12.0-16.2	2.1-2.3	23-41	23-25
1301-1400	12.5-17.0	2.2-2.9	30-42	25-26
Breeding Bulls				
1300-1500	9.3-10.3	2.0-2.2	23-31	22-25
1501-1700	10.3-11.3	1.7-2.2	23-31	22-25
1701-1900	11.3-12.3	2.0-2.2	26-29	26-29
1901-2100	12.3-13.3	2.0-2.3	27-33	27-33

From National Research Council: Nutrient requirements of beef cattle, ed 8, Washington, DC, 1990, National Academic Press.
*Values represent guidelines, and individual variations dictate the constant appraisal of body condition to ensure desirable results.
†Net energy (NE) measured in megacalories (Mcal).
‡Assumes medium- to large-frame steers.

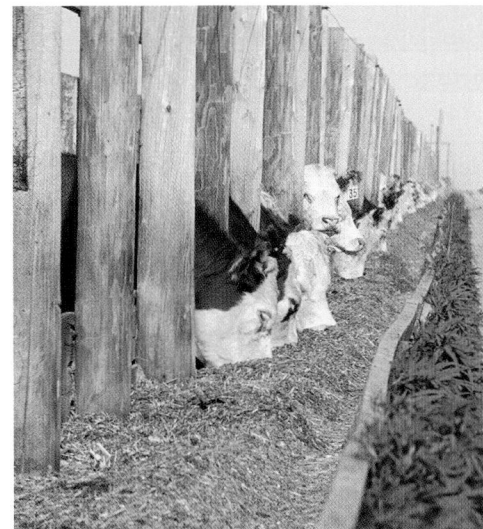

FIGURE 10-6 Large quantities of forage and grain are ingested by finishing cattle on a daily basis; this is paramount to fulfillment of energy requirements.

BOX 10-12	Salt Use in Cattle

Rule 1: Supply
3 to 5 lb in each spring and summer month
1 to 1.5 lb in each fall and winter month

Rule 2: Availability
Make salt available at all times.

Rule 3: Rotation
Continue to rotate salt.
Mangers throughout pasture

vitamin A daily because they contain high levels of grain. Vitamins E and D are added to finishing rations when feed ingredients are devoid of these vitamins, or when production practices merit their inclusion (see Tables 10-3 and 10-4).

SHEEP

Feeding represents the single largest cost of production for all types of sheep operations. Sheep producers control their revenue by offering feed that supports optimal production, is cost-effective, and minimizes nutrition-related problems. Sheep production is divided into two principal areas: the breeding flock and lamb production.

BREEDING FLOCK

Ewes are the foundation of the sheep operation; they produce lambs and generate wool (Box 10-13). These two cash crops can be influenced greatly by feeding management. The mature ewe (3 to 8 years of age) needs only sufficient feed to maintain her normal weight from the time her lambs are weaned until 15 weeks (21-week gestation) into her next

calcium is not required. Grain contains adequate levels of phosphorus to meet the needs of finishing cattle. Finishing rations are balanced to contain a calcium/phosphorus ratio of 2:1 or higher. Salt is added to diets or is fed on a free-choice basis to finishing cattle to meet the sodium requirement (Box 10-12). The less forage that is formulated into the diet, the greater is the need for trace-mineral supplementation.

High-quality forage contains adequate quantities of vitamin A precursors and vitamin E. Generally, finishing rations are supplemented with 20,000 to 30,000 IU of

BOX 10-13	Common Sheep Breeds

Wool Breeds
Rambouillet
Merino
Debouillet
Columbia
Targhee

Meat Breeds
Suffolk
Dorset
Hampshire
Shropshire
Southdown
Oxford

Combination Breeds
Polypay
Texel
Tunis
Leicester
Cheviot

BOX 10-14	Energy Intake Variables in Sheep

- Breed size
- Gender
- Reproductive status
- Weaning age
- Multiple birth
- Age
- Environment
- Stress
- Shearing
- Forage quality

BOX 10-15	Advantages and Disadvantages of Pasture Feeding Livestock

Advantages
- Provides exercise
- Uses land unsuitable for other purposes
- Decreases diseases transmitted through close contact with other animals
- Decreases feed costs
- Good-quality pastures can provide quality feedstuffs.

Disadvantages
- Depends on soil quality (deficiencies result in poorer quality pasture)
- Large acreage often needed to support animal's energy requirements
- Land may be made valuable for other uses.

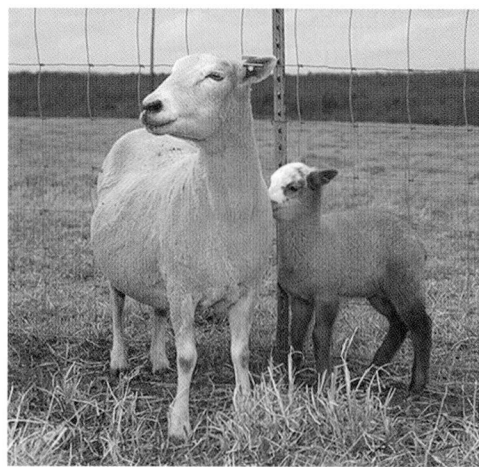

FIGURE 10-7 Ewes serve as the foundation of the sheep operation. Good feeding management ensures healthy lambs and first-class wool production.

pregnancy, assuming that not much weight was lost during lactation. Pasture is adequate to meet her nutrient needs during this period of production (see Figures 10-1 and 10-5 for reviews of the nutrient composition of pasture).

Energy
The energy requirements of the ewe largely depend on the stage of the reproductive cycle (Box 10-14). During the first two-thirds of the pregnancy, energy requirements are close to those required for MNRs, and good pasture or hays can supply all energy needs (Box 10-15). In the last trimester, energy requirements increase, and forage must be supplemented with grains. Poor care during the last trimester of pregnancy leads to lambing problems, lower wool output, and depressed milk production. A common problem attributed to poor nutrition in ewes is lambing paralysis or ketosis. Feeding inadequate forage with little or no grain can create a deficiency of usable carbohydrates during the last trimester of pregnancy in ewes carrying twins or triplets and can lead to paralysis and coma in the mother. Prevention is the least

expensive route to avoid pregnancy disease in the breeding flock. Energy requirements are highest during lactation and are proportional to the number of lambs the ewe is nursing (Figure 10-7 and Table 10-11).

TECHNICIAN NOTE A common problem attributed to poor nutrition in ewes is lambing paralysis or ketosis.

Protein
Adequate protein intake ensures good wool production and reproductive function (Box 10-16 and Table 10-11). The most limiting amino acid for the maturation of wool is methionine; protein ingested by the breeding flock must contain adequate levels of this amino acid. Most often, pasture, silage, and forage contain adequate levels of protein and amino acids to meet the needs of the breeding flock. If low-grade roughage (e.g., cobs, straw, stalks) is fed over extended periods of time, the ration must be supplemented daily with a protein supplement or with a nonprotein nitrogen source (Box 10-17).

TABLE 10-11	Daily Nutritional Considerations in Sheep

WEIGHT, LB	ME, MCAL*	DAILY CONSUMPTION (AS FED), LB/DAY	TOTAL CRUDE PROTEIN, LB/DAY	MINERALS, G CA^{2+}	P	VITAMINS A, 1000 IU	E, IU
Weaned Lambs to Finishing							
20-40	1.3-2.6	1.2-2.9	0.35-0.45	4.9-6.5	2.2-2.9	0.47	12
41-60	2.6-3.2	2.9-3.4	0.45-0.48	6.5-7.2	2.9-3.4	0.95	24
61-80	3.2-3.8	3.4-3.7	0.48-0.51	7.2-8.6	3.4-4.3	1.40	21
81-100	3.8-4.0	3.7-4.1	0.51-0.53	8.6-9.4	4.3-4.8	2.30	25
101-Finish	4.0-4.2	3.8-4.1	0.53	8.2-9.4	4.5-4.8	2.80	25
Ewe Lambs							
Early							
80-100	2.9-3.0	3.4-3.7	0.35-0.36	5.2-5.5	2.7-2.8	3.0-3.1	21
101-120	3.0-3.1	3.7-3.9	0.35-0.36	5.2-5.5	2.8-3.0	3.1-3.4	22
121-140	3.1-3.2	3.7-3.9	0.35-0.36	5.5	3.0-3.3	3.4-3.7	24
141-160	3.1-3.3	3.9-4.1	0.35-0.36	5.5	3.3-3.4	3.4-3.7	26
Late							
80-101	5.0-5.4	3.7-3.9	0.41-0.44	6.4-7.8	5.0-5.4	3.1-3.9	22
101-120	5.4-5.8	3.0-4.1	0.44-0.45	7.8-8.1	5.4-5.8	3.9-4.3	24
121-140	5.8-6.2	4.1-4.4	0.45-0.48	8.1-8.2	5.8-6.2	4.3-4.7	26
141-160	6.2-6.3	4.4-4.7	0.46-0.48	8.1-8.2	6.2-6.3	4.3-4.7	27
Lactation							
80-100	2.9-3.0	5.1-5.7	0.67-0.71	8.4-8.7	5.6-6.0	4.0-5.0	32-34
101-120	3.0-3.1	5.7-6.1	0.71-0.74	8.7-9.0	6.0-6.4	5.0-6.0	34-36
121-140	3.1-3.2	6.1-6.7	0.74-0.77	9.0-9.3	6.4-6.9	6.0-7.0	36-38
Ewes: Maintenance to Early and Mid Gestation							
110-130	2.4-2.6	2.4-2.9	0.21-0.27	2.0-3.2	1.8-2.5	2.35-2.80	18-20
131-150	2.6-2.7	2.5-3.1	0.27-0.29	2.5-3.5	2.4-2.9	2.80-3.30	20-21
151-170	2.7-2.9	2.9-3.7	0.29-0.31	2.8-3.8	2.4-3.3	3.30-3.75	21-22
171-190	2.9-3.1	3.0-3.9	0.31-0.33	2.9-3.9	2.8-3.4	3.75-4.25	22-24
Ewes: Late Gestation (Last 30 Days) and Lactation							
100-130	4.0-6.0	4.1-5.9	0.43-0.45	5.6-6.9	4.8-5.2	4.25-5.10	24-27
131-150	4.2-6.6	4.4-6.1	0.45-0.47	6.9-9.1	5.2-6.6	5.10-5.95	26-28
151-170	4.4-7.0	4.7-6.3	0.47-0.49	7.6-9.5	6.6-7.4	5.95-6.80	28-30
171-190	4.7-7.5	4.9-6.6	0.49-0.51	8.5-9.6	6.8-7.8	6.80-7.65	30-33

*ME (metabolizable energy) is measured in megacalories (Mcal); 1 Mcal = 1000 kcal.

BOX 10-16	Variables in Protein Requirements of Sheep

- Breed size
- Reproductive status
- Age
- Body condition
- Ratio of protein to energy
- NPN availability

BOX 10-17	Feeding Guidelines for Nonprotein Nitrogen (Npn) Use in Sheep

- Balance NPN within total nutritional profile. Feed continuously after 3- to 6-week transition.
- Avoid sporadic availability.
- Maintain nitrogen/sulfur ratio at not more than 10:1.
- Restrict use to not more than 1.0% dry matter, with one-third of total nitrogen ration as NPN.
- Prevent excess intake and possible toxicity.
- Watch NPN levels when they coincide with high roughage intake.

From Ensminger ME, et al: Feeds and nutrition, Clovis, CA, 1990, Ensminger Publishing; Maynard LA, et al: Animal nutrition, ed 7, New York, 1979, McGraw-Hill; McDonald P, et al: Animal nutrition, New York, 1995, Longman Scientific and Technical; Naylor JM, et al: Large animal clinical nutrition, St Louis, 1991, Mosby.

BOX 10-18	Milk Replacement for Lambs

Optimal Requirement
25% to 30% fat
20% to 25% protein derived from milk product
<30% lactose derived from milk product

Feeding
Provide ration immediately.
Ration should be 20% to 24% protein, high in vitamins and minerals, well balanced, and ground fine.
Note: Avoid cow's milk (too high in lactose).

From Ensminger ME, et al: Feeds and nutrition, Clovis, CA, 1990, Ensminger Publishing; Maynard LA, et al: Animal nutrition, ed 7, New York, 1979, McGraw-Hill; McDonald P, et al: Animal nutrition, New York, 1995, Longman Scientific and Technical; Naylor JM, et al: Large animal clinical nutrition, St Louis, 1991, Mosby.

Minerals and Vitamins

Trace-mineral salt blocks and granular salt represent popular methods of offering minerals and salt to ewes on pasture. Sheep store copper well in various organs and tissues and develop toxicity symptoms to copper more rapidly than other livestock. Care should be taken to prevent exposing sheep to high levels of copper in their trace-mineral source.

Good-quality pasture and roughage are adequate in vitamins A and E, with ample levels to meet the needs of the breeding flock. Supplemental vitamin A should be provided when low-grade roughage or long-stored hays are used as a major source of energy in wintering rations (see Table 10-11).

LAMBS

Lambs must be nursed with colostrum milk within the first hour after birth to improve survivability. Colostrum milk provides immunologic protection and energy for the newborn lamb. The lamb must consume at least 6 to 8 oz of colostrum to receive immunologic protection. Lambs are weaned successfully at 8 weeks of age or earlier.

> **TECHNICIAN NOTE** Lambs must receive colostrum within the first hour after birth to have immunologic protection.

Lambs can be successfully weaned from their mother at 1 day of age and offered a milk replacer (Box 10-18). They should be weaned from the milk replacer at 3 to 4 weeks of age and transitioned to a high-quality, palatable solid feed. Post-weaning rations (until lambs reach 50 lb) should consist of high-quality protein (16% to 20% crude protein), should provide high energy, and should be well fortified with vitamins and minerals.

Grower (50 to 85 lb) and finisher (more than 85 lb) rations for lambs are normally formulated to contain 15% to 16% and 13% to 14% protein, respectively. A simple ration of shelled corn, long alfalfa hay, and supplement

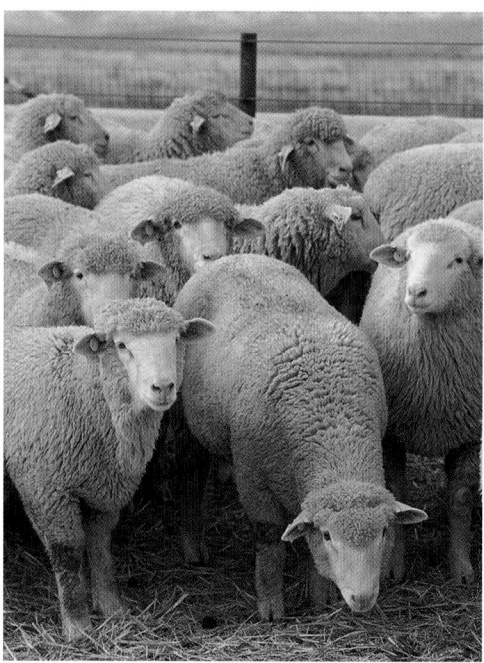

FIGURE 10-8 Optimal feed regimens in sheep will provide excellent results.

(protein, calcium, vitamins, trace minerals) can be fed to growing-finishing lambs (Figure 10-8). Research does not clearly indicate the need for vitamin additions to rations for early lambs, but it has become a common practice to fortify these rations with vitamins A, D, and E (see Table 10-11).

Large, fast-growing lambs are susceptible to overeating disease (enterotoxemia), which can cause death. This disease is caused by toxins produced by *Clostridium perfringens* and appears to be related to overeating by lambs of a ration high in grain. Vaccination with bacterin or toxoid can be used for lambs older than 2 months of age and will virtually eliminate symptoms of overeating disease.

SWINE

The swine industry has changed dramatically over the past 30 years. Most pigs are raised in confinement to reduce labor requirements for the owner and to improve the environment for the animal. The genetic base of the swine industry has changed to a more prolific breeding herd and better-muscled, faster-growing offspring. Feed still accounts for 60% to 70% of the cost of raising swine. Few swine are grazed on pasture; most are fed complete high-grain rations in self-feeders or are limit-fed if in the breeding herd. The production of pigs normally is divided into three distinct areas: the breeding herd, starter pigs, and growing-finishing pigs.

> **TECHNICIAN NOTE** Feed accounts for 60% to 70% of the cost of raising swine.

BREEDING HERD

For profitable production of swine, sows must be bred and must gestate 114 days, nurse a litter for 21 to 35 days, and

TABLE 10-12	Complete Feed Ration Considerations in Swine		
	COMPLETE RATION		
STAGE WEIGHT	PROTEIN, %	FED, LB	COMMENTS
Weaning pigs (12-20 lb)	20-24	Free feed	Use if weaned early and transitioning to solid feed.
Starter pigs (up to 40 lb)	18-20	Free feed	
Feeder and finisher pigs (40 lb to 220-250 lb finishing weight)	13-18	Free feed*	May be limited in feed after 125 lb
Gilts and sows			
Breeding and maintenance	11-14	4-6	Increase amount to maintain body condition and last month of gestation through weaning.
Gestation	11-14	4-6	
Lactation	14-20	10-15	
Boars	14-16	4-7	Increase in breeding season.

*See text on feeding methods.

rebreed within 10 days after weaning; this cycle must be continued for five to seven litters. Nutrition plays a key role in allowing this to occur, especially during lactation (Table 10-12).

Energy

After breeding and for the first two-thirds of gestation, energy intake is limited to 6000 to 7000 kcal ME per day. The total amount of feed is increased during the last third of gestation; 9000 to 10,000 kcal ME is provided per day, and this contributes additional energy to developing fetuses during this last stage of gestation. Overfeeding energy during gestation has a direct negative impact on lactation feed intake; this can impair lactation performance.

In lactation, the goal of the swine producer is to encourage as much energy intake by the lactating female as possible (15,000 to 20,000 kcal ME per day). Sows are often fed twice per day to ensure fresh feed and improved energy intake. Frequently, fat is added to the lactation ration to improve palatability and energy density. Sows peak in milk production between the second and third weeks of lactation, and they should be full fed to support the production of milk. A guideline for feeding lactating sows is to offer 4 to 5 lb of the base ration plus 1 additional pound for every pig nursing (Figure 10-9).

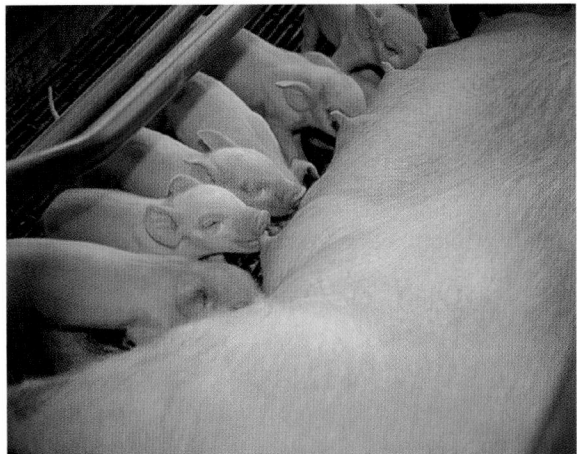

FIGURE 10-9 Sow nursing piglets in containment of farrowing pen.

BOX 10-19	Prevention of Iron Deficiency Anemia in Baby Pigs

- Allow access to soil that has not been in contact with other pigs.
- Inject 100 to 200 mg iron before 72 hours of age.
- Paint sows' teats lightly with iron solution periodically.
- Encourage prestarter ration creep feeding early.
- Provide iron supplementation in creep feeder.

TECHNICIAN NOTE   Sows are often fed twice daily to ensure adequate energy intake.

Protein

Protein requirements during gestation are relatively low (11% to 12% crude protein, 0.5 lb of protein per day). Development of the fetus and of reproductive tissue requires small amounts of protein each day.

During lactation, sows require higher levels of protein intake to support milk production (2 to 3 lb of protein per day); this is accomplished by feeding a ration with higher protein content at a greater intake level. Sows not fed adequate levels of protein or energy during lactation will support milk production with loss of body tissue stores. Sows can lose more than 100 lb in weight during lactation if not fed proper amounts of energy or protein.

Minerals and Vitamins

Minerals and vitamins need to be supplemented throughout the life of pigs. The breeding herd is normally fed a diet fortified with the minerals calcium, phosphorus, salt, zinc, iron, copper, iodine, selenium, and manganese. Calcium and phosphorus are kept at a balance of 1:1 to 2:1 for all stages of production. Low levels of calcium and phosphorus in breeding-herd rations can lead to fracture and lameness in the female.

Sow's milk is virtually devoid of iron, and anemia of nursing pigs will occur unless they are supplemented with another source of iron (Box 10-19). The two most common ways to supply additional iron are as follows:

1. Injection of iron (150 to 200 mg) as iron dextran or other iron-carbohydrate complexes at 3 days of age.
2. Oral iron solution given at 3 days of age or swabbed onto the dam's udder several times during lactation.

The vitamins supplemented in breeding-herd diets are the fat-soluble vitamins A, D, E, and K and the water-soluble vitamins thiamin, riboflavin, niacin, pantothenic acid, B$_6$, B$_{12}$, choline, biotin, and folic acid. Adequate additions of these vitamins ensure proper development of the fetus in gestation and milk production in lactation (Box 10-20).

> **TECHNICIAN NOTE**   Sow's milk is devoid of iron, and nursing pigs will develop anemia unless they are supplemented with iron.

STARTER PIGS

Pigs are commonly weaned at 3 to 5 weeks of age and remain in the starter phase until they weigh 40 to 50 lb (Figure 10-10). The earlier the age at weaning, the more complex is the ration required to help in the transition from mother's milk to solid food. Starter diets (20% to 24% protein) consist of very complex and nutrient-dense complete feed and therefore are often purchased from a commercial feed manufacturer. The highest-quality ingredients are used to make starter diets and include milk products, fish meal,

---

BOX 10-20 | Orphan Piglet Feeding

Homemade Replacer
32 oz whole cow's milk
Water-soluble antibiotics
1 raw egg
16 oz half-and-half

Directions for Feeding Piglets
Give 2 oz per feeding per piglet every 3 hours.
Feed in a shallow, clean feeding pan.
Be sure that all piglets are eating.
Give iron supplementation as needed.
Start creep feeding at 7 days of age.

---

spray-dried blood products, oats, corn, and fat. Vitamin and mineral supplementation levels are high in starter diets. This feed typically is pelleted and costly (see Table 10-12).

As the pig ages, the complexity and nutrient density of the starter ration decrease, leading to a lower-cost formula. In the last 2 or 3 weeks of the starter period, crude protein decreases to 18% to 20%, and the diet is often offered as a ground feed.

GROWING-FINISHING PIGS

Growing-finishing diets have been modified to complement changes in the genetic base of modern swine. Leaner pigs require higher levels of protein and consume less energy than previous generations (see Table 10-12).

Energy

Complete grower-finisher rations are based on cereal grains and frequently have fat added to increase caloric intake. Fibrous feed ingredients often are not used or are used sparingly to prevent depressions in caloric intake. Corn, wheat, sorghum, and barley, the more popular cereal grains used to supply energy, constitute 60% to 85% of the ration.

Protein

Contemporary swine nutrition concentrates not on the protein content of feed, but on amino acid levels. Lysine typically is the first limiting amino acid in swine formulas. Amino acid levels are decreased as a percentage of the diet throughout the growing-finishing phase.

Amino acid levels are matched to muscle growth throughout the growth period to maximize lean tissue growth. Underfeeding of amino acids depresses muscle deposition, and overfeeding of amino acids leads to excess, which is costly.

Typical protein sources in growing-finishing diets include soybean meal, meat and bone meal, and synthetic amino acids. When protein sources are expensive, synthetic amino acids can replace a portion of the protein source with no loss in performance. The most commonly available synthetic amino acids are lysine, methionine, threonine, and tryptophan (Figure 10-11).

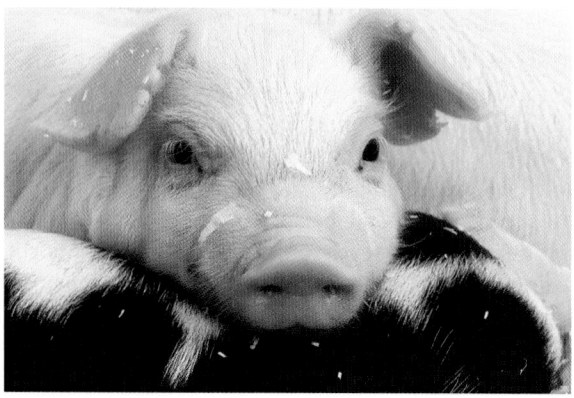

FIGURE 10-10 Young pigs need to be kept in a clean, dry, draft-free environment for optimal health and growth.

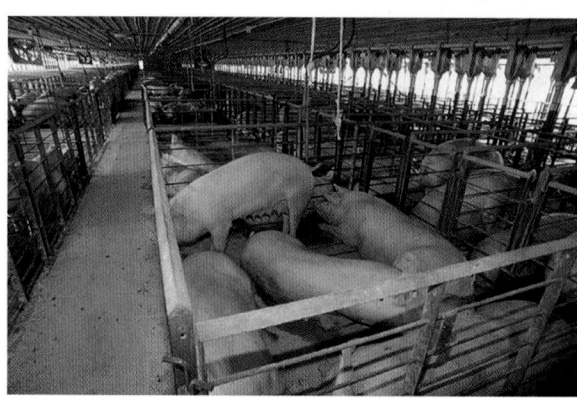

FIGURE 10-11 Grower-finisher pigs are fed large quantities of complete rations to obtain the most desirable carcass quality.

Minerals and Vitamins

Growing-finishing swine are fed diets fortified with the minerals calcium, phosphorus, salt, zinc, iron, copper, iodine, selenium, and manganese. Calcium and phosphorus are kept at a balance of 1:1 to 2:1 throughout this period. Deficiencies of phosphorus will depress growth performance as the animal grows.

Riboflavin, niacin, pantothenic acid, and vitamin B_{12} are the water-soluble vitamins most likely to be deficient in swine diets formulated with grains and plant protein. The fat-soluble vitamins A, D, E, and K also should be added to growing-finishing rations.

HORSES

Horses evolved eating grass and other range forage. Consequently, grass and hays should serve as a foundation for feeding all horses (Figure 10-12). In general, forage intake should be at least 50% of the horse's diet for healthy gut function, and daily forage intake ranges from 1% to 3% of the horse's body weight as dry-matter intake. Feed constitutes the greatest single cost in the horse business, but its economic significance varies more widely than with any other class of livestock. Most horses are kept for recreation, sport, or hobby purposes. Consequently, meeting the nutrient needs of horses is a major factor in determining their efficiency, health, and years of service. As with other animals, the horse needs nutrients for maintenance, growth, reproduction, and production. "Production" with regard to horses is athleticism because unlike other large animal species, they are used primarily for work, competitive sport, and recreation.

> **TECHNICIAN NOTE** Good-quality grass and legume hay are crucial for all horses.

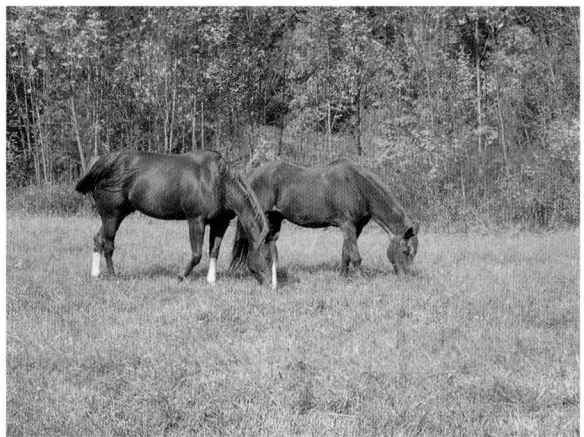

FIGURE 10-12 Horses evolved to forage on grasses and legumes. Good turnout and pasture may serve as the foundation for providing nutrient needs to horses. (Courtesy Dr. Joanna Bassert.)

MAINTENANCE HORSES

Good-quality grass or legume hay, free-choice water, and salt and minerals as needed are the main foods needed by the adult horse during maintenance.

Water

Water is the most important nutrient in the horse's diet. Water could be considered the first limiting nutrient for horses, in that survival depends on water. The amount of water needed on a daily basis will depend on the climate and the horse's activity. Water losses occur through urine, feces, respiratory gases, and water in sweat. During lactation, water is lost through milk. Water intake is proportional to dry-matter intake (DMI). The composition and digestibility of the feedstuffs also affect the intake. Water needs to be supplied to horses in adequate amounts and must have good palatability. Water is involved in the functions of the gut for digestion, for the propulsion of digesta, and for intermediate metabolism, as well as for regulation of body temperature. Water constitutes 65% to 75% of the body weight (BW) of an adult horse and 75% to 80% of a foal's body weight. Voluntary water intake at rest in a moderate or cool environment can range from 25 to 70 ml/kg BW per day. Intake will depend on losses through the kidneys, intestines, skin, lungs, and mammary glands, as well as amounts ingested with ration. A rise in environmental temperature from 15° C to 20° C will increase water requirements by 15% to 20% in horses through sweat losses. Cutaneous fluid losses will increase exponentially when ambient temperatures reach 20° C. Evaporative losses through the skin in horses exercising at low intensity amount to about 70% and respiratory losses about 20% to 30%. Resting horses may lose 0.5 L per hour at 20° C ambient temperature, whereas at 35° C, losses may increase to 1.5 L per hour in heat-unadapted horses at rest and will decrease with heat adaptation.

Energy

Animals that are not pregnant, lactating, growing, or working are considered to be in maintenance status. Depending on the temperament and voluntary activity of the horse, energy requirements will vary between minimum, average, and elevated. Stallions and young adult horses have elevated maintenance requirements. Horses with average voluntary activity have moderate energy requirements, and minimum requirements are applied for rather lymphatic horses. For a 1100-lb horse (500 kg), average energy requirements are about 16.7 Mcal per day (minimum = 30 kcal/kg BW; average = 33.3 kcal/kg BW; elevated = 36.3 kcal/kg BW). The goal for the horse owner is to maintain the horse's weight and condition score (Table 10-13). Horses' body condition score should be assessed regularly (see Table 10-13). The amount of ration offered to a horse is based on the horse's weight. The horse's weight in pounds can be estimated most accurately based on multiplication of the heart girth by the horse's length (from the point of the shoulder to the point of the buttocks), divided by 330. When this number is divided by 2.2, the weight in kg is obtained. When horses are

TABLE 10-13	Equine Body Condition Score	
SCORE	DESCRIPTION	PHOTO
1, Poor	Animal extremely emaciated. Spinous processes, ribs, tailhead, tuber coxae, and ischii projecting prominently. Bone structure of withers, shoulders, and neck easily noticeable. No fatty tissue can be felt.	
2, Very thin	Animal emaciated. Slight fat covering over base of spinous processes, transverse processes of lumbar vertebrae feel rounded. Spinous processes, ribs, tailhead, tuber coxae, and ischii prominent. Withers, shoulders, and neck structures faintly discernible.	
3, Thin	Fat built about halfway on spinous processes, transverse processes cannot be felt. Slight fat cover over the ribs. Spinous processes and ribs easily discernible. Tailhead prominent, but individual vertebrae cannot be visually identified. Tuber coxae appear rounded, but easily discernible. Tuber ischii not distinguishable. Withers, shoulders, and neck accentuated.	
4, Moderately thin	Negative crease along back. Faint outline of ribs discernible. Tailhead prominence depends on conformation, fat can be felt around it. Tuber coxae not discernible. Withers, shoulders, and neck not obviously thin.	
5, Moderate	Back level. Ribs cannot be visually distinguished but can be felt easily. Fat around tailhead beginning to feel spongy. Withers appear rounded over spinous processes. Shoulders and neck blend smoothly into body.	
6, Moderately fleshy	May have crease down back. Fat over ribs feels spongy. Fat around tailhead feels soft. Fat beginning to be deposited alongside of the withers, behind the shoulders, and along the sides of the neck.	
7, Fleshy	May have crease down back. Individual ribs can be felt, but noticeable filling between ribs with fat. Fat around tailhead is soft. Fat deposited along withers, behind shoulders, and along neck.	
8, Fat	Crease down back. Difficult to feel ribs. Fat around tailhead very soft. Area behind shoulder filled with fat. Noticeable thickening of neck. Fat deposited along inner thighs.	

TABLE 10-13	Equine Body Condition Score—cont'd	
SCORE	**DESCRIPTION**	**PHOTO**
9, Extremely fat	Obvious crease down back. Patchy fat appearing over ribs. Bulging fat around tailhead, around withers, behind shoulders, and along neck. Fat along inner thighs may rub together. Flank filled with fat.	

From Henneke DR, Potter GD, Kreider JL, et al: Relationship between condition score, physical measurements and body fat percentage in mares, Equine Vet J 15:371–372, 1983.
Photo 1 courtesy Carreen McCarthy; photo 2 courtesy Amy Bentz.

being treated for a disease or an injury and need to be maintained in stalls, the ration should be adjusted to meet minimum energy requirements. Depending on the disease, dietary adjustments should be made. Once the weight is estimated, the National Research Council (NRC) webpage can be used to estimate all requirements for horses (http://nrc88.nas.edu/nrh/). Information needed includes the horse's body weight in kg and the activity level of the horse.

Protein

Most high-quality forages contain adequate to excessive protein for the nutrient needs of adulthood. Protein requirements will vary according to the activity level and the energy requirements.

Minerals and Vitamins

Horses need free access to salt in the form of blocks or lose salt. Some forages or forage/grain combinations need calcium and phosphorus supplementation. Some forages may be deficient in phosphorus; a source of grain usually is a good supplement. Commercial grains are balanced in the calcium-to-phosphorus ratio. The calcium-to-phosphorus ratio in the whole ration (forage plus grain) should range from 1:1 to 3:1. Excessive phosphorus can lead to calcium reabsorption from bones, resulting in nutritional secondary hyperparathyroidism (NSH). Clinically, NSH is characterized by shifting lameness and enlargement of the upper and lower jaws and facial crests. This can occur in adult horses. Magnesium and potassium are present in good-quality forages. Microminerals such as copper, zinc, iodine, iron, manganese, and selenium may be deficient in forages. Ideally, forage analysis should be performed to assess dietary amounts. If analysis is too expensive, common North American values can be found for forages and legumes at www.Equianalytical.com, under common feed values. Mineral supplements should be added to diets only if deficiencies are known. Adding minerals ad libitum or without knowing ration composition can unbalance intake, even leading to toxicity or reduced absorption of other minerals.

> **TECHNICIAN NOTE** Horses need free access to salt, in the form of blocks or lose salt.

Vitamins

Requirements for vitamins A, D, and E, thiamin, and riboflavin have been determined for horses. Beta carotene is the natural source of vitamin A and is present in forages in various concentrations. Pasture (nondormant) contains the greatest, and mature grass hays the lowest concentrations. Vitamin D is found in plants and is synthesized in the skin. Under normal farm conditions, where horses are worked regularly, no supplementation is necessary. Vitamin E varies in equine feeds. Fresh forages and those harvested at immature stages contain the highest concentrations; grains have lower concentrations. Thiamin is found in high concentrations in cereal grains. Riboflavin is found in high concentrations in legumes such as alfalfa and clover, and in lower concentration in grass hays. Riboflavin is produced in the equine hindgut.

GESTATION AND LACTATION

Broodmares require good-quality, balanced rations, and their nutrient requirements change considerably as they advance from being open (not pregnant) through pregnancy and lactation.

Energy

In general, during the first 7 months of pregnancy, energy requirements are very similar to those for maintenance at the time of breeding. Current estimates of digestible energy requirements for gestating mares are 11%, 13%, and 20% above maintenance for the 9th, 10th, and 11th months, respectively. Mares should be bred at a body condition score of 5 or higher. Mares that have an inadequate body condition score (<5) in early or mid gestation should be fed additional energy to reach a body condition score of at least 5 by the 9th month of gestation. However, ideally, mares should be at a body condition score of 5 to 6 when bred. Mares entering the breeding season with a moderate body condition score (5 or higher) require fewer cycles for conception and have higher conception rates than mares entering breeding season in a thinner condition. Mares kept in environmentally stressful conditions should also receive extra energy. Mares with 400 to 600 kg of body weight need 15.9 to 24 Mcal per day during the last month of gestation. After parturition, energy requirements increase considerably in the first half of lactation for milk production. Energy requirements for early lactation for mares with 400 to 600 kg of body weight range from 25 to 38 Mcal/day (Figure 10-13). Therefore, it is advisable to increase energy intake progressively during the last month of gestation to achieve the requirements for lactation. Introduction of a grain concentrate in the last month of gestation will increase energy density and adapt the mare's gastrointestinal tract. Energy requirements of lactating mares vary according to lactation month; in the last half of gestation, requirements drop as milk production decreases, so energy needs range from 22 to 32.7 Mcal/day in 400- to 600-kg mares. It is estimated that 2 months after foaling, mares may produce 9 to 12 kg of milk daily.

> **TECHNICIAN NOTE** Mares entering the breeding season with a moderate body condition score (≥5) require fewer cycles for conception and have higher conception rates than mares entering breeding season in a thinner condition.

Protein

Early pregnancy requirements for protein are similar to those for idle horses. From the 5th month to parturition, needs depend on body weight and fetal weight gain. Again

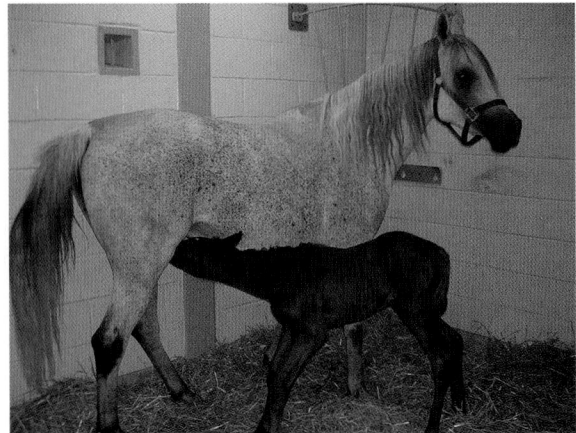

FIGURE 10-13 The mare's nutrient requirements double during lactation. It is estimated that 2 months after foaling, mares may produce 20 to 25 lb of milk daily. (Courtesy Dr. Joanna Bassert.)

from the NRC webpage (http://nrc88.nas.edu/nrh/), this value can be calculated on the basis of nonpregnant body weight in kg and the month of gestation. Restriction of protein during lactation can lead to reduced milk production and increased reproductive problems. Protein is supplied by forage or concentrate and should be added at levels to ensure that minimum protein requirements are met. Most mares are fed high-protein legume hay, such as alfalfa, and grain, which should supply almost all protein needs during lactation. Lactation protein requirements will depend on milk production, which varies between 3% and 2% of the mare's body weight from the 1st to the 5th month of lactation. This calculation can be done on the mentioned webpage; information needed includes the mare's body weight in kg and the month of lactation. Lactating mares have higher intakes for milk production and extra feed intake, leading to a 2- to 3-fold increase in intake over maintenance. Dry-matter intake can be estimated to be around 2.5% to 3% of the mare's body weight.

Minerals and Vitamins

In general, it is important that the ration of the gestating-lactating mare supply sufficient calcium and phosphorus. Calcium and phosphorus requirements increase in the 7th and 8th months and further increase in the 9th to 11th months of gestation. Magnesium requirements also increase during late gestation and lactation. Copper is a micromineral that should be fed to meet requirements in pregnant mares. Low levels of dietary copper have been associated with increased risk for osteochondrosis. However, it is important to feed a ration that is balanced in all nutrients. The zinc-to-copper ratio should be close to 3:1 to decrease the risk for osteochondrosis incidence, particularly in growing horses. Vitamins A and E may enhance reproductive status. Requirements for vitamin A during pregnancy are 60 IU/kg BW, and for vitamin E 2 IU/kg BW.

FOALS

After 2 months of age, the mare's milk does not cover requirements. It is at this time that consideration needs to be given to individual feeding or creep feeding of the foal. Foals will begin to nibble on grain and hay by 3 weeks of age. Creep feeding should be initiated at an early age and with small amounts of creep feed. A general rule of thumb is to offer 450 g (1 lb) of creep feed per month of age per day up to a maximum of 2.7 kg (6 lb). Foals typically are weaned at 6 months of age and then are offered 0.45 to 1.35 kg of grain and 0.7 to 1 kg of hay daily per each 45 kg of live weight. The energy needed for growth is the sum of the energy needed for maintenance and the energy needed for gain. Requirements will vary with age and body weight. Again, the easiest way to calculate requirements is by using the webpage recommended by the NRC. The adult expected weight is needed along with the age of the horse (http://nrc88.nas.edu/nrh/). Growing horses should not be fed above energy requirements because this increases the risk for developmental orthopedic disease. All other nutrients required can be calculated from the same web page. In practical terms, foals should not get overweight. Average daily gain should be monitored. Horses should be weighed or their weight estimated at least on a monthly basis to ensure correct weight gain. Good-quality hay should be part of the diet of the growing horse. Daily intake can be calculated as 2.5% of the horse's body weight on a dry-matter percentage. For example, hay usually consists of about 90% dry matter; a 300-kg colt should ingest 7.5 kg of dry matter or 8.3 kg of ration (hay added with grain or not) as fed. Good-quality alfalfa hay, for example, may provide all needed nutrients for a growing horse. Hay and pasture nutritional analysis should be performed to ensure required nutrients.

> **TECHNICIAN NOTE** Creep feeding should be initiated at an early age and with small amounts of creep feed. Foals typically are weaned at 6 month of age and then are offered 0.45 to 1.35 kg of grain and 0.7 to 1 kg of hay daily per each 45 kg of live weight.

Water

Nursing foals will drink water in addition to milk; therefore, water should be available for the mare and the foal all the time. Intakes have been reported to be about 4 kg of water in suckling foals at 1 month of age, in addition to about 17.4 kg of milk.

Minerals and Vitamins for Growing Horses

Calcium and phosphorus are important for bone formation and diverse metabolic functions. Requirements vary according to the average daily gain. The ratio of calcium to phosphorus should be 1:1 to 3:1. Meeting requirements and maintaining the ratio should be the goals in attaining optimal bone growth. Excessive phosphorus can lead to nutritional secondary hyperparathyroidism, clinical signs of which have already been described. Alfalfa is a good calcium source for the growing horse. If grain is added to the diet, a commercial formula, balanced for calcium and phosphorus, should be used. Copper is an important mineral to consider when feeding growing horses. Low body copper has been associated with osteochondrosis—an abnormal calcification of growing bones. Excessive zinc may reduce copper absorption (zinc toxicosis) or may interfere with copper metabolism. The incidence of osteochondrosis has been reduced when foals are fed a ration containing a zinc-to-copper ratio of 3:1. Selenium deficiency results in myopathy in horses (white muscle disease), leading to weakness, impaired locomotion, difficulty in suckling and swallowing, respiratory distress, and abnormal cardiac function. Deficiency in forages occurs in several regions of the world. Maximum tolerable levels are 2 mg/kg of dry matter (DM). Acute selenium toxicity, also called *blind staggers,* is characterized by apparent blindness, head pressing, perspiration, abnormal pain, colic, diarrhea, increased heart rate and respiratory rate, and lethargy. Chronic intoxication (alkali disease) leads to alopecia (mane and tail) and cracking of the hooves along the coronary band. Blood selenium status can indicate deficiencies. The true requirements are unknown, but a minimum of 1 to 3 mg of selenium should be given to horses each day.

The role of vitamin A during growth has not been well studied; however, 45 IU/kg BW is required. Vitamin D requirements for sun-deprived places are 22.2 IU/kg BW (0 to 6 months of age); 17.4 IU/kg BW (7 to 12 months of age); 15.9 IU/kg BW (13 to 18 months of age); and 13.7 IU/kg BW (19 to 24 months of age). Deficiency of vitamin D is characterized by bone deformities. Bone development and growth were abnormal in ponies deprived of sunlight and dietary vitamin D. Vitamin E requirements for growth have not been established. Muscular dystrophy caused by nutrition has been seen in mares that consumed diets low in vitamin E (6 to 8 IU vitamin E/kg DM); however, these diets were also low in selenium. Current recommendations are for 2 IU/kg/BW per day of vitamin E.

WORKING HORSES

Water

Fluid losses of exercising horses will depend on duration and intensity of exercise, as well as on ambient temperature and humidity. Losses will be greater during higher-intensity exercise and will not decrease with duration of exercise. Sweat losses will be greater at higher ambient temperature and humidity. Heat acclimation takes about 3 weeks and reduces sweat losses, but dehydration will still occur because of sweating. Hydration of working horses should be monitored. Exercised horses may increase requirements by 20% to 300% above maintenance levels through sweat and respiratory losses. Sweat losses during exercise can be as high as 15 L per hour.

Energy

Work can be classified into light, moderate, heavy, and very heavy exercise intensity (Table 10-14), and horses should be fed to reach the requirements for the desired performance (Table 10-15). The amount of daily energy required for working horses will include the energy needed for maintenance plus the energy needed for daily exercise. A strong relationship has been noted between heart rate and oxygen consumption; therefore, energy expenditure can be estimated from heart rate. Based on average weekly exercise, the National Research Council (NRC) has developed different calculations for energy consumption. Information needed to calculate energy requirements on the NRC webpage includes the horse's weight and the type of activity. For growing exercising horses, extra energy will be needed for growth. Sometimes it can be a challenge to maintain the body condition score of horses at very intense work intensity.

Protein

Exercising horses require additional protein to develop and repair muscles. This increased need for protein is met typically by an increase in DMI. If only fat is added as an energy

TABLE 10-14	Exercise Intensity Levels of Horses		
EXERCISE CATEGORY	**MEAN HEART RATE**	**DESCRIPTION**	**TYPE OF EVENT**
Light	80 bpm	1-3 hr/week, 40% walk, 50% trot, 10% canter	Recreational riding Beginning of training, occasion show
Moderate	90 bpm	3-5 hr/week, 30% walk, 55% trot, 10% canter, 5% show jumping, cutting, skill work	School horses, recreational, beginning training, frequent show horses, polo, ranch work
Heavy	110 bpm	4-5 hr/week, 20% walk, 50% trot, 15% canter, 15% gallop, jumping, other skill work	Ranch work, polo, show horses (frequent strenuous events), low-medium eventing, race training (middle stages)
Very heavy	110-150 bpm	Various; 1 hr/week speed work, 6-12 hr/week slow work	Racing (flat + endurance) Elite 3-day event

From National Research Council: Nutrient requirement of horses, ed 6, Washington, DC, 2007, National Academy Press.

TABLE 10-15	Nutrient Supply for Horses*			
ENERGY	**PROTEIN**	**VITAMINS AND MINERALS**		**COMMENTS**
Nursing Foals				
Supplement mare's milk	>16%	Ca/P 1:1 to 3:1 Meet requirements for age Cu >25 mg/kg BW Vitamin A 50 IU/kg BW		At 2 months of age, begin 1 lb creep feeding; concentrate mixture/month of age/day Adequate Ca²⁺, P, trace minerals in grain mix Zn/Cu ratio 3:1 to avoid developmental orthopedic disease Wean at 4 months
Weaning				
Adequate to feel but not see the ribs	15%	Ca²⁺ 0.7% P 0.4% Adequate Ca/P ratio and Zn/Cu ratio Vitamin A 50 IU/kg BW		Dry-matter intake = 3% of BW Free-choice good roughage and trace-mineral salt 1 lb concentrate mix/month of age/day: 7-9 lb mix
Yearling				
Adequate to feel but not see the ribs	13%	Ca²⁺ 0.5% P 0.3% Vitamin A 50 IU/kg BW		Dry-matter intake = 2.5% BW Free-choice good roughage, trace-mineral salt 1 lb concentrate mix/100 lb BW: 7-9 lb max Feed as mature horse at 90% of mature weight Avoid growth spurt and feeding above energy requirements
Adult Maintenance				
Adequate to feel but not see the ribs, BCS 5	8.5%	Ca²⁺ 0.3% P 0.2% Vitamin A 50 IU/kg BW		Dry matter = 1.5%-2% BW ½-1½ lb roughage/100 lb BW Free-choice trace-mineral salt

BW, Body weight; *Ca*, calcium; *Cu*, copper; *P*, phosphorus.
*Free-choice, potable water should be available at all times.
Overeating winter and fall: feed ↑ P, ↓ Ca²⁺ 14 days before parturition. Eliminate or reduce moldy or mycotoxin-laden feed. Thiamin deficiency.
Overgrazing feeding lambs in rich pasture (cause not fully discovered): ↓ grain intake while ↑ roughage quality, 1 week before; ↑ animals' intake of high-energy diets; vitamin A deficiency; ↑ when water is restricted. Rare nontoxic horse.

source, protein needs may not be met. The additional protein for energy can be estimated on the NRC webpage (http://nrc88.nas.edu/nrh/). Body weight and intensity of exercise activity are needed for the calculation. Excessive dietary protein may be deleterious because more water is needed to eliminate excessive protein from the body. An increase in urea occurs; this is deleterious for stalled horses because ammonia will increase in the air. Also, excess protein leads to acidification of blood, which is not wanted in high-intensity exercising horses that have lactic acidosis. Environmental contamination is increased with excessive dietary protein.

Minerals

Calcium requirements increase only with very high levels of exercise. Phosphorus and magnesium requirements increase with exercise intensity. Sodium, chloride, and potassium are the main electrolytes lost in sweat, so replacement strategies are important for sport horses. Free-choice salt should always be available. Sweat losses of sodium, potassium, and chloride are about 3.08 g/L, 1.6 g/L, and 5.54 g/L, respectively. Long-distance exercising horses may benefit from oral electrolyte supplementation before, during, and after exercise. Dietary potassium usually exceeds requirements and is stored in the hindgut, so replacement during exercise is not absolutely necessary and may be deleterious. Potassium lost in sweat should be replaced after exercise has ceased. Electrolyte supplementation should not try to replace all electrolytes lost during exercise, but rather should try to replace about 50% of losses during exercise, and the remainder after exercise. Electrolyte supplementation during exercise maintains thirst and therefore hydration. During exercise, clinical signs associated with sweat electrolyte losses include increased capillary refill time, increased skin pinch return time, reduced gut sounds, increased heart rate recovery time, increased heart rate, heart rate arrhythmias, muscle cramps, loss of impulsion, unwillingness to continue, synchronous diaphragmatic flutter, hyperthermia, and exhaustion syndrome. If the primary cause is not treated, signs may evolve to paralytic ileus, colic, and laminitis. Simple electrolyte replacement strategies can be applied by using about 22 g of NaCl mixed with yogurt or applesauce, supplied every 10 miles or every 16 km of exercise if ambient temperatures are mild. At higher temperatures, the dose can be doubled. This amount will replace electrolyte losses contained in 2.5 L of sweat. After exercise, potassium should be added to replacement formulas. A formula containing about 80 g of Na Cl and 30 g of KCl replaces electrolytes lost in about 10 L of sweat. Additional benefits have been derived by adding calcium or magnesium to electrolyte formulas.

FEEDING SICK HORSES

Hospitalized horses can develop protein-calorie deficits, hypermetabolic stress, or catabolic wasting states. These have negative clinical effects, and early interventional feeding is vital in equine critical care. Horses should be fed 50% of their daily energy requirements initially after surgery or after days of starvation. Energy intake should be increased over several days to meet requirements. Major gastrointestinal tract (colic) surgery is especially challenging in the perioperative period. The animal needs diets rich in protein, calories, and micronutrients despite **reduced gastrointestinal motility.** The veterinarian will focus closely as to when gastrointestinal motility returns to support the sick horse. Often, homogenized, moistened alfalfa pellet mashes are high-protein, high-energy, and nonirritating formulas designed for replenishing nutrients. Such diets may be given as slurries through nasogastric tubes and often are enriched with nutriment modules. Liquid enteral formulas based on the mare's milk replacement and on commercial equine critical care formulas are available and well tolerated. Formulas should be given in small, frequent feedings via indwelling nasogastric tubes.

REFERENCES

1. Ensminger ME: Swine science, Danville, IL, 1990, Interstate Printers and Publishing.
2. McDonald P, Edwards RA, Greenhalgh JFD, et al: Animal nutrition, ed 7, New York, 1995, Longman Scientific and Technical Publishing.
3. Nash MJ: Crop conservation and storage, Oxford, England, 1985, Pergamon Press.
4. Church DC: Livestock feeds and feeding, Corvallis, OR, 1984, O and B Books.
5. Shirley RL: Nitrogen and energy nutrition of ruminants, Orlando, 1986, Academic Press.
6. Neumann AL: Beef cattle, New York, 1977, John Wiley & Sons.

RECOMMENDED READINGS

Cunha TJ: Swine feeding and nutrition, New York, 1977 Academic Press Inc.

Garmsworthy PC: Nutrition and lactation in the dairy cow, London, 1988, University Press.

Haresign DJ: Recent developments of pig nutrition, London, 1985, Butterworth.

Jones DH, Wilson AD: Nutritive quality of forage. In Hacker ED, editor: The nutrition of herbivores, Sydney, 1982, Academic Press.

Kruesi WK: Sheep raiser's manual, Charlotte, VT, 1985, Williamson Publishing.

Linciciome DR: Sheep: applied and basic research information, Scottsdale, AZ, 1983, International Goat and Sheep Research.

Lloyd LE, McDonald BE, Crampton EW: Fundamentals of nutrition, ed 3, San Francisco, 1978, WH Freeman & Sons.

Machlin LJ: Handbook of vitamins, New York, 1984, Marcel Dekker.

Maynard LA, Loosli JK, Hintz JF, et al: Animal nutrition, ed 7, New York, 1979, McGraw-Hill.

Menzies CS: United States sheep and goat industry, Ames, IA, 1982, CAST Report.

National Research Council: Nutrient requirements for beef cattle, ed 7, Washington, DC, 2000, National Academic Press.

National Research Council: Nutrient requirements for dairy cattle, ed 7, Washington, DC, 2001, National Academy Press.

National Research Council: Nutrient requirements for horses, ed 6, Washington, DC, 2007, National Academy Press.

National Research Council: Nutrient requirements for sheep, ed 6, Washington, DC, 1985, National Academy Press.

National Research Council: Nutrient requirements for swine, ed 10, Washington, DC, 1998, National Academic Press.

Naylor JM, Ralston SL: Large animal clinical nutrition, St Louis, 1991, Mosby.

Pond WG: Swine production and nutrition, Westport, CT, 1984, AVI Publishing.

Taylor RE: Beef production and the beef industry, Minneapolis, MN, 1984, Burgess Publishing.

Tribble LG, Stansbury WF: Swine report, Dallas, 1985, Texas Technical University.

Webster J: Calf husbandry: health and welfare, London, 1984, Collins.

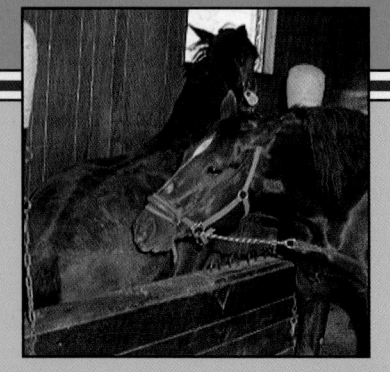

11 | Animal Reproduction (Theriogenology)

Walter R. Threlfall

OUTLINE

Overview of Female Reproduction, *368*
Anatomy, *368*
Physiology, *368*
Overview of Male Reproduction, *370*
Anatomy, *370*
Physiology, *370*
Canine Reproduction, *372*
General, *372*
Estrous Cycle, *373*
Breeding, *378*
Gestation, *378*
Parturition, *378*
Feline Reproduction, *379*
General, *379*
Estrous Cycle, *379*
Gestation, *380*
Parturition, *380*
Equine Reproduction, *380*
General, *380*
Bovine Reproduction, *387*
General, *387*
Estrous Cycle, *387*

Insemination, *388*
Gestation, *389*
Parturition, *389*
Ovine Reproduction, *389*
General, *389*
Estrous Cycle, *390*
Breeding, *390*
Gestation, *391*
Caprine Reproduction, *391*
General, *391*
Camelid Reproduction, *391*
General, *391*
Breeding, *391*
Gestation, *391*
Parturition, *391*
Breeding Soundness Examination of the Male, *392*
Semen Analysis, *393*
Other Diagnostic Tests, *394*
Breeding Soundness Examination of the Female, *394*

LEARNING OBJECTIVES

When you have completed this chapter, you will be able to:

1. Pronounce, define, and spell each of the Key Terms in this chapter.
2. Do the following regarding reproduction:
   • Locate the anatomic parts of the reproductive system, including endocrine organs in the cranium.
   • Describe hormonal changes that occur during the estrous cycle and pregnancy.
   • Compare and contrast the processes of oogenesis and spermatogenesis.
   • Explain the process of fertilization and embryo development, including the anatomic locations of these events.
3. Compare and contrast canine, feline, and equine estrous cycles, gestation, and parturition. Also do the following:
   • Describe the collection process and interpretation of canine vaginal cells, and state the importance of vaginal cytologic examination in breeding dogs.
4. Compare and contrast the bovine, ovine, caprine, and camelid estrous cycles, gestation, and parturition.

KEY TERMS

Allantois
Amnion
Anestrus
Artificial insemination
Chorioallantois
Chorion
Corpus hemorrhagicum
Corpus luteum
Cryptorchid
Embryo
Estrogen
Estrus
Fetal membranes
Follicle
Follicle-stimulating hormone
Gonadotropin-releasing hormone
Luteinizing hormone
Oocyte
Oxytocin
Parturition
Pineal gland
Placenta
Progesterone
Prolactin
Relaxin
Seasonally polyestrous
Superfecundation
Superfetation

The author and the publisher wish to acknowledge the contributions of Carlos R.F. Pinto, Bruce Edward Ellis, and Dale Paccamonti for their previous contributions to this chapter.

5. Identify and put in order the important aspects of a breeding soundness examination in a male.
6. Identify and put in order the important aspects of a breeding soundness examination in a female.

INTRODUCTION

The process of reproduction in domestic animals includes an elegant cascade of physiologic events that result in the birth of a newborn, which carries the genes for the next generation. Offspring are essential to ensure that another generation of animals is available for food and fiber (cows, pigs, and sheep), for companionship (dogs, cats, and horses), and for sport (horses). The efficient management of animal reproduction requires a clear understanding of the anatomy, physiology, and pathology of the reproductive system. The study of animal reproduction is called *theriogenology*, and it is a cornerstone of herd health programs. Although unique differences have been noted between the reproductive systems of various domestic animal species, far more similarities have been observed. Therefore, a basic knowledge of hormones, hormonal interaction, spermatogenesis, breeding, fertilization, pregnancy, and birth is needed for an understanding of the normal aspects of reproduction in all mammalian species. When normalcy is understood, problems and abnormal events are more easily recognized. Furthermore, if normal and abnormal processes are learned for one species, transfer of that knowledge to other species may help solve medical problems. This chapter provides an overview of female and male reproductive systems, followed by a more in-depth review of the most important aspects of reproduction in the canine, feline, equine, bovine, swine, ovine, caprine, and camelid.

OVERVIEW OF FEMALE REPRODUCTION

ANATOMY

The primary anatomic structures involved in the reproductive processes of female mammals include the hypothalamus, the pituitary, the **pineal gland**, the ovaries, and the tubular genitalia: oviducts, uterus, and vagina. The location and function of each of these structures and the effects of the hormones they produce and receive are extremely important toward an understanding of the female reproductive system and the diseases that affect it.

PHYSIOLOGY

Endocrinology

Endocrine glands, located throughout the body, form vital chemical signals called *hormones* that drive many processes in the body, including reproduction. Therefore, to understand reproduction, we must first understand the structure and location of these critical organs and the effects of the hormones they produce.

In female mammals, hormonal changes give rise to a carefully orchestrated, repeating cycle that is designed to bring about mating, pregnancy, and birth. The length of the cycle varies among species, and because it is a cycle, it has no true beginning or ending. However, because of its importance, discussion of the female reproductive process often begins with ovulation.

> **TECHNICIAN NOTE**   **Superfecundation** refers to multiple sires of two or more offspring during a single gestation.

Ovulation

Ovulation is the ejection of an egg (ovum) from a **follicle** in the ovary. The hormonal influences that bring about ovulation begin in the brain of the animal in a region called the *pituitary*, which is located ventral to the larger hypothalamus and is composed of two primary regions: the anterior pituitary or adenohypophysis, and the posterior pituitary or neurohypophysis. Endocrine control of follicular development in the ovary comes from hormones released by the adenohypophysis. Refer to Figure 11-1 for a summary of hormonal control of ovarian activity.

After ovulation, the remaining follicular sac fills with blood that subsequently clots. This clot-filled structure is known as the **corpus hemorrhagicum**, or bloody body (Figure 11-2). The clot serves as a nutritional matrix to support rapid development of surrounding cells. This enables the tissue to develop into a specialized endocrine structure known as the **corpus luteum (CL)** (Figures 11-3 and 11-4). The luteal tissue produces progesterone (P4), and as the CL increases in size, so too does the level of **progesterone** it produces. Progesterone aids in the preparation of tubular genitalia for a possible pregnancy and also assists the maintenance of pregnancy, if it occurs.

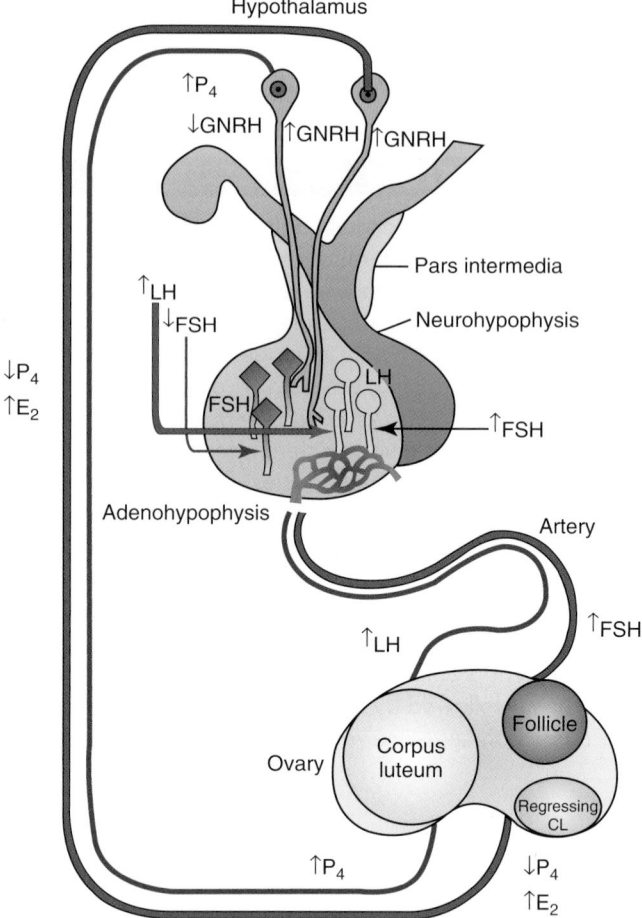

Hormonal Control of Ovarian Activity

FIGURE 11-1 Summary chart of hormonal control of ovarian activity.

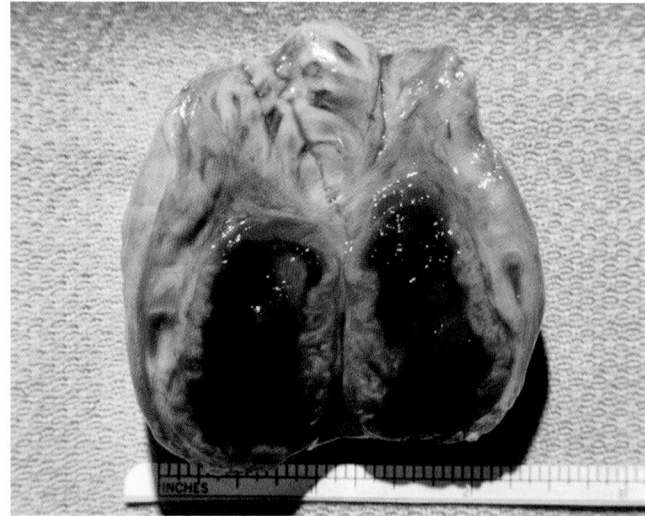

FIGURE 11-2 Corpus hemorrhagicum of the mare.

As the follicle matures and approaches ovulation, the ovum within the follicle also matures. The ovum contains half the genetic material of future offspring, and the sperm contains the other half. If ovulation does not occur within the normal length of time, the ovum within the follicle will

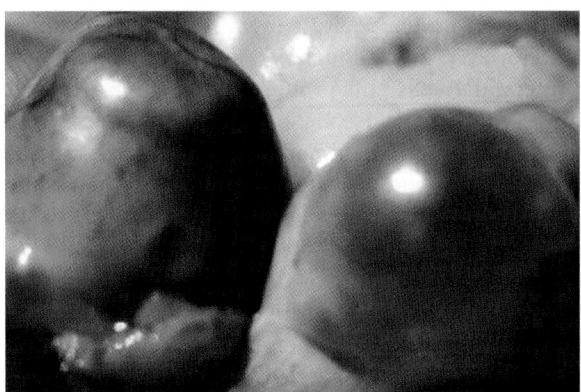

FIGURE 11-3 A bovine corpus luteum (CL) and follicle on an ovary.

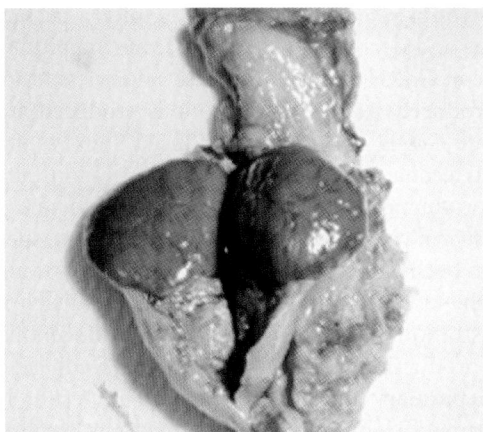

FIGURE 11-4 A cut section of a bovine corpus luteum (CL).

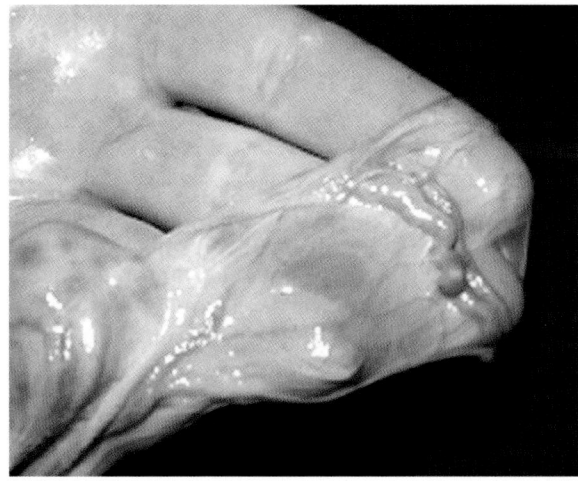

FIGURE 11-5 A bovine oviduct showing fingers inserted into the infundibulum (the first part of the oviduct).

degenerate. Therefore, it loses the capability of being fertilized if it is released late, but usually it is not released at all, and it deteriorates within the follicle. Keep in mind that females are born with a finite number of **oocytes** (immature eggs), most of which do not develop fully and are not ovulated. When the ovum is released, it is covered with the cumulus cells that surrounded it within the follicle. These cells are important in the follicle because they serve as a matrix that helps provide nutrition to the oocyte so that it can mature; after ovulation, the layer of cumulus cells serve as a roughened surface by which the oviduct can move the ovum toward the uterus.

If the ovum is not fully mature at the time of ovulation, as it is in some species, the maturation process is completed in the ampulla—the middle portion of the oviduct. Fertilization, which involves penetration of the ovum by the sperm, occurs in the oviduct near the junction of the ampulla and the isthmus (Figure 11-5). The fertilized ovum eventually passes through the *isthmus* (the last portion of the oviduct) in its passage to the uterus. In some species such as the equine, the ovum if not fertilized remains in the oviduct and degenerates.

The CL is maintained for a predetermined time following ovulation in most species, regardless of whether or not fertilization occurs. If fertilization occurs and an embryo makes its way successfully to the uterus, a chemical signal (early conception factor) is released from the embryo. If the signal is not released, prostaglandin F2alpha is released from the endometrium, and the CL in the ovary regresses. Conception factors are produced by embryos, depending on the species, as early as 12 to 18 hours after conception. With regression of the CL comes a rapid drop in progesterone.

Superfecundation refers to multiple sires of two or more offspring during a single gestation. This is not to be confused with **superfetation**, which occurs when a pregnant dam ovulates and conceives again while pregnant. This can occur in any species, including primate and bipara (animals that have twins), but most frequently occurs in multipara (animals that have litters).

Estrous Cycle

> **TECHNICIAN NOTE** The estrous cycle is determined by the interrelationships of the following endocrine organs: pineal gland, hypothalamus, pituitary gland, ovary, and uterus.

The estrous cycle of various species is determined by hormonal changes occurring in that species. The word *estrous* is an adjective that here relates to what "kind" of cycle. **Estrus**, the noun, describes the period of time that the female is in "heat," or is sexually receptive. Sexual receptiveness in animals is brought about by the ratio of estrogen to progesterone. In some species, **estrogen** alone is not capable of inducing estrus. Some, if only slight, quantities of progesterone must always be present. In the primate, sexual "receptivity," or interest, is driven primarily by nonhormonal factors. *Puberty* in animals is defined as the time when the first ovum is released; it does not signify the first signs of heat.

Embryo

The oocyte is surrounded by the zona pellucida, which must be penetrated by the sperm. Once this process occurs, no additional sperm can enter the oocyte. After formation of the embryo, continued cellular divisions occur, forming a multicellular blastocyst. The blastocyst hatches when the zona pellucida degenerates. The outermost layer of cells of the embryo provides nutrients and support to the inner portions of the embryo. This trophoblastic layer subsequently develops into the placenta. The inner cell mass of the blastocyst is composed of the endoderm, the mesoderm, and the ectoderm. The endoderm will develop into intestine, liver, and lungs. The mesoderm will develop into the cardiovascular system, the musculoskeletal system, and a portion of the reproductive system. The ectoderm will develop into hair, skin, and nervous system. Ectopic pregnancies (fetus developing outside the uterus) occur only in the primate. If a fetus is outside the uterus in our domestic species, the uterus has ruptured, and the fetus will be dead or very soon dead. The placental attachment of each species is unique with regard to the layers of cells present in the endometrium (uterine lining) and the placenta. These species differences account for the varying quantities of maternal antibodies that are transferred from the dam to the fetus via the placenta, and the varying need that newborns have for colostrum.

OVERVIEW OF MALE REPRODUCTION

ANATOMY

The primary anatomic structures involved in the reproductive processes of male mammals include the hypothalamus, the pituitary, the testes, the accessory sex glands (such as the prostate, bulbourethral gland, ampullae, and vesicular glands), and the tubular genitalia—vas deferens and urethra.

PHYSIOLOGY

The male differs greatly from the female in the production of gametes. Whereas in the female, only 1 to 10 oocytes ovulate during an estrous cycle, males are continually producing and excreting millions of sperm cells. Also, testicular anatomy differs significantly from ovarian anatomy. The testis is made up of many tubules, each of which connects to a central collecting duct. Between the tubules are the interstitial cells, which continually produce testosterone (Figure 11-6). Each tubule is lined by primordial germ cells (immature sperm cell precursors) and Sertoli cells. The Sertoli cells surround all developing sperm cells, leaving them with no other contact with the body. This is critical in that the developing sperm are recognized as a foreign substance to the male and would be destroyed by the immune system if they were not protected. As the sperm cells mature, they leave their attachment to the Sertoli cell and are moved through the tubules.

The entire testis is covered by a tight capsule—the tunica albuginea. The paired testes are contained within the scrotum. The scrotum maintains the testes at a lower body temperature than the rest of the body. If the testes are not kept at a lower temperature, sperm cell production will cease. However, even though sperm cell production ceases, the interstitial cells still produce testosterone. A common example of these consequences is seen in a cryptorchid animal. A cryptorchid animal has one or both of the testes retained in the abdomen. If the testes are in the abdomen, the animal is sterile but will still show masculine behavior because testosterone is still produced by the testes.

Although the anatomy of the testes differs from that of the ovary, the control of sperm cell production is similar to that of oocyte production; however, it is more continuous and does not occur in cycles. In the male, **luteinizing hormone** (LH) from the anterior pituitary causes an increase in testosterone production (see Figure 11-6). As testosterone production rises in the testes, it causes a decrease in **gonadotropin-releasing hormone** (GnRH) in the hypothalamus and decreased LH release from the pituitary. The decrease in GnRH and in LH release causes less testosterone to be produced. As less testosterone is produced, it follows that more GnRH and LH are produced, thus resulting in a balanced feedback mechanism and relatively constant testosterone production. Testosterone is essential for the production of sperm cells. If testosterone is not present, sperm cells will not be produced. The concentration of testosterone within the testis is 10 times that in the systemic circulation. Administration of testosterone decreases endogenous testosterone production because of negative feedback on the anterior pituitary and hypothalamus. This results in lower testosterone concentrations within the testis. Because testosterone is needed for sperm cell production, the exogenous testosterone eventually will decrease sperm cell production.

The other hormone involved in sperm cell production is **follicle-stimulating hormone** (FSH). Just as in the female, FSH release is triggered by GnRH from the hypothalamus (see Figure 11-6). The FSH acts on the Sertoli cell to increase the division of primordial sperm cells and to release more sperm cells that are embedded in the Sertoli cells. As sperm cell production rises, the hormone inhibin feeds back on the hypothalamus and the anterior pituitary to decrease GnRH and FSH, respectively. This causes fewer sperm cells to be produced. As fewer cells are produced, the FSH will increase to produce more sperm cells, thereby keeping sperm cell production relatively constant. In general, FSH causes production of the gamete (oocyte in the female and sperm cell in the male), and LH causes production of the dominant hormone (progesterone in the female and testosterone in the male).

After the sperm cells are released, they move through the tubules and into the head of the epididymis. Within the epididymis, the sperm cells attain motility and the ability to fertilize. Movement through the epididymis to the tail of the epididymis is relatively constant and cannot be increased by increasing the number or frequency of ejaculates. The sperm cells are finally stored in the tail of the epididymis, where they may be ejaculated, or voided in the urine if they are not ejaculated (Figure 11-7).

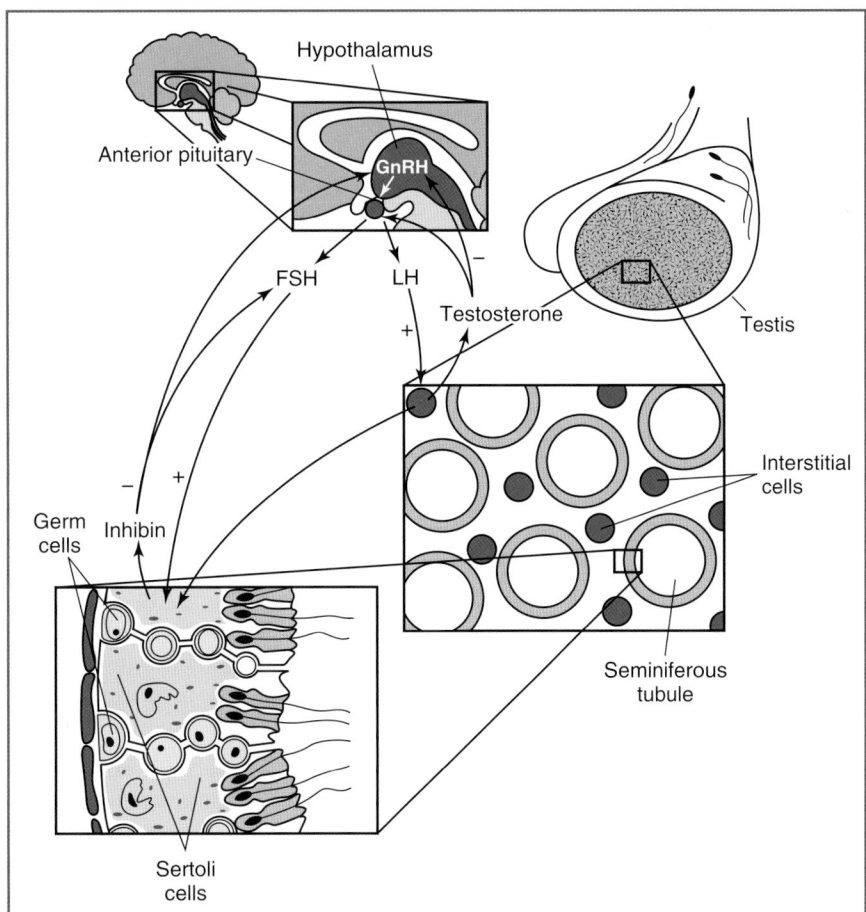

FIGURE 11-6 General hormonal control of male reproduction. Pulsatile gonadotropin-releasing hormone (GnRH) causes follicle-stimulating hormone (FSH) to be released from the anterior pituitary. FSH causes increased sperm growth, maturation, and release. Inhibin from Sertoli cells in the tubules feeds back on the anterior pituitary and causes release of less FSH. GnRH secretion from the hypothalamus also results in luteinizing hormone (LH) release, which causes testosterone production by the interstitial cells of Leydig. The rise in testosterone causes release of less LH and GnRH.

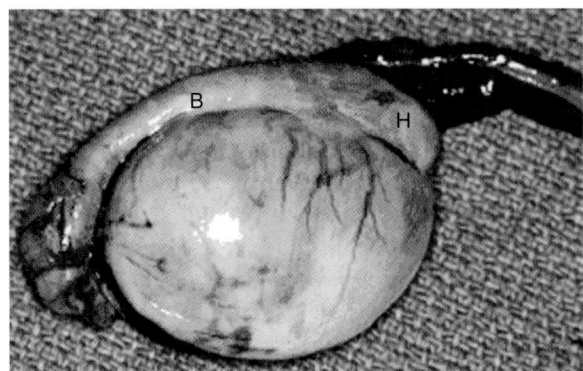

FIGURE 11-7 Lateral view of the right canine testis and epididymis with the head (H), body (B), and tail (T) of the epididymis.

Ejaculation through the penis is the final process in sperm production and delivery. In most domestic species, the penis comprises cavernous blood tissue surrounded by a firm covering, or tunic. An erection occurs when the male is sexually stimulated. During sexual stimulation, parasympathetic innervation causes increased blood flow into the cavernous portions of the penis. As blood flow to the penis is increased, muscles around the proximal penis contract to prevent blood outflow. Because the cavernous portions of the penis are contained within the tunic, pressure increases, resulting in a penile erection. Any disruption of cavernous tissue or the tunic can result in erection failure.

During an erection, the sperm cells in the tail of the epididymis are moved to the end of the ductus deferens into the ampullae through the process called *emission*. Once the sperm cells are present in the ampullae, stimulation to the penis during mating causes ejaculation. Ejaculation is forceful expulsion of the semen through the penis. The force comes from sympathetic nerves causing smooth muscle contractions in the urethra. During ejaculation, sperm cells are mixed with fluid from the accessory sex glands. Accessory sex glands include ampullae, prostate, vesicular glands, and bulbourethral glands. Each species has one or all of these glands, and different glands have different clinical problems in each species. When sperm cells are mixed with accessory sex gland fluid, the result is now termed *semen*. Secretions from accessory sex gland fluid add various components to the ejaculate, increase the volume, and stabilize the sperm cell membrane. Once sperm cells enter the female reproductive tract, the sperm cell membrane undergoes a physical and biochemical change called *capacitation*. Capacitation is required before sperm cells are capable of fertilization. In the uterus, sperm cells are quickly moved to the oviduct, where fertilization occurs. Sperm cells are moved to the oviduct by uterine contractions.

Spermatogenesis

At the level of the seminiferous tubule within the testis, spermatogonia (cells that give rise to mature sperm) are distributed around a basement membrane and are surrounded by Sertoli cells, which provide nutrition and an appropriate environment for developing sperm. Stem cells can undergo many divisions to produce more stem cells, as well as to produce differentiating germ cells that are destined to become mature sperm. The initial differentiated cells are called *primary spermatocytes*; they undergo the first meiotic division to become *secondary spermatocytes*. During this meiotic process, cell divisions occur without duplication of genetic material, resulting in cells with one-half the chromosomal number (haploid) of normal somatic cells. The purpose of this process is to produce germ cells that can result in an embryo with the normal number of chromosomes after fertilization. With completion of the second meiotic division, spermatids have the haploid set of chromatids.

Once the spermatid is formed, many morphologic changes occur. These changes include development of a flagellum (tail) and acrosome, elimination of excess cytoplasm, and chromatin condensation. These unique changes to the cell ultimately make it capable of independent streamlined movement, penetration of the oocyte membrane and surrounding structures, and delivery of genetic material for completion of fertilization. The fully differentiated cell is the *spermatozoan* (sperm) (Figure 11-8). Spermatogenesis is

completed when spermatozoa move into the lumen of the seminiferous tubule.

Within the testis, spermatozoa are continually produced rather than produced in "batches." This is accomplished by staggering, in time and space, the initiation of cells into the differentiated pool. At a given location within a seminiferous tubule, several germ cells are in a specific maturational stage. Several stages occur throughout the length of the seminiferous tubule and over time at a particular location. In the dog, it takes 13.8 days for a location in the seminiferous tubules to contain the same stage again (i.e., the cycle is 13.8 days). It takes approximately 48 to 50 days for spermatogenesis, from start to finish, and thus takes approximately 3.5 cycles to produce a spermatozoan. Sperm production is continual, not sporadic.

Although spermatogenesis is completed within the testis, sperm maturation is not achieved until the spermatozoa pass through the epididymis. In the canine, this takes approximately 12 to 14 days. During this time, sperm have the ability to be motile, then suppressed; motility is returned, and cytoplasmic droplets are eliminated. From start to ejaculation, formation of a mature sperm cell in the dog takes about 62 days. Other species require a similar length of time.

> **TECHNICIAN NOTE**   The canine estrous cycle consists of proestrus, estrus, diestrus, and anestrus, and is usually 6 months in length in that order.

CANINE REPRODUCTION

GENERAL

The female canine is known as the *bitch*, and the male is known as the *dog*, or the *stud*. The delivery of fetuses is known as *whelping*. Offspring are known as *pups* or *puppies* (Table 11-1). The castrated male is called a *neuter ed male*, and the female that has had the gonads removed is called an *ovariectomized bitch*, or a *spayed bitch* if the uterus was also removed. The bitch reaches puberty at approximately 6 to 24 months, dependent on the adult size of the dog.

At puberty, GnRH is released from the hypothalamus and stimulates the release of FSH from the pituitary (see Figure 11-1). This occurs during the last month of the estrous cycle, known as **anestrus**. The canine estrous cycle consists of proestrus, estrus, diestrus, and anestrus, and is usually 6 months in length in that order (Box 11-1). Each stage varies in length. Proestrus and estrus, for example, each last approximately 9 days. Diestrus is usually a few days fewer than 60 days, and anestrus lasts approximately 4 months in most breeds, but may last closer to 9 months in Basenji, wolves, and wolf crosses.

FSH influences early development of the follicle and estrogen production. Ova are released from the follicles approximately 2 days after a spike in LH. However, unlike in

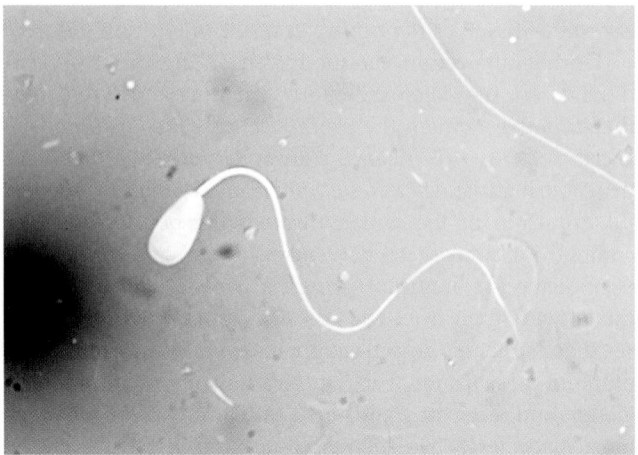

FIGURE 11-8 Photomicrograph of normal sperm.

TABLE 11-1	Reproductive Terminology and Facts for Common Domestic Species						
ANIMAL	ADJECTIVE	IMMATURE	MATURE FEMALE	MATURE MALE	BIRTHING	GESTATION PERIOD	CYCLE
Dogs (Dog)	Canine	Puppy	Bitch, Dam	Dog	Whelping	58-70 days	Two per year for most breeds
Cats (Cat)	Feline	Kitten	Queen	Tom	Queening	58-70 days	Induced ovulation Seasonally polyestrous from spring and early fall
Horses (Horse)	Equine	Foal Weanling Yearling	Mare Female younger than 3 years: Filly	Stallion Castrated: Gelding Male younger than 3 years: Colt	Foaling	330-345 days	Seasonally polyestrous Early spring through early fall
Cattle (Ox)	Bovine	Calf	Cow Younger than 2 years old: Heifer	Bull Castrated: Steer	Calving	279-283 days	Polyestrous all year
Swine (Pig)	Porcine	Piglet	Sow Pre-parous: Gilt Spayed: Yelt	Boar Castrated: Barrow	Farrowing	112-115 days	Polyestrous all year
Sheep (Sheep)	Ovine	Lamb	Ewe	Ram Castrated: Wether	Lambing	144-147 days	Seasonally polyestrous from early spring to early fall
Goats (Goat)	Caprine	Kid	Doe	Buck Castrated: Wether	Kidding	145-155 days	Seasonally polyestrous from early spring to early fall
Llamas/Alpacas (Llama/Alpaca)	Camelid	Cria	Female Dam Hembra	Male Stallion Macho	Unpacking	330-350 days	Induced ovulators Polyestrous

other species, the ova are not fertilizable (not mature) when they are first released. An additional 2 days is required for the ova to become mature enough for fertilization to occur, and once mature, the ova remain fertilizable for 3 days. Hormonal fluctuations occurring throughout the estrous cycle can be used to determine where the bitch is in her cycle. This is especially true of progesterone and luteinizing hormone concentrations.

ESTROUS CYCLE

Proestrus

Proestrus lasts approximately 9 days (range, 3 to 17 days). The beginning of proestrus is designated by the presence of a serosanguineous (bloody) discharge from the vulva. During proestrus, estrogen from the developing follicles continues to increase owing to stimulation of FSH release from the pituitary.

Increasing estrogen causes edema of the vulvar lips, and swelling increases until the vulva is very firm and enlarged. During proestrus, the endometrium, which lines the uterus, becomes highly vascularized and engorged with blood. As blood vessels extend to the surface of the endometrium, they leak blood through the vessel wall (a process called *diapedesis*) and into the uterine chamber. Subsequently, blood emerges from the vulva as a loose, serosanguineous discharge. The male is attracted to the female at this time, but she will not stand to be mated.

Vaginal cytologic examination aids in determining the reproductive status of a bitch. Not only can it assist in determining the stage of estrus, it also gives insight into the reproductive health of the animal. Each stage of the estrous cycle incurs changes in the cells collected from the vagina. The presence or absence of red blood cells, for example, and the appearance of epithelial cells that line the vagina give indications of the estrous stage of the bitch. These cellular changes

BOX 11-1 | Importance of Vaginal Cytologic Examination in Breeding Dogs

Overview

Under the influence of estrogen and other hormones, the epithelial lining of the vagina in the bitch undergoes predictable changes throughout the estrous cycle. These changes occur in response to varying levels of ovarian hormones found in the bloodstream (Figure 1). As estrogen increases, vaginal mucosa thickens, and vaginal epithelial cells become "cornified" and subsequently flake off (desquamate) from the wall of the vagina. During the process of cornification, epithelial cells transition from looking like round, poached eggs (called *parabasal cells*) to large, thin sheets of tissue paper (called *anucleated cells*). This dramatic change is a useful tool for estimating times of maximum fertility in the bitch, and helps veterinarians and breeders identify optimal times for breeding or artificial insemination. It is also an excellent indicator of reproductive health. Although vaginal cytologic examination is widely used in dogs, it is also applicable to breeding programs in the cat and the rat.

Materials Needed

- Examination gloves
- Vaginal speculum (optional)
- Cotton swabs
- Sterile saline
- Glass microscope slides
- Methanol or commercial spray fixative for cytology
- Giemsa, Wright, or Diff-Quik stain

Obtaining and Evaluating the Sample

With the bitch standing, the vulvar lips are gently parted and a cotton-tipped moistened swab is inserted several inches past the vulva (Figure 2) at an angle greater than 45 degrees along the dorsal aspect of the vestibule. This is done to avoid entry into the urethra. A speculum may be used to assist in opening the vestibule and to facilitate passage of the cotton-tipped swab, but this is not recommended. When the swab stops forward progression, it is at the vestibular sphincter (Figure 3).

The swab should be elevated so that it is now parallel to the floor. Gentle pressure is applied to permit passage through the sphincter and progression to the anterior vagina. The swab is rotated in the vagina to collect cells and is subsequently withdrawn from the bitch. The swab is then rolled across a clean microscope slide, forming three parallel lines on the slide. The slide is alcohol-fixed and stained.

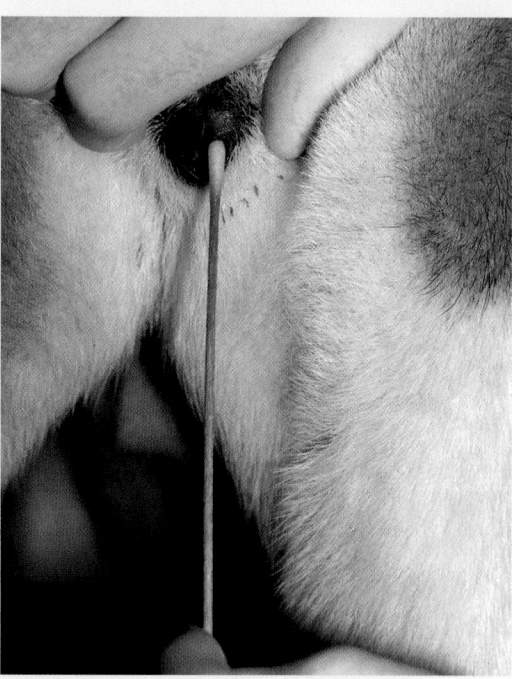

FIGURE 2 A Beagle bitch is placed in standing position for vaginal cytologic examination. The vulvar lips are parted, and a sterile, saline-moistened, cotton-tipped swab is inserted into the vestibule. The swab is redirected at the vestibular sphincter, so it is parallel to the floor, and is advanced to the anterior vagina.

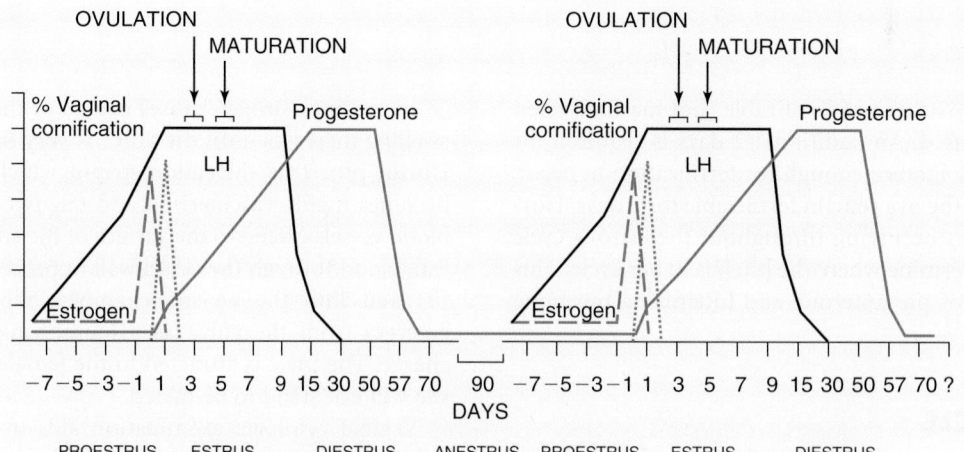

FIGURE 1 The canine estrous cycle. Proestrus lasts about 9 days. During proestrus, vaginal cornification increases about 10% per day; estrogen levels peak near the end of proestrus. Throughout most of a 9-day estrus, 100% cornification is noted. At the beginning of estrus, the luteinizing hormone (LH) peaks. Progesterone starts to rise before the LH spike. About 2 days after the LH peak, ovulation occurs, followed by 2- to 3-day maturation of oocytes. At the start of diestrus, vaginal cornification abruptly declines to less than 50% cornified. Diestrus lasts about 57 days and is characterized by high progesterone. At the end of diestrus, progesterone declines, and the bitch enters a 90- to 150-day anestrus. The cycle then starts again.

BOX 11-1 | Importance of Vaginal Cytologic Examination in Breeding Dogs—cont'd

Even though changes in the appearance of vaginal epithelial cells represent a developmental continuum, only a few fundamental cell types are recognized during cytologic evaluation: parabasal, intermediate, superficial, and anucleated (Figure 4). Fully cornified cells are anucleated superficial cells. However, many epithelial cells will appear to be somewhere in between these types. In addition, white and red blood cells and bacteria are commonly seen in vaginal smears depending on the stage of the estrous cycle. They offer additional clues to technicians and veterinarians regarding the reproductive status of a particular bitch.

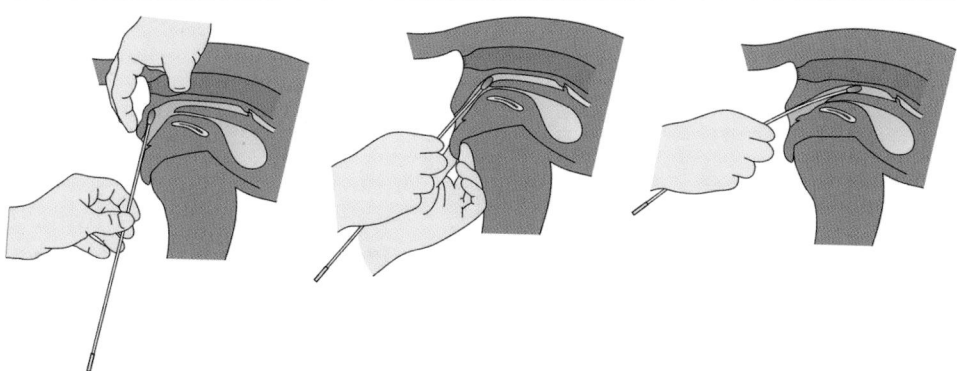

FIGURE 3 A diagram demonstrating cell collection for vaginal cytologic preparation and examination. (From Eilts BE: Determining estrous status, NAVS Clinician's Brief 5:40, 2007.)

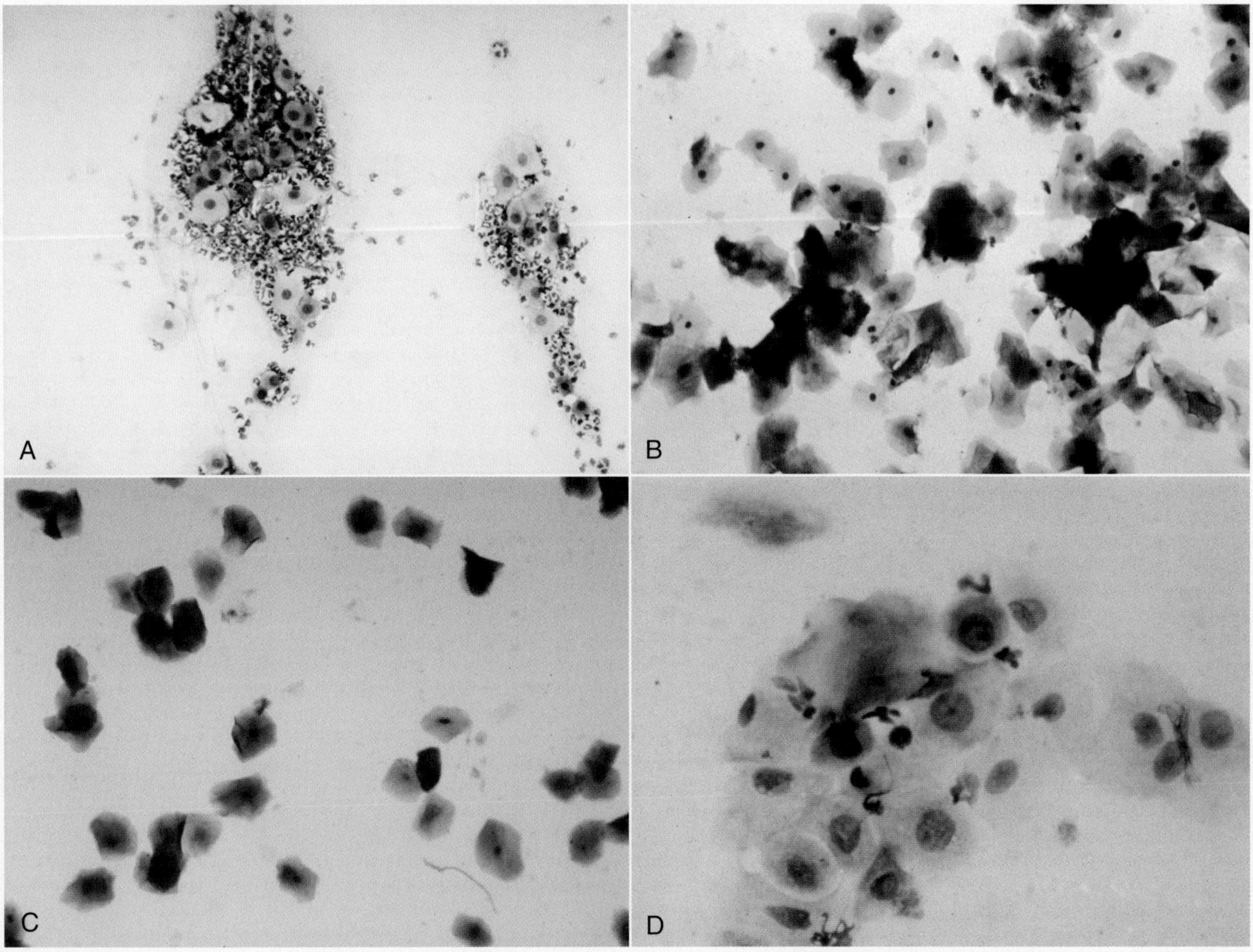

FIGURE 4 **A,** Early proestrus: Vaginal cytologic specimens contain parabasal and a few epithelial cells and a multitude of neutrophils and red blood cells, mucus, and debris. **B,** Late proestrus: Superficial, nucleated epithelial cells predominate, and the amount of mucus is decreased. **C,** Estrus: Nucleated and anucleated superficial cells are visible. Stark absence of all other cell types is evident. **D,** Diestrus: Many parabasal and superficial epithelial cells are visible, with no neutrophils, red blood cells, mucus, or debris.

BOX 11-1	Importance of Vaginal Cytologic Examination in Breeding Dogs—cont'd

Summary of the Canine Estrous Cycle

STAGE IN ESTROUS CYCLE		BEHAVIOR OF BITCH	CLINICAL SIGNS	DURATION	PHYSIOLOGY	PREDOMINANT CELL TYPE	PRESENCE OF DEBRIS AND MUCUS
Follicular Phase (follicle present)	Proestrus	Attracts male, but will not stand for male	• Serosanguineous discharge • Hyperemic, swollen vulva	About 9 days	• Increase in estrogen as follicle develops • Uterus enlarges • Vaginal epithelium proliferates—RBCs leak from capillaries	• Early proestrus: nondegenerate neutrophils • Mixture of parabasal, intermediate, and superficial epithelial cells; variable presence of bacteria (see Figure 11-4, A) • Late proestrus: number of neutrophils decreases and number of superficial cells increases (see Figure 11-4, B)	Yes, abundant
	Estrus	Female seeks out males and will stand for coitus	• Clear discharge • Reduced swelling in vulva	About 9 days	• LH surges • Estrogen decreases • Progesterone increases • Glandular secretions increase; vaginal epithelium becomes hyperemic and ovulation occurs	• 90% to 100% of cells are keratinized, superficial epithelial cells • Many are enucleated • Bacteria often seen attached to superficial cells (see Figure 11-4, C)	Yes, but reduced
Luteal Phase (corpus luteum present)	Diestrus	Stops accepting male	• Small amount of discharge • Little evidence of vulvar edema	70 to 80 days	• CL secretes large amounts of progesterone • Uterine gland hypertrophy • Cervix constricts and vaginal secretions become tacky	• Sudden decrease in superficial cells to 20% • Increase in number of small intermediate cells • Neutrophils present that may contain phagocytized RBCs and bacteria • This stage can look like proestrus cytologically (see Figure 11-4, D)	Scant
	Anestrus	No behavioral signs	• Scant discharge • No vulvar edema	Variable depending upon if pregnant or not	• Reproductive system is at rest • Secretions are scant if present • Cervix is closed • Vaginal mucosa is pale	• Parabasal and intermediate cells predominate • No superficial cells • RBCs and neutrophils present in low numbers or absent	None

From Beimborn VR, Tarpley HL, Bain PJ, Latimer KS: *The canine estrous cycle: staging using vaginal cytological examination*. Available at: http://www.vet.uga.edu/vpp/clerk/beimborn/. Veterinary Clinical Pathology Clerkship Program, Class of 2003, Ross University, School of Veterinary Medicine, St. Kitts, West Indies (Beimborn); and Department of Pathology, College of Veterinary Medicine, The University of Georgia, Athens, GA (Tarpley, Bain, Latimer). Developed from online source.
CL, Corpus luteum; *LH*, luteinizing hormone; *RBCs*, red blood cells.

BOX 11-1	Importance of Vaginal Cytologic Examination in Breeding Dogs—cont'd

Because a luteinizing hormone (LH) peak may occur as long as 2 days after full cornification, vaginal cytologic examination cannot offer a precise prediction of ovulation. Therefore, hormone assays such as the one pictured in Figure 5 can be used to indicate surges in LH, thereby offering a more precise estimate of ovulation (2 days after the LH peak). Other commercially available assays are helpful when performed after rises in progesterone levels leading to an LH peak, or when relaxin is measured to confirm pregnancy (Figure 6).

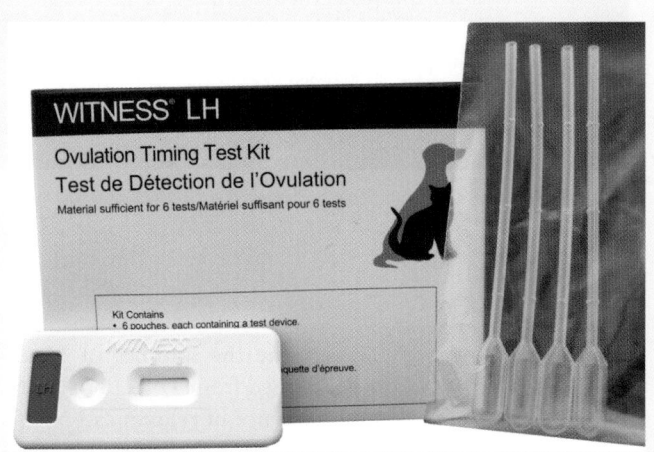

FIGURE 5 A commercially available kit is used to perform quantitative luteinizing hormone (LH) analysis.

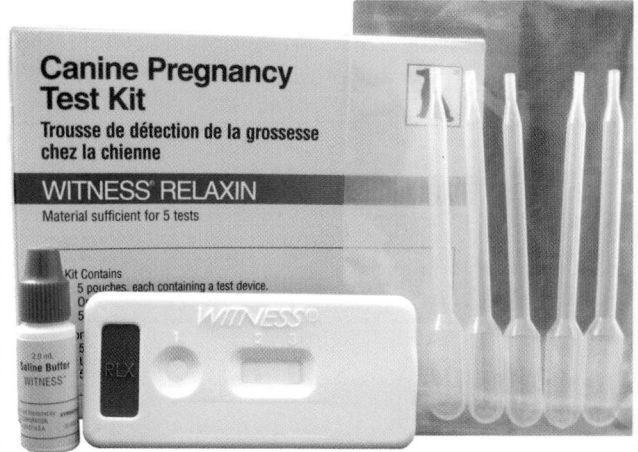

FIGURE 6 A commercially available kit is used to measure canine relaxin to determine pregnancy in a bitch.

assist veterinary personnel to identify particularly fertile periods for insemination. Refer to Box 11-1 for an illustrated discussion of vaginal cytology.

> **TECHNICIAN NOTE** Estrus in most species is due to the relationship of estrogen to progesterone.

Estrus

Estrus lasts approximately 9 days (range, 3 to 18 days). It is suggested that the total time of proestrus and estrus should not exceed 21 days to be considered normal. When in estrus, the bitch will flag, described as the tail raised and held to one side, and will stand for the male. She may, at the beginning of the "courtship," play with the male to establish a behaviorally friendly relationship. If natural breeding or service occurs, the male and the female will be "locked" together (tied) for up to 30 minutes. Vulvar edema decreases rapidly as estrogen is decreasing, such that wrinkles appear in the vulva, and thus the vulva appears smaller than during proestrus. The vulvar discharge generally becomes serous or slightly brownish. In some bitches, the discharge may remain red, but vaginal cytologic examination may not reveal intact red blood cells, indicating that the cells have previously lysed.

It should be remembered that not all bitches demonstrate heat at this time. Some bitches, although in physiologic estrus, will never show signs of standing heat.

In the dog, most ova are released from follicles within 96 hours of the peak in luteinizing hormone (LH). Younger bitches tend to ovulate within 24 hours of the increase, and older bitches ovulate slightly later. The bitch may remain in estrus for 7 or 8 days following ovulation, even though a functional corpus luteum is present. Ova in the bitch are not fertilizable at the time of ovulation and require another 48 hours to become fully mature in the oviduct.

A fertile estrus can be successfully induced in the bitch with ergot products such as cabergoline or bromocriptine if she is at least 4 months from her previous estrus. These products work well and are affordable. Cabergoline offers a slight advantage in that it does not cause the intestinal upset observed many times with bromocriptine.

Diestrus

Diestrus lasts approximately 58 days. Diestrus ends when a pregnant bitch whelps, or when a nonpregnant bitch's progesterone concentration drops to below 1 ng/ml. Prostaglandin F2alpha does not appear to be important as a natural controller of CL regression in the bitch, but it is used frequently to lyse (cause to regress) a CL. **Parturition** occurs within approximately 24 hours after the CL is no longer functional. Progesterone at this time is less than 1 ng/ml. Uterine involution after whelping or in the nonpregnant bitch is not complete until approximately 120 days after ovulation.

Anestrus

This is the period of least reproductive activity. The uterus is regenerating from the previous estrus and diestrus or pregnancy. No ovarian activity occurs until toward the end of anestrus. Anestrus lasts approximately 120 days (range, 60 to 200+ days).

> **TECHNICIAN NOTE** Tests for levels of luteinizing hormone and progesterone can be used to predict when a bitch should be bred.

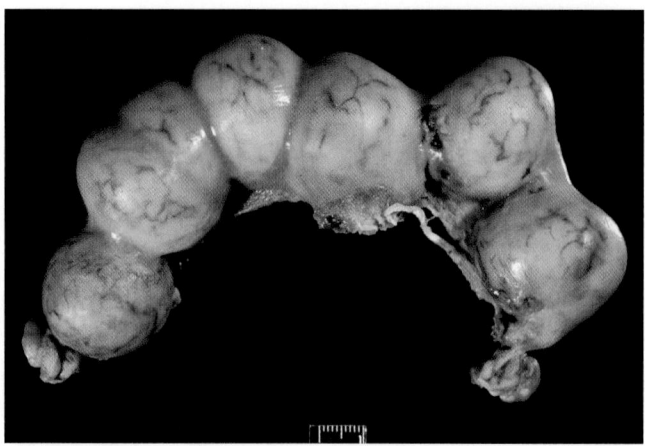

FIGURE 11-9 Amnionic vesicles within the canine uterus.

BREEDING

Insemination of bitches can be done by natural service (the male is breeding the female) or by **artificial insemination**, which can include vaginal, surgical, or transcervical approaches. Timing has to be most precise when cryopreserved (frozen) semen is used. Although frozen semen can be stored for potentially a thousand years in liquid nitrogen at −196° C (−320.8° F), it has the shortest life span of all semen sources once it is thawed. Ideally, fertilization should occur within 12 hours after thaw. Fresh semen delivered by natural service or by artificial insemination remain capable of fertilization in the reproductive tract for up to 5 days, with 3 days expected from all but subfertile males. Insemination ideally should be performed once at the correct time. Natural service can be performed at the 2nd to 4th day after the LH spike, or after progesterone reaches a serum concentration of 2.0 ng/ml. The disadvantage of performing LH assays is that samples require daily obtainment, which is inconvenient and expensive for owners. Therefore, the author would prefer progesterone assays. Progesterone measures approximately 5.0 ng/ml at the time of ovulation, and usually above 10 ng/ml at the fertile period. Progesterone is very valuable at predicting when to inseminate if used before high concentrations are reached. Once concentrations reach greater than 10 ng/ml, their predictive value is lost, and one is better served by using vaginal cytologic examination and observing for the reappearance of white blood cells and noncornified epithelial cells.

GESTATION

Gestation length in the bitch is approximately 60 days from fertilization. Pregnancy examination by palpation is possible in most bitches at 21 to 30 days of gestation (Figure 11-9). Ultrasonographic examination is also very useful for the diagnosis of pregnancy and of the vibrancy of fetuses, but it should not be used to determine the number of fetuses. Ultrasonography may be performed from 17 to 18 days until term. An assay based on the presence of **relaxin** can be used from 21 days to term, but it may yield slightly better results if used after day 23 following fertilization. Radiographs can be used from 43 days until term but provide the most information if used closer to term (2 to 4 days before the expected due date). Determinations of fetal count, size of fetuses in relationship to the pelvis of the dam, and presentation of the first fetus to be delivered all can be determined via radiography.

PARTURITION

Stage I of whelping represents the commencement of uterine contractions without an abdominal component and averages 6 to 12 hours, but can be as long as 36 hours. The bitch is usually restless and may show nesting behavior. She often appears nervous, pants, and may tremble or shiver. Body temperature drops to 37.2° C (99° F) about 24 hours before stage II in approximately 85% of bitches. This temperature drop is related to the abrupt decline in progesterone and can be useful for the dog owner, to signal that whelping is imminent. To be reliable, the temperature should be taken at the same time each day, preferably in the morning before any activity. Stage II, when the bitch pushes the puppies out, lasts approximately 20 to 60 minutes per puppy (Figure 11-10). However, no longer than 2 hours should elapse between deliveries. Stage II usually lasts a total of 3 to 6 hours but may be as long as 24 hours total. The presentation of the puppies is 60% anterior in the bitch. A blackish-green discharge is normal during parturition and comes from the site of placental attachment to the uterus.

The canine placenta is positioned around the fetus like a ring on a finger and serves as a narrow band of attachment of the **chorioallantois** to the endometrium (Figure 11-11). This type of placentation is called *zonary*.

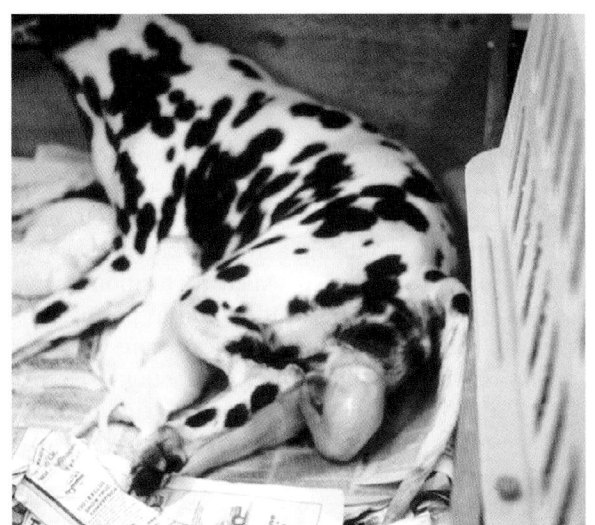

FIGURE 11-10 A puppy delivered during a normal canine parturition.

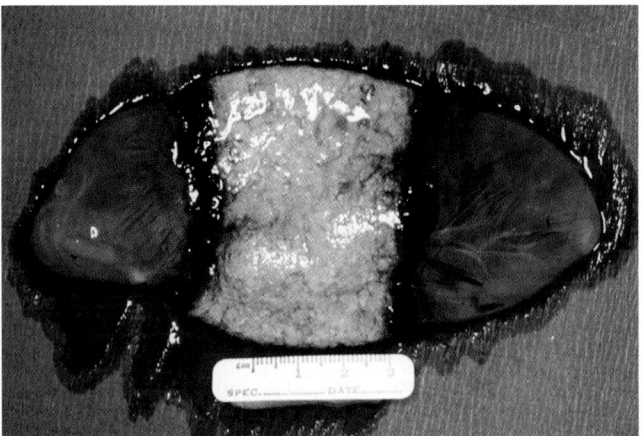

FIGURE 11-11 Zonary placentation of the bitch.

Guidelines for recognizing dystocia (difficult birth) include strong continual contractions for 30 minutes without progress; weak, infrequent contractions for 2 hours without progress; and a prolonged interval between puppies. If any of these criteria is met, veterinary examination is warranted. Ultrasound can be used to assess fetal viability, but radiography is the only reliable method for accurately determining the number of pups in utero, their relative size, and their position.

FELINE REPRODUCTION

GENERAL

The female feline is known as the *queen*. The male is referred to as the *tom*. The offspring are *kittens*. The neutered male is just that. The female that has had the gonads removed is known as *spayed* if the uterus was also removed, or *ovariectomized* if it was not. The delivery of fetuses is known as *queening*. The queen is a **seasonally polyestrous** and cycles from January through October. For this reason, queens are considered long daylight length breeders. These are approximate times and individual variation has been noted, especially if the queen is exposed to artificial lighting. Puberty usually begins at 4 to 12 months of age, depending on the photoperiod at this age. Queens should have had an estrus by 18 months of age. Puberty for queens occurs at a weight of about 2.5 kg. If the length of light is constant at 12 to 14 hours per day, a continuous season can be established and maintained. The anatomy of the reproductive tract of the queen is similar to that of the bitch, with ovaries approximately 1 cm long and uterine horns approximately 10 cm long. The body of the uterus is approximately 2 cm long.

ESTROUS CYCLE

The queen is an induced ovulator, although spontaneous ovulation may occur if triggered by proper visual or pheromone cues. Cycle length is 4 to 30 days (average length, 14 to 19 days), and estrus lasts approximately 10 days. If queens are exposed to constant daylight, ovulation will not occur. Decreasing daylight will lead to a prolonged anestrus. Queens can live to 14 years of age or older, but litter size may decrease with age.

During estrus, increased vocalization is the norm. In addition, the queen may roll, demonstrate lordosis, and tread in place, and this behavior will intensify with handling. Anorexia may be seen, and urine spraying may occur. No vulvar discharge is evident. The behavior may be interpreted as abnormal behavior and assistance requested. Breeding usually is recommended after the 3rd day of estrus for the best probability of impregnation. Luteinizing hormone is the hormone produced and released by the mating stimulus. An increase in this hormone occurs within 10 minutes of copulation. This increase in LH may last up to 24 hours. Less than 50% of all queens ovulate with a single mating. The primary hormones of significance are follicle-stimulating hormone (FSH), luteinizing hormone (LH), progesterone (P4), estradiol (E2), **prolactin**, and relaxin. The outcome of a heat where breeding occurred may include pregnancy (CL formed), nonpregnancy (CL formed), or no ovulation (no CL). Although mating occurs, ovulation is not necessarily induced. If ovulation occurs but there is no pregnancy, the CL is maintained for approximately 5 to 6 weeks. If no CL is formed, the queen will return to estrus in approximately 3 to 14 days.

Progesterone increases 2 to 3 days after breeding and peaks at days 21 to 30 from the increased presence of CLs that form from ovulated follicles. By day 45, the placenta produces progestogens, which gradually decrease until parturition. Without a stimulus to cause ovulation, progesterone will remain at baseline even though the queen shows signs of heat. Estradiol concentrations increase during estrus and decrease after ovulation or regression of unovulated follicles. In the pregnant queen, concentrations of free estrogens increase before parturition, thereby sensitizing the uterus to the effects of **oxytocin**.

Prolactin concentration is increased during the last half of gestation. A significant increase in prolactin is seen 3 days before birth. Prolactin concentrations remain increased during lactation but are at baseline in the nonpregnant state. Relaxin is produced by the fetoplacental unit and is responsible for relaxing the pelvic connective tissue before delivery of offspring. Concentrations are detectable by day 25 of pregnancy and plateau at approximately day 35.

Prostaglandin F2alpha (PGF2alpha) is secreted by most tissues within the body and is a major part of the inflammatory reaction. However, the placenta and the endometrium are major sources within the reproductive tract. Concentrations of PGF2alpha start to rise at day 30 of gestation and plateau at day 45. PGF2alpha concentrations increase greatly before delivery and have beneficial effects on uterine contractility at term. PGF2alpha can induce abortion in queens and was used in this species before it was used in the canine.

> **TECHNICIAN NOTE** Fertilization of oocytes occurs in the oviduct—NOT in the uterus.

GESTATION

Fertilization in the queen as in all species covered within this chapter occurs in the ampule portion of the oviduct—not in the uterus. Fertilized eggs migrate down the uterine horn. This transuterine migration occurs as in all multipara, so spacing between fetuses will permit maximal area for placental attachment. The type of placentation is zonary, like in the dog. Epithelial cells of the fetal **chorion** are in direct contact with maternal chorionic endothelial cells. The average duration of pregnancy is 65 days after breeding. The heartbeat is ultrasonographically detectable at approximately day 16. The range of gestation based on breeding may be varied because of multiple breedings, and because ovulation is not induced when suspected. When parturition occurs before the 60th day of gestation, the fetuses are considered premature and generally do not survive. Observable signs of pregnancy include increased size of the teats by the 2nd to 3rd week, with increased mammary enlargement through term. Weight gain is obvious by mid gestation and will depend on the age of the queen, previous litters, and the size of the litters. Pregnancy can be diagnosed by abdominal palpation of the uterus by approximately 18 days after fertilization; this diagnosis is accurate until approximately day 32 to 35, when all amniotic vesicles coalesce and are no longer discernible. Ultrasonographic imaging is excellent, starting at approximately day 15, and can be used through term. Radiographic diagnosis of pregnancy is used from approximately day 40 until term. The author prefers not to use this technique until nearly 60 days for maximal information and uses it mostly for fetal count.

PARTURITION

Parturition can last from as few as a couple of hours to over a day with survival of the fetuses. Queens usually build nests, resulting in higher survival rates of the fetuses. Queens can return to estrus while nursing a litter of kittens. Depending on the season of the year in which parturition occurred, estrus may occur from 2 weeks to 2 months postpartum.

Stage I of parturition, as in all species, begins with uterine contractions without abdominal contractions. Decreased activity is seen with behavioral changes, including that the queen is more or less social. Fetal movements are increased, lactational secretion is evident, and relaxation around the perineal area is noted. Stage I ends when the chorioallantoic membrane ruptures. Stage II is the period when all fetuses are delivered. Stage III is the time when the placentas are completely passed, and the uterus returns to normal. Uterine size is reduced rapidly, but reepithelialization of the endometrium takes weeks. After parturition, the queen has an anestrus, depending on the time of year.

Dystocias are uncommon in the queen; when they occur, they usually are seen among purebreds. The queen is the only animal commonly seen in a veterinary practice that can assist itself from the outside with a dystocia. It can pull on the fetus by grasping with its teeth if the fetus is exposed through the vulva, and by pulling as well as pushing with uterine and abdominal contractions. Fetal causes of dystocia are primarily large fetuses, lateral deviation of the head, and breech deliveries, which can be delivered, but can reduce the speed, and this can result in fetal death. Maternal causes of dystocia include uterine torsion, primary and secondary uterine inertia, and a small pelvic size due to poor nutrition or young age. If radiographs are performed before the onset of labor, the owner will know how many fetuses to expect. If the most posterior fetus is in the proper presentation, position, and posture, oxytocin (2 IU IM per cat) and, in the case of many delayed deliveries, calcium can be administered. Oxytocin can be repeated at 20- to 30-minute intervals if fetal movement is noted posteriorly in the birth canal.

EQUINE REPRODUCTION

GENERAL

The *mare* is the female of the equine species. A *filly* is a young mare, which usually implies that she is younger than 3 years of age, but this is open to some horse owners' interpretation. A *stallion*, the male of the species, has both testes in the scrotum. If the testes are not in the scrotum, the animal should be called a male horse or **cryptorchid**—not a stallion. A *colt* is, in reality, a young male; the term may be used descriptively up to 3 years of age, but again this is open to interpretation by the owner. Also, to confuse this further, some owners will call all foals, colts! The delivery of the fetus is known as *foaling*. A foal is the newborn of the species and is usually called this until approximately 1 year of age, or January 1 (the universal birthdate of most equine breeds) of the next year, when the foal will be known as a *yearling*. The foal may also be called a *weanling* after separation from its mother, or upon reaching 2 to 3 months of age. Again, this is open to interpretation. A male that has been castrated is called a *gelding*. A mare that has had the ovaries removed is called a *spayed* or *ovariectomized mare*. The uterus is not removed from mares along with the ovaries because this is a much more complicated procedure than removing the ovaries, and removing it provides no advantage in most species. However, it is common to call ovariectomized mares *spayed*. A thick tunic called the *tunica albuginea* covers the ovary in the mare. This prevents ovulation from occurring anywhere on the surface, as occurs in other species, and therefore it can occur only at the ovulation fossa (Figure 11-12). The endometrium consists of approximately 13 folds; this permits expansion of the uterus and attachment of the placenta during pregnancy (Figure 11-13).

Estrous Cycle

The estrous cycle of the filly is initiated at approximately 12 to 24 months of age. Puberty is reached for the colt at approximately the same age, but it is impossible to know the exact day that it was reached. Puberty of colts usually implies that they are capable of impregnating a mare successfully. Most fillies are fertile at 2 years of age, but many stallions are not fertile until they reach the age of 3. There is little reason to be concerned as long as the stallion is examined and no clinical problems are found at 2 years of age. However, if the stallion is 3 years old and is not fertile, one should be suspicious of permanent fertility problems. Reaching puberty in the filly (first ovulation) does not imply that the reproductive tract is mature. Signs of estrus may appear before puberty, but ovulation usually occurs between these ages. Breed variation due to size has been observed in that Miniature horses usually reach puberty before the draft breeds.

Onset of estrus is initiated by production and release of GnRH. In the case of the equine, the influence of light on GnRH concentration is substantial. The equine is a seasonally polyestrous animal and, therefore, is influenced greatly by the increasing length of daylight during spring. The peak of estrous activity occurs near June 21 (the longest daylight day of the year), and the least activity occurs near December 21 (the shortest daylight day of the year). It has been suggested that light entering the eyes of the horse will cause a change in melatonin production through increases or decreases of only 3 to 5 minutes of total light in a day (Figure 11-14). Although humidity has been associated with some species as a controller of estrual activity, it does not appear to be important in the horse. Temperature, although not necessarily beneficial for the induction of estrual activity, can influence the positive effects of light. Extremely cold conditions can override the beneficial effects of increased light and can delay the occurrence of estrus in mares. Nutrition is an important influence in the mare, as it is in all species. If the nutritional requirements of the mare are not met to maintain all body functions adequately, cycling activity will not occur. The reproductive system is the only body system that can cease to function if the animal's nutritional requirements are not met. If mares are pregnant, they will attempt to maintain their pregnancy, possibly to the point of their own death from starvation. Stress can influence estrual activity in that if stress is severe enough, estrual activity will not occur. This does not occur frequently, but it can occur, usually in heavily worked athletes.

The average length of heat in the mare is 5 days, but it can extend from fewer than 2 to 9 days. Length of the estrous cycle on average is 21 days but can range from 19 to 28 days. The fact that a mare has reached puberty does not imply that her reproductive tract is mature. Fillies younger than 2 years old can have a 50% abortion rate; older fillies can have an abortion rate of approximately 25%. Although the filly has ovulated and meets the definition of sexually mature, the uterus in many young female equines requires additional time to reach the point of maintaining a fetus to term. The reason for early breeding in most fillies is that they have proved to be useless for any other purpose. High rates of abortion are good indications that they should not be used

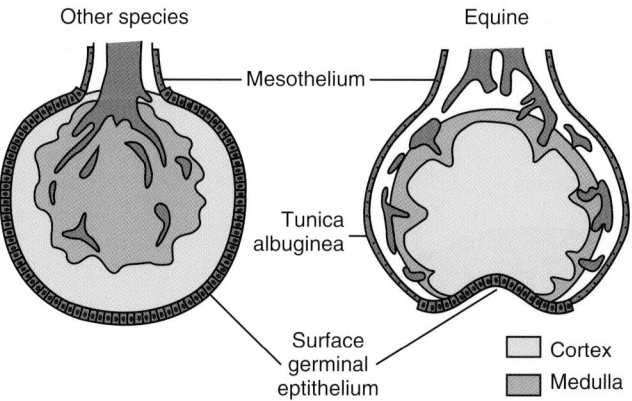

FIGURE 11-12 Comparison of mare ovary with other species.

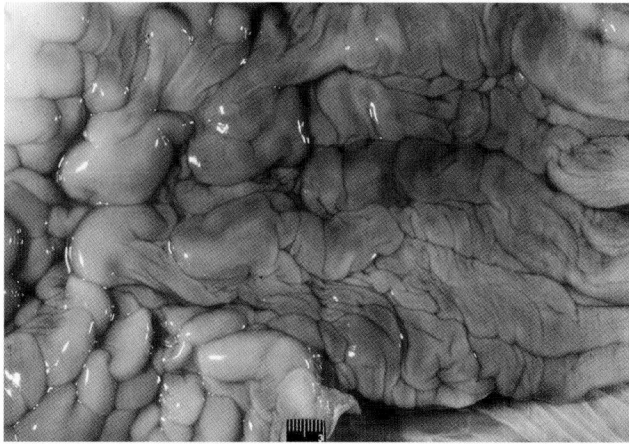

FIGURE 11-13 Endometrial folds.

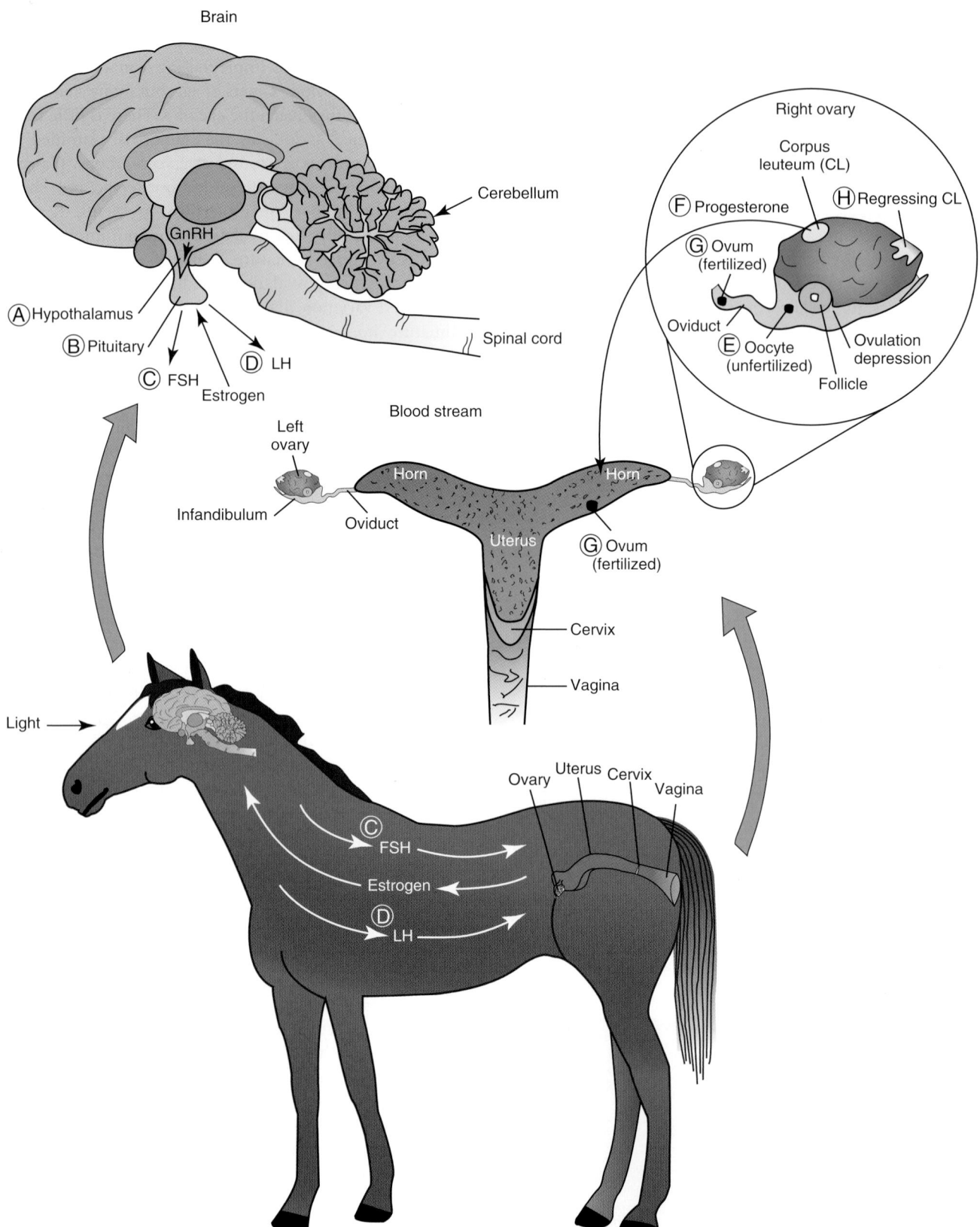

FIGURE 11-14 **A,** For species that are seasonally polyestrous, such as the horse, extended daylight stimulates elevation of gonadotropin-releasing hormone (GnRH) in the hypothalamus. **B,** Rise of GnRH stimulates excretion of follicle-stimulating hormone (FSH) in the pituitary gland. **C,** FSH is carried in the bloodstream to the ovaries, causing the development of a follicle. Each follicle contains one egg or oocyte. As the follicle grows, it produces estrogen. **D,** Increased estrogen levels cause another release of GnRH from the hypothalamus; this in turn causes luteinizing hormone (LH) to be released from the pituitary. **E,** The mature oocyte in the follicle is released suddenly from the follicle through a process called *ovulation*. After ovulation, the ovum (no longer called *oocyte*) passes into the oviduct, where fertilization occurs. After several days in the oviduct, the young embryo moves into the uterine horn, where it implants into the endometrium. **F,** After ovulation, the follicle is transformed into a corpus luteum (CL). The CL produces progesterone, the hormone that maintains pregnancy. **G,** If fertilization does not occur, the uterus (in most species) secretes prostaglandin. Prostaglandin binds to receptors on the CL and lyses it. **H,** Without the CL, progesterone levels drop, and the estrous cycle is repeated.

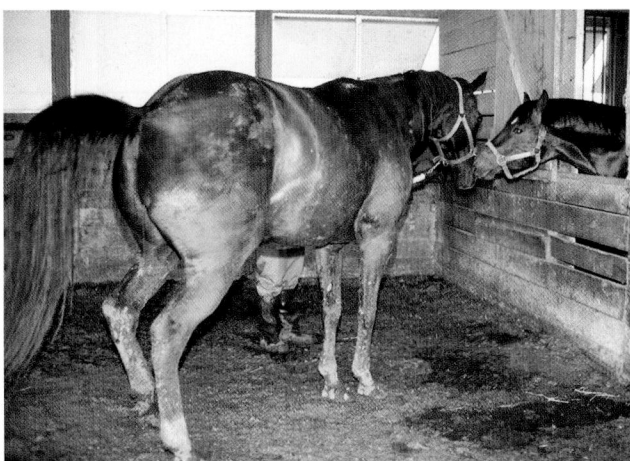

FIGURE 11-15 Stallion *(right)* teasing a mare *(left)* through a dutch doorway.

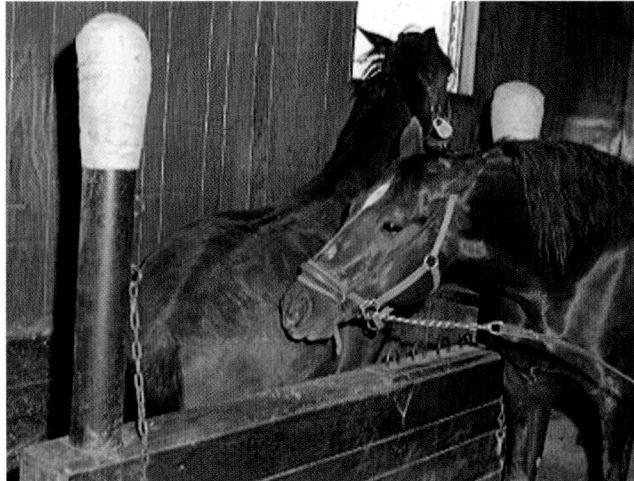

FIGURE 11-16 Stallion *(right)* teasing a mare *(left)* in stocks.

as broodmares. The exception is when the filly is used as an embryo donor.

Estrus

Signs of estrus include frequent urination, tail raised, frequent opening and closing of the vulva, exposing the clitoris, decreased kicking, ear position forward, leaning toward the stallion, and standing for the stallion. The ear position of the horse provides considerable information on the disposition and attitude of that horse. Signs of diestrus (presence of a CL and under the influence of progesterone) include clamping or swishing of the tail, increased kicking, increased striking, increased biting, ears back, and moving away from the stallion.

Some mares will not exhibit signs of heat while in physiologic estrus. This may be precipitated by the presence of a foal or by a teaser that is overly aggressive. Some mares will exhibit signs of estrus when not in physiologic estrus, including standing for the stallion. Various methods may be used for teasing of mares, and the preferred method is determined primarily by the managerial system. These methods include taking the mare to the stallion with the stallion in a stall or in a teasing pen (Figure 11-15). They may also involve taking the stallion to the mares with the mares in a small coral or pen, or chutes, or walking the stallion through a field where the mares are housed (Figures 11-16). Some will tease by permitting the stallion to enter the stall of the mare while the stallion is held on a lead from the outside of the stall. The controllability of the stallion may eliminate some of these possibilities. A pony stallion can be used in some situations, so there is less probability of an accidental breeding. A teasing system that includes actual physical contact of the stallion and the mare will yield the best results. It has been demonstrated that teasing is based on sight, sound, and smell or pheromones. Research conducted by our group at Ohio State has shown that vocalization of the stallion is very important. Inclusion of smell or pheromones with vocalizations will increase the number of mares responding, and even the inclusion of a life-size stallion cardboard cutout

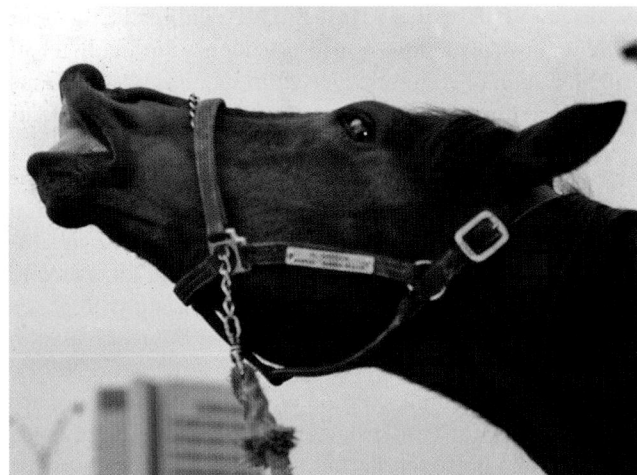

FIGURE 11-17 Flehmen response of stallion.

may lead to additional mare responses. The flehmen response occurs when a stallion approaches a mare that may be in heat and curls the upper lip upward, exposing the vomeronasal organ inside the nose, so the pheromones can more exactly and easily be perceived (Figure 11-17). Physical contact between a mare and a live stallion is preferred if a teasing program is to be used as part of the breeding program. The author prefers to use palpation of the genital tract instead of teasing to determine estrous status.

> **TECHNICIAN NOTE** The flehmen response occurs when a stallion curls the upper lip upward, exposing the vomeronasal organ inside the nose, so the pheromones from the mare can more exactly and easily be perceived.

The mare usually will ovulate during estrus. This generally takes place approximately 48 hours before the end of heat, and the ovum is released into the ovulation fossa. Ovulations generally (80%) occur between 4:00 PM and 8:00 AM.

However, because of the long life span of the sperm in the equine, nighttime breedings offer no advantage. Follicles may range from 2.5 to 12.5 cm in diameter at the time of ovulation but usually fall in the range of 3.5 to 5.0 cm. Ovulation can occur in the mare with no obvious signs of heat. This is especially true in mares that have recently foaled, in maiden mares, and in mares being teased with a very aggressive teaser.

It is very common for mares to show signs of heat without being in a physiologic estrus. This occurs primarily in late winter, early spring, or late fall. Twin ovulations occur frequently in the equine (average, 18%), but some families of horses have higher rates because this is an inherited condition. Because of great variability in length of the estrous cycle and estrus, ovulation time has great variability. In the equine, the fertilizing capability of the ovum is greatest within the 1st 12 hours post ovulation and then decreases rapidly; it is best if sperm are present within the oviduct before ovulation occurs, or if the mare is inseminated within the 12-hour window post ovulation. Sperm usually have a highly fertilizing life span of 72 hours. The ovum requires no additional time for maturation once released, so the process can occur immediately if sperm are present. On some occasions, it may be best to inseminate mares after ovulation to increase the possibility of conception. This usually is associated with a decrease in the quality of the sperm, or a reduction in situations where single breedings are to be made on mares to conserve semen. These postovulation inseminations are highly successful if performed within 12 hours. Ovulation can be induced in the equine when a nearly mature follicle is present by the administration of human chorionic gonadotropin (hCG) or GnRH developed for equine usage, such as deslorelin. Both approaches are approximately the same in terms of their success in inducing ovulation, but hCG may take longer to achieve the same percentage.

Once ovulation occurs, the corpus hemorrhagicum, followed by the corpus luteum, forms very rapidly within the antrum—the space previously filled with follicular fluid. Luteal cells of the follicular wall rapidly increase in number and begin to form progesterone. The CL is fully functional within approximately 5 days post ovulation, or possibly within 8 to 9 days from the onset of heat. It is at this time that the CL can be lysed with the aid of prostaglandin (PGF2alpha), which can be given medically, or can be released naturally within the body if severe tissue trauma has occurred. Under average conditions, the CL will be maintained and will continue to produce progesterone until approximately day 14 post ovulation. The ovaries during the period of the CL will continue to have follicular activity and may actually ovulate around day 8 to 10 after the initial ovulation. The cervix should be closed; if it is not, this may indicate lack of progesterone or a laceration of the cervix. Figure 11-18 shows a relaxed cervix. At 14 days post ovulation, progesterone concentrations begin to decrease. Within 3 days, the progesterone concentration reaches baseline (<1.0 ng/ml), and the mare returns to heat. If conception occurred, the CL will be maintained and progesterone will

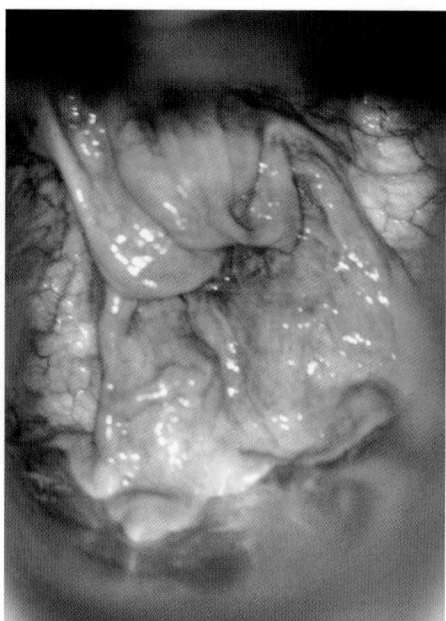

FIGURE 11-18 Relaxed cervix of mare during estrus.

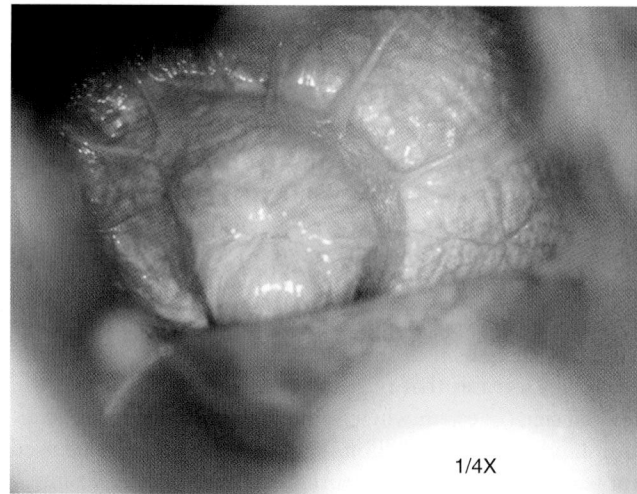

1/4X

FIGURE 11-19 Closed cervix of mare during diestrus.

remain elevated. Under this hormonal influence, the cervix will be closed (Figure 11-19).

The breeding season in North America for most breeds of horses begins approximately February 1st because it is undesirable for offspring to be born before January 1st. Foals born December 31st would be 1 year old the next day. The naturally occurring breeding season occurs during spring and summer, from approximately April 1st to September 1st. During this time, the mare is seasonally polyestrous, implying that multiple estrous cycles are occurring within this segment of the year, and not year round. In winter, however, the mare is naturally anestrus (Figure 11-20). The human imposed breeding season on the equine extends from February 1st through approximately July 15th in many breeds. This creates many of the equine reproductive problems that owners and veterinarians encounter.

Equine Ovary

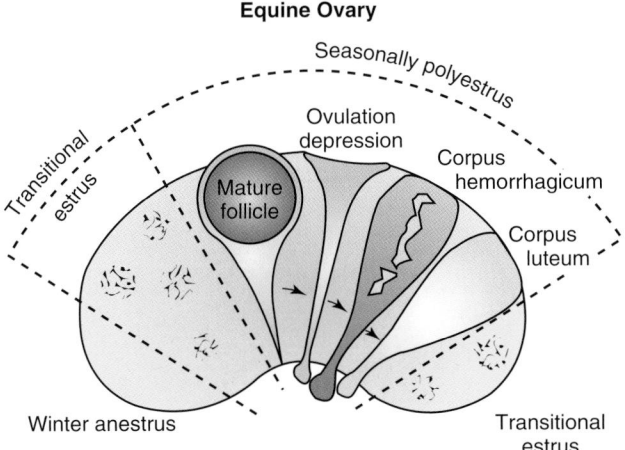

FIGURE 11-20 Annual ovarian activity. The horse is naturally poly-estrous during the spring and summer and is in anestrus during winter months. Some horses are artificially induced to begin estrual cycling during winter months by being exposed to artificial lighting. Under the influence of prolonged light, follicular production is stimulated. Corpora hemorrhagica and corpora lutea follow.

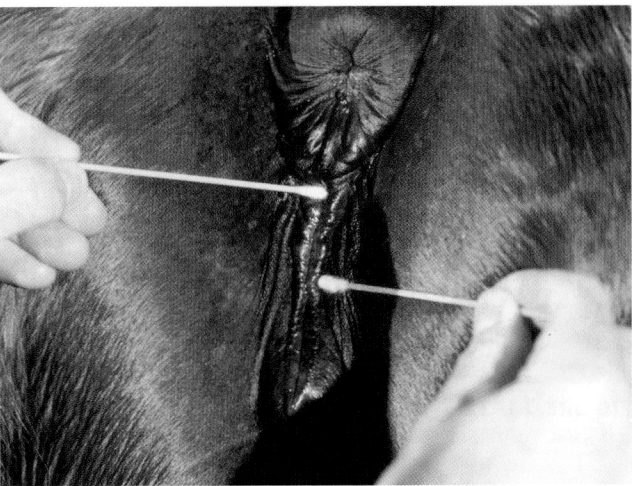

FIGURE 11-21 Vulvar conformation assessment with dorsal opening of the vulva above the pubis.

Mares can be induced into estrus earlier in the year with the use of artificial lighting. The amount of light needed to induce cycling is approximately equal to the amount needed to read fine print in a newspaper in all areas of the horse's stall. This light can be supplied in any light form, such as incandescent, fluorescent, or mercury vapor. It is not about the quality of the light as much as the quantity. Several lighting programs can be used for this purpose, but the author prefers to use the flash system, whereby the lights are on for 2 hours in the window of time between 1:00 AM and 4 AM. The effect is seen on the pineal gland, as previously described. It requires approximately 60 days for this system to initiate follicular activity, and possibly another 30 days for the estrous cycle to become stabilized.

The use of progestogens can shorten the period from follicular development to ovulation. Mares will need to be treated for 10 to 14 days, and this treatment may save 30 to 45 days of reproductive time. Progestogens will work only if sufficient follicular activity is present on the ovaries. Administration of hCG will induce luteinization of follicles if sufficient follicular activity is present to permit CL formation, and if the mare enters into a luteal phase. Other hormonal methods of enhancing follicular development have not been highly successful and therefore are not currently recommended. Melatonin has been fed experimentally to mares and has induced earlier cycling activity. However, this program must be initiated approximately 5 months before the breeding season begins, and for this reason has not been used commercially. Other hormones have been used to initiate follicular development, but these have not been successful in maintenance of CLs following ovulation. Prostaglandin F2alpha is successful in bringing a mare into heat only if a CL is present on the ovary.

Examination of the Reproductive Tract

Palpation of the mare's reproductive tract via the rectum has long been a tool for obtaining more information to use in determination of heat and ovulation status. Important precautions of this technique are to think safety at all times and to position oneself in the safest position. One should remember that palpation stocks are designed only to decrease the movement of the mare from side to side. They are not designed to keep the mare from jumping over the front or from kicking over the rear of the chute. For this reason, in some instances, the best method for positioning the mare is to not have a door on the front or back of the stocks, or to not use stocks. This is possible by palpating the mare around a corner of a building, in a stall doorway, or out in the open, with the palpator up close to the mare. Findings on genital palpation when a mare is in heat include a decrease in uterine tone, relaxation of the cervix, and an increase in the size of follicles present. The body of the uterus is examined, and this is followed by cervical palpation.

A very important anatomic consideration is the conformation of the vulva. This should be examined every time a mare is palpated, and possibly by the owners at other times. The dorsal opening of the vulva should be at or below the pubic bone (Figure 11-21). A decrease in the normal conformation of the vulva permits air and fecal material to enter, resulting in temporary to permanent reduction in conception. It can cause a mare to become sterile owing to chronic irritation and scar tissue formation within the endometrium (lining of the uterus). It can also result in abortion. The surgical repair for this condition is called *Caslick's surgery.*

Vaginal examinations sometimes are done to gain additional information on estrous status. Important considerations of this technique must start with proper preparation of the perineum, so contamination of the reproductive tract will not occur. This would include wrapping the tail and tying it to the side, and washing the perineal area with soap or detergent. Surgical scrubs are not indicated, nor are they

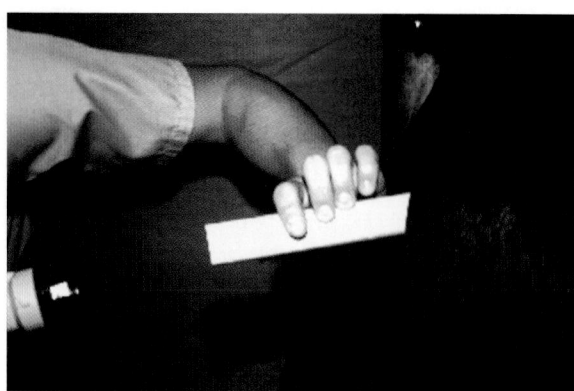

FIGURE 11-22 A vaginal examination is performed on a mare using a disposable speculum.

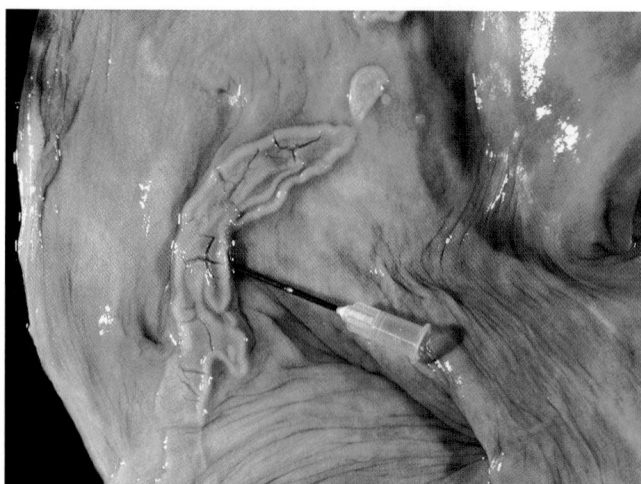

FIGURE 11-23 Endometrial cups of a mare are visible at the end of the needle.

recommended. A sterile vaginal speculum lubricated with sterile lube is inserted into the vestibule by pulling the vulvar lips laterally (Figure 11-22). The speculum is pushed gently upward and forward until the vestibular sphincter is encountered. Once in contact with the sphincter, additional pressure anteriorly and parallel to the ground may be necessary to get the speculum through the lumen of this structure. Forward steady pressure is the best method of dilating this structure. Once in the vagina, the cervix and the vaginal wall should be easily visible.

Insemination

Artificial insemination in the mare is accomplished by first preparing the perineal area as described previously and then placing the artificial insemination rod or tubing into the uterus with sterile gloved hand and arm covered in sterile lubricant. If "deep" intrauterine insemination is performed, special tubing will be carefully threaded up the uterine horn to the opening of the oviduct (papilla). This technique is employed when the sperm concentration is low, or when poorer-quality semen is used. The usual method of inseminating is to place semen in an artificial insemination rod using a syringe. Immediately before placing the rod into the reproductive tract, approximately 2.5 cc of air is drawn into the syringe and is used to push the semen as close to the distal tip of the rod as possible without spilling semen. This is done to remove air from the distal tip of the rod, so that no air enters the uterus, which could have a detrimental effect on the sperm.

Gestation

Pregnancy in the mare is dependent not only on the initial CL of pregnancy, but also on the formation of additional CLs, beginning at approximately day 35 of gestation. Secondary CLs are stimulated to develop by a substance produced by endometrial cups within the endometrium. The source of the tissue that results in endometrial cup formation is the developing fetal membrane (Figure 11-23). A portion of the membrane embeds itself in the endometrium and becomes an endocrine-producing unit from

approximately 35 to 120 days. The substance produced is known as *equine chorionic gonadotropin (eCG)*; in older literature, this was known as *pregnant mare serum gonadotropin (PMSG)*. It has a superovulatory effect in most other species, but not in the equine. CLs are derived from follicles that developed on the ovaries; they may ovulate but more frequently luteinize without releasing the ovum. These secondary CLs will maintain the pregnancy until day 100, and then are no longer required. In some mares, progesterone from the placenta is sufficient by day 68 of pregnancy to maintain pregnancy in the absence of the ovaries. This indicates that the placenta in the mare is a critical source of progesterone and progestogens, which are vitally important to maintain pregnancy. Progesterone begins to decrease by the second trimester; the responsibility for maintaining pregnancy then is transferred to the other progestogen formed from the placenta.

The placenta in the equine is diffuse, indicating that attachments are present throughout the chorioallantoic membrane (chorioallantois), with the only exceptions seen at the isthmus portion of the oviducts and at the cervix. The equine placenta is classified as epitheliochorial, indicating that six layers of tissue are present between the blood of the fetus and that of the dam.

Pregnancy diagnosis in the equine has long been based on palpation of the reproductive tract via rectal examination. Recently, ultrasonographic examination has reduced or eliminated this procedure in many practices. Ultrasonographic examination is more accurate and facilitates the diagnosis of pregnancy earlier than is possible with palpation. Depending on the ultrasound unit, pregnancy can be diagnosed as early as day 10. Most portable units are accurate at 13 to 14 days. However, because it is not known exactly when some mares ovulate, it is better to wait until day 14 to 15. Some ovulations occur later than anticipated, and in the case of twin ovulations, it is best to do an ultrasonographic examination again a few days later, "just in case."

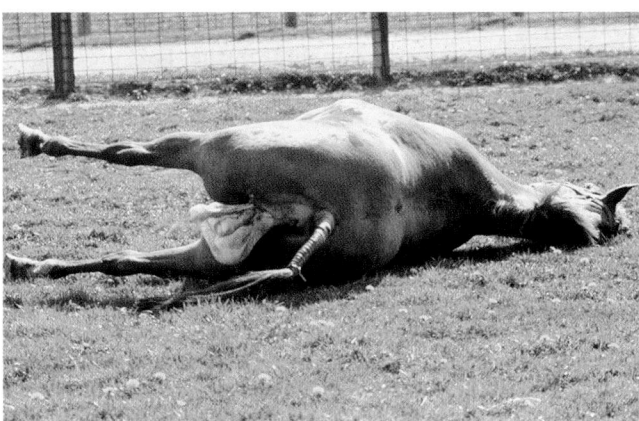

FIGURE 11-24 Parturition in the mare with fetal head, limbs, and amnionic membrane exposed.

Parturition

Induction of parturition in the mare is never based on length of gestation alone. Because of the great variability of normal gestation length (320 to 360 days) in the equine, it is dangerous to the survival of the offspring to induce on the basis of a breeding date. One should always palpate the mare for fetal viability, presentation, position, and posture; these can be determined when the pregnancy reaches approximately 330 days, or when anything appears to be unusual regarding the pregnancy. Important factors to consider before induction include the presence of colostrum, relaxation of vulva and pelvic ligaments, and cervical dilatation of at least 2.5 cm (unless estrogen or another preparation has been used to induce cervical relaxation before induction). Commercially developed tests are available to determine the colostrum electrolytes, which have been related to preparedness for parturition. If the mare does not appear to be at term, the fetus probably is not. Fetuses delivered before they are mature enough will have insufficient surfactant in their lungs and will have difficulty breathing, or may not be able to do so normally and may die. The time to evaluate this is before induction—not afterward. Although other substances can be used to induce parturition, the author has had excellent results inducing parturition without incident with oxytocin.

Parturition in the equine is very rapid and very strenuous. Three stages of parturition have been identified, as in all mammalian species, but the second is short. Stage II begins with rupture of the chorioallantois. Once this occurs, it should be estimated that the fetus will need to be outside the birth canal within 70 minutes for survival. Although exceptions to this are known, as with everything, it is usually not the case. This makes it imperative to be observant and to know immediately when the delivery process is no longer normal, and to give or seek assistance (Figure 11-24).

> *TECHNICIAN NOTE* Foal heat occurs between 2 and 18 days after parturition and can be a fertile heat in many mares.

Foal heat (the first estrus after delivery of the foal) can occur between day 2 and day 18 postpartum. These heats can be fertile, but the likelihood of another pregnancy increases if the uterus has involuted normally. It is beneficial for conception for the mare to ovulate later during this period rather than sooner. Ovarian senility will occur if the mare lives long enough. A female is born with all the ova she will ever have. Each time she has a cycle and/or as she ages, these ova are used and eventually become exhausted. The number of ova in the mare has not been calculated, as it has in the bovine, but it is estimated to be close to 70,000 to 120,000. When these oocytes are gone, the mare will stop cycling but still may exhibit signs of heat related to estrogen and progesterone originating from the adrenals.

BOVINE REPRODUCTION

GENERAL

A *heifer* is a female bovine usually younger than 2 years of age. A *cow* is a female bovine older than 2 years of age. A *bull* is a male bovine. A *steer* is a castrated male bovine. The neonate is known as a *calf*, and the delivery is known as *calving*. The age at puberty, as is the case in most species, is determined by body size. Heifers will be approximately 50% to 60% of their adult body size when puberty occurs. Nutrition (especially carbohydrates) is very important in determining the age at which puberty occurs. The reproductive system is a luxury system, and the ovaries can "shut down" if insufficient nutrition is present. The age range for onset of puberty is 5 to 20 months (average, 9 to 11 months). Beef breeds such as Angus reach puberty earlier than other beef or dairy breeds. Zebu and Zebu crosses generally reach puberty as the latest of the beef breeds. The desired age at first calving is approximately 2 years. Therefore, pregnancy must occur by approximately 15 months of age (gestation is 9 months).

> *TECHNICIAN NOTE* Because cows have a very short estrus heat, barn personnel should check cows for heat 3 times a day.

ESTROUS CYCLE

The cow is a polyestrous animal, indicating that she has cycles year round. Cows demonstrate estrus by being restless, anxious, and bellowing. Sometimes the cow may go off feed, and in the case of dairy cows may demonstrate a related decrease in milk production. Increased walking has been noted, and pedometers, which are linked to computers via telemetry, have been used to detect estrus. Cows mount other cows frequently. However, only those cows that are in heat will stand to be mounted, hence the term "standing heat." Sexual pheromones produced by cows in heat attract other cows and bulls to them. Observation of heat in the herd is best performed 3 times per day when the cows are not eating, being milked, or being moved. It is also best when they are observed from a distance. Observation is based on which cows stand to be mounted by other cows.

The stages of the estrous cycle are follicular and luteal or estrus, metestrus, and diestrus. The cow is a polyestrous animal, indicating that she cycles year round without much seasonal influence. Day 1 of the estrous cycle is designated as the day signs of heat are observed. The cycle length is approximately 21 days. The estrous cycle can range from 18 to 24 days and can be normal. Cows are in heat for approximately 8 to 18 hours. During the follicular phase of the cycle, follicles are increasing in size and luteal tissue is regressing. During the luteal phase of the cycle, the CL is developing and progesterone is increasing. Metestrus occurs immediately after estrus, and the primary significance of this period having its own designation is that metestrous blood may be seen in the vulvar discharge within 3 days following heat. Metestrus is the period of the corpus hemorrhagicum (CH) that occurs immediately after ovulation. This is the period when the former site of the follicle, now known as the *ovulation depression (OVD)*, is filling with blood. In the ruminant, ovulation occurs from anywhere on the surface of the ovary. The CH is sometimes confused with an immature follicle on rectal palpation. As the CL forms, the exact site of oocyte release may (but not always) be palpated as the crown of the CL.

A decrease in progesterone (P4) occurs on day 17 in cows with a 21-day cycle. Estrogen from developing follicles over the next 3 to 4 days is increased in the blood, which has an effect on the uterus and cervix. If the cow is palpated during estrus, uterine tone will be excellent (turgid). This is comparable with the double-walled rubber hose. The uterus will be coiled tightly. Increased estrogen from the mature follicle causes positive feedback on the hypothalamic-pituitary axis, resulting in a surge of luteinizing hormone (LH). This LH surge causes ovulation. The sharp spike in LH occurs at the beginning of estrus, with ovulation occurring approximately 24 hours later. Ovulation occurs about 8 to 12 hours after the cow goes out of standing heat. It is generally desirable to inseminate the cow before ovulation but shortly after estrus. Poor conception rates, especially with cryopreserved semen, occur if cows are bred too early. Oocytes are viable only for about 12 hours after ovulation. Once ovulation occurs, the CL develops. If pregnancy does not occur, the uterus releases prostaglandin F2alpha (PGF2alpha), the CL regresses, and progesterone falls.

Diestrus is the longest portion of the estrous cycle; it is that portion where progesterone dominates. The CL will remain functional until day 17 if the animal is not pregnant. It remains functional longer if conception occurred along with maternal recognition of pregnancy. The uterine luteolysin in the cow is PGF2alpha. The CL is "fully" functional in the cow by day 6 post ovulation. This implies that it is producing maximal quantities of P4 and has the capability to respond to exogenous PGF2alpha by regressing. Follicular wave patterns are seen in cows approximately every 10 days and are controlled by follicle-stimulating hormone (FSH) pulses, which cause the development of new follicles. One follicle becomes dominant and begins to produce a substance called *inhibin*, which inhibits further FSH production and release, thus preventing other follicles from maturing. The dominant follicle continues to grow in response to lowering concentrations of P4. Estrogen increases positive feedback on the hypothalamic-pituitary axis to cause a surge of LH, which in turn stimulates ovulation.

Control of estrus has been most efficient with progestational preparations. These have been administered intravaginally as controlled internal drug release (CIDR) preparations. The progestational preparation is absorbed through the vaginal wall until the CIDR is removed. Injectable implants have been used in the past. Cows will come into estrus when the progesterone is gone unless an abnormality in cyclic activity is present. Artificial insemination has long been restricted in cattle because of the short heat and the failure of observed heats in this species. With the introduction of estrus control has come a steady increase in artificial insemination of beef and dairy cattle.

INSEMINATION

Cows that are observed to be in heat should be inseminated approximately 12 hours later. A major problem, however, arises when cows are not observed for signs of heat at the proper times, and heats are missed. If they are not observed in heat, they are not bred. Unobserved estrus is a major cause of lost reproductive time in dairy cows. Therefore, devices such as heat detector patches were developed. These are dye packets that are placed on the dorsal sacral vertebral area, so if another cow or a teaser bull mounts the cow, the owner will be able to easily know after the fact rather than have to be present at the exact time of mounting.

Vasectomized bulls with lateral deviation of the penis to decrease the spread of venereal disease can be used as the "teaser" animal. This works better than relying on other cows in the herd. These bulls can be equipped with chin ball markers, which will release a chalk-like or dye-like material when they mount a cow. The dye is easily observed, and the amount of dye is related to whether the cow was in heat or the bull was just over zealous! Teaser bulls are used more in beef operations than in dairy operations because of close handling and multiple times per day contact with dairy cows, as well as the potential danger a bull may pose to those involved in a dairy operation by their presence. An additional sign of estrus is a clear mucous discharge, which may extend from the vulva to the ground. If the discharge is not clear, abnormalities should be expected. The single exception is metestrous bleeding, whereby the mucus may contain small amounts of blood after the heat.

Natural mating by bulls usually is very rapid, with mounting and a single thrust forward and ejaculation occurring during the forward movement.

> **TECHNICIAN NOTE** The number of caruncles is determined by birth, and no additional caruncles are formed.

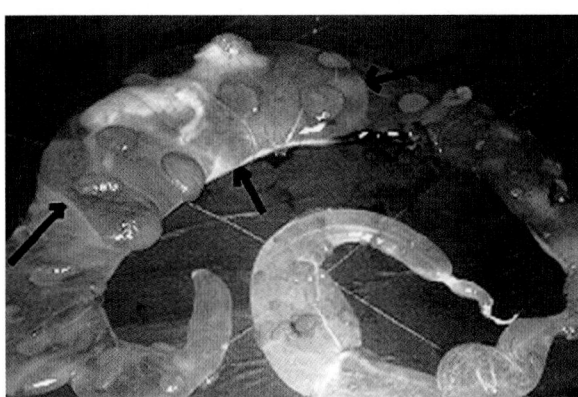

FIGURE 11-25 A bovine fetus is visible within the amnion *(arrows)*, which is within the chorioallantois. Notice the protruding red cotyledons that dot the outside of the chorioallantois. Cotyledons make up the fetal half of the bovine placenta and interlock with caruncles *(not shown)* on the maternal half to provide a passageway (placentome) between the cow and the fetus for the transfer of nutrients.

GESTATION

The gestation of the cow is approximately 279 to 283 days, but some breeds are outside of this average. The placenta is cotyledonary, indicating that the **fetal membranes** are attached to the endometrium at specific areas and not to the entire endometrium, as is the case in the mare and the sow (Figure 11-25). The **placentome** is the name given to the cotyledon (fetal) and caruncle (maternal) portions of the membrane combined. The caruncle looks similar to a mushroom protruding from the endometrium. There is no normal placental attachment between these areas within the uterus. Adventitial placentation occurs when caruncular attachments are insufficient to supply the fetus, and additional attachments are attempted in noncaruncular areas. The cow has an average of 75 to 120 caruncles; once damaged or destroyed, they are not replaced.

Pregnancy is diagnosed primarily by palpation, but replacement of this technique with ultrasonographic examination is steadily increasing. Rectal examination is performed after 28 days, and ultrasonographic examination can be performed a few days sooner with a higher degree of accuracy.

Udder enlargement begins weeks to months prepartum, depending on whether it is a cow or a heifer. Udder edema may be present and if severe should be treated. Colostrum, which is the first secretion of the udder, should be fed to all calves, or they should be permitted to nurse. The pelvic ligaments relax, permitting the tail head and the "hips" to slightly change angles; this permits a greater pelvic opening. The vulva becomes edematous and elongated. None of these changes makes prediction of parturition a science!

PARTURITION

Stage I of parturition consists of cervical relaxation to a width of 6 to 10 cm up to a week or so before delivery. Uterine contractions usually begin about the time the cervix will permit a hand to be passed. These contractions force fetal fluid within the allantoic sac (**allantois**) into the cervix and aid the Ferguson reflex. The Ferguson reflex is a cyclic mechanism by which dilatation of the cervical lumen stimulates a neural response that increases oxytocin release, which further dilates the cervix. The fetus is the final reason for maximal cervical dilatation. Cervical dilatation in the bovine with annular cervical rings is slower than in species with longitudinal cervical folds, but it should continue. Abdominal discomfort is present, with restlessness and weight shifting. Cows attempt to isolate themselves from the rest of the herd. The average length of stage I of labor is 6 hours, but it may go as long as 24 hours.

Stage II begins with rupture of the chorioallantoic membrane. This rupture is not as dramatic as in the mare, where many times a large "gush" of fluid is forcibly expelled up to 30 cm from the mare. Strong abdominal and uterine contractions occur. Dilatation of the cervix by the fetus causes release of oxytocin, and this is followed by release of PGF2-alpha to aid in uterine contractility. The cow will be up and down during stage II. If dilatation does not continue between two examinations during stage II of parturition spaced 30 minutes apart, delivery is slowed significantly or stopped, and a cesarean may be indicated. Although the **amnion** may appear at the vulvar opening during this stage, it will rupture instead of being passed around the fetus, as in the case of the mare, because of hundreds of attachments with the chorioallantoic membrane. Cows may be sternal or in lateral recumbency at the time of delivery. A standing delivery can occur, as sometimes occurs in the mare, but it does not occur as frequently. The fetus is delivered during this stage. The average length of stage II is 2 to 4 hours, but cows can take up to 6 hours, and heifers can take up to 12 hours.

During stage III, the placenta is passed and the uterus begins its return to normal. Major myometrial contractions continue for approximately 3 days postpartum, and continued reduction in uterine size due to contraction persists for weeks. Nursing stimulates continued periodic release of oxytocin, which aids in uterine contraction and return to normal. The effectiveness of oxytocin is of greatest clinical significance during the first 24 hours postpartum. After the first 24 hours, the uterus has reduced sensitization to estrogen, and oxytocin does not have the same clinical effectiveness as when estrogen is present. PGF2alpha will have better effects than oxytocin after the 24-hour period.

OVINE REPRODUCTION

GENERAL

A *ewe* is a female sheep. A *ram* is a male sheep. A *wether* is a castrated male sheep. Ewes and rams younger than 1 year of age are known as *ewe lambs* or *ram lambs*. Delivery of fetuses is known as *lambing*. Puberty in sheep is very dependent on body weight, but because most sheep are seasonally polyestrous, it depends to a great deal on time of year. Body weight should be approximately 60% to 70% that of the adult.

ESTROUS CYCLE

Most breeds are seasonally polyestrous, with cyclic activity occurring during late summer, fall, and early winter owing to the decreasing photoperiod and therefore decreased release of melatonin from the pineal. Sheep have their primary breeding season from September through December. Pygmy goats, because of their very small size, may reach puberty at 4 months if it is the correct time of year. As daylight length becomes shorter, ewes start to cycle. Small ruminants receive light through the eyes, and it travels to the pineal gland. Release of melatonin causes release of GnRH from the hypothalamus, which causes release of FSH and LH from the pituitary, and the ewe begins cycling. The length of the estrous cycle is approximately 16.5 days. Ovulation occurs 24 to 30 hours after the beginning of estrus. The first estrus of the year can be abnormal. Lambs reach puberty by the breeding season after their birth. Ewes remain in heat for approximately 36 hours. The length of gestation usually is between 144 and 151 days but is influenced by the number of fetuses carried. Owing to large fetuses and difficult lambing, some ewe lambs should not be bred as lambs but should be held and bred as yearlings (lambs at 2 years of age). With proper nutrition and parasite control programs, many ewe lambs are bred to lamb as yearlings. The reason for lambing at approximately 1 year of age is the reduced expense of maintaining the ewe lamb for a year with no return on the investment. Body condition scores should be noted before breeding, and those with scores lower than 2.5 on a scale from 1 to 5, with 5 representing "overconditioned," should be *flushed.* This term is used when nutrition to ewes is increased before breeding, because it has been shown that the number of oocytes will be increased. Flushing of ewes with body condition scores above 2.5 serves no useful purpose. Ewes with a body score over 3.5 to 4.0 may have decreased productivity owing to their overweight condition.

Stages of the estrous cycle in sheep include follicular and luteal or estrus and diestrus. Estrus detection in sheep is difficult unless it is a breed with a short tail! Signs to observe include tail raised and frequent movement from side to side. Close examination may reveal slight swelling of the vulva, and in white breeds hyperemia of the vulva and surrounding area. The ewe may urinate a little more frequently in the presence of the ram, but this is subtle. The ewe will seek out the ram when in estrus. The ram will seek out ewes at any time! Vasectomized rams are frequently used as part of an artificial breeding program. The ram wears a breeding harness, which fits around the shoulders and has a crayon between the front legs. When he mounts the ewes, he leaves a mark on their back (Figure 11-26). The degree of marking indicates either that the ewes are in heat, or that the ram is overly zealous! After gestation or the breeding season, ewes become anestrus because of lengthening daylight hours. Ewes respond to the pheromones of the ram, and this can initiate earlier cycling activity than would otherwise occur. It may shorten the anestrus by a few weeks. This will be most successful if no ram is near the ewes until the last 6 to 8 weeks before ram introduction.

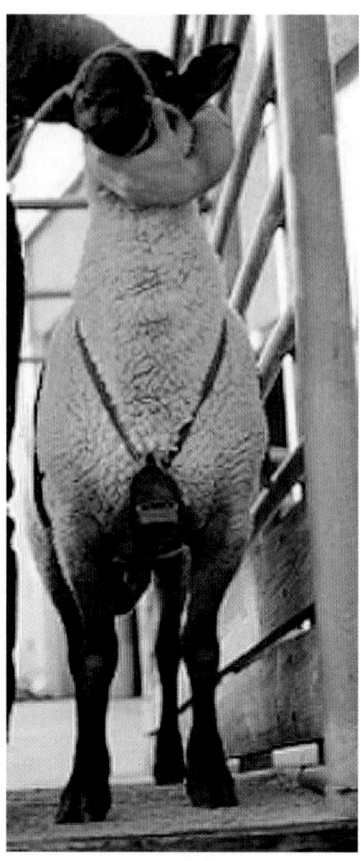

FIGURE 11-26 A ram fitted with a marking harness to detect estrus.

BREEDING

Breeding should occur toward the end of estrus, but if sheep are bred naturally, semen deposited at the beginning of heat will still be capable of fertilizing oocytes when required. Mating behavior of rams, like that of bulls, is short and fast, and includes pawing at the side, a flehmen response, mounting, one or two thrusts forward, and ejaculation. Diestrus begins with formation of the OVD and progresses through the CH. Luteinization continues, and the CL is formed. The CL is fully functional in approximately 5 days. If maternal recognition of pregnancy does not occur, PGF2alpha is released and the CL regresses at approximately the 13th day of the cycle. Under pasture conditions, with ewes cycling naturally, a young ram lamb can be used to breed 10 to 15 ewes. A yearling ram will be able to cover (breed) 25 to 30 ewes, and mature rams are capable of servicing 35 to 50 ewes.

Estrous cycles of ewes can be somewhat synchronized with utilization of prostaglandin F2alpha injected 2 weeks apart. The prostaglandin F2alpha will cause the corpora lutea to regress, and ewes will be in heat within 3 days. A marking harness on the rams will aid in determining which ewes have come into heat and have been bred. The color of the chalk can be changed every 16 to 17 days to determine which ewes have been bred during more than one heat. Use of progesterone sponges and intravaginal progesterone inserts, such as controlled internal drug release (CIDR) inserts, enables synchronization of heats in ewes. Sponges or CIDRs impregnated with progesterone are placed in the vagina of the ewe for approximately 10 to 14 days. After the intravaginal inserts are removed, the ewe enters estrus within 72 hours. When combined with an injection of equine chorionic gonadotropin (eCG), intravaginal inserts can be used in a superovulation program for ewes, or to induce estrus during the nonbreeding season. eCG will induce follicular development when injected shortly before the time of sponge removal. When synchronizing ewes, one must be certain that a sufficient number of rams are available to breed the ewes within a short time. Ewes not synchronized usually have a lambing season of 4 to 5 weeks. This permits some ewes to be bred twice if necessary. However, long lambing seasons are managerially not desirable. Abortions in sheep commonly occur for unknown reasons in up to 5% of the flock. The presence of disease responsible for abortion can greatly increase this percentage.

GESTATION

Pregnancy can be determined by changing marking chalk on the ram and noting which ewes do not return to estrus. Ultrasound can be used to determine pregnancy and provides the added advantage of determining the number of fetuses. This is helpful when determining the nutritional needs of each ewe and of the flock as a whole. Informative ultrasonic examinations are performed rectally at 25 days and transabdominally at 35 days or later in gestation. Serum progesterone levels have also been used to determine pregnancy, but this is not specifically a pregnancy test. The test merely determines whether or not progesterone is elevated (as seen during pregnancy), but it should not be used as a definitive pregnancy test. The ewe's pregnancy is maintained by the production of progesterone, first from the CL and later from the placenta.

CAPRINE REPRODUCTION

GENERAL

A female goat is known as a *doe*, usually of any age. The male is known as a *buck* (not a *ram*). A castrated male is known as a *wether*. The young are known as *kids*, and the birthing process is known as *kidding*. Estrous cycle length in goats is 21 days. Estrus lasts approximately 1 to 1½ days. The first estrus of the year is usually abnormal. Ovulation occurs toward the end of standing heat, as with the ewe. Diestrus is the time when the CL is present and progesterone concentrations are elevated. Male goats have a strong odor because of scent glands located around the horn bases, which are used to mark territory. They also tend to urinate on their own hindlegs and produce copious pheromones. In fact, buck odor and pheromones can stimulate does to cycle earlier than they normally would without the presence of the buck. Does in estrus will congregate around the smell of the buck, whether or not the buck is attached to the smell. Does may urinate a little more often. The vulva may be a little swollen and more hyperemic. Does demonstrate estrus by flipping their tails up and sideways frequently. Mating is the same as

for the ram and includes pawing at the side, a flehmen response, mounting, thrusting, and ejaculation. Goats go into anestrus during the summer as daylight lengthens.

CAMELID REPRODUCTION

GENERAL

Camelids (llama and alpaca) are polyestrous animals. The neonate is known as a *cria*, although this in reality is defined as "birth," or the creation of life. The age of puberty in the female is approximately 10 to 12 months, and the length of estrus is between 1 and 30 days. Waves of follicles develop simultaneously until the dominant follicle is selected. The follicle will increase from 4 to 5 mm to a mature size of 7 to 12 mm in the last 3 to 6 days of development. It may remain this size for another 2 to 8 days until mating and ovulation; if this does not occur, the follicle will regress, and another follicle will develop to take its place. Camelids are induced ovulators; however, matings that occur in the absence of a mature follicle do not result in ovulation.

BREEDING

The male reaches puberty not at the time he is capable of producing sufficient sperm to achieve conception, but at the time that adhesions of the penis to the prepuce are "broken down," usually at 3 years of age. The relationship of testicular weight to body weight is 0.03%, whereas the ratio in bulls is 0.18% and in rams is 1.4%. The orgling sound made by the male during mating may contribute to neural stimuli; this leads to luteinizing hormone release and ovulation. Because follicles mature rapidly over the last 3 to 6 days of development, several ultrasonographic examinations may be necessary to determine the fate of the follicle. Estrous activity may be more dependent on the absence of progesterone than on the presence of estrogen. Females in heat will assume the breeding position when approached by a male. They may also seek out males when in estrus. Mating occurs in a ventrally recumbent position and may last up to 60 minutes but averages 20 minutes.

GESTATION

The length of pregnancy is approximately 344 (330 to 350) days. Although ovulations occur equally from both ovaries, pregnancies are noted predominantly (98%) in the left horn. Placentation is epitheliochorial. The pregnancy is CL dependent, and if the CL is removed, the pregnancy is terminated. Compared with other domestic species, the expected pregnancy termination rate is much higher. The range of embryonic loss is 10% to 50%, most of which occurs within the first 60 days. After the first 2 months, the pregnancy termination rate is only 5%. Although twin ovulations may occur, delivery of twins is rare.

PARTURITION

Parturition in the camelid has been referred to as "unpacking." The first stage lasts approximately 1 to 2 hours. Stage

II, with expulsion of the fetus, lasts approximately 20 to 30 minutes; stage III lasts approximately 1 to 4 hours and includes expulsion of the placenta. Placentas should be passed within 6 hours and if retained should be treated with oxytocin. The placenta should never be removed manually.

Ovulation and fertility return approximately 20 days postpartum. If the female is not bred relatively early postpartum, she may cease to cycle owing to high milk production in relationship to feed supply, or may be producing a hormone during lactation that prevents follicular maturation.

> **TECHNICIAN NOTE** The purpose of a breeding soundness examination (BSE) of the male is to determine his potential fertility without actually breeding females.

BREEDING SOUNDNESS EXAMINATION OF THE MALE

Males of all species should have a breeding soundness examination (BSE) before they are used for breeding. The breeding soundness examination of most species includes a physical examination, notation of potentially inherited defects, external genitalia examination, internal secondary sex gland examination, if possible, and semen evaluation.

The purpose of a BSE of the male is to determine his potential fertility without actually breeding females. Although no available testing is as accurate as fertility trails, the BSE described here does provide a very reliable assessment of fertility. Primary factors involved in the examination include physical reproductive characteristics, semen quality, attitude, disposition, libido, and any system abnormalities that could influence his reproductive performance. An example of a system abnormality includes lack of rear leg soundness, especially in large animals.

The examination begins with identification of the animal. This is best done with permanent markers such as a microchip, a tattoo, a brand, or color markings if distinct. Identification is followed by obtainment of a complete history with emphasis on reproductive performance. This would include age, previous injuries or illnesses, temperament, the reason for the BSE, previous fertility, method of breeding the male (natural service or artificial insemination), number of females serviced over a given time, number of matings per week, and results of any previous BSEs. A complete physical examination is performed, including a detailed examination of the external genitalia. The scrotum would be examined for the presence of two testes, the symmetry of those testes, the normalcy of the epididymis, the presence of vas deferens, free movement of the testes within the scrotum, and the absence of palpable abnormalities within the testes. Refer to Figure 11-27 for an example of an asymmetric scrotum in a bull. The size of the testes or the scrotum should be recorded because a link between size and fertility has been established. Scrotal circumference is used primarily in the ruminant, and testicular size is used primarily in other species.

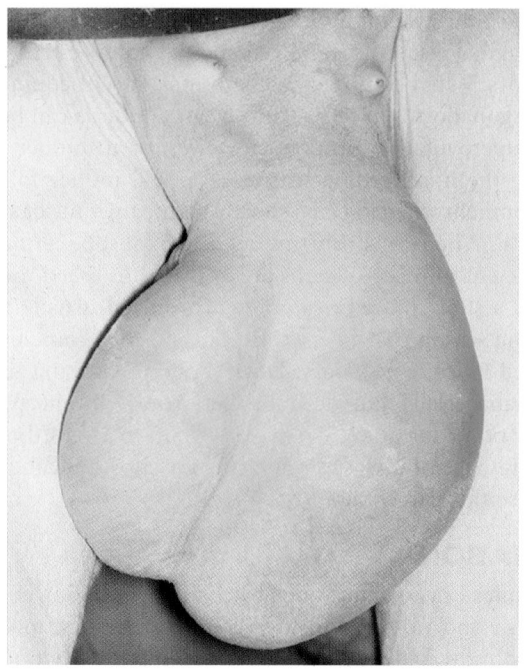

FIGURE 11-27 Bull scrotum indicating enlargement of left testis.

The internal genitalia are examined in species that will permit it. The bull and the stallion have seminal vesicles, a prostate, and a bulbourethral gland; in the dog, only the prostate is examined because this is the only accessory sex gland present in the dog. Seminal vesicles are predominantly important in the bull and stallion because this is the one gland that is responsible for major clinical problems in the two species. The vas deferens and the ampulla are also examined. Other nonreproductive structures are examined during the rectal examination procedure, including internal inguinal rings in the stallion and in the bull. If possible, the male's libido should be assessed. When semen is being collected by an artificial vagina, by a condom, or by electro-ejaculation, the male should be observed for time and difficulty in protruding the penis, obtaining an erection, and ejaculating. Electro-ejaculation is commonly performed in bovine, ovine, and caprine species. Electro-ejaculation can be used in the boar and the stallion but usually is not done because these animals require general anesthesia for the procedure. The process is performed by placing a probe in the rectum of the animal and applying a very low electrical current in pulses (Figure 11-28). One should apply only sufficient current to achieve the desired result of erection and ejaculation; it has been the experience of the author when using this technique on quadriplegic men that all complained about headaches and chest pains as the process was performed. The penis is cleansed thoroughly before semen is collected from the stallion; however, no cleaning is performed in other domestic species. The penis and the prepuce should be visualized during this procedure to ensure that they are normal. When an artificial vagina (AV) is used, bulls, rams, boars, and stallions require a warm water jacket on the AV to increase the likelihood of a successful procedure

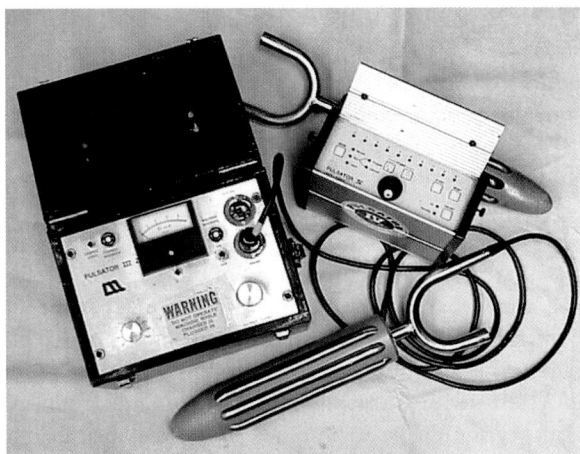

FIGURE 11-28 Two models of ruminant electro-ejaculators and two rectal probes.

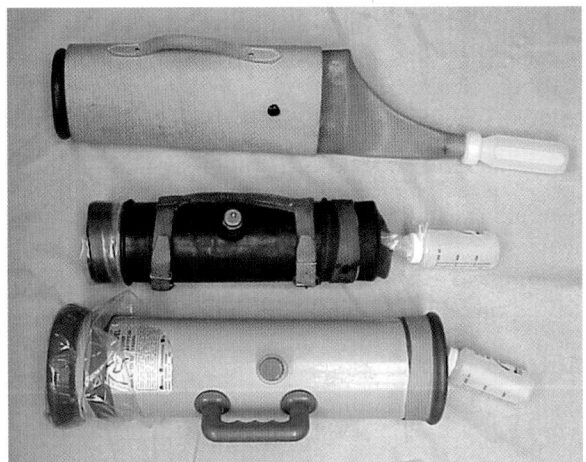

FIGURE 11-29 Three models of equine artificial vaginas from top to bottom: Missouri, Hannover, and ARS/Colorado.

(Figure 11-29). When the AV is used for the dog, no water jacket is required because stimulation of the dog and ejaculation are not dependent on the artificial vagina.

SEMEN ANALYSIS

Once semen has been obtained, it is examined first for motility. This is accomplished by placing a small drop of semen on a warm slide with a warm coverslip if needed using a warm pipet, and evaluating immediately with a 200× or 400× microscope. Cooler than body temperatures can reduce motility very rapidly, and care should be taken to avoid reducing motility by the evaluation technique. Sperm are evaluated individually in most species to assess movement. Looking at large numbers of sperm simultaneously usually does not allow a true assessment of individual sperm movement. Dilution of the sample may be necessary in some species to determine individual sperm movement. This dilution should not be done with a semen extender because an extender may enhance motility, generating false results. At least 100 sperm should be examined, and their relative speed and direction should be noted. Final results for this portion

of the examination will include the percentage of normal mobility. Most species of sperm move rapidly forward in a straight line. The exception is stallion sperm, which often travel via circular movement.

Speed of movement is also reflected in the rotation of the sperm cell. The sperm cell head is flat, not rounded. Therefore, when viewed from the top, it appears wide and long. However, when viewed from the side, the head is narrow and long. Rotation speed is determined by noting whether the sperm appears to be narrow in one plane of view. If so, this is an indication that the sperm has slowed its movement because our eyes are not able to see the extremely rapid rotational movement of sperm. The fact that the rotation is detected visually confirms that the movement of the sperm is slower than normal. Normally, our eyes are incapable of seeing only the wide portion of the cell. Rapid forward progressive movement is ideal and indicates excellent motility. A finding of 70% or more progressively motile sperm is desirable.

The direction of movement is determined by observing the path that sperm cells travel across the field. This is best done by observing a few cells within a field at the same time and recording the percentage of sperm demonstrating normal movement. Sperm that move in a straightforward progressive manner are demonstrating normal sperm movement. Undesirable movements seen in sperm include sideways oscillations of the head, zigzap motility, circular movement, and vibrating or shaking movement. These fruitless movements sap valuable energy from the sperm and inhibit or prevent forward mobility, making it less likely that the sperm will reach the egg. Motility can be determined by visual observation, although experience is necessary to do this, and by use of a computerized motion analyzer. The computer tracks and plots the movement of each sperm and summarizes its speed and direction. This is an excellent method of motility determination, but it has the disadvantage of requiring a costly device.

Once the motility assessment has been completed, the morphologic examination is begun. This is performed by placing a drop of eosin-nigrosin stain on a warm slide and mixing it carefully with a small drop of the ejaculate. It is also permissible to do a wet mount (semen mixed with 10% buffered formalin) and examine it with a phase contrast microscope. The stained slide examination is performed by determining the percentage of normal sperm among 100 cells. A 1000× oil immersion objective is used to visualize the cells. Morphologic abnormalities can be classified as primary or secondary abnormalities. Primary abnormalities are those that occur in the testis; secondary abnormalities occur after the sperm exits the testis. Examples of primary abnormalities include deformities of the head and midpiece, as well as immature sperm that leave the testes prematurely. Secondary abnormalities include detached heads, distal protoplasmic droplets, reversed tails, detachment of the galea capitis, and coiling of the tail. When performing a semen examination, it is imperative to distinguish normal from abnormal sperm. Determination of primary from secondary abnormalities can be made on-site, or the task can be forwarded to a diagnostic laboratory if abnormal sperm are detected at a rate greater than 30%.

Sperm concentration is usually determined using a hemocytometer or a similar sperm-counting device, but it may be estimated in some species. In addition, the volume of the ejaculate should be determined. In the stallion, urethral cultures are routinely collected approximately 2.5 cm proximal to the urethral opening before and after ejaculation. Semen is also cultured. The relative presence and type of microorganisms cultured may have relevance to the reproductive success of the male.

OTHER DIAGNOSTIC TESTS

Endocrine profiles, karyotyping, ultrasonographic examination of the testicles, and testicular biopsy are additional tests that can be performed on the male. Assays of FSH levels provide the most useful information regarding endocrine profiles, but they are not commercially available for most species. Testicular biopsy is performed with a split-needle biopsy instrument after a very small incision is made in the skin. Care should be taken to miss the arteries providing blood supply to the testis. Their location for each species is well described in anatomy textbooks. Depending on the species, this is usually done with little to no sedation and subcutaneous local anesthesia. General anesthesia can be used but is rarely necessary. In smaller species such as the cat and the small dog, a wedge incision can be used if necessary, but trauma to the testicle is increased. All of this information should be recorded onto permanent records, and the owner should be given a copy of the results.

BREEDING SOUNDNESS EXAMINATION OF THE FEMALE

The breeding soundness examination of the female is usually performed when infertility or a subfertility problem is detected. Sometimes in mares, a BSE is performed before a sale, to ascertain fertility status. The examination begins with obtainment of an accurate history, including age, breed, vaccination status, deworming status, housing, feed use, cyclic activity, signs of estrus, interestrus intervals, breedings, methods of breeding, dates of breeding, male fertility status, number of pregnancies, dates of parturitions, any dystocias or retained placentas, any abortions, and all available results of previous BSEs.

In species where it is possible, examination of the reproductive tract begins with palpation and/or ultrasonographic examination. All information obtained should be recorded in the permanent record. The external reproductive tract should be examined for the presence of any abnormalities. Uterine cultures can be obtained easily in the mare and in the cow, but this becomes more difficult as the size of the animal decreases. Any vaginal examination or diagnostic technique to be performed in the mare should be preceded by a thorough cleansing of the perineal area. This is accomplished by wrapping the tail and tying it to the neck of the

mare or the contralateral axillary area. A bucket of clean warm water filled with soaking cotton is used during the scrubbing procedure. Care should be taken during the washing process to avoid contaminating the wash water with soap or dirt from the mare. To accomplish this, the assistant must designate one hand as the "clean" hand, to apprehend the soaking cotton from the bucket. Once removed, the clean cotton is transferred to the "dirty" hand, soap is applied, and the scrub carried out. Because most of the work is performed by the "dirty" hand, it is typically the dominant hand. Only the clean hand obtains the clean cotton from the clean bucket. Once the cotton is used, it is thrown to the ground. This system reduces the possibility of contamination. Also, the bucket should be maintained a safe distance from the mare, so that no contaminants from the mare or from the washing procedure enter the bucket. A thorough rinse is performed to remove all residual soap from the mare. After the mare has been thoroughly scrubbed, transcervical uterine cultures may be acquired. Although transcervical cultures in the canine have been described, this is a more difficult procedure in small animals, making surgical acquisition of cultures necessary. Vaginal cultures should be obtained in the canine with guarded culture rods, because the canine vagina usually is not sterile. Interpretation of culture results therefore should take into account other clinical findings and the patient's history. The uterine lumen of all species is sterile. Once samples are obtained, they should be plated immediately or placed in a transport medium and shadowed from sunlight and other forms of ultraviolet light. The vagina and the external os of the cervix should be evaluated in all species by digital or visual examination.

Although many times referred to as a *uterine biopsy*, it is actually an endometrial biopsy that is of value in most species. The endometrium is that portion of the uterus that is most involved in pregnancy maintenance. The biopsy is of greatest value in diffuse placentation species and is least valuable in cotyledonary species. The two most important indicators of the presence and severity of problems are inflammation and fibrosis. Again, biopsy specimens can be obtained through the vaginal lumen in the mare and in the cow using biopsy forceps (Figures 11-30 and 31). Other

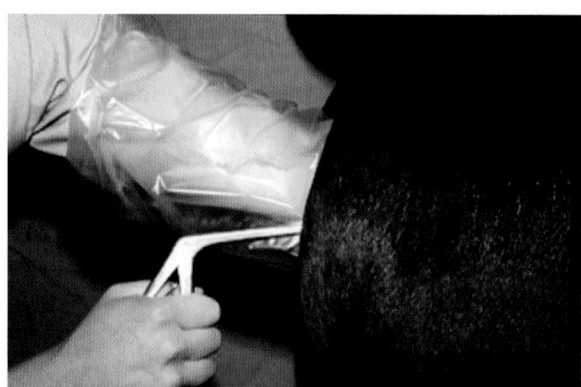

FIGURE 11-30 A uterine biopsy instrument is inserted through the vagina and the cervix into the uterus.

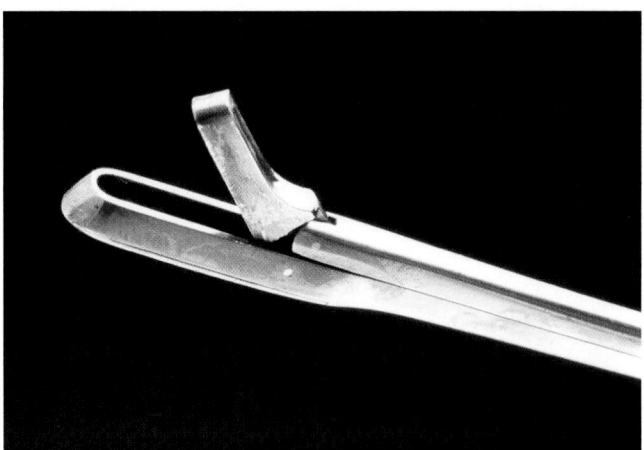

FIGURE 11-31 Equine endometrial biopsy instrument.

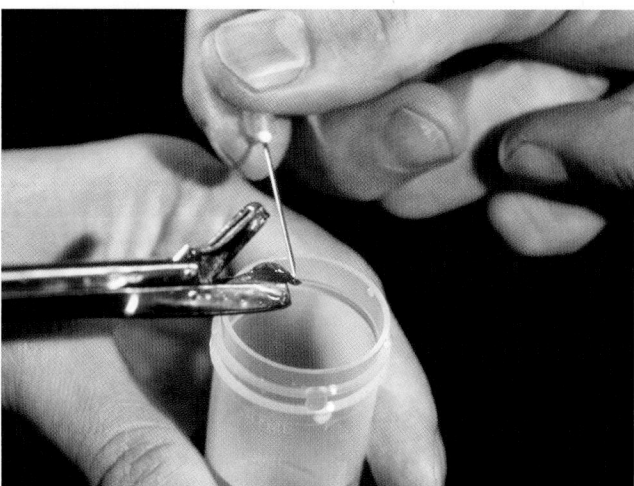

FIGURE 11-32 Endometrial tissue teased from biopsy instrument into fixative.

species require a surgical approach to the uterus similar to a cesarean, but with much less incision length. Once a biopsy sample has been obtained, care should be taken to avoid inadvertently crushing the tissue. The specimen should be immediately teased out of the biopsy instrument using a fine-gauge needle and placed in the fixative of choice (Figure 11-32). Endometrial cytologic examination is also of value, especially when results are needed immediately, because this technique can be performed quickly and results obtained within minutes. Cytology samples are best obtained in all species by gently rolling a saline-moistened swab against the endometrium and onto a glass slide. Samples for cytologic examination are stained with solutions such as Diff-Quik, Wright, and Giemsa stains and are examined immediately.

RECOMMENDED READINGS

Carleton C, editor: Blackwell's five minute veterinary consults: clinical companion—equine theriogenology, New York, 2008, Williams & Wilkins.

Ettinger SJ, Feldman EC, editors: Textbook of veterinary internal medicine, ed 7, St Louis, 2009, Saunders.

Root Kustritz MV: The practical veterinarian: small animal theriogenology, St Louis, 2003, Butterworth-Heinemann.

Youngquist RS, Threlfall WR, editors: Current therapy in large animal theriogenology, St Louis, 2007, Saunders.

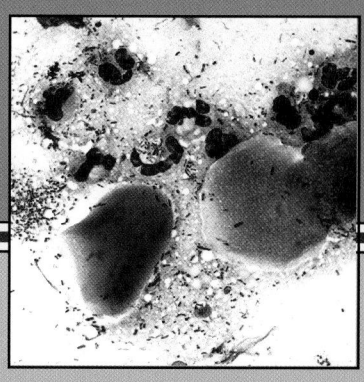

12 Hematology and Cytology

Maxey L. Wellman and M. Judith Radin

OUTLINE

Hematology, *399*
Complete Blood Count (CBC), *399*
Automated Hematology Analyzers, *399*
Packed Cell Volume (PCV), *400*
Red Blood Cell (RBC) Count, *401*
Hemoglobin Concentration, *401*
Red Blood Cell Indices, *401*
Red Cell Distribution Width (RDW), *402*
Plasma Protein Determination, *402*
White Blood Cell (WBC) Count, *403*
Preparation of Blood Smears, *404*
Blood Smear Evaluation, *405*

Coagulation Testing, *417*
Cytology, *418*
Solid Tissue Masses and Enlarged
  Organs, *418*
Thoracic and Abdominal Effusions, *419*
Synovial (Joint) Fluid, *420*
Stains, Immunophenotyping by Flow
  Cytometry, and DNA-Based Testing, *420*
Submission of Samples to a Reference
  Laboratory, *420*
Otic Cytology, *421*

LEARNING OBJECTIVES

When you have completed this chapter, you will be able to:

1. Pronounce, define, and spell all Key Terms in this chapter.
2. Describe proper collection techniques, handling of blood samples, and components of a complete blood count (CBC).
3. Describe advantages, disadvantages, and capabilities of automated hematology analyzers.
4. Do the following regarding blood counts:
   - Compare and contrast procedures used to determine red blood cell mass (packed cell volume [PCV], hematocrit [HCT], hemoglobin, and red blood cell [RBC] count), and discuss the causes and significance of abnormal values.
   - Describe methods used to calculate RBC indices and red cell distribution width (RDW), and discuss the causes and significance of abnormal values.
   - Describe methods used to determine plasma protein concentration, and discuss the causes and significance of abnormal values.
   - Describe methods used to determine the white blood cell (WBC) count and the platelet count.
5. Do the following regarding blood smears:
   - Describe the technique used to prepare a stained blood smear, list factors that influence the quality of the smear, and discuss the process used to evaluate a blood smear.
   - Describe normal and abnormal morphology of RBCs, WBCs, and platelets in each species as they appear on a blood smear.
   - Discuss the causes and significance of RBC, WBC, and platelet abnormalities commonly observed on a blood smear.
   - Describe the procedure used to perform a differential WBC count, and calculate absolute values.

KEY TERMS

Activated clotting time
  (activated coagulation
  time [ACT])
Activated partial
  thromboplastin time
  (APTT)
Agglutination
Anisocytosis
Band neutrophil
Basophil
Blood smears
Coagulation cascade
Complete blood count
  (CBC)
Cytology
D-Dimers
Eosinophil
Fibrin(ogen)
  degradation products
  (FDPs)
Fibrinolysis
Hematocrit (HCT)
Hemocytometer
Hemoglobin
Hemostasis
Heterophil
Left shift
Lymphocyte
Mean corpuscular
  hemoglobin
  concentration (MCHC)
Mean corpuscular
  volume (MCV)
Monocyte
Packed cell volume
  (PCV)
Plasmin
Platelets
Prothrombin time (PT)
Red blood cell indices
Red blood cells (also
  called "erythrocytes")
Refractometer
Reticulocyte
Rouleaux
Segmented neutrophil

KEY TERMS— cont'd

Spherocytes
Toxic Change
White blood cells (also called "leukocytes")

6. Do the following regarding coagulation testing:
   - Explain normal primary and secondary hemostasis, including intrinsic, extrinsic, and common pathways.
   - Discuss bleeding time, activated clotting time (ACT), activated partial thromboplastin time (APTT), and prothrombin time (PT) and the uses and significance of each.
   - Discuss tests used to evaluate fibrinolysis, including fibrin(ogen) degradation products (FDPs), D-dimer tests, and fibrinogen tests.
7. Do the following regarding cytology:
   - Explain uses for and limitations of cytology.
   - Describe procedures used to evaluate the cytology of solid tissue masses, enlarged organs, thoracic and abdominal effusions, and synovial fluid.
   - Discuss procedures used to submit cytology samples to a reference laboratory.
   - Describe collection and preparation of otic cytology samples, and identify common findings on normal and abnormal otic cytology preparations.

INTRODUCTION

Laboratory testing often is an integral component of patient evaluation performed to assess health, establish a diagnosis, and monitor response to disease. Inaccurate results may lead to an incorrect diagnosis, unnecessary testing, and ineffective treatment, so it is critical that laboratory results be accurate. Whether samples are submitted to a reference laboratory or are analyzed in the practice, veterinary technicians should be knowledgeable about proper sample collection and processing, as well as sample requirements, routine maintenance, calibration, and quality control procedures for each instrument being used. Manufacturers' recommendations should be followed to extend the longevity of each instrument and ensure accurate results. A basic understanding of the principles of each instrument is helpful in knowing how to determine when an instrument is not functioning properly, in performing troubleshooting, and in recognizing when sample quality or pathologic abnormalities might interfere with determination of accurate results.

If samples are sent to a reference laboratory, the veterinary technician should contact the reference laboratory for information about proper specimen storage and submission requirements to avoid damage or degradation before arrival to the reference laboratory. Veterinary reference laboratories are recommended over human reference laboratories because veterinary reference laboratories have instruments specifically designed or calibrated for processing blood from animals and are staffed by technicians and pathologists with the appropriate expertise. Accurate interpretation of laboratory results requires species-specific reference intervals, ideally determined by the laboratory performing the test because results may vary depending on the instrument and the reagents used or even the location (e.g., effects of high altitude on red blood cell mass).

The **complete blood count (CBC)** is one of the most commonly performed laboratory tests because it provides information about **red blood cells** (RBCs, or erythrocytes), **white blood cells** (WBCs, or leukocytes), **platelets**, and plasma protein concentration that can be helpful in determining health or disease and in monitoring response to therapy. **Cytology** is being used more frequently by veterinary practices to evaluate superficial masses, abnormal tissues, and fluid accumulations because it is relatively inexpensive, and results are available more quickly than with some other diagnostic tests. This chapter will focus on techniques and methods used for CBC and cytology, rather than on interpretation, although common abnormalities are included for blood smear evaluation.

HEMATOLOGY

COMPLETE BLOOD COUNT (CBC)

Blood samples for a CBC are collected in a tube containing an anticoagulant. The preferred anticoagulant for mammals and most non-mammalian species is ethylenediaminetetraacetic acid (EDTA), which prevents clotting by binding calcium. EDTA preserves cell morphology unless samples are stored for extended periods. For some non-mammalian species, heparin is the preferred anticoagulant because EDTA causes red blood cell (RBC) lysis. However, heparin typically causes artifacts in cell morphology. For those species, it is recommended that a blood film be made from a drop of non-anticoagulated blood at the time of sampling. All samples should be clearly labeled with an identification number or name and the date and time of collection.

Commercially available lavender top blood collection tubes contain EDTA, and green top tubes contain heparin; both are available in several different sizes. The 2-ml blood collection tubes are used most often, and this volume is sufficient for a CBC from all species. It is important to fill the collection tubes with the correct volume of blood because overfilling or underfilling can cause erroneous results. Several types of blood collection tubes and their intended uses are indicated in Table 12-1. It is important to mix the blood by gently inverting the tube several times after collection to make sure all of the blood contacts the anticoagulant. Samples should be inspected grossly for small clots before a sample is processed for a CBC, and if clots are present, a new sample should be collected. The tube should be inverted 10 to 15 times before the blood is processed through an automated hematology analyzer, a microhematocrit tube is filled, or **blood smears** are made, to ensure that RBCs, white blood cells (WBCs), and platelets are evenly distributed throughout the volume of blood.

TABLE 12-1	Blood Collection Tubes	
COLOR OF TOP	**ANTICOAGULANT**	**PURPOSE**
Lavender	EDTA	CBC, platelet count
Green	Heparin	CBC in some non-mammalian species; electrolytes and biochemical profile for some instruments
Blue	Citrate	Coagulation tests
Red	None	Biochemical profile (see Chapter 13); serum protein electrophoresis
Red and black*	None	Biochemical profile (see Chapter 13)

CBC, Complete blood count; *EDTA,* ethylenediaminetetraacetic acid
*Separator gel in these tubes facilitates separation of serum from cellular components.

> **TECHNICIAN NOTE** Blood in EDTA tubes should be mixed after collection and before a packed cell volume is determined, a blood smear is made, or the sample is processed through an automated hematology analyzer.

The CBC typically includes a PCV (**packed cell volume, or hematocrit** [HCT]), RBC count, **hemoglobin** concentration, **mean cell volume** (MCV), **mean corpuscular hemoglobin concentration** (MCHC), RBC distribution width (RDW), platelet count, WBC count, and WBC differential. Newer instruments with direct laser measurement may include RBC hemoglobin content (CH), hemoglobin content of **reticulocytes** (CHr), corpuscular hemoglobin concentration mean (CHCM), hemoglobin concentration distribution width (HDW), mean cell volume of reticulocytes (MCVr), platelet volume distribution width (PDW), and plateletcrit (PCT). The CBC also may include determination of plasma protein concentration and, in many laboratories, examination of a blood smear to evaluate cell morphology and perform a manual differential WBC count. It is important to use species-specific reference intervals for interpretation of results, whether they are generated manually or by automated instruments (Table 12-2).

AUTOMATED HEMATOLOGY ANALYZERS

Newer hematology analyzers designed for processing blood samples from animals are becoming more widely used in practice settings. Automated hematology analyzers count RBCs, WBCs, and platelets; determine hemoglobin concentration; and calculate **RBC indices**. These instruments also determine cell size and evaluate other cell parameters such as granularity of the cytoplasm and shape of the nucleus for WBCs. Compared with manual methods, thousands of cells are counted instead of hundreds of cells. In general, results are accurate and reproducible, and are available in a very short time. Larger instruments can be loaded with multiple samples, allowing the technician time to perform other tests while the samples are being processed.

These instruments use light scatter from a focused laser beam, impedance technology, and various staining methods to count and evaluate cells. Cells are directed through a small aperture, and each cell is individually evaluated. With light scatter methods, cells scatter light from a laser beam in different directions and at different angles, depending on physical properties of the cell. This allows the instrument to count RBCs and determine their size, count WBCs and generate a WBC differential, and count platelets and determine their size. With impedance methods, cells interfere with an electrical current, and the size of the cells is proportional to the deflection of the current. Special stains also can be used to further distinguish different populations of cells.

Instrument settings for the size of each cell type are important and may vary with species, which is why instruments designed for human samples often do not generate accurate results for samples from domestic animals. Newer automated hematology analyzers are manufactured with

TABLE 12-2 | CBC Reference Intervals*

PARAMETER	DOG	CAT	HORSE	COW	LLAMA
Plasma protein, g/dl	5.7-7.2	5.6-7.4	6.5-7.8	7.0-9.0	5.6-7.2
Hematocrit, %	36-54	25-46	27-44	23-35	24-40
Hemoglobin, g/dl	11.9-18.4	8.0-14.9	9.7-15.6	8.3-12.3	10.1-17.7
Red blood cells, $\times 10^{12}$/L	4.9-8.2	5.3-10.2	5.1-10.0	5.0-7.5	8.8-16.1
MCV, fl	64-75	42-53	43-55	43-52	22-32
MCHC, g/dl	32.9-35.2	30.0-33.7	34.4-36.9	34.5-36.3	39.5-46.2
RDW	13.4-17.0	16.0-21.0	19.8-25.4	17.8-23.7	22.8-29.6
Reticulocytes, $\times 10^9$/L	<60	<50	0	0	0
Platelets, $\times 10^9$/L	106-424	150-600	125-310	192-746	310-2800
White blood cells, $\times 10^9$/L	4.1-15.2	4.0-14.5	4.7-10.6	3.0-13.5	7.4-19.9
Segmented neutrophils, $\times 10^9$/L	3.0-10.4	3.0-9.2	2.4-6.4	0.7-5.1	3.5-13.7
Band neutrophils, $\times 10^9$/L	0-0.1	0-0.1	0-0.1	0-0.1	0-0.1
Lymphocytes, $\times 10^9$/L	1.0-4.6	0.9-3.9	1.0-4.9	1.1-8.2	1.3-5.7
Monocytes, $\times 10^9$/L	0.0-1.2	0.0-0.5	0.0-0.5	0.0-0.6	0-0.8
Eosinophils, $\times 10^9$/L	0-1.3	0-1.2	0-0.3	0-1.5	0-3.9
Basophils, $\times 10^9$/L	0	0-0.2	0-0.1	0-0.1	0-0.3

CBC, Complete blood count; *MCHC,* mean corpuscular hemoglobin concentration; *MCV,* mean corpuscular volume; *RDW,* red cell distribution width.
Note: These values were determined in the authors' laboratory using a CellDyn 3500 hematology analyzer and may differ from other published reference intervals. Reference intervals should be generated for each laboratory. Most reference laboratories report species-specific reference intervals with the patient's results.

computer software that makes adjustments for analysis of blood from a variety of animal species. Many of these analyzers are easy to use and provide reliable results, especially for healthy animals with normal CBCs. However, evaluation of a blood smear is strongly recommended if the animal is anemic, thrombocytopenic, or leukopenic, and in cases of moderate to marked leukocytosis. Each instrument should be validated by the laboratory for every species being evaluated, and an adequate quality control program that includes regular analysis of commercially available control material should be established by the user. Reference laboratories and laboratories in academic settings often establish criteria for evaluating blood smears as part of the CBC. In some laboratories, all blood smears are evaluated as part of the quality assurance program, and because important morphologic changes sometimes are detected only by microscopic examination.

PACKED CELL VOLUME (PCV)

PCV (or HCT), RBC count, and hemoglobin concentration are used to evaluate RBC mass, which is an indication of the oxygen-carrying capacity of blood. In veterinary medicine, the PCV is the most commonly used parameter to assess RBC mass because it can be measured manually. Determination of PCV is quick and inexpensive to perform, and it is done often to assess hydration and to monitor fluid therapy, even if a CBC is not performed.

PCV is the percentage (%) of RBCs in a specific volume of blood. PCV is determined by filling a plain microhematocrit tube ⅔ to ¾ full with EDTA anticoagulated blood, sealing one end with a specific kind of clay, and centrifuging the sample in a microhematocrit centrifuge for a specified

length of time and speed according to the manufacturer's recommendations. Longer periods of time for centrifugation may be required for blood samples from cattle, sheep, and goats because their RBCs are smaller than RBCs from dogs and cats. During centrifugation, RBCs are tightly packed toward the sealed end of the microhematocrit tube. After centrifugation, three components of the blood are visible in the microhematocrit tube: a column of packed RBCs at the bottom, a buffy coat layer of WBCs and platelets just above the packed RBCs, and plasma at the top (Figure 12-1). The PCV is determined by using a special wheel or chart with a grid. To measure the PCV, align the bottom of the RBC column with zero and the top of the plasma portion with 100, and determine where the top of the RBC column intersects the grid; this point indicates the PCV as a percentage (%) (Figure 12-2).

Automated hematology analyzers calculate HCT by multiplying the mean cell volume (MCV, see later) by the RBC count (see later). Although values are determined by different methods, the terms *PCV* and *HCT* often are used interchangeably. They should be numerically similar, and both are usually accurate indicators of RBC mass. However, errors in determination of HCT and PCV can occur. If the blood collection tube has been inadequately filled, excess anticoagulant causes RBCs to shrink, falsely decreasing the PCV. When the sample is processed by the automated hematology analyzer, the diluent allows the RBCs to expand to their normal volume, so in this case, HCT is a more accurate indication of RBC mass. If **agglutination** of RBCs is noted, as occurs in immune-mediated hemolytic anemia, the RBC count from the automated instrument will be falsely decreased owing to clumping of RBCs. This falsely decreases the HCT because it is calculated using the RBC count. In this case, the spun PCV is a more accurate indication of RBC mass.

RED BLOOD CELL (RBC) COUNT

RBCs can be counted accurately by automated instruments using laser or impedance technology. The RBC count is reported as the number of RBCs $\times 10^{12}$/L (or $\times 10^6$/μL). Manual RBC counts are not very accurate compared with those determined by automated instruments and are not recommended. Because changes in RBC count usually are proportional to changes in PCV and HCT, most clinicians use PCV and HCT to evaluate RBC mass. However, the RBC count is useful in calculating RBC indices (see later), which may be helpful in classifying anemia.

HEMOGLOBIN CONCENTRATION

Hemoglobin is the protein in RBCs that carries oxygen from lungs to tissues. Hemoglobin concentration, reported as g/dl, is determined by automated analyzers using several different methods. Hemoglobin concentration cannot be measured accurately by manual methods. Changes in hemoglobin concentration usually are proportional to changes in PCV (or HCT). In most species except camelids (camels, llamas, alpacas, vicunas), PCV (or HCT) divided by 3 is a good estimate of hemoglobin concentration. Hemoglobin concentration is useful in determining RBC indices (see later), which are used to classify anemia.

RED BLOOD CELL INDICES

MCV is used as an indicator of the average size of RBCs and is reported in femtoliters (fl; 1 fl = 10^{-15} L). The analyzer measures the volume of each RBC counted and determines the mean volume for the RBC population. MCV also can be calculated from a manually determined PCV and RBC count (Box 12-1), but manual RBC counts are not very accurate. Marked species differences in MCV have been noted (see Table 12-2). RBCs with normal MCV are called *normocytic*, RBCs with an increased MCV are called *macrocytic*, and

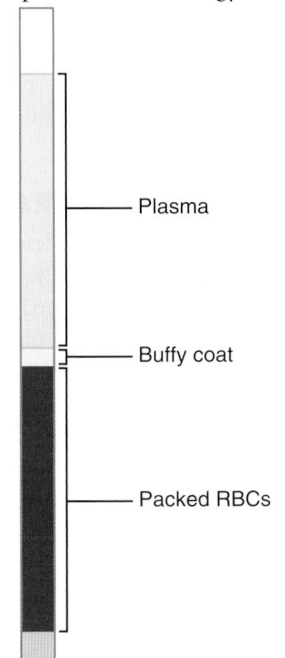

FIGURE 12-1 Microhematocrit tube after centrifugation. The plasma is located in the upper portion and the packed red blood cells (RBCs) are in the lower portion. The buffy coat containing white blood cells (WBCs) and platelets is between the plasma and the packed RBCs. (Illustrated by Tim Vojt, Biomedical Media, The Ohio State University College of Veterinary Medicine. Copyright The Ohio State University.)

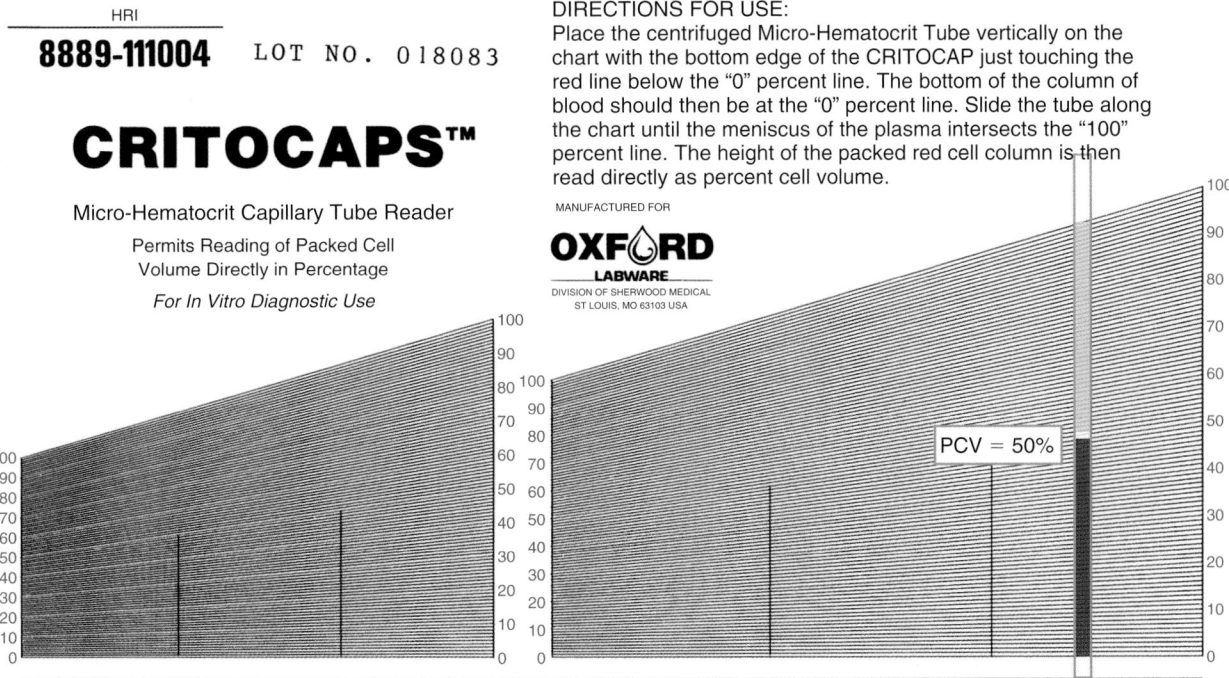

FIGURE 12-2 Determination of packed cell volume (PCV). A card with a grid can be used to determine the PCV from a centrifuged microhematocrit tube by following the instructions indicated on the card. The PCV in this patient is 50%. (Illustration by Tim Vojt, Biomedical Media, The Ohio State University College of Veterinary Medicine. Copyright The Ohio State University.)

BOX 12-1 Calculation of RBC Indices

$$MCV \text{ (fL)} = \frac{HCT \% \times 10}{RBC \text{ count} \times 10^{12}/L}$$

Example: HCT = 42%, RBC count = $6 \times 10^{12}/L$

$$MCV = \frac{42 \times 10}{6} = 70 \text{ fL}$$

$$MCHC \text{ (g/dl)} = \frac{Hemoglobin \text{ g/dl}}{HCT \%} \times 100$$

Example: Hemoglobin = 15 g/dl, HCT = 45%

$$MCHC = \frac{15}{45} \times 100 = 33 \text{ g/dl}$$

HCT, Hematocrit; *MCHC*, mean corpuscular hemoglobin concentration; *MCV*, mean corpuscular volume; *RBC*, red blood cell.

those with a decreased MCV are called *microcytic*. MCV often is increased in regenerative anemias associated with hemorrhage or hemolysis, but usually is normal in nonregenerative anemias associated with inflammation, chronic renal failure, and primary bone marrow disease. MCV may be decreased in iron deficiency anemia resulting from chronic external blood loss.

MCHC is the average amount of hemoglobin in a specific volume of blood and is calculated from the hemoglobin concentration and HCT as determined by the automated instrument (see Table 12-2). In most species, MCHC is 32 to 36 g/dl, but in camelids, MCHC ranges from 41 to 45 g/dl. MCHC is increased if intravascular hemolysis or in vitro hemolysis is associated with sample collection or handling. Lipemia and large numbers of Heinz bodies can interfere with measurement of hemoglobin concentration, resulting in falsely increased MCHC. RBC agglutination may cause a falsely decreased HCT, and thus an increased MCHC. If MCHC is increased, it is helpful to examine the plasma to determine whether hemolysis or lipemia is present, and to evaluate a blood smear to see whether Heinz bodies or agglutinated RBCs are evident. In the absence of hemolysis, lipemia, or Heinz bodies, an increased MCHC may indicate instrument error. RBCs with a normal MCHC are called *normochromic*, and those with a decreased MCHC are called *hypochromic*. RBCs often are normochromic in health and in nonregenerative anemia. Hypochromic RBCs occur in marked regenerative anemia and in some animals with severe iron deficiency.

Mean corpuscular hemoglobin (MCH), the average amount of hemoglobin in each RBC, is reported in picograms. MCH is calculated from the hemoglobin concentration and the RBC count as determined by the automated instrument, but MCH is not used clinically and may not be reported as part of a CBC.

RED CELL DISTRIBUTION WIDTH (RDW)

The RDW is a mathematical index that describes the variation in RBC size or **anisocytosis**. It is the coefficient of variation of the size of the RBCs as determined by the automated analyzer and is calculated by dividing the standard deviation of RBC volume (size) by the MCV. In most species, the distribution of RBC size is seen as a bell-shaped curve with a fairly consistent RDW for each particular species. An increased RDW may indicate regenerative anemia or early iron deficiency anemia. This can be visualized as widening of the bell-shaped curve generated by the analyzer or by evaluation of a blood smear for anisocytosis. A decreased RDW is not clinically relevant.

PLASMA PROTEIN CONCENTRATION

Plasma protein concentration can be determined by refractometry from the plasma portion of the spun microhematocrit tube. Plasma in the microhematocrit tube should be evaluated for clarity and color before plasma protein concentration is determined. Plasma from healthy dogs and cats is clear and colorless, whereas plasma from horses and cows often is clear and light yellow owing to dietary differences. Changes in color and clarity may be important indicators of disease and should be reported as part of the CBC.

> **TECHNICIAN NOTE** Changes in color and clarity of the plasma may be important indicators of disease and should be recorded.

The microhematocrit tube is gently broken slightly above the buffy coat, the tube is inverted, and the unbroken end is used to fill the prism of a **refractometer** by capillary action with the cover on the prism closed. Tapping the end of the microhematocrit tube directly on the face of the prism may scratch the surface and should be avoided. Plasma protein concentration is determined through the eyepiece by visualizing where the distinction between the darker staining region at the top and the lighter staining region at the bottom intersects the scale for plasma protein concentration (Figure 12-3). Many refractometers also are used for urine specific gravity, so it is important to use the correct scale for plasma protein, reported in g/dl.

Plasma protein concentration as determined by refractometry is accurate if the plasma is clear and of normal color for the species. If the plasma is lipemic or excess anticoagulant is present, plasma protein concentration may be falsely increased. Plasma protein concentration also can be falsely increased from marked hyperglycemia or azotemia (increase in blood urea nitrogen [BUN]). Marked hemolysis and bilirubin can falsely increase plasma protein, but often the increase is minimal. Plasma protein concentration usually is slightly higher than serum protein concentration owing to the presence of fibrinogen. Plasma fibrinogen concentration sometimes is used as an indicator of inflammation in horses and cattle, and can be determined semiquantitatively by a heat precipitation method (Procedure 12-1) or quantitatively by coagulation analyzers.

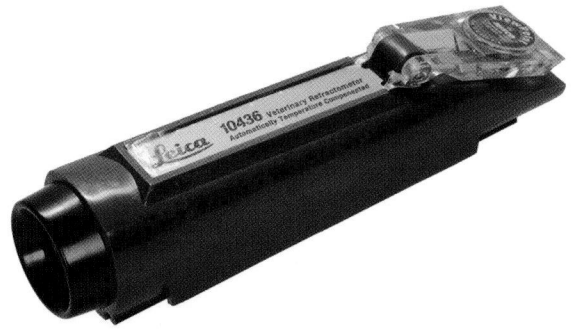

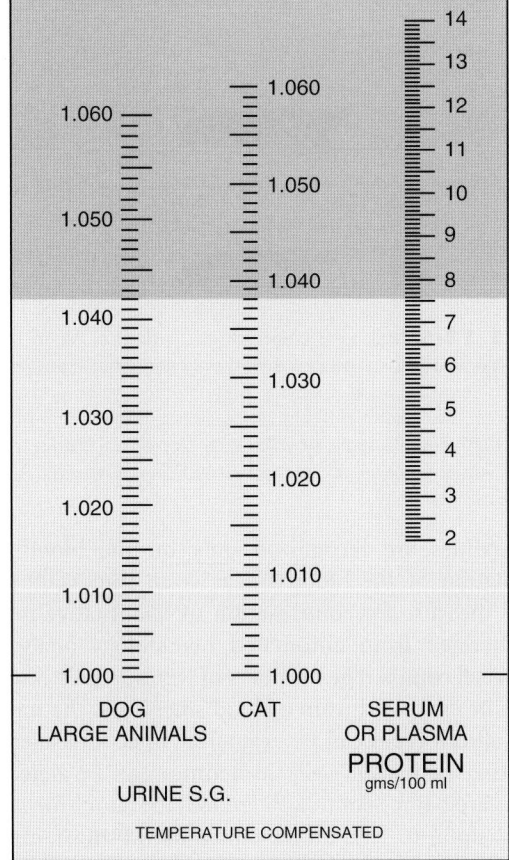

FIGURE 12-3 Plasma protein determination. A refractometer is shown on the top with the scale depicted below. The protein concentration is determined by visualizing where the distinction between the darker portion at the top and the lighter portion at the bottom cross-intersects the scale. In this patient, the total protein concentration is 7.5 g/dl. (Illustration by Tim Vojt, Biomedical Media, The Ohio State University College of Veterinary Medicine. Copyright The Ohio State University.)

WHITE BLOOD CELL (WBC) COUNT

WBCs can be counted manually or by automated instruments, or they can be estimated from the buffy coat layer or blood smear evaluation. For manual WBC counts, a **hemocytometer** and commercially available reagents are used. A hemocytometer (an improved Neubauer hemocytometer is recommended) is a specialized counting chamber with a surface that contains a pair of etched counting grids and a special weighted coverglass (do not discard the coverglass). The Leuko-TIC (bioanalytic GmbH, Umkrich/Freiburg, Germany) reagent system is recommended

PROCEDURE 12-1	Determination of Fibrinogen by Heat Precipitation

- Fill two microhematocrit tubes $\frac{2}{3}$ to $\frac{3}{4}$ full with EDTA anticoagulated blood.
- Centrifuge both tubes in a microhematocrit centrifuge according to the manufacturer's recommendations for determination of PCV.
- Gently break one microhematocrit tube slightly above the buffy coat, and use the unbroken end to fill the prism of a hemocytometer.
- Read the total protein (TP) in g/dl using the scale for plasma protein concentration.
- Heat the second microhematocrit tube in a 56° C water bath for 3 minutes to precipitate fibrinogen.
- Recentrifuge the heated microhematocrit; the precipitated fibrinogen will settle just above the buffy coat.
- Gently break the microhematocrit tube above the buffy coat, and determine the total protein (TP) in g/dl.
- Calculate the fibrinogen concentration:
  (TP of unheated microhematocrit tube − TP of heated microhematocrit tube) × 100 = Fibrinogen concentration in mg/dl

EDTA, Ethylenediaminetetraacetic acid; *PCV,* packed cell volume.

because the Unopette-System is no longer available. Detailed manufacturer's instructions must be followed carefully for accurate results. Briefly, 20 µL of blood is diluted, RBCs are lysed, and a small volume of diluted blood is added to the hemocytometer just beneath the coverslip. WBCs are counted in the four large corner squares of the grid, and the number of WBCs is multiplied by 50 to determine WBCs/µL (Figure 12-4). Diminishing the light by lowering the substage condenser may enhance contrast to make it easier to visualize the WBCs. Both grids of the hemocytometer should be filled with the same sample and counted. WBC counts from each grid should be within 10% of each other if the procedure has been performed accurately. If not, the sample should be reloaded and recounted.

TECHNICIAN NOTE Carefully follow the detailed instructions for using commercially available reagents and a hemocytometer to achieve the most accurate WBC counts by manual methods.

WBC counts as determined by automated hematology analyzers often are more accurate and precise than manual WBC counts because the instrument counts thousands of cells. The WBC count can be estimated by quantitative buffy coat (QBC; Becton Dickinson, Franklin Lakes, NJ) analysis, in which the buffy coat layer is measured in a specialized microhematocrit tube with a float that expands the buffy coat region for optical scanning. The WBC count also can be estimated by evaluation of a stained blood smear (see later). Species-specific reference intervals should be used to interpret the WBC count.

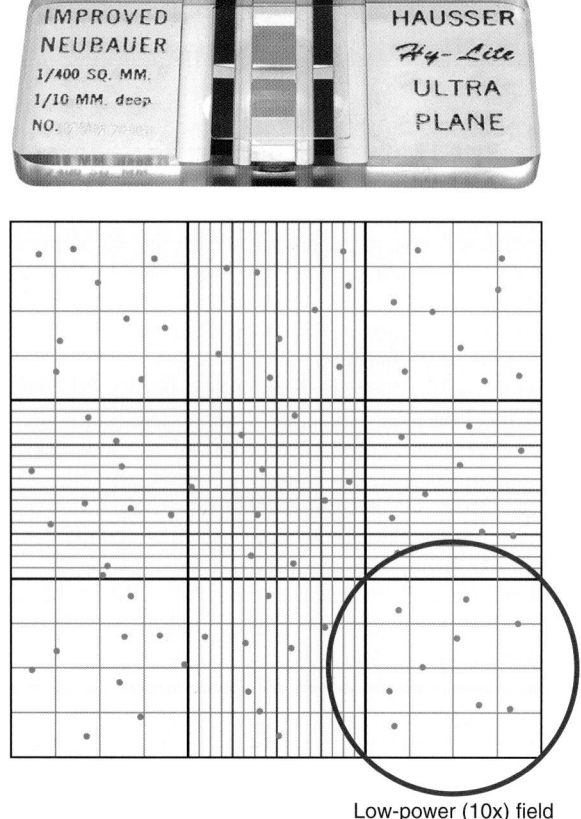

Low-power (10x) field

FIGURE 12-4 Manual determination of white blood cell (WBC) counts. An improved Neubauer hemocytometer is shown on the top and the counting chamber is shown below. The pink circle indicates a corner square, which can be visualized through the 10x objective. In this patient, 36 cells are seen in the 4 corner squares and the WBC count is 36 × 50 = 1800/µL. (Illustration by Tim Vojt, Biomedical Media, The Ohio State University College of Veterinary Medicine. Copyright The Ohio State University.)

Birds and reptiles have nucleated RBCs; this interferes with WBC counts as determined by some instruments and by the manual method described previously for mammalian species. Some newer hematology analyzers are able to determine WBC counts from birds and reptiles, or WBCs can be determined indirectly using a different reagent system (Thrombo-TIC or Ery-TIC; bioanalytic GmbH). Other protocols using methyl violet, Phloxine B dye, or Natt and Herrick solution have been described.

Platelet Count

The platelet count as determined by automated hematology analyzers is accurate for most species unless macroplatelets or platelet clumps are present, which occurs most commonly in cats. The number of platelets can be estimated from the blood smear (see later) or counted manually using commercially available reagent systems (Thrombo-TIC) and a hemocytometer. Marked species differences have been noted in the numbers of circulating platelets (see Table 12-2).

PREPARATION OF BLOOD SMEARS

Microscopic evaluation of a blood smear is an important component of a CBC because some hematologic

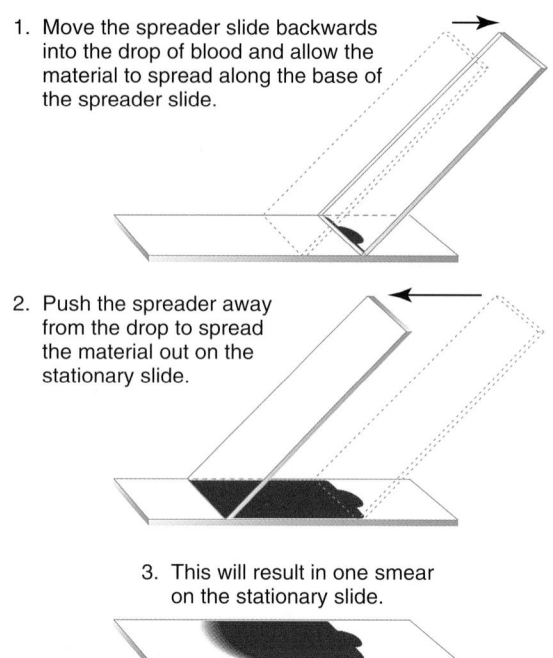

1. Move the spreader slide backwards into the drop of blood and allow the material to spread along the base of the spreader slide.

2. Push the spreader away from the drop to spread the material out on the stationary slide.

3. This will result in one smear on the stationary slide.

FIGURE 12-5 Making a blood smear. A drop of blood is placed on one end of a glass slide that is held stationary on a flat surface, and a second "spreader" slide is used to push the drop forward in a smooth, even motion, resulting in a blood smear that is evenly distributed across the stationary slide. (Illustration by Tim Vojt, Biomedical Media, The Ohio State University College of Veterinary Medicine. Copyright The Ohio State University.)

abnormalities are recognized only on the blood smear. Examination of the blood smear is an important quality control measure for confirmation of quantitative information obtained from automated hematology analyzers or manual cell counts. The numbers of RBCs, WBCs, and platelets can be estimated from a blood smear, and the morphology of all cell types can be evaluated. Infectious agents and circulating neoplastic cells sometimes can be detected. If samples are being sent to a reference laboratory for analysis, it may helpful to send an unstained blood smear, especially if a delay in transit is anticipated, to determine whether any changes are pathologic or are due to sample processing. Smears from samples being processed in the practice should be made immediately after blood is collected, for optimal preservation of cell morphology.

Preparation of high-quality blood smears is a technical skill that requires practice. Blood smears should be made with new, clean microscope slides using one of several methods. Most commonly, a small drop of blood is placed close to one end of a microscope slide that is held stationary on a flat surface (Figure 12-5). A second "spreader" slide is held at a 30- to 45-degree angle near the front of the drop of blood, and is moved backward to contact the front edge of the drop of blood. A short hesitation allows the blood to flow by capillary action along the edge of the spreader slide before the spreader slide is pushed forward in a smooth, even motion with minimal downward pressure until the end of the stationary slide is reached. This should result in a blood smear that is evenly distributed across $\frac{1}{2}$ to $\frac{3}{4}$ of the stationary slide. If the drop of blood is too small, the spreader slide is pushed too slowly, or the angle of the spreader slide is too obtuse, the smear will be too thin or too short. If the drop of blood is too large, the spreader slide is pushed too quickly, or the angle of the spreader slide is too acute, the smear may be too thick or too long.

> **TECHNICIAN NOTE** Making adequate blood smears requires practice but is a skill worth developing because much information can be gained by examination of a blood smear.

Blood smears should be dried quickly before staining to prevent RBC artifacts. Slides should be labeled at one end with the date and the animal's name or identification number. Ideally, slides should be stained within several hours. A lapse longer than 48 hours may result in inadequate staining. Unstained smears being sent to a reference laboratory should be stored at room temperature, not in a refrigerator or freezer because water condensation will damage the cells. Unstained smears should be stored away from formalin fumes and shipped separately from surgical biopsies that have been placed in formalin, because formalin vapors inhibit optimal staining. The reference laboratory should be contacted for instructions about how to properly package and ship blood smears to avoid breakage or damage.

Romanowsky-type stains such as Wright stain or Wright-Giemsa stain provide optimal staining but can be labor-intensive, require distilled water, and may need frequent filtering. Several commercially available staining procedures that mimic Wright or Wright-Giemsa stain have been described. Diff-Quik (Baxter Scientific Products, McGraw Park, IL) is commonly used in veterinary practices, but other similar stains are available. These stains are relatively inexpensive and convenient to use. Although they may overstain nuclei, blur chromatin detail, and fail to stain cytoplasmic granules in some cells, they are adequate for determining a leukocyte differential and for evaluating most morphologic abnormalities, if used properly.

BLOOD SMEAR EVALUATION

A properly maintained, high-quality microscope is a good investment for evaluating blood smears and cytology samples. The microscope should be binocular with adjustable oculars, an adjustable substage condenser, and planachromatic 10×, 40× (high dry), and 100× (oil immersion) objectives. If additional objectives are an option, some microscopists prefer to have 4×, 20×, and 50× (oil immersion) objectives. The technician should be familiar with optimizing the light by adjusting the condenser, iris diaphragm, and diffuser, depending on the sample being evaluated. For evaluation of blood smears and cytology samples, the substage condenser should be in a relatively high position, and the iris diaphragm should be open. The manufacturer's manual often contains instructions for proper light adjustment. Use of the 40× objective requires mounting of a coverslip onto the slide for optimum visualization, but the oil

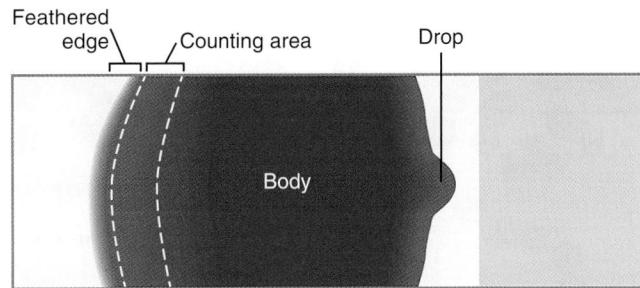

FIGURE 12-6 Regions of a blood smear. The body, the counting area, and the feathered edge are shown. (Illustration by Tim Vojt, Biomedical Media, The Ohio State University College of Veterinary Medicine. Copyright The Ohio State University.)

immersion objective is recommended for blood smear evaluation. For oil immersion objectives, a drop of immersion oil is placed on the slide to achieve optimal optics. Oil immersion objectives should be gently wiped clean after use, as directed by the manufacturer. All other objectives should be kept free of immersion oil.

Accurate evaluation of blood smears requires a systematic procedure for examination and expertise in identifying normal cells, morphologic abnormalities, and artifacts. A blood smear consists of three regions: body, counting area, and feathered edge (Figure 12-6). The body, the largest part, is a homogenous area beginning at the end of the slide where the drop of blood was placed and continuing to the counting area. In the body, the blood smear is thick and cells are piled on top of each other, so it is difficult to identify cells or evaluate cell morphology. The feathered edge is the end of the blood smear farthest away from the drop. At the feathered edge, many of the cells may be broken, distribution of cells may be uneven, and RBCs often lose their central zone of pallor. Cell morphology should not be evaluated at the feathered edge. The counting area is between the body and the feathered edge and appears progressively thinner as it approaches the feathered edge. The counting area contains a monolayer of cells. In this region, RBCs, WBCs, and platelets can be identified, and their morphology can be adequately evaluated. Most of the blood smear evaluation is performed in the counting area.

The blood smear should be evaluated initially with the 10× objective. In the body of the smear, RBCs can be evaluated for **rouleaux** formation or agglutination (Figure 12-7). Rouleaux formation refers to RBCs in chains that resemble a stack of coins. In horses and cats, rouleaux formation is common, whereas in dogs, rouleaux formation may be an indication of inflammation (increased plasma proteins), or it may be an artifact of smear preparation. *Agglutination* refers to irregular, variably-sized clumps of RBCs that form because of excess antibodies bound to the surface of RBCs. This occurs in immune-mediated hemolytic anemia (IHA), which is most common in dogs (Case Presentation 12-1). It may be difficult to distinguish rouleaux formation from agglutination on the blood smear. A saline dispersion test often is performed by adding 10 drops of saline to 1 drop of EDTA anticoagulated blood and gently mixing the sample.

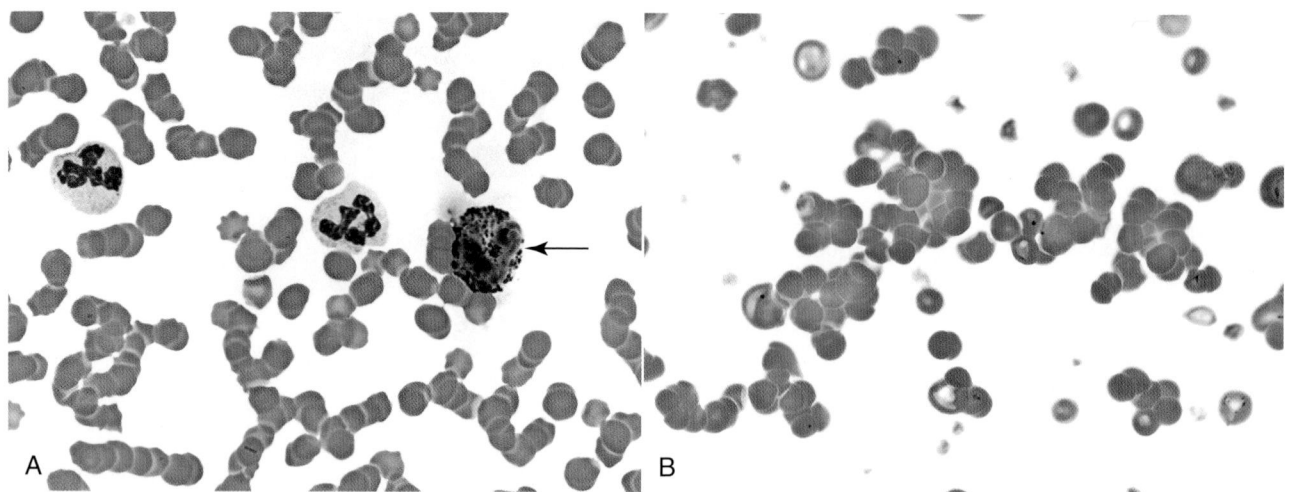

FIGURE 12-7 Rouleaux and agglutination. **A,** Rouleaux formation is normal in horses and is shown at low magnification on the left. The red blood cells (RBCs) appear like a stack of coins. Two neutrophils are present on the left, and a basophil on the right *(arrow)*. **B,** RBC agglutination, as shown on the right, occurs most commonly in dogs with immune-mediated hemolytic anemia. The RBCs are in irregular clumps of various sizes. (Wright stain.)

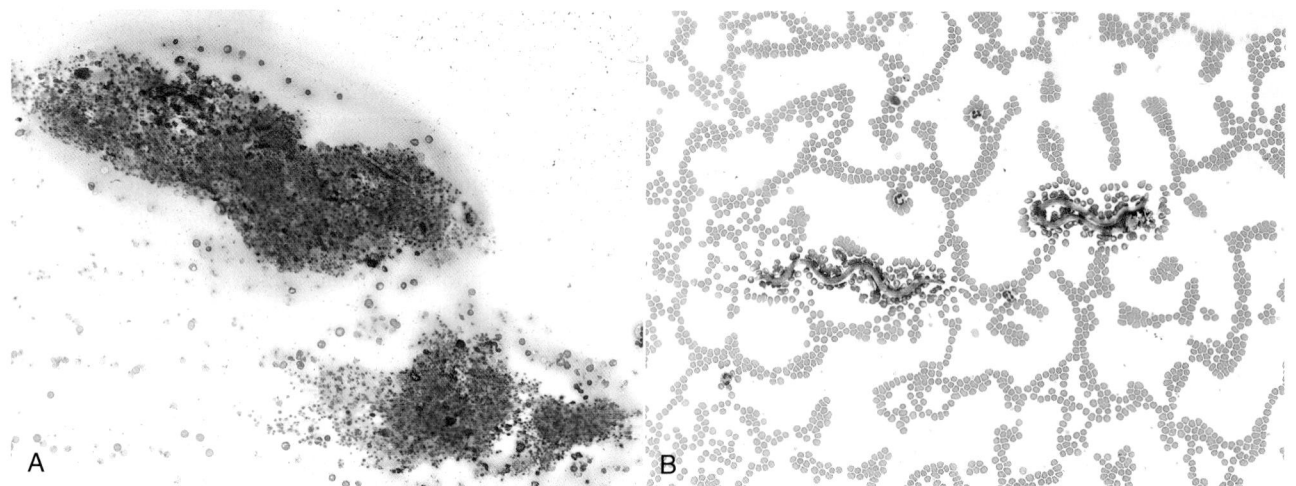

FIGURE 12-8 Scanning the feathered edge. **A,** Large platelet clumps are most often detected on the feathered edge during 10× scan of the blood smear and, if present, may falsely decrease the platelet count or estimate. **B,** Two microfilaria are present in this field. (Wright stain.)

A drop of the diluted blood is added to a clean glass slide, and the sample is observed using 10× or 40× magnification. A coverslip can be added but is not necessary. Saline disperses rouleaux but not agglutination.

The 10× objective also should be used to scan the feathered edge for platelet clumps, microfiliaria, and large, abnormal cells (Figure 12-8). It is important to recognize platelet clumps because platelet clumping may falsely decrease platelet counts as determined manually or by an automated analyzer, or estimated by evaluating the smear at higher magnification. Although more sensitive methods may be used to detect microfilaria, one should not overlook their presence on a blood smear. Recognition of abnormal cells at the feathered edge is helpful because they may be present in low numbers and missed if only the counting area is evaluated. The WBC count can be estimated from several fields in the counting area using the 10× objective. An average of about 10 to 30 WBCs should be present per 10× field for a normal WBC count in most species. The number of WBCs/10× field multiplied by 100 (or the number of WBCs/20× field multiplied by 500) can be used to estimate the number of WBCs/µL. The counting area of the blood smear can be located using the 10× objective by recognizing the region in which a monolayer of evenly dispersed cells can be seen between the body and the feathered edge.

The counting area of the smear should be evaluated with the 100× oil immersion objective using a systematic approach to estimate platelet number, evaluate cell morphology, and perform a differential WBC count. Always evaluate platelets, RBCs, and WBCs in the same order. The order is not critical, but using the same order for each blood smear is an important part of a systematic approach.

CASE PRESENTATION 12-1 IMMUNE-MEDIATED HEMOLYTIC ANEMIA (IHA) AND THROMBOCYTOPENIA (ITP)

Signalment: 6-year-old, spayed female Collie

History: acute onset of severe lethargy

Physical examination: pale, icteric mucous membranes; tachypnea; enlarged spleen

CBC	Patient		Reference Interval
Plasma protein, g/dl	7.6	H	5.7-7.2
Plasma appeared clear and moderately yellow.			
HCT, %	17	L	36-54
Hemoglobin, g/dl	5.0	L	11.9-18.4
RBCs, ×10^{12}/L	2.2	L	4.9-8.2
MCV, fL	80	H	64-75
MCHC, g/dl	29.1	L	32.9-35.2
RDW	19.1	H	13.4-17.0
Reticulocytes, ×10^9/L	477.5	H	<60

RBC morphology: There is marked agglutination that did not disperse with saline. Moderate anisocytosis, marked polychromasia, and numerous spherocytes are observed. Numbers of Howell-Jolly bodies and nRBCs are increased.

Platelets, ×10^9/L	94	L	106-424
WBCs, ×10^9/L	34.6	H	4.1-15.2
nRBCs, ×10^9/L	10.9	H	0
Band neutrophils, ×10^9/L	8.2	H	0-0.1
Segmented neutrophils, ×10^9/L	28.2	H	3.0-10.4
Lymphocytes, ×10^9/L	1.8		1.0-4.6
Monocytes, ×10^9/L	7.3	H	0.0-1.2
Eosinophils, ×10^9/L	0		0-1.2

WBC morphology: Moderate numbers of Döhle bodies and moderate cytoplasmic basophilia and vacuolation are interpreted as toxic change.

Interpretation

RBCs A marked macrocytic, hypochromic anemia is present that is markedly regenerative, based on the increased reticulocyte count. Reticulocytes are less mature RBCs and are characterized by macrocytic, hypochromic indices. The increased numbers of Howell-Jolly bodies and nRBCs likely are part of the regenerative response. Marked agglutination and the presence of numerous spherocytes are hallmarks of immune-mediated hemolytic anemia (IHA), especially when there is no history of blood transfusion. This case illustrates the importance of evaluating a blood smear.

Platelets Platelets appear mildly decreased on the blood smear, and no platelet clumps are noted. Some dogs with IHA also have immune-mediated thrombocytopenia (ITP). However, other causes of thrombocytopenia cannot be excluded. Disseminated intravascular coagulation (DIC) is a serious complication that occurs in some dogs with IHA, resulting in thrombocytopenia secondary to consumption of platelets.

WBCs Moderate to marked neutrophilia with a left shift and monocytosis is typical for dogs with IHA. These animals do not really have inflammatory disease, but likely have increased concentrations of cytokines that stimulate increased production of WBCs as well as RBCs. The toxic changes in the neutrophils are the result of rapidly increased proliferation of neutrophils in the bone marrow. Some dogs with IHA also have lymphopenia, which is due to a superimposed stress leukogram and treatment with corticosteroids, but this dog has normal numbers of lymphocytes.

Summary

Evaluation of the blood smear is important in establishing a diagnosis of IHA. Key features that are present in many (but not all) dogs with IHA include the following:

- RBC agglutination (does not disperse with saline)
- Spherocytes (remember to look only in the counting area)
- Anisocytosis, polychromasia, Howell-Jolly bodies, and nRBCs
- Leukocytosis due to neutrophilia with a left shift and monocytosis
- Thrombocytopenia and macroplatelets in dogs with concurrent ITP

CBC, Complete blood count; HCT, hematocrit; MCHC, mean corpuscular hemoglobin concentration; MCV, mean corpuscular volume; nRBC, nucleated red blood cell; RBC, red blood cell; RDW, red cell distribution width; WBC, white blood cell.

TECHNICIAN NOTE Blood smears should be examined with 10× and 100× oil immersion objectives in a systematic manner for adequate evaluation.

Platelets

In mammals, platelets are non-nucleated fragments of cytoplasm released from megakaryocytes in the bone marrow. In most mammals, platelets are smaller than RBCs. The cytoplasm stains light blue and contains small, light purple granules (Figure 12-9). Platelets may not stain as well in horses, and platelets from llamas and alpacas are very small compared with those from other species. In birds and reptiles, platelets have nuclei and are called *thrombocytes* (see Figure 12-9). Platelets that approach the size of RBCs are called *macroplatelets* and in some species may indicate increased platelet production. Macroplatelets may be normal in cats and in Cavalier King Charles Spaniels. In Cavalier King Charles Spaniels, an estimate of the platelet count from the blood smear may be more accurate than an automated platelet count. Other morphologic abnormalities are unusual but should be noted.

In general, automated platelet counts are more accurate than manual platelet counts. The platelet count can be estimated on the blood smear by determining the number of platelets in several oil immersion fields. On average, 6 to 15 platelets per oil immersion field should be noted. The average number of platelets can be multiplied by 15,000 or 20,000 to

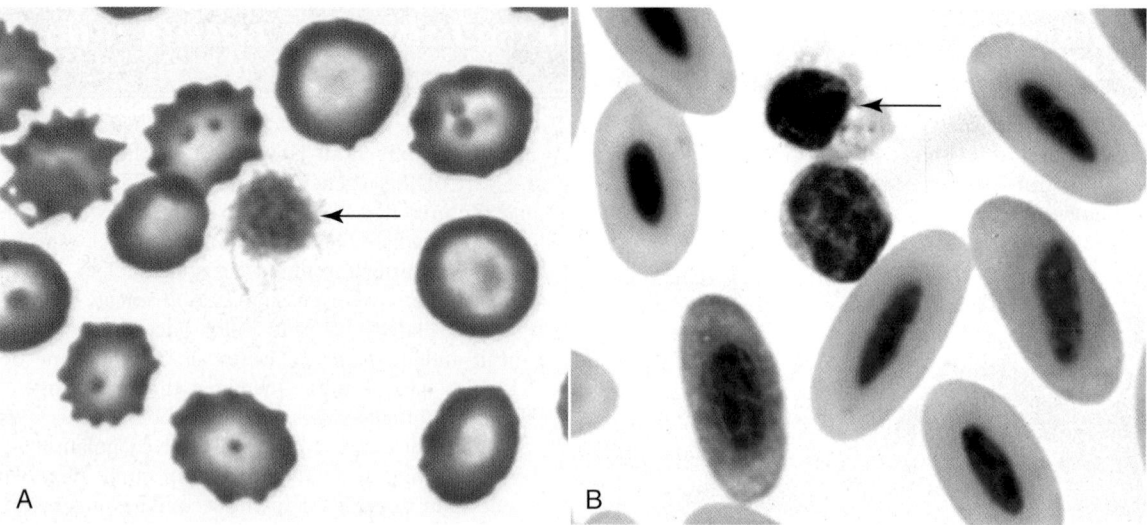

FIGURE 12-9 Platelets and thrombocytes. **A,** A platelet from a dog is shown in the center *(arrow)*. Platelets in mammals do not have nuclei, and the cytoplasm appears granular. **B,** A thrombocyte from a bird is shown in the upper center *(arrow)*, just above the small lymphocyte. In birds and reptiles, thrombocytes often are round to oval and have round nuclei. The cytoplasm may appear vacuolated and may contain several small granules, as shown in this thrombocyte. (Wright stain.)

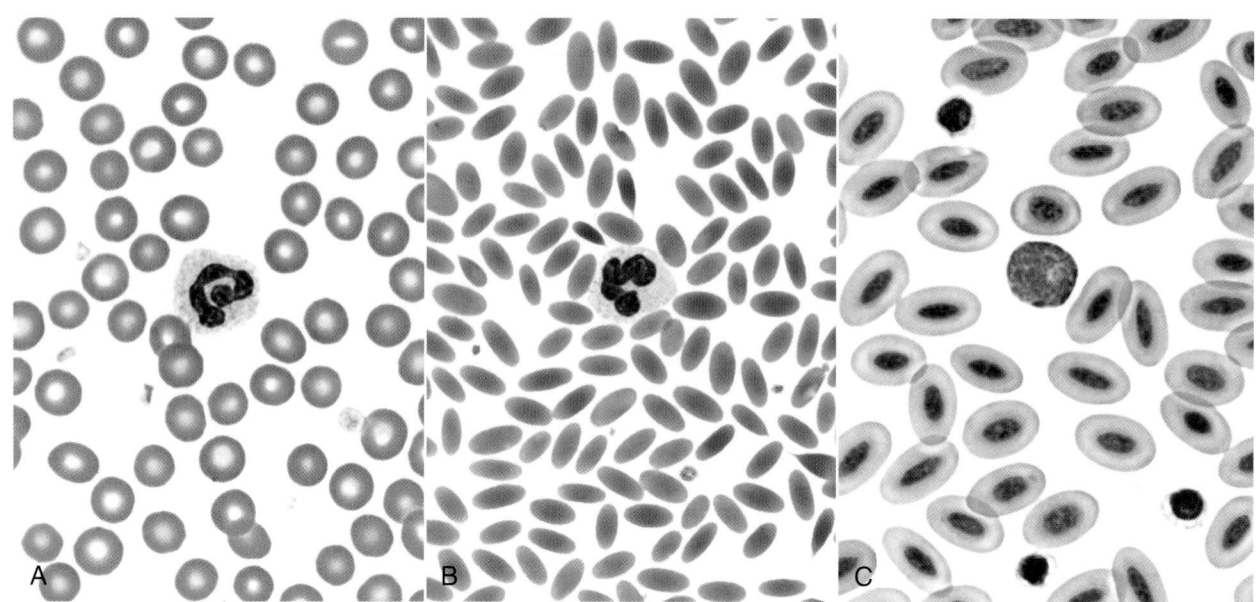

FIGURE 12-10 Red blood cells (RBCs) in various species. **A,** RBCs in dogs have a prominent central zone of pallor. **B,** RBCs in camelids are oval. Several teardrop-shaped RBCs (dacrocytes) are seen in this field. **C,** RBCs in birds and reptiles are oval and have oval nuclei. (Wright stain.)

estimate the number of platelets/μL. If the platelet count is decreased, or if platelets appear decreased on the blood smear, make sure the feathered edge is examined for the presence of platelet clumps. A decreased platelet count is called *thrombocytopenia*; if marked, this condition may be associated with abnormal bleeding. Increased platelet counts, called *thrombocytosis*, are less common and typically do not cause clinical signs, unless the thrombocytosis is marked.

RBCs

RBC morphology varies with species (Figure 12-10). In most mammals, RBCs circulate as biconcave discs and appear round and flat with varying degrees of central pallor on a blood smear. The central zone of pallor is most prominent in RBCs from dogs, and it is least apparent in RBCs from cats, horses, and goats. RBCs from camelids are oval, and RBCs in birds and reptiles are oval and have nuclei. Marked species differences in RBC size have been reported. Of commonly evaluated domestic animals, RBCs from dogs have the largest diameter (7 μ), followed by RBCs from cats (5.8 μ), horses (5.7 μ), cows (5.5 μ), sheep (4.5 μ), and goats (3.2 μ). Species differences have also been observed in the variation of RBC size (anisocytosis). RBCs from cattle have more anisocytosis than those from other species; RBCs from dogs typically have very little anisocytosis. Increased anisocytosis occurs in regenerative anemia as the result of increased numbers of larger, less mature RBCs, and in iron deficiency anemia because of increased numbers of microcytic RBCs. Several breed differences in RBC size have been recognized in dogs. Some poodles have macrocytic RBCs, and some Japanese breeds have microcytic RBCs. Macrocytic RBCs have been reported in some cats infected with feline leukemia virus.

Numerous morphologic changes can occur in RBCs, some of which have clinical relevance (Figure 12-11). Sometimes these changes are subjectively reported as slight or 1+, moderate or 2+, or marked or 3+ or 4+. *Poikilocytosis* refers to variation in RBC shape, but a more specific term should be used if possible. *Leptocytes*, RBCs with increased surface area, often appear as target cells (*codocytes*). Target cells have a round area of hemoglobin in the central zone of pallor and usually have minimal clinical relevance (Figure 12-11, *C*).

Stomatocytes appear to have a mouth-like clear area near the center of the RBC. These often are an artifact of smear preparation, although stomatocytosis has been reported as an inherited defect in several breeds of dogs.

Crenated RBCs, also called *echinocytes*, have evenly distributed, short, blunt to sharply pointed projections from the surface (Figure 12-11, *A*). Echinocytes most often are an artifact of slow drying of the smear, but have been associated with renal disease, lymphoma, rattlesnake envenomation, and chemotherapy in dogs, and have been noted following exercise in horses. Acanthocytes have longer, blunt or club-shaped projections that are unevenly distributed on the RBC surface (Figure 12-11, *B*). Acanthocytes can occur in dogs with hemangiosarcoma and in cats with hepatic lipidosis. If physical or chemical injury to RBCs occurs (e.g., iron deficiency), small vacuoles may form in the RBC membrane. If the vacuole ruptures, these projections resemble horns. If two projections are present, the cell is called a *keratocyte*

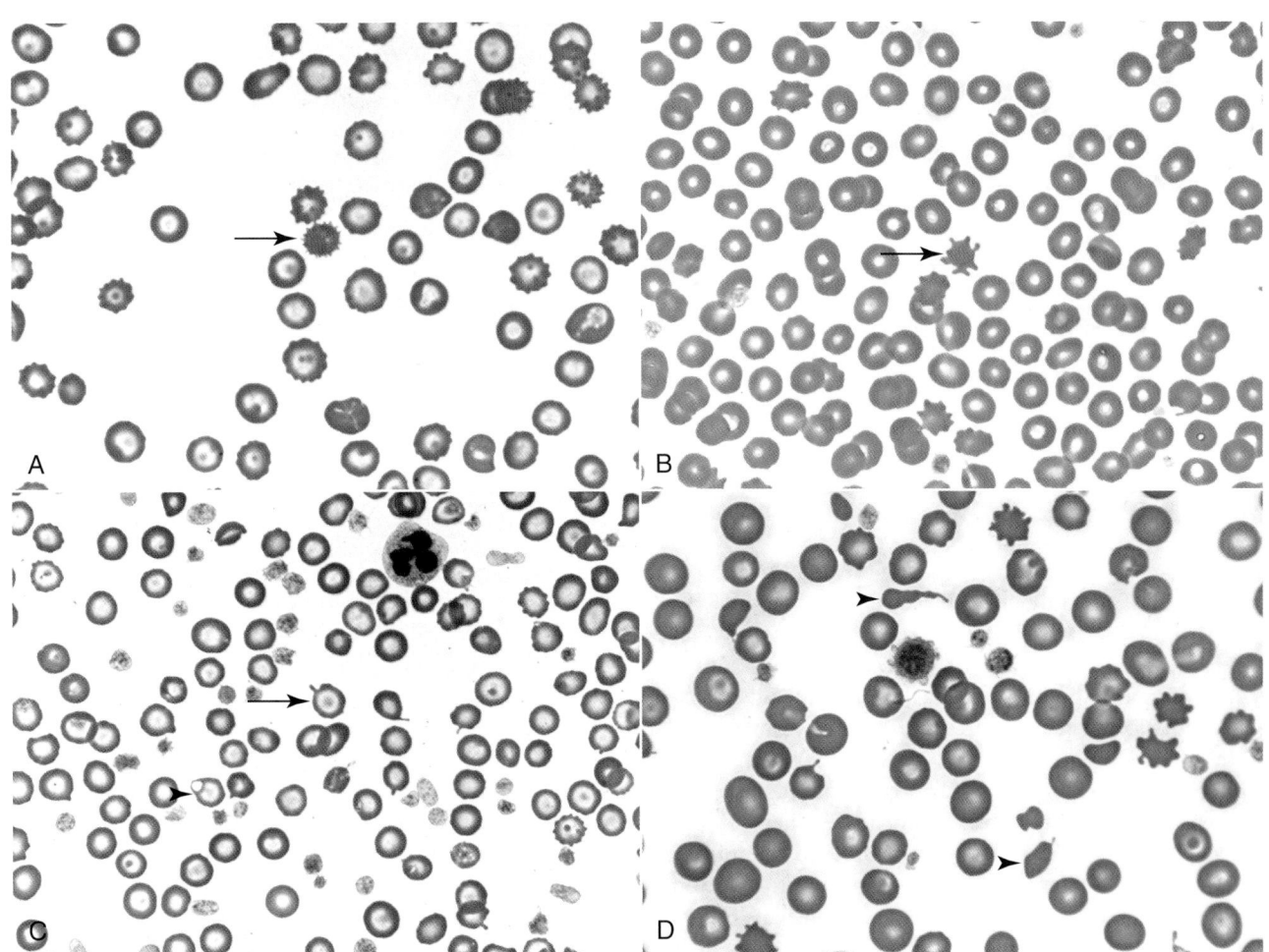

FIGURE 12-11 Red blood cell (RBC) abnormalities. **A,** Crenated RBCs have numerous sharp, evenly distributed projections on the surface and often are an artifact of drying. The cell in the center *(arrow)* shows how sharp the projections can appear, but several echinocytes in this field have projections that are not quite as sharp. **B,** Acanthocytes have several blunt projections that are not evenly distributed on the surface. An acanthocyte can be seen in the center *(arrow)* of this blood smear from a dog with hemangiosarcoma. **C,** Keratocytes have two portions of membrane that project from the surface of the RBC, resembling horns *(arrowhead)*. Several apple stem RBCs have only one projection *(arrow)*. This smear is from a dog with iron deficiency anemia, so the RBCs appear hypochromic and the platelets appear increased. **D,** Several RBC fragments *(arrowheads)* in a blood smear from a dog with hemangiosarcoma.

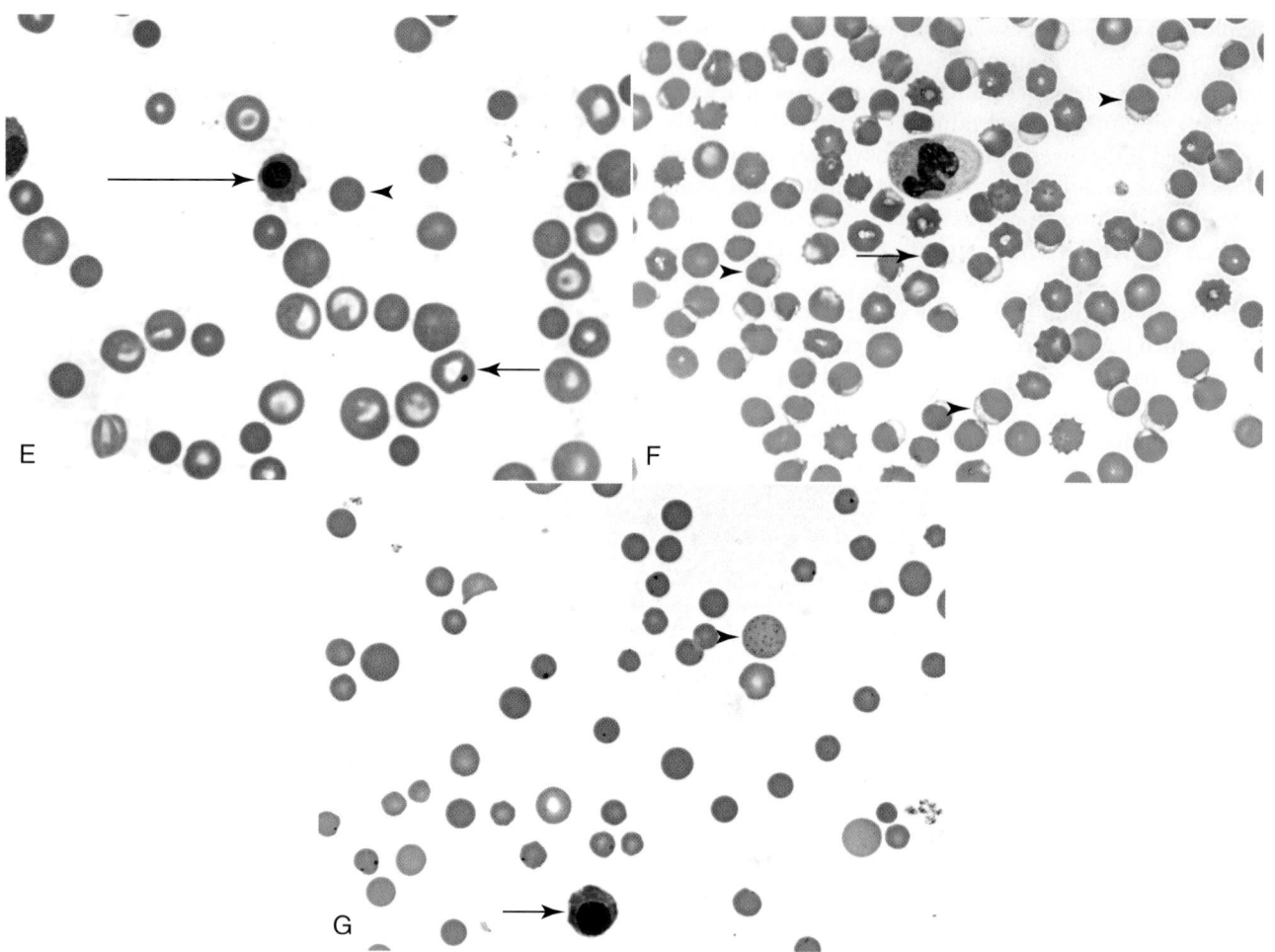

FIGURE 12-11, cont'd E, Spherocytes *(arrowhead)* appear slightly smaller and denser than normal RBCs. Numerous spherocytes and increased numbers of polychromatophilic cells are evident and are characterized by more basophilic cytoplasm in this blood smear from a dog with immune-mediated hemolytic anemia. Both a nucleated RBC *(long arrow)* and a Howell-Jolly body *(short arrow)* can be seen in regenerative anemia. **F,** Numerous eccentrocytes *(arrowheads)* can be seen in this blood smear from a dog. The hemoglobin has been pushed to one side of the cell, leaving a clear portion of the cytoplasm with a thin rim of membrane. A pyknocyte is noted in the center *(arrow)*; this is an eccentrocyte that has lost the portion of cells with minimal hemoglobin, so it appears as a small, dense RBC. **G,** An RBC with basophilic stippling *(arrowhead)* appears as small blue dots throughout the cytoplasm. This blood smear is from a cow with regenerative anemia. Several cells with Howell-Jolly bodies are also present, and a nucleated RBC is evident at the bottom of the field *(arrow)*. (Wright stain.)

(Figure 12-11, *C*); if only one projection is visible, the RBC is called an *apple stem cell.* Fragments of RBCs, sometimes called *schistocytes,* can occur with diseases that cause intravascular trauma to the RBCs such as disseminated intravascular coagulation, hemangiosarcoma, or heartworm disease (Figure 12-11, *D*).

Spherocytes are RBCs that lack a central zone of pallor and often appear slightly smaller and denser than normal RBCs (Figure 12-11, *E*). Spherocytes result from antibody binding to the RBC surface and from removal of a portion of the membrane by macrophages in the spleen. This occurs in IHA, which is most commonly recognized in dogs. It is difficult to recognize spherocytes in horses and cats, but IHA is much less common in these species. Recognizing spherocytes on a blood smear is an important part of the diagnosis of IHA, and care should be taken to evaluate only the counting area of the blood smear. Almost all RBCs resemble spherocytes near the feathered edge, and it is much more difficult

to recognize spherocytes in thicker portions of the smear. Small numbers of spherocytes may be present if oxidative damage or microvascular injury occurs, and after a blood transfusion.

Oxidative damage results in several morphologic abnormalities in RBCs. *Eccentrocytes* are RBCs in which the hemoglobin has shifted to one side of the cell, creating a clear area outlined by a thin rim of membrane (Figure 12-11, *F*). Pyknocytes form if the thin region is disrupted, leaving a slightly irregular, dense portion of RBC (Figure 12-11, *F*). Eccentrocytes occur as a result of oxidative damage to the RBC membrane. Heinz bodies occur with oxidative damage to hemoglobin, which binds to the inner surface of the membrane, creating a pale structure that may protrude from the surface (Figure 12-12, *C*). When stained with NMB, Heinz bodies appear blue and are easier to visualize (Figure 12-12, *D*). Heinz bodies are found in RBCs from healthy cats but are interpreted as abnormal if they are numerous or large,

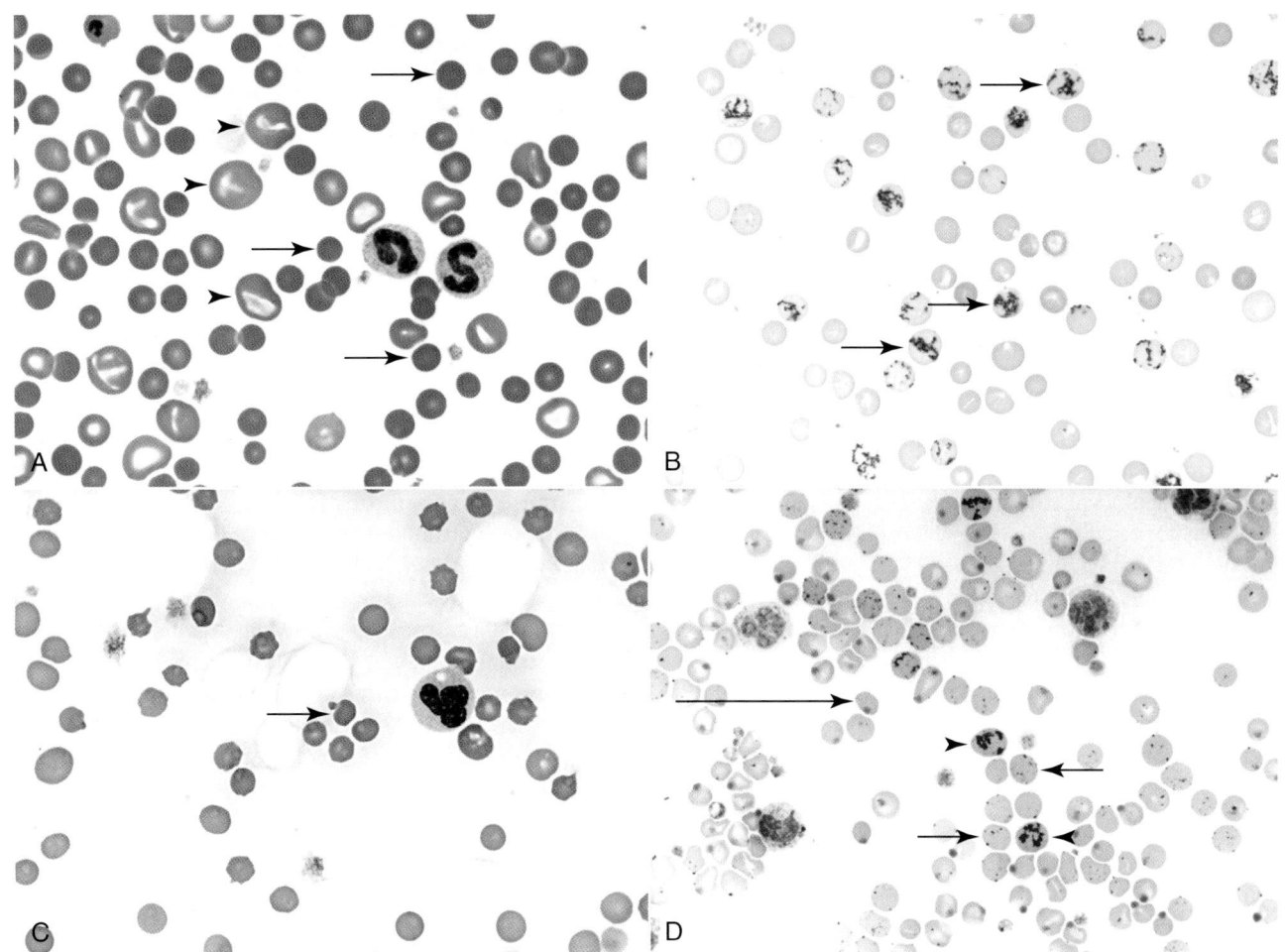

FIGURE 12-12 Polychromatophilic red blood cells (RBCs) and reticulocytes. **A,** Numerous spherocytes *(arrows)* and polychromatophilic RBCs *(arrowheads)* can be seen in this blood smear from a dog with immune-mediated hemolytic anemia. Polychromatophilic RBCs are larger and more basophilic than normal RBCs. Increased numbers of polychromatophilic cells are suggestive of a regenerative response from the bone marrow. These same cells would be reticulocytes if they were stained with new methylene blue. **B,** This blood from a dog with immune-mediated hemolytic anemia has been stained with new methylene blue. Numerous aggregate reticulocytes are shown *(arrows)*. **C,** This blood smear is from a cat. An RBC with a protruding Heinz body is seen in the center *(arrow)*. Heinz bodies are evident in many of the other RBCs. They appear as lighter-staining structures if they do not protrude from the RBC, in which case they are more difficult to see. **D,** This blood, from a cat with Heinz body hemolytic anemia, has been stained with new methylene blue. Aggregated reticulocytes *(arrowheads)* would be counted as reticulocytes to determine whether the anemia is regenerative. Also, numerous punctate reticulocytes *(short arrows)* would not be counted as part of the reticulocyte count. The Heinz bodies are the larger, dark-staining structures that often protrude from the RBC *(long arrow)*. **A** and **C** have been stained with Wright stain. **B** and **D** have been stained with new methylene blue.

or if multiple Heinz bodies are present per RBC. Heinz bodies in other species are abnormal and may be associated with exposure to many different oxidative compounds, including ingestion of onions, garlic, and zinc-containing objects in dogs and wilted red maple leaves in horses.

Occasional nucleated RBCs (nRBCs), or metarubricytes, can be seen in peripheral blood from healthy animals. Increased numbers of nRBCs can occur in markedly regenerative anemia (Figure 12-11, *E*), but increased nRBCs in animals with nonregenerative anemia may indicate primary bone marrow disease. Increased nRBCs along with basophilic stippling (see later) in animals that are not anemic have been associated with lead toxicity. Some splenectomized animals will have increased nRBCs and Howell-Jolly bodies (see later). nRBCs may be erroneously counted as WBCs by manual methods and by some automated

hematology analyzers, resulting in a falsely increased WBC count. If nRBCs are included in the WBC count, this should technically be reported as a total nucleated cell count. The simplest way to enumerate nRBCs is to include them in the differential and report them as nRBCs/μL. However, the WBC count can be corrected for the presence of nRBCs. When a differential leukocyte count is performed, nRBCs are tallied separately and are expressed as nRBCs per 100 WBCs. The corrected WBC count = (Total nucleated cell count × 100) ÷ (# nRBCs + 100). However, this correction is not necessary unless large numbers of nRBCs are present, or unless WBCs are counted using automated hematology analyzers that cannot distinguish nRBCs from WBCs.

Howell-Jolly bodies, which are nuclear remnants that appear as small, round basophilic structures in RBCs, sometimes are increased in animals with regenerative anemia

(Figure 12-11, *E* and *G*). Basophilic stippling appears as numerous small basophilic dots from aggregated ribosomes. Basophilic stippling may occur in lead toxicity and in regenerative anemia in cattle and horses, or in intense regenerative responses in dogs and cats (Figure 12-11, *G*).

Polychromasia is the term used to describe RBCs with cytoplasm that is more basophilic than that of normal RBCs (Figure 12-12, *A* and *C*). These cells usually are larger and have more RNA and less hemoglobin than mature RBCs. Healthy animals may have a few circulating polychromatophilic RBCs, but these usually account for less than 1% of the RBCs. Increased numbers of polychromatophilic RBCs occur in regenerative anemia, indicating an appropriate bone marrow response. The regenerative response by the bone marrow can be more quantitatively evaluated by performing a reticulocyte count (Procedure 12-2). Dogs have only aggregate reticulocytes (Figure 12-12, *B*) but cats have aggregate and punctate reticulocytes (Figure 12-12, *D*). Aggregate reticulocytes have clumps of reticulum and are a more accurate indication of the bone marrow response than punctate reticulocytes, which have small, single dots of reticulum and are not an indication of active regeneration. Only aggregate reticulocytes are counted. Calculating the absolute reticulocyte count, reported as reticulocytes/μL, is recommended, and this value is reported by most large reference laboratories. The percentage of reticulocytes or the corrected reticulocyte percentage (CRP; see Procedure 12-2) can be used to assess regeneration if the RBC count is not available. Reticulocyte counts >60,000/μL (or CRP >1%) in dogs and >50,000/μL (or CRP >0.4%) in cats are compatible with regenerative anemia.

Several RBC parasites can be identified from blood smear evaluation. Many of these parasites cause anemia, but other than the hemotropic *Mycoplasma* species in cats, most are uncommon in the United States. Species-specific hemotropic *Mycoplasma* organisms have been described in dogs, cats, pigs, cows, llamas, and alpacas. Hemotropic *Mycoplasma* organisms appear as small basophilic cocci or rings on the RBC surface or in the surrounding plasma if the organisms have detached from the cell (Figure 12-13). These structures often resemble stain precipitate, so care should be taken to evaluate a blood smear with minimal stain precipitate. *Anaplasma marginale* infects bovine RBCs and appears as a dark, round structure, 1 to 2 μ in diameter, within RBCs, sometimes near the edge. *Babesia* organisms, most commonly seen in dogs, may be single or paired teardrop-shaped structures several microns in diameter, or they may be much smaller, irregularly shaped structures, depending on the species. Additional references can be consulted for identification of other hemotropic parasites. DNA-based and serologic tests are available for many of the hemotropic parasites to confirm infection.

PROCEDURE 12-2 | Reticulocyte Count

1. Add several drops of new methylene blue (NMB) to several drops of EDTA anticoagulated blood in a small test tube.
2. Incubate for 10 minutes at room temperature.
3. Make a conventional blood smear from the NMB-stained blood, and allow the smear to dry in ambient air.
4. Count a total of 1000 RBCs as reticulocytes, which contain clumps of dark-staining aggregated organelles (see Figure 12-12), or as normal RBCs.
5. Calculate the **percentage of reticulocytes** by dividing the number of reticulocytes counted in Step 4 by 1000. A **corrected reticulocyte percentage** (CRP) can be determined if the RBC count is not available to calculate an absolute reticulocyte count (Step 6).

$$CRP = \frac{\% \text{ reticulocytes} \times \text{Patient's PCV}}{45 \text{ (dog) or } 37 \text{ (cat)}}$$

6. Calculate the **absolute number of reticulocytes** by multiplying the percentage of reticulocytes determined in Step 5 by the RBC count as determined by the automated hematology analyzer. Absolute reticulocytes are reported as the number of reticulocytes $\times 10^9$/L, or as the number of reticulocytes per microliter.
   Example: Reticulocyte count = 200
   RBC count = 2.2×10^{12}/L
   Percentage reticulocytes: 200/1000 = 20%
   Absolute reticulocytes: $(0.20) \times (2.2 \times 10^{12}$/L$)$ = 440,000/μL

EDTA, Ethylenediaminetetraacetic acid; *RBC,* red blood cell.

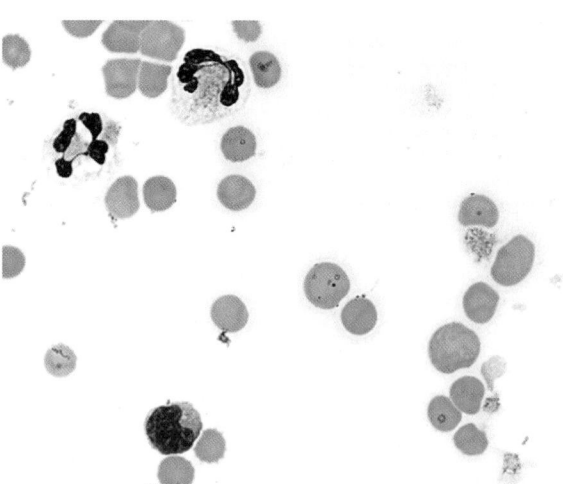

FIGURE 12-13 *Mycoplasma haemocanis.* Although uncommon in dogs, the red blood cell (RBC) in the center shows a small, rod-shaped form on the upper edge, small cocci on the lower edge and in the center, and several ring forms in the cytoplasm. Several other RBCs have similar parasites. In dogs, *M. haemocanis* sometimes forms chains of organisms *(shown in the RBC in the lower left portion of the smear).* (Wright stain.)

> **TECHNICIAN NOTE** Important species differences in RBC morphology have been noted, and RBC morphologic abnormalities can be helpful in establishing a list of differential diagnoses.

WBCs

Most WBCs have distinctive morphologic features that allow them to be identified using routine stains. Marked species variations in morphology may be observed (Figure 12-14). Determination of the numbers of each type of WBC can be helpful in establishing a list of differential diagnoses. A differential WBC count is performed by identifying and enumerating a minimum of 100 leukocytes consecutively encountered in the counting area of the blood smear. At least 200 cells should be counted if the WBC count is increased. Cells are classified as **segmented neutrophils, band neutrophils, eosinophils, basophils, lymphocytes, monocytes,** or abnormal cells, to determine the percentage of each cell type. Neutrophils, eosinophils, and basophils collectively are called *granulocytes* because they have cytoplasmic granules that are visible on routine staining. Percentages of each cell type are relative numbers and have minimal diagnostic utility. The WBC differential should be interpreted based on absolute numbers of each cell type, determined by multiplying the percentage of each cell type (expressed as a decimal) by the total WBC, and reported as the number of each cell per μL of blood (or per liter of blood—the international unit for cell enumeration). For example, if 60% neutrophils (0.6 expressed as a decimal) are present and the total WBC count is 10,000/μL (10.0×10^9/L), the absolute number of neutrophils is 6000/μL (6.0×10^9/L). The morphology of the leukocytes is evaluated, and any abnormalities are noted.

Neutrophils

Neutrophils are the predominant circulating WBCs in dogs, cats, and horses, but in cattle, sheep, and goats, lymphocytes are the predominant circulating WBCs. In pigs, about equal numbers of neutrophils and lymphocytes are present in peripheral blood. An increased number of neutrophils is called *neutrophilia* and often occurs with inflammation. Mature neutrophils, called *segmented neutrophils,* or "segs," are about 12 μm in diameter and are characterized by a segmented nucleus that often has three to five lobes. The condensed chromatin stains darkly, and in most domestic animals, the cytoplasm is relatively clear with poorly visible, neutral-staining granules (Figure 12-14, *A*). The granules are slightly eosinophilic and appear more prominent in neutrophils from cattle (Figure 12-14, *B*). In some species, neutrophils are called **heterophils** because of intense staining of the granules. Heterophils are the most abundant granulocytes in rabbits and in many non-mammalian species. The granules are larger and typically are rod- or seed-shaped, but they may appear oval or round in some species. The granules appear dark orange or reddish-brown with routine stains and may obscure the nucleus (Figure 12-14, *C*).

Less-mature neutrophils sometimes are released from the bone marrow during inflammation. Band neutrophils, often called "bands" or "stabs," have a C- or S-shaped nucleus with parallel sides or minimal nuclear constriction. Bands may be slightly larger than segmented neutrophils, and the cytoplasm may appear slightly more basophilic (Figure 12-14, *A*). In more intense inflammatory reactions, metamyelocytes and occasionally myelocytes can be released from the bone marrow. Metamyelocytes have an indented nucleus and are slightly larger and have more cytoplasmic basophilia than bands. Myelocytes have a round nucleus and are slightly larger and more basophilic than metamyelocytes. The chromatin is progressively less condensed in less-mature cells, so it stains lighter (Figure 12-14, *A*). An increased number of circulating band neutrophils (and metamyelocytes and myelocytes) is called a **left shift** and indicates that the bone marrow is releasing less-mature cells to meet demand. If the number of band neutrophils (and metamyelocytes and myelocytes, if they are present) exceeds the number of segmented neutrophils, this is called a *degenerative left shift* and often indicates a poor prognosis.

Several morphologic abnormalities indicate intense stimulation of neutrophil production and shortened maturation time. These changes are called **toxic changes** but do not necessarily imply an association with a toxin. Döhle bodies are whorls of rough endoplasmic reticulum that appear as grayish-blue, round to irregularly shaped aggregates in the cytoplasm (Figure 12-14, *A*). Small Döhle bodies may be normal in some healthy cats. Cytoplasmic basophilia is the result of retention of rough endoplasmic reticulum, and vacuolation is due to degranulation of lysosomes or disruption of cell membrane integrity. Toxic granules are coarse pink or reddish granules in the cytoplasm; they are primary granules with increased staining permeability. Nuclear features of toxic change may be more subtle and include vacuolation, hyposegmentation, ring formation, and fragmentation. Rarely, formation of giant neutrophils occurs. Toxic changes can be subjectively reported as mild, moderate, or marked, depending on the percentages of cells affected and the severity of the change.

Several other abnormalities in neutrophil morphology sometimes are noted. Hypersegmented nuclei are seen with increased endogenous or exogenous corticosteroids, which prolong the time neutrophils circulate before moving to the tissues. Pelger-Huet anomaly is a congenital or acquired defect in nuclear segmentation of neutrophils and eosinophils; it is most often seen in dogs. With this anomaly, an apparent marked left shift may include bands, metamyelocytes, and myelocytes. Careful inspection of the cells reveals that the chromatin is condensed and the cytoplasm is relatively clear, similar to mature segmented neutrophils. This is an incidental finding in dogs, and most are otherwise healthy; Australian Shepherds are predisposed to Pelger-Huet anomaly. However, Pelger-Huet anomaly should be reported to prevent misinterpretation of the apparent left shift. Birman cats sometimes have neutrophils with prominent granules as a breed variation in otherwise healthy cats. Prominent neutrophil granules also have been reported in some inherited storage diseases, but these are rare. Infectious agents, such as bacteria, fungal elements, viral inclusions, and rickettsial inclusions, occasionally can be observed. Neutrophils with intracellular infectious agents may be easier to detect at the feathered edge than in the counting region.

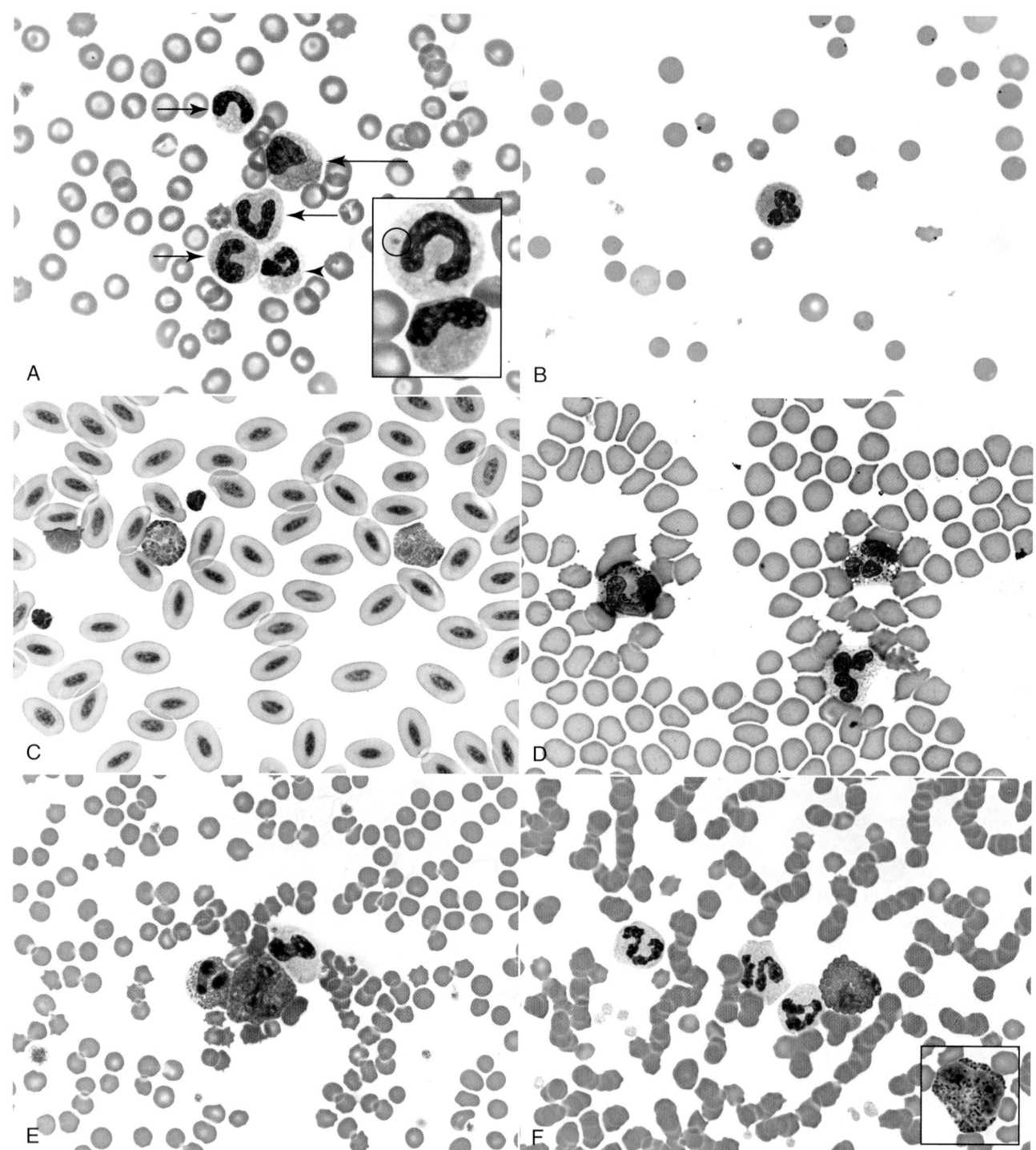

FIGURE 12-14 White blood cells (WBCs) from various species. **A,** This blood is from a dog with a degenerative left shift. A segmented neutrophil *(arrowhead)*, three bands *(short arrows)*, and a metamyelocyte *(long arrow)* can be seen. The bands have C- or U-shaped nuclei with relatively condensed chromatin and basophilic cytoplasm. The metamyelocyte has an indented nucleus with less condensed chromatin, and the cytoplasm is basophilic. *Inset,* The band neutrophil has basophilic cytoplasm that appears vacuolated. The pale blue structures are Döhle bodies *(open circle)*. These toxic changes are associated with marked inflammation. **B,** The granules in this neutrophil from a cow are more eosinophilic than neutrophils from dogs, cats, or horses. **C,** The heterophil on the left has granules that are larger, more irregular or seed-shaped, and darker red than the granules in the eosinophil on the right, which are round and stain brighter red. The two smaller cells with dark nuclei are thrombocytes in this blood smear from a bird. **D,** A basophil can be seen on the left and an eosinophil above a neutrophil on the right in this blood smear from a dog. Basophils in dogs have a few dark granules in the cytoplasm. Basophils appear larger than neutrophils, and the nuclei appear twisted with chromatin that is slightly less condensed than in neutrophil and eosinophil nuclei. **E,** An eosinophil with pink granules can be seen on the left, a basophil with lavender granules in the center, and a segmented neutrophil with inconspicuous granules on the right in this blood smear from a cat. **F,** Three segmented neutrophils and an eosinophil can be seen in this blood smear from a horse. In horses, eosinophils have numerous large granules, so they are easy to identify. *Inset,* Basophils in horses and cows have numerous dark-staining granules that may obscure the nucleus.

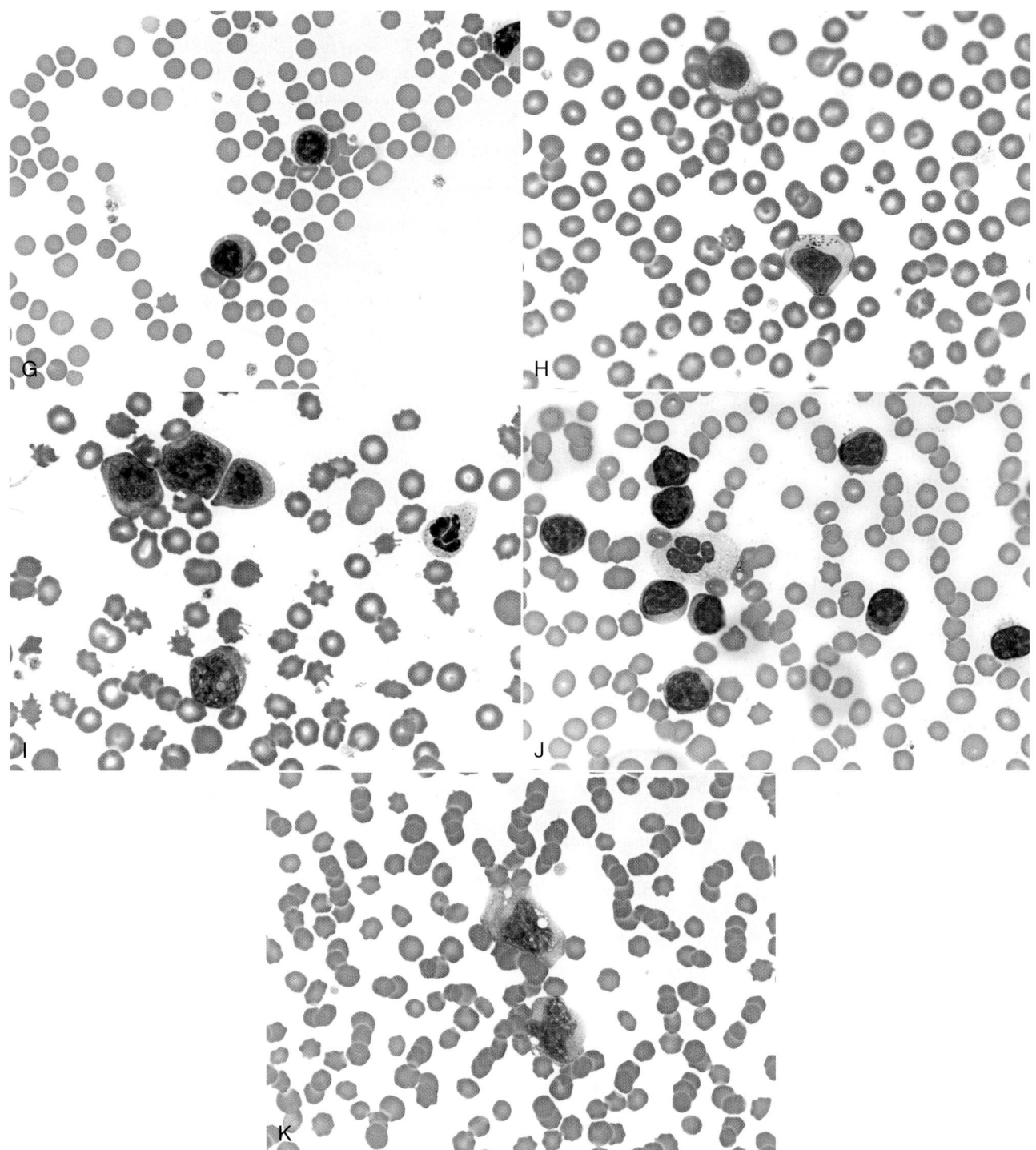

FIGURE 12-14, cont'd G, A normal lymphocyte is shown in the upper portion and a reactive lymphocyte in the lower portion of this blood smear from a cat. The reactive lymphocyte has abundant basophilic cytoplasm with a perinuclear clear area. **H,** Two large granular lymphocytes in a blood smear from a dog with chronic lymphoid leukemia. Large granular lymphocytes have several azurophilic granules in the cytoplasm. **I,** Several neoplastic lymphocytes from a dog with acute lymphoid leukemia. Neoplastic lymphocytes are larger than normal lymphocytes and have abundant basophilic cytoplasm. Nuclei have less condensed chromatin and may have one to several nucleoli. A neutrophil is shown on the right for comparison. Normal lymphocytes are smaller than neutrophils. **J,** Most of the cells are neoplastic lymphocytes in this blood smear from a horse with chronic lymphocytic leukemia. The lymphocytes are smaller than the neutrophils and have minimal cytoplasm and nuclei with condensed chromatin and inconspicuous nucleoli. **K,** Two monocytes can be seen in this blood smear from a horse. Monocytes appear similar in most mammalian species and are characterized by abundant basophilic cytoplasm that often contains clear vacuoles. Nuclei are indented or irregular in shape and have moderately condensed chromatin that appears unevenly dispersed. (Wright stain.)

Eosinophils

Eosinophils circulate in low numbers in health. They are important mediators of hypersensitivity reactions and contain substances that can damage and kill some parasites. Increased numbers, called *eosinophilia*, often occur with allergic reactions and in some parasite infections. Eosinopenia (decreased eosinophils) occurs in response to corticosteroids. Marked species variation in eosinophil morphology has been noted. In most species, nuclei are segmented and have condensed chromatin. The prominent feature is the presence of numerous pink to reddish granules in colorless to pale blue cytoplasm. In dogs, the granules are round and intermediate in size and number. Sometimes variation in granule size is evident within the same cell (Figure 12-14, *D*). In Greyhounds, the granules often do not stain but appear instead as clear structures in the cytoplasm. In cats, the granules are numerous, small, and rod-shaped (Figure 12-14, *E*). Eosinophils in cows have numerous, small, round, brightly staining granules, whereas in horses, the granules are numerous, brightly staining, and much larger than in other species (Figure 12-14, *F*). Eosinophils from most non-mammalian species have numerous round, brightly eosinophilic granules, although in some species, the granules may be oval or elongate. In a few non-mammalian species, the granules stain light blue.

Basophils

Basophils circulate in very low numbers; often none are encountered during routine evaluation of blood smears from healthy animals. Increased numbers of basophils (or *basophilia*) may be present in hypersensitivity reactions or parasite infections, similar to eosinophils. The morphology of basophils is variable, depending on the species. In dogs, basophils appear somewhat larger than neutrophils and have a twisted or irregularly shaped nucleus with chromatin that appears less condensed (Figure 12-14, *D*). The cytoplasm is more basophilic than in neutrophils, and there may be several dark blue granules or no visible granules, in which case the cells are more difficult to identify. In cats, basophils have numerous lavender granules (Figure 12-14, *E*). Basophils from horses and cows typically have numerous dark bluish-purple granules and may resemble mast cells, but the nucleus is segmented (Figure 12-14, *F*). Basophils from most non-mammalian species have round nuclei with numerous dark purple granules that may obscure the nucleus, similar to mammalian mast cells. In some species of turtles, basophils may be the most abundant circulating leukocytes.

Lymphocytes

Lymphocytes are the predominant circulating cell in cattle, sheep, and goats, but they are less numerous than neutrophils in other species. Most circulating lymphocytes are smaller than a neutrophil (9 µ in diameter). A round nucleus with condensed chromatin almost fills the cytoplasm, resulting in a high nuclear-to-cytoplasmic ratio. In many lymphocytes, only a narrow crescent of pale blue cytoplasm is visible (Figure 12-14, *G*). In cows, up to 50% of lymphocytes may be intermediate to large, even in the absence of disease. Lymphocytes from most non-mammalian species resemble lymphocytes from mammals. In most species, a small percentage of circulating lymphocytes have a few azurophilic granules in the cytoplasm. These cells are called *large granular lymphocytes* (LGLs). Increased numbers of LGLs occur with some types of chronic inflammation and in some forms of chronic lymphocytic leukemia (CLL; Figure 12-14, *H*). Lymphocytes can have abnormal granules from inherited storage diseases, but these are rare.

Intermediate to large lymphocytes sometimes circulate secondary to antigenic stimulation. These larger lymphocytes, called *reactive lymphocytes,* have more abundant, more intensely basophilic cytoplasm that may contain a perinuclear clear area (Figure 12-14, *G*). It may be difficult to distinguish reactive lymphocytes from neoplastic lymphocytes that circulate in acute lymphoid leukemia and in some animals with lymphoma. Nuclei in reactive and many neoplastic lymphocytes have less condensed chromatin, but reactive lymphocytes usually do not have visible nucleoli. The number of reactive lymphocytes usually is low, whereas the number of neoplastic lymphocytes may be very high.

A lymphocytosis can occur with antigenic stimulation and often is seen in young animals such as puppies and kittens. A transient lymphocytosis due to epinephrine release is common in cats and young horses that become excited during blood collection. Lymphoid neoplasia is associated with persistent lymphocytosis. Many animals with acute lymphoid leukemia (ALL) have marked lymphocytosis, whereas animals with lymphoma and circulating neoplastic lymphocytes have mild to moderate lymphocytosis. The neoplastic lymphocytes in ALL and lymphoma usually are large and have abundant basophilic cytoplasm, fine chromatin, and prominent nucleoli (Figure 12-14, *I*). In CLL, mild, moderate, or marked lymphocytosis may occur, but the lymphocytes typically are small and appear well differentiated (Figure 12-14, *J*). In dogs with CLL, the most common neoplastic cells are LGLs (Figure 12-14, *H*).

Monocytes

Monocytes usually circulate in relatively low numbers and appear similar in most species, including birds and reptiles (Figure 12-14, *K*). Monocytes are larger than neutrophils and have abundant gray blue cytoplasm. The cytoplasm sometimes contains several clear vacuoles. Nuclei are round, oval, indented, or variable in shape and have less condensed chromatin than neutrophils. It may be difficult to differentiate monocytes from bands or metamyelocytes with toxic changes. Monocytosis can occur with inflammation or hemolysis. Reactive monocytes are characterized by more deeply staining cytoplasm with a perinuclear clearing, and may occur with some types of chemotherapy and in some inflammatory responses. Monocytes in tissues become macrophages, but in blood, it is unusual to see phagocytized material in the cytoplasm.

> **TECHNICIAN NOTE** Evaluation of a blood smear can be very helpful because of marked species differences in the morphology of some of the leukocytes; clinically relevant changes in the WBC differential may not be detected by some automated instruments.

Other Cells

Mast cells sometimes can be detected on blood smears from animals with inflammatory disease or mast cell tumors. Mast cells are large, round cells with round nuclei and abundant basophilic cytoplasm that contains numerous purple granules. Because of their larger size, mast cells may be most readily detected on the feathered edge. Similarly, neoplastic hematopoietic cells often are large compared with normal circulating hematopoietic cells and can be detected at the feathered edge. These cells should be noted, and if questions about cell identification arise, smears can be sent to a reference laboratory for further evaluation. Broken cells, sometimes called *smudge cells*, can occur if too much pressure is used to make the blood smear, or if too much time has elapsed between collecting the blood and making the smear. Poorly preserved cells with pyknotic nuclei may be present if the sample has been exposed to heat, or if a delay between blood collection and smear preparation occurs. Broken or poorly preserved cells should not be counted in the differential; if high numbers are present, a differential will not be accurate, and a fresh sample should be collected.

COAGULATION TESTING

Hemostasis (or blood clotting) requires interaction between blood vessel, platelets, and coagulation factors. When a blood vessel is damaged, endothelial cells lining the inside of the vessel are destroyed, and subendothelial proteins such as collagen are exposed. Platelets then adhere to the subendothelial collagen, forming a platelet plug to slow bleeding. Formation of the initial platelet plug is termed *primary hemostasis*. At the same time, tissue factors are released that activate the **coagulation cascade**, or secondary hemostasis. Coagulation factors are plasma proteins that undergo step-wise activation, ultimately resulting in conversion of prothrombin to thrombin. Thrombin then converts fibrinogen to fibrin. A meshwork of fibrin forms in and around the platelet plug, stabilizing the plug and preventing it from being washed away by the flow of blood. If the fibrin clot does not form, a patient may initially stop bleeding as the platelet plug forms, but may begin to bleed again as the primary platelet plug is dislodged. As the blood vessel heals, fibrinolytic pathways such as **plasmin** are activated and the clot is dissolved. Abnormalities in the hemostatic system can result in bleeding or thrombosis.

A variety of tests can be used to evaluate hemostasis. A coagulation panel typically includes a platelet count and tests used to evaluate coagulation factors. The platelet count is performed on blood collected in EDTA. Using laboratory testing, the coagulation cascade can be divided into two pathways that result in formation of thrombin: *intrinsic* and *extrinsic* pathways. Factors shared by the two pathways are part of the "common" pathway. Depending on clinical indications, tests for **fibrinolysis** and platelet function also may be performed. A few tests can be done within the clinic setting, but others are more specialized, requiring shipping of samples to a reference laboratory. For accurate hemostatic testing, it is critical to strictly follow the procedures indicated by the test kit or the reference laboratory.

Two tests that can be performed in-house are bleeding time and **activated clotting time (ACT)**. Bleeding time measures the time it takes for the primary platelet plug to form. A ⅛- to ¼-inch slit is made using a #11 scalpel blade or a commercially available lancet in a nonhaired area of skin such as the gingiva or the inside of an inverted lip. Filter paper is used to remove blood drops every 30 seconds, making sure not to touch the wound. The time until bleeding stops is recorded. Normal animals should stop bleeding in 1 to 5 minutes. If platelet number is normal, this test may be used to screen for abnormal platelet function. ACT evaluates intrinsic and common pathways of the coagulation cascade and requires a special tube that contains diatomaceous earth to activate clotting factors. The ACT tube must be prewarmed to 37° C before filling with exactly 2 ml of whole blood. The tube is inverted 5 times and is incubated at 37° C for 1 minute. The tube is then checked by inverting every 5 to 10 seconds to determine the time it takes for a clot to form. Abnormalities in the coagulation cascade prolong the time until clot formation. This test should not be done on animals that are severely thrombocytopenic (<10,000 platelets/μl). ACT can also be performed using a point-of-care instrument (iSTAT, Abaxis, Union City, CA).

Two common tests of the coagulation cascade are **activated partial thromboplastin time (APTT)** and **prothrombin time (PT)**. APTT evaluates the intrinsic and common pathways, whereas PT evaluates the extrinsic and common pathways. Instruments that perform these tests measure the time it takes for fibrin to form using optical end-point or electrical impedance methods. These tests will be prolonged when a deficiency of clotting factors results from consumption, decreased production, or genetic abnormalities. Because APTT and PT methods must be specifically adapted for use in animals, it is best to use a veterinary reference laboratory, not a human laboratory. Some small in-house analyzers designed for the veterinary market are becoming available. APTT and PT tests require citrated plasma and careful adherence to collection and processing requirements. Venipuncture must be clean because trauma to the vessel will release tissue factor that can activate coagulation. Likewise, blood samples should not be taken from a heparinized catheter because heparin will interfere with testing. Whole blood must be added to a blue top (citrate) tube in exactly a 9:1 ratio of blood to 3.8% trisodium citrate and well mixed. The vacuum present in the blue top vacutainer tube should result in correct filling of the tube. Underfilling or overfilling of the tube will produce erroneous results. After centrifugation, the plasma is removed and is stored in plastic (not glass) tubes.

Plasma should be refrigerated if samples are to be run within 4 hours for APTT, or within 24 hours for PT. If samples are to be shipped to a reference laboratory, they should be frozen and transported on a sufficient amount of ice to keep them frozen until arrival to the laboratory. It is important to communicate with the reference laboratory before obtaining samples from the patient to ensure compliance with all sampling and shipping requirements. Other tests of the hemostatic system may have additional requirements, which should be determined ahead of time.

> **TECHNICIAN NOTE** Blood must be added to a blue top tube in exactly a 9 : 1 ratio of blood to trisodium citrate. Underfilling or overfilling of the tube will produce erroneous results.

Fibrinolysis can be evaluated by measuring **fibrin(ogen) degradation products (FDPs),** or **D-dimers.** FDPs are formed when fibrin or fibrinogen undergoes proteolysis by plasmin. D-Dimers are specific products of fibrin proteolysis and are considered to be more reflective of active degradation of clots. The Thrombo-Wellcotest (Remel, Lexexa, KS) is used to measure FDPs and may be performed in-house. Blood from a clean venipuncture is added to a tube provided by the test kit that contains a clot accelerator. Serum from the tube is collected and mixed with latex particles that are coated with antibodies against FDPs. The presence of FDPs is indicated by macroscopic agglutination of the latex beads. D-Dimer tests are run in reference laboratories and usually require citrated plasma.

Fibrinogen is the most abundant of the coagulation factors. Decreases in fibrinogen occur when clot formation (consumption) is excessive, or when production is decreased owing to liver failure or genetic factors. Fibrinogen production increases with inflammation. Fibrinogen can be measured using tests of fibrin clot formation (e.g., thrombin time), immunologic methods, or heat precipitation. Although easy to perform in-house (see Box 12-2), the heat precipitation test is not very accurate at low concentrations of fibrinogen; more sensitive methods are recommended if hypofibrinogenemia is suspected.

CYTOLOGY

Cytology refers to the microscopic examination of cells that have exfoliated from tissues or have accumulated in fluid. Cytology may be helpful in establishing a provisional or definitive diagnosis for inflammatory or neoplastic lesions involving many different types of tissues. Sample collection is relatively noninvasive, and the equipment needed for sample collection and processing is inexpensive and readily available in most veterinary practices. Most samples can be collected on an outpatient basis, and results often are available the same day if samples are interpreted in the practice, or within 24 hours if samples are sent to a reference laboratory. Samples can be collected from a wide variety of sites and from many different tissues. However, important limitations include inability to evaluate surgical margins, vascular invasion, organization of cells within the mass, and association of cells with normal tissues—all of which require histopathology. The definitive diagnosis of many neoplasms and the grading of some tumors also require histopathology. High-quality preparations are essential for adequate interpretation of cytology samples, so attention to detail in sample collection and processing should be a high priority. Hemodilution may limit cytologic interpretation, and some tissues do not exfoliate readily when sampled by fine-needle aspiration. Complications are rare but include hemorrhage, infection, injury to adjacent structures, and dissemination of neoplastic cells.

> **TECHNICIAN NOTE** Cytology may be helpful in determining whether inflammation or neoplasia is present and in some cases can be used to establish a definitive diagnosis.

SOLID TISSUE MASSES AND ENLARGED ORGANS

Superficial cutaneous and subcutaneous nodules, peripheral and internal lymph nodes, liver, spleen, kidneys, lungs, thyroid, prostate, and some internal masses are easily sampled by fine-needle aspiration using a 21- to 25-gauge needle of appropriate length for the tissue coupled to a 12- to 20-ml syringe. Preparation of superficial sites is similar to that for venipuncture; however, sterile surgical preparation should always be performed when internal masses and organs are sampled. The mass is identified by palpation, radiography, or ultrasonography and is manually isolated. Ultrasound is useful for guiding the needle for aspiration of focal or diffuse neoplastic infiltrations involving internal organs to increase the likelihood of a diagnostic sample and to decrease the risk of complications. Make sure to minimize the ultrasound gel before sample collection to avoid contamination of the sample, which can interfere with staining and preclude adequate evaluation of the stained smear.

Once the lesion has been identified and isolated, the needle is introduced into the lesion and suction is applied several times. Depending on the tissue and the size of the lesion, the needle is redirected several times and suction is reapplied to ensure adequate sampling. Suction is released before the needle and syringe are withdrawn, to minimize contamination with blood or cells from surrounding tissue. Frequently, only a small volume of aspirated material is present in the needle or hub of the syringe, but this usually is adequate to obtain several smears.

For small skin masses and aspiration of some internal masses, sometimes only the needle is used to repetitively poke the lesion several times without using a syringe to apply negative pressure. The sample is collected only by the cutting action of the needle. The needle can then be attached to a syringe before the smears are made. If only a small amount of material has been collected by this technique or by the more conventional aspiration technique, the needle is detached, air is aspirated into the syringe, the needle is replaced, and a small amount of material is carefully expelled onto several clean glass slides. While working quickly, a spreader slide and a pull or push technique is used to disperse the cells (Figure 12-15). Failure to disperse the cells on the slide results in smears that are too thick for interpretation. This is one of the most common errors in preparation of cytology samples. Too much pressure during slide preparation results in broken cells; this is a relatively common error. Application of minimal pressure during slide preparation usually results in slides that are of acceptable quality (Figure 12-16).

Impression smears can be made from ulcerated masses or from a small portion of a biopsy sample before formalin fixation for histopathology. Before sampling, blood and superficial debris should be gently blotted from ulcerated

1. Place a drop of cytologic specimen close to the center of one of the slides. Invert one slide, touch the slides together, and allow the material to start to spread.

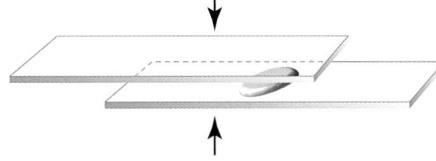

2. The top slide is used to disperse the sample.

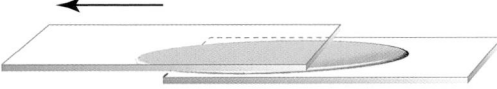

3. This will result in two pull smears of similar appearance.

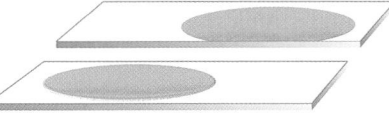

FIGURE 12-15 Technique for making cytology smears. A small drop of aspirated material is placed near the center of one slide. A second slide is used to gently disperse the material. (Illustration by Tim Vojt, Biomedical Media, The Ohio State University College of Veterinary Medicine. Copyright The Ohio State University.)

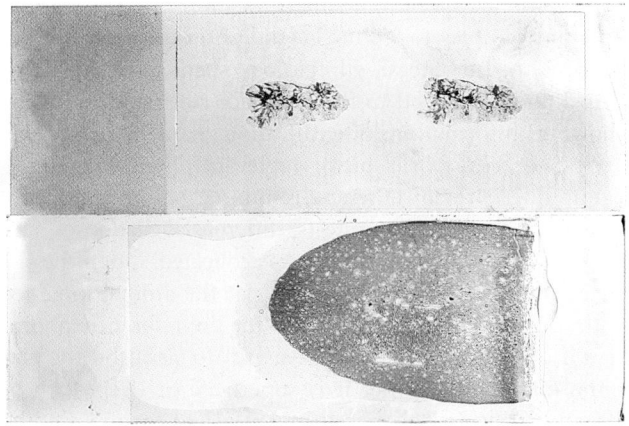

FIGURE 12-16 Impression smear (top) and fine-needle aspirate smear (bottom). Cell density is adequate on both slides.

lesions using absorbent paper. For biopsy samples, tissue fluid should be blotted from a freshly cut surface, taking care not to damage the tissue or disrupt surgical margins. Clean glass slides are touched to the surface of the ulcerated lesion or biopsy sample using minimal pressure. Several touch impressions often can be made on a single slide (see Figure 12-16). For some dense, firm masses that may not exfoliate cells easily, a sterile scalpel blade can be gently scraped across the surface of the lesion and the material spread on a slide, but this often results in broken cells. Using the scalpel to make a cross-hatch pattern on the surface of the tissue before making impression smears is an alternate method that may result in better cell exfoliation with less cell breakage.

Smears made from fine-needle aspirates or impression smears should be labeled with the patient's name or identification number and date, and allowed to dry in ambient air before staining. It is not necessary to fix the slides with heat or acetone for routine staining. Slides should not be exposed to formalin fumes or packaged with samples that have been fixed with formalin. This is important because formalin fumes prevent adequate staining. Slides should not be stored in a refrigerator because water condensation will lyse cells and prohibit adequate staining. Slides can be sent unstained to a reference laboratory or stained for in-house interpretation.

THORACIC AND ABDOMINAL EFFUSIONS

Fluid can be collected from thoracic and abdominal effusions or fluid-filled masses. Sterile technique should be used to avoid infection or sample contamination. Fluid should be placed in collection tubes containing EDTA to prevent clotting in case the sample is contaminated with blood. If the sample clots, cell counts will be inaccurate. EDTA tubes are not sterile, so a separate portion of the fluid should be kept aside and sterile if culture will be performed. Fluid samples can be processed and interpreted in the veterinary practice or sent to a reference laboratory.

The clarity and color of the fluid should be described because they may be important indications of disease processes. Normal thoracic and abdominal fluid is clear and colorless in small animals but may have a yellow tint in large animals. Cloudy samples may indicate increased cells or protein concentration, or the presence of lipid. Samples that are cloudy from lipid may remain cloudy after centrifugation, whereas the supernatant will be clear in samples that are cloudy from increased cells. Hemorrhagic samples or samples contaminated with blood appear pink to red, depending on the amount of blood. If hemorrhage is suspected, a PCV can be performed as an indication of the severity of hemorrhage. Samples that are white or tan often contain lipid or high numbers of inflammatory or neoplastic cells. Fluid may appear brown if there has been previous hemorrhage, or if leakage of bowel contents has occurred. A greenish discoloration may be seen in animals that have a ruptured bile duct. Yellow fluid may be noted if hemolysis and icterus are present, if there has been previous hemorrhage, or if the bladder has ruptured.

Total protein concentration and specific gravity are determined by refractometry, similar to the plasma protein concentration. This information will be used to determine whether the fluid is a transudate, a modified transudate, or an exudate; this may be helpful in establishing a differential diagnosis. Cells should be enumerated manually using a hemocytometer or an automated instrument, or the number can be estimated from a direct smear. Automated instruments provide accurate cell counts if the count is high, but may not be accurate for the low cell counts that often are present in transudates, cerebrospinal fluid, or synovial fluid. If the cell count is >10,000/μL, or if the fluid is turbid or bloody, direct smears should be made using the pull or push technique already described. If the fluid is relatively clear, the cell count will be low; cytologic interpretation is more readily accomplished if the cells are concentrated. Cells can be concentrated using a cytocentrifuge or using techniques similar to those used in preparing urine sediment. Slides are air-dried and are sent to a reference laboratory or stained for in-house interpretation. If a fluid sample is to be sent to a reference laboratory, air-dried direct and sediment smears should be made and submitted with the fluid. Cell degeneration and bacterial overgrowth can occur during transport and inhibit adequate evaluation of cell morphology. Slides made at the time the sample was collected are useful for the clinical pathologist in assessing cell morphology and determining whether any bacteria that are present are clinically significant.

SYNOVIAL (JOINT) FLUID

Synovial fluid is evaluated in animals that have swollen joints, joint pain, or fever of undetermined origin. Samples often are collected in EDTA to prevent clotting. However, EDTA may interfere with evaluation of viscosity and the mucin clot test, so sometimes a portion is placed in a red top tube, which does not contain anticoagulant. Normal joint fluid is clear and colorless, very light yellow, or straw-colored. Normal joint fluid is very viscous because it contains a protein called *mucin*. A mucin clot test is performed to evaluate mucin quality by adding equal volumes of joint fluid to 2.5% glacial acetic acid. If a normal amount of mucin is present, a tight, white clot forms, often reported as "good." If the mucin has been degraded by bacterial or cellular enzymes, or diluted by an effusive process, the clot will be soft or less distinct (fair or poor) or absent.

Viscosity also can be evaluated by subjectively determining how long of a strand forms when a wooden applicator stick is placed in the fluid and withdrawn slowly. A strand of 2 to 3 cm is normal; shorter strands are reported as decreased. Cell counts are very low in normal synovial fluid and can be performed using a hemocytometer or by evaluating a direct smear. Acetic acid cannot be used as a diluent because the mucin will precipitate and the counts will be inaccurate. Automated instruments can be used to determine cell counts, but the results may be inaccurate if the count is very low. When an automated instrument is used for cell counts, synovial fluid samples can be pretreated with hyaluronidase to prevent the sample from clogging the aperture and to ensure accurate cell counts. Most of the cells in normal synovial fluid are large mononuclear cells. Neutrophils are increased in animals with joints infected by bacteria and in cases of immune-mediated polyarthritis.

STAINS, IMMUNOPHENOTYPING BY FLOW CYTOMETRY, AND DNA-BASED TESTING

Wright stain, Wright-Giemsa stain, or commercially available quick stains such as Diff-Quik are most commonly used for cytology smears. Most commercially available quick stains are a modification of Wright or Wright-Giemsa stain and are inexpensive and easy to use. These stains provide good color contrast, cytoplasmic detail is good, nuclear detail is acceptable, and most infectious agents are stained. These stains also are permanent, which is an advantage for practitioners who interpret cytology in-house and want a second opinion from a clinical pathologist. Mast cell granules and granules in some lymphocytes stain purple with Wright and Wright-Giemsa stains, whereas some commercially available quick stains do not consistently stain these granules (Figure 12-17). This is important because cutaneous mast cell tumors are found commonly in dogs, and large granular lymphocytes are the neoplastic cell type in some cats with gastrointestinal lymphoma or dogs with CLL. These tumors may be misdiagnosed by cytology if only commercial quick stains are used. Special stains sometimes are used to determine cell lineage or to identify causative agents. These stains usually are available at commercial reference laboratories or academic institutions. Immunophenotyping by flow cytometry and DNA-based testing may be useful in the diagnosis of some neoplastic diseases and can be performed on cytology samples by some laboratories. The laboratory should be contacted for information on requirements for sample submission.

SUBMISSION OF SAMPLES TO A REFERENCE LABORATORY

The reference laboratory should be contacted to obtain information about sample submission. Many reference laboratories provide special containers for submitting glass slides and fluid samples to minimize slide breakage and sample degradation. In general, all cytology specimens should be labeled and submitted to the reference laboratory with the following information: identification name or number, species, age, sex, a brief history, relevant physical examination findings, previous therapy, a summary of results of previous pertinent diagnostic tests, differential diagnoses, and the site from which the sample was collected. Often the site can be indicated on a line drawing of the animal included on the submission form prepared for the reference laboratory. If a mass is present, it is useful to describe the size of the mass and whether it is superficial or deep, firm or soft, and freely movable or firmly attached to surrounding tissue. Although commonly omitted, this information is very helpful to the clinical pathologist in making an

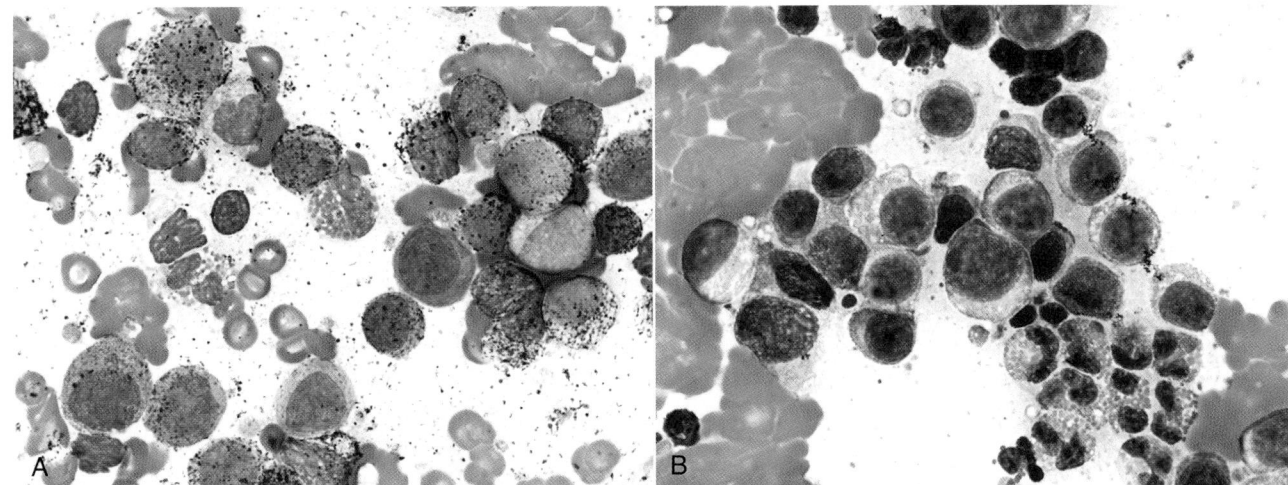

FIGURE 12-17 Anaplastic mast cell tumor stained with Wright stain **(A)** and Diff-Quik **(B)**. Note that purple mast cell granules and eosinophilic granules from the eosinophils in the center are apparent on the slide stained with Wright stain, but only the eosinophil granules are apparent on the slide stained with Diff-Quik. Although the eosinophils are an indication that this could be an anaplastic mast cell tumor, the diagnosis would be much more difficult with the slide stained with Diff-Quik.

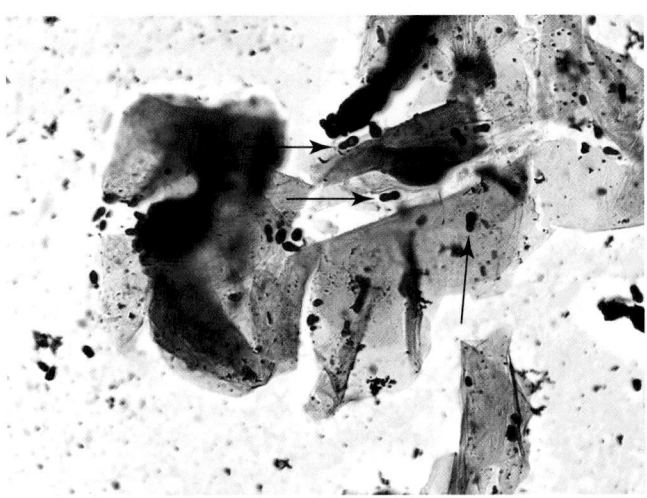

FIGURE 12-18 Swab from the external ear canal of a dog with *Malassezia* overgrowth. Large numbers of *Malassezia* organisms *(arrows)* are present extracellularly and on the surface of the anucleate squamous epithelial cell. No inflammatory cells are present, which is not unusual in some dogs with *Malassezia* overgrowth. (Wright stain.)

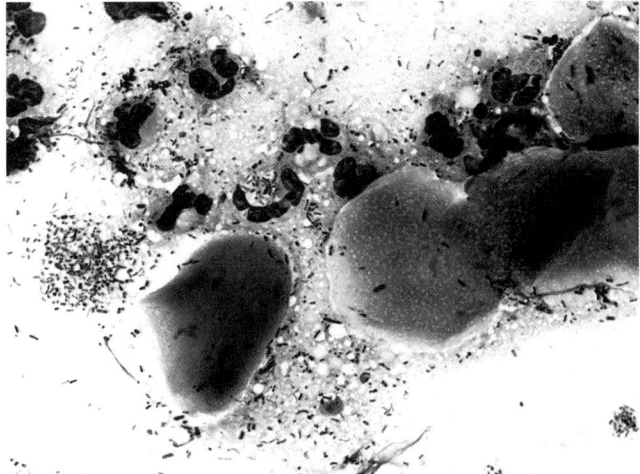

FIGURE 12-19 Swab from the external ear canal of a dog with neutrophilic inflammation due to bacterial infection. Large numbers of bacteria that include rods and cocci are present extracellularly and within the degenerate neutrophil in the center. Several anucleate squamous epithelial cells are present. (Wright stain.)

interpretation and providing the most complete information for optimal patient care.

OTIC CYTOLOGY

Cytology frequently is performed on samples collected from the external ear canal using clean cotton-tipped swabs, which then are rolled onto clean glass slides to prepare a thin layer of material. Samples collected from the horizontal portion of the ear canal should be collected using an otoscope. For evaluation of inflammation, infectious agents, and neoplasia, slides are air-dried and stained routinely. Pathogenic bacteria stain adequately with Wright stain. Samples prepared to check for the presence of mites usually are examined unstained before the slide is allowed to dry. A drop of

immersion oil can be added before a coverslip is applied, to prevent the slide from drying. Some practices keep two sets of stains: one for otic cytology and fecal samples, and one for blood smears and other cytology samples, to avoid contaminating the latter set of stains.

Smears prepared from normal external ear canals are minimally cellular, and often only a small amount of poorly staining cerumen is present. Low numbers of keratinized anucleate squamous epithelial cells (Figure 12-18) and small numbers of cocci or yeasts *(Malassezia pachydermatis)* may be observed. Large numbers of bacteria (>15 to 25/high power field) or yeasts (>10/high power field), mixed populations of rods and cocci, inflammatory cells, and intracellular bacteria (Figure 12-19) support a diagnosis of infection,

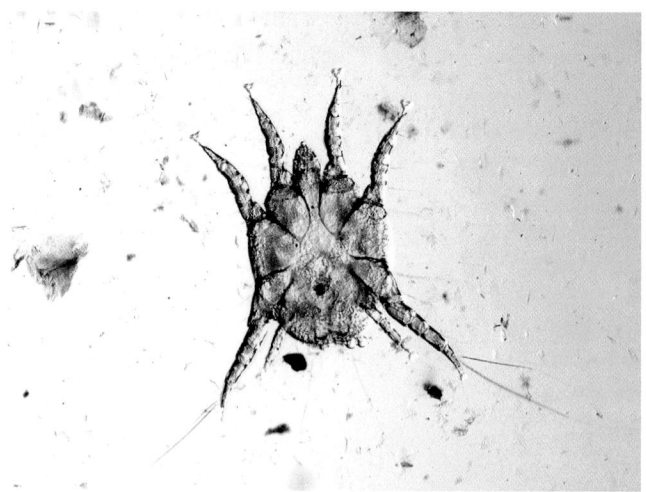

FIGURE 12-20 *Otodectes* mite from a swab from the external ear canal of a cat. (Unstained.)

especially in conjunction with clinical signs, patient history, and culture results. *Malassezia* organisms are 2 to 6 μm by 4 to 7 μm and have a characteristic peanut or footprint shape because of the broad-based budding that occurs during replication (see Figure 12-18). *Otodectes cynotis,* the most

common parasitic infestation of the external ear canal, occurs more commonly in cats than in dogs. Both mites and eggs can be present (Figure 12-20). Numerous benign and malignant neoplasms involving the external ear canal have been described. Fine-needle aspiration may be helpful in a presumptive diagnosis of neoplasia, but biopsy may be required for a definitive diagnosis.

RECOMMENDED READINGS

Hematology
Jain NC: Essentials of veterinary hematology, Philadelphia, 1993, Lea and Febiger.

Thrall MA: Veterinary hematology and clinical chemistry, Baltimore, 2012, Wiley-Blackwell.

Weiss DJ, Wardrop KJ: Schalm's veterinary hematology, ed 6, Ames, IA, 2010, Wiley-Blackwell.

Cytology
Cowell RL, Tyler RD, Meinkoth JH: Diagnostic cytology and hematology of the dog and cat, ed 3, St Louis, 2008, Mosby.

Cowell RL, Tyler RD, Meinkoth JH: Diagnostic cytology and hematology of the horse, ed 2, St Louis, 2002, Mosby.

Raskin RE, Meyer DJ: Atlas of canine and feline cytology, Philadelphia, 2001, Saunders.

13 Clinical Chemistry, Serology, and Urinalysis

M. Judith Radin and Maxey L. Wellman

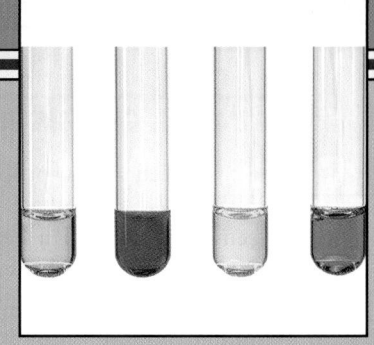

OUTLINE

Clinical Chemistry, *424*
Preanalytical Factors, *425*
Analytical Factors, *426*
Chemistry Analyzers, *426*
Quality Control, *427*
Serology, *428*
Types of Serologic Tests, *429*

Urinalysis, *430*
Equipment and Collection, *430*
Color and Turbidity, *430*
Specific Gravity, *431*
Chemical Evaluation, *431*
Microscopic Examination, *433*

KEY TERMS

Aciduria (aciduric)
Alkaluria (alkaluric)
Azotemia
Calibrator
Control
Crystalluria
Cylindruria
Cystocentesis
ELISA
Hemolysis
Icterus
Isosthenuria
  (Isothenuric)
Levy-Jennings chart
Lipemia
pH
Pyuria
Quality control (QC)
Refractometer
Specific gravity (SG)
Spectrophotometry

LEARNING OBJECTIVES

When you have completed this chapter, you will be able to:

1. Pronounce, spell, and define all of the Key Terms.
2. Do the following regarding clinical chemistry:
   - Explain the purpose of the clinical chemistry profile and list the preanalytical and analytical factors that can affect clinical chemistry testing.
   - Compare and contrast the use of chemistry analyzers in veterinary and human medicine.
   - Define a calibrator and a control, and describe how they are used in quality control.
3. Describe the general principles of serologic testing, and discuss the most common methods of serologic testing.
4. Do the following regarding urinalysis:
   - Describe proper collection techniques and handling of urine samples.
   - List and describe methods for the physical and biochemical evaluation of urine.
   - Describe the preparation of urine for microscopic evaluation, list the cellular elements that can be found in the urine sediment, and identify the three most common urine crystals.

INTRODUCTION

Evaluation of most patients will include a minimal database consisting of complete blood count (CBC; see Chapter 12), chemistry profile, and urinalysis. In addition, serology may be used as an adjunct to routine diagnostic testing, especially if the patient is suspected of having endocrinologic or infectious disease. Chemistry panels, urinalyses, and serologic tests may be run in the clinic or may be sent to an outside reference laboratory for analysis. Regardless of where the samples are analyzed, accurate and reliable results depend on careful attention to preanalytical and analytical factors. It is critical that a veterinary technician has a working knowledge of proper sample collection, sample processing and storage, and **quality control** (QC) to ensure accurate and reliable results.

This chapter provides an overview of common methods and instrumentation employed in biochemical, serologic, and urinalysis testing. Emphasis is on understanding preanalytical and analytical factors that can affect the ability to provide reproducible and accurate test results. Because the veterinary technician is usually responsible for maintaining and troubleshooting instrumentation, an overview of the principles of operation of common instruments is given.

CLINICAL CHEMISTRY

The clinical chemistry profile is an essential part of the basic database used to evaluate most patients. It can be used to screen for disease in a healthy-appearing individual (e.g., geriatric profiles), to assess risk before surgery, to distinguish between differential diagnoses, or to assess severity of disease. With use of serial sampling, it may be possible to monitor the progression of disease or response to therapy, including potential adverse drug reactions. The routine chemistry panel is typically run on serum and often measures 15 to 20 constituents (Case Presentation 13-1). Some calculated values such as anion gap or osmolality may be provided. In addition, indices for common interferences such as **hemolysis**, **lipemia**, or **icterus** may be included. The clinical chemistry profile is most valuable when interpreted in conjunction with other patient information such as the history, physical examination findings, CBC, and urinalysis. It is generally most helpful in making interpretations if samples for the CBC, chemistry profile, and urinalysis are obtained from a patient within a short time of each other.

The chemistry panel is not a direct measure of individual organ or cellular function. However, organ or cellular functional integrity can be inferred by changes in constituents in the blood that reflect leakage from damaged cells, failure to normally clear waste products, or failure to regulate electrolytes or various metabolites. Constituents of a routine chemistry panel can be grouped to look for patterns that suggest specific organ or cellular dysfunction, for example, increases in blood urea nitrogen (BUN) and serum creatinine (SC) indicate **azotemia** (increased nitrogenous wastes in the blood). However, BUN and SC must be interpreted in conjunction with patient hydration status and a concurrent urine **specific gravity** (SG) to distinguish dehydration (prerenal azotemia) from impaired kidney function (renal azotemia). If a dehydrated patient has normally functioning kidneys, increases in BUN and SC should be accompanied by high urine SG, indicating that the kidneys are capable of concentrating urine to conserve as much water as possible. In patients with renal azotemia, the kidneys fail to adequately concentrate urine, and SG is lower than expected to compensate for dehydration.

CASE PRESENTATION 13-1 PRESURGICAL PANEL ON A YOUNG DOG

Signalment: 10-month-old mixed breed male dog
History: a presurgical chemistry panel was run before orthopedic surgery for hip dysplasia

	UNITS	SAMPLE 1		SAMPLE 2		REFERENCE INTERVAL
BUN	mg/dl	13		13		5-20
Creatinine	mg/dl	0.8		0.9		0.6-1.6
Phosphorus	mg/dl	5.2		6.4		3.2-8.1
Calcium	mg/dl	0	L	11.5		9.3-11.6
Sodium	mEq/L	139	L	152		143-153
Potassium	mEq/L	47.3	H	4.7		4.2-5.4
Chloride	mEq/L	98	L	111		109-120
Anion gap	mEq/L	68	H	21		15-25
Osmolality (calculated)	mOsm/kg	277	L	303		285-304
Bicarbonate	mmol/L	20.4		25		16-25
ALT	IU/L	21		25		10-55
AST	IU/L	23		28		12-40
ALP	IU/L	0	L	35		15-120
CK	IU/L	97		131		50-400
Cholesterol	mg/dl	144		166		80-315
Total bilirubin	mg/dl	0.3		0.4		0.1-0.4
Total protein	g/dl	4.9	L	5.4		5.1-7.1
Albumin	g/dl	3.3		3.6		2.9-4.2
Globulin	g/dl	1.6	L	1.8	L	2.2-2.9
A:G ratio		2.1		2.0		0.8-2.2
Glucose	mg/dl	91		112		77-126

A:G, Albumin-to-globulin; ALP, alkaline phosphatase; ALT, alanine aminotransferase; AST, aspartate aminotransferase; BUN, blood urea nitrogen; CK, creatine kinase; H, high; L, low.

Interpretation
This biochemical panel includes a typical menu of constituents for a baseline biochemical panel. When the first sample produced unrealistic results, some of which were not compatible with life, it was noted that the original sample had been submitted in a purple top (ethylenediaminetetraacetic acid [EDTA]) tube. Sample 2 was drawn in a red top tube, and serum was obtained. Most parameters were now within the reference interval. The low globulins may be due to the young age of the dog. This case illustrates the importance of using the correct tubes and samples for analysis, and the critical role of the veterinary technologist in ensuring high-quality laboratory results.

Serum enzymes can be used to detect hepatocellular injury, cholestasis, or muscle damage. In dogs and cats, increases in alanine aminotransferase (ALT) and aspartate aminotransferase (AST) indicate hepatocellular damage, whereas AST and sorbitol dehydrogenase (SDH) are used for that purpose in horses and cattle. AST also may increase with muscle damage, so it is often interpreted with creatine kinase (CK), an enzyme released from muscle but not from the liver. Other enzymes increase with cholestasis, including alkaline phosphatase (ALP) and gamma glutamyltransferase (GGT). Increases in bilirubin usually accompany increases in ALP and GGT if cholestatic disease is present. However, ALP is not specific for cholestasis and may be induced by corticosteroids or other drugs, especially in dogs. Likewise, bilirubin is not specific for cholestasis and may increase with hemolysis. If bilirubin is increased, a hematocrit and blood film should be evaluated to look for anemia and causes of hemolysis.

Increased serum glucose may indicate diabetes mellitus, excitement, or stress. Excitement-induced hyperglycemia should be transient, and glucose should return to normal once the animal is calm. However, with excitable animals, this distinction may be more difficult. Ancillary tests such as serum fructosamine may help distinguish between these causes of hyperglycemia.

Electrolytes include sodium, potassium, chloride, bicarbonate, calcium, and phosphorus. Electrolyte concentration in blood reflects extracellular fluid concentrations but may not be a good indicator of intracellular or total body content. Disturbances in electrolyte concentrations may result from altered function of the gastrointestinal tract, kidney, skin, and endocrine systems. Electrolytes both fluctuate with and play a role in regulating water balance and acid-base status.

Total or serum proteins are composed of albumin and globulin, with albumin being the serum protein normally found in the highest concentration. Typically, total protein and albumin are measured and globulins are determined by subtracting albumin from the total protein concentration. Species differences have been noted in the binding of albumin to the test reagent used by some analyzers, so it is important for reference laboratories to establish reference intervals for individual species. Rabbits often have spuriously high measured albumin compared with total protein owing to enhanced dye binding. Albumin can act as a transporter for various serum constituents, for example, calcium binds to albumin, and hypoalbuminemia (decreased albumin) will be accompanied by a decrease in total calcium (hypocalcemia). Globulins make up the remainder of the total protein and contain immunoglobulins and other factors that can increase with inflammation (acute phase proteins). Increases in both albumin and globulins (hyperproteinemia) occur with dehydration, whereas globulins increase with inflammatory diseases and some lymphoid neoplasms. Hypoalbuminemia may develop from loss through the kidney or gastrointestinal tract, or from decreased production due to liver failure. Both albumin and globulin can decrease with hemorrhage.

Case Presentation 13-1 illustrates some of the constituents found in a basic biochemical panel. Specialty panels of more or fewer analytes are often available from reference laboratories or may be designed for use with in-clinic analyzers to be more cost-efficient, depending on the needs of the patient and the client. Additional specialized tests are becoming increasingly available at reference laboratories, diagnostic laboratories, and universities to further aid in diagnosis.

The veterinary technician is a key player in ensuring high-quality and accurate results of laboratory tests. Accuracy and reliability of biochemistry tests depend on preanalytical and analytical factors. Preanalytical factors are those factors that can affect the quality of the sample before the biochemical tests are actually run. Analytical factors are those factors that are directly involved in performing the biochemical assay.

PREANALYTICAL FACTORS

Preanalytical factors that can affect the quality of test results include collection procedures, sample labeling, sample handling and processing, and shipping procedures. Patient variables such as age, breed, or diet may also affect sample quality. Lipemia due to the presence of circulating triglycerides and hemolysis due to rupture of red blood cells (RBCs) are commonly encountered interferences. Ideally, dogs and cats should be fasted 12 hours before sampling to avoid lipemia that may occur following a meal. Fasting is not required for ruminants because continual digestion in the rumen eliminates significant postprandial changes. Difficult venipuncture, use of a needle of incorrect size, excessive pressure on the syringe, or rough transfer of blood to the collection tube may result in hemolysis of RBCs. Whether tests are performed in-house or are sent to a reference laboratory, minimal equipment needed to obtain a sample for a biochemical profile includes needles, syringes, blood collection tubes, sample storage tubes with caps, and a centrifuge. All equipment should be clean and in working order. Use of the correct sampling tube is essential (see Case Presentation 13-1).

Biochemical profiles are typically performed using serum or heparinized plasma. Serum is often the preferred sample and is obtained by collecting blood in a red top tube, which lacks an anticoagulant. If you are drawing multiple samples through the same needle, it is best to fill the red top tube first, followed by tubes containing anticoagulant. This helps avoid contamination of the serum with anticoagulants, which may interfere with analysis. The tube is set in the upright (vertical) position in a test tube rack, and the blood is allowed to clot for 15 to 30 minutes at room temperature. The tube is then centrifuged for 10 minutes at a relative centrifugal force of 1000 to 2000 g to separate the serum from cellular components and fibrin. A guide should be available with the centrifuge to allow determination of the settings needed to obtain the correct centrifuge speed. When the upper serum layer is removed from the tube, it is important to avoid pulling up cells from the clot into the serum sample. Some red top tubes contain a serum separator to aid in clean removal of the serum. Refrigeration of the sample during the clotting procedure is not recommended because it will delay clot formation. This can result in an incompletely clotted sample at the time of serum removal or formation of a fibrin clot above the cells in the serum portion of the sample. The presence of fibrin in a sample can clog analyzer tubing or can falsely alter the measured amount of an analyte. Serum should be separated as soon as a firm clot has formed. Leaving serum on the clot for longer than 1 hour will result in decreased glucose concentration as a result of utilization by cells in the sample. Alterations in serum electrolytes and enzymes may result from cell leakage or lysis, and hemolysis of RBCs may occur if samples are stored on the clot for prolonged periods of time. When serum is stored, the sample should be capped to prevent evaporation, which would falsely increase the concentrations of serum constituents.

In some cases, it may be preferable to use heparinized plasma collected in a lithium heparin (green top) tube. Heparinized samples are often used when sample size is limited, as from birds or other small pets. Heparinized plasma or whole blood may be the preferred sample type for some benchtop analyzers or point-of-care instruments. It is important that green top tubes be filled to the correct volume to avoid introducing dilution errors. An advantage of heparinized samples is that both hematology and chemistry data can be obtained from a single green top tube. One note of caution is that cell morphology and the staining quality of blood smears made from heparinized samples are not ideal (see Chapter 12). Similar considerations apply for rapid and clean removal of the plasma, as described previously for serum samples. Additional specific sample requirements may apply for some assays performed by reference laboratories, so it is important to contact the reference laboratory before sample collection and submission.

> **TECHNICIAN NOTE**   Serum or heparinized plasma should be removed from the clot as soon as possible to prevent inaccurate results.

Visual inspection of the serum or plasma may indicate the presence of some common interfering substances (Figure 13-1). Normal serum from dogs and cats should be clear and colorless, whereas serum from horses and ruminants will have a light yellow color. Hemolysis is characterized by red discoloration of the sample, whereas bilirubin imparts a yellow to orange color. Lipemia is characterized by increased turbidity of the sample, ranging from haziness to an overtly milky appearance. Lipemia is often accompanied by in vitro hemolysis, giving the sample a pink, milky appearance. Some drugs can interfere with an assay, so it is important to know all medications that the animal has received. Information on the effects of interfering substances on individual biochemical tests should be provided by the reference laboratory or by the test kit instructions supplied by the manufacturer for in-clinic assays.

Every sample should be clearly identified through all steps of the process to avoid mix-up of samples. Information on

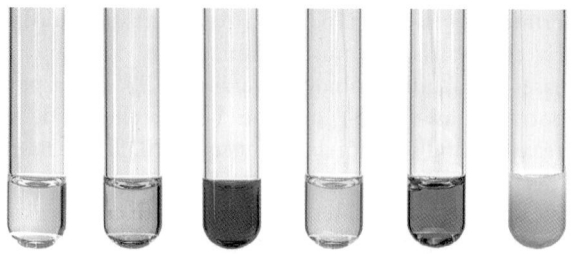

FIGURE 13-1 Examples of normal serum and serum with substances that may interfere with some analyses on a chemistry panel. From left to right are normal cat, normal horse, hemolysis in a dog, hyperbilirubinemia in a dog, hyperbilirubinemia in a horse, and lipemia with mild hemolysis in a dog.

labels might include the names of the owner and the patient, medical record number, age, breed, and sex. When a sample is sent to a reference laboratory, unique identifying information for the patient, as well as the clinic name and phone number, should appear on the tube and submission sheet. Reference laboratories often have standardized submission forms, which should be completely filled out with all requested information. Reference laboratories should provide specific instructions for proper shipping of samples.

ANALYTICAL FACTORS

Analytical factors involve actual performance of biochemical assays and include the analyzer and other equipment, test methods and components, quality control, and operating and maintenance procedures. Proper maintenance of equipment, attention to assay methods, and quality control are essential whether tests are performed in a large reference laboratory or in a veterinary practice setting using benchtop or point-of-care analyzers.

CHEMISTRY ANALYZERS

Chemistry analyzers vary with analytical methods used, speed of sample processing (throughput), cost per sample, and maintenance requirements. In large commercial laboratories, many high-throughput analyzers were designed for use with human samples but have been adapted for use with veterinary samples. Although some tests designed for humans may be used just as they are with animal specimens, others require significant modification owing to variation between human and animal species. As a result, veterinary reference laboratories go through extensive test validation to ensure accurate measurement of analytes and establishment of species-specific reference intervals. If a laboratory that analyzes primarily human samples will be used as a reference laboratory, it is important to check first with the laboratory to determine whether appropriate method validation has been done to ensure accurate results with veterinary samples. Smaller benchtop analyzers are available for use in veterinary hospitals; purchase of these analyzers is an economic decision for the practice. Analyzers that are marketed for veterinary practices often come with manufacturer-established reference intervals. However, it is important to keep in mind that "normal" may be influenced by many factors such as age, breed, or even location (e.g., high altitude vs. sea level).

Most large, high-throughput analyzers found in reference laboratories use liquid reagent–based chemistry and spectro-photometric methods to determine the concentration of an analyte. Addition of the patient sample to the liquid reagent results in a chemical reaction and subsequent development of a colored chemical product. Light of a specific wavelength is passed through the sample, and the change in color is measured by a photodetector. Color development is proportional to enzyme activity or to the concentration of the analyte of interest. Because measurement is dependent on light transmittance, liquid reagent methods are susceptible to interferences that may add color or increase the turbidity of the sample. Common interferences include bilirubin, hemolysis, and lipemia. Some systems use blanking methods to try to minimize the effects of interfering substances. Reports often give a numeric estimation of the level of interference in the patient sample, such as icteric index, hemolytic index, or lipemic index. Manufacturers of tests or the reference laboratory should be able to provide interference guides that relate the index level at which interference becomes significant and the direction of the effect the interference has on an analyte (e.g., Is the analyte falsely increased or decreased?).

Dry reagent systems use reflectance photometry and are more commonly found in small analyzers designed for use in veterinary practices (e.g., Heska DRI-CHEM, Loveland, CO; IDEXX VetTest and Catalyst Dx, Westbrook, ME). This type of analyzer has a lower throughput, but reagent management is simpler. The patient sample is added to a test strip or pad that is impregnated with reagents, resulting in a chemical reaction. Color development is measured by the amount of light reflected off the surface of the reagent pad and is correlated with the amount of the analyte in the sample. These methods are less sensitive to interference by lipemia, hemolysis, or icterus. Reconstituted chemistry systems combine dry reagents with **spectrophotometry** (e.g., Abaxis VetScan, Union City, CA). Reagents are lyophilized in prepackaged assay tubes or rotors. Addition of the patient sample reconstitutes the reagents, and developed color is measured by a photometer.

Total electrolytes, ionized electrolytes, and blood gases are measured using electrochemical methods (potentiometry or amperometry). These methods are used in many blood gas and point-of-care analyzers (e.g., iSTAT, Abaxis). A sample is placed in contact with a semi-permeable membrane that prevents the ion that is being measured from equilibrating across both sides of the membrane. This generates an electrical difference or current that is in proportion to the concentration of the ion and can be measured using electrodes.

> | **TECHNICIAN NOTE** Proper calibration, routine maintenance, and running of daily controls are essential components of good quality control and of production of accurate and reliable results.

QUALITY CONTROL

Good quality control (QC) is essential if a laboratory is to produce accurate and reliable results. A QC system is designed to detect problems before test results are transmitted to the clinician. The veterinary technician needs to have a working knowledge of QC procedures to ensure that all components of a testing system are functioning correctly, and to recognize when something is amiss and take corrective action. Errors may occur if deterioration of reagents is caused by expiration, improper storage, or handling. Components of an analyzer may fail. This can present as a sudden change, as when tubing becomes clogged or breaks. Failure of other components may be more gradual, resulting in a drift of control values over time. Detailed maintenance records are important in tracking issues with an instrument and for making decisions as to when an instrument needs to be repaired or replaced. It is important to have a standard operating procedure (SOP) for each instrument. An SOP is a detailed, step-by-step description of performing a test or operating an instrument. Use of an SOP ensures that the test is performed in a uniform fashion every time, whether the same technician or multiple technicians perform the assay. All reagents, **controls**, and **calibrators** should be dated when opened or reconstituted and properly stored. Reagents and controls should be discarded appropriately on the expiration date.

Most manufacturers provide recommendations for instrument calibration. Instruments should be calibrated every 6 months, or as recommended by the manufacturer. Calibration is the process whereby the instrument is adjusted using a standardized material, called a *calibrator*. A calibrator contains a known, standard amount of a reference material, and the instrument is adjusted so that the instrument reading matches the known amount of reference material in the calibrator. In addition to regularly scheduled calibration, calibration should be done after a major service, or as part of troubleshooting when QC values are out of range. Calibrators are commercially available, usually through the manufacturer of the instrument. For some larger instruments, a representative from the manufacturer may calibrate the instrument as part of a routine maintenance call. For other instruments, the technician will have this responsibility. Careful and current calibration is important because instruments that are not properly calibrated may not yield accurate results. All calibrations should be recorded in an instrument log.

Routinely running controls is an integral part of good QC. A control is a material that contains a known quantity of the analyte that is being tested. Controls are used to monitor the performance of a test to ensure that the instrument and/or test procedure is working correctly and consistently. Controls are different from calibrators. Calibrators are used to set up and adjust the instrument and/or procedure to perform correctly and to desired specifications. In contrast, controls are used on a regular and frequent basis to independently monitor the performance of the instrument or the analytical procedure in its entirety, including the calibration procedure, and to assess consistency over time. With good QC practices, calibrator material that is used to set up an instrument or procedure should not additionally be used as the control material. If the calibrator material is used as a control, errors in the calibration procedure or shifts due to degradation of the calibrator might be missed.

Controls are commercially available and may be provided with test kits or purchased separately. For chemistry instruments, running at least two control levels (normal and abnormal) is recommended. In some cases, low, normal, and high controls may be run if both high and low values of the analyte are clinically important. For small in-house laboratories, a minimum of one abnormal control should be run. Controls should be run at least daily and before patient samples are run. In large reference laboratories, controls are often run more frequently, as at the beginning of each new shift. Even in small laboratories, where an instrument may not be used every day, a control should be run daily. Running controls just before analyzing a patient sample is the absolute minimal requirement. Control values should be recorded in a log and compared with targeted values provided with the individual lot of control material. It is helpful to plot the results on a graph (e.g., **Levy-Jennings chart**) to quickly determine whether an individual control value is out of the acceptable range, or if an unacceptable trend is developing over a 20- to 30-day period (Figure 13-2). Some analyzers come with software to record, graph, and analyze control data. Usually, the acceptable variation in controls is within ±2 standard deviations of the mean. This means that less than 5% of the time, a control may be slightly out of the acceptable range. If this is an isolated incident, no further action is required. In some cases, the control can be repeated immediately, or the technician may choose to wait until the next regularly scheduled time to run the controls. If one or several controls fall significantly outside the acceptable range, immediate action should be taken to troubleshoot and correct the problem. A pattern of controls consistently

falling on one side of the mean, especially if values are near the assay limits, suggests a need for calibration of the instrument. A pattern of control values that are progressing toward the upper or lower acceptable limits suggests deterioration of control materials, reagents, or instrument components. Several good resources for additional information on quality control are listed in the Recommended Readings section.

Some of the small point-of-care instruments (e.g., iSTAT, Abaxis) that use single-use, self-contained cartridges and electrochemical methods for measurement of analytes do not require in-house calibration because each cartridge is calibrated during manufacture. Electronic checks are done to ensure QC. When a patient sample is run, the instrument reads electronic signals from the cartridge to determine whether the sample is correctly loaded, and if each cartridge is functioning properly. These instruments require proper attention to preanalytical factors such as correct shipping and storage of cartridges, handling of cartridges, blood collection, and loading of cartridges.

SEROLOGY

A serologic test uses antibodies to detect an antigen. Serology is commonly used for endocrinology testing, detection of infectious agents, or drug testing. In endocrine and drug tests, the antigen measured by the serologic test usually is the hormone or drug, respectively. For infectious agents, the test may detect antigens from the pathogen. Examples include tests for feline leukemia virus antigen and parvovirus antigen. More commonly, the serologic test detects antibodies produced by the patient as part of the immune response directed against an infectious agent. A single positive serologic test for antibodies will indicate that an animal has been exposed to the infectious agent. With some diseases, this is adequate for diagnosis. For example, equine infectious anemia (EIA) virus results in lifelong infection with ongoing antibody production, so a single test is adequate for diagnosis. The exception to this is an uninfected foal that acquired antibodies to EIA by ingestion of colostrum from an infected mare. Maternal antibodies result in a positive EIA test until the antibodies are cleared by the foal at around 6 months of age. After this time, the foal will become negative if not infected.

When an antibody response is evaluated, paired samples taken 1 to 3 weeks apart are usually needed to diagnose an active infection because of the time it takes for an animal to develop a humoral immune response. The first sample is taken when the patient initially shows clinical signs and is presented for examination. Antibody titers should rise over the next 2 to 3 weeks, after which the second sample is taken. Typically, a 4-fold increase in antibody titer is expected if the patient has an active infection. This contrasts with an animal with antibodies from previous exposure to the pathogen, in which case antibody levels should not rise. Antibodies resulting from vaccination may interfere with some serologic tests. Laboratories conducting the tests or the manufacturer's instructions should provide information concerning the extent of this problem with a particular test.

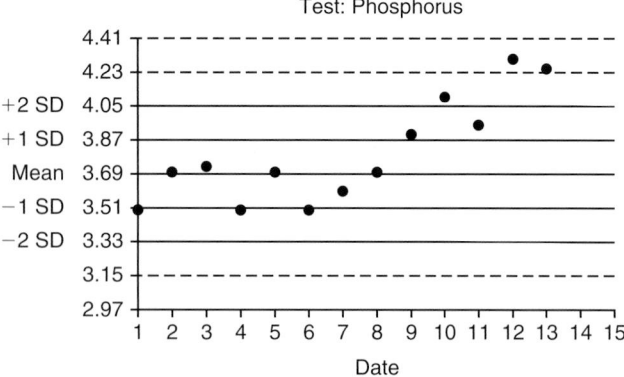

FIGURE 13-2 Levy-Jennings chart illustrating daily control measurements for phosphorus. Information provided with the control lot included the mean, ±1 standard deviation (SD), and ±2SD. An upward trend is noted for the control data, which eventually results in data points greater than 2 SD from the mean. Both the upward trend and the presence of multiple data points above the 2 SD limit indicate the need for immediate troubleshooting of this assay.

TYPES OF SEROLOGIC TESTS

Serology can be performed using a variety of techniques. Methods such as enzyme-linked immunosorbent assay (**ELISA**), radioimmunoassay (RIA), immunoradiometric assay (IRMA), Western analysis, agar gel immunodiffusion (AGID), virus neutralization, hemagglutination inhibition, and complement fixation have been used to detect antigens from, or antibodies against, infectious agents. Many of these tests use serum or plasma, but other types of samples such as saliva or fecal swabs can be used, depending on the organism of interest. Studies have shown that the gel in serum separator tubes may interfere with measurement of some antibodies, drugs, and hormones, so it is best to check with the reference laboratory to determine the ideal collection method. Hormones are more likely to be measured in serum or plasma using RIA, IRMA, or ELISA. With all of these methods, the basic principle is to link binding of antigen and antibody to a detection system (Figure 13-3). Common detection systems result in production of a colored substrate, emission of light (chemiluminescence), or capture of a radiolabeled substance. Because of the requirements for validating and carrying out these types of assays, most are performed in diagnostic laboratories. Diagnostic laboratories can provide necessary information on the type of sample, proper handling, shipping requirements, and interpretation of results.

An example of an ELISA assay is shown in Figure 13-3. Typically, an antibody against the antigen of interest is bound to a solid matrix. The patient sample is mixed with reagent containing an enzyme-labeled antibody against the antigen. The mixture containing the enzyme-labeled antibody/antigen complex is added to a chamber containing the matrix-bound antibody. The matrix-bound antibody captures the enzyme-linked antibody/antigen complex. Unbound antigen and enzyme-labeled antibody are washed away. A colorless chemical substrate is added that is acted on by the enzyme to generate a colored substance. The generated color can be read spectrophotometrically, which allows a quantitative measure of an antigen. Other platforms have the user visually evaluate the test for the presence of a colored spot or line on the test unit; any test of this type is qualitative. Positive and negative controls are included with the assay. When these types of tests are performed, it is critical to follow all QC guidelines and instructions. Variations in temperature, incubation times, and washing can interfere with the accuracy of the test.

ELISA methods can quantify the amount of antigen and can be automated for use in larger laboratories. An example is the Immulite Immunoassay System (Siemens, Deerfield, IL), which uses chemiluminescence as the detection system to measure hormone levels. In this system, the solid matrix is a bead, which captures antigen (hormone)/enzyme-labeled antibody complexes. After washing, a chemiluminescent substrate is added that emits light when acted on by the enzyme. Light photons are read by a photomultiplier to determine the concentration of the hormone in the patient sample. This is a very sensitive method that can

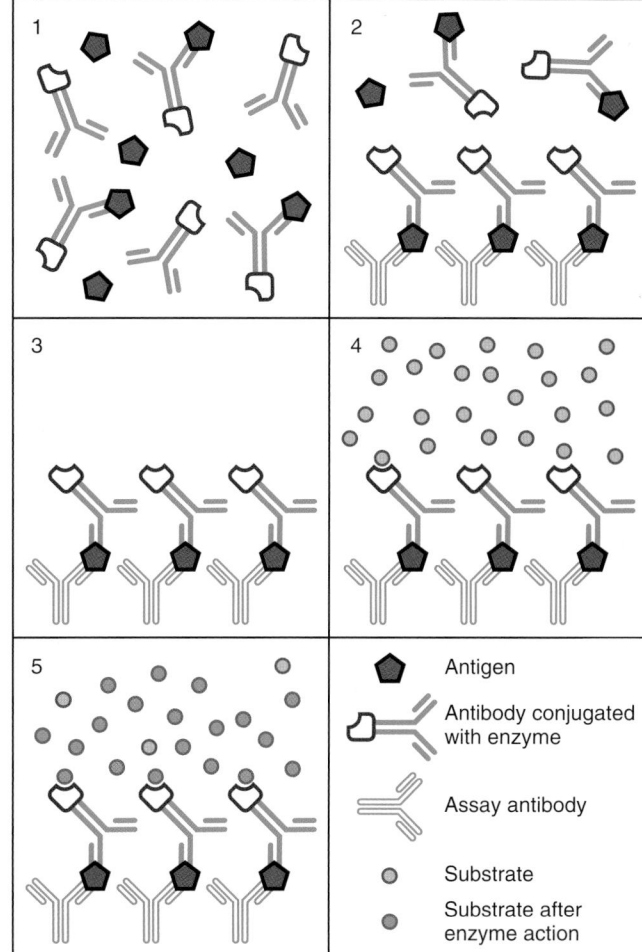

FIGURE 13-3 Example of an enzyme-linked immunosorbent assay (ELISA). (1) An antibody that is conjugated with an enzyme is incubated with the patient sample containing the antigen of interest, allowing binding of the antigen and the labeled antibody. (2) A second antibody against the antigen is fixed to a solid matrix. The sample containing the antigen-labeled antibody complexes is incubated with the fixed second antibody. This fixed antibody binds to the antigen. (3) The sample is washed, removing any unbound labeled antibody, antigen, or other nonspecific materials. (4) A chemical substrate for the enzyme is added. (5) The chemical reaction between the substrate and the enzyme results in a color change that is proportionate to the amount of antigen. (Illustration by Tim Vojt, Biomedical Media, The Ohio State University College of Veterinary Medicine. Copyright The Ohio State University.)

detect hormone concentrations at picogram and femtogram levels.

Serologic testing based on ELISA technology has become increasingly available for in-clinic use (e.g., SNAP tests). These tests are often used to screen for infectious agents and can be designed to detect antigen or antibody. Additionally, tests can be packaged to screen for more than one organism at a time. An example is the SNAP4Dx test (IDEXX), which screens for heartworm antigen, along with antibodies against *Borrelia burgdorferi* (Lyme disease), *Ehrlichia canis*, and *Anaplasma phagocytophyllum*. This type of test gives a qualitative positive or negative result. With tests that detect antibodies to an infectious agent, a positive test indicates that the animal has been exposed to the pathogen and has developed a humoral immune response. Further testing may be needed to confirm an active infection. A positive result for an antigen from an organism usually indicates infection with that organism.

URINALYSIS

Urinalysis is an essential part of the baseline data obtained from most patients. To maximize its usefulness in interpreting all of the patient's laboratory data, a urine specimen should be collected within a short time relative to blood collection for the chemistry panel and CBC. In addition to specimen labeling, which provides important identifying information as described earlier, the method of collection should be noted because this can affect interpretation when bacteria, blood, or epithelial cells are found. Collection methods include free catch, **cystocentesis**, catheterization, or collection from the floor or cage. Collection from the floor or cage is the least desirable method due to the likelihood of environmental contamination of the sample. Samples should be collected in a clean and preferably sterile syringe or glass or plastic container. Sampling for bacterial culture should be done before the rest of the urinalysis is performed, to avoid contamination.

Ideally, urine should be examined within 30 minutes of collection. Because of the potential effects of storage on urine composition, the times of collection and analysis should be included with the sample. If analysis is delayed, the urine should be protected from exposure to UV light because this would result in deterioration of some constituents such as bilirubin. Containers should be tightly capped to prevent evaporation or loss of volatile constituents such as ketones. Urine can be stored in the refrigerator, but the stability of urinary constituents is variable. Recommendations for maximum storage time at refrigeration temperature range from 6 to 24 hours. Initial **pH**, concentration, and the presence of bacteria can significantly affect urine stability. Crystals can form or dissolve depending on length of storage and pH. Before analysis is begun, refrigerated samples should be allowed to come to room temperature.

EQUIPMENT AND COLLECTION

Free catch is a simple method of collecting urine, but it requires that the animal conveniently void spontaneously or in response to gentle manual compression. A disadvantage of this method is that it will include contamination from the urethra and from areas around the urethral opening and the lower genital tract. Contamination may be lessened by catching urine midstream, avoiding early and late portions of the stream. The point of the stream at which the sample is caught should be noted on the specimen. Care should be taken if manual compression is used to induce voiding. If the bladder is fragile, as may occur with an obstructed animal, manual compression may cause additional damage or even rupture of the bladder.

Catheterization of the bladder can be used to collect a urine sample and avoid contamination from the lower urinary tract. The size of the catheter must be matched to the size of the urethra, so that passage of the catheter does not cause damage. Equipment should be sterile, and care must be taken to perform this procedure in a sterile manner to avoid introducing bacteria into the bladder. Catheterized samples often contain squamous epithelial cells from the urethra and may contain blood if the procedure caused trauma to the urethra or bladder. "Traumatic catheterization" is a technique for sampling bladder masses such as transitional cell carcinomas.

Cystocentesis is performed by inserting a needle attached to a syringe through the ventral body wall and into the bladder. Sterile preparation of the body wall should be done before the procedure is begun. Urine is aspirated directly from the bladder, thus avoiding the effects of urethral contamination on cellular and other components. Cystocentesis is the preferred method for obtaining urine samples for bacterial culture. A disadvantage of this method is that often some iatrogenic hemorrhage contributes RBCs and leukocytes to the specimen.

Analysis of the urine specimen requires glass or plastic pipettes, clean conical centrifuge tubes, a centrifuge, a **refractometer**, urine chemical test strips (dipsticks), microscope slides, coverslips, and a microscope. Urine stains, such as Sedi-Stain (BD Diagnostic Systems, Sparks, MD), may be used to assist with microscopic evaluation.

COLOR AND TURBIDITY

Physical examination of the urine includes color and turbidity. This should be done using a mixed sample before centrifugation. Normal urine is yellow to amber in color. The more dilute the urine, the lighter the color will be. Addition of constituents to the urine will alter the color. Red to reddish brown color indicates the presence of RBCs (hematuria), hemoglobin from lysed RBCs (hemoglobinuria), or myoglobin from muscle damage (myoglobinuria). Hematuria and hemoglobinuria may be distinguished grossly by letting the sample sit, or by centrifuging the sample. RBCs settle to the bottom of the tube, whereas hemoglobin remains in solution. Myoglobin will also stay in solution. Additional testing is needed to distinguish myoglobin from hemoglobin because these cannot be distinguished by visual inspection or chemical test strips (Procedure 13-1). Bilirubin imparts a dark yellow, yellow brown, or yellow green color to urine. Unusual discoloration may result from drug treatment.

In most species, normal urine should be clear. Exceptions are equine urine, which is normally cloudy due to the presence of calcium carbonate crystals, and normal rabbit urine, which is densely turbid as the result of mucus and calcium carbonate crystals. Upon sitting or refrigeration, clear urine may become cloudy from precipitation of salts and crystals. Increased turbidity of urine may be due to the presence of epithelial or inflammatory cells, blood, mucus, casts, crystals, or microorganisms. Microscopic inspection will help determine the cause.

PROCEDURE 13-1	Ammonium Sulfate Test to Differentiate Myoglobinuria from Hemoglobinuria

- Centrifuge the urine. Observe the color, or test with a dipstick.
  - Red/brown color in the supernatant or a positive dipstick result for blood/heme indicates the presence of hemoglobin or myoglobin.
  - Red blood cells (RBCs) should be in the sediment.
- Slowly add 2.8 g ammonium sulfate to 5 ml of urine, and mix well.
- Pour the urine through a filter paper.
- Observe the filtrate for color, or test the filtrate with the blood/heme pad on a dipstick.
  - If the filtrate remains red/brown or the dipstick remains positive, this indicates the presence of myoglobin.
  - Hemoglobin should precipitate and be trapped by the filter paper.

TABLE 13-1	Readings from a Medical Refractometer

Readings can be converted to specific gravity (SG) values for cat urine using the following chart or formula: Feline urine SG = $(0.846 \times$ Medical refractometer reading$) + 0.154$

READING ON A MEDICAL REFRACTOMETER SCALE	FELINE URINE SG
1.005	1.004
1.010	1.008
1.015	1.013
1.020	1.017
1.025	1.021
1.030	1.025
1.035	1.030
1.040	1.034

Modified from George JW: The usefulness and limitations of hand-held refractometers in veterinary laboratory medicine: an historical and technical review, *Vet Clin Pathol* 30:201–210, 2008.

SPECIFIC GRAVITY

Specific gravity (SG) is related to the number and molecular weight of particles in the urine and is used as an indicator of the concentrating ability of the kidney. A refractometer is a quick and simple way to measure SG. Refractometry measures the bending of light as it passes through a solution and is related to the density (number of particles) of a fluid. Urine should be obtained before initiation of treatment with fluids, diuretics, corticosteroids, or other drugs that will affect SG. To determine SG, a drop of urine is placed on the window of the refractometer, and the urine SG is read from the appropriate scale (see Chapter 12, Figure 12-3). It is best to use a refractometer designed for veterinary patients because there is a special scale for cats. However, if a medical refractometer is used, a conversion scale can be used for cat urine (Table 13-1). SG can be performed on a turbid sample with or without centrifugation, but sometimes it is easier to use a centrifuged sample because particulate material can obscure the scale on the instrument. Maintenance of the refractometer is straightforward. The window should be cleaned with water and wiped with a soft cloth. Care should be taken to avoid scratching the window because this would interfere with the ability to read the scales. Accuracy of the refractometer should be periodically checked by using distilled water, which should read an SG of 1.000.

Reference intervals are not used for urine SG because an appropriate SG varies with the hydration status of the animal. A healthy kidney should be able to concentrate urine in the face of dehydration or dilute urine to prevent overhydration. SG less than 1.008 indicates that the kidneys are functioning and are able to actively dilute the urine. The SG should reach or exceed minimal levels in dehydrated animals if the kidneys are functioning normally. The minimal SG in dehydration is 1.030 for dogs, 1.035 for cats, and 1.025 for horses and cattle. SG that is lower than the minimal SG for a dehydrated adult animal indicates impaired kidney function. Urine with the SG in the range of 1.008 to 1.012 is considered **isothenuric** and indicates that the urine is being neither concentrated nor diluted compared with plasma. This may be normal in a well-hydrated animal but would be considered evidence of renal dysfunction if the patient is dehydrated or overhydrated.

Quantities of other substances in the urine must be interpreted in conjunction with SG, for example, 4+ protein in urine with an SG of 1.010 represents more severe proteinuria than 4+ protein in concentrated urine with an SG of 1.045.

CHEMICAL EVALUATION

A variety of tests are routinely performed using chemistry reagent strips. Urine should be at room temperature when tested and does not need to be centrifuged unless it is turbid. Urine is placed on reagent pads, or the test strip is dipped in the urine. Chemical reactions result in color changes of the pads. Directions accompanying the reagent strips indicate the appropriate incubation time. The color change of the strips is visually compared with a key usually found on the container of the strips, or the strip may be read by an automated reader. Reagent pads for leukocytes and SG that are designed for use with human samples do not work in animals and should not be used. Reagent strips are sensitive to storage conditions such as temperature, humidity, and light, so the containers should be capped immediately after a strip is taken out for use.

> *TECHNICIAN NOTE* Urine that has been stored in the refrigerator should be brought to room temperature before undergoing chemical analysis.

pH

pH is a measure of the concentration of hydrogen ion. As hydrogen ion concentration increases, pH decreases. A pH of 7 is neutral, whereas a urinary pH below 7 is **aciduric** (increased hydrogen ions), and a pH above 7 is **alkaluric** (decreased hydrogen ions). The pH of urine varies with diet and the acid-base status of the patient. Normal urine pH of carnivores such as dogs and cats is 5.0 to 7.5, whereas that of herbivores, including horses, cattle, sheep, and camelids, is 7.5 to 8.5. Omnivores such as pigs may have acidic or alkaline urine. Because the kidney is responsible for maintaining normal blood pH by regulating hydrogen and bicarbonate excretion, urine pH often reflects acidosis or alkalosis in the patient, although this relationship is not always true.

Urine pH should be measured shortly after the sample has been obtained. As urine stands, the pH will increase due to loss of carbon dioxide. Urease-positive bacteria in the urine as part of a urinary tract infection or from contamination can cause urine pH to increase as the result of ammonia production. Various drugs may alter urinary pH, so it is important to know what medication the patient is currently receiving.

Protein

Reagent strips measure proteinuria from negative to 4+ (1000 mg/dl). Normal urine can have a trace to 1+ reading, especially if the urine is concentrated. Alkaline urine (pH >8) can result in a false-positive protein, whereas acidic or very dilute urine can falsely decrease the amount of protein detected. Reagent strips are most sensitive to albumin and may poorly detect other types of protein such as globulins, Bence Jones proteins, hemoglobin, myoglobin, or mucoproteins. Special tests are needed for accurate measurement of globulins and Bence Jones proteins. Inflammation or hemorrhage in the urinary tract will cause proteinuria. If proteinuria is accompanied by inactive urine sediment, this may help localize the source of the proteinuria to the kidney. Glomerular diseases often result in selective loss of albumin, and sensitive tests are available to measure small amounts of albumin in the urine.

Sometimes it is clinically helpful to quantify urine protein excretion by performing a urine protein-to-creatinine ratio. In this case, protein and creatinine in the urine are measured using a chemistry analyzer. Urine should be obtained by cystocentesis or midstream catch and centrifuged before analysis. The ratio is calculated by dividing protein (mg/dl) by creatinine (mg/dl). In dogs, a urine protein-to-creatinine ratio is normally <0.5, whereas a ratio >1.0 is abnormal, indicating significant proteinuria.

Glucose

Normal urine should not contain glucose. When blood passes through the glomerulus, an ultrafiltrate of the plasma is formed that contains many of the same constituents found in plasma, including glucose. Normally, the tubules are able to reabsorb all glucose from the ultrafiltrate. Glucosuria occurs if glucose in the glomerular ultrafiltrate exceeds the ability of the renal tubules to reabsorb the glucose. This will occur if blood glucose levels exceed renal thresholds of 180 mg/dl for dogs, 300 mg/dl for cats, or 100 mg/dl for horses and cattle. Glucosuria can be transient, as when an animal has stress-related or drug-induced hyperglycemia or

persistent with a metabolic condition such as diabetes mellitus. In general, the chemical reaction is specific for glucose, but the reagent pads are prone to degradation, limiting the shelf life of the reagent strips. If refrigerated, urine should be brought to room temperature to avoid falsely low results. Oxidizing cleaning products such as peroxide and hypochlorite may produce false-positive reactions, whereas formaldehyde or vitamin C may yield false-negative reactions.

Ketones

Ketonuria occurs with metabolic diseases involving increased lipid or impaired carbohydrate metabolism, such as diabetic ketoacidosis in dogs and cats, ketosis in cattle, or starvation. Ketones (acetoacetate, acetone, and beta-hydroxybutyrate) may be detectable in the urine before reaching readily detectable levels in the blood. Reagent test strips are most sensitive to acetoacetate and acetone, whereas beta-hydroxybutyrate is not detected. Thus, it may be possible to miss ketonuria at some stages of diabetic ketoacidosis. Because ketones, especially acetone, are volatile and may be lost on exposure to air, urine samples should be tested right away, or the sample should be tightly capped until testing. Bacteria from infection or contamination can decrease acetoacetate.

Bilirubin

Bilirubin results from the metabolism of hemoglobin and is normally excreted in the bile. Serum bilirubin may increase with hemolytic disease or cholestasis. Dogs, especially males, normally may have small amounts of bilirubin in concentrated urine samples. The renal threshold for bilirubin is low in dogs, so bilirubinuria may be detected before icterus can be discerned clinically. Bilirubin is not detected in normal cat urine, so bilirubinuria in this species indicates disease. Urine should be tested within 30 minutes of sample collection. At room temperature and upon exposure to air, bilirubin will be metabolized to biliverdin, which is not detected by dipstick chemistry. Bilirubin is also light-sensitive, so urine should not be stored in clear containers if analysis will be delayed.

Blood or Heme

The dipstick test for blood (sometimes labeled "heme") is based on the ability of hemoglobin or myoglobin to act as a peroxidase to generate a colored chemical substrate. The test is designed to detect the presence of blood that is not discernible to the naked eye, so the sensitivity of dipsticks is very high, becoming positive with as few as 5 RBCs/ml. This test cannot distinguish between intact RBCs (hematuria), free hemoglobin (hemolysis or hemoglobinuria), and myoglobin, so results must be interpreted in conjunction with microscopic examination of urine sediment for intact RBCs. Urine should be mixed before testing is done with the reagent pad. The presence of RBCs in urine sediment (see later) accompanied by a negative blood dipstick test can occur if the urine is centrifuged or is allowed to settle before testing. Some urinary acidifiers such as ascorbic acid may cause a false-negative result. Oxidizing disinfectants may produce a false-positive. Hemolysis may occur with alkaline urine or with dilute urine (SG <1.008).

MICROSCOPIC EXAMINATION

To aid in interpretation, urine samples should be prepared using a standardized method. Samples should be gently mixed, and 5 or 10 ml should be added to a conical centrifuge tube. The sample should be centrifuged at 1500 to 2000 rpm (relative centrifugal force of 400 to 500 g) for 5 minutes. Remove the supernatant by pipetting or decanting, leaving 0.5 ml of supernatant with the pellet in the tube. Gently re-suspend the pellet and add stain if desired. The sample may be examined with or without staining. If using stain, always add a consistent number of drops of stain to avoid the effects of variable dilution on interpretation. Place a drop of the urine sediment on a microscope slide, and cover with a coverslip. Improved contrast of the wet mount can be achieved by lowering the condenser and partially closing the iris diaphragm. Results are recorded as the number of elements per low power field (LPF, or 100× magnification) or high power field (HPF, or 400× magnification). LPF is used to identify and enumerate casts and to look for crystals, cells, sperm, mucus, and lipid droplets. HPF is used to enumerate RBCs, leukocytes, and epithelial cells, and to identify microorganisms and crystals.

Cellular Elements

The numbers and types of cellular elements depend in part on the sampling method. Squamous epithelial cells are larger polygonal cells with small nuclei that originate from the urethra, vagina, or prepuce (Figure 13-4). Squamous cells are found in free catch or catheterized samples, are absent in cystocentesis, and have no clinical significance. Transitional epithelial cells are medium in size and may be found singly or in clusters (Figure 13-5, A). They can occur in larger numbers or in sheets in samples obtained by catheterization. They appear as round to oval, elongate or caudate in shape and line the renal pelvis, ureters, bladder, and proximal urethra. Atypical-appearing transitional epithelial cells or

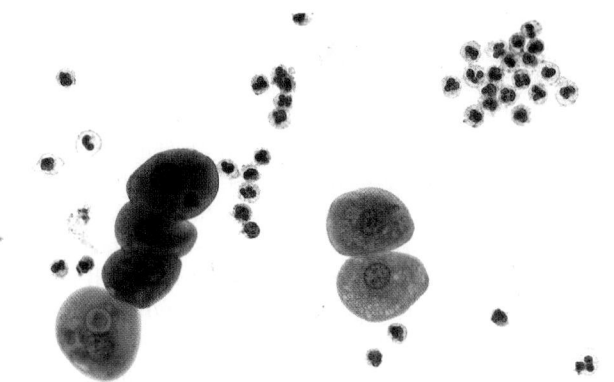

FIGURE 13-4 Urine sample obtained by free catch from a dog, illustrating six noncornified squamous epithelial cells originating from the urethra, as well as many neutrophils. Note the large size of the squamous epithelial cells compared with the neutrophils (Sedi-Stain).

large rafts of cells may be seen with transitional cell carcinoma (Figure 13-5, B). Dry preparation of a sediment smear stained with Wright stain or a quick stain may aid in differentiation between cancer and hyperplasia, especially if inflammation is present (Figure 13-5, C). Renal tubular epithelial cells are small round cells that may be seen with tubular degeneration and in association with casts.

Occasional leukocytes and RBCs are found normally in urine with 0 to 8 each /HPF expected in a voided sample, 0 to 5 each /HPF in a catheterized sample, or 0 to 3 each /HPF in a cystocentesis sample (Figures 13-4 and 13-6). Higher numbers of RBCs can be seen with a traumatic catheterization or with cystocentesis if traumatic hemorrhage has occurred. The presence of leukocytes or RBCs does not localize the regional source of the cells within the urinary tract, and it may not be possible to distinguish between genital and urinary tract origin with voided and catheterized samples. The condition of increased numbers of leukocytes is called **pyuria** and indicates inflammation in the urinary tract. Pyuria is frequently associated with infection, and careful examination for microorganisms and possibly a culture should be performed. The presence of leukocyte casts (see later) indicates inflammation in the kidney. RBCs may lyse in very dilute urine or may shrink (crenate) in highly concentrated urine.

Casts

Casts consist of protein with entrapped cells and debris that typically form in the distal renal tubules, where flow is slowest and acidity and solute concentration are highest, favoring precipitation of protein. The presence of casts localizes the problem to the kidneys, but the number of casts does not reflect the severity of disease. A few hyaline casts (0 to 2/LPF) (Figure 13-7, A) and granular casts (0 to 1/LPF) (Figure 13-7, B) are considered normal, whereas cellular, waxy, and fatty casts are always abnormal. The condition of increased numbers of casts is called **cylindruria**. Hyaline casts are pure protein casts that appear homogenous and colorless, and are difficult to see (Figure 13-7, A). They may be found in healthy animals and with increased protein leakage or tubular protein secretion. Hyaline casts may dissolve in dilute or alkaline urine. Cellular casts contain cells that have been trapped within the protein matrix. Leukocyte casts indicate inflammation, whereas RBC casts occur with hemorrhage (Figure 13-7, C). Tubular epithelial cells can slough and become entrapped in cases of tubular necrosis or pyelonephritis (Figure 13-7, D). Granular casts can be coarsely or finely granular and result from degeneration of cellular casts (Figure 13-7, B). Waxy casts are the result of continued degeneration of granular casts and indicate a chronic renal lesion. Waxy casts are smooth with blunt ends and folds or cracks (Figure 13-7, E). Fatty casts contain lipid droplets that accumulated in cells before becoming part of the cast.

Crystals

The presence of crystals in the urine is termed **crystalluria**. Crystals form or dissolve in urine, depending on pH,

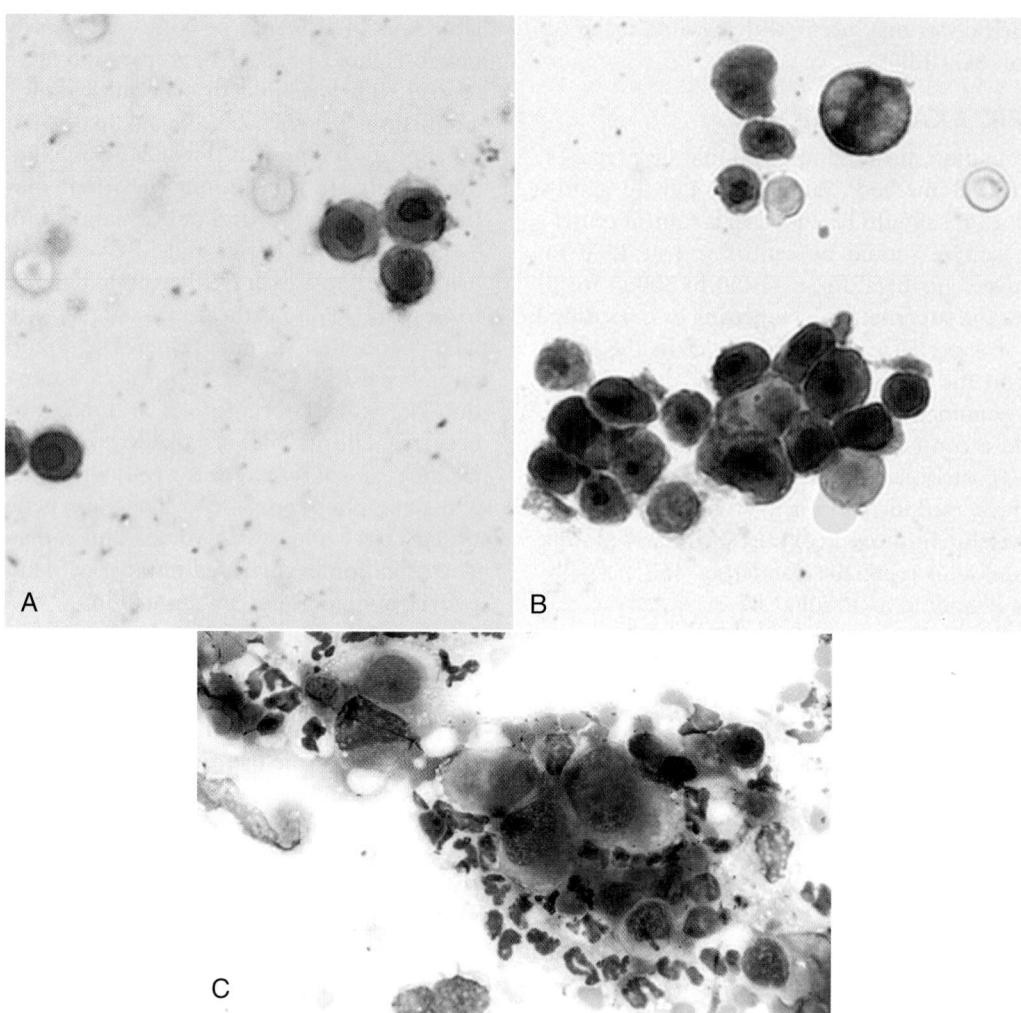

FIGURE 13-5 Urine sediment from a dog with **(A)** normal transitional epithelial cells, and **(B)** a cluster of atypical-appearing transitional epithelial cells, suggestive of transitional cell carcinoma (Sedi-Stain). **(C)** Wright stained smear of urine sediment from a dog with transitional cell carcinoma. Note the variation in nuclear and cellular size, the stippled chromatin pattern, multiple nucleoli, and the basophilic cytoplasm. These characteristics of neoplastic epithelial cells are often easier to see with Wright stain than with Sedi-Stain or unstained preparations. Neutrophils, red blood cells, and bacteria are present in the background.

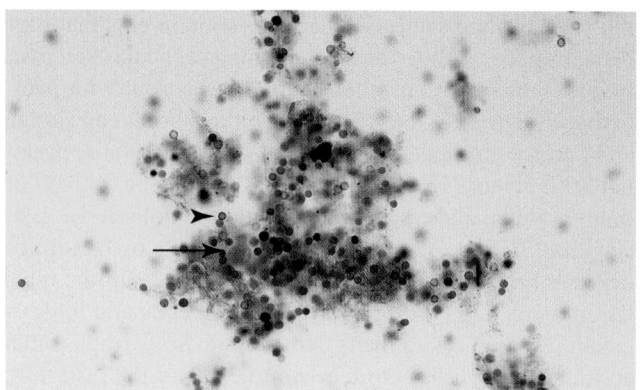

FIGURE 13-6 Urine from a dog illustrating red blood cells (RBCs; *arrowhead*) and white blood cells (WBCs). A transitional epithelial cell is indicated by an arrow (Sedi-Stain).

concentration, and temperature. Crystalluria is often of no clinical significance or it may be associated with risk for urolithiasis (stone formation), or it may indicate abnormal metabolism of a substance or may be a response to composition of the diet. Crystals such as struvite (Figure 13-8, *A*), calcium oxalate (Figure 13-8, *C*), and calcium phosphate are commonly found in the urine of normal dogs and cats. Horses normally have calcium carbonate crystals (Figure 13-8, *B*), especially if they are on forage with high calcium content, such as alfalfa. Dihydrate and monohydrate forms of calcium oxalate (Figure 13-8, *C*) may be normal or may be associated with urolithiasis or increased urinary calcium loss. The hippuric acid–like form of calcium oxalate monohydrate has been associated with ethylene glycol (antifreeze) toxicity (Figure 13-8, *D*). Bilirubin crystals may form in

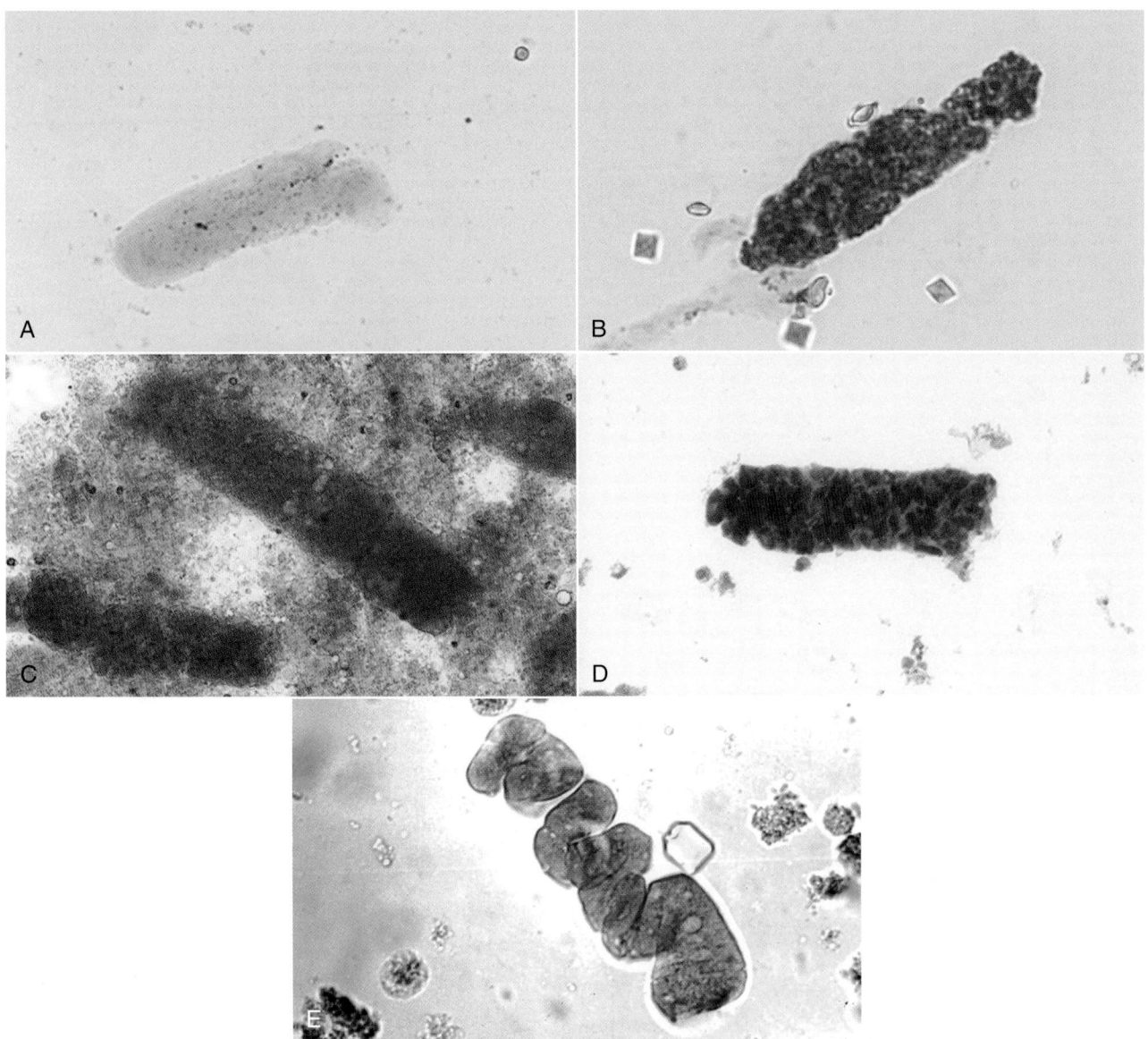

FIGURE 13-7 Urine from dogs. **A,** A hyaline cast (Sedi-Stain). **B,** A granular cast and calcium oxalate crystals (Sedi-Stain). **C,** Three red blood cell (RBC) cellular casts with cellular debris in the background (unstained sediment). **D,** A cellular cast (Sedi-Stain). **E,** A waxy cast with the typical smooth appearance and well-defined edges and folds (Sedi-Stain).

patients with bilirubinuria (Figure 13-8, *E*). Ammonium biurate and other urate crystals may be seen in Dalmatians as the result of an inherited error of metabolism, and in some dogs with portosystemic shunts (Figure 13-8, *F*). Cystine crystals occur in dogs with inherited defects in amino acid transport (Figure 13-8, *G*). Drugs and their metabolites that are excreted by the kidney may form crystals (e.g., sulfonamides).

Microorganisms
The significance of microorganisms in a urine sample must be interpreted in conjunction with the sampling method and whether an associated inflammatory response is seen. Whereas cystocentesis samples should be sterile, voided and catheterized samples may be contaminated from the lower urinary and genital tracts. Contaminants will readily grow at room temperature, causing deterioration of cellular and chemical constituents. It is important to make sure that equipment used for urinalysis, including stains, is free of contamination because this will confound microscopic interpretation and culture results. Bacteria are the more common urinary tract pathogens, but fungal infections also can occur. Failure to find microorganisms in urine sediment does not exclude infection as a cause of urinary tract inflammation.

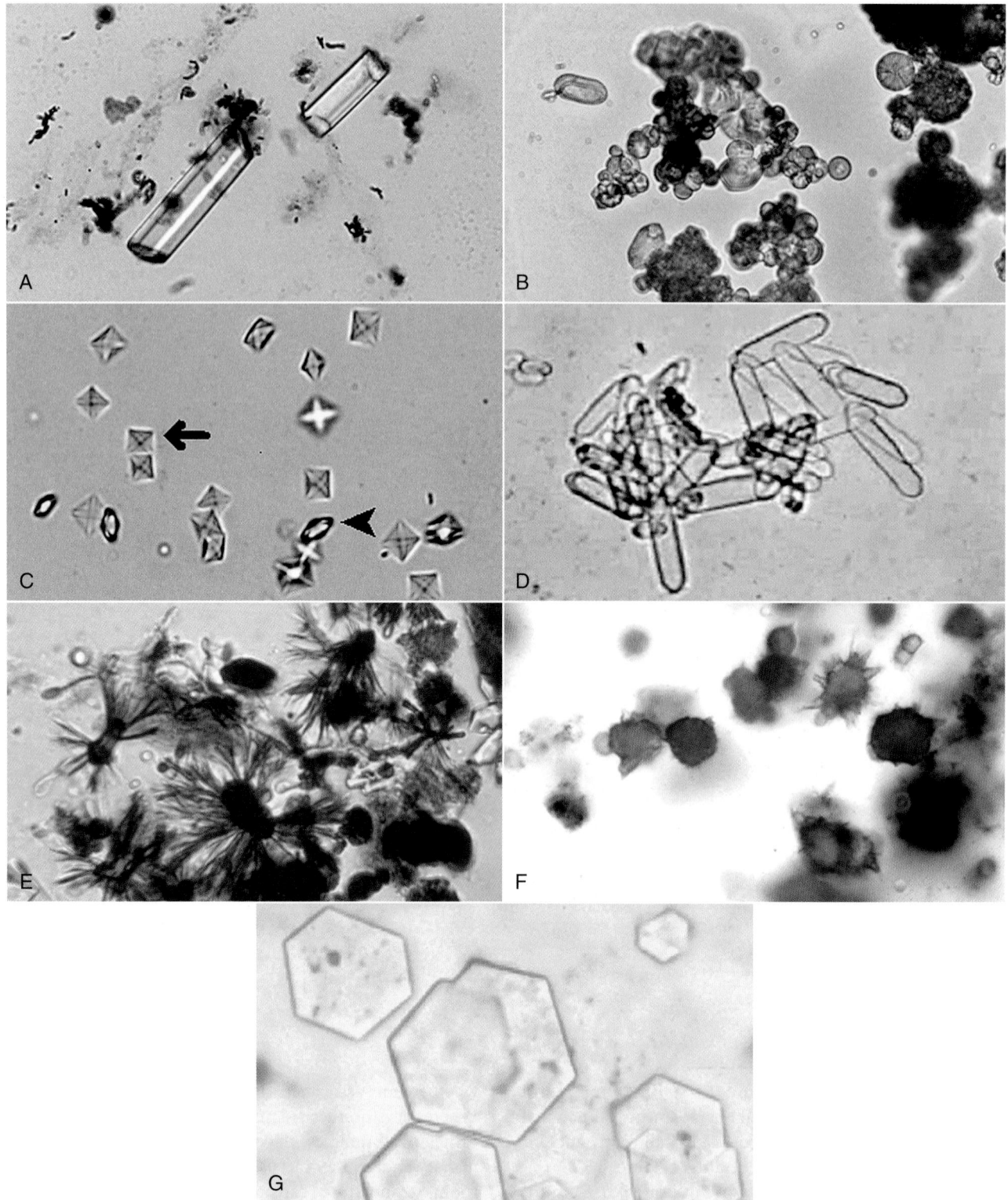

FIGURE 13-8 Urine sediments. **A,** Struvite crystals from a dog. **B,** Calcium carbonate crystals from a horse. These crystals are a normal finding and exhibit a variety of shapes. **C,** Calcium oxalate dihydrate *(arrow)* from a dog. Several calcium oxalate monohydrate "hemp seed" morphology crystals are present *(arrowhead)*. **D,** Calcium oxalate monohydrate crystals with hippuric acid–like morphology. **E,** Bilirubin crystals from a dog. **F,** Ammonium biurate crystals from a dog. **G,** Cystine crystals from a dog (Sedi-Stain).

RECOMMENDED READINGS

Chemistry

Kaneko JJ, Harvey JW, Bruss ML: Clinical biochemistry of domestic animals, Burlington, MA, 2008, Elsevier.

Thrall MA: Veterinary hematology and clinical chemistry, Baltimore, 2012, Wiley-Blackwell.

Tietz NW, Burtis CA, Ashwood ER, et al: Tietz textbook of clinical chemistry and molecular diagnostics, St Louis, 2006, Elsevier Saunders.

Quality Control

The American Society of Veterinary Clinical Pathology: Principles of quality assurance and standards for veterinary clinical pathology. Available at: http://www.asvcp.org (accessed on July 23, 2012).

Westgard QC: Tools, technologies and training for healthcare laboratories. Available at: http://www.westgard.com (accessed on July 23, 2012).

Serology

Zimmerman KL, Crisman MV: Diagnostic equine serology, Vet Clin North Am Equine Pract 24:311–334, 2008.

Urinalysis

Chew DJ, DiBartola SP: Interpretation of canine and feline urinalysis: Nestle-Purina clinical handbook series, Wilmington, DE, 1998, The Gloyd Group.

Chew DJ, DiBartola SP, Schenck P: Canine and feline nephrology and urology, ed 2, St Louis, 2010, Elsevier Saunders.

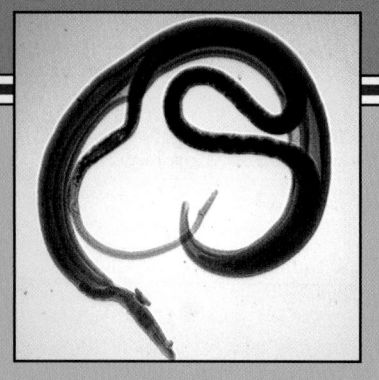

14 Parasitology

Sara-Louise Roberts Newcomer and Charles M. Hendrix

OUTLINE

The Veterinary Technician's Role in Educating Clients Regarding Zoonotic Parasitic Diseases of Small Animals, 441
Trematodes (Flukes) of Zoonotic Importance, 441
Paragonimus kellicotti (Lung Fluke of Dogs and Cats), 441
Avian Schistosomes (Causative Agent of Schistosome Cercarial Dermatitis), 443
Cestodes (Tapeworms) and Metacestodes (Larval Tapeworms) of Zoonotic Importance, 445
Dipylidium caninum (Cucumber Seed Tapeworm, Double-Pored Tapeworm), 445
Echinococcus granulosus/Echinococcus multilocularis, 448
Spirometra mansonoides, 450
Nematodes (Roundworms) of Zoonotic Importance, 451
Toxocara canis, Toxocara cati, and *Toxascaris leonina* (Ascarids/Roundworms)—Visceral Larva Migrans and Ocular Larva Migrans, 452
Baylisascaris procyonis—Neurologic Larva Migrans, 454
Ancylostoma caninum, Ancylostoma braziliense, and *Ancylostoma tubaeforme; Uncinaria stenocephala* (Hookworms)—Cutaneous Larva Migrans (Creeping Eruption, Plumber's Itch, Sandworms), 455
Trichuris vulpis (Whipworms)—Trichuriasis, 457

Strongyloides stercoralis and *Strongyloides cati* (Threadworms)—Strongyloidosis; *Aelurostrongylus abstrusus*, 458
Enterobius vermicularis (Human Pinworm)—Enterobiasis, 460
Dirofilaria immitis (Heartworms)—Human Dirofilariasis, 461
Arthropods of Zoonotic Importance, 462
Acarines (Mites and Ticks), 462
Protozoans of Zoonotic Importance, 467
Giardia Species, 467
Toxoplasma gondii, 471
Cryptosporidium parvum—Cryptosporidiosis, 472
Pentastomes (Snake Parasites) of Zoonotic Importance, 473
Pentastomes, 473
Diagnosis of Endoparasitism, 474
Collection of Fecal Samples, 474
Small Animal Fecal Samples, 474
Examination of Fecal Samples, 474
Gross Examination of Feces, 475
Microscopic Examination of Feces, 475
Examination of Direct Smears, 476
Concentration Methods for Fecal Examination, 477
Examination of Feces for Protozoa, 478
Special Staining for Coccidian Parasites, 478
Antigen Tests, 478
Sample Collection at Necropsy, 478
Shipping Parasitologic Specimens, 479
Miscellaneous Procedures for Detection of Endoparasites, 479

LEARNING OBJECTIVES

When you have completed this chapter, you will be able to:

1. Pronounce, define, and spell all Key Terms in this chapter.
2. Identify the common name, affected species, key clinical signs, methods of diagnosis, life cycle, zoonotic potential, treatment, prevention, and control of the digenetic flukes of zoonotic importance.

KEY TERMS

Aberrant/erratic parasite
Acariasis
Arthropod
Bradyzoite
Cestode
Cutaneous larva migrans
Cysticercoid
Definitive host
Digenetic fluke
Ectoparasites
Egg packet
Endoparasite
Hermaphroditic
Heterogonic life cycle
Homogonic life cycle
Hypobiosis
Intermediate host
Many-host tick
Metacestode
Microfilaria (microfilariae, pl)
Miracidium
Multilocular hydatid cyst
Nematode
Neurologic larva migrans
Ocular larva migrans (OLM)
One-host tick
Oocyst
Operculated egg
Otoacariasis
Paratenic host/transport host
Parthenogenesis
Plerocercoid
Procercoid
Proglottid
Protozoan
Pseudoparasite
Pseudotapeworm
Pyrethrin
Schistosome
Schistosome cercarial dermatitis
Seed ticks

3. Identify the common name, affected species, key clinical signs, methods of diagnosis, life cycle, zoonotic potential, treatment, prevention, and control of the cestodes and metacestodes of zoonotic importance.
4. Identify the common name, affected species, key clinical signs, methods of diagnosis, life cycle, zoonotic potential, treatment, prevention, and control of the nematodes (roundworms) of zoonotic importance. Also do the following regarding nematodes:
   • Describe the origin and clinical signs of *visceral larva migrans*, *ocular larva migrans*, *neurologic larva migrans*, and *cutaneous larva migrans*, including risk factors for and methods of preventing these zoonotic diseases.
   • Identify the common name, affected species, key clinical signs, methods of diagnosis, life cycle, zoonotic potential, treatment, prevention, and control of *Dirofilaria immitis* (heartworms).
5. Identify the common name, affected species, key clinical signs, methods of diagnosis, life cycle, zoonotic potential, treatment, prevention, and control of the arthropods of zoonotic importance.
6. Identify the common names, affected species, key clinical signs, methods of diagnosis, life cycle, zoonotic potential, treatment, prevention, and control of the protozoans of zoonotic importance.
7. Identify the common names, affected species, key clinical signs, methods of diagnosis, life cycle, zoonotic potential, treatment, prevention, and control of the pentastomes of zoonotic importance.
8. Do the following regarding collection and examination of fecal samples for the diagnosis of endoparasitism:
   • Describe the principles of collection, storage, and examination of fecal samples, including safety precautions that must be observed.
   • Describe indications for and procedures used to examine feces by direct fecal smear, fecal flotation, and sedimentation.
9. Do the following additional tasks regarding diagnosis of endoparasitism:
   • List the special procedures used to detect the coccidian parasites *Giardia*, *Cryptosporidium* spp., and *Cystoisospora* spp.
   • Describe how necropsy findings are used to diagnose parasitism after death.
   • Explain how samples are prepared and shipped to an outside laboratory for diagnosis of parasitism.
   • Explain how the Baermann technique is used to detect nematode larvae in feces and tissues.
   • Compare and contrast the blood examination and concentration techniques used to diagnose *Dirofilaria immitis*.

KEY TERMS — cont'd

Simian
Sparganosis
Sparganum
Tachyzoite
Three-host tick
Trematode
Trombicula species
Trophozoite
Two-host tick
Unilocular hydatid cyst
Visceral larva migrans
  (VLM)

INTRODUCTION

Most parasites are capable of causing significant damage to the host. This potential damage may be a function of the number of parasites present, location within the host, production of toxins, and interference with the host's normal physiologic processes. Clinical signs associated with parasitism may include life-threatening anemia, hypoproteinemia, diarrhea, vomiting, and intestinal obstruction; however, damage from most parasites is more insidious, such as interference with normal weight gain or milk production. Parasitism is most severe in animals younger than 1 year, but it may affect animals of any age.

Parasites are divided into two large groups: **endoparasites** (internal parasites), which include nematodes, cestodes, **trematodes,** protozoa, and acanthocephalans; and **ecto-parasites** (external parasites), which include fleas, lice, ticks, mites, chiggers, biting flies, and myiasis-inducing flies. Endoparasites and ectoparasites are found on or in all animals and in every tissue and organ system. Some parasites are host specific, whereas other parasites are capable of infecting a broad range of species. Modes of transmission vary considerably from direct transmission to an extremely complex life cycle involving the use of intermediate hosts or transport hosts. In all modes of parasite transmission, specific environmental conditions play a key role.

Entire textbooks have been written about veterinary parasitology, and it would be impossible in a single chapter to cover all of the parasites that affect animals. Therefore, this chapter will focus on the major parasitic conditions that may be encountered in a small animal practice in North America. It will detail those parasites that are of highest importance in terms of zoonotic potential, and the important points that the veterinary technician must convey to a client. This chapter will specifically emphasize the important role that technicians play in protecting public health by educating clients about the many zoonotic parasitic diseases that may affect the pet, the client, and the client's immediate family.

In this chapter, parasites will be grouped as follows: trematodes (flukes), cestodes and metacestodes (tapeworms and their larval stages), nematodes (roundworms), arthropods (crustaceans, insects, mites, and ticks), and protozoa (one-cell organisms). A comprehensive outline will summarize the following points for each of the parasites: the parasite's common name, name derivation, and pronunciation; the type of parasite; species affected by the parasite; key clinical signs of infected animals; an abbreviated life cycle; laboratory test(s) used to diagnose the infection/infestation; the zoonotic potential for clients; treatment; and prevention and control techniques. Technician Notes highlight important information that is relevant to each zoonotic parasite. The section that focuses on parasites will be followed by a discussion of methods used to diagnose endoparasitism.

THE VETERINARY TECHNICIAN'S ROLE IN EDUCATING CLIENTS REGARDING ZOONOTIC PARASITIC DISEASES OF SMALL ANIMALS

When we consider the various professional responsibilities noted in the Veterinarian's Oath, it is easy to focus on the health and welfare of animals. However, "the promotion of public health" is also mentioned in the oath. The veterinarian's and veterinary technician's role in the promotion of public health is vital but often overlooked until a client is encountered who is relying on them for information about a zoonotic disease with which his or her pet has been diagnosed.

This chapter will cover a number of different parasites, many of which are zoonotic. The veterinary technician plays a vital role in helping to educate clients regarding these parasites. This chapter will detail the life cycle, diagnostics, treatments, and prevention for each zoonotic parasite. It is important to pay close attention to the life cycles of these parasites because they contain important bits of information that are crucial to explaining the risks, methods of prevention, and reasons why the specific treatment intervals are important. For example, understanding the life cycle of *Ancylostoma caninum*, the "canine hookworm," reminds us that a minimum of two consecutive treatments with pyrantel pamoate, 2 weeks apart, is essential to treatment for all the life stages of this hookworm. Treating a puppy or a dog appropriately for this parasite is very important because it causes *cutaneous larva migrans*, a zoonotic condition more often seen in children. *A. caninum* will be discussed in greater detail later in the chapter.

It is also important to keep in mind that when communicating with clients, the use of words or language that clients can understand and comprehend is key to effective communication. Many of today's clients will have performed extensive Internet searches in advance of an appointment, so understanding the details of these parasites will better prepare the veterinary technician for dialogue with clients to ensure that the information they have researched is accurate and relevant. This will also give the veterinary technician an opportunity to help ease clients' concerns and to show them that every member of the health care team is committed to excellent care of their pet, and to the health and well-being of their families too. (See Case Presentation 14-1 for an example of the importance of effective client communication.)

> **TECHNICIAN NOTE** Extensive knowledge of parasites' life cycles is vital, because they contain important bits of information that are crucial in explaining the risks, preventions, and reasons why specific treatment intervals are important.

TREMATODES (FLUKES) OF ZOONOTIC IMPORTANCE

Trematodes (digenetic flukes) are flatworms that parasitize a wide variety of domesticated and wild animals. These parasites are often associated with diseases of the intestinal tract; however, some digenetic flukes parasitize the respiratory passages (e.g., *Paragonimus kellicotti*) or the blood vasculature (e.g., the schistosomes). These flukes usually can be diagnosed by the finding of operculated ova in the feces of infected animals.

> **TECHNICIAN NOTE** Most of the parasitic flukes of domesticated animals are **digenetic flukes**. The prefix "di-" means "two." The suffix "gen-" means "beginning," hence "two beginnings." The digenetic flukes of most domesticated animals have two intermediate hosts—a first intermediate host and a second intermediate host—in addition to the **definitive host**.

PARAGONIMUS KELLICOTTI (LUNG FLUKE OF DOGS AND CATS)

- **Parasite's common name:** The lung fluke of dogs and cats
- **Pronunciation:** "Pear-ah-**gahn**-ee-muss" "kell-ee-**cot**-eye"
- **Derivation:** "Para," from Latin, *to bear* (can reproduce); "gonimus," from Greek, *productive; having generative power* (produces a lot of eggs); "**kellicotti,**" *most probably named for an early researcher or investigator whose last name was Kellicott*
- **Type of parasite:** platyhelminth—trematode (fluke)—digenetic trematode (fluke)

Species Affected

Dogs and cats associated with aquatic environments that might serve as suitable environs for snails and crayfish, the first and second intermediate hosts, respectively. Humans are rarely infected owing to the fact that people seldom ingest raw or poorly cooked crayfish. These parasites are usually found in pairs in fluid-filled cystic spaces within lung tissue. This is an unusual digenetic fluke in that it is found within the respiratory system—most digenetic flukes are associated with the gastrointestinal (GI) tract or some branch of the GI tract (e.g., the bile duct).

Key Clinical Signs of Infected Animals

Chronic, deep intermittent cough, lethargy, or occasionally dyspnea.

Abbreviated Life Cycle

Hermaphroditic flukes (individual worms with both male and female reproductive organs present) produce **operculated eggs** (eggs with a tiny door-like structure at one end). When an egg makes contact with water, the operculum opens, releasing a free-swimming ciliated larva known as a *miracidium*.

CASE PRESENTATION 14-1 HOOKWORM AND ROUNDWORM INFECTION IN A LITTER OF PUPPIES

History

A litter of 5-week-old, American Staffordshire terrier puppies (three males and one female) was presented for evaluation of an acute illness. Two of the four puppies had been lethargic and anorexic for 1 day before presentation. On the morning of the office visit, one male in particular was recumbent and not responsive. There was no history of deworming, and the dam was not on a heartworm preventive or intestinal anthelmintic. The other two puppies were bright and alert and still playful, and had good appetites.

The clients were a young couple with two young children. As far as they were aware, the puppies were fine until the previous day, but when they found one puppy unresponsive that morning, they called to make an appointment right away. They were very concerned but only had $100 to treat the puppies.

Physical Examination of Puppy #1

This puppy was laterally recumbent and unresponsive. His temperature did not register on the thermometer. His pulse was 85 bpm (normal, 100 to 180 bpm), and his respiratory rate was 12 breaths per minute (normal, 18 to 34 breaths per minute). The puppy had white, tacky mucous membranes, his abdomen was severely distended, and he weighed 3 pounds and appeared underweight. His limbs were cold and his hair coat was dull. He was estimated to be 10% dehydrated.

Physical Examination of Puppy #2

This puppy was depressed but responsive. His temperature was 101.2° F (normal, 100.5° F to 102.5° F), his pulse was 180 bpm (normal, 100 to 180 bpm), and his respiratory rate was 48 breaths per minute (normal, 18 to 34 breaths per minute). His mucous membranes were white, and a capillary refill time (CRT) was unable to be determined. His abdomen was severely distended, and his hair coat was dull. He weighed 3 lbs and was estimated to be 8% dehydrated.

Diagnostics

A fecal centrifugation was positive for roundworms and hookworms. While waiting for the fecal results, puppy #2 passed a bowel movement that consisted mostly of roundworms and very little fecal material. His packed cell volume (PCV) was 20% (normal, 26% to 36%).

Diagnosis

- Parasitism—hookworms (*Ancylostoma caninum*) and roundworms (*Toxocara canis*)
- Anemia and dehydration

Outcome

Based on the presentation of puppy #1, his poor prognosis, and the limited financial resources available to pay for treatment of the puppies, it was recommended that puppy #1 be euthanized in the hope of saving the other three. A necropsy was performed on puppy #1. Preliminary results received that day revealed a perforated duodenum, ascites, anemia, intestines filled with roundworms and hookworms, and roundworms penetrating through the perforation and extending into the abdominal cavity.

Treatment

Puppy #2 was given subcutaneous fluids and pyrantel pamoate. Puppy #3 and puppy #4 were also given pyrantel pamoate. All three puppies were sent home with a second dose of pyrantel to be given in 2 weeks.

Discharge

The owners of the puppies were still very concerned and very confused. The puppies had been indoors, and they were unsure where the puppies had contracted these worms. Furthermore, they thought that maybe they just had one or two worms and didn't understand how puppy #1 had gotten so sick so fast. They wondered about the prognosis for the other three puppies, and if there was anything else they should do.

Analysis of the Case

In addition to answering the clients' questions, what important points should you discuss with the owners with regard to this situation?

1. Be mindful of the gravity of the situation by first demonstrating empathy because these owners just had to euthanize one of their puppies. Remember that they did the best they could with the information they had because they had brought the puppies in just as soon as they knew something was wrong.

2. Be thoughtful as you share the life cycle of these parasites with them, explaining that these puppies likely became infected in utero and while nursing. As a result, they had a very large worm burden that caused puppy #1 and puppy #2 to become very sick. Use language that they will understand, avoid medical jargon, and give them small chunks of information a little bit at a time. Pause periodically to check that they have heard you and to answer any questions they may have before you continue.

3. Because the puppies did get the worms from the dam, recommend that she be brought in to be examined and treated for parasites. For subsequent pregnancies, to avoid this situation, it is recommended that she be on a combination monthly heartworm and intestinal worm preventive. In addition, the puppies should be dewormed every other week starting at 2 weeks of age.

4. It is equally important that you inform them that their children are susceptible to these parasites through fecal-oral contamination. Remind them of the importance of good hygiene and of daily removal and disposal of the dam's and puppy's fecal material to decontaminate the environment.

5. Reassure them that you are available if they have other questions, and emphasize their role in helping the puppies to survive.

This case illustrates the value of effective communication and client education concerning parasitic zoonoses, and the important role that veterinary technicians play in protecting public health.

TECHNICIAN NOTE Within the life cycle of a typical digenetic fluke, the **miracidium** is the ciliated, motile stage that emerges from the operculated egg of a digenetic fluke. The miracidium is covered with tiny moving hairs that allow it to swim in the water and to come in contact with the first intermediate host of the fluke, which is usually a snail. The miracidium MUST penetrate the skin of the first intermediate host for the life cycle to continue. Upon penetration, the miracidium develops into a sac-like structure called a *sporocyst.*

The miracidium penetrates an aquatic snail (first intermediate host) in water. Multiplicative reproduction takes place in the snail, eventually releasing many larvae known as *cercarial stages.* These stages penetrate a crayfish (second Intermediate host) Within this host, cercarial stages mature to the encysted metacercarial (infective) stage. A dog or cat eats the crayfish with the metacercariae, which are released in the intestine. Metacercariae penetrate the intestinal wall, penetrate the diaphragm, and then enter the thoracic cavity, eventually penetrating the lung parenchyma. Juvenile flukes pair up and induce the formation of a cystic space, which must connect with a bronchiole, producing a portal through which the operculated eggs will exit the host. Fluke eggs are coughed up and swallowed, and exit the host in feces.

TECHNICIAN NOTE The cercarial stage is the developmental stage that emerges from the first intermediate host (usually a snail) of a digenetic trematode (fluke). The cercarial stage penetrates the second intermediate host, which ultimately will become infective for the definitive host, OR it attaches to vegetation and develops into a metacercarial stage, which ultimately will be ingested by the definitive host, OR it penetrates the skin of the definitive host directly (as in the case of *schistosome cercarial dermatitis*).

Laboratory Test(s) Used to Diagnose the Infection

Whereas the eggs of most digenetic flukes will sink during simple fecal flotation and centrifugation procedures, the operculated eggs of *Paragonimus kellicotti* will float on the surface of most fecal flotation solutions (Figure 14-1).

Zoonotic Potential for Clients

Paragonimus kellicotti is very rarely seen in humans; it would be seen only in hunters or survivalists who consume raw or poorly cooked crayfish from an area endemic for *P. kellicotti.* There is a species of this genus that does infect humans—*Paragonimus westermani*—but this fluke does not infect dogs.

Treatment

Fenbendazole in two divided doses totaling 50 mg/kg or in a single dose of 100 mg/kg of body weight each day for 10 to 14 days.

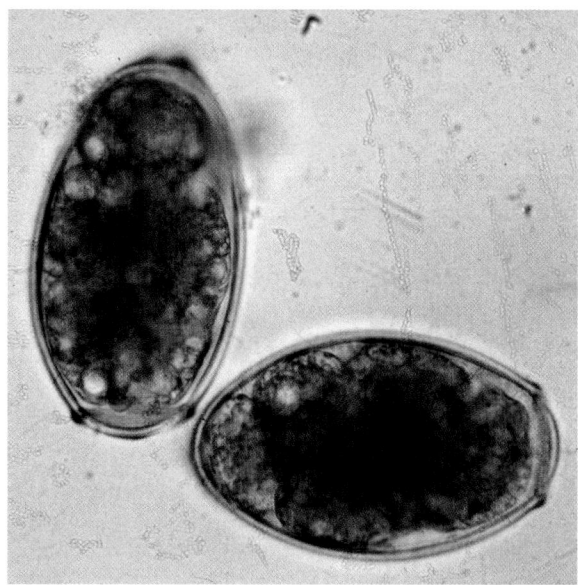

FIGURE 14-1 Operculated eggs of *Paragonimus kellicotti.*

Prevention and Control Techniques

Never allow dogs or cats to roam freely around lakes, streams, and ponds. Never feed raw crayfish to dogs or cats.

TECHNICIAN NOTE *Paragonimus kellicotti* can also be diagnosed using thoracic radiography or tracheal washes, but fecal flotation usually proves to be a simpler and more economical diagnostic procedure.

AVIAN SCHISTOSOMES (CAUSATIVE AGENT OF SCHISTOSOME CERCARIAL DERMATITIS)

- **Parasite's common name:** The blood fluke of wild birds. This parasite produces *schistosome cercarial dermatitis* or "swimmer's itch."
- **Pronunciation:** "**shiss**-toe-sew-em" "sir-**care**-ree-al" "der-muh-**tie**-tiss"
- **Derivation: "schistos,"** from Greek, *split*; "**soma,**" from Greek, *body*; "**kerkos,**" from Greek, *tail. Schistosoma* can also be called *Bilharzia,* after Theodor Bilharz, a German physician who worked with blood flukes.
- **Type of parasite:** platyhelminth—trematode (fluke)—digenetic trematode (fluke)—schistosome—avian schistosome

Species Affected

Aquatic, migratory birds are the primary definitive hosts; however, human beings serve as incidental hosts for this zoonotic skin condition, which can be contracted after humans swim or wade in cercaria-infested waters.

Location of Parasite Within Host

Although these parasites (e.g., *Trichobilharzia* or *Ornithobilharzia* species) are normally found within the blood vasculature of many aquatic or migratory birds, this condition (caused by juvenile stages of the fluke) localizes in the skin of humans.

Key Clinical Signs of Infected Animals

Signs of infection in migratory birds are of greatest concern to wildlife biologists, rather than veterinarians. The skin reaction in humans is characterized by the production of highly pruritic, raised, red papules in the skin, a condition known as *schistosome cercarial dermatitis* or *swimmer's itch*. This condition often causes the closing of recreational areas surrounding streams, lakes, and ponds. This syndrome occurs along flyways of aquatic, migratory birds.

> **TECHNICIAN NOTE** **Schistosome cercarial dermatitis** is a zoonotic condition resulting from repeated penetration of the cercarial stage of blood flukes of birds, usually migratory aquatic birds. This condition manifests as papular or pustular areas in the skin of humans who have come in contact with infested waters containing these cercarial stages of avian schistosomes.

Abbreviated Life Cycle

Adult **schistosomes** are found in blood vasculature supplying the intestinal tract of aquatic, migratory birds. Schistosomes are dioecious, which means that there are separate sexes (adult male and adult female schistosomes).

> **TECHNICIAN NOTE** A schistosome is a "blood fluke" that inhabits the blood vasculature of its definitive host. These blood flukes are unusual in that they are not hermaphroditic (as most digenetic flukes are). They are dioecious, that is, there are male schistosomes and there are female schistosomes. Schistosomes are unusual in that the host becomes infected by means of penetration of the cercarial stage—there is no metacercarial stage in the life cycle of schistosomes.

The term *schistosome* means "split body" (i.e., the male schistosome has a long, deep groove running down its long body). Within this long, deep groove (called the *gynecophoric canal*), the female schistosome will reside (Figure 14-2). Schistosomes mate, and the female schistosome produces eggs, which work their way from the lumen of the blood vasculature to the lumen of the intestine. The eggs pass in feces into the aquatic external environment. Upon contact with water, the eggs hatch, releasing a motile, ciliated miracidium. The miracidium penetrates the first intermediate host, an aquatic snail. Within the snail, asexual (multiplicative) reproduction takes place, ultimately producing the cercaria, which exits the snail. The cercarial stage is a motile, swimming stage; it has a tail that it uses for swimming in water before it penetrates the host (Figure 14-3). This cercarial stage penetrates the skin of the definitive host—an aquatic, migratory bird. From the site of penetration,

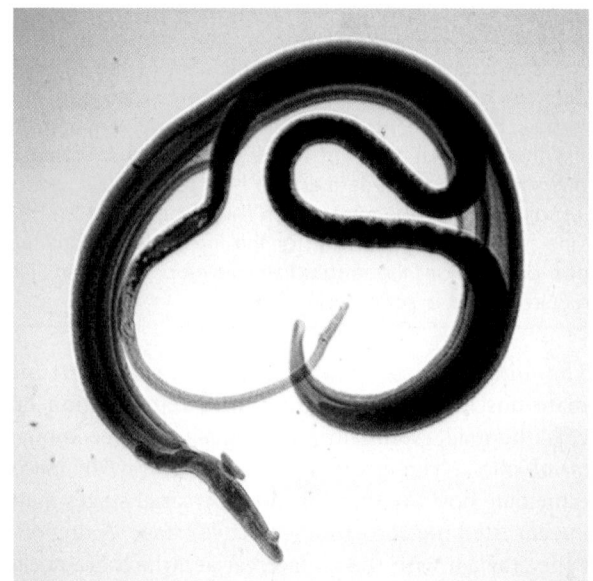

FIGURE 14-2 Adult male and female schistosomes in copula. Female schistosome lies in the gynecophoric canal of the male schistosome's body.

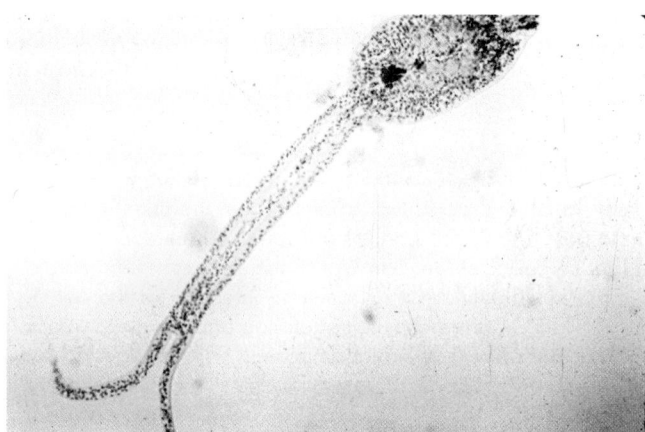

FIGURE 14-3 The motile, fork-tailed cercaria of an avian schistosome. When cercariae repeatedly penetrate the skin of humans, a condition known as *schistosome cercarial dermatitis* results.

cercariae migrate to the blood vasculature, where they develop into male or female avian schistosomes. This is the "normal" life cycle of the avian schistosome. Migratory birds use flyways that run north and south across North America. Along the way are resting areas for these migrating birds—lakes, streams, and ponds. Infected birds will shed eggs in their feces and the life cycle continues in these aquatic environs. However, sometimes the cercarial stage will penetrate the skin of humans who happen to be swimming or wading in these infested waters. With repeated penetration of human skin by these cercarial stages, an allergic reaction will take place. Highly pruritic, raised, red skin papules are produced in a skin condition known as *schistosome cercarial dermatitis* or *swimmer's itch* (Figure 14-4). Recreational areas surrounding streams, lakes, and ponds will often be closed owing to this zoonotic skin condition.

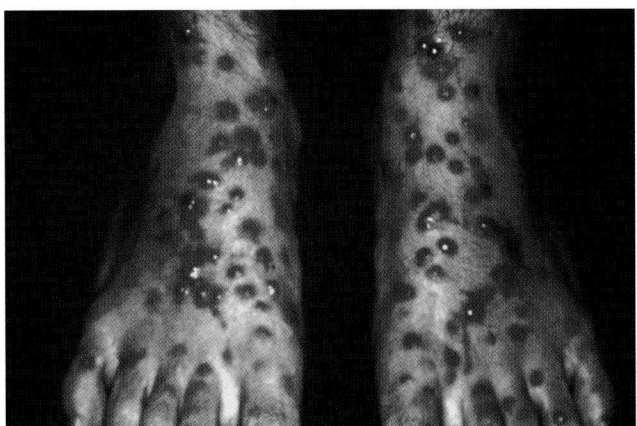

FIGURE 14-4 Gross photograph of schistosome cercarial dermatitis in the feet of a man.

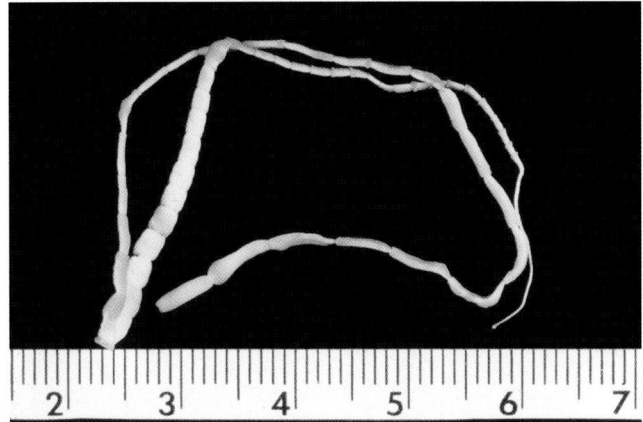

FIGURE 14-5 *Dipylidium caninum*, the cucumber seed tapeworm, from the small intestine of a cat.

Laboratory Test(s) Used to Diagnose the Infection

For aquatic, migratory birds, fecal flotation may reveal the presence of schistosome ova, a concern for wildlife biologists. For infected humans, the observation of highly pruritic, red, raised papules in skin that has contacted cercaria-infested waters may be indicative of infection. If identified, such cases should be referred to a human dermatologist. The veterinarian or wildlife biologist serves as a resource person for the human physician.

Zoonotic Potential for Clients

Schistosome cercarial dermatitis has a seasonal occurrence and is limited to humans exposed in infested lakes and ponds along flyways.

Treatment

Infected clients should be referred to a human dermatologist for treatment.

Prevention and Control Techniques

Observe posted warning notices that are usually posted around lakes, ponds, and streams frequented by migratory aquatic birds and infested with cercarial stages.

> **TECHNICIAN NOTE** Technicians must remember that every state has a practice act that prohibits them from giving medical (not veterinary) advice to clients. Clients exhibiting questionable lesions must always be referred to a physician. It is the veterinary professional's job to educate, but not to treat, humans.

CESTODES (TAPEWORMS) AND METACESTODES (LARVAL TAPEWORMS) OF ZOONOTIC IMPORTANCE

Cestodes are adult tapeworms, and metacestodes are the larval stages of tapeworms. These flatworms parasitize a wide variety of domesticated and wild animals. Adult cestodes are often associated with parasites of the intestinal tract; however, their larval stages may be found in a wide variety of extraintestinal sites. Cestodes usually can be diagnosed by finding characteristic gravid tapeworm proglottids filled with egg packets in the case of *Dipylidium caninum* or typical Taeniid-type ova (hexacanth embryos) in the cases of *Taenia, Multiceps,* or *Echinococcus* species.

> **TECHNICIAN NOTE** A **cestode** is the adult stage of a tapeworm usually found in the intestinal tract of the definitive host. Tapeworms are long and flattened parasites. The three basic parts of a tapeworm are the scolex, the neck, and the strobila. The strobila is composed of proglottids. A **metacestode** is the larval stage of a tapeworm that is usually found in an extraintestinal site (a site outside of the intestinal tract within the intermediate host). Several types of metacestode stages are known, including the cysticercoid, the cysticercus, the coenurus, the hydatid cyst, and the sparganum.

DIPYLIDIUM CANINUM (CUCUMBER SEED TAPEWORM, DOUBLE-PORED TAPEWORM)

- **Parasite's common name:** Double-pored tapeworm, or the cucumber seed tapeworm
- **Pronunciation:** "**Dip**-ah-**lid**-ee-yum" "kay-**nine**-num"
- **Derivation:** "Dipylos," from Greek, *having two entrances* (there are two genital pores); "**eidos**," from Greek, *form or shape* (in its form); "**canis**," from Latin, *dog*
- **Type of parasite:** platyhelminth—eucestode (true tapeworm [adult])

Species Affected

These common tapeworms are found in the small intestine of dogs, cats, and ferrets (Figure 14-5). Humans, especially small children, may also become infected with the adult tapeworm.

Key Clinical Signs of Infected Animals

Dogs and cats are most often asymptomatic but may be described by the owner as frequently dragging their anus

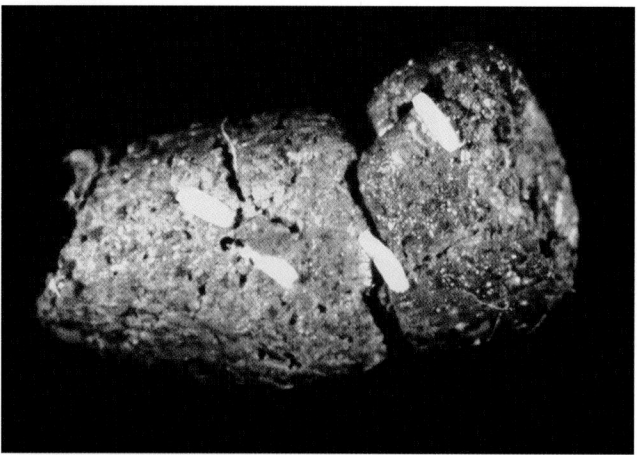

FIGURE 14-6 Segments of *Dipylidium caninum* on fresh dog feces.

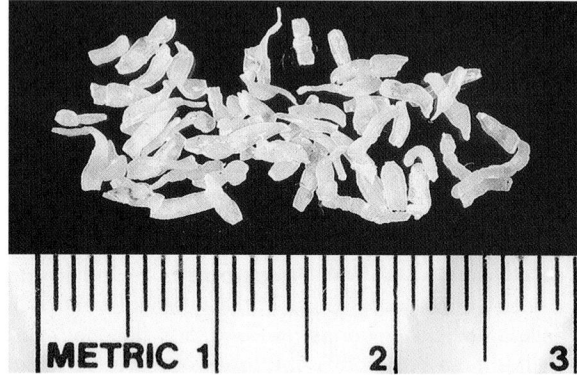

FIGURE 14-7 Dried segments of *Dipylidium caninum* from the bedding of a dog. (From Hendrix CM, Robinson E: Diagnostic parasitology for veterinary technicians, ed 4, St Louis, 2012, Mosby.)

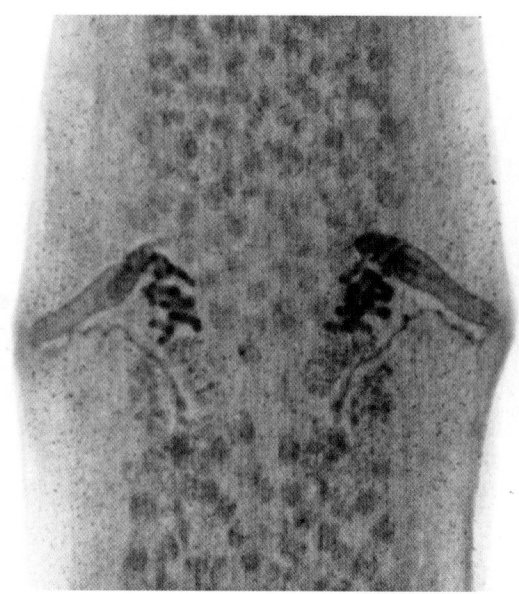

FIGURE 14-8 *Dipylidium caninum*, the double-pored tapeworm, possesses two sets of both male and female reproductive organs, located laterally, next to the two lateral genital pores.

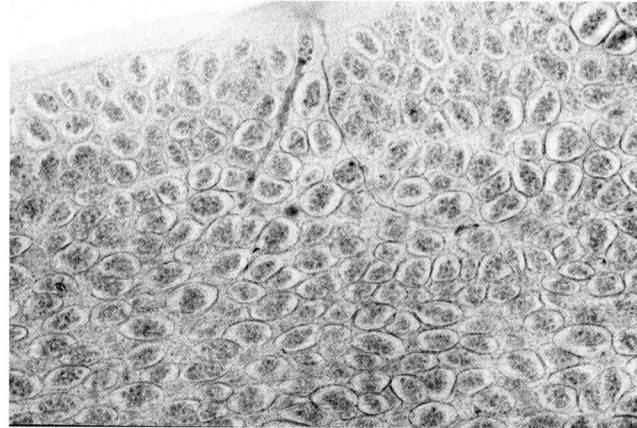

FIGURE 14-9 Microscopic view of a gravid proglottid of *Dipylidium caninum* containing thousands of egg packets.

along the ground as a result of pruritus. The most common sign is the presence of gravid tapeworm proglottids (tapeworm segments) in the feces (on top of or adjacent to the host's voided feces) (Figure 14-6) or around the anus of the infected host. Dried out tapeworm segments resembling dry uncooked white rice (Figure 14-7) may be found within the bedding of the pet or even on the owner's bed sheets, if the pet happens to sleep with the owner.

Abbreviated Life Cycle

Each mature and gravid proglottid of *Dipylidium caninum* possesses two sets of both male and female reproductive organs, located laterally, next to the two lateral genital pores (Figure 14-8).

> **TECHNICIAN NOTE** There are three types of **proglottids**: immature, mature, and gravid. Proglottids are arrayed in a chain-like manner (much like boxcars in a freight train). In this configuration, the immature (youngest) proglottids are closest to the scolex, and the gravid (oldest) proglottids are farthest from the scolex. Mature proglottids are located in the middle of the strobila.

Among tapeworm proglottids, both cross-fertilization and self-fertilization can occur. A mature proglottid has functioning male and female reproductive organs, but older, gravid proglottids contain a uterus filled to capacity with thousands of egg packets (Figure 14-9), each packet containing from 20 to 30 individual hexacanth (six-toothed) embryos (Figure 14-10). Owing to the expanding uterus, both sets of reproductive organs atrophy to the point that the only organ remaining in the segment is the uterus. Individual gravid proglottids are voided in the external environment in host feces, eventually rupturing and releasing egg packets, which in turn break open, releasing the individual hexacanth embryos.

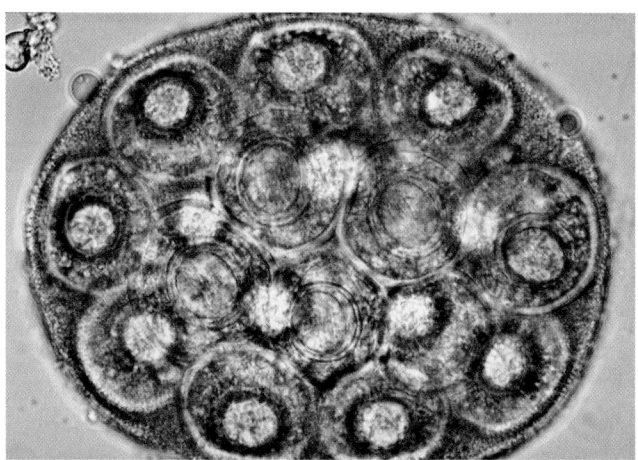

FIGURE 14-10 A single egg packet of *Dipylidium caninum* containing 20 to 30 individual hexacanth embryos.

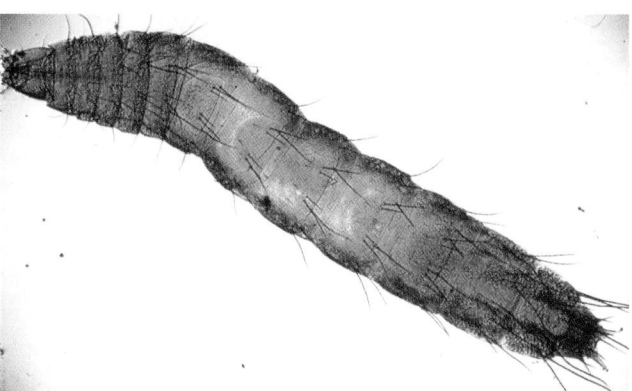

FIGURE 14-11 The maggot-like larval stage of *Ctenocephalides felis* ingests the egg packets and serves as the intermediate host for *Dipylidium caninum* (when it becomes an adult flea).

> **TECHNICIAN NOTE** An **egg packet** is the typical reproductive "offspring" produced by adult *D. caninum*, the cucumber seed or double-pored tapeworm of dogs and cats. Each egg packet consists of 20 to 30 hexacanth embryos surrounded by a thin envelope or eggshell. Thousands of egg packets are found within each gravid proglottid of *D. caninum*. Egg packets are discharged through either of the lateral genital pores of this tapeworm.

The hexacanth embryo is eaten by a maggot-like larval cat flea *Ctenocephalides felis* (Figure 14-11) (pronounced "ten-oh-cef-**al**-ah-dees" "**fee**-lis"), the intermediate host for this tapeworm. Within the larval cat flea, each ingested hexacanth embryo develops into a cysticercoid, the infective stage of the tapeworm (Figure 14-12).

> **TECHNICIAN NOTE** A **cysticercoid** is the infective stage of the tapeworm—an immature tapeworm scolex that is found within a small fluid-filled cavity or vesicle or bladder. Cysticercoids usually are found in invertebrates such as mites or fleas. A very common canine/feline tapeworm that utilizes the cysticercoid stage is *Dipylidium caninum*, the cucumber seed or double-pored tapeworm of dogs and cats.

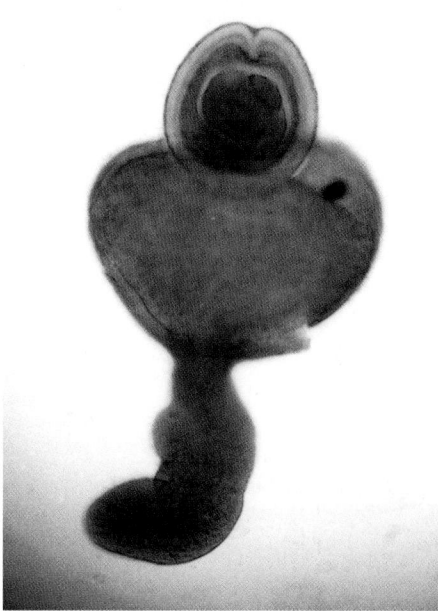

FIGURE 14-12 Cysticercoid, the infective stage of *Dipylidium caninum*, dissected from the flea intermediate host.

Each cysticercoid contains one immature tapeworm scolex that can grow and produce one adult tapeworm. The larval cat flea will continue its metamorphosis, developing through the pupal stage to the blood-feeding adult flea. Infective cysticercoids are found within the body of the adult flea. During the host's grooming process, the dog or cat ingests adult fleas containing cysticercoids. The flea is "digested," releasing the cysticercoids. The scolex within each cysticercoid attaches to the lining of the small intestine, and an entirely new tapeworm begins to grow, producing immature, mature, and gravid proglottids. For each cysticercoid that is ingested by a dog, cat, or child, one adult tapeworm will form.

Laboratory Test(s) Used to Diagnose the Infection

The veterinary technician should be able to identify both motile and dried proglottids of *D. caninum*. If the proglottid has dried out, it may be reconstituted with water to return to its former shape with typical features, the "cucumber seed tapeworm." The pair of characteristic, lateral genital pores gives it the common name of "double-pored tapeworm." (*Note*: *Dipylidium caninum* may be confused with *Taenia pisiformis* ["**tee**-nee-ah **pie**-sah-form-iss"] in the dog, and with *Taenia taeniaformis* ["**tee**-nee-ah" "**tee**-nee-ah-form-iss"] in the cat. *Taenia pisiformis* is commonly found in hunting dogs because the intermediate host is usually a rabbit or a hare. *T. taeniaeformis* is found in cats that frequently consume rodent intermediate hosts. These *Taenia* species of tapeworms have gravid proglottids, similar to those of *D. caninum*; however, each proglottid has only one set of male and female reproductive organs connecting to a single lateral genital pore [Figure 14-13].)

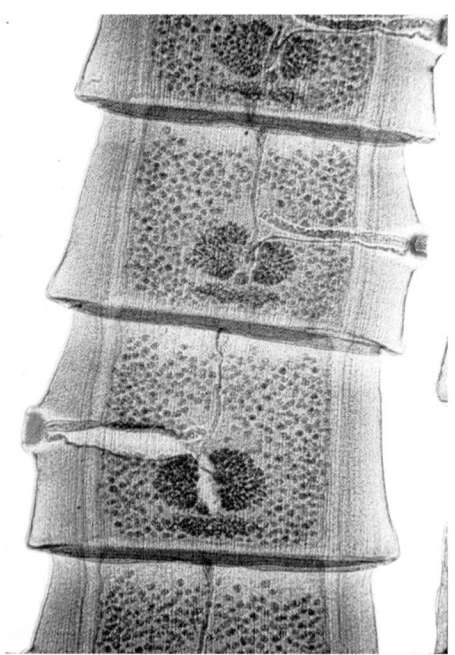

FIGURE 14-13 *Taenia pisiformis*, a canine taeniid, possesses a single set of both male and female reproductive organs, located laterally, next to the single lateral genital pores. Contrast with Figure 14-8.

If gravid proglottids of *D. caninum* are ruptured during defecation by the dog or cat, it may be possible to observe the egg packets on fecal flotation; however, this is a rare occurrence. Egg packets usually are observed when the veterinary technician teases a gravid proglottid open and observes the egg packets using a compound microscope.

Zoonotic Potential for Clients
If small children are in the home, clients should be warned of the zoonotic potential of this parasite. If a child ingests a flea containing the infective cysticercoid, it is possible for the child to harbor adult *D. caninum*. Such cases must be referred to a human physician or pediatrician.

Treatment
For *D. caninum*, praziquantel is the treatment of choice (only one treatment is required). Fenbendazole is effective against *Taenia* species, but not against *D. caninum*. Flea preventive and control techniques are necessary to prevent reinfection. All pets in the home environment must be treated for both tapeworms and fleas.

Prevention and Control Techniques
Administer anthelminthics routinely to all pets in the home environment. Flea populations in the home must be controlled.

> **TECHNICIAN NOTE** *Dipylidium caninum* is rarely diagnosed by examining a fecal sample. It is most commonly diagnosed through astute observation by the technician when obtaining a fecal sample and noticing and identifying the characteristic segments around the pet's anus.

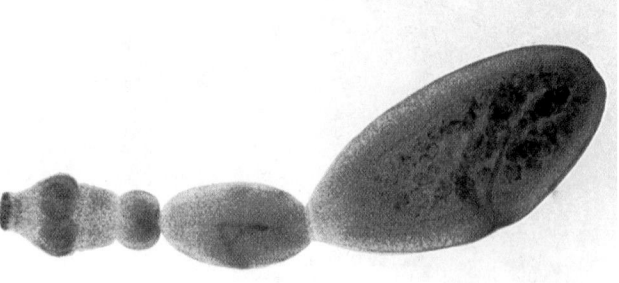

FIGURE 14-14 Tiny, adult tapeworm of *Echinococcus* species. Note that this tapeworm has only three proglottids—immature, mature, and gravid.

ECHINOCOCCUS GRANULOSUS/ ECHINOCOCCUS MULTILOCULARIS

- **Parasite's common name:** *Echinococcus granulosus*—the unilocular hydatid cyst tapeworm of dogs (adult tapeworm); *Echinococcus multilocularis*—the multilocular hydatid cyst tapeworm of cats and foxes (adult tapeworm)
- **Pronunciation:** "Ee-**kine**-oh-**cock**-us" "gran-you-**low**-sus"; "Ee-**kine**-oh-**cock**-us" "mull-tee-**lock**-you-**lair**-riss"
- **Derivation:** "Echino," from Greek, *a prickly husk*; "**coccus**," from Greek, *a berry*; "**granulo**," from Latin, *granules or grains*; "**Echino**," from Greek, *a prickly husk*; "**coccus**," from Greek, *a berry*; "**multi**," from Latin, *many or much*; "**loculus**," from Latin, *cell or cubicle*.
- **Type of parasite:** platyhelminth—eucestode (true tapeworm [adult])—hydatid cyst (metacestode)

Species Affected
For *Echinococcus granulosus*, the definitive hosts, primarily canids, harbor the adult stages of the tapeworm in the small intestine. The intermediate hosts, sheep and cattle, harbor the larval stage of the tapeworm, the unilocular hydatid cyst, in a variety of visceral organs (the liver, the lung, and the brain). For *Echinococcus multilocularis*, the definitive hosts, primarily cats and foxes, harbor the adult stages of the tapeworm. The intermediate hosts, microtine rodents (mice, voles, and rats), harbor the larval stage of the tapeworm, the multilocular hydatid cyst, in the liver and lung. Both *E. granulosus* and *E. multilocularis* are extremely important zoonotic parasites—humans are capable of serving as intermediate hosts for both species.

Key Clinical Signs of Infected Animals
Both species are extremely small tapeworms (approximately 2 to 8 mm) (Figure 14-14) and usually do not produce clinical signs in the canine or feline definitive host. This tapeworm's small innocuous size is not indicative of the severe pathology that its metacestode stages (larval stages) produce.

> **TECHNICIAN NOTE** A unilocular hydatid cyst is a type of metacestode/larval tapeworm that is closely associated with *Echinococcus granulosus*. The unilocular hydatid cyst consists of a large, spherical, fluid-filled vesicle or cyst enclosed by a thick, fibrous cyst wall, which is of host origin. The unilocular hydatid cyst has an innermost lining called a *germinal membrane*. The germinal membrane will bud off thousands of brood capsules. Each brood capsule produces many protoscolices within itself. When ingested by a suitable definitive host, each protoscolex will form one adult tapeworm.

The **unilocular hydatid cyst** for *E. granulosus* is a thick, fibrous cyst wall that contains a single, large, fluid-filled cyst lined by a thin germinal membrane that forms or buds off brood capsules that contain protoscolices. The **multilocular hydatid cyst** for *E. multilocularis* is a very thin cyst wall that contains highly invasive multi-compartmented fluid-filled cysts lined by a thin germinal membrane that forms or buds off brood capsules that contain protoscolices. Clinical signs in the intermediate host will vary from the animal being asymptomatic to having severe symptoms, depending on the organ or organ system in which the hydatid cysts develop.

> **TECHNICIAN NOTE** A multilocular hydatid cyst is a type of metacestode/larval tapeworm that is closely associated with *Echinococcus multilocularis*. The multilocular hydatid cyst consists of many, tiny, spherical, fluid-filled vesicles or cysts; however, these cysts are NOT enclosed by a thick, fibrous cyst wall of host origin, as in the case of *Echinococcus granulosus*.

Abbreviated Life Cycle

Adult tapeworms are found within the small intestine of the respective definitive host. Unlike most other tapeworms, these tiny tapeworms have only a scolex plus three segments: immature, mature, and gravid proglottids. The hermaphroditic flukes produce eggs ("typical Taeniid-type ova"). The eggs have a thick, striated cyst wall and contain a hexacanth (six-toothed) embryo (Figure 14-15).

> **TECHNICIAN NOTE** Hexacanth embryos are tapeworm eggs that usually are produced by Taeniid-type tapeworms—*Taenia*, *Multiceps*, and *Echinococcus* species. They have a striated eggshell, called an *embryophore*, and contain an embryo with six tiny teeth on the inside, hence the six-toothed or hexacanth embryo. These eggs are also referred to as *typical Taeniid-type eggs*.

The ova pass in the feces to the outside environment. A suitable intermediate host (e.g., sheep for *E. granulosus* and mouse for *E. multilocularis*) must ingest the ovum. For every ovum that is ingested by a suitable intermediate host, one hydatid cyst will form. The host reaction to the presence of an entire unilocular hydatid cyst due to *E. granulosus* is the deposition of a thick cyst wall to encase that cyst. With *E.*

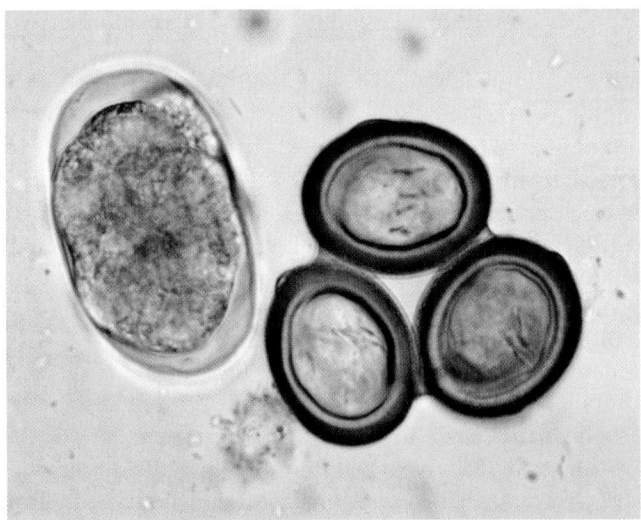

FIGURE 14-15 Typical taeniid-type eggs of *Echinococcus* species. They have a striated embryophore (eggshell) with a single hexacanth (six-toothed) embryo inside. This tapeworm's typical taeniid-type eggs are identical to those of *Taenia* species and *Multiceps* species.

multilocularis, no similar cyst wall is produced, allowing daughter cysts to form outside of the original mother cyst. Daughter cysts will produce granddaughter cysts, granddaughter cysts will produce great granddaughter cysts, and so forth. This type of external budding associated with *E. multilocularis* can go on indefinitely, and without the cyst wall to contain it, the cyst will become invasive, destroying normal host tissues. The host eventually will die, and the hydatid cyst must be ingested by the definitive host. For every protoscolex within the hydatid cyst that is ingested by the definitive host, one adult tapeworm will develop in the small intestine of that host.

Laboratory Test(s) Used to Diagnose the Infection

Identification of adult tapeworms or their proglottids in the definitive host is difficult owing to their extremely small size. Routine fecal examinations do not allow for distinction of *Echinococcus* species from other tapeworm eggs (*Taenia* or *Multiceps* species). A commercial enzyme-linked immunosorbent assay (ELISA) is available.

Zoonotic Potential for Clients

For *E. granulosus*, this tapeworm is most prevalent in areas where sheep are raised. The most common source of human infection is contact with an infected dog (improper handwashing after handling of dog feces). On sheep farms, lack of regular preventive anthelmintic therapy for dogs living on the premises allows them to become infected by consuming infected sheep viscera containing unilocular hydatid cysts. In the United States, most cases of human echinococcosis are seen in immigrants from geographic areas in which cystic echinococcosis is endemic. *E. multilocularis* is found in areas where foxes and wild rodents are plentiful and is often seen in outdoor cats that feed on infected rodents. These parasites are seen in a region extending from eastern Montana to central Ohio, as well as in Alaska and throughout Canada. Most human cases have been found in Alaskan tribes of Native Americans.

Treatment

In dogs, praziquantel is the preferred treatment followed by confinement for 48 hours to collect and destroy feces containing infective eggs. In ruminants, surgical excision of hydatid cysts can be performed followed by long-term albendazole treatment. Owing to the large numbers of wild rodents, therapy is not attempted in these hosts.

Prevention and Control Techniques

Do not feed sheep viscera to dogs or give them access to sheep carcasses. Discourage predation on wild rodents. Test and treat all dogs to eliminate adult tapeworms, especially those that are in frequent contact with sheep. Consider use of vaccination for E. granulosus in sheep. Use proper hygiene when handling dogs, cats, and foxes. Put fences around vegetable gardens to keep these animals away.

> **TECHNICIAN NOTE** *Echinococcus* species are parasites that should be reported to state and federal authorities if an outbreak is suspected. The other reportable parasites are *Cochliomyia hominivorax, Psoroptes* species of large animals (the scabies mite), and *Boophilus annulatus,* the Texas cattle fever tick. The knowledgeable and observant veterinarian and his or her technician serve as the first line of defense against these important reportable parasites.

SPIROMETRA MANSONOIDES

- **Parasite's common name:** "Zipper tapeworm," or the "sparganosis" tapeworm
- **Pronunciation:** "Spy-row-**meet**-tra" "man-sun-**oid**-ees"
- **Derivation: "Spiro,"** from Greek, *coil* (coiled); **"metra,"** from Greek, *womb* (coiled uterus); **"manson,"** *after Sir Patrick Manson, British physician;* **"eidos,"** from Greek, *form.*
- **Type of parasite:** platyhelminth—cotyloda (pseudotapeworm [adult])/metacestode stage (sparganum)

Species Affected

These adult tapeworms are found in the small intestine of both dogs and cats. The first intermediate hosts, crustaceans, harbor the first metacestode (larval) stage, the **procercoid** stage.

> **TECHNICIAN NOTE** The procercoid stage is the developmental stage that parasitizes the first intermediate host in the life cycle of a pseudotapeworm. This host is usually an aquatic crustacean. The first intermediate host containing the procercoid stage must be ingested by the second intermediate host. After ingestion, the procercoid will develop into the plerocercoid/sparganum stage within the tissues of the second intermediate host.

The second intermediate hosts—amphibians, other reptiles, and small mammals including the dog—harbor the second metacestode stage—the **plerocercoid** or **sparganum** stage. Humans are also capable of harboring the plerocercoid stage, producing a condition known as **sparganosis.**

> **TECHNICIAN NOTE** In the life cycle of a pseudotapeworm, the plerocercoid/sparganum stage is the infective developmental stage that parasitizes the second intermediate host in the life cycle of a pseudotapeworm. The plerocercoid/sparganum stage is a solid-bodied metacestode stage that possesses a deeply invaginated acetabular scolex. In the life cycle of *Spirometra mansonoides,* in some second intermediate hosts, the plerocercoid stage is capable of undergoing uninterrupted asexual multiplication. Infection with the plerocercoid/sparganum stage is referred to as *sparganosis.*

Location of Parasite Within Hosts

Adult tapeworms are found within the small intestine of the canine or feline definitive host. The plerocercoid stage or sparganum may be found subcutaneously or intramuscularly within the second intermediate host.

Key Clinical Signs of Infected Animals

Adult tapeworms produce very little pathology (nonspecific gastrointestinal signs). If the metacestode form of this adult tapeworm infects the dog or cat, a single sparganum usually is produced subcutaneously, resulting in very little pathology. If this sparganum begins to multiply asexually, fatal results may ensue (proliferative sparganosis) (see "Abbreviated Life Cycle").

Abbreviated Life Cycle

Adult **pseudotapeworm**s (in this case *Spirometra*) are found in the small intestine of the canine or feline definitive host. This tapeworm is called the "zipper tapeworm" because the proglottids may divide in the middle of the tapeworm and then reunite—much like a zipper coming unzipped. Proglottids seldom break off of this tapeworm's strobila, instead operculated eggs (Figure 14-16) exit the centrally located uterus through the associated uterine pore. Upon contact with water, these operculated eggs "hatch," releasing a motile, ciliated hexacanth embryo stage, the coracidium. The coracidium is covered with tiny moving hairs and spins about in the water. This developmental stage must be ingested by the first intermediate host, a microscopic aquatic crustacean. Within the crustacean, the coracidium develops into the next metacestode stage, the procercoid. In turn, the crustacean is ingested by the second intermediate host, an amphibian (frog), a reptile (snake), or a small mammal (mouse). Within that second intermediate host, the procercoid stage develops into the next metacestode stage, the plerocercoid stage or sparganum, which may be found entwined within the subcutaneous tissues or within the musculature. The canine or feline definitive host becomes infected by ingesting the

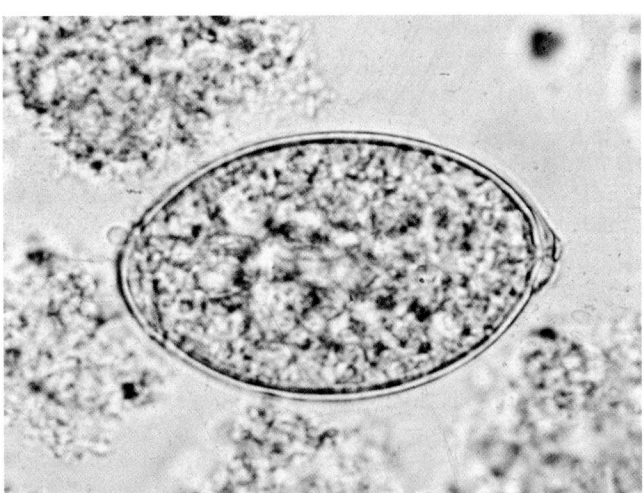

FIGURE 14-16 Operculated egg of pseudotapeworm, *Spirometra mansonoides*, the zipper tapeworm.

second intermediate host containing the plerocercoid stage/sparganum. Within the host's small intestine, the plerocercoid/sparganum emerges from its tissue sites and attaches to the mucosa of the stomach, and a new tapeworm begins to grow. (*Note*: If a dog ingests the aquatic crustacean containing the procercoid or the second intermediate host containing the plerocercoid/sparganum, the plerocercoid/sparganum may migrate to the dog's subcutaneous tissues or muscles. In these sites, the plerocercoid/sparganum may undergo uncontrolled multiplicative asexual reproduction [i.e., one plerocercoid/sparganum becomes two plerocercoids/spargana, two plerocercoids/spargana become four plerocercoids/spargana, four become eight, eight become sixteen, and so on] to the point that these plerocercoids/spargana multiply throughout the dog's body, causing a fatal condition known as *proliferative sparganosis*—the spargana literally overtake the host's body. This condition has been reported in humans also and is a severe zoonotic condition.)

Laboratory Test(s) Used to Diagnose the Infection

Fecal flotation may reveal an operculated egg, which is the characteristic egg type produced by a pseudotapeworm. This egg is very similar in form to that of a digenetic trematode.

Zoonotic Potential for Clients

Humans can become infected in one of three ways. First, humans may become infected by drinking water containing the copepod first intermediate host, which contains the procercoid stage. Humans then would serve as the second intermediate host containing the plerocercoid stage in the human's subcutaneous tissues. Humans also may become infected by ingesting the second intermediate host (e.g., a frog), which contains the plerocercoid stage. This would occur only if humans ate a raw frog. The plerocercoid would migrate to and infest the human's subcutaneous tissues. Finally, human infection could occur if a poultice made from

an infected second intermediate host (e.g., a frog), which contains the plerocercoid or sparganum stage, were applied to a human's open wound. The sparganum could migrate from the frog's tissues to the human's tissues and produce a subcutaneous sparganum.

Treatment

Praziquantel is the anthelminthic of choice for the adult stage of *S. mansonoides*. If spargana are found antemortem in the subcutaneous tissues of a cat or dog, they may be surgically removed from the tissues. No treatment is known for proliferative sparganosis in dogs.

Prevention and Control Techniques

Dogs and cats should be prevented from roaming and drinking water from infected lakes, streams, or ponds. In addition, predation and carrion consumption should be prevented.

> **TECHNICIAN NOTE** Whenever single operculated eggs are observed on fecal flotation, a technician may erroneously conclude that the dog or cat is infected with a digenetic trematode. This most often is not the case. The presence of single operculated eggs on fecal flotation usually means that the dog or cat is infected with *Spirometra mansonoides*.

NEMATODES—ROUNDWORMS OF ZOONOTIC IMPORTANCE

Nematodes are colloquially referred to as *roundworms* because of a unique feature—they are round when observed on cross-section. Nematodes come in all shapes (from cylindrical to round) and sizes (from the tiny *Strongyloides stercoralis* to the giant kidney worm, *Dioctophyma renale*). Roundworms are capable of parasitizing the widest assortment of domesticated and wild animals and are found in a variety of body organs and systems. Nematodes can be found in the gastrointestinal tract, the circulatory system, the respiratory tract, the urogenital system, and the eye. In fact, these parasites can be found throughout the bodies of many of our domesticated animals. These roundworms usually are diagnosed by finding characteristic eggs on fecal flotation, or microfilariae on examination of peripheral blood smears, by the use of ELISA tests, by observation of unique larval stages in tracheal or bronchial washes, or through a variety of other techniques. Knowledge of their complex life cycles is an essential component of veterinary clinical practice.

> **TECHNICIAN NOTE** A nematode is a roundworm. These parasites are called "roundworms" because they are round in cross-section. Many types of roundworms are associated with both dogs and cats. Some common species of canine nematodes are *Toxocara canis*, *Ancylostoma caninum*, *Trichuris vulpis*, and *Dirofilaria immitis*. Some common species of feline nematodes are *Toxocara cati*, *Ancylostoma tubaeforme*, and *Dirofilaria immitis*.

TOXOCARA CANIS, TOXOCARA CATI, AND TOXASCARIS LEONINA (ASCARIDS AND ROUNDWORMS)—VISCERAL LARVA MIGRANS AND OCULAR LARVA MIGRANS

- **Parasite's common name:** canine ascarid/roundworm; feline ascarid/roundworm; and canine and feline ascarid/roundworm
- **Pronunciation:** "**Tocks**-oh-care-ah" "**kay**-niss"; "**Tocks**-oh-care-ah" "**cat**-eye"; "**Tocks**-ass-care-riss" "**lee**-oh-**nine**-ah"
- **Derivation:** "**Toxon,**" from Greek, *a bow* (shaped like a bow or quiver); "**caro,**" from Latin, *flesh*; (infecting flesh-eating mammals); "**canis,**" from Latin, *a dog or hound* (infecting dogs); "**catus,**" from Latin, *the domestic house-cat* (infecting cats); "**toxon,**" from Greek, *a bow* (shaped like a bow or quiver); "**askaris,**" from Greek, *a worm*; "**leonine,**" from Greek, *a lion*
- **Type of parasite:** nematode (roundworm)—ascarid (roundworm)

Species Affected

Adult *Toxocara canis* and *Toxocara cati* are found in the small intestine of dogs and cats, respectively (Figure 14-17). Adult *Toxascaris leonina* are found in the small intestine of dogs and cats. The life cycle of these roundworms is varied and very often these worms may use a variety of mammals as paratenic or transport hosts. A paratenic or transport host is a host in which a parasite does not undergo further development, but in which it remains encysted or in "suspended animation," serving as a source of the definitive host when the definitive host ingests the paratenic host. For example, rats and mice may eat infective eggs of *T. canis*. In these atypical hosts, the infective second stage larva will hatch from the egg and will migrate to some extraintestinal tissue site. At this site, the second stage larva will encyst or rest. If this mouse is ingested by a dog, the larva will excyst in the intestine of the dog and will continue its development to the adult stage in the canine definitive host. When humans act as paratenic hosts, the conditions that result from this infection are known as **visceral larva migrans** (VLM) and *ocular larva migrans* (OLM). These zoonoses most often are associated with the canine ascarid, *T. canis*.

Key Clinical Signs of Infected Animals

T. canis in young puppies most commonly causes diarrhea, vomiting, and an enlarged abdomen. Other signs are constipation, flatulence, and poor growth rate. Clinical signs are not as common in adult dogs but most frequently include diarrhea. *T. cati* infections in young kittens are often asymptomatic, but heavy infections can cause diarrhea, abdominal distention, rough hair coat, and dehydration. Adult cats tend to be asymptomatic. *T. leonina* causes similar signs in kittens and puppies.

Abbreviated Life Cycle

Among these three parasites, the life cycles differ greatly. For the purpose of expediency, only the life cycle of *T. canis* will be discussed here. Adult male and female ascarids are found in the small intestine of the canine host. After copulation, the female produces unembryonated eggs that pass into the external environment in the dog's feces. Under environmental conditions of warmth and humidity, the ascarid egg will begin to embryonate (its dark central mass will begin to divide), until eventually a first stage larva may be found within the ascarid egg. While in the egg, this larva will moult (shed its cuticle or skin) and develop into the second stage larva (Figure 14-18). It is this stage (the egg containing the second stage larva) that is infective for the canine host. A dog must ingest this egg for the life cycle to continue. For a dog younger than 3 months, the larva will hatch in the small intestine, get into the bloodstream, and migrate through the liver and get into the lungs. In the lungs, the developing larva is coughed up and swallowed and eventually returns back to the small intestine, where it eventually matures to the adult stage. (*Note:* This whole series of events is known as *tracheal migration.*) For a dog older than 3 months, the larva will hatch in the small intestine and get into the bloodstream, but it will be carried to somatic sites (e.g., muscles, kidney, mammary gland) throughout the dog's body and become an encysted second stage larva in these extraintestinal sites. At these sites, the encysted larva

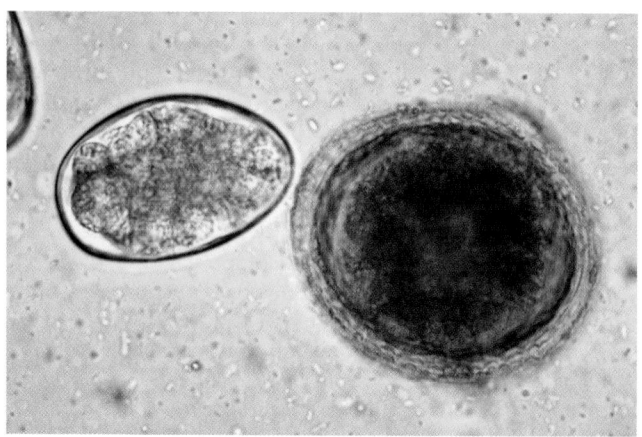

FIGURE 14-17 Unembryonated egg of *Toxocara canis (right)*. Note round silhouette, rough eggshell, and dark pigmented central egg mass.

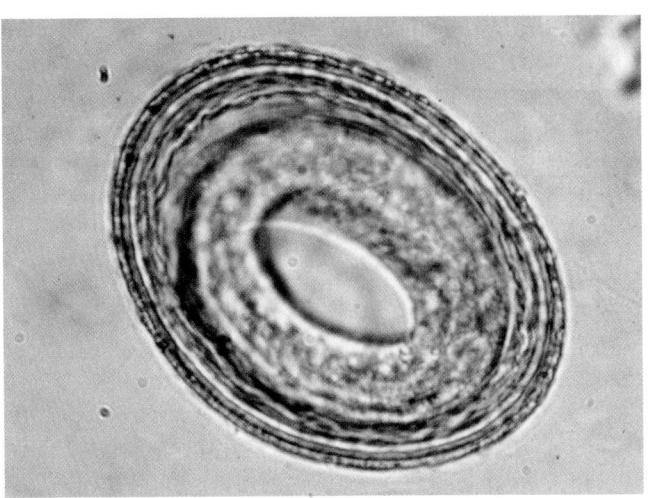

FIGURE 14-18 Infective stage of *Toxocara canis*—an egg containing a second stage larva. This stage is infective for the canine host.

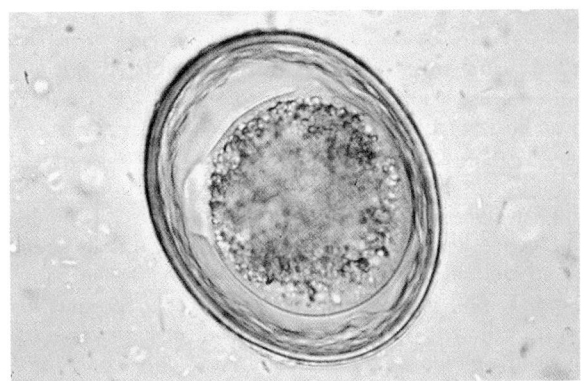

FIGURE 14-19 Unembryonated egg of *Toxascaris leonina*. Note oval silhouette, smooth eggshell, and hyaline (glass-like) central egg mass.

undergoes no further development—it is "sleeping" or in suspended animation, or it is in a state of arrested development (**hypobiosis**). (*Note:* This whole series of events is known as *somatic migration.*)

> **TECHNICIAN NOTE** **Hypobiosis** is a life cycle term that means, "being in suspended animation" or "undergoing arrested development." For example, in the life cycle of *Toxocara canis*, the migrating larvae will not undergo development past the second stage larva until they are ingested by a suitable canine de*finitive host.* These larvae are said to be undergoing hypobiosis or are hypobiotic.

If a female dog older than 3 months ingests the egg containing the second stage larva, the migrating larval stage follows the somatic migration route and becomes encysted within the extraintestinal tissues. During the height of pregnancy, this larva will migrate from the mother to a developing fetus, where it will reside in the liver. Soon after birth, the larva will migrate from the liver to the lungs, where it will be coughed up and swallowed to return to the small intestine to mature to the adult stage. This whole series of development uses somatic migration in the dam and tracheal migration in the puppy. Alternatively, the migrating larva may encyst within the mammary gland (again, somatic migration). During lactation, the encysted larva may become activated and may be passed to the puppy in the milk. This larva develops directly to the adult stage within the puppy's small intestine (somatic migration in the pregnant female, no migration at all in the puppy). Finally, if the egg containing the second stage larva is ingested by a mouse (a paratenic host), the migrating larval stage follows the somatic migration route and becomes encysted within the mouse's extraintestinal tissues. If a dog ingests the mouse paratenic host, the encysted larva will escape and grow to an adult in the small intestine (somatic migration in the mouse paratenic host, no migration at all in the dog that ate the mouse).

Laboratory Test(s) Used to Diagnose the Infection

Ascarid infections in dogs and cats usually are diagnosed using fecal centrifugation/flotation techniques and proper identification of unique egg types (Figures 14-17 and 14-19).

Zoonotic Potential for Clients

These parasites can produce two serious zoonotic conditions known as *VLM* and *OLM*. Young children living in close proximity with kittens or puppies are at risk, especially if they ingest ascarid eggs containing infective second stage larvae. To get either of these conditions, a child must ingest the ascarid egg containing the infective second stage larva (known as *transmission by the fecal-oral route*). After ingestion, the larva undergoes extensive migration through the liver or lung (in the case of VLM) or eye (in the case of OLM) within the child, as if the child were a paratenic host. Parents should be warned to use caution regarding uncovered sandboxes, playgrounds contaminated with dog/cat feces, or other sites where these infective eggs might be picked up and ingested by the child. Dogs or puppies and kittens that are not on a parasite preventive agent can serve as reservoirs for infection.

Treatment

Commonly used anthelminthics include pyrantel and fenbendazole, as well as most monthly heartworm preventive agents such as moxidectin and milbemycin oxime. Selamectin is also approved for use in cats and kittens for this purpose. Begin deworming puppies and kittens at 2 weeks of age, repeating at 2-week intervals to eliminate shedding of *Toxocara* eggs. Deworming dams (or maintaining them on proper monthly heartworm/anthelmintic preventives) before breeding is another important preventive measure. The Companion Animal Parasite Council (CAPC) recommends year-round treatment of all dogs and cats with broad-spectrum heartworm anthelminthics that also have activity against parasites with zoonotic potential.

> **TECHNICIAN NOTE**   **Visceral larva migrans (VLM) and ocular larva migrans (OLM)** are terms that describe zoonotic conditions caused by the ingestion of an egg containing an infective second stage larva of a roundworm (usually *Toxocara canis*). These larvae will hatch from their eggs and migrate from the host's intestine and travel throughout the visceral organs, usually the liver and/or the lung. Visceral larva migrans is usually seen in young children who have ingested these infective eggs of *T. canis*. The infected human serves as a paratenic or transport host for *T. canis*. When liver or lung tissues are involved in the migration pathway, the condition is described as *visceral larva migrans*. When the orbit (eye) is involved in the migration pathway, the condition is described as *ocular larva migrans*. *T. canis* is capable of producing both visceral larva migrans and ocular larva migrans in human beings.

Prevention and Control Techniques

Daily removal of feces and cleaning of kennels is essential in preventing *Toxocara* infection. Sandboxes should be covered when not in use. Furthermore, humans can prevent VLM and OLM by having pets strategically dewormed, removing feces from the environment, enforcing leash laws and collection of feces by owners, practicing proper hygiene, discouraging pica in children, and teaching them the importance of handwashing.

> **TECHNICIAN NOTE**   Ascarids should be considered in any puppy or kitten presenting with gastrointestinal signs. Remember that obtaining an adequate fecal sample is key to a definitive diagnosis by identifying the eggs in that sample. Consider routinely deworming all puppies and kittens that are not on monthly preventive agents, and always warn clients of the zoonotic potential of this parasite, particularly those owners with young children.

BAYLISASCARIS PROCYONIS—NEUROLOGIC LARVA MIGRANS

- **Parasite's common name:** raccoon ascarid
- **Pronunciation:** "Bay-liss-**ass**-care-riss" "pro-sigh-**own**-niss"
- **Derivation:** "**Baylis,**" named after renowned British parasitologist, H.A. Baylis; "**askaris,**" from Greek, *a worm*; **Procyonidae** is a New World family of the order Carnivora. It includes raccoons, coatis, kinkajous, olingos, ringtails, and cacomistles.
- **Type of parasite:** nematode (roundworm)—ascarid (roundworm)

Species Affected

Raccoons, but may also be found on occasion in dogs.

Location of Parasite Within Host

Similar to the ascarids of dogs and cats, adult *Baylisascaris procyonis* may be found within the small intestine of the raccoon definitive host. Just as *T. canis* is associated with VLM and OLM in humans, *B. procyonis* produces a condition called *neurologic larva migrans*, in which the larval stage of this ascarid migrates through neural tissues (e.g., brain and spinal cord) of any mammalian or avian paratenic host that may have happened to ingest an egg containing an infective second stage larva.

Key Clinical Signs of Infected Animals

Baylisascaris procyonis (raccoon roundworm) is a common parasite of raccoons that is similar to *Toxocara* species of dogs and cats; however, it typically does not cause clinical disease in dogs or cats. Adult *B. procyonis* produces little pathology in the small intestine of the definitive host (the raccoon). This nematode produces significant pathology in any animal that might ingest the infective stage of this parasite, an egg containing a second stage larva. These larvae are capable of migrating through the intestinal wall of the paratenic host and then migrating through the brain and other neural tissues such as the spinal cord. Such migration will produce severe neurologic signs and even death.

Abbreviated Life Cycle

Adult male and female *B. procyonis* are found in the small intestine of the definitive host. After copulation, the female parasite will produce unembryonated eggs. These eggs will pass into the external environment in raccoon feces. Under environmental conditions of warmth and humidity, the ascarid egg will begin to embryonate (its dark central mass will begin to divide), until eventually a first stage larva may be found within the ascarid egg. While in the egg, this larva will moult (shed its cuticle or skin) and develop into the second stage larva. It is this stage (the egg containing the second stage larva) that is infective for the definitive host. A raccoon must ingest this egg for the life cycle to continue in its normal manner, ending with adult ascarids being found in the raccoon's small intestine. If a mammalian or avian paratenic host ingests the egg containing the second stage larva, the larval stages migrate through neural tissues (e.g., brain and spinal cord). This paratenic host becomes a dead-end host in that it usually succumbs to this highly pathogenic zoonotic parasite.

Laboratory Test(s) Used to Diagnose the Infection

B. procyonis may be diagnosed in the definitive host using routine fecal flotation.

Zoonotic Potential for Clients

Should a child ingest the *B. procyonis* egg containing the infective second stage larva, a condition similar to VLM or OLM may result; however, the condition specific to this parasite, **neurologic larva migrans**, involves migration of larval stages through the brain and spinal cord of the child, an almost certainly fatal condition.

Neurologic larva migrans is a term that describes a zoonotic condition caused by the ingestion of an egg containing an infective second stage larva of the roundworm *Baylisascaris procyonis*, commonly referred to as the "raccoon ascarid." This zoonotic parasite produces an egg, which if allowed to embryonate to the degree that it contains an infective second stage larva, and which if ingested by almost any mammalian or avian host, the larva will hatch from the egg in the host's intestine and migrate extensively through the host's central nervous system, usually the brain and spinal cord.

Treatment

Keeping raccoons as pets or as captives is not recommended; therefore, treatment is not encouraged. If dogs or cats become infected with the adult *B. procyonis*, the same treatment as for *Toxocara* species is indicated.

Prevention and Control Techniques

For *B. procyonis* in areas where raccoons are prevalent, maintaining the home environment so that raccoons are discouraged from visiting is the best preventive measure (securing areas that commonly attract raccoons such as garbage cans, outdoor cat food containers, and open basements).

Keeping raccoons or other wild animals as household pets or captive fauna, particularly when small children are in the home, should be strongly discouraged.

ANCYLOSTOMA CANINUM, ANCYLOSTOMA BRAZILIENSE, AND ANCYLOSTOMA TUBAEFORME; UNCINARIA STENOCEPHALA (HOOKWORMS)—CUTANEOUS LARVA MIGRANS (CREEPING ERUPTION, PLUMBER'S ITCH, SANDWORMS)

- Parasite's common name: hookworm
- Pronunciation: "An-sea-los-**toe**-mah" "kay-**nine**-num"; "An-sea-los-**toe**-mah" "brazil-ee-**inn**-sea"; "An-sea-los-**toe**-mah" "two-buh-**four**-me"; "Un-sin-**air**-ee-ah" "sten-oh-**cef**-ah-lah"
- Derivation: "**Ankylo**," from Greek, *bent or crooked* (anterior end curves dorsally); "**stomas**," from Greek, *mouth* (this parasite has a large buccal cavity or mouth); "**canis**," from Latin, *a dog or hound*; "**braziliense**," *pertaining to Brazil*; "**tuba**," from Latin, *a trumpet*; "**forma**," from Latin, *form*; "**Uncus**," from Latin, *hook* (anterior end curves dorsally); "**stenos**," from Greek, *narrow* (this parasite has a narrow buccal cavity or mouth); "**kephale**," from Greek, *head*.
- Type of parasite: nematode (roundworm)—hookworm

Species Affected

These hookworms are found in the small intestine of dogs and cats (Figure 14-20). As a group, hookworms may produce

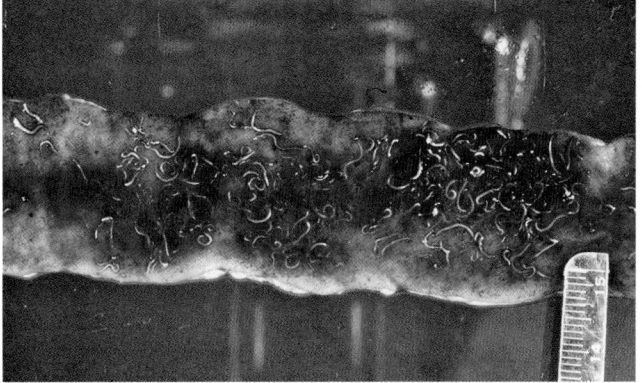

FIGURE 14-20 Adult *Ancylostoma caninum* in the small intestine of a dog.

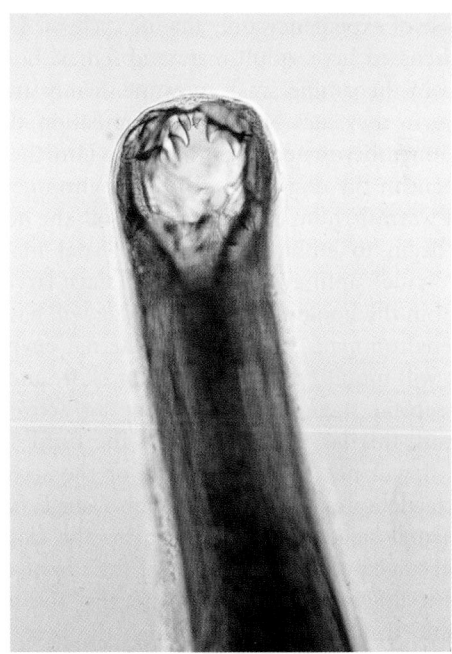

FIGURE 14-21 Anterior end of adult *Ancylostoma caninum*. Note three pairs of ventral teeth and the large buccal cavity.

a zoonotic condition in humans known as ***cutaneous larva migrans* (CLM)**.

Cutaneous larva migrans is a zoonotic skin condition that occurs when an infective third stage larva of a hookworm (usually *Ancylostoma braziliense*) penetrates the skin of a human being and travels within superficial layers of the epidermis, producing highly pruritic, serpentine (twisting) tracts in the skin. Common names for this skin condition include *sandworms*, *creeping eruption*, and *plumber's itch*.

Key Clinical Signs of Infected Animals

Canine hookworms are voracious blood feeders owing to their unique teeth and their large buccal cavity (Figure 14-21). Pale mucous membranes and hydremia (watery blood) may be seen, signaling anemia, particularly in young puppies. Diarrhea may also be observed—blood-tinged or black and tarry. Chronic infections may lead to puppies that are underweight and have a distended abdomen, poor hair coat, and inappetence. Although *Ancylostoma braziliense* causes only mild diarrhea and gastrointestinal upset, this is a significant hookworm because it is the primary cause of CLM, or creeping eruption, in man. With *Ancylostoma tubaeforme*, cats are often asymptomatic unless heavily infected and then may demonstrate regenerative anemia and weight loss. *Uncinaria stenocephala* causes signs similar to those of *Ancylostoma caninum*, but with dermatitis as a result of larval migration in the skin.

Abbreviated Life Cycle

Among these four parasites, the life cycles differ greatly. For the purpose of expediency, only the life cycle of *A. caninum* will be discussed here. Adult male and female hookworms are found in the canine small intestine, firmly attached to the mucosa as they suck blood. After copulation, the female produces unembryonated eggs that pass into the external environment in the dog's feces. Under environmental conditions of warmth, humidity, and moist soil, the hookworm egg will begin to embryonate (the internal morula will begin to divide) until eventually a first stage larva may be found within the hookworm egg. This egg will hatch in the external environment. While in the external environment, this larva will moult (shed its cuticle or skin) and develop into the second stage larva. It will be an active, feeding larva. Again, this larva will moult to the third stage, but this time it will not shed the cuticle of the second stage larva. Instead, it is an ensheathed third stage larva—the developmental stage that is infective for the canine host. This larval stage penetrates the skin of the canine definitive host. For a dog younger than 3 months, the larva will migrate into the bloodstream, through the liver, and into the lungs. In the lungs, the developing larva is coughed up and swallowed and eventually returns back to the small intestine, where it eventually matures to the adult hookworm. (*Note*: This whole series of events is known as *tracheal migration*.) For a dog older than 3 months, the larva will migrate into the bloodstream and will travel to assorted somatic sites (e.g., muscles, kidney, mammary gland) throughout the dog's body and become an encysted second stage in these extraintestinal sites. In these sites, the encysted larva undergoes no further development—it is "sleeping" or in suspended animation, or it is in a state of arrested development (hypobiosis). (*Note*: This whole series of events is known as *somatic migration*.) If the infective larva penetrates the skin of a female dog older than 3 months, the migrating larval stage follows the somatic migration route and becomes encysted within the extraintestinal tissues. During the height of pregnancy, these larvae will migrate from the dam to the developing fetuses, where they will reside in the liver.

Soon after birth, the larvae will migrate from the liver to the lungs, where they will be coughed up and swallowed to return to the small intestine to mature to the adult stage. This whole series of development uses somatic migration in the dam and tracheal migration in the puppy; however, this is a rare sequence of events in the life cycle of the canine hookworm. More commonly, the migrating larva may become encysted within the mammary gland (again, somatic migration). During lactation, the encysted larva may become activated and may be passed to the puppy in the milk. These larvae develop directly to the adult stage within the puppy's small intestine (somatic migration in the pregnant female, no migration at all in the puppy). If the infective larva penetrates the skin of a mouse (a paratenic host), the migrating larval stage follows the somatic migration route and becomes encysted within the mouse's extraintestinal tissues. If a dog ingests the mouse paratenic host, the encysted larva will escape and grow to an adult in the small intestine (somatic migration in the mouse paratenic host, no migration at all in the dog that ate the mouse).

Laboratory Test(s) Used to Diagnose the Infection

Fecal centrifugation/flotation of fresh feces and egg identification (Figure 14-22).

Zoonotic Potential for Clients

Canine hookworms (especially *A. braziliense*) are zoonotic parasites. If an infective hookworm larva penetrates the skin of a human, the migrating larval stage will produce a zoonotic skin condition known as *CLM* (a.k.a. creeping eruption, sandworms, plumber's itch) (Figure 14-23). Skin penetration can occur on contact, so walking barefoot will predispose humans to infection. This condition is typified by raised, erythematous, pruritic, tortuous tracts in the skin. The public health significance must be considered, especially in households with an infected puppy or kitten and young children. This is a similar environmental scenario to that of *T. canis* and the other ascarid infections.

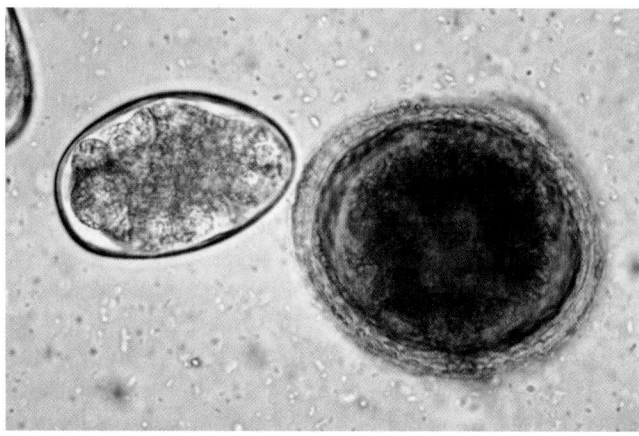

FIGURE 14-22 Unembryonated egg of *Ancylostoma caninum* (left). Note eight-cell morula within smooth oval eggshell.

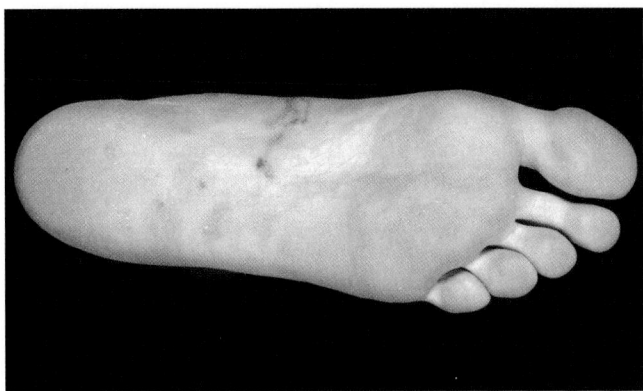

FIGURE 14-23 Cutaneous larva migrans due to *Ancylostoma braziliense* in the sole of a man's foot. This zoonotic skin condition is also known as *creeping eruption, sandworms,* or *plumber's itch.*

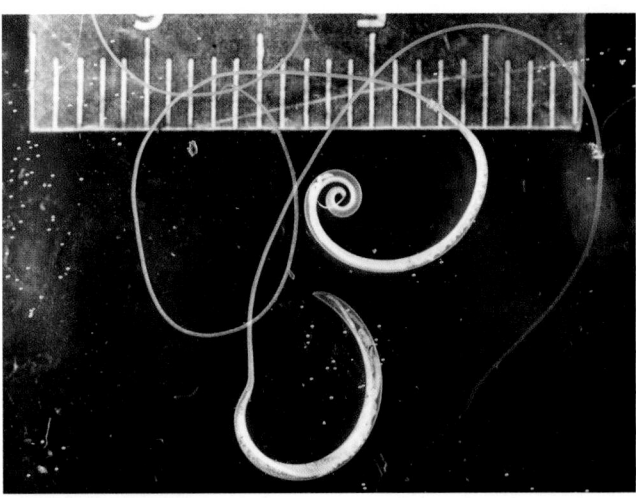

FIGURE 14-24 Whip-shaped adult of *Trichuris vulpis* with its thin anterior end and its fat posterior end.

Treatment

Treatment is the same as for *T. canis* (see treatment of *T. canis* for details). In cases of severe anemia in young puppies, transfusions may be required.

Prevention and Control Techniques

Bitches should be free of hookworms before breeding and should be kept out of potentially contaminated areas during pregnancy. Whelping should always take place in sanitary quarters. Litters should be treated with age-appropriate anthelminthics at 2, 4, 6, and 8 weeks of age. Humans can prevent CLM by avoiding skin-to-soil contact (not walking barefoot) and by deworming pets routinely.

> **TECHNICIAN NOTE** Hookworms should be considered in any puppy or kitten that presents with signs of anemia or gastrointestinal problems. *Ancylostoma caninum* infection can be fatal in young puppies as a result of anemia. Remember that obtaining an adequate fecal sample with proper identification of ova in the sample is key to a definitive diagnosis. Routine deworming should be scheduled for all puppies and kittens not on monthly preventive agents. Clients with children must be warned of the zoonotic potential.

TRICHURIS VULPIS (WHIPWORMS)—TRICHURIASIS

- Parasite's common name: whipworm
- Pronunciation: "Try-**cure**-iss" "**vulp**-iss"
- Derivation: **"Trich,"** from Greek, *hair*; **"oura,"** from Greek, *a tail*; **"vulpis,"** from Latin, *fox-like*. *Trichuris vulpis* resembles a whip, hence its name, the whipworm (Figure 14-24). The genus name of the whipworm *Trichuris* is actually a misnomer. *Trichuris* species do not have a hair-like tail, but rather a long hair-like anterior end and a fat posterior end. So *Trichuris vulpis* is actually a "hair head," as exemplified by its eastern European name, *Trichocephalus vulpis.*
- Type of parasite: nematode (roundworm)—whipworm

> **TECHNICIAN NOTE** *Trichuris vulpis* resembles a whip, hence its name, the whipworm. For both species of whipworms, a very fresh fecal sample is best for diagnosis. The veterinary technician must be able to recognize the whipworm's unique whip-like shape (fat posterior handle with long, filamentous anterior end) and its unique trichinelloid egg type.

Species Affected

Trichuris vulpis is found in members of the canine family such as dogs and foxes. *Trichuris campanula,* the feline trichurid, is found in cats, usually outside of North America. There are also trichurids that parasitize ruminants and pigs, so the only domestic species that does not serve as a definitive host for trichurids is the horse.

Location of Parasite Within Host

Trichurids are associated with the cecum and portions of the large intestine. This parasite is a bloodsucker. It has a tiny mouth on its anterior end, with a tiny stylet just inside the opening. The whipworm "threads" its anterior end through the mucosa, much like a needle and thread passing through cloth. The fat, posterior "handle" of the whipworm is found within the intestinal lumen.

Key Clinical Signs of Affected Animals

T. vulpis is a voracious blood feeder. Adults use the lash-like anterior end to tunnel into the large intestinal mucosa; the whipworm "threads" its anterior end into the tiny blood vessels and uses a stylet-like mouthpart to cannulate the vessel, ingesting whole blood. Dogs are able to tolerate large burdens of whipworms, with little clinical effect. If the worms number in the hundreds or thousands, they may produce diarrhea, weight loss, or unthriftiness. The feces may contain frank blood, producing an anemia.

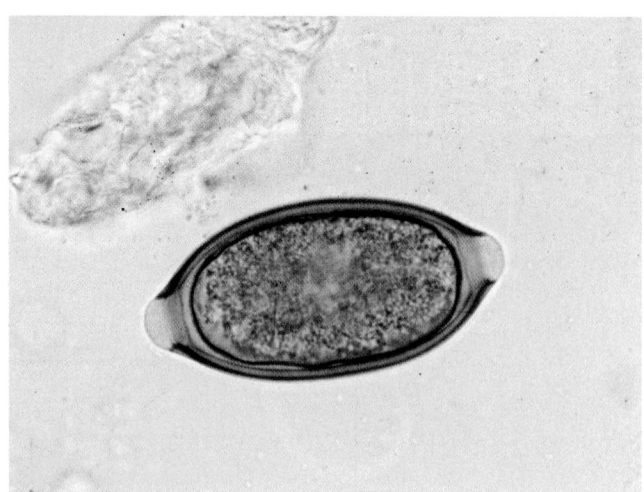

FIGURE 14-25 Bioperculate, symmetric, yellow, football-shaped egg of *Trichuris vulpis.*

Abbreviated Life Cycle

The bioperculate, symmetric, yellow, football-shaped eggs (Figure 14-25) are passed in the feces. Under environmental conditions of warmth and humidity, the whipworm egg will begin to embryonate (its central mass will begin to divide), until eventually a first stage larva may be found within the egg. This larva will moult again within the egg (shed its cuticle or skin) and develop into the second stage larva. The egg containing the second stage larva of *T. vulpis* is the stage that is infective for the canine host. It is important to note that these infective whipworm eggs are extremely resistant to adverse environmental conditions and can remain in the environment for years. The canine host ingests the eggs and the larvae penetrate the anterior small intestine, and then move to the cecum and large intestine where they develop to the adult stage. It takes approximately 12 weeks for the infective larva to develop to the sexually mature, egg-producing adult.

Laboratory Test(s) Used to Diagnose the Infection

Fecal centrifugation/flotation of fresh feces and egg identification.

Zoonotic Potential for Clients

If a child should ingest the infective whipworm eggs, it is possible for the eggs to develop to the adult stage within the cecum and large intestine; however, this is an extremely rare occurrence.

Treatment

Fenbendazole is given initially for 3 days, is repeated in 3 weeks, and is used for a final treatment in 3 months to ensure that all life stages have been treated. Some monthly heartworm preventive agents including milbemycin and moxidectin also treat *T. vulpis* infections.

Prevention and Control Techniques

To adequately control whipworm infection, rigorous hygiene is paramount. Dog kennels and exercise runs should be constructed with concrete flooring and should be cleaned regularly. These eggs can survive in soil for months to years, so access to contaminated areas should be avoided.

> **TECHNICIAN NOTE** Feline trichurids (*Trichuris campanula*) are extremely rare in North America, but sometimes trichurid eggs may be observed on flotation of feline feces. These eggs are probably pseudoparasites, that is, species of trichurids that parasitize a cat's prey—birds, rats, and mice. When these prey are eaten by a cat and digested, the eggs of the prey's trichurids may pass through the intestinal tract and may be found in the cat's feces.

STRONGYLOIDES STERCORALIS AND STRONGYLOIDES CATI; (THREADWORMS)— STRONGYLOIDOSIS AELUROSTRONGYLUS ABSTRUSUS FELINE LUNGWORM

- **Parasite's common name:** intestinal threadworms (*S. stercoralis* and *S. cati*). Feline lungworm (*A. abstrusus*)
- **Pronunciation:** "Stron-gee-**lloyd**-ees" "stir-co-**ral**-iss"; "Stron-gee-**lloyd**-ees" "**cat**-eye." "A-lure-oh-**stron**-gee-lus" "ab-**stru**-sus"
- **Derivation: "Strongylos,"** from Greek, *round* (this is a roundworm); **"eidos,"** from Greek, *form* (in the form of); **"stercora,"** from Latin, *dung;* **"catus,"** from Latin, *the domestic housecat.* **"Aeluro,"** from Greek, *cat;* **"Strongylos,"** from Greek, *round* (this is a roundworm); **"ab-,"** from Latin , "from, off, away from"; **"strus,"** from Latin, *to build*
- **Type of parasite:** nematode (roundworm)—threadworm (*S. stercoralis* and *S. cati*) or lungworm (*A. abstrusus*)

Species Affected

Threadworms (*Strongyloides stercoralis* and *Strongyloides cati*) are found in the small intestine of dogs and cats. (*Note:* This parasite is also seen in horses, cattle, and pigs.)

Key Clinical Signs of Infected Animals

Bloody, mucoid diarrhea leading to dehydration may be seen in very young puppies and kittens. Infection can result in emaciation and stunted growth. *S. cati* is nonpathogenic in adult cats. The human variety of *S. stercoralis* parasitizes human beings; the canine variety of *S. stercoralis* parasitizes dogs. Because these varieties have the same specific epithet, caution should be taken whenever humans are around diarrhea associated with the canine *Strongyloides.* Transmission is possible, so thorough handwashing is recommended. *Aelurostrongylus abstrusus*, the feline lungworm, typically produces a mild, chronic cough in infected cats. These parasites are associated together because they both produce first stage larvae in the feces of infected cats. Many times when these larvae are detected on a feline fecal flotation, a practitioner's first instinct is to make a diagnosis of feline strongyloidosis, which is an uncommon occurrence in cats.

A more common occurrence is lungworm infection with *A. abstrusus*.

Abbreviated Life Cycle

Intestinal threadworms are unusual parasites in that only the female worm is parasitic. There are no parasitic male worms. These parasitic threadworms are very tiny. The parasitic females are triploid (3N) relative to chromosome count. When an organism is triploid, it means that the organism has three times the "normal" number of chromosomes. These triploid female worms are found buried in the mucosa of the small intestine. Because she is triploid, the female is capable of producing eggs, without having been fertilized by the "nonexistent" male worm—this is essentially a "virgin birth" process called *parthenogenesis*.

> **TECHNICIAN NOTE** **Parthenogenesis** is a modified form of sexual reproduction characterized by the formation of an ovum without the fertilization of a male's spermatozoan. The prefix "partheno-" means "virgin," and the suffix "-genesis" means "beginning." The only parasites that undergo parthenogenesis are members of the genus *Strongyloides*. In the life cycle of *Strongyloides*, the adult female worm is the only parasitic stage. There are no parasitic male *Strongyloides*.

The 3N eggs pass to the outside environment and will be dependent upon environmental conditions as to which type of external life cycle will take place. If environmental conditions are extremely cold or hot, the eggs will embryonate (the internal morula will begin to divide), until eventually a first stage larva may be found within the threadworm egg. This egg will hatch in the external environment. While in the external environment, this larva will moult (shed its cuticle or skin), develop into the second stage larva, moult again, and develop into the third stage larva. This larva has the same chromosome count as the parasitic female; it cannot be free-living and MUST reenter its host by penetration. This larva penetrates the oral mucosa, gets into the systemic circulation, and eventually returns to the gut as an adult parthenogenetic female. This type of life cycle as described is called the **homogonic life cycle** (prefix "homo-" meaning "same"; suffix "-gonic" meaning "egg"; hence, "same egg type").

The eggs that are produced have the same chromosome count as the parasitic 3N female worms that produced them.

> **TECHNICIAN NOTE** The **homogonic cycle** is one of two pathways in the life cycle of *Strongyloides stercoralis*. The prefix "homo-" means "same." The suffix "-gonic" means "ovum" or "egg"; hence, "same egg type." The homogonic cycle takes place when environmental temperatures are adverse (harsh weather). In the homogonic cycle, the parthenogenetic female worm produces eggs that will eventually develop into female larvae that ultimately develop in parasitic female worms. These female worms must infect a new host immediately and reestablish the infection to survive.

The parasitic parthenogenetic female is also capable of producing eggs, some of which are haploid (N) and some of which are diploid (2N). These haploid and diploid eggs (which are identical in appearance to the 3N eggs described previously) pass to the outside environment and will also be dependent upon environmental conditions as to which type of external life cycle will take place. If the environmental conditions are fair (not extremely cold or hot), the eggs will embryonate in the environment and develop into a third stage larva, as described for 3N eggs. The larvae that hatch from the N eggs will be free-living male larvae, and the larvae that hatch from the 2N eggs will be free-living female larvae. These larvae mature to free-living adult male and female threadworms. They will copulate, and the free-living female will produce 3N eggs, which will develop as described. Because this larva has the same chromosome count as the parasitic female, it cannot be free-living (like its "parents") and MUST reenter its host by penetration. This 3N larva penetrates the oral mucosa, gets into the systemic circulation, and eventually returns to the gut as an adult parthenogenetic female. This type of life cycle as described (for N and 2N eggs) is called the **heterogonic life cycle**—prefix "hetero-" meaning "different"; suffix "-gonic" meaning "egg"; hence, "different egg type."

> **TECHNICIAN NOTE** The **heterogonic cycle** is one of two pathways in the life cycle of *Strongyloides stercoralis*. The prefix "hetero-" means "different." The suffix "-gonic" means "ovum" or "egg"; hence, "different egg type." The heterogonic cycle takes place when environmental temperatures are fair (not extremely cold or hot). In the heterogonic cycle, parthenogenetic female worms produce eggs that eventually will develop into male worms and female worms. These male and female worms will breed only once and will produce eggs that will produce larvae that must infect a new host immediately.

The eggs that are produced have a different chromosome count (N and 2N) from the parasitic 3N female worms that produced them. *Note*: The parthenogenetic female actually produces three types of eggs, which are morphologically identical: N, 2N, and 3N eggs. With the "adverse environmental" homogonic cycle, only 3N eggs are capable of surviving; with the "optimal environmental" heterogonic cycle, not only do 3N eggs survive, but also 2N and N eggs.

Laboratory Test(s) Used to Diagnose the Infection

Strongyloides larvae (L1 stage) can be detected with a fresh fecal sample using the Baermann technique. Mucosal scrapings may reveal adult female parasites, eggs, and first stage larvae (Figure 14-26). *A. abstrusus* can be diagnosed on fecal flotation, or by using the Baermann sedimentation technique.

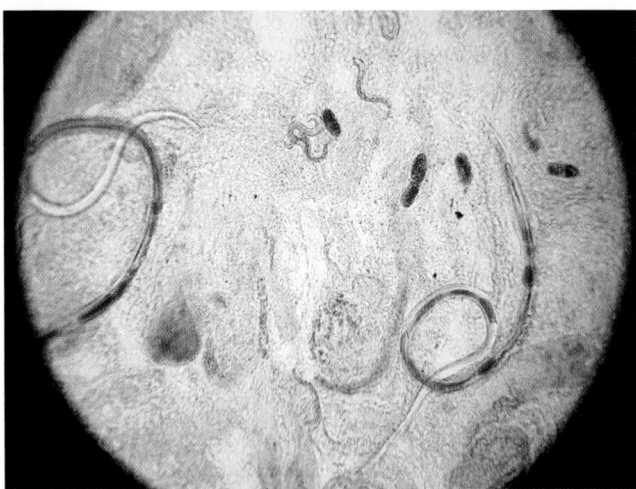

FIGURE 14-26 Small intestinal mucosal scraping, revealing adult females, eggs, and first stage larvae of *Strongyloides stercoralis*. There are no parasitic male *Strongyloides stercoralis*.

Zoonotic Potential for Clients

Strongyloidosis is seen with greater frequency during the hot, humid months of summer. The disease is endemic in the Appalachian United States, especially in eastern Tennessee, Kentucky, and West Virginia. Humans become infected by the fecal-oral route, that is, by handling of infected feces and having that fecal material come in contact with the mouth. The disease can be prevented by proper sanitation and handwashing.

Treatment

Ivermectin and fenbendazole are the drugs of choice for strongyloidosis in dogs; cats may be treated with fenbendazole.

Prevention and Control Techniques

Thorough washing of impervious surfaces with steam or concentrated salt or lyme solutions, followed by rinsing with hot water, effectively destroys *Strongyloides* species. The animal's bedding should be removed or replaced. Humans should avoid skin-to-soil contact by not walking barefoot.

> **TECHNICIAN NOTE**   First stage (L1) larvae of *Aelurostrongylus abstrusus* are often confused with the larvae of *Strongyloides cati*; however, L1 larvae of lungworms possess a prominent dorsal appendage on the tail that distinguishes them from larval *Strongyloides* species.

ENTEROBIUS VERMICULARIS (HUMAN PINWORM)—ENTEROBIASIS

- **Parasite's common name:** human pinworm
- **Pronunciation:** "En-tear-**oh**-bee-us" "ver-mick-you-**lair**-us"

- **Derivation:** "Enteron," from Greek, *intestine*; **"bios,"** from Greek, *life* (living creature in the intestine); **"vermicularis,"** *worm-like in shape or appearance* (this is a worm-like creature that lives in the intestine)
- Type of parasite: nematode (roundworm)—pinworm

> **TECHNICIAN NOTE**   A **pseudoparasite** is an object that is mistaken for a parasite, for example, *Enterobius vermicularis*, the human pinworm, is often a source of infection for humans, especially small children. Dogs and cats are NEVER infected with pinworms but are often incriminated as sources of infection by some pediatricians. Pinworms are parasites of herbivores and omnivores, but never carnivores. Therefore, the pinworm can be described as a pseudoparasite of dogs and cats.

Species Affected

Enterobius vermicularis, the human pinworm, never parasitizes dogs or cats. Parents of children infected with pinworms are frequently advised by physicians to take the family pet to the veterinary clinic and have that pet treated for pinworms. An important rule of thumb to remember is that pinworms are parasites of omnivores (e.g., humans, mice) and herbivores (e.g., horses, cattle), but never carnivores (e.g., dogs, cats).

Location of Parasite Within Host

This parasite is found in the cecum and colon of humans, especially children.

Key Clinical Signs of Infected Animals

None. This is not a parasite of dogs or cats. A common misperception is that dogs and cats spread this infection to children.

Abbreviated Life Cycle

Adult pinworms are found in the cecum and ascending colon of humans, particularly children. During the evening hours, adult female pinworms migrate to the anus and deposit their eggs (with a pruritic glue-like secretion) in the child's perianal or perineal region. Within a day or two, the eggs become infective. Because the glue is pruritic, the child will often scratch the area. Within 2 months after ingestion of the pinworm eggs, mature worms will be found in the cecum, appendix, and ascending colon.

Laboratory Test(s) Used to Diagnose the Infection

Diagnosis of pinworm infection in children should never take place in a veterinary clinic. It is the veterinary team's job to educate and inform the public regarding the intricacies of this common childhood parasite. A physician will perform the National Institutes of Health Scotch tape test to reveal the characteristic asymmetric ovum of *Enterobius vermicularis* (Figure 14-27).

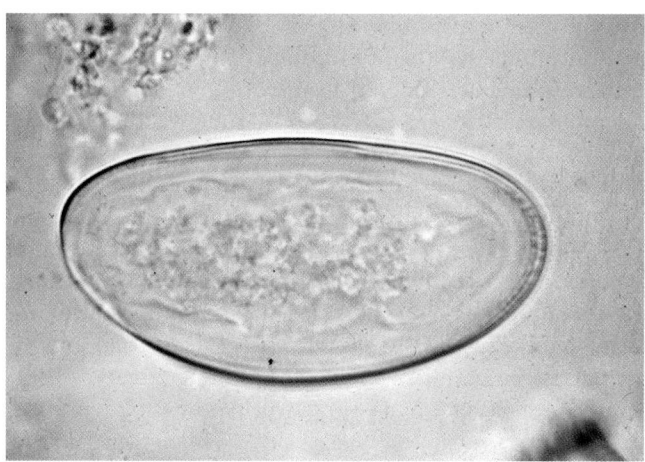

FIGURE 14-27 Characteristic asymmetric ovum of *Enterobius vermicularis.*

Zoonotic Potential for Clients

E. vermicularis may be found in primates, so any client who owns a **simian** should be advised of this malady.

Treatment

Infected primates should be treated with piperazine.

Prevention and Control Techniques

Physicians and pediatricians must be informed of the details of the life cycle of this human parasite.

> *TECHNICIAN NOTE* *E. vermicularis* is the most common worm infection in the United States and may often be incorrectly blamed on the household pet. Humans are essentially the primary means of transmission of *E. vermicularis*; therefore, other humans in the household, as well as children in care centers, are often the actual source of the infection. Clients with concerns about pinworms should be properly educated and redirected so that spread of the infection does not continue in their home.

DIROFILARIA IMMITIS (HEARTWORM)— HUMAN DIROFILARIASIS

- **Parasite's common name:** canine heartworm
- **Pronunciation:** "Dye-row-phil-**air**-e-ah" "**em**-meh-tus"
- **Derivation: "Dirus,"** from Latin, *fearsome, terrible;* **"filum,"** from Latin, *thread;* **"immitis,"** from Latin, *cruel*
- Type of parasite: nematode (roundworm)—filariids

Species Affected

Adult heartworms are usually found within the pulmonary arteries and right ventricle of dogs, cats, and ferrets; however, they are known for being aberrant or erratic parasites, capable of being found in a variety of ectopic sites. **Microfilariae** (Figure 14-28) are usually found within the peripheral blood of the canine host.

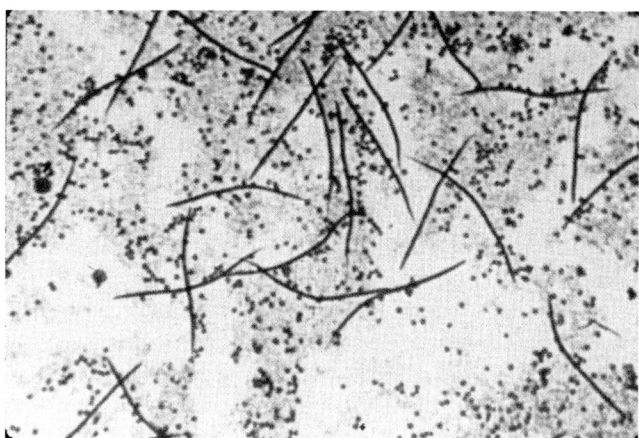

FIGURE 14-28 Microfilariae of *Dirofilaria immitis,* modified Knott's test.

> *TECHNICIAN NOTE* An **aberrant** or **erratic parasite** is a parasite that has wandered into an organ or location in which it is not normally found, for example, *Dirofilaria immitis,* the canine heartworm, usually resides in the canine right ventricle and branches of the pulmonary artery. The canine heartworm becomes an aberrant parasite when it "gets off track" during its migration to the heart and becomes established in the anterior chamber of the canine eye. Such aberrant/erratic infections are usually solitary infections, that is, only a single specimen may be found in these aberrant/erratic sites.

Key Clinical Signs of Infected Animals

Dogs may be asymptomatic early in infection; as disease advances, they show weight loss, decreased exercise tolerance, and cough. In advanced cases, dyspnea, fever, ascites, cyanosis, and periodic collapse may occur. Cats can also be infected but are not good hosts. Ferrets can be infected as well. Cats may be asymptomatic, may have sporadic vomiting, or may show mild signs of respiratory illness such as a chronic cough. They may also develop signs of acute respiratory distress syndrome (ARDS) or may die suddenly. In addition, because cats are not the natural host, they may present with ectopic infection as a result of adult worms in the CNS, eye, or subcutaneous tissues.

Abbreviated Life Cycle

Adult male and female heartworms are found within branches of the pulmonary arteries and in higher worm burdens in the right ventricle. Fertilized adult females produce microfilariae, which are found within the peripheral blood.

> *TECHNICIAN NOTE* **Microfilaria** (microfilariae, pl): This "pre-larval" developmental stage is often associated with *Dirofilaria immitis,* the canine heartworm. Microfilariae usually can be found in the peripheral blood of dogs infected with *D. immitis.* After ingestion of the microfilarial stage by the mosquito intermediate host, larval development takes place. Each microfilaria will ultimately develop into an infective third stage larva.

A female mosquito must take a blood meal, ingesting the microfilariae. Microfilariae (310 microns long, tapered anterior end, straight tail) are initially found in the mosquito's midgut but migrate to the mosquito's kidneys. Here they develop into first stage larvae, which moult to second stage larvae, which molt to third stage larvae. These larvae break out of the kidneys and migrate to the mosquito's proboscis (mouthparts). When the infected adult female mosquito takes a blood meal from an uninfected dog, the third stage larvae will emerge onto the skin surface from the mosquito's proboscis and will penetrate the puncture wound made by the mosquito during the blood feeding process. The larvae migrate through the subcutaneous tissues, moulting to fourth-stage larvae, which eventually migrate to the pulmonary arteries and in higher worm burdens will spill over into the right ventricle, where they moult to fifth stage larvae–the adult stage. The time that it takes for the third stage larva to mature to the adult stage is approximately 6 months. Adult male and female heartworms breed, the female produces microfilariae, and the life cycle begins again. (*Note*: There is another filarial parasite, *Acanthocheilonema* [nee *Dipetalonema*] *reconditum* [A-canth-oh-**kyle**-low-nee-ma {Dye-peh-tal-low-**nee**-ma} reh-con-**dye**-tum], which parasitizes dogs and whose microfilariae [285 microns long, rounded anterior end, buttonhook tail] may be confused with the microfilariae of *D. immitis*. This nematode is found subcutaneously and utilizes the flea, *Ctenocephalides felis*, as its intermediate host.)

> **TECHNICIAN NOTE** Within the life cycle of a parasite, the host that harbors the immature, asexual, or larval stage of a parasite is the **intermediate host**, for example, the intermediate host for *Dirofilaria immitis*, the canine heartworm, is the mosquito. Larval (immature) heartworms are found within the Malpighian tubules (kidneys) of the mosquito intermediate host.

Laboratory Test(s) Used to Diagnose the Infection

A wide variety of commercially available canine and feline ELISA serologic tests can be used to detect both adult and microfilarial antigens. In microfilaremic dogs, the direct blood smear and the modified Knott's test are good techniques to demonstrate the presence of microfilariae, especially when educating clients. Radiography and ultrasonography are often confirmatory.

Zoonotic Potential for Clients

Humans rarely serve as incidental hosts for *D. immitis*. Human dirofilariasis usually manifests as a pulmonary "coin lesion" within the lung. Humans are dead-end hosts (the parasite is incapable of reproducing within people).

Treatment for Animals

For dogs, the treatment of choice is melarsomine for adult stages and a microfilaricide such as ivermectin or milbemycin for microfilariae. Cage rest during and for up to 1 month after treatment is critical. For cats, no effective treatments are available for heartworm, but corticosteroids are often used to treat the interstitial lung reaction.

Prevention and Control Techniques

Mosquito repellents are indicated for humans. All dogs and cats should receive heartworm anthelmintic preventive medication every 30 days, year-round. Because this parasite causes a deadly disease that is difficult and dangerous to treat in dogs and is essentially unable to be treated in cats, prevention must be emphasized when educating clients. Clients should be instructed to give heartworm preventive treatment every 30 days, as opposed to monthly, because instructions to give it monthly may be interpreted as at any time during the month, and the 30-day interval is crucial for effective prevention. Periodic testing and treatment for dogs not on preventive are encouraged.

> **TECHNICIAN NOTE** During the heartworm infection process, the female mosquito does not inject infective third stage larvae of *Dirofilaria immitis* into the puncture wound made during the feeding process. Instead, she deposits the larvae within a pool of hemolymph onto the skin surface, and the larvae make their way into the puncture wound.

ARTHROPODS OF ZOONOTIC IMPORTANCE

> **TECHNICIAN NOTE** An **arthropod** is any member of the phylum Arthropoda. Most of the members of this phylum have jointed appendages in the adult stage. Relative to veterinary parasitology, arthropods include a wide variety of creatures with "jointed feet," such as centipedes, millipedes, crustaceans, insects, and mites and ticks.

ACARINES (MITES AND TICKS)
Sarcoptes scabei

- **Parasite's common name:** the "scabies" mite
- **Pronunciation:** "Sar-**cop**-tes" "**skay**-bee-eye"
- **Derivation:** "Sarkos," from Greek, *flesh*; **"koptein,"** from Greek, *to cut* (this is a mite that tunnels though the epidermis); **"scabere,"** from Latin, *to scratch*
- **Type of parasite:** arthropod—chelicerate—acarine (mite)—sarcoptiform mite (tunneling mite)

Species Affected

Almost every species of mammal has its own variety of this tunneling mite, for example, humans are infested with *Sarcoptes scabei* variety *hominis*, and dogs are infested with *Sarcoptes scabei* variety *canis*. *Sarcoptes scabei* variety *felis* is rare; however, cats are infested with a similar tunneling mite—*Notoedres cati*.

Key Clinical Signs of Infected Animals

Infestation by mites (or ticks) is called **acariasis**, and infestation by *S. scabei* is referred to as *sarcoptic acariasis*. *S. scabei* produces extreme pruritus (itching) and alopecia (loss of hair) in all infested animals. The mite is spread by direct contact, so one infested dog in the household environment is capable of transmitting the parasite to all uninfested dogs in the home.

Abbreviated Life Cycle

Four developmental stages have been noted in the life cycle of *S. scabei*—egg, larva, nymph, and adult. Initially, adult male and female mites are found on the skin surface, but after copulation, the female mite will burrow into the skin, making tunnels within the epidermis. As she tunnels, she will lay her eggs within the tunnel shaft. As the eggs hatch, released larvae will penetrate the wall of the tunnel and will themselves make new tunnels that are perpendicular to the initial main shaft. It is this tunneling that produces the extreme pruritus associated with *S. scabei*.

Laboratory Test(s) Used to Diagnose the Infection

Sarcoptic acariasis is diagnosed by superficial skin scraping using a scalpel blade. The scraped material (crusts from affected areas often are most diagnostic) is transferred to a glass slide containing a drop of mineral oil, and the collected material is examined under a compound microscope. *S. scabei* mites are round to oval in shape, and they possess jointed legs. At the end of some of the legs is a long, unjointed pedicel (straight stalk) with a tiny sucker on its end. This morphologic feature (the unjointed pedicel with tiny sucker) can be best likened to a plumber's friend (plunger) (Figure 14-29). The eggs of *S. scabei* are oval in shape and may contain a developing larval mite.

Zoonotic Potential for Clients

Transmission to humans most commonly occurs from direct contact with an infested dog but can also occur from a contaminated environment and fomites. Mites can be readily transmitted between dogs (and to cats) from direct contact.

Treatment

Selamectin is the drug of choice. Three topical treatments are given at 2-week intervals. All clinically suspected *S. scabei* cases should be treated even if multiple skin scrapings are negative.

Prevention and Control Techniques

Because of zoonotic potential, lesions on affected animals should not be held or touched directly, and the hospital environment should be decontaminated (with pyrethrins). Therapeutic trials with reliable acaricides are essential to confirm or rule out scabies in pruritic dogs with negative skin scrapings.

Otodectes cynotis (Oh-toe-DECK-teez sigh-an-OH-tiss)

Also known as *ear mites*, *Otodectes* organisms are not zoonotic parasites but are mites of great economic importance in small animal veterinary practice. Ear mites usually are observed by using an otoscope—an instrument that is essential to veterinary diagnostics. Ear mites are similar to *S. scabei* in that their size is similar to a grain of table salt, so they are visible to the naked eye. These mites can be easily observed on and collected from the tip of a cotton applicator stick during the ear cleaning process. Collected mites should be transferred to a drop of mineral oil that has been placed on a glass slide, and a cover slip should be applied over the oil. The morphologic details of this common mite can be observed using a compound microscope. As with sarcoptiform mites, ear mites are round to oval in shape, and they possess jointed legs. At the end of some of the jointed legs is a short, unjointed pedicel (stalk) with a tiny sucker on its end. This morphologic feature (the short, unjointed pedicel with a tiny sucker) is diagnostic for *Otodectes cynotis* (Figure 14-30).

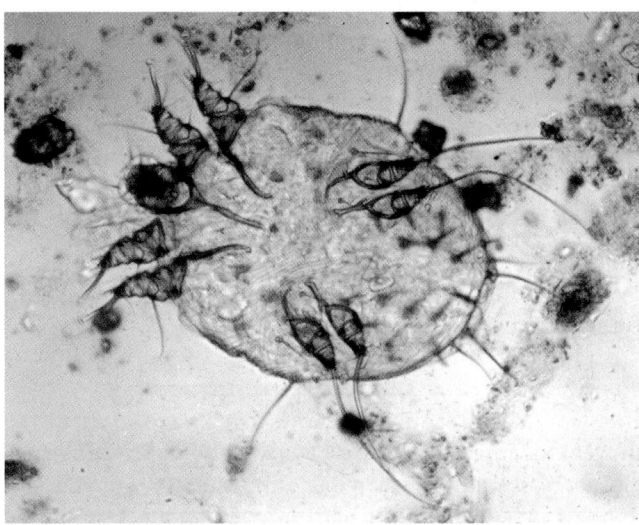

FIGURE 14-29 Deep skin scraping, adult *Sarcoptes scabei* mite.

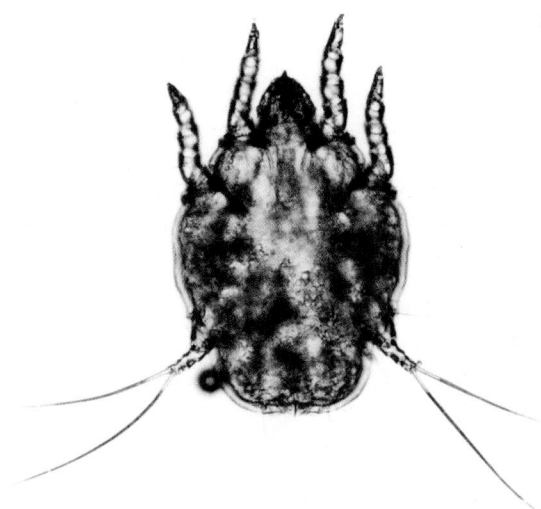

FIGURE 14-30 Adult *Otodectes cynotis* from the external ear canal of a dog.

Demodex canis (DEE-moe-decks KAY-niss)

This is a hair follicle and sebaceous gland dwelling mite, not a sarcoptiform mite. It produces a similar syndrome with localized alopecia or generalized alopecia. This type of acariasis is nonpruritic, unless complicated by secondary bacterial infection, and cannot be spread by direct contact. Canine demodicosis can be spread only by intimate body contact between an infested dam and her puppies during the nursing process. Demodectic acariasis can also be associated with immunodeficiency in infected adult dogs older than 18 months. It can be diagnosed with a deep skin scraping and microscopic identification of its unique morphology. It is long and slender (carrot shaped) and resembles an eight-legged alligator (Figure 14-31). It owes its appearance to its predilection site—the long, thin, confining hair follicle.

Cheyletiella parasitivorax

- **Parasite's common name:** walking dandruff mite
- **Pronunciation:** "Shay-leh-tea-**el**-lah" "pear-ah-sit-ah-**vor**-ax"
- **Derivation:** "Chele," from Greek, *claw* (a claw); "**ella**," *little,* is a diminutive suffix often used in the names of parasites or bacteria; "**parasitos**," from Greek, *parasite*; "**vorare**," from Latin, *to devour.*
- **Type of parasite:** arthropod—chelicerate—acarine (mite)

Species Affected

Dogs, cats, and rabbits.

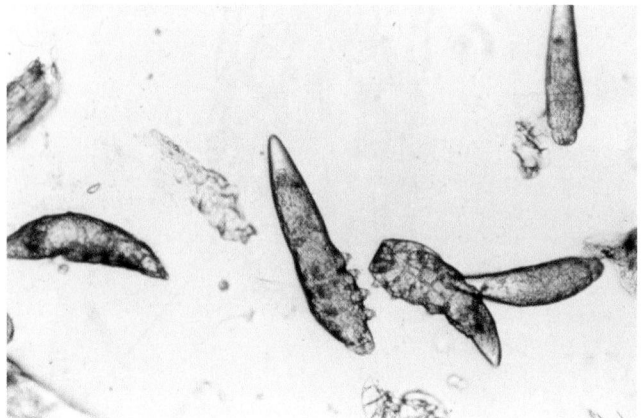

FIGURE 14-31 Deep skin scraping, adult *Demodex canis,* the follicle mite of dogs.

Key Clinical Signs of Infected Animals

Cheyletiella parasitivorax causes intense pruritus in affected animals. It is usually seen in young puppies and kittens. Lesions appear on the dorsum above the tail, and on the neck. Lesions appear as a dry, scaly dermatitis with dandruff, with or without pruritus. Cats may develop miliary dermatitis. Bitches and queens are often asymptomatic carriers of these parasites. With any type of dandruff in rabbits, *Cheyletiella* should be considered. These mites produce a scurfy skin condition, that is, they produce excess keratin debris (dandruff). If the pelage (hair coat) of infested animals is parted with a fine-toothed comb, the observer will be able to detect these mites as they walk along the skin surface. They are tiny, white mites, and when observed grossly (using a hand-held lens or Optivisor), they take on the appearance of "walking dandruff."

Abbreviated Life Cycle

Four developmental stages have been identified in the life cycle of *C. parasitivorax*—egg, larva, nymph, and adult stages.

Laboratory Test(s) Used to Diagnose the Infection

Identification of unique mites can be made on the skin surface or within the hair coat of rabbits through flea combing. *C. parasitivorax* can be removed from the hair coat using a fine-toothed comb, and the debris collected can be transferred to a solid black piece of construction paper. This parasite manifests as "walking dandruff." Mites are approximately 0.5 mm in length and have a unique appearance—a bell pepper shape, with a pair of accessory hooks on its capitulum (head). At the end of each leg is a tiny comb-like structure (Figure 14-32).

Zoonotic Potential for Clients

Owners should be especially concerned if a dog, cat, or rabbit is diagnosed with *Cheyletiella* species because this mite is highly contagious. If the infested animal is in the home or is frequently handled by owners, the mite is readily transferred to humans, even with brief amounts of exposure, or through clothing. Infestation in rabbits may be mild clinically; however, infestation in humans can be severely pruritic and irritating. When this mite is diagnosed in a pet, the zoonotic potential should be stressed to the client.

Treatment

Infested pets should be treated topically with pyrethrins. Systemic treatment with ivermectin, selamectin, or moxidectin for 6 weeks is also recommended.

Prevention and Control Techniques

Infested animals should be isolated and treated to prevent the spread of disease. Owners should wear protective clothing and gloves when handling infested animals. All animals in direct contact with infested animals should be treated.

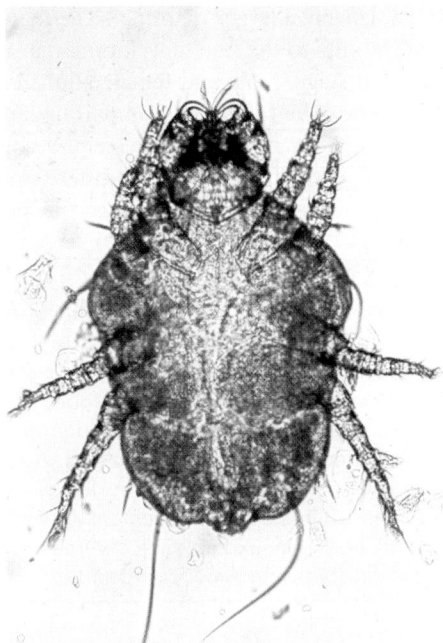

FIGURE 14-32 Adult mite, *Cheyletiella parasitivorax,* "walking dandruff." Mites are approximately 0.5 mm in length, with a unique appearance—a bell pepper shape, with a pair of accessory hooks on its capitulum (head). At the end of each leg is a tiny comb-like structure.

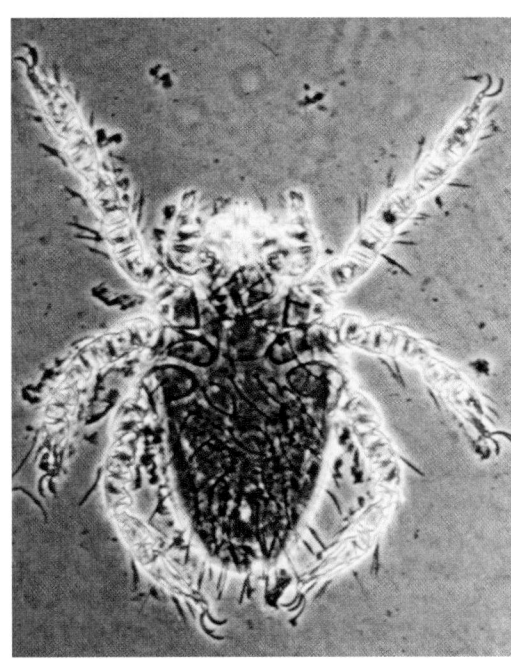

FIGURE 14-33 Six-legged larval *Trombicula* species. The larval chigger is the only parasitic stage in the life cycle of this ectoparasite.

Trombicula Species (Chiggers)

- **Parasite's common name:** chiggers, jiggers, red bugs
- **Pronunciation:** "Trom-**bic**-you-lah"
- **Derivation:** The genus name is derived from the family name, Trombiculidae. An etymologic breakdown is not available.
- **Type of parasite:** arthropod—chelicerate—acarine (mite) —"chigger" (free-living adult mite)

Species Affected

Warm-blooded animals, both avian and mammalian. Some species may feed on reptiles and snakes.

Location of Parasite Within Host

The six-legged larval chigger (Figure 14-33) is the only stage of this mite that is parasitic. Larval chiggers are found attached to the skin of the infested host. They feed and then drop off the host. Contrary to popular belief, these mites DO NOT burrow into the skin.

Key Clinical Signs of Infected Animals

When these larval mites attach to the skin, they inject their saliva into the skin. This saliva liquefies the host's tissues. The chiggers suck up this liquid "food." After the chiggers are filled to capacity, they fall off of the host, where they moult to the free-living eight-legged nymphal stage.

Abbreviated Life Cycle

Four developmental stages have been identified in the life cycle of **Trombicula** species—egg, six-legged larva,

eight-legged nymph, and eight-legged adult. This is an unusual mite in that ONLY the six-legged larval stage is parasitic. All other parasitic stages (nymphal and adult) are free-living in nature and nonparasitic.

Laboratory Test(s) Used to Diagnose the Infection

These mites can be easily observed on and collected from the skin of an infested host. They are firmly attached to the host. Collected mites should be transferred to a drop of mineral oil that has been placed on a glass slide, and a cover slip should be applied over the oil. The morphologic details (the six-legged larval stage) of this common mite can be observed using a compound microscope. Chiggers are round to oval in shape and slightly hairy; they possess six jointed legs.

Zoonotic Potential for Clients

Once attached to a canine host, chiggers are rarely transmitted to a human host; however, it is possible for the chigger to be "riding aboard" the dog or cat host and be mechanically transferred to a human, to whom it may attach and upon whom it may feed.

Treatment

Dogs or cats infested with chiggers should be bathed immediately in **pyrethrin**-based shampoos.

Prevention and Control Techniques

Restrict the pet's access to areas frequented by chiggers (bushes and undergrowth).

TECHNICIAN NOTE Contrary to popular belief, chiggers never burrow into the skin of the infested vertebrate host. They attach to the vertebrate host and then inject saliva into the skin; this liquefies host tissues. The chigger sucks up liquefied host tissues, then drops off of the host.

Ticks (various species)

- **Parasite's common name:** ticks
- **Pronunciation:** Thousands of different species of ticks are known. A few genera affecting small animals include *Dermacentor* (Derma-ah-**cen**-tor) species; *Rhipicephalus sanguineus* (Rip-ah-**cef**-ah-lus san-**gwen**-e-us) species; *Amblyomma* (Am-blee-**oh**-mah) species; *Ixodes* (Ick-**zoo**-dees) species
- **Type of parasite:** arthropod—chelicerate—acarine (tick)—Ixodid tick (hard tick)

Species Affected

Almost every species of warm-blooded animal (mammals and birds) and poikilothermic animals (e.g., snakes, other reptiles) are capable of serving as host for the many genera of ticks. Humans are susceptible, particularly after spending time in the outdoor environment.

Key Clinical Signs of Infected Animals

Infestation by ticks (or mites) is called **acariasis**. As ectoparasites, ticks produce an infestation, inhabiting areas of the skin, both haired and nonhaired, especially the external ear canal (**otoacariasis**). Ticks are voracious blood feeders, capable of producing significant anemia in all species of domestic and wild animals. Ticks are capable of producing tick paralysis, an ascending flaccid motor paralysis affecting all species of mammals, including humans. Tick paralysis may result from a salivary toxin produced in the tick's mouthparts or from an ovarian toxin secreted by a gravid, adult, female tick. Ticks are also very important in that they serve as intermediate hosts for many protozoan parasites, and as vectors for many bacteria, viruses, chlamydial agents, spirochetes, and assorted other pathogens, many of which can be spread from domestic and wild animals to human beings.

Abbreviated Life Cycle

There are four developmental stages in the life cycle of the tick—egg, larva, nymph, and adult stages. Initially, adult male and female ticks are found on the host's skin surface, usually in close proximity to each other (abutting each other). After copulation and incubation, the adult female tick will drop off of the host and lay her eggs in the external environment. Eggs will hatch, producing the six-legged larval stage (often referred to as **seed ticks**). The larval stage will crawl up a blade of grass and attach to its first host, usually a small mammal. It feeds on this host, drops off the host, and moults to the eight-legged nymphal stage. The nymphal stage will crawl up a blade of grass and attach to

its second host, usually a larger mammal. The nymph feeds, drops off, and moults to the final developmental stage—the eight-legged adult stage. Male and female adults crawl up a blade of grass, get on the final host, and pair up, and the life cycle begins again. This narrative is descriptive of a three-host type of life cycle because three different hosts are involved in the progression from the egg to the adult stage.

TECHNICIAN NOTE A three-host tick is an individual tick that will feed on three individual animals or three different species of animal. These three-host ticks often attach to the first host immediately after hatching from the egg—they are in the six-legged larval stage. They feed and drop off this host, moulting to the eight-legged nymphal stage. They find another host and attach to it. Again, they feed and drop off this host and moult to the eight-legged adult stage. The adult stage will eventually attach to the third and final host. An example of a three-host tick is *Dermacentor variabilis*, the American dog tick.

One-host ticks, two-host ticks, three-host ticks, and **many-host ticks** have been identified; the number of hosts varies among the myriad of tick genera that occur throughout the world.

TECHNICIAN NOTE A one-host tick is an individual tick that will feed on a single animal or a single species of animal. One-host ticks often attach to the host immediately after hatching from the egg—they are in the six-legged larval stage. They do not drop off this host, but moult to the eight-legged nymphal stage. Again, they do not drop off this host, but moult to the eight-legged adult stage. An example of a one-host tick is *Boophilus annulatus*, the Texas cattle fever tick. A many-host tick is an individual tick that is capable of feeding on many different hosts. These many-host ticks make frequent visits to the different hosts. These frequent visits are the reason that these ticks may also be classified as periodic parasites. An example of a many-host tick is *Otobius megnini*, the spinose ear tick, a type of soft tick.

Laboratory Test(s) Used to Diagnose the Infection

Most veterinary practices are not interested in the speciation of ticks commonly found on domestic animals. Some diagnostic laboratories have the capacity to render generic or specific identification of ticks should a veterinary practice desire to do so. These laboratories use a dichotomous key to render their diagnoses. These keys use the morphology of the tick mouthparts for identification; however, unengorged male and female ticks must be submitted because it is difficult to identify engorged female ticks.

Zoonotic Potential for Clients

The many genera of ticks are capable of transmitting a variety of zoonotic diseases from animals to humans

TABLE 14-1	North American Ticks Commonly Associated With Zoonotic Diseases		
TICK/COMMON NAME	**DISEASES**	**REGION FOUND (UNITED STATES)**	**HOSTS**
Amblyomma americanum/ Lone star tick	Rocky Mountain spotted fever Tularemia Q fever Ehrlichiosis Tick paralysis	East of central Texas to the Atlantic coast, north to Iowa	Livestock Dogs Deer Birds Humans
Dermacentor andersoni/ Wood tick	Rocky Mountain spotted fever Tularemia Q fever Tick paralysis Cytauxzoonosis	Western states south to Arizona and New Mexico	Dogs Cats Livestock Mammals Humans
Dermacentor variabilis/ American dog tick	Rocky Mountain spotted fever Tularemia Q fever Tick paralysis Ehrlichiosis Cytauxzoonosis	Eastern two-thirds of United States	Dogs Cats Mammals Humans
*Ixodes scapularis/*Blacklegged tick (sometimes called the deer tick)	Lyme disease Ehrlichiosis Babesiosis Tick-borne encephalitis Tick paralysis	Most of the United States, especially the Northeast, upper Midwest, and northern California	Mammals (deer) Birds Humans
Rhipicephalus sanguineus/ Brown dog tick	Tick paralysis Babesiosis Ehrlichiosis Rocky Mountain spotted fever Hepatozoonosis Haemobartonellosis	Most of the United States	Dogs

(Tables 14-1 and 14-2). Clients should be counseled regarding the pathogenicity of many of these zoonotic conditions and the need for rigorous tick control programs.

Treatment

Pyrethrins, permethrins, fipronil, and amitraz are some of the tick treatments and preventive agents that are commercially available for dogs. Fipronil and selamectin are the two main tick preventives that are safe for use in cats. It is imperative to remind clients that most of the tick products available for dogs are toxic to cats, and so dog products should not be applied to cats, nor should cats be housed in close proximity to dogs after the products have been applied.

Prevention and Control Techniques

Dogs are very susceptible to tick bites and tick-borne diseases. Vaccines are not available for many of the tick-borne diseases with which dogs can become infected. It is important to use a tick preventive product on your dog to reduce the chances that ticks may transmit zoonotic disease to you or your other pets. Pets should be checked daily for the presence of ticks, especially after they have been outdoors. If ticks are found on the animal, they should be promptly removed and destroyed, but great care should be taken when doing so. Tick habitats on the premises and in the home can be reduced by proper landscaping and lawn maintenance.

TECHNICIAN NOTE When removing a tick, it is important that residual tick mouthparts never be left in the pet's skin, or secondary infections may result. It is also important to use disposable gloves during the tick removal process because pathogens may be transmitted from the tick to the owner's bare skin.

PROTOZOANS OF ZOONOTIC IMPORTANCE

TECHNICIAN NOTE A **protozoan** is a unicellular (one-cell) organism. Some protozoans are parasitic in human beings and in wild and domestic animals. Based on the means of movement, these protozoans can be broken down into several types: ciliates (moving by means of tiny beating "hairs"), flagellates (having one or more whip-like flagella), amoebae (moving by means of pseudopodia), and apicomplexans (moving by gliding).

GIARDIA SPECIES

- **Parasite's common name:** *Giardia*
- **Pronunciation:** "Gee-**ard**-dee-uh"

TABLE 14-2 Characteristics of Common Tick-Borne Diseases

DISEASE/CAUSE	CLINICAL SIGNS	DIAGNOSIS	TREATMENT	ZOONOTIC POTENTIAL	TECHNICIAN TIPS
Rocky Mountain spotted fever/*Rickettsia rickettsii*	Fever, depression, anorexia, lymphadenopathy, coughing or dyspnea, abdominal pain, and edema of face or extremities	Presumptive through serologic testing with IFA (showing fourfold rise between acute and convalescent titers), along with clinical signs	• Doxycycline is treatment of choice. • Chloramphenicol in pregnant bitches or puppies younger than 6 months	• Direct transmission from dogs to people does not occur. • Dogs are short-term reservoirs and sentinels for the disease.	• Disease occurrence highest from April to September • Ticks removed from pets must not be crushed by unprotected fingers to prevent exposure.
Q fever/*Coxiella burnetii*	• Goats, sheep, and cattle are primary domestic reservoirs, and unapparent infection is typical because clinical signs rarely develop in infected livestock. • Can cause abortion and abortion storms in sheep and goats when infection passes through previously uninfected flock or herd	• Serologic testing is diagnostic tool of choice with complement fixation and ELISA. • Microscopic demonstration of *Rickettsia* in impression smears from placenta also diagnostic	• Tetracycline antibiotic treatment is effective. • Separation of pregnant animals and burning or burying of infective reproductive tissues/fluids can reduce spread.	• *Coxiella burnetii* is transmitted via inhalation, direct or indirect contact with infected animals, or direct or indirect contact with their dried excretions. • Humans are not typically infected by tick bites.	• In the United States, Q fever outbreaks have resulted mainly from occupational exposure involving veterinarians, slaughterhouse workers, sheep and dairy workers, livestock farmers, and laboratory workers.
Tularemia/*Francisella tularensis*	• Varies with species infected • Rabbits, hares, rodents—naturally infected, most often found dead • Sheep—high fever, lethargy, anorexia, rigid gait, diarrhea, polyuria, weight loss, tachycardia, tachypnea, dyspnea • Clinical disease occurs occasionally in cats and rarely in dogs.	• Definitive diagnosis through bacterial culture from clinical specimens such as blood, exudates, or biopsy • Can also be confirmed by demonstration of organism with PCR or IFA	• Streptomycin and tetracycline are antibiotics of choice for treating wild and domestic animals. • Early treatment should prevent death.	• Most cases of tularemia in United States are associated with bites of infected ticks, mosquitoes, and biting flies or with handling of infected rodents, rabbits, or hares. • Another source is contaminated wild rabbit meat.	• Tularemia is extremely infectious and is readily transmitted from infected animals to humans. • Strict protective measures should be used in handling animals, their bedding, and all laboratory samples.

Disease/Organism	Clinical Signs	Diagnosis	Treatment	Zoonotic Potential	Comments
Ehrlichiosis (canine monocytic ehrlichiosis)/*Ehrlichia canis* (rarely caused by *Ehrlichia chaffeensis*)	• Fever, depression, anorexia, lymphadenopathy • Thrombocytopenia, bleeding episodes	• Blood smear and serology using IFA is best. • ELISA can also be used. • Clinical signs and response to therapy can be presumptive diagnosis before definitive diagnostic answers are received.	• Doxycycline is preferred method of therapy. • Early treatment is critical.	• Most *Ehrlichia* spp. may be infectious to humans, but dog-to-dog or dog-to-human transmission does not occur. • Dogs can, however, bring vectors into human environment.	• Low platelet numbers might increase bleeding time after blood sample collection. • Most cases occur during highest tick activity—months of April to September. • Infected dogs pose little to no hazard to humans, so long as ticks are well controlled.
Tick paralysis/salivary neurotoxin produced by certain female ticks	• Hindlimb weakness rapidly progressing to generalized weakness, then complete flaccid paralysis • Dogs become recumbent in 24 to 72 hours, and death can occur as a result of paralysis of respiratory muscles.	Diagnosis rests entirely on finding of ticks on an animal with compatible clinical signs, removal of ticks, and rapid clinical improvement within 24 to 48 hours.	• Tick removal can be curative. • Use insecticide if ticks are not found. • Whole body shave if necessary • Supportive care until clinical signs resolve	Some ticks may cause tick paralysis in humans; animal-to-animal or zoonotic transmission does not occur.	• Delay in finding and removing ticks can affect prognosis significantly. • Remember to remove the entire tick head because toxin resides in salivary gland. • Tick paralysis can also affect cats, lambs, calves, goats, and foals.
Cytauxzoonosis/*Cytauxzoon felis*	• Anorexia, lethargy, dyspnea, icterus and fever, pallor, and death • Anemia and leukopenia	• ID of organism on blood smear or from tissue aspirates in acute cases • PCR can be used to confirm presence of organism in cats that are subclinical.	Atovaquone and azithromycin used in combination are the most current therapy.	No evidence of human infection has been found.	• Clinical suspicion and early diagnosis through identification of organism on blood smear or from tissue aspirates have resulted in successful response to treatment. • Outdoor cats in areas where bobcats roam are at risk for this deadly disease.

ELISA, Enzyme-linked immunosorbent assay; *ID*, identification; *IFA*, immunofluorescence assay; *PCR*, polymerase chain reaction.

- **Derivation:** "Giard," named after the French biologist, Alfred Giard
- **Type of parasite:** protozoan—Mastigophoran (flagellate)

Species Affected

Virtually all domestic species and many wild species of animals are affected. Six species of *Giardia* are recognized: *Giardia lamblia* (a.k.a. *G. intestinalis* or *G. duodenalis*), which infects humans and other mammals; *G. muris*, which is found in mice and other mammals; *G. ardeae* and *G. psittaci* in birds, *G. agilis* in amphibians, and *G. microti* in voles. *Giardia* is the most common intestinal parasite affecting people worldwide.

Key Clinical Signs of Infected Animals

Many infected animals may be asymptomatic. In those that are symptomatic, diarrhea is characteristic and most common in young puppies and kittens, as well as in animals that are stressed, immunosuppressed, or housed in groups. Clinical disease in cats is uncommon. Affected animals may experience weight loss, secondary to diarrhea.

Abbreviated Life Cycle

The life cycle begins with a noninfective cyst being voided in the feces of an infected animal. The cyst is highly resistant to both heat and cold and to drying out. This oval cyst form possesses four prominent nuclei. When a host ingests the cyst, the motile tear-shaped **trophozoite** emerges from the cyst and begins to feed within the gut.

> **▌TECHNICIAN NOTE**   A trophozoite (literally, "a tiny, moving organism") is a term for a tissue stage, for example, a fast growing developmental stage that occurs in cysts in the life cycle of *Toxoplasma gondii* and other similar apicomplexan parasites.

Motile trophozoites cover the tops of intestinal epithelial cells, limiting absorption. The trophozoite multiplies by longitudinal binary fission. The resulting trophozoite and cyst form, then pass through the digestive system in the feces into the external environment. Although the trophozoites may be found in the feces, only the cysts are capable of surviving outside of the host.

Laboratory Test(s) Used to Diagnose the Infection

Finding organisms, both cysts and trophozoites (Figures 14-34 and 14-35, respectively), on direct fecal smear is diagnostic; however, a negative result does not rule out infection. Zinc sulfate flotation medium in combination with centrifugation should be subsequently used. Serial fecal samples may be necessary over a period of 3 to 5 days. ELISA kits can also be used to detect fecal *Giardia* antigens.

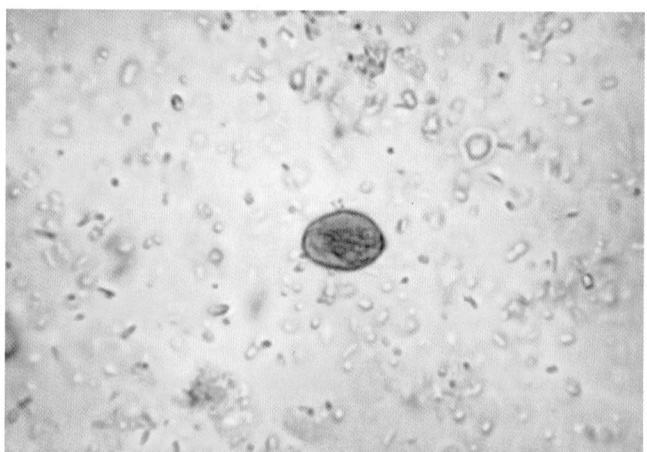

FIGURE 14-34 Cyst of *Giardia* species.

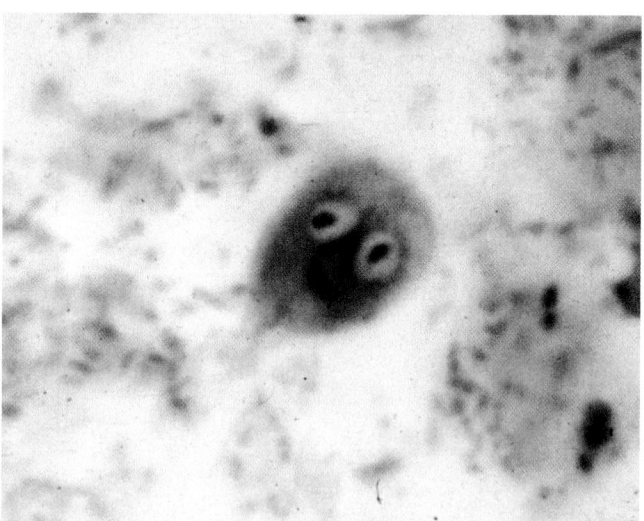

FIGURE 14-35 Trophozoite of *Giardia* species.

Zoonotic Potential for Clients

The veterinary technician should always consider this parasite and its zoonotic potential, especially in a dog or a cat with diarrhea. *Giardia* species have not been shown to be highly host-specific and therefore can likely be spread from dogs and cats to humans. Because this organism is spread by fecal-oral contact, young children are most at risk, along with immunocompromised individuals.

Treatment

Fenbendazole and metronidazole are used to treat giardiasis in dogs and cats. Empirical treatment with fenbendazole is a common prescription for dogs with diarrhea because of its effectiveness against *Giardia*, as well as its effectiveness against *Trichuris vulpis* infection (both of which can be difficult to diagnose).

Prevention and Control Techniques

Promptly removing feces from cages, runs, and yards limits environmental exposure. Cysts can be inactivated by most quaternary ammonium compounds, a 1:32 dilution of household bleach, steam, or boiling water. Grassy areas should be considered contaminated for at least 1 month after infected dogs have left the premises. Cysts contaminating the hair of dogs and cats may be a source of reinfection, making shampooing and rinsing of the animal's coat important in limiting disease spread.

> **TECHNICIAN NOTE** Although *Giardia* species are not highly host specific and can be spread from domestic animals to humans, a much more likely source of infection is contaminated water sources. In addition, infants and children in child care facilities can be at increased risk for infection. So even though a pet is often the primary suspect when humans are diagnosed with giardiasis, other sources of infection must be considered.

TOXOPLASMA GONDII

- **Parasite's common name:** "toxo"
- **Pronunciation:** "Tox-oh-**plaz**-ma" "**gon**-dee-eye"
- **Derivation: "Toxon,"** from Greek, *a bow* (shaped like a bow or quiver); **"plasma,"** from Greek, *anything molded or formed*; **"gondii,"** from the gundi, a small, stocky rodent found in Africa. (Gundis live in rocky deserts across the northern parts of the continent.) The protozoan parasite *Toxoplasma* was first described in the gundi.
- **Type of parasite:** protozoan—apicomplexan

Species Affected
The ONLY host that will harbor the sexual stages of this parasite is the feline. All other warm-blooded mammals are capable of serving as the intermediate host for this protozoan parasite.

Key Clinical Signs of Infected Animals
As definitive hosts, most cats with *Toxoplasma gondii* will be asymptomatic. Kittens infected transplacentally or when nursing are often the most severely affected patients; will show signs of lethargy, depression, ascites, and fever; and can often die suddenly. Older cats with clinical illness may present with a variety of clinical signs from very general ones such as fever and anorexia, to more specific symptoms involving any body system that is affected by the spread of **tachyzoites** or **bradyzoites** throughout the body.

> **TECHNICIAN NOTE** A bradyzoite (literally, "a slow growing, tiny organism") is a term for a tissue stage, for example, a slow growing developmental stage that occurs in cysts in the life cycle of *Toxoplasma gondii*. A tachyzoite (literally, "a fast growing, tiny organism") is a term for a tissue stage, for example, a fast growing developmental stage.

Abbreviated Life Cycle
The life cycle of *T. gondii* has two phases: a sexual phase and an asexual phase. The sexual phase of the life cycle takes place

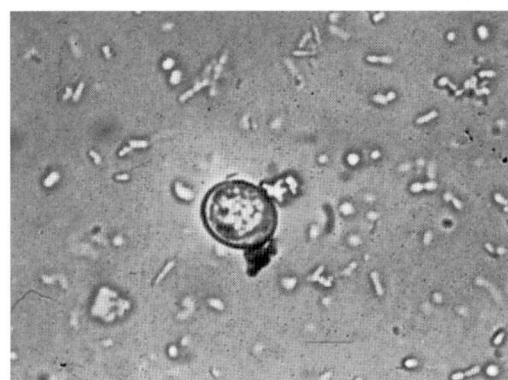

FIGURE 14-36 Oocysts of *Toxoplasma gondii*, fecal flotation. (From Hendrix CM, Robinson E: Diagnostic parasitology for veterinary technicians, ed 4, St Louis, 2012, Mosby.)

only in cats, both domestic and wild (definitive hosts). The sexual stages of *T. gondii* are found within feline intestinal cells. Macrogametes are fertilized by microgametes, and **oocysts** are formed. These oocysts are very tiny and have undergone sporulation. The asexual phase can take place in any warm-blooded animal (intermediate hosts). Both mammals (including the cat) and birds are suitable intermediate hosts. In the intermediate host, the parasite invades cells and forms intracellular cysts containing slow growing (slowly dividing) forms called *bradyzoites*. These cysts are found primarily in muscles and brain. Because the host's immune system does not recognize these cysts as being "foreign," the bradyzoites multiply to the point that the infected cell that they are within bursts open and release tachyzoites (rapidly dividing forms). These tachyzoites may form even more cysts, which may be made up of bradyzoites or tachyzoites. Tissue cysts are ingested by a cat (when it feeds on an infected mouse). The cysts are digested and eventually infect cells of the small intestine, and then undergo sexual reproduction to form oocysts. These oocysts are shed in the feces of the cat (Figure 14-36). Animals and humans that ingest oocysts (e.g., by eating unwashed vegetables contaminated with cat feces) or tissue cysts in improperly cooked meat become infected. The parasites enter macrophages in the lining of the intestine and are distributed via the bloodstream throughout the body.

Laboratory Test(s) Used to Diagnose the Infection
Diagnosis of *T. gondii* is usually presumptive, based on clinical signs consistent with *T. gondii* infection and positive serologic testing (ELISA), combined with a clinical response to medications and exclusion of other causes for the clinical signs. Definitive diagnosis can be confirmed by identification of the organism in tissues or body fluids on necropsy or through a biopsy specimen, but this is not common.

Zoonotic Potential for Clients
Kittens that live outdoors and hunt are generally infected at a very young age. Minimizing the shedding of oocysts into

the environment from infected cats or kittens is important and can be done by feeding cats and dogs only commercial cat food and never feeding them raw or undercooked meat. This parasite usually is of greatest concern to pregnant women because of the possibility of the spread of infection transplacentally to the developing fetus.

Treatment

Clindamycin is the treatment of choice in dogs and cats.

Prevention and Control Techniques

Litter boxes must be cleaned daily because oocysts need a minimum of 1 to 3 days to sporulate and become infective. This time frame is dependent on temperature and gets longer as the temperature gets colder. Disinfect litter boxes with boiling water at least once weekly. Cover outdoor sandboxes. These precautions are often adequate for preventing zoonosis, and immunocompromised individuals need not necessarily be separated from their cats. Pregnant women must avoid contact with soil, cat litter, raw meat, and cats excreting oocysts. All persons should wash hands and surfaces after handling raw meat or cleaning litter boxes.

> **TECHNICIAN NOTE** Although humans can be infected by a cat that is shedding oocysts, people more often are infected by eating raw or undercooked meat containing cysts. This disease can be difficult to confirm antemortem in dogs and cats; because of this, it is important to consider other, more common sources of human infection.

CRYPTOSPORIDIUM PARVUM—CRYPTOSPORIDIOSIS

- **Parasite's common name:** "Crypto," "cryptosporidiosis"
- **Pronunciation:** "Crypt-oh-spore-**rid**-ee-yum" "**par**-vum"
- **Derivation:** "**Kryptos,**" from Greek, *hidden* (this is a very tiny protozoan parasite); "**sporos,**" from Greek, *seed*: "**eidos,**" from Greek, *form* or *shape*; "**parvum,**" from Latin, *small*. This is a very tiny protozoan parasite—the smallest protozoan parasite found in the gastrointestinal tract.
- **Type of parasite:** protozoan—apicomplexan—coccidian

Species Affected

Cryptosporidium species will infect all species of domestic animals—especially calves, dogs, and cats, but also rodents and humans. Cryptosporidiosis usually occurs in dogs that are younger than 6 months.

Location of Parasite Within Host

This tiniest of protozoan parasites is found on the tips of the villi of the small intestine.

Key Clinical Signs of Infected Animals

Cryptosporidiosis can be asymptomatic, or it may cause gastrointestinal symptoms. It produces an acute, watery diarrhea with mucus that may persist for a few weeks. Many dogs recover spontaneously from cryptosporidiosis, having shown no clinical signs. Other dogs may develop only mild diarrhea. However, in dogs with weakened immune systems, cryptosporidiosis can cause chronic diarrhea and extreme dehydration. *Cryptosporidium* can be extremely life threatening in immunocompromised dogs.

Abbreviated Life Cycle

Oocysts of *Cryptosporidium parvum* may be found in untreated surface water, contaminated water supplies, and cattle manure, and on objects that have been contaminated with human feces. If ingested by a suitable host, oocysts pass through the stomach and enter the small intestine. Within the intestine, oocysts will excyst ("hatch"), releasing four motile, arc-shaped sporozoites. The sporozoites adhere to the external cell wall of the intestinal cells. Here they begin to multiply, producing the next parasitic stage—the merozoite stage. Six to eight merozoites are produced from one sporozoite. This is asexual multiplication—there are no male or female parasitic stages. These merozoites break out of the host's cells and invade new cells, repeating this process. Merozoites can continue to invade new intestinal cells and multiply. This results in large numbers of *C. parvum* parasites and infected intestinal cells. At some point, some of these merozoites develop differently into both male and female gametocytes. These male and female gametocytes unite to form gametes, developing between the layers of the cell wall. They become oocysts. These oocysts break out and are carried away with the intestinal contents. At this stage, the host is likely to have symptoms of cryptosporidiosis—a profuse diarrhea will quickly carry these oocysts out of the body. Some of the oocysts mature very quickly. They can release their sporozoites before they are passed into the external environment in the feces. These sporozoites immediately invade intestinal cells and begin to multiply, starting the process of cryptosporidiosis again. When the host's immune system is healthy, the body will eventually fight off the parasite. The intestine will eventually heal, and diarrhea and associated symptoms will subside. For immunocompromised individuals, infection with *Cryptosporidium* will continue on and on, becoming a vicious and deadly cycle. Infective oocysts are passed into the external environment. They are quite resilient, being unaffected by cold, chlorine, and other chemicals added to water to disinfect it. These oocysts can survive long periods of time in moist conditions. They will perish if they dry out. If another suitable host swallows them, a *Cryptosporidium* infection will begin anew.

Laboratory Test(s) Used to Diagnose the Infection

This parasite can be diagnosed using fecal flotation procedures (Figure 14-37). Commercial serologic tests are

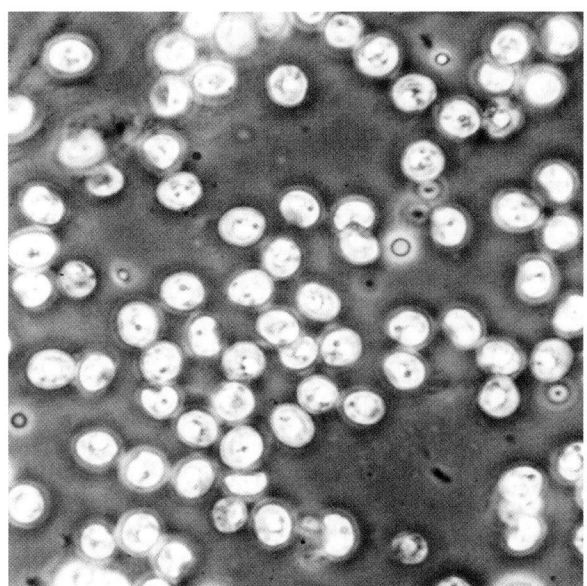

FIGURE 14-37 Oocysts of *Cryptosporidium parvum*, fecal flotation.

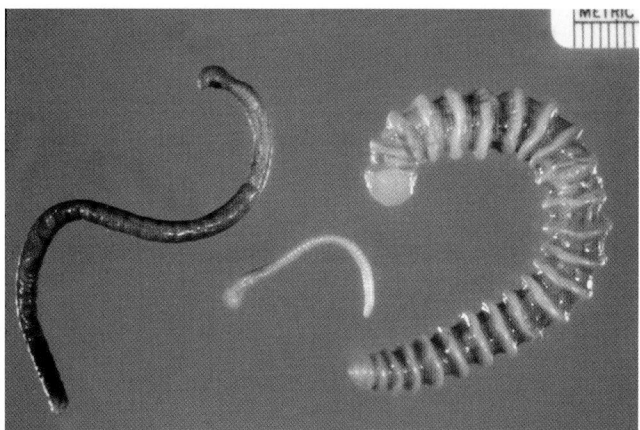

FIGURE 14-38 Assorted pentastomids from the respiratory passages of snakes.

available to identify antibodies against *C. parvum* in the dog's blood. A positive test means that the dog has been exposed to this protozoan, but not that it is currently infected. *Cryptosporidium* exposure rates are high in dogs.

Zoonotic Potential for Clients

C. parvum can cause chronic diarrhea and severe dehydration in humans with HIV or AIDS, and can easily develop into a life-threatening secondary infection in people with compromised immune systems.

Treatment

No reliable treatment is available for enteritis due to *C. parvum* in dogs; in most cases, dogs recover from cryptosporidiosis spontaneously. If treatment is necessary, broad-spectrum antibiotics may be prescribed. A high-fiber diet can help relieve the symptoms of diarrhea associated with this infection. Supportive therapy (e.g., fluid replacement) can help dogs suffering from dehydration.

Prevention and Control Techniques

Contaminated areas in the dog's environment must be disinfected with a 1:10 bleach and water solution. The pet's bedding should be washed in hot water using a quality household detergent in combination with chlorine bleach. The infected dog must be isolated from other pets, children, and individuals with compromised immune systems.

> **TECHNICIAN NOTE** Because of medical privacy issues, members of the veterinary team should never make client inquiries regarding the client's medical information (e.g., infection with HIV/AIDS). However, when confronted with a diagnosis of cryptosporidiosis in dogs, the severity of the zoonotic potential must be communicated to every pet owner or client.

PENTASTOMES (SNAKE PARASITES) OF ZOONOTIC IMPORTANCE

PENTASTOMES

- **Parasite's common name:** pentastomes, tongueworms
- **Pronunciation:** "pen-tah-stomes"
- **Derivation:** "Pente," from Greek, *five*; "**stomum,**" from Greek, *mouths*. On the anterior end of all adult pentastomes is a mouth surrounded by four hooks. Early researchers believed that these hooks were mouths, so they erroneously believed that these strange creatures had five mouths.
- **Type of parasite:** arthropod—pentastomid

Species Affected

Adult pentastomes are primarily parasites of snakes and reptiles (assorted genera and species) (Figure 14-38). Nymphal pentastomes may be found in a variety of internal organs (liver, spleen, lymph nodes, etc.) in mammals. Only one adult pentastome does parasitize mammals—*Linguatula serrata* (pronunciation "Lin-**gwat**-you-lah" "ser-**ah**-tah"), the canine pentastome, found in the nasal passages of the dog.

Location of Parasite Within Host

Adult pentastomes are always associated with some portion of the respiratory tract (e.g., nasal passages, lungs, air sacs), but larval pentastomes are associated with mesenchymal tissues (e.g., liver, spleen, lymph nodes).

Key Clinical Signs of Infected Animals

L. serrata infects the nasal passages of dogs (Figure 14-39). Dogs may sneeze or have a slight to moderate nosebleed. Infected snakes and reptiles are usually asymptomatic. Adult pentastomes in these species are usually incidental postmortem findings at necropsy.

Abbreviated Life Cycle

The life cycle of *L. serrata*, the canine pentastome, will be discussed. Adult male and female pentastomes are found in

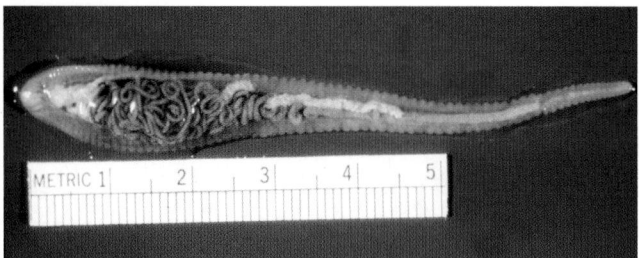

FIGURE 14-39 *Linguatula serrata*, the canine pentastome, from the nasal passages of a dog.

the nasal passages of the dog. Female pentastomes produce eggs that pass out into the environment in the dog's feces. Each egg will contain a mite-like larval stage, with four or six jointed legs with hook-like claws on the end. The intermediate host, usually a rat or a rabbit, must ingest these larvae. Within the intermediate host, the mite-like larval stage migrates to any one of assorted mesenchymal tissues (e.g., liver, spleen, lymph nodes, omentum). At these sites, the larval stage develops into the nymphal stage, a C-shaped, worm-like or grub-like creature. The dog becomes infected with adult pentastomes by ingesting the intermediate host containing the nymphal stages. The nymphal stage will bore through the wall of the intestine and diaphragm, reaching the lungs. It migrates up the bronchial tree until it reaches the nasal passages, where these parasites reside as adults.

Laboratory Test(s) Used to Diagnose the Infection

Diagnosis may be made by fecal flotation and microscopic examination of nasal swabs. Pentastome eggs are unique in that they are round and contain a mite-like larval stage. Within the ovum, the larval stage has jointed legs ending with claws. The nymphal stage within parenchymal tissues often assumes a characteristic C shape in situ. This stage can be identified in a histopathologic tissue section.

Zoonotic Potential for Clients

Clients should be advised that they are capable of serving as the intermediate host for pentastomes, which might infect snakes. Should the client ingest the mite-like larval stage, the nymphal stage may develop within the human's liver, spleen, omentum, or other tissue.

Treatment

Currently, no treatments are available for pentastomes in snakes or reptiles.

Prevention and Control Techniques

Owners of snakes and reptiles should wash their hands after contact with feces or saliva from snake or reptiles. In addition, handling fecal-contaminated water, dishes, and other equipment within the herpetarium may result in accidental transmission. Prey fed to captive snakes and reptiles should be pentastome free.

> **TECHNICIAN NOTE** For the most part, pentastomes are parasites of snakes and reptiles. One species of pentastome does infect domestic animals. *Linguatula serrata* is the canine pentastome found in the nasal passages of dogs.

DIAGNOSIS OF ENDOPARASITISM

Parasites can infect the oral cavity, esophagus, stomach, small and large intestines, and other internal organs of domesticated animals. Detection of the presence of these parasites involves collection and microscopic examination of feces. Diagnosis usually is made by finding life cycle stages of the parasite within the feces. These stages include eggs, oocysts, larvae, segments (tapeworms), and adult organisms. Veterinary technicians may perform the following procedures to detect parasitic infections.

COLLECTION OF FECAL SAMPLES

Fecal samples collected for routine examination should be as fresh as possible. Specimens that cannot be examined within a few hours of elimination should be refrigerated or mixed with equal parts of 10% formalin. The need for fresh feces stems from the fact that eggs, oocysts, and other life cycle stages may be altered by development, making diagnosis extremely difficult.

SMALL ANIMAL FECAL SAMPLES

Several methods are used for collecting feces from companion animals. An owner may collect a fecal sample immediately after the animal has defecated. The feces may be stored in any type of container, such as a zippered plastic bag or a clean, small jar with a tight cap. Veterinary hospitals may dispense containers to their clients for this purpose. In either case, only a small amount of feces (1 teaspoon) is required for proper examination by the technician. All specimens should be properly identified with the owner's name, the animal's name, and the species of animal.

Fecal samples also may be collected directly from the animal at the veterinary hospital, using a gloved finger or a fecal loop. If a glove is used, the feces may remain in the glove, with the glove turned inside out, tied and labeled. Samples collected with a fecal loop should be used for direct examination only because the amount collected is relatively small.

EXAMINATION OF FECAL SAMPLES

Several precautions should be taken during fecal examination:

- Fecal samples are handled with care. The feces may contain parasites, bacteria, or viruses that are zoonotic (i.e., animal diseases that may be transmitted to people). Appropriate clothing, such as a clean laboratory coat or jacket and latex gloves, should be worn during the laboratory examination. If gloves are not worn, hands should be frequently washed with soap and water. No food or drink should be allowed in the examination area. Likewise, workers should refrain from applying makeup or adjusting contact lenses. Laboratory coats should never be worn outside of the veterinary clinic; this reduces the chances of spreading any infection.

- The laboratory area is cleaned thoroughly after fecal examinations have been completed. Spilled materials create a hazardous area in which to work and could pose a serious threat to staff members' health.
- Accurate and thorough records are maintained. Records should contain the date, the owner's name, and any parasites found in the sample. If the sample is negative, it should be recorded as such.

GROSS EXAMINATION OF FECES

Several characteristics of the feces should be recorded and reported to the veterinarian:

- *Consistency.* Fresh feces should be somewhat formed, depending on the species of animal. Diarrhea or constipation could be the result of a parasitic infection.
- *Color.* Fecal color may be affected by the food an animal eats. Also, malabsorption or a parasitic infection may alter the color of feces.
- *Blood.* Blood may impart a dark reddish-brown color to feces, or it may appear as bright red streaks in the feces. In either case, blood may indicate a severe parasitic infection or other serious intestinal disease. Blood in the feces is an important clinical finding and should be brought to the attention of the veterinarian. Digested blood has a dark, tarry appearance.
- *Mucus.* Mucus in the feces can be a result of digestive disorders or a parasitic infection. In either case, its presence should be reported to the veterinarian.
- *Gross parasites.* Adult parasites or tapeworm segments can be found in the feces. Adult roundworms resemble strings of spaghetti, whereas tapeworm segments look more like pieces of cooked rice. Tapeworm segments may be identified by microscopic examination. The segments of two common tapeworms infecting dogs and cats are shown in Figure 14-40.

Figure 14-41 shows common tapeworm segments—*Moniezia* species, found in cattle feces, and *Anoplocephala* species, found in horse feces.

Occasionally, a client may submit a dried tapeworm segment to be identified. To identify the tapeworm species, the dried segments must be soaked in saline for 1 to 4 hours to rehydrate them. Once the segments are rehydrated, they may be identified by their unique size, shape, and morphologic features, and by the eggs contained within.

Segments of some tapeworm species do not contain eggs, and some segments may have expelled their eggs before the examination was conducted. In either case, a tapeworm segment may be identified as such by the finding of small mineral deposits (calcareous bodies) within the segment (Figure 14-42). This is done by crushing the tapeworm-like segment between two glass slides and examining the material with a microscope.

MICROSCOPIC EXAMINATION OF FECES

Microscopic examination of feces is the most reliable method to detect parasitic infection. A compound microscope with

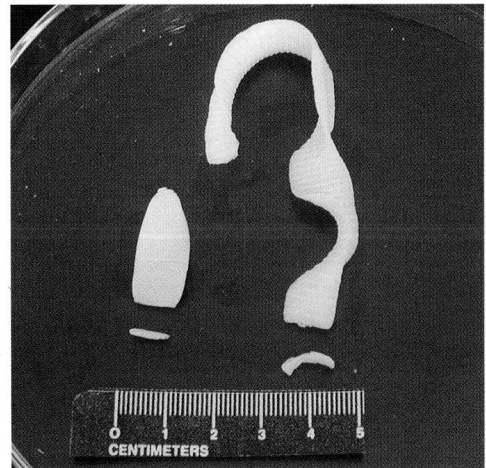

FIGURE 14-41 Chains and individually mature segments of tapeworms of horses, *Anoplocephala (left)*, and cattle, *Moniezia (right)*.

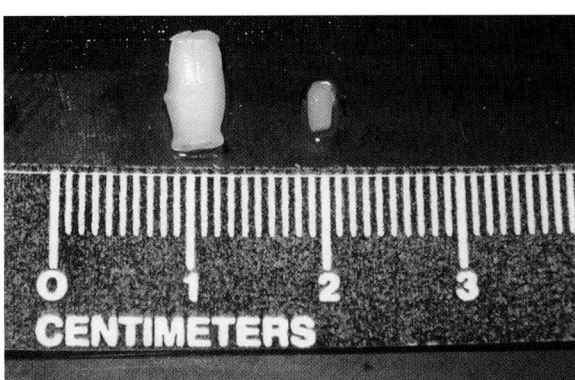

FIGURE 14-40 Mature segments of the most common tapeworms of dogs and cats. *Left, Taenia* spp. *Right, Dipylidium caninum.*

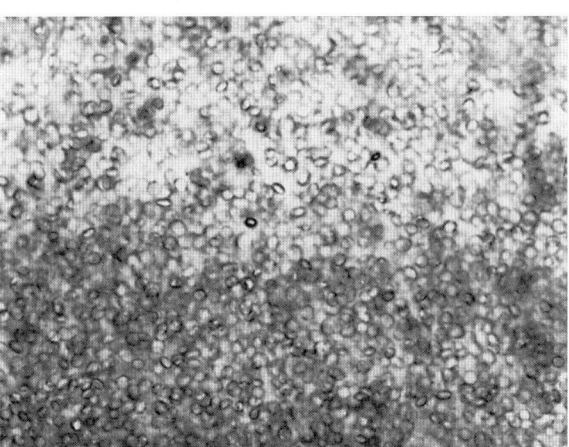

FIGURE 14-42 Microscopic calcium deposits (calcareous bodies) in tapeworm tissue.

4×, 10×, and 40× objectives is required for proper examination of a fecal specimen. A mechanical stage is helpful. A micrometer is also recommended but is not required.

Fecal specimens should be examined routinely using the 10× objective. The examination should begin at one corner of the slide and end at the opposite corner, moving over the slide in a systematic pattern (Figure 14-43). The microscope should be focused continually with the fine-tuning knob during the examination. The initial plane of focus should be that of air bubbles because most helminth eggs are found in this plane. Any material found during the initial scan, including parasite eggs, may be more closely examined using the more powerful objectives.

Calibration of the Microscope

The size of the various stages of many parasites is often important for correct identification. Some examples are *Trichuris* versus *Capillaria* eggs and *Dipetalonema* versus *Dirofilaria* microfilariae. Accurate measurements are obtained easily with the use of a calibrated eyepiece on the microscope. Calibration must be performed on every microscope to be used. Each objective (lens) of the microscope must be individually calibrated.

The stage micrometer is a microscope slide etched with a 2-mm line marked in 0.01-mm (10-μm) divisions (Figure 14-44). The veterinary technician should remember that 1 micron (μ) = 0.001 mm.

The eyepiece scale is a glass disc that fits into and remains in one of the microscope eyepieces. This disc is etched with hash marks spaced at equal intervals. The number of hash marks on the disc may vary with different manufacturers, but the calibration procedure is the same for all.

The stage micrometer is used to determine the distance in microns between the hash marks on the eyepiece scale for each objective lens of the microscope being calibrated. This information is recorded and labeled on the microscope for future reference.

To begin the calibration procedure, the veterinary technician should start on low power (10×) and focus on the 2-mm line of the stage micrometer. Therefore, 2 mm = 2000 μm.

The eyepiece is rotated so that the hash mark scale is horizontal and parallel to the stage micrometer scale. The zero (0) point is aligned on both scales.

The point on the stage micrometer aligned with the "10" hash mark is determined on the eyepiece scale. For example, the 0.125 mm mark might align with the "10" hash mark.

This number is multiplied by 100. In the above example,

$$0.125 \times 100 = 12.5 \, \mu m$$

This means that at this power (10×), the distance between hash marks on the eyepiece scale is 12.5 μm.

These steps are repeated at each magnification (10×, 40×, 100×). The information is recorded on a label that is attached to the calibrated microscope. For example,

Objective	Distance Between Hash Marks, μm
10×	12.5
40×	2.5
100×	1.0

To measure an object such as a parasite egg, one end of the egg is placed on the zero mark of the ocular scale, and the number of divisions to the other end of the egg is counted. The number of divisions counted is multiplied by the calibration factor for the objective being used. For example, a trichostrongyle egg is 24 divisions long and 13.5 divisions wide when measured with the 40× objective. The calibration factor for the 40× objective is 2.5. Therefore, the egg is

$$24 \times 2.5 = 60 \, \mu m \text{ long}$$

and

$$13.5 \times 2.5 = 33.75 \, \mu m \text{ wide}$$

To measure a microfilaria, the head (the anterior end) is aligned with the zero mark of the ocular scale, and the number of divisions to the end of the tail (the posterior end) is counted. To measure round parasite eggs, the technician should measure through the middle of the egg at its greatest diameter. For more accurate measurements, the higher objective is used (40× instead of 10×).

EXAMINATION OF DIRECT SMEARS

A direct smear of feces is used to rapidly estimate an animal's parasite burden. This procedure also is used to detect some of the motile protozoa found in feces.

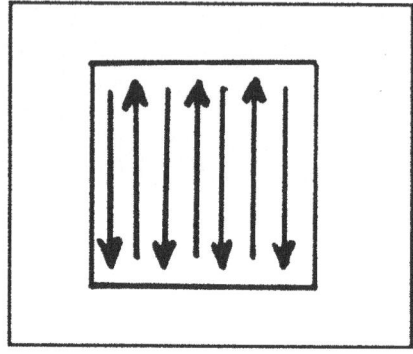

FIGURE 14-43 A scheme of movement of the microscopic field to examine the area under the cover slip thoroughly.

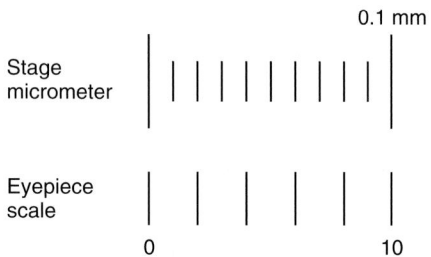

FIGURE 14-44 Stage micrometer *(upper scale)* and eyepiece scale *(lower scale)* used to calibrate the microscope.

Advantages of direct smears include short preparation time and minimal equipment required to run the procedure. Disadvantages include the small amount of feces examined, which may not be sufficient to detect a low parasite burden, and the amount of extraneous fecal debris on the slide, which could be confused with parasitic material.

A fecal sample for a direct smear preparation may be obtained from an animal using a fecal loop or a rectal thermometer (after the animal's temperature is measured). Either way, only a very small amount of feces is needed.

CONCENTRATION METHODS FOR FECAL EXAMINATION

The following methods are used to concentrate parasitic material in feces. A concentration technique makes it possible to examine a large amount of feces in a relatively short time. Also, a low parasite burden can easily be identified. Two types of procedures are used most often in veterinary hospitals: flotation and sedimentation.

Fecal flotation methods are based on the specific gravity of parasitic material and fecal debris. *Specific gravity* refers to the weight of an object as compared with the weight of an equal volume of water. The specific gravity of most parasite eggs is between 1.100 and 1.200 g/mL, whereas the specific gravity of water is 1.000.

To allow for flotation of parasite eggs, oocysts, and other life cycle stages, the flotation solution must have a higher specific gravity than that of the parasitic material. Several salt and sugar solutions work well for flotation. Most have a specific gravity of 1.200 to 1.250. In this range, heavy fecal debris sinks to the bottom of the container, while parasitic material rises to the top of the solution.

Sodium nitrate solution is the most common fecal flotation solution used in veterinary hospitals today. This solution is efficient for floating parasite eggs, oocysts, and larvae. It may be purchased with commercial diagnostic test kits or in individual aliquots. The major disadvantage of using sodium nitrate is the expense. Sodium nitrate also forms crystals and distorts eggs if allowed to sit longer than 20 minutes.

Another solution commonly used for flotation is saturated sugar solution. Sugar solution is inexpensive and does not crystallize or distort eggs. Sugar solution may be made anywhere and has a long shelf life. Although sticky to work with, spilled sugar solution may be removed with warm, soapy water.

Zinc sulfate solution is more commonly used in diagnostic laboratories. Zinc sulfate floats protozoal organisms with the least amount of distortion. It generally is used in combination with one of the previously mentioned solutions.

The least desirable solution used is saturated sodium chloride solution. This solution corrodes laboratory equipment, forms crystals, and severely distorts parasite eggs. Saturated sodium chloride solution is also a poor flotation medium, as the maximum specific gravity obtainable is 1.200, allowing heavier eggs to remain submerged. Several choices of flotation techniques are available.

Standard Fecal Flotation

The standard or simple fecal flotation is one of the most common flotation techniques used in veterinary hospitals. This technique uses a test tube or vial, in which feces and flotation solution are mixed (Figure 14-45). A cover slip or microscope slide is placed on top of the test tube, and the unit is allowed to sit undisturbed. Any parasite eggs in the feces float to the top and adhere to the underside of the cover slip or microscope slide. The cover slip or slide then is removed and microscopically examined for parasitic material. Although the standard flotation technique is easy to perform, it is less efficient at floating parasitic material than the centrifugal technique, described later in this chapter.

Commercial flotation kits use the same principle as the standard flotation technique. These kits contain a vial with a filter; some also include prepared flotation solution. Examples of commercial flotation kits include Ovassay Plus (Synbiotics, San Diego, CA), and Ovatector (BGS Medical Products, Venice, FL) (Figure 14-46). These kits are simple

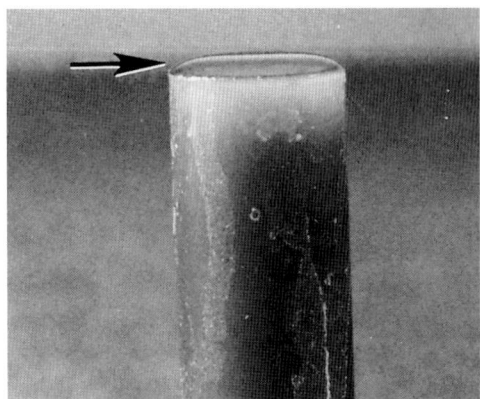

FIGURE 14-45 Vial filled with flotation solution, showing appearance of meniscus.

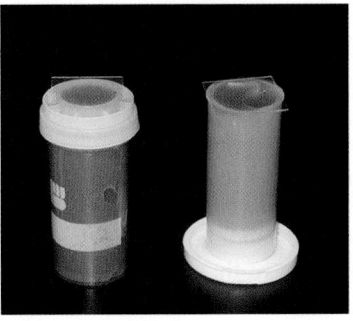

FIGURE 14-46 Ovassay (*left*) and Ovatector (*right*) are two examples of commercial fecal flotation kits.

to use but expensive when compared with the simple flotation technique. Some practices reduce the expense by washing and reusing the vials and filters; this practice should be discouraged.

Centrifugal Flotation

Centrifugal flotation for parasite eggs, oocysts, and other parasitic material is the most efficient method available. It requires less time to perform than the standard flotation method. The only drawback to this procedure is that it requires a centrifuge with a horizontal (nonfixed) rotor that can hold 15-mL centrifuge tubes. If such a centrifuge is available, centrifugal flotation is preferred because it is easy to perform, and samples can be run individually or in batches.

If testing multiple samples, the veterinary technician may want to use a numbering system to keep the samples in order. A number is assigned to the patient, and that number is written on the corresponding centrifuge tube with a marking pen. This minimizes the chances of error.

Fecal Sedimentation

Fecal sedimentation concentrates parasite eggs, oocysts, and other parasitic material by allowing them to settle to the bottom of a tube of liquid, usually water. A disadvantage of this technique is the amount of fecal debris that mixes with the parasitic material, which makes microscopic examination somewhat difficult.

This procedure is used to detect heavy eggs that would not float in flotation solution, or eggs that would become distorted by the flotation solution. Trematode (fluke) eggs are often considered too heavy for flotation and are often found using fecal sedimentation. Although some flotation solutions can be adjusted to a specific gravity of 1.300 to float these eggs, such solutions are not used routinely because some distortion may occur.

EXAMINATION OF FECES FOR PROTOZOA

All of the previously described procedures may be used to detect protozoal cysts. However, some protozoans do not form cysts and pass out of the host in the trophozoite form. Trophozoites are one-cell, motile organisms that lack the rigid wall of a cyst, making flotation without distortion or death of the trophozoite impossible. Therefore, the direct smear technique, using saline and a stain, is the preferred procedure for examination of a fecal sample for protozoal organisms.

In a direct smear, trophozoites may be recognized by their movement. *Giardia* species are tear-shaped and have five to eight flagella. They move with a jerky motion. Trichomonads are long, slender organisms with a single flagellum attached to the dorsal surface, forming a sail-like structure that ripples as the organism glides through debris. Amoebae move with a flowing motion, extending a part of the body (pseudopod) and moving the rest of the body after it.

Stains also may be used to recognize certain structural characteristics of trophozoites and cysts. Lugol's iodine and new methylene blue are stains commonly used with the direct smear procedure. These stains do not preserve the slide but do facilitate examination of the specimen, making identification easier.

If a protozoal parasite cannot be identified on direct smears, fecal smears containing protozoal trophozoites can be dried, stained with Diff-Quik, Wright, or Giemsa stain, and sent to a diagnostic laboratory. Many other procedures are used for staining and preserving protozoal trophozoites. Most of these procedures are used in diagnostic laboratories and are not explained here.

SPECIAL STAINING FOR COCCIDIAN PARASITES

Several coccidian parasites require special staining techniques for identification. Two procedures are discussed in this chapter.

The acid-fast staining technique is used to identify *Cryptosporidium* species in feces. *Cryptosporidium* is a parasite of the gastrointestinal tract of many animals, including people. The oocysts are 2 to 8 µm in diameter and are almost undetectable in flotation solution to the inexperienced eye. Acid-fast staining can aid detection of oocysts in a fecal smear.

The second procedure uses Diff-Quik stain for identification of *Cystoisospora* species. *Cystoisospora* species (*Isospora* = *Cystoisospora*) are coccidia found in the gastrointestinal tract (especially the jejunum) of many animals, but they are of greatest concern in pigs. This parasite can cause the death of many piglets before any oocysts are found in the feces using conventional flotation methods. Therefore, an intestinal mucosal scraping must be stained and examined for other diagnostic stages (schizonts, merozoites) of this parasite. This procedure involves scraping the mucosa of the jejunum and smearing the scrapings onto microscope slides. After the slides have been air dried, they are stained with Diff-Quik and examined with the oil immersion objective.

For accurate results with either of these procedures, several samples should be examined. If such examination is not possible, feces or intestines may be sent to a diagnostic laboratory. Collection and shipping of parasitic specimens are described later in this chapter.

ANTIGEN TESTS

Antigen tests for *Giardia* and *Cryptosporidium* are available and may be used for their detection.

SAMPLE COLLECTION AT NECROPSY

Necropsy (postmortem examination) is an important method of diagnosing many diseases, including parasitism. The types of lesions produced by immature parasites and any adult parasites found in the body cavity and tissues, along with histopathologic examination of infected tissues, are used in diagnosis. Veterinary technicians are responsible for the samples collected, making sure they are contained, preserved, labeled, and shipped properly. Refer to Chapter 17 for more information about necropsy techniques.

Two methods may be used to recover parasites from the digestive tract at necropsy: the decanting method and the sieving method. With either method, the veterinary technician must separate the different parts of the digestive tract and work with the contents of each individually.

Parasites recovered from the digestive tract may be preserved in 70% alcohol or 10% neutral buffered formalin for later identification. Occasionally, bladder worms or cysticerci may be found attached to the viscera of domestic animals. A bladderworm is a fluid-filled, balloon-like structure that is actually a larval tapeworm. These should be handled with care because the fluid within the bladder can be allergenic and may also be zoonotic. To identify the parasites recovered, the veterinary technician should consult the references listed at the end of this chapter. If in-hospital diagnosis is not possible, the samples may be preserved as previously described and sent to a diagnostic laboratory for identification.

SHIPPING PARASITOLOGIC SPECIMENS

Any parasitologic specimen shipped to a diagnostic laboratory should be preserved with alcohol or formalin, unless otherwise directed by laboratory personnel. Specimens should be packaged in a leakproof container and sealed with Parafilm (Fischer Scientific, Pittsburgh, PA) or tape. If specimen containers are found leaking, the shipment will not be delivered. Feces can be sent fresh or mixed at a ratio of 1:3 with 10% formalin. Whole parasites or segments can be preserved in alcohol or formalin and placed in a leakproof container (clean small jar, medicine vial, or clot tube).

All specimen containers should be labeled as to the site from which the specimen was obtained, the owner's name, the animal's species, name, or identification number, and the referring veterinarian (including telephone number and address). The labeled specimen container should be placed in a shockproof shipping container to prevent breakage during shipping. Styrofoam containers filled with shredded newspaper work well for shipping parasitologic specimens.

A cover letter should be included with the specimen and should contain a brief history of the animal, findings upon necropsy, and the reason for submitting the samples to the laboratory (e.g., fecal examination, special staining, species identification). Without this background information, the diagnostic laboratory is unlikely to provide accurate results.

> **TECHNICIAN NOTE** Any parasitologic specimen shipped to a diagnostic laboratory should be preserved with alcohol or formalin, unless otherwise directed by laboratory personnel. Specimens should be packaged in a leakproof container and sealed with Parafilm (Fischer Scientific) or tape. If specimen containers are found leaking, the shipment will not be delivered.

MISCELLANEOUS PROCEDURES FOR DETECTION OF ENDOPARASITES

Baermann Technique

The Baermann technique is used to recover nematode larvae from feces, tissues, or soil. This technique uses warm water to stimulate larvae to move about. As the larvae do so,

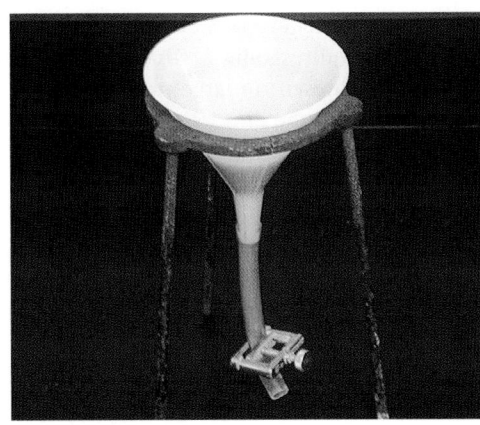

FIGURE 14-47 Baermann apparatus is used to recover larvae of roundworms from feces, soil, or animal tissues. This apparatus is most useful in recovering larvae of lungworms.

they sink to the bottom of the funnel for collection and identification.

This technique is performed with a Baermann apparatus (Figure 14-47). The apparatus consists of a ring stand and a ring holder, a glass funnel with a piece of rubber tubing on the end, a clamp, and a wire net or cheesecloth. The sample is placed on the wire screen or cheesecloth, and warm water is added to barely cover the sample. All air bubbles are allowed to flow from the tube of the funnel by releasing the clamp. The apparatus is allowed to sit undisturbed for 12 to 24 hours.

A drop of fluid from the bottom of the funnel is removed (usually the first drop) and placed on a microscope slide. If any larvae are found swimming on the slide, the slide is heated with a match to render them immobile.

Larvae recovered from fresh feces are almost always those of lungworms. Larvae from *Strongyloides stercoralis* can be found in fresh canine feces. If the feces are not fresh, all sorts of parasitic and nonparasitic larvae and adults may be seen. For more detailed information on the descriptions of larvae, consult the reference by Bowman.

Examination of Blood Samples

Dirofilaria immitis, the canine heartworm, is the most important parasite of the vascular system in domestic animals in the United States. For this reason, in-hospital blood examinations are commonly performed to detect heartworms.

The following procedures can be performed by veterinary technicians to identify *D. immitis*. As mentioned earlier, a clean environment and proper handling of samples are vital to quality control in any laboratory. Improper handling of any sample may result in inaccurate results.

Direct Blood Smear

Direct examination of the blood for microfilariae is the simplest procedure to perform. This procedure detects movement of microfilariae and other parasites among the red blood cells. As with direct examination of feces, direct examination of blood requires only a small sample. However, unless parasites are present in large numbers, they may be missed. For this reason, the direct smear is not a good diagnostic technique for diagnosing microfilariae.

Microfilariae of primary interest are those of *D. immitis*, the canine heartworm, and *Dipetalonema (Acanthochelionema) reconditum*, a subcutaneous parasite of dogs. Differentiation between the two is extremely important because treatment for heartworms is expensive, somewhat stressful, and involves use of arsenical compounds.

In a direct blood smear, microfilariae of *Dirofilaria* species coil and uncoil, whereas those of *Dipetalonema* species may glide smoothly across the slide. However, this is not always the case. Also, the number of *Dirofilaria* species microfilariae in a sample is greater than that of *Dipetalonema* species. Again, this is not always the case. Direct examination of the blood is used only to determine the presence of microfilariae, not the type. For this, a concentration technique that "relaxes" and stains microfilariae is used. These procedures are discussed later in this chapter.

Thin Blood Smear

The thin blood smear is prepared and stained in exactly the same way as a blood smear for a differential white blood cell count. When doing a differential white blood cell count on an animal, the veterinary technician should note any parasitic organisms seen. Occasionally, microfilariae may be found. Because of their size, microfilariae usually are found along the feathered edge. Because differentiation of microfilariae is not possible in a thin blood smear, other procedures must be performed for identification. Trypanosomes, protozoans, and rickettsiae also may be found among or within cells. As with the direct smear procedure, a small blood sample is used, and mild parasitic infections may be missed.

Thick Blood Smear

A thick blood smear examines a slightly greater volume of blood than does a thin blood smear. Again, microfilariae may be seen, but they cannot be differentiated easily using this method.

Concentration Techniques
Buffy Coat Method

The buffy coat method is a concentration technique used on a small volume of blood. When blood is placed in a microhematocrit tube and is centrifuged for determination of the packed cell volume (PCV), it separates into three layers: plasma, white blood cell layer (buffy coat), and red blood cell layer (Figure 14-48). Microfilariae can be found on the surface of the buffy coat layer. This technique is quick and may be performed in conjunction with a PCV and total protein evaluation. However, differentiation of microfilariae is not possible.

The following concentration techniques may be used for differentiating *D. immitis* from *D. reconditum*.

Modified Knott's Technique

The modified Knott's technique is a simple procedure that allows differentiation of microfilariae. This technique concentrates, "relaxes," and stains microfilariae, while lysing red blood cells to make the microfilariae more visible.

Figure 14-49 of *D. reconditum* and Figure 14-50 of *D. immitis* are helpful in identifying microfilariae. Table 14-3

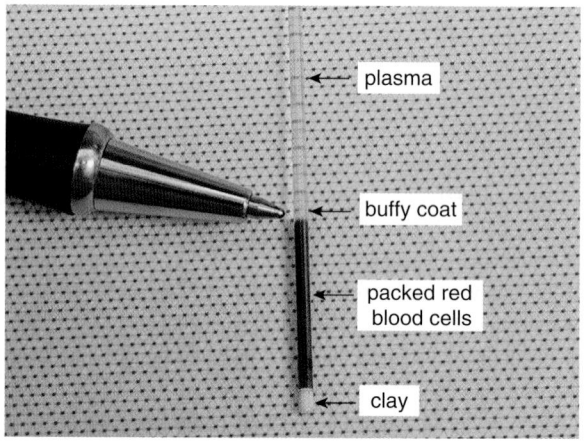

FIGURE 14-48 Buffy coat in a hematocrit tube lies between the plasma above and packed red blood cells below. A plug of clay prevents the blood from escaping the tube during centrifugation.

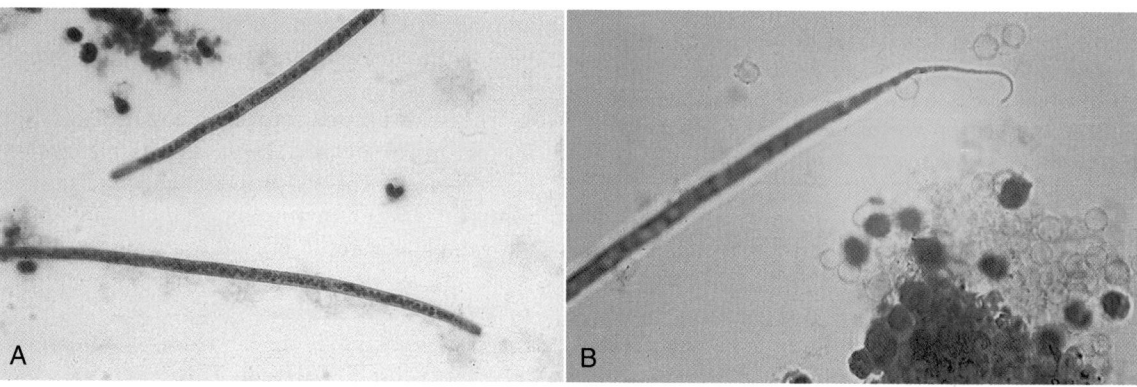

FIGURE 14-49 Cranial (**A**) and caudal (**B**) ends of a *Dipetalonema reconditum* microfilaria.

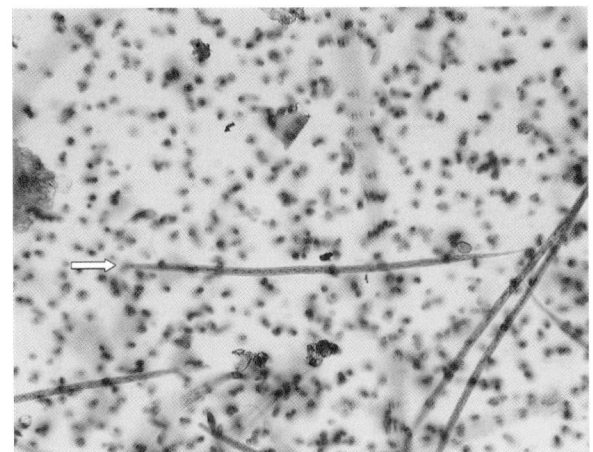

FIGURE 14-50 Microfilariae of *Dipylidium immitis* using the Difil test.

TABLE 14-3	Differentiation of Microfilariae Using the Modified Knott Technique

	DIROFILARIA IMMITIS	DIPETALONEMA RECONDITUM
Body length	310 μm	290 μm
Mid body width	6 μm	6 μm
Head	Tapered	Blunt
Tail	Straight	Hooked*

From Hendrix C, Sirois M: Laboratory procedures for veterinary technicians, ed 5, St Louis, 2007, Mosby.
*Artifact of formalin fixation.

shows the characteristics that may be used when identifying microfilariae. The veterinary technician should always examine as many microfilariae as possible because mixed infections can occur. The most accurate method for differentiation is measuring the length and width of the body. However, with some practice, general characteristics of microfilariae may be used for identification if a means of measuring microfilariae is not available.

Filter Techniques

Filter techniques are the method used most commonly in veterinary practices for detection of microfilariae in the blood. These kits come complete with filters, lysing solution, stain, and directions for use.

Most kits require 1 mL of whole blood to test for heartworms. The blood is mixed with nine parts of lysing solution and is passed through a filter. The filter is rinsed, removed, and placed on a slide. A drop of stain is added, a coverslip is applied, and then the filter is microscopically examined for microfilariae. Differentiation of microfilariae is possible but difficult using the filter technique. If microfilariae are present, it is best to perform other diagnostic procedures for identification purposes.

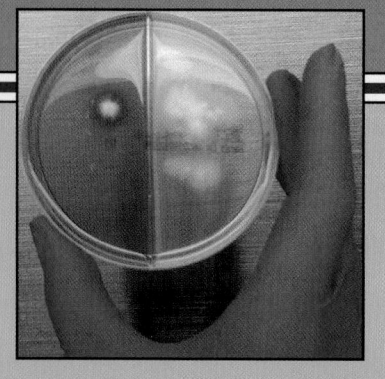

15 Clinical Microbiology

Sara D. Lawhon

OUTLINE

Safety, *485*
Sample Collection, *485*
General Culture Collection
    Information, *485*
Special Collection and Handling
    Procedures, *488*
Sample Processing, *490*
Direct Microscopic Examination, *490*
Gram Stain Procedure and
    Interpretation, *490*
Acid-Fast Stain Procedures, *492*
Bacterial Culture and Identification, *492*
Disposal, *492*
Equipment, *493*
Culture Media, *493*
Preliminary Evaluation of Cultures, *497*
Recording, Interpreting, and Reporting
    Results, *498*
Identification Procedures, *498*
Special Culture Procedures, *501*
Common Bacterial Species, *502*

Antimicrobial Susceptibility Testing, *505*
Indications, *505*
Methods, *505*
**Quality Control Testing and Quality
    Assurance,** *509*
Fungal Culture (Mycology), *509*
Safety, *509*
Standard Dermatophyte Culture, *509*
Microscopic Examination of Dermotophyte
    Cultures, *509*
Microscopic Appearance of Yeasts, *510*
Virology, *510*
Viral Detection, *510*
Molecular Detection of Pathogens, *512*
Polymerase Chain Reaction (PCR), *512*
DNA Sequencing, *513*
Nosocomial Infections, *514*
Agents of Nosocomial Infections, *515*
Recognition and Control of Nosocomial
    Infections, *515*

KEY TERMS

Abscess
Acid-fast stain
Anaerobe
Antimicrobial
  susceptibility test
Catalase
Coagulase
Dermatophyte
Differential medium
Disc diffusion test
Enrichment medium
Fastidious
Gram stain
Hemolysis
Indigenous flora
Minimum inhibitory
  concentration (MIC)
Monoclonal antibodies
Nosocomial infection
Opportunistic infection
Oxidase
Selective medium
Transport medium
Yeast

LEARNING OBJECTIVES

When you have completed this chapter, you will be able to:

1. Pronounce, define, and spell all Key Terms in the chapter.
2. Identify circumstances under which dangerous microorganisms (including those classified as "select") should not be cultured in a private practice setting.
3. Do the following regarding the collection of samples:
   - Describe factors that must be considered to ensure that quality bacterial culture samples are obtained.
   - List the indigenous flora and pathogens commonly recovered from specific anatomic sites, and describe methods used to collect representative samples.
   - Describe the special collection and handling procedures used to culture samples from tissues, urine, the respiratory tract, blood, joints, milk, and feces.
   - Identify appropriate transport media and conditions that must be met for safe transport of culture samples to an outside laboratory.
4. Do the following regarding sample processing:
   - Identify primary stains used to prepare samples for direct microscopic examination and specific organisms identified by each.

The authors and the publisher wish to acknowledge the contribution of Robert L. Jones, whose original works served as the foundation for this chapter.

- Describe the procedure for preparing and staining a sample with Gram stain, acid-fast stain, or modified acid-fast stain, including the appearance of positive and negative reactions for each.
5. Do the following regarding bacterial culture and identification:
   - Describe the principles of bacterial culture, including options for safe disposal of microbiological laboratory waste and basic equipment required to perform routine microbiological cultures.
   - Describe the differences between nutrient, enrichment, selective, and differential media, and identify commonly used plate and tube media in each category.
   - Describe the information derived from the results of biochemical testing with (1) triple sugar iron agar slant, (2) lysine iron agar slant, (3) Christensen's urea agar slant, (4) motility media, (5) indole test media, and (6) citrate test media.
   - Describe the procedures used to inoculate a culture plate for isolation and tube media for biochemical testing.
   - Identify media used for primary isolation of bacterial pathogens and conditions required for incubation of aerobic and anaerobic bacteria.
   - Explain how examination of growth on a culture plate is used to identify pathogens and guide decisions regarding further testing.
   - Describe the roles that catalase, oxidase, and coagulase biochemical tests, as well as hemolysis patterns, play in preliminary grouping of Gram-positive and Gram-negative bacteria.
   - Describe the procedure used to perform, interpret, and report results of a quantified urine culture.
6. List common bacterial flora and pathogens; identify the classification of each and associated diseases caused by each agent.
7. Do the following regarding antimicrobial susceptibility testing:
   - Explain the reasons for susceptibility testing and the guidelines set by the Clinical Laboratory Standards Institute (CLSI) for performing and interpreting antimicrobial susceptibility tests.
   - Describe the procedures for and principles of interpretation of the broth dilution test and the disc diffusion test.
8. Describe the principles of quality control testing.
9. Do the following regarding fungal culture (mycology):
   - Describe the methods used to collect dermatophytes, to inoculate dermatophyte test medium and Sabouraud dextrose agar, and to interpret culture results.
   - List common pathogenic yeasts and dimorphic fungi and associated diseases caused by each agent.
10. Do the following regarding the molecular detection of pathogens:
    - List the methods commonly used to detect viral pathogens in patient samples.
    - Explain principles underlying each of the following methods (enzyme-linked immunosorbent assay [ELISA] testing, virus isolation, electron microscopy, immunohistochemical staining).
    - Explain the difference between monoclonal and polyclonal antibodies as it relates to their use in detecting viral pathogens.
    - Explain the uses for and principles of the polymerase chain reaction test and DNA sequencing.
11. Do the following regarding nosocomial infections:
    - Explain why an understanding of the nature of nosocomial infections is crucial to a veterinary technician's ability to provide quality patient care.
    - List the agents commonly associated with nosocomial infections, factors that predispose a patient to these infections, and methods used to control and prevent them.

INTRODUCTION

The veterinarian looks to the clinical microbiology laboratory to rapidly and accurately provide information about the presence of infectious agents (bacteria, fungi, and viruses) in patient samples and to provide guidance and support for making decisions regarding treatment of infections. As a veterinary technician, you will have a direct impact on the success of identification of infectious agents through collection of appropriate samples, proper labeling and handling of those samples, and culture or timely submission of those samples to a diagnostic laboratory. The goal of this chapter is to help you understand the principles of sample collection, culture, and test interpretation, as well as the prevention of **nosocomial infections** in practice.

Increasingly, veterinary practices rely on diagnostic laboratories (e.g., state veterinary diagnostic laboratories, private laboratories) to culture patient samples for bacteria and fungi. This has several benefits. First, it may not be safe to culture certain samples in a veterinary practice. By sending samples to diagnostic laboratories, the veterinarian reduces the risk to veterinary personnel and clients. Second, it requires some expertise to recognize bacterial and fungal pathogens, and to differentiate them from **indigenous flora.** Additionally, it is necessary to do regular quality control testing on media and antibiotics to avoid erroneous conclusions that could negatively impact patients. Further, if tests or cultures are performed infrequently, it may be more cost-effective to submit the samples to a diagnostic laboratory than to maintain an inventory of media and reagents that may not be used. Finally, regulatory issues such as the need to report select agents to the Centers for Disease Control (CDC) make it advantageous to submit samples to diagnostic laboratories where personnel are familiar with these regulations. Finally, after isolating an organism in a practice, it may be necessary to send an isolate to a laboratory for further identification. Shipping regulations for routine patient samples are usually different from those for isolates, so it is often simply easier to submit all patient samples to an outside laboratory. Although these considerations are significant, some practices routinely perform microbiological cultures. Some examples of frequently performed cultures in private practice include milk cultures in dairy practices and cultures of the reproductive tract in equine practices.

This chapter describes current methods in clinical microbiology with focus on practical application of these methods. This is an exciting time in clinical microbiology. Our understanding of the relationships between bacteria and animals is changing. New studies using DNA sequencing seek to determine the identity of organisms that inhabit the body but cannot be grown or cultured using current methods. These "microbiome" studies are ongoing and will help us better understand both healthy and disease states in animals and people. In the near future though, the standard methods outlined here, namely, bacterial culture, will continue to be the primary way that bacterial and fungal pathogens are identified.

Readers with a strong interest in diagnostic clinical microbiology procedures are encouraged to read the recommended readings at the end of this chapter.

SAFETY

When preparing to culture patient samples, it is important to consider whether or not it is safe to do so. Some bacterial and fungal agents can be dangerous to handle because the cultured organism may be highly infectious. For this reason, it is best to perform cultures in a biological safety cabinet to protect workers who are handling samples and cultures. Highly infectious agents may be classified by governments as "select" agents or agents of interest because of their potential use as biological weapons. Because of the risk to personnel handling these agents, their culture is best left to specialized laboratories that have the appropriate safety equipment and procedures in place. Identification of these agents must also be reported to appropriate regulatory agencies such as the Centers for Disease Control (CDC). Examples of bacterial select agents include *Bacillus anthracis, Brucella abortus, Francisella tularensis*, and *Yersinia pestis*. Examples of fungal select agents include the dimorphic fungi *Coccidioides immitis, Histoplasma capsulatum*, and *Blastomyces dermatididis*. No attempt should be made to culture these agents in private practice.

SAMPLE COLLECTION

GENERAL CULTURE COLLECTION INFORMATION

The results of microbiological culture are dependent on the quality of samples collected. It is important to remember that the skin, mucous membranes, conjunctiva, respiratory tract, urogenital tract, and particularly the gastrointestinal tract are normally inhabited by a variety of bacterial species often called "normal" flora or indigenous flora (Table 15-1). One of the challenges of bacterial culture is determining whether an organism is a pathogen or is present as part of the indigenous flora. Indigenous flora can also cause infection, particularly **opportunistic infection.** This means that although these organisms usually are harmless, they can cause disease under certain circumstances. This typically happens when there is a failure in host defenses. When choosing the sample to collect, one must consider the pathogens likely present at an anatomic site in a specific species (Table 15-2).

The first step in collecting samples for culture is to determine the best sample to collect given clinical signs in the patient and anticipated pathogens. The samples most commonly collected are body fluids such as urine and blood, feces, washes of infected sites such as transtracheal washes or bronchoalveolar lavage fluids, tissues (biopsy and necropsy specimens), and swabs collected from these sites. In collecting samples, it is important to avoid contamination from normal flora (Figure 15-1). This is done by aseptically preparing sample collection sites when possible.

Ideally, it is best to collect samples early in the disease process, before initiation of antimicrobial therapy, because antimicrobials can interfere with isolation of pathogens. If a

TABLE 15-1	Indigenous (Normal) Flora	
AEROBES	**OBLIGATE ANAEROBES**
Skin, Ear	
Staphylococcus, Micrococcus, Streptococcus, and transient environmental and fecal contaminants	
Mouth, Nasopharynx, Oropharynx	
Micrococcus, Staphylococcus, Streptococcus (alpha- and beta-hemolytic), *Bacillus*, coliforms, *Proteus, Pasteurella, Actinobacillus, Haemophilus, Mycoplasma*, and others	*Bacteroides, Prevotella, Porphyromonas, Fusobacterium, Actinomyces*, spirochetes, and others
Trachea, Bronchi, Lungs	
Only transient contaminants	
Stomach, Small Intestine	
Small quantities of alpha-hemolytic *Streptococcus*	*Lactobacillus*
Large Intestine	
Streptococcus, Escherichia coli, Klebsiella, Enterobacter, Proteus, Enterococcus, and others	*Clostridium, Fusobacterium, Bacteroides, Porphyromonas, Prevotella*, spirochetes, *Lactobacillus*
External Genitalia (Vulva, Prepuce)	
Micrococcus, Staphylococcus, Corynebacterium, and fecal organisms	
Conjunctiva, Uterus, Mammary Glands	
These areas occasionally may contain small numbers of insignificant bacteria.	

culture is needed and a patient is receiving antimicrobial therapy, it is best to collect the sample just before the next drug dose, when antimicrobial concentration will be lowest.

If stained slides are to be prepared in addition to culture, be sure to collect sufficient material for both. Anticoagulants such as ethylenediaminetetraacetic acid (EDTA), heparin, and sodium citrate prevent bacterial growth, so samples that contain these anticoagulants should not be submitted for culture.

Although it may seem obvious, it is absolutely critical to correctly label samples. If multiple samples are collected from the same patient, it is important to label each sample with the site from which it was collected.

Blood and joint fluids are often submitted to the laboratory in blood culture bottles that contain broth. This is done to increase the chance of recovery of bacteria that are difficult to grow or are slow growing, and to dilute antimicrobial proteins from the animal that will inhibit bacterial growth.

TABLE 15-2	Bacteria Associated With Infections			
CANINE	**FELINE**	**EQUINE**	**PORCINE**	**RUMINANTS**
Conjunctivitis/Corneal Ulcer				
Staphylococcus	Staphylococcus	Often fungal	Streptococcus	Moraxella bovis/bovoculi
Streptococcus	Pasteurella	Streptococcus	Staphylococcus	Branhamella
Pseudomonas	Chlamydophila	Staphylococcus		Streptococcus
				Staphylococcus
				Mycoplasma
				Escherichia coli
Central Nervous System				
Rare	Rare	Streptococcus	Streptococcus	Histophilus somni
		Actinobacillus	Escherichia coli	Listeria monocytogenes
		Escherichia coli		Escherichia coli
				Pasteurella
Gastroenteritis				
Salmonella	Salmonella	Salmonella	Salmonella	Salmonella
Clostridium perfringens		Clostridium perfringens	Escherichia coli	Escherichia coli
Campylobacter		Clostridium difficile	Clostridium perfringens	Clostridium perfringens
Clostridium difficile		Escherichia coli	Clostridium difficile	Mycobacterium avium subsp. paratuberculosis
		Actinobacillus	Brachyspira hyodysenteriae	
		Rhodococcus equi		
Genital Tract				
Brucella canis	Streptococcus	Streptococcus	Brucella suis	Brucella
Escherichia coli	Pasteurella	Escherichia coli	Streptococcus	Listeria monocytogenes
Streptococcus	Escherichia coli	Klebsiella	Leptospira	Truperella (Arcanobacterium) pyogenes
Staphylococcus		Pseudomonas		Campylobacter
Mycoplasma				Mycoplasma
Mastitis				
Staphylococcus	Staphylococcus	Streptococcus	Streptococcus	Streptococcus
			Staphylococcus	Staphylococcus
			Escherichia coli	Truperella (Arcanobacterium) pyogenes
			Actinobacillus	Mycoplasma
			Truperella (Arcanobacterium) pyogenes	Mycobacterium
				Escherichia coli
				Klebsiella
				Nocardia
Musculoskeletal				
Staphylococcus	Rare	Streptococcus	Streptococcus	Clostridium
Escherichia coli		Actinobacillus	Mycoplasma	Truperella (Arcanobacterium) pyogenes
Pseudomonas		Escherichia coli	Escherichia coli	Escherichia coli
Brucella canis		Rhodococcus equi	Erysipelothrix	Streptococcus
Anaerobes		Staphylococcus	Truperella (Arcanobacterium) pyogenes	Erysipelothrix
		Clostridium		Histophilus somni
				Mycoplasma

TABLE 15-2	Bacteria Associated With Infections—cont'd			
CANINE	**FELINE**	**EQUINE**	**PORCINE**	**RUMINANTS**
Otitis				
Staphylococcus	Rare	Rare	Streptococcus	Streptococcus
Pseudomonas				Pasteurella
Streptococcus				Truperella (Arcanobacterium) pyogenes
Malassezia				Mycoplasma
Corynebacterium				
Actinomyces canis				
Anaerobes				
Upper Respiratory Tract				
Bordetella bronchiseptica	Pasteurella multocida	Streptococcus equi	Bordetella bronchiseptica	Histophilus somni
			Pasteurella multocida	Truperella (Arcanobacterium) pyogenes
Pneumonia				
Bordetella bronchiseptica	Rare	Streptococcus	Bordetella bronchiseptica	Histophilus somni
Pasteurella	Pasteurella multocida	Actinobacillus	Pasteurella multocida	Truperella (Arcanobacterium) pyogenes
Klebsiella	Chlamydia	Rhodococcus equi	Mycoplasma	Mannheimia haemolytica
Escherichia coli	Bordetella	Pasteurella	Haemophilus parasuis	Pasteurella multocida
Mycoplasma		Staphylococcus	Actinobacillus pleuropneumoniae	Truperella (Arcanobacterium) pyogenes
Streptococcus		Klebsiella	Streptococcus	Fusobacterium
Staphylococcus		Pseudomonas		Mycoplasma
Anaerobes		Bordetella bronchiseptica		
Pleuritis				
Anaerobes	Anaerobes	Streptococcus	Actinobacillus	Mannheimia
Actinomyces	Pasteurella	Anaerobes		Pasteurella
	Nocardia			Truperella (Arcanobacterium) pyogenes
Skin Wounds, Abscesses				
Staphylococcus	Pasteurella multocida	Streptococcus	Streptococcus	Truperella (Arcanobacterium) pyogenes
Streptococcus	Streptococcus	Corynebacterium pseudotuberculosis	Staphylococcus	Dermatophilus
Pseudomonas	Staphylococcus	Pseudomonas	Truperella (Arcanobacterium) pyogenes	Actinomyces
Nocardia	Anaerobes	Dermatophilus		Actinobacillus
Actinomyces		Staphylococcus		Staphylococcus
Anaerobes				Corynebacterum pseudotuberculosis
Urinary Tract				
Escherichia coli	Staphylococcus	Streptococcus	Actinobaculum suis	Corynebacterium renale
Proteus	Escherichia coli	Escherichia coli	Streptococcus	Truperella (Arcanobacterium) pyogenes
Staphylococcus	Enterococcus			
Enterococcus				
Streptococcus				
Klebsiella				
Pseudomonas				
Mycoplasma				

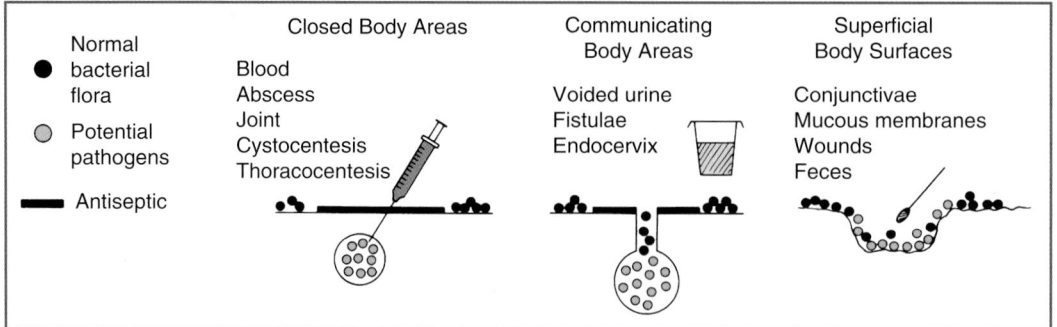

FIGURE 15-1 Methods used to collect bacterial culture specimens with consideration of indigenous flora.

Unfortunately, because it takes only one viable bacterial cell to turn a broth culture positive, it is easy to contaminate these cultures with indigenous flora of the skin such as *Staphylococcus epidermidis* or environmental organisms such as *Bacillus* spp.

> **TECHNICIAN NOTE**   When a sample is placed directly in broth culture, it is relatively easy to contaminate the culture. A broth culture can be contaminated at several different points: when collecting the sample (particularly with indigenous flora from the skin of the patient), during inoculation of the bottle, or in the clinical laboratory. Remember that it takes only one viable bacterial cell to turn a broth culture positive.

SPECIAL COLLECTION AND HANDLING PROCEDURES

Tissues

Tissue samples can be collected aseptically during surgery or biopsy, or they may be collected during necropsy. The conditions surrounding collection dictate how much tissue is collected and how it is submitted. Samples collected at surgery should be placed in a sterile container and submitted. Samples collected at necropsy should contain representative lesions and should be sufficiently large to allow decontamination of the external surface of the tissue using alcohol or flame before culture. If anaerobic culture is desired, an anaerobic swab should be collected or the sample should be placed in a transport container approved for anaerobic culture. Tissue samples should be refrigerated or on ice during shipment to the laboratory.

Aerobic and Anaerobic Swabs

Swabs serve as a convenient method for collecting and submitting cultures. It is important to consider whether indigenous flora present at the site of collection may interfere with culture. At sites such as skin, several different organisms may be present. These may be incidental and not pathogenic. In these cases, biopsy may be preferable to using a swab. When using an anaerobic swab, it is helpful to confirm that the sample is anaerobic before submission. Most commercial anaerobic swab systems have an oxygen indicator that allows the user to confirm that the sample is maintained in an anaerobic environment. Swabs are often used to collect samples from **abscesses** (pockets of infection that contain purulent material composed of bacteria, neutrophils, and macrophages). When collecting samples from abscesses, it is tempting to collect the purulent material, but it is generally better to collect the sample at the leading edge or capsule of the abscess, where bacteria are actively growing.

> **TECHNICIAN NOTE**   When using swabs to prepare both stained slides and bacterial cultures, one can set up cultures first, then prepare the slides, or one should be sure to collect separate swabs for each purpose because glass slides typically are not sterile.

Urine

The ideal sample for urine culture consists of at least 0.5 ml of urine collected by cystocentesis and submitted in a urine transport system. The number of bacteria present in a urine sample is used to determine whether an infection is present or not, and as a measure of severity of infection. Sterile tubes designed for submission of serum (red top tubes) are often used for this purpose. This is acceptable if the tubes are refrigerated until culture media are inoculated. Because bacteria can die during transport, it is preferable to use systems designed for urine that will maintain bacteria without promoting their growth or allowing them to die.

Cystocentesis is the preferred collection method for bacterial culture because the external genitalia have indigenous flora. In some animal species, it is not anatomically possible to perform a cystocentesis. In these cases, it is necessary to catch urine as it is voided (free catch) or to collect it using an indwelling urinary catheter. Ideally, free catch urine samples should be collected after the patient has already begun to urinate (midstream). Free catch urine samples typically include bacteria, so it is important to evaluate the number of bacteria present in the sample to determine whether an infection is present. For appropriate interpretation of culture results, it is important to inform the laboratory staff which collection method was used. Low numbers of organisms present in a free catch urine sample typically reflect indigenous flora on the external genitalia rather than an infection.

Bronchoalveolar Lavage and Transtracheal Wash Samples

Bronchoalveolar lavage and transtracheal wash samples are collected by aseptically introducing a small amount of sterile saline or other sterile wash fluid into the bronchus or trachea and then removing it by aspiration. These samples should be examined directly by microscopy and cultured. The ideal sample consists of at least 0.5 ml of fluid in a sterile container (e.g., a red top tube). Samples should be shipped under refrigeration.

Blood Culture

Patients can have local infections that spread to multiple organs. Infections that affect multiple organs or organ systems (e.g., the respiratory tract and the gastrointestinal tract) are called *disseminated infections* or *systemic infections*. Bacteria are transported from a site of local infection throughout the body by the blood or lymph. For this reason, a blood culture is performed when systemic disease is suspected. Infection of the blood is called *bacteremia*. Because bacteremia is transient, bacteria may or may not be present in the blood at the time that a sample is collected. So to increase the chance that bacteria will be present, a total of three blood samples should be collected from the patient, each collected at a different time (at least 30 minutes apart) and each collected from a different vein over a 24-hour period. The skin over the vein should be aseptically prepared similar to a surgical site because the blood is inoculated into broth blood culture media, and any bacteria on the skin can be inadvertently inoculated into the media, leading to false-positive results. Samples are collected from separate veins because during collection, the vein can be contaminated by bacteria from the skin. This contamination does not usually harm the patient because the patient's immune system clears the infection, but it can cause false-positive culture results. If aerobic and anaerobic cultures are desired, separate samples should be collected.

Joint Fluid

Joint fluid typically is submitted in blood culture media to improve recovery of organisms. Samples may also be submitted in sterile vials (red top tubes) or on swabs. Joint fluid can clot, so anticoagulants are sometimes used. Most anticoagulants such as heparin or EDTA interfere with bacterial culture, so samples with these agents should not be submitted. Sodium polyanethol sulfonate (SPS) is an anticoagulant that does not interfere with bacterial culture and can be used if desired to prevent clotting of joint fluid.

Milk

Collect the sample before milking the animal. Clean and dry the udder just as you would for milking, using individual paper towels to dry the teats before sampling. Wear gloves for sampling. Beginning with the teats on the far side of the udder, scrub the teat opening thoroughly (10 to 15 seconds) with cotton balls or gauze moistened with 70% isopropyl alcohol. It is important not to touch the clean teat end. When collecting milk, start with the closest teats. Discard the first two streams of milk from each teat. Collect 1 to 2 ml of milk in a sterile vial, taking care not to touch the vial with the teat. Label the sample with the animal identifier and with the quarters collected. It is acceptable to combine milk from all teats, but this should be noted on the sample and submission forms. It is also important to collect milk before providing any antibiotic treatment. Samples should be maintained on ice or refrigerated and transported to the laboratory within 24 hours. Samples that will be held for longer periods before culture should be frozen immediately. After sample collection, the udder should be handled as when milking is complete (e.g., teat dipping).

Feces

Collect 1 to 10 g of fresh feces in a clean container, and ship the sample to the laboratory refrigerated or on ice. Because many different bacteria are present in feces, selective media that exclude the growth of most organisms are used when culturing feces. Organisms most commonly sought from feces in cases of diarrhea are *Salmonella*, *Campylobacter*, *Clostridium perfringens*, *Clostridium difficile*, and *Mycobacterium avium* subsp. *paratuberculosis*.

Sample Transportation

Sample transportation often is not adequately considered but is a critical component of getting good results from culture. It is important to use transport systems and media appropriate for the sample. Examples of transport systems are shown in Figure 15-2. In addition to using appropriate media, it is important to consider what will happen to a sample as it is shipped to the laboratory. Samples shipped to an outside laboratory must be shipped in accordance with federal shipping regulations. Other than milk samples, which may be frozen after collection, samples should not be frozen

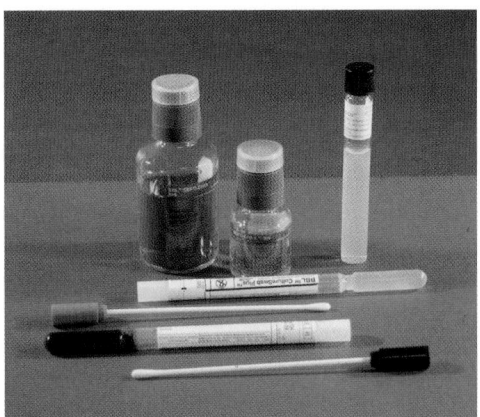

FIGURE 15-2 Culturette swab transport systems with transport media (black medium is Amies **transport medium** with charcoal), Port-a-Cul Anaerobic Transport Tube (BD Diagnostic Systems; BD, Franklin Lakes, NJ), and blood culture bottles. Swabs are used to collect culture inoculum and are placed into transport systems or tubes of medium for preservation of the viability of bacteria during transportation to the laboratory for culture. Blood culture bottles are inoculated with blood to prevent coagulation and contamination during transport to the laboratory for incubation.

because freezing and thawing a sample can kill bacteria. Milk samples are different because the fat in the milk protects the bacteria.

> **TECHNICIAN NOTE** In general, samples should be refrigerated or on ice during shipment, but not frozen. For accurate culture results, samples should be protected from extreme temperatures while in transit.

SAMPLE PROCESSING

DIRECT MICROSCOPIC EXAMINATION

Direct examination of specimens from patients can be helpful when one is making decisions about therapy. It is particularly helpful to directly examine exudates, material from draining tracts, and thoracic fluid from patients with pneumonia. However, it can be difficult to prepare adequate slides from samples that contain a high concentration of protein or large numbers of neutrophils or other leukocytes. Several slides should be prepared and examined because some slide-to-slide variation will be noted. For the quantity of bacteria to be sufficient to allow visualization on a prepared slide, approximately 10^5 bacteria per milliliter of fluid are required. Consequently, examining slides from samples in which bacterial numbers are low can be frustrating, and it is important to remember that infection may be present even when no bacteria are found.

> **TECHNICIAN NOTE** Because they may contain alcohol and other flammable liquids, some stains may need special containment in flammable liquid cabinets. These come in a variety of sizes. Regulations for housing flammable liquids vary by state, so it is recommended that you determine what the regulations are in your area.

Before examining prepared slides, it is important to confirm that the microscope has been properly aligned for Köhler illumination to ensure that stains appear as the correct color. Köhler illumination uses a collector lens, a field diaphragm, a condenser diaphragm, and a condenser lens to provide indirect illumination of samples. This results in an even field of light and prevents artifacts from the light source from interfering with the image. Preparing control slides simultaneously with specimen slides is valuable for evaluating the performance of any stain. Control slides are also helpful because prepared slides from patient fluids or tissues can be difficult to evaluate. Control slides can be purchased or made depending on the skills of the technician.

GRAM STAIN PROCEDURE AND INTERPRETATION

Several different types of stains are used for identification of bacteria. The stain used most commonly is the **Gram stain**, which is named after its developer Hans Christian Gram. This technique uses dyes to distinguish between bacterial cell walls. Gram-positive organisms have a cell wall largely composed of peptidoglycan; Gram-negative organisms consist of a double-lipid bilayer comprising inner and outer cell membranes with a space in between called the *periplasmic space* (Figure 15-3 and Procedure 15-1). In addition to the Gram stain, another commonly used stain is the **acid-fast stain**, which is used to identify organisms such as *Mycobacterium* spp., which have significant amounts of mycolic acid content in the cell wall. Several different procedures are used for acid-fast staining, most commonly, the Ziehl-Neelsen procedure. A variant of the acid-fast stain may also be used; this is often called the *partial* or *modified acid-fast stain*, or the *modified Ziehl-Neelsen stain*, or *Kinyoun's acid-fast stain*.

> **TECHNICIAN NOTE** Microscopic analysis of urine sediment should not be used as a substitute for culture. The presence of rod-shaped bacteria can be readily detected, but cocci are often difficult to identify in urine samples. Inflammation is an important component of urinary tract infection. The presence of bacteria inside neutrophils is typically indicative of phagocytosis rather than contamination of the sample.

The presence of neutrophils, other cells, or protein can alter the pH and other physical and chemical properties that are important for an accurate Gram stain. It is difficult to know in advance how the fluid will stain. In general with fluids, it is advisable to run a control slide with the sample to be tested. This will help you evaluate how well you are performing the staining procedure. It can be difficult to get an adequate slide when working with thick, viscous fluids. Thick, viscous samples can retain stains (such as crystal violet in the Gram stain). Additionally, these fluids tend to dry as a uniform sheet, fail to decolorize adequately, and will wash off the slide during wash steps. No simple solution is known for working with viscous fluids, except to try to dilute them with sterile saline and to make and examine several slides with varying thicknesses of fluid.

> **TECHNICIAN NOTE** It is important that the sample on the slide be thin enough for good visual examination with the microscope. Viscous fluids such as thick exudates may be too thick for adequate examination. Samples can be diluted in sterile normal saline until an appropriate thickness is achieved.

After preparing the Gram stain, examine the slide with a microscope. Scan the slide first at low magnification before switching to the oil immersion lens. Be careful not to get oil on lenses that are not designed for oil, and clean all lenses after examining specimens because organisms can become detached from the slide and can be carried over onto other samples.

When interpreting the sample slide, it is important to consider the control slide and how well it has stained. The control slide will help you interpret the sample slide and will

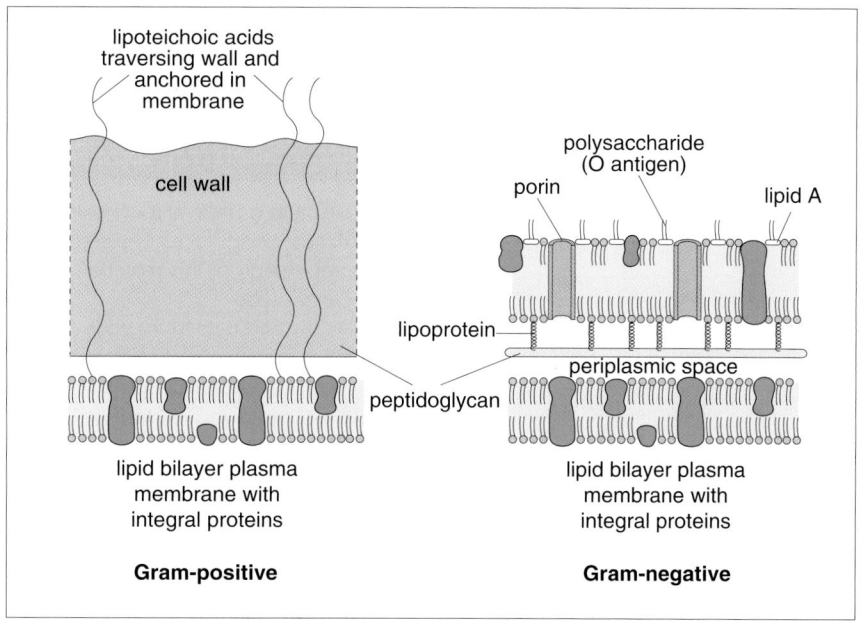

FIGURE 15-3 Structure of the cell walls of Gram-positive and Gram-negative bacteria. Note the difference in composition of the cell wall of Gram-positive bacteria (which is largely made up of peptidoglycan) and the cell wall of Gram-negative bacteria (which has a double-lipid bilayer composed of inner and outer cell membranes with a space in between called the *periplasmic space*). On slides prepared with Gram stain, Gram-positive organisms retain crystal violet stain and appear purple, whereas Gram-negative organisms do not retain crystal violet, but counterstain with safranin and appear pink. (From Goering R, Dockrell H, Zuckerman M: *Mim's medical microbiology*, ed 4, St Louis, 2008, Mosby.)

PROCEDURE 15-1	Gram Stain Procedure and Interpretation*

1. On a glass slide, prepare a thin, air-dried sample of the material to be examined. (This can be a colony from a culture plate, an exudate or fluid collected from a patient, or an impression smear from tissue or fluid from a patient or other sample.)
2. If a sample will also be cultured, be sure to collect separate material for the Gram stain and for the culture (the glass slide is not sterile, so the sample used for the Gram stain cannot subsequently be used to inoculate culture media).
3. Fix the dry specimen by flooding the slide with absolute methanol for 1 minute, or with heat by passing it through the flame of a Bunsen burner for 5 to 10 seconds (until the slide is warm to the touch). Heat fixation can be challenging. Individual users may find it necessary to test heat fixation by trial and error to get a good feel for timing and temperature. Heating to 60°C for 3 minutes should be sufficient to kill the bacteria and fix them to the slide,
although it will be significantly easier to use methanol. Methanol fixation has been reported to provide consistent and accurate results and may be preferable for new users. Methanol is potentially hazardous (toxic if ingested and flammable).
4. Flood the slide with crystal violet solution, and let stand for 1 minute.
5. Rinse the slide briefly with tap water.
6. Flood the slide with Gram iodine solution, and let stand for 1 minute.
7. Rinse the slide briefly with tap water.
8. Decolorize the sample with Gram decolorizer (25% acetone, 75% isopropanol) for 1 to 5 seconds, and immediately rinse the slide with tap water.
9. Flood the slide with safranin counterstain for 30 seconds to 1 minute.
10. Rinse the slide briefly with tap water, blot carefully, and air-dry.

*Note: Perfecting this stain requires trial and error with known positives and negatives. Even experienced users have difficulty with some organisms. When results are inconclusive, it is best to run a control slide side-by-side with the sample.

---

help you decide whether you need to stain another one. It is also important to consider the source of the sample and the organisms likely present at specific anatomic sites. Finally, it can be helpful to stain a slide using a Wright-based stain (e.g., Diff-Quik stain) for comparison with the Gram-stained slide.

TECHNICIAN NOTE It is important to remember that samples stained with Wright stains such as Diff-Quik cannot be used to determine whether an organism is Gram-positive or Gram-negative. Examination of samples stained with both stains is helpful.

PROCEDURE 15-2	Acid-Fast Stain Procedure (for detection of acid-fast organisms like *Mycobacterium* spp.)

1. Suspend a small amount of the sample in saline on a slide. When using feces, tissue, or exudates, make a direct preparation of this material, if possible.
2. Air-dry and heat-fix the slide (set the slide on a slide warmer for a minimum of 5 minutes).
3. Flood the slide with carbol fuchsin for 5 minutes.
4. Rinse the slide with tap water.
5. Decolorize the sample with acid alcohol for 3 minutes.
6. Rinse the slide with tap water.
7. Counterstain the sample with malachite green for 1 minute.
8. Rinse the slide with tap water.
9. Blot the slide dry with bibulous paper, or use a slide dryer.

ACID-FAST STAIN PROCEDURES

Other stain procedures such as acid-fast staining are required to determine the identity of organisms such as *Mycobacterium* spp. and *Nocardia* spp. (Procedure 15-2). After you have prepared an acid-fast stain, examine the control slide first to confirm that positive and negative controls are appropriately stained. Then examine the slides prepared from patient samples. Acid-fast organisms stain bright pink to red. Non–acid-fast organisms and the background should stain green.

With acid-fast stains of fluids, cytologic samples, and feces, it can be difficult to find the *Mycobacterium* spp. because the organisms can be very small and difficult to see. It is important to be absolutely certain before calling a slide positive because consequences for the patient are significant. Negative findings have low predictive value. If test results are questionable and *Mycobacterium* is suspected, additional testing can be performed to confirm the diagnosis.

> **TECHNICIAN NOTE**   With acid-fast stains of fluids, cytologic samples, and feces, it can be difficult to find the *Mycobacterium* spp. because the organisms can be very small and difficult to see. It is important to be absolutely certain before calling a slide positive because consequences for the patient are significant.

Kinyoun's modified Ziehl-Nielsen acid-fast stain is used for identification of partially acid-fast organisms such as *Nocardia* spp. (Procedure 15-3). Examine the Kinyoun's modified Ziehl-Nielsen acid-fast–stained slides prepared from patient samples as described for the acid-fast stain. Partially acid-fast organisms stain bright pink to red. Non–acid-fast organisms and the background should stain blue-green.

Acid-fast–stained samples from pure cultures usually are easy to interpret because the organism must be bright pink to red to be positive. It can be difficult for new technicians to interpret modified acid-fast stains because organisms tend to stain purple rather than green with this stain. Difficulty can arise with partially acid-fast organisms. It can be tempting to interpret as positive those organisms that stain

PROCEDURE 15-3	Kinyoun's Modified Ziehl-Nielsen Acid-Fast Stain Procedure (for identification of partially acid-fast organisms like *Nocardia* spp.)

1. Suspend a small amount of the sample in saline on a slide. When using feces, tissue, or exudates, make a direct preparation of this material, if possible. Always include a control slide.
2. Air-dry and heat-fix the slide (set the slide on a slide warmer for a minimum of 5 minutes).
3. Flood the slide with carbol fuchsin for 3 to 4 minutes.
4. Rinse the slide with tap water.
5. Decolorize the sample with 1% sulfuric acid for approximately 4 minutes.
6. Rinse the slide with tap water.
7. Counterstain the sample with malachite green for 1 minute.
8. Rinse the slide with tap water.
9. Blot the slide dry with bibulous paper, or use a slide dryer.

purple with the modified procedure. This should not be done. If doubt arises, a new sample should be stained and counterstained with malachite green for a longer time (up to 3 minutes). This should allow for proper color development, making the slide easier to interpret. If doubt remains, additional testing is required.

> **TECHNICIAN NOTE**   Acid-fast–stained samples from pure cultures usually are fairly easy to interpret because the organism must be bright pink to red to be positive. Difficulty can arise with partially acid-fast organisms. It can be tempting to interpret as positive those organisms that stain purple with the modified procedure. This should not be done. If doubt arises, a new sample should be stained and counterstained with malachite green for a longer time (up to 3 minutes). This should allow for proper color development, making the slide easier to interpret.

BACTERIAL CULTURE AND IDENTIFICATION

DISPOSAL

It is important to plan how waste will be disposed of before the laboratory is set up and bacteria are cultured. Most large laboratories steam-sterilize (autoclave) laboratory waste materials. In a small practice setting, this may not be possible. Most practices reserve use of the autoclave for sterilizing surgical and other equipment and may prefer not to autoclave bacterial culture material in the same unit. In many locations, commercial contractors will dispose of biological waste for a fee.

> **TECHNICIAN NOTE**   Local, state, and federal regulations on biological waste disposal should be considered before a laboratory is set up. Waste can be disposed of in the laboratory or through a commercial contractor.

EQUIPMENT

The primary item of equipment needed for routine bacterial culture is a good-quality light microscope with low power and oil immersion lenses and an incubator that will maintain culture materials at a constant temperature (usually 35°C to 37.5°C). Some organisms are **fastidious** in their growth requirements and will need specialized atmospheric conditions or nutrients to grow. Typically, clinical microbiology laboratories use incubators supplied with carbon dioxide gas (to provide a 5% carbon dioxide atmosphere) to enhance the growth of fastidious bacteria. This equipment can be expensive and is beyond the routine needs of most veterinary practices.

CULTURE MEDIA

The type of medium used for a culture is dependent on the sample being tested and the pathogens expected, given the anatomic site and the patient species. Obtaining details of the patient's signalment and a brief history is necessary for selection of appropriate media for the culture. Isolation of pathogens from samples collected from anatomic sites that have significant indigenous flora, such as the gastrointestinal tract, relies on the use of selective media that will inhibit the growth of most organisms, as well as **enrichment media** that will inhibit the growth of some organisms while allowing or promoting the growth of likely pathogens. The list of standard media used for routine cultures will vary by laboratory based on the preference of the microbiologist.

Media for culture can be liquid broth or solid agar plates and tubes. For initial isolation of organisms, solid agar plates are typically used because they allow the isolation of individual bacteria. Broth cultures started directly from patient samples usually contain a mixed bacterial population and should be cultured onto agar plates before identification or susceptibility testing is performed. It is important to work from pure cultures derived from individual bacterial colonies. Tests performed on mixed cultures (two or more types of bacteria mixed together) will give erroneous results and may interfere with clinical decision making.

Most laboratories use a combination of a nutrient-rich medium that will allow the growth of most bacteria, such as trypticase soy agar plates with 5% blood added (blood agar plate), and a **selective medium**, such as MacConkey's agar plates, which allow the growth of Gram-negative enteric organisms like *Escherichia coli* but inhibit Gram-positive organisms. Many media options are available for culture depending on the type of culture (Table 15-3). Media can be purchased from a variety of suppliers as ready-to-use prepared media or as dehydrated media that must be reconstituted and prepared for use. For the small laboratory, it is generally more efficient and cost-effective to purchase prepared media that have already been quality control tested.

Isolates that require definitive identification can be subcultured on agar slants and shipped to reference laboratories. It is preferable to ship the isolate on an agar slant rather than a plate because plates are more likely to be broken during

TABLE 15-3	Purposes for Specific Media
MEDIA AND PURPOSE	**REACTIONS AND INTERPRETATION**
Blood agar plate (trypticase soy agar with 5% sheep blood) Primary isolation medium. Streak for colony isolation.	This medium is used for primary isolation of organisms and for subculture of organisms. It is important to observe growth rates, colony morphology, and relative numbers of organisms (the number of quadrants on the primary plate with growth; e.g., 1st, 2nd). Antimicrobial susceptibility tests and biochemical tests should be inoculated from isolated colonies grown on this medium.
Brucella blood agar plate Primary isolation medium. Streak for colony isolation.	Similar to blood agar plates, these plates provide a rich medium for the culture of anaerobic organisms.
MacConkey's agar plate Primary isolation medium for selection of Gram-negative organisms. Streak for colony isolation. Allows differentiation of lactose fermentation.	When lactose is fermented, a local pH drop around the colony causes a color change in the pH indicator. Pink colonies are able to use lactose (*Escherichia coli*), and white or colorless colonies are lactose nonfermenters (*Salmonella, Pseudomonas*).
Hektoen enteric agar Used for direct isolation of *Salmonella* spp. from feces. Streak for colony isolation.	This agar contains lactose and a different pH indicator from MacConkey's agar. When colonies are able to ferment lactose, they will turn orange to yellow to salmon pink. *Salmonella* and *Proteus* will not ferment lactose and will appear as blue-green colonies with black centers from the production of hydrogen sulfide. Such colonies subsequently must be confirmed as *Salmonella*.
Selenite or tetrathionate broth Used to enrich samples for the detection of *Salmonella* spp. Fecal samples are added to these broths and are incubated overnight at 35°C.	Selective agar plates such as MacConkey's agar are struck with the broth and incubated for detection of *Salmonella*. The broth uses sulfur compounds to inhibit the growth of other organisms while permitting the *Salmonella* to grow.

TABLE 15-3 | Purposes for Specific Media—cont'd

MEDIA AND PURPOSE	REACTIONS AND INTERPRETATION
Salt mannitol agar Primarily used to differentiate species of *Staphylococcus* based on mannitol fermentation. Streak for isolation.	Bacteria that grow in the presence of high salt concentration and ferment mannitol produce acid products that turn the phenol red from pink to yellow. Bacteria not utilizing the mannitol, but utilizing peptones, will result in an increase in pH, turning phenol red from pink to bright pink.
Triple sugar iron (TSI) agar slant For determining the ability of organisms to utilize glucose, sucrose, and lactose and to produce hydrogen sulfide. Inoculate the slant and stab the butt once with an inoculating needle.	A yellow color change is indicative of acid production (A), and red is indicative of alkalinization (K). Phenol red is the pH indicator. When the carbohydrates in TSI agar are fermented, the resulting acid production and decrease in pH cause the color change of phenol red to yellow. If proteins are utilized as an energy source instead of carbohydrates, deamination of proteins leads to an increase in pH (alkalinization), and the media will be orange or red. In the butt of the tube, glucose fermentation is detected while the slant detects utilization of lactose and sucrose. Results are recorded as slant/butt: A, Acid production; K, alkaline; NC, no change. Black precipitation indicates production of hydrogen sulfide and is recorded as H_2S^+. (See Figure 15-8 for an example of a TSI reaction.)
Lysine iron agar slant For differentiating microorganisms, especially *Salmonella*, based on lysine decarboxylation/deamination and H_2S production. Inoculate the slant and stab the butt once with an inoculating needle.	L-Lysine hydrochloride is the substrate used to detect lysine decarboxylase and lysine deaminase enzymes. By eliminating lactose and adding lysine, the medium can differentiate enteric bacilli based on their abilities to decarboxylate and deaminate lysine. The result is recorded slant/butt. Purple color in the slant indicates lysine deaminase–negative; portwine color in the slant indicates lysine deaminase–positive and is typically indicative of *Proteus*; purple color in the butt indicates lysine decarboxylase–positive.
Christensen's urea agar slant For determining whether an organism produces urease. Inoculate the slant.	Positive samples will turn the agar pink. Strong positives will be bright pink. Urease breaks the carbon-nitrogen bond of amides to form carbon dioxide, ammonia, and water. Members of genus *Proteus* are known to produce urease. When urea is broken down, ammonia is released and the pH of the medium is increased. This pH change is detected by a pH indicator that turns pink in a basic environment. (See Figure 15-8 for an example of a positive urease reaction.)
Motility media For determining whether an organism has and is able to use flagella. Inoculate by stabbing the media using an inoculating needle. Incubate at 35°C. If *Listeria* is suspected, incubate at room temperature.	The low agar concentration of motility medium allows limited movement of motile bacteria from the area of the stab. Some bacteria will diffuse through the entire media, and others may show only diffusion as nodules off of the stab line. Nonmotile organisms will not grow beyond the stab line.
Indole test media For determining the ability of an organism to split indole from tryptophan. Inoculate the broth, incubate 24 hours, and then add Kovac's reagent.	Positive samples will have a red color form within seconds of addition of Kovac's reagent. Tryptophan is hydrolyzed to indole, pyruvic acid, and ammonia by tryptophanase. Tryptophanase catalyzes deamination or removal of the amine group from the tryptophan molecule producing indole. (See Figure 15-8 for an example of a positive indole test.)
Citrate test media For differentiating Enterobacteriaceae based on the capability of utilizing citrate as the sole source of carbon. Inoculate the slant.	A positive reaction will turn the media blue, and a negative reaction will leave the media green. When the organism utilizes and oxidizes citrate, CO_2 is produced and combines with sodium and water to form sodium carbonate. Alkaline sodium carbonate raises the pH of the media, causing the change in color.

shipping and are more difficult to secure to prevent accidental spills or exposure. Swabs work well for shipping isolates. A key challenge for the veterinarian and the technician in the private practice setting is to decide when cultures should be submitted to an outside laboratory. For a variety of reasons, including employee safety, some practices always submit cultures to an outside laboratory.

> **TECHNICIAN NOTE** It is important to remember that shipping purified bacteria is different from shipping patient samples, and shipping regulations may be different. The reference laboratory and the commercial shipper should be consulted for guidance on shipping bacteria.

Enrichment, Selective, and Differential Media

Enrichment media are used to enhance the recovery of organisms that are difficult to grow, or that occur in low numbers in the presence of indigenous flora. Selective media are media that prevent the growth of some types of organisms and are used to facilitate isolation of organisms from mixed cultures. MacConkey's agar is an example of selective media because the bile salts that it contains inhibit growth of some bacteria. MacConkey's agar is also a **differential medium** because it contains an indicator that allows the user to identify or differentiate between organisms that can use lactose (lactose-positive) and those that cannot use lactose (lactose-negative) (Figure 15-4). Some media can be both enrichment and selective media. Two examples are selenite broth and tetrathionate broth, both of which are used to enhance the growth of *Salmonella*. These media work by inhibiting the growth of organisms that cannot grow in the presence of sulfur compounds. *Salmonella*, unlike many enteric bacteria, is able to grow in these media.

Inoculation of Media

Most microbiological culture work is performed using Petri plates that contain media with agar added as a solidifying agent. Biochemical reactions are tested using differential media in tubes. These media may have agar or may be prepared as broth. Before use, all media should be quality control tested using known organisms to confirm that they work properly. Before any medium is inoculated, it should be inspected to ensure that it is free of contamination, and care should be taken to prevent contamination when media and patient samples are handled. With a permanent marker, the plates for a culture should be labeled with the date, the patient identifier, and the sample. In diagnostic laboratories, each sample is given a unique identifying number (accession number) that allows the culture to be followed from start to finish and allows all culture results to be tracked.

Examples of inoculation of plate media and tube media are shown in Figures 15-5 through Figure 15-7. When plate media are inoculated, the sample should be aseptically placed in the first quadrant of the plate. Then the plate should be struck for isolation using an inoculating loop. To streak a plate for isolation of colonies, the loop is passed 2 or 3 times into the primary quadrant containing the sample. Care should be taken to not go back into the primary quadrant. This is repeated in the second, third, and fourth quadrants until all four quadrants have been used (see Figure 15-5).

Tube media may or may not have a slant. The slant is formed by tilting the tube while the medium is in molten form and keeping it in this position until it hardens. The

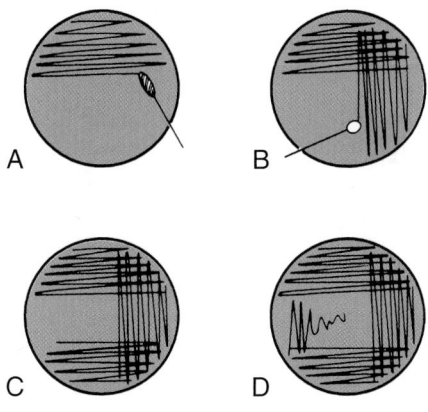

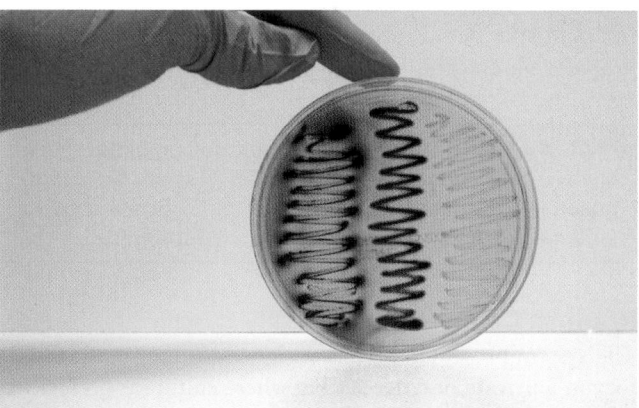

FIGURE 15-4 MacConkey's agar plate inoculated with lactose-positive *Escherichia coli* with bile salt precipitation on the far left *(pink with hazy precipitate)*, lactose-positive *E. coli* in the middle *(pink)*, and lactose-negative *Proteus mirabilis* on the far right.

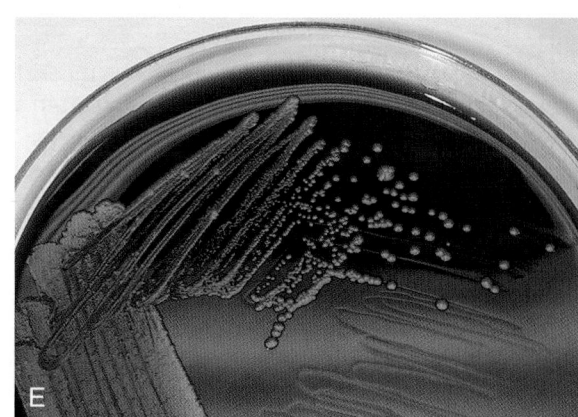

FIGURE 15-5 Inoculation procedure for agar plate media and streaking method for isolation of bacterial colonies. **A,** Inoculate with swab, covering one-fourth to one-third of the plate. **B,** Streak lightly, overlapping the previous area. **C,** Flame loop, allow it to cool, and streak next area. **D,** Repeat as in **C. E,** Photo illustrates well-isolated colonies.

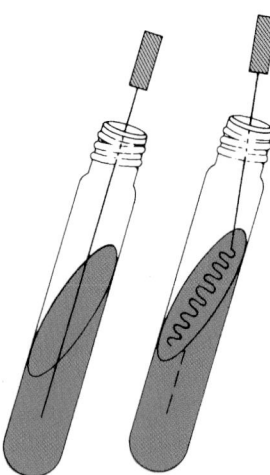

FIGURE 15-6 Inoculation procedure for agar tube media. Inoculation of agar slant and butt, such as triple sugar iron (TSI). The inoculation needle first is stabbed into the butt and then is removed and streaked over the agar slant surface in a back-and-forth motion.

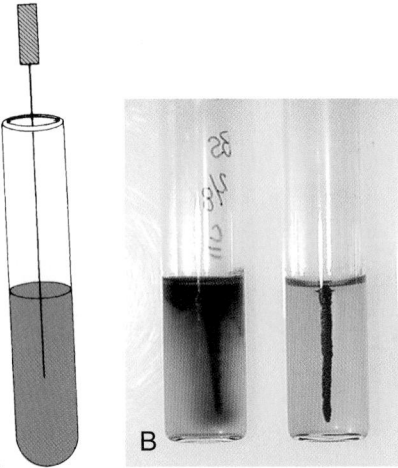

FIGURE 15-7 Inoculation procedure and results for motility media. A, Inoculation of motility test media. The inoculation needle is stabbed into the medium and is withdrawn along the same tract. B, Motile bacterial growth in the left tube and nonmotile growth in the right tube.

slant is struck by carefully passing the loop across the surface in a zigzag pattern. With some media, it is important to stab the butt of the tube (see Figure 15-6). Motility media are inoculated by using an inoculating needle to stab the butt of the tube and carefully withdrawing the needle along the stab line (Figure 15-7, *A* and *B*).

Incubation Conditions

Plates should always be incubated in an inverted position (lid down). If they are not inverted, moisture from the plate collects on the lid and can fall onto the plate surface. This causes contamination of the culture or mixing of bacteria on the plate surface, creating a lawn of bacterial growth rather than isolated colonies. After inoculation, plates and biochemical tests should be incubated overnight at 35°C to 37.5°C. For some susceptibility tests, the length of the incubation time

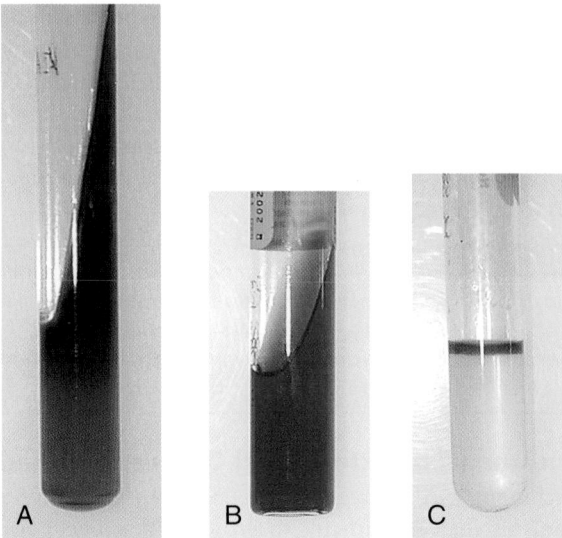

FIGURE 15-8 A, Alkaline slant and acid butt reaction (K/A) in triple sugar iron (TSI). B, Positive urease reaction after slant inoculation. C, Positive indole test.

is critical (see "Antimicrobial Susceptibility Testing," on page 505). Screw-caps for tube media should be left loose during incubation.

Fastidious organisms are organisms with specific growth requirements. Fastidious organisms often grow better in the presence of 5% carbon dioxide. This should be remembered when an incubator without carbon dioxide is used because these organisms will be less likely to grow.

It is important to inspect plates at least once daily. If no bacteria grow from a specimen where organisms were observed on direct microscopy, the plates should be held and examined for 3 days before the final result of "no growth" is reported. Cultures from patients receiving antimicrobial therapeutics may be held for an additional 2 days to allow bacteria weakened by the drugs to grow. It is usually unnecessary to hold cultures beyond this time. Culture of slow-growing organisms should not be attempted in the small laboratory because specialized media are required for both isolation and identification. Contamination is particularly a problem for cultures held for long periods.

> **TECHNICIAN NOTE** After inoculation, plates should always be incubated in an inverted position (lid down), generally overnight at 35°C to 37.5°C. Screw-caps for tube media should be left loose during incubation.

Routine Culture Systems

The system presented here is designed for the small laboratory in a private practice setting where culture is performed to aid in clinical decision making. It is not intended for definitive identification of all organisms. This system is designed to be effective for routine aerobic culture and determination of the presence of anaerobic bacteria.

Culturing anaerobic bacteria and slow-growing or difficult-to-grow organisms requires expertise and the type of equipment found in diagnostic or reference laboratories.

Primary Isolation Media

Selection of media for initial inoculation of samples is dependent on the site from which they are collected. Specifics for urine, milk, feces, and blood culture are listed separately. A sample initially should be struck or plated on a blood agar plate and MacConkey's agar plate. If an anaerobic culture is desired, an additional blood agar plate can be inoculated and incubated in an **anaerobe** jar, from which the oxygen is removed using a commercially available system. The anaerobically cultured plate is periodically compared with the aerobic plate. Suspect anaerobes can be subcultured to plates that are incubated aerobically and anaerobically and then evaluated. Colonies that do not grow on the aerobic plate are anaerobes. Although identification and susceptibility testing of anaerobes are possible, it is generally not cost-effective for the small laboratory to perform these tests.

In some practices, enriching the growth of fastidious organisms is done by inoculating a trypticase soy broth tube or a brain heart infusion broth tube. These are rich media that support the growth of fastidious organisms. Unfortunately, broth enrichment cultures can be easily contaminated, and care must be exercised in detecting the presence of organisms that grow only on the enriched culture.

PRELIMINARY EVALUATION OF CULTURES

Evaluating a culture accurately after 24 to 48 hours of culture is of the utmost importance for accurate and timely completion of the culture. The technician will be able to do this more easily and efficiently as he or she gains experience and skill. The first step in this process occurs before the sample is plated, when the technician evaluates the appropriateness and quality of the sample and decides which media to inoculate. The technician should also consider whether or not indigenous flora is likely present in a sample. Cultures of samples collected from sites that are normally sterile are the simplest to evaluate because only one or two organisms or colony types are present on the culture plates in most cases. It is more difficult to evaluate cultures of samples collected from sites where indigenous flora is present. The skin, the gastrointestinal tract, the external genitalia, and the respiratory tract all have indigenous normal flora (see Table 15-1). In the presence of indigenous flora, it can be difficult to identify pathogens. It is not necessary to identify every organism present in cultures from sites where indigenous flora is likely. In fact, it can be distracting and misleading for the veterinarian or the technician to do so.

> ⌐ TECHNICIAN NOTE   In general, when an appropriate sample is collected and handled properly, the predominant organism is most likely the causative agent. Typically, lesions and infections are caused by a single organism or at most by two organisms.

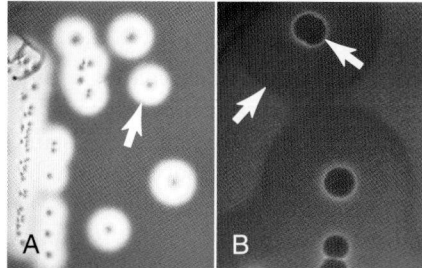

FIGURE 15-9 Patterns of hemolysis observed in blood agar plates. A, Complete hemolysis (also named β-hemolysis if the organism is *Streptococcus*). B, Double-zone hemolysis as produced by *Staphylococcus intermedius*.

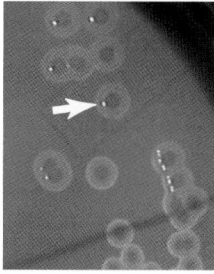

FIGURE 15-10 Alpha-hemolysis produced by some strains of *Streptococcus*.

After overnight incubation of the plates, the next step is to look carefully at the culture plates, taking care not to contaminate them. The technician should determine how many different organisms are present, which of those organisms are the major organisms present (those that make up most of the colonies), how many colonies of each organism are present, the appearance of the colonies, and how the organisms affect surrounding media. Changes to the media can include **hemolysis** (clearing of media around the colony). Hemolysis can be an indication of virulence (Figures 15-9 and 15-10).

Bacteria are identified by their cell wall structure, shape, and growth characteristics. In identifying an organism, it is important to notice first the amount of time that it took to grow and the number of quadrants of the agar plate on which it is present. The level of growth on the blood agar plate can indicate the degree of infection. A common tool for relative quantification of the number of organisms present in a culture is noting the number of quadrants in which the organism grew. The scale typically used is 1+ to 4+, where 4+ indicates that the organism grew on the entire plate, as compared with 1+, which indicates that the organism grew only in the primary or first quadrant of the plate.

A series of questions can help the technician make decisions about an organism. Was it present on the blood agar plate on the first day, or did it take longer to grow? Is the organism also present on the MacConkey's agar plate? Is the organism hemolytic? If so, is the hemolysis complete or partial? What is the Gram staining reaction of the organism? Questions like these can help the technician decide the next steps needed to identify the organism. It is imperative that the information provided on each plate be considered in the context of the whole culture and the site where the sample was collected. Sometimes a single colony is important, and sometimes it is not. For example, *Pseudomonas aeruginosa* is a virulent pathogen that tends to be resistant to several classes of antimicrobial agents, but it can also be present in feces as indigenous flora. A single colony of *P. aeruginosa* in a urine sample collected by cystocentesis is important to note and test for susceptibility to antimicrobial drugs, whereas a single colony of this organism from a fecal sample is not important.

> **TECHNICIAN NOTE** Culture results should be evaluated with consideration of potential pathogens and indigenous flora. Relative numbers of bacteria should be noted.

New technicians will find it necessary to perform biochemical tests to adequately identify organisms. With experience, it becomes easier for the technician to recognize pathogens on the basis of their growth characteristics and to evaluate cultures. However, even experienced technicians find it helpful to routinely perform some biochemical tests for bacterial identification.

RECORDING, INTERPRETING, AND REPORTING RESULTS

It is important to record all observations about a culture and the results of biochemical and susceptibility tests performed on a culture. These results become part of the patient's medical record and are legal documents that should be carefully maintained. In general, a worksheet that follows a consistent format and is used for all cultures can be helpful and can make it easier for anyone in the laboratory or the practice to evaluate a culture that is in progress. This worksheet should briefly summarize initial findings and daily observations about the progress of each step until the culture is complete.

IDENTIFICATION PROCEDURES

After preliminary evaluation of the culture is complete, the next step is to isolate and identify significant organisms. If isolated colonies are present on initial culture plates, it may be possible to work directly from these plates. In general though, it is helpful to subculture organisms to a new blood agar plate for further workup. The first step in identifying an organism is to determine its Gram staining reaction and morphology. The next steps are summarized in flow charts based on colony morphology and Gram reaction results (Figure 15-11).

The Gram staining reaction is based on the ability of the bacterial cell wall to retain crystal violet stain. Organisms that can retain this stain appear purple under light microscopic examination and are called Gram-positive organisms. Organisms that cannot retain crystal violet are counterstained with safranin in the Gram stain procedure. These Gram-negative organisms appear pink under light microscopic examination.

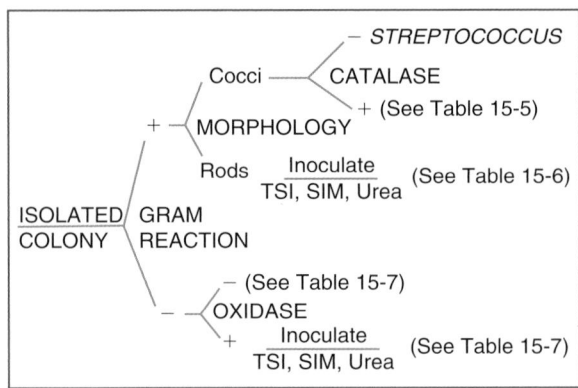

FIGURE 15-11 Flow chart for bacterial identification procedure.

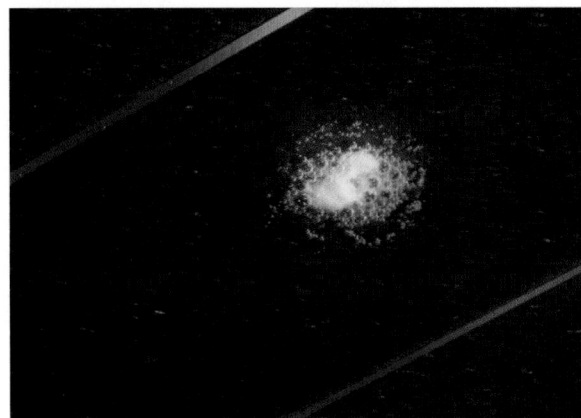

FIGURE 15-12 Positive catalase test. Catalase produces bubbles in the presence of hydrogen peroxide.

Biochemical Tests for Identification
Catalase Test

The **catalase** test, which is based on the ability of bacteria to convert hydrogen peroxide to water and oxygen gas, tests for the presence of the enzyme catalase. To perform this test, place a sample of an isolated colony on a glass slide with an inoculating loop or with a sterile wooden stick; then place a small drop of hydrogen peroxide on the bacteria, and observe. Formation of bubbles indicates a positive test (Figure 15-12); absence of bubbles indicates a negative test. This test is commonly used to differentiate staphylococci (which are catalase-positive) from streptococci and enterococci (which are catalase-negative). The test uses 3% hydrogen peroxide, which can be purchased at the grocery store or pharmacy.

> **TECHNICIAN NOTE** Hydrogen peroxide degrades over time, so it is best to put a small amount in a glass dropper bottle (preferably a brown or dark bottle that will protect it from light) and store it in the refrigerator. The hydrogen peroxide should be tested periodically with a known *Staphylococcus* isolate to confirm that it is working.

Oxidase Test

This test is used to identify bacteria containing the respiratory enzyme cytochrome oxidase. The **oxidase** test is commercially available in several different types. A colony is picked from a blood agar plate and is tested with the oxidase reagent. Iron from inoculating loops or needles can give a false-positive, so it is best to use wood, plastic, or a cotton swab for this test. A positive test is indicated by the formation of a blue color; a negative test result is colorless (Figure 15-13). Generally, the color change is seen in less than 30 seconds. It can take up to a minute for some organisms like *Pasteurella* to turn positive. This test is commonly used to differentiate Gram-negative bacteria.

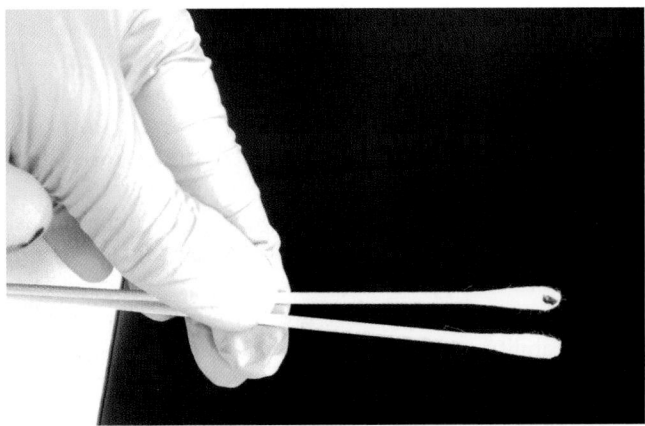

FIGURE 15-13 Oxidase test. Oxidase reagent turns blue in the presence of bacteria with cytochrome oxidase.

Presumptive Identification

Once the Gram reaction and morphology have been determined and subsequent preliminary tests such as oxidase and catalase tests have been performed, an organism can be grouped and appropriate differential tests chosen and performed (see Figure 15-11).

Gram-positive cocci are divided between catalase-negative (*Streptococcus* and *Enterococcus*) and catalase-positive (*Staphylococcus* and *Micrococcus*) organisms (Tables 15-4 and 15-5). Streptococci are differentiated by the pattern of hemolysis that they produce (see Figures 15-9 and 15-10). Although α-hemolytic *Streptococcus* isolates are generally considered to be normal flora unless found at a normally sterile anatomic site, β-hemolytic streptococci are generally considered pathogenic. Beta-hemolytic streptococci such as *Streptococcus agalactiae* are also differentiated on their ability to produce a synergistic hemolysis with *Staphylococcus aureus* in the CAMP test (Figure 15-14). Enterococci were previously categorized as fecal α-hemolytic streptococci and typically grow in the presence of bile and salt. Enterococci usually are considered pathogenic only when found at a normally sterile site. They are commonly found in urinary tract infections and, unlike α-hemolytic streptococci, are positive for bile esculin and the ability to grow in the presence of 6.5% sodium chloride.

Catalase-positive, Gram-positive cocci include *Staphylococcus* and *Micrococcus* isolates. *Micrococcus* is usually

TABLE 15-4	**Identification of Gram-Positive, Catalase-Negative Cocci**						
ORGANISM	**HEMOLYSIS**	**LANCEFIELD GROUP**	**BILE ESCULIN**	**6.5% SODIUM CHLORIDE**	**LACTOSE***	**TREHALOSE***	**SORBITOL***
Streptococcus agalactiae	Beta	B	−	−	+	+	−
Streptococcus canis	Beta	G	−	−	+	−	−
Streptococcus dysgalactiae	Alpha	A, C, G, L	−	−	V	+	−
Streptococcus equi subsp *equi*	Beta	C	−	−	−	−	−
Streptococcus equi subsp *zooepidemicus*	Beta	C	−	−	+	−	+
Enterococcus spp.	Alpha	D	+	+	V	V	V
Streptococcus viridans group	Alpha	NA	−	−	V	V	V
Streptococcus bovis group	Alpha	D	+	−	V	V	V

Key: +, positive test result; −, negative test result; *NA*, not applicable; *V*, variable.
*Lactose, trehalose, and sorbitol are sugars. These sugars are added to media such as cysteine tryptic agar with a pH indicator such as phenol red. If the *Streptococcus* isolate is able to ferment the sugar, the media will change color (from red to yellow). Most rapid test kits include a version of sugar fermentation for distinguishing streptococci.

TABLE 15-5	**Identification of Gram-Positive, Catalase-Positive Cocci**			
ORGANISM	**HEMOLYSIS**	**COAGULASE**	**GLUCOSE FERMENTATION**	**MANNITOL FERMENTATION**
Staphylococcus aureus	+ (double zone)	+	+	+
*Staphylococcus pseudintermedius/ S. intermedius**	+	+	+	±
Staphylococcus (coagulase-negative species)	±	−	+	±
Micrococcus	−	−	−	

*Note that canine isolates are now *S. pseudintermedius*, but isolates from many other animal species are still called *S. intermedius*.
Key: +, positive test result; −, negative test result; ±, test result may be positive or negative.

TABLE 15-6	Identification of Gram-Positive Rods						
ORGANISM	MOTILITY (22°C)	CATALASE	HYDROGEN SULFIDE IN TSI	UREASE	COMPLETE HEMOLYSIS	COLONY MORHPOLOGIC CHARACTERISTICS
Listeria monocytogenes	+	+	−	−		Very small
Erysipelothrix rhusiopathiae	−	−	+	−	Slow	Very small
Truperella (Arcanobacterium) pyogenes	−	−	−	−	V	Very small
Corynebacterium renale	−	+	−	+	V	Medium-sized, white
Corynebacterium pseudotuberculosis	−	+	−	+	−	Dry, waxy, white
Rhodococcus equi	−	+	−	+	V	Large, mucoid, pink

Key: +, positive test result; −, negative test result; V, variable.

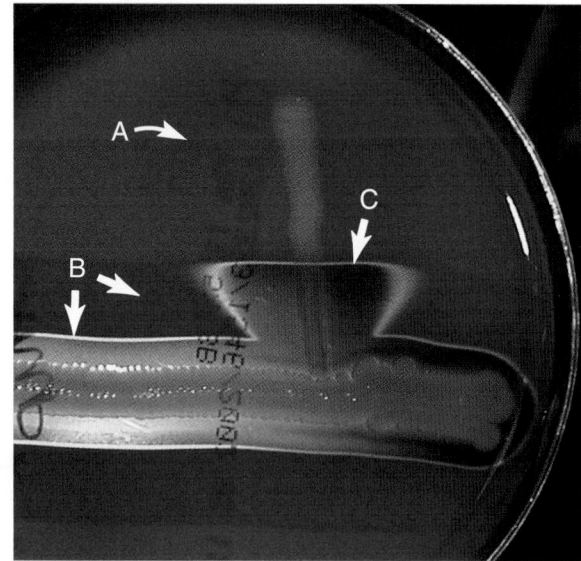

FIGURE 15-14 CAMP test for *Streptococcus agalactiae*. The isolate (A) to be tested is inoculated perpendicular to a stock strain of double-zone hemolytic *Staphylococcus* (B), producing a synergistic triangle of hemolysis (C) as a positive CAMP test.

nonpathogenic and oxidase-positive and is unable to ferment glucose on triple sugar iron (TSI) slants. *Staphylococcus* isolates are differentiated on the basis of their production of **coagulase**. Coagulase converts fibrinogen in rabbit plasma to fibrin and has historically been a measure of virulence. Coagulase-negative staphylococci are typically indigenous floras and often are considered nonpathogenic unless they are transferred to normally sterile sites during procedures such as hip replacement and intravenous catheter placement.

> **TECHNICIAN NOTE** Recently, *Staphylococcus schleiferi* subsp. *schleiferi* (which is coagulase-negative) was associated with pyoderma in dogs. This fact, combined with new knowledge about drug resistance in *Staphylococcus* isolates, is changing interpretation of the presence of coagulase-negative *Staphylococcus* in patient samples.

Small Gram-positive rods are differentiated by catalase activity, colony morphology, and use of TSI slants, urea agar, and motility testing (Table 15-6). These organisms will be discussed individually. Gram-positive branching rods should be tested for catalase production and stained with acid-fast stain to determine whether they could be *Mycobacterium* spp. or *Nocardia* spp.

Gram-negative organisms are sub-grouped according to their ability to produce oxidase (Table 15-7). Oxidase-negative, Gram-negative bacteria are typically members of the family Enterobacteriaceae. They can be identified using a handful of biochemical tests and are readily identified with most commercial identification systems. Oxidase-positive, Gram-negative organisms of veterinary importance can be differentiated using colony morphology, as well as TSI slants, urea agar, and motility testing. Weakly oxidase-positive organisms such as *Pasteurella* spp. can be difficult to recognize and to identify.

Definitive Identification

Definitive identification of organisms often requires extensive testing and can be labor-intensive. It is not practical for the small laboratory. Isolates requiring definitive identification can be forwarded to reference laboratories. Additionally, the advent of inexpensive sequencing makes this technology attractive for definitive identification of bacteria; this method is offered by a variety of laboratories. Sequencing is discussed later.

Commercial Identification Kits

Development of commercially available identification kits has significantly changed microbiology and has simplified identification of isolates in the small laboratory. Most kits consist of a series of biochemical tests provided as a single unit. These tests are inoculated with an isolated organism (called an "isolate") and are incubated for a set period of time under specific conditions. Results are recorded and are compared with a database of biochemical test results from known bacteria to determine the identity of the isolate.

For the small, low-volume laboratory, these kits can be an accurate, cost-effective alternative to prepared media, because they have a long shelf life, require minimal storage space, and provide results that are easy to interpret. The manufacturer's

TABLE 15-7 Identification of Gram-Negative Rods

ORGANISM	OXIDASE	GROWTH ON MACCONKEY'S AGAR	TSI	HYDROGEN SULFIDE	MOTILITY	UREASE	INDOLE	CITRATE UTILIZATION
Escherichia coli	−	G	A/A, K/A	−	+	−	+	−
Enterobacter spp.	−	G	A/A, K/A	−	+	+	−	+
Klebsiella spp.	−	G	A/A, K/A	−	−	+	±	+
Citrobacter spp.	−	G	K/A	+	+	+	+	+
Proteus mirabilis	−	G	K/A	+	+	+	−	+
Proteus spp.	−	G	K/A	−	+	+	V	+
Salmonella spp.	−	G	K/A	+	+	−	−	+
Actinobacillus spp.	+	G or NG	A/A	−	−	+	−	−
Aeromonas spp.	+	G	A/A	−	+	−	+	V
Mannheimia haemolytica	+	G or NG	A/A	−	−	−	−	−
Pasteurella multocida	+	NG	A/A	−	−	−	+	−
Pasteurella spp.	+	NG	A/A	−	−	−	−	−
Bordetella bronchiseptica	+	G (w)	K/NC	−	+	+	−	+
Brucella canis	+	NG	K/NC	−	−	+	−	−
Moraxella bovis	+	NG	K/NC	−	±	−	−	−
Pseudomonas aeruginosa	+	G	K/NC	−	+	±	−	+
Pseudomonas spp.	+	G	K/NC	−	+	V	−	+

Key: +, positive test result; −, negative test result; ±, test result may be positive or negative; A, acid; G, growth; K, alkaline; NC, no change; NG, no growth; V, variable; w, weak reaction. The letter before the slash refers to the condition of the media in the slant of the test tube; the letter after the slash refers to the condition of the media in the butt of the test tube.

directions should be strictly adhered to because failure to do so can lead to inaccurate identification of organisms. It is important to remember that these commercial kits are typically designed for isolates collected from humans and may not have an adequate database for veterinary isolates. This is primarily true for oxidase-positive, Gram-negative bacteria and catalase positive, Gram-positive rods. In general, oxidase-negative, Gram-negative enteric bacteria are adequately identified by commercial identification kits.

TECHNICIAN NOTE Development of commercially available identification kits has significantly changed microbiology and has simplified identification of isolates in the small, low-volume laboratory. These kits can serve as an accurate, cost-effective alternative to prepared media.

SPECIAL CULTURE PROCEDURES
Fecal Culture
Feces are often cultured to identify pathogens that cause diarrhea. Of these, the most common are *Salmonella*, *Campylobacter jejuni*, *Clostridium perfringens*, and *Clostridium difficile*. In the case of *C. perfringens* and *C. difficile*, disease correlates with the presence of toxins produced by these agents rather than with the presence of the organisms. Enzyme-linked immunosorbent assay (ELISA) tests are typically used to detect the presence of these toxins. Additional causes of diarrhea include *Yersinia enterocolitica*, *Mycobacterium avium* subsp. *paratuberculosis*, and *Lawsonia*

intracellularis. Isolation of pathogens from fecal material typically requires enrichment and selective media. To isolate *Salmonella*, enrichment for these organisms is usually performed using overnight incubation in selenite or tetrathionate broth. The following day, the broth enrichment cultures are subcultured onto Hektoen enteric agar or a similar selective agar and MacConkey's agar. These agar plates are then incubated overnight at 35°C. Subsequently, they are examined for the presence of suspect colonies, which then are confirmed using biochemical tests. These may include TSI agar slants, lysine iron agar slants, urease agar, and indole test media. Other media such as xylose tergitol agar can also be employed for the recovery of *Salmonella*. *C. jejuni* can be difficult to culture. This organism requires an oxygen-reduced environment for growth and may require specialized *Campylobacter* medium, which incorporates antimicrobial agents to reduce the growth of other organisms. *Campylobacter* cultures are typically incubated at higher temperatures such as 42°C for up to 48 to 72 hours. Suspect *Campylobacter* colonies are flat, nonhemolytic, and gray with an irregular edge. Gram stain of suspect *Campylobacter* colonies should reveal Gram-negative small curved bacteria.

Blood Cultures
Blood culture media are inoculated immediately upon collection (see "Sample Collection" on page 489). Care must be taken not to contaminate blood cultures. As discussed previously, a single organism can result in a positive culture. Aerobic samples are typically vented using a blood culture

venting needle. Bottles should be incubated at 37°C. A sample from the culture bottle should be subcultured onto agar plates at least twice over a 10-day period. Blood cultures are typically held up to 14 days before they are reported as negative. In human hospitals, blood cultures are performed using an automated incubator system that alerts the user when a bottle turns positive. These systems are expensive and typically are beyond the needs of the average veterinary practice.

Quantified Urine Cultures

When urine is cultured, the number of organisms is important for determining the likelihood and severity of infection. The number of organisms present in a 1-milliliter (mL) urine sample can easily be quantified using commercially available, disposable calibrated inoculating loops. Typically, two loops are used—one that holds a 1-μL sample and another that holds a10-μL sample.

> **TECHNICIAN NOTE** When urine is cultured, the number of organisms is important for determining the likelihood and severity of infection. This is done by performing a quantified urine culture.

These are inoculated onto separate blood agar plates in a pattern that makes it easy to count the colonies (Figure 15-15). Each plate should be labeled with the patient information and the dilution. The 1-μL loop holds the equivalent of a 1:1000 dilution of urine because 1000 μL of urine is present in every milliliter. In contrast, the 10-μL loop holds the equivalent of a 1:100 dilution of urine because every milliliter of urine contains one hundred 10-μL samples. To determine how many bacteria are present in each milliliter of urine, the number of colonies on the plate is multiplied by the dilution factor of the plate. For example, if 54 colonies of *E. coli* are present on the 1:1000 plate, this represents 54,000 *E. coli* per milliliter of urine (54 × 1000). By convention, this number would be reported as 54,000 colony-forming units (CFUs) of *E. coli* per milliliter of urine. The term "CFU" is used to describe the number of bacteria because it is not possible to know whether more than a single bacterium formed the colony that grows on the plate. If more colonies are present than can reasonably be counted, or more than 100 colonies are seen on the 1:1000 dilution plate, the culture is reported as "greater than 100,000 CFU/ ml." The 1:1000 dilution plate should have approximately $\frac{1}{10}$ as many bacteria as the 1:100 dilution plate. If it does not, the technician should evaluate whether proper technique was used.

A MacConkey's agar plate should also be inoculated because enteric Gram-negative organisms that grow on MacConkey's agar are common causes of urinary tract infection. Inoculation of the MacConkey's agar will aid in rapid isolation and identification of these organisms. All plates should be incubated overnight at 37°C. Urine cultures should be held for 3 days before they are reported as negative.

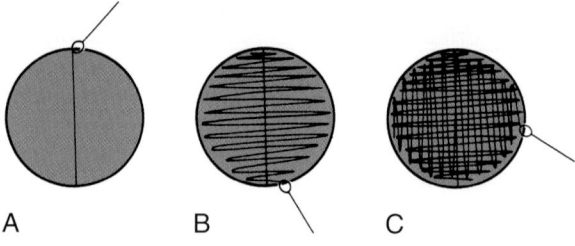

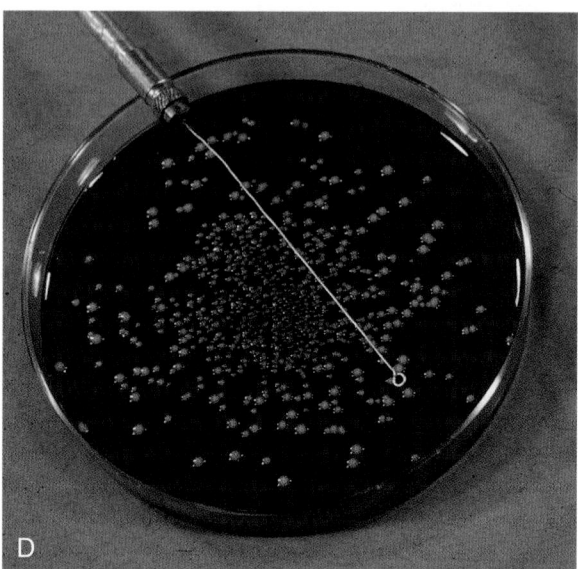

FIGURE 15-15 Procedure for inoculating media for semi-quantitative bacterial colony counts when culturing urine or milk. **A,** Primary inoculation with calibrated loop. **B,** Streak at right angles to primary inoculation. **C,** Streak at right angles to previous streak. **D,** Photo illustrates a plate with more than 100 colonies resulting from inoculation with a 1-μl loop indicating more than 10^5 bacteria/ml of urine.

Milk

A milk culture is similar to a urine culture in that the organisms present must be quantified. Plates are inoculated using calibrated inoculation loops and are labeled accordingly. The most significant organisms are the agents of contagious mastitis such as *Staphylococcus aureus*, *Streptococcus agalactiae*, and *Mycoplasma* spp. Mastitis caused by environmental organisms such as coliforms and alpha-hemolytic streptococci also occurs; these organisms should be quantified as well. Ideally, separate samples from each quarter of the udder should be prepared.

> **TECHNICIAN NOTE** The most significant organisms found in milk are the agents of contagious mastitis such as *Staphylococcus aureus*, *Streptococcus agalactiae*, and *Mycoplasma* spp.

COMMON BACTERIAL SPECIES
Gram-Positive Cocci

Staphylococcus spp. are catalase-positive, Gram-positive cocci that normally inhabit the skin and mucous membranes. *Staphylococcus aureus* is a normal skin inhabitant of people, cats, and large animals. *Staphylococcus pseudintermedius* (formerly *S. intermedius*) is a normal inhabitant of the skin of dogs. Please note that *S. intermedius* is still an appropriate name, and this organism is found in species other than dogs (birds, horses, etc.). For practical purposes, *S. pseudintermedius* and *S. intermedius* are identical by commonly used biochemical tests and there is little clinical benefit in attempting definitive identification.

Streptococcus spp. are catalase-negative, Gram-positive cocci that normally inhabit the mouth and skin. These organisms cause infection in these sites and can cause generalized infections, including septicemia. In rare but serious cases, these organisms can cause necrotizing fasciitis.

Enterococcus spp. (previously the group D streptococci) are catalase-negative, Gram-positive cocci that can grow in the presence of bile salts. Members of this genus are normal inhabitants of the gastrointestinal tract and are associated with opportunistic infections, particularly urinary tract infections.

Gram-Positive Rods

Bacillus spp. are Gram-positive rods. These organisms are ubiquitous and are commonly found as culture contaminants, although some are associated with diseases such as mastitis. The most important member of this genus is *Bacillus anthracis*, the causative agent of anthrax. This organism should not be cultured because it is easily aerosolized and is potentially lethal. It is also a select agent regulated by the U.S. government.

Corynebacterium spp. are pleomorphic in shape and cause a variety of diseases. *Corynebacterium pseudotuberculosis* is an important veterinary pathogen that causes caseous lymphadenitis in sheep and goats and both abscesses and ulcerative lymphangitis in horses (commonly called "pigeon fever"). The colonies of this organism are typically small, with a dry, waxy appearance. It typically takes 48 hours for colonies 1 mm in diameter to form. *Corynebacterium renale* and related organisms cause renal disease and pyelonephritis in cattle. This genus consists of many organisms, a number of which are indigenous floras.

Trueperella (Arcanobacterium) pyogenes was previously classified as a *Corynebacterium* and subsequently as *Actinomyces* before it was assigned to the genus *Arcanobacterium*. In 2011, this organism was reclassified as *Trueperella*. A common inhabitant of the skin and mucous membranes of cattle and other ruminants, this organism is an opportunist. It is catalase negative and produces a small hemolytic colony (less than 1 mm in diameter) after 48 hours of culture.

Erysipelothrix rhusiopathiae causes disease in swine, turkeys, and marine mammals. This small, catalase-negative rod forms pinpoint colonies with partial hemolysis on blood agar plates. It can be difficult to distinguish this organism from alpha-hemolytic streptococci. This organism produces hydrogen sulfide along the stab line when inoculated into TSI agar.

Listeria monocytogenes is a cause of foodborne illness and a causative agent of listeriosis in ruminants. It is a small catalase-positive rod that is motile at room temperature. It can cause septicemia in neonatal animals, abortion, and encephalitis. Isolation of this organism can be difficult, but because of its zoonotic potential, this should be left to reference laboratories.

Rhodococcus equi is an aerobic, nonmotile, CAMP-positive, Gram-positive rod. It causes pneumonia in foals and, rarely, disseminated disease in adult horses. It is a common soil-borne organism, and the presence of a virulence plasmid is required for disease.

Actinomyces spp. are branching rods typically found in the mouth and the upper respiratory tract. These organisms are associated with bony lesions of the head and neck and can cause wound infection. This genus includes both aerobic and anaerobic members.

Acid-Fast Bacteria

Mycobacterium spp. have cell walls that include mycolic acid, which does not retain Gram stain but stains positively with carbol fuchsin. Organisms in this genus are typically slow-growing, sometimes taking weeks to grow sufficiently for colonies to be seen. Their culture is best left to reference laboratories, but the ability to stain specimens such as fluids, impression smears, and feces can aid in the presumptive diagnosis of mycobacterial infection. It is important to evaluate staining technique by staining a control slide simultaneously with the sample being tested (see section on acid-fast staining). Culture for identification of *M. tuberculosis* should be performed only in a reference laboratory with appropriate safety equipment.

Colonies of *Nocardia* spp. have an appearance of white chalk. Gram stain reveals the presence of long, branching, Gram-positive rods. These rods are partially acid-fast when stained with Kinyoun's acid-fast staining procedure, and the rods have a "beaded" appearance on the slide. They may be described as rough or dry and take up to 5 days to grow under standard culture conditions.

> **TECHNICIAN NOTE** Culture of *Mycobacterium* spp. is best left to reference laboratories, particularly culture for identification of *M. tuberculosis*, which requires appropriate safety equipment.

Gram-Negative Bacteria

Gram-negative bacteria typically are divided on the basis of their production of cytochrome oxidase and their ability to grow on MacConkey's agar. The oxidase test is usually the first test performed when these organisms are identified. Members of the family Enterobacteriaceae, which includes *E. coli*, are oxidase-negative. Coliforms (*E. coli*, *Klebsiella*, *Enterobacter*) are found as normal inhabitants of the gastrointestinal tract and frequently are opportunistic pathogens. These bacteria are frequently the cause of urinary tract and wound infections. They also cause infection in neonatal animals, including enteritis and septicemia. These organisms vary in their susceptibility to antimicrobials, so if they are isolated, it is valuable to perform susceptibility testing. They can also be present in infections of the respiratory tract and the reproductive tract.

Salmonella causes diarrhea and septicemia in a variety of animal species and is commonly isolated from feces of reptiles and amphibians. This organism is particularly important as an agent of nosocomial and zoonotic infections, making it important to practice good hand hygiene and to disinfect equipment, cages, and stalls when this organism is suspected.

Proteus spp. cause urinary tract infections but can also be present as opportunists in wounds, in ears, and on skin.

> **TECHNICIAN NOTE** *Proteus* spp. can readily swarm a plate, overgrowing other, more slowly growing organisms. The potential presence of this organism makes it advisable to use selective media in initial cultures.

Other enteric organisms *(Serratia, Citrobacter, Edwardsiella, Hafnia)* can also be present as opportunists and as indigenous flora. They are less commonly isolated but can be significant because of potential antimicrobial resistance.

Aeromonas is frequently found in infections from aquatic animals, including fish and amphibians. These oxidase-positive Gram-negative rods are commonly found in soil and water. They are occasional causes of septicemia in mammals.

Actinobacillus spp. are oxidase-positive, small, Gram-negative rods that typically grow on MacConkey's agar. They are similar to *Pasteurella* and are often isolated from foals with septicemia or joint infection. They can also be present as normal respiratory flora in adult horses.

Pasteurella spp. are part of the indigenous flora of the mouth and upper respiratory tract. They are oxidase-positive, short, fat rods (also called *coccobacilli*). They can ferment glucose but may not do this well on TSI agar slants. Often they do not grow on MacConkey's agar. *Pasteurella multocida*, one of the most commonly isolated members of this genus, is associated with cat bites and abscesses in cats, and with infection in most other mammals. Although many animals carry *P. multocida*, strains are not typically passed between species. *P. multocida* can cause rapidly progressing cellulitis in people who have been bitten by cats. For this reason, it is imperative that people bitten by cats seek medical attention without delay; in addition, they should act in accordance with legal requirements pertaining to the rabies vaccination status of any cat that has bitten a person and should present their related concerns to appropriate regulatory officials.

> **TECHNICIAN NOTE** *Pasteurella* strains often do not grow on MacConkey's agar and are slow to convert the oxidase reagent to positive. Absence of growth on MacConkey's agar does not indicate the absence of Gram-negative organisms.

Haemophilus spp. are oxidase-positive, small coccobacilli that commonly inhabit the oronasal mucosa and can be important respiratory pathogens. They may be difficult to cultivate because they require enriched media such as lysed blood cells and additional carbon dioxide for growth. Their culture is best left to diagnostic or reference laboratories with specialized equipment. They are included in this discussion because they can grow as satellite colonies around colonies of *Staphylococcus* spp., and may be encountered on initial culture of samples collected from the respiratory tract. They often fail to grow when subcultured, unless appropriate conditions are provided.

Pseudomonas spp. are oxidase-positive rods commonly found in soil and water. These bacteria are generally opportunists but are significant pathogens because they usually are resistant to several classes of antimicrobial agents. They are often hemolytic and secrete a green pigment called *pyocyanin* into media surrounding colonies. They may have a metallic appearance on blood agar plates, and they are lactose-negative on MacConkey's agar.

Bordetella spp. are small, oxidase-positive coccobacilli that cause infection of the respiratory and reproductive tracts. They are rapidly urease-positive (within 4 hours). They can be associated with reproductive failure and abortion. *Bordetella bronchiseptica* is a causative agent of canine tracheobronchitis (commonly referred to as "kennel cough").

Brucella spp. are small, oxidase-positive coccobacilli. They are rapidly urease-positive (within 10 minutes). These bacteria are usually associated with abortion and reproductive failure. They typically grow over several days and require increased atmospheric carbon dioxide. Some members of this genus are select agents, and their culture is best left to reference laboratories with appropriate safety equipment and procedures.

Other Gram-Negative Rods

Many Gram-negative organisms of clinical importance have not been discussed here. Only the organisms of greatest importance for the small laboratory have been discussed. For further information, readers are directed to the recommended reading list.

Anaerobes

Many important anaerobic pathogens have been identified. In general, the culture of obligate anaerobes is challenging and is best left to reference laboratories with specialized equipment and media. Anaerobic pathogens can be Gram-negative or -positive rods or cocci. They are part of the indigenous flora of the gastrointestinal tract and often are found in abscesses or mixed infections. Some of the common Gram-negative anaerobic rods are members of the genera *Bacteroides, Dichelobacter, Fusobacterium, Porphyromonas,* and *Prevotella*. Among the anaerobic Gram-positive cocci, *Peptostreptococcus* is probably the most common genus. The most important anaerobic Gram-positive rods are of the *Clostridium* spp. Most *Clostridium* of veterinary significance can be directly detected in tissues using serologic techniques that are best left to reference laboratories. The two organisms of greatest importance for the small laboratory are *C. perfringens* and *C. difficile,* which were previously discussed under fecal culture (see page 501). Both of these agents are readily cultured using anaerobic techniques, but both are part of the indigenous flora of the gastrointestinal tract, so their presence does not necessarily indicate disease. Diagnosis of *Clostridium*-induced enteritis requires identification of certain toxins.

Spirochetes and Curved Bacteria

Several significant veterinary pathogens are spirochetes, or curved bacteria. Although these organisms are important, they are difficult to culture and are potentially zoonotic. Indeed, the diseases caused by these organisms are diagnosed primarily through alternate methods including serologic or molecular testing rather than culture. Among the most important spirochetes are *Leptospira* spp., *Borrelia burgdorferi, Brachyspira hyodysenteriae,* and *Campylobacter* spp. *Leptospira* spp. are shed in the urine of affected animals and cause febrile illness, renal disease, abortion, and infertility. *B. burgdorferi* is the causative agent of Lyme disease and of lameness and arthritis in dogs. *B. hyodysenteriae* causes diarrhea and dysentery in pigs and typically is diagnosed by identification of large spirochetes in Gram-stained, direct smears made from colonic mucosa of affected animals. *Campylobacter* spp. may cause gastroenteritis and abortion.

> **TECHNICIAN NOTE** Several significant veterinary pathogens are spirochetes or curved bacteria. Diseases caused by these organisms are diagnosed primarily through alternate methods including serologic or molecular testing rather than culture.

Mycoplasma

Mycoplasma spp. lack cell walls and therefore are not visible on Gram stain. They are associated with mucous membranes and can cause urinary tract infection in dogs and cats, joint and respiratory infections in cattle, pigs, and sheep, and mastitis in cattle. These bacteria are difficult to culture and require specialized transport media.

Obligate Intracellular Organisms

Obligate intracellular bacteria will not grow on standard culture media. Like viruses, they require cultured animal cells to grow. Infections with these organisms are often diagnosed using serologic or molecular testing. Important genera include *Anaplasma, Chlamydia, Chlamydophila, Coxiella, Ehrlichia, Rickettsia,* and *Neorickettsia.*

ANTIMICROBIAL SUSCEPTIBILITY TESTING

INDICATIONS

Antibiotics are agents produced by bacteria or fungi that inhibit microbial growth. Antimicrobial agents include both antibiotics and synthetic agents that inhibit microbial growth. **Antimicrobial susceptibility testing** is performed to guide the veterinarian in selection of appropriate antimicrobial drugs to treat bacterial infections. (See Case Presentation 15-1 for an example of how susceptibility testing is used to guide treatment.) Several methods are available to determine whether bacteria are susceptible or resistant to antimicrobial drugs. Performance of these tests is highly standardized, and they should be performed in accordance with the guidelines put forth by the Food and Drug Administration (FDA) and the Clinical Laboratory Standards Institute (CLSI; formerly NCCLS). It is important to use the appropriate concentrations of bacteria for these tests because using too many bacteria can lead to the conclusion that the bacteria are resistant to a drug when they are not, and vice versa. In microbiology laboratories, the McFarland concentration standards are used to estimate bacterial numbers. The 0.5 McFarland standard is typically used in susceptibility testing and is equivalent to approximately 1.5×10^8 bacteria per milliliter of diluent.

Quality assurance testing is essential in susceptibility testing to ensure that all tests and reagents perform appropriately. Drugs and media that exceed the expiration date may not work. Testing with reagents that do not work will lead to erroneous results and could result in inappropriate treatment of patients. Testing a drug that is inactive because it was not stored properly, or that is inactive for other reasons, may lead to the erroneous conclusion that an isolate is resistant. It is also important to know what the result of a test means. Interpretive criteria are used to evaluate the results of a test and to determine whether bacteria are susceptible or resistant to specific drugs (Table 15-8). The guidelines put forth in the CLSI M31-A3 document should be consulted when these tests are performed. The CLSI Subcommittee on Veterinary Antimicrobial Susceptibility Testing meets several times a year to discuss and update guidelines. New guidelines are generally approved every 3 years. At the time of this writing, an updated version is imminent.

METHODS
Broth Dilution or Microbroth Dilution

This method of susceptibility testing uses dilution of antimicrobial agents in liquid culture (broth) to determine the lowest amount of antimicrobial that will inhibit growth of the bacterium being tested (**minimum inhibitory concentration**, or **MIC**). Commercial systems are available for this type of susceptibility testing. The manufacturer's instructions should be followed when a commercial system is used. A pure culture must be used. For microbroth dilution methods, cultures are adjusted to a final concentration of 1×10^5 bacteria per milliliter. For each drug tested, a series of 2-fold dilutions of antimicrobial encompassing a clinically relevant range of concentrations is prepared. Following inoculation, the dilutions are incubated overnight at 37° C, and the MIC is then determined (Figure 15-16, *A* and *B*).

CASE PRESENTATION 15-1 URINARY TRACT INFECTION

History

Bailey, a 6-year-old female, mixed breed dog was presented for inappropriate urination. The owner reported that during the previous week, Bailey had several "accidents" in the house, and seemed to need to go outside more frequently. After she was housetrained as a puppy, Bailey had never urinated indoors until the onset of this problem. The owner also reported that when cleaning up the urine from the "accidents," she noticed that it smelled bad. Physical examination revealed no abnormalities, although Bailey tensed when abdominal palpation was attempted; consequently, it was not possible to do a thorough abdominal examination. Acute cystitis with a possible bacterial infection was suspected, and urine was collected by cystocentesis for urinalysis, culture, and sensitivity testing.

Laboratory Results

The urine was cloudy, and urinalysis indicated the presence of leukocytes, red blood cells, and glucose. Knowing that β-lactam antibiotics concentrate in the urine and are effective against most of the organisms that commonly cause urinary tract infection (UTI), the attending veterinarian prescribed amoxicillin with clavulanate for 10 days while waiting for culture results. Three days later, culture results arrived from the laboratory. *Enterobacter cloacae* was cultured from the urine at greater than 100,000 CFUs/ml. The minimum inhibitory concentrations (MICs) of the antibiotics tested were as follows: amoxicillin with clavulanate, >32 μg/ml; ampicillin, >16 μg/ml; ceftiofur, 1 μg/ml; cephalexin, >16 μg/ml; enrofloxacin, <0.5 μg/ml; tetracycline, <2 μg/ml; and trimethoprim with sulfonamide, <0.5 μg/ml. Based on evaluation of the MIC of each drug, the organism was considered resistant to β-lactam antibiotics (amoxicillin with clavulanate, ampicillin, ceftiofur, and cephalexin), but was considered susceptible to the other three (enrofloxacin, tetracycline, and trimethoprim with sulfonamide).

Outcome

In view of these results, the veterinarian decided to prescribe enrofloxacin and directed the owner to discontinue amoxicillin with clavulanate and to start giving the new antibiotic instead. After the change in therapy, Bailey's urinary tract infection quickly resolved. Additional testing indicated that she also had diabetes mellitus, which may have predisposed her to the urinary tract infection. With careful management of her diabetes, she had no repeat occurrences.

Conclusion

This case illustrates the value of bacterial culture and sensitivity testing in selecting appropriate antimicrobial treatment for patients with bacterial infections. Without data provided by these tests, Bailey's infection probably would not have been eliminated, and she would have continued to have ongoing or recurrent urinary tract infections. By using these data to guide treatment, the attending veterinarian was able to quickly and effectively eliminate Bailey's UTI, thereby relieving her discomfort and decreasing the likelihood of complications from this infection.

Disc Diffusion (Kirby-Bauer Method)

This method uses bacterial growth in the presence of antimicrobial-saturated paper discs on agar plates to determine whether an organism is susceptible to an antimicrobial agent. Mueller-Hinton agar plates are inoculated with the bacterium being tested, and a paper disc impregnated with the antimicrobial agent at a specific concentration is placed on the surface of the inoculated plate. The plate is incubated for 18 to 24 hours at 37° C. Some organisms require a full 24 hours of incubation. If the bacterium is inhibited by the antimicrobial agent, a clear zone will be present around the paper disc, where the bacterium does not grow. This is called the *zone of inhibition* (Figure 15-16, *C* and *D*; Procedure 15-4). The diameter of the zone is measured using a caliper or ruler, and this value is then compared with the breakpoints for that drug to determine whether the organism is susceptible or resistant or somewhere in between (intermediate).

PROCEDURE 15-4	Basic Protocol for Performing Disc Diffusion Testing

1. Using a sterile swab, pick three to five isolated colonies that are less than 48 hours old, and that ideally are cultured on a tryptic soy agar plate supplemented with 5% sheep's blood (blood agar plate).
2. Mix the bacterial colonies in tryptic soy broth until a concentration equivalent to a 0.5 McFarland standard is achieved.
3. Within 15 minutes of adjusting the bacterial suspension to the appropriate concentration, dip a sterile swab into the solution. Rotate the swab against the wall of the tube to remove excess liquid from the swab.
4. Inoculate the dry surface of a Mueller-Hinton agar plate by streaking the swab over the entire surface. Repeat the streaking process 2 more times, rotating the plate 60 degrees each time.
5. Discs should be placed on the agar surface using a commercially available dispenser or sterile forceps. Gently press on the discs with sterile forceps to ensure their adherence to the agar surface. (A maximum of 12 discs can be applied to the 150-mm plates.)
6. Invert the plate and place in an incubator. Incubate the plate for 18 to 24 hours at 37° C. Some organisms, including staphylococci, require a full 24 hours of incubation. Guidelines established in the CLSI M31-A3 document should be consulted when performing these tests.
7. Remove the plate from the incubator, and measure the zones of inhibition using a rule or a caliper (Figure 15-18, *D*).
8. Compare the diameter with the guidelines (breakpoints) established in CLSI M31-A3.

Note: Streptococcus spp. and other fastidious organisms are inoculated onto Mueller-Hinton agar with blood. When *Streptococcus* spp. are tested, no more than nine discs should be placed on each 150-mm plate.

| TABLE 15-8 | Summary of Antimicrobial Susceptibility Testing Interpretive Criteria |

ANTIMICROBIAL AGENT	DISC CONTENT	ZONE DIAMETER, mm	
		SUSCEPTIBLE	RESISTANT
Ampicillin*†, Enterobacteriaceae	10 μg	≥17	≤13
Ampicillin*†, Staphylococci	10 μg	≥29	≤28
Ampicillin*†, Enterococci	10 μg	≥17	≤16
Ampicillin*†, Streptococci (not *Streptococcus pneumoniae*)	10 μg	≥26	≤18
Amoxicillin/Clavulanic acid*, *Staphylococcus* spp.	20/10 μg	≥20	≤19
Amoxicillin/Clavulanic acid*, Other organisms	20/10 μg	≥18	≤13
Cefazolin*	30 μg	≥18	≤14
Cephalothin*‡	30 μg	≥18	≤14
Cefovecin§	30 μg	≥23	≤19
Ceftiofur, Bovine/Swine (respiratory disease)	30 μg	≥21	≤17
Clindamycin, Dogs (skin and soft tissue infections)	2 μg	≥21	≤14
Enrofloxacin, Cats (dermal)/Dogs (dermal/respiratory/UTI)	5 μg	≥23	≤16
Enrofloxacin, Bovine (respiratory disease)	5 μg	≥21	≤16
Florfenicol, Bovine (respiratory disease)	30 μg	≥19	≤14
Florfenicol, Swine (respiratory disease)	30 μg	≥22	≤18
Gentamicin, Dogs/Equine Enterobacteriacae, *Pseudomonas aeruginosa*	10 μg	≥16	≤12
Oxacillin*¶ *Staphylococcus aureus*	1 μg	≥13	≤10
Oxacillin*¶ Staphylococci other than *S. aureus*	1 μg	≥18	≤17
Penicillin*, Staphylococci	10 μg	≥29	≤28
Penicillin*, Enterococci	10 μg	≥15	≤14
Penicillin*, Streptococci–β-hemolytic group	10 μg	≥24	≤24
Tetracycline*#, Organisms other than streptococci	30 μg	≥19	≤14
Tetracycline*#, Streptococci	30 μg	≥23	≤18
Tilmicosin, Bovine (respiratory disease)	15 μg	≥14	≤10
Tilmicosin, Swine (respiratory disease)	15 μg	≥11	≤10
Trimethoprim-sulfamethoxazole*¶, Enterobacteriaceae, and Staphylococci	1.25/23.75 μg	≥16	≤10
Tulathromycin, Bovine (respiratory disease)	30 μg	≥18	≤14

Modified from Clinical Laboratory Standards Institute (CLSI) document M31-A3, Table 2, pp. 65-72, 2008. Inclusion of drugs in this table does not constitute a therapeutic recommendation. Numbers in this table are provided for educational purposes only. Serious consequences can arise from inappropriate use of antimicrobial agents. Breakpoints are continually updated by the CLSI Subcommittee on Veterinary Antimicrobial Susceptibility Testing. Veterinary technicians and veterinarians are strongly cautioned that inappropriate susceptibility testing can lead to increased therapeutic failure. Current CLSI guidelines should be consulted before any testing of patient samples is conducted. There are regulatory concerns regarding use of antimicrobial use in food animals. Presentation of interpretive criteria here is for educational use and does not represent a therapeutic recommendation.
*Breakpoints have not been validated for veterinary species.
†Ampicillin is used to test for susceptibility to amoxicillin.
‡Cephalothin is used to test for susceptibility to all first-generation cephalosporins, such as cephapirin and cefadroxil. Cefazolin should be tested separately with the Gram-negative enteric organisms.
§Cefovecin breakpoints are provided by manufacturer.
¶Oxacillin is used to test for susceptibility to methicillin. Caution should be used in interpretation of this test. An additional secondary method, such as polymerase chain reaction (PCR), should be used for confirmation.
#Tetracycline is used to test for susceptibility to chlortetracycline, oxytetracycline, and doxycycline.
¶Trimethoprim/sulfamethoxazole is used to test for susceptibility to trimethoprim/sulfadiazine.

> **TECHNICIAN NOTE** Several methods are available for determining whether bacteria are susceptible or resistant to antimicrobial drugs. Broth dilution (microbroth dilution) is used to determine the minimum inhibitory concentration (MIC) of various antimicrobials. **Disc diffusion** (Kirby-Bauer Method) is used to determine susceptibility based on **zones of inhibition**.

Breakpoints

The CLSI M31-A3 document establishes breakpoints for each organism and each drug. A breakpoint is the number—either MIC or diameter of the zone of inhibition—at which an organism should be called *susceptible* or *resistant* to a drug. These breakpoints are determined from clinical studies of organisms in specific disease conditions (e.g., respiratory disease in cattle). In cases where there are no veterinary breakpoints, breakpoints determined for humans are used. For some organisms, no breakpoint has been determined.

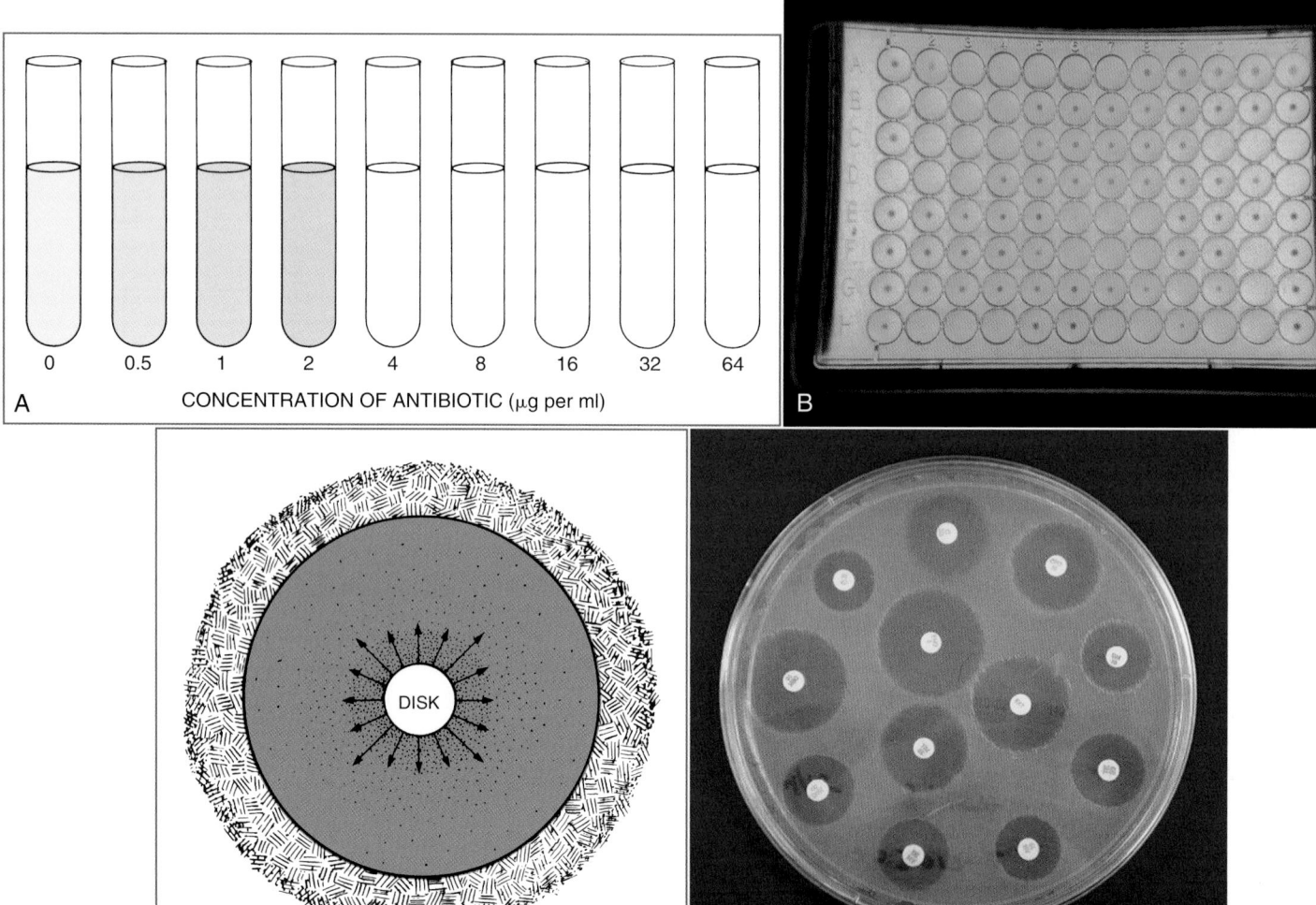

FIGURE 15-16 Antimicrobial susceptibility testing. **A,** Broth dilution susceptibility test. The organism grew in broth containing antibiotic in the amounts of 0.5, 1, and 2 μg/ml, but growth was inhibited in the tube containing 4 μg/ml. Therefore, the minimum inhibitory concentration is 4 μg/ml. **B,** Picture of broth dilution test results using a 96-well plate format; wells A1 through 7 contain a 2-fold dilution series consisting of 0.25, 0.5, 1, 2, 4, 8, and 16 μg/ml of ampicillin. Growth was noted in wells 1 and 2, but not in well 3, so the minimum inhibitory concentration is 1 μg/ml. **C,** As antibiotic diffuses from the disc, the concentration of antibiotic is highest near the disc and is logarithmically diluted as it diffuses radially into a larger area. At some point, the antibiotic is diluted below the minimal inhibitory concentration for the test organism; this allows the organism to grow. **D,** Resulting zones of inhibition are measured and interpreted with the use of Table 15-8.

QUALITY CONTROL TESTING AND QUALITY ASSURANCE

One of the most important aspects of laboratory testing is ensuring that tests are accurately performed. This requires periodic testing of known organisms or samples followed by comparison with standard results. It also involves ensuring that laboratory equipment is functioning accurately. Equipment should be tested and test results should be recorded and maintained, so that when a problem arises with a test, it is possible to identify the source of the problem. Simple things like keeping a thermometer in an incubator and recording the temperature each day can help prevent erroneous test results from affecting patient care.

FUNGAL CULTURE (MYCOLOGY)

SAFETY

It is best to perform fungal cultures in a biological safety cabinet to protect workers who are handling samples and cultures. The only fungal cultures likely to be performed in a veterinary practice are **dermatophyte** cultures. Even when a culture is performed, it is common for the veterinarian to ship the inoculated media to a diagnostic laboratory for identification of any fungi that have grown, to minimize the risk of handling these agents in the practice. Of particular concern would be handling dimorphic fungi such as *Coccidioides immitis*, *Histoplasma capsulatum*, and *Blastomyces dermatididis*. These fungi are highly infectious. They occur as **yeasts** in the veterinary patient, but the more infectious mycelial or hyphal form of the fungus grows at room temperature. Samples from patients suspected of having these infections should be submitted to a diagnostic laboratory with the risk clearly stated on the submission form, so that appropriate precautions are taken in handling the sample. Culture of these agents should not be performed in the veterinary practice.

STANDARD DERMATOPHYTE CULTURE

Specimen Collection and Media Inoculation

Dermatophytes are fungi that invade hair, nails, and superficial layers of the skin. The patient is sometimes examined with a Wood's lamp because some dermatophytes (usually less than 50%) will fluoresce when exposed to long-wavelength ultraviolet light.

To culture dermatophytes, hair should be gently plucked or collected by brushing the lesion or the patient's hair coat with a new toothbrush. Nails can be collected using nail clippers. Gently push plucked hairs or nails into the surface of the agar. Inoculate a dermatophyte test medium (DTM) and Sabouraud dextrose agar.

> **TECHNICIAN NOTE** To culture dermatophytes, hair should be gently plucked or collected by brushing the lesion or the patient's hair coat with a new toothbrush. Nails can be collected using nail clippers. Gently push plucked hairs or nails into the surface of the dermatophyte test medium (DTM) and Sabouraud dextrose agar.

These media are commercially available in a variety of forms. A popular system involves a plate containing both media. This plate should be labeled with patient information and the date collected. The plate should then be contained in a loosely sealed plastic bag and incubated at room temperature for up to 3 weeks. DTM agar contains phenol red, which turns the media red as dermatophytes grow. The red color may be observed as early as 3 to 5 days after inoculation. Dermatophytes are not the only organisms that will alter the color of the media, so microscopic examination is required to identify the organism involved. The Sabouraud dextrose agar is also inoculated because dermatophytes that are inhibited from sporulating on the DTM agar will sometimes sporulate on this medium. Most dermatophyte colonies will be white to yellowish tan (Figure 15-17). Darkly pigmented colonies are likely to be contaminants.

MICROSCOPIC EXAMINATION OF DERMATOPHYTE CULTURES

Place a thin line of lactophenol aniline blue on a clean glass slide. Tear off a piece of clear adhesive tape; press the tape onto the surface of the colony, and pull it away. Gently place the tape over the line of stain, and observe under high dry (40×) magnification. Discard slides in an antifungal disinfectant. Identify the organism by comparing the conidia with pictures in a reference manual. (See "Recommended Reading List.")

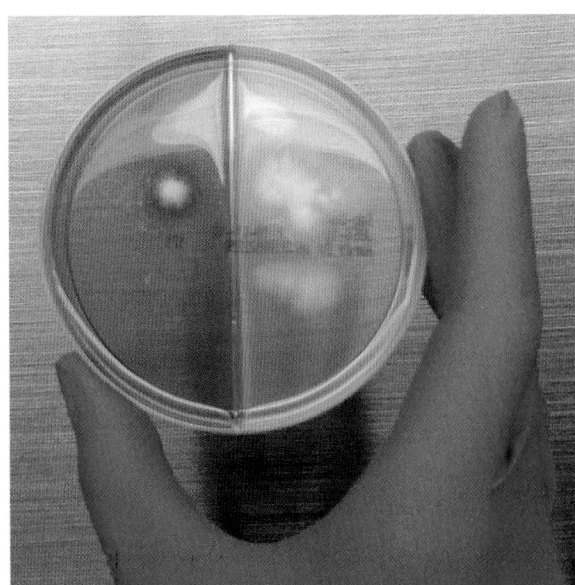

FIGURE 15-17 *Microsporum canis* growing on dermatophyte test medium (orange medium) and Sabouraud dextrose medium (tan).

MICROSCOPIC APPEARANCE OF YEASTS

Yeast can be easily observed in patient samples. In most cases, yeasts will be identified during cytologic examination of an exudate from a patient sample. The most important yeasts identified are listed below. Again, the dimorphic fungi should be cultured only in a reference laboratory with appropriate safety equipment and protocols.

Malassezia pachydermatis

Malassezia pachydermatis is frequently found in patients with otitis externa, but it can also be seen in dermatitis, particularly in patients with underlying diseases that may cause immunosuppression such as diabetes mellitus or hypothyroidism. This organism is readily observed in Diff-Quik–stained slides prepared from swabs of the external ear. The organism is often described as looking like a "footprint" or a "snowman" (Figure 15-18, *A*) and can be identified by cytologic examination; culture is not required.

Candida albicans

Candida albicans is an opportunistic fungal organism associated with vaginitis in people and present in a variety of veterinary clinical specimens, including samples from the avian respiratory and gastrointestinal tracts, canine and feline skin, and the equine reproductive tract. Cytologic examination of this organism reveals a single-celled, ovoid organism approximately 4 to 6 µm in size that may be budding (Figure 15-18, *B*). The yeast will stain positive with Gram stain. Definitive identification of this organism requires culture, which can readily be performed by inoculating Sabouraud dextrose agar and incubating it at room temperature or at 37°C.

Coccidioides immitis

Coccidioides immitis is a dimorphic fungus typically found in the San Joaquin valley in California. The related *Coccidioides posadasii* is found throughout the desert southwestern United States. Both organisms cause respiratory lesions, draining tracts, and osteomyelitis in dogs and horses, as well as in other animals. In the mammalian host, the reproductive form or arthroconidium enlarges and forms a spherule (20 to 100 µm in diameter), which can be visualized in cytologic specimens (Figure 15-18, *C*).

Cryptococcus neoformans

Cryptococcus neoformans is identified by the abundant capsular material surrounding a yeast cell approximately 2 to 20 µm in diameter. India ink is often used to stain impression smears of lesions taken from animals suspected of having this infection (e.g., cats with rhinitis) (Figure 15-18, *D*). Identification can be confirmed by culture on Sabouraud dextrose agar, but this is best left to a reference laboratory.

Histoplasma capsulatum

Histoplasma capsulatum is a dimorphic fungus that is diagnosed by visualization of the yeast in tissues or fluids from exudative lesions (Figure 15-18, *E*). The yeast may be found in circulating leukocytes or urine sediment.

Blastomyces dermatididis

Blastomyces dermatididis is a dimorphic fungus presumptively diagnosed by cytologic examination of prepared patient specimens. The presence of broadly budding yeast measuring approximately 5 to 20 µm is indicative of infection (Figure 15-18, *F*). In dogs, this infection is multisystemic and clinical signs may include dyspnea and cutaneous lesions such as draining tracts, anorexia, and lameness with osteomyelitis.

Sporothrix schenckii

Sporothrix schenckii is a dimorphic fungus that grows on decaying plant material and causes cutaneous and disseminated lesions in cats and people; it can be zoonotic. In cats, cutaneous lesions are more common, although these can become disseminated infections. Sporotrichosis in cats is typically diagnosed by cytologic evaluation of impression smears made from exudates from ulcerated lesions or from aspirates of abscesses or nodules.

> **TECHNICIAN NOTE**   *Malassezia pachydermatis* is frequently found in patients with otitis externa. This organism is readily observed in Diff-Quik–stained slides prepared from swabs of the external ear. The organism is often described as looking like a "footprint" or a "snowman."

VIROLOGY

VIRAL DETECTION

Several methods may be used to detect viruses in patient samples. Antibody-based tests that detect viral antigen and molecular methods that detect viral nucleic acid are the most commonly used diagnostic methods in veterinary practice. In most in-house laboratories, virus detection is limited to antibody-based tests such as the enzyme-linked immunosorbent assay (ELISA), which do not require specialized equipment to perform or interpret the test. In diagnostic laboratories, viruses may be detected by a variety of techniques, including ELISA, virus isolation, demonstration of viral particles by electron microscopy, immuohistochemical staining of histopathologic samples, and molecular tests.

Antibody-Based Tests

ELISAs can be used for detection of antibodies or antigens. To detect a virus, an antibody specific for a viral protein or viral antigen (known as a *primary antibody* or a *capture antibody*) is bound to a solid carrier such as plastic (e.g., a plastic well in a 96-well plate) or a cellulose or nylon membrane. Because a solid carrier is used, these tests are sometimes called *solid phase immunoassays*. The patient sample (e.g., blood, serum, feces) is incubated on the membrane or in the well, allowing the primary antibody to bind with the

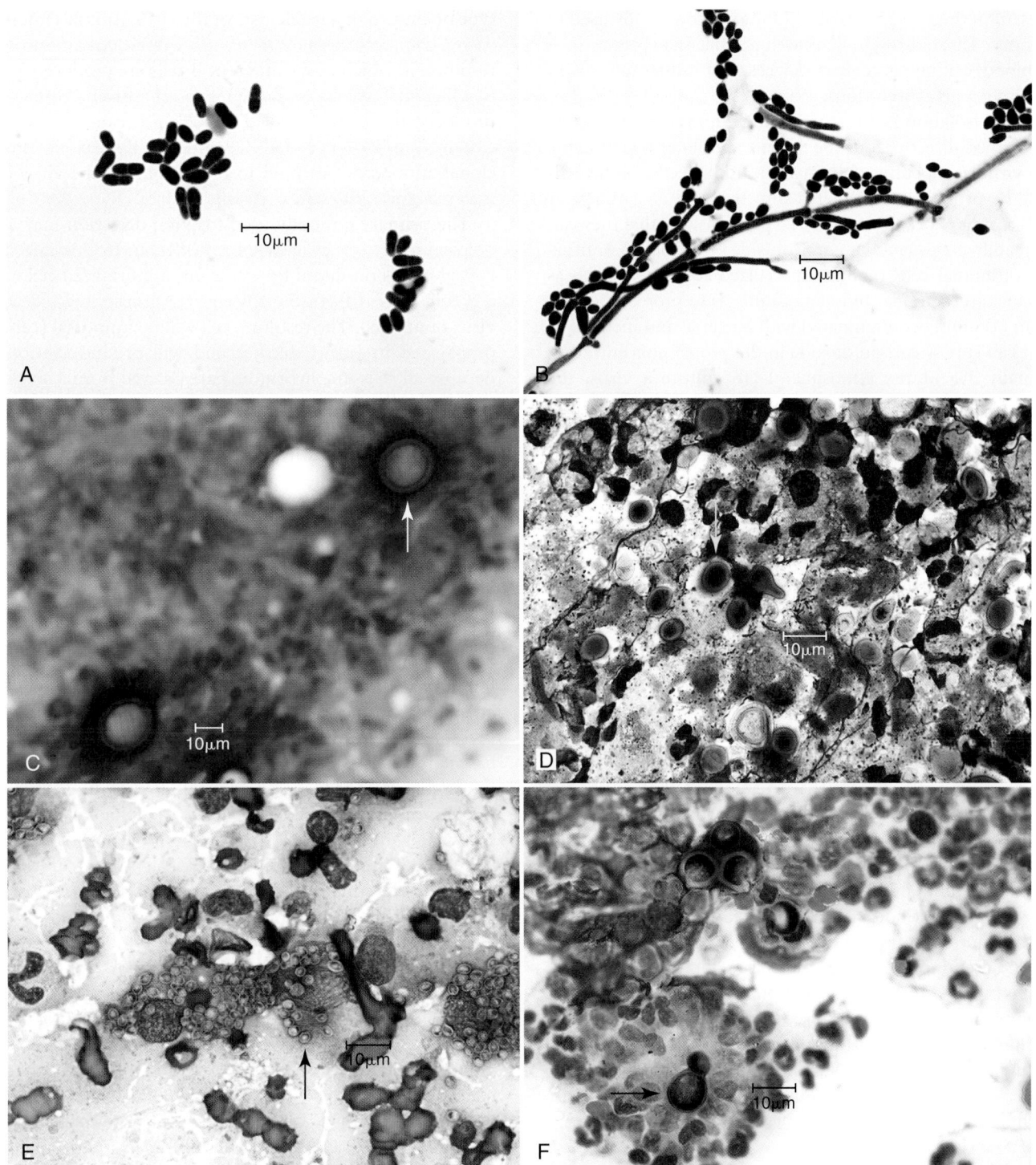

FIGURE 15-18 Cytologic pictures of yeasts in patient specimens stained with Wright's-based stain. **A,** *Malassezia pachydermatis.* Note the characteristic "footprint" or "snowman" shape. **B,** *Candida albicans.* Note the single-celled, ovoid organism measuring approximately 4 to 6 μm that may be budding. **C,** *Coccidioides* spp. Note the spherule (20 to 100 μm in diameter). **D,** *Cryptococcus neoformans* (2 to 20 μm in size). **E,** *Histoplasma capsulatum.* **F,** *Blastomyces dermatididis.* (Photos generously provided courtesy Dr. Gwendolyn Levine.)

viral antigen present in the patient sample. The membrane or well is washed, and then a labeled secondary antibody also specific for the viral antigen is added to the well or membrane and is incubated for a time to allow binding. The secondary antibody is usually labeled with an enzyme such as horseradish peroxidase. The well or membrane again is washed, and substrate for the enzyme is added. The enzyme acts on the substrate, producing a visible color change. The amount of enzyme activity (reflected by the intensity of the color change) is directly related to the amount of virus present in the patient sample. ELISAs are commonly used in in-house laboratories to detect feline leukemia virus antigen in blood, canine parvovirus in feces, and influenza virus in respiratory tract secretions.

Virus isolation from tissue or body fluid samples may be performed directly from the patient sample or by culturing the virus using cultured human or animal cells. These cells may be primary cells isolated directly from an animal, or cells that have been immortalized previously so that they can be readily propagated *in vitro* (outside of the body). Culturing of animal cells requires specialized equipment such as tissue culture hoods (biosafety cabinets) to protect the cells from becoming contaminated with bacteria, and incubators that can supply carbon dioxide in the proper concentration (usually 5% of the atmosphere). To culture a virus, the patient sample is usually passed through a filter that will remove bacteria but not viruses (often a filter with pores that are 0.2 μm in diameter). The sample is then inoculated onto cultured cells and is incubated for a few days. After incubation, changes in the cells are noted.

Electron microscopy is used to examine infected cultured cells or patient samples for the presence of viruses. These samples may be filtered or tested directly. The sample is stained with a heavy metal and sprayed onto a grid (small metal disc). The grid with the sample is placed in the electron microscope and is examined for the presence of viruses. The viral family can often be identified by the virus structure.

Immunohistochemical staining is similar to ELISA in that both rely on the use of antibodies that bind only the virus in question with subsequent detection of that antibody-antigen complex either directly or indirectly through the use of another antibody. The antiviral antibodies used in diagnostic tests are typically called *primary* antibodies because they are the antibodies that directly bind the virus or antigen. The primary antibody is then detected using a labeled secondary antibody that binds to the primary antibody. The secondary antibody usually binds a region of the antibody that is highly similar or is "evolutionarily conserved" between individuals of an animal species. In immunohistochemical staining, the secondary antibody can be labeled with a compound that is detected with a fluorescent microscope, or with an enzyme or dye that will precipitate and will be visible with light microscopy.

> **TECHNICIAN NOTE** Direct and indirect viral detection is commonly performed in practices using solid phase enzyme-linked immunosorbent assay (ELISA) tests such as the SNAP test. These tests are simple to use and are generally sensitive and specific.

The primary antibody used for virus detection can be derived by injecting animals with the virus or antigen and then purifying resulting antibodies from the serum of the animal. Antibody that is generated by a single B lymphocyte (B cell) or its progeny (called *clones*) will recognize a single type of antigen or a single part of the virus. Animals injected with a complete virus or bacterium will mount an immune response in which many different B cells are produced, each of which may recognize a different viral antigen. Antibodies produced this way are called *polyclonal* because the serum contains antibodies produced by multiple B cell clones. Polyclonal antibodies can bind to or "recognize" the virus but may recognize different parts of the virus.

The primary antibody used for viral detection may also be produced from cells called *hybridomas*. In this case, the hybridoma is produced by fusing an immortalized cell with a B cell derived from the spleen of a mouse injected with virus or antigen. The resulting cell will be immortal (can be propagated in tissue culture) and will produce antibody. Because all cells in a hybridoma are derived from a single B cell, antibodies produced by a hybridoma recognize a single antigen and are called *monoclonal*. **Monoclonal antibodies** are preferred because it is possible to identify the specific antigen that they detect, and cross-reactivity with nonviral proteins can be reduced or eliminated.

MOLECULAR DETECTION OF PATHOGENS

In general, bacterial and eukaryotic genetic material comprises two linear strands of deoxyribonucleic acid (DNA) held together by hydrogen bonds. Each strand consists of four nucleotide bases: adenine, thymine, cytosine, and guanine. Adenine and guanine are purines; cytosine and thymine are pyrimidines. The nucleotides form base pairs. A base pair consists of two nucleotides—one on each strand of the double-stranded DNA, held together by hydrogen bonds. In Watson-Crick DNA base pairing, adenine (A) forms a base pair with thymine (T), and guanine (G) forms a base pair with cytosine (C). In ribonucleic acid (RNA), uracil (U) substitutes for thymine. A short segment of DNA is often called an *oligonucleotide* or an "oligo."

POLYMERASE CHAIN REACTION (PCR)

The **polymerase chain reaction** (PCR) allows rapid, exact duplication of short pieces of DNA (generally between 100 and 2000 base pairs in length, copied multiple times within 3 hours) (Figure 15-19). In a PCR reaction, DNA from the patient sample or bacteria (DNA template) is mixed with two different short oligonucleotide primers (17 to 25 nucleotides in length). Sample DNA is called a DNA template to distinguish it from the DNA product of the PCR reaction, which is called PCR product. One primer binds specifically to one DNA strand, and the other primer binds specifically to the other DNA strand. In addition to the DNA template and the primers, DNA polymerase, reaction buffer, and magnesium chloride are mixed within the PCR tube. This tube is then placed in a special piece of equipment, called a *thermocycler*. The thermocycler is essentially a metal block that is heated and cooled repeatedly under the control of a microchip processor. In the first step of PCR, the hydrogen bonds holding the two strands of the DNA template together are broken by heating the DNA to about 94°C. This is called

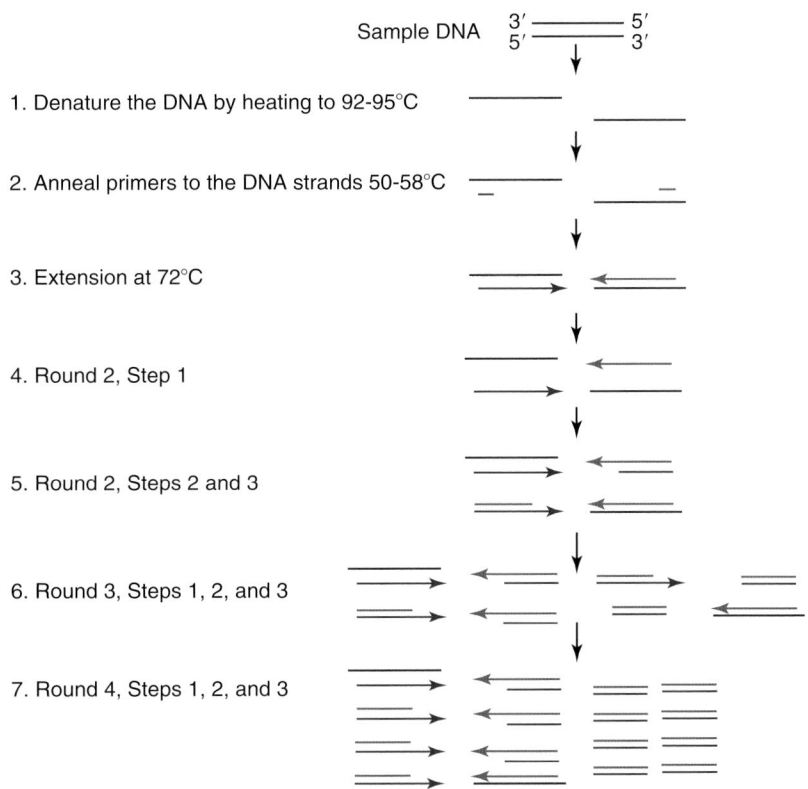

Sample DNA

1. Denature the DNA by heating to 92-95°C

2. Anneal primers to the DNA strands 50-58°C

3. Extension at 72°C

4. Round 2, Step 1

5. Round 2, Steps 2 and 3

6. Round 3, Steps 1, 2, and 3

7. Round 4, Steps 1, 2, and 3

FIGURE 15-19 Depiction of polymerase chain reaction (PCR) process and products. PCR consists of making multiple copies of a DNA template by using a three-step process. This process is commonly called *amplifying* DNA, because it can be used to detect a small amount of DNA by making more copies. These DNA copies are called *PCR products*. In this graphic depiction of the three-step process, original sample (template) DNA is shown in blue, and primers and PCR products are shown in pink and green. PCR reactions are typically run as 35 to 45 cycles with three repeating steps that consist of denaturing the template DNA at 94°C, annealing (binding) the primers at a lower temperature (50°C to 58°C), and extending the PCR product at 72°C.

denaturing the template DNA. The reaction is then cooled to a lower temperature, called the *annealing temperature*. At this temperature, the primers can bind to the DNA template. The temperature is then raised to 72°C, and the DNA product is extended by the DNA polymerase. This increase in temperature helps to ensure that the replicated DNA is copied exactly, that is, the higher temperature helps to prevent the occurrence of DNA base pair mismatches. After this extension step, the whole process of denaturing, annealing, and extension is repeated approximately 40 times (40 cycles). As the steps are repeated, the DNA is copied exponentially (amplified). The resultant PCR product may be detected during "real time," while the DNA is amplified, or after all PCR cycle steps are complete.

PCR has revolutionized pathogen detection and phylogenetic analysis. Many of the techniques discussed here use PCR as their foundation. With the advent of PCR, it is no longer necessary to actually grow a bacterium or virus in culture to obtain sequence information. This has a variety of practical consequences. PCR can be used to identify obligate intracellular bacteria or viruses (such as *Ehrlichia canis*, or *Rickettsia rickettsii*) that cannot be cultured using standard methods. PCR can also be used to rapidly detect slow-growing organisms like *Mycobacterium avium* subsp. *paratuberculosis*. PCR makes it possible to perform diagnostic

tests without the need to maintain viral or bacterial stock. Instead, DNA from a pathogen or a fragment of DNA from a pathogen (such as a PCR product) can be used as the control for a molecular test, thereby making it possible for a greater number of diagnostic laboratories to test for foreign animal diseases without maintaining hazardous bacteria and viruses. In the event of a foreign animal disease outbreak, this capability should increase the speed at which the outbreak can be identified and stopped.

TECHNICIAN NOTE DNA testing is a valuable tool for detection of obligate intracellular organisms, viruses, and difficult to culture bacteria. PCR-based tests provide rapid results and are highly sensitive. It is important to remember that it is not possible to distinguish between live and dead organisms. Also, some body fluids contain inhibitors of PCR, which can lead to false-negative results.

DNA SEQUENCING

In addition to PCR, **DNA sequencing** can be used to identify pathogens. Although it is not performed in most veterinary practices, sequencing may be used to rapidly identify bacteria, fungi, and viruses. Sequencing is still an expensive test and is not yet routinely performed, but it provides a way to definitively identify most organisms. For most bacterial organisms, the 16S ribosomal DNA (rDNA) is the segment of the genome that is sequenced because this gene is evolutionarily highly conserved (very similar) among bacterial species but is usually different enough to allow identification of a specific species. Within some genera of bacteria, it is necessary to sequence different genes because the 16S rDNA is highly conserved with little variation between species. Within fungal organisms, the D1-D2 spacer region of the ribosomal DNA is used as the target that is sequenced. With viral agents, it is necessary to know whether the viral nucleic acid is DNA or RNA. When the nucleic acid is RNA, additional procedures are needed to isolate and convert the RNA to complementary DNA, or cDNA, so that the target can be sequenced.

TECHNICIAN NOTE Not all bacteria can be differentiated using 16S rDNA, and other gene targets may be necessary to differentiate between species in which the 16S rDNA is highly conserved.

New methods of sequencing are changing the ways that complex populations of bacteria such as those found in the gastrointestinal and respiratory tracts, and in the soil, are evaluated. It is now possible to identify the families of bacteria present in these complex samples by sequencing. This is called determining the *microbiome* of a sample. As this technology improves and matures, it will undoubtedly be applied to patient samples.

TECHNICIAN NOTE Because sequencing does not require viable bacteria, DNA from isolates needing further identification can be submitted instead of bacteria. DNA does not have the same shipping regulations as bacterial isolates, thus it can be easier to submit.

NOSOCOMIAL INFECTIONS

Nosocomial infections are infections that hospitalized patients acquire from the hospital environment, another patient, or a health care provider. Clearly these infections are undesirable, and every effort should be made to prevent them. Infections that the patient is incubating at the time of admission but that become apparent while the patient is hospitalized are called *community-acquired*. In addition to patient-to-patient transmission of pathogens, in veterinary practice, organisms can be transmitted from patients to human personnel (zoonotic transmission). These infections can be serious, and precautions must be taken to protect hospital personnel. In addition, clients must be advised if their animal has or contracts a potentially zoonotic organism.

Many factors contribute to pathogen transmission to hospitalized patients. These factors can be related to the patient, the pathogen, or the physical surroundings of the patient, or

to contact with veterinary personnel. Hospitalized patients typically are stressed by their illness or by the fact that they are not in their normal surroundings. Underlying disease conditions such as diabetes mellitus or hypothyroidism and therapies such as chemotherapy can suppress the patient's immune system, making the patient more susceptible to infection. Ironically, antimicrobial therapy can predispose the patient to infection by altering or reducing the normal floras that prevent pathogen colonization.

In some cases, the patient's vaccination status can affect its susceptibility to infection. Dogs that have been vaccinated previously against canine parvovirus and canine distemper are at less risk for contracting these diseases when they are encountered, whereas puppies that have not received vaccines or have not completed the series of inoculations have less protection. It is frequently common practice to require certain vaccinations (e.g., the respiratory pathogen *B. bronchiseptica*) before boarding otherwise healthy animals to prevent transmission of these agents.

Nosocomial transmission can result from both virulent pathogens and opportunistic organisms. Opportunistic infections are often associated with nosocomial transmission because of increased patient susceptibility for the reasons previously noted. Nosocomial agents can also be transmitted on physical items such as food bowls, cage mats, clippers, thermometers, and any other item in close contact with the patient. These and other inanimate objects capable of carrying infectious agents are called *fomites*. It is important to clean and disinfect or sterilize these items to prevent possible transmission of organisms between patients. Additionally, hospitalized patients are housed in close proximity to one another, increasing the opportunity for potential spread of organisms directly from patient to patient. This is particularly true for nosocomial transmission of airborne respiratory pathogens.

Finally, hospital personnel can transmit pathogens between patients, from a fomite to a patient, or occasionally zoonotically. Although it is more common for a person to acquire a zoonotic agent from a patient, a patient can acquire a zoonotic agent from a person. Transmission of a zoonotic agent is usually by direct contact, so handwashing is an important method of reducing pathogen transmission. Wearing gloves is another important way to protect both personnel and patients from spread of agents, but it is important to wash hands or use hand sanitizer every time gloves are removed. It is also important to wear protective clothing and to change lab coats or coveralls after treating patients with infections caused by organisms that are easily spread.

TECHNICIAN NOTE Good hygiene is critical in patient care. Simple acts such as consistent hand hygiene can significantly reduce the risk of transmission of pathogens between patients and between patients and caregivers.

AGENTS OF NOSOCOMIAL INFECTIONS

Bacteria are commonly associated with nosocomial infections, but viruses, fungi, and some parasites can also be transmitted from patient to patient. Bacterial agents that infect the respiratory tract, gastrointestinal tract, and skin are common causes of nosocomial infections. For instance, bacterial pathogens such as *Streptococcus equi* subsp. *equi* (*S. equi*), *Salmonella* spp., *C. perfringens*, and *C. difficile* are frequently implicated. This is due in part to the types of disease that they cause. *S. equi* is a respiratory pathogen of horses, but the other three agents all can cause diarrhea in susceptible patients. Diarrhea readily spreads pathogens across a large surface area. Drug-resistant organisms are frequently transmitted to patients, often through contact with health care providers. The most common of these organisms are methicillin-resistant staphylococci, vancomycin-resistant enterococci, and multidrug-resistant Gram-negative organisms such as *E. coli*, *Salmonella*, *Klebsiella*, *Enterobacter*, and *Pseudomonas*. These agents can colonize a patient and cause disease while the patient is hospitalized or at a later date.

Viruses are the second most likely cause of nosocomial infections. Among the most common viral nosocomial infections are canine distemper, canine parvovirus, feline panleukopenia, equine influenza, and equine herpesvirus. Respiratory viral pathogens are frequently implicated because they are readily transmitted between healthy patients by aerosols.

RECOGNITION AND CONTROL OF NOSOCOMIAL INFECTIONS

The most common indicators of nosocomial infection in a hospital include an increased number of patients with clinical signs specific to the suspected agent and increased isolation of a single agent from multiple patients. Early recognition of possible nosocomial infection is the key to reducing patient morbidity and preventing further spread of the pathogen. Once the technical staff believes that transmission is occurring, the next step is to identify potential or likely sources of the infection (e.g., fomites, inadequate handwashing, faulty sterilization of equipment, patient-to-patient spread) and to intervene. Most commonly, several interventions are implemented simultaneously. Although intervention is important, of even greater importance is having a sound plan for routine disinfection of animal housing areas, equipment, and treatment areas and having a monitoring system in place to ensure that procedures are consistently and correctly followed. For a detailed discussion on specific disinfectants, antiseptics, and sterilization, please see Chapter 30.

> **TECHNICIAN NOTE** Increased numbers of patients with clinical signs specific to the suspected agent and increased isolation of a single agent from multiple patients may be indicators of nosocomial transmission and should be investigated. All practices and potential sources must be thoroughly analyzed.

RECOMMENDED READINGS

Anonymous: Difco and BBL manual, Sparks, MD, 2007, BD Diagnostic Systems.

Clinical and Laboratory Standards Institute (CLSI): Performance standards for antimicrobial disk and dilution susceptibility tests for bacteria isolated from animals, approved standard, ed 3, CLSI document M31-A3, Wayne, PA, 2008, Clinical Laboratory Standards Institute.

Giguère S, Prescott JF, Baggot JD, et al: Antimicrobial therapy in veterinary medicine, ed 4, Ames, IA, 2006, Blackwell Publishing.

Greene CE: Infectious diseases of the dog and cat, ed 4, Philadelphia, 2012, WB Saunders.

Hirsch DC, MacLachlan NJ, Walker R: Veterinary microbiology, ed 2, Ames, IA, 2004, Blackwell Publishing.

Jones R: Clinical microbiology. In McCurnin DM, Bassert JM, editors: McCurnin's clinical textbook for veterinary technicians, ed 7, Philadelphia, 2006, WB Saunders.

Quinn PJ, Carter ME, Markey B, et al: Clinical veterinary microbiology, London, 2006, Mosby.

Sellon D, Long M: Equine infectious diseases, Philadelphia, 2007, WB Saunders.

Songer JG, Post KW: Veterinary microbiology: bacterial and fungal agents of animal disease, Philadelphia, 2004, Saunders Elsevier.

St. Germain G, Summerbell R: Identifying fungi, Belmont, CA, 2010, Star Publishing Company.

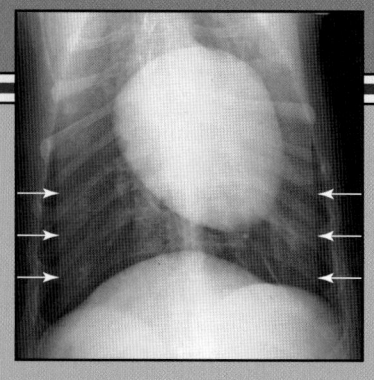

16 Diagnostic Imaging

Lorrie Gaschen

OUTLINE

Radiology, 518
Legal Records and Film
 Identification, 518
Filing of the Radiograph, 519
Production of X-Rays, 519
X-Ray Equipment, 523
Image Quality in Digital
 Radiography, 527
Digital Radiography Artifacts, 527
Exposure Factors, 529
Image Formation With Film-Screen
 Systems, 532
The Darkroom, 537
Radiographic Film Quality, 539
Radiation Safety, 541

Radiographic Contrast Agents, 547
Positioning, 550
Restraint, 550
Ultrasonography, 551
Ultrasonography Basics, 551
Ultrasound-Tissue Interaction, 551
Ultrasound Display Modes, 553
The Ultrasound Image, 554
Ultrasound Artifacts, 554
The Ultrasound Examination, 555
Nuclear Medicine, 556
Alternative Imaging Modalities, 556
Computed Tomography, 557
Magnetic Resonance Imaging, 558

LEARNING OBJECTIVES

When you have completed this chapter, you will be able to:

1. Pronounce, define, and spell all Key Terms in this chapter.
2. List and describe methods for labeling and filing radiographic films.
3. Do the following regarding the production of x-rays:
   - Describe the properties of x-radiation.
   - Describe the parts of the x-ray tube and machine, and discuss the role each part plays in generation of x-radiation.
   - Explain the production of the useful x-ray beam and scatter radiation, and discuss the negative consequences of scatter radiation.
4. Do the following regarding x-ray equipment:
   - Describe the features of and uses for portable, mobile, stationary, and fluoroscopic x-ray equipment.
   - Describe the features, advantages and disadvantages of, and uses for computed radiography and digital radiography equipment.
5. Do the following regarding image quality and exposure factors:
   - Describe common digital radiography artifacts, including how to identify and prevent each one.
   - Define *DICOM, PACS, RIS,* and *teleradiography,* and explain the role of each in the production and management of digital radiographs.
   - Define *milliamperage, exposure time, kilovoltage,* and *focal-film distance,* and explain how each of these exposure factors is set to produce a quality diagnostic radiograph.
   - Explain the purpose for a technique chart, and describe the procedure used to formulate a technique chart.

The authors and publisher wish to acknowledge Beth Paugh Partington for her contributions to previous editions of this textbook.

6. Do the following regarding image formation with film-screen systems:
   - Explain the principles of image formation using nonscreen x-ray film and film-screen cassette-based systems.
   - Describe the structure and characteristics of grids and the Potter-Bucky diaphragm, and explain the roles they play in the production of a diagnostic image.
7. Do the following regarding film processing and radiographic film quality:
   - Discuss the design, features, and organization of an x-ray darkroom.
   - Describe use and maintenance of the equipment used to process x-ray film, including operation of the automatic processor.
   - Define *radiographic detail*, *contrast*, and *density*, and explain how these factors are controlled by changing milliamperage and kilovoltage to optimize image quality.
   - List common technical errors and artifacts, and steps that can be taken to minimize them.
8. Do the following regarding radiation safety:
   - Describe the hazards of x-radiation, and explain the role of beam filtration in minimizing its damaging effects.
   - Discuss the units of measurement used to quantify x-radiation, and the methods used to monitor x-radiation exposure.
   - Define *maximum permissible dose*, and explain the principles and practices used to minimize exposure to x-radiation, including the use of personal protective equipment.
9. Do the following regarding radiographic contrast agents:
   - List commonly used positive and negative radiographic contrast agents, and explain how they are used in the production of a diagnostic contrast study.
   - Describe the contrast procedures used to image the gastrointestinal system, urinary system, and spinal cord.
10. Explain the principles of patient positioning for radiographic studies, including the importance of appropriate restraint.
11. Do the following regarding ultrasonography:
    - Describe the indications for and characteristics of ultrasonography in diagnostic imaging.
    - Describe the basic principles of production of an ultrasound image, including the appearance of various tissues and organs on a finished image.
    - Describe how a patient is prepared for ultrasound imaging, and the procedure used to conduct an ultrasound examination.
    - Discuss the equipment used to produce a B-mode, M-mode, or Doppler ultrasound image.
    - Describe the appearance of an ultrasound image, as well as the appearance and cause of common artifacts.
12. Describe indications for and characteristics of therapeutic and diagnostic nuclear medicine, computed tomography, and magnetic resonance imaging.

INTRODUCTION

Radiology and ultrasonography are the primary diagnostic imaging techniques available to the veterinarian. However, for the veterinarian to arrive at the correct diagnosis on the basis of a radiographic or ultrasound examination, images of high quality must be available. The responsibility to provide useful diagnostic images usually falls to the veterinary technician.

This chapter deals with the basic but essential information needed to produce x-ray films and sonograms of diagnostic quality. It is not the intent of this chapter to offer a course in radiation physics, ultrasound physics, and proper positioning of animals for examination. Excellent textbooks on these subjects have been written and should provide the veterinary technician with the detailed information needed (see Curry et al, 1990; Douglas et al, 1987; Han and Hurd, 2005; Lavin, 2006; Morgan, 1993; and Ticer, 1984). These books should be consulted when the need arises. This chapter discusses the basic information needed to support and assist the veterinary technician in the areas of radiology and diagnostic ultrasonography. A short introduction to the use of nuclear imaging, computed tomography, **digital radiography, computed radiography,** and magnetic resonance imaging is included. Every effort is made to simplify radiation and ultrasound physics.

RADIOLOGY

LEGAL RECORDS AND FILM IDENTIFICATION

Radiographs are part of the legal medical record and should be clearly labeled as to which animal has been examined. Identification should include name of the patient and owner or patient identification number, date of examination, and name of the practice.

> **TECHNICIAN NOTE** Radiographs are part of the legal medical record and must be correctly identified and carefully labeled.

Several methods of film labeling are available. In one method, leaded numbers and letters are placed on the cassette at the time of exposure (Figure 16-1, *A*). These show up as white markings on a finished radiograph. Also available is a special graphite-impregnated tape on which the desired information can be written or typed and placed on the cassette, or the information can be taped on a special filter at the time of exposure (Figure 16-1, *B*). One of the better film identification methods is a light flasher system (Figure 16-2). It is simple and inexpensive. The required information is typed on a card that is placed in the imprinter. This system requires placement of a small, leaded blocker in the upper left-hand corner of the film cassette, which will prevent exposure to that part of the film. The card is placed in the light flasher in the darkroom. The unexposed, left-hand corner of the exposed radiograph is placed underneath the card, and the light is flashed through the card. The information recorded on the card is transferred to the x-ray film and will be processed when the radiograph is developed (Figure 16-3).

One final identification method requires both a film identification camera and special windowed film cassettes.

This method allows an individual to type the required information on a 3 × 5-inch card and to place the card into the ID camera. The windowed corner of the cassette then is automatically opened and "flashed" by the camera, and the information is exposed on the x-ray film. The benefits of this system are that the camera will automatically identify the date and time of the examination; this can be done in daylight, and the area on the film in which the identification information is placed is constant (Figure 16-4).

In digital radiography, the patient information is part of the **DICOM** tag (see page 528 for more information concerning the DICOM tag). The owner's name, animal's name, clinic name, examination date, species, breed, weight, gender, region examined (e.g., thorax or skull), and other pertinent information are introduced into the study using vendor software; this information is ultimately linked to the digital information that forms the radiograph and is visible on each radiograph taken for that patient to make it a part of the permanent record for legal purposes.

In addition to the legal identification imprinted on the film, it is necessary to identify the body part x-rayed at the time of exposure. Leaded right and left markers should be placed on the cassette at the time of exposure to identify the extremity being examined or the side on which the animal is positioned for examination (i.e., right or left lateral recumbency). Additional specialty film markers include Mitchell markers, each of which consists of a plastic bubble containing two to four tiny lead balls that fall toward gravity. These are used primarily in standing radiography of the equine head to assist in identifying fluid levels in paranasal sinuses. Timing markers are used in contrast studies, such as upper gastrointestinal studies and excretory urography, to indicate when the film was obtained in relation to when the **contrast** medium was administered (Figure 16-5). Front leg versus hindleg and medial versus lateral side identification markers are critical for proper interpretation of equine lower extremity radiographs.

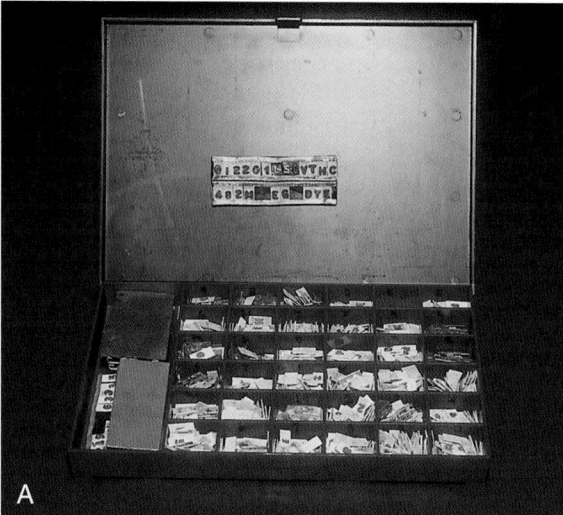
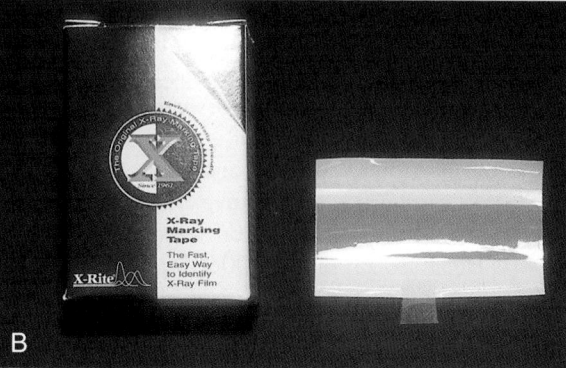

FIGURE 16-1 Film labeling. **A,** Leaded letters and numbers placed on the cassette at the time of exposure. **B,** Radiographic label tape.

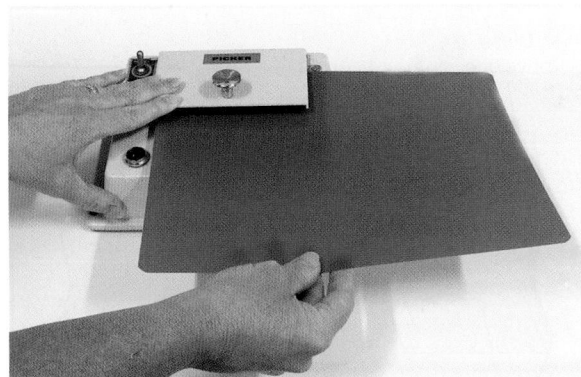

FIGURE 16-2 Light flasher. Patient information is printed onto a radiograph with an identification printer.

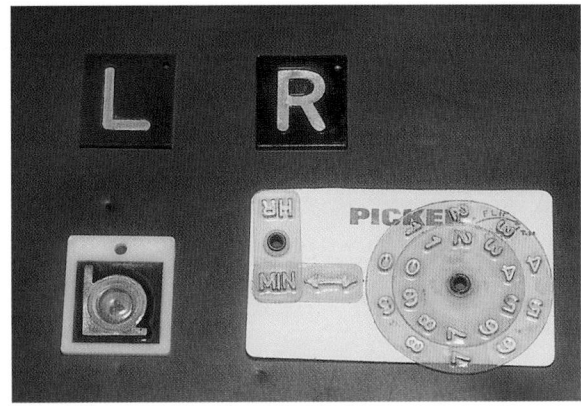

FIGURE 16-5 Leaded letters for film labeling. Left and right markers are used to label extremities and the side of recumbency. The Mitchell marker *(lower left)* is used to identify gravitational direction, and the timer marker *(lower right)* is used with contrast studies to identify the length of time since contrast medium administration.

Louisiana State University		
Veterinary Teaching Hospital & Clinics		
No. 46478	Date 3/20/97	
DOB 9/24/84	Owner Partington	
Spec. Feline	Sex F/S	Breed Somali
Animal's Name Emmy		
Baton Rouge, Louisiana		

FIGURE 16-3 Film identification as it appears on a radiograph. The identification is flashed onto the film after x-ray exposure with a light flasher system or a film identification camera.

FILING OF THE RADIOGRAPH

Because a radiograph is part of the medical record, one must be able to retrieve it when needed. The radiographs from each examination should be placed in an x-ray envelope and filed according to the filing system used for other hospital records (i.e., by last name or case number). The following information should be recorded on the envelope: owner's address, animal identification, date, and type of examination. In addition, the radiographic technique used for the examination can be recorded on the envelope to provide an easy reference for follow-up studies. Many veterinary practice software programs have radiograph and film folder labels automatically available for printing when the patient information is entered. These film labels are convenient, but because they are printed and added to the radiograph after it is exposed and developed, use of this system increases the risk for radiograph misidentification.

It would be most advantageous to the veterinarian if the envelope could be coded for use as a self-teaching file. Several color tape systems have been devised to code cases for specific purposes. The system chosen could be refined to include a combination of colors to identify species, breed, system examined, and so on. Morgan (1993) outlined an excellent color-coded system for x-ray retrieval purposes.

PRODUCTION OF X-RAYS

Basic Principles

A basic understanding of x-ray production, radiologic image formation, interactions of radiation with tissue, and radiation protection is essential. For those with little knowledge of physics or mathematics, the idea of having to learn basic radiation physics may seem like a large undertaking. However, the aim is not to teach radiation physics but rather to present basic concepts that are useful for those who use x-ray equipment. **X-rays** can be defined as nonluminous electromagnetic radiation that is similar to visible light and to radio and television signals but of much shorter wavelengths. The shorter the wavelengths, the greater is the energy

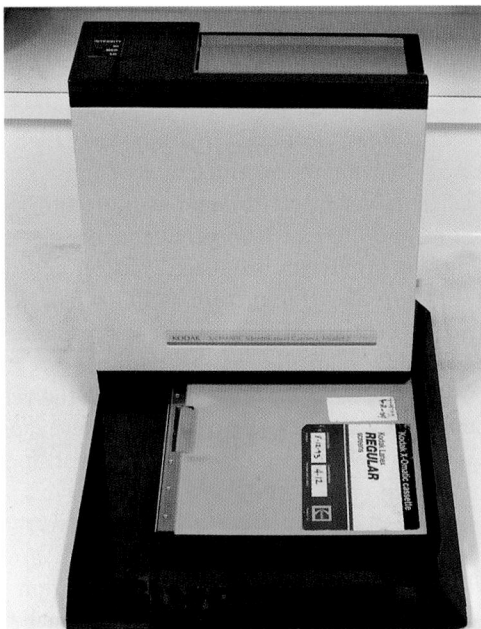

FIGURE 16-4 Film identification camera and special windowed x-ray cassette. Patient information is typed onto a 3 × 5-inch card and is inserted into the top of the camera. The special cassette slides into the camera, which opens the window and flashes the identification onto the film.

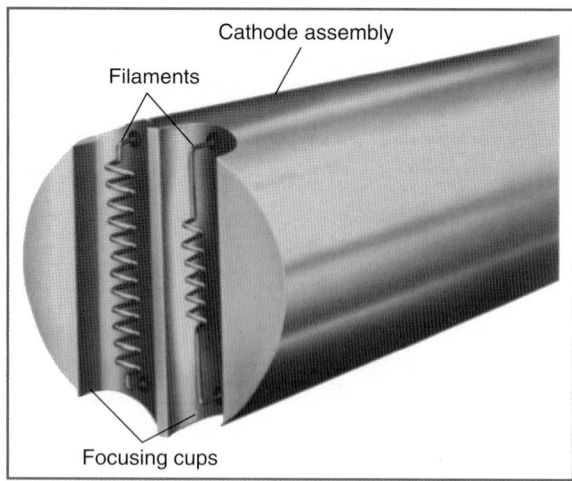

FIGURE 16-6 Cathode assembly showing focusing cups and filaments of two different sizes. Their arrangements produce electron beams that are focused onto narrow rectangles on the target. The smaller filament produces an electron stream of a smaller cross-sectional area and therefore a smaller focal spot. (From Eastman Kodak Company: The fundamentals of radiography, ed 12, Rochester, NY, 1980, Eastman Kodak, Radiographic Markets Division.)

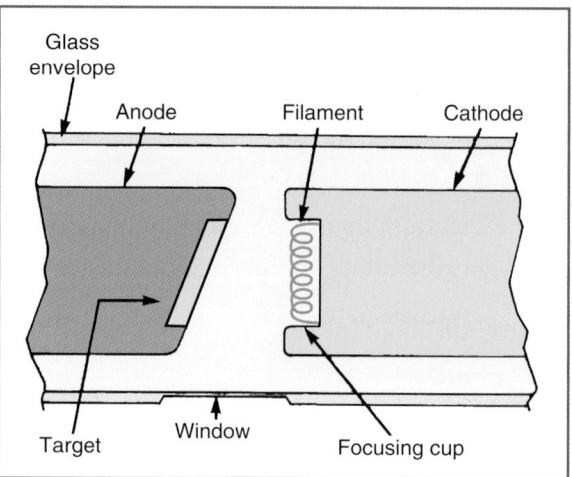

FIGURE 16-7 Stationary-anode x-ray tube. Diagram shows the relationship of the anode to the cathode. (From Eastman Kodak Company: The fundamentals of radiography, ed 12, Rochester, NY, 1980, Eastman Kodak, Radiographic Markets Division.)

of the x-ray beam. The greater the energy of the x-ray beam, the greater is its penetration.

X-rays are capable of penetrating tissues through which they pass and affecting x-ray detectors and fluorescent screens. Because of these characteristics, x-rays are widely used in medicine for the study, diagnosis, and treatment of certain disorders, especially those of internal structures of the body.

Unfortunately, because of their short wavelengths, x-rays are not visible. As a consequence, many veterinarians, physicians, x-ray technologists, and veterinary technicians tend to become careless in their day-to-day use of x-rays by neglecting to use protective equipment or to apply basic radiation safety rules.

The X-Ray Tube
Filament and Focusing Cup
The source of x-rays used in diagnostic radiology is the x-ray tube. Generators and transformers are used in radiology only for the purpose of providing and controlling the amount of electricity reaching the x-ray tube. The x-ray tube is composed of a positively charged **anode** (+) and a negatively charged **cathode** (−) enclosed in a vacuum within a glass envelope surrounded by lead housing. The cathode contains one or two coiled wire filaments within hollowed-out wells or focusing cups. The filaments provide a source for electrons (e−) that are used to produce x-rays (Figure 16-6). The filament is heated to a critical temperature, and the electrons are boiled off and form an electron cloud within the focusing cup. The electrons then are accelerated rapidly toward the positively charged anode. The collision of the speeding electrons into the anode results in the production of heat and x-rays. The oncoming electrons eject orbital electrons from the atoms of the anode, and the release of energy resulting from this interaction takes the form of

x-rays. X-rays are directed downward or vertically through the window of the tube by the angle of the anode and the lead shielding of the x-ray tube (Figure 16-7). Two electrical circuits are present in every x-ray tube: a high-voltage, or **kilovoltage**, circuit and a low-voltage, or **milliamperage**, circuit. The kilovoltage circuit controls the electrical potential between the anode and the cathode. This controls the speed of electron acceleration and the energy level or penetrability of the resulting x-ray beam. Thus the energy of the x-ray beam is a function of the energy of the electrons striking the anode. The milliamperage circuit controls the electrical potential across the filament and affects the volume of electrons created, and thus the number or volume of x-rays created. The filament must produce electrons without melting. Toward this effect, an alloy of tungsten is used because it is less brittle and more efficient than pure tungsten for the production of electrons. This alloy has a high melting point and is used for the manufacture of most x-ray tube filaments. The larger filament contains more tungsten than the small one and therefore can produce more electrons. As a result, the electron beam produced is larger and does not produce as sharp an x-ray picture as the smaller filament. Unfortunately, because of its size, the small filament may melt more rapidly than the larger one, if an excess load is placed on it. As a result, the veterinarian and the veterinary technician must always be aware of the limits and capabilities of the equipment when selecting which filament (focal spot) to use for a given procedure.

Focal Spot
The smaller filament provides a small target region or focal spot for electrons at the anode. In general, the small filament is used to obtain images of higher quality. However, because of the limited number of electrons provided by a small filament, its use is generally restricted to the lower mAs (milliamperage × time in seconds) settings used primarily in tabletop (nongrid) extremity radiography. When higher tube

current and shorter exposure time are desired, the larger filament must be used, although loss of detail will result from the larger focal spot.

The size of the focal spot is determined by the size of the electron beam that is accelerated within the tube when high-voltage potentials are applied between the anode and the cathode. Thus electrons traveling at an extremely high speed in the vacuum tube are suddenly stopped on the "target" area of the anode. As has been mentioned, the anode target is usually composed of an alloy of tungsten. Tungsten is used because it has the following special properties as a target material:

- High atomic number for efficient production of x-rays
- High melting point to withstand the large amount of heat generated by the electron beam
- High capacity to transfer heat from the area in which electrons are absorbed
- High **density** to absorb the electron beam in a small surface area
- Low vapor pressure to maintain the vacuum inside the x-ray tube
- Relatively easy machinability into the appropriate shape at a reasonable cost

Stationary Anode

In early x-ray equipment, **stationary anodes** were used in most x-ray tubes. This type of x-ray tube is still prevalent in some veterinary practices in which older equipment is used, in dental equipment, and in small portable units used extensively in large animal extremity radiology.

In x-ray tubes with stationary anodes, the target area is a small tungsten block about 3.18 mm thick embedded in a large block of copper. The copper is used to absorb and diffuse the tremendous amount of heat generated by the interaction of the electron beam with the target areas. This type of tube is popular and effective in radiography of the extremities of horses and dogs. However, it has limited application for the abdomen and thorax because the stationary anode x-ray tube cannot produce a sufficiently powerful x-ray beam to penetrate thicker body parts. It is also limited in its ability to produce short x-ray exposure of sufficient strength for chest radiography to eliminate respiratory motion artifact (see Figure 16-7).

Rotating Anode

Rotating anodes became popular with the advent of more powerful x-ray machines and the requirement for radiologists to obtain x-ray images of higher quality. Rotating anode tubes can use much higher tube currents, shorter exposure times, and focal spots as small as 0.1 mm, because the electrons deposit their energy over a larger target region as the anode rotates (Figure 16-8).

The target of a rotating anode is a tungsten alloy bonded to molybdenum or graphite to help diffuse the tremendous heat generated by a high-powered x-ray machine. Rotating anodes are 7.5 to 12.5 cm in diameter. These tubes must dissipate enormous amounts of heat. The apparatus used to

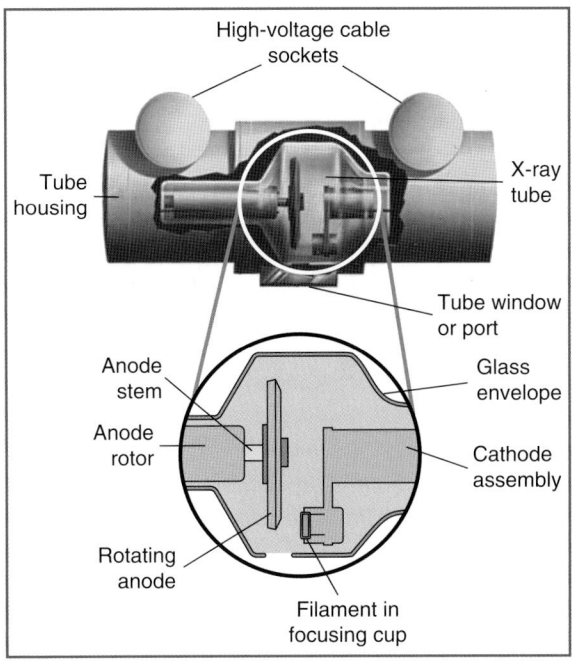

FIGURE 16-8 Modern rotating-anode radiographic tube. Exploded schematic view demonstrates the relationship of the filament to the rotating target. (From Eastman Kodak Company: The fundamentals of radiography, ed 12, Rochester, NY, 1980, Eastman Kodak, Radiographic Markets Division.)

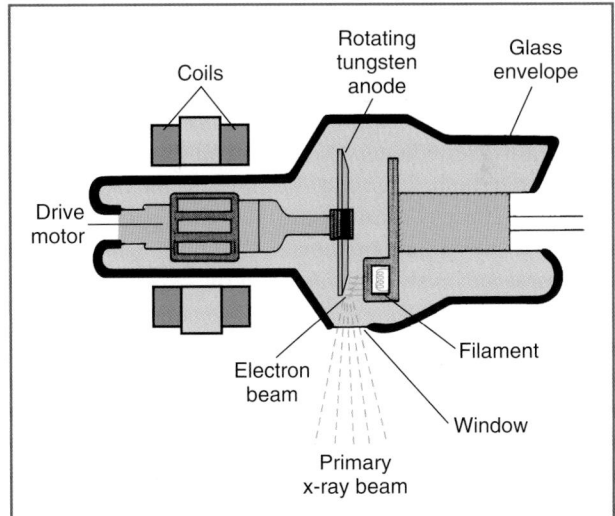

FIGURE 16-9 Rotating-anode tube. Heat is better dissipated by placing the target material at the circumference of a high-speed rotating disc.

rotate the anode and dissipate the heat must be of the highest quality and perfectly balanced to prevent the tube from wobbling. Any imbalance causes the anode to wobble, leading to loss of image quality and eventual tube destruction. Figure 16-9 shows a diagram of a rotating anode tube. Some tubes may rotate at speeds varying from 3600 revolutions per minute (rpm) to 10,000 rpm. Rotating anode x-ray machines generally have a two-step exposure switch. The first step of the switch starts the anode rotating, and the second step of

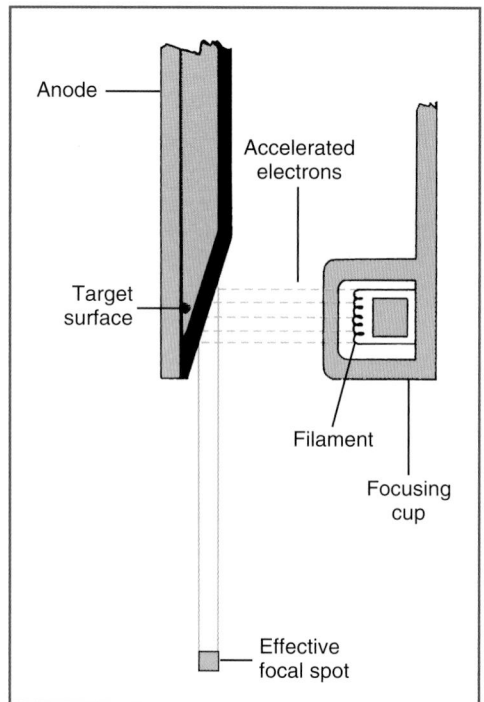

FIGURE 16-10 Effective focal spot. The surface area is decreased when the target area is constructed at a 20-degree angle to the electron beam.

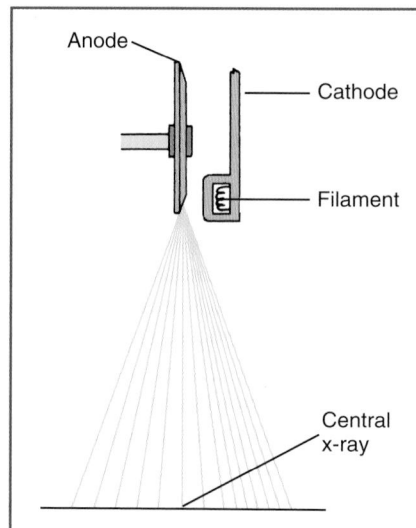

FIGURE 16-11 Heel effect, produced by uneven intensity of the primary beam. Intensity decreases rapidly toward the anode.

the switch activates the high-voltage circuit, resulting in x-ray production. The anode is angled for two reasons. One, the angle directs the x-ray beam vertically to exit the tube window; and two, it creates a smaller, more compact effective focal spot to create better resolution and produce a higher-quality radiograph. The actual focal spot is the target on the anode. The effective focal spot is the tightly packed focused primary x-ray beam that exits the tube window. The actual focal spot is always larger than the effective focal spot (Figure 16-10).

Heel Effect

When an x-ray beam leaves the tube, it has an uneven x-ray photon distribution. This phenomenon is related to the angle of the target areas and to absorption by the anode and target material. As a result of this engineering feature, the x-ray beam is more intense at the side of the cathode than in the center of the beam or on the anode side. This phenomenon is called the **heel effect** (Figure 16-11).

This feature can be used to great advantage in veterinary radiology when x-raying parts of uneven thickness—a common problem in thoracic and abdominal radiography of deep-chested dogs. By placing the thickest part of the patient toward the cathode side of the x-ray tube, a more uniform density can be obtained on the radiograph.

> **TECHNICIAN NOTE**   Always place the thickest part of the area being x-rayed toward the cathode side of the x-ray tube.

Tube Rating Chart

A rating chart is provided by all manufacturers of x-ray tubes. The tube rating chart provides important information on the maximum safe exposure time that can be used with specific milliamperage and kilovoltage settings. If longer-than-designated exposure times are used, tube damage may occur. The size of the anode focal spot determines the rating of the tube because size controls the amount of energy it can absorb and convert into x-rays and heat.

The Physics of X-Ray Production

X-rays are produced when all the energy packed in extremely rapidly moving electrons comes to an abrupt stop on encountering the target in the x-ray tube. Most of the energy of the electrons is not converted into x-rays but is dissipated as heat. In fact, more than 99% of the energy dissipated in the target is lost as heat, and less than 1% is converted to x-ray energy. This explains the elaborate system of heat dissipation built into the x-ray tube (described in the previous section).

Two events may occur when electrons approach the atoms of the target: (1) Electrons may miss the atoms and their orbital electrons and go through the entire target and eventually be absorbed by the backing material of the target or the lead shielding of the x-ray tube, or (2) incoming electrons may interact with the electron cloud of the atoms in the target material and produce x-rays by transferring their energy to these atoms. Both of these events produce x-ray photons, most of which are produced by slowing of the electrons as they are absorbed into the target. The faster the electrons travel, the greater is their energy and, therefore, the greater is the energy, as well as the penetrating power, of the resulting x-ray beam.

Scatter Radiations

In passing through a patient, an x-ray beam becomes attenuated; in other words, its energy decreases gradually. Scatter

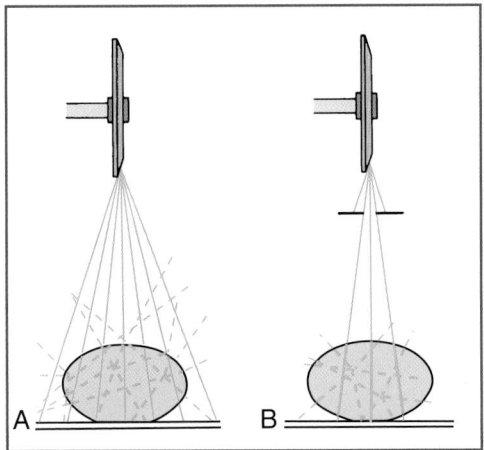

FIGURE 16-12 Scatter radiations. **A,** Scatter radiations are produced when the primary beam is redirected after interacting with structures in the patient's body. **B,** Reduction in the amount of radiation produced when the primary beam is restricted by a diaphragm or a collimator.

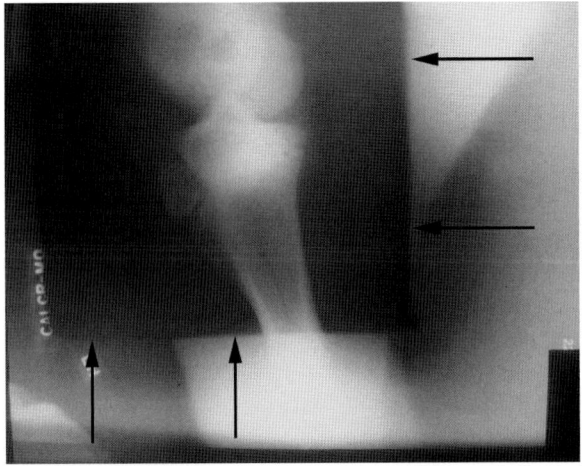

FIGURE 16-13 Lateral radiograph of an equine stifle. Note the close collimation on the joint *(arrows)* and that the scatter radiation from this area was of sufficient strength to penetrate the rest of the horse's leg, creating an underexposed image of the leg on the rest of the radiograph.

radiations are lower-energy x-ray photons that have undergone a change in direction after interacting with structures in the patient's body (Figure 16-12).

Scatter radiation is of concern because it decreases film quality and increases radiation exposure for personnel involved in restraining the patient as the radiograph is taken. Most scatter radiations contribute to overall film blackness or radiographic density, but do not contribute to the useful image. This results in reduced subject contrast. Scatter radiations are the primary source of radiation exposure for technicians who manually restrain patients. Scatter radiations are directly increased with increases in the following three factors: kilovoltage, thickness of the part being x-rayed, and size of the field (Figure 16-13).

Careful collimation with beam-limiting devices and close attention to technical factors to avoid the need for retakes

are the best ways to decrease radiation exposure from scatter radiations. Several techniques are used to reduce scatter radiations and their effects on the radiograph. Use of beam-limiting devices, correct kilovolt peak (kVp) settings, compression radiography, and **grids** are a few ways to control scatter radiations. They are discussed later in this chapter.

> **TECHNICIAN NOTE** Scatter radiations coming from the area of the patient exposed during radiography are the main source of radiation exposure for the veterinary technician.

X-RAY EQUIPMENT

The type of x-ray unit encountered in a veterinary practice will vary according to the caseload and the type of practice. Because one may be working with a large or small animal practitioner, in a large corporate practice, or in a veterinary teaching hospital, it is necessary to be familiar with the various types of x-ray units found in such practices.

Regardless of type and model, most x-ray machines share many features. For small animal radiology, an x-ray machine must have a table on which the animal can be positioned (Figure 16-14). For larger animals, hand-held or stationary cassette holders are used most often (Figure 16-15). All x-ray machines must have a control panel to select kilovoltage, milliamperage, and time of exposure. An x-ray machine may have numerous auxiliary meters, buttons, dials, or switches, but kilovoltage, milliamperage, and time of exposure are the three primary factors in x-ray production (Figures 16-16 and 16-17). Many x-ray machines have a common selector control for milliamperage and time of exposure. This mAs dial or setting automatically sets the highest milliamperage station and the fastest time to provide the requested mAs. Milliamperage × time in seconds (mAs) controls the volume or number of x-ray photons produced. In older machines, milliamperage and time (in fractions of a second) must be set manually to produce a given mAs. The amperage (A) in mAs is always capitalized because it refers to Andre M. Ampere, the physicist credited with the discovery of electric currents.

Three types of x-ray machines are generally used in veterinary practice: portable units, mobile units, and stationary units. Please refer to Chapter 34 for a discussion of dental radiographic units.

> **TECHNICIAN NOTE** Kilovoltage, milliamperage, and time of exposure are the three factors that must be set correctly for production of a properly exposed radiograph.

Portable Unit

As the name implies, portable units can be carried "easily" from one location to another. Weight varies from 6.75 to 20.25 kg or more. These units are generally used on blocks or on custom-made stands. From a safety perspective, they

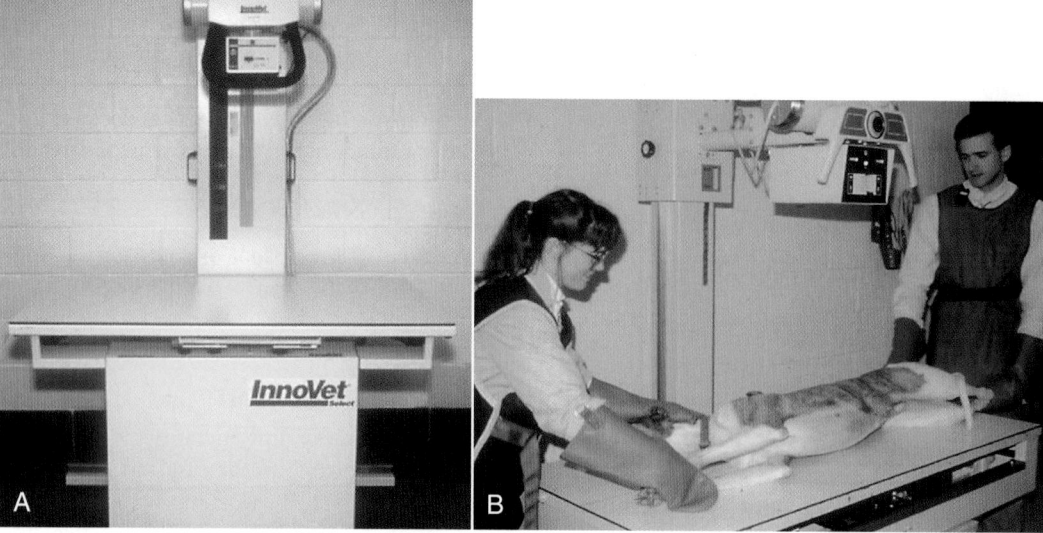

FIGURE 16-14 A, A 300-mA x-ray machine commonly used in small animal practice. B, Canine patient correctly positioned on an x-ray table for a lateral thoracic radiograph.

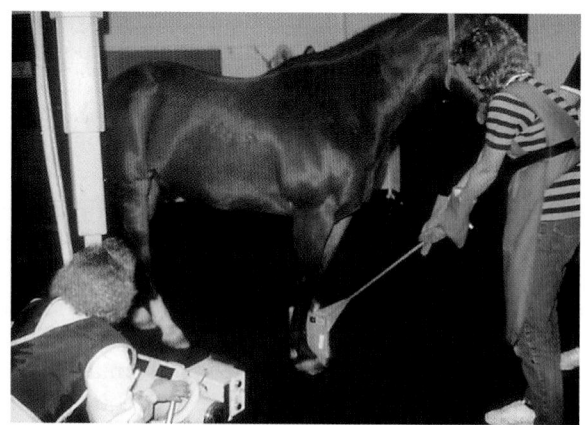

FIGURE 16-15 Large animal radiography unit with special film cassette holders for equine extremities.

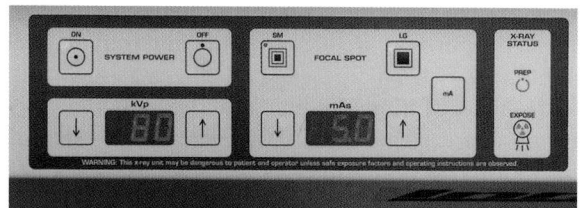

FIGURE 16-16 Typical instrument panel of an x-ray machine used by veterinarians showing digital panels with buttons for selection of milliamperage, time, and kilovolt peak (kVp).

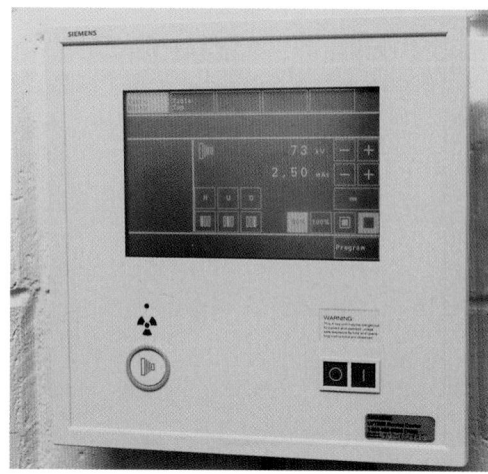

FIGURE 16-17 Wall-mounted operator control console used in some of the larger veterinary clinics and several veterinary teaching hospitals.

should never be hand-held. This recommendation applies especially to lighter models that have less shielding. Hand holding an x-ray machine not only places the operator close to the x-ray tube but also decreases film quality because of tube motion during exposure.

Common characteristics of portable units include the following:

- A single focal spot of about 1.2 mm, a stationary anode tube, and a single filament, although a few models have two filaments and focal spot sizes
- Collimation varying from lead plate adaptable to the film size to lighted collimator with adjustable field size
- Tube output up to 90 kVp at 10 mA, usually with settings at 10, 20, and 30 mA, and at 70, 80, or 90 kVp
- Electronic timer ranging from 0.01 to 10 seconds
- Electrical input of 110 V with an adapter to 220 V

Some models may use 12 DC (direct current) or operate on an automobile battery with converter (Figure 16-18).

Mobile Unit

Mobile units are medium-powered, wheel-mounted units that can be moved around the hospital. In many small animal practices, these units are used as fixed units and remain in one room. They are also popular in mixed practices, in which the same unit can be used for both large and small animals.

These units are powered by 220-V or 110-V outlets. The 220-V units require more extensive electrical wiring, especially if the same units must be used at several locations. These units are equipped with a long, heavy power cord that can be a problem when working with large animals. The 110-V units usually are lighter and therefore easier to move around, and the power cord is smaller; these can be advantages when x-rays of equine extremities are taken. However, these units are usually less powerful than 220-V units.

Stationary Unit

Stationary units are more powerful and are found in most small and large animal hospitals. A typical stationary small

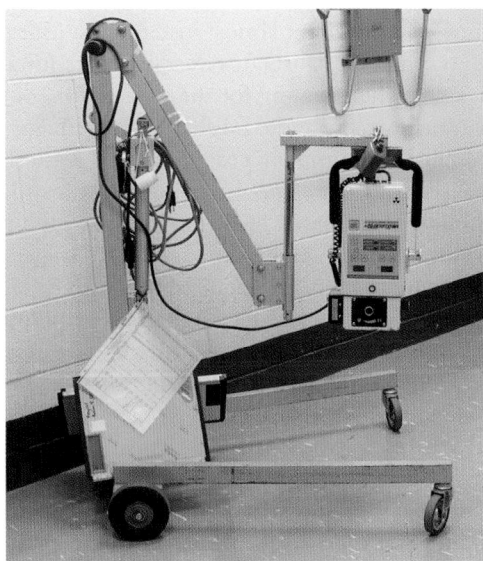

FIGURE 16-18 Portable x-ray unit. Such units are commonly used in large animal practices, mostly for examination of extremities. This particular unit has a lighted collimator and a mobile operating stand.

animal unit is shown in Figure 16-14. Custom large animal units and radiography/fluorography rooms are found in all veterinary teaching hospitals. Some of these units are among the most powerful diagnostic x-ray units installed in the United States. They vary in size from 300 mA, 100 kVp up to 2000 mA, 150 kVp. They can be powered by single-phase or three-phase generators. The x-ray tube may be suspended from the ceiling or attached to a floor-stand support. The tube can rotate 90 degrees in all directions and usually has a heavy duty collimator (Figure 16-19).

Stationary units commonly seen in small animal veterinary practices are of the 300 to 500 mA type with an exposure time of $\frac{1}{60}$ second to $\frac{1}{120}$ second. All of these units can hold a cassette tray under the table with or without a Potter-Bucky grid. Some units have an image intensifier unit for fluoroscopic study or a fixed fluoroscopic screen.

Fluoroscopy

Fluoroscopic units are better suited to the study of moving structures and dynamic processes than are x-ray films. Although films exposed close together in time provide some information about these structures and processes, an image that is continuous in time is required for maximum information. The presentation of a continuous image is called **fluoroscopy**; it involves directing the x-ray beam through the patient and onto an image intensifier. The image intensifier amplifies the x-rays coming through the patient, thus reducing the amount of radiation needed for continuous exposure. The resulting images can be videotaped for analysis, and the tapes can be stored as part of the permanent medical record. The use of fluoroscopy is usually confined to gastrointestinal studies, tracheal studies, and myelography, and is essential for heart and vascular studies. Fluoroscopy is commonly used to view the changing diameter of the trachea during inspiration and expiration that occur in patients with tracheal collapse, and to view the motility of the esophagus in animals that have regurgitation. Fluoroscopic equipment

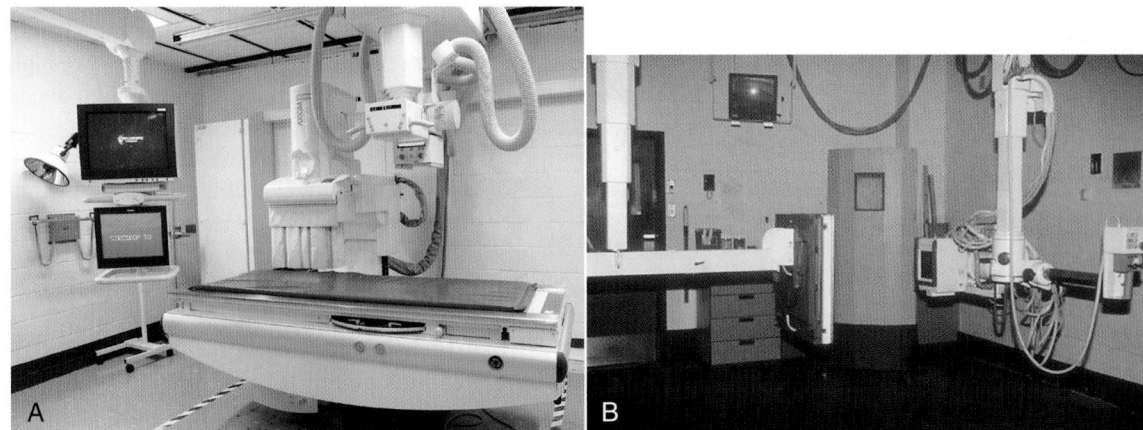

FIGURE 16-19 Stationary units. **A,** Radiography/fluorography unit used for special procedures, such as angiography. This type of unit may be encountered in a few large and small animal hospitals and is found in all veterinary teaching hospitals. **B,** High-powered stationary large animal unit that includes a ceiling-suspended x-ray unit and a Potter-Bucky suspension system. The two units can be interlocked when needed for a fixed focal spot-film distance.

is available only in larger veterinary specialty hospitals and referral centers. For a more extensive discussion of fluoroscopy, review the chapters that cover this subject in Curry et al (1990), Douglas et al (1987), Eastman Kodak Company (1980), Lavin (2006), and Morgan (1993).

Digital Radiography

Medical imaging is currently undergoing rapid and revolutionary changes. Digital imaging techniques are now used for computed tomography (CT), diagnostic ultrasound, nuclear medicine, magnetic resonance imaging (MRI), digital radiography (DR), computed radiography (CR), and digital fluoroscopy (DF). CR and DR are different. In DR, an x-ray tube coupled to a specialized detector panel that changes x-rays into electrical signals is used. The analog image is digitalized and displayed on the integrated computer screen (Figure 16-20). Creating an image in this manner allows postproduction digital enhancement. This enhancement can allow the operator to alter the image using software that has functions similar to conventional image-processing software such as magnification, rotation, annotation and measurement of images, contrast, brightness, and zoom. The main advantage of this ability to alter the image is the decrease in retakes, which saves time and reduces the technician's exposure to harmful radiation. CR uses very similar equipment to that used in conventional radiography, except that in place of a film to create the image, an imaging plate is used. In this manner, all chemical exposure, expense, and darkroom time are eliminated because the imaging plate is run through a computer scanner to read and digitize the image. Both CR and DR images can be printed onto film with a dry laser camera and will closely resemble typical radiographs, or they can be printed onto a variety of imaging printers that process digital data. In most practices, the images are read on the computer screen, and data are downloaded onto digital videodiscs (DVDs), compact discs (CDs), or external hard drives for permanent archiving.

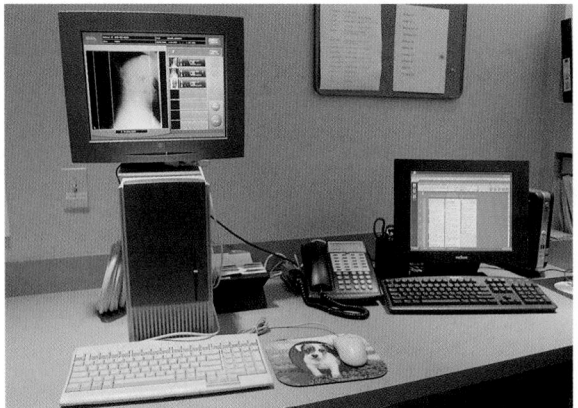

FIGURE 16-20 Digital radiology control system. Computer on the left is the digital radiography workstation where images are viewed, optimized, and then stored or printed. Computer on the right is an RIS, or radiology information system, used to couple patient data with images.

The advantages of these systems over traditional film-screen systems are numerous. They require no film, screens, or processing. The images can be manipulated after acquisition to adjust brightness and contrast, so exposure parameters do not have to be as precise. In equine practices, exposures can be repeated as many times as needed. This provides a major advantage in field work because the study is not limited by the number of cassettes available, and each image can be seen almost immediately. This prevents the need to return to the farm to repeat exposures and to make trips to the hospital to develop films. Portions of an image often can be magnified, which improves visualization of small parts and enhances image interpretation in orthopedics and imaging of exotic animals. Because images can be downloaded to CD, DVD, or external hard drives, physical storage space is not required for archiving, as it is for film. Another major advantage is that because the data are digitalized, images can be sent almost instantly via Internet connections to other specialists or referral centers for a second opinion, rather than waiting for the mail or for courier services to transport the radiographs. Disadvantages include increased initial equipment cost, problems typical of any computer system such as power failures and lost data, and the possibility of increased radiation exposure as a result of overuse. Although film archiving space is no longer needed, hard drive storage units are required to store the large data files that are generated on a daily basis. Furthermore, the data must also be stored on a remote hard drive as a backup mechanism. This is referred to as a *picture archival computing system* and is discussed later.

The dynamic range of an image consists of the number of shades of gray that can be represented. The maximum number of shades of gray in a digital system is related to the numeric range of each pixel. The larger the dynamic range, the more shades of gray there are between white and black, providing a more gradual scale. The dynamic range of the x-ray beam is 2^{10}. It is impossible to appreciate this large dynamic range because the human eye can see only 2^5 or 32 shades of gray from white to black. However, a computer can display a much broader dynamic range. The dynamic range of a digital system is a function of computer and software capacity. Images with low dynamic range have high contrast but only in some portions of the image. High dynamic range allows for wider image latitude.

Poor spatial resolution is a main disadvantage of digital radiography compared with film radiography. Conventional screen-film systems can image structures measuring 100 μm, whereas DR structures are typically limited to 500 μm. Resolution is controlled by the design of the detector array.

Computed Radiography

Computed radiography (CR) is similar to DR except that an x-ray detector similar to a cassette is used and must be processed in a special machine (Figure 16-21). The special cassette contains a photostimulable phosphor that changes x-ray photons into a latent electronic image that is "read" by the processor and transferred to the computer. This makes

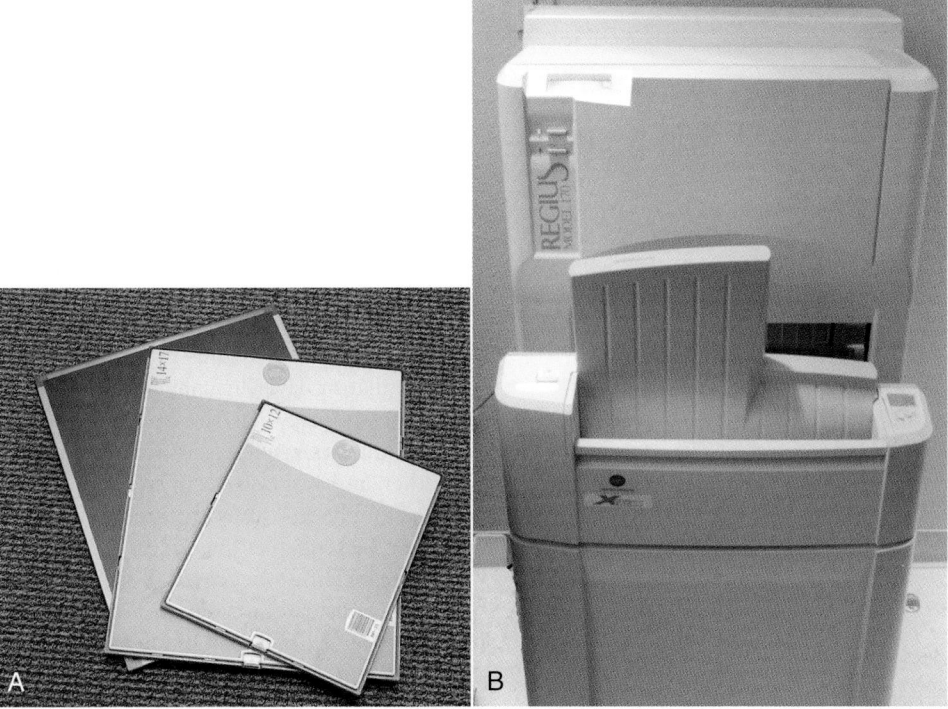

FIGURE 16-21 Computed radiology. **A,** Special cassettes containing a photostimulable phosphor instead of film to capture the latent x-ray image. **B,** Computed radiology reader that takes the specialized cassette and downloads the latent image into a computer.

the time required for image acquisition with CR slightly longer than with DR. However, image data have all the advantages and disadvantages of DR.

The same radiographic equipment is used for CR and DR as for film systems, and similar principles of operation apply. For instance, grids and collimation to limit scatter radiation are used in the same manner as with film radiography. However, some systems do not use a grid because the vendor software can digitally reproduce the effects of a grid (digital grid compensation).

CR and DR do not use less radiation to produce an image compared with film radiography, and the same principles of radiation protection apply. Technique charts for CR and DR are much simpler than for film radiography, and so allow a wide range of object types and sizes to be exposed with a small range of kVp and mAs settings. Also, CR and DR systems are not as sensitive as conventional film-screen systems to underexposures and overexposures.

IMAGE QUALITY IN DIGITAL RADIOGRAPHY

The technician must be familiar with several issues regarding image quality in digital radiography. Currently, a minimum of 2.5 line-pairs/mm is recommended for adequate spatial resolution (the ability to distinguish two adjacent structures) in digital imaging detector panels and imaging plates. The wide latitude (large dynamic range or many shades of gray) in digital images allows both bone and soft tissues to be seen at the same exposure setting; this is not possible with film systems. The mAs is not related to film blackening in digital imaging because digital systems automatically compensate

for overexposures and underexposures. However, severe underexposure will result in too few x-ray photons striking the detector panel (in the case of DR) or the imaging plate (in the case of CR), leading to production of a grainy image with poor resolution (an effect known as "quantum mottle" or "noise"). Monitor resolution also plays an important role in image quality. The brightness (luminescence) of the monitor is important for proper image viewing (minimum 50-foot lambert), as is the pixel density (minimum of 2000 × 2000, or 2 mega-pixels, is recommended). Magnification of an image will result in pixelation (loss of quality due to the visibility of individual pixels), which becomes more apparent than in the nonmagnified image. The magnitude of this effect is related to the original pixel density or line-pair rating of the detector panel or imaging plate.

DIGITAL RADIOGRAPHY ARTIFACTS (BOX 16-1)

Digital radiography has its own types of artifacts that are different from those seen in film radiography, but malpositioning, patient movement, geometric distortion, double exposures, and other classical technical errors still occur, as they do with traditional film-screen systems. Although film radiographs are viewed with a backlight on a view box, digital images are viewed on a computer screen. Digital system software uses a "look-up table" (LUT) to determine the brightness of pixels in the image. Different body regions (e.g., thorax, extremity) have different LUTs that are adjusted by the manufacturer of the DR equipment to make each digital image look a certain way, which maximizes its diagnostic value. Images that are too dark or that are lacking in

BOX 16-1	Digital Artifacts

Lucent halo around metal implants
- Uberschwinger artifact, or rebound effect (an artifact of digital processing that may be mistaken for bone lysis)

Linear striations seen in the background of the image
- Planking artifact (due to plate saturation, i.e., overexposure)

Disappearance of thin tissues or soft tissues surrounding bone
- Overexposure

Grainy appearance (Quantum mottle or "noise")
- Underexposure

Nonuniform appearance to the image
- Inhomogeneous tabletop
- Contrast media on table or detector

Ghost images
- Taking an image quickly after a previous image that required a very high exposure (e.g., an equine stifle)
- Double exposures (computed radiography [CR] only)
- Failure to erase a CR plate

Fogging
- CR plate exposed to radiation from any source: through wall if storage room adjacent to x-ray room or cassette left in x-ray room while exposure made

White spots
- Scratches on CR imaging plate
- Hair, dirt, or other particles trapped in the CR cassette

contrast should have the LUT re-adjusted, so that the raw data are not lost and all diagnostically important parts of the body region are seen on the image. The vendor's technical support team makes adjustments to LUTs in almost all instances.

The Uberschwinger artifact, or rebound effect, appears like a lucent halo around metal or areas with large density differences between adjacent objects (bone and metal). This is caused by computer image processing that is used to determine how much edge enhancement is used to make bone borders appear sharp in the digital image. This artifact can be mistaken for lysis around a bone screw or pin.

Exposure artifacts can be due to both overexposure and underexposure. If the image appears grainy, mottled, or pixelated, even though the image "appears" to be properly exposed, it is really underexposed. Overexposure occurs when more x-rays than required are used; in a digital system, which is more sensitive to x-ray exposure, the detector panel can quickly become saturated to a point where it cannot respond correctly to more x-rays. Pixels in the overexposed region of the image get set to a maximum value; consequently thin areas of the anatomy appear completely black and therefore are not visible. The user can brighten the image in the software viewer, but the overexposed anatomy will never be visible. Most commonly, the skin and soft tissues appear burnt away from the bone in images of the extremities. Sometimes, linear striations can be seen in the

background of the image as the result of plate saturation (normally, air is uniformly black); this is called *planking*.

The heel effect is not seen in DR because the software compensates for the heterogeneity of the x-ray beam so that the finished image appears uniform. This is not the case for CR because the image plate is separate from the detector and is put through a reader. Inhomogeneous x-ray machine tabletops and contrast media on the table or detector will interfere with calibration of the detector, preventing the image from having a uniform appearing exposure.

Ghost images occur with DR systems. This happens when images from a previous exposure stay on the detector panel scintillating layer, usually when objects that require a very high exposure (e.g., the equine stifle) are imaged. This artifact appears when exposures are made quickly one after the other, and can also occur in CR systems.

Double exposures are possible in CR systems because they use a cassette, like the one used in film radiography. Also, if the plate fails to be erased in the reader, the image of a previous exposure can remain in subsequent images. Other CR-specific artifacts include fogging, as is seen in film radiography. CR plates are very sensitive to radiation compared with film. The outer portions of the image will appear darker compared with the more central areas because of radiation entering the periphery of the cassette that contains the imaging plate.

As with film-screen systems, scratching the surface of the imaging plate or allowing hair or other particles to be trapped in the CR cassette will lead to white artifacts on the image. When this is noticed, the cassette, image plate, and light guide in the reader have to be inspected and cleaned.

DICOM, PACS, RIS, and Teleradiology

Medical image dissemination (distribution to other locations) and archiving (storage) has been revolutionized since the transition from analog (film-based) to digital imaging, and since introduction of the DICOM (digital imaging and communications in medicine) standard. DICOM is a universal digital image format. Images produced from equipment using the DICOM standard can communicate with another vendor's software. This makes **teleradiology** (electronically sending an image to another location) possible, because images can be sent electronically from one hospital workstation to the workstation of another hospital, even though it may not possess the same imaging equipment or software. Specifically, DICOM 3.0 is the current standard and is universally accepted, but connectivity between workstations and modalities (ultrasound [US], MRI, CT, radiography, etc.) can still be difficult because vendors sometimes use proprietary methods that other systems cannot read.

Each DICOM image file contains image information and patient identification, modality used (CT, US, MRI, etc.), date and time of the examination, and display formats. Imaging modalities that operate on the DICOM standard include CT, digital or computed radiography, MRI, US, and SC (secondary capture such as from a film scanner). DICOM functionality enables image storage, query (searching), retrieval, display, and manipulation. The term "DICOM service object" refers to any image produced from any modality. DICOM roles are sender and receiver functions. A service class provider (SCP) and service class users (SCUs) allow DICOM communications to happen. DICOM service classes specify types of communications, such as store, print, send, and retrieve.

When images are acquired from any modality, DICOM standard arranges them as images, studies, and series. Each patient has a number of images that are part of a study. Each study may consist of one or more series of images. A series can consist of a single image or several images. The imaging software reads the tags of each image so that it recognizes which images belong to which series and study. Therefore, when a patient's record is pulled up with the hospital's software, the images are organized automatically into groups according to date, modality, study, and series. DICOM functions also allow generation of a worklist and print functions. A worklist can communicate with the hospital information system (HIS) or the radiology information system (RIS) so that the images become part of that patient's digital hospital record. DICOM print allows digital images to be printed out onto a medium. This is often done on film produced from a dry laser printer.

PACS

PACS, or picture archival computing systems, are used to move images around to different computer workstations within a single hospital or between hospitals and as a method of storing imaging data permanently. They use the DICOM standard. Benefits of PACS include the following: (1) They eliminate the need to generate and store film hard copies, (2) communication with other veterinarians for information dissemination is improved, (3) tracking down lost films is no longer an issue, and (4) multiple users can view the images at the same time. As with any computer system, however, there are inherent disadvantages. When computer systems go down, become blocked, or lose connectivity, decreased productivity may occur, and data can become lost (like a film radiograph). Furthermore, users must have good, preferably excellent, working knowledge of computer systems or must have a consultant or department at the hospital that can troubleshoot and maintain the PACS at all times.

A PACS consists of various imaging modalities, a server for archiving images, and viewing stations connected to the local area network (LAN). Each imaging modality is "told" where to send the DICOM image information by IP address, application entry (AE) title, and port number of the recipient of the images. In turn, the archive server has the same information about the modality, so that the two can communicate. The AE title, assigned by the technologist, is a name, such as "Ultrasound Room One." The port is the electronic route that the information will travel, and the IP address is the computer's individual address, similar to a street address.

Three components of the PACS with which the technologist may work are the server, the workstation, and the monitor. The server receives the images and catalogs them into a database. The imaging software searches this database using the patient's name and identification number, the date, the modality, the veterinarian's name, and so forth.

The workstation consists of a computer with imaging software to display the DICOM information as an image (radiographic, ultrasound, CT, MRI, etc.). This workstation allows images to be sent (exported), received, and manipulated (contrast, brightness, magnification, etc.); measurements (length, width, circumference, angle, etc.) to be made; and images to be viewed on dual monitors, printed, and copied onto a CD-ROM with a DICOM viewer embedded.

Monitors are critical to image quality. Numerous combinations of monitor size, resolution, luminosity, graphics card quality, type (liquid crystal vs. cathode ray tube), and cost are available. A high-quality graphics card is necessary for viewing cine-loops, as with ultrasound studies. Ultrasound, CT, MRI, and nuclear medicine (NM) images are of inherently low resolution and do not require high-resolution monitors for adequate viewing. Digital radiographic images, however, do require high-resolution monitors. Minimally, monitors should have 1024×768 at 32-bit resolution for all digital imaging viewing.

RIS

RIS, or radiology information systems, are computer software programs that allow all patient data to be made available and coupled with digital imaging data. The advantage of the RIS is that when patient identification information or results of a test are entered by any individual in the hospital, this information is "coordinated" with all other hospital forms and records, for instance, when patient identification and details are entered into the digital file, that information is automatically transferred to radiology forms. There is no need for redundant entry of patient IDs by each secretary, technologist, or veterinarian. These systems are fairly new and are just now being integrated into the veterinary marketplace. For more information on computerized medical records, please read Chapter 3, "Veterinary Medical Records."

Teleradiology

Teleradiology allows the transmission of digital data across the Internet from private practices to referral centers around the world. Specialists can receive images almost instantly, interpret them, and quickly send back a written report. There is no longer the need to package and label films to be sent by mail carriers, which also delays response time. This has dramatically improved patient care and continuing education for the practitioner. Any digital data (MRI, CT, ultrasound, digital, and CR) can be sent directly, and analog data (regular radiographs and laboratory data) can be digitized or scanned into a computer and sent as well.

EXPOSURE FACTORS

The veterinary technician is responsible for selecting an x-ray technique that will produce a diagnostic radiograph.

Factors that must be selected include time of exposure, milliamperage, and kilovoltage. As has been mentioned, most recent x-ray machines have a common dial for time of exposure and milliamperage, called the *mAs setting*. Selection of each factor is based on an accurate technique chart. Preparation of a technique chart is discussed later in this chapter.

Other factors that enter into the production of a diagnostic radiograph are focal-film distance, type of intensifying screen, type of x-ray film, and tabletop versus grid technique. All of these variables are discussed in greater detail.

Milliamperage

The milliamperage setting controls the quantity of electrons boiled off the filament in the x-ray tube. It is a quantity factor because it controls the quantity of x-rays that will be produced at the target area. Most diagnostic units used in small animal radiology are operated at settings from 50 to 300 mA. The smallest portable x-ray unit commonly used in large animal practices may use current flow as low as 10 or 20 mA, whereas larger units used in small animal hospitals and veterinary teaching hospitals may have a current flow of up to 2000 mA.

Adjustments of the milliamperage setting control on an x-ray machine allow control of the quantity of x-rays produced. When one increases the milliamperage setting, radiographic density—or film blackness—is increased; conversely, when one decreases the milliamperage setting, a reduction in radiographic density—or a lighter film—results.

Exposure Time

Exposure time is the time in fractions of a second during which the anode is positively charged. The longer the exposure time, the greater is the number of electrons that flow from the cathode to the anode, and the greater is the number of x-ray photons that are produced. Because both exposure time and milliamperage affect the number of photons created, and because you want the shortest exposure time possible to decrease patient motion blur, you should always use the highest milliamperage setting and the lowest time setting to arrive at the desired mAs. By using the highest milliamperage setting, you are maximizing the number of electrons in the focusing cup, so you have to charge the anode only for a short period (exposure time) to get the number of electrons needed to the anode to create the desired number of x-ray photons.

> **TECHNICIAN NOTE**   Always use the highest milliamperage setting and the lowest time setting to arrive at a particular mAs. This will decrease motion blur on the radiograph.

To understand this concept, consider the following example: An exposure made at 100 mA and at $\frac{1}{10}$ second should produce a film of equivalent density as an exposure made at 200 mA and $\frac{1}{20}$ second. In both cases, the mAs factor (milliamperage × time) is the same and is equal to

10 mAs. Shorter exposure times reduce the problem of motion; this may result in loss of detail. For this reason, a thoracic radiograph on a dog or cat should be taken at $\frac{1}{20}$ to $\frac{1}{60}$ second to prevent blurring of the radiograph as a result of respiratory motion.

Kilovoltage

Kilovoltage is a quality factor that regulates the energy of the x-ray beam. This setting regulates the voltage differential applied between the anode and the cathode in the x-ray tube. The higher the voltage, the faster the electrons are accelerated, and the greater is the energy of the x-ray beam. The greater the energy, the greater is the amount of patient tissue that can be penetrated. Increasing the kilovoltage will also increase radiographic density, or film blackness, because of increased x-ray photons passing through the patient. The kilovoltage setting most often used in diagnostic radiology varies from 40,000 to 150,000 V (40 to 150 kV).

The kilovoltage setting affects the scale of contrast on a radiograph. Contrast is necessary to differentiate anatomic structures in an image. The *scale of contrast* refers to the number of shades of gray that can be seen. If no contrast existed, everything would have the same radiographic opacity. Using low kVp settings produces a higher-contrast image (more black and white in appearance with few grays) because the beam is more discriminating than a beam with a high kVp. Use of high kVp settings results in a darker image, which shows little difference in opacity between bone, soft tissue, and fat (low contrast). The kVp setting must be high enough to penetrate the patient, but not so high as to decrease contrast. If a radiograph is too light because of exposure problems, and mAs is increased with no resulting increase in film density or blackness, x-ray photon energy may be insufficient (too low a kVp) to penetrate the patient.

> **TECHNICIAN NOTE**   You can increase radiographic density or film blackness by increasing the energy level of x-ray photons (kVp) or the total number of x-ray photons (mAs).

Focal-Film Distance

The *focal-film distance* refers to the distance between the target in the x-ray tube and the surface of the x-ray detector. This factor is normally kept constant from one exposure to another. It is usually kept at a distance of 70 to 85 cm (28 to 34 inches) for large animal radiology and 90 to 105 cm (36 to 42 inches) for small animal radiology.

It is important to keep the focal-film distance constant from one exposure to the next because it has a significant influence on exposure factors. An increase in distance decreases the number of x-rays reaching the film. This is not a linear relationship. If you double the focal-film distance, the number of x-rays reaching the film will be reduced by a factor of four. This is often referred to as the *inverse square law*, which states that the intensity of the x-ray beam at a given point is inversely proportional to the square of the distance from the x-ray source.

> **TECHNICIAN NOTE** If you double the film distance from the x-ray source, you will decrease the x-ray beam intensity to one-fourth of the original strength. Small changes in focal-film distance can result in big changes in radiographic density.

It sometimes is necessary to change the focal-film distance to obtain proper positioning. The following simple calculation will help you choose the new mAs setting when the distance is changed:

$$\frac{\text{Old mAs} \times \text{New distance}^2}{\text{Old distance}^2} = \text{New mAs}$$

For example, if an x-ray taken at 10 mAs at 100 cm must be taken at 50 cm, by using the formula given, the new mAs setting can be calculated as follows:

$$\frac{10 \text{ mAs}}{100^2} \times 50^2 = 2.5 \text{ mAs}$$

This new mAs setting should produce an image of similar radiographic density as is produced by the original setting of 10 mAs.

Technique Chart

A technique chart is an essential component for obtaining diagnostic x-ray examinations in a consistent way. A technique chart must be formulated for each x-ray machine because differences in output are seen with each machine (even those made by the same manufacturer). Therefore, you should never use an x-ray chart formulated for another x-ray machine without making appropriate changes. If you select exposure factors from a good technique chart, consistent radiographic examinations of diagnostic quality will be obtained. In addition, x-ray film will be saved because waste from repeated exposures will be avoided.

Several types of technique charts can be formulated. Each type must be formulated with the goal of using the maximum potential of a particular x-ray machine. Perhaps the most popular type of technique chart used by veterinarians is a variable kilovoltage chart. A variable mAs chart probably is more appropriate for the most powerful x-ray machines. However, a combination of variable kilovoltage and mAs technique charts is best. Such charts take into consideration the need to adapt a technique chart for different body systems, such as a thoracic and abdominal study and examinations involving the musculoskeletal system.

This chapter cannot discuss appropriately every type of technique chart. The principle of how to prepare a variable kilovoltage technique chart, along with an example of such a chart (Table 16-1), is given. For a more extensive discussion of how to prepare different technique charts and examples of each, please refer to discussions of this topic by

TABLE 16-1	Variable kV Technique Chart for an X-Ray Machine of 300 mA, 125 kV, $\frac{1}{120}$-Second Timer With FFD of 40 Inches				
THICKNESS, CM	**KV**	**MA**	**SECONDS**	**MAS**	**GRID**
4	48	300	$\frac{1}{120}$	2.5	No
5	50	300	$\frac{1}{120}$	2.5	No
6	52	300	$\frac{1}{120}$	2.5	No
7	54	300	$\frac{1}{120}$	2.5	No
8	56	300	$\frac{1}{120}$	2.5	No
9	58	300	$\frac{1}{120}$	2.5	No
10	63	300	$\frac{1}{60}$	5	Yes
11	65	300	$\frac{1}{60}$	5	Yes
12	67	300	$\frac{1}{60}$	5	Yes
13	69	300	$\frac{1}{60}$	5	Yes
14	71	300	$\frac{1}{60}$	5	Yes
15	73	300	$\frac{1}{60}$	5	Yes
16	75	300	$\frac{1}{60}$	5	Yes
17	77	300	$\frac{1}{60}$	5	Yes
18	79	300	$\frac{1}{60}$	5	Yes
19	81	300	$\frac{1}{60}$	5	Yes
20	84	300	$\frac{1}{60}$	5	Yes
21	87	300	$\frac{1}{60}$	5	Yes
22	90	300	$\frac{1}{60}$	5	Yes
23	93	300	$\frac{1}{60}$	5	Yes
24	96	300	$\frac{1}{60}$	5	Yes
25	99	300	$\frac{1}{60}$	5	Yes
26	102	300	$\frac{1}{60}$	5	Yes
27	105	300	$\frac{1}{60}$	5	Yes
28	99	300	$\frac{1}{30}$	10	Yes
29	102	300	$\frac{1}{30}$	10	Yes
30	105	300	$\frac{1}{30}$	10	Yes

FFD, Focal-film distance; *kV*, kilovolts; *mA*, milliamperes; *mAs*, milliamperes per second.
Radiographs were taken with Kodak Lanex Regular screens and Kodak TML x-ray film.

Han and Hurd (2005), Lavin (2006), Morgan (1993), and Ticer (1984).

Formulation of a Technique Chart

A technique chart is formulated by a series of trial-and-error exposures. It is necessary, however, to standardize as many variable factors as possible before starting trial exposures. Factors such as type of cassette and intensifying screen, type of x-ray film, and focal-film distance must be constant, and a grid should be used if available. Darkroom procedures must be standardized to include fresh solution and the developing time recommended by the manufacturer based on the temperature of the solution. All of these factors should be constant because the technique chart will be valid only under conditions of formulation. If, for example, cassettes and intensifying screens in a veterinary practice are of different age or speed, the film density for a given technique will be different from one study to the next, even though the same factors are used.

To begin making a variable kVp chart for the abdomen, one must use the following technique. For trial exposure, a normal dog with a lateral abdominal measurement (measuring over the liver) of approximately 15 cm should be selected. A trial exposure at a setting of 80 kVp at 7.5 mAs is suggested. Two exposures are made at this setting. In selecting the mAs setting, the shortest possible time of exposure for a given mAs setting is selected. The two films are then developed according to standard technique and are examined for proper "diagnostic" density. If the films are overexposed or underexposed, a second series of exposures is made. Use the 15% rule for kVp. If the radiograph is too dark, decrease the kVp by 15%. If the radiograph is too light, increase the kVp by 15%. Once you are close to a properly exposed radiograph, use the 15% rule to keep increasing and decreasing the kVp in 5% increments until your exposure is just right. All films should be examined and compared with each other for consistent density between exposures. Once the best film is selected, you can begin to formulate the technique chart. Start with the factors that produced the "diagnostic" film. Then, subtract 2 kVp for each centimeter decrease from the original measurement. Add 2 kVp to the original kVp for each centimeter increase from the original measurement up to 80 kVp. Add 3 kVp for each centimeter increase when the kVp is above 80 until you get to 100 kVp. Add 4 kVp for each centimeter increase when the kVp is above 100 kVp until you reach a maximum of 125 kVp.

Because scatter radiation is increased with increased thickness of a part to be x-rayed, it is recommended that a grid be used for thicknesses greater than 10 cm. If you are creating a technique chart for extremities or for areas smaller than 10 cm, a grid will not figure into your technique formula.

Table 16-1 shows a variable kilovoltage technique chart formulated for an x-ray machine of 300 mA, 125 kV, and $\frac{1}{120}$ second minimum time of exposure. Remember, however, that this is only an illustration of how to formulate a technique chart. This chart should not be used with any single x-ray machine without adaptation to that particular machine.

> **TECHNICIAN NOTE**   Technique charts are developed for a specific focal-film distance, film, cassette screen, and development process. If you change any one of these factors within your practice, the technique chart will need to be updated.

IMAGE FORMATION WITH FILM-SCREEN SYSTEMS

When an x-ray beam penetrates a body system and reaches an x-ray film, a latent image is produced that will be revealed when the film is processed chemically. Several factors are involved in the formation of a high-quality latent image. This section discusses factors that enter into the formation of an x-ray image.

X-Ray Cassette

Cassettes (film holders) used in veterinary medicine are of two types. The nonscreen type is a direct-exposure cassette in which the film is placed in a cardboard cassette or a plastic film holder (Figure 16-22). This nonrigid system must be light-proof and is used when great detail is needed for an examination. The disadvantage of this type of cassette is that it requires an exposure time in excess of 26 times the normal exposure time of a regular par screen cassette system. Nonscreen exposures should be used only when the animal is under general anesthetic or heavy sedation to stop motion, and when no personnel are required for restraint in the radiology room. Nonscreen exposures are used primarily for intraoral occlusal studies of the nasal cavity and dental arches.

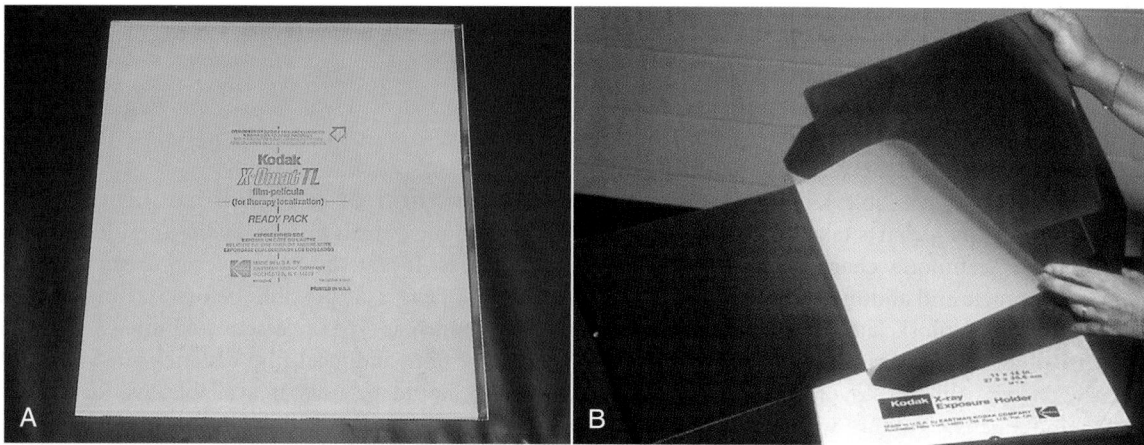

FIGURE 16-22 Nonscreen film. **A,** Ready pack film with a special emulsion for direct exposure. **B,** X-ray exposure holder for regular screen film. Use of a soft cassette such as this necessitates exposure time in excess of 26 times the normal exposure time of a regular par screen cassette system. (From Eastman Kodak Company: The fundamentals of radiography, ed 12, Rochester, NY, 1980, Eastman Kodak, Radiographic Markets Division.)

The second type is the more conventional image-intensifying screen, which is placed in a rigid cassette (Figure 16-23). It is important that the hinges of the cassette be of the highest quality to ensure excellent and uniform contact between the x-ray film and the intensifying screen, and to prevent light leakage that could fog or darken the film. Various materials are used in the manufacture of x-ray cassettes. Most cassettes have a solid front made of plastic or light metal. Recently, carbon fiber (mostly graphite) has also been used. Such cassettes are excellent and may reduce by as much as 20% the quantity of x-rays needed to make an exposure. The cassette back may be made of steel and can sustain moderate patient weight without being damaged. Sometimes a small area of about 7 × 3 cm is shielded from the primary beam for the purpose of film identification (see Figure 16-4).

Cassettes are expensive and should be handled with care. When dropped, they may warp, or if the cover is forced, the hinges may be damaged, resulting in a cassette that does not close properly. If film contact is not perfect along the surface of the cassette, distortion of the x-ray image will occur. The surface of the cassette should be kept clean at all times to prevent the creation of film artifacts.

Intensifying Screens

Intensifying screens are the smooth, shiny white inner surfaces of the film cassette. They are made of layers of tiny crystals bonded together on a plastic support and covered with a protective coating. These crystals fluoresce, or emit light, after exposure to x-rays. The screens are placed into the inner surfaces of the cassette, and the x-ray film is sandwiched between. Because film is more sensitive to light exposure than to radiation exposure, the use of fluorescent intensifying screens dramatically decreases the amount of radiation needed to produce a film of diagnostic radiographic density. Thus, screens allow much lower mAs settings, which decrease loss of detail as a result of motion,

decrease patient radiation exposure, and help to prolong the life of the x-ray tube. In addition, intensifying screens increase radiographic contrast and therefore improve radiographic detail.

Intensifying screens are mounted in pairs in an x-ray cassette (Figure 16-24). They are made of the following four components:

1. Backing of cardboard or plastic, most commonly a Mylar material.
2. Reflecting layers, such as titanium dioxide, that reflect light from the active layer back toward the x-ray film.
3. An active layer of light-emitting phosphor, such as calcium tungstate or rare earth material, that produces fluorescence, exposing the film after absorption of x-rays.
4. A plastic coating that reduces static electricity and provides a protective covering that can be cleaned.

The screens must be cleaned on a regular basis—at least monthly, or whenever screen artifacts are noted on a radiograph. It is best to use a cleaning product recommended by the manufacturer for this purpose. If such a product is not available, a 70% alcohol solution will work (Figure 16-25). The surface of the screen must be thoroughly dry before an

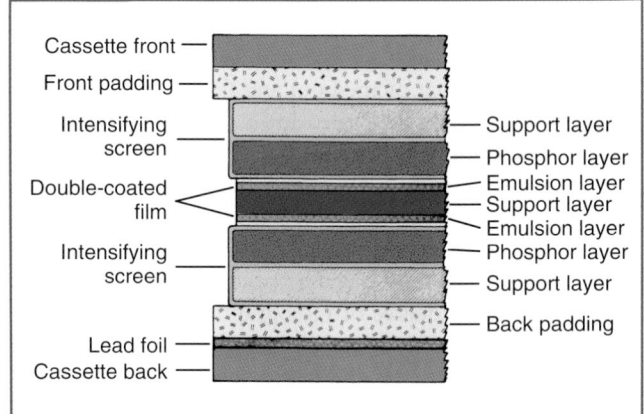

FIGURE 16-24 Cross section of a cassette-intensifying screen system.

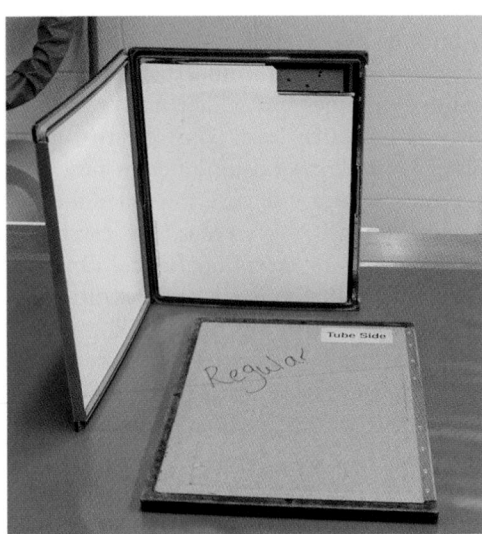

FIGURE 16-23 Open and closed rigid film cassette with image-intensifying screens.

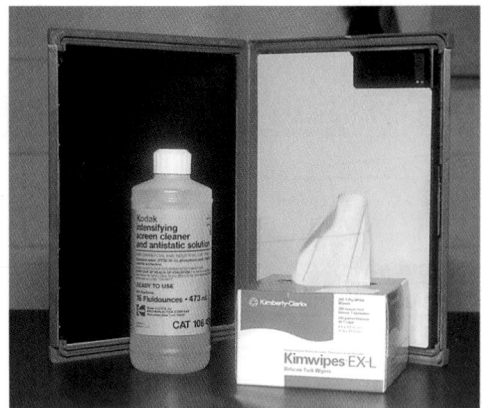

FIGURE 16-25 Open film cassette with a single intensifyin[g] (shiny white surface), used for detailed extremity radiograph[y] should be handled carefully and cleaned regularly wit[h] solutions.

x-ray film is inserted or the cassette is closed; otherwise, the film will stick to the screens and will permanently ruin them. Any stain on the surface of the screen will interfere with transmission of light from the screen to the film, causing an artifact. The technician must be careful not to spill or splash darkroom chemicals onto the surfaces of the screens, or they may be ruined. For this reason, emphasis is placed on the maintenance and cleanliness of screens.

Screen Speed

The speed of a screen pertains to its ability to convert absorbed x-ray energy into visible light. *Screen speed* is a relative term that refers to the amount of radiation required by that screen to produce a film of diagnostic radiographic density. A fast screen requires less radiation than a regular, medium, or par screen to produce the same degree of blackness on the radiograph. The faster the screen, the poorer is the radiographic detail or resolution. Fast screens have a thicker phosphor layer and larger crystals to increase x-ray absorption and light production. Slower or detail screens have smaller crystals and are less efficient at light conversion but produce a radiograph of greater detail and resolution. Detail screens are also called *fine screens* and generally require 4 times the amount of radiation required by a medium or par screen. These are best for obtaining radiographs of birds and small exotic animals. Regular screens are intermediate in speed between par or medium and fast screens.

The original phosphor used in intensifying screens was calcium tungstate. This phosphor produces light in the blue spectrum and is commonly found in veterinary hospitals that have acquired used cassettes and screens from local human hospitals. Improved rare earth phosphors introduced in 1975 emit light in the green spectrum and are able to produce the same degree of radiographic detail as calcium tungstate screens with less radiation exposure. Table 16-2 shows the relative speed of various calcium tungstate and rare earth screens. Rare earth screens are more efficient because they absorb more x-ray photons per crystal and produce more light per absorbed photon. These properties of rare earth screens have definite advantages in veterinary medicine, including the following:

- Reduced exposure time
- Reduced motion artifacts
- Decreased tube voltage, resulting in improved contrast
- Decreased tube current, which prolongs the life of the tube
- Reduced production of heat in the x-ray tube
- Reduced patient radiation dose

> **TECHNICIAN NOTE** Rare earth screens are advantageous for veterinary radiography because they require fewer x-rays to produce a diagnostic radiograph. Lower exposures mean lower radiation doses to the patient and technician, fewer retakes because of patient motion, and longer x-ray tube life.

The main disadvantage of rare earth screens at this time is their cost, which is much greater than that of regular calcium tungstate screens. They have a definite place in large animal radiology because of their speed. This is an important factor when they are used with smaller, low-capacity portable x-ray units. Table 16-3 presents an example of a technique chart that can be used with a small, portable x-ray unit in combination with the rare earth screen.

There is a misconception in veterinary medicine that intensifying screens last forever. This is not true. Screens have a predictable lifetime and gradually wear out with repeated use. Most rare earth screens are worn out after 10 to 12 years of regular use. The radiograph produced with an old screen will have a white speckled pattern, most notably in black areas on the film. This artifact is called *screen craze*. Most screens have a company name and a screen number printed on the edge. By calling the manufacturer, the technician can find out the age of the screen, as well as the best type of film to use with that particular screen.

X-Ray Film

Because the recording medium for film-based x-ray examinations is photographic film, some basic principles of photography must be understood.

An x-ray film is prepared from a suspension of light- and x-ray–sensitive granules embedded in a gelatin emulsion coated over a polyester base. The sensitive granules are usually silver bromide crystals of different sizes. The gelatin matrix is protected by a thin covering called the *T coat*. Just like the image-intensifying screens, the crystals come in various sizes. Images of exceptional detail can be recorded on films containing small crystals. In faster films, the crystals are larger, which results in loss of detail; however, this may be compensated for by shorter exposure times. Because they have shorter exposure time, faster films sometimes provide better image detail because the images contain fewer motion artifacts.

X-ray film can be separated into two categories: screen film (Figure 16-26) and nonscreen film. Screen film is sensitive primarily to wavelengths of light emitted from intensifying screens. Nonscreen films are designed for direct exposure

TABLE 16-2	Relative Speed of Calcium Tungstate* and Rare Earth† Screens
SCREEN TYPE	**ASA FILM SPEED**
detail calcium tungstate	30
tungstate	100
th	150
	200
	250
	300
	400
	600

to x-rays and are relatively insensitive to visible light from screens. Nonscreen films provide superb detail and are especially good for intraoral examination of the nasal cavity, dental studies, and examination of bony extremities. Because this type of x-ray film is exposed by x-rays only, it provides the disadvantage of needing long exposure times to obtain necessary film density (Figure 16-27). Patients should be under general anesthetic and no personnel should be in the room during nonscreen film exposures.

Screen film is less sensitive to direct **ionizing radiation**, but is sensitive to visible light. This type of film requires less exposure to produce a radiograph because of its sensitivity to the fluorescence emitted by intensifying screens. Remember that screens produce a specific color or spectrum of light. The film used should be matched in sensitivity to the light spectrum of the screen.

Rare earth screens do need special x-ray films to produce an optimal radiograph. Every x-ray film manufacturer produces a rare earth type of x-ray film. The endless names and types of combinations of x-ray film and image-intensifying screens available on the market have led to great confusion. Again, please refer to Douglas et al (1987) and Morgan (1993) for more elaborate discussion of this important topic.

> **TECHNICIAN NOTE** Be sure that the x-ray film you are using is maximally sensitive to the spectrum of light that the screens are emitting.

Grids

When x-rays enter a patient, some pass straight through to the film cassette, but a great many are scattered or redirected along a different path before exiting the patient. The purpose of a grid is to control the scatter radiation before it reaches the x-ray cassette. A grid is constructed of a sheet of lead

TABLE 16-3	Technique Chart for Portable X-Ray Unit of 10 mA at 90-kV, 15 mA at 80-kV, and 20 mA at 70-kV Capacity Kodak Cassette When Rare Earth Screen of Regular Speed* Is Used				
EXAMINATION	**SIZE**	**VIEW**	**KVP**	**TIME, SEC**	**DISTANCE, CM**
Fetlock	Foal	DP or obliques	80	0.02	60
	Large adult		80	0.04	70
Carpus	Foal	DP or obliques	80	0.02	70
	Large adult		80	0.04	70
Tarsus	Foal	Lat	80	0.02	70
		DP	80	0.04	70
	Adult	Lat	80	0.04	70
		DP	80	0.08	70
Stifle	Adult	Lat	80	0.1	70
		CdCa	90	0.25	70

CdCa, Caudocranial; *DP*, dorsoplantar or dorsopalmar; *kV*, kilovolts; *kVp*, kilovolt peak; *Lat*, lateral; *mA*, milliamperes.
*For more complete treatment of cassette- and image-intensifying screens, refer to Douglas et al (1987) and Morgan (1993). Both have excellent discussions of all types of screens available on the market today.

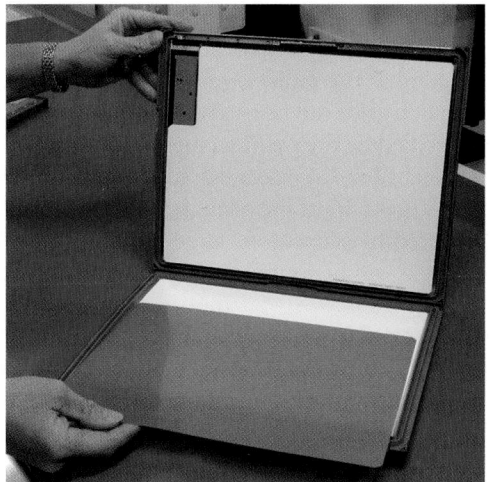

FIGURE 16-26 Screen film manufactured for the special purpose of being used with image-intensifying screens. Such film, when used with the proper screen, will drastically reduce x-ray exposure time.

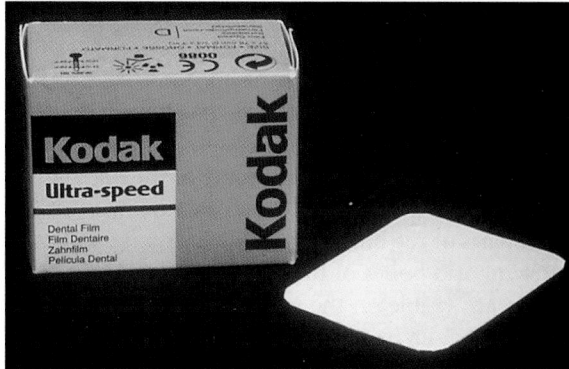

FIGURE 16-27 Prepackaged nonscreen film that can be used for dental and occlusal intraoral radiographic examinations. This type of film requires long exposure times because of the lack of intensifying screens. When this type of film is used, patients should be under general anesthetic, and the technician should take the exposure from outside the room or behind a radiation safety barrier.

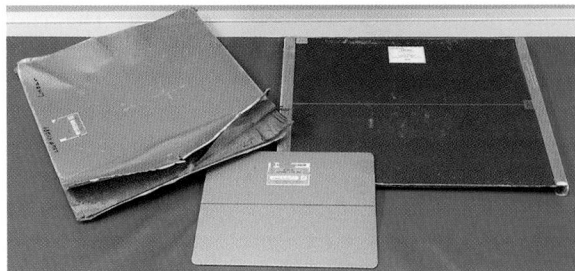

FIGURE 16-28 Three grids commonly used in veterinary radiology of large and small animals. The upper left grid has been damaged and opened, allowing visualization of hundreds of thin layers of metallic strips used to stop scatter radiation.

strips interfaced with radiolucent spacers made of plastic or aluminum. These strips are encased in an aluminum protective cover for durability. Grids come in various sizes, similar to x-ray cassettes, and are placed directly over the cassette between the animal and the cassette or, more commonly, in a special tray just under the x-ray table above the cassette tray (Figure 16-28).

The purpose of a grid is to allow only the primary x-ray beam to pass through, thereby preventing scatter radiation from reaching the film. The grid is constructed in such a way as to absorb all radiation that does not pass between the lead strips. This arrangement may absorb most scatter radiation if grids of high ratios are used. However, it has the disadvantage of absorbing part of the primary x-ray beam and therefore requires greater exposure time to obtain a given film density. Figure 16-29 shows how a grid absorbs scatter and secondary radiation and prevents it from reaching the film.

Grids are made of different ratios and numbers of strips per 2.5 cm. The ratio varies from 5:1 to 16:1 and from 60 lines (strips) per 2.5 cm to 120 lines per 2.5 cm. The higher the ratio and the greater the number of lines per 2.5 cm, the more radiation is absorbed by the grid. The *ratio of a grid* refers to the relation between the height of the lead strips and the width of the radiolucent spaces. For example, if the height of the lead strip is 12 times greater than the thickness of the space, the grid ratio will be 12:1, and if it is 10 times greater, the ratio will be 10:1. The greater the ratio, the more efficiently the grid absorbs scattered radiation. Figure 16-29, *A*, shows the ratio of a 5:1 grid. For veterinary work, a grid with a ratio of 8:1 at 103 lines per 2.5 cm is recommended.

The grid is most useful when parts of the body in which scattering is considerable are x-rayed; this in practice includes all thick parts of the body (e.g., thorax, abdomen, skull) and those joints and bones of thickness in excess of 10 cm. The grid lines are visible on the resulting film, but this is made up for by the increased resolution of the image on the radiograph.

Grids may be parallel or focused. A parallel grid is constructed with strips that are parallel to each other. A focused grid is one in which the lead strips and spacers are gradually angulated from the center to the periphery of the grid. The distance from the point of convergence, or the focal point,

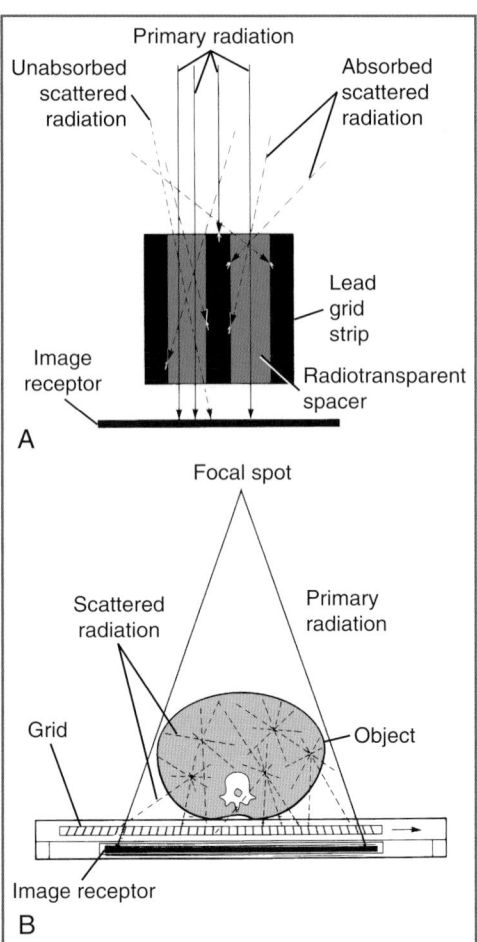

FIGURE 16-29 Cross section of a grid. **A,** Diagram of a small section of a grid showing how a large proportion of the scatter radiation is absorbed and image-forming primary radiation passes through to the image detector. **B,** Diagram of focused Potter-Bucky diaphragm being moved toward the right. (Modified from Eastman Kodak Company: *The fundamentals of radiography,* ed 12, Rochester, NY, 1980, Eastman Kodak, Radiographic Markets Division.)

is referred to as its *focal distance,* or *radius.* The advantage of a focused grid is that it allows unobstructed amounts of radiation to pass through it at the center and at the edge of the grid as long as the radiation is parallel to the axis of the lead strips. Such grids can be used only at a specific focal-film distance specified by the manufacturer. If distances above or below the focal-film distance are used, grid cutoff will occur, which means that part of the primary beam will be absorbed by the grid. With grid cutoff, large areas that are incompletely exposed will be found on the resulting radiograph.

Potter-Bucky Diaphragm

One other type of grid encountered in veterinary hospitals is the Potter-Bucky diaphragm. This is simply a movable grid. The movement of the diaphragm is timed to suit a particular exposure, and the grid moves across the film during the exposure so that the grid lines are not visible on the resulting film. When a movable grid is used, the exposure time must be increased by a factor of four, or the kilovoltage must be increased by about 20%. Usually, Potter-Bucky diaphragms are positioned under the table and are electronically linked to the timer of the x-ray machine (Figure 16-29, *B*).

Another method of reducing scatter radiation is the air gap technique. This simple technique consists of increasing the distance between the patient and the surface of the cassette. With this technique, the amount of scatter radiation produced is not reduced, but less scatter radiation reaches the film because of the increased distance between patient and film. With the air gap technique, it is not necessary to increase exposure factors, as must be done with a grid. However, this technique will decrease the sharpness of the image because of increased subject-to-film distance. It is less effective at high kilovoltage settings because higher-energy scatter occurs in a forward direction. This technique is used most commonly in veterinary radiology for magnification purposes.

> **TECHNICIAN NOTE** Always use a grid between the patient and the film cassette when the body part being x-rayed is greater than 10 cm thick.

THE DARKROOM

The importance of the darkroom in radiography cannot be overemphasized. Radiography unquestionably begins and ends in the darkroom, in which films are loaded into cassettes ready for exposure and are returned for processing into a finished radiograph. Most mistakes made in veterinary radiography are related to the processing of radiographs. It is necessary to keep the darkroom clean and light-proof. It is essential for the technician to have thorough knowledge of x-ray darkroom technique and of conventional or automatic processing. The chemicals should be changed, replenished, maintained, and mixed according to the strict directions of the manufacturer.

Equipment

A darkroom need not be spacious. For most veterinary practices, a small room of about 240 × 240 cm (8 × 8 feet) is adequate. However, it is essential that this room be made totally dark. If there is a window in the room, there is no reason not to open it for ventilation when the darkroom is not in use; however, the window should be light-proof when closed. One can easily determine whether a darkroom is light-proof by turning off all lights, including the safelight, closing the door tightly, and slowly turning around in the center of the darkroom while looking for any light leaking into the room. It is also important that a lock or a light-proof cylindrical entrance be placed on the door to prevent its being opened while films are being processed. A darkroom need not be completely dark because a safelight can be used during film processing. A safelight is a light bulb shielded by a plastic filter that stops any light to which the film is sensitive from penetrating the filter and entering the room. It is important that the safelight bulb not exceed the wattage recommended for the type of filter used; otherwise, the exposed films will be "fogged," or partially exposed, and the quality of the radiographs will be compromised. The proper type of light filter must be used in the darkroom. Orange, red, or yellow filters may be used with most x-ray films; but with the rare earth type of x-ray film, a special red filter must be used (Figure 16-30). No films should be exposed to the safelight any longer than is necessary. It is important to work rapidly but carefully when processing x-ray films and loading and unloading films in the cassettes.

A worktable should be placed in the darkroom for loading and unloading cassettes; it should be located as far away from the processor as possible, so that liquid or dry chemicals will not be spilled on it. Above or below the bench, shelves should be placed to store unexposed films and cassettes. X-ray film must be kept in a cool, dry place, protected from extraneous x-rays.

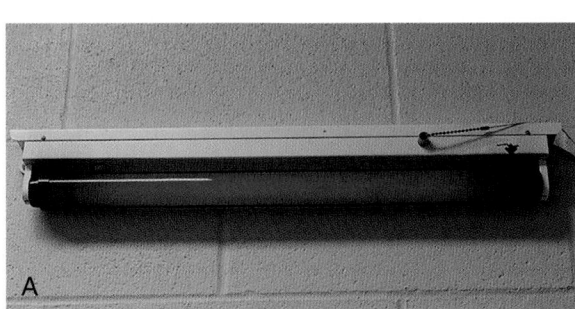
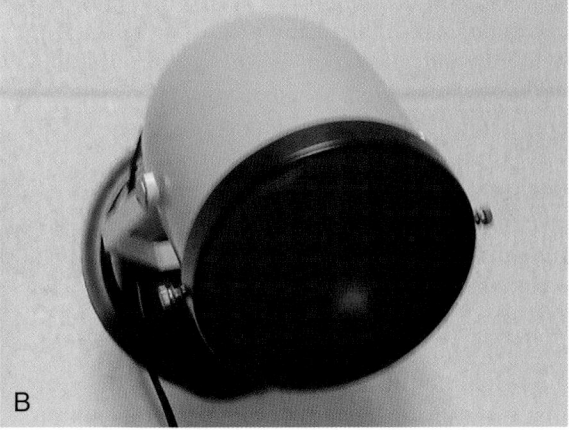

FIGURE 16-30 A and B, Two examples of darkroom safelights. The filters must be matched to the light sensitivity of the film being used in the darkroom and must not be cracked or incompletely sealed by the filter holder.

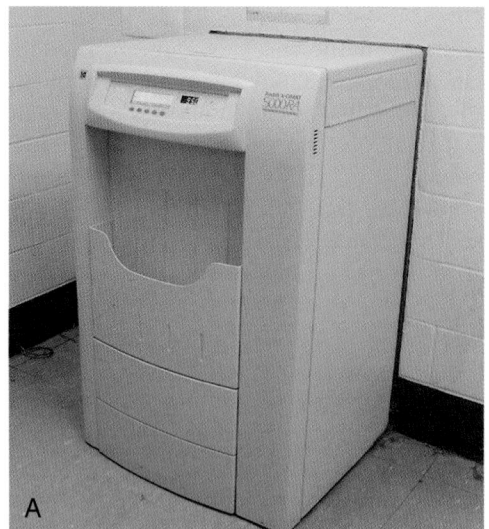

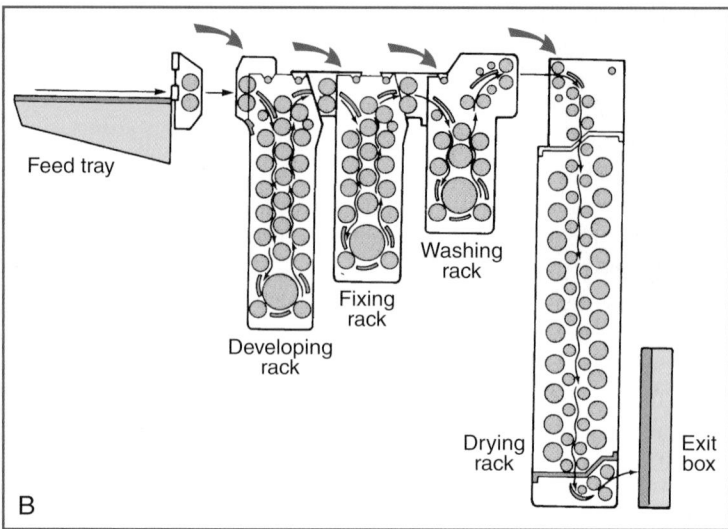

FIGURE 16-31 Automatic processor. **A,** Kodak X-OMAT processor (a 90-second processor). **B,** Diagram of the mechanism inside a typical automatic x-ray processor.

> *TECHNICIAN NOTE* Remember that all film and safelights are not created equal. Make sure the wavelength or color of light to which your film is sensitive is completely blocked by your safelight filter.

Automatic Film Processors

Several makes and sizes of automatic processors are available on the market. In recent years, most veterinary hospitals have invested in automatic processing systems, and hand developing methods have become outdated. Small-capacity, 90-second processor units can be installed in most darkrooms without remodeling. Larger processor units necessitate some remodeling because the input tray must be in the darkroom and the output side must be outside of the darkroom. Their use usually requires structural and plumbing modifications (Figure 16-31).

With automatic film processors, it is necessary to maintain fresh solution and to ensure that solutions are flowing properly within the processor. Automatic processors may speed up and standardize film processing but require similar, if not more, maintenance than hand processing tanks. It is important to provide ventilation in the darkroom when automatic processors are used. Usually, a good-quality, light-tight exhaust fan installed in the ceiling is adequate.

Film Storage

X-ray films must be handled and stored properly for maximum usefulness. The film must be protected from light, x-radiation, gamma radiation, heat, moisture, and pressure. All these hazards may result in film fogging and decreased radiograph quality. As has been mentioned, the darkroom can fulfill this function if the room is kept clean and free of moisture. It may be helpful if x-ray films are kept in their original boxes and placed in a cabinet. Special bins can be purchased to store x-ray films, but they

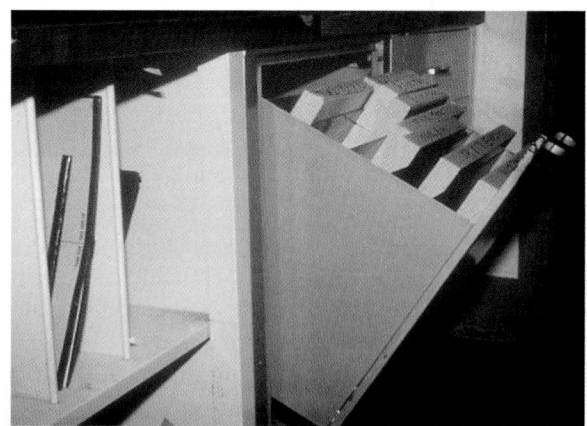

FIGURE 16-32 Film storage bin commonly used in a darkroom; it is designed to store open x-ray box films to load x-ray cassettes. This bin is wired to a switch that will automatically turn off the darkroom lights when opened.

are an unnecessary expense if proper care is used in storage (Figure 16-32).

Cassette Loading and Unloading

Care must be taken to prevent static electricity, bending, creasing, or scratching when x-ray film is transferred from its box to the x-ray cassette. The film should be handled carefully, held only by the corners, and pulled from the box using a slow and continuous motion (Figure 16-33). The film should be placed carefully into the cassette, and the edges should not extend over the edge of the film cassette. Great care should be taken to prevent damage to or soiling of the intensifying screen when x-ray film is removed from the cassette.

Handling X-Ray Film

When exposed films are placed in the automatic processor tray, they must be handled carefully. X-ray film is more

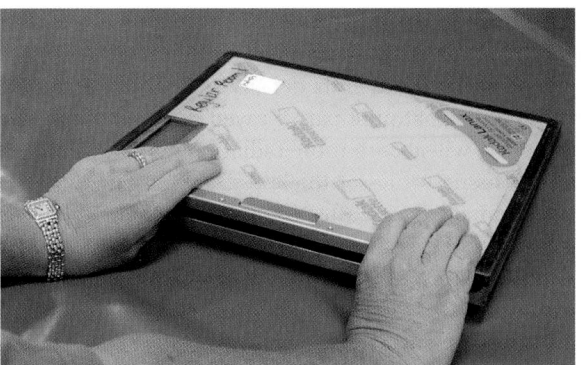

FIGURE 16-33 When loading a cassette, use both hands to prevent kink marks, and carefully place the film into the cassette. The cassette must be closed and latched gently.

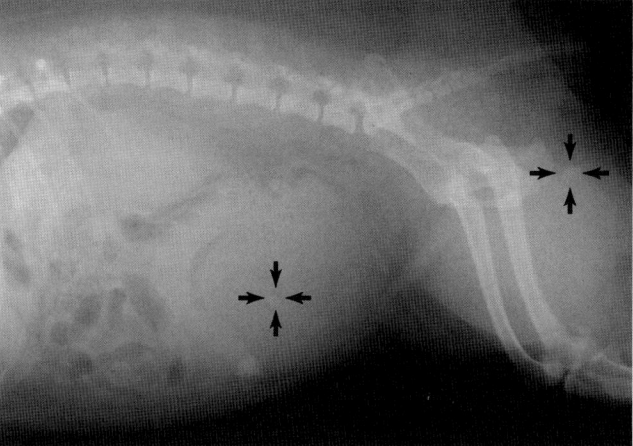

FIGURE 16-34 Lateral radiograph showing good radiographic detail and contrast. Round, mineral opaque structures (uroliths) are seen within the urinary bladder *(arrows near the middle)*. The urinary bladder is large as the result of obstruction by another stone within the urethra *(arrows on the right)*.

sensitive after exposure and before development than at any other time. The films should be handled only by the corners before and after processing. It is most important to have dry hands when handling exposed, nonprocessed films. Any developer or fixer solution that touches the film before processing will create an artifact on the processed film; however, this usually is not an issue with automated processors.

Silver Recovery

In larger veterinary practices, the silver contained within the x-ray film emulsion may be removed and recovered. Most of the silver that is not exposed to x-rays is not converted to metallic silver and accumulates within the fixer solution. Silver recovery units can be attached to the fixer solution to remove the silver by an electrolytic process. However, this practice is economical only for the larger-volume veterinary hospital. Silver can also be recovered from exposed and nonexposed x-ray film. A few companies specialize in recycling x-ray film for silver recovery. This could result in a small cost savings at the time an x-ray archive is purged of the old cases on file.

RADIOGRAPHIC FILM QUALITY

It is of utmost importance to produce radiographs of excellent quality to arrive at a radiographic diagnosis. A film of good diagnostic quality should provide excellent detail, correct scale of contrast, and optimal density (Figure 16-34). Each of these film characteristics is briefly discussed.

Detail

Radiographic detail refers to the degree of sharpness that defines the edge of an anatomic structure. It represents the best possible reproduction of an organ. Detail is influenced by every possible factor, but geometry and motion factors are more influential than others.

The focal-film distance (aka: source image distance, or SID) is one important factor in the loss of detail. If the focal spot is too close to the part x-rayed, magnification and lack of distinction will be noted at the margins of the structures. Therefore, it is important to keep the focal-film distance as long as possible without significantly reducing x-ray beam intensity. Most veterinary hospitals have radiographic technique charts that use a focal-film distance of 36 to 48 inches (80 to 110 cm). Furthermore, the object film distance (OFD) should be kept as short as possible to prevent image distortion due to magnification. This is why the goal is to have the object that is being examined as close to the x-ray detector as possible.

Movement in veterinary radiology is a constant problem, especially with older units that have a minimum exposure time of $\frac{1}{10}$ second. Movement can be due to respiration, intestinal movement, and patient movement. Sedation is necessary to prevent unsharpness due to patient movement, and mAs settings are adjusted to prevent blurring due to respiratory and bowel movement. It is difficult to produce diagnostic films of the thorax with a unit that does not have a minimum time of exposure of at least $\frac{1}{30}$ second and ideally $\frac{1}{120}$ second. With large animals, movement is a constant problem with a small, portable unit. This is why rare earth screens are becoming so popular in veterinary medicine; they offer the advantage of a much shorter required exposure time.

The size of the focal spot is another important factor that influences detail. The larger the focal spot, the poorer is the detail. Because most equipment in veterinary medicine has a rather large focal spot of 0.8 mm or greater, loss of detail may be significant, especially with older units that have focal spots of 1.2 to 2 mm. Therefore, it is important to place the part to be x-rayed as close as possible to the x-ray film. If the part is too far from the film, magnification and distortion will result in loss of detail. This is especially important in large animal radiology.

Other exposure factors that affect detail are poor filmscreen contact and overexposed or underexposed radiographs that often result from an improper technique chart or from carelessness. Poor radiographic processing causes more ruined radiographs than all other factors combined.

All processing errors affect detail. It is therefore important to standardize the developing process by following exactly the instructions of the manufacturer.

Radiographic Contrast

Radiographic contrast refers to the density or opacity difference between two areas on a radiograph. High contrast means that opacity differences are large and fewer shades of gray are present. High-contrast radiographs are very black and white. *Latitude* refers to the range of different opacities on the radiograph. Long-latitude radiographs have a much larger number of shades of gray, but the difference or contrast between shades is small. High-contrast radiographs are preferred for spine and extremity films. Long-latitude, low-contrast radiographs are preferred for thoracic films.

Kilovoltage is the exposure factor that has the greatest influence on radiographic contrast. The higher the kilovoltage, the greater the latitude, and therefore the greater the number of shades of black, gray, and white (lower contrast) (Figure 16-35). Absorption of the x-ray beam at high kilovoltage is more uniform among the various tissues in the body, resulting in less contrast. Therefore for thoracic examinations, a high-kilovoltage technique is recommended. For skeletal studies, a lower-kilovoltage technique is recommended to produce a higher-contrast image.

Other factors that reduce contrast are scatter radiation (which can be greatly decreased by the use of a grid), light leakage, and rapid, high-temperature processing techniques.

Radiographic Density

Radiographic density refers to the degree of blackness of the film. It is the result of the amount of light that was transmitted to the x-ray film after interaction of the crystals in intensifying screens with the x-ray beam. When a film is properly exposed, the anatomic part x-rayed will have good contrast with good differential absorption of the x-ray beam by various tissue densities. Therefore, the part should be seen clearly but should not be so dark as to overexpose anatomic structures to the degree that they are difficult to differentiate from the background film density. The thickness and the density of the anatomic part x-rayed do affect density. The thickest part will absorb more radiation, sometimes as much as denser tissues of lesser thickness.

The primary factor affecting density is the mAs setting. As has been discussed, the mAs factor is a quantity factor that regulates the quantity of x-rays produced. If more x-rays reach the film, more light will be emitted by the screens, and the film will be darker. Therefore, it can be stated that high mAs settings will increase film density, and low mAs settings will reduce film density.

Another factor that affects film density is the kilovoltage setting. At a higher kilovoltage, the x-ray tube is more efficient in producing x-rays and therefore increases the energy level of x-rays produced. If all other exposure and development factors are kept constant, increasing the kilovoltage will increase the radiographic density. This effect is more apparent at lower-kilovoltage settings for a given part than at higher-kilovoltage settings.

The distance from the focal spot to the surface of the film is another important factor in film density. If everything remains constant except the distance, a given radiograph could be substantially overexposed if the distance is reduced, or it could be underexposed if the distance is increased. This effect can be dramatic because the intensity of the radiation is reduced or increased as the square of the distance is changed. This effect is discussed in the section regarding inverse square law (see page 530) and does emphasize the need for consistency and for accurate measurement of the focal-film distance.

Magnification

Magnification is a technique that is rarely used in veterinary practices, but it is popular in veterinary teaching hospitals. Magnification is based on the principle that a larger image of an anatomic structure can be obtained if the distance

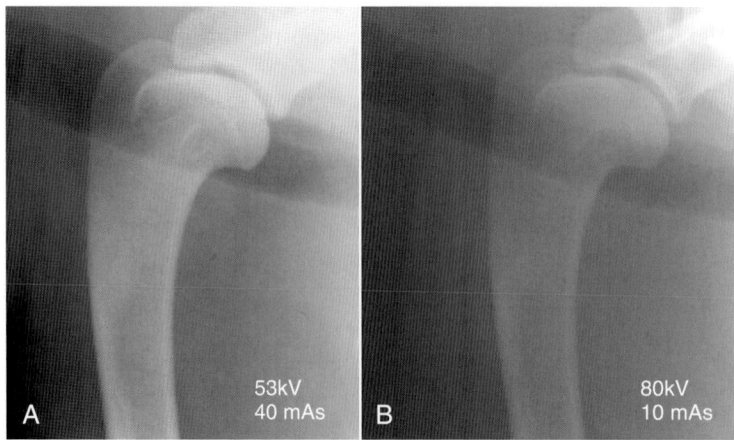

FIGURE 16-35 Mediolateral radiograph of the shoulder showing high (**A**) and low (**B**) contrast. In **A**, the kilovolt peak (kVp) is set at 53, whereas in **B**, it is set at 80. In **B**, little difference in opacity between bone and soft tissue leads to a low-contrast image, caused by nondiscriminating absorption of the higher-energy x-ray beam.

between the object and the film is increased. Generally, the object to be magnified is placed halfway between the film cassette and the focal spot of the x-ray tube. This results in an x-ray image that is twice as large as the actual anatomic structure. However, to obtain diagnostic films, it is necessary to have a small focal spot. A focal spot of 0.3 mm or smaller is needed for radiographic magnification. If larger focal spots are used, the advantage of direct magnification is lost because of blurring at the margin of an organ produced by the larger focal spot. This technique would be useful for veterinarians, especially for studies of extremities in small dogs and cats and for studies of the skull.

Technical Errors and Artifacts

Several errors can be made in handling x-ray films or in setting up a technique for an examination. In general, these errors will reduce the quality of the radiograph and in certain cases may nullify its diagnostic value. Boxes 16-2 and 16-3 are intended to help the technician identify causes of errors and take corrective measures. Box 16-2 summarizes technical errors other than those that occur as a result of film processing. Box 16-3 summarizes errors caused by poor film processing. See Case Presentation 16-1 for analysis of a thoracic radiographic study of a patient that had been hit by a car; this account illustrates how radiographic artifacts can confound accurate diagnosis.

The advent of automatic processing equipment has helped tremendously in eliminating many errors made in hand tank processing techniques. It has standardized film processing and has made it easier to trace the causes of processing mistakes, which usually are mechanically related. Even with automatic processors, many mistakes can be made; these must be recognized and corrected for the best possible radiographs to be obtained.

Several other mechanical failures may occur with automatic processors. It is important to keep the processor clean at all times. It is especially important to wash the roller assembly thoroughly at least once each week. Processors are sophisticated machines that must be serviced regularly by professionals. It is unreasonable and cost-ineffective for a veterinarian to expect the technician to service the processor. However, it is the responsibility of the technician to be able to recognize processor problems and correct them when possible. It is also the technician's responsibility to keep the processor clean at all times and to ensure that fresh developer and fixer solutions are provided as needed.

RADIATION SAFETY

Few diagnoses in medicine or surgery cannot be aided by the use of diagnostic radiology. Therefore, it behooves technicians to be aware of the hazards of using x-rays or any other type of ionizing radiation. It is the responsibility of the veterinarian to ensure that proper radiation safety measures are observed in the hospital. It is also the veterinarian's responsibility to instruct the technician in proper use of the equipment and to ensure that the design of the x-ray room meets state regulations.

BOX 16-2	Technical Errors

Increased Film Density
    Too high mAs or kV settings
    Too short focal-film distance
    Wrong measurement of anatomic part
    Equipment malfunction
    Speed of intensifying screen too fast

Decreased Film Density
    Too low mAs or kV settings
    Too long focal-film distance
    Wrong measurement of anatomic part
    Speed of intensifying screen too slow

Black Marks or Artifacts
    Film scratches
    Crescent mark from rough handling
    Static electricity (linear dots or tree pattern)
    Top of film black, resulting from exposure to light while still in box
    Defective cassette that does not close properly, exposing margins of film to light

White Marks (Artifacts)
    Dirt or debris between film and screen
    Defect or crack in screen
    Contrast medium on tabletop, skin, or cassette

Gray Film
    Film accidentally exposed to radiation (scatter, secondary, or direct)
    Lack of grid for examination of a thick part
    Outdated film
    Film stored in a too hot or too humid place

Distorted or Blurred Radiograph
    Motion: patient, cassette, or machine
    Too great object-film distance, causing magnification and distortion
    Poor film-screen contact
    Poor centering of primary x-ray beam

Linear Artifacts
    Gridlines
    Grid out of focal range
    Primary beam not centered
    Grid upside down
    Grid damage, causing distorted gridlines

Miscellaneous Artifacts
    Cone cut, causing underexposed margins
    Target damage, resulting in inconsistent film density: requires tube replacement
    Double exposure
    Blank film: faulty equipment, nonexposed film processed

---

kV, Kilovolts; *mAs,* milliamperes per second.

All animal tissues are sensitive to radiation, that is, absorption of radiation doses above a certain minimum roentgen value will change or alter the tissue. The following tissues (not in order of sensitivity) are most readily affected by ionizing radiation: skin, lymphatics, hematopoietic and

BOX 16-3	Common Technical Errors With Automatic Processors

Increased Density
Temperature of developer too high
Overreplenishment
Light leak from cover or in darkroom
Speed too slow
Faulty thermostat

Decreased Density
Temperature of developer too low
Underreplenishment
Exhausted developer, necessitating thorough cleaning of tanks every 6 months
Faulty thermostat

Processing Streaks
Crossover rollers dirty
Dirty wash water
Air tubes need cleaning

Scratches on Film
Guide shoes misaligned or dirty
Dryer air tubes malpositioned

Wet or Damp Film
Thermostat malfunction
Dryer temperatures too low
Insufficient air venting
Film not hardened sufficiently

Film Overlap
Film fed too rapidly into processor
Tension on rollers too high

leukopoietic (blood-forming) tissues, breast, thyroid, bone (especially the epiphysis or growing centers), and the germinal epithelium or gonads. These tissues are sensitive to all forms of ionizing radiation. All animal species are affected, including humans, even though different degrees of sensitivity have been noted among species. The more rapidly dividing tissues are affected most by radiation.

Technicians should remember that one of the best means of protection at their disposal is to take care to avoid retakes. Careful attention to patient positioning, thickness measurements, setting techniques, and film processing will decrease the need for radiograph retakes and will reduce technician and patient radiation exposure. See Chapter 4 for additional radiation safety information.

Radiation Filtration

The x-ray beam is a composite or spectrum of x-ray photons of various energy levels. The kVp setting is the highest energy level within the beam, but there are photons of all levels from the kVp setting on down. The useful portion of the x-ray beam (the portion that passes through the patient to interact with film and screens) is the upper two-thirds of the energy levels. The lower third of the x-ray beam energies is too weak to pass through the patient. This radiation is called *soft radiation*. It is of no use for image formation and only causes increased radiation exposure for the patient. Aluminum has a marked effect on filtration of softer (lower energy level) x-rays. Insertion of 1 or 2 mm of an aluminum filter into the path of the primary beam at the portal of the x-ray tube is essential to filter out or absorb the soft x-rays that are a component of all x-ray beams in the diagnostic range. By absorbing this soft radiation, the filter reduces the amount of radiation absorbed by the patient. Increased aluminum filtration also generally improves latitude and detail by improving the quality of the x-ray beam.

Radiation Measurement

To understand radiation safety and radiation dose units of measurement, it is necessary to define a few terms commonly used in the measurement of radiation exposure.

Roentgen

The *roentgen* (R) is defined as a unit of radiation exposure that will liberate a charge of 2.58×10^{-4} coulombs per kilogram of air. Roentgens are a measure of radiation exposure or x-ray machine output and generally are evaluated with an ionization chamber placed below the primary x-ray beam. As an example, 1 R is the approximate exposure to the body surface for an anteroposterior radiograph of the abdomen for an average adult human.

Rad

The unit of absorbed dose of ionizing radiation is called a **rad**. It is the energy imparted by ionizing radiation to a unit mass of irradiated material and is equal to 100 ergs/g of tissue. The number of rads deposited in tissue per roentgen of radiation exposure varies with the energy of the x-ray beam and with the composition of the absorber.

Rem

Rem is an abbreviation for rad equivalent man; it is the product of the dose in rads and the relative biological effectiveness of the radiation used. This unit of measurement makes allowance for the fact that the effect of radiation on different tissues varies with the type of radiation or the relative biological effectiveness. A rem is equal to the absorbed radiation dose in rads multiplied by a quality factor:

$$Rem = Rads \times Quality\ factor$$

Because the quality factor for diagnostic radiation is 1, for all practical purposes in veterinary practice, 1 rem = 1 rad. For larger particles of radiation, such as neutrons, protons, and alpha particles, the quality factor increases from 3 to 20. These larger, more dangerous particles of radiation are not emitted from diagnostic x-ray machines.

Old units such as rad, roentgen (R), and rem have been replaced with SI units. Box 16-4 lists conversions to the new units of gray (Gy), coulomb/kg (C/kg), and sieverts (Sv).

CASE PRESENTATION 16-1 RADIOGRAPHIC STUDY OF A PATIENT RECENTLY HIT BY A CAR

A 6-year-old, male, intact Labrador retriever was presented for examination and diagnostic workup after being hit by a car. The patient was ambulatory and alert on presentation but had a respiratory rate of 60 breaths per minute (N 10-30 breaths per minute). The attending veterinarian ordered routine thoracic radiographs to rule out pulmonary contusions, rib fractures, and pneumothorax. Ventrodorsal (VD) and lateral thoracic radiographs were taken to assess the heart and lungs (Figure 1). Evaluation of the VD view reveals sharply margin-ated lines that appear on the right and left sides of the thorax (see arrows). What do you think could cause the linear mark-ings? What could be done to determine whether this radio-graphic finding is significant?

Answer

These markings are compatible with an air/lung interface resulting from a pneumothorax (presence of air in the pleural space due to leakage from a damaged lung) or an artifact due to the presence of prominent skin folds between the caudal aspect of the forelimbs and the chest wall. The attending veterinarian was uncertain whether this finding was significant and requested an additional view to differentiate these causes.

The technician acquired a VD oblique view by tilting the dog's sternum approximately 15 to 20 degrees to the left (Figure 2). (Note that when this view is acquired, the sternum may also be tilted to the right.) If pneumothorax were present, the lines would remain and would represent the retracted lung lobes caused by the presence of air in the pleural space. The lines in this case are due to superimposition of skin folds over the chest cavity, and so are not indicative of disease. This artifact is commonly seen in dogs, is sometimes seen in cats, and is commonly mistaken for pneumothorax. This case illustrates the importance of identifying and preventing radiographic artifacts to maximize the diagnostic value of a radiographic study.

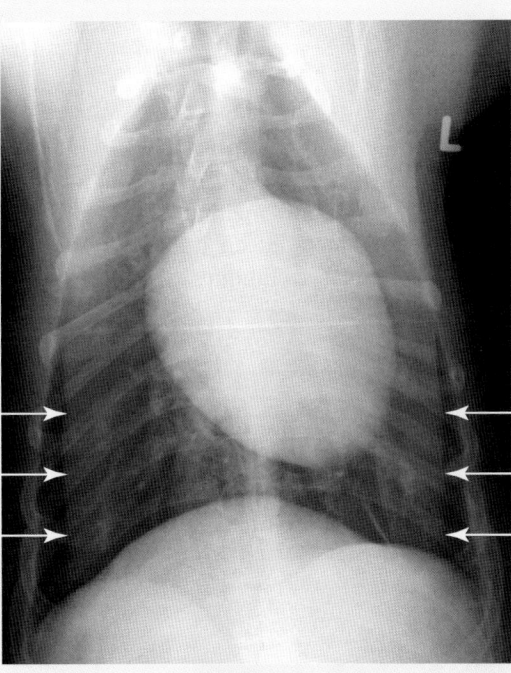

FIGURE 1

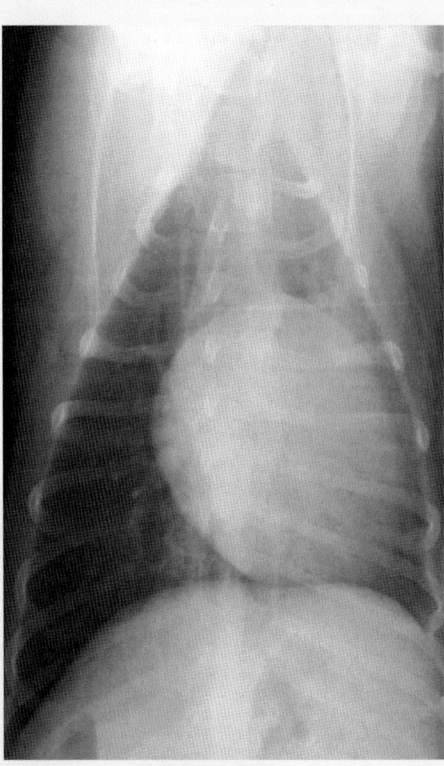

FIGURE 2

Maximum Permissible Dose

The maximum permissible dose (MPD) should be of great interest to the veterinary technician because it is the maximum dose of radiation a person is allowed to receive during occupational exposure over a specified time. This dose is not to exceed 5 rem per year or 1.25 rem in a quarter (13 weeks). The maximum accumulated dose is calculated as: 1(N − 18) rem, where *N* is age in years. N 18 indicates that an individual should not have occupational exposure to radiation before the age of 18. The technician should remem-ber that the MPD is the dose that the U.S. Nuclear Regula-tory Commission has determined should not harm the person receiving it during her or his lifetime. The MPD is maximum occupational exposure allowed by law; techni-cians should try to keep radiation exposure as low as possible by carefully following radiation safety practices.

BOX 16-4	Conversions to New Units of Gray (Gy), Coulombs/kg (C/kg), and Sieverts (Sv)

The rad (rad) is replaced by the gray (Gy): 1 kilorad (krad) = 10 gray (Gy), 1 rad (rad) = 10 milligray (mGy), 1 millirad (mrad) = 10 microgray (μGy), 1 microrad (μrad) = 10 nanogray (nGy)

The gray (Gy) replaces the rad (rad): 1 gray (Gy) = 100 rad (rad), 1 milligray (mGy) = 100 millirad (mrad), 1 microgray (μGy) = 100 microrad (μrad), 1 nanogray (nGy) = 100 nanorad (nrad)

The roentgen (R) is replaced by coulombs/kg (C/kg): 1 kiloroentgen (kR) ≈ 258 millicoulomb/kg (mC/kg), 1 roentgen (R) ≈ 258 microcoulomb/kg (μC/kg), 1 milliroentgen (mR) ≈ 258 nanocoulomb/kg (nC/kg), 1 microroentgen (μR) ≈ 258 picocoulomb/kg (pC/kg)

Coulomb/kg (C/kg) replaces the roentgen (R): 1 coulomb/kg (C/kg) ≈ 3876 roentgen (R), 1 millicoulomb/kg (mC/kg) ≈ 3876 milliroentgen (mR), 1 microcoulomb/kg (μC/kg) ≈ 3876 microroentgen (μR), 1 nanocoulomb/kg (nC/kg) ≈ 3876 nanoroentgen (nR)

The rem (rem) is replaced by the sievert (Sv): 1 kilorem (krem) = 10 sievert (Sv), 1 rem (rem) = 10 millisievert (mSv), 1 millirem (mrem) = 10 microsievert (μSv), 1 microrem (μrem) = 10 nanosievert (nSv)

The sievert (Sv) replaces the rem (rem): 1 sievert (Sv) = 100 rem (rem), 1 millisievert (mSv) = 100 millirem (mrem), 1 microsievert (μSv) = 100 microrem (μrem), 1 nanosievert (nSv) = 100 nanorem (nrem)

Personal Monitoring

To protect staff members from overexposure, the radiation that each person receives can be measured on a film badge. A film badge is a container that holds a special film designed to record a wide range of exposures. The film holder incorporates several different types of metal filters that permit differentiation of types of ionizing radiation exposures. This badge should be worn outside the apron on the collar at the level of the thyroid gland (Figure 16-36). Film badges can be exposed by heat, pressure, and chemical fumes. The film badge should be taken care of and stored outside the radiology area so that the amount of radiation it detects is actually the amount to which the person is occupationally exposed.

Radiation monitoring badges come in several forms: rings, clips, and wrist badges. Several companies offer a badge service. These badges are mailed back to the company and are analyzed on a monthly or quarterly basis.

Film badge readings are reported in millirem (mrem), or $\frac{1}{1000}$ rem. The annual MPD equals 5000 mrem. Technicians using x-ray machines should insist that the veterinarian for whom they work provide them with a radiation monitoring device.

Protection Officer

Every veterinary hospital should have an employee who is in charge of radiation safety. His or her responsibilities should include maintaining badges, ensuring that the x-ray machine is properly calibrated, and maintaining a good exposure control system that includes an updated technique chart system. Low-exposure techniques that provide quality

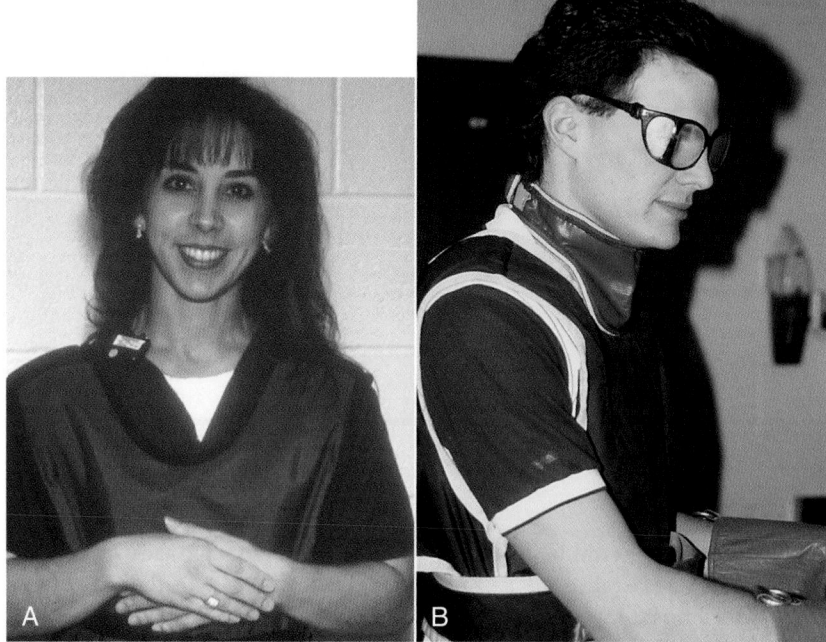

FIGURE 16-36 Each technician working in radiology should have a film badge to measure occupational radiation exposure. **A,** The film badge should be worn outside the lead apron at the level of the upper neck. This technician also wears a ring badge inside her lead gloves to measure the dose to the hands. **B,** This technician, who works in a busy radiology department, wears leaded glasses and a thyroid shield, in addition to gloves and an apron.

diagnostic radiographs should be the ultimate goal. Safe, reliable radiography equipment that is clean and, in the case of digital equipment, calibrated correctly, with software that is regularly updated, and with a server that can handle the quantity of data necessary to efficiently operate the veterinary practice is imperative. A reliable shielding program *requiring* all staff to follow the ALARA (as low as reasonably achievable) principle whenever they are creating an image is equally important. The employee in charge of this essential part of the veterinary practice must ensure that compliance with all government regulations is a priority.

Protection Practices

- Always use a collimator and always use the smallest possible aperture that will cover the anatomic area of interest (Figure 16-37).
- Make sure that an aluminum filter is present at the portal of the x-ray tube. This is needed to protect the patient, not the technician.
- Make sure that proper exposure factors are used, to prevent the need for retakes.
- Make sure the animal is positioned properly the first time—again, to prevent the need for retakes. This is even more important with increased use of digital imaging, which allows rapid image acquisition and viewing and lends itself to abuse through frequent reexposures and patient positioning readjustments.
- Never permit any part of your body to be in the path of the primary x-ray beam, even if it is covered by lead shielding. Protective equipment is designed to protect your body from scatter radiation. It is of no use if the body part is placed in the primary beam.
- Protection includes use of your well-maintained lead gloves, apron, thyroid shield, and lead glasses, if your practice provides them. If this basic safety equipment is not provided, you have three choices: Purchase your own, ask the practice managers to make the purchase, or change jobs!

- Always wear an apron, a thyroid shield, and gloves when holding an animal, or if you must be in the room when an exposure is made. The apron, gloves, and thyroid shield should have a 0.5-mm lead equivalent minimum to ensure good protection from secondary and scatter radiation. Lead eyewear is becoming commonplace in veterinary practice as more technicians and veterinarians become aware of the damage that long-term radiation exposure can cause to the lenses of their eyes (Figures 16-38 and 16-39).

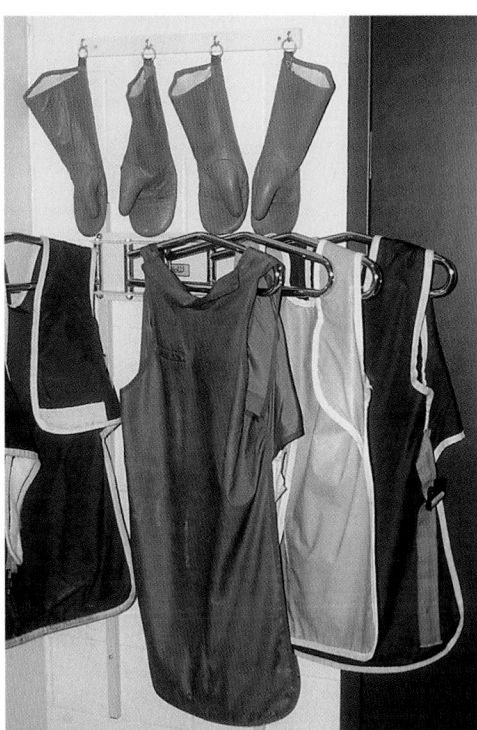

FIGURE 16-38 Aprons and gloves on a stand. It is important to keep the apron on a stand and the gloves well aerated when not in use, to increase the useful life of these items. The apron should have a minimum of 0.5 mm of lead equivalent.

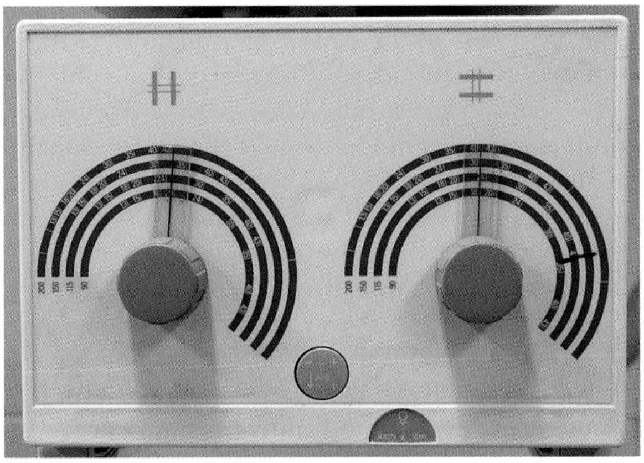

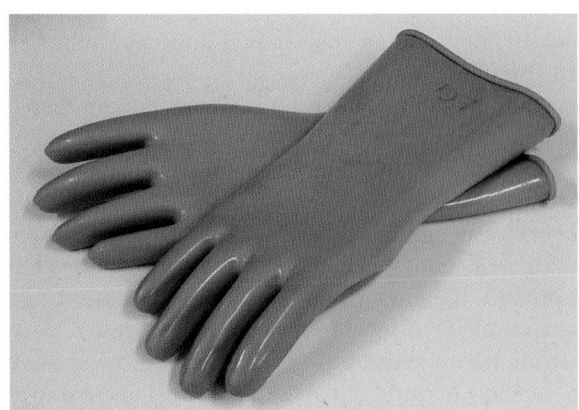

FIGURE 16-37 A collimator is used to limit the size of the x-ray beam to the part to be examined. By coning down on the area of interest, the amount of scatter and secondary radiation can be drastically reduced, improving image quality and decreasing technician exposure.

FIGURE 16-39 Lead gloves should have a minimum of 0.5 mm of lead equivalent; 1 mm of lead equivalent is ideal. They should always be worn when restraint is needed for examination.

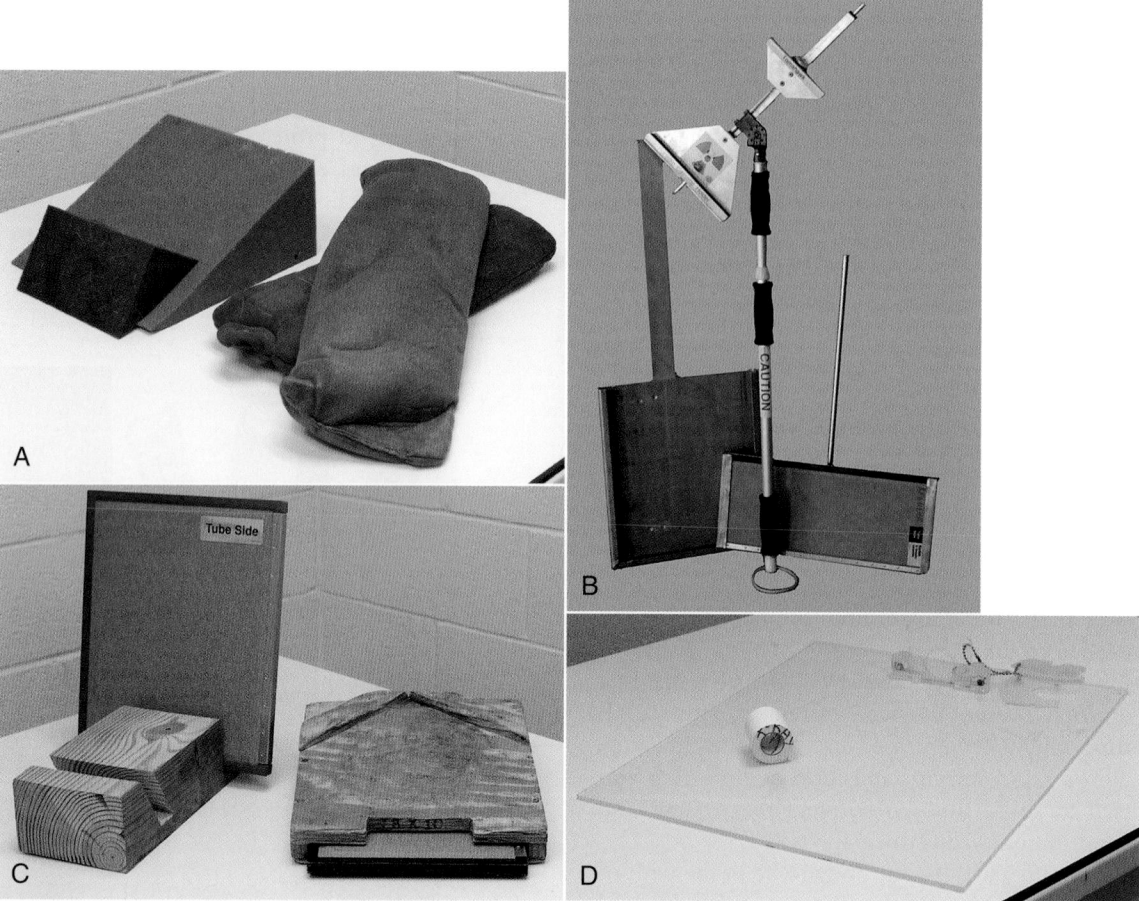

FIGURE 16-40 Several commercially available positioning devices can be used to help position animals and reduce the time needed to perform the examination. **A,** Various foam wedges and sandbags used to position small animals. **B,** Cassette holders for large animal examinations. **C,** Wood blocks for examination of large animal feet. **D,** Lucite tray with neck restraint holder for avian radiology. Porous tape is used to position wings on anesthetized birds.

- Use accessory equipment designed to reduce radiation exposure, such as cassette holders, restraining devices, and positioning devices (Figures 16-40 and 16-41).
- Anesthesia or tranquilization of the patient should be provided every time an animal cannot be controlled easily and adequately for a given examination.
- Only required personnel should be in the examining room at the time of exposure. A pregnant woman should not be in the room, nor should anyone younger than 18 years.
- If you have to restrain manually, and you are therefore unable to leave the room, *always look away* and lean back as far as possible from the x-ray table when you are taking an exposure.
- *Dose creep* is a term used in digital radiography to describe the incremental increases in technique made in an attempt to reduce the amount of "noise" adversely affecting the quality of the image. Technicians should never increase technique and therefore personal and patient exposure to potentially harmful radiation in an effort to cut down on noise.
- Use good, fast screens to reduce the milliamperage settings as much as possible.

> **TECHNICIAN NOTE** When working in radiology, always remember the "big three" of radiation safety: time, distance, and shielding.

Radiation safety is a frame of mind. It is a habit, and it requires awareness of the danger of radiation. It is easy to become careless with radiation because it is invisible, tasteless, and odorless and produces no external stimulation at diagnostic levels. Technicians should always remember that although invisible, radiation is dangerous to one's health. X-ray effects are cumulative. The ionization that results from continued exposure to x-rays and other high-energy rays constitutes the cumulative effect. These rays can destroy all living tissue if absorbed doses are high enough. Secondary radiation is less harmful than primary radiation but is still extremely harmful. Therefore, carelessness has no place in radiology. Remember the big three methods of radiation protection: time, distance, and shielding. Time means avoiding retakes; do it right the first time. Lower the time of exposure; keep the mAs as low as possible to still produce diagnostic radiographs. Distance means staying as far away

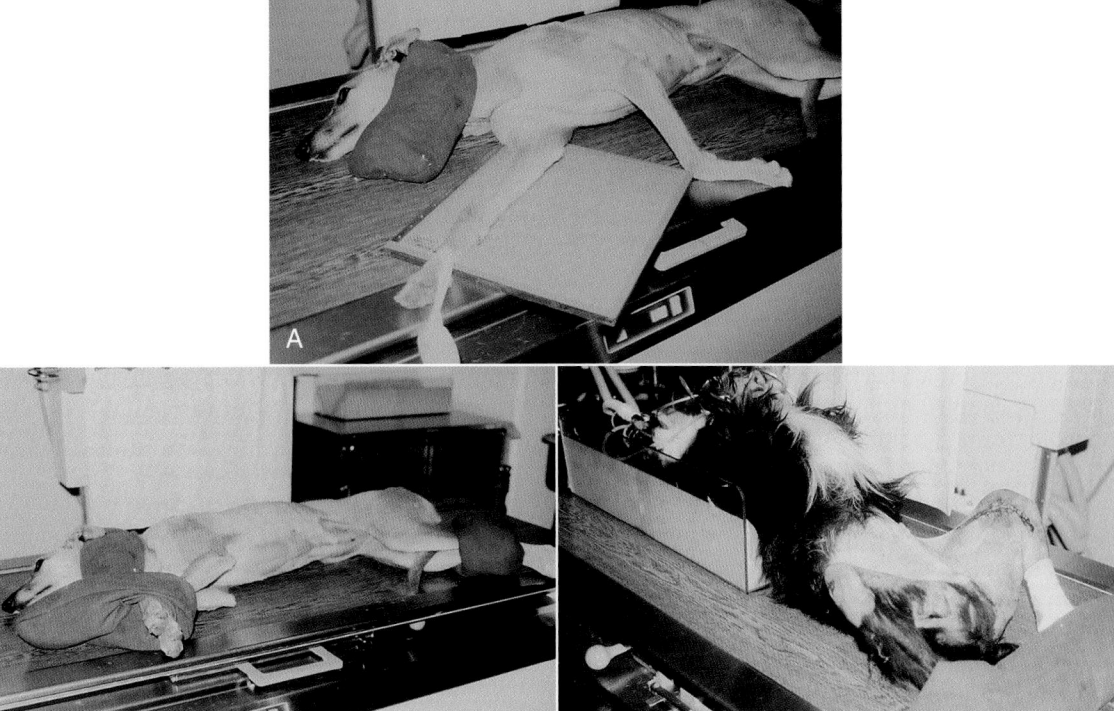

FIGURE 16-41 A, Sandbags and porous tape can help position tranquilized patients for some extremity radiographs. B, Sandbags can take the place of manual restraint for lateral thoracic and abdominal radiographs. C, The use of lucite positioning trays and sandbags can often take the place of manual restraint in postoperative radiography.

as possible from the patient and the x-ray beam. Shielding means always wearing an apron and gloves. It is important to take care of your apron and gloves. Hang them carefully after use, and do not allow the apron to be folded. Careless handling causes creases and cracks to develop in the gloves and aprons, reducing their effectiveness.

RADIOGRAPHIC CONTRAST AGENTS

In radiology, contrast means density difference. In many radiographic examinations, natural or inherent contrast of the anatomy is insufficient for a diagnosis to be made; this is especially true in gastrointestinal, urogenital, and spinal cord disease. The addition of positive or negative contrast medium can increase the radiographic density difference between anatomic structures, increasing the likelihood of correct image interpretation. In veterinary medicine, the following four types of contrast media are used (Figure 16-42):

1. Radiolucent gases: air, nitrous oxide, carbon dioxide
2. Insoluble inert radiopaque medium: barium sulfate
3. Soluble ionic radiopaque medium: iothalamate, diatrizoate
4. Soluble nonionic radiopaque medium: iohexol, iopamidol

Radiolucent gases absorb small amounts of radiation, resulting in images of greatly reduced radiographic opacity. These agents are used primarily in double-contrast gastrograms, double-contrast cystograms, and, rarely, pneumoperitoneography. Contraindications for their use are noted

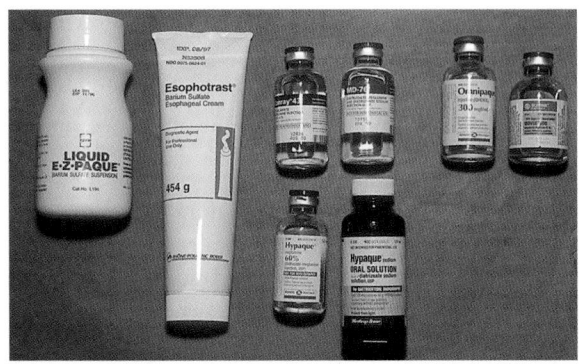

FIGURE 16-42 Positive-contrast medium used in veterinary radiology. The first two containers are barium to be used orally or rectally only. The next four contain ionic iodinated contrast, and the last two on the right hold nonionic iodinated contrast.

primarily in patients with severe hemorrhagic cystitis, in which the likelihood for gas absorption into the circulation is increased. Nitrous oxide and carbon dioxide are considered safer than room air because their increased solubility is less likely to cause serious air embolization.

Barium sulfate has a high atomic number and absorbs a large amount of radiation, resulting in greatly increased radiographic opacity. It is used almost exclusively for upper and lower gastrointestinal examinations. Barium sulfate is inert, nonabsorbed, and fairly soothing to the gastrointestinal tract. It coats the gastrointestinal mucosa better than organic iodides, improving visualization of the luminal surface. Barium sulfate is available in powder, paste, or liquid form. Micropulverized, solubilized barium sulfate solutions are vastly superior to powdered barium sulfate products because of increased uniformity of the mucosal coating. Contraindications for use include severe constipation and upper or lower bowel perforations. As with all oral contrast media, care should be taken when treating patients with known aspiration pneumonia or a high likelihood of aspiration.

Soluble radiopaque ionic contrast media include iothalamate and diatrizoate. The negatively charged iothalamate and diatrizoate are benzoic acid derivatives with three iodine molecules. They are coupled with positively charged sodium or meglumine to form a soluble salt. The high atomic number of iodine increases radiation absorption and increases radiographic opacity. These products can be used orally for gastrointestinal examinations; intravascularly for venous or arterial studies and excretory urography; in the peritoneal cavity, bladder, and urethra; intra-articularly; in draining wounds for fistulography; and in salivary ducts for sialography. Ionic organic iodides should not be used in the respiratory tract, nor should they be used intrathecally for myelography. Because ionic iodides are essentially hyperosmolar salt solutions, when used intravascularly they can result in an increase in intravascular fluid volume followed by an osmotic diuresis. The hyperosmolarity can cause diarrhea when ionic iodides are administered orally. Because of these properties, these agents are contraindicated in dehydrated patients and in patients with known iodine sensitivity.

The newest class of positive contrast agents includes the nonionic organic iodides, represented by iohexol, iopamidol, and iotolan. These agents can be used similarly to ionic organic iodides but offer the advantage of not dissociating into positively and negatively charged ions in solution. This allows the agents to be used intrathecally (in the cerebrospinal fluid space around the spinal cord) for myelography and everywhere ionic iodides can be used. These contrast agents are still hyperosmolar but much less so than the ionic organic iodides. They appear to have a lower incidence of adverse effects and contrast reactions but with the disadvantage of increased costs.

Organic iodides (both ionic and nonionic) may cause serious contrast reactions or adverse effects when given intravenously, intra-arterially, or intrathecally. These reactions are much less likely when the agents are used orally. Contrast reactions include nausea and vomiting, hypotension, cardiac arrest, and anaphylaxis. These reactions occur infrequently, but it is advisable to have a catheter in place as well as rapid access to fluids, oxygen, endotracheal tubes, and cardiopulmonary resuscitation drugs during organic iodide contrast procedures. Do not leave these patients unattended after contrast administration. For a thorough discussion of contrast media and contrast procedures, see Douglas et al (1987), Han and Hurd (2005), Lavin (2006), Morgan (1993), and Thrall (2007).

Common Contrast Media and Applications
Esophagus
Contrast agents. Barium sulfate, 100% weight/volume (wt/vol) suspension, is used alone and diluted to evaluate an enlarged esophagus or as a thick paste if the esophagus is not enlarged. Barium mixed with food may be more appropriate for diagnosis of esophageal strictures. Oral organic iodides (ionic or nonionic) are used when perforation of the esophagus is suspected.

Procedure. No special preparation is needed. Ideally, the study is done by using fluoroscopy. If this is not available, the exposure must be made when the animal swallows. Barium is administered with a syringe into the buccal pouch.

Stomach and Small Bowel (Upper Gastrointestinal Studies)
Contrast agents. Three types of contrast agents are used for upper gastrointestinal studies: barium sulfate 25% to 30% (wt/vol), oral iodides, and negative contrast, including air, carbon dioxide, and nitrous oxide. Barium sulfate is the most commonly used agent for upper gastrointestinal studies when perforation is not suspected. Negative contrast media are used in combination with barium sulfate for double-contrast studies. Oral iodinated products are given when perforation is suspected because barium sulfate will not be resorbed once it leaks into a body cavity.

Procedure. Food should be withheld for 24 hours, and warm water enemas should be administered about 2 to 3 hours before the gastrointestinal study is performed. Acepromazine can be used without adverse effects on gastrointestinal motility.

Dosage. The dosage for barium sulfate is 10 ml/kg, and for oral Hypaque or Gastrografin, 3 ml/kg.

Film sequence. The survey film consists of a ventrodorsal and a lateral view. Immediately after administration of contrast medium, four films should be taken to completely evaluate the stomach: a ventrodorsal view, a dorsoventral view, and both right and left lateral views. At 15, 30, and 60 minutes, the film sequence consists of ventrodorsal and right lateral views. These same views are taken at various intervals until contrast reaches the large bowel. The timing sequence will vary with the patient and the suspected disease process.

Large Bowel (Lower Gastrointestinal Study, Barium Enema)
Contrast agents. Barium sulfate 10% to 15% (wt/vol) or iodinated preparations, such as Gastrografin or oral Hypaque, are used for lower gastrointestinal studies.

Precautions. Barium sulfate should not be used when a perforation is suspected. A barium enema should not be performed within 48 hours after a biopsy specimen of the colon or rectum has been obtained.

Preparation. The patient is fasted for 24 to 48 hours and may be given a gastrointestinal cleansing agent such as Golytely (Braintree Labs, Randolph, Massachusetts). Warm water enemas must be given before the examination because it is essential that the entire large bowel be cleansed before a barium enema is performed. A Bardex (French; Bard Hospital Division, C.R. Bard, Covington, Georgia) catheter and a barium container are needed for the study.

Procedure. The animal should be anesthetized. The balloon-tipped catheter is inserted into the rectum, and the cuff is inflated to form a firm seal against the colonic wall. Barium or iodine is placed in the colon by gravitational flow. A 15% (wt/vol) barium sulfate solution is used for barium enemas. The dose is 5 to 10 ml/0.45 kg of body weight. Ideally, the study is done by using fluoroscopy. Radiographic views needed are lateral, ventrodorsal, and right and left ventrodorsal oblique. After completion, the barium is evacuated and air is injected to obtain a double-contrast study of the large bowel.

Urinary Tract
Contrast agents. Several kinds of contrast studies are available for evaluation of the kidneys. However, this discussion is limited to the intravenous pyelogram (IVP), which is most often used in practice.

An IVP, or excretory urogram, is performed by injecting contrast medium intravenously. Ionic organic iodide products are most commonly used. A meglumine diatrizoate and sodium diatrizoate preparation is probably the most popular contrast product used for IVP examinations. The standard dose of contrast is 800 mg of iodine per kilogram, which may be increased by 50% in patients with poor renal function.

Complications. The most common complications encountered with an IVP are vomiting, anaphylactoid reactions, and hypotension. Vomiting is a transient reaction of short duration and is not serious in nature, but care should be taken that the animal does not aspirate during the procedure. Anaphylactoid reactions are rare but must be attended to immediately. For this reason, it is necessary to have epinephrine available for immediate administration whenever an IVP is done. Hypotension is rare, but when it occurs, it can be life threatening and may lead to renal failure.

Contraindications. The only serious contraindication is dehydration or iodine sensitivity.

Procedure. The animal should be fasted for 24 hours, but water should be available to prevent dehydration. Enemas should be given when needed, at least 2 to 3 hours before the IVP. Ventrodorsal and lateral films should be taken before examinations. Films should be taken with the patient in ventrodorsal and lateral positions immediately after injection of contrast medium and at 5 and 15 minutes after injection. When needed, follow-up studies may be performed at 20 or 25 minutes after injection.

> **TECHNICIAN NOTE** The intravenous pyelogram (IVP) is the most commonly used contrast study of the kidneys.

Urinary Bladder
Contrast agents. Ionic organic iodide contrast materials are most desirable for retrograde cystography. Nonopaque contrast materials, such as air, carbon dioxide, and nitrous oxide, are used in addition to organic iodides for double-contrast cystography. Barium sulfate is not used.

Procedure. The colon should be cleansed. Depending on the breed and size of the animal, different catheters may be used. A Foley catheter, a tomcat catheter, or a soft flexible male catheter is needed. In addition, a syringe and a three-way valve are needed. Two types of cystography are commonly performed in veterinary practice: positive-contrast cystography and double-contrast cystography. Positive-contrast cystography is used to detect leaks or rupture of the lower urinary tract after trauma. Ionic organic iodide contrast at concentrations of 10% to 15% is injected retrograde into the urinary bladder at a dose of 5 to 15 ml/kg of body weight. Double-contrast cystography is used to detect all other forms of urinary bladder disease. A catheter is placed into the urinary bladder, and all urine is removed. Next, 3 to 10 ml of organic iodide contrast is injected, followed by carbon dioxide or room air at a dose of 5 to 15 ml/kg of body weight. Because of the variability of urinary bladder volume, it is best to fill the bladder to palpable turgidity. Lateral and oblique ventrodorsal radiographic views are most helpful.

Urethrography
Contrast agents. Ionic organic iodide compounds at 20% concentration are best for urethrography.

Procedure. A balloon-tipped catheter (Foley type) is placed into the distal urethra. The cuff is inflated for a snug fit to prevent contrast from leaking around the catheter, and 10 to 20 ml of contrast is hand-injected rapidly into the catheter. X-rays are taken during injection of the last few milliliters. A lateral view and two oblique views should be taken during separate injections of contrast material.

Spinal Cord
Myelography is the contrast examination most frequently performed to localize and characterize spinal cord lesions. Myelograms are always performed with the animal under general anesthetic. Nonionic iodinated contrast medium is injected into the subarachnoid space (cerebrospinal fluid space) at the cisterna magna (skull-C1 space) or into the caudal lumbar spine area (L4-L6). Myelography is most commonly performed before surgical intervention.

Contrast agents. Two nonionic contrast agents are currently in wide use in veterinary medicine: iopamidol (Isovue; Bracco Diagnostics, Princeton, New Jersey) and iohexol (Omnipaque; Sanofi Winthrop, Malvern, Pennsylvania). The dose of contrast medium ranges from 0.25 ml/kg for cervical evaluation with a cisternal injection to 0.45 ml/kg for cervical evaluation with a lumbar injection. The concentration of iodine should be between 240 and 300 mg/ml, and injection volume should not exceed 15 ml.

Contraindications. Contraindications for myelography include infection of the spinal cord and meninges. If the veterinarian should choose to treat spinal disease medically rather than surgically, myelography would be contraindicated.

Procedure. Survey films should be taken first. The site of injection should be aseptically prepared. Spinal needles of 20 to 22 gauge and 3.75 to 8.75 cm should be available because the size of the animal may vary considerably, and some dogs are so obese that even an 8.75-cm needle may be too short. Carefully collimated films are taken in the ventrodorsal and lateral positions immediately after administration of contrast medium.

POSITIONING

Proper positioning is essential to obtain diagnostic radiographs. It is again the responsibility of the veterinary technician to properly position the animal. It is not the intent of this chapter to discuss positioning at length. Please refer to excellent treatment of this topic by Butler et al (2000), Douglas et al (1987), Han et al (2005), Lavin (2005), Morgan (1993), and Ticer (1984).

> **TECHNICIAN NOTE** Proper positioning is essential if diagnostic radiographs are to be obtained.

Principles of Positioning

To achieve proper positioning, the technician should remember that two views at right angles are necessary to obtain a diagnostic study. This principle applies to all examinations in small animals and to extremities in large animals. Exceptions to this rule include thoracic and spinal examinations in the horse, and examinations in traumatized or debilitated animals when only lateral views can be taken without causing undue stress.

Another principle that should be remembered is the importance of centering the primary beam on the lesion itself, when known. This is especially important in orthopedic cases in both small and large animals. For example, fracture healing may look different when the x-ray beam is centered over the fracture line as opposed to a short distance away from it. Costly errors have been made by veterinarians who removed supporting devices before the correct time. These errors occurred because fractures may have appeared healed when the primary beam was centered away from the fracture line itself.

It is important when performing a radiographic examination to use an x-ray film that is sufficiently large to completely cover the system to be examined. When x-raying large dogs, it may be necessary to use two films for the abdomen: one for the cranial abdomen and one for the caudal abdomen, which is generally taken at a lower kVp setting. For extremities, the primary beam should be directed at the lesion. It is good to have an x-ray detector large enough to include proximal and distal portions of the joint, to make it possible to visualize the spatial anatomic relationship of the lesion to adjacent structures.

These principles are basic but essential. Proper positioning is achieved through practice. These topics are well illustrated and discussed in the references mentioned. A positioning reference textbook should be available in the radiology room of every veterinary practice.

RESTRAINT

The importance of restraint to achieve proper positioning cannot be overemphasized. It is also an essential part of radiation safety. Without proper restraint, many examinations should not be undertaken. In some cases, attempting to perform examinations without adequate restraint would be life threatening with large animals and dangerous with certain small animals.

Many types of restraint may be used; some are mechanical or manual, and some are chemical. For the purpose of radiation safety, manual restraint should be avoided as a routine procedure. When it is essential to be in the room with the animal, a protective lead apron, a thyroid shield, gloves, and preferably lead glasses should be worn, and the x-ray beam should be limited to the area to be examined by coning devices or by adjustment of the collimator.

Mechanical restraint is available in various forms. Several commercial devices designed for animal positioning are available, varying in price from a few dollars to several hundred dollars. One of the most useful and inexpensive devices for use with dogs is a simple muzzle, which often has a calming effect on an animal (see Chapter 6). Sandbags and sponges can also be used to obtain excellent positioning. Once the animal is positioned properly, it is most important to take the radiograph rapidly because one can hope for only a few seconds of adequate restraint before the animal moves.

Chemical restraint can be achieved with tranquilizers, analgesics, or anesthetics (see Chapters 28 and 29). Chemical restraint has contributed greatly to the progress made in radiology by allowing positioning that otherwise would be impossible to achieve. For example, complete examination of the skull should not be attempted without anesthesia. Every time total immobility or relaxation is required for proper positioning, anesthesia should be used. Most spinal examinations will prove nondiagnostic unless they are done with the animal under anesthesia. In several circumstances, tranquilization is adequate to control most animals. Tranquilizers are excellent for control of frightened or aggressive dogs and cats. They are most useful for controlling large animals.

Again, good positioning is essential in producing diagnostic x-ray films. It takes time to learn and become proficient in achieving every position needed for a variety of examinations in large and small animals. However, most organs can be x-rayed with the use of proper techniques, equipment, and accessory devices, along with mechanical or chemical restraint or both.

ULTRASONOGRAPHY

Ultrasound imaging is becoming an essential diagnostic tool in veterinary practice. It is portable; does not require the use of ionizing radiation; and is noninvasive, well tolerated by patients, and accepted by clients. As ultrasound equipment becomes affordable, the only problem with its introduction into practice as a routine diagnostic imaging modality is the long learning curve associated with its use. Recent veterinary graduates are more familiar with the uses and indications for ultrasonography because veterinary schools have integrated ultrasonography into the curriculum. All new veterinary technicians are encouraged to familiarize themselves with the basics of diagnostic ultrasonography but must remember that ultrasonography is user dependent. In other words, image quality and interpretation are only as good as the skills of the person doing the examination.

ULTRASONOGRAPHY BASICS

Sound is a mechanical pressure wave made up of a series of compressions and rarefactions transmitted through a medium. Sound waves are characterized by wavelength or distance between compressions, frequency in cycles per second, and velocity or speed of transmission (Figure 16-43). These characteristics are integrated by the following formula:

$$\text{Velocity} = \text{Wavelength} \times \text{Frequency}$$

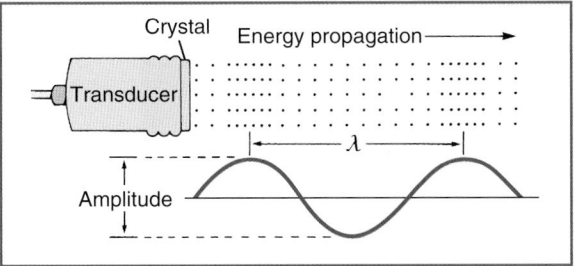

FIGURE 16-43 Sound wave with wavelength = λ. *Closely spaced dots*, compressions; *widely spaced dots*, rarefactions. The amplitude is proportional to the loudness.

For simplicity, assume that the speed of sound in the body is 1540 m/second. Therefore, as the frequency of sound increases, the wavelength decreases. Shorter sound waves produce increased image resolution but decreased patient penetration. The frequencies used in veterinary diagnostic ultrasound examination generally range from 2.5 to 12 megahertz (MHz). A **hertz (Hz)** is 1 cycle per second. Therefore, typical ultrasound frequencies range from 2.5 million to 12 million cycles/second. Audible sound ranges from 20 to 20,000 Hz.

Real-time, gray-scale ultrasonography is based on the pulse-echo principle. A short pulse of sound, usually 2 or 3 cycles long, is produced from the transducer and transmitted into the patient. The sound wave strikes an echogenic surface in the patient and returns some of the sound to the transducer. The strength of the returning sound wave determines the brightness of the image, and the time it takes for the sound to travel into the patient and back to the transducer determines where the echo will be seen on the screen. Remember that the time it takes for a sound wave to traverse a distance and be reflected back is a function of the distance between the sender and the reflector and the speed of the sound wave in that medium. For all practical purposes, the speed of sound in small animal tissues is constant at 1540 m/second.

Ultrasound production and reception are based on the piezoelectric effect. A piezoelectric crystal will change shape or thickness when subjected to a voltage pulse. Rapid pulses of electrical energy are converted into mechanical energy or sound waves by the vibrating crystal. Returning sound waves cause the crystal to vibrate, and that mechanical energy is converted into electrical energy by the transducer. This electrical signal is transformed into the gray-scale image on the screen. The transducer acts as both the sound transmitter and the receiver. The operating frequency of the transducer is partially determined by the thickness of the piezoelectric crystal. The thinner the crystal, the higher is the transducer frequency. The transducer transmits sound 0.01% of the time. It receives returning sound waves 99.9% of the time.

ULTRASOUND-TISSUE INTERACTION

To better understand the ultrasound image, it is important to understand the interaction of ultrasound within tissue. As the sound wave proceeds through the body, it is progressively attenuated or weakened. This attenuation limits the depth of penetration of the sound wave and therefore limits the depth of structures that can be effectively imaged. The ultrasound beam is attenuated or weakened by absorption, reflection, scattering, refraction, and diffraction. Reflection is a redirection of the sound beam back to the transducer and is the basis for the diagnostic image. Absorption is sound energy converted to heat within the tissues. Scattering is the intertissue microreflection of sound, which is responsible for much of the echo texture of various organs. Refraction and diffraction are the result of bending of the sound beam as it crosses areas of differing tissue densities. Refraction attenuation is important in the generation of several ultrasound artifacts.

Sound reflection or echo production forms the basis of the ultrasound image. An echo is produced whenever the ultrasound beam crosses an acoustic interface. An acoustic interface is the boundary between two tissues of differing acoustic impedances, or Z. See the following equation:

$$\text{Acoustic impedance (Z)} = \text{Density (P)} \times \text{Speed of sound}$$
$$\text{transmission (C), or } Z = P \times C$$

If we assume that the speed of sound in soft tissue is constant at 1540 m/second, then the main factor that influences acoustic impedance is the density or composition of tissue. Thus the more different two adjacent tissues are, the greater will be the echo reflection between them. This is why homogeneous populations of cells (lymphomas, lymph nodes, regenerative liver nodules) produce few echoes and are generally hypoechoic (darker). If the acoustic interface difference is small, only a small percentage of sound will be reflected. If the difference is large, a large portion of sound will be reflected. Most soft tissues have a Z, or acoustic impedance, within 1% to 2% of the liver.

INTERFACE	% REFLECTION
Fat/muscle	0.94
Fat/bone	49.00
Tissue/air	100.00

By looking at this list, one can see that the acoustic impedance (Z) between fat and muscle is low, whereas the acoustic impedance between fat and bone and between soft tissue and air is high. This property is the reason why ultrasound cannot be used to image through bone or gas. Too much of the sound beam is reflected back from bone and gas interfaces because of the large change in tissue density.

Patient Preparation

Patient preparation is important because 100% of the sound is reflected when the ultrasound beam intersects air. Hair traps air, and this is how it insulates the animal, but if one tries to pass an ultrasound beam through hair, most of the beam is reflected before it ever enters the animal. A careful close clip of the area to be examined and removal of dirt and scales will improve the ultrasound image. A generous volume of ultrasound gel is beneficial for displacing air and coupling the transducer to the skin (Figure 16-44). Small animals are placed in a padded V-trough table on their backs or in lateral recumbency for abdominal examination, and in lateral or sternal recumbency for cardiac examination. Most small animals tolerate abdominal and cardiac examinations well and rarely require tranquilization. A special cardiac table

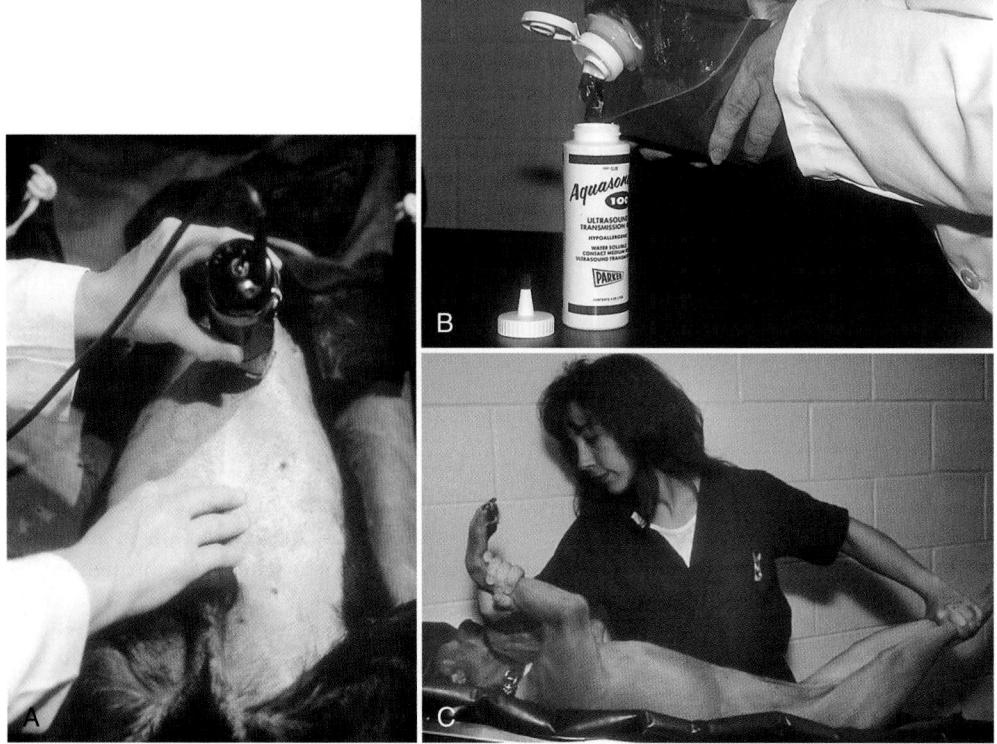

FIGURE 16-44 Patient preparation for abdominal ultrasound examination. **A,** Careful close clip of entire abdomen. **B,** Clean the skin surface, and use a generous volume of coupling gel. **C,** Place the animal in dorsal recumbency on a padded V-trough, and gently restrain during the examination.

with large and small holes in it is helpful for echocardiography. The animal is placed in lateral recumbency with the chest area over the hole of appropriate size; this allows better ultrasound transducer access (Figure 16-45). Large animal examinations are done in the standing tranquilized animal. Again, close clipping, especially for tendon examinations, is critical for an optimal examination.

> **TECHNICIAN NOTE** Hair traps air, and if not clipped, most of the beam would be reflected before it ever enters the animal. This is why good patient preparation is so critical.

ULTRASOUND DISPLAY MODES

The returning echo can be displayed in several ways. **A-mode**, or amplitude mode, displays returning echoes as spikes from a baseline. Echo depth is determined by its location along the baseline. Echo intensity is displayed by the height of the spike. A-mode ultrasound machines are used predominantly in ophthalmology and have little value in veterinary practice.

B-mode, or brightness mode, forms the basis for two-dimensional imaging. Returning echoes are displayed as dots on the image screen. The brightness of the dot is a function of the strength of the returning echo. The placement of the dot is a function of the time it took for the echo to return to the transducer. The cross-sectional image is formed through data storage. The sound beam is automatically swept across the patient while the transducer is held steady and is moved slowly over the area of interest. Rapid collection of images is called *real time*. This permits direct observation of moving structures, such as a beating heart or the movement of a puppy in a pregnant female. With B-mode real-time equipment, images are displayed in gray scale. Gray scale is a technique in which various echo strengths are displayed in numerous shades of gray from black to white, similar to a black and white television picture.

M-mode, or time-motion (TM) mode, is produced by passing a narrow sound beam across a body part. Each echo interface is presented as a dot. The motion of the body part is displayed by sweeping the image across the screen or image recorder. M-mode can be thought of as a thin sector of B-mode displayed as a function of time. M-mode is used primarily for echocardiography (ultrasonic examination of the heart). Ideal ultrasound equipment for veterinary practice would include a real-time B-mode scanner with M-mode capabilities (Figure 16-46).

The selection of appropriate transducers is critical when ultrasound equipment is purchased. Transducers vary in type, size, style, shape, and frequency. Linear array transducers are made with several piezoelectric crystals stacked side by side. The crystals are fired in rapid sequence to produce a rectangular cross-sectional image. It is difficult to use these transducers for intercostal cardiac studies and for subcostal studies in the cranioabdominal area in small animals. Linear array transducers are used primarily for transrectal reproductive examinations in cattle and horses. Newer, small-footprint convex array transducers are used most commonly for small animal imaging.

Sector scanners produce a triangular field. The crystal is swept across the area by mechanical or electronic means, and the transducer generally has a small contact area. Newer, more expensive transducers may incorporate annular array and dynamic focusing technology. These transducers form the ultrasound beam by adding together many small beams from an array of small crystals. Dynamic focusing allows the operator to place any portion within the beam into maximum resolution without having to change transducers.

Deciding which frequency of transducer to use is easy. Use a transducer with the highest possible frequency to maximize resolution while still allowing penetration to the needed depth. Remember that the higher the frequency of the transducer, the shorter is the sound wavelength and the better is the resolution. However, as the frequency increases, the depth of sound beam penetration decreases. For

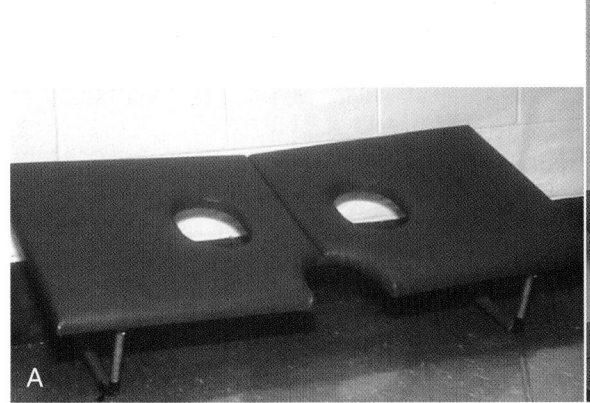
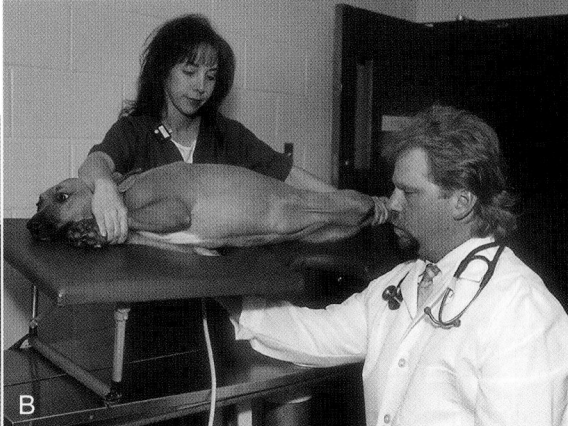

FIGURE 16-45 A, Small animal cardiac ultrasound table. B, Patient properly positioned and restrained for echocardiography. The dog's cardiac notch is placed over the table hole, so the sonographer can access the chest from beneath the table.

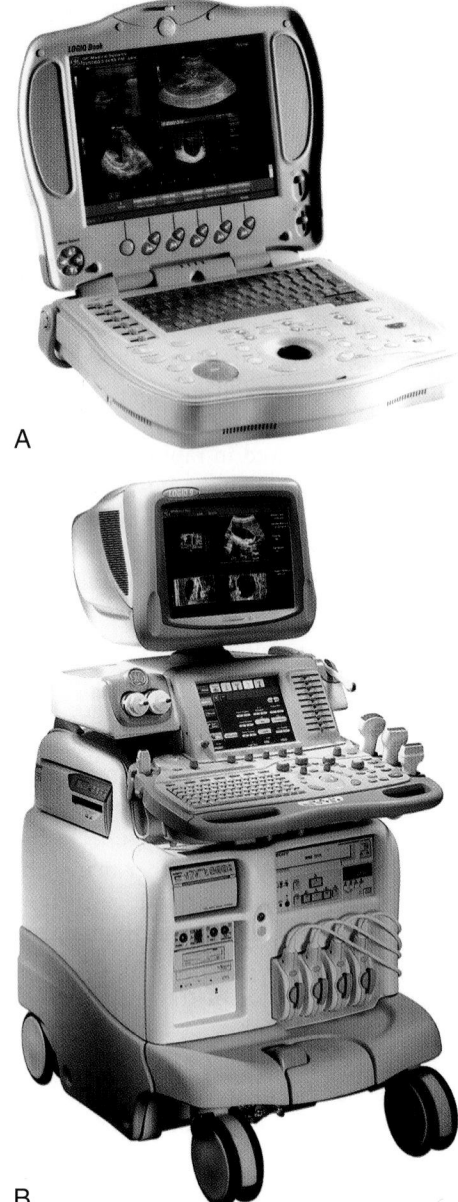

A

B

FIGURE 16-46 A, Portable notebook-style, real-time B-mode, M-mode, and color Doppler dedicated veterinary ultrasound unit that can be used on both large and small animals. **B,** Larger mobile veterinary ultrasound unit most commonly used in small animal practices. (Courtesy Sound Technologies, Inc., Carlsbad, CA.)

abdominal ultrasonography in small dogs (15 kg or less) and cats, a 7.5-MHz transducer is ideal. For medium-size to large breed dogs, a 5-MHz transducer works well. A guide for selecting a transducer is shown in Box 16-5.

> **TECHNICIAN NOTE** Use a transducer with the highest possible frequency to maximize resolution while allowing penetration to the necessary depth.

Ultrasound equipment controls vary from machine to machine, but a time-gain compensation (TGC) control is fairly universal. The echoes coming from acoustic interfaces

---

BOX 16-5 | Guide for Selecting a Transducer

High Frequency
Increases resolution
Increases attenuation
Decreases penetration

Low Frequency
Decreases resolution
Decreases attenuation
Increases penetration

---

close to the transducer are stronger than those returning from farther away from the transducer. Time-gain amplification compensates for progressive attenuation of the ultrasound beam with increasing depth. TGC is operator dependent and is set for the best-looking uniform image. TGC controls most often consist of a series of slide pods on the front of the machine. The top pod is the near field of the image, and the lowest pod is the far field, or bottom, of the image.

THE ULTRASOUND IMAGE

As one begins to use ultrasound, a greater appreciation for detailed anatomy is required. The ultrasound image is a thin cross-sectional slice through the body in a new or different orientation. It helps to use a standard image orientation, which places the head or the front of the animal on the left in the sagittal or longitudinal view, and the animal's right on the left of the screen on the transverse or axial view.

Ultrasound terminology is easy to remember. *Echogenicity* refers to the strength or amplitude of the returning echoes. A structure that is sonodense or echogenic (bright) produces echoes. A structure that is **anechoic** or sonolucent (dark) produces few or no echoes. A structure is **hyperechoic** (brighter than) if it produces more echoes than adjacent structures. A structure is **hypoechoic** (darker than) if it produces fewer echoes than surrounding structures. An **isoechoic** (same as) structure has a level of echogenicity similar to that of adjacent structures. Remember that *echogenicity* is a relative term. Any structure can be made bright by adjusting machine control settings. Compare organs at the same depth and control settings to prevent misinterpretation of relative echogenicities.

ULTRASOUND ARTIFACTS

Most people fail to take the time to fully understand ultrasound artifacts. They ignore artifacts because, by definition, an artifact does not contribute useful image information. This is not true of ultrasound artifacts, however; they provide accurate clues to what makes up the ultrasound image.

Reverberation Artifact

A reverberation artifact occurs when the ultrasound beam hits gas or air. Because of the large drop in acoustic impedance (soft tissue/air interface), the entire ultrasound beam is

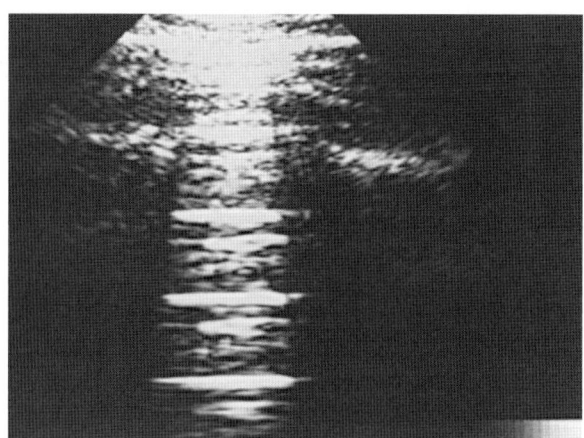

FIGURE 16-47 Reverberation artifact from the air-filled lung of a normal horse. Parallel, evenly spaced echogenic bands represent reverberation between the transducer and the pleural surface.

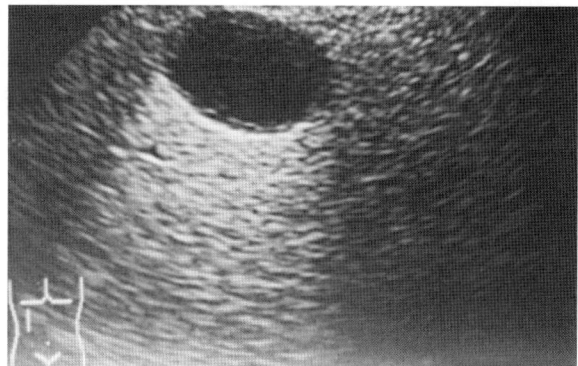

FIGURE 16-48 Bright echogenic band beneath the gallbladder represents acoustic enhancement. The ultrasound beam is not attenuated as much as it traverses the fluid-filled gallbladder as it is in the surrounding liver.

reflected back to the transducer. A portion of the reflected beam bounces off the transducer surface and reenters the patient. It hits the air interface a second time, and the same thing happens again. This occurs repeatedly and appears on the screen as a set of bright parallel lines that are the same distance from each other. Each parallel line represents the distance between the transducer and the gas interface. Reverberation artifacts can also be referred to as *dirty shadowing* or *comet tails* (Figure 16-47).

Shadowing

A shadowing artifact occurs because of inadequate sound beam penetration through a highly reflective or sound-absorptive substance. Acoustic shadowing is an area of darkness or hypoechogenicity that occurs deep to dense material, such as bone, calcium, or calculi. Small objects cast an acoustic shadow only if they are within the focal zone or narrow portion of the ultrasound beam.

Acoustic Enhancement

If the ultrasound beam passes through an area with few tissue interfaces (low-attenuation region), the emerging ultrasound beam will have greater intensity than would be expected and will be brighter or more echogenic distal to the nonattenuating structure. The best example of this is the normal gallbladder surrounded by the hepatic parenchyma. Liver tissue distal or deep to the gallbladder appears brighter than adjacent hepatic tissue (Figure 16-48). This artifact is seen deep to fluid-filled structures and is also referred to as *through-transmission*.

Refraction, or Edge Artifact

Refraction is a hypoechoic band or stripe at the margin of a curved structure caused by refraction or bending of the sound beam. The sound beam is deflected from its true path and never returns, with an effect similar to shadowing. An edge artifact is helpful in identifying smooth round structures, such as early pregnancy vesicles.

Mirror-Image Artifact

The ultrasound machine places the returning echo on the viewing screen as a function of the time it took the echo to return. If the sound wave reverberates within a highly echogenic structure before returning to the transducer, the image will be duplicated on the screen distal to the original image. This is most commonly seen as a duplication of the gallbladder in mirror image on the other side of the diaphragm.

Slice-Thickness Artifact

If the width of the ultrasound beam cuts through the edge of a cystic structure and solid tissue, the solid tissue may look as if it is layered within the cyst. This artifact is responsible for the erroneous appearance of debris within the urinary bladder and gallbladder, although no debris may be present. The erroneous appearance is the result of volume averaging of tissue by the ultrasound machine.

THE ULTRASOUND EXAMINATION

Performing a complete ultrasound examination requires at least 20 to 30 minutes. When ultrasound is used for a quick answer to a question such as whether a female patient is pregnant or has a pyometra, the examination will be shorter. When ultrasound is used for diagnosis of abdominal disease, a complete examination should be performed every time.

It is important to have a thorough understanding of the normal appearance of various abdominal organs before trying to identify abnormalities associated with disease. Ranking of small animal abdominal organs from least echogenic (darkest) to most echogenic (brightest) is given in Box 16-6.

Remember that echogenicity is a relative term, and one must compare organs at similar control settings and similar depths to avoid misinterpretation.

TECHNICIAN NOTE It is important to have a thorough understanding of the normal appearance of various abdominal organs before trying to identify abnormalities associated with disease.

BOX 16-6	Ranking of Small Animal Abdominal Organs from Least Echogenic to Most Echogenic

Renal medulla (least echogenic)
Liver
Renal cortex
Spleen
Prostate
Renal sinus fat (most echogenic)

BOX 16-7	Uses of Ultrasound in Large and Small Animals

- Tendon injury evaluation and response to surgery or therapy
- Diagnosis of tendon sheath infections, adhesions, and foreign bodies
- Evaluation of joint effusions, intra-articular injury, osteomyelitis, and neoplasms
- Evaluation of congenital and acquired cardiac disease and response to therapy
- Diagnosis of pleural effusion, pleuritis, and pleuropneumonia
- Evaluation of lung and mediastinal masses
- Evaluation of soft tissue, neck, thyroid, parathyroid, tongue, and mediastinal disease
- Evaluation of hepatic, renal, splenic, adrenal, urinary bladder, gallbladder, and biliary disease
- Diagnosis of abdominal and peripheral vascular malformations
- Peritoneal and pleural fluid assessment and sampling
- Evaluation of abdominal masses of unknown origin
- Diagnosis of intestinal foreign bodies, intussusceptions, infiltrative disease, and neoplasia
- Testicular and prostate evaluation and location of retained testicles
- Pregnancy diagnosis, fetal evaluation, twin removal, and complete fertility evaluations
- Evaluation of soft tissue neoplasia, granulomas, abscesses, and foreign bodies
- Diagnosis of umbilical infections and persistent and patent urachus
- Ocular and orbital evaluation
- Vascular thrombosis and catheter foreign body evaluation
- Guidance for fine-needle aspiration, drain placement, biopsy, and culture

Clinical Use

Ultrasonography is now a mainstay of veterinary diagnostics and is used almost as frequently as radiography. Equipment designed for use in humans is readily adaptable for use in veterinary medicine, and several companies are producing dedicated veterinary ultrasound machines. Both 5- and 7.5-MHz transducers are popular for small animal and non-reproductive large animal imaging. The 3- and 5-MHz linear array transducers are used extensively for transrectal large animal reproductive ultrasonography. Traditional cardiac and solid abdominal organ examinations remain the mainstay, but ultrasound is used to answer hundreds of clinical questions in a wide variety of species. Box 16-7 lists common ultrasound applications in both large and small animals.

NUCLEAR MEDICINE

ALTERNATIVE IMAGING MODALITIES

Many veterinary schools and some progressive specialized veterinary practices have nuclear medicine capabilities. Nuclear medicine can be divided into therapeutic and diagnostic procedures. Currently, veterinary therapeutic nuclear medicine involves administration of radioactive iodine (^{131}I) for the treatment of hyperthyroidism and thyroid tumors. Diagnostic nuclear medicine involves administration of radionuclides and detection of the electromagnetic radiation emitted from the animal with a gamma scintillation camera. Radionuclides are atoms with unstable nuclei that undergo radioactive decay. Radioactive decay is the transformation or disintegration of an unstable nucleus by spontaneous emission of electromagnetic radiation. Electromagnetic radiation that is of nuclear origin is termed *gamma rays*, in contrast to diagnostic radiation (x-rays), which originates from the electron cloud that surrounds the nucleus.

> **TECHNICIAN NOTE** Currently, veterinary therapeutic nuclear medicine involves the administration of radioactive iodine (^{131}I) for the treatment of hyperthyroidism and thyroid tumors.

Diagnostic nuclear medicine does not generate visual images equivalent to those of diagnostic radiology, but it detects functional or physiologic, pharmacologic, and kinetic data from the patient in image or numeric data form. Figure 16-49 shows a standard gamma scintillation camera, control panel, and nuclear medicine computer. Common clinical uses of veterinary nuclear medicine include bone scanning for detection of tumor metastasis to bone and radiographically undetectable bone injury or infection, lung scanning for detection of pulmonary embolism and as a pulmonary function test, renal scanning for assessment of kidney perfusion and function, and thyroid scanning for characterization of hyperthyroidism and detection of metastasis. Other, less common nuclear medicine studies include hepatobiliary scanning, brain scanning, labeled white blood cell scanning for detection of occult infection, lymphoscintigraphy, nuclear angiography, and scanning for detection of an unknown focus of blood loss.

The most commonly used radionuclide is technetium 99m (^{99m}Tc). This agent is commercially available from a disposable technetium generator. Technetium is administered in an ionic form as ^{99m}TcO$_4$ (pertechnetate) or is bound

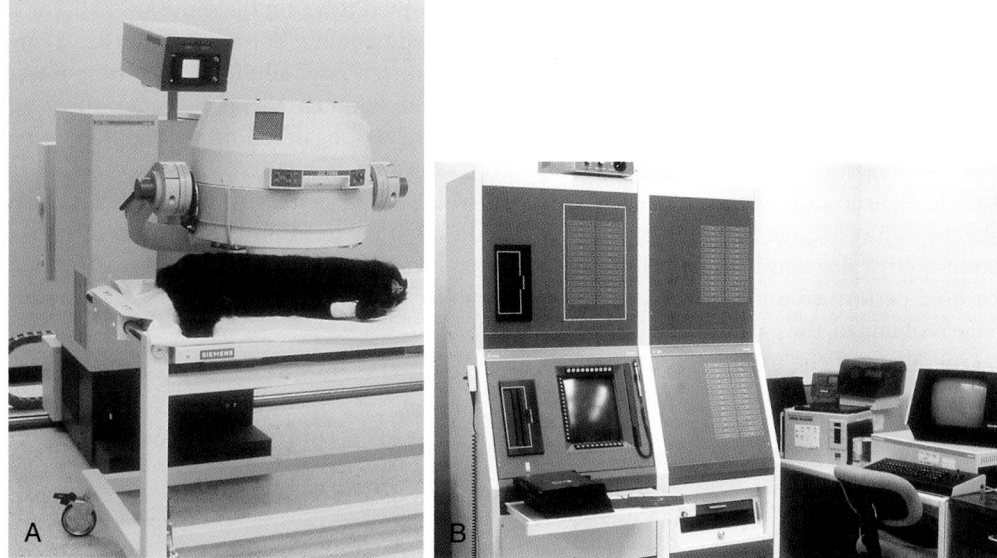

FIGURE 16-49 A, Gamma scintillation camera in position over a dog during a whole body bone scan to check for metastatic neoplasia. B, Control panel monitor, nuclear medicine computer, and matrix camera.

to a specific organ-localizing pharmaceutical agent before administration. Technetium is the radiopharmaceutical of choice because it has a 6-hour physical half-life and emits a 140-keV gamma ray, which is appropriate for most imaging studies. The radioactive or physical half-life of a radionuclide is the time required for the number of radioactive atoms to decrease by 50%.

Radiation safety practices are important with nuclear medicine. When working in a practice that uses nuclear medicine, one should insist on receiving comprehensive instruction in radiation principles and safety. This chapter is meant only as an introduction.

The primary route of radionuclide administration to veterinary patients is intravenous. Latex examination gloves should be worn and careful injection techniques should be used to ensure that the entire dose is delivered intravenously and not perivascularly. This is especially important in equine bone scans for which a large dose of radionuclide is administered. Routes of excretion of radioactive imaging agents vary with the agent used. Technetium is excreted primarily in urine, with a lesser amount excreted in feces. Animals should be housed in a separate restricted area of the hospital, and their stool and urine should be carefully collected and held for decay until levels are below exempt quantities. Always wear latex examination gloves, and limit contact with patients to only that necessary for their care. Never eat or bring eating utensils (coffee cups, spoons, etc.) into a nuclear medicine area. The dose of radiation to the patient is small, but repeated physical contact or accidental ingestion of radionuclides may be harmful to the nuclear medicine technologist. Animals should be held in the restricted area until they pose no radiation threat to their owners or to the population at large. This involves generally 3 to 10 physical half-lives of the radiopharmaceutical, depending on specific state regulations.

> **TECHNICIAN NOTE**   The primary route of radionuclide administration to veterinary patients is intravenous. Latex examination gloves should be worn and careful injection techniques should be used to ensure that the entire dose is delivered intravenously and not perivascularly.

COMPUTED TOMOGRAPHY

Over the past 15 years, diagnostic imaging techniques available to veterinary patients have expanded. Most veterinary schools and some specialty practices have access to CT scanning. A CT scan is obtained by passing a thin x-ray beam transaxially through the patient and measuring the x-ray attenuation at multiple sites in a thin slice of the patient's anatomy. The computer then reconstructs the transmitted x-ray data into a cross-sectional image on a monitor. Images are in digital format and are stored on a PACS; they can be printed out on film for storage using a dry laser printer. Advantages of CT over standard radiography include greatly improved radiographic contrast, spatial resolution, and cross-sectional anatomic presentation, all of which eliminate the problem of superimposition of structures, as occurs in radiography. The most common uses of CT in veterinary medicine include head and spinal examinations for neurologic disease and radiation treatment planning. CT allows the veterinarian a noninvasive look inside the patient's skull (Figure 16-50).

When a CT scan is performed, the patient is placed in the ventrodorsal or dorsoventral position on the long, narrow, movable CT table. The table then moves the patient through the circular gantry that houses the x-ray tube and detectors (Figure 16-51). In older units, the table moves in a measured stepwise fashion. During each table step, the CT scanner obtains a single cross-sectional slice of data. Modern scanners have what is called a *helical scan mode* such that the x-ray tube turns 360 degrees around the patient, while the patient bed moves slowly through the gantry. This results in spiral or helical acquisition of the images, which then are reconstructed instantaneously by the computer to appear as conventional transverse images. The advantage of the helical CT scanner is speed. Helical scanners are excellent for moving regions like the thorax because they are fast, and the entire thorax of even a large dog can be scanned during a single short breath-hold performed under anesthesia.

When a CT image is obtained, the patient must be heavily sedated or under general anesthetic to prevent any motion and must be positioned perfectly straight. Most studies are

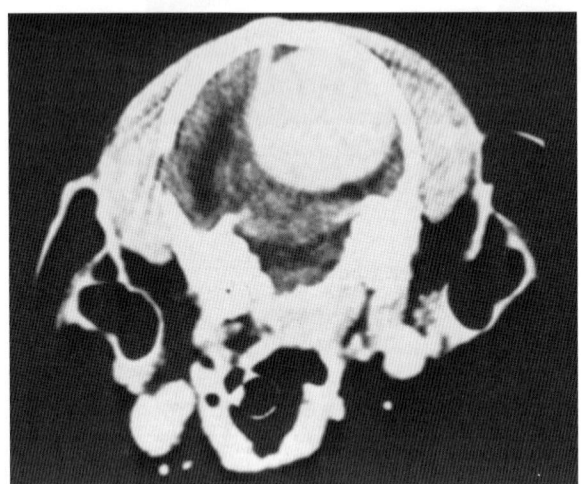

FIGURE 16-50 Computed tomogram of a dog brain showing a large contrast-enhancing brain tumor (meningioma) in the central cerebrum.

performed twice on the same animal. The first study is performed without contrast, and the second is performed after intravenous administration of iodinated contrast. Urographic contrast agents are commonly administered at a dose of 800 mg of iodine per kilogram of body weight. Contrast will highlight vascular structures, and some neoplasms will have a characteristic contrast enhancement pattern. In addition to examination of the brain, CT can be used to identify and characterize musculoskeletal, thoracic, and abdominal disorders, as well as vascular anomalies.

> **TECHNICIAN NOTE**   When CT studies are performed, the same contrast agents are used as for radiographic contrast procedures, but at a much lower concentration, because CT is much more sensitive than radiography for detecting the presence of contrast agents.

MAGNETIC RESONANCE IMAGING

The newest imaging modality to be used in veterinary medicine is magnetic resonance imaging (MRI). MRI is similar to CT in that the image is a thin slice of cross-sectional anatomy made up of a matrix of volume elements. MRI differs from CT in that it uses no ionizing radiation to create the image. Instead, MRI represents the intensity of a radio wave signal from tissue in which hydrogen nuclei have been disturbed by a characteristic radiofrequency pulse. MRI is superior to CT in image resolution, anatomic definition, and sensitivity to tissue composition differences. Because of this, MRI is vastly superior to CT for imaging of the brain and spinal cord and is currently used primarily for head and

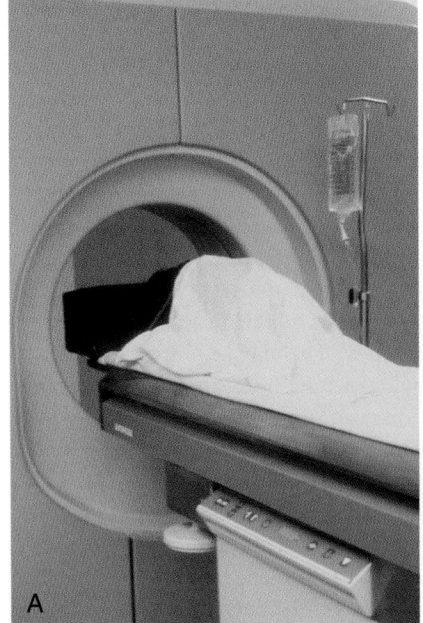
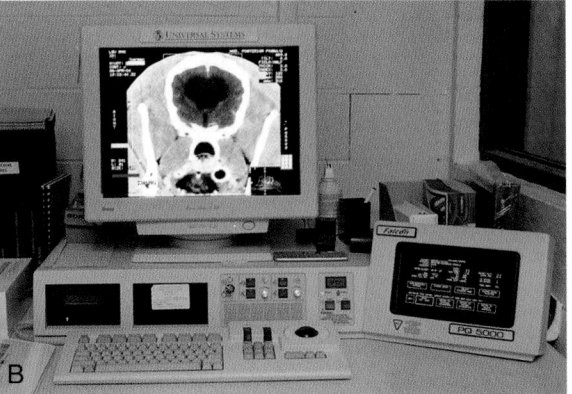

FIGURE 16-51 A, Dog in position for a brain computed tomogram. The large circular gantry houses the x-ray tube and detectors. The table moves the patient through the gantry in precise, measured, incremental steps. B, Computed tomography (CT) control panel located outside the shielded CT room.

spine evaluation. One disadvantage of MRI is the much longer scan time required compared with CT. Figure 16-52 shows a sagittal canine brain magnetic resonance image of a patient with a large, contrast-enhancing pituitary tumor.

> **TECHNICIAN NOTE** MRI differs from CT in that it uses no ionizing radiation to create the image. MRI is superior to CT in image resolution, anatomic definition, and sensitivity to tissue composition differences. Because of this, MRI is vastly superior to CT for imaging of the brain and spinal cord and is currently the state of the art modality for head and spine evaluation.

Two general types of MRI units (also called *magnets*) are used in veterinary imaging: low field strength open magnets (Figure 16-53, *A*) and high field strength, or

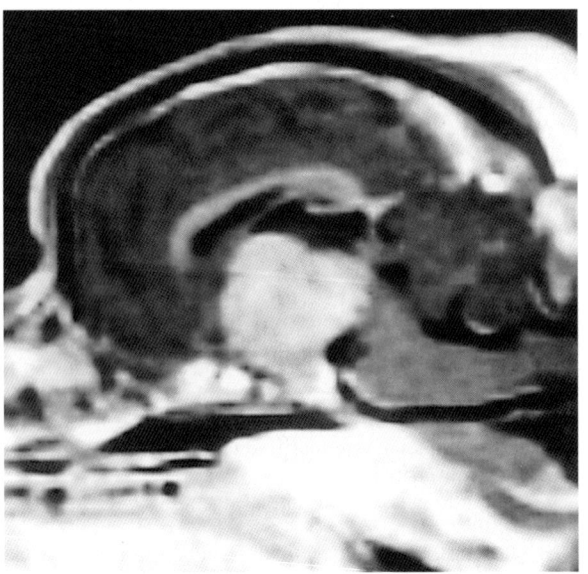

FIGURE 16-52 Sagittal T1 post–gadolinium contrast magnetic resonance image of a dog with a large enhancing pituitary macroadenoma.

superconductive, magnets (Figure 16-53, *B*). Magnetic field strength is measured in tesla (T). Low field strength magnets are 0.4 T or less, and high field strength magnets are 0.6 T and above. The most typical superconducting magnet has field strength of 1 or 1.5 T. Regardless of the type of magnet used, the technician needs to be aware of several safety measures and patient management concerns peculiar to MRI.

About half of all veterinary teaching hospitals have in-house MRI units. In most private veterinary practices, CT and MRI examinations are often done off the practice premises in an imaging center; a mobile, truck-based MRI unit; or a human hospital. Therefore, everything needed to anesthetize, resuscitate, and recover a patient needs to be taken to the imaging site. Most practices that perform off-site imaging have a large tackle box or a physician's bag filled with all necessary drugs, fluids, catheters, intravenous access lines, syringes, needles, tape, gauze, and endotracheal tubes. It often helps to do a mock run or a pretend case before a clinical case to ensure that everything is correctly packed. Imaging centers and hospitals appreciate clean, odor-free, and flea- and tick-free veterinary patients. It is a good idea to bathe the patient within 24 hours before the examination if possible and to ensure that the patient's bowels and bladder have been evacuated before the patient enters the hospital or imaging center.

A serious problem with MRI is the strong magnetic field in the vicinity of the machine (Figure 16-54). One cannot use anything made of ferromagnetic metal in or around the magnet. The magnetic field will rapidly and forcefully pull these objects into the magnet, potentially injuring anyone in its path. Such objects include gas anesthetic machines, oxygen tanks, intravenous poles, clipboards, ink pens, leashes, collars, and beepers. Nonmagnetic products are available for use during MRI, but they are generally prohibitively expensive for most veterinary hospitals. The exception is an aluminum oxygen tank. Because of this limitation, anesthesia generally is provided with injectable drugs and heavy tranquilization. Plugging the animal's ears with cotton is essential for maintaining sedation and protecting hearing because

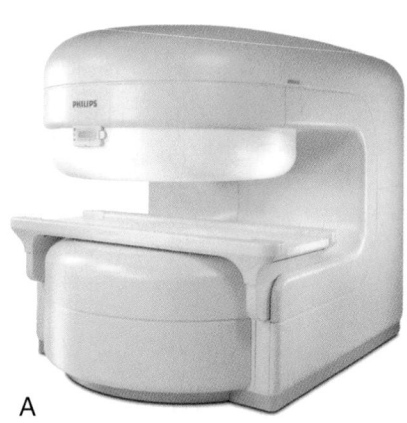
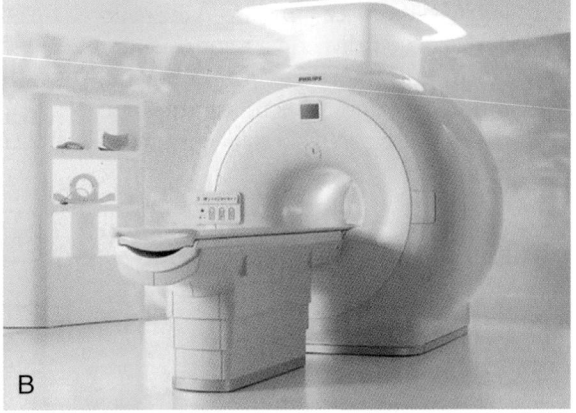

FIGURE 16-53 A, An open or low field strength magnetic resonance imaging (MRI) scanner. These machines make it easier to position and monitor the patient but may require longer scan times. **B,** Superconductive or high field strength MRI scanner. The circular closed MRI gantry can make patient positioning difficult.

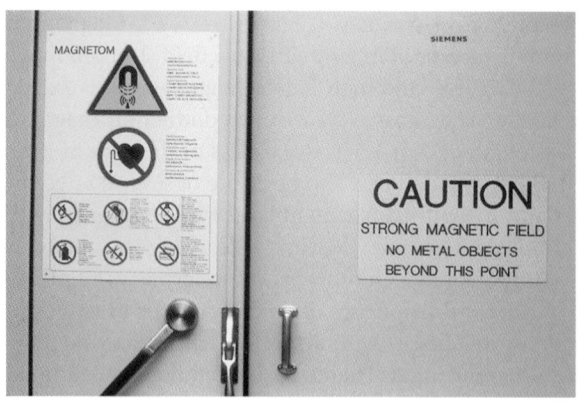

FIGURE 16-54 Warning signs positioned at the entrance to a magnetic resonance imaging (MRI) scanner. The technician must realize that the MRI magnet is always turned on and that the high magnetic field may extend beyond the scanner room door. Never bring anything metallic into the MRI suite.

of the loudness of the magnet during scanning. Personnel remaining in the room to monitor anesthesia must use ear protection. Patients must be absolutely still for MRI. Any motion will severely degrade the image, so they must be in a fairly deep anesthetic plane. This is sometimes complicated because it is often difficult to carefully monitor animals during the examination because of the narrow tubular shape of some magnets and the inability to use mechanized monitoring devices. Patients that cannot tolerate deep injectable general anesthetic with minimal monitoring are not good candidates for out-of-clinic MRI. MRI examinations generally take 45 to 60 minutes to perform and are done with and without intravenous contrast, similar to CT examinations, but with a paramagnetic contrast agent (usually gadolinium pentetic acid). Organic iodide contrast will not work for MRI examinations.

In addition to anesthesia and monitoring difficulties created by the high magnetic field, personal safety is a concern, and precautions must be taken. It is important to remember that even though no images are being produced and the MRI technician is not at the controls, the magnet is still on at full power at all times. Credit cards and watches may be permanently damaged if carried too close to the high magnetic field. Any device that delivers a radiofrequency signal cannot be close to an MRI unit; these include but are not limited to televisions, radios, and pager transmitters. In addition, technicians with cardiac pacemakers, aneurysm or intracranial hemoclips, neural stimulators, metallic fragments within the orbits, or hearing aids should not be in charge of patient care during an MRI. If you ever have any questions regarding what can and cannot be brought into the MRI room, ask the MRI technician in charge before entering.

> **TECHNICIAN NOTE**   The high magnetic field in an MRI unit is always on. It is never safe to bring anything made of a ferromagnetic metal close to the machine.

RECOMMENDED READINGS

Barr F, Gaschen L: BSAVA manual of canine and feline ultrasonography, Gloucester, UK, 2011, British Small Animal Veterinary Association.

Butler JA, et al: Clinical radiology of the horse, ed 3, Oxford, England, 2008, Blackwell Scientific Publications.

Curry TS, Dowdey JE, Murry RC: Christensen's introduction to the physics of diagnostic radiology, ed 4, Philadelphia, 1990, Lea & Febiger.

Douglas SW, Herrtage ME, Williamson HD: Principles of veterinary radiology, ed 4, East Sussex, England, 1987, Bailliere Tindall.

Drost WT, Reese DJ, Hornof WJ: Digital radiography artifacts, Vet Radiol Ultrasound 49(Suppl 1):S48, 2008.

Eastman Kodak Company: The fundamentals of radiography, ed 12, Rochester, NY, 1980, Eastman Kodak.

Hall EJ: Radiobiology for the radiologist, ed 4, Philadelphia, 1993, Lippincott-Raven.

Han CM, Hurd CD: Practical guide to diagnostic imaging for veterinary technicians, ed 3, St Louis, 2005, Mosby.

Kealy JK, McAllister H, Graham J: Diagnostic radiology and ultrasonography of the dog and cat, ed 5, St Louis, 2011, Saunders.

Lavin LM: Radiography in veterinary technology, ed 4, St Louis, 2006, Saunders.

Morgan JR: Techniques of veterinary radiography, ed 5, Ames, IA, 1993, Iowa State University Press.

Nyland TG, Mattoon JS: Small animal diagnostic ultrasound, ed 2, St Louis, 2002, Saunders.

O'Brien TR: O'Brien's radiology for the equine practitioner, Jackson, WY, 2005, Teton NewMedia.

Rantanen NW, McKinnon AD: Equine diagnostic ultrasonography, Baltimore, 1998, Williams & Wilkins.

Sirois M, Anthor E: Handbook of radiographic positioning for veterinary technicians, Independence, KY, 2009, Delmar Cengage Learning.

Stashak TS: Adam's lameness in horses, ed 5, Plymouth, UK, 2002, Plymbridge Distributors Ltd.

Thrall DE: Textbook of veterinary diagnostic radiology, ed 5, St Louis, 2007, Saunders.

Ticer JA: Radiographic technique in veterinary practice, ed 2, Philadelphia, 1984, Saunders.

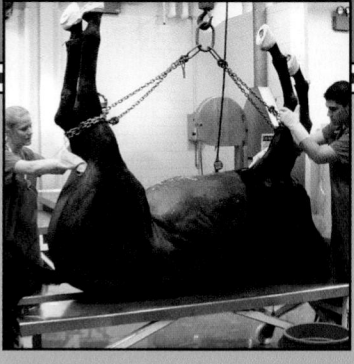

17 Basic Necropsy Procedures

Thomas J. Van Winkle and Perry L. Habecker

OUTLINE

Necropsy Reports, *564*
Fixatives, *566*
Facilities and Instruments, *566*
Ancillary Procedures, *567*
Shipping Diagnostic Specimens, *569*
Necropsy Procedure for a Small
  Mammal, *569*
Tissue Collection, *569*
Dissection, *570*
Preliminary Observations, *570*
External Examination, *570*
Reflection of Skin and Limbs and
  Examination of Superficial Organs and
  Body Cavities, *570*
Examination of Skull and Brain, *573*
Dissection and Examination of Neck and
  Thoracic Viscera, *574*
Dissection and Examination of Abdominal
  Cavity, *576*

Dissection and Examination of Female
  Reproductive Tract, Urinary Tract, and
  Accessory Male Reproductive
  Organs, *577*
Dissection and Examination of Intestinal
  Tract, *577*
Dissection and Examination of Abdominal
  Aorta, Rectum, and Anal Glands, *578*
Dissection and Examination of Vertebral
  Column and Spinal Cord, *578*
Necropsy Variations, *578*
Ruminants, *578*
Horse, *580*
Pig, *580*
Fetus, *581*
Birds, *581*
Laboratory Animals, *581*
Cosmetic Necropsies, *582*

LEARNING OBJECTIVES

When you have completed this chapter, you will be able to:

1. Pronounce, define, and spell all Key Terms in the chapter.
2. List the indications for a necropsy.
3. Explain how to prepare for a necropsy, including record keeping and handling of the body.
4. Describe the techniques used to preserve tissues, including specific uses for various tissue fixatives.
5. Describe the facilities, instruments, and supplies needed to perform a necropsy, including protective clothing.
6. Do the following regarding collection of specimens and shipping procedures:
   - Explain the collection techniques and shipping procedures for microbiological, parasitologic, toxicologic, and cytologic specimens.
   - Explain the special procedures used and precautions observed when performing a necropsy on a rabies suspect.
7. Do the following regarding the necropsy procedure for a small mammal:
   - Describe the procedures used to collect tissues for histologic examination.
   - Explain the principles of tissue dissection, including external examination of the carcass.
   - Describe the initial steps of a necropsy dissection, including reflection of the skin and limbs, and examination of superficial organs and body cavities.
   - Describe the steps for dissection and examination of the skull and brain, neck and thoracic viscera, abdominal cavity, genitourinary tract, intestinal tract, vertebral column, and spinal cord.

KEY TERMS

Abomasum
Appendicular skeleton
Atlas
Atrioventricular (AV)
  valve
Autolysis
Axis
Diaphragm
Duodenum
Foramen magnum
Forestomach
Gross pathology
Histopathology
Hydronephrosis
Hyoid bone
In situ
Laminae
Lesions
Mediastinum
Meninges
Myocardium
Necropsy
Omentum
Pathogenesis
Pathology
Pituitary gland
Prosector
Pulmonary artery
Sciatic nerve
Sternum

8. Do the following regarding necropsy variations:
   • Describe variations in the necropsy procedure specific to ruminants, horses, and pigs, as well as to fetuses and placental tissues.
   • Explain the differences between a complete necropsy and a cosmetic necropsy.
   • Explain the role of the technician in prion disease surveillance.

INTRODUCTION

Necropsy is the examination of an animal after it has died to determine abnormal and disease-related changes that occurred during its life. The term *necropsy* originated from the Greek language and means "viewing the dead." Necropsy is also known as *autopsy*, which is Greek for "seeing with one's own eyes."

Before beginning our discussion of necropsy, it is important to understand the meaning of terms that are used frequently in this chapter. **Pathology,** for example, is the science and study of disease, especially the causes and development of abnormal conditions. **Gross pathology** refers to pathologic changes in tissue that are visible with the unaided eye, whereas **histopathology** refers to pathologic changes in tissue that are microscopic and can be seen with the use of a microscope. **Lesions** are alterations or abnormalities in a tissue (pathologic changes), and the **pathogenesis** is the sequence of events that leads to or underlies a disease.

Necropsies are done for a variety of reasons. A necropsy is often done on an animal for the following reasons:

- To determine the disease process or processes that led to the animal's death
- To determine the accuracy of the clinical diagnosis
- To evaluate the positive and negative effects of therapeutic measures

In situations in which more than one animal is at risk, as in multiple-animal households, farms, and laboratory animal facilities, the necropsy is helpful in determining whether other animals are at risk for infection, inherited conditions, or injury caused by toxins or environmental hazards. An additional and sometimes unexpected benefit of a necropsy is that it gives the technician the opportunity to increase his or her knowledge about animal anatomy each time one is performed. (See Case Presentation 17-1 for an example of

how a necropsy can be used to determine the disease process that led to the animal's death.)

Successful performance of a necropsy requires knowledge of anatomy and gross pathology and a systematic technique for examination of the animal's body. Well-trained technicians, working with appropriate supervision, perform necropsies in many diagnostic laboratories and in most laboratory animal facilities (Figures 17-1 and 17-2). In practice situations, technicians trained in necropsy techniques and supervised by a veterinarian familiar with the case can and should perform necropsies. Necropsies should be performed frequently enough that the techniques are familiar to the technician and to the supervising veterinarian. During the necropsy, all abnormalities and disease processes should be exposed and described. If necessary, appropriate samples are collected for histopathology, cytology, bacteriology, virology, parasitology, and toxicology. Descriptions of gross findings should be recorded and included in a report, together with the animal's species, age, sex, and breed (signalment); the history; and the clinical findings. Samples that are submitted to the laboratory for further testing should be packaged with a copy of the report. The report should be added to the animal's record, together with the histopathology and other reports. Digital photos of lesions are helpful and can be sent to the laboratory, along with the reports, or as separate electronic files by e-mail.

CASE PRESENTATION 17-1

Boots, a 3-year-old male, neutered, domestic shorthair cat, was presented for necropsy after he died suddenly and unexpectedly. The owners asked their veterinarian if she would examine the body because this was their second cat that had died unexpectedly within the previous month. The owners had several cats that lived mostly outdoors, and they were worried that a neighbor (who was hostile to the cats because of predation of birds at his bird feeder) might have "done something bad" to them. Other than the owners' perception that Boots was sluggish for 2 days before death, no significant historical findings were reported.

Methodical dissection of the cadaver revealed no evidence of trauma such as bruising or fractured bones. Tissues were fresh. Abdominal viscera were grossly normal. No stomach contents were found. When the chest cavity was opened, 5 ml of cloudy gray-green fluid was noted in the right pleural space. A culture swab was inserted into the fluid to obtain a sample before proceeding further. The lungs and heart were then extracted. Pleural surfaces on the right side retained a thin sheet of velvety yellow fibrin. Right lung lobes were compressed and firmer than the normal appearing left lung lobes. Samples of lung were placed in a biopsy bottle containing 10% buffered formalin, and culture swab and tissue samples were forwarded to a reference laboratory. Bodily remains were bagged and frozen.

Test results were received in less than a week. The histopathology report stated that the lung samples showed evidence of a severe acute pleuropneumonia with bacteria. *Pasteurella multocida* was recovered from the aerobic culture.

This case demonstrates how a necropsy can be used to determine the cause of death. In this case, the necropsy, coupled with two simple tests (histopathology and culture), showed that a natural disease process (severe bacterial pleuropneumonia) caused this patient's death. Although it was not clear how the patient got this infection, *Pasteurella pleuropneumonia* is a documented disease entity that could not have been the result of the neighbor's actions. A visit to the veterinarian when the signs were first evident might have saved Boots' life.

> **TECHNICIAN NOTE** The owner's permission must be obtained before the necropsy is performed, and the animal for necropsy must be correctly identified.

Before we begin to describe the necropsy procedure, several important things must be considered. First, confirm that the owner's permission has been obtained before the necropsy is performed. Second, make sure that the animal for necropsy is correctly identified. The species, breed, sex, age, and identifying tags or tattoos should be carefully matched with the information on the owner's permission form and the medical record. This step is critical to prevent performing the necropsy on the wrong animal. If the animal has a radiofrequency identification device (RFID, aka microchip), the device can be collected for verification. In addition, the owner's preference for disposition of the body (e.g., cremation, private cremation, burial) should be determined before the necropsy, if possible. It is important to perform the necropsy as soon as possible after the animal's death to avoid decomposition (**autolysis**). If the necropsy must be delayed, the body should be refrigerated as soon as possible. Small animals should be placed in thin plastic bags with identification tags secured on both the body and the outside of the bag. Decomposition occurs most rapidly in large, obese animals at high temperatures. It is particularly troublesome in large animals that rely on gut fermentation for their nutrients because the rumen continues to generate heat long after the animal's death. The body should not be frozen

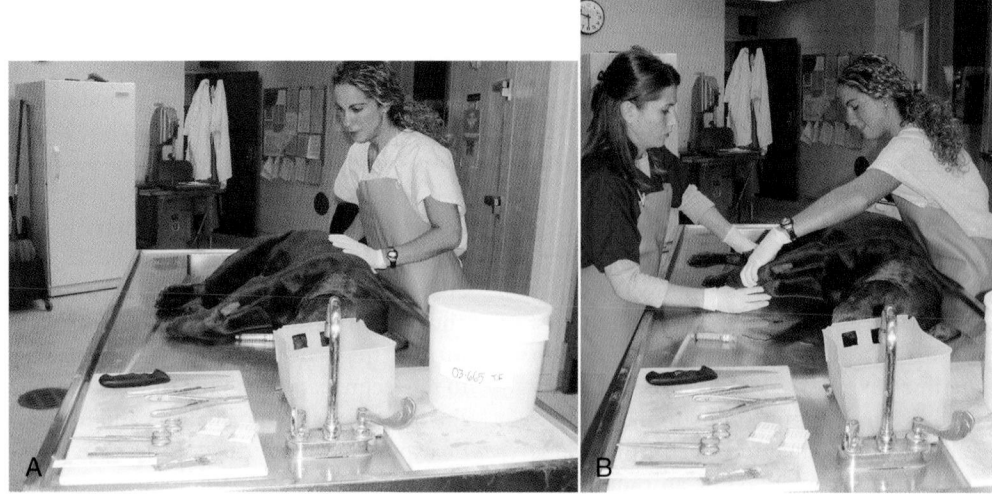

FIGURE 17-1 Prosectors ready to begin a small animal necropsy.

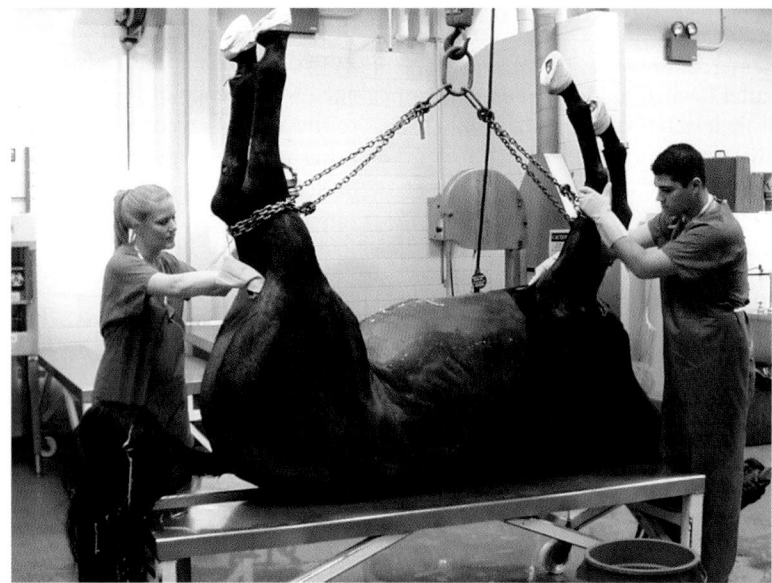

FIGURE 17-2 Prosectors ready to begin a large animal necropsy.

because freezing and subsequent thawing cause many postmortem artifacts.

> **TECHNICIAN NOTE** If the necropsy must be delayed, the body should be refrigerated as soon as possible. The body should not be frozen because freezing and subsequent thawing cause many postmortem artifacts.

The signalment, history, and clinical findings should be reviewed before the necropsy is begun. The record should include the owner's name, address, and telephone numbers; names of other veterinarians involved with the case; the animal's species, breed, age, sex, and name or identification; and the hospital record number. The history should include vaccination history, owner's observations of the clinical signs, length of illness, and a list of other animals at risk.

The clinical findings should include results of the physical examination and clinical tests (e.g., complete blood count [CBC], clinical chemistries, radiographs), surgical procedures, and the date and time of death or euthanasia.

NECROPSY REPORTS

While the necropsy is performed, all abnormalities should be described and recorded. A report in which the findings are described should be written after the necropsy has been completed. Tentative conclusions (diagnoses) may be made at the end of the report (Figure 17-3).

All lesions are described and recorded by using the following criteria (examples are given in parentheses):

- Location (caudal dorsal left lung lobe, left ventricle, cornea)
- Number (one, two, hundreds)

Owner: Brown
Clinic #: 01-34567
Animal name: Ralph
Clinician: Smith
Date/time of death: 01/17/11 (9 AM)
Date/time of necropsy: 01/17/11 (11 AM)

This is a 3.0-kg, 7½-year-old, spayed, female seal-point Siamese cross cat in adequate postmortem and emaciated nutritional condition. There is a clipped area on the distal aspect of the right front leg with an electrocardiogram (ECG) lead taped in place. The left antebrachium is clipped, and a catheter is in the left cephalic vein. The ventral cervical area and the ventral and lateral abdomen are clipped. There is little body fat, and the muscle mass is reduced.

There is approximately 100 ml of yellow stringy fluid in the abdomen. There are multifocal, 2- to 10-mm, yellow-tan clots of fibrin throughout the abdomen and loosely adherent to abdominal organs. There are white-tan, multifocal to confluent, 1- to 5-cm diameter plaques on the surface of the liver, spleen, small intestine, omentum, mesentery, diaphragm, and body wall. The small intestine and colon are dilated (1 to 2 cm in diameter), and the wall of the small intestine is multifocally thickened. In the most severely affected area, at the jejunoileal junction, the serosa is corrugated and the wall is 3 to 5 mm thick. The abdominal and sternal lymph nodes are enlarged (0.5 to 2.0 cm in diameter) and white on the capsular surface. On section, they have a normal lymph node architecture with a thick white cortex.

The lungs are heavy, wet, and red-purple, and they sink in formalin. There is approximately 5 ml of serosanguineous fluid in the pericardium.

Gross Findings

Lungs: moderate to severe acute pneumonia, presumptive
Abdomen: severe fibrinous peritonitis
Small intestine and colon: severe chronic enteritis and colitis, presumptive
Pericardium: moderate serosanguineous effusion
Abdominal and sternal lymph nodes: severe reactive hyperplasia, presumptive

Gross Diagnosis

- Euthanasia
- Feline infectious peritonitis (FIP)
- Severe enteritis and colitis, presumptive
- Severe pneumonia, presumptive

Comment

I am not sure if the changes in the small intestine and colon are due to FIP or some other process. The lung lesion is also not typical for FIP. Impression smears of the peritoneal surface lesions reveal a mixed population of inflammatory cells, including neutrophils, lymphocytes, plasma cells, and macrophages, consistent with the diagnosis of FIP.

Samples of lung and small intestine are submitted for bacterial culture. Samples of lymph nodes, small intestine, colon, lungs, liver, and spleen are submitted for histologic-examination.

FIGURE 17-3 Sample necropsy report.

- Color (red, green, yellow-tan)
- Size (either measurements, such as 3 × 5 × 4 cm, or weights for liver and heart)
- Shape (round, flat, spherical, stellate)
- Distribution (focal, multifocal, diffuse)
- Consistency (soft, firm, hard, rubbery)
- Odor (sweet, sour, ammonia)

Findings are usually recorded in the order in which they were encountered in the necropsy. Either the present or the past tense should be used (not both), and the descriptions should be as specific as possible without drawing conclusions. For example, "there are multiple dark red 1- to 4-mm-diameter soft nodules in all lung lobes" rather than "hemangiosarcoma." On the basis of the descriptions, the veterinarian formulates a morphologic diagnosis, which includes severity, time, distribution, lesion, and anatomic site. An example of a diagnosis might be "severe acute multifocal interstitial pneumonia."

FIXATIVES

Ten percent buffered formalin is the most widely used fixative for the preservation of tissues. Slices of tissue (generally, no thicker than 1 cm) should be placed in large volumes of formalin. Generally, there should be 10 times as much formalin solution as tissue (by volume). This solution may be purchased from a variety of sources and is also easily prepared. It is made by mixing nine parts of water with one part of commercially available formaldehyde solution (37% to 40% HCHO). The addition of 6.5 g of dibasic anhydrous sodium phosphate and 4 g of monobasic sodium phosphate per 1000 ml of solution creates neutral buffered 10% formalin. This is an excellent general purpose fixative and is somewhat more desirable than plain (acidic) 10% formalin. The addition of buffers is important because it eliminates the formation of undesirable hematin pigment in tissue sections. Formalin (and all fixatives) should be handled with care. Formalin is a contact irritant and a carcinogen. Protective plastic gloves, preferably of nitrile composition, should always be worn when fixatives or fixed tissues are handled. Containers with fixatives should be kept closed except when placing tissues in them, and fixatives should be handled and used in a well-ventilated space.

> **TECHNICIAN NOTE** Ten percent buffered formalin is the most widely used fixative for the preservation of tissues. Tissues should be placed in large volumes of formalin (10:1 formalin-to-tissue ratio).

For the preservation of whole brains, intact spinal cords, and bones, 50% formalin, made by mixing one part 10% buffered formalin with one part of commercial formaldehyde (37% to 40% HCHO), is superior to the 10% solutions. The stronger 50% solution penetrates and fixes the large tissue mass more rapidly and more thoroughly than 10% formalin. Formalin fixation is usually complete within 24 hours (large brains may take 48 hours). Tissues fixed in 10% formalin are traditionally stored in 10% formalin, but storage in 70% alcohol is superior.

Bouin's fixative is less widely used than 10% formalin, but it is preferred in some instances because it produces less tissue shrinkage and better preservation of cellular detail. Fetal tissues, intestinal epithelium, eyes, testes, endocrine glands, and the inclusion bodies associated with viruses are particularly well preserved with this fixative. Bouin's fixative may be purchased from a variety of sources.

> **TECHNICIAN NOTE** All containers of fixed tissue samples should be clearly labeled. Appropriate caution should be used in handling, shipping, and disposing of all fixatives.

FACILITIES AND INSTRUMENTS

Necropsies should be performed in a well-lit, well-ventilated space, ideally outside the usual surgical and treatment areas. The area should be easy to clean and disinfect, have adequate drainage for fluids and water, and be large enough to comfortably move around in (Figure 17-4). When necropsies are performed in the field (outdoors), appropriate disposal of tissues and inadvertent spread of disease become particular concerns.

The person performing the necropsy (called the **prosector**) should wear protective clothing, such as a plastic apron, a laboratory coat, or scrubs, which can be removed and either discarded or cleaned after the necropsy (Figure 17-5). Latex or other protective plastic gloves should be worn at all times, and a mesh glove should be worn on the nondominant hand when cutting large animals. In addition, a surgical mask should be worn when dealing with animals that have died from infectious diseases that can be spread through aerosolization. Protective footwear (boots or booties) is appropriate when dealing with larger animals.

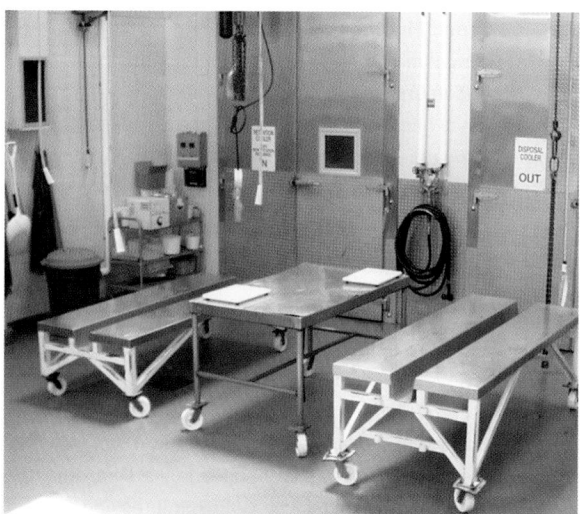

FIGURE 17-4 View of a large animal necropsy room.

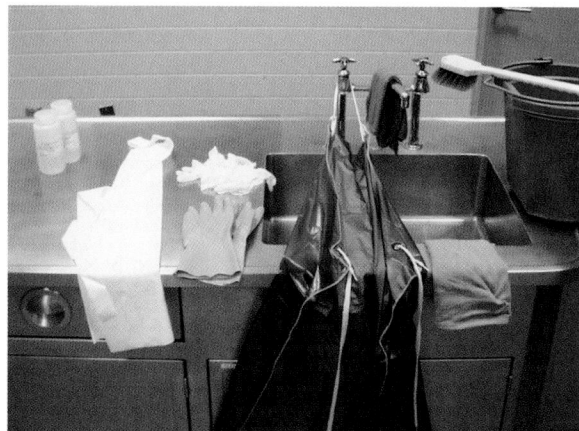

FIGURE 17-5 Personal protective clothing and equipment commonly used in a large animal necropsy.

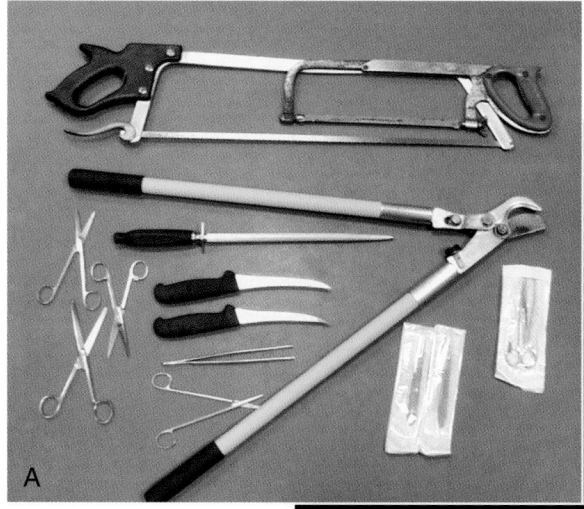
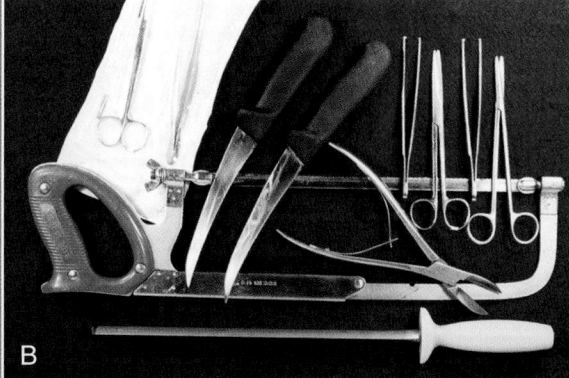
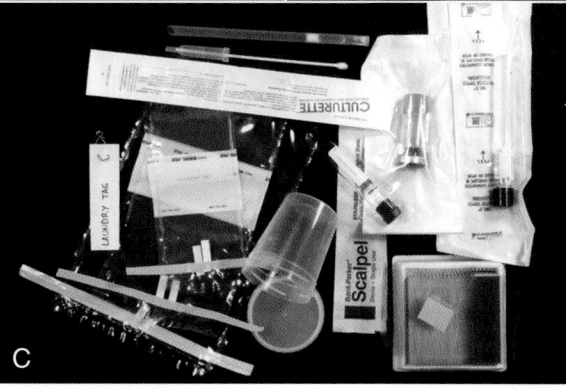

FIGURE 17-6 A and B, Instruments commonly used in a large animal necropsy. C, Equipment commonly used in a large animal necropsy.

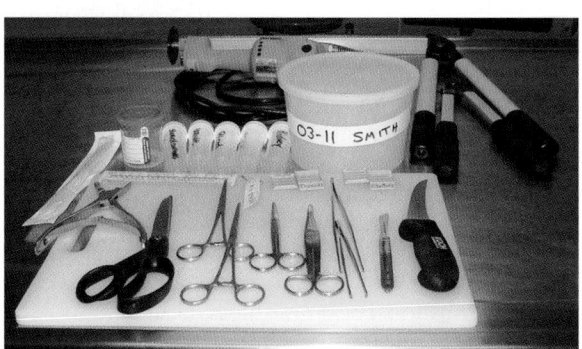

FIGURE 17-7 Instruments and equipment commonly used in a small animal necropsy.

BOX 17-1	Instruments Used in Typical Necropsy Procedure

- Necropsy knives (sturdy ones that can be sharpened) and honing steel
- Scalpel handle and blades
- Scissors (large and small operating, Mayo, or Metzenbaum scissors work well)
- Forceps (large- and small-toothed)
- Serrated, all-purpose, plastic-handled utility scissors
- Bone-cutting forceps
- Hacksaw, meat saw, or Stryker saw (for brain removal)
- Lopping (pruning) shears for cutting ribs and bones
- String or hemostats for closing off bowel ends
- Labeled plastic buckets or screw-top plastic containers containing formalin
- Tissue cassettes (for small tissues) and clip-on laundry tags for identifying tissues
- Labeled, sealable, plastic bags and plastic vials or bottles for refrigerated and frozen samples
- Culturettes for aerobic and anaerobic cultures

Necropsies do not require specialized equipment or instruments. Most instruments can be obtained from surgical suppliers and hardware stores (Figures 17-6 and 17-7). Box 17-1 lists the instruments used in a typical necropsy.

TECHNICIAN NOTE All equipment and instruments should be thoroughly cleaned and disinfected after the necropsy. Instruments should be dedicated for necropsy use only to prevent the spread of pathogens.

ANCILLARY PROCEDURES

Before samples are collected for examination in the microbiology, parasitology, and toxicology departments, the diagnostic laboratory should be contacted for specific advice on which samples should be collected, how they should be collected, and how they should be packaged and submitted. This minimizes potential errors and provides the laboratory with the best possible specimens.

> **TECHNICIAN NOTE**   Contact the diagnostic laboratory for specific advice on which samples should be collected, how they should be collected, and how they should be packaged and submitted.

Tissues and specimens for bacteriology, mycology, and mycoplasma cultivation are collected aseptically, placed in Culturettes or sterile containers without preservatives, and submitted to the laboratory without delay. Frozen specimens should not be submitted. Sterilized instruments should be used to collect samples for microbiological testing. If the surface of the tissue is contaminated, it can be seared with a flamed spatula, the surface can be cut with a sterile blade, and a Culturette or needle attached to a sterile syringe can be inserted to swab or aspirate the tissue for testing.

Specimens collected for microbiology always should include the primary site of disease. Other samples may include heart blood, lung, liver, spleen, stomach contents of aborted fetuses, placenta, exudates, synovia, brain, and small intestine. When intestine is submitted, a 10-cm segment of intestine is tied off at each end to prevent excessive contamination by the internal contents. The instruments used to do this are heavily contaminated by the microbes exposed at the cut ends. For this reason, intestine should be collected last and placed in a separate container to prevent contamination of other tissue samples. Tissue sections of $2 \times 3 \times 1$ cm and fluid specimens of 3 to 5 ml are desirable.

Tissues for virus isolation are collected aseptically and may be refrigerated in a sterile container or immersed in sterile 50% buffered glycerol in sterile containers and preserved by freezing. Fresh, refrigerated tissue immersed in virus transport medium (available from the virology laboratory) is the preferred method of tissue submission. Lung, liver, spleen, kidney, and brain are prime specimens. Sections need to measure $5 \times 5 \times 10$ mm. Contact the virology laboratory for the appropriate technique.

For toxicology, blood, liver, stomach contents, kidney, fat, brain, and urine may be saved. Blocks of tissues $10 \times 5 \times 4$ cm (approximately 200 g), 10 to 20 ml of blood, and 50 to 100 ml of fluid are desirable. They may be frozen.

If rabies is suspected, the animal's head should be sent to the appropriate laboratory for testing, according to the guidelines and laws of the state (Procedure 17-1). In cases in which rabies is suspected, decapitation or other necropsy procedures should not be attempted unless the technician has been specifically trained to perform this procedure. A necropsy should be performed on the rest of the carcass only if a rabies test result for the brain is negative.

For cytologic examination, smears are made (after gentle blotting on absorbent paper) either by scraping the cut surface of the specimen with a new scalpel blade and then spreading the scraped material onto a slide or by lightly

---

PROCEDURE 17-1 | Rabies Procedure

Technicians and clinicians should be familiar with the rabies policies and guidelines of your state.

In all cases where rabies is suspected, the animals should be handled only by clinicians and technicians who are preimmunized against rabies and have a serum titer greater than 1:5. For small animals, prosectors should double-glove and wear protective masks and goggles. For animals larger than large dogs, personnel should wear rubber boots, a scrub suit, an apron, double gloves (the outer glove is heavy vinyl with gauntlets), and a face shield for splash protection. Pathology personnel who decapitate and extract brains must use the additional protection of a Tyvek coverall or alternatively a surgical gown and apron. A HEPA-filtered helmet and face shield are suggested when working on equine species because of concerns about aerosolization of West Nile virus.

In cases where rabies is the primary or only differential diagnosis, the head should be carefully removed by disarticulation at the atlantooccipital junction using a disposable scalpel or knife, double-bagged, placed in a refrigerated container (with ice packs, not dry ice), and sent to the appropriate laboratory for fluorescent antibody (FA) testing. The remaining carcass should be double-bagged in a red biohazard bag, labeled as a rabies suspect, and disposed of as a biological hazard.

Some states require removal of the brain before submission to the laboratory for animals larger than a large dog (horses, cattle, etc.). To remove the brain of a large animal for rabies testing, use a special head vise or hold the head on the table (eyes may be removed to facilitate head holding). Remove as much hide and flesh over the calvaria as safely possible. The rostral transverse cut through the skull is made behind an imaginary line connecting the lateral canthi of the eyes. Lateral saw cuts start at the dorsolateral notch of the occiput and just miss the dorsal projection of the coronoid process. A small hatchet, inserted into the saw cuts, can be used to lever the calvaria. Then, cranial nerves and meningeal attachments can be severed and the brain removed. Hemisection, parasagittal section, or selective subsection of the brain should be performed for the rabies laboratory submission, as directed by the state testing laboratory.

In cases where a person has been bitten or exposed to saliva through open wounds, and rabies is not on the differential list or the animal did not have neurologic signs, either the whole head or two transverse slices of the brain (one involving the medulla and cerebellum bilaterally and the other involving the hippocampus bilaterally) should be submitted for rabies testing. The necropsy can be performed in the usual manner.

In all cases, tables and instruments must be carefully disinfected and cleaned. Disposable scalpels are placed in a sharps container, and other instruments must be cleaned and disinfected.

All submitted tissues must be accompanied by a completed state rabies questionnaire.

pressing small pieces of tissue against the surface of a clean slide. Several impressions are made across the slide. Slides are generally submitted unstained to the laboratory, or they can be stained and examined at the time of the necropsy.

> **TECHNICIAN NOTE** If rabies is suspected, the animal's head should be sent to the appropriate laboratory for testing, according to the guidelines and laws of the state.

SHIPPING DIAGNOSTIC SPECIMENS

The rules for shipping diagnostic samples, technically referred to as "clinical specimens," have changed in recent years. Senders can be fined if containers break or specimens leak during normal transit conditions. Correct labeling is important, and a special packaging symbol (UN 3373) might be required. A computer search of the web reveals many helpful sites (e.g., www.fedex.com/us/services/pdf/PKG_Pointers_Specimens.pdf). Most courier companies abide by International Air Transportation Association (IATA) rules, which impose the highest packaging and labeling standards. The simplest advice is to contact the courier to request specific packaging requirements.

In general, all clinical specimens must be shipped in rigid primary containers that cannot leak. Excess formalin can be removed if the specimen has been fixed. The primary container is enclosed by a secondary container, usually a sturdy sealable plastic bag. Primary and secondary containers should be labeled. The plastic bag should contain absorbent material in case the primary container leaks. This package then goes inside a rigid shipping box. Cushion the contents of the shipping box. Styrofoam shipping boxes with outer cardboard shells are ideal. Formalin-fixed material does not need refrigeration, but bacterial cultures and fresh or frozen tissues might need freezer packs. Never use ice. Submission forms should not be placed next to primary containers, and, if condensation is likely, the submission form should be in its own plastic bag.

NECROPSY PROCEDURE FOR A SMALL MAMMAL

The following procedure is appropriate for dogs, cats, ferrets, rodents, and rabbits. A brief outline of this procedure is provided in Procedure 17-2.

TISSUE COLLECTION

Tissues collected for histologic examination must be handled carefully before fixation and must be properly labeled for identification. Tissue sections should not be squeezed, stretched, or rinsed with water, and epithelial surfaces should not be rinsed or rubbed with fingers or instruments before samples are obtained for histopathologic examination. Tissues become rigid with fixation, so if there is a need to retain the flatness of the tissue (such as a nerve or a section

---

PROCEDURE 17-2 | Necropsy Procedure Outline

1. Before you begin dissection, make sure you have the owner's permission, the correct animal, disposition instructions, body weight, labeled formalin container, instruments, cassette for bone marrow, tag for brain, cardboard for nerve and skin, and an understanding of the clinical history.
2. All routine tissues and all lesions are collected, all lesions are described (measured and weighed if appropriate), and all necessary microbiological, cytologic, and toxicologic samples are collected for every necropsy.
3. Weigh the animal and do the external examination, remove the eyes, then place the body in left lateral recumbency, and make a midline skin incision extending into axillary and inguinal areas to reflect limbs; extend the incision rostrally to the mandibular symphysis and caudally to the perineum.
4. Dissect and examine, section, and collect (DESC) skin, lymph nodes, salivary glands, and testes or mammary glands. Open coxofemoral, stifle, and scapulohumeral joints. DESC synovium, skeletal muscle, sciatic nerve, and bone marrow.
5. Open abdomen (midline), puncture diaphragm, open chest (bilateral, cutting ribs) and pericardium, collect microbiological samples, and examine organs and vessels in situ. (*Note:* Discuss the case with the clinician at this time.) DESC thyroid, parathyroids, and adrenal glands.
6. Remove tongue from oral cavity, and reflect tongue, tonsils, larynx, and esophagus caudally. Cut spinal cord and vertebral column at atlantooccipital joint, remove skin and muscle from calvaria, cut calvaria with Stryker saw in hood, and remove caudal-dorsal calvaria and dorsal meninges. Transect cranial nerves, and remove brain and pituitary. Open tympanic bullae. Section head longitudinally, and examine nasal and oral cavities.
7. Remove tongue, tonsils, esophagus, trachea, lungs, heart, and thoracic aorta together. Serially section tongue, open esophagus, and trachea. Open right atrium, then right ventricle, then follow pulmonary arteries, isolate heart, and open left atrium, left ventricle, and thoracic aorta. Weigh the heart. Collect whole heart in cats and small dogs, three sections of heart in larger animals. Serial section lungs, saving one section from each lobe.
8. Remove distal duodenum, jejunum, ileum, colon, and mesenteric lymph nodes together by stripping from mesentery (open later unless critical). Remove liver, duodenum, pancreas, stomach, and spleen en bloc. Serial section spleen, open stomach and duodenum, express gallbladder, weigh liver, and serial section liver (collect one section of each lobe). Open gallbladder, stomach (collect fundus and pylorus), duodenum, and pancreas (one section of right lobe with duodenum and one section of left lobe). Collect samples from all tissues.
9. Remove floor of pelvis, and DESC right kidney and ureter, left kidney and ureter, urinary bladder, urethra, prostate, ovaries and uterus, cervix and vagina, rectum, anal glands, and abdominal aorta. DESC small intestine, colon, and mesenteric lymph nodes.
10. Remove spinal cord if necessary.

of skin), it can be placed on a piece of cardboard. The tissue will remain adhered to the cardboard after immersion in formalin.

Sections from paired organs may be trimmed differently from one another to distinguish them from one another. For example, the left kidney may be sectioned longitudinally, and the right kidney may be cut transversely. In addition, sections can be labeled with clip-on laundry tags for identification purposes. If there is any possibility that a section of tissue may lose its identity (i.e., be difficult to distinguish) when mixed with other specimens, the sections should be tagged with clip-on laundry tags. If tissue samples are small, they may be placed in separate labeled containers, such as tissue cassettes. The **pituitary gland** of a small animal, for example, is well differentiated from other tissues when placed in a small tissue cassette.

> **TECHNICIAN NOTE** Tissues collected for histologic examination must be handled carefully before fixation and must be properly marked for identification.

In all cases, it is desirable to save sections of critical tissues for histopathologic examination. These include lung, **myocardium,** liver, spleen, pancreas, stomach, small intestine, kidneys, lymph nodes, whole brain, endocrine organs, urinary bladder, colon, and muscle.

DISSECTION

The method of dissection described here is a standard technique that can be applied to all mammalian species and is based on the following two precepts:

1. In stepwise fashion, each part of the carcass is examined **in situ** (as it first appears in the carcass); it is then isolated from the carcass and examined as a whole; finally, it is dissected and examined.
2. Once a part has been taken from the body, it is dissected to completion (exceptions include tissues from the gastrointestinal tract, brain, spinal cord, and eyes). Sections for histologic or laboratory examination are collected before further dissection is undertaken.

This method is the opposite of those that call for evisceration now and dissection later—methods that disrupt the entire carcass all at once, and that lead to forgotten or lost tissues. Immediate complete dissection of one part at a time reduces the possibility of lost or forgotten parts and leaves the remainder of the carcass intact. In this way, if the findings in one organ suggest that another part or parts of the carcass should be explored in situ, this is still possible and has not been precluded by previous dissection.

PRELIMINARY OBSERVATIONS

Before the necropsy is begun, the prosector should review the signalment (species, breed, color, sex, age, weight, animal identification), the clinical history, and available laboratory data. It is important that the time of death and the time of necropsy be recorded. The animal should then be weighed,

and the weight should be recorded in grams or kilograms. All organs that are abnormal in size or shape should be measured and/or weighed.

> **TECHNICIAN NOTE** Before the necropsy is begun, the prosector should review the signalment (species, breed, color, sex, age, weight, animal identification) of the animal, the clinical history, and any available laboratory data.

EXTERNAL EXAMINATION

The exterior of the animal is examined: body conformation, hair coat, skin, nose, mouth (lips, cheeks, gums, teeth, tongue), eyes (eyelids, conjunctiva, cornea, sclera, anterior chamber, iris, lens), ears, mammae, penis, prepuce, scrotum, vulva, anus, and feet. Because the retina undergoes rapid decomposition after death, dissection begins with the eyes. The upper and lower eyelids are examined and excised. The membrana nictitans is grasped with tissue forceps, the globe is lifted, and soft tissue attachments to the bony orbit are incised with scissors or a scalpel in a 360-degree arc. As the globe is freed from the orbit, care must be taken to avoid application of excessive tension to the optic nerve. The optic nerve is carefully severed at the optic canal. The excised globe is examined, and then extraocular muscles, fascia, fat, conjunctiva, and membrana nictitans are dissected from the globe. The interior of the eye can be examined by immersing the globe in clear, cool water. The sclera is examined, and the unopened globe is immersed in Bouin's fixative or formalin.

REFLECTION OF SKIN AND LIMBS AND EXAMINATION OF SUPERFICIAL ORGANS AND BODY CAVITIES

The animal is placed in left lateral recumbency (left side down). A midline incision is made beginning at the right axilla and extending cranially to the mandibular symphysis (Figure 17-8). The incision is continued in the opposite direction caudally as a median or paramedian incision, passing between the mammae and around the penis, prepuce, and scrotum to the perineum (Figure 17-9). The upper forelimbs are reflected by dissection between the scapula and the ribs. Fat, fascia, and superficial muscles are reflected back, together with the skin. Skin of the ventral aspect of the neck and throat is reflected. Abdominal skin is reflected, and hindlimbs are reflected by extending the incision into the coxofemoral (hip) joints. The animal is now placed in dorsal recumbency (on its back) (Figure 17-10).

Skin incisions are extended down the cranial medial aspects of both rear legs, and the skin is reflected. As they are exposed during dissection, superficial organs are examined and samples from these organs are collected: lymph nodes (mandibular, superficial cervical, prescapular, axillary, inguinal, popliteal), mammary glands, testes, and skin.

In all necropsy examinations, several joints are examined before the body cavities are opened. The coxofemoral joints

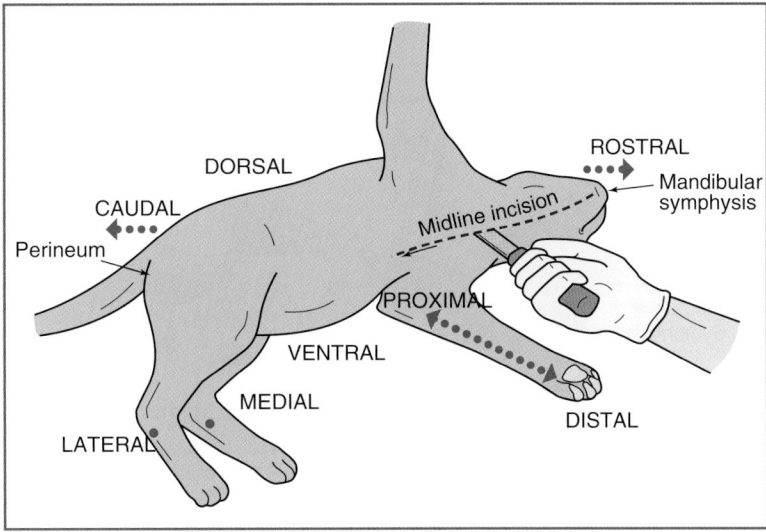

FIGURE 17-8 The necropsy begins with the animal placed on its left side. A midline incision is made from the mandibular symphysis.

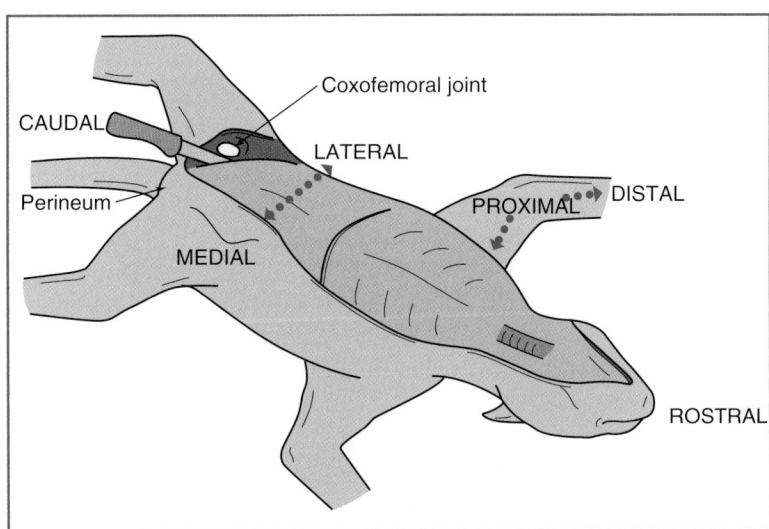

FIGURE 17-9 The front limbs are reflected by making incisions between the ribs and the scapulae. The hind legs are reflected by incising the coxofemoral (hip) joints.

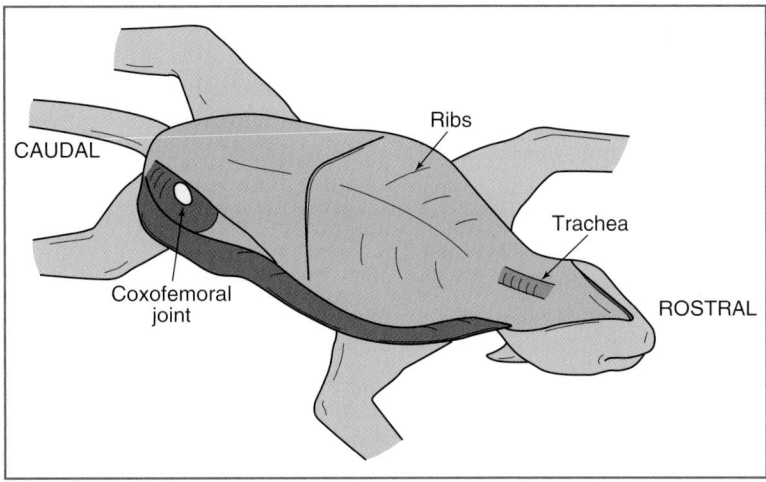

FIGURE 17-10 After all four limbs have been reflected, the animal is positioned in dorsal recumbency (on its back).

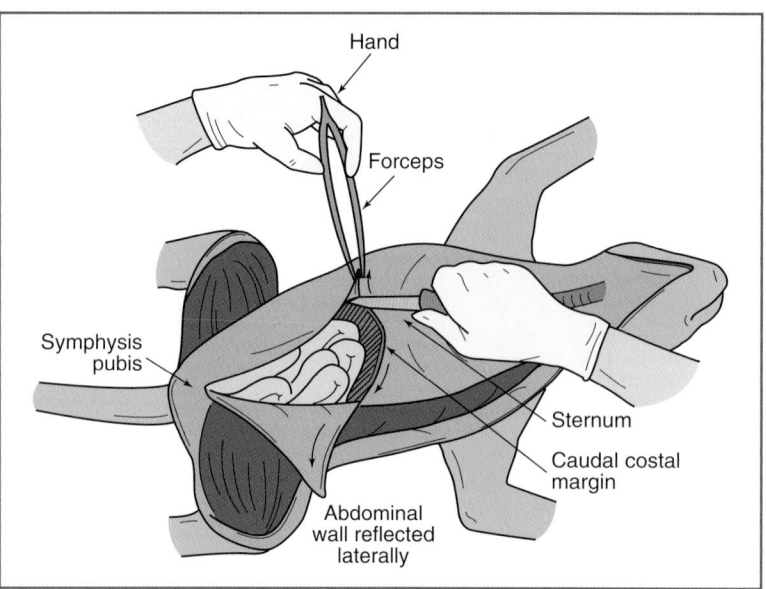

FIGURE 17-11 The abdominal wall is incised with a midline incision. The right and left halves of the abdominal wall are reflected laterally by making incisions from the sternum along both right and left caudal costal margins.

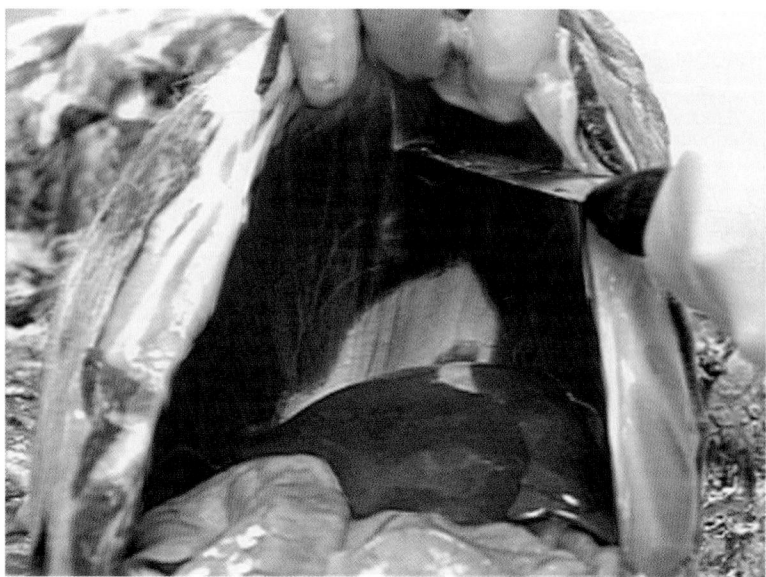

FIGURE 17-12 The diaphragm is punctured to test for negative pressure in the pleural cavity.

are opened and examined during the initial incision. The scapulohumeral and stifle joints are also examined during all routine necropsies. The atlantooccipital joint will be examined when the head is removed.

Samples of the **sciatic nerve,** synovium with patella, and skeletal muscle are collected. Bone marrow samples for impression smears or histopathologic examination should be collected at this time. Generally, marrow is obtained by cracking the upper midshaft femur with pruning shears.

You should, at this point, have already collected the following: eyes, lymph nodes, testes or mammary glands, skin, synovium, sciatic nerve, skeletal muscle, and bone marrow.

Next, the three major body cavities (peritoneal, pleural, pericardial) are opened. All organs are examined in situ, and

any abnormalities are noted. The abdomen is opened by making a midline incision from the **sternum** to the symphysis pubis and by making incisions laterally from the sternum along both caudal costal margins. The abdominal wall is then reflected laterally to expose the abdominal cavity (Figure 17-11).

The **diaphragm** is now punctured to check for negative pleural pressure (Figure 17-12), and the diaphragm is cut away from the ventral and lateral rib cage. The ventral rib cage is removed by cutting the ribs bilaterally (on both sides) midway between the costochondral junction and the vertebral column (Figure 17-13). This should be done with utility scissors or pruning shears. Examine the pleural surface of the rib cage. In young animals, the costochondral growth plate

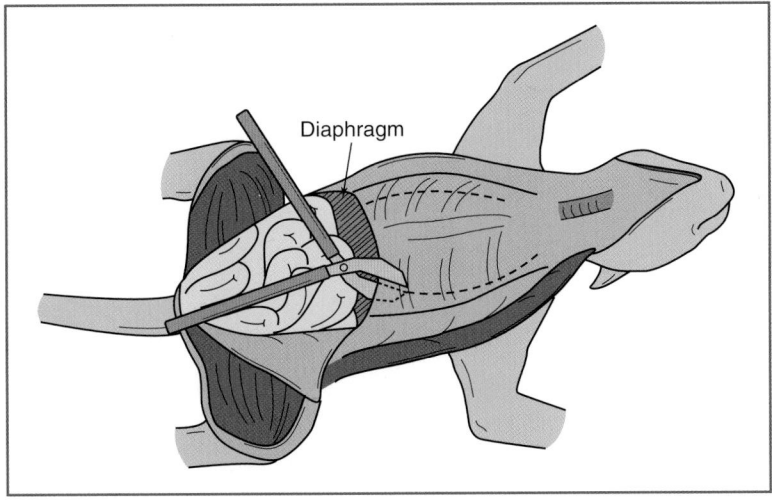

FIGURE 17-13 The ventral portion of the rib cage is removed by cutting the ribs bilaterally (on both sides) with heavy pruning shears.

may be examined and saved for histopathologic examination. Next, the pericardial sac is opened, and the exterior of the heart is examined.

> **TECHNICIAN NOTE** The history and preliminary findings are reviewed with the clinician after all body cavities have been opened.

The thyroid, parathyroids, and thymus should be identified at this time and removed. The adrenal glands should then be identified and removed. The adrenal glands are sectioned, and the corticomedullary ratio is noted. The mandibular salivary glands, parotid salivary glands, parotid lymph nodes, jugular veins, and parapharyngeal and retropharyngeal lymph nodes are examined.

EXAMINATION OF SKULL AND BRAIN

Remove the tongue from the oral cavity, and reflect the tongue, tonsils, larynx, and esophagus caudally (Figure 17-14). An incision is made through the intermandibular muscles, along the medial surface of the ramus of each mandible, from the angle to the symphysis. The frenulum of the tongue is incised, and the tongue is pulled (or pushed) ventrally between the rami. The tongue is used as a handle, and right and left paramedian incisions are extended from the larynx to the thoracic inlet, exposing the length of the trachea and esophagus. It is necessary to cut or disarticulate the **hyoid bones** dorsal to the pharynx to free the tongue, larynx, pharynx, trachea, and esophagus as a unit.

The spinal cord is transected by an incision into the ventral atlantooccipital joint. Atlantooccipital membranes, ligaments, and joint capsule are transected, disarticulating the head from the vertebral column (Figure 17-15, A and B). The skin is removed from the head by leaving it attached to the skin of the body and peeling the head forward out of the skin. The superficial muscles of the head are removed. External ears are opened and examined. Temporal

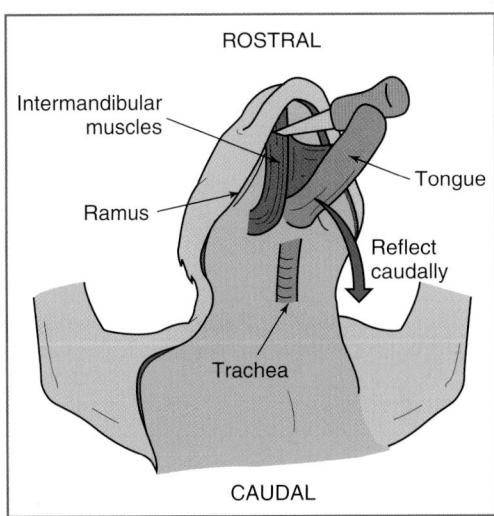

FIGURE 17-14 Examination of the tongue, tonsils, larynx, and esophagus. These are reflected caudally after the intermandibular muscles have been incised.

muscles are removed, exposing the calvaria (skull cap) (Figure 17-16).

The calvaria and caudal wall of the cranial cavity are removed from the skull as a unit, exposing the dorsum of the brain. Three cuts are made with a Stryker saw, a hacksaw, or a meat saw to accomplish this. The first is a transverse cut through the frontal bones. This cut is usually made immediately caudal to the orbits. Care is taken to make the cut just deep enough to transect bone, but not deep enough to engage the brain beneath.

The second and third cuts are made through the side walls and the caudal wall of the cranial cavity. At 45-degree angles to the longitudinal **axis** of the skull, they extend from the lateral ends of the transverse cut to the medial faces of the occipital condyles (Figure 17-17). In small animals, the bone may be broken away piecemeal, progressing cranial from the **foramen magnum** with scissors, bone-cutting forceps, or

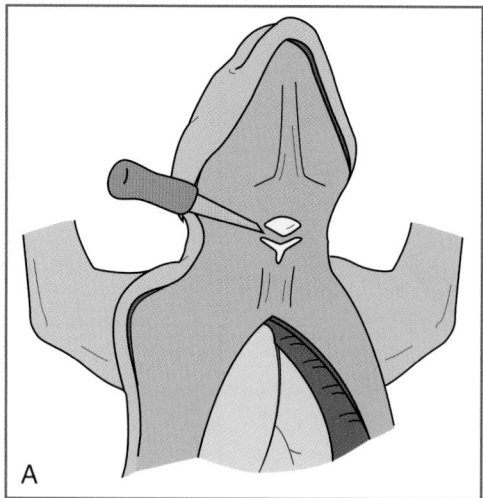 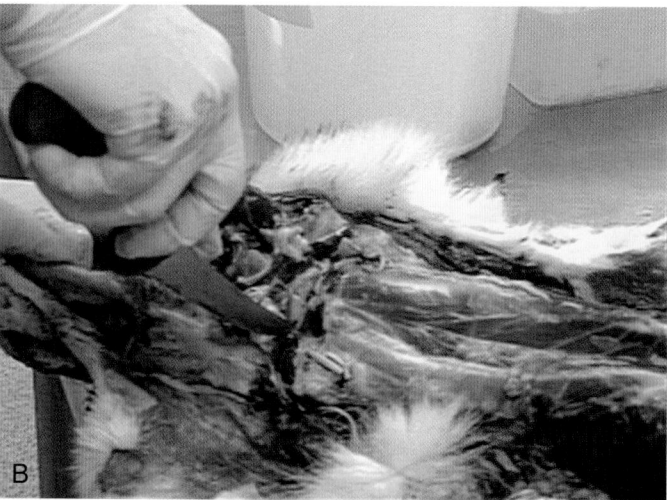

FIGURE 17-15 A and B, The spinal cord is transected ventrally by first making an incision into the atlantooccipital joint. The head is disarticulated from the vertebral column.

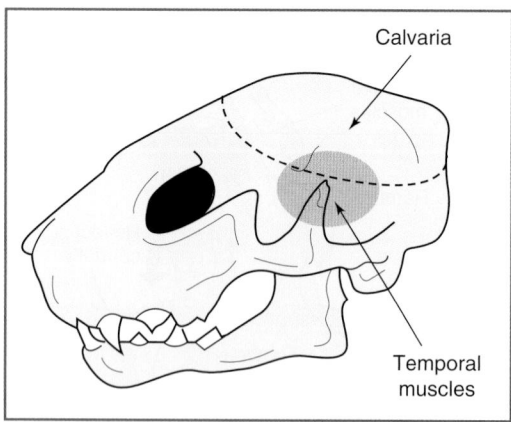

FIGURE 17-16 The temporal muscles are removed to reveal the skull cap, or calvaria.

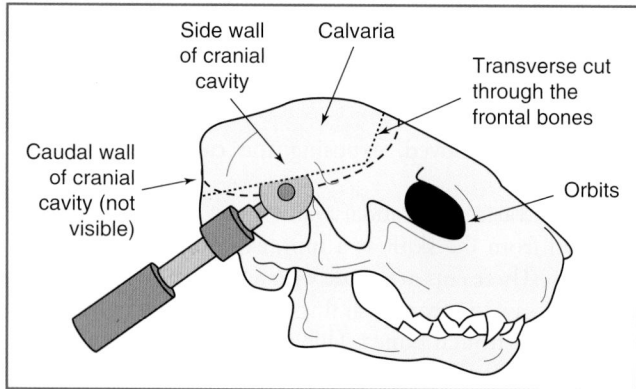

FIGURE 17-17 The cranial cavity is opened by removing the calvaria and the caudal wall as a unit.

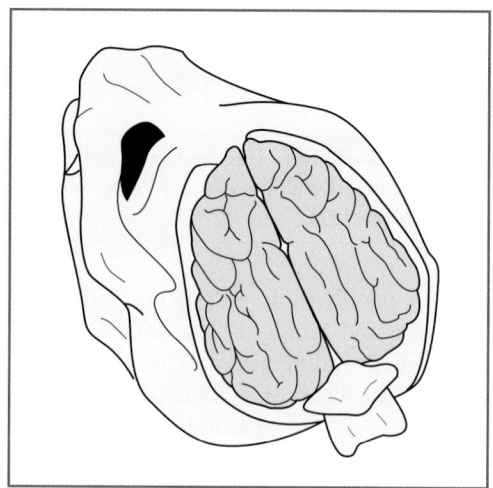

FIGURE 17-18 The meninges and the surface of the brain are examined in situ.

For removal of the brain, the dorsal meninges are removed and the cranial nerves are transected, progressing rostrally from the foramen magnum. The brain is examined, tagged, and then immersed in 50% formalin. Brain slicing is postponed until after the brain has been thoroughly fixed in formalin.

The pituitary gland is removed from its fossa with the brain and examined. The middle ears (tympanic bullae) are opened ventrally by using rongeurs. For examination of the nasal septum, turbinates, and frontal or maxillary sinuses, the skull is sectioned longitudinally with a saw. The oral cavity is examined.

DISSECTION AND EXAMINATION OF NECK AND THORACIC VISCERA

The cervical and thoracic viscera are removed from the body and examined. The trachea and the esophagus are used as a handle, and the thoracic organs are removed from the body by cutting between the dorsal **mediastinum** and

postmortem shears. The calvaria and the caudal wall as a unit are pried loose from surrounding bones and removed. The **meninges** (the three membranes that cover the brain) and the surface of the brain are examined in situ (Figure 17-18).

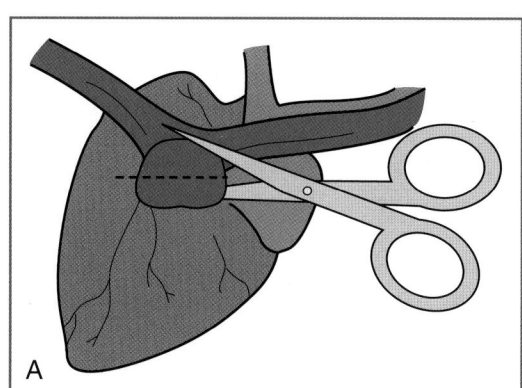

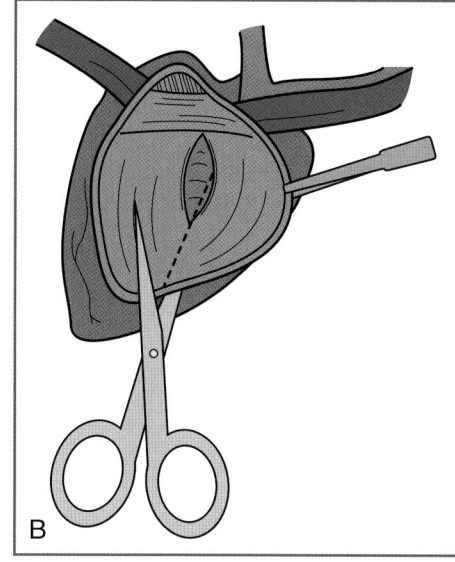

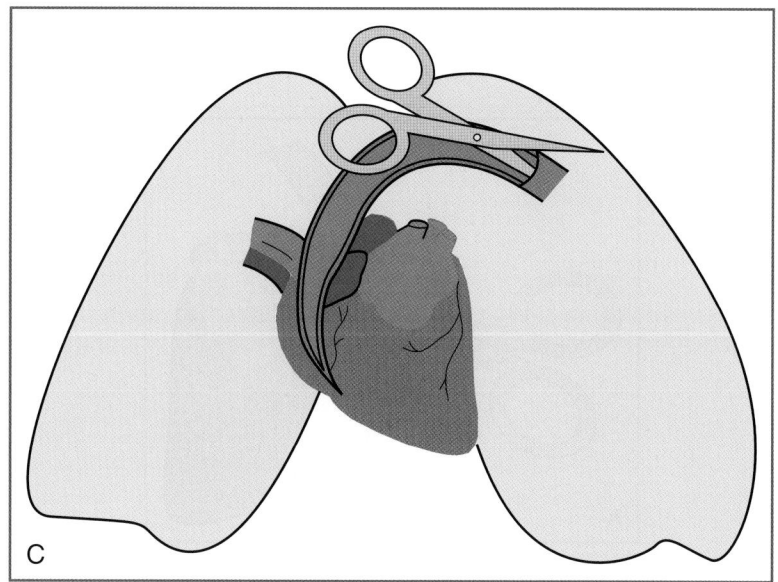

FIGURE 17-19 A, Dissection of the heart begins with an incision into the right auricle. B, The heart is incised through the right atrium and ventricle following the interventricular septum. The incision is then continued into the pulmonary artery. C, The pulmonary artery is incised, and the incision is continued into each lung lobe.

the vertebral column from the thoracic inlet back to the diaphragm. The dorsal incision is carried above the aorta. At the diaphragm, the aorta, the postcava, and the esophagus are transected, and the throat, neck, and thoracic viscera are removed as a unit. This unit is dissected and examined from tongue to aorta. The tongue is examined and is sliced transversely. The pharynx is opened middorsally with scissors, and the pharynx and tonsils are examined. The esophagus is opened longitudinally by a middorsal incision. The larynx is opened middorsally with utility scissors or a knife, and the incision is extended through the trachea to the lungs. The lungs are examined and palpated (for fine fixation, the lung may be "inflated" with 10% formalin, gravity fed into the trachea or bronchi).

The right side of the heart and the pulmonary arteries are examined before the lungs are cut. The heart is held

so that the right side is on the prosector's left and the left side is on the right. The right auricle is incised, and the incision is extended away from the prosector to the far end of the right atrium (Figure 17-19, *A*). The incision is then directed downward through the right **atrioventricular (AV) valve** and along the interventricular septum to the apex of the right ventricle. The incision is continued up along the interventricular septum through the pulmonic valve into the **pulmonary artery** (Figure 17-19, *B*). The right free wall of the heart is reflected, and the valves and endocardial surfaces are examined. The pulmonary arteries are opened into each lung lobe (Figure 17-19, *C*). Air passages and transected lung tissue are examined. Sections of lung are squeezed gently to assess fluid content. Bronchial lymph nodes are examined and sliced longitudinally.

The heart and major vessels are then removed from the lungs. The heart is again held so that the right side is on the prosector's left and the left side is on the right. The left auricle is incised, and the incision is extended away from the prosector to the far end of the left atrium (Figure 17-20, *A*). The incision is then directed downward through the left AV valve and along the center of the left ventricular free wall to the apex of the left ventricle (Figure 17-20, *B*). The aortic valve and aorta are examined by cutting up through the septal leaflet of the left AV valve and into the aorta (Figure 17-20, *C*). The valves, endocardium, and endothelial surfaces are then examined. The heart may be weighed after all major vessels have been removed at the base of the heart. Next, the myocardium is sliced longitudinally for examination, and samples are collected. Small hearts should be fixed whole after they have been opened.

DISSECTION AND EXAMINATION OF ABDOMINAL CAVITY

Examination of the abdominal cavity begins with examination of the portal vein as it enters the liver and removal of the intestinal tract. The intestine is removed by stripping the mesentery from the small intestine and colon. The **duodenum** is clamped or tied and transected distal to the tail of the pancreas. The colon is transected at the pelvic inlet, and the intestinal tract is removed and set aside for later examination. If the animal is thought to have intestinal disease, the intestines are examined at this time.

The stomach, liver, spleen, pancreas, and duodenum are removed by cutting the attachments between these organs, the diaphragm, and the ventral body wall. The spleen is examined and sectioned. The stomach is opened along the greater curvature, and the duodenum is opened. The gallbladder is squeezed to determine patency of the bile duct, the gallbladder is opened, and the stomach, duodenum, and pancreas are dissected from the liver, examined, and sectioned. A section of the right side of the pancreas is collected with the duodenum, and a section of the left side is collected separately. The liver is then examined and sectioned. Multiple slices (approximately 1 cm apart) are made in the liver, and samples are collected from each lobe.

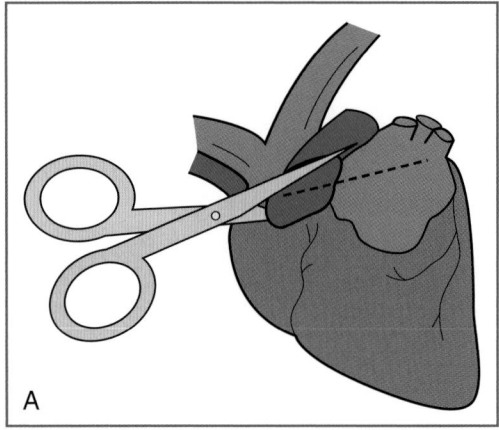

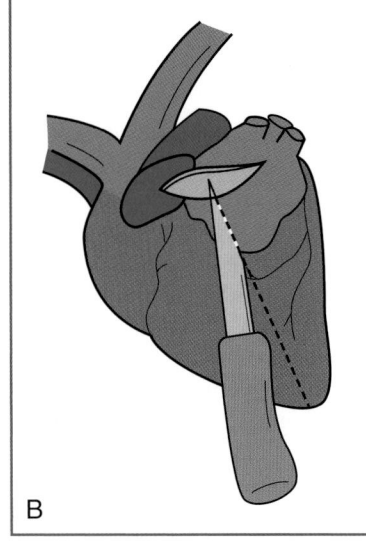

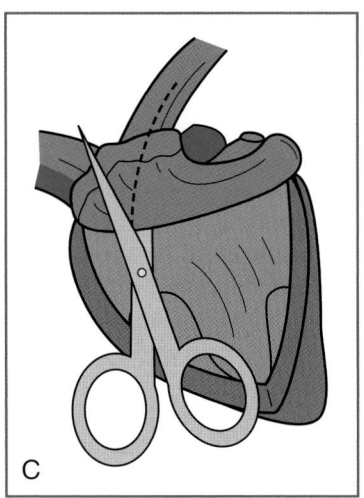

FIGURE 17-20 A, The second half of the heart is dissected by incising the left auricle and continuing the incision into the left atrium. B, From the left atrium, the incision is continued through the left atrioventricular (AV) valve into the left ventricle to the apex. C, The incision is then continued into the aorta.

DISSECTION AND EXAMINATION OF FEMALE REPRODUCTIVE TRACT, URINARY TRACT, AND ACCESSORY MALE REPRODUCTIVE ORGANS

The floor of the pelvis should be removed to facilitate examination and removal of the urogenital tract. This is accomplished by making paramedian cuts through the obturator foramina on the floor of the pelvis. The mesovarium, mesosalpinx, and mesometrium are examined. Ovaries, oviducts, and uterus are freed from mesentery and reflected toward the pelvis.

The left kidney is dissected free from the abdominal wall but remains attached to the ureter. It is sliced longitudinally, and the capsule is peeled from one-half of the kidney (Figure 17-21). The surface, cortex, medulla, and pelvis are examined. The ureters are examined and palpated. If the ureters or renal pelvis is dilated, the ureters are opened from kidney to bladder with a scissors. The ureter is cut near the bladder, and the kidney is removed. Sections are taken from the middle of both halves—one with the capsule intact and one with the capsule removed. Samples are also collected from any other renal lesions. The right kidney is then examined in the same manner.

The urinary bladder is incised and opened (Figure 17-22). Serosa, mucosa, and cut surfaces are examined. Care should be taken to avoid rubbing mucosal surfaces. The urethra is opened and examined, and the prostate is examined and sectioned.

> **TECHNICIAN NOTE** Care should be taken to avoid rubbing the mucosal surfaces of examined tissues.

Ovaries, oviducts, uterus, cervix, vagina, and vulva are removed from the carcass as a unit. Large ovaries are sliced longitudinally, oviducts are examined and palpated, and uterus, cervix, vagina, and vulva are opened with scissors or a knife. Serosa, contents of the uterus, endometrium, cut surfaces, cervical folds, and luminal surfaces of vagina and vulva are examined.

DISSECTION AND EXAMINATION OF INTESTINAL TRACT

The intestinal tract is examined by laying it out on the table and examining the serosal surface. The tract is then opened from the duodenum through the colon by using scissors. The mucosa is examined, and sections are taken from the jejunum, ileum, and colon, including lesions. The mucosa should be handled carefully to prevent creation of artifacts. Once sections have been taken, the mucosa can be gently rinsed with water to reveal mucosal details.

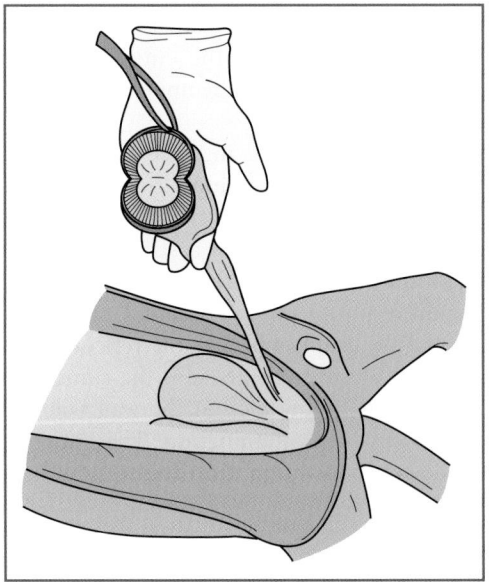

FIGURE 17-21 The kidney is dissected with a longitudinal incision. The renal capsule is then peeled away to reveal the renal surfaces.

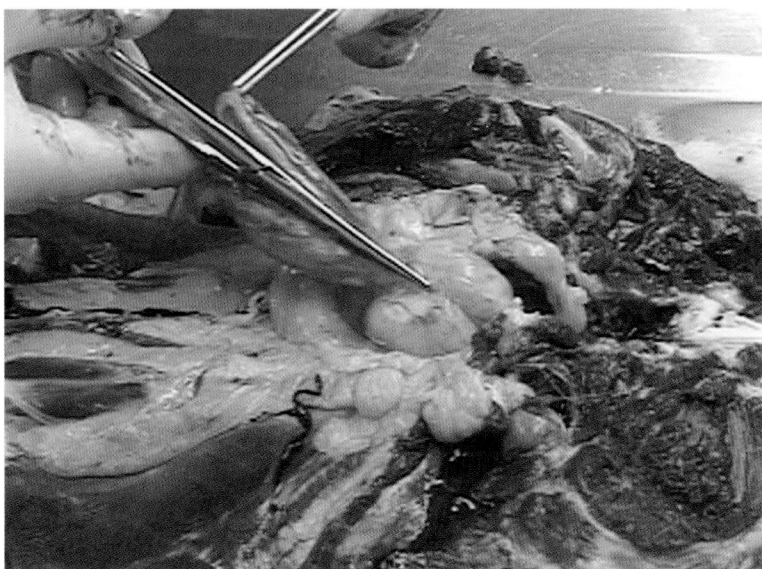

FIGURE 17-22 The urinary bladder is incised and opened in situ, and the incision is continued through the prostate and urethra.

DISSECTION AND EXAMINATION OF ABDOMINAL AORTA, RECTUM, AND ANAL GLANDS

The abdominal aorta is opened longitudinally and examined, and a section is taken for histologic examination. The rectum is opened, and the anal sacs are examined.

DISSECTION AND EXAMINATION OF VERTEBRAL COLUMN AND SPINAL CORD

The manner and extent to which the vertebral column is dissected will depend on the history and size of the animal. For more extensive examination of the vertebral column and spinal cord, the remaining rib cage, the four limbs, and most of the dorsal spinal musculature are removed from the vertebral column and pelvis. A dorsal laminectomy is performed to demonstrate ventral or lateral impingements on the spinal cord of small animals. The spinal cord is covered dorsally by the vertebral arches; each arch consists of a right and a left lamina, which unite to form the dorsal spinous process (spine). Beginning at the **atlas,** the right and left **laminae** of each vertebra are cut with bone shears or, in larger specimens, with the Stryker saw. The laminae of atlas and the axis are broad and difficult to cut, but the remainder of the vertebrae present little difficulty. Once several dorsal arches have been freed, the connected arches are held as a handle and are used to reflect succeeding arches dorsally and caudally. When the entire roof of the vertebral canal has been removed, meninges, spinal cord, and vertebrae are examined in situ. Spinal cord and meninges are removed by cutting spinal nerve roots, and the floor of the vertebral canal and the intervertebral discs are examined.

NECROPSY VARIATIONS

The following sections describe variations on the basic small mammal necropsy procedure that are useful in dealing with ruminants, horses, pigs, fetal farm animals, birds, and laboratory animals.

RUMINANTS

Necropsy of a ruminant is done with the animal in left lateral recumbency. This positions the rumen on the down side, which facilitates removal of the abdominal organs (Figure 17-23).The right inguinal area is incised, and the coxofemoral joint is penetrated. Muscles near the pelvis are severed, and the right hindlimb is reflected away from the body. Each mammary gland is undermined at its body wall attachment and retracted caudally. The mammary glands should remain attached to the body by the perineal skin, so that gland position can be identified when they are serially sectioned. The right axilla is incised so that the entire forelimb can be reflected away from the body. The upper half of the trunk is then skinned.

Entry into the abdomen is initiated by cutting the body wall behind the last rib. Cuts along the midline and upper flank permit exposure of the cavity (Figure 17-24). After an in situ inspection, the **omentum** is stripped from the **forestomachs;** double-string ligatures are placed on the duodenum (near the pylorus) and rectum, and a single ligature is placed around the esophagus near the reticulum. This prevents excessive leakage of contents. If the rumen is severely distended with gas, a tiny nick in the wall will release the gas without excessive contamination. The entire intestinal tract is removed by severing the mesenteric root, and the

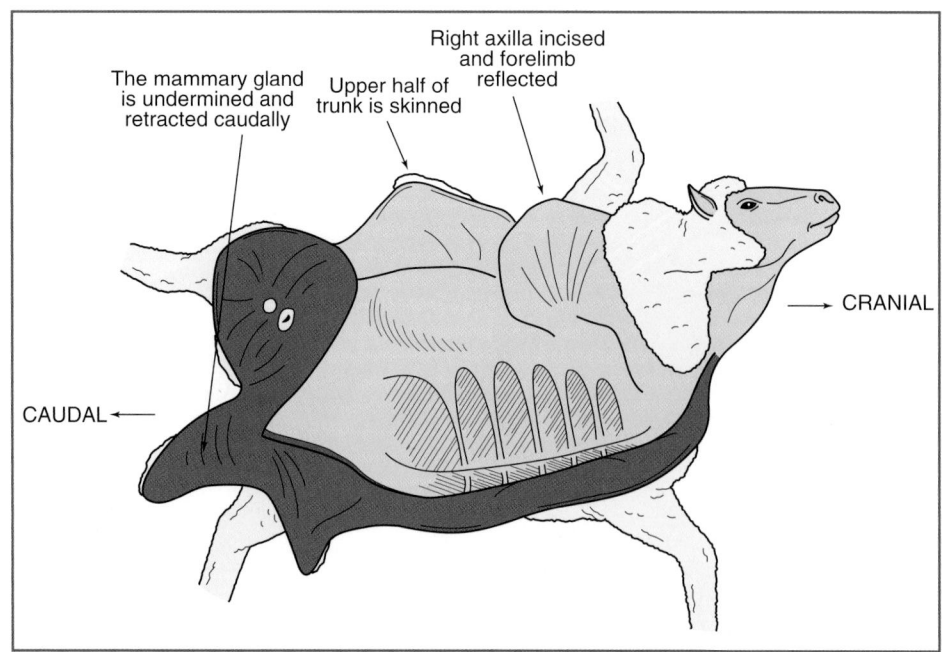

FIGURE 17-23 The ruminant is positioned in left lateral recumbency; this positions the rumen on the "down side" and facilitates access to the abdominal organs.

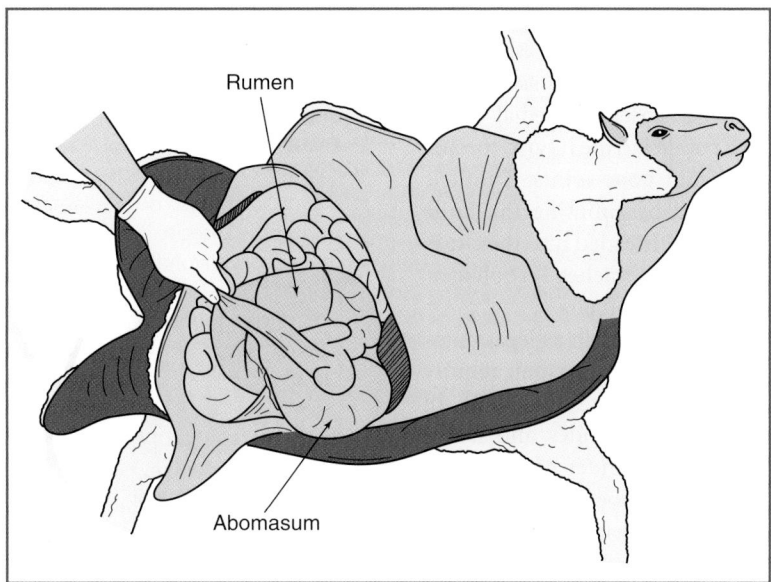

FIGURE 17-24 Access to the abdominal cavity is achieved by making an incision along the midline, followed by cuts along the last ribs.

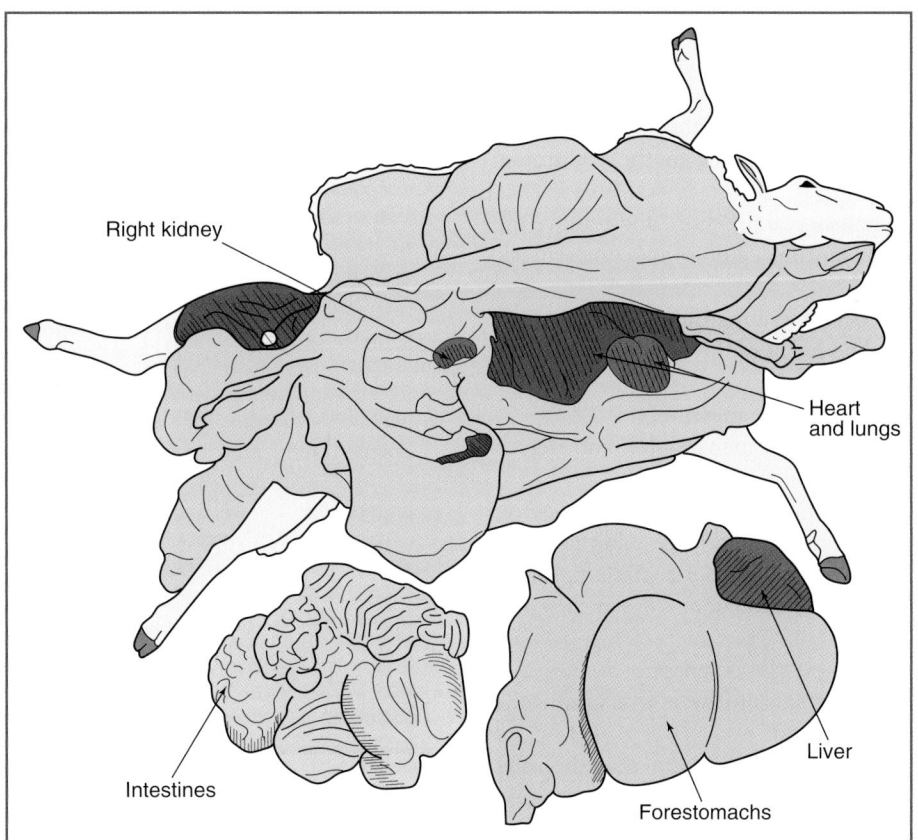

FIGURE 17-25 After the omentum is examined in situ, it is stripped from the forestomachs. The duodenum, rectum, and esophagus are ligated, and the entire intestinal tract is removed by severing the mesenteric root.

intestines are opened, examined, and sampled while still attached to the mesentery (Figure 17-25). The dorsal attachments to the rumen are cut, and the forestomachs and **abomasum** are rolled onto the floor. Ruminoreticular contents should be examined for foreign objects or undesirable plant material.

Thoracic contents are readily removed via an abdominal cavity approach. The large size of the chest cavity, coupled with the difficulty of cutting ribs of mature animals, encourages use of this procedure. The diaphragm is incised along its costal attachment, and the caudal and ventral mediastinal attachments are severed. The tongue, larynx, trachea, and esophagus are then freed of their attachments. Disconnecting the hyoid-laryngeal apparatus can be difficult. Bold knife cuts medial to the mandible expose the lateral surfaces of hyoid bones. The knife can then be inserted medial to the hyoid bones and pulled forward parallel to the larynx, forcing the knife through one of the hyoid bone joints. Thoracic inlet connective tissues are severed by rimming the knife medial to the first ribs. The tongue is threaded into the chest, and the entire unit—tongue, larynx, trachea, esophagus, lungs, and heart—is pulled into the abdomen.

In ruminants, various circumstances (such as legal mandates or the presence of neurologic disease) may require sample collection for prion disease testing (Box 17-2). In these cases, brainstem, pharyngeal lymph nodes, and sometimes the tonsils are collected. The remainder of the ruminant necropsy is similar to that described for the small mammal.

HORSE

Left lateral recumbency is the preferred body position for necropsy of a horse. Reflect the right forelimb and the right hindlimb as described for the ruminant. Skin the trunk, and enter the abdomen. The intestines are removed in the following multistep process:

1. Retract and drape the free portion of the large colon over the horse's body to facilitate access to the abdominal viscera.
2. Sever the ileum at the ileocecal junction, and remove the small intestine by cutting along the mesenteric insertion.
3. Cut the duodenum where it wraps around the mesenteric root; a string ligature here will reduce contamination by digesta.
4. Next, remove the small intestine mesentery.
5. Sever the small colon near the pelvic inlet, and detach along the mesocolon.
6. With careful blunt dissection, peel the soft connective tissue and pancreas adhering to the large colon near the mesenteric root. When your hand can encircle the mesenteric root, advance the knife to cut as close to the aorta as possible.
7. Obtain samples from the large colon and cecum, and empty them of their contents. Rinse and examine the mucosal surfaces.

The remainder of the necropsy is similar to the procedure done on ruminants and small mammals. Special attention should be given to the guttural pouches and jugular veins.

All joints of the **appendicular skeleton** should be opened. Joints are best approached from the medial and cranial aspects after the skin has been reflected. The coffin joint is the most difficult joint to access, but access is easier if the foot can be split (with a saw). Splitting the foot also facilitates examination of the hoof wall lamina. Spinal cord removal is extremely tedious without access to a meat cutter's band saw. Alternatively, the cervical cord can be extracted by disarticulating the cervical vertebrae, one by one. Remove as much muscle as possible before disarticulating at the facets and

annulus fibrosus. Sever the nerve roots by advancing a pair of thin, long-handled scissors along the wall of the spinal canal. Grasp the cord by its dura mater, and make every effort to avoid crushing the soft central nervous system tissue.

PIG

For necropsy of a pig, small mammal procedures apply. Because enteric disease is a frequent reason for necropsy, attention should be focused on collecting the freshest possible gut tissues. It is customary to examine the nasal

---

BOX 17-2	Prion Disease Surveillance

Abnormal prions are the cause of fatal neurodegenerative diseases collectively known as transmissible spongiform encephalopathies (TSE). Species-specific diseases include chronic wasting disease (CWD) of deer, scrapie of sheep and goats, and bovine spongiform encephalopathy (BSE; "mad cow disease"), which affects cattle and humans. Prions are unconventional infectious agents that are proteins (i.e., neither bacterial nor viral) with an insidious mode of transmission. State departments of agriculture and state wildlife agencies rely upon technicians to collect tissues from the heads of targeted species. Because testing is regulated by state and federal entities, technicians must be certified by demonstrating that they can properly document and collect the required specimens.

Pharyngeal lymph nodes and brainstem are required samples. Procedural details are beyond the scope of this text because sample collection is not as straightforward a task as it might initially seem. For example, the brainstem is typically harvested with a "brain spoon," which is a modified tablespoon with sharpened edges. This spoon is inserted through the foramen magnum, advanced, and twisted and retracted, pulling out an intact brainstem. A skilled technician can collect brainstems with the "spoon" more quickly than by any other technique. Lymph nodes are concealed in the loose connective tissue and fat around the pharynx. Species variability in lymph node location has been noted, and salivary glands are occasionally collected in error because of their similar size, shape, and color. Tonsils are included in some sampling protocols. They are not always distinctive anatomic structures, and anatomic landmarks are needed for consistent site selection. Skill is required to collect samples efficiently and intact, without undue crushing or slashing. Samples are fixed in formalin. Some surveillance programs also include fresh tissues. A Web search will generate numerous sources of information about TSE, and some of these sites provide detailed instructions and photos for sample collection. Here is one website that is well developed and easily understood:

http://www.michigan.gov/emergingdiseases /0,1607,7-186-25806_26402-65642-,00.html

Basic personal protection equipment (examination gloves and apron) is usually sufficient. However, animals known to have neurologic disease, or that otherwise appear to have been unhealthy, should be handled as though they are rabies suspects.

turbinates of market-weight pigs. This is accomplished with a transverse saw cut of the snout at the level of the second and third premolars. Mature swine have sinus bone covering much of the calvaria. Brain removal is best accomplished by hemisectioning the head.

FETUS

Fetuses are often severely autolyzed, sometimes mummified, because of in utero retention after death. Nevertheless, sample collection is justified. Fetal membranes (placenta) should be carefully examined, and all abnormal appearing sites should be sampled. Equine fetal membranes are examined for completeness. Fetuses from cattle and horses are measured (weighed if possible) to estimate gestational age. Standardized charts are available in many veterinary textbooks. Crown-to-rump length (the distance from the poll to the tail base along the dorsum) is determined with a flexible tape measure.

The fetus is placed in right lateral recumbency because fetal abdominal organs are more easily sampled from the left side. The left limbs are removed, and the body wall is skinned. The abdominal wall is incised behind the rib, and the incision is extended along the ribs, sublumbar flank, and midline without touching the underlying viscera or allowing the body wall to drop onto the viscera. The left hemidiaphragm and costosternal cartilage are cut with the tip of the knife, and, similar to the abdominal approach, the rib cage is retracted without touching the underlying tissues. The ribs usually break along the vertebral column.

Organs are sampled in situ with sterile tools and aseptic technique. The organs of greatest interest for viral cultures are lungs, liver, kidneys, and lymphoid tissue (e.g., spleen, thymus). Samples for bacterial culture are usually taken from stomach fluid, lungs, and liver. The body can now be routinely examined for anatomic correctness, and samples collected for histologic examination. The umbilical stump and brain should always be examined and collected.

BIRDS

Birds suspected of having infectious or zoonotic disease (psittacosis) should be submitted to a diagnostic laboratory for necropsy. If avian necropsies are done, the prosector should wear protective clothing, gloves, and a mask. The carcass should be wetted by immersing it in warm, soapy water or disinfectant to decrease the spread of infectious agents and reduce the quantity of irritating, aerosolized dander and feathers. After external examination, the bird is placed in dorsal recumbency, and the feathers are parted along the ventral midline. For small birds, one wing may be pinned to a corkboard or cardboard for easier dissection. A skin incision extending from the beak to the vent is made, and the skin is reflected. The legs are reflected laterally by cutting into and exposing the coxofemoral joint. The abdomen is opened, as in the small mammal necropsy technique, and the sternum and lateral ribs are removed by cutting through the sternum, ribs, coracoid bones, and clavicles with scissors, utility scissors, poultry shears, or pruning

shears, depending on the size of the bird. Air sacs and abdominal and thoracic contents are examined, and samples are taken for examination by a microbiologist if necessary.

> **TECHNICIAN NOTE** Birds suspected of having infectious or zoonotic diseases (psittacosis) should be submitted to a diagnostic laboratory for necropsy.

For small birds (e.g., hummingbirds, finches), the entire carcass can be fixed after the body cavities have been opened. For larger birds, the joints, nerves, muscles, eyes, brain, and spinal cord can be examined as in the small mammal necropsy technique. The spinal cord in small birds is difficult to remove without damaging it. The entire vertebral column with the spinal cord inside should be collected and fixed after the limbs, head, and muscles surrounding the vertebral column have been removed. The vertebral column and the spinal cord can be submitted whole and decalcified and trimmed by the pathology laboratory.

In larger birds, the thyroid and parathyroid glands, located at the thoracic inlet adjacent to the carotid arteries, are removed. The heart is removed and examined. The entire gastrointestinal tract, liver, pancreas, and spleen are removed, beginning with the esophagus. The spleen, liver, and gastrointestinal tract are examined, and specimens are collected as in the small mammal necropsy. The tongue, trachea, and lungs are then removed and examined, and samples are collected. The gonads (only the left ovary is present in birds) and adrenal glands are removed and fixed whole in small birds, and then the kidneys are removed, examined, and sampled.

LABORATORY ANIMALS

The necropsy technique for small mammals can be used for most laboratory animals, including rodents; however, for evaluation of the health status of laboratory animal colonies, more extensive testing is required. Complete health monitoring includes serology, bacteriology, parasitology, and genetic monitoring, in addition to gross pathology and histopathology. It is beyond the scope of this chapter to include techniques for blood collection for serology, bacteriologic sampling techniques, techniques for ectoparasite and endoparasite examination, and genetic monitoring. Many laboratories provide complete diagnostic services and health monitoring for laboratory animals; such laboratories should be contacted before specimens (either from live animals or from necropsies) are submitted to them.

> **TECHNICIAN NOTE** The necropsy technique for small mammals can be used for most laboratory animals. However, for evaluation of the health status of laboratory animal colonies, more extensive testing is required.

The technique for small mammals is followed, except for the following variations for small rodents. An entire hindlimb can be removed at the coxofemoral joint, the skin can be removed, and the limb can be fixed whole for bone, bone marrow, synovium, nerve, and skeletal muscle samples. For small rodents (e.g., mice, hamsters, gerbils), the lungs should be inflated with formalin after the thorax has been opened but before the lungs and heart are removed from the thorax. A 5- to 10-ml syringe with a small- to medium-bore needle is filled with formalin. The needle is threaded caudally for a few millimeters from the middle of the trachea, and the trachea is clamped with a hemostat rostral to the needle insertion site. The lungs are gently inflated until they fill the thorax. The trachea is then clamped or tied below the needle insertion site, and the lungs and heart are removed from the chest as described on p. 574. The heart is often too small to open easily; before fixation, it can be cut longitudinally through the middle of the right and left ventricles.

The intestinal tract can be opened in a few places and then infused with formalin by using a 5-ml syringe and a small-bore needle, or the entire tract can be opened up and pinned to cardboard before fixation. The kidney and adrenal gland on each side can be removed as a unit and left together for fixation after the kidney has been incised longitudinally to evaluate the pelvis for **hydronephrosis.** The uterus and ovaries or the testes and seminal vesicles and coagulating gland can be removed, along with the urinary bladder, and fixed whole without sectioning.

The spinal cord in small animals is difficult to remove without damaging it. The entire vertebral column with the spinal cord inside should be collected and fixed after the limbs, head, and muscles surrounding the vertebral column have been removed. The vertebral column and the spinal cord can be submitted whole and decalcified and trimmed by the pathology laboratory.

COSMETIC NECROPSIES

Cosmetic necropsies, although of more limited value than complete necropsies, can be performed when disease processes are limited to the abdomen and chest. A midline incision is made in the ventral abdomen from the xiphoid to the pubis. The abdominal organs are examined in situ, and the diaphragm is cut away from the ventral rib cage. The colon and the urethra are tied off at the pelvic inlet and are transected caudal to the tie. By reaching up through the diaphragm, the prosector can grasp and transect the trachea and esophagus at the thoracic inlet. Thoracic and abdominal contents are removed as a unit and are dissected and described as in a noncosmetic necropsy. Body cavities are examined. Cavities are filled with paper towels, and the ventral abdominal incision is sutured.

> **TECHNICIAN NOTE**   Cosmetic necropsies, although of more limited value than complete necropsies, can be performed when disease processes are limited to the abdomen and chest.

RECOMMENDED READINGS

King JM, Dodd DC, Roth L, et al: The necropsy book, ed 5, Gurnee, IL, 2003, Charles Louis Davis DVM Foundation.

Latimer KS, Rakich PM: Necropsy examination. In Richie BW, Harrison GJ, Harrison LR, editors: Avian medicine: principles and application, Lake Worth, FL, 1994, Wingers Publishing.

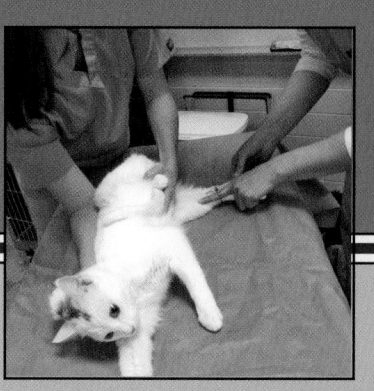

PART FOUR
Medical Nursing

18 | Diagnostic Sampling and Therapeutic Techniques

Harold Davis, Darlene L. Riel, Marika Pappagianis, and Kristin Miguel

OUTLINE

Basic Guidelines, *586*

ADMINISTRATION OF MEDICATION IN THE SMALL ANIMAL, *586*
Oral Administration, *586*
Orogastric Intubation, *587*
Transdermal Administration, *588*
Topical Ophthalmic Administration, *588*
Aural Administration, *588*
Intrarectal Administration, *588*
Intranasal Administration, *589*
Intradermal Administration, *589*
Subcutaneous Administration, *589*
Intramuscular Administration, *590*
Intravenous Administration, *590*
Intravenous Catheter Placement, *591*
Intravenous Catheter Maintenance, *596*
Intravenous Chemotherapy Administration, *596*
Intratracheal Administration, *598*
Intraosseous Administration, *599*
Intraperitoneal Administration, *599*

SAMPLING TECHNIQUES IN THE SMALL ANIMAL, *599*
Blood Sample Collection, *599*
Cephalic Venipuncture, *601*
Jugular Venipuncture, *601*
Lateral Saphenous Venipuncture, *601*
Medial Saphenous or Femoral Venipuncture, *602*
Marginal Ear Venipuncture, *602*
Arterial Blood Sample, *603*
Urine Sample Collection, *604*
Voided Collection, *604*
Manual Bladder Expression, *605*
Cystocentesis, *605*
Catheterization, *606*

Fecal Sample Collection, *609*
Thoracocentesis, *609*
Abdominocentesis, *610*
Diagnostic Peritoneal Lavage, *611*
Transtracheal Wash, *611*
Percutaneous Technique, *612*
Sample Handling, *613*
Cytologic Sample Interpretation, *613*
Arthrocentesis, *614*
Joint Fluid Collection of Distal Joints in the Dog and Cat, *614*
Joint Fluid Analysis, *616*
Bone Marrow Aspiration, *616*
Iliac Aspiration, *617*
Humeral Aspiration, *619*
Femoral Aspiration, *619*
Fine-Needle Aspiration, *619*

ADMINISTRATION OF MEDICATION IN THE LARGE ANIMAL, *620*
Oral Administration, *620*
Syringes, *620*
Balling Guns (Pilling), *621*
Nasogastric and Orogastric Intubation, *621*
Nasogastric Intubation, *622*
Orogastric Intubation, *624*
Intravenous Administration, *624*
Equine, *624*
Bovine, *627*
Camelid, *628*
Ovine and Caprine, *629*
Porcine, *629*
Intramuscular Administration, *630*
Equine, *631*
Bovine, *632*
Ovine and Caprine, *633*
Porcine, *633*
Camelid, *634*

KEY TERMS
Abdominocentesis
Anorexia
Arthrocentesis
Coupage
Cystocentesis
Diagnostic peritoneal lavage
Extravasation
Foley catheter
Hematoma
Hemolysis
Inflammation
Intraosseous
Leukocytosis
Neutropenia
Osmolality
Pancytopenia
Percutaneous
Phlebitis
Pleural effusion
Pneumothorax
Polymerase chain reaction (PCR)
Rumen
Thoracocentesis
Thrombocytopenia
Thrombophlebitis
Thrombosis
Vasodilatation

Subcutaneous Administration (SQ, SubQ, SC), *634*
Intradermal Administration, *635*
Intraperitoneal Administration, *636*
Equine, *636*
Bovine, *637*
Caprine and Ovine, *637*
Porcine, *638*
Intranasal Administration, *638*
Intramammary Administration, *638*
Topical Ophthalmic Administration, *638*
Epidural Administration, *639*
Equine, *640*
Bovine, *640*
Camelid, *640*
Ovine and Caprine, *641*
Porcine, *641*
Transdermal Administration (Cutaneous, Topical), *641*
Intrasynovial Administration, *641*
Rectal Administration, *641*
Rectal Medications, *641*
Enema Administration, *642*

SAMPLING TECHNIQUES IN THE LARGE ANIMAL, *642*
Venous Blood Sample Collection, *642*
Equine, *644*
Bovine, *645*
Camelid (Llama, Alpaca, Lamoid, South American Camelid), *647*
Ovine and Caprine, *648*
Porcine, *648*
Arterial Blood Sample Collection, *651*
Equine, *652*
Camelid, *654*
Bovine, Ovine, and Caprine, *654*
Urine Sample Collection, *654*

Equine, *654*
Camelid, *655*
Bovine, *656*
Ovine and Caprine, *657*
Porcine, *657*
Fecal Sample Collection, *657*
Milk Sample Collection, *658*
Sterile Milk Sample, *658*
Nonsterile Milk Sample, *658*
Colostrum Sample, *659*
Rumen Fluid Collection, *659*
Oral Gastric Tube (Orogastric Tube, Ororumen, Stomach Tube) Method, *659*
Bovine, *659*
Small Ruminant, *660*
Rumenocentesis, *660*
Thoracocentesis (Thoracentesis, Pleurocentesis, Chest Tap, Pleural Tap), *660*
Equine and Bovine, *660*
Camelid, *661*
Transtracheal Wash (Tracheal Wash, Trach Wash), *662*
Equine Transtracheal Aspiration, *662*
Bronchoalveolar Lavage (BAL), *663*
Abdominocentesis, *664*
Equine Abdominocentesis, *665*
Equine Abdominocentesis (Foal), *665*
Camelid Abdominocentesis (Adult), *667*
Camelid Abdominocentesis (Neonatal), *668*
Bovine Abdominocentesis (Adult), *668*
Bovine Abdominocentesis (Neonatal), *668*
Ovine and Caprine Abdominocentesis, *668*
Cerebrospinal Fluid Collection (Spinal Tap, CSF Tap), *669*
Equine, *669*
Camelid, *671*

LEARNING OBJECTIVES

When you have completed this chapter, you will be able to:

1. Pronounce, define, and spell each of the Key Terms in this chapter.
2. List and describe general guidelines for the collection of samples for laboratory testing, and do the following regarding the administration of medication in the small animal:
   - Describe indications and methods for administration of medication to cats and dogs using each of the following approaches: oral, orogastric, transdermal, ophthalmic, aural, intrarectal, intranasal, intradermal, subcutaneous, intramuscular, intravenous, intratracheal, intraosseous, and intraperitoneal.
   - Compare and contrast placement of IV catheters in the peripheral and jugular veins in cats and dogs. Describe the specific steps to carry out placement of through-the-needle (TTN), over-the-needle (OTN), and multi-lumen catheters.
3. Compare and contrast the patient's preparation, positioning, and procedures for blood collection using venipuncture and arterial blood sampling techniques.
4. List and describe procedures for collection of urine samples in cats and dogs. Provide advantages and limitations of each method.

5. Describe the indications, materials needed, and procedures for performing fecal sample collection, thoracocentesis, and abdominocentesis.
6. Describe diagnostic peritoneal lavage (DPL) and list its indications and contraindications. Compare and contrast percutaneous and endotracheal lavage techniques.
7. Define arthrocentesis and list indications for performing it in the cat or the dog. List materials needed, and explain the procedure.
8. Explain the procedure of collecting bone marrow aspirate samples. List indications, contraindications, and potential complications. Compare and contrast the procedure if the sample is obtained from the ilium, humerus, or femur, and explain how the procedure of fine-needle aspiration differs.
9. Describe the methods of orally administering medication to large animal species.
10. Compare and contrast the procedures for administering large volumes of medication via nasogastric tubes in the horse and orogastric tubes in ruminants and swine.
11. Do the following regarding intravenous administration of medication in the large animal:
    - Describe the procedure for intravenous administration of medications in the horse using the jugular vein, intravenous catheterization, the cephalic vein, and the lateral thoracic vein.
    - List indications for use of specific veins for intravenous administration of medication in ruminants and swine.
    - Compare and contrast the materials needed and procedures for placing IV catheters in camelids and food animal species.
12. List possible sites of intramuscular administration for each large animal species, and describe limitations and contraindications if food animal species.
13. Compare and contrast the methods used for administration of medication to horses and food animal species using each of the following approaches: subcutaneous, intradermal, intraperitoneal, intranasal, intramammary (cows only), ophthalmic, epidural, transdermal, intrasynovial, and rectal.
14. Compare and contrast venous and arterial blood collection techniques in equine, camelid, and food animal species.
15. List and describe procedures for collection of urine and fecal samples in equine, camelid, and food animal species. List advantages and limitations of each method.
16. Describe procedures for collection and evaluation of milk samples from dairy animals.
17. Describe procedures for collection of rumen fluid in large animals.
18. Describe the indications, materials needed and procedures for performing a thoracocentesis, transtracheal wash, bronchoalveolar lavage, abdominocentesis, and cerebrospinal fluid collection in equine, camelids, and food animal species.

INTRODUCTION

The veterinary technician plays a vital role in the preparation, collection, and submission of diagnostic samples. Following diagnosis, therapeutic interventions may be required of the veterinary technician. Veterinary technicians commonly begin their careers by first developing their skills in basic techniques such as administering medications, and then progress to more advanced sampling techniques. For this reason, this chapter discusses the administration of medication first, followed by sample collection for both small animal and large animal sections. Given the advances in veterinary nursing, it is incumbent on the veterinary technician to have the knowledge, skills, and ability to collect diagnostic samples and perform therapeutic techniques. When performing or assisting in performing procedures, veterinary technicians should be aware of the indications for performing the procedure, equipment needed, correct technique to be used, potential complications of the procedure, and postprocedure nursing care. Technicians should have expertise in a diverse range of procedures, such as blood and urine sample collection, IV and arterial catheter placement, and fluid and medication administration. These procedures and others will be addressed in this chapter.

BASIC GUIDELINES

All supplies needed for medicating patients, collecting diagnostic samples, and performing therapeutic procedures should be gathered ahead of time. Samples should be collected and stored in appropriate containers with the patient's name and hospital identification number and date printed on each label.

Whenever a needle is inserted through the skin as a part of a treatment (e.g., subcutaneous injection) or a sampling procedure (e.g., bone marrow aspiration), the skin should be properly prepared and free from obvious **inflammation** and infection. Microbes and other contaminants present on the skin surface may be introduced into the underlying tissue when the needle is inserted. Needles and IV catheters from which the protective coverings have been removed should remain sterile and should be handled only at the hub (e.g., the shaft should not be touched or set down on a nonsterile surface).

Having knowledge of potential risks or complications will place the veterinary technician in a position to be proactive rather than reactive to problems. The technician should be able to assess the patient and recognize when problems are occurring and should have a "game plan" in mind for addressing problems. For example, a technician who is knowledgeable in IV catheter complications is performing IV catheter care and notices that the catheter insertion site is erythematous, swollen, painful, and warm to the touch. The veterinary technician assesses the problem as **thrombophlebitis**, determines that a new catheter is needed, and removes the old one.

Pretreatment blood and urine samples should be obtained before administration of fluids and/or medications. Administration of fluids and recent ingestion of a high-fat or high-protein meal may alter blood or urine laboratory values.

> **TECHNICIAN NOTE**   Pretreatment blood and urine samples should be obtained before administration of fluids or medications.

Administration of Medication in the Small Animal

Multiple routes are available for administration of fluids and medication. The route used depends on many factors, including, but not limited to, the patient's condition and temperament, types of medication or fluid, urgency involved in administering fluid or medication, cost, ease of administration, and whether a systemic or local effect is desired.

ORAL ADMINISTRATION

The administration of medication by direct placement into the oral cavity is frequently and easily performed. Technicians should be adept at administering oral medications to animals and capable of demonstrating techniques for pet owners.

> **TECHNICIAN NOTE**   Technicians should be adept at administering oral medications to animals and able to demonstrate techniques for pet owners.

Oral medications usually are administered in liquid, capsule, or tablet form. Liquids are easy to administer through a dropper or syringe. Pulverized tablets and the contents of capsules can be mixed with a small volume of food, water, or flavored liquid. When liquids must be administered with a syringe or dropper, the patient's lower lip is pulled out at the commissure. The tip of the syringe or dropper is placed between the cheek and the gums, and small volumes of liquid are injected. The muzzle should be held at a neutral angle and not elevated. Hyperextension of the neck or movement by the patient during administration may result in fluid aspiration into the trachea. If the patient struggles or coughs, or if fluid spills out of the mouth, the patient should be allowed to rest before further administration attempts are made. Flavored liquid compounds are also a viable method, especially for cats that may react with hypersalivation because of the unpleasant tastes or bitterness of some medications.

A tablet or capsule is most easily administered to a dog if it is hidden in meat, cheese, or a chunk of canned pet food. There are also commercially available flavored treats in which tablet and capsule medications can be hidden. Cats rarely consume pills hidden in food. Cats will meticulously eat the food that surrounds the pill and leave the medication. If a patient has a diminished appetite, it may not consume the entire amount of medication-laced food and will not receive a sufficient dose of medication.

An animal that will not consume baited food is medicated by tilting the head back, prying open the jaws, and placing the pill far back on the base of the tongue (Figures 18-1 and 18-2). The tablet will be expelled if it is not placed far enough back in the pharynx. The technician holds the muzzle closed, rubs under the animal's chin, taps the tip of the nose, or blows air into the nostrils to stimulate the animal to swallow. When the animal licks its nose, it can be assumed that the tablet has been swallowed. However, some dry pills or capsules, such as doxycycline, can take minutes to hours to travel the length of the esophagus before reaching the stomach. This prolonged contact between medication and the delicate lining of the esophagus can cause irritation and esophageal strictures. Therefore to avoid complications, it is beneficial to follow dry pills with administration of liquid via a syringe. Flavored liquids such as chicken broth or tuna juice may be welcomed by the patient.

A specially designed device is available for administering tablets to fractious cats and dogs. The tablet is secured in the flexible tip of a plastic rod that is inserted into the back of the mouth. The rod plunger is quickly depressed, and the pill is propelled down the esophagus. Technicians can

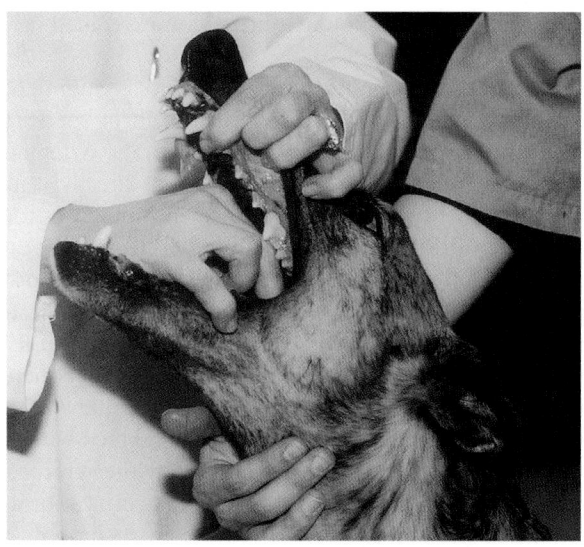

FIGURE 18-1 A dog's muzzle held open as a tablet is placed in the back of the mouth.

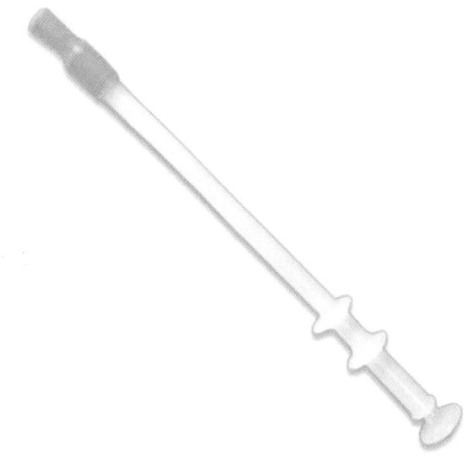

FIGURE 18-3 A pilling device used to administer pills to the back of the oral cavity. The flexible tip accepts tablets or capsules and is activated by depressing the syringe-like plunger.

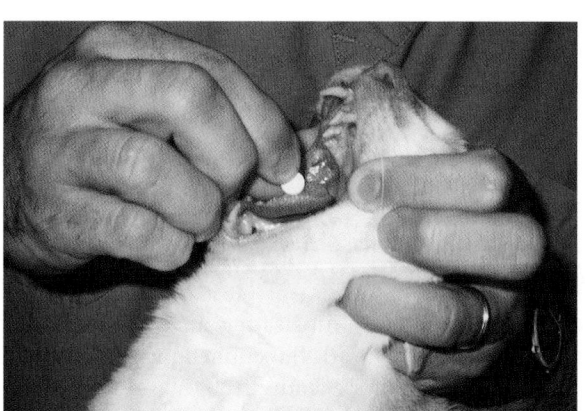

FIGURE 18-2 A cat's neck is hyperextended so its nose points toward the ceiling. The lower jaw is open as a tablet is placed in the back of its mouth.

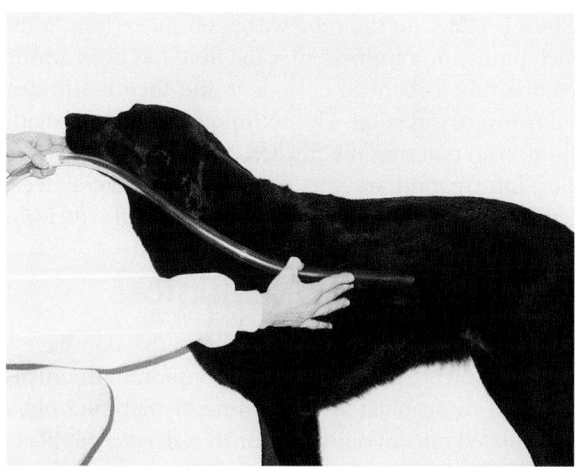

FIGURE 18-4 A length of stomach tube is measured from the nose to the 13th rib. It is marked with tape.

demonstrate use of the "pill gun" to owners for administration of medication at home (Figure 18-3).

OROGASTRIC INTUBATION

Sometimes it is necessary to administer medication, food, or fluids through a tube passed through the mouth and directly into the stomach. This technique is used to administer activated charcoal solutions or to lavage the stomach to treat animals that have ingested toxins. Orphan or weak neonates who cannot nurse can be fed milk replacer via a tube passed through the mouth and into the distal esophagus or stomach. An orogastric tube (OGT) is also passed in an attempt to decompress a patient with gastric dilatation (bloated stomach). Dogs usually permit OGT placement with moderate resistance. Cats, with the exception of neonates, usually require sedation.

The length of 10- to 22-French plastic or rubber tube required to extend from the tip of the nose to the 13th rib is measured and marked on the tube with tape or ink (Figure 18-4). If the tube is to be placed in the distal esophagus to feed an animal, the distance between the tip of the nose and the 8th rib is marked. Water-soluble gel is used to lubricate the tip of the tube. The animal is restrained in sternal recumbency or in a standing or seated position. A roll of tape, a plastic or wooden speculum with a hole in the middle, or a plastic syringe case with smooth ends is placed behind the canine teeth to hold the mouth open. The muzzle is kept in a normal position and is held so that the mouth speculum does not become dislodged.

The tube is slowly passed through the speculum (Figure 18-5). Swallowing will be noted as the tube passes over the base of the tongue and into the esophagus. If the animal coughs, the tube may have entered the trachea and should

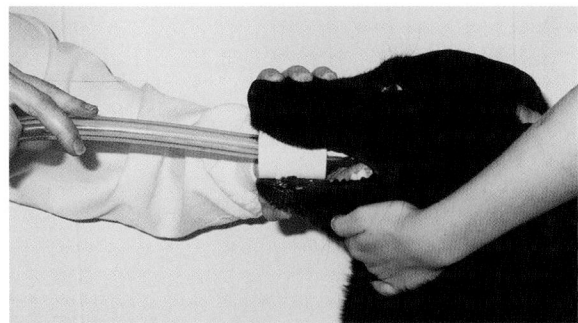

FIGURE 18-5 A roll of tape holds the mouth open as a stomach tube is passed through the roll and into the oral cavity.

be removed. Once the tube is in the esophagus, it is advanced the premeasured length until it enters the stomach.

Correct placement of the tube in the gastrointestinal tract should always be verified before the introduction of any medications or fluids. Refer to the discussion of nasoesophageal tubes and nasogastric tubes (NGTs) for instruction on how to check tube placement.

Fluid is added to the tube with a 60-ml syringe, a metal drench pump, or a funnel. After the fluid has been administered, the tube is bent to occlude it and then is withdrawn in a downward direction. This technique prevents a backflow of fluid from entering the trachea.

For information on the placement of enteral feeding tubes, refer to Chapter 9, "Companion Animal Nutrition."

TRANSDERMAL ADMINISTRATION

Certain medications applied topically to the skin have systemic and local effects. Many drugs commonly administered by the oral route, such as prednisone or methimazole, can be formulated into an ointment for transdermal application. Other medications, such as nitroglycerin, are manufactured as a cream to be applied directly to the skin.

Medications, such as nitroglycerin, may be absorbed by the individual making the application; therefore, disposable gloves should be worn to prevent absorption. A small quantity of ointment is applied to a sparsely haired region, such as the pinna of the ear, the groin, or a shaved area on the ventral thorax. If gloves are unavailable, the ointment can be applied to a small piece of wax paper and wiped onto the skin. The treated area is covered with a light bandage so it will not be accidentally touched. A note is placed on the front of the patient's cage specifying the medication used, the site to which the medication has been applied, and the duration of time that must pass before the application site can be safely touched.

Many topical medications are dispensed in a liquid or aerosol form to control fleas, ticks, mites, heartworms, and intestinal parasites. Depending on the product, the medication may be sprayed on the hair on the entire body or applied to the skin between the shoulder blades. Manufacturers' directions regarding application should be followed closely. Gloves are worn during the application, and the site of administration should not be touched for a specified period after the application.

The transdermal application of analgesics is gaining popularity. One analgesic manufactured in a form specifically for transdermal application is fentanyl citrate. A fentanyl-impregnated self-adhesive patch is placed directly onto a shaved, dry region of skin. The technician should not touch the adhesive side of the patch containing the fentanyl because the medication is absorbed topically. Gentle pressure is applied with the palm of the hand over the patch application site for 1 minute to help the patch adhere to the skin. Each patch can be applied only once because it may not adhere to the skin and deliver the complete dose of fentanyl if it is removed and reapplied. The patch can be covered with tape on which the date and time of placement have been recorded.

It is important to place the fentanyl patch in a location from which the animal cannot remove it, such as on the intrascapular region. It should not be applied to skin that will be in contact with a heating pad, a heat lamp, or another external heat source. The rate of drug delivery is increased when the skin beneath the patch warms and the cutaneous vessels vasodilate.

Topical application of creams (e.g., EMLA cream, lidocaine, prilocaine) desensitizes the skin so that a venipuncture is more comfortable for the patient. This topical anesthetic must be in contact with the skin for at least several minutes (ideally 30 to 60 minutes) for it to reach its maximal effectiveness.

AURAL ADMINISTRATION

The key to successfully medicating an ear is to have the medication in contact with the epithelium of the ear canal to enhance its absorption and effectiveness. Therefore, the ear must be cleared of debris before the medication is applied.

When medication is placed into the ear canal, the pinna is grasped and pulled upward and slightly out laterally, similar to the motion of introducing an otoscope cone for an otoscopic examination. This helps to straighten the vertical ear canal. The tip of the medication dispenser is placed into the vertical ear canal, and the dispenser is squeezed. The base of the ear is massaged to distribute the medication.

INTRARECTAL ADMINISTRATION

The mucosa of the large intestine is capable of absorbing medications delivered intrarectally. Medications delivered by this route may have both local and systemic effects. Absorption is most effective when the intestine is free of fecal material. Antiemetic tablets or suppositories can be administered intrarectally to vomiting patients that cannot be medicated orally. A gloved, lubricated finger is used to insert the tablet into the rectum a distance of at least 5 cm. The medication is then gradually absorbed.

Antiseizure drugs, such as diazepam, can be given intrarectally if an IV or intranasal administration is difficult to perform. A lubricated short rubber feeding tube or a urinary catheter is inserted 8 to 10 cm into the rectum. Diazepam is placed into a syringe and is injected through the catheter. Several milliliters of warm water are then flushed into the catheter to disperse the drug. Diazepam can also be injected directly into the rectum with a needleless syringe.

Enemas are also administered per rectum. A syringe containing the enema is lubricated and inserted into the rectum. After the enema has been injected, the animal should be placed in an area where it can defecate, such as outdoors or near a litter box.

Warm-water enemas are administered through lubricated plastic tubing inserted through the rectum and into the large intestine. Water is funneled or injected into the end of the tube held in a raised position. The tube is moved back and forth and is slowly advanced up the intestinal tract as fecal material is expelled.

When a medication, such as lactulose, is added to the enema solution, it must be retained within the large intestine for a specified length of time. The solution is injected into a urinary catheter or feeding tube placed into the descending colon. The rectum is held closed with a gloved hand to prevent the enema from exiting. After the allotted time has passed, the catheter is removed and the intestine is evacuated.

INTRANASAL ADMINISTRATION

Certain vaccines—such as those given for feline infectious peritonitis, feline viral rhinotracheitis-calici-panleukopenia, and *Bordetella bronchiseptica*—are formulated for intranasal (and/or intraocular) administration. The patient's muzzle is held in one hand and is elevated slightly. The tip of the vaccine dispenser is placed into the nostril, and the dispenser is compressed. Alternatively, the patient's head can be tilted back, and the pipette containing the vaccine can be squeezed to dispense the liquid onto the plane of the nose. The vaccine runs into each nostril as the animal inhales. This method frequently results in less sneezing after the administration than when the dispenser tip is placed directly into the nostril.

Diazepam can be administered intranasally for the immediate treatment of status epilepticus if intravascular access cannot be obtained. Diazepam is absorbed more rapidly into the systemic circulation by the intranasal route than by the intrarectal route.

INTRADERMAL ADMINISTRATION

Intradermal (ID) injections are performed to desensitize the skin with a local anesthetic or to perform allergy skin testing. Most animals will not tolerate skin testing unless they are sedated. The hair on the lateral aspect of the trunk is shaved with a #40 clipper blade. The skin is carefully wiped with a water-moistened gauze sponge. Vigorous scrubbing or use of an antimicrobial cleaning solution is contraindicated because skin irritation that may occur interferes with testing. For an ID injection, a fold of skin is lifted, and a 25- to 27-gauge needle attached to a 1-ml syringe is inserted with the bevel up into the dermis. A 0.1-ml volume of allergen is injected. The injection site will look like a translucent lump if the injection is performed correctly. The skin is then examined for tissue reaction.

SUBCUTANEOUS ADMINISTRATION

The subcutaneous (SC) injection is easily and frequently performed and is the most common route for administering vaccines, isotonic fluids, and some types of antibiotics. With the exception of delayed absorption in obese animals, the SC route for injection, in general, offers relatively rapid absorption rates for most injectables. However, the SC route is not recommended in severely dehydrated or critically ill patients when immediate absorption is required. In an emergency situation, the IV or **intraosseous** route provides much faster absorption. The IV route is preferred when large volumes of fluid must be administered.

Moderate volumes of isotonic fluids can be injected under the skin to rehydrate animals if IV or intraosseous access is unavailable. Approximately 50 to 100 ml of body-temperature fluids can be injected per site, depending on the patient's size. Owners of patients that may require long-term fluid supplementation at home (e.g., those with chronic renal disease) can be instructed on how to administer SC fluids.

The preferred site for most SC injections is the dorsolateral region from the neck to the hips. The dorsal region of the neck and back should be avoided because of the difficulty involved in treating any abscesses or masses that may occur after an injection. When vaccinations are administered, especially to feline patients, the intrascapular region should be avoided because of the incidence of vaccine-induced tumors. Feline vaccinations should be administered in as distal a portion of an extremity as possible. The following sites are recommended for feline vaccination: right front leg, rhinotracheitis-calici-panleukopenia; right rear leg, rabies; and left rear leg, feline leukemia. The intrascapular area should also be avoided for insulin injections because of the relatively poor absorption of insulin from that site and the fibrosis that may occur as a result of repeated injections. Insulin should be injected into alternating sites along the dorsolateral or ventrolateral aspect of the trunk.

When an SC injection is administered, a fold of skin is tented, and the needle is inserted at the base of and parallel to the long axis of the fold. If the needle is inserted perpendicular to the long axis, the needle may penetrate both sides of the skin, and the syringe contents may be accidentally deposited onto the patient's hair. The syringe plunger is retracted slightly, and the needle hub is checked for blood before injection. If blood appears in the hub, a vessel has been penetrated, and the needle should be removed and reinserted in another location. After the injection, the skin is briefly massaged to facilitate drug distribution. If multiple vaccinations or medications are administered, injection sites should be a minimum of several centimeters apart.

INTRAMUSCULAR ADMINISTRATION

The intramuscular (IM) route is appropriate for the injection of small volumes of medication. Drugs are most often administered in the lumbosacral musculature lateral to the dorsal spinous processes or in the semimembranosus or semitendinosus muscles of the rear leg. Deep lumbar injections in the third to fifth lumbar region are used to administer heartworm treatment. Placement of the needle in the lumbosacral muscles is not recommended in very thin animals. When injections are made into the semimembranosus or semitendinosus muscles, the needle should enter the lateral aspect of the muscle and be directed caudally to prevent penetration of the sciatic nerve. Contact of the needle with the sciatic nerve may cause pain and lameness. In well-muscled animals, the cranial thigh and even the gastrocnemius are used. Occasionally, the triceps muscles on the caudal aspect of the front legs are used as injection sites. The neck is never used as a site for intramuscular (IM) injection.

When an IM injection is performed, the muscle is isolated between fingers and thumb, and a 22- to 25-gauge needle attached to a syringe is embedded in the muscle. As with SC injections, the needle hub is checked for blood before medication is administered, to make certain a vessel is not inadvertently penetrated. If blood is observed, the needle is removed and is inserted into another site. Once placement within the muscle has been verified, the drug is slowly injected. The site is massaged for a few seconds after the injection to help distribute the substance.

INTRAVENOUS ADMINISTRATION

Many medications are administered directly into a vein. Intravenous (IV) injection is used for drugs or fluids that must rapidly reach high blood levels or that would be irritating to tissue or insufficiently absorbed if given by another route (Procedure 18-1). Certain anesthetics, chemotherapeutic agents, anticonvulsant drugs, and drugs used in cardiopulmonary resuscitation are given IV. If an extremely rapid onset of action is required, the IV or intraosseous route is chosen.

The most frequently used sites for IV injection in the dog are the cephalic and lateral saphenous veins. Cats are most often given IV injections in the cephalic, medial saphenous, and femoral veins. The jugular vein is used to administer injections in both large and small animals if an IV jugular catheter is in place.

When an IV injection is administered, the vessel is occluded with a tourniquet or with digital pressure. Air bubbles are expelled from the syringe before the needle is inserted into the vein. The skin and hair over the vein are swabbed with alcohol, and the needle is inserted into the vein. Blood will appear in the needle hub when the needle penetrates the vein, but IV placement is confirmed by aspirating blood back into the syringe. Pressure is released from the vein, and the syringe contents are injected. The needle is

PROCEDURE 18-1	Intravenous Injection

- Occlude the vessel with digital pressure or a tourniquet.
- Grasp the extremity and pull the skin tautly in a distal direction.
- Wipe an alcohol-soaked cotton ball over the hair and skin covering a distal section of a peripheral vein.
- Insert a 22- to 25-gauge needle attached to a syringe with the bevel facing up through the skin and into the vein.
- Aspirate a small volume of blood into the syringe to ensure that the needle is within the vein.
- Release the pressure from the vein.
- Inject the contents of the syringe into the vein.
- Remove the needle and apply digital pressure to the needle insertion site for 30 to 60 seconds until hemostasis occurs.
- If a hematoma occurs when the needle is inserted, remove the needle and apply digital pressure over the hematoma until the bleeding subsides. Make another injection attempt proximal to the initial site or in a different vein.

withdrawn, and firm pressure is applied to the venipuncture site until hemostasis occurs.

TOPICAL OPHTHALMIC ADMINISTRATION

If it is necessary to administer topical ophthalmic medications to treat ocular diseases or specific vaccines, such as feline rhinotracheitis-calici-panleukopenia, a formulation may be used that is designed for intranasal and/or intraocular administration. To successfully place a medication onto the surface of the eye, the technician must ensure good restraint of the patient. Control of the front limbs of the patient is essential, along with minimizing movement of the animal, to prevent the medication from being inadvertently placed on the eyelids or the face. Eye medication dispensed to a patient should be used exclusively on that patient and on no other patients, to prevent transmitting ocular infection. The tip of the medication dispenser should not come into direct contact with any surface of the eye, including the cornea, to prevent contamination and scratching of the cornea. If an ophthalmic medication is a solution that appears cloudy, contains particulate matter, or has a color change, it should not be used.

Ophthalmic medications should be administered slightly warm or at room temperature. The technician can take refrigerated medications and place them in the palm of his or her hand for 1 to 2 minutes before administration because this makes it more comfortable for the patient. The eyelids are held open with the thumb and index finger of one hand, and the hand holding the medication is rested on the patient's head as 1 drop of the medication is deposited onto the sclera (Figure 18-6). For medications that are ointments, the lids are held open with the thumb and index finger of one hand, and a 3- to 5-mm strip of ointment is squeezed onto the upper sclera or the lower palpebral border. The ointment dissipates across the cornea when the animal blinks.

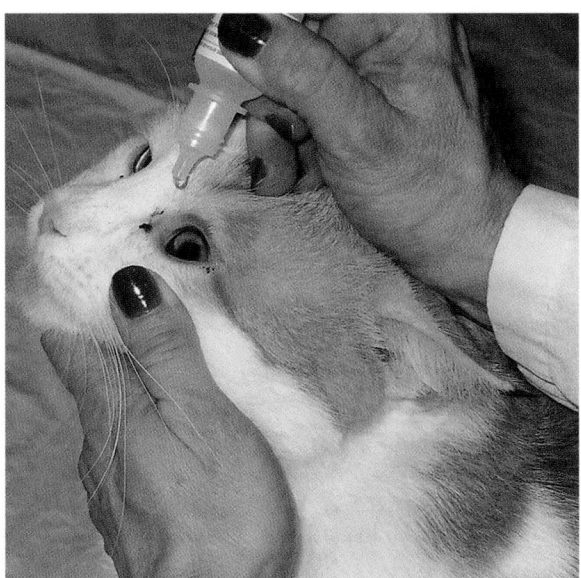

FIGURE 18-6 Ophthalmic drop is directed onto the sclera of a cat.

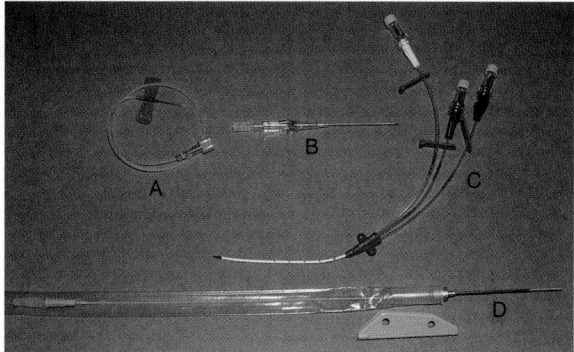

FIGURE 18-7 Examples of four types of IV catheters. Catheter A is a butterfly; catheter B is an OTN; catheter C is a multi-lumen (triple-lumen) catheter; and catheter D is a through-the-needle catheter.

If the patient requires multiple topical ophthalmic medications in the same eye, these should be applied 3 to 5 minutes apart to allow sufficient absorption. In the scenario of needing to administer both a solution and an ointment, the solution should be placed in the eye 3 to 5 minutes before the ointment. If the ointment is applied first, it may coat the cornea and interfere with absorption of the solution.

INTRAVENOUS CATHETER PLACEMENT

Patients often require temporary venous access for medications, fluids, and electrolyte replacement therapy or for transfusion of blood products. Medications and fluids with osmolalities less than or equal to 600 mOsm may be safely administered via a peripheral vein. Site selection depends on available vessels, the condition of the vessels and the patient, expense, and the urgency of the situation. The veterinary technician should be familiar with types of catheters, placement techniques, and catheter maintenance.

A variety of catheters are commercially available. The length and gauge (diameter) of the catheter to be used are dependent on the species and size of the patient and the veins available and their condition. Four general categories of IV access devices are available: winged needle (butterfly), over-the-needle (OTN), through-the-needle (TTN), and multi-lumen catheter (Figure 18-7).

The winged needle is for short-term use when the animal is not moving around very much. Applications might include blood collection or administration of nonirritating medications. It is easy for the indwelling sharp needle to puncture the vessel wall, allowing for SC infiltration of fluids or medications. The needles have plastic wings on the shaft to facilitate placement or taping in place. Plastic tubing of various lengths extends from the needle to the syringe connector port. The OTN catheter is the most common type of catheter used today. It is used primarily for peripheral vein catheterization. This type of catheter is fitted outside or over a steel needle. The needle point extends a millimeter or so beyond the catheter tip for entry into the vein. Catheters passed through the needle are called through-the-needle (TTN) catheters. TTN catheters are usually longer than OTN catheters (8 inches to 12 inches) and are used primarily in the jugular vein. A plastic sleeve to prevent contamination protects the catheters. Once the catheter is placed and the needle has been withdrawn from the insertion site, a needle guard is placed. The needle guard protects the needle from sticking the animal and shearing the catheter, but can be fairly bulky in the small animal. Multi-lumen catheters have two to three separate lumina in one catheter. Multi-lumen catheters allow simultaneous infusions at a single catheter site. Although one catheter is placed, the multi-lumen catheter provides the same functions as two or three separately introduced single-lumen catheters. Catheter placement is usually completed **percutaneously** with a guide wire. Multi-lumen catheters are more expensive than commonly used IV catheters.

Although slight variation may be noted, the setup for venous (peripheral and jugular) or arterial catheterization is essentially the same, no matter what type of catheter is being placed. The veterinary technician will gather a catheter (butterfly, OTN, TTN, or multi-lumen); a syringe filled with heparinized saline flush; an injection cap or T-connector; tape and/or nonabsorbable suture; bandage material; clippers; and antiseptic scrub and solutions. Refer to Case Presentation 18-1 for an example of a case requiring placement of a multi-lumen jugular catheter to accommodate the needs of a critically ill dog.

Peripheral Vein Catheterization

Common peripheral insertion sites include the cephalic, medial (cat), and lateral (dog) saphenous veins. There is a tendency to insert a lateral saphenous catheter into the vessel as it traverses the hock; as an alternative, it might be preferable to insert the catheter into the lateral saphenous vein on the caudal surface of the leg because it is easier to secure in this location.

The area of the insertion site is generously shaved. Surgical preparation is performed with antiseptic scrub and solution. Aseptic technique is important to prevent indwelling

CASE PRESENTATION 18-1 PATIENT WITH DIABETIC KETOACIDOSIS AND ASPIRATION PNEUMONIA

History

Jojo, a 26-kg, 10-year-old, male, castrated Labrador Retriever presents to the clinic with a 2-week history of vomiting. The owner reports that he vomited 2 to 3 times per day for the first week but was showing no lethargy at the time. However, vomiting continued, and Jojo became lethargic 2 to 3 days before presentation. He progressively became worse and developed partial anorexia 4 days before and complete anorexia 2 days before admission. The owner reported increased water consumption and increased frequency of urination before the onset of vomition. He is not given any medications and is up to date on his immunizations.

Significant Physical Examination Findings

The veterinarian performed an initial physical examination and found the following:

Patient was depressed but responsive; temp = 103.8, respiratory rate = 60, body condition score is 3/9 with diffuse and symmetric muscle atrophy, decreased skin elasticity, and tacky mucous membranes; estimated level of dehydration is 8%. The clinician auscultated quiet lung sounds except in the left cranioventral region. Abdominal palpation revealed large, firm intestines and a painful mid abdomen. The patient's breath had an acetone smell. Reading of the pulse oximeter was 92%.

Veterinarian's Orders

Based on the history and physical examination findings, the veterinarian ordered the following:

1. Complete blood count (CBC) to evaluate evidence of an infectious or inflammatory process.
2. Serum chemistry panel (including electrolytes) to rule out metabolic and electrolyte derangements.
3. Urinalysis and culture to rule out glucosuria, ketonuria, and infection.
4. Arterial blood gas sample to assess oxygenation, ventilation, and acid-base status.
5. Chest radiographs to rule out pulmonary parenchymal disease.
6. Abdominal ultrasound to further define the source of abdominal pain.
7. Placement of a multi-lumen jugular catheter and initiation of fluid therapy.

Nursing Care Plan

It is the technician's responsibility to carry out the veterinarian's orders and to independently develop a nursing plan of care. This plan should include the following interventions:

1. Perform physical assessment of hospitalized patient. Do this regularly.
2. Place multi-lumen jugular catheter using aseptic technique. The technician will want to be sure to take steps to minimize the risk for bacterial contamination when placing and caring for any indwelling catheter.
3. The doctor said to develop a fluid plan using lactated Ringer's (see Box) assuming 8% dehydration; correct the dehydration over 8 hours and replace abnormal losses as they occur.

Calculation of Jojo's Fluid Therapy Plan

Replacement volume (26 kg × .08) = 2.1 L
Maintenance volume = 1.5 L
Total volume = 3.6 L or 3600 ml
2100 ml × 8 hours = 263 ml/hour lactated Ringer's
1500 ml/24 hours = 63 ml/hour lactated Ringer's
- Administer 326 ml/hour (263 ml + 63 ml) over 8 hours; then decrease to 63 ml/hour for remaining 16 hours.
- Make up abnormal losses (vomiting, diarrhea, and polyuria) by adding previous hours' abnormal losses to next hours' fluid input.
- Reevaluate patient at frequent intervals to determine desired end-point.

---

4. Obtain laboratory samples. Steps are taken to avoid unnecessarily stressing the patient and gathering samples using proper sample collection techniques to avoid preanalytical error.
5. Obtain an arterial blood gas sample, making sure to minimize the risk of preanalytical error such as an anticoagulant-dilutional problem, introduction of air into the sample, or improper storage of the sample.
6. Take diagnostic thoracic radiographs while minimizing stress to the patient.

Diagnostic Test Results

1. Serum chemistry profile:
   Demonstrated an elevated serum glucose of 741 mg/dl. In addition, patient was hypokalemic (2.1 mEq/L) and hypophosphatemic (2.9 mg/dl) and had metabolic acidosis (pH 7.32, HCO_3 14.1 mEq/L).
2. Arterial blood gas analyses:
   Revealed that the patient was hypoxemic; Jojo's PaO_2 was 74.7 mm Hg while breathing room air.
3. Complete blood count:
   Showed leukocytosis (37,500 μl) with left shift (750 μl metamyelocytes and 9750 band) and marked toxicity and hemoconcentration (HCT 50%, TP 9.6 g/dl).
4. Urinalysis:
   Showed glycosuria and ketonuria.
5. Thoracic radiographs and abdominal ultrasound:
   Were consistent with aspiration pneumonia (Figure 1, *A* and *B*) and pancreatitis, respectively.

Veterinarian's Problem List

1. Diabetic ketoacidosis
2. Pancreatitis
3. Aspiration pneumonia
4. Hypoxemia

Veterinarian's Second Set of Orders

- Initiate regular insulin therapy—5.2 units IM initially, then 2.6 units IM q2hours. Measure blood gas (BG) q2hours, supplement fluids with dextrose to 2.5% when BG approaches 250 mg/dl, and notify clinician.

CASE PRESENTATION 18-1 PATIENT WITH DIABETIC KETOACIDOSIS AND ASPIRATION PNEUMONIA—cont'd

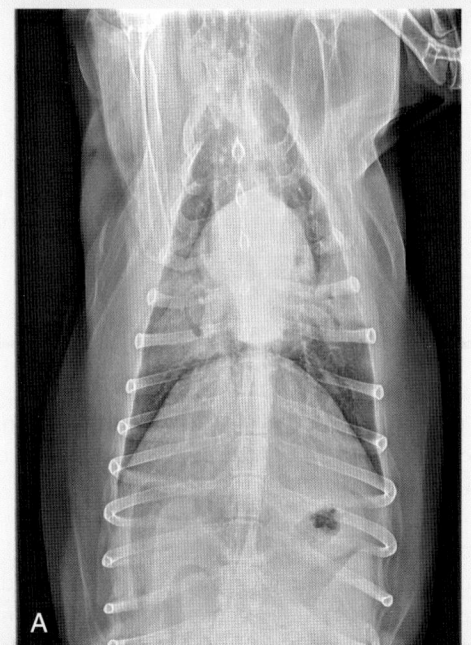

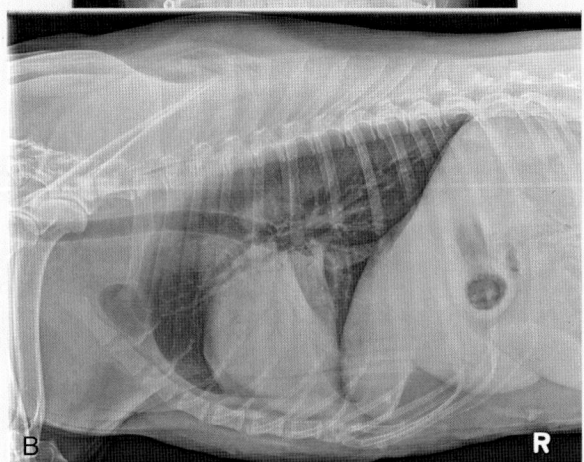

FIGURE 1 A, Dorsoventral thoracic radiograph. **B,** Lateral thoracic radiograph. A focal alveolar pattern is seen in the caudal portion of the left cranial lung lobe. An alveolar pattern is also present in the right middle lung lobe associated with a lobar sign. These radiographs are consistent with aspiration pneumonia. (Radiographs courtesy Radiology Service, William R. Pritchard Veterinary Medical Teaching Hospital, University of California-Davis, CA.)

- Supplement lactated Ringer's solution (LRS) with 40 mEq/L of K^+ (split ½ with KCL and ½ with K_2PO_4); based on serum potassium measurements, adjust potassium concentration per protocol; split ½ with KCL and ½ with K_2PO_4.
- Place nasal prongs for oxygen supplementation (Figure 2) with oxygen flow rate of 50 to 200 ml/kg/min; adjust to maintain SpO_2 or PaO_2 greater than 95% or 85 mm Hg, respectively.
- Check serum electrolytes every 4 hours; notify clinician if potassium is <2.0 or >5.5 mEq/L.

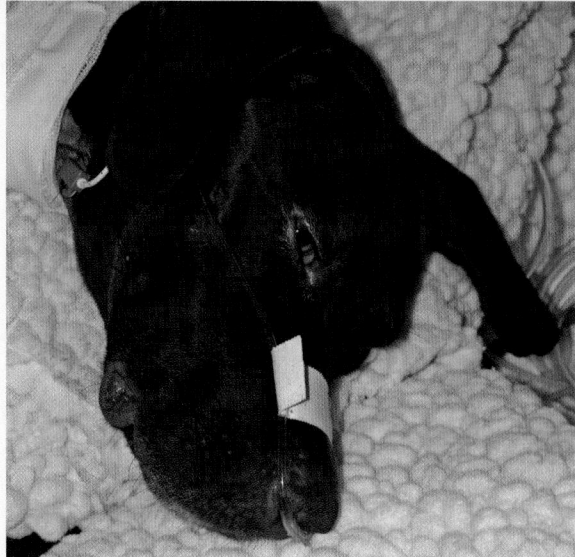

FIGURE 2 Nasal prongs placed for oxygen supplementation.

- Check arterial blood gases every 24 hours.
- Check venous blood gases at 1600 and 2400.
- Obtain temp, pulse, and respiration rates q4hours × 6, then q6hours if vitals are within normal limits.
- Measure SpO_2 q4hours.
- Nebulize and coupage patient q4hours.
- Post patient NPO status.
- Administer ampicillin 22 mg/kg IV q8hours.
- Administer enrofloxacin 10 mg/kg q24hours.
- Administer famotidine 3 mg IV q24hours.
- Administer 0.05 mg/kg oxymorphone IM q4hours for pain.

Nursing Concerns and Plans
- Administer proper dose of insulin using the correct insulin syringe. Have dose verified by a colleague before administration.
- Verify compatibility of various drugs, and take steps to ensure that they are not mixed in the intravenous line during administration.
- Ensure that those drugs that require dilution are diluted correctly, and that all drugs are administered at the proper rate.
- Verify that potassium orders do not exceed the maximum safe administration rate of 0.5 mEq/kg/hour; inform the clinician if it does.
- Monitor patient for resolution of dehydration and restoration of intravascular blood volume.
- Monitor patient for resolution of hyperglycemia and ketonuria.
- Monitor and document fluid "in's and out's." Does input (IV fluids) exceed output (urine production), or vice versa?
- Provide IV catheter care as per protocol.
- Assess patient regularly and monitor specifically for development of the following complications. Consider possible interventions for these complications:

Continued

CASE PRESENTATION 18-1 PATIENT WITH DIABETIC KETOACIDOSIS AND ASPIRATION PNEUMONIA—cont'd

1. Pain.
2. Fluid overload (skin elasticity—"jelly-like," acute increase in body weight, increase in respiratory rate and/or effort, auscultation of crackles, urine output should not exceed 2 ml/kg/hour [assuming no renal disease]).
3. Hypoglycemia.
4. Evidence of infection.
5. Hypokalemia or hyperkalemia.
6. Catheter-related problems (phlebitis, thrombosis, perivascular fluid infiltration).

Outcome

Jojo's glucose reached 220 mg/dl within 12 hours, and ketonuria subsequently resolved. Dextrose (50%) was added to the patient's fluids to make a 2.5% solution. Jojo was started on long-acting insulin. Metabolic acidosis resolved by day 2. Aspiration pneumonia resolved based on thoracic radiographs taken on day 4 and normal arterial blood gas readings. Oxygen therapy was therefore discontinued on day 4. The patient was discharged on day 6 and was prescribed NPH insulin to be administered twice daily by owner.

---

catheter-related infection. A facilitative incision or a relief hole reduces skin tension and friction against the catheter. The relief hole may be made with a #11 blade or a 20-gauge needle. A 0.5- to 1-mm incision is made directly over the vessel extending through the dermis.

> **TECHNICIAN NOTE**   A facilitative incision or a relief hole reduces skin tension and friction against the catheter; it is indicated in severely dehydrated patients and in patients with tough skin.

A facilitative incision is indicated in severely dehydrated patients and in patients with tough skin. Care should be taken to avoid the vessel when making the relief incision. Local anesthetic blocks are rarely needed. The vein is occluded upstream of the insertion site by a tourniquet or an assistant. The distal portion of the leg is grasped in the palm of the hand of the veterinary technician, and the leg is extended to tense and immobilize the vein. It is not recommended to use the thumb to stabilize the vein because this compresses and collapses the vein. Flexion of the carpus will increase stretch on the vessel and improve vessel immobilization in achondroplastic breeds. With the bevel up, the catheter is inserted through the skin or relief hole at approximately a 15-degree angle.

The catheter is advanced into the vessel; when blood appears in the flash chamber (hub), the needle and the catheter are advanced together as a unit for an additional 1 to 4 mm. This ensures that the end of the catheter is entirely inside the lumen of the vessel. Then while holding the needle steady and maintaining longitudinal tension on the leg, the catheter is advanced off of the needle and into the vessel lumen. The catheter is capped with an injection cap or a T-connector and is flushed with heparinized saline. A $\frac{1}{2}$-inch (1.3-cm) strip of adhesive tape is wrapped around the circumference of the hub of the catheter and leg to secure the catheter. A 2 × 2 gauze pad is placed over the insertion site. A 1-inch (2.54-cm) second piece of tape is placed sticky side down underneath the catheter and then is wrapped around the leg. Roll gauze is wrapped around the catheter

and leg proximal and distal to the insertion site. Finally, tape is applied to the top and bottom of the gauze where it interfaces with the skin.

Jugular Vein Catheterization

Placement of a jugular catheter provides several advantages over use of a peripheral catheter: (1) allows administration of fluids that have **osmolality** greater than 600 mOsm/L and constant rate infusions of drugs known to cause **phlebitis**, such as diazepam, pentobarbital, and mannitol; (2) enables measurement of central venous pressure (CVP); (3) facilitates frequent aspiration of blood samples; and (4) is necessary for the administration of total parenteral nutrition (TPN).

> **TECHNICIAN NOTE**   Fluids or drugs that have an osmolality greater than 600 mOsm/L should be administered through a jugular vein.

The key to a successful jugular catheter insertion is the patient's positioning and vessel immobilization. If the patient is not positioned properly, it can be difficult to visualize and immobilize the vein. Jugular catheters are placed antegrade with the tip of the catheter always directed toward the heart. Placement of the jugular catheter is best done with the patient in lateral recumbency. The patient's head is extended and its forelimbs positioned caudally by an assistant. Sedation of uncooperative patients is recommended. Placement of a bag of fluids, a sandbag, roll gauze, or rolled towels under the neck may be helpful (Figure 18-8). This flexes the neck and helps to make the vessel more accessible. The assistant should hold off the vein by pressing into the thoracic inlet; this should cause the vein to engorge and "stand up." The other end of the vein is immobilized by extending the head.

> **TECHNICIAN NOTE**   Placement of a bag of fluids, a sandbag, or rolled towels under the neck helps to make the vessel more accessible for a jugular catheter placement.

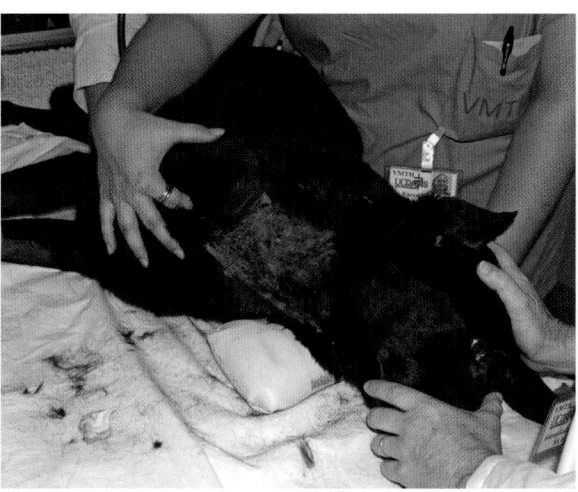

FIGURE 18-8 A sandbag placed under the neck facilitates jugular catheter placement by flexing the neck and providing better access to the vessel.

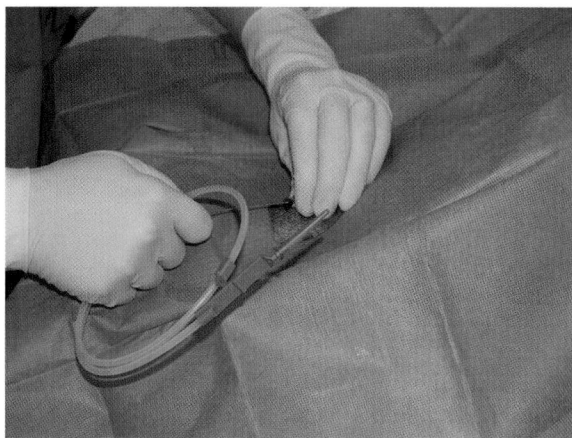

FIGURE 18-10 When the Seldinger technique is used, the guide wire is threaded through the over-the-needle (OTN) catheter; care should be taken to avoid contaminating the flimsy wire.

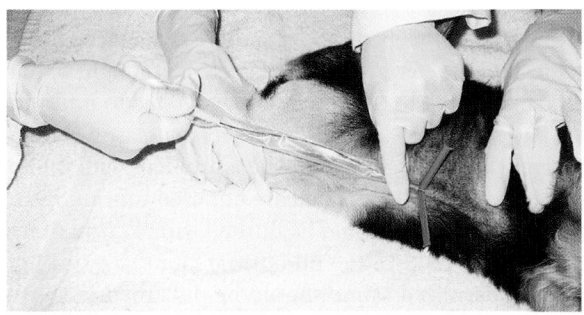

FIGURE 18-9 The catheter is threaded into the jugular vein through a protective sleeve.

The area of the insertion site is generously shaved. A surgical preparation is performed with antiseptic scrub and solution. To place a through-the-needle catheter, the catheter needle should be introduced SC. The needle tip is positioned over the vein and is aligned as close as possible to the longitudinal axis of the vein. The needle tip is inserted into the vein; it may be necessary to angle the needle somewhat to pick up the superficial vein wall. Once it is estimated that the entire needle tip is within the lumen of the vein, the needle is stabilized, and the catheter is threaded into the vein (Figure 18-9). Once the catheter is fully advanced into the vein, apply pressure over the venous puncture site, and back the needle out. Once the bleeding has stopped, secure the needle guard around the needle. The plastic protective bag and stylet are removed; the catheter is aspirated to confirm its proper placement and to clear the catheter of air. It is then flushed with heparinized saline. The catheter should be capped with an injection cap or a T-connector and again is flushed with heparinized saline. The catheter is sutured or stapled close to the insertion site. The insertion site is then covered with a sterile 2 × 2-inch gauze pad, and the catheter site is bandaged.

The Seldinger guide wire technique facilitates placement of a multi-lumen catheter. The Seldinger technique uses a smaller introducing catheter, or trocar, and a guide wire to safely gain venous access. Before the procedure is begun, the required distance for catheter insertion is premeasured. The aim for a jugular catheter is to have the tip of the catheter lying within the thoracic cavity, just cranial to the right atrium. This distance is commonly estimated by measuring the distance from the intended insertion site to the caudal edge of the triceps muscle. The insertion site is widely clipped and surgically prepared in a routine manner. Infiltration of the intended insertion site with local anesthetic is recommended in awake animals. The technician wears sterile gloves; in some circumstances, a hat, a mask, and a sterile gown may also be appropriate. The distal port of the multi-lumen catheter is identified; this is the port that terminates at the very tip of the catheter and is the one through which the guide wire will be passed. All ports of the multi-lumen catheter are flushed with heparinized saline, and all ports with the exception of the distal port are capped. The insertion site is draped; this is important because the guide wire is long and flimsy and the risk for guide wire contamination is high if draping is not sufficient.

> **TECHNICIAN NOTE** The required distance for a jugular catheter insertion is estimated by measuring the distance from the intended insertion site to the caudal edge of the triceps muscle.

A small relief incision is made through the dermis with a scalpel blade at the site of the intended insertion. The introducing needle or short OTN catheter enters the skin through the relief incision and is inserted into the underlying vessel. The guide wire is threaded through the inserting needle or catheter into the vein (Figure 18-10). The distal end of the wire has a flexible J-tip to prevent puncturing through the vessel wall. In some instances when it is difficult to pass the J-tip along the vessel, it may be advantageous to use the straight end of the guide wire instead. To prevent embolism of the guide wire, the technician should retain a hold of the

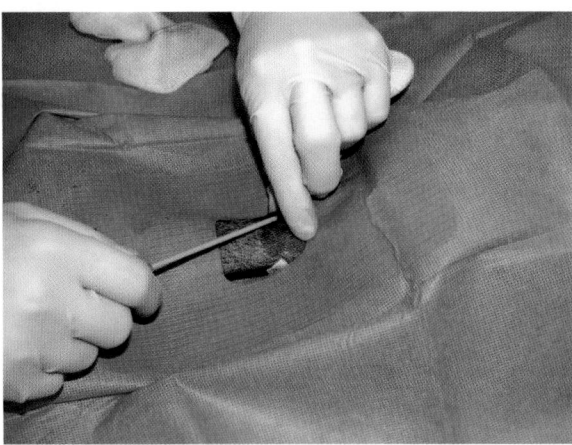

FIGURE 18-11 The dilator is used to enlarge the insertion site. The dilator is grasped near the distal tip; using a forward twisting motion, the dilator is advanced into the vessel.

wire at all times. Once the guide wire has been inserted approximately ⅔ to ¾ of its length into the vessel, the introducing needle or catheter is removed, and a vessel dilator is threaded over the wire, the skin entry site may need to be enlarged with a #11 blade to accommodate the dilator. The dilator is grasped near the distal tip, and, using a forward twisting motion, the dilator is advanced into the vessel (Figure 18-11). To minimize blood loss, pressure is applied over the insertion site with aseptic gauze pads as the dilator is removed, leaving the guide wire in place. In the case of a sheath introducer, the dilator is incorporated into the sheath and is removed once the sheath is in place. The multi-lumen catheter is threaded over the guide wire until the proximal end of the guide wire protrudes from the hub of the catheter. If an excessive length of the guide wire was advanced into the vessel, it will be necessary to back the guide wire out of the vessel to achieve this. Finally, while the proximal end of the guide wire is held, the catheter is advanced into the vessel the desired distance as determined by premeasurement (Figure 18-12). The wire is removed, and all ports are aspirated to remove any air and to ensure that blood is easily drawn through the catheter. If necessary, the catheter may be repositioned to allow effective aspiration of blood; aseptic technique must be maintained throughout this time. All ports are then flushed with heparinized saline. The catheter is sutured in place, and the insertion site is covered by aseptic gauze and bandaged appropriately.

INTRAVENOUS CATHETER MAINTENANCE

IV catheter care should be performed every 48 hours or on an as-needed basis. The catheter dressing should be removed and the site inspected. The veterinary technician looks for signs of phlebitis, infection, or **thrombosis**. Signs of phlebitis may include erythema, swelling, tenderness upon palpation, and an apparent increase in skin temperature over the vein. Signs of infection include those seen with phlebitis and may include a purulent discharge. Thrombosis is characterized by a vein that "stands up" without being held off and a

thick cord-like feeling to the vein. When signs of phlebitis or thrombosis are apparent, the catheter should be removed and a new one placed at a different site. While the catheter is flushed with heparinized saline, the insertion site should be observed for leaking of fluid at the insertion site and pain upon injection. If either is observed, the catheter should be removed and replaced with a new one. If any portion of the catheter is exposed, it should not be reinserted, and this should be documented in the medical record. If the catheter site looks good, the site should be cleaned with an iodophor or chlorhexidine solution. When the catheter site is dry, cover the insertion site with a sterile 2 × 2-inch pad. Then rebandage the catheter. Traditionally, it has been recommended to leave a catheter in place no longer than 72 hours. These recommendations come from human medicine. It has been our experience that as long as routine catheter care is performed and the catheter is removed when problems are first noticed, one can often exceed the 72-hour rule.

IV catheters should be observed several times a day. If the catheter bandage is found to be wet, the reason should be identified, and the bandage should be changed. Swelling distal to the catheter is usually indicative of a tight bandage. Swelling proximal to the catheter may be due to infiltration. If the patient is molesting its bandage, the reason should be investigated; there may actually be a problem with the catheter or bandage. Catheters that are not used continuously for fluid administration should be flushed with 4 U/ml of heparinized saline (1000 U/250 ml normal saline) every 4 hours. Bags of heparinized saline should be discarded every 12 to 24 hours to minimize the risk of contamination. If a catheter is not going to be used for a prolonged time, a heparin lock should be considered. The dead space of the catheter is filled with 100 U/ml heparin every 12 hours. The concentrated heparin solution is never flushed into the patient; it is aspirated before medication is administered or before the heparin lock is renewed. The catheter should be clearly labeled so as to prevent inadvertent flushing of concentrated heparin into the patient.

INTRAVENOUS CHEMOTHERAPY ADMINISTRATION

The use of chemotherapeutic agents to treat neoplasia is becoming more common in companion animal practices. The veterinary technician should be familiar with chemotherapy administration protocols and safety precautions. Refer to Chapter 4 for information regarding safe handling of chemotherapeutic medications. Because many chemotherapeutic agents are carcinogens, it is advisable to minimize exposure to these drugs during administration. Latex gloves, safety glasses, masks, and nonpermeable, long-sleeved, elastic-cuffed gowns should be worn by technicians at the time of administration. For maximal protection, chemotherapeutic material should be drawn up in an oncology hood, and a needleless administration system should be used to avoid inadvertent human exposure (Figures 18-13 and 18-14, *A* through *D*). Materials used for chemotherapy administration should be gathered in advance

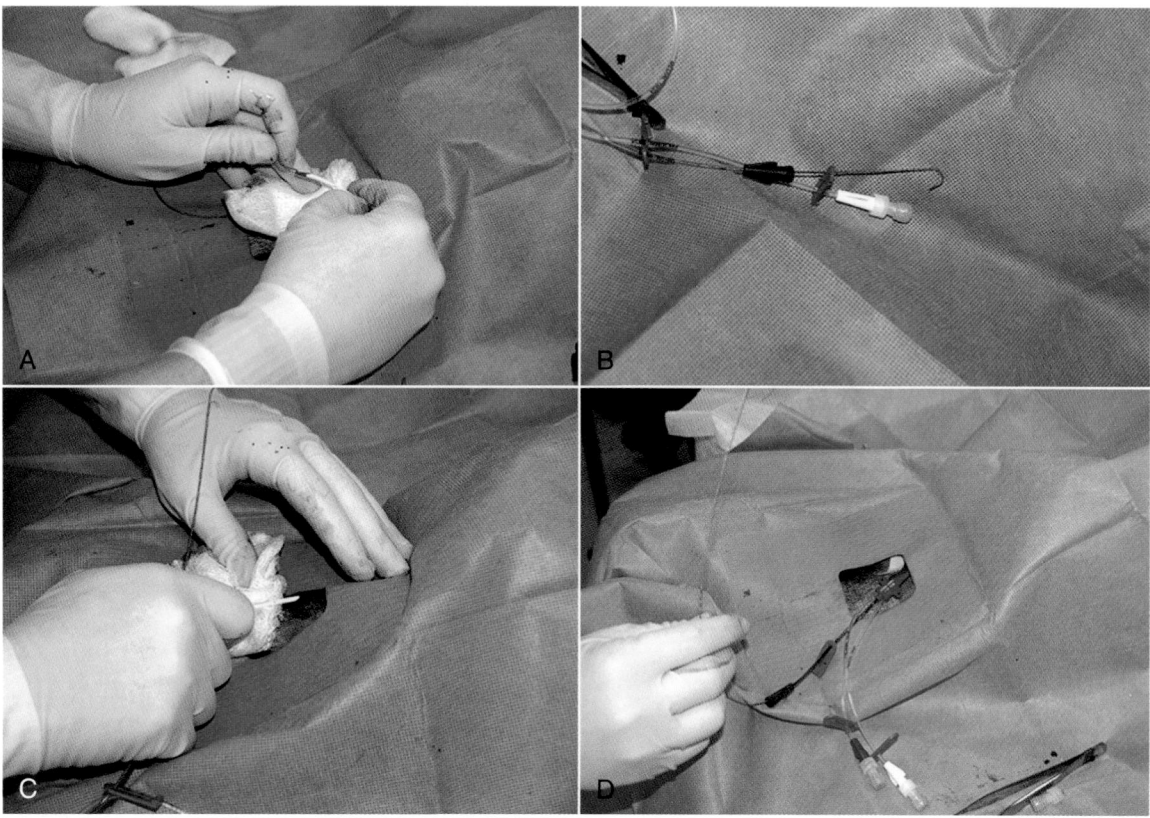

FIGURE 18-12 The proximal end of the guide wire is threaded up the catheter (**A**) until it comes out at the distal catheter hub (**B**). The wire is then grasped and the catheter is threaded into the vessel (**C**). The wire is then removed from the catheter (**D**).

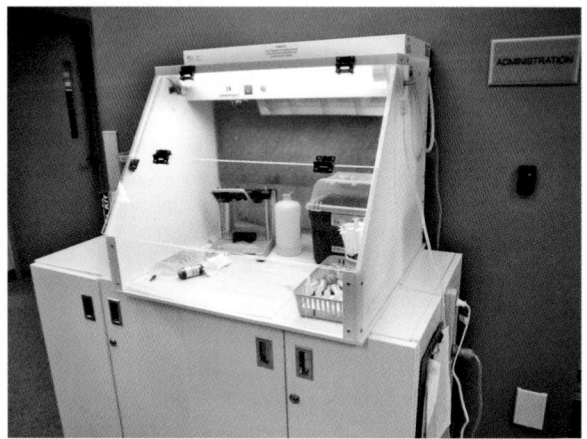

FIGURE 18-13 Example of an oncology hood used by veterinary technicians to safely draw up chemotherapeutic products.

of administration, and afterward should be discarded in leakproof hazardous waste containers. If a regular needle system is to be used, drug aerosolization can be minimized by placing an alcohol-soaked gauze sponge over the injection cap during administration.

IV catheters are used to administer cytotoxic solutions, especially those that cause tissue irritation when injected extravascularly. Examples of such drugs, which are termed *vesicants*, include doxorubicin, vincristine, vinblastine, and actinomycin D.

IV chemotherapy catheters must be placed with extreme care. The catheter should be placed in a peripheral vein, and the vessel must be punctured only once during placement. If a "clean stick" is not achieved on the first placement attempt, a different vein should be used. This prevents tissue irritation caused by drug leakage from the previous puncture site. It is permissible, but not advisable, to place the catheter in the same vein at a more proximal site if the initial site has been given time to seal with a clot. Non-heparinized 0.9% sterile saline solution should be used to flush the catheter when specific chemotherapy drugs, such as doxorubicin, that precipitate when mixed with heparin are used.

Catheters used for drug administration should be frequently evaluated for patency. The area proximal to the catheter site should be freely visible so that **extravasations** may be observed. Signs that the chemotherapeutic agent has leaked out of the vein include loss of catheter patency, redness or swelling at or proximal to the injection site, and vocalization or signs of discomfort by the patient.

If extravasations occur, as much of the drug should be removed from the site as possible by aspirating 5 ml of blood back through the catheter. The tissue surrounding the site should be infused with saline solution, corticosteroids, or 2% lidocaine, and warm or cold compresses should be applied, depending on the chemotherapy drug used.

When chemotherapy administration is complete, the catheter is flushed with several milliliters of sterile,

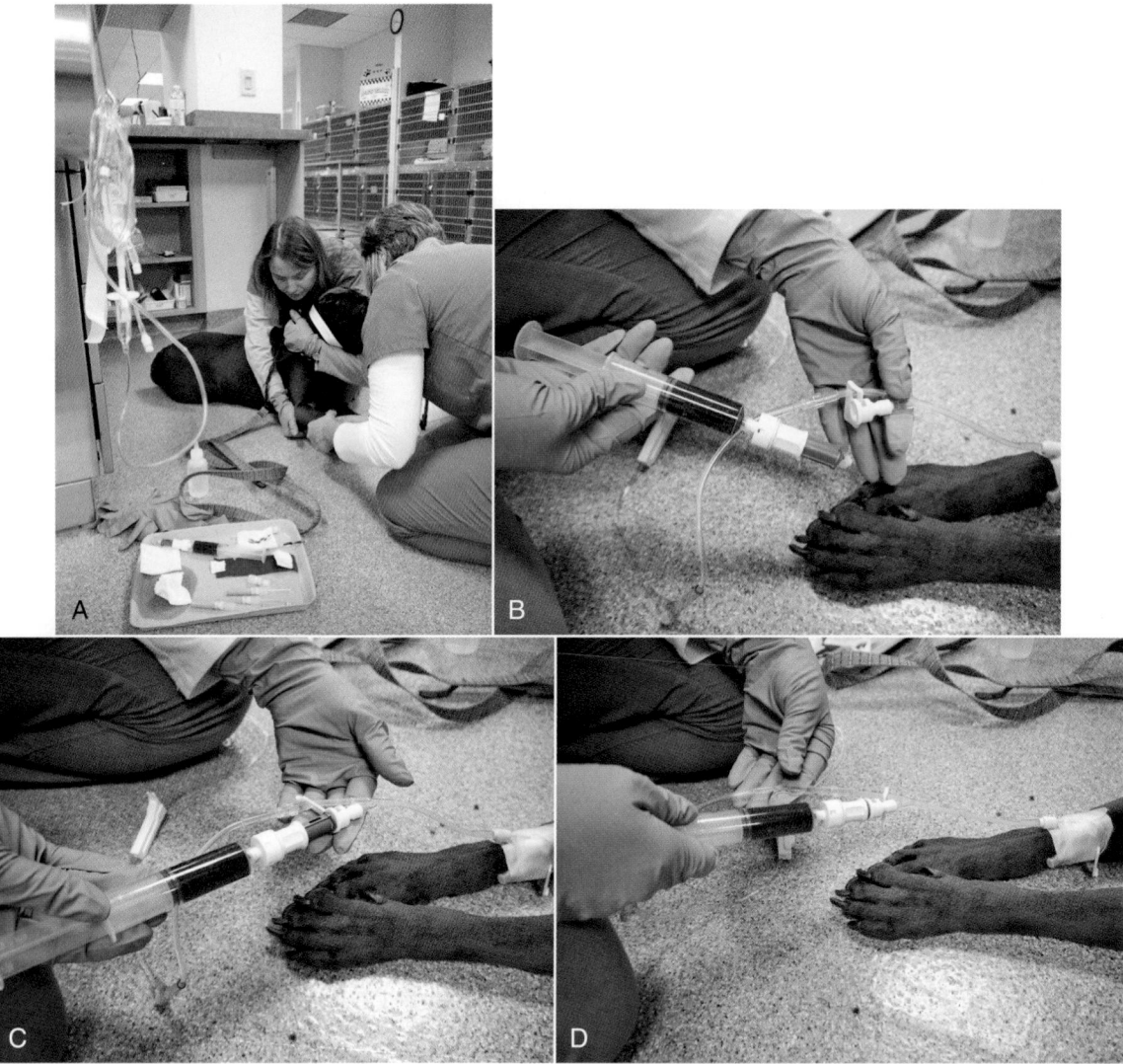

FIGURE 18-14 A, All materials needed to administer chemotherapy to a patient are gathered before administration is attempted. Veins are examined. B, A needleless connection system is used to administer chemotherapeutic agents safely. C, A locking system allows the syringe to be attached to the injection hub. The connecting system allows for administration of medication without the risk of inadvertent self-injection by the technician. D, Forward pressure advances the white "female" portion of the connector system over the blue "male" portion. Injection of the chemotherapeutic agent is then safely administered. (A, Courtesy Dr. Joanna Bassert.)

nonheparinized 0.9% saline solution. An alcohol-soaked gauze sponge covers the catheter as it is removed from the vein.

The skin puncture site is covered with an antibiotic-treated gauze pad and is securely bandaged.

When less than 2 ml of a chemotherapeutic drug, such as vincristine, is injected IV, a 23- or 25-gauge butterfly catheter is often used. After the drug has been administered, the catheter is flushed with several milliliters of saline solution. The tubing is crimped to prevent fluid from leaking back out of the catheter, and the needle is removed from the vein. The needle is covered with an alcohol-soaked gauze pad as it is removed from the skin, and the venipuncture site is bandaged.

INTRATRACHEAL ADMINISTRATION

In an emergency situation, such as during cardiopulmonary resuscitation, drugs can be injected directly into the trachea of an unconscious animal. The absorption by this route is extremely rapid.

> **TECHNICIAN NOTE** In an emergency situation, such as during cardiopulmonary resuscitation, medications can be injected directly into the trachea because absorption of the drug by this route is extremely rapid.

When an intratracheal injection is performed, a polypropylene urinary catheter or rubber feeding tube is inserted into the trachea, either directly or through an endotracheal tube. The drug contained in a syringe is forcefully injected through the urinary catheter or feeding tube. Approximately 10 ml of air or 3 to 10 ml of sterile saline solution is injected through the catheter or tube immediately afterward to disperse the drug. The acronym ALE (e.g., atropine, lidocaine, or epinephrine) is useful in helping to remember which drugs can be administered via the endotracheal tube. The intratracheal dosage is usually twice the IV dosage.

INTRAOSSEOUS ADMINISTRATION

Needles are placed directly into the bone marrow cavity to deliver fluids, drugs, and blood products when IV catheterization is not possible or cannot be performed rapidly. The intraosseous route is often overlooked and may be useful in emergency situations. Medications and fluids quickly enter the central circulation via intramedullary vessels in the marrow cavity. Intraosseous placement of a needle or catheter allows rapid fluid delivery to neonates, small animals, and patients with circulatory collapse. Intraosseous needles are removed as soon as IV access can be established.

Placement of an intraosseous needle or catheter is contraindicated in patients with sepsis. Catheters are not placed in bones that are fractured or infected. Skin overlying the insertion site should be free of infection so that skin surface pathogens are not introduced into underlying tissue during intraosseous needle placement. If the bone cortex is punctured multiple times during insertion attempts, a different bone should be used; fluid that is administered may leak from the bone into SC tissue.

Sites for intraosseous administration include tibia, femur, humerus, and occasionally iliac wing or ischium. The intraosseous catheter or needle should have a stylet that helps prevent the needle from bending or becoming occluded with a core of bone as it is inserted. Needles used include 15- to 18-gauge bone marrow needles specially designed for intraosseous access. If intraosseous access is needed in a neonate, an 18- to 22-gauge hypodermic needle can be used. If the hypodermic needle plugs with a core of bone, it sometimes can be flushed out with saline solution. A 22-gauge, 3.75-cm needle can be nested inside an 18-gauge, 2.5-cm needle to serve as a stylet during placement.

When an intraosseous catheter or needle must be placed into the femur, the hip region is shaved and aseptically prepared. The patient is placed in lateral recumbency, and the technician stands at the dorsum of the patient. The trochanteric fossa of the femur of the upside leg is identified on the medial aspect of the greater trochanter of the proximal femur.

Approximately 0.5 to 1.0 ml of 2% lidocaine is injected into the skin, the SC tissue, and the periosteum over the trochanteric fossa to provide local anesthesia. A stab incision is made through the skin. The femur is grasped, and the hip is held in a flexed position. The intraosseous needle is introduced medial to the greater trochanter and parallel to the femoral shaft. This needle is inserted through the skin

incision and into the femur by using firm, steady pressure as the wrist is rotated back and forth. Insertion of the needle through a skin incision helps decrease the likelihood that skin contaminants will be carried into the bone. During needle insertion, care is taken to prevent piercing the sciatic nerve, which is posteromedial to the greater trochanter of the femur. When the needle enters the marrow cavity, the needle will feel firmly embedded. Placement can be ascertained through aspiration of bone marrow into a syringe attached to the needle hub.

Once placed, the needle is secured by wrapping a "butterfly" tab of tape around it as it exits the skin. The tape is sutured to the skin. A povidone-iodine ointment–treated gauze pad is applied to the skin entry site. A bulky gauze bandage is placed around the needle for further stabilization. Patency of the intraosseous needle is maintained by flushing every 6 hours with 1 to 2 ml of heparinized 0.9% saline solution. The needle may remain in place for up to 3 days but is difficult to maintain in an ambulatory patient.

INTRAPERITONEAL ADMINISTRATION

The intraperitoneal (IP) route involves placement of substances directly into the abdominal cavity. This route is used occasionally to administer noncaustic fluids, blood products, or medications. It may be used in neonates when intravascular or intraosseous access is difficult to obtain. Specific chemotherapy drugs, such as asparaginase, can be given IP. Body-temperature fluids may be infused into the abdominal cavity to lavage the abdomen in animals with peritonitis or pancreatitis. Warm or cool fluid IP lavage may be used to help treat patients with severe hypothermia or hyperthermia.

Substances injected into the peritoneal cavity are absorbed more rapidly than those administered SC but more slowly than those given by the intravascular or intraosseous route. When a drug or fluids must be administered into the peritoneal cavity, the ventral abdomen between the umbilicus and the bladder is shaved and aseptically prepared. An 18- to 22-gauge needle or catheter is inserted into the abdominal cavity on the ventral midline, a few centimeters caudal to the umbilicus.

A syringe is attached and aspirated. If the needle is in the proper location in the peritoneal cavity, no blood or fluid will be aspirated into the syringe. If blood or fluid enters the syringe tip, the needle may have punctured a vessel or an abdominal organ. The needle is removed, and a new needle is inserted into a different site. If the syringe remains empty when negative pressure is applied, the medication or fluids have been injected.

Sampling Techniques in the Small Animal

BLOOD SAMPLE COLLECTION

Veterinary technicians perform venipuncture on a routine basis to collect blood samples for laboratory tests or to inject a drug or medication. Proper animal restraint is as important as the venipuncture technique. Refer to Chapter 6 for additional information about restraint and handling of small animals. Blood samples must be collected with minimal trauma to the vessel and minimal stress and discomfort to the patient (Procedure 18-2). Patients' stress can affect several laboratory tests (e.g., leukogram, cortisol and glucose concentrations).

A venipuncture is performed with a needle and syringe or with a Vacutainer collection system. The Vacutainer system consists of a double-pointed needle, a plastic holder, and collection tubes with and without anticoagulants (Figure 18-15). The method and needle gauge selected depend on the vessel size, the amount of blood required, the intended use of the sample, and the technician's preference.

Most venipunctures in cats and small dogs are performed with 22-gauge needles. Larger-gauge needles, such as 20- and 18-gauge, may be used in large breed dogs and in most farm animals. For any venipuncture technique, the needle should always be inserted into the vein with the bevel facing upward.

PROCEDURE 18-2 | Venous Blood Collection

- Attach a 20- to 25-gauge needle to a 1- to 6-ml syringe.
- Occlude the vein with a tourniquet or digital pressure.
- Wipe the skin and hair on top of the vein with an alcohol-soaked cotton ball to help identify the vein.
- Insert the needle with the bevel facing up through the skin and into the vein at a 25-degree angle.
- Slowly retract the syringe plunger and collect a blood sample.
- Release the pressure on the vein and release the syringe plunger when a sufficient volume of blood has been collected.
- Remove the needle from the vein.
- Apply digital pressure to the venipuncture site as soon as the needle is removed until hemostasis occurs.

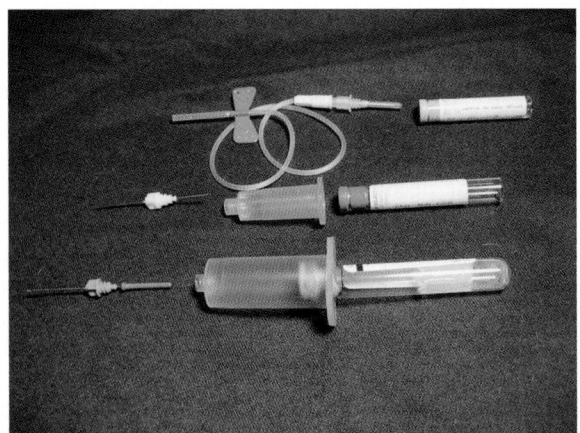

FIGURE 18-15 The Vacutainer blood collection system is used to collect blood samples directly into the collection tubes. The system consists of a needle, a holder, and collection tubes. (From Hendrix CM, Sirois M, editors: Laboratory procedures for the veterinary technician, ed 5, St Louis, 2007, Mosby Elsevier.)

> **TECHNICIAN NOTE**   For venipuncture, the needle should be inserted with the bevel facing upward.

Blood collected for coagulation profiles (i.e., activated clotting time, prothrombin time, activated partial thromboplastin time) should be collected carefully with minimal tissue trauma and venous stasis. The needle ideally should penetrate the vessel on the first attempt to minimize the amount of tissue fluid that enters the sample; tissue fluid (thromboplastin) may initiate the clotting cascade.

Smaller, 25- to 28-gauge needles are used with smaller vessels, fragile vessels, or multiple venipunctures. Frequent sampling to establish a blood glucose curve is a situation in which the use of a small-gauge needle is appropriate. The amount of negative pressure applied to aspirate the blood into the syringe must not be excessive. Forceful retraction of the syringe plunger may result in **hemolysis** of red blood cells as they pass through the needle, yielding erroneous laboratory values. Application of excessive negative pressure may also cause the vein to collapse.

Just before a venipuncture, hair and skin over the vessel are wiped with a cotton ball saturated with 70% isopropyl alcohol. This helps to remove some superficial skin contaminants, causes **vasodilatation**, and improves visualization of the vein. In animals with a dense hair coat, the vessel may be easier to identify if the hair over the vessel is parted with the use of an alcohol-soaked cotton ball or shaved with a clipper. When blood is drawn for bacterial culture, the region on top of the vein is shaved and aseptically prepared. Sterile gloves are worn when blood is collected for a culture.

The most important aspects of any venipuncture technique are proper restraint of the animal and proper distention and immobilization of the vessel. These objectives are most easily accomplished when the procedure is done as a two-person project. The veterinary technician should attempt the venipuncture only when the vessel can be clearly delineated. Blind venipuncture attempts are doomed to failure and unnecessary patient discomfort. If the technician is unable to locate the vessel by visual inspection or digital palpation, the manner in which the vessel is distended and immobilized must be changed.

> **TECHNICIAN NOTE**   The most important aspects of any venipuncture technique are proper restraint of the animal and proper distention and immobilization of the vessel.

When blood is collected, excessive restraint should be avoided because it may incite greater resistance from the animal than is caused by the venipuncture procedure itself.

To collect blood from a peripheral vein, introduce the needle into the occluded vessel as far distally as possible. If the initial venipuncture attempt is unsuccessful, reinsert the needle more proximal to the previous entry site. For a jugular venipuncture, the initial attempt is made in the caudal region of the jugular vein. Subsequent venipuncture attempts can be made in a more cranial region. If the vessel is damaged in the distal portion of the vein, a more proximal region is still patent and usable for blood collection.

After blood is collected, the needle is detached from the syringe and the stopper is removed from the collection tube before blood is transferred into the tube. This reduces the hemolysis that may occur if blood is forcefully ejected through the narrow lumen of a needle. If blood is transferred into a tube containing an anticoagulant, such as lavender-topped ethylenediaminetetraacetic (EDTA) tubes, the stopper is quickly replaced, and the tube is gently inverted a few times to mix the blood with the anticoagulant. Vigorous shaking can cause hemolysis. The tube containing the anticoagulant should be at least half filled with blood to achieve the appropriate blood-to-anticoagulant ratio.

The most frequently used sites for canine blood collection are the cephalic, jugular, and lateral saphenous veins. The cephalic, jugular, femoral, and medial saphenous veins are used for feline venipunctures.

CEPHALIC VENIPUNCTURE

The patient may be positioned in sternal or lateral recumbency. The restrainer leans over the top of the animal and grasps the leg of interest at the elbow. The other hand and arm can be used to restrain the animal's head if the animal is awake, to prevent an aggressive response to the skin puncture. If the animal is in sternal recumbency, the restrainer should lean on his or her elbow to help prevent the animal from withdrawing its leg at some critical time during the procedure. A tourniquet or a thumb or forefinger is wrapped around the forearm at the level of the elbow. Pressure at this point occludes the cephalic vein. The skin then is rotated outward to roll the vein to the top (anterior) of the forearm.

The veterinary technician grasps the leg with one hand at the level of the metacarpus and further extends the leg. In "loose-skinned" animals, it may be necessary to flex the carpus. The objective is to tether the vein between the two points of traction (at the elbow and at the carpus) so that the vein is distended and does not roll from side to side.

The needle is directed, as much as possible, along the longitudinal axis of the vein. The needle is inserted through the skin with the bevel facing up. The skin puncture is the painful part, and animals often will move in response to it. Once the animal has settled down, the needle can be directed into the vein.

If blood does not spontaneously flow into the hub of the needle, gently aspirate to determine whether the needle is or is not in the vein. If it is not, the needle should be advanced a bit farther and the process repeated. The needle can be advanced to its full length. If at this point the venipuncture has not been successful, the needle will have to be withdrawn to its subcutaneous (SC) position (do not remove it entirely because another skin puncture will then be necessary). It is most important to withdraw the needle slowly, while gently aspirating. The deep wall of the vein may have been inadvertently penetrated, thus the lumen will be found as the needle is withdrawn.

Once the blood sample is taken or the drug is administered, the needle is withdrawn from the vein, and digital pressure is applied over the venipuncture site for at least 30 seconds. The site should be monitored for bleeding or **hematoma** formation for an additional several minutes.

JUGULAR VENIPUNCTURE

The patient may be positioned in sternal or lateral recumbency. Some large breed dogs prefer to remain seated on the floor (Figure 18-16). Alternatively, the patient is restrained on a table in sternal recumbency (Figure 18-17). One hand grasps the legs at the carpal joint and stretches the legs over the edge of the table. In any position, the head will have to be extended. The restrainer or the veterinary technician occludes the vein by applying occlusive pressure at the thoracic inlet. Care must be taken to avoid compressing the trachea or impairing breathing. Vein distention and immobilization can be maximized by pressing into the thoracic inlet in a caudal direction and by further extending the head. Extensive longitudinal traction, however, can collapse the vein. With optimal positioning, the vein is easy to palpate (or visualize) and does not roll much from side to side. In sternal positioning, venipuncture is usually done in a cephalad direction; in lateral positioning, venipuncture is generally done in a caudal direction; the procedure is performed as previously described.

LATERAL SAPHENOUS VENIPUNCTURE

The patient is usually positioned in lateral recumbency (Figure 18-18). The restrainer grasps the upper leg at the

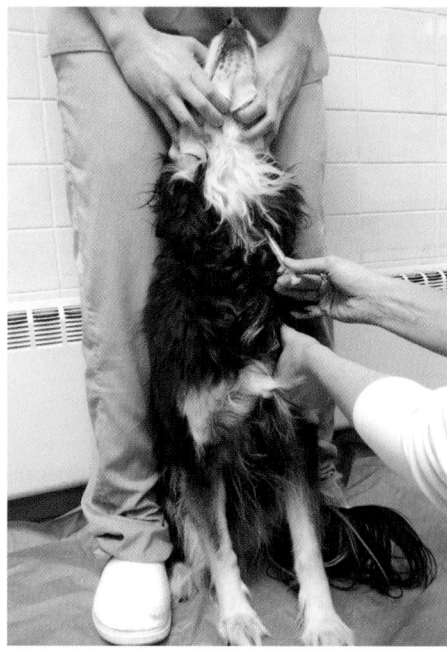

FIGURE 18-16 Dog positioned for jugular vein venipuncture in a sitting position while backed against a wall.

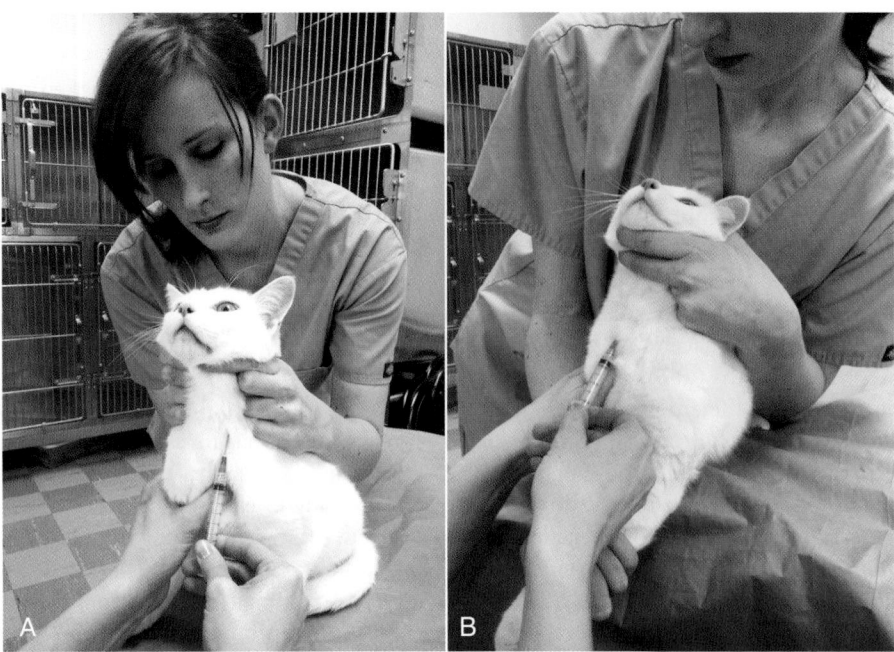

FIGURE 18-17 A, Cat positioned in a sitting position for jugular vein venipuncture. **B,** Cat positioned in a stretched position for jugular vein venipuncture. (**A,** Courtesy Dr. Joanna Bassert.)

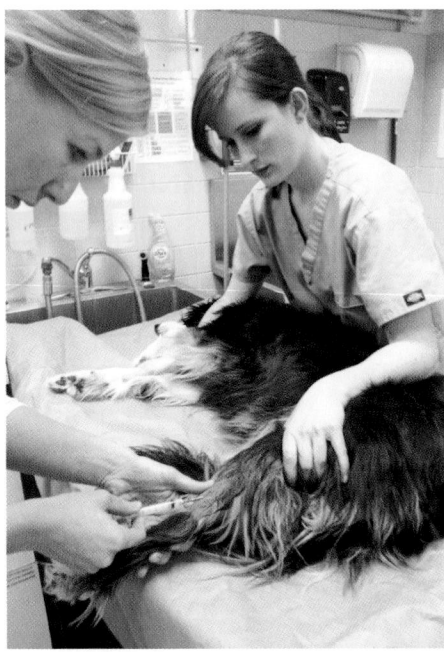

FIGURE 18-18 Dog positioned in right lateral recumbency for venipuncture of the lateral saphenous vein. (Courtesy Dr. Joanna Bassert.)

stifle. The other hand and arm can be used to restrain the animal's forelegs and head if the animal is awake. Circumferential pressure is applied at the stifle to occlude and distend the vein. The veterinary technician grasps the leg with one hand at the level of the metatarsus. It should not be necessary for the veterinary technician to use his or her thumb to help immobilize the vein. Venipuncture is performed as previously described.

MEDIAL SAPHENOUS OR FEMORAL VENIPUNCTURE

The medial saphenous or femoral vein is used to collect small volumes of blood. The canine patient is usually positioned in lateral recumbency. The restrainer grasps the lower leg at the stifle while reflecting the upper leg caudally with the forearm. The other hand and arm can be used to restrain the animal's forelegs and head if the animal is awake. Circumferential pressure is applied at the stifle to occlude and distend the vein.

The feline patient is grasped by the scruff of the neck and is placed in lateral recumbency (Figure 18-19). The upper hind leg is abducted and flexed to expose the medial surface of the bottom leg. Applying pressure with the edge of the hand that abducts and extends the upper leg distends the vein. The veterinary technician grasps the leg with one hand at the level of the metatarsus. Venipuncture is performed as previously described.

MARGINAL EAR VENIPUNCTURE

On occasion, the technician will collect blood from a peripheral capillary bed to check for erythroparasitic organisms, such as *Babesia* spp. or *Haemobartonella* spp. Also, a small drop of capillary blood is collected by clients who monitor their diabetic pets' blood glucose levels at home. A peripheral capillary blood sample can be obtained by clipping the quick of a toenail or lacerating the buccal mucosa. A more desirable, less painful alternative is to collect a sample from the marginal ear vein, which is most easily visualized as it courses around the periphery of the dorsal aspect of the pinna.

When a capillary sample is collected, the pinna of the ear is warmed with a heated cloth, a light source, or the

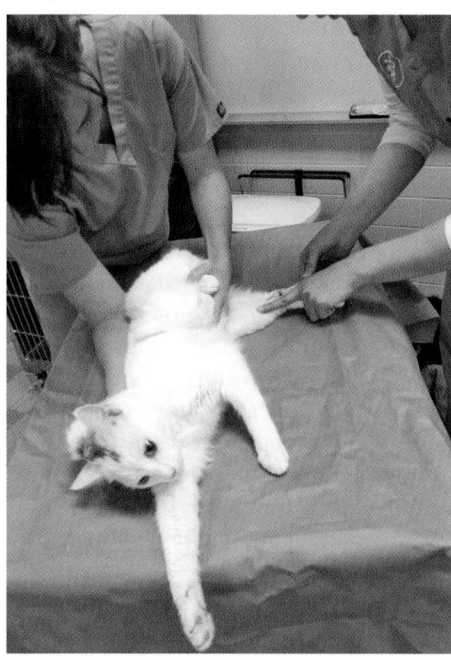

FIGURE 18-19 Cat in a right lateral stretch position for venipuncture of the medial saphenous vein.

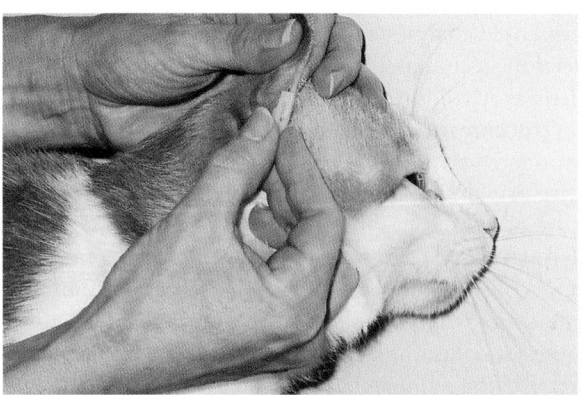

FIGURE 18-20 Collection of a peripheral capillary blood sample from the marginal ear vein of the cat with a lancet.

technician's hands to help vasodilate the marginal ear vein; it is then wiped with a small amount of alcohol. A 25-gauge needle or lancet is used to nick the vein, and the pinna is massaged until a sufficient drop of blood is obtained (Figure 18-20).

When a sample must be examined for erythroparasites, blood is collected into a heparinized capillary tube and is later smeared onto slides for a microscopic examination. If blood is collected for measurement of blood glucose, a Glucometer test strip is placed alongside the drop of blood on the pinna, and the blood is wicked directly onto the test strip. The test strip should be designed to measure a capillary, not venous, blood sample. The technician must make certain that the patient does not move its head or flick its ear, or the blood sample may be lost. After the blood sample has been obtained, firm pressure should be applied to the puncture site for approximately 15 seconds.

ARTERIAL BLOOD SAMPLE

One of the best ways to assess pulmonary function is through arterial blood gases. Blood gases tell us about the patient's ability to ventilate and oxygenate. Blood gases measure the partial pressure of carbon dioxide ($PaCO_2$—ventilation) and oxygen (PaO_2—oxygenation) in the blood. Blood gas measurements are performed on a pH and blood gas analyzer. Over the past few years, new, inexpensive point-of-care instruments have been developed to measure pH and arterial blood gases. These analyzers are cost-effective and easy to use.

> **TECHNICIAN NOTE** One of the best ways to assess pulmonary function is through measurement of arterial blood gases.

Collection of a blood sample for blood gas analysis entails percutaneous puncture of an artery, such as the dorsal metatarsal or femoral artery. In the unconscious or anesthetized patient, the sublingual artery may be used. The dorsal metatarsal artery is smaller, but the interstitial connective tissues around it are "tighter" (compared with the femoral artery); this facilitates vessel positioning and minimizes postpuncture hematoma formation. The dead space of a 1- or 3-ml syringe (with a 25-gauge needle) is coated with lithium or sodium heparin (1000 U/ml); excess heparin is expelled from the syringe. In addition, a Vacutainer tube cork, an alcohol swab, and a thermometer will be needed. When the sample is collected, care should be taken to avoid introducing air or applying excessive negative pressure, both of which can affect your PaO_2 measurement. Once the sample collection is complete, withdraw the needle and apply digital pressure over the puncture site for at least 1 minute; monitor for bleeding or hematoma formation for another 4 minutes. Air is expelled from the syringe, and the syringe is capped with the cork and placed in an ice water bath if the laboratory test cannot be performed immediately. Blood gas samples may stay in an ice water bath for several hours before metabolism alters pH or blood gas values.

Dorsal Metatarsal Artery Sample

An arterial puncture is usually done with the animal in lateral recumbency; however, it can be accomplished when the animal is standing if it resents the lateral recumbent positioning. If the patient is in lateral recumbency with the hock extended, it may be helpful to tape the paw to a table or sandbag. The pulse is palpated with one or two fingers of one hand (Figure 18-21). With the bevel up, the skin and the arterial wall may be punctured in a single motion while following the path of the artery, or in a two-step fashion: skin first then artery. Watch for a backflash of blood in the needle hub, then gently aspirate a 1- to 1.5-ml sample. If the arterial puncture is unsuccessful, the needle can be inserted a bit farther. As for a venipuncture, when the needle is withdrawn, this should be done slowly and with gentle aspiration applied to the plunger in case the deep wall of the artery was

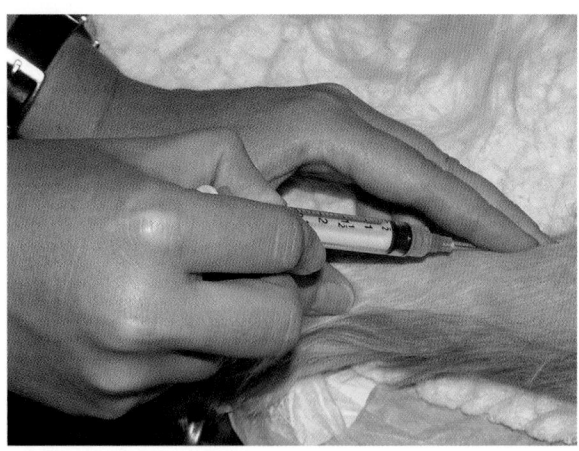

FIGURE 18-21 Palpating the dorsal metatarsal artery for arterial blood sampling.

inadvertently punctured during the introduction. The needle is withdrawn to its SC position, and the arterial puncture is reattempted.

Femoral Artery Sample

Arterial puncture is performed with the animal in lateral recumbency with the down leg extended caudally. The top leg should be positioned so that it is out of the way. After the puncture site has been prepared properly, the first and middle fingers of one hand locate the artery, and the leading edge of the same hand can be used to slide the skin and underlying SC tissues toward the inguinal region. The femoral artery must be immobilized properly to prevent it from rolling away from the needle. The syringe is held at a 45-degree angle over the site where the pulse is strongest. The needle is advanced through the skin as previously described and the sample collected.

Arterial Catheter Placement

Arterial catheters are inserted for continuous measurement of direct arterial blood pressure and for collection of multiple arterial blood samples. The most common artery selected for catheterization is the dorsal metatarsal artery. The dorsal metatarsal offers many advantages over the femoral artery. The cylindrical nature of the tarsus allows the catheter to be taped rather than sutured. Risk of hematoma formation and hemorrhage is reduced because of the tight SC tissues. It is easier to maintain the catheter position because the catheter does not move and kink in the SC tissues.

A 20- or 22-gauge OTN catheter may be placed in the dorsal metatarsal artery. The patient is placed in lateral recumbency with the hock extended; it may be helpful to tape the paw to a table or sandbag. The insertion site is clipped and aseptically prepared. The catheter is flushed with heparinized saline. The artery to be catheterized is palpated with one or two fingers of one hand. A relief hole is made completely through the dermis with the beveled edge of the needle (without entry into the artery). The catheter is

positioned SC above the artery with the bevel up. The needle tip and the artery are palpated simultaneously with the finger(s) of the opposite hand. The catheter is inserted into the artery steeply at first just so that the tip of the needle penetrates the upper wall of the artery, and then flat against the skin surface and parallel to the longitudinal axis of the artery so that the bevel of the needle and the end of the catheter lie in the lumen of the artery. A "flash back" of blood should be seen in the hub of the needle; the catheter is gently advanced into the artery to its full length. The needle is replaced with a T-connector and stopcock. The catheter is taped in place and flushed with heparinized saline. Refer to "Peripheral Vein Catheterization" for further details.

The catheter may be attached to a continuous flush system or flushed with heparinized saline every 2 hours. The toes should be checked for warmth every 2 to 4 hours. If the toes are cool, the catheter will have to be removed. Catheter care is performed every 48 hours.

URINE SAMPLE COLLECTION

A urine sample may be obtained by several methods. The veterinary technician should be familiar with the various techniques. Urine is most often collected for gross and microscopic analyses and for culture if indicated. Common collection techniques include obtaining urine from the patient as it voids, from manual expression of the bladder, by **cystocentesis**, and from catheterization of the bladder. Most references advocate a volume of 7 to 10 ml for a quantitative urinalysis; however, smaller samples are sufficient for culture or spot assays for ketones or glucose.

Urine collected is stored in clean, dry containers. Urine that is collected for culture is collected and submitted in sterile containers. Samples that are not analyzed within 30 minutes of collection are refrigerated in secured sealed containers. Urine samples are returned to room temperature before analysis.

VOIDED COLLECTION

A naturally voided sample is easy to collect. It is most commonly obtained from canine patients by walking the dog outdoors and catching a midstream sample. These samples are adequate for routine urinalysis. These free catch samples are not acceptable for culture because they contain bacteria, cells, and debris from skin, hair, and the genitourinary tract. The initial void of urine contains the greatest concentration of contaminants and should be excluded from collection. Innovative collection devices can be easily made to catch the urine of a voiding dog because most dogs stop urinating if a person gets too close. Examples are devices made of a log rod or a straightened clothes hanger with a loop at one end for holding a disposable cup or container.

> **TECHNICIAN NOTE** Urine is most easily obtained from a dog by walking it outdoors and catching a voided midstream sample.

Hospitalized patients can be elevated on a raised grate in a clean cage. Urine is collected from the cage floor with a syringe after the animal urinates.

Fresh voided urine samples of cats are obtained from litter boxes that are clean and empty. Lining the litter box with a plastic bag or with clear plastic food wrap facilitates collection of the sample. For cats that prefer litter in boxes, shredded wax paper and specialty nonabsorbent litter made of plastic beads, such as NOSORB (Catco, Inc., Cape Coral, Florida), are options. After the cat urinates in the litter pan, urine is collected by a syringe or is poured into a clean container.

MANUAL BLADDER EXPRESSION

Urine collected by manual expression of the bladder can be used for routine urinalysis but should not be used for culture because urine obtained by this method will contain contaminants from the lower urinary tract, skin, and hair. Bladder expression can be difficult to accomplish in some patients because transabdominal compression causes pressure inside the bladder to increase, but the urethral sphincter may not relax simultaneously. Manual expression of the urinary bladder is warranted in patients with neurologic impairment when the animal cannot initiate voluntary urination or does not have the ability to completely empty the bladder.

To perform manual expression of the urinary bladder, place a hand on either side of the caudal abdomen of a patient that is standing or in lateral recumbency. Isolate the bladder between the palmar surfaces of the fingers, and apply firm and steady pressure until urine is produced. In small breed dogs and in cats, it is possible to use only one hand.

If urine cannot be produced by manual expression with moderate compression, an alternate method of emptying the bladder or obtaining a sample must be employed. Do not overexert pressure. Extreme caution is exercised in patients with an overly distended bladder in the presence of urethral obstruction, such as that seen in obstructed male cats. Urethral or vesicular rupture may occur in these patients.

CYSTOCENTESIS

Cystocentesis is the percutaneous aspiration of urine from the bladder. A cystocentesis procedure is indicated to obtain a sterile urine sample for analysis and/or culture and sensitivity testing. The sample is free of bacteria, cells, and debris from the lower urinary tract. This procedure also minimizes iatrogenic urinary tract infection caused by catheterization, especially in patients with preexisting disease of the urethra and/or urinary bladder. Cystocentesis sampling can also aid in localization of hematuria, pyuria, and bacteriuria. Cystocentesis is used as a last resort to empty an overly distended bladder when a urethral obstruction prevents urinary catheterization. The common contraindication for cystocentesis is attempting to perform the procedure when urine in the bladder is inadequate, or when the patient resists restraint and abdominal palpation. It is recommended to wait until sufficient urine is present in the bladder or to seek ultrasound guidance along with proper physical and chemical restraint, if necessary. Although statistically rare, laceration of the bladder and laceration of the bowel resulting in peritonitis are additional complications. Patients having recent abdominal surgery or trauma, suspected bleeding disorders, pyometra, or suspected caudal abdominal or bladder tumor should not undergo cystocentesis procedures.

> **TECHNICIAN NOTE** Cystocentesis is the percutaneous aspiration of urine from the bladder.

Supplies needed to perform a cystocentesis in canine and feline patients include a 22-gauge, 1- to 1.5-inch needle attached to a 12-ml or larger syringe. The patient can be standing, in lateral recumbency, or in ventral recumbency. The site allows ventral or ventrolateral insertion into the bladder wall, depending on the patient's positioning. When cystocentesis is performed, most (but not all) of the urine should be removed from the bladder. Excessive pressure from a full bladder might lead to extravasation of urine from the puncture site when the needle is withdrawn. On the other hand, removal of the entire volume of urine increases risk of contact between the needle and the bladder wall, which may result in damage to the bladder. Thus it is ideal to insert the needle a short distance cranial to the trigone region of the bladder. Having the needle a short distance cranial to the junction of the bladder with the urethra, rather than at the apex of the bladder, permits removal of urine and decompression of the bladder, without the need for reinsertion of the needle into the bladder lumen. If the needle is placed into or adjacent to the apex of the bladder, it may not remain in the bladder lumen because the bladder progressively decreases in size following aspiration of urine. Furthermore, the technician should position the needle at about a 45-degree angle through the bladder wall, creating an oblique needle tract. When the needle is directed in this fashion, the elasticity of the vesicle musculature and the interlacing arrangement of individual muscle fibers will provide a better seal of the small pathway created by the needle when it is removed. Use of ultrasound as an imaging tool to identify the location and the size of the bladder is becoming common practice. Ultrasound-guided cystocentesis also offers visualization of the needle as it enters the bladder wall. Procedures for ventrolateral (Figure 18-22) and ventral cystocentesis (Figure 18-23) are outlined in Procedure 18-3. Note that in male dogs, the prepuce and the penis are diverted laterally, and the needle is inserted on the ventral midline or slightly paramedian. If blood enters the needle, another cystocentesis attempt is made with a different needle and syringe. The needle should never be redirected once it is in the abdominal cavity because accidental laceration of viscera may occur. Last, the technician needs to remember to always release negative aspiration pressure on the plunger of the syringe before withdrawing the needle and syringe apparatus.

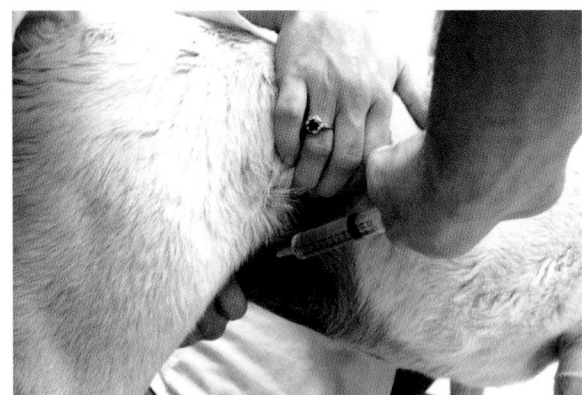

FIGURE 18-22 Performing a cystocentesis using a ventrolateral approach.

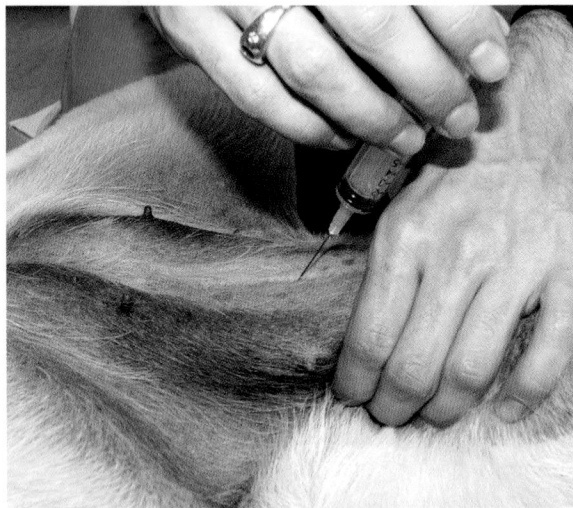

FIGURE 18-23 Performing a ventral cystocentesis with the patient in dorsal recumbency.

> *TECHNICIAN NOTE* Remove negative aspiration pressure on the plunger of the syringe before withdrawing the needle when performing any paracentesis procedure, such as a cystocentesis.

CATHETERIZATION

Indications for urinary catheterization include collecting a urine sample, emptying the bladder, relieving a urethral obstruction, allowing access to the urinary tract for radiographic studies, and treating patients with conditions for which an indwelling urinary catheter is indicated. Complications of urinary catheterization include urinary tract infection, particularly with indwelling catheters or in patients with immunosuppression. Even though aseptic techniques are used while the catheter is placed, these approaches may induce urethral inflammation or a bacterial urinary tract infection. Urethral and bladder irritation and trauma are other possible complications. Trauma from catheterization may cause increases in red blood cell count, protein, and transitional epithelial cells in the sample. Urine samples

---

PROCEDURE 18-3 | Procedure for Cystocentesis

Ventrolateral Cystocentesis
- Patient is placed in lateral recumbency or standing.
- Palpate abdomen to determine size and location of bladder.
- Hold the syringe with the needle in one hand, and stabilize the bladder from below with the free hand. The bladder should be pressed dorsally and caudally to immobilize it against the pelvis.
- Wipe area of insertion with alcohol.
- Insert the needle into the abdominal cavity and bladder, angling caudomedially at a 45-degree angle to the bladder wall and toward the trigonal region, as previously described.
- Aspirate urine in the syringe. After the desired sample volume is obtained, stop aspiration or release negative pressure on the plunger of the syringe before withdrawing the needle from the bladder and abdominal cavity.

Ventral Cystocentesis
- Patient is placed in dorsal recumbency. This may take two assistants to accomplish this, especially in large breed or deep-chested dogs.
- Palpate abdomen to determine size and location of bladder.
- Wipe the area of insertion with alcohol. Stabilize the bladder against the pelvis with one hand.
- Insert the needle into the abdomen, staying on midline, into the bladder. The needle should be positioned at a 45-degree angle and directed caudally.
- Aspirate desired sample. Release negative pressure on the syringe plunger before withdrawing the needle.

---

may contain contaminants from the genital region and the urethra. However, urine obtained by catheterization is acceptable for bacterial culture if a sample cannot be obtained by cystocentesis.

Indwelling urinary catheters are placed in patients at risk for urethral obstruction, such as male cats that have recently had urethral calculi removed, and in patients with neurologic impairment or traumatic conditions that interfere with normal urination. Catheterization is also an important part of quantizing urinary output.

The prepuce or vulva is gently rinsed twice with a warm antimicrobial solution and water and is then dried. Sterile gloves are worn to detach the catheter or connect it to extension tubing or a collection system. A closed system is created by connecting the catheter to IV extension tubing that is connected to a sterile collection bag. Commercial urinary collection bags are available on the market, or an empty sterile fluid bag can be used. The collection bag serves as a urine reservoir. Its contents must be measured and emptied periodically.

Indwelling urinary catheters should be inspected for occlusion. The patient is also monitored for adequate urine output. A normotensive, normovolemic patient with intact renal function should produce 1 to 2 ml of urine per

TABLE 18-1	Sizing Chart for Urethral Catheter Selection: General Guidelines for Selection of Urethral Catheters		
ANIMAL	**SEX**	**WEIGHT**	**URETHRAL CATHETER SIZE**
Canine	Male	<9 kg	3.5-French
	Male	9-23 kg	5- or 8-French
	Male	>23 kg	10- or 12-French
	Female	<9 kg	5-French
	Female	9-23 kg	8- or 10-French
	Female	>23 kg	10- or 12-French
Feline	Male	All weights	3.5-French
	Female	All weights	3.5-French

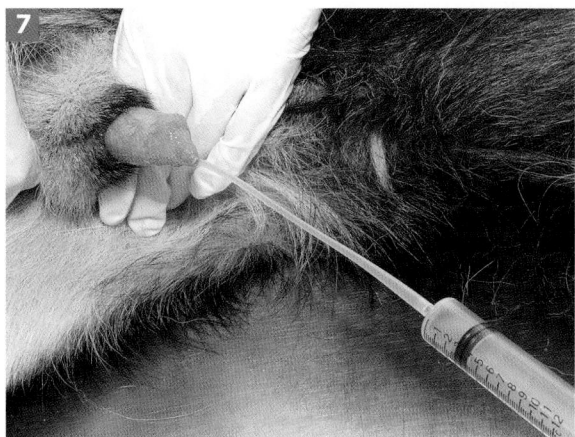

FIGURE 18-24 Urinary catheterization of a male dog. Once the catheter is placed in the urethra, a sterile syringe is attached and urine is gently aspirated. (From Taylor SM: Small animal clinical techniques, St Louis, 2010, Saunders.)

kilogram of body weight per hour. If urine in the reservoir bag is not adequate, the patient's urinary bladder should be palpated for distention. The urinary catheter should be inspected for obstructions or kinks. The bladder can be gently compressed to determine whether urine will flow through the catheter. A small volume of sterile 0.9% saline solution can be flushed through the catheter in an attempt to relieve obstruction.

Indwelling urinary catheters should be removed as soon as possible to reduce inflammation of the urinary tract and catheter-induced infections. If catheterization is required on a long-term basis, a new catheter should be placed every 4 to 5 days.

Urinary catheters are available in French sizes. See Table 18-1 of general guidelines for catheter selection. Note the length of available urinary catheters on the market. Many catheters that are manufactured for the human market do not possess the length needed for large breed canine male anatomy.

Likewise, long catheters should be premeasured externally on the patient and excessive lengths not advanced in smaller patients because the catheter can tie itself in a knot within the urinary bladder, making withdrawal impossible without surgical intervention. Measurement therefore is made to the caudal portion of the bladder.

Male Dog

Placement of a urinary catheter in a male dog is not difficult unless a urethral obstruction is present. Polypropylene urinary catheters are rigid and easy to pass into the urinary bladder for a sample collection or for emptying of the bladder. If the catheter is to remain indwelling, a softer, flexible feeding tube or a silicone self-retaining **Foley catheter** is more desirable and comfortable for the patient.

The dog is placed in lateral recumbency with the upper leg abducted. Carefully clip any long hairs around the preputial orifice. Flush the prepuce with a dilute antiseptic solution, and rinse with warm sterile saline solution or water. An assistant retracts the prepuce so that the tip of the penis is exposed and maintains this position. The tip of the penis is gently washed with an antiseptic solution and is rinsed with warm saline solution or water. Sterile gloves are donned. The catheter is taken aseptically out of the packaging, and the distal tip of the catheter is lubricated with a sterile water-soluble lubricant or sterile lidocaine ointment. If sterile gloves are not worn, the catheter should be kept wrapped so that it can be handled aseptically as it is advanced through the urethra. Sterile scissors can be used to cut a movable "butterfly" tab at the end of the packaging. The tab is then used to feed the catheter into the bladder; this allows the operator to avoid touching the sterile catheter.

Insert and advance the catheter into the urethra. The catheter should never be forced. If the catheter cannot be passed, a smaller catheter should be used. It is common to feel some resistance at the level of the os penis—the portion of the urethra that curves around the ischial arch—and at the level of the prostate gland in older intact males. Steady gentle pressure should overcome this slight resistance. The catheter can be guided around the curvature at the ischial arch by applying digital pressure on the perineum externally or by pressing the catheter with an index finger placed in the rectum.

Urine should flow into the catheter as it enters the neck of the bladder. The catheter is then advanced 1 cm farther, or to the predetermined measurement. A sterile syringe is attached to the catheter, and urine is slowly aspirated from the bladder (Figure 18-24). The first few milliliters of urine suctioned from the catheter should be discarded because it may contain contaminants and should not be submitted for urinalysis or culture.

The catheter may be withdrawn from the bladder when the desired procedure is completed. If the catheter is to remain in the bladder, it must be secured. If the catheter is a self-retaining Foley catheter, the appropriate volume of sterile saline or water is injected into its distal balloon cuff via the one-way valve at the proximal end of the catheter. The catheter must be secured in the following fashion (optional for a Foley catheter): Two stay-suture loops are made through the skin on two sides of the distal prepuce with 3-0 or 4-0 nylon suture material. An adhesive tape "butterfly" tab is folded around the catheter and over on itself at the location where the catheter exits the penis. A suture is passed through one side of the tape and then through the nylon loop in the prepuce. This is repeated on the other side of the tape and with the other nylon loop in the prepuce. This secures the catheter to the prepuce so that it remains in place. Stay-suture loops remain in place in the prepuce and allow catheter adjustments or changes without the need to pass another needle through the prepuce.

Female Dog

Urinary catheterization is more challenging in the female dog than in the male. Catheterization can be accomplished with the patient in a standing position, in lateral recumbency, or in sternal recumbency with the hind legs dangling from the end of the table. With a conscious dog, it is preferred that the dog stand with its hindquarters positioned at the end of an examination table. The assistant should support the patient under the abdomen to prevent lowering of the hindquarters during catheterization. Excessive long hairs are clipped from the vulvar area. The vulvar and perineal areas are gently washed with a dilute, warm antiseptic solution and rinsed with sterile saline solution or water. The ventral vaginal floor is instilled with 1.0 ml of sterile 2% lidocaine jelly. The two techniques required to pass the catheter include (1) visualization with a speculum and a light source and (2) a blind technique in which a digit is used to palpate and guide the catheter. A sterile speculum is used for visualization of the urethral orifice. Examples of a speculum include a lighted vaginal speculum, a Killian nasal speculum, an otoscope fitted with a large-diameter speculum, and a laryngoscope blade. The speculum of choice is gently inserted into the vagina. Exercise caution to avoid the clitoral fossa. After donning sterile gloves, insert the speculum vertically, and straighten to horizontal when the pelvic canal is entered. With the aid of a light, locate the urethral papilla and the urethral opening, and insert a lubricated catheter. The papilla and the urethral orifice can be found 2 to 4 cm into the vagina in most dogs (Figure 18-25). Advance the catheter until urine is obtained or at the premeasured length. If a speculum is not available, the blind technique can be performed. While wearing sterile gloves, place a lubricated finger into the vagina and slides it 2 to 5 cm along the ventral floor until the papilla and the external urethral orifice are located. Introduce the catheter into the vagina and guide it into the urethral orifice by the finger in the vestibule. Acknowledge proper placement by palpating the catheter within the urethral orifice, not in the cranial vestibule (Figure 18-26). Advance the catheter until urine is obtained or until the premeasured length is reached. Attach a sterile syringe to the catheter, and apply gentle negative pressure for the desired sample. If the catheter is to remain in place, it is ideal to select a self-retaining Foley catheter. Once the catheter is placed in the bladder, inflate the balloon cuff with the appropriate volume of sterile saline or water to prevent the

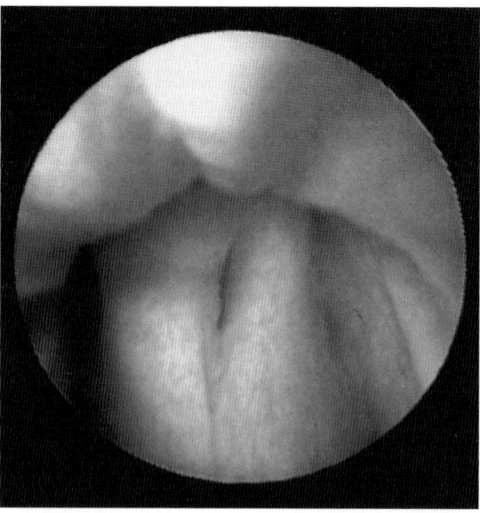

FIGURE 18-25 Urethral orifice on the ventral floor of the vagina in a female dog. (From Ettinger SJ, Feldmen E, editors: Textbook of veterinary internal medicine, ed 6, Philadelphia, 2005, Elsevier Saunders.)

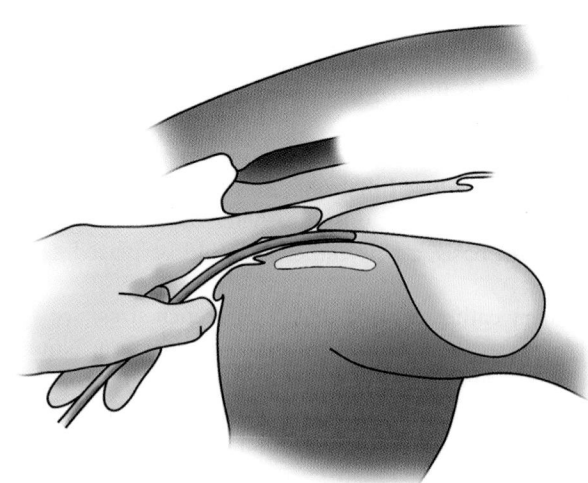

FIGURE 18-26 Urinary catheterization of a female dog. The finger in the vestibule over the urethral orifice guides the urinary catheter ventrally into the urethra. (From Taylor SM: Small animal clinical techniques, St Louis, 2010, Saunders.)

catheter from slipping out of the bladder. Then tape the catheter to the tail to prevent the dog from stepping on it. Place a closed collection system on the free end of the Foley catheter.

> **TECHNICIAN NOTE** The most common reason for catheterizing a male cat is to relieve a urethral obstruction.

Male Cat

Routine catheterization of male cats for urine collection is rare. The most common reason for catheterizing a male cat is to relieve a urethral obstruction. Catheterization of male cats often warrants the use of sedation or a general anesthetic. Exercise extreme caution when sedating obstructed

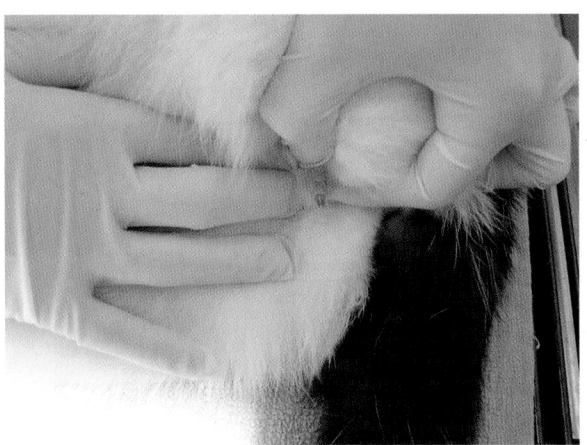

FIGURE 18-27 Retraction of the prepuce to expose the penis for feline urinary catheterization.

cats. Cats that have been obstructed long term are often obtunded and hyperkalemic and therefore should be carefully evaluated and monitored before anesthetic agents are administered. The cat is placed in lateral or dorsal recumbency with its hind legs drawn cranially. The prepuce is retracted to expose the glans of the penis (Figure 18-27). The perineum is prepared aseptically as described for the male canine catheterization, and the penis is extended dorsally so that the urethra is parallel to the vertebral column. An evaluation of the tip of the penis of an obstructed cat should be done at this time. Wearing gloves, first palpate the tip of the penis to check for the presence of a distal urethral plug or calculus. If an obstruction is present in the tip of the penis, gently massage the penis between the thumb and the forefinger to attempt to dislodge the plug. If this is unsuccessful, proceed with catheterization. With sterile gloves, lubricate a 3.5-French polypropylene or silicone tomcat catheter, and pass it into the urethra. If resistance is met, slightly withdraw the catheter and with slight rotation, re-advance it. If the catheter cannot be easily advanced, inject a small volume of sterile saline or water through the catheter. Exercise extreme care when attempting retropulsion of a urethral calculus. Avoid excessive force or volume of fluid that could result in significant urethral trauma or rupture of the urinary bladder. Once the catheter has been placed and urine flow is good, secure the catheter in place in the same fashion described for the male dog. The cat should be fitted with an Elizabethan collar to prevent removal of the catheter and the urine collection system.

Female Cat

Routine catheterization of female cats for urine collection is also rare. Just as in male cats, this procedure is not often done because of difficulty and sedation requirements. The cat is placed in sternal recumbency, and the perineal region is prepared aseptically. The technician dons sterile gloves, the lips of the vulva are pulled caudally, and a sterile 3.5-French catheter is inserted into the vagina. Keeping midline, the catheter is advanced. The urethra papilla is located about 0.7 to 1.0 cm within the vagina. The catheter should pass into the urethra with little resistance. When urine flows out of the catheter, attach a syringe. Discard the first 1 to 2 ml of urine that flows, and obtain a second sample for analysis. Remove the catheter or secure the catheter in place, and attach a closed urine collection system as previously described.

FECAL SAMPLE COLLECTION

Fecal samples are commonly collected from the ground, floor, cage bottom, or litter box after the animal defecates. Alternative methods include a lubricated fecal loop or a gloved finger inserted into the rectum to remove feces. Gross and microscopic examinations of feces for mucus, blood, intestinal parasites, and ova are commonly performed in veterinary practices. Fresh fecal samples are placed in a sealed container or bag. If samples are to be checked for parasites but are not examined for several hours, they should be refrigerated. Refer to Chapter 14 for additional information about sample collection for a parasitologic examination.

THORACOCENTESIS

Thoracocentesis is a procedure that may be used to diagnose or treat pleural filling defects (**pneumothorax** or **pleural effusion**). Air and fluid, which may compress the lungs within the pleural cavity, can be removed via thoracocentesis, allowing the lungs to reexpand. Pleural filling defects should be considered when the patient has tachypnea; short, shallow breaths; respiratory distress; open-mouth breathing; and cyanosis. Chest auscultation may reveal diminished or absent breath sounds and muffled heart sounds. If a pneumothorax or a pleural effusion is suspected, oxygen should be administered, and a thoracocentesis should be performed to stabilize the patient before stressing the patient while taking radiographs.

> **TECHNICIAN NOTE** Pleural filling defects should be considered when the patient has tachypnea; short, shallow breaths; respiratory distress; open-mouth breathing; diminished breath sounds; and cyanosis.

Materials Needed

- Sterile gloves
- Over-the-needle catheter: 2 inch (5.08 cm) to 5 inch (12.7 cm)
- Intravenous extension tubing
- Three-way stopcock
- Syringe
- Scalpel blade #15
- Lidocaine 2%
- Clippers
- Antiseptic scrub and solution
- Vacutainer blood tubes: lavender-top EDTA and red-top clot tubes
- Culture transport media

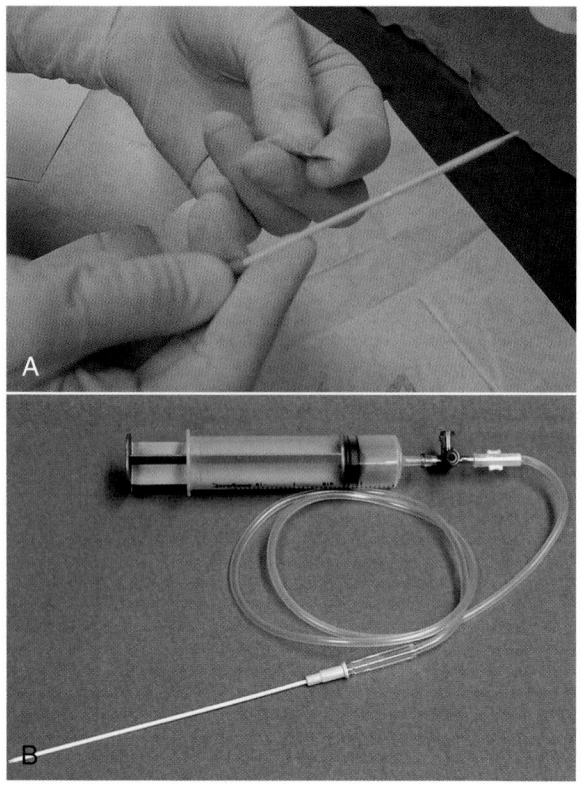

FIGURE 18-28 **A,** Using a blade to place two to three fenestrations in an over-the-needle (OTN) catheter. **B,** The setup for a thoracocentesis using a syringe, a stopcock, extension tubing, and an OTN catheter.

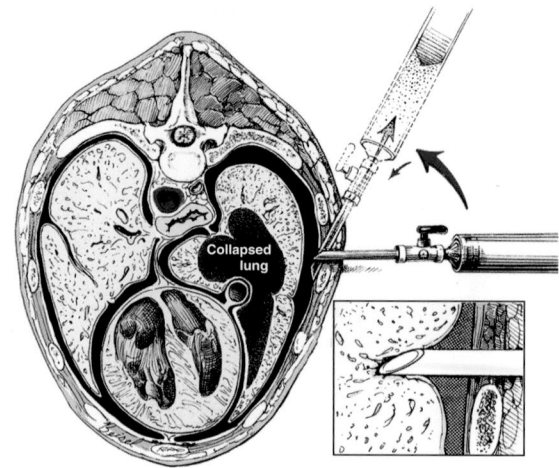

FIGURE 18-29 An over-the-needle (OTN) catheter is used to perform a thoracocentesis. (From Tobias KM, Johnston SA: *Veterinary surgery small animal*, St Louis, 2012, Saunders.)

Procedure

Thoracocentesis is performed at the 7th to 8th intercostal space. An area several inches in diameter is clipped and surgically prepared. It is best to prep an area on the thorax dorsally for collection of air and ventrally for fluid. Lidocaine (1 to 2 ml) is injected into and around the intended insertion site.

After putting on surgeon's gloves, assemble the equipment. It is helpful to add two or three small fenestrations to the catheter with the scalpel blade. Attach the stopcock to the syringe, and attach the extension tubing to the stopcock (Figure 18-28). An additional extension tube can be added to the free port of the stopcock and the end of the tube placed in a bowl or a graduated cylinder to collect the pleural fluid.

The patient may stand or be placed in sternal or lateral recumbency. Intercostal vessels and nerves run along the caudal aspect of each rib; therefore, the catheter will be inserted just cranial to the rib, and in the caudal aspect of the intercostal space. With the catheter perpendicular to the chest wall, the catheter is advanced gradually through the chest wall until a flash of fluid is seen in the hub or a pop is felt. Once in the thoracic cavity, the catheter is advanced over the needle a few millimeters so that the needle no longer extends beyond the catheter; the needle and the catheter together are then directed ventrally staying close to the thoracic wall to avoid lung tissue. When in position, the catheter

alone is advanced and the needle is subsequently removed. Extension tubing is quickly attached to the catheter (Figure 18-29). In cats, a butterfly catheter can be used instead of extension tubing and catheter. In this instance, the needle is inserted in a direction that is parallel to the long axis of the rib with the bevel facing the thoracic cavity. If the thoracocentesis is nonproductive, it may be necessary to withdraw a few millimeters and redirect the catheter or needle. Using gentle pressure, aspirate until you achieve slight negative pressure, or until the patient's condition improves. Ultrasound can be useful for determining the end-point for the procedure.

Complications include pneumothorax, lung laceration, and laceration of an intercostal vessel or internal thoracic artery leading to hypovolemia secondary to hemothorax.

Post-thoracocentesis nursing care includes close observation, respiratory rate measurement, auscultation of lung sounds, and measurement of oxygen saturation with a pulse oximeter. Laboratory samples may be submitted for cell count, total protein, cytologic examination, biochemical analysis (e.g., triglycerides, glucose, lactate), and culture and sensitivity.

ABDOMINOCENTESIS

Abdominocentesis is the aspiration of fluid from the abdominal cavity. The procedure is considered diagnostic and therapeutic. It can aid in the diagnosis of hemoabdomen or uroabdomen, peritonitis, or ascites (from cardiac or hepatic causes). It is not indicated when the patient has suffered a penetrating abdominal injury or is suspected of having a pyometra.

The veterinary technician sets up for the procedure by gathering sterile gloves, two to four 20- or 22-gauge needles, a syringe, clippers, antiseptic scrub and solution, and laboratory tubes (EDTA and clot tubes and culture transport media). The abdominocentesis is performed at the right, midabdominal region so as to avoid the liver, spleen, and urinary bladder. An area several inches in diameter is clipped and surgically prepped. A local anesthetic is not usually necessary. The patient may be standing or may be placed in sternal or lateral recumbency. Using aseptic technique, the needle is gently introduced into the peritoneal cavity. Gently aspirate or allow fluid to flow from the hub into the test tubes. Rotation of the needle or placement of a second needle into the abdomen 2 cm from the first can stimulate fluid flow. If no fluid is retrieved, the procedure should be repeated in one or two other locations. As an alternative, abdominocentesis can be performed with an 18- to 20-gauge OTN catheter.

This procedure has a high incidence of false-negative results. Large volumes (5 to 7 ml/kg) of peritoneal fluid are necessary for detection by this method. Use of a syringe can increase the likelihood of false-negative results as a result of occlusion of the needle with omentum or viscera. If the abdominocentesis result is negative, a **diagnostic peritoneal lavage** may be indicated.

Postprocedure nursing care includes monitoring of vital signs and observation for pain, abdominal distention, and continued bleeding or bruising of the centesis site. Laboratory samples may be submitted for cell count, packed cell volume, total protein, cytologic examination, biochemical analysis (e.g., creatinine, potassium, bilirubin, lactate), and culture and sensitivity.

DIAGNOSTIC PERITONEAL LAVAGE

Diagnostic peritoneal lavage (DPL) consists of infusion of fluid into the abdomen followed by retrieval of the fluid for laboratory analysis. This procedure has greater diagnostic accuracy than abdominocentesis. Indications are the same as for abdominocentesis or when the abdominocentesis result is negative. DPL has the same contraindications as abdominocentesis and is not indicated when historical, physical, or radiographic evidence suggests the need for an exploratory laparotomy. Caution should be exercised in patients with respiratory distress because instilled fluid will place pressure on the diaphragm, potentially impairing ventilation.

Materials Needed
- Peritoneal lavage catheter or a long OTN catheter
- Intravenous administration set
- Isotonic crystalloid
- Basic surgical set
- Sterile gloves
- Vacutainer blood tubes: lavender-top EDTA and red-top clot tubes
- Culture transport media
- Lidocaine 2%
- Surgical prep materials
- Vacutainer blood tubes: lavender-top EDTA and red-top clot tubes
- Culture transport media

Procedure
The bladder is emptied, and the patient is placed in lateral recumbency. The skin of the ventral abdomen is clipped and prepared caudal to the umbilicus. The skin and the abdominal wall are infiltrated with lidocaine. If a peritoneal lavage catheter is used, the veterinarian may make a small midline incision just caudal to the umbilicus through the skin, SC tissue, and superficial abdominal fascia. As an alternative, the veterinarian may make the incision just to the right of the umbilicus so as to minimize risk of trauma to the spleen and descending colon. If an OTN catheter is used, the veterinarian will make a stab incision. The catheter is inserted through the incision and is directed caudally and dorsally. The catheter is gently aspirated; if a diagnostic sample is obtained, there is no need to perform the lavage. If a diagnostic sample is not obtained, approximately 20 ml/kg of warmed crystalloid solution is infused into the abdomen. The patient is gently rocked from side to side. The fluid is allowed to flow freely from the catheter, or it is gently aspirated. If the fluid is clear, the catheter is removed; otherwise, it is sutured in place temporally for serial evaluations.

Post-DPL nursing care is the same as for abdominocentesis.

TRANSTRACHEAL WASH

It has been proved that culture swabs of the pharynx and the tonsil region are unreliable in evaluating lower respiratory tract disease because of contamination of the samples with oral flora (*Bordetella* may be an exception). Appropriate sampling is obtained more consistently by using techniques that completely bypass the mouth and oropharynx. Transtracheal lavage and aspiration provide a means of obtaining from the tracheobronchial tree material that is uncontaminated by the oral cavity for culture and cytologic examination. The technique is simple and clinically useful, and can be accomplished within a relatively short time.

The veterinarian makes the decision to perform a transtracheal lavage based on clinical, radiographic, and hematologic findings. Patients often have a chronic productive cough and the examiner can often elicit a cough easily by external palpation of the laryngeal area. There are many pulmonary conditions in which this procedure is indicated, because it can identify a wide spectrum of diagnostic clues such as inflammation and inflammatory cells (eosinophils, neutrophils, etc.), parasitic eggs and larvae, infectious agents (bacteria, fungi), and abnormal tracheobronchial cells such as neoplastic cells. Culture and sensitivity studies are frequently performed on the fluid extracted from transtracheal lavages. Patients that are not ideal candidates for a transtracheal lavage procedures are those with severe respiratory distress and those that are compromised when manipulated. Patients with coagulopathy conditions may require plasma transfusions before the procedure or may be best suited for a tracheal lavage procedure through a sterile endotracheal tube (see endotracheal lavage).

Risks and complications relative to the procedure include postprocedural hemorrhage, SC emphysema, acute dyspnea, pneumomediastinum, pneumothorax, and iatrogenic infection.

Note that it is best to have the patient awake with a cough reflex present. Therefore, heavy sedation or a general anesthetic is not advised for the procedure. An oxygen source, including a face mask, should be at hand at all times. Preoxygenation of the patient via a face mask is advised, even in eupneic animals. Common procedural techniques and approaches to tracheal lavage are described in the following sections.

PERCUTANEOUS TECHNIQUE

Method 1: Two-Catheter System
Materials Needed
- Over-the-needle (OTN) catheter: firm, 16-gauge × 2-inch indwelling OTN catheter
- Polypropylene urinary catheter: 3.5-French (Fr) catheter*
- 20-ml or 35-ml syringe filled with sterile nonbacteriostatic saline (approximately 0.5 to 1.0 ml/kg of body weight)
- Three-way stopcock (optional)
- Scalpel blade #11 (optional)
- Sterile gloves
- Lidocaine 2% drawn up in a syringe
- Bandage material: sterile 2 × 2-inch gauze with antiseptic gel, gauze roll, and tape

Procedure
1. *Positioning.* Restrain the animal in sitting or sternal recumbency. Large breed dogs are managed better on the floor and in a corner of a room. Extend the animal's head dorsally so that the nares point toward the ceiling.
2. *Site.* Cricothyroid ligament or intertracheal membrane (through trachea between cartilage rings). For the latter approach, it is generally practiced to use a lower site near the thoracic inlet in large breed dogs to ensure that the catheter tip will reach the tracheal bifurcation (dependent on catheter length).
3. *Preparation.* Standard clipping of hair and surgical prep over the area. Infiltrate with 2% lidocaine to level of ligament.
4. *Incision.* Stab incision 2 to 3 mm is optional. No suturing is required. Alternatively, tenting of the skin and introduction of the catheter through the skin before positioning and advancing through the cricothyroid ligament or intertracheal membrane is advised.
5. *Placement of catheters.* Rigid 16-gauge indwelling catheter with stylet in place is placed through SC tissues to the level of the ligament. Steady the trachea with one hand, and with the other hand hold the catheter. With

*Alternatively, you can use a 14-gauge OTN catheter and a 5-Fr urinary catheter.

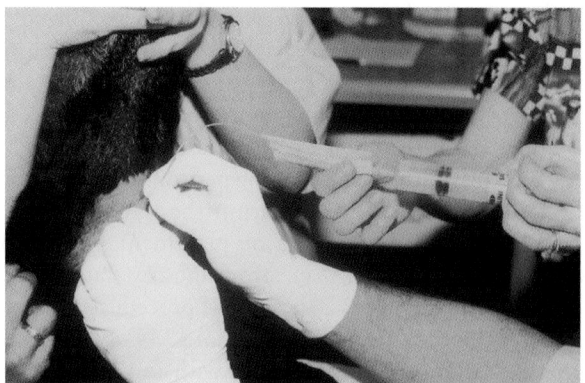

FIGURE 18-30 Percutaneous transtracheal lavage in a dog using a two-catheter system.

firm action, pass through the ligament and into the lumen of the trachea. The catheter should be placed at 45 degrees once inside the tracheal lumen, pointing down toward the tracheal bifurcation. Advance the catheter over the stylet and remove the stylet. Keep a hand on the hub of the catheter at all times. Next, verify placement by attaching a syringe to the catheter in place in the trachea. Air should be easily aspirated. Pass the urinary catheter through the indwelling catheter to a predetermined level (measure from larynx to caudal border of the scapula to approximate distance to tracheal bifurcation; Figure 18-30).

6. *Obtaining sample.* Attach to the urinary catheter a sterile 20-ml or 35-ml syringe containing no more than 10 ml of nonbacteriostatic saline. Rapidly infuse the saline and aspirate while slightly moving the urinary catheter back and forth within the trachea gently. It may be helpful to **coupage** the animal's chest at this time because the greatest amount of material will be aspirated if suction is applied while the animal coughs. Repeat this procedure until the fluid in the syringe is cloudy or contains visible clumps of mucus. The presence of the optional stopcock allows air to be evacuated from the syringe without disrupting the assembly. If desired, repeat aspiration procedure with a new syringe for two samples: one for a culture and one for cytology. When the procedure is complete, cap the syringe containing the laboratory samples with a new needle. *Note:* Do not expect to retrieve all of the saline infused through the catheter. A yield of 20% to 25% is common.
7. *Patient monitoring.* Monitor the patient closely during sample collection. Oxygen can be delivered directly through the catheter or by face mask, if necessary.
8. *Removal of catheters.* Remove the urinary catheter first, then the indwelling catheter. This will prevent contamination of soft tissues with the catheter tip.
9. *Bandage placement.* A light pressure wrap with a sterile 2 × 2-inch gauze square with antiseptic dressing applied to the entry site is sufficient. This may prevent excessive bleeding or SC emphysema.

Method 2: Through-the-Needle Catheter
Materials Needed
- Through-the-needle (TTN) catheter, 19-gauge × 12 inches
- 20-ml syringe filled with 10 ml of nonbacteriostatic saline
- Three-way stopcock
- Scalpel blade #11 (optional)
- Sterile gloves
- Lidocaine 2% drawn up in a syringe
- Bandage material: sterile 2 × 2-inch gauze with antiseptic gel, gauze roll, and tape

Procedure
1. *Positioning, site preparation, and incision* (Steps 1 to 4) are the same as in Method 1.
2. *The trachea is stabilized* with one hand while the catheter is held with the other hand. The needle of the catheter is placed through the SC tissues until it contacts the ligament. The angle of the needle is perpendicular to the trachea with the bevel pointing down. With a firm action, introduce the needle through the ligament; then change the angle of the needle to 45 degrees, pointing downward toward the tracheal bifurcation. Advance the catheter through the needle, sliding the catheter down the enclosed plastic housing. Make sure that the needle is pointing down toward the bifurcation. If not, the catheter may feed back up through the larynx, causing the animal to chew or gag. After the catheter is advanced to its full length, withdraw the needle from the trachea and skin, leaving the catheter in place. If the needle is left in the trachea and the animal begins to move, the catheter may be severed off by the needle tip, leaving the catheter as a foreign body in the trachea. The needle guard provided with the catheter should be placed over the needle at this point to prevent injury to the animal or cutting of the catheter with the exposed sharp tip.
3. *Obtain the sample and monitor the patient* as described in Method 1 (Steps 6 and 7).
4. *Withdraw the catheter.* Remove the catheter from the trachea and skin, making sure to avoid cutting the catheter with the needle.
5. *Bandage placement.* Same as described in Method 1 (Step 9).

Endotracheal Lavage
Materials Needed
- Sterile endotracheal tube suitable for the patient's size
- Polypropylene urinary catheter: 5-Fr or larger
- 20-ml syringe filled with sterile nonbacteriostatic saline
- Three-way stopcock
- Sterile gloves
- Lidocaine 2% (for feline patients to facilitate intubation and reduce laryngeal spasms)
- Laryngoscope
- Gauze roll to secure endotracheal tube
- Anesthetic agents necessary to achieve intubation with endotracheal tube

Procedure
1. *Anesthetic plan.* Should be established for the patient. It is necessary to induce anesthesia in the animal just to the depth necessary to cleanly place a sterile endotracheal tube. Care should be taken not to contaminate the tip of the endotracheal tube within the oral cavity. Laryngeal spasms may be reduced, especially in the feline patient, with the use of a few drops of 2% lidocaine placed on the arytenoids before intubation. Anesthetic agents commonly used include ketamine hydrochloride and diazepam, propofol, and thiopental. Monitor the animal closely. Apnea is a common finding with propofol and barbiturate induction agents. Once the endotracheal tube has been placed and secured with roll gauze, the animal can be allowed to recover from the induction dose to a lighter plane of anesthesia so that a cough response is elicited when the procedure is performed. It is necessary to hold the head of the patient in case the animal begins to chew the endotracheal tube. It is ideal to position the patient in ventral recumbency.
2. *Placement of catheter.* With sterile gloves, advance the polypropylene urinary catheter to a predetermined distance to the tracheal bifurcation (measure from larynx to the caudal border of the scapula to approximate the distance to tracheal bifurcation).
3. *Obtain the sample* as described in Method 1, Step 6.
4. *Remove the polypropylene catheter.*
5. *Monitor and recover the patient.* Provide supplemental oxygenation through the endotracheal tube as needed. Monitor the patient's respiratory effort and signs for distress. Thickened mucous secretions may occlude the airway. Suction the endotracheal tube with an aspiration catheter, if necessary. Remove the endotracheal tube when patient regains swallowing reflex and no longer tolerates the tube in place. Continue to monitor the patient until ambulatory.

SAMPLE HANDLING
Tracheal lavage samples are commonly submitted for both culture and cytologic examination. Aerobic and anaerobic cultures are often requested by the clinician. If a reference laboratory is used, check with the laboratory for its protocols on sample handling. Laboratory staff may provide transport media for your samples. If samples are submitted in a syringe, the needle should be sealed with a rubber stopper and the sample refrigerated and cultured within 12 hours. If smears for cytologic examination are made before shipment, they should be made from both supernatant and sediment after centrifugation. Be sure to make monolayer smears and to air dry. Smears may then be packaged in a protective container for shipment. If an on-site cytology examination is preferred, suitable stains include Romanovsky's and Giemsa-type stains.

CYTOLOGIC SAMPLE INTERPRETATION
Material obtained from deep transtracheal lavage procedures includes cellular elements normally lining the

tracheobronchial tree; cells infiltrated from inflammatory, hemorrhagic, congestive, neoplastic, or other pathologic processes; and background material derived from mucus, proteinaceous exudate, or cellular fragments. Causative agents, including bacteria, fungi, or parasites, may be observed.

ARTHROCENTESIS

Arthrocentesis is the aspiration of fluid from a joint. Disorders involving joints are etiologically diverse, ranging from congenital, developmental, and acquired disorders to various infections and immunologic diseases. Depending on the specific disorder, joint disease may be a primary or a secondary symptom. For the veterinarian to establish and differentiate the diagnosis of joint disease in the dog or cat, synovial fluid analysis is essential.

Indications for joint fluid analysis include persistent or cyclic fever, especially fever of unknown origin (FUO). Indications also include generalized stiffness or limb lameness, especially associated with systemic signs of illness, fever, **leukocytosis**, neutrophilia, hyperfibrinogenemia, malaise, and **anorexia**. Arthrocentesis may be indicated in patients with definite lameness. Palpation of localized pain and/or joint swelling may be detected, along with a change in stability or range of motion involving the affected joint or joints.

Contraindications for joint fluid collection include moderate to severe pyoderma or lick granuloma. The risk is too great for potential inoculation of the joint from the infected skin. Risks and complications include trauma with or without hemorrhage into the joint, especially when degenerative changes involving the joint are present, making access difficult, and when patients are uncooperative and are not immobilized. Iatrogenic contamination or inoculation of the joint is a complication prevented by good aseptic technique.

JOINT FLUID COLLECTION OF DISTAL JOINTS IN THE DOG AND CAT

Equipment needed for arthrocentesis includes the following: $\frac{3}{4}$-inch or 1-inch, 25-gauge needles and 3-ml syringes; 1-inch or $1\frac{1}{2}$-inch, 22-gauge needles and 3-ml syringes; clean microscope slides and coverslips; sterile gloves; clippers; and aseptic surgical preparation supplies.

Patient restraint is essential. Joint fluid sometimes can be obtained from the distal joints without sedation or any type of anesthetic if the patient is not painful. However, sedation or light tranquilization and the use of analgesics are necessary for uncooperative patients and/or for those experiencing pain.

Patient preparation includes placing the animal in lateral recumbency. Prepare the sites by clipping the animal's hair and proceeding with aseptic surgical preparation.

> **TECHNICIAN NOTE** A steady hand is essential in performing arthrocentesis.

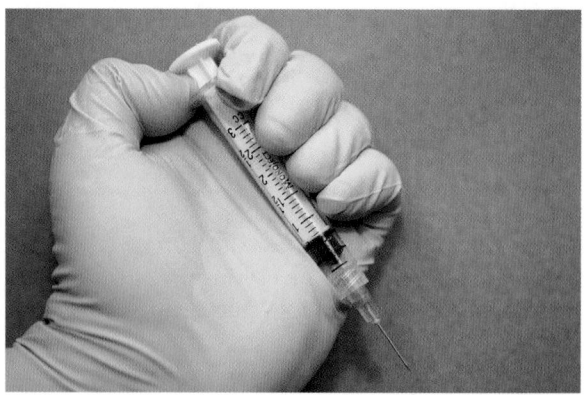

FIGURE 18-31 Hold the syringe in such a manner that you can easily aspirate back on the plunger, and you do not have to reposition your hands. The shown "dart" technique is favorable with many clinicians and technicians.

With sterile gloves donned, palpate the joint space to be entered with the index finger. Introduce the needle attached to the syringe. Hold the syringe in such a manner that you can easily aspirate back on the plunger without having to reposition your hands on the syringe. A steady hand is essential to minimize joint trauma and to produce a noncontaminated (bloody) sample (Figure 18-31). Slight negative pressure is applied to the syringe upon entry into the joint. The suction should always be released before the needle is withdrawn. This prevents contamination (blood) from the skin, SC tissues, and synovium. An adequate sample often includes just enough fluid to fill the needle hub.

Common sites for arthrocentesis in the dog and cat include the distal joints, including carpus, tarsus, and stifle (Figure 18-32). Techniques for these sites are described next.

Carpus

The joint is held in flexion. The needle can be inserted into any palpable intercarpal space. The medial radiocarpal joint is most commonly used to avoid the cephalic vein, which courses over the carpal joint. The needle is inserted perpendicular to the skin to avoid articulating surfaces.

Tarsus

The jock is held in partial flexion at 90 degrees with the metatarsals and the tibia. The joint may be approached medially or laterally. During a lateral approach, care must be taken to avoid the caudal branch of the saphenous vein. The needle is inserted just caudal to the lateral malleolus and dorsal to the tibial tarsal bone. The needle is directed under the lateral malleolus, where it forms a lip over the fibular tarsal bone. One should keep the syringe and the needle parallel (flat) with the metatarsal bones, heading in the direction of the animal's toes. A $\frac{3}{4}$-inch, 25-gauge needle is often inserted and advanced to its full length before fluid is obtained from a medium-size or large dog.

Stifle

The stifle joint is partially flexed during the procedure. The patella, the straight patellar ligament, the tibial tuberosity,

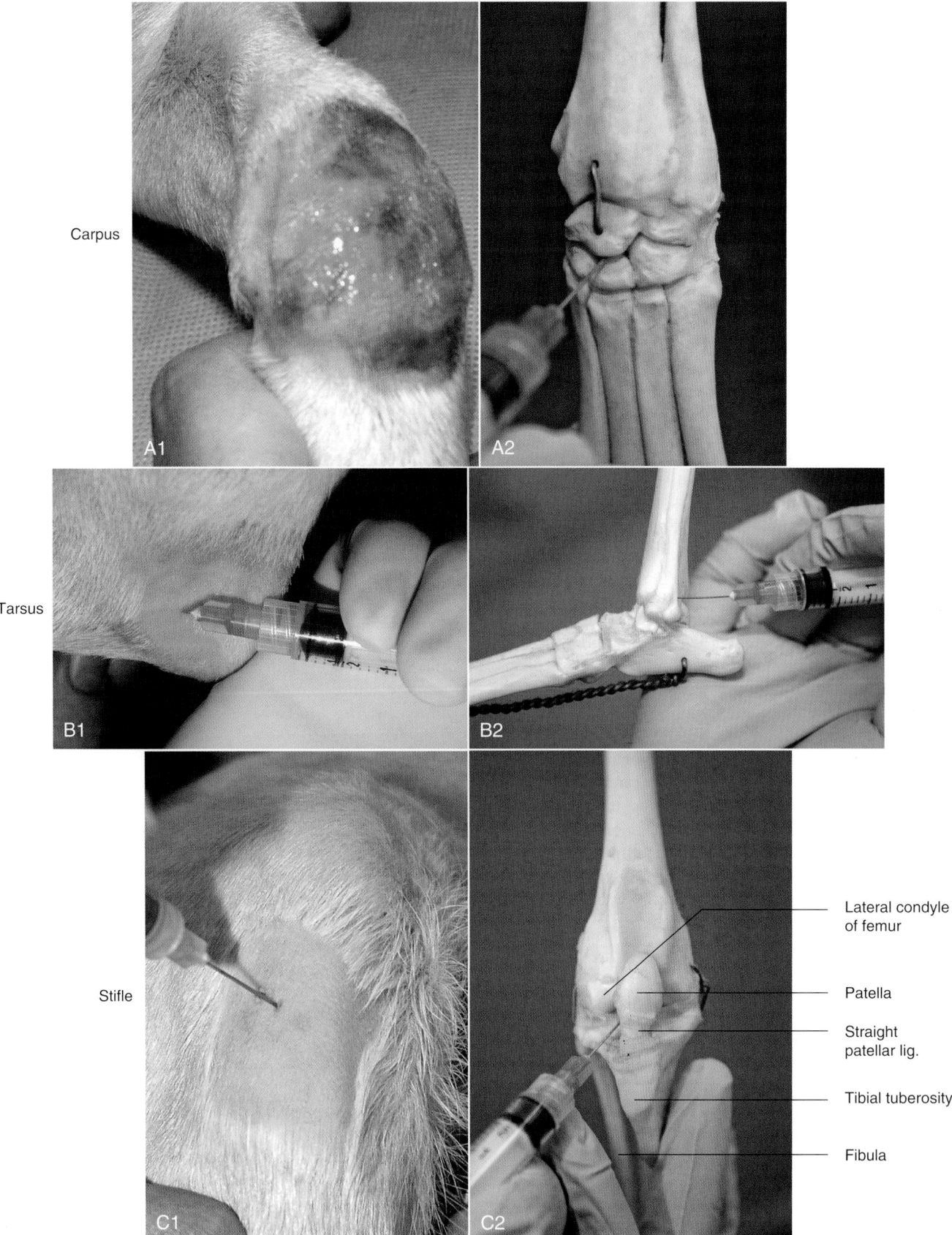

Carpus

A1

A2

Tarsus

B1

B2

Stifle

C1

C2

Lateral condyle
of femur

Patella

Straight
patellar lig.

Tibial tuberosity

Fibula

FIGURE 18-32 The carpus (**A1** and **A2**), tarsus (**B1** and **B2**), and stifle (**C1** and **C2**) are common sites for arthrocentesis in the dog and cat. Illustrations show the skeletal joint anatomy and a patient. The carpus can be approached perpendicular at any intercarpal space (**A1** and **A2**). The tarsus can be approached laterally with the needle directed caudal to the lateral malleolus and keeping the syringe and needle parallel with the metatarsal bones (**B1** and **B2**). Reference landmarks for the stifle joint are the patella, the straight patellar ligament, the tibial tuberosity, and the lateral condyle of the femur (**C2**).

and the lateral condyle of the femur provide landmarks for tapping the stifle. These landmarks form a triangle that aids in entering the joint space. The needle is inserted just lateral to the straight patellar ligament and is directed medially (approximately 35-degree to 45-degree angle) and slightly upward into the origin of the cruciate ligaments between the femoral condyles. A longer 1-inch to $1\frac{1}{2}$-inch needle is usually necessary for tapping the stifle.

JOINT FLUID ANALYSIS

A single drop of synovial fluid is sufficient for gross and histologic appearance. The synovial joint analysis is complete with an additional drop of synovial fluid for a bacterial culture (aerobic, anaerobic, and *Mycoplasma*). If samples are submitted to a reference laboratory, synovial fluid can be placed in a small EDTA tube. When synovial fluid is minimal, excess EDTA should be decanted from the EDTA collection tube to minimize a diluting effect.

Gross Appearance

A normal synovial fluid sample consists of a small volume of about 0.05 to 0.3 ml. It is colorless, clear, and viscous. An increased volume of synovial fluid can be observed in both noninflammatory and inflammatory joint diseases. A bloody tap as a result of trauma during the collection procedure can usually be distinguished from hemarthrosis because blood is incompletely mixed with the synovial fluid. Blood can be aspirated from inflamed (septic; acutely traumatized coagulation defects) joints. Yellow-tinged fluid is a result of previous hemorrhage with release of hemoglobin pigments into the joint fluid (inflammatory, degenerative, and traumatic joint disease). If red blood cells (RBCs) or white blood cells (WBCs) or both are present in excess, an increase in turbidity or lack of clarity is observed. Viscosity can be subjectively evaluated by observing the fluid exiting the needle and moving onto a microscope slide. A normal joint sample will form a long string between the needle and the slide. In addition, the drop on the slide should remain global rather than dispersing over the slide. A thin, runny consistency is a frequent, consistent finding in inflammatory disorders. Occasionally, poor viscosity is observed in degenerative or traumatized joints.

Culture

Aerobic, anaerobic, and *Mycoplasma* cultures are most often negative in polyarthritis. A negative culture therefore supports a noninfectious inflammatory polyarthritis disorder.

Histologic Appearance

Normal values are noted in Box 18-1. Absolute cell counts can be done with a hemocytometer. Joint fluid samples are often small, and cell counts are estimated. Estimated counts are more often obtained in a clinical setting. This can be accomplished by recording the number of nucleated cells per microscopic field and comparing the counts with a peripheral blood smear of known concentration of nucleated blood cells.

BOX 18-1	Normal Values of Synovial Fluid

Cell count
    Red blood cells—Rare
    Nucleated cells/mm^3—250 to 3000
Differential for nucleated cells
    Mononuclear—94% to 100%
    Neutrophils—0% to 6%

Examples of Joint Fluid Analysis

1. Blood smear = 6 WBCs/high power field (hpf) from a blood sample containing 18,000 WBCs/µl
   Synovial fluid smear = 0 to 1 WBC/hpf
   Estimated count = 0 to 3000/mm^3
   The estimated count and zero to an occasional observed WBC suggest a normal joint.
2. Blood smear = 6 WBCs/hpf from a blood sample containing 20,000 WBCs/µl
   Synovial fluid smear = 12 WBCs/hpf
   Estimated count = 40,000/mm^3
   The estimated count and frequent appearance of WBCs on the smear suggest a markedly elevated nucleated cell count.

Differential

Normal synovial fluid contains a mixture of small and large mononuclear cells. The absolute number of mononuclear cells varies considerably. Therefore, the subclassification and absolute count of mononuclear cells provide limited diagnostic information. Elevations tend to occur with traumatized or degenerative joints, chronically inflamed joints, and joints with osteochondrosis.

Polymorphonuclear Neutrophils (PMNs)

Polymorphonuclear neutrophils are generally absent; if present, they should account for less than 10% of the nucleated cell count. An increase in the relative (normal cell count) or absolute number of PMNs indicates inflammation of the synovial joint lining. Generally, more severely inflamed joints will contain a greater concentration of WBCs with a greater percentage of PMNs.

TECHNICIAN NOTE   Common sites for bone marrow aspiration include the iliac wing, femur, and humerus.

BONE MARROW ASPIRATION

Bone marrow aspiration is performed to evaluate the cells in the bone marrow. Bone marrow aspirations for cytologic examination or a core biopsy are safe, easily performed techniques that may yield valuable information regarding the cause or pathogenesis of many disease processes.

Indications for bone marrow aspiration include patients with nonresponsive anemia, **thrombocytopenia**, **neutropenia** without suspicion of infection (i.e., sepsis),

pancytopenia, suspected hematopoietic malignancies (i.e., myelogenous leukemia), polycythemia, and inappropriate RBC response, such as the presence of nucleated RBCs in peripheral blood without the presence of reticulocytes or without anemia. Patients that are suspected to have neoplasia, such as lymphoma or multiple myeloma, undergo bone marrow aspiration procedures. Clinical staging of lymphoma and the presence of mast cell tumors are also indications.

Contraindications include clotting factor abnormalities as well as severe thrombocytopenia, which is a relative contraindication and may require the administration of plasma or platelet-rich plasma before the procedure is begun.

Complications include infection at the site if aseptic technique is not maintained, especially in leukopenic patients; damage to soft tissue structures; and hematoma formation if a coagulopathy or thrombocytopenia is present.

> **TECHNICIAN NOTE** Stainless steel Rosenthal bone marrow aspirate needles are manufactured with a matched stylet. The stylet and the needle have matching identification numbers that identify them as a unit.

Supplies needed to perform bone marrow aspiration include a bone marrow aspiration needle. This needle may be purchased from a variety of manufacturers, but types commonly used in a small animal practice are 18-gauge, 1-inch Rosenthal needles with a matched stylet and 16-gauge, $^{15}/_{16}$-inch Illinois needles with a matched stylet and depth stop (Figure 18-33). Other equipment required consists of a #11 scalpel blade, a 12- or 20-ml syringe, sterile gloves, a sterile drape, local anesthetic such as 2% lidocaine in a

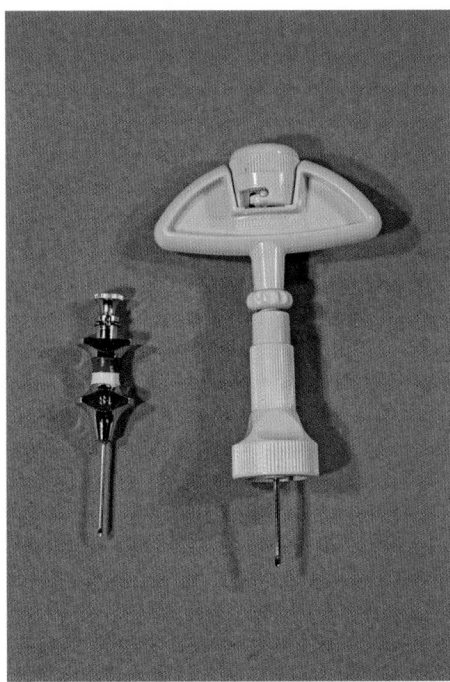

FIGURE 18-33 Bone marrow aspiration needles: 18-gauge stainless steel Rosenthal needle; 16-gauge Illinois-style needle with depth stop.

syringe with a needle, clean glass slides, and an EDTA collection tube. A complete blood count (CBC) with reticulocyte count is done within 24 hours before or after the aspirate so that peripheral and marrow cell populations can be composed. The bone marrow aspiration procedure is a very painful procedure. Heavy sedation with good analgesic agents in combination with a local infiltrate anesthetic or general anesthetic is warranted.

Bone marrow aspirations are most commonly performed in the ilium, humerus, and femur in small animal patients (Figure 18-34). The patient's size, age, and conformation determine which site is used. It is important to remember that the bone marrow of aged patients is less active in long bones than in flat bones; therefore in geriatric patients, a higher success rate for a cellular diagnostic sample is attained with a flat bone, such as the ilium. Bone marrow aspiration procedures are performed using strict aseptic technique. The hair over the site is clipped, and the skin is surgically prepared. Sterile gloves are worn by the person performing the aspiration. Patient positioning for the dorsal iliac crest is sternal or lateral recumbency; lateral recumbency for the humeral head; and lateral recumbency for the intratrochanteric fossa of the femur.

ILIAC ASPIRATION

The patient is placed in sternal or lateral recumbency with its legs drawn forward for better palpation of the wings of the ilium. The hair is clipped from the procedure site, and the skin is prepared for aseptic surgery. Local infiltration of 2% lidocaine is done by injecting into the skin, the SC tissue, and periosteum of the bone. A stab relief incision is made into the skin over the iliac crest with a #11 scalpel blade. The stylet of the bone marrow needle is inspected to confirm that the stylet is perfectly occluding the distal tip and is in place, or the needle may become plugged with cortical bone. If a Rosenthal needle style is used, the operator must hold the needle in such a fashion that the stylet does not back out by placing counter pressure on the stylet with an index finger or the palm of the hand. One hand is placed on the ilium to stabilize it. The bone marrow needle with its stylet in place is advanced through the skin incision and onto the bone. The needle is advanced into the bone by rotary motion while the wrist is twisted only in a clockwise, counterclockwise motion. The goal is to keep a single axis and to avoid wobbling of the needle. This is accomplished by keeping the elbow immobilized and using wrist action only. Considerable force is typically required. The needle is advanced into the bone 1 to 1.5 cm, or until the needle is well seated.

Once the needle is well seated and stabilized in the bone, the stylet is removed from the needle and is placed on a sterile field. A 12- or 20-ml syringe is firmly attached to the bone marrow needle, and negative pressure is applied to the syringe plunger. Aspiration should be very quick, and negative pressure should be immediately discontinued once 0.1 to 1.0 ml of sample is obtained. Actual aspiration of the marrow fluid is most painful for the patient, and the conscious, sedated patient may show signs of discomfort.

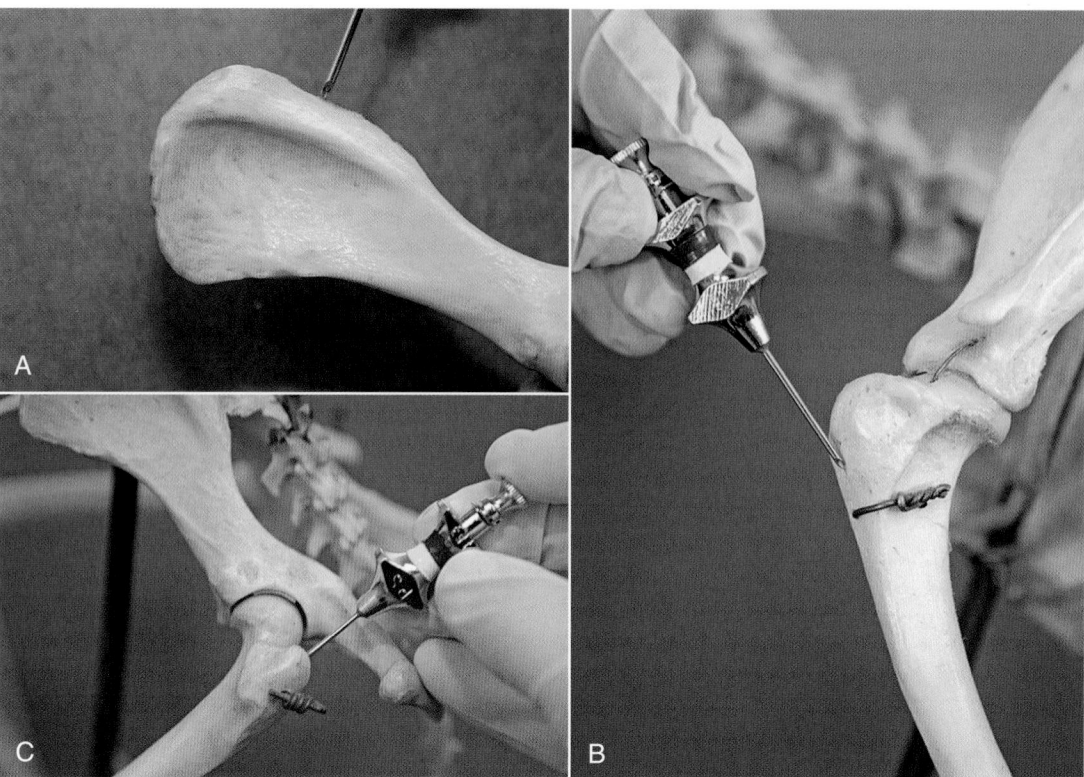

FIGURE 18-34 Common sites for bone marrow aspiration in dog and cat patients. **A,** Wing of the ilium. **B,** Greater tubercle of the proximal humerus. **C,** Trochanteric fossa of the femur.

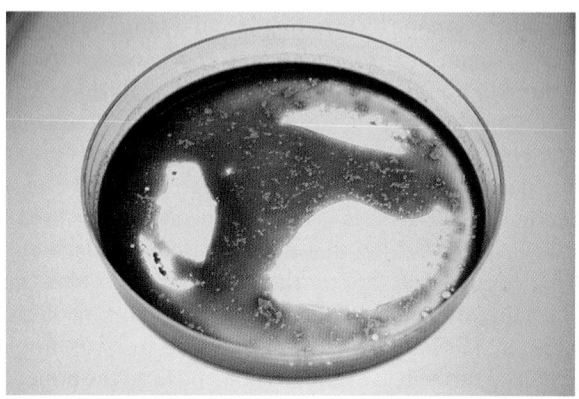

FIGURE 18-35 Bone marrow aspirate sample displayed in a Petri dish. Note the bone spicules.

Restrainers of unanesthetized patients should be prepared for the patient to react with a yelp, a cry, or movement.

Once the bone marrow enters into the syringe and negative pressure is released, the syringe is removed from the bone marrow needle. The sterile stylet is replaced into the needle. Six to eight fresh smears are made immediately. This is accomplished by placing a drop of the sample on tilted microscope slides or by putting some of the sample into a Petri dish and tilting the dish so that the blood separates from the marrow particle. Bone marrow is usually more viscous than blood, contains bony spicules, is a deeper red, and contains fat globules (Figure 18-35). Bone marrow

particles can be picked up with the tip of a hypodermic needle or a microhematocrit tube and transferred to a microscope slide. A pull slide is made with each sample. A pull slide is made by placing a clean glass slide on top of the slide containing the sample and pulling the slides apart to create two slides for cytologic analysis. The excess bone marrow sample should be immediately placed in an EDTA collection tube. It is helpful to do this exercise simultaneously, with someone making the slides and another pair of hands placing the excess sample into the anticoagulant EDTA collection tube. If this collaboration cannot be done, it is recommended to have the collection syringe precoated with an anticoagulant, such as 2.5% to 3.0% EDTA solution.

While the patient still has the bone marrow aspiration needle in place, quickly take one of the pull slides and examine it to determine whether bone marrow elements are present (Figure 18-36). This screening can be done with a drop of new methylene blue stain and a coverslip. If the sample is not adequate, another sample can immediately be obtained. In this way, the patient will not have to be rescheduled for another invasive procedure, and the veterinarian will not be delayed in getting a result and a diagnosis.

Once the sample has been determined to be adequate, the bone marrow needle is removed in the same fashion it was placed, by clockwise, counterclockwise motion to pull it out.

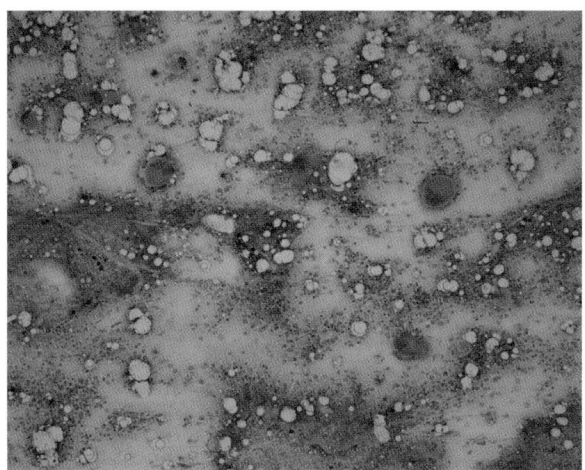

FIGURE 18-36 Microscopic view of a bone marrow aspirate under low 10x power stained with new methylene blue. Note nucleated precursor cells and large megakaryocytes.

Once removed, pressure is held on the site until hemostasis occurs.

The dried unstained smears, along with the excess sample in the EDTA collection tube, are packaged in a protective container for a reference laboratory.

HUMERAL ASPIRATION

The humerus is an excellent bone site for marrow aspiration. The craniolateral aspect of the greater tubercle of the proximal humerus is the insertion site. The advantage of this site is that it consists of less tissue, fat, and muscle overlying the bone. When a patient is heavily muscled or overweight, the dorsal iliac crest is difficult to palpate; this site is always palpable and superficial in animals with this conformation. The humerus is advantageous to use in animals with narrow iliac wings, such as small toy breed dogs and cats.

The patient is placed in lateral recumbency, and the presenting proximal humerus is clipped, surgically prepped, and infiltrated with a local anesthetic. The bone marrow needle is placed perpendicular to the humeral shaft as the elbow is flexed, and the shoulder is rotated or abducted externally. The assistant holding the limb in position should concentrate on using pressure points, such as the elbow and the blade of the scapula, as the operator advances the needle with constant pressure and force. Squeezing the soft tissues while trying to maintain the position of a limb often results in severe bruising of the thrombocytopenic patient. Techniques for site preparation, needle placement, bone marrow aspiration, and slide preparation are identical to those described for iliac bone marrow aspiration.

FEMORAL ASPIRATION

The femur can be used in small breed dogs and cats for bone marrow aspiration. Site preparation, needle placement, marrow aspiration, and slide preparation procedures are identical to those described for bone marrow aspiration from the ilium.

The patient is placed in lateral recumbency, and the presenting hip region is surgically prepared over the palpable greater trochanter of the femur. The needle is placed within the trochanteric fossa of the femur on the medial aspect of the greater trochanter of the proximal femur. Once aseptically prepped, 2% lidocaine is injected into the skin, SC tissue, and periosteum over the trochanteric fossa. A stab incision is made through the skin. The operator grasps the femur, and the hip is held in a flexed position. The bone marrow aspiration needle is introduced medial to the greater trochanter and parallel to the femoral shaft. Once the needle is well seated within the shaft of the femur, the sample is taken and is processed as described previously.

FINE-NEEDLE ASPIRATION

Fine-needle aspiration is a quick procedure performed routinely in veterinary practices to acquire a sample of fluid or tissue cells from an accessible mass in the dermis, viscera, or lymph node. These cytologic samples aid in differentiating between inflammation and hyperplasia of structures, such as lymph nodes or mammary glands. They also help to differentiate between inflammation, neoplasia, and hyperplasia of the skin, SC, or other superficial masses. Complications of fine-needle aspiration procedures include minor hemorrhage, tissue damage, and infection.

Supplies needed to perform a fine-needle aspiration include 25- to 22-gauge needles. Needle lengths are determined by the depth of the mass to be sampled. Other supplies include 3- to 6-ml syringes, clean glass microscope slides, and surgical scrub or alcohol for skin preparation.

The animal is restrained so that the mass to be aspirated is accessible. The skin over the underlying mass may be surgically prepped (for visceral aspirates) or wiped with alcohol to remove superficial contaminants. Secure the mass with a free hand and introduce a 22-gauge needle into the mass with the other. With large masses, the needle is directed into peripheral parts of the lesion to avoid the necrotic center. The needle is redirected within the tissue once or twice and is removed. A syringe containing at least 1 ml of air is attached to the needle. Depress the syringe plunger quickly because expulsion should be rapid and forceful to remove all material from the needle lumen onto a clean microscope slide. If the aspirated material is liquid, a push slide can be made; if the material is more viscous, a pull smear is made.

An alternate technique for performing fine-needle aspiration involves the use of a 3- to 12-ml syringe attached to the needle. After the needle has been inserted into the mass, suction is applied to the syringe plunger to aspirate cells into the needle. During this process, the needle may be redirected once or twice; however, negative pressure is released before the needle is withdrawn from the mass. The needle is then detached from the syringe, and the operator aspirates 1 to 2 ml of air into the syringe and reattaches the air-filled syringe onto the needle. The syringe plunger is then forcefully depressed as described before to expel the contents of the needle onto a clean microscope. Slides can be made by a push or a pull technique.

Administration of Medication in the Large Animal

ORAL ADMINISTRATION

Medications to be administered orally (per os, PO) are available in a variety of forms, including tablets, capsules, powders, pastes, and liquids.

The simplest way to administer oral medications to all large animal species is by placing them in food or water. For a variety of reasons, this route may not always be feasible (patient is NPO, patient detects bitter substance in food or water and refuses to consume, decreased appetite is associated with the illness, multiple animals are housed and fed communally). It is also extremely unreliable because it may be difficult to determine the amount that is actually ingested. The oral route allows slower absorption than IV or IM administration, but it is the only route that can be used for certain medications.

Oral medications are administered by a variety of methods, including syringes, drenching, balling guns, and nasogastric and orogastric intubation.

SYRINGES

Many commercially available products come in a paste form in premeasured dosing syringes, which make accurate dosing and administration easy. Other oral medications are provided in tablet form and need to be crushed and mixed with water or simply dissolved in water over time. The easiest way to do this is by placing the tablets in a 60-ml catheter tip syringe, adding water, and letting the tablets dissolve. The technician should always be aware of the medications that are in use, and should use safe handling practices. For some medications (e.g., chloramphenicol), a mask, safety glasses, and gloves are advised while preparing and while administering the medication. It is a good practice to assume that oral medications will be unpalatable to the patient and to add molasses, Karo, maple syrup, or thin applesauce to the mixture. Proper restraint of the head should be used with the syringe method, with the free arm cradling the head and reaching around so that the hand is up over the muzzle. The technician then inserts the syringe into the mouth at the commissure of the lips near the interdental space, between the cheeks and teeth, and advances it as far back into the mouth as possible (Figure 18-37). With firm pressure, the medication is given, and the syringe can be withdrawn. Lifting the head slightly may encourage the animal to swallow rather than spit out the medication. The medication should not be injected too rapidly because it may be lost from the other side of the mouth, or it may be aspirated.

The technician should be conscious of the probability of the patient's spitting out the material and getting it on the skin or mucous membranes of personnel. Always wash

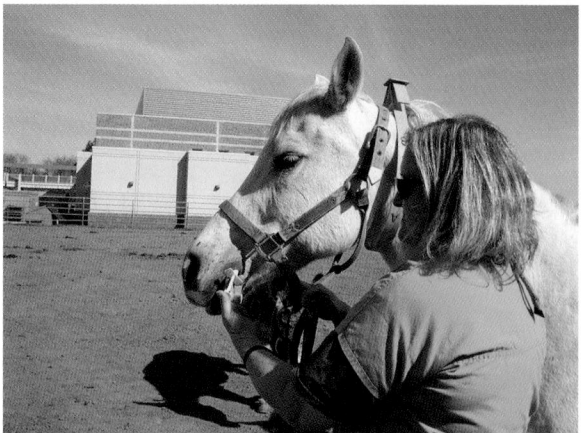

FIGURE 18-37 Administering oral medication via syringe to an adult.

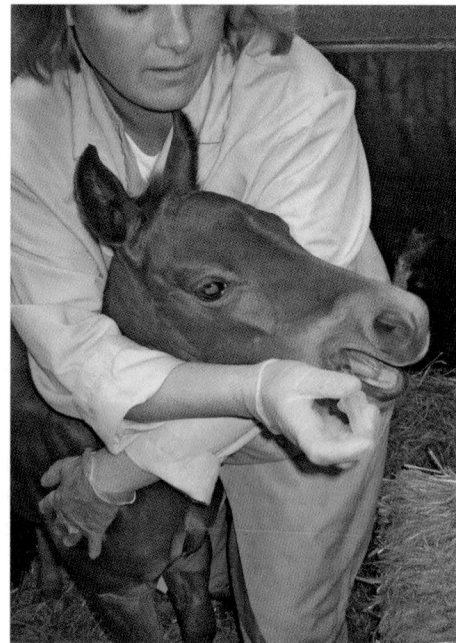

FIGURE 18-38 Administering oral meds to a foal.

hands and skin that have been in contact with the medication.

Oral medications should be administered carefully to neonatal equines to prevent squirting the medication out the other side of the foal's mouth, and to prevent squirting the medication into the trachea. If the patient is laterally recumbent, it should be moved into a sternal position to ensure that medication administered into the mouth gets past the epiglottis and into the esophagus. The patient should be kept in a sternal position for at least a minute to reduce the possibility of aspiration. The technician should restrain neonates that are ambulatory and standing by holding them close to his or her own body, with one arm around the patient's chest and the other arm reaching over the neck, and placing the syringe into the side of the mouth opposite the technician (Figure 18-38). The technician should use caution, making sure not to place his or her own face close to the

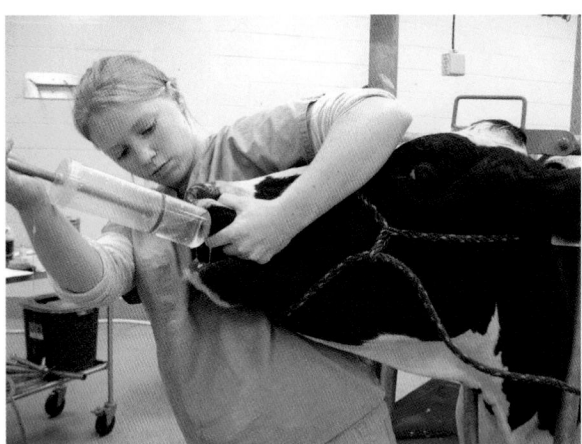

FIGURE 18-39 Bovine drench with dose syringe.

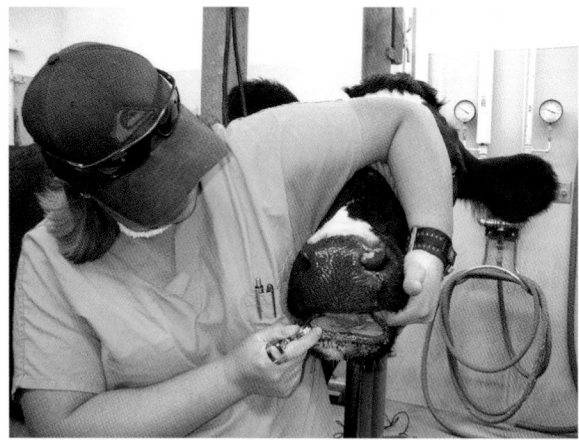

FIGURE 18-40 Using balling gun to administer medication in pill form to a cow.

foal's head to avoid getting hit in the face or head if the foal tosses its head. No pressure should be placed on the poll of the foal because the foal may push back against the pressure and rear up. This is very risky for foals because they can fall backward and suffer severe injury or death from hitting their head on the ground.

Drench (Dose Syringe)

Liquid medication or small volumes of fluid can be administered using a dose syringe. For calves, sheep, and goats, a catheter tip syringe can be used, whereas a large dose syringe is appropriate for adult cattle. Drenching in sheep and goats should be limited to small volumes of fluid (no greater than 30 ml). The animal is held with the nose slightly elevated and pulled toward the handler; the tip of the dose syringe is inserted into the interdental space, and the fluid is slowly dribbled onto the tongue (Figure 18-39).

> **TECHNICIAN NOTE** Mineral oil should never be given via drench. Inhalation of mineral oil can be fatal.

BALLING GUNS (PILLING)

For cattle, sheep, and goats, balling guns are commonly used to accomplish oral tablet administration. Several sizes are available, and the appropriate size should be selected in accordance with the size of your patient. Using a large balling gun on a small calf, goat, or sheep can result in splitting of the soft palate and rupture of the pharynx. The balling gun should have a smooth end, preferably made of rubber to limit the trauma that can be caused to the back of the mouth, including the soft palate, pharynx, and esophagus. The gun should be inspected before each use to make sure that no sharp edges have formed. All food should be removed from the patient's mouth before dosing. For cattle, placing the patient in a head gate will help restrain the animal for the procedure. The technician should stand next to the animal's

head while facing the same direction as the animal. The arm nearest the animal reaches over and grasps the mouth at the interdental space and opens the animal's mouth by pressing on the hard palate. Alternatively, placing a finger in one nostril and the thumb in the other, then pulling the nose dorsally, will encourage cattle to open their mouth, making insertion of the gun easier. The balling gun is inserted into the mouth and is gently worked back to the pharynx. Once the thumb rings of the gun are at the commissure of the lips, the plunger is depressed (Figure 18-40). The animal's head should be kept down to prevent loss of medication. Cattle will lick their nostrils once they swallow the pill.

When working with sheep and goats, back them up to a wall and straddle the shoulders as stated before. Insert a hand into the interdental space at the commissure of the lips, open the mouth, and insert the balling gun to the back of the throat before depressing the plunger. If the balling gun is not inserted far enough, the medication may be chewed by the animal and spit out. If the balling gun is inserted too far, serious damage to the pharynx and larynx may occur. To decrease the chance of aspiration of the medication, the head of the animal should not be overly elevated, and the neck should not be overextended.

> **TECHNICIAN NOTE** Read labels carefully because certain medications can cause severe complications for staff members if they are mishandled. For example, chloramphenicol tablets should not be crushed because inhaling the powder has been shown to increase the risk of fatal aplastic anemia in humans.

NASOGASTRIC AND OROGASTRIC INTUBATION

When large volumes of an oral medication need to be given (mineral oil, fluids, bismuth), or when oral fluid therapy or

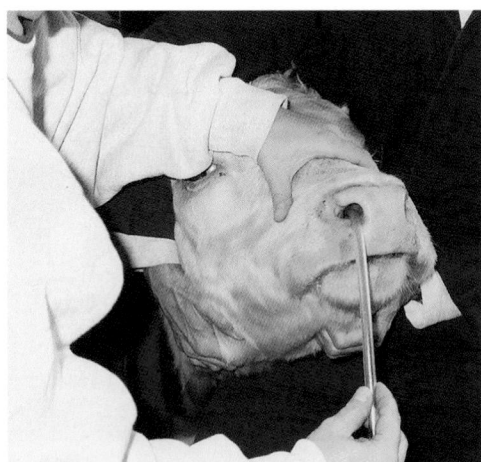

FIGURE 18-41 Nasogastric intubation of bovine with a foal stomach tube.

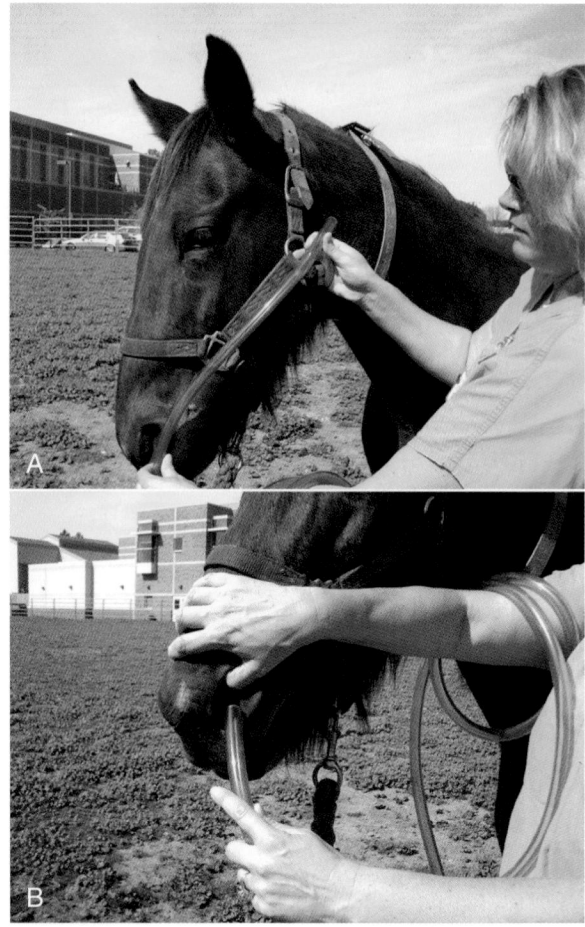

FIGURE 18-42 A, Estimating the length of tube required to reach the pharynx of the horse. **B,** Inserting a nasogastric tube (NGT) in the horse. Technician stands to the side of the horse for safe positioning.

enteral feedings are required for extended periods, an oro-gastric tube (OGT for cattle, sheep, goats, pigs, and camelids) or a nasogastric tube (NGT for horses, cattle, adult sheep and goats, neonatal camelids) should be used.

Nasogastric intubation is a procedure that is commonly used in equine patients. Cattle, sheep, goats, and camelids have small nasal passages, and although nasogastric intubation (with small-diameter tubes) can be done (Figure 18-41), the usual method for these species is placement of an OGT.

NASOGASTRIC INTUBATION

Many different sizes of tubes can be used; choosing one is dependent on the size of the patient and the thickness of the solution that needs to be given (or retrieved, if that is the intent of the procedure). An estimation should be made of the length of the tube required from the entrance of the nostril to the point of the stomach or **rumen**. For horses, it is helpful to mark the tube at a point where the tube should reach the pharynx (Figure 18-42). This is helpful because the tube can be rotated upward when it reaches the pharynx to deflect it into the esophagus rather than down the trachea. If the tube is cold, soaking it in warm water will make it more pliable for insertion. The tube should be lubricated with water-soluble lubricant or warm water to aid in easy passage. The patient is restrained as outlined earlier and, with a hand over the muzzle and thumb placed into the nostril, the tube is passed in a ventral manner through the ventral nasal meatus and nasopharynx. Resistance is felt when the tube passes into the esophagus.

Once the tube has passed into the esophagus and traveled down to the rumen or stomach, the premeasured mark made on the tube should be checked, and presence in the rumen or stomach, not the trachea, confirmed. Most patients will cough if the tube is placed into the trachea, but at times a cough will not be elicited (small-diameter tubes; flexible, soft tubes used in neonates; comatose patients that are lacking cough reflex, etc.); therefore it is essential that proper placement is confirmed before medication is administered. When the tube is passing through the esophagus, it is often possible

to visualize tube advancement and feel the tube. This view can be enhanced by moving the tube in and out a bit and looking at the neck for the movement. For all patients, blowing into the tube should elicit gurgles from the tube or rumen or stomach fluid smell, and if an assistant places a stethoscope over the area of the rumen or stomach, he or she should be able to hear bubbling as air passes over the fluid. Aspirating on the tube should reveal negative pressure (but this should not be the only check because the opening of the tube may be up against tissue). Placing one's mouth on the distal end of the tube and sucking back may result in an unpleasant mouthful of gastric fluid; this has the potential for causing illness in the person if enteric bacteria are present.

Once the position of the tube has been verified, the patient is checked for gastric reflux. If no abnormal amount of gastric fluid is noted, medication, fluids, and so forth can be administered using a stomach pump, a dose syringe, or gravity flow (Figure 18-43). For neonates, a 60-ml syringe is placed on the end of the tube and is aspirated to check for reflux. For some patients requiring repeated administration of medications or food, the NGT should be left in place. This can be accomplished in adult equines by coiling and then

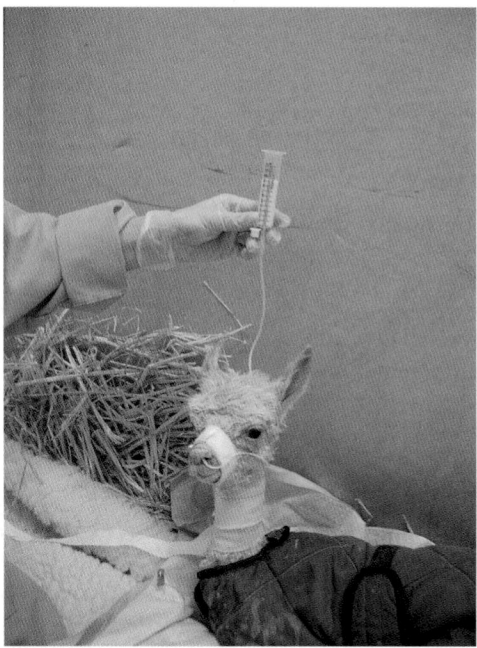

FIGURE 18-43 Technician administering enteral feeding via gravity flow into nasogastric tube (NGT) in alpaca cria.

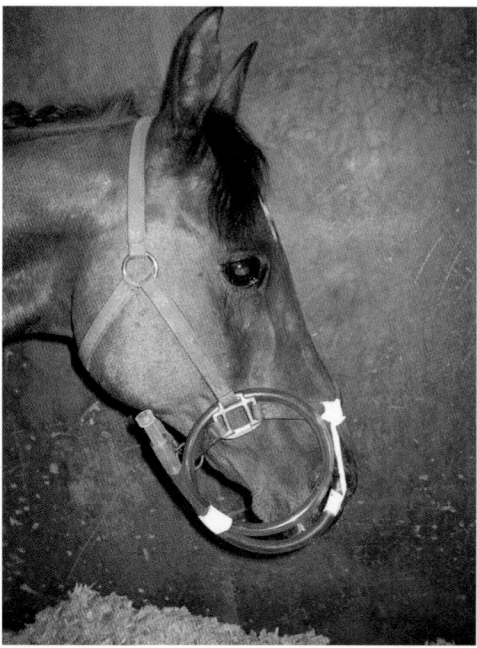

FIGURE 18-44 Nasogastric tube (NGT) secured to halter of horse for repeated NGT procedures.

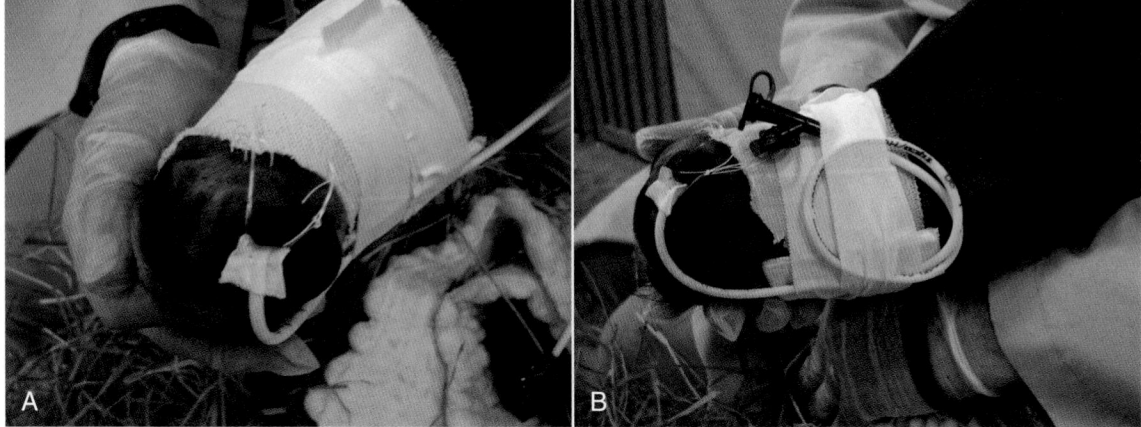

FIGURE 18-45 **A,** Placing suture loops in tape that is adhered to the muzzle of a foal allows the tube to be secured without causing irritation to the nares, as occurs when sutures are placed directly through the skin. **B,** Nasogastric tube (NGT) well secured to foal, easily accessible, and very likely to stay in place, even with movement of the foal.

taping the tube to the halter of the patient (Figure 18-44). A syringe case, a tube cap, or another adaptor should be placed on the end of the tube. In neonatal patients, tubes can be secured into place by using elastic tape around the muzzle of the patient and then coiling the tube off to the side of the mouth (while making sure it does not interfere with the action of the mouth). A 1-inch piece of butterflied tape can be secured to the tube at the base of the nostril; then, by using suture material, the tape can be affixed to the elastic tape around the muzzle (Figure 18-45, *A* and *B*). This method of securing the tube is preferred over suturing the tube directly to the nostril because direct suturing is irritating to the patient, causing it to rub at the tube and pull it out.

> **TECHNICIAN NOTE** When placing "stay" tape around the muzzle of a neonate, care must be taken to keep the tape loose enough to allow for opening of the mouth and to keep it secured well above the nostrils to prevent occlusion of the nostrils.

Once the process is complete, the pump is removed from the end of the tube, and the tube is held up above the patient's head to deliver any remaining medication from the tube into the stomach/rumen. A small amount of water or air can be pumped into the tube to clear the tube. Care should be taken to avoid aggressively or forcibly pumping it in. The end of the tube is then covered with the technician's thumb and kinked, and in gentle, long motions, the tube is pulled out. Complications from removal of the tube can include nosebleed or aspiration of any residual fluid or medication. The patient should be closely monitored after medication is delivered in this fashion for colic symptoms, bloat, or respiratory problems.

NGTs are routinely passed in horses to relieve gastric distention. The tube is passed as described earlier, and once placement in the stomach has been established, a known amount of water is pumped into the tube, causing a siphon, and gastric fluid and contents are collected back from the tube into a bucket. The tube is manipulated as needed, and the procedure repeated while fluid is collected. If significant gastric fluid is retrieved, the tube can be secured in place by coiling it and taping it to the halter. This is less stressful for the patient than repeated passing of the tube, and it is more time efficient for the staff. If a syringe casing is placed in the end of the tube, gastric reflux can be very accurately quantified. If a large amount of gas is present, the veterinarian may decide it is prudent to leave the tube in place with no cap so as to provide continuous decompression and relief to the patient.

NGTs may also be inserted to provide gastric lavage. This may be helpful in relieving feed impactions. Water is pumped into the tube, and gastric contents collected as described earlier. As long as the water that is inserted is being retrieved, more water can be inserted and so on, to attempt to dilute the impacted material.

OROGASTRIC INTUBATION

As a result of small nasal passages, OGT is the routine choice for food animals and camelids (Figure 18-46). Medications and oral fluids can be administered, transfaunation of rumen contents can be accomplished, enteral feeding can be administered, and some bloats can be relieved. Using the restraint techniques described earlier, an OGT can be passed into a large animal patient. OGTs can be passed in sheep restrained while set up on their rumps. Piglets can be lifted by the back of the head and neck. A $\frac{5}{8}$- to 1-inch-diameter tube can be passed in adult cattle, whereas a 9.54-mm-diameter tube is appropriate for adult sheep and goats. Small-diameter 10-Fr to 18-Fr tubes are useful for neonatal kids, lambs, and crias. The technician should hold the tube next to the animal and place a mark at the point estimated to reach the rumen (from mouth to last rib). A speculum should be used in the animal's mouth to prevent the patient from biting down on the tube, although neonatal kids, lambs, and crias do not require use of a speculum. A wide assortment of items can be used as speculums, ranging from a roll of tape for small patients to polyvinyl chloride (PVC) pipe or a piece of garden hose to a metal Frick speculum for cattle. The speculum needs to be inserted over the tongue root in the middle of the mouth. In cattle, "popping" or "give" will be felt when the speculum passes into the pharynx. At this point, the tube is passed through the speculum and down the esophagus into the rumen. Slight resistance should be felt when the tube enters the esophagus. It is essential to make sure that you are in the rumen, not in the trachea, before any medication is administered. This can be done by blowing on the end of the tube and listening for gas crackles, feeling negative pressure, and noting the smell of rumen fluid. In ruminants, placing a tube into the rumen may stimulate regurgitation through and around the tube.

Once placement has been confirmed, medication can be pumped into the patient or gravity flow used for smaller patients and neonates. Do not forcibly pump or administer medications, to prevent rupture of the rumen or damage to the esophagus. When finished, the end of the tube is covered with the technician's finger and kinked; it is then pulled out using gentle motions.

> **TECHNICIAN NOTE** Occluding the end of the tube and kinking it prevents any residual fluid from entering the trachea when the tube is removed from the patient.

INTRAVENOUS ADMINISTRATION

Intravenous (IV) injections are commonly performed on large animal patients. Drugs administered via the IV route are very rapidly absorbed. Some medications are quite caustic, and injecting them into the vein dilutes the drug, making it less caustic than it would be if it were administered IM or SC.

EQUINE

With most horses, minimal restraint (halter and lead rope) can be used to successfully administer medication by this route. If the patient is uncooperative, aggressive, or sensitive to needles, placing the animal in the stocks or using a second person and a twitch may make the procedure easier and may reduce the likelihood of injury to personnel and complications associated with misdirected puncture.

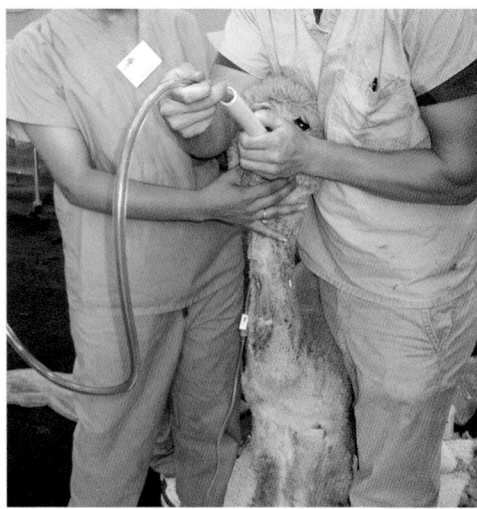

FIGURE 18-46 Passing an orogastric tube (OGT) in an alpaca patient.

Jugular Vein

The jugular vein is the most common site for IV administration in equine patients.

The right or left jugular vein is chosen, using the most cranial half of the neck. This is preferred because of the muscle layer that lies in the upper half of the neck and protects the underlying carotid artery from potential puncture. The preference is the right jugular vein because in most horses, the esophagus lies within the left jugular furrow and could potentially be tapped with an aggressive venipuncture. The site is then wiped down with alcohol, and digital pressure is applied to the jugular furrow below the intended puncture site to distend the vein. For adult horses, a 1.5-inch needle is used (18-, 19-, or 20-gauge is adequate). With the free hand, the needle is inserted into the vein in an upward direction (toward the head). Once blood drips from the hub of the needle, the needle is advanced all the way until just the hub is visible. It is critical to identify that the needle is in a vein, not in an artery, because medication accidentally injected into the artery goes directly to the brain, and this can result in a serious, violent reaction that may even prove fatal. Certain substances that are injected perivascularly (e.g., phenylbutazone) can cause severe necrosis to tissue with which they come in contact. When a large-bore needle is inserted, arterial blood will forcibly pulse out of the hub of the needle and tends to be bright red, whereas venous blood will steadily drip from the hub of the needle and tends to be darker red.

> **TECHNICIAN NOTE** Arterial blood will forcibly pulse out of the hub of the needle and tends to be bright red, whereas venous blood will steadily drip from the hub of the needle and tends to be darker red.

The syringe with medication can now be attached to the needle, making sure not to inadvertently move the needle perivascularly. Before any substance is injected, confirmation of placement needs to be reestablished. Gently aspirate the plunger of the syringe to confirm that blood enters the syringe and that it is not bright red in nature (indicating arterial puncture). Remove digital pressure from the jugular furrow, and administer the medication in a slow and continuous fashion. Once all medication is administered, remove the needle and syringe and apply digital pressure over the site for a couple of minutes to reduce potential hematoma formation.

IV injection of a medication may result in an anaphylactic reaction (mild to severe). Reactions may include sweating, urticaria (hives), anxiety, agitation, difficulty breathing, and even collapse. If the technician notes any of these responses, the remainder of the drug in the syringe should not be given, the technician should move safely away from the animal, and the veterinarian should be notified of the situation. An injection of epinephrine may be necessary, and the technician should have prior arrangements with the veterinarian regarding the amount to administer in the event that an anaphylactic emergency occurs when the veterinarian is not immediately present.

> **TECHNICIAN NOTE** Administration of a drug by any route can result in an anaphylactic reaction.

Other sites for IV injection include the cephalic vein and the lateral thoracic vein, but these sites are usually reserved for catheter placement instead of routine injection of medications because they are more awkward to access on the patient.

Equine IV Catheterization

For repeated IV drug injections or when large volumes of IV fluids are required, an indwelling catheter should be placed in the jugular vein. If either jugular vein is not accessible as a result of thrombosis or trauma, or if the horse pesters the jugular catheter, it may be necessary to catheterize the cephalic vein or the lateral thoracic vein. Many different types of catheters are available; selection should be made based on the length of time the catheter will be in place and the number of ports that may be necessary. For adult equine patients when OTN catheters are used, 14 gauge × 5.25 inches is sufficient, but for neonates, small ponies, or miniature horses, 16 gauge × 3.25 inches may be preferred. Miniature horse neonates may require a smaller catheter, and an 18- to 20-gauge × 3-inch catheter may be used, with the realization that the size of the catheter will dictate the fluid administration rates that can be achieved.

> **TECHNICIAN NOTE** Polyurethane and Silastic catheters are less thrombogenic than catheters made of Teflon and can be maintained in veins for longer periods.

The site chosen is shaved and surgically scrubbed to remove all debris. A final wipe with Betadine solution is then placed over the area and is left to dry. A "bleb" of lidocaine (ID administration using a 25-gauge needle and approximately 2 ml of lidocaine) should be administered over the intended injection site, including above the site, to desensitize an area for suturing the catheter in place. A sterile field is created by opening up a package of sterile gloves and aseptically laying the desired catheter on the gloves. All necessary items should be placed on the sterile field or kept readily accessible nearby.

While wearing sterile gloves, the technician grasps the catheter with the dominant hand and uses the other gloved hand to apply digital pressure to the jugular furrow. The catheter is inserted through the skin (into the "bleb") at approximately a 45-degree angle and should be inserted toward the heart, with the direction of blood flow. Once the lumen of the vein has been accessed (identified by the "flash" of blood at the hub of the catheter), the catheter is aligned more perpendicular to the vein and is advanced 1 cm more.

If the catheter is still in the vein (as indicated by flash back blood coming from the catheter), the hand applying digital pressure releases and then grasps the top of the stylet portion of the catheter. The catheter is then slid all the way into the vessel, and the stylet is removed at the same time. Recheck to make sure that the vein is still catheterized by applying digital pressure yet again (below the tip of the catheter), and watch for blood to drip from the hub. Once this has been confirmed, attach an intermittent infusion plug (PRN) or T-port, and suture the catheter into place (Figure 18-47, *A* through *E*).

> **TECHNICIAN NOTE**   Once the stylet has been withdrawn from the catheter, it should not be reintroduced because the sharp tip may cut through the catheter, causing a small piece to be dislodged into the vein, or may make a very jagged edge on the catheter.

If the carotid artery is catheterized, bright red blood will forcibly pulse out of the catheter. If this should occur, immediately remove the catheter and apply digital pressure over the sight for a minimum of 5 minutes to prevent the

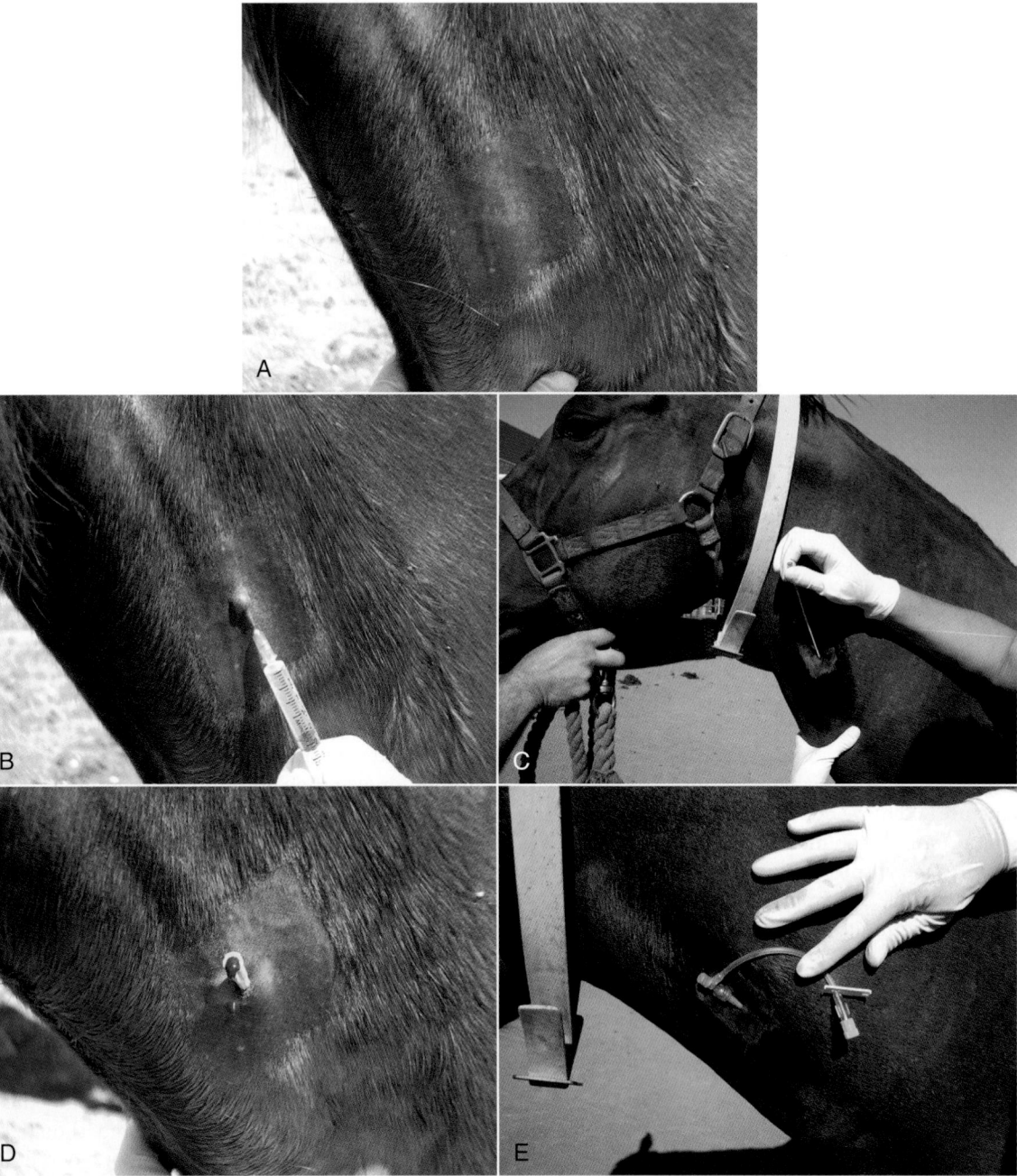

FIGURE 18-47 **A**, Distending the vein by placing pressure on the vein for IV catheter placement in equine jugular vein. **B**, Injecting ID lidocaine as local anesthetic. **C**, Inserting a catheter. **D**, Catheter in the vein; blood dripping from the catheter confirms placement in the vein. **E**, T-port attached to the catheter.

formation of a hematoma. Neck wraps or stents can be placed over catheters to stabilize them and to prevent the patient from rubbing them out. A common practice is to apply a small amount of antibacterial ointment before placing a wrap over the catheter. If the catheter remains in place long term, the ointment used can be alternated (e.g., Nolvasan, Betadine, triple antibiotic) in an attempt to reduce the chance of a resistant *Staphylococcus* infection taking hold. Foals and adult horses that spend a considerable amount of time in recumbency should have wraps placed over the catheter to protect the site from bedding, urine, and manure. When IV catheters are placed in recumbent neonatal foals, it is helpful to place a rolled-up towel under the neck to enhance the view of the jugular vein and stretch the skin. Making a small nick in the skin at the insertion site with a needle or a blade will facilitate insertion of the catheter. It is extremely helpful to have an assistant stretch the skin while digital pressure is applied, thus maintaining distention while the catheter is advanced.

When administering fluids or medications into an IV catheter, the technician should always first clean the injection port with isopropyl alcohol to prevent bacterial contamination.

If the technician wishes to use a guide wire–type catheter, the same steps as for preparing and placing the catheter are used, but use of guide wire–type catheters entails a few extra steps (refer to Seldinger guide wire technique as described for small animals, or read directions on individual packages). The most important point to remember when placing these types of catheters is to NEVER let go of the guide wire until the catheter has been successfully placed and the guide wire fully removed.

Cephalic Vein

For IV catheterization of the cephalic vein (Figure 18-48), the standard preparation is made, and the catheter is inserted proximal to the carpus and upward. A 14- to 16-gauge × 3.25- to 5.25-inch catheter is an appropriate choice for an adult equine. Placement of a T-port is beneficial; in some

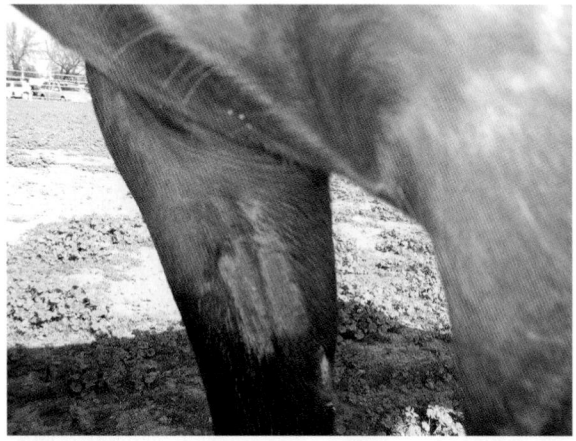

FIGURE 18-48 Site shaved for IV catheterization of equine cephalic vein.

cases, a piece of IV extension tubing is connected to the catheter so that IV infusions can be made without disturbing the catheter wrap. The catheter can be covered with sterile gauze and elastic wrap.

Lateral Thoracic Vein

The site is shaved, and standard preparation is performed. The IV catheter is inserted in a cranial direction (toward the front of the horse). This large-diameter vein can accommodate a large-bore catheter, if necessary. The vein is deeper than other veins used for IV catheterization. A wrap is placed over the catheter and around the body of the horse.

BOVINE

Jugular Vein

For administration of IV medication or fluids to a bovine patient, the jugular vein is the most feasible route to use. Proper restraint of the animal is critical for the safety of the animal and of the staff. For adult bovines, the head should be haltered; ideally the animal should be placed into a head gate or stanchion. The head is lifted slightly and is pulled away from the side to be used and tied with a quick-release knot. This will give the technician a good visual of the area and will prevent the animal from knocking its head into the technician. Calves may be restrained while standing, with the handler holding the calf up against his or her body or in recumbency. Once the animal has been sufficiently restrained, the injection site is cleaned with 70% isopropyl alcohol until all organic material and debris are removed. Using fingers or a fist placed into the jugular groove, the technician occludes the vessel with one hand and performs a venipuncture with the other. Ballottement of the vessel (stroking with a finger over the vein in a downward direction) will help to make the vein more prominent and will assist with visualization. For the jugular vein, a 16- to 18-gauge × 1½-inch needle should be used. The technician will introduce the needle into the skin at a 45-degree angle, using strong committed motion because the skin of cattle is relatively tough. Once the vein has been accessed, blood should exit the needle hub. Placement in the vein, not in an artery, is confirmed, and the needle is inserted all the way to the hub. At this time, the syringe containing the medication to be administered can be attached to the needle. By aspirating back, the technician can reconfirm that the needle is still in the vein. If no blood is obtained, the needle should be redirected without being completely removed from the skin. Once in the vein, pressure applied to the jugular groove for occlusion can be removed, and the medication can be administered. After the entire amount has been administered, the needle and syringe are removed, and digital pressure is applied over the access site to prevent hematoma formation.

Coccygeal Vein

For small volumes (up to approximately 5 ml) of nonirritating (xylazine, acepromazine, oxytocin) medication, the coccygeal vein can be used.

> **TECHNICIAN NOTE**   Administering irritating drugs into the coccygeal vein can cause thrombosis of the vein and sloughing of the tail.

Dairy cows are fairly accepting of tail vein injections because holding the tail up vertically to access the vein also provides restraint ("tail jack"). Beef cattle may need to be placed in a chute for the safety of personnel. An 18- to 20-gauge × 1.5-inch needle is appropriate for tail vein injections. Palpate the midline of the ventral surface of the tail to determine the location of the second or third coccygeal vertebra. The site is cleaned with 70% isopropyl alcohol. The needle is inserted, the syringe is attached (the needle may be inserted independent of the syringe or with a syringe attached), and the plunger is withdrawn slightly to check for placement in the vein. Once in the vein, the medication is injected (Figure 18-49).

Subcutaneous Abdominal Vein

The SC abdominal (milk or mammary) vein is rarely used to administer IV injections; use of this vein is strongly discouraged, as noted in the section on blood sample collection. It is hazardous to the animal and dangerous for the technician.

Auricular Vein

This vein is not typically used for IV injections but could be used for IV injections of very small amounts of medications. To limit movement, the head should be tied.

Bovine IV Catheter

When large volumes of fluids are to be administered or repeated IV injections are performed, a catheter should be placed in the jugular vein to avoid trauma to the vessels from repeat venipuncture. To place an IV catheter, the restraint techniques outlined previously should be used. The site that is clipped and surgically prepared, and an antiseptic, such as Betadine solution, is wiped onto the site and left to dry. Because of the thickness of cattle skin, a cutdown using a #15 scalpel blade or a puncture with a needle of the same size as the catheter will allow easier insertion of the catheter. If a blade is used to cut the skin before catheter insertion, a local anesthetic bleb should be placed. A 12- to 16-gauge × 5¼-inch catheter is used on adult cattle, while a smaller size, such as 15- or 18-gauge × 3¼ inch, can be used for calves (Figure 18-50).

The cephalic vein can be used for catheter placement if the jugular veins are inaccessible. In addition, the caudal auricular vein (ear vein) may be used for small-gauge catheters, but these are difficult to maintain because the animal often has a propensity to rub the catheter and displace it (Box 18-2).

CAMELID

Although the jugular vein is the most common site of catheterization and IV injection in llamas and alpacas, it is not as easily accessed as it is in other large animal species. Injections can be given high on the neck or low on the neck, but

BOX 18-2	Materials Needed for Catheter Placement

Catheter of choice
Heparinized saline (flush) with syringe and needle
T-port
PRN adaptor (intermittent infusion plug)
Razor
Surgical soap
Suture material
Sterile gloves
Betadine-soaked gauze
Alcohol-soaked gauze
Wrap materials (antibiotic ointment, Elastikon, gauze)

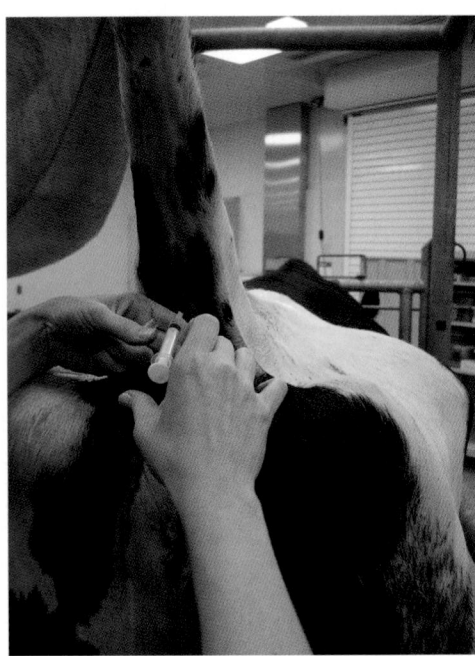

FIGURE 18-49 IV injection into the coccygeal vein of a cow.

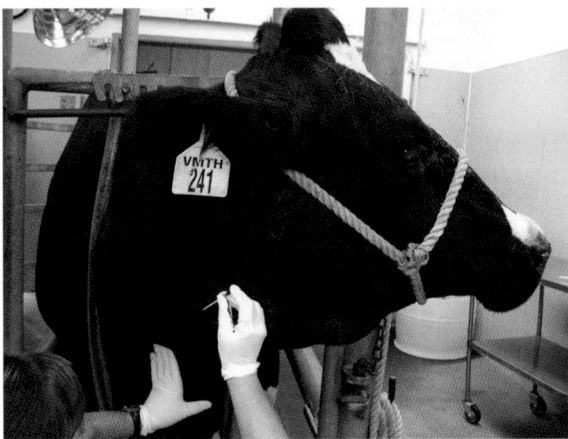

FIGURE 18-50 Jugular catheter placement in adult bovine.

not in the middle portion of the neck. Each of these sites (high or low) has potential for complication. Refer to Camelids in the forthcoming section on venus blood sampling techniques for details about locating the high and low landmarks around the jugular vein.

Camelid IV Catheterization

To complicate matters further, camelids have very thick skin (up to 1 cm in adult males), and the large transverse processes of the cervical vertebrae help to protect the underlying jugular vein. To place a catheter in the jugular vein, use the upper or lower third of the neck, and not the middle third. A 14 gauge × 5¼ inch catheter is acceptable for adults, and a 16- to 20-gauge × 3¼-inch catheter can be used for crias. The process outlined earlier for the bovine should be used to place a catheter in the camelid. In adult animals, it is beneficial to make a cut in the thick skin where the catheter will be inserted. The cephalic vein can also be used, but placement and maintenance may be difficult because of the camelid's propensity to lie down in sternal recumbency ("kushed").

> **TECHNICIAN NOTE** The thick skin and large transverse processes of the cervical spine help to protect camelids from exsanguination caused by bites from fighting males.

OVINE AND CAPRINE

As with the other large animal species already discussed, the most common route for IV administration in the goat or sheep is the jugular vein. Proper restraint is essential for administering medication efficiently and effectively. It is possible for one person to perform the procedure, but the procedure will go more smoothly with assistance. For both sheep and goats, after backing the animal up against a wall, the technician straddles the patient over the shoulders facing the head and gently grasps under the mandible and lifts the head up and away from the vein to be punctured. The technician should not underestimate the strength of these animals. If caught off guard, the technician may end up "riding" the neck of the animal. For sheep, the wool should be parted for visualization of the skin. Sheep can be set up on their rump and veins accessed as described for blood collection. The area is wiped down with isopropyl alcohol, digital pressure is applied in the jugular furrow to distend the vein, and then a needle is inserted into the vessel (20 gauge × 1 inch for adults; 22 gauge × 1 inch for kids and lambs). Once the vein has been punctured and it has been established that it is venous blood, attach the syringe with medication, aspirate back for confirmation, and slowly inject the substance. After all medication has been delivered, remove the needle, and apply digital pressure for a couple of minutes to prevent hematoma formation.

Ovine and Caprine IV Catheterization

The jugular vein is the most suitable site for placing a catheter, but the cephalic vein can be used if jugular access is not an option. The procedure for placing a catheter in the goat or sheep is the same as that described previously. For adults, 14- to 18-gauge × 3.5- to 5.25-inch catheters are appropriate, and for lambs and kids, 18- to 22-gauge × 1.5- to 3.25-inch catheters are used. It is helpful to nick the skin at the insertion site with a needle to ease insertion of the catheter through the skin.

PORCINE

IV administration to pigs is accomplished using the auricular veins, located on the dorsal aspect of the pinna. Three veins are present, and the one used most commonly for injection is the lateral vein. The pig should be restrained by using a snare or a chute, or, if small enough, an assistant can hold the animal against his or her body. Pigs have very sharp teeth and strong jaws. Without sufficient restraint, a bite is a serious possibility. The ear should be cleaned with alcohol-soaked gauze and the base of the ear occluded with digital pressure. A small-gauge needle is inserted into the vessel at a very shallow angle. The needle should be attached to the syringe at the time of insertion because of the very fragile nature of these vessels. Aspirate very gently to confirm venous placement, release occlusion, and then inject the substance with steady pressure. Remove needle and syringe, and apply digital pressure. The cephalic vein can also be used, but in small piglets, the jugular vein should be used because of the small diameter and difficulty involved in accessing the cephalic and ear veins at that age.

Porcine IV Catheterization

To catheterize the ear vein, a 19- or 21-gauge butterfly catheter or an 18-gauge OTN catheter is used. The base of the ear is occluded with digital pressure or by using a rubber-band tourniquet, and the dorsal aspect of the pinna is surgically prepared. The catheter is then inserted toward the base of the ear into the vein as described previously for injecting into the vein, and the tourniquet or pressure is released. The catheter is then capped with a PRN and is secured to the ear using glue. To provide support, a roll of gauze is placed against the inside of the pinna, and the margins of the ear are bent around the roll of tape and secured with strips of adhesive tape (Figure 18-51).

Complications of IV catheterization include phlebitis, thrombophlebitis, and local cellulitis. Septicemia may result if a venipuncture is made through dirt or fecal material. This can occur in veins that have been injected or catheterized, and thrombophlebitis can result in life-threatening conditions for the animal. Animals that are highly compromised may develop these conditions, even when excellent cleanliness and technique are used. If veins are rendered unusable, it may become impossible to administer needed fluids and medications. The technician should be attentive to any changes in the appearance of the vein, including such things as swelling, heat, pus, a thick-corded feel to the vein, or the appearance of fluid from the catheter site, and should promptly inform the veterinarian when any of these is noticed.

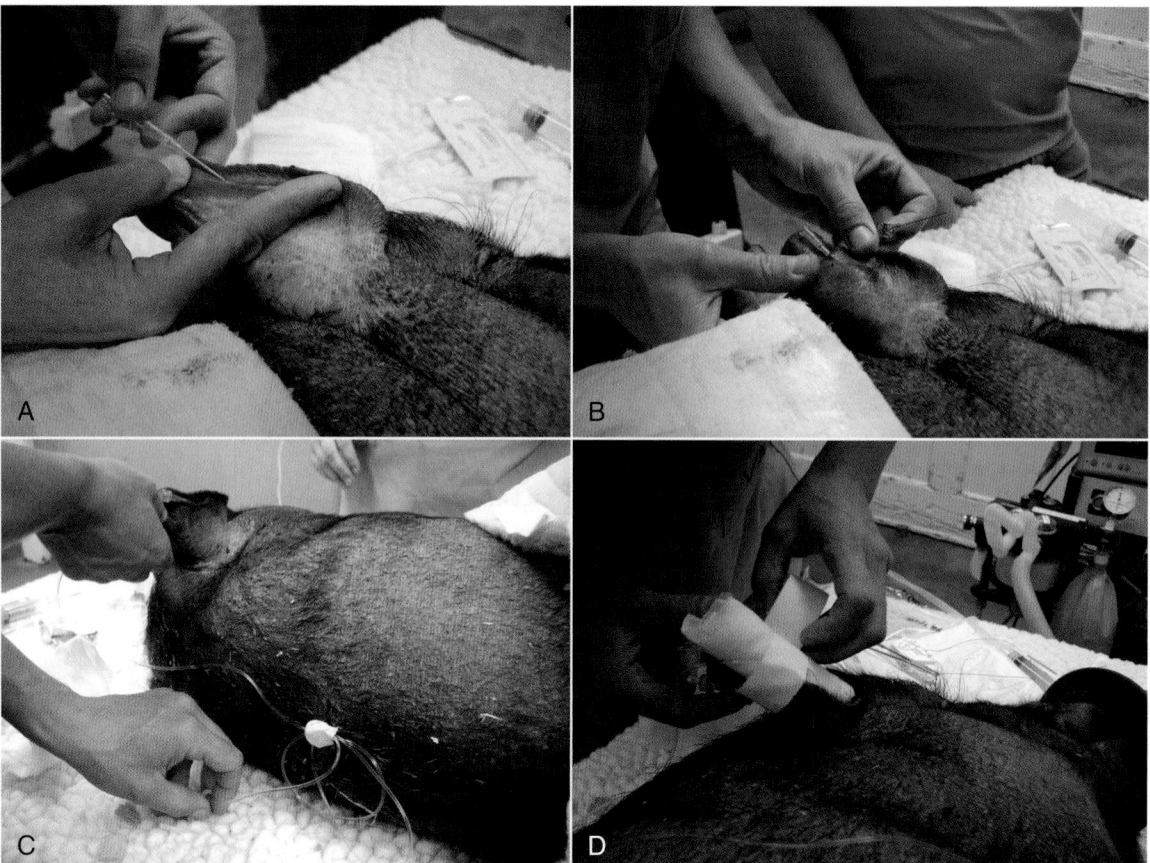

FIGURE 18-51 A, Inserting an IV catheter into the auricular vein of a pig. B, Removing a stylet. C, Attaching an IV line to the back of a pig. D, Wrapping the ear with gauze and tape to secure the catheter.

INTRAMUSCULAR ADMINISTRATION

Drugs that are administered directly into the muscle are absorbed relatively quickly. The intramuscular (IM) route provides more rapid drug absorption than the SC route and slower absorption than the IV route. The standard procedure for IM injection is to restrain the animal as needed based on its size and temperament, and clean the injection site with 70% isopropyl alcohol or another appropriate disinfectant until dirt and debris are removed. Selection of needle size is determined by the viscosity of the drug, the size of the muscle, and the volume to be administered. The needle is inserted into the muscle all the way to the hub, making sure to touch only the hub, not the shaft. Inserting the needle without the syringe attached is useful so that if the animal moves, the needle is likely to remain in place. If the needle is inserted with the syringe attached, the added weight of the syringe may cause the needle to come out of the muscle if the animal moves. Attach the syringe containing the drug to be delivered, and gently aspirate back to identify that you are in a muscle and have not hit a vessel. If you have punctured a vessel, remove the needle, start with a new needle, and repeat the process.

TECHNICIAN NOTE If the technician, when aspirating back on the second attempt, uses the same needle that hit a vessel on the first attempt, residual blood will travel into the syringe, causing the technician to believe that yet again a vessel has been struck.

Once you have confirmed that the needle is in the muscle, inject the substance with steady pressure. Do not aggressively force the solution into the muscle because the pressure may make the syringe detach from the needle, causing medicine to spray everywhere. The technician would be unable to determine the exact amount of drug actually delivered to the patient. Some substances that are injected can prove harmful to personnel if they come in contact with mucous membranes (eyes, mouth, etc.). Once the medication has been delivered, remove the syringe and needle. Apply pressure if any blood comes from the injection site, and massage the area gently.

If repeated IM injections are required, various sites should be used in an attempt to minimize muscle damage and pain.

EQUINE

Several locations can be used for IM administration of therapeutics to equine patients. These sites include lateral cervical (neck), semimembranosus and semitendinosus, and pectoral and gluteal muscles on both the left and the right side of the animal. When choosing the location for IM injections, the technician should consider the volume to be delivered, the viscosity of the solution, potential injury to personnel, and the potential for complications with the muscle chosen. Restraint with a halter and lead rope as the minimum must be used whenever an injection is given. Placing a horse in stocks will greatly reduce the likelihood that the animal will move once the needle is introduced and will prevent injury to personnel, although getting caught in the stocks can be detrimental to a patient that has a reaction to the medication given. Individual horses respond differently to needles. Some respond only slightly or not obviously at all. Others can respond violently. One method used to desensitize the injection site just before a needle insertion consists of rubbing the site very firmly and rapidly back and forth 100 times using an alcohol-soaked cotton swab or piece of gauze, and then immediately inserting the needle. Some people like to tap the horse firmly with the edge of the fist just before inserting a needle into the muscle. This is also thought to desensitize the area before insertion of the needle. Other people are convinced that tapping in this manner before a needle insertion simply lets the horse know what is about to happen. The technician should use whatever method proves to be a good approach for him or her.

Lateral Cervical (Neck) Muscles

IM injections into the neck protect the safety of personnel. Small volumes (less than 10 ml in an adult horse) should be delivered into the lateral aspect of the neck. Choose a spot in the triangular space that is bordered dorsally by the nuchal ligament, ventrally by the cervical vertebrae, and caudad about 1 handwidth in front of the cranial border of the scapula (Figure 18-52). An 18- to 22-gauge needle is

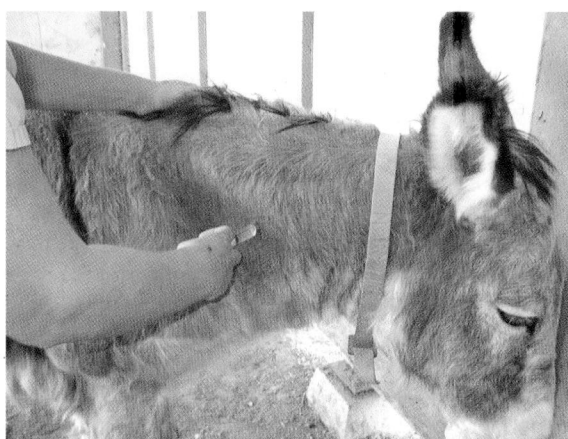

FIGURE 18-52 IM injection in the neck of a donkey. Needle is placed in an imaginary triangular area of the lateral neck to avoid the cervical vertebrae, the scapulae, and the ligamentum nuchae.

appropriate for most horses. The needle is inserted with a quick thrust directly into the muscle. Some technicians make a point of grasping the skin next to the injection site between the fingers and pulling up. The injection is administered, and the skin is released back into place. This method results in a needle hole in the skin a few inches away from the needle hole in the muscle. When the skin is released, it acts as a barrier, preventing leakage of the drug. The neck muscles are not recommended for IM injections in foals because soreness caused by the injections may make the foals reluctant to position themselves for nursing.

Semimembranosus/Semitendinosus Muscles

Semimembranosus and semitendinosus muscles are located on the caudal aspect of the hindlimb between the point of the buttock and the hock. These muscles are often used with minimal complications. Particular attention needs to be paid to the sciatic nerve that runs down the lateral aspect of the leg because an inadvertent injection into the nerve can cause paralysis. The technician should stand facing toward the tail end of the animal with his or her body next to the hip of the horse. Positioning with the body closely pressed into the horse's hip will lessen the impact if the animal chooses to kick. If the technician is tall enough, he or she can reach across the horse and insert the needle into the opposite leg (Figure 18-53, A and B). This reduces the chance of being kicked because a horse that kicks in response to insertion of the needle will usually kick with the leg that has received the needle.

An 18- or 19-gauge × 1.5-inch needle should be inserted with swift action into this muscle group. Once the animal has stopped moving, attach the syringe and proceed as described previously. If injecting large volumes of medication, it is preferential to detach the syringe from the needle after 15 ml has been administered, withdraw the needle slightly, and redirect the needle within the muscle. There is no need to remove the needle completely, but care should be taken to avoid side-to-side movement, because moving the needle can cause trauma to the tissue. Once the needle has been redirected, reattach the syringe, aspirate, and inject as described earlier. Continue this process until all of the solution has been administered.

Excessive distention caused by injection of large volumes of medication can result in tissue necrosis. When repeatedly injecting into these muscle groups, it is advisable to rotate between right and left sides to minimize muscle soreness and decrease the likelihood of puncturing a vessel. The large size of the muscles in this area makes them a good choice for IM injections in foals. This approach can be used with the foal standing and restrained, or when recumbent. Repeated IM injections in the hind legs may cause soreness that appears as lameness, which usually lasts for only a few days after the last injection. Repeated injections may lead to increased vascularization in the area, making it more difficult to insert the needle without encountering blood.

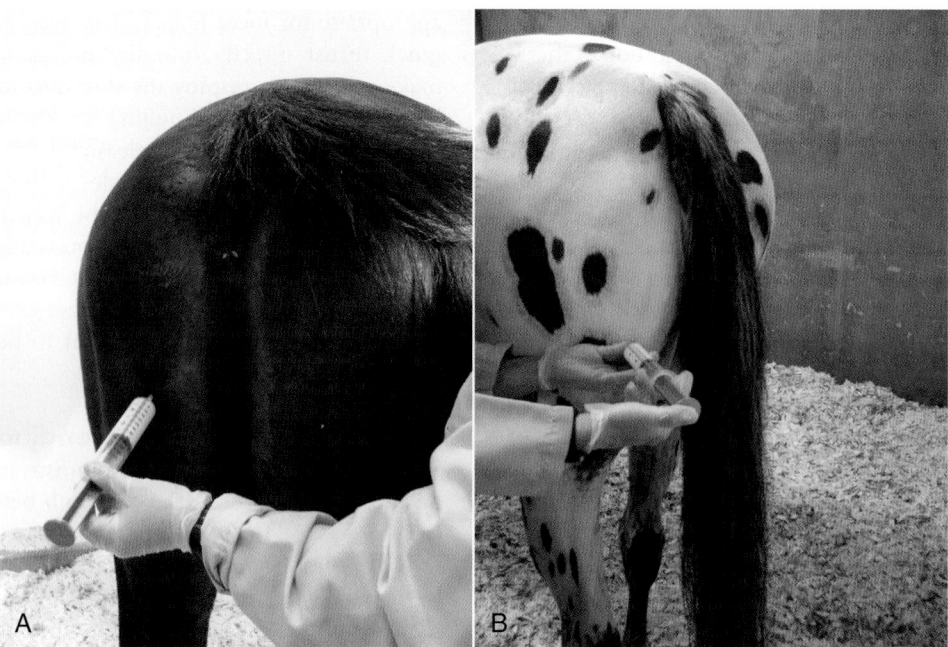

FIGURE 18-53 A, Technician positioned on the opposite side of the injection for an IM injection into the semitendinosus muscle group of a horse. B, Technician positioned on the same side as the injection.

Pectoral Muscles

The pectoral muscles are located between the front legs. As with the hind end, safety needs to be considered when this site is chosen. A needle insertion at this site usually elicits less of a reaction than an injection into the hind legs, but the technician should assess the temperament of the animal and be prepared for the horse to move forward, jump to the side, strike, or rear. The technician should stand next to the shoulder of the horse facing the head. Reaching around with the hand farthest from the horse, insert the needle all the way to the hub. An 18- to 20-gauge × 1- to 1.5-inch needle is appropriate (Figure 18-54). The pectoral muscles are relatively small, and repeated IM injections at this site may cause pain and swelling. Resultant edema that may be seen after an IM injection at this site can be temporarily unsightly and may be of consideration, depending on the planned use of the horse.

Gluteal Muscles

The gluteus, or rump, of the horse is the largest muscle mass on the hindquarters. It is located high on the rear limb, lateral to the spine, and caudal to the point of the hip (Figure 18-55). It can accommodate large volumes and repeated injections but is not often chosen as the site for IM injections because it is difficult to detect inflammation caused by IM injections in the gluteus, and if an abscess forms, adequate drainage from this area can be very difficult. If the gluteus is used, the technician should stand close to the hip of the horse and insert the needle with a quick thrust, as for other IM sites.

BOVINE

Because most cattle are eventually consumed, IM injections are highly discouraged to prevent muscle damage. If it is

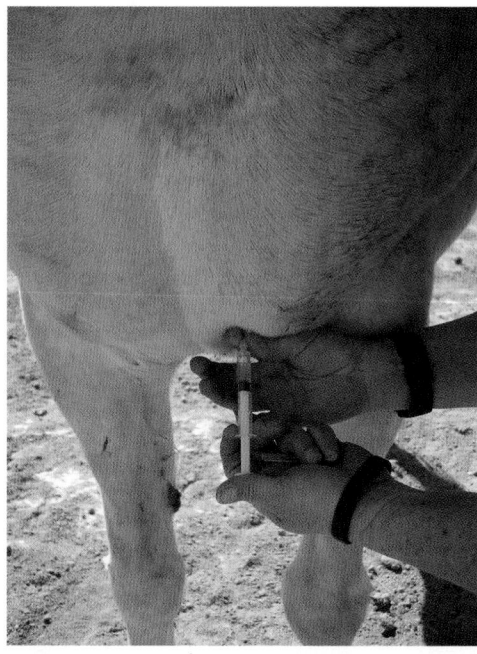

FIGURE 18-54 IM injection into pectoral muscles of the horse.

absolutely necessary to give an IM injection, the muscles of the neck should be used. The animal should be restrained in a head gate or a squeeze chute. The technician should approach the animal from the forequarters and stay close and, while leaning in to the animal, should place a halter on the head and tie it securely to the side. The borders are the same as those described for equine patients (spine, nuchal ligament, and scapula). The needle should be inserted with a quick thrust into the muscle. In accordance with beef quality assurance guidelines, the needle must be clean and

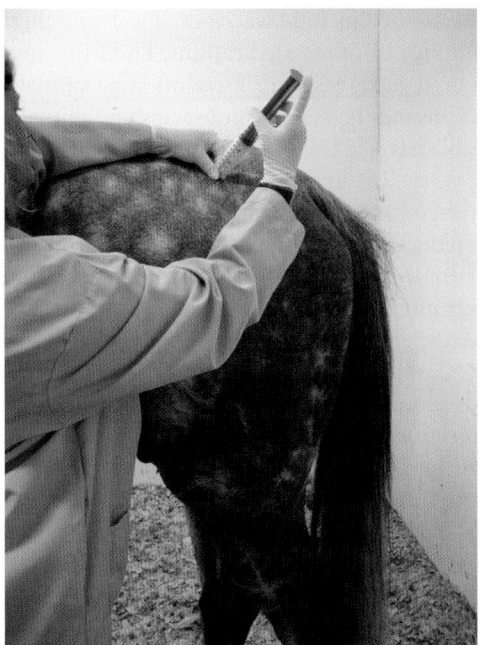

FIGURE 18-55 IM injection into equine gluteals.

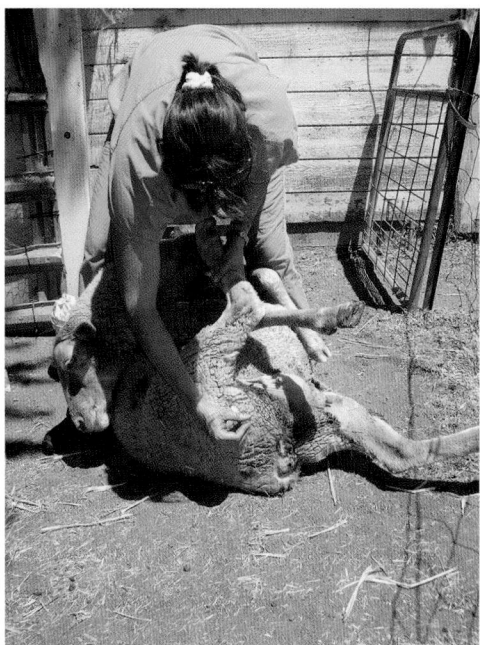

FIGURE 18-56 Technician administering IM injection to sheep.

sharp, the injection should be smooth so as not to cause too much muscle damage, and no more than 10 ml of substance should be administered in one spot at any one time.

Semitendinosus, semimembranosus, shoulder, and gluteal muscles should not be used for IM injections in cattle. Damage to these muscles renders the areas condemned. Because these muscles are included in the higher-valued cuts of meat, IM injection into them can result in expensive losses.

OVINE AND CAPRINE

Sheep and goats have small muscle masses. As with cattle, semitendinosus, semimembranosus, and shoulder muscles should not be used for meat animals. If the semitendinosus and semimembranosus muscles are used for IM injection, the technician must avoid the sciatic nerve, which runs caudal to the femur down the back of the hind legs (Figure 18-56). The neck is commonly used for IM administration (Figure 18-57). The gluteals and triceps can be used for very small volumes. IM injections into the neck may cause significant soreness, and the animal may be reluctant to raise its head. This can be particularly problematic in kids and lambs because they may become too sore to nurse. Once the muscle to be used has been identified, the standard procedure described for large animals is followed. For adult sheep and goats, an 18- to 20-gauge × 1-inch needle should be used. A 20- to 22-gauge × 1-inch needle is appropriate for lambs and kids.

PORCINE

IM injections in pigs can prove complicated because of the thickness of the skin, the tendency to store a thick layer of SC body fat, the difficulty involved in restraining them, and

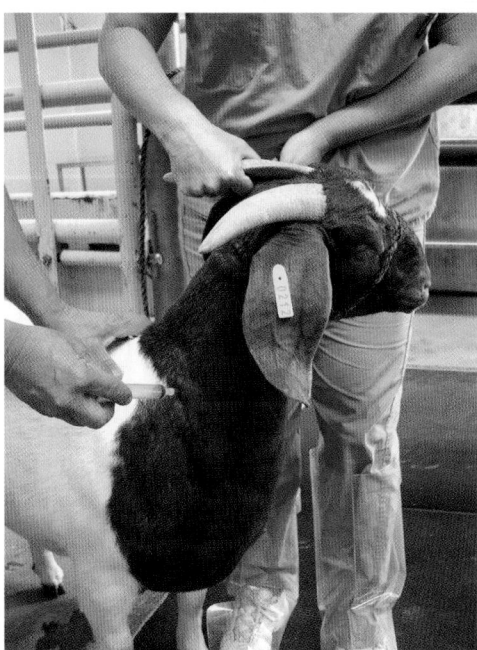

FIGURE 18-57 Site for IM injection in the neck of a goat.

the potential for damage to muscle (meat). Generally, the cervical neck muscles just caudal and ventral to the ear are used. In adults, a maximum volume of 5 to 10 ml per site is recommended. Piglets can receive 1 to 2 ml per site. For adults, a long needle (at least 1.5 inches) should be used to avoid the fat because injecting into the fat will delay drug absorption. Depending on the size of the animal, the needle gauge can be anywhere from 20 gauge for piglets to 16 gauge for larger stock. Drug residues in various muscles will reduce the market value of the animal. The gluteal,

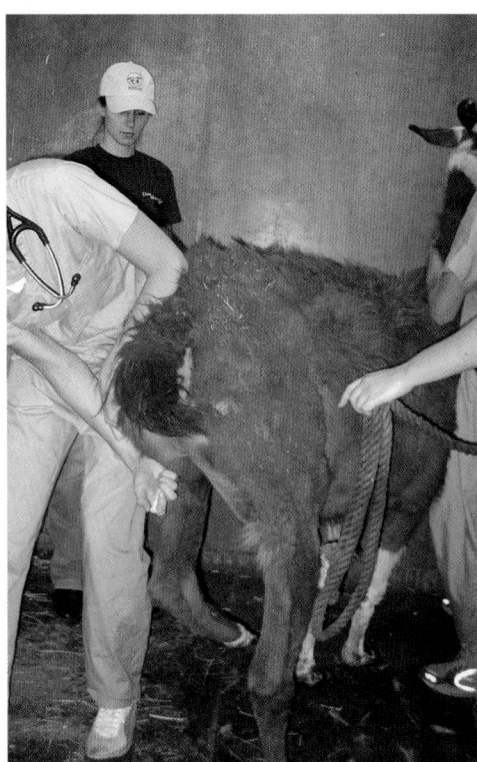

FIGURE 18-58 Llama receiving IM injection into the semitendinosus.

semimembranosus, and semitendinosus muscles can be used, but not in animals destined to be used for meat. In accordance with the same meat quality assurance guidelines identified earlier for cattle, the technician will grasp the skin in this area and will pull cranially. With a firm motion, insert the needle at a perpendicular angle to the skin. Once the needle is in, attach the syringe, aspirate back, and inject the medication.

CAMELID

IM injection sites for llamas and alpacas are generally the same as for other large animal species. They do not have a large muscle mass in any one place, so SC is the preferred route for administration of large volumes or potentially irritating substances. The neck should not be used because of the potential for soreness in the area. The semimembranosus and semitendinosus muscles are good choices for IM injection in these animals (Figure 18-58). For adults, an 18- to 20-gauge × 1-inch needle is appropriate. Twenty-gauge to 22-gauge × 1-inch needles are recommended for crias.

SUBCUTANEOUS ADMINISTRATION (SQ, Subq, SC)

In all species, subcutaneous (SQ, Subq, SC) injections can be given anywhere that the skin is able to be lifted and tented. Medications that are administered SC are absorbed less rapidly than IV or IM injections, but more rapidly than those given orally or intradermally. Therapeutic agents that are

administered SC include vaccines, local anesthetics, and small volumes of other medications. Fluid therapy may be administered via an SC route for some large animal patients. SC injections may be desired for use in show animals because a noticeable adverse reaction is less likely at the injection site with SC versus IM injections. The meat animal production industry recommends that drugs be administered SC in an effort to reduce tissue damage (damage to the meat) that can occur with IM injections. Strict regulatory requirements have been put forth for administration of pharmaceuticals to cattle; the medications must be administered per label, and most of those used in cattle are labeled for SC administration.

SC injections are done by inserting a needle between the skin and the body of the animal. The site selected should have loose skin that is easily grasped. It is wiped with 70% isopropyl alcohol, the skin is grasped and pulled away from the body of the animal, and then the needle is inserted into the base of the tented skin. The needle size used will depend on the viscosity of the substance to be administered, the size of the animal, and the thickness of its skin. A 20- to 25-gauge needle no longer than 1 inch should be used for SC injections in horses. An 18- to 22-gauge × 1.5-inch needle is a common choice for calves, sheep, goats, and pigs. Adult cattle may require a 16- to 18-gauge needle. Before injecting the substance from the syringe, aspirate back to make sure that the vessels have not been punctured. Once needle placement in the SC space has been confirmed, gently inject the medication. The solution should be ejected easily from the syringe, and a bleb, or bump, is often visible under the skin. A slow flow of solution may indicate that the needle is ID rather than SC. If this resistance is felt, the needle should be repositioned before the injection is continued. After the needle and syringe have been removed, the injection area should be gently rubbed to lessen the bump that has been created and to increase circulation in the area, which promotes absorption of the medication. If an SC injection into edematous tissue is performed, a bump is not likely to be observed.

For equines, the loose skin on the side and at the base of the neck is the easiest spot for SC injection (Figure 18-59).

For bovines, the loose skin of the neck and just behind the elbow is most easily used as the site for SC injection. Large volumes of drugs may be injected SC behind the elbow. Veterinarians perform SC injections on cattle in the loose skin on either side of the ischiorectal fossa for administration of leptospirosis vaccines. The technician should not tent the skin when injecting *Brucellosis* vaccines, to ensure that no drug is accidentally injected into the person who is administering it.

For llamas, a common site for SC injection is just behind the elbow (Figure 18-60).

In goats, injection sites for SC administration include just behind the elbow (Figure 18-61), which can be done with the goat restrained in a standing position, and the axillary region where the forearm meets the body, which can be reached easily by lifting a front leg and the lateral chest, caudal to the shoulder (Figure 18-62).

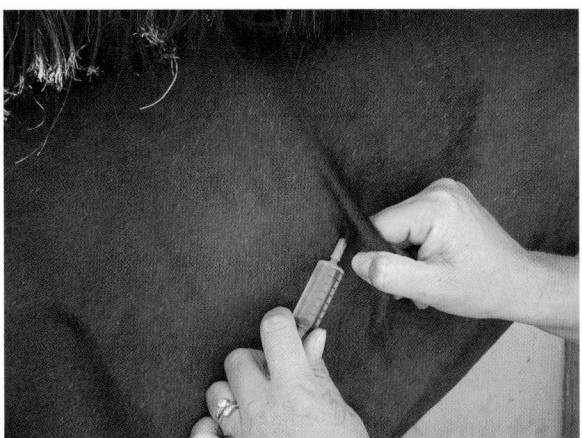

FIGURE 18-59 SC injection into loose skin on the lateral neck of a horse.

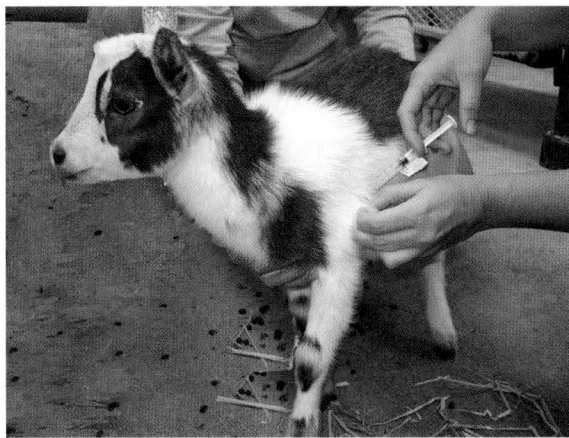

FIGURE 18-61 Goat kid receiving SC injection behind the elbow.

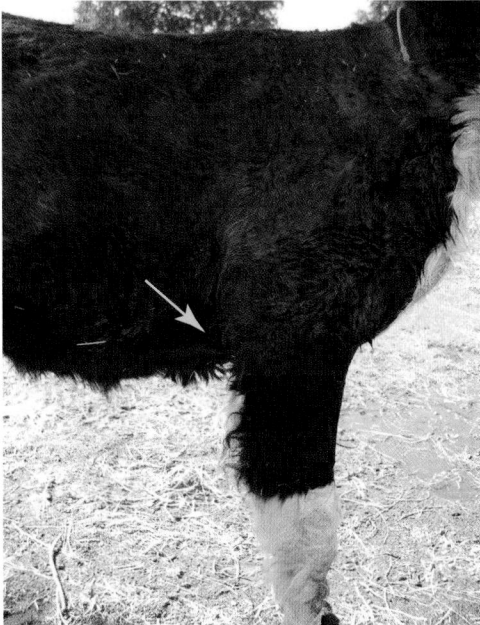

FIGURE 18-60 Loose skin located behind the elbow in llamas can be a site for SC injection.

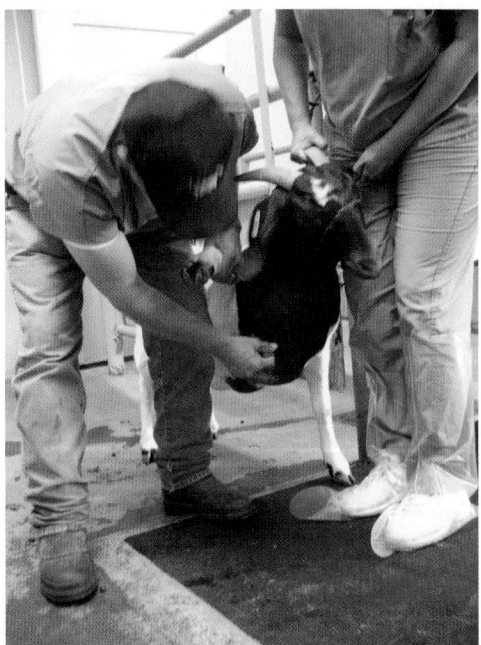

FIGURE 18-62 Lifting the front leg of a goat provides access to the axillary area for SC injection.

For sheep, the sites chosen should be free of wool. SC injections can be done with the animal restrained in a standing position but are facilitated by restraining the sheep while set up on its rump. This provides easy access to the most wool-free site, including the axillary area where the forearm meets the body and the inguinal area and the flank fold (Figures 18-63 and 18-64).

In pigs, it is challenging to find loose skin. Possible SC injection sites include the axillary and inguinal regions and the skin caudal to the base of the ear. The size of the animal will determine where the injection can be given. Holding piglets up by the hind legs will expose an injection site on the inside of the flank along the abdominal wall. Grasp the skin and pull dorsally, and make sure the injection is shallow. The needle should be inserted at an approximately 10-degree angle. Larger pigs should be restrained using

a hog snare or chute to access the loose skin just caudal to the ear.

INTRADERMAL ADMINISTRATION

Intradermal (ID) administration is the injection of a substance between the dermis and the epidermis (skin layers). This route results in very slow absorption. ID injections are performed primarily for the purposes of skin testing, allergen identification, and provision of local anesthesia. Cattle, goats, and sheep are tested for tuberculosis by means of an ID injection into the caudal tail fold (Figure 18-65). ID injections in swine can be given at the base of the ear. For allergy testing in horses, the side of the neck is commonly used. ID injections are also used to treat nodular skin lesions and sarcoid (a common tumor affecting the skin of horses).

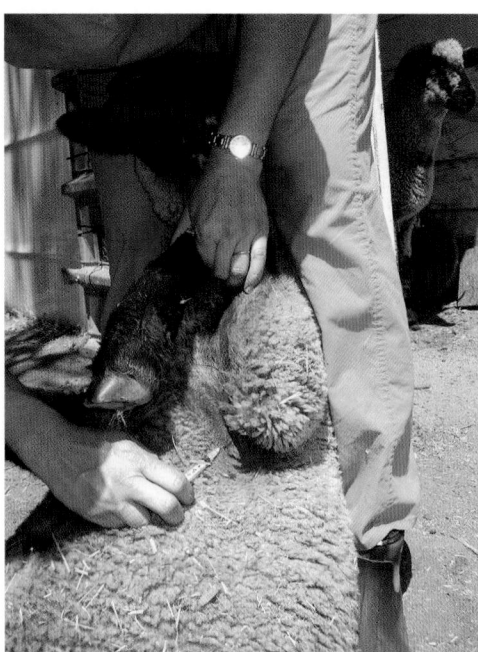

FIGURE 18-63 Technician administering SC injection in the axillary area of a sheep while restraining in setup position.

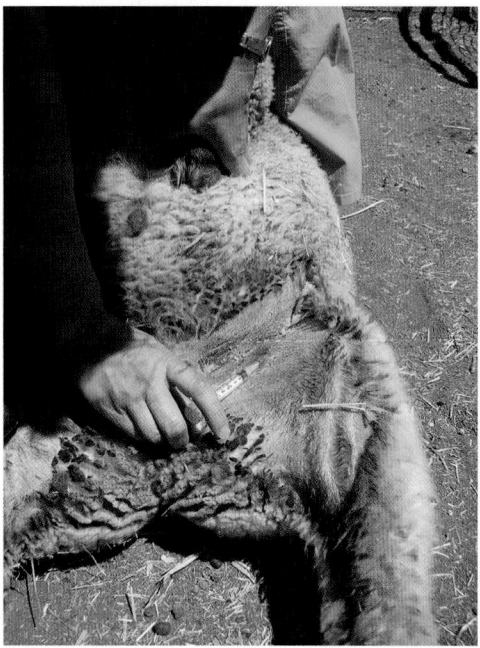

FIGURE 18-64 Administration of SC injection into the inguinal area of a sheep.

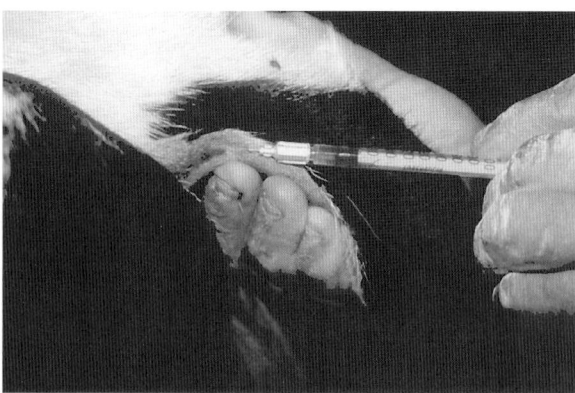

FIGURE 18-65 ID injection is made into the caudal skin fold to test for tuberculosis in the cow.

syringe plunger is withdrawn slightly to aspirate and to make sure that no vessels have been penetrated. The solution is slowly injected. Resistance should be felt if the needle is correctly placed in the dermis. A noticeable bleb should appear as the injection is made. If no bleb is visible, the needle has been placed too deep. Massaging the site (as is suggested with SC injections) is not done following ID injections because the solution is intended to remain localized.

For goats, sheep, and swine, a 25- to 22-gauge × $\frac{1}{5}$- to 1-inch needle is used. Cattle have very thick skin, and a 20- to 22-gauge × 1.5-inch needle is more appropriate.

INTRAPERITONEAL ADMINISTRATION

EQUINE

In the equine patient, intraperitoneal (IP) administration of fluids and medication is usually accomplished through an abdominal lavage system. The drain system is inserted surgically by the veterinarian during abdominal surgery or in a standing position when peritonitis is suspected and general anesthesia is not necessary. The technician will not be involved with the surgical procedure but will be responsible for care and maintenance afterward. To lavage the abdomen, latex tubing is attached to the desired fluids and is connected to the drain system using a 5-in-1 connector. The desired amount of fluid (routinely 10 L for an adult equine patient, adjusted for smaller patients) is administered along with any medication (heparin, antibiotics, etc.), the latex tubing is clamped off, and the patient is walked. This is done to attempt to distribute the fluid and medication throughout the abdominal cavity while washing internal organs and breaking up any adhesions. The latex tubing is then unclamped, and fluid is allowed to drain out of the abdomen back into the original fluid bag (Figure 18-66, *A* through *C*). Ideally, the amount returned is equal to the amount originally administered. This process can be repeated several times per day. When the drain system is handled, gloves should be worn, and the technician should pay careful attention to keeping the system clean while not introducing any contaminants during administration.

For horses, the selected site should be clipped, cleaned, and allowed to dry. Depending on the purpose of the injection, use of an antiseptic agent may be contraindicated because it may interfere with test results, so the technician preparing for the procedure should be clear on the intent of the veterinarian. The skin is grasped between the thumb and the forefinger and is pulled up from the body. A small needle (25 to 27 gauge × $\frac{5}{8}$ inch) is placed parallel to the site with the bevel directed up and inserted at a slight angle. The

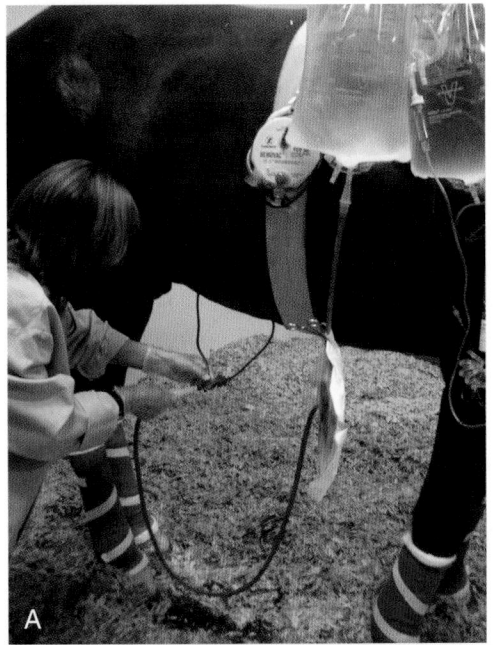

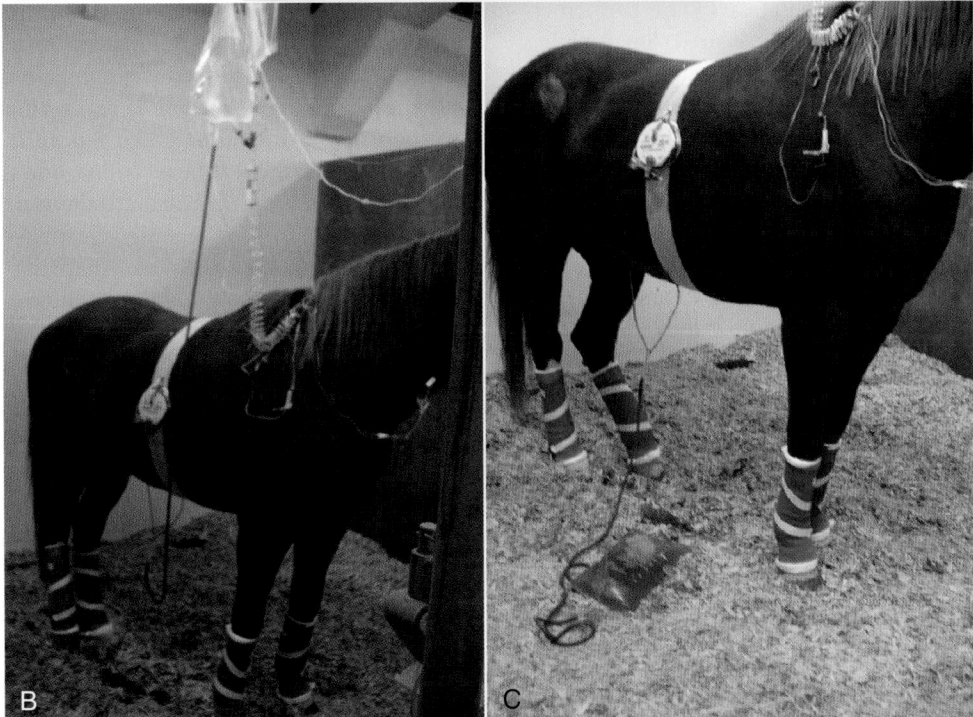

FIGURE 18-66 A, Technician attaches latex tubing from the IV fluid bag to abdominal drain tubing from an animal for equine abdominal lavage. B, Fluid bag is raised to allow fluid to flow through tubing and into the abdominal cavity. C, The empty fluid bag is lowered to the ground to retrieve peritoneal fluid from the abdominal cavity.

BOVINE

IP injections may be indicated if IV administration is not possible and for treatment of peritonitis. If an IP injection is administered in cattle, the site selected is usually in the paralumbar fossa. Care must be taken when on the left side to prevent puncturing the rumen and when on the right side to prevent puncturing the intestine or dilated or displaced internal organs.

CAPRINE AND OVINE

IP injections are usually reserved for neonatal kids and lambs with umbilical infection or hypoglycemia. Lift the neonate by its front legs; use a 20-gauge needle attached to the syringe filled with medication, inserting it just to the left of the umbilicus up to a depth of 1 cm. Aspirate back to verify that you have not hit a vessel or an internal organ. Once placement is sonfirmed, inject medication into the peritoneal cavity. Remove the needle and syringe.

PORCINE

In neonatal pigs, fluids are generally administered IP because of the impracticality of placing IV catheters and administering fluids by that route. Fluids should be given at body temperature and should be nonirritating and isotonic. The site used needs to be prepared using aseptic technique to ensure that contaminants are not introduced. The piglet is held up by the rear legs, and an 18-gauge × ¾- to 1-inch needle is inserted paramedially between the midline and the flank. The needle is stabilized to prevent damage to internal organs. To perform this procedure in a mature, standing pig, follow the preparation guidelines and insert a 16- to 18-gauge × 3-inch needle through the paralumbar fossa.

Complications from IP administration include peritonitis, abscess, and injury to internal organs.

INTRANASAL ADMINISTRATION

Certain vaccines and local anesthetics are administered intranasally. Intranasal anesthetics may be used before other procedures involving the nasal cavity are performed. The head of the patient needs to be secured. Small piglets can be held, whereas a hog snare should be used to restrain larger pigs. A halter and lead rope (and a head gate for adult cattle) may provide sufficient restraint for most large animals. The technician uses his or her free hand to steady the head.

An easy method is to bring the free arm under the mandible and reach around while placing the hand on top of the muzzle area. Any nasal discharge should be wiped away from the nares using damp gauze sponges. While the head is slightly lifted, a needleless syringe containing the medication is introduced into the nostril, and the substance is injected, preferably when the animal inspires. The patient may sneeze afterward, causing the medication to spray. The technician should take precautions to prevent having his or her own mucous membranes sprayed from the sneeze.

Oxygen can be administered intranasally to help with certain conditions, such as pneumonia or hypoxic ischemic encephalopathy. Oxygen may be administered to preparturient females that are considered to have a high-risk pregnancy in an attempt to increase the oxygen content of circulating blood in both the dam and the fetus.

While using a commercially available product (AirLife O_2 catheter; Cardinal Health, Dublin, Ohio) or a small rubber feeding tube, determine the distance from the medial canthus of the eye to the entrance of the nostril. This is how far the catheter will be inserted into the nostril. Gently insert the catheter ventrally into the nasal passage to the point that was measured. To maintain the catheter in the nostril for the long term, it is beneficial to first wrap adhesive tape (Elastikon [Johnson & Johnson, New Brunswick, New Jersey] works very well) loosely around the muzzle. Then the catheter, with a piece of butterflied 1-inch adhesive tape attached, can be secured using suture material to connect the butterfly to the Elastikon. The end can be hooked up to an oxygen source, providing the desired oxygen flow in liters per minute.

INTRAMAMMARY ADMINISTRATION

Intramammary infusion of antibiotics is used routinely to treat or control mastitis in cows and is also performed on goats and sheep. Because of the high risk of introducing contaminants (organic debris, yeast, or other opportunistic organisms) during this process, the procedure must be performed aseptically. Minimal restraint is usually required, but a tail jack restraint may be necessary for some cows.

The udder is completely milked out and manually stripped. Residual milk present will dilute the medication. The teats are cleaned with a teat dip and then are thoroughly dried using a separate cloth for each teat. Each teat is wiped with an alcohol-soaked sponge and air dried. The teats on the far side from the technician are cleaned before those on the near side. This will prevent transmission of contaminants from the dirty teats to the clean teats.

Teats on the near side are infused first. The teat is grasped at the base, and a sterile teat cannula or disposable mammary infusion cannula on an antibiotic syringe is partially inserted into the teat (up to 4 mm); the antibiotic is injected slowly into the canal. For goats and sheep with a very small teat orifice, a sterile tomcat catheter can be used. Proceed to the next teat with the new cannula and syringe, and then move to the teats on the far side and repeat. It is recommended that the end of the teat be occluded, and the teat and udder be gently massaged to distribute the medication. After the teats have been infused, teat dip is reapplied and is left to dry. In very cold (0° C) conditions, chapping and frostbite can occur, so the animal should not be moved outside while the udder is wet.

> *TECHNICIAN NOTE* Partial insertion of the cannula into the teat canal delivers fewer contaminants to the udder than would occur with full insertion.

TOPICAL OPHTHALMIC ADMINISTRATION

To treat ocular diseases or conditions (ulcers, abrasions, lacerations, keratitis), topical ophthalmic ointment and solutions are routinely administered. When treatment is provided in an ointment form, a small amount is applied directly into the eye. To deliver the intended amount successfully into large animal patients (both adults and neonates), proper restraint of the head must be employed. Hands should be well cleaned or gloved. The lower eyelid of the particular eye that needs medicating is pulled down slightly, and the ointment is applied without touching the surface of the eye. The lid is then let go, and the blinking action distributes the medication. Another method of ointment application involves wearing sterile gloves and placing a small ribbon of ointment on a gloved finger. The ointment on the finger is then touched directly to the eye. This eliminates the risk of scratching the eye with the end of the ointment tube.

Ophthalmic solution can be applied by gently pulling the lower eyelid out slightly and placing drops into the lower conjunctival sac. Drops may come directly from a plastic bottle with dispenser or may be administered using a small sterile syringe—with no needle attached.

When both ointment and solution are applied, the technician should apply the solution before applying the ointment. This will prevent the solution from running over the ointment without being absorbed directly into the eye.

Most patients become resentful of repeated applications into the eye, and many eye conditions are quite painful, so it may be necessary to place a long-term lavage system to properly treat the disease or condition.

> **TECHNICIAN NOTE** Eye conditions may require aggressive treatment with administration of ophthalmic medication as often as every hour.

Two types of lavage systems are available to supply medication. The subpalpebral lavage system is inserted through incisions made into the upper or lower eyelids (Figure 18-67). The narrow rubber tubing is inserted through the incision(s) of the eyelid to open directly in the conjunctival sac and away from the cornea. Because the tubing is very narrow, liquid solutions are delivered through the system instead of ointments. Once the tubing is placed, the system is secured to the skin above the eye and is extended over the poll (IV extension tubing is attached to make the appropriate length to extend up and over the head). A PRN (intermittent infusion plug) is attached to the end of the system and should be changed every 24 hours, or more often if it becomes friable from repeated injections. The medication to be delivered should be warm enough so as not to cause discomfort to the patient, and the lines should be cleared after

the administration using a very slow bolus of air (1 to 2 ml). The injections should be given very slowly. If resistance is felt when solution is injected into the lavage system, the veterinarian should be notified so that the tube can be cleared of any debris. If air is used, the patient may startle when air hits the eye, so the technician should be prepared for any adverse reactions.

The second type of lavage system is placed through the nasolacrimal duct (tear duct). The tubing is inserted into the nasal punctum, and a small stab incision is created through the nostril to pass the tubing through and attach it to the skin. This will prevent the tubing from moving inside the nostril and will prevent the patient from rubbing it out. The method of medication delivery described previously is used. This approach requires a greater volume of medication than is given by the subpalpebral lavage method.

The veterinarian may choose to provide protection to the eye in the form of protective eye cups or hoods (Eye-Saver, JorVet, Jorgensen Labs, Loveland, Colorado; Guardian Mask, Guardian Mask Company, Burnet, Texas) (Figure 18-68). These provide protection from sunlight and serve as a mechanical barrier, preventing the horse from rubbing the eye and keeping it free of debris.

EPIDURAL ADMINISTRATION

Epidural administration deposits drugs into the epidural space. This procedure may be done to provide anesthesia or for pain control. Epidural injection of analgesics or local anesthetics provides complete analgesia and muscle relaxation caudal to the block. For all species, proper restraint is required for the success and safety of this procedure. Two locations may be used for epidural administration. The

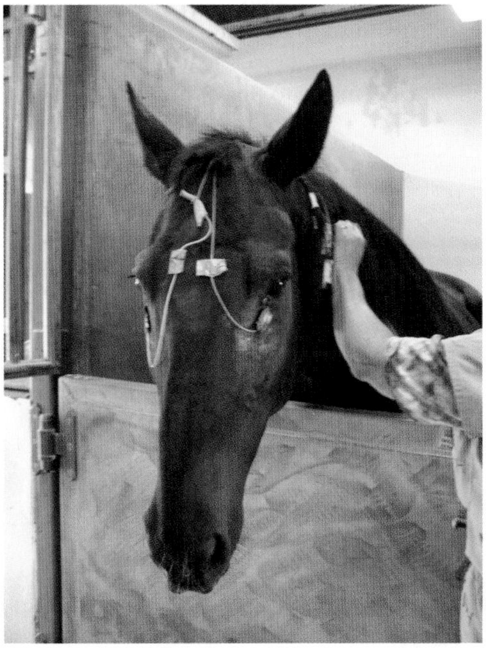

FIGURE 18-67 Subpalpebral lavage system in an equine patient.

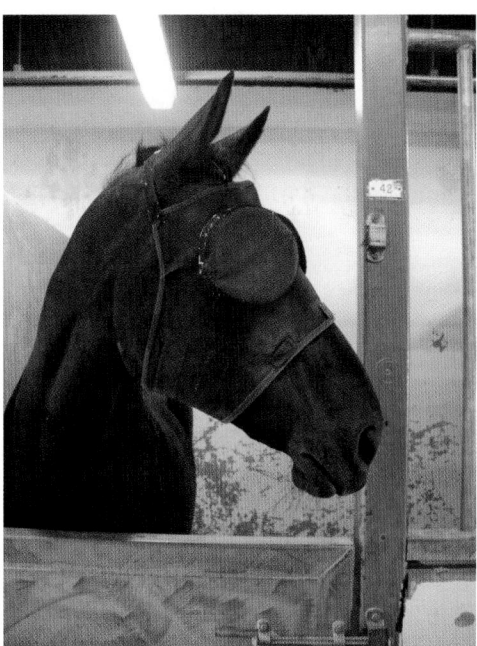

FIGURE 18-68 Guardian Mask (Guardian Mask Company, Burnet, Texas) placed on the head to provide protection to the eyes of a horse.

cranial epidural is located at the lumbosacral junction (between L6 and S1), and the caudal epidural is located between S5 and C1 or C1 and C2. The veterinarian will choose the location for the epidural, depending on the effect that he or she wishes to achieve.

EQUINE

The horse should be restrained in stocks and a twitch applied. Some horses will require the administration of a sedative. The technician will clip, shave, and aseptically prepare a 3-inch square (approximately) area over the first and second coccygeal vertebrae. This site can be identified by lifting the tail up and down with one hand while feeling for the vertebral space with the other hand (Figure 18-69). This area is usually close to where the coarse tail hairs originate. An SC bleb of local anesthetic is placed. The technician should attempt to have the horse stand still and squarely upon its legs. If the animal is not standing squarely, an uneven distribution of the drug will occur because more will run into one side of the epidural space.

The technician should prepare the supplies necessary, including sterile gloves, local anesthetic, a sterile 12-ml syringe, and a 19-gauge × 1.5-inch needle (3.5 inches for very large horses) or an 18-gauge epidural catheter with stylet.

> **TECHNICIAN NOTE** To hand the sterile syringe to the veterinarian, open the plastic syringe casing and gently slide the syringe into the sterile gloved hand of the veterinarian without touching the outer casing to the glove. To provide the veterinarian with a sterile needle, remove the needle cap, and while holding the needle cover tightly, point the hub toward the veterinarian, so that he or she may use sterile gloved fingers to pull the needle from the cover.

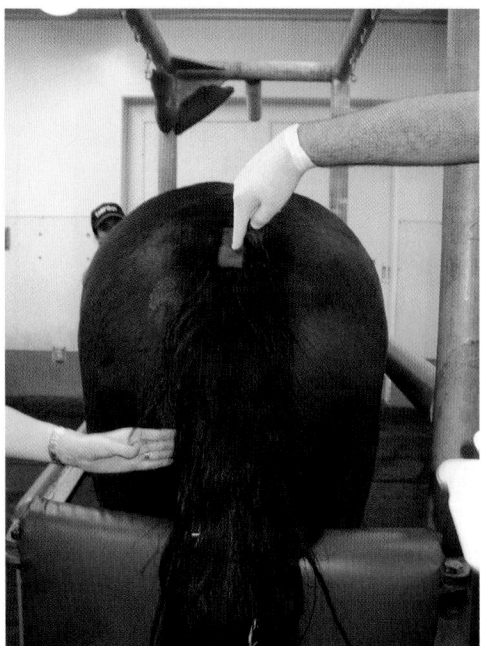

FIGURE 18-69 Locating the site for equine epidural injection.

Directing the needle slightly cranially and ventrally into the epidural space at an approximately 45-degree angle to the rump, an 18- to 19-gauge × 1.5-inch needle is inserted about 1 inch in adult horses. When the needle enters the epidural space, a slight "pop" is felt, and resistance to the passage of the needle is lessened. The drug is injected, and the needle may be left in place to facilitate an additional injection. An epidural catheter may be placed and secured to the skin to facilitate repeated drug administration. When the needle or catheter is removed, antibiotic ointment is applied to the site.

The technician should be aware that hind leg instability may occur following epidural anesthesia. Lidocaine, carbocaine, xylazine, and morphine are commonly administered as epidurals.

BOVINE

The technician first must ensure that the animal is sufficiently restrained. To locate the site, move the tail up and down using one hand while using the other hand to feel the top of the vertebrae to find the first movable joint (S1 and S2). Clip, shave, and aseptically prep a 3 × 3-inch area (approximately). An 18-gauge × 1.5- to 3-inch needle is inserted perpendicular to the spine and into the vertebral space between S1 and S2 (Figure 18-70). A "pop" is felt when the space is entered. The epidural space is a relative vacuum compared with atmospheric conditions, and the medication will be sucked into the space. (A drop from the syringe into the hub of the needle should quickly be drawn into the needle.) Three milliliters of 2% lidocaine is commonly used for bovine epidurals.

CAMELID

The tail is moved up and down to locate the intervertebral space between S5 and C1. In most llamas and alpacas, this will be the first movable joint because the five sacral vertebrae are usually fused. The site is clipped and surgically prepared. Owners may object to clipping of the fiber, so efforts should be made to shave only a small site and to

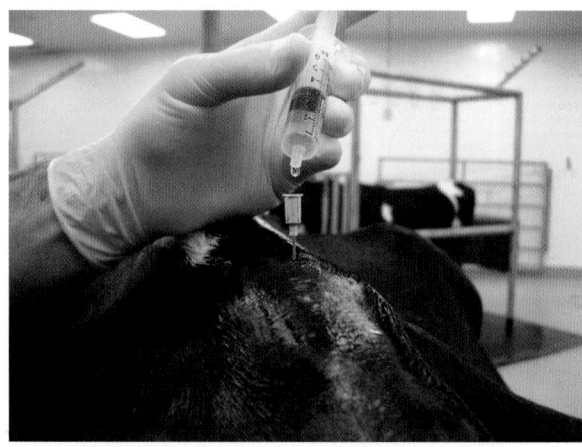

FIGURE 18-70 Technician performing epidural injection in a bovine patient.

secure surrounding fibers away from the site with adhesive tape. A 20-gauge × 1.5-inch needle is inserted. The veterinarian will confirm a successful insertion as described for other large animals.

OVINE AND CAPRINE

According to the procedure guidelines for cattle, an 18- to 21-gauge × 1- to 1.5-inch needle is inserted at a 45-degree angle. Sheep and goats are very sensitive to local anesthetics.

PORCINE

The site used for epidural injection in pigs is different from the site described earlier for other large animal species. The lumbosacral junction (between L6 and S1) is accessible for porcine epidurals. This is considered a cranial epidural, whereas sites commonly described for other species are used for caudal epidurals. To locate the site, an imaginary line is drawn vertically up from the patella to the back, and a dorsal midline site is clipped and surgically prepared. An 18- to 20-gauge spinal needle may be used; the length is determined by the size of the animal.

TRANSDERMAL ADMINISTRATION (CUTANEOUS, TOPICAL)

Application of medication through the skin is done primarily in the form of an impregnated patch that is placed directly on the skin and is left there to be absorbed. Fentanyl, scopolamine, nitroglycerin, and estrogen are common medications that can be delivered in this fashion. When any type of impregnated patch is applied to the skin, gloves should be worn, so that the technician does not medicate himself or herself. The location that is chosen to place the patch should be shaved and the area cleaned with alcohol-soaked gauze. After the area has dried, the patch can be applied.

When it is time to remove or replace the patch, gloves need to be worn in case any residual medication is left on the patch. The patch should then be disposed of according to local guidelines (fentanyl has strict legal disposal requirements). The area should be wiped with a gauze sponge to remove any excess product.

Caution needs to be applied when any product is administered transdermally, so that the technician or other personnel do not come in contact with the substance and absorb it through their own skin.

Many other ointments, solutions, and creams may be applied topically without the need to bandage the area. With these treatments, gentle application of the desired medication via gauze sponges, swabs, or directly from the gloved hand to the affected area will be effective. Before application, the area should be cleared of any debris. In some instances, such as severe burns or wounds, the outer perimeter will be débrided first. The technician should wear gloves at all times when using topical or transdermal products to limit the potential for contaminants to be added to the medication

and for personal safety (to prevent inadvertent absorption of the substance).

INTRASYNOVIAL ADMINISTRATION

Patients may require administration of medication, such as antibiotics or anesthetic agents, directly into a joint. Intrasynovial administration affords high drug levels localized in the joint compared with levels that would result from systemic drug administration. Veterinarians commonly perform intrasynovial injection on equine patients, but the procedure may be performed on other large animal species as well. Although the technician usually does not perform the injection, he or she may be asked to prepare the joint that will be infused and to assist with the procedure.

The site that is to be injected needs to be surgically scrubbed and cleaned to minimize the chance of introducing a contaminant into the joint. The technician lays out sterile gloves of appropriate size, several needles of the requested gauge and length (18 or 19 gauge × 1.5 inches is common for adult horses), and the syringe with the solution to be injected. All of these items must be handled in an aseptic fashion.

Proper restraint of the patient is necessary to ensure the safety of personnel and of the patient. Using a twitch in addition to a halter and lead rope lessens the likelihood of movement during the procedure. In addition, chemical sedation should be used to prevent movement and subsequent trauma while the needle is introduced into the joint.

Once the injection is complete, the needle and the syringe are withdrawn, and pressure can be applied to the site to prevent seepage. The patient should be monitored for pain, heat, or swelling over the joint.

Joint flushing (joint irrigation, joint lavage) is commonly performed with the animal given a general anesthetic, but it is also performed on young animals that have received injectable anesthetics or very heavy sedation (because of the risk involved, heavy sedation is not commonly used). Two needles are placed at different sites on the affected joint capsule, and sterile flush forced through one needle exits through the other. Joint lavage may be followed by intrasynovial injection of antibiotics after the exit needle is removed.

RECTAL ADMINISTRATION

Rectal administration of therapeutics in large animals is used as a method of delivering medication to a patient that cannot tolerate oral medication as a result of ileus or regurgitation, or to deliver an enema to a constipated patient.

RECTAL MEDICATIONS

To deliver medication per rectum, a tube of appropriate size should be selected based on the size of the patient. A Harris enema tube (24-French) or a fenestrated tube (multiple holes along the distal end) is appropriate for adult animals, foals, and calves, whereas smaller-diameter soft rubber tubes can be used for lambs, kids, and crias. The fenestrated tube may provide better distribution of the medication, but the fenestrations on some tubes may be rough and may cause irritation to the rectal mucosa. The technician should always check the tube for any rough edges and should avoid using any tube that is not smooth. The distal end of the tube is lubricated with a water-soluble solution (such as KY Jelly), and the tube is inserted 1 to 12 inches into the rectum. This distance is determined by the size of the patient. Appropriate restraint, tailored to the individual species and age of the animal, is used. For standing animals, the technician should take precautions to stand to the side of the animal to avoid getting kicked.

Medications are dissolved in a small amount of water (or at the veterinarian's request, in another solution, such as DMSO) and are injected gently via a catheter tip syringe into the tube; this is followed by a small "chaser" of water (or air) to ensure that all medication is administered and none remains in the tube. The tube is then gently removed. It may be necessary to remove feces from the rectum before medications are administered. The technician must discuss this with the veterinarian in advance because it may or may not be necessary, and risk for injury to the animal is increased when a hand is inserted into the rectum. Rectal tears can be fatal. If instructed to do so, the technician must have fingernails clipped short and must wear no rings or watches. With a well-lubricated rectal sleeve, the technician will gently insert the hand a short distance into the rectum and will gently remove obvious feces present before the tube is inserted.

The veterinarian may administer 2% lidocaine per rectum to facilitate performance of a rectal examination by reducing patient straining. A 60-ml syringe containing lidocaine is attached to rubber tubing or to IV extension tubing that is inserted into the rectum, and the drug is injected. Sedation may be given via the epidural route for patients that are straining, to prevent potential problems, such as rectal tears, during the examination.

ENEMA ADMINISTRATION

Enemas are administered to constipated animals to assist defecation. They can be administered to animals of any age or species. The tube used and the volume and composition of fluid administered will vary with the size and condition of the animal. Fluids should be nonirritating and warmed to room temperature, but should not be warmed above body temperature.

> **TECHNICIAN NOTE** Administration of cold enema solutions can lead to hypothermia in young patients.

Neonates

A common practice of many horse owners is to routinely administer a prepackaged human enema to newborn foals to facilitate passage of meconium (feces that has accumulated in the foal while in utero). Warm-water enemas and enemas containing other agents, such as gentle soap, mineral oil, or other lubricants, are administered using a tube and gravity flow. Retention enemas are routinely used in hospitalized neonatal patients. Excessive enema volume and repeated enemas can be harmful to the patient. The technician must be aware of variation in patient size. The standard 120 to 180 ml of fluid delivered for an equine neonate would be far too much for a cria.

The tip of the tube is well lubricated with a water-soluble lubricant, and the tube is gently advanced into the rectum. Once the tube is inserted the desired distance into the rectum, a 60-ml catheter tip syringe, a funnel, or an enema bucket can be attached to the end and the desired amount of solution delivered. Gravity flow is preferred to pumping of fluid because it is possible to tear the rectum. If a syringe is used, gentle pressure is applied until all of the enema solution has been delivered. After all solution has been administered, cap off the end of the tube with the thumb, and gently remove the entire length of tubing.

Retention Enemas

Retention enemas involve insertion into the rectum of a well-lubricated Foley catheter with balloon. The tube is inserted a few inches (usually 2 to 4 inches) into the rectum, and the balloon is inflated using a syringe containing air or water. The enema solution (often Mucomyst [acetylcysteine]) is infused. The catheter is then clamped off using a hemostat, and the tube is left in place for at least 15 minutes. The hemostat is then removed, the balloon deflated, and the catheter removed (Figure 18-71, *A* through *D*).

Enema Administration to Adult Animals

Enemas can be administered to adult animals. With the animal properly restrained, the technician stands to the side of the patient, inserts a well-lubricated tube (an NGT can be used for enema administration to large animals), and delivers the enema solution. The technician administering the enema may derive benefit from preparing in advance of the procedure by cutting one hole in the center of the bottom of a large plastic trash bag (for head) and cutting a hole on either side of the bottom of the bag (for arms). Wearing the bag as a protective covering may be desirable because some enemas may result in a rapid projectile expulsion of fluid and feces.

Sampling Techniques in the Large Animal

VENOUS BLOOD SAMPLE COLLECTION

Blood sampling is a simple method that is used routinely to gather a large quantity of diagnostic data. The choice of blood collection tube (or syringe with anticoagulant added) will determine which laboratory parameters can be evaluated. Some tests require serum (obtained after clotting of a whole blood sample), some require plasma (serum plus fibrinogen) obtained by using an anticoagulant, and some require whole blood for analysis. Blood sample tubes containing an anticoagulant should be filled to capacity to

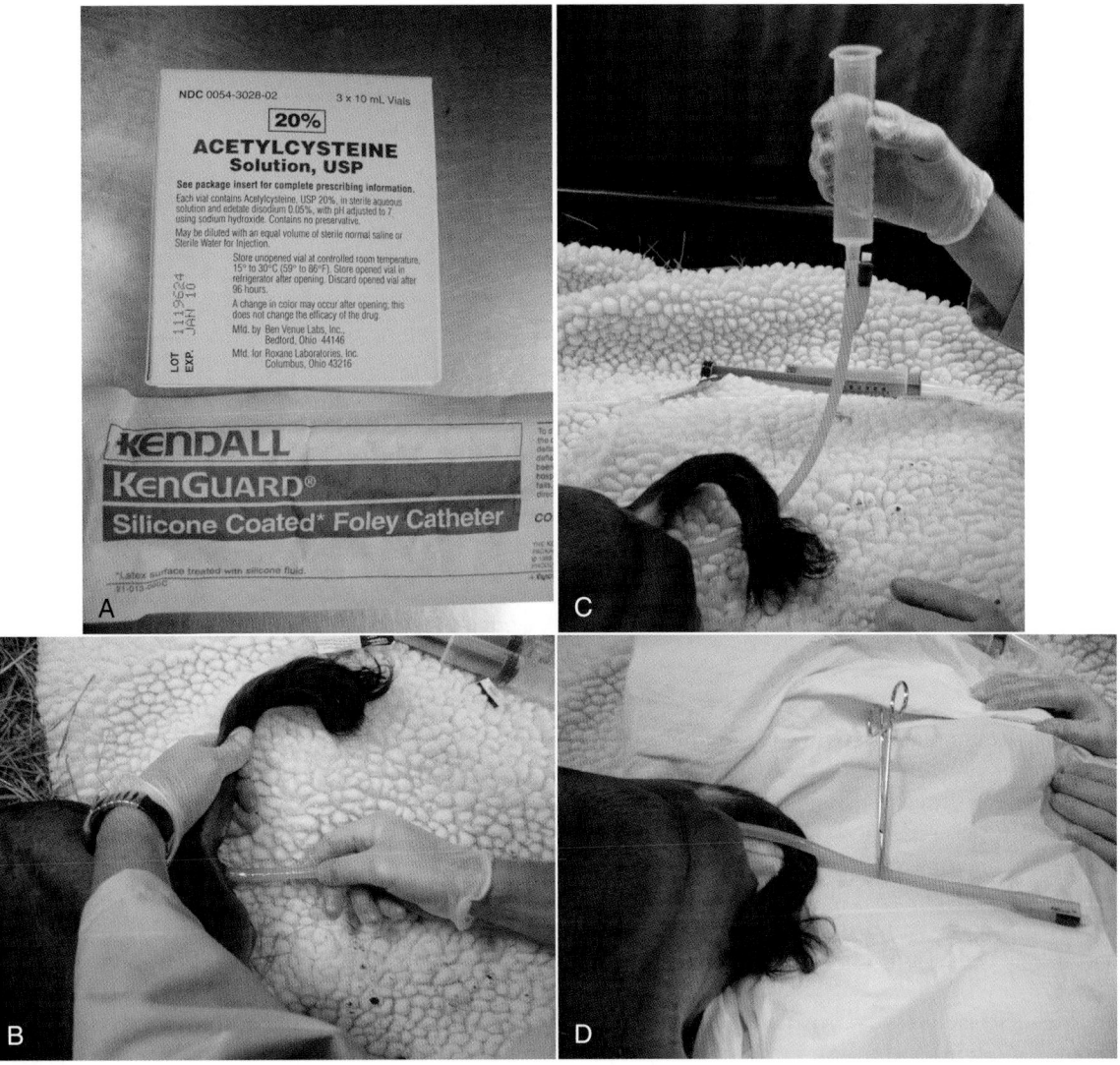

FIGURE 18-71 A, Acetylcysteine and Foley catheter for retention enema in equine neonate. B, Inserting well-lubricated Foley catheter into the rectum. C, Administering an enema solution via gravity flow. D, Foley catheter is clamped off to allow for retention of enema.

ensure the correct blood-to-anticoagulant ratio. Insufficient blood mixed with the anticoagulant may lead to erroneous laboratory results. Once collected, the sample should be gently inverted several times to ensure adequate mixing of the blood with the anticoagulant.

For all sites and species, the hair and/or skin should be cleaned with isopropyl alcohol to remove any obvious debris. In addition to providing antibacterial activity, alcohol facilitates visualization of the vein and acts as a local vasodilator. If blood cultures are desired, a full sterile prep (as described earlier) is required.

> **TECHNICIAN NOTE**   Cleaning the hair and/or skin with isopropyl alcohol provides antibacterial activity and facilitates visualization of the vein.

The choice of vein depends on the appearance of the vessels, the position of the animal, and the disposition of the animal. If repeated samples will be required, the technician should start first with a more distal venipuncture site, with subsequent samples taken progressively more proximal on the vein. The bevel-up position of the needle facilitates venipuncture and is less traumatic to the skin and vein on puncture. If the need to collect multiple samples is anticipated, placement of an IV catheter should be considered.

A syringe and needle or a Vacutainer needle and collection tube may be used. When a needle and syringe are used, the needle may be inserted first and then the syringe attached, or, in some cases, the needle may be attached to the syringe before insertion. The Vacutainer system can be used by inserting the long end of the double-ended needle into the vein and then slipping a blood collection tube over the exposed needle. Alternatively, the tube may be placed on the double-ended needle before injection by inserting the tube into the holder and pressing the rubber stopper against the metal end of the needle until the top of the rubber stopper is aligned with the circumferential score on the tube

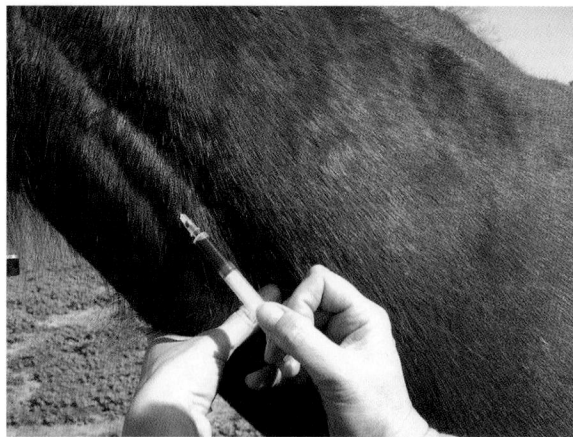

FIGURE 18-72 Venipuncture of equine jugular vein.

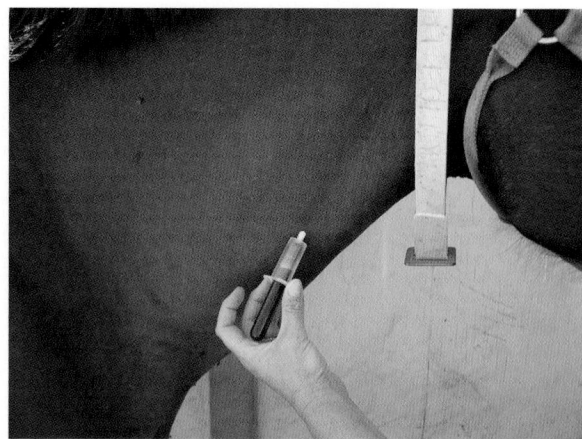

FIGURE 18-73 Blood collection from equine jugular vein using the Vacutainer system.

holder. Do not push it farther until the needle is inserted into the lumen of the vein. Once in the lumen, the tube is pushed fully onto the needle. If the tube is pushed fully onto the needle before the other needle end is in the vein, the vacuum is broken, and blood will not flow into the tube.

EQUINE

Veins commonly used for blood sampling in the adult equine include the jugular, the cephalic (located on the medial aspect of the forelimb), the transverse facial (runs transversely beneath the facial crest and above the transverse facial artery), and the lateral thoracic (located in the cranial ventral third of the thorax caudal to the point of the elbow).

Additionally, for recumbent equine neonates, the saphenous vein (on the medial aspect of the hindlimb) can be safely used.

Restrain the horse as necessary, depending on its behavior. A halter and lead rope may be the only restraint required, but additional restraint is necessary in some horses.

Jugular Vein

To occlude and distend the vein, pressure is placed on the jugular furrow in the lower third of the neck. With an alcohol-soaked sponge or cotton ball, ballottement of the vessel is performed (stroked several times in a downward direction). A 19- to 25-gauge × ⅝- to 1.5-inch needle is inserted into the lumen of the vessel, and blood is aspirated using a syringe or a Vacutainer tube (Figures 18-72 and 18-73).

Some animals object *vehemently* to the needle insertion. For these patients, if the needle is inserted first and the animal jumps, twitches, or otherwise moves, the needle is more apt to remain in place without the weight of the syringe. Once the animal settles, the syringe is attached and the blood sample is aspirated.

Transverse Facial Vein

The transverse facial vein runs transversely beneath the facial crest and above the transverse facial artery and can be located midway between the medial canthus of the eye and the rostral end of the facial crest (Figure 18-74).

> **TECHNICIAN NOTE** To locate the site, the technician may place the thumb at the medial canthus and the index finger at the lateral canthus and draw an imaginary V shape diagonally down to the facial crest.

This vein is commonly used in nonfractious horses to collect small volumes of blood. There is no need to occlude the vein. A 22- to 25-gauge × ⅝- to 1-inch needle is inserted perpendicular to the skin beneath the facial crest and is advanced until bone is felt. The syringe is then attached, and the needle is withdrawn slowly during aspiration. When blood enters the syringe, placement is maintained until collection is complete (see Figure 18-74, *B* and *C*). A very minimal risk for hematoma formation or bleeding from this site has been noted. Horses rarely object to needle insertion at this site. Caution must be used when handling needles around the face of the horse because carelessness can lead to puncture of the eye. The hand that holds the needle should always be cupped, protecting the eye from the needle.

Cephalic Vein

The cephalic vein is located on the medial aspect of the forelimb and can be safely accessed in many horses. The site is cleaned with a rubbing alcohol wipe, which also enhances visibility of the vein. The vein is occluded above the needle insertion site (as with all veins, blood flows back toward the heart). A 20- to 22-gauge × 1- to 1.5-inch needle is inserted (Figure 18-75). Horses may quickly lift up the foot when the needle is inserted, so it is beneficial to insert the needle first and then attach the syringe when the horse has placed the foot back on the ground, to reduce the likelihood of the needle coming out of the horse when the foot is lifted. Because this site is low on the animal, the risk for hematoma formation is enhanced, so after removal of the needle, the technician must make a concerted effort to apply pressure to the site. If the technician is completing other work on the patient, a cotton ball may be placed on the site and adhesive tape wrapped around the limb, but this can be left on only

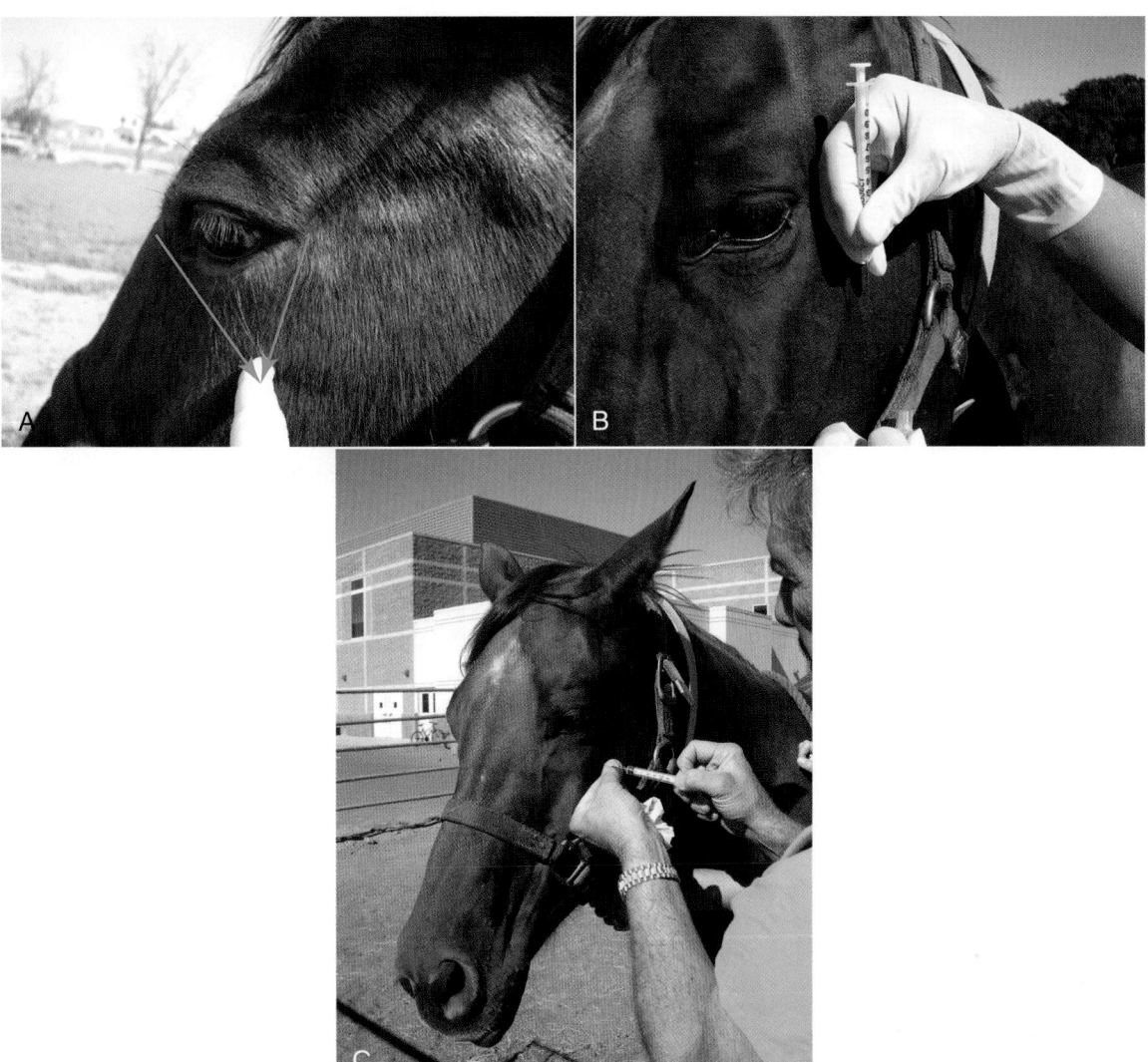

FIGURE 18-74 A, Needle insertion site for a transverse facial blood sample can be located by drawing imaginary lines from the medial canthus and the lateral canthus, intersecting them at the facial crest, and inserting the needle just below the facial crest. **B,** Holding the syringe to protect the eye in case the horse moves while the technician is preparing to insert the needle. **C,** Blood collection from the transverse facial vein.

very briefly because circulation can be compromised. The technician must remove the tape before leaving the patient.

Saphenous Vein
The saphenous vein is located on the medial aspect of the hindlimb. It is unsafe for the technician to use this site in nonanesthetized adult horses. It can be used successfully in recumbent neonates. Care needs to be taken to apply sufficient digital pressure after removal of the needle.

BOVINE
Jugular Vein
Restrain the animal with its head elevated slightly and tied securely. If necessary, nose tongs may be applied for additional restraint. Distend the jugular vein by placing pressure low in the jugular furrow. The bovine jugular vein is very large, and the palm of the hand should be used to occlude the vessel. Firmly wiping the jugular groove several times in

a downward direction with an alcohol-soaked sponge facilitates visualization of the vein. Thrust the needle (16 to 18 gauge × 1.5 inch) into the vein with the needle tip directed cranially at about a 45-degree angle (Figure 18-76). Maintain distention of the vein while collecting the blood; then apply digital pressure at the site when the needle is removed.

Coccygeal Vein (Tail Vein)
The tail vein is commonly used when a large number of cattle are bled and when the jugular vein of an individual patient is thrombosed or inaccessible. The animal should be restrained in a chute or stanchion, and a tail jack restraint applied. This provides restraint and positions the tail for venipuncture. With one hand, the tail is lifted up and toward the back of the animal until it is vertical. The ventral surface of the tail is cleaned with 70% isopropyl alcohol to remove dirt and fecal material. An 18- to 21-gauge × 1.5-inch needle is attached to a syringe. The diameter of the coccygeal vein

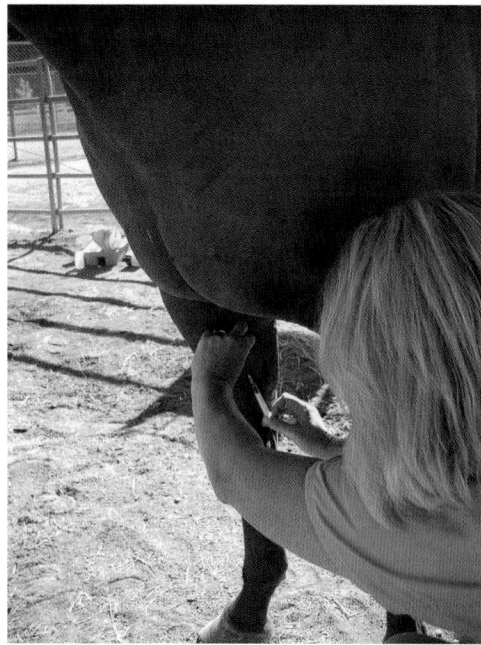

FIGURE 18-75 Venipuncture of equine cephalic vein.

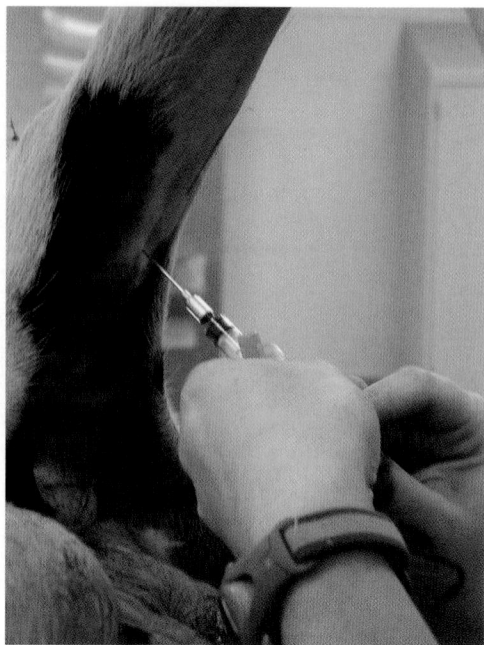

FIGURE 18-77 Venipuncture of bovine coccygeal vein.

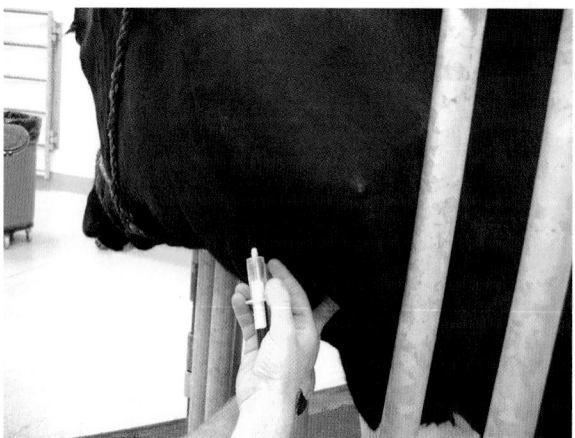

FIGURE 18-76 Blood collection from bovine jugular vein.

is considerably smaller than that of the jugular vein, so larger needles are inappropriate. Locate the soft space between two vertebrae by palpating between two bony prominences. These are hemal processes, which are bony canals on the ventral aspect of the vertebral bodies that protect the artery and vein. Insert the needle perpendicular to the midline until bone is felt, and then slowly back the needle out slightly from the bone while applying suction to the syringe. Blood should flow freely into the syringe. If preferred, a Vacutainer needle and tube can be used instead of a needle and syringe (Figure 18-77).

After sample collection is complete, withdraw the needle, lower the tail, and apply pressure to the site for approximately 15 seconds to discourage hematoma formation. The coccygeal artery lies in close proximity to the coccygeal vein and may be inadvertently punctured. If this is done, digital pressure should be applied to the site for at least 1 minute to prevent hematoma formation.

Subcutaneous Abdominal Venipuncture (Milk Vein)

The right and left milk veins are located along the ventro-lateral body wall of the thorax and abdomen. These provide major venous drainage of the udder. Use of these veins for venipuncture can result in life-threatening conditions for the cow. Milk veins are very large and are prone to prolonged and pronounced bleeding and large hematoma formation; they are at great risk for infection because they are easily contaminated by feces, dirt, and other material when the animal is recumbent. Thrombosis of the milk vein may lead to insufficient circulation to the udder, and collateral circulation is inadequate to overcome the problem. **It is recommended that these veins never be used for venipuncture.**

On very rare occasions and as a last resort, a veterinarian may direct the technician to collect a blood sample from the milk vein. In the event that no other vein is available for sampling and the veterinarian has deemed it necessary to collect a sample from the milk vein, the animal must be restrained adequately in a chute or stanchion with a tail jack or a leg restraint applied. The technician should stand next to the shoulder of the cow facing the tail, or should stand close to the flank facing the head. The technician then should bend just enough to insert the needle while keeping his or her head up to avoid contact when the cow kicks (there is a strong likelihood that the animal will kick when the needle is inserted).

Select an accessible site. Clean with isopropyl alcohol, stabilize the vein with one hand, hold the skin taut, and insert the needle (18- to 22-gauge × 1.5-inch needle) in either direction (the blood flows cranially) with the syringe attached. Alternatively, a Vacutainer collection needle may be inserted and a Vacutainer collection tube attached. After the

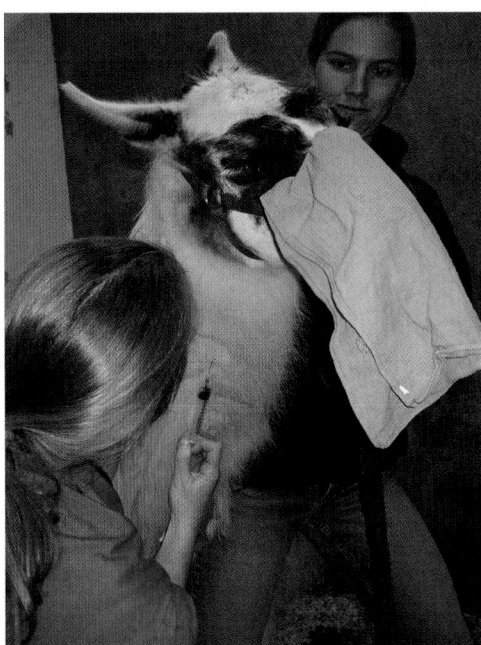

FIGURE 18-78 Blood collection from llama jugular vein. A towel can be draped loosely through the halter on the bridge of the nose to protect personnel from being spit upon if the animal objects to the procedure.

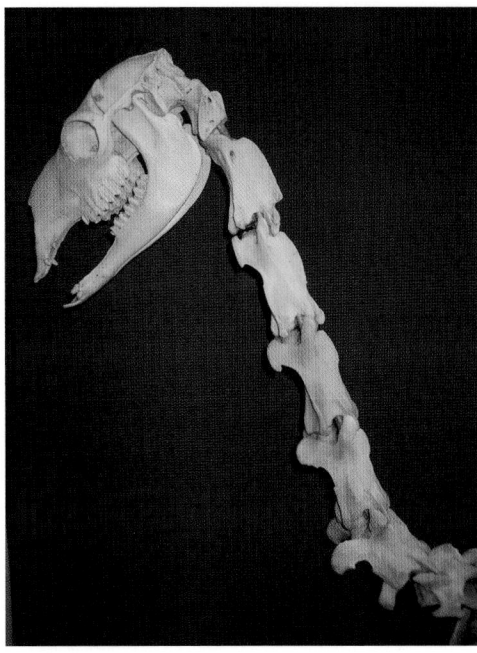

FIGURE 18-79 Cervical vertebrae of llama. The 6th cervical vertebra is used as a landmark for low neck venipuncture.

needle has been removed, prolonged digital pressure must be applied over the puncture site (for several minutes).

CAMELID (LLAMA, ALPACA, LAMOID, SOUTH AMERICAN CAMELID)

Jugular Vein

Llamas and alpacas provide challenges in jugular venipuncture. In adult animals, visualization of the jugular vein is not possible. No jugular groove is visible, the skin over the jugular vein is thick (in males it can be 1 cm thick), and fibers are long. The transverse process of a cervical vertebra has a ventral projection that curves around the jugular furrow, and llamas and alpacas have valves in the jugular vein that function to keep blood flowing toward the heart rather than allowing backflow when the head is lowered.

A jugular venipuncture can be performed at a high or a low site. The high site can be located by creating an imaginary line along the ventral border of the mandible and dropping an imaginary line vertically down from just in front of the ear. The intersection of these two lines provides a guide for locating the vein. In some animals, a fluid wave may be visualized by occlusion and ballottement of the vein (stroking the vein toward the occluding hand). The skin is thickest at this point, but the jugular vein is separated here from the carotid artery by a muscle, making the likelihood of arterial penetration at this site less than at the low neck site (Figure 18-78).

The low position is located by palpating the ventral projection of the transverse process of the sixth cervical vertebrae (this is close to the thorax and prominent) and occluding the vein just above the transverse process (Figure 18-79). As

with the high neck site, ballottement of a fluid wave can help to identify the vein. The skin is thinner at this location, and movement of the head is less of a problem than with the high neck site, but the fiber is thicker. The carotid artery and the jugular vein are in close proximity in this area; this increases the chance of arterial penetration.

Saphenous Vein

The saphenous vein is superficial and is found on the medial aspect of the stifle. This vein can be used in recumbent animals. The vein lies in close proximity and cranial to the artery.

Auricular (Ear) Vein

The ear vein can yield small amounts of blood, sufficient for many laboratory tests. Digital pressure is usually sufficient to raise the vein, but if necessary, an elastic band can be wrapped temporarily around the base of the ear as a tourniquet.

Middle Coccygeal Vein

The middle coccygeal vein is located as in cattle but is more superficial in camelids—just under the skin.

Cephalic Vein

The cephalic vein lies similar in placement to that of dogs and can be accessed in adults when the animal is in sternal recumbency (kushed position).

Neonatal Camelids (Crias)

Veins commonly used in neonates include the jugular, cephalic, and saphenous veins, and occasionally the ear vein.

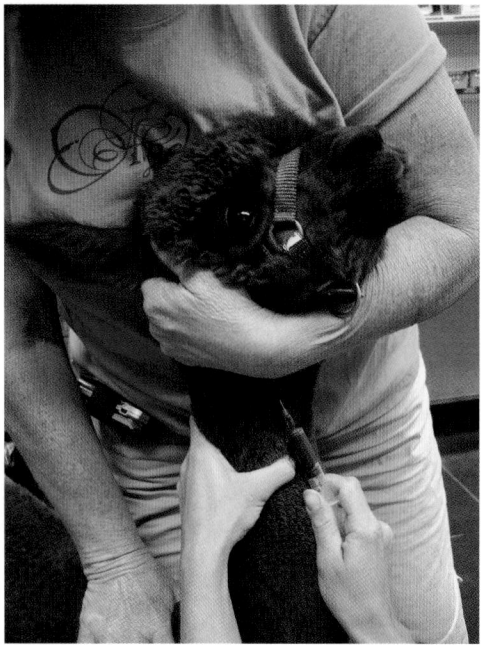

FIGURE 18-80 Blood collection from the jugular vein in alpaca cria.

The jugular vein is much easier to use in the neonate than in the adult because the skin is thin, and the jugular vein can be easily distended and visualized (Figure 18-80).

OVINE AND CAPRINE

Jugular, cephalic, and femoral veins are commonly used in sheep and goats. The ear vein also provides an accessible site for blood sampling.

Most sheep will be restrained in a "set-up" position on the rump with the back side leaning up against the handler (Figure 18-81). Jugular, cephalic, femoral, and ear samples can be taken from this position. Jugular, cephalic, and ear samples can be obtained from some sheep while they are standing, but having sheep "set up" on the rump will drastically reduce the amount of effort required to carry out most procedures (Figures 18-82 through 18-85). The jugular, cephalic, and ear veins can be easily accessed in goats while they are standing. The handler can restrain the animal by backing it into a corner and then straddling the goat with the handler's legs tight on either side of the neck, or can push the goat up against a wall. When straddling the animal, the handler should not underestimate the strength of the animal, and must be prepared so that an inadvertent ride is avoided. The femoral vein is accessible when the goat is in lateral recumbency.

PORCINE

Blood collection from swine is more difficult than from other large animals. These animals are challenging to restrain; have thick jowls, short legs, and tough skin; and are fat. Sampling can be done with the animal restrained or with the animal under anesthetic. The technician should be aware that in addition to commercial hogs, many pigs that are receiving veterinary care are beloved pets, and the handling

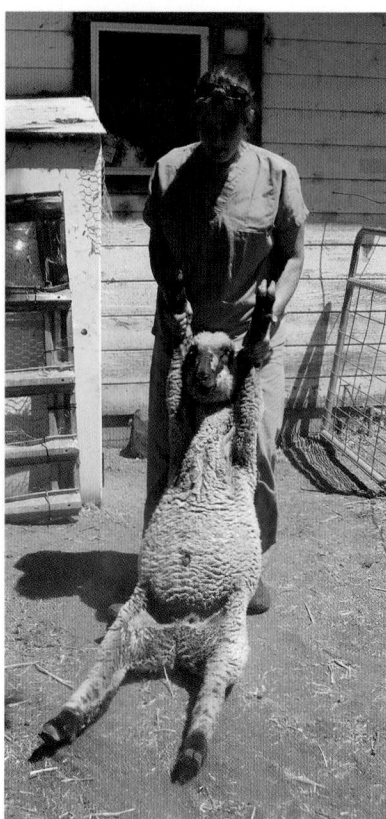

FIGURE 18-81 Setting sheep on the rump is an effective method of restraint for venipuncture and many other procedures.

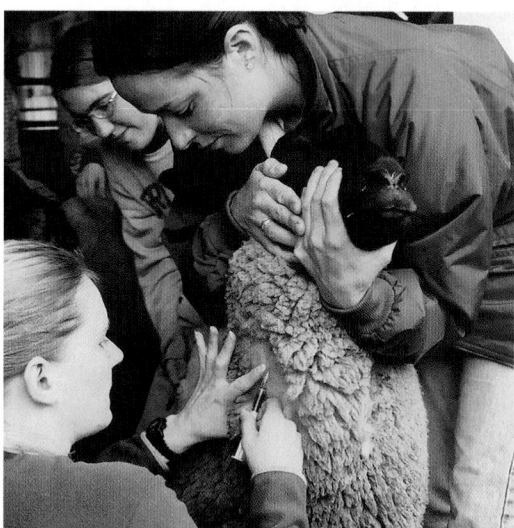

FIGURE 18-82 A technician crouches in front of a standing sheep to collect blood from the jugular vein. Note that the assistant at the rear of the sheep prevents the sheep from backing away from the technician.

and restraint required for venipuncture and other procedures should be explained well to the owner.

Veins commonly used for venous blood collection in pigs include cranial vena cava, jugular, auricular, cephalic, and peripheral leg veins, and occasionally the orbital sinus or tail vein.

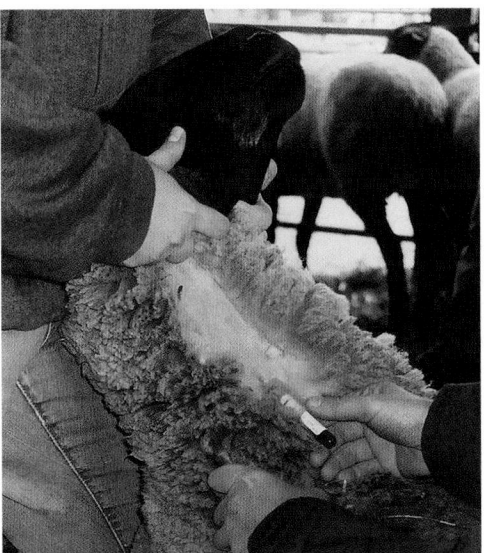

FIGURE 18-83 Sheep placed in a seated position to allow blood to be collected from the jugular vein.

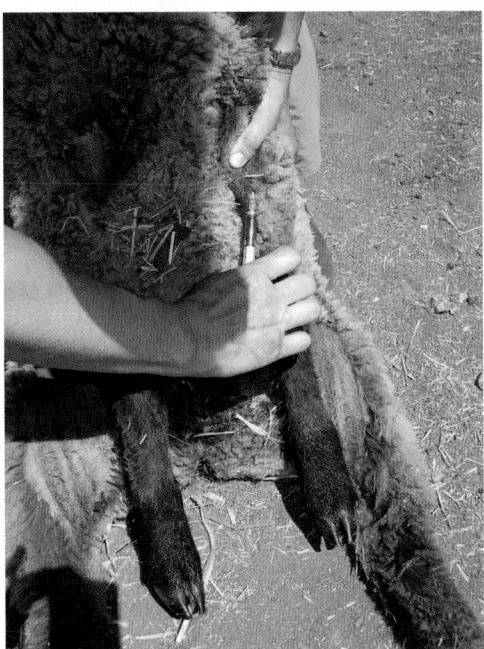

FIGURE 18-84 Collecting blood sample from cephalic vein while sheep is set up on the rump for restraint.

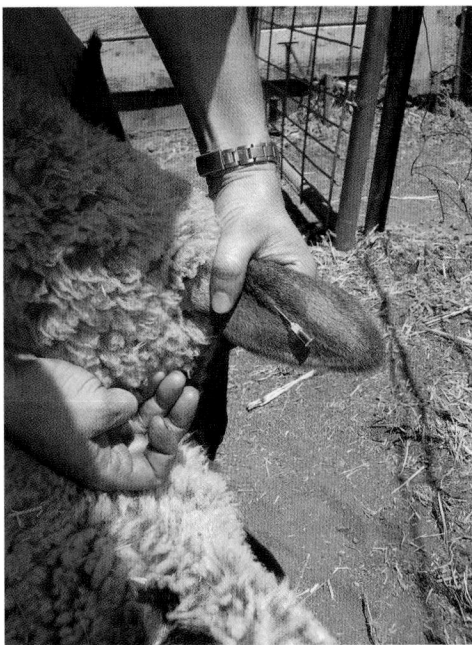

FIGURE 18-85 Blood samples can be obtained from the auricular vein in sheep.

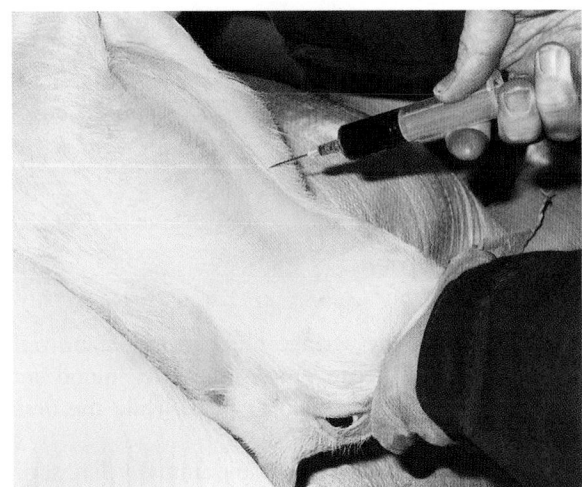

FIGURE 18-86 Venipuncture of right anterior vena cava in a small pig in dorsal recumbency.

Cranial Vena Cava

The cranial vena cava may be used for collection of blood from commercial pigs when a large volume of blood is desired, for example, for collection of blood to be used in transfusions or for health certificates. It is not used on pot-bellied or other pet pigs because of risk of death from the procedure. The cranial vena cava is located in the thoracic inlet between the first pair of ribs. The right side of the animal should be used to prevent damage to the phrenic nerve, which is anatomically more protected on the right side of the animal than on the left. Hitting the phrenic nerve may alter the function of the diaphragm and can result in

life-threatening cardiac or respiratory problems. For piglets, a 20-gauge × 1.5-inch needle is used. An 18- to 20-gauge × 1- to 1.5-inch needle is appropriate for small pigs (up to approximately 25 kg). For pigs weighing more than 25 kg, an 18- to 20-gauge × 1.5- to 3.5-inch needle is used. Large adults require a 16- to 18-gauge × 4- to 4.5-inch needle.

When blood is collected from a small pig, the animal is placed on its back (dorsal recumbency) on a 45-degree incline, with the head lower than the hips. The head is extended and the front legs pulled caudally. The jugular furrow is visualized, and the needle with a syringe attached is inserted into the furrow lateral to the manubrium of the sternum. The needle is pointed toward the caudal aspect of the top of the opposite shoulder blade (Figure 18-86). As the

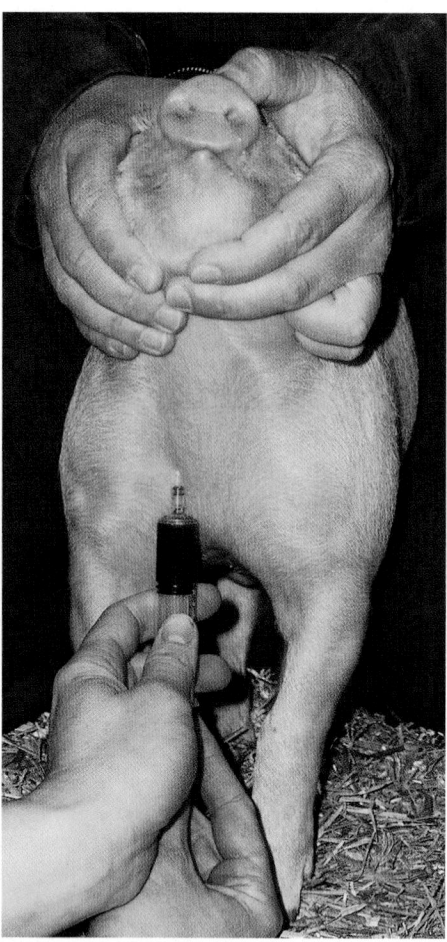

FIGURE 18-87 A blood sample from the right anterior vena cava is taken with the needle directed into the jugular fossa just lateral to the manubrium sterni.

needle is inserted, the syringe plunger should be pulled slightly to maintain negative pressure. When blood enters the syringe, the needle is held in place while the desired amount of blood is aspirated.

Blood can also be collected with the animal well restrained in a standing position with the head slightly elevated. Larger hogs are restrained with the use of a hog snare. The person with the syringe crouches in front of the right side of the pig facing the body of the pig, or can crouch to the side of the right shoulder facing the neck. The needle is inserted into the right jugular furrow lateral to the manubrium (Figure 18-87), directed toward the shoulder. The cranial vena cava in large pigs is deep (4 inches may be required to reach the lumen).

Jugular Vein

The jugular vein can be used for blood sample collection in commercial pigs of any age. It is not recommended for collection from pot-bellied or other pet pigs because of the risk of death from the procedure. It is located in the jugular furrow. It is not as deep as the vena cava, so fewer potential complications are associated with its use. The jugular vein has a smaller diameter than the vena cava and is more

difficult to access, especially in large or heavy pigs. The needle size selected depends on the size of the animal. A jugular venipuncture in piglets can be done with a 20-gauge × 1.5-inch needle. Large pigs may require 16-gauge × 3- to 3.5-inch needles. To prevent puncture of the phrenic nerve, the right side of the animal should be used when possible. The needle should be inserted cranial to the manubrium where the jugular furrow appears deepest. The animal is restrained as for a vena cava venipuncture. An imaginary horizontal line that passes through the shoulders and the manubrium sterni is visualized. A second line is visualized that extends from the manubrium sterni to the scapula at an angle of 45 degrees to the first line. The needle is inserted perpendicular to the skin at the intersection of the second line with the deepest part of the right jugular fossa. The needle is directed caudodorsally and should not be angled toward either scapula. Because the vein is superficial, the syringe plunger should be retracted slightly as soon as the needle penetrates the skin. The needle is advanced until blood is aspirated into the syringe. Once a sufficient volume of blood has been collected, the needle is removed.

The technician should be aware that fewer complications and lower risk for incidental injury to the animal are associated with venipuncture of the more distal veins discussed next.

Auricular Vein

The auricular vein is located near the lateral border of the pinna of the ear. It is easily visualized on the dorsal side of the ear and can be seen even more clearly by placing digital pressure at the base of the lateral surface of the ear. The ear is held and digital pressure (or rubber-band tourniquet) applied at the base of the ear to distend the vein. A needle with a syringe attached can be inserted into the vein while gently pulling back on the plunger. To prevent collapse of the vein with aspiration, some people prefer to insert the needle and allow the blood to drip from the needle hub directly into the uncapped collection tube. For most pigs, a 20-gauge × 1-inch needle is appropriate. For large adult pigs, an 18- to 19-gauge × 1-inch needle may be used. Vacutainer collection needles and tubes may apply too much suction, and, as in the case of excess pressure on the syringe plunger, they tend to cause the vein to collapse. When an adequate blood sample has been collected, pressure is released from the base of the ear, the needle removed, and pressure applied to the insertion site. For repeated sampling, placement of an IV catheter should be considered.

Peripheral Leg Veins

The cephalic vein on the front leg, the saphenous vein on the hind leg, and branches of veins located on the lower limbs are accessible in small pigs and can be used for venous sampling. These veins can be visualized and are readily accessible in anesthetized pigs. To prevent collapse of the vein, the needle is inserted, and blood is allowed to drip from the hub of the needle into the open collection tube (Figure 18-88). Collection of blood from the standing and restrained pig can

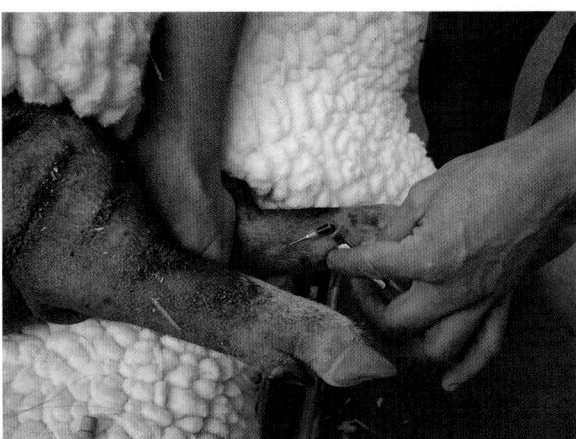

FIGURE 18-88 Collecting blood from the peripheral leg vein in a pig. Blood dripping from the needle hub into the collection tube prevents vein collapse.

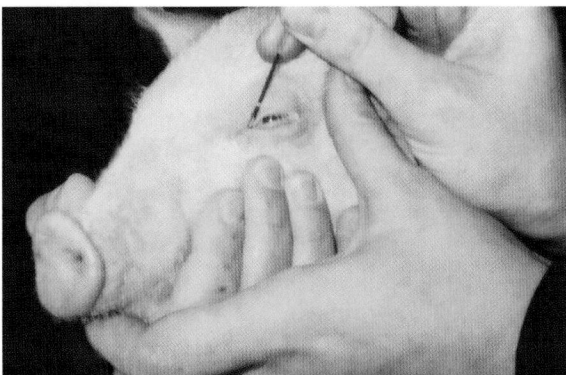

FIGURE 18-89 Small quantities of blood can be collected from the orbital sinus of the pig.

be done by placing hand pressure or a tourniquet above the collection site to distend the vein. A 20-gauge × 1- to 1.5-inch needle is inserted at approximately a 45-degree angle to the skin in the direction of the body.

Coccygeal Vein

Although this site is not commonly used in commercial pigs, it is frequently used for blood sample collection from pot-bellied pigs. It can be used for venipuncture in adult pigs with intact (not docked) tails. A 20-gauge × 1-inch needle is inserted at the ventral midline of the tail perpendicular to the skin.

Orbital Sinus (Medial Canthus of the Eye)

The orbital sinus is adjacent to the medial canthus of the eye and can be used for collection of small volumes of blood. A 20- to 22-gauge × 1-inch needle can be used for piglets. Sampling on larger pigs may require a 16- to 18-gauge × 1.5-inch needle. The needle is inserted into the medial canthus deep into the third eyelid (nictitating membrane) and is advanced at a 45-degree angle toward the opposite jaw until bone is felt. The needle is then rotated between the fingers until blood enters the hub. The syringe is attached and blood collected with gentle aspiration. When collection is complete, the needle is removed and digital pressure applied over the medial canthus with the head elevated. A microcapillary tube with the end broken to form a rough point can be used in lieu of a needle (Figure 18-89).

ARTERIAL BLOOD SAMPLE COLLECTION

Arterial blood samples are commonly obtained for blood gas analysis. This analysis usually provides information on oxygen and carbon dioxide content, pH, base deficit, and bicarbonate in the sample. This information is used to evaluate respiratory status. If the data include base deficit and bicarbonate, the analysis is also used to assess metabolic (acid-base) status. Arterial blood reflects the ventilation status of an animal more accurately than venous blood because arteries carry freshly oxygenated blood from the heart to the body. Veins carry blood back to the heart for circulation to the lungs, where oxygen is replenished and carbon dioxide released. Arterial blood gas samples are frequently obtained intraoperatively from animals under a general anesthetic. Arterial catheters are commonly placed in anesthetized animals to facilitate sequential blood sampling. Values obtained from the sample analysis allow close anesthesia monitoring.

Arterial samples are routinely collected in nonanesthetized foals and crias, and are less frequently taken from adult equines and camelids. Arterial sampling in cattle, sheep, goats, and pigs is rarely done on nonanesthetized animals.

The smallest gauge needle possible should be used to minimize trauma to the vessel. For most sample sites, a 25-gauge needle and a 1- or 3-ml syringe are used. A very small amount of heparin (enough to fill the needle and appear in the hub) is aspirated into the needle, and the plunger is pulled back on the syringe to coat the syringe. The needle is removed, and a new 25-gauge needle is placed on the syringe; the heparin is then expelled from the syringe through the new needle. In this way, the needle being used for the injection is as sharp as possible, because it was not dulled by puncturing the rubber stopper of the heparin vile. The heparin residue that remains in the syringe is sufficient to prevent coagulation but is not enough to alter laboratory results. Some veterinarians prefer to use commercially prepared blood gas syringes containing powdered heparin (Figure 18-90).

Some veterinarians prefer to have sites for arterial puncture shaved before cleaning with alcohol (this is often the case with arterial samples on neonatal patients). The area is palpated to determine the location of the artery. Arteries pulsate; veins do not. The selected artery site is given a surgical prep or is at least cleaned well with 70% isopropyl alcohol before insertion of the needle. It is not necessary to occlude arteries as is done with venous blood sampling. Depending on the patient's behavior and the site selected, the needle may be inserted first and the syringe attached when blood comes from the hub, or the needle may be inserted with a

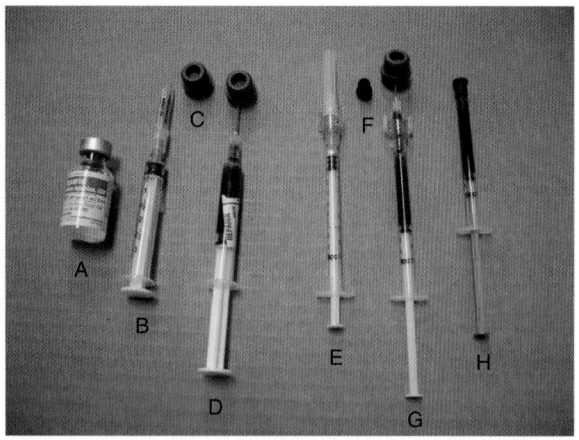

FIGURE 18-90 Syringes for blood gas sample collection. *A*, Sodium heparin (1000 U/ml). *B*, 3-ml syringe with barrel coated with heparin. *C*, Rubber stopper. *D*, Blood sample in syringe. *E*, Commercial preheparinized syringe (Micro ABG, Marquest, Englewood, Colorado). *F*, Stopper. *G*, Micro ABG syringe with needle inserted into the rubber stopper. *H*, Micro ABG syringe with cap.

syringe attached. When the needle enters the artery, bright red blood pulses from the needle hub into the syringe. With most arterial samples, blood will rapidly fill the syringe. Very little force is placed on the plunger of the syringe because the blood in the artery is under pressure and will spurt out. Do not expect blood to spurt from the needle as would be expected with a large-gauge needle. A minimum of 1 ml of blood should be collected into the syringe that has been prepared with liquid heparin to ensure results with diagnostic value. Smaller volumes can be taken using commercial blood gas syringes because these syringes are designed to eliminate dilutional errors. When the needle is withdrawn, firm digital pressure should be applied immediately to the puncture site and should be maintained for several minutes. Arteries are far more susceptible to hematoma formation than veins. The technician must make sure to apply sufficient pressure long enough to stop bleeding and prevent formation of a hematoma. If care is taken with this step, the artery will be preserved and will be able to handle repeated sampling. If insufficient pressure and time are taken to hold off the collection site, the artery will become damaged and may become unusable for future sampling; the related area may suffer from impaired circulation, thus compromising the condition of the patient.

> **TECHNICIAN NOTE** Following the collection of arterial blood samples, firm digital pressure should be applied immediately to the puncture site and maintained for several minutes.

Any bubbles present in the syringe are expelled, and the tip of the needle is inserted into a rubber stopper to occlude the needle tip and prevent air from entering the syringe. Samples for blood gas analysis must remain anaerobic (not contaminated by atmospheric air) because exposure to air

will modify oxygen and carbon dioxide values. The syringe should be rolled between the palms to ensure distribution of anticoagulant throughout the sample. If the sample is not analyzed promptly, it should be placed in an ice water bath. Placing the sample in a freezer or on ice (with no water added) can damage the sample and affect the results of the analysis.

> **TECHNICIAN NOTE** Samples for blood gas analysis must remain anaerobic (not contaminated by atmospheric air) because exposure to air will alter the laboratory values obtained.

EQUINE

Arteries commonly used for blood sampling in horses include facial (most often used in anesthetized animals), transverse facial, carotid, and metatarsal (in recumbent foals and anesthetized animals). In addition to these sites, arterial sampling on foals can include brachial and palmar (digital) arteries.

The facial artery is accessible in the area under the mandible to the facial crest. This site is commonly used for arterial catheterization in anesthetized animals (Figure 18-91, *A* through *D*).

The transverse facial artery lies caudal to the lateral canthus of the eye (Figure 18-92). Some people prefer to inject 0.25 ml of 2% lidocaine into the skin over the artery before a sample needle insertion, but often there is little or no objection from horses when this site is used without a lidocaine block.

The carotid artery is accessible in the lower third of the neck, in the dorsal aspect of the jugular groove, and is deeper than the jugular vein. The artery feels like a cord, and a pulse is not usually palpable. An 18- to 19-gauge × 1.5-inch needle is directed into the artery at a 90-degree angle.

The dorsal metatarsal artery is located on the lateral aspect of the third metatarsal bone (cannon bone on hindlimb) and is the preferred site of sampling in recumbent foals (Figure 18-93). A pulse is usually quite palpable. If a pulse is not obvious, the technician may put firm digital pressure proximal to the selected site, slowly release pressure, and feel for the pulse; this often enhances the pulse quality distally. In very sick neonates with poor blood pressure, the pulse may not be felt. In these patients, it is helpful to place a warm-water bottle or compress over the artery to enhance the feel of local pulsation of the artery. The technician sits with the foal's hind hoof secured between the technician's knees. The artery is palpated with one hand, and the needle inserted with the other hand. The foal's leg can be secured by holding it between the technician's legs (Figure 18-94). Some patients require that another handler restrain the foal; the technician should make use of available help because procedures can be done more quickly and with less stress to the patient and less risk for injury to personnel when sufficient restraint is used. The behavior and condition of some foals allow the procedure to be done by the technician with

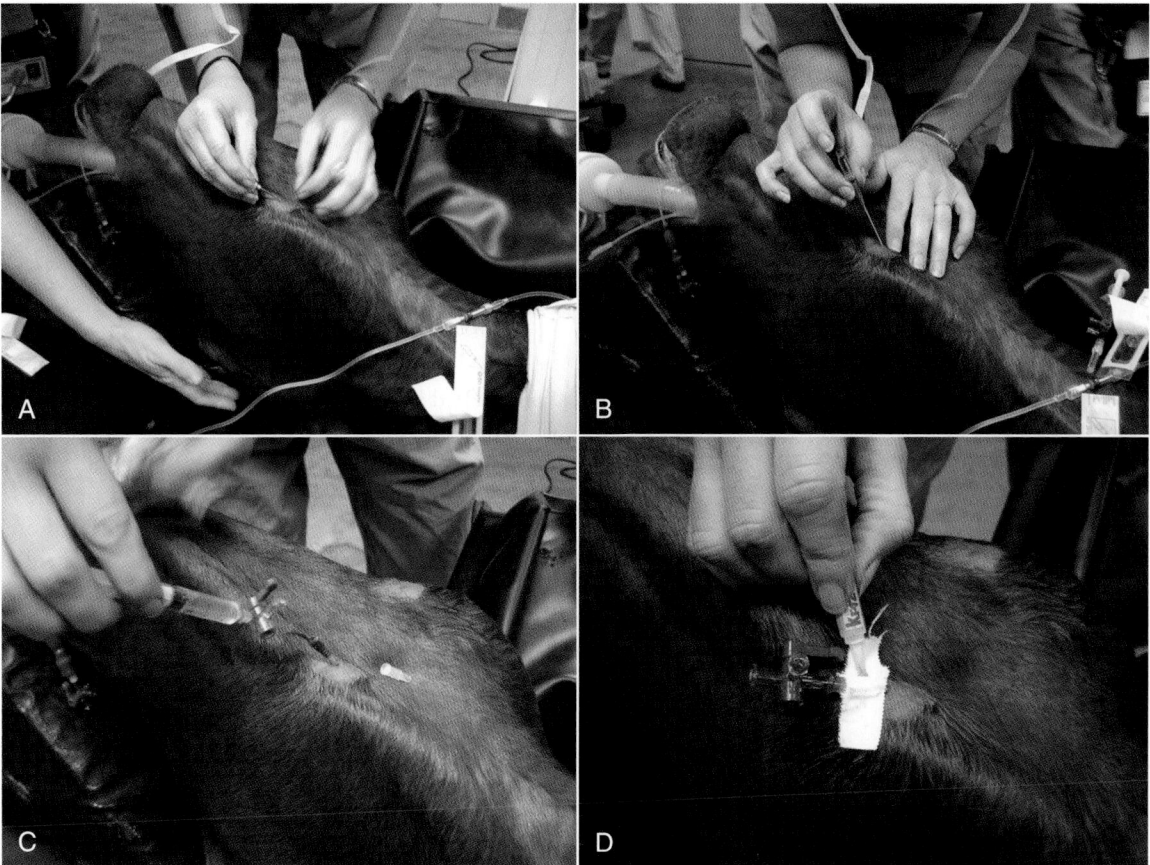

FIGURE 18-91 **A,** Nicking skin with a needle to ease insertion for placing the arterial catheter in the facial artery. **B,** Inserting the catheter. **C,** Placing stopcock on the catheter. **D,** Securing the arterial catheter with glue.

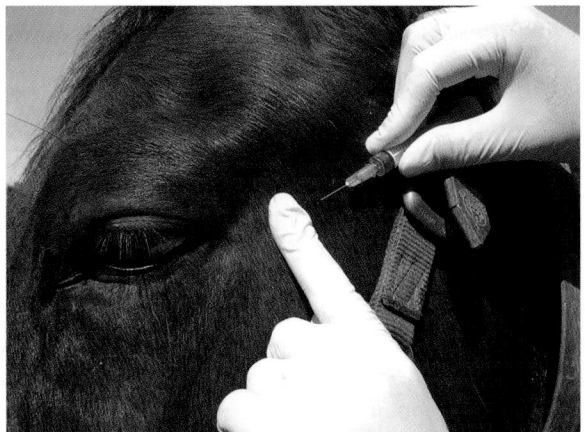

FIGURE 18-92 Collecting an arterial sample from the facial artery in an awake equine.

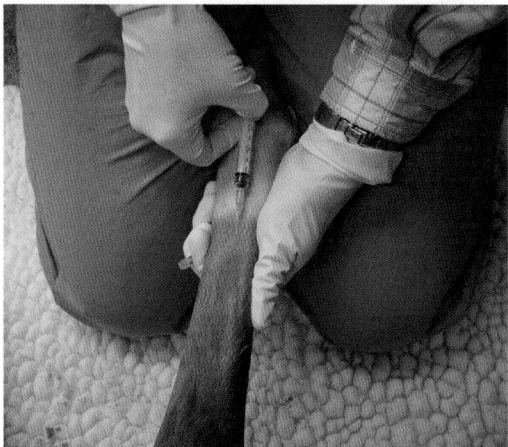

FIGURE 18-93 Restraining the foal's hind leg between the technician's knees facilitates collection of arterial samples from the metatarsal artery in foals.

no additional restraint. This decision depends on the patient and the experience and skill of the technician. Many foals will accept this procedure if the needle is slowly and smoothly inserted into the skin. Some foals (even though very sick) will vehemently object to the needle insertion and will jerk and kick the leg. In these foals, the needle is quickly inserted, and the syringe is attached after the foal's leg is again secured in place.

The palmar (digital) artery is palpable on the abaxial surface of the fetlock. This site is more difficult to access because the artery moves around quite a bit, and the location precludes restraining the foal's leg between the technician's legs.

The brachial artery may be palpated where it crosses the medial aspect of the proximal forearm and may

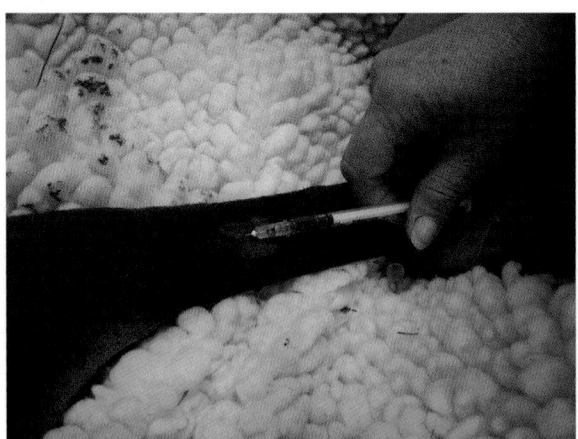

FIGURE 18-94 Collecting an arterial sample from the metatarsal artery in a recumbent foal.

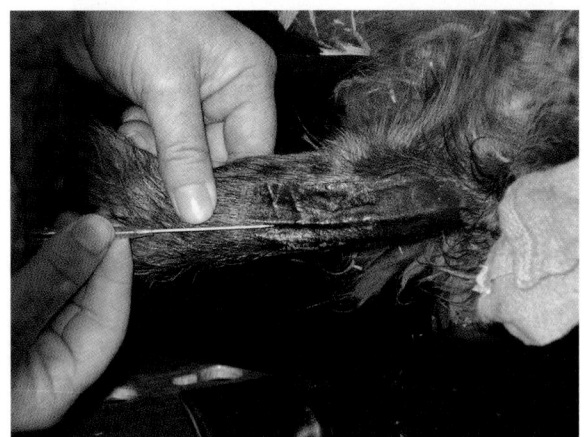

FIGURE 18-95 Placing an arterial catheter in the ear of a llama.

yield a sample when attempts at other sites have been unsuccessful.

CAMELID

The auricular (ear) artery is often used in llamas and alpacas for arterial sampling (Figure 18-95).

BOVINE, OVINE, AND CAPRINE

Arteries used for sampling in these animals include the transverse facial, carotid, auricular, and dorsal metatarsal. As noted previously, collection of arterial samples from these animals is usually restricted to anesthetized individuals or neonatal patients.

Arterial Catheterization

A short OTN catheter can be placed in the artery of an anesthetized patient.

Arteries commonly catheterized in the horse include transverse facial and dorsal metatarsal. Arteries commonly catheterized in food animals include transverse facial, dorsal metatarsal, and auricular.

URINE SAMPLE COLLECTION

Urine is collected from patients to screen for systemic (e.g., rhabdomyolysis, azoturia) or urinary tract disease. Urine is routinely analyzed in race and performance horses for drug detection purposes. Urine can be collected for urinalysis from all large animal species in a free catch midstream sample. Catheterization is recommended for samples that will be cultured, but, as is described later, bladder catheterization is not always possible. Cystocentesis is not practical in horses because of the inability to stabilize the bladder and the risk for intestinal perforation with the needle. It may be performed by some veterinarians on small ruminants.

For all urine samples, the sample should be collected in a dry, clean container (sterile if a culture is desired and catheterization is performed). A midstream sample should be collected because the initial stream contains more bacteria, mucus, and cell debris than the rest of the urine and does not as accurately reflect the actual content of the urine. Bacterial contamination in free catch samples is significant. Urine samples degrade rapidly, so samples should be analyzed promptly (within 20 minutes) or refrigerated for no longer than 2 days.

> **TECHNICIAN NOTE** Urine samples degrade rapidly, so they should be analyzed promptly or refrigerated for no longer than 2 days.

Complications of urinary catheterization include infection of the urinary tract if sterile technique is not followed, mucosal irritation, slow and painful urination, and bacterial contamination of the sample.

EQUINE
Free Catch Method

Urination may be encouraged by placing the horse in a freshly bedded stall. Sometimes standing the horse on a grassy area will encourage urination. Other suggestions include running water on cement and tickling the prepuce with a piece of straw. Some race and performance horses have been conditioned to urinate when whistled to. Recumbent neonates frequently will urinate when they are assisted to stand. The technician should be prepared by having a urine collection container within reach when helping a foal to rise or supporting it in a standing position.

> **TECHNICIAN NOTE** A midstream sample should be collected.

Cleansing of the external genital area is not necessary when urine is collected for drug testing.

Urinary Catheterization
Materials Needed

- Urinary catheter: use the tube with the smallest outer diameter possible to minimize trauma to the urethra (Figure 18-96)

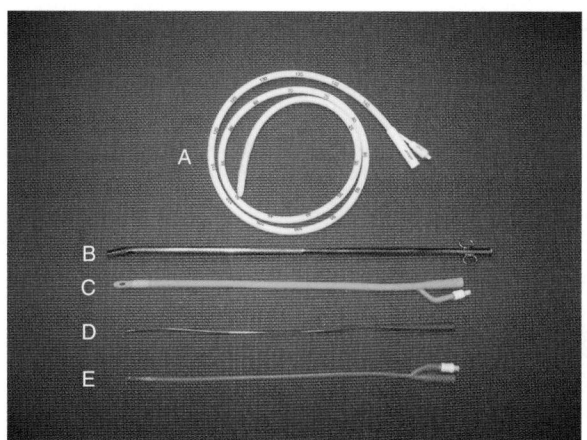

FIGURE 18-96 Urinary catheters. **A,** Stallion catheter. **B,** Mare Chambers catheter. **C,** 28-French Foley catheter. **D,** 12-French Foley catheter. **E,** 12-French red rubber feeding tube.

- Adult males: urinary (Foley) catheter 24-French to 28-French with 6- to 9-mm outer diameter and approximately 140 cm long
- Colts: red rubber feeding catheter 12-French
- Adult females: Chambers catheter or Foley catheter 30-French
- Fillies: Foley catheter 12-French
- Sixty-milliliter catheter tip syringe
- Sterile gloves
- Gentle antimicrobial soap and 70% rubbing alcohol or other disinfectant cleanser (povidone-iodine solution and scrub)
- Soft cotton
- Sterile lubricant
- Sterile collection containers (for urinalysis, cytologic examination, and culture)
- Sedation

Male Horses

Sedation is usually required when stallions and geldings are catheterized for restraint and extension of the penis from the prepuce. The technician should be positioned cranially to avoid being kicked. Retract the prepuce, grasp the penis gently but firmly caudal to the glans penis (hold steady as the horse may attempt to retract the penis), and wash the penis with dilute antibacterial soap. Care must be taken to cleanse the urethral process and the urethral diverticulum (a blind pouch located dorsal to the urethral opening), making sure to remove any smegma "bean" present in the diverticulum. Then rinse with water. This must be done to prevent introduction into the bladder of bacteria that are present at the urethra and prepuce, and to prevent bacterial contamination of the urine sample. While wearing sterile gloves, apply sterile, water-soluble lubricant to the tip of a flexible urinary catheter. Hold the penis with one hand, and use the other hand to gently advance the catheter through the urethra and into the bladder. A curvature is present in the area of the ischial arch (just ventral to the anus), and

slight force may be necessary to advance the catheter past this point. The horse characteristically will raise its tail when the catheter passes over the ischial arch just before it reaches the bladder.

If urine does not flow from the catheter, a syringe can be attached to gently aspirate the sample. Excessive negative pressure must not be used because it may cause minor hemorrhage and can alter the sample composition. A small volume of air can be injected into the catheter, or the catheter can be repositioned, if necessary, to encourage flow.

Female Horses

Wrap the tail and tie it out of the way to prevent hair from entering the vagina or touching the glove or catheter, thus introducing contaminants.

Thoroughly clean the vulva and the perineum. Using sterile gloves with sterile, water-soluble lubricant, locate the urethral orifice on the ventral aspect of the vaginal vault. The orifice is approximately 10 to 12 cm from the ventral commissure of the vulvar lips. A small Chambers catheter, stallion catheter, or Foley catheter can be used. Lubricate the catheter, and use a finger to slide the catheter in and down into the urethral orifice; advance the catheter 5 to 10 cm (2 to 4 inches) until it enters the bladder (Figure 18-97, *A* through *D*). The flow of urine can be promoted as described earlier.

CAMELID

Free Catch Method

Llamas and alpacas urinate and defecate on communal dung piles, so, if possible, the animal should be led to a dung pile. Attaching a collection cup to the end of a broom or dowel facilitates collection without requiring personnel to be close enough to distract the animal. Both males and females urinate in a caudal direction while in a squatting position. Complete urination usually takes 30 to 60 seconds.

Urinary Catheterization of Llamas and Alpacas

In addition to the sigmoid shape of the penis, which makes passage of urinary catheters extremely difficult, male llamas and alpacas have a membranous flap at the ischial arch that prevents passage of urinary catheters into the bladder, so this procedure cannot be done in male patients.

Materials Needed for Urinary Catheterization of Female Llamas and Alpacas

- Sterile gloves
- Sterile, water-soluble lubricant
- Sixty-milliliter catheter tip syringe
- Red rubber tube or polypropylene catheter 5-French
- Gentle antimicrobial soap or other cleanser
- Soft cotton
- Sample collection containers (sterile if culture desired)
- Sedation, if necessary

Restrain the llama or alpaca. Clean the lips of the vulva and dry the area. While wearing sterile gloves, place a small

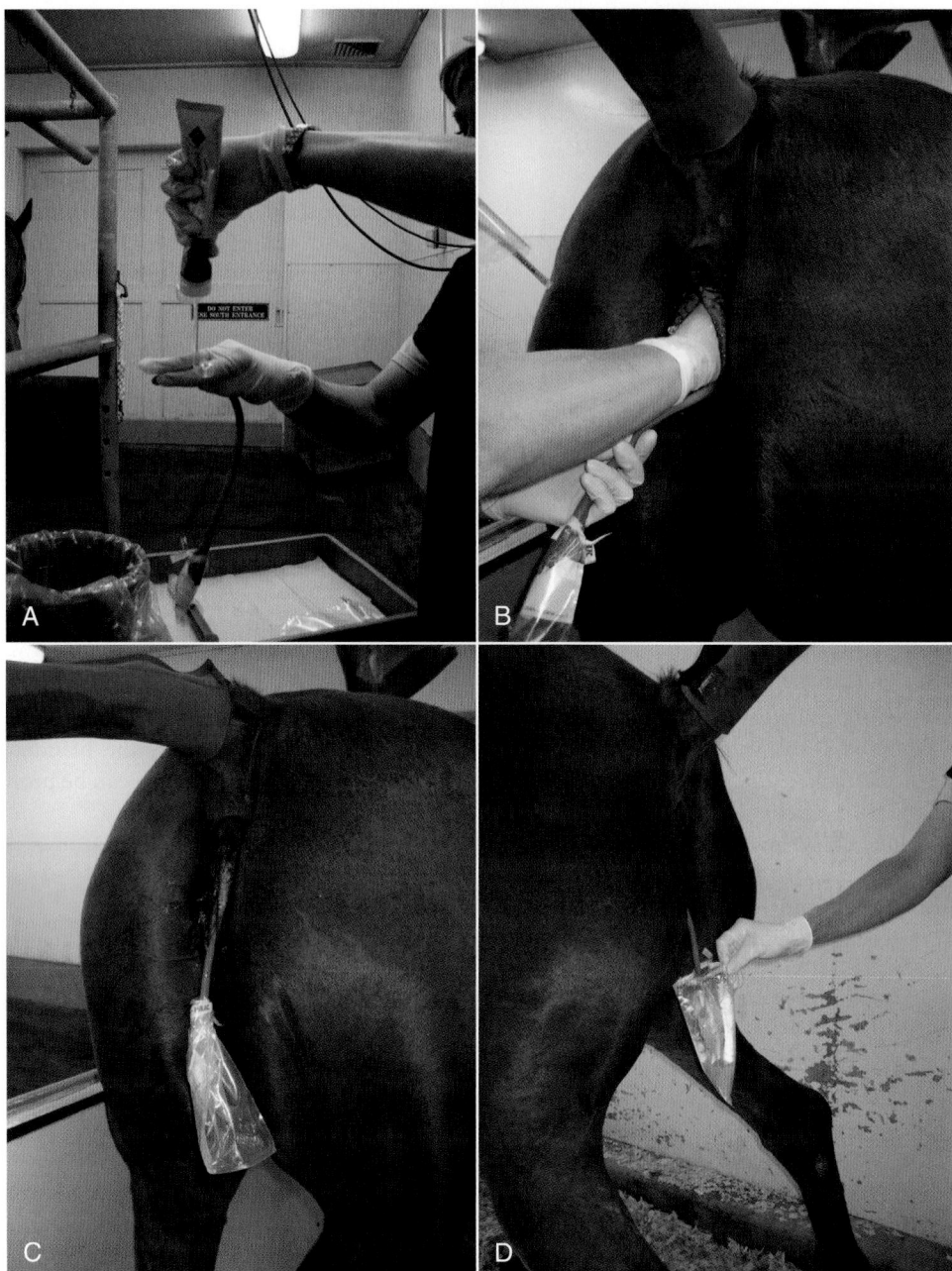

FIGURE 18-97 Urinary catheterization in the mare. **A,** Applying sterile, water-soluble lubricant to the back of a sterile gloved hand holding a urinary catheter. **B,** Inserting a urinary catheter. **C,** Urinary catheter with a small plastic bag on the end for sample collection. **D,** Collecting a urine sample from a catheter.

amount of lubricant on the glove. Insert a finger into the vulva and locate the external urethral orifice. This is felt as a groove on the floor of the vulva. When located, withdraw the finger slightly, and slide the catheter along the dorsal aspect of the index finger into the orifice. Sliding the catheter along the finger in this manner avoids insertion into a blind ventral urethral diverticulum, which is located just caudal to the orifice of the urethra. Slowly advance the catheter. For most adult llamas or alpacas, the catheter is inserted about 25 cm from the vulvar lips to enter the bladder. Collect a free-flowing sample into a sterile container, or attach a syringe and gently aspirate the fluid.

BOVINE
Free Catch Method
Place the animal in a chute or stanchion, and allow the animal to relax. Urination in cows may be encouraged by lightly stroking the vulvar tip and the skin beneath the vulva. The technician may try repeated parting of the lips of the vulva to elicit urination. Steers and bulls may oblige with urination if the prepuce is massaged and splashed with warm water. Urine is collected into a container, or, depending on the required analysis, a urine dipstick (litmus paper test strip) can be held directly in the stream of urine. This technique is often used to monitor urine pH and ketones.

Urethral to bladder catheterization in male cattle is virtually impossible because of the anatomy and therefore is not performed by the technician.

Cows can be catheterized with a small-diameter (0.5-cm) catheter with techniques similar to those used for mares. The perineal region is gently scrubbed with an antiseptic solution and is rinsed well with warm water. A sterile gloved and lubricated hand is inserted into the vagina and is slid forward along the floor of the vagina (approximately 10 cm in an adult), where a finger is inserted into the suburethral diverticulum; the catheter tip is then guided over the diverticulum and into the external urethral orifice. Urine will flow through the catheter when it has reached the bladder.

OVINE AND CAPRINE
Free Catch Method

Both ewes and does tend to urinate immediately after rising following a period of recumbency. The technician should be prepared to collect a urine sample when the animal rises. This is the easiest approach and causes the least stress to the animal.

Urination may be induced in ewes by occluding the nostrils for up to 45 seconds while the animal is standing. This causes stress to the animal and may be unpleasant for the owner to view. This should be taken into consideration and explained to the owner clearly before the method is attempted. The animal will indicate discomfort by struggling, and as the nostrils are released and the animal is allowed to breathe again, she will urinate. Holding the nostrils of does seldom results in urination. Providing clean bedding/a newly cleaned pen may elicit urination and may be an easy way to encourage urination. Male ruminants may respond to manual stimulation of the prepuce; the technician should be prepared with a collection container and should make every effort to collect a sample when the animal obliges.

Urinary Catheterization
Males

As with male cattle, male sheep (rams) and male goats (bucks) have anatomic obstacles that make catheterization of the bladder extremely difficult, and the procedure is not commonly attempted. Catheterization of the urethra (not completely into the bladder) is commonly performed on blocked goats (urinary passage is blocked with urinary stones). The urethra opens 1 to 2 cm beyond the tip of the glans penis through the urethral process. It is difficult to enter this narrow structure with a catheter. The S-shaped curvature of the penis (sigmoid flexure) provides another obstacle to passage of a catheter. In addition, a urethral diverticulum (a blind sac) near the ischial arch prevents the catheter from entering the bladder. Male goats can be catheterized directly into the bladder from the body wall through an ultrasound-guided procedure. This is done to allow the urethra to heal or to release pressure caused by accumulation of urine.

Females

Properly restrain the animal and hold or tie the tail out of the way during the procedure to prevent contamination. Cleanse the vulva. While wearing sterile gloves, apply sterile, water-soluble lubricant to the fingers, and pass the fingers into the vagina. The urethral opening is found midline on the ventral surface within 5 to 10 cm of the vulva (depending on the size of the animal). The vulvae of ewes and does are quite small. A small animal vaginal speculum may be helpful in allowing visualization of the urethral opening. A 5-French to 12-French urinary catheter is inserted. Female ruminants have a small suburethral diverticulum (blind sac) that extends from the ventral aspect of the urethra. If the catheter is inadvertently fed into the diverticulum, resistance will be felt, and the catheter should be pulled out slightly and redirected more dorsally. When the catheter is in the bladder, urine is likely to flow spontaneously, but if necessary, gentle aspiration can be placed on the catheter with a sterile syringe.

PORCINE

The technician should be ready with a collection cup because free catch urine is necessary for a urinalysis in swine. It is common for adult swine to urinate 2 or 3 times a day.

Males should be confined and observed; when quiet, the prepuce may be stroked with a warm wet towel or a soft brush. Titillating the vulva by stroking with the fingers, a soft brush, or dry straw can be attempted in females.[1] Male pigs cannot be catheterized because of the inaccessibility of the penis and the small diameter of the urethra.

Females can be catheterized with the aid of a vaginal speculum and a canine catheter, but this procedure is not routinely performed.

FECAL SAMPLE COLLECTION

Fecal samples are collected for gross visual inspection; to check for the presence of mucus, sand, or blood (frank or occult); for microscopic examination to check for intestinal parasites; and for microbiological culture or **polymerase chain reaction (PCR)** assay. Occasionally, feces may be evaluated for osmolality and electrolyte concentration (to determine the presence of an osmotic diarrhea). The technician should be familiar with the normal character (content, consistency, color, and odor) and volume of feces for each species.

Feces contain a variety of bacteria that are normal and nonpathogenic. Fecal samples are cultured for specific microorganisms (such as *Salmonella*) by inoculating the feces into an enrichment medium that is designed to inhibit growth of many normal bacteria while encouraging growth of the specific bacterium to be identified. Some PCR assays that are now available are more sensitive and provide quicker results than microbial culture for specific pathogens. If the animal is not producing feces, the technician may be asked to collect a rectal swab for a laboratory culture.

Fresh feces should be collected and placed in a clean container. Fresh feces will yield more accurate diagnostic information for parasite identification and an accurate culture result. Feces may be collected from the ground or from the rectum with a gloved hand.

> **TECHNICIAN NOTE**   Fresh feces will yield more accurate diagnostic information for parasite identification and culture.

If feces are to be collected directly from the rectum, the person must have fingernails clipped short and should be wearing no rings or watches. The horse is restrained (preferably in stocks) and an obstetric sleeve worn with generous amounts of lubrication gel applied to the sleeve. The person will stand slightly to the side of the horse, touch fingertips together, and slowly and gently insert the hand just far enough into the rectum to collect a handful of feces. The glove or sleeve can be turned inside out and tied in a knot to store the sample. The utmost care must be taken by the technician because rectal tears can occur and may be life threatening.

If sand colic is suspected in a horse, fecal sedimentation may be used as a diagnostic test. Feces can be mixed in the glove or sleeve with water and the sleeve hung up to allow solid material to settle in the sleeve. Sandy material may be seen or felt through the fingers of the glove.

MILK SAMPLE COLLECTION

Milk samples are routinely collected from dairy animals to test for the presence of mastitis. Mastitis is an inflammation of the mammary gland that is commonly caused by bacterial infection. Inflammation may be present without a bacterial component if the teat or udder has received a traumatic injury (kicked, stepped on, cut). Clinical mastitis refers to the presence of obvious clinical signs, including a hard, hot udder; abnormal appearance or smell of the milk; and pain. Subclinical mastitis must be confirmed by diagnostic testing of the milk.

Colostrum samples are frequently collected from mares and cows and tested to determine the quality of colostrum present.

STERILE MILK SAMPLE

Thoroughly wash and dry hands. Clean the teat end with an alcohol-soaked cotton swab. Repeat until the cotton is clean after rubbing the end of the teat. Allow the alcohol to dry. Using clean, dry hands, remove the top of a culture tube. Each quarter of the cow's udder (each half in small ruminants) is considered individually. If milk from more than one teat is collected, the teats nearest the milker should be sampled first to prevent contamination of the far-side teats by the arm of the milker. Hold the tube so that no dirt or debris will fall into the tube, and do not allow anything to touch the opening of the tube. Discard the first few squirts of milk, then squirt a stream of milk directly into the collection tube and replace the top.

Refrigerate the sample for up to 24 hours before laboratory processing.

NONSTERILE MILK SAMPLE
Samples for California Mastitis Test

The California mastitis test (CMT) is commonly used to identify the presence of mastitis in cows (or does and ewes). This test involves the use of a white plastic test paddle with four cups labeled A to D and a reagent fluid (Figure 18-98).

The teats are cleaned and dried. It is not necessary to clean the entire udder. If washed completely, the risk of introducing contaminants from the udder into the teat orifice is increased. Strip a small amount of milk, and discard the first stream before collecting the sample to avoid a false-positive result. Strip a small amount from one teat into one well of the paddle. Do the same for the remaining teats, and note which teat was milked into each well (Figure 18-99). An

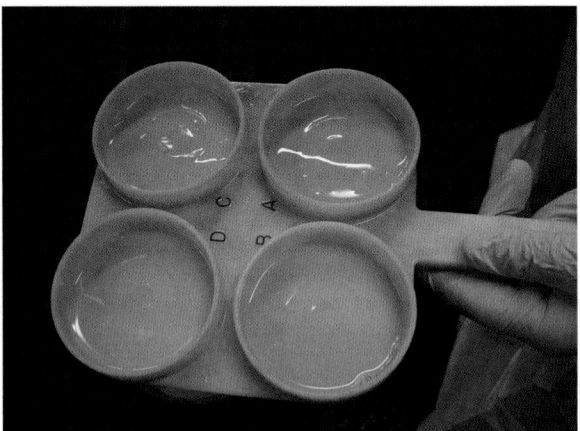

FIGURE 18-98 CMT (California Mastitis Test) paddle.

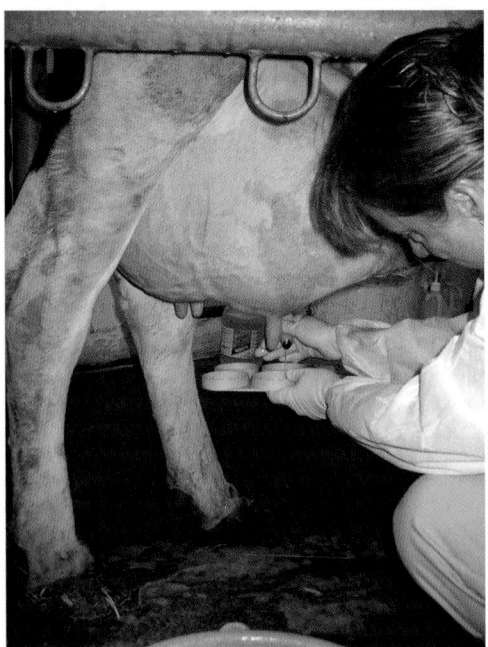

FIGURE 18-99 Collecting milk samples into a California Mastitis Test (CMT) paddle. Milk from each teat is collected separately into a cup on the paddle.

equal volume of CMT reagent solution (one part milk to one part reagent solution) is added to each well, the paddle is gently moved to swirl the milk, and the resultant solution is graded on the basis of gel formation.

0 = No gel

Trace = Precipitate disappears with continued movement of the sample

1 = First visible precipitate does not disappear

2 = First visible gel—mixture moves toward the center of the cup, leaving the bottom of the outer edge of the cup exposed

3 = Egg yolk–type clot sticks to the bottom of the plate and may have the appearance of cottage cheese

The number indicates the severity of inflammation.

COLOSTRUM SAMPLE

Colostrometers provide a specific gravity assessment of the sample. Colostrum may be submitted for laboratory analysis, including immunoglobulin (Ig)G content and an antierythrocyte alloantibody determination. Sterile samples are not required.

The mare's udder should be washed well with soft cotton saturated with gentle soap and warm water and rinsed well before milking after foaling. The technician should be familiar with the use of a colostrometer and should collect the appropriate volume (usually 5 to 10 ml) of colostrum. Samples can be milked directly into a collection tube or poured from another container into the necessary tubes.

RUMEN FLUID COLLECTION

Rumen fluid is collected and analyzed for diagnosis of diseases of the forestomachs (the reticulum, rumen, and omasum) in large and small ruminants. Characteristics of interest include color, pH, odor, microbial organisms and numbers, and electrolyte levels. Rumen fluid may also be collected for therapeutic purposes. When collected from a healthy animal, it may be used for transfaunation (inoculation of the sick animal's rumen with normal rumen flora needed to aid digestion).

ORAL GASTRIC TUBE (OROGASTRIC TUBE, ORORUMEN, STOMACH TUBE) METHOD

Tubes are inserted orally (through the mouth) in cattle. The nasal passages of cattle have a smaller diameter than those of horses; this significantly limits the diameter of tube that can be placed nasally.

Materials Needed

- Stomach tube—For adult cattle: medium to large diameter with internal diameter no less than 1.5 cm because smaller size is more likely to become obstructed with ingesta. For calves, sheep, and goats, small and medium foal stomach tubes can be used.
- Water-based lubricant
- Frick speculum (cattle)
- PVC pipe "speculum," block of wood with hole cut in center, roll of tape (sheep, goats)
- Dose syringe
- Sample collection container

TECHNICIAN NOTE A Frick speculum is commonly used on cattle to pass OGTs. For small ruminants, a short piece of polyvinyl chloride (PVC) pipe may be used as a mouth speculum.

BOVINE

Restrain the animal to sufficiently limit movement of the head. Do not overly elevate the head during this procedure. Ruminants may regurgitate fluid around the tube, and having the head overly elevated increases the likelihood of aspiration of the fluid.

Estimate the length of tube needed to reach the rumen by extending the tube outside the animal from the mouth to the rumen. The restrainer wraps one arm around the muzzle and places nose tongs (or places one finger into one of the animal's nostrils and a thumb into the other nostril) and pulls the nose upward to open the mouth. Standing to the side of the animal, insert the speculum (to prevent biting of the tube) over the root of the tongue in the center of the mouth. Popping or "give" is felt as the speculum passes over the root of the tongue and into the pharynx.

Lubricate the tip of the tube with a water-soluble lubricant or with water. Insert the tube through the speculum. Resistance is usually felt when the tube reaches the back of the pharynx. As the animal swallows, the tube is advanced down the esophagus. If the tube is not easily advanced, it may be necessary to slightly withdraw and rotate the tube and try again. Blowing into the tube dilates the esophagus and may ease passage of the tube. Proper placement of the tube in the esophagus is confirmed by palpating (the trachea and tube may be felt as two distinct tubular structures) or visualizing the tube in the esophagus and feeling mild resistance as it is passed. Coughing may indicate that the tube is in the trachea, and feeling air pass out of the tube upon exhalation may indicate placement into the trachea (these are not always reliable).

Placement of the tube within the rumen can be confirmed by blowing into the tube and listening for gurgling from the end of the tube, or by blowing into the tube with an assistant auscultating the abdomen with a stethoscope over the rumen (left paralumbar fossa) while listening for gurgles. Air should be heard bubbling in the rumen. Additional confirmation of placement is done by smelling the exposed end of the tube (Figure 18-100). The distinctive odor of fermented gas may be detected coming from the tube. Aspiration of rumen fluid (rumen juice) clearly confirms placement of the tube.

A dose syringe is used to collect the rumen fluid sample. The initial fluid is discarded because it often contains an excessive amount of saliva, which may erroneously elevate the pH of the fluid. When the process is complete, the tube is kinked and withdrawn with a smooth downward motion.

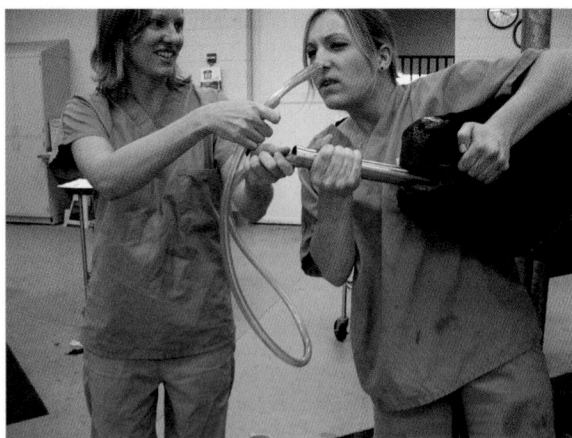

FIGURE 18-100 Checking for rumen smells to confirm placement of an orogastric tube (OGT) in the cow.

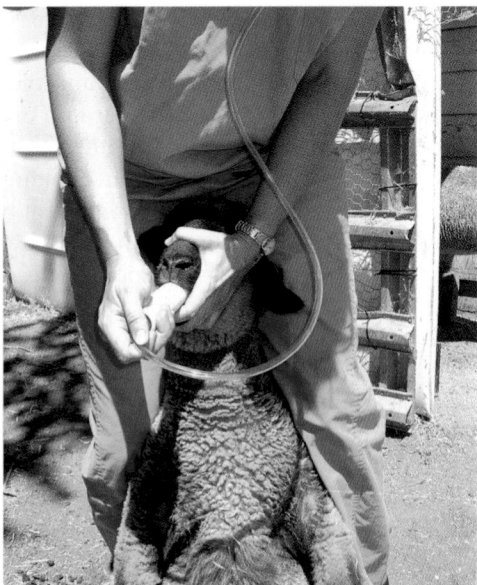

FIGURE 18-101 Polyvinyl chloride (PVC) pipe used as a mouth speculum in sheep for orogastric tube (OGT) insertion. The speculum prevents the animal from biting the tube.

This prevents rumen contents from leaking out of the tube and entering the trachea as the tube is withdrawn. The pH of the sample should be measured immediately after the sample is obtained.

SMALL RUMINANT

Restrain as necessary. Sheep may be backed into a corner and straddled or "set up" on their rump; goats may be pushed against a wall or backed into a corner and straddled. A speculum is placed between the lower incisors and the dental pad. A short piece of PVC pipe or a block of wood with a hole in the center or even a roll of tape may be used as a speculum (Figure 18-101). Whatever is used must be long enough to reach the back of the mouth so that the tube is not deflected to the side, where it can be bitten or chewed by the animal.

Select a tube of suitable size and length (approximately $\frac{3}{8}$ to $\frac{1}{2}$ inch in outside diameter), and estimate the necessary

length as described for cattle; proceed with tube passage as described previously.

RUMENOCENTESIS

This method is seldom used because of the ease and safety of the stomach tube method described earlier.

The ventral abdomen caudal to the xiphoid process and left of the ventral midline is clipped and surgically prepared. The veterinarian inserts a needle with a syringe attached (14-gauge needle for cattle, 16- to 18-gauge needle for small ruminants) through the skin and into the rumen. Rumen fluid is aspirated into the syringe.

THORACOCENTESIS (THORACENTESIS, PLEUROCENTESIS, CHEST TAP, PLEURAL TAP)

Thoracocentesis is the aspiration of fluid from the thoracic cavity. It is performed in large animals to obtain pleural fluid samples for diagnostic purposes and therapeutically to drain fluid, air, or exudate from the pleural cavity. Pleural fluid is produced by the cells of the pleura, which line the pleural cavity and the surface of the lungs. Fluid volume and character change with the presence of disease in the pleural cavity or lungs. In the normal animal, little or no fluid is obtained from the thorax. When disease is present, large volumes of fluid may be obtained from the thorax. Gross analysis of the fluid ascertains color, opacity, and the presence of fibrin material, pus, and odor. Laboratory analysis includes cytologic and microbiological examinations, and often determination of pH, lactate, and glucose. Occasionally, PCR analysis is done to identify certain pathogens.

This procedure is generally performed by the veterinarian, and the technician is called upon to set up, prep, and assist with the procedure. If facilities allow, the technician may perform the laboratory analysis of the sample. When an indwelling chest drain is placed, the technician will be expected to maintain the drain and monitor the patient (Figure 18-102).

EQUINE AND BOVINE
Materials Needed
- Sterile gloves
- Ample collection tubes
  - EDTA (for cytologic examination)
  - Serum (for microbiological examination)
  - Heparin (for pH, lactate, and glucose determination) or fluoride (for pH and glucose assessment), depending on specific laboratory analyzer requirements
- Instrument of veterinarian's choice
  - Needle (minimum 3 inches) with large gauge
    or
  - 14- to 16-gauge IV catheter
    or
  - Sharp trocar and cannula
    or

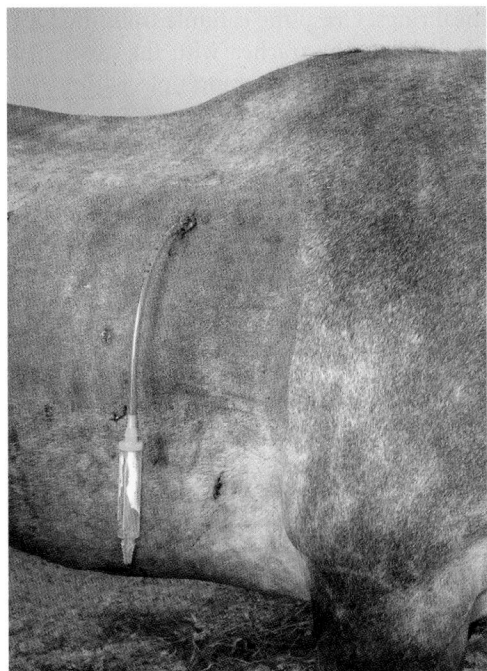

FIGURE 18-102 Indwelling chest drain with Heimlich valve.

- Teat cannula
  or
- Bitch catheter
- Two percent lidocaine 3 to 5 ml
- Six-milliliter syringe with 20- to 22-gauge × 1-inch to 1.5-inch needle
- Scalpel blade #15
- Sterile 35- to 60-ml luer tip syringe
- Three-way stopcock
- IV extension tubing
- Suture material, needle drivers, and scissors
- Ultrasound machine, if available and requested by veterinarian

Restrain the horse and administer sedation as needed. The veterinarian will select the appropriate site on the right or left lateral thorax and may use ultrasound to identify the most appropriate site. The patient may require thoracocentesis on both left and right sides. Each side of the thorax may yield different laboratory results because diseases of the plural cavity may cause blockage of normal communication between right and left sides. It is possible that abnormal fluid may be present on one side, while the other side remains essentially normal.

> **TECHNICIAN NOTE** A patient may require thoracocentesis on both left and right sides because each may yield different laboratory results.

Shave and aseptically prepare a large area from the olecranon back to the 10th intercostal space and from the point of the shoulder to well below the olecranon. The needle will be inserted into the ventral portion of the 6th and 7th

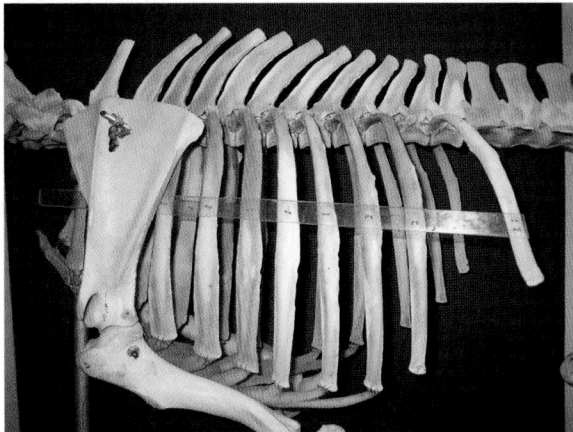

FIGURE 18-103 Side view of alpaca ribs.

intercostal (between the ribs) space 10 to 12 cm dorsal to the olecranon, above the lateral thoracic vein, and below the anticipated level of fluid. The site can also be determined with the use of ultrasonography, if indicated. Inject 5 ml of 2% lidocaine into the skin and SC to make a bleb on the cranial aspect of the rib, and deep enough into the intercostal muscles to include the parietal pleura. A stab incision is made into the anesthetized bleb with a scalpel blade. Avoid allowing the entrance of air during the procedure. A teat cannula (12- to 14-gauge × 3 inches) can be used to remove small volumes of air or fluid. A wider-bore sterile metal bitch catheter or a human thoracic drainage cannula may be needed if a large volume of fluid is present or if the fluid is thick. The needle, catheter, or cannula with extension tubing and three-way stopcock attached is inserted cranial to the rib border and is advanced through the parietal pleura. This approach is done to prevent damage to the intercostal vessels and nerves that run along the caudal border of the ribs. The heart, pericardial sac, and lateral thoracic vein must be avoided. Once in the pleural cavity, a syringe is attached to the stopcock, and fluid is aspirated. When the fluid has been collected, the veterinarian may stitch a purse-string suture around the stab incision and tighten the suture as the cannula is removed.

CAMELID

The preferred site for thoracocentesis is at the 6th or 7th intercostal space 10 to 15 cm dorsal to the sternum (Figure 18-103). The area is clipped and surgically prepped. Any long fiber that may contaminate the shaved site should be taped back out of the way. Local anesthetic is injected as described for equines. A 14- to 16-gauge × 2-inch needle or teat cannula with a syringe attached is inserted near the cranial border of the rib. The pleural space is entered approximately 2 to 3 cm under the skin. The sample is aspirated into the syringe, and the needle is withdrawn and antibiotic ointment applied to the centesis site.

Thoracocentesis in other large animals is similar to the procedures described for camelids and equines; the cannula size is dependent on the size of the animal.

Complications of thoracocentesis include pneumothorax, dyspnea, and iatrogenic infection.

TRANSTRACHEAL WASH (TRACHEAL WASH, TRACH WASH)

Transtracheal aspiration is the collection of fluid from the lower respiratory tract (bronchi, bronchioles, and alveoli) for cytologic and microbiological analyses; it is performed to assist the diagnosis of lower airway and lung disease. The fluid is a mixture of secretions and cellular material that has collected in the distal portion of the trachea.

EQUINE TRANSTRACHEAL ASPIRATION

The two methods used for this procedure are percutaneous and endoscopic. Both procedures are also carried out in bovine and other large animal species by the same method.

Percutaneous Method

Restrain the horse appropriately. A horse may require mild sedation (heavy sedation should be avoided because it may suppress the cough reflex). Select a site on the midline of the neck directly over the trachea about one-third of the way down the neck. Clip or shave an area approximately 4 × 4 inches, perform a sterile prep, and set up necessary materials.

> **TECHNICIAN NOTE** A horse may require mild sedation when a transtracheal wash is performed, but heavy sedation should be avoided because it may suppress the cough reflex.

Materials Needed

- Sterile gloves
- Surgical blades: #20 to #30 for adults; #15 to #20 for foals a few months old
- Syringes of NaCl: one or two 60-ml syringes containing 30 ml of 0.9% NaCl (do not use bacteriostatic saline). Place the syringe back into the case.
- Commercially available equine tracheal wash kit (Jorgensen Labs)
- Needles: one or two 25-gauge needles for capping the collection syringe after the sample is obtained

Procedure

1. Inject approximately 1 to 2 ml of 2% lidocaine ID and SC over the selected site on the trachea, and apply a final prep.
2. Open the tracheal wash kit, and while wearing sterile gloves, remove the long catheter. Tie the long catheter in a loose half-hitch knot. This will allow the catheter to stay completely on the sterile field (created by the open sterile glove package) and will make it easier to control the distal tip to prevent contamination by accidental touching of something before or during insertion.
3. After the sterile prep procedure, make a stab incision with the scalpel blade through the skin between the tracheal rings. Grasp the cannula from the kit with one hand. Stabilize the trachea with the other hand, palm side up; use fingers and thumb placed on each side of the trachea, and hold firmly.
4. Insert the distal tip of the needle with bevel side down through the incision, and advance it into the tracheal lumen. If resistance is felt, redirect the tip of the needle between the tracheal ring spaces, then advance into the trachea. A burst of air will exit the needle when it penetrates the lumen of the trachea.
5. Remove the stylet. This prevents possible laceration and loss of catheter tubing. Place on a sterile field in case it is needed again.
6. Insert the catheter until it reaches the thoracic inlet.
7. Attach the 60-ml syringe and retract the plunger. Air is aspirated if the catheter is in the tracheal lumen. If no air is aspirated, reposition the catheter because it may be bent or occluded against the tracheal wall.
8. Once air has been aspirated, infuse 30 ml of NaCl, and immediately try to aspirate a 5-ml or larger fluid sample (only a small portion of the fluid that is instilled will be retrieved). A 5-ml sample should be sufficient for microbiological and cytologic examination.
9. Continue aspirating while slowly withdrawing the catheter. Stop withdrawing when fluid for aspiration is evident, and collect as much as possible with a catheter at that location.
10. Withdraw again as needed to continue the collection of fluid (do not reinsert the catheter). If fluid is not obtained, infuse 10 ml of NaCl, and aspirate again (Figure 18-104, A through D). The total volume of saline infused (first and second attempts) should not exceed 50 ml.

Some horses will cough while saline is infused, which may have the positive effect of increasing the yield of mucopurulent material. Unfortunately, coughing may also cause the catheter to kink cranially, which may prevent collection of any sample. With a sample syringe, remove the catheter while keeping the cannula in place. This helps to prevent an SC infection, because otherwise the contaminated catheter would come into direct contact with tissue at the insertion site when removed. Remove the cannula, apply pressure to the site, control any bleeding, and place a 4 × 4-inch piece of gauze with antiseptic ointment over the incision for 24 hours. Use a sterile needle to cap the syringe containing the sample for transport to the laboratory.

Cellulitis or SC abscessation at the tracheal puncture site is the most common complication. If swelling occurs, warm compresses are applied. Other complications include SC emphysema around the trachea, pulmonary foreign body as a result of the presence of a catheter piece in the airway, acute dyspnea, tracheal laceration, minor SC hemorrhage, and iatrogenic infection.

Endoscopic Method

Use of an endoscope is considered noninvasive and allows visual examination of the upper airways, trachea, carina, and

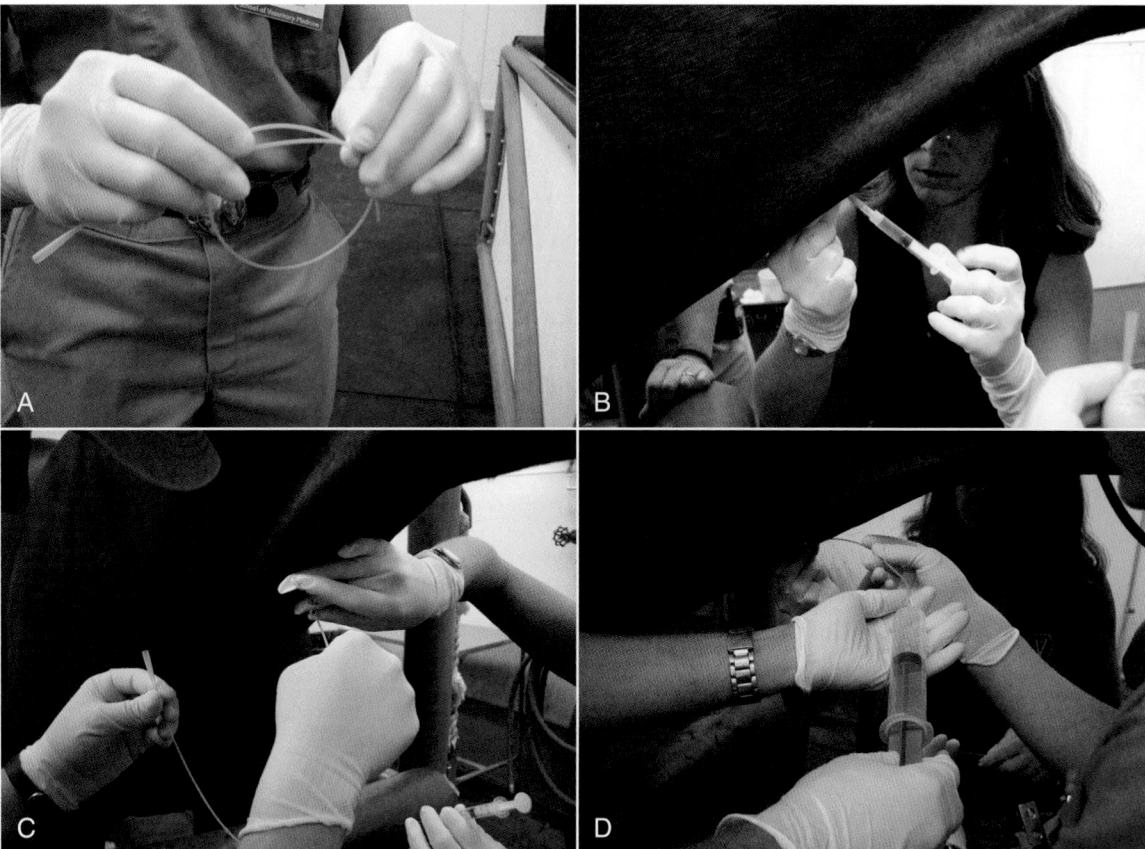

FIGURE 18-104 Transtracheal aspiration of equine patient. **A,** Coiling catheter to keep sterile and easily controlled. **B,** Aspirating air to confirm placement in the tracheal lumen. **C,** Inserting a catheter into the trachea. **D,** Aspirating a sample.

primary and secondary bronchi; however, the presence of the endoscope leads to questionable accuracy of the microbial samples recovered with this technique. An endoscope is inserted through the nasal cavity to the tracheal lumen. Special tubing (polyethylene tubing or endoscopic microbiological aspiration catheter) is placed through the biopsy channel of the endoscope, and fluid is injected and aspirated for collection of the sample. Use of these specialized sample collection items decreases the likelihood of contamination from the pharynx or the endoscope, which would otherwise occur with the endoscopic approach. It is usually necessary to infuse saline, as described for the percutaneous approach, to aspirate a fluid sample from the trachea.

BRONCHOALVEOLAR LAVAGE (BAL)

Bronchoalveolar lavage is a procedure used to collect fluid samples from the lower airway. BAL provides fluid samples that are better for cytologic assessment than samples obtained by transtracheal aspiration, but the fluid samples are representative of only a limited area of the lung and are subject to contamination caused by passing the tube through the nares. BAL is performed by inserting a sterile tube into the nares and trachea. To prepare for the procedure, the technician should have sterile BAL tubing, a syringe containing 50 ml of 2% lidocaine, and three syringes, each containing

60 ml of sterile saline (not bacteriostatic saline). The veterinarian may choose to use more or less saline, so the technician should check before the procedure to be sure of the desired amount of saline that should be ready in syringes.

The horse should be sufficiently restrained and may require sedation. While the tube is passed into the trachea, 2% lidocaine is injected into the tube whenever the horse coughs. This acts as a local anesthetic to the bronchi and helps to decrease the cough reflex. It is not uncommon to use the entire 50 ml of lidocaine before the procedure is complete. Sterile saline (previously drawn up into three separate 60-ml syringes) is injected and aspirated (as is done through the transtracheal aspiration procedure) (Figure 18-105).

> **TECHNICIAN NOTE** While the BAL tubing is passed into the trachea, 2% lidocaine may be injected into the tube whenever the horse coughs to decrease the cough reflex.

This procedure can also be done with the use of an endoscope, with sterile tubing passed through the biopsy channel of the scope so that saline can be injected and fluid samples aspirated. This method is preferred for sample collection when bronchial and/or alveolar disease is suspected. Use of the endoscope allows sampling from specific areas of the

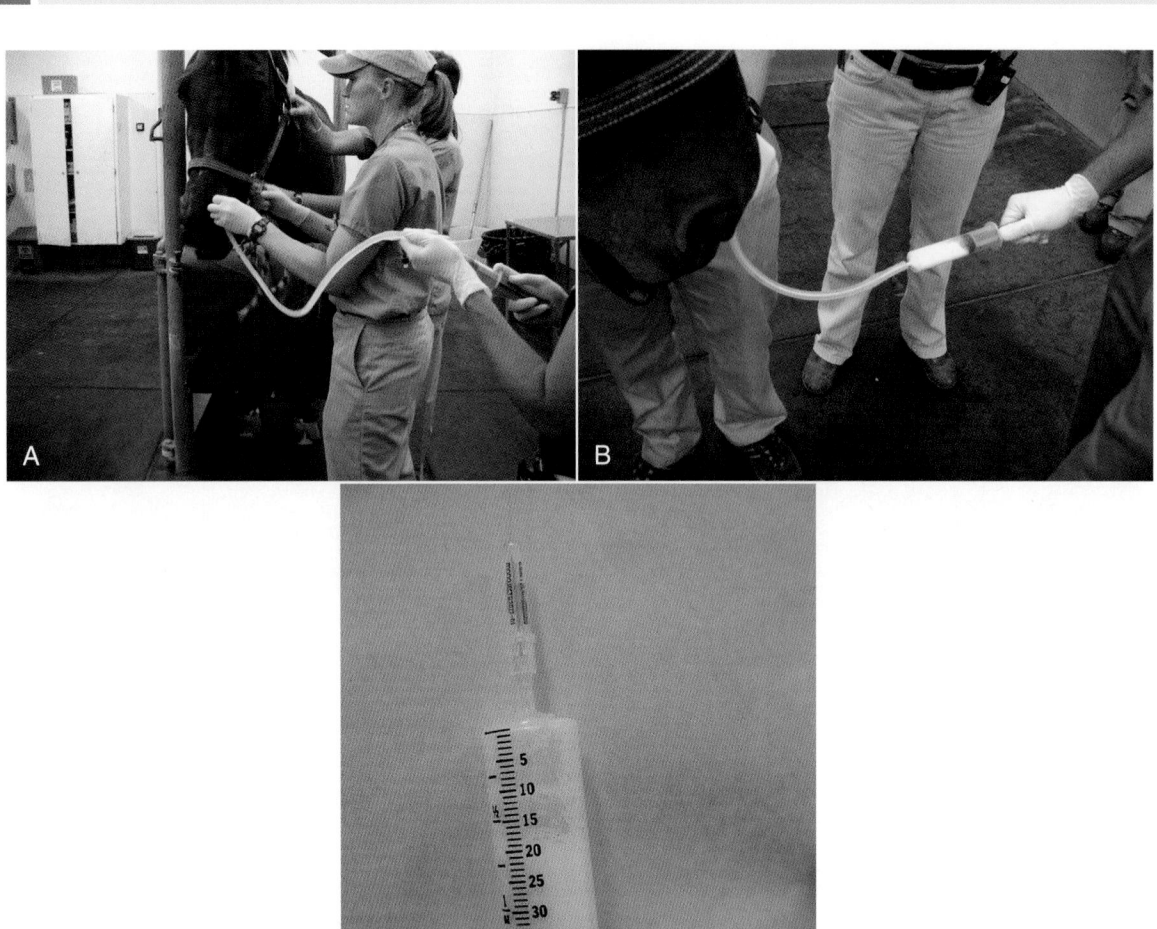

FIGURE 18-105 Bronchoalveolar lavage (BAL) of an equine patient. **A,** Inserting BAL tubing with a syringe containing lidocaine attached to the end of a tube. **B,** Collecting a BAL sample. **C,** Syringe containing BAL sample is capped before transport to the laboratory.

lung, but a limited sample is obtained rather than the pooled secretions that are obtained when a transtracheal aspiration is done.

If the veterinarian intends to perform both a percutaneous transtracheal aspiration and a BAL, the transtracheal aspiration should be performed first. This will allow fluid samples to be obtained before any contamination may be introduced with passage of the BAL tubing (or endoscope). Often the cough reflex is intentionally suppressed for the BAL, whereas a cough may be desirable during the transtracheal aspiration procedure.

ABDOMINOCENTESIS

Peritoneal fluid obtained by abdominocentesis (abdominal tap, peritoneal tap, paracentesis, belly tap) can provide

valuable diagnostic information. Peritoneal fluid is produced by the cells of the peritoneum. These cells line the abdominal cavity and the outer surfaces of abdominal organs. The composition of this fluid is determined by the condition of the abdominal organs. Analysis focuses on gross appearance, laboratory results, and the volume of fluid present. Accumulation of fluid in the abdominal cavity is abnormal.

> **TECHNICIAN NOTE**   The composition of peritoneal fluid is determined by the condition of the abdominal organs.

Abdominocentesis is commonly performed on horses, camelids, cattle, sheep, and goats. The veterinary technician may be asked to prepare for and assist with the procedure or to perform the procedure. Several variations on the procedure may be performed, and the technician will be directed by the veterinarian as to which approach is preferred. With any of these techniques, consideration should be given to ensuring that the sample is not contaminated, that no contaminants are introduced into the patient, that as little trauma as possible is inflicted upon the patient, and that personnel are not injured while the sample is obtained.

Indications for abdominocentesis include colic, suspected peritonitis, weight loss, abdominal distention, chronic diarrhea, signs of internal hemorrhage, abnormal ultrasound findings, and FUO.

For all species:
- Gather all required supplies (include alternates in case use of first-choice instruments is unsuccessful).
- Appropriately restrain the patient.
- Clip or shave the area chosen.
- Perform sterile prep.
- Wear sterile gloves and maintain sterility throughout the procedure.

EQUINE ABDOMINOCENTESIS

Many horses require minimal restraint for the procedure. If possible, the horse should be restrained in standing stocks. A handler should remain at the horse's head, and twitch should be applied or sedation administered, depending on the nature of the horse and the degree of discomfort the horse is exhibiting.

When preparing the site and when performing the procedure, the person should squat next to the horse adjacent to the forelimbs and facing the rear of the horse. This position reduces the likelihood of the person being kicked with the horse's hind leg. The person should take care to keep the head up and safely away from the belly and legs of the horse and should be prepared to move back quickly if necessary to remain safe. If the technician is assisting with the procedure and will be collecting the fluid into tubes, he or she should be positioned similarly on the opposite side of the animal (if space permits) or should wait until the instrument has been inserted, and then should squat or bend over next to the veterinarian (being prepared to step back quickly, if necessary) and with outstretched hand place the collection tube under the needle or cannula.

Determine the site for the tap. Locate the lowest portion of the abdomen, and locate the ventral midline. This is usually 2 to 4 inches caudal to the xiphoid. Abdominocentesis can be performed at the ventral midline, but use of a paramedian site 1 to 2 inches to the right of midline reduces the likelihood of tapping the spleen (in horses) or the rumen (in ruminants). Abdominocentesis should not be performed through skin abrasions or surgical lesions, and whenever possible, tapping through edema should be avoided. The clinician may perform ultrasonography to assist in determining the most desirable site for abdominocentesis and to prevent penetration of organs.

> **TECHNICIAN NOTE** Abdominocentesis can be performed at the ventral midline, but use of a paramedian site to the right of the midline reduces the likelihood of tapping the spleen (in horses) or the rumen (in ruminants).

Teat Cannula or Female Canine Urinary Catheter (Bitch Catheter) Method

Use of a blunt-tipped bovine teat cannula or stainless steel female canine urinary catheter reduces the risk of bowel penetration; therefore this method may be chosen over the needle method for animals with abdominal distention or bowel distention (as identified by rectal examination performed by a veterinarian). This method requires the use of local anesthetic.

Shave an area approximately 2 inches square. Perform a sterile prep. Aspirate 2 ml of 2% lidocaine into a 3-ml syringe. Perform local anesthesia by infusing the skin and SC tissue with approximately 1 ml of lidocaine, using a 25-gauge needle. Insert the needle into the center of the shaved area (avoid any obvious cutaneous vasculature), aspirate to check for blood, and then infuse the lidocaine. Remove the 25-gauge needle, and place a 19-gauge × 1.5-inch needle directly into the center of the SC bleb. Insert the needle completely to the hub, and inject the remaining 1 ml of lidocaine while slowly removing the needle from the patient. This is done to block the parietal peritoneum.

Complete the sterile prep with a final swab of Betadine solution (or alternate antiseptic).

Materials Needed
(Figure 18-106)
- Four-inch teat cannula or bitch catheter
- #15 scalpel blade
- Two-milliliter EDTA tube
- Three-milliliter serum tube

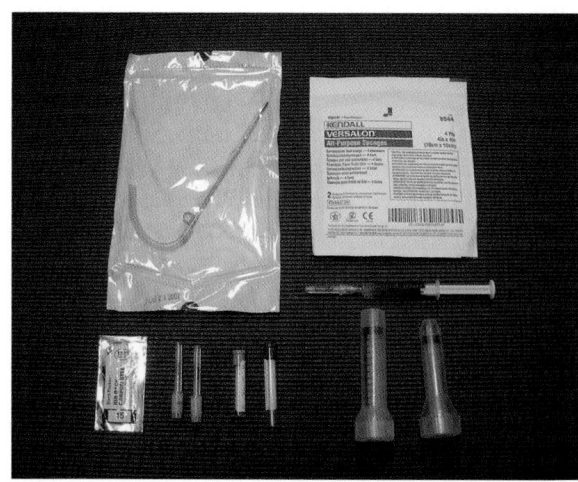

FIGURE 18-106 Supplies for abdominocentesis. Bitch catheter, 4 × 4-inch sterile gauze sponges, #15 scalpel blade, 19-gauge × 1.5-inch needles, 2-ml EDTA tube, 3-ml plain tube, 3-ml syringe with 25-gauge × 1-inch needle containing 2% lidocaine, 12-ml syringe, and 6-ml syringe.

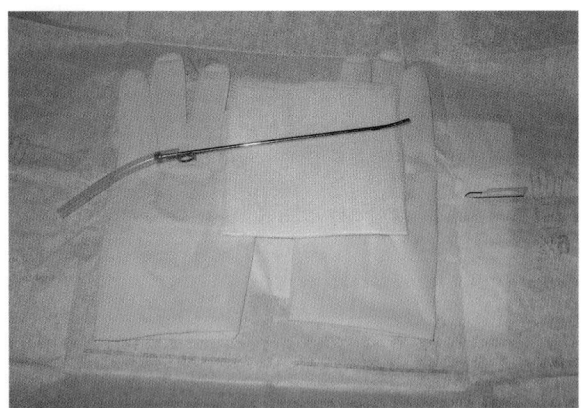

FIGURE 18-107 Sterile field with sterile supplies for abdominocentesis.

- Heparin tube or syringe (depending on laboratory capabilities)
- Sterile 4 × 4-inch gauze sponges

Create a sterile field by opening a pair of sterile gloves and placing the teat cannula (or bitch catheter or needle), scalpel blade, and sterile gauze (4 × 4 inches) onto the field (Figure 18-107).

Put on sterile gloves.

Puncture the center of one gauze 4 × 4-inch sponge with the scalpel blade, and put the teat cannula through the gauze. This will help prevent contamination of the sample with blood or dust.

Using the scalpel blade, make a stab incision through the skin. Hold the blade with about ⅜ inch exposed. Using the back of the gloved hand, gently touch the horse's belly, then insert the scalpel blade straight into the bleb and pull it straight out. Avoid cutting the musculature. Slowly but firmly insert the teat cannula through the incision perpendicular to the musculature. The muscle will feel "gritty," and a slight "pop" will be felt when the peritoneum is punctured. A decrease in resistance is felt when the abdomen has been entered. If firm resistance is felt at this point, it may indicate contact with an organ, and care must be taken if further manipulation on the cannula is required. Once the cannula is in, expect to wait while the horse takes a few breaths before fluid begins to flow from the cannula. If fluid does not immediately flow, the cannula can be gently "flicked" with a finger in an effort to encourage flow, and the cannula can be moved around slightly, rotated, or redirected. If necessary, a syringe may be attached to the cannula, and aspiration may be attempted (Figure 18-108).

The first few drops of fluid may contain contaminants, so these drops should not be included in the sample. Collect the sample by gravity flow into collection tubes. The EDTA tube should be collected first because most of the desired laboratory tests will require this sample. The tube should be filled as much as possible to ensure the correct ratio of EDTA to abdominal fluid. If less than 1 ml of abdominal fluid is collected, results of the laboratory analysis may be inaccurate. A common practice is to remove the rubber stopper

from the EDTA tube and shake the tube to remove a bit of the EDTA before the fluid sample is collected. This is useful when a small sample volume is obtained. When refractometry is performed, excessive EDTA in relation to sample size will falsely elevate the protein reading. EDTA samples are used for cytologic analysis, protein measurement, and packed cell volume (PCV) (if fluid appears bloody). A serum (plain, clot) tube should be collected for bacterial culture (as little as 1 drop of fluid is sufficient for this purpose). Some facilities have the capability to perform pH, gas, lactate, and glucose analyses. The technician should be familiar with laboratory capabilities and with appropriate anticoagulant requirements. For many analyzers that perform these additional tests, heparin is the choice of anticoagulant. Some facilities will require a sodium fluoride tube for glucose and lactate measurements.

> **TECHNICIAN NOTE** The technician should be familiar with laboratory capabilities and should be knowledgeable about appropriate anticoagulant requirements.

When removing the cannula, the technician should be aware that some omentum may have attached to the cannula and can follow it out when the cannula is pulled from the site. To prevent it from being exteriorized, care should be taken to use fingers to guard close to the site when the cannula is removed. As a result of incidental perforation of skin vessels, slight bleeding is common after removal of the cannula. Manual pressure applied to the site usually stops the bleeding. If necessary, the veterinarian will suture or staple the site. The centesis site can be cleaned gently and antibiotic ointment applied daily for a couple of days.

18- to 22-Gauge × 1.5-Inch Needle Method

Local anesthetic is usually not required for this method, but this varies depending on the horse.

The needle is held midway between thumb and forefinger and is inserted through the skin while superficial veins are avoided. The fingers are moved slightly to grasp the hub of the needle for gradual advancement. The needle should be inserted at slight intervals, pausing before each interval of advancement to notice (by feel) whether a scratching sensation is present. The scratching sensation indicates that bowel is rubbing over the tip of the needle. The fingers should be removed from the needle periodically to watch for rotary or "flicking" movement of the needle, which is also indicative of bowel contact. Periodic back and forth movement of the needle in time with respiration is normal. The needle is advanced slowly to the hub if no bowel is encountered, or until fluid is obtained. If abdominal fluid is not seen in the needle hub, the needle can be repositioned and rotated, and a syringe may be used to try to aspirate a sample. If fluid is not obtained, 1 to 2 ml of air (in a sterile syringe) may be injected in an effort to dislodge any material that might be occluding the needle. Another option to encourage the flow of fluid is to insert a 2nd or 3rd needle a few centimeters

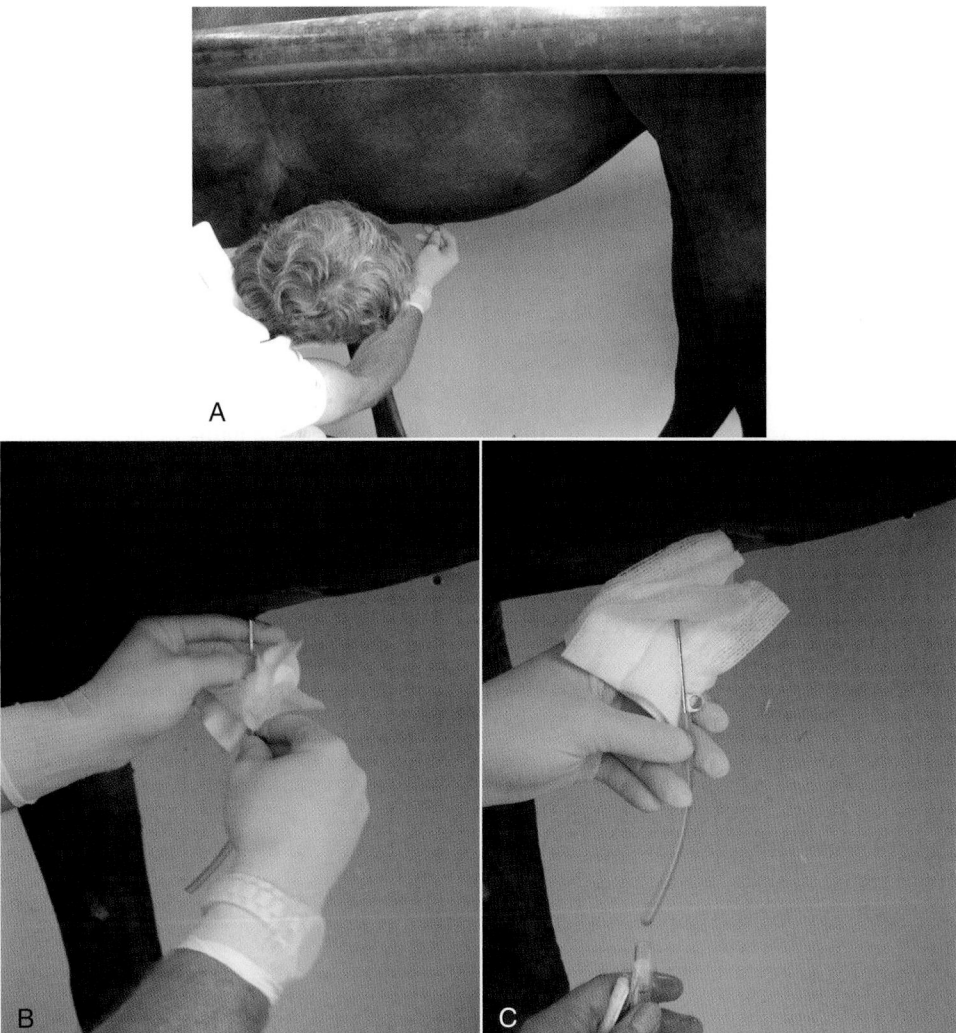

FIGURE 18-108 A, Incision on prepped and blocked ventral midline area for an equine abdominal tap. B, Insertion of a bitch catheter through an incision. C, Collection of abdominal fluid through a bitch catheter into collection tubes.

from the first (while leaving the 1st needle in place) to release negative pressure in the abdomen.

> **TECHNICIAN NOTE** Periodic back and forth movement of the needle in time with the animal's respiration is normal.

18-Gauge × 3.5-Inch Spinal Needle Method

This long needle may be required in very large horses, draft horses, and obese individuals. Some clinicians report that this long needle is also useful in Arabian horses to facilitate penetration beyond the abdominal wall and the subperitoneal fat layer.

Local anesthetic is not usually necessary for this method, but this varies depending on the horse.

With the stylet in place, the needle is inserted to a depth of approximately ¼ inch. The stylet is removed before further advancement and the procedure is continued, as is done with a standard needle.

EQUINE ABDOMINOCENTESIS (FOAL)

Sedation is usually indicated. The procedure is safer for the patient and for personnel if sufficient human assistance is provided for physical restraint and positioning of the foal.

For neonates younger than 1 month or for actively colicky foals, abdominocentesis can be done with the sedated foal restrained in lateral recumbency. A 20-gauge × 1- to 1.5-inch needle is inserted caudal to the xiphoid midline or the right paramedian (off center but near the midline). Foal intestine is thin and fragile, and care must be taken to avoid contacting the bowel. A blunt-ended, small-diameter teat cannula or a canine bitch catheter can be used and poses less risk for intestinal laceration than a needle, but local anesthetic and a stab incision are needed before the cannula is inserted. Lack of subperitoneal fat in foals increases the risk for laceration of the bowel with a scalpel blade when a stab incision is made. The blade must be held with the fingers up near the tip of the blade to maintain control and ensure that it is not inserted too deeply. For foals older than 1 month, an 18- to 20-gauge × 1.5-inch needle, a teat cannula, or a bitch catheter would be appropriate, and the procedure would be performed as for younger foals.

> **TECHNICIAN NOTE** Foal intestine is thin and fragile, and care must be taken to avoid contacting the bowel.

CAMELID ABDOMINOCENTESIS (ADULT)

Two sites are commonly used for abdominocentesis in camelids: a ventral midline site and a right paracostal (near the ribs) site. The paracostal site is easier to tap because camelids frequently choose to drop to sternal recumbency ("kushed" position) when they object to a procedure, making the ventral midline site unavailable. The midline site is also complicated by a thick subperitoneal fat layer on either side of the linea alba, and visualization may be obscured by a long-fiber coat hanging from the sides of the animal.

Provide appropriate restraint by using a camelid chute or by having a handler push the left side of the animal up against a wall or fence. Chemical sedation may be required for some animals.

The paracostal abdominal tap site is located on the right side of the animal about 4 inches behind the caudal-most curve of the ribs (approximated by placing the palm of the hand behind the last rib) about one-third of the way up between the ventral abdomen and the spine (Figure 18-109). Clip or shave a 3- to 4-inch square area. It is helpful to keep long fibers in the surrounding area clear of the site by taping them back.

Perform a sterile prep. Using a 22- to 25-gauge needle, inject 1 to 3 ml of 2% lidocaine into the skin and SC tissue. Perform a final sterile prep of the site. Using a #11 or #15 scalpel blade, make a stab incision. Using a quick, controlled thrust, insert a 4-inch blunt-ended teat cannula perpendicular to the abdomen. Advance it slowly into the abdomen. If fluid does not flow, the tip of the cannula can be gently repositioned, a syringe may be attached, and negative

pressure may be applied, or a few milliliters of air can be injected into the abdominal cavity.

For the ventral midline approach, select the lowest site, which is just caudal to the umbilicus. To avoid the retroperitoneal fat pads on either side of the linea alba (which will obstruct the cannula and prevent a sample collection), the site chosen should be directly on the linea alba. Clip a 3- to 4-inch area, perform a sterile prep, and inject a small amount of local anesthetic (as described earlier). Using a scalpel blade, create a small stab incision and insert a teat cannula as described for an equine abdominal tap.

CAMELID ABDOMINOCENTESIS (NEONATAL)

The cria (neonatal llama or alpaca) can be mildly sedated as needed and should be restrained in lateral recumbency. A teat cannula or a 20-gauge × 1-inch needle may be used at the same site as for the standing adult camelid.

BOVINE ABDOMINOCENTESIS (ADULT)

The animal is placed in a head gate, stocks, or a chute that will allow access to the right side of the animal. A tail jack restraint may be sufficient, but chemical sedation may be necessary depending on the behavior of the animal and the site used.

An 18-gauge × 1.5-inch needle is sufficient for abdominocentesis in most adult cattle, although some very large individuals may require a 3-inch needle. A teat cannula can be used instead of a needle. If "hardware disease" (traumatic reticulitis from ingestion of heavy foreign objects) is suspected, the site selected should be just caudal to the xiphoid and to the right of the midline, as described for horses. The person performing the tap should stand by the animal's forelimbs facing backward and should be aware of the risk of being kicked. If general effusion or widespread disease is suspected, alternate sites can include the flank fold on the right side of the animal or the ventral abdomen at the lowest point approximately 2 to 4 inches to the right of the umbilicus. Tapping the abdomen through the flank fold can be done successfully without local anesthetic.

BOVINE ABDOMINOCENTESIS (NEONATAL)

Abdominal taps on calves can be done with the animal standing or in left lateral recumbency. Appropriate restraint is necessary, and sedation may be required to keep the animal still. A ventral midline site about 4 cm (approximately 1.5 inches) cranial to the umbilicus or a paramedian site approximately 4 cm to the right of the umbilicus can be used. As described earlier, a needle or a teat cannula can be used for the centesis.

OVINE AND CAPRINE ABDOMINOCENTESIS

Abdominocentesis in sheep and goats may be performed to investigate abdominal distention, poor forestomach motility, and suspected uroabdomen (caused by urinary tract obstruction or ruptured bladder). A ruptured bladder is common in male goats (bucks) secondary to obstructive urolithiasis and leads to the accumulation of urine in the abdominal cavity.

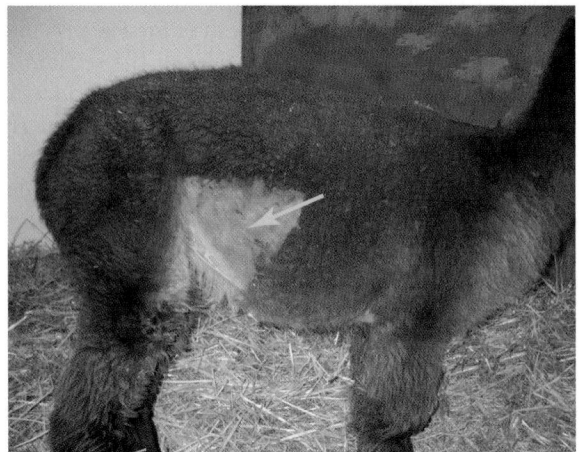

FIGURE 18-109 Paracostal site on an alpaca for abdominocentesis.

Manually restrain the animal, and sedate it, if necessary. A local anesthetic may be indicated, even if a needle is used for abdominocentesis. The procedure can be done with the animal standing.

Select a site at the lowest point of the abdomen 2 to 4 cm to the right of the ventral midline (to prevent tapping the rumen). Avoid the mammary veins (milk veins or SC abdominal veins) of females and the penis and prepuce in males. An 18- to 20-gauge × 1.5-inch needle or teat cannula can be used. Local anesthetic is necessary for the stab incision required with the use of a teat cannula and may be desirable even if a needle is used. If peritonitis is suspected, the veterinarian may choose to tap multiple sites to increase the chance of confirming a diagnosis. Additional sites include those caudal to the xiphoid, medial to the right and left milk veins, and slightly cranial to the mammary gland on the right and left of the midline.

The most common complications associated with abdominocentesis are failure to obtain a sample and slight skin hemorrhage. Protrusion of omentum through the site of puncture in the abdominal wall can also occur. More serious complications of abdominocentesis in large animals include penetration of the bowel, penetration of the spleen, damage to the xiphoid process if the centesis site is too cranial, and introduction of bacteria leading to peritonitis or cellulitis. SC abscessation and cellulitis are uncommon when an unremarkable abdominocentesis procedure is performed, but risk for these complications increases markedly when the intestine has been punctured, when abdominocentesis is done through edematous tissue, and when animals have septic peritonitis.

CEREBROSPINAL FLUID COLLECTION (SPINAL TAP, CSF TAP)

Cerebrospinal fluid may be collected from patients when central nervous system disease is suspected. CSF fluid analysis includes gross visualization of color, clarity, and the presence of particulate matter. Total protein, cytologic examination, and chemistry are performed on the fluid. The technician will be expected to prepare the site, restrain the patient, and assist the veterinarian while the veterinarian performs the procedure.

EQUINE

Atlantooccipital Site (AO Tap)

This site is located at the dorsal midline just caudal to the poll. Collecting spinal fluid from this site requires a general anesthetic. With the animal anesthetized, it is placed in lateral recumbency. The area is clipped and shaved, and a complete sterile prep is performed. When all preparations have been made, the nose is directed down toward the front feet to flex the head. The head should be at a right angle to the neck. The veterinarian inserts an 18-gauge × 3-inch spinal needle into the atlantooccipital space (about 5 to 7 cm deep) and, once in, removes the trocar (stylet) and places it onto a sterile field. A sterile syringe is attached to the needle, and a sample is gently aspirated. Alternatively, fluid may be collected directly into a tube by free flow. If the fluid is blood-tinged, aspirate a few milliliters, and then attach a new syringe. The technician should be prepared with additional syringes in case multiple samples can be obtained. The trocar (still sterile) is replaced in the needle, and the needle is withdrawn. Following removal of the needle, any blood present can be cleaned from the site, and a Betadine-soaked gauze sponge can be placed at the site.

The AO tap in neonates is done with a 20-gauge × 1.5-inch needle directed at the mandible. Fluid should drip from the needle hub. Normally, 3 to 6 ml of fluid is obtained.

Lumbosacral Site (LS Tap)

This site can be located by making an imaginary line across from the caudal edge of each tuber coxae and another line at the dorsal midline. A slight depression can be palpated using firm pressure at the intersection of these imaginary lines, just caudal to the 6th lumbar spinal process (L6). A large area is clipped and shaved, and a sterile prep is performed. Sedation is required, and use of a twitch for restraint is indicated because the animal must remain very still for the procedure. The horse should be placed in stocks. Local anesthetic is injected into the skin and SC. The patient should be standing as squarely as possible (the best that its condition will allow) because an asymmetric stance makes collection more difficult (Figure 18-110, A through F). If sufficient personnel are available, it is helpful to have someone stand behind the horse to comment to the veterinarian regarding placement of the needle, so that small errors in the direction of insertion can be noted and corrected. The veterinarian inserts a 6-inch (15-cm) × 18-gauge spinal needle perpendicular to the midline (about 11 to 15 cm, or 4.5 to 6 inches). For some draft horses and warm-blooded animals, longer needles (up to 8 inches) may be needed. When the needle reaches the subarachnoid space, the patient may respond with movement. The trocar is removed from the needle and is placed onto a sterile field. The technician places a sterile syringe in the veterinarian's still sterile, gloved hands. The initial sample may be contaminated with blood, so a second or third syringe may be collected if sufficient fluid is aspirated. The veterinarian may instruct assistants to occlude both jugular veins in an attempt to increase intracranial pressure. The trocar (still sterile) is replaced into the needle, and the needle is removed.

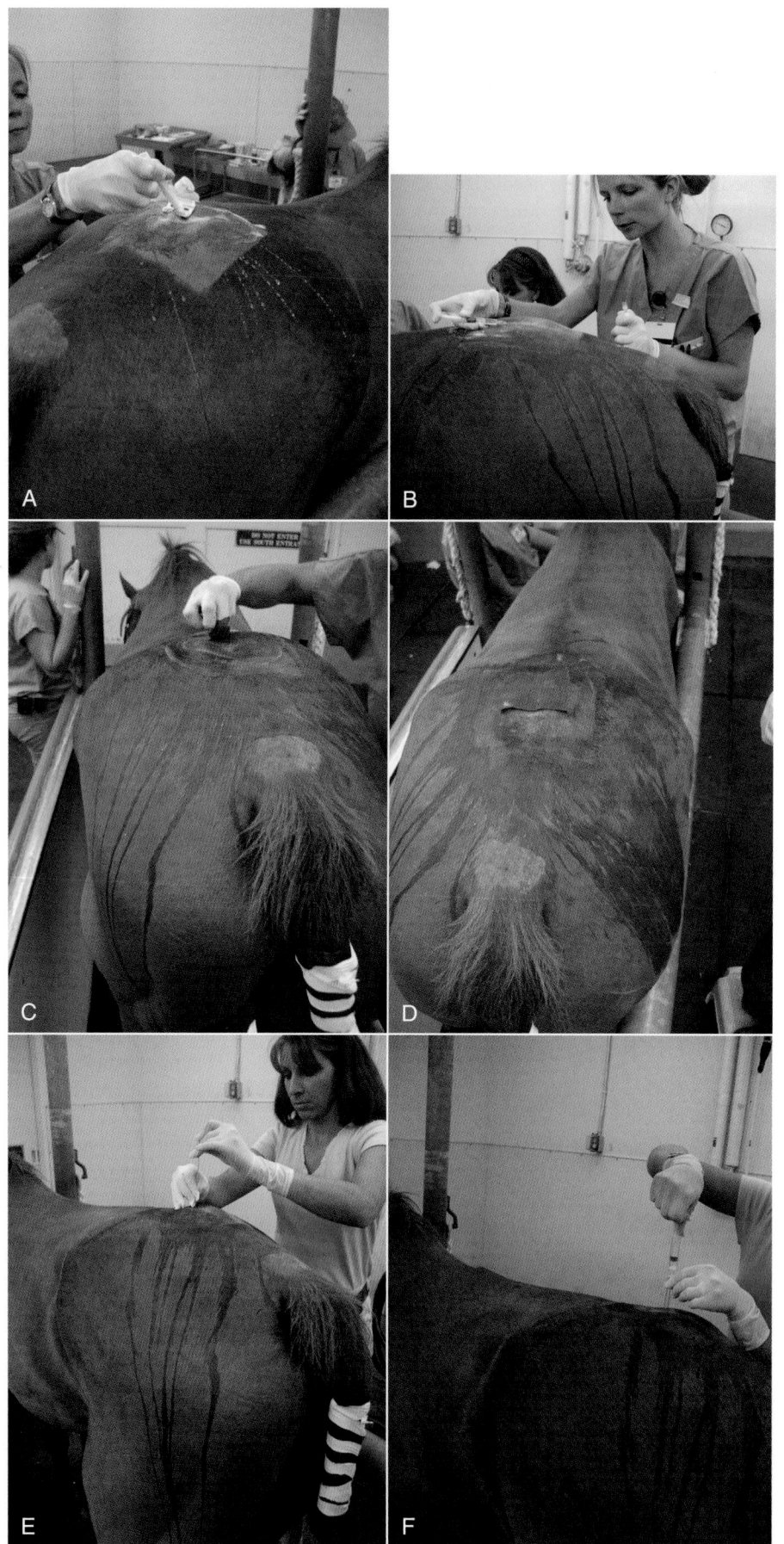

FIGURE 18-110 A, Shaving the area for lumbosacral (LS) spinal tap. B, Injecting 2% lidocaine for local anesthetic block. C, Prepping the site with Betadine solution. D, Site covered with Betadine-soaked gauze. E, Inserting a spinal needle. F, Aspirating a spinal fluid sample.

TECHNICIAN NOTE The patient should stand as squarely as possible for an lumbosacral tap.

The lumbosacral CSF tap in neonates can be done with the foal standing, in sternal recumbency, or in lateral recumbency, using a 3-inch × 20-gauge spinal needle.

Complications that may result from CSF taps include trauma to the spinal cord during needle placement, herniation of the cerebellum (can occur with high intracranial pressure or as the result of aggressive aspiration), and infection of the meninges. These can lead to the death of the patient. Chances of these complications occurring are minimized by having the patient sufficiently restrained to remain still and by following strict sterile technique throughout the procedure.

CAMELID

CSF collection from llamas and alpacas follows the same procedure guidelines as described for horses.

The atlantooccipital site is located midline as it intersects the wings of the atlas. In adults, a 20-gauge × 2.5-inch spinal needle is used, and the subarachnoid space is usually reached at a depth of 4 cm.

The lumbosacral site is midline about 2 cm caudal to the dorsal spinal process of the 7th lumbar vertebra. Landmarks used to locate the site include the tuber sacrale of the pelvis and the dorsal spinal process of the last lumbar vertebra. The site is cranial to the tuber sacrale. An 18- or 19-gauge × 3.5-inch spinal needle is appropriate for most adult llamas and alpacas.

ACKNOWLEDGMENTS

The authors wish to acknowledge the faculty, residents, technical staff, and students at the William R. Pritchard Veterinary Medical Teaching Hospital of the University of California, Davis. Particular appreciation goes to Monica Aleman, MVZ, PhD; Lisle George, DVM, PhD; Fred Librach, Equine Clinical Instructor; Debbie Donaldson, RVT; Sarah Hayes, RVT; and Teri Joseph, RVT.

REFERENCE

1. Hanie EA: Large animal clinical procedures for veterinary technicians, St Louis, 2006, Mosby.

RECOMMENDED READINGS

Bowden C, Masters J, editors: Textbook of veterinary medical nursing, London, 2003, Butterworth Heinemann.

Busch SJ, editor: Small animal surgical nursing, St Louis, 2006, Mosby.

Colville T, Bassert JM, editors: Clinical anatomy and physiology for veterinary technicians, St Louis, 2002, Mosby.

Ettinger SJ, Feldmen E, editors: Textbook of veterinary internal medicine, ed 6, Philadelphia, 2005, Saunders.

Fowler ME: Medicine and surgery of South American camelids, Ames, IA, 1998, Iowa State University Press.

Frandson RD, Wilke WL, Fails AD: Anatomy and physiology of farm animals, Baltimore, 2003, Lippincott Williams & Wilkins.

Hanie EA: Large animal clinical procedures for veterinary technicians, St Louis, 2006, Mosby.

Hendrix CM, Sirois M, editors: Laboratory procedures for the veterinary technician, ed 5, St Louis, 2007, Mosby.

House JK, Smith BP, Van Metre DC, et al: Ancillary tests for assessment of the ruminant digestive system, Vet Clin North Am Large Anim Pract 8:203, 1992.

Kopcha M, Schultze AE: Peritoneal fluid. II. Abdominocentesis in cattle and interpretation of nonneoplastic samples, Compend Contin Educ Pract Vet 13:703, 1991.

Lawhorn B: A new approach for obtaining blood samples from pigs, J Am Vet Med Assoc 192:781, 1988.

Macintire DK, Drobatz KJ, Haskins SC, et al: Manual of small animal emergency and critical care medicine, Baltimore, 2005, Lippincott Williams & Wilkins.

McKenzie EC: Abdominocentesis in large animals: methods and interpretation of results, Proceedings of the 25th Forum of the American College of Veterinary Internal Medicine, Seattle, 2007, ACVIM, p 27.

Orsini JA, Divers TJ: Manual of equine emergencies, ed 3, St Louis, 2008, Saunders.

Radostits OM, Gay CC, Blood DC, et al, editors: Veterinary medicine, a textbook of the diseases of cattle, sheep, pigs, goats and horses, ed 10, Oxford, 2007, Saunders.

Rockett J, Bosted S: Veterinary clinical procedures in large animal practice, Clifton Park, NY, 2007, Thomson Delmar Learning.

Rose RF, Hodgson DR: Manual of equine practice, ed 2, Philadelphia, 2000, Saunders.

Sirois M, editor: Principles and practice of veterinary technology, ed 3, St Louis, 2011, Mosby.

Smith BP, editor: Large animal internal medicine, ed 4, St Louis, 2009, Mosby.

Smith MC, Sherman DM, editors: Goat medicine, Philadelphia, 1994, Lea & Febiger.

Taylor FGR, Hillyer MH, editors: Diagnostic techniques in equine medicine, Philadelphia, 1997, Saunders.

Terry C, Rashmir-Raven A, Linford RL: Placing an intravenous catheter in horses, Vet Tech 4:207–212, 2000.

Williams CSF: Routine sheep and goat procedures, Vet Clin North Am Large Anim Pract 6:737–758, 1990.

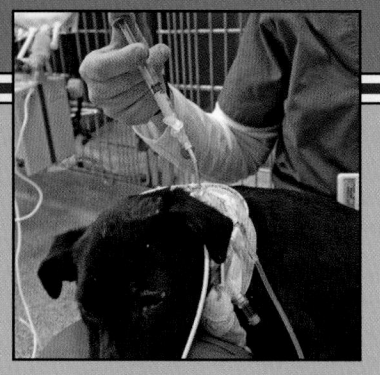

19 Small Animal Medical Nursing

Kathianne Komurek

KEY TERMS

Anorexia
Azotemia
Barrier nursing
Cachexia
Dyspnea
Eclampsia
Etiology
Galactostasis
Hematemesis
Hematochezia
Hemoptysis
Hepatic encephalopathy
Hypoxemia
Hypoxia
Mastitis
Melena
Metritis
Orthopnea
Pathogenesis
Pleural effusion
Polydipsia
Polyuria
Regurgitation
Stridor
Technician assessment
Tenesmus
Zoonoses

OUTLINE

The Veterinary Technician Practice Model: A Nursing Process, *674*
Step 1: Gather Patient Data, *674*
Step 2: Identify and Prioritize Technician Evaluations, *674*
Step 3: Develop Nursing Care Plan, *675*
Step 4: Re-Evaluate Patient, *679*
The Medical Record, *681*
Small Animal Diseases, *681*
Respiratory Disease, *682*
Cardiovascular Disease, *685*
Digestive and Hepatobiliary Diseases, *689*
Urinary Disease, *695*
Endocrine Disease, *698*
Reproductive Disease, *699*
Immune-Mediated Disease, *700*
Joint Disease, *701*
Disease of the Eyes, Ears, and Skin, *701*
Infectious Disease, *701*
Cancer, *705*

LEARNING OBJECTIVES

When you have completed this chapter, you will be able to:

1. Pronounce, define, and spell all Key Terms in this chapter.
2. Explain the relationship between the "Five Freedoms of Animal Welfare" and the responsibilities of the veterinary technician.
3. List in order the four steps that constitute the veterinary technician practice model, and describe what is involved in carrying out each step of the nursing process.
4. Explain the relationship between etiology, pathogenesis, lesions, and clinical signs.
5. Do the following regarding respiratory disease and cardiovascular disease in the small animal:
   - Compare and contrast the clinical relevance of upper versus lower respiratory disease in dogs and cats, and describe how inflammation might be related to nasal discharge, coughing, dyspnea, and hypoxia.
   - Discuss the etiology and pathogenesis of cardiovascular disease in dogs and cats and list and describe the most common cardiovascular diseases.
6. Discuss the etiology and pathogenesis of digestive and hepatobiliary diseases in dogs and cats and list and describe the most common digestive and hepatobiliary diseases.
7. Do the following regarding urinary, endocrine, and reproductive disease in dogs and cats:
   - Discuss the etiology and pathogenesis of urinary disease and list and describe the most common urinary diseases.
   - Discuss the etiology and pathogenesis of endocrine disease and list and describe the most common endocrine diseases.
   - Discuss the etiology and pathogenesis of reproductive disease and list and describe the most common reproductive diseases.
8. Do the following regarding immune-mediated disease, joint disease, and diseases affecting the eyes, ears and skin of dogs and cats:
   - Discuss the etiology and pathogenesis of immune-mediated disease and list and describe the most common immune-mediated diseases.

The authors and publisher wish to acknowledge Jody Rockett, Susan M. Eddlestone, Glenna E. Mauldin, and G. Neal Mauldin whose original work served as the foundation for portions of this chapter.

- Discuss the etiology and pathogenesis of joint disease and list and describe the most common joint diseases.
- List common diseases affecting the eyes, ears and skin.
9. Do the following regarding infectious disease in dogs and cats:
   - Discuss the etiology and pathogenesis of infectious disease.
   - List and describe special protocols needed to provide nursing care for dogs and cats with infectious diseases.
   - Explain how to educate clients about stopping the spread of infectious disease.
10. Do the following regarding the development, detection, and treatment of cancer in small in small animals:
    - Discuss the biology of cancerous tumors in dogs and cats, and explain how tumors are classified.
    - Explain the clinical manifestations of cancer in small animals, how it is diagnosed, and the treatment options available.
    - Describe the safe handling of chemotherapeutics and complications of cancer therapies in dogs and cats.

INTRODUCTION

The veterinary technician has many responsibilities in clinical practice that can broadly be divided into three categories: managerial, technical, and nursing duties. As a manager, the veterinary technician serves as a leader and may be in charge of training and supervising others. Technical responsibilities may include collecting diagnostic samples, testing those samples, and carrying out imaging studies. As a nurse, the veterinary technician provides direct care to patients and instructs owners to provide continued care at home. The overarching goal of these diverse duties is to protect and provide for the veterinary patient. Indeed, veterinary technology and the practice of veterinary technicians exemplify the tenets of animal welfare, which are succinctly classified by the Farm Animal Welfare Council of the United Kingdom as the "Five Freedoms of Animal Welfare." These include the following:

1. **Freedom from Hunger and Thirst:** by ready access to fresh water and a diet to maintain full health and vigor.
2. **Freedom from Discomfort:** by providing an appropriate environment, including shelter and a comfortable resting area.
3. **Freedom from Pain, Injury, or Disease:** by prevention or rapid diagnosis and treatment.
4. **Freedom to Express Normal Behavior:** by providing sufficient space, proper facilities, and company of the animal's own kind.
5. **Freedom from Fear and Distress:** by ensuring conditions and treatment that avoid mental suffering.

The first two freedoms constitute what is often referred to as "basic patient care" in veterinary technology and are provided to all patients (healthy and sick) at all times. In addition to basic patient care, the veterinary technician, together with the veterinarian, is responsible for the prevention and treatment of animal pain, injury, and disease, and, in the course of providing this care, minimizes levels of fear and distress as much as possible.

To ensure that excellent care is provided consistently, veterinary technicians practice a disciplined, planned approach to each and every patient. This discipline is known as the veterinary technician practice model and is relevant to all veterinary patients, but particularly those that are hospitalized.

THE VETERINARY TECHNICIAN PRACTICE MODEL: A NURSING PROCESS

The veterinary technician practice model is a cyclic nursing process that involves gathering subjective and objective data on the patient (known as the database), identifying and prioritizing technician evaluations based on these data, developing a nursing care plan and implementing specific interventions to address identified problems, and, last, evaluating the patient's response to interventions and therapies provided in the plan. The evaluation process requires patient data to be gathered again, the patient reassessed, new technician evaluations identified, and the plan of care adjusted to include new interventions if needed. Thus, the cyclic nursing process is repeated until all goals of the nursing care plan are met.

Detailed information pertaining to patient care, such as interpretation of a complete blood count (CBC), for example, or placement of a urinary catheter, is found throughout this textbook. Refer to the Table of Contents at the front of the textbook for direction to specific nursing topics.

> **TECHNICIAN NOTE** The Veterinary Technician Practice Model provides a structured nursing process to ensure that consistently excellent care is provided to each and every patient.

STEP 1: GATHER PATIENT DATA

The veterinary technician gathers subjective and objective patient data, known as the database, in the following ways:

1. Gathers the initial medical history from the owner, or reviews this information in the patient's chart if the initial history has been gathered by the veterinarian or another veterinary technician.
2. Reviews the medical record for past historical information.
3. Performs a physical examination.
4. Reviews laboratory results and diagnostic, surgical, and medical reports.
5. Consults with the attending veterinarian regarding any questions about the case not mentioned in the medical record.

STEP 2: IDENTIFY AND PRIORITIZE TECHNICIAN EVALUATIONS

Based on patient information gathered in the first step of the nursing process, the veterinary technician makes a clinical judgment regarding the physiologic and psychological needs of the patient. This judgment is called a *technician evaluation* and is based on the technician's independent critical thinking and analysis of the gathered data. For easy reference regarding common patient evaluations gathered during the physical examination, refer to Chapters 3 and 28 (Tables 19-1, 19-2, and 19-3).

As an example, a patient with tachypnea, cyanosis, and dyspnea (the data) would be given a technician evaluation

TABLE 19-1	Physical Parameters of the Cat and Dog	
PARAMETER	**ADULT CAT**	**ADULT DOG**
Rectal temperature, °F (T)	100.0-102.2	100.0-102.2
Heart rate, beats/minute (HR)	140-220	60-160 (smaller breeds may have higher rate)
Respiratory rate, breaths/minute (RR)	20-42	16-32
Mucous membrane quality	Moist	Moist
Capillary refill time, seconds (CRT)	<2	<2
Skin turgor/SNAP, seconds	Immediate/<2	Immediate/<2
Systolic blood pressure, mm Hg (BP)	120-160	130-160
Intraocular pressure, mm Hg (IOP)	15-25	15-25
Oxygen saturation (SaO$_2$)	>95%	>95%
Urine volume, ml/kg body wt/day	10-20	20-100

TABLE 19-2	Mucous Membrane Color Assessment
COLOR	**PHYSIOLOGY**
Pink/Pale Pink	Normal
Pale/White	Inadequate blood volume or low hemoglobin concentration
Blue/Purple (cyanotic)	Inadequate oxygenation of tissues
Yellow (icteric)	Hyperbilirubinemia
Brick Red (injected)	Endotoxemia, shock

TABLE 19-3	Lung Auscultation Sounds and Their Associations
SOUND	**ASSOCIATION**
Wheeze (musical, high or low pitched)	Bronchial disease
Crackles (popping)	Pleural disease, pulmonary disease
Absent lung sounds/muffled heart sounds	Space-occupying problem: effusions, diaphragmatic hernia

of hypoxia. This assessment is separate from the medical diagnosis made by the veterinarian, which focuses on the cause of the problem, such as congestive heart failure. The technician is observing the patient's physiologic response to congestive heart failure and assigns technician evaluations independently based on the data gathered. Additionally, technician evaluations may include information on the owner's level of knowledge regarding care of the pet and the owner's ability to cope with the responsibility. Technician evaluations fall into three broad categories: identification of actual problems, risk of future problems, and level of client knowledge and/or coping abilities that may or may not impair at-home care of the pet. Tables 19-4, 19-5, and 3-1 provide a selection of technician evaluations.

Once a list of technician evaluations has been generated, each evaluation is prioritized in terms of importance to the livelihood of the patient. For example, let's imagine that a cyanotic, dyspneic patient has a body condition score of 5/5. At that moment, it is more important for the livelihood of the patient to breathe than it is to have an ideal body weight, so the technician evaluation of "hypoxia" takes precedence over the technician evaluation of "overweight" when the

nursing plan is devised and implemented. Refer to Table 3-2 in Chapter 3 for a list of technician evaluations.

> **TECHNICIAN NOTE** A technician evaluation is a clinical judgment that the veterinary technician makes regarding the physiologic and psychological needs of the patient.

STEP 3: DEVELOP NURSING CARE PLAN

Once technician evaluations have been identified and prioritized, each should have a desired outcome associated with it. In our patient with hypoxia, for example, the desired outcome is adequate oxygenation, which would be evidenced by resolution of the dyspnea and the return of mucous membranes

TABLE 19-4	Selection of Technician Evaluations and Interventions			
TECHNICIAN EVALUATION AND DEFINITION	**POTENTIAL PHYSIOLOGIC CONSEQUENCES**	**CLINICAL FINDINGS**	**DESIRED PATIENT OUTCOME**	**TECHNICIAN INTERVENTIONS**
Anorexia Complete or partial loss of appetite	Poor immune function Decreased wound healing Dehydration Electrolyte imbalance Hypoalbuminemia Hepatic lipidosis Cachexia Hypoglycemia Hypothermia Seizures Death	Loss of appetite for >2 days Prolonged diminished appetite	Sustained return of appetite and intake of appropriate number of daily calories	Administer doctor-prescribed appetite stimulant, antiemetics, antacids Encourage patient to eat on its own: • Coax/socialization • Novel, odoriferous foods • Stress-free eating area • Patient hygiene • Assisted feeding: syringe, orogastric tube Feeding tube management and meal administration Monitor calorie intake Basic patient monitoring*
Dehydration Loss of total body water	Decreased renal perfusion Electrolyte imbalance Hypothermia	Tacky/dry mucous membranes Delayed skin turgor Enophthalmos Decreased urine output Increased PCV and TP Hyperalbuminemia Increased urine concentration	Restoration of normal hydration: • Moist mucous membranes • Normal skin turgor • Normal urine output	Administer fluid therapy per doctor's orders Basic patient monitoring Monitor fluid intake and output Monitor for signs of fluid overload: • Presence of lung crackles • Presence of new heart murmur • Presence of edema • Increasing body weight • Increased serous nasal discharge • Increased central venous pressure Treat/prevent electrolyte imbalance

Continued

TABLE 19-4	Selection of Technician Evaluations and Interventions—cont'd

TECHNICIAN EVALUATION AND DEFINITION	POTENTIAL PHYSIOLOGIC CONSEQUENCES	CLINICAL FINDINGS	DESIRED PATIENT OUTCOME	TECHNICIAN INTERVENTIONS
Hypovolemia Loss of intravascular fluid	Decreased perfusion of vital organs: kidneys, heart, and brain Hypothermia Shock End-organ failure Death	Dry mucous membranes Pale to white mucous membranes Prolonged CRT Tachycardia Weak pulses Altered mentation Hemorrhage Increased or decreased PCV Hypoalbuminemia Hypotension	Restoration of normovolemia: • Pink/moist mucous membranes • Normal CRT • Normotensive • Normal cardiac function	Administer fluid therapy per doctor's orders Basic patient monitoring Monitor fluid intake and output Monitor for signs of fluid overload: • Presence of lung crackles • Presence of new heart murmur • Presence of edema • Increasing body weight • Increased serous nasal discharge • Increased central venous pressure Administer blood transfusion per doctor's orders Monitor for signs of transfusion reaction: • Anxiety • Nausea, vomiting, diarrhea • Fever • Pruritus • Skin erythema • Urticaria
Hyperthermia Elevated body temperature	Increased metabolism Dehydration Electrolyte imbalance Shock Coagulopathies CNS abnormalities Death	Temperature >103° F Panting (dog) Warm skin Tachypnea Tachycardia Altered mentation	Restoration and maintenance of normal body temperature/ Thermoregulation	Cool patient: • Provide cool environment • Apply alcohol to foot pads • Apply ice packs to groin, foot pads • Cool-water bath Basic patient monitoring* Treat/prevent dehydration Administer doctor-prescribed antipyretics
Hypothermia Decreased body temperature	Decreased metabolism Decreased tissue perfusion Ischemia Shock Death	Temperature <99° F Shivering Altered mentation Prolonged CRT Bradycardia Decreased respirations Cyanosis	Restoration and maintenance of normal body temperature/ thermoregulation	Provide heat support: • Warm-water circulating blanket • Bair Hugger blanket (Arizant Healthcare, Inc., Eden Prairie, Minnesota) • Incubator • Warmed IV fluids Severely hypothermic patients must be warmed slowly Basic patient monitoring Oxygen therapy

TABLE 19-4	Selection of Technician Evaluations and Interventions—cont'd			
TECHNICIAN EVALUATION AND DEFINITION	**POTENTIAL PHYSIOLOGIC CONSEQUENCES**	**CLINICAL FINDINGS**	**DESIRED PATIENT OUTCOME**	**TECHNICIAN INTERVENTIONS**
Pain Unpleasant sensation	Increased stress response leading to: • Increased metabolism • Tachycardia • Hypertension • Nausea • Vomiting • Anorexia • Immunosuppression	Refer to pain scales Changes in behavior, posture, and reaction to palpation Symptoms of *acute* pain also include: • Tachycardia • Tachypnea • Hypertension	Resolution or reduction of pain as evidenced by decreasing pain score	Administer doctor-prescribed analgesics Monitor for breakthrough pain Basic patient monitoring Monitor for signs of adverse reaction to analgesics: • Vomiting and diarrhea • Melena • Decreased respiratory rate • Constipation • Agitation (cats) Physical therapy Provide comfortable environment Educate owner on changes to patient lifestyle and environment (chronic pain)
Electrolyte imbalance Abnormal plasma electrolyte levels	Dehydration Nausea, vomiting Polyuria/polydipsia Muscle weakness Seizures/tremors Cardiac abnormalities Altered mentation Coma Death	Depending on specific electrolyte, may see: • Bradycardia • Tachycardia • Arrhythmias • Muscle weakness • Muscle tremors • Seizures	Normal electrolyte concentrations	For deficiencies: • Administer doctor-prescribed supplementation For elevations: • Administer doctor-prescribed medications • Fluid diuresis Basic patient monitoring Monitor ECGs Provide padded bedding for patients with muscle tremors, seizures
Urethral obstruction Unable to void a normal stream of urine because of occlusion of urethra	Buildup of toxins in the bloodstream Dehydration Electrolyte imbalance Bladder rupture and urine peritonitis Coma Death	Stranguria Full, turgid bladder on palpation with inability to express urine Vomiting Altered mentation	Normal elimination of urine	Urinary catheterization per doctor's orders Administer doctor-prescribed medications Monitor urine output, urine stream Manual bladder expression (neurologic patients) Basic patient monitoring Treat/prevent dehydration Treat/prevent electrolyte imbalance Educate client on technique for manual bladder expression (neurologic patients)

Continued

TABLE 19-4	Selection of Technician Evaluations and Interventions—cont'd			
TECHNICIAN EVALUATION AND DEFINITION	**POTENTIAL PHYSIOLOGIC CONSEQUENCES**	**CLINICAL FINDINGS**	**DESIRED PATIENT OUTCOME**	**TECHNICIAN INTERVENTIONS**
Cardiac insufficiency Inadequate cardiac output necessary for tissue perfusion	Ischemia Necrosis Fluid accumulation Hypoxia Hypovolemia End-organ failure Death	Tachypnea Tachycardia Abnormal heart sounds Prolonged CRT Pale or cyanotic mucous membranes Weak or asynchronous pulses Exercise intolerance Syncope Signs of ATE[†] (cats) Signs of CHF[†] ECG abnormalities Hypotension or hypertension	Adequate cardiac output: • Normal CRT • Pink mucous membranes • Normal heart rate • Normal respirations • Normotensive	Oxygen therapy Basic patient monitoring Monitor for signs of CHF/ATE Monitor ECG, oxygen saturation Monitor blood pressure Monitor fluid intake and output Administer doctor-ordered medications Monitor for adverse effects of medications Low-sodium diet
Hypoxia Inadequate oxygenation	Tissue ischemia Death	Cyanotic mucous membranes Dyspnea Tachypnea Altered mentation Decreased oxygen saturation (SaO_2) Altered arterial blood gas (ABG) values ($\downarrow PaO_2$)	Adequate oxygenation: • Pink mucous membranes • Normal respirations • Normal oxygen saturation • Normal ABG values	Oxygen supplementation Basic patient monitoring Monitor oxygen saturation with pulse oximetry and arterial blood gas analysis
Overweight Excessive intake of nutrients	Obesity is a predisposing factor to a wide variety of small animal diseases	Body condition score of 4+ out of 5	Body condition score of 3/5, ideal body weight	Determine ideal body weight and daily calorie requirement Develop a nutritional weight loss and exercise plan for patient Educate owner on health consequences of obesity and importance of plan implementation Monitor patient's progress to ensure appropriate degree of weight loss
Underweight Inadequate intake or absorption of nutrients to meet metabolic demands	Malnutrition leads to: • Multi-systemic organ dysfunction • Dehydration • Electrolyte imbalance • Vitamin deficiency	Body condition score of 1 to 2 out of 5	Body condition score of 3/5, ideal body weight	Determine ideal body weight and daily caloric requirement Develop nutritional plan for weight gain Treat electrolyte imbalance Treat vitamin deficiency Treat anorexia, if present Client education regarding feeding plan Monitor patient's progress to ensure appropriate degree of weight gain

TABLE 19-4	Selection of Technician Evaluations and Interventions—cont'd			
TECHNICIAN EVALUATION AND DEFINITION	POTENTIAL PHYSIOLOGIC CONSEQUENCES	CLINICAL FINDINGS	DESIRED PATIENT OUTCOME	TECHNICIAN INTERVENTIONS
Vomiting Forceful expulsion of contents from the stomach and/or intestines	Anorexia Dehydration Electrolyte imbalance Malnutrition Weight loss	Nausea Vomiting Abdominal pain	Resolution of vomiting	Isolate patient if contagion is suspected Administer doctor-prescribed medications Fast the patient Provide nutritional support/dietary therapy (e.g., small, frequent meals of bland food) Basic patient monitoring Decrease smell of strong odors (trigger nausea/vomiting) Prevent/treat dehydration Treat electrolyte imbalance Treat anorexia
Diarrhea Frequent passage of loose, unformed stool	Dehydration Electrolyte imbalance Malnutrition Weight loss	Diarrhea Abdominal pain	Passage of normally formed stool	Isolate patient if contagion is suspected Administer doctor-prescribed medications Prevent/treat dehydration Basic patient monitoring Ensure patient hygiene: • Clip away matted fur • Clean perineal area with warm water and a mild soap • Thoroughly dry patient after bathing Provide nutritional support/dietary therapy
Constipation Infrequent and often difficult passage of hard stool	GI toxin buildup Anorexia Vomiting Electrolyte imbalance Rectal prolapse	Abdominal distention Abdominal pain Altered mentation Palpation of large amounts of hard stool in colon	Easy passage of normally formed stool at least once a day	Ensure adequate hydration Administer enema Basic patient monitoring Treat anorexia Feed high-fiber or low-residue food

ATE, Arterial thromboembolism (saddle thrombus); *CHF*, congestive heart failure; *CNS*, central nervous system; *CRT*, capillary refill time; *ECG*, electrocardiogram; *PCV*, packed cell volume; *TP*, total protein.
*Basic patient monitoring as listed in Box 19-1.
†See text for clinical signs.

to a normal pink color. Each technician evaluation is accompanied by one or more interventions, or actions, to help achieve the desired patient outcome. Technician interventions number in the hundreds; Box 19-1 gives some examples of common technician interventions employed in the course of small animal medical nursing. A technician intervention can be something seemingly simple, such as a nail trim, but when taken in the context of a feline patient with forelimb paralysis who cannot use the scratching post to maintain healthy nails, a nail trim is an integral part of patient care because it prevents the nails from growing into the pads, causing an infection.

The nursing care plan refers to the entire list of interventions specific to each technician evaluation for a particular patient. Tables 19-4 and 19-5 provide examples of technician interventions for select technician evaluations.

STEP 4: RE-EVALUATE PATIENT

The care plan is continuously revised as the patient responds (beneficially or adversely) to the interventions, and new technician evaluations are identified based on changes in patient status. In some cases, additional data such as laboratory and imaging studies are required to fully assess the patient's response to nursing interventions and to the

TABLE 19-5	A Selection of "At-Risk" Technician Evaluations	
TECHNICIAN EVALUATION	**CHARACTERISTICS OF AN AT-RISK PATIENT**	**TECHNICIAN INTERVENTION**
Risk of aspiration	Loss of gag and swallow reflexes • Patient is sedated or anesthetized • Altered mentation • Damage to cranial nerves • Megaesophagus	Feed gruel-consistency foods Elevate food and water bowls Maintain elevation of head and forelimbs for 10 minutes after eating Feeding tube meals Do not feed patients recovering from anesthesia until they can swallow
Risk of infection	Compromised immune system function • Naïve • Immature • Suppressed • Deficient Break in physiologic barriers to infection • Skin lacerations, burns • Change in acidity of GI tract • Change in normal GI tract flora • Decreased urine concentration	Monitor for signs of infection, including: • Fever • Swelling, discharge, erythema • Pain • Change in lung sounds (pneumonia) • Decreased blood glucose (sepsis) • Increased white blood cell count Administer doctor-prescribed prophylactic antibiotic therapy Prevent both contagious and nosocomial infections • Reverse isolation • Proper aseptic technique when handling patient
Risk of infectious disease transmission	History of exposure Symptoms of a potential contagious disease • Fever • Cough • Vomiting/diarrhea • Sneezing, nasal discharge, conjunctivitis Any patient with confirmed contagious infectious disease	Treat as outpatient when possible Institute standard hospital isolation protocols Educate owner regarding at-home isolation procedures and disease transmission to other household animals
Risk of self-trauma	Patients with pruritic or inflammatory disease Patients with localized pain (e.g., feline declaw) Patients with: • IV catheter • Urinary catheter • Feeding tubes • Chest tubes Patients with skin sutures or staples	Administer doctor-prescribed medications to alleviate pruritus, inflammation, and pain and to treat underlying disease process (e.g., topical corticosteroids) Administer doctor-prescribed medications to treat underlying disease process (e.g., topical flea control) Sedate patient Deter patient from area: • Bandage site (catheters, tubes) • Sweater/t-shirt (pruritus) • E-collar • Bite-not collar
Risk of pain	Patients needing an invasive medical procedure known to be painful (chest tubes, bone marrow aspirate) Patients with severe inflammatory disease (acute pancreatitis) Patients undergoing surgical procedures	Preemptive analgesia as prescribed by doctor Monitor for breakthrough pain

BOX 19-1 Examples of Technician Interventions (Relevant to Internal Medicine)

Basic Patient Care
Ensure patient can breathe
Provide access to proper amounts of food and water
Provide access to clean litter box/frequent walks outside
Provide adequate, comfortable, clean housing
Provide patient hygiene—grooming, bathing, clipping
Provide exercise for mobile patient
Provide patient safety
Provide relief from pain and discomfort

Medication Administration and Catheter Placement
Medication/fluid administration: oral
Medication/fluid administration: subcutaneous
Medication/fluid administration: intravenous
Medication/fluid administration: intraosseous
Medication administration: intramuscular
Medication administration: topical—eye
Medication administration: topical—ear
Medication administration: topical—nose
Medication administration: topical—skin
Catheter placement: intravenous
Catheter placement: intraosseous
Catheter placement: urinary

Tube Management
Tracheostomy tubes
Chest tubes
Feeding tubes

Patient Monitoring
Basic patient monitoring: temperature, pulse, respiration, CRT, mucous membranes, skin turgor, body weight, mentation, appetite, urination, defecation
Advanced monitoring of critical patient may include thoracic auscultation, pulse oximetry, capnography, arterial blood

gases, measurement of fluid losses/output, central venous pressure, ECG, blood pressure
Monitor laboratory values as they pertain to the disease process and medical therapies
Monitor for pain
Monitor for desired effects of medical therapies
Monitor for adverse effects of medical therapies
Monitor for desired effects of fluid therapy
Monitor for adverse effects of fluid therapy
Monitor for desired effects of electrolyte replacement
Monitor for adverse effects of electrolyte replacement

Client Education (addressing client knowledge deficit)
Pet selection
Kitten and puppy care and training
Reproduction and neonatal care
Nutritional recommendations
Grooming care
Problem behavior management
Preventive care: vaccinations, parasite control, dental care
Drug therapies: indications, dosing, side effects
Drug therapies: handling and storage
Drug therapies: importance of compliance
Drug therapies: importance of follow-up diagnostics
Medication administration techniques
Subcutaneous fluid administration
Feeding tube management and meal administration
Wound management/bandage care
Disease pathophysiology
Infectious disease control
Chronic pain management

Client Support
Hospice care
Grief counseling

CRT, Capillary refill time; *ECG*, electrocardiography.

treatment prescribed by the attending veterinarian. In this way, the first phase of the veterinary practice model is repeated, demonstrating the its cyclical pattern. Case Presentation 19-1 provides an example of a nursing care plan.

THE MEDICAL RECORD

All patient data, technician evaluations, interventions, and nursing care plans are recorded in the medical record using the SOAP (subjective, objective, assessment, and plan) format; please refer to Chapter 3 for detailed information. Specific flow sheets for hospitalized patients may be used for ease of recording technician interventions, such as administration of medication and fluid therapy and monitoring of vital signs.

SMALL ANIMAL DISEASES

Etiology is the study of the causation or origination of disease. For example, the etiologic agent or cause of heartworm disease is the bloodborne parasite *Dirofilaria immitis*.

Many causes of disease are known, including infectious agents, toxins, physical trauma, nutritional deficits, genetic defects, aging, and psychological stress. If the cause of a disease is unknown, it is termed *idiopathic*. **Pathogenesis** is the mechanism of development of a disease; it can be acute or chronic. Regardless of whether the pathogenesis of a disease is acute or chronic, complex or simple, it ultimately leads to injury to cells and body tissues, which may be visible as gross and microscopic lesions. Examples of common pathologic mechanisms that lead to disease include inflammation, cell injury (such as infectious, toxic, and physical), cell growth abnormalities (such as neoplasia, hypertrophy, and hyperplasia), metabolic disturbances, and immune system dysfunction. The body's response to these pathologic events may be evident to the veterinary technician as clinical signs.

The overall process for disease may be summarized as follows:

Etiology → Pathogenesis → Lesions → Clinical Signs

CASE PRESENTATION 19-1 AN EXAMPLE OF A NURSING CARE PLAN

Signalment: California Sunset (Cal), 3-year-old, male castrated red and white tabby DSH

Chief Complaint: Owner reports that Cal is acting lethargic and has not been eating well since yesterday.

Pertinent History: Owner has three cats and one litter box, so it is difficult to know whether Cal is urinating and defecating normally. Litter box is cleaned every other day. Owner is unaware of any inappropriate urination or defecation. Owner meal-feeds appropriate amount of high-quality commercial dry and wet food.

Physical Examination:

Body weight: 13 pounds; Body condition score: 3/5; Temperature: 101.5° F; Heart rate: 160 bpm, sinus rhythm; Synchronous and strong pulses; Respiration: 22 bpm, lungs clear; Mucous membranes: pink and moist; CRT: <2 seconds; Skin turgor: normal; Skin and hair coat: normal; Ears, eyes, and nose: normal; GI system: large amounts of firm stool in colon, no reaction to palpation; Urogenital system: normal; Musculoskeletal system: normal.

Medical Diagnosis (by veterinarian): Uncomplicated constipation

Technician Evaluations: Constipation; Client knowledge deficit

Nursing Care Plan

1. Constipation

INTERVENTION	RATIONALE
Administer 100 ml Normasol SC, per doctor's orders	Prevent dehydration that may occur because of fluid loss from enema and/or vomiting that may occur following enema
Prepare and administer enema	Soften stool and allow for passage of stool
Place patient in large cage with two litter boxes	Allows patient movement, which helps stimulate bowel evacuation
	Allows for ample places to defecate
Basic patient monitoring (rectal temperature avoided)	Enemas can precipitate a vagal response, which may cause vomiting and bradycardia
	Palpation of abdomen to ensure that all stool was passed
Patient hygiene: Bathe perineal area and back legs	Enema liquid and stool typically stain these areas

2. Client knowledge deficit

INTERVENTION	RATIONALE
Litter box management • Four litter boxes for three cats is ideal • Cleaned every day	Patient's constipation is secondary to inadequate access to clean litter boxes for normal, daily elimination

Part of the pathogenesis of heartworm disease, for example, involves the physical presence of the heartworm, which irritates the lining of the pulmonary vessels, causing inflammation. Continued inflammation of the pulmonary vasculature leads to coughing—a well-known clinical sign of heartworm disease. Keep in mind that the technician evaluation consists of the technician's observation of the patient's physiologic response to disease. This is why it is important for the technician to have a basic grasp of the pathogenesis of common small animal medical diseases. The information presented in this chapter on pathogenesis is, by necessity, very brief and focuses on the most common diseases seen in cats and dogs. The reader is referred to the recommended reading list at the end of the chapter for more extensive information.

It is worth noting that not all patients with disease show outward signs of illness. Heart disease is an example of this. In patients with heart disease, the body compensates to maintain proper heart function, and the patient appears outwardly healthy. When these homeostatic mechanisms fail, congestive heart failure results, and only then does the patient show overt signs of illness. The same is true for a patient with well-controlled disease, such as diabetes mellitus, that is not ill.

In small animal veterinary medicine, some diseases are more prevalent in dogs than in cats, and are more common in certain breeds and at certain life stages than others. Table 19-6 provides a quick reference on patient signalments associated with various common diseases discussed in this chapter.

RESPIRATORY DISEASE

Most diseases of the respiratory tract ultimately result in inflammation, irritation, and obstruction or restriction of the airway. Each of these processes causes an array of clinical symptoms. It is important for the veterinary technician to be familiar with all of the symptoms because they help direct the nursing process. A technician familiar with the signs of respiratory disease, for example, will be more focused when taking a history, completing a physical examination, performing technician evaluations, and carrying out diagnostic and therapeutic interventions.

Nasal discharge results from inflammation or irritation of the nasal mucosa and can be serous (clear liquid), mucoid (opaque and sticky), mucopurulent (green-yellow and mucoid), or hemorrhagic (bloody). It is important to note whether the discharge is unilateral or bilateral. When a medical history is obtained, the duration and progression of the nasal discharge are important to ascertain. Nasal and sinus congestion is caused by inflammation of the epithelial tissue that lines the nasal and sinus passages. Vasodilatation of capillaries, leakage of fluid from these vessels into surrounding parenchyma, and increased production of mucus by epithelial cells lead to narrowing of the nasal and sinus passages, causing partial or, in severe cases, complete obstruction. Clinically, the patient presents with a "stuffy nose." Both nasal discharge and edema can compromise airflow, leading

TABLE 19-6	Common Signalments Associated With Selected Small Animal Diseases					
	PEDIATRIC	**YOUNG ADULT**	**MATURE ADULT**	**SENIOR**	**GERIATRIC**	**BREED PREDISPOSITIONS**
	CAT <7 MO **DOG <7 MO**	**CAT 1-6 YR** **DOG 1-5 YR**	**CAT 7-10 YR** **DOG 6-8 YR**	**CAT 11-14 YR** **DOG 9-11 YR**	**CAT 15+ YR** **DOG 12+ YR**	
Disease						
Degenerative atrioventricular (AV) valve disease		d		d	d	Cavalier King Charles spaniel, Dachshund, and most small breed dogs
Hypertrophic cardiomyopathy	c	c	c	c	c	Maine Coon, Ragdoll, American and British shorthair, Bengal, Norwegian Forest cat, Persian, Sphynx, Turkish Van
Dilated cardiomyopathy		d	d	d		Boxers, Cocker spaniel, Doberman, Great Dane, Irish Wolfhound, Newfoundland, Portuguese water dog, Retriever, St. Bernard, Scottish Deerhound
Inflammatory bowel disease			c, d	c, d		German Shepherd dog, Siamese cat
Idiopathic megacolon			c	c		Domestic shorthair, Domestic longhair, Siamese
Exocrine pancreatic insufficiency		d	c, d	c, d		German Shepherd dog, Rough Coated Collie
Chronic hepatitis			d	d		Bedlington Terrier, Dalmatian, Labrador Retriever, West Highland White Terrier, Doberman Pinscher, English Springer spaniel, American and English Cocker Spaniel
Congenital portosystemic shunt	c, d	c, d				Terrier-type dogs, Irish Wolfhound, Old English Sheepdog, Labrador Retriever, Golden Retriever, Himalayan, Persian
Chronic renal failure			c, d	c, d	c, d	
Struvite urolithiasis		c, d	c, d	c, d	c, d	
Calcium oxalate urolithiasis		c, d	c, d	c, d	c, d	Miniature Schnauzer, Lhasa Apso, Yorkshire Terrier, Bichon Frise, Shih Tzu, Miniature Poodle, Persian, Himalayan
Urate urolithiasis		d				Dalmatian, Siamese
Cystine urolithiasis		d	d			Basset Hound, Chihuahua, Dachshund, English Bulldog, Irish Terrier, Newfoundland Yorkshire Terrier
Diabetes mellitus			c, d	c, d	c	Miniature Poodle, Dachshund, Cairn Terrier, Beagle, Schnauzer
Hyperadrenocorticism			d	d	d	Poodle, Dachshund, Beagle, Boxer
Hypoadrenocorticism		d	d	d		Bearded Collie, Great Dane, Portuguese water dog, Rottweiler, Standard Poodle, West Highland Terrier, Soft-Coated Wheaten Terrier
Hyperthyroidism			c	c	c	
Hypothyroidism		d	d	d		Airedale Terrier, Cocker Spaniel, Dachshund, Doberman Pinscher, Golden Retriever, Irish Setter, Miniature Schnauzer

to open-mouth breathing in some patients. Additionally, the diminished sense of smell may cause **anorexia**, particularly in cats. Nursing care for these patients includes providing airway humidification, relieving nasal congestion through administration of pediatric nasal decongestants, keeping the patient's face clean of nasal discharge, and treating anorexia.

A *sneeze* is defined as an involuntary, spasmodic, forcible expulsion of air from the mouth and nose in an effort to expel respiratory irritants. Frequent, rapid bouts of sneezing are abnormal. In dogs, sneezing is most commonly seen with inhalation of foreign material; with cats, it is most often associated with upper respiratory viral infection. Until proven otherwise, sneezing patients, particularly cats, should be treated as if they are contagious, and isolation procedures should be instituted.

A patient with nasal discharge, congestion, and/or sneezing should be closely examined for facial swelling that can accompany the causative disease, such as a tooth root abscess, migration of nasal foreign bodies, neoplasm, or fungal infection.

Obstruction of the pharynx or larynx can cause *stertor*, a loud snoring or snorting sound, or **stridor**, a high pitched inspiratory wheeze. The presence of either sound justifies a thorough examination of the upper airways, and steps must be taken to ensure an open airway.

A *cough* is a forceful expulsion of air from the lungs through the mouth. It may be a reflexive or conscious action resulting from irritation or inflammation to the pharynx, larynx, trachea, bronchi, or pleura. A cough may be productive, meaning that mucus, fluid, or blood is brought up from the airway (and usually swallowed), or nonproductive, sometimes called a "dry cough." **Hemoptysis**, the coughing up of blood, is most often seen with heartworm disease. The owner often confuses a productive cough, particularly in cats with asthma, with retching or vomiting, so careful questioning is indicated when a medical history is gathered (Table 19-7). Palpation of the trachea may elicit a cough in patients with tracheal irritation. Thorough auscultation of the thoracic cavity is necessary to detect abnormal lungs sounds or heart abnormalities (coughing in dogs can be seen with congestive heart failure). Nursing care of the coughing patient includes providing airway humidification, decreasing pressure to the trachea (harness vs. collar, weight management), and in dogs, decreasing excitement.

Pleural effusion is the accumulation of excessive fluid within the thoracic cavity. Causes include fluid overload, infection, lymphatic obstruction, coagulopathies, and trauma. Pleural effusion restricts normal breathing because the presence of fluid in the thoracic cavity causes compression of the lung tissue and inadequate lung expansion. Clinically patients often present in respiratory distress with increased inspiratory effort. On examination, lung sounds are decreased and heart sounds are muffled. Cats may have noticeable decreased chest compliance if significant amounts of fluid are present. The presence of pleural effusion is confirmed via thoracocentesis or radiography. For a patient in respiratory distress, thoracocentesis is performed before

TABLE 19-7	Coughing vs. Retching/Vomiting in the Cat	
	COUGHING	**RETCHING/VOMITING**
Head and neck position	Extended straight out (parallel to the floor)	Head hanging over neck
Body position	Crouched down on all four legs	Sitting or standing up
Fluid	Small amount of clear foam, often swallowed immediately	Variable
Accompanying abdominal contractions	No	Yes
Accompanying wheezes	Yes	No
Signs of nausea (lip-smacking, hypersalivation, vocalization) before episode	No	Oftentimes

radiographs, to relieve pressure on the lungs. Nursing care for patients with pleural effusion includes providing oxygen supplementation, decreasing stress, performing therapeutic thoracocentesis, and monitoring for hypoxia.

Dyspnea, or respiratory distress, is difficulty breathing characterized by increased respiratory effort, often with an abdominal component to the breath. Patients often exhibit **orthopnea**, the inability to breathe except in an upright position; dogs tend to stand with their necks extended and their elbows abducted, while cats prefer sternal recumbency. Cats do not pant, so the presence of open-mouth breathing with noticeable chest movement equates to dyspnea. Any interruption of normal airflow (e.g., upper or lower respiratory tract obstruction), adequate lung inflation (e.g., pleural effusion, pneumothorax), or alveolar gas exchange (e.g., pneumonia) can cause dyspnea.

The respiratory pattern can yield some clue to the location of the problem. Patients with upper airway disease tend to exhibit increased inspiratory effort and take slow, deep breaths; patients with lower airway disease typically exhibit increased expiratory effort and have shallow, rapid breaths. Dyspneic patients are in critical condition, and demonstration of a patent airway and provision of oxygen are required immediately (refer to Chapter 25, "Emergency and Critical Care Nursing"). If pleural effusion or pneumothorax is present, thoracocentesis is performed as quickly as possible to help stabilize the patient. Stressing a dyspneic patient can result in death. Therefore, thorough examination and diagnostic tests begin once the patient's condition has stabilized. Additionally, patients need to be closely monitored by the veterinary technician during these procedures for signs of hypoxia and commonly need oxygen support throughout the diagnostic procedures.

Hypoxia is defined as deficient oxygenation of tissues. Hypoxia can result from reduced blood flow (e.g., congestive heart failure), decreased oxygen-carrying capacity (e.g., anemia), hypoventilation (e.g., pleural effusion), or ventilation/perfusion mismatch (e.g., pneumonia). Pulse oximetry yields an estimate of tissue oxygen saturation, which in a normal patient is greater than 95%. Hypoxia manifests clinically as tachypnea, cyanosis or pallor, and dyspnea. Nursing care for the hypoxic patient is presented in Table 19-4.

Hypoxemia refers to a decrease in arterial oxygen partial pressure (PaO_2) as measured by arterial blood gas analysis.

> **TECHNICIAN NOTE** Unduly stressing a dyspneic patient can cause respiratory arrest. Ensure a patent airway, provide oxygen immediately, and do not perform diagnostic tests until the patient is stable.

Diagnostic procedures for respiratory diseases include rhinoscopy, bronchoscopy, radiography, ultrasonography, computed tomography (CT) and magnetic resonance imaging (MRI) scans, cytologic examination and cultures of secretions, exudates and effusions, biopsies, blood gas analysis, capnography (measurement of exhaled carbon dioxide), serum fungal titers, and parasitologic tests. Table 19-8 summarizes the general therapeutic approach to a patient with

respiratory disease. Table 19-9 lists common respiratory diseases and their specific treatments.

CARDIOVASCULAR DISEASE

Heart Disease, Heart Failure, and Congestive Heart Failure

Heart disease is a pathologic abnormality that affects the myocardium, the valves, rhythm conduction, or the overall structure of the heart (shunts). In cats, myocardial disease accounts for more than 80% of heart disease cases; in dogs, valvular disease accounts for more than 75% of cardiac cases. The body has incredible compensatory mechanisms to maintain cardiac output when faced with an abnormally functioning heart; therefore, most patients are asymptomatic at home. Early detection of heart disease is reliant upon thorough annual physical examinations and, for predisposed breeds, screening echocardiograms. On physical examination, a patient with heart disease may have tachycardia; a weak, bounding, or asynchronous femoral pulse; a heart murmur; and/or an arrhythmia. Diagnosis of heart disease relies on diagnostic imaging of the heart—radiography and echocardiography—and electrocardiography. In recent years, serum cardiac biomarkers such as B-type natriuretic peptide (BNP) have become available to aid in diagnosis. With the notable exception of some congenital disorders that may be corrected with surgery (e.g., patent ductus arteriosus), no efficacious treatments are currently available to slow

TABLE 19-8	Therapeutic Approach to Patients With Respiratory Disease	
TREATMENT	**RATIONALE**
Ensure open airway • Intubate • Position patient to alleviate pressure on airway • Administer bronchodilators • Remove foreign body	Prevent respiratory arrest
Ensure adequate patient oxygenation • Provide supplemental oxygen	Treat/prevent hypoxia
Decrease stress in dyspneic patients • Minimal handling • Quiet environment • Sedation	• Stress causes an increased demand for oxygen, which a dyspneic patient may not be able to meet • Leads to respiratory decompensation and possible respiratory arrest
Thoracocentesis	Immediate removal of pleural effusion will allow for proper lung inflation
Airway humidification • Vaporizer • Nebulization • Steam therapy (outpatient) • Saline nasal drops • Systemic hydration	• Mucous membranes lining respiratory tract must be moist to function properly • Dry mucous membranes promote inflammation, increase mucus, decrease mucociliary clearance, and decrease local immune function and barrier protection
Antitussives	Control nonproductive cough
Expectorants	Thin mucous secretions and encourage productive cough
Prophylactic antibiotics	Prevent bacterial infection secondary to compromised respiratory tract function
Anti-inflammatories	Reduce inflammation of the airways
Antibiotics	Treat primary infection
Antiparasitics	Treat primary infection
Antifungals	Treat primary infection

TABLE 19-9	Small Animal Respiratory Diseases			
DISEASE	**PATHOGENESIS**	**CLINICAL SIGNS**	**DIAGNOSTICS**	**TREATMENTS**
Rhinitis/sinusitis	Inflammation of the mucosa of the nasal passages and sinuses caused by viral, bacterial, or fungal infection; foreign bodies, allergies, neoplasia, or tooth root abscess	Nasal discharge Nasal/sinus congestion Sneezing Facial swelling Open-mouth breathing	History and clinical signs Determination of infectious agent Radiograph Computed tomography (CT)/magnetic resonance imaging (MRI) scans	Airway humidification Treat underlying cause: • Foreign body removal • Antifungal therapy • Tooth extraction • Allergy relief • Antibiotics • Anti-inflammatories
Brachycephalic airway syndrome	Upper airway obstruction seen in brachycephalic breeds caused by a constellation of anatomic deformities, including stenotic nares, elongated soft palate, hypoplastic trachea, and laryngeal collapse	Voice change Stertor Stridor Exercise intolerance Hypoxia	Signalment Physical examination Direct visualization of upper airway Radiographs	Emergency treatment of dyspnea Weight management Avoid overheating Exercise restrictions Surgical correction of anatomic deformities
Laryngeal paralysis	Damage to the recurrent laryngeal nerves resulting in paralysis of the arytenoid cartilage	Change in voice Stridor Exercise intolerance Gagging or coughing with eating or vocalization Dyspnea	Direct visualization of larynx	Maintain open airway (intubation) Emergency treatment of dyspnea Surgery—laryngoplasty
Feline bronchitis (feline asthma)	Irritation and inflammation of the bronchi causing bronchial constriction, hypertrophy of bronchial smooth muscle, and increased production of mucus. Varied causes: allergic, fungal, bacterial, parasitic, idiopathic	Cough Wheezing Dyspnea	Radiographs Cytologic examination and culture of fluid from tracheal wash or bronchoalveolar lavage Fecal analysis for lung parasites Heartworm test	Emergency treatment of dyspnea Maintenance: • Bronchodilators • Corticosteroids • Improve indoor air quality to decreased inhaled allergens • Treat infections/parasites
Pneumonia	Inflammation of the lung caused by bacterial, viral, fungal infection or by aspiration of a foreign body or stomach contents	Cough Hypoxia Crackles heard on lung auscultation Fever Anorexia Weight loss	Radiographs Bronchoscopy Cytologic examination and culture of tracheal wash Viral and fungal serology	Oxygen therapy Airway hydration Frequently changing patient positioning Coupage Bronchodilators Antibiotics Antifungals
Diaphragmatic hernia	A congenital or acquired rent in the diaphragm, allowing abdominal organs to enter the thoracic cavity	Dyspnea Tachypnea Lethargy Anorexia Decreased lung sounds Muffled heart sounds	Radiographs	Emergency treatment of dyspnea Surgical hernia repair

TABLE 19-9	Small Animal Respiratory Diseases—cont'd			
DISEASE	**PATHOGENESIS**	**CLINICAL SIGNS**	**DIAGNOSTICS**	**TREATMENTS**
Pyothorax	Pus in the pleural cavity caused by bacterial infection secondary to foreign bodies (grass awns in dogs), penetrating wound to the chest wall (bite wounds in cats), or progression of lung infection	Hypoxia Cough Fever Lethargy Anorexia Decreased lung sounds Muffled heart sounds Pleural effusion	Pleural fluid analysis, cytologic examination	Oxygen therapy Drainage of effusion • Thoracocentesis • Chest tubes Antibiotics Analgesia for patients with chest tubes
Chylothorax	Accumulation of chyle in the pleural cavity, resulting from decreased lymphatic drainage (obstructed thoracic duct) or increased lymphatic flow	Cough Hypoxia Decreased lung sounds Muffled heart sounds Pleural effusion	Pleural fluid analysis, cytologic examination	Oxygen therapy Thoracocentesis Treatment of underlying disease Feed low-fat diet Benzopyrone medication Thoracic duct ligation
Pneumothorax	Air in the pleural cavity caused by trauma to the thoracic cavity (blunt force, penetrating wounds) or secondary to underlying pulmonary disease; can be idiopathic	Hypoxia Decreased lung sounds Muffled heart sounds	Radiographs	Oxygen therapy Drainage of air • Thoracocentesis • Chest tubes with continuous suction Treatment of underlying disease Analgesia for trauma cases, patients with chest tubes

the progression of heart disease toward heart failure, so it is recommended that asymptomatic patients should be closely monitored. This includes periodic echocardiograms and, perhaps more importantly, education of owners to monitor the resting respiratory rate at home for tachypnea—one of the earliest signs of heart failure. As time progresses, the compensatory mechanisms sustaining cardiac output eventually fail, causing *heart failure*, which results in inadequate tissue perfusion. A patient with heart failure has clinical signs referable to the perfusion deficit: tachypnea, exercise intolerance (dogs), syncope, weakness, prolonged capillary refill time (CRT), and pale mucous membranes. Sudden death can also occur. In cats with heart failure, clinical signs more often are nonspecific and include anorexia, depression, and weight loss. Patients diagnosed with heart failure are treated with medications to restore cardiac output, such as angiotensin-converting enzyme (ACE) inhibitors, beta blockers, positive inotropes, calcium channel blockers, antihypertensives, and antiarrhythmic drugs. Low-sodium diets, stress reduction, and exercise restrictions are recommended.

> **TECHNICIAN NOTE** The first sign that heart disease has progressed to heart failure is tachypnea. Teaching the owner to monitor the resting respiratory rate of the patient at home therefore is an important tactic of early detection.

Congestive heart failure (CHF) results when decreased cardiac output and tissue hypoxia cause poor venous return, leading to fluid overload (congestion). If the left side of the heart is damaged, this condition is classified as left-sided congestive heart failure. In this condition, fluid backs up into the lungs (pulmonary edema) and, in cats, into the pleural space (pleural effusion). Clinical signs are consistent with respiratory compromise and hypoxia; dyspnea, tachypnea, cyanosis, and abnormal respiratory sounds, including crackles, wheezes, and decreased lung sounds, are heard on thoracic auscultation. Coughing is commonly seen in the dog, but not in the cat. If the right side of the heart is damaged, this condition is classified as right-sided CHF, with congestion occurring in the abdominal and thoracic cavities. Clinical signs include edema, jugular distention, abdominal distention due to ascites, hepatomegaly, and pleural and pericardial effusions. It is common for cardiac patients to first present in congestive heart failure. These are critical cases requiring oxygen therapy, diuretics, and removal of any effusion that is present. Once the patient is stable, diagnosis and treatment of the underlying heart disease are pursued. Nursing care for patients with CHF is presented in Table 19-4 under the associated **technician assessments** of hypoxia and cardiac insufficiency.

> **TECHNICIAN NOTE** Coughing is a common sign of congestive heart failure in the dog, but not in the cat.

Cardiomyopathy

Cardiomyopathy is a disease of the heart muscle. Cardiomyopathy can be primary or secondary. Primary cardiomyopathies are not caused by any other cardiovascular or systemic disease. They are classified as hypertrophic, dilated, arrhythmogenic right ventricular (Boxer cardiomyopathy), and restrictive/unclassified. Hypertrophic, and to much lesser degrees restrictive and dilated, cardiomyopathies are seen in cats; the most commonly seen form in dogs is dilated cardiomyopathy. Secondary cardiomyopathies are the result of an underlying disease process, for example, ventricular hypertrophy secondary to feline hyperthyroidism, or dilated cardiomyopathy secondary to canine parvovirus infection.

Hypertrophic cardiomyopathy (HCM), the most common form of feline cardiomyopathy, is characterized by increased thickness of the left ventricle wall and a small ventricular lumen. The presence of these abnormalities on echocardiogram confirms the diagnosis. Treatment commences once the patient is in heart failure and may include the use of diuretics, ACE inhibitors, beta blockers, and/or calcium channel blockers. Cats with HCM (or any cardiomyopathy) are at risk for arterial thromboembolism (ATE), wherein blood clots form in the heart and lodge in the aortic trifurcation, disrupting the blood supply to the hindlimbs. Clinical signs of ATE include hindlimb paresis/paralysis and severe pain, cyanotic toe pads, absent or poor femoral pulses, and coolness of the affected limb. Cats with undiagnosed HCM may first present with signs of arterial thromboembolism. Prevention of thromboemboli is an important goal when feline cardiomyopathy is treated, but unfortunately is difficult to achieve because no single drug has proved effective; however, many new antithrombolytic medications are being researched for prevention of this life-threatening complication.

Dilated cardiomyopathy (DCM), the most common canine cardiomyopathy, is characterized by extreme atrial and ventricular dilatation with decreased contractility. Primarily the left side of the heart is damaged; however, right-sided DCM can be seen. Diagnosis is confirmed by radiography, electrocardiography, and echocardiography. Treatment commences once the patient is in heart failure and may include the use of diuretics, ACE inhibitors, and positive inotropes.

Degenerative Atrioventricular Valve Disease

This disease affects the cardiac valve leaflets or cusps and is characterized by thickening of the tissue. It primarily affects dogs, with approximately 60% of cases involving only the mitral valve and 30% involving both mitral and tricuspid valves; only the tricuspid valve is affected in 10% of patients. Degenerative changes lead to insufficient functioning of the valves; therefore, these diseases are referred to as *mitral valve* or *tricuspid valve insufficiency*. Mitral valve insufficiency has been documented in cats, but it is uncommon. On physical examination, localizable heart murmurs are evident. Diagnosis is made on the basis of valvular changes seen via echocardiography. Treatment commences once the patient is in heart failure and may include the use of diuretics,

---

BOX 19-2	Clinical Signs of Heartworm Disease

DOG	CAT
• Coughing	• Coughing
• Exercise intolerance	• Vomiting
• Dyspnea	• Dyspnea
• Syncope	• Lethargy
• Hemoptysis	• Anorexia
• Epistaxis	• Weight loss
• Signs of right-sided CHF	• Collapse
	• Sudden death

CHF, Congestive heart failure.

ACE inhibitors, positive inotropes, and antihypertensives. Arrhythmias are common sequelae in advanced stages of this disease; if present, an antiarrhythmic medication is added to the treatment regimen.

Heartworm Disease

Heartworm disease is a mosquito-borne infectious disease that affects both cats and dogs. (See Chapter 14 for information regarding the life cycle of *Dirofilaria immitis* and diagnostic testing.) Clinical signs of heartworm disease differ between the cat and the dog (Box 19-2). This difference in clinical signs is a reflection of worm burden and the longevity of the adult worm. In dogs, large numbers (30 or more) of adult worms can be present in the pulmonary arteries, the right atrium and ventricle, and the caudal vena cava, and they can live up to 7 years. In the cat, heartworm infection generally consists of one to three worms that survive up to 3 years; they tend to reside primarily in the pulmonary arteries but can migrate to the right atrium. Diagnosis of canine heartworm disease is based on a positive serum test result for heartworm antigen. Diagnosis of feline heartworm disease via antigen testing alone is unreliable because unisex infection is common in cats. A positive heartworm antibody titer, the presence of basophilia and eosinophilia on a complete blood count, and enlarged pulmonary vessels on radiography support the diagnosis; the presence of a worm on echocardiography confirms it.

Treatment of canine heartworm disease consists of adulticide therapy, with microfilaricide therapy starting 3 to 4 weeks later. In some cases, surgical removal of worms from the right atrium is necessary as a lifesaving procedure; adulticide therapy usually is started a few weeks postoperatively, once the patient's condition has stabilized. Adult heartworms die slowly over a period of 2 to 30 days. During this time, patients are at risk for pulmonary thromboembolism (PTE). Clinical signs of PTE include fever, coughing, and, in more severe cases, dyspnea and hemoptysis. To minimize the development of PTE, it is important to restrict exercise for 3 to 4 weeks after administration of adulticide therapy. Patients with a high worm burden and severe cardiopulmonary disease are at high risk for PTE and must be stabilized before the adulticide is administered. Treatment with prednisone, heparin, and oxygen, as well as cage rest for 1 week, is recommended before the patient is treated with the adulticide.

Treatment for feline heartworm disease is unrewarding because a safe and effective adulticide protocol has yet to be found. Treatment focuses on supporting the patient through the natural course of the infection and eventual self-cure, which occurs in about 80% of patients. Prednisolone is given to stave off the inflammatory response caused by worm death. The death of just one heartworm can trigger anaphylactic shock or can cause pulmonary thromboembolism, both of which can result in sudden death.

For both dogs and cats, the key to treating heartworm disease is preventing infection; this is achieved by the use of any one of several approved macrolide preventive agents.

Systemic Hypertension

Systemic hypertension is defined as an increase in systemic blood pressure. In small animals, repeated demonstration of systolic blood pressure greater than 180 mm Hg in a calm patient qualifies as systemic hypertension; however, a systolic blood pressure of 160 to 179 mm Hg is suspicious and warrants further investigation. Systemic hypertension may be classified as primary (idiopathic) or secondary. Although primary hypertension is more frequently recognized in small animals now than in years past, hypertension secondary to another disease process is still the most commonly diagnosed form, representing more than 80% of cases. Chronic kidney disease, hyperthyroidism, hyperadrenocorticism, and diabetes mellitus most often are associated with secondary systemic hypertension. Most hypertensive patients are asymptomatic; therefore, early detection is important, and routine blood pressure screening is recommended for patients with predisposing disease. In cats, because of the high incidence of both chronic kidney disease and hyperthyroidism, routine screening of patients 10 years of age and older is encouraged. It is not unusual for the diagnosis of systemic hypertension to be made first, leading to the diagnosis of the primary disease.

Additionally patients presenting with cardiac disease should have their blood pressure monitored. Routine fundic examinations are performed in at-risk patients because enlarged retinal vessels and retinal hemorrhage are early warning signs of impeding retinal detachment due to hypertension. Unfortunately, the most common presenting sign in a patient with undiagnosed severe hypertension is acute blindness caused by retinal detachment. Once hypertension has been diagnosed, treatment with antihypertensive medication (calcium channel blockers, ACE inhibitors) is begun immediately. The goal is to gradually lower blood pressure into the normal range, avoiding a dramatic drop. Frequent blood pressure monitoring takes place early on to help titrate the medication dose and to ensure normotension. The successful treatment plan also includes diagnosing, treating, and monitoring underlying disease in patients with secondary systemic hypertension.

> **TECHNICIAN NOTE** System hypertension is often secondary to another disease such as chronic kidney disease, hyperthyroidism, or hyperadrenocorticism.

DIGESTIVE AND HEPATOBILIARY DISEASES
Gastrointestinal Tract

Most diseases of the stomach and small intestine ultimately result in local inflammation, irritation, and/or obstruction of the gastrointestinal (GI) tract, with each of these pathologic processes causing a finite array of clinical symptoms. It is important for the veterinary technician to be familiar with each of these symptoms because they help to focus medical history questions, localize the anatomic location of the problem, develop technician evaluations, and direct diagnostic and therapeutic approaches.

Regurgitation is the passive expulsion of material from the mouth, pharynx, or esophagus. Nausea and abdominal contractions are not typically seen. Patients can exhibit difficulty eating (dysphagia), hypersalivation, and gagging. Regurgitated material typically consists of undigested or partially digested food. Patients are at risk for aspiration of stomach contents and development of pneumonia. Nursing care includes elevating food and water bowls, keeping the patient's head and forelimbs elevated for 10 minutes after a meal, changing the form of food (gruel, meatballs), and monitoring for signs of aspiration.

Vomiting is defined as the forceful expulsion of contents from the stomach and the upper small intestine; it is an active process that requires abdominal contraction (retching). Nausea often precedes vomiting, with patients exhibiting anxiety, hypersalivation, vocalization, and lip-smacking. Vomitus can comprise any combination of undigested or digested food, hair, mucus, bile, and gastric secretions. Patients may vomit intestinal parasites (e.g., roundworms) or pieces of foreign material that they ingested (yarn, ribbon, tennis balls, plastic bags, etc.). If the patient is vomiting fresh or digested blood, this is termed **hematemesis**. When a medical history is obtained, it is important to question the owner regarding the amount and content of the vomitus, and the duration, severity, and frequency of vomiting. Questions must also be asked to confirm the presence of vomiting at home. Owners may present the pet for vomiting when in reality the patient is experiencing regurgitation, particularly with dogs. With cats, owners need to be carefully questioned to help distinguish "trying to bring up a hairball" (retching) from coughing. It must be remembered that vomiting can have non-GI causes, and a full system review is always indicated. Vomiting patients are prone to dehydration and electrolyte imbalance; monitoring for and treating these secondary problems is of importance in ensuring complete patient care. Nursing care for the vomiting patient is summarized in Table 19-4.

TECHNICIAN NOTE   It is important to distinguish between vomiting and regurgitation, which often appear the same to the owner. When a medical history is taken, careful questioning regarding these episodes is necessary to make the distinction.

Diarrhea is characterized by the frequent passage of loose, unformed, often watery stool. When a medical history of a patient with diarrhea is obtained, it is important to question the owner regarding the duration, severity, frequency, amount, and quality. This information can assist in localizing diarrhea as involving the small or large bowel (Table 19-10). Knowing the duration of the problem—acute versus chronic—helps the clinician to direct diagnostic testing. Patients with diarrhea are prone to dehydration, so monitoring for and treating dehydration is of importance in ensuring complete patient care. Nursing care for the patient with diarrhea is summarized in Table 19-4.

Constipation is characterized by the infrequent and often difficult passage of hard stool. In establishing the history of constipation, questioning the owner regarding when the last normal bowel movement was observed is important. Constipation can be a primary GI problem caused by bowel obstruction or diminished bowel motility; however, it can also occur secondary to orthopedic pain (cannot posture to defecate), environmental stressors (e.g., poor litter box management), and dehydration. It is essential to complete a full systems review when obtaining a medical history, to evaluate all potential causes. Nursing care for the constipated patient is summarized in Table 19-4.

Hematochezia is the presence of blood in the feces. It can be seen with diarrhea or as streaks of blood on the outside of normally formed stool. Hematochezia usually indicates a problem with the colon or rectum.

Melena is defined as the presence of digested blood in the feces. The stool is characteristically a tarry black color. Melena may be seen in patients with upper GI bleeding caused by, for example, endoparasites, ulcerations, neoplasms, or coagulopathies.

Tenesmus is defined as painful straining at urination or defecation. A thorough medical history and physical examination must be completed to determine which body system is involved. Tenesmus of GI origin is usually the result of colonic disease, often accompanying diarrhea or constipation.

The diagnostic approach to a patient with stomach or intestinal disease primarily involves fecal analyses (e.g., flotation, cytologic examination, virus detection, cultures), plain and contrast radiography, ultrasonography, endoscopy, surgical exploration, and biopsies of the GI tract. A minimum database (CBC, serum chemistry, urinalysis [UA]) is helpful in documenting secondary problems, such as electrolyte imbalance and inflammation, but often in itself does not lead to a definitive diagnosis.

Treatment of a patient with GI disease is multimodal; it involves medical management of symptoms and treatment of the primary cause and can include medical and/or surgical approaches. Table 19-11 summarizes common symptomatic medical therapies. Table 19-12 provides a summary of common diseases and disorders of the GI tract in cats and dogs.

Exocrine Pancreas
Pancreatitis

Pancreatitis occurs when the digestive enzyme trypsin is prematurely activated within the pancreatic tissue instead of within the duodenum, as is normal. The presence of trypsin in the pancreas causes autodigestion of pancreatic tissue, resulting in local inflammation and necrosis, as well as focal peritonitis. Pancreatitis may be acute or chronic in nature; acute disease is seen more commonly in dogs, and chronic disease is more common in cats. Most cases of acute pancreatitis are idiopathic; however, risk factors for developing acute pancreatitis include dietary indiscretion (dogs), particularly a high-fat meal, blunt force trauma, pancreatic hypoperfusion, and use of pancreotoxic drugs. In most cases, the cause of chronic pancreatitis is unknown. However, because cats have only one pancreatic duct, which joins the common bile duct before emptying into the duodenum, an association with concurrent bile duct/liver inflammation (cholangiohepatitis) and/or inflammatory bowel disease has been noted in this species. Clinical signs associated with canine pancreatitis include anorexia, vomiting, abdominal pain, diarrhea, and fever. Clinical signs associated with feline pancreatitis include anorexia, lethargy, weight loss, hypothermia, and vomiting. Patients with severe acute disease may go on to develop hypotension, disseminated intravascular coagulation, renal failure, and multi-organ failure. Definitive diagnosis requires pancreatic biopsies. A presumptive diagnosis is commonly made and relies upon a constellation of laboratory work (minimum database and pancreatic lipase immunoreactivity concentrations) and diagnostic imaging findings. Treatment of acute pancreatitis includes administration of intravenous fluid therapy, analgesics, antiemetics, mucosal protectants, and antibiotics to prevent secondary sepsis,

TABLE 19-10	Small Bowel vs. Large Bowel Diarrhea	
	SMALL BOWEL DIARRHEA	**LARGE BOWEL DIARRHEA**
Volume of feces	Increased	Normal or decreased
Mucus in feces	Uncommon	Common
Blood in feces	Melena may be seen	Hematochezia may be seen
Frequency of bowel movements	Normal	Increased
Tenesmus	Rare	Common
Weight loss	Common	Rare

TABLE 19-11	Medical Management of Gastrointestinal Symptoms
TREATMENT	**RATIONALE**
Limited fasting	24 to 36 hour fast will lessen clinical signs by allowing the GI tract to rest; indicated for vomiting and/or diarrhea
Fluid therapy	Treat or prevent secondary dehydration Ensure patient hydration in patients with chronic constipation Treat electrolyte imbalances
Dietary therapy	Bland diets: easier to digest, gentler on the GI tract. Generally fed as small, frequent meals. Ideal for patients with nonspecific vomiting or diarrhea. Hypoallergenic diets: novel proteins and carbohydrates for patients with food allergies or intolerance. Reduce inflammation. Fiber-rich diets: helpful in patients with diarrhea or constipation. Fiber helps normalize colonic health. Low-residue diets: helpful for patients with chronic constipation Feeding tube placement: to feed around the problem (e.g., esophagitis, pancreatitis) and/or to treat severe anorexia Total parental nutrition: reserved for patients with severe malabsorption disease
Probiotic therapy	Helps to normalize proper concentration and composition of GI bacterial flora
Antiemetics	Control vomiting
Antacids	Decrease gastric acidity. Indicated for patients with or at risk for ulcerative diseases. Can also help decrease nausea.
Mucosal protectants	Protect the mucosal lining of the GI tract. Used in patients with or at risk for ulcerative disease.
Promotility drugs	Used to promote stomach emptying and intestinal peristalsis, which is helpful for reducing vomiting in select patients. Used to increase colonic motility for feline patients with idiopathic megacolon.
Antidiarrheal drugs	Decrease GI transit time, which is helpful in the treatment of diarrhea.
Enemas, laxatives, stool softeners	For the treatment of constipation
Antibiotics	For patients with specific antibiotic-responsive diseases or for patients at risk for sepsis or aspiration pneumonia.
Anthelminthics	For patients with diagnosed or suspected endoparasites.
Anti-inflammatories	Reduce GI inflammation.

and feeding a bland, low-fat diet through a feeding tube as soon as possible.

Patients with chronic pancreatitis have a history of recurrent, intermittent, milder episodes of clinical symptoms, making diagnosis more difficult. Chronic pancreatitis can lead to exocrine pancreatic insufficiency (EPI) or diabetes mellitus (DM). Symptomatic treatment of GI symptoms, identification and treatment of concurrent disease, and treatment of EPI or DM, if present, are the mainstays of the therapeutic plan.

Exocrine Pancreatic Insufficiency

Exocrine pancreatic insufficiency is caused by insufficient production and secretion of pancreatic digestive enzymes. In dogs, this is most commonly the result of pancreatic acinar atrophy. In cats, EPI is commonly caused by chronic pancreatitis. Loss of digestive enzymes leads to maldigestion and malabsorption of ingested nutrients, causing clinical signs of polyphagia, weight loss, and chronic diarrhea that is pale, fatty, and voluminous. A greasy hair coat may result from poor absorption of fatty acids from the diet. EPI also leads to cobalamin (vitamin B_{12}) deficiency, particularly in cats, which contributes to weight loss and diarrhea.

Documentation of low serum trypsin-like immunoreactivity (TLI) concentration confirms the diagnosis of EPI. Treatment consists of oral replacement of pancreatic digestive enzymes given at mealtimes and parenteral supplementation of cobalamin.

Hepatobiliary System

Disease of the liver and gallbladder leads to varied physical and laboratory abnormalities (Table 19-13) dependent on the location, chronicity, and severity of the disease process. Patients with severe hepatobiliary disease may develop **hepatic encephalopathy** (HE). Hepatic encephalopathy results when the brain is exposed to GI toxins, such as ammonia, as a consequence of decreased liver function or portosystemic shunts, which compromise the normal functioning of liver detoxification or the enterohepatic circulation. Clinical signs of HE include altered mentation, head pressing, hypersalivation, circling, ataxia, seizures, blindness, behavior changes, lethargy, and coma. Symptomatic treatment of HE focuses on decreasing the amount of ammonia in the systemic circulation; this can be achieved by decreasing ammonia production in the intestines. Therapies include oral lactulose, which decreases ammonia absorption; small,

TABLE 19-12 | Small Animal Gastrointestinal Diseases

DISEASE	PATHOGENESIS	CLINICAL SIGNS	DIAGNOSTICS	TREATMENTS
Esophagitis	Inflammation of the esophagus caused by administration of certain medications, gastroesophageal reflux, chronic vomiting, ingestion of caustic agents May lead to ulcers and stricture	Regurgitation Excessive drooling Anorexia Vomiting	History and clinical signs Plain and contrast radiographs are helpful Endoscopy ± biopsy is definitive	Antacids Promotility drugs Mucosal protectants Antibiotics Gastrostomy feeding tube
Acute gastritis	Inflammation of the stomach mucosa often caused by ingestion of spoiled food, toxic plants, foreign objects, or irritating drugs	Acute vomiting Hematemesis Abdominal discomfort Anorexia	History and clinical signs Radiographs Minimum database	Appropriate symptomatic therapies Removal of foreign body Treatment of toxicity
GI obstruction	Obstruction of the stomach or intestines Potential causes include intussusception, foreign body, neoplastic mass	Acute, severe, intractable vomiting Abdominal pain Diarrhea Sepsis Shock	History and clinical signs Plain and contrast radiographs Ultrasound Minimum database	Appropriate symptomatic therapies Treatment of shock Surgical correction of cause
Gastrointestinal ulcers	Defect in the mucosal layer caused by NSAID administration, neoplasia, and liver disease	Anorexia Vomiting Hematemesis Melena	History and clinical signs Endoscopy, direct visualization, and biopsies	Appropriate symptomatic therapies Eliminate underlying cause
Acute enteritis	Inflammation of the intestinal mucosa often caused by infectious agents (viral, bacterial, parasitic), dietary changes, or indiscretions	Small bowel diarrhea ± vomiting Abdominal pain Fever Anorexia	Fecal analyses Serum viral testing	Appropriate symptomatic therapies
Canine antibiotic-responsive enteropathy (ARE)	Abnormal host immune response to an elevated number of bacteria in the small intestines	Diarrhea Weight loss	History, clinical signs, and response to treatment Routine fecal analysis to rule out parasites	Empirical broad-spectrum antibiotic therapy
Inflammatory bowel disease	Idiopathic intestinal inflammation; antigenic hypersensitivity is currently believed to the main cause	Chronic, recurrent pattern of weight loss, vomiting, diarrhea, and/or anorexia Thickened bowel loops on palpation	Exclude all other causes of symptoms Full-thickness biopsies of the intestines	Appropriate symptomatic therapies Cobalamin supplementation in cats Immunosuppressant therapy for severe cases
Colitis	Inflammation of the colon caused by parasites, diet, bacteria	Large bowel diarrhea	Fecal analyses Endoscopy and biopsies for severe and/or prolonged cases	Appropriate symptomatic therapies
Feline idiopathic megacolon	Dysfunction of the colonic smooth muscle that results in a dilated and hypomotile colon Cause unknown	Chronic constipation Tenesmus Vomiting Abdominal pain Weight loss	Radiographs demonstrate megacolon	Appropriate symptomatic therapies Subtotal or total colectomy

NSAID, Nonsteroidal anti-inflammatory drug.

TABLE 19-13	Functions of the Hepatobiliary System and Consequences of Dysfunction	
NORMAL HEPATOBILIARY FUNCTION	**CONSEQUENCE OF HEPATOBILIARY DYSFUNCTION**	**ASSOCIATED CLINICAL SIGNS**
Detoxification of GI toxins via enterohepatic circulation	Buildup of toxins in bloodstream	Anorexia, vomiting, lethargy, depression, hepatic encephalopathy
Production of albumin	Hypoalbuminemia	Ascites
Production of clotting factors	Coagulopathy	Hemorrhage, petechiation
Protein metabolism and conversion of ammonia to urea (urea cycle)	Malnutrition, hyperammonemia, decreased blood urea nitrogen (BUN)	Weight loss, hepatic encephalopathy
Carbohydrate metabolism: gluconeogenesis and glycogenolysis	Hypoglycemia	Altered mentation, seizures
Fatty acid metabolism and synthesis of cholesterol	Hypercholesterolemia or hypocholesterolemia	
Vitamin storage/activation	Deficiencies of vitamins D, E, A, K, C, and B	Varies—relates to specific vitamins (e.g., vitamin K deficiency = coagulopathy)
Bilirubin metabolism and excretion	Hyperbilirubinemia, bilirubinuria	Icterus, anorexia, vomiting, lethargy, depression
Bile acid metabolism	Elevated serum bile acids	

frequent meals of a diet that contains a moderately restricted amount of highly digestible proteins; antibiotic therapy to reduce ammonia-producing bacteria; and administration of probiotics to encourage growth of beneficial intestinal bacteria. Management of acute HE also includes fluid therapy, treatment of electrolyte imbalances, patient fasting, administration of lactulose enemas, and treatment of seizures.

Diagnosis of hepatobiliary disease involves laboratory analyses, diagnostic imaging (radiography and ultrasonography), and histopathologic examination. Serum assays may reveal increases in liver enzymes, bilirubin (hyperbilirubinemia), ammonia (hyperammonemia), and bile acids, and decreases in glucose (hypoglycemia), albumin (hypoalbuminemia), and blood urea nitrogen. Abnormal urinalysis findings include bilirubinuria and the presence of bilirubin crystals and ammonia biurate crystals. Treatments are specific to the diagnosed disease and often include nutritional support, antioxidant therapy, antibiotics, and/or anti-inflammatories.

Feline Hepatic Lipidosis

Feline hepatic lipidosis (FHL) is characterized by an accumulation of lipids or fats within the cytoplasm of more than 80% of hepatocytes. As hepatocytes swell, cholestasis and hepatic damage result. Hepatic lipidosis is caused by a derangement of lipid metabolism associated with anorexia of approximately 7 days. Obese cats are predisposed to FHL; however, any cat experiencing prolonged anorexia is at risk for developing the disease. Feline hepatic lipidosis is seen secondary to environmental stressors or to concurrent diseases (such as other hepatobiliary diseases, pancreatitis, or inflammatory bowel disease [IBD]) that promote prolonged anorexia. FHL can also be idiopathic in nature. In addition to anorexia, clinical signs of FHL include recent, dramatic weight loss; lethargy; vomiting; icterus; dehydration; and palpable hepatomegaly. Some patients develop hepatic encephalopathy. Definitive diagnosis of FHL requires liver biopsies; however, most patients are not stable enough to withstand this procedure. A presumptive diagnosis is made on the basis of history, physical examination, diagnostic imaging, and serum chemistry results. Additional diagnostics may be necessary to diagnose a concurrent disease process. FHL is a potentially lethal disease; however, early and aggressive treatment (Table 19-14), particularly nutritional support, greatly improves patient survival.

> **TECHNICIAN NOTE** Hepatic lipidosis is caused by a derangement of lipid metabolism associated with anorexia of approximately 7 days.

Canine Chronic Hepatitis

Hepatitis is defined as inflammation of the liver parenchyma. Chronic hepatitis (CH) indicates a history of liver disease for a prolonged period—usually longer than 4 to 6 months. Causes of CH include viral infection, leptospirosis, copper storage disease, and hepatotoxic drugs. However, most cases are idiopathic with a suspected autoimmune component. Progression of the disease is characterized by hepatocyte swelling and necrosis, loss of hepatic mass and subsequent loss of liver function, hepatic fibrosis, portal hypertension (high blood pressure in the portal veins), and cirrhosis (fibrosis of the liver). Clinical signs are generally nonspecific and include vomiting, diarrhea, anorexia, weight loss, and **polyuria/polydipsia**. Icterus is occasionally seen. Patients with portal hypertension often have ascites, evidence of GI ulcerations, and/or hepatic encephalopathy. Clinical signs usually are not apparent until 75% of the liver mass is lost, which makes early detection of liver dysfunction imperative. Routine screening of liver enzymes, particularly for predisposed breeds, at annual examinations is the best approach. Definitive diagnosis of chronic hepatitis is made on the basis of liver biopsy; however, clinical signs, persistently elevated serum liver enzymes, abnormal liver function assays, and

TABLE 19-14	Therapeutic Approach to Feline Hepatic Lipidosis
THERAPY	**RATIONALE**
Fluid therapy	Treat dehydration Treat electrolyte imbalance (hypokalemia and hypophosphatemia)
Administration of parenteral antiemetics	Control vomiting
Nutritional support: • Syringe feeding or nasogastric or orogastric tube feeding until patient is stable for anesthesia • Placement of esophagostomy or gastrostomy feeding tube • Tube-feed patient calorie-dense, high-protein diet for 4 to 6 weeks (outpatient) • Nutritional supplementation may include: • ʟ-Carnitine • Arginine	Treat anorexia Resolve altered lipid metabolism; this will reverse lipid accumulation in the hepatocytes (will mobilize fats)
Antioxidant therapy: • S-Adenosylmethionine • Vitamin E • Silymarin (milk thistle)	Protect cells from oxidative damage
Parenteral vitamin supplementation: • B-vitamins • Vitamin K	Correct B-vitamin deficiency resulting from anorexia and from concurrent pancreatitis or inflammatory bowel disease (IBD) if present Correct vitamin K deficiency coagulopathy seen secondary to decreased dietary fat intake and cholestasis

TABLE 19-15	Therapeutic Approach to Canine Chronic Hepatitis
THERAPY	**RATIONALE**
Glucocorticoids	Reduce inflammation and fibrosis in early stages of the disease process
Antioxidant therapy: • S-Adenosylmethionine • Vitamin E • Silymarin (milk thistle)	Protect cells from oxidative damage
Ursodiol	Increase bile flow Decrease toxic effects of bile on hepatocytes Anti-inflammatory and antioxidant properties
Small, frequent meals of prescription diets: • High-quality, digestible protein • Vitamins E and K and B-vitamins	Resolve secondary malnutrition issues and vitamin deficiencies Provide support for liver regeneration
Antibiotics	For treatment of primary bacterial infection, if present
Feed low-copper, high-zinc diet Copper chelation therapy	For treatment of copper storage disease, if present

Diagnosis of a PSS is based on elevated serum postprandial bile acids, hyperammonemia, and direct visualization of shunting vessel(s) via ultrasonography or contrast radiography, or during surgery. Congenital PSSs generally are diagnosed in cats and dogs younger than 2 years of age. Acquired PSSs are typically seen in older dogs as sequelae of chronic hepatitis. For extrahepatic PSSs, surgical ligation of the shunt is the treatment of choice. Medical management of HE is required immediately before and for 2 months after surgery. Surgical ligation of intrahepatic shunts is not achievable, so treatment relies on medical management of hepatic encephalopathy.

Feline Cholangitis
Cholangitis refers to inflammation of the bile ducts. In some cases, inflammation spreads to the liver; this is termed *cholangiohepatitis*. Cholangitis/cholangiohepatitis can be acute or chronic. Acute cholangitis is caused by an ascending bacterial infection from the small intestines and is characterized by neutrophilic inflammation. Clinical signs include fever, vomiting, lethargy, icterus, and abdominal pain. Chronic cholangitis is characterized by lymphocytic-plasmacytic inflammation, and the cause is unknown. Possible causes include immune-mediated disease, progression of acute cholangitis, and liver fluke infection. Clinical signs include anorexia, weight loss, lethargy, and icterus. Diagnosis and differentiation between the two forms relies upon history,

diagnostic imaging of microhepatica support a presumptive diagnosis. Table 19-15 outlines medical therapy for chronic hepatitis.

Portosystemic Shunt
Portosystemic shunts (PSSs) are extrahepatic or intrahepatic vascular abnormalities that connect portal and systemic circulations. Extrahepatic shunts are congenital and typically involve one or two vessels that connect the portal vein to the vena cava. Intrahepatic shunts can be congenital or acquired secondary to portal hypertension and are multiple small shunts within the hepatic parenchyma. Clinical signs include hepatic encephalopathy, polyuria/polydipsia, and signs of bladder irritation secondary to urate stone formation.

BOX 19-3	Causes of Chronic Kidney Disease

Renal inflammation
- Glomerulonephritis
- Interstitial nephritis
- Pyelonephritis

Amyloidosis

Structural damage to the kidney
- Polycystic kidney disease
- Congenital renal dysplasia
- Hydronephrosis

Acute renal failure

Renal toxicity

Renal neoplasia

Systemic disease
- Hypertension
- Infectious diseases (various)

Idiopathic

TABLE 19-16	Functions of the Kidney and Consequences of Kidney Disease	
RENAL FUNCTION	**CONSEQUENCES OF RENAL DYSFUNCTION**	**ASSOCIATED CLINICAL SIGNS**
Filtration and excretion of metabolites and toxins	Buildup of toxins in the bloodstream: azotemia	Nausea, vomiting, oral ulcers, anorexia, altered mental status
Maintenance of water balance and blood pressure	Inadequate urine-concentrating ability, dehydration, hypertension	Polyuria/polydipsia, tacky or dry mucous membranes, skin tenting, constipation
Filtration and conservation of plasma albumin	Proteinuria, hypoalbuminemia	Weight loss, ascites, edema
Maintenance of electrolyte balance	Hypokalemia, hyperphosphatemia	Muscle weakness, myopathy, nausea, vomiting
Production of erythropoietin hormone	Hormone deficiency causing anemia	Pale mucous membranes, exercise intolerance, lethargy
Metabolism of vitamin D to active form	Hormone deficiency contributing to calcium and phosphorus imbalance	Bone abnormalities (rare) and soft tissue mineralization

clinical signs, blood work, diagnostic imaging, bile culture, and liver biopsies. Treatment is largely the same for both forms of the disease: fluid therapy, antioxidants, antibiotics, ursodiol, nutritional support, and vitamin supplementation. Glucocorticoid therapy is added for the treatment of chronic cholangitis.

URINARY DISEASE

Chronic Kidney Disease

Chronic kidney disease (CKD) is characterized by an irreversible, progressive loss of functioning renal tissue. The causes of CKD are varied (Box 19-3), and a large number of cases are idiopathic. Clinical signs relate to impairment of fluid homeostasis, the buildup of toxins in the bloodstream, and electrolyte abnormalities that result from diminishing kidney function (Table 19-16). Diagnosis of CKD is based on serial documentation of **azotemia** with concurrent inadequate urine specific gravity in a well-hydrated patient. *Azotemia* refers to serum elevations of the protein metabolites creatinine and blood urea nitrogen (BUN). Urine specific gravity (USG) measures the concentration of urine and is a reflection of patient hydration status and of kidney function. Less than adequate USG in a well-hydrated patient is indicative of impaired urine concentrating ability by the kidney.

> **TECHNICIAN NOTE** Diagnosis of chronic kidney disease is based on serial documentation of azotemia with concurrent inadequate urine specific gravity in a well-hydrated patient.

The International Renal Interest Society (IRIS) has proposed a four-tier system for staging chronic kidney disease based on serum creatinine concentration. This system also provides for substages of CKD based on the presence and severity of proteinuria and systemic hypertension. Table 19-17 summarizes the staging system and provides a correlation with USG, percent remaining kidney function, and clinical signs. Staging of CKD helps in directing patient treatment and monitoring plans and in determining prognoses. Additional clinical pathologic abnormalities include nonregenerative anemia, decreased serum potassium (hypokalemia) in cats, increased serum phosphorus (hyperphosphatemia), metabolic acidosis, hypoalbuminemia, proteinuria, and hematuria. Radiography and ultrasonography can provide valuable diagnostic information on the primary cause of CKD, for example, neoplasms or cysts. Secondary disease processes are common in CKD patients and include systemic hypertension and bacterial urinary tract infection. Curative treatment can be accomplished in select patients with renal transplantation; however, not every patient meets the clinical qualifications for this procedure, and its cost is prohibitive for most clients. Palliative treatment and nursing care are the norm and focus on slowing progression of the disease, treating concurrent disease, correcting electrolyte imbalances, ameliorating clinical signs, and providing nutritional support (Table 19-18). Periodic patient monitoring (about every 3 months) consists of physical examination, blood pressure measurement, complete blood count, serum chemistry panel, urinalysis, and urine culture. These steps are essential for documenting response

TABLE 19-17	Staging and Clinical Signs of Chronic Kidney Disease

STAGE	PLASMA CREATININE LEVEL, MG/DL		URINE SPECIFIC GRAVITY		REMAINING KIDNEY FUNCTION	TYPICAL PROGRESSION OF CLINICAL SIGNS
	DOG	CAT	DOG	CAT		
1. Nonazotemic	<1.4	<1.6	>1.030	>1.035	100%	None
2. Mild renal azotemia	1.4-2.0	1.6-2.8	Variable	Variable	33%	Polyuria/polydipsia
3. Moderate renal azotemia	2.1-5.0	2.9-5.0	1.008-1.029	1.008-1.034	25%	Vomiting, nausea, lethargy, weight loss, anorexia, dehydration
4. Severe renal azotemia	>5.0	>5.0	1.008-1.029	1.008-1.034	<10%	Muscle wasting and weakness, oral ulcerations, constipation/diarrhea, pale mucous membranes, cervical ventroflexion (cats), hypothermia, altered mental status, seizures

Based on 2009 IRIS Guidelines for the Staging of Chronic Kidney Disease (CKD). Available at: www.iris-kidney.com.

TABLE 19-18	Conservative Medical Management of Chronic Kidney Disease (CKD)

TREATMENT	RATIONALE
Hydration: Increase water intake: canned foods, water fountains, multiple water bowls, flavored water, etc. Subcutaneous fluids Intravenous fluids	1. Prevent dehydration caused by loss of urine concentrating ability. 2. Treat dehydration caused by polyuria, vomiting, diarrhea, anorexia. 3. Treat electrolyte imbalances.
Specialized diet: Lower in protein Lower in sodium Lower in phosphorus Higher in potassium Higher in B-vitamins Higher in omega-3 and -6 fatty acids	1. Slow disease progression. 2. Protein restriction decreases proteinuria and protects the kidney. 3. Lower dietary sodium helps combat/treat hypertension. 4. Lower dietary phosphorus intake. 5. Patients with CKD are often deficient in the water-soluble B-vitamins because of the polyuria that they experience. Supplementation is helpful. 6. Omegas fatty acids reduce renal inflammation.
Prophylactic potassium supplementation (cats)	1. Combat increased urinary losses of potassium.
Appetite stimulants and antiemetics	1. Patients with CKD can experience anorexia, nausea, and vomiting because of increased toxins in the bloodstream and dehydration.
Antacids	1. Treat increased stomach acidity seen in patients with CKD.
Intestinal phosphate binders	1. Decrease absorption of dietary phosphorus.
Erythropoietin supplementation	1. Treat anemia caused by deficiency of this kidney hormone in patients with CKD.
Calcitriol supplementation	1. Slow progression of the disease (dogs).
Antihypertensive medications	1. Treat hypertension. 2. Some drugs reduce proteinuria and provide protection for the kidney.

to treatment, making therapeutic adjustments, and screening for secondary complications, all of which help to provide patients with a high quality of life.

> **TECHNICIAN NOTE** Medical management of chronic kidney disease focuses on slowing progression of the disease, treating concurrent disease, correcting electrolyte imbalances, ameliorating clinical signs, and providing nutritional support.

Urolithiasis

A *urolith* is a pathologic stone formed from mineral salts found in the urinary tract. Formation of uroliths is dependent upon urine pH, urine concentration, and urine saturation. Clinical signs depend on location, number, size, and shape, and whether concurrent urinary tract infection is present. Urolith classification is generally based on the predominant mineral component, such as struvite, calcium oxalate, or urate. Naming of uroliths is based on anatomic location: nephrolith, ureterolith, urocystolith, and urethrolith. The term *calculus* is also used, for example, a bladder stone is often called a *cystic calculus*. Clinical signs are dependent on urolith location. If the urolith is located in the bladder, no clinical signs may be present, but more commonly, stranguria (straining to urinate), pollakiuria (abnormally frequent urination), and hematuria are seen. If the urolith is in the urethra, frequent attempts may be made to urinate, and dribbling of urine may be noted. If the urethra is completely obstructed by the stone(s), abdominal pain, anorexia, depression, and vomiting will be observed. Uroliths seen on plain or contrast radiographs or on ultrasound establish the diagnosis. Generally, treatment of uroliths consists of surgical removal and/or medical dissolution (typically prescription diets), depending on anatomic location and stone composition. Lithotripsy and urohydropulsion may also be used. In the case of uroliths causing urethral obstruction, immediate relief of the obstruction via urinary catheterization and correction of electrolyte imbalances that result from the obstruction are required. (See Chapter 25 for detailed information on the treatment of urethral obstructions.) Retrieved uroliths are sent to an outside laboratory for quantitative analysis. Additionally, determination of concurrent urinary bacterial infection and subsequent antibiotic therapy is important. The overall recurrence rate for uroliths is high—up to 50%; therefore, prevention of future stone formation is very important. Specific dietary therapy is initiated to modify urine pH on the basis of stone type. Switching to canned food, or otherwise increasing water intake, is recommended to decrease urine concentration and increase urine output. Client education is extremely important because long-term therapeutic compliance is essential in decreasing recurrence of uroliths.

Bacterial Cystitis

Bacterial infections of the bladder are common in the dog and are rare in the healthy cat. Lower urinary tract infections (UTIs) can be caused by a variety of bacteria; the most common pathogen in small animals is *Escherichia coli*. Female dogs are more prone to infection than male dogs. UTI is a common secondary complication in cats and dogs with diabetes mellitus, chronic kidney disease, or hyperadrenocorticism, and in patients with indwelling urinary catheters. Clinical signs result from inflammation of the urethra and bladder and include dysuria (painful urination), hematuria, pollakiuria, and urinating in inappropriate places. Diagnosis is made on the basis of the presence of white blood cells, red blood cells, and bacteria found during microscopic examination of urine. Urine culture and sensitivity is performed to identify the causative agent and its antimicrobial sensitivities. Treatment consists of appropriate antimicrobial therapy for 1 to 2 weeks. Seven to 10 days after completion of the antibiotic course, a urine culture is performed to confirm resolution of the UTI. If the UTI is still present, it is important to ascertain from the owner whether failure to give the patient the entire course of antibiotics occurred. In truly resistant or recurrent cases, a 4-week course of antibiotics is required. Additionally, abdominal radiography and

ultrasonography are performed to look for other sources of UTI, such as a urolith. If not done previously, full screening for and treatment of underlying systemic disease are pursued at this time.

Feline Lower Urinary Tract Disease

Feline lower urinary tract disease (FLUTD) is a clinical term used to describe the constellation of signs indicating irritation of the bladder and urethra in the cat, such as stranguria, dysuria, hematuria, pollakiuria, and inappropriate urination. FLUTD is most common in adult cats between 2 and 6 years of age. FLUTD may be classified as nonobstructive or obstructive. In more than half of patients with nonobstructive FLUTD, the underlying cause is feline idiopathic cystitis (FIC). The other common cause of nonobstructive FLUTD is the presence of uroliths. The most common causes of obstructive FLUTD are urethral plugs and FIC. Urethral plugs comprise a mucoprotein matrix and crystalline material, commonly, struvite crystals. Obstructive FLUTD, commonly referred to as *urethral obstruction*, is a medical emergency. Patients present with abdominal pain, vomiting, altered mental status, and the inability to pass a normal stream of urine. Immediate relief of the obstruction and correction of electrolyte imbalances that result from the obstruction are required. (See Chapter 25 for detailed information on the treatment of urethral obstruction.) Although no gender preference has been noted for nonobstructive FLUTD, because of the unique anatomy of their urethra, obstructive FLUTD is seen primarily in males.

> **TECHNICIAN NOTE** Feline lower urinary tract disease can be nonobstructive or obstructive.

Diagnosis of FLUTD requires a very thorough approach because no one sign or combination of signs is pathognomonic. A detailed history is critical to establish a time course of symptoms and to elucidate any triggers. A thorough diagnostic approach includes a complete urinalysis, urine culture and sensitivity, radiography, and ultrasonography. Patients may require bladder contrast studies or may be referred to veterinary specialty centers for cystoscopy. If uroliths, UTI, neoplasia, or any other causative disease process is ruled out, feline idiopathic cystitis is diagnosed; this is a diagnosis of exclusion. (Please refer to the previous section for information regarding diagnosis and treatment of uroliths and bacterial urinary tract infections.)

Clinically, FIC is a self-limiting disease, with symptoms lasting 3 to 5 days and spontaneous resolution occurring in most patients. It is not uncommon for the only sign to be inappropriate urination. A recurrent pattern is seen in about half of patients. FIC is a multifactorial disease with a complex pathogenesis that involves disorders of the hypothalamic-pituitary-adrenal axis, the nervous system, and the bladder itself. Environmental stressors, behavioral disturbances, and dietary factors play a large role in this disease process. Treatment of FIC is equally complex and multifaceted (Box 19-4),

BOX 19-4	Treatment for Feline Idiopathic Cystitis

Environmental Modification
- Litter box management
- Provide appropriate number of litter boxes
- Provide suitable type and amount of litter in the litter boxes
- Place litter boxes in a quiet, safe area of the house
- Clean frequently
- Reduce overcrowding and bullying
- Pheromone therapy
- Avoid punishing the cat
- Environmental enrichment
- Increase water intake
- Increase amount of canned cat food fed
- Use water fountains

Pharmacologic Intervention for Severe/Recurrent Cases
- Analgesics
- Glucosamine therapy for the health of the bladder lining
- Antispasmodics to reduce urethral spasms
- Antidepressants, antianxiety medications for diagnosed behavioral disorders

with overriding goals of stress reduction, increased water intake, and, for severe and recurrent cases, targeted drug therapy for pain management, bladder health, and diagnosed concurrent behavioral disorders. Client education and support are critical in managing this chronic disease.

ENDOCRINE DISEASE

Hyperthyroidism

Hyperthyroidism is a disease that affects cats in which the thyroid gland is overactive, producing abnormally large amounts of the thyroid hormones thyroxine (T_4) and triiodothyronine (T_3), resulting in an increased basal metabolic rate. In 98% of patients, hyperthyroidism is caused by a unilateral or bilateral benign functional thyroid adenoma; 2% of patients have malignant thyroid carcinoma. Clinical signs are related to the increased metabolic rate and include weight loss, increased appetite, increased activity level, polyuria and polydipsia, vomiting, and diarrhea. Approximately 10% of cats present with weight loss, anorexia, vomiting, and depression; this is termed *apathetic hyperthyroidism*. On physical examination, tachycardia, a heart murmur, an enlarged thyroid gland, and hypertension may be seen. Elevated serum T_4 concentration confirms the diagnosis of hyperthyroidism in most patients. Additional diagnostics include free T_4 concentration, T_3 suppression tests, and thyroid scintigraphy. Three-view chest radiographs are recommended to rule out the possibly of a metastatic thyroid carcinoma. Secondary thyrotoxic hypertrophic cardiomyopathy and systemic hypertension are commonly seen, as well as concurrent CKD. These disease processes must be monitored for, diagnosed, and managed as part of overall patient care. Treatment of hyperthyroidism falls into two categories: curative and palliative. Palliative treatment consists of antithyroid medication, typically methimazole, which is given once or twice a day. Antithyroid medication blocks thyroid hormone synthesis, thus decreasing the levels of circulating thyroid hormones. The dose is titrated to effectiveness based on frequent monitoring of T_4 levels and resolution of clinical signs. Curative treatment consists of surgical removal of the thyroid gland or radioactive iodine (^{131}I) treatment. A thyroidectomy may involve the removal of one or both thyroid lobes. Radioactive iodine treatment is provided at specialized, licensed treatment centers and consists of a single subcutaneous injection of ^{131}I, which is preferentially absorbed into abnormal thyroid tissue and destroys it. Radioactive iodine therapy is considered the treatment of choice for patients with healthy renal function.

Hypothyroidism

Hypothyroidism is a disease that primarily affects dogs, although a rare congenital form can be seen in kittens. Patients with this disease have an underactive thyroid, resulting in subnormal circulating levels of thyroid hormones; this causes a subsequent decrease in metabolic rate. In dogs, the most common cause of hypothyroidism is immune-mediated destruction of the gland. Clinical signs are varied and many. The most common signs are weight gain, exercise intolerance, altered mentation, and lethargy caused by the decreased metabolic rate. On physical examination, hypothermia, bradycardia, truncal alopecia, and seborrhea may be noted. Diagnostic confirmation includes documenting low serum T_4 and free T_4 levels and elevated thyroid-stimulating hormone (TSH) levels, as well as evaluating complete blood count and a full serum chemistry panel. Treatment of hypothyroidism consists of oral thyroxine replacement therapy. The dose is titrated to effectiveness based on frequent monitoring of T_4 levels and resolution of clinical signs.

Diabetes Mellitus

Diabetes mellitus (DM) may result from insufficient production of insulin by pancreatic beta cells (type 1, or insulin-dependent), or from insulin resistance characterized by the body's inability to respond properly to endogenous insulin (type 2, or non–insulin dependent). Dogs tend to develop insulin-dependent DM, but cats are more prone to non-insulin dependent DM. Clinical signs include increased appetite, weight loss (generally in a previously obese patient), polyuria, and polydipsia. Feline patients with an advanced form of the disease often present with a plantigrade stance; dogs may present with cataracts. Diagnosis consists of documenting elevated blood glucose (hyperglycemia) with concurrent glucose in the urine (glucosuria). Cats are particularly prone to stress-induced hyperglycemia, so elevated fructosamine levels are often used to help confirm diabetes mellitus in this species.

TECHNICIAN NOTE   Clinical signs of diabetes mellitus include polyuria, polydipsia, weight loss, and increased appetite. Cats may have a plantigrade stance; dogs may have cataracts.

Treatment of patients with diabetes mellitus is achieved through subcutaneous insulin injections, generally given once or twice a day, dietary changes, and maintenance of a healthy body condition score. As with many other hormone therapies, the dose of insulin must be titrated to effectiveness. This is achieved by monitoring glucose levels, which can be done through various methods, including serial blood glucose curves in hospital or at home, periodic fructosamine testing, and urine glucose monitoring. Based on these results, the veterinarian will make changes to the insulin dose. In most newly diagnosed cats, immediate and aggressive treatment with insulin is associated with spontaneous remission within 3 to 4 months and subsequent discontinuation of insulin therapy. Dogs, on the other hand, need lifelong treatment. Recommendations for dietary change vary, but in general, cats are given a high-protein/low-carbohydrate diet, and dogs are given a higher-fiber diet. The technician plays a vital role in client education and support of diabetic patients. Owners must be taught how to properly handle and administer insulin and perform glucose curves; they also must be educated on monitoring for and treating hypoglycemia.

Uncontrolled or undiagnosed diabetes mellitus will progress to a condition called *diabetic ketoacidosis (DKA)*. As the patient's body continues to be unable to use glucose, an alternative pathway for carbohydrate metabolism is used. By-products of this pathway are ketones, which are toxic metabolites. The presence of ketones in the urine (ketonuria) is a hallmark finding of DKA, as is the fruity order to the breath that ketones impart. Patients with DKA are critically ill and can present with anorexia, depression, polyuria, polydipsia, weight loss, and vomiting. On physical examination, they are often dehydrated and hypothermic, have altered mental status, and may have cardiac arrhythmias. Clinical pathologic abnormalities include hyperglycemia, glucosuria, ketonuria, metabolic acidosis, and decreased serum potassium, phosphorus, and sodium. Treatment of a patient with DKA is very complex and focuses on insulin therapy, fluid replacement therapy, and correction of electrolyte abnormalities and acidosis.

Hyperadrenocorticism

Hyperadrenocorticism (HAC), or Cushing's syndrome, is a disease that primarily affects dogs and is characterized by elevated circulating levels of cortisol (hypercortisolemia) produced by the adrenal cortex. The cause can be a functional anterior pituitary tumor, which secretes large quantities of adrenocorticotropic hormone (ACTH), or a functional adrenal tumor, which secretes large quantities of cortisol. In some patients, both types of tumors are present. Pituitary-dependent HAC is the most common form of the disease. Feline Cushing's is rare and when diagnosed is almost always seen with concurrent diabetes mellitus. Clinical signs are a result of the hypercortisolemia and include increased appetite, weight gain, lethargy, muscle weakness, polyuria, polydipsia, skin and hair coat abnormalities, and a pot-bellied appearance. The patient often is prone to secondary skin and urinary infection. Diagnosis of HAC is multifactorial, taking into consideration findings on physical examination, the minimum database, specialized endocrine function tests, and diagnostic imaging of the brain and adrenal glands. Specialized tests that assess adrenal gland function include the ACTH stimulation test, the low-dose dexamethasone suppression test, the high-dose dexamethasone suppression test, and endogenous ACTH levels. (Refer to Chapter 13 for more information on these tests.)

Treatment of patients with pituitary-dependent HAC consists of pharmacologic intervention aimed at decreasing the amount of cortisol being produced by the adrenal glands. This can be achieved by using a drug that promotes the complete or partial destruction of adrenal cortex tissue (mitotane) or one that inhibits the synthetic pathway of cortisol production (trilostane). The treatment of choice for adrenal-dependent HAC is surgical removal of the adrenal tumor(s). The patient is placed on glucocorticoid (in some cases, mineralocorticoid) replacement therapy immediately after surgery. If both adrenal glands were removed, this therapy is lifelong. If only one gland was removed, replacement therapy usually can be discontinued within 3 months as the remaining adrenal gland regains normal functioning. Adrenalectomy is the treatment of choice in feline patients with either form of the disease.

Hypoadrenocorticism

Hypoadrenocorticism is caused by adrenal gland atrophy or destruction, resulting in inadequate secretion of glucocorticoids and mineralocorticoids, primarily cortisol and aldosterone. Hypoadrenocorticism, or Addison's disease, primarily affects dogs. Common historical information on these patients includes episodic events of anorexia, vomiting, diarrhea, polyuria, polydipsia, weakness, and collapse—especially during periods of stress. Weight loss, bradycardia, weak femoral pulses, altered mentation, and prolonged capillary refill time can be seen on physical examination of a patient experiencing an Addisonian crisis. Common clinical pathologic abnormalities seen in these patients include anemia, azotemia, hypoglycemia, and elevated serum potassium (hyperkalemia), with a concurrent decrease in sodium (hyponatremia). Definitive diagnosis is made with an ACTH stimulation test that reveals low cortisol levels before and after administration of ACTH. Treatment of the acute patient is a medical emergency and focuses on treating dehydration and electrolyte imbalance, managing gastrointestinal symptoms, and administering glucocorticoids. Long-term management of the disease is achieved through mineralocorticoid supplementation, with some dogs also requiring glucocorticoid replacement therapy.

REPRODUCTIVE DISEASE

Postpartum Disorders of the Dam

Mastitis refers to inflammation of one or more mammary glands. It is common in bitches but rare in queens. Clinical signs include fever, anorexia, depression, lethargy, and warm, swollen, painful mammary glands. In less severe cases, the dam may not be symptomatic; however, neonates show signs of neglect. Diagnosis is made on the basis of history and clinical signs and culture of the milk. Treatment consists of systemic antibiotics (preferentially those safe for the neonate) and ensuring adequate hydration and caloric intake for proper milk production.

Galactostasis is stasis of milk in the mammary glands, resulting in enlarged, painful mammary glands. Unlike mastitis, patients with galactostasis are not systemically ill. Treatment is not indicated during the first 1 to 3 weeks of the postpartum period. Treatment, which is begun if galactostasis occurs during the weaning period, focuses on decreasing milk production (reducing food and water intake and preventing nursing) and decreasing inflammation with gentle application of warm compresses. Massage of the mammary gland is contraindicated.

Metritis is a bacterial infection of the uterus. Signs usually develop within the first week of parturition. Metritis is associated with retained placentae, retained fetuses, and dystocia. Clinical signs suggestive of metritis include fever, depression, foul-smelling uterine discharge, and neglect of the neonates. Patients may present in endotoxemic or septicemic shock. Diagnosis is based on history, physical examination, diagnostic imaging, and culture of uterine discharge. Initial therapy consists of replacing fluid deficits, treating shock, if present, and initiating antibiotic therapy. Upon stabilization of the patient, removal of the uterus or administration of medication to promote evacuation of the uterus is performed.

Eclampsia (hypocalcemia) usually occurs 2 to 3 weeks postpartum in bitches with large litters but occasionally can occur before birth. Eclampsia is rare in queens. Presenting signs include weakness and trembling and may proceed to tonic convulsions. Diagnosis is based on clinical signs in a lactating female and low serum calcium levels. Emergency treatment involves administration of intravenous 10% calcium gluconate to effect. Outpatient treatment includes ensuring that the dam receives oral calcium lactate or calcium gluconate and vitamin D, and preventing the puppies from nursing. Puppies are hand-fed with nursing bottles and milk replacer until 4 weeks old.

Canine Prostatic Disease

Prostatic disease is occasionally seen in older intact male dogs. Clinical signs include straining to stranguria, dysuria, hematuria, and/or difficulty in defecation. Conditions that affect the prostate include benign prostatic hyperplasia, bacterial prostatitis, prostatic abscess, prostatic cyst, and prostatic neoplasia.

The following noninvasive techniques are used to evaluate the prostate: rectal palpation, routine radiology, sonography (ultrasound), urethrography, cytologic studies, and bacterial cultures of prostatic washes or the prostatic fraction of the ejaculate. Frequently, it is difficult to differentiate neoplasia, infection, and hyperplasia with these noninvasive techniques. Consequently, surgical exploration and biopsy may be required to establish a definitive diagnosis.

Treatment varies, depending on the specific process. Dogs with benign prostatic hyperplasia respond to castration. Medical treatment for benign prostatic hyperplasia involves administration of medications that inhibit or depress testosterone synthesis. Prostatic abscesses and cysts require surgical drainage. Bacterial prostatitis and prostatic abscesses are treated with antibiotics. Prostatic neoplasia is generally highly malignant, and treatment is directed toward palliation rather than cure. Some dogs with prostatic cancer may benefit from castration because the tumors possess testosterone receptors.

IMMUNE-MEDIATED DISEASE

Immune-mediated diseases are those in which the immune system has lost tolerance of self and perpetuates damage to the body's organs. Autoimmunity may be primary (idiopathic) or secondary, that is, the result of an underlying disease process. Secondary immune-mediated disease can result from infection, cancer, vaccine administration, or exposure to certain drugs or toxins.

> **TECHNICIAN NOTE**   Immune-mediated diseases are those in which the immune system has lost tolerance of self and perpetuates damage to the body's organs.

Immune-Mediated Hemolytic Anemia

Hemolytic anemia is characterized by red blood cell (RBC) destruction. One cause of hemolytic anemia, and the most common cause in dogs, is immune-mediated destruction of RBCs. *Immune-mediate hemolytic anemia (IMHA)* may be primary or secondary. Most cases in the dog are primary, whereas IMHA secondary to blood parasite infection is more common in the cat. In primary IMHA, the immune systems targets the RBC as foreign (an antigen) and develops autoantibodies against red blood cell membrane components. In secondary IMHA, the immune system attacks the pathogen that is adhered to the RBC membrane, as is normal, but it also indiscriminately destroys normal RBCs. Clinical signs of IMHA include lethargy, exercise intolerance, pale or yellow mucous membranes, tachycardia, heart murmur, splenomegaly, hepatomegaly, fever, and abdominal pain. Diagnosis is based on CBC findings consistent with hemolytic anemia and evidence of autoimmunity: autoagglutination and a positive Coombs test (see Chapter 12 for detailed information). Once the diagnosis of IMHA is made, the search for an underlying disease is undertaken. If no underlying disease can be documented, primary IMHA is diagnosed. Treatment for IMHA includes immunosuppressive therapy, judicious use of blood transfusions, fluid therapy, and treatment of any underlying disease. Patients with acute, severe anemia will be hypoxic and likely will require oxygen supplementation. Thromboembolism is a common and often fatal complication of IMHA; therefore, treatment with anticoagulants is also instituted.

Acquired (Immune-Mediated) Myasthenia Gravis

Myasthenia gravis (MG) is a disorder of neuromuscular transmission that causes muscle weakness. Acquired MG is caused by an immune system dysfunction that produces autoantibodies against acetylcholine receptors (AChRs) in the postsynaptic membrane. This is differentiated from congenital MG, which is an inherited deficiency of these receptors. Acquired MG is more common in dogs than in cats. The main clinical sign is generalized weakness that is worsened with exercise and resolves with rest. If the patient has megaesophagus (large, dilated esophagus) as a result of the disease, presenting signs include hypersalivation and regurgitation. The presence of autoantibodies against AChRs in the serum confirms the diagnosis. The presence of megaesophagus is determined by radiographs. Treatment includes administration of anticholinesterase inhibitors, which prolong the action of acetylcholine at the synapses, thereby improving muscle strength, and immunosuppressive drugs. Patients with megaesophagus and regurgitation are at risk for aspiration (see Table 19-5); appropriate nursing care for regurgitation is instituted (see previous section on regurgitation).

JOINT DISEASE

Osteoarthritis

Osteoarthritis (OA) is a chronic, progressive deterioration of the articular cartilage of the joint caused by joint laxity (e.g., cranial cruciate ligament rupture, hip dysplasia) and/or abnormal load bearing of the joint (e.g., hip dysplasia, obesity). As articular cartilage deterioration continues, it triggers an inflammatory response leading to joint capsule changes and effusion and to subchondral bone hypertrophy with formation of osteophytes (abnormal bony outgrowths, sometimes called "bone spurs"). OA affects both dogs and cats and can be found in the axial and appendicular skeleton. Historical information on a patient with osteoarthritis points to orthopedic pain and reduced mobility as evidenced by decreased ability to navigate stairs or to jump, difficulty rising after sleeping, a change in walking habits or in willingness to play (exercise intolerance), trouble getting into and out of the litter box, uncharacteristic aggression, and/or obvious lameness.

> **TECHNICIAN NOTE** Historical information on a patient with osteoarthritis points to orthopedic pain and reduced mobility.

Palpation of affected joints reveals pain, swelling, crepitus, decreased range of motion, and joint laxity. Confirmation of OA is based on radiographs; however, early arthritic changes often are not seen, so a presumptive diagnosis may be made on the basis of history and clinical signs. Prevention of osteoarthritis is ideal. This entails early detection and correction of predisposing orthopedic deformities such as hip dysplasia. Treatment of any underlying disease process is necessary but does not generally stop the progression of joint changes if OA is already present. Management of osteoarthritis is multimodal. Dietary management is necessary to maintain the patient's optimal body weight, thereby reducing stress on the joints. Administration of chondroprotective medications and supplements promotes synovial joint health. Control of joint inflammation helps decrease joint pain; veterinary-specific nonsteroidal anti-inflammatory (NSAIDs) drugs and omega-3 fatty acids are frequently given. Patients on long-term NSAID therapy need to be closely monitored for deleterious side effects such as gastrointestinal ulcerations and kidney or liver disease. Complementary medicine modalities, such as acupuncture, may be employed to address inflammation and pain. Physical therapy can help the patient regain range of motion and can promote muscle strength. Moderate controlled exercise is important in maintaining muscle strength and joint mobility. The veterinary technician must counsel owners on the many environmental and lifestyle changes that need to be implemented to decrease painful stimuli and accommodate the pet's reduction in mobility. These often include use of pet stairs and ramps to reach elevated locations such as the bed or a cat tree, instruction on proper technique for lifting a dog into and out of a car, moving cat bowls off of high surfaces, changing to low-profile litter boxes, and using deep foam bedding to provide cushioning and comfort for arthritic joints.

DISEASE OF THE EYES, EARS, AND SKIN

It is beyond the scope of this chapter to provide an in-depth discussion of the many diseases that affect the eyes, ears, and skin of small animals. Table 19-19 provides a summary of some of these clinically relevant diseases.

INFECTIOUS DISEASE

Infectious diseases are those diseases caused by pathogenic microorganisms that invade and colonize within the tissues and fluids of an individual animal (host). Infectious diseases are prevalent in the cat and dog and involve many different pathogens, such as viruses, bacteria, fungi, and rickettsiae (endoparasites are covered in Chapter 14). Infectious diseases can be transmissible, such as kennel cough, or nontransmissible, such as a cat bite abscess. This chapter focuses on transmissible infectious diseases. Required components and steps of infection are as follows (Figure 19-1):

1. The pathogen: must be able to avoid host defense systems, reproduce in the host, and cause disease.
2. Reservoir: can be an animal, insect, or fomite (inanimate objects such as water, bowls, cages, clipper blades, instruments, towels, scrubs, etc.) in which the pathogen can survive.
3. Portal of exit (from the animate reservoir): where/how the pathogen leaves the reservoir, often related to clinical signs of the disease process (e.g., sneezing).
4. Mode of transmission: how the pathogen travels to the next host:

TABLE 19-19	Small Animal Diseases of the Eyes, Ears, and Skin			
DISEASE	**PATHOGENESIS**	**CLINICAL SIGNS**	**DIAGNOSTICS**	**TREATMENT**
Conjunctivitis	Inflammation of the conjunctiva caused by infectious agents, allergies, environmental irritation, foreign bodies, dry eye	Ocular discharge, chemosis, hyperemia, ocular discomfort, pawing at the eye	Based on clinical signs Demonstration of infectious agents on cytologic examination and culture of conjunctival scrapings	Treat underlying cause Eye irrigation Topical antibiotics/ antivirals/ antihistamines Prevent self-trauma
Corneal ulcer	Ulceration of corneal epithelium caused by mechanical abrasion, infectious agents, keratoconjunctivitis sicca Secondary bacterial infection ensues Complete perforation possible	Pain indicated by blepharospasm, photophobia, and epiphora Corneal edema Concurrent conjunctivitis	Ulceration may be evident on gross examination Demonstration of ulcer with fluorescein stain	Treat underlying cause Topical antibiotics Topical atropine for pain Topical antivirals Prevent self-trauma Contact lens or collagen shield placement Third eyelid or conjunctival flap
Cataracts	Pathologic lens opacity caused by inherited disorder or secondary to various underlying diseases	Cloudy lens, pupil dilated, vision loss Ocular pain	Ophthalmic examination demonstrates loss of tapetal reflex and visual confirmation of cataract Ocular ultrasound	Treat underlying cause Surgical removal of lens with or without placement of artificial lens
Glaucoma	Reduced drainage of aqueous humor through the anterior chamber and ciliary body, causing increased intraocular pressure (IOP) Can be primary (inherited) or secondary to underlying ocular inflammation	Dilated or fixed pupil, buphthalmia, conjunctival hyperemia, corneal edema, vision loss	Tonometry reveals increased IOP Gonioscopy to measure iridocorneal drainage angle	Early detection in predisposed breeds with routine tonometry Medical treatments aimed at reducing aqueous humor production and increasing aqueous drainage
Anterior uveitis	Inflammation of the anterior uvea caused by infectious disease, corneal ulceration, trauma, immune-mediated disease	Blepharospasm, epiphora, photophobia, aqueous flare, decreased intraocular pressure	Based on clinical signs Centesis of aqueous fluid for culture Serologic examination for infectious disease	Treat underlying cause Topical atropine Topical antibiotics/ antivirals Topical anti-inflammatories Prevent self-trauma
Aural hematoma	Blood-filled swelling on the inner surface of the pinna Associated with excessive head shaking and ear scratching, often seen with otitis externa or media	Focal swelling noted on physical examination	Based on history and clinical signs Fine-needle aspirate of mass reveals blood	Surgical drainage and flushing and topical and systemic anti-inflammatories Prevent self-trauma

TABLE 19-19	Small Animal Diseases of the Eyes, Ears, and Skin—cont'd			
DISEASE	**PATHOGENESIS**	**CLINICAL SIGNS**	**DIAGNOSTICS**	**TREATMENT**
Otitis externa	Inflammation of the external ear canal caused by atopy, food sensitivities, ectoparasites, foreign bodies, neoplasia Secondary bacterial and yeast infections common Dogs with pendulous ears predisposed	Aural hyperemia, discharge, exudate, and odor Excoriations on pinna Crusts and scales and hyperpigmentation Pawing, scratching at ear Local pain	Based on clinical signs Thorough otoscopic evaluation for deformities, neoplasms, foreign bodies, parasites Cytologic examination and culture of exudate to determine underlying cause	Treat underlying cause Flush and dry ear canals Topical ceruminolytics Topical and/or systemic anti-inflammatories Topical and/or systemic antibiotics Prevent self-trauma
Otitis media/ interna	Inflammation of the middle or inner ear structures Generally a progression of otitis externa	Head shaking, pawing at ear, head tilt, circling, facial nerve paralysis, Horner's syndrome May also have signs of otitis externa	Visualization of bulging or ruptured tympanum on otoscopic examination Radiographs, computed tomography (CT) and magnetic resonance imaging (MRI) of tympanum and bullae	As for otitis externa Extended course of systemic antibiotics generally indicated Severe cases require surgical intervention
Nasopharyngeal polyp	Inflammatory polyp that originates in the middle ear and extends into the nasopharynx and external ear canal Believed to be caused by feline herpesvirus and feline calicivirus	Sneezing, nasal discharge, stertor, voice change Digital palpation of mass under soft palate Mass in external ear canal May see signs of otitis media	Direct visualization under sedated examination Diagnostic imaging is helpful in severe cases	Removal of polyp Ventral bulla osteotomy in severe cases
Bacterial pyoderma	Primary or secondary infection of the epidermis and hair follicles May be superficial or deep	Scaling, pruritus, papules, pustules, crusts, erythema, swelling, exudation of blood and pus, draining tracts, odor, and pain	Clinical signs Impression smears Culture and sensitivity of swabs or biopsied skin	Treat underlying cause Prevent self-trauma Systemic antibiotics Topical antibiotics Mediated baths Clip hair coat
Allergic skin disease	Hypersensitivity reaction secondary to atopy, food sensitivity, ectoparasites, skin infection	Pruritus, erythema, papules, crusts, alopecia, military dermatitis, pododermatitis, eosinophilic ulcers, plaques, and granulomas	History and clinical signs Diagnostics of underlying cause are extensive	Treat underlying cause Prevent triggers Prevent self-trauma Antihistamines Topical and systemic anti-inflammatories Medicated baths

a. Direct transmission is immediate and requires direct contact of skin or mucous membranes with infected animal or its secretions or excretions (e.g., nose-to-nose contact can transmit feline herpesvirus), ingestion of virus (e.g., ingestion of parvovirus-laden feces), or inhalation of virus (e.g., inhalation of aerosolized canine parainfluenza virus).

b. Indirect transmission is delayed and requires contact with a contaminated fomite (e.g., transmission of ringworm through contaminated clipper blades) or is

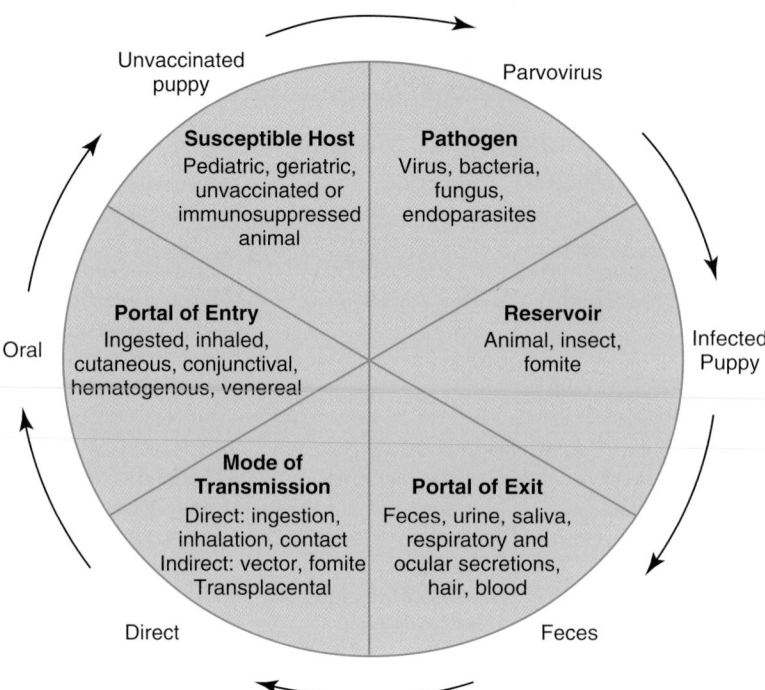

FIGURE 19-1 Required steps for infection of transmissible diseases.

transmitted via a biological vector, usually an insect (e.g., heartworm disease transmitted via mosquito bite). Hands of veterinary personnel can also be considered a vector.

   c. Transplacental transmission.

5. Portal of entry (route of infection): where/how the pathogen gains entry into the new host.

6. Host susceptibility: exposure to a pathogen does not guarantee infection and disease. The host must be susceptible to the pathogen. Specifically, this means that the host has a naïve, immature, suppressed, or deficient immune system and cannot kill the pathogen. However, other considerations could be listed here, such as species specificity (dogs cannot contract feline herpesvirus), opportunity for exposure (a city-dwelling dog is less likely to be exposed to *Leptospira*), and geographic location of the host (certain tick vectors are found only in particular areas).

It is useful to classify transmissible infectious diseases. Infectious diseases that are transmitted directly between animals or indirectly through fomites contaminated with animal secretions are considered contagious (e.g., feline calicivirus). Infectious diseases that require a biological vector are termed *vector-borne* (e.g., *Borrelia burgdorferi*). **Zoonoses** are infectious diseases that are transmitted directly from animals to humans (e.g., rabies virus). Infectious agents that can infect a human or an animal via a common vector (fleas, ticks) are called *shared-vector zoonoses*. *Reverse zoonoses* are infectious diseases that are transmitted from humans to animals (e.g., dermatophytosis).

Control of transmissible infectious diseases involves interrupting the process of infection:

1. Kill the pathogen while it is in the host or animate reservoir: antibiotic, antiviral, antiparasitic medication.

2. Kill the pathogen while it is living on a fomite: sanitation, disinfection, sterilization.

3. Kill the pathogen while it is living in/on a vector: preventive antiparasitic medication, environmental pesticide, soap and water. (Wash your hands between patients!)

4. Strengthen host defense systems:
   a. Administer vaccination (see Chapter 8).
   b. Maintain proper health and nutrition.

5. Decrease host exposure:
   a. Limit exposure of immunodeficient and immunosuppressed individuals, for example, by a change in lifestyle (e.g., keep cats with feline immunodeficiency virus indoors).
   b. Follow proper isolation protocols for contagious animals to prevent spread of disease.

Isolation Facilities and Procedures

Recognition by the veterinary technician of a patient with a potentially contagious disease, based on history and clinical signs, is an important front-line defense of hospital-wide infectious disease control. Patients suspected to have a contagious disease should not be made to wait in the receiving area, but instead should be brought immediately into an examination room, preferably one designated for such cases. Depending on the disease and on whether the patient is stable, the recommended course of action is to discharge the patient, with at-home care provided by the owner. In critical cases, or in cases where the owner is unable to provide care, patients are admitted into an isolation ward separate from the main population of patients and boarders. An isolation ward designed with a separate, negative-pressure air ventilation system, double-door entryways with an anteroom, its own water supply, and a single wall of cage banks is ideal. Placement of wall-mounted hand sanitizer dispensers in multiple locations is desirable. The isolation ward should have its own clinical equipment and cage supplies. The number of staff entering isolation wards on any given day should be limited. Personnel should thoroughly wash their hands and don shoe covers, a gown, and examination gloves before entering the ward (this is termed **barrier nursing**). Barrier nursing is the most effective management approach against contracting a zoonotic disease. Hands are washed and new gloves are put on before the next patient is nursed. All supplies, tabletops, and countertops should be properly disinfected after each use.

> **TECHNICIAN NOTE** Barrier nursing is a method that creates a "barrier" between a contagious patient and the nurse, in an effort to reduce transmission of an infectious pathogen to other patients. Wearing shoe covers, gloves, and a gown during nursing care and isolating the patient when able are components of barrier nursing.

It is recommended that patients are not moved into new cages as part of the disinfection process but instead are returned to their original, cleaned cage. This helps to decrease disease transmission and decreases stress to the animal by minimizing handling. When one is readying to leave the isolation ward, shoe covers, gowns, and gloves are removed and hands are thoroughly washed; ideally this is done in the anteroom, if present. Waste and laundry are bagged in isolation, brought out, placed in another bag, and properly disposed of or washed. Some patients may have their own individual biohazard bags for waste and laundry cage-side. When washing laundry from infected patients, care must be taken to provide proper sanitation; this includes using dilute bleach and hot water and refraining from overfilling the laundry machine, so that linens are thoroughly washed.

Nursing Care

Patients with infectious diseases often require extensive nursing care and support while the patient's body fights the infection. This is especially true of infections for which there is no direct way to destroy the pathogen (e.g., antibiotics), as occurs with viral infections. Supportive care requires attending to the patient's basic needs and treating symptoms of the disease, such as nasal discharge, vomiting, or dehydration. Many infectious diseases compromise the function of patients' immune system, putting them at risk for secondary infection. Monitoring these patients for signs of secondary infections (see Table 19-5) while administering prescribed prophylactic antibiotic therapy is important.

Client Education

Veterinary technicians have a critical role in educating and supporting the owner of a pet with a transmissible infectious disease. Because the preference is to treat most infectious disease cases on an outpatient basis, the bulk of care falls to the client. The veterinary technician must provide oral and written instructions on patient care, demonstrate medication administration techniques, educate the owner on isolation procedures to control spread of the disease to other animals in the household, educate the owner about zoonotic potential (e.g., ringworm), and provide information about household disinfection protocols. The veterinary technician must support owners throughout this process, which can be overwhelming and at times frustrating for them. A classic example is a patient with ringworm infection: the months-long duration of treatment, the unpleasant nature of the treatment (odoriferous lime-sulfur baths), the expensive oral antifungal medication, the intense disinfection protocols, the zoonotic potential, and the high rate of recurrence are all extremely stressful and frustrating for the owner. Frequent phone calls and in-office visits are often necessary to ensure owner support and compliance, thereby completing patient care.

Small Animal Infectious Diseases

It is beyond the scope of this chapter to provide detailed information on all infectious diseases seen in small animals; instead, focus is placed on clinically relevant contagious diseases and important zoonotic diseases seen in the clinical setting. These are summarized in Tables 19-20 through 19-25.

CANCER

Oncology is the study of cancer. Cancer is a disease of uncontrolled growth of abnormal cells. The process of uncontrolled cell growth and subsequent formation of a tissue mass is called *neoplasia*. These masses are called tumors or neoplasms, and in addition to uncontrolled growth, they may have the ability to invade and destroy tissue and spread to other parts of the body (see tumor classification in the following section). Tables 19-26 and 19-27 provide a brief overview of select feline and canine cancers.

Tumor Biology

Virtually any type of normal cell may undergo neoplastic changes that result in tumor formation. *Carcinogenesis* is a multifactorial process by which normal cells are transformed into tumors. Classically, three events must take place before malignant transformation can occur: initiation, promotion, and progression. During initiation, the cell is exposed to a factor or factors (carcinogens) that rapidly and irreversibly alter its DNA, giving it the potential to replicate unchecked. An initiated cell is not a cancerous cell yet but requires further mutations caused by an agent or event that stimulates proliferation of the cell to grow into a neoplasm. This stage is called *promotion*. Additional cellular mutations occur over time during the third phase of carcinogenesis—progression—which is characterized by continued growth of the tumor that ultimately leads to clinical disease. Factors with carcinogenic potential include inherited genetic

TABLE 19-20	Contagious Diseases of the Respiratory Tract				
DISEASE AND PATHOGEN	**MODE OF TRANSMISSION**	**PATHOGENESIS**	**CLINICAL SIGNS**	**DIAGNOSTICS**	**TREATMENTS**
Feline upper respiratory tract disease Feline herpesvirus-1 (FHV-1)	Direct: contact with mucosal secretions Indirect: contaminated fomites	Viral replication in the mucosal lining of the upper respiratory tract, conjunctiva, and tonsils Secondary infections ensue Infection usually leads to asymptomatic carrier state with chronic flare-ups	Rhinitis Conjunctivitis Anorexia Fever Corneal ulcers	History and clinical signs Virus isolation and detection can be performed but is generally reserved for chronic cases	Relieve nasal congestion Airway humidification Treat anorexia Treat corneal ulcers Treat conjunctivitis Treat dehydration Antibiotics for secondary infection Decrease stress
Feline upper respiratory tract disease Feline calicivirus (FCV)	Direct: contact with mucosal secretions Indirect: contaminated fomites	Viral replication in the epithelial lining of the upper respiratory tract, conjunctiva, and tongue Secondary infections ensue Infection usually leads to asymptomatic carrier state with chronic flare-ups	Rhinitis Conjunctivitis Fever Gagging, hypersalivation due to lingual and oral ulcers Anorexia Joint pain	History and clinical signs Virus isolation and detection can be performed but is generally reserved for severe cases	Airway humidification Treat conjunctivitis Treat anorexia Relieve oral ulcer pain: • Systemic analgesics • Topical diluted lidocaine Antibiotics for secondary infection Decrease stress
Canine infectious tracheobronchitis (kennel cough) Canine adenovirus type 2 (CAV-2); canine parainfluenza; *Bordetella bronchiseptica*	Direct: contact with mucosal secretions Direct: inhalation of airborne virus Note: cats are susceptible to kennel cough also	Viral replication in the respiratory epithelium	Acute, harsh cough Gagging/retching Nasal discharge	History and clinical signs	Avoid exercise and excitement Decrease pressure on trachea: harness vs. collar Maintain hydration ± Antibiotics ± Antitussives

defects, hormones, viruses, diet, immune system dysfunction, trauma, chronic inflammation, radiation, and a wide variety of chemicals. However, establishing a simple cause-and-effect relationship between a specific carcinogenic factor and subsequent tumor development in an exposed or affected individual is extremely difficult.

Tumor Classification

Tumors can be benign or malignant. Benign tumors do not invade or destroy surrounding normal tissues or spread to a new site. However, they can still impair tissue function, causing significant problems through their physical presence. For instance, even though most meningiomas (tumors of the meninges that surround the brain and spinal cord) are histologically benign, they can cause severe neurologic dysfunction and death as a result of compression of the brain or spinal cord. Malignant tumors are capable of invasion and destruction of local tissue and of metastasis. *Metastasis* is the process by which cancer cells spread from a primary tumor to secondary locations, such as lungs, lymph nodes, and visceral sites (e.g., liver). The mechanisms of metastasis are not fully understood, but the metastatic process involves a series of basic steps that are similar regardless of the tumor type. First, cancer cells of the primary tumor must detach themselves from the mass and invade the vascular or lymphatic vessels. Once in the circulation, these cells are transported to distant tissues, where they eventually reach the metastatic site. The cells then leave the circulation and invade tissue. A metastatic tumor is established when these cells are able to survive and grow at the new site. It should be noted that some tumor cells can spread directly along serosal surfaces.

Text continued on p. 712

TABLE 19-21	Contagious Diseases of the Digestive and Hepatobiliary Systems				
DISEASE AND PATHOGEN	**MODE OF TRANSMISSION**	**PATHOGENESIS**	**CLINICAL SIGNS**	**DIAGNOSTICS**	**TREATMENTS**
Feline panleukopenia Feline parvovirus (FPV)	Direct: ingestion of feces (fecal-oral) Indirect: contaminated fomites Transplacental	Replication of the virus within the intestinal crypts, bone marrow, and lymphoid tissue Secondary sepsis common	Anorexia Lethargy Fever Vomiting Dehydration Abdominal pain ± Diarrhea Septic shock Cerebellar hypoplasia	History Clinical signs CBC: leukopenia Fecal parvovirus antigen ELISA test	Control vomiting Treat dehydration and electrolyte imbalance Treat anorexia Treat hyperthermia Antibiotics to treat/ prevent secondary bacterial infections Monitor for sepsis
Canine parvoviral enteritis Canine parvovirus (CPV-2)	Direct: ingestion of feces Indirect: contaminated fomites	Replication of the virus within the intestinal crypts, bone marrow, and lymphoid tissue Secondary sepsis and protein-losing enteropathy common	Anorexia Lethargy Fever Vomiting Diarrhea, often bloody Dehydration Abdominal pain Septic shock	History Clinical signs CBC: leukopenia Fecal parvovirus antigen ELISA test	Control vomiting Treat dehydration and electrolyte imbalance Treat anorexia Administer plasma to treat hypoalbuminemia Antibiotics to treat/ prevent secondary bacterial infection Monitor for sepsis
Canine infectious hepatitis Canine adenovirus type 1 (CAV-1)	Direct: ingestion of saliva, feces, urine	Infection begins in the tonsils and spreads to the liver, spleen, kidneys, lungs, and vascular endothelial cells	Fever Injected mucous membranes Petechiation Enlarged tonsils Anorexia Dehydration Prolonged bleeding Signs of hepatitis	History and clinical signs Virus isolation	Treat dehydration Administer blood products Prophylactic antibiotic therapy

CBC, Complete blood count; *ELISA*, enzyme-linked immunosorbent assay.

TABLE 19-22	Polysystemic Contagious Diseases				
DISEASE AND PATHOGEN	**MODE OF TRANSMISSION**	**PATHOGENESIS**	**CLINICAL SIGNS**	**DIAGNOSTICS**	**TREATMENTS**
Feline leukemia Feline leukemia virus (FeLV)	Direct: contact with saliva, nasal secretions Iatrogenic transmission though blood transfusion or contaminated needles	Virus replicates in oropharyngeal lymphoid tissue, then spreads to the spleen, thymus, lymph nodes, and bone marrow Patients may become latent carriers	Anorexia Weight loss Fever Generalized lympadenopathy Signs of severe anemia Evidence of immunosuppression: gingivitis, chronic viral respiratory disease, etc. Evidence of lymphoma	FeLV Antigen testing (ELISA and IFA) on blood, bone marrow	Maintain good husbandry and nutritional health Keep indoors Semiannual physical examinations, preventive medicine and routine laboratory work to monitor for anemia Routine dental prophylaxis Antiviral therapy Immunomodulators Blood transfusion Chemotherapy (for lymphoma)

Continued

TABLE 19-22 | Polysystemic Contagious Diseases—cont'd

DISEASE AND PATHOGEN	MODE OF TRANSMISSION	PATHOGENESIS	CLINICAL SIGNS	DIAGNOSTICS	TREATMENTS
Feline immunodeficiency Feline immunodeficiency virus (FIV)	Direct: inoculation of saliva through bite wounds Transplacental Iatrogenic transmission though blood transfusion	Virus replicates in the salivary glands and lymphoid tissue Patients may become latent carriers	Weight loss Generalized lymphadenopathy Fever Anterior uveitis Evidence of immunosuppression: gingivitis, chronic viral respiratory disease, etc. Evidence of lymphoma	FIV antibody testing (ELISA and Western blot) on blood	Maintain good husbandry and nutritional health Keep indoors Semiannual physical examinations, preventive medicine, and routine laboratory work Routine dental prophylaxis Antiviral therapy Immunomodulators Treatment of secondary disease
Feline infectious peritonitis (FIP) Feline coronavirus (FCoV)	Direct: ingestion of feces (fecal-oral) Indirect: contaminated fomites	Virus replicated in the intestinal tract, a portion with mutated and infected macrophages, thus disseminating throughout the body and causing the clinical disease	Effusive Form • Ascites • Pleural effusion • Weight loss • Fever • Anorexia Noneffusive Form • Uveitis • CNS signs • Signs of organ failure as granulomas form in the liver, spleen, kidneys, and GI tract	History and clinical signs Serum globulin and albumin concentrations Cytologic examination and analysis of effusions Antigen detection in effusive fluid Tissue biopsies	Thoracocentesis or abdominocentesis Corticosteroids to reduce immune overreaction Immunomodulators
Canine distemper Canine distemper virus (CDV)	Direct: inhalation of airborne virus Direct: contact with urine, feces, mucosal secretions	Infection starts in lymphatic system of the respiratory tract and spreads to the GI and urogenital tracts, and to CNS and optic nerves. Progression of clinical signs often follows progression of infection	Nasal discharge Ocular discharge Cough Fever Diarrhea Anorexia Lethargy Hyperkeratosis of foot pads, nasal planum CNS signs: • Seizures • Head tilt • Ataxia • Paralysis	Clinical signs Antibody titers Virus isolation	Treat dehydration Antibiotics Anticonvulsants Antipyretics Analgesics Anti-inflammatories
Leptospirosis Leptospira spp.	Direct: contact with urine Indirect: contaminated fomites Note: Cattle and wildlife are reservoirs	Bacterial infection ensues in multiple tissues, particularly liver and kidneys	Anorexia Fever Joint pain Vomiting Diarrhea Evidence of hemorrhage Evidence of hepatitis Evidence of kidney disease	History and clinical signs Leptospira antibody serology	Antibiotics Treat dehydration Treat kidney disease Treat liver disease

CNS, Central nervous system; ELISA, enzyme-linked immunosorbent assay; IFA, indirect fluorescent antibody test.

TABLE 19-23	Contagious Diseases of the Nervous System and Skin				
DISEASE AND PATHOGEN	**MODE OF TRANSMISSION**	**PATHOGENESIS**	**CLINICAL SIGNS**	**DIAGNOSTICS**	**TREATMENTS**

Rabies
Rabies virus
(RV)
	Direct:
	  inoculation of
	  saliva into
	  skin, usually
	  through a bite
	  wound
	Note: Reservoir
	  is usually
	  wildlife
		The virus travels from
		  peripheral nerves
		  to spinal cord and
		  brain, and then
		  from brain to
		  salivary glands via
		  peripheral nerves
		Rapid progression of
		  neurologic signs
		  ensues
			Apprehension
			Nervousness
			Hyperexcitability
			Aggression
			Seizures
			Paralysis
			Hypersalivation
			Inability to
			  swallow
				Postmortem virus
				  isolation in
				  brain tissue
					No therapeutic
					  protocols for
					  infected patients
					Infection is lethal

Ringworm
  (dermatophytosis)
Microsporum spp.
  and Trichophyton
  spp.
	Direct: contact
	  with skin,
	  hair, claws
	Indirect:
	  contaminated
	  fomites
		Dermatophytes infect
		  growing hairs,
		  penetrating the
		  hair shaft and hair
		  follicle and
		  causing a local
		  inflammatory
		  response
			Alopecia
			Erythema
			Crusting, scaly
			  skin
			Hyperpigmentation
			Folliculitis
				Dermatophyte test
				  medium culture
				Direct
				  microscopic
				  evaluation of
				  hair or skin
				  scraping
					Topical antifungals:
					• Ointments
					• Bath/dip
					  Oral antifungals

TABLE 19-24	Vector-Borne Pathogens				
DISEASE AND PATHOGEN	**VECTOR**	**PATHOGENESIS**	**CLINICAL SIGNS**	**DIAGNOSTICS**	**TREATMENTS**

Lyme disease
Borrelia
  burgdorferi
	Ixodes spp. tick	Bacterial infection and
		  subsequent
		  inflammation of
		  various tissues,
		  including skin, joint
		  capsule, lymph
		  nodes, kidney,
		  liver, and heart
			Fever
			Anorexia
			Lameness
			Swollen joints
			Lymphadenopathy
			Signs of kidney
			  failure
				History and clinical
				  signs
				Serology for
				  antibodies
				Analysis of joint
				  effusion
					Antibiotics
					Treatment for
					  specific organ
					  damage

Rocky Mountain
  spotted fever
Rickettsia rickettsii
	Dermacentor
	  spp. tick
		Rickettsial infection of
		  the vascular
		  endothelium,
		  causing vasculitis
		  and secondary
		  thrombocytopenia
			Fever
			Depression
			Cough/dyspnea
			Vomiting/diarrhea
			Evidence of
			  hemorrhage
			Central nervous
			  system (CNS)
			  signs
			Shock
				History and clinical
				  signs
				Laboratory data
				Antibody titers
				Isolation of
				  pathogen in
				  body fluids and
				  tissue
					Antibiotics
					Fluid therapy
					Treatments aimed
					  at managing
					  organ-specific
					  damage

Canine ehrlichiosis
Erhlichia spp.
	Rhipicephalus
	  spp. tick
		Rickettsial infection of
		  the vascular
		  endothelium,
		  causing vasculitis
		  and, of
		  macrophages,
		  which disseminate
		  throughout the
		  body, particularly
		  to the liver and
		  spleen
			Fever
			Depression
			Lymphadenopathy
			Splenomegaly
			Hepatomegaly
			Evidence of
			  hemorrhage
			Lameness, swollen
			  joints
				History and clinical
				  signs
				Laboratory data
				Antibody titers
				Isolation of
				  pathogen in
				  body fluids and
				  tissue
					Antibiotics
					Fluid therapy
					Blood transfusion
					Treatments aimed
					  at managing
					  organ-specific
					  damage

TABLE 19-25 | Selection of Small Animal Zoonoses

DISEASE/PATHOGEN	PORTAL OF EXIT	PORTAL OF ENTRY	PATIENT PRESENTATION	MANIFESTATION IN HUMANS	PREVENTION IN CLINICAL SETTING
Rabies	Saliva	Skin: through bite wound Skin: open wound or abrasion	See Table 19-23.	Fever Lethargy Central nervous system (CNS) signs, including paresis and seizures	Barrier protection when handling alive or deceased rabid patients Wash hands
Plague: *Yersinia pestis*	Respiratory secretions Pus from lymph nodes *Note:* Shared vector = Rodent fleas	Inhalation Mucous membranes Abraded skin	Cough Enlarged tonsils, mandibular and cervical lymph nodes, often draining pus	Fever Headache Swollen, draining lymph nodes	Barrier nurse patients Wash hands Disinfect surfaces
Cat-scratch fever: *Bartonella* spp.	Flea feces *Note:* Shared vector = Cat fleas	Skin: inoculation through cat scratch or bite	May be asymptomatic Direct correlation with clinical signs still under investigation Associated with gingivitis, uveitis, fever, lymphadenopathy	Lympadenopathy Fever Signs of infection at scratch site	Avoid being scratched by cat (good restraint, no rough play, wear protective gloves when handling fractious cats) Cat-associated wounds should be washed immediately with soap and water
Ringworm	Hairs	Skin	See Table 19-23.	Pruritic, raised, red, circular skin lesions	Barrier nurse patients Wash hands
Bacterial enteritis: *Campylobacter, Salmonella*	Feces	Oral	Diarrhea	Diarrhea Headache Joint and muscle aches	Barrier nurse all patients with diarrhea Wash hands Disinfect surfaces Follow personal safety protocol when performing fecal analysis Wash hands
Toxoplasmosis: *Toxoplasma gondii*	Aerosolized spores from dried (old) feces	Oral	Fever Diarrhea Uveitis Ascites	Fever Lethargy Lympadeonpathy Infection of fetus: CNS damage, abortion, stillbirth	Barrier nurse patients Follow personal safety protocol when performing fecal analysis Wash hands
Leptospirosis	Urine	Mucous membranes Abraded skin	See Table 19-22.	Fever Rash Meningitis Hemorrhage Liver disease Kidney disease	Barrier nurse patients Wash hands Disinfect surfaces Follow personal safety protocol when performing urinalysis

TABLE 19-26	Feline Cancers			
NAME	**LOCATION**	**PREDISPOSING FACTORS**	**METASTASES**	**TREATMENT**
Squamous cell carcinoma (SCC)	Skin: nasal planum, ear tips, eyelids Oral: sublingual	Sun exposure + Unpigmented skin Papillomavirus infection	Not common	Surgical excision Radiation Laser therapy
Mast cell tumor (MCT)	Skin	Breed: Siamese prone to malignant form of these tumors	Not common, but malignant MCTs can spread to spleen, liver, and lymph nodes	Surgical excision
Injection site sarcoma (ISS)	Skin Muscle	Use of adjuvanted vaccines + Abnormal local immune response	Lungs	Surgical excision
Lymphoma	Alimentary tract Mediastinum Liver Spleen	Breed: Siamese and oriental breeds (mediastinal form) Viral infection: feline leukemia virus (FeLV), feline immunodeficiency virus (FIV) Chronic inflammation (alimentary form)	Regional lymph nodes Neighboring abdominal organs	Chemotherapy
Mammary gland adenocarcinoma	Mammary glands	Breeds: Siamese, domestic shorthair Intact females Females spayed later than 1 year of age	Lymph nodes Lungs Liver	Surgical excision Chemotherapy

TABLE 19-27	Canine Cancers			
NAME	**LOCATION**	**PREDISPOSING FACTORS**	**METASTASES**	**TREATMENT**
Mast cell tumor (MCT)	Skin, subcutis	Breeds: Boxer, Boston Terrier, Beagle, Labrador Retriever, Schnauzer Sites of chronic inflammation or injury	Regional lymph nodes Spleen Liver	Surgical excision Chemotherapy Radiation
Multicentric lymphoma	Lymph nodes Liver Spleen Bone marrow	Breeds: Golden Retriever, Cocker Spaniel, Rottweiler, Boxer, English Bulldog	Lung CNS	Chemotherapy
Osteosarcoma	Appendicular or axial skeleton	Breeds: large and giant breed dogs, Greyhound (racing)	Lung	Surgical amputation Limb-sparing procedure Chemotherapy
Hemangiosarcoma (HSA)	Vascular endothelium • Spleen • Heart • Subcutis	Gender: male Breeds: Golden Retriever, German Shepherd dog	Lung	Surgical excision Chemotherapy
Perianal adenoma	Sebaceous glands of the perineum	Gender: intact male (hormonally driven) Breeds: Cocker Spaniel, Beagle, Bulldog, Samoyed	None	Castration Surgical excision

> **TECHNICIAN NOTE**   Benign tumors do not invade or destroy surrounding normal tissues or spread to a new site. However, they can still impair tissue function, causing significant problems through their physical presence.

In addition to being classified as benign or malignant, tumors are categorized according to their tissue of origin and their histologic features (Table 19-28). Carcinomas, for example, arise from epithelial tissues, including skin, mucous membranes, glandular structures, and organs, such as the liver or kidneys. Carcinomas generally spread through both the lymphatic system and the bloodstream, so regional lymph node and lung metastases are commonly seen. Sarcomas, on the other hand, arise from mesenchymal tissues, such as cartilage, connective tissue, or bone. These tumors spread through the bloodstream and less frequently through lymphatics. Because of this, pulmonary metastases are relatively more common with sarcomas, and local lymph node involvement is rarer. The prefix of a tumor's name indicates the specific tissue of origin. For example, an osteosarcoma is a sarcoma originating from bone. The suffix of the name generally indicates whether the tumor is benign or malignant, with "-oma" designating a benign tumor (e.g., fibroma) and "-sarcoma" or "-carcinoma" designating a malignant tumor (e.g., fibrosarcoma). Exceptions to this rule include lymphoma, melanoma, and insulinoma, all of which are malignant tumors. More than 100 histologic types of cancer are known; each requires individualized treatment and carries a different prognosis. It is important to realize that the incidence and behavior of cancer in dogs are often quite different from its incidence and behavior in cats, even though tumor names and histologic types may be the same.

Other methods used to classify tumors and help predict behavior and prognosis include tumor grade and stage. Tumors of the same histologic type are graded by the histopathologist according to defined microscopic features, for example, the cells in a low-grade soft tissue sarcoma have close to normal cellular architecture (well differentiated) and few mitotic figures (slow cell division) and exhibit minimal invasion of surrounding normal tissue. In contrast, the cells in a high-grade soft tissue sarcoma have abnormal cellular architecture (undifferentiated) and numerous mitotic figures (rapid cell division) and exhibit aggressive invasion of surrounding normal structures. Well-established and reliable grading systems have been used for some types of tumors, such as canine mast cell tumors and soft tissue sarcomas. Tumor staging is performed by the veterinarian according to physical characteristics of the tumor and results of diagnostic tests that assess the extent of malignant disease. The World Health Organization's tumor staging system, known as the TNM system, categorizes tumors according to features of the tumor at the primary site (T), whether involvement of regional lymph nodes (N) is evident, and whether the

TABLE 19-28	Classification of Tumors in Animals	
TISSUE TYPE	**BENIGN**	**MALIGNANT**
Connective Tissue		
Bone	Osteoma	Osteosarcoma
Cartilage	Chondroma	Chondrosarcoma
Fibrous tissue	Fibroma	Fibrosarcoma
Fat	Lipoma	Liposarcoma
Smooth muscle	Leiomyoma	Leiomyosarcoma
Skeletal muscle	Rhabdomyoma	Rhabdomyosarcoma
Blood vessels	Hemangioma	Hemangiosarcoma
Hemolymphatic Tissue		
		Lymphoma
		Multiple myeloma
Epithelial Tissue		
Skin	Papilloma	Squamous cell carcinoma
Sebaceous gland	Adenoma	Adenocarcinoma/carcinoma
Sweat gland	Adenoma	Adenocarcinoma/carcinoma
Ceruminous gland	Adenoma	Adenocarcinoma/carcinoma
Mammary gland	Adenoma	Adenocarcinoma/carcinoma
Nasal mucosa	Adenoma	Adenocarcinoma/carcinoma
Gastrointestinal mucosa	Adenoma	Adenocarcinoma/carcinoma
Biliary tract	Adenoma	Adenocarcinoma/carcinoma
Urinary tract	Adenoma	Adenocarcinoma/carcinoma

Modified from Ehrhart EJ, Powers BE: The pathology of neoplasia. In Withrow SJ, Vail DM, editors: Withrow and MacEwen's small animal clinical oncology, ed 4, St Louis, 2007, Saunders.

tumor has metastasized to distant sites (M). Defined subclassifications, represented by numbers following T, N, and M (e.g., $T_3N_1M_0$), describe the size and extent of the tumor at each of these locations.

Clinical Manifestations of Cancer

Tumor growth can cause clinical signs in several ways. As in the earlier example of the meningioma, the physical presence of a tumor can disrupt normal bodily functions. Certain types of tumors, such as those of the central nervous system (CNS), bone, eyes, and GI and urinary tracts, are particularly painful. Highly vascular or ulcerated tumors can contribute to significant blood loss. Ulcerated tumors can lead to secondary local infection. Tumors of endocrine glands cause abnormal hormone secretion and subsequent disruption in body function. Cancer **cachexia** is a syndrome characterized by weight loss and muscle wasting. It is caused by the physical presence of the tumor (e.g., oral or gastric neoplasm preventing intake or digestion of food) and/or by the secondary problems of nausea, anorexia, and vomiting that accompany the cancer or its therapy. Paraneoplastic syndrome is caused by hormones or other substances synthesized by the tumor, which circulate systemically and affect multiple organ systems or tissues (Box 19-5). The disease of cancer, as a whole, can suppress the immune system, leaving the patient susceptible to infectious diseases (see "Risk of Infection" section, Table 19-5).

Nursing care of the cancer patient requires symptomatic management of all clinical signs.

Pain must be recognized and treated. Treatment includes pharmacologic intervention, complementary medicine modalities, and husbandry and environmental changes to ensure patient comfort. Nutritional support for cancer patients is a priority and focuses on providing proper hydration, meeting caloric needs and other nutrient requirements (proteins, vitamins, fatty acids), and ensuring intake of the diet. Control of nausea and vomiting is achieved with antiemetics. Preventive measures are taken to limit the risk of secondary infection. Signs of paraneoplastic syndrome are managed accordingly.

Diagnosis and Treatment of Cancer

Because cancer can affect almost any cell in the body, diagnosing and staging of cancer employs a wide variety of diagnostic tools, which are summarized in Box 19-6. Once a definitive diagnosis has been made, available therapeutic options can be identified. The clinician, the technician, and the client should discuss together the various choices with respect to the goal of treatment (palliative vs. curative), prognosis, benefits, potential complications, and cost. When speaking to the client, it is important to use simple terms that are easily understood. Information handouts are helpful to explain commonly performed procedures, such as amputation and mastectomy, as well as the care and monitoring of incisions and bandages. Handouts can also be used to explain the nature, method of action, and expected side effects of common chemotherapy drugs and radiotherapy.

BOX 19-5 | **Examples of Paraneoplastic Syndromes and Associated Tumors**

Cancer cachexia
- Multiple tumor types

Hypoglycemia
- Hepatocellular carcinoma
- Insulinoma
- Leiomyosarcoma

Hypercalcemia
- Lymphoma
- Apocrine gland adenocarcinoma of the anal sac
- Parathyroid tumor
- Multiple myeloma

Polycythemia
- Renal carcinoma

Disseminated intravascular coagulation
- Hemangiosarcoma
- Mast cell tumor
- Lymphoma
- Thyroid carcinoma

Anemia
- Multiple tumors

Hyperproteinemia
- Multiple myeloma
- Lymphoma

Fever
- Multiple tumors

BOX 19-6 | **Methods of Diagnosing Cancer**

Diagnostic imaging
- Plain and contrast radiography
- Ultrasound
- Magnetic resonance imaging (MRI) and computed tomography (CT) scans
- Nuclear medicine scans

Cytologic examination
- Fine-needle aspirates
- Thoracocentesis, abdominocentesis fluid
- Bone marrow aspirates
- Skin scrapings
- Tissue swabs
- Blood smears
- Urine sediment

Histopathologic examination of tissue samples obtained by:
- Punch biopsy
- Needle core biopsy
- Incisional biopsy
- Excisional biopsy

Molecular tests of fluids and tissues
- Polymerase chain reaction (PCR)
- Western blots
- Immunohistochemistry

Three primary treatment options are available for dogs and cats with cancer: surgery, chemotherapy, and radiotherapy. A single modality is recommended for some animals, whereas multimodality protocols combining more than one type of treatment are preferred for others.

Surgery

Surgery is the treatment of choice for localized cancer in dogs and cats: it is practical and cost effective and will be curative in many cases. Successful surgical resection of malignant cancer requires an aggressive approach. The tumor must be removed completely with a minimum of cosmetic and functional loss for the animal. A concerted attempt is made during resection to avoid incising the tumor and contaminating the surgical field with neoplastic cells: cells released in this manner may implant in the wound, resulting in local recurrence. Instead, surgical resection should be performed in the normal tissues surrounding the mass, so that a generous margin of normal tissue is removed together with the tumor. The primary limitations of surgery include its potential for damage to surrounding normal structures and its inability to address systemic spread of tumor. Animals whose tumors have metastasized generally undergo surgery as a diagnostic or palliative procedure only. Aggressive and complex resection and reconstruction surgeries should not be performed if long-term disease control is not possible; in such instances, surgery should be combined with other modalities (adjuvant therapy), if it is done at all. The oncologic surgeon must be familiar with all potential therapy options if he or she is to provide the best care for an individual animal.

Another type of surgery used to treat cancer is cryosurgery. A cold source (usually liquid nitrogen) is used to freeze superficial cancers that are smaller than 2 cm in diameter. After freezing, the treated tissue dies and sloughs away, leaving a wound that later heals. Permanent discoloration or loss of hair may be associated with this process. Cryosurgery is useful for small, superficial lesions, such as eyelid, skin, and anal masses. A disadvantage of cryosurgery is that the completeness of tumor removal cannot be determined because no tissue can be submitted for margin evaluation. Cryosurgery should not be used to treat large, invasive masses, or in cases in which a definitive histologic diagnosis has not yet been made.

Radiotherapy

Ionizing radiation can be used to treat cancer. Radiation causes cell death by disrupting the DNA of the cell or by destroying important molecules required for normal cell function. Death occurs when the cell is so injured that it can no longer repair itself or divide. Radiotherapy is most appropriately prescribed for the treatment of localized cancers and will not address systemic disease. It can be used alone or in combination with surgery or chemotherapy. Most radiotherapy protocols involve the administration of multiple small doses (fractions) on a Monday, Wednesday, and Friday or a Monday through Friday schedule, usually for 15 to 21 fractions. Because radiation targets DNA, it is most effective against tumor cells with rapid rates of proliferation. Similarly, adverse effects of radiotherapy are seen in normal tissues within the irradiated field that have a high rate of cell turnover, such as the gastrointestinal tract, the bone marrow, the epidermis, and hair follicles.

Potential adverse effects of radiation are divided into late-phase and acute effects. Late-phase effects of radiotherapy develop months to years after treatment and usually involve permanent changes, such as necrosis or fibrosis of normal tissues. Acute effects are usually seen during the latter stages of a course of radiotherapy and, although they may require additional nursing care, are temporary. The most common acute effects of radiation occur because rapidly dividing normal cells in tissues, such as the skin and mucosal linings of the intestinal tract, have growth characteristics that are similar to those of cancer cells and thus are extremely sensitive to radiation. This means that damage to acutely responding normal tissue in the radiation field actually mimics damage to neoplastic tissue. For this reason, acute toxicities of radiotherapy should never be permitted to limit the dose delivered: if radiotherapy is temporarily discontinued to provide time for repair of acutely injured normal tissue, tumor tissue will be allowed to repair.

A frequent acute adverse effect of irradiation of oral or nasal tumors is mucositis of the oral cavity. Flushing the animal's oral cavity with prescription veterinary mouthwashes can decrease the discomfort associated with this condition. Irradiation of skin may also induce a desquamative dermatitis or loss of superficial layers of the epidermis. With regular cleaning and use of analgesics as needed, these conditions generally resolve within 2 to 3 weeks. Oil-based or occlusive topical creams should be avoided, and self-trauma, such as licking, must be prevented. Elizabethan collars are especially useful because they prevent self-trauma while still allowing access to the radiation field for topical treatments. Hair loss or change in color within the radiation field may be permanent, and the owner should be made aware of this possibility before radiotherapy is begun.

> **TECHNICIAN NOTE** Surgery and radiotherapy are preferred treatment modalities for local cancers; chemotherapy is the preferred treatment for systemic cancers. Depending on the cancer, a single modality may be best, whereas for others, a multimodal approach is ideal.

Chemotherapy

Chemotherapy is the treatment of cancer with chemical agents. Chemotherapeutic agents are cytotoxic and cause tumor cell death by injuring the DNA or protective cellular membrane of the cancer cell. Chemotherapy provides a means of delivering antitumor therapy to the whole body and therefore is most appropriate for animals that have systemic, as opposed to local, neoplastic disease. Indications for chemotherapy include (1) primary treatment for known chemotherapy-sensitive tumors, to "shrink" the tumor before surgery for more effective resection, to prevent local tumor recurrence after surgical resection, and to sensitize neoplastic tissue before radiotherapy; and (2) palliative (vs. curative) treatment, to provide temporary relief from clinical signs caused by cancer and to maintain the animal's quality of life for as long as possible. Chemotherapy drugs can be given orally, intramuscularly, and intravascularly. Many chemotherapy protocols are used in veterinary medicine; most involve multiple agents that are given on rotating schedules, for example, every other day or weekly or every 3 weeks.

Administration and Safe Handling of Chemotherapeutics

Chemotherapeutic agents have the potential to be teratogens (they may cause defects in a developing fetus), mutagens (they may cause injury to chromosomes), and carcinogens. No safe level of occupational exposure has been identified; therefore, every effort must be put forth to reduce accidental exposure when handling chemotherapeutic agents. The veterinary community must recognize, promote, and institute policies and procedures that facilitate the safe mixing, handling, and administration of these drugs. Procedure 19-1 summarizes protocols for safe handling and administration of chemotherapy drugs.

Some chemotherapeutic drugs are administered orally and are given by the owner at home. Owners need to be thoroughly informed regarding handling these drugs and must be instructed to wear examination gloves during their administration.

> **TECHNICIAN NOTE** There is no safe level of occupational exposure to chemotherapy drugs. Safe handling and administration protocols must be followed to limit exposure and protect the staff.

Complications of Chemotherapy

Nursing considerations for the chemotherapy patient are summarized in Box 19-7. Chemotherapy drugs can cause immediate reactions upon administration and can cause toxic reactions during the days and weeks after administration. Table 19-29 lists potential side effects of select chemotherapy drugs. The veterinary technician must be aware of and monitor for these complications.

Local Tissue Necrosis

Some intravascular (IV) chemotherapy agents are potent vesicants and irritants, which, if accidentally given perivascularly, can cause local tissue necrosis potentially severe enough to require limb amputation. It is important when administering IV chemotherapy drugs that the IV catheter is confidently and properly placed and secured. It is also important that the patient cannot disturb the catheter during infusion of the drug. If, despite all precautions, the chemotherapy agent is given perivascularly, do not remove the IV catheter. Irrigate the area with sterile saline both through the catheter and subcutaneously to dilute the drug.

PROCEDURE 19-1	Safe Handling and Administration of Chemotherapy Drugs

To minimize the risk of topical contamination
1. Wear approved chemotherapy administration gloves. Latex examination gloves are not impermeable to chemotherapeutic agents. If chemotherapy administration gloves are not available, double-glove with latex examination gloves.
2. Wear a nonabsorbent chemotherapy administration gown, or, at minimum, wear a buttoned-up laboratory coat.
3. Do not push air bubbles out of the syringe.
4. Use of commercially available chemotherapy dispensing systems (e.g., PhaSeal) can decrease the risk of exposure.
5. Use safety goggles or other protective eyewear.

To avoid the oral route of contamination
1. Never eat or drink in the chemotherapy administration room.
2. Never smoke or apply makeup in the chemotherapy administration room.
3. Never store chemotherapeutic drugs with food or other drugs.
4. Caution clients (and veterinary staff) always to wear gloves when administering chemotherapeutic drugs by the oral route.

Chemotherapy Waste Disposal
1. Separate chemotherapy waste from other sharps and biohazards, including needles, syringes, catheters, gloves, and masks.
2. Contact a local human hospital for aid in disposal of all chemotherapy-associated waste.

Precautions for Patient Care and Cleanup (Although the amount of active drug eliminated from the patient may be minimal, it is prudent to take precautions.)
1. Chemotherapeutic drugs are excreted in feces and urine: wear chemotherapy gloves when cleaning up after patients for 48 hours after drug administration.
2. No guidelines have been established for the disposal of pet waste; however, caution clients about cleaning up after their pets. If the patient urinates or defecates inside the home within 48 hours of receiving chemotherapy, owners should wear gloves to clean up the waste and should double-bag all waste.

From Withrow SJ, Vail DM: Withrow and MacEwen's small animal clinical oncology, ed 5, St Louis, 2013, Saunders.

Subcutaneous administration of dexamethasone in the area is often recommended. Apply cold compresses to the area for the next 72 hours. Close monitoring for redness, swelling, pain, and skin sloughing is instituted. The veterinarian may need to intervene and débride the necrotic tissue.

Hypersensitivity Reactions

Administration of chemotherapy drugs may elicit an allergic reaction. Hypersensitivity reactions are more common in

---

BOX 19-7 Nursing Considerations for Administration of Chemotherapy Drugs

Concerns Before Drug Administration

Admitting
1. Patient status
   a. History since last chemotherapy
   b. Physical examination
2. Appropriate diagnostics submitted
   a. Blood work
   b. Radiographs

Treatment Plan
1. Verification
   a. Drug and dosage
   b. Blood work
2. Appropriate catheterization
   a. Necessary equipment assembled
   b. Vein selection
   c. Aseptic technique
   d. Completely clean stick
   e. Intravenous challenge with nonheparinized saline bolus before and after drug administration
3. Appropriate protective equipment for person mixing and administering drugs
4. Appropriate protective equipment for person restraining animal

5. Knowledge of drug toxicities
6. Emergency protocols established
   a. Treatment for extravasation
   b. Treatment for anaphylaxis
   c. Treatment for chemical spill
7. Client informed of potential toxicities

Concerns During Drug Administration
1. Extravasation of drug
2. Anaphylactic reaction
3. Patient comfort

Concerns After Drug Administration
1. Hematologic toxicity
2. Nonhematologic toxicity
3. Appropriate medications prescribed
   a. Chemotherapy drugs
   b. Antibiotics
   c. Other medications (e.g., antiemetics)
4. Treatment documentation
   a. Patient medical record
   b. Future treatment plan
   c. Client information handouts

TABLE 19-29 Toxicities and Reactions Associated With Chemotherapy Drugs

AGENT	VESICANT OR IRRITANT	HYPERSENSITIVITY	BONE MARROW TOXICITY	GI TOXICITY	ALOPECIA, DELAYED HAIR GROWTH
5-Fluorouracil	+	None	++	+	+
Actinomycin	++	None	++	++	None
Chlorambucil	Not applicable (oral drug)	None	+	+	None
Cisplatin	+	None	++	+++	None
Cyclophosphamide	None	None	++	++	+
Doxorubicin	+++	++	+++	++	+
L-Asparaginase	None	++	+	None	None
Vincristine	++	None	+	+	None

+, Mild; ++, moderate; +++, severe.

---

dogs than in cats. The degree of reaction ranges from a local allergic response to anaphylaxis. Close monitoring of the patient during drug infusion for pruritus, which often manifests as head shaking from itchy ears, as well as for restlessness, urticaria, skin erythema, vomiting, and diarrhea, is critical. In rare cases, hypovolemic shock may ensue. Treatment for a hypersensitivity reaction requires immediate discontinuation of the chemotherapy infusion and administration of antihistamines and glucocorticoids. If severe, epinephrine and fluids are also given. Patients that have a history of an allergic reaction to a chemotherapy drug are often pretreated with antihistamines and glucocorticoids 30 minutes before chemotherapy administration to prevent anaphylaxis. Dilution and slow administration of IV

chemotherapy drugs will minimize the risk of a repeat hypersensitivity reaction.

Toxicities

Chemotherapy targets cells undergoing rapid proliferation, such as neoplastic cells. However, chemotherapeutic agents cannot differentiate between cancer cells and normal cells that have high proliferation rates, such as cells of the bone marrow, the gastrointestinal tract, and hair follicles. Damage to these cells accounts for some of the toxicities seen with chemotherapy.

Bone marrow suppression, or myelosuppression, usually is noted 5 to 7 days post administration. Although any blood cell line can be affected, neutropenia is the most clinically relevant. Periodic complete blood counts are necessary to monitor for this toxicity. If myelosuppression is evident, administration of the next round of chemotherapy is typically delayed, and the patient is closely monitored for signs of secondary sepsis (see "Risk of Infection" section, Table 19-5). If fever ensues, the patient is started on prophylactic antibiotics, and diagnostics are performed to find the location of the infection and treat it appropriately.

Gastrointestinal toxicity manifests as anorexia, nausea, and vomiting. In rare cases, hemorrhagic diarrhea may be seen. Management of gastrointestinal symptoms generally involves administration of antacids, antiemetics, and appetite stimulants (see Table 19-11). For patients with significant anorexia, feeding tubes are placed.

Alopecia and delayed hair growth, although certainly not life-threatening effects, can be very disconcerting to owners; clients should be counseled ahead of time about this particular chemotoxicity.

> **TECHNICIAN NOTE** Chemotherapeutic drugs cannot differentiate between cancer cells and normal cells that have high proliferation rates, such as cells of the bone marrow and gastrointestinal tract, and hair follicles. Damage to these cells accounts for some of the toxicities seen with chemotherapy.

After each treatment, the animal is monitored for signs of chemotoxicity. Clients should be given detailed handouts describing known toxicities for each chemotherapeutic agent and associated clinical signs. If the client detects any abnormalities, the animal should be reevaluated. If chemotherapeutic agents are administered properly and the client is carefully educated regarding potential risks, toxicity can be minimized, and the animal should maintain an excellent quality of life during therapy.

CASE PRESENTATION 19-2 THE NURSING PROCESS IN ACTION

Signalment: Dempsey, 14-year-old, male castrated black and white DSH

Chief Complaint: Dempsey is urinating a lot.

Pertinent History: Upon further questioning, it is revealed that Dempsey is drinking more, and that the litter box is "flooded" with urine. His appetite has been slightly less than normal over the past few weeks. The owner characterizes it as "finicky" and has been offering different foods in an attempt to get him to eat enough.

STEP ONE: Gather data.

Subjective Appearance: Patient is bright, alert, and reactive.

Physical Examination:

Body weight: 9 pounds 2 ounces (previous weight 6 months ago was 10 pounds 1 ounce); Body condition score: 2.5/5; Temperature: 100.2° F; Heart rate: 186 bpm, sinus rhythm; Pulses are synchronous and strong; Respiration: 32 bpm, lungs clear; Mucous membranes: pink and tacky; CRT: <2 seconds; Skin turgor: delayed; Skin and hair coat: normal; Ears, eyes, and nose: normal; GI system: normal; Urogenitary system: kidneys are small, smooth, and rounded; Musculoskeletal system: muscle wasting noted over epaxials; Systolic blood pressure: 150 mm Hg.

Abnormal Laboratory Values:

- Elevated creatinine: 3.5 mg/dl
- Elevated blood urea nitrogen: 62 mg/dl
- Decreased potassium: 3.5 mEq/L
- Increased phosphorus: 8.1 mEq/L
- Increased albumin: 4.6 g/dl
- Increased total protein: 9.6 g/dl
- Increased packed cell volume (PCV): 49%
- Decreased urine specific gravity: 1.020
- 3+ protein on urine dipstick and elevated urine protein : creatinine ratio

STEP TWO: Identify and prioritize technician evaluations.

Summary of Problems:

- Polyuria and polydipsia
- Diminished appetite over a period of weeks
- Weight loss
- Body condition score 2.5/5
- Tacky mucous membranes
- Delayed skin turgor
- Small kidneys
- Muscle wasting
- Azotemia
- Hypokalemia
- Hyperphosphatemia
- Dilute urine
- Proteinuria
- Increased total protein and albumin
- Increased packed cell volume

Critical Thinking: Group problems together to arrive at technician evaluations:

Tacky mucous membranes + Delayed skin turgor + Increased packed cell volume + Increased total protein and albumin = DEHYDRATION

Weight loss + Body condition score 2.5/5 + Muscle wasting = UNDERWEIGHT

Diminished appetite over a period of weeks = ANOREXIA

Hypokalemia + Hyperphosphatemia = ELECTROLYTE IMBALANCE

At the same time, the doctor is arriving at a medical diagnosis:

Stage 3 chronic kidney disease: Small kidneys + Azotemia + Dilute urine + Proteinuria

- Which is causing anorexia, electrolyte imbalance, weight loss, dehydration, and polyuria/polydipsia

Continued

Prioritize technician evaluations:
1. Dehydration
2. Electrolyte imbalance
3. Anorexia (although important, the anorexia Dempsey is experiencing is secondary to dehydration and electrolyte imbalance, so correcting these will help resolve the anorexia)
4. Underweight
5. Client knowledge deficit

STEP THREE: Develop a nursing care plan.

1. Dehydration
   A. Desired outcome: restoration of hydration as evidenced by moist mucous membranes, normal skin turgor, normal serum protein levels, and normal PCV at recheck examination.
      i. Plan: Administer 100 ml subcutaneous fluids (SQF) of Normasol per doctor orders.
2. Electrolyte imbalance
   A. Desired outcome: normal electrolyte concentrations at recheck examination.
      i. Dispense oral potassium supplement per doctor's orders.
      ii. Dispense oral phosphate binder per doctor's orders.
3. Anorexia
   A. Desired outcome: sustained return of normal appetite and intake of appropriate quantity of daily calories within 3 days as evidenced by owner's report on patient's appetite.
      i. Dispense oral appetite stimulant per doctor's orders.
      ii. Also see under "Client knowledge deficit."
4. Underweight
   A. Desired outcome: Total weight gain of 1 pound. Goal of 5 to 8 ounces by next examination.
      i. Calculate daily caloric needs and quantity in cups/cans of his new diet that the owner should feed Dempsey (see later).
5. Client knowledge deficit
   A. Explain CKD
      i. Answer all of owners' questions regarding the disease.
      ii. Counsel owners on progressive nature of this disease.
      iii. Impress upon owners the importance of compliance with treatments.
      iv. Give owners a list of signs to watch for that would indicate an emergency.
      v. Explain link between CKD and polyuria and polydipsia and that this will persist. Recommend extra litter boxes to prevent episodes of inappropriate urination.
   B. Instruct owners how to assemble SQF bag, line, and needle, and how to administer prescribed amount of SQF once a week.
      i. Provide link to clinic's website, where a video of this is posted for owners to refer to if they need a reminder.
   C. Instruct owners on proper needle disposal.
   D. Instruct owners on oral administration of medications.
   E. Explain any side effects of medications.
   F. Provide owners with samples of prescription kidney diets.
   i. Explain the importance of feeding a kidney diet.
   ii. Explain that Dempsey must eat, and remind owners to contact you if Dempsey does not eat the new food in the next 2 days.
   G. Explain what Dempsey's caloric requirements are, how much food he should be fed, and that owners should ensure that he is eating.
      i. Provide owners with measuring cup.
      ii. Encourage owners to weigh Dempsey at home once a week on a baby scale.
   H. Schedule Dempsey for a follow-up visit per the doctor's recommendation.
   I. Provide owners with written summary of plan.

STEP FOUR: Re-evaluate patient and assess patient's response to interventions.

1. Call owner in 3 days' time for an update:
   The owner is glad you called because Dempsey has not eaten very much at all, not even the meat baby food that you suggested on your list. As you question the owner, you discover that Dempsey seems interested in the food but starts lip-smacking and rapidly swallowing, then walks away after smelling it. You consult with the veterinarian regarding your concern that Dempsey is nauseous, and that it is contributing to his anorexia. The veterinarian agrees with your new technician evaluation (nausea) and prescribes an antacid and a drug that is both an antiemetic and an appetite stimulant. You fill the prescription and call the owner to come pick it up, and you discuss how to administer the new medicines.
2. Call the owner 4 days later (1 week from diagnosis):
   The owner reports that Dempsey is doing much better. He is eating the prescription diet well and tolerated his first SQF dose at home. The owner is very confident that Dempsey is receiving all of his medications. The owner weighed Dempsey yesterday, and his weight was 9 pounds 4 ounces. You remind the owner of the scheduled follow-up visit where Dempsey will be reexamined and will have laboratory work performed to evaluate his response to treatment.
   The desired outcome for anorexia has been met.
3. One month follow-up visit from date of diagnosis (summarized):
   Owner reports that Dempsey's appetite is back to normal, and that he seems friskier than before. He is taking all his meds.
   Physical examination was normal with the exception of small, smooth, rounded kidneys (not expected to change) and persistent mild muscle wasting over the epaxials. Body weight was 9 pounds 8 ounces.
   Abnormal Laboratory Values*:
   Elevated creatinine: 2.9 mg/dl
   Elevated blood urea nitrogen: 46 mg/dl
   Urine specific gravity: 1.020
   2+ proteinuria
   Desired outcomes for dehydration, electrolyte imbalance, and anorexia have been met.
   The short-term goal for underweight has been met.

---

*Resolution of these abnormal values is not expected with chronic kidney disease. The goal is to maintain levels as close to normal for as long as possible.

RECOMMENDED READINGS

Brooks HB: General pathology for veterinary nurses, Oxford, 2010, Wiley-Blackwell.

Cheville NF: Introduction to veterinary pathology, ed 3, Ames, IA, 2006, Blackwell.

The Merck veterinary manual, ed 10, White House Station, NJ, 2010, Merck & Co.

Merrill L: Small animal internal medicine for veterinary technicians and nurses, Ames, IA, 2012, Wiley-Blackwell.

Moore F: Principles of barrier nursing in the veterinary hospital, Vet Nurse 2:258, 2011.

Nelson RW, Couto CG: Small animal internal medicine, ed 4, St Louis, 2009, Mosby.

Norsworthy GD, Grace SF, Crystal MA et al: The feline patient, ed 4, Ames, IA, 2011, Wiley-Blackwell.

Orpet H: The nursing process. In Orpet H, Welsh P, editors: Handbook of veterinary nursing, ed 2, Oxford, 2011, Wiley-Blackwell.

Rockett J, Lattanzio C, Anderson K: Patient assessment, intervention and documentation for the veterinary technician: a guide to developing care plan and SOAPs, Clifton Park, NY, 2009, Delmar Publishing.

Withrow SJ, Vail DM: Withrow and MacEwen's small animal clinical oncology, ed 4, St Louis, 2007, Saunders.

WEBSITES

Feline Interstitial Cystitis and Environmental Modification: The Ohio State University College of Veterinary Medicine: The Indoor Pet Initiative: http://indoorpet.osu.edu/.

Infectious Diseases

The European Advisory Board on Cat Diseases (ABCD): http://www.abcd-vets.org

Center for Disease Control, Healthy Pet, Healthy People: http://www.cdc.gov/healthypets/index.htm

Kidney Disease

International Renal Interest Society (IRIS): http://www.iris-kidney.com/

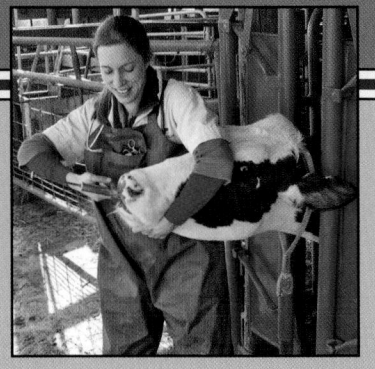

Amy I. Bentz, Laura H. Javsicas, Jonathan R.O. Garber,
and Matthew L. Stock

OUTLINE

**The Importance of Physical
   Examination,** 722

EQUINE MEDICINE, 722
**Common Diseases and Conditions of
   Horses,** 722
Respiratory Disease, 722
Cardiovascular Disease, 727
Hemolymphatic Disease, 727
Gastrointestinal Disease, 728
Liver Disease, 732
Neurologic Disease, 732
Urinary Tract Disease, 735
Dermatologic Disease, 736
Ophthalmologic Disease, 737
**Care of the Hospitalized Equine
   Patient,** 737
Patient Monitoring, 737
Therapeutics, 744
Laboratory Studies, 744

FOOD ANIMAL MEDICINE, 747
**Common Diseases and Conditions of
   Ruminants,** 747
Care of the Neonate and Neonatal
   Diseases, 747
Digestive System, 750
Respiratory System, 756

Reproductive System/Mammary Gland, 758
Metabolic Disorders, 761
Hemolymphatic System, 762
Cardiovascular System, 763
Nervous System, 764
Ophthalmologic Disease, 767
Musculoskeletal System, 768
Diseases of the Skin, 770
Urinary System, 770
**Common Diseases and Conditions
   of Swine,** 771
Care of the Neonate, 771
Multisystemic Diseases, 772
Gastrointestinal System, 773
Respiratory System, 773
Reproductive System, 773
Nervous System, 777
Musculoskeletal System, 777
Behavior, 777
Potbellied Pigs, 778
**Common Diseases and Conditions of
   Camelids,** 779
Care of the Neonate and Neonatal
   Diseases, 780
Conditions of the Digestive System, 782
Metabolic Conditions, 782
Nervous System, 784
Health Maintenance, 785

LEARNING OBJECTIVES

When you have completed this chapter, you will be able to:

1. Pronounce, define, and spell all Key Terms in the chapter.
2. Explain the importance of a thorough physical examination and medical record for large
   animal patients.
3. List and describe the most common diseases and conditions of the horse for each body
   system, including the causes and pathogenesis of each: respiratory, cardiovascular,
   hemolymphatic, gastrointestinal, neurologic, urinary tract, dermatologic, and
   ophthalmologic.
4. Explain how to care for a hospitalized equine patient.

*The authors and publisher wish to acknowledge the contribution of Marjorie S. Gill, whose original
work served as the foundation for the food animal portion of this chapter.*

5. List and describe the most common diseases and conditions of ruminants for each body system, including special care and conditions of the neonate: digestive, respiratory, reproductive/mammary gland, metabolic, hemolymphatic, cardiovascular, nervous, ophthalmologic, musculoskeletal, dermatologic, and urinary.
6. Do the following regarding common diseases and conditions of swine:
   - Discuss common diseases and conditions of swine, including neonatal care, multisystemic diseases, gastrointestinal disease, and diseases of the respiratory, nervous, and musculoskeletal systems.
   - Discuss normal and abnormal behaviors of swine.
   - Discuss the special care and concerns of potbellied pigs.
7. Do the following regarding common diseases and conditions of camelids:
   - Discuss common diseases and conditions of camelids, including special care and conditions of the neonate.
   - List and describe the most common diseases of camelids for each of the following body systems: digestive, metabolic, and nervous.
   - List preventive health measures in the management of camelids.

INTRODUCTION

As in small animal practices, veterinary technicians employed in equine and food animal practices carry out a four-step practice model while caring for hospitalized patients. A database is gathered first on the large animal patient, including a thorough physical examination. Using independent, critical thinking, the veterinary technician develops a list of pertinent technician evaluations and prioritizes them on the basis of physiologic and psychological needs of the patient. Subsequently, technician interventions are developed and carried out. At regular time intervals, the veterinary technician reevaluates the patient and assesses the efficacy of the nursing care plan. As the status of the patient changes, the veterinary technician keeps the attending veterinarian informed and makes adjustments to the nursing care plan. In this way, the technician practice model helps to ensure that each and every large animal patient is given consistently excellent nursing care.

Working with horses and food animals requires a solid knowledge of herd and prey species behavior and safe methods for restraining and handling them. These topics are covered in detail in Chapter 5, "Animal Behavior" and in Chapter 6, "Restraint and Handling of Animals," respectively. Herbivorous farm animals, for example, instinctively react to danger by running away. A quiet, calm voice and slow movement are essential for reassuring large animal patients. However, animals are unpredictable, and large animals because of their size can be particularly dangerous. Therefore, it is important to be practical and alert when nursing large animals to avoid being kicked, bitten, or pushed. Dress appropriately, and be sure to wear protective leather boots so that feet are properly protected from injury under the weight of a large and heavy hoof.

This chapter provides an overview of medical conditions commonly encountered in equine and food animal species.

THE IMPORTANCE OF PHYSICAL EXAMINATION

A thorough physical examination is an integral part of the diagnostic assessment and monitoring of large animals. Because veterinary technicians play an important role in the day-to-day monitoring of hospitalized patients, learning to perform a thorough physical examination is vital. Refer to Chapter 7 for a detailed description of how to complete a physical examination on large animal species. Review the normal parameters for a horse (Box 20-1). It is crucial to record all observations and findings of the physical examination in the medical record. The medical record provides the only record of the patient's progress or deterioration and is a legal document. Refer to examples of medical records in Chapter 3.

Equine Medicine

COMMON DISEASES AND CONDITIONS OF HORSES

Infectious diseases are discussed under the specific body systems that they affect. Refer to Tables 8-5 and 8-6 in Chapter 8, "Preventive Health Programs," for a summary of diseases against which commercial vaccines are available in horses. Immunization guidelines established by the American Association of Equine Practitioners and detailed descriptions of ways to administer all types of vaccines are included in Chapter 8.

RESPIRATORY DISEASE

Horses with respiratory disease may have increased respiratory rate (tachypnea) and effort (dyspnea), nasal discharge, and cough, as well as decreased performance, fever, and lymphadenopathy. Horses with problems in the upper respiratory tract, larynx, pharynx, guttural pouches, nasal passages, and sinuses may have unilateral or bilateral nasal discharge or decreased airflow from one or both nostrils, and may make a noise when breathing (stridor or stertor). However, abnormalities in the upper respiratory tract typically are not heard during auscultation, even during rebreathing examinations. Horses with problems in the lower respiratory tract (lungs and trachea) may have bilateral nasal discharge, but abnormal lung sounds are often audible during rebreathing examination. Abnormal sounds may include crackles, wheezes, decreased airflow, and prolonged

BOX 20-1	Normal TPR Parameters for an Adult Horse at Rest

Temperature (T): 99°F to 101.5°F
Pulse (P): 28 to 44 beats/minute (bpm)
Respiration (R): 6 to 16 breaths/minute (bpm)

recovery from the rebreathing examination. Table 20-1 summarizes diseases of the respiratory tract.

Diagnostic tests that can be used to assess the upper airway include endoscopy, radiography, and computed tomography (CT) or magnetic resonance imaging (MRI). Diagnostic tests performed to assess the lower airway include bronchoscopy, bronchoalveolar lavage (BAL), transtracheal wash (TTW), ultrasonography, radiology, and pulmonary function testing. Refer to Chapter 18, "Diagnostic Sampling and Treatment Techniques," for more information on performing some of these techniques. Hematology can help to determine whether a disease is due to an infectious cause. Figure 20-1 illustrates the flow of events during the diagnostic workup of a horse with lower respiratory tract disease.

Strangles

Strangles is a common, highly contagious respiratory disease of horses caused by the bacterial pathogen *Streptococcus equi equi*. Strangles typically produces swelling and abscesses of the submandibular and retropharyngeal lymph nodes. Affected horses have fever, depression, poor appetite, and painful swellings under the mandible. The abscesses under the mandible enlarge, rupture, and drain purulent exudate. The retropharyngeal lymph nodes may rupture into the guttural pouches, resulting in guttural pouch empyema and purulent nasal discharge. Diagnosis of strangles is based on culture of the bacteria from nasal secretions, a nasopharyngeal wash, or guttural pouch wash. Horses may develop abscesses within the thorax, abdomen, and central nervous system (CNS). The development of an abscess in abnormal locations is termed *bastard strangles*. These cases are particularly difficult to treat successfully. Diagnosis of bastard strangles is based on measuring serum antibody levels via an SeM protein titer. Horses with complicated cases of strangles and those with abscesses that have already ruptured should be treated with antibiotics. *S. equi equi* is typically sensitive to penicillin. Horses with strangles should be maintained under a strict isolation protocol. Recovered horses remain contagious and represent a threat to susceptible horses for approximately 6 weeks after recovery from clinical disease. Horses may become asymptomatic carriers of strangles, posing a great risk to other horses, as the result of **persistent infection (PI)** of the guttural pouches. Detection of carriers is based on polymerase chain reaction (PCR) testing of a guttural pouch wash and guttural pouch endoscopy.

Immunization against *S. equi* does not completely prevent infection in horses but minimizes clinical signs. The modified live-virus intranasal vaccine induces mucosal immunity, providing better protection and fewer side effects, compared with the killed intramuscular vaccine. However, it is not approved for use in pregnant mares and young foals.

Guttural Pouch Diseases

The guttural pouches are two large symmetric dilatations of the eustachian tube that are present in all Equidae. They are located just above the pharynx and larynx and can be accessed during an endoscopic examination through small

TABLE 20-1	Common Equine Respiratory Diseases			
DISEASE/ETIOLOGIC AGENT	**PATHOGENESIS**	**CLINICAL SIGNS**	**DIAGNOSIS**	**TREATMENT**
Infectious				
*Equine influenza	• Contagious viral respiratory disease • Transmitted via aerosolization of virus during coughing • Incubation period: 2 to 3 days • Duration of illness: 3 to 4 days • Damage to clearance mechanisms of the lung predisposes to bacterial pneumonia	• Fever • Cough • Depression • Nasal discharge	• Not typically performed • Polymerase chain reaction (PCR) • Serology • Virus isolation	• No specific antiviral therapy • Nonsteroidal anti-inflammatories • Rest for at least 3 weeks • Isolate horses
*Equine herpes virus-1 (EHV-1, rhinopneumonitis), and *equine herpes virus-4 (EHV-4)	• EHV-1 and EHV-4 are contagious viruses that cause respiratory disease • EHV-1 also causes abortion and neonatal and neurologic disease (discussed elsewhere) • Transmitted via respiratory secretions and fomite transmission • Incubation period: 2 to 10 days • Duration of illness: 4 to 5 days	• Fever • Cough • Depression • Nasal discharge • Typically more mild signs than influenza	• Not typically performed • PCR • Serology • Virus isolation	• No specific antiviral therapy for respiratory cases • Nonsteroidal anti-inflammatories • Rest for at least 3 weeks • Isolate horses
*Equine viral arteritis	• Contagious virus causing respiratory disease, limb swelling, conjunctivitis, and abortion in horses • Stallions infected after puberty develop persistent infection in the accessory sex glands and transmit the viral infection to mares during breeding	• Often asymptomatic • Fever • Anorexia • Serous nasal discharge • Coughing • Limb edema • Abortion	• Serology	• No specific antiviral therapy for respiratory cases • Nonsteroidal anti-inflammatories • Isolate horses
*Strangles (*Streptococcus equi* subsp. *equi*)	• Contagious bacterial disease • Transmitted in nasal secretions • Causes swelling and abscesses of the submandibular and retropharyngeal lymph nodes • Recovered horses remain contagious for 6 weeks after recovery from clinical disease • Asymptomatic carriers harbor the bacteria in their guttural pouches	• Fever • Depression • Anorexia • Painful swellings under the mandible • Purulent nasal discharge • Guttural pouch empyema • Airway obstruction due to swollen lymph nodes	• Culture or PCR of guttural pouch or nasopharyngeal wash	• Supportive care (anti-inflammatories, fluids) until abscesses have ruptured • Penicillin following rupture of abscesses • Tracheostomy if severe airway obstruction

Continued

TABLE 20-1	Common Equine Respiratory Diseases—cont'd			
DISEASE/ETIOLOGIC AGENT	**PATHOGENESIS**	**CLINICAL SIGNS**	**DIAGNOSIS**	**TREATMENT**
Bacterial pneumonia	• Colonization of the lungs by opportunistic bacteria due to compromise of natural defense mechanisms • Risk factors: long-term transportation, dysphagia, aspiration following esophageal obstruction (choke)	• Exercise intolerance • Fever • Tachypnea • Cough • Mucopurulent nasal discharge • Anorexia • Chest pain	• Hematology: increased white blood cell count and fibrinogen • Transtracheal wash (TTW) cytology and culture • Thoracic radiographs • Thoracic ultrasound	• Broad-spectrum antibiotics based on culture and sensitivity of TTW samples • Nonsteroidal anti-inflammatories • Anti-endotoxin therapies
Inflammatory				
Heaves/recurrent airway obstruction (RAO)	• Allergic airway disease of older horses • Airway inflammation, bronchoconstriction, and excessive mucus production occur in response to allergen exposure	• Cough • Nasal discharge • Flared nostrils • Tachypnea • Dyspnea • Wheezing	• Hematology: normal • Bronchoalveolar lavage (BAL) or TTW cytology • Thoracic radiographs	• Environmental management • Systemic or inhaled corticosteroids • Systemic or inhaled bronchodilators
Inflammatory airway disease (IAD; small airway inflammatory disease)	• Hyperreactive response to allergens, pollutants, and infectious agents, resulting in airway inflammation, bronchoconstriction, and mucus production	• Normal at rest • Exercise intolerance • Poor performance • Chronic cough, especially during exercise • Excess secretions in the airways after exercise	• Hematology: normal • BAL or TTW cytology • Thoracic radiographs • Pulmonary function testing	• Environmental management • Systemic or inhaled corticosteroids • Systemic or inhaled bronchodilators
Exercise-induced pulmonary hemorrhage	• Unknown. May be due to rupture of capillary vessels during strenuous exercise • May be aggravated by inflammatory airway disease or upper airway obstruction	• Observation of blood in airways via endoscopy • Epistaxis • Poor performance	• Endoscopy 30 to 90 minutes after exercise • BAL or TTW cytology • Thoracic radiographs	• Furosemide • Treatment of inflammatory airway disease if present

*Vaccine is available.

openings in the dorsal lateral nasopharynx. The internal and external carotid arteries and several cranial nerves travel superficially under the surface of the guttural pouch lining and are vulnerable to damage from pathologic conditions. The purpose of the guttural pouches may be to lower the temperature of blood to the brain (internal and external carotid arteries) during exercise. Bacterial infection of the guttural pouch is termed *guttural pouch empyema* and is often associated with strangles. Fungal infection of the guttural pouch is termed *guttural pouch mycosis*, and the causative agent is often *Aspergillus* spp.

A bacterial infection of the guttural pouch (empyema) usually is a sequela to strangles or retropharyngeal lymph node abscesses. Clinical signs include swelling in the throat-latch region and bilateral mucopurulent nasal discharge. Horses with guttural pouch empyema can be treated conservatively with antimicrobials and guttural pouch lavage; this may be effective in many horses that are treated early in the course of the disease. However, in more chronic cases, the mucopurulent material becomes inspissated and forms gelatinous concretions (chondroids) that lie on the floor of the guttural pouches. Resolution of empyema requires removal of the chondroids using endoscope-guided instruments or surgical removal.

During guttural pouch mycosis, a fungal plaque usually forms over the internal carotid artery, adjacent to nerves that control swallowing. Horses may have life-threatening blood loss from rupture of the internal carotid artery or dysphagia

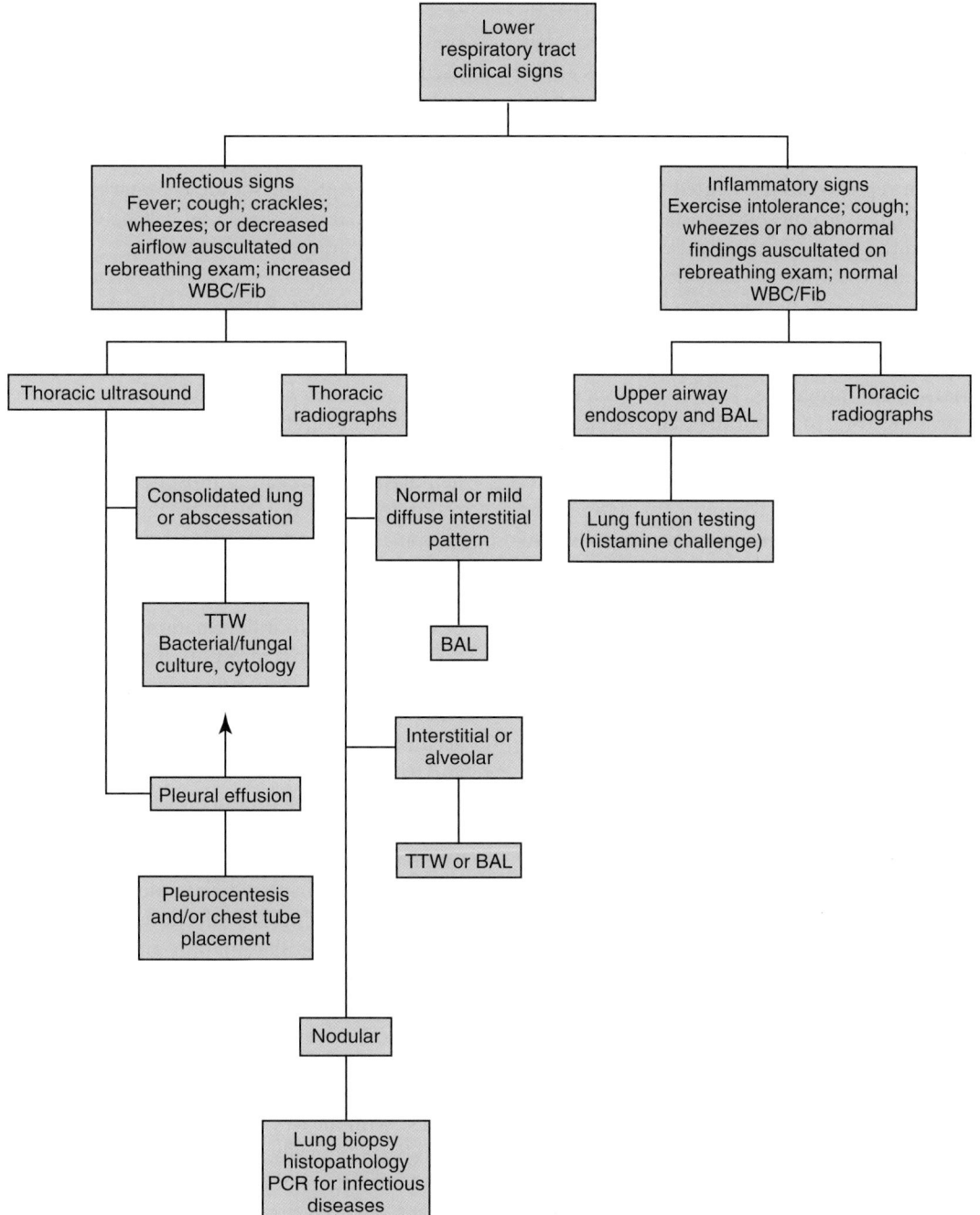

FIGURE 20-1 Sample flow chart for diagnostic assessment of horses with lower airway disease. *BAL,* Bronchoalveolar lavage; *Fib,* fibrinogen; *TTW,* transtracheal wash; *WBC,* white blood cell count.

from damage to the nerves. The most effective treatment is surgical occlusion of the internal carotid artery, which deprives the fungus of nutrients and prevents fatal hemorrhage.

The accumulation of air in guttural pouches (guttural pouch tympany) occurs in foals and weanlings and is usually associated with an abnormality of the opening to the pouches. It can occur unilaterally or bilaterally and is characterized by a fluctuant, nonpainful swelling in the throat-latch region. Surgical treatment is available.

Herpes

Equine herpesvirus (the causative agent of rhinopneumonitis) is a contagious virus that produces respiratory disease, abortion, and neonatal and neurologic disease (ascending paralysis) in horses. It is a reportable disease in some states. Clinical signs of respiratory disease caused by equine herpesvirus are milder but hardly distinguishable from equine influenza. The incubation period is longer (2 to 10 days), and horses may remain ill for 4 to 5 days. Equine herpesvirus is transmitted through the herd by aerosol transmission, respiratory secretions, and fomite transmission. Abortion secondary to equine herpesvirus occurs in the 7th to 11th month of gestation, and the mare does not appear sick at the time of abortion. Vaccination is recommended for performance horses and broodmares. Neurologic disease caused by equine herpesvirus is not common; however, a few large outbreaks have been reported in the United States over the past few years with high morbidity and mortality. Horses are often febrile early in the course of the disease, and the fever may have resolved by the time of examination. Affected horses demonstrate signs of incoordination, inability to urinate, and poor tail tone. Recumbency due to weakness and incoordination in the hindlimbs can occur in severe cases and carries a poor prognosis. Recovery in surviving horses can be prolonged (2 to 3 months), and horses may not return to completely normal neurologic function. Use of standard quarantine protocols (e.g., quarantine all new horses for 30 days) and of individual equipment with proper disinfecting techniques is important in minimizing disease transmission.

Protection against respiratory disease following equine herpesvirus vaccination is inconsistent and relatively short-lived. None of the currently available vaccines claims to provide protection against the neurologic form of herpesvirus in horses, although studies suggest that certain vaccines may decrease nasal shedding and the severity of disease. Sedentary adult horses not exposed to other horses may not be vaccinated or may be vaccinated only once or twice per year, whereas young horses and horses engaged in performance activities should be vaccinated every 3 to 4 months. Inactivated univalent vaccines should be administered to broodmares during the 3rd, 5th, 7th, and 9th months of pregnancy to prevent abortion. Although 100% protection against abortion is not achieved, the incidence of abortion caused by equine herpesvirus is significantly decreased by adherence to a proper vaccination program.

Heaves

Heaves or recurrent airway obstruction (RAO) is an allergic airway disease caused by airway inflammation, narrowing of small airways (bronchoconstriction), and excessive production of mucus. Heaves typically affects horses 15 years of age and older. Clinical signs of heaves include cough, nasal discharge, flared nostrils, increased respiratory rate, increased expiratory effort, and wheezing. The severity of clinical signs may range from exercise intolerance and an increased respiratory rate at rest to severe respiratory distress (dyspnea) at rest. Clinical signs often fluctuate seasonally. Most affected horses are allergic to dust and molds present in hay and straw. Horses cannot be "cured" of heaves but can often be controlled with appropriate management practices. Environmental management to remove offending allergens is the most important intervention. This consists of maintaining horses at pasture, soaking hay or eliminating hay from the diet, using low-dust bedding and grain, and removing horses from the barn when stalls are being cleaned. Medical therapy of horses with heaves may be necessary in moderately to severely affected horses. Corticosteroids to reduce inflammation and bronchodilator therapy to relax small airways are used. They may be administered systemically (IV, IM, PO) or by inhalation using a special mask (e.g., Aeromask, Trudell Medical International, London, Ontario, Canada; AeroHippus, Trudell Medical International; Equine Haler, Equine Healthcare ApS, Hørsholm, Denmark). Many horses require only seasonal treatment and can be weaned off of medications when antigen levels are low.

Inflammatory Airway Disease

Inflammatory airway disease (IAD) is a common cause of poor performance in horses of all ages, although young horses may be predisposed. The exact cause of IAD is unknown. Possible predisposing factors include deep inhalation of particulate matter, exercise-induced pulmonary hemorrhage (EIPH), atmospheric pollutants, and prior respiratory infection with bacteria or viruses. The airways mount a rapid and aggressive defense against inhaled foreign particular matter called *inflammation*. Some horses appear to develop a more profound inflammatory response than others. Although inflammation is an important defense mechanism against infection, it may cause more harm than good when the response is excessive. Pathologic changes observed in the small airways of affected horses consist of accumulations of various inflammatory cells surrounding and within the airways. This inflammatory response not only results in excessive production of mucus, but also is responsible for the bronchoconstriction observed in the disease. The narrow, inflamed airways of affected horses are "hyperreactive," meaning that their tendency to constrict in response to allergens, pollutants, infectious agents, and inert particles is exaggerated. Inflammation and constriction of bronchi impair gas exchange within the lungs, thereby limiting athletic performance.

Clinical signs of IAD include exercise intolerance or poor performance, chronic cough especially during exercise, and excessive secretions in the airways after exercise. Unlike in horses with heaves, the respiratory rate at rest and lung sounds are typically normal. IAD can be distinguished from infectious causes of cough such as bronchitis or pneumonia by lack of fever, normal complete blood count (CBC), and lack of severe abnormalities on thoracic radiography or ultrasonography. Cytologic examination of a bronchoalveolar lavage or transtracheal wash is important, to characterize the type of inflammation and rule out infectious causes. Endoscopy typically reveals increased mucus in the trachea. Pulmonary function testing is a sensitive test to detect airway hyperreactivity.

Treatment of IAD consists of environmental management to decrease exposure to dust and allergens and inhaled or systemic corticosteroids and bronchodilators.

Bacterial Pneumonia and Pleuropneumonia

Bacterial pneumonia occurs as the result of aspiration of bacteria that normally inhabit the oral cavity and upper respiratory tract. Horses of all ages can be affected, although young horses are predisposed. Colonization of the lungs by opportunistic bacteria occurs when natural defense mechanisms are compromised or overwhelmed by large numbers of bacteria. Long-term transportation is a risk factor for the development of bacterial pneumonia because clearance of debris and bacteria from the trachea is decreased when horses are trailered. Dysphagia and aspiration of feed material following esophageal obstruction (choke) can result in bacterial pneumonia. When bacterial infection spreads from lung tissue to the pleural space, called *pleuropneumonia*, pleural effusion can occur.

Clinical signs of pneumonia include exercise intolerance, fever, tachypnea, cough, bilateral mucopurulent nasal discharge, inappetence, and chest pain (pleurodynia). Rebreathing examination may reveal crackles and/or wheezes over affected areas and a tracheal rattle if large quantities of secretions are present in the trachea. If pleural effusion is present, lung sounds may be markedly decreased ventrally. Most horses with bronchopneumonia cough when the rebreathing bag is applied, whereas normal horses do not.

Diagnosis of bacterial pneumonia is based on physical examination, blood work abnormalities, diagnostic imaging (ultrasound and thoracic radiographs), and culture and cytologic examination of transtracheal wash fluid. Initial treatment consists of broad-spectrum antibiotics until culture and sensitivity results are available to direct therapy and anti-inflammatory agents. In horses with pleural effusion, pleural drainage may help remove exudates and debris and may facilitate reexpansion of the lungs. Drainage of pleural fluid can be accomplished with intermittent thoracocentesis or indwelling chest tubes. See Chapter 25, "Emergency and Critical Care Nursing," for information on performing thoracocentesis.

CARDIOVASCULAR DISEASE

Horses with cardiac disease are often asymptomatic, and examination of the cardiac system may be prompted by auscultation of a heart murmur or arrhythmia. When clinical signs do occur, they may include exercise intolerance, tachycardia, weakness, syncope (fainting), and respiratory crackles on auscultation. Diagnostic assessment may include electrocardiogram (ECG), echocardiogram, and measurement of blood levels of cardiac enzymes (troponin I).

Second-Degree Atrioventricular Block

Second-degree atrioventricular (AV) block is a common arrhythmia in horses, particularly fit, athletic horses. The arrhythmia occurs as the result of altered conduction through the AV node in the heart, resulting in contracture of the atria without the ventricles. This can occur because of high vagal tone, electrolyte imbalances, and the effects of medications such as alpha$_2$-agonists (xylazine, detomidine). When the horse is auscultated, a regularly irregular rhythm is heard, often described as "dropped beats." This arrhythmia usually is not clinically significant, and a few minutes of exercise, which stimulates the heart rate to increase, results in return to normal sinus rhythm. If the arrhythmia does not

go away, and the heart rate does not increase with exercise, it is considered significant, and further diagnostics are warranted.

Atrial Fibrillation

Atrial fibrillation is the most common clinically relevant arrhythmia in horses. Horses are predisposed because of the large size of their atria and their high vagal tone. Clinical signs include exercise intolerance or poor performance. Auscultation of horses with atrial fibrillation reveals an irregularly irregular rhythm. Although most horses with atrial fibrillation do not have underlying heart disease, if heart disease is present, the prognosis for treatment is poor. Therefore, a complete cardiac workup, including echocardiography, is warranted.

Horses without underlying cardiac disease can be converted to normal sinus rhythm with the use of quinidine or electrical conversion. Quinidine is administered via nasogastric tube until conversion occurs or signs of toxicity develop. Electrical conversion can be performed under general anesthesia by placing electrodes directly into the heart under ultrasound guidance.

HEMOLYMPHATIC DISEASE
Viral Arteritis

Equine viral arteritis is a contagious viral disease that produces limb swelling, conjunctivitis, abortion, and respiratory disease in horses. Limb swelling is painful and results from vasculitis (inflammation of blood vessels). Stallions infected after puberty develop persistent infection in the accessory sex glands (ampullae) and transmit the viral infection to mares during breeding. Abortion can occur at any point during gestation and results from viral damage to blood vessels of the placenta. The vaccine for equine viral arteritis is approved for use in stallions and nonpregnant mares under the supervision of the U.S. Department of Agriculture (USDA). Pregnant mares should not be vaccinated against equine viral arteritis. Vaccination induces seropositivity and may interfere with testing requirements for export. Therefore, a negative status should be confirmed before vaccination.

Equine Infectious Anemia

Equine infectious anemia (EIA) is a persistent viral disease of horses that causes anemia, fever, and weight loss; some horses are inapparent carriers that may appear healthy. The virus is transmitted from infected horses by large biting flies (tabanids). Once infected, horses become permanently infected and become carriers of the virus for the rest of their lives. Infected horses produce antibodies to the virus, so they will have a positive test result in the agar gel immunodiffusion test (AGID; Coggin's test) or the enzyme-linked immunosorbent assay (ELISA) for EIA virus. Horses must have a negative (Coggin's) test result for EIA within 6 to 12 months for the issuance of health certificates for interstate travel, international travel and show, and sale. A USDA-accredited veterinarian must draw blood for testing and provide a detailed description of the horse on specified forms. The health certificate for interstate travel cannot be issued until a negative test result is returned from a state or federally recognized laboratory. Horses not traveling or sold should still be tested on a yearly basis. If a positive test result is obtained, the entire herd is quarantined until all horses on the premises are tested (usually 60 days). Only the state veterinarian can release the quarantine. Because horses that have a positive test result for EIA are persistent carriers, they serve as a reservoir of the virus. Therefore, infected horses must be quarantined for life (at a distance greater than 200 yards from other horses) or euthanized.

Anaplasmosis

Anaplasmosis, also known as *equine granulocytic ehrlichiosis*, is caused by infection with the bacteria *Anaplasma phagocytophilum*, formerly called *Ehrlichia equi*. These bacteria are transmitted by biting ticks of the genus *Ixodes*. Clinical signs include fever, anemia, icterus, lethargy, stiffness, and limb edema. Diagnosis is based on observation of the organism within white blood cells on a peripheral blood smear, PCR, or serology. The treatment of choice is intravenous (IV) oxytetracycline for 5 to 7 days. A rapid response to treatment is expected.

Lyme Disease

Lyme disease is caused by infection with the bacteria *Borrelia burgdorferi*. Lyme is transmitted by biting ticks of the genus *Ixodes*. Lyme disease occurs only in areas where both ticks and reservoir mammalian hosts (typically small rodents) coexist. In North America, Lyme disease is predominantly seen along the Eastern Seaboard, in the upper Midwest, in Texas, and on the Pacific Coast (California). Most horses exposed to Lyme disease do not have clinical signs. The most common clinical signs attributed to Lyme disease include stiffness, mild to moderate lameness in multiple limbs, and behavioral changes (e.g., dullness). Other signs include chronic weight loss, skin hypersensitivity and resentment to being touched, uveitis, and joint swelling.

Diagnosis of Lyme disease is challenging because of the nonspecific clinical signs and the limitations of available tests. Therefore, it is important to always rule out other possible causes of the clinical signs. Diagnostic tests that identify antibodies against the bacteria include a Western Blot, ELISA, multiplex assay, and the C-6 ELISA SNAP test. Treatment should be considered in horses with positive test results and consistent clinical signs. Treatment with IV oxytetracycline or oral doxycycline for at least 1 month is typically required. No vaccine has been approved for use in horses, but the recombinant outer surface protein A (rOspA) canine vaccine is safe for use in horses. Tick prevention is recommended.

GASTROINTESTINAL DISEASE

The most common signs of gastrointestinal disease in the adult horse include colic, weight loss, anorexia, diarrhea, and fever. Diagnostic assessment of gastrointestinal disease may include hematology and serum chemistry, oral examination, rectal examination, abdominocentesis, ultrasonography, radiography, endoscopic examination of the stomach (gastroscopy), and fecal diagnostic testing.

Colic

Refer to the "Colic" section in Chapter 25, "Emergency and Critical Care Nursing," and the "Abdominal Surgery" section in Chapter 33, "Large Animal Surgical Nursing."

Gastric and Colonic Ulceration

Young horses are particularly prone to development of gastric ulceration. Stress, a high-grain diet, musculoskeletal pain, and administration of nonsteroidal anti-inflammatory drugs (NSAIDs) are common predisposing factors. Gastric ulcers are common in performance horses of all disciplines. Clinical signs of gastric ulceration include bruxism (grinding of teeth), hypersalivation, abdominal pain after eating, and anorexia. Foals with gastric ulceration often lie still in dorsal recumbency with their forelimbs over their head or extended out straight. Gastric ulcers are diagnosed via gastroscopy—examination of the stomach with a 3-meter endoscope. Antiulcer medications, such as histamine H_2 blockers, intestinal protectants, and proton pump inhibitors, can be used to treat gastric ulceration. The proton pump inhibitor omeprazole (GastroGard, Merial Limited, Duluth, Georgia) has been shown to be superior to other medications for the prevention and treatment of gastric ulceration in horses. Management practices that can help prevent and treat gastric ulcers include having hay or grass available at all times, feeding alfalfa hay, feeding grain as small frequent meals, and decreasing stress (increasing turnout, providing a companion).

Phenylbutazone (NSAID) toxicosis in horses can produce renal insufficiency and oral, gastric, and colonic ulceration in horses. Colonic ulcers occur in the right dorsal colon and are difficult to treat. Colonic ulcers secondary to phenylbutazone toxicity can produce abdominal pain, marked protein loss, melena (blood in manure), peritonitis, colonic stricture, or colonic rupture—a syndrome known as *right dorsal colitis* (Table 20-2). Dehydration and excessive dosages are the most important predisposing factors for the development of phenylbutazone toxicosis, although some horses are more sensitive to the effects and may develop the syndrome after administration of appropriate doses. Phenylbutazone should be given at the minimal effective dose, with no more than 4 gram per day administered to a horse of full size. Hydration status, protein levels, and renal values should be monitored in horses receiving prolonged treatment with NSAIDs.

Colitis

Colitis in horses can result in rapid, life-threatening fluid loss (hypovolemia), shock, **endotoxemia**, electrolyte loss, and acid-base imbalance as a result of diarrhea. Some horses may develop hypovolemic shock and electrolyte imbalance before the appearance of diarrhea. In addition to diarrhea, clinical signs of colitis include depression, inappetence, abdominal

TABLE 20-2	Common Causes of Acute Colitis in the Adult Horse			
DISEASE/ETIOLOGIC AGENT	**PATHOGENESIS**	**CLINICAL SIGNS**	**DIAGNOSIS**	**TREATMENT**
Infectious Salmonellosis/ *Salmonella* spp.	• Bacterial infection caused by exposure to contaminated environment, feed, water, or animals that are actively shedding the bacteria • Risk factors: stress; history of surgery, transportation, or change in feed; concurrent disease, particularly colic; treatment with antibiotics	• Diarrhea • Depression • Anorexia • Colic • Tachycardia • Injected mucous membranes • Prolonged capillary refill time (CRT)	• Fecal culture • Fecal polymerase chain reaction (PCR)	• Appropriate symptomatic treatment* • Isolate horses until five consecutive negative fecal samples are obtained
Clostridiosis/*Clostridium perfringens, Clostridium difficile* (clostridial diarrhea)	• Anaerobic bacteria that produce toxins, resulting in profound inflammation and secretion from the GI tract • Overgrowth of *C. difficile* is the most common cause of antibiotic-associated diarrhea	• Diarrhea • Depression • Anorexia • Colic • Tachycardia • Injected mucous membranes • Prolonged CRT	• Fecal PCR or enzyme-linked immunosorbent assay (ELISA) for toxins • Fecal culture	• Appropriate symptomatic treatment* • Metronidazole • Isolate horses
Potomac horse fever[†]/*Neorickettsia risticii* (equine monocytic ehrlichiosis)	• Bacterial infection caused by ingestion of infected freshwater insects	• Diarrhea • Depression • Anorexia • Colic • Tachycardia • Injected mucous membranes • Prolonged CRT • Laminitis	• Serology • Whole blood PCR • Response to oxytetracycline	• Appropriate symptomatic treatment* • Oxytetracycline
Larval cyathostomiasis/ Small *Strongyle* infection	• Reemergence of encysted larvae from large colon disrupts mucosal barrier, resulting in fluid and protein loss • Most common in horses younger than 6 years of age that have not developed immunity	• Diarrhea • Depression • Anorexia • Colic • Tachycardia • Injected mucous membranes • Prolonged CRT • Weight loss • Ventral edema	• Fecal flotation • Intestinal biopsy	• Appropriate symptomatic treatment* • Fenbendazole 10 mg/kg for 5 days or moxidectin
Toxic Right dorsal colitis	• Inhibition of normal mechanisms that help maintain the normal GI mucosal barrier, resulting in ulceration, particularly in the stomach and right dorsal colon • Kidney damage occurs because of decreased blood flow • Toxicity can occur within a few days if administered at excessive doses • Some horses are more sensitive and develop toxicity at recommended doses • Toxicity is exacerbated by dehydration	• Oral ulceration • Anorexia • Lethargy • Weight loss • Colic • Ventral edema	• History of treatment with nonsteroidal anti-inflammatory drugs (NSAIDs) • Hypoproteinemia • Abdominal ultrasound: thickening of the right dorsal colon • Gastroscopy: gastric ulcers • Urinalysis: abnormal urine specific gravity, hematuria suggestive of NSAID-induced kidney damage	• Appropriate symptomatic treatment* • Colloid therapy—hypoproteinemia • Low bulk, easily digested diet • Antiulcer medications • Sucralfate—gastric and colonic ulceration • Misoprostol inhibits the effects of NSAIDs on the mucosa

Continued

TABLE 20-2	Common Causes of Acute Colitis in the Adult Horse—cont'd			
DISEASE/ETIOLOGIC AGENT	**PATHOGENESIS**	**CLINICAL SIGNS**	**DIAGNOSIS**	**TREATMENT**
Blister beetle toxicity/ Cantharidin	• Blister beetles contain cantharidin, a highly irritating compound • Ingestion of cantharidin causes direct irritation of the gastrointestinal tract and urinary tract as it is excreted through the kidneys • Exposure occurs through ingestion of alfalfa hay contaminated with blister beetles	• Diarrhea • Depression • Anorexia • Colic • Tachycardia • Injected mucous membranes • Prolonged CRT • Hematuria • Stranguria	• Hypocalcemia • Hypomagnesemia • Hyposthenuria • Detection of toxin in GI contents or urine	• Appropriate symptomatic treatment* • Mineral oil to evacuate GI tract • Activated charcoal to bind toxin • Calcium and magnesium supplementation
Antibiotic administration	• Alteration of normal GI flora allowing proliferation of pathogenic organisms such as *C. difficile, C. perfringens,* and *Salmonella* • Oral administration of TMS, erythromycin, metronidazole and parenteral administration of tetracycline and ceftiofur are most common causes	• Diarrhea • Depression • Anorexia • Colic • Tachycardia • Injected mucous membranes • Prolonged CRT	• History • Test for *C. difficile, C. perfringens,* and *Salmonella*	• Appropriate symptomatic treatment* • Stop antibiotic administration • Isolate horses

*Refer to Table 20-3 for treatment guidelines for all causes of colitis. Specific treatments are noted.
†Disease for which vaccines are available.

pain, tachycardia (increased heart rate), injected (brick red) mucous membranes, and prolonged capillary refill time. Agents that produce colitis in horses are listed in Table 20-2. The most common life-threatening causes of colitis include *Salmonella* spp., *Clostridium* spp., and *Neorickettsia risticii* (formerly *Ehrlichia risticii*). Horses with colitis should be considered contagious and maintained under an isolation protocol. The approach to treatment of horses with colitis is consistent regardless of the cause (Table 20-3). IV fluid therapy is crucial to support the cardiovascular system, replace fluid losses, and correct electrolyte and acid-base imbalance. Colloid therapy (plasma, hetastarch, dextran) may be necessary because of protein loss, which can lead to peripheral edema as blood leaks from blood vessels into surrounding tissue (Figure 20-2). Complications of colitis include laminitis (founder), cardiovascular collapse, cardiac arrhythmias, and thrombophlebitis.

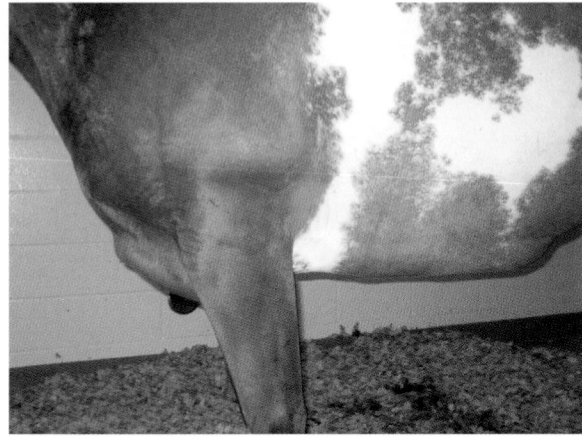

FIGURE 20-2 Ventral edema secondary to protein loss in horse with colitis.

Potomac Horse Fever

Potomac horse fever (PHF) is caused by *N. risticii* and produces diarrhea, fever, abortion, and laminitis. The life cycle of this organism is complicated. The bacteria infect a parasite, which lives in fresh water snails. The snails are ingested by fresh water insects, such as caddis flies and mayflies. Horses become infected when they accidentally ingest the fresh water insects, snails infected with the flukes, or feces from birds and bats that are infested with the fluke. Therefore, cases are most often seen near fresh water. Geographically, clinical disease is observed predominantly in states east of the Mississippi and in California. Diagnosis of PHF is based on serum testing for antibodies or PCR analysis of whole blood samples. *N. risticii* is very sensitive to treatment with oxytetracycline, and a favorable response to treatment is supportive of the diagnosis. Inactivated bacterin vaccines are commercially available. Although the vaccine is not effective at preventing infection, it may minimize clinical signs, and horses living in affected areas may be vaccinated. Vaccination should precede the months of peak disease incidence (June through October).

TABLE 20-3	Medical Management of Colitis in Adult Horses
TREATMENT OR THERAPY	**RATIONALE(S)/SPECIFIC TREATMENTS**
Crystalloid fluid therapy	1. Treat dehydration and hypovolemia caused by increased loss, diarrhea, and decreased intake. 2. Replace sodium, chloride, and potassium lost via the GI tract. • Addition of specific electrolytes to fluids may be required. 3. Correct acid-base abnormalities. • Addition of sodium bicarbonate to fluids may be required. *See Chapter 24 for discussion of fluid therapy.*
Colloid fluid therapy	1. Treat hypoproteinemia caused by protein leakage through inflamed intestine and catabolism due to negative energy balance. • Crystalloid fluids will decrease protein levels further; therefore, hypoproteinemia can limit the quantity of crystalloids that can be given. 2. Maintain oncotic pressure. 3. Plasma *See Chapter 24 for discussion of fluid therapy.*
Endotoxemia therapy	1. Cardiovascular resuscitation with intravenous crystalloid ± colloid fluids to prevent organ damage. • Laminitis prevention • Cryotherapy • Neutralize circulating endotoxin and inhibit endotoxin-induced inflammation (see below) 2. Neutralize circulating endotoxin. • Hyperimmune plasma and serum: may bind endotoxin, contains anticoagulants and anti-inflammatory proteins • Polymixin B: binds endotoxin; risk of kidney damage warrants monitoring urine output and kidney values 3. Inhibit endotoxin-induced inflammation. • NSAIDs: inhibit inflammation • Pentoxyfilline: inhibits inflammation; increases deformability of red blood cells • Heparin: may inhibit intravascular coagulation; low-molecular-weight heparin preferable because of fewer side effects • Dimethyl sulfoxide (DMSO): scavenges free radicals, little evidence of efficacy in horses
Antibiotics	1. Antibiotics are indicated for certain causes of colitis, such as Potomac horse fever (PHF) and clostridiosis (see Table 20-3). 2. Use of antibiotics in other cases is controversial and is typically reserved for cases with signs of septicemia, including profound and persistent neutropenia and persistent fevers.
Probiotic agents	1. Reestablishment of normal GI flora may discourage colonization of pathogenic bacteria.
Antisecretory agents	1. Bismuth subsalicylate: may decrease secretion of fluid from GI tract but the requirement of very large volumes in adult horses limits efficacy 2. Di-tri-octahedral smectite (Biosponge): adsorbs toxins, specifically clostridial toxins
Nutrition	1. Oral intake often is not sufficient to meet energy requirements because of anorexia, malabsorption of nutrients, and increased caloric demand due to sepsis and inflammation. 2. Horses should be encouraged to eat good-quality hay, fresh grass, and easily digestible grain. 3. Partial or total parenteral nutrition is warranted in horses that remain inappetent for longer than 3 days. *See Chapter 10 for discussion of nutrition.*

Choke

Choke indicates obstruction of the esophagus. Chronic dental disease and retained deciduous caps are common predisposing conditions for the development of choke. Horses in overcrowded environments may eat feed too quickly and choke. Removing the competition usually alleviates this behavior. The esophagus is usually obstructed by grain or hay. Many horses will continue to attempt to eat despite their inability to swallow. Clinical signs include anxiety, gagging, excessive salivation, and feed and saliva coming from the nostrils. The obstruction can be visualized via an endoscopic examination. In some instances, the obstruction can be relieved by sedation and time, although manipulation and hydropulsion using a nasogastric tube may be required. Horses must be heavily sedated to lower their head during manipulation of the nasogastric tube to prevent water and feed from entering the trachea. Aspiration pneumonia is a significant complication; therefore, preventive treatment with antibiotics is warranted, and horses should be closely monitored for signs of infection. Feed restriction and/or feeding as a mash is often required for a few days to allow the esophagus to heal and to prevent recurrence of the obstruction. An esophageal stricture is a less common complication and occurs in horses with circumferential damage to the esophageal mucosa. In cases with prolonged obstruction, esophageal rupture may occur.

> **TECHNICIAN NOTE**   *Choke* refers to obstruction of the esophagus, usually as a result of impacted food in the esophagus.

Gastrointestinal Neoplasia

Lymphosarcoma is the most common neoplasia in horses and most commonly affects the gastrointestinal tract. Infiltration of the intestine may result in chronic weight loss, diarrhea, and hypoalbuminemia. A presumptive diagnosis is supported by exclusion of other causes of weight loss, thickening of the intestinal wall on ultrasound, and palpation of enlarged mesenteric lymph nodes on rectal examination. Definitive diagnosis is made by biopsy of the intestine (via gastroscopy, rectal mucosal biopsy, laparoscopy, or laparotomy) or identification of neoplastic cells in abdominal fluid. The liver, spleen, and kidney may also be affected.

Squamous cell carcinoma is the most common neoplasia of the stomach. Horses often present with weight loss and anorexia. Diagnosis is made by gastroscopy. The prognosis for gastrointestinal neoplasia is grave, and treatment typically is not attempted.

LIVER DISEASE

Liver disease in horses can result from toxic, infectious, inflammatory, metabolic, obstructive, and neoplastic causes. Clinical signs of liver disease vary depending on the cause but may include weight loss, anorexia, jaundice, fever, colic, photosensitivity (e.g., sunburn seen in areas of nonpigmented skin), and neurologic symptoms (e.g., hepatic encephalopathy). Serum chemistry analysis is critical for diagnosis of liver disease or failure and for monitoring of response to treatment. Transabdominal ultrasound examination of the liver can be helpful in the diagnosis and allows for selection of a site for transabdominal liver biopsy. Liver biopsy is the best way to determine the cause of liver disease. Treatment of liver disease depends on the cause but may include anti-inflammatories, antibiotics, and nutritional management.

NEUROLOGIC DISEASE

Brain and Brainstem Disorders

The four most common disorders of the brain and brainstem in horses are rabies, equine viral encephalitis (alphaviruses: Eastern, Western, Venezuelan; flavivirus: West Nile), leukoencephalomalacia (moldy corn toxicity), and head trauma. Damage to the cerebrum (forebrain) may produce altered mentation, altered states of consciousness, head pressing, and seizures (Figure 20-3). Damage to the brainstem may damage the cranial nerves, which control the muscles of facial expression, facial sensation, mastication (chewing), swallowing, balance, vision, taste, and ocular position (Figure 20-4). Brainstem lesions also lead to incoordination of the limbs and altered breathing patterns.

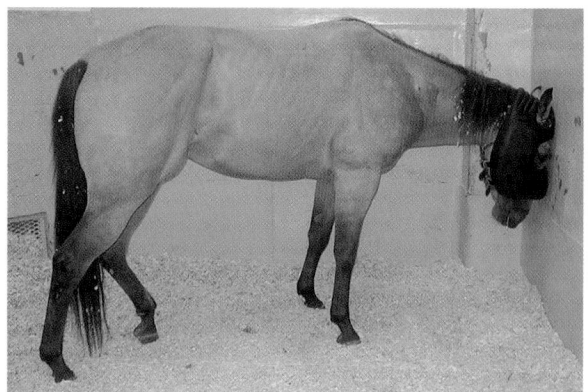

FIGURE 20-3 Horse head pressing as a sign of cerebral dysfunction.

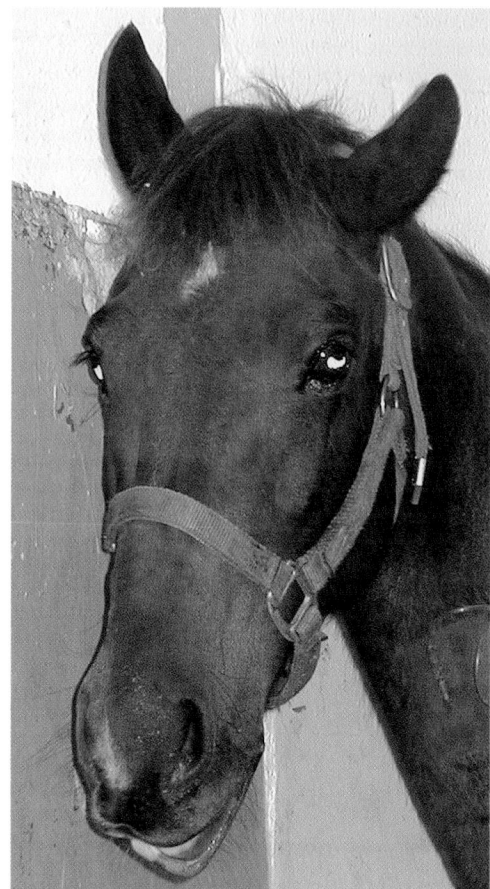

FIGURE 20-4 Horse with facial nerve paralysis (flaccid facial musculature, droopy ear and eyelid on the affected side) as a sign of brainstem dysfunction.

Diagnostic aids for the evaluation of horses with cerebral or brainstem dysfunction include cerebrospinal fluid (CSF) analysis, skull radiographs, and CT or MRI.

Rabies

Rabies is a zoonotic infection that is universally fatal. Horses usually acquire the infection by a bite wound from a wild animal. Skunks, foxes, raccoons, and bats are the most common reservoirs in North America. Clinical signs are highly variable but often begin as fever, hindlimb ataxia, and hyperesthesia (hyperresponsiveness to touch). Neurologic signs rapidly progress to involve the brain and brainstem. The duration of neurologic signs before death is relatively short, ranging from 3 to 10 days.

Horses should be vaccinated against rabies on an annual basis. Vaccinated horses that have been exposed to a rabid animal should be revaccinated promptly and observed for 90 days. Unvaccinated horses with known rabies exposure should be observed for 6 months and should not be vaccinated.

No accurate antemortem test for rabies is available; it is important to be cautious when handling horses with suspected rabies. The diagnosis of rabies is confirmed by fluorescent antibody stain of brain tissue. People handling potentially rabid horses should avoid contact with saliva; should wear gloves, protective eyewear, and disposable outerwear; should wash hands thoroughly; and should avoid contact with CSF. A list of individuals who have had contact with the potentially rabid horse must be kept, and these individuals must be informed of the result of the test (generally within 24 to 48 hours). A postexposure rabies vaccination should be administered to humans in contact with rabid animals. Individuals with occupational exposure to livestock and wildlife should undergo a prophylactic rabies vaccination series.

Viral Equine Encephalitis

Four main types of viral equine encephalitis are known: Eastern, Western, Venezuelan, and West Nile. The viral equine encephalitides produce rapidly progressive, highly fatal neurologic disease in horses. Mosquitoes transmit the infection to horses; therefore, disease incidence is seasonal in most geographic regions. Clinical signs of Eastern, Western, and Venezuelan encephalitis are practically indistinguishable and include profound depression, fever, ataxia, head pressing, dementia, and multiple cranial nerve abnormalities. Clinical signs of West Nile encephalitis include weakness, ataxia, muscle fasciculations, and cranial nerve deficits (such as droopy lip). Hyperesthesia (extreme sensitivity to touch) around the head and neck is a common clinical sign. The mortality rate is extremely high with Eastern equine encephalitis (75% to 100%), moderate with Venezuelan (40% to 80%), and lower with Western (30% to 50%) and West Nile (36% to 44%). Treatment consists of supportive care to provide hydration, nutrition, and a clean, dry environment. The prognosis is poor with Eastern equine encephalitis and guarded with Western, Venezuelan, and West Nile encephalitides. Diagnosis is confirmed by serologic testing (a high titer or a fourfold increase in antibodies to Eastern, Western, and Venezuelan viruses identified by complement fixation, neutralization, or hemagglutination inhibition assays, or a positive immunoglobulin [Ig]M capture ELISA for West Nile and Venezuelan). Fluorescent antibody or virus isolation in brain tissue is used to make a diagnosis from postmortem samples.

Vaccines for Eastern, Western, and West Nile equine encephalitis are highly efficacious, and clinical disease in vaccinated horses is rare. Horses in the United States should be vaccinated against Eastern and Western equine and West Nile encephalomyelitis viruses before the mosquito season in the spring. Horses living in southern states with a year-round mosquito season should be vaccinated 2 to 3 times per year. Broodmares should receive a booster of their vaccination in the 10th month of gestation (use only killed-virus vaccines in pregnant animals) to ensure adequate colostral antibody protection for the foal. Vaccination against Venezuelan equine encephalomyelitis is not routinely recommended because the disease has not been reported recently in the United States and does not currently pose a threat to the U.S. horse population, except those near the Mexican border.

Leukoencephalomalacia

Equine leukoencephalomalacia (moldy corn toxicity) is caused by ingestion of a fungal toxin produced by *Fusarium moniliforme*. This mold has a predilection for corn, and affected kernels are usually pink to brown. The fungal toxin causes liquefactive necrosis of the cerebral cortex. Clinical signs include profound depression, head pressing, altered states of consciousness, incoordination, and aimless wandering. Treatment consists of supportive care, and the prognosis for recovery is poor. Horses often die within 24 hours of manifesting neurologic signs.

Head Trauma

Horses most commonly acquire two types of skull fractures depending on the nature of the traumatic injury. Horses that suffer a frontal impact with a solid object develop depression fractures of the frontal and parietal bones. Common neurologic signs observed in horses with this type of fracture are due to cerebral damage and include depression, seizure, stupor, and aimless wandering. Horses that flip over backward develop fractures of the petrous temporal bone and of the junction of the basisphenoid and basioccipital bone. Neurologic signs associated with these fractures include abnormalities of balance, incoordination of limbs, nystagmus (rhythmic eye movement), abnormal respiratory patterns, and coma. Diagnosis is confirmed by radiographic examination of the skull. Treatment consists of supportive care and anti-inflammatory therapy (corticosteroids, dimethyl sulfoxide [DMSO]). Surgical decompression of frontal and parietal fractures may improve the neurologic status of some horses.

Temperohyoid Osteoarthropathy

Temperohyoid osteoarthropathy (THO) is a syndrome of adult horses that results from arthritis at the junction of the stylohyoid bone and temporal bones in the head, just below the inner ear. Some cases may be due to extension of infection from the middle ear. Clinical signs may be due to the arthritis itself or to fracture of bones surrounding the joint. Horses in early stages of the disease may have no clinical

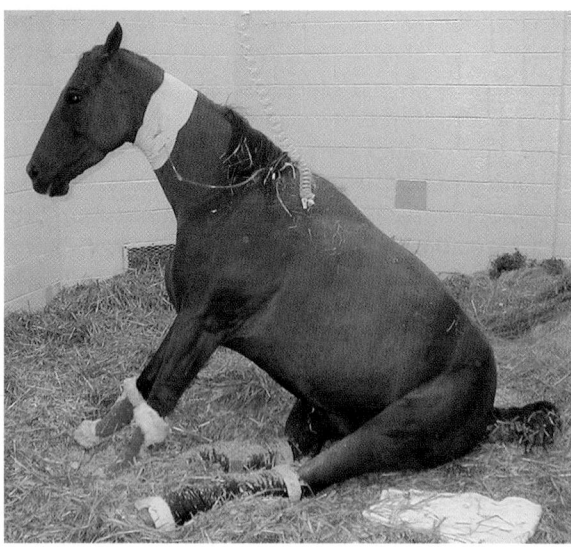

FIGURE 20-5 Horse in dog-sitting position as a result of a spinal cord dysfunction.

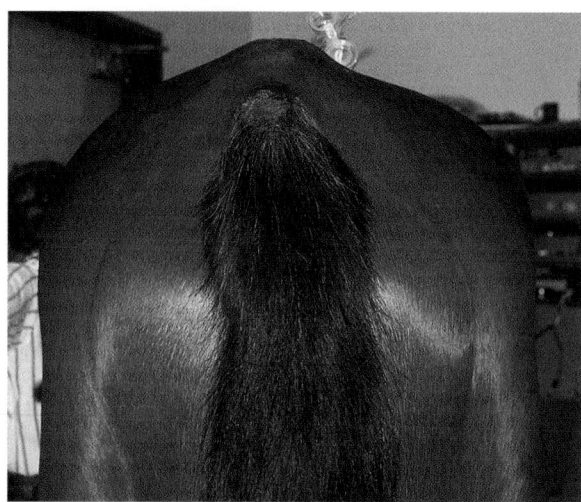

FIGURE 20-6 Asymmetric gluteal muscle atrophy in a horse with spinal cord dysfunction involving a lower motor neuron.

signs or may exhibit difficulty chewing, pain on palpation of the parotid region, and head shaking. Once the joint has fused as a result of the arthritis, sudden jerking of the head may fracture the petrous temporal bone, resulting in damage to the vestibular and facial nerves that lie near the joint. This results in sudden onset of head tilt, ataxia, nystagmus, facial paralysis, and difficulty swallowing. Certain events such as dental work, passing a nasogastric tube, or head trauma may precipitate fracture. Diagnosis is based on endoscopy of the guttural pouches and/or radiographs, allowing observation of the thickened stylohyoid bone. Treatment consists of anti-inflammatories and antibiotics. If cases are identified before significant nerve damage has occurred, surgery can be performed to remove a portion of the stylohyoid or ceratohyoid bone to decrease pressure at the joint and prevent fracture.

Spinal Cord Disorders

The five most common disorders of the spinal cord are cervical vertebral malformation caused by stenotic or dynamic compression of the spinal cord (wobbler syndrome), equine protozoal myelitis, equine herpesvirus myeloencephalopathy (rhinopneumonitis), equine degenerative myeloencephalopathy, and vertebral fracture. Damage to the spinal cord causes spinal ataxia (incoordination of the limbs without abnormalities of the brain and brainstem), which may progress to dog sitting and recumbency (Figure 20-5). Muscle atrophy from a lower motor neuron disorder can indicate a spinal cord disorder (Figure 20-6). Diagnostic aids to differentiate these diseases include neurologic examination, cervical radiographic examination, myelographic examination, and CSF analysis.

Wobbler Syndrome

Cervical vertebral malformation is a manifestation of developmental orthopedic disease characterized by compression of the cervical spinal cord by malformed or unstable cervical vertebrae. Males are affected 4 times more frequently than females, and Thoroughbreds appear to be predisposed. Clinical signs of symmetric incoordination usually begin between 6 months and 3 years of age. The hindlimbs usually are more severely affected than the forelimbs. The likelihood of disease is determined by evaluation of plain film cervical radiographs, and the diagnosis is confirmed by myelographic examination. Surgical stabilization improves the neurologic status of some patients.

Equine Protozoal Myelitis

Equine protozoal myelitis (EPM) is a common cause of neurologic disease in horses. Horses are dead-end, aberrant hosts of the protozoan parasites. *Sarcocystis neurona* is the most common protozoan parasite that causes spinal cord disease in horses; opossums are the primary hosts of this parasite, and horses are likely infected via fecal-oral transmission. Birds are secondary hosts and do not appear to be infectious for horses. Clinical signs of EPM are directly referable to the location of the organism in the CNS. Therefore, EPM should be considered in a horse demonstrating neurologic signs. Most horses with EPM (85%) demonstrate signs such as ataxia, weakness, and muscle atrophy as a result of spinal cord damage. Clinical signs are often asymmetric. Other signs such as cranial nerve deficits may occur. Diagnosis is confirmed by identification of antibodies to the organism in CSF. Treatment of EPM consists of administration of antiprotozoal drugs; the most common and effective treatment for EPM is ponazuril. Another treatment is a combination of two antibiotics that inhibit folic acid metabolism: sulfadiazine and pyrimethamine, with treatment given for an average of approximately 90 to 120 days.

Herpes

Equine herpesvirus can produce respiratory disease, abortion, and neonatal and neurologic disease in horses. The neurologic form is characterized by ascending paralysis, with hindlimbs more severely affected than forelimbs. Horses often demonstrate urinary incontinence, poor tail tone, and penile prolapse. Diagnosis is confirmed by PCR testing of whole blood for the neurologic form of the virus. Administration of the antiviral medication valacyclovir may improve recovery and decrease nasal shedding if administered early in the disease process. The prognosis for return to normal neurologic function is approximately 80%. Recently, a number of outbreaks have been reported in the United States with higher mortality than in the past. Cases are now considered reportable to the state veterinarian. Isolation of suspect and confirmed cases is essential to prevent spread of infection through the barn or hospital.

Equine Degenerative Myelopathy

Equine degenerative myelopathy results in symmetric spinal ataxia that is more severe in the hindlimbs than in the forelimbs. Clinical signs appear between 6 months and 2 years of age. The disease appears to be familial in some breeds. No definitive antemortem diagnostic test is available, and the diagnosis is usually made on the basis of neurologic examination, CSF analysis, cervical radiographs, and myelographic examination. Dietary supplementation with vitamin E may prevent progression of disease and may result in improvement in clinical signs in some instances. The prognosis for return to normal neurologic function is poor.

Vertebral Fracture

Cervical vertebrae, caudal thoracic vertebrae, and the thoracolumbar junction are the most common sites of vertebral fracture. A cervical vertebral fracture leads to tetraparesis (weakness in all four limbs), whereas fracture of thoracic and lumbar vertebrae produces paraparesis (weakness of hindlimbs) or paraplegia (paralysis of hindlimbs). Diagnosis is confirmed by radiography. If the fracture is nondisplaced, nuclear scintigraphy may aid in identification of the fracture site. Surgical correction may be attempted for fractures of the cervical vertebrae, but repair of thoracic or lumbar vertebrae is not attempted.

Tetanus

Tetanus is a highly fatal neurologic disease in horses characterized by a stiff, stilted gait, hyperexcitability, seizure, and coma. The causative organism is commonly present in the environment. The most common portals of entry for disease in horses include a subsolar abscess, a penetrating wound, or an infected intramuscular injection site. Tetanus **toxoid** (inactivated) is a safe and efficacious vaccine for preventing clinical disease. Healthy horses without risk factors should be vaccinated annually for tetanus. Unvaccinated horses at high risk for development of tetanus (wounds, subsolar abscess, surgery) should receive tetanus **antitoxin** in addition to tetanus toxoid to provide immediate protection against disease. Tetanus antitoxin is associated with fatal serum hepatitis; its administration should be limited to patients at high risk for disease.

> **TECHNICIAN NOTE** Different neurologic diseases can have similar clinical signs in horses. It is important to take proper precautions, such as the use of gloves and eye protection, when working with these patients. Rabies is zoonotic (infectious to humans) and is fatal.

Botulism

Botulism is a rapidly progressive, often fatal neurologic disease in horses characterized by profound weakness, muscle fasciculations, and dysphagia (inability to swallow). The causal organism produces a neurotoxin that may gain entry to the body by colonizing the intestinal tract (foals), infected wounds, or contaminating feedstuff. Colonization of the intestinal tract in foals occurs in particular geographic regions of the United States, especially in Pennsylvania, Ohio, and Kentucky. This is a preventable disease, and it is imperative to vaccinate for botulism in affected areas. The vaccine is effective, and unvaccinated horses can die quickly after an infection. The initial series is administered monthly for 3 months, then once a year.

URINARY TRACT DISEASE

Urinary tract disease is relatively uncommon in horses compared with other species. Diagnostic investigation of renal disease may include hematology and serum chemistry, urinalysis, rectal examination (the left kidney can be palpated per rectum), ultrasonography, and cystoscopy (endoscopic examination of the bladder and urethra).

Acute Renal Failure

Acute renal failure in horses is most often the result of toxic causes. Aminoglycoside antibiotics (gentamicin, amikacin), oxytetracycline, polymyxin B, an antibiotic used in the treatment of endotoxemia, and NSAIDs are commonly implicated. Dehydration exacerbates renal damage caused by these drugs. Excretion of hemoglobin, a breakdown product of red blood cells, and myoglobin, a breakdown product of muscle, by the kidneys (hemoglobinuria and myoglobinuria) can also result in acute renal failure because these pigments damage the tubules in the kidneys. Hemoglobinuria is secondary to hemolytic anemia, and myoglobinuria is secondary to rhabdomyolysis (see muscle disease section). Signs of acute renal failure include oliguria (decreased urination), anorexia, and changes in urine concentration. Serum chemistry testing reveals increased blood urea nitrogen (BUN) and creatinine levels. Electrolyte abnormalities may also be present. Urinalysis should be performed (see urinalysis section). The mainstay of treatment for acute renal failure is IV fluids for diuresis. Frequent monitoring of renal values is necessary to determine the response to fluid therapy and the length of time that fluid therapy is required. Urine output should be closely monitored.

Urinary Calculus

Uroliths, urinary stones, are most commonly found in the bladder but can also be found in the kidney, ureter, and urethra. Stones are composed of calcium carbonate or calcium phosphate. Bladder stones are more common in geldings than in mares. The most common clinical sign is blood in the urine after exercise. Other signs include straining to urinate, passing small amounts of urine frequently, and incontinence. Diagnosis is confirmed by palpation of the bladder per rectum. Cystoscopy, endoscopy of the urinary bladder, allows direct visualization of the stones. Ultrasonography of the bladder can also be used to visualize the stone. The treatment of choice is surgical removal of the stone.

Polyuria/Polydipsia

Horses normally drink between 4% and 6% of their body weight daily (20 to 30 liters for a full-size horse). *Polydipsia* in horses is defined as drinking more than 10% of their body weight daily. Horses normally urinate 1% to 3% of their body weight daily (5 to 15 liters for a full-size horse) because most water is lost via feces. *Polyuria* is defined as urinating more than 5% of body weight daily.

Polyuria/polydipsia (PU/PD) can be due to physiologic causes, including lactation, heat, exercise, diarrhea, and glucocorticoid administration. Certain diseases can also result in PU/PD. PU/PD is a common sign of equine pituitary pars intermedia syndrome (Cushing's disease; see Chapter 35 for more information) in older horses. PU/PD can also result from psychogenic water drinking, a behavioral problem, diabetes, or chronic renal failure. A water deprivation test may be performed to help differentiate the causes.

DERMATOLOGIC DISEASE

Ringworm

Equine dermatophytosis (ringworm) is a fungal infection of the superficial layer of skin. Fungi commonly involved include *Trichophyton* and *Microsporum* spp. Transmission of fungal infection occurs by direct contact between affected animals. Younger animals (younger than 4 years of age) are more likely to be affected. Infected areas of skin have a bull's-eye appearance with circular patches of hair loss and a circle of inflammation at the periphery of the lesion. Diagnosis is confirmed by fungal culture on commercially available dermatophyte culture medium. Although infection is usually self-limited, application of topical antifungal drugs will speed recovery.

Rain Rot

Dermatophilosis (rain scald, rain rot) is a common bacterial infection caused by *Dermatophilus congolensis* that produces crusting lesions. The crusts can be pulled out with a tuft of hair, and the remaining lesion is a glistening yellow crater. The organisms readily colonize wet, macerated skin; therefore, the disease is common in winter and spring. An impression smear of the tuft should be stained with Wright stain. Organisms are identified as a double chain of cocci with a "railroad track" appearance. The organisms usually are easily cultured and form an applesauce-like colony on specialized growth medium. Affected horses should be bathed with an iodine-based or chlorhexidine shampoo and placed in a dry environment. Administration of penicillin will speed recovery in severely afflicted horses.

Culicoides Hypersensitivity

Culicoides hypersensitivity is a syndrome characterized by mane and tail rubbing whereby affected horses develop an allergic pruritic skin condition secondary to the bite of *Culicoides* flies. Body regions classically affected include the face, ears, mane, withers, rump, base of the tail, and ventral abdomen. Dermatitis usually begins as a seasonal condition, but its severity and duration increase as the horse ages. Pruritus usually is noted during the fly season but will vary in length depending on geographic location. The condition is diagnosed by correlating the time of year with physical evidence of self-mutilation, especially in the mane and tail areas. Intradermal skin testing can be useful in confirming the diagnosis. Treatment involves reduced insect exposure and concomitant use of anti-inflammatory medication. Because *Culicoides* breeds in stagnant waters, affected horses should be moved away from ponds, lakes, or irrigation canals. Water troughs and barrels should be cleaned frequently and the water kept fresh to prevent use as breeding sites by the flies. Because *Culicoides* feed primarily at dusk, night, and dawn, horses should be kept stabled during these times. Stabling is most effective if the doors and windows can be closed, and if the stall is lined with a fine-mesh screen. Frequent application of insecticide to the screen may be useful. Fans are helpful to reduce exposure because *Culicoides* cannot fly well in brisk breezes. Application of insecticides and repellents is a necessary part of disease control. The most effective products are those containing pyrethrins with synergists and repellents. Frequent bathing not only decreases scale and crust but also seems to decrease pruritus. Corticosteroid therapy is often necessary in these cases to control pruritus.

Sarcoid

Equine sarcoid, a benign, locally invasive tumor of the skin, is the most common tumor in horses. These tumors may produce raised, hairless lesions with a corrugated surface that often bleed when traumatized, known as *fibroblastic sarcoids*, or a flattened form known as *verrucous sarcoids*. The cause of sarcoid is unknown, but a viral agent is suspected. Surgical resection, cryotherapy (freezing), laser therapy, immunotherapy (intralesional mycobacterial cell wall extract), radiotherapy (iridium 191), and chemotherapy (intralesional cisplatin) are accepted treatment modalities with variable success. It is difficult to predict the response to a given treatment modality, and combination therapy is often necessary.

Melanomas

Melanomas are relatively common skin tumors, particularly in gray horses. They occur most commonly in the perineal region but can occur on other areas of the body. Melanomas appear as darkly pigmented nodules in the skin. They usually are benign but tend to enlarge, causing mechanical problems, such as interfering with defecation. Most clinicians believe that it is better not to attempt surgical removal unless they are located in an area that interferes with tack, or unless they are so large that they interfere with normal body functions. Administration of cimetidine has been reported to be effective in many horses to reduce the size of melanomas. Once cimetidine is discontinued, the tumors usually enlarge. Autologous vaccines (vaccines made from the horse's tumor) have been used with some success.

OPHTHALMOLOGIC DISEASE

Equine Recurrent Uveitis

Equine recurrent uveitis (moon blindness) is the most common cause of blindness in horses. It is an immune-mediated condition, and many factors (heredity, parasites, leptospirosis) have been implicated in its development; however, the inciting cause is often unknown. Affected horses experience episodes of intraocular inflammation characterized by swelling of the eyelids, corneal edema, and hypopyon (inflammatory cellular exudate in the anterior chamber). Over time, the episodes become more frequent and severe and produce permanent ocular damage, including retinal degeneration, cataracts, and synechiae (adhesions of the iris to the lens or to the anterior chamber). One or both eyes may be affected. Recurrent uveitis cannot be cured but often can be controlled with long-term anti-inflammatory therapy. Acute episodes are treated with ophthalmic preparations containing atropine and corticosteroids if no corneal ulceration is noted. Systemic anti-inflammatory therapy (e.g., flunixin meglumine) is beneficial. Horses with end-stage uveitis are blind and have small, collapsed ocular globes (*phthisis bulbi*). If a corneal ulcer is present, antimicrobials and NSAIDs are used. Once the ulcer completely resolves, a topical steroid may be used. These cases require diligent observation and long-term treatment.

Corneal Ulceration

Corneal ulceration commonly results from ocular trauma. Fluorescein stain is used to detect corneal abrasions because it adheres to abnormal cornea (Figure 20-7). Defects in the corneal surface will stain an apple-green color. Corneal ulceration in most horses responds readily without complications to the administration of ophthalmic antibacterial ointment (bacitracin, neomycin, polymyxin B). In some instances, the ulcer will be colonized by fungus (e.g., *Pseudomonas* or *Aspergillus* spp.). These organisms produce collagenase, which destroys the cornea and creates a "melting" corneal ulcer. These ulcers are rapidly progressive, and the eye is prone to rupture. Frequent antimicrobial dosage regimens may require the placement of a subpalpebral lavage system (Figure 20-8) to allow frequent medication administration for a painful eye. Aggressive topical antimicrobial therapy may be successful, but suturing a conjunctival pedicle flap to provide blood supply to the affected area may be necessary to save the globe in some instances. Deep, melting corneal ulcers often heal with a fibrous scar that may impair vision in the future.

> **TECHNICIAN NOTE** Recurrent uveitis (moon blindness, periodic ophthalmia) is the most common cause of blindness in horses.

CARE OF THE HOSPITALIZED EQUINE PATIENT

In the equine hospital setting, veterinary technicians are responsible for primary patient monitoring, administration of medications, general daily care of horses, and supervision of lay technical support. This section provides an overview of the daily management of equine patients in the hospital setting. The nursing process is an integral part of caring for hospitalized equine patients. Table 20-4 describes some technician assessments and interventions that may be encountered when treating equine patients. Refer to Case Presentation 20-1, which demonstrates use of the technician practice model.

PATIENT MONITORING

The level of patient monitoring required for a hospitalized horse depends on the severity and nature of the disease.

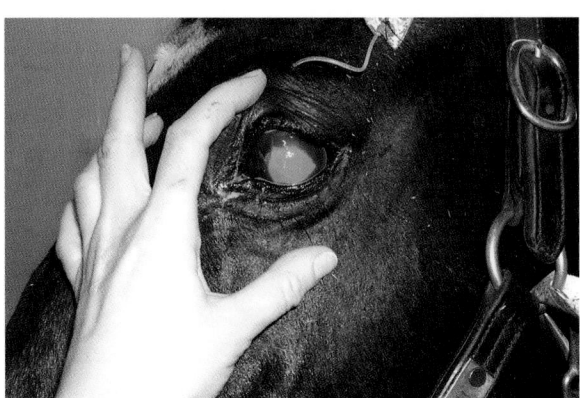

FIGURE 20-7 Patient with corneal ulceration stained with fluorescein. (Courtesy Dr. Amy Bentz.)

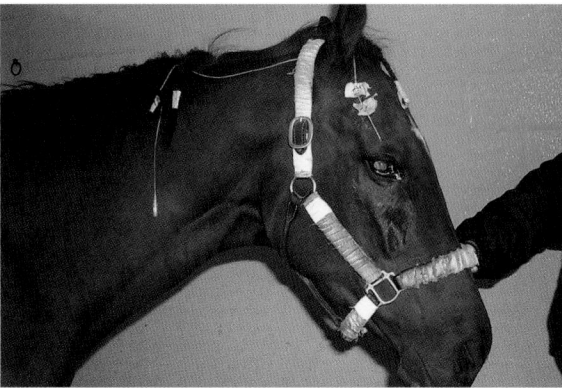

FIGURE 20-8 Subpalpebral catheter placement used to administer topical ocular medication. (Courtesy Dr. Amy Bentz.)

| TABLE 20-4 | Selection of Technician Evaluations and Interventions Applicable to the Equine Patient |

TECHNICIAN EVALUATION AND DEFINITION	POTENTIAL PHYSIOLOGIC CONSEQUENCES	CLINICAL FINDINGS	TECHNICIAN INTERVENTIONS
Anorexia Complete or partial loss of appetite	Poor immune function Decreased wound healing Dehydration Electrolyte imbalances Hypoalbuminemia Hepatic lipidosis (particularly in animals with concurrent illness or pregnancy) Cachexia Hypoglycemia Seizures Death	Loss of appetite for longer than 2 days Prolonged diminished appetite Increased total bilirubin Increased liver values (hepatic lipidosis)	Administer doctor-prescribed treatment for primary disease and antacids Encourage patient to eat on its own: • Novel, odoriferous foods • Coax/socialization Enteral feeding via nasogastric tube Parenteral supplementation of dextrose, amino acids, and lipids
Dehydration Loss of total body water	Decreased renal perfusion Electrolyte imbalance	Tacky/dry mucous membranes Skin tenting Increased packed cell volume (PCV) and total protein (TP) Increased renal values (creatinine, blood urea nitrogen [BUN])	Administer fluid therapy per doctor's order Monitor fluid intake and urine output
Hypovolemia Loss of intravascular fluid	Decreased perfusion of kidneys, heart, and brain Shock	Dry mucous membranes Pale to white mucous membranes Prolonged capillary refill time (CRT) Tachycardia Weak pulses Hemorrhage Increased PCV and TP Normal or decreased PCV and decreased TP (blood loss) Decreased jugular fill	Administer fluid therapy per doctor's orders Administer blood transfusion per doctor's orders Monitor for signs of transfusion reaction: • Increased heart rate, temperature, or respiratory rate from baseline • Hives
Endotoxemia Group of clinical signs due to endotoxin in bloodstream	Hypovolemia Shock Systemic inflammation Coagulopathies Laminitis GI hypomotility	Fever Tachycardia Hyperemic mucous membranes Leukopenia Laminitis Depression	Administer doctor-prescribed treatments (see Table 20-3 for specific treatments)
Pain	GI hypomotility Hyperthermia Anorexia Weight loss Depression Decreased milk production Recumbency	Pawing, rolling, looking at flank Tachycardia Tachypnea Decreased locomotion Decreased response to human interaction Postural changes	Administer doctor-prescribed analgesics Monitor for breakthrough pain Monitor for signs of adverse reaction to pain meds: • Decreased GI motility resulting in decreased fecal output and borborygmi and/or colic (opioids, alpha2-agonists) • Increased renal values and/or decreased protein (nonsteroidal anti-inflammatory drugs [NSAIDs]) Provide comfortable environment: • Deep bedding • Pad feet for laminitis

TABLE 20-4	Selection of Technician Evaluations and Interventions Applicable to the Equine Patient—cont'd			
TECHNICIAN EVALUATION AND DEFINITION	**POTENTIAL PHYSIOLOGIC CONSEQUENCES**	**CLINICAL FINDINGS**	**TECHNICIAN INTERVENTIONS**

Hypoxia
Decreased
  oxygenation
	Death	Cyanotic mucous membranes
		Dyspnea
		Tachypnea
		Altered mentation
		Decreased oxygen saturation
		Altered arterial blood gases
		  (ABGs)
			Oxygen therapy
			Monitor vitals, watch for changes in
			  respiration
			Monitor oxygen saturation and
			  ABGs
			Administer doctor-prescribed
			  treatments for primary disease

Recumbency
Inability to stand
	Pneumonia
	Pressure sores
	Colic
	Urinary tract infection
		Recumbency	Keep in sternal position if possible
			Change position at least every 6
			  hours
			Sling if possible
			Deep bedding or pad, head
			  bumper, leg wraps
			Feed soft feed, mineral oil to keep
			  feces soft
			Evacuate rectum twice daily if
			  needed
			Place indwelling urinary catheter or
			  catheterize periodically to drain
			  bladder

See Chapter 19 for a discussion of technician evaluations and development of a nursing care plan.

Horses with infectious disease require frequent patient monitoring (e.g., every 4 to 6 hours). Any critically ill patient needs constant IV fluid administration and intensive care monitoring. Most such patients will be monitored frequently for signs of discomfort, heart rate, respiratory rate, hydration, capillary refill time, abdominal pain, respiratory distress, shock, laminitis, and gastrointestinal motility. An increased heart rate (tachycardia) is indicative of pain. A rate of 60 beats per minute (bpm) or greater indicates serious pain in an adult horse.

Patient monitoring forms are designed to identify trends in physical signs. Patient treatment forms coordinate treatment periods when several individuals may be responsible for administering medications. Treatment sheets and monitoring forms may be combined for low-maintenance, elective patients. However, for intensive care patients, monitoring should be more detailed, and many hospitals use a flow sheet. It is important to recognize that monitoring and treatment forms are a permanent part of the medical record, which represents a legal document or record of all events during hospitalization.

Isolation Procedures

Horses with contagious diseases should be hospitalized in isolation facilities. The most common diseases that require an isolation protocol are colitis (salmonellosis), strangles (*S. equi equi*), and the neurologic form of equine herpesvirus (EHV)-1. Personnel wear disposable gloves, boots, and body suits while attending to isolation cases. A disinfectant foot dip should be used when entering and exiting each stall. Protective boots, gloves, and suits should be discarded when

exiting the isolation area. Horses in isolation should not be walked in areas where other horses are grazing. Waste from the stall should be disposed of in an inaccessible area, and dedicated equipment should be used to clean the stall. If possible, personnel attending to isolation cases should not attend to foals or immunocompromised patients. Please see the American Association of Equine Practitioners (AAEP) Biosecurity Guidelines for more information on isolation protocols (see recommended websites).

Recumbency

Recumbent horses are particularly challenging to manage effectively in a hospital setting. Neurologic and musculoskeletal diseases are the most common problems resulting in recumbency in horses. Figure 20-9 presents a basic flow chart of nursing care for the recumbent horse. Recumbent horses and foals quickly develop pressure sores (decubital ulcers) over the pelvis (tuber coxae), elbows, and head if not properly managed (Figure 20-10). Manure- and urine-soaked bedding must be removed frequently because horses develop irritated skin and sores. Pressure sores rapidly become deep and may infect underlying bony structures. Muscle damage can occur as the result of pressure and decreased circulation. In addition, recumbent horses may have decreased intestinal motility and may fail to void urine. Therefore, soft feed, such as fresh grass, should be offered to recumbent horses to facilitate fecal evacuation and prevent impaction. Horses unable to defecate should have feces manually removed twice daily. Placement of an indwelling urinary catheter or periodic catheterization of the urinary bladder is often necessary when recumbent patients are managed. Recumbent horses

CASE PRESENTATION 20-1 NURSING CARE PLAN: BACTERIAL PNEUMONIA

Signalment: Patches, 5-year-old Paint gelding

Chief Complaint: Owner reports that Patches has had a decreased appetite for 2 days and has been coughing.

Pertinent History: Patches was shipped last week from Oklahoma to Florida. Patches was vaccinated routinely 2 months ago. The owner reports no previous health problems.

Physical Examination: Body weight: 1100 pounds; Body condition score: 5/5; Temperature: 103.5° F; Heart rate: 48 bpm, sinus rhythm; Synchronous and strong pulses; Respiration: 28 bpm, wheezes dorsally, quiet ventrally; Mucous membranes: pink and slightly tacky; CRT 2 to 3 seconds; Skin turgor: slightly decreased; Ears, eyes, and nose: serous discharge both nostrils; Gastrointestinal borborygmi: within normal limits; Musculoskeletal system: normal.

Problem List: Fever; Decreased lung sounds in ventral quadrant, history of cough, tachypnea; Mild dehydration

Initial Diagnostic Plan: Lower respiratory disease is suspected on the basis of thoracic auscultation, cough, and tachypnea. A rebreathing exam is performed to further assess the lungs. Crackles are auscultated cranioventrally and wheezes dorsally. The patient coughs during the exam and has a prolonged recovery. CBC and serum chemistry are run and reveal leukocytosis and hyperfibrinogenemia (inflammatory leukogram) and increased PCV and TP.

Based on these findings, an infectious cause of lower respiratory disease is suspected (refer to Figure 20-1). The history of the patient shipping over a long distance makes bacterial pneumonia likely. Thoracic radiographs are performed and reveal an alveolar pattern in the cranioventral lung fields. A transtracheal wash is performed to obtain a sample for culture and sensitivity to guide antibiotic therapy and for cytologic examination to confirm infection.

Medical Diagnosis (by veterinarian): Pleuropneumonia

Treatment Plan (by veterinarian):

TREATMENT	RATIONALE
Potassium penicillin IV q6hours	Broad-spectrum antibiotics are warranted pending culture
Gentamicin IV q24hours	and sensitivity results from TTW, which will allow selective
Metronidazole PO q12hours	therapy.
Flunixin IV q12hours	Decrease inflammation and relieve fever.
Intravenous fluids	Correct dehydration.

Technician Evaluations: Altered ventilation; Hypovolemia; Hyperthermia; Abnormal eating behavior; Exercise intolerance; Risk of altered gas diffusion; Risk of sepsis and endotoxemia

Nursing Care Plan:

1. Altered ventilation

TECHNICIAN INTERVENTION	RATIONALE
• Monitor respiratory rate and effort	• Animals with compromised lung function due to infection may have elevated respiratory rates and increased respiratory effort
• Monitor mucous membrane color	
• Auscult thorax for abnormal lung sounds	• Intensity and quality of abnormal lung sounds may indicate severity of pulmonary disease
• Monitor nasal discharge: describe quantity, quality, and color	• Blue discoloration of mucous membranes is indicative of compromised gas diffusion and low levels of circulating oxygen (hypoxia). Refer to Table 20-5.
	• Nasal discharge is an abnormal finding and should be monitored
• Monitor heart rate and signs of discomfort	• Heart rate may increase when the patient experiences pain. Pleural pain is common in horses with bacterial pneumonia and pleuritis
	• Heart rate may also increase as a compensatory mechanism to improve oxygenation of tissues if the patient is hypoxic
Improve air quality	• Dust may aggravate the respiratory system because normal clearance mechanisms are compromised
• Decrease dust in environment	
• Feed low dust hay and grain	• Administration of oxygen increases oxygen saturation in the blood
• Remove horse from barn when stalls are being cleaned	
If condition worsens and patient becomes hypoxic, consider giving nebulized nasal oxygen	

CASE PRESENTATION 20-1 NURSING CARE PLAN: BACTERIAL PNEUMONIA—cont'd

2. Hypovolemia

TECHNICIAN INTERVENTION

- Place jugular intracatheter
- Administer intravenous fluids, per doctor's orders
- Maintain catheter
  - Check for patency and thrombosis
  - Heparinize catheter
- Monitor hydration status via PCV/TP
- Monitor pulse rate, quality, and intensity
- Monitor capillary refill time

- Monitor urine output and water consumption
  - Monitor urine specific gravity

RATIONALE

- IV fluids correct hypovolemia caused by dehydration by increasing the liquid portion of blood
- Increased blood volume increases perfusion of kidneys and helps prevent damage due to use of aminoglycoside (gentamicin) and the NSAID flunixin
- Blood pressure decreases with dehydration because blood volume is reduced. Pulses become weaker as blood pressure drops
- Whenever a patient is on IV fluids, it is important to regularly monitor the patient's hydration status, so clinicians are sure that the patient is not being overhydrated or underhydrated
- Heart rate may increase as the body compensates for decreased tissue perfusion during hypovolemia
- CRT is slowed during hypovolemia because blood pressure is reduced and perfusion of gum tissue is reduced

Indication of adequate kidney perfusion
Compromised kidneys lose their ability to concentrate and dilute urine. Specific gravity reflects the concentration of the urine

3. Hyperthermia

TECHNICIAN INTERVENTION

Administer flunixin IV q12hours as per order

Monitor body temperature regularly

Monitor for signs of endotoxemia (see Table 20-5)

RATIONALE

Flunixin meglumine is an NSAID that decreases inflammation and reduces fever

- The veterinary technician monitors whether or not treatment is effective in reducing fever
- Infection can worsen if antibiotic therapy is not effective, and body temperature may rise if infection spreads to bloodstream (sepsis)
- Gram-negative organisms are a cause of bacterial pneumonia

4. Abnormal eating behavior

TECHNICIAN INTERVENTION

Treat primary disease
Administer antibiotics as per order:
- Potassium penicillin IV q6hours
- Gentamicin IV q24hours
- Metronidazole PO q12hours
Encourage patient to eat by feeding novel, odoriferous feeds
- Offer food by hand, if effective
- Allow to graze if possible
- Feed low-dust hay and grain

- Monitor GI function:
  - Auscult all four quadrants of the abdomen and record manure production and manure quality
  - Monitor for signs of abdominal pain

RATIONALE

Appetite will likely improve with resolution of fever and infection

- Providing appetizing foods and encouragement increases the likelihood that the patient will eat. Patients need energy for immunologic health
- Dust may aggravate the respiratory system because normal clearance mechanisms are compromised

- Peristalsis can be altered when patients are stall-bound and inactive
- Illness, such as sepsis, can cause an ileus

5. Exercise intolerance

TECHNICIAN INTERVENTION

Hand-walk patient if possible
Allow access to grass

RATIONALE

Activity and pasture improve peristaltic activity

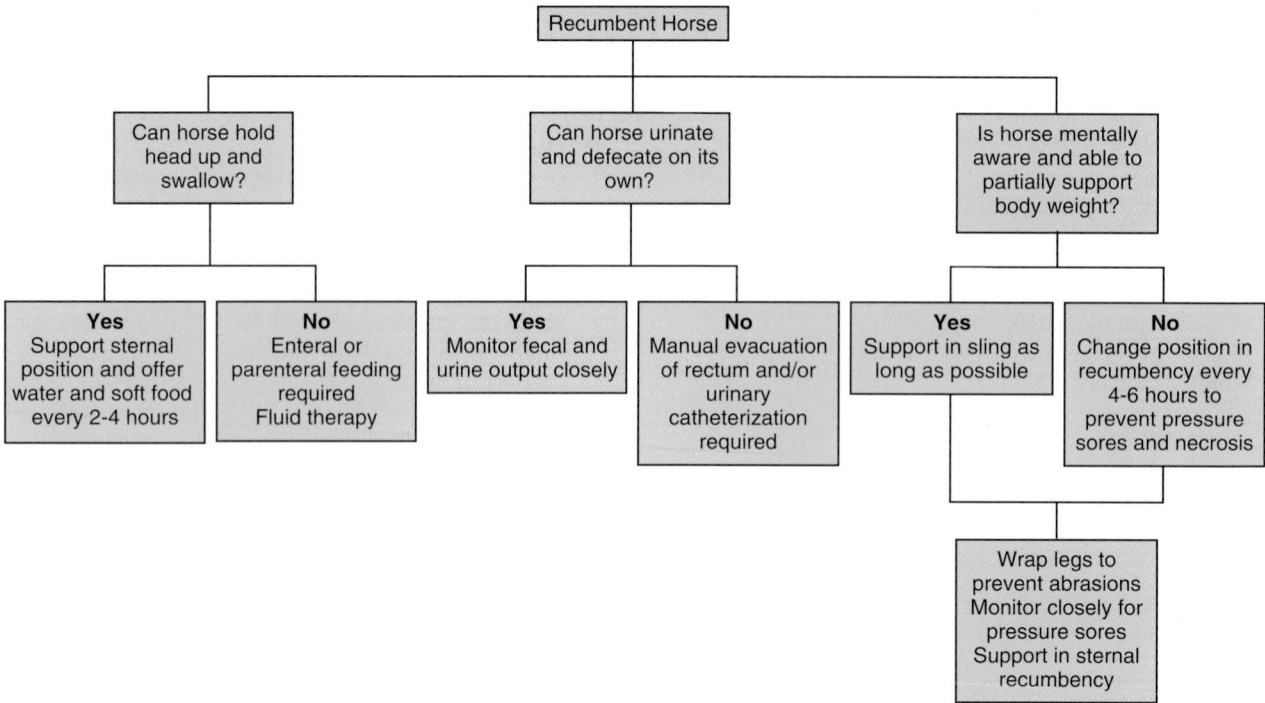

FIGURE 20-9 Flow chart for nursing approach to the recumbent patient.

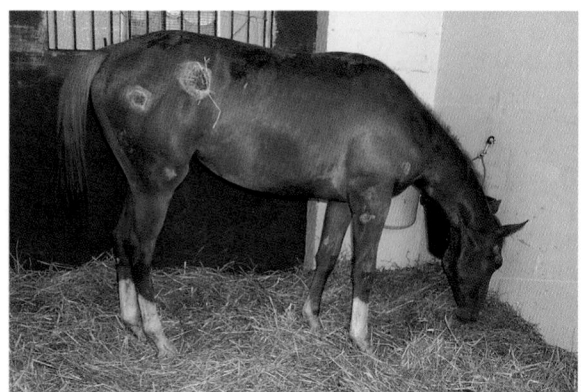

FIGURE 20-10 Recovered botulism patient with decubital ulcers. (Courtesy Dr. Amy Bentz.)

should be deeply bedded on straw, placed on a padded mat, or placed on a mattress to prevent the development of pressure sores (see Figure 20-10). The position of the horse should be changed every 6 hours; multiple attendants are required to move an adult recumbent horse. A sling can be used only in horses that can partially support their own weight but are not able to stand on their own (Figure 20-11, *A* through *D*). Horses cannot be supported solely by a sling because of constriction of breathing and development of sling-induced pressure sores. Recumbent adult horses can rarely be managed for longer than 1 or 2 weeks without the development of life-threatening complications (pneumonia, urinary tract infection, colic, pressure sores).

Endotoxemia

Endotoxin is a component of the cell wall of Gram-negative bacteria. Endotoxemia refers to the group of clinical signs caused by endotoxin circulating through the bloodstream. Clinical signs associated with endotoxemia include fever, tachycardia, hyperemic mucous membranes (Figure 20-12), leukopenia, laminitis, and depression. The most common cause of endotoxemia in horses is gastrointestinal disease that compromises the intestinal wall (such as diarrhea or colic due to small intestinal obstruction), allowing translocation of bacteria across the intestinal wall and into the bloodstream. Other causes of endotoxemia include retained placenta, metritis (uterine infection), pneumonia, peritonitis, and large wounds. Horses are extremely sensitive to the effects of endotoxin, and aggressive treatment is required. In addition to the specific treatments provided in Table 20-3, removal of the source of endotoxin is important. This may include surgical excision of compromised intestine, uterine lavage, and drainage of pleural or peritoneal fluid. Early recognition and treatment of signs of endotoxemia are critical to a positive outcome, and technicians should monitor at-risk patients closely for these signs.

> **TECHNICIAN NOTE** Horses with infectious contagious diseases should be hospitalized in isolation facilities. The most common infectious diseases requiring isolation are colitis (Salmonellosis), strangles *(S. equi equi),* and the neurologic form of equine herpesvirus (EHV)-1.

Feeding and Anorexia

Whenever possible, hospitalized patients should be offered feed similar to what they are fed at home. Sudden changes in diet predispose horses to colic or diarrhea. When a horse is admitted to the veterinary hospital, it is imperative to ask

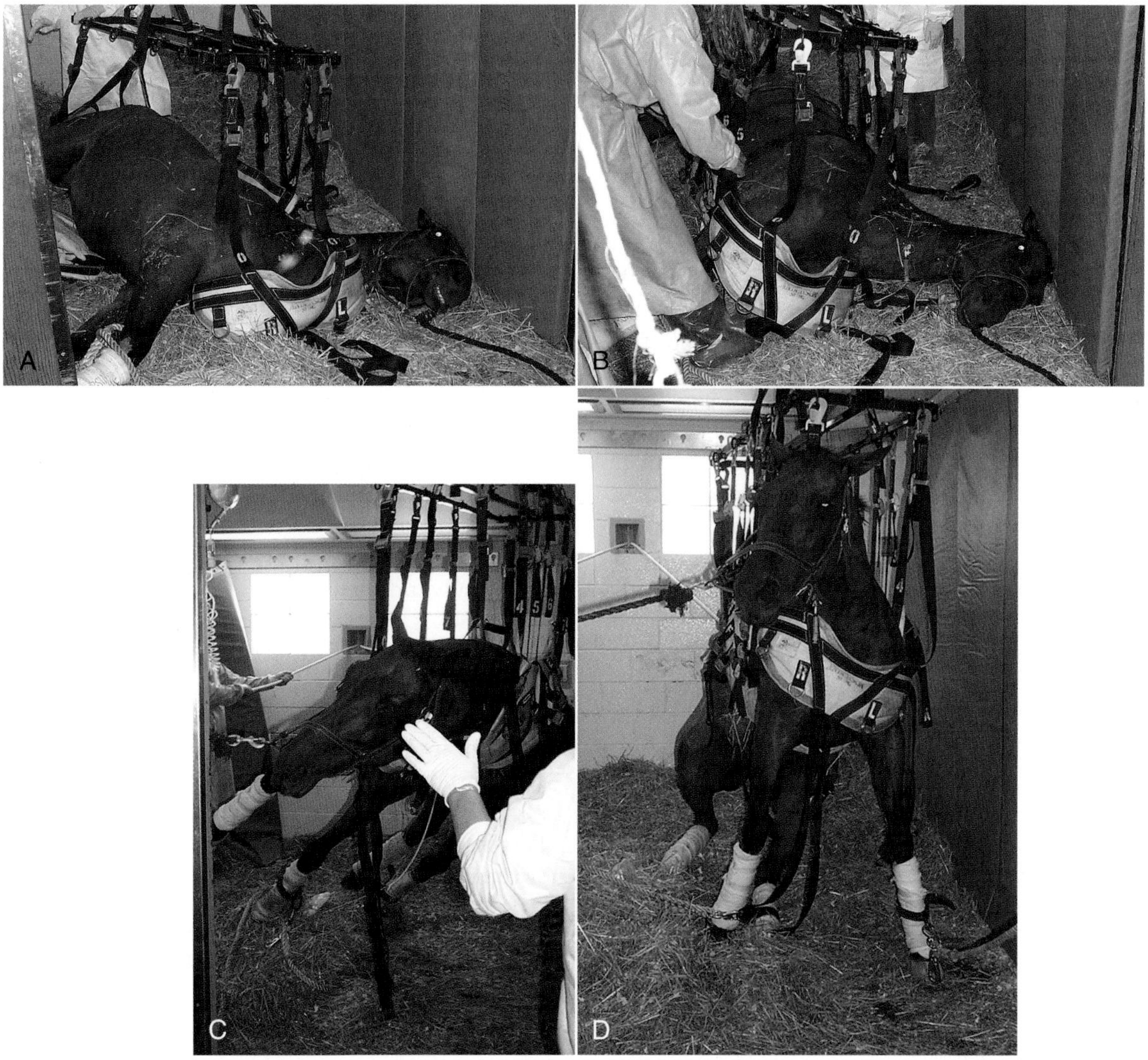

FIGURE 20-11 A, Placing sling over horse's head. B, Securing sling on recumbent horse. C, Slowly lifting recumbent horse in a sling using a mechanized pulley system. D, Recumbent horse brought to a standing position. (Courtesy Dr. Amy Bentz.)

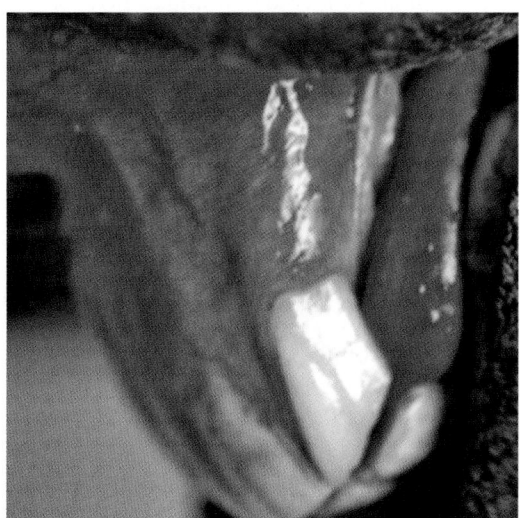

FIGURE 20-12 Hyperemic mucous membranes—an indication of endotoxemia.

the owner or trainer for details on the horse's typical diet. In some instances, feeding must be specialized to accommodate the patient's disease. After medical resolution of colic, horses should be offered soft feed, such as bran mash, fresh grass, and small amounts of good-quality hay. Feed should be offered frequently in small quantities to horses with gastrointestinal tract disease rather than two large daily meals. Horses with heaves (recurrent airway obstruction) should be offered water-soaked hay and a dust-free complete pelleted diet. Inappetent horses should be offered highly palatable, calorie-dense feed to increase energy intake. In horses that are dysphagic, enteral nutrition, consisting of a commercial formula or blended pelleted feed, can be provided via a small-bore nasogastric feeding tube. Parenteral (intravenous) nutrition, consisting of IV dextrose, amino acids, and/or lipid, can be used in horses that cannot tolerate sufficient enteral feeding to meet caloric requirements. Catheter care is critical when parenteral nutrition is provided because of the risk for septic thrombophlebitis. A dedicated line and strict aseptic technique are recommended.

THERAPEUTICS

An IV catheter can be placed for repeated administration of medications or continuous fluid infusion. IV catheters should be flushed with heparinized saline flush (2 to 10 U/ml) every 6 hours and monitored twice daily for heat, swelling, and pain. Infection at the catheter site may occur in the subcutaneous tissue or in the vein (septic thrombophlebitis). Septic thrombophlebitis can be life threatening in horses and is more likely to occur in horses with endotoxemia, systemic infection, and those being treated with parenteral nutrition.

The ideal antimicrobial is effective against a wide range of bacterial organisms (broad spectrum), easy to administer, and nontoxic. Penicillin has good efficacy against common Gram-positive pathogens in the horse (*Streptococcus zooepidemicus, S. equi equi*) and is relatively safe. It is frequently administered intramuscularly (procaine penicillin) and intravenously (potassium penicillin). Procaine penicillin should never be administered intravenously. Life-threatening anaphylactic reactions are reported with IV procaine penicillin administration and should be treated with epinephrine. Aminoglycoside antimicrobials (gentamicin, amikacin sulfate) are efficacious against Gram-negative pathogens and can be administered intramuscularly or intravenously. These antimicrobials are nephrotoxic, so renal function should be monitored during therapy. Trimethoprim-sulfa antimicrobials have a moderate Gram-positive and Gram-negative spectrum and are administered orally. Ceftiofur sodium has a good Gram-positive and Gram-negative spectrum and may be administered intramuscularly or intravenously. Metronidazole is administered orally or per rectum to treat anaerobic bacterial infection. Specific indications are known for the administration of other antimicrobials, but some are not widely used because of the risk of antimicrobial-induced colitis. Chloramphenicol is used sparingly in horses because of the human health risk for idiosyncratic, fatal aplastic anemia from exposure during patient administration.

Many analgesic medications are available for horses. Phenylbutazone, flunixin meglumine, and firocoxib are NSAIDs that provide mild to moderate pain relief. NSAIDs also reduce fever (antipyretic) and inflammation. Phenylbutazone is most effective for the treatment of musculoskeletal pain. Ketoprofen, meclofenamic acid, and naproxen are less commonly used drugs that provide mild to moderate analgesia for musculoskeletal pain. Flunixin meglumine is more effective for soft tissue and visceral (abdominal) pain. In addition, flunixin meglumine may combat the effects of endotoxemia in horses with gastrointestinal tract disease. Lidocaine given as a continuous rate infusion provides analgesia and may have anti-inflammatory properties as well. Care must be taken to give lidocaine at appropriate rates because overly rapid administration can result in seizure. Sedatives that also provide analgesia include xylazine and detomidine (alpha$_2$ agonists). Xylazine provides

approximately 20 minutes of sedation and analgesia. Detomidine provides up to 1 hour of sedation and analgesia. Butorphanol is a narcotic agonist that provides up to 1 hour of sedation and analgesia for moderate to severe pain. Acepromazine has no analgesic properties and provides only moderate tranquilization. Acepromazine also causes hypotension and can cause persistent paraphimosis in stallions.

Corticosteroids have potent anti-inflammatory properties and are administered for allergic airway disease, allergic skin conditions, immune-mediated disease, and joint inflammation. Corticosteroids are administered topically, orally, parenterally (intravenously or intramuscularly), and intra-articularly. Adverse effects of corticosteroid administration include immunosuppression, polyuria or polydipsia, poor hair coat, muscle wasting, poor wound healing, laminitis, and progression of degenerative joint disease. Therefore, corticosteroids are administered with caution and only when specifically indicated.

DMSO is an anti-inflammatory drug that is used occasionally in horses to relieve swelling and edema associated with CNS trauma, traumatic musculoskeletal injuries, laminitis, and **myositis**. DMSO may be administered topically, orally, or intravenously (diluted in crystalloid fluids as a 10% solution). Nitrile gloves are used when the product is handled because it can be absorbed when latex gloves are worn. Rapid IV administration may result in hemolysis, hematuria, and sweating in horses.

> **TECHNICIAN NOTE** The veterinary technician plays a central role in the day-to-day monitoring and care of hospitalized patients; therefore, the abilities to be observant and to perform a thorough physical examination are vital.

LABORATORY STUDIES

Clinicopathologic testing provides important information for the veterinarian to identify an impairment of an organ system, confirm a clinical diagnosis, assess patient response to therapy, and formulate a prognosis. The normal values of many clinicopathologic tests vary among species. In addition, species-specific characteristics are associated with diseases and the significance of abnormal findings. This section concentrates solely on equine-specific alterations in clinicopathologic values in health and disease. Refer to Chapters 12 and 13 for additional information.

Hematology

A complete blood count (CBC) provides information pertaining to red blood cell (RBC) count, RBC morphology, total white blood cell (WBC) count, WBC differential (including neutrophils, lymphocytes, eosinophils, and monocytes), WBC morphology, and fibrinogen concentration. RBCs are most easily estimated using the packed cell volume (PCV). The normal range of the PCV depends on the breed but generally is between 32% and 45%.

Hot-blooded breeds (Thoroughbreds, Arabians, Quarter horses) have higher resting RBC counts compared with ponies and draft horses. Low PCV (less than 30%) is indicative of anemia. Horses have a large muscular spleen that normally contains up to one-third of the circulating RBC volume. With excitement and exercise, the PCV in horses can increase by as much as 50% secondary to splenic contraction. Therefore, the resting PCV is highly variable and must be serially evaluated in excitable patients. In addition, the response of the spleen to massive hemorrhage precludes use of the PCV to estimate the magnitude of blood loss for at least 24 hours. Total protein levels will decrease and lactate levels will increase in horses with acute blood loss.

Evaluation of the total and differential WBC count is important to identify the presence of infection. In most instances, bacterial infection will manifest as an increase in WBC count (leukocytosis) characterized by an increase in the number of mature neutrophils (mature neutrophilia). Fibrinogen is a coagulation factor and an acute phase protein in horses, produced by the liver in response to inflammation. Fibrinogen concentrations remain increased until infection has resolved.

Horses are particularly sensitive to circulating endotoxins released from the cell walls of Gram-negative bacteria. Endotoxins cause margination and sequestration of WBCs. Therefore, a profoundly low WBC count (leukopenia) characterized by low neutrophil count (neutropenia) and immature band neutrophils (left shift) is indicative of Gram-negative **septicemia** or gastrointestinal disease, with inflammation allowing mucosal absorption of Gram-negative bacteria. High eosinophil counts (eosinophilia) are indicative of a massive parasite infestation or possibly allergic disease. Low lymphocyte counts (lymphopenia) may be observed in horses with early viral infection.

Serum Chemistry

A serum chemistry panel provides specific information pertaining to the liver, kidney, muscle, and serum electrolyte concentrations. Horses normally have a yellow tint to the serum as a result of increased serum bilirubin levels because horses do not have gallbladders. Serum bilirubin concentrations will increase dramatically if feed is withheld for longer than 24 hours as a result of a normal physiologic response; this does not indicate liver disease. Most species develop low serum albumin levels with chronic liver disease because of decreased production; however, horses maintain production of albumin even with marked impairment of liver function. Reliable indicators of liver dysfunction in horses include high serum γ-glutamyltransferase (GGT) activity, high serum sorbitol dehydrogenase (SDH) activity, high serum bile acid concentrations, low blood urea nitrogen (BUN) concentrations, and increased ammonia levels.

In most species, renal failure produces low serum calcium and high serum phosphorus concentrations. Horses are obligate calcium excreters, and chronic renal failure often produces a marked increase in the serum calcium concentration.

Reliable indicators of renal failure in horses include high serum creatinine and BUN and electrolyte abnormalities, including low sodium and chloride and high potassium and calcium levels. The large colon of horses exchanges vast quantities of electrolytes and fluids on a daily basis. Horses with colonic inflammation may develop marked electrolyte abnormalities before diarrhea occurs. Low serum sodium, chloride, and potassium levels in horses with abdominal pain or depression often indicate loss of electrolytes into the lumen of the colon and impending diarrhea.

Serum creatine phosphokinase (CK) is an indicator of muscle damage in all species. Horses have large muscle masses in comparison with ruminants and small animals. Moderate increases in serum CK levels (2 to 4 times normal) readily occur in horses after prolonged transport, prolonged recumbency, exercise in an unconditioned horse, or rolling from abdominal pain. Moderate increases do not usually indicate primary muscle disease. Horses with primary muscle disease, such as exertional rhabdomyolysis (tying up, azoturia, Monday morning sickness), have increases in serum CK activity of up to 200 times normal values. Aspartate aminotransferase (AST) is an enzyme found in muscle tissue and liver tissue. Increases are expected when primary muscle disease or liver disease is present.

Lactate

Lactate, or lactic acid, is produced by cells undergoing anaerobic metabolism owing to lack of oxygen. Lactate levels in the blood therefore increase (hyperlactatemia) in conditions of decreased oxygen delivery to tissues. This most commonly occurs as the result of hypovolemia. In horses, severe hypovolemia is seen with colic and diarrhea. Lactate levels in venous blood can provide an objective measurement of the magnitude of hypovolemia and can help in monitoring the response to fluid therapy. In adult horses, normal lactate levels are lower than 1.5 mol/L. Other causes of increased blood lactate levels include anemia, cardiac disease, and respiratory disease.

In colic cases, comparison of the lactate level in peripheral blood with an abdominal fluid sample obtained via abdominocentesis (see later) can be useful in determining the viability of the intestine. Causes of colic in which the blood supply to the intestine is compromised, such as a large colon volvulus or a strangulating small intestinal lesion, result in local production of lactate by the ischemic bowel. In such cases, the lactate level in the abdominal fluid will be higher than that in the peripheral blood.

Blood Gas Analysis

Blood gas analysis provides information on oxygen and carbon dioxide content, pH, base deficit, and bicarbonate levels in the sample. Arterial samples are indicated to evaluate patients with respiratory disease; venous samples are indicated in patients with diseases affecting metabolic acid-base status, such as diarrhea and kidney disease. See Chapter 18 for a discussion of sampling techniques for arterial blood gas samples.

Urinalysis

Urinalysis is essential for evaluation of primary renal disease. Refer to Chapter 18 for information about obtaining urine samples in horses. Normal horse urine is usually alkaline (pH 7 to 9) and contains many calcium carbonate crystals. Alkaline urine usually produces a false-positive reaction for protein on urine dipsticks. Horses have a large number of mucous glands located within the renal pelvis; therefore, normal horse urine may appear thick and mucoid. Red urine is abnormal and results from the presence of frank blood (primary urinary tract disease), hemoglobin (hemolytic anemia), or myoglobin (myositis). Differentiation of these sources of red urine requires special testing of urine and serum samples. Urine specific gravity and urinary electrolyte excretion ratios should be obtained to investigate primary renal function. Urine specific gravity indicates the ability of the kidney to concentrate urine; normal values in resting horses should be greater than 1.030. Urinary electrolyte excretion ratios indicate the ability of the kidney to conserve electrolytes. Identification of WBCs and numerous bacteria indicates a urinary tract infection. Protein in the urine (proteinuria), glucose in the urine (glucosuria), and casts indicate renal disease.

Evaluation of Body Fluids

Evaluation of cerebrospinal, synovial (joint), and abdominal cavity fluid provides important information pertaining to inflammation, infection, or neoplasia within that particular body cavity. These body fluids can be analyzed for total protein, total cell count, differential cell count, and bacterial culture, and in testing for specific infectious diseases.

Some neurologic diseases in horses require CSF analysis for diagnosis. Because some neurologic diseases, such as rabies, have zoonotic potential, CSF must be collected and handled with caution (e.g., protective eyewear or face shields, lab coats, and gloves) to prevent exposure to the infectious agent. In horses with spinal cord disease, CSF is collected under sedation from the lumbosacral space. With brain and brainstem disease, CSF is collected in anesthetized horses from the atlantooccipital space. See Chapter 18 for more information on sampling techniques. Normal nucleated cell counts are less than five cells per microliter (predominantly lymphocytes). The normal total protein concentration is variable depending on the laboratory but usually is less than 80 mg/dl (higher than in other species). Abnormalities in protein and cell counts can identify an inflammatory, infectious, or neoplastic process, but CSF analyses are often nonspecific. Antibodies to the agents of several equine neurologic diseases (equine protozoal myelitis, herpes myeloencephalopathy, equine encephalomyelitis) can be detected in CSF and provide specific information regarding the cause of neurologic signs. Complications associated with a CSF tap include iatrogenic (operator-induced) spinal cord trauma and the introduction of bacteria into the CNS.

Abdominal pain, an abnormal rectal examination, abdominal distention, and fever of unknown origin are indications for abdominocentesis in horses. See Chapter 18 for more information on sampling techniques. Normal abdominal fluid is straw yellow colored and clear, has a total protein of less than 2.5 mg/dl, and has a normal total nucleated cell count less than 5000/ml (50% neutrophils). Analysis of abdominal fluid can reveal devitalized bowel in horses with acute abdominal pain (colic), an abdominal abscess, a tumor in horses with a mass in the abdomen identified via rectal palpation or abdominal ultrasound, and a ruptured bladder in foals with abdominal distention. Complications of abdominocentesis include traumatic bowel rupture, intra-abdominal hemorrhage from trauma to the spleen, and iatrogenic septic peritonitis.

Bacterial Culture and Susceptibility Testing

The veterinary technician often plays an important role in bacteriologic testing of specimens collected from patients with infectious disease. Specimens (blood, joint fluid, abdominal fluid, feces, urine, wound exudate, infected bone, etc.) are frequently collected from horses with infectious disease for culture. Following proper procedures during collection and transport of these specimens to the laboratory for culture and susceptibility testing improves the chances of growing the causative organism. Specific guidelines must be followed for the collection and transport of different types of specimens. For example, blood is usually placed in a special enhancement medium immediately after collection for transport to the laboratory. Special methods are used for the collection and transport of samples submitted for aerobic and anaerobic culture. Identifying the causative agent in an infectious process and determining the in vitro susceptibility pattern to antibiotics are often critical in choosing the appropriate antibiotic regimen. Fecal samples are often submitted for *Salmonella* spp. or *Clostridium* spp. cultures from horses with diarrhea. Fecal samples for *Salmonella* spp. culture should be submitted at least 12 hours apart for five samples. If culture results are negative for these five samples, the horses are not shedding *Salmonella* organisms. Fecal samples may be tested for *Clostridium* toxins and *Clostridium* spp. culture; samples should be submitted daily for 3 consecutive days. Fecal samples may be submitted for other diagnostic tests, such as ELISA for rotavirus, or PCR for *Salmonella* or *Clostridium*.

Polymerase Chain Reaction Testing

Polymerase chain reaction (PCR) is a laboratory technique that identifies and amplifies a specific segment of genetic material (DNA) from bacteria, viruses, or animals. Because DNA samples are unique, this technique allows very sensitive and specific diagnostic testing for bacterial and viral pathogens, as well as for heritable genetic diseases. The sample tested depends on which test is being performed. For example, PCR is the diagnostic test of choice for the neurologic form of EHV-1. Because the virus circulates within the white blood cells, the sample of choice is whole blood, specifically the buffy coat containing white blood cells. PCR detects a DNA sequence that is unique to the neurologic form of EHV-1 and differentiates it from respiratory forms.

PCR is also useful in the diagnosis of PHF by detecting *N. risticii* in whole blood samples, salmonellosis and clostridiosis by identifying specific species of the bacteria in fecal samples, and strangles by identifying *Streptococcus equi* subsp. *equi* in samples from the guttural pouch.

PCR can be used to diagnose genetic disorders by identifying the segment of DNA specific to the disease. PCR is used for the diagnosis of a number of inherited disorders, including hyperkalemic periodic paralysis (HYPP), polysaccharide storage myopathy (PSSM), glycogen branching enzyme deficiency, malignant hyperthermia, and hereditary equine regional dermal asthenia. For example, HYPP is caused by a point mutation (a single nucleotide difference in the DNA sequence) in the sodium channels of muscle cells. PCR analysis of blood or hair samples from the patient allows diagnosis of the disease. Because PCR allows detection of animals that are carriers of a genetic defect, it can be used to screen animals before breeding to eliminate the risk of passing on the disorder.

> **TECHNICIAN NOTE** Horses normally have yellow serum as a result of a high serum bilirubin level compared with other species because they do not have gallbladders. Serum bilirubin concentrations increase dramatically if feed is withheld for longer than 24 hours. This condition, which is called *fasting hyperbilirubinemia*, is a normal physiologic response in horses and does not indicate liver disease.

Food Animal Medicine

With fewer veterinarians choosing food animal practice, practice owners have found it increasingly difficult to hire a veterinary associate. For these individuals, optimizing the use of veterinary technicians is of great importance. Capitalization of technician skills can help meet client and patient needs and can improve practice productivity and efficiency, as well as increasing revenue by leveraging the veterinarian. As is done in small animal and equine hospitals, veterinary technicians working in well-managed food animal practices perform a wide variety of tasks and take on all nursing responsibilities. Veterinarians focus on those tasks that they alone can do by law (surgery, diagnosis, prognosis, and prescription) and delegate all nursing and support care tasks to veterinary technicians. Thus in fiscally savvy food animal practices, veterinary technicians perform laboratory procedures, diagnostic tests, diagnostic imaging (Figure 20-13), anesthesia, preparation of pharmacologic and biological agents, and administration of injections or other treatments. They assess and monitor hospitalized patients using the technician practice model and carry out the orders of the attending veterinarian by completing medication and treatment orders. On a herd level, veterinary technicians can assist with ration balancing, body condition scoring, metabolic profiling of herds or flocks, monitoring of health, and planning of herd consultation visits. Veterinary technicians

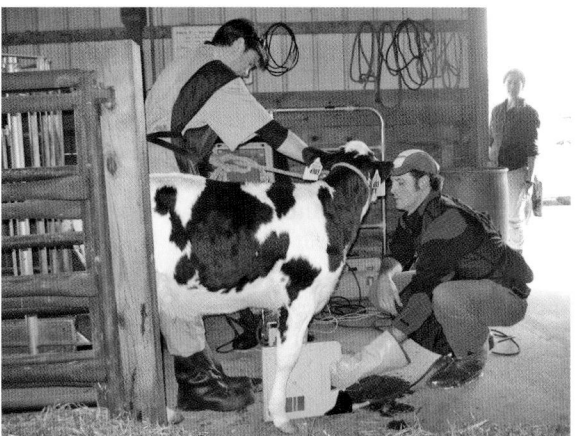

FIGURE 20-13 Veterinary technicians in food animal practice may assist with a variety of procedures. Here, veterinary technicians work collaboratively to obtain digital radiographs on a calf.

can perform necropsies and collect tissue specimens. During necropsy, the veterinary technician may record findings and take digital pictures for subsequent review by the veterinarian. Technicians may also possess special talents or training, such as expertise in artificial insemination or corrective foot trimming. A cognizant, well-trained, and knowledgeable technician can anticipate the needs of the food animal patient and producer, thereby enhancing the productivity of the food animal medical team.

> **TECHNICIAN NOTE** Capitalization of veterinary technician skills in food animal practice can help meet client and patient needs and can improve practice productivity, efficiency, and revenue.

COMMON DISEASES AND CONDITIONS OF RUMINANTS

CARE OF THE NEONATE AND NEONATAL DISEASES

Calves

Food animal veterinarians often assist cows and heifers that have difficulty calving. Calves that are born via forced fetal extraction or cesarean section (C-section) are frequently compromised. Although the veterinarian attends to the dam, especially in the case of a C-section, the veterinary technician can provide intensive care to the neonate, if necessary. The most important first steps are to place the newborn calf into sternal recumbency and ensure that it is breathing. All mucus should be cleared from the nose, mouth, and upper airway. The calf may be briefly hung upside down with the head off the ground to allow drainage of these fluids, and then the calf should be replaced to a sternal recumbency position. A piece of straw or hay may be used to tickle the nose and stimulate respiration. Additionally, placement of digital pressure on or a small-gauge needle into the nasal septum is often a successful respiratory stimulus. Hypothermic stimulation, or pouring cold water over the head and ears, can induce a gasp reflex and stimulate respiration. For difficult cases, doxapram hydrochloride, a respiratory stimulant, may be injected under the tongue to induce respiration. If these techniques fail, artificial respiration can be provided by mouth-to-nose resuscitation, or by raising and lowering the upper forelimb while simultaneously pressing and releasing the rib cage. Once the calf is breathing, it should be vigorously rubbed dry with a towel, and the umbilical cord should be dipped in iodine or chlorhexidine solution.

Colostrum ingestion soon after birth is critically important for neonatal survival and prevention of infectious disease. The placenta in cattle and other ruminants prevents in utero transfer of immunoglobulins (antibodies) from the dam to the fetus. As a result, these species are essentially **agammaglobulinemic** at birth and rely on ingestion and absorption of colostrum antibodies and nonantibody immune factors to protect newborns from infection during the first few months of life. Transfer of immunity can be compromised by colostrum deficiencies, ingestion failure, or absorption failure. Specialized epithelial cells in the jejunum and ileum absorb antibodies by pinocytosis. These cells are replaced soon after birth by normal intestinal epithelial cells, and absorption of antibodies terminates within 24 hours of birth. Therefore, it is important that the neonate receives an appropriate dose of colostrum within the first 6 hours of life. The calf should receive colostrum at the rate of 10% of its body weight within the first 4 to 6 hours.

Several laboratory tests are available for direct or indirect detection of **failure of passive transfer (FPT)** of maternal antibodies, including single radial immunodiffusion (SRID), sodium sulfite precipitation, zinc sulfate turbidity, and serum total solids (STS) analysis. Most laboratory tests are considered impractical or too expensive for routine use. However, STS can be measured inexpensively using a hand-held refractometer. An STS concentration greater than 5.5 g/dl, in the absence of dehydration, is indicative of successful passive transfer. Primarily, STS testing is useful for monitoring the overall success of a farm's colostrum feeding program. If at least 80% of calves have STS greater than 5.5 g/dl, the farm is considered to have an adequate colostrum feeding program. Veterinary technicians may play a valuable role in monitoring a farm's colostrum feeding program by collecting blood samples (Figure 20-14) once weekly from newborn calves (1 to 7 days old) and analyzing each calf's STS concentration.

Partial or total FPT can make a calf susceptible to a variety of disease conditions. For valuable calves, treatment of FPT may be achieved by plasma transfusion. Compromised calves are more likely to develop umbilical infection (omphalophlebitis), which may lead to any combination of the following problems: septicemia, septic arthritis, anterior uveitis, meningitis, vegetative endocarditis, pneumonia, and diarrhea. Calves experiencing these problems should immediately be given broad-spectrum antimicrobial agents, supportive therapy, such as fluids with dextrose and electrolytes, and other treatments specific to the problems encountered. If omphalophlebitis is present and does not respond

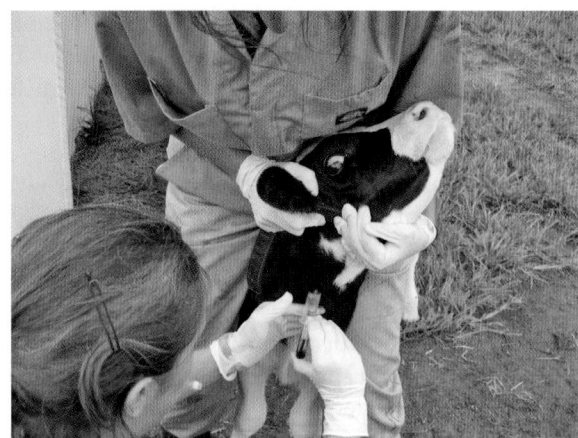

FIGURE 20-14 Blood collected from a newborn calf is used to monitor the farm's colostrum feeding program.

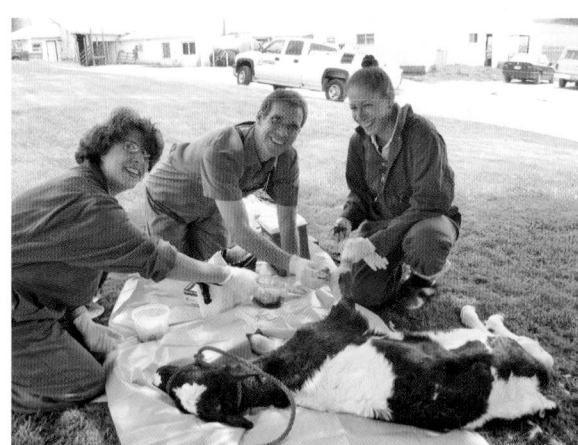

FIGURE 20-15 Delicate procedures, such as joint lavage in this Holstein calf, may be performed in the field with the assistance of a veterinary technician.

to antimicrobial therapy, surgical removal of infected umbilical remnants should be considered if the patient is a good surgical candidate. Septic arthritis should be treated with broad-spectrum systemic antibiotics and one of the following treatments: IV regional antibiotic perfusion, joint lavage (Figure 20-15), or arthrotomy.

> **TECHNICIAN NOTE**   Colostrum ingestion soon after birth is an important part of the prevention of infectious disease in neonates, and veterinary technicians may play a valuable role in monitoring a farm's colostrum feeding program.

Calf Scours

Diarrhea or scours, a common problem among young dairy and beef calves, is associated with multiple infectious and noninfectious causes. Viral causes include rotavirus, coronavirus, and bovine viral diarrhea (BVD) virus. Bacterial enteritis (Figure 20-16) may result if the calf is infected with *Escherichia coli*, *Salmonella* spp., *Clostridium* spp., and

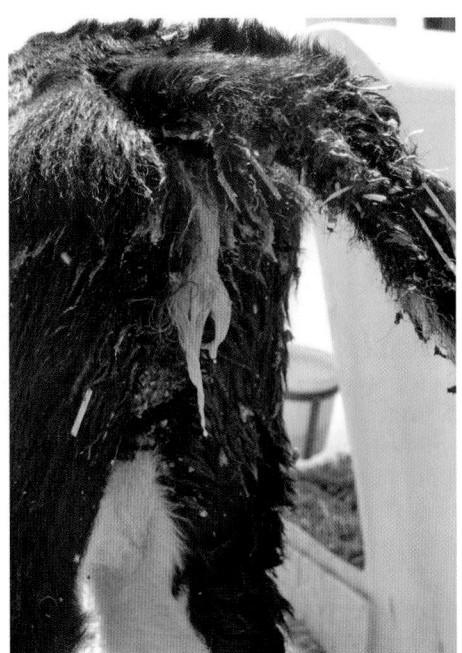

FIGURE 20-16 Bacterial enteritis in a young Holstein calf.

protozoal pathogens, such as coccidia or *Cryptosporidium*. In addition, a variety of management conditions, including poor nutrition and improper sanitation, may cause or contribute to the development of diarrhea. Regardless of cause, affected calves often develop watery diarrhea, rapidly leading to severe dehydration, metabolic acidosis, **hypoglycemia**, shock, and hypothermia. Treatment is aimed at rapid replacement of lost fluids and correction of acidosis and electrolyte abnormalities. Sick, weak calves should be started on warm, balanced IV fluids supplemented with dextrose and bicarbonate. Oral electrolyte solutions may be administered to replace lost fluids, but it is important that the calf's normal milk or milk replacer feedings also be offered. On farms where calf diarrhea is a persistent problem, it is very important to ensure adequate colostrum feeding, and it may be necessary to vaccinate cows and heifers before calving.

White Muscle Disease

White muscle disease (WMD), also known as *nutritional myodegeneration*, occurs in young calves, lambs, and kids born to dams receiving diets deficient in selenium during gestation. Dietary deficiency of selenium and/or vitamin E may cause degeneration of cardiac or skeletal muscle. If skeletal muscles are affected, muscular weakness or stiffness followed by eventual recumbency and death may occur. If the heart is primarily involved, sudden death can occur. On necropsy, skeletal and cardiac muscles appear pale and may have the white streaks that give the disease its name.

Early cases of the skeletal form of WMD may respond to injections of vitamin E and selenium. Prevention includes ensuring that the dam's ration has adequate amounts of vitamin E and selenium and administering supplements of selenium to the dam before parturition in areas of the country where soil is deficient in selenium. Selenium can be toxic, so the manufacturer's recommendations must be followed carefully.

Lambs and Kids

A successful lambing and kidding season begins with a ewe or doe health check at least 1 month before parturition. Dams should be vaccinated annually during this time with *Clostridium perfringens* type C and D toxoid and *Clostridium tetani* toxoid. This is usually available as a single combination vaccine. By boostering the animal before lambing or kidding, colostral antibodies will be improved for the neonate. As with calves, young small ruminants are born with an immature immune system and rely on colostral antibodies for disease protection. Subsequently, passive transfer of antibodies to lambs and kids will help to provide protective immunity against these specific clostridial diseases while the young are still nursing. Once weaned, these animals will be given their primary vaccination series for these diseases, usually at around 2 to 3 months of age.

One of the most important components of successful rearing of lambs is establishment of a strong ewe-lamb bond. Sheep are gregarious and stay together as a group, even during lambing; this may result in lamb "stealing" by late-pregnant ewes. Lambing in individual pens (lambing jugs, 4 feet square and 30 inches high) helps to prevent this from happening. Licking of amniotic fluid from the lamb by the ewe clears the lamb's airway, stimulates breathing, and allows the ewe to identify that lamb as her own. Intervention provided during or right after parturition by the owner or veterinarian might confuse the ewe as to whether or not the lamb is hers. Ewes are capable of identifying their own lamb(s) after only a few hours of contact, whereas lambs require several days before they can identify their mothers. This is another reason for using individual lambing pens. Treatment of the lamb for hypoglycemia, chilling, or illness should be provided in the lambing pen if at all possible because separation of the lamb for longer than 1 hour may result in rejection of the lamb by the ewe.

The first week of life, especially the first 48 hours, is the most critical time for lambs and kids; as much as 50% of lamb and kid mortality occurs during this time. Two major problems that may occur are hypothermia and hypoglycemia. The relatively large body surface of a lamb (vs. body mass) can serve as a significant drain of body heat and energy. Lambs and kids are born with minimal body fat stores; therefore, hypoglycemia can develop if newborns do not ingest colostrum (high in fat) within the first 12 to 24 hours. The dam's udder should be checked immediately postpartum to ensure that it is producing milk and that mastitis is not present. Ewes tend to have a thick wax plug that blocks the end of the teat before initial nursing. Occasionally, the lamb is unable to remove the plug when it begins to nurse, and this results in unsuccessful nursing. Lambs and kids should be examined for congenital problems that might affect nursing, such as cleft palate.

Hypothermia and hypoglycemia usually can be prevented with good management practices. Pens should be built to prevent drafts and may even be designed with a supplemental heat source (heat lamp) for lambs. Securing a corner of the pen and providing a heat source in that area attracts lambs away from the ewe, so that they may rest safely from possible accidental trauma from the dam. It is helpful to have frozen sheep or goat colostrum on-hand, but cow colostrum may also be used. A small percentage of lambs have developed neonatal isoerythrolysis-type syndrome around 10 days after ingesting cow colostrum. Commercial lamb and kid milk replacers are available for orphan rearing or to supplement lambs or kids of poor-producing mothers. Lambs and kids need to be fed 10% to 15% of their body weight daily divided into three to four feedings during the first few days after birth. Later, twice-a-day feeding is adequate. They should be offered hay and starter grain early, but milk should be the major energy source until they are at least 6 weeks old. If a lamb or kid is hypoglycemic and hypothermic, it is best to rewarm the animal before providing any oral therapy. During a hypothermic crisis, the lower esophageal sphincter relaxes, and milk or oral supplements may be regurgitated, potentially resulting in aspiration. Rewarming when the core body temperature is low is best achieved by immersing the neonate in warm water (100° F to 105° F) while taking care to support the head. Veterinary technicians may be instrumental in herd or flock management during the kidding or lambing period.

> **TECHNICIAN NOTE** The key to successful rearing of lambs is the establishment of a strong ewe-lamb bond; lambing in individual pens (lambing jugs) helps establish this bond.

Enterotoxemia

Enterotoxemia caused by *C. perfringens* is recognized worldwide as a common, frequently fatal disease of young sheep and goats. Aspects of enterotoxemia in small ruminants include severe enterocolitis, sudden death, diarrhea in goats, and neurologic signs in lambs. The main cause of enterotoxemia is *C. perfringens* type D, a Gram-positive anaerobic rod that produces toxins. Many outbreaks of enterotoxemia involve dairy goats raised under intensive management conditions, whereas the greatest losses in sheep occur among lambs in feedlots receiving concentrated rations. Although outbreaks have occurred in situations where feeding practices were consistent, sudden feed changes such as accidental exposure to grain, turnout to lush pasture, feeding of bran or molasses mash to recently fresh animals, and feeding of bakery goods have been associated with enterotoxemia epidemics. In ruminant species, it is believed that commensal *C. perfringens* type D organisms reside in the intestines, but sudden ingestion of readily fermentable carbohydrate-rich feed serves as a nutrient substrate for rapid proliferation of the organism. Death of the animal is due to damage to vital neurons, generalized toxemia, and shock. Clinically, lambs show lethargy, overt neurologic signs, minimal diarrhea, and death, as opposed to kids, which show more prominent diarrhea and colic and fewer neurologic signs followed by death.

Treatment of enterotoxemia consists of IV fluids, *C. perfringens* type C and D antitoxin, anti-inflammatories, and antibiotics. In addition, cathartics and absorbents, such as activated charcoal, magnesium sulfate, and kaolin-pectin, have been used. In the face of an outbreak, previously vaccinated animals should receive a booster vaccination, and unvaccinated animals should be vaccinated and given antitoxin. Rations containing high-carbohydrate feeds should be adjusted immediately. Small ruminants are considered highly susceptible to enterotoxemia and should be vaccinated every 6 months. In herds with a history of disease, 4-month vaccination intervals may be more appropriate. Initial vaccinations should be followed 3 to 4 weeks later by booster vaccinations; semiannual or triannual vaccinations should be followed 3 weeks before parturition by booster vaccinations for maximal benefit for the newborns. Kids should be vaccinated at 4 to 6 weeks of age and again at weaning. Vaccines with *C. perfringens* type C and D with or without tetanus are preferable to polyvalent clostridial vaccines available for cattle.

> **TECHNICIAN NOTE** Small ruminants are considered highly susceptible to enterotoxemia and should be vaccinated every 6 months.

DIGESTIVE SYSTEM

Disorders of the gastrointestinal system that require medical management are common in ruminants and are frequently addressed by veterinarians and food animal producers. A summary of common infectious and noninfectious diseases of adult ruminants is included in Table 20-5. Several of these conditions are considered an emergency, and rapid assessment by a veterinary technician improves the likelihood of a positive outcome. Other gastrointestinal diseases are more chronic and may negatively affect the productivity of the animal.

Analysis of rumen fluid is useful to establish the cause of rumen dysfunction, such as occurs with grain overload. Evaluation of a rumen fluid sample includes assessment of color, consistency, odor, pH, microscopic examination, rumen chloride, and redox potential. The normal color of rumen fluid is olive or brownish green. Grain overload results in fluid that is milky gray, whereas prolonged stasis or decomposition in the rumen changes the color to dark green or black. The consistency of normal rumen fluid is slightly viscous, and salivary contamination increases viscosity. The odor of normal rumen fluid is aromatic and strong, but it develops an acidic smell with grain overload and a putrid odor with stasis and decomposition.

The pH of rumen fluid is normally 6.5 to 6.8 (5.5 to 6.5 with high-grain diets). Rumen fluid pH less than 5.5 is suggestive of grain overload. Microscopic examination is performed to assess the types of bacteria present and protozoal

TABLE 20-5	Common Medically Managed Gastrointestinal Conditions of Ruminants				
DISEASE/ETIOLOGIC AGENT	**SPECIES AFFECTED**	**PATHOGENESIS**	**CLINICAL SIGNS**	**DIAGNOSIS**	**TREATMENT**
Infectious Actinomycosis (lumpy jaw)/*Actinomyces bovis*	Bovine	• Normal bacterial flora of ruminant mouth • Entry via mouth wounds • Infection results in osteomyelitis of the mandible or maxilla	• Hard, immovable bony mass on mandible or maxilla • Inability to masticate • Subsequent anorexia and weight loss	• Oral examination • Radiography • Isolation of organism from infected tissues	• Sodium iodide and antibiotics • Surgical débridement • Anti-inflammatories
Actinobacillosis (wooden tongue)/*Actinobacillus lignieresii*	Bovine, ovine	• Normal bacterial flora of ruminant mouth • Entry via mouth wounds	• Cattle: tongue is hard with diffuse nodular swellings • Sheep: swellings around lips and face • Excessive salivation • Inability to masticate • Subsequent anorexia and weight loss	• Oral examination • Biopsy and isolation of the organism	• Sodium iodide and antibiotics • Anti-inflammatories
Winter dysentery/ Coronavirus	Bovine	• Fecal-oral transmission	• Explosive diarrhea • Mild depression • Partial anorexia	• Fecal samples for laboratory diagnostics	• Supportive treatments • Usually spontaneous recovery within a week
Bovine viral diarrhea (BVD) virus	Bovine	• Natural exposure to the virus • Persistently infected (PI) animals may have mucosal disease if they are exposed to a cytopathic strain of virus	• Fever • Weight loss • Diarrhea • Mucosal ulceration • Blunted oral papillae • Highly variable clinical presentation	• Physical examination • Identification of virus in blood by laboratory testing • Serology (acute and convalescent)	• Supportive fluid therapy • Prophylactic antibiotics
Parasitism	Bovine, caprine, ovine	• Ingestion of infective larvae	• Chronic diarrhea • Weight loss • Unthriftiness • Pale mucous membranes	• Fecal float	• Anthelmintics
Johne's disease/ *Mycobacterium paratuberculosis*	Bovine, caprine, ovine	• Oral ingestion during perinatal period • In utero transmission	• Cattle: chronic diarrhea • Weight loss	• Fecal samples for laboratory diagnostics • Serology	• None • Prevention important
Salmonellosis	Bovine, caprine, ovine	• Fecal-oral transmission	• Severe diarrhea, which may include blood or mucus • Fever • Anorexia	• Fecal samples for laboratory diagnostics	• Supportive fluid therapy • Anti-inflammatories • Prophylactic antibiotics

Continued

TABLE 20-5	Common Medically Managed Gastrointestinal Conditions of Ruminants—cont'd				
DISEASE/ETIOLOGIC AGENT	**SPECIES AFFECTED**	**PATHOGENESIS**	**CLINICAL SIGNS**	**DIAGNOSIS**	**TREATMENT**
Enterotoxemia/ *Clostridium perfringens* types C and D	Bovine, caprine, ovine	• Normal inhabitant of GI tract • Sudden diet change—increased carbohydrates • Rapid overgrowth and subsequent toxin production	• Sudden death • Hemorrhagic diarrhea • Fever • Glucosuria	• Fecal samples for laboratory diagnostics	• Antibiotics • Supportive fluid therapy • Anti-inflammatories • Antitoxin • Prevention with vaccine
Noninfectious Pharyngeal abscessation	Bovine	• Trauma associated with improper oral administration of treatments	• Pharyngeal swelling • Anorexia • Excessive salivation • Malodorous breath • Extension of head and neck • Mild bloat • Fever	• Careful digital palpation of the pharynx per os • Endoscopy • Radiography	• Antibiotics • Anti-inflammatories • Supportive therapy if animal cannot eat or drink
Rumen indigestion	Bovine, caprine, ovine	• Rapid feed changes • Moldy or spoiled feeds • Change in rumen environment	• Acute anorexia • Decreased rumen motility • Malodorous diarrhea	• History • Physical examination • Rumen fluid analysis	• Transfaunation • Supportive fluid therapy
Grain overload (carbohydrate engorgement, lactic acidosis)	Bovine, caprine, ovine	• Excessive intake of carbohydrates • Increased volatile fatty acids (VFAs) and lactic acid • Decreased rumen pH and motility • Increased rumen osmolarity leading to severe dehydration	• Depression • Anorexia • Bloat • Diarrhea • Dehydration • Incoordination • Recumbency • Death	• History • Physical examination • Rumen fluid analysis	• Lavage rumen or rumenotomy surgery • Oral antacids • Antibiotics • Supportive fluid therapy • Anti-inflammatories
Rumen tympany (bloat)	Bovine, caprine, ovine	• Free gas bloat: obstruction of eructation • Frothy bloat: consumption of legumes or grains leading to stable rumen froth	• Severe abdominal distention • Dyspnea • Depression • Anxiety	• History • Physical examination • Passage of orogastric tube	• Passage of orogastric tube • Oral administration of detergent • Supportive fluid therapy • Anti-inflammatories
Traumatic reticuloperitonitis (hardware disease)	Bovine	• Indiscriminate eating habits leading to accidental ingestion of sharp foreign body • Penetration of reticulum and subsequent peritonitis	• Fever • Anorexia • Reluctance to rise or move • Cranial abdominal pain • Kyphosis	• Radiography • Ultrasonography • Blood work (complete blood work [CBC], plasma fibrinogen) • Abdominocentesis	• Oral magnet • Antibiotics • Surgical intervention to remove foreign body

activity. In healthy animals, Gram-negative bacteria predominate in the rumen. The rumen chloride concentration is normally less than 25 mEq/L but may be elevated in cases of ileus or obstruction. The redox potential test uses new methylene blue (NMB) to evaluate anaerobic fermentation. To perform the test, 1 ml of 0.03% NMB is mixed with 20 ml rumen fluid (control sample is untreated rumen fluid). The rumen microflora, if active, reduces NMB, and the mixture returns to the color of rumen fluid. This usually takes about 3 minutes (1 to 3 minutes if on a grain diet; 3 to 6 minutes if on a hay diet).

Pharyngeal Trauma and Abscessation

Pharyngeal trauma occurs relatively frequently in cattle and may result in cellulitis, abscess, or hematoma formation. It is almost always caused by trauma associated with improper use of a balling gun, long-dose syringe, speculum, paste dewormer gun, or rigid stomach tube. Less commonly, a foreign body (sharp stick or wire) may penetrate the pharynx. Clinical signs include anorexia, salivation, malodorous breath, extension of the head and neck, feed coming from the nares, and mild bloat. In more severe cases, fever, obvious pharyngeal swelling, dysphagia, coughing, and aspiration pneumonia may occur. Careful digital palpation of the pharynx per os is often diagnostic. Always wear gloves during palpation of the mouth or pharynx in cattle because of the concern of rabies. Endoscopy and radiography may be of great benefit in diagnosing the site of the lesion, the extent of the cellulitis, and the presence of a foreign body.

Treatment requires aggressive use of antimicrobial drugs for 10 to 14 days. Anti-inflammatories may help reduce inflammation in early stages of the disease. Supportive therapy is also important, especially if the animal cannot eat or drink. Feed and water may be administered with a soft stomach tube or via a temporary rumenostomy. The best way to prevent this condition is to exercise caution when using balling guns, dose syringes, and stomach tubes. It is critical that the animal's head is adequately restrained to prevent excessive movement and subsequent injury (Figure 20-17). The veterinary technician can play an important role in educating food animal producers about proper use of this equipment.

> **TECHNICIAN NOTE** Pharyngeal trauma in cattle can be prevented by careful use of oral dosing equipment.

Rumen Indigestion

In ruminants, the term *indigestion* describes the disruption of normal reticulorumen function; this condition is very common in ruminants. It results from a rapid feed change or introduction of feed materials that rapidly change the rumen environment. Moldy or overheated feeds are typically implicated. Clinical signs include acute anorexia, reduced rumen motility, and potentially malodorous diarrhea. The disease is self-limiting, and affected cattle return to normal

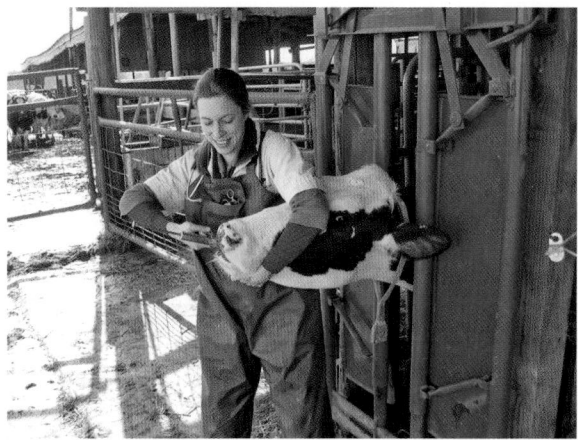

FIGURE 20-17 This veterinary technician is demonstrating proper restraint of a cow's head during administration of medicine with the use of a balling gun.

function in a few days. Diagnosis is usually based on history and clinical signs. Rumen fluid analysis may be useful in confirming the diagnosis. Rumen transfaunation is the single best way to return normal rumen function. Additionally, oral fluids and probiotics may supplement treatment.

> **TECHNICIAN NOTE** Indigestion is a very common disease in ruminants. It is usually self-limiting.

Grain Overload (Carbohydrate Engorgement, Lactic Acidosis)

Grain overload in ruminants results from consumption of excessive amounts of highly fermentable carbohydrate feed and subsequent production of large quantities of lactic acid in the rumen. Excess carbohydrate ingestion leads to increased production of volatile fatty acids by rumen microflora; this lowers rumen pH and decreases rumen motility. *Streptococcus bovis* organisms then proliferate and produce large amounts of lactic acid, which further lowers rumen pH (4.0 to 5.0). Additionally, *Lactobacillus* spp. are acid-resistant, and this allows them to proliferate and produce more lactic acid. The result is an increase in rumen fluid osmolarity, and so fluid is drawn into the rumen. This creates characteristic "splashy rumen" sounds and leads to severe dehydration and metabolic acidosis. If affected animals are not treated early, they may develop severe metabolic acidosis leading to shock and acute death. Animals that do not die from acute acidosis may develop secondary problems, such as rumenitis, liver abscess, laminitis, and/or **polioencephalomalacia.**

Ruminants with grain overload rapidly develop clinical signs of depression, anorexia, bloat, diarrhea, dehydration, incoordination, and recumbency leading to death. The diagnosis is based on a history of sudden exposure to large amounts of grain, typical clinical signs, and a rumen pH of less than 5.0. Rumen fluid analysis can confirm the diagnosis.

Medical treatment involves rapid removal of rumen contents. In cattle, this may be achieved by lavaging the rumen with a large-bore stomach tube or by performing rumenotomy surgery. In small ruminants, rumen lavage is not possible with a large-bore tube, and rumenotomy is required. In addition, animals are given oral antacids, antibiotics, anti-inflammatories when rehydrated, and thiamine, all of which help to prevent liver abscess, polioencephalomalacia, and laminitis. In more severe cases, IV fluids with sodium bicarbonate should be administered to correct dehydration and acidosis. Whether an animal is treated medically or surgically, rumen transfaunation is often helpful to reestablish normal rumen microflora and improve appetite.

> **TECHNICIAN NOTE**   Grain overload is an emergency situation in ruminants and may lead to death if rapid patient assessment and subsequent treatment are not provided.

Rumen Tympany (Bloat)

Gas production is a normal occurrence during rumen fermentation, and healthy animals are capable of eructating the gas that the rumen produces. However, in some cases, abnormal distention of the rumen with gas may occur, resulting in bloat. Bloat is described as free gas bloat or frothy bloat depending on the cause. Free gas bloat results from failure to eructate normally and may be associated with esophageal foreign bodies (choke); motor function abnormalities of the rumen, such as vagal indigestion; body position (lateral recumbency); hypocalcemia; or pharyngitis. Frothy bloat occurs when large quantities of legumes or certain grains are ingested, resulting in development of froth in the rumen that blocks eructation. Clinical signs of bloat include distention of the left paralumbar fossa, discomfort, dyspnea with open-mouth breathing, anorexia, salivation, anxiety, depression, and sudden death.

Treatment of free gas bloat involves passing an orogastric tube. If hypocalcemia is the underlying problem, administration of calcium is therapeutic. Forced exercise stimulates rumen motility and eructation. In addition, rumen stimulants improve motility and normal belching. If an animal is critically bloated and passing a stomach tube is too stressful, an emergency procedure called *rumen trocarization* should be performed.

Frothy bloat requires different treatment because the froth must first be dissipated before gas can be expelled from the rumen. To reduce surface tension of the froth, several products may be used, including poloxalene, household detergent, mineral oil, or dioctyl sodium sulfosuccinate (DSS). Once the frothy bloat becomes a free gas bloat, it can be eructated or relieved via an orogastric tube.

Traumatic Reticuloperitonitis

Traumatic reticuloperitonitis (TRP), or hardware disease, results from penetration of the reticulum by a foreign body and is one of the most common gastrointestinal problems affecting the forestomach compartments of mature dairy

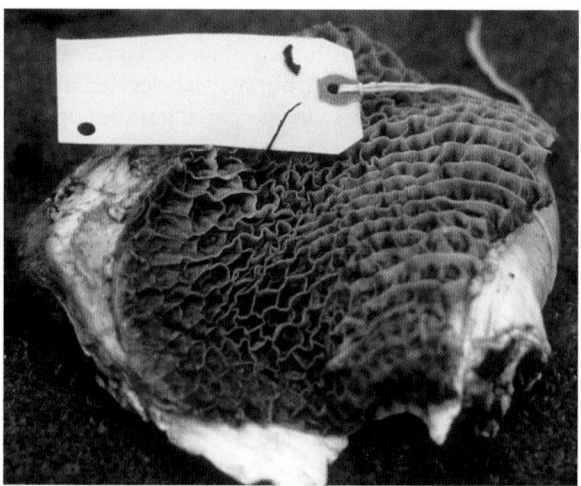

FIGURE 20-18 Cattle are indiscriminant eaters. Hardware disease in cattle is the result of metallic foreign bodies unknowingly being swallowed. These objects will settle in the reticulum and eventually may penetrate through the wall of the reticulum. In this photo, a thin metal wire protruding from the wall of the reticulum is visible against the light colored luggage tag.

cattle. The indiscriminate eating habits of cattle, in contrast to small ruminants, can lead to accidental ingestion of foreign materials that settle in the reticulum (Figure 20-18). Foreign bodies ingested by cattle, like wires and nails, are usually ferromagnetic. Subsequent to ingestion of a foreign body, four outcomes are possible:

1. Attachment of the object to a magnet without further disease problems.
2. Penetration of the reticular wall with acute inflammation and mild clinical disease if no penetration into the peritoneal cavity occurs.
3. Perforation of the reticular wall into the peritoneal cavity with acute localized TRP.
4. Migration of the foreign body with penetration into the peritoneal or thoracic cavity and resulting abscessation (thoracic, reticular, hepatic), vagal indigestion, **pericarditis**, myocarditis, or other secondary problems.

Acute cases of TRP result in anorexia, a sharp decrease in milk production, reluctance to rise or move, cranial abdominal pain, and kyphosis. Uncomplicated cases may improve in 3 to 5 days, but progression of the severity of signs may indicate failure to contain localized peritonitis or extension of the infection to other organs. A heart rate greater than 90 bpm or a high fever generally indicates more severe disease, such as diffuse peritonitis or pericarditis. A heart rate less than 60 bpm is suggestive of vagal indigestion. Cranioventral abdominal radiography or ultrasonography can offer valuable assistance in the diagnosis of TRP.

Peritoneal fluid analysis may be helpful in the diagnosis of TRP, especially in chronic cases, when WBC changes are infrequently observed. It may be necessary to sample multiple sites because of the size of the rumen, and cattle are capable of localizing an infection by depositing a large amount of fibrin. Failure to obtain a fluid sample does not rule out TRP. A relatively accurate diagnosis of peritonitis can be made if the nucleated cell count of peritoneal fluid is greater than 6000 cells/µl and the total protein is greater than 3 g/dl.

Medical treatment of TRP is often successful and is geared toward treating reticulitis and/or peritonitis by the use of systemic broad-spectrum antimicrobials and preventing further perforation of the reticulum by oral administration of a magnet. Even if a foreign body has perforated the reticular wall, a magnet may return the foreign body to the lumen. Surgical intervention may be necessary if TRP fails to respond to medical treatment.

> **TECHNICIAN NOTE** Traumatic reticuloperitonitis (TRP) or hardware disease is caused by the ingestion of sharp metallic objects, such as wire. Sharp objects can perforate the wall of the reticulum, causing peritonitis and liver and reticular abscesses, and can perforate the pericardium, causing pericarditis.

Endoparasitism

Endoparasitism is a severe problem for small ruminants. Although sheep and goats differ in terms of feeding behavior, where sheep graze and goats browse, they can be infected with the same internal parasites. Typical internal parasites include *Haemonchus contortus*, *Ostertagia ostertagi*, and *Trichostrongylus* spp. The most important parasite of small ruminants in North America is *Haemonchus contortus*, also known as *the barber poll worm*, aptly named for the spiraling of blood-filled intestines around the white-colored ovary and uterus. These parasites have developed multi-drug resistance after years of indiscriminant anthelmintic administration. As a result, parasite control has been a major problem in small ruminant flocks and herds.

Severe parasitism results in anemia, pale mucous membranes, subcutaneous edema ("bottle jaw") caused by hypoproteinemia, ill thrift with poor fleece or wool, and weight loss. Feces may be soft, but diarrhea is rarely observed. Sudden death may be observed in animals that have a severe, acute parasite infection.

In severe cases, immediate anthelmintic administration using an effective dewormer is recommended. Fecal flotation and McMaster fecal egg count can be performed before anthelmintic administration and can be repeated 10 to 14 days after treatment to determine the therapeutic effectiveness of the dewormer. It is recommended that a greater than 90% reduction in fecal egg count per gram of feces occurs when an effective dewormer is used. Blood transfusions may be required in animals with a PCV less than 10%. Animals should be kept in a quiet, confined environment with good-quality forage with high protein content and with water easily accessible. Prevention of severe parasitism includes pasture rotation, strategic deworming protocols using effective anthelmintics, and selective culling of animals with heavy parasite burden.

Salmonellosis

Salmonellosis typically manifests as acute diarrhea, but in rare cases, individuals become chronically infected and have

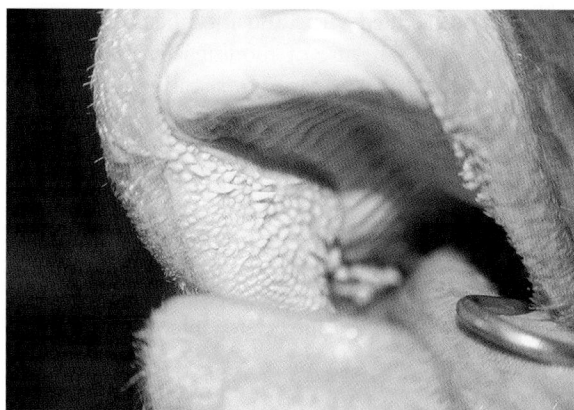

FIGURE 20-19 Blunted oral papillae seen in a calf with chronic bovine viral diarrhea (BVD)–mucosal disease.

recurring bouts of diarrhea with or without fever, anorexia, and dehydration. Severe acute cases may progress to endotoxemia, shock, and subsequent death. Animals that survive may continue to carry and shed the organism, posing a threat to other animals. Submission of multiple fecal samples for culture is necessary to establish a diagnosis. Because of the recent isolation of multi-drug–resistant strains, the use of antibiotics for treatment of salmonellosis is controversial. Treatments include anti-inflammatories, fluid therapy, particularly in young animals with septicemia and/or endotoxemia, and potentially antibiotics, depending on the condition of the animal and the strain isolated.

Bovine Viral Diarrhea Virus

Bovine viral diarrhea (BVD) is a common viral pathogen affecting all ages of cattle. BVD can manifest as sudden onset of fever, depression, anorexia, oral and GI ulcers and erosions, and diarrhea (sometimes with blood and mucus). The disease may progress rapidly through a group of animals. BVD also plays an important role in respiratory diseases in cattle by causing immunosuppression and susceptibility to secondary bacterial pathogens. The virus is responsible for abortions, in utero infections, and birth defects. Exposure of pregnant cattle to the noncytopathic strain of BVD between days 80 and 125 of gestation may result in an infected fetus, which becomes persistently infected (PI) and immunotolerant to the virus. Later in life, a PI calf may be exposed to cytopathic strains of BVD; this results in mucosal disease (MD) in these calves. Clinical signs of BVD-MD include intermittent or persistent diarrhea, weight loss, anorexia, unthriftiness, crusty eyes or muzzle, blunting of oral papillae (Figure 20-19), and chronic coronary band lesions. MD has nearly a 100% mortality rate. Diagnosis of BVD is made by physical examination, identification of characteristic necropsy findings, virus isolation from tissues or the buffy coat of whole blood samples, and serology (paired samples 2 to 4 weeks apart are most helpful).

No treatment is available for BVD, but antimicrobials are often used to prevent secondary bacterial infection. Vaccination of dairy and beef animals is important to help prevent the disease. Both killed virus and modified live-virus vaccines are available. The use of modified live-virus vaccines should be avoided in pregnant cows, calves, nursing pregnant cows, and immunosuppressed animals. Vaccination of calves experiencing chronic BVD using the modified live-virus vaccine may result in the death of the animal.

> **TECHNICIAN NOTE** Bovine viral diarrhea (BVD) may cause gastroenteritis, respiratory tract disease, immunosuppression, abortion, in utero infection, and birth defects in cattle.

Johne's Disease (Mycobacterium paratuberculosis)
Cattle

Johne's disease, characterized in cattle by chronic diarrhea and weight loss, is caused by *Mycobacterium paratuberculosis*, a slow-growing, acid-fast organism (Case Presentation 20-2). The bacterium is transmitted from infected cows to their calves via the fecal-oral route, with calves younger than 6 months most susceptible to infection. Although infection occurs early in life, clinical signs do not usually develop in cattle until the animal is at least 2 years of age (Figure 20-20). Often the diagnosis is made on the basis of history, clinical signs, and lack of response to conventional treatments, such as antimicrobial and anthelmintic therapy.

Johne's disease is a terminal disease for which no effective treatment is available. Control programs in cattle have been outlined for producers who wish to eliminate the disease from their herd. These programs involve the use of repeated serologic testing, fecal cultures, culling of positive or clinically ill animals, and maintenance of separate disease-free and infected herds. These programs are costly and labor intensive, so most producers choose to live with the disease, culling clinically affected cows and exposed offspring. A cattle vaccine, the use of which is state controlled, is available and is used to control the development of clinical disease in herds with a high incidence of Johne's disease.

Small Ruminants

Johne's disease in small ruminants has several unique features compared with the disease in cattle. The most important difference is that Johne's disease in small ruminants is not characterized by diarrhea. Second, although Johne's disease is more infective for younger animals, exposed adults can develop clinical signs of the disease. Agar gel immunodiffusion on a serum sample is fairly accurate and serves as a good screening test. Also, recent notable advancements have been made in fecal diagnostic testing for Johne's disease in small ruminants.

RESPIRATORY SYSTEM

Diseases of the respiratory system in ruminants are important because they are very common (Table 20-6). As a result, these pathogens are frequently an important part of the ruminant vaccination program. Many multivalent vaccines protect against both viral and bacterial respiratory pathogens. Veterinary technicians may play an important role in ensuring appropriate administration of these vaccines on farms.

Bovine Respiratory Disease Syndrome (BRDS)

Bovine respiratory disease syndrome (BRDS) affects cattle of all ages, but particularly beef calves during the first 45 days in the feedlot and dairy calves younger than 6 months of age. The syndrome is caused by a complex interaction of respiratory viruses, bacteria, and stress. Transportation, cold weather, close confinement, and exposure to viral

---

CASE PRESENTATION 20-2 CHRONIC WEIGHT LOSS AND DIARRHEA

A 4-year-old cross-bred beef cow with a 4-month history of weight loss and diarrhea was seen. She had been treated with LA200 (Liquamycin, Pfizer Animal Health, New York City) every other day for three treatments, and she had been dewormed twice with IvomecPlus (ivermectin and clorsulon, Merial, Duluth, Georgia) at monthly intervals beginning 3 months before she was seen, with no response. Clinical findings included emaciation (BCS of 2/9), submandibular edema, diarrhea, and good appetite. Differentials for chronic weight loss and diarrhea included Johne's disease, GI parasites, chronic salmonellosis, chronic renal disease, chronic liver disease, chronic BVD, and BLV. Clinical findings, chronicity of the disease, and failure to respond to conventional treatments made Johne's disease likely. A rectal mucosal biopsy was taken, and acid-fast organisms were found within the rectal mucosal cells. The cow was humanely euthanized, and gross and histopathologic findings resulted in a definitive diagnosis of Johne's disease. The owner was counseled to cull this cow's offspring, and education of the client concerning the disease impact on his herd was provided by the attending veterinary technician.

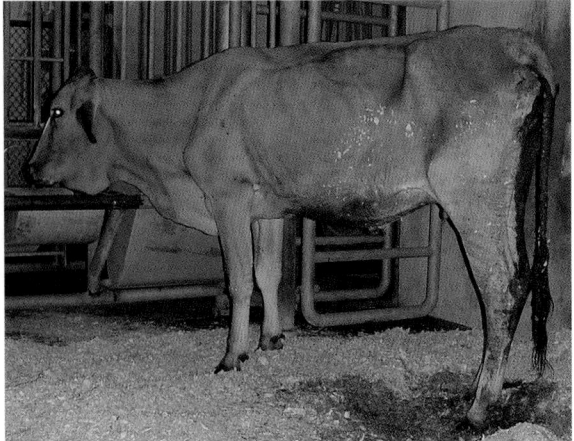

FIGURE 20-20 Severe emaciation, intermandibular edema, and chronic diarrhea in a cow with Johne's disease (*Mycobacterium paratuberculosis*).

TABLE 20-6	Common Respiratory Pathogens of Ruminants				
DISEASE/ ETIOLOGIC AGENT	**SPECIES AFFECTED**	**PATHOGENESIS**	**CLINICAL SIGNS**	**DIAGNOSIS**	**TREATMENT**
Bacterial Pathogens					
Pasteurella multocida	Bovine, Caprine, Ovine	• Normal inhabitant of upper respiratory tract • Stress or concurrent viral infection leads to pneumonia	• Fever • Dyspnea • Cough • Nasal discharge • Ocular discharge	• History • Clinical signs • Transtracheal aspirate for bacterial isolation	• Antibiotics • Anti-inflammatories
Mannheimia haemolytica	Bovine, Caprine, Ovine	• Normal inhabitant of upper respiratory tract • Stress or concurrent viral infection leads to pneumonia	• Fever • Dyspnea • Cough • Nasal discharge • Ocular discharge	• History • Clinical signs • Transtracheal aspirate for bacterial isolation	• Antibiotics • Anti-inflammatories
Histophilus somnus	Bovine	• Stress or concurrent viral infection leads to pneumonia	• Fever • Dyspnea • Cough • Nasal discharge • Neurologic signs	• History • Clinical signs • Transtracheal aspirate for bacterial isolation	• Antibiotics • Anti-inflammatories
Mycoplasma bovis	Bovine	• Ubiquitous in the environment on some farms	• Variety of clinical syndromes • Relatively mild respiratory signs: mild cough, low fever • Otitis media in calves: head tilt	• History • Clinical signs • Transtracheal aspirate for bacterial isolation	• Antibiotics • Anti-inflammatories
Viral Pathogens					
Infectious bovine rhinotracheitis (IBR)/Bovine herpesvirus-1	Bovine	• Recent herd additions • Stress • Inhalation	• High fever • Dyspnea • Nasal discharge • Cough • White mucosal plaques • Abortion • Conjunctivitis	• Physical examination and identification of characteristic plaques • Serology (acute and convalescent)	• Prophylactic antibiotics • Anti-inflammatories • Prevention: vaccination
Parainfluenza virus (PI3)	Bovine, Caprine, Ovine	• Exposure to the virus • Stress	• Fever • Coughing • Nasal discharge • Ocular discharge	• Isolation of virus • Serology (acute and convalescent)	• Prophylactic antibiotics • Anti-inflammatories • Prevention: vaccination
Bovine viral diarrhea (BVD) virus	Bovine	• Natural exposure to the virus • Recent herd additions • Stress	• High fever • Depression • Mucosal lesions • Diarrhea	• Physical examination • Serology (acute and convalescent)	• Prophylactic antibiotics • Anti-inflammatories • Prevention: vaccination
Respiratory syncytial virus (RSV)	Bovine, Caprine, Ovine	• Spread via infected respiratory secretions	• Subcutaneous emphysema • High fever • Coughing • Dyspnea • Nasal discharge	• Physical examination • Serology (acute and convalescent)	• Prophylactic antibiotics • Anti-inflammatories • Prevention: vaccination
Coronavirus	Bovine	• Natural exposure to the virus	• Fever • Coughing • Nasal discharge • Ocular discharge	• Nasal swab for identification of virus • Serology (acute and convalescent)	• Prophylactic antibiotics • Anti-inflammatories

and bacterial pathogens predispose to the development of respiratory disease. BRDS in feedlot cattle is often referred to as shipping fever.

Generally, infection with one or more of the respiratory viruses occurs first, followed by bacterial infection of the lower respiratory tract or bronchopneumonia. A number of viruses, including infectious bovine rhinotracheitis (IBR), BVD, parainfluenza virus (PI3), bovine respiratory syncytial virus (BRSV), and coronavirus, may cause primary pneumonia or may predispose cattle to secondary bacterial infection. These bacteria include *Pasteurella multocida*, *Mannheimia haemolytica*, and *Histophilus somni*. Each of these bacterial pathogens may also produce respiratory disease in susceptible, immunocompromised animals.

Cattle with BRDS experience depression, standing with their heads lowered, anorexia, fever (104° F to 107° F), mucopurulent ocular and nasal discharge, cough, and dyspnea (Figure 20-21). Morbidity and mortality within a group may be quite high, depending on the immune status of the group and the pathogens involved. The diagnosis of BRDS is based on a history of the cattle undergoing stress, typical clinical signs of pneumonia, and the presence of bronchopneumonia on necropsy. Samples from a transtracheal aspirate can be submitted for cytologic examination, bacterial and viral isolation, and antimicrobial sensitivity.

Successful treatment of cattle with BRDS hinges on early diagnosis and the institution of appropriate antimicrobial therapy. Individual sick animals should be isolated from the rest of the group and treated with broad-spectrum antimicrobial therapy for at least 5 days. Antimicrobial agents typically used for the treatment of shipping fever include ceftiofur, florfenicol, tilmicosin, tulathromycin, tetracycline, and enrofloxacin. When large numbers of animals are ill, antimicrobial agents may be added to the water or feed to simplify treatment. In addition, fresh water, hay, and adequate shelter should be provided.

Metaphylaxis, which involves the mass treatment of animal populations before onset of overt disease, is commonly employed by feedlots and involves the treatment of cattle with long-acting antimicrobial agents.

Preconditioning (castration, dehorning, deworming, and vaccination) of calves before weaning and vaccination before transport from stocker to feeder operations decrease stress on cattle during these transitions and may prevent the development or lessen the severity of disease.

> **TECHNICIAN NOTE** BRDS, which affects primarily feedlot calves and dairy calves younger than 6 months of age, is caused by a complex interaction of respiratory viruses, bacteria, and stress.

Ovine Progressive Pneumonia (OPP)

OPP manifests as progressive respiratory failure but also causes mastitis ("hard bag"), neurologic signs, and arthritis. The pulmonary form is predominant in the United States, and clinical signs include exercise intolerance, open-mouth breathing, exaggerated expiratory effort, and an occasional dry cough. In the later stages of the disease, weight loss occurs despite a good appetite. The disease causes an interstitial pneumonia, and affected animals usually die within 3 to 8 months of onset of clinical signs. Diagnosis is based on clinical signs, necropsy, and serology testing.

REPRODUCTIVE SYSTEM/MAMMARY GLAND

Diseases of the reproductive system and the mammary gland are extremely common in ruminants, especially dairy animals. Therefore, veterinary technicians may be involved in programs designed to monitor or control these diseases. For example, veterinary technicians may collect aseptic milk samples for culture and then may perform the laboratory procedures required to identify common mastitis pathogens (Figure 20-22). These procedures provide veterinarians and food animal producers with valuable information that can aid in the treatment of clinical cases and the design of control strategies on a farm.

Mastitis
Cattle

Mastitis is inflammation of the mammary gland caused by invasion of the streak canal of the teat by a variety

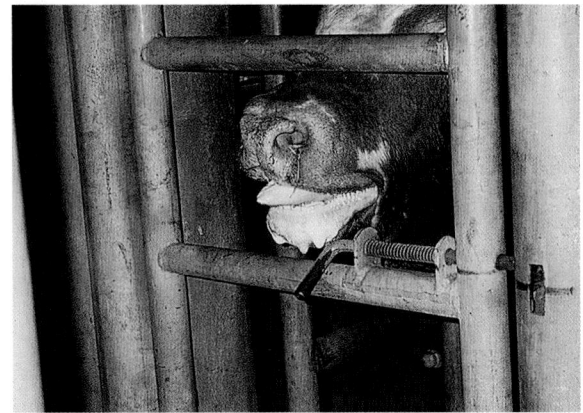

FIGURE 20-21 Severe dyspnea and open-mouth breathing in a heifer with bovine respiratory disease syndrome (BRDS).

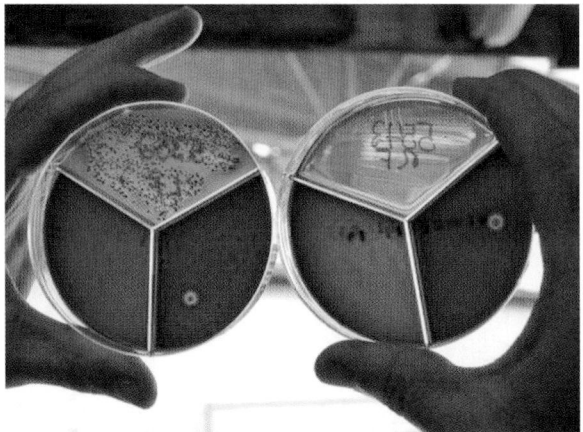

FIGURE 20-22 Veterinary technicians may be required to perform laboratory procedures to identify common mastitis pathogens of dairy cattle.

of pathogens. Economically, mastitis is one of the most important diseases in the dairy industry, and it is the single most common disease syndrome in adult dairy cows. Anatomically, the mammary gland is relatively resistant to infection, but severe environmental contamination of the teats, injury to the streak canal, or improperly functioning milking machine equipment may predispose the udder to infection.

Mastitis may be categorized in several different ways. First, there is the distinction between subclinical and clinical mastitis. Subclinical mastitis refers to an infection of the mammary gland resulting in elevation in somatic cell count (SCC) but no clinical change in milk from the affected quarter. Clinical mastitis refers to an infection resulting in elevated SCC and a clinical change in milk from the affected quarter. Second, mastitis can be subdivided into two broad but overlapping categories based on the source of the infection: contagious and environmental. Contagious mastitis is spread from an infected mammary gland to a healthy one via contaminated milking equipment, through nursing calves, or by the milker's hands. *Streptococcus agalactiae* and *Staphylococcus aureus* are examples of bacteria causing contagious mastitis. Environmental mastitis results when bacteria from the cow's environment gain access to the mammary gland and cause infection. Organisms characteristically associated with environmental mastitis cases include the coliform bacteria, like *Escherichia coli* and *Klebsiella pneumoniae*. Other mastitis-causing organisms that fall between these two broad categories, maintaining alternate niches in the host or in the environment, include *Streptococcus dysgalactiae*, *Streptococcus uberis*, and *Staphylococcus* spp.

Clinical mastitis is diagnosed by clinical examination of the milk and udder (Figure 20-23), but diagnosis of subclinical mastitis relies primarily on use of the California mastitis test (CMT). Refer to Figure 20-24 for an example of the CMT paddle. Notice that there is one cup for each quarter and teat. For more information about the CMT and instructions for completing the test, refer to Chapter 18, "Diagnostic Sampling and Treatment Techniques." Depending on the pathogen and various physiologic factors, mastitis may produce a wide range of abnormal secretions, from milk with flakes or clots to purulent material or blood. Aseptic collection of a milk sample for culture often provides important information on the cause of mastitis and may guide treatment decisions. The degree of inflammatory response varies depending on the pathogen. Cows with *toxic mastitis* are suffering from endotoxemia and usually have a watery or **serous** secretion from the affected gland. **Gangrenous mastitis** causes gangrene of the gland with a distinct blue line of demarcation separating normal and affected tissues. Secretions from affected glands are watery, gangrenous portions are cold to the touch, and these portions of the gland will eventually slough. Toxic and gangrenous mastitis may cause the death of the cow.

Depending on the causative agent, mastitis can be successfully treated if recognized early. Treatment of mastitis involves the use of appropriate antimicrobial therapy—systemic and/or intramammary. Cows with toxic mastitis usually require intensive treatment with anti-inflammatories, IV or oral fluids, and supplemental calcium. Only antibiotics approved for use in dairy cows should be administered for the treatment of mastitis. In addition, antibiotic milk withdrawal times must be closely monitored. The veterinary technician should be familiar with these approved drugs and withdrawal times and can serve as an important resource for education of the dairy farmer.

Prevention of mastitis is of paramount importance in the dairy industry. Control may be achieved by the implementation of the five-point plan for mastitis control, which includes the following:

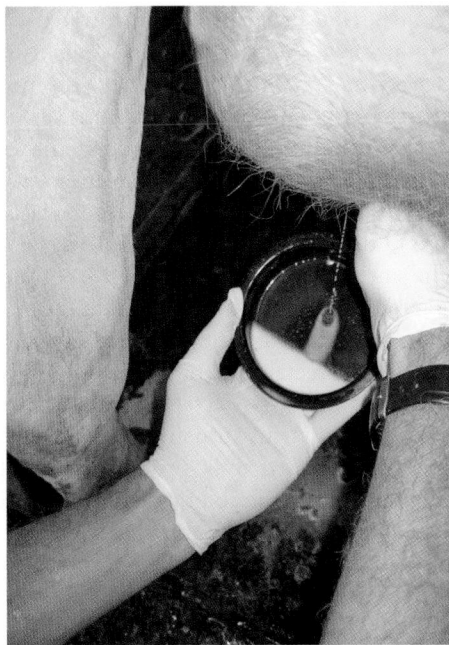

FIGURE 20-23 For diagnosis of clinical mastitis, examination of the mammary gland involves evaluation of milk stripped from the gland onto a strip cup plate.

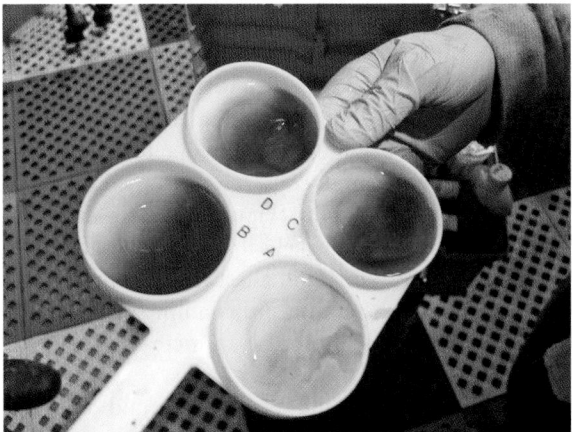

FIGURE 20-24 Subclinical mastitis in dairy cattle is often identified by using the California Mastitis Test (CMT). Testing involves stripping milk from each quarter into a corresponding well of the CMT paddle seen in this photo. A reagent is then mixed with the milk, and the degree of coagulation of the mixture is recorded.

1. Hygiene: Perform premilking and postmilking teat dipping and try to keep cows clean and dry between milkings.
2. Use proper milking procedures with well-functioning equipment when milking.
3. Practice dry cow treatment of every quarter of every cow and develop a veterinary-prescribed therapeutic plan for clinical cases.
4. Cull cows as necessary based on economics.
5. Maintain good records on each cow in terms of production, reproduction, milk quality, and clinical mastitis.

> **TECHNICIAN NOTE** Control of mastitis in cattle may be achieved by implementation of the five-point plan for mastitis control.

Small Ruminants

Mastitis in sheep and goats can be caused by a variety of bacteria, including coliforms, *Staphylococcus* spp., *Pseudomonas* spp., *Streptococcus* spp., and *Pasteurella haemolytica*. Blue bag mastitis, caused by *S. aureus* or *P. haemolytica*, is of much concern to sheep and goat producers. *S. aureus* is associated with the gangrenous form of mastitis and may be severe enough to cause death of the animal. *P. haemolytica* infection may lead to abscess formation in the udder. Treatment of mastitis is similar to that provided for cattle.

Additionally, ovine progressive pneumonia (OPP) can result in mastitis. With this disease, the ewe's udder and milk will appear normal; however, the udder will feel firm when palpated as a result of the presence of fibrous connective tissue that occurs with OPP. Development of fibrous tissue in the udder results in markedly decreased milk production.

> **TECHNICIAN NOTE** Infection with *S. aureus*, which is most likely to be associated with the gangrenous form of mastitis in sheep and goats (blue bag), may progress rapidly, resulting in death of the animal.

Retained Placenta (Fetal Membranes)

Retained placenta is a common postpartum disease affecting dairy cattle. After calving, the placenta usually is passed within 2 to 4 hours and is considered retained if it has not been expelled by 12 hours (Figure 20-25). The cause is unknown, but it is more likely to occur after the birth of twins, after abortion during the last half of pregnancy, and in cases of **dystocia**. Selenium and vitamin A and E deficiencies have been suggested to cause an increased incidence of retained placenta.

Manual removal of the placenta should be avoided because this may result in endometrial damage and infection with prolonged uterine involution and delayed breeding. Although uterine infusion is controversial, most veterinarians agree that cows with signs of systemic illness resulting from retained placenta should receive systemic antibiotic

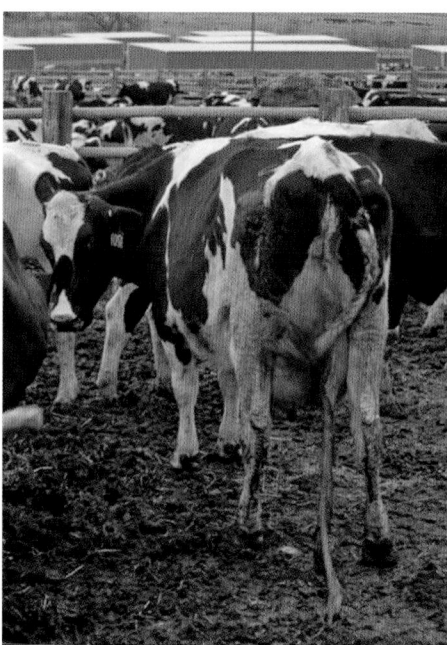

FIGURE 20-25 Holstein first calf heifer with retained fetal membranes.

therapy. If nutrition is suspected as a predisposing factor, the ration should be evaluated to ensure that it contains recommended levels and ratios of energy, protein, calcium, vitamins A and E, and selenium.

Metritis

Postpartum uterine infection, or metritis, is common in dairy cattle and is less common in beef cattle and small ruminants. Uterine infection in ruminants is associated with retained placenta, dystocia, delivery of twins, and unbalanced prepartum diets. Many bacterial species have been isolated from bovine uterine infections, but the organism most commonly associated with bovine metritis is *Arcanobacterium pyogenes*. *Endometritis* refers to infection of only the endometrial layer of the uterus, and is very common. Primarily, these infections do not cause systemic effects but may reduce fertility. *Septic metritis* (acute puerperal metritis) refers to severe uterine infection of the endometrium and deeper layers of the uterus during the 1 to 10 day postpartum period. The most severe manifestation—perimetritis—is relatively rare and involves infection of all uterine layers.

Diagnosis of metritis in cattle is done primarily by physical examination and rectal palpation. Detection of abnormal uterine discharge after transrectal palpation is diagnostic. Cows with septic metritis usually have fever, anorexia, depression, and decreased milk production. Treatment of metritis involves systemic antibiotic therapy and use of anti-inflammatories. If a dairy farm is experiencing high levels of metritis, it may be important to review dry cow nutrition and evaluate the farm's calving management.

Pseudopregnancy

Pseudopregnancy is a common pathologic condition in goats that may develop in does with or without exposure to a buck. The condition is characterized by accumulation of fluid in the uterus and one or more corpora lutea (CL) on the ovaries. Adult goats seem to be more prone than yearlings to development of the condition. Out-of-season breeding or breeding delayed until after the first or second estrous cycle during the fall breeding season appears to cause a higher incidence of pseudopregnancy. Treatment involves the use of luteolytic products, such as prostaglandin (PG) F2alpha. Successful lysis results in uterine evacuation of fluid.

METABOLIC DISORDERS

Periparturient Hypocalcemia (Milk Fever)

Milk fever is a common metabolic disease affecting periparturient dairy cows and is the result of a severe decline in serum calcium, usually occurring within 48 hours of calving. This disease rarely occurs in first-calf heifers, and the incidence of the condition increases with the age of the cow. Hypocalcemia results from feeding dry cows a high-calcium diet, which causes lack of response by the parathyroid gland and a decrease in vitamin D levels. As a result, the cow is slow to mobilize calcium reserves from the bone when there is a sudden demand for calcium at the beginning of lactation.

Cows with hypocalcemia develop muscle tremors, weakness, and a staggering gait, eventually leading to recumbency. Cows with milk fever often lie in sternal recumbency with their head turned into the flank. Affected cows have a dry nose, rumen atony with bloat, and no urine or feces production. Unless the cow is treated quickly, she may die from the effects of low serum calcium. Cows in the early stages of milk fever (before recumbency) often respond to the administration of oral calcium. For recumbent cows, slow administration of IV calcium gluconate is the treatment of choice. Cows often respond rapidly to calcium therapy and will begin to lacrimate, eructate, urinate, and defecate during treatment. Additional calcium gluconate should be administered subcutaneously for more prolonged calcium supplementation.

Prevention of milk fever is achieved by providing a well-balanced, low-calcium diet during the dry period. Total dietary intake of calcium should be restricted during the dry period. It is important to keep dry cows separate from the rest of the herd, so they can be fed appropriately.

> **TECHNICIAN NOTE** Milk fever is a common metabolic problem in periparturient dairy cows resulting from a severe decline in serum calcium level.

Ketosis

Ketosis occurs in high-producing dairy cows during the first few months of lactation if they are unable to meet the energy demands of lactation. To provide energy for milk production, the cow begins to mobilize fat, the breakdown of which results in the formation of ketone bodies that accumulate in the blood. Ketosis in dairy cows may result from a primary deficiency in energy intake, or it may be secondary to a disease process, such as abomasal displacement, mastitis, or metritis, that causes anorexia.

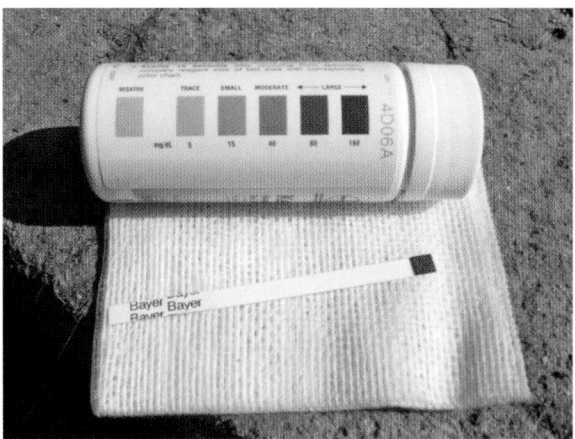

FIGURE 20-26 Cow-side diagnostic test used to detect ketosis in cattle.

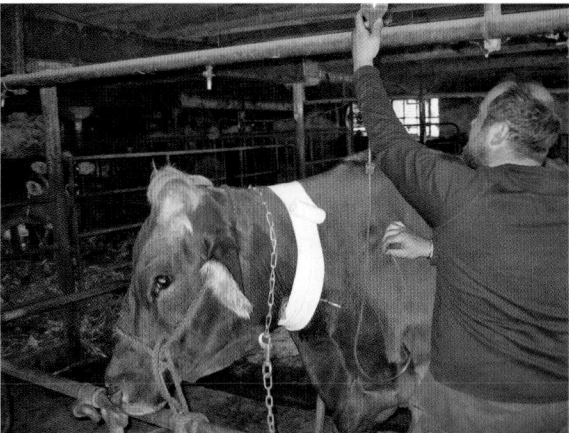

FIGURE 20-27 Cattle diagnosed with clinical ketosis must have their negative energy balance corrected. Administration of intravenous glucose solution by way of simplex tubing, as seen in this picture, aids in the correction of ketosis.

Ketones have a characteristic odor that can be detected on the cow's breath; they may be detected in the milk, urine, and blood of affected cows using a variety of cow-side diagnostic tests (Figure 20-26). Excessive quantities of ketones and a low blood glucose level may cause the cow to display central nervous system signs known as *nervous ketosis*.

Ketosis usually responds to administration of energy sources, such as IV glucose (Figure 20-27) or oral propylene glycol. It is important to determine the cause of ketosis and to correct the underlying problem. The cow's ration should be examined to make certain it contains adequate digestible energy to meet requirements for maintenance and lactation.

Pregnancy Toxemia

Pregnancy toxemia is a metabolic disease that commonly affects pregnant ewes and does during late gestation. Clinical signs can occur in pregnant animals that are overconditioned or thin, or are in normal body condition. Affected animals generally are pregnant with multiple fetuses and are in the last month of gestation. The condition is uncommon

BOX 20-2	Body Condition Score for Sheep

0   Absence of lumbar musculature and subcutaneous fat, leaving a profound depression between tips of dorsal and transverse spinous processes

1   Moderate concavity between dorsal and transverse spinous processes

2   Mild concavity between dorsal and transverse spinous processes

3   No depression (straight line) between dorsal and transverse spinous processes

4   Slight bulging (convexity) between dorsal and transverse spinous processes

5   Profound convexity between dorsal and transverse spinous processes (cannot palpate spinous processes)

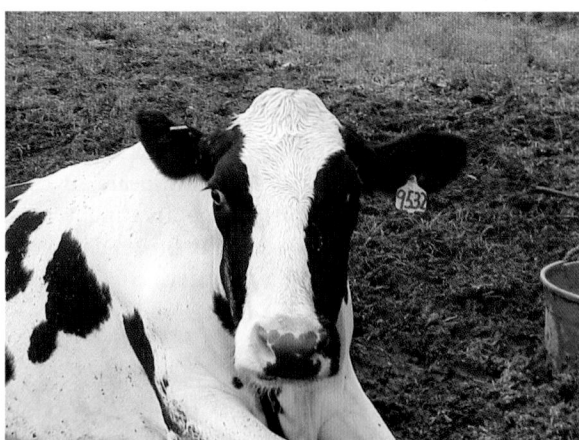

FIGURE 20-28 Clinical signs of lymphosarcoma vary greatly depending on which body system is affected. The cow in this picture depicts an alert down cow unable to rise because of a tumor mass within the spinal column. Also, note the bulging appearance of the animal's right eye.

in dams carrying a single fetus or in yearlings bred for their first pregnancy. Clinical cases usually follow a period of negative energy balance resulting in hypoglycemia, increased fat catabolism, and ketosis in susceptible animals.

A diagnosis of pregnancy toxemia should be considered whenever late-pregnant ewes or does appear weak or recumbent. Clinical signs include anorexia, hypoglycemia, ketonemia, ketonuria, weakness, depression, incoordination, mental dullness, and impaired vision, followed by recumbency and death. Urine or blood ketones can easily be checked using commercially available portable meters. Recumbency is generally indicative of a poor prognosis. Treatment often includes intravenous dextrose, propylene glycol, B-vitamins, and supplemental calcium. In addition, corticosteroids may be used to promote gluconeogenesis, increase appetite, induce parturition or abortion, and assist lung maturation in the fetus. Furthermore, it is critical to evaluate the remaining herd/flock for evidence of disease and to prevent additional cases. Preventive measures include slowly increasing the grain ration to provide additional energy weeks before parturition, deworming pregnant ewes, and decreasing stress.

Body condition scoring of ewes or does 4 to 6 weeks before the expected date of parturition allows detection of problems and subsequent time for correction. Late gestation body condition scores (BCSs) should increase to a 3 to 3.5 level at parturition. Palpation of the lumbar epaxial musculature is a rapid and relatively simple means of evaluating the BCS in sheep (Box 20-2). Although goats distribute fat deposits slightly differently than sheep, this BCS scoring system can be used in goats as well to estimate body condition.

HEMOLYMPHATIC SYSTEM

Lymphosarcoma

The adult form of lymphosarcoma is associated with bovine leukosis virus (BLV) and is the most common neoplastic disease of cattle. Lymphosarcoma is mostly likely to affect cattle between the ages of 2 and 6 years. Although many cattle are exposed to BLV and any given herd may have a high incidence of cattle with titers to BLV, the actual number of cattle that develop neoplastic disease is small (less than 5%). Malignant tumors may develop in lymph nodes, lymph tissue behind the eye or around the spinal cord (Figure 20-28), abomasum, heart, kidney, uterus, or other organs; therefore, clinical signs may vary greatly depending on the organ(s) or system(s) involved. A positive titer to BLV only suggests exposure to the virus but does not confirm neoplastic disease. No treatment or vaccine is available. Because the virus is spread by infected lymphocytes, every effort should be made to prevent the transfer of blood between infected and noninfected animals (i.e., changing needles and disinfecting surgical instruments between animals).

> **TECHNICIAN NOTE** Malignant lymphosarcoma tumors associated with BLV may develop in peripheral or deep lymph nodes, in lymph tissue behind the eye, or around the spinal cord, abomasum, heart, kidney, uterus, or other organs; therefore, clinical signs may vary greatly depending on the organ(s) or system(s) involved.

Caseous Lymphadenitis

Caseous lymphadenitis (CL) is the most common cause of lymph node abscess in small ruminants and is a major cause of carcass condemnation in sheep. This highly contagious disease is caused by *Corynebacterium pseudotuberculosis*. The disease is readily spread from animal to animal by contact with contaminated purulent material. The bacterium usually gains entry through broken skin, but the organism may also invade intact skin or may enter the body via inhalation or ingestion. Then, it infects the lymphatic system, where characteristic abscesses develop. The disease can become endemic in a herd or flock and is difficult to eradicate because of its poor response to therapeutics and its ability to persist in the environment for long periods (up to 8 months in soil).

Abscessed lymph nodes have a thick capsule and central cores of dry, green-white caseous material that may displace remnants of lymphoid tissue peripherally. The presence of external abscesses is highly suggestive of CL, particularly in an endemic herd or flock, but a culture is needed to confirm the diagnosis. Weight loss may be observed in cases of chronic, generalized infection.

In general, aggressive culling is recommended in herds or flocks with CL outbreaks because affected animals serve as reservoirs of infection. Kids and lambs should be separated from infected adults at birth and raised on pasteurized goat or cow colostrum and milk. Vaccination may be helpful in reducing the incidence of abscess; however, undesirable side effects can occur. Treatment techniques include surgical removal of unopened abscesses; lancing, draining, and flushing of opened abscesses; long-term antimicrobial therapy (4 to 6 weeks), and intra-abscess formalin or antimicrobial injection.

> **TECHNICIAN NOTE** Caseous lymphadenitis, a highly contagious disease caused by *C. pseudotuberculosis*, is the most common cause of lymph node abscess in small ruminants.

Copper Toxicity

Sheep are more prone than goats to the development of copper toxicity. Sheep absorb copper from the diet in proportion to the amount offered rather than according to the body's need. Copper accumulates in the liver, causing liver damage that precedes the onset of clinical signs. Usually, stress, such as shipping, handling, traveling to shows, and feed changes, will trigger the release of copper from the liver. Sudden release of copper from the liver causes an acute hemolytic crisis. Sources of copper that have been responsible for toxicity in sheep include trace mineralized salt, cattle mineral blocks, copper oxide wire particles, and copper sulfate foot baths. Clinical signs include depression, anorexia, weakness, hemoglobinuria, anemia, and icterus (Figure 20-29).

Although the prognosis is typically poor, therapy with D-penicillamine and ammonium molybdate helps to eliminate stored copper. Additional treatments may include diuresis with IV fluids, oxygen therapy, and potentially a blood transfusion. Even if lambs live through the acute hemolytic crisis, significant, irreversible renal damage often results from the hemoglobinuria and may result in death or necessitate humane euthanasia.

Anaplasmosis

Anaplasmosis caused by the intraerythrocytic organism, *Anaplasma marginale*, is primarily a disease of adult cattle. Red blood cells infected with the organism are removed from the blood by the liver and spleen and subsequently are destroyed, resulting in severe anemia. Associated clinical signs include pale mucous membranes, icterus, weakness, and depression or aggressive behavior resulting from anoxia

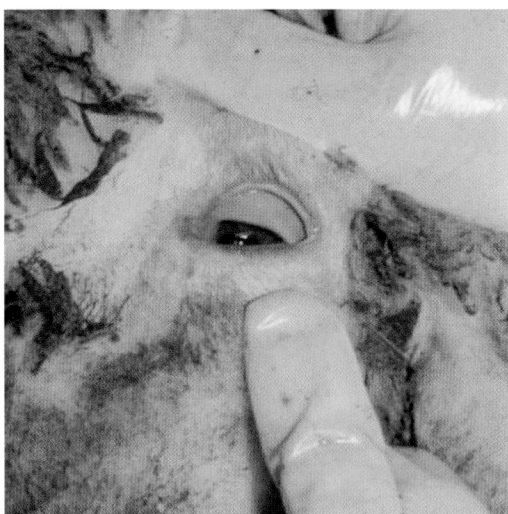

FIGURE 20-29 Icterus in animals can result from acute hemolytic crisis and is diagnosed by astute assessment of the sclera. The sheep in this picture is icteric as the result of copper toxicity.

to the brain. Anaplasmosis often causes sudden death without obvious clinical signs, and it must be differentiated from other causes of sudden death, such as anthrax, clostridial disease, bloat, and lightning. The organism is sensitive to tetracycline, so this drug is used for treatment and prevention of the disease. No commercial vaccine is currently available for the prevention of anaplasmosis.

Anthrax

Bacillus anthracis is the causative agent of this acute disease, which results in sudden death in animals and humans. Anthrax is endemic in many areas of the southern United States. Because people can easily contract the disease, it is important to not perform a necropsy on any animal suspected of dying from anthrax. Exposure of anthrax bacilli to the air, as in the case of necropsy, results in spore formation by the organism and permanent contamination of the surrounding environment. If anthrax is strongly suspected as the cause of death, the area federal veterinarian should be notified immediately. Anthrax-contaminated carcasses should be buried in lime or incinerated. A live-virus vaccine is available, and its use should be considered in high-risk areas. The organism is sensitive to penicillin, but in most cases, treatment cannot be initiated quickly enough to save the animal. In recent years, anthrax has become an important issue in cases of bioterrorism.

> **TECHNICIAN NOTE** Anaplasmosis, anthrax, clostridial disease, lightning, and bloat are causes of sudden death in cattle.

CARDIOVASCULAR SYSTEM
Vegetative or Valvular Endocarditis

Vegetative or ulcerative lesions may develop on the heart valves of cattle, in particular the right atrioventricular (AV)

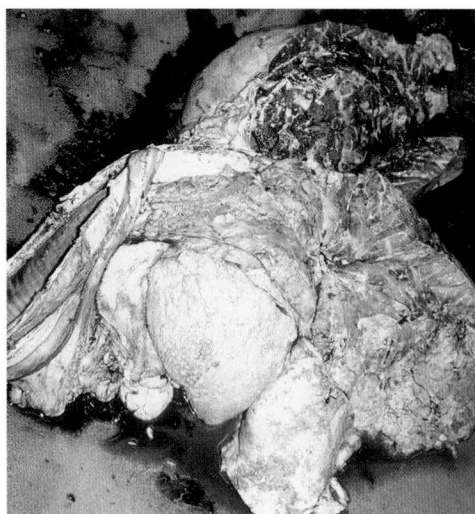

FIGURE 20-30 Severe fibrin formation with purulent exudate on the heart of a cow that died of pericarditis caused by traumatic reticuloperitonitis (hardware disease).

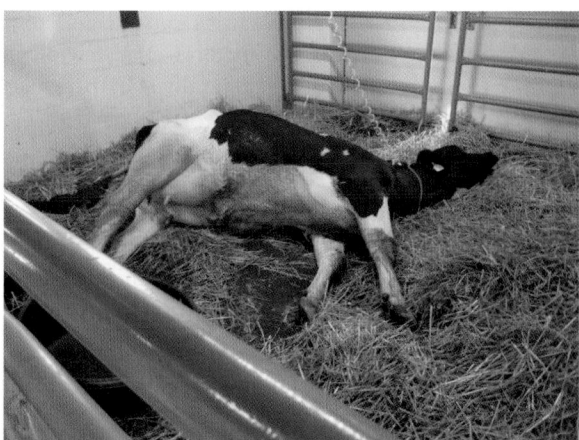

FIGURE 20-31 Although rabies in cattle is rare, any animal that presents with abnormal clinical neurologic signs (e.g., pharyngeal paralysis, opisthotonus, head pressing) should be considered a suspect, and extreme care should be taken to prevent exposure. (Courtesy Dr. Amy Johnson.)

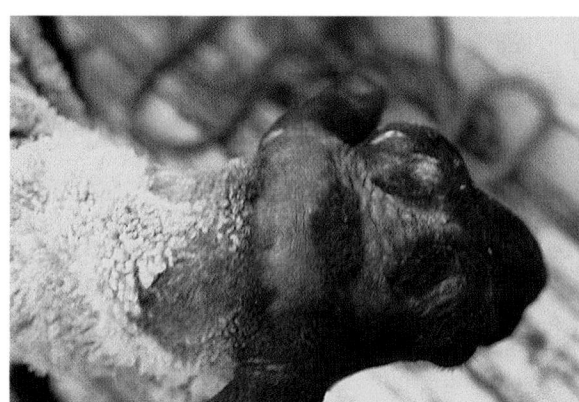

FIGURE 20-32 A ewe with scrapie exhibiting pruritus and wool loss over the poll.

valve, as a result of septic emboli from other sites. Treatment often is not successful because of inadequate penetration of the lesions with antibiotics and irreversible damage to the valves. Penicillin given at high levels for long periods has yielded the best results.

Pericarditis

Pericarditis is inflammation of the pericardial membrane surrounding the heart. In cattle, it is usually due to traumatic pericarditis, an extension of traumatic reticuloperitonitis. Pericarditis develops after penetration of the pericardial sac by a metallic foreign body. It results in a mixed bacterial infection that causes severe local inflammation and deposition of fibrinous exudates, leading to a friction rub (Figure 20-30). Effusion then develops, creating splashing sounds around the heart, especially if the fluid is mixed with gas. Fluid accumulation compromises heart function and can lead to heart failure. Clinical signs include fever, kyphosis, abduction of the elbows, shallow abdominal respirations, and characteristic heart sounds on auscultation. Signs of heart failure occur late in the course of the disease, and death is usually due to toxemia or heart failure. Treatment is difficult and requires long-term use of antibiotics and supportive therapies.

> **TECHNICIAN NOTE** Pericarditis in cattle usually is due to penetration of the pericardial sac by a metallic foreign body.

NERVOUS SYSTEM

Many disorders in ruminants affect the nervous system. Table 20-7 summarizes principal information about the most commonly seen neurologic disorders in these species.

Rabies

Rabies is a fatal, viral, neurologic disease of mammals. Rabies most often is transmitted by the bite of an infected wild animal, with skunks, raccoons, and foxes being the greatest threat to domestic livestock. Two forms of rabies may occur: the furious form, in which the affected animal demonstrates hyperexcitability, fear, or rage; or the dumb form, in which extreme depression, paresis, or paralysis manifests (Figure 20-31). Definitive diagnosis of rabies is made by examination of the suspected animal's brain on necropsy. Several vaccines are available for use in ruminants. Rabies poses a serious human health concern; therefore, care should be taken when handling animals suspected of having rabies.

Scrapie

Scrapie is a transmissible spongiform encephalopathy (prion protein) that manifests primarily as weight loss. Other clinical signs include pruritus with wool loss (Figure 20-32), ataxia, fine muscle tremors of the face, head pressing, abnormal gait, and disorientation. Scratching of the sheep's back usually will elicit nibbling or licking of the lips. An antemortem diagnosis may be attempted by immunohistochemistry on biopsy of lymphoid tissue of the third eyelid,

TABLE 20-7	Common Neurologic Diseases of Ruminants				
DISEASE/ETIOLOGIC AGENT	**SPECIES AFFECTED**	**PATHOGENESIS**	**CLINICAL SIGNS**	**DIAGNOSIS**	**TREATMENT**
Bacterial Pathogens					
Listeriosis/*Listeria monocytogenes*	Bovine, Caprine, Ovine	• Widely distributed in environment • Ingestion of contaminated feed • Organism invades the host through breaks in mucosa	• Depression • Circling • Head tilt • Facial desensitization and asymmetry • Ataxia • Nystagmus • Dysphagia • Recumbency • Death	• Neurologic examination • Cytologic evaluation of cerebrospinal fluid (CSF) • Isolation of organism • Necropsy	• High doses of antibiotics • Anti-inflammatories • Supportive care (fluids, transfaunation, reduce musculoskeletal injury)
Tetanus/*Clostridium tetani*	Bovine, Caprine, Ovine	• Infection of deep wounds by spores • Toxin produced during bacterial growth	• Stiff gait • Saw-horse stance • Erect ears • Lock-jaw • Recumbency • Death	• History • Clinical signs	• Antitoxin • Antibiotics • Anti-inflammatories • Supportive care (fluids, sedation to relax muscles, transfaunation, reduce musculoskeletal injury)
TEME/*Histophilus somni*	Bovine	• Inoculation of respiratory/ genital mucous membrane • Blood clot formation with infection/ bacteremia	• Respiratory signs may precede neurologic signs • Recumbency • Blindness • Cranial nerve deficits • Star-gazing (opisthotonus) • Retinal hemorrhage • Death	• History • Clinical signs • Isolation of causative organism from infected tissues • Necropsy	• High doses of antibiotics • Anti-inflammatories • Supportive care (fluids, transfaunation, reduce musculoskeletal injury)
Viral Pathogens					
Rabies	Bovine, Caprine, Ovine	• Inoculation with contaminated saliva • Migration of virus through peripheral nervous system to central nervous system (CNS) • Zoonotic	• Paralytic form more common than furious form in ruminants • Depressed • Dull • Recumbency • Ataxia • Vocalization • Excessive salivation	• History • Clinical signs • Necropsy	• No treatment • Prevention: annual vaccination

Caprine arthritis encephalitis (CAE)	Caprine	• Ingestion of contaminated colostrum
		• Close or direct contact with infected animals
		• Recent herd additions
			• Locomotor deficits
			• Progressive weakness and paralysis
			• Cranial nerve deficits
			• Weight loss
			• Arthritis
			• Respiratory disease
				• Serology
				• Polymerase chain reaction (PCR) on whole blood
					• No treatment
					• Prevention:
					  ○ Heat-treat colostrum
					  ○ Feed colostrum from negative does
					  ○ Conduct periodic serologic testing of herd and cull or separate positive animals

Continued

TABLE 20-7	Common Neurologic Diseases of Ruminants—cont'd				
DISEASE/ETIOLOGIC AGENT	SPECIES AFFECTED	PATHOGENESIS	CLINICAL SIGNS	DIAGNOSIS	TREATMENT
Parasitic Pathogens					
Meningeal worm/ *Parelaphostrongylus tenuis*	Caprine, Ovine	• Ingestion of snail or slug with infective larvae • Close proximity to white tail deer population	• Ataxia • Weakness • Recumbency • Tetraplegia • Cranial nerve deficits	• History • Clinical signs • CSF analysis is suggestive • Necropsy	• High doses of anthelmintics • Anti-inflammatories • Supportive care (transfaunation, fluids, reduce musculoskeletal injury)
Metabolic					
Polioencephalomalacia	Bovine, Caprine, Ovine	• Rumen insult leading to decreased thiamine, producing rumen microflora • Increased sulfur consumption in diet or water	• Depression • Anorexia • Blindness • Dorsomedial strabismus • Ataxia • Head pressing • Recumbency • Star-gazing (opisthotonus) • Nystagmus	• Clinical signs • Thiamine level determination • Necropsy • Cerebral cortex fluorescence under ultraviolet (UV) light	• Thiamine • Anti-inflammatories • Supportive care (transfaunation, reduce musculoskeletal injury)
Nervous ketosis	Bovine	• Severe ketosis leading to central nervous system signs	• Excessive licking or chewing • Excitement • Hypersensitive • Ataxia	• Clinical signs • Large quantity of ketones detected in urine or blood	• Treatment of ketosis, including dextrose and propylene glycol • Anti-inflammatories

TEME, Thromoembolic meningoencephalitis.

submandibular lymph node, and rectal mucosa. Postmortem confirmation can be achieved by histopathologic examination or immunohistochemistry of the brain. Scrapie is a reportable disease, and no known treatment is known. Genetic testing can be performed to predict the susceptibility of individual sheep to the scrapie prion. A scrapie eradication program is currently in place in the United States. Veterinary technicians play an important role in this regulatory work.

Tetanus

Spores of the bacterium *Clostridium tetani* may infect wounds, resulting in tetanus. In an anaerobic environment, such as a wound, the organism produces several potent neurotoxins that are responsible for the typical clinical signs. The disease commonly occurs after puncture wounds or surgical procedures, such as castration, tail docking, and dehorning. Animals with tetanus develop progressive muscle tetany characterized by a "sawhorse" stance with stiff, erect ears, rigid extension of the limbs (Figure 20-33), and prolapse of the third eyelid. Affected animals are hyperresponsive to external stimuli, such as loud noises. Death is usually due to respiratory failure or aspiration pneumonia in bloated animals.

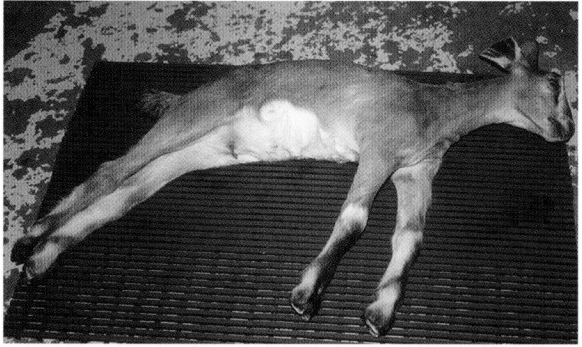

FIGURE 20-33 Severe extensor rigidity ("sawhorse" position) in a kid with tetanus.

Treatment involves removal of toxin-producing bacteria by débriding and disinfecting wounds or surgery sites. In addition, high doses of penicillin and tetanus antitoxin should be administered. Affected animals should be kept in a quiet environment and provided supportive care.

Tetanus can be prevented by administering tetanus toxoid at least 1 month before parturition. Vaccination of kids and lambs should be initiated by 6 to 8 weeks of age. Tetanus toxoid and/or antitoxin should be given to small ruminants any time surgery is performed or injury occurs.

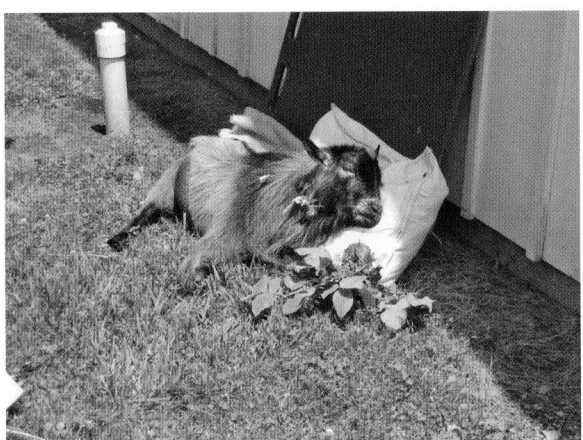

FIGURE 20-34 Goats diagnosed with listeriosis must be provided with supportive care over an extended period. (Courtesy Dr. Amy Johnson.)

> **TECHNICIAN NOTE** Small ruminants are extremely susceptible to tetanus; therefore, tetanus toxoid and/or antitoxin should be given to small ruminants any time surgery is performed or injury occurs.

Polioencephalomalacia (Polio)

Polioencephalomalacia is a CNS disease that results from an underlying defect in thiamine metabolism. This disease may occur after sudden ration changes or secondary to grain overload or excessive sulfur consumption. Animals with polio show CNS neurologic signs, including blindness, ataxia, depression, opisthotonus, convulsions, coma, and death. Early in the course of the disease, affected animals respond well to treatment with thiamine; however, the longer the animal has been affected, the longer recovery takes.

Listeriosis

Listeria monocytogenes is responsible for three different clinical syndromes in ruminants: septicemia, abortion, and neurologic disease. Neurologic involvement produces fever, anorexia, depression, **proprioceptive** deficits, head tilt, circling, and recumbency. Cranial nerve dysfunction causes unilateral drooping of the ear, eyelid, nose, and lips with excessive salivation. Although ingestion of contaminated corn silage is frequently blamed, consumption of any rotting contaminated vegetation can lead to infection.

The organism is sensitive to tetracycline and penicillin, but treatment of listeriosis often is unrewarding. Supportive care is important for a successful outcome (Figure 20-34). No vaccine is available for protection against this disease. The organism has zoonotic potential and poses a serious human health risk when contaminated milk, milk products, or meat has entered the human food supply.

Caprine Arthritis Encephalitis

Caprine arthritis encephalitis (CAE) most often affects dairy goats and causes nonresponsive arthritis (usually carpi) in adults and acute leukoencephalomyelitis in young goats. It may also cause chronic pneumonia (interstitial), chronic encephalomyelitis, chronic weight loss, and mastitis. The arthritic form is seldom seen before 1 to 2 years of age. No treatments for CAE are known. Transmission occurs primarily through infected colostrum and the milk of infected dams. Positive serology and polymerase chain reaction (PCR) are used to help diagnosis CAE. Only about 15% of seropositive goats ever develop clinical disease. Positive serology tests in kids younger than 90 days old may reflect colostral transfer of antibodies; likewise, a negative serologic test result cannot be used to exclude a diagnosis of CAE because the time required for seroconversion is variable. Control and prevention consist of periodic serology testing and aggressive culling of positive animals, separating kids from CAE-positive dams at birth, providing colostrum to kids from CAE negative does, and heat-treating colostrum before feeding.

OPHTHALMOLOGIC DISEASE

Pinkeye

Pinkeye, or infectious **keratoconjunctivitis**, usually is caused by *Chlamydia psittaci* in sheep and *Mycoplasma conjunctivae* in goats, although either organism can cause pinkeye in both species. Carrier animals and apparently uninfected animals in a herd or flock serve as an important source of infection. Both organisms may persist for months in ocular tissue and are spread by contact with infected ocular secretions. Clinical signs, regardless of the cause, include conjunctival hyperemia, ocular discharge, light sensitivity, blepharospasm, corneal edema, and vascularization of the cornea. Severe cases may result in corneal ulceration or corneal abscessation. Both infections are self-limiting, and recovery can be expected in a few weeks; however, systemic and/or topical treatment with tetracycline is recommended to prevent spread of infection and development of severe eye lesions with loss of sight.

> **TECHNICIAN NOTE** Pinkeye, or infectious keratoconjunctivitis, usually caused by *C. psittaci* in sheep and *M. conjunctivae* in goats, often is treated with tetracycline in both species.

Infectious Bovine Keratoconjunctivitis

Infectious bovine keratoconjunctivitis (IBK), or bovine pinkeye, is an infectious and contagious ocular disease of cattle characterized by conjunctivitis and corneal ulceration (Figure 20-35). Ultraviolet light and mechanical irritants, such as dust and weeds, may disrupt the corneal epithelium, allowing entry of *Moraxella bovis*, the causative agent of pinkeye. Flies have been shown to act as vectors for the bacteria. Initial clinical signs include lacrimation, blepharospasm, and photophobia. If ulceration becomes deep, the cornea may rupture, and vision will be lost.

Individual treatment of pinkeye involves subconjunctival injection of antibiotics, usually penicillin (Figure 20-36). Eye

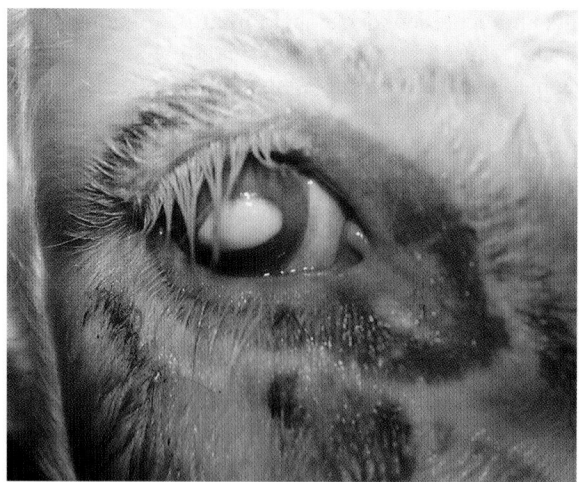

FIGURE 20-35 A large central corneal ulcer in a bull with infectious bovine keratoconjunctivitis (IBK) (pinkeye).

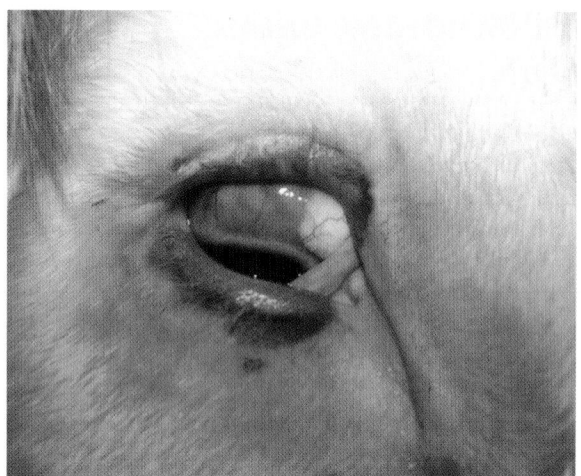

FIGURE 20-36 Penicillin injected subconjunctivally for treatment of infectious bovine keratoconjunctivitis (IBK) (pinkeye).

patches may be applied to affected eyes to decrease photophobia and protect the eye from flies. More severe cases may require surgery, such as a third eyelid flap or tarsorrhaphy (suturing the lids closed) to protect deeper ulcers as they heal. In the case of herd outbreaks, it may be impractical to treat each animal with local therapy, so systemic antibiotics, such as long-acting tetracycline, can be administered to the group.

MUSCULOSKELETAL SYSTEM

Lameness is commonly encountered in ruminants and most often is caused by lesions or problems in the foot. Upper leg problems, such as anterior cruciate ligament rupture, coxofemoral (hip) luxation, fractures, and arthritis, account for remaining cases of lameness. When foot problems occur, they most often are seen in the claws that bear the most weight—front medial and hind lateral claws. It is important to examine all foot problems early because many conditions can quickly lead to osteomyelitis and/or septic arthritis if not

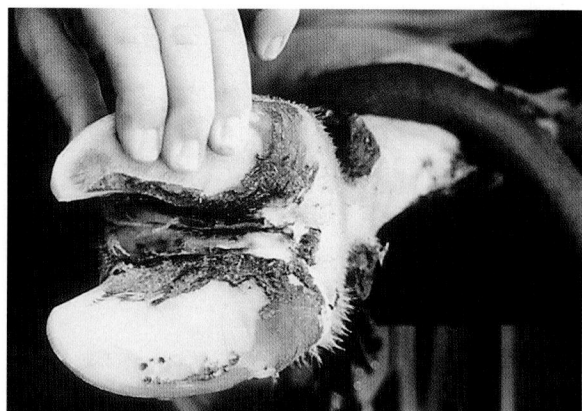

FIGURE 20-37 Interdigital necrobacillosis or foot rot in a cow.

properly treated. Regardless of the cause of lameness, it can lead to loss of production as a result of decreased milk production, weight loss, delayed breeding or anestrus, and culling. Intensive housing and feeding of large groups of animals have led to an increased incidence of lameness.

> **TECHNICIAN NOTE**   Lameness is commonly encountered in ruminants and most often is caused by lesions or problems in the foot.

Interdigital Necrobacillosis
Cattle

Interdigital necrobacillosis, or foot rot, is an infection of the interdigital skin and underlying tissues. In cattle, it is caused by *Fusobacterium necrophorum*. Infection results in an ulcerated, foul-smelling area between the claws (Figure 20-37). Swelling may be apparent above the coronary band, and in severe cases, cellulitis up to the carpus or hock may occur. The disease is particularly prevalent when ruminants are kept in wet, muddy conditions. If left untreated, foot rot can invade deeper tissues of the foot, causing septic arthritis, osteomyelitis, and chronic lameness.

Treatment for foot rot can be successfully provided as aggressive topical treatment and systemic antibiotics, such as tetracycline or ceftiofur. In some cases, it may be necessary to débride necrotic tissue and even bandage the foot with antimicrobial agents to promote healing. Preventive measures, such as foot baths, are commonly employed on farms.

Small Ruminants

Lameness in multiple animals in a herd or flock usually is due to contagious foot rot caused by *Dichelobacter nodosus* and *F. necrophorum*. Initial signs occur 10 to 20 days after exposure and include inflammation of interdigital skin, followed by slight undermining of the sole at the heels. Undermining eventually involves the sole and wall. Some sheep are resistant to infection, some improve with spontaneous clearing of infection, and others become chronic carriers of the disease. The usual source of bacteria is chronic carrier sheep or surfaces previously contaminated.

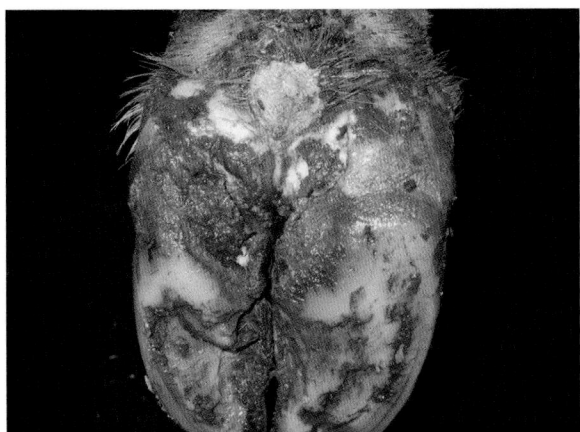

FIGURE 20-38 Papillomatous digital dermatitis or hairy heel warts of the hind feet cause severe lameness in affected dairy cattle.

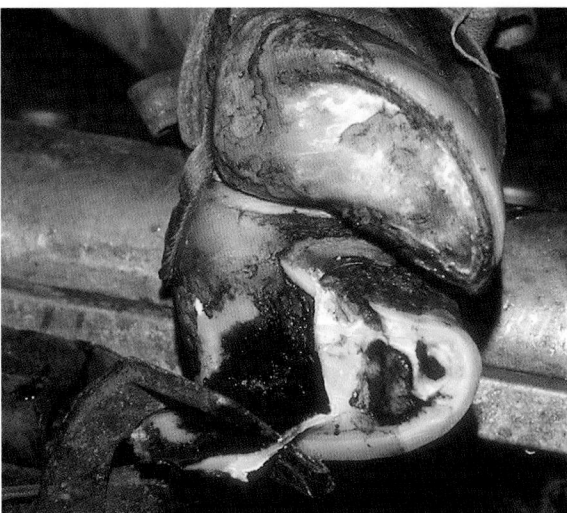

FIGURE 20-39 Debris packed between layers of sole in a bull with laminitis and subsequent underrun heel and sole.

Successful treatment involves thorough inspection of all animals and trimming and treatment of all affected animals. Animals should be divided into affected and unaffected groups and placed on clean pastures after treatment. Foot baths are useful for treatment after trimming and may contain copper sulfate, zinc sulfate, or formalin. Zinc sulfate may be the best choice because it is less irritating. Copper sulfate poses a threat if sheep can drink the bath, and formalin is a carcinogen and an environmental hazard. Once a treatment program has been initiated, all sheep should be checked weekly, trimmed if needed, and placed in the foot bath. Segregation of infected sheep and goats and culling of chronic carriers are essential for successful foot rot control.

Papillomatous Digital Dermatitis

Papillomatous digital dermatitis (PDD), or hairy heel wart, has become an important cause of lameness in dairy cattle worldwide. Initially, PDD appears as superficial inflammation of the skin of the bovine digit, but it progresses to a circumscribed, erosive, and proliferative lesion on the hind feet, adjacent to the interdigital ridge and heel bulbs (Figure 20-38). Granulation tissue develops with outgrowths of dermal tissue that grossly resemble hair, thus the common name, hairy heel wart. The disease is contagious with fairly high morbidity within any given herd. At this time, the origin of PDD is still being researched; it is believed that spirochete bacteria are involved, and *Treponema* spp. are most commonly identified. Topical antibiotics, such as oxytetracycline, are highly effective in curing individual cases. Routine use of foot baths with copper sulfate or formalin is effective for controlling this disease within a herd.

Laminitis

Laminitis, or founder, is a diffuse, aseptic inflammation of the corium (sensitive lamina) of the feet. Acute laminitis occurs sporadically and may be due to sudden excessive grain ingestion, or it may occur secondary to other diseases that occur during the postparturient period. Chronic laminitis is more often associated with constant feeding of high-grain diets, as occurs commonly in high-producing dairy cows, feedlot cattle, and show cattle.

Clinical signs include stiffness, pain, reluctance to walk, and difficulty rising. Affected animals spend a lot of time lying down, and when they do stand, they may stand with their backs arched, front legs crossed, or kneeling on the front legs in an attempt to redistribute body weight because of the pain. Acute cases of laminitis are treated by correcting any existing underlying problems and by administering anti-inflammatories. Laminitis often leads to serious sequelae, including sole ulcers, white-line disease, abnormal hoof growth with horizontal or vertical hoof-wall cracks, underrun heel and sole (Figure 20-39), and even osteomyelitis or septic arthritis. Frequent foot trimming helps to prevent these problems.

> **TECHNICIAN NOTE** Acute laminitis may be due to sudden excessive grain ingestion or may occur secondary to other diseases that occur during the postparturient period.

Blackleg and Malignant Edema

Infections by *Clostridium chauvoei* (blackleg) and *Clostridium septicum* (malignant edema) are two important causes of lameness and sudden death in young cattle. These bacteria produce spores that enter the animal through the digestive tract or through skin wounds, producing severe necrotizing myositis and cellulitis. The swollen muscle mass often contains gas pockets that are palpable as subcutaneous emphysema. Animals with these infections usually are found dead, but if they are found alive, high fever and lameness typically result from severe muscle damage. Animals identified in early stages of an infection may be treated with high doses of penicillin and surgical débridement of wounds; however, the prognosis for recovery is poor. The best way to prevent these clostridial diseases is to vaccinate calves with a multivalent bacterin; pregnant cows should be vaccinated to provide colostral antibody protection to calves.

DISEASES OF THE SKIN
Cutaneous Papillomas (Warts)

Cutaneous papillomas are a benign neoplasia caused by papillomavirus. They are common in young cattle and appear as tan, white, or gray protruding masses with a dry, horny surface. Small warts may be crushed or surgically removed to stimulate development of natural immunity and to hasten healing. Because warts are usually self-limiting, no treatment may be necessary. However, in long-standing, severe, or non-responsive cases, the immune status of the patient must be considered.

Dermatophytosis (Ringworm)

Trichophyton verrucosum is the fungus responsible for ringworm in cattle. Ringworm is most likely to occur in calves housed in crowded conditions during winter. Multiple circular lesions develop, particularly around the head and neck (Figure 20-40). If left untreated, most lesions resolve on their own in 2 to 3 months. If treatment is desired, especially in the case of show animals, topical agents, such as iodine, bleach (1 : 10 in water), chlorhexidine, or 5% lime sulfur, may be useful. The immunocompetency of the animal should be questioned in cases that do not respond spontaneously or with treatment.

Contagious Ecthyma (Orf)

Contagious ecthyma (sore mouth, orf), a common viral disease of small ruminants, causes crusty, proliferative lesions around the mouth and nose of lambs and kids and similar lesions on the teats and udder of ewes and does (Figure 20-41). The infection is self-limiting, taking 4 to 6 weeks to run its course. Because it is a viral disease, no treatment is known; however, antimicrobials may be given to prevent secondary bacterial infection. Supportive therapy may be administered to those lambs and kids too painful to nurse.

A live-virus vaccine is available, but its use should be limited to those flocks or herds already experiencing a problem. The virus is zoonotic (transmissible to humans), so care should be taken when infected animals are handled or the live-virus vaccine administered (gloves should be worn).

> **TECHNICIAN NOTE** Contagious ecthyma (sore mouth, orf), a common viral disease of small ruminants, is zoonotic (transmissible to humans), so care should be taken when infected animals are handled.

URINARY SYSTEM
Pyelonephritis

Pyelonephritis, caused most commonly by *Corynebacterium renale* or *Escherichia coli*, is an ascending urinary tract infection that often affects females because of their short, wide urethra. This infection occurs more often in the periparturient period, when animals are more stressed and the urogenital tract is more susceptible to entry of bacteria.

Clinical findings include hematuria, pyuria, straining (**stranguria**) and discomfort during urination, and frequent urination (pollakiuria). Affected ruminants may have a fluctuating fever, a variable appetite, and decreased milk production. In cattle, if the left kidney is affected, rectal palpation may reveal an enlarged, fluctuant, painful kidney.

Treatment is often unrewarding but may be attempted with high doses of penicillin given over long periods. In valuable animals in which only one kidney is affected, nephrectomy may be indicated.

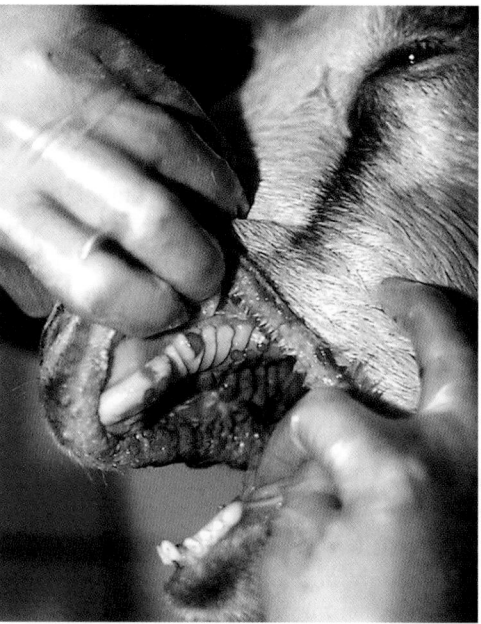

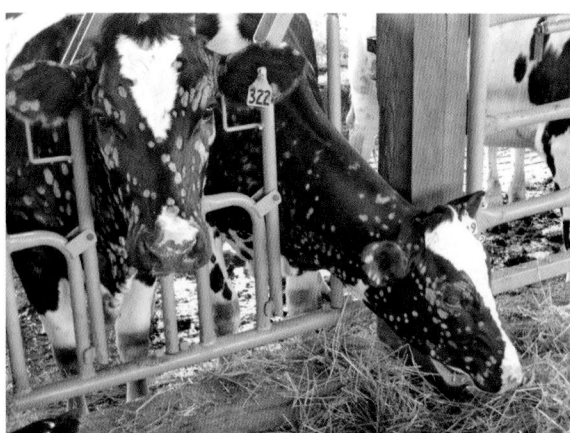

FIGURE 20-40 This picture depicts extensive lesions associated with dermatophytosis in cattle.

FIGURE 20-41 Ulcerative and proliferative lesions in and around the mouth of this doe are due to contagious ecthyma, or orf.

Urolithiasis

Urolithiasis is a common disease of small ruminants. Pets and young, castrated male animals fed a diet of grain and high-calcium forage (e.g., alfalfa, clover) are most commonly affected. The composition of the calculus is reflective of the diet. Grain-fed animals are more likely to have urinary calculi (uroliths) with struvite (magnesium ammonia phosphate) composition, and animals fed forage that is high in calcium have calculi composed of calcium carbonate.

Clinical signs, such as anorexia, weakness, or depression, may be nonspecific. More telling signs include dysuria, stranguria with dribbling of urine, vocalization, tail flagging, abdominal distention, and bruxism indicative of discomfort. Common locations for obstruction include the urethral process, which is an appendage at the distal end of the penis that is used in reproduction, and the urethra at the level of the distal sigmoid flexure.

This condition is an emergency. Treatment involves relieving the urinary tract obstruction (Figure 20-42). Excision of the urethral process under sedation might initially relieve the obstruction but typically is only a temporary solution. The urethra can be flushed to dislodge any other calculi, but these cases frequently require surgery for complete removal of the obstruction. See Chapter 33 ("Large Animal Surgical Nursing") for further information. Because of multiple electrolyte abnormalities that result from urinary obstruction, as well as the risk of cystitis or ascending infection, animals are treated with appropriate fluid and electrolytes, broad-spectrum antimicrobials, and anti-inflammatories.

Prevention of this disease is multifactorial. Urine output should be increased by stimulating water consumption by adding salt to the ration. It is recommended to acidify the urine to help increase the solubility of uroliths produced by adding ammonium chloride to the ration. Reduce or eliminate from the diet feeds such as grain and high-calcium forage.

COMMON DISEASES AND CONDITIONS OF SWINE

CARE OF THE NEONATE

Neonatal pigs have few fat stores and therefore require supplemental heat during the first few weeks of life. During the first week, the temperature of the sleeping area should be 92°F to 95°F (33.3°C to 35°C), the second week 89°F to 92°F (31.7°C to 33.3°C), and the third week 86°F to 89°F (30°C to 31.7°C). Colostrum intake soon after birth is important in this species. Adequate nutrition is also important because hypoglycemia can quickly develop in the undernourished piglet. If piglets appear hungry, the sow should be examined for mastitis or metritis, which can cause hypogalactia (low milk production) or agalactia (absence of milk production). Hypoglycemia may lead to a weakened piglet that is susceptible to a variety of diseases or crushing by the dam when she lies down. Frequent observation of the sow or gilt and of the piglets will help the clinician determine whether nursing behavior is normal. If hypoglycemia is detected, piglet(s) may be treated with 5 to 10 ml of 5% dextrose injected intraperitoneally by aseptic technique. Pigs that are rejected or orphaned, or that are not receiving adequate nutrition from the mother, may be supplemented with a milk replacer designed for pigs. Young pigs quickly learn to drink from shallow pans and therefore do not usually require bottle feeding, which can be labor intensive. These piglets can also be offered prestarter feed at an early age. Pigs are curious by nature, and by exploring their environment, they learn to eat solid feed quickly.

Processing of piglets raised in confinement includes iron dextran injections at 3 days of age (Figure 20-43), and clipping needle teeth prevents injury to the dam's udder and to other piglets in the litter (Figure 20-44). Castration may also be performed, and tails may be docked (Figure 20-45) to prevent tail biting, which can result in an ascending infection

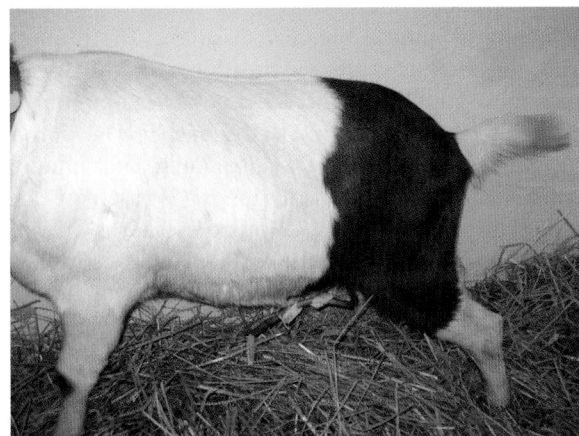

FIGURE 20-42 Urolithiasis is common in small ruminants. This is a castrated male goat that has undergone a surgical procedure to correct urinary obstruction.

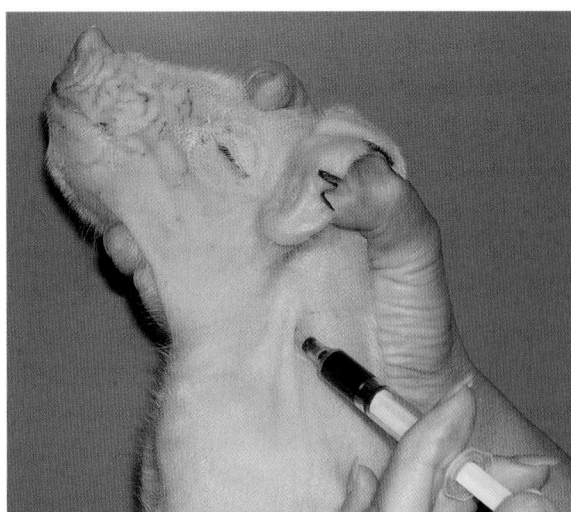

FIGURE 20-43 Baby pigs raised in confinement require iron dextran supplementation by 3 days of age.

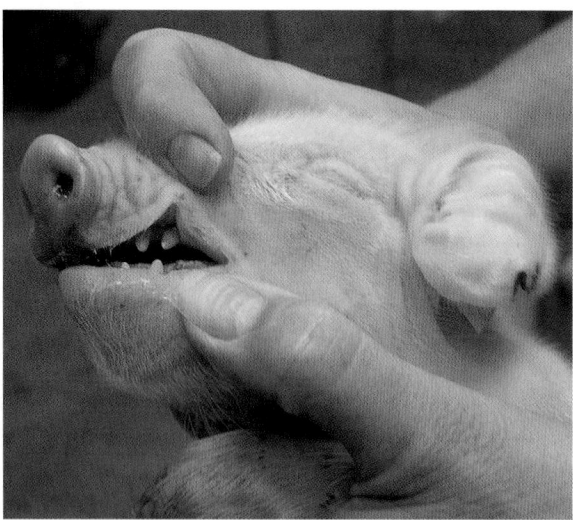

FIGURE 20-44 Needle teeth in neonatal pigs should be clipped to prevent bite injuries to the dam and littermates.

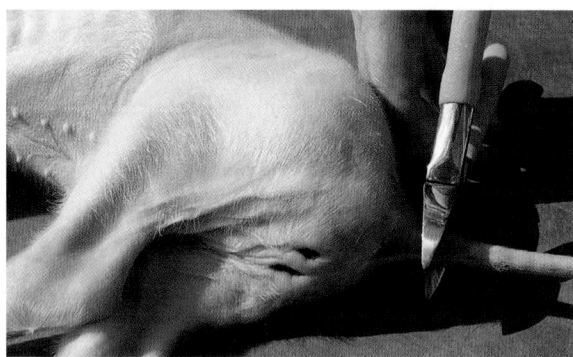

FIGURE 20-45 Tail docking is often performed at several days of age to prevent tail biting in pigs kept in confinement. Also note recent castration incisions.

of the spinal cord or spinal abscesses. These are common pig-processing techniques that are much less stressful to piglets if they are performed at a few days of age; they are important for disease prevention.

> **TECHNICIAN NOTE** Prevention of hypothermia and hypoglycemia in the neonatal period is important for successful pig rearing.

MULTISYSTEMIC DISEASES

Erysipelas

Erysipelas is caused by a bacterium that enters the body through lymphoid tissue, such as tonsil or intestinal lymph tissue, or via breaks in the skin. Up to 50% of healthy swine may carry and shed the organism. Septicemia quickly develops after infection, and the organisms tend to localize in the skin, heart, and joints. Infection causes high fever and may produce characteristic diamond skin lesions. This form often results in death if not recognized early. The chronic form of the disease is more likely to result in vegetative endocarditis

or chronic, nonsuppurative polyarthritis with lameness. The treatment of choice for the acute form is penicillin, but nothing is effective for treatment of the chronic form. Immunization against erysipelas is effective and inexpensive and should be provided at weaning and repeated every 6 months.

Pseudorabies Virus (Aujeszky's Disease, Mad Itch)

Swine are considered the natural host of pseudorabies virus (PRV), and although many other species are affected by this virus, most are dead-end hosts. Infection in baby pigs results in development of neurologic signs and in some cases vomiting and diarrhea. Mortality in this age group is high. Weaning and growing pigs exhibit fever, pneumonia, a dry, nonproductive cough, and flu-like signs. Loss to death can be high in nursery-age pigs, but fairly low in finishers. Infection in adults may cause reproductive problems, including early embryonic death, abortion, or stillbirth in pregnant sows or gilts. Serologic tests (ELISA) are used for screening herds for PRV. No treatment for PRV is known, and vaccination for the disease is closely regulated by state officials. A pseudorabies eradication program is currently in place in the United States.

> **TECHNICIAN NOTE** PRV is responsible for the development of neurologic signs in baby pigs, flu-like signs in growing pigs, and embryonic death, abortion, or stillbirth in pregnant sows or gilts.

Porcine Reproductive and Respiratory Syndrome (PRRS)

Infection with PRRS is prevalent in U.S. swine herds. The virus enters the body through the respiratory tract, replicates in the pulmonary cells, and results in pneumonia. A viremia follows, and the virus may cross the placenta to infect embryos or fetuses. General clinical signs include fever, lethargy, inappetence, and cyanosis of the ears, vulva, tail, abdomen, and snout ("blue ear disease"). The respiratory syndrome manifests as labored breathing, increased secondary respiratory infection, increased post-weaning mortality, and decreased rate of gain and feed efficiency. The reproductive syndrome includes abortion, stillbirth, fetal mummies, and the birth of weak piglets. Diagnosis is based on clinical findings, histopathologic examination, virus isolation, immunofluorescence, and/or PCR. Serology is also available, but because seroprevalence is high in U.S. swine herds, the presence of antibodies does not necessarily mean that the herd is experiencing clinical disease as a result of PRRS. No treatment for PRRS is known, but antimicrobials may be administered in the event of secondary bacterial infection. A modified live-virus vaccine is available. Control measures are variable and are dependent upon the current herd status and the goals of the producer.

GASTROINTESTINAL SYSTEM

Diarrhea in Young Pigs

Common causative agents for baby pig diarrhea include enterotoxigenic *E. coli* (ETEC) or colibacillosis, rotavirus, coronavirus or transmissible gastroenteritis (TGE), clostridial enteritis, coccidiosis, and parasites such as *Strongyloides ransomi* or threadworms (Table 20-8).

Regardless of the cause of diarrhea in young pigs, good nursing care is important for survival. Free-choice oral electrolyte solutions should be provided in shallow pans. Antimicrobials may be used if risk of secondary bacterial infection is present. Additionally, it is important to keep the piglets warm, at least at 32.2° C (90° F), to prevent loss of energy and rapid wasting.

> **TECHNICIAN NOTE** Baby pig diarrhea may be caused by enterotoxigenic *E. coli* (ETEC) or colibacillosis, rotavirus, coronavirus or transmissible gastroenteritis (TGE), clostridial enteritis, coccidiosis, and parasites (*Strongyloides ransomi* or threadworms).

Diarrhea in Grower and Finisher Pigs

Swine dysentery, salmonellosis, proliferative enteropathy (ileitis), and whipworms are common causes of diarrhea in growing and finishing swine (Table 20-9). Most treatment is aimed at prevention of these diseases by reducing pathogen exposure with good sanitation, use of all-in, all-out pig facilities, segregated early weaning, and stress reduction.

RESPIRATORY SYSTEM

Pneumonia in pigs is a common disease process that can significantly affect growth performance. Clinical signs typically include coughing, "thumping" or shallow rapid breathing, depression, and weight loss. Common causes of respiratory disease include atrophic rhinitis, swine influenza, *Mycoplasma* pneumonia, pleuropneumonia, and *Pasteurella* pneumonia (Table 20-10). These diseases have a propensity to decrease growth rate and feed efficiency. Prevention of disease is the goal of treatment, but antimicrobials can be used to help treat the causative agent or secondary pathogens.

REPRODUCTIVE SYSTEM

The typical length of gestation for swine is 114 days, or 3 months, 3 weeks, 3 days. Reproductive efficiency and improved economic return are critical for the production of swine in a commercial operation. Subsequently, it is important to optimize the number of piglets weaned per sow throughout the animal's lifetime. Therefore, it is important to minimize abortions and reproductive failure in sows. Several infectious agents are responsible for poor reproductive efficiency in swine, including PRRS, porcine parvovirus (PPV), brucellosis, and leptospirosis.

Porcine Parvovirus

PPV is present in nearly 100% of swine herds worldwide. If the virus infects a male or a nonpregnant female, the pig seroconverts and eliminates the virus with no clinical signs. If a pregnant female becomes infected, the virus crosses the placenta and infects rapidly dividing fetal cells. If the pregnancy lasts less than 30 days, the embryo is killed and is resorbed by the dam. Between 30 and 70 days of gestation, the fetus is killed and mummified, and after 70 days of gestation, the fetus mounts an immune response and survives to term, although it may be born weak or dead. The only clinical signs of PPV include reproductive problems in pregnant sows or gilts. Mummies of different sizes, stillbirths, and live

TABLE 20-8	Common Infectious Causes of Diarrhea in Young Pigs				
DISEASE/ ETIOLOGIC AGENT	**AGE AFFECTED**	**PATHOGENESIS**	**CLINICAL SIGNS**	**DIAGNOSIS**	**TREATMENT**

Colibacillosis/ Enterotoxigenic *E. coli* (ETEC)	• 0 to 6 days	• Ingestion of organism in environment after birth
		• Most often K88 virulence factor
		• Poor sanitation
			• Profuse diarrhea
			• Affects single piglets or the entire litter
			• Dehydration
			• Depression
			• Emaciation
				• Antemortem: clinical signs and age of affected piglets
				• Necropsy: isolation of organism with virulence factors
					• Supportive care (oral electrolyte solution containing glucose)
					• Antibiotics sensitive against organism
					• Prevention:
					  ○ Provide good hygiene in farrowing pens
					  ○ Pre-farrowing vaccination with Köhler milk culture (oral vaccination with live culture of farm-specific strain of ETEC)

Continued

TABLE 20-8		Common Infectious Causes of Diarrhea in Young Pigs—cont'd			
DISEASE/ ETIOLOGIC AGENT	**AGE AFFECTED**	**PATHOGENESIS**	**CLINICAL SIGNS**	**DIAGNOSIS**	**TREATMENT**
Transmissible gastroenteritis (TGE)/ Coronavirus	• 6 to 21 days	• Ingestion from contaminated environment • Poor sanitation • Dogs, cats, starlings, houseflies, and carrier pigs have all been implicated in spread of the virus • Typically in winter months	• Diarrhea • Vomiting • Inappetence • Dehydration	• Detection of viral antigen in epithelial cells of small intestine	• Provide warm, draft-free, dry environment • Make water and nutrient solution freely accessible • Prevention: ○ All-in, all-out farrowing and nursery units ○ Reduce exposure to animal vectors ○ Vaccination for sows
Enterotoxemia/ Clostridium perfringens type C	• 3 to 4 days	• Ingestion of spores from the environment	• Sudden death • Hemorrhagic enteritis with intestinal mucosal shedding	• Antemortem: clinical signs and age of affected piglets • Necropsy: isolation of organism	• Supportive care (oral electrolyte solution containing glucose) • Antitoxin • Prevention: ○ Pre-farrowing vaccination ○ Good hygiene
Coccidiosis/ Isospora suis	• 7 to 10 days	• Fecal-oral route • Observed in continuous farrowing units • Poor sanitation	• Diarrhea • Dehydration • Emaciation	• Fecal float • Small intestinal impression smears	• Amprolium • Trimethoprim-sulfonamide • Prevention: ○ All-in, all-out farrowing units ○ Provide good hygiene in farrowing and nursery pens
Parasites/ Strongyloides ransomi (threadworms)	• 2 to 14 days	• Routes of infection: prenatal, percutaneous, oral, colostrum • Larvae from the sow can accumulate in the fetus during late gestation and can migrate to the small intestine after birth	• Diarrhea • Dehydration • Unthriftiness • Poor weight gain	• Fecal float • Necropsy: detection of adult worms in small intestine	• Anthelmintics • Prevention: ○ Good sanitation
Rotavirus	• 3 to 5 weeks	• Ingestion from contaminated environment	• Same as TGE but less severe	• Electron microscopy of feces	• Same as TGE

TABLE 20-9	Common Infectious Causes of Diarrhea in Grower and Finisher Pigs			
DISEASE/ETIOLOGIC AGENT	**PATHOGENESIS**	**CLINICAL SIGNS**	**DIAGNOSIS**	**TREATMENT**

Swine dysentery/ *Brachyspira hyodysenteriae*	• Fecal-oral route	• Colitis
		• Diarrhea
		• Emaciation
		• Dehydration
			• Isolation and identification of bacteria in colon
			• Fluorescent antibody test on fecal smears
				• Antibiotics sensitive to the organism
				• Prevention:
				  ○ Maintain a closed herd
				  ○ Cull affected animals
				  ○ Good sanitation
				  ○ Segregated early weaning

Salmonellosis	• Sow to piglet via placenta
	• Ingestion of contaminated feed or water
	• Stress due to overcrowding can increase shedding of organism
		• Enterocolitis leading to profuse watery diarrhea
		• Dehydration
		• Emaciation
		• Septicemia leading to pneumonia or hepatitis
			• Isolation of causative agent via culture or polymerase chain reaction (PCR) assay	• Supportive care (oral fluids, anti-inflammatories)
				• Antibiotics may decrease severity of disease but should be used with caution because of multiple resistant strains
				• Prevention:
				  ○ Isolate or cull affected animals
				  ○ Practice good hygiene in pens, feeding areas, and water sources
				  ○ Enforce strict biosecurity protocols
				  ○ Decrease overcrowding of pens
				  ○ Improve pig comfort

Proliferative enteropathy (ileitis)/ *Lawsonia intracellularis*	• Fecal-oral route
	• Feces can be transmitted on boots and rodents
		• Intermittent diarrhea
		• Hemorrhagic diarrhea in older pigs
		• Anorexia
		• Weight loss
		• Melena
		• Anemia
			• Isolation of bacteria from feces via PCR assay
			• Necropsy:
			  ○ Thickened ileum
			  ○ Silver staining techniques will show presence of intracellular bacteria
				• Antibiotics
				• Prevention:
				  ○ Vaccinate young pigs
				  ○ Segregated early weaning
				  ○ All-in, all-out facilities
				  ○ Good sanitation

Whipworms/*Trichuris suis*	• Fecal-oral route	• Anorexia
		• Mucoid to bloody diarrhea
		• Dehydration
		• Death
			• Fecal float
			• Necropsy:
			  ○ Adult worms in cecum
				• Anthelmintics
				• Prevention:
				  ○ Good sanitation

TABLE 20-10	Common Infectious Causes of Respiratory Disease in Pigs			
DISEASE/ ETIOLOGIC AGENT	**PATHOGENESIS**	**CLINICAL SIGNS**	**DIAGNOSIS**	**TREATMENT**

Atrophic rhinitis (AR)/*Bordetella bronchiseptica* and *Pasteurella multocida*	• Sow-to-piglet and pig-to-pig contact via nasopharyngeal route
	• Chronic, progressive disease causing nasal turbinate atrophy
	• Environmental factors: high ammonia levels, stress, concurrent disease, suboptimal nutrition can contribute to lesions
		• Early signs:
		  ○ Sneezing
		  ○ Mucopurulent nasal discharge
		• Later signs:
		  ○ Twisted or shortened snouts
		  ○ Excessive tearing
		  ○ Epistaxis
		  ○ Decreased growth rate
		  ○ Decreased feed efficiency
			• Necropsy:
			  ○ Degree of nasal atrophy by cross sectioning the snout at level of 2nd premolar
				• Antibiotics
				• Prevention:
				  ○ Pre-farrowing vaccines
				  ○ All-in, all-out farrowing units
				  ○ Improved ventilation
				  ○ Eradication by depopulation and repopulation with AR-negative animals

Continued

TABLE 20-10	Common Infectious Causes of Respiratory Disease in Pigs—cont'd			
DISEASE/ ETIOLOGIC AGENT	**PATHOGENESIS**	**CLINICAL SIGNS**	**DIAGNOSIS**	**TREATMENT**

Swine influenza	• Pig-to-pig contact via nasopharyngeal route
	• Zoonotic
		• Fever
		• Conjunctivitis
		• Rhinitis
		• Nasal discharge
		• Sneezing
		• Coughing
		• Weight loss
			• Virus isolation from nasal or pharyngeal swabs
			• Necropsy:
			  ○ Virus isolation from trachea or lung tissues
				• Supportive care
				• Antibiotics for secondary infection
				• Prevention:
				  ○ Vaccination
				  ○ Good biosecurity protocols

Mycoplasma pneumonia/ Mycoplasma hyopneumoniae	• Pig-to-pig contact via nasopharyngeal route
	• Aerosol transmission
	• Most common cause of chronic pneumonia in swine
		• Dry, nonproductive cough
		• Fever
		• Decreased appetite
		• Dyspnea
			• Isolation of organism from nasal swabs
			• Serology
				• Antibiotics
				• Prevention:
				  ○ Provide adequate ventilation
				  ○ Avoid overcrowding
				  ○ Segregated early weaning
				  ○ All-in, all-out facilities
				  ○ Vaccination reduces lesions and improves weight gain

Pleuropneumonia/ Actinobacillus pleuropneumoniae	• Pig-to-pig contact via nasopharyngeal route
	• Aerosol transmission
		• Peracute:
		  ○ Death
		• Acute:
		  ○ High fever
		  ○ Dyspnea
		  ○ Coughing
		• Chronic:
		  ○ Intermittent cough
		  ○ Reduced appetite
		  ○ Decreased weight gains
			• Isolation of organism from nasal swabs
			• Serology
			• Necropsy:
			  ○ Characteristic firm, well-demarcated abscesses associated with pericarditis and pleuritis
				• Antibiotics
				• Prevention:
				  ○ Monitor herds with serology and cull positive animals
				  ○ Quarantine replacement animals before introduction to the herd
				  ○ Metaphylactic antibiotics
				  ○ Provide adequate ventilation
				  ○ Avoid overcrowding
				  ○ Segregated early weaning
				  ○ All-in, all-out facilities
				  ○ Vaccination reduces lesions and improves weight gain

Pasteurella pneumonia/ Pasteurella multocida	• Normal inhabitant of upper respiratory tract • Stress or concurrent infection leads to pneumonia	• Fever • Dyspnea • Moist, productive cough • Anorexia	• Isolation of organism • Serology • Necropsy: ○ Bronchopneumonia	• Treat primary disease • Antibiotics • Anti-inflammatories

pigs may be present in the same litter. Abortions are not typical of parvovirus infection in swine. Because the virus is ubiquitous, a single positive titer is not useful in confirming a diagnosis of reproductive failure caused by PPV. Prevention may be achieved by natural exposure of gilts to sows before breeding. Natural infection usually results in lifelong immunity. Vaccines are available, but immunity lasts only 4 to 6 months, so vaccination must be repeated before each breeding. Also, vaccination may interfere with development of natural immunity.

Leptospirosis

Leptospira pomona and *Leptospira bratislava* are the primary serovars adapted to swine, although other serovars may incidentally infect pigs. Bacteria are shed through the urine and reproductive discharge of infected animals and enter susceptible animals through mucous membranes or broken skin. Once infected, bacteremia develops, and the organism localizes and multiplies in the kidney, and in pregnant females may cross the placenta and infect and kill the fetuses. Aborted, weak, and stillborn pigs may be the only obvious clinical signs. Diagnostic tests include demonstration of high antibody titers in the dam (interpreted in light of vaccination status) or in fetal fluids, culture of the organism, darkfield microscopy of urine or fetal fluids, fluorescent antibody of fresh tissue, and PCR techniques. Treatment may be accomplished with tetracycline given in the feed or administration of parenteral tetracycline. Many monovalent and multivalent vaccines are available for the protection of breeding stock; however, the immunity is short-lived, so animals should be vaccinated every 6 months at breeding.

> **TECHNICIAN NOTE** Pathogens responsible for abortion and reproductive failure in swine include pseudorabies virus (PRV), brucellosis, porcine reproductive and respiratory syndrome (PRRS), porcine parvovirus (PPV), and leptospirosis.

NERVOUS SYSTEM
Salt Poisoning

Salt poisoning, also known as *sodium ion toxicosis* or *water deprivation*, occurs in commercial and pet swine as the result of overconsumption of excessive sodium (direct salt poisoning) or inadequate water intake (indirect salt poisoning) or possibly both. Water deprivation causes hyperosmolarity within the CNS, so that when water is consumed, osmotic pressure draws fluid into the CNS, causing cerebral edema. Affected pigs show signs of restlessness, pruritus, constipation, and thirst, followed by depression, blindness, convulsions, and death. Salt toxicity is a well-recognized entity in commercial swine, but descriptions of medical treatment of affected animals are limited because it usually is not economically feasible to treat individual commercial pigs. Successful treatment of pet pigs has been reported. Treatment consists of slow rehydration with fluids that gradually return sodium to a normal level.

MUSCULOSKELETAL SYSTEM
Porcine Stress Syndrome

Porcine stress syndrome (PSS) is also known as *malignant hyperthermia*. Susceptibility to PSS is caused by a single autosomal recessive gene, and disease is manifested only in pigs that are homozygous recessive for this gene. However, this defective gene is closely associated with desirable characteristics, such as good feed conversion and high percent lean. The gene for PSS has been identified in almost every breed of swine but is especially prevalent in the Pietrain breed. Stress, halothane, and other anesthetics may precipitate the development of PSS. Severity of clinical signs is related to degree of stress, and signs include muscle and tail tremors, dyspnea, alternating blanched and reddened areas of skin, elevated body temperature (hyperthermia), cyanosis, muscle rigidity, and death. At slaughter or on postmortem examination, the musculature is pale, soft, and watery. Susceptibility to stress can be diagnosed with a DNA probe test, which will identify both homozygous and heterozygous carriers. Once clinical signs develop, the affected animal may be treated by removing the stress, applying external cooling, and administering dantrolene sodium, if available. It is important to prevent this condition through genetic selection of breeding stock that is not stress susceptible.

> **TECHNICIAN NOTE** Porcine stress syndrome (PSS), or malignant hyperthermia, is a genetic disease that results in muscle tremors, hyperthermia, and death. Stress, halothane, and other anesthetics may precipitate the development of PSS.

BEHAVIOR

The pig's normal response to fear includes vocalization and attempts to escape. Pigs are naturally curious and spend a great deal of time exploring their environment. The prehensile organ of the pig is the snout, and in general, they have a keen sense of smell. Pigs have poor eyesight and therefore are reluctant to venture into areas with unusual odors and changes in light intensity. Once familiar with their surroundings, they begin to investigate by rooting with their snout, which may lead to destructive behavior. Rooting is a normal foraging behavior. Pigs are sensitive to heat and as a result will wallow in mud to better thermoregulate (Figure 20-46). Additionally, swine maintain clean sleeping and feeding areas.

Swine have a strong social hierarchy that is established by aggressive behavior. This begins as early as birth, when teat order is established. Because more milk is produced in the cranial mammary glands, stronger, more assertive piglets will fight to claim these teats. Co-mingling of pigs, as occurs at weaning, leads to reestablishment of this hierarchy. This reordering usually occurs within 12 to 24 hours, with the dominant pig establishing itself first. Some changes in rank may occur within the middle members, but the top and bottom of the order remain fairly stable. In established hierarchies, the dominant pig assumes a recumbent position,

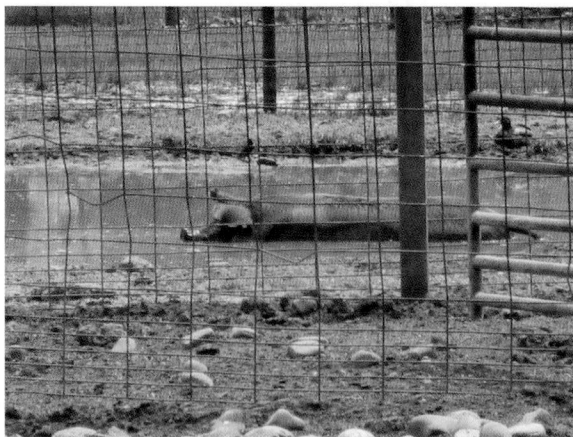

FIGURE 20-46 Pigs are sensitive to heat and will wallow in the mud to better thermoregulate.

BOX 20-3	Recipe for Milk Replacer Used to Raise Piglets

Thoroughly mix the following three ingredients. Administer orally via nursing bottle.
1. 1 quart whole cow's milk
2. 1 oz white corn syrup or honey
3. 1 oz cream or corn oil

and its belly is nuzzled by subordinates, possibly as an allogrooming ritual.

Abnormal behavior is likely to develop because of stressful living conditions, as occur during weaning, poor ventilation, overcrowding, or an imbalanced diet. Behaviors such as poor manure habits, having dirty sleeping and feeding areas, extreme aggression, tail biting, ear biting, and flank biting can be a valuable indicator of environmental (physical, climatic, or social) or managerial deficiencies. These behaviors can be controlled by providing diversions, such as toys (e.g., bowling balls, inner tubes), for pigs to play with within the pen.

Mature boars have well-developed tusks for slashing and will bite each other as part of normal aggressive behavior. Boars raised together undergo a dominance procedure but typically do not violently fight each other; however, boars from different litters can fight and may seriously injure each other. Sows and weaned pigs will also fight, and even though they do not have large tusks, they will bite.

A dam's aggression toward piglets (hysteria) or savaging of baby pigs usually is exhibited by gilts. These same gilts may be normal during subsequent farrowings. Possible causes of hysteria include stress resulting from the inability of the gilt to make a "nest," human interference during farrowing, and perhaps genetic predisposition. Piglets can be removed at birth and reintroduced once parturition is complete because initiation of nursing often calms the gilt.

POTBELLIED PIGS

Ownership of potbellied pigs has increased in recent years, with a growing number of people keeping these animals as pets. It is important to remember that these animals are pets first and pigs second, and they should be treated accordingly. Veterinary technicians can play a critical role in educating clients about nutrition and husbandry needs of these animals.

Nutrition and Husbandry

Without proper knowledge of potbellied pig husbandry and nutritional needs, health and behavior problems are inevitable. According to one report, approximately 50% of potbellied pigs are abandoned or rehomed before they are 1 year of age. This occurs because of unrealistic expectations of the owners and their unwillingness or inability to provide for the pig's environmental needs. The most common misconception held by pet pig owners is that their potbellied pig will weigh only 40 to 50 lb when fully grown. Although a few pigs remain small, most of them will weigh closer to 120 lb when mature, and they do not reach full size until they are 2 to 3 years old. Breed standards set by the North American Potbellied Pig Association describe a pig weighing no more than 95 lb and having a maximum height of 18 inches at the shoulder at 1 year of age. The most common nutritional disease of potbellied pigs is obesity; however, many stunted and malnourished pigs are seen because of their owner's misguided attempts to keep them small. Several companies have developed diets specifically for miniature pigs. Miniature pigs should never be fed commercial swine feed; feed for miniature swine is lower in protein and fat and has a higher fiber content than commercial swine rations. Miniature pig feed is generally classified as starter, grower, breeder, or maintenance. A homemade milk replacer can be used to raise piglets (Box 20-3). Starter rations are intended for newly weaned pigs. The most appropriate ration for the average potbellied pig is the maintenance ration, which contains 12% protein, 2% fat, and 12% to 15% fiber. Most potbellied pigs are adopted by owners at 6 to 8 weeks of age and are spayed or neutered during the first few months. They begin to lead sedentary lifestyles early, so maintenance rations are probably the best choice for these pigs. If the pig is not spayed or neutered and/or it leads an active life, grower rations may be a better choice. Some commercially available potbellied pig feed has urinary acidifiers to help prevent cystitis, so if this seems to be a problem, this specialty ration may be considered. Recommendations concerning the amount to feed potbellied pigs vary; some references suggest 2% to 2.5% of body weight, others suggest 1 cup of feed per 50 to 80 lb. These are general guidelines, and owners must be advised to feed their pets according to body condition.

Although potbellied pigs should have a rotund potbelly, they should never have turgid, fat-filled jowls or rolls of fat hanging over the hocks. They should have ribs that should easily be palpated but not seen (Figure 20-47). Appropriate treats for the pig include low-fat, low-salt (see salt poisoning under swine) snack food, such as popcorn (air popped without salt or butter), and small amounts of dried or fresh

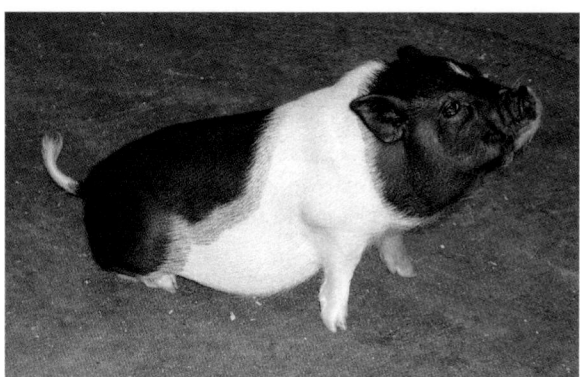

FIGURE 20-47 A healthy potbellied pig of appropriate size for its age.

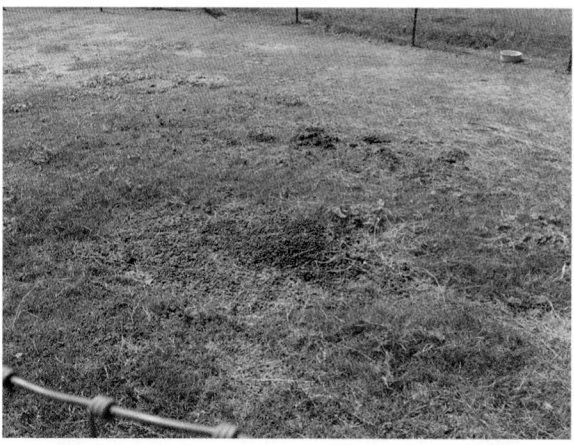

FIGURE 20-48 South American camelids have pelleted feces and use communal dung piles. .

fruit. Requiring that the pig earn its treats is one way of continually reinforcing the pig's position as a subordinate member of the family. Obesity is likely to be the leading cause of health problems and decreased life span in pet pigs. Arthritis, heart disease, and kidney failure are just a few possible geriatric diseases, all of which may be hastened by obesity. Sometimes entropion and corneal damage occur in morbidly obese pigs. Water intake in pigs is important for prevention of cystitis, urolithiasis, and salt poisoning. Pigs have a habit of alternating between eating and drinking and may make a mess at feeding time. Owners should be advised to not restrict water for this reason. Food and water should be provided in an easy-to-clean environment, such as a shower stall, or by placing the food and water in a large shallow pan to try to make cleanup easier. Pigs are particular about the temperature of drinking water, so water should not be allowed to get too cold in the winter or too hot in the summer because this may restrict intake and cause problems. Pigs are foraging animals that normally spend much of the day in search of food or at rest. When kept as pets, pigs are fed two to three small meals a day and spend little time looking for food or eating. Mealtime can be extended in a variety of ways; this increases exercise for pigs and makes them more active participants in the acquisition of food. In good weather, the pig's ration may be spread over the yard. A rooting box can be constructed out of wood or by using a plastic wading pool. The box is filled with large, smooth stones, and food can be spread among the stones. This not only extends feeding time but also allows the pig to fulfill its rooting needs in an acceptable place. Other useful techniques include the use of a Manna Ball or a Buster cube, which allows the pig to slowly acquire its food while exercising at the same time.

TECHNICIAN NOTE Obesity is the most common nutritional disease of potbellied pigs and is likely to be the leading cause of health problems and decreased life span in pet pigs.

COMMON DISEASES AND CONDITIONS OF CAMELIDS

In general, camelids may be classified as Old World or New World camelids. Old World camelids include dromedary, or one-humped, camels, and bactrian, or two-humped, camels. New World camelids, also called *South American camelids (SACs)*, include the llama (*Lama glama*), the alpaca (*Lama pacos*), the guanaco (*Lama guanicoe*), and the vicuña (*Vicugna vicugna*).

TECHNICIAN NOTE New World camelids, also called *South American camelids (SACs)*, include the llama (*Lama glama*), the alpaca (*Lama pacos*), the guanaco (*Lama guanicoe*), and the vicuña (*Vicugna vicugna*).

All SACs have 74 chromosomes and therefore have produced fertile hybrids. Camelids may live to be 15 to 20 years old or older. SACs originated from the South American Andes; thus they became accustomed to dry, cooler climates and high altitudes. Camelids have a complex, three-compartment stomach with digestion similar to ruminants. Whereas llamas tend to browse, alpacas prefer to graze. Camelids regurgitate and rechew food, as do ruminants, but they more efficiently extract protein and energy from poor-quality forage than do ruminants. SACs have pelleted feces and use communal dung piles (Figure 20-48). Llamas are typically used for meat, leather, and fiber, and as pack animals. Alpacas are known for their superior fiber, but they are also used as a source of meat and leather. Two breeds of alpacas—the huacaya and the suri—have gained popularity in the United States. The huacuya breed is the most common; its fiber is crimped and shorter than that of the suri. The suri has a hair coat that consists of long fibers with no crimp that hangs from the body in ringlets.

Llamas and alpacas are herd animals and therefore need to live with at least one other llama or alpaca. Gelded male llamas or adult female llamas can be used as guardians for sheep, goats, alpacas, cattle, and miniature horses.

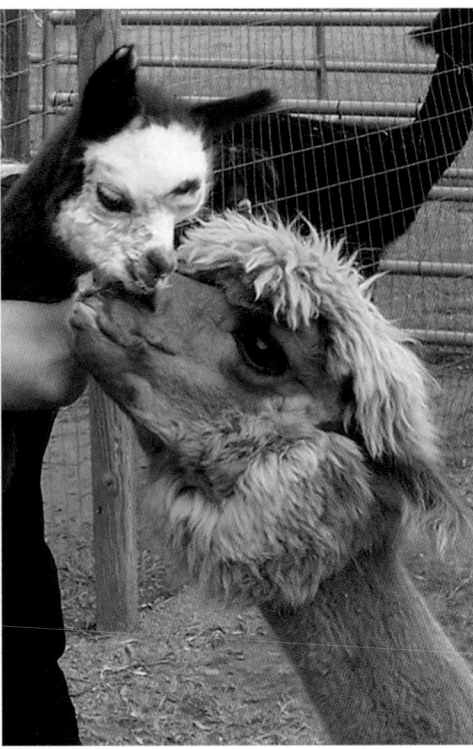

FIGURE 20-49 The neonatal camelid is referred to as a *cria*. The dam and the cria form strong family bonds. (Courtesy Ms. Vida Palmer.)

> **TECHNICIAN NOTE** Llamas and alpacas are herd animals and therefore need to live with at least one other llama or alpaca. Gelded male llamas or adult female llamas can be used as guardians for sheep, goats, alpacas, cattle, and miniature horses.

As camelid popularity increases, veterinary technicians can participate in client education, as well as in recognition of disease, herd management, and care of sick or debilitated animals.

CARE OF THE NEONATE AND NEONATAL DISEASES

Neonatal camelids are referred to as *crias*, and the newborn and its dam form a strong family bond (Figure 20-49). The newborn alpaca cria should weigh at least 12 lb at birth, and the normal llama cria should weigh more than 15 lb. The neonate is covered with an epidermal membrane that attaches at the mucocutaneous junctions, the coronary bands, and the umbilicus and will flake off shortly after birth. Crias are born with the eyelids open and the incisors erupted. Camelid mothers do not lick the cria dry, nor do they stimulate the baby to stand. The mother may stand over the cria and vocalize with a humming sound.

> **TECHNICIAN NOTE** The camelid fetus is covered with an epidermal membrane that will dry and flake off shortly after birth.

After birth, crias should attempt to stand within 30 to 60 minutes and should actively try to nurse the dam within the first hour. If nursing has not occurred by 6 hours after birth, intervention is essential. Observation of nursing and assessment of passive transfer are of great importance in neonatal care. Similar to other food animal species, veterinary technicians can aid in delivery and management of neonatal cria.

To prevent FPT, the newborn should be observed closely for the first 3 to 4 hours to ensure that it nurses. It is desirable to get colostrum from the dam into the cria; however, if this is not possible, cow, goat, or sheep colostrum can be substituted. The cria should receive 20% of its body weight in colostrum in four to six feedings during the first 24 hours after birth. It may be beneficial to feed colostrum to premature or sick crias for 3 to 4 days after birth. In the event that the cria will not nurse, orogastric intubation should be performed to make certain that the cria receives adequate colostral immunity. If colostrum is not available, an IV plasma transfusion is strongly recommended. Passive transfer can be evaluated using serum radial immunodiffusion, serum total solids, and sodium sulfite turbidity. These tests are most beneficial in crias that are between 36 hours and 7 days of age.

Orphaned crias may be bottle-fed kid or lamb milk replacer, or whole cow's milk. The cria should receive milk at 10% to 15% of its body weight per day. Initially, this amount can be divided into four to six feedings per day, but feedings can be reduced gradually to two to four feedings per day. Weighing the bottle-fed cria to document adequate weight gain is important.

Newborns should be carefully watched, especially during the first 48 hours of life. Crias that are considered "at risk" include premature crias, crias born to mothers with dystocia, newborns with congenital defects, crias that suffer excessive umbilical bleeding, crias born to the same mating that experienced problems in previous years, and crias that develop FPT. At-risk crias often show abnormalities in vital signs, labored respirations, weakness, depression, failure to nurse, failure to stand, and straining with failure to pass meconium. Meconium should be passed within 18 to 24 hours after birth. It is not necessary to administer enemas to every neonate; however, if the cria is straining, a warm soapy water enema can be administered.

As with other neonates, the newborn cria should be examined thoroughly, the umbilicus dipped in disinfectant, and the cria weighed daily. The newborn should be alert and should have clear eyes and erect ears. Typically, body temperature is 100° F to 102° F (37.8° C to 38.9° C); heart rate, 70 to 100 bpm; and respiratory rate, 20 to 30 breaths/minute. Compare with the adult camelid in Box 20-4.

> **TECHNICIAN NOTE** Typically, the temperature, pulse, and respiration (TPR) of a normal cria is as follows: T = 100° F to 102° F (37.8° C to 38.9° C); P = 70 to 100 bpm; and respiratory rate is 20 to 30 breaths/minute.

Temperature (T): 99°F to 102.5°F
Pulse (P): 60 to 90
Respiration (R): 10 to 30

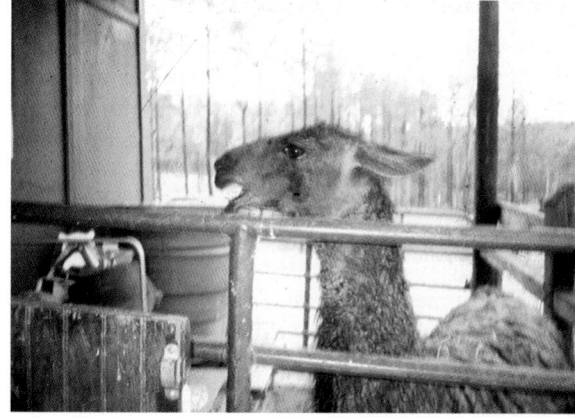

FIGURE 20-51 Monitoring of camelids during the hot summer months for signs of heat stress, such as open-mouth breathing, is important. (Courtesy Dr. David Pugh.)

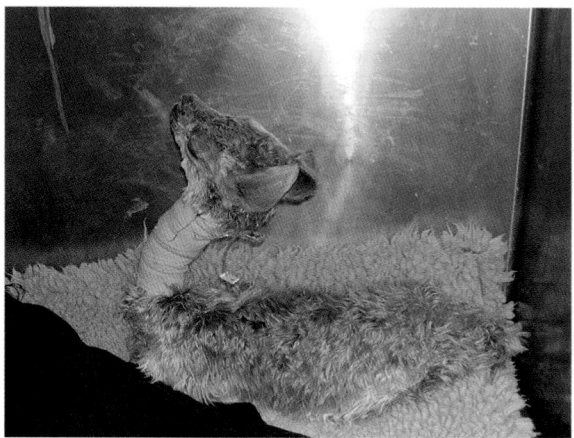

FIGURE 20-50 Premature crias often have nonerect or curled ears as a result of immature cartilage in the ears.

Considerable variation in the length of gestation of alpacas and llamas has been noted (330 to 360 days), with some pregnancies lasting longer than 1 year. This variation makes it difficult to determine prematurity based on length of gestation. Prematurity is not based entirely on gestational length. Signs of prematurity in the newborn are of greater importance than time in utero. Low birth weight may be the most obvious sign, but premature crias also show signs such as weakness and inability to stand or hold the head up to nurse. Affected crias have excessive laxity of tendons and ligaments and may walk on their fetlocks; they have nonerect or curled ears as a result of immature cartilage in the ears (Figure 20-50), the hair coat is especially silky, and the rubbery covering of the toe persists for 1 to 2 days in premature crias (disappears in 6 to 12 hours in full-term crias). The incisors are not erupted in premature crias, and the mucous membranes may be dark red from decreased oxygenation as a result of undeveloped lungs. Prematurity is life threatening and requires immediate and intensive therapy.

TECHNICIAN NOTE Considerable variation in gestation has been noted in alpacas and llamas (330 to 360 days), with some pregnancies lasting longer than 1 year. Therefore, it may be difficult to determine prematurity based on length of gestation.

Once the condition of prematurity has been established, the cria should be provided supplemental heat and oxygen. Most premature crias are incapable of nursing the dam, so

it is suggested that a warm plasma transfusion using camelid plasma be administered. After plasma transfusion, IV fluids with dextrose can be given to meet any existing fluid deficits and to prevent hypoglycemia. A common sign of hypoglycemia in crias is an inability to lift the head to nurse (Figure 20-51). Premature crias are susceptible to infection, so administration of broad-spectrum antibiotics is usually initiated. If the cria is strong enough to nurse, it should be fed milk at the rate of 10% to 15% of its body weight divided into four feedings a day. If the cria is incapable of nursing, tube feeding via an orogastric tube may be necessary (a stallion urinary catheter works well). Intensive care is continued until the cria matures appropriately or is capable of survival without additional support. Maturation is evident by eruption of the incisors and straightening of the ears. Any angular limb deformities may be addressed by application of light support splints; often these deformities improve as the neonate matures. Daily weights are helpful in assessing the health of the neonate and in ensuring adequate oral nutrient intake.

TECHNICIAN NOTE Most premature crias are incapable of nursing the dam, so it is suggested that a warm plasma transfusion using camelid plasma be administered.

Congenital abnormalities are relatively common among camelids. This high prevalence is blamed on the narrow genetic pool available to breeders before importation of native South American camelids during the 1980s. Even with greater genetic diversity, congenital defects continue to plague breeders. Common congenital defects include choanal atresia, atresia ani, wry face, patent urachus, and cleft palate. Choanal atresia is the presence of a membranous or osseous separation of the nasal and pharyngeal cavities. Because camelids are obligate nasal breathers, the primary clinical sign in affected newborns is open-mouth breathing. This condition is probably hereditary and the prognosis for life is poor; therefore, euthanasia is recommended.

CONDITIONS OF THE DIGESTIVE SYSTEM

Diarrhea is an important cause of morbidity in neonatal camelids. Many factors may be involved in the cause of neonatal diarrhea, including management and nutritional factors and a variety of pathogens. The most common pathogens causing diarrhea in neonates are *E. coli, Clostridium perfringens* (types A, C, and D), coronavirus, *Cryptosporidium* spp., *Giardia* spp., and coccidia (Table 20-11). If diarrhea in the young is not treated effectively, it may lead to the development of chronic diarrhea, which may ultimately result in chronic renal failure.

> **TECHNICIAN NOTE** Diarrhea is an important cause of morbidity in neonatal camelids; if not treated effectively, it may lead to the development of chronic diarrhea, which may ultimately result in chronic renal failure.

Diarrhea in crias younger than 7 days of age is likely due to nutritional factors in bottle-fed crias or to colibacillosis infection, especially in cases of inadequate colostrum ingestion. It should be kept in mind that diarrhea may be multifactorial and can involve more than one pathogen. Numerous diagnostic tests are available to help determine the cause of neonatal diarrhea, so that the clinician can initiate appropriate treatment for affected individuals and can control the spread of disease through the rest of the group.

> **TECHNICIAN NOTE** Diarrhea may be multifactorial and can involve more than one pathogen. Numerous diagnostic tests are available to help determine the cause of neonatal diarrhea, so that the clinician can initiate appropriate treatment for affected individuals and can control the spread of disease through the rest of the herd.

METABOLIC CONDITIONS

Hepatic Lipidosis

When excessive fat accumulates in liver cells, the disease process is termed *hepatic lipidosis, fatty infiltration,* or *fatty liver disease.* This syndrome has been well defined in cats, cows, sheep, goats, ponies, and humans. Although there are differences in conditions that initiate hepatic lipidosis between these species, usually a period of inadequate energy intake (i.e., negative energy balance) initiates body fat mobilization. Unfortunately, in camelids, the disease outcome is nearly always fatal if not recognized early and treated aggressively.

Middle-aged, pregnant, or lactating females are most likely to be affected. Typical histories of these affected camelids include recent significant loss of appetite or severe weight loss varying from a couple of days to several weeks. Affected animals have various types of body conditioning (i.e., thin to obese). In some cases, other medical problems or changes in social or environmental conditions were noted, such as uncharacteristically hot weather or movement of animals into or out of certain pastures or pens, evident around the time the condition developed.

Therapy must be focused on increasing energy intake immediately. Offering a variety of appetizing feeds such as grass clippings or blackberry leaves can help stimulate feed intake. Injections of B-vitamins can be beneficial for appetite stimulation. If more aggressive oral supplementation is required, a liquid gruel can be administered via orogastric tube. Soaking alfalfa pellets in hot water and mixing in calf electrolytes, calcium propionate, propylene glycol, and other ingredients can provide energy sources and fermentable material. Transfaunation can be used to repopulate the microbial fauna and restimulate fermentation. Collected rumen fluid from cattle, sheep, or goats can be used in llamas or alpacas.

In more severe cases, intensive supportive care and dietary management, including total parenteral nutrition (TPN), may be required. The prognosis is always guarded in severe cases of hepatic lipidosis, even with aggressive nutritional support. All sick camelids should be considered at risk for developing hepatic lipidosis, especially those with anorexia or metabolic demands of pregnancy and lactation. Close monitoring of feed intake in sick animals is absolutely essential to prevent death.

> **TECHNICIAN NOTE** Deficient energy intake is a hallmark factor in initiating hepatic lipidosis; therefore, therapy must be focused on increasing energy intake immediately.

Prevention of hepatic lipidosis is based on ensuring adequate energy and protein intake, especially in pregnant and lactating females, by feeding good-quality forage and appropriate supplementation. Lactating dams have the highest nutrient requirements and should be fed the best-quality forage and supplemented with a grain product containing energy and protein sources. Given the strong association between significant weight loss and hepatic lipidosis, one can use routine (monthly or bimonthly) weight or body condition evaluation to determine potential risk. Veterinary technicians can assist with on-farm herd management programs to assess adequate nutrition by assigning body condition scores using a 5- or 9-point system. Refer to Chapter 10, Large Animal Nutrition, for more information about these two BCS systems.

> **TECHNICIAN NOTE** The best and easiest method of evaluating a camelid nutritional program is by body condition scoring.

Heat Stress

Heat stress is a common occurrence in llamas and alpacas during the summer season. Because these animals originate from the Andes Mountains of South America, where high heat and humidity are not as common as in many areas of the United States, llamas and alpacas are not adapted to

TABLE 20-11	Common Infectious Causes of Diarrhea in Young Camelids				
DISEASE/ ETIOLOGIC AGENT	**AGE AFFECTED**	**PATHOGENESIS**	**CLINICAL SIGNS**	**DIAGNOSIS**	**TREATMENT**
Colibacillosis/ *Escherichia coli*	Less than 7 days	Ingestion of organism from the environment Umbilical infection Usually thin, undernourished animals Failure of passive transfer (FPT) Poor sanitation	Profuse diarrhea Abdominal distention Weight loss Pica Fever	Isolation of organism	Supportive care (anti-inflammatories, IV fluids, total parenteral nutrition [TPN] ±) Antibiotics
Enterotoxemia/ *Clostridium perfringens* types A, C, and D	8 to 35 days	Ingestion of organism from the environment Usually fast-growing, large animals Poor sanitation	Sudden death Fever Abdominal distention Central nervous system (CNS) involvement Diarrhea	Isolation of the organism	Typically unrewarding Broad-spectrum antibiotics Supportive care (anti-inflammatories, IV fluids, TPN ±) Prevention: ○ Vaccinate dams 1 month before parturition, then crias by 1 month of age
Coronavirus	Less than 10 days	Fecal-oral route	Dark green diarrhea Dehydration Possible death if untreated	Electron microscopy of feces	Supportive care (anti-inflammatories, IV fluids, TPN ±)
Cryptosporidiosis/ *Cryptosporidium* spp.	Less than 7 days	Ingestion of organism from the environment Zoonotic	Fecal material watery to pasty	Direct smear with acid-fast stain Enzyme-linked immunosorbent assay (ELISA) test for antigen in feces	Supportive care (anti-inflammatories, IV fluids, TPN ±)
Giardiasis	Longer than 7 days	Fecal-oral route with contaminated water Zoonotic	Chronic diarrhea Weight loss	Direct smear ELISA test in feces	Fenbendazole
Coccidiosis/ *Eimeria lamae, E. alpacae, E. macusaniensis*	Longer than 21 days	Ingested from contaminated feed, water, milk Poor sanitation	Profuse diarrhea Dehydration Weight loss	Fecal float with sugar solution	Amprolium Sulfadimethoxine Supportive care (anti-inflammatories, IV fluids, TPN ±) Prevention: ○ Supplemental anticoccidial drugs in grain or water (decoquinate) ○ Good management and maintenance of hygienic facilities

handle these conditions. It is critical to manage them in a way that protects them from heat stress because it can lead to illness and even death of the animal.

During warmer months of the year, there are many ways to keep animals cool. Shade is an easy way to keep them from getting too hot. Trees, barns, and shelters that provide shade are great places for camelids to relax and stay cool during the heat of the day. Fans are an excellent way to keep the air moving and keep the animals cool. Small pools have been used for camelids to alleviate heat stress. If available, an air-conditioned room or area of the barn can help keep animals cool or can be used as a place to which animals that begin to show signs of heat stress can be moved. Giving llamas and alpacas plenty of fresh water helps to prevent heat stress. Multiple sources of cool, clean water should be available so that all animals have a place to drink.

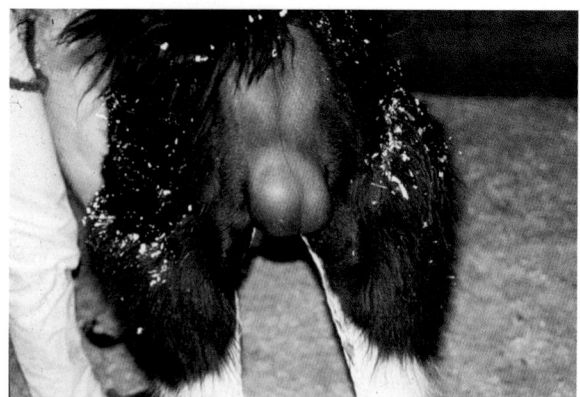

FIGURE 20-52 Another sign of heat stress in camelids is scrotal swelling in intact males. (Courtesy Dr. David Pugh.)

> **TECHNICIAN NOTE** Providing plenty of fresh water, shade, air movement, and small pools will help keep camelids cool and will prevent heat stress.

Management of camelids during warmer months is critical in alleviating heat stress. Shearing is one of the most important ways to help llamas and alpacas keep cool. Because the fibers work to trap heat close to the animal's body, shearing helps the animal lose body heat more effectively through evaporation. If possible, shearing from head to toe (leaving about 1 to 3 inches of fiber on the body) is most effective, but barrel cuts (e.g., abdomen and thorax only) also help. Work that needs to be performed on animals should be performed early in the morning, when temperatures are cooler.

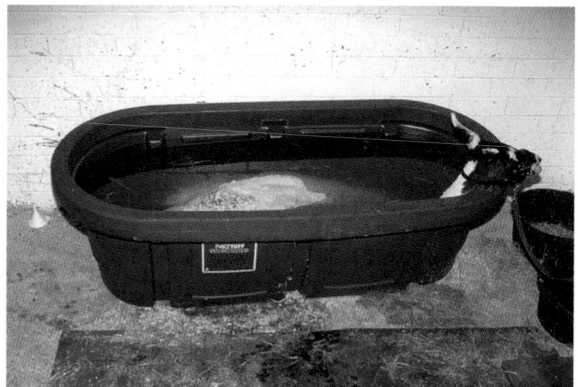

FIGURE 20-53 Animals that are recumbent as a result of heat stress may benefit from the use of water flotation tanks. (Courtesy Dr. Christine Navarre.)

> **TECHNICIAN NOTE** Shearing of camelids before the onset of hot weather and careful monitoring of the animals during summer months are important for the prevention of heat stress.

It is important to know when llamas and alpacas are most in danger of heat stress. Monitoring the animals is important during summer months, so that any signs of heat stress may be detected early. Signs to watch for include nasal flaring, open-mouth breathing, tachypnea, dyspnea, drooling, depression or dullness, not eating feed, scrotal swelling in intact males (Figure 20-52), weakness, trembling, rectal temperature greater than 104°F (40°C), heart rate greater than 90 bpm, and respiratory rate greater than 40 breaths/minute.

Treatment of llamas and alpacas with heat stress should first consist of cooling the animal down using water or alcohol. Additional cooling with a fan or an air conditioner may be useful. If the animal has not been shorn, this may be considered in the treatment regimen, but only if it does not cause further stress. Other therapies include cool IV fluids with electrolytes, anti-inflammatories, and good nursing

care, including lifting the animal periodically if it is unable to stand. Water flotation tanks are especially useful for this purpose (Figure 20-53). The most important aspect of heat stress is prevention.

NERVOUS SYSTEM

Meningeal Worm (*Parelaphostrongylus tenuis*)

One parasite that is of great importance to llama and alpaca producers is the meningeal worm, *Parelaphostrongylus tenuis*. Llamas and alpacas and other animals, such as domestic small ruminants, are aberrant hosts of this parasite, whereas the white-tailed deer is the normal host. This parasite does not cause clinical disease in white-tailed deer, but in camelids, it causes high morbidity and mortality. *P. tenuis* larvae migrate through the spinal cord of aberrant hosts, causing neurologic deficits such as ataxia, stiffness, and paralysis (Figure 20-54). Additionally, gradual weight loss, depression, and death can occur. Neurologic signs generally begin in the hind limbs and progress to the front limbs. The course of disease may be acute to chronic, ranging from death within days to ataxia that lasts months to years.

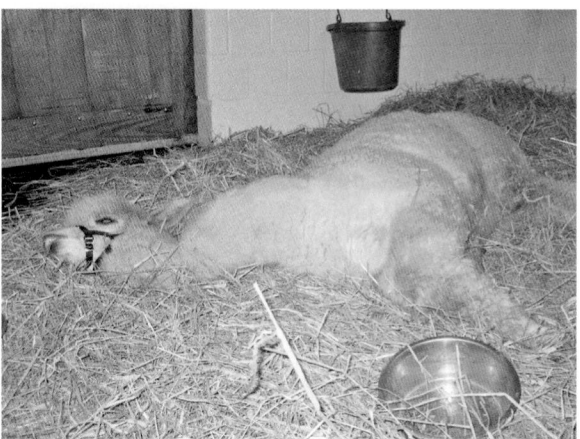

FIGURE 20-54 Neurologic llama.

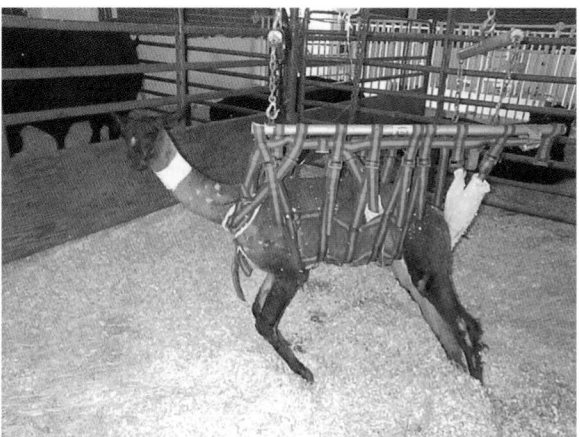

FIGURE 20-55 Camelids that are unable to stand may benefit from the use of slings and physical therapy. (Courtesy Dr. Christine Navarre.)

> **TECHNICIAN NOTE** *P. tenuis* larvae migrate through the spinal cord of aberrant hosts, such as llamas and alpacas, causing neurologic deficits that may be acute or chronic in nature.

Dewormers are used for treatment of meningeal worm. Anti-inflammatories are important to reduce inflammation associated with aberrant spinal cord migration and to prevent further clinical signs. Dexamethasone should not be administered to pregnant females because this drug may induce abortion. Supportive care, including slings, physical therapy, and hydrotherapy, will aid recovery, especially if the animal is recumbent (Figure 20-55).

The prognosis for survival depends on the severity of clinical signs. A decreased prognosis is given if the animal is recumbent. Many animals suffer permanent neurologic deficits but may remain productive members of the herd for breeding and as pets.

> **TECHNICIAN NOTE** The prognosis for survival depends on how severe the clinical signs become. A decreased prognosis is given if the animal is recumbent.

Rabies

Similar to all mammals, camelids are susceptible to rabies. The reservoir host varies with geographic location. Annual vaccination is recommended. Initial signs include lameness, ataxia, and posterior paresis progressing to an aggressive or paralytic form of the disease. Typically, the aggressive syndrome manifests itself as frequent biting, attacks on pen mates, vocalization, and eventually recumbency. Depression, anorexia, circling, salivation, flaccid muscles, and recumbency are signs of the paralytic form.

> **TECHNICIAN NOTE** Similar to all mammals, camelids are susceptible to rabies, demonstrating an aggressive or paralytic syndrome. Therefore, annual vaccination is recommended.

HEALTH MAINTENANCE

Veterinary technicians may be important in helping with camelid herd health maintenance using veterinary-derived protocols. Camelids are routinely vaccinated for *C. perfringens* types C and D and tetanus. Vaccination for these diseases may be started as early as 2 to 3 days of age and repeated at 2 to 3 weeks of age. A booster vaccination is suggested at 6 and 12 months of age. From that point, annual revaccination is recommended. Other vaccines that can be used in camelids include rabies, equine rhinovirus, equine influenza, equine herpesvirus, West Nile virus, leptospirosis, and *E. coli*, depending on the herd location and the potential threat of these diseases within a given herd.

Camelids may acquire a great variety of internal and external parasites, some of which are common to sheep, goats, cattle, and horses. Parasite control programs are most effective if customized to the individual farm because recommendations from other farms or other areas of the country are of little use. Parasite control strategies should be developed through a local veterinarian who has knowledge of fecal parasite egg counts. The sugar flotation method is recommended for fecal egg counting because this method is more precise than traditional salt flotation methods. Fecal egg counts should be performed periodically and should include all animals if fewer than 10 animals live on the farm. If more than 10 animals are included in the herd, 10% of the herd should be tested. Fecal egg counts performed approximately 2 weeks after deworming medication has been administered are useful for evaluating the efficacy of the dewormer used and may facilitate evaluation of the development of anthelmintic resistance.

Dental disease is a common condition affecting camelids. Common diseases include tooth root abscesses, malocclusion, and normal aging changes. Additionally, all camelids have canine teeth ("fighting teeth") that are particularly well developed in the intact male. These include two maxillary canine teeth on each side and one mandibular tooth on each side. It is a common practice in North America to blunt these teeth in some manner to prevent serious lacerations of the ears, throat, limbs, and scrotum when males fight. Routine teeth trimming using rotary tools, gigli wire, and small equine dental instruments can help control overgrown teeth caused by malocclusion.

Foot trimming is a routine part of health maintenance in camelids. The camelid foot has two digits on each foot. The plantar surface is covered with a soft, cornified layer of epithelium similar to the heel bulb in small ruminants. This structure is called the *slipper*. A small, non–weight-bearing nail is located at the extremity of each digit and is closely attached to the distal phalanx (P3) via the corium or sensitive lamina. The nail may require periodic trimming.

Body condition scoring is a method that subjectively grades animals by determining the quantity of subcutaneous fat stores. A 10-point system is used, with 1 being emaciated, 5 being desirable, and 10 being severely obese. Late-pregnant animals should have a slightly higher body condition with reserves to support impending lactation. Lactating animals will lose body condition rapidly as they produce milk. Important times to assess BCS include early to mid pregnancy, early to mid lactation, and periodically (4 to 6 times per year) for other animals of the herd to assess energy status.

> **TECHNICIAN NOTE** Veterinary technicians play a vital role in camelid herd health management through programs such as vaccination, parasite control, dental examinations, foot trimming, and body condition scoring.

RECOMMENDED READINGS

Anderson DE, Rings DM: Current veterinary therapy—food animal practice, ed 5, St Louis, 2009, Saunders.

Anderson DE, Whitehead CE: Alpaca and llama health management, Vet Clin North Am Food Anim Pract 25:xi, 2009.

Cooper VL: Diagnosis of neonatal pig diarrhea, Vet Clin North Am Food Anim Pract 16:117, 2000.

Cowart RP: An outline of swine diseases, ed 2, Ames, IA, 2001, Iowa State University, Blackwell Science.

Divers TJ, Peek SE: Rebhun's diseases of dairy cattle, ed 2, St Louis, 2008, Saunders.

Evans CN: Alpaca field manual, ed 2, Manhattan, KS, 2005, Able Publishing and Ag Press.

Fowler ME: Medicine and surgery of South American camelids, ed 3, Ames, IA, 2010, Wiley-Blackwell Publishing.

Fubini SL, Ducharme NC: Farm animal surgery, ed 1, St Louis, 2004, Saunders.

Hanie EA: Large animal clinical procedures for veterinary technicians, St Louis, 2006, Mosby.

Koterba AM, Drummond WH, Kosch PC, editors: Equine clinical neonatology, Philadelphia, 1990, Lea & Febiger.

Orsini JA, Divers TJ: Manual of equine emergencies, ed 3, St Louis, 2009, Saunders.

Pugh DG: Sheep and goat medicine, St Louis, 2002, Saunders.

Radostits OM, Gay CC, Hinchcliff KW, et al: Veterinary medicine, ed 10, New York, 2007, Saunders.

Reed S, Bailey W, Sellon D, editors: Equine internal medicine, ed 3, St Louis, 2009, Saunders.

Robinson NE, editor: Current therapy in equine medicine, ed 2, Philadelphia, 1987, Saunders.

Robinson NE, editor: Current therapy in equine medicine, ed 3, Philadelphia, 1991, Saunders.

Robinson NE, editor: Current therapy in equine medicine, ed 4, St Louis, 1997, Saunders.

Robinson NE, editor: Current therapy in equine medicine, ed 5, St Louis, 2003, Saunders.

Robinson NE, editor: Current therapy in equine medicine, ed 6, St Louis, 2009, Saunders.

Scott PR: Sheep medicine, London, 2007, Manson Publishing/The Veterinary Press.

Smith BP, editor: Large animal internal medicine, ed 4, St Louis, 2009, Mosby.

Smith GW: Bovine neonatology, Vet Clin North Am Food Anim Pract 25:xi, 2009.

Smith MC, Sherman DM: Goat medicine, ed 2, Ames, IA, 2009, Wiley-Blackwell Publishing.

Straw BE, Zimmerman JJ, D'Allaire S, et al: Diseases of swine, ed 9, 2006, Blackwell Publishing.

Tynes VV: Potbellied pig husbandry and nutrition, Vet Clin North Am Exot Anim Pract 2:193, 1999.

Tynes VV: Preventive health care for pet potbellied pigs, Vet Clin North Am Exot Anim Pract 2:495, 1999.

Van Amstel S, Shearer J: Manual for treatment and control of lameness in cattle, ed 1, Ames, IA, 2006, Blackwell.

Wills RW: Diarrhea in growing-finishing swine, Vet Clin North Am Food Anim Pract 16:135, 2000.

RECOMMENDED WEBSITES

American Association of Equine Practitioners: Vaccination guidelines. Available at: http://www.aaep.org/vaccination_guidelines.htm (accessed on August 22, 2012).

American Association of Equine Practitioners: Biosecurity guidelines. Available at: http://www.aaep.org/pdfs/control_guidelines/Biosecurity_instructions%201.pdf (accessed on August 22, 2012).

21 Neonatal Care of the Puppy, Kitten, and Foal

Margret L. Casal and Amy I. Bentz

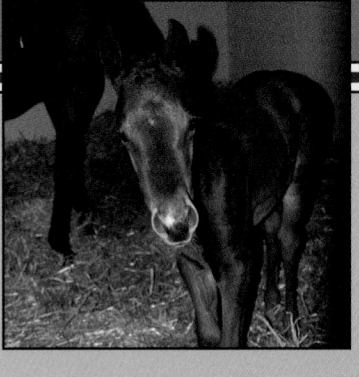

OUTLINE

Neonatology of Puppies and Kittens, *789*
Definition, *789*
History, *789*
Physical Examination, *789*
Normal Development, *790*
Diagnostics, *791*
Routine Maintenance, *791*
Common Concerns and Disorders in
  the Puppy and Kitten, *793*

Neonatology of Foals, *797*
The Perinatal Period and the High-Risk
  Mare, *797*
The Neonatal Period: The Normal
  Foal, *799*
The Neonatal Period: The Sick Foal, *802*
Nutrition of the Neonatal Foal, *808*
Summary, *809*

KEY TERMS

Congenital
Dehydration
Foal
Genetic
Hypoglycemia
Hypothermia
Mare
Neonatal period
Thermogenesis

LEARNING OBJECTIVES

When you have completed this chapter, you will be able to:

1. Pronounce, define, and spell all Key Terms in this chapter.
2. Define the neonatal period for puppies and kittens, obtain an accurate and thorough clinical history for all littermates and parents, and describe the procedure for physical examination of a neonate, including equipment needed and potential abnormalities.
3. Explain the timeline of normal development in neonatal puppies and kittens.
4. Do the following regarding performance of diagnostic procedures and routine maintenance in neonatal puppies and kittens:
   - Discuss how to perform diagnostic procedures on a neonatal puppy or kitten, including obtaining blood and urine samples, performing an ultrasound, and taking radiographs.
   - Discuss appropriate times to give medical treatments to neonatal puppies and kittens, including deworming and health examinations; be able to explain to the owner proper nutrition, preventive medicine, and behavior issues.
5. Do the following regarding common concerns and disorders in the puppy and kitten:
   - Explain common concerns and disorders of neonatal puppies and kittens, such as hypothermia, hydration status, hypoglycemia, malnutrition, fading puppy or kitten syndrome, and neonatal isoerythrolysis in kittens.
   - Discuss proper care of an orphaned neonatal puppy or kitten, including appropriate ambient temperatures and diet and common complications involved with orphaned neonates.
6. Do the following regarding the perinatal period and the high-risk mare:
   - Differentiate between normal and abnormal perinatal periods in the mare, and explain how to care for a high-risk mare.
   - Identify the stages of labor in a mare, and describe how to treat any complications that may arise at each stage.
7. Describe the normal development of a neonatal foal that occurs during the first 24 hours, and identify normal vital signs and behavior.
8. Do the following regarding care of the sick foal:
   - List the signs of a critically ill foal, including symptoms of prematurity and dysmaturity and classic early clinical signs of disease.
   - Identify common sites and procedures for venous and arterial blood collection, as well as appropriate needles, syringes, and restraint techniques to be used in the neonatal foal.

- Identify parameters that should be monitored in the hospitalized foal, and describe complications that may arise during hospitalization.
- Describe proper nursing care for the foal to prevent contamination, including washing of hands and injection sites, changing of IV fluid lines, and maintenance of IV and jugular catheters.
- Explain appropriate physical therapy for the recumbent foal, the necessity for being kept in sternal position and rotated, and proper restraint techniques that can be used for the ambulatory foal.

9. Explain alternative methods that can be used to ensure that nutritional needs are met if a foal is unable to nurse from the mare.

INTRODUCTION

Human medicine is rich with volumes of books containing tables, graphs, and guidelines, such as the "Denver scores," which detail normal and abnormal development of babies and are readily available to clinicians for assessment of human pediatric patients. In contrast, veterinary medicine is challenged by diversity among species and breeds of animals and by the far broader ranges of what constitutes "normal" and "abnormal." Relatively speaking, veterinary personnel must rely on far fewer reference resources, making empirical experience and the observations of breeders critically important. Because the development of body systems continues well after birth, young animals are particularly vulnerable to age-related problems. A thorough history and physical examination are important for detecting developmental complications and illnesses. This chapter addresses normal neonatal development and the most common reasons for illness in the puppy, kitten, and **foal.**

NEONATOLOGY OF PUPPIES AND KITTENS

DEFINITION

The **neonatal period** in puppies and kittens is characterized by complete dependency on the bitch or queen for survival. The first 2 to 4 weeks of a puppy's or kitten's life is considered, by most sources, to be the neonatal period. During this time, neonates fully depend on their mothers for nutrition, warmth, and care. The following information pertains to puppies and kittens during this highly vulnerable time of their life.

HISTORY

Because of the unusual or nonspecific clinical signs associated with ill puppies and kittens, it is important to obtain a comprehensive history not only of the patient, but also of the littermates, parents, and other relatives. The history should include the number of ill animals, the method by which they were raised, their normal environment, the behavior of each puppy or kitten within the litter, body weight curves, duration and types of clinical signs, and medications given. The queen's or bitch's history should include vaccination dates, estrous cycle (intervals and duration), breeding practice, medications or supplements given during pregnancy, and problems during pregnancy or birth. Has the disorder that the patient is experiencing been seen in previous litters or in any of the relatives? In certain cases, clients are advised to bring the whole litter or at least one healthy littermate, including the mother, so that the patient can be compared with its littermate(s). If the patient or its littermates have not been vaccinated, it may be better to have them come in the back door to prevent exposure to all the infectious diseases that may linger in the waiting room.

> **TECHNICIAN NOTE** Because of the unusual or non-specific clinical signs associated with ill puppies and kittens, it is of great importance to obtain a comprehensive history not only of the patient, but also of the littermates, parents, and other relatives.

PHYSICAL EXAMINATION

Physical examination of the neonate (younger than 3 to 4 weeks of age) and the juvenile patient can be challenging. Owners and littermates that were brought in for comparison can be quite distracting. Usually, one cannot expect cooperation from the youngest of our patients, especially those that are already aware of their surroundings. They are so distracted by the new environment that something as simple as a menace reflex is difficult to elicit. If more than one neonate is being examined, it is important to properly identify each individual. Several methods of doing this may be used, such as painting toenails with different colors of nail polish, applying collars made of yarn of different colors, and drawing pictures of unique markings. Refer to Figure 21-1 for an example of a newborn medical record that includes

Newborn Record

Name: _____ Date of birth: _____

Species: _____ Breed: _____ Sex: _____

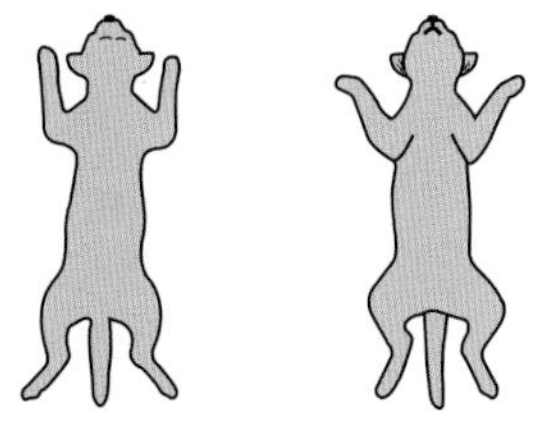

Dorsal   Ventral

Identifying marks: _____

Newborn checklist	
Dew claws	Murmurs
Fontanel	Diarrhea staining
Palate	Persistent urachus
Hernias	Sucklling reflex
Malformations	Righting reflex

FIGURE 21-1 An example of a newborn medical record that includes schematics on which to draw identifying features of the patient.

schematics on which to draw identifying features of the patient. Although it is common practice to perform a physical examination on an adult, it is less common to perform an examination on a tiny puppy or kitten. The following paragraphs, therefore, are devoted to the examination of neonates. Some specific examples are given, but keep in mind that the list is not complete. Some of the developmental landmarks described later may be helpful in detecting abnormalities.

A pediatric stethoscope with a 2-cm bell is a helpful tool when neonatal animals are examined. In addition, a digital thermometer allows rapid measurement of body temperature without causing great discomfort. Because the neonate can have a body temperature lower than 94° F (34.4° C), a digital thermometer that measures as low as 85° F (29.4° C) is necessary. Neonates cannot regulate their body temperature during the first 2 weeks of life. Therefore, they should be examined on a warm, clean surface rather than on a cold metal table. To evaluate the hydration status of a neonate, the oral mucous membranes must be examined and not skin turgor, because turgor is not developed in the integument of neonates as it is in adults (Figure 21-2). Moist mucous membranes are present in an adequate state of hydration. The neonate is born with hair that covers most of the body except the ventral abdominal skin. Lack of hair or a sparse hair coat may indicate a **genetic** abnormality of the skin or premature birth (Figure 21-3). The neonate normally has hairless, dark-pink ventral abdominal skin. Bluish or dark-red discolorations are indicative of a neonate in distress (cyanosis or sepsis, respectively). Other than urine and feces, a discharge from any orifice is abnormal in the neonate. The neonate's

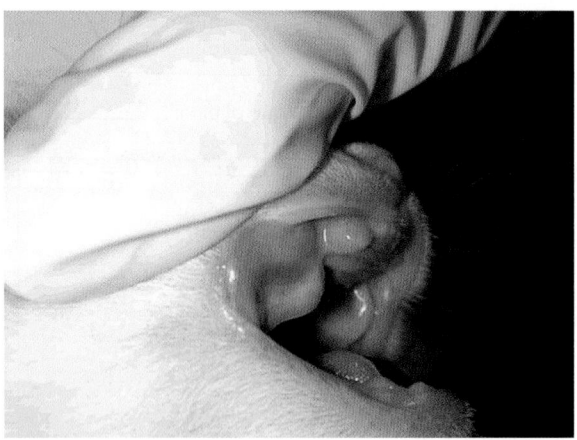

FIGURE 21-2 Mucous membranes in the mouth of a newborn kitten. Note the pale pink appearance, which shows the normal color at this age.

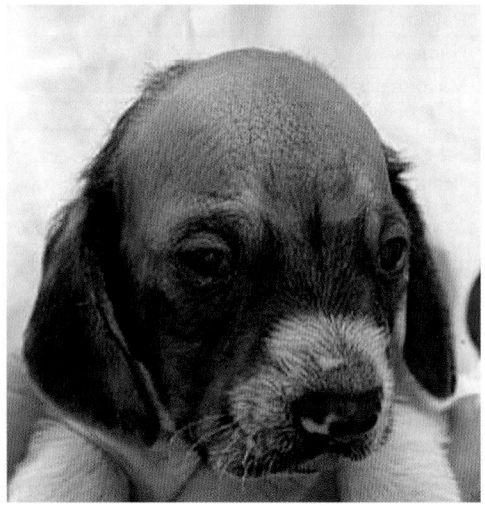

FIGURE 21-3 Two-week-old abnormal puppy displaying hairlessness and cloudy, slightly crusty eyes.

head, body, limbs, and tail are examined for symmetry and normal conformation. The head is specifically examined for open fontanelles, cleft palate, bulging eyes from behind closed eyelids (infection behind closed eyelids), and formation of the nose and external ears. Flattening or malformations of the chest are noted and are suggestive of swimmer syndrome (pectus excavatum). Bulges in the neck area are also abnormal and may be attributed to gas in the esophagus, ectopic heart, or goiter. Neonatal puppies are mildly pudgy, and neonatal kittens are generally on the lean side. Neither of them should ever be bloated, which would be a sign of distress. The abdomen and the urachus are specially examined for defects of the abdominal wall and ventral urine scalding, such as cannibalism as a result of an overzealous mother, ventral closure defects, and a persistent urachus. The genitals and the anus are checked for patency by stimulating urination and defecation using a moistened cotton ball. The presence of hair coat anomalies over the dorsum may indicate the presence of spina bifida. The tail is examined for

muscle tone, length, curliness, and kinks. Abnormalities in tone may indicate neurologic problems such as abnormal innervation of the distal pelvis.

> **TECHNICIAN NOTE**   Neonatal puppies and kittens should be examined in a room in which no other animals with infectious diseases were recently present. Freshly washed, clean towels and blankets should be available and examination gloves worn to minimize the spread of infectious agents because neonates do not have a mature immune system.

NORMAL DEVELOPMENT

During the first week of life, newborn kittens and puppies sleep throughout most of the day (80%) and nurse vigorously for a short time every 2 to 4 hours. Because the brain is not completely developed at birth, neuromuscular reflexes are missing, and the only motor skills present are crawling, suckling, and distress vocalization. Neonates only respond to stimuli such as odor, touch, and pain. The queen or bitch initiates urination and defecation by licking the urogenital area. At 3 days of age, kittens and puppies should be able to lift their head, and by 1 week, they can crawl in a coordinated manner. Puppies and kittens are unable to maintain their body temperature during the first few days of life, and the shiver reflex does not develop until after the first week of life. Body temperature at birth (94.5°F to 97.3°F [34.5°C to 36.3°C]) is lower than in adults and rises to 94.7°F to 100.1°F (34.8° to 38.3°C) during the first week of life. Heart and respiratory rates may be irregular at birth (pulse [P] = 160 to 200 beats/minute [bpm], respiration [R] = 10 to 20 breaths/minute), and respiration has no abdominal component. During the first week, neonates begin to adjust to the new extrauterine environment, and their respiratory and heart rates increase (P = 200 to 220 bpm, R = 16 to 35 breaths/minute). The umbilical cord dries during the first day of life and typically falls off by day 2 to 3. The flexor tone present at birth switches over to extensor tone after the 4th day of life (Box 21-1). Although sex determination in normal newborn puppies is unambiguous, it can be challenging in kittens. The sex of kittens can be determined at birth by evaluating the anogenital distance, which is shorter in females (7.6 ± 1 mm) than in males (12.9 ± 1.5 mm). Male kittens are born with descended testicles, which are able to move freely into and out of the scrotum until 5 to 7 months of age. In dogs, the testicles do not descend until 6 weeks of age.

During the 2nd week of life, kittens and puppies begin to crawl, and their body temperature slowly rises toward normal adult levels. Kittens and puppies will have doubled their birth weight by 7 to 10 and 10 to 12 days, respectively. They begin to open their eyes at 7 to 12 days of age, and the external ear canals open at 14 to 16 days of age. The iris is not well pigmented and has a blue-gray color, and the cornea is slightly cloudy as a result of increased water content. Kittens may have divergent strabismus. By 3 weeks of age, puppies

BOX 21-1	Neurologic Examination of the Very Young Pediatric Patient

- Suckling reflex: should be present at birth; puppy or kitten will try to suck or chew on a finger.
- Pressing reflex: should be present at birth; puppy or kitten will press its head against a bowed hand.
- Flexor tone: present until 3 to 4 days of age; when a puppy or kitten is held by the head, it will "roll up" and adduct its hind legs.
- Extensor tone: after 4 days of age, a puppy or kitten held by its head will stretch its back and hind legs.
- Lumbar reflex: forcefully rubbing a healthy puppy or kitten in the lumbar region will result in vocalization and great activity.
- Extensor reflex: patient is placed in dorsal recumbency, and the toe of a hindlimb is pinched. If the puppy or kitten is younger than 3 weeks of age, it will adduct the other hindlimb. Normal!
- Magnus reflex: patient is placed in dorsal recumbency, and its head is bent toward one side. Before 3 weeks of age, it will stretch its legs on this side and bend the legs on the other side.
- Tonic neck reflexes: patient is held by the thorax, and its neck is bent toward one side; it should stretch the limbs on this side. The head is bent dorsally; the front limbs should be stretched and the hindlimbs adducted. Present until 3 weeks of age.
- Hopping reflex: is already present at 2 to 4 days of age.
- Anogenital reflex: if the patient's anogenital region is stimulated with a moist cloth or cotton, it should urinate or defecate. Present until 3 to 4 weeks of age.
- Palpebral and corneal reflexes: should be present as soon as the eyes are open.
- Menace reflex: can be present as early as 2 weeks of age but usually not until 10 to 14 weeks of age.

and kittens are able to stand and have good postural reflexes. Refer to Box 21-2 for details about the development of specific organ systems.

TECHNICIAN NOTE Although sex determination in normal newborn puppies is unambiguous, it can be challenging in kittens. The sex of kittens can be determined at birth by evaluating the anogenital distance, which is shorter in females (7.6 ± 1 mm) than in males (12.9 ± 1.5 mm).

DIAGNOSTICS

Blood can be easily obtained from the jugular vein in neonates. However, no more than 10% of the circulating volume should be drawn over the course of a week. In other words, if a neonate weighs 250 grams, no more than 2.5 ml of blood should be drawn in 1 week. If a neonate remains in the hospital for several days, it may be worthwhile posting a chart next to the patient, where every nurse can record the amount of blood drawn to prevent the patient from becoming

anemic. This is especially helpful in neonates that cannot maintain proper blood glucose levels and need to be subjected to multiple blood draws (1 drop of blood equals about 0.1 ml). Because of the small amount of sample drawn at any given time, a collection tube of appropriate size should be used to ensure that the anticoagulant ethylenediaminetetraacetic acid (EDTA) does not dilute the sample, resulting in false laboratory data.

To obtain urine samples, the neonate can simply be stimulated to urinate by gently rubbing the genital area with a moistened cotton ball. Alternatively, the bladder can be carefully expressed. It is rarely necessary to obtain sterile urine samples by cystocentesis, which should be avoided because of the fragility of neonates' skin and organs.

Imaging techniques include radiography and ultrasonography. An ultrasound examination is best performed using a 7.5-MHz transducer, and neonates generally tolerate this imaging technique better than radiography. Radiography of neonates requires high-detail intensifying screens and single-emulsion films. For optimal contrast, no whole body radiographs should be taken, and the kilovoltage should be reduced to half that of an adult because little body fat and poor mineralization are present at this age. If possible, a normal littermate should be radiographed for comparison.

TECHNICIAN NOTE Because neonates have immature kidneys, it is normal to find urine specific gravities between 1.012 and 1.020, as well as glucose in the urine of puppies and kittens younger than 2 weeks of age.

ROUTINE MAINTENANCE

Healthy neonatal puppies and kittens born to healthy mothers with good maternal instincts require almost no care during the first weeks of life. If neonates were born via cesarean section, the umbilical remnant should be treated with iodine (1%), and they should be encouraged to nurse as quickly as possible to ensure uptake of colostrum. Beginning at 2 weeks of life, kittens and puppies should be dewormed with pyrantel pamoate (4.54 mg/kg PO) at 2-week intervals for at least three doses. Treatment is aimed mainly at eliminating roundworms. Once puppies and kittens are past the neonatal stage, that is, between 6 and 8 weeks of age, they should be seen at a veterinarian's office for their first official health examination. This visit will include a thorough physical examination, a fecal examination, vaccines, and "The Talk." It is of utmost importance to make sure that the new owner of a kitten or puppy understands the following basic concepts:

- Proper nutrition in young animals contributes to the pet's overall well-being and may decrease joint and other orthopedic problems in later years.
- Preventive practices such as administration of deworming medications and vaccines are important in ensuring pet health. Many of the diseases against which we vaccinate are fatal.

BOX 21-2 | Select Organ Development

- **Heart:** At birth, the right and left ventricles have approximately the same mass, changing to an ultimate adult ratio of 1:2 to 1:3 throughout puberty, and changing in cardiac axis and shape. During this time, the canine heart changes from ellipsoid at birth to more globoid in adulthood. At 1 month of age, puppies and kittens still have lower blood pressure, stroke volume, and resistance in the peripheral vasculature than adults, but they have higher heart rate, cardiac output, and central venous pressure. Responses to cardiovascular drugs during the first weeks of life are less intense than in the adult. Development of the heart has been well studied in the dog, and it has been shown that normal adult values of the aforementioned parameters are reached by 7 months of age. It is important to keep these differences in mind when evaluating chest radiographs, electrocardiograms (ECGs), and echocardiograms.

- **Immune system:** Virtually no antibodies are transferred in utero to canine and feline fetuses, and they are born immunologically immature. Puppies and kittens are dependent on the colostral transfer of antibodies (passive immunity) for postnatal protection against infectious diseases. In puppies and kittens, colostrum needs to be ingested within the first 24 and 16 hours of life, respectively, whereby mainly immunoglobulin (Ig)G and IgA are absorbed. Thereafter, the gut seems to be closed for further absorption. Depending on the type of maternally derived antibodies, these may last from 6 to 16 weeks after birth. Relative to the size of the puppy, the greatest size of the thymus is noted at birth, but its absolute size will be greatest at puberty, after which it begins to atrophy. Although the thymus and the immune system are thought to be mature by 3 to 4 months of age, puppies and kittens have the ability to produce functional IgM shortly before birth. Lymph node structure is normal at birth, but few lymphocytes are present; these increase in number during the first months of life. Lymph nodes should be palpable at birth, but facial nodes are easier to palpate because of their increased reactivity.

- **Liver:** Drugs that require hepatic metabolism should be carefully administered to neonatal patients because the liver does not reach full metabolic capacity until well after the neonatal period. Neonatal albumin and plasma protein levels are significantly lower than in adults. Dosages of drugs that are bound to albumin or plasma proteins must be adjusted accordingly. The liver is the site of the production of most coagulation factors. Because of its immaturity, many coagulopathies may be exacerbated during the neonatal age. Because growing requires rapid bone turnover, serum concentrations of alkaline phosphatase (ALP) are often elevated, but they should never be increased more than twofold to threefold in healthy, growing animals. Serum ALP and gamma-glutamyl transferase (GGT) are not reliable indicators of liver disease during the first 2 weeks of life because both are present in colostrum and are absorbed through the gut, increasing ALP and GGT levels greatly in the neonate. Lack of an increase in ALP and GGT in a puppy younger than 2 weeks can be used as an indicator of not having received colostrum.

- **Kidney:** The neonate is particularly susceptible to dehydration because water makes up 82% of body weight, and water turnover is about twice that of an adult. Because of the neonate's limited ability to conserve fluid and the immaturity of the kidney, fluid requirements are high at 13 to 22 ml/100 g body weight per day. Nephrons are not completely formed until the 3rd week of life, and glomerular filtration rates increase from 21% at birth to 53% by 8 weeks of age. Whereas tubular secretion generally is thought to be mature by 8 weeks of age, some reports indicate that it takes 6 months for tubular function to be complete. Either way, this explains the low urine specific gravity until 8 weeks of age (1.006 to 1.017), increased concentrations of amino acids and proteins, and glucosuria—a common finding in neonates up to 2 weeks of age. Given the immaturity of renal function, medications that affect kidney development should be avoided, and dosages of those that are excreted through the kidney must be adjusted to the patient's age.

- **Thyroid:** Serum thyroid hormones differ between puppies and kittens and their adult counterparts and also differ significantly with time during the first 12 weeks of life. Therefore, it is critical to know the exact age of puppies or kittens and to not use the standard reference range for adult normal dogs or cats, respectively. Lack of thyroid hormones in the neonate leads to much more serious disease than in the adult because of involvement of the thyroid in development. Clinical signs in affected puppies and kittens may be as mild as apathy and failure to thrive or as severe as joint and bone abnormalities, complete dullness, extremely stunted growth, and, in cats, constipation. Serum thyroid hormones should be determined at the slightest suspicion of hypothyroidism because the earlier treatment is initiated, the better the outcome. Therapy is performed as in adults, but thyroid levels should be checked frequently in young patients and results compared with normal values for the corresponding age group.

- **Gastrointestinal system:** The neonate is born with a sterile GI system, which will develop its own flora to assist digestion during the first few days of life. GI peristalsis is weaker (slower), intestinal blood flow is reduced, and gastric fluid has a higher pH. It is clear that medication, changes in the environment, or disease will cause upset to this yet fragile system, which is most commonly apparent in the form of diarrhea. The most common causes of diarrhea in the orphaned neonate are overfeeding and inappropriate dilutions of milk replacer.

- Behavior issues need to be addressed as early as possible to avoid the development of entrenched undesirable behavior that could lead to euthanasia of the pet later in life.

Undesirable behavior is one of the most common reasons for abandonment of dogs and cats younger than 1 year of age. Discussing proper behavior and suggesting puppy classes will contribute to a long-lasting, happy owner/pet relationship. Microchipping should be recommended at this time. Because the needle for placing a microchip is fairly large and the procedure may be painful, the skin can be numbed using lidocaine gel at the injection site, which should be carefully cleaned before placement. Please wear gloves when using lidocaine gel because you do not want to numb your own fingers!

> **TECHNICIAN NOTE** Have puppy and kitten care kits handy that describe whom to call in an emergency, vaccination plans, whom to contact for behavior issues, and what to feed the pediatric pet.

COMMON CONCERNS AND DISORDERS IN THE PUPPY AND KITTEN (BOX 21-3)

Hypothermia

When puppies and kittens are born, they have almost no subcutaneous fat and thus little insulation. Initially, body heat is produced by brown fat metabolism, which is under the control of the sympathetic nervous system (nonshivering **thermogenesis**). Because of their relatively large surface area when compared with older animals, heat loss is much greater in neonates. As long as neonates are close to their dams and the mammary glands, little heat loss occurs, so they can maintain thermal balance. However, as the neonate begins to take up food, its metabolic rate increases, which in turn elevates its body temperature. Shivering and vasoconstrictive mechanisms may begin at around 6 to 8 days, but by about 6 weeks, puppies and kittens are good homeotherms and have a body temperature that is similar to that of adults.

Hypothermia in the neonate is a serious problem. Gut motility slows with decreasing body temperature, ultimately causing an ileus. When hypothermic neonates are tube-fed, the milk replacer may be regurgitated and aspirated, resulting in pneumonia, or the ingesta may ferment, leading to bloat. This causes increased pressure on the thorax, which in turn causes labored breathing. Most neonates in pain or respiratory distress swallow air, which exacerbates a bloated

BOX 21-3	Neonatal Illness That Needs Immediate Attention

- Hypothermia
- Dehydration
- Hypoglycemia
- Neonatal isoerythrolysis
- Malnutrition

condition. In this way, a downward spiral forms that ultimately results in circulatory collapse and death. Hypothermia also inhibits cellular immune functions, which may lead to increased susceptibility to infection. A neonate is considered hypothermic if its body temperature drops below 94° F (34.4° C) at birth, below 96° F (35.6° C) at 1 to 3 days of age, or below 99° F (37.2° C) at 1 week of age. Clinical signs in a chilled neonate with a body temperature above 88° F (31.1° C) include restlessness, continuous crying, red mucous membranes, and skin that is cool to the touch. However, muscle tone is still good, respiratory rate is greater than 40 breaths/minute, and heart rate is greater than 200 bpm. When body temperatures fall into the range of 78° F to 85° F (25.5° C to 29.4° C), the neonate appears lethargic and uncoordinated but responsive. Moisture is seen around the corners of the lips, heart rate drops to below 50 bpm, and respiratory rate is between 20 and 25 breaths/minute. No abdominal sounds are heard, and metabolism is impaired, resulting in hypoglycemia (see later discussion). Below 70° F (21.1° C), the neonate appears to be dead. If extreme measures of arousal result in a response, treatment may be attempted. Hypoxia also contributes significantly to hypothermia. Therefore, the neonate should be provided with proper ventilation or oxygen administration whenever possible.

Treatment consists of slowly ($\approx$2° F/hour) reheating the patient by providing appropriate ambient temperature and humidity. Heating pads, heat lamps, warm water gloves, rice bags, and incubators can be used, but it is essential that the temperature be controlled and monitored carefully, especially when heating lamps or heating pads are used, because the neonate cannot escape if the temperature is too warm. Warm air and oxygen in a human neonatal incubator or a veterinary oxygen cage is optimal for rewarming the hypothermic neonate. Warm IV fluids can also be given, but at no more than 2° F above body temperature. Do not give anything orally until the patient has audible gut sounds and is moderately rewarmed. Rapid rewarming will result in heat prostration with increased respiratory rate and effort. Eventually, the patient will become cyanotic and will have diarrhea and seizures. Raising the neonatal body temperature by more than 4° F is usually fatal because of delayed organ failure. Thermal burns may occur if the surrounding temperature is not properly monitored.

> **TECHNICIAN NOTE** Hypothermia in the neonate is a serious problem. Gut motility slows with decreasing body temperature, ultimately causing ileus. When hypothermic neonates are tube-fed, the milk replacer may be regurgitated and aspirated, resulting in pneumonia, or the ingesta may ferment, leading to bloat.

Dehydration

Any disease process or imbalance of fluids or electrolytes will quickly lead to **dehydration** in the neonate because of increased body water, increased water turnover, and immaturity of the renal system. As indicated before, checking the oral mucous membranes assesses hydration in the neonate because the skin turgor is not yet developed, as it is in adults. Moist mucous membranes are present in an adequate state of hydration, but tacky to dry mucous membranes indicate 5% to 7% dehydration. At 10% dehydration, the mucous membranes are dry, and the decrease in skin elasticity is noticeable.

Fluid requirements are high in neonates, but total volumes that can be given are low. All fluids should be warmed to 98° F to 99° F (36.6° C to36.7° C) before administration unless the neonate is substantially colder. In that case, fluids should be warmed to 2° F higher than current body temperature. Boluses can be given at 3.3 ml per 100 grams of the neonate's weight over 5 to 10 minutes. The maintenance dose is 6 ml/kg/hour. To this, 50% of the deficit is added over 6 hours (Deficit = Body weight [BW] × % dehydrated). Fluids can be given intravenously (IV), intraosseously (IO), intraperitoneally (IP), or subcutaneously (SQ). It is often easiest to place a short 23- or 25-gauge catheter into the jugular vein for fluid administration. Another option is IO fluid delivery: the bone is still soft enough that an 18- or 19-gauge needle can be placed into the proximal tibia or the proximal femur, and fluids are given at the same rate as IV fluids. It is important that each bone not be punctured more than once because fluid will leak out of the other hole. Administering fluids at a constant rate is best accomplished by using a syringe pump or a pediatric drip (60 drops/minute). If IV or IO access is not available, fluids are given IP or SQ. However, absorption rates are slow with both routes, and they are not ideal for long-term fluid therapy. When fluids are given IP or SQ, the volume should be divided into 2 to 3 boluses per day. In many cases, the neonate is acidotic, but because of limited liver function, the neonate has difficulty metabolizing lactate into bicarbonate. In most cases, lactated Ringer's with 20 mmol/L of maintenance potassium is sufficient.

> **TECHNICIAN NOTE** Dehydration occurs very quickly in neonates because their fluid requirements are much greater than those of adults, and they are less able to conserve fluids. Therefore, fluid replacement therapy is a key element in nursing a neonate back to health.

Hypoglycemia

The risk of **hypoglycemia** is great because the neonate is born with few glycogen stores and has poor gluconeogenesis in the liver. As long as the neonate is healthy, it can maintain normal blood glucose concentrations for up to 24 hours without nursing. However, failure to suckle will result in hypoglycemia after 24 to 36 hours as a result of depletion of hepatic stores. A variety of clinical signs may occur in the hypoglycemic (serum glucose less than 30 mg/dl) neonatal patient, including tremors, crying, irritability, increased appetite, dullness, lethargy, coma, stupor, and seizures.

Treatment consists of giving dextrose slowly IV or IO at 0.5 to 1 g/kg as part of a 5% to 10% dextrose solution in normal saline. Care should be taken when giving 5%

dextrose mixed with lactated Ringer's solution because the mixture will become hypertonic, and volume replacement will have to be monitored carefully. Higher concentrations of IV dextrose should be avoided because of its irritant nature (phlebitis). Dextrose can be given at higher concentrations directly to the mucous membranes of the mouth if the neonate is not dehydrated or hypothermic (1 to 2 ml of a 5% to 15% dextrose solution). Dextrose solutions should never be given SQ because they may cause tissue damage. After treatment, blood glucose levels should be monitored because of the risk of hyperglycemia as a result of poor regulatory mechanisms in the neonate.

> **TECHNICIAN NOTE** Hypoglycemia is one of the most common causes of seizures in neonatal puppies and kittens.

Neonatal Isoerythrolysis in Kittens

Cats with blood type A have low titers of naturally occurring antibodies against blood type B red blood cells. Therefore, blood type B kittens born to blood type A queens do not show any clinical signs of incompatibility reactions after ingestion of colostrum-containing alloantibodies. However, all blood type B cats have high titers of naturally occurring antibodies against type A red blood cells. This may lead to incompatibility reactions when blood type A kittens receive colostral antibodies from a blood type B queen. Clinical signs are variable and range from jaundice and death within the first 2 days of life to no signs at all (which is rare). Sometimes the tail tip becomes necrotic and falls off at 10 to 14 days of life. Studies at the University of Pennsylvania indicate that kittens at risk for neonatal isoerythrolysis must be removed from their queens only during the first day of life.

Kittens can be tested at birth using handy blood-typing cards (e.g., DMS Laboratories, Flemington, New Jersey), and if blood type B kittens are born to blood type A queens, they can be fostered to a blood type B queen or hand-raised during the first 24 hours of life. If kittens have neonatal isoerythrolysis during the first day of life, they should be removed from the queen for 24 hours and given supportive care.

Malnutrition

Many milk replacers can easily cover the daily caloric requirements of both puppies and kittens. However, it seems that the fluid requirements are not easily met. Regular feeding is important to maintain good hydration in the neonate. If only three feedings per day can be provided, then a commercial milk replacer with a formulation that comes closest to the bitch's or queen's milk should be used (Table 21-1) and extra fluids provided SQ. Overfeeding or a high lactose content in the milk replacer often cause diarrhea. Nothing is better than mother's milk; it contains bile salt–activated lipase, which is necessary for proper digestion. After each meal, the neonate should be encouraged to urinate and defecate by stimulating the anogenital region with a moistened

TABLE 21-1	Overview of Requirements and Milk Comparison		
AGE	**PUPPIES, kcal/100 g/day**	**KITTENS, kcal/100 g/day**	**FLUIDS FOR BOTH, ml/100 g**
Week 1	13-15	<38 at birth; 28 thereafter	18 ml average
Week 2	15-20	28	Range, 13-22
Week 3	20	27	Same
Week 4	≥20	25	Same

	BITCH'S MILK	**QUEEN'S MILK**	**COW'S MILK‡**	**GOAT'S MILK‡**
Fluid content	77	79	88	87
Fat, %	9.5	8.5	3.5	4.1
Protein, %	7.5	7.5	3.3	3.6
Lactose, %	3.4	4.0	5.0	4.7
Calcium*	0.24	0.18	0.12	0.13
Phosphorus*	0.18	0.16	0.10	0.16
ME†, kcal/100 ml milk	146	121	70	69

*g/100 ml.
†Metabolizable energy.
‡When mixing cow's or goat's milk as a milk replacer for neonates, be aware that to cover the fat or protein requirements, the lactose concentrations will be far too high and will cause diarrhea. Commercial milk replacers are a better choice.

cotton ball. Neonates should be weighed daily on a suitable scale until 3 weeks of age to ensure proper weight gain.

Occasionally, a neonate will not nurse from a bottle or will not gain the expected weight because of illness or malformations. Tube feeding is necessary in these cases. However, a puppy or a kitten should never be tube-fed if its body temperature is lower than normal for its age. If the body temperature is too low, the gut shuts down and the ingested material starts to form a gas, which in turn will bloat the neonate, leading to serious distress. Tube feeding is performed by first measuring the distance from the tip of the neonate's nose to the end of the chest (Figure 21-4). Using a felt-tip pen or a piece of tape, a mark is made at 75% of this distance on the feeding tube, measuring from the distal end of the feeding tube. Insert this length of a clean and dry feeding tube gently into the mouth of the neonate while holding the patient upright. No force is needed because most neonates will swallow the feeding tube easily. The syringe with the milk replacer is connected to the tube, and the plunger is pulled back gently. Negative pressure indicates that the feeding tube is indeed in the lower esophagus, not in the lungs. When milk replacer alone is fed to puppies or kittens, a 5-French feeding tube is used. As a rule of thumb, about 5 ml of milk replacer can be given per feeding to a 160-gram puppy or kitten.

TECHNICIAN NOTE Tube feeding is a safe and efficient method of supplementing neonates, especially when more than one neonate needs to be fed. Risk of aspiration is less than with syringe or bottle feeding.

Fading Puppy or Kitten Syndrome

The fading puppy or kitten syndrome is characterized by anorexia, lethargy, emaciation, death, and birth defects in cats and dogs. Kittens or puppies may be stillborn or may be born small, weak, and unable to nurse, resulting in dehydration, hypothermia, hypoglycemia, and death within the first few days of life. Other neonates appear healthy during the first weeks of life; become weak, depressed, and anorexic; or die of starvation at the time of weaning.

Causes of neonatal death include poor management, malnutrition, inappropriate environmental conditions, **congenital** and genetic defects, and infection. Management and environmental problems can be easily detected by obtaining a detailed history or inspecting the facility. Problems may include poor hygiene, inappropriate temperature and humidity, overcrowding, frequent introduction of new animals, inappropriate use of medication, or exposure to chemical toxins. Nutritional deficiency can be caused by an inadequate diet for the mother or the neonate. Treatment involves supportive care for the sickly neonate and removal of inciting causes. If causes are not immediately apparent, necropsies of neonates that have died are recommended.

TECHNICIAN NOTE Fading puppy or kitten syndrome is not a diagnosis but rather a clinical description and requires further workup to find a cause.

Orphan Care

Fostering neonatal kittens and puppies is time-consuming, given that the neonate is completely helpless and requires almost 24-hour care. It is rewarding, however, once the happy, healthy puppy or kitten is ready for its new home. Materials needed include warm and clean bedding, milk bottles with a variety of different rubber nipples, feeding tubes, syringes, a gram scale, cotton balls, hand sanitizers, and fur clippers; it may be necessary to isolate the orphan

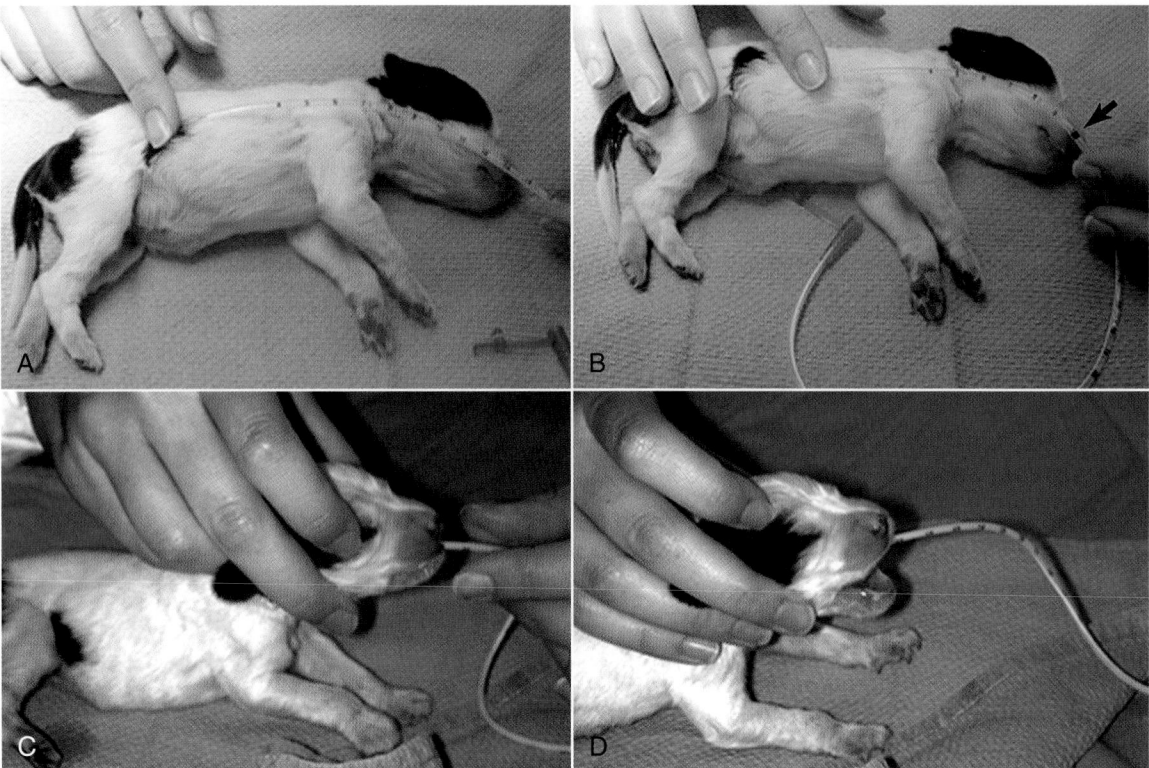

FIGURE 21-4 Tube feeding. **A,** Measure from the tip of the nose to the last rib. **B,** Make a mark at 75% of length *(arrow)*. **C,** Insert tube gently to the mark. **D,** Check for negative pressure and give milk slowly.

from the other animals. Kittens or puppies need to be hand-raised because of maternal death or abandonment, lack of milk in the mother, maternal aggression, large litter size, malformation, or trauma. When more than one neonate is taken care of, it is essential that each patient be uniquely identified so that progress can be assessed. Each orphan must be weighed daily, and records should be kept. Ambient temperature and humidity of 84°F to 90°F (29°C) and 55% to 60%, respectively, should be provided during the 1st week of life, if possible. During the 2nd week, ambient temperature can be lowered to 79°F to 84°F (26.1°C to 29.0°C), and to 73.4°F to 79°F (23°C to 26.1°C) during the 3rd week. Shivering reflexes will set in during the 2nd week of life and will contribute to an increase in body temperature. The neonate must be kept warm and well hydrated at all times, in keeping with the principles outlined earlier. Proper nutrition or supplementation (Box 21-4) and clean and dry housing should be provided. After feeding, the orphan must be stimulated to urinate and defecate.

Common pitfalls are overfeeding and underfeeding. Overfeeding milk replacers often results in diarrhea, and underfeeding in dehydration and lack of weight gain. Homemade formulas are often deficient in growth factors, amino acids, and other nutrients essential for growth. Many of the commercial milk replacers are made using cow's milk as a base; therefore, they are not always complete. The energy density of the formula might be too high, and fluid requirements will not be fulfilled, or vice versa, the energy density is too low, and the stomach capacity is too small for the

BOX 21-4	Overview of Neonatal Nutrition

- Puppies and kittens should be able to take up their daily requirements in 4 or 5 meals per day during the first few weeks of life.
- Puppies should gain 1 g for every 2 to 5 g of milk intake.
- Kittens are born at 80 to 120 g and should gain between 70 and 100 g weekly.
- During the first week of life, kittens will ingest only 10% to 15% of their body weight in milk. Thereafter, this volume increases to 20% to 25% of their body weight in milk (weeks 1 to 4).
- Puppies get their energy from fat during the first weeks of life, whereas kittens get theirs from protein. Therefore, milk replacer contents should be carefully reviewed before use.
- Many milk replacers can easily cover the daily caloric requirements of both puppies and kittens. However, it seems that the fluid requirements are not easily met. If only three feedings per day can be provided, then use one of the milk replacers, as outlined earlier, and provide the extra fluids SQ.

required amount. Therefore, commercial milk replacers should be carefully evaluated, and homemade milk replacers should be made only by using proven recipes (Table 21-2). Other problems that may arise include housing sick animals in the same room with orphans; overcrowding; improper hygiene (not washing hands between patients); too many fosters per person; damp blankets; and a cold, drafty

TABLE 21-2	Recipes for Homemade Milk Replacers		
	PUPPIES		KITTENS
INGREDIENT	RECIPE 1	RECIPE 2	RECIPE 1
Skim milk	43.8 g	64 g	70 g
Low-fat curd	40 g	15 g	15 g
Egg yolks	10 g	15 g	3 g
Vegetable oil	6 g	3 g	3 g
Lactose			0.8 g
Lean ground beef			8 g
Vitamin/mineral mix	0.2 g	2.5 g	0.2 g
Calcium carbonate		0.5 g	

BOX 21-5	Considerations When Using Medication in the Pediatric Patient

- Total body water higher (up to 82% of body weight)
- Less fat
- Less muscle mass
- Muscle not well vascularized
- Plasma protein lower
- Gastric pH higher
- GI peristalsis weaker (slower)
- Lower intestinal blood flow
- Better intestinal absorption of proteins
- Not fully developed intestinal flora
- Blood-brain barrier not fully developed
- Liver: some enzymes need up to 4 months to develop
- Kidney: glomerular filtration developed by 3 to 4 weeks
- Kidney: tubular secretion developed by one-half year
- Energy (calories) obtained through digestion of fat
- Sixty-five percent of fat is digested in the stomach
- No lipase in milk—lower weight gain
- Milk curdles in stomach = normal!
- High energy requirements—never fast a puppy or a kitten!

environment. Last, because of differences in physiology, medications will not be taken up and metabolized at the same rate as in adults. Care should be taken when choosing medications and administering them. Box 21-5 outlines the main physiologic differences between neonates and adults.

> **TECHNICIAN NOTE** Weight loss, or lack of weight gain, is the first indication that a neonate is not doing well. Therefore, proper identification and accurate daily weight recordings for each orphan ensure that a problem will be identified before it is too late for therapy.

NEONATOLOGY OF FOALS

Breeding a **mare** and delivering a foal are exciting times for many horse owners. Some clients breed mares that they have owned for years because they want a foal that will be used for pleasure riding. Other owners breed mares to obtain foals that will be used in competition such as racing. The goals are the same in both instances: to deliver a healthy foal and to recognize when problems arise in the neonatal period. This section focuses on two critical areas: the perinatal period, because the late-term pregnant mare is preparing to deliver a foal, and the neonatal period, when the foal is vulnerable to disease. The normal development of foals will be discussed; this will be followed by a discussion of potential diseases and treatment of foals that require intensive care. It takes a team of veterinary personnel to manage the care of sick and debilitated foals. Veterinary technicians play a critical role on this team. That role will be highlighted in this chapter.

THE PERINATAL PERIOD AND THE HIGH-RISK MARE

Many mares have routine pregnancies and deliver healthy foals. However, sometimes the mare develops problems in late-term pregnancy and requires treatment. These mares, referred to as *high-risk mares*, often exhibit early warning signs, indicating a problem with the pregnancy.

The average length of gestation in a mare is 340 days, but normal gestation can range from 320 days to 400 days. When mares have multiple pregnancies, they often deliver around the same time of day with each pregnancy, so this is an important part of the history to obtain. When a mare is bred and becomes pregnant, she is evaluated at regular intervals by a veterinarian early in the pregnancy. The veterinarian performs a rectal examination and transrectal ultrasound around 15 days, 30 days, and then 90 days. These examinations ensure that the mare is retaining the embryo, identify the presence or absence of twins, and evaluate amniotic and allantoic fluid levels surrounding the embryo. As long as the mare is maintaining the pregnancy and findings are within normal limits, she is monitored closely for any changes but often is not evaluated again until the end of her pregnancy. In late-term pregnancy (7 to 10 months), the mare is reevaluated by a veterinarian and is closely watched for any abnormal signs. During this time, the mare should be comfortable, bright, alert, and eating readily. Exercise is important to maintain the mare's physical condition because delivery (parturition) is explosive in horses, and the foal should be delivered within 30 minutes of stage 2 labor (water breaking). She should have no vaginal or udder discharge. If a vaginal discharge is present, this may indicate a problem, such as placentitis or urine pooling, and the mare needs to be evaluated by a veterinarian. Toward the end of gestation, the mare's udder slowly enlarges, and before delivery, beads of milk appear on the end of her teats. This is called *waxing*. Unless delivery is imminent, the mare should <u>not</u> have milk dripping or streaming from her udder. Dripping occurs unexpectedly for three reasons: twins are present, the mare has placentitis, or the owner has calculated the wrong delivery date.

A veterinarian needs to evaluate the mare to determine the cause of dripping milk. The most common reason is that the mare has an ascending placentitis, and subsequent inflammatory changes cause premature lactation. Older mares are especially prone to this problem as a result of poor vulvar conformation as they age. Performing a transrectal ultrasound allows the veterinarian to evaluate placental thickness near the cervical star (the area of the placenta next to the cervix that is most often affected by ascending placentitis) and fetal fluid volume and appearance. The veterinarian can also evaluate gross fetal movement and can measure the eye orbit to estimate fetal age. A transabdominal ultrasound will aid in evaluating the foal and placenta and can provide valuable information.

Vaginal examination in a late-term pregnant mare is not recommended unless delivery is imminent because this can actually induce ascending placentitis. If the placenta appears thickened or detached, and/or the fetal fluid is more hyperechoic (increased whiteness is noted on ultrasound from the presence of cellular debris), the mare has placentitis and requires treatment. Typical treatment includes the use of broad-spectrum antimicrobials, such as trimethoprim-sulfa, and nonsteroidal anti-inflammatory medications, such as flunixin meglumine and progesterone (Regu-Mate is most commonly used in mares). This treatment is designed to kill any bacteria present, decrease inflammation associated with placentitis, and help maintain the pregnancy until term. Many mares respond to this treatment quickly, and abnormal clinical signs, such as premature udder development and dripping milk, will resolve. If left untreated, most of these mares will deliver premature foals that have a poor chance for survival. If diagnosed and treated early enough, no long-term effects on the foal may be noted, but this depends on how long the foal was affected and the extent of damage to the placenta. These mares are classified as "high risk" and need to be monitored closely for foaling. An attended foaling is important to ensure that the foal has the best chance for survival, and to treat the foal quickly if any problems are noted. Other reasons for mares to be classified as "high risk" include the presence of twins and a history of foaling problems.

> **TECHNICIAN NOTE**   Unless delivery is imminent, the mare should <u>not</u> have milk dripping or streaming from her udder. Dripping occurs unexpectedly for three reasons:
> 1. Twins are present.
> 2. Placentitis is present.
> 3. The owner has miscalculated the delivery date.

High-risk mares may be referred to a foaling facility or a veterinary hospital to have an attended foaling and prompt delivery of medical care. Methods used to monitor high-risk mares include a video camera placed in the stall to observe the mare's behavior without human interaction and telemetry to monitor heart rates of the mare and the foal. It is important for the mare to feel as comfortable as possible. Labor consists of three stages: stage 1, stage 2, and stage 3. Mares can begin stage 1 of labor (exhibit behavioral changes indicating impending labor), but if they feel threatened, they can stop the labor and resume later. A video camera offers

the optimal way to unobtrusively observe the mare's behavior. Telemetry used to measure heart rates of the foal and the mare is a noninvasive way to assess fetal and maternal health. In late-term pregnancy, the foal has a heart rate between 40 to 150 bpm. During some periods, the foal's heart rate is low (e.g., 40 bpm) because the foal is sleeping; at other times, the foal's heart rate is 120 bpm or higher, for instance, during periods of exercise. The important point to note is that the foal should have a range of heart rates over time, not a sustained low or high heart rate, which can indicate that the foal is stressed in utero. Over the course of gestation, the resting fetal heart rate will gradually decrease and often will stay around 40 to 80 bpm during periods of rest. A late-term pregnant mare should have a heart rate around 40 to 50 bpm, with higher rates during periods of exercise (e.g., pasture turnout).

It is often difficult to predict exactly when a mare will foal. As parturition (foaling) approaches, the mare's udder slowly enlarges and fills with milk, her vulva lengthens, and pelvic ligaments relax. Many mares develop "wax" (drops of dried milk) on the tips of their teats. Often mares foal at night, when the stable is quiet, but some mares readily deliver a foal in the afternoon while surrounded by noise. Knowing when a multiparous mare has foaled in the past is helpful; they often foal around the same date during each pregnancy. Also, knowing her prior behavior changes will provide clues to when she might foal. A maiden mare (primiparous: mare has never foaled) can be more challenging, but checking her vulvar relaxation, her udder development, and the presence of wax on her teats will aid in predicting delivery. Commercial kits are available that measure the rise in calcium in the mare's first milk (colostrum) and accurately predict foaling in some normal mares. A rapid rise in colostral calcium represents one of the most consistent and significant changes before parturition. Calcium levels in colostrum samples can be rapidly measured in nearly every diagnostic laboratory and with the use of simple hard-water test kits. Colostral calcium levels above 10 to 12 mmol/dl are considered significant enough to predict parturition within the ensuing 24 hours. However, parturition in high-risk mares often is not reliably predicted by these kits. Despite the different methods that are available, the best approach for determining when a mare will foal is to have a well-trained staff member monitor the mare's behavior 24 hours a day (especially by video camera in the stall) and note any changes. A docile mare may become cranky; an aggressive mare may become docile. Some mares drip milk from their udders just before foaling.

During stage 1 of labor, many mares show obvious behavior changes, such as agitation, pacing, nickering, lifting the tail head (as a result of oxytocin release), turning and biting at her sides, and kicking her abdomen. If sweating around her shoulders is observed, the mare will foal within 30 minutes. For veterinary technicians, this time is crucial. It is best to notify the veterinarian, stay near the mare, ensure that all necessary equipment is present, and wrap the mare's tail with brown gauze to keep it clean and out of the way.

BOX 21-6	Necessary Equipment for a High-Risk Attended Foaling

- Towels
- Stainless steel bucket
- Warm water
- Chains
- J-lube (lubricant to aid in foal's delivery)
- 1% iodine solution to dip foal's umbilicus
- Electrocardiography (ECG) machine to check foal's heart rate and rhythm
- Capnograph to measure foal's CO_2 level
- Endotracheal tubes (7, 8, and 9 mm) and 10-ml air syringe
- Ambu bag
- Oxygen supply
- IV catheter, prepared sterile scrub, sterile gloves, and suture
- IV fluids (5% dextrose in water [D_5W], Normosol R, or Plasma-Lyte)
- Blood gas syringe (heparinized 3-ml syringe)
- Blood tubes, syringes, and needles
- Glucometer

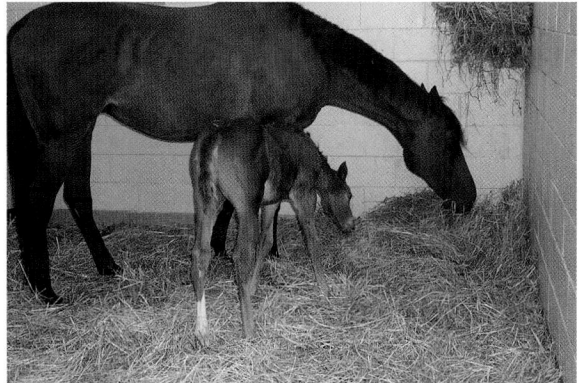

FIGURE 21-5 Mare and foal bonding in the stall. (Courtesy Dr. Amy Bentz.)

Box 21-6 lists equipment needed when one is attending a high-risk foaling.

Stage 2 of labor is explosive in mares and starts when the placenta ruptures and allantoic fluid escapes (water breaking). The foal should be delivered within 30 minutes, but many foals are delivered within 10 to 15 minutes. If the foal is not delivered within 30 minutes, the foal will experience hypoxemia (low oxygen blood levels) and consequently may develop neurologic deficits or may die. Therefore, this is an emergency, and if the foal is unable to be delivered vaginally, a cesarean section is needed. If the foal's nose is protruding from the vulva, an endotracheal tube can be placed into the foal's trachea and breaths delivered via an Ambu bag. This will meet the foal's oxygen needs and will provide time to prepare for a cesarean section.

Stage 3 of labor occurs when the mare passes her placenta. This can be painful, and many mares lay down to expel the placenta. The placenta should be collected, weighed, and evaluated to ensure that it is completely intact. If a piece is missing (often the tip of the placenta), the mare needs to be treated for a retained placenta. When the foal is delivered, the mare should show immediate interest in the foal by nickering and cleaning him. Before she stands, it is best to strip the umbilical cord of blood and gently break it near the foal's body, leaving a 2- to 3-inch remnant.

The mare will be thirsty and will need fresh, clean water. Additional bedding should be added to the stall because it will be slippery from fetal fluids. Many mares show mild discomfort (looking at her sides, kicking her abdomen), and a dose of a nonsteroidal anti-inflammatory drug (NSAID), such as flunixin meglumine, will often provide analgesia. Mares are often protective of newborn foals, so intervention should be minimized, and they should be left alone as much

as possible to permit bonding (Figure 21-5). However, during the postpartum period, if the mare is not interested in the foal or appears to be in pain (e.g., rolling in the stall), intervention is necessary. Occasionally, mares develop complications postpartum that require immediate treatment, or the foal may be rejected by the mare. Examples of complications include mild colic, large colon volvulus, uterine artery hemorrhage, retained placenta, and peritonitis. Depending on the problem, the foal may be able to stay with the mare or may need to be removed and raised as an orphan (called a "bucket baby") or "grafted" onto a nurse mare.

> **TECHNICIAN NOTE** High-risk mares should have an attended foaling at a veterinary hospital to ensure optimal survival of the mare and the foal. Foaling equipment should be assembled and kept close to the mare's stall for easy access. Once stage 2 has started, sweating is often noted around the mare's shoulders, and the mare normally will deliver a foal within 30 minutes.

THE NEONATAL PERIOD: THE NORMAL FOAL

When a foal is born, many changes occur within the first 24 hours of life. In the wild, a foal must be able to stand, nurse, and run from predators within a short time, or their survival will be in jeopardy. Domesticated equine patients are similar, and a neonatal foal develops rapidly. If not, the foal is often ill and requires treatment. Initial milestones for a foal after parturition include a suckle reflex shortly after birth (curling the tongue and seeking to nurse), standing within 1 to 2 hours, and nursing successfully within 6 hours (often by 2 to 3 hours old). The first urination normally occurs around 12 hours. Foals pass meconium (black, sticky fecal material) within a few hours after birth, but some foals have difficulty and become uncomfortable, so they may require a warm-water, soapy enema. A typical enema for a 50-kg foal consists of 500 ml of warm water mixed with a small amount of Ivory soap. Within 24 hours of birth, the foal should be strong, alert, and capable of running. A nursing neonatal foal will urinate frequently. Urine will be dilute (specific gravity, 1.001 to 1.006) because mare's milk is mostly water. Fecal

CASE PRESENTATION 21-1 PREMATURE FOAL

A 20-year-old Thoroughbred mare delivered a foal at day 318 of gestation—earlier than the owner expected. She exhibited stage 1 signs of labor, which included restlessness and pacing for a few hours. She advanced to stage 2 and delivered a foal within 10 minutes. The mare's placenta was delivered completely, but it seemed thick and heavier than normal (13 lb). The filly was small (85 lb; 39 kg) with a domed head, a silky hair coat, and floppy ears (Figure 1). The foal had difficulty standing and was not able to nurse, so the owner shipped the mare and the foal to an equine referral veterinary hospital. On physical examination, the mare appeared healthy with no problems noted and did not require treatment. On physical examination, the 15-hour-old foal was depressed and recumbent. She was tachycardic (HR = 140 bpm) and tachypneic (60 breaths/minute) with mildly cool limbs and bounding pulses. As a result of her history and presentation, the foal was diagnosed as premature, and an ascending placentitis in the mare was considered a likely cause.

An IV catheter was placed in the foal's right jugular vein, and blood samples were taken for CBC, chemistry profile, IgG, and blood culture. An arterial blood gas was also taken from the left great metatarsal artery. Blood work abnormalities included a low IgG (400 mg/dl), hypoglycemia (20 mg/dl), and hypoxemia (PaO_2 = 65 mm Hg). Initial treatment included intranasal oxygen insufflation at 3 L/minute, a 2-L bolus of Normosol-R fluid IV, 5% dextrose at 188 ml/hour to provide dextrose, antimicrobial medication (400 mg ceftiofur sodium IV q6hours), and 1 L of HiGamm-Equi plasma IV to provide antibodies because the foal was unable to nurse.

The foal became bright and alert a few hours after treatment and attempted to stand. Because she was premature, radiographs were taken to assess the ossification of her cuboidal bones (carpi and hocks). Her cuboidal bones were not completely ossified, so she was permitted to stand only briefly when changing position. During the first 48 hours of hospitalization, the foal responded quickly to treatment. Repeat blood work demonstrated resolution of the initial abnormalities, and no bacteria grew on the blood culture. The foal tolerated a few feedings of her mare's colostrum via nasogastric intubation with no reflux. The foal developed a normal suckle and was fed a few ounces of her mare's milk every 2 hours by bottle. She tolerated the feedings well with no sign of discomfort, so the amount was gradually increased.

Over the next week, the filly gradually became stronger, and IV fluids and oxygen therapy were discontinued. Her antimicrobial medication was changed to oral trimethoprim-sulfa. The filly was allowed to stand for 10 to 20 minutes at a time, and repeat radiographs showed increased ossification of her cuboidal bones. By 4 weeks after delivery, the foal was healthy, required no medication, and had normal ossification of her cuboidal bones (Figure 2). Her grateful owners took her home, and the filly and the mare were placed in a small paddock every day, slowly increasing turnout time over 2 weeks. The filly and the mare had no subsequent problems.

The owners were instructed to send the mare to a hospital for an attended foaling in the future because the mare's age predisposes her to placentitis and delivery of a premature foal.

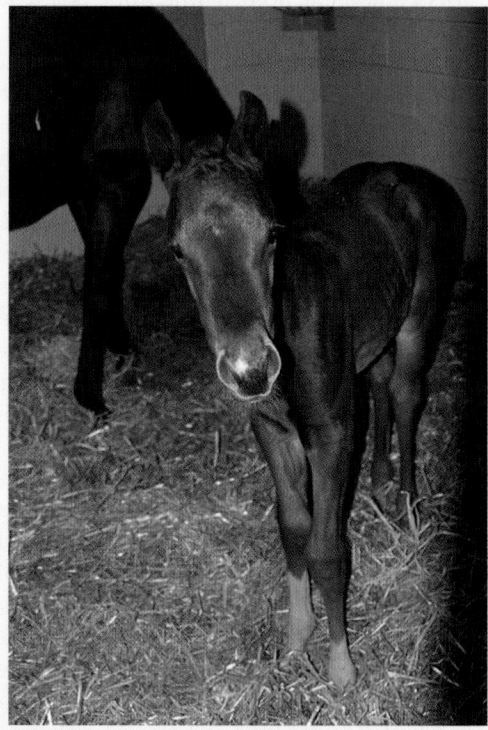

FIGURE 2 Healthy foal after treatment for prematurity. (Courtesy Dr. Amy Bentz.)

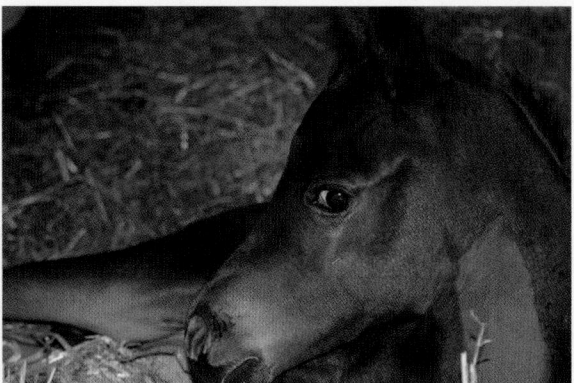

FIGURE 1 Premature foal with domed head and silky hair coat. (Courtesy Dr. Amy Bentz.)

material will be soft and yellow, and foals will defecate 1 or 2 times per day.

Observing the foal's behavior for a few minutes without human interaction is important to assess the foal's attitude and energy level. On physical examination, a neonatal foal should be bright, alert, and responsive. Normal temperature, pulse, and respiration (TPR) at birth is as follows: T = 99°F to 100°F (rectal temperature), P = 60 to 80 beats/minute (bpm), and R = 10 to 20 breaths/minute. The foal's heart rate will gradually increase to 120 bpm, and respiratory rate will gradually increase to 40 to 60 breaths/minute. Mucous membranes are pink and moist with a capillary refill time (CRT) less than 2 seconds. Eyes should be open and bright with no redness or discharge. Foals are born without a menace response, and it often takes a few weeks for a menace response to develop. The heartbeat should be strong and regular with a synchronous pulse. A quiet systolic murmur may be present (often a flow murmur) but disappears over time. Respiratory rate and effort should be frequent and steady. Thoracic auscultation may initially sound moist, but will resolve over time. The foal's abdomen should not be swollen, and the umbilical remnant should be clean and dry. The foal's legs are weak initially, but after 24 hours, the foal should be able to stand readily and run quickly. No joint swelling should be evident on palpation. A foal will quickly bond to its mother and follow at her flank. Neonatal foals will sleep about 10 to 20 minutes, then will stand and nurse for 5 minutes, play, and sleep again. Normal nursing behavior includes the foal facing the mare's tail, bumping the udder to encourage milk let-down, then nursing for about 5 minutes. The foal should readily use both teats. Palpating the mare's udder after observing the foal as it nurses is important, to ensure that the foal is nursing successfully from both sides of the udder. A healthy foal nurses equally from both teats, such that the mare's udder contains minimal milk. A sick foal may appear to nurse, but when the udder is palpated, it is found to be engorged and painful to the touch. Healthy foals gain an average of 2 to 4 lb (1 to 2 kg) daily and grow rapidly.

The neurologic system of a newborn foal is different from that of an adult horse. When the foal is standing for the first time, a basewide stance and exaggerated steps when walking are considered normal. Increased response to visual, auditory, and tactile stimuli and jerky movements are also normal. When the normal standing foal is restrained, it struggles initially, then falls limp, as if sleeping, into the arms of the handler. Loosening the restraint causes the foal to support its weight again. This specific behavior must be kept in mind by people who are restraining standing foals for procedures, as during placement of an IV catheter.

Routine Neonatal Therapy

Routine care for all foals includes applying 1% iodine to the foal's umbilical remnant at birth, then 3 or 4 times daily for 2 days, while monitoring the foal's attitude, appetite, urination, and fecal production. Foals from mares not vaccinated with tetanus toxoid in the last 4 to 6 weeks of gestation should receive 1500 international units (IU) of tetanus antitoxin intramuscularly. On some farms, an enema is routinely administered after birth.

It is important to measure the foal's antibody levels (immunoglobulin [Ig]G) approximately 12 hours after delivery. Foals are born without antibodies and need to drink colostrum within 12 to 24 hours after birth to gain antibodies. Colostrum contains antibodies from the mare, other proteins, growth factors, and opsonins to protect the foal

from bacterial infection. High-quality colostrum has a specific gravity of 1.080 or higher, and a sample taken shortly after parturition can be measured using a colostrometer. Within the first 12 to 24 hours of life, the foal's gastrointestinal (GI) tract is able to absorb antibodies from colostrum. After 24 hours, the foal can no longer absorb the mare's antibodies. The IgG level should be greater than 800 mg/dl after 12 hours of age. Failure of passive transfer (FPT) of antibodies occurs when the foal's IgG level is less than 800 mg/dl after 24 hours old. Reasons include poor-quality colostrum from the mare, lack of colostrum as a result of milk dripping before parturition, or the foal is too weak or has a limb deformity such as carpal contracture, which prevents the foal from standing to nurse. FPT is associated with increased susceptibility to infection or sepsis, and foals must be monitored carefully (e.g., daily weight and TPR assessed) so problems can be identified quickly.

Several tests may be used to measure IgG levels; each has advantages and disadvantages. The radial immunodiffusion test is accurate but expensive and has limited availability for routine screening. The commercial IgG screening kit with an enzyme-linked immunosorbent assay (ELISA), such as SNAP ELISA (produced by Idexx Inc., Portland, Maine), is the most commonly used test because it is quick, accurate, easily performed, and readily available. Of the many rapid test methods available, including zinc sulfate turbidity, latex agglutination, the glutaraldehyde coagulation test, and SNAP ELISA, only SNAP ELISA has sensitivity (and specificity) in the 800-mg/dl range.

FPT before 24 hours is treated by giving the foal high-quality colostrum from another mare via nasogastric intubation. After 24 hours, it is treated with IV administration of plasma from an appropriate donor. Commercial plasma is available (e.g., HiGamm-Equi, Lake Immunogenics, Ontario, New York), and although expensive, it is the safest and most reliable product. This plasma is harvested from hyperimmunized donors; it has been shown to have IgG levels that far exceed normal plasma and is tested for anti-equine antibodies. If fresh plasma is given from an on-site donor, a cross-match should be performed to lessen the risk of a significant transfusion reaction. Plasma is administered via a sterile IV catheter. It is paramount to use a blood administration IV line with a filter to strain out any large particles from the plasma. As a general rule, 1 L of commercial plasma raises the IgG level of a 45-kg foal by 200 mg/dl.

> **TECHNICIAN NOTE** A neonatal foal needs to be monitored closely for appropriate developmental milestones. An immunoglobulin (Ig)G level should be measured by 12 hours of age to ensure that passive transfer of maternal antibodies has occurred.

Laboratory Evaluation

The laboratory parameters (hematology and serum chemistry values) of neonatal foals are distinctly different from those of adult horses. Coagulation values are initially different from those of adult horses. Published references are available from the University of Florida, College of Veterinary Medicine, in Gainesville, but because of variations in technique and equipment between different laboratories, reference ranges for values need to be established individually at each facility that examines samples from veterinary patients. As foals age, many of their blood values reach typical adult levels, so by 1 month, the levels of many parameters are similar to those of adult horses.

When a complete blood count (CBC) is evaluated, the packed cell volume of the normal foal during the first 24 hours of life (e.g., greater than 40%) is greater than that of an adult horse. Subsequently, a fall into the low normal range of an adult can be observed over the ensuing 2 weeks to 1 year. Band neutrophils are not normal in the healthy foal. Values greater than 100 to 150 band cells/dl are considered abnormal and usually indicate acute infection, such as sepsis. Measuring plasma fibrinogen concentration can be helpful, to evaluate the presence of active inflammation. Fibrinogen is an acute phase protein that is produced by the liver in response to active inflammation. Fibrinogen levels vary between laboratories but in general do not exceed 420 mg/dl in foals up to 1 week of age. At birth, before the foal has nursed from the mare and when it has not absorbed IgG from the mare's colostrum, the plasma protein concentration of an equine neonate is considerably lower than that of an adult horse (e.g., between 4 and 4.5 mg/dl). After successful passive transfer of immunoglobulins from the mare's colostrum, the foal's total protein increases to approximately 5.6 mg/dl, which is below the normal range for an adult horse.

The activities of various serum enzymes are distinctly different in foals than in adult horses. Alkaline phosphatase, gamma-glutamyl transferase, sorbitol dehydrogenase, alanine transaminase, and glucose levels should be consistently higher in foals than in adults. An increase in alkaline phosphatase has been attributed to increased metabolic activities in bone, intestine, and liver. Increased gamma-glutamyl transferase and sorbitol dehydrogenase activities are attributed to greater activity in the liver in foals and may be associated with greater mass of the liver in relation to total body mass. Changes in alanine transaminase levels are of questionable clinical significance because this enzyme has not been shown to be specific for a particular organ system in the horse. The serum glucose concentration in normal foals ranges from 60 to 120 mg/dl. A decrease in serum glucose concentration to below the normal reference range is a concern and is indicative of insufficient caloric uptake of the foal or metabolic derangements in the critically ill foal. In normal foals, serum levels of creatinine and blood urea nitrogen often are above reference values for adults for the first 36 to 72 hours of life but gradually decrease to adult values.

THE NEONATAL PERIOD: THE SICK FOAL

Foals are born with minimal energy reserves, such as stored fat, and can quickly deteriorate with infection. They need to drink good-quality colostrum from the mare within 24 hours of delivery. If FPT of maternal antibodies occurs because of lack of nursing or because poor-quality colostrum is ingested, foals are prone to infection. Three main sites of entry for bacteria and viruses have been identified: GI tract, respiratory tract, and umbilicus. The foal is born with sterile GI and respiratory tracts. During the 1st week of life, foals eat their mother's manure to colonize their GI tracts with proper bacteria. Because horses live in a dirty environment, foals are exposed to many pathogens. If foals are compromised for any reason, they are more likely to develop bacteremia (bacterial infection in the bloodstream) and sepsis.

Some foals develop infection as a result of their contaminated environment. Other foals are predisposed to developing infection from abnormal conditions in utero. Risk factors for compromised foals include prematurity, twin foals, a history of placentitis, the mare is sick and is not producing much milk, or the foal is exhibiting abnormal behavior after delivery, such as weakness and inability to nurse, resulting in FPT. Premature foals are born before they reach 320 days of gestational age. Signs of prematurity include low birth weight, weakness, silky hair coat, floppy ears, domed forehead, flexor tendon laxity, and angular limb deformities (e.g., incomplete ossification of cuboidal bones in the carpus and tarsus on radiographs). This incomplete ossification can result in crushing injuries of cuboidal bones from simple weight bearing, so these foals require extensive care for weeks and restrictive standing until the bones are completely ossified. The term *dysmaturity* usually refers to a large foal (e.g., greater than 65 kg) with longer than expected gestation (e.g., 400 days). The foal's hair coat will be coarse and long, and the incisor teeth will be erupted through the mucous membranes. The foal may be weak, may be unable to nurse correctly, and may have angular limb deformities. Both of these types of foals are often a product of their mare's abnormal placenta and have increased susceptibility to disease and injury, requiring veterinary care.

Some foals have minor problems, such as orthopedic problems or an inguinal hernia, and require mild to moderate diagnostics and intervention. However, classic early clinical signs of disease in critically ill foals include lethargy, depression, decreased suckle reflex, decreased nursing, and increased periods of recumbency and sleeping. Unfortunately, foals can become critically ill quickly and can rapidly deteriorate, so they need to be monitored closely, especially in the 1st week of life. If a foal is developing any of these signs on the farm, the veterinarian needs to evaluate the foal and determine whether a referral is needed for additional care. It is difficult to manage sick neonatal foals on the farm. They often require 24-hour care and extensive monitoring for optimal recovery. Sometimes, even despite the best care, critically ill foals do not survive. Because intensive care is expensive, the owner needs to choose among treatment options with the veterinarian's guidance and in keeping with long-term goals for the foal.

Early clinical signs of disease in critically ill foals include lethargy, depression, decreased suckle reflex, decreased nursing, and increased periods of recumbency and sleeping. Foals can become critically ill quickly and can rapidly deteriorate, so they need to be monitored closely for attitude, appetite, activity, urination, and defecation, especially in the 1st week of life.

Admitting the Critically Ill Foal

A neonatal team consisting of a veterinarian, a veterinary technician, and assistants is vital to the initial evaluation and treatment of the critically ill foal. Many foals may require supportive care and may recover quickly, but some will not survive without intensive management. A skilled veterinary technician plays an important role in treating these cases and recognizing when complications develop. Numerous foal neonatal intensive care units (NICUs) provide quality care for these foals; spending time in a NICU to gain experience is invaluable.

When a foal is admitted, triage by the veterinarian and the veterinary technician is important in determining the initial diagnostic evaluation and treatment. A foal that is able to walk into the NICU receives less intensive care than a hypothermic, recumbent foal. Initial triage includes obtaining a foal's history and weight, and performing a quick assessment of attitude, condition, TPR, and the cardiovascular system (heart rate, rhythm, pulse, and limb temperature, all of which indicate perfusion). Ambulatory foals should be gently restrained during the examination to minimize stress and are usually stabled with their dams to permit normal nursing.

A comatose, recumbent foal should be evaluated and treated rapidly, so many NICUs have standard protocols. Box 21-7 lists common diseases of neonatal foals. The foal is placed on a padded surface, and its eyes are protected from trauma. At least three people are needed to restrain the foal: one person holding the head, the 2nd holding the front legs, and the 3rd holding the hind legs. The foal's attitude is assessed, and lack of response to stimuli indicates poor brain perfusion. Mucous membranes are often dark purple with prominent vessels (injected mucous membranes). Icterus (yellow color of mucous membranes and sclerae) is commonly noted in foals with sepsis. Petechiae (small areas of hemorrhage) may be noted on oral mucous membranes or on the foal's pinna (outer ear). The eyes may be sunken and entropion present (lower eyelids rolled inward) as a result of hypovolemia (decreased blood volume). Pupil size should be noted and eyes stained with fluorescein to check for corneal ulceration. Miotic (constricted) pupils often indicate sepsis. The foal may have tachycardia (e.g., greater than 150 bpm) or bradycardia (e.g., less than 70 bpm), and pulse may be bounding or difficult to palpate. Respirations may be fast (more than 60 breaths per minute) or slow (fewer than 20 breaths per minute). The ribs should be carefully palpated, especially over the heart, to detect the presence of rib fractures. Auscultation of the GI tract may reveal audible

---

BOX 21-7 | Common Diseases of Neonatal Foals

- Neonatal encephalopathy: "dummy foal" or neonatal maladjustment syndrome resulting in abnormal behavior, poor nursing ability, and weakness, and associated with other problems, such as sepsis, neonatal gastroenteropathy, and neonatal nephropathy.
- Neonatal gastroenteropathy: abnormal GI tract motility and absorption leading to intolerance of enteral nutrition, such as reflux noted after feeding.
- Neonatal nephropathy: renal insufficiency that may resolve or may be too severe for recovery.
- Neonatal isoerythrolysis: acute, severe anemia caused by destruction of the foal's red blood cells due to maternal antibodies causing an incompatibility reaction.
- Sepsis or septic shock: acute, severe bacterial infection causing multiorgan dysfunction, including poor perfusion of the limbs, cardiovascular collapse, and metabolic derangements, such as profound hypoglycemia.
- Meconium retention: meconium is retained in the colon, and the foal will display abdominal discomfort, such as tail flagging and rolling.
- Colitis: foal develops acute diarrhea, often caused by an infectious organism, such as rotavirus, *Salmonella* spp., or *Clostridium* spp., and requires immediate treatment in an isolated stall.
- Patent urachus: foal's urachus is not closed and leaks urine.
- Ruptured bladder: foal's urinary bladder or associated structures (e.g., ureters) develop a tear, and urine leaks into the abdomen.
- Septic arthritis or septic physitis: foal develops an infected joint or an infected growth plate.
- Failure of passive transfer (FPT): foal does not receive maternal antibodies from the mare's colostrum within 24 hours of age.
- Musculoskeletal abnormalities (e.g., flexural deformities, angular limb deformities): foal has tendon contracture, valgus, or varus problems causing deviated limbs.
- Prematurity: foal is born before 320 days of gestational age and exhibits typical signs, such as low birth weight, soft hair coat, floppy ears, domed head, and incomplete ossification of cuboidal bones.
- Dysmaturity: very large foal is born at longer-than-expected gestational age (e.g., 400 days), with long hair coat and erupted incisors; often has limb deformities.
- Entropion: Lower eyelid rolls inward to the cornea, causing corneal abrasion or ulceration.

---

borborygmi or the absence of GI sounds. The abdomen should be evaluated for distention, and the umbilical remnant examined for discharge. Joints should be carefully palpated for swelling. Urine should be caught for dipstick and specific gravity. Fecal matter should be examined, especially if diarrhea is present, because isolation of the patient may be required. Limb temperature is important to assess. Often, these foals will be hypothermic (T less than 99° F) and will have poor perfusion to their limbs. Consequently, the foal's legs will be cold, and pulses in the limbs will be difficult to feel. The median artery (on the medial upper forelimb near the elbow) and the great metatarsal artery (on the lateral distal hindlimb) are frequently used to assess pulses and to obtain arterial blood gas samples. The foal's blood pressure should be assessed.

Initial blood samples include an arterial blood gas drawn from the great metatarsal artery to assess oxygen and carbon dioxide levels. A venous sample for CBC, chemistry profile, glucose level, and blood culture can be taken at the time of catheter placement. Typical blood work abnormalities of these critically ill foals include IgG less than 800 mg/dl, low white cell count (e.g., less than 5000 cells/μl), increased fibrinogen concentration, profound hypoglycemia (less than 40 mg/dl), increased lactate, low oxygen concentration, and increased carbon dioxide levels.

Initial treatment often entails administration of intranasal oxygen (oxygen insufflation), sterile placement of an IV catheter in the jugular vein, fluid therapy using crystalloid fluids (e.g., Normosol-R), fluids containing dextrose (e.g., D_5W), and broad-spectrum antimicrobials. Placement of a jugular catheter requires aseptic technique. The area over the vein is clipped, and sterile scrub and sterile gloves are used to clean the area for 5 minutes. Masks worn by foal handlers are helpful in preventing contamination of the area. Placement of an IV catheter is an ideal way to draw the first sample for blood culture while using a sterile syringe and sterile gloves. Whereas many critically ill foals may have sepsis, blood cultures are positive only about 30% of the time. In the past, sepsis usually was caused by a Gram-negative organism, but in recent years, Gram-positive sepsis is on the rise. Antimicrobial therapy should be based on isolation of infecting organisms and antimicrobial sensitivity testing. Special attention should be paid to physiologic features of the neonate, such as reduced hepatic activity and renal immaturity. Antimicrobial therapy must be instituted as soon as sepsis is suspected, without waiting for culture results, which take a few days to finalize. In general, using ceftiofur sodium or a combination of penicillin and an aminoglycoside (e.g., amikacin) provides appropriate coverage. Shock therapy fluids can be administered at 20 ml/kg/hour for short periods, so many critically ill foals (e.g., a 50-kg foal) receive 3 L of fluid within the first 2 hours of admission.

Often after administration of a few liters of IV crystalloid fluids and dextrose, the foal's perfusion will improve. The foal will appear more alert, will sit up, and will seek to nurse. To prevent corneal ulceration, ophthalmic ointment is placed in both eyes, and entropion is corrected if present. A hypothermic foal should be gradually warmed using blankets or forced-air warming units (Bair Hugger, Arizant Healthcare Inc., Eden Prairie, Minnesota). It is imperative that the foal is warmed slowly, or increased metabolic demand will cause cardiovascular collapse. Blood pressure is monitored closely; decreased blood pressure is one of the first signs that the foal is not responding to treatment. A foal's recumbency is changed every few hours to prevent decubital ulcers and to permit expansion of the down lung. Glucose measurements are frequently obtained using a glucometer to ensure that the foal's glucose concentrations are within normal limits. If the foal remains hypoglycemic or hyperglycemic, malmetabolism may be present as a result of sepsis, and close monitoring is required. Performing frequent urine dipsticks and assessing specific gravity will ensure that the foal is not losing glucose in the urine (glucosuria), and that the kidneys are responding appropriately to fluid therapy.

> **TECHNICIAN NOTE** Once a neonatal foal is admitted to a veterinary hospital, blood pressure should be monitored closely because decreased blood pressure is one of the first signs that the foal is not responding to treatment.

Once the foal's cardiovascular system has stabilized, additional diagnostics can be performed. Thoracic radiographs and/or ultrasonographic examination may be needed to assess for pneumonia or the presence of rib fractures. Ultrasonographic evaluation of the abdomen is often used to better assess the GI tract for meconium retention, to evaluate the bladder to ensure that it is intact, or to examine the internal remnant of the umbilicus. The external umbilical remnant is outside of the abdomen. It contains remnants of the urachus (which connects to the urinary bladder); two umbilical arteries, which travel caudally and insert into the bladder wall; and one umbilical vein, which courses cranially to the liver. Sick foals often develop a patent urachus and omphalitis (inflammation of the umbilicus). Externally, the umbilical remnant will be moist and enlarged, and the foal will strain or will dribble small streams when urinating. Examination of the urogenital system includes palpation of the umbilical, inguinal, and scrotal areas for hernias and distention. If the foal has mild colic, it will often flag its tail when defecating. The foal may roll onto its back and fold its front legs over the chest to indicate abdominal pain. When the foal's temperature is taken, fecal matter should be detected on the thermometer. If this does not occur and the foal exhibits signs of abdominal discomfort, the possibility of a nonpatent GI system caused by an anatomic abnormality (atresia ani, atresia coli) should be considered.

When additional venous blood samples are required, the cephalic and saphenous veins are ideal for collection; the smallest needle and syringe possible should be used, or a tuberculin syringe or a 22-gauge, 1-inch needle and a 3-ml syringe may be selected. Adequate restraint is paramount for successful performance of venipuncture in recumbent foals; this usually requires three people. Figure 21-6 depicts correct restraint of the recumbent neonatal foal to obtain a blood culture from the saphenous vein. Restraining the foal using bony areas, such as joints, offers the best approach for preventing harm to soft tissue areas, such as the foal's abdomen. A foal's veins tend to roll, so clipping the area over the vein is helpful. After alcohol is applied to the area, the needle should be gently inserted at a 45-degree angle so a blood sample can be obtained. If additional arterial blood gas samples are required, the procedure is similar. Three persons

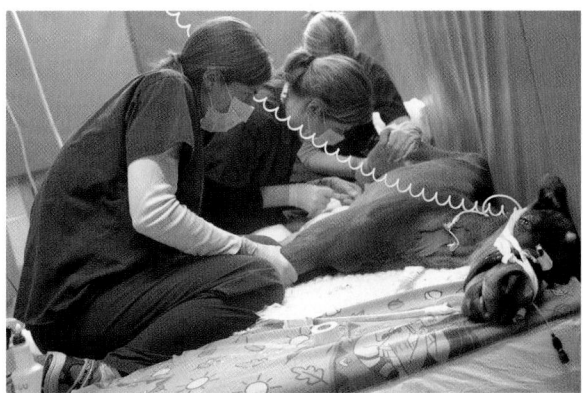

FIGURE 21-6 Correct restraint of the recumbent neonatal foal to obtain a blood culture from the saphenous vein. (Courtesy Sabina Louise Pierce, University of Pennsylvania.)

are needed to restrain the foal. One person holds the foal's head and ensures that the eyes are protected from abrasion, the second holds the front legs, and the third person holds the hind legs. An area over the great metatarsal artery is clipped, and alcohol is applied. Arterial samples are painful, so infusing 0.1 to 0.2 ml of lidocaine into the area using a tuberculin syringe and needle is vital when the sample is collected. It is important to use a specialized blood gas syringe to collect an arterial sample. Draw back on the plunger to 0.5 ml before taking the sample, to ensure that arterial blood can flow into the syringe. Palpate the arterial pulse and insert the needle gently at a 45-degree angle. Blood should immediately flow into the syringe and should appear bright red. If blood flows slowly and appears dark, it may be a venous sample. However, if the foal is comatose and has extremely cold limbs and poor pulses, the sample may indeed be an arterial sample.

Over the course of hospitalization, the foal may require additional treatment, including maintenance fluids, nutritional support, blood pressure support, treatment for orthopedic conditions, and a ventilator. Maintenance fluid rates can range from 90 to 150 ml/hour for the average 50-kg foal. Each case varies depending on the foal's illness and clinical course. Some foals with mild to moderate illness are hospitalized only for a few days and are discharged on medication. Critically ill neonatal foals are often hospitalized for a few weeks, and treatment is often expensive. Figure 21-7 depicts a typical IV fluid setup for a critically ill foal. The best outcome for a neonatal foal is early detection of disease on the farm followed by rapid intervention before the foal becomes critically ill.

> **TECHNICIAN NOTE** A critically ill neonatal foal should be evaluated and treated quickly by a veterinary team at a referral hospital for optimal outcome.

Monitoring and Nursing Care

Once the foal has been admitted to the veterinary hospital and initially examined, diligent monitoring is critical. Tables

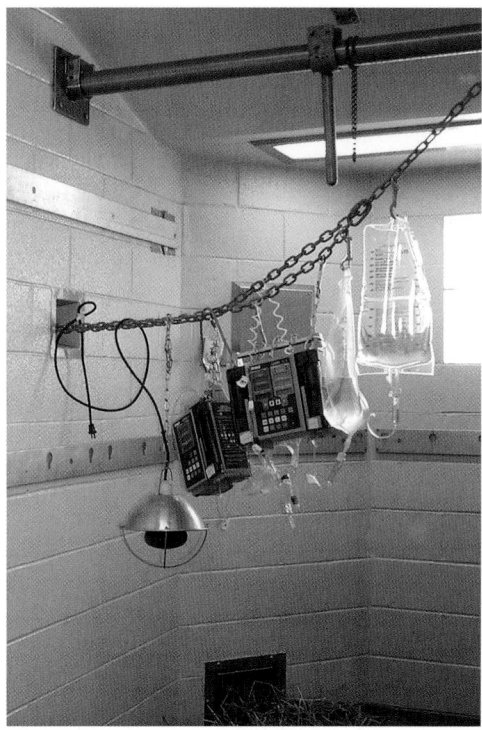

FIGURE 21-7 Typical IV fluid setup for a critically ill foal. (Courtesy Dr. Amy Bentz.)

21-3 and 21-4 list important considerations for evaluating the critically ill foal. The objective of frequent monitoring is to detect subtle changes signifying improvement or deterioration in the foal's condition. Complications during hospitalization include resistant nosocomial (hospital-acquired) infection, additional sites of infection (septic arthritis, osteomyelitis, thrombophlebitis, pneumonia), corneal ulcers, and decubital ulcers. The severity of the patient's illness will dictate the required frequency of monitoring. Parameters are recorded on a flow sheet for easy comparison at different time points. As a foal deteriorates, one of the earliest changes noted is decreasing blood pressure. Monitoring blood pressure frequently aids in detecting deterioration in the foal's condition and permits treatment changes before the case spirals downward. Performing regular TPRs will also aid in assessing the foal. A recumbent foal's temperature is often between 99° F and 101.5° F (37.2° C to 38.6° C). A hypothermic foal often is unable to maintain a normal body temperature and may have a temperature less than 99° F (37.2° C), despite the use of warming methods. A recumbent foal with a temperature greater than 102° F (38.9° C) is febrile and may not respond to the antimicrobial of choice.

Hallmarks of nursing care for the foal include strict attention to asepsis and close observation of minor details. An experienced veterinary technician is invaluable and often will note changes in the foal before they are noticed by the veterinarian. If more than one foal is being treated by the technician, techniques such as handwashing between patients should be used to prevent cross-contamination. Skin injections should be made only after the area has been cleaned with alcohol and dried. Intramuscular injections are limited

TABLE 21-3	Key Aspects of Medical History and Nursing Assessments Regarding the Neonatal Foal	
MEDICAL HISTORY	**WHAT TO ASK THE OWNER**	**NURSING ASSESSMENT AND ACTION**
Delivery, attitude, appetite, and weight gain	• "Was the foaling attended? If so, any problems noted?" • "Is the foal bright, alert, and nursing periodically?" • "Have there been any changes in the foal's attitude or activity level?"	• Assess whether the foal is bright and alert or dull and depressed • Monitor the foal's attitude, appetite, and weight gain • Check the mare's udder after foal nurses to ensure that the foal is nursing well
Urination and manure production	• "Is the foal urinating and defecating readily?" • "Is the foal straining?" • "Have there been any changes in urination (amount, effort, or frequency)?"	• Assess whether the foal is urinating readily or if the foal strains to urinate • Assess amount and consistency of the foal's manure
Medication administration	• "Is the foal receiving any medication or supplements?"	• If so, check the medications to ensure that they are stored and administered correctly

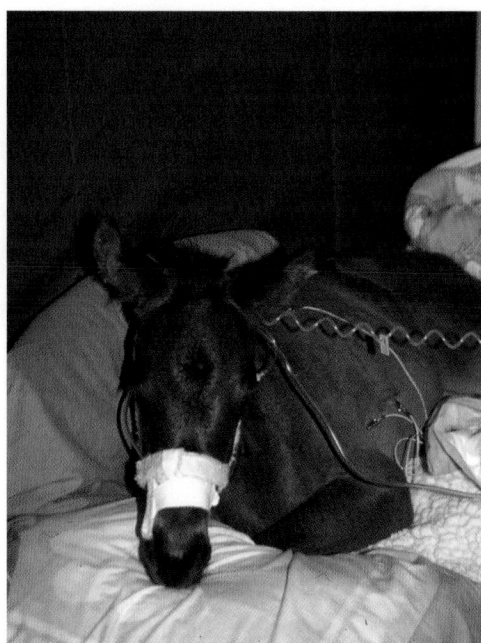

FIGURE 21-8 Correct sternal recumbency of a foal with a pillow placed at the foal's shoulder. (Courtesy Dr. Amy Bentz.)

removed and replaced within 72 hours. Silastic or polyurethane catheters are less thrombogenic and may remain in place for several weeks, but the catheter site should be monitored closely for swelling or thickening of the jugular vein. These catheters are expensive but quickly become cost-effective when compared with Teflon because of the extended time that they can remain in place and the decreased likelihood that thrombophlebitis will develop.

The foal should be kept clean, dry, and warm. Milk should be warmed to a tepid (not hot) temperature before it is fed to the foal. Physical therapy (passive range of motion) can be a helpful modality for recumbent foals, especially when one joint (often the fetlock joint) has a mild contracture. Foals should be kept in a sternal position to permit adequate expansion of the lungs. This position can be attained by using pillows at the shoulder or wedge-shaped pads. Figure 21-8 shows correct positioning of a foal in sternal recumbency using a pillow at the foal's shoulder. The recumbent foal will require frequent turning from side to side (every 2 hours) to encourage complete ventilation of the lungs and to prevent decubital ulcers. Foals should be encouraged to stand and ambulate, when possible. This effort may range from the handler suspending the foal for a few minutes to the foal standing on its own once assisted.

Restraint should be safe for the foal, mare, and handlers. Ambulatory foals usually are restrained with one hand under the neck and the other surrounding the rump. It is not recommended to restrain a foal by its tail because the handler may inadvertently break the foal's tail. Bracing the foal against a wall provides greater security and better control during a struggle. To lead a foal behind the mare, one person should walk the mare with a chain over her nose. The second person places a long cotton lead around the foal's chest and

to the semimembranosus region and should not be given in the neck, pectorals, or gluteal region. Fluid lines should be changed daily to prevent contamination (see Figure 21-7). Major line changes should be performed every 3 days. If a fluid line is accidentally disconnected, it should be considered contaminated and must be replaced. All IV ports should be capped with injection caps and cleaned with alcohol swabs before a needle is inserted. Multidose vials of injectable drugs and injection caps or ports must be disinfected with an alcohol swab before needle insertion. Needles and syringes are not reused. If IV fluids are not attached continuously, catheters should be flushed with 3 ml of heparinized saline solution every 6 hours. It is important to avoid administering too much heparinized saline too frequently, or the foal may become heparinized. If IV fluids are attached continuously, 3 ml of sterile saline without heparin may be used to flush the catheter between medications. The interval for catheter changes depends on the type of catheter material used and the status of the vein. Teflon catheters should be

TABLE 21-4	Key Physical Assessments and Self-Guiding Questions Regarding a Neonatal Foal	
PHYSICAL ASSESSMENT	**WHAT TO CHECK**	**NURSING ASSESSMENT QUESTIONS**
Mentation and walking	• Observe the foal for signs of dullness, depression, and reluctance to move	• Is the foal quiet and depressed or reluctant to move?
Body condition and hair coat	• Evaluate the foal's size and body condition; many foals are about 100 pounds (45 kg). • Foals should have an adequate body condition and a soft hair coat. • If possible, it is ideal to weigh the foal every day for the first few weeks.	• Is the foal smaller or larger than expected? • Does the foal have adequate body condition? • Or is the foal thin with a silky or overlong hair coat?
Vital signs	• Temperature, pulse, and respiration	• Does the foal have a fever (>101.5° F [38.6° C]) or hypothermia (<99° F [37.2° C])? • Is the foal's heart rate increased (>150 beats/minute) or decreased (<70 beats/minute)? • Is respiratory rate increased (>60 breaths/minute) or decreased (<20 breaths/minute)?
Hydration status and cardiorespiratory system	• Mucous membrane color and quality • Capillary refill time (CRT) and jugular vein refill time • Pulse quality • Thoracic auscultation to assess heart rate and rhythm, detect heart murmurs, or assess pulmonary sounds • Assess whether the foal's respiratory rate and effort are within normal limits or are changing to faster/slower rates and deeper or more shallow efforts. • Assess whether periods of apnea are occurring (>20 seconds of breath-holding).	• Are the foal's oral mucous membranes pink and moist with CRT<2 seconds, or dark red, injected, and icteric with petechiae? • Are the foal's heart rate and rhythm consistent and within normal limits or changing frequently? • Are pulses strong or weak? • Does the foal have stable blood pressure or consistently low blood pressure values? • Is nasal discharge, coughing, or any abnormalities noted on thoracic auscultation of the respiratory system?
Abdomen, urination, and defecation	• Check for signs of abdominal pain such as pawing or rolling. • Auscult both sides of the abdomen to determine whether borborygmi are present and to note distention. • Note whether the foal is urinating and defecating and how often, or if the foal strains, flags its tail, or has diarrhea or skin scalding.	• Is the foal comfortable or painful? • Are borborygmi or any abdominal distention present? • Are there wet spots in the stall caused by urine? • Do you see any fecal material from the foal? • Is the external umbilical remnant small and dry or moist and large?
Integument and eyes	• Check for decubital ulcers, urine, and/or fecal scalding, linear dermal necrosis over hocks, generalized edema, presence of entropion, corneal ulceration, hyphema, miotic pupil, injected or icteric sclerae.	• Do the foal's jugular veins at the site of catheter placement have any signs of swelling or jugular vein thickening? • Is the foal clean and dry, or does it have urine or fecal scalding around the hind legs? • Are the foal's eyes open and comfortable, or do they appear closed and painful?
Thermoregulation and metabolic derangements	• Assess whether the foal is able to maintain body temperature or if it is consistently abnormal (hypothermic or febrile). • Check whether the foal's glucose levels are within normal limits or are consistently abnormal.	• Does the foal have a normal body temperature, or is the foal hypothermic (<99° F [37.2° C]) or febrile (>101.5° F [38.6° C])?
Musculoskeletal assessment	• Check the foal for joint swelling (effusion), acute lameness, joint contracture, incomplete ossification of cuboidal bones, and tendon and ligament laxity.	• Is the foal walking comfortably, or does he appear lame and reluctant to move?

the remaining rope around the rump. While holding the rope at the foal's withers, the person walks on the left side of the foal.

> **TECHNICIAN NOTE** A critically ill neonatal foal should be monitored closely for any changes in condition and treated appropriately. Blood pressure monitoring is vital to assess the foal's stability. A foal with decreasing blood pressure requires immediate attention.

NUTRITION OF THE NEONATAL FOAL

The healthy foal will nurse readily from the mare and will receive adequate nutrition. Ideally, a hospitalized foal is able to nurse from the mare to receive adequate nutrition. Some foals are unable to nurse because of different problems (e.g., neonatal encephalopathy, abnormal esophageal motility leading to aspiration pneumonia, cleft palate). Figure 21-9 shows a foal with neonatal encephalopathy incorrectly seeking to nurse on a wall. An indwelling nasogastric tube can be placed and taped to the foal's halter to permit feeding every 2 hours. It is an acquired skill to place these slender tubes because they can be difficult to palpate in the esophagus. These tubes can remain in place for weeks (or until the foal rubs them out and requires a new one). It is imperative to check a hospitalized foal's tongue daily. When foals are unable or reluctant to swallow and are treated with antimicrobials, they are prone to develop oral candidiasis. This yeast infection coats the tongue with a white plaque and requires daily treatment or debulking of the plaque using a dry 4 × 4 gauze sponge to apply potassium permanganate topically and/or oral fluconazole.

To ensure that adequate nutrition is offered, the foal should be weighed daily. Foals with mild disease usually will gain 1 to 2 lb/day (0.5 to 1 kg). Alternate options for feeding foals include bottle feeding, bucket feeding, and bonding the foal to a nurse mare. Bottle feeding of foals is labor intensive and must be done properly, or the foal may develop aspiration pneumonia. This method is often used when a foal temporarily is unable to nurse from his mare. Orphan foals

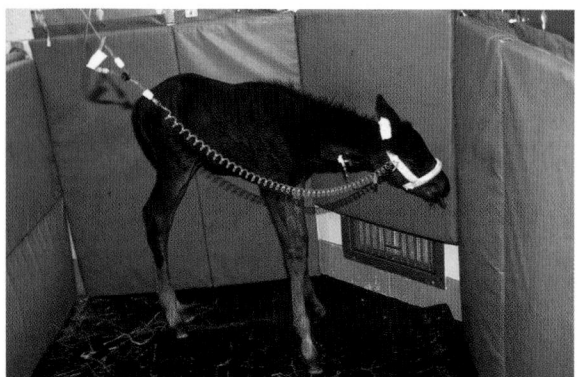

FIGURE 21-9 A foal with neonatal encephalopathy incorrectly seeking to nurse on a wall. (Courtesy Dr. Amy Bentz.)

are raised by giving milk in a bucket. Although this method is fine initially for many foals, behavioral problems often develop; these foals need to be handled properly to prevent problems.

The accepted energy requirement for the compromised equine neonate is 130 to 150 kcal/kg/day. To meet this requirement, a foal consumes approximately 20% of its body weight per day. Often critically ill foals lack a normal suckle reflex and have an abnormal GI tract. These foals do not tolerate large amounts orally, so small, frequent feedings such as 60 ml every 2 hours via a nasogastric tube are ideal initially for an average foal (100 pounds; 45 kg). If the foal tolerates these feedings, the volume of milk may be gradually increased to 5% to 10% of its body weight, divided into 12 feedings every 2 hours. If the foal does not have reflux when a nasogastric tube is passed, an indwelling nasogastric tube can be placed to feed the foal. Tube placement must be checked before each feeding to ensure proper positioning. If the tube has moved, aspiration pneumonia may result. The recumbent foal is placed in sternal recumbency, is fed, and is kept sternally for 20 minutes after feeding to prevent aspiration of milk.

Many critically ill foals do not tolerate enteral nutrition initially; feeding should be discontinued if regurgitation, abdominal distention, colic, or severe diarrhea occurs. Additional calories are administered IV (parenteral nutrition) to offer a sufficient energy intake for the critically ill foal. Two sources may be used for parenteral nutrition: commercial products and recipes using glucose, amino acids, lipids, trace minerals, and vitamins prepared for each foal individually. Because parenteral nutrition contains lipids and glucose, it is an optimal medium for bacterial growth. The IV bag and line must remain sterile at all times and IV line changes performed every 3 days to eliminate problems with contamination.

Fresh mare's milk is the ideal source of oral nutrition for foals and is easily digestible. When available, mare's milk should be used to feed healthy and critically ill neonatal foals. If the foal's mare is in the hospital, she can be milked every 2 hours (with or without giving oxytocin before milking) to obtain milk for the foal. The mare's udder and the caretaker's hands should always be cleaned before milking to prevent mastitis. Proper restraint of the mare is important during milking. Lubricating the hand or udder with sterile lubricating jelly helps decrease chafing. Gentle massage or application of warm compresses before milking helps soften the udder and assists in milk expression. Milk can be collected by hand or with the use of an inverted 60-ml dosing syringe. Several alternatives to mare's milk are available, but all have their drawbacks. Milk replacers are readily available, but they have high salt content, can be difficult for the foal to digest, and can cause diarrhea. Preparations formulated for enteral nutrition of other species generally are not suitable for the foal. Goat's milk is palatable but causes some metabolic abnormalities and should not be used alone for extended periods. All utensils used in feeding foals should be thoroughly cleaned and disinfected before and after use because

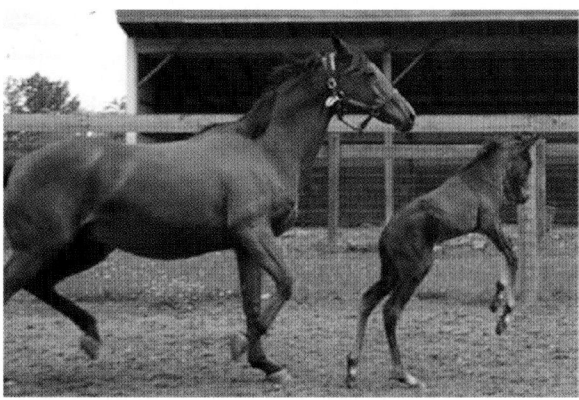

FIGURE 21-10 The ultimate desired outcome for a neonatal intensive care unit (NICU) foal. (Courtesy Dr. Amy Bentz.)

the GI tract is a potential portal for infection. Once reconstituted, milk replacers should be kept refrigerated. These preparations should be discarded after 2 hours at room temperature.

> **TECHNICIAN NOTE** Fresh mare's milk is the ideal source of oral nutrition for foals and is easily digestible. When available, mare's milk should be used to feed healthy and critically ill neonatal foals. Milk replacers formulated for foals can also be used, but they must be prepared correctly because of high salt content and can be difficult for neonatal foals to digest.

SUMMARY

Working with neonatal foals can be rewarding. It is especially enjoyable to watch a pregnant mare deliver a healthy foal, see them bond, and eventually observe them running in the pasture together. When a foal becomes ill and requires intensive care, it can be challenging for the owner and the neonatal veterinary team to care for the foal. Figure 21-10 depicts the ultimate desired outcome for an NICU foal. Although some of these foals do not survive, many foals recover and lead normal lives as athletes, in great part because of the tremendous effort of many dedicated veterinary technicians. It is a privilege to work with many of these caring people who continue to move the veterinary profession forward.

RECOMMENDED READINGS

Puppies and Kittens

Casal ML: Feline paediatrics. In Raw ME, Parkinson TJ, editors: The veterinary annual, London, UK, 1995, p 210.

Davidson AP: Approaches to reducing neonatal mortality in dogs. In Concannon PW, England G, Verstegen J III et al, editors: Recent advances in small animal reproduction, Ithaca NY, 2003, International Veterinary Information Service.

Gunn-Moore D: Small animal neonatology: they look normal when they are born and then they die, Prague, Czech Republic, 2006, WSAVA Proceedings.

Hoskins JD: Veterinary pediatrics: dogs and cats from birth to six months, Philadelphia, 2001, Saunders.

Hotston Moore P, Sturgess CP: Care of neonates and young animals. In Simpson GM, England GC, Harvey MJ, editors: BSAVA manual of small animals, Cheltenham, UK, 1998, British Small Animal Veterinary Association.

Neonatology in the Foal

Axon J, Palmer JE, Wilkins PA: Short and long term athletic outcome of neonatal intensive care unit survivors, Lexington, KY, 1999, Proceedings of the Annual American Association of Equine Practitioners Convention, vol 45.

Barton MH, Morris DD, Crowe N, et al: Hemostatic indices in healthy foals from birth to one month of age, J Vet Diagn Invest 7:380, 1995.

Barton MH, Morris DD, Norton N, et al: Hemostatic and fibrinolytic indices in neonatal foals with presumed septicemia, J Vet Intern Med 12:26, 1998.

Bentz AI, Palmer JE, Dallap BL, et al: Prospective evaluation of coagulation in critically ill neonatal foals, J Vet Intern Med 23:161, 2009.

Bentz AI, Wilkins PA, MacGillivray KC, et al: Thrombocytopenia in two thoroughbred foals with sepsis and neonatal encephalopathy, J Vet Intern Med 16:494, 2002.

Marsh PS, Palmer JE: Bacterial isolates from blood and their susceptibility patterns in critically ill foals: 543 cases (1991-1998), J Am Vet Med Assoc 218:1608, 2001.

McClure JT, Miller J, Deluca JL: Comparison of two ELISA screening tests and a non-commercial glutaraldehyde coagulation screening test for the detection of failure of passive transfer in neonatal foals, Lexington, KY, 2003, Proceedings of the Annual American Association of Equine Practitioners Convention, vol 49.

McKenzie HC III, Furr MO: Equine neonatal sepsis: the pathophysiology of severe inflammation and infection, Compend Contin Educ Pract Vet 23:661, 2001.

Paradis MR: Equine neonatal medicine: a case-based approach, St Louis, 2006, Saunders Elsevier.

Peek SF, Semrad S, McGuirk SM, et al: Prognostic value of clinicopathologic variables obtained at admission and effect of antiendotoxin plasma on survival in septic and critically ill foals, J Vet Intern Med 20:569, 2006.

Pierce SW: Foal care from birth to 30 days: a practitioner's perspective, Lexington, KY, 2003, Proceedings of the Annual American Association of Equine Practitioners Convention, vol 49.

Vaala WE, Lester GD, House JK: Initial management and physical examination of the neonate. In Smith BP, editor: Large animal internal medicine, ed 4, St Louis, 2009, Mosby.

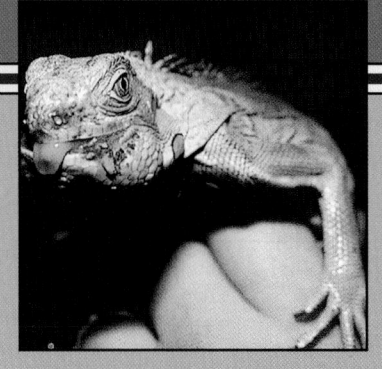

22 Care of Birds, Reptiles, and Small Mammals

Thomas N. Tully, Jr.

OUTLINE

Birds, *812*
Taking the Clinical History, *812*
Behavior Considerations During the
  Examination Process, *813*
Sample Collections and Diagnostic
  Procedures Commonly Used in
  Birds, *814*
Anesthesia, *817*
Husbandry and Treatment in the
  Hospital, *818*
Avian Nutrition, *820*
Managing the Hospitalized Avian
  Patient, *822*
Zoonoses and Common Clinical
  Problems, *823*
Reptiles, *823*
Taking the Clinical History, *824*
Sample Collection and Diagnostic
  Procedures, *824*
Radiography, *826*

Anesthesia, *826*
Husbandry in the Hospital, *827*
Nutrition, *828*
Skin, *832*
Feces, *832*
Sputum, *832*
Zoonoses and Common Clinical
  Problems, *832*
Small Mammals, *833*
Ferrets, *833*
Rabbits, *835*
Rodents, *838*
Guinea Pigs, *839*
Hamsters, *840*
Gerbils, *841*
Mice, *841*
Rats, *842*
Prairie Dogs, *842*
Hedgehogs, *842*
Sugar Gliders, *843*

KEY TERMS

Basilic vein
Capillaria
Chelonian
Cloaca
Colonic wash
Conjunctivitis
Crop
Dysbiosis
Ecdysis
Giardia
Glottis
Heterophil
Medial metatarsal vein
Palpebral edema
Perineum

LEARNING OBJECTIVES

When you have completed this chapter, you will be able to:

1. Pronounce, define, and spell all Key Terms in this chapter.
2. Do the following regarding the intake process and examination of birds:
   - Explain how to properly transport an avian patient to the veterinary hospital.
   - List the information included in an accurate and thorough clinical history for an avian patient, and explain proper capture and restraint techniques for an effective and timely examination with minimal stress for the patient.
3. Explain the sample collections and diagnostic procedures commonly used in birds, as well as proper anesthetic induction techniques and intubation procedures.
4. Do the following regarding management and care of a hospitalized avian patient:
   - Discuss the proper husbandry of avian patients, including the purpose and procedure of wing trimming and toenail clipping.
   - Explain the dietary and water requirements for pet birds.
   - Describe the care of a hospitalized avian patient, including common routes for administering medication, housing requirements, cage cleaning, monitoring appetite, crop emptying, and basal metabolic rate.
   - List zoonoses and other common clinical problems associated with avian patients, and explain how to prevent transmission to humans.
5. List the materials needed to properly treat and handle reptile species in the veterinary hospital, and discuss the information needed for an accurate and thorough clinical history of a reptile patient.

6. Do the following regarding the collection of samples, diagnostic procedures, radiography and anesthesia in reptiles:
   - Explain sample collections and diagnostic procedures commonly used in reptiles.
   - Describe proper restraint and handling techniques when obtaining radiographs of reptilian patients, and anesthesia and intubation recommendations for the chelonian, snake, and lizard.
7. Do the following regarding management and care of a hospitalized reptile patient:
   - Describe husbandry requirements for the reptilian patient, including temperature, humidity, and substrate preferences.
   - Explain the dietary and light requirements, as well as nutritional deficiencies, of chelonians, snakes, and lizards.
   - Discuss diagnostic sampling of skin, feces, and sputum in reptile patients.
   - List common zoonoses associated with reptiles and explain how to prevent their transmission to humans.
8. Explain the proper care of a ferret, including nail trimming, blood collection techniques, anesthesia procedures, and nutritional requirements. Also, list common presenting complaints in this species.
9. Explain the proper care of a rabbit, including nutritional requirements, anesthesia techniques, and general care procedures. Also, list common presenting complaints in this species.
10. Discuss the use of antibiotics, anesthesia, and antiparasitic agents in pet rodents.
11. Describe the special dietary and housing requirements of guinea pigs, including substrate preferences and problems with delivery of young.
12. Describe the proper care of hamsters, gerbils, mice, rats, prairie dogs, hedgehogs, and sugar gliders, including husbandry requirements, dietary requirements, and common disease conditions.

INTRODUCTION

The veterinary field of exotic or nondomestic pet medicine is expanding in the areas of pet ownership, and many owners are willing to pay for excellent health care for their animals (Figure 22-1). Caged and aviary birds are now the 3rd most common small animal pet. The 2011-2012 National Pet Owners Survey of the American Pet Products Manufacturers Association (APPMA) reported that 5.7 million households owned a total of 16.2 million birds. Pet bird owners are using veterinary care for their animals according to the *U.S. Pet Ownership and Demographics Source Book* of the American Veterinary Medical Association (Wise, 2007). This chapter discusses avian and nondomestic pet species, with particular attention paid to individual requirements of birds, reptiles, and small mammals. It is important to note that approximately 85% of the presenting disease problems of companion exotic animals result from pet owners' lack of basic nutritional and husbandry information for that particular species. New owners of companion exotic species have relatively little knowledge about what is required to maintain a healthy animal. It is imperative that the veterinary community, in particular veterinary technicians, take the lead in being the information resource for owners of companion exotic species. With proper education of pet owners, all species covered in this chapter will have a greater chance of living long and healthy lives. For information on handling and restraint of the animals described in this chapter, see Chapter 6.

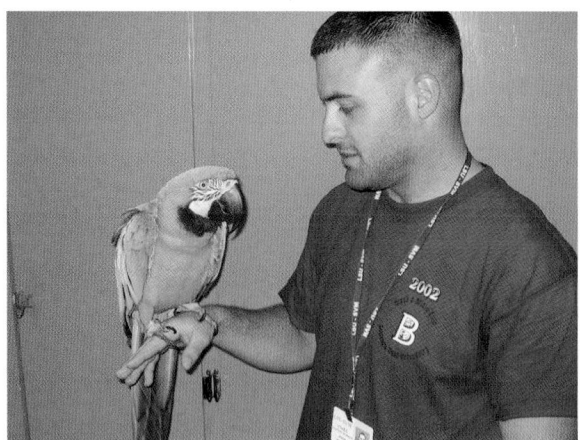

FIGURE 22-1 A bird is an attractive, popular companion.

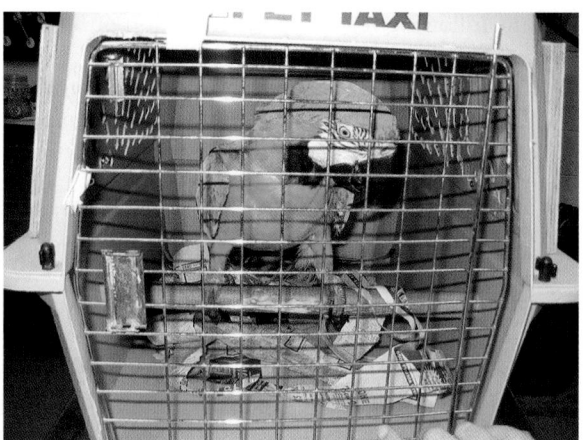

FIGURE 22-2 A pet carrier is recommended for transport of companion birds to the veterinary hospital.

> **TECHNICIAN NOTE** It is important to note that approximately 85% of presenting disease problems of companion, exotic animals result from lack of basic nutritional and husbandry requirements for that particular species.

BOX 22-1	Common Pet Birds

Psittacines
Budgerigar
Cockatiel
Amazon parrot
Macaw
Conure
Lovebird
African gray parrot

Passerines
Canary
Zebra finch
Java rice bird

BIRDS

The veterinary technician may, on occasion, be involved in telephone communication with a bird owner. When owners call regarding transport of their bird to the veterinary hospital, it is important to give specific instructions to reduce patient stress and injury. If at all possible, the owner should bring the bird in its own cage or carrier. If the bird is large and its cage will not fit in the vehicle, the animal should be transported in a plastic small animal carrier. Small animal carriers work well for birds, particularly carriers with a front door opening. Newspaper or a towel can be used to cover the bottom, which is easily cleaned when removed. Wooden dowels can be placed in the carrier as perches and secured in place from the outside with screws and washers (Figure 22-2). Owners should be advised to never bring their bird to the veterinary hospital unsecured; the bird should be brought in a pet carrier or, if small, in its cage. Before leaving their residence, owners should not clean the bird's cage, except to empty the water dish. Good evaluation of the bird's environment is helpful to the veterinarian, and clean papers and cage do not provide that information.

> **TECHNICIAN NOTE** Owners should be advised to never bring their bird to the veterinary hospital unsecured; the bird should be brought in a carrier or, if small, in its cage. The cage should <u>not</u> be cleaned before the visit other than to empty the water dish. This enables the veterinarian to examine the environment in which the bird lives.

All grit should be removed because some birds tend to gorge themselves on grit, particularly when ill. The cage should be covered with a towel or a blanket to protect it from

the weather, and the owner should be instructed to bring along any medication and vitamin supplements that the bird is taking, as well as a sample of food. Most avian telephone inquiries should be considered emergencies because most owners are unfamiliar with early signs of illness, the bird's inherent ability to mask clinical problems, and the rapid speed with which avian species succumb to disease.

TAKING THE CLINICAL HISTORY

Following is a suggested list of questions to ask owners regarding their pet bird:
- What is the chief complaint?
- Obtain the signalment (includes species, gender, and age): Box 22-1 lists common pet species.
- Origin: Where was the bird obtained? How long has it been owned by the presenting party?
- Environment: What is the construction and design of the cage? Is it painted? If so, what type of paint has been used? What is the design and composition of the water and food bowls, substrate (newspaper, wood shavings, corncob, etc.), and perches? Where is the bird kept (indoors or outdoors)? In what room of the house is it kept (e.g., kitchen or garage, where potential toxins may be located)? Is it kept close to a window? Are insecticides, household

TABLE 22-1	Recommended Psittacine Diet	
FOOD GROUP	**WHAT IT SUPPLIES**	**WHAT IT LACKS**
Cereals and grains, 45%-50%	Proteins, fats, B-vitamins	Vitamins A, D, and K and calcium (high phosphorus)
Vegetables, 45%-50%	Vitamins A and K, fiber, carbohydrates ± calcium	Proteins, fats, vitamin D$_3$
Fruit, approximately 5%	Sugars, simple carbohydrates	Proteins, vitamins, minerals
Meats (in combination with dairy products), about 5%	Proteins, fats, calcium	

Mineral supplements (e.g., cuttlebone, oyster shell, mineral blocks, avian vitamins) may be added to the above diets.
Commercial pelleted diets are primarily cereal-and-grain-based with vitamin and mineral supplementation added.

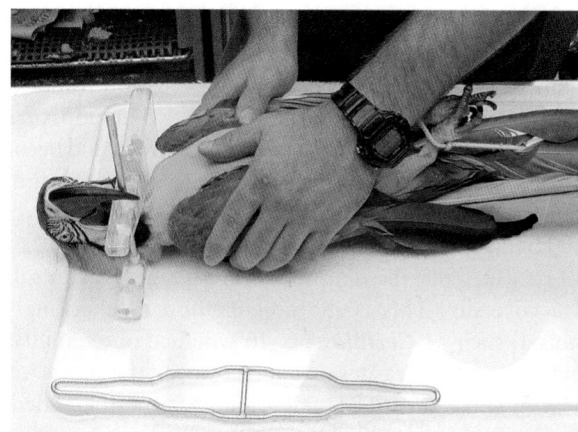

FIGURE 22-3 Once the bird is restrained, an avian examination board may be used to easily examine the patient and obtain diagnostic samples. Care should be taken to prevent chest compression by the handler.

cleaners, or other chemicals used around the house in the vicinity of the cage? Is the bird allowed out of the cage? If so, is it allowed to fly freely, and how well is it supervised?

- Diet: What is the bird being fed (e.g., pellets, seed, fruits, vegetables, grain)? Who manufactures the pellets? How often is the bird fed? Are vitamins and minerals added to the food? How often is the water changed? How is the food prepared and stored? Table 22-1 lists a recommended psittacine diet.
- Appetite: Notes should be made regarding the bird's overall appetite and daily food consumption.
- Feces: Questions regarding the consistency, color, and number of droppings per day are all important. The client should be asked whether feces have been previously submitted for parasite evaluation.
- Cagemates: Are there other animals in the collection in the same cage or in the household? If so, how many, what species, and what degree of contact do they have with the patient? Does the owner maintain a quarantine policy?
- Moulting cycle: When did the bird go through its last general moult? Are any abnormalities in the feather coat or feather growth evident?
- Behavior: What is the overall attitude and behavior of the bird, including voice quality and changes in vocalization? Have behavior-related problems been reported in the past (e.g., feather picking, screaming, other abnormal behavior)?
- Previous medical history: Has the bird been ill before? Is there a history of disease in other pets in the house? If so, what illnesses have been diagnosed and treated in the past? Has the pet visited a veterinarian before? Previous records from other veterinary visits would be helpful in gaining a complete overview of the patient's health history.

BEHAVIOR CONSIDERATIONS DURING THE EXAMINATION PROCESS

As recommended, all birds should be brought to the practice in a carrier or a cage (see Figure 22-2). Although a carrier may be recommended, some avian patients will arrive unrestrained. However, the owner brings a bird into the room, it should be understood that the patient is in an unfamiliar, stressful environment. To reduce behavior complications that may arise as a result of the examination, certain considerations are recommended. Capture and restraint is necessary for an examination, but pain and stress should be reduced as much as possible. To achieve this goal, capture and restraint should be accomplished using a towel that covers the hand being used to grasp the bird. The bird should be in a standing position with the towel in full view as the hand approaches the patient's head. Most birds will allow the hand within the towel to grasp behind the neck with very little resistance if the towel is slowly advanced in full view. All diagnostic testing materials and medications should be ready before the bird is restrained. Examination, diagnostic sample collections, treatments, and procedures must be performed quickly to reduce stress and adverse psychological effects of the hospital visit (Figure 22-3). Once the examination has been completed, positive reinforcement provided by scratching the bird behind its head and communicating with it will aid in transitioning the bird back to the owner.

If the avian patient has to be hospitalized, placing the bird's cage within a hospital cage will help with accommodation to the unfamiliar surroundings. If the cage is too big to be placed in the hospital cage, familiar food and toys will help promote psychological well-being. Pet bird owners should understand that returning the bird to its familiar home surroundings as soon as possible not only will enhance the animal's psychological comfort but may facilitate the healing process as well.

SAMPLE COLLECTIONS AND DIAGNOSTIC PROCEDURES COMMONLY USED IN BIRDS

Diagnostic plans in avian species are no different from clinical approaches to other domestic pets. Evaluation of the stool is an important first step. The technician should become familiar with normal stool presentation to determine differences between polyuria (excessive urine output) and diarrhea (change in fecal consistency and amount) (Figure 22-4). Fecal parasites may be detected on fresh smears with saline and a coverslip. This is the best method of checking for protozoa, such as *Giardia* spp. To enhance one's ability to detect protozoan parasites on a direct smear, the slide should be warm, and a drop of Lugol's iodine should be added to the saline for contrast. Fecal flotation will allow parasite ova (e.g., ascarids, *Capillaria* spp.) to float to the slide surface. Fecal sedimentation is an important procedure for the diagnosis of flukes, which may be seen in wild avian species, including raptors. Fecal specimens that are Gram-stained may provide information regarding the microbial flora (e.g., bacteria, yeast) of the patient's digestive tract. Although the fecal Gram stain has been advocated for many years as a helpful diagnostic test, its usefulness has been recently questioned. It appears that the fecal Gram stain does not provide a valid assessment of bacterial flora within the digestive system. The disease condition for which the fecal Gram stain would be most helpful in diagnosis is gastrointestinal candidiasis *(Candida albicans)*. Most cage-bird species have preponderantly Gram-positive organisms inhabiting the digestive system.

> **TECHNICIAN NOTE**   To enhance one's ability to detect protozoan parasites on a direct smear, the slide should be warm, and a drop of Lugol's iodine should be added to the saline for contrast.

Cloacal Swab

A cloacal swab is often performed on a psittacine species to identify the bacterial flora of the lower gastrointestinal tract.

A cotton swab is moistened, inserted into the **cloaca**, and gently rotated. Cloacal swabs are useful for cytologic evaluations and in looking for inflammatory cells (e.g., **heterophils**). Commercially manufactured culturette swabs are also used to obtain samples for microbial culture and for *Chlamydia psittaci* or viral isolation.

Oral Examination and Crop Wash

The technician should become adept at assisting in the performance of an oral examination and crop wash by the veterinarian. Good restraint technique is essential (see Chapter 6). An avian beak speculum is placed in the bird's mouth parallel to the commissure and is rotated to open the beak (Figure 22-5). A choanal culture is recommended when birds are exhibiting upper respiratory disease signs. The culturette is placed in the rostral area of the choana to prevent cross-contamination with microbial flora in the oral cavity (Figure 22-6).

Another important diagnostic technique is the crop wash, which permits examination of the upper gastrointestinal tract. A sterile or clean tube is passed through the mouth into the **crop** or into the esophagus in birds with an underdeveloped crop. A syringe of sterile saline is connected to the tube, and a simple flush is performed (Figure 22-7). Tubes may be made of plastic, rubber, or metal and have a ball tip (Figure 22-8). The crop wash is important in performing a direct microscopic examination in which a wet mount technique is used to evaluate the sample for protozoan parasites (e.g., *Trichomonas* spp.), megabacteria *(Rhabdus ornithogaster)*, and yeast *(Candida albicans)*. Slides may be prepared for cytologic examination with Diff-Quik or Wright stain, which is used to look for inflammatory cells, such as heterophils. A Gram stain is often performed on crop wash samples from psittacine species, or the sample may be submitted for culture and sensitivity. A culturette may be passed into a bird's crop and submitted for culture and sensitivity diagnostics. When a culturette is passed into a bird's crop, extreme caution must be observed to prevent the patient from biting the culturette and swallowing the tip. Young psittacine species readily accept culturettes into the crop through normal feeding responses.

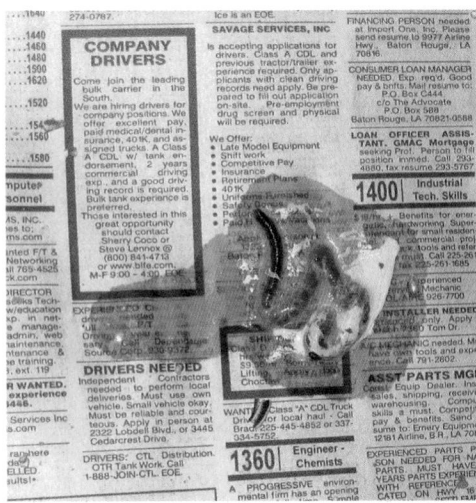

FIGURE 22-4 Normal psittacine stool. Note the dark solid feces, white solid urates, and liquid urine.

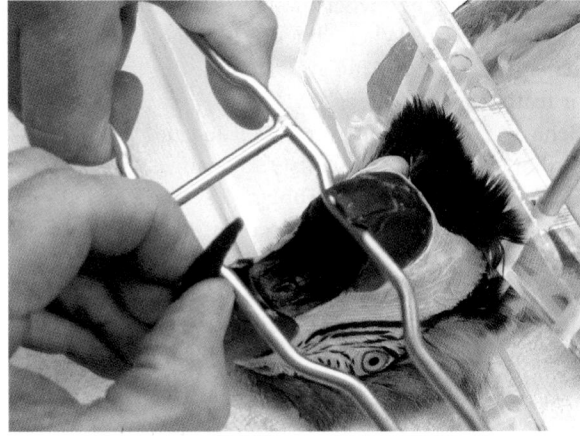

FIGURE 22-5 Oral examination demonstrating the use of a beak speculum on a macaw.

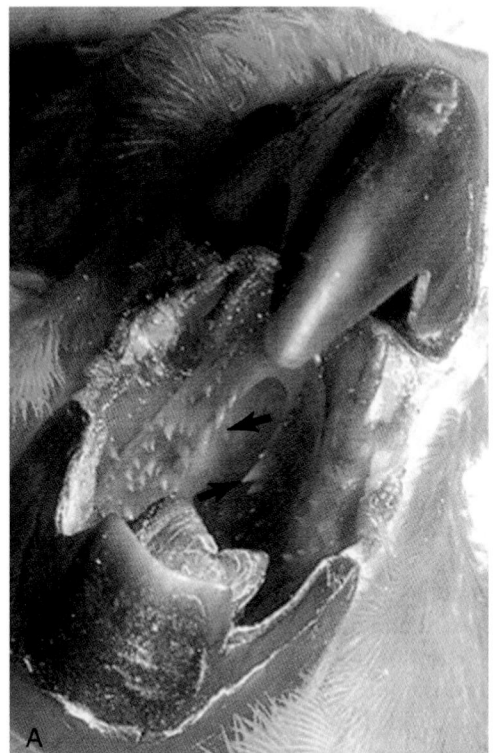

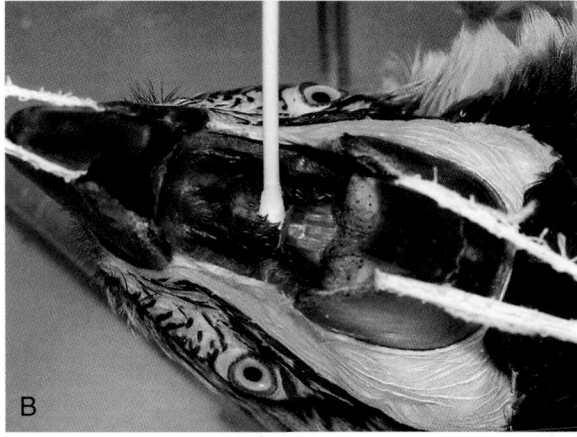

FIGURE 22-6 *A,* Arrow indicates correct placement of culturette. *B,* Culturette placement in the rostral aspect of the choana.

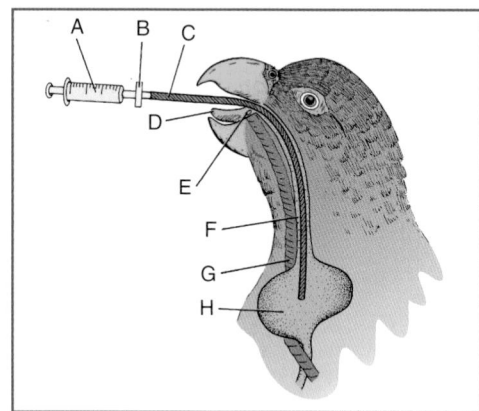

FIGURE 22-7 Proper tube placement for a crop wash or for tube-feeding a bird. The bird's neck should be gently stretched. *A,* Syringe. *B,* Adaptor, if necessary. *C,* Tube. *D,* Tongue. *E,* Tracheal opening. *F,* Proximal esophagus. *G,* Trachea. *H,* Crop.

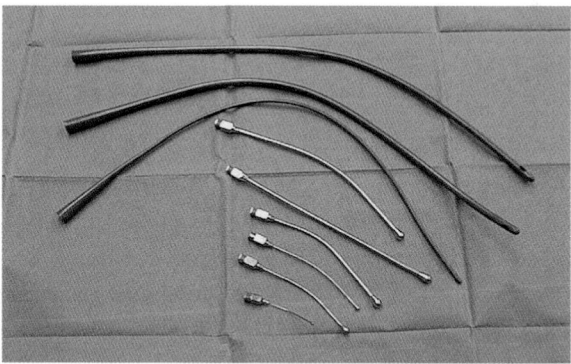

FIGURE 22-8 Various tubes used for tube-feeding and crop washes.

> **TECHNICIAN NOTE** Young psittacine species readily accept culturettes into the crop through normal feeding responses.

Passing a tube into the crop of the psittacine bird is an important technique to learn because tube-feeding is often necessary to administer medications and/or nutritional supplementation (see Figure 22-7). The tube should be passed over the trachea at the base of the tongue down the esophagus and palpated in the crop at the level of the thoracic inlet. Food that is administered using a feeding tube must have a lower temperature than the bird. Most psittacine species have a body temperature of 102° F to 104° F, therefore the food should be fed between 98° F and 101° F. The feeding formula must be thoroughly mixed before uptake into the syringe. Many baby birds develop thermal burns from hot feeding formula (hotter than the bird's body temperature), usually on the weight-dependent ventral surface area of the crop. This injury can be prevented by careful preparation of food by the attending technician. The one rule of thumb to remember when a tube is used for feeding or performing a crop wash is to try to pick a tube with a diameter larger than the **glottis** (Figure 22-8).

> **TECHNICIAN NOTE** Thermal burns to the crop of young birds can be easily prevented by proper preparation of food and feeding at recommended temperatures.

The glottis of the bird is located at the base of the tongue and is easy to visualize. The tube may be passed into the crop easily by positioning the tube in the side of the bird's mouth (see Figure 22-7). The tube is easily palpated through the wall of the crop and the skin. While doing a crop wash or a tube-feeding, the handler should watch the back of the bird's mouth to ensure that food or water does not begin to accumulate. If the crop is overfilled, the bird may aspirate. If the crop overfills, put the bird down, and let it attempt to clear its airway. The bird itself has a better chance of clearing its airway than does the technician or the veterinarian using cotton-tipped applicators. Never handle a bird after placing oral medications into the crop or filling the crop, unless the bird is experiencing respiratory difficulty.

> **TECHNICIAN NOTE** Never handle a bird after placing oral medication into the crop or filling the crop, unless the bird is experiencing respiratory difficulty.

Hematology

Hematology is an important part of the diagnostic evaluation of avian patients. Common venipuncture sites include the **basilic vein**, the right jugular vein, and the **medial metatarsal vein**, but other sites may be used, depending on the avian species and the experience of the phlebotomist. Each blood collection location has its own advantages and disadvantages; the veterinarian and the technician will often choose their own sites of preference, but the right jugular vein is the recommended site for most, if not all, pet bird species. Never try to collect blood from an avian vein unless it is visualized. Avian blood vessels are too mobile and the vessel walls too elastic to collect from this location alone.

The right jugular vein is large and is easily found in most birds on the right dorsolateral aspect of the neck (Figure 22-9). However, it is highly mobile and therefore difficult to stabilize. In most birds, the right jugular vein is located in a featherless tract lateral to the trachea. With minimal practice and proper restraint, avian jugular venipuncture becomes an easy procedure to perform. An avian restraint board is recommended for blood collection from larger psittacine patients (see Chapter 6). Small psittacine and passerine patients can be hand-held when blood is being drawn for diagnostic tests.

> **TECHNICIAN NOTE** The right jugular vein is the recommended site for most, if not all, companion avian species.

In general, the basilic vein is accessible but is difficult to completely immobilize in the psittacine patient because of the tremendous strength of the pectoral muscles (Figures 22-10 and 22-11). In most avian patients, the basilic vein is the easiest vein to use for intravenous injections. Unfortunately, although the basilic vein is easy to visualize, when a needle is removed from this vein, an obvious hematoma will form. When collecting blood from the basilic vein, it is important for the technician to apply digital pressure to the site for at least a minute after the needle has been removed to reduce the size of hematoma formation. The owner should be informed of the hematoma when the bird is returned after the examination. In larger parrot species and other birds, the basilic vein is a good choice for placement of intravenous catheters.

The medial metatarsal vein is easy to immobilize and secure, even in an awake, fractious patient. However, if large volumes of blood are to be collected, the medial metatarsal vein may not be a good choice in psittacine patients. In larger parrot species and other birds, the medial metatarsal vein is a good choice for placement of intravenous catheters.

A blood sample may be obtained from a clipped claw "toenail," but this is painful for the patient and often causes

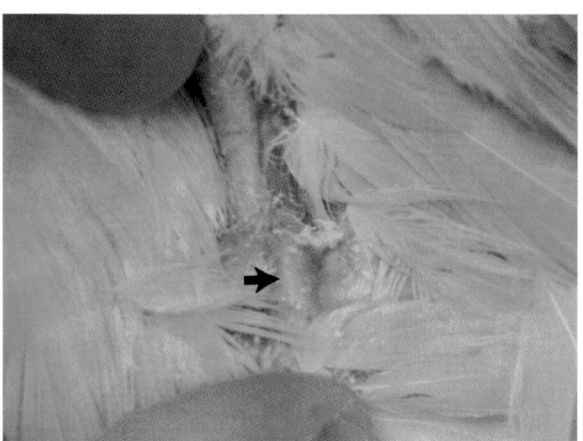

FIGURE 22-10 Location of the basilic vein (black arrow). Ventral view of humerus, radius, and ulna.

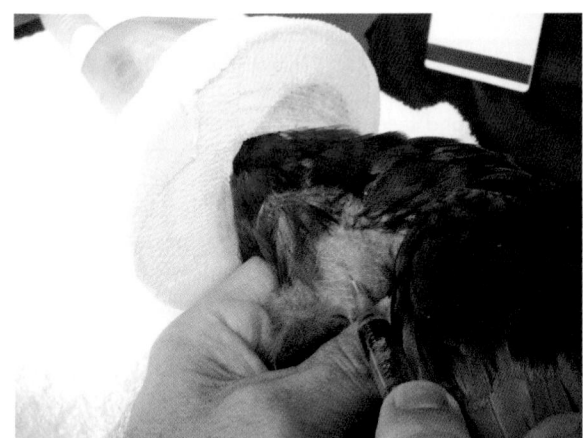

FIGURE 22-9 Location of the right jugular vein, the most common site of blood collection in pet avian species.

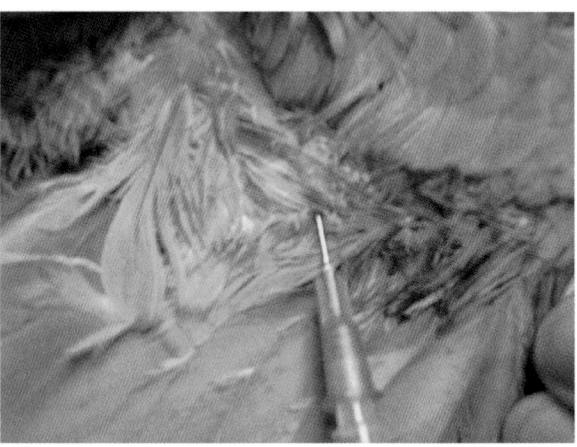

FIGURE 22-11 Intravenous injection using the basilic vein.

lameness for several days after the procedure. It may result in poor blood flow, low yield, and invalid results. Therefore, blood obtained from toenail clipping is recommended only for DNA-based gender determination testing.

Blood may be collected in syringes, microhematocrit tubes (Figure 22-12), or blood collection tubes from the hub of the needle. A 3-ml syringe with a 26-gauge needle should be used to collect blood in most avian patients. In extremely small psittacine and passerine patients, a 1-ml syringe with a 30-gauge needle may be used. The technician should learn to proficiently perform a complete blood count (CBC) on avian blood.

Radiography

Radiography is an important diagnostic tool in avian patients. Typically, lateral and ventrodorsal views of the whole body or selected extremities may be taken (Figure 22-13). Technique charts must be developed using the equipment available. Contrast films may be made with standard contrast agents, including iohexol and barium

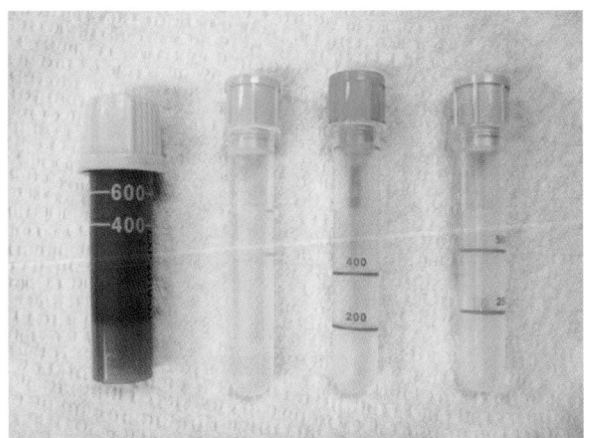

FIGURE 22-12 Microtainer tubes used to transport blood samples for diagnostic testing.

sulfate. Because good positioning and absence of motion are important for high-quality radiographs, it is generally recommended that all avian patients must be sedated or anesthetized, except those that may be too ill. Proper positioning is important, and an avian restraint board is essential (Figure 22-14). Other diagnostic procedures, such as laparoscopy, endoscopy, tracheal or air sac washes, biopsies, cytologic examinations, and bone marrow aspirates, may be performed on the patient. The technician's role may be to secure the animal with good restraint during the more sophisticated procedures.

ANESTHESIA[1]

Once it has been determined that the avian patient is in good condition for the anesthetic protocol, induction occurs. In most avian cases, isoflurane gas with oxygen is used. Use of sevoflurane and desflurane has increased in recent years, but the higher price of these products and the small difference in their overall advantage over isoflurane keeps their usage at a low level.

A mask or induction chamber may be used to induce the patient and prepare for intubation. For gas induction, it is generally recommended to provide 5% flow of isoflurane with 2 L flow of oxygen.[1] It is extremely important to have an anesthetist specifically monitor the patient's response to the anesthetic agent. At 5% flow of isoflurane, most avian patients undergo rapid induction and are ready for intubation in less than a minute.

For intubation, all material should be prepared and ready to use before the procedure is performed. Materials needed for intubation include the endotracheal tube (noncuffed, 2.0 to 5.0 interior diameter for most companion avian species) and hemostats. A noncuffed tube is used to prevent pressure necrosis from developing on the mucosal surface of the trachea. Hemostats are used to grasp the tongue and extend it to expose the glottis. The tube from the anesthesia machine is then disconnected from the face mask and is placed on the end of the endotracheal tube. The tube should be secured by

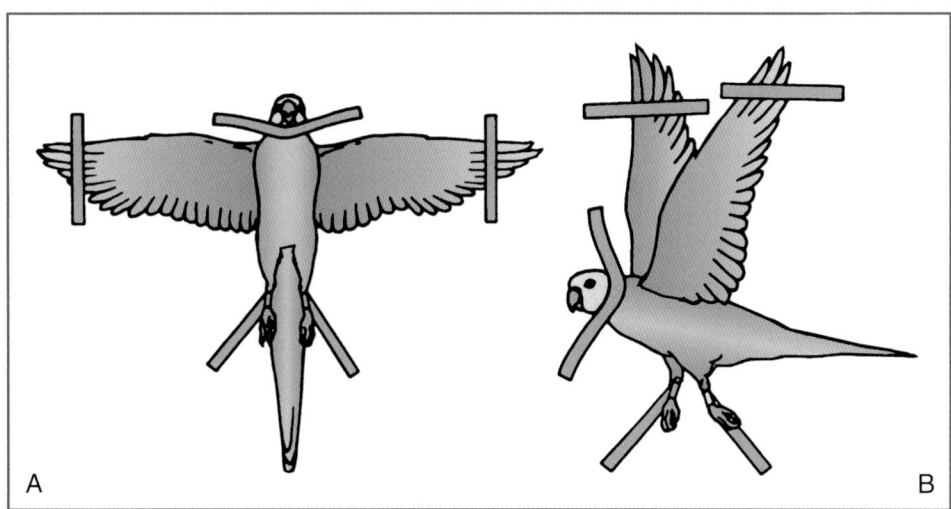

FIGURE 22-13 Positioning of a budgerigar for radiographs using masking tape. **A,** Ventrodorsal and **(B)** lateral positions.

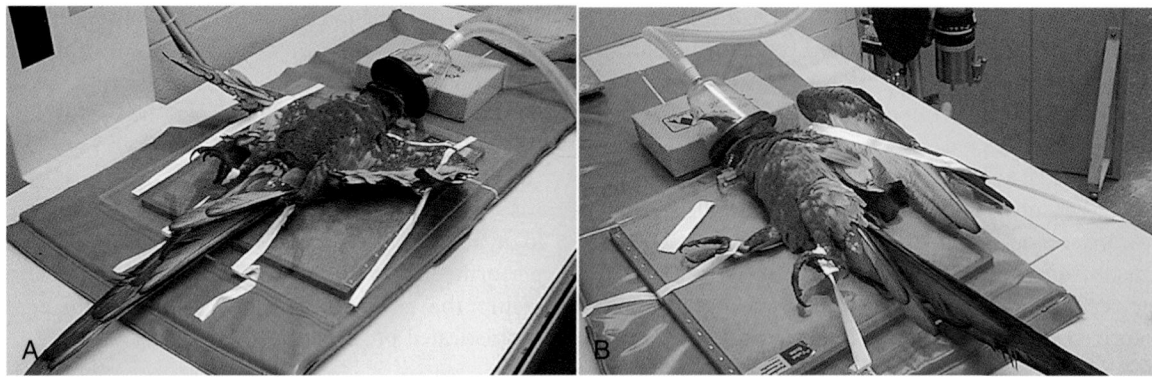

FIGURE 22-14 Ventrodorsal **(A)** and lateral **(B)** positioning of a macaw with the use of adhesive tape. The bird is on a Plexiglas avian restraint board for uniform positioning of patients. A face mask is used for administration of inhalant isoflurane anesthesia.

attaching a strip of white cloth tape to the tracheal tube and wrapping it around the back of the bird's head. The patient should be monitored, as is required for all patients under general anesthesia.

HUSBANDRY AND TREATMENT IN THE HOSPITAL

Generally speaking, medication administered in food or water will not reach adequate therapeutic levels in the avian patient. This is an unreliable way to administer most medications because of inconsistent intake of water by most birds. Direct oral absorption is inconsistent with tablets, but most liquid suspensions tend to work well. With the advent of compounding pharmacies, many medications can be formulated into oral suspensions that are flavored to enhance palatability. Other than oral administration, common methods of providing medication to avian patients are intramuscular, intravenous, intraosseous, and subcutaneous routes. Intramuscular injection of medication in birds is best accomplished in the large pectoral muscle mass. Drugs injected into the caudal half of the animal (e.g., the legs) may result in the agent's absorption into the bloodstream and its being shunted toward the kidneys by way of the renal portal system. Potentially nephrotoxic drugs, such as aminoglycosides, should never be administered by injection into the legs, except in ostriches, emus, and rheas, and only when patients are adequately hydrated. The basilic vein is recommended for intravenous drug treatment; the distal ulna is the best location for placement of an intraosseous catheter to treat birds with medication (Figure 22-15). Subcutaneous fluid therapy should be provided in the featherless areas of the axillary and inguinal regions.

> **TECHNICIAN NOTE** Intramuscular injection of drugs into birds is recommended in the large pectoral muscle mass.

Procedures that the veterinary technician often performs include nail trims and clipping of the wing feathers. Figure 22-16 illustrates one technique for clipping the flight feathers of pet birds. Both wings should be clipped for a symmetric

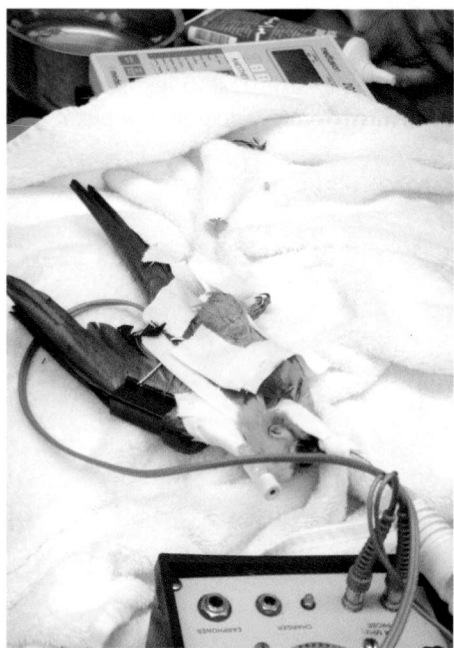

FIGURE 22-15 Placement of an intraosseous catheter in the distal ulna of a bird's wing.

effect, but owners request many different feather-clip variations. Typically, the primary flight feathers are cut for heavier birds, and both primary and secondary feathers are cut for lighter birds, to achieve maximal flight restriction. If only one wing is clipped, the bird cannot control its flight and will be prone to injury. Feather clipping is flight restriction, not prevention. Find out what the owner wants to achieve through the feather trim and how the owner wants the feathers clipped. No technique for trimming wing feathers will prevent the bird from some degree of flight. In the end, both the owner and the technician or the veterinarian must be happy with the look and flight restriction of the trim.

Nails should be trimmed in larger psittacine species with a Dremel motor tool (Dremel, Inc., Racine, Wisconsin). For small psittacine species and passerines, human nail clippers or an electrocautery unit can be used. Cautery units can be

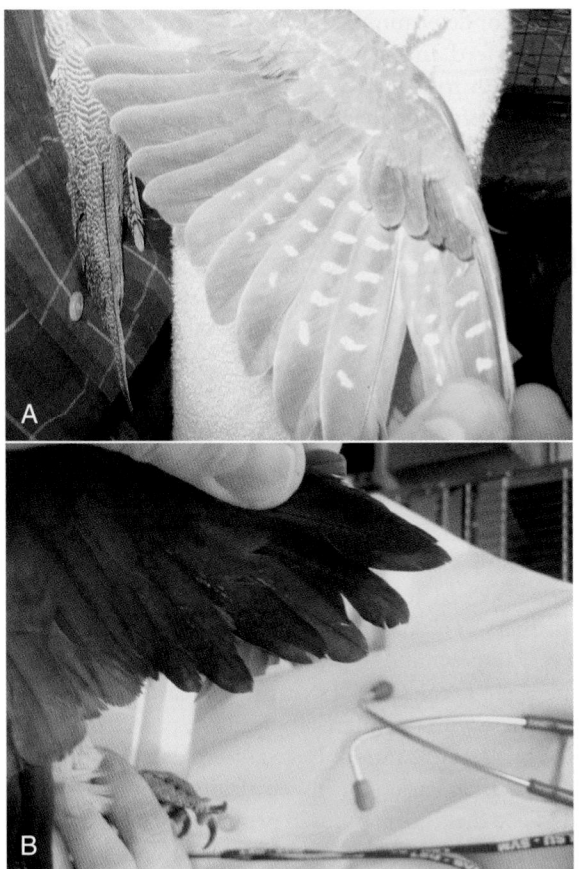

FIGURE 22-16 A, Ventral view of extended wing (when a proper feather trim is performed, a symmetric cut of the 10 outermost feathers is made below the level of the dorsal coverts). **B,** Proper feather trim of wing on African gray parrot.

used on the nails of birds of all sizes, but they work especially well on smaller species (Figure 22-17).

> **TECHNICIAN NOTE** No technique for trimming wing feathers will prevent the bird from some degree of flight.

Grinding with a Dremel motor tool cauterizes as it reduces the length of the nails (Figure 22-18). Chemical cautery (as with silver nitrate sticks) should be available if bleeding occurs, especially in younger birds.

Dietary management and nutritional support are particularly important in the compromised avian patient. Table 22-1 provides basic feeding guidelines for psittacine species and other seed-eating birds. It is important to remember to keep the cage as clean as possible. Food and water dishes should be cleaned at least daily and occasionally more often. Fresh fruits, vegetables, and meats should be left in a food dish only for short periods of time. Food consumption should be closely monitored. New foods, especially pelleted avian diets, should be introduced gradually. Some foods, such as peeling vegetables, fruits, and nuts, may serve as a source of activity for the bird while eating. Tube-feeding in psittacine birds is an important nursing procedure. Generally, a commercially available cereal-based baby avian formula (Exact, Kaytee Inc., Chilton, Wisconsin) is recommended for hand raising young psittacine species. Tube-feeding should begin with small amounts given frequently and slowly increased in volume and administered over shorter time intervals. The bird should be weighed 1 or 2 times per day to chart weight gain. It is essential that a gram

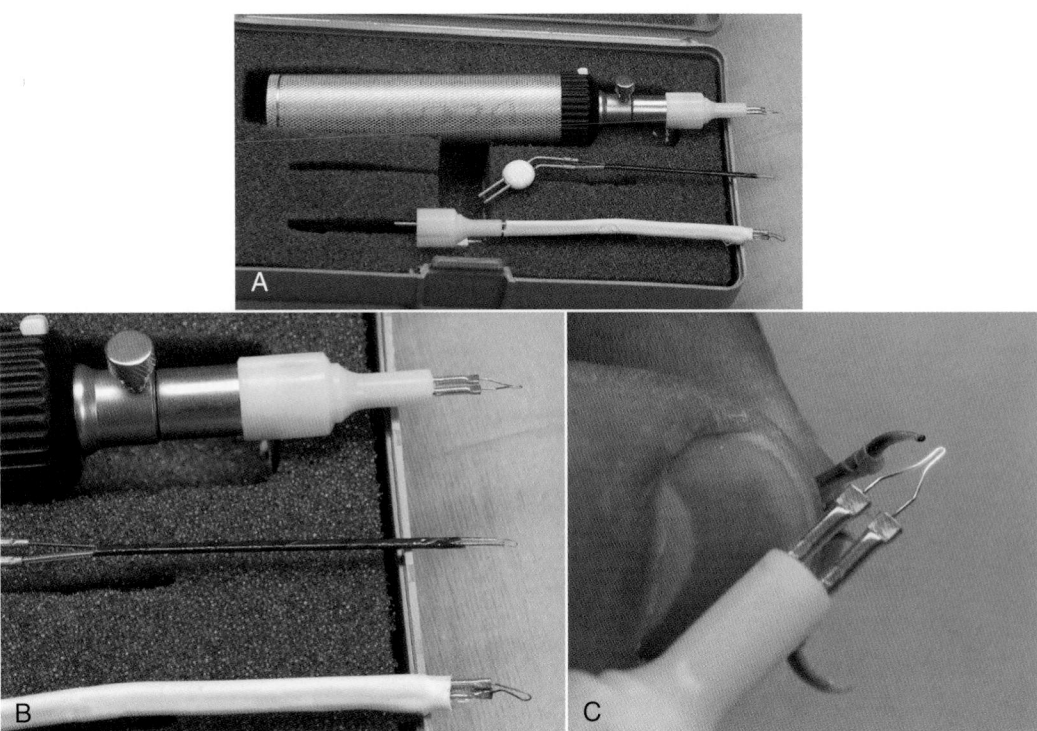

FIGURE 22-17 A, Electrocautery unit for trimming small birds' nails. **B,** Different electrocautery tips. **C,** Trimming bird nails with cautery unit.

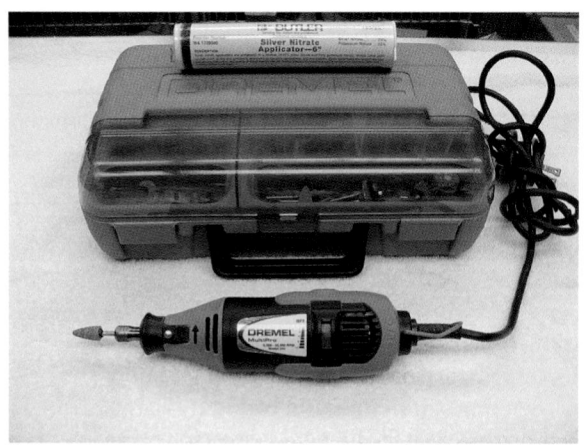

FIGURE 22-18 Motor tool for grinding larger birds' nails and grooming beaks.

scale that weighs in at least 1-gram increments should be used for all avian and exotic animal patients; no substitutions are acceptable. The crop should be monitored for prompt emptying, and stools should be examined for consistency. The basal metabolic rate (BMR) may be calculated as a rough approximation of energy requirements using the formula $K(W^{0.75})$. The normal K value for a nonpasserine species, such as parrots, is approximately 78, and W is the weight of the bird in kilograms. This value should be doubled for an ill bird. For passerine species, 130 times the body weight raised to the power of 0.7 should be used.

> **TECHNICIAN NOTE** It is essential that a gram scale that weighs in at least 1-gram increments should be used for all avian and exotic animal patients; no substitutions are acceptable.

For carnivorous birds, such as raptors, a high-quality carnivore critical care diet (Lafeber Co., Ordell, Illinois) may be given to meet energy requirements.

AVIAN NUTRITION

Nutritional problems encountered in avian medicine include inadequate diets and poor feeding practices. It is generally accepted that nutritional disease is common in pet birds. Although nutritional disease historically has been common, the development and general acceptance of pelleted diets for companion avian species have reduced its occurrence in recent years. Many hospitalized avian patients need nutritional support that may differ from their normal diet. Excessive or inadequate energy intake, imbalance of nutritional supplements, and ingestion of toxic substances (e.g., heavy metal) will create additional challenges for the veterinary professional.

Diet-induced diseases frequently occur in psittacine and passerine bird species as a result of diverse nutrient requirements unknown to the owner. Unfortunately, each species of bird has different nutritional needs, and few or no data are

available for determining the specific quantities of a particular diet to feed. In the past, all-seed diets, seed diets supplemented with fruits and vegetables, and other human foods have been recommended as "the diet" for companion avian species. This antiquated recommendation has led to nutritionally induced disease presentations and death of pet birds.

> **TECHNICIAN NOTE** Unfortunately, each species of bird has different nutritional requirements, and few or no data are available for determining the specific quantity of a particular diet to feed.

Small birds have high metabolic rates and high energy requirements; therefore, a continuous supply of food should always be available. However, most commercially available seed diets are deficient in certain limiting nutrients such as specific amino acids, vitamins, trace minerals, and macrominerals, like calcium and sodium. In addition, seeds are not the primary or natural diet of most companion avian species. It is very important that owners are aware of the natural diet of the avian species they are caring for, and that they try to mimic these with commercially available products. Although many birds are commonly fed seed diets, natural diets contain a wide variety of insects, fruits, plant material, and seeds. Seed diets are composed primarily of sunflower seeds, which are high in fat but low in calcium and vitamin A. A diet high in sunflower seeds therefore gives rise to obesity and nutritional deficiencies.

Although recommended to diversify avian diets, the practice of adding fruits and vegetables sold for human consumption introduces foods composed primarily of water, carbohydrates, and fiber. Many fruits and vegetables are deficient in protein, vitamins, and minerals needed for many avian species. Birds may select food items based on water and sugar content, texture, color, and taste rather than their nutrient content. Too often, the result is imbalanced nutrient intake, which over time can lead to illness or death.

Captive birds develop nutritional deficiencies by habitually selecting specific food items from a diversified diet. It is important to always ask the owner what the bird is eating and what foods the owner is offering. In most cases, what the owner offers and what the pet ingests are two different diets. Because many malnourished birds often overeat certain food items offered to them, it is unclear whether this is a cause or an effect of malnutrition. Unfortunately, this eating behavior leads to the popular misconception that birds are able to preferentially balance their own diets.

> **TECHNICIAN NOTE** It is important to always ask the owner what the bird is eating and what foods the owner is offering. In most cases, what the owner offers and what the pet ingests are two different diets.

All birds have similar nutritional requirements, including water, proteins and amino acids, carbohydrates, fats, vitamins, inorganic elements, and minerals. Although similar in basic nutritional requirements, it is the often subtle difference in nutrients between species that is important for their health. An important requirement for calcium in the avian diet is similar to that for all animals. The calcium requirement for psittacine species has not been determined, but the maintenance requirement for chickens is 0.1% of the diet. Many of the seeds consumed by companion birds make up less than 0.03% of the diet, suggesting that the requirement is larger than 0.05%.

Proteins required by companion birds are composed of approximately 20 amino acids. Ten of these amino acids are essential: arginine, histidine, isoleucine, leucine, lysine, methionine, phenylalanine, threonine, tryptophan, and valine. In the infant bird, glycine and proline are very important. In the United States, methionine and lysine are often absent from the avian diet. Evidence suggests that increased protein may be needed during certain points in the reproductive cycle. In the wild, insects may supply these increased protein requirements. It is difficult, if not impossible, for bird owners to meet protein requirements of birds by feeding only seed mixtures. Although insect larvae and insects are commercially available, it is difficult and often not practical for avian owners to provide this food to birds. Owners should be informed of insect availability when the species they are keeping require such offerings.

White worms (*Enchytraeus* larvae), ant pupae, water shrimp (*Daphinia* spp.), aphids, waxworms, and mealworms are commercially available insects that may be used in avian diets to supply extra protein and fat. This is especially important at the beginning of breeding season.

Food appropriately balanced between carbohydrates, protein, fats, vitamins, minerals, and water is essential for all birds. The stewardship of confined birds must address good nutrition at several levels: the daily satisfaction and health of the bird, and long-term contributions to growth, maturation, defense against disease, and reproductive health (the hallmark of good nutrition).

The major benefits of commercially prepared foods (e.g., pelleted diets) are nutrient balance and convenience (Figure 22-19). Manufacturers commonly formulate commercial food using sound scientific principles in accordance with established nutrient recommendations. Although adherence to these recommendations and quality of ingredients may vary among manufacturers, an extruded or pelleted diet supplies all nutrients in a single particle. Such formulations help prevent alteration of nutrient balance by uninformed owners who feed imbalanced seeds or human foods, or by birds that consume different quantities of imbalanced foods that are fed separately.

Although seeds are a popular, convenient, and inexpensive method of providing nutrients to companion birds (Figure 22-20), they are not necessarily the best food for pet birds. The seeds found in most commercial mixes are not native to the areas where most companion avian species originate.

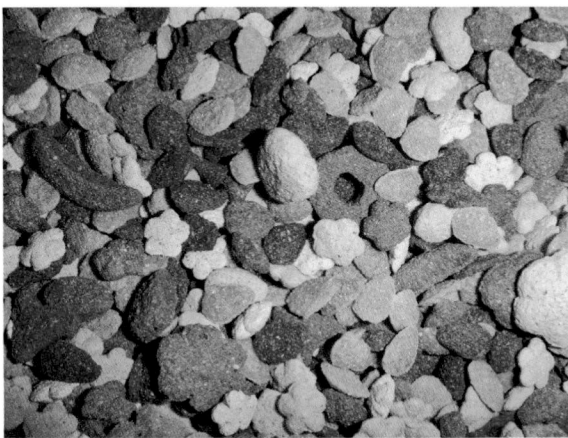

FIGURE 22-19 A commercial-based pelleted diet is recommended as the base diet for most companion avian species.

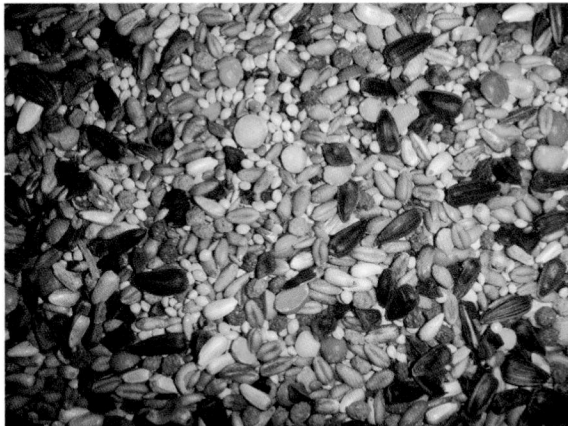

FIGURE 22-20 A typical commercial avian seed diet that can be used to supplement a pet bird's diet in which seed is part of the natural food selection.

A well-balanced seed mixture can supply essential nutrients such as fats, carbohydrates, and some minerals. However, seeds are rarely, if ever, an appropriate sole nutritional source because they provide inadequate levels of protein, vitamins, and minerals. Commercially available seed mixtures vary greatly in type and quality. Individual types of seeds are sold in most stores; thus formulating seed mixtures is a common practice. Unfortunately, the availability of individual types of seeds promotes nutrient imbalance when uninformed owners create a mixture based primarily on the price and physical appearance of the seeds.

At this time, it is recommended that a base commercially pelleted diet be provided for companion avian species. Pelleted diets have vitamins and minerals incorporated into the product. Supplementation with a high-quality seed mixture, vegetables, and, to a lesser extent, fruits in measured amounts rounds out the diversified diet. First and foremost, owners should be aware of the natural diet of the particular avian species they are keeping. The natural diet should be followed as closely as possible with commercially available products. The addition of a high-quality vitamin and mineral supplement is controversial, but it may be added if instructions are closely followed.

Insoluble and soluble mineral grit is often provided to birds as a dietary supplement. Insoluble grit (e.g., quartz, silica) is used in the ventriculus (gizzard) to mechanically break down food. Soluble grit (e.g., oyster shell, cuttlebone, mineral block) is completely digested and serves as a source of minerals (e.g., calcium, phosphorus). Oversupplementation of insoluble mineral grit may be harmful to companion avian species and may lead to gastrointestinal disease. It is recommended that all caged birds have a source of soluble grit, preferably in the form of a cuttle bone (Figure 22-21, *A*) or, for bigger birds, a mineral block (Figure 22-21, *B*).

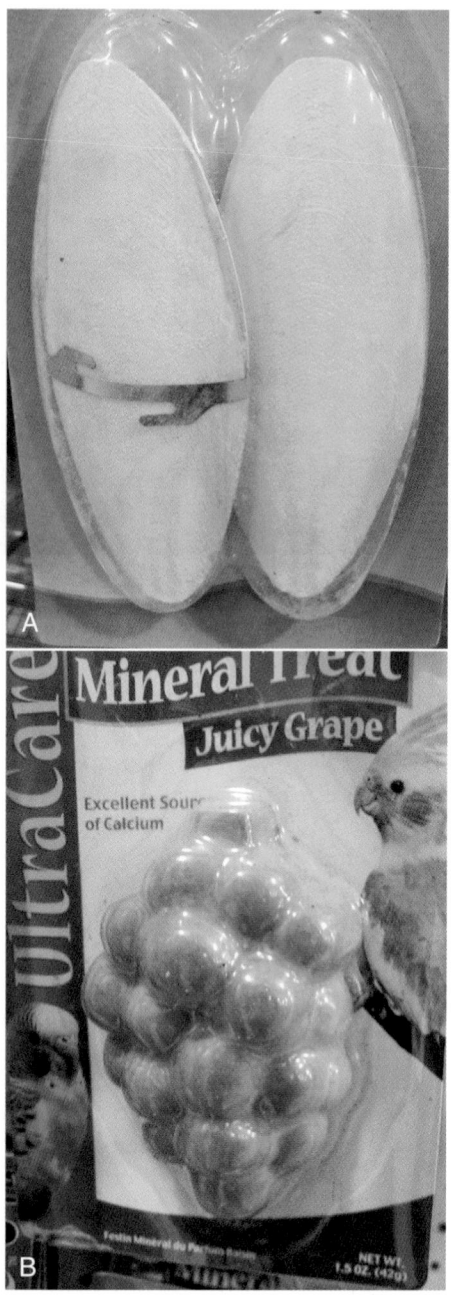

FIGURE 22-21 **A,** All companion avian species should have calcium supplement in their cage. **B,** Mineral blocks provide a calcium source for pet birds.

> **TECHNICIAN NOTE** It is recommended that all caged birds have a source of soluble grit, preferably in the form of a cuttle bone or, for bigger birds, a mineral block.

Although feeding a well-balanced food diet is essential, it is easy to overlook the single most important dietary component: water. Water makes up more than 50% of a bird's body weight. Because birds have no sweat glands, water intake plays an important role in thermoregulation. Breeding females may require increased amounts of water for egg production and for heat regulation while incubating eggs.

Even though some food is high in water content, free water may be required for efficient digestion and absorption of other ingested offerings. Some avian species have an enhanced physiologic ability to extract water from their food. As a general rule, birds should always have access to fresh, clean water. Studies have shown that canaries will die within 48 hours if water is withheld.

Water should be provided in containers that are easily accessible, but not in a location that will allow feces, feathers, or food particles to accumulate. For this reason, water bowls should be attached to the walls of enclosures, near or above food bowls. In addition, use of large water bowls should be discouraged because they may invite bathing.

> **TECHNICIAN NOTE** Water should be provided in containers that are easily accessible, but not in a location that will allow feces, feathers, or food particles to accumulate.

MANAGING THE HOSPITALIZED AVIAN PATIENT

Hospital facilities must be appropriate for the species that are housed. Bird cages should be kept in a separate room, if possible, to minimize the stress of sounds and sights of other species. Isolation of birds also prevents contamination with potentially pathogenic bacteria. For example, psittacine birds have a mostly Gram-positive gut flora. Housing birds near animals with Gram-negative gut flora, such as dogs, cats, reptiles, and carnivorous birds, could result in Gram-negative enteric infection. A visual barrier, such as a cage cover or a hide box in the cage, should be provided for the hospitalized bird. Large parrots may do well in standard dog or cat cages if adequate perches and water and food bowls are provided. Plexiglas custom cages are an excellent alternative and are easily cleaned. Perches should be disposable, simple to disinfect, and sized according to the individual patient. An isolation area is required for avian psittacosis suspects. Cleanliness is one of the most important details in the hospital.

Temperature control is important, particularly with sick birds. In general, birds tolerate cold better than heat. Sudden changes in temperature and drafts should always be prevented. Sick birds have difficulty maintaining and regulating their own body temperature, as do birds with poor feather coats, oil-damaged feathers, or plucked feathers. Therefore, these birds should be kept warm, but not hot. Temperatures between 80° F and 90° F are best. The bird should be observed for signs of heat stress or shivering. Common signs of heat stress in avian patients include panting, extended wings, flushed (reddish) facial patches on macaws, and depression. An environmentally controlled cage or unit should be available for intensive care avian patients.

ZOONOSES AND COMMON CLINICAL PROBLEMS

Chlamydophila psittaci is commonly diagnosed in pet bird species. Avian chlamydiosis is considered a top differential diagnosis for a sick bird that has nonspecific clinical illness (e.g., signs of diarrhea, vomiting, or just not doing well). Patients that have recently been through quarantine or pet shops and have been exposed to other birds are most suspect.

Avian chlamydiosis is a disease transmissible to humans that is caused by the bacterium *C. psittaci*. Patients suspected of potentially being infected with *C. psittaci* should be treated with appropriate antibiotics. The bird should be isolated, gloves and masks should be used, and feces should be disposed of through cleaning of the cage and bagging of disposable substrate. Transmission occurs primarily through respiratory inhalation of the infectious elementary body. Psittacosis is a potentially fatal disease in humans. Many wild birds may carry *C. psittaci* organisms without showing clinical signs. It is important that the veterinary technician working with birds become familiar with this disease.

REPTILES

It is estimated that 13 million pet reptiles are kept in the United States according to the 2011-2012 pet survey of the American Pet Products Manufacturers Association (APPMA). Although the number of pet reptiles does not match dog and cat populations, a significant population of animals requires veterinary health services. The diversity of reptile species maintained in captivity requires education of owners on health, nutritional, and environmental management (Box 22-2). With excellent owner care, most reptile species live long, healthy lives. In many cases, it is the responsibility of the technician to handle and collect diagnostic samples and to educate owners about their captive reptile.

Once a veterinary hospital decides to treat reptile species, a few pieces of specialized equipment are needed to provide an adequate hospital environment and to aid the technician and veterinarian. Required medical equipment includes an electronic gram scale, an incubator, a heating pad, tuberculin and microliter syringes, an exotic animal formulary (see "Recommended Readings"), microhematocrit tubes, rubber mouth specula (spatula), snake cloacal probes, and metal feeding tubes (Figures 22-22 to 22-24).

Materials commonly used for turtle-shell repair include epoxy, resin, and fiberglass patches. There has been a move

| **BOX 22-2** | Reptiles Commonly Maintained as Pets |

Snakes
Boa constrictor *(Boa constrictor)*
Ball python *(Python regius)*
Corn snake *(Elaphe guttata guttata)*
Burmese python *(Python molurus)*

Chelonia
Box turtle *(Terrapene spp.)*
Red-eared slider *(Trachemys scripta elegans)*
Mud turtle *(Kinosternon spp.)*

Lizards
Bearded dragon *(Pogona vitticeps)*
Common tegu *(Tupinambis teguixin)*
Green iguana *(Iguana iguana)*
Green anole *(Anolis carolinensis)*
Jackson's chameleon *(Chamaeleo jacksonii)*
Panther chameleon *(Chamaeleo pardalis)*
Leopard gecko *(Eublepharis macularius)*
Tokay gecko *(Gekko gecko)*
Savannah monitor *(Varanus exanthematicus)*
Water dragon *(Physignathus lesueurii)*

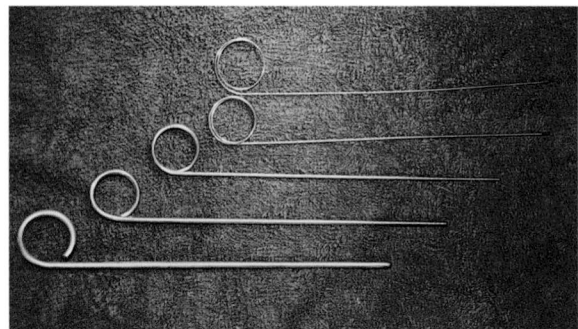

FIGURE 22-22 Snake cloacal probes for sexing.

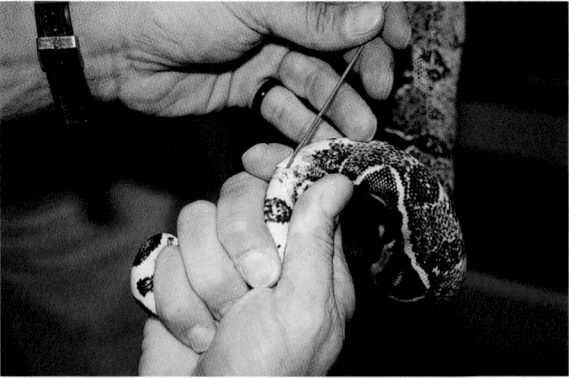

FIGURE 22-23 Snake sexed with cloacal probe.

away from using epoxy resins, dental acrylics, and patches for turtle-shell repair and toward fracture fixation using cerclage wire and open wound healing (Figure 22-25). We have found that a combination of cerclage fixation of fragments and protection of the fracture site with epoxy resin leads to faster healing and release. Surgical equipment used for

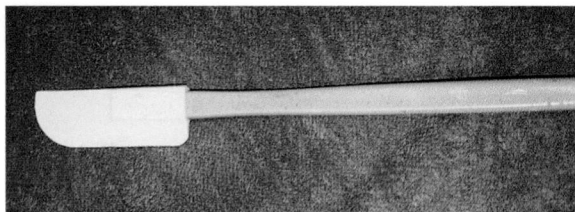

FIGURE 22-24 A spatula is often used as a reptile oral speculum.

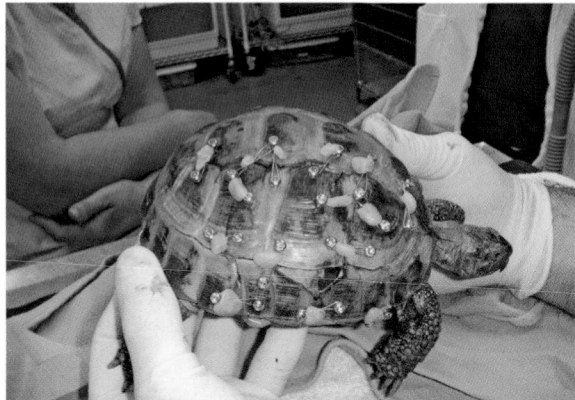

FIGURE 22-25 Turtle shell injury associated with various traumatic injuries is a common presentation.

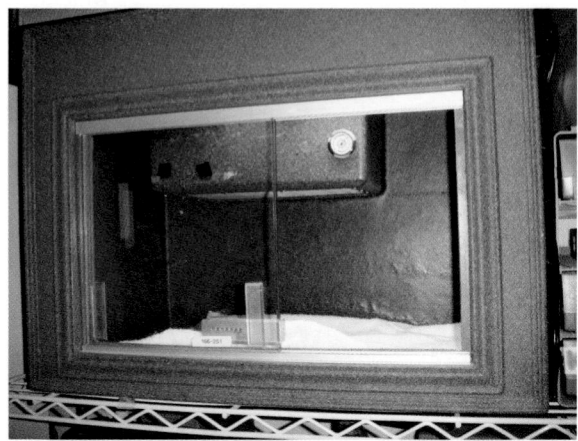

FIGURE 22-26 An example of a reptile hospital cage.

reptiles and available in most exotic animal practices includes a Dremel motor tool, stainless steel suture material, transparent surgical drapes, and a magnifying surgical headset.

Reptile housing equipment must be adaptable to the different species that may be hospitalized. Examples of hospital caging and equipment include fluorescent light tubes (regular and full spectrum), a humidifier, fiberglass cages, small aquaria with secure ventilated tops, a heated room, and heat lamps and pads (Figure 22-26). To aid in capture and restraint, a snake hook, tongs, Plexiglas tubes, and a pole snare should be available. As with other exotic species, proper restraint reduces stress on client, animal, and health care personnel. Once a practice is properly equipped and personnel are trained, interesting patients and cases will begin to receive quality health care.

TAKING THE CLINICAL HISTORY

Following is a list of questions to ask clients regarding reptile patients:
- Chief complaint: Why does the owner want the pet examined?
- Signalment (including species—identification as specific as possible): What is the age and gender of the animal, and how long has the client owned the animal?
- Origin: Where did the animal come from?
- Environment: Factors such as cage design, construction materials, substrates, perches, and branches are of critical importance in determining the health of these species. Temperature and humidity and photo period and exposure to sunlight or full-spectrum artificial light may have a significant impact on the animal's health. The owner should be questioned regarding the location of the cage in the house, the type of heat source used, and the usual temperature gradient within the cage. For aquatic species, questions pertaining to water quality control, filter systems used, sources of water, and frequency of water change are important. Owners need to list types of cleaning agents and disinfectants used and frequency of use.
- Food: How often is food offered? How much is consumed? What is the source of the food? How is the food stored, and how is it presented to the animal?
- Water: How often is the water cleaned or changed? How is it offered to the animal? If a water bowl is used, how large is it? For many species, it is important to offer water in a bowl large enough for animals to completely submerge.
- Feces: How often does the animal defecate in relation to feeding? What is the color and consistency of the stool? Has the owner previously submitted a fecal sample for a parasite evaluation?
- Cagemates: Does the client have other animals in his or her collection or in the same cage? If so, what species are they, and where are they kept? Does the owner maintain a quarantine policy? If so, for how long?
- Behavior: What is the current attitude and behavior of the patient, and have any recent changes been noted?
- Shedding: For lizards and snakes, how often does the animal shed? When was the last period of shedding, or **ecdysis**?
- Previous medical history: Has the animal been ill previously? If it has, it is important to get the owner to describe the illness and any treatments that were provided. It is often helpful to include the attending veterinarian's name. Have other animals in the collection ever been ill?

SAMPLE COLLECTION AND DIAGNOSTIC PROCEDURES

Diagnostic approaches to reptiles are often similar to those of other small animal species. As with any diagnostic procedure, ability through experience and confidence determines who will collect the sample needed from the patient. Any of the procedures listed in this section can be mastered by the technician who has the proper sampling equipment and desire.

Colonic Wash

Fecal samples may be collected and examined for gastrointestinal parasites. A fresh sample should be examined under a wet mount for protozoan parasites. Other tests performed on the fecal sample include flotation and sedimentation. If a fecal sample is not available at the time of examination, specimens may be collected by performing a colonic wash; this is done by passing a lubricated tube or catheter through the cloaca into the colon. A syringe of sterile saline is attached, and a typical flush is performed. The recommended volume of saline for a **colonic wash** is 1% or less of the animal's weight. Samples from the colonic wash may be examined for parasites or parasite eggs or prepared for cytologic examination and/or culture and sensitivity.

Bone Marrow

Large lizards, crocodilians, and other **chelonian** species yield adequate diagnostic bone marrow specimens from their femoral cavities.[2] Bone marrow from turtles and tortoises may be obtained by drilling a hole between outer and inner layers of the bony shell and by using a biopsy needle (Vim-Silverman, Becton-Dickinson Primary Care Diagnostics, Franklin Lakes, New Jersey) to obtain the sample.[2] The hole should be patched with epoxy or acrylic resin.[2] Snake diagnostic bone marrow specimens may be obtained from marrow cavities in the ribs.

Stomach Lavage

To examine the upper gastrointestinal tract, especially for identification of cryptosporidiosis, a stomach wash is often performed. This procedure is well tolerated by most reptiles and is quick and easy to execute in the practice. A lubricated soft rubber catheter is advanced through the mouth into the stomach after premeasuring alongside the animal. The stomach area is in the midcranial body area; this location should be used as a reference point for tube placement length. A syringe containing sterile isotonic saline is attached to the catheter, and a simple flush is performed after the stomach is agitated with external palpation. Samples obtained are used for direct microscopic examination for parasites, to prepare slides for cytologic examination, or to perform Gram stain for culture and sensitivity.

Urine Samples

Urine samples may be collected from those species that produce a large volume of urine. Many turtles and lizards have urinary bladders. All reptiles have a cloaca into which the reproductive, gastrointestinal, and urinary tracts empty. Routine urinalysis may be performed on fresh urine samples obtained via cystocentesis. Cystocentesis may be performed on turtles by advancing a needle cranial to the hindlimb. Turtles typically void when stressed; thus handling the patient may yield a urine sample. Green-stained solid urates

rehydrated with saline may reveal amoebic cysts or fluke ova when examined under a microscope.

Blood Samples

Depending on the species, considerable variation is seen when blood samples are collected from reptiles. Do not withdraw more blood than is necessary. If you are not sure of the volume needed, contact your diagnostic laboratory. Direct cardiocentesis and venipuncture can be achieved using the ventral and lateral caudal veins; jugular, brachial, popliteal, periorbital, and pterygopalatine veins; and dorsal postoccipital sinuses, depending on the species and size of the animal.[2] Toenail clipping is not recommended for blood sample collection because of the inability to obtain reliable hematologic results from this site.

Venipuncture techniques in snakes depend on the experience of the handler. Recommended blood collection locations include the caudal or coccygeal vein of the tail, cardiac puncture, and the ventral abdominal vein or palatine vessels. For blood collection at any site, proper restraint of the reptile patient is necessary. For lizards, the caudal tail vein is often most accessible; however, cardiac puncture and the ventral abdominal vein may be used (Figures 22-27 and 22-28). In turtles, large jugular veins are present and are easily used for venipuncture sites (Figure 22-29).

In large crocodilians, turtles, and tortoises, the occipital sinus and the caudal tail vein are acceptable locations. The

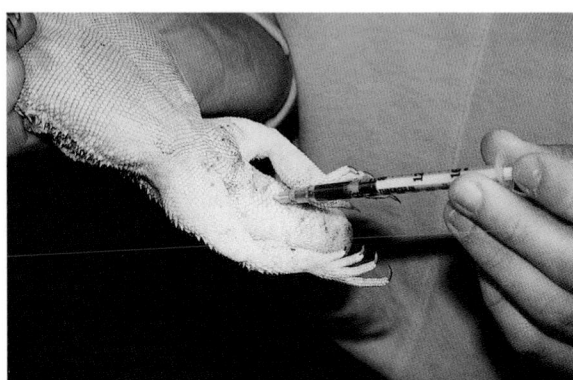

FIGURE 22-27 Restraint of a bearded dragon for venipuncture using the tail vein.

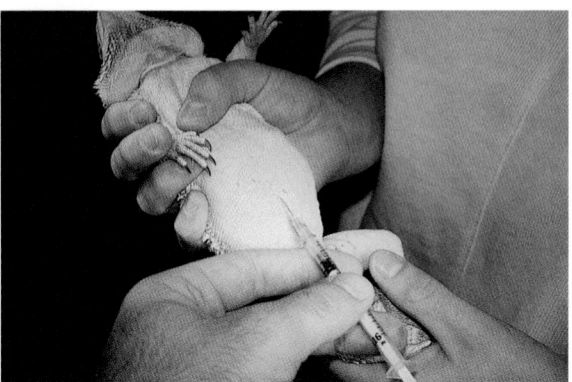

FIGURE 22-28 Venipuncture from the ventral abdominal vein.

TABLE 22-2	Anesthetic Agents: Chelonians[3]		
DRUG	**DOSAGE**	**ROUTE**	**COMMENTS**
Ketamine	10-20 mg/kg	Intramuscular	Mild sedation
Ketamine	20-40 mg/kg	Intramuscular	Moderate sedation
Tiletamine	5-10 mg/kg	Intramuscular	Mild sedation
Propofol	10-15 mg/kg	Intravenous	General anesthesia
Ketamine (K) + Medetomidine (M)	5-10 mg/kg (K) 0.075-0.1 mg/kg (M)	Intramuscular	Mild sedation
Ketamine (K) + Medetomidine (M)	10-15 mg/kg (K) 0.1-0.15 mg/kg (M)	Intramuscular	Moderate sedation
Isoflurane	5%/1 L oxygen	Inhalant	Induction
Isoflurane	3%/1 L oxygen	Inhalant	Maintenance

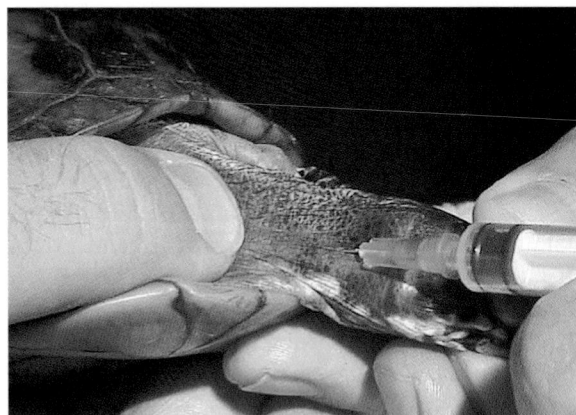

FIGURE 22-29 Jugular venipuncture in a box turtle. The jugular veins are located dorsally at the 10 o'clock and 2 o'clock positions.

site chosen will depend on the veterinarian and the technician and their experience with the particular species that is tested. In small lizards, the peribulbar and retrobulbar plexus may be used for blood samples by inserting a heparinized microhematocrit tube between the eyelids and directing it to the inner edge of the orbit. Rotating the tube will damage the plexus, yielding enough blood to fill the collection device.

RADIOGRAPHY

Radiography often is useful to aid in the diagnosis of reptile patients. For many species, radiographs may be taken on unsedated animals by restraining them in shallow boxes, acrylic tubes, or canvas bags. It is important to remember to take at least two views. With turtles, a third (frontal) view should also be taken. Contrast studies may be done, and barium sulfate is easily administered; however, gastrointestinal transit times are long, and it may take 1 week to complete a gastrointestinal barium study. Other diagnostic procedures may be used, according to the preference of the veterinarian. The technician's knowledge of restraint and of reptile behavior will aid in any immobilization process.

ANESTHESIA
Chelonians[3]

Induction using a gas anesthetic agent is not recommended for chelonians because of their propensity to not breathe for

long periods of time. Injectable anesthetic agents are often used in chelonians for induction and placement of endotracheal tubes (Table 22-2). Because of the lack of available resources for pharmacokinetic studies on anesthetic agents in reptiles, it is very important to remember that many of the drug dosages used by clinicians have been developed anecdotally. Considering the prolonged drug clearance that has been noted in chelonians, drugs with reversible antagonistic agents should be used as frequently as possible.

Intubation with assisted ventilation is recommended, with the glottis located at the base of the tongue. As with birds, chelonians have complete cartilaginous rings; therefore, uncuffed tracheal tubes should be used. A very small amount of topical lidocaine can be applied to the glottis on a cotton-tipped applicator to reduce the incidence of laryngospasm.

Positive-pressure ventilation is recommended throughout the procedure at 4 to 6 breaths per minute. Dorsal recumbency adversely affects a chelonian's ability to breathe; therefore, large chelonians should not be maintained in dorsal recumbency for prolonged periods of time.

Lizards[4]

Table 22-3 lists common protocols in which injectable anesthetic agents are used on lizard patients. Although propofol is a popular anesthetic choice among veterinarians anesthetizing lizards, one must be aware of the common side effects of apnea and cardiovascular depression. Adverse side effects associated with propofol administration are primarily dependent on dose and rate of delivery, with high dose and fast rate increasing the chance of occurrence.

Isoflurane and sevoflurane are the gas anesthetic agents of choice for lizard species. As with chelonians, it is difficult to induce certain lizard species using gas anesthesia alone because of their ability to stop breathing. Therefore, lizards should be induced with an injectable anesthetic agent, then intubated and maintained on gas anesthesia. Intubation, ventilation, and monitoring of the lizard patient are similar to approaches used for chelonians.

Snakes[3]

Dissociative agents, including ketamine and tiletamine, are frequently used to anesthetize snakes to collect diagnostic

TABLE 22-3	Anesthetic Agents: Lizards[4]	
DRUG	**DOSAGE**	**COMMENTS**
Ketamine	5-10 mg/kg	As preanesthetic followed by inhalant anesthesia
Ketamine (K) Medetomidine (M)	5-10 mg/kg (K) 0.1-0.2 mg/kg (M)	Start with low dose of ketamine; medetomidine is reversible with antipamezole
Antipamezole	0.5-1.0 mg/kg	Reversal for medetomidine; can split amount of SC and IM or IV
Propofol	10-15 mg/kg	Give IV at a slow rate to avoid apnea; allows enough relaxation for endotracheal intubation; provides 20-30 minutes of anesthesia
Tiletamine/Zolazepam	5-10 mg/kg	Severe respiratory depression possible; good for muscle relaxation before intubation
Butorphanol	0.05-1.5 mg/kg	Used in combination with other protocols for analgesia

samples and perform minor surgical procedures. Because concern has arisen about the ability of dissociative agents to provide adequate visceral analgesia in snakes, they are not recommended for use in invasive surgical procedures. Although inexpensive and easily administered through the intramuscular route, another disadvantage of using this class of drugs in snakes is the extended recovery time.

Inhalant anesthetics (e.g., isoflurane, sevoflurane) are recommended for general anesthetic procedures. A noncuffed tube similar to that described for chelonians and lizards should be placed in the snake patient. Positive-pressure ventilation is recommended for snake patients under gas anesthesia, with ventilation occurring 4 to 6 times/minute. The snake should be placed in a darkened, heated environment to decrease recovery time and reduce external stimuli.

HUSBANDRY IN THE HOSPITAL

Reptiles require a controlled microenvironment in a hospital setting. It is important to remember that temperature and humidity are important because these animals are poikilothermic (i.e., they depend on their environment to regulate their body temperature). A temperature gradient should be provided, whenever possible, by using a thermostat at each end of the cage, resulting in a cooler end and a warmer end. For most species, temperature should not exceed 32°C (90°F) or dip below 24°C (75°F). Humidity is the other important environmental consideration that is determined by species-specific requirements. In general, most captive reptile species respond well to humidity ranges of 50% to 70%. The technician must remember that jungle species usually require higher humidity, whereas desert species do better in lower humidity ranges.

> *TECHNICIAN NOTE* In general, most captive reptile species accommodate well in humidity ranges of 50% to 70%. The technician must remember that jungle species usually require higher humidity, whereas desert species do better in lower humidity ranges.

It is important that hospitalized reptiles are maintained at the upper end of their temperature gradient during convalescence to assist recovery. For many species, a variety of

aquaria are sufficient for short-term hospitalization. Any substrate used should be one that is easily cleaned and disinfected or disposable, such as newspaper. It is important to house reptiles separately from psittacine birds, in particular, to prevent contamination of birds from the normal Gram-negative flora of most reptiles. Cages should be provided with hide boxes or areas of seclusion and perching for some species, such as iguanas and some snakes.

> *TECHNICIAN NOTE* It is important that hospitalized reptiles are maintained at the upper end of their temperature gradient during convalescence to assist recovery.

Tube-feeding is an important technique for the veterinary technician to learn. Supplemental feed administration using a tube is easily accomplished, even by technicians without much experience with reptiles. A tube should be well lubricated and passed the distance necessary to place it in the stomach. The glottis of reptiles is adjacent to the base of the tongue and is easily avoided. The glottis of snakes may actually be extended by the animal outside the mouth to accommodate large prey items. The tube is gently passed all the way to the stomach, and food is injected. Fluids may also be administered by this route. For patients that are anorexic, supplemental tube-feeding may be accomplished by using a blended formula of food that is appropriate for the species. Commercial critical care supplements (Carnivore Critical Care, Lafeber Co., Ordell, Illinois; Critical Care for Herbivores, Oxbow Animal Health, Murdock, Nebraska) are also available that can be tube-fed to herbivorous, carnivorous, and insectivorous species after reconstitution with water. Dietary references for reptile species are listed in the "Recommended Readings." It is imperative that the technician become familiar with proper reptile diets to maintain healthy animals and supplement sick patients.

Injections are usually administered to reptiles in the cranial half of the animal's body, primarily the epaxial muscles and the muscles of the forelimbs (e.g., biceps brachii, long heads of triceps brachii) (Figure 22-30), because the renal portal system routes blood from the caudal third of the body through a capillary network into the kidneys before

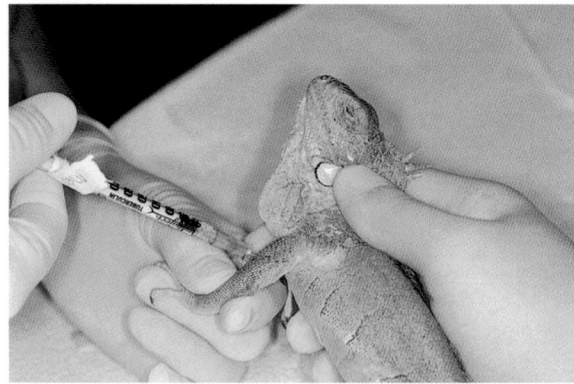

FIGURE 22-30 Injection into the forelimb of an iguana.

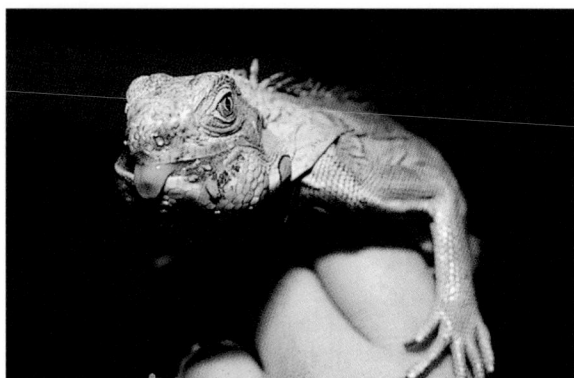

FIGURE 22-31 Metabolic bone disease in a lizard caused by an improper diet.

BOX 22-3	Recommended Daily Diets for Chelonians

- Eighty-five percent vegetables, such as collards, radish, turnip greens, dandelions, kale, cabbage, bok choy, broccoli, cauliflower, and summer and winter squash
- Ten percent fruit, such as grapes, apples, oranges, pears, peaches, plums, dates, melons, strawberries, raspberries, mangoes, and tomatoes
- Greater than 5% high-protein food, such as dry maintenance dog food, parrot chow, cereals, mice, and scrambled eggs

returning it to the general circulation. It is important to refrain from giving nephrotoxic drugs in the caudal third of the reptile patient's body. Injection sites are easily found in all reptile species, either in the forelimbs or in the epaxial musculature of the snake. Oral medications are easily given using a stomach tube. Liquids are preferred over tablets, which are not consistently absorbed.

> **TECHNICIAN NOTE** It is important to refrain from giving nephrotoxic drugs in the caudal third of the reptile patient's body.

NUTRITION

Dietary requirements vary tremendously from species to species and may be an important factor in the disease of the patient. Dietary deficiencies are not commonly seen in snakes, which eat a whole animal diet; however, a variety of dietary deficiencies are commonly seen in lizards, turtles, and crocodilians. One of the most common is metabolic bone disease, which is caused by inappropriately low calcium intake, low vitamin D_3 intake, or excessive phosphorus intake (Figure 22-31). This may be prevented by feeding a suitable diet and by exposing the animal to ultraviolet (UV) light, either naturally or artificially. It is essential that reptiles, especially lizards, have full-spectrum light available during

normal daylight hours. Sunlight through glass does not provide the needed light supplementation because of the blocking ability of glass; direct sunlight or appropriate artificial lighting is needed. Animals with metabolic bone disease must be treated very gently because their bones are subject to pathologic fracture. Vitamin A deficiency is commonly diagnosed in turtles and tortoises and usually manifests as an overgrown beak, **palpebral edema**, and **conjunctivitis**. This underscores the importance of thoroughly researching the dietary history of the reptile patient.

> **TECHNICIAN NOTE** It is essential that reptiles, especially lizards, have full-spectrum light available during normal daylight hours.

Chelonians

Land tortoises are primarily herbivores but occasionally eat insects and small rodents. In captivity, diets should be composed primarily of vegetables (mainly dark leafy greens, red and yellow produce, and grasses), some fruits, and limited quantities of high-protein food. Typical tortoise diets are listed in Box 22-3.

Successfully caring for captive tortoises relies heavily on varying the diet. A shallow water dish should be provided to allow consumption, although caution should be taken not to overfill with water because the tortoise and the box turtle cannot swim and will drown if submerged. The water should be changed daily because turtles may defecate in the water dish.

Sunlight or ultraviolet light should be provided to allow cholecalciferol (vitamin D) synthesis for shell formation and repair and to stimulate the appetite and basking behavior. Multivitamins containing vitamin D may be added to the diet every 1 to 2 weeks.

Aquatic turtles need a variety of foods to achieve a balanced diet. Most of the diet should be composed of whole animals, such as mice, earthworms, chopped goldfish or guppies, and slugs. Small quantities of insects, such as crickets, mealworms, flies, and grasshoppers, are acceptable options. It is not recommended to feed such meats as hamburger or shellfish. Vegetables, such as dark leafy greens, carrots, bell peppers, cabbage, or romaine lettuce, may be offered in small amounts. Commercial diets are available in floating stick forms, but supplementing these diets with natural foods (e.g., earthworms, small fish) should be considered. Some tropical fish food products can be used to vary a turtle's diet. Note that aquatic turtles will feed only if they are in the water.

The most common nutritional deficiency in captive turtles is vitamin A deficiency. Clinical signs include respiratory infection, edematous eyes, urogenital tract obstruction, and beak overgrowth. Hypovitaminosis A can be prevented by providing a proper diet that supplies beta carotene, found in such foods as earthworms, small fish, and green leafy vegetables. The most common clinical disease presentations of sick turtles are associated with anorexia and dehydration. Anorexia and dehydration are primarily husbandry related; causes include stress, lack of food, improper ambient temperature, improper diet, parasitic infection, or metabolic disorders.

> **TECHNICIAN NOTE** Successfully caring for captive tortoises relies heavily on varying the diet.

Snakes

Snakes are carnivores and need a varied diet. Specific dietary needs depend on the species of snake, although staples generally include rodents. The size of the rodent fed should be about the same diameter as the snake's body and about $\frac{1}{8}$ of the animal's length. Typical rodents used for snake food include rabbits, rats, mice, gerbils, chickens, lizards, and/or other snakes. It is usually prudent to feed frozen or freshly killed rodents to prevent injury or infection caused by prey bites to the snake (Figure 22-32).

Most species of snake are fed once every 1 to 2 weeks, but the size of the prey and the frequency of feeding depend on both time of year and signalment of the snake. If the snake is fed more often than once a week, the environment needs to be warm enough to facilitate digestion. The incidence of nutritional deficiency in the captive snake is rare because most are fed whole prey. Note that snakes eat infrequently, and inappetence or weight loss may go undetected. Periodic weighing is recommended to prevent nutritional deficiency. Although water requirements are low, water should be supplied on a daily basis.

Lizards

Most captive lizards are omnivores, eating such foods as mealworms, crickets, grasshoppers, and waxworms. Most insects are calcium deficient; therefore, to improve their nutritional composition, they should be fed a nutritionally supplemented diet (see Case Presentation 22-1). How much these nutritionally supplemented insect diets improve their nutritional composition is debatable. Lizards in the wild are primarily carnivores, eating invertebrate or vertebrate prey. In general, captive lizards require vitamin and mineral supplementation with an emphasis on a variety of food. Juvenile lizards should be fed 1 to 2 times a day and the adults, 2 to 3 times per week. Most lizards are diurnal and require day feedings and time to bask in natural or ultraviolet light.

Herbivorous lizards, such as the green iguana, require a varied diet to ensure adequate nutritional balance. Recommended diets for herbivores include leafy greens (e.g., romaine lettuce, collard greens), mustard greens, and clover. Vegetables, including green beans, okra, carrots, and squash, are also adequate dietary substances. It is important to note that certain vegetables, such as spinach, cabbage, peas, and potatoes, contain substances that bind calcium and other trace minerals, inhibiting their absorption.

Commercial iguana food is available to provide a base diet for these animals. Commercial diets do not require additional supplementation if the captive lizard is fed a diet based primarily on such purchased food. Homemade diets of vegetables and fruit should always be supplemented with appropriate vitamins and minerals. Technicians can advise lizard owners to purchase a quality reptile vitamin, containing vitamin D_3, to be administered 1 to 2 times a week if a good diet is provided.

> **TECHNICIAN NOTE** Captive lizards require vitamin and mineral supplementation with an emphasis on a variety of food.

Common iguanas also require protein for normal growth and development. Juvenile iguanas in captivity generally need more protein and calcium than do adults. Common protein sources include dark green leafy vegetables such as collards, turnip greens, kale, bok choy, and broccoli with leaves. Iguanas should never be fed a meat-based diet or any commercial food other than iguana food. Commercial dog and cat food will cause renal disease and death.

Water should be provided in a bowl for bathing and drinking. Note that some lizards (e.g., chameleons) will drink water only if it is in the form of droplets on plant leaves, similar to dew. Therefore, it is important to spray or mist the animal's enclosure several times a day. In addition, most

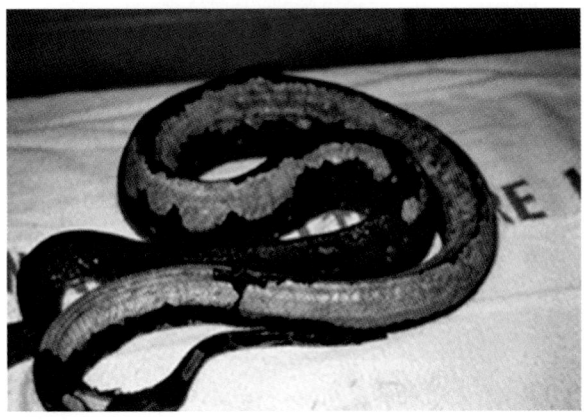

FIGURE 22-32 Snake injury due to live prey bites.

CASE PRESENTATION 22-1

Dragontale, an 18-month-old bearded dragon *(Pogona vitti-ceps)*, came to the veterinary practice with a 3- to 4-week history of lethargy and anorexia (Figure 1). The bearded dragon had been owned for about 14 months and was maintained in a 10-gallon glass aquarium with wood shavings as substrate. The habitat was located on the floor and had a single 60-watt bulb as a heat source. When cleaned, the shavings were removed, the inside was wiped down with a kitchen cleaner of unknown brand, and new substrate was placed in the bottom of the enclosure. One time a day, the animal was fed lettuce, carrots, and crickets that had been dusted with a calcium-rich powder. Tap water was used as the water source and was provided in a bowl. The owners had observed Dragontale becoming lethargic and nonmobile, sleeping more often, and looking anorexic. Another concern was that the tongue always seemed to be sticking out, and a dark red lesion could be seen on the tip. The reluctance of their pet to eat had resulted in the owners force-feeding crickets to the sick animal.

On physical examination, the patient was responsive but depressed, exhibited very limited voluntary movement, and did not hold its head in a normal position. The lesion on the tip of the tongue was determined to be a slight irritation of the surface as a result of exposure from reluctance to retract it into the oral cavity. Anatomic swellings were noted in several locations (e.g., tibia, carpus, pelvis, proximal dorsal tail), and the mandible was extremely flexible (Figures 2 and 3). Dehydration was estimated at 8% based on corneal moisture, the tackiness of oral mucous membranes, and skin tenting. Radiographs indicated low bone density based on the radiolucent skeletal structure (Figure 4). Evidence of a fracture involving the proximal tail vertebra was also noted (Figure 5). Blood was collected from the ventral tail vein for a complete blood count and plasma chemistry panel (Figure 6). The only abnormality noted in the hematology results was an approximate 1:1 calcium-to-phosphorus ratio (7.9 mg/dl calcium, 7.1 mg/dl phosphorus). The normal calcium-to-phosphorus ratio in bearded dragons should average 2.2:1.1. Based on the history,

physical examination findings, and diagnostic test results, the top differential diagnosis was nutritional secondary hyperparathyroidism (NSHP), or "rubber jaw."

Nutritional secondary hyperparathyroidism is a form of metabolic bond disease (MBD). *Metabolic bone disease* is a descriptive term used to describe a collection of medical disorders that affect the integrity and function of bones.[2] Husbandry effects, including chronic nutritional deficiencies of calcium and/or vitamin D_3, an imbalance of the calcium-to-phosphorus ratio (feeding crickets as a primary food source), or inadequate exposure to ultraviolet (UV) radiation in diurnal animals, will predispose reptiles to MBD. Although many reptile species are susceptible to NSHP, lizards and aquatic turtles seem to be most commonly affected.[2] If the animal is not receiving enough calcium in the diet or has an

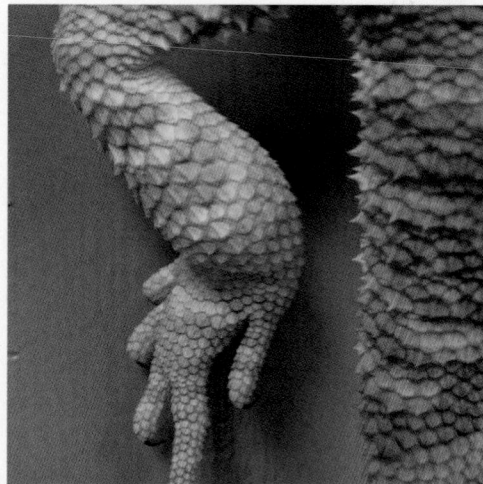

FIGURE 2 Swelling of the tibia—a clinical sign linked to metabolic bone disease in lizard species.

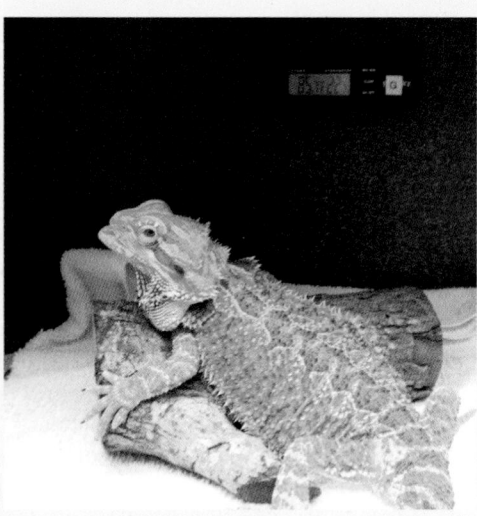

FIGURE 1 Dragontale, a bearded dragon that presented with a 3- to 4-week history of lethargy and anorexia.

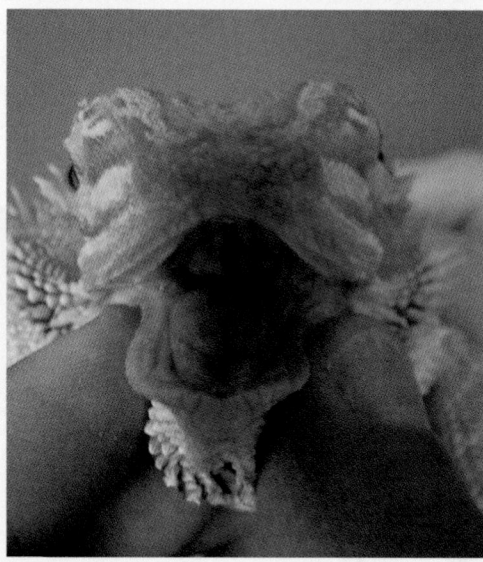

FIGURE 3 The mandible was extremely flexible upon examination.

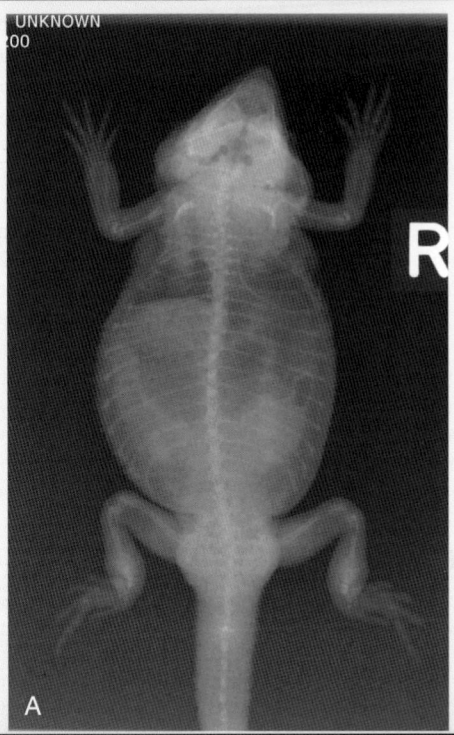

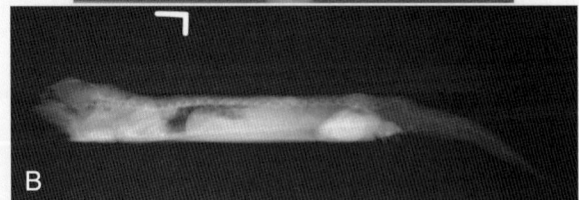

FIGURE 4 A, Dorsoventral and lateral (B) radiographic images reveal general lack of bone density.

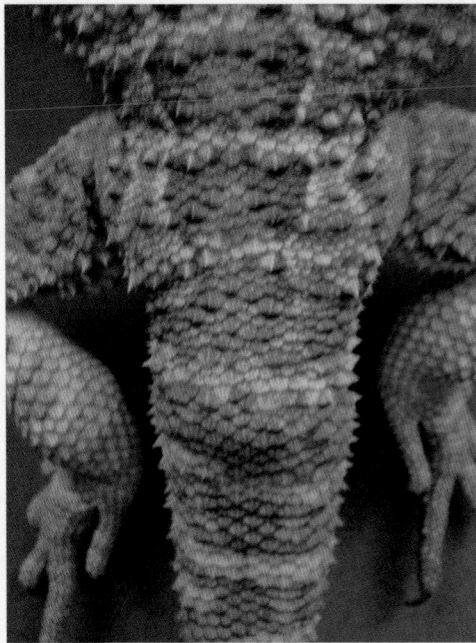

FIGURE 5 An elevated area of the proximal tail that resulted from a fracture associated with general lack of bone density.

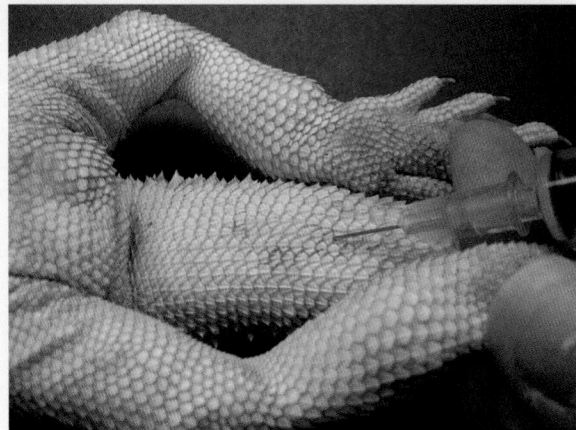

FIGURE 6 Blood collection from the ventral tail vein.

inability to absorb calcium from the gastrointestinal tract as a result of lack of vitamin D_3, the body will resorb calcium stores from the bone. Although serum calcium levels remain within normal limits to maintain life, the bones become weaker with loss of the stabilizing mineral. To compensate for loss of calcium and subsequent bone instability, affected skeletal structures stimulate immature bone cell development that increases the diameter of the bones. This gives the false impression of large "muscles." Instead of showing muscle tissue, the increased size of the extremities or jaw actually reflects underdeveloped bone.

In lizards that have a history of depression, anorexia, and reluctance to move, as with Dragontale, NSHP should be considered a top differential diagnosis. Other signs of NSHP include an enlarged and/or "rubber-like" mandible, evidence of fracture, and enlargement of long bones. Radiographs of clinically affected animals will reveal thin bone cortices, pathologic fractures, or evidence of recently or partially healed fractures.[2]

The most important part of the treatment plan involves communicating with, informing, and educating the owner on proper nutritional and dietary requirements for the species. For bearded dragons, the diet should be supplemented with calcium and vitamin D_3, and the environment must have the proper temperature range with animal exposure to natural sunlight and ultraviolet light in the 290- to 320-nm wave length. For bearded dragons, the preferred optimal temperature range (day, 84°F to 88°F; night, 68°F to 74°F; winter cool down, 62°F to 69°F) with a 50- to 75-watt sun spotlight bulb and natural spectrum lighting is required.[3] Artificial UV light and sunlight are needed to convert vitamin D in the body to vitamin D_3 (cholecalciferol), which is active and facilitates calcium uptake in the intestinal tract. Two commercially available lights—Vitalite (Durotest Corp., Lyndhurst, New Jersey) and Colortone 50 (Westinghouse, Somerset, New Jersey)—are recommended for proper UV wavelength exposure for reptile species.[2] To aid in UV ray exposure for lizard species, a black light bulb and natural sunlight are encouraged.

Treatment for Dragontale consisted of calcium supplementation with calcium gluconate 50 mg/kg given subcutaneously, q24hours once, and repeated weekly for 4 to 6 weeks as needed

(American Pharmaceutical Partners, Schaumburg, Illinois); calcium glubionate 10 mg/kg given orally, q24hours, until the condition had resolved (Calcionate Syrup, Rugby Laboratories, Inc., Duluth, Georgia); fluid therapy, consisting of replacement of dehydration deficit followed by maintenance of 25 ml/kg/day for 5 days, then a switch to oral administration until the animal was drinking on its own (Normasol, Hospira, Inc., Lake Forest, Illinois); vitamins A, D₃, and E 0.1 ml given IM once and repeated in 1 week (Northwest

Pharmacy and Compounding Center, Houston, Texas); dietary supplementation of 10% of body weight up to 5 ml given orally q24hours (Carnivore Care, Oxbow Company, Murdock, Nebraska); offer of Herbivore Critical Care (OxbowAnimal Health, Murdock, Nebraska), fresh vegetables with a calcium-to-phosphorus ratio greater than 1.5:1 (e.g., watercress, kale, broccoli tops, carrots, oranges, cantaloupe, raisins), and a mealworm dusted with calcium supplementation; and pain medication—meloxicam 0.2 mg/kg given orally, q24hours, until pain had resolved (Metacam, Boehringer Ingelheim Vetmedica, Inc., St Joseph, Missouri). To supplement the therapeutic treatment regimen, the lizard was placed in a heated environment within its physiologic optimal temperature range, was provided artificial UV light, and was exposed daily to direct sunlight (Figure 7). Dragontale recovered from NSHP and, with proper diet and husbandry, has maintained excellent health.

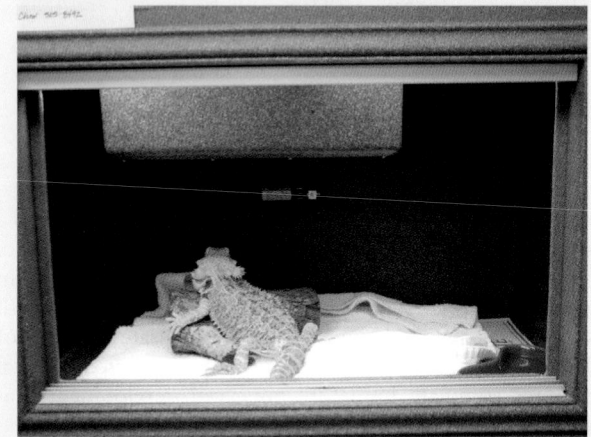

FIGURE 7 Proper hospital enclosure for reptiles with patient inside.

REFERENCES

1. Eliman MM: Hematology and plasma chemistry of the inland bearded dragon, *Pogona vitticeps*, Bull Assoc Reptile Amphibian Vet 7:10, 1997.
2. Mader DR: Metabolic bone disease. In Mader DR, editor: Reptile medicine and surgery, ed 2, St Louis, 2006, Saunders, p 841.
3. Rossi JV: General husbandry and management. In Mader DR, editor: Reptile medicine and surgery, ed 2, St Louis, 2006, Saunders, p 25.

lizards should be sprayed with water or allowed to bathe to prevent skin problems associated with low humidity.

SKIN

Clinical dermatologic diseases have been noted in reptilian species, as in other animals. Proper diagnostic techniques are needed to identify the problem to implement appropriate treatment.

Skin specimens may be cultured for bacterial and fungal organisms. For fungal identification, dermatophyte test medium (DTM), fungal growth medium, or Sabouraud culture medium may be used. Bacterial organisms may be isolated on blood agar or subcultured in a thioglycollate-containing medium. Samples for skin culture may be taken by using cotton-tipped culturettes or pieces of affected skin, scales, or dermal scutes.

FECES

Fecal material can be very useful in diagnosing parasite infestations, bacterial infections, pancreatic enzyme levels, and the presence of blood in the gastrointestinal tract. The fecal specimen should be as fresh as possible. If a fresh voided sample is not available, fecal material may be removed from the terminal alimentary tract by gentle palpation or by insertion of a fecal extractor or a cotton-tipped applicator stick through the cloacal vent.[5] A warm-water enema may stimulate defecation in difficult cases. As with the colonic wash,

1% or less of the animal's body weight is recommended as the fluid volume to use for enemas in most captive reptile species.

SPUTUM

To obtain a sample of sputum, insert a cotton-tipped applicator into the discharge. Roll the sample applicator across a microscope slide, add a drop of coloring agent, apply a coverslip, and examine for parasite ova.[6] Parasites commonly diagnosed in sputum samples are *Rhabditis* spp., *Entomelas* spp., and *Strongyloides stercoralis*. When handling diagnostic samples, proper hygiene is essential because of the zoonotic potential of many animal diseases and parasites.

ZOONOSES AND COMMON CLINICAL PROBLEMS

The technician should be aware of common zoonotic infections and clinical problems associated with reptiles. *Salmonella* spp. are considered part of the normal gastrointestinal flora of reptile species. If infected, humans will develop severe gastrointestinal disease. In most cases, reptiles will shed *Salmonella* spp. in the feces if immunosuppressed. To reduce exposure to this infectious bacterium, the reptile should be maintained in good health with reduced stress. Individuals handling reptiles should practice excellent hygiene and should always wash their hands once the animal has been placed back into its enclosure.

SMALL MAMMALS

FERRETS

Ferrets have been gaining in popularity as a companion animal, thus it is imperative that technicians become familiar with these pets.

"Nail" Trims

Ferrets do not have retractable claws, but they do have a vascular "quick" delineation that can be used as a landmark to trim. Small nail-trim scissors or human nail clips are recommended for ferret nail trims. If bleeding occurs after a nail trim, silver nitrate sticks can be used for chemical cautery. Ferret nails are sharp, and owners often request nail trims to blunt the claws.

Blood Collection

When sample collections of blood are obtained, physical restraint alone is often inadequate. Chemical restraint or general anesthesia using isoflurane or sevoflurane is commonly employed. Common locations for collecting blood samples include the jugular vein, the cranial vena cava, and the cephalic vein. When blood is collected from a ferret, the head must be securely restrained, with the technician grasping around the neck with thumb and fingers resting on the mandible. To position an animal for jugular venipuncture, it is often best to stretch the animal out, using the other hand to grasp the hindlimbs. The ferret's thick skin and subcutaneous fat make blood collection from the jugular vein difficult. For drawing adequate blood samples, the cranial vena cava may be preferred (Figure 22-33).

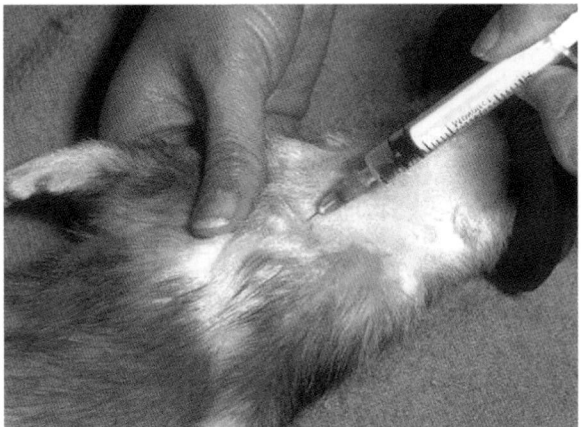

FIGURE 22-33 Cranial vena cava venipuncture of an anesthetized ferret with its head in an anesthetic mask.

Anesthesia

Ketamine hydrochloride or gas anesthetic agents, such as isoflurane or sevoflurane, may be used for chemical restraint. When a gas anesthetic is used, an induction chamber is recommended for induction. The patient may be removed from this chamber because it loses the ability to right itself. The anesthetic may then be continued with the use of a face mask. For longer procedures, the animal should be intubated. Use of gas anesthetic agents on ferret patients is very similar to the techniques and procedures applied for cats. Sample collection on the anesthetized animal is much easier and safer than on the animal not anesthetized, and is less stressful to the animal. Urine may be obtained by cystocentesis because the bladder is easily palpated. If desired, for prolonged anesthesia, ferrets are easily intubated with small standard endotracheal tubes or Cole tubes. Ferrets should be fasted for at least 5 hours before anesthetic induction because they commonly regurgitate if food or water is inside the stomach.

Strategies for treating ferrets in the practice revolve around the handler's ability to restrain the animal and perform treatment in the most efficient and the quickest manner possible. For oral drug administration, Nutrical, dairy products, and sweets are useful for bribing animals and hiding medications. Most ferrets will do almost anything for yogurt or ice cream. Liquid medications are much easier to administer than pills.

Nutrition

Ferrets are strict carnivores, with general dietary requirements of roughly 30% protein and 25% fat. High-fiber diets are not recommended. Several commercially available ferret-specific diets will provide the proper nutrition for these animals. If ferret diets are not available, a high-quality cat food may be used, but this is not preferred. Although a cat food diet may be slightly low in protein for the pregnant or lactating ferret, few problems have been reported in ferrets eating high-quality cat food diets. Small quantities of apples, cooked meat, or dried fruit can also be offered, although consistency in the diet is generally recommended because the ferret may resent dietary changes. Body weight may exhibit seasonal fluctuation, with summer and autumn months showing possible weight reduction. Fresh water should be provided on a daily basis.

General Information and Common Presentations

A potentially fatal clinical problem of the ferret is estrogen toxicity in females caused by prolonged estrus. Female ferrets are induced ovulators and occasionally will not cycle out of heat unless bred. These animals become severely anemic and thrombocytopenic because of toxic effects of estrogen on the bone marrow. Ferrets often are brought into the practice with signs of lethargy, dyspnea, petechial hemorrhage, vomiting, and diarrhea. These signs are best treated by prevention and education of the client. Female ferrets not intended for breeding should be spayed before their first heat. Because most ferrets in the United States have been spayed and descented before purchase, this is not a concern for most owners. Ferrets that have been spayed or neutered and descented by a breeding facility at an early age will have one or two tattooed blue dots on the surface of the pinna (Figure 22-34). When an owner would like the ferret descented, the procedure involves surgically removing the two anal scent glands of the animal. The two anal scent gland openings are located at the 4 o'clock and the 8 o'clock position when the anal mucocutaneous junction is slightly everted (Figure 22-35). Most ferrets have had the anal scent glands removed before purchase (look for the ear tattoo) but still have a musky odor. Shampooing the ferret on a regular basis will reduce the musky smell but will not eliminate the odor. Ferret-specific shampoo and cologne products are recommended and can be purchased at most large retail pet outlets.

> **TECHNICIAN NOTE** Ferrets that have been spayed or neutered and descented by a breeding facility at an early age will have one or two tattooed blue dots on the surface of the pinna.

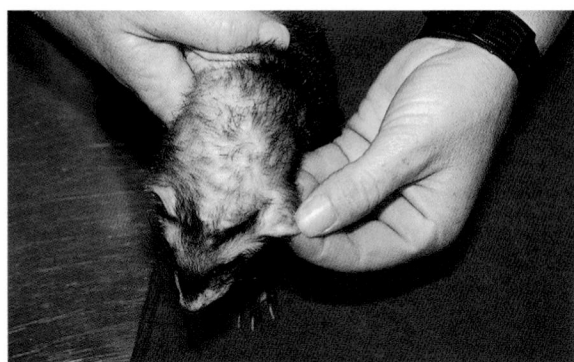

FIGURE 22-34 A tattoo (two dots) indicates that this is an early spayed or neutered, descented ferret.

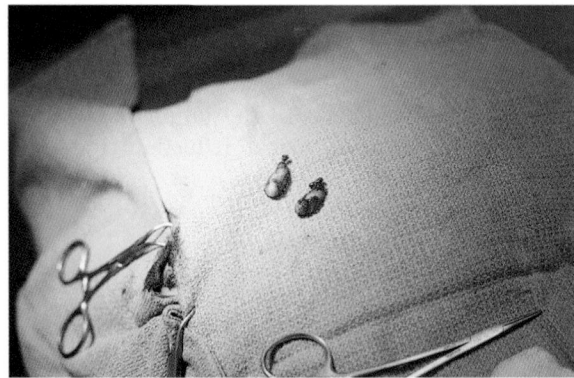

FIGURE 22-35 Anal sacs removed from a ferret.

Clinical signs similar to those of prolonged estrus (e.g., hair loss, swollen vulva) may be caused by adrenal hyperplasia (Figures 22-36 and 22-37). Female ferrets that have been spayed at an early age are extremely susceptible to this clinical condition. This condition also affects male ferrets that have been neutered at an early age. An adrenal hyperplasia workup should be performed on an older spayed female ferret exhibiting signs of vulvar swelling. Adrenal hyperplasia can be treated by partial adrenalectomy and/or administration of therapeutic agents (e.g., leuprolide acetate). The response to therapy and to surgery has been varied. In most ferret cases in which adrenal hyperplasia has been confirmed, treatment is effective in resolving overt clinical signs. Owners must be aware that a ferret diagnosed with adrenal hyperplasia will never be cured of the disease no matter how effective the treatment may be at resolving clinical disease signs.

Ferrets are susceptible to human influenza, and clients should be counseled that when members of the family have influenza, the ferret should not be handled. Human influenza in a ferret must be differentiated from canine distemper and bacterial pneumonia, to which ferrets are also susceptible. All have similar signs of respiratory disease: nasal and ocular discharges, coughing, and sneezing. In most cases, the ferret with influenza will recover from infection on its own in 5 to 10 days. A treatment protocol that includes antihistamines and decongestants may be of benefit. The nonvaccinated ferret will not survive canine distemper infection,

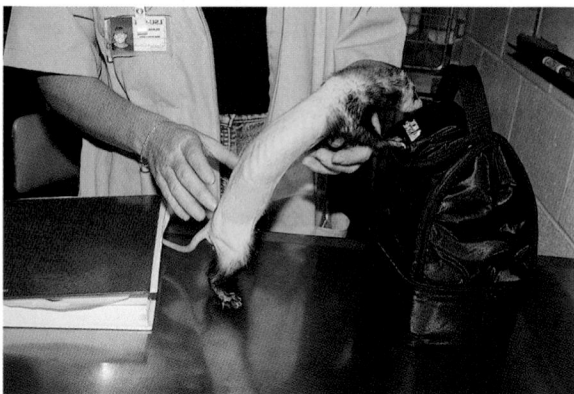

FIGURE 22-36 Hair loss in a ferret as a result of adrenal gland disease.

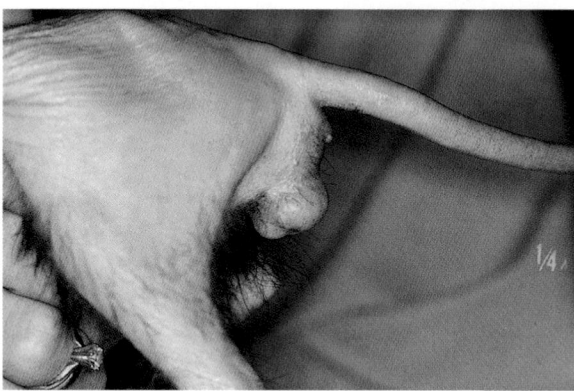

FIGURE 22-37 Swollen vulva in a ferret as a result of adrenal gland disease.

and signs usually progress to severe dyspnea, anorexia, and sometimes involvement of the central nervous system.

> **TECHNICIAN NOTE** A potentially fatal common clinical problem of the ferret is estrogen toxicity in females caused by prolonged estrus.

Parasites are a problem that must be understood by the ferret owner. Heartworm prevention is required in animals that are maintained in an outdoor enclosure where they are exposed to mosquitoes. In the author's opinion, ferrets are more susceptible than dogs to heartworm disease. Fleas commonly plague ferrets, even if maintained within a household setting. Feline flea control products generally are safe to use on flea-infested animals. Ear mite treatment and control and heartworm prevention are also important issues that need to be addressed with the owner (see Chapter 14).

> **TECHNICIAN NOTE** In the author's opinion, ferrets are much more susceptible than dogs to heartworm disease.

Ferrets are fond of chewing on objects, preferably soft rubbery toys, and should be watched closely for foreign body ingestion. A ferret that has signs of anorexia should be considered to have a potential gastrointestinal obstruction. Toys for ferrets should be limited to objects that they cannot bite or "ferret tubes" in which they can crawl. Ferrets have very strong jaws and sharp teeth; there are few leather or rubber objects that they cannot bite, chew, and eventually swallow. Many reports have described various neoplastic diseases in ferrets, including insulinomas, osteomas, lymphosarcomas, and fibrosarcomas. If a ferret is depressed or moribund, a blood serum glucose test should be performed because hypoglycemia is a common event.

Ferrets should be vaccinated for canine distemper using the PUREVAX ferret canine distemper vaccine (Merial, Duluth, Georgia). The American Ferret Association, Inc. (AFA) recommends that 1 ml of the vaccine should be injected subcutaneously in healthy ferrets at 8, 11, and 14 weeks of age, and then annually. If ferrets are older than 14 weeks of age or have an unknown or outdated vaccine history, a series of two vaccines should be given 2 weeks apart, then annually on the anniversary of the first booster. In cases where kits are exposed, the vaccine may be given as young as 6 weeks of age. Ferrets are not susceptible to feline panleukopenia and therefore should not be vaccinated. In many jurisdictions, ferrets are required to have a rabies vaccine and tag, although often they are not required to wear the tag. It is unlikely that an indoor ferret will be exposed to the rabies virus, but the IMRAB-3 rabies vaccine (Rhone Merieux, Inc., Athens, Georgia) will protect the ferret in the event of exposure and will support its quarantine if a person is bitten. The AFA recommends that all ferrets should be vaccinated against the rabies virus. At the present time, the general trend is to modify these recommendations for distemper and rabies vaccinations in ferrets, similar to dogs and cats. The prudent technician should monitor AFA updated vaccine recommendations for initial protection and booster. Ferrets are highly susceptible to vaccine reactions. Signs most commonly associated with vaccine reactions are swelling and redness at the vaccine site, drooling, rapid breathing, and increased body temperature. Ferrets that are scheduled to receive vaccines should be fasted before injection (for both distemper and rabies inoculation) and monitored for at least 30 minutes after the procedure is completed. Other preventive medicine measures regarding ferrets include good dental care and surveillance for gastrointestinal parasites.

> **TECHNICIAN NOTE** Ferrets should never be vaccinated against canine distemper using a vaccine of ferret cell origin.

Fluids may be administered per os or subcutaneously in a ferret that is less than 5% dehydrated, whereas an indwelling intravenous catheter should be placed in any animal that is more than 5% dehydrated. Subcutaneous fluids may be administered in the subcutaneous space between the shoulder blades. The cephalic and lateral saphenous veins are routine sites for intravenous catheter placement.

Fecal samples are often given voluntarily by patients before or during an examination. If a fecal sample needs to be obtained, a lubricated, small, feline fecal loop often provides a sufficient sample for a test evaluation.

RABBITS

The rabbit is not a rodent, but rather is a lagomorph of the family Leporidae. Rabbits may be housed indoors or outdoors and fed primarily a grass-based diet (Oxbow Animal Health, Murdock, Nebraska) with supplemented grass-based pellets. Rabbits come in many sizes, ranging from the Flemish Giant (6 to 7.5 kg) to Dutch and Polish breeds (1 to 2 kg). If proper husbandry practices are maintained, a pet rabbit should live a long, healthy life (5 to 6 years). Rabbits are sensitive to extremely hot and cold conditions, primarily to heat.

Rabbits defend themselves by using their long incisors to bite and by kicking with their hind legs. When kicking, their sharp claws can seriously injure the handler. Owners often inquire about "declawing" their rabbit, but this surgical procedure is strongly discouraged. Regular nail trims and/or nail caps (Soft Paws Inc., Lafayette, Louisiana) are recommended to owners who complain of their rabbit's sharp claws. In sexing the rabbit, stretching the **perineum** while the animal is in dorsal recumbency will reveal the anogenital area. Males have a round urethral opening; females have a slit opening.

Nutrition

Dietary requirements vary according to the age and use of a rabbit. For example, a balanced mixture of timothy grass, grass hay, and vegetables is the recommended diet for most pet rabbits, wherein show and production rabbits typically do better on commercially produced pellets. In general, however, rabbits are herbivores with high fiber requirements.

The recommended pet rabbit diet consists of a timothy (or other grass) hay in conjunction with a grass-based pellet as a regulated supplement. Pellets are fed at the rate of 0.25 cup/2.27 kg (5 lb) body weight divided into two meals. During gestation and lactation, the amount of protein and available energy should be increased. This may require increasing the number of pellets in the diet. Sugary treats should not be fed. "Treats" of fresh greens or other vegetable supplements are encouraged only as occasional rewards. Food items recommended as treats include carrots, small pieces of ripe banana, rice cakes, dry wheat bread, and dandelion leaves. It is important to remove any uneaten portion because spoilage can cause gastrointestinal upset. The rabbit should be offered good-quality grass hay (e.g., Bermuda grass, timothy grass, oat hay, marsh grass, orchard grass) ad libitum. Alfalfa hay is considered to contain an excess of protein and calcium and is thought by some to contribute to urinary calculi and improper function of the gastrointestinal tract. Fresh, dark leafy greens should be fed at a rate of 1 cup/0.45 kg (1 lb) body weight.

Regular feeding schedules are important for the rabbit. Because rabbits are nocturnal in nature and consume most of their feed during the night, hay should be given in the morning and pellets in the afternoon or evening. Adequate fresh water is essential to ensure proper feed intake. Water delivery systems (e.g., sipper bottles) are superior to water bowls that may tip or become contaminated with feces. Syrup or molasses applied to the tip of the sipper tube may induce use and encourage water consumption.

> **TECHNICIAN NOTE** Rabbits are nocturnal and consume most of their feed during the night. Hay should be given in the morning and pellets in the afternoon or evening.

Other components of rabbit nutrition include vitamin supplementation. Vitamin A deficiency can result in infertility and other reproductive complications, central nervous system defects, and increased neonatal mortality. Most fresh commercial grass–based pellets contain adequate vitamin A to prevent such deficiencies; adding a supplement to a diet already fortified with vitamin A can cause toxic complications. Technicians should advise rabbit owners to buy fresh commercial grass hay and commercial grass–based pelleted diets and to monitor the rabbit's appetite.

All commercial feed should have a mill location and date of manufacture clearly printed on the bag; it is recommended to purchase feed within 90 days of production. Feed older than 6 months has poor nutritional quality. In addition, feed that contains antibiotics generally is not recommended. Antibiotic medication impregnated in the feed may disrupt the intestinal flora, resulting in **dysbiosis** and causing diarrhea, anorexia, or death.

Pellets high in calcium or excessive vitamin D can occasionally produce chalky-white or cream-colored urine. Termed *dystrophic calcification*, excess calcium causes urinary lithiasis or excessive excretion of calcium "sand" and may even cause calculi to form in the kidney and in the ureter. Normal urine color in the rabbit varies from straw to reddish brown.

Anesthesia

The rabbit that is a candidate for anesthesia should have food withheld for 8 to 12 hours and should be free from respiratory disease. Some breeds of rabbits have atropinesterase, which inactivates atropine. Atropine may be given subcutaneously as a preanesthetic agent to decrease salivation. If a rabbit has atropinesterase, it may be necessary to increase the dose of atropine. Although it is recommended, intubation is not required for the stable rabbit patient when anesthetized because they rarely regurgitate and are extremely difficult to intubate. To aid in intubation of a rabbit, both endoscopic observation of the laryngeal opening and use of an intubation aid (BAAM, Great Plains Ballistics, Inc., Lubbock, Texas) are helpful. Recommended endotracheal tubes in rabbits have inside diameters of 2 to 4 mm. A medium laryngoscope or rigid endoscope will aid in passing the tube into the rabbit's glottis to near the thoracic inlet. To prevent laryngospasm, do not use a topical anesthetic on rabbits.

> **TECHNICIAN NOTE** Although it is recommended, intubation is not required for the stable rabbit patient when anesthetized because they rarely regurgitate and are difficult to intubate.

Injectable anesthetic agents used in rabbits include ketamine, xylazine, and acepromazine; isoflurane is the inhalation anesthetic agent of choice. Movement of the nictitating membrane over approximately one-third of the cornea, a respiratory rate of 18 to 24 respirations per minute, abdominal musculature relaxation, and loss of ear, mouth, toe pinch, and palpebral reflexes indicate a suitable plane of surgical anesthesia in the rabbit.

By placing a rabbit in dorsal recumbency and gently stroking its ventrum, one causes hypnosis to occur. Hypnosis is a good technique for restraint for injections and radiographic procedures.

General Procedures

When intravenous injections are given to rabbits, the dorsal surface of the ear should be shaved to expose the marginal ear vein. Visibility of this vein will increase if alcohol is rubbed on the area. The central artery of the ear or the cephalic or lateral saphenous vein can be used for bleeding (Figure 22-38, *A*). Caution should be applied when the ear vein or artery is used in rabbit patients. If the blood supply is disrupted, necrosis of the ear tissue can occur. Other blood collection sites, including the lateral saphenous vein, the

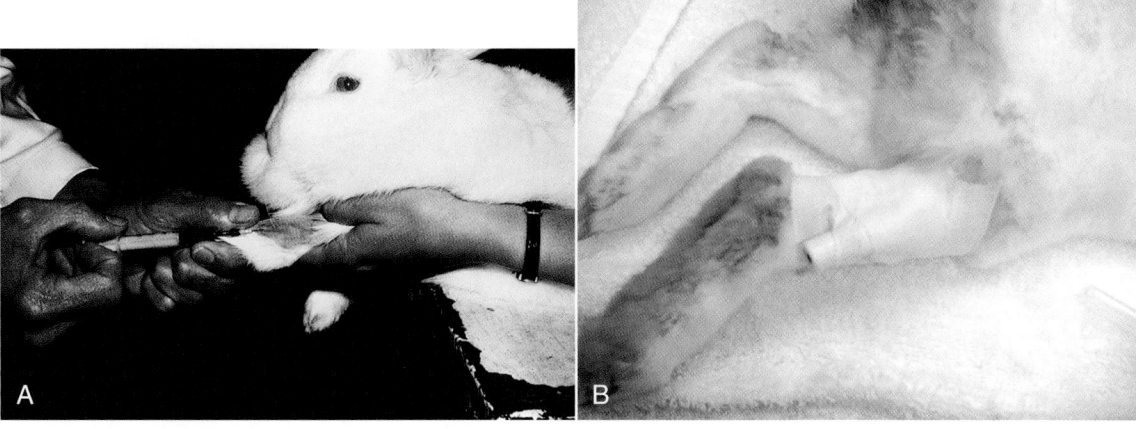

FIGURE 22-38 A, Blood collection from the cephalic vein of a rabbit. B, The lateral saphenous vein of a rabbit is readily accessed in most patients for blood collection and treatment.

cephalic vein, and the cranial vena cava, are recommended in rabbit patients. The cranial vena cava should be used for blood collection only under strict professional supervision. The lateral saphenous vein, which is located higher on the leg than in dogs, may be used to place an indwelling catheter and is often the preferred site for blood collection (Figure 22-38, *B*).

> **TECHNICIAN NOTE** The lateral saphenous vein, which is located higher on the leg than in dogs, may be used to place an indwelling catheter and is often the preferred site for blood collection.

Common Presentations

Rabbits may be affected by various infections and parasitic organisms. A pet rabbit may have hair loss caused by self-trauma, nutritional deficiencies, bacterial dermatitis (*Pasteurella multocida, Pseudomonas aeruginosa, Staphylococcus aureus,* and *Fusobacterium* spp.), parasites (e.g., ear mites [*Psoroptes cuniculi*; Figures 22-39 and 22-40] fur mites [*Cheyletiella parasitovorax*]), and rabbit lice *(Haemodipsus ventricosus)*. Flea prevention and control are needed for rabbits, especially for animals that are maintained outside (see Chapter 14). Ulcerative lesions on the ventral surface of the rear hocks are usually due to poor husbandry or to environmental pressures. Fungal organisms that have been noted to cause dermatopathy in rabbits are *Microsporum gypseum* and *Trichophyton mentagrophytes.*

An anorexic pet should be examined for malocclusion, hairballs, trauma, dietary changes, stress, dysbiosis, or poor feed. Heat stress (stroke) is common when adequate cooling is not provided in the summer. Diarrhea may be caused by colibacillosis, rotavirus infection, *Clostridium* infection, mucoid enteropathy, antibiotic intake, or Tyzzer's disease *(Bacillus piliformis)*. A high-fiber diet that includes timothy hay has been shown to improve digestive tract function and reduce the incidence of hairballs.

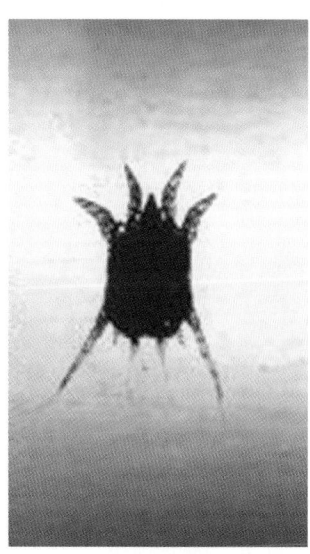

FIGURE 22-39 Microscopic view of *Psoroptes cuniculi,* the rabbit ear mite.

One of the main disease problems in rabbits is *P. multocida* infection (snuffles). Clinical signs include nasal discharge, torticollis, abscesses, conjunctivitis, and respiratory distress. Venereal spirochetosis should always be considered when rabbits are exhibiting infertility. *Eimeria stiedae* is a hepatic coccidium that may affect attitude and eating habits.

Encephalitozoon cuniculi is a protozoan parasite that will cause torticollis. Both *E. cuniculi* and *P. multocida* can be diagnosed with the use of serologic testing (Sound Diagnostics Inc., Woodinville, Washington).

Rabbits are territorial and fight when sexual maturity is reached, or when a male is placed in a female's cage for breeding. Neutering or an ovariohysterectomy is recommended to prevent unwanted offspring.

Malocclusion often leads to elongated incisors and sharp enamel points on molars. Rabbit-specific dental instruments should be used (Jorgensen Laboratories, Loveland,

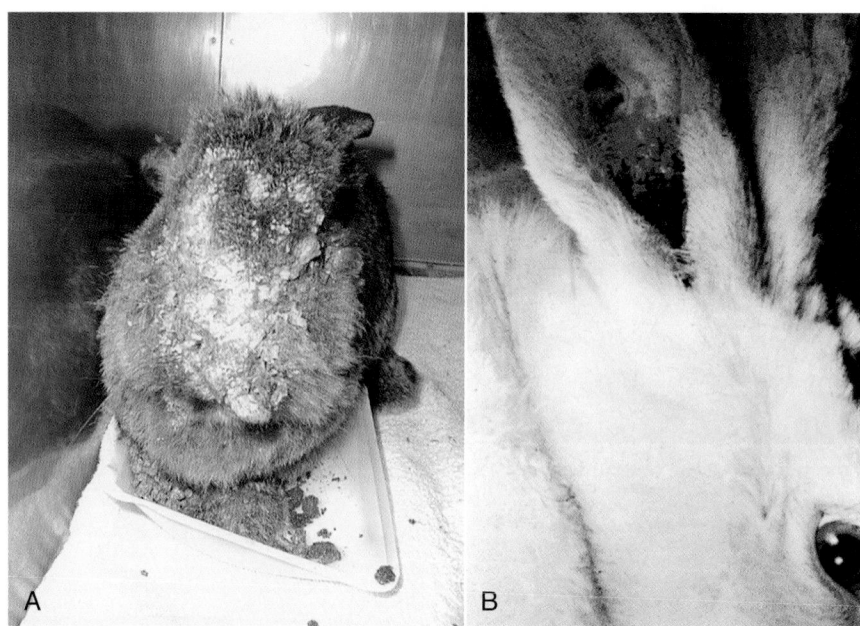

FIGURE 22-40 A, Rabbit exhibiting severe clinical signs of *Psoroptes cuniculi* infestation, extending to the face. B, *P. cuniculi* infestation in the external ear canal of a rabbit.

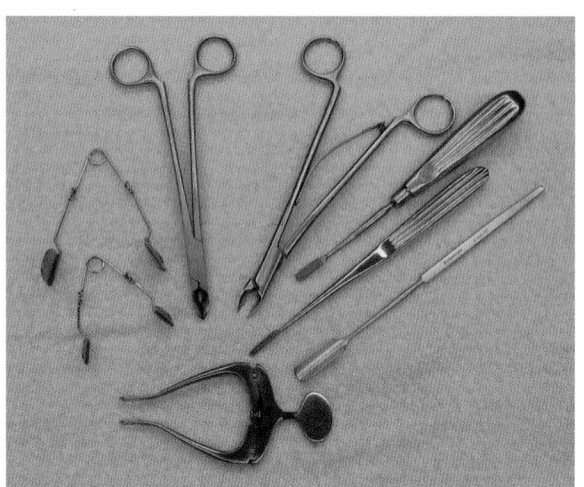

FIGURE 22-41 Rabbit dental instruments.

Colorado) to reduce tooth fracture and other complications associated with dental procedures (Figure 22-41). Most tooth-trimming procedures are done with the patient under general anesthesia, particularly when a Dremel motor tool (Dremel Inc., New York City, New York) is used. Gingival, lingual, and buccal lacerations are primary complications when trimming molars. To access the oral cavity when trimming molars, a nose cone is used to maintain gas anesthesia, and buccal specula are recommended.

RODENTS

Rodent species commonly seen in the veterinary hospital include guinea pigs, hamsters, gerbils, rats, and, to a lesser extent, mice. Although all of these animals are rodents, each species has particular anatomic characteristics, dietary requirements, and diseases. Blood collection in most rodent species can be accomplished using the anterior vena cava while the patient is under general anesthesia.

Antibiotic Therapy

Care must be taken when prescribing antibiotics to rodents. Guinea pigs, rabbits, and hamsters are extremely sensitive to the penicillin class of antibiotics, which may cause severe intestinal flora changes (dysbiosis); penicillins, streptomycin, and dihydrostreptomycin are drugs that may cause this problem. Tetracyclines work well in cases that require antibiotic therapy. An exotic animal formulary is essential in an exotic animal practice, to obtain specific information and dosage.[7]

> **TECHNICIAN NOTE** Guinea pigs, rabbits, and hamsters are extremely sensitive to penicillin antibiotics.

Anesthesia

Ketamine hydrochloride, pentobarbital sodium, and thiamylal sodium are injectable anesthetic agents that may be used in rodents. Isoflurane and sevoflurane are the anesthetic agents of choice, providing quick induction and recovery along with an adequate plane of anesthesia. Most rodents are induced in a chamber in which the anesthetic gas (e.g., isoflurane, sevoflurane) and oxygen are fed. Once the animal has been induced in the chamber, it is removed and fitted with a mask of appropriate size. Rodents are rarely intubated while being maintained under anesthesia.

Antiparasitic Agents

Carbaryl powder, dichlorvos, and ivermectin can be used to treat ectoparasites. Dichlorvos, thiabendazole, and ivermectin are adequate for treating internal parasites. See Chapter 14 for additional information on parasitology.

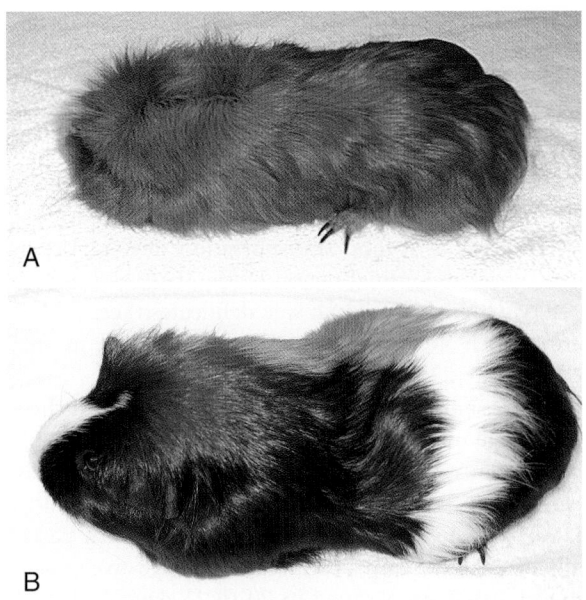

FIGURE 22-42 **A,** The Abyssinian guinea pig and **(B)** the English guinea pig are common house pets.

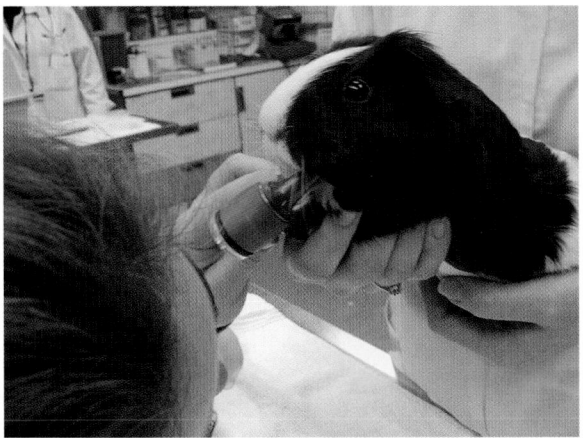

FIGURE 22-43 An otoscope with a disposable head may be used to examine a guinea pig's premolars and molars.

GUINEA PIGS

The cavy, or guinea pig, is a rodent related to porcupines and chinchillas. Guinea pigs have a long gestation that leads to the birth of large, precocious young. The most common guinea pig species kept as pets are the English or American, Abyssinian, and Peruvian long hair types (Figure 22-42, *A* and *B*). The guinea pig has open-rooted teeth that may become malocpcluded (Figure 22-43). The overgrown teeth will irritate the gingiva, causing excessive salivation. Although the female has only two mammary glands, it can successfully raise litters of three or more offspring.

Nutrition

Guinea pigs are notoriously fastidious eaters. They are herbivores with normal coprophagous behavior. Abrupt changes in feed or feeding systems can result in refusal to eat or drink for extended periods.

The recommended diet is a grass-based commercial guinea pig pellet and ad libitum grass hay. A high-fiber diet will reduce the incidence of hairball formation. As a result of specific nutrient and vitamin requirements, guinea pigs *should not* be fed rabbit or any other diet designed for another species. Guinea pigs should be provided hard food diets that promote gnawing because malocclusion can prevent eating and drinking.

Feed and water are best placed in bowls that cannot be chewed (e.g., stainless steel or ceramic crocks). A vitamin C supplement such as Tang (Kraft Foods, Inc., East Hanover, New Jersey) may be added to the water. Food should consist of a freshly milled, complete guinea pig ration. Storage in a freezer or refrigerator will extend the life of the food. All food and water containers should be placed above the substrate to prevent soiling.

Unlike other pet rodents, guinea pigs require dietary vitamin C supplementation. Guinea pigs lack an enzyme in glucose to the vitamin C pathway, thus requiring a daily dietary ascorbic acid supplement. Commercially prepared guinea pig diets generally contain minimal vitamin C concentrations, as well as depleted concentrations with a shelf life longer than 3 months. Vitamin C is highly unstable in the feed, especially when exposed to heat. Use of old feed is one of the primary reasons vitamin C deficiencies are seen. Fresh fruit can be used to supplement commercial diets; to prevent gastrointestinal upset, avoid abrupt changes in diet. Diets supplemented with produce high in ascorbic acid, including spinach, kale, parsley, chicory, bell peppers, and oranges, are recommended.

> **TECHNICIAN NOTE** Unlike other pet rodents, guinea pigs require dietary vitamin C supplementation because they lack an enzyme in glucose to the vitamin C pathway.

The cavy requires 0.5 mg/kg body weight of dietary ascorbic acid per day because it lacks L-gulonolactone oxidase. Absolute requirements of 10 mg/kg/day of ascorbic acid are recommended, with increases up to 30 mg/kg/day if pregnant. If supplementation is not provided in the feed, 1 g/L may be added to the water, or one small handful of cabbage or kale or ¼ of an orange may be given daily. Guinea pigs must be fed species-specific food within 90 days of milling. Fruit and vegetable supplementation is discouraged because of the possibility of disturbing the normal gut bacterial flora. To ensure that the guinea pig is receiving adequate doses of vitamin C daily, oral supplementation in the form of tablets specifically manufactured for these animals is recommended (Oxbow Animal Health, Murdock, Nebraska). Clinical signs of vitamin C deficiency include alopecia, anorexia, dehydration, and poor wound healing, along with eventual periodontal disease such as brown discoloration of teeth and temporomandibular joint (TMJ) inflammation.

Fresh water is essential for the guinea pig and should be provided daily. Water bottles or other water delivery systems are recommended to prevent water contamination or spillage. Note that the guinea pig has a propensity for chewing and gnawing; water valves should be located outside the cage to prevent destruction.

A female guinea pig that is bred past 7 or 8 months of age may have trouble separating the pubic symphysis, causing a nondeliverable dystocia. Fat pads may occlude the pelvic canal, complicating parturition. These problems usually lead to dystocia or death. If the sow is experiencing dystocia, cesarean retrieval of the young can often save the babies. Food preferences are established within a few days after birth for the young. Hand rearing of the young requires regular stimulation of the anus for defecation and the urethral opening for urination, as with most neonatal mammals. Females usually allow foster nursing of other young.

Guinea pigs rarely become excited or bite when handled. Through their gentle nature, they become conditioned to their surroundings. However, if a group is contained in an enclosure, subordinate animals may be traumatized (as by hair loss and bite wounds) by dominant cagemates.

Foot pad dermatitis resulting in ulcers may develop in animals placed on wire (Figure 22-44). Metal, plastic, and glass make excellent cages for guinea pigs. The substrate may consist of paper (shredded), wood shavings, or hay. Chewing the substrate is a vice commonly associated when animals develop a submandibular abscess. Hard fibrous splinters penetrate the oral mucosa, inoculating the tissue with bacteria (usually *Streptococcus zooepidemicus*) that develop into abscesses. Changes in the substrate may be indicated to stop this problem, although it may be difficult to find an adequate alternative substrate, which must have absorptive qualities for opaque, pale yellow, crystalline urine.

To sex a guinea pig, the handler must observe the urethral orifice and the anus. The male has no break in the ridge between the openings, but the female has a shallow U-shaped break.

One boar will service up to 10 sows beginning at 8 weeks of age. The sow becomes sexually mature around 5 to 6 weeks of age. Gestation length on average is 63 to 68 days, with litter size ranging from one to six precocious offspring.

HAMSTERS

The golden hamster is a native of Syria and comes in many different color varieties (Figure 22-45). Cheek pouches that extend along the head and neck to the proximal dorsum of the back serve as a food transportation device. Along the caudal lateral abdominal region lie the flank glands. A dark brown patch of skin on each side delineates these sebaceous glands, which are used to mark territory and in mating rituals (Figure 22-46).

Hamsters have a tendency to bite and are good at chewing through cage material. To accommodate the animal's physical nature, an exercise wheel should be placed in the cage.

Female hamsters often attack newly introduced males and females. Hamsters live 18 to 24 months, have a gestation length of 16 days, and produce on average five offspring. Young hamsters are weaned in 20 to 25 days. If disturbed, the female may cannibalize her litter or hide them in her cheek pouches. When the young are hidden in the cheek pouches, they may suffocate. Hamsters can be picked up by holding the nape skin at the base of the neck or by cupping the hands under the hindlimbs.

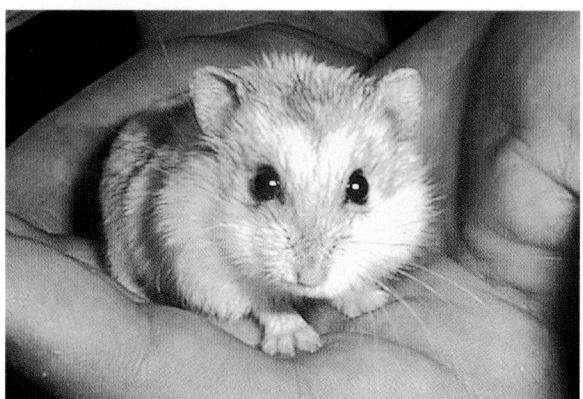

FIGURE 22-45 Dwarf hamsters are popular pets.

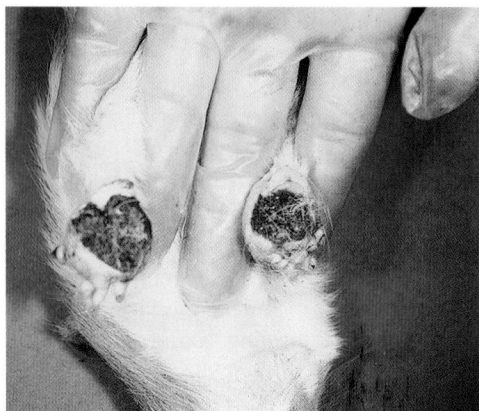

FIGURE 22-44 Foot pad dermatitis is a problem that commonly affects guinea pigs.

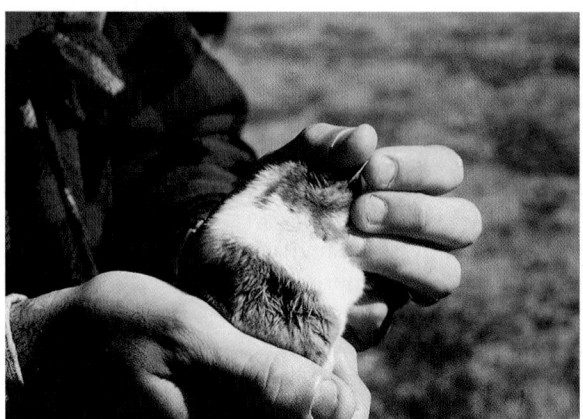

FIGURE 22-46 Flank glands on hamsters, noted in this figure by the moistened area in the caudodorsal region of the animal.

TECHNICIAN NOTE Hamsters on average live 18 to 24 months and have a gestation period of 16 days.

Several hamster habitats are commercially available. An aquarium with a mesh top may be used to house a hamster, with hardwood shavings as the substrate of choice. Aromatic shavings, such as cedar or pine, may cause ocular and respiratory irritation, severe dermatitis, and allergic reactions. Sipper bottles are perfect for water dispensing, and non-chewable bowls should be used for food containers, or food should be placed on the floor of the enclosure. All food and water should be made available to the young.

A commercial pelleted hamster diet is preferred over a seed-based product. Treats, including small amounts of seed, may be given to hamsters, but the base diet should consist of the pelleted product.

Males have a greater anogenital distance than females. Hamsters may be mated monogamously or in a harem. It is important that females with young are not disturbed, so that cannibalism or abandonment of the litter does not occur.

Wet tail is a general term used to refer to diarrhea in the hamster. Bacterial infection, cestodiasis, and antibiotic administration are a few causes of diarrhea in these rodents.

GERBILS

The Mongolian gerbil is a popular pet native to Mongolia and northeastern China. It is an active burrowing animal adapted to a desert environment.

TECHNICIAN NOTE Under no circumstances should gerbils be grabbed by the tail. As a defense mechanism, the tail skin will deglove, necessitating a tail amputation.

The gerbil has a life span of 3.5 years, along with gestation length of 25 days without lactation and 24 to 48 days with lactation. Litter sizes average five offspring that wean in approximately 25 days (Figure 22-47). Certain gerbil lines are prone to epileptiform seizure activity. Gerbils are friendly rodents that may be housed in hamster units (Figure 22-48).

These animals are good at escaping; therefore, the cage should be designed to prevent chewing.

The gerbil's diet may be similar to that of the hamster, and water can be supplied in a sipper bottle. Sexing is accomplished by measuring the urogenital distance, which is much longer in the male than in the female. Males assist with care of the young.

Gerbils commonly have a nasal dermatitis caused by a bacterial infection initiated by their burrowing activity. Topical antibiotic treatment is recommended for resolution of this infection.

Tyzzer's disease may be diagnosed in gerbils and is caused by *Bacillus piliformis*. Dietary change and colibacillosis also may cause diarrhea in these animals.

MICE

Mice are small rodents that are used most often in the research setting but are maintained as pets. Mice usually are aggressive and bite. They are territorial animals that quickly develop a hierarchy when placed in groups (Figure 22-49). These small animals require small quantities of food and water but are escape prone and may develop an unpleasant odor.

Clinical conditions commonly affecting mice include ectoparasites, neoplasia, and trauma. Most mice have a life

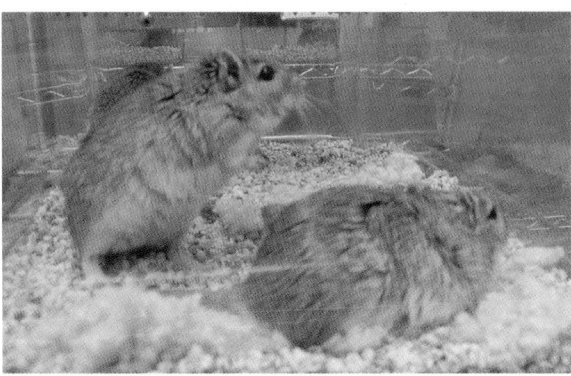

FIGURE 22-48 Typical small rodent cage containing gerbils.

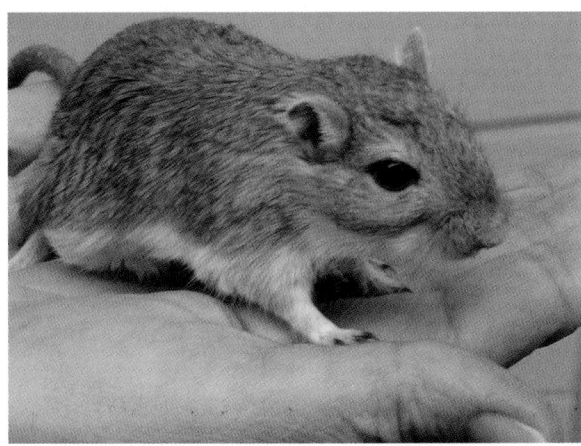

FIGURE 22-47 Young gerbil.

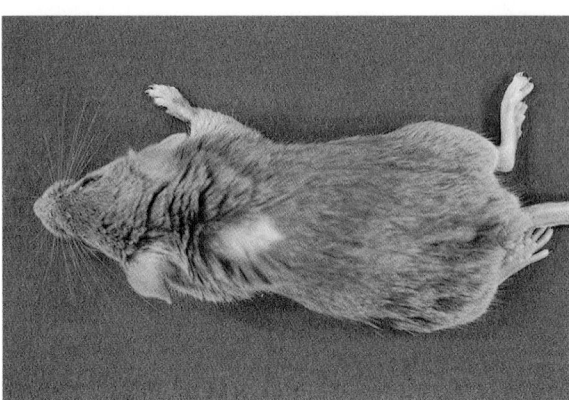

FIGURE 22-49 Trauma (cagemate-inflicted hair loss) in a mouse. This is commonly referred to as *barbering*.

span of 2 years and are prone to geriatric disease conditions within a relatively short time of ownership. One of the most common geriatric disease conditions is neoplasia. Tumors of various types have been identified in mice, making educating owners particularly important to aid in early detection and treatment.

Housing should be similar to that of gerbils and hamsters. Hardwood shavings or chips are recommended instead of aromatic softwood chips (cedar and pine) because of potential liver damage and epithelial damage.

Housing should be cleaned regularly to prevent odor and health problems. Pelleted rodent feed and fresh water in sipper bottles are recommended to be supplied free choice.

Male mice have a greater urogenital distance than females. Female mice become sexually mature at 50 days of age and are best bred in the harem scheme, with one male combined with two to six females.

RATS

Rats are clean and unassuming and can be trained to be good pets (Figure 22-50). These animals may live up to 3 years or longer and become sexually mature at 1.5 to 2 months of age.

As with mice, rats are relatively short-lived, predisposing them to geriatric disease. Rats are also highly susceptible to neoplasia, particularly mammary gland tumors. In addition, *Mycoplasma* spp. respiratory infections are commonly diagnosed and clinically may appear as dyspnea with signs of nasal discharge, which is commonly tinged with a red color as a result of the pigment of harderian gland secretions. Enrofloxacin and tetracycline have been used to treat *Mycoplasma* spp. infections in rats.

> **TECHNICIAN NOTE**   Rats seldom bite, but caution must be used in a stressful situation.

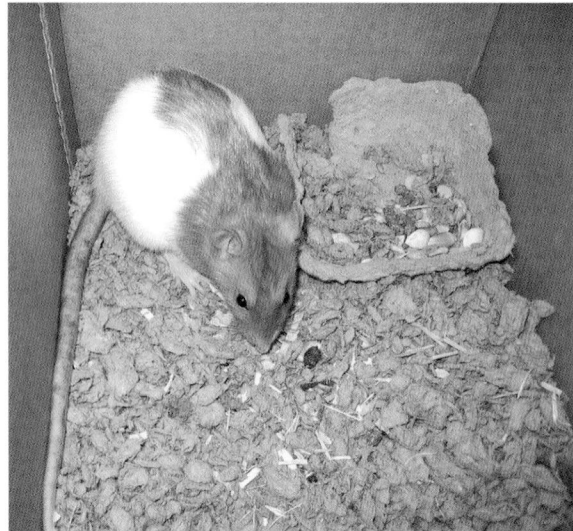

FIGURE 22-50 *Rats make one of the best companion animals of all rodent species.*

Commercial rodent cages can be obtained for proper housing. The substrate should be similar to that provided for other rodents. A rodent pellet or cube diet is the recommended base diet for rats. Several excellent rodent pellet or cube diets are available at pet stores. Treats (e.g., vegetables, fruit, yogurt drops) may be provided in small, regulated quantities.

Males have a longer anogenital distance than females. Gestation length is 22 days, and nesting material should be provided before birth.

PRAIRIE DOGS

The black-tailed prairie dog *(Cynomys ludovicianus)* may be brought to a veterinary practice, even though it is illegal to keep wild North American species as pets. Wild prairie dogs may be infected with zoonotic diseases, including hantaviruses, rabies, ectoparasites, *Salmonella* spp., the plague bacteria, and monkeypox. Some prairie dogs have been raised in captivity and therefore are unlikely to carry dangerous zoonotic diseases. Nevertheless, it is recommended that all prairie dogs remain where they belong—in their natural habitat.

Prairie dogs may live up to 10 years and can survive on rodent chow and timothy grass hay. They are, however, susceptible to obesity, making it essential to monitor food intake, especially in adult animals. Digging and tunneling are important parts of their daily activity. Deep bedding enables this type of exercise and allows them to hide and feel secure. Prairie dogs can be managed very similarly to rats with regard to their management and care. The scrotal sac is the identifying characteristic of male prairie dogs when sex determination is required. Venipuncture is best accomplished using the lateral saphenous or cephalic vein. Jugular venipuncture or cranial vena cava collection should be attempted only when the patient is under general anesthesia.

Disease problems commonly identified in captive prairie dogs include obesity, respiratory disease, malocclusion, infectious pododermatitis, trauma, and neoplasia. The most difficult situation to overcome for most prairie dogs raised in captivity is obesity. Obesity usually complicates concurrent disease states, making it difficult at times to differentiate the primary disease problem from complications caused by excess body fat. To reduce the incidence of obesity in prairie dogs, a primary diet of grass hay supplemented with grass-based pellets is recommended. The pellets should be regulated and the animal's dietary intake monitored to prevent overfeeding.

HEDGEHOGS

The African hedgehog *(Atelerix albiventris)* has become an increasingly popular pet in recent years. These nocturnal spinal animals often adapt best to captivity when left alone. Hedgehogs like to hide, like dark quiet areas, and will burrow to escape. Hedgehogs may be maintained very similarly to rodents. For example, enclosures that are 20 gallons or larger and are lined with absorbable paper bedding make excellent habitats.

The life span of hedgehogs is 3 to 5 years. The most common disease conditions are neoplasia and external parasites. Yearly physical examinations are needed for teeth cleaning, nail trimming, and tumor checks. Hedgehogs are not rodents, and they rely on an insectivore-omnivore diet such as the one listed in Box 22-4.

One feature of hedgehog medicine is that hedgehog patients must be anesthetized simply to be examined. Their spines are very sharp, so caution must be taken during handling; gloves are necessary, particularly before anesthesia is administered (Figure 22-51).

Blood collection sites include cranial vena cava, jugular vein, cephalic vein, and lateral saphenous vein, with the cranial vena cava as the site of choice. Diseases commonly diagnosed in hedgehogs are neoplasia, obesity, otitis externa, dermatitis, external parasites, and respiratory disease (Figure 22-52).

SUGAR GLIDERS

Sugar gliders are nocturnal marsupials from Australia (Figure 22-53). Like hedgehogs, they are unusual pets with unique qualities that should be considered carefully by a potential owner before a purchase is made. They are very social animals. If maintained as a single pet, a glider will require

BOX 22-4	Recommended Daily Diet for Hedgehogs

- 3 tsp high-quality cat or kitten chow
- 1 tsp fruit vegetable mix
- Four to eight small mealworms or two to three small crickets

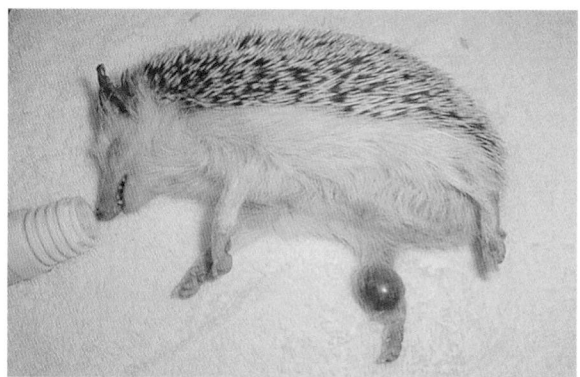

FIGURE 22-52 This hedgehog has a tumor on its rear leg. Tumors are common in hedgehogs.

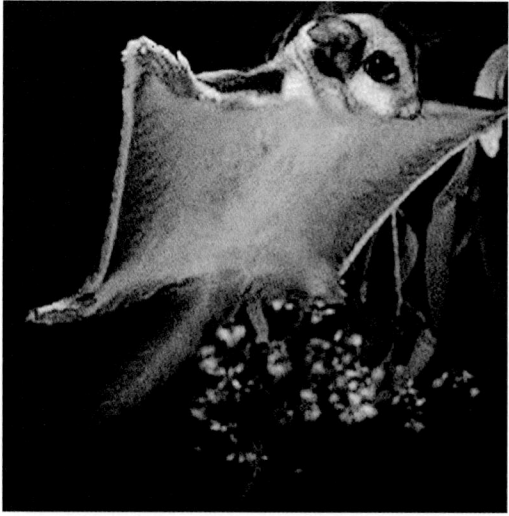

FIGURE 22-53 A sugar glider with its skin stretched out, giving it the ability to "fly" and also its name.

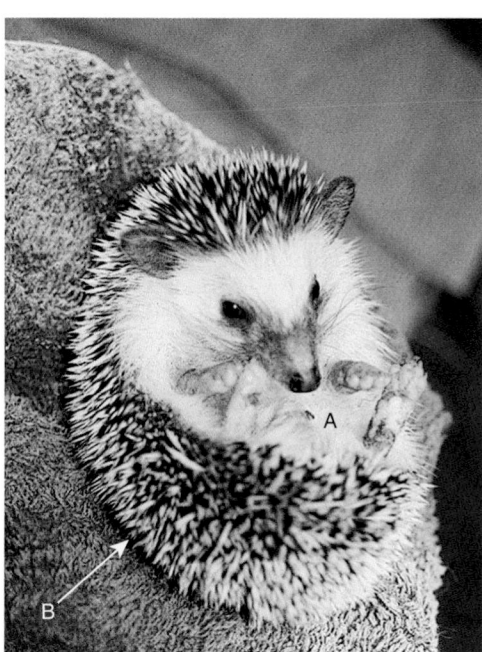

FIGURE 22-51 The ventral surface of hedgehogs is devoid of spines (A), but the dorsal aspect is covered with sharp spines (B).

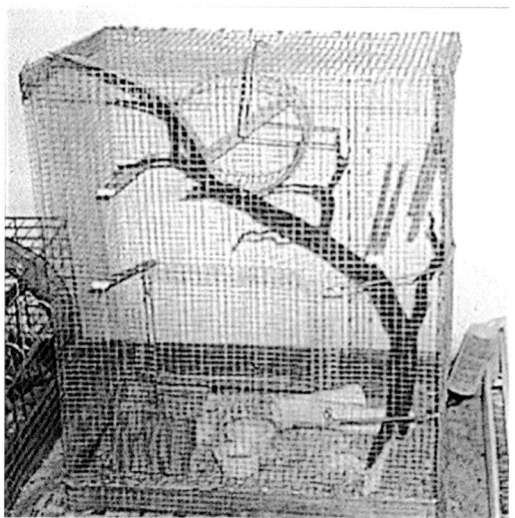

FIGURE 22-54 A typical sugar glider enclosure.

BOX 22-5 | Daily Sugar Glider Diet[8]

Diet 1

NutriMax (VetsPride, Nashville, Tennessee)—Formulated and manufactured specifically for sugar gliders
- Recommended feeding using NutriMax
  - Ad libitum—approximately 2-3 ounces available at all times
  - NutriMax—about 75% of sugar gliders' daily diet
  - Remaining 25%—fruits, vegetables, along with VitaMax (VetsPride) multivitamin supplement, as directed on the label

Diet 2

Glide-R-Chow (PocketPets, Cape Coral, Florida)
- Manufactured to meet the daily nutritional needs of sugar gliders
- Recommended feeding using Glide-R-Chow
  - 2 ounces available at all times to sugar gliders
  - Primary food—75% of daily diet
  - 25% diet—fruits, vegetables, along with Glide-A-Mins (PocketPets) multivitamin supplement, as directed on the label

REFERENCES

1. Tully TN: Birds. In Mitchell MA, Tully TN, editors: Manual of exotic pet practice, St Louis, 2009, Saunders, p 250.
2. Frye FL: Reptile clinician's handbook, Malabar, FL, 1995, Krieger.
3. Kirchgessner M, Mitchell MA: Chelonians. In Mitchell MA, Tully TN, editors: Manual of exotic pet practice, St Louis, 2009, Saunders, p 207.
4. Nevarez J: Lizards. In Mitchell MA, Tully TN, editors: Manual of exotic pet practice, St Louis, 2009, Saunders, p 164.
5. Mitchell MA: Snakes. In Mitchell MA, Tully TN, editors: Manual of exotic pet practice, St Louis, 2009, Saunders, p 136.
6. Boyer TH: Essentials of reptiles: a guide for practitioners, Lakewood, CO, 1998, American Animal Hospital Association.
7. Carpenter JW: Exotic animal formulary, ed 3, St Louis, 2005, Saunders.
8. Brust DM: Sugar gliders: a complete veterinary care guide, Sugar Land, TX, 2009, Veterinary Interactive Publications, p 65.

RECOMMENDED READINGS

2011-2012 American Pet Products Manufacturers Association's (APPMA) National Pet Owners Survey. Available at: http://www.americanpetproducts.org/pubs_survey.asp (accessed on August 1, 2011).

Campbell TW, Ellis CK: Avian and exotic animal hematology and cytology, Ames, IA, 2007, Blackwell Publishing Ltd.

Eliman MM: Hematology and plasma chemistry of the inland bearded dragon, *Pogona vitticeps*, Bull Assoc Reptile Amphibian Vet 7:10, 1997.

Fox JG: Biology and diseases of the ferret, ed 2, Philadelphia, 1998, Lippincott Williams & Wilkins.

Frye FL: Reptile clinician's handbook, Malabar, FL, 1995, Krieger.

Harcourt-Brown F: Textbook of rabbit medicine, Oxford, UK, 2002, Butterworth-Heinemann.

Harkness JE, Wagner JE: The biology and medicine of rabbits and rodents, Philadelphia, PA, 1995, Lea & Febiger.

Johnson CA, Harrison LR: Exotic companion medicine handbook for veterinarians, Lake Worth, FL, 1996, Wingers Publishing.

Journal of Avian Medicine and Surgery, Lawrence, KS, Association of Avian Veterinarians, Allen Press (published quarterly).

Journal of Exotic Pet Medicine, Philadelphia, Elsevier (published quarterly).

Journal of Herpetological Medicine and Surgery, Lawrence, KS, Association of Reptilian and Amphibian Veterinarians, Allen Press (published quarterly).

Journal of Zoo and Wildlife Medicine, Lawrence, KS, American Association of Zoo Veterinarians (published quarterly).

Lewington JH: Ferret husbandry, medicine and surgery, Edinburgh, Scotland, 2000, Butterworth-Heinemann.

Mader DR: Metabolic bone disease. In Mader DR, editor: Reptile medicine and surgery, ed 2, St Louis, 2006, Saunders, p 841.

Quesenberry KE, Carpenter JW: Ferrets, rabbits and rodents: clinical medicine and surgery, ed 2, St Louis, 2004, Saunders.

Spadafori G, Speer BL: Birds for dummies, Foster City, CA, 1999, IDG Books.

Tully TN, Dorrestein GM, Jones AK: Handbook of avian medicine, ed 2, Oxford, UK, 2009, Saunders/Elsevier.

additional attention from the owner to meet its psychological needs. In addition, their nocturnal habits give rise to much activity throughout the night, which can be annoying to those who wish to sleep.

Housing needs to consist of a tall wire enclosure with fresh branches and places to hide, such as a bird box (Figure 22-54). The wire mesh should have spacing no larger than 1 inch square to prevent escape. The bottom tray should be lined with shredded paper or pelleted paper products for easy cleaning and optimal absorption of urine, food, and water.

Malnutrition (e.g., hypocalcemia, hypoglycemia) is one of the most common disease conditions diagnosed in sugar gliders. To assess the sugar glider's condition through blood testing, blood collection is best performed while the animal is under general anesthesia. The location of choice for venipuncture in sugar gliders is the cranial vena cava.

Commercial pelleted glider diets are available, but they are not actively marketed in most areas. One source of information worth exploring is the Internet. Websites that focus on these animals can be found via most search engines. An example of a complete sugar glider diet is listed in Box 22-5.[8]

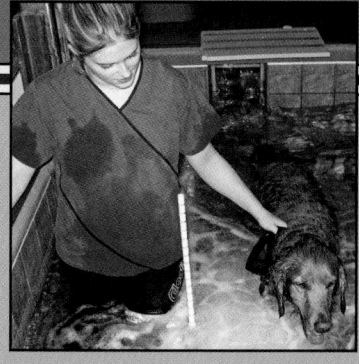

23 | Physical Therapy, Rehabilitation, and Alternative Medical Nursing

Laurie McCauley and Christine Jurek

OUTLINE

Alternative Concepts in Nutrition, 847
Nutraceuticals, 848
Glandulars, Cell Therapy, and Glandular-like Products, 848
Herbal Medicine, 850
Western Herbs, 851
Chinese Herbal Medicine, 851
Ayurvedic Herbs, 852
Aromatherapy, 853
Homeopathy, Homotoxicology, and Flower Essences, 853
History and Principles, 853
Practice, 855
Flower Essences, 857
Acupuncture, 858
Terminology and Record Keeping, 858
Acupuncture Theories, 859
Techniques, 859

Veterinary Spinal Manipulative Therapy (Chiropractic), 860
History, 860
Philosophy and Theory, 861
Treatment, 861
The Technician's Role, 862
Applied Kinesiology, 862
Physical Therapy and Rehabilitation, 865
Exercise-Based Therapy, 866
Therapeutic Exercises, 866
Hydrotherapy, 867
Land Treadmill, 868
Manual Therapies, 868
Passive Range of Motion, 870
Electrical and Magnet-Based Therapies, 871
Light and Sound–Based Therapies, 873
Assistive Devices, 875

LEARNING OBJECTIVES

When you have completed this chapter, you will be able to:

1. Pronounce, define, and spell all Key Terms in this chapter.
2. Do the following regarding alternative concepts in nutrition:
   - Describe considerations in the development of home-prepared diets for dogs and cats.
   - List commonly used nutraceuticals and glandulars and describe their therapeutic uses.
3. Do the following regarding the use of herbal medicine:
   - List commonly used Western herbs, Chinese herbs, and Ayurvedic herbs and describe their therapeutic uses.
   - Describe the principles of aromatherapy and list common aromatherapy oils and their uses.
   - Explain the basic principles of homeopathy and list forms of homeopathic preparations and considerations for storage and administration.
   - Describe the principles of flower essence therapy and list common flower essences and their uses.
4. Explain the principles and techniques of acupuncture and describe the role of the veterinary technician in acupuncture therapy.
5. Describe how chiropractic and applied kinesiology can benefit animal patients and explain the role of the veterinary technician in each discipline.
6. List common indications for veterinary rehabilitation.

KEY TERMS

Acupuncture
Applied kinesiology
Aromatherapy
Ayurvedic medicine
Chiropractic therapy
Cryotherapy
Glandular therapy (glandulars)
Goniometry
Holistic
Homeopathy
Hydrotherapy
Massage
Modality
Myotherapy
Neuromuscular electrical stimulation (NMES)
Nutraceutical
Passive range of motion (PROM)
Pulsed electromagnetic field therapy (PEMF)
Rehabilitation
Thermal agents
Traditional Chinese medicine (TCM)
Ultrasound (therapeutic)

The authors and publisher wish to acknowledge the contributions of Caroline Adamson Adrian and Robert A. Taylor to the "Physical Therapy and Rehabilitation" chapter in previous editions of this textbook.

7. Compare and contrast the physical therapeutic modalities used in veterinary rehabilitation, including exercise-based therapies, electrical and magnet-based therapies, light and sound–based therapies, and superficial thermal therapies.
8. List supportive and assistive devices commonly used for animal patients and explain the importance of podiatric care in the overall health of dogs.

INTRODUCTION

Complementary and alternative therapy can be an exciting and rewarding part of veterinary medicine. Whether you work at a completely nonconventional practice or at a surgical referral center, you will have clients who seek a more natural approach to their pet's care than standard veterinary medicine provides. Often, clients feel more comfortable speaking with a technician about less mainstream ideas than they do with a veterinarian.

The term **holistic** refers to a "whole animal" approach to health care. It focuses on wellness as an ongoing, dynamic process with great variability in the state of health. On one end of the spectrum is perfect health, and on the other end is disease. Most patients fall somewhere in between. Holistic medicine seeks to bring the patient to an ever greater state of general health and well-being compared with the conventional approach of simply treating disease.

An animal in perfect health has bright eyes and a shiny coat and is muscular and fit, energetic, and robust. Not only is this animal in balance internally, it also has a much greater capacity to adapt to its environment. It is able to rebalance and heal easily after it receives an external insult such as exposure to an infectious agent or trauma. Anything less than perfect health leaves room for improvement.

It may seem strange to include **rehabilitation** with complementary medicine, but it fits perfectly with the concept of "holistic." Although some practitioners limit rehabilitation therapy to traditional techniques, it is common to see **acupuncture** and chiropractic treatments, as well as any of the other listed therapies, included in veterinary rehabilitation practice. They all fit smoothly together for the purpose of healing the whole animal. The technician contributes to holistic health care of veterinary patients both as an assistant and as a therapist under the supervision and direction of the veterinarian.

This chapter offers an overview of the complementary modalities most commonly used in veterinary practice today, including veterinary rehabilitation concepts and therapies. The following modalities will be discussed: nutrition; herbal medicine; **homeopathy,** homotoxicology, and flower essences; acupuncture and traditional Chinese medicine (TCM); physical modalities, including chiropractic **applied kinesiology** (AK); and rehabilitation. Case reports will illustrate the principles and practice of various therapies. For additional information about complementary medicine practices, refer to the list of "Recommended Readings and Resources" at the end of the chapter.

ALTERNATIVE CONCEPTS IN NUTRITION

One of the most commonly asked questions in veterinary practice is, "What should I feed my pet?" Often, the technician is the staff member responsible for educating clients about nutrition. A solid understanding of basic nutrition is essential for every veterinary technician in every practice, with no exceptions. Even in a surgical referral practice, counseling clients on proper nutrition to optimize surgical recovery is an important aspect of providing the best and most complete health care. This section is meant to expand upon basic knowledge of animal nutrition and to introduce some novel concepts in companion animal nutrition.

Excellent nutrition is a particularly important part of holistic practice because it is fundamental in attaining optimal health. Many clients who seek alternative medical care for their pets are already educated about nutrition, sometimes even more educated than the veterinary health care team. On the downside, misinformation and hype abound, especially in the Internet age. It can be difficult to convince a client that a vegetarian diet is inappropriate for cats when the lady at the health food store swore it cured her Fluffy's cancer. Therefore, nutrition is becoming an important issue in any practice because clients need sound nutritional advice from well-informed veterinary professionals.

A good holistic diet is based on using whole, natural ingredients in a balanced ration. For small animals, the most wholesome healthy diet is a balanced, home-prepared diet. In the case of herbivores, the best diet is pasture provided on a soil with balanced minerals, supplemented with hay and grain only when necessary. The term *balanced* is an important one because an improperly prepared or unbalanced diet can cause disease or minimally can be a hindrance to attaining ideal health. Balance can be achieved with each meal, as it is with commercial pet food, or it may be achieved on a daily to weekly basis, as with our own diets.

> **TECHNICIAN NOTE** Not every client is willing or able to provide a balanced home-prepared diet for his or her pet. Many excellent nutritious and wholesome commercially prepared pet foods are readily available for purchase.

It is important to note that a healthy water source, such as spring water, is significant for the patient's overall health. Water can be a source of healthy vitamins and minerals, or it can contain harmful toxins and additives. A good rule of thumb is that if you would not drink your tap water, neither should your pet.

Some recommendations may simply be unattainable for large animal patients, but we can do our best to optimize the resources that are available such as proper pasture management and using sources of good-quality hay and grain, along with supplementation to balance the mineral and vitamin components of the diet. Soil testing and hay analysis for nutrient content are reasonably accessible and should be done regularly as food sources change.

We will now discuss in greater depth home-prepared diets. Meat used in the home-prepared diet for carnivores may be raw or cooked, depending on the owner's preference and the pet's constitution. Raw diets are controversial, and a great deal of information is available on this topic. The theory behind raw diets is that a wild carnivore (feline or canine) catches prey and eats it; no cooking is involved. Raw meat contains more enzymes and is "what nature intended." It is more digestible and contains greater quantities of unspoiled nutrients than are found in cooked meat (consider raw vs. cooked vegetables). The difficulty is that most people are unable to provide a fresh catch for their domestic cat or dog. Also, commercial raw meat is processed and packaged. This introduces the problem of bacterial contamination, which carnivores are generally (but not always) well equipped to handle because they have a more acidic environment in their stomach and intestines. The risk is increased with ground meat because it has a greater surface area and therefore offers increased risk for bacterial growth. Bacterial contamination of veterinary raw diets is of even greater concern for pet owners, who handle the food, than it is for the pet itself. Care must be taken to educate clients about the health risks posed by handling raw meat. This is particularly true for immunosuppressed and elderly clients. The same procedures and precautions should be followed when raw meat intended for cooking is handled: immediately clean and disinfect any surface that the raw food touches, including your hands.

Where raw bones are concerned, it is true that they do not readily splinter or break teeth as cooked bones do, but they are not without their dangers.

> **TECHNICIAN NOTE** Many dogs, when introduced to raw bones, are very enthusiastic about their new diet, and in their eagerness, they may consume large pieces of bone that subsequently can cause gastrointestinal (GI) obstruction. This is a less common occurrence in cats than in dogs, but bone obstructions can occur. Bones must be introduced carefully, and if the pet is overzealous, the bones may be ground, or a calcium powder may be substituted. Powders are not helpful for dental health as are bones, but it is best to err on the side of caution to ensure the safety of the patient.

Vegetables should be cooked (lightly steamed) and chopped or minced or grated because carnivores have difficulty breaking down plant cell walls to obtain intracellular nutrients. In the wild, one of the most substantial sources of plant-based nutrients is the gastrointestinal tract of herbivorous prey. Plant material processed by the adept gastrointestinal tract of prey species serves as a substantial source of nutrients not otherwise available to the predator. Overall, raw diets, if properly prepared and balanced, can enhance an animal's health, but they are not ideal for every patient, and they are not a cure for all diseases and disorders.

Holistic commercial diets are becoming more readily available to pet owners. Many pet food companies that produce standard dry and canned foods are including a holistic product line, and some small pet food companies focus exclusively on providing holistic diets for animals. Balanced raw commercial diets are available in frozen, freeze-dried, and dehydrated forms.

> **TECHNICIAN NOTE**   It is important to realize that just because a company labels a diet "holistic" or "natural" does not mean that it is. Careful research is important before the determination is made of whether a diet meets the nutritional needs of a particular patient. Be sure to inspect not only the guaranteed analysis and ingredient list, but also information on sources of the ingredients.

It is important to assess the processing of a commercial food as well as the quality of its ingredients, but this can be a challenging task. As a rule of thumb, stick with companies that are helpful and willing to offer tours of the food processing plant (some may be limited because of contamination concerns). It may be best to steer clients toward diets that obtain all ingredients from the United States, Canada, and New Zealand (for lamb).

A new product in the pet food industry is the limited-grain or grain-free diet. This mimics the nutrient profile of a raw diet without concern for contamination. In addition, many of these diets are dry, which makes the convenience appealing. Some other dry diets are baked rather than extruded, providing a more natural nutrient profile with better digestibility.

Supplementation of the diet with probiotics and digestive enzymes may be beneficial, particularly for those pets and breeds (such as the German Shepherd) that tend to have sensitive digestive systems. Addition of plain yogurt is a simple way to help balance the GI flora, but many commercially prepared products that provide this balance are available.

Each patient is assessed to find a diet option best suited to the pet's particular nutritional needs. The diet must be feasible for the client and must meet the demands of the pet owner's financial limitations, lifestyle, time constraints, and capabilities. An acceptable alternative to home-prepared meals may involve choosing several (three to four) commercial diets and rotating them to provide an overall balance in nutrients. For example, one diet may give an animal less than an ideal (although meeting minimum requirements) amount of a certain micronutrient. When diets are rotated, this will likely balance out in the long run because another diet may have more of that nutrient (Case Presentation 23-1).

> **TECHNICIAN NOTE**   Remember that holistic medicine is about treating each patient as an individual. With that in mind, there is no "best" diet for every animal. Each patient must be assessed to find the optimal diet for him or her that is feasible for the caretaker to provide.

NUTRACEUTICALS

The use of **nutraceuticals** is quickly becoming mainstream in both human and veterinary medicine. The term refers to nutritional supplements that are not herbs and are not approved for use as drugs but are thought to convey therapeutic benefit to the patient. Many types of nutraceuticals are available. They are used to treat many conditions and assist in maintaining the general health and well-being of the patient. Following is a brief discussion of the more commonly used nutraceuticals (Table 23-1).

GLANDULARS, CELL THERAPY, AND GLANDULAR-LIKE PRODUCTS

As the name implies, this type of supplement uses animal products to supply nutrients (steroids, enzymes, and raw materials of some organs, such as liver) to the patient. The theory behind use of **glandular therapy (glandulars)** is that

TABLE 23-1	Commonly Used Nutraceuticals	
NUTRIENT	**PRIMARY TARGET AREA(S)**	**FUNCTION**
Glucosamine chondroitin Perna mussel Hyaluronate Cetyl myristoleate	Joints	Promote joint lubrication Reduce progression of or prevent arthritis Reduce pain and improve mobility
Shark and bovine cartilage	Joints Cancer	Reduce pain and improve mobility Anticancer function (shark cartilage is significantly more potent)
Methyl sulfonyl methane (MSM)	Muscle	Supports muscle function and metabolism
S-Adenosyl methionine (SAM-e)	Liver	Antioxidant
Coenzyme Q10	Heart, gingiva	Antioxidant: reduces free radical damage
Taurine	Heart, eye	Amino acid—used when deficiency occurs
L-Carnitine	Heart	Antioxidant/free radical scavenger
Superoxide dismutase Vitamin E/Selenium Vitamin C Vitamin A	Whole body	Antioxidants/free radical scavengers
Essential fatty acids	Skin (also other tissues)	Inhibit inflammation

CASE PRESENTATION 23-1 FELINE GASTROINTESTINAL DISEASE

Signalment: Ivy, a 1-year-old spayed female domestic medium-hair cat, 5½ lb

Chief Complaint: Soft stool and diarrhea of 6 weeks' duration

Pertinent History: Ivy was rescued from an animal shelter 6 weeks before presentation and had always had soft stool. She had been vaccinated and dewormed 3 times while at the shelter. When she was spayed, she was found to have two mummified kittens in utero with a pyometra. She recovered nicely after surgery, but her stool became worse. The diarrhea was soft-serve consistency, foul-smelling, and voluminous. Fortunately, normal frequency without straining was evident, and she consistently used her litter box.

A fecal examination was negative for parasites. Her diet initially consisted of dry and canned premium brand cat food. Although she ate voraciously in a large quantity for her size (½ cup dry plus 2 tbsp canned bid), she had not gained weight since she had been rescued. A prescription diet (canned and dry, then canned only) for GI sensitivity had been tried for 3 days, but no improvement was noted, and Ivy began vomiting (partially digested food). Ivy had not been adopted to a permanent home because of her ongoing GI issues.

Significant Examination Findings: Ivy was quite thin (body condition score 3/9), and her hair coat was unthrifty (dull and brittle). Her intestines were palpably thickened. No further abnormalities were found.

PROBLEM LIST	DIFFERENTIAL DIAGNOSIS
Chronic small intestinal diarrhea (localized based on volume, frequency)	Parasites, small intestinal bacterial overgrowth (SIBO), inflammatory bowel disease, food allergy, foreign body, infection, exocrine pancreatic insufficiency (EPI), neoplasia
Thickened intestinal walls	Parasites, inflammatory bowel disease, infection, neoplasia
Vomiting	Parasites, small intestinal bacterial overgrowth (SIBO), inflammatory bowel disease, food allergy, foreign body, infection, EPI, neoplasia
Thin body condition	Secondary to GI disease

Client Communication: Ivy's initial presentation made a definitive diagnosis difficult. A thorough workup would be pursued, and diet change and treatment would be initiated while results were pending. A fasting blood sample was drawn for a CBC and chemistry panel, with additional serum saved for further testing if indicated.

Initial Treatment Plan: Ivy was started on GI Encaps (Thorne Research Inc.; contains plantain, slippery elm, marshmallow, licorice), ½ capsule daily to soothe her GI tract; and Prozyme Plus (Prozyme Products; contains rice starch, lipase, amylase, protease, cellulase, and lactase), ⅛ tsp added to each meal. Her diet was transitioned to a limited ingredient canned food with duck protein source over a period of 3 days.

Initial Diagnostic Plan and Results (in order):
- Fecal parasite examination: negative
- CBC, comprehensive chemistry profile: within normal limits, except borderline low albumin
- Fecal culture: negative
- *Giardia* titer: negative
- TLI (trypsin-like immunoreactivity, a test for EPI): within normal limits
- Cobalamin and folate levels: slightly low cobalamin, folate levels normal (diagnostic for SIBO)
- Abdominal radiographs: within normal limits, except for thickening in the walls of the small intestine

Working Diagnosis: SIBO of unknown cause

Progress and Revised Treatment Plan: Ivy responded favorably to her initial therapy (she stopped vomiting), but her stool remained soft, and she did not gain weight. Rather than pursue an immediate exploratory surgery with biopsies, we elected to transition Ivy to a raw diet. She was adopted to a home (mine) where her special dietary needs could be met consistently. Ivy was initially fed 2 tbsp of raw chicken breast 3 times daily and was monitored for adverse reactions (vomiting, worsening diarrhea). She was enthusiastic about her new diet and tolerated it well. Her stool started to become firmer after 3 days. At that point, chicken wings were introduced to try to transition her to whole food. This also was well tolerated. Because we would keep Ivy on a limited ingredient diet for several weeks, she was started on Thorne Feline Basic Nutrients Multivitamins (1 capsule daily), which she ate readily. GI Encaps were discontinued, but she remained on Prozyme Plus.

Two weeks later, Ivy had normal stool and had gained 1 lb. She regained a healthy weight within 2 more weeks and was transitioned to a more balanced diet, including a small quantity of pureed vegetables. After several months, an "accidental" trial of commercial dry cat food resulted in no adverse effects, and she currently maintains a healthy to generous weight on a dry food and raw chicken diet (fed at separate meals). Her diarrhea never recurred, and she has no health problems to date (6 years later).

Discussion: Ivy's GI issues likely were caused by a combination of a significant diet change (she was found as a stray on the streets of Milwaukee) and chronic infection (pyometra). Her workup, as with so many small animals with diarrhea, ruled out some problems but never resulted in a definitive diagnosis. Although exploratory surgery with an intestinal biopsy likely would have yielded more information and possibly a definitive pathologic and histologic diagnosis, the cause would likely remain unknown. Traditional practice and therapy would have possibly included antibiotic therapy, metronidazole, or steroids and a limited or single-ingredient diet (food trial). Fortunately, a simple diet change with a single, highly digestible protein was enough to help Ivy's body rebalance her GI tract and heal (Figure 1). It is interesting to note that cats, unlike dogs, are obligate carnivores, meaning that they must have meat in their diet and can lead a healthy life without grains or even vegetables as long as vitamins and minerals are properly supplemented.

Whereas cooked, nonprocessed meat may have been a reasonable alternative, raw meat is more digestible. Part of

Continued

CASE PRESENTATION 23-1 FELINE GASTROINTESTINAL DISEASE—cont'd

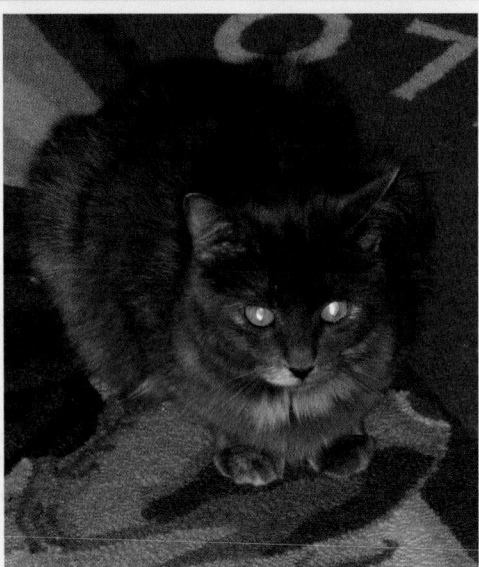

FIGURE 1 Ivy is now the picture of perfect health.

my motivation to try a raw versus cooked diet with this cat was that my staff was quite skeptical about it at the time, and because she was kept at our clinic throughout this entire period, they were aware of the remarkable improvement in her health in a short time after more conventional approaches had led to more problems (vomiting). The most significant change, and the one most indicative of a "cure," was that Ivy is now able to eat just about anything (including stolen strawberries and asparagus) and thrives on a diet now full of variety, including the dry food that she originally ate.

Principle components of the veterinary technician plan of care included:

1. Provision of prescribed dietary supplements and diets as per order.
2. Monitoring stool appearance and consistency, appetite, body condition and weight changes.
3. Monitoring for vomiting and changes in hydration status.
4. Collection, submission and analysis of blood and stool samples as per order.
5. Collection of radiographs as per order.

If Ivy had been adopted by a client, nutritional counseling and follow-up communication would have been carried out by the veterinary technician as part of the technician plan of care.

---

if sources of whole tissue are provided to a patient with a dysfunctional or suboptimally functioning organ or gland, the patient will receive the necessary substances to improve function and in some cases heal his or her own diseased tissue. A good example of this is providing a product that contains bovine thyroid gland for a patient with a borderline low thyroid level.

As with any food ingredient, it is important to have a reputable source for these products because they are made from animal products. A handful of companies in the United States use human grade ingredients in their products and have rigorously standardized and tested their products. These companies often provide guidelines for dosing and administration to animals. One company is now making products specifically for dogs and cats, using a powdered form that is highly palatable. This type of therapy sometimes presents a moral and ethical dilemma for holistic practitioners because of animal use, but the more reputable companies try to be as ethical and humane as possible in their formulations.

Veterinary technicians should be familiar with the glandular-type and nutraceutical products used within the practice. In addition, technicians should be aware of the various types of commercial and home-cooked diets that are appropriate and inappropriate for patients. Finally, technicians should understand and be prepared to explain the veterinarian's recommendations and the rationale for them.

HERBAL MEDICINE

Herbal or botanical medicine refers to the practice of using plant materials (including flowers, stems, leaves, bark, seeds, roots) to treat patients. Herbal medicine is the most ancient known medicine and the foundation of modern medicine. Using plants as medicine predated written communication, and evidence of the use of plants in ancient cultures is widespread. Herbal medicine is still a large practice in the world today, with an estimated 80% of the world's population using this form of therapy as a primary means of health care. Even today, about 20% of our drugs are derived from a plant source. The technician should become familiar with the herbal pharmacy, just as he or she knows about the drugs on the shelf.

Information about the medicinal use of herbs can be found in the *Materia Medica*, which is similar to a drug formulary.

> **TECHNICIAN NOTE**   Herbs tend to be less toxic than drugs because the therapeutic substances are not as concentrated. Plants also contain other substances that can act synergistically with the active compound. However, herbs are not to be used carelessly. Many herbs are extremely safe at many times the therapeutic dose, but others, similar to some drugs, have a low margin of safety.

Many medicinal herbs have not been proven safe in pregnancy, and some are toxic to cats. This is important to remember because many clients equate herbs with complete safety; they need to be educated on their proper use and side effects, just as they should with any medication prescribed.

In the United States, herbs are regulated as a food because they are natural substances and cannot be "owned." Currently, we rely mainly on testing based in Europe and Asia to substantiate the effects of individual herbs, although one company researches and markets *combinations* of herbs, which may be patented under U.S. Food and Drug Administration (FDA) regulations. Unfortunately, this does nothing to assure us of the quality or purity of the products because of the lack of FDA regulation. Therefore, the herbal practitioner must be cautious about the source of prescribed herbs. This is another issue that must be emphasized to clients, who often do not understand the difference between medication purchased at the practice and the bottle they buy at the local supercenter.

If practicing with a veterinarian who uses therapeutic herbs, the veterinary technician should be familiar with commonly used preparations and should be able to properly prepare and dispense them. As with all practices, veterinary technicians are responsible for client education and for reviewing home-care instructions with the pet owner.

WESTERN HERBS

Western herbs are now more commonly used in veterinary medicine. With the holistic movement in human medicine, most people are now familiar with products such as echinacea, ginseng, and St. John's wort. In fact, one company has patented a milk thistle and *S*-adenosyl methionine (SAM-e) combination product for use in dogs and cats with liver disease. Proper dosing and administration for animals have not been scientifically proven in most cases, but doses for the more commonly used herbs have been fairly well established.

Herbs come in many different forms (Figure 23-1), and each has advantages and disadvantages when used in animal species. Bulk herbs are the most commonly used preparation

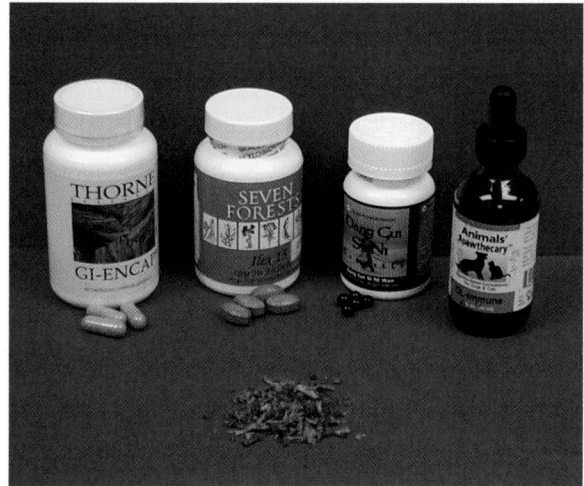

FIGURE 23-1 Commonly used herbal preparations. *Clockwise, left to right:* capsules, tablets, tea pills, liquid, dried herbs (foreground).

for herbivores. The product is often dried and prepared (chopped or powdered). Some of the tastier herbs are administered to carnivores in this form. Capsules and tablets are often used for carnivores because they are more easily disguised. Teas are prepared by straining the herbs into water. Herbs are fairly easy to prepare but are not always readily accepted by animals (depending on the patient and the herb). Extracts are made by concentrating the herb in alcohol or glycerin. A standardized extract is much like a drug in that a specific amount of active ingredient is measured rather than measurement of the herb itself. Milk thistle, for example, is often sold as a standardized extract containing 70% silymarin. Poultices and compresses are used topically for short periods. They are made by soaking the herb or extract in hot water, then allowing it to cool. The product is then held in place manually or with gauze for a short period. Ointments are used topically and generally are left in place. Essential oils may be used topically; some can be taken internally in extremely dilute form. They are concentrated and must be used cautiously.

Many herbs can be useful in combination. Some companies produce excellent and safe herbal combination products for animals. Be cautious, however, of combination formulas listed as "proprietary blend" because you do not know the exact dose of each herb in the formula, and patient safety could be at risk. Another precaution involves using herbals and medications that achieve the same effect (i.e., anti-inflammatory), because of increased risk for adverse effects.

> **TECHNICIAN NOTE** The use of herbs is not limited to symptomatic treatment.

Herbs may be used to support the general health of the patient (known as *tonification*). When used in this way, herbs are taken over a long time. Ginkgo is often used in this way to support mental function in geriatric patients. Herbs may be used in detoxification, as when milk thistle is used to help protect and support the liver after steroid therapy (Table 23-2).

Most herbs are generally best administered on an empty stomach. For herbivores, this may be impossible. The next best way to administer herbs is with a small amount of water. Sometimes salt-free broth or clam juice works well for small animals. If food is the only way to get the herb to the patient, try to avoid giving the herb with a full meal. It is also best to avoid any food with strong flavor, such as peppermint, near the time of administration.

CHINESE HERBAL MEDICINE

Chinese herbs actually consist of many substances, including minerals and animal tissue. Individual botanical herbs may be used in the same way that Western herbs are used. Some overlap has been noted between Chinese and Western herbs. The main difference between the two is the use of **traditional Chinese medicine** (**TCM**) in a patient's diagnosis and treatment with Chinese herbs.

The Chinese herbal practitioner must have a clear TCM diagnosis when prescribing an herbal therapy. The TCM

TABLE 23-2	Commonly Used Western Herbs and Their Therapeutic Uses		
COMMON NAME	**SCIENTIFIC NAME**	**ACTIVE PARTS**	**INDICATIONS/AFFINITY**
Aloe	*Aloe vera*	Gel layer of leaf	Skin irritation (topical)
Cranberry	*Vaccinium macrocarpon*	Fruit	Urinary tract infection
Dandelion	*Taraxacum officinale*	Root (whole plant)	Diuretic
Echinacea	*Echinacea purpurea*	Whole plant	Immune support
Eyebright	*Euphrasia officinalis*	Whole plant	Eye irritation (topical)
Ginkgo	*Ginkgo biloba*	Leaves	Promotes mental alertness
Hawthorn	*Crataegus laevigata*	Leaves, berries, blossoms	Supports heart function
Milk thistle	*Silybum marianum*	Seeds, fruit, leaves	Liver support, detoxification
Slippery elm	*Ulmus fulva*	Bark	Soothes the GI tract
Valerian	*Valerian officinalis*	Root	Anxiety, sleep disorders

TABLE 23-3	Common Ingredients in Chinese Herbal Preparations			
CHINESE NAME	**COMMON NAME**	**SCIENTIFIC NAME**	**INDICATIONS TCM**	**INDICATIONS WESTERN**
Sheng jiang	Ginger	*Zingiber officinale*	Regulates stomach qi	Nausea
Ma huang	Ephedra	*Ephedra sinica*	Dispels wind cold	Bronchitis, asthma
Huang lian	Coptis	*Coptis japonica*	Clears damp heat	Inflammation
Sheng di huang	Rehmannia	*Rehmannia glutinosa*	Nourishes yin	Adrenal, liver support
Chi shao	Red peony	*Paeonia rubra*	Invigorates blood	Pain
Tang kuei	Angelica	*Angelica sinensis*	Nourishes blood	Itching
Wu rong	Maitake	*Grifola frondosa*	Enhances qi	Cancer (immune stimulation)
Yunnan paiyao	(Proprietary blend)		Stops bleeding	Hemorrhage

TCM, Traditional Chinese medicine.

examination includes a detailed history and tongue and pulse diagnosis. The diagnosis is more descriptive of the condition of the body than of anatomic disease or causes of disease. For example, an exterior cold excess pattern would describe the common cold, which in Western terms would be referred to as a viral upper respiratory tract infection.

For example, the herb ma huang, or ephedra, is used to "disperse congestion in the lung" and "release the exterior." In terms of TCM, the patient may be diagnosed with an exterior cold excess pattern of disease. In terms of our knowledge of pharmacology, this substance dries mucous membranes, and derivatives are used to treat the common cold, which is an exterior pathogen.

Herbal medicine is considered "stronger" than acupuncture. Practitioners often use the properties and taste of the herbs to choose the most appropriate herb or formula. Most TCM practitioners in China use acupuncture only in acute cases and prescribe herbs along with it to bring about more thorough treatment. Often for more chronic conditions or to help patients maintain health, herbs alone are used.

The formulas are named for their function or their main ingredients. Unlike Western herbs, each herbal formula is generally a combination of several products that work together to bring about an effect. It is a much more complex system than the Western approach. Certain herbs are found in many common formulas (Table 23-3). For this reason, the practitioner using Chinese herbs should undertake formal training. Forms are similar to Western preparations (see Figure 23-1), including tablets and pills, powders, granules,

liquid teas and extracts, and topical preparations (ointments, plasters, and liniments). Many of the formulas come in tiny tablets known as *tea pills.* These are handy for use in treating cats, but large dogs may require 10 or more pills per dose.

As with Western herbs, and perhaps even more important, herbs must come from a reputable source that ensures quality control. The use of animal products in many formulations makes this a more serious concern. Several companies in the United States distribute products of uniform quality that are produced under the most ethical circumstances possible (e.g., some animal products from endangered species are substituted with a similar product from a related domestic animal). For some holistic practitioners, the use of animal products may result in a moral dilemma, and these veterinarians may choose to avoid having these products in their pharmacy.

AYURVEDIC HERBS

Ayurveda means "the science of life." Similar to TCM, it emphasizes health and wellness, not just treatment of disease. It originated in India and is believed to predate TCM and even to have contributed to its foundation. It includes not only herbal prescriptions, but also diet, **massage**, exercise, and meditation as part of a patient's therapy. The goal of **ayurvedic medicine** is to balance the three elements of nature, known as *Doshas,* which exist in every living organism.

As with Chinese herbs, ayurvedic herbs may be prescribed on the basis of pharmacology (similarly to Western herbs), according to the three Doshas (similar to TCM yin, yang, and

TABLE 23-4	Common Ingredients in Ayurvedic Herbal Formulas		
COMMON NAME	**SCIENTIFIC NAME**	**INDICATIONS AYURVEDA**	**INDICATIONS WESTERN**
Ashwagandha	*Withania somnifera*	Balances vata and kapha	Fatigue, skin disease
Boswellia	*Boswellia serrata*	Balances vata and kapha	Arthritis (anti-inflammatory)
Cinnamon	*Cinnamomum zeylanicum*	Reduces vata and kapha	Digestive disorders
Licorice	*Glycyrrhiza glabra*	Pacifies vata and pitta	Soothes urinary and GI tracts
Neem	*Azadirachta indica*	Antiseptic	Wounds, rashes
Shatavari	*Asparagus racemosus*	Balances vata and pitta	Bladder infection
Turmeric	*Curcuma longa*	Reduces kapha	Arthritis, liver support

qi), or on the basis of taste and temperature. For example, licorice is considered a sweet herb. Sweet herbs are considered to be cold and wet and are used to nourish and soothe. In terms of pharmacology, licorice reduces the breakdown of prostaglandin, which protects the stomach from excess acid. Thus it is a treatment for stomach ulcers, which cause a burning sensation. Ayurvedic herbs tend to be provided in formulations of multiple ingredients and, like Chinese herbs, some ingredients are commonly found in multiple formulations (Table 23-4).

> **TECHNICIAN NOTE** The veterinary technician who works with a veterinarian who treats patients using herbal therapies should be familiar with the more commonly used herbs: indications, contraindications, precautions, and appropriate dosing. Awareness of common herb-drug interactions is also important.

The veterinary technician may be asked to prepare the herbal formula, to administer, to dispense, and to explain a prescribed formula to the client. This requires thorough knowledge of the herbal pharmacy.

AROMATHERAPY

Aromatherapy is the therapeutic use of volatile essential oils to obtain a physiologic or psychological effect (Table 23-5). Oils are distilled or extracted from plants and are considered the "last possible and most sublime" parts of the plant. Flowers, buds, fruits, peels, leaves, bark, wood, roots, and seeds can be used. Oils can be applied topically by themselves or in a massage oil, ingested (not common), or administered by nebulization (the oil is made into a mist and inhaled). The effect of inhalation is most likely due to rapid absorption by both nasal and lung mucosae. Plants or parts of plants can be burned and the smoke inhaled. Potential uses of aromatherapy include antibacterial and antifungal uses (tea tree oil and thyme oil), relaxation or sedation (lavender oil), behavior modification (positive or negative), conditioning (citronella bark collars), and medicinal purposes.

> **TECHNICIAN NOTE** The role of the veterinary technician in aromatherapy is to apply oils at the recommendation of the veterinarian while having a basic knowledge of their treatment purpose and being able to discuss their use and benefits.

> **TECHNICIAN NOTE** Lavender is a commonly used essential oil. It can be applied topically to the head for calming effects and on cuts, burns, insect bites, and abrasions to speed healing.

HOMEOPATHY, HOMOTOXICOLOGY, AND FLOWER ESSENCES

Homeopathy is a system of medicine that is based on the principle that "like cures like." It involves treating each patient as an individual based on his or her group of symptoms. Practitioners use extremely diluted versions of herbs and other substances, which are called *remedies*, to treat patients. It is sometimes difficult to understand, but this system can generate amazing results when used by a skilled practitioner. Homotoxicology and flower essence therapies are similar in practice but often can be easily practiced by a veterinarian with basic knowledge and understanding.

HISTORY AND PRINCIPLES

Samuel Hahnemann, a German physician, first used and developed homeopathy in the late 1700s. At that time, medications were given to patients with no assurance of safety. The scientific process as we know it did not exist, and trial and error determined which substances would be good medications. Quinine was being used to treat patients with malaria but often caused as much harm as good. Hahnemann ultimately recognized that symptoms of disease were expressions of the body's attempt to restore homeostasis in response to an imbalance or insult.

The initial postulate was that giving a patient a medication that simulates the disease would stimulate the body's own defenses, and the patient would heal. This is similar to, although not completely the same as, the principle of vaccination. It is the reverse of allopathic (or Western or modern) medicine, which uses drugs to counteract symptoms, thereby suppressing them. For example, if cortisone is used to treat a rash, the symptoms will return, sometimes with greater intensity, if the treatment is not repeated for many days. Later, a more serious disease, such as a stomach ulcer, may develop. Western medicine would consider the two conditions to be unrelated, but a homeopath considers them both to be signs of disorder in the body.

TABLE 23-5	Common Aroma Therapy Oils and Their Uses			
HOW APPLIED	**ACTION**	**INDICATIONS**	**CHEMICAL CONSTITUENTS**	**CONTRAINDICATIONS**
Basil Temples, navel and chest, insect stings and bites, inhale or add to food	Antispasmodic, anti-infectious, antiviral, anti-inflammatory, antibacterial, and decongestant	Gastroenteritis, lethargy, relax muscle, soothe insect bites, stimulate sense of smell, may help bronchitis	Methyl chavicol, linalool, terpene alcohol, terpene esters, phenols, ketones, camphor, oxides	Epilepsy, skin test for sensitivity
Birch Dilute with oil for massage, add to bath water	Analgesic, antispasmodic, anti-inflammatory, liver stimulant, supports bone function	Arthritis, inflammation, muscular pain, tendonitis, hypertension, cramps, cystitis	Esters, methyl salicylate	Topical use only, do not use in cats, skin test for sensitivity, epilepsy
Chamomile (German) Diffuse topical, dietary supplement	Sedating, calming, antispasmodic, anti-inflammatory, decongestant; supports digestive, liver, and gallbladder function; reduces scarring, relieves allergies	Insomnia, nervous tension, bursitis, tendonitis, dermatitis, liver and gallbladder disease, inflammatory bowel disease	Sesquiterpenes, sesquiterpenols, sesquiterpene oxides, sesquiterpene lactones, coumarins, ethers	Nontoxic
Cinnamon Diffuse topical, dietary supplement	Antimicrobial, anti-infectious, antiviral, antifungal *(Candida)*, antibacterial, circulatory stimulant	External parasites, dental problems, pneumonia	Ethers, eugenols, cinnamaldehyde	Repeated topical use can result in extreme contact sensitization; diffuse with caution because it may irritate the nasal membrane
Cypress Topical	Improves circulation, supports nerves and intestines, anti-infectious	Arthritis, bronchitis, intestinal parasites, pulmonary infection, spasms	Monoterpenes, sesquiterpenols, diterpenols	Nontoxic
Lavender Diffuse topical, dietary supplement	Antiseptic, analgesic, antitumoral, anticonvulsant, sedative, anti-inflammatory	Burns, cuts, and abrasions; allergies, seizures, insomnia, inflammatory skin lesions, depression, hives, insect bites, nervous tension	Monoterpenes, sesquiterpenes, esters, lavandula, ketones, sesquiterpenones, aldehydes, lactones	Nontoxic
Lemon Diffuse or add a few drops to water and spray air; dietary supplement	Anti-infectious, disinfectant, antibacterial, antiseptic, antiviral, vitamin C–like action to improve microcirculation, enhance immune function	Anemia, asthma, promote leukocyte formation, digestive problems, respiratory infection, strengthens nails, insect repellent	Monoterpenes, sesquiterpenes, aldehydes	Very photosensitizing (avoid applying to skin that will be exposed to the sun)

TABLE 23-5	Common Aroma Therapy Oils and Their Uses—cont'd			
HOW APPLIED	**ACTION**	**INDICATIONS**	**CHEMICAL CONSTITUENTS**	**CONTRAINDICATIONS**
Peppermint Diffuse topical (massage on stomach for upset or temples for headache), dietary supplement	Anticarcinogenic, supports digestion, expels worms, decongestant, anti-infectious, antibacterial, antifungal, mucolytic, stimulant, stimulates gallbladder, expectorant, stimulates sense of taste	Gastroenteritis, colic, inflammatory bowel disease, diarrhea, fever, motion sickness, bronchitis, asthma, headaches when applied topically, cough	Monoterpenes, monoterpenols, monoterpenones, terpene oxides, terpene esters, coumarins	Avoid contact with the eyes, mucous membranes, or sensitive skin areas. Do not apply to a fresh wound or burn. Neurotoxic (respiratory depressant, convulsant), cardiac dysrhythmias
Rosemary Diffuse topical, dietary supplement	Mucolytic, expectorant, antispasmodic, antibacterial, antiseptic, neurologic stimulant	Respiratory infection, bronchitis, nervous tension, cystitis, arthritis, dry or erythematous skin	Monoterpenes, sesquiterpenes, monoterpenols, terpene esters, terpene oxides, monoterpenones	Epilepsy
Thyme Dilute topical	Antimicrobial, antifungal, antiviral	Pneumonia, asthma, gastroenteritis, skin and oral infections	Monoterpenols, terpene esters	Dermal and mucous membrane irritant
Valerian Diffuse topical, dietary supplement	Sedative to the central nervous system	Restlessness, sleep disturbances, nervousness, tension	Monoterpenes, sesquiterpenes, monoterpenols, terpene esters, sesquiterpenols, sesquiterpenones	Repeated use can result in contact sensitization

Note: If the animal is pregnant or is nursing, oils should be used only with the veterinarian's consent. Many of these oils have not been tested on pregnant or nursing animals. Cats are more sensitive to most oils, and caution should be used when applying. Some oils that are therapeutic for dogs are toxic to cats.

Hahnemann discovered that the more he diluted medicine, the stronger the beneficial effects became, whereas the harmful effects diminished or disappeared altogether. Although most physicians were concerned with treating one symptom, the "chief complaint" as we know it, he astutely observed that these medications had multiple effects on the body (some beneficial, some harmful, and some neutral). He decided to try his medications on healthy patients to see if they caused the symptoms of illness. For example, a healthy patient who took cold medicine might experience dry nose and throat, in addition to drowsiness or even inability to sleep, depending on the drug combination given. Hahnemann recorded the effects that his medicines had on healthy patients and noted in detail all physical and emotional changes. This practice is known today as a *proving*.

One of Hahnemann's beliefs was that medication should closely match the specific symptoms of each patient. No two persons exhibit the same symptoms, even though they may have the same virus. Many people exhibit the same cold symptoms each time they are sick, regardless of the strain of

the virus. Hahnemann therefore chose medications that mimicked his patients' specific emotional and physical symptoms and in this way was able to establish a precise method of choosing a medicine for each individual patient. Because of the safety and efficacy of his highly diluted preparations, others sought to learn how to treat patients in this manner. Hahnemann recorded his philosophy and findings in a book entitled *The Organon of Medicine*. Homeopathy is still widely practiced today in Europe, although less so in the United States. The earliest mention of veterinary homeopathy came from Hahnemann himself, when he stated in a lecture in the early 1800s that a similar approach could be applied to animals. Today, organizations and courses are available worldwide for veterinarians who would like to practice homeopathic medicine.

PRACTICE

When a patient is seen by a homeopathic practitioner, a clear and detailed history is essential for a successful outcome. The owner is asked many questions, some of which may seem minute and unimportant. Any previous diagnostics and therapies (and responses) should be noted, even for minor problems. The patient is observed, and details about his or her physical status and personality and reactions to certain situations are noted and recorded. This should always include a thorough "Western" physical examination because these findings may lead to symptoms not discovered by the owner (such as a fast heart rate). The veterinarian may also note something of a serious nature that may need a "Western" approach before using homeopathy. For example, an older patient in congestive heart failure that comes to the hospital dyspneic and cyanotic needs to be stabilized first. Once out of a life-threatening situation, the patient can be evaluated, and a more long-term approach can be taken.

Minute details can be important when patients are treated homeopathically. Even the way the patient greets the veterinarian can be important in finding the correct remedy. All details are recorded, and a list of remedies that are appropriate for each sign or symptom is compiled. This is called *repertorizing*. From this list, the most appropriate remedy is prescribed. In modern times, much of this work can be done by computer, although some practitioners still do all of their research by hand. The remedy is then dispensed to the owner with specific instructions on dosage and administration.

> **TECHNICIAN NOTE** It is important that the remedy be handled properly and given exactly as directed.

Homeopathic remedies are available in several strengths, called *potencies*. Potency is inversely proportional to dilution: the less actual substance present, the stronger the medicine. In general, it is best to use the lowest potency (or least dilute) necessary to bring about a cure. Sometimes the dose will be given only once, sometimes multiple times. The remedy should be discontinued when symptoms cease or the patient shows improvement. Occasionally, a patient will experience an exacerbation of symptoms, called an *aggravation*. This usually passes within a few hours and generally is not a matter of concern. Usually, it indicates that the correct remedy was chosen, but if the patient becomes weaker, an "antidote" (another remedy) to the prescribed remedy can be given. Antidotes to each remedy are listed in the *Materia Medica*.

Homeopathic remedies are fragile compared with Western medications and are available in several forms (Figure 23-2, Table 23-6). They should not be touched and should be administered away from food, whenever possible. The remedy is effective as soon as it gets into the mouth; as long as it touches the lips, gums, or tongue, it does not need to be swallowed. Remedies should never be returned to the bottle. They should be stored at room temperature away from moisture (keep container sealed) in a dark place, preferably in a cabinet away from strong herbs, Western medication, and magnetic fields (microwaves, computers, stereo speakers).

Homeopaths believe that things that suppress symptoms actually drive disease deeper into the body, or create greater

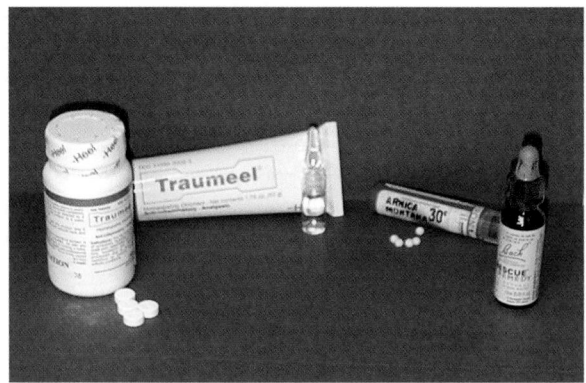

FIGURE 23-2 Homeopathic preparations. *Clockwise, left to right:* tablets, ointment, injectable (foreground), pellets, liquid (flower essence).

TABLE 23-6	Homeopathic Preparations
FORM	**ADMINISTRATION**
Pellets (sugar) or tablets	Use whole (dispense from cap into the patient's mouth, avoiding contaminating the cap) or crush between a folded sheet of paper
	Pour into patient's mouth or drop between lips and gum
	Can also be dissolved in distilled or spring water and administered by dropper
Liquid	Use dropper and apply on tongue or between cheek and gum
Topical injections	Apply to affected area
	May be used SQ, IM, intralesion
	Often used at acupuncture points

imbalance. Depending on how "deep" or serious the disorder is, a succession of several remedies may be required to restore a patient to health. Changes in symptoms are noted, and a new remedy is chosen until the patient is healthy.

> **TECHNICIAN NOTE** A disorder that may seem minor by traditional medicine may actually be quite serious from a homeopathic perspective. Similarly, a patient may be considered healthy by Western standards but may still be imbalanced and thus in need of further treatment when undergoing homeopathic treatment.

Homeopathy can be used at many levels. The least complex is as treatment for acute disease, which should quickly restore health to a vital, strong patient. An example of this is the use of *Arnica montana* to treat a patient with bruising from trauma. Several remedies are fairly easily used in acute situations, even without extensive training (Table 23-7). Next is treatment on a constitutional level, which takes into account the nature (physical traits, personality, emotions) of the patient and the "disease" symptoms, past and present. The goal is to help the patient recover and maintain a state of health. The most complex is miasmic treatment, in

TABLE 23-7	Commonly Used Single Homeopathic Remedies for Acute Use
REMEDY	**SYMPTOMS**
Arnica	Bruising, bleeding
Calendula	Topical for skin irritation
Ledum	Hives, stings
Nux Vomica	Vomiting
Pulsatilla	Purulent discharge
Thuja	Vaccine reaction

TABLE 23-8	Commonly Used Homotoxicology Products and Their Indications	
PRODUCT	**INDICATIONS**	**MAIN INGREDIENTS**
Discus Compositum	Sciatica, hindlimb weakness	*Berberis, cimifuga, colocynthis*
Spascupreel	Muscle spasm	*Aconitum, colocynthis, atropinum*
Traumeel	Inflammation, pain	*Arnica, aconitum, belladonna*
Vertigoheel	Vestibular issues	*Cocculus, coneum*
Zeel	Arthritis	*Silicea, arnica, Rhus tox*

which the ultimate goal of therapy is to prevent disease by addressing genetic weaknesses. This is very challenging in the veterinary patient and therefore is not often undertaken.

Homeopathy can be further divided into classical homeopathy, in which the patient is treated with one remedy at a time, and modern homeopathy, in which the patient is given a combination of remedies to match his or her given set of symptoms. Homotoxicology is the most commonly used form of combination homeopathy in veterinary medicine. The remedies are compounded using the most commonly indicated remedies to treat a specific set of symptoms, such as low back pain. This alleviates the need to repertorize and choose one remedy (Table 23-8).

The combination therapy can be used in a more "Western" approach. For example, Traumeel (see Figure 23-2) is a commonly used treatment for bruising, trauma, inflammation, and arthritis. It comes in several forms (oral tablets and liquid, injectable, and cream) and contains arnica, calendula, echinacea, and several other individual remedies that work together to provide the desired effect.

From a scientific standpoint, much research has investigated the use of homeopathy. The individualized nature of the treatments can make effectiveness difficult to "prove" from a Western standpoint, but many double-blind placebo-controlled studies have been conducted. Research on the biphasic nature of medication has assisted our understanding of how diluted forms of medication can have the opposite effect of the therapeutic dose of the same medicine on the body. For example, a clinical dose of atropine causes drying of mucous membranes, but a tiny dose has been shown to increase secretions of mucous membranes. Both in vitro and clinical studies have shown homeopathic remedies to be effective, but thus far we do not understand exactly how they work.

FLOWER ESSENCES

Flower essence therapy, developed by Edward Bach in the 1930s, uses an approach similar to that of homeopathy to treat patients. Bach believed that all substances used to treat patients should be completely nontoxic, even in undiluted form. He developed 37 essences derived from plants (flowers, bushes, trees) and 1 derived from water (rock water) for a total of 38 remedies (Table 23-9). These essences are not diluted to the extent that homeopathic remedies are.

Use of flower essences is based more on a psychological or emotional than physical level. Bach himself described 12 pathologic emotional states that he believed would lead to physical disease if left untreated. For example, the remedy Aspen is used to treat patients with fear of the unknown, and holly is used to treat patients exhibiting jealousy or suspiciousness. Of course, the emotional nature of animals can be difficult to determine, but this approach is not unreasonable and can be highly rewarding. Flower essences may, like homeopathy, be used in acute situations as well as to treat patients on a constitutional basis.

All individual essences are provided as a liquid. The remedy most commonly used is called *Rescue Remedy* (see Figure 23-2), and it is a combination of five flower essences (rock rose, cherry plum, star of Bethlehem, clematis, impatiens). The preparation may also be found in a cream. It is used to treat animals in times of stress, anxiety, or trauma. For those interested in using flower essences, Rescue Remedy is an excellent starting point and can be used in such situations as trauma or surgery recovery, or even for the frightened and panic-stricken boarding patient. These remedies are administered similarly to homeopathic remedies, but they are generally sold in stock bottles. The stock flower remedy should be diluted in spring water or in a combination of water and alcohol (increases shelf life) to make a treatment bottle. Generally, 2 drops of each stock remedy (4 if using Rescue Remedy) are placed in a 1-ounce glass amber vial with a dropper. Up to five remedies may be combined in a single treatment bottle (Rescue Remedy counts as a single remedy). Remedies are given by dropper directly into the mouth. They may also be added to drinking water (from a few drops in a bowl for a cat to 15 drops per gallon for a horse). Another method is to give the remedy in a spray bottle as a mist (usually into the environment), which is an effective and stress-free means of treating birds and small mammals. It can also be used topically. Administration is generally repeated at various intervals. In an acute situation, this may be as often as every 30 seconds. For a less urgent situation, it may be daily for several days or weeks. Flower essences and homeopathic remedies should be stored similarly.

These flower remedies, like their homeopathic counterparts, are safe to use and can have a profound effect on a

TABLE 23-9	Basic Flower Essences and Their Uses
ESSENCE	**INDICATIONS**
Rescue Remedy	Shock, trauma, stress
Cherry plum	Panic, loss of control
Clematis	Lack of responsiveness
Impatiens	Impatience, irritability
Rock rose	Extreme fear
Star of Bethlehem	Shock, trauma
Agrimony	Prolonged grief, moping, and withdrawing
Aspen	Fear of unknown things (strangers)
Beech	Intolerance, rigidness
Centaury	Submissiveness, timidness
Cerato	Indecisiveness (need constant reassurance)
Chestnut bud	Repetitive actions (helps break bad habits)
Chicory	Possessiveness (separation anxiety)
Crab apple	Detoxification
Elm	Overwhelming stress (of working, competing, travel)
Gentian	Depression
Gorse	Hopelessness
Heather	Attention-seeking behavior (constant barking, whining)
Holly	Jealousy, especially when aggressive or spiteful
Honeysuckle	Grief, homesickness
Hornbeam	Helps adjust to changes
Larch	Lack of confidence
Mimulus	Fear of known things (thunderstorms)
Mustard	Mood swings, depression, gloom
Oak	Workaholic (overworks to exhaustion)
Olive	Lack of energy, exhaustion
Pine	Excessive grief, rejection, guilt
Red chestnut	Worry, overprotectiveness
Rock water	Inflexibility
Scleranthus	Indecision with mood swings, motion sickness
Sweet chestnut	Extreme stress, mental anguish
Vervain	Excessive enthusiasm, hyperactivity
Vine	Aggression, dominance
Walnut	Stress as a result of change
Water violet	Aloofness, withdrawal
White chestnut	Restlessness, repetitive thoughts
Wild oat	Frustration, boredom, lack of concentration
Wild rose	Apathy, resignation
Willow	Resentment, sulkiness

patient when the correct remedy is given. They are often used as an adjunct to other therapies that do not do as much to address the emotional aspect of healing. As you can imagine, the technician can be of great value to the veterinarian who practices homeopathy. By assisting in observation of the

patient and in client education, the technician can have a substantial impact on the success of treatment.

ACUPUNCTURE

The term *acupuncture* comes from the Latin words *acus*, meaning "needle," and *pungere*, meaning "to pierce." It is the technique of piercing the skin with a needle at specific, predetermined "acupuncture points." It is now known that these points can be stimulated by more than just needles; they can also be stimulated by pressure, injection of fluid, laser, **ultrasound (therapeutic)**, surgically implanted material, and electricity.

Acupuncture has been used longer than 4000 years in the East as one medical method within traditional Chinese medicine (TCM). TCM is a system of medicine that includes herbology, massage, and nutritional and lifestyle management. Early Chinese veterinary applications of acupuncture started with the domestication of animals. Veterinary acupuncture came to the United States in the early 1970s, and in 1974, the International Veterinary Acupuncture Society (IVAS) was organized, with the aim of fully integrating acupuncture into Western veterinary science. Acupuncture is used to treat all species from ferrets and birds to dogs and cattle to elephants and killer whales.

In the United States, acupuncture is increasingly used as a **modality** in the treatment of musculoskeletal, neurologic, cardiovascular, respiratory, GI, reproductive, and dermatologic disorders. Although it has the ability to help many areas of the body, pain management is probably the most common use of acupuncture today. Because it is considered a medical procedure, in most states only a licensed veterinarian may treat an animal with acupuncture. Currently, several certification courses are available to veterinarians, typically consisting of more than 100 hours of lecture followed by a comprehensive written and practical examination at the end of the course.

TERMINOLOGY AND RECORD KEEPING

Acupuncture points are connected through pathways called *meridians* or *channels*. In TCM, it is believed that the body's vital energy or life force (bioelectricity) circulates in a cyclic predetermined course through the meridians. Most species have 14 classical meridians: 12 are associated with specific organ systems on which they have a primary influence, and 2 run on the midline of the body. Paired organ-related meridians are named *lung (LU)*, *large intestine (LI)*, *stomach (ST)*, *spleen (SP)*, *heart (HT)*, *small intestine (SI)*, *bladder (BL)*, *kidney (KI)*, *pericardium (PC)*, *triple heater (TH)*, *gallbladder (GB)*, and *liver (LV)*. The unpaired channels are the conception vessel (CV), which runs on the ventral midline, and the governing vessel (GV), which runs on the dorsal midline. Individual acupuncture points are named and recorded by pairing the meridian with a number (e.g., LV3 is the third point on the liver meridian, SP6 is the sixth point on the spleen meridian). In addition, there are "extra" points that do not lie on meridians and trigger points; these are temporarily tender areas that can move on and off the meridians during episodes of pathologic conditions.

> **TECHNICIAN NOTE** Acupuncture points are connected through pathways called *meridians* or *channels*.

ACUPUNCTURE THEORIES

According to TCM theory, energy circulates through each meridian every 24 hours. Meridians run on the surface of the body, where acupuncture points can be accessed and manipulated. Blockage of energy circulation manifests as dysfunction or disease. Medical conditions that can be helped result from stagnant energy circulation or lack of sufficient energy to function optimally. Stagnant energy manifests as painful spasms or swelling, whereas deficient energy manifests as atrophy or weakness. To bring the body into balance and to facilitate healing, it is necessary to stimulate or sedate energy levels at acupuncture points. Many theories about how acupuncture works have been put forth. The most current acupuncture theories discussed in the human literature are as follows: gate theory, endogenous opioid theory, autonomic nervous system input theory, humoral theory, and bioelectrical theory.

The gate theory explains the analgesic effects of acupuncture. It has been shown that different types of neurons transmit pain. When an acupuncture needle is inserted, thin myelinated nerve fibers carry a message to the spinal cord. Neurotransmitters are released and are taken up by interneurons. When the impulse from unmyelinated pain nerve fibers causes the release of neurotransmitters, the receptors are full and the "gate" is closed to that signal, with little to no message of pain reaching the brain.

The endogenous opioid theory explains how acupuncture causes release of beta-endorphins, met-enkephalins, and leu-enkephalins in both blood and cerebrospinal fluid (CSF). These endogenous opioids reduce pain similarly to morphine and torbutrol, and their effects can be reversed with naloxone (an injectable agent used in veterinary medicine to reverse the effects of morphine). Opiates are also known to have systemic effects that can be produced by acupuncture. For example, opiate receptors in the gut are responsible for decreasing peristalsis and increasing segmental contractions, thus effectively controlling diarrhea.

The autonomic nervous system theory looks at how needles inserted into the skin can have an effect on muscles and organs of the body. Numerous viscerosomatic (relating organs to muscles) relationships have been studied, and it has been found that visceral and somatic fibers have adjacent tracts in the spinal cord and distribution in the dorsal gray matter. Examples of this relationship include muscle cramping seen secondary to inflammation of the intestines and the phenomenon of *referred pain*, which is seen when pain is felt in one part of the body, but it is different from the part of the body that was stimulated.

The humoral theory was first postulated after studies showed that transfer of blood, CSF, or brain tissue from an animal under acupuncture analgesia to an animal not receiving acupuncture resulted in analgesia of the recipient. Beta-endorphins are released by acupuncture and may contribute to analgesia, but they are not the only important component. Serotonin is also important and increases by 30% to 40% in the systemic circulation after acupuncture. Acupuncture has been shown to cause systemic increases in growth hormone, prolactin, oxytocin, luteinizing hormone, white blood cells, immunoglobulins, antibodies, and interferons, depending on which points are stimulated.

> **TECHNICIAN NOTE** The humoral theory was first postulated after studies showed that transfer of blood, cerebrospinal fluid (CSF), or brain tissue from an animal under acupuncture analgesia to an animal not receiving acupuncture resulted in analgesia of the recipient.

The bioelectrical theory states that healing and analgesic properties of acupuncture are based on a direct current (DC) system. In this system, electrical signals are generated and propagated by Schwann cells, satellite cells, and glial cells. Acupuncture points, like amplifiers, would boost the DC signal along the nerve pathways. Insertion of a metal acupuncture needle would, in effect, short-circuit the system and block pain perception. In this system, acupuncture points boost the DC signal along the meridian, similar to the way an amplifier boosts electricity along a high-power tension wire.

TECHNIQUES

Dry needling is performed with the use of stainless steel acupuncture needles (Figure 23-3). These needles are 25 to 36 gauge and range from ½ inch to 2 inches long when used with companion animals, or up to 4 inches long when used

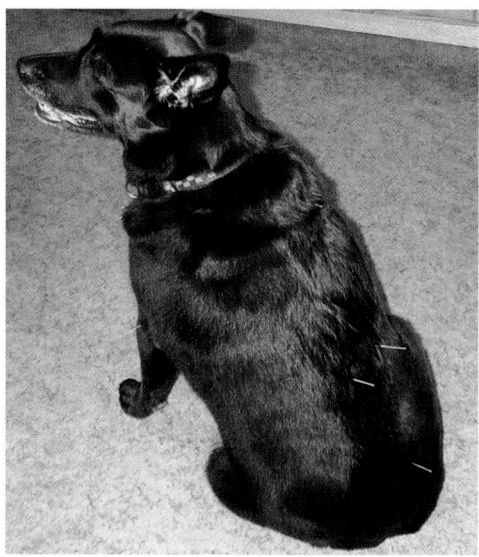

FIGURE 23-3 Dakota is receiving acupuncture treatment for spondylosis.

with large animals. Large animal practitioners often use hypodermic needles in their patients.

Moxibustion is the burning of dried leaves of the *Artemisia vulgaris* or mugwort plant. The moxa stick can be moved slowly over an acupuncture point or can be placed on an inserted needle. This is often done for animals with degenerative changes that do better in warm dry climates than in cold or damp settings. In TCM, this adds energy to a deficient area.

Aquapuncture is the injection of a solution into an acupuncture point. The most commonly used substance is vitamin B_{12}, although electrolyte solutions, saline, dimethyl sulfoxide (DMSO), vitamin C, antibiotics, herbal extracts, homeopathics, and local anesthetics can be used. It is thought that pressure on the point or the solution itself will stimulate nerve fibers.

Electroacupuncture is the passing of electrical energy through acupuncture points. Stimulation is accomplished by connecting an electronic device to the inserted needles. Indications include paralysis or paresis, severe and chronic painful conditions, and conditions not responsive to dry needling. Microcurrent therapy is the use of a machine that generates a microcurrent of electricity that can be used on acupuncture points or directly over areas of pain or muscle spasm.

To achieve continuous stimulation of an acupuncture point, various materials may be surgically implanted at acupuncture points; this is called *implantation*. Although catgut, stainless steel, and silver can be used, the most common implant is gold in the form of solid beads or wires. This technique is most commonly used for young dogs with painful hip dysplasia, older dogs with coxofemoral arthritis, and dogs of any age with epilepsy. This is considered a surgical procedure.

Low-intensity or "cold" lasers have been used to stimulate acupuncture points. Laser puncture is a noninvasive form of intense light therapy that uses various frequencies and wavelengths to promote positive physiologic changes within cells (Figure 23-4).

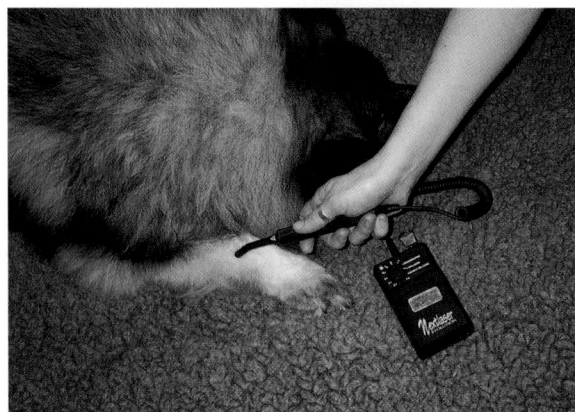

FIGURE 23-4 Laser acupuncture can be used for painful or swollen areas or with animals that are sensitive to needling.

Acupressure is simply the stimulation of an acupuncture point by means of physical pressure. Because it is considered noninvasive, it is not legally as tightly restricted and often is used during massage therapy. It does not have as intense an effect because it does not stimulate deeper levels of the point, but it can be quite effective. The technician with knowledge of commonly used points can provide additional benefit to patients and can give the veterinarian feedback about any reactive (tender) points a patient may have.

Acupuncture needles can be placed into tissue perpendicularly or at an angle. When the needles are removed, they should be gently pulled in the same direction in which they were inserted. If resistance is felt when the needle is removed, tapping around the needle, rolling it back and forth, or gently holding down the skin on either side of the needle while pulling the needle gently will ease it from the tissue. Occasionally, the needles will come out crooked, which is not unusual because they bend easily. All needles should be accounted for and placed into a sharps container.

The technician's role in acupuncture includes having a general understanding of how and why acupuncture works to be able to discuss it with clients; charting the points in the record; assisting if patient restraint or diversion is required; helping to ease a patient's anxiety, if needed; and removing and counting the needles.

TECHNICIAN NOTE If resistance is felt when the needle is removed, tapping around the needle, rolling it back and forth, or gently holding down the skin on either side of the needle while pulling the needle gently will ease it from the tissue.

VETERINARY SPINAL MANIPULATIVE THERAPY (CHIROPRACTIC)

Chiropractic, also referred to as veterinary spinal manipulative therapy (VSMT), is used to manually restore reduced motion in the spine and limbs, thereby improving patient mobility and comfort, and in many cases nervous system function. The term is derived from the Greek *cheir* ("hand") and *praxis* ("practice"). A. E. Homewood defined chiropractic medicine as "that science and art which uses the inherent recuperative powers of the body and deals with the relationship between the nervous system and the spinal column, including its immediate articulations, and the role of this relationship in the restoration and maintenance of health."

HISTORY

Manipulation of the spine is an ancient practice. References were made to this form of treatment as early as 2700 BC in China. Even Hippocrates noted the effects of this type of therapy because he noted, "Look well to the spine for the cause of disease." Chiropractic began in the United States in 1895 with D. D. Palmer, who began to treat the spine as a primary method of healing his patients. His son, B. J. Palmer, further developed chiropractic into a system of medicine, and founded the first school of chiropractic in Davenport, Iowa. He claimed to have treated animal patients and people in his hospital at the school.

Currently in most states, veterinary chiropractic adjustments must be performed by a trained professional (a veterinarian or a chiropractor). Training leading to certification in veterinary chiropractic is available for both groups of professionals through postgraduate courses, typically consisting of at least 200 hours of lecture and hands-on labs, a certification examination (written and practical), and completion of several case reports. To remain certified, a veterinarian must complete 30 hours of continuing education every 3 years.

> **TECHNICIAN NOTE** Proper chiropractic technique requires a great deal of time and effort to learn. This is why human chiropractors go to school for 3 to 4 years before practicing. It is important that only a thoroughly trained professional adjust an animal patient.

PHILOSOPHY AND THEORY

Chiropractic is much more than the stereotyped "bone out of place." A chiropractic problem, known as a *subluxation* or a *vertebral subluxation complex (VSC)*, involves an abnormal relationship between two adjacent vertebrae. This is an anatomically complex area known as the *motor unit* (Figure 23-5). It consists of muscles, ligaments, connective tissue, a spinal nerve and other smaller nerves, blood vessels, lymphatics, and CSF. The hallmark or "triad" of signs that occur with a subluxation includes altered mobility, pain on palpation, and abnormal tension in the surrounding (paraspinal) muscles.

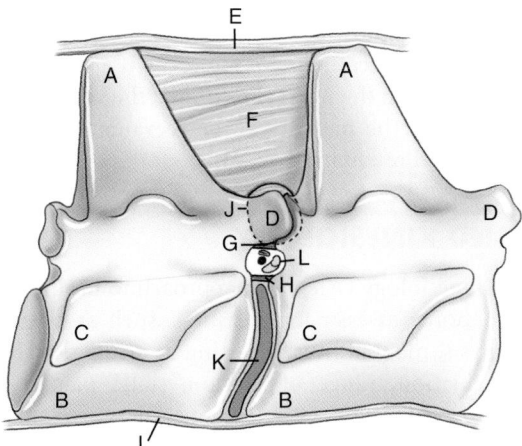

FIGURE 23-5 The motor unit is a complex anatomic and dynamic area that consists of two adjacent vertebrae and the tissues in between. *A,* Dorsal spinous process. *B,* Vertebral body. *C,* Transverse process. *D,* Articular facet joint. *E,* Supraspinous ligament. *F,* Interspinous ligament. *G,* Ligamentum flavum. *H,* Dorsal longitudinal ligament. *I,* Ventral longitudinal ligament. *J,* Joint capsule. *K,* Intervertebral disc. *L,* Intervertebral foramen.

> **TECHNICIAN NOTE** A chiropractic subluxation is much more subtle than a partial luxation, or dislocation. It is a description more of function than of anatomic position; thus the disrelationship is not always apparent radiographically. Most often, it is discovered by palpation.

Many explanations about how subluxations occur have been validated by scientific research. The causes of subluxation can vary from overt trauma to minute repetitive stress to the area, such as abnormal spinal movement secondary to left forelimb lameness. Clinical signs range from mild discomfort to reduced reflexes to serious organ dysfunction. By determining where abnormal motion occurs and correcting reduced motion in the spine, we can restore normal biomechanics to the body and reset normal neurologic pathways, thus aiding proper nervous system function. Restoration of full motion to joints of the limbs can be equally important in maintaining spinal health because the body functions as a whole and all segments are connected.

TREATMENT

The chiropractic appointment begins with a clear and detailed history. It is helpful if the patient has previously received a thorough "Western" medical workup before the chiropractic appointment, but this is not always the case. Examination proceeds with observation of posture and gait, palpation of the spinal column and the extremities (limbs and tail), neurologic evaluation, and review of diagnostic images and lab work. It is as detailed (or more) as a typical general physical examination. Problem areas are recorded using a consistent system of terminology (several are available).

Once problem areas have been identified, the veterinarian determines whether a chiropractic adjustment is an appropriate therapy for the patient at that time. Sometimes additional diagnostics may be required, either in the future or before any adjustment is performed. For example, a horse may have neurologic deficits consistent with equine protozoal myelitis (EPM), and a spinal fluid analysis and an EPM test may be indicated. In this case, chiropractic may help and could be an appropriate therapy to perform at the initial visit, but other primary therapies are warranted. In some cases, as when patients have acute paralysis secondary to intervertebral disc disease, it may be more appropriate to obtain further diagnostics (such as radiographs and a myelogram) before adjusting the patient, to ensure that areas of active disc disease are avoided.

The next step is for the veterinarian to adjust the patient. Although treatment principles are similar, each veterinarian has a unique technique that he or she has developed. Certification courses teach basic techniques, but advanced techniques and variations may also be learned. Often it is easiest to treat patients in a standing position. However, sometimes a sitting or sternal recumbent position may work better for small animal patients. Cats, in particular, are easier to treat while lying on the treatment table than when they are forced to stand.

The veterinarian will check the motion between two spinal segments by applying pressure aligned with the way the joint surface glides. If reduced mobility is found in a given area, the veterinarian takes the motion as far as it will go and applies a short, quick motion in the plane of motion of the joint. Sometimes a popping noise (like someone cracking a knuckle) will accompany the adjustment, although this is more common in people than in animals. The adjustment should generally be painless for the patient, although sometimes a problem area may present some momentary mild discomfort. If a seriously painful area is found, the veterinarian will likely avoid treating that area altogether, at least until further diagnostics have been done. It is important to keep the patient relaxed and to make the treatment a positive experience (for both the patient and the client); therefore, all problem areas may not be corrected in a single visit. After treatment, the veterinarian will instruct the client on aftercare and follow-up visits and will provide additional recommendations. Usually, some period of rest or reduced exercise is recommended, and massage and stretching may have to be done at home.

THE TECHNICIAN'S ROLE

Restraint is particularly important for first-time patients because they are unsure about the process and may be nervous or frightened. Restraint can be simple, such as gentle petting, kind words, or a food distraction (Figure 23-6). Often a patient may have to be repositioned so that the veterinarian is in the best position to perform the necessary adjustment. Most patients accept and enjoy the treatment, so generally, only gentle physical restraint is necessary. It may, however, be necessary to use more rigorous methods of restraint if the situation warrants. Some canine or feline patients may need to be muzzled (especially if they are regular patients at a general practice—they may be expecting a blood draw or a vaccine rather than a relaxing and comfortable treatment). Some horses will require twitching or hobbling, especially if they are not used to being routinely

handled. Cattle may be restrained in a chute. Occasionally, although most veterinarians avoid it, chemical restraint is necessary for some patients to relax enough to receive a safe and effective treatment. This is much more likely to happen early in the treatment program, and most patients will not need to be sedated more than once or twice.

In a large animal practice, sometimes the technician may be required to stabilize nearby segments so that an adjustment may be more effective or specific. For example, when a veterinarian adjusts T6 in the horse, the technician must stand on the opposite side of the horse in a specific position (both body and hands) to stabilize T5 and T7. Proper technique is required to provide the most effective treatment and to ensure the assistant's safety.

> **TECHNICIAN NOTE**   Thorough knowledge of skeletal anatomy is important if one is to provide assistance with stabilization.

The technician should become comfortable with all anticipated restraint techniques before using them because any unfamiliarity or nervousness may contribute to patient anxiety, and it is important for the patient to be as relaxed as possible. Practicing on the staff's pets is often a good method of developing proficiency in this important role. The technician thus takes a very active role in restraint and stabilization and may be asked to record examination findings and treated areas during the session. Thus it is important to be familiar with what abbreviations or chiropractic notations are used at the practice.

Immediately after treatment, the technician may be asked to massage the patient, apply essential oils, or walk the patient for several minutes to help the patient "hold" the adjustment. Another active role for the technician is client communication. It is important to be familiar with expected results and the veterinarian's recommendations for aftercare and to be able to answer commonly asked questions about the examination, treatment, or aftercare. If a situation arises that deviates from the normal response, the veterinarian can be alerted, and the patient can be reevaluated in a timely fashion (Case Presentation 23-2).

APPLIED KINESIOLOGY

Applied kinesiology (AK) is an approach to health care that uses functional assessment measures, such as posture and gait analysis, manual muscle testing as a functional neurologic evaluation, range of motion, static palpation, and motion analysis, to diagnose patients. These assessments are used in conjunction with standard methods of diagnosis, such as clinical history, physical examination, and laboratory testing, to develop a clinical impression of the unique physiologic condition of each patient. Thousands of professionals, including chiropractors, physicians, osteopaths, dentists, podiatrists, psychologists, and veterinarians, belong to the International College of Applied Kinesiology (ICAK).

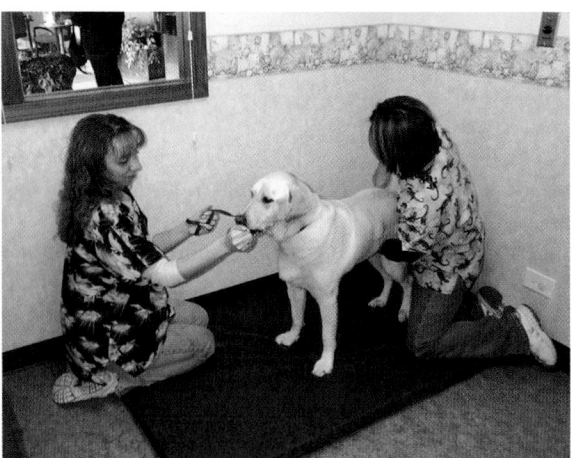

FIGURE 23-6 Chiropractic adjustment. A technician uses food to gently restrain a patient in a standing position while the veterinarian performs an adjustment.

CASE PRESENTATION 23-2 EQUINE HINDLIMB LAMENESS

Signalment: Anna, a 6-year-old Trakehner thoroughbred mare in training as a hunter and jumper

Chief Complaint: Right hindlimb lameness of 3 weeks' duration

Pertinent History: Anna was purchased 3 months before and had been completely sound until she came in from turnout. She was placed on stall rest for 1 week, with 10-minute hand walks twice daily. Initially, her lameness appeared to be in the left rear limb; 5 days later, it was noted in the right rear limb. Previous examination had resulted in no localization of the lameness. Current supplements included glucosamine and MSM.

Significant Examination Findings: Right rear limb lameness with a pronounced hip hike and somewhat shortened stride. Significant back pain was noted with muscle tightness and tenderness in the lumbar spine. No pain was noted in the limb itself, and a thorough examination of her unshod foot revealed no pain or injury.

Problem List:
- Right rear limb lameness
- Back pain with muscle tightness and tenderness
- Reduced spinal mobility, particularly in the lumbar region and pelvis

Initial Therapy Plan: A chiropractic adjustment was performed to address the back pain and decreased mobility in the pelvis and lumbar spine, with follow-up pending response. No further treatment was provided as a result of an inability to definitively localize the lameness.

Client Communication: The owner was instructed to hand walk Anna for 10 minutes after her adjustment to help loosen her muscles and stimulate her nervous system to "reset" her now improved posture and motion to "normal." She would be allowed short turnout (1 to 2 hours) in a small paddock for 3 days after adjustment, and if sound at that point, could do some walking and trotting on a loose rein for 20 minutes each day until her next visit 7 days later.

Progress: Anna responded favorably to her adjustment, showing significantly reduced lameness the following day. Lameness recurred 3 days later, so she was not ridden but was still allowed turnout.

The following week, Anna's lameness remained unchanged, and no significant findings were noted in the limb itself. Her back was still a bit tender but was notably improved. Reduced mobility was still significant. Acupuncture was performed before chiropractic adjustment to try to alleviate some of the discomfort and to loosen tight muscles. An aquapuncture technique using ½ ml of 50 mcg B_{12} inserted to a depth of ¾ inches at each tender-reactive point (local points around the pelvis: GBBDTC reactive and treated bilaterally; GB 27 and 28 reactive on the right, treated bilaterally; points along the back: BL 20 reactive on the right, treated bilaterally along with BL 21) was elected because of ease of use and continued pain-reducing effects. Ting points (which are strong points in the feet at the ends of the channels that are used to unblock energy: BL 67 reactive on the right, treated bilaterally) were bled using a 25G ¾-inch hypodermic needle inserted to a depth of ¼ cm. After chiropractic adjustment (pelvis: RPI—right side posterior inferior; lumbar spine: L7 posterior, L6 posterior,

L4 posterior left; thoracic spine: T9 posterior left; cervical spine: C6 body left, APL—atlas posterior left), the mare was still lame but had a less pronounced hip hike. The same plan was followed for aftercare, with the understanding that further diagnostics (nerve blocks, possibly nuclear scan) would be indicated if Anna failed to respond favorably to combined therapy.

A follow-up report from the owner indicated that Anna was still sore the day after treatment but appeared completely sound on the third day. She maintained soundness all week so was lightly ridden at the end of the week with no relapse. On examination, she trotted soundly with an occasional short stride in the right rear limb, so the lameness was not completely resolved. Far fewer reactive acupuncture points were found (GBBDTC reactive on the right, treated bilaterally; BL 20 reactive on the right, treated bilaterally), and her spinal mobility was much improved. She exhibited minimal back pain, and her muscles were relaxed and supple. After chiropractic adjustment (RPI, L7P, L6P, L1PR, T8PL), Anna trotted off with excellent balance and symmetry. Her owner was instructed to increase the duration of exercise, with some collected activity at the walk and trot and canter work on a loose rein. She was also taught some stretching exercises to use before riding. Another treatment was scheduled the following week.

By week 3, Anna was working soundly under saddle as recommended. On examination, she walked and jogged without lameness and appeared nicely balanced. Her back was supple and pain free. No reactive acupuncture points were found. A chiropractic examination and adjustment was performed (L7P, L6PL, L3PR). At this point, because her lameness had resolved completely, further exercises were recommended to help her maintain balance and to strengthen her back (Cavaletti poles, leg yields).

Anna has maintained soundness since her second treatment. Her trainer remarked about how balanced and

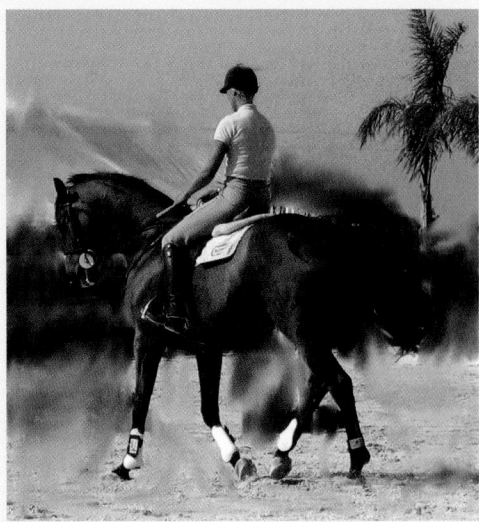

FIGURE 1 Anna exhibits excellent balance and strength with the help of regular chiropractic maintenance.

Continued

CASE PRESENTATION 23-2 EQUINE HINDLIMB LAMENESS—cont'd

supple she had become, working much better after her treatments than before the lameness had appeared. She is now adjusted monthly to maintain mobility and help prevent injury and is competing successfully in hunters and equitation (Figure 1).

Discussion: Anna's rapid and complete response to acupuncture and chiropractic is fairly typical of a young horse without significant structural problems. Of greatest significance is that her lameness would have been quite a mystery if she were diagnosed and treated with a Western perspective: there was absolutely no sign of pain in the right rear limb itself. Anti-inflammatory therapy may have resulted in temporary soundness, but prolonged use while she was in training could have resulted in permanent structural changes that would have caused further and more serious lameness over time. Early intervention with pain management and restoration of joint mobility throughout her spine has given her not only relief from her lameness but also better balance and symmetry than she had initially. This should lead to a longer career and a reduced likelihood of injury as long as this mobility is maintained.

The technician's involvement in Anna's case was comprehensive and included assisting with the examination and restraint, preparation of acupuncture materials, segment stabilization for chiropractic adjustment, communication with the client, and demonstration of stretching techniques.

Veterinarians can take a basic 100-hour certification course through the ICAK.

> **TECHNICIAN NOTE** Applied kinesiology (AK) is a diagnostic system that uses manual muscle testing to augment normal examination procedures.

George Goodheart, DC, is recognized as the creator of the field of AK. As early as 1964, he recognized that dysfunction of muscle and tendon receptors in a particular muscle could affect the strength of that muscle and have a negative effect on the stability of a related joint. Whereas most practitioners were treating musculoskeletal problems by addressing hypertonic muscles, Dr. Goodheart saw that most of the time, problems were related to muscle paresis. He came to discover that muscle weakness could be caused by a large number of factors affecting output from the ventral horn; this discovery has since been supported by research. Dr. Goodheart investigated the effects of many different existing techniques on the efficiency of muscle function, including the following:

- Manipulative therapy
- Neurologic relationships
- Chapman's reflexes, which are known in AK as *neurolymphatic reflexes*
- Bennett's reflexes, which are known in AK as *neurovascular reflexes*
- Cranial sacral therapy
- Meridian therapy
- Nutritional and biochemical therapy
- Organ-muscle relationships
- Psychological relationships
- Electrical and magnetic relationships

One of the tools used in AK is manual muscle testing for functional neurologic assessment. It can be used to evaluate and correct functional imbalances in the structural, chemical, mental, and energetic systems of the patient. It is important to note that manual muscle testing is only a small part of AK, and these terms are not mutually interchangeable. In

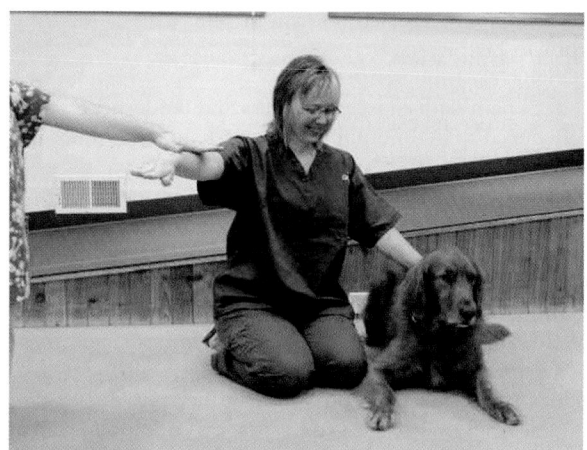

FIGURE 23-7 Applied kinesiology (AK). A dog diagnosed with manual therapy.

muscle testing, the professional places pressure against a certain muscle, and the patient tries to resist the motion caused by this pressure. For example, if one person held an arm out to the side parallel to the ground, the major muscle holding it there would be the deltoid muscle. If the professional put pressure downward and the deltoid muscle was weak, the arm would go down relatively easily. If the deltoid muscle was strong, it would take much greater force to bring the arm down.

It was discovered early on in AK that babies and quadriplegic individuals could be tested indirectly by having a third person touch them while the physician tests the surrogate's muscle for changes in strength. The same tests or challenges are applied to the patient, but the muscle testing response is received through the surrogate. This same principle has been applied with great success to animals. Because it is hard to tell an animal to resist a given motion, the technician can act as the surrogate third person for the animal by touching the muscle in question. The tester tests the corresponding muscle in the surrogate and can gain information about the patient's muscle (Figure 23-7). How surrogate testing works is not really known at this time. It is hypothesized that neurologic information, which is conveyed electrically, is transferred to the mostly salt and water surrogate by contact with the patient.

Once the physician using AK finds a muscle that is unbalanced, he or she attempts to determine why that muscle is not functioning properly; possible reasons include improper facilitation and neuromuscular inhibition. On the basis of response to therapy, it appears that in some of these conditions, the primary dysfunction is due to deafferentation—loss of normal sensory stimulation of neurons as a result of functional interruption of afferent receptors. It may occur under many circumstances but is best understood by the concept that with abnormal joint function (subluxation or fixation), the uncharacteristic movement causes improper stimulation of the local joint and muscle receptors. This changes the transmission from these receptors through the peripheral nerves to the spinal cord, brainstem, cerebellum, and cortex, and then to the effectors from their normally expected stimulation. Symptoms of deafferentation arise from numerous levels, such as motor, sensory, autonomic, and conscious levels, or from anywhere throughout the neuraxis. The physician works out the treatment that will best balance the patient's muscles. Treatment may involve specific joint manipulation or mobilization, various myofascial therapies, cranial techniques, meridian and acupuncture skills, clinical nutrition, dietary management, evaluation of environmental irritants, and various reflex procedures.

The technician usually is highly involved in kinesiology and is often responsible for the important task of acting as a surrogate, as well as for writing down examination findings and treated areas and assisting with restraint and communication with clients. The technician should have a basic knowledge of the procedure and should know what abbreviations or AK notations are used at the practice.

> **TECHNICIAN NOTE** In some cases, the examiner may test for environmental or food sensitivity by using a previously strong muscle to find what weakens it.

PHYSICAL THERAPY AND REHABILITATION

Physical rehabilitation is a relatively new practice in both human and animal realms. Although evidence that various physical therapeutic modalities were used on people dates back to Hippocrates, physical therapy as we know it today originated in Great Britain in the late 1800s. By the early 1900s, physical therapy and rehabilitation had been established as a profession in the United States. It has been used with horses and then with companion animals for approximately 25 years. As with human medical practice, rehabilitation is transitioning from "alternative" to mainstream therapy. In fact, in 2010, the American Veterinary Medical Association (AVMA) recognized the American College of

Veterinary Sports Medicine and Rehabilitation as the first established specialty board for veterinarians.

Rehabilitation can be defined as relief of pain and restoration of mobility and function. Whereas the term *physical therapy* (or *physiotherapy*) is more specific, referring mainly to the physical aspects of a disability or disorder, *rehabilitation* is a broader term that may encompass lifestyle management, as well as physical intervention. Rehabilitation by nature is a team effort. Patients do best when a collaborative effort is made between the primary veterinarian, the specialist (surgeon, neurologist), and the therapy team. The therapy team may consist of a veterinarian and/or a physical therapist, who can direct and oversee the therapy program, as well as one or several veterinary technicians and physical therapy assistants. Every team must be dynamic in roles and responsibilities. Good communication and feedback are essential to a successful rehabilitation program.

The role of the veterinary technician in a rehabilitation program is often extensive. Training and certification programs are available for technicians who wish to increase their skill level in this rapidly growing field. (Refer to the list of references at the end of this chapter.) In many rehabilitation practices, the veterinary technician is the primary care-giver, performing all exercise-based and assistive therapies, as well as most manual and modality-based treatments. Providing primary care often becomes the veterinary technician's full-time responsibility in rehabilitation practices.

> **TECHNICIAN NOTE** Patient assessment and client communication are much more demanding for a rehabilitation therapist because of the intense nature of the practice, so these skills must be developed along with technical skills.

Many indications for rehabilitative intervention are known, ranging from complete paralysis to athletic management and training (Box 23-1). Most commonly, we tend to see a variety of postsurgical orthopedic patients, as well as geriatric patients with chronic musculoskeletal and neurologic disorders.

So now that we know that rehabilitation is appropriate for a given patient, how can we determine the most appropriate therapy program to provide? This is determined through thorough patient evaluation, including a comprehensive history, a general physical examination, and orthopedic and neurologic examinations tailored to the individual patient. A healthy, athletic dog recovering from tibial plateau leveling osteotomy (TPLO) surgery may have no disorder except for the surgical limb, whereas a geriatric horse may have both osteoarthritis and neurologic weakness. Generally, the entire patient is examined briefly, and problem areas are targeted for more comprehensive examination, including measurement of muscle girth and range of motion of compromised joints (**goniometry**), as well as of contralateral healthy joints.

BOX 23-1	Common Conditions Seen at Rehabilitation Facilities

Musculoskeletal
Osteoarthritis
Developmental orthopedic disease (hip dysplasia, elbow dysplasia, OCD)
Joint injuries
Sprain, strain, muscle tears
Muscle contractures
Tendonitis and bursitis
Anterior cruciate ligament injuries (partial or full tears)
Joint replacement
Fracture repair
Arthrodesis
Amputation

Neurologic
Intervertebral disc disease
Fibrocartilaginous embolism
Peripheral neuropathy
Degenerative myelopathy
Wobbler's disease

Other
Weight management
Wound healing
Athletic conditioning

OCD, Osteochondrosis.

TECHNICIAN NOTE Depending on your practice, all or some of the evaluation may be done by a veterinarian, a physical therapist, a veterinary technician, or a physical therapy assistant. It is important for any technician involved in rehabilitation practice to have thorough knowledge of the evaluation process.

After evaluation, the therapist must devise a therapy plan. Goals may be established by both the client and the therapist, and they may be both general (return to agility competition at the previous level) and specific (strengthen the quadriceps muscle and restore full stifle flexion). The approach to the therapy plan is somewhat different from that used in general medicine, where we seek the cause of pathology before treating the disease. In rehabilitation, treatment is based on a problem list of dysfunctions (Box 23-2). These are often grouped into primary and secondary, or compensatory problems. Additionally, (incidental) problems may be noted but are not directly related to the presenting complaint. These may or may not need to be addressed in the treatment plan. Once a plan of action is presented and is agreed upon by the client, therapy can begin.

TECHNICIAN NOTE The rehabilitation technician can play a major role in providing treatment, often directing a patient's therapy under supervision of a qualified veterinarian and/or physical therapist. The technician can deliver most if not all of the therapeutic modalities described in this section under supervision of a qualified veterinarian, as long as he or she is properly educated.

BOX 23-2	Common Problems of Physical Dysfunction

Pain
Inflammation (swelling, heat)
Reduced range of motion
Hypermobility
Muscle atrophy
Muscle tightness
Muscle spasm and trigger points
Fibrosis and scarring
Abnormal gait (lameness, pacing)
Neurologic dysfunction (CP deficits)
Ataxia
Weakness
Exercise intolerance

Modalities discussed in this section include the following: exercise-based therapy (therapeutic exercises, **hydrotherapy**, land treadmill), manual therapy (**passive range of motion [PROM]** and massage), electrical and magnet-based therapy (neuromuscular stimulation, bioelectrical therapy, magnetic and electromagnetic therapy), light and sound–based therapy (laser and ultrasound), superficial **thermal agents**, and assistive devices. Acupuncture and chiropractic are often provided as part of a rehabilitation program; they are discussed in detail in the previous section.

EXERCISE-BASED THERAPY

Exercise is essential in any rehabilitation program. Intensity level and duration are dependent on the patient's strength and pain level. For a geriatric patient who is arthritic and neurologically weak, exercise may be very gentle and may be performed with a great deal of assistance. Sessions would be short and frequent (three or four 5- to 10-minute sessions throughout the day). For an athletic animal at the end stage of returning to competition, exercise may be very rigorous and demanding (two to three 20- to 30-minute sessions per day, with cardio, strength, and sport-specific activity intermixed). As a rule, it is best to start out conservatively, so that the patient does not experience an initial setback. By assessing the response to initial sessions, the therapist can better tailor a program that challenges a patient without causing excessive fatigue or pain.

THERAPEUTIC EXERCISES

Exercises are used for strengthening and stretching specific muscles or muscle groups, building endurance, enhancing balance and proprioception, and reeducating about normal posture and gait. Examples of exercises and their purposes are provided in Table 23-10. Many of these exercises are custom-made for the individual patient and condition.

Strengthening exercises can target specific muscle groups, such as hamstrings and gluteals. They are used when atrophy is present or when increased strength in specific areas is desired. Some exercises target a broader range of muscles, such as abdominals and paraspinals (diagonal limb

TABLE 23-10	Exercises	
EXERCISES	**TYPE**	**USED FOR**
Sit to stand	Strengthening	Rear limbs
Walking on a hill	Endurance	
Zigzag	Proprioception	Whole body
Parallel to top	Strengthening	Side closest to the top
Balance board	Balance Proprioception	Limbs on the board
	Strengthening	Limbs not on the board
Goosing (abdominal contractions)	Strengthening	Core, posture
Cavaletti poles	Proprioception	Gait training
Sit up and wave	Strengthening	Core, forelimbs

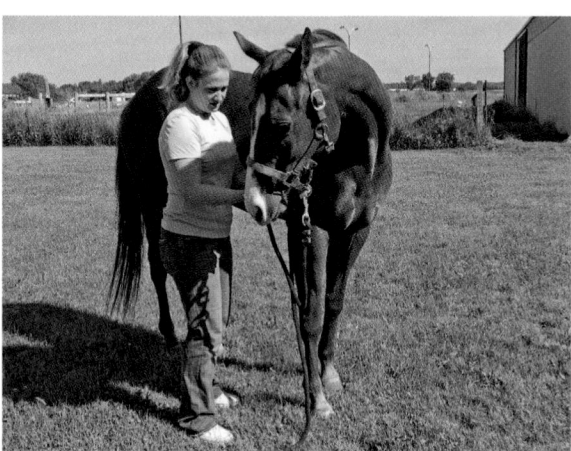

FIGURE 23-8 A technician performs a carrot stretch exercise to improve lateral cervical flexion in a horse.

lift). These are core-strengthening exercises, and they are appropriate at some level for every rehabilitation patient. Stretching exercises can also be targeted at a specific muscle or group of muscles and can be active or passive (Figure 23-8).

Proprioceptive exercises help a patient develop better awareness of where his or her body is. Balance exercises improve overall stability (Figure 23-9). Both of these types of exercise help patients who are weak and ataxic, but they also help improve athletic performance when seconds count. These exercises are also crucial for rehabilitation of a patient with an injured joint because ligaments contain proprioceptive fibers, which often are damaged with joint injury.

Endurance exercises emphasize the cardiovascular system and are whole body exercises. They may include walking, jogging, and swimming. Neuromuscular reeducation exercises involve posture and gait corrections that vary in degree of therapist assistance. The weaker the muscle or the more abnormal the gait pattern, the more assistance is needed. As a general rule, the patient is asked to do as much as physically possible, and the therapist assists as needed to attain correct posture and gait.

An exercise plan is generally developed by the attending veterinarian or physical therapist. The rehabilitation technician performs the exercises, modifying them as needed on the basis of patient response. He or she may also be responsible for teaching clients how to do exercises at home (home exercise plan, or HEP).

HYDROTHERAPY

Hydrotherapy was used in 400 BC by Hippocrates to treat rheumatism and paralysis. In the United States in the 1970s, it was found that when racehorses swam after an injury, they were able to return to the track faster than their comrades who did not have access to water. Unfortunately, it was also found that their muscle mass increased without the benefit of strengthening the bone (which is done when there is a compressive force), so they were also more likely to fracture a limb shortly after returning to the track. To address this, the underwater treadmill was invented. In 1998, the first

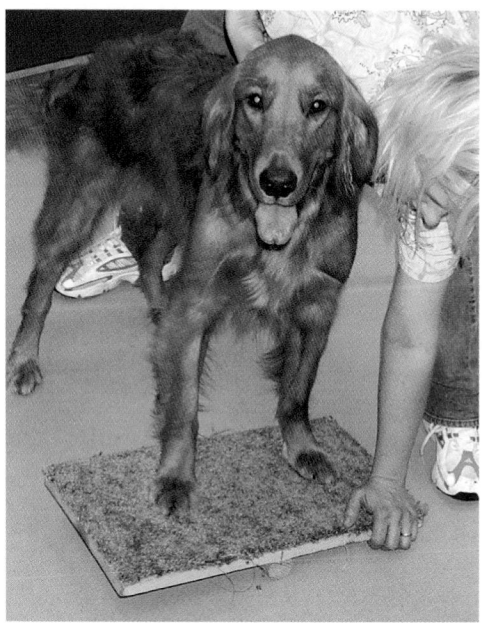

FIGURE 23-9 Rudy increases his forelimb balance and proprioception on the rocker board.

underwater treadmill was designed for use specifically in companion animals. Now, so many different units are available on the market for both canine and equine treadmills that we could devote an entire chapter to them!

Walking on an underwater treadmill in a warm-water environment provides the benefits of increased joint range of motion, improved muscle flexibility and mobility, enhanced circulation, and facilitation of front-to-rear and side-to-side balance. Because it can relieve pain and increase muscle strength while putting decreased weight on the joints, this activity is extremely beneficial in the treatment of osteoarthritis. It is also an invaluable tool when working with patients with neurologic deficits because many patients can take steps in water before they can perform voluntary motion on land. Swimming, without an underwater treadmill, also provides many of these benefits. However, dogs most commonly swim with stronger strokes in the forelimbs compared with the rear limbs. This may not be the best treatment if the goal is to strengthen the rear limbs. Also, paralyzed patients tend to improve more quickly with walking on the underwater treadmill.

For companion animals, massage, stretching, and exercises can also be done in the water before, during, or after swimming or walking on the underwater treadmill. It is generally more difficult and even dangerous to be in a therapy tank with horses, so generally, this is not done for them.

> **TECHNICIAN NOTE** Athletic dogs and horses can benefit from underwater treadmill and swimming for conditioning and for improving athletic performance.

Dynamic variables in the aquatic environment include buoyancy, resistance, flexion and extension of the limbs, speed, and patterning. Buoyancy can be added if a life vest is worn; this makes swimming easier. Resistance can be increased with the use of jets (Figure 23-10). To maximize flexion, balloons/waterwings can be used, or the water level can be lowered to just above the joint you want to flex. When the depth of the water is changed, resistance, buoyancy, and flexion/extension are affected. The deeper the water, the greater the buoyancy, and the easier movement is for the patient. Slightly above shoulder depth creates the greatest buoyancy without loss of flexion of the limbs. If decreased flexion is warranted, the water level should be above the shoulder because this results in a gait in which the animal walks on its toes. The greatest resistance with the least buoyancy occurs when the patient walks at about elbow depth. Altering treadmill speed will affect the speed of the patient, and will thereby change the intensity of the workout. *Patterning* can be defined as teaching the body to act in a certain way without conscious thought (an example for people would be riding a bicycle or skiing). With animals, we can work on proper gait by moving their limbs or stimulating their limbs to move in a certain pattern (walk, trot, or pace).

Although the physician determines the variables associated with hydrotherapy, the technician plays a very

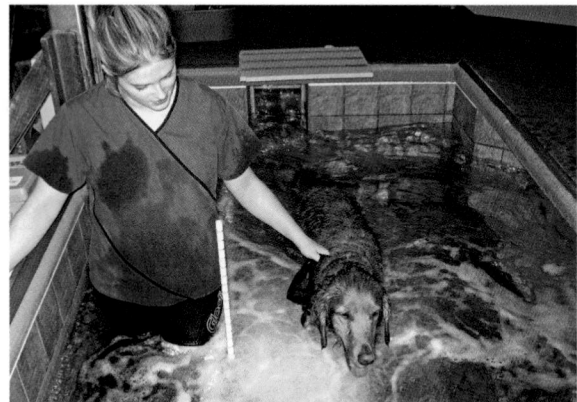

FIGURE 23-10 Underwater treadmill therapy. Jets can increase resistance for a more intense workout.

important role. In addition to keeping detailed records of each session, the technician stays in the pool with the canine patient, facilitates correct motion, monitors the patient, and provides massage, stretching, or exercises as needed. Before getting into the pool, if the patient is fecal incontinent, the technician can use a cotton swab to rectally stimulate the patient to defecate outside. When the patient is done with the pool, the technician may towel dry and/or blow the patient dry. Technicians should also be responsible for pool care (testing the water and adding any chemicals that may be needed). For equine patients, training the horse to safely enter and exit the treadmill (whether an in-ground or tank system is used) while monitoring and adjusting variables, and holding the lead, would be the technician's responsibility.

LAND TREADMILL

Land treadmills are used for increasing strength and endurance and for reeducating on front-to-back balance and normal foot placement. Walking either just uphill or just downhill can alter habitual compensations after an injury. By walking uphill, a patient with nonclinical hip dysplasia can strengthen the muscles around the hip, decreasing laxity and delaying the onset of clinical signs. When a patient places a limb laterally after surgery, the patient will often place it back in normal position when walking on a treadmill, especially if the treadmill is set at an angle that decreases weight on that limb. Although treadmills re-create the same motion as walking on land, fewer muscles are used because the belt movement reduces the body's need for self-propulsion. Therefore, the benefits of the treadmill are maximized when the treadmill is used to go uphill or downhill.

The goal of teaching patients to use the treadmill is to have them be comfortable getting on at one end and off at the other end when done, and enjoying the workout in between. Horses, in particular, adapt well because this movement is similar to entering a trailer. To make the transaction easier, have the patient walk across the treadmill 3 times (sitting and then standing on the third pass for canine patients). On the fourth pass, start the treadmill. Do not start too slowly because this is awkward. Quickly go to a normal pace with no hesitation between steps. Keep patients looking forward to avoid habits of side winding.

The technician's role is to teach the patient to use the treadmill without fear, to monitor the patient for gait changes and weariness while on the treadmill, and to record time, speed, angle, and progress of the patient.

MANUAL THERAPIES
Massage
Massage is defined as a systematic and scientific manipulation of soft tissues of the body for the purpose of obtaining or maintaining health. Massage has been performed for thousands of years. More than 70 types of human massage philosophy are known, many of which can be applied to animals.

Types

Shiatsu is a Japanese form of massage that literally means "finger pressure." Shiatsu practitioners use finger pressure at specific points in the body (correlating with acupuncture points) to promote circulation and stimulate the nervous system.

In trigger-point massage, or **myotherapy**, the therapist feels for taut bands or knots that have a point of maximal tenderness. Pressure on this point can cause local pain, referred pain, and muscle spasms in humans and animals. The manual technique for deactivating a trigger point is ischemic compression. When direct pressure is applied over the point, the tissue becomes ischemic (blood is pushed out of the tissue), and when the pressure is removed, the tissue becomes hyperemic (blood quickly infiltrates the tissue). This often relieves the tension, band, or knot, and the pain. This pressure is usually held for 8 to 15 seconds, and if a spasm is felt during application of pressure, pressure should be maintained until the muscle stops firing.

Sports massage can be broken into event massage and maintenance massage. Event massage (related to a massage done on an athlete before, during, or after competing) can be broken down into pre-event, inter-event, and post-event. The goal of pre-event massage is to leave the animal relaxed and ready for the event. Inter-event massage keeps the patient tuned up and ready for the next event, and post-event massage flushes out metabolic waste and reduces muscle spasms and soreness. The goal of maintenance massage is to help prevent injury and expedite the healing of injured tissue.

TTEAM is a system of massage used to teach physical awareness of the body. It is a form of massage that is devoted to nonhabitual motion to reeducate the nervous and musculoskeletal systems. TTEAM has an impact on an emotional level, in addition to aiding focus, coordination, and balance. A major difference between TTEAM and other forms of massage is that massage works on deeper tissue, and TTEAM manipulates only the skin.

Swedish massage is the most commonly used massage system in North America. These techniques began in the late 1700s and will be discussed here for use with animals. Studies have shown that massage is beneficial in reducing stress, enhancing blood and lymph circulation, decreasing pain, promoting sleep, reducing swelling, enhancing relaxation, and increasing oxygen capacity of the blood.

Techniques

Effleurage is the most commonly used stroke in animals. It is a gliding stroke that follows the contour of the body. Hand over hand, thumb over thumb, and one hand on either side of the body are the most common variations. It is repeated several times at the beginning and at the end of the massage to evaluate the tissue and enhance blood flow (warm it up, then aid in flushing lactic acid). Animals usually prefer these strokes flowing with the hair. Although effleurage is often thought of as a light stroke, deeper strokes are used to lengthen muscles and assist stretching.

Pétrissage, or kneading, consists of rhythmic lifting, squeezing, and releasing of tissue. It assists in removing metabolic waste and promoting circulation. The hands form a C shape and can be alternated in a circular motion, can "roll" the skin, or can spread up and out to help widen or broaden the muscle (Figure 23-11).

Friction is the manipulation of tissue done to promote circulation. It is commonly used over tendons when tendonitis is present, over knots and trigger points, and over joint capsules with excessive fibrous tissue. It is also used to break up skin adhesions and scar tissue (wait 3 to 4 weeks after injury or surgery before applying this technique). When friction is applied to deep tissue, one finger or thumb is placed on the skin and either rubs the skin or is attached to the skin and rubs the tissue underneath. This can be done longitudinally (with muscle fibers), across fibers (perpendicular to the muscle fibers), circularly, diagonally, or in a J pattern.

Tapotement is a tapping motion of the hands or fingers. When done for a short time, it stimulates nerve endings (pre-event sports massage or for toning of atrophied muscles). When done longer, it has a more sedative effect. Coupage, which is used to loosen phlegm congestion in the lungs, is a form of tapotement. The hands are cupped, and strokes start at the caudal aspect of the ribs and move forward. Proper positioning using wedges or pillows can help maximize the effectiveness of coupage. This stroke may be continued for 5 to 10 minutes on each side (Figure 23-12).

Vibration is rapid shaking or slower rocking of the tissue. The speed of vibration affects the outcome: faster vibrations are stimulatory, whereas slower speeds are inhibitory. It differs from tapotement in that the therapist's hands do not leave the patient's skin. It can aid in relaxing muscles and

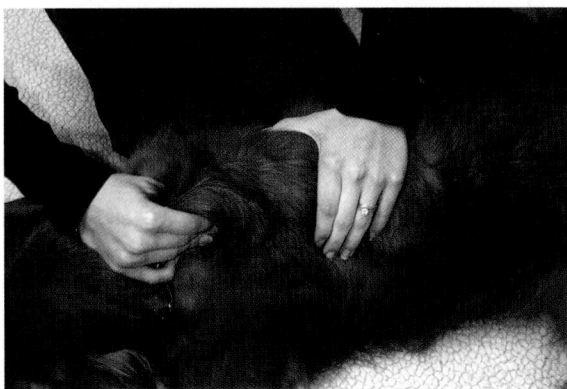

FIGURE 23-11 Bandit receiving pétrissage. Notice the C shape of the hands and the alternating pattern of the hands.

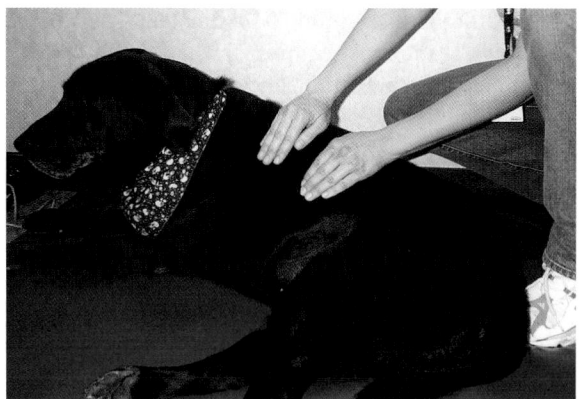

FIGURE 23-12 Coupage, a form of tapotement, is performed on Shadow. Note that the hands are cupped and alternating. Motion starts at the base of the ribs and moves forward.

reducing trigger-point activity, and when used over a joint capsule in the proper position, it can act as joint mobilization.

Swedish Massage

Swedish massage breaks down the massage into several elements, including intention, touch, pressure and depth, excursion, speed, rhythm and continuity, duration, and sequence. Intention is the consciously sought out goal of the therapist. Therefore, the massage outcome is different if the therapist wants to create relaxation versus invigoration. Touch is the vehicle of massage and conveys the intention. Pressure is the force applied to the surface, usually through the therapist's hands. Depth is the distance traveled into the patient's tissue. The therapist controls the force, but the patient has greater control over the depth. Often, applying less pressure slowly will increase depth, whereas fast, higher pressure will cause splinting (muscle contracting in a protective reflex) to occur. Excursion is the length of one massage stroke. In a cross-friction massage, meant to relieve tendonitis, the excursion may be only 1 to 2 cm, but in a beginning effleurage stroke, the excursion may extend from the head all the way to the tip of the tail. Speed refers to how fast the hand moves over the patient. In an invigorating pre-event sports massage, the speed will be much faster than if the therapist's goal is to achieve relaxation. Repetition or regularity of the stroke defines its rhythm, similar to music. The concept of continuity in massage refers to the uninterrupted flow of strokes and to the unbroken transition from one stroke to the next. It is difficult for the patient to relax if the rhythm is not smooth, or if the continuity is not fluid. Duration is the length of time devoted to one area. In humans, a relaxing massage does not usually last longer than 1 hour without creating muscle soreness. The duration of a small animal massage is usually 30 minutes, and for a large animal, as with humans, it is approximately 1 hour long. A sequence is the arrangement of massage strokes.

A typical example of a sequence would be as follows:
- Start with effleurage on the face and head.
- Continue down the back and sides.
- Use pétrissage over the paraspinal muscles (including kneading, circles, or strokes going with or perpendicular to the muscle fibers).
- Apply ischemic compression on trigger points if found.
- Move on to one side of the neck.
- Carry on down the forelimb.
- Perform effleurage, with strokes running from the toes to the heart to flush toxins.
- Continue by using skin rolls along the body wall.
- Apply the same techniques you used in the forelimb to treat the rear limb.
- Gently flip the patient over if a canine, or walk around to the other side if an equine.
- Repeat your techniques on the other side.
- Finish up with a final effleurage.

Signs of relaxation include sighing, yawning, licking the lips, hanging the head (equine), burping, and flatulence. Signs that the pressure is too great include increased respiratory rate, opening the eyes (if previously closed), fidgeting, and incessant licking (canine) or swishing of the tail (equine).

Contraindications

Several contraindications to massage are known, and areas of the body called *endangerment sites* are too delicate to support massage and should be avoided. Contraindications include massage over bacterially or virally infected lesions, over open wounds, over the area of an acute injury or an inflammatory condition, over an area of hemorrhage, or after a recent high fever. Endangerment sites include the throat, eyeballs, brachial plexus, abdomen (deep, near the aorta), and over the kidneys, among others.

Precautions should be taken when massaging a patient with heart disease or over a neoplastic area.

TECHNICIAN NOTE Effleurage is the most commonly used stroke in animals. It is a gliding stroke that follows the contour of the body.

PASSIVE RANGE OF MOTION

Passive range of motion (PROM) is the use of stretching to prevent the loss of normal range of motion, to return normal range of motion if absent, to increase cartilage nutrition in the joint, and to stimulate cartilage regeneration. Most of the nutrition received by the chondrocytes (cartilage cells) comes from the capillary-rich synovial capsule, which then bathes the cartilage via the synovial fluid. If the joint is stationary, the joint fluid is not circulated, and less nutrition is available to the chondrocytes.

If PROM is to be done postsurgically or in a joint with restricted motion, each joint that is stretched should be worked on separately. However, when PROM is performed on a patient with a neurologic disorder, where it will be used to prevent loss of motion and to increase cartilage nutrition and regeneration, each limb is approached as a whole (Figure 23-13). Rules of PROM include the following:

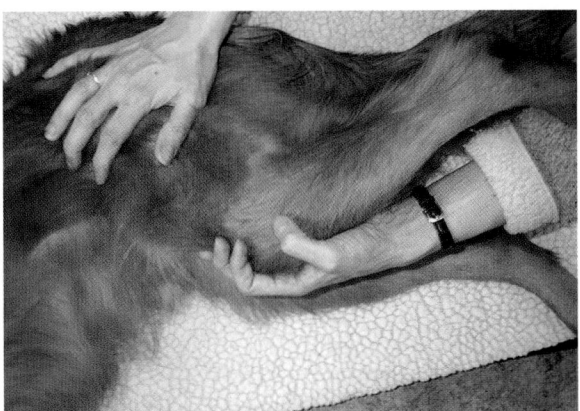

FIGURE 23-13 A technician performs passive range of motion (PROM) on a neurologic patient.

Over heart or cardiac pacemakers
Use on animals with seizure disorders
Over areas of peripheral vascular disease or thrombophlebitis
Over areas of decreased pain/temperature sensation
Over infection
Over neoplasms
Over the carotid sinus
Any time active motion is contraindicated

1. It should never hurt.
2. If the patient is lying in lateral recumbency, keep the worked limb parallel to the ground to prevent torque of the joints.
3. Flex the most proximal joint first and work distally.
4. Do not let the stifle go under the rib cage.
5. Hold the limb flexed for 10 seconds, hold it in extension for 10 seconds (to the front, then 10 seconds to the back), and repeat this 10 times.
6. Massage the muscles you are stretching.
7. Guide the limb, do not pull it.
8. Do not hyperextend the carpus or tarsus because permanent tendon or ligament damage may occur. These joints are flexed and relaxed, unless a contracture issue involves these joints.
9. If the case is postsurgical, set up your hands on either side of the joint on which you are working (each joint is worked one at a time), and then move your eyes too and keep them on the surgery joint to prevent inadvertent motion of this joint.
10. Hip and shoulder joints have rotation and flexion and extension. Start with small circles and gradually increase the motion while performing 10 rotations. Stabilize the distal joints.

The technician can take an active role in PROM, performing this modality under a veterinarian's direction. This can be done successfully in equine and canine patients.

ELECTRICAL AND MAGNET-BASED THERAPIES

Neuromuscular Stimulation

Neuromuscular electrical stimulation (NMES) is the application of electrical current to elicit a muscle contraction. The main purpose of NMES in rehabilitation is to attain muscle strengthening. Clinical uses include reducing disuse atrophy (post surgery or injury), reversing muscle atrophy (the patient that is not using a limb post surgery or injury), and strengthening selected muscles (neuromuscular reeducation). Although NMES is an effective treatment, it is not

done without risk. Refer to Box 23-3 for a list of contraindications when NMES stimulation is used.

A voluntary muscle contraction recruits small-diameter, slow-twitch, type I, fatigue-resistant fibers first. Constant tension of the muscle is maintained by asynchronous recruitment of those fibers—some are relaxing as others are contracting. An electrically induced muscle contraction first recruits large-diameter, fast-twitch, type II fibers because of their low threshold for electrical excitation. These fibers tend to be recruited simultaneously, and as they fatigue, tension in the muscle begins to decrease. With continued NMES therapy, studies have revealed that properties of fast-twitch, type II muscle fibers begin to resemble those of slow-twitch, type I muscle fibers and decrease the fatigability of the muscle.

In treating a patient, pads are placed over the motor point of the muscle (the area in which the least electricity is needed to produce a contraction—usually where a nerve enters the muscle) and over a distal point (usually just proximal to the musculotendinous junction) on the muscle (Figure 23-14). If a solid contraction cannot be created, the proximal pad should be rearranged to make sure it is truly over the motor point.

Treatment parameters usually are determined by the attending veterinarian or physical therapist and include frequency (pulses per second, measured in Hertz [Hz]), pulse duration (in microseconds), intensity, duty cycle (contraction time vs. relaxation time), ramp (time to full contraction), and treatment time. Waveform or current type (alternating current [AC] vs. direct current [DC]) may be determined by the type of machine used.

The technician's role in NMES is to shave and clean the skin with alcohol, apply the gel and pads, and use the NMES machine to obtain a strong yet pain-free contraction. The patient should be monitored throughout the session because pads sometimes migrate, causing reduced effectiveness or even discomfort if placed incorrectly. Finally, the session should be recorded in the patient's record, with details on all treatment variables described previously, as well as any unusual reactions noted. Knowledge of anatomy is essential for performing this task. Muscles and muscle groups that are routinely stimulated include triceps muscles, paraspinal

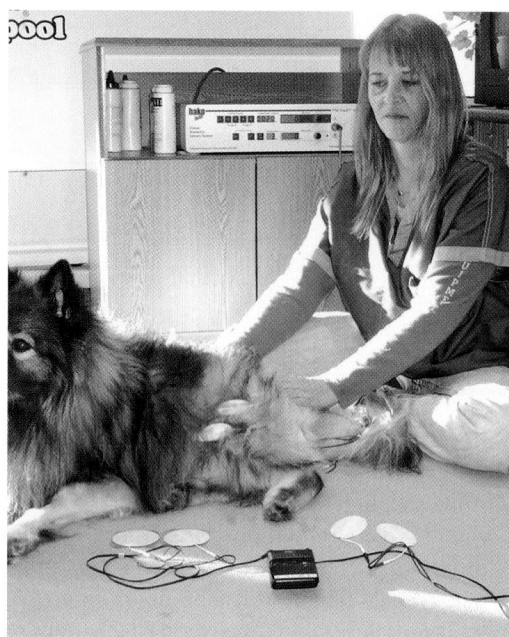

FIGURE 23-14 A dog receives neuromuscular electrical stimulation (NMES) from the Hako-Med unit, which is visible in the background. A smaller, hand-held NMES unit is visible on the floor in the foreground.

muscles, gluteal muscles, hamstring muscles, quadriceps muscles, and cranial tibial muscles. Forelimb flexor muscles, forelimb extensor muscles, deltoid muscles, and gastrocnemius muscles also may be stimulated.

Bioelectrical Stimulation

Electricity is found naturally in all of us. In ancient Greece, physicians used electric eels in footbaths to relieve pain and enhance circulation. It is known that certain electrical impulses facilitate bodily functions, including actions needed for healing. Two types of devices that can deliver electricity through the patient are transcutaneous electrical nerve stimulation (TENS) units and interferential units.

TENS units most frequently use frequencies of 75 to 100 Hz for pain relief. The down side of using TENS units is that the pain often returns relatively quickly.

Interferential therapy can be used with one frequency in one direction and another in a perpendicular direction, so that where they are superimposed, summation is followed by cancellation of the current. It can also be used with two pads on one side for topical treatment or muscle stimulation. This therapy is most effective in treating deep, aching, and chronic pain, but it can also be used for acute pain and electroanalgesia. Frequencies used are usually 4000 Hz in one direction and 4001 to 4100 Hz in the other direction. This puts the frequency in the periphery at a 4000-Hz range and between 1 and 100 Hz (often scaling up and down) where the frequencies cross.

Most units have attached leads that are placed on either side of the area to be treated or, in the case of interferential, on all four sides. Typically, before the leads are attached, the patient is shaved and the skin is cleaned with alcohol to remove hair and dead skin. Reusable or carbon pads are attached to the unit's leads with gel to increase conductivity. The frequency is set and the amplitude is adjusted so the patient feels a sensation but has no pain.

The technician's role in bioelectrical stimulation is to administer and record the treatment. This includes shaving if needed, applying gel and pads, and setting the machine to the proper frequency and intensity. Additional training with individual units will be needed before this can be done effectively.

Magnetic and Electromagnetic Stimulation

Magnets have been used for centuries in medicine. Magnetism can be separated into stationary magnets, which have north and south poles, and electromagnetic therapy, which uses electricity of different frequencies along with magnets to create an electromagnetic field. Units of measurement for magnetism are gauss (G) and tesla (T). Most therapeutic magnets range from 1000 to 3000 G. Below 500 G has been deemed ineffective. The north and south poles of a magnet are reported to have different effects. Effects of using the north pole end of the magnet include pain relief, stimulation of bone healing, enhanced vasoconstriction, decreased blood pressure, and decreased rate of mitosis, which in turn slows the growth rate of cancer cells and bacterial cells. Effects of using the south pole side of the magnet include strengthening and promoting growth by stimulating cell multiplication (therefore should not be used with bacterial or viral infection or close to tumors), enhanced vasodilatation, slowed bone healing, and increased ascites, edema, and inflammation. Some therapeutic magnets have both north and south poles that may be held on a given area or wrapped over an area. Products are available that place magnets in horse blankets or leg wraps and in dog and cat beds and collars.

In electromagnetic therapy, pulsating electromagnetic waves are produced by electrical charges undergoing acceleration. These waves can be generated with different frequencies and can create different physiologic changes in the body. For instance, it is known that an electrical field surrounding each joint plays a part in the continual regeneration of cartilage and connective tissue. A disturbance in this field occurs if osteoarthritis or inflammatory joint disorders are present. Pulsed signal therapy (PST) is one type of **pulsed electromagnetic field therapy (PEMF)** that allows reconstruction of the disturbed electrical field (Figure 23-15). This returns the natural regeneration capabilities and reactivates the chondrocytes (cartilage cells) and connective tissue to increase production of proteoglycan and collagen, which aids in repairing cartilage defects. In addition to osteoarthritis, this unit has been shown to aid repair of tendon and ligament injuries (do not use for partial cranial cruciate tears because it removes the early scar tissue critical for stabilization) and wound healing. A battery-operated unit, the Assisi device, uses different frequencies from those used in PST. It increases nitric oxide, which reduces pain and inflammation, reduces edema, improves blood flow, and has been shown to increase angiogenesis (development of new blood vessels),

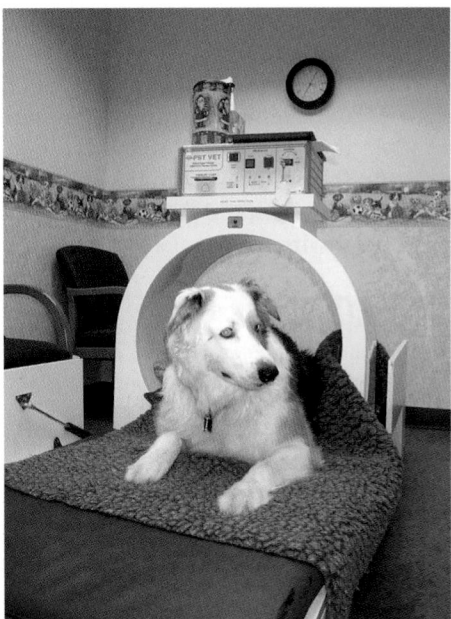

FIGURE 23-15 Pulsed signal therapy (PST) has an 80% to 85% success rate in treating osteoarthritis with good to excellent results. Because the treatment area measures 13 inches, feet, hocks, stifles, hips, and lower back often can be treated at the same time.

BOX 23-4 | Clinical Applications of Ultrasound

Joint contracture and scar tissue: heats and stretches to improve range of motion
Tendonitis and bursitis: increases blood flow, decreases pain
Pain and muscle spasm: increases pain threshold and reduces muscle spindle activity
Wound healing: use at low intensity 2 weeks post injury
Calcium reabsorption: still to be substantiated
Chronic wounds: stimulates production of wound factors

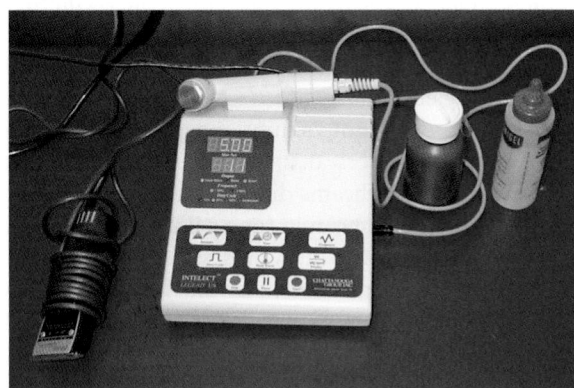

FIGURE 23-16 Setting up the ultrasound is one of the technician's responsibilities.

as well as improve tissue regeneration and tendon tensile strength after surgery. PEMF has been used extensively in equine sports medicine for musculoskeletal and neurologic conditions as well. It has been used successfully to treat navicular disease, tendon injuries, arthroses, spavins, delayed wound healing, and diseases of the thoracolumbar spine. Artificial insemination centers also use PEMF to extend the productive capacity of bulls that suffer from degenerative lumbosacral disease.

> **TECHNICIAN NOTE** Most therapeutic magnets range from 1000 to 3000 G. Magnets below 500 G have been deemed ineffective.

LIGHT AND SOUND–BASED THERAPIES
Therapeutic Ultrasound

Therapeutic (vs. diagnostic) ultrasound is the use of sound waves to treat tissue. It works by producing heat, but it also has some nonthermal effects that are not fully understood. The therapeutic value of ultrasound includes increased collagen extensibility, increased blood flow, increased range of motion due to changes in contractility of muscle, decreased pain and muscle spasm, increased enzyme activity, changes in nerve conduction velocity, accelerated wound healing due to facilitation of the inflammatory process, and enhanced transdermal delivery of medication (phonophoresis). Refer to Box 23-4 for a list of clinical applications for therapeutic ultrasound.

Variables that determine the amount of heat produced by the sound wave include frequency, intensity, duty cycle, duration of exposure, and size and type of the tissue to be treated. At a frequency of 1 MHz, the depth of penetration is 4 to 5 cm, whereas at a frequency of 3 MHz, penetration depth is only 1 cm. The proximity of the bone and the thickness of the tissue determine the frequency that is used. Intensity determines whether thermal or nonthermal effects will be seen. Intensities over 1.0 W/cm^2 produce thermal effects that increase circulation and help reduce joint contractures. Intensities less than 1.0 W/cm^2 produce nonthermal effects that enhance wound healing. The duty cycle is the fraction of time that the sound wave is emitted during a pulse period. In a continuous mode, intensity is constant and may cause "unstable cavitations," which can be destructive to tissue but may be beneficial for stretching scar tissue. In a pulsed mode, most commonly 20% or 50%, the wave is interrupted in an on/off pattern. Pulsed ultrasound is used to enhance healing and eliminate swelling. Time is determined by the size of the area being treated, as well as by the size of the therapeutic device. Generally, we treat an area twice the size of the sound head for about 5 minutes. As sound increases the temperature in the tissue, it is important to continuously move the sound head. If it is held stationary, burns of the skin, muscle, or periosteum may result.

The technician's role in ultrasound is to shave the area, clean the area with alcohol, and perhaps administer ultrasound treatment under the physician's supervision (Figure 23-16). Treatment is also charted after the therapy session; charting includes details on areas treated, duration, duty cycle, frequency, and intensity.

Laser

Laser stands for *light amplification by stimulated emission of radiation*. Albert Einstein first introduced this concept in 1917. Low-level laser therapy (LLLT, also known as "cold" laser) is the stimulation of tissue with low-energy lasers to achieve a therapeutic effect. The most common indications for LLLT include treating pain associated with degenerative joint disease (arthritis) and intervertebral disc disease (IVDD), postoperative pain, and soft tissue injuries. It is also used to stimulate healing of wounds and ulcers, to stimulate acupuncture points (see Figure 23-4), to relieve trigger points, and to reduce edema, stomatitis, gingivitis, and temporomandibular joint dysfunction. Lasers most commonly used in LLLT are visible red helium-neon (HeNe) lasers that have a wavelength in the 600- to 700-nm range, invisible infrared (IR) gallium-arsenide (GaAs) lasers that have a wavelength in the 900-nm vicinity, and gallium-aluminum-arsenide (GaAlAs) lasers that have a wavelength in the 800-nm vicinity. Laser beams differ from conventional light in that they are monochromic (one color creates a narrow spectrum) and coherent (the waves stay together and are consistent). Most lasers have polarized light (light waves oscillate in the same plane), small divergence (nearly parallel beam), and high mean output power (MOP), indicating that many watts are put out. LLLT may be indicated for soft tissue trauma, wounds, tendonitis, and pain relief (Figure 23-17). Some of the biological effects seen with LLLT include accelerated cell division, increased leukocyte phagocytosis, stimulation of fibroblasts and collagen formation, and degranulation of mast cells (it is interesting to note that mast cell degranulation may also occur when a needle is placed in an acupuncture point).

Precautions

Lasers may induce retinal lesions and therefore are classified by their irradiation properties. Class I lasers have 0.4 mW output (MOP) or less. Class II lasers have 0.5 to 1.0 mW MOP, and if they shine in your eyes, a blink reflex is usually adequate to prevent retinal damage. A Class IIIa laser has 1 to 5 mW MOP, which means that caution must be used near the eyes because retinal damage may occur if the laser is

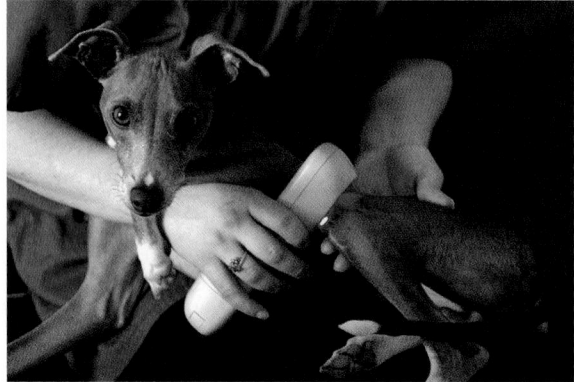

FIGURE 23-17 Laser Q-1000. A dog receives laser therapy for a stifle injury.

directed into the eye (even if the lid is closed). Class IIIb lasers have 5 to 500 mW MOP and are considered dangerous to the eyes. A class IV laser has greater than 500 mW MOP and is dangerous to the retina (special glasses must be worn at all times when the laser is in use) and is a potential fire hazard. Generally, the more powerful the laser, the greater is the risk of adverse reactions, and the more likely it is that use of the laser would be limited to veterinarians.

> **TECHNICIAN NOTE**   Some of the biological effects seen with LLLT include accelerated cell division, increased leukocyte phagocytosis, stimulation of fibroblasts, collagen formation, and degranulation of mast cells.

Superficial Thermal Therapy

Cold and heat therapies affect physiologic change in the body. Although fairly simple to apply, cold and heat therapies can be extremely beneficial for the rehabilitation patient.

Cryotherapy, or cold therapy, when applied to the body, removes heat. Actions include vasoconstriction, which reduces postsurgical bleeding and bruising (when the cooling agent is removed, a rebound vasodilatation occurs—red coloration may be seen in the skin), slows nerve conduction (thereby decreasing pain sensation), and decreases enzyme activity (decreasing inflammation). The larger the animal, the longer it takes to cool the deep tissue. A small dog may need 5 to 8 minutes for a stifle and a medium dog 10 to 12 minutes for a stifle, while a full-coated giant breed may need 15 minutes of cryotherapy to sufficiently bring the internal temperature down for therapeutic effect. Multiple rounds of cryotherapy can be beneficial. An example would consist of 10 minutes of cold and 10 minutes without cooling, followed by 10 minutes of cold up to 3 times daily. Horses do not need cryotherapy on their limbs for longer than 15 minutes. Cryotherapy is most commonly delivered to large animal patients via cold hosing, but various commercial products such as ice boots are available.

Postsurgically, cold can be applied by filling a Dixie cup three-fourths full and freezing it. The paper is unraveled, and gauze can be placed at the incision to prevent water from contaminating the incision. Commercial CoolPacks are easy to keep in the freezer. Frozen peas can also be used because they are moldable and hold the cold fairly well, but because air surrounds the individual peas, and air is a poor conductor, gel packs are superior. A mixture of alcohol and water in a Ziploc freezer bag at a ratio of 1:2 stays cold and malleable. Double bagging is recommended to prevent cold leaks. If the patient is shaved or short-coated, wrapping the alcohol bag in a towel may be required. Machines are made for cooling that can either spray liquid nitrogen on the affected area or use a flowing ice bath in conjunction with compression to decrease swelling and pain. In large animal patients, running a cold hose over an injury is also effective. Therapeutic ice boots are available for equine extremities.

Actions of heat include increasing circulation, increasing muscle contractility, increasing the ability of collagen to stretch, and decreasing pain. The recommended method is wet heat. A hand towel for small areas or a bath towel for larger areas may be folded into thirds and rolled (to be unrolled around a joint) or accordion-folded (to be placed over a flat surface). Run the towel under warm to hot water and apply to the area. If you cannot keep your hand on the towel because it is too hot for you, it is also too hot for the patient. A big, thick towel or plastic wrap may be placed over the wet towel to keep the heat in.

Heat can be applied for 10 to 15 minutes over areas of chronic arthritis, preceding exercises to warm up muscles and joints, or if an area is cold to the touch on examination (signifying a chronic condition with decreased blood perfusion). Heat can also be used over an area of infection once the patient is taking antibiotics to enhance penetration of the drug into the area. Sweat wraps can be used on equine extremities and commonly contain DMSO, (nitrofurazone) or dexamethasone, surrounded by plastic and a quilted wrap. This is thought to decrease inflammation and swelling.

Contraindications

Do not use cryotherapy and heat therapy over areas that do not have sensory sensation, because tissue damage may occur.

ASSISTIVE DEVICES

Sometimes patients cannnot reach a previous level of function or do not achieve an acceptable level of function or comfort without an assistive device. These devices range from simple protective devices such as boots and nail covers to complex custom orthotics, prosthetics, and wheelchairs. Not only do these devices help the patient recover or adapt physically, but many patients benefit from the emotional lift gained from increased mobility and independence.

Wheelchairs

Wheelchairs allow a dysfunctional patient the freedom of movement and a means of performing regular exercise (Figure 23-18). If properly introduced to a patient, they are not only accepted but are fully enjoyed by both patient and client. Although they offer greater freedom of movement for the patient, wheelchairs can tip or become stuck on surrounding obstacles, so supervision is important. Initially, they should be used for very short (5- to 10-minute) periods to allow the patient to adjust to them. Some dogs may have difficulty eliminating, but most do adapt with time. For all but very small dogs, carts are not recommended for indoor use and are generally used only for periods of supervised exercise.

Wheelchairs range from fully adjustable aluminum frames with two wheels, a neoprene seat, and a harness to complex four-wheeled "quad" carts with head and neck support. It is important that each wheelchair or cart be properly fitted for the individual's balance and comfort. If the balance is not quite right, it may be difficult or uncomfortable for the patient to move in the apparatus. Sometimes it takes 30 to 45 minutes to adjust the cart to fit properly, introduce the patient to walking confidently, and teach the client the basics of cart care and troubleshooting.

Harnesses and Slings

Harnesses and slings are often used for the same patients that would benefit from the use of wheelchairs, but harnesses and slings may be used instead if full independence is expected to return shortly. They allow clients to assist their dog via weight and balance support without injuring their own back in the process. Some slings are simple, with a fabric support that slides under the abdomen, and some harnesses are fully adjustable, with support for both front limbs and hindlimbs. The more complex the harness, the more instruction owners will need on how to apply, fit, and adjust the harness to their pet and on how to use it properly on a regular basis. Large animals that need weight-bearing and balance assistance can benefit from a harness and sling system attached to a ceiling beam. Although stall confinement is necessary for these patients, the benefits of being upright tremendously reduce complications that may occur when a horse or cow is recumbent. Because of their massive size and body weight, pressure sores and life-threatening gastrointestinal stasis can develop rapidly in large animal patients that must endure prolonged recumbency.

Protective Devices

Paws and nails may be traumatized when patients are unable to lift their feet properly because of paresis and instead may knuckle and drag their paws. Nail caps can be applied to protect nails from wear as long as enough nail is present at the base to allow proper attachment of the cap. Nail caps are extremely helpful to wear when knuckling is seen because they allow the foot to continue direct contact with the ground. Boots can be helpful in protecting not only nails but the entire paw. Although boots reduce tactile ground contact, they can be useful if a patient traumatizes the side or dorsum of the foot. They can be heavy and durable or light and disposable. Elastic bands may be attached to some boots, providing assistance with dorsiflexion to help reduce knuckling.

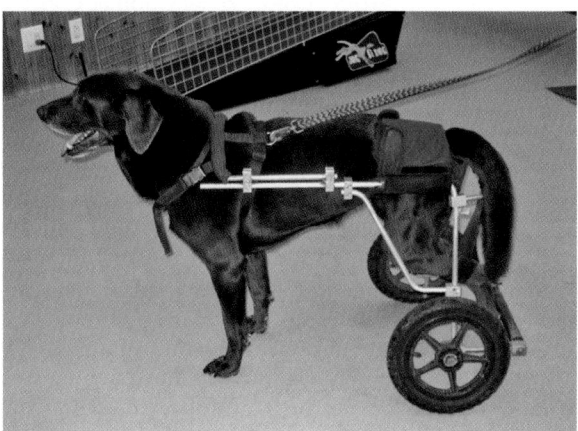

FIGURE 23-18 After suffering paralysis, Lucy is able to be independently mobile in her custom cart.

CASE PRESENTATION 23-3 CANINE INTERVERTEBRAL DISC DISEASE

Signalment: Sebastian, a 7-year-old neutered male Beagle, 40 lb

Chief Complaint: Quadriplegia 5 days after ventral slot for IVDD at C5-C6

Pertinent History: Sebastian initially became painful 2 days before surgery. He cried when he lifted his head and was reluctant to move. He was examined by his regular veterinarian, who took radiographs (which were unremarkable) and started him on prednisone (10 mg bid 3 days, then sid 4 days). That evening, he was more painful, so tramadol was prescribed (50 mg bid). The following morning, he was swaying while walking, so he was referred to the local emergency clinic, which monitored him over the weekend. Over the weekend, he lost voluntary motion. An MRI was performed by a neurologist, who found a compression at C5-C6. Sebastian was taken immediately to surgery and underwent a ventral slot procedure at the site of disc rupture with fenestration from C2 to C6. He was managed at the emergency clinic for 5 days, with pain control consisting of a fentanyl patch and tramadol 50 mg tid. He was released for rehabilitation 5 days after surgery. His pain patch was removed before transfer. Additionally, he had undergone a femoral head ostectomy (FHO) on his right hip 3 months before presentation (as a result of hip dysplasia).

Significant Examination Findings: Contusion along ventral neck with heat and tight, tender, spastic muscles along the cervical spine; quadriplegia with no weight-bearing ability; crepitus at the right hip with moderate muscle atrophy in the right rear limb. Sebastian was able to maintain a sternal position when assisted to rise from lateral recumbency but was unable to lift his head more than 2 inches off the floor.

Problem List:
- Quadriplegia
- Cervical pain post IVDD and decompressive surgery
- Muscle spasm, tightness, and tenderness along the cervical spine
- Heat and inflammation along the cervical spine
- Contusion along the incision line
- Crepitus at the right hip secondary to previous FHO

INITIAL THERAPY PLAN	PURPOSE
Acupuncture daily for 3 days, then every other day for 1 week, tapering further as pain subsides	Pain control, stimulation of healing, nervous system support
Spascupreel	Reduce muscle spasm
Cryotherapy 2 times daily	Reduce inflammation and pain
Massage 30 minutes daily	Relieve pain and tightness in the muscles, increase circulation to promote healing, stimulate nerve endings
Passive range of motion daily	Maintain range of motion, stimulate nerve endings

INITIAL THERAPY PLAN	PURPOSE
Neuromuscular electrical stimulation (NMES)—both triceps and supraspinatus muscles every other day	Promote muscle strengthening passively
Supplements:	
Vitamin C 250 mg bid	Antioxidant support
Vitamin E 400 IU/day	Antioxidant support
Vitamin B complex 50 mg/day	Nervous system support
Traumeel 1 tab tid	Reduce bruising and pain
Discus Compositum 1 tab tid	Promote neurologic strengthening
Hako-Med electrical current therapy daily for 3 days, then every other day for 1 week	Pain relief
Therapeutic exercises with weekly consultation to revise exercise plan	Neurologic stimulation, strengthening, reeducation on ambulation

Client Communication: The recommended therapy plan was presented to the client and was immediately approved.

Treatment: Acupuncture was performed with a dry needle technique (GV 14, tip of tail; BL 17, BL 27 to facilitate movement of qi down the governing vessel and bladder meridians that run through the spine; GB 20 and 39 to facilitate qi movement through the gallbladder meridian to the back legs; LI 10 and SI 3 to facilitate qi movement down the front legs) using Hwato needles (22G 1 inch) inserted to a maximum depth of ½ inch. Spascupreel (0.5 ml) was injected subcutaneously at gallbladder 21 bilaterally to reduce muscle spasms near the surgery site (lower cervical spine). Sebastian's urinary bladder was expressed manually until empty. He did not attempt or appear to be able to urinate on his own.

Progress: By the next morning, Sebastian was able to lift his head and support some weight in all four limbs for about 10 seconds. An exercise consultation was done with a physical therapist to determine what exercises would be appropriate for him. He still needed assistance to attain a sternal position from lateral recumbency but did make an attempt. He needed assistance to attain and maintain sitting and standing positions. He continued to progress daily his first week, by the end of the week was able to move from a lateral to a sternal position unassisted and to stand with only balance support for 1 minute, and was attempting to take steps with all four limbs (although he lacked coordination). Irritation at the pain patch site and at his incision was resolved, but muscle spasms persisted, and his neck was sore at the end of the day. He had started to urinate on his own, with excellent bladder awareness and control.

   The following week, Sebastian continued to progress to increased weight-bearing activity, improved coordination to the point where ambulation training could be initiated, and improved comfort; muscle spasms had resolved. Pain

CASE PRESENTATION 23-3 CANINE INTERVERTEBRAL DISC DISEASE—cont'd

management was greatly reduced (Tramadol, Traumeel, and Spascupreel were discontinued; Hako-Med therapy was also discontinued). After surgical staple removal, hydrotreadmill therapy was initiated with great success: Sebastian moved all four limbs independently with reasonable coordination.

At the beginning of week 3, Sebastian was able to transition from a down position to standing and could walk for several minutes with balance support. His right rear limb was the weakest, partly as a result of his already present atrophy after FHO surgery, so neuromuscular stimulation was changed to work on his right quadriceps, hamstrings, gluteals, and digital extensors. By the end of week 3, Sebastian was able to walk unassisted and negotiate a course of weave cones, small stairs, poles on the ground, and gentle hills.

Sebastian continued to progress with ongoing acupuncture, hydrotreadmill therapy, and a home exercise program. Within 6 weeks after the initial injury, he was running and playing with no restrictions. After 3 months, he had regained enough strength in his right rear limb to be almost completely balanced and symmetric.

Discussion: Sebastian's remarkable progress was due largely to compassionate holistic care. His response to therapy was dramatic and fairly rapid, but the treatments themselves only partly contributed to the speed of his recovery. He received intensive pain management and appropriate exercise to facilitate neurologic healing. He was kept in a nurturing environment, where he received extra attention, got sufficient rest, and was given a healthy diet. He was taken outside to eliminate at least 4 times daily and was

encouraged with his favorite treats and toys. Sebastian was treated as an individual with specific needs that we strived to meet each day, and this holistic focus was what made the difference in his successful recovery (Figure 1). Technicians played a fundamental role in Sebastian's therapy and general care. In addition to assisting with the examination and acupuncture treatments, they took a primary role in performing cryotherapy, Hako-Med, massage, PROM, NMES, and exercises. They also were responsible for communication with the client and nursing care. This is an excellent example of how crucial technician care can be in returning a critically ill or injured patient to health and mobility.

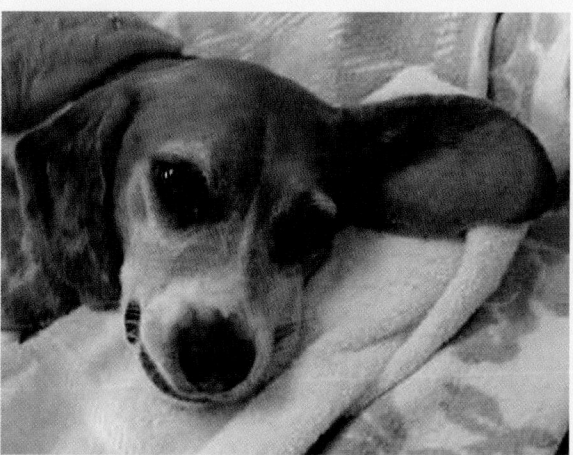

FIGURE 1 Sebastian, the little Beagle that could.

For large animals, boots are used to assist recovery from hoof injuries and are available in a variety of configurations. Some are fastened by straps and levers and are removable (these are beneficial when medication needs to be applied); others are more like a glue-on shoe and are semi-permanent.

Braces and Orthotics

Sometimes patients cannot bear their full weight on a weak or injured limb. Commercially available braces and wraps may provide light to moderate support for recovery while strengthening exercises are carried out. These braces are commonly available for the carpus and hock in dogs, and for the hock and fetlock in horses. Neoprene braces are available for stifles, shoulders, and elbows in dogs. When a patient requires rigid support or needs support in a joint that is not commonly braced, such as the equine stifle, a custom orthotic is indicated. An orthotic device may be used not only to provide support but also to limit range of motion. This is important in joints in which hypermobility is seen. Braces may provide assistance with limb alignment and may help to reduce the adverse effects of having legs of different lengths. A hock brace with a foot lift, for example, is helpful in a canine patient with a limb length discrepancy that causes

carpal hyperextension in the affected (shorter) limb. The brace limits extension in the affected limb to 160 degrees while allowing full flexion; the lift neutralizes the effects of the limb length discrepancy so the patient is able to work and strengthen muscles needed for greater mobility. Orthotics are commonly used in horses suffering from traumatic injury, typically on the lower limb. Prosthetics are used to replace a part of the limb that is missing. These must be custom-fashioned to prevent pain and ensure correct balance and stability. The technician can be involved in cast molding the affected limb so that a model limb can be generated for use by the orthotist or the prosthetist.

It is important that the introduction of assistive devices be progressive and positive, and that their use is limited initially, if possible. Complications resulting from use of assistive devices include skin irritation and ulceration, chewing, breakdown and wear, and lack of patient acceptance. Careful monitoring and excellent client education increase the likelihood of success.

TTouch Wrap or Anxiety Wrap

TTouch is part of TTEAM, which is mentioned in the massage section of this chapter. TTouch for small animals includes a variety of techniques that positively affect animals

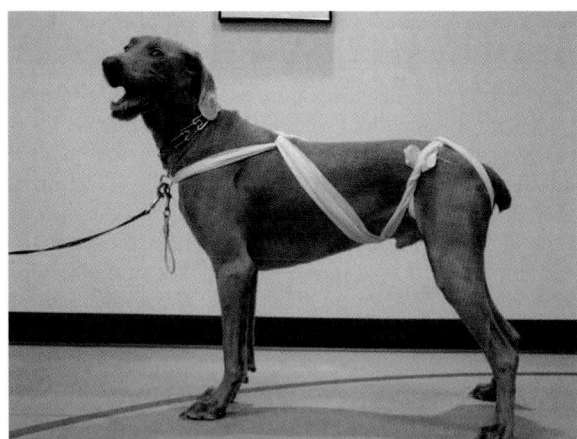

FIGURE 23-19 Sterling wears a TTouch wrap to assist calming.

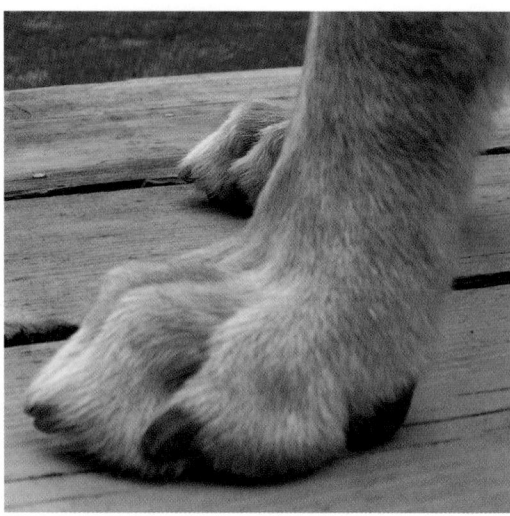

FIGURE 23-20 Example of a dog's foot with toenails of proper length. Note that nails do not contact the ground.

and give a sense of well-being. A certification course in these techniques is offered to both veterinary technicians and laypeople. One method used to calm anxious dogs involves application of an ace bandage that is wrapped and tied in a continuous pattern around the ventral neck, rib cage, abdomen, and hind legs (Figure 23-19). Remarkably, the calming effects of this application are usually seen within 5 to 10 minutes. The ace bandage can be applied to anxious dogs before potentially stressful activities or events, such as the arrival of guests and thunderstorms.

A Word About Podiatry

An old adage states: "No hoof, no horse." If a hoof is trimmed improperly, the horse (or cow) cannot balance properly, and if shod, a horse is not able to "wear into" a normal hoof shape and angulation. Although wild ungulates wear their hooves continually, domestic ungulates require regular hoof care. It takes a great deal of knowledge, skill, and experience to correctly trim and balance a hoof.

Unlike horses, which bear all of their weight on their hooves, the dog toenail is NOT a weight-bearing structure; therefore, the most important goal of a proper nail trim in canines is to shorten the toenail so that it is off the ground. A rule of thumb is that on a hard, smooth surface, you should be able to slide a panel from a small cardboard box under the nail. Not only do excessively long nails ache from pressure that they were never meant to bear, they can also alter a dog's posture and contribute to injury. If the quick is excessively long, the patient can be sedated and the nail trimmed back into the quick (ouch!), or the nail can be trimmed away from the quick. This is a *corrective* toenail trim. Starting at the tip of the nail, the trimmer is angled upward toward the top of the nail base, and the top "shelf" of the nail is removed. Then the sides are trimmed to match. The nail can also be ground back until the nub of quick, surrounded by cuticle, is uncovered, looking much like a pencil point. This will recede and is not painful. The technique takes some practice, but it is amazing how short a nail can get even when a long quick is present. A general rule of thumb is to make the nail itself the ideal length

(Figure 23-20), and the quick will follow suit. This allows for a more comfortable trim and more dramatic results and therefore better client compliance.

SUMMARY

Rehabilitation and complementary veterinary medicine encompass a vast amount of material. This chapter offers an overview of some of the more common modalities used today and is not a comprehensive guide to alternative medicine or rehabilitation. Many of the individual subjects discussed in this chapter have their own texts written on the subject and are taught in courses lasting months to years. The veterinary technician may become skilled in many of these modalities, such as massage and flower essences, and can serve as an excellent source of information for clients regarding other modalities such as acupuncture and **chiropractic therapy**. As clients experience the benefits of physical therapy and alternative medicine in their own health care, they are increasingly interested in pursuing the same care for their pets. As the demand for complementary veterinary medicine, physical therapy, and rehabilitation grows, more veterinarians are pursuing advanced certification and are seeking veterinary technicians with training and expertise in these areas.

RECOMMENDED READINGS

Books

Gersh MR: Electrotherapy in rehabilitation, Philadelphia, 1992, FA Davis.

Graham H, Vlamis G: Bach flower remedies for animals, Forres, Scotland, 1999, Findhorn Press.

Michlovitz SL: Thermal agents in rehabilitation, ed 3, Philadelphia, 1996, FA Davis.

PDR People's desk reference for essential oils, Orem, UT, 1999, Essential Science Publishing.

Pitcairn R, Hubble Pitcairn S: Dr. Pitcairn's complete guide to natural health for dogs and cats, ed 3, New York, 2005, Rodale Books.

Pontinen PJ: Low level laser therapy as a medical treatment modality, Tampere, Finland, 1992, Art Urpo.

Salvo SG: Massage therapy principles and practice, St Louis, 2003, Saunders.

Schoen AM: Veterinary acupuncture: ancient art to modern medicine, St Louis, 1994, Mosby.

Schoen AM, Wynn SG: Complementary and alternative veterinary medicine: principles and practice, St Louis, 1998, Mosby.

Schwartz C: Four paws five directions: a guide to Chinese medicine for cats and dogs, Berkley, CA, 1996, Celestial Arts Publishing.

Tisserand R, Balacs T: Essential oil safety: a guide for health care professionals, Philadelphia, 1995, Churchill Livingstone.

Wulff-Tilford M, Tilford G: All you ever wanted to know about herbs for pets, Irvine, CA, 1999, Bowtie Press.

Wynn SG, Marsden SM: Manual of natural veterinary medicine: science and tradition, St Louis, 2002, Mosby.

Wynn SG, Marsden SM: Manual of natural veterinary medicine: science and tradition, St Louis, 2002, Mosby.

Journals

Haussler KK: Chiropractic evaluation and management, Vet Clin North Am Equine Pract 15.1:195, 1999.

Videos

Schreiber M: Sports massage for the equine athlete, Equissage, Round Hill, VA (telephone: 800-843-0224). Available at: http://www.equissage.com/

Vaughn L: Body works for dogs, Animal Healing, Pound Ridge, NY (telephone: 877-929-1515). Available at: www.animalhealing.com

Whalen-Shaw P: Canine massage: an instructional guide, Integrated Touch Therapy, Circleville, OH (telephone: 800-251-0007). Available at: http://www.integratedtouchtherapy.com/

Contacts

Musculoskeletal therapies for animals, Madison, WI (telephone: 866-646-8684). Available at: www.MTAvet.com

Professional Organizations

Academy of Veterinary Homeopathy: www.theavh.org

American Association of Rehabilitation Veterinarians: www.rehabvets.org

American College of Veterinary Sports Medicine and Rehabilitation: www.vsmr.org

American Holistic Veterinary Medical Association: www.ahvma.org (telephone: 410-569-0795).

American Physical Therapy Association: www.apta.org

American Veterinary Chiropractic Association: www.animalchiropractic.org (telephone: 918-784-2231).

International Association of Veterinary Rehabilitation and Physical Therapy: www.iavrpt.org

International College of Applied Kinesiology: www.icak.com

International Veterinary Acupuncture Society: www.ivas.org

Veterinary Botanical Medicine Association: www.vbma.org

Massage Schools

Equissage: Round Hill, VA, www.equissage.com (telephone: 800-843-0224).

fur30TTEAM training Canada, 5435 Rochdell, Vernon, British Columbia, Canada (telephone: 604-545-2336).

Healing Oasis: Sturtevant, WI, www.thehealingoasis.com (telephone: 262-878-9549).

Integrated Touch Therapy, Inc.: Circleville, OH, www.integratedtouchtherapy.com (telephone: 800-251-0007).

TTEAM training USA, PO Box 3793 Santa Fe, NM (telephone: 800-854-TEAM).

Rehabilitation Certification Training

Canine Rehabilitation Institute, Inc., Wellington, FL, www.caninerehabinstitute.com (toll-free phone and fax: 888-651-0760; outside the U.S.: 561-651-0760; e-mail: info@caninerehabinstitute.com).

Northeast Seminars, East Hampstead, NH, www.neseminars.com

The Healing Oasis, Sturtevant, WI, www.thehealingoasis.com

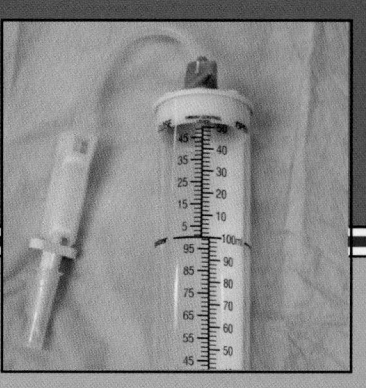

24 | Fluid Therapy and Transfusion Medicine

Courtney Beiter, Edward Cooper, Olivia M. Holt Williams, and Margaret Mudge

OUTLINE

Fluid Therapy, *883*
Indications for Fluid Therapy, *883*
Body Fluid Compartments, *883*
Types of Intravenous Fluids, *883*
Specifics of Fluid Administration, *885*
Fluid Additives, *891*
Monitoring Fluid Therapy, *893*
Complications of Fluid Therapy, *894*

Transfusion Medicine, *895*
Indications for Blood and Plasma
  Transfusion, *895*
Blood Donors, *896*
Pretransfusion Testing, *896*
Blood Collection, *898*
Blood Products, *900*
Blood Product Administration, *901*

LEARNING OBJECTIVES

When you have completed this chapter, you will be able to:

1. Pronounce, define, and spell all Key Terms in the chapter.
2. Explain the indications for fluid therapy and describe the body fluid compartments, including movement of fluids between these compartments.
3. Compare and contrast crystalloid and colloid fluids, and describe the uses for and characteristics of each.
4. Do the following regarding the administration of fluids and fluid therapy additives:
   • Discuss the objectives of each phase of fluid therapy and the specific products and administration rates used during each phase.
   • Compare and contrast the indications for and techniques used to administer fluids by the intravenous, subcutaneous, intraosseous, and enteral routes.
   • Explain the indications for and techniques used to administer potassium chloride, dextrose, and sodium bicarbonate.
5. Do the following regarding monitoring and complications of fluid therapy:
   • Describe the methods used to monitor the effectiveness of fluid therapy.
   • Discuss common complications of fluid therapy, including appropriate interventions.
6. Do the following regarding transfusion medicine:
   • Describe the indications for blood, plasma, and blood component transfusion.
   • Discuss the selection and care of blood donors.
   • Explain pretransfusion testing, including blood typing, antibody screening, and cross-matching.
7. Do the following regarding collection techniques, blood products and product administration:
   • Describe the techniques used to collect blood from a dog, cat, or horse.
   • List blood products, including the indications for and benefits provided by each.
   • Describe the technique used to administer blood products to a patient, including calculating administration rates.
   • Discuss patient monitoring during blood transfusions and recognition and management of transfusion reactions.

KEY TERMS

Agglutination
Anaphylaxis
Anemia
Blood type
Coagulopathy
Colloid
Cross-match
Cryoprecipitate
Crystalloid fluid
Dehydration
Hemolysis
Hypersensitivity
Hypertonic
Hypotonic
Hypovolemia
Isotonic
Maintenance rate
Oncotic pressure
Packed cell volume
  (PCV)
Platelet concentrate
Platelet-rich plasma
Resuscitation (fluid)
Replacement
Transfusion reaction

INTRODUCTION

Fluid therapy is an extremely important aspect of patient care, especially in the setting of emergent and critical illness. The optimal fluid type, the amount to be given, and the route of administration can vary considerably depending on the patient's clinical picture. Despite extensive research, no single approach to fluid administration has been proven to consistently offer clear advantage. Furthermore, fluids are not without potential risks and complications. Consequently, formulating a fluid therapy plan (that addresses what type, how much, and how fast to give the fluids) can offer considerable challenge. The key, very simply stated, is to give an appropriate fluid and give enough of it, but try not to give too much. To develop and implement an appropriate fluid therapy plan, it is important to understand body fluid compartments and characteristics of different fluid types, consider rates and routes of administration, monitor effectiveness of achieving fluid therapy goals, and recognize potential complications. The first part of this chapter provides a systematic approach to fluid therapy, for large and small animals, that is intended to guide these decisions.

Along with effective fluid therapy, blood product transfusions can be a life-saving or life-prolonging component of treatment, and the veterinary technician plays an integral role in the collection, processing, and transfusion of blood and blood products. The technician should be able to recognize severe hemorrhage and life-threatening **anemia,** and should be aware of available blood products. In many practices, the veterinary technician will be responsible for collection of blood from donor animals, as well as for separation and storage of blood components. Proper blood product administration and monitoring of transfused patients are also important technician responsibilities because blood transfusion is not without risks and adverse effects. The second part of the chapter provides information on indications for blood transfusion, pretransfusion testing, blood donors and blood collection, processing of blood components, blood product storage, transfusion administration, and **transfusion reactions.**

FLUID THERAPY

INDICATIONS FOR FLUID THERAPY

The decision to initiate fluid therapy is often based on various clinical and practical considerations. Generally speaking, fluids are used to replace that which has been lost, to replace that which is being lost, or to keep up with the basic physiologic need for water when the patient cannot do so for itself. Some related indications, among others, are provided in Box 24-1.

BODY FLUID COMPARTMENTS

To understand the effects of different fluid types after they are administered, a general understanding of body fluid compartments is extremely important. The body is made up of approximately 60% water (referred to as "total body water," or TBW). TBW is spread across the intracellular fluid (ICF) and extracellular fluid (ECF) spaces (Figure 24-1). The primary barrier between these spaces is the cell membrane. ICF accounts for ⅔ of TBW (or about 30% to 40% of body weight) and ECF makes up ⅓ of TBW (or about 16% to 20% of body weight). ECF is further divided into interstitial (ISF) and intravascular (IVF) fluid spaces. The primary barrier between these spaces is the vascular endothelium. The ISF constitutes approximately ¾ and the IVF (the blood plasma) approximately ¼ of the ECF. From these percentages, it can be determined that dogs, cats, and horses have a circulating

| BOX 24-1 | Clinical Indications for Fluid Therapy |

- Maintaining hydration
- Replacing fluid deficit (dehydration)
- Replacing ongoing losses
- Treating decreased oncotic pressure
- Treating hypovolemia
- Treating shock states
- Improving/increasing urine production
- Correcting acid-base or electrolyte disorders
- Maintaining IV access and delivering other medications

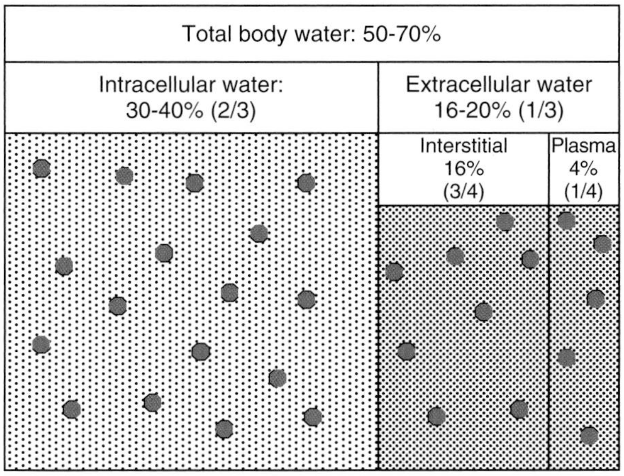

Total body water: 50-70%	
Intracellular water: 30-40% (2/3)	Extracellular water 16-20% (1/3)

FIGURE 24-1 Diagram of body fluid compartments.

blood volume of approximately 80 to 90 ml/kg, 40 to 60 ml/kg, and 80 ml/kg, respectively.

TECHNICIAN NOTE Dogs, cats, and horses have a circulating blood volume of approximately 80 to 90 ml/ kg, 40 to 60 ml/kg, and 80 ml/kg, respectively.

These fluid compartments are important to consider because of differences in permeability of barriers to assorted substances provided in intravenous (IV) fluids (water, electrolytes, **colloids**, etc.). For example, water is able to move across all barriers (vascular endothelium and cell membrane) based entirely on concentration gradient. Therefore, the volume of distribution for water is the TBW. Electrolytes, however, can move freely across the vascular endothelium but cannot move across the cell membrane, so they will distribute throughout the ECF based on relative proportions of ISF and IVF. Said another way, when an electrolyte solution is administered, approximately ¼ will remain in the vascular space and ¾ will move into the interstitium. Large molecules, such as colloids, do not readily move across the vascular endothelium and so are relatively confined to the vascular space. This means that IV administration of colloids will result primarily in expansion of the vascular volume. Furthermore, colloids may have the ability to move fluid from the interstitium into the vascular space by increasing the **oncotic pressure** of blood.

TYPES OF INTRAVENOUS FLUIDS

Intravenous fluids typically are classified on the basis of their composition and physiochemical properties. Two main categories are crystalloids and colloids.

Crystalloids

Crystalloid solutions contain various electrolytes in water and are further characterized on the basis of their osmolality compared with the osmolality of blood (Table 24-1).

Hypotonic fluids have an osmolality less than that of blood (normal plasma osmolality is approximately 280 to 310 mOsm/L) and by definition provide water in greater proportion than electrolytes. Examples of hypotonic fluids include dextrose 5% in water (D_5W), 0.45% sodium chloride (NaCl), and "maintenance" fluids such as Normosol M and Plasmalyte 56. It is important to note that although the osmolality of D_5W is close to that of blood, dextrose is quickly metabolized, leaving free water. The purpose of D_5W is to provide free water without causing osmotic injury to red blood cells or to the endothelium at the time of administration. Hypotonic fluids may be used to replace a free water deficit and to treat hypernatremia (high blood sodium). Given the decreased tolerance for sodium load in patients with heart disease, hypotonic fluids are ideally suited to replace deficits or maintain hydration in these patients. It should be emphasized that these fluids should never be used in **resuscitation** or administered rapidly as a bolus because they are highly ineffective for expanding

TABLE 24-1	Assorted Crystalloid Solutions and Electrolyte Compositions						
FLUID	**Na**	**K**	**Cl**	**Ca**	**Mg**	**OSMOLALITY, mOsm/kg**	**BICARB PRECURS**
Dextrose 5% in water	0	0	0	0	0	287	0
0.45% NaCl	77	0	77	0	0	154	0
0.9% NaCl	154	0	154	0	0	308	0
Lactated Ringer's solution (LRS)	130	4	109	3	0	278	28 lactate
Plasmalyte 148	140	5	98	0	3	294	27 acetate
Normosol R	"	"	"	"	"	"	23 gluconate
3% NaCl	513	0	513	0	0	1026	0
7% NaCl	1198	0	1198	0	0	2396	0

All values in mEq/L unless otherwise indicated.

vascular volume and could cause overly rapid changes in blood osmolality.

> **TECHNICIAN NOTE** Given the decreased tolerance for sodium load in patients with heart disease, hypotonic fluids are ideally suited to replace deficits or maintain hydration in these patients.

Isotonic crystalloids have an osmolality approximately equal to that of blood and provide water in equal proportion to electrolytes. Examples of isotonic crystalloids include 0.9% NaCl (normal saline) and balanced electrolyte solutions (BES) such as Plasmalyte 148, Normosol R, and lactated Ringer's solution. Because these fluids have applications in resuscitation, rehydration, and **replacement** of ongoing losses, they are by far the most commonly used crystalloids. As previously indicated, IV administration of an isotonic crystalloid will result in rapid redistribution to the interstitial space so that only 25% to 35% will remain in the vascular space after 20 to 30 minutes.

In addition to providing water and electrolytes, isotonic crystalloids can affect acid-base balance. Owing to its relatively high chloride content, 0.9% NaCl has acidifying effects, and BES contain bicarbonate precursors and have alkalinizing effects. This might make normal saline an ideal choice for the vomiting patient with hypochloremic metabolic alkalosis, or BES an ideal choice for a patient with severe acidemia. Isotonic crystalloids are not without potential adverse effects, especially if given in very large quantities. For example, these fluids have the potential to cause tissue edema and create acid-base disturbances.

> **TECHNICIAN NOTE** 0.9% NaCl has acidifying effects, and balanced electrolyte solutions contain bicarbonate precursors and have alkalinizing effects.

Hypertonic crystalloids have an osmolality greater than that of blood and provide electrolytes in greater proportion than water. Examples of hypertonic fluids include 3% and 7% hypertonic NaCl. It is important to note that 23% NaCl

solutions are available but must be diluted to a concentration no greater than 7.5% to avoid osmotic injury. The high osmolality of hypertonic saline will cause a shift of fluid from the interstitium to the intravascular space, promoting rapid expansion of vascular volume (volume expansion) to aid in resuscitation. However, because electrolytes readily redistribute across the endothelium, the effects are fairly transient, lasting only 20 to 30 minutes. Another therapeutic application of hypertonic saline is treatment of head trauma/traumatic brain injury. The osmotic effects of this fluid help draw fluid out of the cerebral interstitium, thereby decreasing intracranial pressure while simultaneously increasing blood volume and blood pressure. Hypertonic saline should not be administered any faster than 0.5 to 1 ml/kg/minute because rapid volume expansion can trigger a reflex bradycardia. In addition, hypertonic saline should be used with caution in dehydrated patients. Although volume expansion will still occur, worsening of interstitial or intracellular **dehydration** may be noted.

Colloids

Colloid solutions contain high-molecular-weight molecules suspended in an isotonic crystalloid. As was previously discussed, these larger molecules tend to remain within the vascular space, thereby conferring oncotic pressure (the portion of total osmotic pressure contributed by colloids). Colloids can be classified as natural (such as plasma or albumin solutions) or synthetic (such as hetastarch, hydroxyethyl starch in sodium chloride injection [VetSarch, Abbott Inc.], dextrans, etc.). Given the tendency to remain within the vascular space and provide relatively efficient and prolonged volume expansion, colloids are well suited for use in resuscitation. In addition, they are used to provide oncotic support for patients with hypoproteinemia. Synthetic colloids have been associated with the potential to cause **coagulopathy**. Administration of hetastarch at doses greater than 20 ml/kg/day can result in prolonged clotting times and impaired platelet function. However, this has not been shown to be associated with increased risk of bleeding or need for transfusion, and doses up to 40 ml/kg/day are likely acceptable. A relatively newer synthetic colloid, VetStarch, has been formulated to decrease impact on coagulation with minimal

TABLE 24-2	Fluid Resuscitation Guidelines				
FLUID	**EFFICIENCY**	**SHOCK DOSE, ml/kg**		**INITIAL BOLUS, ml/kg**	
Isotonic crystalloid	0.25-0.33	Dog/Horse*	80-90	Dog	20-30
		Cat	40-60	Cat	10-15
Hypertonic Crystalloid	5-10	Dog	3-6	Dog	2-3
		Cat	2-4	Cat	1-2
Colloid	1-1.5	Dog	20-30	Dog	5
		Cat	10-15	Cat	3-4
"Turbostarch" Hypertonic/Colloid	5-10	Dog	3-6	Dog	2-3
		Cat	2-4	Cat	1-2

Efficiency reflects the increase in vascular volume for each milliliter administered.
*Horse is the same as dog for all categories.

effects at doses of 50 to 100 ml/kg/day. Other reported adverse effects associated with synthetic colloids include renal injury and anaphylactic reactions.

> **TECHNICIAN NOTE** Given the tendency to remain within the vascular space and provide relatively efficient and prolonged volume expansion, colloids are well suited for use in resuscitation.

SPECIFICS OF FLUID ADMINISTRATION
Phases of Fluid Therapy
Resuscitation Phase

Fluid resuscitation is aimed at restoration of vascular volume in an effort to reverse **hypovolemia** and/or a shock state. The amount administered during resuscitation is determined on the basis of the amount of vascular volume lost and the relative efficiency with which fluid expands the intravascular space (Table 24-2). Generally speaking, it is expected that patients in hypovolemic shock have lost approximately 30% of their blood volume. This equates to 25 to 30 ml/kg in dogs and horses, and 12 to 18 ml/kg in cats. As was previously discussed, it is necessary to give 3 to 4 ml of an isotonic crystalloid for each desired 1-ml increase in vascular volume. Therefore, the "shock dose" for isotonic crystalloid is 80 to 90 ml/kg for dogs and horses, and 40 to 60 ml/kg for cats. For hypertonic saline, the vascular volume increases 5- to 10-ml for every 1 ml given. With the desired increase in vascular volume, this translates into a hypertonic "shock dose" of 3 to 6 ml/kg in dogs and 2 to 4 ml/kg in cats. Synthetic colloid solutions such as hetastarch increase vascular volume by 1 to 1.5 ml for every 1 ml of solution administered. As such, "shock doses" for hetastarch are 20 to 30 ml/kg in dogs and 10 to 15 ml/kg in cats.

Mixed resuscitation using different types of fluids in the same patient has several potential benefits. By combining the beneficial effects (e.g., profound expansion from hypertonic saline, prolonged effects of colloids), total doses of each fluid are reduced, and side effects are diminished. One particular type of combination therapy involves the use of a colloid (e.g., hetastarch or VetStarch) and 23.4% NaCl in a 2:1 ratio to dilute hypertonic saline to a 7% solution. This combination, sometimes referred to as "turbostarch," is dosed in a similar manner to hypertonic saline alone.

Volumes determined as "shock doses" for these different fluids are meant to serve as a guideline. Fluid administration should be titrated to effect based on clinical response. This is typically achieved by giving some fraction of the shock dose over some period of time (such as $\frac{1}{4}$ over 10 to 15 minutes) and then reassessing for improvement in perfusion parameters. It is important that blood pressure not be used as the sole means of determining response to therapy. Generally speaking, arterial blood pressure is highly preserved and therefore decreases only in advanced stages as the patient decompensates. Along these lines, it is also the first parameter to normalize even though hypovolemic shock may continue. Therefore, improvement in heart rate (HR), capillary refill time (CRT), mucous membrane color, warmth of distal extremities, etc., should be noted and used to guide therapy (see "Monitoring Fluid Therapy," on page 893). If perfusion parameters have not improved with the initial bolus, it should be repeated. If a full shock dose has been administered, but the patient is not stable, investigation should be conducted into sources of ongoing loss or causes of shock unrelated to hypovolemia.

> **TECHNICIAN NOTE** Volumes determined as "shock doses" for these different fluids are meant to serve as a guideline. Fluid administration should be titrated to effect on the basis of clinical response.

In large animals that require immediate resuscitation, it is difficult to deliver "shock doses" of isotonic **crystalloid fluids** or colloids within 10 to 15 minutes. Instead, hypertonic saline can be delivered quickly because of the small volume required, and can be followed by isotonic crystalloids. Placement of a second jugular catheter can be helpful for delivery of the large volumes needed, and high-volume oscillating pumps can be used to increase the speed of fluid delivery; however, high delivery pressures may cause damage to the jugular veins, so this method should be used only when absolutely necessary.

Replacement Phase

Once resuscitation has been achieved (or in cases in which it was not necessary), the next phase of fluid therapy is replacement. Replacement fluid therapy involves correction of dehydration, replacement of ongoing losses, and provision of maintenance fluid requirements. It is generally assumed that fluid losses are isotonic in nature (vomiting, diarrhea, blood loss, etc.); therefore, an isotonic crystalloid is most commonly used during replacement.

> **TECHNICIAN NOTE** Replacement rate = Dehydration + Ongoing losses + Maintenance

To determine the contribution of dehydration to the replacement rate, calculate the fluid deficit by multiplying the patient's body weight in kilograms by the estimated percent dehydration expressed as a decimal (please see Chapter 7 regarding assessment of hydration). For example, a 30-kg dog with 8% dehydration would have a fluid deficit of 2.4 L (30 × 0.08). The length of time over which the deficit will be replaced must then be determined. Depending on the clinical situation, replacement over 4 to 24 hours may be acceptable, with chronic loss replaced more slowly. The argument is made that rapid rehydration with high fluid rates equates to pouring water over a dry sponge. If water is poured faster than the sponge can absorb, most of it will run off. When a patient is rehydrated, rapid delivery of IV fluids to correct dehydration will result in loss through the kidneys (like overflow of the sponge) and will not result in effective rehydration. Once the time frame for replacement is determined, the fluid deficit is divided by the number of hours over which fluids will be administered. In the previous example, if the fluid deficit related to dehydration is replaced over 12 hours, the rate of administration will be 200 ml/hour (2400 ml divided by 12 hours).

Provision for ongoing loss is determined by quantifying or estimating fluid losses over a period of time and then increasing the fluid administration rate accordingly. Examples of ongoing losses include vomiting, diarrhea, bleeding, cavitary effusions (effusion into body cavities), increased insensible losses (panting), and inappropriate urinary losses. It is important to not include appropriate urinary losses (1 to 2 ml/kg/hour) in a calculation of ongoing losses because appropriate urinary losses are accounted for in the **maintenance rate**. Quantifying water losses can be accomplished by using collection devices (catheters, drains, etc.) or by weighing fluids (e.g., vomiting diarrhea, urination) collected in absorbable pads. This is achieved by weighing the soiled pads and subtracting the weight of the pads themselves. Then, every gram of weight measured is equal to 1 ml of fluid loss. If it is not possible to measure losses because they are on the floor or outdoors, volumes can be estimated (although it is generally recommended to double the perceived or estimated volume to more accurately reflect the loss). In either case, the volume of losses that occur over a given period (e.g., 4 to 8 hours), should be divided by the number of hours over

which they occurred, and the resulting rate (in ml/hour) should be added to the fluid administration rate for the next period of time. For example, if a dog has multiple episodes of vomiting and diarrhea totaling 200 ml over a 4-hour period, the administration rate should be increased by 50 ml/hour to replace these losses, and the patient should be reassessed 4 hours later.

The maintenance rate is meant to supply the basic physiologic need for water lost through urine, the GI system, and insensible losses (as from the respiratory tract). Various guidelines have been used to determine the daily maintenance fluid requirement (expressed in ml/day), including the formulas 40 to 60 ml/kg/day, 30 ml/lb/day, 2 to 4 ml/kg/hour, and 30 × Body weight (kg) + 70. Although fairly straightforward, these guidelines assume a linear relationship between body weight and daily fluid requirement. Unfortunately, because of differences in body surface area-to-volume ratios, these calculations can underestimate the needs of small patients and can overestimate the needs of large patients.

An allometric scale, as represented by the formula 132*Body weight (kg)$^{(3/4)}$ for dogs, and the formula 80*Body weight (kg)$^{(3/4)}$ for cats, may be better suited to determine daily fluid maintenance requirements in these species. The major obstacle to using these formulas is the need to calculate a $\frac{3}{4}$ exponent. However, this can be overcome by using a multifunction calculator to perform the following calculations: (1) multiply body weight expressed in kilograms (BW) by itself twice (BW*BW*BW), (2) press the square root button twice, and (3) multiply the result by 132 (for dogs) or 80 (for cats). The final result is then divided by 24 to obtain the hourly maintenance fluid rate expressed in ml/hour. In horses, a maintenance rate of 40 to 60 ml/kg/day is typically used. Larger (draft breed) horses are given maintenance fluids at a lower rate (40 ml/kg/day), and neonatal foals are given maintenance fluids at a higher rate (up to 90 ml/kg/day).

> **TECHNICIAN NOTE** To calculate the hourly maintenance rate (expressed in ml/hour) using the formula 132*Body weight (kg)$^{(3/4)}$ for dogs and the formula 80*Body weight (kg)$^{(3/4)}$ for cats, perform the following calculations: (1) multiply body weight expressed in kilograms (BW) by itself twice (BW*BW*BW), (2) press the square root button twice, (3) multiply the result by 132 (for dogs) or 80 (for cats), and (4) divide the final result by 24.

The replacement rate determined by this process should serve as a good starting point, provided that it is followed up by periodic reassessment of hydration status and revision of the fluid therapy plan (see "Monitoring Fluid Therapy" on page 894).

Maintenance Phase

Once dehydration has been corrected and losses are not ongoing, the patient can be moved to the maintenance phase of fluid therapy. Patients that present without dehydration or ongoing losses may start out on a maintenance rate during hospitalization if they are unwilling or unable to drink adequately on their own. Maintenance rates are determined as described previously. Isotonic crystalloids are often used for maintenance fluid therapy. However, these fluids (intended for replacement) provide sodium and chloride well in excess of what is needed for maintenance purposes (because patients normally drink water, not salt solution, to maintain fluid balance). Hypotonic, or "maintenance," crystalloids (Table 24-3) better match true maintenance requirements, but for reasons of availability and ease, isotonic fluids are most often used. For most patients with normal cardiac and renal function, the excess electrolyte load is easily handled and excreted by the kidneys, thereby justifying this common practice. (See Case Presentation 24-1 and Case Presentation 24-2 for examples of fluid rate calculations and fluid administration in a dog and a horse, respectively.)

Routes of Administration

Several factors should be considered when the optimal route for fluid administration is decided. These factors include the nature of the disease process, the stability of the patient, the magnitude of the fluid deficit and ongoing losses, the characteristics of the fluid loss, the decision of whether to treat the animal as an inpatient or an outpatient, the expected length of the hospital stay (if needed), the equipment and technical expertise required, and the ultimate goal of fluid therapy for that patient. Possible routes of administration in small animals include IV (central or peripheral), subcutaneous, and intraosseous; in large animals, routes include IV and enteral via nasogastric tube.

Intravenous

The IV route offers several advantages, especially for acutely and/or critically ill patients (those requiring urgent or immediate attention). The IV route offers the ability to administer fluids rapidly for volume expansion. In addition, multiple different fluid types can be given IV, including hypotonic, isotonic, and hypertonic crystalloids, as well as colloids and blood products. Because of the ability to rapidly titrate fluid administration, the IV route is preferred for fluid resuscitation, intraoperative fluid therapy, anesthetized patients, replacement of significant dehydration and ongoing loses, and critically ill patients in general.

> **TECHNICIAN NOTE** Because of the ability to rapidly titrate fluid administration, the IV route is preferred for fluid resuscitation, intraoperative fluid therapy, anesthetized patients, replacement of significant dehydration and ongoing loses, and critically ill patients in general.

Multiple sites are available for IV catheter placement, including cephalic, medial and lateral saphenous, lateral thoracic (in horses), and jugular veins. One should take into consideration the reason for IV catheter placement when choosing which vein to use. If a catheter is placed for routine fluid therapy or for correction of dehydration, a peripheral vessel such as the cephalic, saphenous, or lateral thoracic vein can be used. If a catheter is placed in a critical patient, such as one that may need serial blood sampling or multiple medication constant rate infusions (CRIs), a central line should be placed. Central line catheters are also useful when simultaneous medications that may not be compatible are administered because they have multiple lumina through which medications can be administered (Figure 24-2). Usually this is done through the jugular vein, but central line catheters can be placed in the lateral or medial saphenous vein and advanced into the caudal vena cava.

Care should be taken to use aseptic technique when placing an intravenous catheter. This is especially true for central venous catheters. The catheter site should be clipped and enough hair removed from the area to ensure that there will be no contamination from the surrounding fur. A surgical scrub, such as chlorhexidine, should be used to clean the

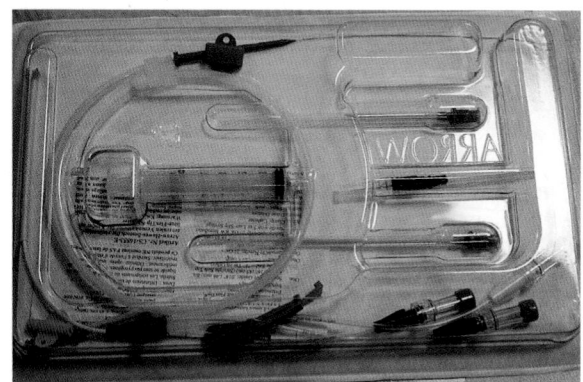

FIGURE 24-2 A multi-lumen central catheter.

TABLE 24-3	Maintenance Fluids							
FLUID	**Na**	**K**	**Cl**	**Ca**	**Mg**	**OSMOLALITY, mOsm/kg**	**EFFECTIVE OSMOLALITY, mOsm/kg**	
0.45% NaCl	77	0	77	0	0	154	154	
0.45% NaCl + 2.5% Dex	77	0	77	0	0	297	154	
Normosol M	40	13	40	0	3	100	100	
Plasmalyte 56	40	13	40	0	3	100	100	

All values in mEq/L unless otherwise indicated.

CASE PRESENTATION 24-1

A 10-kg Miniature Schnauzer presented with a history of severe vomiting, diarrhea, lethargy, and anorexia over the previous 3 to 4 days. On initial physical examination, heart rate (HR) was 200 beats per minute (bpm) (normal, 80 to 120 bpm), pulses were weak, mucous membranes were pale pink, capillary refill time (CRT) was 4 seconds (normal <2 seconds), and the patient was depressed. Systolic arterial blood pressure as measured with a Doppler monitor was 60 mm Hg (normal, 110 to 140 mm Hg). The patient was estimated to be 10% dehydrated.

Resuscitation Phase

Plasmalyte was started IV at a rate of 20 ml/kg (200 ml total) over 10 minutes. The patient was then reassessed. Systolic arterial blood pressure increased to 100 mm Hg, HR was 180 bpm, CRT was 3 seconds, and a slight improvement in mentation was evident, along with an increase in pulse quality.

Because physical parameters were improved, but not normal, a repeat bolus of 200 ml Plasmalyte was administered IV over 15 minutes. A second reassessment revealed further improvement as evidenced by systolic arterial blood pressure of 120 mm Hg, HR of 140 bpm, CRT of 2 seconds, and increased responsiveness. At this point, the resuscitation phase was complete.

Replacement Phase

Because the patient was determined to be 10% dehydrated on presentation, 1000 ml of fluid (0.1*10 kg) was needed to correct the fluid deficit. The attending veterinarian elected to replace this deficit over 18 hours, using an administration rate of 55 ml/hour (1000 ml/18 hour).

The maintenance rate for this patient was calculated as 31 ml/hour ($[132*10^{3/4}]/24$), so replacement fluids were started at a rate of 86 ml/hour (55 ml/hour + 31 ml/hour). During the first 6 hours at this rate, the patient was estimated to have had 300 ml in ongoing losses from vomiting and diarrhea (50 ml/hour*6 hours). So the maintenance rate for the next 6 hours was increased to 136 ml/hour (86 ml/hour + 50 ml/hour) to replace this loss.

During this time, estimated ongoing losses decreased to 120 ml (20 ml/hour*6 hours). So the maintenance rate for the subsequent 6 hours was adjusted to 106 ml/hour (86 ml/hour + 20 ml/hour) to reflect this decrease. After this, no further losses occurred, and upon reassessment, the patient was determined to be rehydrated. At that point, the replacement phase was complete.

Maintenance Phase

At the onset of the maintenance phase, the fluid administration rate was reduced to the maintenance rate of 31 ml/hour. Shortly thereafter, the patient started to eat and drink. The maintenance rate was gradually reduced and then discontinued, at which point the maintenance phase was complete.

CASE PRESENTATION 24-2

A 500-kg Quarterhorse gelding was presented with a 48-hour history of diarrhea, inappetence, and lethargy. On initial physical examination, heart rate (HR) was 70 beats per minute (bpm) (normal, 28 to 40 bpm), pulses were weak, mucous membranes were congested and dark pink, capillary refill time (CRT) was 4 seconds (normal <2 seconds), and the patient was depressed. The patient was estimated to be 10% dehydrated.

Resuscitation Phase

Lactated Ringer's solution (LRS) was administered IV at a rate of 20 ml/kg (10 L total) over 20 to 30 minutes. The patient was reassessed. At that point, HR was 60 beats/minute, CRT was 3 seconds, and slight improvement in mentation and increased pulse quality were noted. Because physical parameters were improved, but not normal, a repeat bolus of 10 L LRS was given IV over the next 20 to 30 minutes. A second reassessment revealed HR of 50 bpm and CRT of 2 seconds, and the patient was responsive and urinated. At this point, the resuscitation phase was complete.

Replacement Phase

Because the patient was determined to be 10% dehydrated on presentation, 50 L (0.1*500 kg) was needed to correct the fluid deficit. The attending veterinarian elected to replace this deficit over 18 hours using an administration rate of 2.5 to 3 L/hour (50 L/18 hours).

The maintenance rate for this patient was calculated as 1.25 L/hour (500 kg*60 ml/kg/day divided by 24 hours). So replacement fluids were started at a rate of approximately 4 L/hour (2.5 to 3 L/hour + 1.25 L/hour). During the first hour, the patient continued to have watery diarrhea with estimated losses of 1 L/hour. Therefore, the maintenance rate was increased to 2.25 L/hour (1.25 L/hour + 1 L/hour) to replace this loss. The patient was reassessed by physical examination every 4 hours, and packed cell volume and total protein were checked every 6 hours while large losses were ongoing.

site by starting in the center and gradually moving outward, until the gauze is clean. The site can then be wiped clean with alcohol or Zephiran (sanofi-aventis) solution. Proper restraint is key for catheter placement. The holder should occlude the vessel above the patient's elbow for catheters being placed in the cephalic vein, and above the knee for catheters being placed in the medial or lateral saphenous vein. If a catheter is being placed into the jugular vein, the vessel should be occluded at the thoracic inlet. Once placed, the catheter should be secured using tape for those placed in a peripheral vessel. Central line catheters should be sutured in place to ensure that they do not slip or back out of the vein. All catheters should then be wrapped using Kling (Johnson and Johnson, New Brunswick, New Jersey) and Vetwrap (3M, Maplewood, Minnesota). This will help to keep the catheter site clean and will keep the catheter more secure.

All catheters should be closely monitored daily for any complications. For peripheral venous catheters, this includes checking the patient's foot for swelling or the presence of phlebitis, and flushing the catheter to check for patency. The catheter tape and wrap should be monitored for excessive tightness or slipping. Any concerns should be addressed immediately. If a patient's foot is swollen, the catheter tape or wrap may need to be loosened or replaced. If the catheter is no longer patent when flushed, or if evidence of phlebitis (pain or irritation when the catheter is flushed) is found, the catheter should be removed and replaced. All catheters should be closely monitored for signs of infection, including swelling, irritation of or discharge from the catheter site, and fever. If a patient acquires a fever of unknown origin while in the hospital, any intravenous catheters should be removed and replaced in a different vein as a precaution.

> **TECHNICIAN NOTE** If a patient acquires a fever of unknown origin while in the hospital, any intravenous catheters should be removed and replaced in a different vein as a precaution.

Central venous catheters should always be unwrapped at least once a day. The site should be cleaned using a surgical scrub and wiped with an alcohol or Zephiran solution. The site should then be rewrapped with bandage material. Gloves (sterile or nonsterile) should always be worn when central venous catheters are handled, so that the possibility of introducing infection can be minimized. Patients with jugular catheters should be monitored closely for facial swelling. This can result from the bandage being placed too tightly, or from jugular vein thromboses.

Intravenous fluids are administered one of two ways: by using a gravity-fed system, or by using a fluid pump. With a gravity-fed system, fluids are kept elevated above the patient and flow into the body by gravity. The fluid rate is manually adjusted by opening or closing the roller clamp on the administration set. The rate is largely dependent on the patient's position and therefore should be closely monitored to avoid fluid overload or insufficient flow. A Buretrol (Baxter, Deerfield, Illinois) is placed between the fluid bag and the administration set (Figure 24-3) to decrease the risk of fluid overload. The Buretrol holds a maximum of 150 ml and can be clamped off just below the fluid bag so that no more than 150 ml can be administered unless it is refilled. It is extremely important to properly calculate the fluid rate based on the delivery rate of the drip set (the number of drops/ml) to avoid fluid overload or insufficient flow. To perform the fluid rate calculation, you will need to know the desired fluid infusion rate and the size of the drip set you will be using (10 drops/ml or 60 drops/ml). See Box 24-2 for sample calculations. Whenever possible, a fluid pump should be used to administer intravenous fluids because this will help to ensure the accuracy of the fluid administration. Two main types are available for use in veterinary patients. The first is a volumetric pump (Figure 24-4), which can be

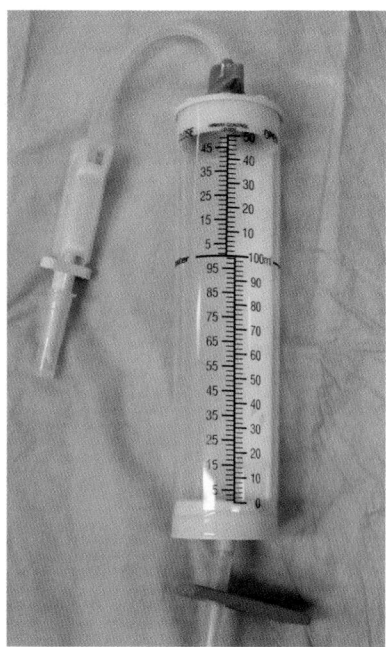

FIGURE 24-3 Example of a buretrol.

BOX 24-2	Calculation for Fluid Drips Sets

Example #1: The prescribed fluid infusion rate is 100 ml/hour, and the drip set has a delivery rating of 10 drops/ml.

$$\frac{100\ ml}{hour} \times \frac{1\ hr}{60\ minutes} = \frac{1.66\ ml}{minute} \times \frac{1\ min}{60\ seconds}$$

$$= \frac{0.02\ ml}{second} \times \frac{10\ drops}{ml}$$

$$= \frac{0.2\ drops}{second} = \frac{1\ drop}{5\ seconds}$$

In this example, the drip rate would be 1 drop every 5 seconds.

Example #2: The prescribed fluid infusion rate is 20 ml/hour, and the drip set has a delivery rating of 60 drops/ml.

$$\frac{20\ ml}{hour} \times \frac{1\ hr}{60\ minutes} = \frac{0.33\ ml}{minute} \times \frac{1\ min}{60\ seconds}$$

$$= \frac{0.0055\ ml}{second} \times \frac{60\ drops}{ml}$$

$$= \frac{0.33\ drops}{second} = \frac{1\ drop}{3\ seconds}$$

In this example, the drip rate would be 1 drop every 3 seconds.

programmed to deliver any volume of fluid over a set amount of time. The other type of fluid pump uses a photoelectrical eye to count the drops of solution as they are being administered. A sensor that is placed over the drip chamber adjusts the rate based on the number of drops per minute programmed into the machine. For large animals, large volumes

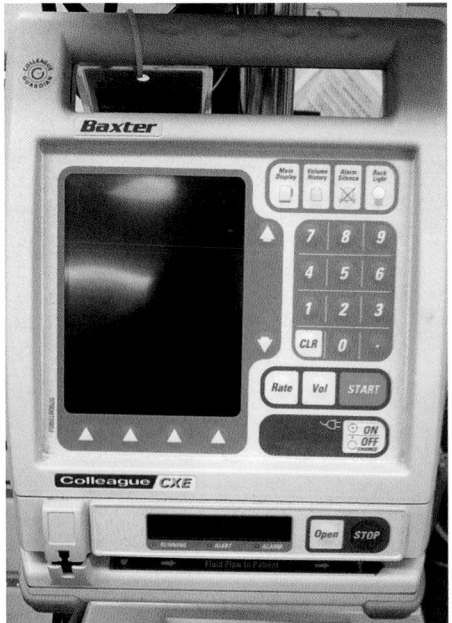

FIGURE 24-4 A volumetric fluid pump.

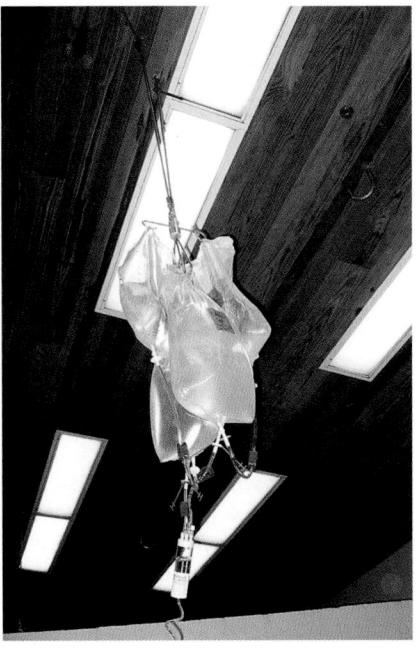

FIGURE 24-5 A total of 20 L of crystalloid fluids can be administered to large animal patients using transfer sets and a large-bore coil administration set. The coiled extension and swivel hanger allow the horse to move freely in the stall while IV fluids are administered.

of IV fluid are often required and are usually delivered by gravity. An example of a large animal fluid administration setup is shown in Figure 24-5.

Subcutaneous

The subcutaneous route can be used to administer large volumes of fluid for slow absorption over time and gradual fluid replacement. This route can be used to help reverse mild to moderate dehydration or to help prevent the development of dehydration in patients that are not eating or

drinking. Subcutaneous fluids can also be helpful for patients that need fluids but cannot be hospitalized, or that require intermittent fluid therapy that the client can provide at home (e.g., renal failure patients). This route of administration should not be chosen for patients with severe compromise from dehydration or significant electrolyte imbalances that need to be corrected. Subcutaneous fluids certainly should not be used for patients that are hypovolemic or hypotensive because volume expansion will not be rapid enough, and the peripheral vasoconstriction associated with shock will result in significantly impaired absorption of fluid from the subcutaneous space.

> **TECHNICIAN NOTE** The subcutaneous route of administration should not be chosen for patients with severe compromise from dehydration, hypotension, or significant electrolyte imbalance.

Subcutaneously administered fluids should be isotonic (LRS or 0.9% NaCl) and should have an osmotic pressure approximately equal to that of extracellular fluid. Dextrose solutions greater than 2.5% should never be given subcutaneously because skin sloughing and abscess formation may occur. The volume of subcutaneous fluid to be administered can be calculated at approximately 30 to 60 ml/kg/day. Subcutaneous fluids usually are absorbed in 6 to 8 hours. Therefore, the dose can be divided accordingly. The total volume administered should be divided into as many spots as possible so as not to cause discomfort. Although useful in small animals, subcutaneous fluids are not typically administered to large animals because of the large volume of fluids needed and the lack of adequate subcutaneous space in these patients.

Subcutaneous fluid administration is relatively safe and easy and can be done at home when appropriate. However, potential complications may occur. Subcutaneous administration of Plasmalyte 148 can cause discomfort because of the acidic pH. Owners should be instructed to use a new needle for each fluid administration; otherwise microbes might be introduced, and abscess formation could occur. Pressure necrosis is possible if too much is administered into one spot on the patient. Despite the relatively slow absorption of subcutaneous fluids, it is possible to cause fluid overload in a patient with underlying heart disease.

Intraosseous (IO; Intramedullary)

The intraosseous (IO) route offers an alternative for patients in which IV access is not possible, such as neonatal patients or small or young patients with cardiovascular collapse. Bone marrow does not collapse in hypovolemic patients, and so this space may be easier to access than a vein in some patients. This route provides rapid dispersion of fluids through the bone marrow and medullary venous channels, and so essentially has the same effect as administering fluids IV. The dosage calculations used for IV resuscitation and replacement can be used when fluids are given by the intraosseous route. In addition, any medication that is given IV is safe to administer IO. This route lends itself best to short-term use because IO catheters can be difficult to maintain. Once the patient has been resuscitated, an intravenous catheter should be placed.

TECHNICIAN NOTE Dosage calculations used for IV resuscitation and replacement can also be used when fluids are administered through an intraosseous (IO) catheter.

Various sites, including the tibial tuberosity, the trochanteric fossa of the femur, the wing of the ilium, and the greater tubercle of the humerus, can be used for IO catheterization. Before catheterization is attempted, the periosteum should be anesthetized using a 1% lidocaine solution, to prevent pain during needle placement. Many different types of needles can be used depending on the patient and the availability of supplies. Options include bone marrow needles, spinal needles, commercial intraosseous needles, and hypodermic needles. The insertion site should be aseptically clipped and prepared to avoid introducing infection and causing osteomyelitis. Aspiration of bone marrow or radiographs can help to confirm proper placement. Potential complications of IO catheter placement include infection at the insertion site and development of osteomyelitis.

Enteral

Enteral fluids are often used in large animal patients, particularly equids. Enteral fluids may be indicated for various reasons. They are typically used when large colon impaction is treated, may be used simultaneously with intravenous fluids, and may include osmotic agents. Enteral fluids can also be a good cost-effective way to maintain hydration status because they are delivered via nasogastric tube and do not require the use of costly fluids, fluid lines, and catheters. Enteral fluids may be administered at scheduled hourly intervals, or they can be given as a constant rate infusion. Deciding between these two methods of administration may ultimately depend on the intensive care unit (ICU) staff and how well the patient tolerates nasogastric intubation. When enteral fluids are delivered as a constant rate infusion, the nasogastric tube should be placed and secured to the halter with tape. A "Christmas tree" adaptor (Figure 24-6) is then placed on the end of the nasogastric tube, and a carboy (Figure 24-7) containing fluids and an administration set are then connected to the adaptor. The carboy is raised above the patient, and fluid is administered by gravity. For the average adult 500-kg horse, a rate of 1 L/hour should be used for maintenance. When enteral fluids are being administered at scheduled hourly intervals, boluses of no more than 8 L at a time should be given to the average adult 500-kg horse.

TECHNICIAN NOTE Enteral fluids are not to be used for patients in shock—they should be used only in patients with a normally functioning GI tract.

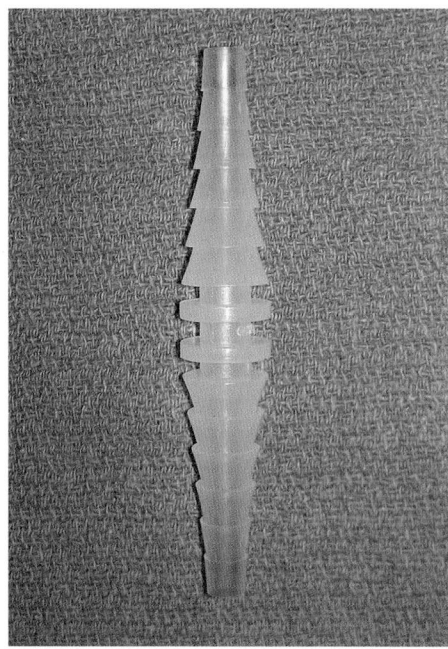

FIGURE 24-6 An example of a "Christmas tree" adaptor used to connect a nasogastric tube to the fluid line.

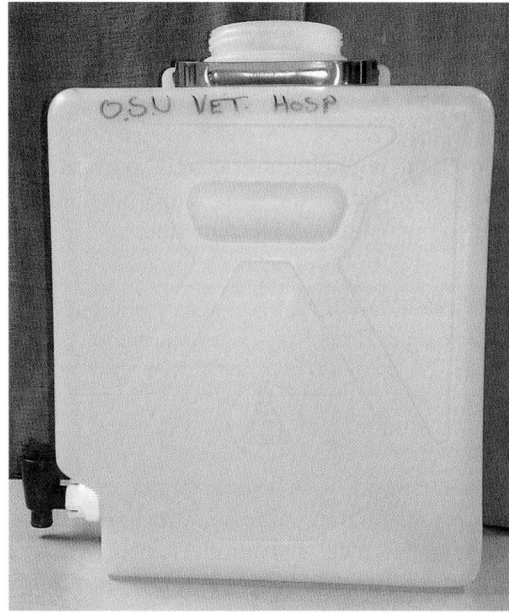

FIGURE 24-7 An example of a carboy used to serve as a container for the administration of large amounts of nonsterile enteral fluid.

FLUID ADDITIVES
Potassium Chloride (KCl)

Patients may present with hypokalemia or may develop hypokalemia in the hospital for a variety of reasons. Hypokalemia can be seen with gastrointestinal losses, such as vomiting or diarrhea, and with urinary losses. Specific causes include chronic renal failure, postobstructive diuresis, dialysis, hyperadrenocorticism (Cushing's disease), diabetic ketoacidosis (DKA), and primary hyperaldosteronism.

TABLE 24-4	Guidelines for Routine Intravenous Supplementation of Potassium in Dogs and Cats		
SERUM POTASSIUM CONCENTRATION, mEq/L	KCl TO ADD TO 250-ml FLUID BAG, mEq	KCl TO ADD TO 1-L FLUID BAG, mEq	MAXIMAL FLUID INFUSION RATE, ml/kg/hour
<2	20	80	6
2.1-2.5	15	60	8
2.6-3.0	10	40	12
3.1-3.5	7	28	18
3.6-5.0	5	20	25

Medications such as loop diuretics, thiazide diuretics, amphotericin B, and pencillins can also cause hypokalemia.

Signs of hypokalemia vary and depend on the severity of the condition. Some patients have no clinical signs. Patients with serum potassium values lower than 3.0 mEq/L may exhibit signs such as polyuria/polydipsia (PU/PD), decreased ability to concentrate urine, and muscle weakness. Patients may exhibit cardiovascular signs, including the development of ventricular and supraventricular arrhythmias. When serum potassium is less than 2.0 mEq/L, prolongation of the QT interval may be seen, and the patient may become unresponsive to antiarrhythmics. These patients are at risk for severe muscle weakness and even respiratory paralysis.

Patients with hypokalemia should be placed on intravenous potassium supplementation. This can be done using potassium chloride (2 mEq/ml KCl) or potassium phosphates (4.36 mEq/ml K^+). To avoid adverse cardiac effects, potassium should not be administered IV at a rate faster than 0.5 mEq/kg/hour (potassium maximum). See Table 24-4 for guidelines to potassium supplementation.

> **TECHNICIAN NOTE**　To avoid adverse cardiac effects, potassium should not be administered IV at a rate faster than 0.5 mEq/kg/hour (potassium maximum).

Dextrose

Patients can present with hypoglycemia or can become hypoglycemic for a variety of reasons, including neonatal or juvenile hypoglycemia, starvation, hepatic insufficiency, hypoadrenocorticism (Addison's disease), insulin overdose, sepsis, insulinoma, non–islet cell tumors, glycogen storage disease, pregnancy, and hunting dog hypoglycemia. Hypoglycemia should be suspected and blood glucose should be checked in patients that show clinical signs such as weakness, seizures, ataxia, collapse, stupor, or muscle tremors. Once a patient is found to be hypoglycemic, treatment should be started immediately. Dextrose (50%) can be administered slowly at a dose of 0.5 to 1 ml/kg IV. It is recommended that dextrose be diluted 1 : 1 (to a 25% solution) to avoid phlebitis that may occur with administration of 50% dextrose. If hypoglycemia does not resolve, an additional bolus can be given. The patient should then be placed on intravenous fluids containing dextrose. If indicated, a balanced electrolyte solution can be used and dextrose can be added to make a concentration of 2.5% to 10%. To avoid osmotic injury and phlebitis, hypertonic solutions (those containing more than 5% dextrose) should be administered only via a central vein.

Sodium Bicarbonate

Sodium bicarbonate can be administered for the treatment of metabolic acidosis; however, its use is controversial and depends largely on the nature and severity of the disturbance. In most cases of metabolic acidosis (e.g., lactic acidosis, diabetic ketoacidosis, renal failure), direct treatment of the underlying cause is recommended because sodium bicarbonate provides only temporary improvement in acid-base balance. For example, patients with diabetic ketoacidosis often have resolution of acidosis with fluid and insulin therapy alone. It has been recommended that sodium bicarbonate should be used in the treatment of metabolic acidosis associated with a shock state. However, because poor tissue perfusion and lactic acidosis usually occur in these patients, volume restoration and shock reversal are best suited to address the metabolic acidosis. Furthermore, administration of sodium bicarbonate has not been shown to result in improved outcomes in patients with metabolic acidosis. Because severe acidemia (pH <7.1) can lead to life-threatening cardiovascular complications such as impaired cardiac contractility, impaired pressor (blood pressure) response to catecholamines, and sensitization to ventricular arrhythmias, sodium bicarbonate should be used only in extreme cases in which the pH is below 7.1 and other directed therapy is not available or has not served to successfully restore acid-base balance. If bicarbonate therapy is indicated, the dosage can be calculated as indicated in Box 24-3.

> **TECHNICIAN NOTE**　Sodium bicarbonate should be used only in extreme cases in which the pH is below 7.1 and directed therapy is unavailable or has not served to restore acid-base balance.

Sodium bicarbonate can also be administered to patients with hyperkalemia because it helps to promote a shift of potassium (K^+) into cells in exchange for hydrogen ions (H^+). Because of the potential for adverse effects, its use is reserved for cases with severe hyperkalemia (K^+ >8 mEq/L). For this purpose, bicarbonate can be administered intravenously at a dose of 1 to 2 mEq/kg over 5 to 10 minutes.

BOX 24-3	Calculations for Bicarbonate Deficit and Isotonic Bicarbonate

Total Bicarbonate Deficit

Base deficit × 0.3 × Body weight (kg) = Deficit in mEq

In cases of acute metabolic acidosis, administer $\frac{1}{3}$-$\frac{1}{2}$ of the calculated dose rapidly (over 5-10 minutes) with the rest administered over the next 12 to 24 hours

Preparing Isotonic Bicarbonate

Remove 150 ml of water from a 1-L bag of sterile water, then add 150 ml *8.4% $NaHCO_3$

or

Remove 250 ml of water from a 1-L bag of sterile water, then add 250 ml †5% $NaHCO_3$

---

*8.4% = 1 mEq/ml; †5% = 0.595 mEq/ml.

Finally, oral bicarbonate supplementation may be indicated for large animal patients with chronic metabolic acidosis (like those with diarrhea).

Several potential adverse effects are associated with sodium bicarbonate administration. It is extremely important to note that bicarbonate should never be administered to a patient with respiratory acidosis (hypoventilation, or high partial pressure of carbon dioxide [$PaCO_2$]) because bicarbonate is rapidly converted to carbon dioxide (CO_2) and so could worsen this condition if ventilation is inadequate. Administration of bicarbonate can also result in paradoxical central nervous system (CNS) acidosis. This means that acidosis in the brain actually worsens despite improvement in peripheral acid-base balance, because CO_2 generated from bicarbonate can readily move into the brain, whereas the bicarbonate itself cannot. "Overshoot alkalosis" is also a possibility. This condition occurs when therapeutic intervention causes the original acidosis to resolve before administered bicarbonate is excreted, leading to a metabolic alkalosis. Finally, administration of oral bicarbonate may cause ulcers to form on the gums of some patients. Therefore, care should always be taken to wipe excess bicarbonate from around the mouth.

MONITORING FLUID THERAPY
Resuscitation Phase

As was previously stated, the primary goal of the resuscitation phase is to restore vascular volume and tissue perfusion. Therefore, monitoring fluid therapy during this phase is geared toward assessing cardiovascular stability, blood volume, and perfusion parameters.

TECHNICIAN NOTE Monitoring fluid therapy during the resuscitation phase is geared toward assessing cardiovascular stability, blood volume, and perfusion parameters.

Perfusion parameters include heart rate, pulse quality, capillary refill time (CRT), mucous membrane color, warmth of distal extremities, and mentation. The presence of tachycardia represents the compensatory sympathetic response to decreased blood volume or blood pressure. The pulse quality of any patient should be strong and synchronous. Patients in compensatory shock may have hyperkinetic (bounding) pulses, whereas those that have significant peripheral vasoconstriction or hypotension will have a weak pulse quality. CRT reflects how quickly blood flow returns to an area after the vessels have been blanched. Compensatory vasoconstriction will result in delayed or prolonged CRT. Pale mucous membranes, which can reflect vasoconstriction or anemia, are most commonly evaluated in the gums. However, tissue on the vulva, penis, or conjunctiva can also be used. Decreased mental status can reflect impaired/diminished blood flow to the brain. Monitoring of fluid therapy during the resuscitation phase should involve close attention to these parameters and ultimately their return to normal.

Tissue perfusion and cardiovascular stability can also be monitored by measuring arterial blood pressure. Complete discussion of blood pressure monitoring is beyond the scope of this chapter, but it is important to note that it is a relatively insensitive marker for blood flow. As was previously mentioned, the compensatory response is aimed at sustaining blood pressure even though perfusion to some tissues may be impaired. In other words, low blood pressure is bad, but normal blood pressure does not mean that everything is okay. Therefore, when fluid therapy is monitored and resuscitation is gauged, it is very important that perfusion parameters and other data are assessed in conjunction with blood pressure. Under most circumstances, efforts should be made to normalize and maintain systolic blood pressure between 110 and 140 mm Hg (or mean blood pressure between 80 and 100 mm Hg).

One potential exception to this is fluid therapy in the face of ongoing hemorrhage (e.g., hemoabdomen). For these patients, aggressive fluid therapy may result in exacerbation of bleeding and worsening of the clinical condition. Therefore, it is argued that targeting a lower "minimally acceptable" blood pressure (90 to 100 mm Hg systolic, 60 to 70 mm Hg mean) may be beneficial in these cases.

TECHNICIAN NOTE When fluid therapy is monitored and resuscitation is gauged, it is very important that perfusion parameters and other data are assessed in conjunction with blood pressure.

Measurement of blood lactate levels has also received a great deal of attention as a potential guide to fluid therapy. Lactate, a by-product of anaerobic metabolism, accumulates when tissues do not receive enough oxygen. Successful fluid resuscitation should result in significant reduction in elevated lactate levels (normal blood levels should be lower than 2 mmol/L). However, some causes of hyperlactemia are unrelated to perfusion and other factors that can affect lactate clearance; this can sometimes limit the usefulness of blood lactate levels as a guide to fluid therapy.

Central venous pressure (CVP) can be a good monitoring tool to help guide fluid therapy. Measurement of CVP is meant to approximate cardiac preload and thereby blood volume. Therefore, CVP can be used to help determine whether a patient may benefit from additional fluid administration or is at risk for volume overload. This is especially true for patients with significant renal and/or cardiac disease because their ability to handle fluids is significantly decreased. What follows is a brief overview of how CVP is measured.

CVP should be measured through a central line placed in the jugular vein and positioned just outside of the right atrium. The measurement can be taken with a pressure transducer and a specialized hemodynamic monitor, or with a water monometer. No matter which method is used, the patient should be placed ideally in lateral recumbency (with the same side down each time CVP is measured), and a minimum of three readings should be obtained to ensure the accuracy of the readings. A normal CVP reading is 0 to 10 cm H_2O. The optimal range is 5 to 8 cm H_2O. Patients with values lower than 5 cm H_2O may be volume depleted, and those with values greater than 14 cm H_2O may have significant volume overload or right-sided heart failure. One should also remember that the trend of CVP measurements (i.e., whether they are going up or down)—not each individual number—should be monitored and used to guide therapy.

> **TECHNICIAN NOTE** It is the trend of CVP measurements (i.e., whether they are going up or down)—not each individual number—that should be monitored and used to guide therapy.

Replacement Phase

As was previously mentioned, assessment of hydration status is an important component of determining replacement fluid rates. Therefore, it stands to reason that frequent monitoring of hydration is an equally important component of determining when the replacement phase should end. What follows is a brief overview of the key components of assessment of hydration and response to replacement fluid therapy. For a complete review of hydration assessment, please refer to Chapter 7.

Hydration status can be monitored in various ways. Indicators of dehydration evident on physical examination include decreased skin turgor, tackiness of mucous membranes, sunken eyes, and, if severe enough, signs of cardiovascular compromise. Other data that can be useful include **packed cell volume (PCV)**/total protein (TP), urine output, urine specific gravity, and changes in body weight. Unfortunately, numerous other factors can potentially affect these parameters and can obscure the assessment of dehydration/rehydration. For example, skin turgor tends to be less accurate in obese or geriatric patients. Panting dogs typically have dry mucous membranes regardless of hydration status, and

kidney disease will impair the usefulness of urine specific gravity. Perhaps the single best way to track changes in hydration and body water is through frequent monitoring of body weight. Generally speaking, a change in body water is the major reason for a short-term change in body weight (over the course of a day or less), with the exception of loss of a substantial amount of body tissue, as would occur after limb amputation, splenectomy, or another similar surgery. In patients that have not had a short-term change in body weight related to surgery, a change in body weight of 1 kg signifies a change in body water content of 1 L. Therefore, weighing a patient at least 1 or 2 times per day, or sometimes more often, can be helpful in determining whether a fluid deficit has been corrected, or if the patient is becoming overhydrated. For example, a 20-kg dog believed to be 5% dehydrated (which corresponds to a 1-L fluid deficit) should weigh 21 kg after correction of the deficit.

> **TECHNICIAN NOTE** Perhaps the single best way to track changes in hydration and body water is through frequent monitoring of body weight.

COMPLICATIONS OF FLUID THERAPY

Although fluid therapy is often the cornerstone of treatment, it is important to realize the potential complications that can arise from fluid administration. Perhaps the biggest concern is the potential to administer an excessive quantity of fluids, causing volume overload. Most patients with normal heart and kidney function are able to tolerate a large volume of fluids, but compromised patients, especially cats, are at greater risk. Volume overload is manifested in various ways. Of greatest concern is the development of pulmonary edema from overload of the left side of the heart. Therefore, respiratory rate and pattern should be closely monitored in patients receiving fluids. If the respiratory rate increases by more than 20%, if respiratory effort increases, or if the patient develops pulmonary crackles, fluids should be stopped until a veterinarian can be reached. Patients with volume overload can develop cavitary effusion (effusions into a body cavity) or peripheral edema, and, as has been mentioned, aggressive volume expansion in the face of uncontrolled hemorrhage can result in worsening of bleeding.

Certain types of fluids can result in coagulation abnormalities. Synthetic colloids such as hetastarch have been implicated in causing prolonged coagulation times and impaired platelet function. In addition, administration of large volumes of fluid, especially in the face of major blood loss, can result in a dilution coagulopathy. This involves a decrease in coagulation factors and platelets when blood is replaced by fluids that do not contain these components.

Although fluid therapy is often used to treat electrolyte and acid-base disturbances, it can also be responsible for causing these problems. For instance, patients can develop major changes in both sodium and chloride depending on the type of fluid given; significant fluid-induced diuresis can be associated with the development of hypokalemia unless the patient is supplemented appropriately; and certain fluid types (e.g., 0.9% NaCl) are acidifying, while others (e.g., Plasmalyte, LRS) are alkalinizing.

TRANSFUSION MEDICINE

INDICATIONS FOR BLOOD AND PLASMA TRANSFUSION

Indications for blood transfusion include acute hemorrhage, chronic anemia, and hemolytic anemia. Causes of acute hemorrhage include trauma, surgical bleeding, coagulopathy, and intracavitary bleeding (bleeding into the abdomen or thorax). Physical examination findings, such as pale mucous membranes, tachycardia, tachypnea, and lethargy, may indicate a need for blood transfusion, especially when blood loss is estimated to be greater than 30% of blood volume. Acute blood loss can result in hypovolemic shock, in addition to loss of red cell mass, so findings may include cold extremities, hypotension, and increased blood lactate concentrations. Additional physical examination findings in horses include sweating and colic. It is important to remember that PCV can still be normal during severe, acute hemorrhage, but PCV and TP will decrease as fluid redistributes from the interstitial to the intravascular space over the first 12 hours after hemorrhage. If intravenous fluids are given for resuscitation, PCV and TP will decrease more quickly. TP will decrease before PCV decreases substantially, especially in horses and dogs, because splenic contraction increases the PCV. Blood transfusion is likely to be necessary if PCV drops to below 20% to 25% during an acute bleeding episode. In cases of acute hemorrhage, whole blood (WB) or packed red blood cells (PRBCs) and plasma, often in conjunction with crystalloids or colloids, are most commonly used to restore oxygen-carrying capacity and circulating volume.

> **TECHNICIAN NOTE** Blood transfusion is likely to be necessary if packed cell volume (PCV) drops to below 20% to 25% during an acute bleeding episode.

In patients with chronic and hemolytic anemia, PCV and TP can be more useful indicators of the need for blood transfusion. Although no universally accepted threshold has been reached in veterinary medicine, generally speaking in chronic cases, PCV of less than 12% to 15%, especially in conjunction with previously mentioned physical examination findings (pale mucous membranes, tachycardia, tachypnea, and lethargy), indicates a need for blood transfusion. Patients with PCV above this level may need a transfusion if they have concurrent disease such as a respiratory condition or sepsis. Because animals with hemolytic or chronic anemia are normovolemic, PRBCs are indicated for transfusion, although WB may also be used.

For both acute and chronic anemia, the primary goal of blood transfusion is to enhance the oxygen-carrying capacity of the blood. Although blood transfusion will temporarily enhance oxygen-carrying capacity, it is essential to diagnose and treat the underlying cause of the anemia.

Platelet transfusions are indicated for patients with severe thrombocytopenia and life-threatening hemorrhage or thrombocytopenia and a need for surgical intervention. In the presence of risk factors for bleeding, a platelet count of 10,000/µl in a cat or 20,000/µl in a dog indicates the need for a platelet transfusion. Values such as these, which indicate the need for transfusion, are sometimes referred to as a *transfusion trigger*. Platelet transfusion may be less beneficial for patients with immune-mediated thrombocytopenia because transfused platelets will be rapidly destroyed and so are reserved for emergency treatment in extreme circumstances.

Plasma transfusions are indicated for treatment of coagulopathy, hypoalbuminemia, and failure of passive transfer of immunity (in large animal neonates). Fresh plasma and fresh frozen plasma contain clotting factors (II, V, VII, VIII, IX, X, XI, XII) and anticoagulant proteins (antithrombin, protein C, protein S), as well as immunoglobulins. Plasma can also be used for colloid support when the total protein is less than 4.0 g/dl, or the albumin is less than 2.0 g/dl. However, a very large volume of plasma is needed to significantly raise blood albumin levels (see later). If clotting factors and albumin are not needed, synthetic colloids such as hydroxyethyl starch are preferred for colloid support. In large animal neonates (such as foals, crias, and calves) with failure of transfer of passive immunity (from the colostrum), hyperimmune plasma is used to increase the serum immunoglobulin concentration. In foals an immunoglobulin (Ig)G concentration less than 800 mg/dl, and in calves a total protein concentration less than 5.5 g/dl, is an indication for plasma transfusion if the animal is more than 12 hours old (Box 24-4 lists commercial sources of fresh frozen equine plasma). For animals with von Willebrand disease, **cryoprecipitate** may be used because it contains more concentrated von Willebrand factor (as well as factor VIII, fibrinogen, factor XIII, and fibronectin). Cryoprecipitate typically would be administered to a patient with known deficiency that needs to undergo a surgical procedure or is having life-threatening bleeding associated with primary hemostatic dysfunction.

> **TECHNICIAN NOTE** Plasma transfusions are indicated for treatment of coagulopathy, hypoalbuminemia, and failure of passive transfer of immunity (in large animal neonates).

BOX 24-4	Commercial Sources of Fresh Frozen Equine Plasma

Veterinary Immunogenics (Cumbria, United Kingdom): www.veterinaryimmunogenics.com
Lake Immunogenics, Inc. (Ontario, New York): www.lakeimmunogenics.com
Mg Biologics (Ames, Iowa): www.mgbiologics.com
EquiPlas (Templeton, California): www.plasvaccusa.com

In addition to plasma, albumin transfusions can be performed to augment blood albumin levels. These transfusions can be performed if colloid administration is insufficient to sustain oncotic pressure, or if the albumin level falls below the minimum critical threshold (<1.5 g/dl) necessary for it to perform its other important functions (wound healing, carrier function, free-radical scavenger, etc.). Available products include 25% human albumin solution (25 g/dl) and 10% canine albumin solution (10 g/dl; Animal Blood Resources International, Dixon, California). Although the human albumin product generally is more cost-effective, it does have significant antigenic potential. Approximately 80% similarity has been noted between canine and human albumin, but administration of the human product has been shown to reliably stimulate antibody production and carries with it the potential for both acute and delayed **hypersensitivity** reactions. The decision to use human albumin in a canine patient should be based on careful consideration of risks and benefits.

BLOOD DONORS

Healthy animals with a good temperament and adequate PCV and body weight may be selected as blood donors. Recommended body weight, PCV, and TP for blood donors are shown in Table 24-5. Some referral hospitals will choose to house donors; others may collect and bank blood from "volunteer" donors or client-owned animals. Blood products (discussed on page 900) are also commercially available and can be stored on-site. All donors should be current on vaccinations and free of intestinal parasites at the time of donation. A thorough physical examination, complete blood count (CBC), and chemistry profile should be performed on animals being considered as blood donors.

Canine and feline donors should be between 1 and 7 years of age and should have good jugular vein access. Feline donors should be housed indoors only. Donor animals should not be on medication, except that used for prevention of heartworms, fleas, or ticks, and should be tested for blood-borne infectious disease. Canine donors should test negative for heartworm antigen, babesiosis, leishmaniasis, ehrlichiosis, anaplasmosis, neorickettsiosis, and brucellosis. Feline blood donors should test negative for feline leukemia virus (FeLV), feline immunodeficiency virus (FIV), hemoplasmosis, and bartonellosis. Equine donors should test negative for equine infectious anemia and should be vaccinated for rhinopneumonitis, tetanus, eastern and western encephalitis, rabies, and West Nile virus. Additional testing may be needed depending on the travel or exposure history of the animal. PCV should be determined for all donor animals before each blood collection.

PRETRANSFUSION TESTING
Blood Typing

Animals used as blood donors should be blood-typed, and any stored blood products should be clearly labeled with donor information and **blood type**. Horses have eight major blood systems, as well as 34 blood factors within 7 of these systems. Based on the vast numbers of blood systems and factors, no true "universal" equine blood type is known. The ideal donor horse is Aa and Qa negative because these blood types appear to be the most immunogenic and have been commonly associated with neonatal isoerythrolysis. A horse of the same breed is more likely to have a similar blood type, so choosing a donor of the same breed may increase the likelihood of having a compatible donor. It would be preferable to blood-type the horse that will receive the transfusion, so that the best blood match can be selected. However; blood must be sent to an equine blood-typing laboratory (Box 24-5), so this is not a practical method of selecting a donor horse in an emergency situation. A rapid equine blood-typing method identifies Aa and Ca antigens; however, this test is not commercially available. Cattle have more than 70 recognized blood group factors, but factor J is the only factor for which naturally occurring antibodies have been identified. Therefore, donor cattle should be negative for factor J.

> **ⅠTECHNICIAN NOTE**　Based on the vast numbers of blood systems and factors, no true "universal" equine blood type is known.

Numerous dog erythrocyte antigens (DEAs) have been identified for canine patients. Among these systems, DEA 1.1, 1.2, and 7 have been shown to be the most immunogenic and, therefore, the most important in canine transfusion medicine. The presence of circulating anti-DEA 1.1 antibody in a recipient will cause **agglutination** and **hemolysis** if DEA

TABLE 24-5	Blood Donor Recommendations		
DONOR SPECIES	**MINIMUM WEIGHT**	**MINIMUM PCV**	**TP**
Canine	25 kg	45%	Within reference range
Feline	5 kg	35%	Within reference range
Equine	450 kg	35%	≥6.0 g/dl

PCV, Packed cell volume; TP, total protein.

BOX 24-5	Equine Blood-Typing Laboratories

Hematology Laboratory
Room 1012, Veterinary Teaching Hospital
One Garrod Drive
University of California, Davis
Davis, CA 95616
Phone: 530-752-1303

University of Kentucky
Equine Parentage Testing and Research Lab
102 Animal Pathology Building
Lexington, KY 40546-0076
Phone: 859-257-3656
www.ca.uky.edu/gluck/ServEPVL.asp

1.1–positive blood is transfused. Therefore, rapid blood-typing cards are used to detect DEA 1.1 (Figure 24-8), and many clinicians rely strictly on the 1.1 typing system.

Some testing laboratories and blood banks can provide extensive canine blood typing for a number of other erythrocyte antigens. Currently, typing is available for DEA 1.1, 1.2, 3, 4, 5, and 7. When blood banks test for all of these antigens, the universal donor is one that is positive for only the DEA 4 antigen (because this antigen occurs in 98% of dogs) and negative for all other DEAs. Ideally, only these dogs would be included in the blood donor program; however, only 15% of the population falls under this category. To broaden the donor pool, dogs positive for DEA 1.1 may be used as donors for DEA 1.1–positive recipients.

In any case, dogs do not have naturally occurring antibodies; therefore, a transfusion reaction is less likely after a first transfusion of red blood cells. However, once exposed to a foreign DEA, a canine patient will develop antibodies through alloimmunization (development of immunity against DEAs of another dog) and thereby will become sensitive. Therefore, it is recommended that blood types of all donors and recipients should be known before transfusion (for at least DEA 1.1), so that type-specific blood can be administered.

The blood group system in cats consists of blood types A, B, and AB. A is the most common blood type, especially for domestic shorthair (DSH) and domestic long-hair (DLH) breeds (which represent 95% to 99% of cats in the United States). Type B is far less common but is seen with greater frequency in some breeds (e.g., 40% to 50% of Devon Rex and British Shorthair; 10% to 20% of Abyssinian, Persian, Himalayan, and Sphinx). Feline blood-typing cards are commercially available and involve a standard agglutination reaction with antitype antibodies (Figure 24-9).

Unlike dogs, cats have naturally occurring circulating alloantibodies (antibodies to antigens of another cat) to the blood type they do not have. In other words, type B cats have high levels of anti-A antibodies, so transfusion of type A blood into a type B cat could result in severe, potentially fatal hemolytic transfusion reaction. If type B blood is transfused into a type A cat, the life span of the transfused cells will be significantly reduced, but overall the transfusion reaction will not be nearly as severe, because circulating anti-B antibodies are weaker by comparison. Type AB cats can receive blood from a donor with any blood type. Because of the risk

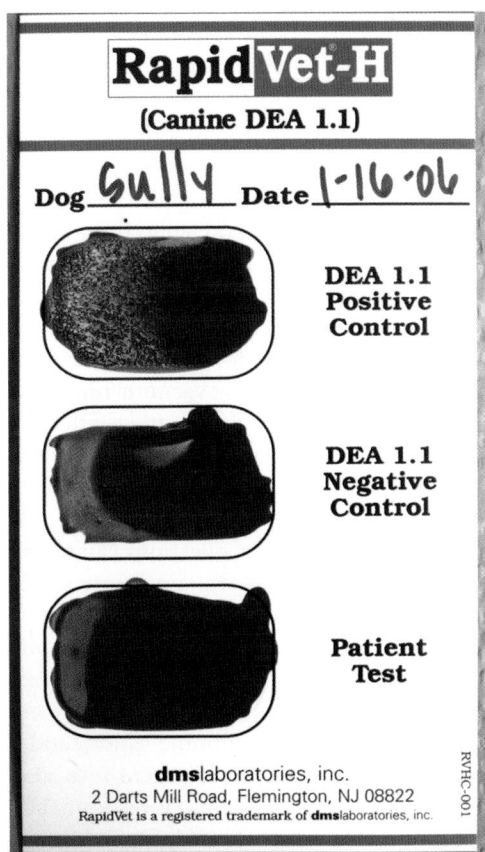

FIGURE 24-8 A canine blood-typing card (Rapid Vet-H, DMS Laboratories, Flemington, New Jersey) is shown. The patient sample does not agglutinate, indicating that the pet is dog erythrocyte antigen (DEA) 1.1 negative.

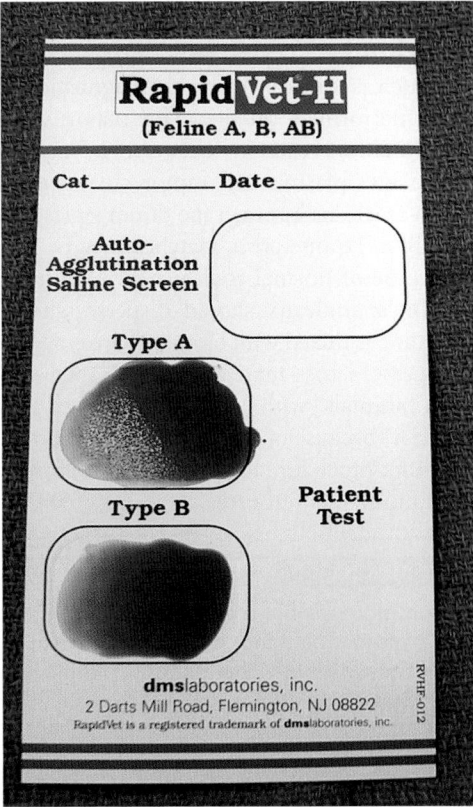

FIGURE 24-9 A feline blood-typing card (Rapid Vet-H, DMS Laboratories, Flemington, New Jersey) is shown. Note the agglutination that indicates this cat is blood type A.

for transfusion reaction, no universal donor is known, and all cats should be blood-typed before transfusion. If typing cards are not available, a **cross-match** (see later) can be used to help determine whether patients are compatible.

In addition to A and B antigens, evidence indicates the presence of another erythrocyte antigen that can result in acute hemolytic reaction. Circulating alloantibodies against this antigen (called the *Mik* antigen) have been detected. Currently, no way to directly test for the presence of *Mik* antigen is known, so a cross-match may be advisable, even if the cat has not been previously transfused.

Antibody Screen

Donor animals ideally should be screened yearly for alloantibodies. Recipients may also be tested for red blood cell (RBC) antibodies; however, such testing is not widely available, so this is not usually practical in the emergency setting. Antibody screens are most commonly performed in mares that may be at risk of having anti-RBC antibodies to the foal's blood type (leading to neonatal isoerythrolysis if the foal ingests colostrum).

In horses and dogs, an initial emergency transfusion may be given without pretesting because the likelihood of naturally occurring RBC antibodies is low. It is important to check for a history of previous transfusion or foaling (horses) because the likelihood of sensitization to RBC antigens is high in these cases. Development of RBC antibodies occurs 5 to 7 days after transfusion, so it is imperative that a cross-match be performed before any subsequent transfusions.

Cross-matching

The cross-match is a readily available diagnostic procedure that can be performed on-site. The major cross-match detects agglutination reactions between the donor's RBCs and the recipient's plasma. The minor cross-match detects agglutination reactions between the donor's plasma and the recipient's RBCs. Equine cross-matches may be difficult to interpret because of normal rouleaux formation (stacking) of equine RBCs; rouleaux should disperse when a small amount of saline is mixed with blood, whereas agglutination will not disperse. Cross-matching can also be difficult to interpret in animals with immune-mediated hemolytic anemia (IMHA) because of the autoagglutination of patient RBCs. The exact procedure for performing a cross-match is described in numerous resources.

> **TECHNICIAN NOTE** The major cross-match detects agglutination reactions between the donor's RBCs and the recipient's plasma. The minor cross-match detects agglutination reactions between the donor's plasma and the recipient's RBCs.

The routine cross-match evaluates agglutination reactions but does not test for hemolytic reactions. Rabbit serum can be used for hemolytic testing, but this is not routinely performed as part of the cross-match. Cross-match testing

also does not accurately predict the life span of the transfused red cells or the development of antibodies to transfused RBCs, and transfusion reactions have been reported even with a compatible cross-match.

BLOOD COLLECTION

The recommended maximum blood donation for dogs is 15% to 20% of blood volume, or approximately 13 to 17 ml/kg. Commercially available blood bags have a standard unit volume of 450 ml, so donor animals should be at least 25 kg if they are to donate 1 unit of blood. Commercially available 450-ml collection bags have a 16-gauge needle attached to the collection line. The donor is usually restrained in lateral recumbency. After a clip and sterile preparation of the jugular area, the needle is inserted into the jugular vein. Specific step-by-step instructions for blood collection in dogs are provided in Procedure 24-1.

The recommended maximum blood donation for cats is 11 to 15 ml/kg, and the standard blood volume collected is 50 to 70 ml. Cats usually need to be sedated or anesthetized for the blood collection procedure. Blood collection in cats is performed using an 18- to 19-gauge needle or a butterfly catheter attached to a syringe or a collection bag containing anticoagulant. Specific step-by-step instructions for blood collection in cats are provided in Procedure 24-2. The ratio of anticoagulant solution to blood should be 1:7. Pediatric (75 ml) transfer packs are commercially available and are good options for storage of feline blood.

The recommended maximum blood donation for horses is 20% of blood volume, or approximately 16 ml/kg body weight. Donor horses should be weighed and should have PCV/TP measured before blood collection. Ideally, PCV should be greater than 35%. Blood is collected from the jugular vein, and both jugular veins may be used if a large volume of blood is needed immediately (Figure 24-10). Specific step-by-step instructions for blood collection in horses are provided in Procedure 24-3. Vacuum canisters may be used to speed collection, but glass bottles with vacuum are not recommended because glass inactivates the platelets and can damage the RBCs. Commercially available 450-ml blood collection bags may be used in horses, as can 2-L bags with sodium citrate anticoagulant. Collections can also be made by the addition of anticoagulant to an empty sterile collection bag.

For all species, the maximum blood collection volume should be calculated based on *lean* body weight. During blood collection from any animal, the donor's heart rate, respiratory rate, mucous membrane color, and attitude should be monitored. Volume replacement with 20 to 40 ml/kg of an intravenous crystalloid fluid is recommended when 20% of the blood volume is collected. For smaller collection volumes that are tolerated with no clinical signs of hypovolemia, the donor does not require intravenous fluids. All donors should have access to fresh water and food after the blood collection.

PROCEDURE 24-1	Protocol for Canine Whole Blood Collection

1. Perform a pre-donation physical examination, including body weight measurement and blood chemistry.
2. Take temperature, pulse rate, and respiratory rate.
3. Evaluate jugular vein quality and location.
4. Place the donor on the examination table in a lateral recumbent or sternal position. Make the animal as comfortable as possible.
5. Shave a 1-inch-square area of skin over the jugular vein.
6. Perform a standard three-pass sterile prep on the phlebotomy site.
7. Place a collection bag on a gram scale and set the scale to zero.
8. Clamp the collection line 3 to 4 inches distal to the needle, using a plastic hemostat to avoid damage to the collection line.
9. Have an assistant apply pressure to the jugular vein at the thoracic inlet to allow for distention and clear identification of the vessel.
10. Remove the needle cap. Insert the needle, bevel up, into the jugular vein.
11. Release the clamp from the collection line.
12. Collect 405 to 480 g of whole blood, carefully rocking the blood bag back and forth to mix blood and anticoagulant (each time an additional 50 to 75 ml has been collected).
13. Have the assistant release pressure over the vein.
14. Clamp the collection line with plastic hemostats.
15. Apply a 4 × 4-inch gauze sponge against the phlebotomy site.
16. Remove and cap the needle while holding pressure on the phlebotomy site with the sponge.
17. Wrap the phlebotomy site with 4-inch-wide Vetrap. Gauze and wrap should be left in place for 30 minutes to avoid bruising or hematoma formation.
18. Apply a hemoclip to the collection line, or heat-seal the collection line at least 2 inches above the bag to imprint a unique identifying line number on the bag.
19. Carefully agitate the collection bag to thoroughly mix the blood and anticoagulant.
20. Label the collection bag with donor identification, date, time, and amount collected.
21. Record the donation in the donor record, including the donor's weight, TPR, as well as blood chemistry, PCV, and TP results. Make sure to note the vessel and patient position used, as well as any problems encountered during the donation.

From Lucas RL, Lentz KD, Hale AS: Collection and preparation of blood products, Clin Tech Small Anim Pract 19:55, 2004.
PCV, Packed cell volume; *TP,* total protein; *TPR,* temperature, pulse, and respiration.

> **TECHNICIAN NOTE** For all species, the maximum blood collection volume should be calculated based on *lean* body weight.

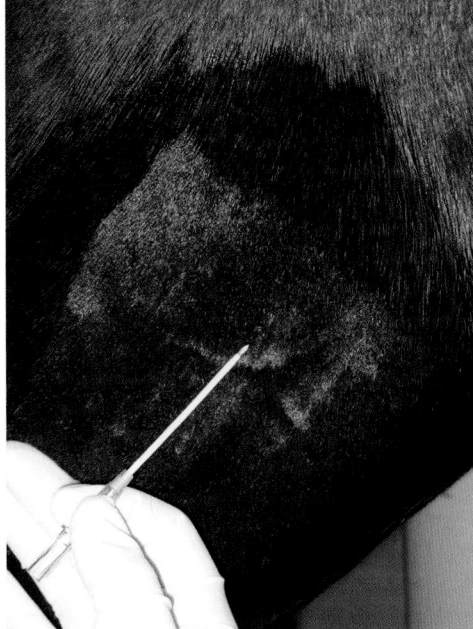

FIGURE 24-10 A 14-gauge, 2-inch intravenous catheter is directed toward the horse's head to optimize blood flow during collection.

Several anticoagulant options may be used for blood collection. If the blood will be transfused immediately, the anticoagulant sodium citrate is acceptable, but it will not support RBC metabolism during storage. If the blood is going to be stored, citrate-phosphate-dextrose (CPD) or citrate-phosphate-dextrose-adenine (CPDA) should be used. When free blood is collected from cavitary hemorrhage (e.g., bleeding into the abdominal or thoracic cavity), less anticoagulant is needed because the blood is already defibrinated. Commercially available devices will collect, wash, and filter free blood. Free blood may be collected into a blood bag with a reduced amount of anticoagulant and then filtered before administration. Recommendations for the ratio of anticoagulant to free blood range from 1:7 to 1:20.

To achieve optimal RBC viability during storage, blood bags should be weighed to ensure adequate fill (blood-to-anticoagulant ratio). Sterility is very important during collection and processing of blood for storage because bacterial contamination and growth may cause a significant transfusion reaction. To minimize bacterial contamination, a closed collection system should be used, and tube sealer should be used to seal the collection tubing, which can be sealed in several increments for later testing or cross-matching.

Whole blood and PRBCs are refrigerated at 1°C (33.8°F) to 6°C (42.8°F), ideally in a dedicated blood bank refrigerator with an alarm system that signals temperature breaches. Donor name, date of collection, blood type, and intended recipient (if known) should be clearly indicated on each blood bag. Blood from different species should be stored in separate refrigerators, or at least on separate shelves, with clear labeling (Figure 24-11).

| **PROCEDURE 24-2** | Protocol for Feline Whole Blood Collection |

1. Perform a pre-donation physical examination, including a body weight measurement and a mini profile.
2. Prepare the anesthesia machine or a sedative as ordered by the attending veterinarian.
3. Prepare the 60-ml feline blood collection system by adding 6 ml of CPDA-1 or ACD anticoagulant solution via the injection port nearest the syringe, making sure to clamp the line to the bag just below the injection port. *If you are using a syringe and butterfly catheter only, use a separate needle to draw up the anticoagulant into the syringe, and then switch to the butterfly catheter.*
4. Place the donor in a cat bag restraint (optional), and make it comfortable.
5. Induce general anesthesia with isoflurane, using a mask, until the patient is in stage III, or administer the sedative.
6. Place the donor in lateral recumbency and remove the restraint bag (if used) to expose the jugular furrow.
7. Shave a 1-inch-square area of skin over the jugular vein.
8. Perform a standard three-pass sterile prep on the phlebotomy site.
9. Close the port of the three-way stopcock nearest the collection bag, and release the clamp.
10. Have an assistant apply pressure at the thoracic inlet to distend the vein.
11. Remove the needle cap.
12. With the bevel up, insert the butterfly catheter into the jugular vein.
13. Collect 54 ml of whole blood by slowly and steadily pulling back the syringe plunger.
14. Gently rock the syringe to mix blood and anticoagulant.
15. Have the assistant release pressure over the vein.
16. Close the port of the three-way stopcock nearest the butterfly catheter.
17. Apply a 4 × 4-inch gauze sponge against the phlebotomy site.
18. Remove the needle while holding pressure on the phlebotomy site with the sponge.
19. Wrap the phlebotomy site with 2-inch-wide Vetrap. The gauze and the wrap should be left in place for at least 30 minutes.
20. Transfer blood from the syringe to a collection bag. *If you are using just a syringe and a butterfly catheter, you will need to transfer the whole blood to a transfer pack for storage. Fresh whole blood may be administered to the recipient directly from the collection syringe, if administered immediately after collection.*
21. Carefully agitate the collection bag to thoroughly mix the blood and anticoagulant.
22. Discontinue the anesthetic. Monitor the anesthetic recovery carefully.
23. Once the donor is awake, remove the neck wrap and return the donor to a holding cage.
24. Record the donation in the donor record, including the donor's weight, the TPR, and blood chemistry, PCV, and TP results. Make sure to note the vessel and the patient position used, as well as any problems encountered during the donation.

From Lucas RL, Lentz KD, Hale AS: Collection and preparation of blood products, Clin Tech Small Anim Pract 19:55, 2004.
ACD, acid-citrate-dextrose; *CPDA,* citrate-phosphate-dextrose-adenine; *PCV,* packed cell volume; *TP,* total protein; *TPR,* temperature, pulse, and respiration.

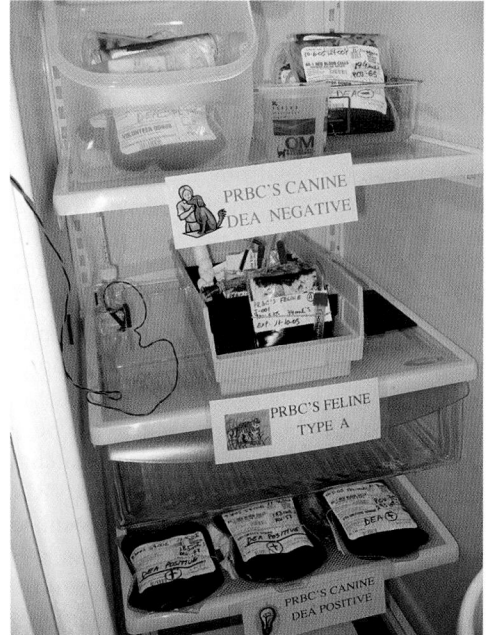

FIGURE 24-11 This refrigerator has been converted into a dedicated blood bank refrigerator. A temperature monitor is provided, and the shelves are clearly labeled.

BLOOD PRODUCTS

Whole blood can be given directly or can be processed to make PRBCs and plasma. To separate the components, blood is centrifuged (at 4° C; 39.2° F) at a relative centrifugal force of 5000× *g* for 5 minutes. Plasma is transferred to a satellite bag using a plasma extractor, and an additive solution is mixed with the PRBCs. Plasma that is used within 8 hours of collection is considered to be fresh plasma, and plasma that is placed in a freezer within 8 hours of collection and that is less than 1 year old is considered to be fresh frozen plasma (FFP). FFP is stored at temperatures less than or equal to −18° C (0° F). FFP should be used within 1 year of freezing to ensure optimal clotting factor activity. If plasma is thawed but is not needed, it can be refrozen within 1 hour of thawing and will maintain coagulation factor activity. Plasma that is frozen longer than 8 hours after collection, or FFP that is older than 1 year of age, is considered frozen plasma (FP). Labile clotting factors (factor V and factor VIII) will be decreased in FP as compared with FFP.

Equine hyperimmune plasma is a U.S. Department of Agriculture (USDA)-regulated product, and the shelf life for immunoglobulin efficacy is 2 to 3 years. Equine hyperimmune plasma ideally is collected by plasmapheresis

PROCEDURE 24-3 | Protocol for Equine Whole Blood Collection

1. Perform a pre-donation physical examination, including body weight measurement and PCV/TP.
2. Take temperature, pulse rate, and respiratory rate.
3. Evaluate jugular vein quality.
4. Restrain the donor horse in stocks, if available. Sedate the patient with xylazine or detomidine, if needed, as ordered by the attending veterinarian.
5. Shave or clip a 1-inch-square area of skin over the jugular vein.
6. Perform a standard three-pass sterile prep on the phlebotomy site.
7. Administer 2 ml of carbocaine subcutaneously at the insertion site of the catheter.
8. Place an IV catheter (3-inch, 10-gauge or 2-inch, 14-gauge), directing the catheter against the flow of blood (see Figure 24-10). Flush the catheter with heparinized saline to maintain patency. Alternatively, the needle from the collection kit may be inserted directly into the jugular vein if only one bag of whole blood is needed.
9. Place a collection bag on a gram scale and set the scale to zero.
10. Clamp the collection line 3 to 4 inches from the catheter/needle, using a plastic hemostat to avoid damage to the collection line.
11. If using a Vet Dynamics 2-L blood collection system (Plasvacc, Templeton, California): a 14-gauge needle with collection line is attached to the collection bag. This is to be used only when blood is needed immediately and is drawn by direct venipuncture instead of from an IV catheter. When not being used, this line should be tied off securely.
12. Squeeze the entire bag of the sodium citrate anticoagulant solution into the large collection bag, and clamp off the line to prevent the solution from flowing back.
13. Insert the 10-gtt/ml solution administration set into the large collection bag via the unused port, and prime it with the sodium citrate anticoagulant solution.
14. Connect the male end of the 10-gtt/ml solution administration set to the donor horse's IV catheter extension line.
15. Place the collection bag lower than the IV catheter to increase flow rate.
16. Open the solution administration set line. Blood should quickly flow into the collection bag.
17. Be sure to continuously and gently rock the collection bag during the collection process to keep the blood and anticoagulant mixed.
18. When the collection bag is full (2 L), remove the 10-gtt/ml solution administration set and insert it into your next collection bag (only if more blood is needed). The blood administration set included with the bag can then be inserted into the full collection bag port to which the 10-gtt/ml solution administration set was previously connected. The blood is now ready to be administered to the recipient horse. Approximately 2 L of blood can be collected in 12 minutes.
19. Apply a hemoclip to or heat-seal the collection line.
20. Carefully agitate the collection bag to thoroughly mix blood and anticoagulant.
21. Label the collection bag with donor identification, date, time, and amount collected.
22. Record the donation in the donor record, including the donor's weight, the TPR, and blood chemistry, PCV, and TP results. Make sure to note the vessel and patient position used, as well as any problems encountered during the donation.

PCV, Packed cell volume; TP, total protein; TPR, temperature, pulse, and respiration.

to minimize any RBC contamination. In horses, up to 20 ml/kg of plasma can be collected every 30 days.

> **TECHNICIAN NOTE** Plasma that is used within 8 hours of collection is considered to be fresh plasma, and plasma that is placed in a freezer within 8 hours of collection and that is less than 1 year old is considered to be fresh frozen plasma.

Canine PRBCs have been shown to have a shelf life of 20 days when stored in CPDA-1, and 35 days when stored in an additive solution such as Nutricel (ProNature Laboratories, Canterbury, NSW, Australia). Other blood products that can be processed from whole blood include **platelet-rich plasma**, cryoprecipitate, and **platelet concentrate**. Cryoprecipitate has a shelf life of 1 year. Platelet concentrate must be stored at room temperature and should be used within 5 to 7 days. Plateletpheresis, another option for preparation of platelet concentrate, has been described for canine platelet transfusions.

In horses, washed RBCs are needed in cases of neonatal isoerythrolysis in foals. The mare is the ideal blood donor for the foal; however, the mare's plasma contains antibodies directed against the foal's RBCs. A technique of centrifugation—removal of plasma supernatant and washing with saline 3 times—is used to prepare washed RBCs.

BLOOD PRODUCT ADMINISTRATION

Refrigerated blood can be transfused directly because warming may cause deterioration of RBCs. In hypothermic patients, or in those receiving large volumes of blood, the blood should be warmed at least to room temperature (22° C; 71.6° F) but no warmer than body temperature (37° C; 98.6° F). Blood products are administered using a commercial blood delivery set with an in-line filter (Figure 24-12). Standard filters have a pore size of 170 to 260 μm, and the filter and administration set should be changed after

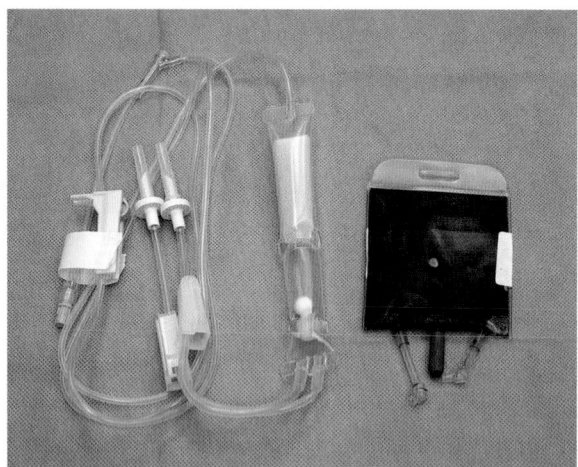

FIGURE 24-12 Commercially available blood administration set with in-line filter to prevent inadvertent infusion of clots.

BOX 24-6	Calculation for Blood Transfusion Volume for Chronic or Normovolemic Anemia

$$\text{Blood transfusion volume (ml)} = \frac{\text{Wt (kg)} \times \text{Blood volume (ml/kg)} \times [(\text{Desired PCV} - \text{Actual PCV})]}{[\text{Donor PCV}]}$$

PCV, Packed cell volume.

BOX 24-7	Equation to Use if Plasma Is Given for the Purpose of Increasing Blood Albumin Levels

$$\text{Volume of plasma administered (L)} = \frac{0.3 \text{ L/kg} \times (\Delta\text{Alb}_{desired}) \times \text{Body weight in kg}}{[\text{Alb}]_{infused}}$$

$\Delta\text{Alb}_{desired}$ = Desired increase in albumin (g/dl); $[\text{Alb}]_{infused}$ = Albumin concentration in the infused solution.

Based on this equation, and assuming an average albumin concentration of 4 g/dl in fresh frozen plasma (FFP), the amount of plasma that would be needed to raise the patient's albumin by 1 g/dl is approximately 75 ml/kg (or about 1.5 L for a 20 kg dog)!

$$\text{e.g., Volume of plasma administered (L)} = \frac{0.3 \text{ L/kg} \times (1 \text{ g/dl}) \times 20 \text{ kg}}{4 \text{ g/dl}} = 1.5 \text{ L}$$

administration of 2 to 4 units of blood. Blood should not be given concurrently with hypertonic or hypotonic solutions, and should not be given with calcium-containing solutions (such as lactated Ringer's solution [LRS]) because calcium in the fluids can serve to overwhelm the citrate anticoagulant, resulting in activation of the coagulation cascade.

> **TECHNICIAN NOTE** Blood should not be given concurrently with hypertonic or hypotonic solutions and should not be given with calcium-containing solutions (such as lactated Ringer's solution [LRS]).

Determination of Volume and Rate

Blood products should be given slowly for the first 10 to 20 minutes so the animal can be monitored closely for signs of transfusion reaction (see page 903), and the transfusion can be stopped, if needed. Approximately 0.3 ml/kg is given over 20 to 30 minutes initially; the rate can then be increased, if needed. The rate of transfusion will depend on the patient's volume status and can be as high as 20 to 40 ml/kg/hour if volume resuscitation is needed. It is not recommended to exceed 2 to 4 ml/kg/hour in patients with significant cardiac disease. The transfusion should be completed within 4 hours to prevent bacterial growth and ensure platelet functionality (in the case of fresh whole blood).

The total volume of blood to be transfused can be calculated based on estimated blood loss (for acute blood loss) or PCV (for chronic or normovolemic anemia). See Box 24-6 for specific guidelines and Case Presentation 24-3 for a clinical example. An estimate of the patient's blood volume is needed to determine the transfusion volume. For horses, blood volume can be estimated as 8% of body weight, so a 500-kg horse would have a blood volume of 40 L. Once blood loss and blood volume have been estimated and PCV of the donor animal (or PCV of the stored blood) is known, the volume of the transfusion can be calculated. In general, the goal should be to replace 25% to 50% of the blood lost.

A useful guideline is that 2 ml/kg of whole blood or 1 ml/kg of PRBCs will raise the PCV by 1%.

Before FFP is administered, the plasma should be thawed in a water bath at 30°C to 37°C. Generally speaking, the amount of plasma required to correct a coagulation abnormality is approximately 10 to 15 ml/kg in dogs and 5 to 8 ml/kg in cats. Although this can serve as a guideline, coagulation times (activated partial thromboplastin time [aPTT] and prothrombin time [PT]) ideally would be assessed after the transfusion is completed to ensure that the values have normalized. Box 24-7 shows the equation to use if plasma is given for the purpose of increasing blood albumin levels.

As the figures in Box 24-7 show, administration of plasma is an inefficient and potentially very expensive way to augment albumin levels. In adult horses, plasma usually is given in 1-L increments "to effect," to treat coagulopathy. "To effect" means that treatment is continued until the desired effect is achieved. In neonatal foals with failure of passive transfer, hyperimmune plasma is given at a dose of approximately 20 to 40 ml/kg. IgG concentration should be rechecked after transfusion of hyperimmune plasma in these patients.

> **TECHNICIAN NOTE** Administration of plasma is an inefficient and potentially very expensive way to augment albumin levels.

CASE PRESENTATION 24-3 EQUINE BLOOD TRANSFUSION

History and Signalment

A 4-year-old Friesian mare (600 kg) was presented to the hospital with acute onset of lethargy and pale mucous membranes. No treatments had been administered before admission to the referral hospital.

Initial Examination

On presentation, the mare appeared lethargic and mildly anxious. Her heart rate was 88 beats per minute (bpm) (normal, 28 to 40 bpm), her respiratory rate was 36 breaths/minute (normal, 8 to 18 breaths/minute), and her temperature was 99.0° F (normal, 98.5° F to 100.5° F). Her mucous membranes were very pale and slightly tacky, and her extremities were cold. Basic blood work showed packed cell volume (PCV) of 18% (normal, 28% to 40%), total protein (TP) of 5.5 g/dl (normal, 5.5 to 7.5 g/dl), and blood lactate of 15 mmol/L (normal <2 mmol/L). Abdominal ultrasound showed a large amount of free fluid and a large mass in the right side of the abdomen. Rectal examination confirmed the right abdominal mass (possible ovary), and pain was associated with palpation. An abdominocentesis was performed. The sample was red and had a PCV of 14% and TP of 5.8 g/dl (results similar to the peripheral blood sample taken on admission). Cytologic examination confirmed that it was consistent with peripheral blood with no evidence of neoplasia or infection. Preliminary diagnosis was intra-abdominal hemorrhage and shock secondary to blood loss from the mass.

Fluid Therapy and Transfusion Plan

The mare was housed in the intensive care unit (ICU) and was started on lactated Ringer's solution (LRS) at a rate of 10 ml/kg/hour. In the meantime, 8 L of whole blood was collected from a donor horse into citrated bags and transfused immediately.

Based on signs of shock, blood loss was estimated to be at least 30%.

$$\text{Total blood volume} = 600 \text{ kg} \times 80 \text{ ml/kg} = 48 \text{ L}$$
$$30\% \text{ of } 48 \text{ L} = 14.4 \text{ L blood lost}$$

Four hours post transfusion, blood work was repeated. The mare's PCV was 12%, TP 4.1 g/dl, and lactate 6.0 mmol/L, and her heart rate remained high, at 80 bpm. Because the mare did not show adequate clinical improvement, a second transfusion was indicated. Two other donor horses were cross-matched and were found incompatible on both major and minor matches. Because these horses did not match, the owner elected to bring in a related Fresian horse for donor blood. An additional 8 L whole blood was transfused over 2 hours. After the second transfusion, PCV increased to 14%, TP increased to 6.0 g/dl, lactate was <2 mmol/L, and heart rate decreased to 54 bpm.

Given the potential for reaction, administration of albumin solutions (whether canine or human albumin) should be approached as with any other transfusion. The volume of albumin to be administered is determined using the equation indicated previously for plasma. However,

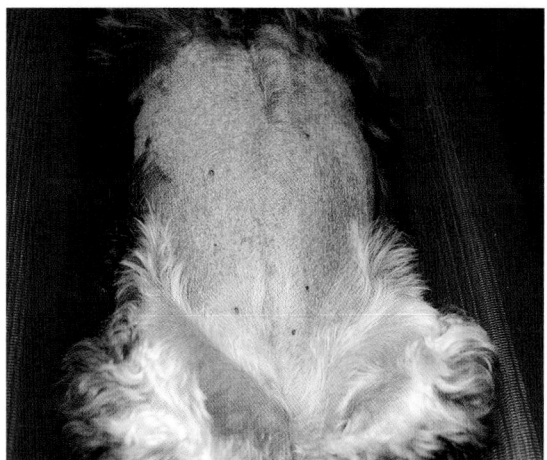

FIGURE 24-13 Transfusion reactions can include many signs. This image depicts cutaneous erythema.

because 25% human albumin has a concentration of 25 g/dl (as opposed to 4 g/dl for FFP), the volume needed to raise the recipient's albumin level by 1 g/dl is 12 ml/kg (rather than 75 ml/kg). The volume of 10% canine albumin (concentration 10 g/dl) needed to raise the albumin level by 1 g/dl is 30 ml/kg.

Monitoring and Transfusion Reactions

The recipient's heart rate, temperature, respiratory rate, and attitude should be monitored every 15 minutes during a transfusion, with particular attention during the first 15 minutes. Transfusion reactions from acute allergic (type I) hypersensitivity can include erythema, urticaria, and pruritus or **anaphylaxis** (Figure 24-13). In horses, sweating and piloerection and muscle fasciculation may be components of an allergic reaction. In canine and feline patients, these reactions tend to be more severe when plasma-containing blood products are used. If an allergic reaction is suspected, the transfusion should be stopped immediately (if severe) or slowed (if mild). Most allergic reactions will resolve on their own; however, some will require administration of corticosteroids or antihistamines, and severe anaphylactic reactions may require administration of epinephrine.

> **TECHNICIAN NOTE** Most allergic reactions will resolve on their own; however, some will require administration of corticosteroids or antihistamines, and severe anaphylactic reactions may require administration of epinephrine.

Acute hemolytic transfusion reactions occur during or within hours of transfusion. This reaction occurs when there is incompatibility between donor and recipient blood, resulting in rapid destruction of transfused RBCs (e.g., when type A blood is administered to a type B cat). This process typically occurs when preexisting antibodies are present and is classified as cytotoxic (type II) hypersensitivity. Clinical signs include hemoglobinemia, hemoglobinuria, and progressive anemia or lack of increase in PCV. In addition, the highly inflammatory nature of this reaction can lead to signs of systemic inflammatory response, disseminated intravascular coagulation (DIC), shock, cardiovascular collapse, and death. Severity of signs is directly related to the volume of transfused blood. When acute hemolytic transfusion reactions occur, the transfusion should be stopped immediately and supportive care initiated.

Delayed hemolytic transfusion reactions can occur longer than 24 hours after transfusion and can result in RBC lysis. Hemolysis of donor blood may occur before transfusion as the result of improper handling. Improper storage, excessive warming of the blood, administration with hypertonic solution, and administration using pumps are examples of improper handling that can lead to RBC destruction.

Nonhemolytic immune reactions such as fever may also occur with blood or plasma transfusion and are the most common reactions seen in veterinary patients. Fever is thought to be caused by donor leukocytes and accumulation of pyrogenic cytokines over time. Therefore, older units of blood products are more likely to cause this response. Decreasing the rate of infusion and possibly administering diphenhydramine are typically all that is needed to treat nonhemolytic immune reactions. Another potential immunologic response is transfusion-related acute lung injury (TRALI). This reaction occurs when leukocyte antibodies from the donor interact with recipient leukocytes. The result is a marked increase in vascular permeability in the lungs and the development of protein-rich edema fluid. Clinical signs include an increase in respiratory rate and effort, development of pulmonary crackles and dyspnea, and fever. The reaction is self-limiting but may last 2 or 3 days. No direct therapy is available (diuretics are not beneficial), but rather intervention is largely supportive (supplemental oxygen or ventilator).

Perhaps the most significant nonimmune acute reaction is transfusion-associated circulatory overload (TACO). This can occur with large or rapidly delivered volumes of blood products, especially in patients that are euvolemic (e.g., those with IMHA or chronic anemia). Cats and patients with cardiac disease are particularly at risk. Clinical signs typically are related to pulmonary congestion and include increased respiratory rate and effort, development of pulmonary crackles, and dyspnea. These signs can be very difficult to distinguish from TRALI, although the clinical circumstances may help (e.g., large volume administered to a small patient would support TACO). If a patient develops TACO, the transfusion should be slowed or discontinued, supplemental oxygen provided, and a single dose of furosemide possibly administered. Other potential complications of blood transfusion include transmission of infectious disease, bacterial contamination, citrate toxicity (leading to ionized hypocalcemia and hypomagnesemia), and hypothermia associated with high-volume transfusions.

In horses, the incidence of adverse reactions with plasma is 10% and the incidence of adverse reactions with whole blood transfusion has been reported as 16%. The incidence of transfusion reactions in dogs has been reported to be approximately 10% to 15%. In cats, the incidence of reactions to red cell transfusion has been reported to be approximately 5% to 10% when type-specific blood is given. No reports have described plasma transfusion in cats. Compatibility on cross-match does not guarantee lack of transfusion reaction and does not accurately predict RBC life span.

It is important to assess the response to transfusion. Physical examination, PCV, blood lactate, and oxygen extraction are among the parameters that should be monitored. It is important to remember that with acute or ongoing hemorrhage, PCV may not increase after transfusion. The primary goal of blood transfusion is to improve oxygen delivery to the tissues, so that all of the information from physical examination and laboratory data should be considered before an additional transfusion is performed.

RECOMMENDED READINGS

Barfield D, Adamantes S: Feline blood transfusions: a pinker shade of pale, J Feline Med Surg 13:11, 2011.

Battaglia AM: Small animal emergency and critical care: a manual for the veterinary technician, Ithaca, NY, 2001, Elsevier.

Bracker KE, Drelich S: Transfusion reactions, Compend Contin Educ 2005, July.

DiBartola SP: Fluid, electrolyte, and acid-base disorders in small animal practice, St Louis, 2006, Elsevier.

Divers TJ: Blood component transfusions, Vet Clin North Am Food Anim Pract 50:615, 2005.

Driessen B, Brainard B: Fluid therapy for the traumatized patient, J Vet Emerg Crit Care 16:276, 2006.

Eddlestone SM: Small animal medical nursing. In McCurnin's clinical textbook for veterinary technicians, ed 7, St Louis, 2010, Elsevier.

Gonzales GL: How to establish an equine blood donor protocol, Proceedings of the Annual Convention of the American Association of Equine Practitioners (AAEP) 47:262, 2001.

Lucas RL, Lentz KD, Hale AS: Collection and preparation of blood products, Clin Tech Small Anim Pract 19:55, 2004.

Perkins GA, Boatwright C: How to rapidly administer intravenous fluids to critically ill equine patients on the farm, Proceedings of the 51st Annual Convention of the American Association of Equine Practitioners 51:246, 2005.

Schott HC: Fluid therapy: a primer for students, technicians, and veterinarians in equine practice, Vet Clin North Am Equine 22:1, 2006.

Slovis NM, Murray G: How to approach whole blood transfusions in horses, Proceedings of the Annual Convention of the American Association of Equine Practitioners 47:266, 2001.

Tocci LJ: Transfusion medicine in small animal practice, Vet Clin North Am Small Anim Pract 40:485, 2010.

Tocci LJ, Ewing PJ: Increasing patient safety in veterinary transfusion medicine: an overview of pretransfusion testing, J Vet Emerg Crit Care 19:66, 2009.

Wardrop KJ, Reine N, Birkenheuer A, et al: Canine and feline blood donor screening for infectious disease, J Vet Intern Med 19:135, 2005.

Ann M. Peruski, Michelle E. Goodnight, Richard E. Cober,
Jarred Matthew Williams, and Andrew J. Niehaus

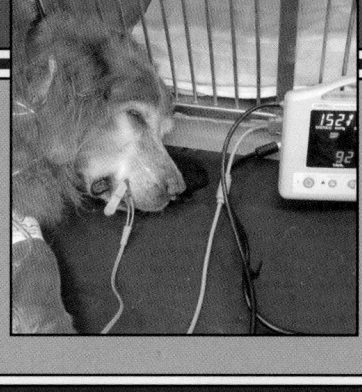

OUTLINE

EMERGENCY AND CRITICAL CARE
  NURSING: SMALL ANIMAL, *908*
Triage, *908*
Telephone Triage, *908*
In-Hospital Triage, *908*
Assessment of Hydration and
  Hypovolemia, *911*
Initial Diagnostics, *912*
Basic First Aid, *913*
The Emergency Care Station and
  Resuscitation Area, *914*
Crash Cart, *914*
Shock and the Systemic Inflammatory
  Response Syndrome, *914*
Reperfusion Injury, *916*
Advanced Emergency Techniques, *916*
Abdominocentesis, *916*
Thoracocentesis, *916*
Thoracic Drain Placement, *917*
Tracheostomy Tube Placement, *917*
Respiratory System Support and Oxygen
  Therapy, *917*
Cardiopulmonary Arrest, *921*
Cardiopulmonary Cerebral
  Resuscitation, *921*
Basic Life Support, *922*
Advanced Life Support, *924*
Care of the Post-Arrest Patient, *926*
Patient Monitoring, *927*
Central Venous Pressure Monitoring, *927*
Arterial Blood Pressure Monitoring, *928*
Care of the Recumbent Patient, *930*
Airway and Endotracheal or Tracheostomy
  Tube Care, *930*
Appropriate Bedding and Patient
  Comfort, *930*
Appropriate Level of Anesthesia or
  Analgesia, *930*
Intravenous Catheter Monitoring and
  Care, *931*

Monitoring and Adjusting Fluid Balance
  (Ins and Outs), *931*
Nutrition, *931*
Ocular Care, *931*
Oral Care, *931*
Range of Motion, *931*
Urinary Catheter Placement and Care, *931*
Standards of Care and Emergency
  Protocols, *931*
Common Toxicities and Emergencies, *931*

CANINE AND FELINE
  ELECTROCARDIOGRAPHY, *933*
Indications for the
  Electrocardiogram, *933*
Principles of Electrocardiography, *935*
Acquisition of the
  Electrocardiogram, *935*
Basic Cardiac Conduction and ECG
  Waveforms, *935*
Electrocardiographic Analysis, *936*
General Rhythm Evaluation, *936*
Cardiac Arrhythmias, *938*
Normal Rhythms, *938*
Disturbances of Supraventricular Impulse
  Formation, *939*
Disturbances of Ventricular Impulse
  Formation, *940*
Disturbances of Impulse Conduction, *942*
Disturbances of Impulse Formation and
  Conduction, *944*
Escape Rhythms, *944*

EQUINE EMERGENCY NURSING, *944*
Gastrointestinal Tract, *944*
General Physical Examination, *945*
Nasogastric Intubation, *946*
Abdominal Palpation Per Rectum, *947*
Abdominal Ultrasound, *947*
Abdominocentesis, *947*

The authors and publisher wish to acknowledge Kirk Ryan, Lee Ann Eddleman,
and Charles T. McCauley for their contributions to previous editions of this textbook.

KEY TERMS

Abdominocentesis
Acidosis
Arrhythmia
Asystole
Atrial fibrillation
Atrial premature
  complexes
Azotemia
Borborygmi
Capillary refill time
Cardiopulmonary
  cerebrovascular
  resuscitation
Chest tube
Choke
Colic
Defibrillation
Disseminated
  intravascular
  coagulation
Down animals
Dystocia
Electrocardiogram
Emesis
Endometrial
Eructation
Fetatome
Fetotomy
Flail chest
Hypovolemia
Hypoxemia
Hypoxia
Ileus
Ischemia
Jugular vein
Mastitis
Metritis
Multiple organ
  dysfunction syndrome
  (MODS)
Pericardiocentesis
Perineal
Pneumothorax
Pulse oximeter
Regional nerve block
Reperfusion injury

KEY TERMS—cont'd

Rumen tympany
Rumenostomy
Sepsis
Stridor
Syncope
Systemic inflammatory
  response syndrome
  (SIRS)
Tachycardia
Tachypnea
Thoracocentesis
Thromboembolism
Toxin
Tracheostomy
Tracheotomy
Transfaunation
Triage
Tube cystostomy
Tympany
Urethral process
Urethrostomy
Urolithiasis
Uterine prolapse
Uterine torsion
Ventricular premature
  complexes
Ventricular tachycardia

Abdominal Radiography, *948*
Specific Conditions, *948*
Abdominal Exploration, *948*
Respiratory Tract, *949*
General Physical Examination, *949*
Thoracic Ultrasound, *950*
Radiography, *950*
Upper and Lower Airway Endoscopy, *950*
Thoracocentesis, *950*
Transtracheal Wash, *951*
Oxygen Administration, *951*
Tracheotomy, *952*
Musculoskeletal System, *953*
Fractures, *954*
Soft Tissue Injury, *955*

EMERGENCY AND CRITICAL CARE
  NURSING: FOOD ANIMAL, *957*
Patient Restraint and Safety, *957*
**Considerations for Food-Producing
  Animals,** *957*
Gastrointestinal System, *958*
General Physical Examination, *958*
Emergency Intervention, *958*
Specific GI Conditions, *959*
Emergencies Involving the Rumen, *959*

Rumen Fluid Analysis and
  Transfaunation, *960*
Respiratory System, *961*
Respiratory Distress, *961*
Choanal Atresia, *962*
Tracheostomy, *962*
Musculoskeletal Injuries, *962*
Orthopedic Emergencies and Downer
  Animals, *962*
Fractures and Joint Luxations, *962*
Down Animals, *963*
Dog/Wild Animal Attacks, *963*
**Dystocia and Obstetrical
  Emergencies,** *964*
Dystocia Box and Equipment, *964*
Examination, *965*
Epidural Anesthesia, *965*
Vaginal Delivery, *965*
Cesarean Section, *966*
Uterine Torsion, *966*
Small Ruminant Dystocias, *966*
Uterine Prolapse, *966*
Toxic Metritis and Toxic Mastitis, *967*
Urolithiasis in Small Ruminants, *967*
History and Physical Examination, *967*
Treatment, *967*

LEARNING OBJECTIVES

When you have completed this chapter, you will be able to:

1. Pronounce, define, and spell all Key Terms in this chapter.
2. Triage a patient over the phone and upon arrival at the veterinary hospital.
3. Do the following regarding emergency and critical care assessment, initial diagnostics, and first aid:
   - Assess hydration and recognize hypovolemia in critical care patients.
   - Identify the diagnostic tests most commonly used in emergency and critical care settings.
   - Explain the principles of basic first aid.
   - Identify the ideal location for an emergency care station and/or resuscitation area, and explain how to set up and stock a crash cart.
4. Compare and contrast the different types of shock, explain how each is treated, and identify and explain advanced emergency techniques most commonly performed on small animals.
5. Discuss disorders of the respiratory system seen in critically ill small animal patients.
6. Do the following regarding cardiopulmonary cerebral resuscitation:
   - List the common causes of cardiopulmonary arrest, and explain the principles of cardiopulmonary cerebral resuscitation (CPCR).
   - Describe the principles of basic and advanced life support in small animals and care of the post-arrest patient.
7. Describe methods used to monitor critically ill patients and the principles of effective patient monitoring.
8. Identify key aspects of recumbent patient care.
9. List common small animal toxicities and emergencies, and discuss appropriate patient stabilization and treatment.

10. Do the following regarding canine and feline electrocardiography:
    - List the indications for and discuss the principles of electrocardiography.
    - Explain the processes used to acquire, analyze, and interpret an electrocardiogram.
    - Identify and explain the significance of common cardiac arrhythmias.
11. Describe initial management, assessment, diagnostic, and treatment procedures for common equine emergencies.
12. Describe initial management, assessment, diagnostic, and treatment procedures for common food animal emergencies.

INTRODUCTION

As the field of veterinary medicine continues to evolve, so does the important role of veterinary technicians in the field of Emergency and Critical Care. Veterinary technicians are often the first medical professionals to evaluate patients. They provide hands-on care and monitoring, administer medications, and provide appropriate nursing care. Organizations such as the American College of Veterinary Emergency and Critical Care (ACVECC) offer certification for veterinarians and technicians who complete additional training and pass an examination covering topics crucial to providing outstanding patient care in this specialty.

This chapter reviews many of the topics that a well-educated critical care technician must understand to provide exemplary care to critically ill or injured patients. The art of telephone triage is often where the technician's job begins, in helping the owner determine whether a condition is truly an emergency warranting immediate treatment. Once complete, telephone triage should lead to an emergency visit, a routinely scheduled visit, or a follow-up phone call. Triage and initial treatment once the patient arrives at the veterinary hospital (or as is often the case with large animals, once the veterinarian arrives at the farm) are discussed.

Basic trauma stabilization, patient assessment and monitoring, and care of the critical patient are also important aspects of the critical care technician's responsibility. Discussion includes how to approach common emergencies in dogs, cats, horses, and food animals, as well as proper techniques for performing **abdominocentesis, thoracocentesis,** and placement of thorocostomy and **tracheostomy** tubes. Treatment for acute **toxin** ingestion is described. Use of the electrocardiograph (ECG) for detection and treatment of common **arrhythmias** is discussed as well.

Completion of this chapter will leave the reader with a solid basis for additional study of emergency and critical care nursing, the capability for recognizing situations that require immediate intervention, and the tools necessary to care for and monitor critical cases.

Emergency and Critical Care Nursing: Small Animal

TRIAGE

The term **triage** is derived from the French word *trier*, meaning "to sort." The modern practice of triage was developed on the French battlefields of World War I. There it served to funnel resources to those who might be saved with intervention while not using precious time and limited supplies of bandages on those who would either survive without intervention or die regardless of the efforts or resources used for treatment. In veterinary medicine, the triage practices used in human military and civilian settings have been tailored to meet our unique needs.

TELEPHONE TRIAGE

Frequently, the first contact that veterinary professionals have with clients whose animals are traumatically injured, exposed to a toxin, or critically ill is via the telephone. Thus it is crucially important that the veterinary technician is able to quickly differentiate patients with injuries and illnesses that are life threatening and may require immediate intervention by the owner and transport to the nearest veterinary clinic, patients that should be seen as soon as possible, and patients that can wait until the caller's family veterinarian is next available. An established system for asking pertinent questions can aid the technician in determining how to advise clients over the phone and ensure that important information is obtained.

Initially, the person answering the phone should obtain a name and phone number, so the caller can be contacted if the call is disconnected. Next, the veterinary technician should determine whether the animal is in respiratory distress or is experiencing life-threatening bleeding. If either of these situations is evident, the caller should be referred to the closest veterinary facility for immediate attention. Other situations that may require immediate care include, but are not limited to, changes in mucous membrane color, acute changes in neurologic status, and potential heat or cold exposure.

> **TECHNICIAN NOTE** Owners call to speak with veterinary professionals because they are worried about their pet. Every call is worthy of your full attention, and callers should know that the veterinary staff is always willing to see their pet.

When appropriate, provide first aid advice. For instance, an owner can be instructed to place a clean dressing over an open wound in preparation for transport to the clinic. If the pet has consumed a noncorrosive toxin, the owner can be instructed to administer hydrogen peroxide (1 teaspoon per 10 lb of body weight) as a single dose to induce vomiting, but only if the pet is awake and is able to swallow. If the pet

has ingested a caustic or corrosive substance (e.g., drain cleaner, ammonia, quaternary ammonium cleaners), never recommend that vomiting be induced because this could worsen esophageal damage. It is important to remind clients to bring any packaging material, vomitus, or remaining toxin with them, if possible, for identification at the clinic. Although it is important to provide and obtain time-sensitive information over the phone, do not delay transport of an animal that is critically ill, injured, or exposed to a toxin just to obtain routine historical information (e.g., monthly deworming program) because this could worsen the outcome.

IN-HOSPITAL TRIAGE

The initial in-hospital triage functions to sort patients into three groups: those needing immediate care or stabilization, those that need to be taken to the treatment area for other reasons (bleeding, vomiting, diarrhea, potential contagion, etc.), and those who can wait with their owner until registration is complete or their scheduled appointment time arrives. One special circumstance is that of cats, because they typically do better if immediately taken to a secluded, dedicated waiting or holding area, even if they do not require immediate treatment. The initial triage should include a *brief* history, a quick physical examination, and targeted discussion with the owners about resuscitation status and initial treatment if necessary.

> **TECHNICIAN NOTE** Animals assessed as unstable, potentially infectious, or disturbing to other clients because of the nature of their illness should be immediately taken to the clinic's treatment or holding area.

The initial triage examination is a short (generally less than 1 to 2 minutes), systematic evaluation of essential organ systems (respiratory, cardiovascular, and neurologic). Although the examination for each essential system is detailed individually, it is important to recognize that these assessments occur simultaneously, and identification of a life-threatening change in any system requires immediate treatment. The remainder of the initial examination is completed once the life-threatening problem has been addressed. Once the stability of these systems has been assessed and a brief abdominal palpation performed, a more thorough secondary examination should be conducted to identify other, non–life-threatening problems. This secondary examination is often conducted once the patient is fully registered, and a more detailed history has been obtained.

Respiratory

As you approach the patient, take note of its respiratory rate, effort, and pattern. An increased respiratory rate (**tachypnea**) may reflect decreased oxygen in the blood (*hypoxemia*), thoracic trauma, or shock, or may be related to a nonrespiratory source such as pain, stress, increased body temperature, traumatic brain injury, or metabolic **acidosis**.

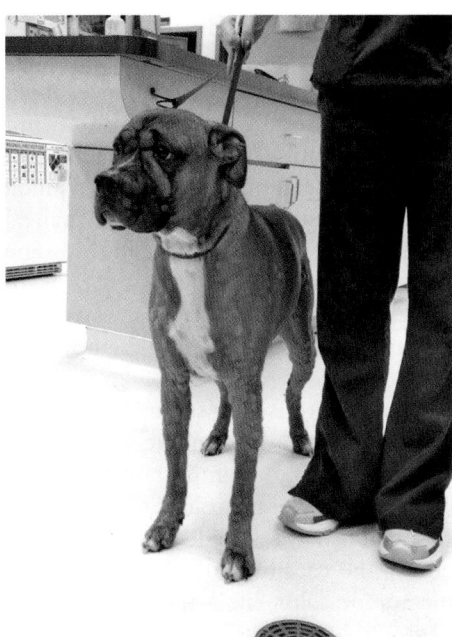

FIGURE 25-1 A cutaneous hypersensitivity reaction. This dog has diffuse urticaria (hives) visible as numerous pink plaques on the limbs, chest, and face. Edema of the muzzle and periorbital area is evident. (Courtesy Dr. Jessica Hamilton.)

A decreased respiratory rate *(bradypnea)* is most commonly associated with elevated intracranial pressure secondary to swelling of the brain, as can occur with traumatic brain injury. The effort involved in breathing may provide clues as to the origin of the problem. For instance, inspiratory dyspnea results in long, slow inspirations with short exhalations and can indicate an extrathoracic airway obstruction such as laryngeal paralysis, or swelling associated with an acute hypersensitivity reaction (Figure 25-1). In contrast, expiratory dyspnea with increased abdominal effort on expiration often develops if an intrathoracic airway obstruction, such as a mass compressing the airway or an inhaled foreign body, is present. The term *labored breathing* is often used to describe breathing that is prolonged and deep. This is seen early often in diseases involving the lung tissue or pleural space. Fast, short, and shallow breaths are the hallmark of a restrictive breathing pattern and reflect impaired ability to expand the lungs. Restrictive breathing is often seen with rib fractures, with pleural space disease (pleural effusion or tumors), or late in diseases of the lung tissue. *Orthopnea* is a term used to describe the condition of maintaining a specific posture to ease breathing. This occurs when dyspnea is so severe that the patient is "air hungry" and does everything it can to keep the airway open. Typically, orthopneic veterinary patients will extend their neck and stand or crouch with their elbows slightly away from their sides (Figure 25-2), and will become extremely distressed and combative or aggressive when placed in any other position.

In evaluation of the patient's respiratory pattern, specific changes indicate the need for immediate intervention. An apneustic pattern is characterized by deep inhalation with an

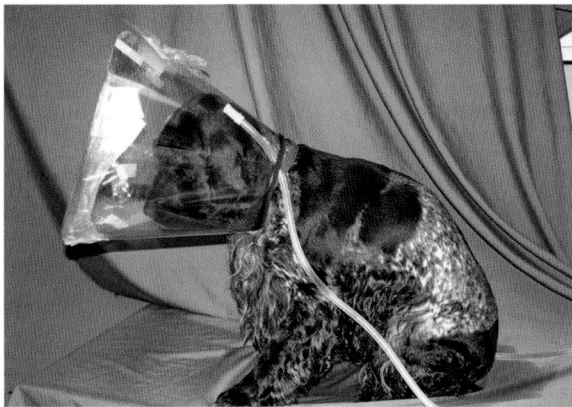

FIGURE 25-2 This dog is sitting in an orthopneic posture, with neck extended, elbows abducted, and hunched posture.

abnormally long pause before exhalation. This typically indicates damage to the pons or upper medulla and can be associated with traumatic brain injury. The term *Cheyne-Stokes breathing* refers to a pattern of alternating tachypnea and bradypnea that occurs when carbon dioxide regulation of respiration is interrupted. It often indicates increased intracranial pressure and occurs as pressure elevates enough to place the patient at risk for herniation. A slow, deep, regular respiratory pattern, called *Kussmaul breathing*, typically indicates respiratory compensation for a metabolic acidosis, such as diabetic ketoacidosis. Paradoxical chest excursion occurs when a segment of the thoracic wall, either soft tissue alone or an unattached section of ribs (a flail segment), moves in the opposite direction in relation to the rest of the chest wall during respiration. This results from changes in intrathoracic pressure and indicates severe trauma to the chest. When paradoxical abdominal breathing is noted, meaning that the abdomen moves inward during inspiration rather than outward as is normal, it is likely that the diaphragm is paralyzed, and the animal may need immediate intervention to control its breathing.

> **TECHNICIAN NOTE** If in doubt about a patient's respiratory status, *always* start supplemental oxygen until further assessment can be completed.

The next part of assessing the respiratory system is the hands-on examination. First, quickly check the mucous membrane color. Blue is bad, but pink is not necessarily good! Any patient whose mucous membranes are blue, purple, or dusky should be immediately taken to the treatment area and provided supplemental oxygen. Similarly, patients with brick red, brown, or injected (mottled pink, purple, or red) mucous membranes warrant a closer look because these colors could indicate situations such as carbon monoxide poisoning, heat stroke, or **sepsis**, which require immediate intervention. Icteric (yellow) mucous membranes indicate high levels of bilirubin. Patients that are icteric may wait if they are otherwise stable. White mucous membranes, although striking, may or may not mean that a patient needs immediate intervention. If mucous membranes are white as a result of anemia that is long-standing, this is less of a concern than if lack of color is related to vasoconstriction during compensated shock.

The final component of the respiratory section of the initial triage examination is thoracic auscultation. Decreased or dull lung sounds can indicate a diaphragmatic hernia, severe pulmonary contusions, **pneumothorax** (if decreased dorsally), or pleural effusion (if decreased ventrally). Increased or harsh bronchovesicular sounds or crackles can indicate pulmonary edema or contusions. **Borborygmi** in the thorax might indicate a diaphragmatic hernia, but it can also be referred from the abdomen. Any absence of lung sounds warrants further investigation in the treatment area.

Cardiovascular

The initial triage examination of the cardiovascular system involves assessment of mentation, heart rate and rhythm, pulse quality, **capillary refill time** (CRT), extremity temperature, and mucous membrane color. Mentation is an important component of the cardiovascular examination because significantly decreased mentation can indicate a shock state, in which the brain is not getting enough blood to maintain normal function. This is sometimes difficult to differentiate from traumatic brain injury or a primary neurologic disorder. To determine the underlying cause, the shock state must be corrected. If the mentation remains altered after the patient is no longer in a shock state, other causes should be pursued.

Heart rate and rhythm may be assessed by digital palpation of the pulse, or through thoracic auscultation using a stethoscope. An abnormally fast heart rate, called **tachycardia**, can indicate compensation for a shock state, pain, fear, anxiety, or any combination of those factors. An inappropriately slow heart rate, termed *bradycardia*, can indicate a life-threatening arrhythmia or, in animals with urethral obstruction, an extremely elevated potassium level. It is important to note that cats in a shock state are often bradycardic, rather than tachycardic. If an arrhythmia is detected, the animal should be taken to the treatment area for an **electrocardiogram** (ECG) to determine the cause of the arrhythmia. Interpretation of ECGs is discussed later in the chapter.

> **TECHNICIAN NOTE** Cats in a shock state often present with bradycardia, rather than with tachycardia (as is seen in dogs).

Pulse quality can provide a great deal of information about the patient's cardiovascular state. Pulse pressure is the difference between systolic and diastolic pressures, and pulse quality is a description of how quickly pulse pressure changes, and how long each pulse lasts. A normal pulse has moderate pulse pressure, a gradual rise and fall, occurs regularly, and is called strong and synchronous. A weak or thready pulse is one in which the pulse pressure is lower than normal and

typically occurs with tachycardia. It can indicate hypotension or decompensated shock. A pulse that is "snappy" has a very large pulse pressure with an extremely rapid rise and fall. This type of pulse often occurs with anemia or with severe aortic regurgitation. If you are unable to palpate the dorsal metatarsal arterial pulse in a dog, this indicates that the mean arterial pressure is likely to be less than 80 mm Hg. If you cannot palpate a femoral pulse in the dog or the cat, this means that the mean arterial pressure is likely less than 60 mm Hg. Both of these situations warrant immediate intervention and, in most cases, fluid therapy.

Evaluation of mucous membrane color is another important part of the cardiovascular system assessment. Possible causes of abnormal mucous membrane color were discussed in the respiratory section. It is important to recognize certain abnormal mucous membrane colors, such as red or injected, because these colors may reflect derangements in the respiratory system or the cardiovascular system. While assessing mucous membrane color, check the CRT. A normal CRT is 1 to 2 seconds. Prolonged CRT may indicate that the patient needs fluid resuscitation or other interventions. A shortened CRT is most commonly associated with the hyperdynamic stage of sepsis, and may not reflect increased perfusion to the tissues.

Neurologic

The focus of the initial triage neurologic examination is to determine whether evidence of traumatic brain injury (TBI) is present. Findings that may support TBI include abrupt changes in mentation; changes in pupil size, symmetry, and responsiveness; altered gait or posture; and altered proprioception or evidence of trauma to the head, such as cuts, scrapes, jaw fractures, proptosis (the globe of the eye protruding from the socket), or epistaxis (nosebleed). Any of these findings should trigger immediate intervention or a more thorough neurologic evaluation.

Mentation can be categorized as normal, dull, obtunded, stuporous, or comatose. A normal animal is alert and interactive with its environment. A dull or depressed animal is interactive with its environment, but does not seem bright and eager to interact. An obtunded animal reacts appropriately to stimuli, but at a much lower level or slower pace than a normal animal. A stuporous animal is completely disconnected from the environment and reacts only to noxious stimuli such as needle sticks for catheter placement. A comatose animal is completely disconnected from the environment and does not react to any stimuli at all. These changes in mentation can be due to neurologic changes such as TBI, but they also can occur with shock or major cardiovascular disturbance.

> **TECHNICIAN NOTE** Elevated carbon dioxide levels can be extremely bad for a patient with increased intracranial pressure and traumatic brain injury (TBI). Reassess breathing frequently with any patient who is experiencing symptoms of TBI.

Evaluating the pupils can provide insight into the extent and location of brain injury in traumatized or acutely ill patients. Unresponsive big (mydriatic) pupils are called "fixed and dilated." This is often very bad because it can indicate an irreversible mid-brain lesion. Caution should be used when this finding is interpreted in very frightened animals, particularly cats, because a high sympathetic drive can dilate the pupils, making them appear nonresponsive to light. Taking the mentation into consideration can be helpful in this situation. For instance, if a cat is laterally recumbent and is nonresponsive, with mydriatic unresponsive pupils, after being hit by a car, TBI is the likely cause. However, if a cat presents for vomiting and has a dull mentation but is interacting appropriately and has mydriatic unresponsive pupils, this is likely due to increased sympathetic output. Unresponsive mid-range pupils are suggestive of a lesion in the medulla and support brain injury. Anisocoria (one big pupil and one little pupil) may indicate an acute cerebral injury, such as blood clot, hemorrhage, or brain injury. Other possible causes of anisocoria are conditions such as Horner's syndrome, in which the nerves controlling the pupil are affected but the brain is not injured. Very rarely, anisocoria is normal for an animal and may not reflect any disease process.

Once overall mentation and pupils have been evaluated, the animal's posture should be more closely evaluated. Three classic postures are related to neurologic injury: decerebrate posture, decerebellate posture, and Schiff-Sherrington posture. Decerebrate posture indicates a complete disconnect between the forebrain and the brainstem. It is characterized by extreme rigidity of all four legs and may involve *opisthotonus* (arching of the neck and back). It is accompanied by a stuporous to comatose mentation and carries a grave prognosis. Decerebellate posture signifies severe injury to the cerebellum. Typically, animals present with rigid forelimbs and flexed hindlimbs, although rigidity may be noted in all four limbs. The main difference between this and decerebrate posture is that animals will have normal mentation. Finally, the Schiff-Sherrington posture can look like decerebrate or decerebellate posture. Typically, the forelimbs are rigid and the hindlimbs are flaccid when the animal is on its side. However, the animal has a normal mentation and often can ambulate when picked up and placed on its feet. The Schiff-Sherrington posture is associated with a chronic T3-L3 spinal cord lesion.

Completing the Initial Triage Examination

Once the respiratory, cardiovascular, and neurologic systems have been initially assessed, a quick abdominal palpation should be conducted to check for pain, **tympany**, or a fluid wave. Individual organs are not assessed during the initial triage examination. If significant pain is detected, this may indicate a problem that requires surgery or a disease such as pancreatitis. Animals with severe abdominal pain often adopt a posture with an arched back and hind legs moved backward (Figure 25-3); others repeatedly stretch into a "praying" posture, with the forelimbs down and stretched in

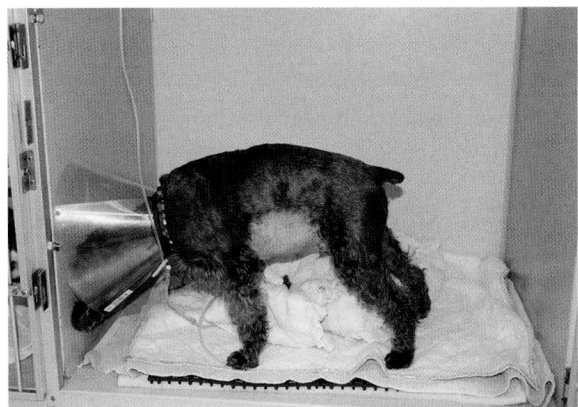

FIGURE 25-3 This dog displays the classic abdominal pain posture: arched back, weight shifted forward, and hind legs shifted backward.

front of them, while the hindlimbs remain standing in a normal position. Tympany raises concern that an intestinal structure is gas-filled, such as the stomach in a gastric dilatation-volvulus, or a loop of small intestine with complete obstruction. A fluid wave could indicate hemorrhage from an internal organ, fluid buildup from inflammation or heart failure, or another cause of ascites.

> **TECHNICIAN NOTE** Appropriate pain control is always important when a critically ill or injured patient is treated.

ASSESSMENT OF HYDRATION AND HYPOVOLEMIA

Part of the initial assessment of every patient presented on an emergency basis is hydration status. Dehydration is a decrease in the water component of blood. Common causes of dehydration in veterinary patients include increased loss of water through vomiting, diarrhea, excessive panting, or polyuria. Decreased water intake also occurs with many disease processes, as well as lack of access to water and other environmental factors. Mild dehydration is clinically undetectable. Most animals are at least 5% dehydrated when clinical signs are noted. Unfortunately, no precise ways are available to quantify dehydration, although several subjective measures may be used (Box 25-1).

The earliest clinical signs of dehydration include tacky or dry mucous membranes. This is most easily assessed in the oral cavity and can be difficult to interpret in animals that are panting excessively or are hypersalivating from nausea or other causes. Capillary refill time is normal until severe dehydration leading to shock develops. As dehydration progresses, lack of skin turgor is noted by tenting the skin of the animal. In a hydrated pet, the skin will return to its original position after it is released. Dehydrated animals will have a persistent skin tent. This test can be misleading in certain animals, however. Puppies and certain dog breeds naturally have excessively pliant, loose skin. They can be severely

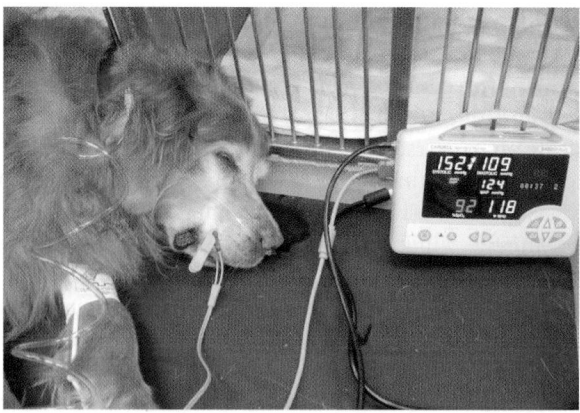

FIGURE 25-4 A pulse oximeter provides a convenient and reliable means of monitoring oxygenation in critical or anesthetized animals. Note the pulse rate (118 bpm) and the blood oxygen saturation (SpO$_2$) (92%) reported on the monitor.

dehydrated and still appear to have fairly normal skin turgor. Conversely, geriatric animals, especially cats, tend to be thinner and have naturally decreased skin turgor. These animals can have a prolonged skin tent despite normal hydration status. In advanced stages of dehydration, the eyes become sunken and appear dry. Mental status is also affected by dehydration. With moderate to severe dehydration, agitation and restlessness can be seen. As dehydration progresses, the animal becomes apathetic and eventually comatose. Body weight can be used to provide an objective measure of dehydration. If a normal weight for the animal is known, dehydration can be estimated by subtracting the current weight from the normal weight. For example, if a dog that normally weighs 25 kg is presented to the hospital for severe vomiting, and its current weight is 23.75 kg, the dog would be estimated to be about 5% dehydrated, based on an acute loss of 5% of its body weight.

Common laboratory abnormalities in dehydrated animals include hemoconcentration, **azotemia**, hypernatremia, and elevated albumin. If azotemia is noted, urine specific gravity should be checked. If urine specific gravity is greater than 1.050, azotemia can be considered prerenal (i.e., due to decreased renal blood flow) and secondary to dehydration in most cases. Isosthenuria (urine specific gravity, 1.012 to 1.018 in the dog, 1.012 to 1.022 in the cat) in the face of dehydration and azotemia suggests that renal disease is present.

During patient assessment, it is important to differentiate a dehydrated animal from a hypovolemic animal. **Hypovolemia** is loss of blood volume and commonly occurs with shock, trauma, hemorrhage, or profuse vomiting and diarrhea. Animals with hypovolemia tend to present with tachycardia and prolonged CRT. Because hypovolemia is an acute process, skin turgor can be normal. In severe cases, hypovolemic shock can be recognized by tachycardia, weak pulses, hypotension, and prolonged CRT. Hypovolemic shock is a true emergency that should be addressed immediately.

TECHNICIAN NOTE   Differentiating dehydration from hypovolemia is very important. Hypovolemic shock is a true emergency and should be addressed immediately.

Treatments for hypovolemia are aimed at restoring the blood volume quickly and include IV catheterization, administration of IV fluids, and possibly blood transfusion for hemorrhaging patients. Identification of the source of the hypovolemia is important. Many times, a history of trauma or illness is reported, but sometimes additional tests such as radiography or ultrasonography are needed to identify the cause. In some cases, emergency surgery is required to address a source of bleeding. Intensive monitoring and nursing care are imperative for a successful outcome in patients with hypovolemia.

In contrast, treatment for dehydration involves replacement of the fluid deficit over several hours. If the patient is severely hypernatremic, rehydration should be even more gradual, sometimes over as long as 48 to 72 hours, because rapid rehydration of a hypernatremic patient can lead to cerebral edema and neurologic signs. During rehydration, patients should be monitored for ongoing sources of fluid loss such as vomiting, diarrhea, or polyuria, and their fluid therapy plans adjusted accordingly (see Chapter 24).

INITIAL DIAGNOSTICS

The initial treatment area should be equipped to perform limited, high-yield diagnostics. These diagnostics are performed after the initial triage examination to help determine the overall stability of the patient. The most commonly used initial diagnostics include packed cell volume (PCV), total protein (TP), blood glucose, venous or arterial blood gas analysis, blood pressure, pulse oximetry (Figure 25-4), ECG, and focused assessment with sonography in trauma (FAST) (ultrasound performed to determine whether fluid or air is present in the abdomen or thorax). PCV and TP provide information about the red blood cell and protein content of the blood. An animal with high PCV and TP may be very dehydrated, and an animal with low PCV may be experiencing red blood cell (RBC) loss or destruction. The color of the serum can also lend clues to the underlying disease process. Icteric or hemolytic serum could indicate extravascular or intravascular hemolysis.

Blood gas analysis provides a great deal of information about the acid-base and respiratory status of the patient. The normal blood pH for veterinary patients is 7.4. If the pH is low, this indicates a buildup of acid in the system, as occurs in diabetic ketoacidosis. If the pH is high, this indicates excess base or loss of acid, as occurs with severe vomiting. An elevated carbon dioxide (CO_2) level indicates an upper airway obstruction such as laryngeal paralysis or hypoventilation, as can occur with TBI, high spinal cord injury, and use of certain medications, such as opioids. A decreased CO_2 level indicates hyperventilation, which can be related to **hypoxemia**, pain, stress, anxiety, or hyperthermia, or can occur as compensation for a metabolic acidosis. The partial pressure of oxygen in arterial blood (PaO_2) can be used to assess pulmonary function. When breathing room air at sea level, a normal patient will have a PaO_2 between 80 and 100 mm Hg. It is a matter of concern when a patient's PaO_2 falls below 60 mm Hg. If a patient cannot maintain a PaO_2 above 60 mm Hg with supplemental oxygen, mechanical ventilation may be required. Many blood gas analyzers also provide a blood lactate level. A lactate level that is above 2.0 mg/dl can indicate poor perfusion and should lead to further evaluation of the patient's fluid status.

The ability to monitor blood pressure is crucial for proper stabilization and management of a critically ill animal. The most common methods are indirect Doppler measurement, oscillometric measurement, and direct arterial catheterization. Normal arterial blood pressure values for dogs and cats are in the range of 80 to 140 mm Hg (systolic), 50 to 80 mm Hg (diastolic), and 60 to 100 mm Hg (mean). Reasonable initial reference points for blood pressure comparison vary by species and breed (in dogs). Most dogs should have an arterial blood pressure of 140/80 mm Hg with a mean pressure of 100 mm Hg. Sighthounds may normally have a slightly higher blood pressure than other breeds. Cats typically have an arterial blood pressure of 130/80 mm Hg with a mean of 100 mm Hg. Hypertension should be suspected if blood pressure readings are consistently above 150/95 mm Hg. Consistency of measurement technique, cuff size, and location are important when trends in blood pressure changes are identified.

Pulse oximetry can be a key part of determining a patient's overall stability. The **pulse oximeter** uses a red light to determine the percent saturation of red blood cells detected by the light source. Normal animals should have a pulse oximetry reading between 97% and 100%. Readings lower than 92% are matters of extreme concern and should be addressed immediately with supplemental oxygen. It is important to remember that a pulse oximeter requires pulsatile blood flow to function, so if the patient's perfusion is poor, or if the mucous membranes are highly pigmented, you might not be able to obtain a reading. Hemoglobin bound to carbon monoxide registers as saturated on pulse oximetry, so pulse oximeters are not reliable in cases of smoke inhalation.

TECHNICIAN NOTE The initial treatment area should be equipped for packed cell volume (PCV)/total protein (TP), blood glucose, blood pressure, pulse oximetry, and electrocardiographic (ECG) monitoring. Blood gas analysis and focused assessment with sonography in trauma (FAST) ultrasound capabilities are also helpful.

An ECG is useful for monitoring the stability of a patient and response to treatment. Specific ECG rhythms and appropriate treatments are discussed later in this chapter. The FAST ultrasound scan is used to quickly assess body cavities for the presence of fluid. Four sites in the abdomen (the subxiphoid area, around each kidney, and at the bladder) are imaged for an abdominal FAST; the heart is imaged from both sides, and each half of the thorax is imaged dorsally and ventrally during a thoracic FAST examination. If any fluid or free air is detected, a sample can be obtained by thoracocentesis or abdominocentesis.

BASIC FIRST AID

Once the patient has been assessed for primary life-threatening conditions, lifesaving measures have been taken, and initial diagnostics have been conducted, the focus moves to the secondary survey and application of basic first aid. During this phase of patient care, a more detailed physical examination is conducted, and non–life-threatening problems are addressed. The spine should be gently palpated. Any step defects or points of tenderness may indicate a spinal problem such as luxation, fracture, or intervertebral disc herniation. Diffuse spinal pain may indicate problems such as meningitis. A complete neurologic examination can help the clinician determine whether a concurrent neurologic deficit is present, requiring further treatment and evaluation.

Examine the head for additional signs of trauma not detected on the initial examination. Evaluate the eyes for corneal ulceration, lacerations, or developing anisocoria. It is important to recheck the pupils during the secondary examination because increased intracranial pressure can develop quickly in both traumatically injured and critically ill patients. Perform a full cranial nerve examination and look in the oral cavity for broken teeth, bleeding, or swelling. Examine the ears for fluid and foreign material.

Wounds should be clipped, thoroughly cleaned, and flushed with sterile saline. After the area has been cleaned, appropriate bandages should be applied. Carefully palpate each limb for pain, swelling, lacerations, or malformations. A splint should be applied to stabilize any fracture or joint instability. Provide additional pain control and/or sedatives if necessary to properly clean wounds and apply bandages or splints. Throughout the initial stabilization, diagnostic, and secondary treatment phases, fluid therapy should be provided as discussed in Chapter 24.

EMERGENCY CARE STATION AND RESUSCITATION AREA

Patient treatment areas should be easily accessible (but out of the main traffic flow of the hospital), clean, and well stocked. Keeping equipment organized and clearly labeled allows new staff members to help in emergency situations in which additional hands may make the difference. Intravenous (IV) catheters, IV fluids, administration sets, and needles and syringes constitute some of the basic equipment that should be available in the emergency treatment area. An oxygen source, suction apparatus, and a crash cart should be placed in close proximity. It is important that functional clippers with working blades, surgical scrub, and tape to secure catheters are kept in the area. In addition, an easily readable **cardiopulmonary cerebrovascular resuscitation** (CPCR) flow chart can be prominently displayed.

CRASH CART

The place where emergency drugs are kept is colloquially termed the *crash cart*. Depending on the size and focus of a clinic, the crash cart may range from a tackle box to a full, rolling cart with attached defibrillator (Figure 25-5). The crash cart should contain emergency medications, needles, syringes, a laryngoscope, endotracheal tubes of various sizes, and an Ambu bag. Larger carts should also contain instrument packs to be used in emergency procedures such as a tracheostomy or open-chest cardiopulmonary cerebrovascular resuscitation.

> **TECHNICIAN NOTE** All items in the emergency crash cart should be inspected for proper function; expiration dates should be checked a minimum of once a week and immediately after any supplies are used. After inspection or use, the crash cart should be restocked.

Red rubber catheters of various sizes may have multiple uses in the treatment and resuscitation area. They may be used to suction airways or wounds, placed as nasotracheal catheters for oxygen administration, placed as urethral catheters, or used to administer medications through an endotracheal tube in a patient that is in cardiopulmonary arrest without the benefit of an IV catheter.

In situations where the upper airway is completely obstructed, disrupted, or otherwise inaccessible to orotracheal intubation, a large-bore IV catheter can be placed percutaneously into the trachea to allow administration of oxygen while the equipment needed for an emergency tracheostomy is prepared.

SHOCK AND THE SYSTEMIC INFLAMMATORY RESPONSE SYNDROME

Shock is a complex syndrome that results from altered blood flow or impaired delivery of oxygen to the tissues. This syndrome is characterized by varying degrees of cardiovascular collapse (despite its name, "shock" does not refer to electrocution). Shock results in a progressive imbalance between the tissue oxygen supply and demand. Left untreated, shock may lead to death or serious complications. Prompt recognition of shock and adequate treatment are crucial for patient survival. Early stages of shock are easily overlooked because animals have various compensatory mechanisms to preserve blood flow and oxygen delivery. Patients with early or compensated shock can be depressed or anxious, and they are often tachycardic and tachypneic. Pulse quality can be normal, decreased, or increased. As shock progresses, more severe alterations such as severe tachycardia, altered mental status, hypotension, pale mucous membranes, and weak pulses occur. Hyperglycemia is common during initial stages of shock but rapidly progresses to hypoglycemia if shock is

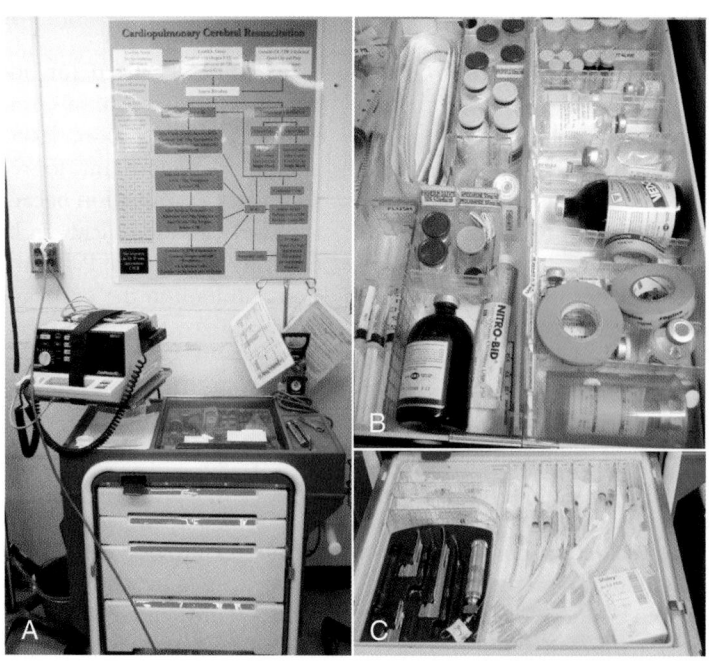

FIGURE 25-5 An effective "crash cart" is easily accessible and is spacious enough to contain an array of emergency supplies.

left untreated. The terminal stages of shock result in massive vasodilatation, hypotension, and cardiac arrest. Early recognition and intervention may prevent development of these signs of decompensated shock.

Shock can be caused by several underlying conditions; animals in shock can have different physical examination findings, depending on the cause. The type of shock most commonly seen in cats and dogs is *hypovolemic shock*. This condition occurs as the result of decreased circulating blood volume. Common predisposing events for hypovolemic shock include trauma, hemorrhage, and severe vomiting and diarrhea. Patients in hypovolemic shock may have delayed capillary refill time, weak pulses, pale mucous membranes, and altered mentation. Treatment for hypovolemic shock is aimed at restoring intravascular volume. Treatment with IV crystalloids, colloids, or hypertonic solutions may be indicated. In animals with severe blood loss, transfusions are often necessary to restore oxygen-carrying capacity. *Distributive shock* occurs from maldistribution of blood flow, from inappropriate vasodilatation, and from pooling of blood in the capillaries. This type of shock is seen in cases of anaphylaxis, heat stroke, and envenomation. Fluid therapy is essential in the treatment of distributive shock; oftentimes, vasopressors are needed to restore normal vascular tone. Weak or bounding pulses and pink mucous membranes are generally seen. *Obstructive shock* occurs when venous return to the heart is impaired. In veterinary medicine, this type of shock can occur with gastric dilatation-volvulus (GDV; when the distended stomach impairs venous return from the abdomen) or with pericardial tamponade (when increased intrapericardial pressure causes collapse of the right atrium). This type of shock is best treated by addressing the underlying cause, with trocarization or surgery for GDV, or **pericardiocentesis**. *Cardiogenic shock* occurs with impaired cardiac output secondary to problems with the heart itself. Common underlying causes include cardiomyopathy, valvular heart disease, and arrhythmias. Animals with cardiogenic shock have weak pulses, hypotension, and pale mucous membranes. Other signs of cardiac failure such as pulmonary edema or ascites are often present. Treatment relies on improving heart function with antiarrhythmics, positive inotropes, vasopressors, or even a pacemaker in certain cases. Diuretics are often needed to promote resolution of pulmonary edema.

Septic shock occurs after a severe infectious insult to the animal. In dogs and cats, common causes of septic shock are pneumonia, parvovirus, gastric or intestinal perforation, and infected bite wounds. Septic shock can also occur as a sequela to severe tissue damage, such as after heat stroke or pancreatitis. Translocation of bacteria from the gastrointestinal (GI) tract into the bloodstream and damaged organs can occur during any form of shock, and can be difficult to treat because altered blood flow may impair systemic antibiotic delivery to the damaged organ. The inflammatory response associated with sepsis causes increased vasodilatation, so septic animals initially present with bright red mucous membranes (Figure 25-6) and bounding pulses. Sometimes

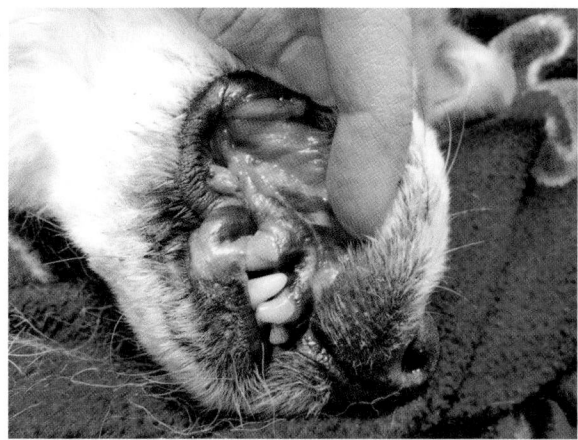

FIGURE 25-6 Hyperemic (injected) mucous membranes are seen in this dog suffering from sepsis secondary to pyometra.

BOX 25-2	Common Causes of the Systemic Inflammatory Response Syndrome

Trauma
Surgery
Shock
Cardiopulmonary arrest and cardiopulmonary cerebral resuscitation (CPCR)
Pancreatitis
Heat stroke
Envenomation
Immune-mediated disease
Neoplasia—solitary tumor or metastatic disease
Infection (sepsis)

generalized erythema occurs, and often fever is present. As septic shock progresses, hypotension worsens, and the patient becomes pale with weaker pulses. Therapy for septic shock involves treating the source of infection (medically and surgically if needed) and providing fluid therapy and broad-spectrum antibiotics.

> **TECHNICIAN NOTE** Animals that present with septic shock often have bounding pulses, bright red mucous membranes, and fever.

During shock, an inflammatory response develops, even if no infection is initially present. Normally, the body's inflammatory response is contained to discrete areas of infection or tissue damage. However, shock results in widespread tissue **hypoxia** and damage, and as a result, the inflammation can progress from a local to a systemic response (Box 25-2). This widespread inflammatory phenomenon is called the **systemic inflammatory response syndrome (SIRS)**. Sepsis is merely the presence of a source of active infection during SIRS. The SIRS response results in widespread vasodilatation (which leads to hypotension), tachycardia, tachypnea, fever, and sometimes marked increases or decreases in white blood cell count (Box 25-3).

During SIRS, inflammatory mediators are released into the circulation; this causes recruitment and activation of white blood cells and platelets. Activated white blood cells cause additional tissue damage and help spread the inflammatory response throughout the body. As the endothelial lining of blood vessels and organs becomes damaged, platelets are activated and the clotting cascade is initiated. Microscopic clot formation occludes capillaries, resulting in even greater impairment of blood flow to the organs and worsening of the inflammatory response. As platelets and clotting factors are consumed by this inappropriate clotting process, normal physiologic clotting mechanisms become impaired, and spontaneous bleeding can occur. This pattern of concurrent thrombosis and bleeding is referred to as **disseminated intravascular coagulation** (DIC) and is among the most serious complications of shock. Despite treatment, DIC is often fatal. Another important and devastating complication of shock and sepsis is the **multiple organ dysfunction syndrome** (MODS). As the SIRS response progresses and microvascular clotting takes place, enough organ damage can occur to result in organ failure. Without timely and aggressive intervention, MODS can lead to permanent organ failure and death. Organs most often affected by MODS include kidney, liver, lung, and heart. Treatment is focused on maintaining blood flow with fluid therapy and vasopressors if needed, antibiotic therapy, and often transfusions of blood and plasma or mechanical ventilation. The prognosis for SIRS that has progressed to DIC and MODS is poor.

REPERFUSION INJURY

Once shock has been identified, and appropriate steps have been taken to improve tissue blood flow and oxygenation, the focus shifts to minimizing the effects of the shock event on the body. During shock or cardiopulmonary arrest, cells become starved for oxygen and begin to use anaerobic respiration. This results in elevated levels of lactate and other cellular by-products in the tissues, which can promote tissue damage. As blood flow and oxygen delivery to the tissues are

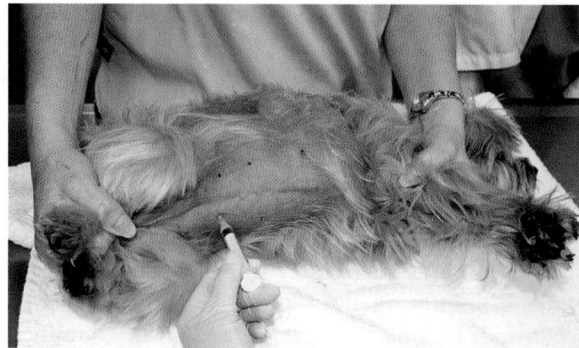

FIGURE 25-7 Abdominocentesis is performed by gently inserting a needle into the abdomen at four locations around the umbilicus until a sample of effusion is obtained.

restored (reperfusion), lactate and free radical molecules can be released into the systemic circulation. White blood cells are also drawn to the damaged tissues, where they become activated and release additional inflammatory mediators, contributing to free radical production. Risk for SIRS follows all episodes of shock and reperfusion.

> **TECHNICIAN NOTE** After treatment for shock, patients are still at risk for complications and organ failure caused by reperfusion injury.

ADVANCED EMERGENCY TECHNIQUES

ABDOMINOCENTESIS

Abdominocentesis is performed primarily as a diagnostic technique. Place the animal in left lateral recumbency. Clip and aseptically prepare the ventral abdomen around the umbilicus. While wearing sterile gloves, place a 20- or 22-gauge needle or an over-the-needle catheter in four quadrants around the umbilicus: cranially and to the left of, cranially and to the right of, caudally and to the left of, and caudally and to the right of the umbilicus (Figure 25-7). Gently and slowly advance the needle or catheter through the skin and abdominal musculature until you feel the tip "pop" into the peritoneal cavity. Then continue to slowly advance the needle or slide the catheter off the stylet. Each needle should be left in place while the others are being inserted. Sometimes fluid will drip freely from one or more of the needles. Should this happen, collect samples in red top and purple top tubes for analysis. Sometimes, a 3-ml or 6-ml syringe is needed to obtain fluid for analysis or culture. At other times, no fluid is obtained, and an ultrasound-guided abdominocentesis or a diagnostic peritoneal lavage should be considered. If the fluid obtained is hemorrhagic in appearance, observe it for clotting. If the fluid develops a clot, it is fresh blood rather than free fluid from within the abdomen.

THORACOCENTESIS

Thoracocentesis is a technique that is both diagnostic and therapeutic. Clip and aseptically prepare the lateral thorax on both sides of the patient. Gather the necessary supplies: a needle or IV catheter, collection tubing, a three-way stopcock, and a syringe that is of appropriate size for the patient. Locate the 7th to 9th intercostal spaces. Using sterile technique, insert the needle or catheter. If thoracocentesis is performed to address pneumothorax, the needle or catheter should be inserted at the level of the division between the top one-third and the bottom two-thirds of the thorax. If thoracocentesis is performed because of effusion, the needle or catheter should be inserted at the level of the division between the top two-thirds and the bottom one-third of the thorax. A local lidocaine block may be helpful if the patient is very agitated but typically is not necessary. Advance the needle or catheter near the cranial aspect of the rib and into the pleural space. Quickly attach the collection tubing and the three-way stopcock to the needle or catheter, and apply suction with the syringe. Some of the sample should be transferred into red top and purple top tubes for analysis and culture. Hemorrhagic samples should be monitored for clotting.

> **TECHNICIAN NOTE** Thoracic drain placement is warranted if thoracocentesis must be performed multiple times over a 12-hour period, if a tension pneumothorax is present, if continuous re-effusion is anticipated, or if a penetrating chest injury has occurred.

THORACIC DRAIN PLACEMENT

The following procedure should be performed when a thoracic drain is placed. Use strict aseptic technique to prevent bacterial contamination of the pleural cavity. Clip and aseptically prepare the skin on the affected side. Identify the 7th, 8th, or 9th intercostal space at the junction of the upper one-third and the lower two-thirds of the thorax. To create a subcutaneous tunnel to help prevent air leakage into the thorax, have an assistant gently pull the skin cranially and keep it in this position until the procedure is complete.

Estimate the proper length of tube by measuring from the desired insertion site cranially to the 2nd rib. Note the distance or mark the appropriate spot on the tube with a sterile marker. Infuse lidocaine into the subcutaneous tissue and the intercostal musculature down to the level of the pleural surface. Make a small stab incision as wide as the tube through the skin and subcutaneous tissue overlying the selected location. Occlude the free end of the tube throughout the placement procedure until a drainage system is connected.

Use the tip of the trocar to bluntly tunnel through the intercostal muscles. To minimize the risk of damaging vasculature and nerves, keep the trocar in contact with the cranial aspect of the rib behind the insertion point. Briefly halt mechanical ventilation when advancing the trocar through the pleural layer and into the pleural space to minimize the risk for iatrogenic trauma. Once the trocar is in the pleural space, slowly advance the tube off the trocar to the

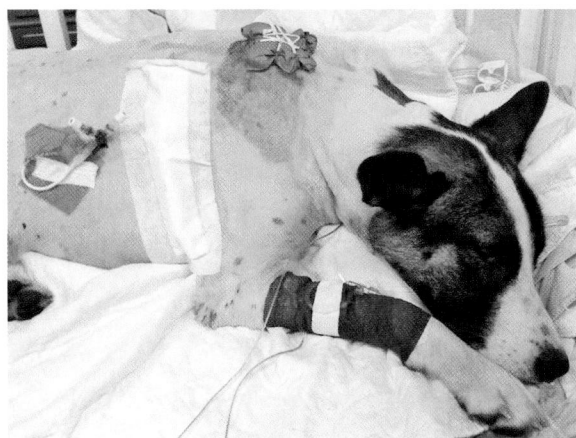

FIGURE 25-8 A thoracic drainage catheter (a small-bore chest tube) is visible in this patient after emergency thoracotomy to remove an arrow from its chest.

predetermined position. Carefully remove the trocar, leaving the tube in place.

Gently move the skin back into its normal anatomic position, creating a short subcutaneous tunnel around the tube. Suture the tube in place using a finger-trap suture pattern. Use a syringe to evacuate the pleural space until negative pressure is detected. Once negative pressure is detected, the thoracostomy tube can be sealed with a cap or attached to a continuous suction device (Figure 25-8).

TRACHEOSTOMY TUBE PLACEMENT

Emergency placement of a tracheostomy tube is indicated in life-threatening upper airway obstruction. The patient should be anesthetized, preferably with an endotracheal tube in place, and positioned in dorsal recumbency. Clip and aseptically prepare the ventral neck. Make an incision from the level of the cricoid cartilage caudally 2 to 5 cm. Gently separate the sternohyoid muscles until the trachea is exposed. Use blunt dissection to pass a hemostat dorsal to the trachea, taking care to avoid disrupting the recurrent laryngeal nerve. Two accepted methods may be used to insert a tracheostomy tube into the trachea. The first is to incise horizontally between the 3rd and 4th or the 4th and 5th trachea rings. Take care to avoid incising more than 50% of the diameter of the trachea. Place stay sutures around the rings above and below the incision. Be sure to label the stay sutures "top" and "bottom" to facilitate changing of the tube. The second technique is to incise vertically through two to four tracheal rings along the ventral midline. Stay sutures are placed on either side of the incision. Once in place, the tube should be secured around the neck using a tie (Figure 25-9) and cleaned as needed, but no less than twice a day.

RESPIRATORY SYSTEM SUPPORT AND OXYGEN THERAPY

Disorders of the respiratory system are common in critically ill animals. These patients can suffer from structural

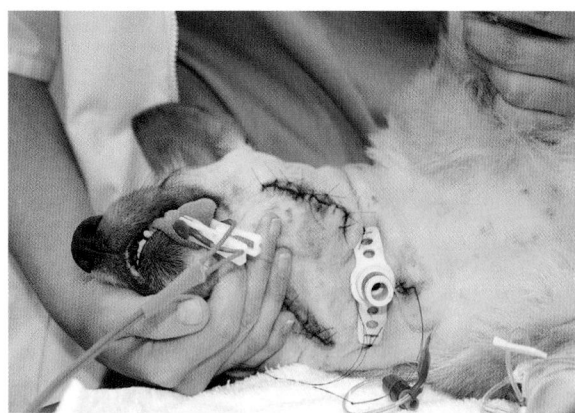

FIGURE 25-9 A properly placed tracheotomy tube allows this patient that is in respiratory distress to breathe until its upper airway obstruction can be addressed.

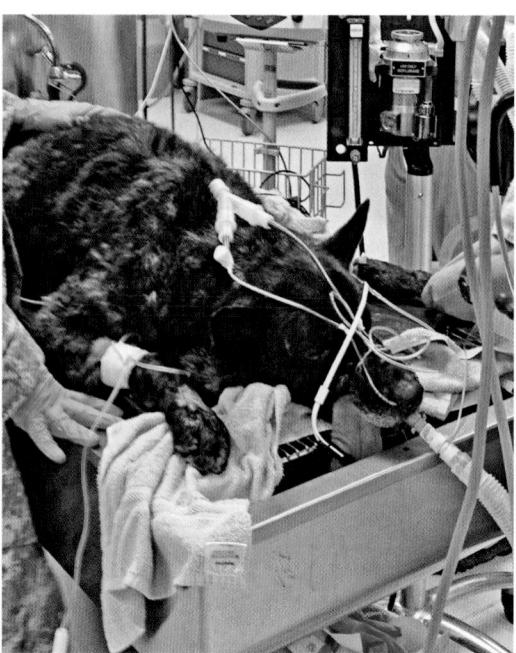

FIGURE 25-10 This Labrador Retriever is receiving supplemental oxygen through bilateral nasal catheters.

problems such as brachycephalic syndrome or collapsing trachea; problems with the lung tissue itself such as pneumonia, hemorrhage, edema, or cancer; or even extrapulmonary problems that lead to respiratory distress such as pleural effusion, pneumothorax, or metabolic disorders. Assessment of the patient's respiratory effort and breathing pattern can indicate which portion of the respiratory system is involved. Animals with obstructive upper airway disease (such as laryngeal paralysis, elongated soft palate, or tracheal foreign bodies) often take very deep, slow breaths. Referred upper airway noises or **stridor** can often be heard. Cats affected by feline asthma (obstructive lower airway disease) have a pronounced expiratory effort and wheezes on auscultation. Animals with pleural space disease such as pneumothorax or with lung disease often breathe rapidly and shallowly. Decreased pulmonary sounds are noted in animals with significant pleural space disease. Thoracic percussion can be used to help determine whether pleural effusion is present. Animals with pulmonary disease (edema, pneumonia, etc.) may have crackles on inhalation and exhalation.

> **TECHNICIAN NOTE** Observing the respiratory pattern and performing careful auscultation can provide clues to the underlying cause of dyspnea.

Mucous membrane color can also be an indicator of respiratory function. Normal animals have pink mucous membranes, whereas animals with poor respiratory function can have pale, gray, or cyanotic mucous membranes.

Animals with respiratory difficulty or distress (dyspnea) should be handled very carefully. These patients are highly stressed and are at risk for decompensation and cardiopulmonary arrest. Common procedures such as restraint and examination, IV catheter placement, and radiography can cause a dyspneic animal to develop cardiac arrest; these procedures should be avoided if possible until the patient is less distressed. Upon identification of a patient with respiratory difficulty, supplemental oxygen should be administered. Common ways of providing oxygen support to conscious

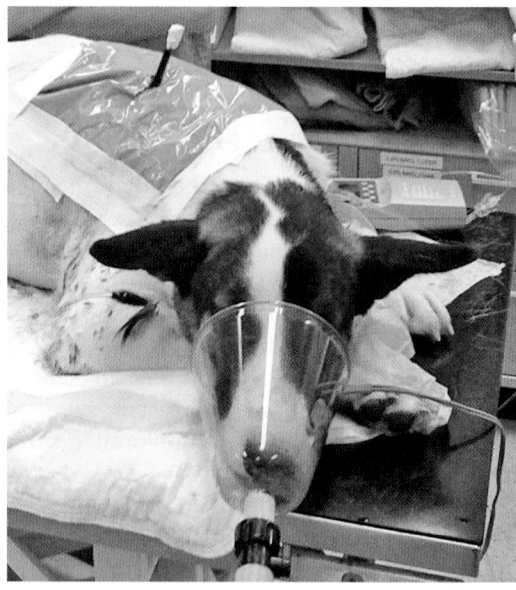

FIGURE 25-11 Administration of supplemental oxygen via face mask in a Beagle.

animals include nasal prongs or cannulas, flow-by, face mask, and oxygen cage or oxygen hood (Figures 25-10 through 25-12). Some animals become increasingly stressed with application of nasal oxygen or with restraint for oxygen delivery by mask; these animals may do better with an oxygen hood or an oxygen cage. Dyspneic animals can also benefit from sedation before handling or procedures. Sedation is used to relax the patient and relieve some of the distress the patient is experiencing. Careful monitoring is important when sedatives are given to distressed patients because certain drugs can interfere with respiration, and the patient

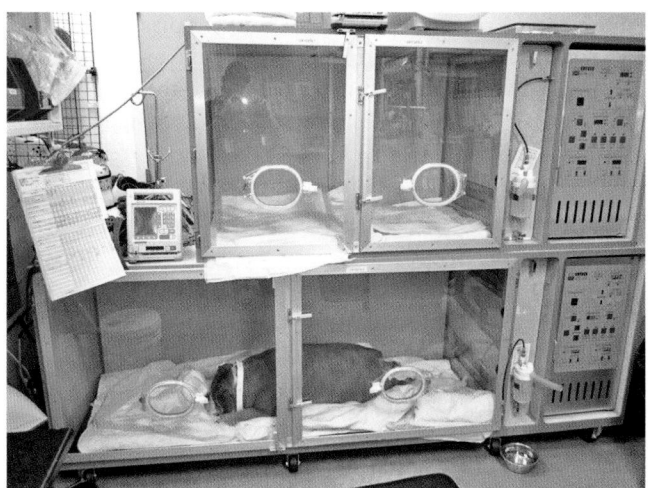

FIGURE 25-12 An oxygen cage can be a very effective means of delivering supplemental oxygen to selected patients.

may require intubation. If pleural effusion or pneumothorax is suspected on the basis of the physical examination, thoracocentesis is indicated to allow the lungs to inflate properly. The technique for thoracocentesis is described on page 916. It is important to remember that thoracocentesis is both a diagnostic and a therapeutic procedure because removal of pleural fluid or air helps relieve the patient's distress, and the fluid can be analyzed to determine the cause of the effusion. Performing thoracocentesis before thoracic radiographs are taken is helpful because pleural fluid causes the lungs to collapse, making radiographic identification of tumors and other lesions much more difficult. Lesions may become apparent on radiographs once the fluid is removed and the lungs are inflated. Some animals will need to return to the oxygen cage to relax in between procedures such as examination, catheter placement, and radiography.

> **TECHNICIAN NOTE** In severely dyspneic animals, handling should be minimized and stressful procedures such as radiographs should be postponed until the animal is more stable.

Pulse oximetry and arterial blood gas measurement can provide valuable information about a patient's respiratory status. The pulse oximeter probe emits light-emitting diode (LED) light at two different wavelengths, which is absorbed selectively by oxygenated and deoxygenated hemoglobin. Pulse oximeters come with a clip-like probe, which is designed to attach to a vascular, poorly haired area such as the tongue, lip, ear flap, or toe webbing. Some models come with a rectal probe and cover, which can be used in recumbent and anesthetized animals in place of the conventional probe. Pulse oximeters measure the percentage of hemoglobin that is saturated with oxygen in arterial blood. Because arterial flow is pulsatile, the pulse oximeter can be used to count pulse rate and should display a pulsating waveform. Normal oxygen saturation values for cats and dogs range from 95% to 100%.

Although the pulse oximeter is a very useful tool, it has some major limitations. It is very important to note that the pulse oximeter measures only the percent of hemoglobin molecules that are saturated with oxygen. It does not reflect the oxygen content of the blood, or the partial pressure of oxygen (PaO_2) in the blood. As long as pulmonary function is normal, even severely anemic animals can have normal pulse oximetry readings (because although they are distressed from having severely decreased hemoglobin levels, saturation of remaining hemoglobin molecules will be normal). Abnormal forms of hemoglobin such as those that result from smoke inhalation or carbon monoxide poisoning can produce normal pulse oximeter readings, even though the patient may be severely hypoxemic.

If the pulse oximeter displays an abnormal reading, immediate evaluation of the patient is warranted. Heart rate, pulse quality, mucous membrane color, and respiratory rate and effort should be noted. An abnormal reading may result from machine error. Common causes of machine error include poor perfusion to the probe site, hypothermia, interference from hair or oral pigmentation, and patient movement. Depending on the patient's status, an arterial blood gas analysis may be performed to confirm hemoglobin saturation and to evaluate the blood oxygen content. However, during troubleshooting of a pulse oximeter that is sounding an alarm that indicates an abnormal value, supplemental oxygen should be provided to the patient until it is determined whether the abnormal value is real or was caused by machine error.

Capnography, or measurement of carbon dioxide levels, can also provide information about respiratory system function. A capnometer can be inserted into the breathing circuit of an intubated patient and connected to an electronic monitor. End-tidal carbon dioxide ($etCO_2$) levels reflect the amount of carbon dioxide present in expired air at the end of exhalation. Increased $etCO_2$ readings may indicate that the patient is hypoventilating, and that assisted ventilation may be needed. Rebreathing of carbon dioxide (as with exhausted soda lime) in an anesthesia circuit will result in increased $etCO_2$ levels. Decreased $etCO_2$ readings may indicate that the patient is hyperventilating or has decreased cardiac output. A leak in the anesthesia system or a poorly inflated endotracheal tube cuff can also result in decreased $etCO_2$ values.

Arterial blood gas monitoring provides a wealth of information about respiratory function. Arterial blood samples are commonly obtained from the dorsal metatarsal artery or femoral artery. To obtain a sample from the dorsal metatarsal artery, the patient is restrained in lateral recumbency. The fur in the area is clipped, and alcohol is used to remove small hairs from the site. The pulse is palpated with a finger, and the other hand gently guides the needle into the artery. Specialized arterial draw syringes are often used; they are vented and fill on their own because of high arterial blood pressures. The angle used for arteriopuncture is steeper than for venipuncture, and the syringe is often nearly perpendicular to the artery (Figure 25-13). To obtain a sample from the

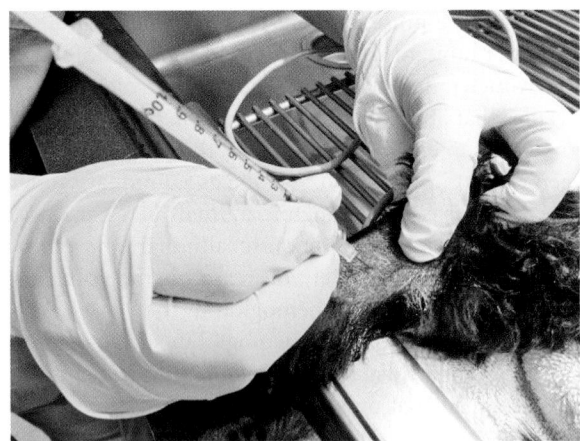

FIGURE 25-13 Proper technique for obtaining an arterial blood gas sample from the dorsal metatarsal artery.

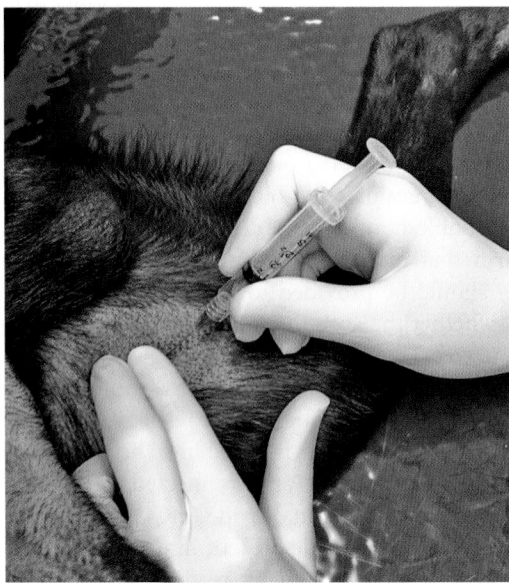

FIGURE 25-14 Proper technique for obtaining an arterial blood gas sample from the femoral artery.

femoral artery, the area is prepped similarly, and two fingers are used to palpate the femoral pulse. The syringe is inserted and is directed toward the artery (Figure 25-14). Acquiring arterial blood samples in cats and distressed patients may be too stressful. The procedure should be delayed if the animal's condition worsens with restraint.

Arterial blood gas interpretation is difficult to master at first and requires practice. Values examined most closely when the respiratory system is assessed are arterial hemoglobin saturation (SaO_2) and partial pressure of oxygen (PaO_2) and carbon dioxide ($PaCO_2$). The SaO_2 is roughly equivalent to values obtained with a pulse oximeter. The $PaCO_2$ is used to assess ventilation status. Hypoventilation (increased $PaCO_2$) can occur from airway obstruction, lung disease, brain disease, sedation or anesthesia, and certain toxicities. Acidemia (decreased blood pH) can occur with elevated $PaCO_2$. Hyperventilation (decreased $PaCO_2$) occurs for a

multitude of reasons. In patients with respiratory distress, hyperventilation is a response to hypoxemia and reflects the body's attempts to get as much oxygen into the lungs as possible. Pain, stress, and anxiety can also result in hyperventilation. In addition, hyperventilation occurs in response to metabolic acidosis, which is a common sequela to many systemic illnesses.

> **TECHNICIAN NOTE** When an arterial blood gas is interpreted, the $PaCO_2$ is used to assess ventilation, and the PaO_2 is used to assess oxygenation.

Oxygenation is reflected in the PaO_2, which is a measure of the amount of oxygen that is dissolved in arterial blood (not including oxygen bound to hemoglobin, as measured by the SaO_2). Decreased PaO_2 indicates hypoxemia. Common physical examination findings in this situation include pale or cyanotic mucous membranes, rapid heart rate, tachypnea, altered pulse quality, and abnormal respiratory effort.

Pulmonary function (the transfer of oxygen molecules from the alveolar gas to the arterial blood) can be approximated by calculating the difference in oxygenation between the two sites. An equation used to calculate the A-a gradient is used in patients that are not receiving supplemental oxygen to assess oxygen exchange. The capital "A" represents the oxygen content of alveolar gas and is determined by the following formula:

$$A = [(P_{atm} - 47) \times 0.21] - PaCO_2/0.8$$

In this equation, P_{atm} is the local barometric pressure (which is 760 mm Hg at sea level), 47 is a constant (water vapor pressure), and 0.21 is the fraction of inspired oxygen (atmospheric air contains 21% oxygen). The $PaCO_2$ is obtained from the arterial blood gas, and 0.8 is a constant. At normal conditions near sea level, this equation can be simplified as follows:

$$A = 150 - PaCO_2/0.8$$

From this value, the PaO_2 (obtained from the arterial blood gas, and represented by the lowercase "a") is subtracted, and the resulting number is the A-a gradient. The normal A-a gradient is 10 to 15; values higher than this indicate that oxygen exchange is impaired, likely as the result of a pulmonary problem (such as pneumonia, edema, blood clots, etc.). Animals with an elevated A-a gradient generally benefit from supplemental oxygen. Unfortunately, the A-a gradient is valid only while the animal is breathing room air. Once the animal is on supplemental oxygen, a different equation is used to assess oxygenation status—the PaO_2/FiO_2 ratio. Once again, the PaO_2 is obtained from the arterial blood gas. The FiO_2 is the fraction (percent) of inspired oxygen in decimal form. For example, a dog receiving 50% oxygen would have an F_iO_2 of 0.5, and a dog breathing room air would have an FiO_2 of 0.21. Normal PaO_2/FiO_2 ratio

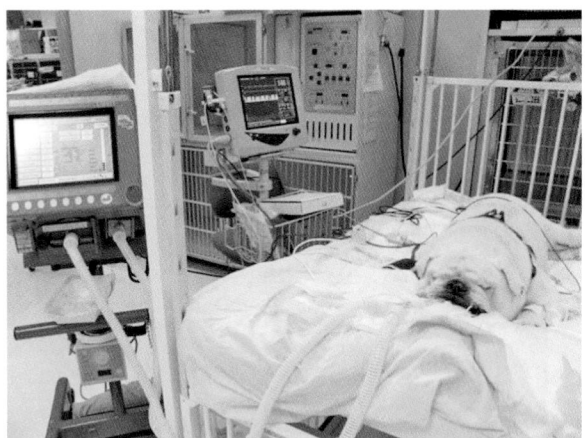

FIGURE 25-15 Patients on mechanical ventilation require intensive, around-the-clock nursing care and monitoring.

values range from 400 to 500, and the PaO_2 is approximately 4 to 5 times higher than the FiO_2. The lower the PaO_2/FiO_2 ratio, the worse is the patient's oxygenation. Mechanical ventilation usually is indicated when the PaO_2/FiO_2 ratio falls below 200.

Mechanical ventilation is a means of providing long-term intensive respiratory support to critically ill dogs and cats. Many veterinary practices have specialized critical care ventilators, which allow for fine alterations in breath support and oxygen delivery. Short-term mechanical ventilation can be accomplished by using a standard anesthesia ventilator. Ideally, the ventilator is used to deliver oxygen mixed with room air, and the patient is sedated with IV drugs during ventilation (Figure 25-15).

Typical monitoring of a ventilator patient includes a central line catheter and central venous pressure (CVP) measurement (see p. 927), an arterial catheter and continuous direct blood pressure monitoring, continuous $etCO_2$ monitoring, continuous pulse oximetry, temperature monitoring, and indwelling urinary catheter placement. Patients require a dedicated nursing staff to ensure that the ventilator and monitors are functioning properly, as well as to perform nursing care of the ventilated patient. Nursing care of the ventilator patient is a highly labor-intensive process. Every 4 to 6 hours, the patient should receive eye lubricant, swabbing of the oral cavity to remove secretions, inspection of all catheters, inspection and maintenance of the endotracheal or tracheostomy tube, passive range-of-motion exercises, and repositioning to prevent pressure ulcers. Ventilator patients are prone to pressure ulcers because of their recumbency. They often develop peripheral edema, especially of the face and legs, after 24 hours of recumbency. In some cases, the tongue becomes edematous, and a temporary tracheostomy must be performed before the animal is allowed to wake up. Pneumonia, a common complication during mechanical ventilation, can lead to sepsis and organ failure. Unfortunately, the prognosis for animals that require mechanical ventilation to maintain oxygenation or ventilation is very guarded.

TECHNICIAN NOTE Patients undergoing mechanical ventilation require extensive monitoring and intensive nursing care.

CARDIOPULMONARY ARREST

Cardiopulmonary arrest consists of cessation of spontaneous respirations and lack of a perfusing heart rhythm. In veterinary medicine, cardiopulmonary arrest most often occurs as the terminal event in a chronic disease process. However, previously healthy animals can experience cardiopulmonary arrest after trauma, critical illness, or anesthetic complications. Resuscitative efforts after cardiopulmonary arrest are referred to as *cardiopulmonary resuscitation (CPR)* or *cardiopulmonary cerebral resuscitation (CPCR)*, which reflects the importance of restoring blood flow to the brain, as well as to the heart and lungs.

Identifying patients that are at high risk for cardiopulmonary arrest is essential because time is crucial for successful CPCR. These patients are likely to have underlying cardiac disorders, respiratory disease, severe trauma, or shock as their main presenting complaint. Other patients at risk for cardiopulmonary arrest include those with acid-base and electrolyte disorders, seizures, anemia, or increased vagal stimulation (vagal tone), and those under general anesthesia. Vagally mediated arrest occurs most commonly in vomiting animals but can also occur after urination, defecation, or restraint. This happens because of reflex bradycardia mediated by the vagus nerve. In critically ill animals, this bradycardia can lead to marked decreases in cardiac output and cardiac arrest. Some animals will have respiratory arrest before a full cardiopulmonary arrest. This most commonly occurs in animals with neurologic or respiratory disease. In these cases, the animal stops breathing, but the heart continues to beat for a short time before complete cardiopulmonary arrest occurs. Identifying these patients as soon as possible after respiratory arrest is crucial for survival. Other indications that a patient may undergo cardiopulmonary arrest include sudden tachycardia or bradycardia, pallor, changes in pulse strength, increased respiratory rate or effort, and even acute agitation or depression. Recognizing these signs of potential impending cardiopulmonary arrest and alerting the other team members is imperative for maximizing the chances for successful CPCR.

TECHNICIAN NOTE The first step in the resuscitation effort is to alert other team members to the crisis and move the patient to a centralized area where the crash cart and oxygen are accessible.

CARDIOPULMONARY CEREBRAL RESUSCITATION

Once a cardiopulmonary arrest occurs, resuscitative measures need to begin immediately. Resuscitation is commonly

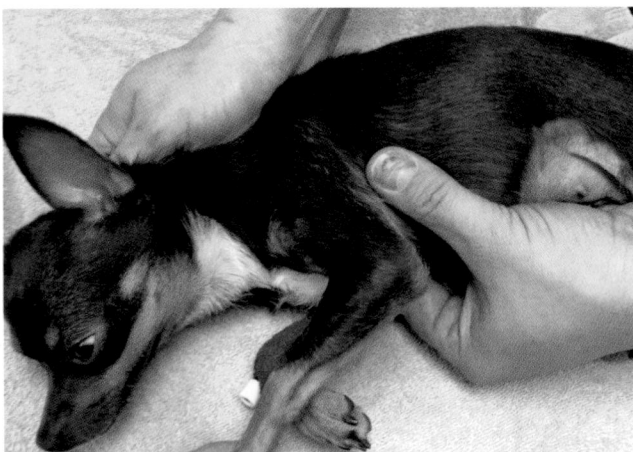

FIGURE 25-16 Proper hand placement for cardiopulmonary cerebrovascular resuscitation in a cat or small dog.

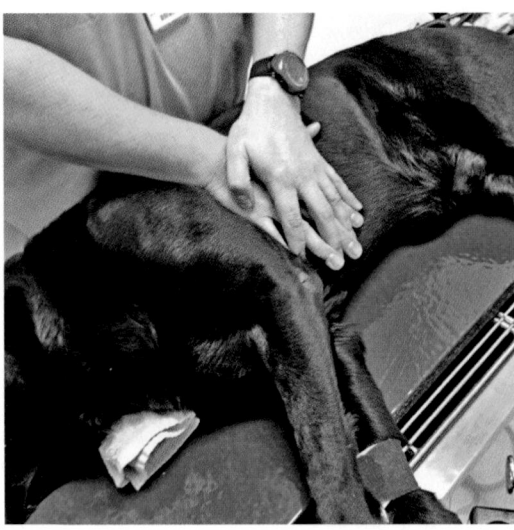

FIGURE 25-17 Proper hand placement for cardiopulmonary cerebrovascular resuscitation in a medium-size to large dog.

classified as basic life support (chest compressions and ventilation) or advanced life support (medications, **defibrillation**, open-chest procedures). Previously, priorities in CPCR were designated "the ABCs" of airway, breathing, and circulation. In recent years, however, controversy has surrounded this approach, and many critical care veterinarians now advocate "the CABs" to reflect the extreme importance of chest compressions and restoring perfusion during the resuscitative effort.

BASIC LIFE SUPPORT

Once a potential cardiopulmonary arrest occurs, first responders should check to see whether a heartbeat is present, and if the animal is breathing. The heart should be auscultated because pulse quality and even an ECG tracing may not reliably reflect cardiac activity. If no heartbeat is heard, chest compressions should begin immediately.

Positioning and technique for delivering chest compressions depend on patient size and conformation (narrow vs. deep chested, etc.). In cats and small dogs (weighing less than 15 pounds), the "cardiac pump" method of chest compression is used. With this technique, blood flow occurs by direct compression and relaxation of the heart. This method does not work well in larger animals because the chest is too large to permit effective direct compression of the heart. Proper technique is very important when compressions are performed by the cardiac pump method. To perform this maneuver, the animal is placed in lateral recumbency, and the care-giver's hand encircles the ventral chest. Compressions are performed directly over the heart. The care-giver should be very careful to use the whole hand, not just the fingertips, to administer compressions (Figure 25-16). The cardiac pump method does not work well in larger animals because the chest is too large to permit effective direct compression of the heart. In larger patients, compressions are applied to the widest part of the chest, with the animal in lateral recumbency (Figure 25-17). With this technique, the heart functions passively, and blood flow is determined by

changes in intrathoracic pressure that occur with each compression and recoil. When the chest is compressed, blood is forced out of the heart, and venous return to the right atrium occurs when pressure is released. To generate adequate pressure to cause this passive blood flow, each thoracic compression should compress the thoracic wall by 30% to 50%. It is extremely important to allow enough time for the wall to recoil back to the normal position before beginning the next compression.

Regardless of the technique used, successful CPCR depends on performing quality chest compressions. In cats and small dogs, a rate of 120 to 130 compressions per minute is recommended. Medium-size to large breed dogs receive compressions at a rate of 100 per minute. Performing chest compressions properly can be very tiring for the care-giver; it is recommended to switch places with another team member every 2 to 3 minutes.

Monitoring the effectiveness of chest compressions can be accomplished by placing a lubricated Doppler blood pressure probe on the cornea; this provides auditory feedback as each adequate compression causes perfusion of the brain and eye. Another way to monitor the effectiveness of chest compressions is to use an end-tidal carbon dioxide (etCO$_2$) monitor. In cardiopulmonary arrest, etCO$_2$ initially falls to zero because no blood flow is available to transport carbon dioxide from the tissues to the lungs for exhalation. As chest compressions begin to restore perfusion, etCO$_2$ should rise. Values above 10 to 15 mm Hg indicate that the compressions are adequate. Assessing chest compressions by palpating pulses is not recommended because venous pulses occur commonly during CPCR and are indistinguishable from arterial pulses. Similarly, mucous membrane color is a poor reflector of cardiac output and tissue perfusion.

In some cases, interposed abdominal compressions are used to enhance venous return to the heart during CPCR. With this technique, the abdomen is compressed during the

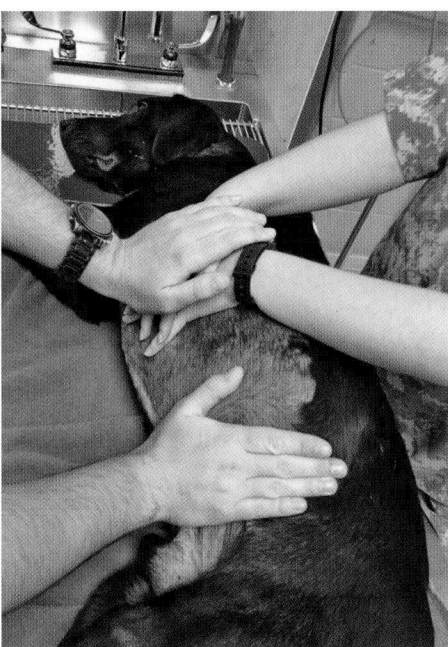

FIGURE 25-18 Proper hand placement for interposed abdominal compressions.

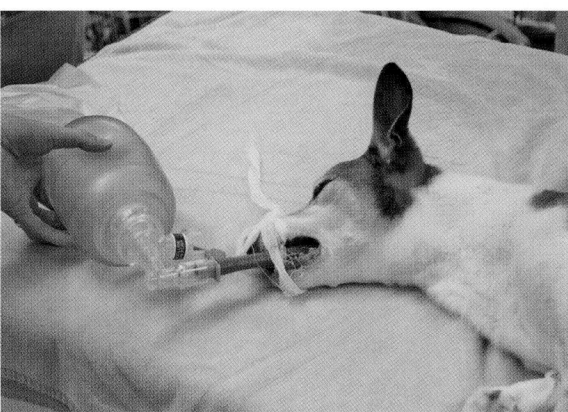

FIGURE 25-19 An Ambu bag is being used to ventilate a dog experiencing respiratory arrest.

recoil phase of the chest compression. Increased abdominal pressure can facilitate blood flow toward the heart. Proper hand placement for this technique is shown in Figure 25-18. Complications of interposed abdominal compressions include organ contusions (especially of the liver) and hemoabdomen.

Recent evidence in human medicine has strongly linked good chest compressions with a greater likelihood of survival and neurologic recovery. Current recommendations are to minimize any interruptions in chest compressions. Chest compressions should be performed continuously while the airway is being secured, catheters placed, and other interventions provided during CPCR. They can be stopped briefly every few minutes to allow inspection of the ECG tracing and to listen for a heartbeat; they should then be resumed immediately.

> **TECHNICIAN NOTE** Care should be taken to minimize any interruptions in chest compression, even for intubation and catheter placement.

In some cases, closed-chest compressions are not adequate to generate blood flow during CPCR. This may be encountered with patients who are suffering from pleural or pericardial effusion, pneumothorax, diaphragmatic hernia, **flail chest**, or penetrating chest trauma. The clinician may decide to perform open-chest CPCR on these animals. Some clinicians also elect open-chest CPCR in giant breed dogs, or in patients that have suffered witnessed traumatic or anesthetic arrest. Open-chest CPCR involves making an incision in the left 5th intercostal space, freeing the heart from its attachments, and directly massaging the heart from apex to

base, mimicking normal contraction. If desired, the descending aorta can also be gently occluded for several minutes by another team member's hand. This promotes preferential delivery of blood to the brain and the heart. The decision to pursue open-chest CPCR should be made early in the resuscitation attempt—ideally after the first or second cycle of resuscitation—to maximize the chances of success.

Once a cardiopulmonary arrest has been identified and chest compressions are under way, the animal's airway needs to be secured. This is achieved with intubation, with an endotracheal tube in most cases, or by emergency tracheostomy in patients with upper airway obstruction. While the animal is prepared for intubation, the oral cavity is quickly inspected for foreign material, vomitus, blood, and obstructive mass lesions (hematomas, neoplasia, etc.). The animal generally is kept in lateral recumbency during intubation. If the airway is too narrow for a standard orotracheal tube to pass, a red rubber catheter can be fed into the trachea as a temporary conduit for oxygen. It is a good idea to have suction ready during intubation to remove mucus or foreign material from the oropharynx. Many patients in cardiopulmonary arrest develop pulmonary edema, and suction is necessary to clear the froth from the endotracheal tube. Once the tube has been placed, it should be secured with a gauze tie, and the patient connected to an oxygen source. Assisted breathing is then begun. Several methods may be used to provide ventilatory support during CPCR. An Ambu bag is a portable, easy-to-use device (Figure 25-19). Some Ambu bags have adaptors to deliver 100% oxygen, but others can deliver only room air, which contains 21% oxygen. An anesthetic machine or ventilator can also be used to deliver 100% oxygen to the animal during CPCR. If a pressure manometer is present (as on most anesthesia machines), a target of 10 to 20 cm H_2O for each breath is appropriate. Regardless of the patient's size, 8 to 12 respirations per minute should be administered in most situations. Rapidly breathing for the animal leads to hyperventilation, which causes constriction of cerebral blood vessels and decreased perfusion of the brain.

TECHNICIAN NOTE Excessive ventilation of the patient during cardiopulmonary cerebral resuscitation (CPCR) causes cerebral vasoconstriction and decreased blood flow to the brain.

Acupuncture is a complementary technique that can be helpful in stimulating respiration when other measures have failed. This acupuncture point is Governor Vessel 26 (GV 26), which is located at the nasal philtrum at the level of the ventral edge of the nares (Figure 25-20). A 25-gauge needle

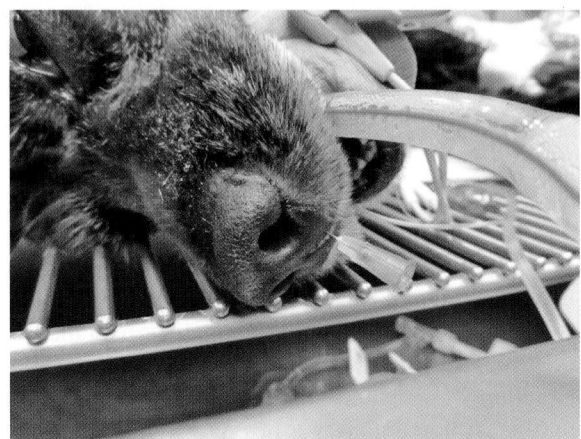

FIGURE 25-20 A needle inserted at the Governor Vessel 26 (GV 26) acupuncture point.

is applied to the bone at this point and then is twirled to stimulate respiratory centers in the brainstem.

ADVANCED LIFE SUPPORT

During CPCR, compressions and ventilations are administered for 2 to 3 minutes at a time before the patient is reassessed (one cycle of CPCR). If the patient is still in cardiopulmonary arrest after the first cycle, advanced life support techniques are often employed. Several drugs are available to assist in CPCR, and it is important for the clinician to be able to properly interpret an ECG to determine which drug is indicated. Three main arrest rhythms in dogs and cats are easily identifiable on ECG: **asystole**, pulseless electrical activity (PEA), and ventricular fibrillation. Asystole ("flatline") is complete cessation of all mechanical and electrical activity in the heart (Figure 25-21). This rhythm is commonly treated with epinephrine, vasopressin, or atropine. Pulseless electrical activity occurs when the electrical system of the heart is functioning (as evidenced by complexes on the ECG), but no mechanical heartbeat occurs in response to electrical stimulation. The appearance of this rhythm can be diverse, but it often mimics ventricular arrhythmia, with wide bizarre QRS complexes occurring at a slow rate (Figure 25-22). This rhythm is treated with epinephrine, vasopressin, or naloxone in certain cases. Ventricular fibrillation is highly disorganized contractile activity of the heart (Figure 25-23). It is often preceded by rapid **ventricular tachycardia**. This is the most common arrest rhythm

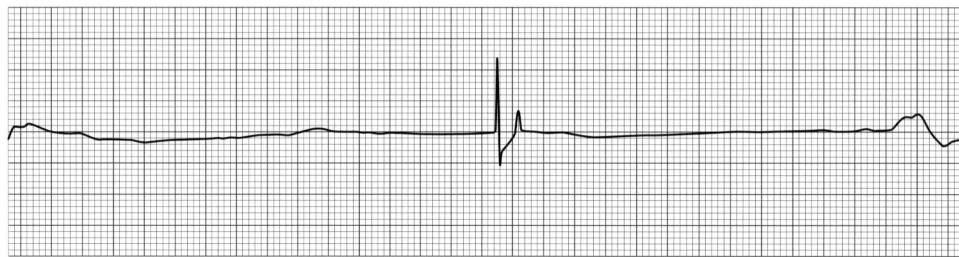

FIGURE 25-21 A single ventricular complex followed by asystole.

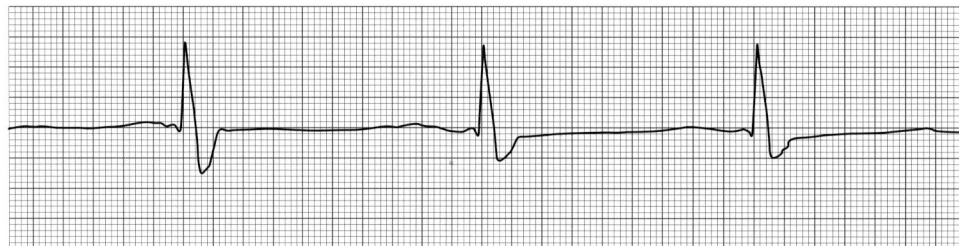

FIGURE 25-22 Pulseless electrical activity.

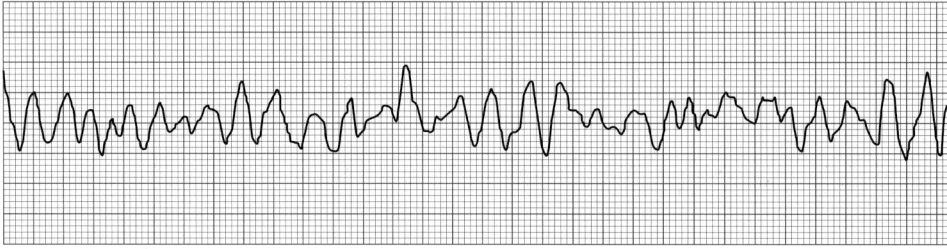

FIGURE 25-23 Ventricular fibrillation.

in humans, but it occurs only occasionally in dogs and cats. The treatment of choice for this arrhythmia is defibrillation. After the first cycle of CPCR, an electrical defibrillator is used to attempt conversion back to a perfusing rhythm. Immediately after the shock is administered, another team member resumes chest compressions and completes the 2-minute cycle of CPCR. If defibrillation was not successful, it can be repeated at a higher setting during the next CPCR cycle. The defibrillator should be used only by trained personnel. Tips for appropriate use of an electrical defibrillator include the following:

1. Apply adequate pressure to the chest with the paddles.
2. Use the largest paddle surface area. The crash cart ideally should contain a set of small, medium, and large external paddles, as well as small and large internal paddles.
3. Use a proper conducting gel or saline solution–soaked gauze to enhance conduction from the paddles to the patient; clip fur if needed.
4. Make sure that all staff members are clear of the patient and the table. (This includes the person operating the defibrillator.)

Alcohol should never be used near defibrillator paddles because of the risk for fire. The recommended initial dose is 2 to 4 J/kg. Initially, use a setting at the lower end of the dose range. The clinician may decide to increase the dose with each subsequent shock. Open-chest defibrillation requires specific paddles and a modified dose of electricity (0.2 to 0.4 J/kg).

In certain cases, additional medications such as magnesium, amiodarone, calcium, or sodium bicarbonate may be indicated during the CPCR attempt. See Table 25-1 for a listing of common CPCR drugs and their indications.

The IV route is preferred for drug administration during CPCR. If a catheter was not placed before the cardiopulmonary arrest episode, it is placed as the patient is being intubated. Because animals have very poor blood pressure during an arrest, a cutdown may be needed to secure venous access. The veins most commonly used for cutdown are the jugular, cephalic, and medial/lateral saphenous veins. In small or young patients, an intraosseous catheter can be used to deliver medications during CPCR. When drugs are administered intraosseously or through a peripheral vein, a large volume (10 to 15 ml) of saline flush should be used to force medication toward the heart and lungs. Sometimes, IV access cannot be achieved during CPCR. In these situations, certain drugs can be administered through the endotracheal tube. To do this, a red rubber catheter is threaded down the endotracheal tube, and the medication is injected into the red rubber catheter. Generally, the dose used is twice the IV dose. A saline flush is then administered to ensure that all drug has passed out of the tube. Only certain medications are safe to administer through an endotracheal tube. They are easily remembered by the acronym NAVEL (*n*aloxone, *a*tropine, *v*asopressin, *e*pinephrine, *l*idocaine). Drugs that are caustic to the lungs such as magnesium sulfate or sodium bicarbonate should never be administered through an endotracheal tube. Drug uptake by the pulmonary circulation is impaired by conditions such as pulmonary edema, which negates this as a suitable route. Good communication between team members performing CPCR is imperative because a vigorous chest compression delivered at an inopportune moment may result in exhalation of medications administered intratracheally. The last route used for drug administration is intracardiac. This method is not routinely recommended because of the risk of damaging the heart muscle or lacerating the coronary arteries, and because of the need to stop chest compressions to administer the drug. This route is used rarely during open-chest CPCR, when the care-giver can guide the needle into the left ventricle.

> **TECHNICIAN NOTE** Drugs that are safe to administer through an endotracheal tube are easily remembered by the acronym NAVEL (*n*aloxone, *a*tropine, *v*asopressin, *e*pinephrine, *l*idocaine).

TABLE 25-1	Dosages of Drugs Commonly Used During CPCR		
DRUG NAME	**CPCR DOSE**	**INDICATIONS**	**ADVERSE EFFECTS**
Epinephrine	0.1 mg/kg IV (1 ml/10 kg)	Asystole, PEA	Arrhythmias, hypertension
Atropine	0.04 mg/kg IV (1 ml/10 kg)	Bradyarrhythmias, vagally mediated arrests, AV block	Arrhythmias, tachycardia, decreased GI motility
Vasopressin	0.8 mU/kg IV (0.4 ml/10 kg)	Asystole, PEA. Can be used in place of second dose of epinephrine	Arrhythmias, hypertension
Lidocaine	2-4 mg/kg IV	Ventricular tachyarrhythmias	Vomiting, neurologic signs (especially in cats; use with caution in this species)
Magnesium sulfate, 200 mg/ml	0.25 mEq/kg IV over 10-15 minutes to effect	Refractory unstable ventricular tachycardias	Bradycardia, hypotension
Calcium gluconate, 10%	0.5-1 ml/kg over 10 minutes to effect	Hyperkalemia	Arrhythmias, hypercalcemia
Amiodarone	5 mg/kg IV over 5-10 minutes	Refractory unstable ventricular tachycardias	Arrhythmias, hypotension, anaphylaxis (rare)

AV, Atrioventricular; *CPCR,* cardiopulmonary cerebral resuscitation; *GI,* gastrointestinal; *PEA,* pulseless electrical activity.

If the patient has arrested from hypovolemic or hemorrhagic shock, fluid boluses should be given during the CPCR attempt to restore vascular volume. Small-volume resuscitation with fluids such as synthetic colloids or hypertonic saline will achieve faster volume expansion than is achieved by resuscitation with crystalloids alone. Small crystalloid boluses of 10 to 15 ml/kg can be given at the start of CPCR; however, it is important to remember that excessive fluid administration can be detrimental because it will reduce cardiac filling and will predispose the animal to fluid overload.

During CPCR, a lot of activity occurs and intervention is performed on the patient over a short period. It is ideal to have a designated team member record the quantity and route of drugs administered and details of defibrillation attempts and circumstances that led to the patient's cardiopulmonary arrest. This ensures that the medical record remains as complete as possible.

Finally, it is important to present the owner with realistic expectations when facing a cardiopulmonary arrest. In hospitalized animals, death often occurs as the final process of a chronic or overwhelming disease. The odds of surviving to hospital discharge are very poor in these patients, with up to 82% undergoing another cardiopulmonary arrest within 12 hours. Dogs and cats undergoing arrest from trauma or anesthesia complications have a greater chance of survival, but the overall rate of survival for all causes of witnessed in-hospital cardiopulmonary arrest is 4% to 9%. If interventions are performed while the animal is in respiratory arrest only, approximately 30% of dogs and 58% of cats are expected to survive. Given these grim statistics, it is reasonable to discuss CPCR with owners of critically ill animals, and to determine their wishes should the pet experience cardiopulmonary arrest. "Do not resuscitate" orders can be written if the owner and the clinician agree that this is the best strategy for the patient. Fortunately, some animals will survive and recover from a cardiopulmonary arrest, and their chances of survival can be maximized by intensive monitoring and care after CPCR.

CARE OF THE POST-ARREST PATIENT

After a successful CPCR attempt, the patient will require intense nursing care and monitoring. For the patient to have the best chance of survival, treatment should be focused on resolving the underlying cause of cardiopulmonary arrest (if possible) and anticipating and treating the systemic effects of cardiopulmonary arrest and resuscitation.

After resuscitation, the cardiovascular system is subjected to the effects of local **ischemia** and **reperfusion injury** of the heart muscle (see page 916 for a discussion of reperfusion injury). Cardiac function is further compromised by the effects of inflammatory mediators and other substances released by peripheral tissues as reperfusion occurs throughout the body. Even the medications used during the CPCR attempt itself, such as epinephrine and atropine, can contribute to ongoing cardiac stress by potentiating reperfusion injury and increasing the oxygen demands of an already stressed heart. In the post-arrest period, patients often develop severe arrhythmias and systemic hypotension, which predispose them to another episode of cardiopulmonary arrest. Continuous ECG monitoring and frequent blood pressure monitoring are imperative in the post-arrest patient. These animals generally require treatment with antiarrhythmic medications and medications given to support cardiac contractility and blood pressure.

The respiratory system is very fragile after cardiopulmonary arrest and CPCR. Oftentimes, patients will have underlying respiratory disease such as pneumonia, thoracic trauma, or pulmonary edema; this makes the lungs especially vulnerable to ongoing injury in the post-arrest period. After CPCR, the patient is at risk for pulmonary edema (cardiogenic or noncardiogenic), atelectasis, pulmonary **thromboembolism**, and acute respiratory distress syndrome (ARDS), as well as for injuries resulting from the CPCR attempt itself. The force used to generate adequate chest compressions can inadvertently result in pulmonary contusion, hemorrhage, or even rib fractures. One hundred percent oxygen is administered during CPCR, and most patients require ongoing oxygen support for hours to days after an arrest. Mechanical ventilation is often needed in the immediate post-arrest period.

The GI tract is also subject to severe insult during cardiopulmonary arrest. Hypoxia and hypotension can lead to microscopic breakdown of the GI mucosal barrier, which permits translocation of intestinal bacteria into the systemic circulation. Patients are at high risk for sepsis secondary to bacterial translocation after cardiopulmonary arrest. Many patients will develop severe, sometimes bloody diarrhea as well. GI hemorrhage can occur after shock and reperfusion from direct injury to the tissues, as well as secondary to coagulopathy. It is important to monitor fluid balance very carefully and to account for ongoing losses due to diarrhea. Most clinicians treat empirically with antibiotics after CPCR, in the hope of killing translocated bacteria before severe sepsis occurs.

Acute kidney injury (AKI) is also common after cardiopulmonary arrest. In health, the kidney has several protective mechanisms to prevent extreme alterations in perfusion. These mechanisms are overcome in severe shock and cardiac arrest, leaving the kidney vulnerable to hypotension and hypoxia. Electrolytes, kidney parameters, and urine output should be monitored closely in the post-arrest period. An indwelling urinary catheter will allow precise monitoring of urine output and will help keep the patient clean. Changes in urine output (polyuria or oliguria) can reflect significant renal injury even if laboratory values are normal. Careful monitoring of fluid "ins and outs" is essential for maintaining fluid balance in the post-arrest patient. Often AKI results in azotemia and altered urine production. With time and supportive care, however, many patients can recover a significant amount of renal function.

The central nervous system is also dramatically affected by cardiopulmonary arrest. Similar to the kidney, the brain normally has autoregulatory mechanisms to ensure a constant supply of oxygen and nutrients, while avoiding intracranial hypertension and fluid overload. When these mechanisms are lost during cardiopulmonary arrest, hypoxic brain injury occurs rapidly. After CPCR, the brain is highly susceptible to reperfusion injury, which can manifest as cerebral edema. Alterations in mental state and nerve function are common in the post-arrest period. Serial neurologic examinations provide the best means of assessing the patient's progress. Initially, evaluation of neurologic function is performed at least hourly. Recording the patient's pupillary light response (PLR), pupil size and symmetry, spontaneous respiratory efforts, response to stimulus, and motor responses is imperative. Common neurologic abnormalities in the post-arrest period include coma or stupor, anisocoria, miosis, altered PLRs, and decreased or absent corneal reflexes. A positive prognostic indicator is recovery of these basic reflexes. Dilated or mid-range nonresponsive pupils can signify a severe brainstem injury, and carry a worse prognosis than anisocoria or miosis. Other poor prognostic indictors for neurologic recovery include failure to resume spontaneous ventilation, seizures, and loss of the ability to regulate basic body functions such as temperature and heart rate. After cardiopulmonary arrest, blindness from hypoxia of the visual cortex (cortical blindness) is very common. If the animal recovers, it often will regain vision, although permanent blindness is possible.

Blood glucose concentrations should also be monitored closely in the post-arrest period. Patients commonly develop hyperglycemia as a result of stress, as well as exposure to exogenous catecholamines such as epinephrine. Hyperglycemia can be detrimental to neurologic function and should be avoided. Some patients will develop hypoglycemia, which often is due to sepsis and reperfusion.

> **TECHNICIAN NOTE**   After successful CPCR, patients should receive frequent neurologic assessments and should be monitored for the development of organ failure.

Many drugs are used to support the patient in the immediate post-arrest period. Controversy surrounds the best approach to these patients, and very few studies in veterinary medicine have evaluated the effects of certain treatments on outcome after cardiopulmonary arrest. Following is a brief description of some of the medications most commonly used, as well as the rationale for their use in the post-arrest period.

Lidocaine is an antiarrhythmic medication that is used to treat rapid or unstable ventricular tachycardias. It is commonly given as a bolus, which may convert the patient's heart back to a normal sinus rhythm. Lidocaine can then be administered as a constant rate infusion (CRI) to control ventricular arrhythmias. When used as a CRI, lidocaine also provides systemic analgesia. It has free-radical scavenging properties as well, which may be beneficial in patients with ischemia-reperfusion injury.

Mannitol is an osmotic diuretic that remains in the intravascular space and draws water from the interstitial space between cells. This causes a shift of fluid from the tissues into the bloodstream, thereby expanding vascular volume, promoting diuresis, and decreasing cerebral edema in the post-arrest patient. Like lidocaine, mannitol has free-radical scavenging properties that may be useful following reperfusion. Because of its diuretic properties, mannitol should be used judiciously in patients with existing renal failure, and fluid balance should be monitored closely.

Dopamine is a synthetic catecholamine administered as a CRI. This medication improves blood pressure by causing peripheral vasoconstriction. A related drug, dobutamine, increases cardiac output by enhancing cardiac contractility. These drugs may have decreased efficacy in acidemic animals. Monitoring of blood gases and pH is recommended after cardiopulmonary arrest because most animals will have a moderate to severe metabolic acidosis. Both of these catecholamine medications can predispose the animal to tachycardia and arrhythmias, so continuous ECG monitoring and frequent monitoring of blood pressure are essential when these drugs are used.

Vasopressin is a medication that is used in hypotensive patients to improve blood pressure. This drug is newer than the catecholamines and has the advantage of working well in an acidemic environment. Vasopressin is given as a CRI. As with the catecholamines, cardiac arrhythmias can occur, so continuous ECG monitoring is needed.

Furosemide is a loop diuretic that is used occasionally in the post-arrest period. Its diuretic effects increase urine output and cause volume contraction. This can help resolve cardiogenic pulmonary edema or fluid overload. This medication should not be used in patients who are hypovolemic.

Cardiopulmonary arrest has severe consequences for all organ systems. Because of this, post-arrest patients are critically ill, and care of these patients is labor-intensive. A positive outcome depends on anticipating and being prepared to handle the common complications of cardiopulmonary arrest. The best approach to these patients is a team approach because these animals often require around-the-clock care and monitoring to minimize the chances of another arrest event. The prognosis for cardiopulmonary arrest is guarded to poor for survival and return to function, and most survivors require several days of intensive care.

PATIENT MONITORING

CENTRAL VENOUS PRESSURE MONITORING

At any given time, approximately 70% to 80% of a patient's total blood volume resides in the venous circulation. Tiny venules collect blood after it passes from the arterial circulation through the capillary beds. The venules drain into the larger systemic veins, which empty into the venae cavae. Although most discussions of blood pressure monitoring involve arterial blood pressure measurement, venous pressure monitoring can also be very useful. Central venous pressure (CVP) is the pressure in the cranial vena cava, just before its entry into the right atrium. Normal CVP is 0 to 5 cm H_2O in the dog. Because so much of the intravascular volume is located in the venous system, CVP is used to evaluate volume status and to assess response to fluid therapy. Decreased CVP may indicate hypovolemia, dehydration, or excessive venodilation. With fluid therapy, CVP can rise to 8 to 10 cm H_2O. Marked increases in CVP may indicate fluid overload, cardiac disease or heart failure, or increased intrathoracic pressure.

> **TECHNICIAN NOTE**   Central venous pressure (CVP) refers to the blood pressure in central veins, such as the cranial vena cava. CVP monitoring can reflect the efficacy of fluid therapy.

CVP values are generally interpreted in light of other hemodynamic parameters such as heart rate, capillary refill time, and arterial blood pressure. Limited value is derived from a single CVP measurement; rather, CVP measurement seems to be most useful clinically when performed repeatedly and monitored for trends in the values. CVP can be used to monitor response to fluid administration, especially in patients at high risk for fluid overload such as animals with oliguric renal failure or heart failure.

Measurement of CVP requires placement of a long central venous catheter. The catheter is placed into the **jugular vein**, is advanced through the cranial vena cava, and is positioned with the tip resting just outside the right atrium. Care should be taken to pre-measure the catheter before insertion, and to avoid intracardiac placement of the catheter. A radiograph can be taken to confirm catheter location after placement; alternatively, if clinicians are experienced with hemodynamic waveforms, they may attach the catheter to a pressure transducer to verify the location. After catheter placement, a water manometer can be used to manually measure CVP. The setup for this procedure includes a three-way stopcock that separates the manometer and a saline or sterile water-filled syringe from an extension set (Figure 25-24). Saline is

used to flush the system, and the manometer is filled with saline. The extension set is then connected to the most distal available port on the central line catheter. During CVP measurement, the animal should be maintained in sternal or lateral recumbency, and the manometer apparatus should be held at the level of the patient's heart, where the tip of the catheter is located (Figure 25-25). The water column of the manometer will gradually equilibrate with the pressure at the end of the catheter over several seconds; this value is the CVP. Alternatively, the central catheter can be attached to a pressure transducer and an electronic monitor. Several anesthesia and critical care monitors have the capacity to continuously measure CVP by using the same monitor as is used for direct arterial blood pressure monitoring (see later section).

ARTERIAL BLOOD PRESSURE MONITORING

During each cardiac cycle, blood pressure varies from a maximum (systolic pressure) to a minimum (diastolic pressure). Blood pressure is generally expressed as a fraction (systolic/diastolic), and mean blood pressure is calculated from those two values. Normal blood pressure values in dogs and cats range from systolic pressures of 80 to 140 mm Hg to diastolic pressures of 50 to 80 mm Hg. This reflects a mean arterial blood pressure of 60 to 100 mm Hg. Several physiologic mechanisms maintain mean arterial pressure within this narrow range to protect the organs from the effects of hypertension and hypotension. Maintaining adequate mean arterial pressure is especially important in the brain and kidney because these organs are highly sensitive to alterations in blood pressure.

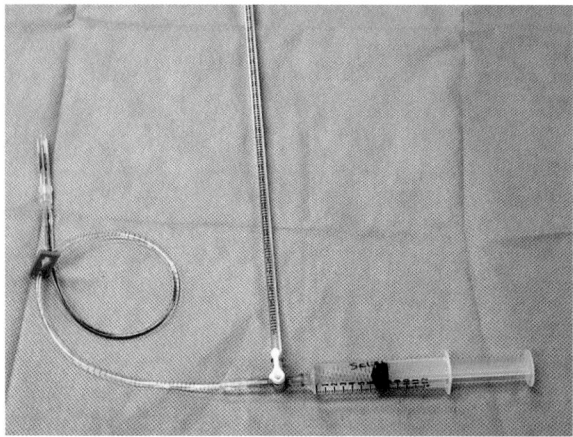

FIGURE 25-24 A water manometer attached to a syringe filled with sterile saline, a three-way stopcock, and an extension set.

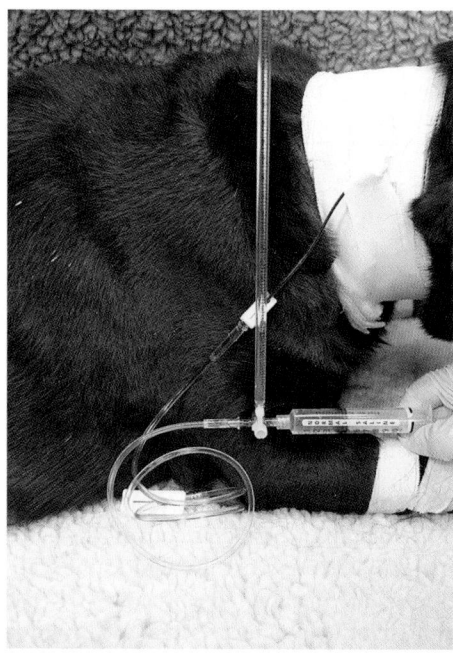

FIGURE 25-25 The base of the water manometer should be held at the level of the tip of the catheter (generally at the level of the heart) for an accurate reading.

Indirect or noninvasive blood pressure monitoring is used most often in veterinary practices and is performed with a Doppler or oscillometric device (Figure 25-26). Oscillometric devices are often paired with other monitoring equipment in the same machine, such as ECG, pulse oximetry, and CO_2 monitors. They can be programmed to measure systolic and diastolic pressure, and to calculate the mean arterial pressure from these values. Oftentimes, these machines can be set to automatically measure and record blood pressure at preset intervals, which makes them especially useful during anesthesia or in the intensive care unit (ICU).

Doppler blood pressure monitoring relies on an auditory signal to determine the arterial blood pressure (Figure 25-27). With this technique, hair is clipped over an appropriate artery (usually the dorsal metatarsal, ventral

digital, or tail artery), and conductive gel is applied to enhance sound transmission. A blood pressure cuff is applied proximal to the artery. The Doppler crystal is positioned directly over the artery and is maneuvered until a clear pulse is heard. A sphygmomanometer is used to inflate the cuff until the pulse sound disappears. The cuff is then slowly deflated until the pulse is heard again. The point where the pulse becomes audible again is the systolic pressure. Unfortunately, this technique cannot be used to reliably assess diastolic or mean arterial pressure in animals. Because the Doppler measurement must be taken manually, this technique is subject to operator error and should be done by a trained individual. Regardless of the method chosen, using the proper blood pressure cuff is imperative for accurate indirect blood pressure monitoring. As a general rule, the cuff width should approximate 40% of the circumference of the limb at the site of cuff placement.

> **TECHNICIAN NOTE** The blood pressure cuff width should approximate 40% of the circumference of the limb at the site of cuff placement.

Direct or invasive blood pressure measurement is the gold standard for blood pressure monitoring. This technique requires catheterization of an artery and the use of specialized monitoring equipment. The most common sites for arterial catheter placement are the dorsal metatarsal and femoral arteries, although the tail artery can also be used. The femoral artery should be catheterized only in anesthetized or recumbent patients because of the risk for hemorrhage if the catheter is dislodged. Unlike veins, arteries usually cannot be visualized under the skin, and catheter placement is accomplished by digital palpation of the artery. Before the arterial catheter is placed, the fur is clipped circumferentially around the limb, and the site is prepped with surgical scrub and wiped with alcohol. Ideally, sterile gloves should be worn during placement of arterial catheters. The insertion angle for arterial catheterization is generally steeper than for venous catheter placement (Figure 25-28). Arteries

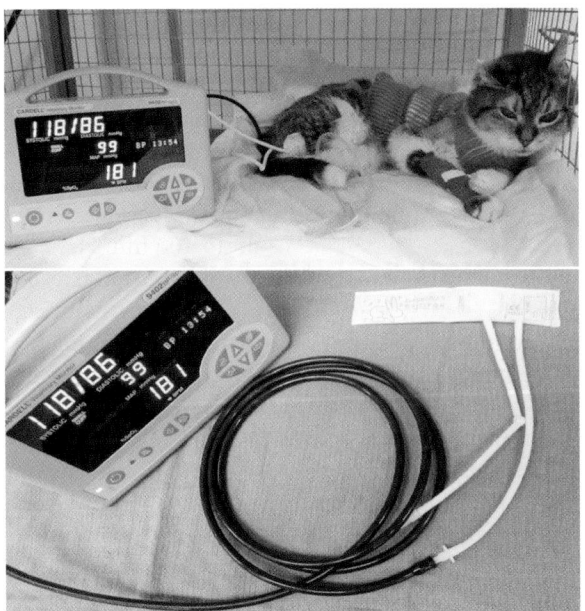
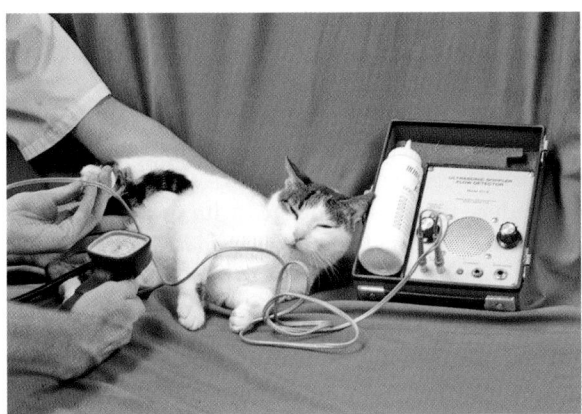

FIGURE 25-26 An oscillometric blood pressure monitor. Note that this patient's arterial pressures are as follows: systolic, 118 mm Hg; diastolic, 86 mm Hg; mean, 99 mm Hg.

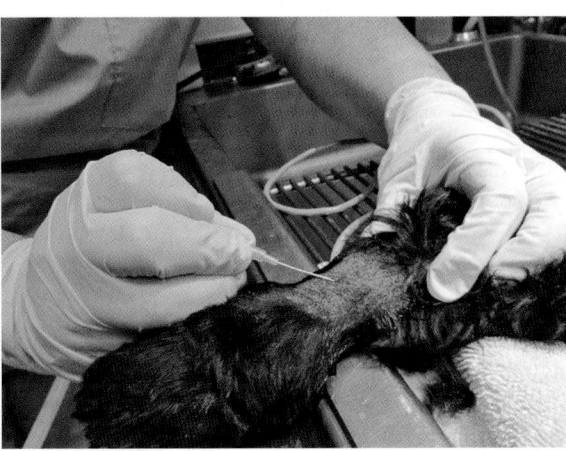

FIGURE 25-27 Obtaining a Doppler blood pressure measurement in a cat.

FIGURE 25-28 A direct arterial catheter is placed in the dorsal metatarsal artery of this dog.

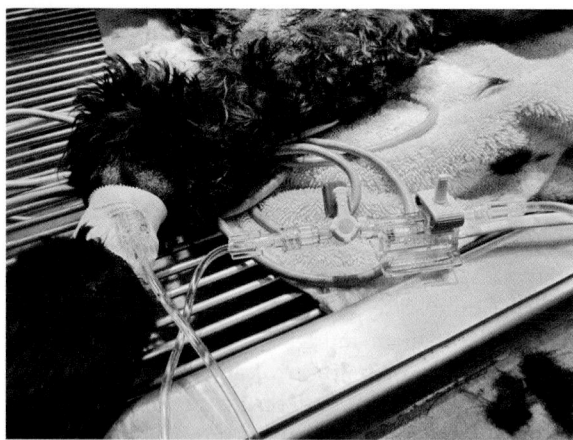

FIGURE 25-29 An electronic transducer is connected to the arterial catheter and is maintained at the level of both the catheter and the patient's heart for direct blood pressure measurement.

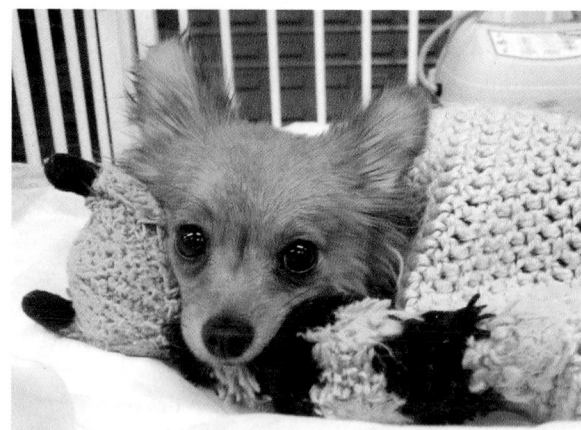

FIGURE 25-30 A patient often is more relaxed if familiar objects are nearby. This puppy is comforted after neck surgery with the aid of his own toy and blanket.

contain more smooth muscle than is found in veins. Consequently, arterial puncture often results in vasospasm, which can make threading the catheter into the artery very challenging. Pausing for a few seconds after getting a flash of arterial blood in the catheter will allow much of the spasm to subside. The catheter should be slowly advanced into the artery and then securely taped in place. To monitor blood pressure, the arterial catheter is connected to a pressure transducer, which generates a waveform on the electronic monitor. A wave is generated with each heartbeat and can be compared with the ECG to see the effects of arrhythmias on blood pressure. These monitors will display systolic, diastolic, and mean blood pressure. It is important to keep the transducer at the level of the tip of the catheter to obtain the most accurate measurements (Figure 25-29). Arterial catheters should be labeled very clearly to prevent accidental intra-arterial injections. No medications should ever be given through an arterial catheter. To prevent blood clots from forming on the end of the catheter, arterial catheters should be flushed every 2 hours unless they are attached to a continuous monitor. Care should also be taken to avoid flushing air bubbles into the artery.

> **TECHNICIAN NOTE** Arterial catheters should be labeled clearly to prevent accidental intra-arterial administration of medications.

CARE OF THE RECUMBENT PATIENT

AIRWAY AND ENDOTRACHEAL OR TRACHEOSTOMY TUBE CARE

Airway care on the recumbent patient includes humidification, sterile suctioning, cuff deflation and repositioning, changing the location of ties, changing the endotracheal (ET) tube daily, and performing cytologic examination of the tip. This is important to prevent pressure damage to the tracheal endothelium and damage from desiccation of the sol layer (the watery portion of the respiratory secretions)

and the mucosa, which decreases mucociliary clearance, and to ensure removal of airway secretions that may clog the tube (if present) and contribute to respiratory distress. Monitoring the cytology of the airway allows identification of any changes in flora and signals the need to improve sterile technique or change antibiotic treatment.

APPROPRIATE BEDDING AND PATIENT COMFORT

Patient comfort is an important component of caring for the recumbent pet. Prolonged recumbency can lead to the development of decubital ulcers. Appropriate bedding (absorbent, easily cleaned) with adequate padding (thick enough to provide support) reduces this complication and maintains the patient in a position conducive to more effective ventilation; it also prevents atelectasis of the down lung. Personal toys and blankets can reassure pets when they are in an unfamiliar, stressful environment (Figure 25-30).

APPROPRIATE LEVEL OF ANESTHESIA OR ANALGESIA

Many recumbent patients suffer from disease processes associated with a fair amount of discomfort or pain (intervertebral disc disease, neurologic dysfunction, tetanus, etc.). Maintaining an appropriate level of pain control is vital for their return to function. Recumbent patients that require mechanical ventilation have additional considerations. Mechanical ventilation is most effective when the patient is anesthetized to a depth that allows complete control of its ventilatory process by the machine. In addition, it is important to reduce the stress associated with the patient's awareness of being intubated and on a mechanical ventilator.

> **TECHNICIAN NOTE** Patient comfort is an important component of caring for the recumbent pet. Personal toys and blankets can reassure pets when they are in an unfamiliar, stressful environment.

INTRAVENOUS CATHETER MONITORING AND CARE

Intravenous catheters should be monitored for patency, evidence of infection, and phlebitis at the placement site at least once a day. This reduces the risk of septic foci developing around the catheters.

MONITORING AND ADJUSTING FLUID BALANCE (INS AND OUTS)

Fluid balance is very important in all patients, especially in those that are unable to respond to changes in intravascular volume, such as those under general anesthesia (because of decreased ability of the body to respond to changes in blood pressure and a blunted response to catecholamine release). Animals with tracheostomy tubes or high levels of anxiety due to recumbency and those that are undergoing mechanical ventilation may experience increased airway free water loss leading to dehydration and peripheral edema. Additionally, overhydration may be secondary to inappropriate antidiuretic hormone secretion, use of medications such as opioids, or alterations in the body's ability to maintain or decrease its own blood volume. Monitoring fluid balance allows adjustment of fluid therapy accordingly.

NUTRITION

Many recumbent patients do not eat appropriately because of their medical condition. Adequate enteral or parenteral nutrition (enteral is preferred) is important to support metabolism, albumin production, immune function, and GI integrity, and to prevent catabolism and complications such as refeeding syndrome (abnormalities in electrolyte balance that occur when the patient is fed after an extended period of anorexia).

OCULAR CARE

Animals with neurologic disease, animals under general anesthesia, and those that lack a palpebral reflex can develop corneal ulceration. Proper ocular care, which includes periodic examinations and frequent application of sterile eye lubricant, is important to prevent ophthalmic complications. Applying fluorescein stain to the corneas every day or every other day will reveal potential ulcers at the earliest stage possible, allowing for appropriate treatment.

ORAL CARE

Keeping the oral mucosa moist using glycerin-soaked gauze and preventing pressure sores on the tongue are important nursing care items for comatose or anesthetized patients. Cleaning the oropharynx with dilute chlorhexidine solution and suctioning debris helps prevent pulmonary aspiration during repositioning of the tracheostomy or endotracheal tube, and decreases bacterial growth.

RANGE OF MOTION

Performing range-of-motion exercises at least 4 times a day will help decrease the amount of peripheral edema that develops by increasing venous drainage and stimulating lymph flow and will prevent contracture and wasting of muscles if the patient is recumbent for a long time.

URINARY CATHETER PLACEMENT AND CARE

Urinary catheters are important to keep the patient clean and reduce risk of urine scald, and to monitor urine output and specific gravity to ensure that the patient is appropriately hydrated. This also allows changes in the appearance of the urine and the composition of the sediment to be monitored. Cleaning the prepuce or vulvar vestibule with dilute chlorhexidine solution 3 times a day reduces the bacterial load and decreases risk for catheter-related urinary tract infection.

STANDARDS OF CARE AND EMERGENCY PROTOCOLS

COMMON TOXICITIES AND EMERGENCIES

Respiratory Distress

The mainstay of treatment for animals in respiratory distress is to minimize stress. Oxygen supplementation should be provided as soon as possible. Patients in respiratory distress often benefit from some sedation. Butorphanol has relatively little effect on the cardiovascular system and can be considered safe for most patients at a dose of 0.2 mg/kg (0.1 mg/lb). If thoracic auscultation supports pneumothorax or pleural effusion, diagnostic thoracocentesis should be performed as previously described. Animals with suspected heart failure should receive furosemide, and cats with suspected asthma should receive two puffs from an albuterol inhaler. After the patient has been stabilized with oxygen, sedation, and medications as appropriate, additional diagnostics such as thoracic radiographs can be performed.

> **TECHNICIAN NOTE** Animals in respiratory distress, especially cats, can die from even small amounts of stress. Do not "strong-arm" them to obtain diagnostic samples. Instead, use oxygen, sedation, and time to decrease their stress enough to allow safe handling.

Trauma

For the traumatically injured patient, perform an appropriate triage examination and address all life-threatening injuries immediately. Intravenous access must be established as early as possible to allow administration of medications if cardiopulmonary arrest should occur. As soon as reasonable, pain control should be initiated. During the secondary exam, all non–life-threatening problems should be addressed: wounds should be cleaned and bandaged, lacerations repaired, and fractures splinted. Operate under the presumption that pulmonary contusions and traumatic brain injury occur, and treat the patient accordingly (provide oxygen for patients with suspected pulmonary contusions,

CASE PRESENTATION 25-1

Murphy, a 2-year-old castrated male Golden Retriever, was presented to the emergency clinic after being hit by a car. The owners witnessed the accident and believe the car was going around 35 mph. Murphy was hit on his right side. After the accident, he tried to walk but collapsed. He began panting heavily on the way to the clinic. He had no previous health problems and took no medication other than heartworm preventive and prescription flea control.

On physical examination, Murphy was alert but appeared uncomfortable. His gums were pale pink and his femoral pulses were weak. He was tachycardic (200 beats/minute) and tachypneic (60 breaths/minute). Harsh lung sounds were heard on thoracic auscultation. A palpable right femoral fracture was noted, and pelvic fractures were suspected on rectal examination. An IV catheter was placed, and samples were taken for PCV/TP (45%/4.2 g/dl) and lactate measurement. The lactate level was 5.6 (high). His blood pressure was 90/60 mm Hg (decreased).

The clinician identified Murphy's cardiovascular status as hypovolemic shock with suspected pulmonary contusions from blunt force trauma. He was given a bolus of lactated Ringer's solution and an injection of hydromorphone (0.05 mg/kg [0.025 mg/lb]) for pain control. An ECG showed sinus tachycardia. Pulse oximetry was performed and was 93% on room air. Supplemental oxygen was given with nasal prongs, and the value increased to 98%. After fluid resuscitation, Murphy's gums were pink, his pulse quality improved, and he was alert and responsive. His blood pressure now measured 130/83 (normal). Radiographs were obtained and showed pulmonary contusions, a comminuted fracture of the right femur, luxation of the left sacroiliac joint, and fractures of the right ilium and ischium.

Murphy was hospitalized on IV fluids, a continuous infusion of fentanyl, and supplemental oxygen. Routine monitoring of blood pressure, urine output, vital signs, and PCV/TP was performed. Appropriate nursing care included use of thick, padded bedding and placement of a urinary catheter. Two days later, his pulmonary contusions had improved, and Murphy underwent surgery to repair the fractures.

Murphy was discharged from the hospital the following afternoon with instructions for strict exercise restriction until the fractures healed. At his recheck visit, the owners reported that Murphy had made a full recovery.

and position the whole body at a 30-degree angle so the head is elevated for patients suspected to have elevated intracranial pressure) until these conditions are ruled out with advanced diagnostics. The trauma patient should be reassessed continuously during the initial stabilization period and then a minimum of once every 3 to 5 minutes until the patient's condition is completely stable. (See Case Presentation 25-1 for an example of emergency management of a trauma patient.)

Acute Abdomen

The term *acute abdomen* refers to sudden onset of abdominal pain that is often severe and of unknown cause. When

BOX 25-4 | Relevant Information When a Patient With Acute Abdomen Is Assessed

- Is the patient vomiting? If so, describe its character.
- Is the patient having diarrhea? If so, include a description.
- Have periodic episodes of pale mucous membranes and collapse been reported?
- Is vaginal or preputial discharge present?
- (For male patients) Is the patient intact? If so, is it cryptorchid?

assessing a patient that presents with an acute abdomen, it is important to obtain a complete history by asking questions about the onset of signs, previous health problems, and any other relevant information (Box 25-4). Answers to these questions help focus the examination and diagnostic workup when the acutely painful patient is approached. Patients with a history of collapse with pale mucous membranes should be closely monitored because this could indicate intermittent abdominal hemorrhage. Any patient with a history of vomiting should be evaluated for risk for aspiration pneumonia. Many causes of diarrhea are infectious, and some can be zoonotic, so it is important to wear gloves when handling patients with severe diarrhea.

Gastric Dilatation-Volvulus

Patients with gastric dilatation-volvulus (GDV) present with acute signs ranging from a single episode of vomiting and agitation to profuse vomiting, retching, and lateral recumbency. Abdominal distention is often a feature of this condition. However, dogs with a very long thorax may not appear to have abdominal distention because the stomach may remain within the thoracic cage in these patients. Initial stabilization requires placement of large-bore IV catheters in the front legs, decompression of the stomach by trocarization or orogastric intubation, and confirmation of the GDV. Once the patient has been stabilized, a surgical abdominal exploratory and gastropexy are recommended.

Urethral Obstruction

Upon presentation, animals with complete urethral obstruction may strain to urinate, or they may be stuporous from hypovolemic shock and hyperkalemia. If a patient suspected of urethral obstruction presents with bradycardia, it should be immediately evaluated for hyperkalemia. Calcium gluconate should be administered (at a dose of 1 ml/kg or 0.5 ml/lb) if hyperkalemia is confirmed. Once the calcium gluconate has been administered, additional measures such as fluid therapy, dextrose administration, and possibly insulin with dextrose should be initiated. Appropriate sedation and urethral de-obstruction should be performed as soon as possible to stabilize the patient.

Toxin Exposure

Essential information must be obtained by asking questions concerning possible toxin exposures (listed in Box 25-5).

BOX 25-5	Relevant Information When a Patient With Possible Toxin Exposure Is Assessed

- What did the animal ingest? OR What product was applied to the skin?
- Did you bring the package with you?
- When do you think the animal ingested it? OR When was it applied?
- Is the animal showing any clinical signs? If so, for how long?
- Was the ingestion or application witnessed, or is it suspected?
- Could other pets or people have been exposed? Are they showing any signs?

BOX 25-6	Systemic Diseases That Cause Cardiac Arrhythmias

- Electrolyte abnormalities such as hyperkalemia, hypercalcemia or hypocalcemia, and hyponatremia that are related to renal or endocrine disease (e.g., Addison's, diabetic ketoacidosis)
- Diseases causing myocarditis (e.g., pancreatitis, pyometra, uremia)
- Shock
- Sepsis
- Neoplasia (e.g., splenic, myocardial)
- Gastric dilatation-volvulus

Answers to these questions will help determine the level of toxicity, ways to provide proper treatment, and how to advise the owner about other animals in the household.

The basic tenet of treating toxicity is decontamination: surface decontamination if it is a topically applied toxin, GI decontamination if it was ingested. Topical decontamination entails copious lavage of the eyes with water or eyewash, generous lavage of the mouth with water, or washing the animal thoroughly in soapy water, depending upon the toxin. GI decontamination starts with induction of **emesis** for any noncaustic toxins. Do *not* induce emesis if the toxin is potentially caustic. Dogs sometimes can be induced to vomit by administering 1 teaspoon of fresh 3% hydrogen peroxide orally for every 10 lb of body weight. Owners may perform this step at home but should not repeat the dose and should still bring their pet in for examination, whether it vomits or not.

> **TECHNICIAN NOTE** Do not use hydrogen peroxide to induce emesis in cats.

Once at the hospital, emesis can be induced by administering apomorphine (0.03 mg/kg [0.015 mg/lb]) subcutaneously to dogs, and xylazine (0.44 mg/kg [0.22 mg/lb]) intramuscularly to cats. Hydromorphone can be given subcutaneously at preanesthetic doses if apomorphine does not induce vomiting in dogs. If these methods do not work, a fast IV bolus of cefazolin (20 mg/kg [10 mg/lb]) will often initiate vomiting.

Depending on the specific toxin, gastric lavage may be warranted. Gastric lavage should be performed only under general anesthesia using an endotracheal tube with an inflated cuff to reduce the risk for aspiration pneumonia. Upon cessation of emesis or completion of gastric lavage, administer activated charcoal if indicated. Some toxins undergo enterohepatic recycling and require administration of multiple doses of activated charcoal. Enterohepatically recycled toxins are often cleared faster if enemas or cathartics are administered. Some common toxins, the system affected,

and general treatment recommendations are listed in Table 25-2.

Canine and Feline Electrocardiography

The electrocardiogram (ECG) is a cardiac diagnostic tool that records electrical impulses generated by the specialized conduction system of the heart that cause coordinated contraction and relaxation of the heart muscle. The waveforms on the ECG indicate specific stages of myocardial depolarization, repolarization, and conduction.

INDICATIONS FOR THE ELECTROCARDIOGRAM

The most common reason to perform an ECG is for detection of an arrhythmia heard on physical examination or suspected on the basis of historical findings. This may include an irregular rhythm, bradycardia, or tachycardia. An ECG should also be performed on any animal with a history of **syncope** (fainting) or episodic weakness (weakness appearing at irregular intervals) because these conditions are commonly caused by cardiac arrhythmias. Arrhythmias are commonly present in patients with advanced cardiac disease such as advanced degenerative valve disease, dilated cardiomyopathy, and hypertrophic cardiomyopathy. Cardiac arrhythmias are also commonly caused by drugs (e.g., cardiac glycosides such as digoxin), toxins, and a variety of systemic diseases (see Box 25-6 for a partial list of systemic diseases that cause arrhythmias).

Analysis of specific waveforms may indicate cardiac chamber enlargement. However, this finding is more specific than sensitive, in that an ECG may be completely normal in an animal with advanced cardiac disease. The ECG can be useful in the diagnosis of pericardial effusion because tracings from these patients may exhibit QRS complexes of decreased amplitude (height), sinus tachycardia, or electrical alternans (alternating height of the QRS complexes between beats). It is also useful for monitoring complications during pericardiocentesis (e.g., ventricular arrhythmias). Monitoring drug therapy for antiarrhythmic and proarrhythmic

TABLE 25-2 Common Toxins by System and Treatment

	SYSTEM AFFECTED								TREATMENT				
TOXIN	CARDIOVASCULAR	GASTROINTESTINAL	HEPATIC	BLOOD COMPONENTS AND COAGULATION	NEUROLOGIC	METABOLIC	RENAL	RESPIRATORY	SURFACE DECONTAMINATION	GASTROINTESTINAL DECONTAMINATION	ACTIVATED CHARCOAL	INTRAVENOUS FLUIDS	OTHER
Acetaminophen			◆	◆						◆	1 dose	Maintenance	N-Acetylcysteine
Alcohol					◆			◆		◆		Maintenance	
Amphetamine	◆				◆					◆		Diuresis	Sedation, treat arrhythmias
Amphibian toxins	◆								Oral cavity			Maintenance	Treat arrhythmias
β-Adrenergic agonists	◆											Diuresis	Sedatives, beta blockers
Caffeine	◆	◆			◆					◆	1 dose	Diuresis	Sedatives, beta blockers
Chocolate	◆	◆			◆					◆	4 doses	Diuresis	Indwelling urinary catheter
Ethylene glycol		◆				◆	◆			◆	4 doses	Diuresis	4-MP or grain alcohol
Grapes and raisins (dogs)		◆					◆			◆	4 doses	Diuresis	Treat renal failure
Ivermectin		◆			◆				Skin if topical	◆	1 dose	Diuresis	
Lily (cat)		◆					◆		Brush pollen off, then wash	◆	1 dose	Diuresis	Prognosis poor if renal failure
Marijuana					◆					◆	4 doses	Maintenance	
Metaldehyde					◆	◆				◆	1 dose	Maintenance	Methocarbamol
NSAIDs		◆	◆				◆			◆	4 doses	Diuresis	Misoprostol
Onion, garlic, chives		◆		◆						◆	1 dose	Diuresis	Blood transfusion may be needed
Pyrethrins					◆				Bathe with dish soap		4 doses	Maintenance	Methocarbamol
Rodenticide (anticoagulant)				◆						◆	1 dose		Vitamin K if PT prolonged
Rodenticide (bromethalin)					◆					◆	12 doses	Maintenance	Methocarbamol
Rodenticide (cholecalciferol)		◆					◆			◆	1 dose	Diuresis	Treat hypercalcemia
Xylitol			◆			◆				◆	1 dose	Diuresis	Dextrose if needed

NSAIDs, Nonsteroidal anti-inflammatory drugs; PT, prothrombin time.

effects and monitoring during anesthesia for the development of arrhythmias and anesthetic depth are other indications for performing an ECG.

PRINCIPLES OF ELECTROCARDIOGRAPHY

The surface ECG measures the electrical activity of the heart by using a positive electrode and a negative electrode attached to the skin. A positive waveform (one that is above the baseline) is generated when the net electrical impulse is directed toward the positive electrode, a negative waveform (one that is below the baseline) is generated when the net electrical impulse is directed toward the negative electrode, and when the net electrical impulse is perpendicular to an imaginary line drawn between the electrodes, no waveform is generated, so the tracing appears as a flat (isoelectric) line on the ECG.

A *lead* is the term applied when the electrical impulses detected at both a positive electrode and a negative electrode are used together to measure the electrical activity of the heart. A standardized lead system is used to measure electrical activity traveling in different directions in a coordinated manner. The leads most commonly used in veterinary medicine are I, II, III, aVR, aVL, and aVF.

Leads I, II, and III are bipolar leads that record electrical activity between two electrodes placed in specific locations. Lead I is generated by placing the positive electrode on the left forelimb and the negative electrode on the right forelimb. Lead II is generated by placing the positive electrode on the right forelimb and the negative electrode on the left hindlimb. Lead III is generated by placing the positive electrode on the left hindlimb and the negative electrode on the left forelimb.

Leads aVR, aVL, and aVF are augmented leads. Augmented leads are different in that they combine the average of the electrical impulses detected at two contact points to generate a negative electrode. Augmented leads then record electrical activity between this negative electrode and a single positive electrode. Lead aVR is generated with the positive electrode on the right forelimb and the negative electrode as the combined average of the left forelimb and the left hindlimb. Lead aVL is generated with the positive electrode on the left forelimb and the negative electrode as the combined average of the right forelimb and the left hindlimb. Lead aVF is generated with the positive electrode on the left hindlimb and the negative electrode as the combined average of the right and left forelimbs.

ACQUISITION OF THE ELECTROCARDIOGRAM

The ECG should be recorded in a standardized manner in a quiet environment where no other electrical devices are being used, to avoid electrical and mechanical interference. The patient should be placed in right lateral recumbency with the limbs perpendicular to the body. Dyspneic patients may need to be recorded in sternal recumbency.

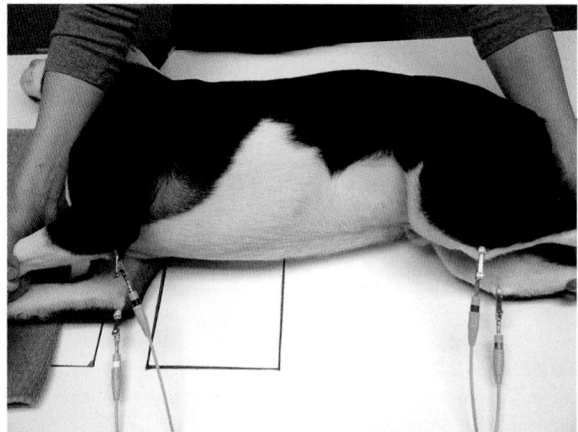

FIGURE 25-31 Example of correct positioning and lead placement for performing electrocardiography (ECG). Note that the dog is in right lateral recumbency, the limbs are perpendicular to the body, and the white electrode is on the right forelimb, the black electrode on the left forelimb, the green electrodes on the right hindlimb, and the red electrode on the left hindlimb.

> **TECHNICIAN NOTE** Patient movement and panting should be prevented as much as possible to minimize mechanical artifacts on the electrocardiogram (ECG). Respiratory artifact typically is reduced by placing the electrodes more distally on the limb.

The white electrode is attached to the right forelimb, the black electrode to the left forelimb, the green electrode to the right hindlimb, and the red electrode to the left hindlimb (Figure 25-31). Electrodes (attached to alligator clips or adhesive patches) may be placed proximal or distal to the elbow or stifle. Alcohol or conductive gel should be applied to the electrodes to allow conduction of electrical activity. The ECG is then recorded using a 50 mm/second or a 25 mm/second paper speed and 10 mm/mV calibration in most circumstances.

BASIC CARDIAC CONDUCTION AND ECG WAVEFORMS

The specialized cardiac conduction system is composed of the sinoatrial node (SA), the atrioventricular node (AV), the bundle of His, left and right bundle branches, and Purkinje fibers (Figure 25-32). Pacemaker cells in the SA node initiate an impulse that propagates quickly through the atrial myocardium causing atrial depolarization (corresponding to the P wave on the ECG). The initial SA impulse is conducted more slowly through the AV node to allow complete atrial depolarization to occur before ventricular depolarization. Conduction through the AV node corresponds to the PR interval on the surface ECG. After conduction through the AV node, the impulse conduction velocity increases dramatically, traversing the bundle of His, left and right bundle branches, and Purkinje fibers to cause coordinated, nearly simultaneous left and right ventricular contraction,

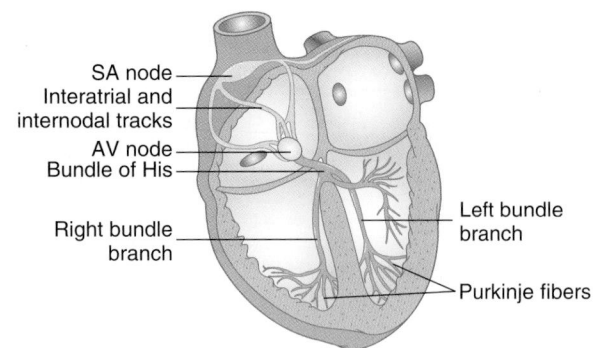

FIGURE 25-32 The cardiac conduction system. (From Thomas J, Lerche P: Anesthesia and analgesia for veterinary technicians, ed 4, St Louis, 2011, Mosby.)

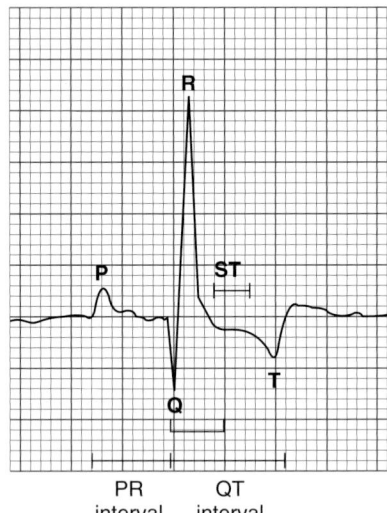

FIGURE 25-33 A normal P-QRS-T complex labeled and with intervals. Note the lack of an obvious S wave. It is not uncommon for normal QRS complexes to have neither a Q wave nor an S wave. Lead II: paper speed, 50 mm/second; sensitivity, 10 mm/mV.

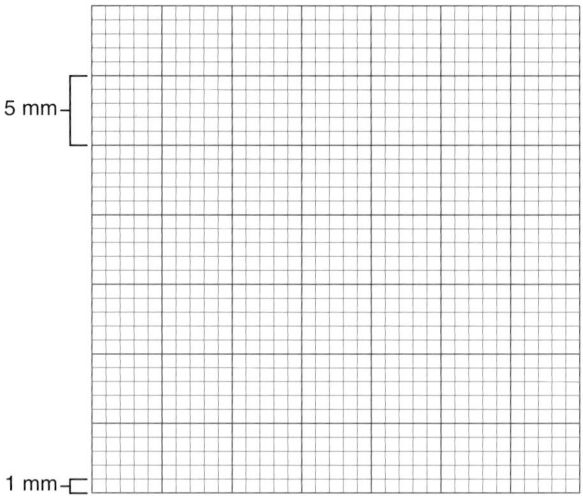

FIGURE 25-34 Standardized electrocardiography (ECG) paper. Each thin line represents 1 mm, and each thick line represents 5 mm.

visualized on the ECG as the QRS complex. The Q wave (initial depolarization of the interventricular septum) is the first negative wave, the R wave (ventricular depolarization) is the first positive wave, and the S wave (basilar ventricular depolarization) is the first negative wave following the R wave. After initial depolarization, the ventricle repolarizes (corresponding to the T wave on the ECG) (Figure 25-33).

ELECTROCARDIOGRAPHIC ANALYSIS

The ECG should be evaluated in a systematic and repetitive manner to avoid misinterpretation and incorrect diagnosis. Four basic features are evaluated on every ECG: heart rate (HR), heart rhythm, P-QRS-T complexes and intervals, and the mean electrical axis. Evaluation of the ECG also requires an understanding of standard ECG paper. All standard ECG paper is composed of narrow vertical and horizontal lines 1 mm apart, creating a grid of 1- mm boxes. The paper is further subdivided every 5 mm by thicker and darker lines,

creating a grid of 5-mm boxes (Figure 25-34). Vertical measurements represent the strength of the electrical impulse expressed in millivolts (mV), and horizontal measurements represent time expressed in seconds. Standard calibration is 10 mm/mV, making each vertical 1-mm box equivalent to 0.1 mV, and each 5-mm box 0.5 mV. Paper speed is typically recorded at a paper speed of 50 mm/second or 25 mm/second, making each horizontal 1-mm box 0.02 second or 0.04 second, respectively, and each 5-mm box 0.1 second or 0.2 second, respectively.

The two most common methods for calculation of HR are average and instantaneous HR. Average HR is determined by counting the number of QRS complexes in a predetermined time period (usually 3 seconds) and multiplying the number of complexes by a factor (20 when 3 seconds is used) to calculate the number of beats per minute (bpm). At 50 mm/second, 30 large (5-mm) boxes are 150 mm in horizontal length, and equal 3 seconds. At 25 mm/second, 15 large boxes are 75 mm in length and also equal 3 seconds. The instantaneous HR is usually used when the rhythm is regular (similar distance between R waves). It is calculated by counting the number of millimeters between two R waves and dividing into 3000 when a paper speed of 50 mm/second is used, or 1500 when a paper speed of 25 mm/second is used.

Evaluation of heart rhythm requires a systematic approach to correctly identify the underlying rhythm and the presence of arrhythmias. This is typically a four-step procedure: (1) general rhythm evaluation, (2) identification of P waves, (3) identification of QRS complexes, and (4) interpretation of the relationship between P waves and QRS complexes.

GENERAL RHYTHM EVALUATION

The first step is to evaluate the overall rhythm and determine whether it is *regular* or *irregular*. If irregularity is present, it should be noted whether there is a pattern to the irregularity (i.e., *regularly irregular* or *irregularly irregular*). This will help the clinician to determine whether an arrhythmia is present, or if the rhythm is of sinus origin (originating from the SA node).

Identification of P Waves

Identification of P waves indicates whether normal coordinated atrial activation, abnormal (ectopic) atrial activation, or no activation is present. Measuring P wave height and width reveals the presence of atrial enlargement.

Identification of QRS Complexes

Identification of QRS complexes allows detection of ventricular depolarization; they should be characterized as normal or abnormal (wide and bizarre). A normal QRS complex likely indicates an electrical impulse of supraventricular origin (arising from above the ventricles and AV node), whereas a wide and bizarre complex could reveal a ventricular ectopic impulse (an electrical impulse arising from the ventricle), ventricular chamber enlargement, or a bundle branch block.

Relationship Between P Waves and QRS Complexes

The relationship between P waves and QRS complexes indicates whether coordinated atrial and ventricular depolarization is present, and must be evaluated to allow the clinician to discern whether the underlying rhythm is of sinus origin or is an arrhythmia. When this relationship is evaluated, it is most important to identify all of the P waves and then to determine whether the PR interval is consistent.

> **TECHNICIAN NOTE** It sometimes is useful to double the calibration to 20 mm/mV, and to look at multiple leads to more easily identify P waves.

Each waveform and interval on the ECG should be correctly identified, both amplitude in millivolts and width in seconds should be measured, and a determination should be made concerning whether or not chamber enlargement is evident (see Figure 25-33 and Table 25-3). All waveform and interval measurements should be performed using lead II.

The P wave documents atrial depolarization and reveals the presence of atrial enlargement. A tall P wave (P-pulmonale) indicates right atrial enlargement, and a wide P wave (P-mitrale) indicates left atrial enlargement. Width is measured from the beginning of the P wave to the end of the P wave. Height is measured from the isoelectric (flat) baseline to the top of the P wave.

The PR interval indicates conduction time through the AV node. Variation in the PR interval may occur with changes in vagal tone or with atrioventricular dissociation. It is measured from the beginning of the P wave to the beginning of the QRS complex (the beginning of the R wave if no Q wave is present).

The QRS complex indicates ventricular depolarization and may reveal abnormalities of ventricular activation. A tall

TABLE 25-3	Normal Canine and Feline Waveform and Interval Measurements	
	CANINE	**FELINE**
Heart rate (HR), bpm	Puppy: 70-220 Toy breed: 70-180 Standard: 70-180 Giant breed: 60-140	120-240
Rhythm	Sinus rhythm Sinus arrhythmia Wandering pacemaker	Sinus rhythm
P wave		
Height	Max: 0.4 mV	Max: 0.2 mV
Width	Max: 0.04 s (giant breed, 0.05 s)	Max: 0.04 s
PR interval	0.06-0.13 s	0.05-0.09 s
QRS		
Height	Small breed: 2.5 mV Large breed: 3.0 mV	Max: 0.9 mV
Width	Small breed: 0.05 s Large breed: 0.06 s	Max: 0.04 s
ST segment		
Depression	No more than 0.2 mV	None
Elevation	No more than 0.15 mV	None
QT interval	0.15-0.25 s	0.12-0.18 s
Electrical axis	+40 to +100	0 to +160

mV, Millivolts; *s*, seconds.

R wave is associated with left ventricular enlargement, and a deep S wave indicates right ventricular enlargement. A wide QRS complex may indicate ventricular enlargement, a bundle branch block, or a ventricular ectopic beat. Width is measured from the beginning of the Q wave (the beginning of the R wave if there is no Q wave) to the end of the S wave. The ST segment indicates the time interval from ventricular depolarization to repolarization. Myocardial ischemia may cause elevation or depression of the ST segment. Width of the ST segment is measured from the end of the S wave to the beginning of the T wave. The T wave indicates ventricular repolarization and may be positive, negative, or biphasic (partly above and partly below the baseline). The QT interval represents total electrical systole and varies inversely with HR. It is measured from the beginning of the Q wave (R wave if no Q wave is present) to the end of the T wave.

The mean electrical axis (MEA) is the net direction of all potentials involved in ventricular depolarization and is related only to the QRS complex. Because the left ventricle has the greatest mass and is the dominant ventricle, the normal MEA is directed toward the left ventricle. If right ventricular hypertrophy or right bundle branch block is significant, the MEA may shift to the right. The MEA can be calculated in a variety of ways. The most common method is to use a six-lead system, determine the isoelectric lead, and find the lead perpendicular to the isoelectric lead. The MEA is in the same direction as the perpendicular lead (positive or negative position). However, a fast method of measuring the MEA is to find the most positive QRS complex in a standard six-lead system, which roughly equates to the MEA.

CARDIAC ARRHYTHMIAS

An *arrhythmia* refers to an irregularity or abnormality in normal cardiac rhythm. Arrhythmias that originate above the AV node (junctional or atrial arrhythmias) are classified as supraventricular arrhythmias, whereas arrhythmias originating below the AV node are ventricular arrhythmias. Arrhythmias can also be categorized on the basis of heart rate (HR). Those with a slow HR are termed *bradyarrhythmias*, and those with a fast HR are *tachyarrhythmias* (see Box 25-7 for a list of common cardiac arrhythmias, including classifications).

NORMAL RHYTHMS
Normal Sinus Rhythm

Normal sinus rhythm (Figure 25-35) is a normal rhythm in the dog and cat, in which each beat is initiated by SA nodal discharge. It is characterized by a regular rhythm with a normal HR, P waves conducted to QRS complexes, and a normal association between P waves and QRS complexes.

Sinus Arrhythmia

Sinus arrhythmia (Figure 25-36) is a normal rhythm in the dog that typically is associated with high vagal tone and/or with breathing. It is not, however, a normal finding in a cat and may indicate high vagal tone caused by underlying central nervous system (CNS), respiratory, or GI disease. When associated with breathing, HR increases with inhalation and decreases with exhalation. It is a *regularly irregular*

BOX 25-7	Classification of Cardiac Arrhythmias

Normal Sinus Impulse Formation
Normal sinus rhythm (a normal rhythm in dogs and cats)
Sinus arrhythmia (a normal rhythm in dogs)
Wandering pacemaker (a normal rhythm in dogs)
Sinus tachycardia
Sinus bradycardia

Disturbances of Supraventricular Impulse Formation
Atrial premature complexes
Atrial tachycardia
Atrial flutter
Atrial fibrillation
Junctional rhythm

Disturbances of Ventricular Impulse Formation
Ventricular premature complexes
Ventricular tachycardia
Ventricular asystole
Ventricular fibrillation

Disturbances of Impulse Conduction
Sinoatrial block
Persistent atrial standstill (silent atrium)
Atrial standstill (hyperkalemia)
First-degree atrioventricular (AV) block
Second-degree AV block
Third-degree (complete) AV block
Bundle branch block

Disturbances of Impulse Formation and Conduction
Sick sinus syndrome

Escape Rhythms
Junctional escape rhythms
Ventricular escape rhythms

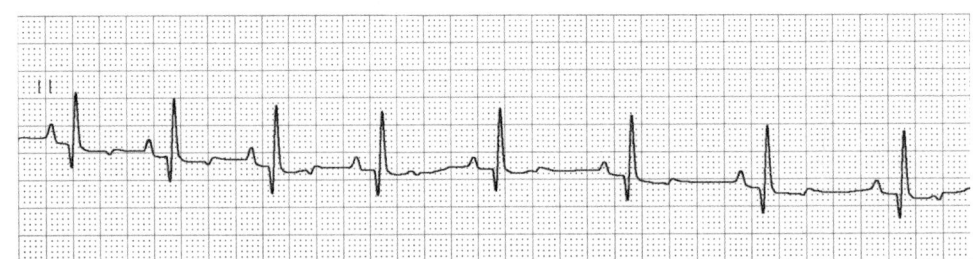

FIGURE 25-35 Normal sinus rhythm (dog, lead II: 50 mm/second, 1 cm/mV). (From Thomas J, Lerche P: Anesthesia and analgesia for veterinary technicians, ed 4, St Louis, 2011, Mosby.)

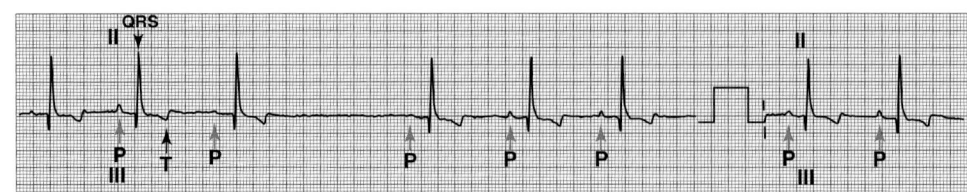

FIGURE 25-36 Example of a normal sinus arrhythmia with a wandering pacemaker. Note the rhythmic increase and decrease in heart rate (HR), as well as the change in amplitude of the P waves with increasing and decreasing HR. Lead II: paper speed, 50 mm/second; sensitivity, 10 mm/mV.

rhythm and is commonly associated with a wandering pace-maker, which is characterized by an increase in the height of the P wave when the HR increases, and a smaller, isoelectric, or negative P wave when the HR decreases.

Sinus Bradycardia

Sinus bradycardia is a rhythm that originates from the SA node, is slower than the normal HR, and has a regular R-R interval (the distance between adjacent R waves). Typically, it is a normal physiologic response to high vagal tone, drugs (e.g., anesthetics, calcium channel inhibitors, beta blockers), or systemic disease (hypothermia or hypothyroidism). Specific therapy is not warranted unless the patient is symptomatic (e.g., is experiencing weakness or collapse).

Sinus Tachycardia

Sinus tachycardia originates from the SA node, is faster than the normal HR, and has a regular R-R interval. It typically occurs as a normal physiologic response to high sympathetic tone caused by pain, excitement, stress, anxiety, or drugs (e.g., atropine, methylxanthines, catecholamines), or as a response to systemic disease such as fever, shock, hyperthyroidism, anemia, hypoxia, or congestive heart failure. Specific therapy typically is not warranted, except for treating the underlying systemic disease.

DISTURBANCES OF SUPRAVENTRICULAR IMPULSE FORMATION

Atrial Premature Complexes

Atrial premature complexes (APCs) (Figure 25-37) are abnormal impulses originating from the atrial myocardium as opposed to the SA node. On an ECG tracing, an APC appears as a premature QRS complex (one that occurs too soon) of identical or nearly identical shape as the normal sinus QRS. Each APC is associated with a premature P wave, which may have an abnormal appearance, and which may be superimposed on the previous T wave. APCs are most commonly associated with left atrial enlargement secondary to structural cardiac disease. Other causes include atrial neoplasia, hyperthyroidism or oversupplementation of thyroid hormone, and hypoxia. Therapy typically is not indicated, but APCs may be a precursor to other atrial arrhythmias.

> **TECHNICIAN NOTE** Atrial premature complexes (APCs) are differentiated from ventricular premature complexes (VPCs) by QRS shape and by the presence or absence of a P wave. APCs have a normally shaped QRS and are associated with a P wave, whereas VPCs have an abnormal, "wide and bizarre" QRS and are not associated with a P wave.

Atrial Tachycardia

Atrial tachycardia (Figure 25-38, *A*) is defined as four or more APCs in succession. Atrial tachycardia usually appears on an ECG tracing as an abrupt or sudden onset and termination of tachycardia with supraventricular (normal or nearly normal) QRS complexes. P waves typically are present but are buried in the previous T wave or ST segment and may be difficult to identify. It is usually a regular rhythm with HR in excess of 200 to 300 bpm. Causes are similar to those of APCs. Therapy may be indicated, especially if the patient experiences weakness, hypotension, or collapse.

Atrial Flutter

Atrial flutter is an uncommon rhythm. It appears on an ECG tracing as a fast rhythm (HR >250 bpm) with supraventricular QRS complexes and saw-toothed flutter waves (F waves—waves similar in appearance to wide P waves, but without a return to an isoelectric baseline between waves) instead of P waves. It may be a regular or irregular rhythm, usually occurs secondary to severe left atrial enlargement, and commonly degenerates into **atrial fibrillation**. Drug therapy typically is warranted, although conversion to a normal rhythm (pharmacologic or electrical cardioversion) may be attempted.

Atrial Fibrillation

Atrial fibrillation (Figure 25-39) is common in dogs, but uncommon in cats.

> **TECHNICIAN NOTE** Atrial fibrillation is identified by lack of P waves and the presence of fibrillatory waves (f waves), and is usually a fast, *irregularly irregular* rhythm with supraventricular (normal or nearly normal) QRS complexes.

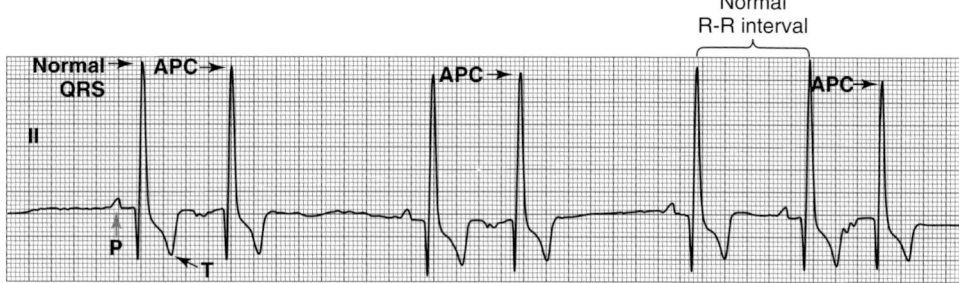

FIGURE 25-37 Example of atrial premature complexes (APCs) (complexes #2, #4, and #7). Note that the QRS complex has a supraventricular (normal) appearance, occurs early compared with a normal R-to-R interval, and has a negative P wave. Lead II: paper speed 50 mm/second; sensitivity, 10 mm/mV.

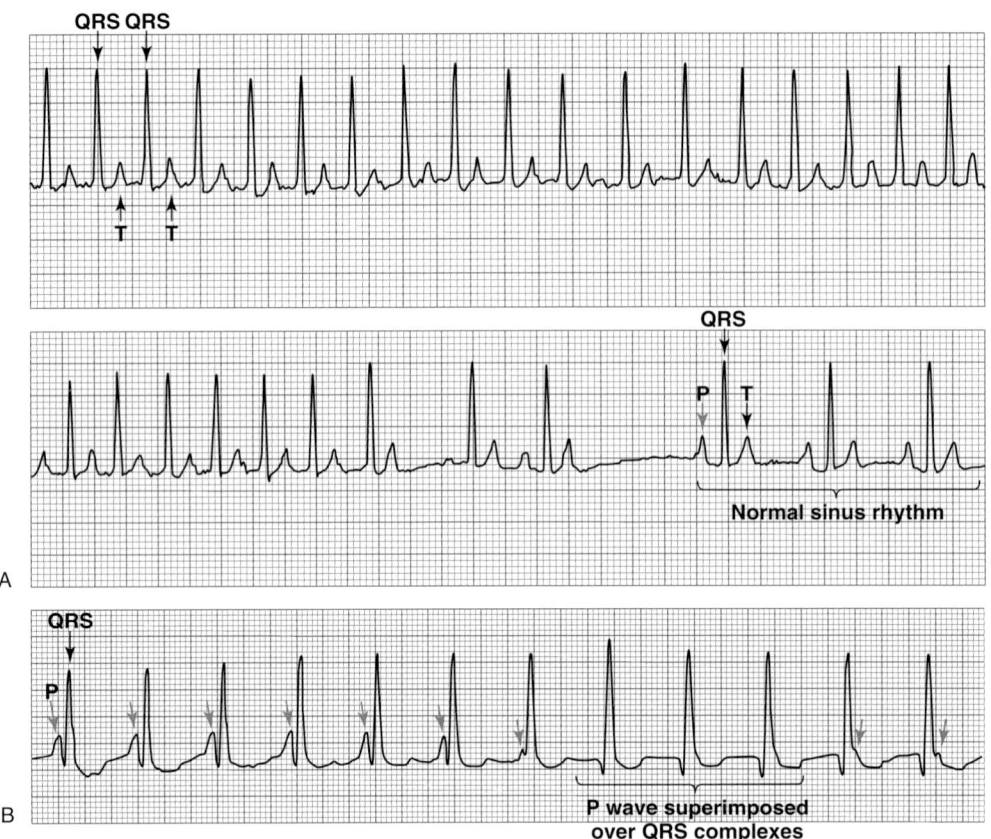

FIGURE 25-38 Examples of supraventricular tachycardias. **A,** Example of an atrial tachycardia. Note the regular tachycardia with supraventricular complexes that abruptly terminates into a normal sinus rhythm. The P waves are buried in the T waves of the preceding complexes. Lead II: paper speed, 25 mm/second; sensitivity, 10 mm/mV. **B,** Example of a junctional tachycardia. Note the regular rhythm, the supraventricular QRS complexes, and the P waves occurring before, superimposed on, and occurring after the QRS complexes. Lead II: paper speed, 50 mm/second; sensitivity, 10 mm/mV.

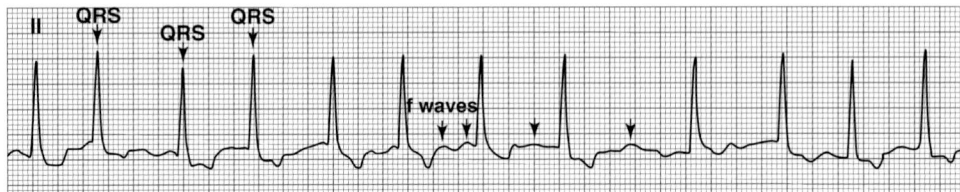

FIGURE 25-39 Example of atrial fibrillation. Note the irregularly irregular rhythm, the lack of obvious P waves, the undulating baseline (f waves), and the supraventricular QRS complexes. Lead II: paper speed, 50 mm/second; sensitivity, 10 mm/mV.

Atrial fibrillation typically is caused by severe left atrial enlargement secondary to underlying structural cardiac disease (e.g., advanced degenerative valve disease, dilated cardiomyopathy). Less commonly, it occurs in giant breed dogs with structurally normal hearts (referred to as *lone atrial fibrillation*) or as the result of high vagal tone. In patients with advanced cardiac disease, therapy is usually indicated.

Junctional Tachycardia

Junctional tachycardia (Figure 25-38, *B*) is a rhythm that originates at the junction of the AV node or from AV nodal tissue. The ECG appearance is similar to that of atrial tachycardia, with supraventricular QRS complexes and a fast,

regular rhythm with abrupt onset and termination; however, P waves may occur before, may be superimposed on, or may occur after the QRS complex. The term *supraventricular tachycardia (SVT)* is commonly used to describe both atrial and junctional tachycardias because they may be indistinguishable. Therapy is similar to that provided for atrial tachycardia.

DISTURBANCES IN VENTRICULAR IMPULSE FORMATION

Ventricular Premature Complexes (VPCs)

Ventricular premature complexes (VPCs) (Figure 25-40) are abnormal beats originating from the ventricular myocardium. The typical appearance is a "wide and bizarre" QRS

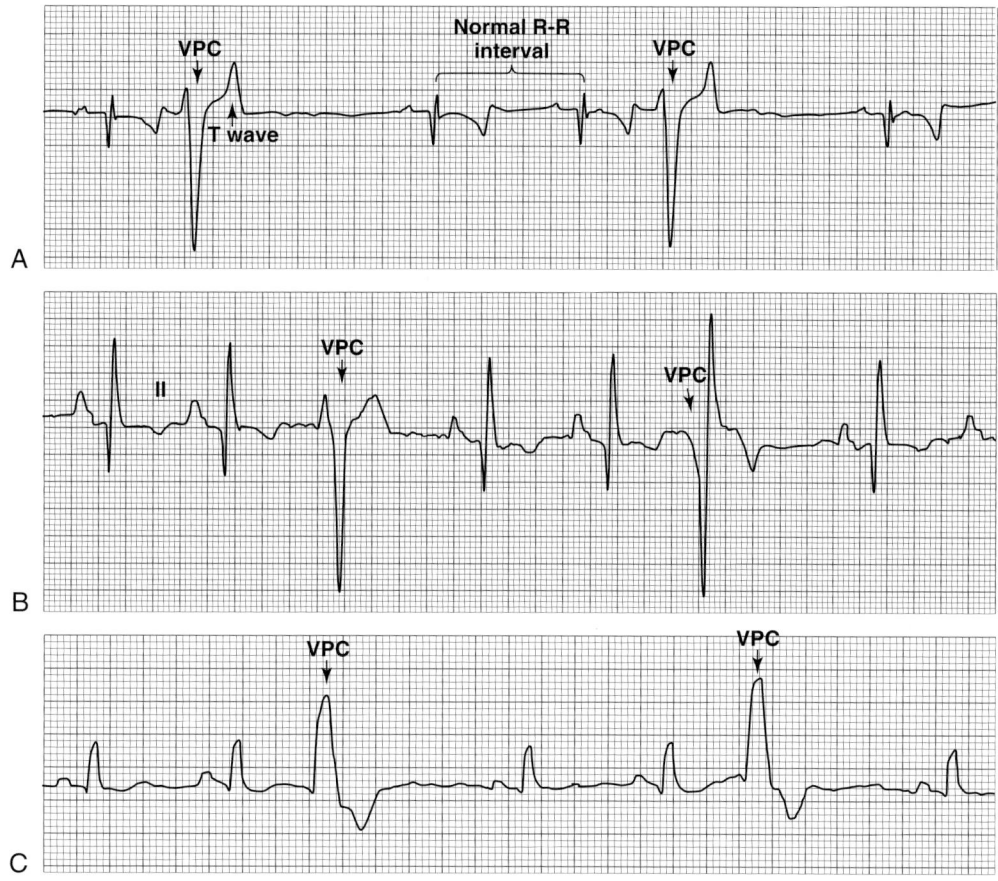

FIGURE 25-40 Examples of single ventricular premature complexes (VPCs). Note the prematurity of the abnormal QRS complexes as compared with the normal sinus R-R interval, the wide and bizarre appearance of the QRS complexes, and the lack of association with P waves. **A,** Examples of single, uniform VPCs (complexes #2 and #5) originating from the left ventricle (as evidenced by the negative QRS complex shape in lead II). **B,** Example of multiform VPCs (complexes #3 and #6). Note the varying shapes of the abnormal QRS complexes. **C,** Example of two VPCs (complexes #3 and #6) originating from the right ventricle (as evidenced by the positive QRS complex in lead II). Lead II: paper speed, 50 mm/second; sensitivity, 10 mm/mV.

complex, indicating that the QRS originated from outside the normal conduction system. There is no association with a P wave, and the QRS occurs earlier than normal. VPCs may occur as single, uniform beats (in which all abnormal QRS complexes are identical), or as multiform beats (in which abnormal QRS complexes differ in appearance). The appearance of two sequential VPCs is called a *couplet*, and of three VPCs in a row is called a *triplet*. A rhythm in which every other beat is a VPC is called *bigeminy*, and one in which every third beat is a VPC is called *trigeminy*. A variety of causes of VPCs are known, including structural cardiac disease, arrhythmogenic right ventricular cardiomyopathy (ARVC), gastric dilatation-volvulus, splenic disease (neoplasia, hematoma), trauma, sepsis, drugs/toxins (e.g., digoxin, digitalis glycosides), electrolyte abnormalities, hyperthyroidism or oversupplementation of thyroid hormone, and excessive catecholamines. Occasional, single, uniform VPCs are not typically treated.

Ventricular Tachycardia

Ventricular tachycardia (Figure 25-41) is a run of four or more VPCs in succession. Ventricular tachycardia may be

sustained (>30 seconds) or paroxysmal (<30 seconds), uniform or multiform. HR may be fast (>160 bpm) or normal (60 to 160 bpm).

> **TECHNICIAN NOTE** R-on-T phenomenon (see Figure 25-41, *B*) is a life-threatening form of ventricular tachycardia characterized by the QRS complex of the VPC originating on the T wave of the preceding beat; it is thought to predispose the patient to ventricular fibrillation.

When HR is normal and the ventricular rhythm competes with the normal sinus rhythm, this may be termed *accelerate idioventricular rhythm (AIVR)*, or slow ventricular tachycardia. Causes of ventricular tachycardia are the same as those of VPCs. Therapy is not always indicated for AIVR. However, therapy is indicated for any rhythm causing weakness, hypotension, or collapse, the presence of R-on-T phenomenon, or HR in excess of 160 bpm.

Ventricular Fibrillation

Ventricular fibrillation (Figure 25-42) is a life-threatening rhythm characterized by chaotic, irregular waves due to lack

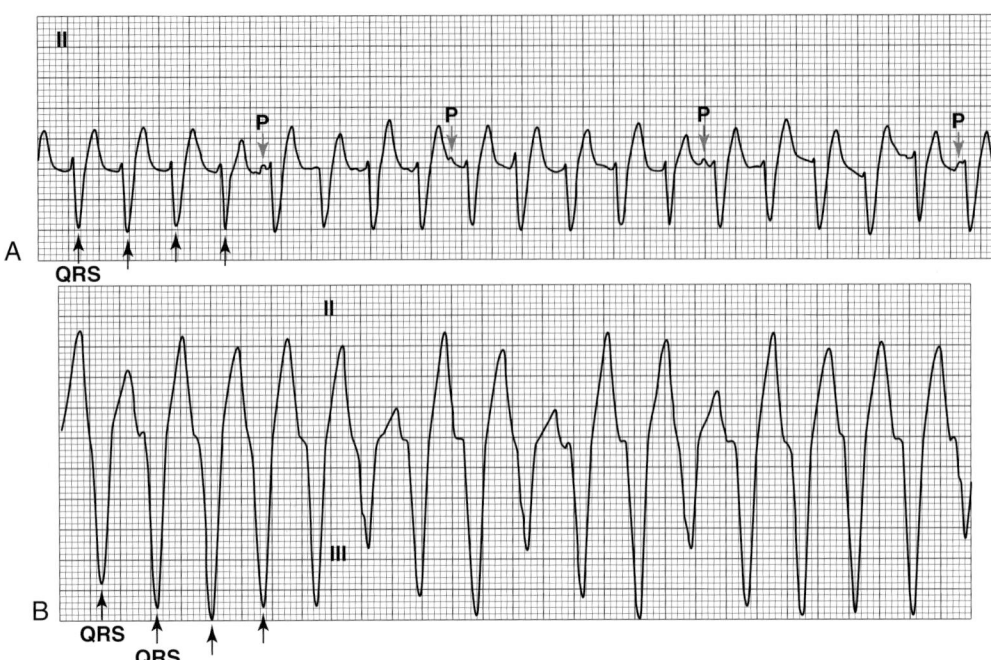

FIGURE 25-41 Examples of ventricular tachycardia. **A,** Uniform ventricular tachycardia. Note the regular rhythm, wide and bizarre QRS morphology, and atrioventricular (AV) dissociation (P waves variably appearing throughout the rhythm not associated with QRS complexes). Lead II: paper speed, 50 mm/second; sensitivity, 10 mm/mV. **B,** Polymorphic ventricular tachycardia R-on-T phenomenon. Note the different morphologies (shapes) of the ventricular complexes with some QRS complexes starting on the preceding T wave with no isoelectric shelf between complexes. Lead II: paper speed, 50 mm/second; calibration, 10 mm/mV.

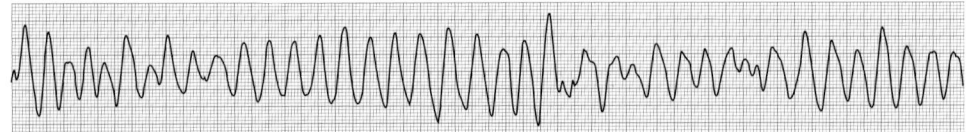

FIGURE 25-42 Example of ventricular fibrillation. Note the lack of coordinated ventricular activity and the chaotic baseline. Lead II: paper speed, 25 mm/second; sensitivity, 10 mm/mV.

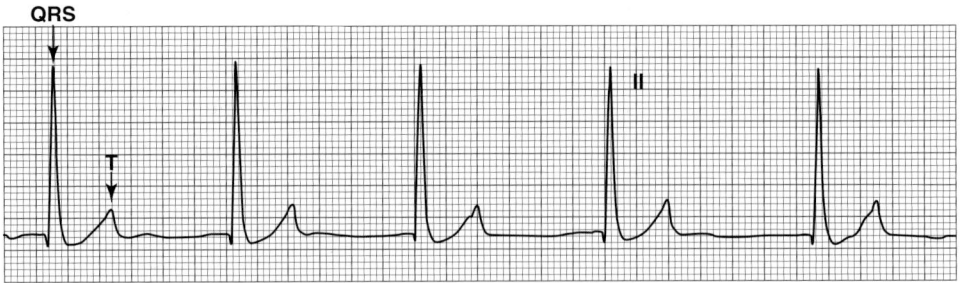

FIGURE 25-43 Example of atrial standstill. Note the lack of P waves, flat baseline, bradycardia, and supraventricular QRS complexes. Lead II: paper speed, 50 mm/second; calibration, 10 mm/mV.

of organized ventricular activity. Electrocardiographically, no evidence of organized cardiac activity (no P-QRS-T complexes) is present. Instead, ventricular fibrillation appears as an unorganized, chaotic baseline. Therapy should be performed immediately with electrical defibrillation.

Ventricular Asystole
Ventricular asystole occurs as the result of lack of ventricular activity and appears as a flat baseline. Therapy should be immediate and should center on restoring a rhythm.

DISTURBANCES OF IMPULSE CONDUCTION
Atrial Standstill
Atrial standstill (Figure 25-43) is a rhythm in which atrial depolarization does not occur when the SA node discharges. It is characterized by lack of P waves, a flat baseline, supraventricular QRS complexes, and bradycardia. The most common cause of atrial standstill is hyperkalemia (typically, serum potassium >8.0 mEq/L) associated with systemic disease (e.g., Addison's disease, urethral obstruction, renal failure, diabetic ketoacidosis).

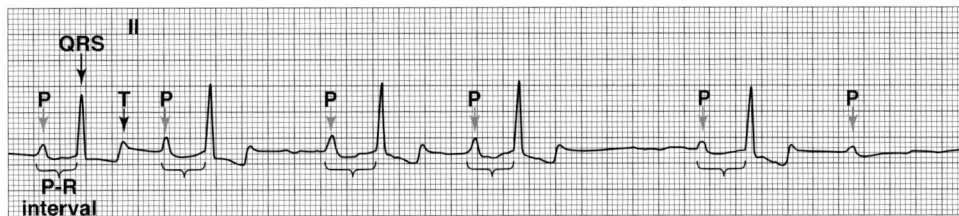

FIGURE 25-44 Electrocardiographic (ECG) example of second-degree atrioventricular (AV) block, Mobitz type I. Note the progressive prolongation of the PR interval before AV block occurs (P wave without a QRS complex). Lead II: paper speed, 50 mm/second; sensitivity, 10 mm/mV.

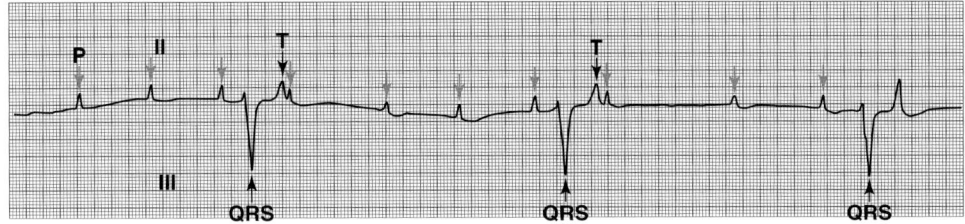

FIGURE 25-45 Electrocardiographic (ECG) example of third-degree (complete) atrioventricular (AV) block. Note the lack of association of P waves with QRS complexes, the wide and bizarre QRS complexes, and the regular atrial and ventricular rhythms, as well as the normal atrial heart rate (HR) (≈140 bpm) and the slow ventricular HR (≈35 bpm). Lead II: paper speed, 50 mm/second; sensitivity, 10 mm/mV.

However, certain breeds of dogs such as English Springer Spaniels may develop a disease referred to as *silent atrium* or *persistent atrial standstill*, in which the atrial myocardium is replaced by fibrous tissue that impairs atrial depolarization. Treatment of atrial standstill secondary to hyperkalemia is aimed at reducing serum potassium and protecting the myocardium. Pacemaker implantation is necessary for treatment of persistent atrial standstill not due to electrolyte disturbances.

First-Degree AV Block

First-degree AV block occurs when conduction through the AV node is delayed, causing a prolonged PR interval on the ECG. First-degree AV block is typically idiopathic, due to AV nodal fibrosis, drug induced, or due to vagal stimulation. Therapy is not indicated, although first-degree AV block may be a precursor to more advanced AV conduction disease.

Second-Degree AV Block

Second-degree AV block (Figure 25-44) is a rhythm characterized by intermittent disruption of AV nodal conduction. On an ECG tracing, some P waves are associated with QRS complexes, and other P waves are not followed by a QRS complex. Second-degree AV block is further subdivided into Mobitz type I and Mobitz type II second-degree AV block. Mobitz type I (Wenckebach periodicity) is due to high vagal tone and is characterized by progressive prolongation of the PR interval until AV nodal conduction is blocked. Mobitz type II is considered more serious and is characterized by a consistent PR interval before AV block. The term *high-grade second-degree AV block* indicates that multiple P waves in a row are not conducted to a QRS complex. It is categorized by the number of P waves occurring in a row before a coordinated P-QRS-T complex. For instance, a 2:1 block means

that there are two P waves for every one QRS complex. High-grade second-degree AV block that causes symptoms such as weakness, lethargy, or collapse is treated with pacemaker implantation.

Third-Degree AV Block

Third-degree AV block (complete AV Block) (Figure 25-45) occurs when there is no conduction of sinus impulses through the AV node. P waves and QRS complexes are completely disassociated. P wave morphology and rate are normal, but QRS complexes are wide and bizarre because of a ventricular escape rhythm, and the ventricular rate is slow (≈40 to 60 bpm). Usually, this rhythm occurs as the result of degeneration and fibrosis of the AV node; however, drugs (e.g., digoxin or beta blocker toxicity), infiltrative myocardial disease, and myocarditis are other possible causes. This condition is treated with pacemaker implantation.

Bundle Branch Block

Bundle branch block (Figure 25-46) is a conduction disturbance that occurs when the sinus impulse is blocked at the level of the left or right bundle branch but is conducted normally through the opposite bundle branch. The ventricle associated with the blocked impulse then is depolarized by cell-to-cell conduction from the normal depolarized ventricle. The ECG appearance of a left bundle branch block consists of wide QRS complexes that are positive in leads I, II, III, and aVF, and that are associated with P waves. The ECG appearance of a right bundle branch block reveals wide QRS complexes with deep S waves in leads I, II, III, and aVF, and that are associated with P waves. Bundle branch blocks may be congenital or idiopathic. Other causes include fibrosis, cardiomyopathy, trauma, and neoplasia. No therapy is indicated.

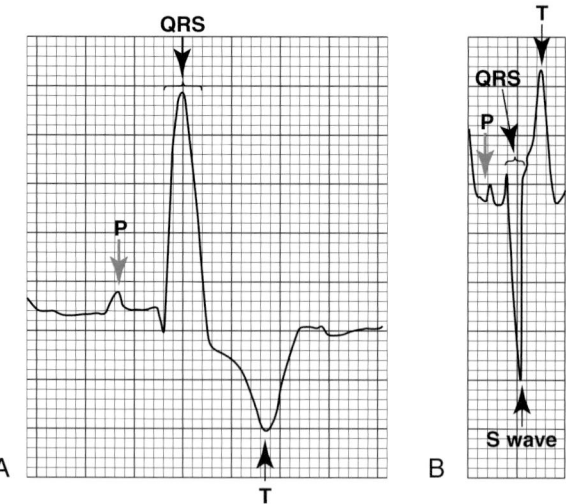

FIGURE 25-46 Electrocardiographic (ECG) examples of left and right bundle branch blocks. Note the wide QRS complexes associated with a normal P wave. **A,** Example of left bundle branch block. Note the wide QRS complex that is positive in lead II. Lead II: paper speed, 50 mm/second; sensitivity, 10 mm/mV. **B,** Example of right bundle branch block. Note the wide QRS complex with a deep S wave in lead II. Lead II: paper speed, 25 mm/second; sensitivity, 10 mm/mV.

> **TECHNICIAN NOTE**   A bundle branch block and a ventricular premature complex (VPC) have wide QRS complexes and can be distinguished from each other by the presence of an associated P wave. Bundle branch blocks have an associated P wave, but VPCs do not.

DISTURBANCES OF IMPULSE FORMATION AND CONDUCTION

Sick Sinus Syndrome

Sick sinus syndrome (SSS) is characterized by abnormal sinus impulse formation and conduction causing a combination of arrhythmias: sinus arrest, sinus bradycardia, atrial tachycardia (bradycardia-tachycardia syndrome), AV nodal conduction block, and intermittent ventricular or junctional escape beats. The underlying cause is unknown. SSS occurs most commonly in older female Miniature Schnauzers, Cocker Spaniels, West Highland White Terriers, and Dachshunds. Clinical signs are related to weakness and collapse. Medical therapy typically is unsuccessful, with most patients requiring pacemaker implantation.

ESCAPE RHYTHMS

Junctional Escape Beats and Junctional Escape Rhythm

Junctional escape beats and junctional escape rhythm occur when the AV node acts as a subsidiary pacemaker in the event that a sinus impulse is not generated. The ECG appearance of a junctional escape beat is a supraventricular QRS complex that occurs after a pause of more than two normal R-R intervals, with a negative or retrograde P wave occurring before, on, or after the QRS complex. A junctional escape rhythm is a sequence of junctional escape beats. The rate of

a junctional escape rhythm is approximately 60 bpm. Junctional escape beats and junctional escape rhythms should not be suppressed.

Ventricular Escape Beats and Ventricular Escape Rhythm

Ventricular escape beats and ventricular escape rhythm occur when the bundle of His and/or Purkinje fibers act as a subsidiary pacemaker when a normal sinus or junctional impulse is not generated. A ventricular escape beat appears as a wide and bizarre QRS complex without a P wave that occurs after a pause of more than two normal R-R intervals. A ventricular escape rhythm is a succession of ventricular escape beats with a rate of approximately 30 to 40 bpm. This rhythm should not be suppressed because it is the only means of maintaining cardiac output.

Equine Emergency Nursing

In equine practice, emergencies make up a large portion of the caseload. The most common emergencies are directly related to the GI system (e.g., **colic**), the respiratory system (e.g., respiratory distress), and the musculoskeletal system (e.g., fractures, wounds). When emergencies occur, there are two potential waves of action: the field response and the referral. The field veterinary team is on the front line of triage, action, and care. Actions of team members may be immediately curative, thus eliminating the need for referral; rapid and stabilizing, thus allowing improved outcome with early and efficient referral; or humane and compassionate, thus allowing elimination of prolonged pain and suffering through euthanasia. For these decisions to be made efficiently and effectively, the veterinary staff needs to be organized, prepared, and thoughtful. These three attributes are characteristics of a great veterinary technician and are essential for success. A well-trained veterinary technician is the backbone of an efficient response to an emergency, especially initial assessment and triage, secured safety of the environment for clients and patients, organization of all supplies, and facilitation of procedures and diagnostics.

The purpose of this section of the chapter is to reflect on the most common equine emergencies seen in the field and the referral clinic, and to specifically address core points that will prepare a veterinary technician to be a valuable and efficient member of the veterinary team.

GASTROINTESTINAL TRACT

One of the most common emergencies in equine practice is colic. The term *colic* refers to any condition that causes abdominal pain. Horses exhibiting signs of colic in the field can be broadly divided into two categories: those that will resolve with minimal or no treatment, and those that will not. The former group encompasses the vast majority of cases. The recommendation is for all colicky patients to receive professional medical attention, but many patients will improve before a veterinarian arrives. In cases that improve, it is impossible to determine the exact cause of the discomfort, although it is believed that gas or spasmodic colic is the most common cause. This type of colic is due to cramping of the GI tract or excessive accumulation of air within the lumen of the bowel. A large percentage of patients will respond to administration of analgesics (e.g., flunixin meglumine), hand walking, sedation with xylazine or detomidine, and laxatives (specifically mineral oil) given through a nasogastic tube. When cases of colic do not respond to this minimal level of treatment, they fall into the smaller percentage of horses, which require intensive treatment (medical or surgical) to correct the condition. It is important to remember that GI pain that is unresponsive to treatment is a potentially life-threatening condition; therefore, early recognition and referral to a tertiary medical center capable of aggressive therapy are essential for the survival of these patients.

For the veterinary hospital staff to be successful in dealing with these acute, often dramatic emergencies, staff members must be prepared with proper supplies and technical support. To be prepared, it is incumbent upon the veterinary technician to have a basic knowledge of supplies and of the technique of the colic workup, as well as knowledge of conditions that commonly cause colic in the horse. When setting up for the emergency, the technician should envision the events that may transpire. However, it is not uncommon for an emergency to arrive that is not routine; therefore, a minimum colic setup should consist of the supplies listed in Box 25-8.

GENERAL PHYSICAL EXAMINATION

Once the doors of the trailer are opened after arrival of the patient to the hospital, an immediate visual assessment of pain and the severity of the condition should commence. This visual triage is essential for maintaining the safety of the patient, the client, and medical personnel. It is important for veterinary staff members to assume control and ensure safety of the environment, while keeping themselves in an uncompromised position. Once unloaded from the trailer, the patient should be moved to the designated examination area, which was previously prepared by the veterinary technician. It is in this area that the general physical examination and most of the diagnostic procedures will occur. The examiner needs a thermometer, a stethoscope, and a keen sense of observation to perform a thorough physical examination. The importance of observation cannot be overstated.

The typical colic examination should include assessment of pain, attitude, temperature, pulse, respiration, mucous membrane color, capillary refill time, and GI motility. The degree of pain can be related to the severity of GI disease.

> **TECHNICIAN NOTE** Horses that are stoic can be very difficult to assess accurately because their level of pain may not reflect the severity of their disease.

Mild pain is recognized by pawing, stretching out—with or without attempts to urinate, curling the upper lip (flehmen

---

BOX 25-8 List of Supplies for a Colic Workup

Nasogastric (NG) Intubation
NG tube, two or more buckets, pump, towels, elastic adhesive tape or nonelastic adhesive tape, and 3-ml syringe case

Standard Blood Work
20-Gauge needle, 12-ml syringe, and purple (ethylenediaminetetraacetic acid [EDTA]), red, and blue top tubes

Sedation
Xylazine, detomidine, butorphanol, romifidine, and acepromazine

IV Catheter
14-Gauge × 5¼″ catheter or smaller (based on patient size), short extension with injection port, suture, normal saline flush, clippers, chlorhexidine or povidone-iodine scrub, 3 ml mepivacaine, examination gloves, and sterile gloves

Ultrasound
Ultrasound machine, 70% isopropyl alcohol, ultrasound gel, and clippers

Rectal Examination
Palpation sleeve, water-soluble lubricant, towels, hyoscine butylbromide (if requested by the attending veterinarian), and lidocaine in a syringe with a long extension tubing connected (if requested by the attending veterinarian)

Abdominocentesis
Clippers, chlorhexidine or povidone-iodine scrub, 3 ml mepivacaine, examination gloves, sterile gloves, 18-gauge × 1.5″ needles, teat cannula, metal bitch catheter, Tuohy needle, sterile 4 × 4-gauge sponges, #15 scalpel blade, purple top tube with the EDTA shaken out, and red top tube

---

response), or standing quietly without a desire to move or eat. Horses frequently respond to light sedation or mild exercise, such as walking. Those with moderate pain can exhibit similar signs, but usually in combination with an elevated heart rate (>50 bpm). They may attempt to repeatedly lie down and stand up, and even occasionally roll while recumbent. Horses with moderate pain often remain comfortable for only short periods (<1 hour), or not at all, despite sedation. Severe abdominal pain is manifest in these horses as violent attempts to throw themselves to the ground, inability to stand for long periods, constant rolling while down, and banging of the side of the head on the ground. Sedation may have no effect, despite the type or amount. A history of severe pain before arrival is often confirmed by the presence of abrasions over the head, face, eyes, and bony prominences of the body (Figure 25-47), as well as a large amount of dirt, hay, or mud in the hair coat.

> **TECHNICIAN NOTE** Abdominal distention can be difficult to assess in a large horse; therefore, it is always important to question the owner regarding the horse's normal abdominal contour.

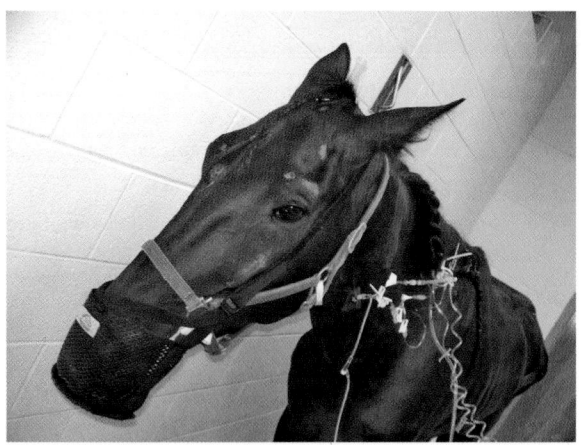

FIGURE 25-47 Colic patients can present with external trauma from pain. Note the periorbital swelling and abrasions.

TABLE 25-4	Relative Sizes of Nasogastric Tubes Used in Equine Patients of Different Sizes		
PATIENT SIZE	OD, INCHES	ID, INCHES	LENGTH, FEET
Miniature horse	¼ (6.4 mm)	⅛ (3.2 mm)	5
Foal	⅜ (9.5 mm)	¼ (6.4 mm)	10
Yearling	⁷⁄₁₆ (11 mm)	¼ (6.4 mm)	12
Small horse	½ (12.7 mm)	⁵⁄₁₆ (7.9 mm)	12
Large horse	⅝ (15.9 mm)	⅜ (9.5 mm)	12
Extra-large horse	¾ (19.1 mm)	½ (12.7 mm)	10

ID, Inner diameter; *OD,* outer diameter.

GI motility can be estimated by auscultation of the abdomen with a stethoscope, beginning in the paralumbar fossa and proceeding along the caudal edge of the costal margin toward the xiphoid. This should be performed on both sides of the abdomen. Sounds typically heard may be the result of large intestinal motility (borborygmi). Normal large intestinal motility is perceived as prolonged fluid rushing that occurs every 2 to 4 minutes. In addition, high-pitched tinkling sounds can be auscultated in the right paralumbar fossa every 2 to 4 minutes and are routinely associated with cecal motility. Always note that the complete absence of GI sounds in a colicky patient is a significant finding. When GI sounds are documented in the record, it is common practice to record the auscultation by abdominal quadrant (upper right, upper left, lower right, and lower left) and by intensity of the sounds (absent, decreased, normal, or increased). Frequently, a very large volume of gas will accumulate in the lumen of the bowel, severely stretching the wall of the large bowel and cecum. To detect this accumulation, simultaneous auscultation and percussion of the abdomen is necessary. This is achieved by percussing or "flicking" the area of the flank circumferentially around the head of the stethoscope and listening for a characteristic "ping."

> **TECHNICIAN NOTE** Various medications can alter heart rate, respiratory rate, attitude, degree of pain, and GI motility; therefore, it is always beneficial to assess these parameters before administration.

Many colic workups include submission of blood for complete blood count (CBC), biochemical profile, packed cell volume (PCV), total protein (TP), lactate, and fibrinogen; therefore, red top, purple top, and blue top blood tubes should be available. After the physical examination and blood work, the complete colic workup may include the following procedures, which are described in detail.

NASOGASTRIC INTUBATION

Passage of a nasogastric tube is an incredibly important and common procedure that may be performed by a veterinarian or an experienced veterinary technician. This procedure is important because horses will not typically vomit, and therefore excessive accumulation of gas and fluid within the stomach can lead to gastric rupture if it is not removed. When very full and possibly on the verge of rupture, an engorged stomach can be the cause of pain, and removal of this fluid and gas can lead to temporary or permanent resolution of pain. Usually, reflux of fluid or gas out of the nasogastric tube indicates that the horse is unable to pass fluid or air through the GI tract in an oral-to-aboral direction. Typically, but not exclusively, the reason for this is a small intestinal functional disorder (**ileus**) or mechanical obstruction (intraluminal or extraluminal lesion). With these problems, the ingesta will eventually back up into the stomach, causing severe distention and pain. Excess fluid that is removed is termed *gastric reflux,* and the amount should be noted.

> **TECHNICIAN NOTE** Because of the consequences of gastric rupture, nasogastric intubation should be performed in all patients examined for abdominal pain.

Nasogastric tubes are available in a variety of sizes and materials (Table 25-4). In general, the size of the patient determines the size of the tube, and in very small horses, such as miniatures and foals, a stallion catheter is oftentimes used. To perform the procedure, the patient may need to be restrained with a twitch, sedated, or both. The smooth end of the tube is lubricated with water or a water-soluble lubricant and is passed through the nose, ventral meatus, and pharynx until the epiglottis is reached. Before it can be advanced farther, the horse must swallow to promote movement of the tube down the esophagus and into the stomach. Waiting for this to happen requires patience on the part of the operator. Once the tube is in the stomach, fluid or air may be readily evacuated, or it may be necessary to pump in 1 to 2 L of water to create a siphon effect that will promote emptying. Evacuation of stomach contents in this fashion should continue until the veterinarian or the veterinary technician is satisfied that the stomach is sufficiently empty. The total amount of water that was introduced to create the siphon should be subtracted from the total amount of gastric reflux; the result is considered the net amount of reflux and should be recorded. If no reflux is obtained, the veterinarian should be consulted before the tube is removed because introduction of various therapeutic agents (e.g., mineral oil, water, electrolytes) may be indicated. The normal stomach contents are light green to yellow, may be foamy, have minimal odor, and usually are less than 2 L in volume. If more than 2 L of reflux is obtained, the tube may be left in place and secured for future attempts at fluid retrieval.

> **TECHNICIAN NOTE** Epistaxis (nosebleeding) is a common occurrence after removal or passage of a nasogastric tube. This is rarely a serious complication and generally resolves within minutes.

ABDOMINAL PALPATION PER RECTUM

It can be very difficult to identify the cause of colic based on the physical examination and nasogastric intubation alone; therefore, rectal palpation is performed by a veterinarian to help identify what section of the GI tract, if any, is responsible for the signs of colic. Major questions to answer during a rectal examination include the following: (1) Are the normally palpable structures in the correct location? (2) Is an abnormal amount of gas distention noted? (3) Is the small intestine distended and palpable? (4) Is a palpable impaction present in the colon, cecum, or ileum? (5) Are any masses present in the abdominal cavity or in surrounding organs? and (6) Is the bowel located in the inguinal rings?

> **TECHNICIAN NOTE** Remember to take the temperature before performing the rectal examination because air introduced into the rectum during palpation can decrease the accuracy of the measurement.

Rectal tears are by far the most serious complication of rectal examination, and they can be absolutely life threatening. To minimize the risk for this complication, the horse should be restrained, ideally in a standing stock whenever possible, and sedated and/or twitched whenever necessary. A plastic rectal sleeve is used to protect the veterinarian's arm from fecal contamination, and copious amounts of water-soluble lubricant are essential. For horses that strain, hyoscine butylbromide can be administered intravenously, or 2% lidocaine can be administered intrarectally or, less frequently, by caudal epidural injection to relax the GI tract. Upon completion of the examination, it is important to examine the sleeve for evidence of blood.

> **TECHNICIAN NOTE** Rectal examination on a colicky patient should be performed only by a veterinarian and in a horse that is adequately restrained.

ABDOMINAL ULTRASOUND

Because of the size of a horse, it is impossible to evaluate the entire abdomen by rectal palpation. Therefore, when it is available, transabdominal ultrasound can be a valuable tool for performing a more thorough evaluation. Ultrasound is a noninvasive, nonpainful technique that is used to identify the normal appearance of and abnormalities associated with the GI tract, other abdominal organs, the thoracic cavity, and the peritoneal cavity, such as abdominal fluid. It may be necessary to clip long or thick hair to obtain an acceptable image; however, efforts should first be made to obtain an image by saturating the hair and skin with isopropyl alcohol. The best images are obtained with probes that are 2.5 to 10.0 MHz in frequency.

Common abnormalities that can be identified by transabdominal ultrasound include distention of small and large intestine, increased wall thickness of GI viscera, and abnormal motility of specific portions of the GI tract. Transabdominal ultrasound can also be used to assess the appearance of the kidneys, liver, spleen, and reproductive tract, and to determine the amount and appearance of abdominal fluid. It is important to remember that thoracic problems can lead to signs of colic; therefore, the chest should also be examined for abnormalities such as diaphragmatic hernia, pneumonia, pleural fluid, or neoplasia.

ABDOMINOCENTESIS

Evaluating the abdominal fluid, which bathes the GI tract, is a very important method of assessing the health of the bowel. This procedure is known as *abdominocentesis* or a "belly tap." The abdominal cavity should be a sterile environment, although this can change in the presence of devitalized or ruptured bowel. Therefore, it is essential to maintain aseptic technique when performing a belly tap. A 10 × 10-cm area of the most dependent part of the abdomen, usually centered 3 to 5 cm caudal to the xiphoid and 3 to 5 cm to the right of the midline, is clipped. The area is cleaned with an initial surgical prep, followed by a sterile surgical prep, and then is blocked with 2 to 5 ml of 2% lidocaine infused into the skin and subcutaneous tissues at the intended site for centesis. A variety of instruments may be used to collect abdominal fluid (Figure 25-48). Once the abdomen has been entered, the fluid should be allowed to drip into purple top (ethylenediaminetetraacetic acid [EDTA]) and red top tubes. The fluid is examined visually for color and clarity. Additional information may be obtained by measuring total protein, glucose, and lactate, and by submitting a sample to the laboratory for cell count, cytologic examination, Gram stain, and culture. Normal peritoneal fluid values are found in Table 25-5.

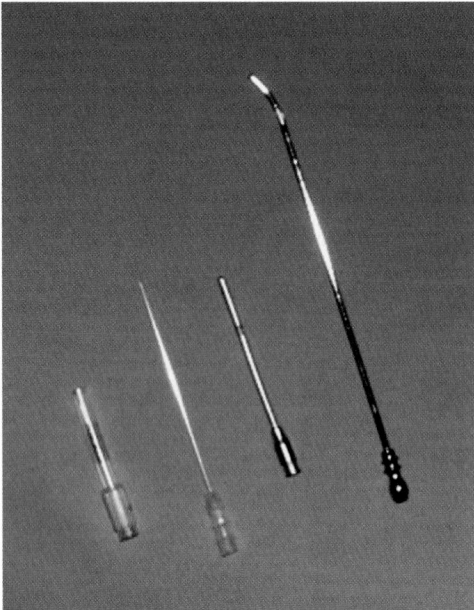

FIGURE 25-48 Common instruments used to perform abdominocentesis. From left to right: 18-gauge × 1.5-inch needle, 20-gauge × 3.5-inch needle, sterile teat cannula, and sterile metal bitch catheter.

TABLE 25-5	Normal Peritoneal Fluid Values	
GROSS APPEARANCE	**CELLULARITY**	**MOLECULAR COMPONENTS**
Clear or straw/ yellow colored	WBC ≤5000 cells/μl ≈50% neutrophils	TP ≤2.5 g/dl Lactate ≤2.0 mmol/dl Glucose >50 mg/dl OR <50 mg/dl difference from blood glucose pH >7.3

TP, Total protein; *WBC,* white blood cell.

ABDOMINAL RADIOGRAPHY

Although not a standard diagnostic procedure for most colic examinations, radiography can be valuable for a few specific conditions. Generally, images of the abdomen reveal low detail because of the large size of a horse's abdomen and the limited ability of the equipment to produce enough radiation to create highly detailed images. It is important to remember that images of the abdomen require a lot of radiation, so personnel should be fully protected to minimize exposure. Radiography is most useful for identifying enteroliths (stones within the GI tract), for examining foals and small horses, such as American miniature horses (in which a rectal examination is not possible), and for performing contrast studies to identify gastric emptying delay.

SPECIFIC CONDITIONS

The goal of the aforementioned examination and diagnostic testing is to decide on a diagnosis and formulate an effective therapeutic plan, whether medical or surgical. Unfortunately, an absolute diagnosis often is not possible after a workup, yet appropriate management of the condition is

BOX 25-9	Common Lesions of the Gastrointestinal Tract

Esophagus
• Obstruction (choke)
Stomach
• Impaction
• Ulceration
• Neoplasia
Small intestine
• Intraluminal obstruction
    • Ascarid impaction
    • Intussusception
    • Ileal impaction
• Extraluminal obstruction
    • Lipoma
    • Herniation
        ■ Epiploic foramen entrapment
        ■ Scrotal hernia
        ■ Umbilical hernia
        ■ Mesenteric rent
        ■ Congenital abnormality
        ■ Diaphragmatic hernia
    • Volvulus
• Ileus
    • Duodenitis/proximal jejunitis (DPJ)
Large intestine
• Intraluminal obstruction
    • Cecal impaction
    • Large colon impaction
    • Small colon impaction
    • Cecocolic intussusception
    • Enterolithiasis
• Extraluminal obstruction
    • Large colon displacement
    • Large colon volvulus
• Ileus
    • Right dorsal colitis
    • Salmonellosis

necessary. To help formulate a plan in the absence of a diagnosis, it is important to have an idea of common conditions affecting each part of the GI tract. Listed in Box 25-9 are common lesions that affect each section of bowel. It is important to remember that each condition may be associated to some degree with the region of the country the horse is in, the age and breed of the horse, the diet and function of the horse (broodmare, racehorse, etc.), and its medical history.

ABDOMINAL EXPLORATION

After examination and workup, surgical intervention may be necessary. When a preoperative diagnosis is accurate, abdominal exploratory surgery is undertaken for therapeutic purposes; however, most colic surgeries are actually the final and most invasive diagnostic step and are therapeutic as well. When this occurs, it is important to remain efficient because the patient will require preoperative preparation to minimize anesthetic time and to ensure the best chance for a positive outcome. In all cases, an IV catheter should be placed, through which perioperative antibiotics, fluids, anti-inflammatories, sedatives, and anesthetic induction drugs can be administered.

> **TECHNICIAN NOTE** The most common reason for surgical intervention in the colic patient is continual pain despite sedation. A tetanus toxoid may have to be given at the discretion of the veterinarian if the patient has not been vaccinated within the past 4 to 6 months, or if the vaccination history is not known.

If it is safe to do so, the ventral abdomen should be clipped from the xiphoid to the inguinal region and from flank to flank, and an initial surgical prep should be performed to remove all gross contamination. The hooves should be picked out and debris removed. Once the patient is anesthetized, a final touchup of the clipping and another initial scrub can be performed. When the patient is in the final location for surgery, a final surgical prep should be performed using chlorhexidine or povidone-iodine scrub.

RESPIRATORY TRACT

The primary purpose of the respiratory tract is oxygen exchange. More specifically, it is to take oxygen into the blood for delivery to tissues and cells and to eliminate carbon dioxide produced by tissues and cells. Failure of oxygen exchange can lead to respiratory distress, which is an emergency. Most commonly, but not exclusively, respiratory emergencies present as the result of an inability of oxygen to diffuse across the alveoli because of lung disease (e.g., pneumonia), an inability of the lungs to expand enough to take in oxygen (e.g., because of pneumothorax), or an inability of oxygen to reach the lungs (e.g., because of upper airway or trachea obstruction). It is important to remember that a horse can present with respiratory distress, or to a lesser degree tachypnea, if it is unable to deliver oxygen to the tissues (e.g., because of anemia). When a patient presents with respiratory distress, it is important to quickly identify the cause. The most efficient way to do this is to divide respiratory emergencies into two broad categories: upper airway and lower airway.

Upper respiratory tract emergencies are among the most common types of respiratory emergencies in general. They are almost always the result of obstruction of airflow to the lungs; are easily recognized as severe distress, anxiety, and a loud noise on inspiration (inspiratory stridor); and should be associated with normal lung sounds on auscultation. In contrast, conditions of the lower respiratory tract are usually due to lung disease (pneumonia or chronic obstructive pulmonary disease [COPD]) or failure to inflate the lungs (due to pneumothorax). Pneumonia is characterized by the presence of abnormal lung sounds, including crackles and wheezes, and COPD is characterized by rapid shallow breaths, expiratory stridor, and abnormal lungs sounds. Pneumothorax is commonly secondary to external trauma to the chest cavity that allows influx of air into the pleural space, which collapses the lung and prevents reexpansion. A patient with this condition will present with rapid, shallow breathing and expiratory stridor; however, lung sounds characteristically will be absent. It is important to remember that severe pneumonia can lead to pleuropneumonia, and severe external trauma can lead to thoracic bleeding. Both conditions can cause an accumulation of fluid into the chest cavity that can present in a similar manner to a pneumothorax.

> **TECHNICIAN NOTE** The mediastinum of the horse is incomplete, and so a pneumothorax can be bilateral; however, in many horses, the mediastinum becomes imperforate and the pneumothorax is unilateral. Consequently, it is important to evaluate both sides of the chest and to never assume that the condition is unilateral.

GENERAL PHYSICAL EXAMINATION

A respiratory emergency is readily identifiable, even at a distance from the patient, because the most common signs of respiratory distress include an increased respiratory rate (tachypnea), flaring of the nostrils, exaggerated thoracic or abdominal movements while breathing, inspiratory or expiratory noise (stridor), and blue to pale blue coloration of the mucous membranes (cyanosis). Affected horses are frequently anxious, panicky, weak, depressed, sick, or reluctant to move their body or chest because of pain. As with painful colicky patients, horses in severe respiratory distress, especially due to upper airway obstruction, may be so painful, anxious, or hypoxic that they may be uncontrollable, unpredictable, and at risk for sudden death. Therefore, it is essential that the veterinarian and the veterinary technician secure the environment and maintain the safety of clients, staff, themselves, and, whenever possible, the patient.

Oxygen is vital to life, and the absence of it, even for brief moments, can be devastating. Therefore, the respiratory examination should be conducted with great efficiency and careful preparation. For all respiratory emergencies, oxygen, supplies for a temporary **tracheotomy**, and an IV catheter should be prepared and ready. If the patient, either at the farm or upon referral, is in severe respiratory distress because of upper airway obstruction, a temporary tracheotomy should be performed immediately before the physical examination. If the patient is not in severe respiratory distress because of upper airway obstruction, or after placement of a tracheotomy tube in a patient with an obstruction, a thorough physical examination should occur. Auscultation of the lungs and trachea is incredibly important for differentiating between upper and lower airway disease, and for characterizing the severity of the disease. Examination of mucous membranes for color is very important because cyanotic (blue) membranes lend a tremendous amount of insight into the degree of hypoxia. As with any physical examination of a horse, evaluation of heart rate, temperature, and gastrointestinal sounds is very important.

Once an airway has been secured and the physical examination is complete, it is important to perform diagnostics in an attempt to find and correct the inciting cause of the distress. However, it is very important to remember that the patient may be unstable and may need oxygen therapy during the diagnostic procedures, or that the patient may need time to become more stable before diagnostic tests are performed. If the patient is stable and is amenable to testing, the diagnostics listed below are the most common and valuable tests for finding the source of the disease.

THORACIC ULTRASOUND

As mentioned earlier, ultrasonography is a noninvasive, non-painful method of evaluating the thoracic cavity. When a transthoracic ultrasound is performed, it is important to saturate the hair with isopropyl alcohol, or to clip the hair and apply ultrasonographic gel to obtain an acceptable image. The best images are obtained with probes that are 2.5 to 10.0 MHz in frequency. When performing an ultrasound, it is good practice to be methodical and thorough. This is usually achieved by moving the probe in a dorsal-to-ventral direction in the intercostal spaces, starting at the cranial aspect of the chest wall and moving in a caudal direction. Thoracic ultrasound can be used to evaluate the amount and appearance of the pleural fluid, the serosal surface of the lungs, and, in diseased lungs that are not properly aerated, the deeper parenchyma. Common abnormalities that can be identified include pneumonia, pleuropneumonia, lung abscesses and tumors, and the presence of air in the pleural space, which would indicate a pneumothorax.

> **TECHNICIAN NOTE** It is important to remember that thoracic problems can lead to signs of colic, as well as to respiratory distress. Therefore, patients with colic should have a thoracic ultrasound examination performed to rule out a diaphragmatic hernia, pneumothorax, and pleuropneumonia.

RADIOGRAPHY

Radiography of the upper and lower respiratory tract is both possible and effective. Radiographs of the head and neck can help to identify pharyngeal swelling, tracheal swelling or compression, foreign bodies, or guttural pouch abnormalities leading to an upper airway obstruction (Figure 25-49). Although the thoracic cavity of the horse is thick, it can be radiographically evaluated effectively because of the amount of air within it. Thoracic radiographs are excellent for identifying a collapsed lung, pleural fluid, pneumonia, COPD, lung abscesses, neoplasia, and pulmonary edema.

UPPER AND LOWER AIRWAY ENDOSCOPY

Endoscopic evaluation of the upper airway is an invaluable diagnostic tool when an upper airway obstruction is suspected. The meatus, pharynx, and guttural pouches can be visualized for evidence of swelling, mass-occupying lesions (neoplasia, abscesses, etc.), and foreign bodies. This is also

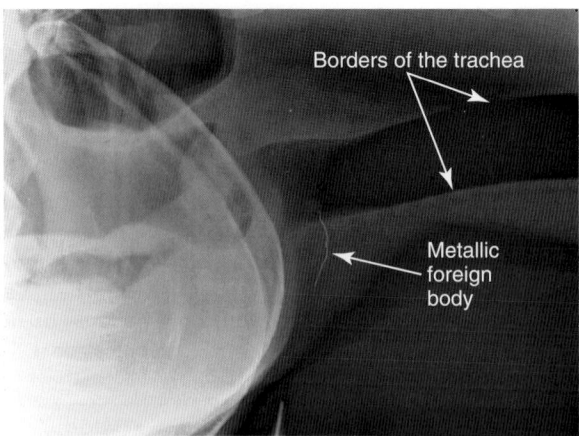

FIGURE 25-49 Radiographs can be an excellent method of identifying upper airway foreign bodies. Note the linear metallic foreign body located in the proximal trachea.

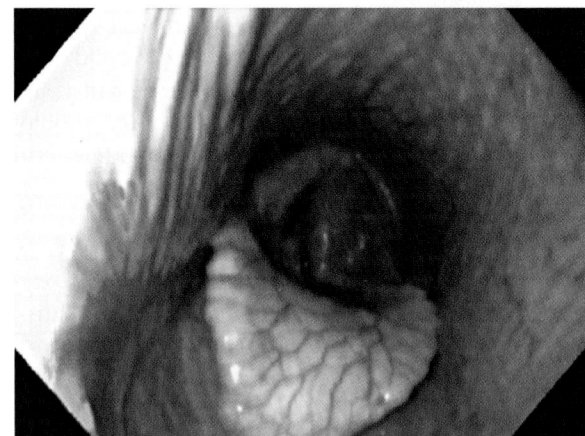

FIGURE 25-50 Patients in respiratory distress can present with an upper airway obstruction. Note the marked decrease in the size of the opening of the trachea.

an excellent opportunity to identify the size of the opening to the trachea and to assess whether a tracheotomy tube should be placed in patients that are not yet in respiratory distress, but are certainly in danger (Figure 25-50). After a complete examination of the pharynx and upper airway has been performed, the endoscope can be moved into the trachea to the bifurcation of the bronchi. This area should be evaluated for swelling or thickening, which can occur with severe COPD or bronchitis. As the endoscope is slowly removed, the trachea can be evaluated for swelling or compression, increased or abnormal secretions or discharge, and laceration of the tracheal mucosa.

THORACOCENTESIS

Horses with lower airway conditions that limit expansion of the lungs, such as pneumothorax or pleural effusion, need the pleural space reduced to its normal volume. This can be done through a procedure known as a *thoracocentesis* or a "chest tap." This is a potentially lifesaving procedure in which the pleural cavity is entered with a needle, catheter, teat cannula, or large **chest tube**. As with an abdominocentesis,

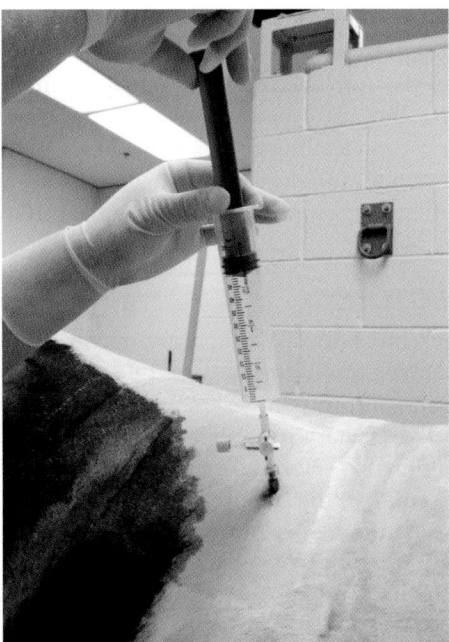

FIGURE 25-51 Example of a teat cannula, a three-way stop cock, and syringe evacuation of air from a pneumothorax.

a thoracocentesis must be performed aseptically and by a veterinarian trained to do this procedure. Unlike abdominocentesis, the location for thoracocentesis is very important and is based on the need to remove pleural fluid or air.

For removal of pleural fluid, ultrasonographic guidance is most helpful to identify an area of the thorax that has a large amount of effusion (typically, a ventral, dependent area). With the horse properly sedated and restrained, the area in which the centesis will be performed, as determined by ultrasound examination, should be clipped and prepared as for an abdominocentesis. The skin, subcutaneous tissue, and intercostal muscle should be blocked with 10 to 20 ml of mepivacaine. The vein, artery, and nerve complex is located along the caudal aspect of each rib; therefore, a stab incision into the skin should be made with a #10 or a #15 scalpel blade along the cranial aspect of the rib. The desired instrument (needle, catheter, cannula, or chest tube) should then be placed through the stab incision and intercostal muscle, and into the pleural space. For removal of air from the pleural space, this procedure is identical, except that the incision generally is made dorsally between the 12th and 15th ribs (because air rises to this location), and ultrasonographic guidance is not as helpful because sound is unable to penetrate a tissue/air interface.

Temporary evacuation of fluid or air can be accomplished using the teat cannula, IV catheter, or needle. Because of the risk of introducing air into the chest cavity, evacuation should be performed with a three-way stopcock and syringe, with active suction for correction of a pneumothorax, or with a one-way valve (i.e., Heimlich valve) for removal of pleural effusion (Figure 25-51).

> **TECHNICIAN NOTE** If the pneumothorax is the result of a laceration of the thoracic wall, the wound should be repaired or sealed before, and along with, evacuation of the air to restore negative intrathoracic pressure.

If it is necessary for fluid to be evacuated continuously or over a prolonged time, a chest tube can be placed and sutured into position with a purse-string suture at the point of entry and a Chinese finger-trap suture pattern to secure the tube. As would be expected, patients should be monitored very closely for respiratory distress because of possible recurrence of pleural effusion or pneumothorax. Patients that have indwelling chest tubes should have these tubes regularly checked to ensure patency, and to confirm that the valve is in place and functional.

TRANSTRACHEAL WASH

If a diagnosis of pneumonia is made, it may be necessary to obtain a bacterial culture and cytologic preparation of respiratory secretions before antimicrobial therapy is begun. This is best performed with a transtracheal wash (TTW). To perform a TTW, the skin over the cranial one-third of the trachea should be clipped and aseptically prepared. A site located in the middle of this clipped area, directly on midline and between the tracheal rings, should be identified. Skin and subcutaneous tissue at this site should be anesthetized with 3 to 5 ml of mepivacaine, and a stab incision made through the skin with a #15 blade. A sharp trocar with a sleeve is placed into the trachea, between two cartilaginous rings, and the trocar is removed. A TTW tube is passed through the sleeve and down into the trachea. Approximately 20 to 30 ml of sterile saline is injected into the tube and flows into the trachea. This fluid is then re-collected via the tubing with a new syringe, and the infusate (infused and subsequently collected fluid) is submitted for cytologic examination and culture. The tube is then removed, and a small amount of antimicrobial can be injected into the sleeve and subcutaneous opening as the sleeve is removed.

OXYGEN ADMINISTRATION

Oxygen supplementation can be beneficial for patients suffering from any respiratory tract disease (upper or more commonly lower) that leads to a decrease in blood oxygen content. Blood oxygen is most accurately determined by measuring the partial pressure of arterial oxygen (PaO_2) through blood gas analysis. Patients with a PaO_2 less than 100 mm Hg should receive oxygen supplementation, although for patients with a PaO_2 less than 60 mm Hg, the need is especially critical. Other parameters that can be used to evaluate for hypoxia when a blood gas analysis is not readily available are heart rate, respiratory rate, mucous membrane color, and lactate concentration. In patients in which oxygen intake by the lungs is adequate, but delivery to or uptake by the tissues is inadequate (e.g., anemia), oxygen supplementation will have only a very modest benefit, because the oxygen-carrying capacity of the red blood cell is at its maximum or is "saturated," and so the extra oxygen given by supplementation cannot be fully used by tissue cells.

To supplement a patient with oxygen, three items are needed: (1) a source of oxygen, (2) a method of measuring and regulating the amount to be given, and (3) a means of delivering the oxygen. Oxygen canisters (tanks) come in a variety of sizes, from small and portable to large and fixed (for whole hospital distribution). The oxygen in these canisters is under a tremendous amount of pressure and therefore must be regulated with a pressure regulator or a pressure-reducing valve. Once oxygen is reduced in pressure (usually from 2000 psi to 50 psi), it is ready for delivery to the patient. A flowmeter is used as a variable-flow valve to enable the veterinary staff to visualize and set the rate at which oxygen will be delivered. The rate of oxygen flow that the patient needs is dependent on its size and the degree of hypoxia. Adults may need at least 15 L/minute for effective therapy; smaller patients such as foals and miniature horses may require as little as 5 L/minute.

It is also important to remember that the oxygen that comes out of the tank is dry and is devoid of humidity, unlike the ambient oxygen that we breathe. Therefore, to avoid drying out the mucous membranes of the respiratory tract, a bubble humidifier is attached to the oxygen delivery tubing (Figure 25-52).

For the standing, awake horse, oxygen typically is delivered passively via a nasal cannula. A nasal cannula with multiple small fenestrations is placed so that the tip of the catheter is positioned in the nasopharynx, and the cannula is secured to the halter or is sutured to the skin of the nostrils by placing adhesive tape in a "butterfly pattern" over the catheter, and suturing the tape to the skin. To determine the

approximate distance to the nasopharynx, the cannula is measured from the opening of the nares to the medial canthus of the eye. The measured length of the cannula is passed into the nasal passages. Oxygen delivery tubing is then used to connect the oxygen source at the bubble humidifier to the nasal cannula. This tubing usually is long, and it is typically hung from a position above the stall, such as a fluid hook.

TRACHEOTOMY

As has been mentioned, a temporary tracheotomy is essential for relieving respiratory distress due to an upper airway obstruction. This procedure is frequently lifesaving, and it is one that all veterinary professionals must be familiar with. A tracheotomy is performed most commonly as an emergency procedure in the standing horse, although if the situation arises, it can be performed on an elective basis, or on a patient that is under general anesthesia. When it is performed on the standing and awake patient, sedation and restraint should be used *if possible* without compromising the patient. The most commonly used and desirable location for the tracheotomy is along the ventral midline, where the trachea can be clearly identified and isolated under the skin and subcutaneous tissue. Usually, this is in the area between the cranial and middle third of the neck. In situations in which the obstruction is below the larynx, the tracheotomy site must be below the obstruction. If time permits, this area should be clipped, aseptically prepared, and infiltrated with 10 to 20 ml of lidocaine or mepivacaine.

It must always be remembered that horses in severe respiratory distress can be unpredictable, dangerous, and panicked. When situations such as this arise, a tracheotomy may have to be performed without clipping, aseptic preparation, local analgesia, sedation, or even much restraint. Always maintain an exit strategy, minimize the number of people needed to be near the patient, and proceed with caution, speed, and efficiency. A well-trained, experienced, and prepared staff is paramount to the safety and success of this procedure under these extreme circumstances. See Case Presentation 25-2 for an example of emergency management of a horse with an upper airway obstruction.

> **TECHNICIAN NOTE** A tracheotomy is a lifesaving procedure that should be familiar to all veterinarians and technicians.

The tracheotomy procedure begins with an 8- to 10-cm vertical incision made in the skin and subcutaneous tissue directly over the trachea. The trachea is then visualized, oftentimes after blunt dissection of the subcutaneous tissue, and a horizontal incision (perpendicular to the trachea) is made through the annular ligament between two tracheal rings. The incision into the trachea should be no longer than one-third of the circumferential diameter of the trachea. Once the tracheal lumen has been entered, the horse will immediately become less distressed.

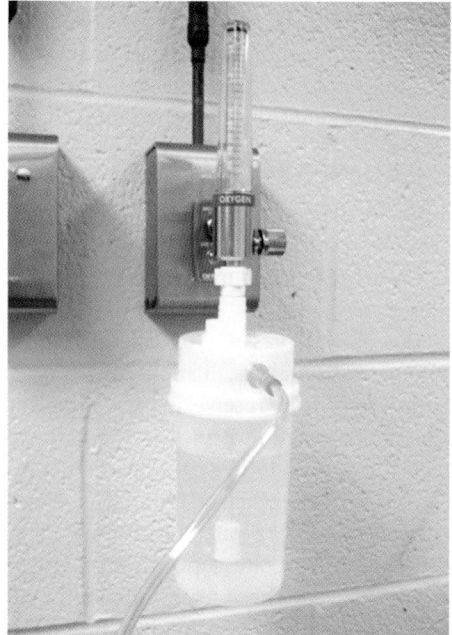

FIGURE 25-52 O₂ source, flowmeter, bubble humidifier, and outflow tubing.

CASE PRESENTATION 25-2 EQUINE

History and Signalment

A 2-year-old quarter horse gelding was presented with a 2-hour history of moderate inspiratory stridor and tachypnea. A presumptive diagnosis of an upper airway obstruction was made by the referring veterinarian, and the horse was immediately referred to the hospital. No treatment had been provided before referral. Three yearlings were moved to the farm 2 weeks ago, and two of them had bilateral mucopurulent nasal discharge.

Initial Physical Examination

On presentation, the horse was in respiratory distress, exhibited severe inspiratory stridor, and was panicky. His temperature was 101°F 38.3°C (normal, 98.5°F [36.9°C] to 100.5°F [38.1°C]), pulse rate was 60 beats per minutes (bpm) (normal, 28 to 40 bpm), respiratory rate was 54 breaths per minute (normal, 8 to 18 breaths per minute), and breath sounds were present in all lung fields. Mucous membranes were cyanotic and tacky, and CRT was normal at less than 2 seconds. Weight was estimated to be approximately 1000 lb (450 kg). Submandibular lymphadenopathy (enlargement of the lymph nodes) was present.

Diagnostic Workup

Results of CBC, chemistry profile, and arterial blood gas revealed elevated PCV (45%; normal, 28% to 40%), normal TP (6.5 g/dl; normal, 5.5 to 7.5 g/dl), elevated white blood cell count (13,000 cells/μl; normal, 4700 to 10,600 cell/μl) with normal differential, and decreased PaO_2 (60 mm Hg; normal, 80 to 100 mm Hg) indicating hypoxemia. Endoscopy revealed compression of the pharynx from both left and right sides, although the left side appeared to be more severely compressed. Guttural pouch endoscopy revealed a large swelling along the floor of both pouches. Moderate to severe lymphoid hyperplasia was evident surrounding the larynx. A guttural pouch wash was performed to collect a sample for bacterial culture. The culture was positive for *Streptococcus equi*. The organism was sensitive to penicillin.

Therapeutic Intervention

Upon completion of the initial physical examination, a self-retaining tracheotomy tube was placed to relieve this patient's respiratory distress. An IV catheter was placed in the left jugular vein. Oxygen insufflation through the tracheotomy tube was initiated at 1 L/minute. Oxygen insufflation was discontinued after 1 hour, when a repeat arterial blood gas revealed PaO_2 of 200 mm Hg. The presumptive diagnosis was acute upper respiratory obstruction resulting from pharyngeal obstruction caused by enlarged retropharyngeal lymph nodes. Infection with *S. equi* (strangles) was believed to be the cause of the lymphadenopathy.

The horse was started on IV potassium penicillin every 6 hours for 5 days, IV flunixin meglumine every 12 hours for 5 days, and IV fluids for 24 hours at maintenance rate. Food was introduced after 24 hours and was gradually increased to free-choice hay over the next 24 hours. The tracheotomy tube was intermittently occluded to determine whether pharyngeal swelling persisted. The horse was able to breathe normally after 4 days. The tube was removed after the fifth day, the catheter was also removed, and the horse was switched to IM procaine penicillin and oral flunixin meglumine for another 5 days.

Outcome

The horse was discharged 7 days after admittance, and the owners were instructed to give the remaining penicillin and flunixin meglumine at home. They were also instructed to isolate the horse, to have the referring veterinarian inspect all other horses at the barn for strangles, and to disinfect all supplies, water buckets, and water sources that came in contact with the new horses, this patient, and all other horses exposed to the new horses. This case illustrates how a rapid, efficient, and coordinated response to this life-threatening emergency by an organized, prepared, and thoughtful veterinary team resulted in a positive outcome for both patient and owners.

The choice of a tracheotomy tube may vary a lot from patient to patient and is based on personal preference. Several different sizes and styles of silicone or stainless steel tubes are available. The size of the tube is dictated by the size of the patient, but as a general rule, the largest tube possible, that will not cause damage to the tracheal rings, should be placed. Indwelling tracheotomy tubes can induce production of a variable amount of mucus and discharge that can clog the tube, causing recurrence of respiratory distress if the tube is not regularly cleaned and maintained. Therefore, close attention to tube maintenance is paramount. The tube should be cleaned as necessary (which may be as frequently as 2 to 4 times a day) and should remain in place until the source of the upper airway obstruction is gone. Once the condition has resolved, the tube can be removed and the tracheotomy incision left to heal by second intention.

MUSCULOSKELETAL SYSTEM

Musculoskeletal injuries are the second most common emergencies in equine medicine (gastrointestinal conditions are the most common). These injuries can be categorized as fractures, lacerations, infections (of the joint, soft tissue, or foot), or luxations. Because of the size and temperament of horses, these injuries, especially fractures, can be severe and life threatening. Many of these injuries are not observed by the owner at the time they occur (e.g., when a horse found at pasture is unable to bear weight on a limb), but other common injuries are readily identified (e.g., when a Thoroughbred racehorse sustains a condylar fracture during a race). Despite the underlying reason for the injury, immediate veterinary attention to the injury is essential for maximizing the chance of a positive outcome. Diagnosing an orthopedic injury, although not always easy, is typically less difficult than diagnosing conditions of the gastrointestinal and respiratory tracts. This fact is especially true when the injury involves the distal limb, which is defined as any area below the carpus or tarsus, because of the minimal amount of soft tissue covering this area. In general, the extent of the procedures necessary to diagnose most injuries is limited to physical examination (for lacerations, open fractures, cellulitis, and foot abscesses), radiographs (for fractures, osteomyelitis, and luxations), ultrasound (for tendon or ligament injuries), and arthrocentesis (for joint infections).

FRACTURES

Like many acute and severe injuries in horses, bone fractures can cause great distress and pain. It is always important to perform a general assessment of the horse first, to ensure that the horse is stable, and to control the environment. Controlling the environment usually means calming the horse, oftentimes with sedation, and minimizing the number of people that need to be involved and at risk. It is important to remember that it may be very difficult to adequately sedate a horse that has a large sympathetic surge (e.g., a racehorse). It is also important to remember that it is possible to oversedate this type of patient and worsen the injury as a result of increased weight bearing. Therefore, an experienced and conscientious team is important for managing these emergencies. Once the horse and the environment have been secured, a swift and accurate assessment of the injured limb should commence. Accurate identification of the region of injury should lead to one of two scenarios. If radiography equipment is readily available without moving the horse, x-rays can be taken to accurately evaluate the injury before transport. If radiography equipment is not available without moving the horse, the limb should be stabilized on the basis of the region of suspected injury. Goals of stabilization should be to decrease pain, minimize or eliminate further injury, minimize damage to soft tissues and vasculature, minimize swelling, and enable some degree of weight bearing. Box 25-10 outlines important steps in the first aid of a fracture. The next sections detail recommended fracture stabilization techniques for achieving these goals.

> **TECHNICIAN NOTE** Appropriate fracture stabilization and immediate medical attention are the most important ways to maximize the likelihood of a successful outcome.

BOX 25-10 | Guidelines for Fracture Stabilization

1. Stabilize the patient and control hemorrhage.
2. Relieve pain and anxiety.
3. Control wound infection.
4. Prevent neurovascular trauma.
5. Prevent trauma to muscle and skin adjacent to fracture site.
6. Minimize trauma to fractured bone ends.

Distal Forelimb Fracture

This region includes the distal metacarpus, proximal and middle phalanges, and sesamoid bones. The goal of stabilizing this area is to align the boney column and protect the soft tissues of the fetlock and pastern from excessive compression. A bandage of moderate thickness is applied from the coronary band to the proximal metacarpus. A rigid splint (PVC, wood, etc.) is then secured to the dorsal aspect of the limb with nonelastic tape and is extended all the way to the ground to include the foot. A commercially available splint called the Kimzey Leg Saver (Kimzey, Inc., Woodland, California) is an acceptable alternative (Figure 25-53). This form of external coaptation is acceptable for fracture of the aforementioned bones, as well as for luxation of the fetlock joint, laceration of the flexor tendons, and disruption of the suspensory apparatus due to fracture through both proximal sesamoid bones.

Distal to Mid Forelimb Fracture

This region includes the mid to proximal metacarpus and carpus. The goal of stabilizing this area is to align the bony column and prevent the lower limb from moving. A bandage is applied from the coronary band to the highest point of the elbow. This bandage can be a Robert Jones bandage, which is composed of multiple layers of sheet cotton or similar material compressed by gauze. The final diameter of the completed bandage should be approximately 3 times the diameter of the limb. A caudal splint, extending from the ground to the point of the elbow, is secured with nonelastic tape. A second splint is secured laterally, again from

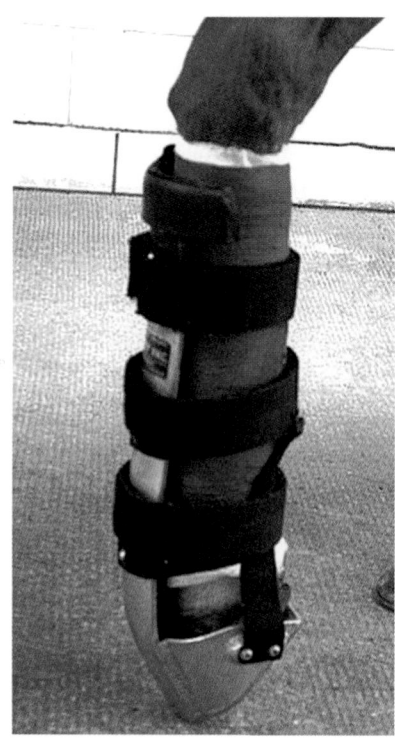

FIGURE 25-53 Kimzey Leg Saver splint applied to the distal limb of a horse with a fracture.

the ground to the point of the elbow. This form of external coaptation is used most commonly for mid to proximal metacarpal fractures.

Mid Forelimb Fracture

This region includes the radius and the elbow. The goal of stabilization is to realign the bony column and prevent movement of the radius in any direction, especially abduction. Bandaging and stabilization are the same as those described previously for fractures of the mid to proximal metacarpus, except that the lateral splint should be long enough to traverse from the ground, across the shoulder joint, and to the proximal margin of the scapula. The most proximal portion of this splint should be secured by wrapping bandage material around the neck and chest, between the forelimbs, over the withers, and under the girth in a figure-eight pattern (Figure 25-54). This form of external coaptation is used most commonly for radial fractures.

Elbow Fracture

If the patient is able to extend, plant, and move the limb, splint stabilization is not necessary. With some olecranon fractures, the triceps apparatus is disrupted, and the patient is unable to extend and fix the leg. In these cases, the goal of stabilization is to lock or fix the carpus in extension. A bandage of medium thickness is applied from the coronary band to the highest point of the elbow, and a caudal splint extending from the ground to the point of the elbow is secured with nonelastic tape.

Proximal Forelimb Fracture

This region includes the humerus and the scapula. It has a large amount of muscle mass and is unable to be properly

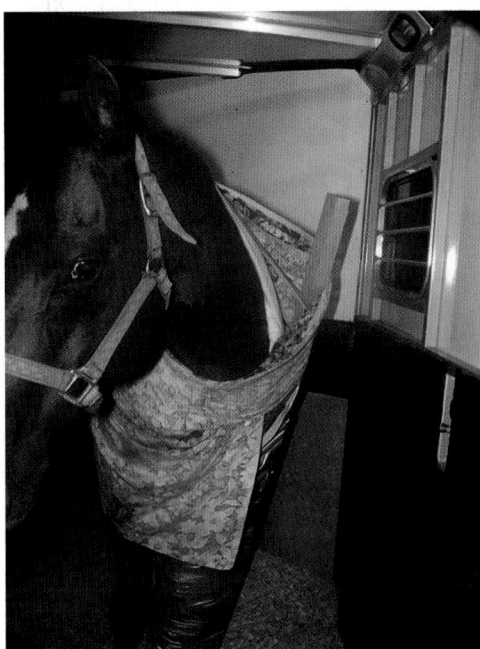

FIGURE 25-54 Full limb Robert Jones bandage with a caudal and lateral splint extending to the withers for transport of a patient with a suspected distal radial fracture.

stabilized; attempts should not be made. The only exception is the case of the distal humeral fracture in which the triceps apparatus has been compromised. In these scenarios, a light bandage with caudal splint can be applied to lock the carpus in extension.

Distal Hindlimb Fracture

As per the distal forelimb fracture, except that the rigid splint is applied along the plantar aspect of the limb. A Kimzey Leg Saver (Kimzey, Inc.) is an acceptable alternative.

Distal to Mid Hindlimb Fracture

This region includes the mid to proximal metatarsus. Fractures in this region are treated as described for the forelimb, except that a moderate bandage is placed and a plantar splint is applied up to the point of the calcaneus (proximal extent of tarsus).

Mid Hindlimb Fracture

This region includes the tarsus, tibia, and stifle. The goal of stabilization is to realign the bony column and prevent collapse and movement of the bones. A Robert Jones bandage is placed from the coronary band to the stifle. A lateral splint extending from the ground to the hip is secured with nonelastic tape. The most proximal end of the splint is secured by wrapping bandage material over the hip, between the hindlimbs, under the flank, and over the lumbar spine in a figure-eight pattern. This form of external coaptation is used most commonly for tibial fractures.

Proximal Hindlimb Fracture

This region includes the femur and the pelvis. The area is heavily muscled; further stabilization is not possible and actually is contraindicated because it could further increase trauma to the fracture site.

SOFT TISSUE INJURY

All other musculoskeletal injuries commonly seen in the horse involve the soft tissues in some fashion. These injuries are usually visible (e.g., lacerations); however, their extent can be misleading because punctures, abscesses, or tendon injuries may also be present. The remainder of this section discusses common soft tissue injuries encountered as emergencies.

Wounds

Lacerations and punctures can occur on any part of the body but are most frequent on the distal limb. These injuries usually result from contact with loose metal, wire, wood, or other horses. Because of the minimal soft tissue covering of the distal limb, minor skin wounds can become life-threatening events when joints, tendon sheaths, or vessels are involved; therefore, all wounds should be evaluated with the idea that the injury could be worse than it appears. Initial triage and evaluation of soft tissue injuries can have a profound influence on the prognosis of the patient.

General Examination

As with other injuries, initial examination should include a general assessment of the patient, with particular attention to blood loss. The vein, artery, and nerve complex of the distal limb is very superficial and is commonly involved. Blood loss can be very difficult or impossible to accurately quantify; therefore, heart rate, respiratory rate, mucous membrane color, packed cell volume (PCV), total protein (TP), and lactate levels are important factors to evaluate. If ongoing hemorrhage is occurring, it is vital that an attempt is made to slow it down or stop it. When you are advising the owner over the phone, or when you are in the field with limited supplies available, be aware that ordinary materials such as towels wrapped tightly over the wound and secured with duct tape can be effective. It is likely that a bandage of this type will become soaked quickly with blood; however, leaving it in place may allow a clot to form and may slow the hemorrhage (although the clot may be unstable). Each time the bandage is changed, the clot may be disrupted, causing bleeding to resume. If the limb is still bleeding upon presentation to the veterinary medical staff, hemostatic forceps (Kelly or mosquito) are used to isolate and ligate the vessel, producing hemostasis.

When the hemorrhage has been controlled, the physical examination performed, and the patient systemically stabilized, a more thorough evaluation of the limb should follow. For examination of the limb with the necessary level of detail, the patient may have to be sedated and the wound desensitized by **regional nerve block** or direct infiltration of the wound with mepivicaine or lidocaine. The wound should be covered with a water-soluble gel, and the hair surrounding the region and the wound should be clipped.

The size of the area clipped depends on the location of the wound. If a synovial structure (joint or tendon sheath) is clearly distant from the wound, and hence is not involved, only the wound needs to be clipped. If there is any possibility that the wound (a laceration or puncture) could involve a joint or tendon sheath, the area should be clipped widely and circumferentially.

Arthrocentesis

For injuries suspected of synovial involvement, a site away from the wound that allows needle access to the suspected joint or sheath should be identified and aseptically prepared. The introduction of a needle into a joint is called *arthrocentesis* or a "joint tap." This procedure should be performed by a veterinarian because many possible sites are unique to each synovial structure. Depending on the structure that is to be entered, an 18- or 20-gauge, 1.5-inch needle is introduced under sterile conditions after the skin overlying the tap site is aseptically prepared. Once the structure has been entered, a small volume of synovial fluid should be obtained (1 to 3 ml), evaluated for color and viscosity, and placed into a purple top (EDTA) tube for cytologic examination and lactate, glucose, and total protein evaluation. Normal values for joint fluid are listed in Table 25-6. Extra fluid can be

TABLE 25-6	Normal Synovial Fluid Values	
GROSS APPEARANCE	**CELLULARITY**	**MOLECULAR COMPONENTS**
Clear or straw/ yellow colored, viscous	WBC ≤500 cells/μl ≈10% neutrophils	TP ≤2.5 g/dl Lactate ≤2.0 mmol/dl Glucose >50 mg/dl OR <50 mg/dl difference from blood glucose pH >7.3

TP, Total protein; *WBC*, white blood cell.

obtained for bacterial culture; however, this infrequently yields bacterial growth and is not commonly useful.

> **TECHNICIAN NOTE**   When an arthrocentesis is performed, the needle should NEVER be introduced through a wound. A site distant from the wound should ALWAYS be used to assess the integrity and involvement of a synovial structure.

After the synovial fluid sample is obtained, sterile normal saline should be injected into the synovial structure, and an assistant should evaluate the wound for evidence of leakage of saline from the synovial structure; this would indicate communication of the wound with the joint or tendon sheath. If the synovial structure distends with saline and nothing exits out of the wound, it is likely (but not guaranteed) that the structure is not involved. Excess fluid should be evacuated and a small amount of antibiotic may be injected into the joint before the needle is removed. If it is determined that the synovial structure is involved, the owner should be informed that a more aggressive approach may be necessary that would involve lavage of the joint and prolonged use of antibiotics (regionally and systemically). These cases are often associated with a potentially worse prognosis and increased cost. If it was clear that the synovial structure was not involved, the workup should focus on the wound.

Wound Management

Once the surrounding skin has been clipped, the wound can be cleaned with an antiseptic soap and rinsed with saline. Wound care is then focused on decreasing further contamination, débriding necrotic tissue, and removing foreign material from the wound. This can be achieved best by irrigating or lavaging the wound with saline under pressure. Saline can be pressurized by using a pressure infusion bag to force saline from a 1-L bag into the wound, by using a 60-ml syringe with a 16- or 18-gauge needle to spray saline into the wound, or by punching multiple holes into the cap of a saline bottle and squeezing saline into the wound. Once the wound has been cleaned and all debris removed, further diagnostics can be performed to assess damage to deeper structures such as bone or tendons.

> **TECHNICIAN NOTE** Wounds, especially deep ones, should not be lavaged with saline under pressure until it has been ensured that a synovial structure is not involved.

Radiography

Radiographic evaluation of the wound provides the best assessment of boney structure involvement. More specifically, radiographs can be used to detect early hairline fractures, fractures of the small bones (e.g., splint bones), or foreign bodies (such as metal or gravel), and to evaluate the risk of developing a bone sequestrum. A sequestrum is a nonviable segment of bone that develops as a result of trauma to the periosteum and disruption of blood supply to the surface of the bone. The nonviable section of bone acts as a foreign body and frequently prevents full wound healing until it is removed.

> **TECHNICIAN NOTE** A sequestrum is a nonviable segment of bone that acts as a foreign body and frequently prevents full wound healing until it is removed.

Ultrasonography

Ultrasonography is helpful for evaluating the structure of tendons and ligaments and for identifying foreign bodies without mineral content (e.g., glass, wood, other organic matter). Portable ultrasound machines are sufficiently powerful to be used in the field for evaluation of most distal limb injuries.

Wound Closure

The decision of how to treat a wound is usually multifactorial and takes into account the anticipated future use of the patient, the level of financial commitment by the owner, and the extent of the injury. As has been mentioned earlier, if a synovial structure is involved, recommended therapy may include surgery under general anesthesia and joint lavage with or without arthroscopic evaluation. When the wound clearly does not involve a synovial structure, management often involves suturing the laceration. This requires the use of standing sedation or general anesthesia. The temperament of the horse, the severity of the injury, and the veterinarian's and owner's preferences will factor into the decision about whether anesthetics should be used.

In most situations, a general surgical pack of instruments that includes a scalpel handle, hemostatic forceps (mosquito and Kelly), thumb forceps (Brown-Adson and rat-tooth), needle drivers (Mayo-Hegar or Olsen-Hegar), and scissors (Mayo and Metzenbaum) is sufficient for suturing a laceration. A selection of Penrose drains of varying sizes is useful to ensure proper drainage when necessary. Preoperative and postoperative care generally consists of administration of antibiotics, anti-inflammatories, analgesics, and prophylactic tetanus toxoid if the vaccination history is unknown, or if the tetanus vaccine was given more than 4 to 6 months before the injury occurred.

Emergency and Critical Care Nursing: Food Animal

It is commonplace to think of farm animal species as being used only to produce food or to make a profit; however, it is becoming increasingly common for farm animal species to be viewed as companion animals or "pasture pets." Consequently, some of these animals have a value or a perceived value rivaling that of any house pet. Other farm animals are used for exhibition purposes or may possess superior genetics, and have market values exceeding $100,000. Regardless of the reason, many farm animal owners are willing to seek emergency veterinary care when necessary.

Emergency treatment requires prompt action on the part of the owner, the veterinarian, and the veterinary support staff. The veterinary technician provides an invaluable service to the veterinarian when performing emergency procedures, but to be fully prepared to assist, the veterinary technician must be familiar with the emergency condition and the procedure at hand, and should be able to anticipate the veterinarian's next step.

> **TECHNICIAN NOTE** The veterinary technician must be familiar with the emergency condition and the procedure at hand, and should be able to anticipate the veterinarian's next step.

PATIENT RESTRAINT AND SAFETY

Emergency situations are not an excuse to compromise the safety of the veterinary team, the client, or the patient. Farm animal species pose a unique set of challenges compared with other domesticated animals. Many farm animals outweigh their owners and handlers by more than 10 times; this increases the level of danger when handling even the mildest mannered patients.

CONSIDERATIONS FOR FOOD-PRODUCING ANIMALS

Certain regulations apply to the use of specific pharmaceuticals in food-producing animals that do not apply to the use of these drugs in non–food-producing species. Some drugs are prohibited from being used in an extralabel manner, and use is strictly forbidden in food-producing animals for many others. The entire veterinary team should be aware of these drug regulations, and attention should be paid to withdrawal times to avoid drug residues in meat and milk. The Food Animal Residue Avoidance Databank (www.farad.org) should be consulted regarding current drug regulations and prohibitions.

GASTROINTESTINAL SYSTEM

GENERAL PHYSICAL EXAMINATION

Before providing emergency treatment, the veterinarian will perform a thorough physical examination on the patient. This is critical for making an accurate diagnosis and for initiating appropriate treatment. The physical examination should include measurement of heart rate and respiratory rate, assessment of body temperature, and evaluation of lung and heart sounds. The technical staff can provide a valuable service to the veterinarian if staff members are trained to help the veterinarian assess these parameters. Auscultation and percussion of the lateral abdominal wall should be performed to listen for hyperresonate sounds referred to as *pings*. Pings represent gas pockets within the viscera and can be a sign of displaced abdominal viscera.

Most veterinarians perform rectal palpation as part of a typical physical examination when assessing a patient for abdominal disease. In cattle, rectal palpation is very useful for assessing caudal abdominal structures, including the uterus, cecum, small intestines, caudal sac of the rumen, and left kidney. A large, distended abomasum can also be palpated rectally in some cases. The veterinarian should be provided with an arm-length plastic rectal sleeve and copious amounts of lubricant. If the veterinarian is palpating several cows, a new, clean sleeve should be provided for each cow.

Ancillary Diagnostics

Other diagnostic tests that can be very useful for assessment of abdominal disease include abdominal ultrasound, abdominocentesis, abdominal radiography, and blood work. If the veterinarian wishes to perform other diagnostics, the veterinary technical staff should be familiar with these procedures and with the necessary equipment.

EMERGENCY INTERVENTION

The veterinary team must be prepared to act quickly to stabilize the patient and prepare for emergency surgery. If the cow is severely compromised, an IV catheter should be placed in the jugular vein, and the cow should be started on IV fluids. Classic biochemical abnormalities include hypokalemic, hypochloremic, metabolic alkalosis. Administration of a nonalkalinizing balanced electrolyte solution (Ringer's solution) is best. If the cow is in hypovolemic shock, a liter of hypertonic saline (7% NaCl) can be administered IV to quickly increase the circulating blood volume. Although hypertonic saline results in rapid expansion of the circulating volume, this effect is transient because hypertonic saline is a crystalloid and consequently will eventually leave the vascular space.

The bovine abdomen is susceptible to various emergency conditions. Among the most acute and life threatening are volvulus of the abomasum and volvulus of the cecum. These conditions can result in colic and may require emergency surgery. Intestinal obstruction can also result from a volvulus of some or all of the intestinal structures. A volvulus

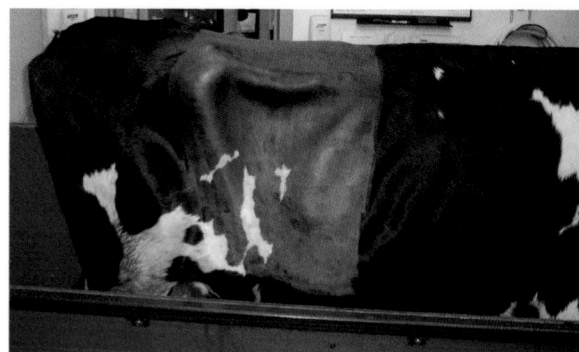

FIGURE 25-55 Cow prepared for right flank surgery. Abdominal surgery in cattle is commonly performed in the right paralumbar fossa. The surgical prep should extend from the tuber coxae cranially to the 12th intercostal space, and from the dorsal midline ventrally to the flank fold.

is especially serious because in addition to causing an obstruction to the flow of ingesta, it may cause compromise of the vascular supply to the affected viscera. Abomasal ulcers can result in focal or diffuse peritonitis (another emergency condition). The rumen produces extremely large amounts of gas on a daily basis, predisposing ruminants to **rumen tympany** (bloat) if there is failure to expel this gas. Bloat can be life threatening if it leads to respiratory compromise. Vagal indigestion is a condition that results in dysfunction of the forestomachs and abomasum caused by dysfunction of the vagus nerve. It can also lead to profound ruminal and abdominal distention.

> **TECHNICIAN NOTE**   Volvulus of the abomasum and volvulus of the cecum are among the most acute and life-threatening conditions of the bovine abdomen.

Abdominal surgery to correct an abomasal volvulus, a cecal volvulus, or another GI abnormality is typically performed in the right flank region (paralumbar fossa) with the animal standing. As soon as the cow is adequately restrained in a headgate and chute system, the right side of the cow is clipped and aseptically prepared. The prepped area should extend from the tuber coxae (point of the hip) cranially to the 12th intercostal space, and from the dorsal midline (spine) ventrally to the flank fold (Figure 25-55). The surgical site is desensitized by performing a regional or local nerve block (options include a paravertebral nerve block, an inverted-L block, or a line block). After desensitization, final surgical prep should be done, and the cow should be moved to the operating room or to the area prepared for sterile abdominal surgery.

> **TECHNICIAN NOTE**   Abdominal surgery to correct an abomasal volvulus, a cecal volvulus, or another GI abnormality is typically performed in the right flank region (paralumbar fossa) with the animal standing.

BOX 25-11	Surgical Equipment for Abdominal Surgery in Cattle

- Large drape
- Towel clamps (qty = 10)
- Hemostats (qty = 10 Kelly, 5 mosquito)
- Scalpel
- Mayo scissors
- 4 × 4 gauze sponges
- Basin with warmed isotonic saline
- Sterile palpation sleeves
- Suture and needles
- Suction and decompression set

The necessary equipment will vary, depending on the surgeon's preference. A list of common surgical equipment for performing abdominal surgery in cattle is provided (Box 25-11).

SPECIFIC GI CONDITIONS
Diarrhea

Diarrhea is a nonobstructive gastrointestinal problem that can result in profound dehydration and hypovolemic shock within hours after onset of diarrhea. Young animals are especially vulnerable to the negative effects of diarrhea, which can result from dietary, parasitic, bacterial, or viral causes; successful treatment depends on an accurate diagnosis. Patients should have a jugular IV catheter placed for administration of IV fluids. Animals that are suffering from hypovolemic shock may benefit from an IV bolus of hypertonic saline to help temporarily restore circulating blood volume. Oral fluids and electrolytes may also help to restore hydration in a dehydrated animal.

Parasitism

Farm animal species are expected to have at least some gastrointestinal parasites, and parasitism is not usually considered an emergency. Parasite overload can result in malabsorption and can account for the diarrhea and dehydration mentioned previously. Some parasites, namely, *Haemonchus contortus*, are avid blood feeders and can cause profound anemia. These problems are especially common in small ruminants (sheep and goats). The presenting complaint is usually weakness and weight loss, and this condition can be fatal if not treated. Mucous membrane color should be assessed as a part of the physical examination, and PCV/TP should be performed. A blood transfusion is often necessary to stabilize these patients until the parasitism can be treated. A suitable blood donor or a supply of homologous red cells should be available. These animals should have an IV catheter placed in a jugular vein for administration of blood or other emergency therapeutics. Owners can be educated on how to monitor their animal's mucous membrane color to assess anemia status, so that treatment can be administered before anemia becomes life threatening.

EMERGENCIES INVOLVING THE RUMEN
Ruminal Tympany

Ruminal tympany, which is commonly referred to as *bloat*, is a condition in which an excessive amount of gas accumulates within the rumen. The rumen is the largest of the forestomach compartments and functions as a fermentation vat. Microbes that live in the rumen normally produce a large amount of gas, which should be expelled periodically through the esophagus in a process called **eructation**. Bloat occurs because of an inability to properly expel this gas. One type of bloat termed *frothy bloat* occurs because a foam-like substance forms within the rumen. This foam is not expelled like normal gas and will lead to bloat. Free gas bloat occurs because of a physical blockage (**choke**) or decrease in rumen motility that prevents eructation so that gas is not expelled.

Bloat becomes life threatening when the distended rumen pushes cranially on the diaphragm and inhibits normal respirations. Emergency decompression is necessary in these cases. In cases of free gas bloat, an esophageal tube is usually sufficient to relieve excessive gas accumulation. Frothy ruminal contents do not pass well through a tube, and pharmacologic therapy is frequently necessary to break down the foam. Poloxalene is a surfactant that is used to relieve frothy bloat in cattle. The dose for poloxalene is 50 g for cattle weighing more than 500 kg. It can be administered via stomach tube or oral drench.

> **TECHNICIAN NOTE**   Bloat becomes life threatening when the distended rumen pushes cranially on the diaphragm and inhibits normal respirations.

Rumenostomy

Surgical decompression of the rumen may also be indicated. **Rumenostomy** is a surgical procedure that is performed to create a permanent hole in the rumen to allow gas to escape. Surgery is performed on the left side of the patient in the flank area (paralumbar fossa region) with the patient under local or regional anesthesia. This procedure provides a more permanent outlet for escape of gas in animals that chronically bloat.

As a last resort, rumen trocars (Figure 25-56) are available to puncture the rumen and allow escape of rumen gas. These devices are inserted directly through the left flank into the rumen. Most modern devices have a tapered, threaded shaft that holds the rumen onto the trocar to prevent the rumen from falling away from the device. Use of these devices is discouraged by the author because leakage of rumen contents around the trocar invariably results in peritonitis. However, in certain instances of severe respiratory depression, it may be the only option available for decompression.

In some cases, solid ingesta must be removed from the rumen. Indications for this include grain overload and rumen acidosis. Standard size esophageal tubes are easily plugged with rumen contents and are not effective for

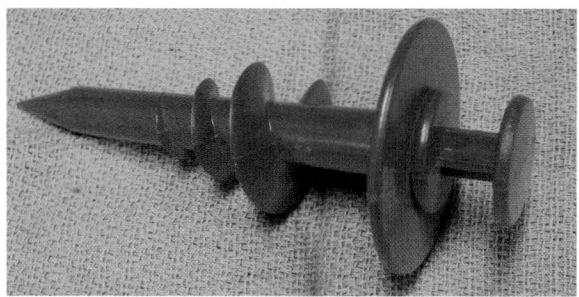

FIGURE 25-56 Rumen trocar used to relieve severe bloat in cattle. The main risk with the use of this device is leakage of rumen fluid around the trocar, which will cause peritonitis. Therefore, use of this device is discouraged except in emergency situations.

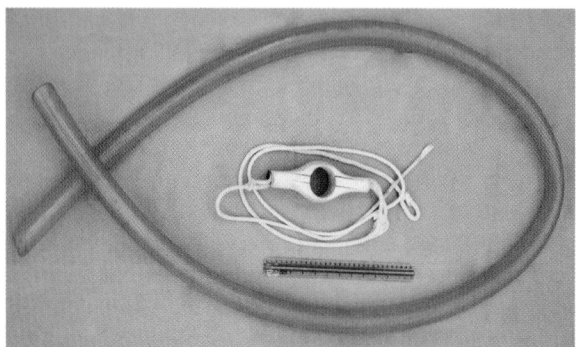

FIGURE 25-57 Kingman tube with mouth gag. This tube is used to remove ingesta, liquid, and gas from the rumen of cattle with severe rumen distention. (*Note:* For size comparison, the ruler is 30 cm in length.)

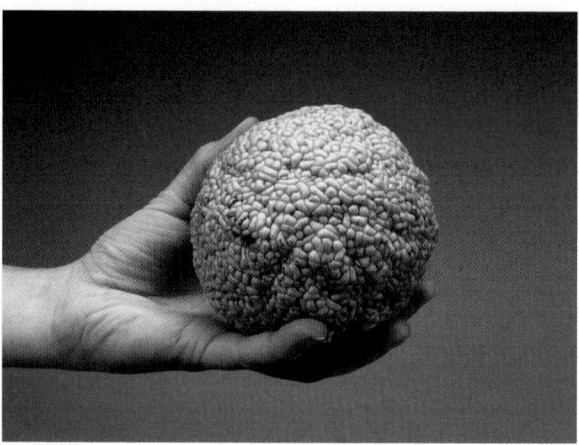

FIGURE 25-58 Photo of a hedge apple. These firm fruits frequently cause esophageal obstruction (choke) when swallowed by cattle. (Courtesy Dr. Bruce Hull, Columbus, Ohio.)

removing solid ingesta. A Kingman tube is a large-bore esophageal tube that can be used for removal of ingesta, liquid, and gas from the rumen (Figure 25-57). To pass a Kingman tube, the patient's head must be securely restrained. A mouth gag that is designed to be used with the Kingman tube is placed in the mouth and securely tied around the head. A thin layer of lubricant or mineral oil can be applied to the tube to aid in passage. With the head extended, the tube is passed through the center hole of the mouth gag until the pharyngeal area is reached. Gentle pressure should be exerted on the tube until the tube passes the pharyngeal region and begins to travel down the esophagus. The tube occasionally will encounter some resistance before entering the rumen, so slightly withdrawing the tube, rotating the tube 90 degrees, and advancing the tube will often enable it to pass. To assist in recovery of rumen contents, the cow's head and the end of the tube should be held as low as possible. Filling the tube with water and allowing the water to drain will create a siphon, which may aid in draining rumen contents. Flushing the tube with water can also overcome blockage of the tube by fibrous rumen material. If the Kingman tube is not sufficient for emptying the rumen contents, a rumenotomy may be indicated.

Choke

Choke is the common name given to an esophageal obstruction caused by swallowing a foreign body. Clinical signs include gagging or retching and excessive drooling. Typically, animals can still breathe, but the condition can be very frightening to watch as the animal retches for long periods without relief. If the animal cannot eructate and expel gas produced in the rumen, severe bloat can result. In cattle, choke is often due to swallowing apples or, frequently, hedge apples (Figure 25-58). It is also a common problem in camelids and is usually due to rapid consumption of pelleted feed material. A palpable ball of feed material or a foreign body may be felt over the cervical esophagus but may not be palpable if the obstruction is at the thoracic inlet. Often the choke will resolve spontaneously, but veterinary intervention may be necessary to relieve the obstruction. If the animal is choking on feed material and the obstructing ball of feed material can be palpated, the area should be gently massaged to facilitate breakup of the mass. If massage is unsuccessful, or if a large foreign body is present, the mass should be moved into the rumen or first stomach compartment. An esophageal tube usually can be used to push the obstructing mass into the stomach. The veterinarian will need a tube of adequate size to pass down the esophagus to relieve the obstruction. Tube size varies with the size of the animal, but the esophagus is very distensible, and a typical large animal nasogastric tube works well for most adults. Adult cattle usually require a more rigid tube than is needed for sheep and goats. Coating the tube with some obstetrical lube or mineral oil may aid in passage and decrease esophageal or pharyngeal trauma.

RUMEN FLUID ANALYSIS AND TRANSFAUNATION

In certain cases, especially cases of grain overload, analysis of rumen contents is beneficial. Analysis of rumen contents includes measurement of rumen pH, a methylene blue reduction test, and microscopic examination of ruminal fluid. The pH should be measured with a pH meter or with pH paper. Normal rumen pH should be roughly 7, but animals that are accustomed to high-grain diets may have a

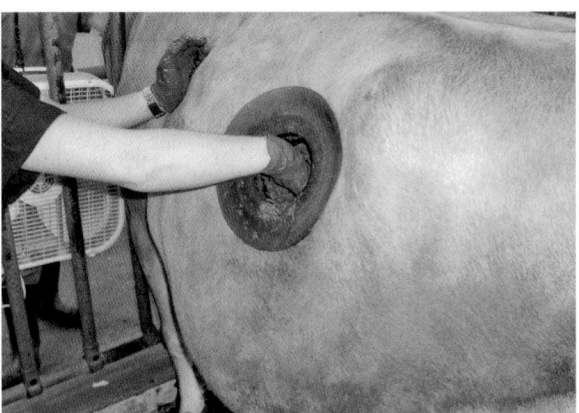

FIGURE 25-59 Collection of rumen contents from a rumen cannulated cow.

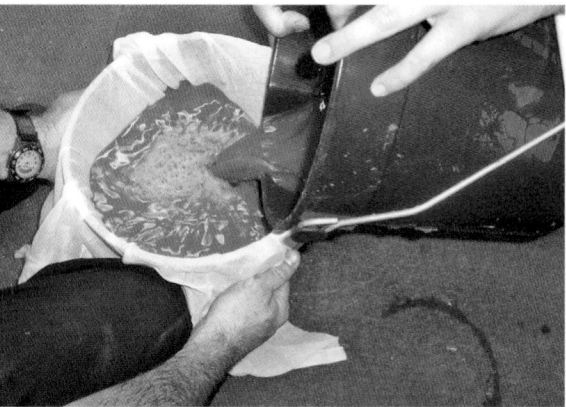

FIGURE 25-60 Rumen fluid being strained with cheesecloth to remove particulate matter before it is pumped through an esophageal tube.

rumen pH as low as 5.5. The methylene blue reduction test is an assay that is used to determine microbial function. One-half milliliter (ml) of 0.03% methylene blue is added to 9.5 ml of strained ruminal fluid to make a total of 10 ml in a clear glass tube. A second tube of ruminal fluid serves as a color control. Methylene blue will color all ruminal contents blue, but the ruminal flora will reduce methylene blue, and the contents of the tube will change back to their natural color within 5 minutes if the ruminal flora is normal. Delayed return to normal rumen fluid color indicates decreased rumen flora activity.

> **TECHNICIAN NOTE** Normal rumen pH should be roughly 7.

A drop of ruminal fluid should be placed on a microscope slide and viewed under low power (10× objective). Many motile protozoa should be seen per low power field. It is normal to see organisms of different sizes, and they should appear active. If the slide or the rumen contents are allowed to cool, the protozoa will appear less active.

If a patient's ruminal contents are abnormal, a ruminal **transfaunation** will be beneficial. Transfaunation is the transfer of ruminal microbes from one healthy individual to another. The purpose of a transfaunation is to enhance rumen function by repopulating rumen microbes. Rumen transfaunation can be performed in any ruminant species, and the rumen flora is similar across species (therefore, bovine rumen contents can be given to another ruminant species). Ruminal fluid typically is collected from a rumen cannulated cow (Figure 25-59). The cap of the rumen cannula is taken off, and rumen contents are removed. Rumen contents are squeezed, and the resultant fluid is collected in a bucket. The resulting dry ball of fibrous rumen contents typically is discarded but may be placed back into the rumen if the donor cow is considered low on rumen contents. The amount of rumen fluid that needs to be collected will depend on the size of the patient. Invariably, fibrous ruminal ingesta will fall into the bucket of rumen

fluid, and this will obstruct the pump that is used for administering rumen fluid to the patient. To avoid this problem, rumen fluid should be strained with cheesecloth (Figure 25-60), so that rumen fluid free of large particulate material can be obtained. Once collected, rumen fluid should be used as soon as possible because its effectiveness decreases with time. Rumen fluid is administered via an esophageal tube similar to the one used for administration of oral fluids.

> **TECHNICIAN NOTE** Once collected, rumen fluid should be used as soon as possible because its effectiveness decreases with time.

RESPIRATORY SYSTEM

RESPIRATORY DISTRESS

Respiratory distress can be a life-threatening condition that is frightening for both the animal and the owner. These cases must be dealt with promptly. Animals that are air-hungry may act unusually aggressive or delirious. Safety precautions should be followed at all times to avoid placing the veterinarian, veterinary staff, owner, or patient in unnecessary danger. A thorough physical examination should be performed to make a diagnosis, but in some situations, it must be abbreviated until the animal is stabilized.

If the patient is in severe respiratory distress, stabilization should be a higher priority than the physical examination. The veterinary team should be prepared to administer oxygen if necessary. This can be accomplished via nasal cannula, face mask, or endotracheal tube. The equipment necessary to achieve safe and effective oxygen delivery should be readily available.

> **TECHNICIAN NOTE** When dealing with patients in respiratory distress, the veterinary team should be prepared to administer oxygen if necessary.

CHOANAL ATRESIA

Choanal atresia (CA) is a congenital condition in which the entrance into the nasopharynx (choana) is blocked; this is frequently seen as an emergency condition in alpaca crias. Alpacas are semi-obligate nasal breathers, meaning that they cannot efficiently pass air through their mouths. Crias born with CA are in severe respiratory distress. Although surgical correction has been attempted, humane euthanasia typically is recommended because of quality of life concerns. Crias should be given oxygen through a face mask, so that the small volume of inspired air has higher oxygen content. A small (8 to 10 French) red rubber catheter should be available to determine the patency of the nasal passage. Radiography may be useful in confirming the diagnosis, and iodinated contrast media can be used to define the caudal limit of the nasal passage.

> **TECHNICIAN NOTE** Alpacas are semi-obligate nasal breathers, meaning that they cannot efficiently pass air through their mouths.

TRACHEOSTOMY

If a patient is presented with an upper airway obstruction, then a tracheostomy can be performed to permit the animal to breathe. The technique is similar to that used in horses. First, the animal should be adequately restrained; cattle should be placed in a chute and headgate. The head should be elevated with a halter. Two halters, one coming off of either side of the head, are helpful to keep the head from being pulled to one side. An approximately 10 × 10-cm area should be prepared for aseptic surgery. This area should be centered on the ventral midline over the palpable trachea at the junction of the cranial third and the middle third of the trachea (Figure 25-61). A tracheostomy tube of adequate size for the patient should be provided. Adult cattle can accommodate tubes with a 10- to 20-mm internal diameter (ID). Calves and small ruminants will require 5- to 10-mm-ID tubes. Young lambs, kids, and crias may require smaller sizes. If the technician is unsure which tube would be best for the specific application, multiple tubes should be prepared.

> **TECHNICIAN NOTE** If the technician is unsure which tracheostomy tube would be best for the specific application, multiple tubes should be prepared.

MUSCULOSKELETAL INJURIES

ORTHOPEDIC EMERGENCIES AND DOWNER ANIMALS

Orthopedic problems can be more problematic in large animal species than in small animal species for several reasons. Fractures and other musculoskeletal problems can be more difficult to repair in these species because of increased forces applied to the fixation. Physical therapy and rehabilitation can be labor-intensive, time-consuming, and

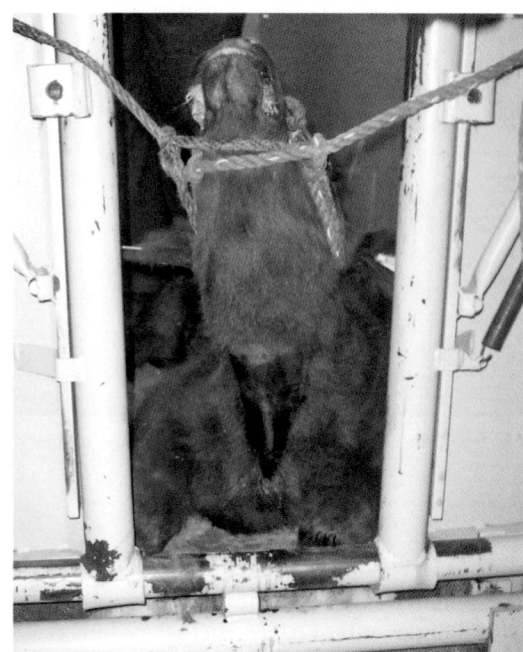

FIGURE 25-61 Calf positioned for a tracheostomy. Two halters are placed on the head, one coming off of either side to keep the head and neck elevated and straight. The mid to cranial cervical region is prepped for surgery.

dangerous. Animals that cannot stand or ambulate are at great risk for secondary problems such as sores and muscle damage due to compression. Ruminants generally make good orthopedic patients because of their calm nature and willingness to lie down, but larger patients are at greater risk than smaller ones for complications. This discussion will be limited to orthopedic emergencies in bovine patients.

> **TECHNICIAN NOTE** Animals that cannot stand or ambulate are at great risk for secondary problems such as sores and muscle damage due to compression.

FRACTURES AND JOINT LUXATIONS

Another common emergency situation for farm animal patients is fracture or joint luxation. Animals with either of these conditions may present with hemorrhage or variable degrees of shock that must be dealt with before the fracture is fixed or the luxation is reduced. If an unstable fracture is present, it should be stabilized so that it does not get worse or cause additional soft tissue damage. Distal fractures (of the metacarpus, radius, metatarsus, or tibia) should be stabilized immediately with a splint or heavy bandage to confer stability. Proximal fractures (of the humerus or femur) are not easily stabilized with splints, but typically have enough surrounding muscle that they are more inherently stable than distal fractures. In smaller patients, slings may afford some support for proximal fractures.

Joint luxation is another musculoskeletal injury that results from trauma and should receive prompt veterinary care. Although it may not be apparent that luxations are emergency situations, the prognosis for successful treatment depends on the rapidity with which they are treated. Joint luxations that are presented, diagnosed, and treated within a few hours after injury have a good chance for successful resolution. Many of these luxations can be corrected by closed (nonsurgical) techniques. This is especially true with shoulder and hip luxations. After several hours, muscle contracture around the limb and debris that accumulates within the joint increase the difficulty with which the joint luxation can be reduced; usually, surgical techniques are necessary for correction.

> **TECHNICIAN NOTE** The prognosis for successful treatment of joint luxation depends on the rapidity with which it is treated.

Animals should be triaged, and any life-threatening problems should be corrected before the joint luxation is treated. Radiographs may be useful for assessing the luxation and formulating a treatment plan. The operating room should be prepared in case surgery is necessary. Traction is often needed in cases of joint luxation or displaced fracture in large animals.

DOWN ANIMALS

Animals that cannot stand are referred to as **"down animals,"** or "downers." Reasons for an animal being down include sepsis and shock; metabolic causes such as hypocalcemia and hypokalemia; orthopedic problems such as fractures, dislocations, and ligament tears; and neurologic diseases. In many cases, the cause remains unknown, but it is important for the veterinary team to try to make an accurate diagnosis so the underlying disease process can be treated. Regardless of the reason the patient is down, secondary skin, muscle, and nerve damage can result, and supportive therapy as well as physical therapy is a mainstay of treatment.

Exceptions may be made for certain orthopedic and neurologic situations, but ideally, down animals should be assisted to help them stand. Several devices can be used to help down cattle stand. A hip lifter is an apparatus that is clamped down tightly over the wings of the ileum. A hook in the center of the device allows attachment of a hoist to assist the cow to stand (Figure 25-62). Hip lifters are relatively lightweight, easy to apply, and easy to use. The disadvantage of using them is that they lift only the rear end of the animal and will allow the cow to tip forward if it cannot bear weight on its front end. Also, because the device concentrates the lifting force on one area, prolonged use can result in skin sores and musculoskeletal trauma over the hip area. Slings may be used to lift cattle more evenly, and can lift front and back ends of the animal simultaneously. Once standing, slings do a better job of distributing the cow's weight more evenly; however, they are designed only to assist an animal to stand, and animals that are completely unable or unwilling to stand will develop complications from prolonged use of slings. In addition, slings are more difficult to

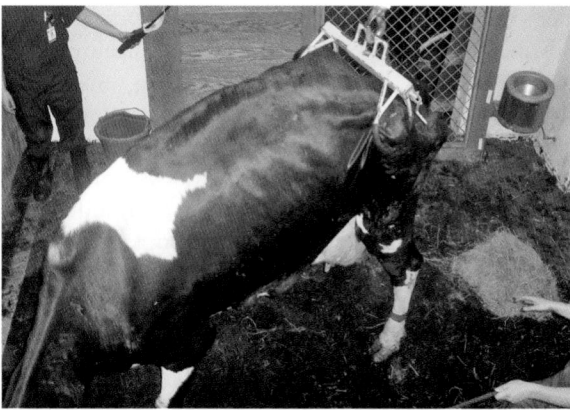

FIGURE 25-62 Cow being lifted in hip lifters. The hip lifters are clamped down around the wings of the ileum, and a hook connected to a hoist is attached to the center of the device and is used to lift the hind end of the cow.

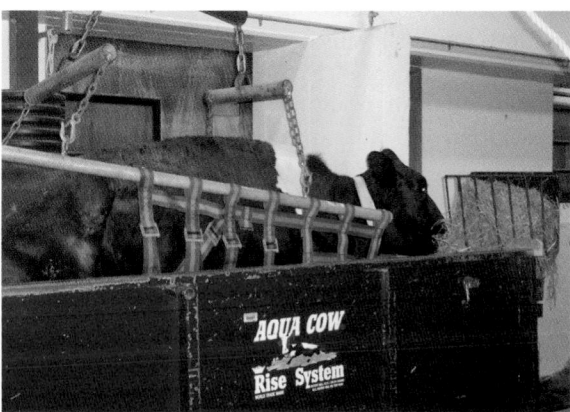

FIGURE 25-63 Down cow supported in a combination of a sling and a float tank. Although each method of support is designed to work independently, the sling offers a level of protection against the cow going down and drowning in the float tank. The sling is actually supporting very little weight of the cow because she is being supported by the water.

apply; it usually takes a team of several experienced people to properly fit a large cow into a sling. Hydroflotation is another option for assisting down cows to stand; it is the best option for supporting cattle for long periods. Hydroflotation of cattle requires specialized float tanks and a team of experienced personnel. Compared with previously described methods of assisting down cows to rise, this method is associated with the least trauma to the animal, and is likely to produce the most favorable outcome. It does, however, carry some unique risks, including drowning of the animal, hypothermia, and infection due to submergence in dirty water (Figure 25-63).

> **TECHNICIAN NOTE** Hydroflotation is another option for assisting down cows to stand; it is the best option for supporting cattle for long periods.

DOG/WILD ANIMAL ATTACKS

Sheep and goats are frequent targets of animal attacks, the most common being dog attacks. Most commonly, the owner's own dog is responsible, and it is important to inform the owner that the attack is likely to occur again if precautions are not taken. If an unknown animal is responsible for the attack, greater concern is raised about infectious disease such as rabies. Although rabies is not common in sheep and goats, it can occur in these species. Attacks can occur anywhere on the body but commonly occur around the head, neck, or extremities. In these locations, serious life-threatening injury can result and may require emergency therapy.

If arterial involvement has resulted in severe blood loss, the animal may need a blood transfusion. The color of the mucous membranes should be noted and PCV/TP should be measured as part of the examination; blood donors or homologous blood should be available. If the animal is still bleeding, hemostasis should be of primary concern. Animals may be in shock after the attack because of the traumatic event or because of blood loss. An IV catheter should be placed in the jugular vein for administration of fluids (for shock) or blood if needed. Neck wounds may directly involve the jugular vein, or resulting cellulitis may make jugular catheterization difficult. In these cases, other peripheral vessels may be used for catheterization.

Although puncture wounds may look superficial, they usually involve deeper structures; this trauma often is not directly obvious. Bite wounds are always contaminated. The depth of these wounds should be explored with a narrow sterile probe. Tissue with questionable viability may be left undébrided until it is known for certain that it is not viable. Other equipment and supplies that should be made available include sterile normal saline for lavage and a 20-ml syringe. A 10 to 12 French red rubber catheter is also useful for lavage of deep wounds. Animal attacks should be considered emergencies and may have fatal consequences, but with proper veterinary care, many of these cases have a successful outcome.

DYSTOCIA AND OBSTETRICAL EMERGENCIES

Obstetrical emergencies must be dealt with in a prompt manner to ensure the health of the dam and the fetus. **Dystocia** (difficult birth) represents the majority of obstetrical emergencies. The cause of the dystocia must be ascertained to ensure proper veterinary treatment and a successful outcome. Management of these cases often requires two or more people. A trained assistant or technician is of utmost importance to the veterinarian and should be proficient in the art of fetal extraction. Often the veterinary assistant or technician will play a lead role in fetal extraction because he or she possesses physical traits that the veterinarian may be lacking. For instance, for managing bovine dystocias, good upper body strength and long arms are an advantage, but for managing dystocias in small ruminants, camelids, and pigs, small hands are invaluable. The veterinary technician should learn the veterinarian's particular style of obstetrical management because many techniques are available, and every veterinarian has his or her personal preferences.

DYSTOCIA BOX AND EQUIPMENT

A dystocia box or a dystocia kit is useful to keep in one centralized location all equipment needed to manage dystocias. Ideally, the kit should be mobile so that it can be moved quickly to the patient (Figure 25-64). Suggested equipment for a farm animal dystocia kit is listed in Box 25-12.

> **TECHNICIAN NOTE** A dystocia box or a dystocia kit is useful to keep in one centralized location all equipment necessary to manage dystocias.

Some veterinarians prefer to use sterile sleeves to perform vaginal examinations; others prefer to scrub their hands and arms carefully before examining the cow. In addition to protecting the uterine environment, sleeves protect the arms of

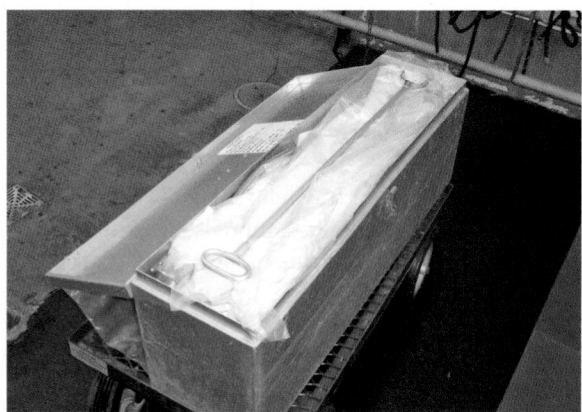

FIGURE 25-64 Dystocia box. Box contains all commonly used equipment for management of a bovine dystocia. The box is kept on a wagon so that it is easily moved around the clinic.

BOX 25-12	Suggested Items to Be Included in a Farm Animal Dystocia Kit

- Obstetrical chains
- Chain handles
- Head snare
- Eye hooks
- Cray hook
- Finger knife
- Sterile water-based lubricant
- Bucket
- Pump
- Soft tube
- Fetatome
- Obstetrical wire
- Wire introducer
- Wire passer
- Wire cutters
- Calf jack
- Soft rope (clothesline)

the veterinarian. If the veterinarian prefers to use sterile sleeves, these should be available, along with sterile lubricant. Certain lubricants can be very toxic if introduced into the abdominal cavity. For this reason, some lubricants are not recommended if a cesarean section (C-section) is a possibility, or if uterine trauma is extensive.

Sterile obstetrical chains should be available for assisting in vaginal extraction of calves. Each chain should be accompanied by at least two handles, so the assistant can help with the delivery. Proper placement of obstetrical chains should be ensured to prevent injury to the calf. The chain should be wrapped around the calf's leg proximal to the fetlock, and a half-hitch should be placed below the fetlock. A calf-jack is a winch that is used to apply traction on obstetrical chains; it can be very useful in helping to extract a large fetus, especially when help is limited. The operator must be very careful that too much force is not applied, or trauma to the fetus or dam may result.

> **TECHNICIAN NOTE** Sterile obstetrical chains should be available for assisting in vaginal extraction of calves. Each chain should be accompanied by at least two handles, so the assistant can help with the delivery.

A **fetatome** is a device that uses obstetrical wire to perform a **fetotomy** (cutting a fetus into smaller parts that can be extracted more easily). Operation of a fetatome requires two people—one to place the fetatome and hold it in position, and an assistant to make the cut.

A Krey-hook is a device that can be used to grab fetal parts when a fetotomy is performed. It is designed so that when traction is applied, it clamps down harder onto the fetus. Eye hooks can also be used in cattle to attach directly under the medial canthus of the eyes to help apply traction to the head. Because of the orbital anatomy of cattle, they can even be applied to live calves without causing severe trauma. A finger knife is a useful tool for making cuts in a fetus while protecting maternal tissues.

A bucket, a pump, and a uterine lavage tube are also recommended for inclusion in a dystocia kit. Access to clean water is important, and plenty of lubricant should be available. Frequently, it is useful to pump water and lubricant into a contracting uterus to distend it and lubricate the birth canal.

EXAMINATION

Every case of dystocia should begin with a thorough examination. In addition to obtaining a history and performing a physical examination, vaginal and/or rectal examination should be performed. A rectal examination can allow the veterinarian to feel the outside of the uterus and may be useful for diagnosis of **uterine torsion**. Most other information can be obtained by performing a vaginal examination.

The **perineal** area should be prepped before the vaginal examination, so manure and dirt are not carried into the vagina. The tail should be tied out of the way to prevent contamination of the area once it has been cleaned. The perineal scrub is not intended to achieve asepsis, but to decrease uterine and vaginal contamination. This reduces the incidence of metritis and keeps the uterine environment cleaner, so the risk for abdominal contamination is lessened if a C-section is performed. If a rectal examination is performed, do not clean the perineal area until after the rectal examination has been completed. Some veterinarians prefer to begin by cleaning out the rectum, so the cow does not defecate on the clean field.

> **TECHNICIAN NOTE** The perineal scrub performed before vaginal examination is not intended to achieve asepsis, but to decrease uterine and vaginal contamination.

EPIDURAL ANESTHESIA

Epidural anesthesia can be useful for reducing the pain associated with vaginal manipulation and for decreasing the force of uterine contractions, so that vaginal manipulation of the fetus can be accomplished. However, if vaginal delivery is to be performed, epidural anesthesia may be contraindicated because the dam will no longer be able to assist in the delivery process. Also, overzealous epidural anesthesia can cause the animal to become recumbent.

> **TECHNICIAN NOTE** Epidural anesthesia can be useful for reducing the pain associated with vaginal manipulation and for decreasing the force of uterine contractions, so that vaginal manipulation of the fetus can be accomplished.

VAGINAL DELIVERY

It is the goal of most veterinarians to deliver the fetus vaginally. In most cases, vaginal delivery affords many advantages over C-section, including faster delivery of the fetus, faster recovery of the dam, and fewer postparturient complications. The veterinary technician must be familiar with the procedure and the equipment needed for it, to provide the greatest help to the veterinarian.

Vaginal delivery can be successfully performed with the fetus presented head first or hind legs first. If the fetus is presented in anterior presentation (front legs first), the head and both front legs must be extended into the pelvis of the dam. If the fetus is delivered in posterior presentation (back legs first), both hind legs are extended and presented in the birth canal. If the fetus is in posterior presentation and the hind legs are retained so that the rump of the fetus is presented first, the presentation is termed *breech*. Breech fetuses must be repositioned before successful vaginal delivery can be performed.

> **TECHNICIAN NOTE** Vaginal delivery can be successfully performed with the fetus presented head first or hind legs first.

CESAREAN SECTION

The incision for a C-section may be made in the flank, on the ventral midline, or paramedian. The surgeon should be asked which approach will be used for each case. Adequate restraint is important for any animal undergoing C-section. A headgate and chute system with a removable side panel is preferred for standing C-sections. C-sections can be performed in small ruminants that are awake; however, because of increased difficulty in keeping the animal restrained, the surgeon will often elect to place these animals in right lateral recumbency. In cattle, the tail is tied to prevent contamination of the surgical site. An epidural is recommended to keep the cow from straining during the procedure, but as noted previously, too much local anesthetic can cause the cow to become weak and recumbent during the procedure.

Before surgery is performed, the appropriate area should be clipped and aseptically prepared. Most commonly, C-sections in ruminants are performed on the left flank with the animal awake. A liberal area should be prepared from caudal to the tuber coxae (the point of the hip) to the 12th intercostal space, and from the dorsal midline to the flank fold, to decrease the risk for abdominal contamination during surgery.

Regional nerve blocks are recommended to anesthetize the flank for standing surgery. Proximal paravertebral or distal paravertebral nerve blocks are preferable over line blocks because the presence of local anesthetic at the surgical site makes surgery more difficult and increases the likelihood of complications of wound healing.

Before a cesarean section is begun, the surgeon's table should be set up with the equipment listed in Box 25-13.

In cattle, assistance is almost always required to extract the calf. The assistant need not scrub but should wear a sterile gown and gloves. The assistant usually assumes the role of neonatologist after extraction of the calf, and therefore should be well versed in care of the neonate.

| BOX 25-13 | Equipment for Bovine Cesarean Section |

- Surgery pack
  - Towel clamps (qty = 10)
  - Hemostats (10 Kelly, 5 mosquito)
  - Mayo scissors
  - Needle holders
  - 2 scalpels
  - 4 × 4 gauze sponges
  - Uterine forceps
- Drapes
- Suture with needles
  - Uterus (absorbable, #2 Chromic gut)
  - Body wall (absorbable, #3 Chromic gut)
  - Skin (nonabsorbable, #3 Braunamid)
- Obstetrical chains
- Sterile sleeves
- Basin with sterile saline

TECHNICIAN NOTE   When a C-section is performed in cattle, assistance is almost always required to extract the calf.

UTERINE TORSION

Uterine torsion is a condition in which the pregnant uterus twists in relation to the maternal pelvis. Uterine torsion is a cause of dystocia in cattle, and it can also occur in camelids. It usually can be corrected by rolling the animal to correct torsion. Rolling a cow to correct uterine torsion usually requires multiple people. The direction of the torsion is important to determine because this will influence the direction in which the animal will need to be rolled to correct the twist. The uterus is immobilized while the animal is rolled. In cattle, this is usually accomplished by the "plank-in-the-flank" method. The cow is cast onto the desired side with a long rope. Other ropes are used to tie the legs together. A long 2 inch × 12 inch board is placed in the flank directly in front of the tuber coxae. An assistant (usually the largest person in the group) stands on the plank near the flank end. The cow is slowly rolled in the desired direction while the assistant bounces up and down on the board. The cow then is palpated and rolled again if necessary. For severe twists, multiple rolls may be necessary to fully correct the torsion. A detorsion rod can also be used to untwist the uterus of a cow. This method requires an open cervix and the ability to pass the rod and a hand into the uterus. The calf's legs are secured to the rod, and the rod is used to flip the calf and the uterus.

Camelids can also suffer from uterine torsion, and similar principles apply. Conservative therapy for correction involves rolling the llama or alpaca. Typically, an assistant will palpate the uterus through the abdomen and will stabilize the uterus while the animal is rolled. Surgical correction is another option for correcting uterine torsion in cases refractory to conservative management and in animals that have had a previous torsion.

SMALL RUMINANT DYSTOCIAS

The same principles apply to dystocias in small ruminants. In these cases, the limiting factor for vaginal manipulation is commonly the size of the veterinarian's hands. If the assistant has smaller hands, he or she is frequently called upon to manipulate the fetus vaginally. It must be remembered that the uterus of small ruminants is more easily ruptured than the uterus of cattle. Therefore, care must be taken when vaginal manipulation is performed.

UTERINE PROLAPSE

Another emergency condition associated with parturition is prolapse of the uterus. **Uterine prolapse** occurs when the uterus folds inside-out through the cervix and the vulvar lips. Variable degrees of uterine prolapse can occur; the most serious are those that involve the entire uterus. Sequelae of uterine prolapse include uterine trauma with potential tearing of the uterine wall, and damage to the uterus due to restriction of the blood supply (ischemia). If the weight of the uterus applies too much traction on the vasculature of the uterus, the uterine artery can rupture, causing fatal hemorrhage. For this reason, caution must be used if a cow with a uterine prolapse is transported over a long distance in a trailer before correction.

> **TECHNICIAN NOTE** Caution must be used if a cow with a uterine prolapse is transported over a long distance in a trailer before correction.

The external environment can be very detrimental to the **endometrial** (inner uterine) lining. A drape or a large plastic bag makes a good surface for protecting the uterus against further contamination and trauma during correction. Before correction of the prolapse, the endometrial surface should be gently cleansed. Warm water or saline is sufficient. Antiseptic solutions should be used with caution because of the potential for chemical damage to the endometrial surface. An epidural should be administered to the cow to decrease straining and to allow the uterus to be replaced with less force. Elevation of the uterus above the vulva can help with reduction (replacement of the uterus). After the uterus has been replaced, the veterinarian typically will perform another procedure to keep the uterus from re-prolapsing. The technician or assistant should learn and be familiar with the specific style of the veterinarian, so that maximal assistance can be provided.

TOXIC METRITIS AND TOXIC MASTITIS

Cattle that develop severe **metritis** and **mastitis** can develop endotoxemia from absorption of endotoxins. These animals may present with signs of toxic shock (tachycardia and tachypnea), they may present with weakness or neurologic deficits, or they may be down. A blood sample should be taken for a complete blood count and a biochemistry profile, so therapy can be specifically tailored to the patient's needs. Cattle usually require IV fluid support and should have an IV catheter placed in a jugular vein. Hypertonic saline may be used to help restore circulating blood volume. If the animal is down on presentation, supportive therapy should be provided to avoid severe nerve and muscle damage.

UROLITHIASIS IN SMALL RUMINANTS

Urethral obstruction due to **urolithiasis** (urinary calculi or stones) is a common disease in ruminants, especially small ruminants (sheep and goats), and is seen almost exclusively in males. Predisposing factors for development of urinary calculi include high-grain diets (diets high in phosphorus), legume forages, and dehydration.

> **TECHNICIAN NOTE** Formation of most stones is associated with ingestion of high-phosphorus diets such as those high in concentrates (grain).

Complete urethral obstruction from urolithiasis is the most common presentation; these cases should be treated as emergencies. Failure to treat these animals in a timely fashion can result in bladder rupture, urethral rupture, or death of the animal. Several treatment options are known; the best option will depend on use of the animal; the age of the animal; concurrent problems such as urethral rupture, bladder rupture, or severe metabolic derangements; and the veterinarian's experience and preferences. (See Case Presentation 25-3 for an example of emergency management of urethral obstruction due to urolithiasis.)

HISTORY AND PHYSICAL EXAMINATION

The veterinarian usually can diagnose urethral obstruction with data obtained from a good history and physical examination. The owner should be questioned about the animal's presenting signs, the duration of the problem, when the animal was last observed to urinate, the quality of the urination (full stream vs. dribbling), access to water, any drugs or other treatments administered, and dietary history.

These animals are usually in pain when presented, and so additional restraint may be necessary to perform a good physical examination. Sedation may be necessary, and acepromazine is a better choice than xylazine because xylazine has diuretic properties and can increase urine production. The veterinarian may wish to perform a rectal examination to palpate the penis and urethra, so supplies needed for a rectal examination should be available. If available, ultrasonography can be a very useful diagnostic tool to evaluate the size of the bladder and the presence of any free fluid (urine) within the abdomen. A $5\frac{1}{2}$ MHz convex probe is ideal for transabdominal ultrasound of most small ruminants. If the animal has formed radiopaque stones, radiography may be useful to determine the quantity and location of the stones (Figure 25-65). Unfortunately, many urinary calculi (e.g., struvite stones) are not radiopaque and will not be visible on survey radiographs. Therefore, the absence of visible stones on radiographs does not rule out a diagnosis of urolithiasis. In cases of chronic obstruction, metabolic derangements are common with potentially fatal consequences, so a biochemistry profile is useful under these circumstances. In particular, electrolytes that can contribute to metabolic abnormalities (sodium, chloride, and potassium) should be measured. Measuring blood urea nitrogen and creatinine is also useful in assessing the severity of azotemia.

> **TECHNICIAN NOTE** The absence of visible stones on radiographs does not rule out a diagnosis of urolithiasis.

TREATMENT

Severe metabolic derangements should be addressed before the obstruction is relieved. This is especially important if the animal is to undergo general anesthesia. Although somewhat counterintuitive, obstructed animals generally will benefit

CASE PRESENTATION 25-3 FOOD ANIMAL

Brutus, a 4-year old male castrated pygmy goat, was presented to the clinic with a history of constipation. The goat was straining, was not eating, and was uncomfortable for 3 days before admission. The owner administered three enemas (one a day since the signs started) and offered a mild laxative with his daily grain, but Brutus refused to eat it. He was fed grain and given "treats" at home.

On physical examination, Brutus appeared uncomfortable and was straining. Digital rectal examination revealed no feces in the rectum, but the urethra was palpated ventrally to the rectum and was found to be pulsating. The prepuce was dry, and a few crystals were found on the hair of the prepuce. The owners were questioned about the last time the goat was observed to urinate; they indicated that this occurred about 4 days before.

A presumptive diagnosis of obstructive urolithiasis was made, and an abdominal ultrasound was performed. The bladder measured approximately 10 cm, but no free fluid was found in the abdomen. The technician placed an IV catheter in the jugular vein and drew blood for a biochemistry profile. 0.9% saline was started at maintenance rate before laboratory results were received. The profile revealed extreme azotemia with BUN and creatinine of 105 mg/dl and 8 mg/dl, respectively. Potassium was 6.9 mEq/L (high). The veterinarian ordered dextrose to be added to the fluids to help lower blood potassium.

After 60 minutes on the new fluid regimen (0.9% NaCl with 5% dextrose at 1.5 times the maintenance rate), the goat was taken to surgery to undergo a tube cystostomy. The goat was anesthetized and was maintained under general anesthesia with isoflurane. Multiple uroliths (stones) were cleaned from the bladder, and a 20 French Foley catheter was placed through the abdominal wall into the bladder. Surgery, anesthesia, and recovery were uneventful.

After surgery, Brutus was offered free-choice hay, but no grain. He was given ammonium chloride to acidify his urine and dissolve any stones in the urethra. Seven days after surgery, the tube was clamped off, and the goat was observed to urinate through his urethra. The clamp was left on the tube for 24 hours, and after a night of successful urinations with the tube clamped, the bulb of the tube was deflated and the tube was pulled.

The owners were given information about urolithiasis in goats. They were told that it is a common problem in male goats, especially those that receive grain in their diets. They were advised to feed no grain at all and were told that good-quality grass hay serves as a sufficient diet for pet goats. They were advised to monitor the goat closely at home for urination because recurrence may occur, and most straining in male goats is due to urinary blockage, not to constipation.

The owners changed Brutus's diet as recommended and stopped feeding grain entirely. They reported that Brutus was doing well after surgery and discharge from the clinic, and they were very pleased with the service provided by the veterinary team.

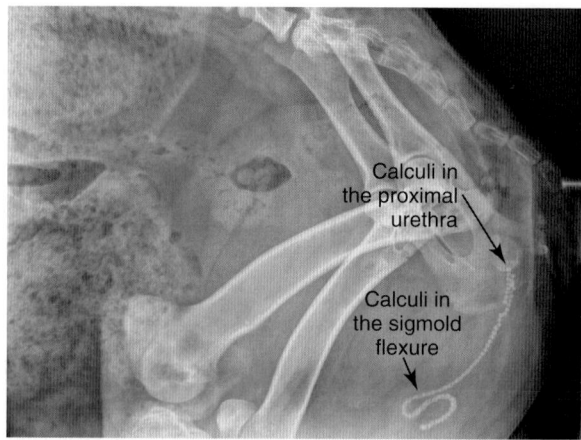

FIGURE 25-65 Radiograph of a male goat with multiple urinary calculi. Calculi line the proximal urethra, including the sigmoid flexure.

from IV fluid therapy before the obstruction is resolved. An IV catheter should be placed in the jugular vein. For most small ruminant patients, a 16-gauge, 3¼-inch catheter should be used. Hyperkalemia (high potassium), hyponatremia (low sodium), and hypochloremia (low chloride) are the most common electrolyte abnormalities. Hyperkalemia is the most dangerous electrolyte disturbance because it may lead to fatal cardiac arrhythmias. These animals should not receive IV fluids containing potassium. Normal strength saline (0.9% NaCl) is the ideal fluid because affected animals are frequently deficient in sodium and chloride, and the fluid does not contain potassium. Sodium bicarbonate and dextrose can also be given IV to help drive potassium into the cells, thus decreasing blood potassium levels.

Treatment objectives for patients with obstructive urolithiasis are to stabilize the patient; to allow for urine drainage, diuresis, and waste removal; and to restore patency to the urinary tract.

The most common place for calculi to lodge and cause an obstruction in goats is the **urethral process**. The urethral process is a small, funnel-shaped appendage on the distal end of the penis. If the urethral process can be visualized, it can be amputated. The most difficult part of this procedure is exteriorization of the penis. Acepromazine at a dose of 0.05 mg/kg given intravenously will allow the animal to relax and will make it more tolerant of penile exteriorization. The goat should be positioned on its rump with its hind legs pulled forward. This positioning will facilitate penile exteriorization. One person should hold the goat in this position, while another attempts to retract the prepuce. Once the penis is visualized, a third person should roll a gauze square into a strip and place it transversely around the shaft of the penis just proximal to the glans penis. The gauze strip should be twisted firmly around the penis to keep the penis from retracting back into the prepuce. The urethral process can now be visualized and amputated.

Urethrostomy is a process that involves creating an opening in the urethra proximal to the obstruction. A urethrostomy can be performed rapidly and typically does not require general anesthesia. Sedation, epidural anesthesia, or a local nerve block is usually sufficient. The procedure may be performed with the animal standing, but positioning the animal on a table with the hind legs hanging over the edge, or elevating the rear quarters of the animal with the legs spread apart, may facilitate the procedure. The procedure can be performed in the perineal region (referred to as *perineal urethrostomy*), or it can be performed in a more ventral location. For urethrostomy, the area from the tail head (dorsal margin) to the area of the scrotum (ventral margin) and laterally from one thigh to the other should be clipped and prepped for surgery. The prepped area may be modified slightly depending on the intended placement of the incision. A vertical incision will be made on the midline ventral to the anus. The penis will be exteriorized in this location and the urethra opened to provide urine drainage. Complications of this procedure include hemorrhage from the penile stump and stricture of the urethra at the surgery site. This is a quick procedure, but it often is not associated with a good long-term outcome because of the possibility of stricture. It is also not an option for breeding animals.

> **TECHNICIAN NOTE** Urethrostomy is a process that involves creating an opening in the urethra proximal to an obstruction by a urinary stone. A urethrostomy can be performed rapidly and typically does not require general anesthesia.

A **tube cystostomy** involves placement of a Foley catheter in the bladder to provide temporary diversion of urine while urinary stones are dissolved or passed. This procedure involves a ventral abdominal approach and is performed under general anesthesia. The following equipment should be prepared: a general surgery pack, a basin and sterile saline, a bulb syringe for lavaging the open bladder and the abdomen, equipment to provide sterile suction, a bladder spoon for removing uroliths from the bladder (Figure 25-66), electrocautery, and a Foley catheter. The appropriate size of the Foley catheter varies from patient to patient, but catheters smaller than 16 French are not recommended because they are easily plugged with blood clots or calculi. The Foley catheter is left in place for about 1 week to allow urine to drain. During this time, the animal is medically managed to dissolve the stones and to relax the urethra, so that any stones trapped in the urethra will pass. After this time, the tube is clamped off, and the patient is observed to confirm passage of urine through the urethra. If the patient can urinate

successfully, the tube is removed. This procedure is more involved than the urethrostomy technique or the urethral process amputation; however, it is associated with a better long-term outcome and is the recommended procedure for breeding animals.

> **TECHNICIAN NOTE** Foley catheters smaller than 16 French are not recommended because they are easily plugged with blood clots or calculi.

Bladder marsupialization involves the creation of a permanent opening from the skin into the bladder to allow drainage of urine directly out of the bladder instead of through the urethra. As with the tube cystostomy, this procedure involves making a ventral abdominal incision with the patient under general anesthesia. Patient preparation and surgical equipment needed to perform a marsupialization are similar to those for a tube cystostomy.

Prevention is a very important aspect of urolithiasis management. Most cases of urolithiasis can be prevented by management changes on the farm—most important, dietary changes. The most important recommendation for owners of pet male goats is to feed **NO** grain. Urine acidifiers like ammonium chloride can be fed to help dissolve phosphatic calculi that form preferentially in alkaline urine. It is very important to have adequate fresh water available at all times because dehydration can predispose to stone formation. A salt and mineral block may be made available to increase thirst and thus water intake.

> **TECHNICIAN NOTE** Prevention is a very important aspect of urolithiasis management. The most important recommendation for owners of pet male goats is to feed **NO** grain.

RECOMMENDED READINGS

Anderson DE, Rings M: Current veterinary therapy: food animal practice, ed 5, St Louis, 2009, Saunders Elsevier.

Auer JA, Stick JA, editors: Equine surgery, ed 3, St Louis, 2006, Saunders.

Ford RB, Mazzaferro EM, editors: Kirk and Bistner's handbook of veterinary procedures and emergency treatment, ed 8, St Louis, 2006, Elsevier.

Fowler ME: Medicine and surgery of South American camelids: llama, alpaca, vicuña, guanaco, Ames, IA, 1998, State University Press.

Fubini SL, Ducharme NG: Farm animal surgery, St Louis, 2004, Saunders.

Mason DE, Ainsworth DM, Robertson JT: Respiratory emergencies in the adult horse, Vet Clin North Am Equine Pract 10:685, 1994.

Mudge MC, Bramlage LR: Field fracture management, Vet Clin North Am Equine Pract 23:117, 2007.

Orsini JA, Divers T, editors: Equine emergencies, ed 3, Philadelphia, 2008, Saunders.

Peterson ME, Talcott PA, editors: Small animal toxicology, ed 2, St Louis, 2006, Elsevier-Saunders.

Silverstein D, Hopper K, editors: Small animal critical care medicine, St Louis, 2009, Elsevier.

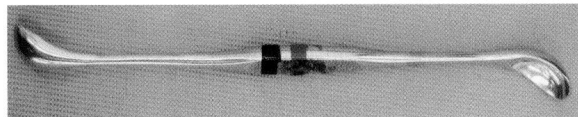

FIGURE 25-66 Bladder spoon. This double-ended spoon is used during a cystotomy procedure to clean the bladder of uroliths.

Smith BP: Large animal internal medicine, St Louis, 2009, Mosby.

Stashak TS, Theoret CL, editors: Equine wound management, ed 2, Ames, IA, 2008, Wiley-Blackwell.

RECOMMENDED WEBSITES

American College of Veterinary Emergency and Critical Care. Available at: www.acvecc.org (accessed on September 12, 2012).

Food Animal Residue Avoidance Databank. Available at: www.farad.org (accessed on September 12, 2012).

Mortimer R: Abnormal calving—pulling the calf. Available at: www.cvmbs.colostate.edu/ilm/proinfo/calving/notes/abnormalcalving.htm (accessed on September 12, 2012).

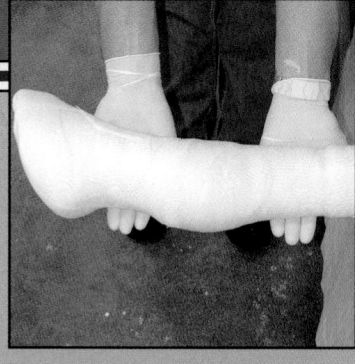

26 Wound Management and Bandaging

Bianca F. Hettlich and Daniel J. Burba

OUTLINE

Wound Healing, *973*
Phases of Wound Healing, *973*
Factors Influencing Wound Healing, *974*

**SMALL ANIMAL WOUND
   MANAGEMENT,** *975*
Wound Management, *975*
Immediate Wound Care, *975*
Wound Débridement, *976*
Wound Closure, *976*
Wound Drainage, *978*
Wound Infection, *978*
Types of Wounds, *978*
Principles of Bandaging, *979*
Adherent Primary Layer, *980*
Nonadherent Primary Layer, *981*
**Bandage, Cast, Splint, and Sling
   Application in Small Animals,** *981*
Distal Limb Bandages, *981*
Casts and Splints, *986*

Slings, *987*
Bandages for Other Locations, *988*
Aftercare for Bandages, Splints, Casts, and
   Slings, *990*

**LARGE ANIMAL WOUND
   MANAGEMENT,** *992*
Wound Care in Horses, *992*
Preparing the Wound, *993*
**Bandage, Splint, and Cast Application
   Techniques for Horses,** *994*
Bandages, *995*
Splint Application, *996*
Cast Application, *997*
Cast Removal, *1002*
**Bandage, Splint, and Cast Application
   Techniques for Cattle,** *1002*
Application of a Claw Block, *1002*
Modified Thomas Splint, *1003*

LEARNING OBJECTIVES

When you have completed this chapter, you will be able to:

1. Pronounce, define, and spell all Key Terms in the chapter.
2. Identify the phases of wound healing, and describe patient, wound, and treatment factors that adversely affect wound healing.
3. Do the following regarding wound management in the small animal:
   • Describe the objectives of and principles of immediate wound care, including wound lavage.
   • Describe the goals of wound débridement and methods used to débride wounds.
   • Differentiate between primary, delayed primary, and secondary wound closure, and between primary, second, and third intention healing.
   • Compare and contrast methods of managing wound drainage and wound infection.
   • Explain the nature of and appearance of abrasions, lacerations, degloving injuries, bite wounds, burns, decubitus ulcers, and pressure sores, and discuss the methods used to treat each.
4. Identify the principles of bandaging, and discuss the purpose of the primary, secondary, and tertiary layers of a bandage, including the specific materials used for each.
5. Do the following regarding application of bandages, casts, splints and slings in small animals:
   • Discuss uses for and characteristics of limb bandages and the technique used to place a Robert Jones bandage or a modified Robert Jones bandage on a small animal limb.

The authors and publisher wish to acknowledge the previous contributions of Giselle Hosgood.

KEY TERMS

Abrasions
Carpal flexion sling
Collagen
Contralateral
Dead space
Débridement
Decubitus ulcers
Degloving injury
Ehmer sling
Epithelialization
External coaptation
Extracellular matrix
Exuberant granulation
   tissue
Fibroblasts
Granulation tissue
Hydrophilic
Hypertonic
Inflammatory phase
Isotonic
Lacerations
Maturation phase
Modified Robert Jones
   bandage
Modified Thomas splint
Moist wound healing
Myofibroblast
Nonadherent dressing
Occlusive
Primary closure
Primary intention
   wound healing
Proliferative phase
Reepithelialization
Robert Jones bandage
Second intention healing
Secondary closure
Semi-occlusive
Spica splint
Third intention wound
   healing
Velpeau sling

- Discuss uses for and characteristics of casts and splints and the technique used to place a cast or splint on a small animal limb.
- Discuss uses for and characteristics of small animal slings and the technique used to place hobbles, or an Ehmer, 90/90 flexion, Velpeau, and carpal flexion sling on a small animal.
- Discuss techniques used to bandage the head, chest, abdomen, tail, and areas that are difficult to bandage such as the pelvis and the axilla.
- Explain aftercare of bandages, splints, casts, and slings, including complications that may occur.

6. Discuss the principles of equine wound care, including treatment of exuberant granulation tissue.
7. Do the following regarding application of bandages, splints, and casts in horses:
   - Discuss uses for, characteristics of, and the technique used to place a lower limb wound bandage or a support bandage on an equine limb.
   - Discuss uses for and characteristics of equine casts and splints and techniques used to place a cast or a splint on an equine limb.
   - Describe the technique used to remove a cast.
8. Discuss uses for and characteristics of bandages, splints, and casts used for cattle and describe technique used to place a claw block or a modified Thomas splint on a ruminant limb.

INTRODUCTION

The veterinary technician plays a crucial role in performing effective wound care, monitoring different phases of healing, and helping to apply and maintain a variety of different forms of bandages and **external coaptation.** Recognizing how wounds heal and what factors alter normal healing will allow the reader to understand the most appropriate form of wound management, whether that may be manual wound care or bandaging. It will also help the reader identify complications of wound healing, enabling early intervention.

WOUND HEALING

PHASES OF WOUND HEALING

The skin forms an important protective barrier against insults from the environment. When injured, either by a traumatic event or by a purposeful insult such as a surgical incision, the physiologic phases of wound healing begin. Wound healing is a continuous process that starts at the moment of injury and lasts up to months thereafter. It can be divided into three phases: inflammatory, proliferative, and maturation, which are distinct in their characteristics but overlap in the time line of healing (Box 26-1). These phases are best observed in a wound left to heal by **second intention healing** (Figure 26-1).

The **inflammatory phase**, the first phase of wound healing, begins immediately. As the injury occurs, blood is released into the wound via injured blood vessels. Platelets aggregate and form a fibrin clot within the wound, which aids in control of bleeding and stabilizes the wound edges. The clot also allows growth factors to be released as part of the clotting cascade. Within a few hours, wound macrophages and neutrophils are recruited and modulate wound

---

BOX 26-1 | Phases of Wound Healing

Inflammatory (lag)
- Begins immediately and lasts 3 to 5 days
- Characterized by formation of a blood clot within the wound, release of growth factors, and recruitment of macrophages and neutrophils to clean up the wound and modulate healing
- The wound is at its weakest during this phase.

Proliferative
- Begins after 2 to 3 days
- Characterized by invasion of fibroblasts, formation of granulation tissue, deposition of collagen, epithelialization across healthy granulation tissue, and wound contraction by myofibroblasts
- Wound strength increases considerably during this phase.

Maturation
- Begins after about 3 weeks and lasts weeks to months
- During this phase, collagen fibers remodel and align, and a final gain in wound strength occurs.

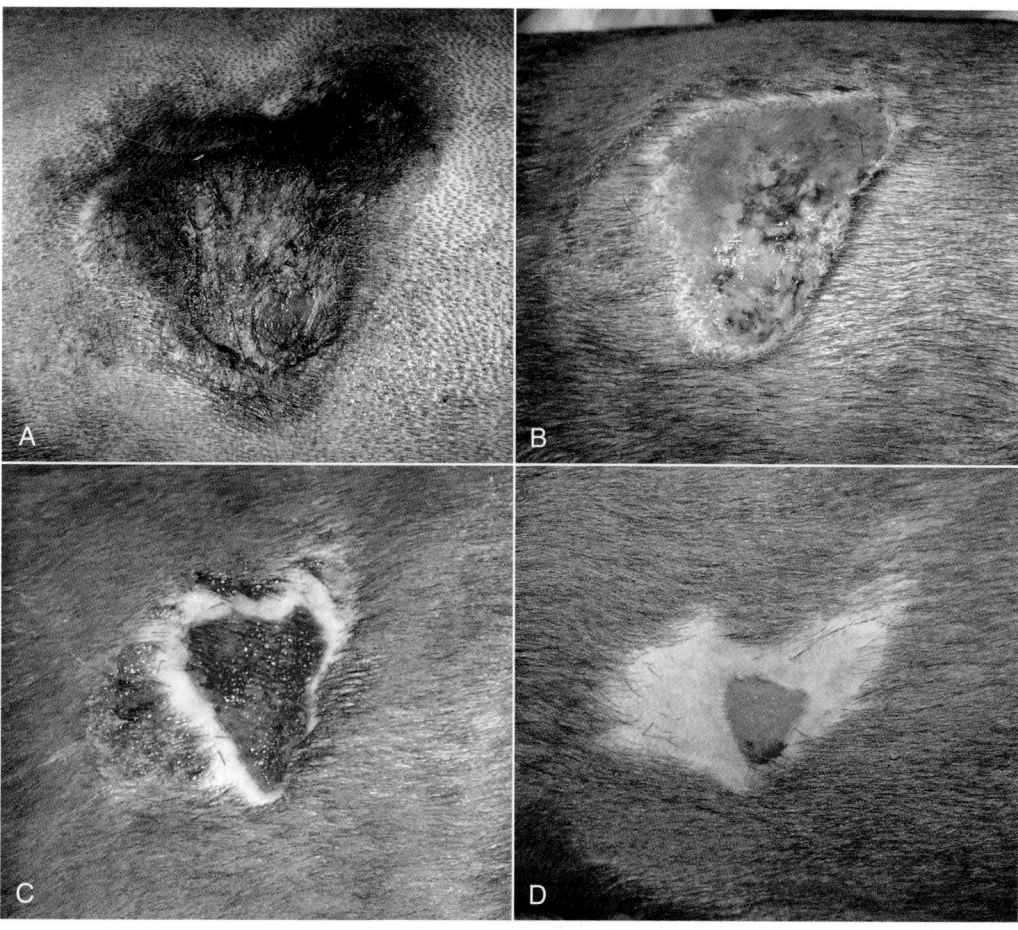

FIGURE 26-1 Phases of wound healing. **A,** The inflammatory phase. Contamination and nonviable tissue have to be eliminated. **B,** Beginning of the proliferative phase. Granulation tissue begins to cover the wound. **C,** Wound contraction. Epithelial cells begin to migrate across the wound. **D,** Epithelialization is well advanced; once complete, the maturation phase will begin.

healing by releasing more growth factors. They also help to remove bacteria and cellular debris from the wound. Wound exudate is the combination of white blood cells and fluid leaked from blood vessels and lymphatics. The inflammatory phase lasts for 3 to 5 days and is often called the *lag phase* because wound strength is at its lowest during this phase.

> **TECHNICIAN NOTE**   During the inflammatory phase of wound healing (the first 3 to 5 days), wound strength is minimal and dehiscence may occur.

The **proliferative phase** overlaps with the inflammatory phase. It begins 2 to 3 days after injury and can continue for several weeks depending on the type and size of the wound. It is marked by **fibroblasts** and endothelial cells entering the wound. Growth factors released into the wound stimulate proliferation and recruitment of these cells, as well as production of an **extracellular matrix**. As cells migrate into the wound, new vessels are formed by angiogenesis to supply oxygen and nutrients to newly forming tissue. **Granulation tissue** begins to fill the wound 3 to 5 days after injury, creating a barrier against infection and a surface for **reepithelialization**. It consists of fibroblasts and **myofibroblasts**, endothelial cells, inflammatory cells, and new blood vessels, all connected by extracellular matrix. Healthy granulation tissue is pink in appearance because of the abundance of capillaries; poor quality granulation tissue is pale because of lack of appropriate blood supply. Fibroblasts then begin to deposit **collagen** into the wound, which finally increases wound strength. Once the wound bed is covered by granulation tissue, fibroblasts decrease in number and are replaced by tissue rich in collagen. Epithelial cells can now migrate across healthy granulation tissue to reestablish a barrier between the wound and the environment. **Epithelialization** usually begins 4 to 5 days after the injury and occurs from the wound edges, moving toward the center. Epithelial cells can also arise from surviving hair follicles and sweat glands. Cells advance in a single layer across the wound until they meet in the middle when migration stops as the result of contact inhibition. New epithelial cells are formed at the wound margins to replace keratinocytes and supply more cells for migration, thereby thickening the epithelial layer. Any scabs covering a wound are epithelialized underneath until the scab falls off. A **moist wound healing** environment enhances cell migration and cleanup and is preferred over allowing a wound/scab to dry out. Once the wound is covered by keratinocytes, a new basement membrane is formed, and cells begin to differentiate to reepithelialize skin. New epithelium tends to be friable and to bleed easily. Wound contraction of the full-thickness skin edges occurs as the result of contractions of myofibroblasts within the granulation tissue. It helps reduce the size of the wound, sometimes considerably. Contraction begins about 1 week after injury and can last for several weeks. Wounds in areas with tight skin will not contract well, and in some areas (e.g., over a joint), wound contraction can lead to poor function.

The final phase of wound healing is the **maturation phase**, which begins approximately 3 weeks after injury and continues for weeks to months—sometimes for years. It is characterized by remodeling and realignment of collagen fibers along tension lines. During this phase, the wound gains the most strength, although it will never be as strong as normal tissue.

A surgically closed wound with direct apposition of wound edges can heal by primary wound healing. The wound will still undergo the three different phases of wound healing; however, in the proliferative phase, granulation tissue does not form because no defect is present between wound edges. Epithelialization begins after a few days and crosses the incision directly. Because of poor wound strength during the inflammatory (lag) phase, wound edges depend entirely on surgical closure during this time. This is why dehiscence is usually seen within the first 3 to 5 days after surgery. Thereafter, wound strength gradually increases, taking a load off sutures or staples.

FACTORS INFLUENCING WOUND HEALING

Wound healing is influenced by many factors such as the health of the animal, the status of the wound, and concurrent treatment of the patient. It is important to consider these factors because they can considerably delay the phases of wound healing or predispose to infection.

Patient Factors

Although age is not a disease, older animals often have concurrent health problems that may alter their healing capabilities. Endocrinopathies such as Cushing's disease and hypothyroidism delay wound healing, as do chronic viral infections such as feline leukemia virus (FeLV) and feline immunodeficiency virus (FIV). Diabetes alters tissue perfusion and release of oxygen, and hyperglycemia interferes with defense against infection. Orthopedic or neurologic problems may lead to periods of prolonged recumbency with increased pressure on certain body parts causing decreased wound healing. Poor nutritional status such as emaciation or diseases that cause low protein and albumin levels (e.g., certain liver diseases) will delay wound healing and alter wound strength. Conversely, obesity is associated with increased risk of wound infection and dehiscence because decreased vascularization of fatty tissue leads to a decreased capacity for healing.

Wound Factors

The origin of a wound has an important influence on wound healing; a surgically created wound tends to have much more predictable healing compared with a traumatically induced wound. Contamination of a wound does not necessarily lead to clinical infection but does require the body to eliminate intruding organisms. If soft tissues are badly injured, they are not able to fight off infection. Local wound defenses cannot be effective if foreign material is present, especially if this material is also contaminated. Even the presence of suture material or drains can interfere with normal healing.

If bacteria are able to multiply beyond a critical number (10^5 organisms per gram of tissue), they will infect tissue, which will stop wound healing. Increased production of wound exudate due to inflammation can lead to fluid accumulation within tissues and separation of tissue planes, further hindering wound healing. Tension on wound edges or movement of surrounding tissues will interfere with the proliferative phase. With proper care, many of these factors can be eliminated.

Concurrent Treatment Factors

Radiation therapy can lead to tissue fibrosis and vascular scarring, both of which negatively affect wound healing. Certain types of chemotherapy can suppress bone marrow function and decrease resistance to infection, thereby contributing to wound healing difficulties. Corticosteroids, especially with long-term use, decrease the body's inflammatory response (thereby increasing risk for infection) and delay all phases of wound healing.

> **TECHNICIAN NOTE** Infection stops the progression of wound healing, and corticosteroids delay all phases of wound healing.

Small Animal Wound Management

WOUND MANAGEMENT

Many animals present with wounds after a traumatic event such as a vehicular accident or a bite. Stabilization of the patient must take precedence over any definitive wound care. A temporary clean bandage should be applied quickly to protect the wound until it can be properly managed. Once stabilized, the animal can receive appropriate wound care (Box 26-2).

IMMEDIATE WOUND CARE

When presented with a wound, the first objective must be to prevent further contamination of the wound, while avoiding contamination of the environment with pathogens from the wound. Gloves must be worn when handling patients with open wounds, and a sterile bandage should be placed when appropriate. The wound can be covered with moist sterile gauze or with sterile, water-soluble lubricant such as K-Y Jelly (Johnson & Johnson Medical, Arlington, Texas). As the hair around the wound is clipped, any hair that falls into the wound will be caught by the sterile lube and can be flushed out after clipping. A scalpel blade or scissors can be used to carefully shave hair from the wound edges. The surrounding skin should then be gently cleaned with an antiseptic such as chlorhexidine or povidone-iodine scrub, but care must be taken to avoid applying soap to the wound because it is cytotoxic to wound cells. The wound is lavaged with a warm **isotonic** crystalloid fluid (e.g., lactated Ringer's solution, 0.9% NaCl) to remove the water-soluble lubricant and, more important, any foreign and loose necrotic debris. Open saline bottles must not be reused because bacterial growth occurs within 24 hours unless an antiseptic is added. Recommended wound lavage pressure is between 8 and 12 psi, which is strong enough to assist debris removal without damaging viable tissue. To achieve this, a 35-ml syringe and a 19-gauge hypodermic needle or over-the-needle catheter are used. These can be connected to a sterile fluid bag via a fluid extension line and a three-way stop-cock, which provides a closed wound lavage system (Figure 26-2).

> **TECHNICIAN NOTE** A 19-gauge catheter and a 35-ml syringe generate the appropriate amount of pressure for effective wound lavage.

Effective wound lavage requires copious amounts of fluid; in highly contaminated wounds, tap water can be used initially instead of sterile isotonic fluids because the main benefit in such a wound comes from the volume of lavage solution rather than the type of fluid used. A dilute antiseptic can be added to lavage fluid, but the cytotoxic potential must be kept in mind. Common mixtures include a 0.05% dilution (1/40) of chlorhexidine solution and a 0.1% dilution (1/10) of povidone-iodine solution.

> **TECHNICIAN NOTE** Copious amounts of a warm isotonic crystalloid fluid (e.g., lactated Ringer's solution, 0.9% NaCl) are best for effective wound lavage.

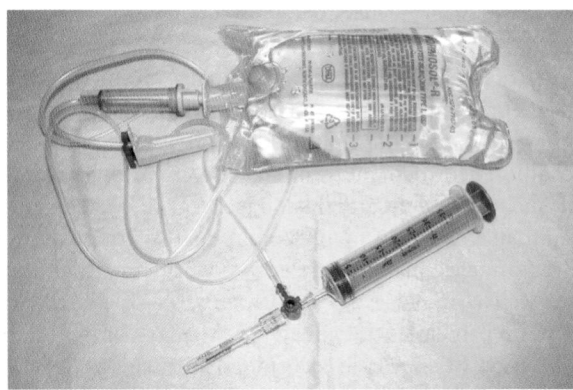

FIGURE 26-2 Setup of a wound lavage system using a 35-ml syringe, a 19-gauge needle or catheter, an extension set, and a bag of sterile isotonic fluid. A three-way stopcock eliminates the need to connect/disconnect.

BOX 26-2	Steps in Proper Wound Management

1. Prevent further contamination.
2. Remove foreign debris and contamination.
3. Débride nonviable tissue.
4. Manage wound drainage.
5. Protect the wound through the inflammatory and proliferative phases.
6. Select appropriate wound closure.

BOX 26-3 | Types of Wound Débridement

Staged Surgical Débridement

Obviously compromised tissue is removed while tissue of questionable health is preserved and removed at a later stage if needed. Used for larger wounds with substantial trauma.

En Bloc Excision

If surrounding skin allows, small wounds can be excised completely and closed primarily.

Enzymatic

Enzymes are used to slowly digest necrotic tissue. Use only in small, contaminated wounds. This technique is not a substitute for surgical débridement.

Mechanical

An adherent primary bandage layer is used to nonselectively débride heavily contaminated wounds. Use only in the inflammatory phase.

Biological

Maggots can be used to ingest necrotic tissue. Used for chronic wounds with poor tissue health.

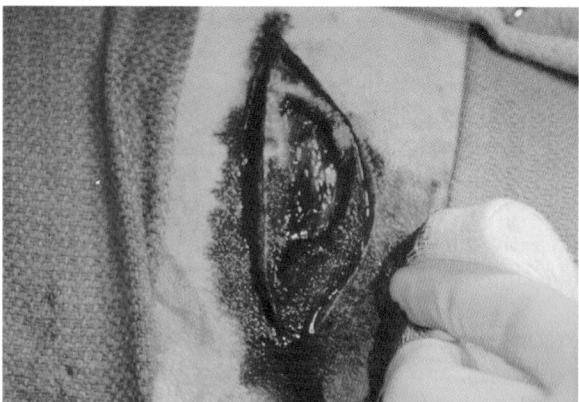

FIGURE 26-3 En bloc resection of a small laceration. The wound is small enough with loose surrounding skin to allow primary closure of the newly created, fresh wound.

BOX 26-4 | Wound Classification

Clean

A wound made under aseptic conditions; a nontraumatic, uninfected operative wound that does not enter a hollow viscus such as the gastrointestinal or urinary tract.

Clean-Contaminated

A surgical wound into which a hollow viscus is entered (respiratory, gastrointestinal, or urogenital tract) without significant contamination; a naturally occurring wound with minor contamination; or a surgical wound with a minor break in sterile technique.

Contaminated

An open traumatic wound; a surgical wound with a major break in sterile technique; or a surgical wound into contaminated areas such as the colon or inflamed/contaminated skin.

Dirty and Infected

An old traumatic wound or an infected wound or perforated viscera; a wound with a high bacterial count (>100,000 organisms per gram of tissue).

WOUND DÉBRIDEMENT

The goal of débridement is removal of obviously contaminated, devitalized, or necrotic tissue and elimination of foreign debris from the wound (Box 26-3). Surgical débridement is usually performed with the patient under general anesthesia in the operating room under aseptic conditions. It is the fastest and most effective way to clean up a heavily contaminated or necrotic wound. Careful wound exploration will aid in overall assessment of the wound to check for complications such as concurrent bony or joint injuries or penetration into a body cavity such as the chest or abdomen. Obviously necrotic tissues are excised, but those with questionable viability may have to be reassessed later to determine whether they will live or die. This staged débridement allows better preservation of viable tissues. Smaller wounds or wounds with little contamination and with viable tissue may be débrided en bloc (as one unit) and closed primarily at this stage (Figure 26-3). Enzymatic agents such as collagenase or trypsin can be used to help break down necrotic debris in small wounds with tenuous blood supply or in patients at high risk for receiving anesthetics. Enzymatic débridement must not be used as a substitute for surgical débridement of wounds with extensive necrosis. Mechanical débridement using an adherent primary bandage layer such as a wet-to-dry bandage can be performed for initial management of highly contaminated wounds. A wet-to-dry bandage causes nonselective débridement; although it is effective, it causes several undesirable side effects (see section on principles of bandaging). Maggots of a special fly can be used to selectively débride dead tissue by ingesting debris and liquefied tissue.

WOUND CLOSURE

Wounds are classified on the basis of whether they are surgically created or are traumatic, as well as according to their level of contamination and the expected number of organisms within the wound (Box 26-4). Degree of contamination (or infection) and chronicity of the wound among other factors dictate the type of wound management and closure to be used (Box 26-5).

Surgically created wounds can be closed by direct apposition and will heal by **primary intention wound healing** across the incision (Box 26-6). Clean traumatic cuts may also undergo **primary closure** after wound lavage. Small wounds with contamination can be excised en bloc and closed primarily. Wounds with a questionable degree of contamination or excess drainage may require a 2- to 3-day period of open wound management before they undergo delayed primary closure (Figure 26-4). This short period of open wound management allows elimination of contamination and improved wound health. Wound closure has to occur before granulation tissue has formed to be called *primary closure*.

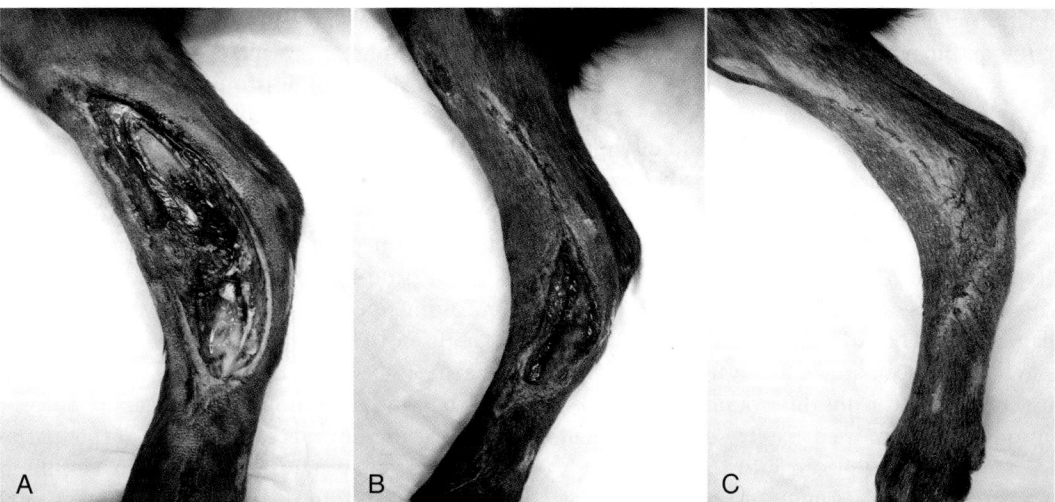

FIGURE 26-4 **A,** Degloving injury to the medial hock of a 1-year-old Labrador. Bones and joints are exposed. The wound has been surgically débrided where safe. After placement of an occlusive, nonadherent dressing for 2 days, delayed primary closure of the most proximal part of the wound was performed. **B,** Day 6: the proximal incision is healing by primary intention and the distal wound is developing healthy granulation tissue. Secondary closure of the distal part of the wound is performed by apposing skin edges over healthy granulation tissue. **C,** Day 18: both aspects of the wound have healed completely. Delayed primary and secondary closure significantly reduced the wound management period compared with second intention wound healing.

BOX 26-5	Factors Influencing Choice of Wound Closure

- Time since the injury
- Extent of foreign body contamination
- Degree of bacterial contamination
- Viability of the tissues
- Damage to the neurovascular supply
- Location of the wound
- Availability of skin for closure
- Tension on the wound

TECHNICIAN NOTE In mildly contaminated wounds that are otherwise amenable to primary closure, the wound can be managed for 2 to 3 days before closing. This method of wound management is known as *delayed primary closure.*

In wounds requiring a longer period of open wound care such as heavily contaminated wounds, **secondary closure** can be performed. These wounds are allowed to form a healthy bed of granulation tissue, which is then folded onto itself with closure of the skin. This type of healing is also referred to as **third intention wound healing.**

Second intention wound healing refers to the process of healing by contraction and epithelialization. Except for surgical débridement, surgical closure is not performed. It is indicated for heavily contaminated wounds for which delayed closure or en bloc excision is not possible. This form of wound healing is often employed in areas with little skin, to close a wound such as the distal limb. The newly epithelialized wound is often friable and easily traumatized. Unfortunately, second intention healing in the distal limb can

---

BOX 26-6	Methods of Wound Closure

Primary Closure With Primary Intention Wound Healing

Surgical apposition of wound edges with sutures or staples. Can be performed in fresh, clean wounds with little loss of soft tissue, such as surgically created wounds. Primary intention wound healing occurs. Epithelialization begins within 1 or 2 days because cells can cross over the incision. Granulation tissue is not needed. En bloc débridement can convert a small, contaminated wound into a clean wound, which then can be closed primarily.

Delayed Primary Closure

Appropriate for wounds older than 6 to 8 hours, with some contamination and questionable ability to heal with primary closure. The wound is treated as an open wound for 2 or 3 days to allow drainage and elimination of infection, and then is surgically closed primarily. Closure occurs before granulation tissue appears.

Secondary Closure

Appropriate for wounds older than 6 to 8 hours, for infected necrotic wounds, and for failed primary wound closure. The wound is allowed to form healthy granulation tissue and then is closed by apposition of granulation surfaces or by excision of granulation tissue and primary closure. This is also known as third intention wound healing.

Second Intention Wound Healing

Appropriate for wounds older than 6 to 8 hours, or for infected, necrotic wounds. The wound is allowed to heal by granulation tissue formation and epithelialization. Disadvantages of this type of healing are the length of time required for complete healing, the cost associated with prolonged treatment, the fragility of the newly epithelialized wound, loss of function due to excessive scarring or contraction, and poor cosmetic results.

produce contraction over joints, muscles, or tendons with impaired function and may not be desirable.

WOUND DRAINAGE

Depending on the quantity of wound exudate and disrupted soft tissues causing **dead space**, passive or active wound drains may be used in conjunction with wound closure. The location of the wound and the amount of drainage will dictate which type of drain can be used. Passive drains function by allowing fluid flow along the drain surface as the result of capillary action. These drains must exit in a dependent location, so that fluid can gravitate toward the exit skin incision and can be removed from the wound. The Penrose drain is the most commonly used passive drain in small animal practice. It is generally placed into smaller wounds with dead space. Passive drains provide a direct avenue for ascending infection and must be covered with a sterile bandage while in place. Active drains, commonly referred to as *closed-suction drains*, work by creating a vacuum within the wound and allowing wound fluid to be removed via a rigid fenestrated drain into an external collection container. Although more expensive than passive drains, closed-suction drains play an important role in the management of more extensive wounds. Drains are removed when the amount of wound fluid decreases (usually after 3 to 5 days) because the simple presence of a drain will stimulate some fluid production.

WOUND INFECTION

A wound is considered infected when the bacterial count is greater than 100,000 (10^5) organisms per gram of tissue. Signs of a wound or incisional infection include swelling, heat, and redness of surrounding tissues. Wound drainage itself is not a sign of infection and should not be used by itself as the determining factor for treatment.

> **TECHNICIAN NOTE** Signs of a wound or incisional infection include swelling, heat, and redness of surrounding tissues. Wound drainage itself is not a sign of infection.

Healthy wounds may exude serosanguineous clear fluid. Discharge from infected wounds can be copious and of varying consistency, color, and odor. With severe infection, systemic signs such as lethargy, pain associated with the wound, and changes in appetite and drinking may occur. The use of antimicrobials depends on the severity of infection and the type of organism, as well as the health of the wound and the patient (see section on factors influencing wound healing). If the overall status of the wound is favorable (good blood supply, superficial infection, minimal foreign body contamination), antimicrobials may not be needed because local wound defenses can often eliminate infection. Wounds with healthy granulation tissue are inherently resistant to infection and do not require antimicrobial use. If infection involves deeper tissues and is well established, oral antimicrobials are appropriate for stable patients; however, if infection is severe and the patient is compromised, intravenous drug administration is indicated. Antibiotics are often chosen empirically on the basis of efficacy against common skin pathogens such as *Staphylococcus* and *Streptococcus* species. Signs of infection should resolve within 2 to 3 days of treatment if the correct antimicrobial was chosen. If infection persists, a resistant organism is present in the wound, and microbial culture and susceptibility testing are recommended to appropriately target antimicrobial therapy. The use of topical antimicrobial drugs such as silver sulfadiazine (Silvazine, Smith & Nephew, Fort Washington, Pennsylvania) is often not effective against deep tissue infection because these agents cannot reach deeper parts of the wound. However, they may be effective in eliminating superficial infection without the use of systemic antimicrobials. Other topical agents such as Aloe vera, honey, and sugar can be used to treat wound infection. Honey and granulated sugar create a **hypertonic** environment, thereby producing an antimicrobial effect, and are able to draw fluid and debris away from the wound. They can be incorporated as the contact layer within a bandage but require frequent bandage changes because especially the sugar is diluted with wound fluid and loses its hypertonic effect.

TYPES OF WOUNDS

Abrasions and Lacerations

Abrasions are partial-thickness dermal wounds that are common in animals after vehicular injury. Because of the preservation of parts of the dermis, these wounds heal well by reepithelialization. Maintaining a moist wound environment (see section on principles of bandaging) will speed epithelialization and is preferred over allowing the wound to dry out and scab over.

Lacerations are produced by tearing of skin and deeper tissues. Tissues are relatively sharply incised, and trauma to the surrounding area is minimal. If such an injury is fresh with minimal contamination, it can be lavaged, débrided, and closed primarily. If small enough, more chronic lacerations can be excised en bloc and then closed primarily. Secondary closure may be performed if the wound is heavily contaminated.

Degloving Injuries

A **degloving injury** is one in which a large section of skin is torn off the underlying tissue in a glove-like fashion. Degloving injuries are common in dogs that jump off or fall out of a moving vehicle and are dragged along the pavement. They can lead to severe loss of tissue, usually involving the distal limbs. Abrasion of bones and exposure of joints are common. These wounds often require weeks to months of wound care. Because of the nature of the injury, degloving wounds tend to be heavily contaminated with foreign debris and have varying amounts of devitalized tissue. Aggressive wound lavage and wound débridement precede granulation tissue formation. Because of lack of loose skin for wound contraction, large defects require skin grafting.

Bite Wounds

Bite wounds can be challenging to assess because they often cause extensive injury to deeper tissues that is not apparent on inspection of the skin. Because of the skin's elasticity, teeth may create only small puncture wounds in the skin, but subcutaneous tissues, muscles, even bone and neurovascular structures can be severely damaged. Along with having tissues crushed and lacerated, bite victims are often shaken, which adds to separation of tissues and creation of dead space. Because of the nature of this injury, these wounds are always considered contaminated. This type of wound is often compared with an iceberg, with the visible wound representing only the tip of the damage. Management of these wounds includes exploration, lavage, and **débridement**. The type of closure depends on the ability to remove contaminated and damaged tissue. Drains are commonly used in bite wounds with extensive dead space. Other penetrating wounds such as projectile injuries (gunshot) and impalement injuries (sticks) are treated similarly.

> **TECHNICIAN NOTE** Bite wounds can be challenging to assess because they often cause extensive injury to deeper tissues that is not apparent on inspection of the skin.

Burns

Burns are classified on the basis of how deep into the tissues the injury reaches and how large the affected area is. Although burns can be caused by accidental or deliberate injury in the animal's environment (barn fire, car muffler, electrical cord, hot liquid, etc.), they are more often caused by accidental inappropriate use of heating blankets and lamps, hair dryers, or poorly grounded electrocautery units. First-degree burns are superficial and are confined to the outermost layer of the skin (epidermis). Affected skin will be reddened and painful but recovers in a few days without treatment. Second-degree burns are the result of partial-thickness dermal injury. These wounds may form fluid-filled blisters across the surface but can also show discoloration of part of the dermis, similar to third-degree burns. The full extent of the damage may not be known until several days after the injury. If enough loose skin is available, second-degree burns can be managed by second intention healing with reepithelialization. Third-degree burns are full-thickness injuries characterized by a thick, leathery, often black layer of dead dermis (eschar). Treatment requires removal of the eschar and débridement of the wound. If left to heal by second intention, these wounds must contract and reepithelialize. Larger burns may require skin grafts to cover the defect. Fourth-degree burns involve deeper tissues apart from the dermis and require surgical reconstruction if large. Animals with extensive burns are critically ill and require intensive care to survive.

Decubitus Ulcers and Pressure Sores

Decubitus ulcers develop over bony prominences as the result of skin compression on hard flooring during long periods of recumbency. Patients with orthopedic and neurologic problems, extremely obese animals, and large and giant breed dogs with little soft tissue coverage over these bony prominences are at particular risk. The most common location for a decubitus ulcer is the elbow, where sores develop on the lateral or caudal surface of the olecranon. These ulcers can be frustrating to eliminate, and efforts must be focused on prevention. Animals must be housed on soft surfaces, which are kept clean and dry. Pressure-relieving sleeves are commercially available and are useful for superficial ulcers. Surgical closure can be attempted after limited débridement but usually fails if the wound continues to be exposed to surface pressure. Advanced reconstructive surgery is required in large ulcers that have failed to respond to more conservative treatment.

Inappropriate or prolonged periods of bandaging (especially with a splint or a cast) can lead to pressure necrosis of the skin, particularly over the olecranon, the calcaneus, and bony prominences of the feet. As with decubitus ulcers, the best treatment for bandage-associated pressure sores is prevention. Susceptible areas must not be padded more (because more padding will cause increased pressure once compressed) but must be protected with the use of doughnut-shaped bandage material such as rolled up stockinette or cast padding. Reddening of the skin with hair loss is an early sign of pressure on the skin. White, purple, or black color changes indicate severe damage to the dermis, which usually leads to sloughing of the affected area and a resultant open wound. Most pressure sores are treated by second intention healing and are left to granulate and epithelialize after the splint or the cast has been modified or removed.

PRINCIPLES OF BANDAGING

Bandages are applied for two main reasons: for management of soft tissue wounds and for stabilization of bone and joint injuries. Additionally, bandages are of benefit after surgery to help decrease hemorrhage and edema, eliminate dead space, increase patient comfort, and protect the wound from the patient and the environment (Box 26-7).

Most bandages consist of three distinct layers: (1) the primary layer, which is in direct contact with the wound, (2) the secondary layer, and (3) the tertiary protective layer (see Table 26-1 for a list of bandage materials, including their use and function). The primary layer is most important for wound protection and healing because it directly influences the wound environment. It may be adherent or nonadherent and may be **semi-occlusive** or **occlusive**. The type of primary layer depends on the phase of wound healing and the amount of exudate present. The secondary layer absorbs and holds exudate (if present) and provides some immobilization and support. If a large amount of exudate is produced, the secondary layer must be thicker to allow absorption of fluid into the bandage without causing strike-through into the tertiary layer. The tertiary layer is the outer, protective layer, which keeps the other layers in place, determines the appropriate amount of pressure and support to be applied, and protects

BOX 26-7	Functions of a Bandage

Soft Tissue Wounds
- Protects the wound from the environment and from the patient
- Aids in débridement of the wound surface
- Manages exudate
- Creates an environment for wound healing
- Provides hemostasis
- Decreases hematoma/seroma formation
- Provides support and comfort
- Delivers topical agents

Orthopedic Injuries
- Stabilizes fractures or joints
- Maintains splints or casts in position
- Restricts motion
- Prevents weight bearing
- Protects soft tissues from further injury
- Decreases swelling

the bandage from the environment. This final layer must not be occlusive, or moisture will accumulate within the bandage.

> **TECHNICIAN NOTE** Most bandages consist of three layers. The primary layer contacts the wound, the secondary layer provides padding, and the tertiary layer holds and protects the other two.

ADHERENT PRIMARY LAYER

A wet-to-dry bandage uses an adherent primary layer for nonselective débridement. It should be used only in inflammatory and débridement stages of heavily contaminated wounds. When a wet-to-dry bandage is applied with an adherent primary layer, moist sterile gauze is placed in contact with the wound bed and then is covered by a relatively thick absorptive secondary layer. Moisture on the wound surface helps to dilute exudate and debris, which then are wicked into the dry secondary layer. This movement of

TABLE 26-1	Types of Primary, Secondary, and Tertiary Bandage Layers	
BANDAGE LAYER	**USE AND FUNCTION**	**PRODUCT EXAMPLES**
Primary Adherent	Nonselective débridement	Sterile wide-mesh gauze
Hypertonic/hyperosmolar	Draws fluid and debris away from wound, antimicrobial effect due to hypertonicity and low water content within wound; some enhance wound healing; use on highly exudative, contaminated, and infected wounds	Hypertonic sodium chloride dressing (20%) (e.g., CURASALT*), granulated sugar, honey
Nonadherent semi-occlusive	*Moderately to Highly Exudative Wounds* Maintains moist wound environment, draws fluid and debris away from wound	*Hydrophilic* Variety of hydrogels (e.g., Curagel*) and hydrocolloids (e.g., Ultec Hydrocolloid Dressing*), absorptive foam (e.g., Hydrosorb Plus Foam*) *Nonhydrophilic* Polyurethane film (e.g., Bioclusive†)
Nonadherent occlusive	*Minimally Exudative Wounds* Maintains moist wound environment, promotes epithelialization, protects new epithelium	*Hydrophilic* Variety of hydrogels (e.g., NU-GEL†) andhydrocolloids (e.g., Tegaderm Hydrocolloid‡) *Nonhydrophilic* Tegaderm Transparent Dressing‡
Nonadherent nonocclusive	Covers surgical incisions, protects recently epithelialized surfaces	Teflon pads (e.g., Telfa pads*), petrolatum-impregnated gauze (e.g., Adaptic†)
Secondary Padding	Absorbs exudate, provides support	Cast padding,‡ rolled cotton†
Tertiary Conforming gauze	Conforms and holds secondary layer	Kling†
Nonocclusive elastic bandage	Holds and protects secondary layer	Vetrap§
Nonocclusive elastic adhesive tape	Holds and protects secondary layer	Elastikon†

*Kendall/Covidien, Mansfield, Massachusetts.
†Johnson & Johnson Medical, Arlington, Texas.
‡3M Skin and Wound Care, St Paul, Minnesota.
§3M Animal Care Products, St Paul, Minnesota.

fluid pulls exudate and dissolved debris with it and away from the wound. As the gauze dries, it adheres to the wound bed, at which time the bandage should be changed. Mechanical débridement occurs when the adhered dried primary layer is pulled away from the wound, taking with it superficial tissue and foreign material. Although such débridement is effective, it is nonselective and will remove not only diseased but also healthy tissue such as new granulation tissue, thereby delaying the healing process. Wet gauze can macerate intact skin if improperly placed, and dried gauze creates a dry environment that is not conducive to wound healing. If fluid strike-through of the tertiary layer occurs, bacteria from the environment can penetrate the bandage and contaminate the wound. In addition, this technique often causes bleeding and pain when the gauze is removed, necessitating proper analgesia or sedation. Because of these undesirable consequences of the wet-to-dry bandage, it has largely been replaced by nonadherent primary layers.

NONADHERENT PRIMARY LAYER

This type of primary layer is in direct contact with the wound bed but does not firmly adhere to it. It is imperative to use a nonadherent primary layer once granulation tissue has formed or epithelialization has begun, to protect and promote second intention wound healing. A semi-occlusive nonadherent primary layer is permeable to air and fluid and allows exudate to be absorbed by the secondary layer. An occlusive nonadherent primary layer is impermeable to air and retains moisture. Materials such as hydrogels and hydrocolloids can be used in different forms as semi-occlusive or occlusive. Moisture-retaining primary layers provide many benefits during wound healing such as maintaining a warm and moist environment, aiding in selective débridement, and improving epithelialization; therefore, they are preferred over adherent primary layers.

> **TECHNICIAN NOTE** Moisture-retaining primary layers provide many benefits, including improved epithelialization, and have become the preferred primary layer for most wounds.

A great variety of nonadherent primary layers are available for the veterinary patient. Highly absorptive primary layers such as hypertonic saline or calcium alginates may be required for very exudative wounds. Materials such as hydrogels, hydrocolloids, and polyurethane film or foam allow absorption of wound fluid while creating a moist wound healing environment. They are best used on wounds with minimal exudate but can be applied throughout the inflammatory and repair phases. This type of layer is much less painful when changed and allows longer intervals between bandage changes once the wound is in the proliferative phase. The moist wound healing environment enhances cell activity and improves granulation tissue formation and epithelialization. A lower infection rate is seen with moist wound healing; however, bacteria may be trapped underneath the occlusive layer if it is not applied correctly and changed at appropriate intervals. Petrolatum-impregnated sterile gauze is an example of a nonadherent, nonocclusive layer commonly used in the proliferative phase. Teflon pads are nonadherent and are frequently used to cover surgical incisions and epithelialized skin. Case Presentation 26-1 illustrates the principles of bandage material selection for management of an open wound.

BANDAGE, CAST, SPLINT, AND SLING APPLICATION IN SMALL ANIMALS

A variety of bandages, splints, casts, and slings are available for use in cats and dogs—each with its own indications for when and where it should be used. Distal limb bandages are often used to protect wounds and to stabilize bone or joint injuries. Splints, casts, and slings are used to provide further stability to orthopedic injuries or to prevent weight bearing. It is important to remember that only injuries below the elbow or stifle joint can be effectively immobilized, and that even with splints or casts, movement of joints and bones is possible. For other body parts, bandages need to be modified. Proper sedation or anesthesia greatly facilitates the application of any bandage and should be employed for every patient. In nonsedated animals, proper restraint is paramount to avoid movement during bandage application.

DISTAL LIMB BANDAGES

The **Robert Jones bandage** can be used to temporarily immobilize limbs distal to the elbow or stifle joint. This bandage relies on an extremely thick secondary layer such as cast padding or cotton, which is tightly compressed by the tertiary layer to cause uniform compression of the distal limb (Figure 26-5). Because of the large amount of padding, little risk of causing vascular compromise is introduced by tightening the outer protective layer. If applied properly, the finished bandage should sound like a ripe melon when tapped. Because of the large amount of bandage material necessary and the resultant cumbersome bandage, the traditional Robert Jones bandage is not often used anymore in small animals.

The **modified Robert Jones bandage** is the most commonly applied distal limb bandage in small animals (Figure 26-6). It uses a much thinner secondary layer and often is referred to as a *soft-padded bandage*. Because less padding is used, the tertiary layer must not be overly tightened, or pressure necrosis may occur. Splints and casts can easily be incorporated into the bandage. The tips of the toes or toe nails are often excluded from the bandage to allow for daily inspection. Care must be taken to avoid leaving too much toe exposed because this will lead to swelling and constriction of blood flow. Because of its frequent use, application of a modified Robert Jones bandage is discussed in detail.

> **TECHNICIAN NOTE** The modified Robert Jones bandage is the most commonly applied distal limb bandage in small animal medicine.

CASE PRESENTATION 26-1

A 2-year-old male, intact German shepherd dog suffered from a degloving injury of the medial aspect of the left rear foot after jumping out of a moving car. Three days later, the dog presented with a large, full-thickness skin wound involving the dorsomedial aspect of the metatarsals (Figure 1) with visible foreign body contamination and areas of nonviable tissue. Parts of metatarsal bones 2 and 3 were exposed. The wound was lavaged with copious amounts of fluid, and some tissue was carefully surgically débrided. A wet-to-dry bandage was applied for additional, nonselective débridement. After placement of sterile, saline-soaked sponges into the wound (Figure 2), several dry sponges were placed over the wet sponges (Figure 3), followed by a thick secondary, absorptive layer of cast padding (Figure 4). Elastic gauze and an outer protective

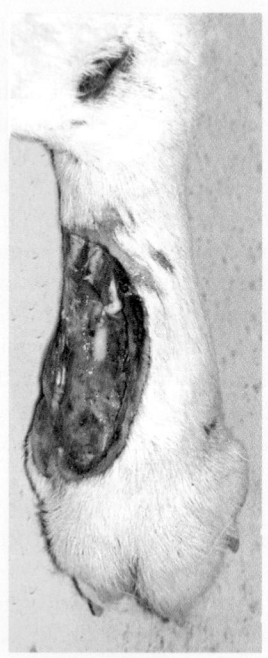

FIGURE 1

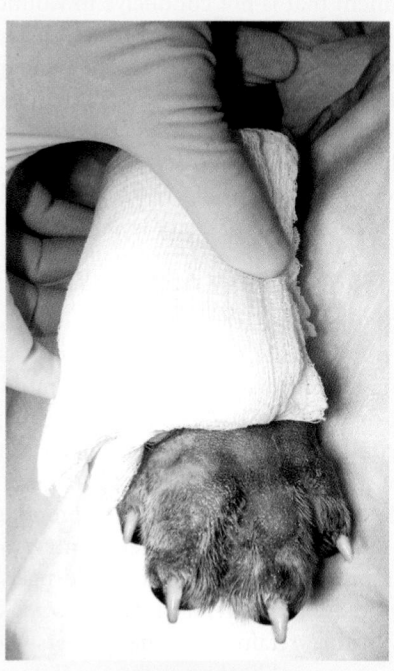

FIGURE 3

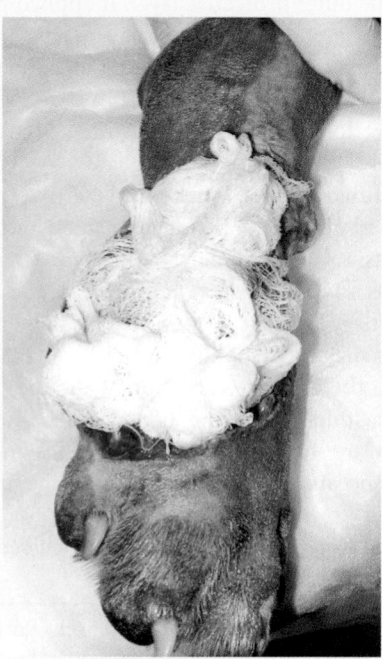

FIGURE 2

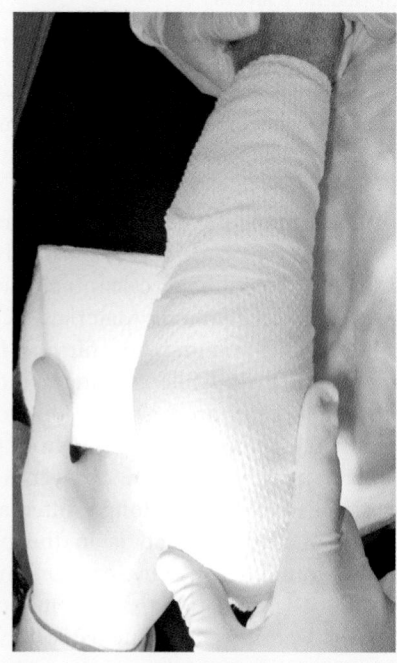

FIGURE 4

layer followed. Bandage changes were performed daily. Wet-to-dry bandages were discontinued on day 3 because the wound did not require further aggressive débridement (Figure 5). Hydrogel, a nonadherent semi-occlusive primary layer, was applied (Curagel, Kendall/Covidien, Mansfield, Massachusetts) and was changed every 2 to 3 days. On day 14, healthy granulation tissue covered the wound bed except the metatarsal bones (Figure 6). On day 21, previously exposed metatarsal bones were covered with granulation tissue, and some wound contraction had occurred (Figure 7). The primary layer was switched to petrolatum-impregnated gauze (Adaptic, Johnson & Johnson Medical, Arlington, Texas), covered by a few dry gauze sponges to help absorb wound fluid. Bandage changes occurred every 2 to 3 days. By day 36, wound size had been reduced by more than 60% because of wound contraction, and healthy granulation tissue was present (Figure 8);

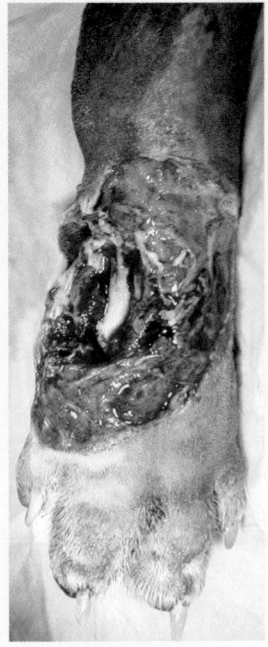

FIGURE 5

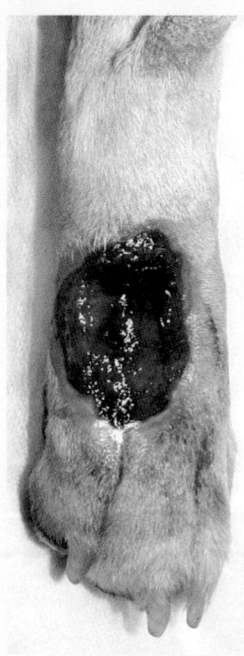

FIGURE 7

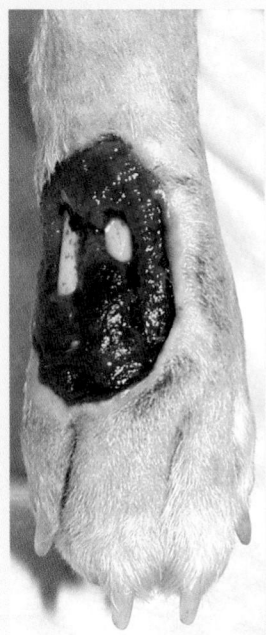

FIGURE 6

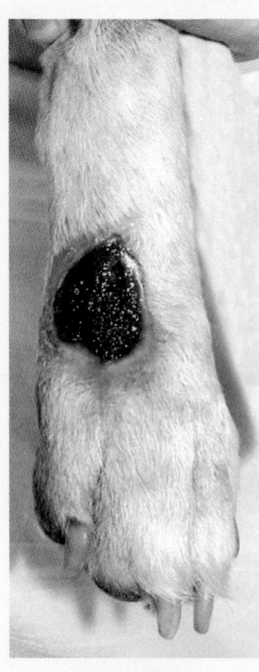

FIGURE 8

Continued

CASE PRESENTATION 26-1—cont'd

epithelialization was noted at the wound edges and continued to cover 50% of the remaining wound by day 42 (Figure 9). The primary layer was switched to a Teflon pad (Telfa pad, Kendall/Covidien, Mansfield, Massachusetts), and bandage changes were reduced to every 4 to 5 days. Epithelialization was complete by day 60 (Figure 10).

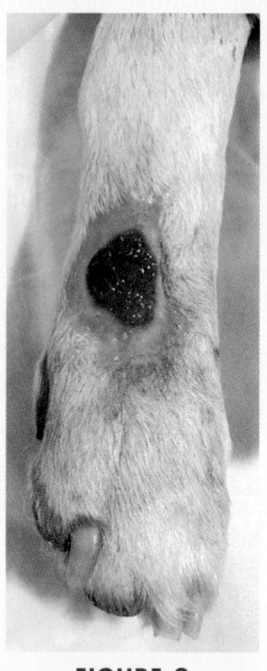

FIGURE 9

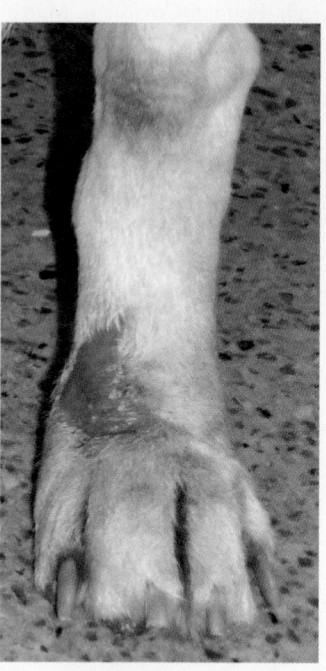

FIGURE 10

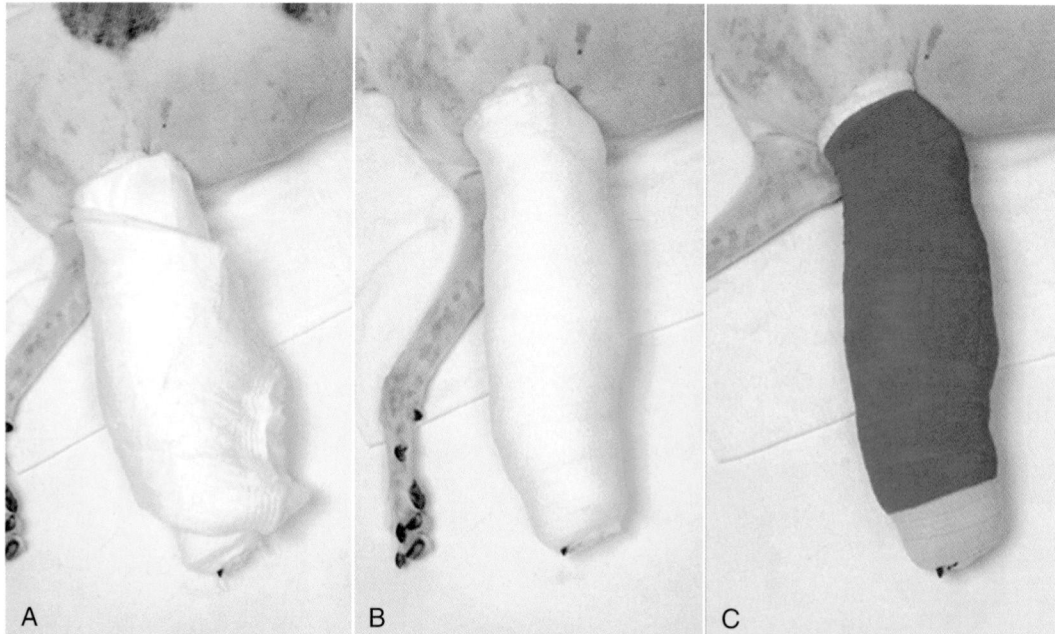

FIGURE 26-5 Robert Jones bandage. **A,** Large amounts of rolled cotton are applied to the forelimb reaching above the elbow. **B,** The thick layer of rolled cotton is evenly compressed with elastic gauze to provide stabilization of the fracture beneath. **C,** A tertiary protective layer has been applied and the distal part of the bandage has been reenforced with elastic adhesive tape. Note how the toenails of the middle two toes are still visible for assessment of swelling.

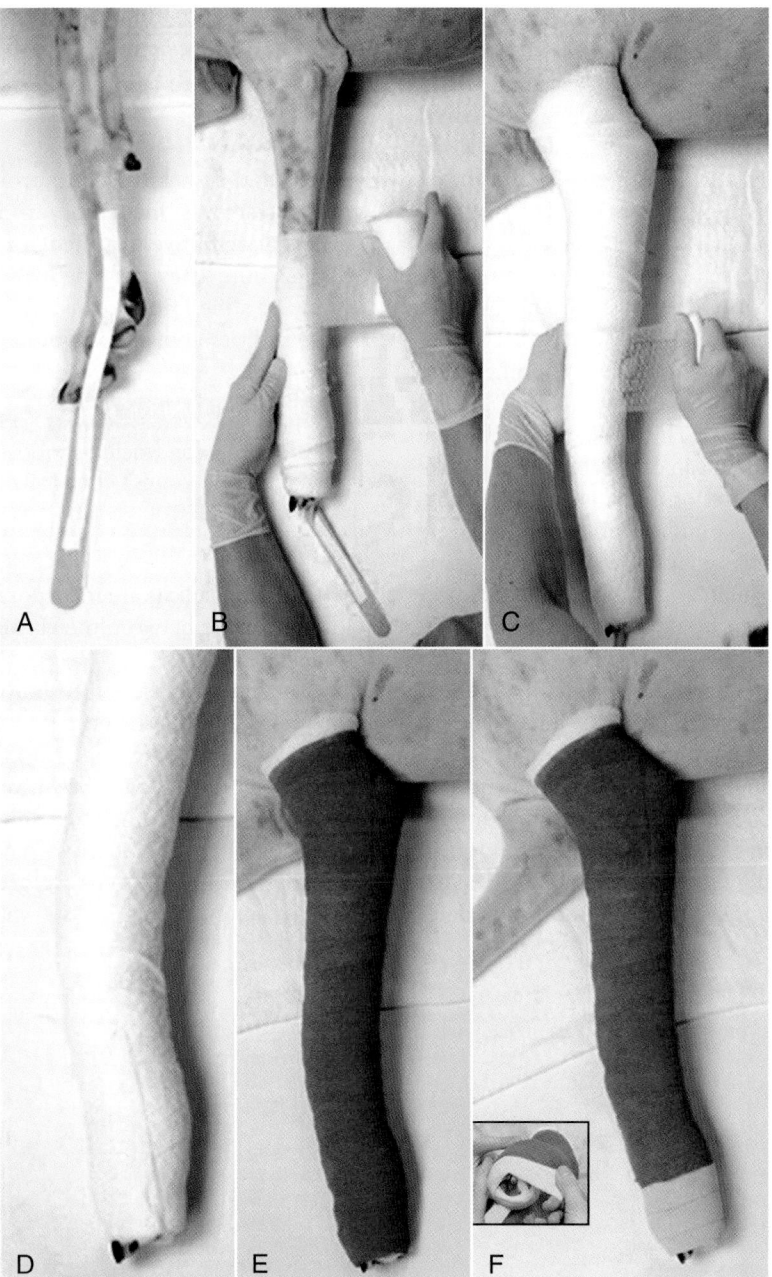

FIGURE 26-6 Modified Robert Jones bandage. **A,** Two thin strips of adhesive tape can be applied to the foot to form stirrups. **B,** Cast padding is applied from distal to proximal with each pass overlapping about 50%. Note how the tips of the middle toenails are visible. None of the subsequent layers must contact the skin, to avoid chafing. **C,** After sufficient padding has been applied, the secondary layer is gently compressed with elastic gauze. Gauze is evenly applied from distal to proximal. **D,** The stirrups are now pulled up to adhere to the outer gauze layer. **E,** The outer, protective layer is placed. Care must be taken to avoid applying this layer too tightly. Note how a thin rim of cotton is visible at the proximal extend of the bandage. **F,** Strips of nonocclusive elastic tape are used to reinforce the distal end of the bandage for walking. Note how the middle two toes can easily be assessed for swelling.

First, the appropriate primary layer is selected on the basis of whether a wound, an incision, or intact skin is present. "Doughnuts" (doughnut-shaped pads) made of soft, nonabrasive material can be placed over bony protuberances or compromised tissue to decrease pressure on these areas. The secondary layer consists of cast padding; different widths are available and should be chosen according to the size of the animal and the extent of the area to be bandaged. The thickness of the secondary layer depends on the amount of

exudate (if present) and compression desired (thicker if more compression is needed). Cast padding is unrolled smoothly without folds or wrinkles, starting at the level of the toenails and proceeding proximally. Padding should be 50% overlapping as the material is unrolled. To avoid placing a secondary layer that is too thin and will slip easily, at least two to three layers of cast padding are applied. If the elbow or the stifle joint needs to be included, cast padding must be applied as far proximal to the elbow or stifle as possible because it is easy for the bandage to slip down and over these high-motion joints. Larger dogs require a surprising amount of cast padding to thicken the secondary layer enough to avoid collapse of the bandage by slippage. Once the desired thickness of padding has been applied, elastic gauze or Kling (Johnson & Johnson Medical) is used to gently tighten the secondary layer. This gauze is applied from distal to proximal and should also overlap 50%. As it is unrolled, the flat surface of the thumb can be used to tighten each pass around the limb. Compression of the secondary layer should be even from distal to proximal. If a splint or a cast is used, it is applied at this point and can be held in place by another layer of elastic gauze or Kling. Finally, the outer protective layer is applied from distal to proximal. This layer should not be touching skin directly because it can cause abrasions. Unlike large animals, cats and dogs do not tolerate excessive tightness of a bandage unless large numbers of secondary layers are used. Therefore, the tertiary layer—especially if elastic material is used—must not be too tight. If properly applied, this bandage will not need to be taped to the limb at the proximal extent. Tape can be used over the foot to provide greater resistance against wear. If slippage of the bandage is a concern, small strips of adhesive tape can be applied to the lateral and medial aspects of the foot before bandaging and used as stirrups. For prolonged bandaging, the portion of adhesive tape on the foot itself can be left for several bandage changes while new thin strips of tape are applied on top of it to form new stirrups. Many times, stirrups are not needed and should not serve as a substitute for poor bandaging technique. If necessary, small strips of cotton can be placed between the toes to decrease abrasions from toenails rubbing against skin or to help absorb moisture.

CASTS AND SPLINTS

Splints and casts are used to provide stability for joint injuries or fractures, for temporary support until surgery, as a means of definitive treatment, or as an adjunct after surgical stabilization. They must be used only for injuries below the elbow or stifle joint because they cannot effectively immobilize injuries above those joints.

> **TECHNICIAN NOTE** Distal limb bandages are not appropriate for fractures above the elbow or the stifle because they cannot effectively immobilize injuries above those joints.

Casts and splints are incorporated into a modified Robert Jones bandage between the elastic gauze layer and the outer protective layer.

Casts encircle the entire limb. Fiberglass casting tape is the preferred material because it produces a lightweight yet very rigid cast (Figure 26-7). A modified Robert Jones bandage is placed over the distal limb, except for the outer protective layer. The bandage must not be too thick to avoid cast loosening, and it must have an even surface free of wrinkles or creases. While gloves are worn, the fiberglass casting tape is immersed in water to activate setting, and

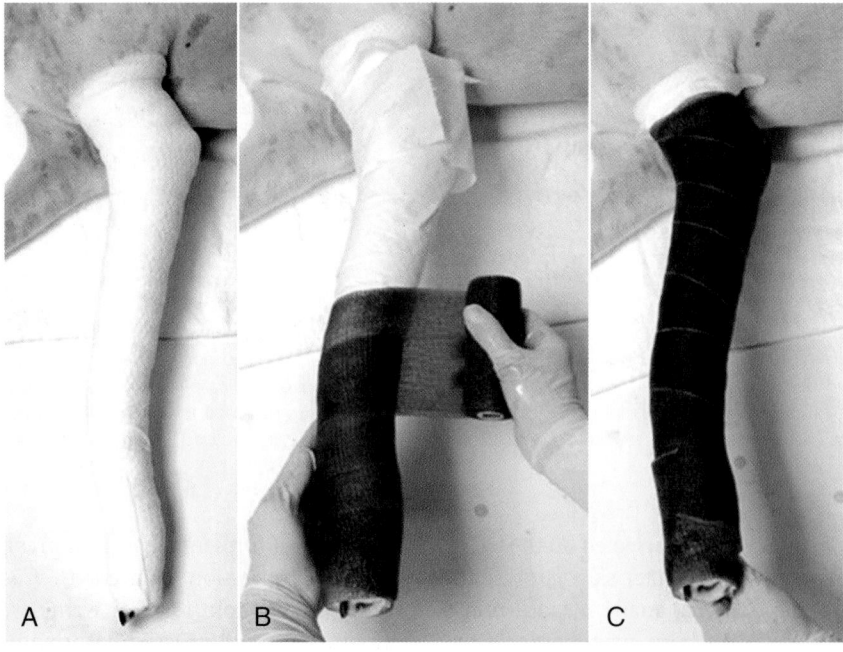

FIGURE 26-7 Forelimb cast. **A,** Casts and splints are applied over a modified Robert Jones bandage before the outer protective layer is applied. This bandage must not be too large, to prevent loosening of material underneath and rubbing of the cast or splint. **B,** A thin layer of toilet paper or paper towels is applied over the elastic gauze to prevent the casting material from sticking to it. The fiberglass tape is applied from distal to proximal with up to 50% overlap. Care must be taken to prevent indentations with fingers or creases, folds, and wrinkles because these can cause pressure points on the skin. **C,** Several layers of fiberglass tape are applied, taking care to avoid having casting material touch the skin. This material is allowed to harden and then is covered by a protective layer unless bivalved.

excess water is shaken out. The tape is then unrolled over the soft-padded bandage from distal to proximal. Care must be taken to avoid folds, wrinkles, or indentations in the cast because these can cause pressure necrosis underneath. The casting material must not contact skin at the ends of the bandage. While the casting tape is overlapped by 30% to 50%, two to three layers are applied to the limb. Once hardened, an outer protective layer can be applied to prevent excessive soiling of the cast. Casts are often bivalved (cut on both sides from top to bottom) with an oscillating cast saw to create two halves, which then are kept together by a layer of elastic gauze or Kling and the outer protective layer (Figure 26-8). Although bivalving a cast weakens its stability, it allows for fast removal of the cast in an emergency situation and is generally recommended.

A variety of prefabricated splints made of plastic or aluminum are available (lateral and spoon splints). Alternatively, fiberglass casting tape or thermoplastic material can be used to make custom splints (Figure 26-9). Using fiberglass tape allows great flexibility because it can be applied in any fashion desired. Most forelimb splints are applied to the caudal limb surface, and rear limb splints are applied laterally, unless only the metatarsi and the foot are splinted, in which case a caudal splint is used.

The original indication for the Schroeder-Thomas splint was to immobilize distal femoral fractures that otherwise were not able to be bandaged. This splint suspends the pelvic limb in a rigid metal frame fashioned to match the outline of the leg. This splint is not recommended anymore because it causes muscle contracture with permanent loss of limb function if used to treat fractures.

A **spica splint** maintains the forelimb or the pelvic limb in extension through application of a soft-padded bandage and addition of a strong lateral support splint that curves over the shoulder or pelvis. This type of splint is most commonly used in the forelimb after elbow luxation reduction when the elbow must be kept in extension and overall mobility of the affected limb must be reduced. Prolonged immobilization must be avoided to prevent muscle contracture and joint damage.

SLINGS

An **Ehmer sling** is a non–weight-bearing sling applied to the pelvic limb to protect the hip joint after injury. It is used primarily after closed reduction of craniodorsal hip luxation or after surgery associated with the coxofemoral joint (such as open reduction of a craniodorsal luxation or acetabular fractures). On principle, a properly applied Ehmer sling will internally rotate and abduct the femur, thereby forcing the femoral head into the acetabulum and maintaining reduction. Broad elastic tape is used to make a figure-8 loop around the stifle and hock while both joints are held in flexion and the hock is externally rotated (Figure 26-10). The tape can then be wrapped around the abdomen to further reduce movement at the hip joint. The abdominal portion of this sling is not placed unless absolutely necessary however, because it can cause increased skin irritation. This is especially true in male dogs because the close proximity of this part of the bandage to the prepuce leads to urine soiling. If only the limb is encircled, care must be taken to apply adhesive tape as far proximally on the femur as the flank fold will allow, to prevent slippage of the sling over the cranial aspect

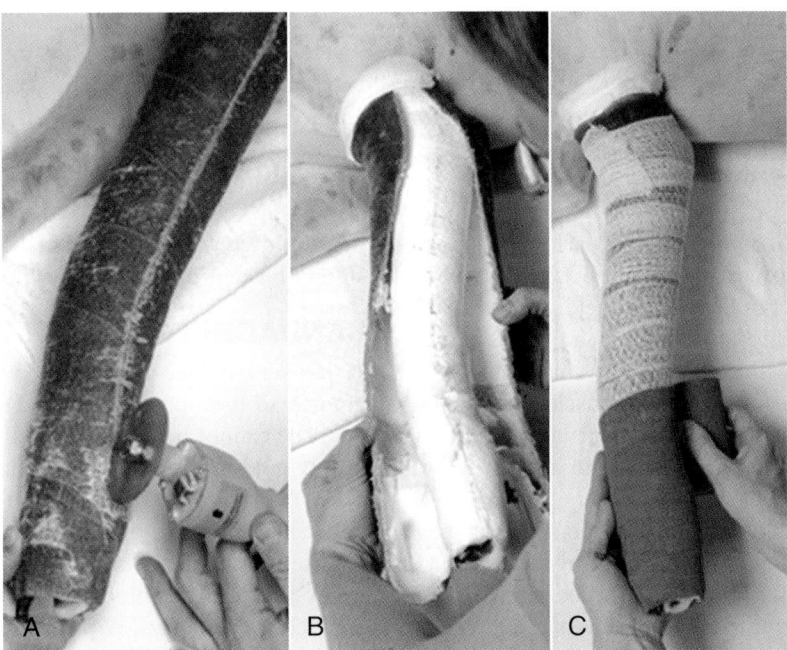

FIGURE 26-8 Bivalving a forelimb cast. **A,** An oscillating saw is used to cut the cast on both sides and create two halves. This saw will not injure the patient. **B,** The bivalved cast is removed. The layer of toilet paper between the casting material and the elastic gauze prevented the two layers from adhering and making it difficult to remove. **C,** The bivalved cast is reapplied to the bandaged limb. Elastic gauze is used to firmly hold both halves together. The tertiary layer is applied.

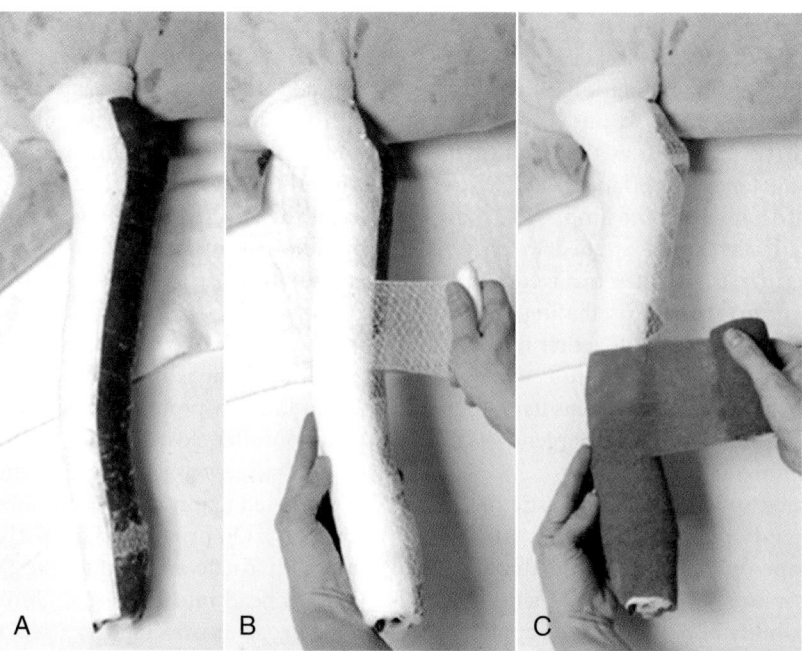

FIGURE 26-9 Caudal forelimb splint. **A,** A prefabricated splint can be used or custom-made out of fiberglass tape. Splints generally are applied to the caudal surface of the forelimb and the lateral surface of the pelvic limb over a modified Robert Jones bandage. **B,** Elastic gauze is used to secure the splint to the bandage. Because the splint does not encircle the entire limb, this gauze must not be tightened too much, to avoid constriction of tissues beneath. **C,** A routine outer layer is placed and the end nearest to the foot is reinforced with elastic tape.

of the stifle joint. Most patients develop skin irritations around the flank fold and **inguinal** area because of the tape, but they can often be treated conservatively for the duration of sling application (typically no longer than 2 to 3 weeks). The foot must be inspected daily because the sling can alter blood flow, leading to significant swelling of the foot. If this occurs, the sling must be altered or removed. Non–weight-bearing slings should not be maintained for longer than 2 to 3 weeks, to prevent muscle and joint contracture.

> **TECHNICIAN NOTE** Non–weight-bearing slings should not be maintained for longer than 2 to 3 weeks, to prevent muscle and joint contracture.

The 90/90 flexion sling is a non–weight-bearing sling that consists of a simple loop of adhesive tape wrapped around the stifle and hock while both joints are held at about 90 degrees of flexion. Use of this sling is critical in puppies after repair of distal femoral fractures, to prevent quadriceps tie-down or contracture by keeping affected muscles stretched. The sling is applied immediately after repair and is maintained for 2 to 3 days until postoperative pain and swelling have decreased.

The **Velpeau sling** is a non–weight-bearing sling for the forelimb that is used to immobilize all joints of the affected leg. It is mainly applied after reduction of medial shoulder joint luxation or after reconstruction of tenuous fractures. The entire forelimb is flexed and brought up against the thoracic wall, and a soft-padded bandage is applied to keep it in place (Figure 26-11). Care must be taken to not impair breathing as this bandage encircles the chest.

A **carpal flexion sling** is a simple non–weight-bearing forelimb sling that is applied with the carpus in flexion (Figure 26-12). It can be used in any situation where weight bearing should be avoided but some movement of the elbow and shoulder joints is acceptable. It can also be used to relieve tension on carpal flexor tendons after injury or surgical repair. If used for an inappropriate length of time, contracture of the carpal flexor tendons is possible.

Hobbles prevent abduction of the pelvic limbs and are used after reduction of ventral hip luxations. They can be applied at the level of the stifle joints or at the metatarsi (Figure 26-13). Because of the vast amount of mobility that cats and dogs have in their hip joints, hobbles may not protect entirely against reluxation. Therefore, patients should be supported with an abdominal sling when ambulating and should be kept on nonslippery flooring.

BANDAGES FOR OTHER LOCATIONS

A tie-over bandage is a versatile wound bandage that can be applied to locations on the body where a traditional limb bandage cannot be used or would be impractical. It is commonly used in the axillary area, around the pelvis, or in any other location that is difficult to bandage. This type of bandage uses suture loops that encircle the wound edges and are used as anchor points for bandage material. The wound is covered in the desired fashion with appropriate primary and secondary layers. A protective tertiary layer such as a paper drape cut to size is used to cover the bandage. These layers are held in place by strands of umbilical tape that criss-cross over the bandage from one suture loop to another. When a tie-over bandage is changed, skin suture loops are

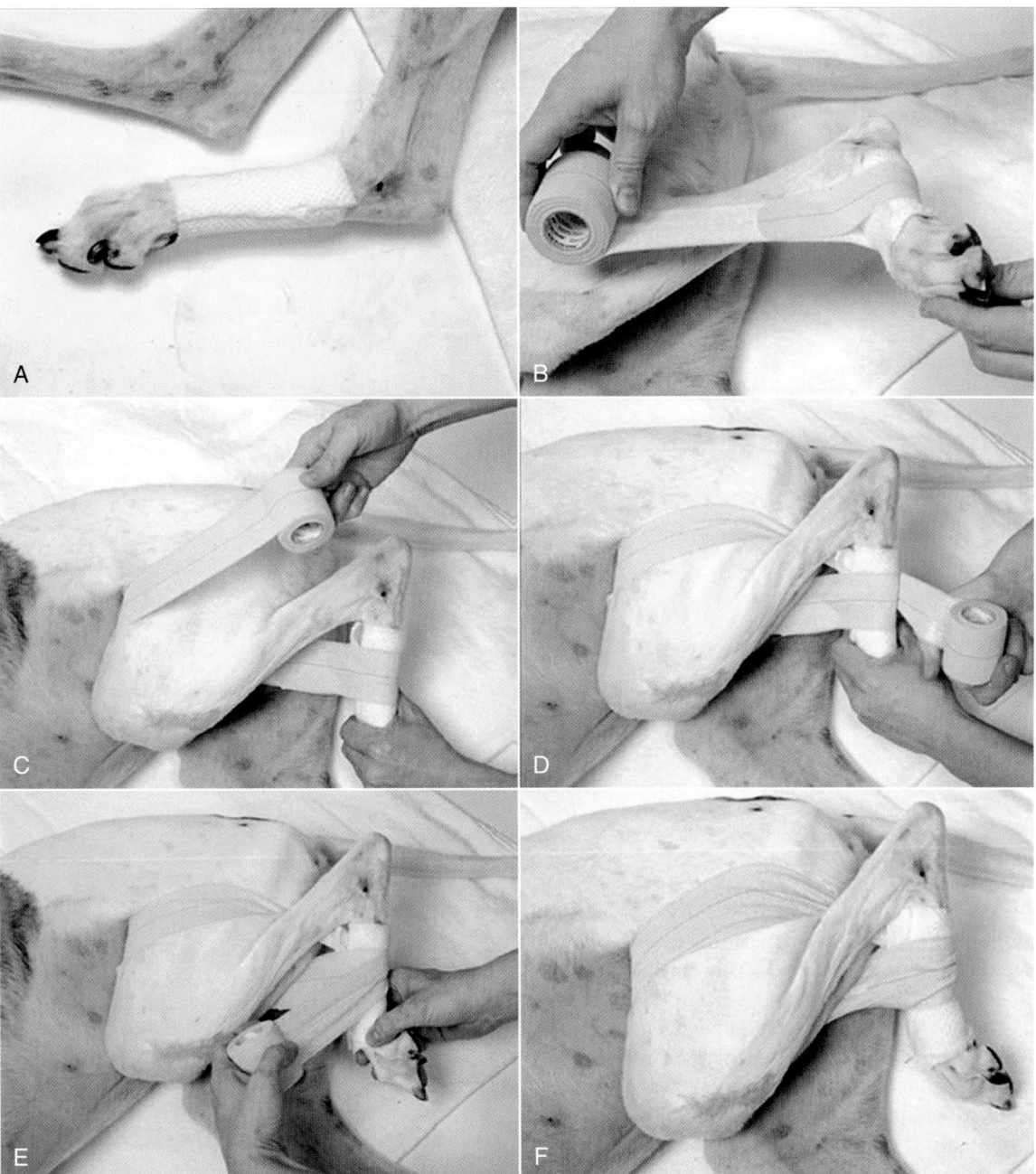

FIGURE 26-10 Ehmer sling. **A,** A thin layer of cast padding is wrapped around the metatarsals. **B,** Adhesive tape is applied around the metatarsals and is taped back onto itself to prevent constriction of soft tissues. **C,** With the hock and the stifle held in full flexion, the tape is passed medially around the thigh as far proximally as possible. This prevents slippage of the tape over the stifle joint. **D,** The tape is then passed over the caudal thigh and medially around the hock. **E,** The tape is passed 1 or 2 more times as necessary. **F,** A properly placed Ehmer sling results in internal rotation and abduction of the femur.

maintained while the umbilical tape is cut for removal of the bandage.

Adhesive drapes can be used instead of tie-over skin sutures to hold primary and secondary bandage layers in place. A tertiary layer is not necessary because the adhesive drape will act as the outer protective layer. These types of bandages are useful for wounds on relatively flat surfaces such as the chest wall or the abdominal wall because in these locations, drapes adhere properly to the skin.

Three-layer soft-padded bandages that encircle the respective body part are usually used for the head, chest, abdomen, and tail. Instead of a tertiary layer such as Vetwrap, more elastic materials such as stockinette can be used to hold primary and secondary layers in place. Head bandages are often applied to the ear after injury or surgery to absorb wound drainage, to provide compression against dead space, or simply to protect the ear from injury caused by head shaking. The affected pinna or both pinnae are often

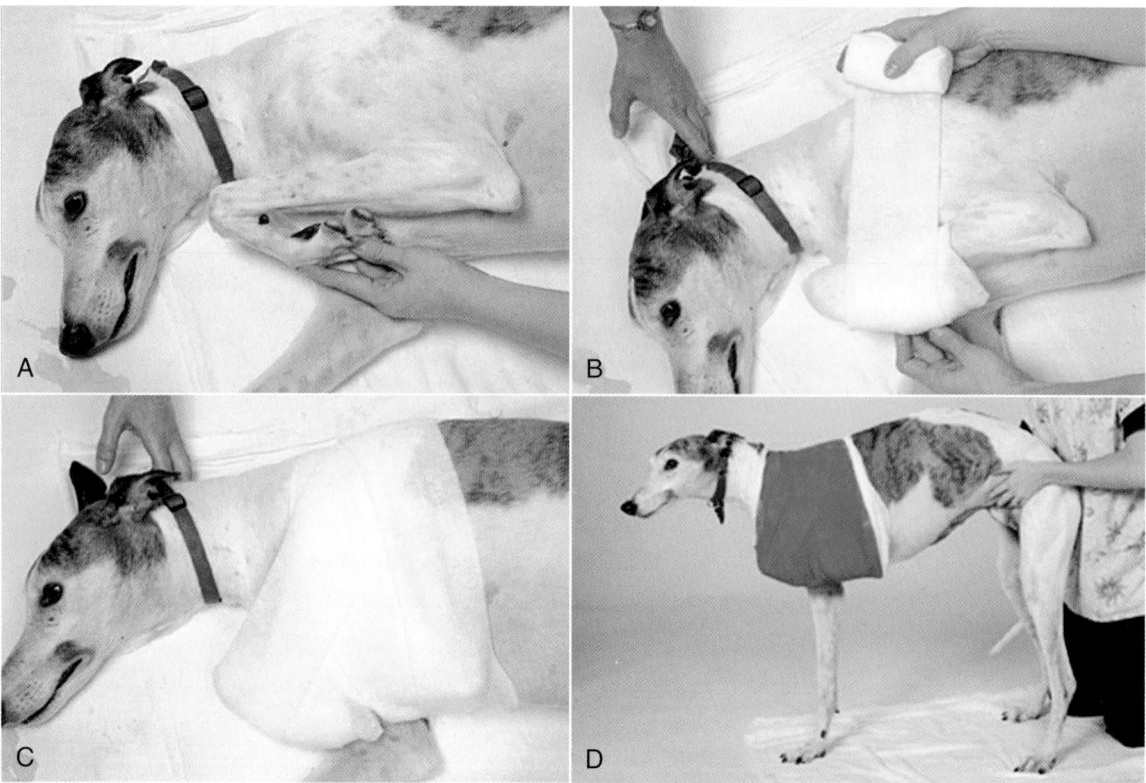

FIGURE 26-11 Velpeau sling. **A,** The entire forelimb is bandaged in flexion. **B,** A soft-padded bandage is applied, beginning with the carpus held in flexion. **C,** The secondary layer is continued over and around the chest. **D,** Elastic gauze and a tertiary layer complete the Velpeau sling. This sling prevents weight bearing on the forelimb.

incorporated into the bandage, so great care is required when the bandage is cut off, to avoid accidentally cutting into the ear (Figure 26-14). A head bandage is often applied immediately after surgery with the animal still under general anesthesia. In these patients, the bandage may be placed too tightly, leading to life-threatening respiratory compromise once patients are extubated. Thus, these animals must be closely monitored during the recovery period. Other complications include corneal abrasions if the bandage is placed too close to the eye.

Bandages around the chest are often applied in a figure-8 pattern around the forelimbs, to prevent slippage (Figure 26-15). Again, care must be taken to avoid restricting respiratory function by applying the bandage too tightly. Figure-8 bandages can be difficult to place around the caudal abdomen or pelvis (especially in male dogs) because urination and defecation must not be impaired by the bandage, and soiling of the bandage is common.

Tail bandages often require a small strip of adhesive tape applied to the skin at the proximal end to keep the bandage from slipping off (Figure 26-16). Syringe casing or other additional protection can be added to the tip of the tail if needed. Avoid placing an excessive amount of secondary layer when placing these bandages.

> **TECHNICIAN NOTE** Head bandages can cause life-threatening respiratory compromise, especially when placed while the patient is still under general anesthesia. Thus, patients must be closely monitored during the recovery period.

AFTERCARE FOR BANDAGES, SPLINTS, CASTS, AND SLINGS

The length of time that a bandage should be kept on depends on the underlying condition. Prolonged immobilization leads to muscle atrophy, contracture of soft tissues, and joint changes; therefore, any type of bandage should be left on only as long as absolutely necessary. Bandage changes are required on a regular basis because complications under the bandage are not obvious to the observer. Wound bandages may have to be changed once or sometimes even twice a day if a large volume of exudate is present. Once healthy granulation tissue has formed, or the wound is in the epithelialization phase, bandage changes can be decreased to every 2 to 3 days. If no wound is evident (e.g., closed fractures, joint injuries), bandages should be changed once a week to allow assessment of the limb for bandage-associated complications.

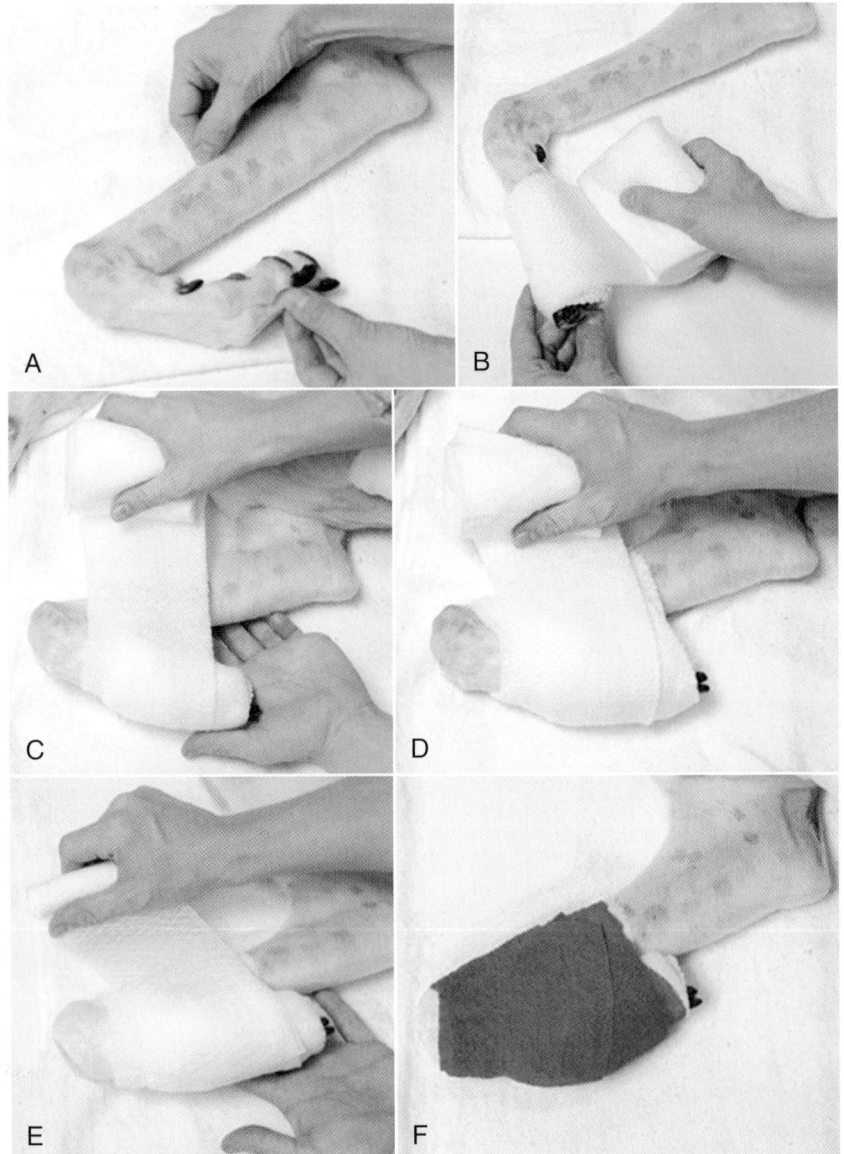

FIGURE 26-12 Carpal flexion sling. **A** through **D,** The carpus is bandaged in flexion. The soft-padded bandage begins around the foot then continues over the distal forelimb with the carpus in flexion. **E** and **F,** Elastic gauze and a protective outer layer are applied. This sling prevents weight bearing on the forelimb.

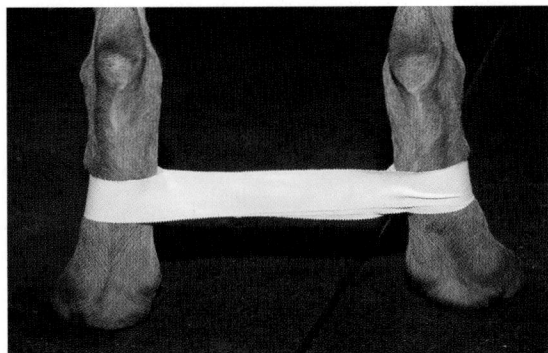

FIGURE 26-13 Hobbles. A strip of adhesive tape is applied around the metatarsal bones of both pelvic limbs. The tape must not be too tight, to avoid swelling and constriction of blood flow. The width of the hobbles should not be greater than the width of the animal's pelvis. Hobbles are used to prevent abduction of the hip joints after ventral coxofemoral luxation.

It is important to limit exercise to short leash walks only for the purpose of elimination until the bandage is removed; activity will increase risks for shifting of the bandage material (if used for fractures), development of chafing and sores, and complications during healing.

Monitoring of distal limb bandages includes daily inspection of the toes for swelling (indicated by increased distance between the toenails) or decreased viability (decreased warmth or abnormal color). The bandage must be kept dry and clean and must be protected when the animal goes outside. Plastic, ziploc, and empty IV fluid bags are simple, water-proof coverings; however, they must not be kept in place for longer than the time required for the patient to eliminate because they cause accumulation of moisture from the foot, which can lead to soft tissue maceration. Most cats and dogs require an Elizabethan

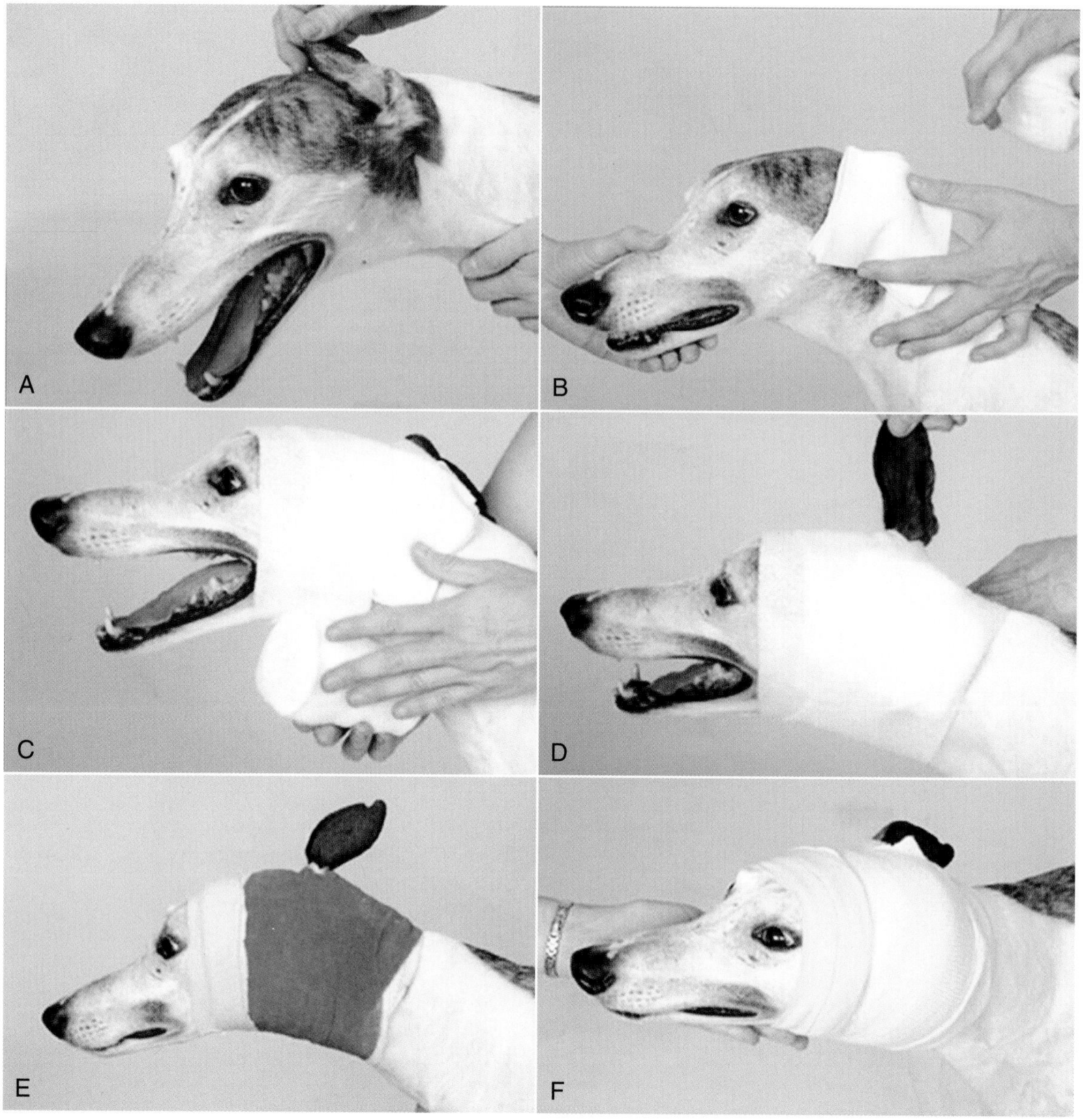

FIGURE 26-14 Head bandage. **A** and **B,** The affected ear is laid across the top of the head, and a primary layer can be applied if indicated. **C** and **D,** Cast padding is applied while the unaffected ear is spared. If desired, elastic gauze can be used to cover the padding; however, care must be taken to not tighten the bandage too much. **E** and **F,** The tertiary layer can consist of material such as Vetwrap or a more elastic layer such as stockinette. Both are held in place by a strip of elastic tape.

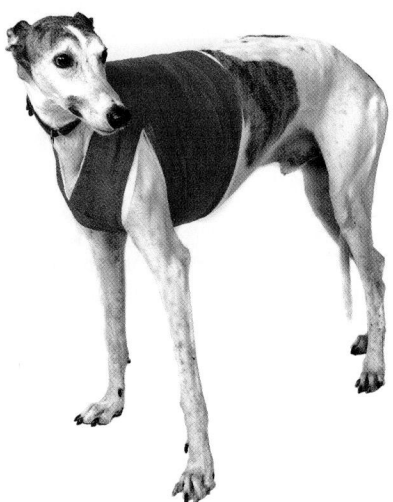

FIGURE 26-15 Chest bandage. A soft-padded bandage with cast padding, elastic gauze, and a protective outer layer has been placed by criss-crossing between the two forelimbs. This helps to keep the bandage in place. Care must be taken to avoid applying this bandage too tightly to prevent respiratory compromise.

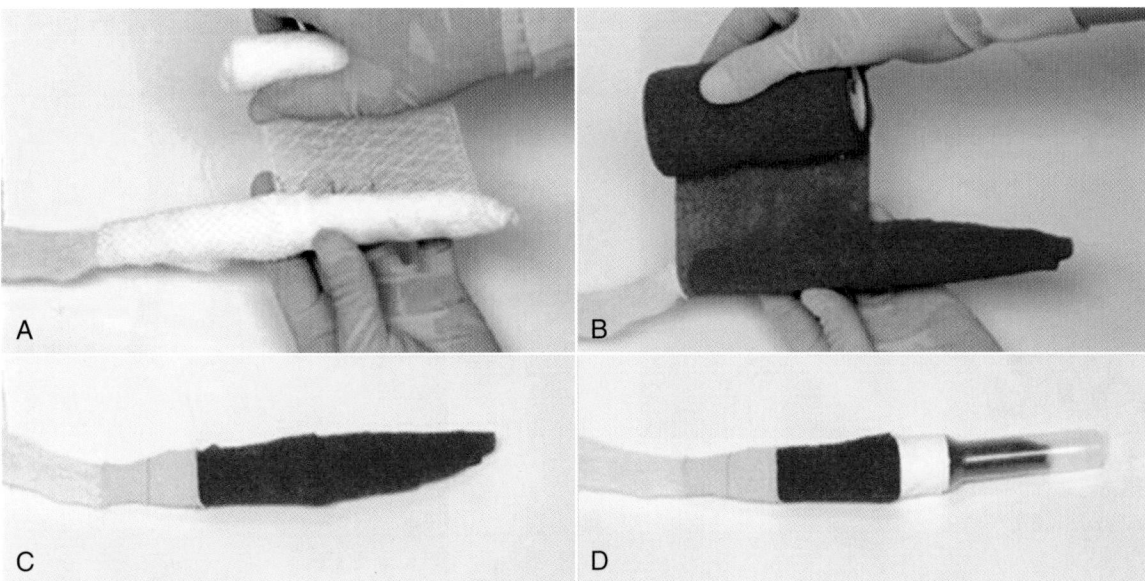

FIGURE 26-16 Tail bandage. **A** and **B**, A small amount of cast padding is used, followed by elastic gauze and a tertiary layer. **C**, Adhesive tape at the proximal end helps to prevent slippage of the bandage. **D**, A rigid covering (e.g., syringe casing) can be added to the tip of the tail to provide further protection.

collar to protect the bandage from damage caused by chewing or licking. A bandage, splint, cast, or sling that is inappropriately tight or that slips may impair blood flow, leading to swelling and possible tissue necrosis. Foul odor from the bandage or a sudden behavior change in the animal such as increased lameness or biting at the limb is a further indication that complications are occurring underneath the bandage. Good client education regarding bandage care required at home and associated complications to watch for is paramount.

Large Animal Wound Management

WOUND CARE IN HORSES

Wound management in horses starts with basic wound care and is no different from that provided for small companion animals. However, the size and nature of the animal and the location of the injury may dictate the way a wound is approached. Ultimately, regardless of the way a wound is managed, the initial care is essentially the same. This includes clipping hair from around the wound, cleansing and débriding, and preparing the wound for closure (if applicable).

PREPARING THE WOUND

When a wound on a horse is first treated, hair from around the edges of the wound is removed with clippers. A water-soluble lubricant or saline solution–soaked gauze should be used to fill the depths of the wound to prevent hair from falling into the wound because hair can act as a foreign body. However, if clippers are not available, wound edges can be

lathered with antiseptic scrub, and a straight-edge razor or a #22 scalpel blade can be used to shave the hair (Figure 26-17).

Methods used to lavage a wound are similar to those described earlier in this chapter for small companion animals. It is important that lavage is performed under pressure because this will dislodge debris and bacteria from the wound. A water hose with a spray nozzle is strongly discouraged because water pressure in this system will actually drive dirt and bacteria into the tissue. The author's preference is to use a small measure of disinfectant in the lavage solution.

Local vs. General Anesthesia

One important step in treating a wound in any horse is providing appropriate restraint. If the wound is to be closed, local anesthesia with tranquilization or general anesthesia may be needed. If tranquilization is used, local or regional anesthetic is also necessary for débridement and closure of the wound. Local infiltration is performed by injecting a local anesthetic (mepivacaine or lidocaine) approximately 1 cm from the wound edge, subcutaneously around the entire wound. A 22-gauge hypodermic needle is used in most situations and is reinserted repeatedly through the skin, each time at the end of the bleb formed by the preceding injection of local anesthetic (Figure 26-18). In this way, the patient will not react to successive injections. If the wound is located on the distal portion of a limb, a ring block or a nerve block (e.g., a palmar nerve block) can be performed, and the portion of the limb distal to the block will be anesthetized (Figure 26-19). If a wound is to be sutured, the same considerations for wound closure in small companion animals apply to large animals.

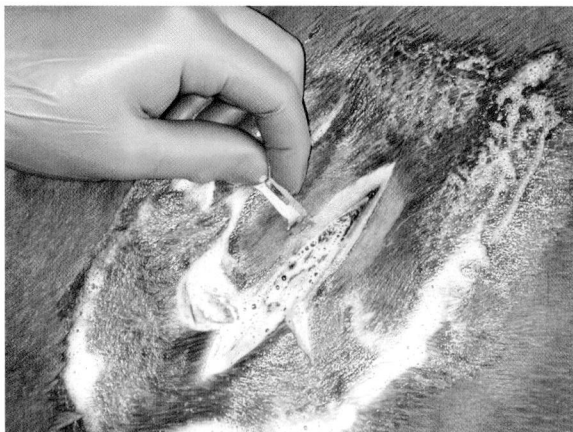

FIGURE 26-17 Once the hair has been lathered with antiseptic (such as povidone-iodine scrub), a #22 scalpel blade can be used to shave away hair from the wound edges.

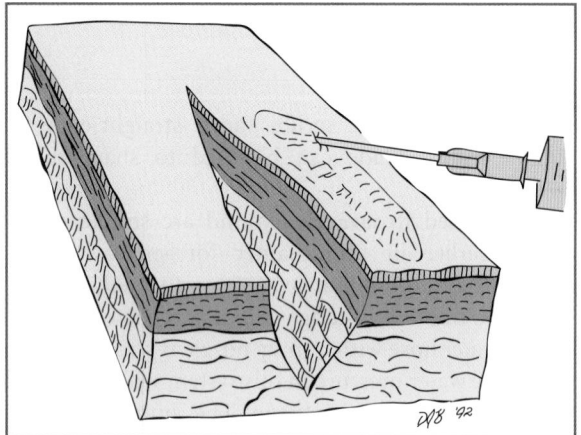

FIGURE 26-18 Proper technique for infiltration of a wound edge with local anesthetic. The needle should enter through the skin at the point of the last injection.

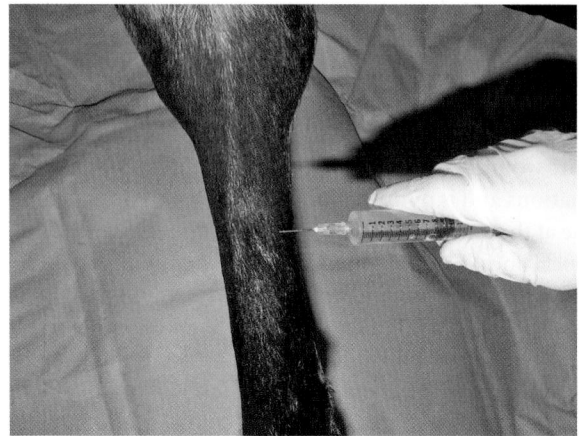

FIGURE 26-19 A ring block using a local anesthetic is infiltrated subcutaneously around the limb of a horse to triage a distal limb wound.

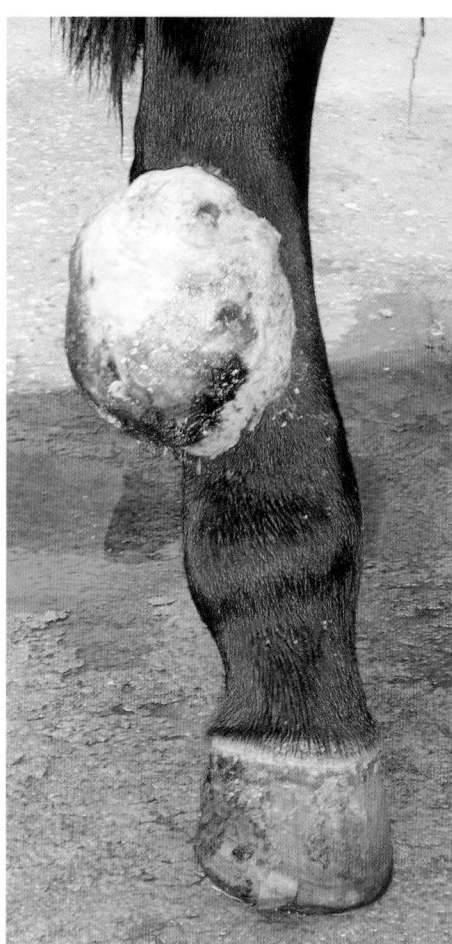

FIGURE 26-20 Exuberant granulation tissue on the metatarsus of a horse.

Exuberant Granulation Tissue in Open Wounds

Open wounds on the distal aspect of the limb (below the carpus or tarsus) of the horse are notorious for developing **exuberant granulation tissue**. Exuberant granulation tissue (EGT), commonly referred to as "proud flesh," can form rapidly in horses. Various measures must be undertaken to keep exuberant granulation tissue in check, or it can become excessive (Figure 26-20). Methods of controlling granulation tissue include immobilization of the limb (as with a cast), wound bandaging, caustic agents such as equal parts of copper sulfate and boric acid powder, cryotherapy, electrocautery, and topical corticosteroids. Surgical excision appears to be the best method of removing and controlling EGT (Figure 26-21). Regardless of the decision to close a wound or allow healing by second intention, bandaging should be part of the wound care provided.

BANDAGE, SPLINT, AND CAST APPLICATION TECHNIQUES FOR HORSES

Bandages and casts serve many purposes and are named for the location that they cover and the purpose that they serve. Various materials are available for use in a bandage or cast, but the most important aspect for selection is their proper application and function. Development of good bandaging and cast application skills is important in ensuring proper function of the bandage or cast. Application and purposes of different types used with horses are discussed.

BANDAGES

Lower Limb Wound Bandage

A lower limb wound bandage covers a wound on a limb distal to the carpus or tarsus. As discussed previously, after a wound has been cleaned and débrided, sutured, or left open, a topical antimicrobial preparation is usually applied.

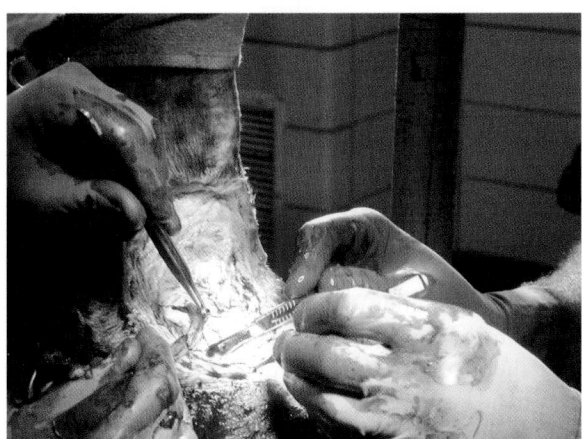

FIGURE 26-21 Exuberant granulation tissue being excised from the dorsum of a horse's tarsus.

A *nonadherent dressing* is then placed directly over the wound. The wound dressing is secured to the limb with *rolled conforming gauze*, which is wrapped around the limb with light pressure, with overlapping, and without wrinkles, to prevent formation of pressure lines, which may cause skin necrosis if applied too tightly. It is wrapped approximately 2 to 4 cm proximal and distal to the wound edges (Figure 26-22).

The *padded layer* is applied next. Sheets cut from a combine cotton roll, rolled cotton, layered cotton sheets, quilted leg wraps, or a military field bandage can be used (Figure 26-23). If cotton sheets are available, five are used. Four sheets are folded in half and neatly rolled. The fifth sheet is folded in the opposite direction over the other sheets to conceal the edges. The padded layer is secured to the limb with a roll of conforming gauze. Pressure is applied during wrapping to compress and conform the padding to the limb. The *outer shell* of the bandage is finished with elastic wrap (Vetrap Bandage Tape, 3M Animal Care Products, St Paul, Minnesota; or an Ace bandage), adhesive elastic tape (Elastikon, Johnson & Johnson Medical, Arlington, Texas), or a flannel track wrap. If an Ace bandage or track wrap is used, it is secured with white tape cut into strips or placed around the bandage in a "barber pole" fashion (Figure 26-24). Elastikon is placed around the top and bottom of the bandage, with half of the tape sticking to the wrap and half to the skin, to prevent slippage and to keep debris (e.g., bedding shavings) from getting inside the bandage (Figure 26-25).

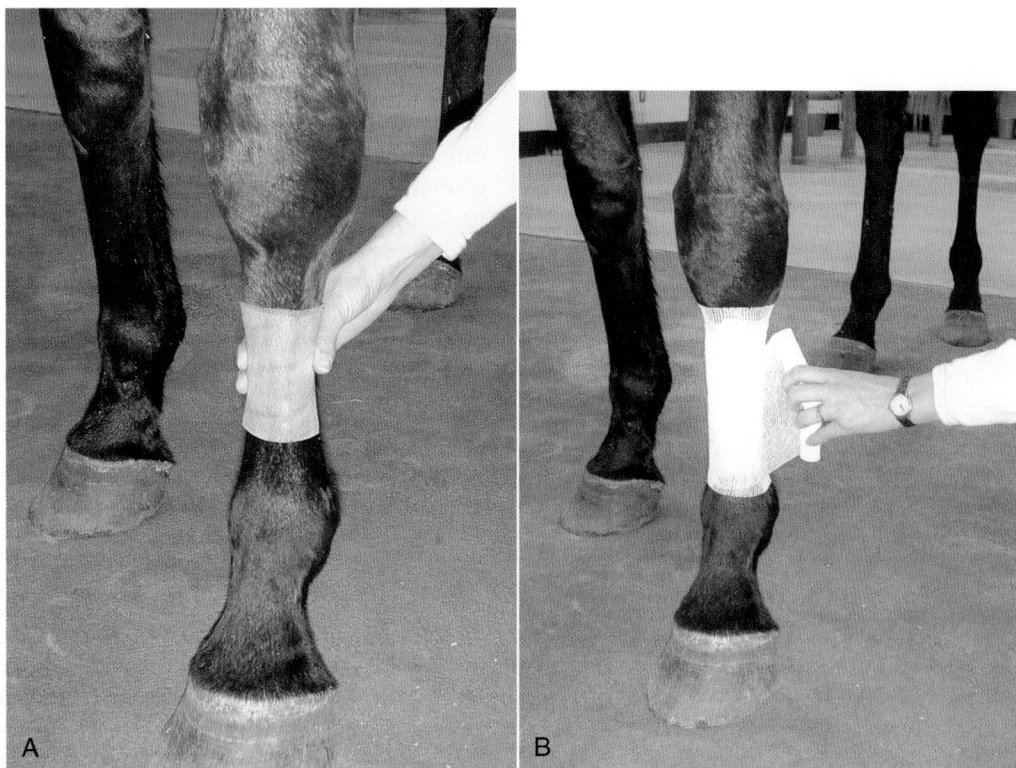

FIGURE 26-22 Application of wound dressing to the distal region of the limb of a horse. **A**, Nonadherent dressing is applied directly over the wound. **B**, Conforming gauze is applied to hold the nonadherent dressing over the wound.

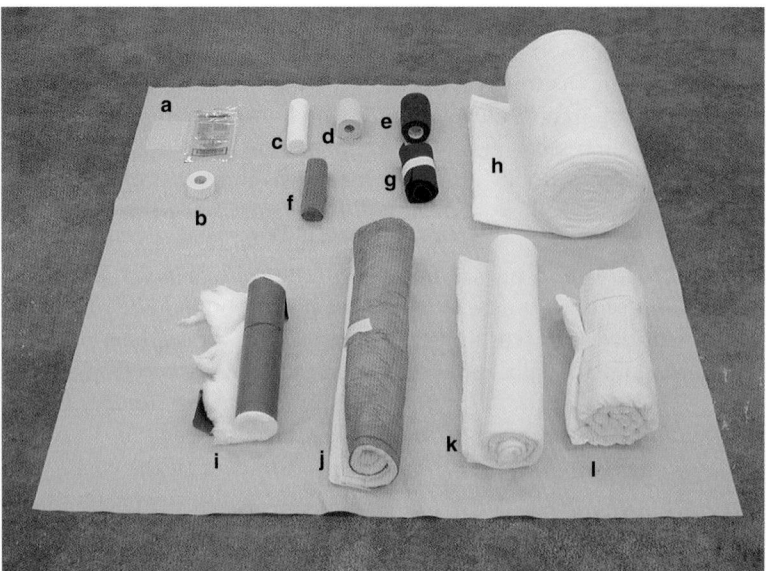

FIGURE 26-23 Various materials can be used in a leg bandage for large animals: nonadherent wound dressing *(a)*, white tape *(b)*, white roll gauze *(c)*, Elastikon (Johnson & Johnson Medical) *(d)*, Vetrap bandage tape (3M Animal Care Products) *(e)*, brown gauze *(f)*, track wrap *(g)*, combine cotton roll *(h)*, rolled cotton *(i)*, military field bandage *(j)*, layered cotton sheets *(k)*, and quilted leg wraps *(l)*.

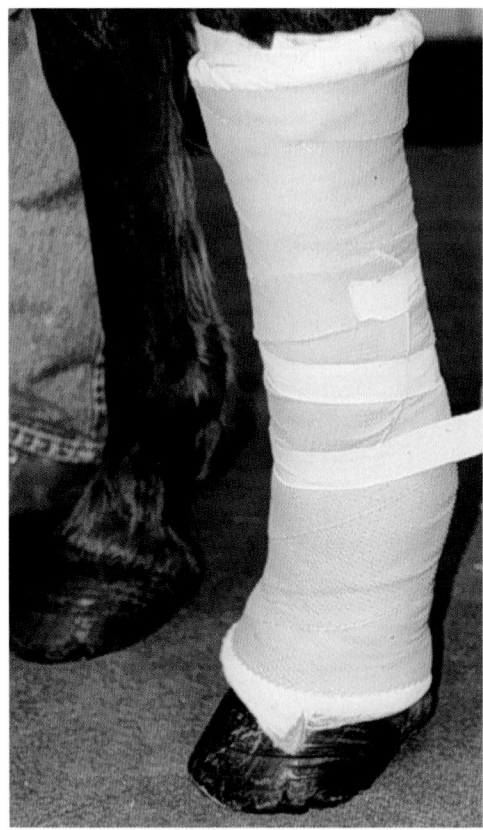

FIGURE 26-24 If white medical tape is used to secure the outer layer of the bandage on a horse's limb, it is secured in a barber-pole fashion to reduce the chance of a tourniquet effect.

Lower Limb Support Bandage

A lower limb support bandage is used to provide support for soft tissues (e.g., ligaments, tendons) of the limb **contralateral** to the injured leg, which is bearing excessive weight because of decreased weight bearing on the injured limb.

The bandage also minimizes static limb edema in a confined, inactive horse. A support bandage is placed on the lower limb in the manner previously described for the lower limb wound bandage *except* that the underlying wound dressing and inner conforming gauze layer are not used. It is unnecessary to place wide adhesive elastic tape around the top and bottom.

SPLINT APPLICATION

A splint is rigid material added to a limb bandage to reinforce immobilization of a particular part of a limb. Various materials, including wooden slats, metal bars, low-temperature thermoplastic material, and casting material, can be used as reinforcement. However, the material most commonly used is polyvinylchloride (PVC) pipe because of its light weight and strength. A 10-cm-diameter pipe split into thirds is ideal. It can be bent by heating with a cutting torch to conform to the fetlock angulation. Length and width of the splint vary with the size of the leg and the area splinted. Depending on the amount of immobilization required, splints can be placed the full length of the forelimb or from just below the carpus or tarsus all the way to the ground surface. In most situations, they are placed on the flexor surface (back) of the limb. Splints are used in situations such as cases of extensor or flexor tendon lacerations and flexure deformities in foals or for needed limb support (as in radial nerve paresis).

A thick support bandage is placed on the limb first. It should be long enough to cover the limb above and below the ends of the splint. This is very important because it will prevent the development of pressure sores. Once the bandage is in place, the splint is secured to the limb with adhesive tape (Figure 26-26). Splints should be reset frequently (at least once per day) in foals, if needed for long periods of time. Because of advances in limb splinting for large animals,

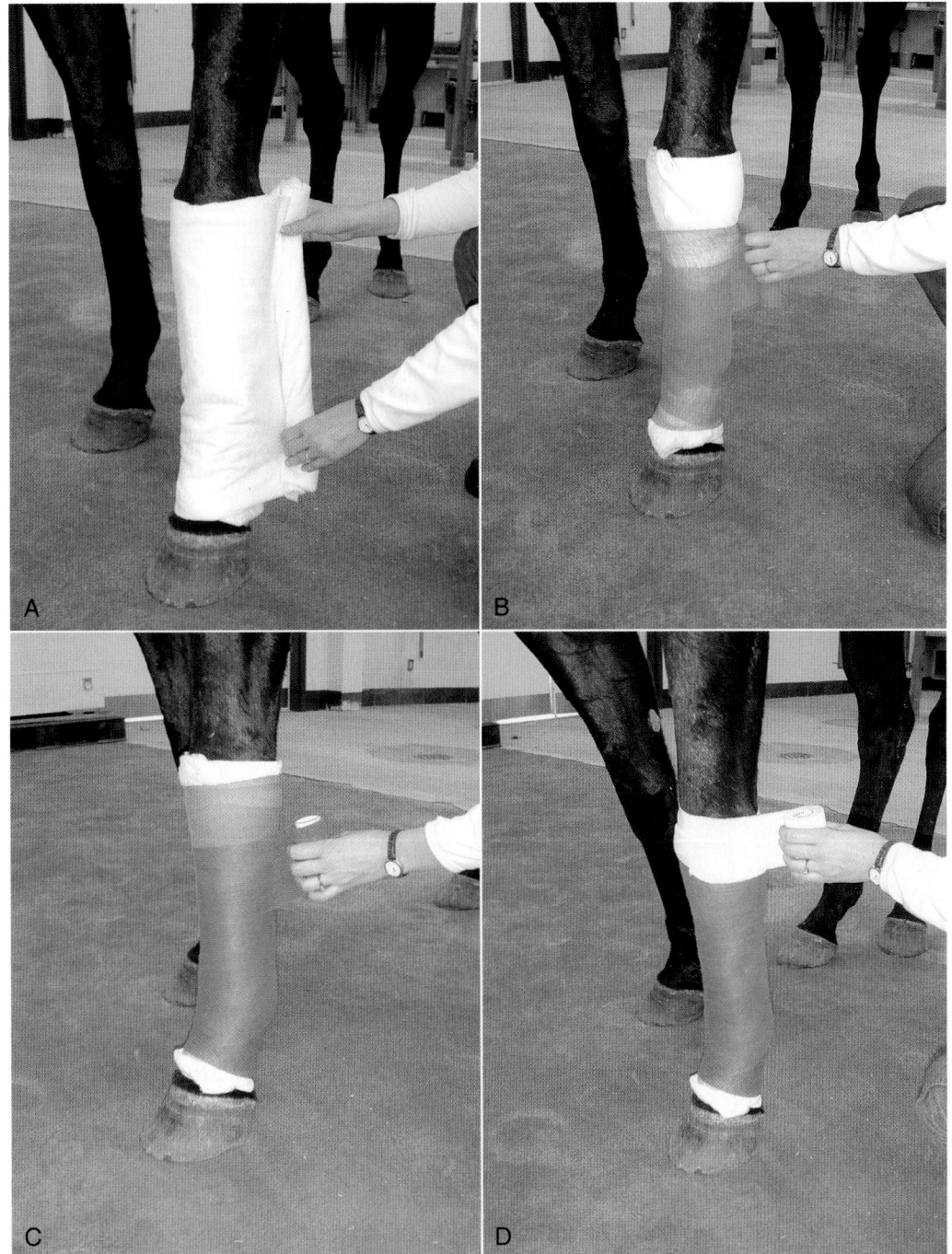

FIGURE 26-25 Application of padded layer of wound bandage. **A,** Cotton wrap is applied snugly around the limb. **B,** Conforming gauze is used to secure the padded layer to the limb. **C,** Vetrap bandage tape (3M Animal Care Products) is applied as the outer shell of the bandage. **D,** Wide adhesive tape is used to provide a seal between skin and bandage.

specially designed splints are now available (DynaSplint, Severna Park, Maryland).

> **TECHNICIAN NOTE** A bandage should cover the limb well above and below the ends of a splint to prevent pressure sores.

CAST APPLICATION

A cast is the external coaptation most frequently used to manage various orthopedic injuries or problems when maximum support and immobilization are required. Casts are commonly used for lower limb problems; however, full limb application is sometimes indicated in large animals. Indications for use of a cast include lower limb fractures, tendon lacerations, support of the lower limb during recovery from orthopedic surgery, heel bulb lacerations, and luxations of the tarsus, fetlock, or pastern. A cast may also be used as an adjunct to internal fixation.

For optimal effectiveness in immobilization, a cast must immobilize the joint proximal and distal to the injury. Full limb casts must extend up to the elbow or stifle as far as possible. The most frequently used material today is fiberglass. Fiberglass (e.g., Delta-Lite, Johnson & Johnson Medical) is appealing because it is lightweight, strong, and relatively easy to apply. However, some veterinarians prefer to use an initial layer of traditional plaster of Paris under the fiberglass. Plaster conforms well to the contour of the limb, reducing the risk for pressure sores.

Before cast application is begun, several things must be considered. A limb cast must be applied properly, or serious problems, such as pressure necrosis, can occur. It is important to remember that applying excessive padding under a cast can result in compression of the padding and loosening of the cast, leading to the development of cast sores. Because of its importance, application of a limb cast is described here in detail.

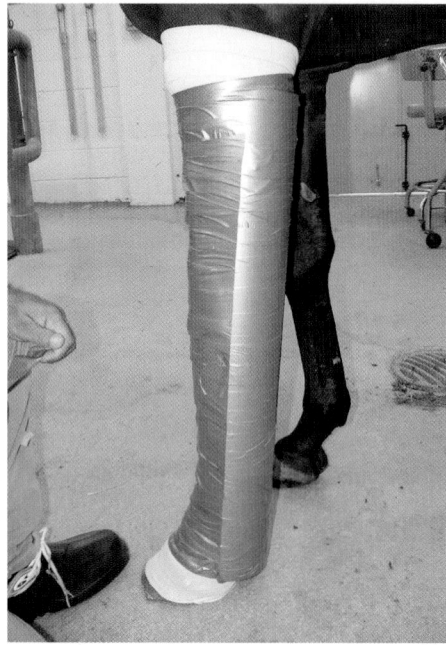

FIGURE 26-26 Application of a full limb splint. A thick bandage is placed on the limb. The splint (polyvinylchloride [PVC] pipe) is positioned along the flexor surface and is secured to the bandage with duct tape.

> **TECHNICIAN NOTE** Excessive padding under a cast can result in compression of the padding and loosening of the cast, leading to the development of cast sores.

Before the procedure is begun, all needed materials should be collected: orthopedic stockinette (3-inch), orthopedic felt, towel clamps, white tape (1-inch), wire (approximately 30 cm), ⅛-inch drill bit and hand drill, broom handle, hoof-trimming equipment (hoof rasp, trimmers, hoof knife), bandage scissors, and cast material (Figure 26-27). Proper application of a cast is essential, especially if it is to remain on the limb for a prolonged period (4 to 6 weeks).

Preparation of the Foot

In general, it is best to apply the cast with the horse under general anesthesia. The horse is positioned in lateral recumbency so the limb to which the cast will be applied is uppermost. Debris is cleaned from the sole, the horseshoe is removed, and the hoof is trimmed. The limb is placed in an extended position perpendicular to the body. Effective support of the leg is essential to maintain the limb in alignment. Traction achieved by using wire looped through holes drilled in the hoof can be helpful. Two holes are drilled in the hoof wall, 5 cm apart near the toe, in the same direction as that in which a horseshoe nail is driven. The ends of the wire are twisted together to form a loop through which a broom handle is placed to apply traction (Figure 26-28).

The frog (the central soft tissue of the hoof) can be packed with povidone-iodine, especially if thrush is present. If a wound is present, a three-layer bandage consisting of a non-adherent dressing, conforming gauze, and adherent elastic tape is used to cover it.

Placement of the Stockinette

The skin must be clean and dry. It can be powdered with talcum or boric acid to help keep the area under the cast dry. The limb is then covered with a double layer of stockinette.

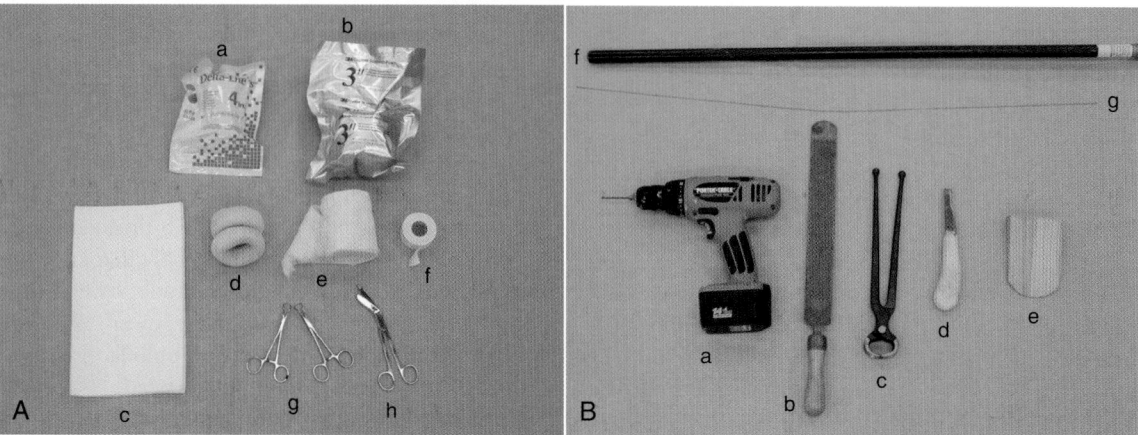

FIGURE 26-27 Materials needed to apply a limb cast to a large animal. **A,** Cast material *(a)*, support foam *(b)*, orthopedic felt *(c)*, orthopedic stockinette (3-inch) *(d)*, cast padding *(e)*, white tape (1-inch) *(f)*, towel clamps *(g)*, and bandage scissors *(h)*. **B,** ⅛-Inch drill bit and hand drill *(a)*, hoof rasp *(b)*, shoe pullers *(c)*, hoof knife *(d)*, wooden wedge block *(e)*, broom handle *(f)*, and wire (approximately 30 cm) *(g)*.

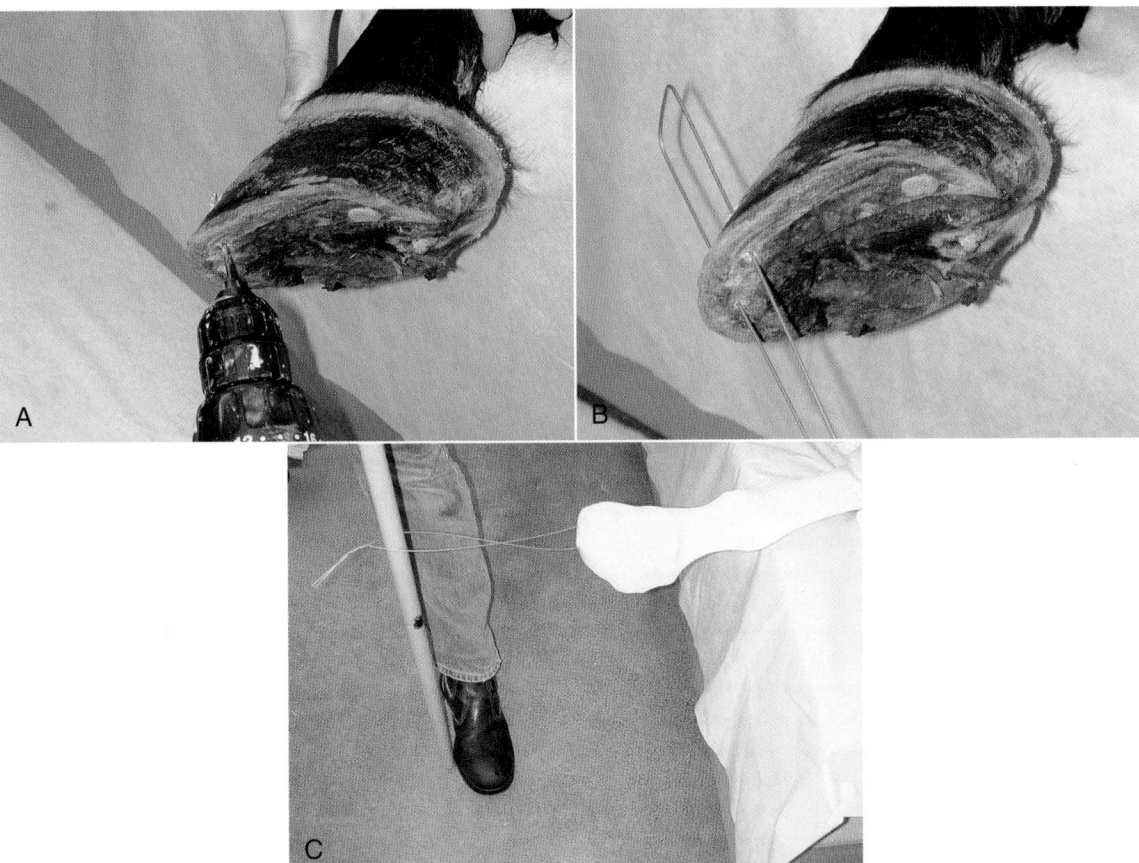

FIGURE 26-28 Traction can be applied to a limb before cast application by drilling two holes in the toe of the hoof **(A)** and threading a loop of wire through the holes **(B)** with a broomstick placed in the loop to apply traction **(C)**.

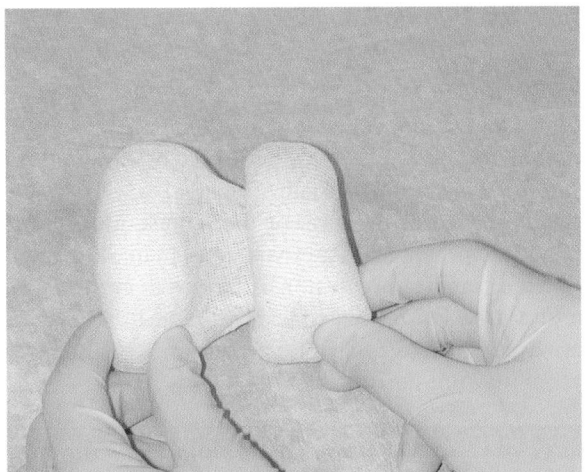

FIGURE 26-29 Orthopedic stockinette used under a cast is pre-rolled. One end is rolled outward and the other end is rolled inward until they meet at the midpoint of the stockinette.

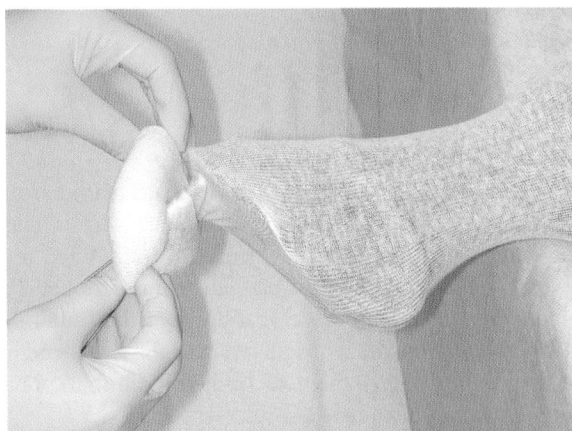

FIGURE 26-30 A twist is placed in the stockinette just beneath the toe, and the inward roll is unrolled up the leg.

The length of the region that the cast will cover is measured, then doubled, and approximately 20 cm is added to this to determine the length of stockinette needed. One end is rolled outward and the other is rolled inward until they meet at the midpoint of the stockinette (Figure 26-29).

Traction wire is threaded through the opening in the stockinette. A broom handle is placed through the wire loop, and traction is applied. The outward roll is first unrolled up the leg. A twist is placed in the stockinette just beneath the toe, and the inward roll is unrolled up the leg (Figure 26-30). Any wrinkles are smoothed out, and towel clamps are used to secure the stockinette to the medial and lateral aspects of the limb above the area to which the cast will be applied (Figure 26-31).

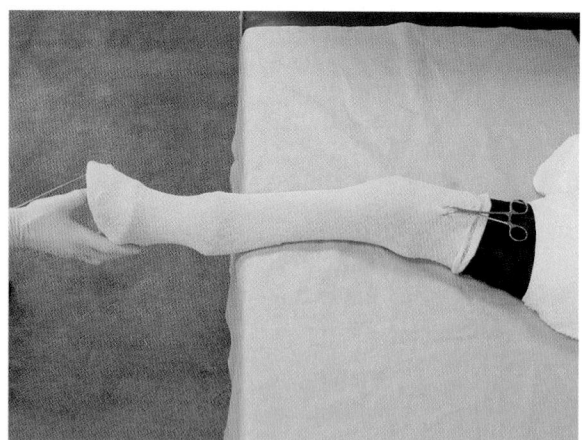

FIGURE 26-31 Before cast material is applied, the orthopedic stockinette is secured with towel clamps to the medial and lateral aspects of the limb above the area to which the cast will be applied.

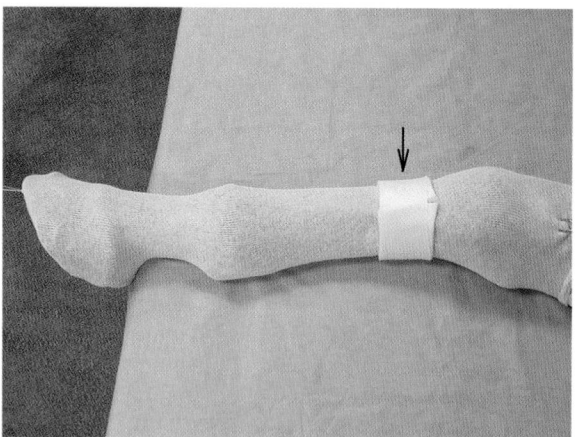

FIGURE 26-32 A strip of orthopedic felt (5 to 7 cm wide) *(arrow)* is placed around the leg at the most proximal limit of the cast. The ends are held in place with 1-inch white tape.

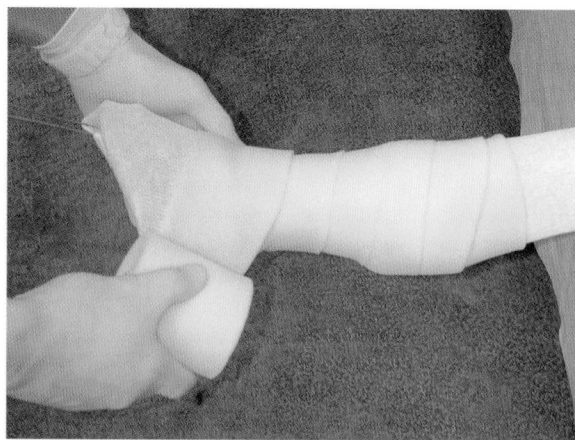

FIGURE 26-33 A roll of support foam can be applied over the stockinette to provide padding under the cast to prevent formation of pressure sores.

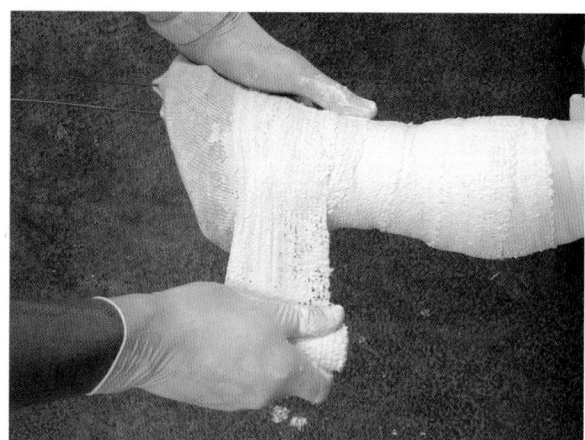

FIGURE 26-34 Application of plaster of Paris.

Application of Orthopedic Felt

A strip of orthopedic felt (5 to 7 cm wide) is placed around the leg at the most proximal limit of the cast. This is held in place with 1-inch white tape (Figure 26-32). When a full limb cast is used, a doughnut pad cut from orthopedic felt is placed over the accessory carpal bone of the forelimb. A thin strip of orthopedic felt is placed over the gastrocnemius tendon and the point of the hock of the hindlimb to prevent the development of pressure sores.

Application of Support Foam

A roll of support foam can be applied next. It is applied over the stockinette, and its purpose is to provide padding under a cast to reduce the development of pressure sores (Figure 26-33). Additional padding on the leg should be avoided because this can become compressed, thus allowing the leg to move within the cast, causing sores.

Application of the Cast Material

To begin, two layers of 3-inch plaster material are carefully and snugly applied to the limb. These layers should be applied without wrinkles to prevent the development of pressure sores. Application of the cast material is usually started at the proximal or distal aspect of the limb. (The author prefers to start distally [Figure 26-34].) A roll of plaster is started at the level of the fetlock and is worked distally, then proximally. Approximately 1 cm of orthopedic felt is left exposed above the top of the cast to prevent formation of a sore. Plaster material is not used in all casts. The veterinarian in charge may prefer that it not be used, or the material may not be available.

> **TECHNICIAN NOTE** It is important that the initial layer of casting material be applied to the limb without wrinkles or finger imprints, which may create pressure sores.

Gloves should be worn when casting material is applied. To save time in identifying the end on a wetted plaster roll, unroll 2 to 3 inches of the plaster material, and hold onto it while wetting the roll in a bucket of warm water (Figure 26-35). Excess water is removed by shaking and gently squeezing the roll. Do not squeeze excessively, or much of the plaster will be lost.

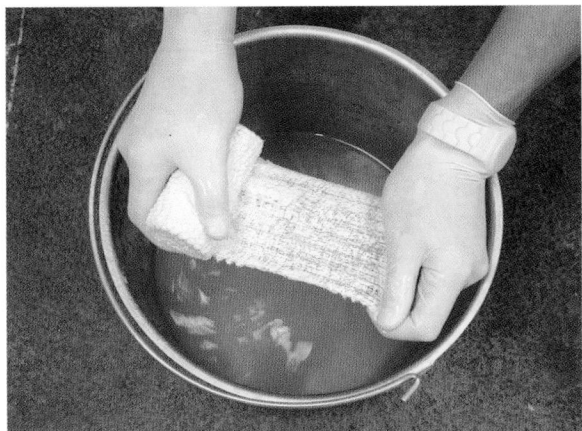

FIGURE 26-35 The end of plaster of Paris cast material is held away from the roll while it is moistened.

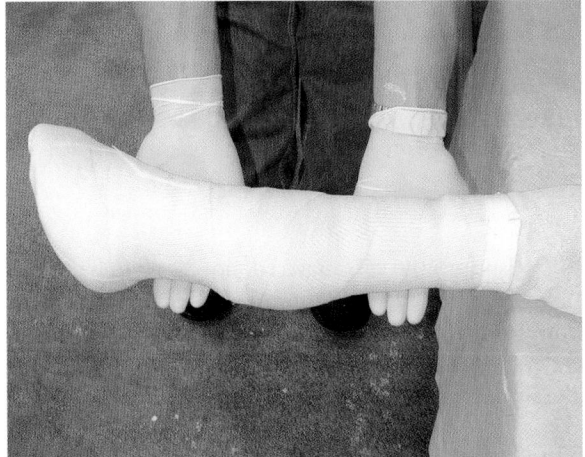

FIGURE 26-36 As the fiberglass cast material is applied, an assistant holds the leg out by resting it on the palms of his or her hands under the metacarpus or metatarsus region. This method prevents finger impressions in the uncured cast material.

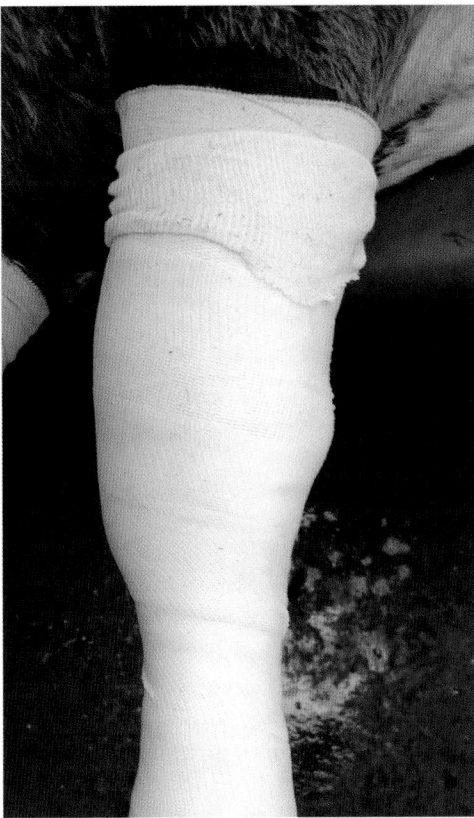

FIGURE 26-37 Approximately 4 cm of orthopedic stockinette left exposed on top of a cast is pulled down over the cast top and is incorporated into the last layers of the cast.

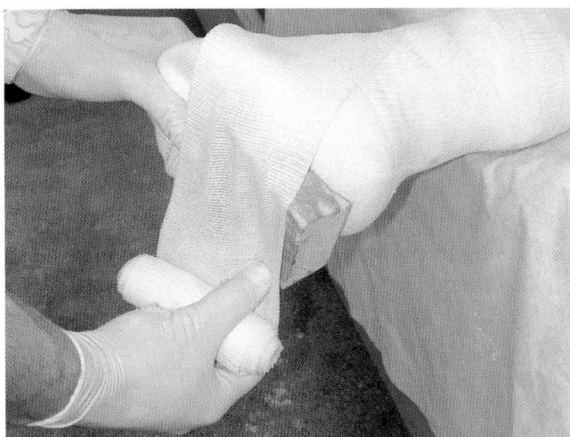

FIGURE 26-38 A wooden wedge block is placed underneath the heel and is incorporated with the last layers of cast material.

Next, the fiberglass cast material is applied. Fiberglass material is held in a bucket of clean water until it is thoroughly wet, and the excess water is shaken out. The author recommends that room-temperature water be used because warm water will speed up the curing process of the resin, resulting in premature hardening of the fiberglass cast material. Usually, it is easier to begin with 3-inch material because it conforms to the limb better. The cast material is overlapped by one third to one half. As the fiberglass casting material is worked toward the foot, the traction wires are cut, and an assistant (technician) holds the leg out by placing a hand under the upper limb region and grasping the tip of the horse's toe with the other hand, or by resting the cast on the palms of the assistant's hands, which are placed under the metacarpus or metatarsus region (Figure 26-36). It is imperative to prevent formation of finger imprints in the cast because they could cause pressure sores to develop.

More pressure is applied to the succeeding layers of fiberglass. This will allow them to laminate better and improves the strength of the cast. Generally, two layers (three to four

rolls) of 3-inch fiberglass cast material are applied, followed by two or three layers (three to four rolls) of 4- or 5-inch fiberglass. At the time the last roll of cast material is applied, the stockinette is unclamped and the excess is cut off, leaving approximately 4 cm. This 4-cm excess is turned down over the top of the cast and is incorporated in the last layer (Figure 26-37). A wooden wedge block is placed underneath the heel and is also incorporated with the last layers (Figure 26-38). A heel wedge allows the horse to walk more easily while wearing a cast because it decreases the breakover force,

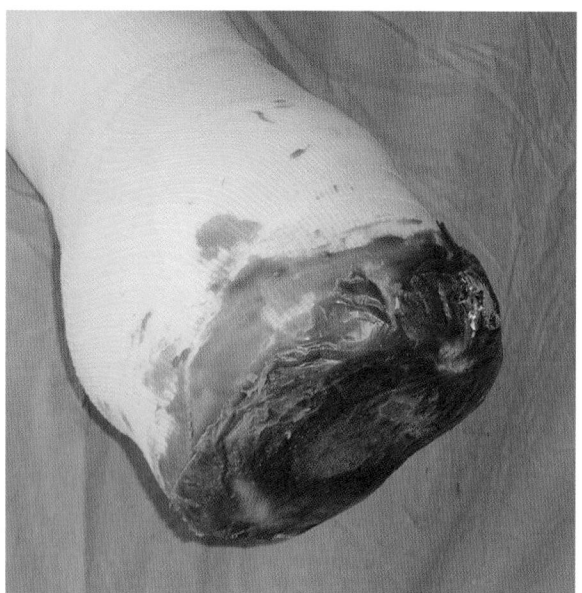

FIGURE 26-39 The bottom of the cast is protected from wear by capping it with hard acrylic. (Technovit, Jorgensen Laboratories, Loveland, Colorado.)

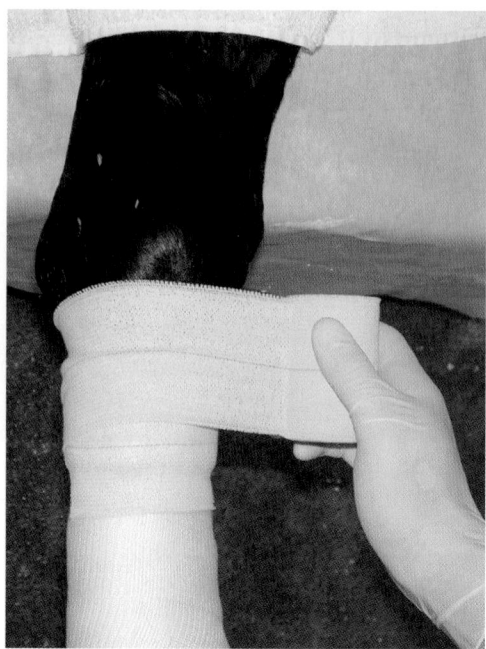

FIGURE 26-40 Elastic adhesive tape is placed on top of the cast to form a seal between skin and cast that prevents debris from getting inside the cast.

reduces pressure on the dorsal proximal limits of the cast at the metacarpus or metatarsus, and allows more even axial weight bearing down through the cast. If a wooden wedge block is not available, a 4-inch roll of fiberglass cast material can substitute as a heel wedge.

When application of the cast is completed, the outer layer is smoothed by running wetted, gloved hands up and down the cast. The bottom of the cast is protected from wear by capping it with hard acrylic (e.g., Technovit, Jorgensen Laboratories, Loveland, Colorado) (Figure 26-39). Finally, elastic adhesive tape is placed around the top of the cast and is attached to the skin (Figure 26-40), or a piece of stockinette is pulled over the top and is taped to the cast and the limb above the cast to prevent debris (wood shavings) from getting inside the cast.

Stall confinement is mandatory after cast application. The patient must be monitored daily. Indications for cast change or removal include breakage, increased lameness, swelling, and exudates coming out of the top of the cast. Horses vary in their reaction and tolerance to a cast. If there is any doubt, a cast should be removed and the limb evaluated.

CAST REMOVAL

A cast is best removed with the animal standing, unless another cast is to be applied. If cast removal is performed under general anesthesia, the limb may be reinjured when the animal is trying to recover from anesthesia. However, general anesthesia is used if the cast is changed. With a Stryker saw, the cast is split on the medial and lateral surfaces, and the cut is continued under the foot (Figure 26-41, *A*). Through this approach, injury to flexor and extensor tendons with the cast saw can be prevented. When cutting over bony prominences, one should be careful to avoid lacerating the skin. Cast cutters are made to oscillate, so it is

best to push into the cast material, not along it, because this will reduce the chance of lacerating the skin. Once the cast is completely cut, the two halves are separated with cast spreaders (Figure 26-41, *B*). A support wrap is then placed on the limb.

> **TECHNICIAN NOTE** A cast is split on the medial and lateral surfaces to prevent injury to flexor and extensor tendons with the cast saw.

BANDAGE, SPLINT, AND CAST APPLICATION TECHNIQUES FOR CATTLE

Principles applied to limb bandaging and cast application are the same in cattle as in horses, but specific techniques are used for cattle. Cattle often are not as cooperative as horses, and they require more restraint.

With cattle, a cast can be applied directly over the dewclaws without causing major problems. However, sores caused by motion of the cast can occur in this area because of an inability to closely fit the cast. This can be remedied by trimming the dewclaws as short as possible and placing a pad of orthopedic felt with holes cut out for the dewclaws between them (Figure 26-42).

APPLICATION OF A CLAW BLOCK

A wooden block is applied to an unaffected claw to alleviate weight bearing on an adjacent claw if it is fractured or injured, or to protect a postsurgical area by raising it higher off the ground (e.g., after amputation of an adjacent claw). The block usually is made from a piece of wood 5 cm thick

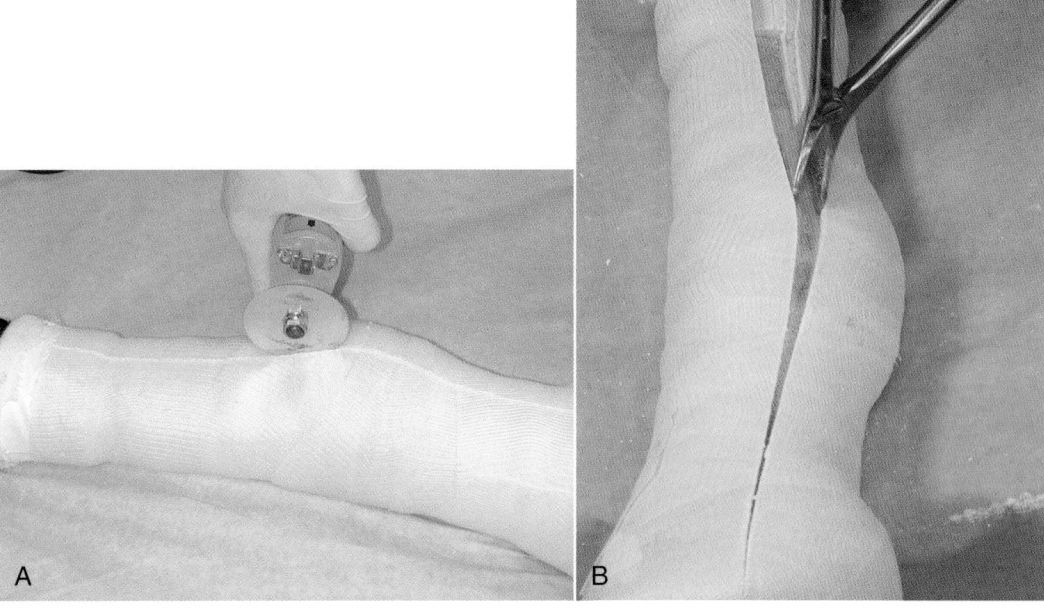

FIGURE 26-41 Removal of a limb cast from a horse. **A,** With a Stryker saw, the cast is split on the medial and lateral surface, and the cut is continued under the foot. **B,** Once the cast is completely cut, the two halves are separated with cast spreaders.

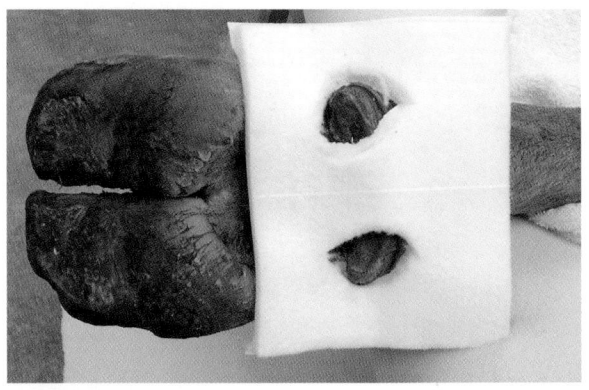

FIGURE 26-42 A piece of orthopedic felt with holes cut out can be placed between the dewclaws to reduce motion under a cast and to help prevent development of pressure sores.

FIGURE 26-43 A claw block made from wood. Grooves are cut on both sides of the block to improve traction and bonding.

and is cut to the shape of the sole surface of the claw. Grooves are cut in the ground surface for traction (Figure 26-43).

The claw is trimmed first, and debris is removed by means of an electric sander or rasp. This is an important step for effective bonding of adhesive to the claw. The block is then bonded to the horny surface of the claw with acrylic cement, such as Technovit (Jorgensen Laboratories) or polyurethane hoof cement (Vettec, Vettec Hoof Care Products, Oxnard, California) (Figure 26-44).

MODIFIED THOMAS SPLINT

Despite advances in external and internal skeletal fixation, **modified Thomas splints** are often used in cattle and small ruminants as a means of external skeletal fixation. The modified Thomas splint is often used in combination with internal fixation or a cast. Indications for its use include fractures

of the tibia or radius and ligamentous injuries of the stifle. Pressure sores in the inguinal or axillary region are a problem when a Thomas splint is used, despite padding of the metal ring part of the splint that fits into that area.

Application of a modified Thomas splint in large ruminants does require special equipment, such as a conduit bender, to bend the round rod iron used to construct the splint. For small farm animals, a beehive and an aluminum rod are used (Figure 26-45). The design of the splint varies somewhat among clinicians, but the purpose is the same—to apply traction and maintain alignment of the limb.

The animal is placed in lateral recumbency first, with the affected leg uppermost. A template to fit the individual animal, devised from a nasogastric tube or other similar flexible tubing, is used to construct the ring that will encircle the proximal part of the leg (Figure 26-46). The ring should be large enough that it does not impinge on any bony prominences. The rod is bent in a ring the same size as the template. The ring is then padded with cotton

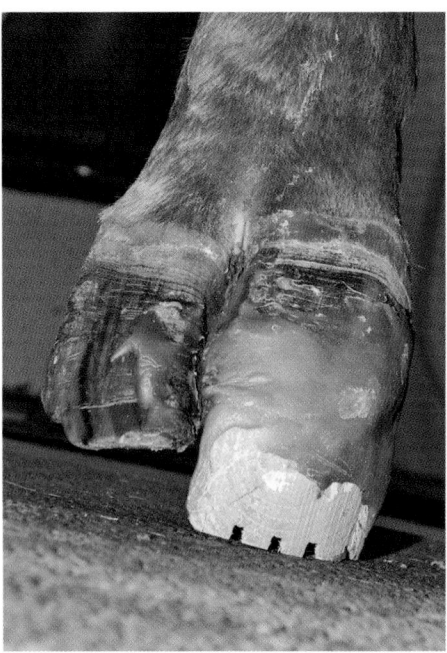

FIGURE 26-44 A wooden block is cemented to the unaffected claw with acrylic (viewed from the dorsal aspect of the foot).

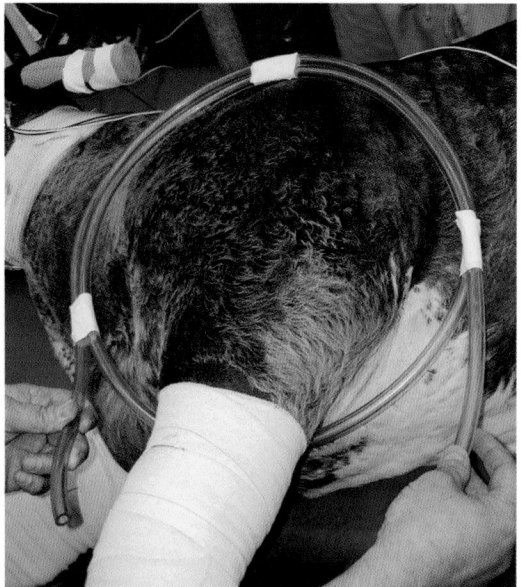

FIGURE 26-46 A template, devised from a nasogastric tube or other similar flexible tubing, is used to construct the metal ring of a modified Thomas splint that will encircle the proximal part of the leg.

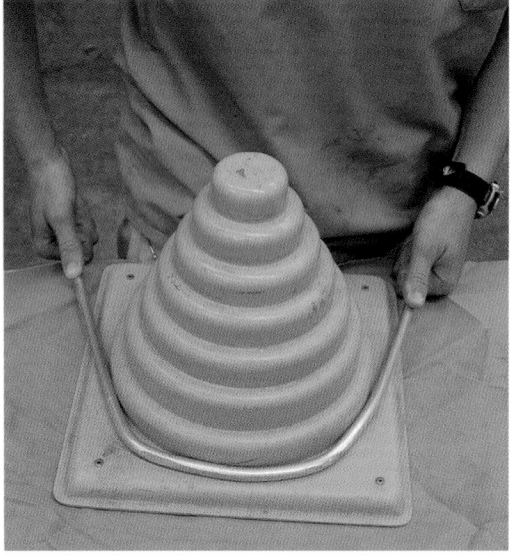

FIGURE 26-45 A ¼-inch aluminum rod is bent with a beehive to construct a modified Thomas splint.

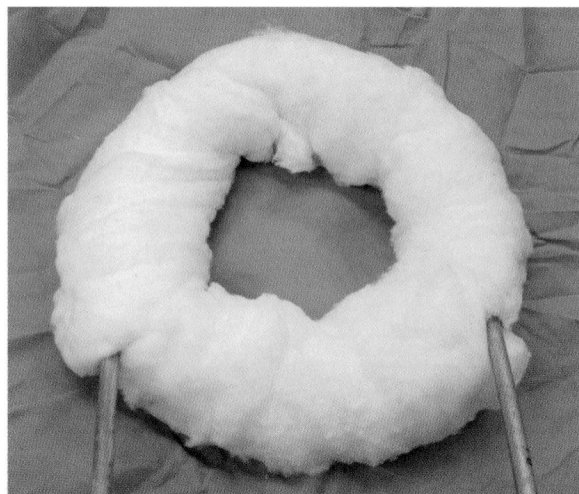

FIGURE 26-47 A metal rod is bent into a ring to construct the proximal part of a modified Thomas splint. Once the ring is constructed, it is padded with cotton.

(Figure 26-47). This is important to reduce pressure sores in the axillary or inguinal region. Variation in design occurs with extensions that come off the ring to support the animal's limb.

One design has the extensions coming off the ring cranially and caudally to the leg (Figure 26-48). Extensions of the splint must be shaped to conform to the angles of the hock and stifle. For the front limb, the extensions are kept straight and are not bent into any shape. These extensions are also bent away (lateral) from the flat plane of the ring to allow the ventral part of the ring to fit into the axillary or inguinal region (Figure 26-49). Another design has the

extensions coming off the ventral aspect of the ring. The ring is then bent so that the extensions are positioned medial to the limb, and so that the ring itself fits the contour of the upper limb (Figure 26-50). This design is used for large animals.

The next portion to be constructed is the distal part of the splint (footplate). A footplate can be constructed in various ways. With one method, two threaded rods are attached to the extensions of the splint. The splint is devised with these types of extensions so that the length of the splint can be adjusted. This design is most useful in large ruminants. Another construct has a piece of metal rod that is bent

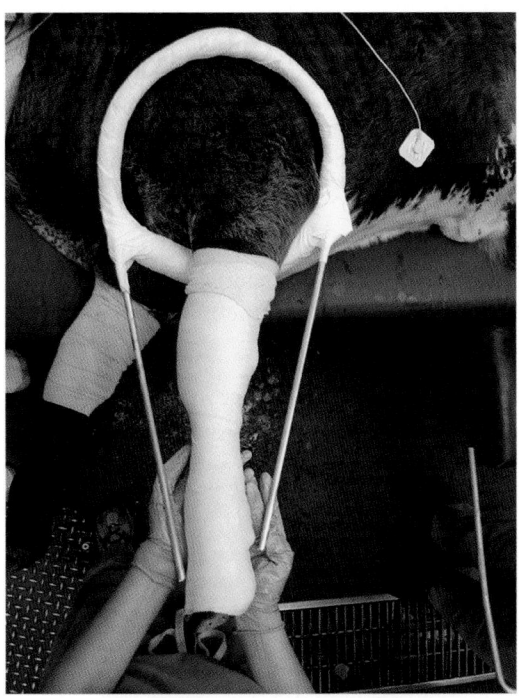

FIGURE 26-48 Construction of a modified Thomas splint. Extensions of the splint come off the edge of the ring and are positioned cranial and caudal to the limb.

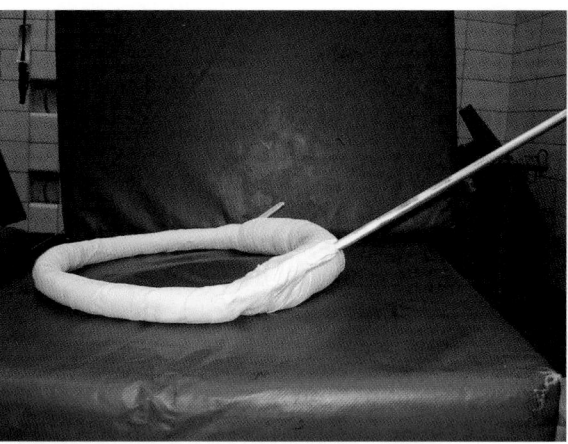

FIGURE 26-49 Construction of a modified Thomas splint. Extensions come off the ring at an angle to allow the ring to properly fit under the axillary or inguinal region.

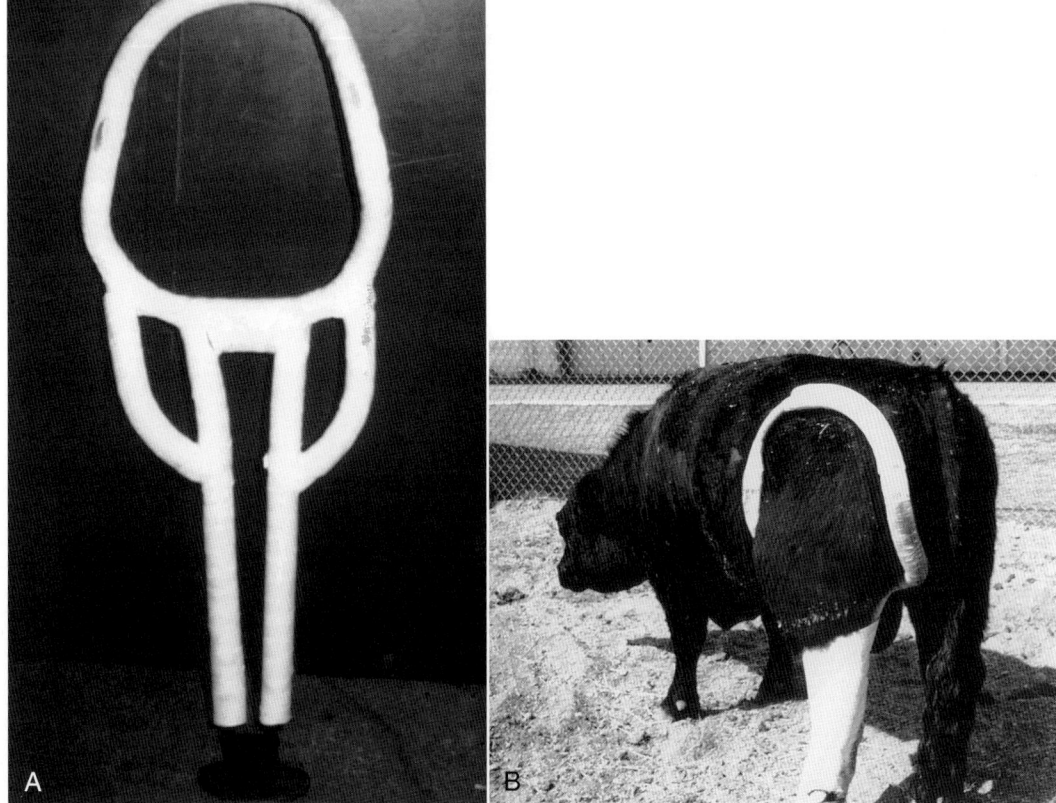

FIGURE 26-50 A modified Thomas splint. This design has the extensions coming off the ventral aspect of the ring. The ring is then bent so that the extensions are positioned medial to the limb, and so that the ring itself fits the contour of the upper limb **(A)**. This design is used for large animals **(B)**. (Photograph courtesy Dr. Dwight F. Wolfe.)

in a flat U shape, positioned under the foot, and connected to the ends of the extensions of the splint with a combination of twisted wire loops and lots of tape (Figure 26-51). This type of design is used in small farm animals. Next, holes are drilled into the hoof walls near the toes and wired to the bottom of the splint (Figure 26-52). Slight traction is placed on the limb as the splint is applied. Traction should be minimal within the splint so as not to create excessive pressure in the axillary or inguinal region, which could interfere with venous drainage or distract the fracture fragments.

> **TECHNICIAN NOTE** When the hoof is secured to a modified Thomas splint, it is important to avoid applying excess traction, because this will create too much pressure in the axillary or inguinal region, which could interfere with venous drainage or distract the fracture fragments.

Once the splint is in position, the limb and splint are covered with layers of cast material (Figure 26-53). Casting tape is applied by "weaving" the material around the limb

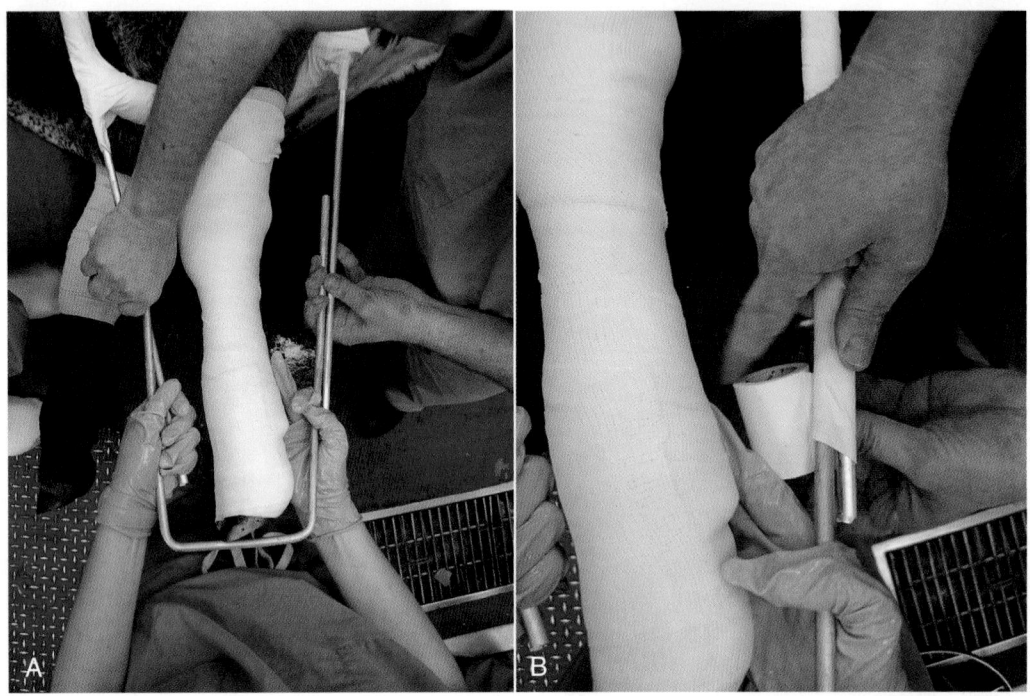

FIGURE 26-51 The footplate in this design of a modified Thomas splint is constructed from a piece of metal rod that is bent into a flat U shape (A) positioned under the foot, and is connected to the ends of the extensions of the splint with a combination of twisted wire loops and lots of tape (B).

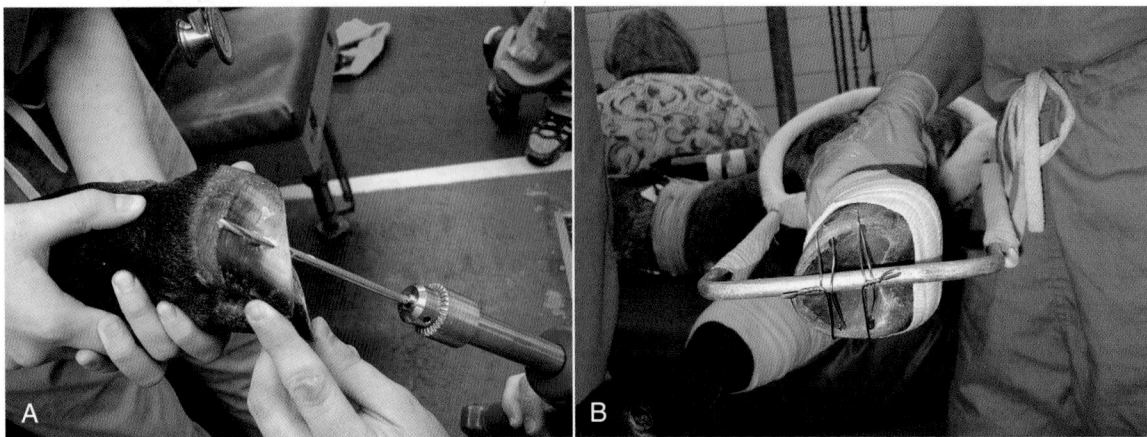

FIGURE 26-52 A, Holes are drilled into the hoof walls near the toes and are wired to the bottom of the splint (B) when a modified Thomas splint is applied.

and extensions of the splint in a figure-eight pattern (Figure 26-54, *A*). The casting tape is twisted 180 degrees with each passage of the material (Figure 26-54, *B*). The cast material should be applied as proximally as possible (Figure 26-55). The bottom of the splint is protected from wear by application of a polyurethane hoof-bonding material (Figure 26-56).

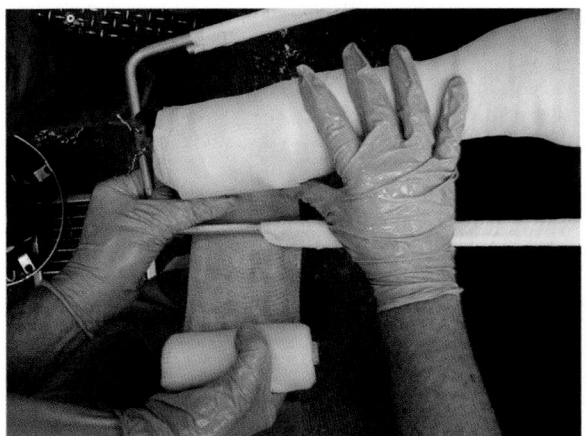

FIGURE 26-53 The limb and the modified Thomas splint are covered with layers of cast material to stabilize the limb.

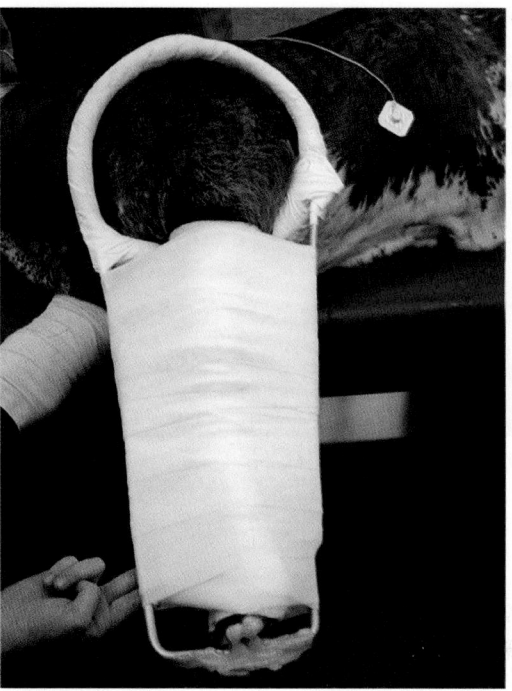

FIGURE 26-55 The cast material is applied as proximally as possible when a modified Thomas splint is applied.

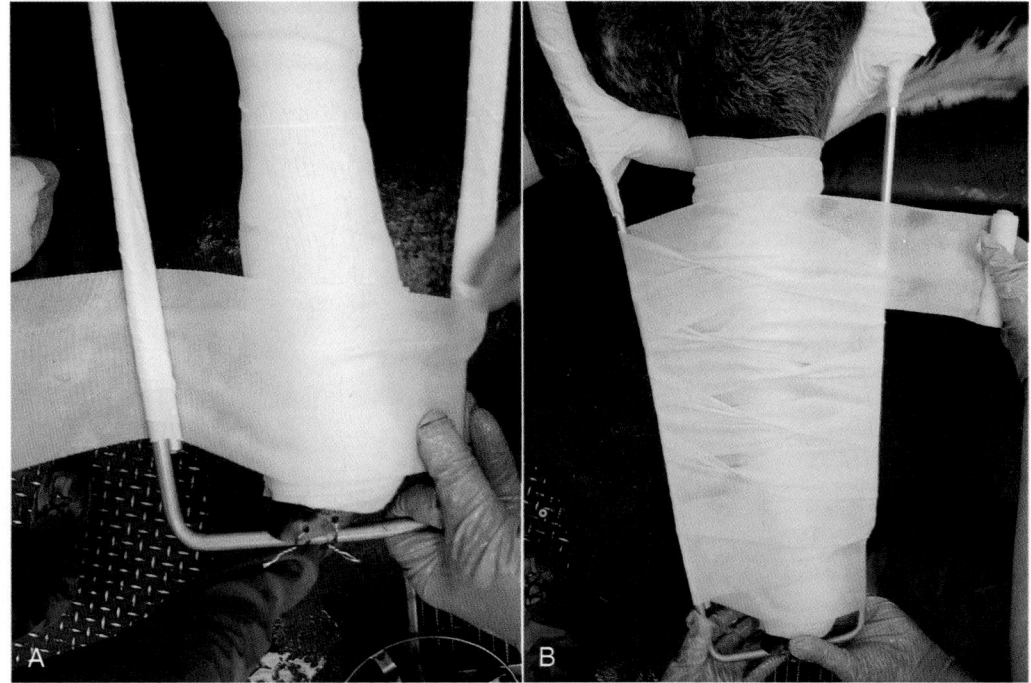

FIGURE 26-54 A, A modified Thomas splint is secured to the limb by "weaving" casting tape around the limb and extensions of the splint in a figure-eight pattern. **B,** The casting tape is twisted 180 degrees with each passage of the material.

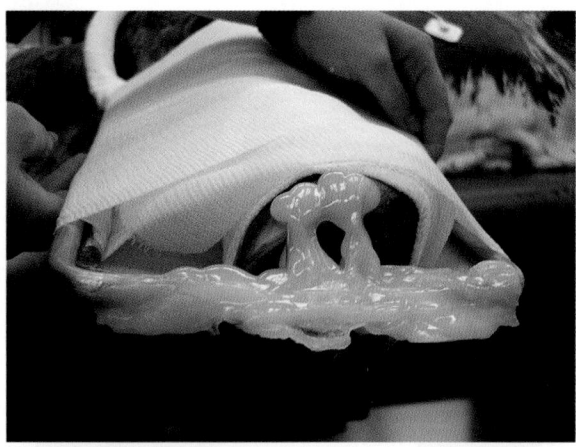

FIGURE 26-56 The bottom of a modified Thomas splint is protected from wear by applying a polyurethane hoof-bonding material.

RECOMMENDED READINGS
Small Animal

Amalsadvala T, Swaim SF: Management of hard-to-heal wounds, Vet Clin North Am 36:693, 2006.

Campbell BG: Dressings, bandages, and splints for wound management in dogs and cats, Vet Clin North Am 36:759, 2006.

Dernell WS: Initial wound management, Vet Clin North Am 36:713, 2006.

Hedlund CS: Surgery of the integumentary system: general principles and techniques. In Fossum TW, editor: Small animal surgery, ed 3, St Louis, 2007, Mosby, p 159.

Hosgood G: Stages of wound healing and their clinical relevance, Vet Clin North Am 36:667, 2006.

Krahwinkel DJ, Boothe HW: Topical and systemic medications for wounds. Vet Clin North Am 36:739, 2006.

Liptak JM: An overview of the topical management of wounds, Austr Vet J 75:408, 1997.

Pavletic MM: Basic principles of wound management. In Atlas of small animal reconstructive surgery, ed 2, St Louis, 1999, Saunders, p 21.

Pavletic MM, Trout NJ: Bullet, bite, and burn wounds in dogs and cats, Vet Clin North Am 36:873, 2006.

Piermattei D, Flo G, DeCamp C: Immobilization (fixation). In Handbook of small animal orthopedics and fracture repair, ed 4, St Louis, 2006, Saunders, p 48.

Pope ER: Head and facial wounds in dogs and cats, Vet Clin North Am 36:793, 2006.

Simpson AM, Radlinsky MA, Beale BS: Bandaging in dogs and cats: basic principles, Compendium 23:12, 2001.

Simpson AM, Radlinsky MA, Beale BS: Bandaging in dogs and cats: external coaptation, Compendium 23:157, 2001.

Swaim SF, Hinkl e SH, Bradley DM: Wound contraction: basic and clinical factors, Compendium 23:20, 2001.

Large Animal

Adams SB, Fessler JF: Treatment of radial-ulnar and tibial fractures in cattle, using a modified Thomas splint-cast combination, J Am Vet Assoc 183:430, 1983.

Auer JA: Drainings, bandages, and external coaptation. In Auer JA, Stick JA, editors: Equine surgery, ed 3, St Louis, 2006, Saunders.

Hendrickson DA: Wound care for the equine practitioner, Jackson, WY, 2005, Teton NewMedia.

Stashak TS: Bandaging and casting techniques for wound management. In Stashak TS, Theoret CL, editors: Equine wound management, ed 2, Ames, IA, 2008, Wiley & Blackwell.

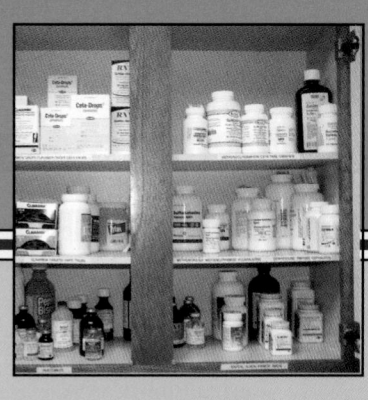

27 Pharmacology and Pharmacy

Katrina R. Viviano

OUTLINE

Basic Pharmacokinetics, *1011*
Drug Absorption, *1011*
Drug Distribution, *1012*
Drug Metabolism, *1012*
Drug Elimination, *1013*
Basic Pharmacodynamics, *1013*
Mechanism of Action, *1013*
Side Effects (or Adverse Reactions), *1014*
Impact of Disease on Drug Pharmacokinetics, *1014*
Cardiovascular Disease, *1014*
Kidney Disease, *1015*
Liver Disease, *1015*
Aging and Drug Pharmacokinetics, *1015*
Adverse Drug Reactions, *1015*
Dose-Dependent Drug Reactions, *1016*
Idiosyncratic Drug Reactions, *1016*
Therapeutic Drug Monitoring, *1016*
Target Organ/Organ Systems Approach to Drug Classification, *1016*
Immune-Mediated Disease, *1016*
Infectious Disease, *1017*
Endocrine Disease, *1020*
Gastrointestinal Disease, *1023*

Liver Disease, *1023*
Cardiovascular Disease, *1024*
Neurologic Disease, *1027*
Neoplastic Disease, *1027*
Parasitic Disease, *1027*
Regulatory Pharmacology, *1031*
Drug Laws and Regulations, *1031*
Definitions and Approval Categories of Drugs, *1031*
Controlled Substances, *1033*
Extra-Label Drug Use, *1034*
Drug Residues in Food-Producing Animals, *1035*
Adverse Drug Event Reporting, *1035*
Drug Compounding, *1036*
Drug Supplements/Nutraceuticals, *1037*
The Veterinary Pharmacy, *1037*
Drug Procurement, *1037*
Drug Dosage Forms, *1037*
Drug Storage and Disposal, *1038*
Prescription Drugs, *1038*
Prescription Writing and Dispensing, *1038*
Drug Calculations, *1040*

LEARNING OBJECTIVES

When you have completed this chapter, you will be able to:

1. Pronounce, define, and spell all Key Terms in this chapter.
2. Describe the principles of basic pharmacokinetics and pharmacodynamics.
3. Describe the impact of cardiovascular, kidney, liver disease and aging on drug pharmacokinetics.
4. Compare and contrast dose-dependent drug reactions and idiosyncratic drug reactions, and explain the role of therapeutic drug monitoring in maximizing drug efficacy and minimizing drug toxicity.
5. Do the following regarding target organ/organ systems approach to drug classification:

The author and publisher wish to acknowledge the contributions of Marvene Augustus and Sonya Bremer Boss to previous editions of this textbook.

KEY TERMS

Adverse drug event
Agonist
Animal Medicinal Drug Use Clarification Act (AMDUCA)
Antagonist
Ascites
Bioavailability
Biotransformation
Center for Veterinary Medicine
Chelate
Controlled Substance Act
Dose-dependent drug reaction
Drug clearance
Drug compounding
Drug distribution
Efficacy
Endogenous substrate
Environmental Protection Agency
Extra-label drug use
Federal Food, Drug, and Cosmetic Act
Food and Drug Administration
Glucocorticoids
Half-life
Hydrophilic
Idiosyncratic drug reaction
Legend drug
Lipophilic
Lyophilized
Mineralocorticoids
Nonionic
Nutraceutical
Over-the-counter drug
Parenteral administration
Pharmacodynamics
Pharmacokinetics
Prescription drug
Steady state

KEY TERMS—cont'd

Targeted therapy
Therapeutic blood level
Therapeutic drug
  monitoring
Therapeutic range
U.S. Department of
  Agriculture (USDA)
U.S. Pharmacopoeia
  (USP)—National
  Formulary (NF)
Veterinarian-client-
  patient relationship
Veterinary feed directive
  drug
Volume of distribution

- List the major diseases affecting the endocrine, gastrointestinal, cardiovascular, and neurologic systems that are treated with pharmaceuticals; and the major immune-mediated, infectious, liver, and neoplastic diseases that are treated with pharmaceuticals.
- List the main drug classes used to treat major animal diseases, and give examples of drugs in each class, including their mechanism of action and common side effects.
- List the main classes of antimicrobial agents used in veterinary patients, and give examples of each, including their spectrum of activity and common side effects.

6. Do the following regarding regulatory pharmacology:
  - Summarize state and federal laws regulating drug use, and explain how they work together to ensure that available drugs are safe and effective, and are used appropriately to treat and prevent animal diseases.
  - List approval categories of drugs, and compare and contrast prescription drugs, over-the-counter drugs, and veterinary feed directive drugs.
  - Explain the concept of a valid veterinary-client-patient relationship, and explain how it affects the use of prescription drugs.
  - Discuss laws affecting the use of controlled substances, and list commonly used drugs that are classified as controlled substances.
  - Define extra-label drug use, and discuss circumstances under which drugs may or may not be used in this manner, including special restrictions on extra-label drug use in food-producing animals.
  - Discuss the significance of drug residues in food-producing animals and the importance of observing withdrawal times to keep the human food supply safe.
  - Define drug compounding and explain legal issues related to compounding of medications.

7. Describe regulatory issues related to procurement, storage, dispensing, and administration of pharmacologic agents; and, list the dosage forms of medications, the routes by which medications may be administered, and factors that affect route selection.

8. Perform dosage calculations required to dispense drugs and to administer drugs to patients.

INTRODUCTION

Pharmacology is the study of drugs used in the diagnosis, treatment, or prevention of disease in man and animals. Pharmacology is a diverse discipline that encompasses the study of the fundamentals of drug movement in the body (or **pharmacokinetics**), the biochemical and physiologic effects of drugs (or **pharmacodynamics**), and the effective use of drugs in a clinical setting (or clinical pharmacology). Topics important to the clinical pharmacology of drugs include therapeutic drug monitoring, the impact of disease and aging on drug disposition (or pharmacokinetics), and adverse drug reactions. Also included in the field of pharmacology are the regulatory requirements governing drug use.

The veterinary technician plays an important role in the veterinary pharmacy and is typically responsible for inventory control, drug administration, patient monitoring, and client communication. The purpose of this chapter is to provide an introduction to pharmacology for the veterinary technician, and to provide practical guidelines for effective drug use in veterinary patients. Emphasis is placed on the knowledge and skills necessary to safely handle, administer, and dispense drugs, monitor for effectiveness and side effects, and educate clients regarding proper use. Some of the classes of drugs more commonly used in veterinary patients are briefly reviewed using a target organ/organ systems approach.

BASIC PHARMACOKINETICS

Pharmacokinetics (PK) is the study of the movement of drugs in the body (i.e., absorption, distribution, metabolism, and excretion). Figure 27-1 provides a schematic diagram used to describe the movement of drugs in the body. Knowledge of a drug's PK is important because it is used to determine appropriate drug doses, dosing regimens, and withdrawal times in food animals. In addition, PK is used during drug development to establish effective and safe dosage forms and regimens. Clinically relevant pharmacokinetic parameters include half-life ($t_{1/2}$), volume of distribution (Vd), clearance (Cl), and bioavailability (F).

DRUG ABSORPTION

Absorption is the uptake of a substance through a surface of the body into fluids and tissues. For drugs, absorption takes place from the site of administration (gastrointestinal tract, muscle, subcutaneous tissues, respiratory tract, or skin) to the circulating blood and plasma. Once the drug is in the blood, absorption continues from the blood to the tissues, with the drug distributed to the site of action and finally to the organs of metabolism and elimination. For a drug to be absorbed and distributed in the body, a concentration gradient (a higher drug concentration outside the cell than inside the cell) is required along with chemical properties that enable the drug to cross multiple cell membranes. Cell membranes are composed of lipids; therefore, drug absorption across cell membranes is most effective for drugs that are lipid soluble (or lipophilic) and uncharged (or **nonionic**), and present at a higher concentration outside the cell than inside the cell. Examples of lipophilic drugs include fluoroquinolones, chloramphenicol, **glucocorticoids**, and cyclosporine. Water-soluble (or hydrophilic) drugs often are poorly absorbed and distributed, and therefore require administration by injection (**parenteral administration**) to achieve effective **therapeutic blood levels** (the blood level at which the drug will have the desired effect). Examples of hydrophilic drugs include aminoglycosides and heparin. In general, drugs that are lipophilic diffuse more readily into tissue than do **hydrophilic** drugs but require more extensive metabolism for elimination.

Bioavailability refers to the fraction of a drug dose that reaches the bloodstream. When administered intravenously, a drug is 100% bioavailable. In contrast, only a fraction of a drug administered outside of a vein reaches the bloodstream. For example, butorphanol (an opioid analgesic that undergoes significant liver metabolism after absorption from the gastrointestinal tract) is only 20% bioavailable when administered orally, but it is 100% bioavailable when administered intravenously. Bioavailability is a function of both absorption and metabolism.

The most common extravascular route used for drug administration is the oral route. The bioavailability of an orally administered drug is dependent on a healthy, functional gastrointestinal (GI) tract. The primary intestinal site of drug absorption is the small intestine because of its high surface area and more alkaline pH. Factors that limit the bioavailability of drugs given orally include binding to food and minerals, metabolism by resident microorganisms (especially in ruminants), intestinal **biotransformation** by enzymes, and metabolism of drugs after transport to the liver via the portal vein. For example, common drugs such as opioids, budesonide (an orally administered locally acting glucocorticoid), and lidocaine are extensively metabolized after oral administration, leading to poor oral bioavailability.

> **TECHNICIAN NOTE** Bioavailability refers to the fraction of a drug dose that reaches the bloodstream. When administered intravenously, a drug is 100% bioavailable. In contrast, only a fraction of a drug administered outside of a vein reaches the bloodstream.

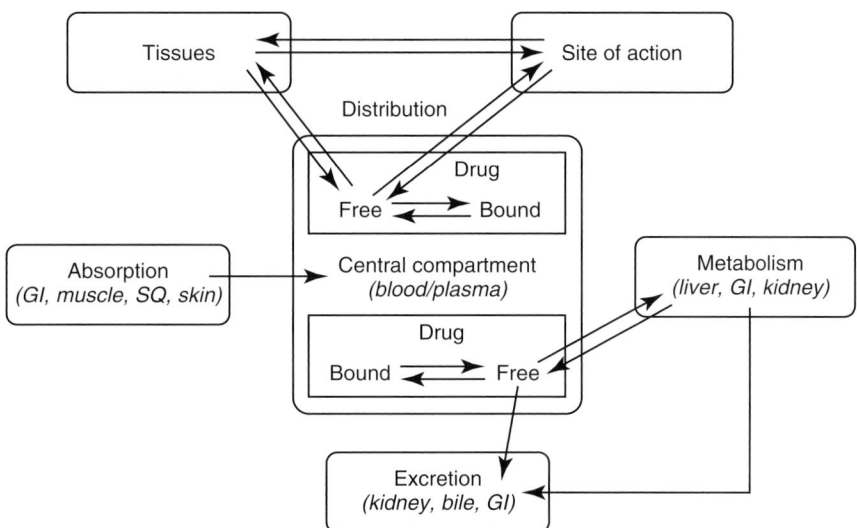

FIGURE 27-1 A schematic diagram used to describe the compartmental movement of drug in the body.

DRUG DISTRIBUTION

Distribution is the movement of an absorbed drug from the blood to various tissues of the body. However, movement out of the blood does not guarantee that the drug will reach the target tissue and the site of action. The **volume of distribution** (Vd) is an estimate of the distribution of a drug in the body (the relationship between the amount of drug in the body and the drug plasma concentration). Drugs that are widely distributed to tissues (lipid-soluble, nonionic drugs), including to extracellular (≈0.3 L/kg) and intracellular (≈0.6 L/kg) fluid compartments, have relatively high volumes of distribution (>0.6 L/kg). For example, when administered orally, enrofloxacin (a fluoroquinolone antibiotic) has a Vd of about 2.8 L/kg. These drugs are distributed throughout the body primarily by passive diffusion across cell membranes. The distribution of water-soluble drugs is limited to the extracellular fluid compartment, resulting in distribution volumes between 0.1 and 0.3 L/kg.

In addition to chemical properties of the drug (lipid solubility, pH, and molecular weight), factors that influence the distribution of drug to tissues include (1) relative tissue blood flow (because highly perfused tissues achieve higher drug concentrations), (2) degree of protein binding (because a protein-bound drug is unavailable to distribute out of the vascular space), (3) degree of tissue binding (because a drug with high affinity for tissue binding will tend to concentrate in tissues), and (4) physical anatomic barriers (blood-brain barrier, epidural barrier, blood-testis barrier).

The most important physical barrier to drug movement is the blood-brain barrier (BBB), which limits entry of drugs into the central nervous system. An important component of the BBB is the P-glycoprotein pump (a protein that protects the brain from exposure to various drugs and substances by actively pumping them out of the cells). The P-glycoprotein pump is also present in other key barrier locations in the body, including gastrointestinal tract, biliary tract, kidney, placenta, and testis. The way in which tissue barriers influence **drug distribution** can be observed in individuals that have a genetic mutation producing a nonfunctional P-glycoprotein pump (condition affecting Collies and a few other breeds). When given ivermectin (a drug that is normally prevented from entering the central nervous system [CNS] by the BBB), dogs carrying the genetic mutation are at increased risk for CNS toxicity because ivermectin is able to enter the brain.

Other drugs affected by the P-glycoprotein pump include milbemycin, selamectin, moxidectin, vincristine, ketoconazole, loperamide, digoxin, and cyclosporine. Many of these drugs also alter drug metabolism, creating complex but important drug interactions.

DRUG METABOLISM

Metabolism (or biotransformation) is the chemical modification of a drug to an active, inactive, or toxic metabolite. Metabolism most commonly inactivates or detoxifies drugs and/or makes them more water soluble for elimination in urine or bile. In contrast, prodrugs (drugs administered in an inactive form) are metabolized to their active form. Examples of prodrugs include benzodiazepines, enalapril, and codeine. In addition, some drugs such as acetaminophen and cyclophosphamide are changed into toxic metabolites.

Drugs are metabolized or biotransformed by enzyme systems. Enzyme systems central to the metabolism of substances are located primarily in the gastrointestinal tract, liver, and kidney but are also present in other tissues. The liver is considered the major site of drug metabolism in the body. Drug metabolism generally occurs in two steps or phases. The major drug-metabolizing enzyme systems are listed in Table 27-1.

During phase I, enzymes metabolize drugs by oxidation (loss of electrons), reduction (addition of electrons), or

| TABLE 27-1 | Major Phase I and Phase II Drug-Metabolizing Enzyme Systems* |

Phase I Metabolizing Enzyme Systems

	METABOLIZED DRUGS	ENZYME INHIBITORS
Microsomal cytochrome P450 enzymes	Numerous	Numerous
Alcohol dehydrogenase	Alcohol	4-Methylpyrazole
Aldehyde dehydrogenase		Antabuse (disulfiram)
Monoamine oxidases	Epinephrine Norepinephrine Dopamine Serotonin	ʟ-Deprenyl Monoamine oxidase inhibitors (MAOIs) and serotonin reuptake inhibitors (SRIs)
Plasma esterases		Pancuronium

Phase II Metabolizing Enzyme Systems

	METABOLIZED DRUGS	COMMENTS
Glucuronide conjugation	Morphine Acetaminophen Salicylic acid	Cats—deficient
Glutathione conjugation	Acetaminophen Acrolein	
Sulfonation	Terbutaline Methimazole Acetaminophen	Pigs—deficient
N-Acetylation	Sulfonamides Hydralazine Procainamide Dapsone	Dogs—absent (lack N-acetyltransferase)
Methylation	Azathioprine 6-Mercaptopurine	Thiopurine methyltransferase Dogs—many variations Cats—deficient

*Including drugs commonly metabolized by each system and clinically significant enzyme inhibitors of phase I enzyme systems, as well as species differences for phase II enzyme systems.

hydrolysis (addition of water). Enzymes responsible for this step are called *cytochrome P450 (CYP 450) enzymes.* The highest concentration of these enzymes is found in the liver.

Each species and individuals within each species have variable quantities of specific CYP 450 enzymes. These differences cause variations in the metabolism of drugs among patients. In addition, some drugs can induce or inhibit CYP 450 enzymes, causing interactions between drugs given concurrently. For example, when ketoconazole (a CYP 450 inhibitor) is given with cyclosporine (a drug metabolized by CYP 450), the plasma level of cyclosporine is significantly higher than when cyclosporine is given alone.

During phase II, various enzymes conjugate (add) a substance to the drug to inactivate it and facilitate its elimination. Glucuronide and glutathione are examples of compounds conjugated to various drugs by these reactions. Species differences have been noted in the presence of these enzymes. For instance, cats are deficient in glucuronyl transferase, decreasing their ability to add glucuronide to drugs metabolized by this enzyme. Also, dogs lack N-acetyltransferase activity and pigs are deficient in sulfate conjugation. Table 27-1 includes the major phase II enzyme systems, drugs commonly metabolized by each system, and species differences.

> **TECHNICIAN NOTE** Drugs are metabolized or biotransformed by enzyme systems. Enzyme systems central to the metabolism of substances are located primarily in the gastrointestinal tract, liver, and kidney but are also present in other tissues. The liver is considered the major site of drug metabolism in the body.

DRUG ELIMINATION

Elimination is the removal of a drug from the body. Routes available for drug elimination include urine, bile, feces, expired air, milk, sweat, saliva, and tears. Relative to other sites, the kidneys eliminate many drugs and their metabolites from the body. Drugs can be excreted into the urine unchanged, or after they have been metabolized. Factors that influence drug elimination through the kidneys include water solubility, protein binding, urine pH and flow rate, and renal blood flow. Because of the significant role that the kidneys play in drug elimination, loss of kidney function will cause drugs to accumulate in the body. Pharmacokinetic values that describe drug elimination are clearance and half-life.

Drug clearance (Cl) is the rate at which a drug is removed from an organ or from the body expressed as the volume of plasma cleared of drug per unit time (ml/minute). It is used to measure the efficiency of drug elimination. Factors that influence the clearance of a drug include protein binding, organ perfusion, drug-metabolizing enzymes, and renal elimination. Clearance is used to determine the dosage regimen necessary to achieve a stable concentration in the blood, called **steady state.** Steady state is reached when the amount of drug administered equals the amount of drug eliminated.

Half-life ($t_{1/2}$) is the time required for the amount of a drug in the body to decrease by one-half, or 50%. Half-life is dependent on the volume of distribution and clearance and provides an estimate of the duration of effect of a drug. Therefore, the half-life of drug is used to estimate the dosing interval. The time needed to reach steady state plasma concentration, or for 97% of a drug to be removed from the body, is approximately 5 times the half-life.

> **TECHNICIAN NOTE** The time needed to reach steady state plasma concentration, or for 97% of a drug to be removed from the body, is approximately 5 times the half-life.

BASIC PHARMACODYNAMICS

Pharmacodynamics (PD) is the study of the biochemical and physiologic effects of drugs and is commonly referred to as "what the drug does to the body." Clinically relevant PD parameters include mechanism of action (MOA), relationship between drug concentration and effect, and side effects or adverse reactions.

The pharmacodynamics of a drug is a function of the concentration of drug at the site of action. For drugs to produce a clinical effect, an adequate concentration of drug needs to reach the site of action for a sufficient period of time. Drug absorption and distribution are PK factors that influence the drug's ability to reach the sight of action; metabolism and elimination affect the period of time that the drug is in the body.

MECHANISM OF ACTION

The biochemical effect of a drug (or MOA) requires that the drug have direct physical interaction with cellular components, or that it interact with specific target cellular proteins, resulting in alteration of the cell's normal physiology. Exceptions to this rule are drugs that produce effects on the basis of their physical characteristics alone. An example of this is the osmotic diuretic, mannitol. Mannitol is a large sugar molecule that is relatively inactive in the body and is excreted by the kidney. The large mannitol molecule in the tubular fluid of the kidney draws water into the renal tubule, thereby increasing excretion of water. Another example is inhalant gas anesthetics. These highly lipophilic drugs readily dissolve in the cell membrane of nerve cells. It is this direct disruption of the cell membrane that is responsible in part for their anesthetic properties.

More commonly, the action of a drug involves interaction with a target protein within a specific cell type. Target proteins can include a variety of cellular components, including enzymes, carriers, ion channels, and receptors. Receptors are specific regulatory proteins that activate a cascade of cellular events when triggered by interaction with a natural substance that is specific to the receptor, called an **endogenous substrate.** Cell receptors are a key component of intracellular communication and cell function. Many pharmacologic compounds (natural and synthetic) are used to activate (act as an **agonist**) or block (act as an **antagonist**) the action of an endogenous substrate at its receptor. An agonist is a drug that produces a physiologic or pharmacologic effect characteristic of the receptor to which it binds. An antagonist, despite binding to its target receptor, does not activate the receptor, but rather blocks activation of the receptor by its agonists (including the endogenous substrate of the receptor). Table 27-2 provides examples of drugs commonly used in veterinary patients and their cellular target proteins.

SIDE EFFECTS (OR ADVERSE REACTIONS)

Side effects or adverse reactions are the undesired effects associated with a drug; they are commonly linked to its MOA. Side effects can result from interaction of a drug with multiple tissue types or multiple cellular targets, or from alteration of the patient's physiology and/or drug pharmacokinetics. Clinically important adverse reactions can occur at standard or inappropriate doses, can arise when other drugs are given concurrently—resulting in interaction between two or more drugs, or can occur as the result of altered drug PK (absorption, distribution, metabolism, or elimination). During illness, a drug's PK can significantly change in patients with underlying liver or kidney dysfunction, and for some drugs, dosage adjustment may be necessary.

IMPACT OF DISEASE ON DRUG PHARMACOKINETICS

Diseases that most commonly affect drug PK include liver disease, kidney disease, and cardiovascular disease. A decrease in major organ function is seen with age, and this influences drug PK in geriatric patients. The effect of aging on drug PK is discussed in the next section.

> *TECHNICIAN NOTE* Diseases that most commonly influence drug absorption, distribution, metabolism, or elimination include liver disease, kidney disease, and cardiovascular disease.

CARDIOVASCULAR DISEASE

Cardiovascular disease alters the distribution of blood flow to tissues through changes in water and sodium balance and long-term activation of the sympathetic nervous system. More blood is distributed to the brain and heart, increasing risk for toxicity to these organs. For example, the risk for arrhythmias and nausea caused by digoxin toxicity is increased in patients with congestive heart failure.

Alternations in gastrointestinal, hepatic, and renal blood flow resulting from cardiovascular disease can affect drug absorption, distribution, metabolism, and elimination. For example, total absorption and rate of absorption of the

TABLE 27-2	Drugs Commonly Used in Veterinary Patients*			
PROTEIN TYPE	**CELLULAR TARGETS**	**EXAMPLE DRUGS**	**ACTION**	**EFFECT**
Enzymes	Cyclooxygenase	NSAIDs Aspirin	Inhibition	Suppress prostaglandin synthesis
	Acetylcholinesterase	Neostigmine Physostigmine	Inhibition	Prevent metabolism of acetylcholine
	Dihydrofolate reductase	Trimethoprim	Inhibition	Prevent folate synthesis (by bacteria)
	Angiotensin-converting enzyme	Enalapril Benazepril	Inhibition	Prevent synthesis of angiotensin II
Carriers	$Na^+/K^+/2Cl^-$ transporter (kidney; loop of Henle)	Furosemide	Inhibition	Prevent sodium and water reabsorption
	Na^+/K^+-ATPase (heart, muscle cells)	Digitalis	Inhibition	Increase intracellular calcium, increase strength of contraction
	Na^+/H^+-ATPase (stomach, parietal cells)	Omeprazole	Inhibition (irreversible)	Decrease stomach acid production (increasing pH)
Ion Channels	Voltage-gated Na^+ channels (sensory neurons)	Lidocaine Procainamide	Inhibition	Decrease sensory input to CNS
Receptors	Opioid receptors μ-Receptors (CNS)	Morphine Fentanyl Naloxone	Agonist Agonist Antagonist	Analgesia (except for the antagonist naloxone)
	κ-Receptors (CNS)	Butorphanol	Agonist	
	Histamine (H2) receptors (parietal cells)	Histamine Famotidine	Agonist Antagonist	Stimulate acid secretion Inhibit acid secretion
	Histamine (H1) receptors (vestibular system)	Histamine Diphenhydramine	Agonist Antagonist	Induce vomiting Prevent vomiting

CNS, Central nervous system; *NSAIDs*, nonsteroidal anti-inflammatory drugs.
*Grouped by cellular target protein. Includes drug's action on cellular target protein and resulting cellular effect.

diuretic furosemide are decreased in patients with congestive heart failure. In addition, patients with heart disease or heart failure are often taking multiple drugs that alter the activity of the sympathetic nervous system, control heart rate and rhythm, and influence electrolyte and fluid balance. This increases the risk for adverse drug effects or drug interactions. For example, low potassium concentrations resulting from furosemide administration can increase the risk for digoxin toxicity and can decrease the **efficacy** of the antiarrhythmic lidocaine.

KIDNEY DISEASE

The kidney is the major organ involved in drug elimination. Kidney disease or failure can cause decreased drug elimination, increasing plasma drug concentrations and the risk for adverse drug reactions or toxicity. Therefore, dose adjustments are recommended for drugs primarily excreted by the kidney (fluoroquinolones, aminoglycosides, enalapril, digoxin, and chloramphenicol in cats). Dose adjustments also may be necessary for drugs associated with increased risk for side effects in these patients (cephalosporins, sulfonamides, tetracycline, furosemide, cimetidine, metoclopramide, and nonsteroidal anti-inflammatory drugs [NSAIDs]). For example, NSAIDs have a negative impact on renal blood flow, especially when blood flow to the kidney is already compromised by decreased blood volume (hypovolemia), because NSAIDs inhibit prostaglandins, including those essential for maintenance of renal blood flow and autoregulation.

The kidney also plays a significant role in maintaining the body's fluid and electrolyte balance. Increased fluid retention associated with kidney disease can alter the volume of distribution of drugs, especially drugs primarily distributed to the vascular compartment or to plasma (penicillins, cephalosporins, and aminoglycosides).

Potential drug interactions in patients with kidney disease are associated with the use of antacids and phosphate binders, which may reduce absorption of orally administered antibiotics, including fluoroquinolones, tetracyclines, and sulfonamides.

LIVER DISEASE

The liver is the primary site of drug metabolism. The liver houses the metabolic enzymes that convert lipophilic drugs to more water-soluble metabolites for elimination by the kidney. Unless liver failure is present, it is difficult to accurately predict the need for dosage adjustment in patients with liver disease. However, dosage adjustment should be considered in the presence of liver failure for drugs metabolized by the liver, including metronidazole, chloramphenicol, and benzodiazepines.

> **TECHNICIAN NOTE** The kidney is the major organ for drug elimination, and the liver is the primary site of drug metabolism.

AGING AND DRUG PHARMACOKINETICS

Normal aging leads to a change in body composition (decreased lean body mass and total body water, and increased fatty tissue) and redistribution of blood flow to the brain and heart, in part as the result of decreased cardiac output. This altered distribution of tissues and blood in geriatric patients influences the distribution of drugs. For example, the distribution of water-soluble drugs is limited to the plasma. Therefore, these drugs (e.g., aminoglycosides, digoxin) should be dosed on the basis of lean body weight to avoid excessive plasma concentrations. Additional changes in physiology associated with aging include decreased drug absorption from the gastrointestinal tract, decreased hepatic metabolism, and decreased renal excretion.

Reduced kidney function associated with aging has the most clinically significant impact on drug disposition. Loss of the ability of the body to eliminate drugs through the kidney results in increased drug plasma concentrations and decreased elimination when standard doses are given. Therefore, drugs excreted primarily by the kidneys often require dosage adjustment to minimize the risk for toxicity in geriatric patients. Table 27-3 summarizes some of the drugs commonly used in geriatric veterinary patients for which a dosage adjustment is recommended.

ADVERSE DRUG REACTIONS

Adverse dose-dependent drug reactions can be subdivided into two types: dose dependent and idiosyncratic.

TABLE 27-3	Drugs Commonly Used in Geriatric Veterinary Patients for Which Dosage Adjustment Is Recommended		
Antimicrobials	NSAIDs	Diuretics	Anticonvulsants
• Aminoglycosides	• Carprofen	• Furosemide	• Potassium bromide
• Fluoroquinolones	• Deracoxib	Cardiac drugs	• Phenobarbital
• Sulfonamides	• Etodolac	• Digoxin	
• Cephalosporins	• Meloxicam	• Enalapril	
• Tetracyclines	• Tepoxalin	• Atenolol	
(exception: doxycycline)		• Lidocaine	

NSAIDs, Nonsteroidal anti-inflammatory drugs.

DOSE-DEPENDENT DRUG REACTIONS

Dose-dependent drug reactions are predictable, affect all members of a species, and often affect multiple species. The likelihood of these reactions increases as the drug dose increases. Dose-dependent drug reactions are a result of the drug itself or a metabolite, and may or may not be associated with the action of the drug. Because these reactions are dose-dependent, **therapeutic drug monitoring** can help to prevent them, and can help to confirm whether the drug is the cause of a suspected reaction. A **dose-dependent drug reaction** often responds to dose reduction or to brief drug withdrawal.

IDIOSYNCRATIC DRUG REACTIONS

Idiosyncratic drug reactions are unpredictable, affect only a small portion of treated animals, and may or may not affect multiple species. These reactions are not dose-dependent, but the risk for a reaction increases with the dose. As with dose-dependent drug reactions, idiosyncratic drug reactions result from the drug itself or from a toxic drug metabolite, but they are not related to the action of the drug. They do not occur immediately, but rather after several days of treatment, and they are often associated with an immune system response (such as fever, antibody production, or T-cell sensitization). Therapeutic drug monitoring is not helpful in identifying or avoiding these reactions. Treatment requires drug withdrawal and drug avoidance in the sensitized patient. Examples of dose-dependent and idiosyncratic drug reactions are listed in Table 27-4.

TABLE 27-4	Dose-Dependent and Idiosyncratic Adverse Drug Reactions Known in Veterinary Species	
DRUG	**SPECIES**	**TARGET ORGAN AFFECTED**
Dose-Dependent		
Acetaminophen	Dog	Liver
	Cat	Red blood cells
Phenobarbital	Dog	Liver
Azathioprine	Dog, Cat	Liver, bone marrow
Ketoconazole Itraconazole	Dog	Liver
Chloramphenicol	Cat, Dog	Bone marrow
Potentiated sulfonamides	Dog	Bone marrow (anemia), eye (dry eye)
Aminoglycosides	Dog, Cat	Kidney
Idiosyncratic		
Potentiated sulfonamides	Dog	Liver, skin, bone marrow, joints
Diazepam	Cat	Liver
Carprofen	Dog	Liver
Methimazole	Cat	Liver, bone marrow, skin (facial excoriations), and neuromuscular junction (myasthenia gravis)
Phenylbutazone	Dog	Bone marrow
Phenobarbital	Dog	Bone marrow

> **TECHNICIAN NOTE**   Dose-dependent drug reactions are predictable and often respond to dose reduction or to brief drug withdrawal. Idiosyncratic drug reactions are rare and unpredictable, and require drug withdrawal and drug avoidance in sensitized patients.

THERAPEUTIC DRUG MONITORING

Therapeutic drug monitoring (TDM) is the periodic measurement of the amount of a drug in the blood. TDM is recommended when the pharmacokinetics of a drug varies significantly among individuals, or when a drug has a narrow **therapeutic range** (a small difference between the amount that is effective and the amount that is toxic). For example, in any group of patients, inherent differences may be noted in drug absorption, drug elimination, and the potential for interaction between drugs that can significantly influence an individual's drug plasma concentrations. The goal of TDM is to optimize drug plasma concentrations to maximize efficacy and minimize toxicity. TDM can be used to determine toxicity, establish a patient's drug levels at a given dose, monitor owner compliance, establish efficacy, detect treatment failure, or determine the pharmacokinetics of a drug in a particular patient.

The reliability of TDM is dependent on the timing and number of blood samples collected, as well as on appropriate sample collection and handling. The difference in timing and number of blood samples collected is dependent on the drug being monitored and what questions the veterinarian wants to answer. In some instances, efficacy may need to be determined; in others, toxicity may be a concern; and for yet others, it may be important to establish the drug concentration for a given patient at a given dose. The drug being tested will dictate the type of sample that must be collected (serum, plasma, or whole blood). The type of tube used for blood collection is of equal importance because some drugs interact with the surface or contents of blood collection tubes, falsely decreasing the drug concentration. For example, serum-separator tubes are best avoided for TDM because the gel within the tube will adsorb drugs like digoxin and phenobarbital, falsely lowering the drug serum concentration. Table 27-5 summarizes the type of sample, recommended blood collection tube, and sample collection time(s) for commonly used veterinary drugs requiring TDM.

TARGET ORGAN/SYSTEMS APPROACH TO DRUG CLASSIFICATION

In the sections that follow, drugs commonly used in veterinary patients will be presented on the basis of the primary diseases they are used to treat. Diseases will be organized according to major organ systems that they affect.

IMMUNE-MEDIATED DISEASE

Immune-mediated diseases are treated with immunosuppressive drugs. The immunosuppressive drugs commonly used

TABLE 27-5	Summary of Sample Collection Guidelines for Commonly Used Veterinary Drugs Requiring Therapeutic Drug Monitoring (TDM)			
DRUG	**SAMPLE**	**TUBE**	**COLLECTION TIME DURING DOSING INTERVAL**	**COMMENTS**
Phenobarbital	Serum Plasma	Red top EDTA	Anytime	Initially at 2-4 weeks, at 3 months, and then every 6 months
Potassium bromide	Serum	Red top	Anytime	Initially post loading dose, at 3 weeks, 3 months, then every 6 months
Digoxin	Serum	Red top	Anytime, generally 4-6 hours post dose	To detect toxicity, especially in patients with kidney disease
Cyclosporine	Whole blood	EDTA	Trough level (immediately before the next dose)	Potential drug interactions
Aminoglycosides	Serum Plasma	Red top EDTA	1, 2, and 4 hours post dose	To check for therapeutic efficacy and to avoid nephrotoxicity
Theophylline	Serum	Red top	Peak and trough concentrations	
Levothyroxine	Serum	Red top	4-6 hours post dose	

EDTA, Ethylenediaminetetraacetic acid.

in veterinary patients are summarized in Table 27-6. These drugs target the immune system (primarily lymphocytes) via different mechanisms of action, and are used either alone or in combination to treat a variety of immune-mediated diseases (hemolytic anemia, thrombocytopenia, skin disease, polyarthritis, systemic lupus erythematosus, and many others). The goal when these agents are used is to control the disease without producing significant side effects. This is achieved by stabilizing the underlying disease process using immunosuppressive doses (generally higher doses), and then by gradually decreasing (or tapering) the amount of each drug given to the lowest dose necessary for long-term control.

Glucocorticoids are the most commonly used immunosuppressive agents. They are available in a variety of formulations differing in chemical structure, and are classified as short acting (hydrocortisone), intermediate acting (prednisone/prednisolone, methylprednisolone, triamcinolone), or long acting (dexamethasone, betamethasone). Long-acting glucocorticoids are eliminated from the body very slowly. This causes three problems. First, it significantly suppresses production of natural glucocorticoids by the adrenal gland. Second, it prolongs the duration of side effects because once the drug is given, it stays in the body until it is naturally eliminated. Third, the slow rate of elimination makes it difficult to taper the dose effectively. For these reasons, use of long-acting agents is best avoided. Glucocorticoid dosage forms include oral, injectable, topical, otic, and ophthalmic.

Cyclosporine A, azathioprine, and chlorambucil are other immunosuppressive agents used for those animals that do not respond to glucocorticoids alone, or that experience significant side effects.

TABLE 27-6	Immunosuppressive Drugs Commonly Used in Veterinary Patients*	
DRUG	**CELL TARGETED**	**SIDE EFFECTS**
Glucocorticoids (GCs)	Neutrophils	Polydipsia Polyuria Polyphagia
	Macrophages	Panting Adrenal gland suppression Gastrointestinal bleeding/ulceration
	Lymphocytes	Steroid hepatopathy Diabetes mellitus Catabolic—muscle/ connective tissue Delayed wound healing Behavior changes
Cyclosporin A	Lymphocytes	Anorexia Vomiting Diarrhea Increased liver enzymes Gingival hyperplasia
Azathioprine	Lymphocytes	Diarrhea Bone marrow suppression (severe in cats) Liver toxicity Pancreatitis
Chlorambucil	Lymphocytes	Bone marrow suppression

*Including cell type targeted and side effects.

> **TECHNICIAN NOTE** Use of glucocorticoids concurrently with nonsteroidal anti-inflammatory drugs (NSAIDs) is contraindicated because of increased risk for gastrointestinal bleeding, ulceration, or perforation.

INFECTIOUS DISEASE

Antimicrobials are a large class of drugs (including antibacterial and antifungal compounds) that are used to kill or inhibit the growth of microorganisms.

Bacterial Infection

The term *antibacterial* is used in reference to substances that kill or inhibit the growth of bacteria, including both substances naturally produced by microorganisms and those manufactured by chemical synthesis. The term *antibiotic* is used to refer only to those antibacterial compounds produced naturally by microorganisms. All antibiotics are considered antibacterial compounds, but not all antibacterial compounds are antibiotics. Often the terms *antibacterial* and *antibiotic* are used interchangeably.

The goal of antibacterial therapy is to assist the body's natural defenses in the elimination of bacterial pathogens while minimizing the risk for toxicity to the patient and selection of antimicrobial-resistant bacteria. Important factors to consider in an effort to maximize the efficacy of antibacterial therapy are (1) establishing a preliminary or definitive diagnosis, including identification of the primary site or organ system affected, and (2) collecting appropriate samples for bacterial culture and sensitivity testing. The choice of starting antibacterial therapy while waiting for bacterial culture and sensitivity testing results is based on considering the most likely infecting organism, the antimicrobial's spectrum of activity (Gram-positive, Gram-negative, or anaerobic organisms), the site of infection, and the risk for toxicity. This method of choosing a specific antibacterial based on observation and experience is called *empirical antibacterial therapy*.

Table 27-7 provides a summary of some of the classes of antibacterial agents most commonly used in veterinary patients, including information on spectrum of activity and clinically important side effects. The most common side effects associated with antimicrobial therapy across all classes of antibacterial drugs are vomiting and diarrhea, which can occur for two reasons. First, antibacterial compounds affect not only the bacterial pathogen but also the normal bacterial flora of the gastrointestinal tract, producing vomiting or diarrhea. Second, some antibacterial drugs can directly irritate the stomach, triggering vomiting and diarrhea. For example, the oral antimicrobial, amoxicillin/clavulanate, commonly makes cats lose their appetite and/or vomit.

Antibacterial-associated vomiting can be mild and self-limiting, but in some cases it can be frequent and severe, requiring the administration of an alternative antibacterial or discontinuation of antibacterial therapy.

> **TECHNICIAN NOTE**   The most common side effects associated with antimicrobial therapy across all classes of antibacterial drugs are vomiting and diarrhea. Many antibiotics have important dose-dependent and idiosyncratic drug toxicities that need to be communicated with the owner at the start of therapy.

Fungal Infection

Fungal infection can arise from a variety of fungal organisms (*Blastomyces, Histoplasma, Cryptococcus, Coccidioides, Aspergillus*), yeasts (*Candida, Malassezia*), and dermatophytes (*Microsporum* spp., *Trichophyton* spp.). Skin and ear infections generally are treated with topical antifungals, and disseminated infections are treated with systemic antifungals. Table 27-8 summarizes the antifungals more commonly used in veterinary patients.

Common antifungal drugs are subdivided into two groups based on their chemistry: polyenes and azoles (imidazoles and triazoles). Antifungals are selectively toxic to fungal organisms by binding to or inhibiting synthesis of ergosterol in the cell membrane. Lack of ergosterol in the fungal cell membrane alters the membrane's function, leading to fungal cell death. Side effects associated also with antifungal therapy occur when the antifungal drug targets the major sterol in mammalian cell membranes—cholesterol (a substance similar to ergosterol).

The duration of treatment with antifungal therapy for patients with systemic fungal infection is weeks to months. For the duration of therapy, each patient must be monitored closely for drug side effects, including decreased appetite, anorexia, and vomiting. Routine monitoring of liver and/or kidney chemistries is recommended in patients being treated with systemic antifungal therapy because of the potential for development of significant organ toxicities in association with specific antifungal therapies.

TABLE 27-7	Classes of Antibacterial Agents Commonly Used in Veterinary Patients*		
CLASS	**EXAMPLES**	**PRIMARY SPECTRUM OF ACTIVITY**	**SIDE EFFECTS AND NOTES REGARDING USE**
Beta-lactams	Penicillins: narrow spectrum • Penicillin G • Penicillin V	• Gram-positive aerobes • Obligate anaerobes	• Diarrhea • Hypersensitivity reactions
	Penicillins: aminopenicillins • Ampicillin • Amoxicillin	• Gram-positive aerobes • Obligate anaerobes	
	Penicillins: potentiated aminopenicillins • Amoxicillin + Clavulanate	• Gram-positive aerobes • Obligate anaerobes • Penicillinase-producing *Staphylococcus* • Gram-negative aerobes	

TABLE 27-7	Classes of Antibacterial Agents Commonly Used in Veterinary Patients*—cont'd		
CLASS	**EXAMPLES**	**PRIMARY SPECTRUM OF ACTIVITY**	**SIDE EFFECTS AND NOTES REGARDING USE**
Beta-lactams— cont'd	Cephalosporins: first generation • Cefazolin • Cephalexin • Cefadroxil Cephalosporins: second generation • Cefotetan • Cefoxitin Cephalosporins: third generation • Cefotaxime • Cefpodoxime • Cetfiofur • Ceftriaxone • Cefovecin	• Gram-positive aerobes • Penicillinase-producing *Staphylococcus* • Penicillinase-producing *Staphylococcus* • Gram-positive aerobes • Gram-negative aerobes • Obligate anaerobes • Gram-negative aerobes • Obligate anaerobes • Penicillinase-producing *Staphylococcus*	
Aminoglycosides	Gentamicin Amikacin Neomycin	• Gram-negative aerobes	• Kidney toxicity • Otic toxicity
Sulfonamide/ dihydrofolate reductase (DHFR) inhibitors	Sulfonamides • Sulfadiazine • Sulfamethoxazole DHFR inhibitors • Trimethoprim • Pyrimethamine	• Gram-positive aerobes • Gram-negative aerobes • Some protozoa	• Diarrhea • Bone marrow suppression • Hypersensitivity reactions in dogs involving joints, bone marrow, skin, liver, and dry eye • Teratogenic
Fluoroquinolones	Enrofloxacin Orbifloxacin Marbofloxacin Ciprofloxacin Difloxacin	• Gram-negative aerobes • *Brucella* • *Chlamydia* • *Mycobacterium* • *Mycoplasma* • *Rickettsia*	• Diarrhea • Young animals—cartilage damage • Cats—blindness • Seizures (in patients with history of seizures) • Should not be used during pregnancy • Ciprofloxacin contraindicated in horses
Amphenicols	Chloramphenicol Florfenicol	• Gram-positive aerobes • Gram-negative aerobes • Obligate anaerobes • *Rickettsia* • *Chlamydia* • *Mycoplasma*	• Diarrhea • Bone marrow suppression • Significant absorption across human skin—wear gloves when handling tablets • Chloramphenicol use illegal in food-producing animals • Florfenicol approved for use in cattle
Macrolides	Erythromycin Clarithromycin Tilmicosin Azithromycin Tylosin	• Gram-positive aerobes • Obligate anaerobes • Penicillinase-producing *Staphylococcus* • *Mycoplasma*	• Diarrhea
Lincosamides	Clindamycin Lincomycin	• Gram-positive aerobes • Obligate anaerobes • *Mycoplasma*	• Diarrhea • Contraindicated in horses
Tetracyclines	Doxycycline Tetracyclines Oxytetracycline	• Gram-positive aerobes • *Chlamydia* • *Rickettsia* • *Borrelia* • *Mycoplasma*	• Diarrhea • Esophageal strictures in cats • Decreased oral absorption when given with calcium- and iron-containing products, antacids, and sucralfate • Doxycycline (IV) contraindicated in horses
Nitroimidazoles	Metronidazole Ronidazole	• Obligate anaerobes • Protozoa	• Neurotoxicity (dose related) • Use illegal in food-producing animals

*Including spectrum of activity and clinically important side effects.

TABLE 27-8	Antifungals Commonly Used in Veterinary Patients			
DRUG	**TYPE**	**SYSTEMIC VS. TOPICAL**	**INDICATIONS**	**SIDE EFFECTS**
Amphotericin B	Polyene	Systemic	Disseminated fungal infection • Blastomycosis • Histoplasmosis • Cryptococcosis • Coccidioidomycosis	Kidney toxicity (toxic to renal tubules) Phlebitis Fever Nausea Vomiting
Ketoconazole	Imidazole	Systemic	Dermatophytes Yeasts Disseminated fungal infection • Blastomycosis • Histoplasmosis • Coccidioidomycosis	Nausea Vomiting Increased liver enzymes Liver toxicity Drug interactions
Fluconazole	Triazole	Systemic	Disseminated fungal infection • Blastomycosis • Histoplasmosis • Cryptococcosis • Coccidioidomycosis	Nausea Vomiting Increased liver enzymes
Itraconazole	Triazole	Systemic	Disseminated fungal infection • Blastomycosis • Histoplasmosis • Cryptococcosis • Coccidioidomycosis • Aspergillosis	Anorexia Vomiting Liver toxicity Drug interactions
Clotrimazole	Imidazole	Topical	Fungal rhinitis Yeast otitis	
Nystatin	Polyene	Topical	Yeast otitis	

ENDOCRINE DISEASE

Thyroid Disease

The prevalence of thyroid disease in veterinary patients varies with species. Hypothyroidism, a condition associated with low circulating thyroid hormone concentrations, is a relatively common disease in dogs and occurs frequently in horses. Hyperthyroidism, a condition associated with increased circulating thyroid hormone concentrations, is the endocrine disease most commonly diagnosed in cats.

Thyroid hormones are produced by the thyroid gland and are essential throughout the body for normal growth, organ function, and metabolism. Thyroid hormones are used by multiple body systems; therefore, alterations in normal thyroid hormone concentrations result in a diverse set of clinical signs. Common clinical signs and recommended therapies associated with thyroid dysfunction in domestic veterinary species are summarized in Table 27-9.

Hypothyroidism is diagnosed on the basis of clinical signs and low serum thyroid hormone concentrations. This condition is treated with thyroid hormone supplementation (most commonly, synthetic L-thyroxine). L-Thyroxine (T_4) is started at standard doses, and patients are monitored for resolution of clinical signs and normalization of serum thyroid hormone concentrations. Thyroid serum concentrations are measured 4 to 6 hours after dosing to assess response to L-thyroxine therapy. Once the disease is controlled, routine monitoring of serum thyroid levels every 6 to 12 months is

recommended. Side effects (signs of hyperthyroidism) are usually due to oversupplementation.

> **TECHNICIAN NOTE** Thyroid serum concentrations are measured 4 to 6 hours after dosing to assess response to L-thyroxine therapy. Once the disease is controlled, routine monitoring of serum thyroid levels every 6 to 12 months is recommended.

Hyperthyroidism is most common in middle-aged to geriatric cats and is diagnosed on the basis of clinical signs and elevated serum thyroid hormone concentrations. Medical therapies for hyperthyroidism include the drug methimazole and radioactive iodine (^{131}I) therapy. Methimazole interferes with the synthesis of thyroid hormone and is available as an oral formulation or a compounded transdermal gel. After methimazole is started, circulating thyroxine levels decrease in most cats within 2 to 3 weeks. Side effects associated with methimazole therapy include anorexia, facial/neck excoriations, lethargy, and vomiting. Serious side effects, including increased liver enzymes and/or decreased blood cell counts, also may occur. Routine blood work every 3 to 6 months is recommended for cats treated long term with methimazole, to screen for changes in blood cell counts or organ function caused by the drug.

TABLE 27-9	Summary of Common Clinical Signs and Recommended Therapies Associated With Thyroid Dysfunction in Veterinary Species		
SPECIES	**THYROID DYSFUNCTION**	**CLINICAL SIGNS**	**THERAPIES**
Dog	Hypothyroidism	Lethargy, weakness Weight gain (normal/decreased appetite) Poor hair growth/hair loss Poor reproductive performance Recurrent infection (skin)	L-Thyroxine (T_4)
Cat	Hyperthyroidism	Hyperactivity Weight loss (increased appetite) Polydipsia, polyuria Increased respiratory rate (intermittent open-mouth breathing) Diarrhea/vomiting	Methimazole Radioactive iodide (^{131}I)
Horse	Hypothyroidism	Decreased appetite Exercise intolerance Muscular problems Scaly hair coat	L-Thyroxine (T_4)

Radioactive iodine (^{131}I) therapy is the definitive therapy for hyperthyroidism in cats. Abnormal thyroid tissue selectively takes up ^{131}I and is slowly destroyed by the beta radiation emitted by radioactive iodine. Treatment with ^{131}I requires referral to a specialty center that is able to properly handle the drug and observe radiation precautions. Cats generally are hospitalized for 3 days to 4 weeks, depending on the dose of ^{131}I used and the state's radiation safety regulations. Within 2 months after treatment with ^{131}I, most cats have normal thyroid hormone concentration. Side effects are uncommon but include the development of clinical hypothyroidism ($\approx$2%) or persistent hyperthyroidism (0.5%).

Diseases of the Adrenal Gland

Diseases of the adrenal gland occur as the result of an increase in function (hyperadrenocorticism) or a decrease in function (hypoadrenocorticism). Hyperadrenocorticism is most commonly associated with excessive production of glucocorticoids or of cortisol by the adrenal gland. Hyperadrenocorticism may result from overproduction of the pituitary hormone adrenocorticotropic hormone (ACTH), with a secondary increase in cortisol (pituitary-dependent hyperadrenocorticism), or from overproduction of cortisol by an adrenal tumor (adrenal-dependent hyperadrenocorticism). Hyperadrenocorticism occurs in dogs and horses; pituitary-dependent disease occurs most commonly.

Medical therapy with mitotane or trilostane is used most commonly for the treatment of hyperadrenocorticism in dogs and horses. Both mitotane and trilostane decrease production of cortisol but through different mechanisms. Mitotane is directly cytotoxic to the adrenal cortex (the region of the adrenal gland that produces cortisol), but trilostane reversibly inhibits the enzymatic conversion of steroid hormones to cortisol.

The goal of either therapy is to decrease cortisol levels and resolve clinical signs of hyperadrenocorticism (i.e., increased eating, drinking, and panting, and weight gain). The efficacy of therapy is evaluated using an ACTH stimulation test, to evaluate the level of circulating cortisol. When treatment with trilostane is provided, the ACTH stimulation test should be performed 4 to 6 hours after a pill is given.

Side effects associated with mitotane or trilostane (signs of hypoadrenocorticism, including lethargy, anorexia, vomiting, and diarrhea) are due to low cortisol levels. Any dog treated with mitotane or trilostane that develops these signs needs to be evaluated by a veterinarian because hypoadrenocorticism can be a life-threatening disease. See Case Presentation 27-1 for an example of management of a patient with mitotane toxicity.

Hypoadrenocorticism refers to decreased production of the steroid hormones cortisol (a glucocorticoid) and aldosterone (a **mineralocorticoid**) by the adrenal gland. Hypoadrenocorticism can be a spontaneous disease (most common in dogs) or can occur in association with treatment of hyperadrenocorticism. Hypoadrenocorticism can be treated with fludrocortisone or with prednisone and desoxycorticosterone.

Fludrocortisone is a synthetic steroid hormone that has both mineralocorticoid (aldosterone) and glucocorticoid (cortisol) activity. Therefore, fludrocortisone can be used alone. The half-life of fludrocortisone is relatively short; thus daily administration is required. As an alternative, desoxycorticosterone can be used, but it provides only mineralocorticoid activity; therefore, concurrent therapy with a glucocorticoid (prednisone) is required to effectively treat hypoadrenocorticism. Prednisone is short-acting and must be administered every day. Desoxycorticosterone pivalate (DOCP) is a long-acting mineralocorticoid that must be given by injection approximately every 25 days. These agents are compared in Table 27-10.

Patients treated with fludrocortisone or with desoxycorticosterone/prednisone require monitoring for normalization of serum sodium and potassium (which generally are abnormal in animals with hypoadrenocorticism) and for resolution of clinical signs (lethargy, vomiting, and

CASE PRESENTATION 27-1

Lucky, a 9-year-old female, spayed, 6.4-kg Miniature Schnauzer was diagnosed 2 months ago with pituitary-dependent hyperadrenocorticism. She was initially treated with a standard induction dose of mitotane 250 mg (40 mg/kg/day) orally once a day. Her ACTH stimulation test 14 days after the start of mitotane induction consistent with pre-cortisol and post-cortisol levels of 2.1 and 2.6 µg/dl, indicating good control of her hyperadrenocorticism and the end of induction therapy. Pre-cortisol and post-cortisol levels between 1 and 5 µg/dl in a dog being treated with mitotane indicates good control. Clinically, Lucky was doing well and subsequently began maintenance mitotane therapy at 125 mg orally twice a week.

Over the next month, despite continued weekly mitotane therapy, her clinical signs of hyperadrenocorticism (increased eating, drinking, and urination) returned, requiring a second induction with mitotane, 250 mg orally once a day. Fourteen days into her second mitotane induction, the owners called Dr. Smith and reported that Lucky was lethargic and inappetent. She was noted to be shaking intermittently. The owners were advised to bring Lucky in for reevaluation. Upon presentation, Lucky was quiet, alert, responsive, and 7% dehydrated. Bloodwork indicated that she was hyperkalemic (7.5 mmol/L), hyponatremic (127 mmol/L), and hypochloremic (97 mmol/L) with an associated metabolic acidosis (total carbon dioxide was 17 mmol/L). These findings support the hypothesis that Lucky's current clinical signs were consistent with the diagnosis of hypoadrenocortism secondary to mitotane therapy.

Mitotane is cytotoxic to adrenal tissue, making it an effective therapy for patients with hyperadrenocorticism (or excessive adrenal function). In dogs, mitotane primarily targets portions of the adrenal cortex (zona fasciculata and zona reticularis) that produce steroid hormones. Excessive production of steroid hormones results in the classic clinical signs of hyperadrenocorticism. In some patients treated with mitotane, the portion of the adrenal gland that produces aldosterone (zona glomerulosa) can also be destroyed by mitotane, resulting in hypoadrenocorticism. All patients treated with mitotane need to be monitored for hypoadrenocortism (lethargy, inappetence, vomiting, or diarrhea) because this can be a life-threatening condition if left untreated; therefore, owners should be counseled that if any of these signs arise in association with mitotane therapy, their dog should be evaluated by a veterinarian. In addition to low cortisol levels, classic electrolyte changes associated with hypoadrenocorticism and low aldosterone levels are high potassium (hyperkalemia), low sodium (hyponatremia), and low chloride (hypochloremia).

Long-term treatment for hypoadrenocortism includes replacement of physiologic levels of cortisol with prednisone, as well as aldosterone replacement with desoxycorticosterone pivalate (DOCP). However, initial therapy includes aggressive fluid therapy with 0.9% NaCl and a physiologic dose of a short-acting corticosteroid (e.g., dexamethasone sodium phosphate). Lucky responded well to fluid diuresis with 0.9% NaCl and 0.5 mg of dexamethasone sodium phosphate IV within the first 24 hours of hospitalization. Lucky was discharged with instructions to discontinue mitotane therapy and to begin treatment with prednisone (5 mg orally every 24 hours) and DOCP (14 mg subcutaneously every 25 days).

TABLE 27-10	Different Pharmacologic Approaches (Monotherapy vs. Combination Therapy) Used in Treatment of Hypoadrenocortism			
STEROID HORMONE	**STEROID ACTIVITY**	**DURATION OF ACTIVITY**	**ROUTE OF ADMINISTRATION**	**DOSING FREQUENCY**
Monotherapy				
Fludrocortisone acetate	Mineralocorticoid and glucocorticoid	18-36 hours	Oral (PO)	Daily
Combination Therapy				
Desoxycorticosterone pivalate (DOCP)	Mineralocorticoid	21-30 days	Intramuscular (IM) Subcutaneous (SQ)	Every 25 days
Prednisone	Glucocorticoid	12-36 hours	Oral (PO)	Daily

diarrhea). The most common side effects may be associated with steroid hormone excess (increased eating, drinking, and urination; panting; and weight gain) or with subtherapeutic mineralocorticoid and/or glucocorticoid levels (lethargy, vomiting, diarrhea, increased serum potassium levels, and decreased serum sodium levels).

> **TECHNICIAN NOTE** Any dog with hyperadrenocorticism treated with mitotane or trilostane that develops signs of hypoadrenocorticism needs to be evaluated by a veterinarian because hypoadrenocorticism can be a life-threatening disease.

Diabetes Mellitus

Diabetes mellitus (DM) is a disease of impaired carbohydrate, protein, and fat metabolism associated with an absolute or relative insulin deficiency. Insulin is a hormone produced in the beta cells of the pancreas that is responsible for cellular uptake of glucose by most tissues (tissues not dependent on insulin for glucose uptake include liver, brain, and red blood cells).

DM occurs in many species but is most commonly diagnosed in dogs and cats. Although the cause of diabetes mellitus in dogs is different from the cause in cats, patients of both species have lost significant beta-cell mass and are insulin deficient at the time of diagnosis. Therefore, insulin administered by injection is necessary to treat DM in both species.

Insulin is made up of a series of linked amino acids (AAs) specific to each species, but with little variation. For example, human insulin has only one AA difference relative to porcine insulin, and the AA sequence of canine insulin is identical to that of porcine insulin. Feline insulin has only one AA sequence difference when compared with bovine insulin. Because insulin is well conserved across species, available therapeutic insulin products may be animal derived (porcine or bovine), human derived, genetically engineered (human recombinant), or synthetic. In practice, the source of insulin can be best matched to the species to be treated on the basis of AA sequence similarities.

Other differences between insulin products include their biological activity (or ability to decrease blood glucose) and the action of the insulin. The biological activity of insulin is expressed as units of activity per milliliter (U/ml). The activity determined for each type of insulin corresponds to the type of syringe needed to administer the appropriate dose (insulin with a bioactivity of 40 U/ml requires a U-40 insulin syringe, and bioactivity of 100 U/ml requires a U-100 insulin syringe). The action of available insulin products is characterized by their speed of onset and anticipated duration of action. Available types of insulin are subdivided into those that are fast, intermediate, or long-acting. Both intermediate-acting insulin and long-acting insulin are administered subcutaneously; fast-acting (regular insulin) can be given intravenously, intramuscularly, or subcutaneously. Table 27-11 summarizes differences among currently available types of insulin.

Standard treatment for DM in dogs and cats involves optimization of diet and administration of insulin injections. Insulin therapy needs to be individualized for each patient because of significant species and individual variations in the action profile (the clinical response to insulin will vary among patients and within a patient from day to day). Therefore, regulation and treatment of a patient with DM requires monitoring of clinical signs (appetite, water consumption, and activity), body weight, and blood glucose levels using glucose curves and/or serum fructosamine levels.

> **TECHNICIAN NOTE** The biological activity of insulin is expressed as units of activity per milliliter (U/ml). The activity determined for each type of insulin corresponds to the type of syringe needed to administer the appropriate dose. Insulin with bioactivity of 40 U/ml requires a U-40 insulin syringe, and insulin with bioactivity of 100 U/ml requires a U-100 insulin syringe.

GASTROINTESTINAL DISEASE

Therapeutic strategies used in the treatment of gastrointestinal disease include nonspecific supportive therapies and targeted therapies based on the primary underlying disease process. Symptomatic supportive care is often necessary before a definitive diagnosis is established, at the onset of **targeted therapy**, or during periods of clinical relapse. Table 27-12 compares common symptomatic and supportive therapies used in the treatment of gastrointestinal disease, including antiemetics (drug used to stop vomiting), prokinetics (drugs used to increase gastrointestinal motility), and drugs used to suppress gastric acid production (antacids) and to aid in ulcer healing.

LIVER DISEASE

Few controlled studies have documented the efficacy and optimal doses of medications and nutritional supplements used to treat liver disease. Drug groups commonly used in the treatment of liver disease include hepatoprotectants, choleretics (drugs that stimulate bile flow), antifibrotics, chelating agents, and targeted therapies for the treatment of hepatic encephalopathy (neurologic signs associated with liver failure).

Hepatoprotectants

S-Adenosylmethionine (SAMe) and silymarin (milk thistle) are considered generally protective of hepatocytes (liver cells), in part because of their antioxidant properties and their support of normal cellular function. Oral absorption of SAMe is greatest when it is given on an empty stomach because food significantly decreases the amount of drug absorbed. SAMe is available as enteric-coated tablets (to prevent the release of active ingredients before it reaches the

TABLE 27-11	Differences Among Types of Insulin Currently Available							
TYPE	**SOURCE**	**ACTIVITY, U/ML**	**SYRINGE**	**ACTION PROFILE**	**ONSET, HOURS**	**DURATION, HOURS**	**TARGET SPECIES**	**ROUTE**
Regular insulin	Human recombinant	100	U-100	Fast	0.5	2-5	Dog Cat	IV IM SQ
NPH	Human recombinant	100	U-100	Intermediate	2-4	12-24	Dog Cat	SQ
Glargine	Synthetic analogue	100	U-100	Long	4-6	12-24	Cat	SQ
PZIR*	Human recombinant	40	U-40	Long	4-6	12-24	Cat	SQ

IM, Intramuscular; *IV*, intravenous; *NPH*, Neutral Protamine Hagedon; *PZIR*, Protamine Zinc Insulin Recombinant; *SQ*, subcutaneous.
*FDA approved for use in cats.

TABLE 27-12	Common Symptomatic and Supportive Therapies Used in Treatment of Gastrointestinal Disease*	
DRUG	**MECHANISM OF ACTION**	**SIDE EFFECTS**
Antiemetics		
Dolasetron and ondansetron	Serotonin receptor antagonist	Arrhythmias
Maropitant	Neurokinin 1 receptor antagonist	
Prochlorperazine and chlorpromazine (phenothiazines)	Dopamine receptor antagonist Histamine receptor antagonist Cholinergic receptor antagonist Adrenergic receptor antagonist	Restlessness, involuntary movement Sedation Seizures Low blood pressure
Prokinetics		
Cisapride	Serotonin receptor agonist	Arrhythmias
Antiemetics/Prokinetics		
Metoclopramide	Dopamine receptor antagonist Serotonin receptor agonist (5-HT4)	Restlessness, involuntary movement
Antacids (increase stomach pH)/Ulcer Therapy		
Famotidine	Histamine antagonism	
Ranitidine	Histamine antagonism Anticholinesterase (prokinetic)	Hypotension (if given IV)
Omeprazole	Proton pump inhibitor	
Sucralfate	Promotes gastric ulcer healing: inactivates pepsin, absorbs bile acids, and increases gastric mucosal prostaglandin synthesis	

*Drug categories include antiemetics, prokinetics, and antacids/ulcer therapy.

small intestine); therefore, tablets should not be broken or crushed. SAMe and silymarin are regarded by the U.S. Food and Drug Administration (FDA) as nutritional supplements; therefore, no standards have been established by any regulatory bodies regarding potency, purity, safety, or efficacy. In addition, bioequivalence between products cannot be ensured. In animals, no known clinically significant side effects have been reported in association with administration of SAMe or silymarin.

Choleretic Drugs

Ursodiol (ursodeoxycholic acid) is the primary choleretic used in veterinary patients. In addition to stimulating bile flow, ursodiol is thought to function as a cytoprotective agent and an antioxidant. Ursodiol is well tolerated in animals. Oral absorption of this drug is enhanced in the presence of food.

Antifibrotic Therapy

Antifibrotic therapy is often indicated in patients diagnosed with liver cirrhosis (or other diseases associated with scarring of the liver). Colchicine is used as an antifibrotic in veterinary patients. Colchicine functions as an antifibrotic in part through its stimulation of collagenase enzyme activity, minimizing collagen deposition in liver tissue. Side effects reported in association with colchicine use include anorexia, vomiting, diarrhea (including hemorrhagic diarrhea), and bone marrow suppression.

Metal Chelation Therapy

Chelating agents, D-penicillamine, and zinc are used to **chelate** (or bind) excessive quantities of metals (commonly copper) that accumulate in association with some types of liver disease. Specifically, D-penicillamine forms a stable water-soluble complex with copper, enabling excessive amounts of copper to be excreted by the kidneys. Side effects reported in association with D-penicillamine use include anorexia, lethargy, and vomiting. Zinc prevents intestinal absorption of copper, decreasing the amount of copper available to the liver. Few side effects have been reported in association with zinc therapy, although excessive supplementation may inhibit iron absorption.

Treatment for Hepatic Encephalopathy

Standard therapy for a patient in liver failure that is exhibiting clinical signs of hepatic encephalopathy (lethargy, dullness, ataxia, or seizures) consists of administration of lactulose and in some cases concurrent administration of antibiotics (e.g., neomycin). Lactulose shortens gastrointestinal transit time and decreases absorption of ammonia (a known toxin that contributes to clinical signs of hepatic encephalopathy). Neomycin helps to decrease the quantity of ammonia-producing bacteria in the gut. The side effect most commonly associated with lactulose and/or neomycin therapy is diarrhea. The goal of treatment is soft stool consistency, but not diarrhea. If diarrhea develops, it is generally responsive to dose reduction.

CARDIOVASCULAR DISEASE

Heart disease is associated with structural damage to or rhythm disturbances of the heart; it may result from damaged cardiac muscle, valvular disease, pericardial disease, rhythm abnormalities, or altered coronary circulation. Heart disease can progress to clinical heart failure, resulting in

TABLE 27-13	Summary of Site of Action, Specific Action, and Side Effects Associated With Diuretics Commonly Used in Veterinary Patients			
DIURETIC	**SITE OF ACTION**	**SPECIFIC ACTION**	**SIDE EFFECTS**
Furosemide	Kidney—loop of Henle	Inhibits $Na^+/K^+/2Cl^-$ reabsorption	Hypokalemia Hypochloremia Metabolic alkalosis
Hydrochlorothiazide	Kidney—distal tubule	Inhibits Na^+/Cl^- reabsorption	Hypokalemia
Spironolactone	Kidney—distal tubule Kidney—collecting duct	Inhibits aldosterone	Hyperkalemia (due to the potassium-sparing effect)

accumulation of fluid in tissues (edema). Treatment of patients with heart failure is dependent on the nature of the underlying problem but often involves the use of multiple drugs, including diuretics (to reduce fluid accumulation), inotropic agents (to improve the contractility of cardiac muscle), antihypertensives (to modulate blood pressure), and antiarrhythmics (to control heart rhythm abnormalities).

Diuretics

Diuretics are used to mobilize edema (fluid in tissues). Significant edema accumulates most commonly in cases of congestive heart failure. Diuretics are also used for some disease processes that affect the kidney, liver, and gastrointestinal tract, to reduce associated fluid retention. The therapeutic goal of diuretic therapy is to increase sodium and water excretion. Sites of action, specific actions, and side effects associated with the diuretics commonly used in veterinary patients are summarized in Table 27-13.

Furosemide is the most potent and the most commonly prescribed diuretic. It is commonly referred to as a *loop diuretic* because of its site of action. Furosemide blocks the key sodium transport mechanism (the Na/K/2Cl symporter) in the portion of the kidney known as the *loop of Henle*. This action inhibits reabsorption of approximately 25% of sodium filtered by the kidney. Consequently, the net effect of furosemide administration is increased sodium and water excretion. Low potassium levels are associated with the use of furosemide; therefore, monitoring of serum potassium levels is recommended. Furosemide is the diuretic of choice for the treatment of edema caused by heart disease. Other uses in large animal patients include therapy for exercise-induced pulmonary hemorrhage (EIPH) in athletic horses and for chronic obstructive pulmonary disease (COPD) in ponies.

Hydrochlorothiazide is a thiazide diuretic that produces a more modest diuresis because it acts farther down the renal tubule. Thiazides block the reabsorption of sodium and chloride in the distal part of the renal tubule. Hydrochlorothiazide is the only veterinary-approved thiazide diuretic (for use in cattle).

Spironolactone works in the distal part of the renal tubule and blocks the action of aldosterone, which is the key hormone responsible for the reabsorption of sodium and the excretion of potassium. Administration of spironolactone results in diuresis by preventing the reabsorption of sodium. Its clinical use is recommended for conditions known to be associated with high aldosterone levels and edema formation, including heart failure, hepatic cirrhosis, nephrotic syndrome, and **ascites**.

> **TECHNICIAN NOTE** Diuretics mobilize edema in the body by altering the reabsorption of sodium with secondary effects on water and potassium levels in the body. Monitoring hydration and electrolyte levels in patients treated with diuretics is essential.

Inotropic Agents

Drugs used to improve the contractility of cardiac muscle fibers are known as *inotropic agents*. The two main inotropic agents used in veterinary patients are digoxin and pimobendan. Digoxin is a naturally derived drug that is used in patients in congestive heart failure (CHF) to improve the ability of the heart to pump blood. Digoxin increases the calcium concentration in cardiac muscle cells, thereby increasing the strength of muscle contractions. In addition, digoxin inhibits ongoing activation of the sympathetic nervous system that results from CHF.

Digoxin has a narrow therapeutic index (low ratio between therapeutic plasma levels and toxic plasma levels). To evaluate its effectiveness and minimize side effects, therapeutic drug monitoring is recommended. Clinical signs associated with toxicity include gastrointestinal signs (anorexia, vomiting, or diarrhea) and life-threatening arrhythmias, which are detected by electrocardiographic monitoring. Treatment for digoxin toxicity requires drug withdrawal.

Pimobendan is both a positive inotrope and a balanced vasodilator (combination venous and arterial dilation) used in the treatment of dogs with CHF. Positive inotropic effects result from its inhibition of an enzyme, phosphodiesterase III, which is located in cardiac muscle cells and blood vessels. Inhibition of phosphodiesterase III increases intracellular calcium levels, which strengthens cardiac muscle contractions and dilates blood vessels. Pimobendan does not increase the risk of developing cardiac arrhythmias and does not require therapeutic drug monitoring. Overall, pimobendan is well tolerated in dogs. Reported side effects include low blood pressure, gastrointestinal upset, nervousness, and kidney failure.

Antihypertensives

Antihypertensives (drugs that lower blood pressure) are used in the treatment of patients with heart failure and other conditions associated with hypertension, including kidney disease, diabetes mellitus, and hyperthyroidism. Antihypertensive drugs dilate blood vessels and are subdivided on the basis of their MOA and the vessels they dilate (venous, arterial, or pulmonary).

Angiotensin-converting enzyme (ACE) inhibitors such as enalapril and benazepril function as vasodilators through inhibition of the angiotensin-converting enzyme. Clinical effects of ACE inhibitors include systemic vasodilatation and decreased circulating levels of aldosterone, which facilitate sodium excretion and diuresis. ACE inhibitors are commonly used in the treatment of congestive heart failure, hypertension, and proteinuria. Enalapril is excreted predominantly by the kidneys, whereas benazepril is excreted by both kidneys and liver. Consequently, benazepril rather than enalapril is recommended in patients with kidney disease.

The calcium channel blocker amlodipine is a vasodilator used to treat cats and dogs with hypertension. Amlodipine suppresses calcium movement into the cells through slow calcium channels. Decreased intracellular calcium in vascular smooth muscle cells produces peripheral vasodilatation and reduced blood pressure. The primary side effect of amlodipine is hypotension (low blood pressure).

Hydralazine is an arteriolar dilator that directly acts on vascular smooth muscle. The MOA of hydralazine is not completely understood but is thought to target calcium metabolism. The primary clinical use of hydralazine is for treatment of congestive heart failure associated with mitral insufficiency and for secondary treatment of hypertension. Side effects most commonly associated with hydralazine include hypotension, reflex tachycardia, and gastrointestinal upset.

Sildenafil is a phosphodiesterase V inhibitor used in veterinary patients for the medical management of canine pulmonary hypertension. The concentration of phosphodiesterase V is high in the lungs and is elevated in patients with pulmonary hypertension. Few side effects have been reported in dogs treated with sildenafil.

Antiarrhythmics

Antiarrhythmics are used to treat disturbances in heart rhythm (arrhythmias), including changes in heart rate and rhythm and in the site of impulse origin or conduction. Arrhythmias can originate from the atria (referred to as *supraventricular*) or from the ventricles (referred to as *ventricular*). Antiarrhythmics are subdivided into classes I through IV on the basis of their pharmacologic effects on the action potential of cardiac cells. Table 27-14 summarizes the antiarrhythmics based on class, MOA, and side effects.

Class I antiarrhythmics block fast sodium channels, providing membrane stabilization and slowing the conduction velocity of the action potential (AP). The two most common class I antiarrhythmics used in veterinary patients are lidocaine and quinidine. Lidocaine is used in the treatment of ventricular tachycardia. Lidocaine has poor oral absorption and a short duration of action, requiring intravenous administration as a constant rate infusion. Quinidine is used in the treatment of horses with atrial fibrillation.

Class II antiarrhythmics consist of beta-adrenergic blocking agents such as propranolol and atenolol. Beta blockers decrease sympathetic input to the heart, decreasing heart rate, contractility, and oxygen requirements of the heart muscle. Class II antiarrhythmics are used in the treatment of both supraventricular and ventricular tachycardias. However, the use of beta blockers is contraindicated in patients in heart failure. Beta-adrenergic blockers cause an increase in the number of beta receptors in the heart muscle (a phenomenon known as *upregulation*). Because of upregulation, patients treated with beta blockers require a gradual dose reduction before discontinuation of therapy, to prevent the development of fatal arrhythmias. Consequently, clients should be advised to follow instructions carefully as the drug is being withdrawn.

The class III antiarrhythmic most commonly used in veterinary patients is sotalol, which also functions as a beta-adrenergic blocker. Sotalol is used to treat ventricular arrhythmias, specifically, boxer ventricular tachycardia and syncope (fainting). Sotalol is eliminated primarily by the kidneys; therefore, dose reduction is recommended in patients with decreased kidney function.

TABLE 27-14	Antiarrhythmics Commonly Used in Veterinary Patients			
CLASS	**MECHANISM OF ACTION**	**EXAMPLES**	**CLINICAL USE**	**SIDE EFFECTS**
I	Slows action potential conduction (blockade of fast sodium channels)	Lidocaine Quinidine	Ventricular tachycardia Supraventricular and ventricular tachycardias Atrial fibrillation (horses)	GI, CNS Urticaria, nasal inflammation, GI, laminitis
II	Beta-adrenergic blockade	Propranolol Atenolol	Supraventricular tachycardia Ventricular tachycardia	Cardiovascular depression
III	Prolongation of action potential (beta-adrenergic blockade)	Sotalol	Ventricular tachycardia (Boxer ventricular tachycardia and syncope)	Cardiovascular depression
IV	Calcium channel blockade	Diltiazem	Supraventricular tachycardia (atrial fibrillation)	Cardiovascular depression

CNS, Central nervous system; *GI*, gastrointestinal.

Class IV antiarrhythmics include the calcium channel blocker diltiazem. Calcium channel blockers slow impulse conduction through the atrioventricular junction (AV node), effectively slowing the ventricular rate. Diltiazem is used to treat supraventricular tachycardias such as atrial fibrillation in dogs.

> **TECHNICIAN NOTE** Because of upregulation of beta receptors, beta-adrenergic blockers require a gradual dose reduction before discontinuation of therapy to prevent the development of fatal arrhythmias. Consequently, clients should be advised to follow instructions carefully as the drug is being withdrawn.

NEUROLOGIC DISEASE

The most commonly used anticonvulsants in veterinary patients are phenobarbital (PB) and potassium bromide (KBr). Their mechanisms of action are considered synergistic through the enhancement of inhibitory neurotransmission. PB is used commonly as a first-line anticonvulsant, except in patients with evidence of hepatotoxicity or an underlying hepatopathy, in which case KBr may be used as first-line therapy. Side effects associated with either anticonvulsant include dose-dependent sedation and/or ataxia, increased drinking and urination, and increased eating with weight gain. Clinical use of both PB and KBr requires therapeutic drug monitoring.

PB therapy can be associated with the development of hepatotoxicity. It is often recommended that liver enzymes be monitored because, if recognized early, hepatotoxicity is reversible with discontinuation of PB. Also, PB is a potent inducer of the hepatic microsomal P450 enzyme system (CYP 1A, 2B, 2C, and 3A), inducing the metabolism of many endogenous and exogenous substances (including itself), which may result in clinically significant drug interactions. Known PB drug interactions associated with commonly used drugs because of their increased metabolism include digoxin, glucocorticoids, antipyrine, and some anesthetics. In addition, PB alters the metabolism of thyroid hormones. Therefore, testing a dog with normal thyroid function that is treated with phenobarbital may result in a misdiagnosis of hypothyroidism. Finally, with chronic therapy, PB serum concentrations decrease and dosage adjustments are often necessary.

Use of KBr in cats is not recommended because 40% of cats treated with KBr develop asthma-like symptoms associated with eosinophilic bronchitis. PB is the anticonvulsant of choice is cats.

> **TECHNICIAN NOTE** Routine therapeutic drug monitoring is necessary for patients receiving anticonvulsants such as phenobarbital or potassium bromide.

NEOPLASTIC DISEASE

Neoplastic diseases (cancer) are treated most often with a combination of surgery, chemotherapy, and radiation therapy. It is common practice to use multiple chemotherapy drugs in the same patient because this more effectively kills tumor cells and decreases drug resistance and toxicity.

Chemotherapy drugs can be subdivided into different groups on the basis of their chemistry and pharmacologic action (alkylating agents, platinum compounds, antimetabolites, natural products, and hormones). These drugs generally target tumor cells (which are actively dividing) but often are associated with significant side effects because of their effects on other rapidly dividing cells of the body, including cells of the gastrointestinal tract, bone marrow, and hair follicles (in humans). Side effects can be anticipated and monitored with knowledge of the expected effects of a particular agent on the species being treated. Table 27-15 summarizes the chemotherapy agents commonly used in veterinary patients, their associated group, toxicities associated with particular tissues and species, and side effects.

Chemotherapeutic agents by definition are cytotoxic (toxic to cells) and consequently require special handling precautions and disposal because of potential hazards to personnel, including the veterinary technician. Personal protective equipment such as chemotherapy safety gloves, eye protection (safety glasses/goggles), and disposable gowns or lab coats should always be used when these agents are handled. In addition, drug preparation should be performed in an exhaust fume hood. Equipment that has come in contact with chemotherapeutic drugs (catheters, syringes, needles, and gloves) needs to be disposed of in accordance with U.S. Department of Labor, Occupational Safety and Health Administration (OSHA) requirements.

Many parenterally administered drugs (e.g., doxorubicin, mitoxantrone, vincristine, vinblastine) cause significant tissue irritation and necrosis if administered outside the vein (extravasation). For this reason, careful catheter placement is critical. The general rule is that any catheter placed for chemotherapy delivery should be placed with a single clean stick and checked for correct placement. When the clinician is uncertain about whether the catheter is in the vein, it should be removed and placed in a different vein.

> **TECHNICIAN NOTE** Personal protective equipment, including gloves, eye protection, and disposable gowns or lab coats, should always be worn when chemotherapeutic agents are handled and administered.

PARASITIC DISEASE
Endoparasites

Endoparasites can be subdivided into three classes: nematodes (roundworms, including stomach worms, hookworms, whipworms, lungworms, heartworms), cestodes (tapeworms), and trematodes (flukes). Available antiparasitic drugs target these different classes of parasites using a variety of mechanisms of action. Antiparasitic compounds are often used in combination to broaden their spectrum of activity. Table 27-16 summarizes the more common antiparasitic drugs used to treat endoparasitic infection in

TABLE 27-15	Chemotherapeutic Agents Commonly Used in Veterinary Patients					
			TOXICITY		**SIDE EFFECTS**	
DRUG (ROUTE)	**DRUG GROUP**	**SPECIES**	**TISSUE**	**TIME FRAME**	**CLINICAL SIGNS**	
Cyclophosphamide (IV)	Alkylating agent	All	Bone marrow	7-10 days	Lethargy Fever Low WBC Low platelets	
			Bladder		Blood in urine	
Chlorambucil (PO)	Alkylating agent	All	Bone marrow	7-14 days	Mild	
Lomustine (PO)	Alkylating agent	All	Bone marrow	7-10 days	Lethargy Fever Low WBC Low platelets	
			Liver Kidney Gastrointestinal			
Cisplatin (IV)	Platinum compound	All*	Kidney toxicity	7-9 days	Lethargy Vomiting High BUN High creatinine	
			Gastrointestinal	≈2 hours	Nausea Vomiting Mild	
			CNS toxicity Bone marrow	7-20 days		
Carboplatin (IV)	Platinum compound	All	Bone marrow	14 days	Lethargy Fever Low WBC Low platelets	
			Gastrointestinal	≈2 hours	Nausea Vomiting	
Vincristine (IV) Vinblastine (IV)	Natural products (microtubule)	All	Bone marrow Tissue irritant (if administered extravascularly) Neurotoxicity	5-10 days	Low WBC Tissue necrosis	
Doxorubicin (IV)	Natural product (antibiotic)	All	Allergic reaction	Minutes	Skin blushing Head shaking Vomiting Diarrhea Collapse	
			Tissue irritant (if administered extravascularly)		Tissue necrosis	
			Bone marrow	7-10 days	Low WBC Low platelets Anemia	
			Gastrointestinal		Nausea Vomiting	
			Cardiotoxicity (dose dependent)		Heart failure Arrhythmias	
Mitoxantrone (IV)	Natural product (antibiotic)	All	Tissue irritant (if administered extravascularly)		Tissue necrosis	
			Bone marrow	7-10 days	Low WBC Low platelets Anemia	
			Gastrointestinal		Nausea Vomiting	
			Cardiotoxicity (dose dependent)		Heart failure Arrhythmias	
L-Asparaginase (IM or SQ)	Natural product (enzyme)	All	Anaphylaxis	<1 hour	Pruritus Vomiting Diarrhea Collapse	

TABLE 27-15	Chemotherapeutic Agents Commonly Used in Veterinary Patients—cont'd					
		TOXICITY			**SIDE EFFECTS**	
DRUG (ROUTE)	**DRUG GROUP**	**SPECIES**	**TISSUE**		**TIME FRAME**	**CLINICAL SIGNS**
Prednisone (PO)	Hormone	All	Gastrointestinal			Vomiting (V) Diarrhea (D) Bloody V/D
			Steroid excess			Increased eating, drinking, and urination Panting Weight gain Muscle loss

BUN, Blood urea nitrogen; *CNS,* central nervous system; *WBC,* white blood cell count.
Note: Cisplatin is contraindicated in cats because of a species-specific, dose-related, fatal primary pulmonary toxicity.

TABLE 27-16	Common Antiparasitics Used in Treatment of Endoparasites In Veterinary Species			
DRUG	**MECHANISM OF ACTION**	**TARGET SPECIES**	**ACTIVITY**	**SIDE EFFECTS AND OTHER COMMENTS**
Fenbendazole Albendazole Netobimin Febantel	Bind parasitic β-tubulin	Cattle Goats Sheep Horses Poultry Pigs Dogs Cats	Nematodes Lungworms Cestodes	High safety margin Teratogenic (some)
Pyrantel Morantel	Agonist at parasitic nicotinic acetylcholine receptors	Sheep Cattle Swine Horses Dogs Cats	Nematodes	Use not recommended in horses intended for food consumption
Praziquantel	Alter parasite intracellular calcium concentration	Dogs Cats Cattle Sheep Goats Pigs Horses	Cestodes Trematodes	Wide safety margin Vomiting at high doses (dogs)
Avermectins Milbemycins	Agonist at invertebrate glutamate-gated chloride channels, causing flaccid paralysis	Cattle Sheep Horses Swine Dogs Cats	Nematodes Arthropods	Genetic predisposition for central nervous system (CNS) toxicity in Collies and related breeds Restricted use in lactating dairy cows (except some topical formulations)

veterinary patients, including target species, antiparasitic activity, and side effects. In addition to broad-spectrum antiparasitics with activity against trematodes, various specific antitrematodal compounds are available for use in cattle and sheep.

Widely used macrocyclic lactones (avermectins [ivermectin, doramectin, and selamectin] and milbemycins [milbemycin oxime and moxidectin]) are considered broad-spectrum antiparasitics with activity against nematodes (gastrointestinal nematodes, lungworms, and heartworms), as well as arthropods (mites, lice, ticks, and fleas). In dogs, macrocyclic lactones are commonly used as heartworm preventive agents, whereas in ruminants, horses, and pigs, they are used primarily to treat gastrointestinal nematodes and arthropod infestations. Limited use of macrocyclic lactones in dogs may be due in part to increased sensitivity of some dogs (Collies and other breeds) to the higher doses of macrocyclic lactones needed to treat gastrointestinal nematode or arthropod infection. The sensitivity of Collies to macrocyclic lactones is associated with genetic alteration of gene coding of an important drug efflux pump, P-glycoprotein. Dogs with the P-glycoprotein mutation are at increased risk for CNS toxicity when macrocyclic lactones (e.g., ivermectin) are used at higher concentrations.

Macrocyclic lactones are highly **lipophilic** drugs with wide tissue distribution, including liver, fat, and skin, enabling a prolonged effect. In food-producing animals, a significant portion of the drug is eliminated through the mammary glands, restricting the use of macrocyclic lactones (except for some of the topical formulations) in lactating dairy cows. Each of the macrocyclic lactones used in food-producing animals (cattle and sheep) requires a withdrawal period post administration.

Ectoparasites

Ectoparasites include insects (flies, lice, fleas) and ascarines (ticks and mites). Strategies for ectoparasite control include preventing host-parasite interaction through the use of contact insecticides such as organophosphates and pyrethrums (pyrethrins/pyrethroids) and/or controlling ectoparasitic infestation with insecticide/adulticide therapy. The most common means of drug delivery for ectoparasite control is topical application.

Ectoparasiticides have a variety of mechanisms of action and include those that function as repellents, others that target the parasite's nervous system, and yet others that target growth and development of the parasite. Toxicity is a risk associated with ectoparasiticide use, and signs of toxicity must be closely monitored during use. Table 27-17 compares the MOA of the ectoparasiticides commonly used in veterinary patients and clinical signs associated with toxicity.

TABLE 27-17	Ectoparasiticides Commonly Used in Veterinary Patients			
ECTOPARASITICIDE	**MECHANISM OF ACTION**	**TARGET HOST**	**TARGET PARASITE**	**CLINICAL SIGNS OF TOXICITY**
Contact Insecticide				
Organophosphates Carbamates	Inhibitor of acetylcholinesterase (AchE)	Cattle Dogs Cats	Fleas Ticks Mites Flies Lice Grubs	Salivation, urination, defecation, depression, twitching, tremors
Pyrethrins Pyrethroids	Target voltage-gated sodium channels of the axonal cell membrane	Cattle Swine Dogs	Mosquitoes Ticks Fleas Mites	Hyperexcitability, tremors, salivation, weakness. Not safe in cats
Agents That Target Parasite's Nervous System				
Amitraz	Monoamine oxidase inhibitor	Dogs Cattle Swine	Ticks Lice Mites	CNS depression (via α_2-adrenergic agonist activity in mammals)
Avermectins	Target invertebrate glutamate-gated chloride channels. Cross-reactivity with mammal GABA and glycine-gated chloride channels	Cattle Swine Dogs Cats	Lice Mites Flies Grubs Ticks	CNS depression Ataxia Some dogs breeds (Collies) susceptible to CNS toxicity
Imidacloprid (neonicotinoids)	Competitive inhibition of invertebrate nicotinic acetylcholine receptors	Dogs Cats	Fleas (larvae, adults)	Tremors
Nitenpyram (neonicotinoids)	Competitive inhibition of invertebrate nicotinic acetylcholine receptors	Dogs Cats	Fleas	Well tolerated
Fipronil	Noncompetitive blockade of chloride ions through GABA and invertebrate glutamate-gated chloride channels	Dogs Cats	Fleas Ticks	Hyperactivity Convulsions
Agents That Target Parasite's Growth and Development				
Insect growth regulators	Arrest developing stages of insects and arthropods	Cattle Dogs Cats	Ticks Fleas Flies	None known
Methoprene Pyriproxifen	Juvenile hormone analogues (maintain insect development in immature egg or larval stages)			
Lufenuron Diflubenzuron	Insect development inhibitors (inhibit chitin synthesis and deposition, interfering with development of insect's exoskeleton)			

CNS, Central nervous system; *GABA,* gamma-aminobutyric acid.

With the development of safe and effective ectoparasiticides that preferentially target the nervous system of invertebrates or their growth and development, use of more toxic repellents is relatively infrequent in veterinary medicine. The pyrethrums are associated with significant toxicities in cats. Organophosphates and carbamates were developed because of their toxic effects on many internal parasites (e.g., roundworms, including hookworms and whipworms) and external parasites (e.g., flies, fleas, ticks, mites, lice), but these agents have a narrow margin of safety. Overall, their use in small animals has significantly decreased, but they still may be used occasionally in equine or swine medicine.

REGULATORY PHARMACOLOGY

DRUG LAWS AND REGULATIONS

State and federal laws regulating drug use in the United States are designed to work in conjunction with one another. Federal laws are the fundamental regulations for drug approval and use, enacted to ensure that available drugs are safe, effective, and prepared in accordance with manufacturing standards. State laws are in place to control the distribution of drugs within the state. For example, state laws address individuals authorized to prescribe and dispense drugs, required record keeping, and licensing of drug distributors. State laws vary, thus each licensed practitioner is required to know the laws for the state in which he or she practices. Veterinarians found to be in violation of federal or state laws regulating the transport, sale, or use of drugs may be subject to any of the following: warning letters, fines, temporary or permanent loss of state veterinary license, or imprisonment.

> *TECHNICIAN NOTE* Federal laws are the fundamental regulations for drug approval and use, enacted to ensure that available drugs are safe, effective, and prepared in accordance with manufacturing standards. State laws address individuals authorized to prescribe and dispense drugs, required record keeping, and licensing of drug distributors.

Federal regulation of drugs began in the mid-1800s, with the Import Drug Act (1848), which was the first federal law to guarantee the quality of medications. Since that time, the federal government has continued to enact laws and regulations to ensure the potency, purity, and quality of drugs. However, it was not until passage of the **Federal Food, Drug, and Cosmetic Act** (FFD&C Act) in 1938 that manufacturers were required to provide evidence of safety under conditions prescribed on the label. The FFD&C Act also required product labeling to include directions for use, warnings, active ingredients, and shelf life. The FFD&C Act remains the law regulating drug approval, use, safety, and efficacy, but it has undergone a series of amendments to address some of its initial pitfalls. Significant changes to the FFD&C Act that

have directly affected drug use in veterinary medicine are outlined in Table 27-18.

In addition to drug laws and regulations derived from the FFD&C Act, the official legal drug compendium for the United States is the **U.S. Pharmacopoeia (USP)–National Formulary (NF)**. The USP is a compilation of all drug substances and products; the NF is focused on providing the active ingredients.

Federal regulating bodies that oversee veterinary products include the **Food and Drug Administration** (FDA), the **U.S. Department of Agriculture** (USDA), and the **Environmental Protection Agency** (EPA). The FDA's **Center for Veterinary Medicine** (CVM) is the governing body that regulates the manufacture and distribution of drugs, food additives, and medical devices used in veterinary species under the FFD&C Act. The CVM oversees regulations regarding approval, safety, efficacy, and post-approval monitoring. The USDA's Animal and Plant Health Inspection Service, Center for Veterinary Biologics, oversees veterinary biologics (vaccines, antitoxins, and diagnostics used to prevent, treat, or diagnose animal diseases) under the Virus Serum Toxin Act of 1913. The EPA's Pesticide Regulation Division, acting under the Federal Insecticide, Fungicide, and Rodenticide Act, oversees pesticides, including those used on inanimate objects, rodenticides, and insecticides.

> *TECHNICIAN NOTE* The amended Federal Food, Drug, and Cosmetic Act (FFD&C Act) of 1938 remains the law regulating drug approval, use, safety, and efficacy in the United States.

DEFINITIONS AND APPROVAL CATEGORIES OF DRUGS

A *chemical* is defined as a drug if it meets at least one of the following criteria: (1) it is recognized by at least one of the official drug compendia (the US Pharmacopoeia/National Formulary or the Homeopathic Pharmacopoeia of the United States) or their supplements; (2) it is used in the diagnosis, treatment, or prevention of disease in either man or animals; or (3) it is a nonfood chemical that affects the structure or function of the body. A *new animal drug* is defined as a drug intended for use in animals other than man; this includes any drug intended for use in animal feed that is not generally recognized as safe and effective. Thus, new drugs intended for use in animal feeds also fall under the category of new animal drugs. Approval and legal use of a new animal drug requires review by the FDA in accordance with the FFD&C Act via a new animal drug application (NADA) or an abbreviated new animal drug application (ANADA).

Each new animal drug is approved by the FDA as a **prescription drug** (also known as a **legend drug**, or an Rx drug), an **over-the-counter drug** (OTC drug, or nonprescription drug), or a **veterinary feed directive** (VFD) drug. Use of prescription and VFD drugs by a veterinarian requires

TABLE 27-18	Time Line of Significant Changes to the Federal Food, Drug, and Cosmetic Act That Have Influenced Drug Use in Veterinary Medicine
YEAR: AMENDMENT	**COMMENTS**
1951: Durham-Humphrey Amendment	Defined prescription drugs in humans (upheld by courts for animal drugs, although prescription animal drugs were not included in the law until 1988 by the Generic Animal Drug Patent Term Restoration Act).
1954: Pesticide Amendment	
1958: Food Additive Amendment	Introduced premarket clearance of food additives, which required manufacturers to demonstrate safety of drug residues in animal products consumed by humans. For the first time, drugs used in food animals were now considered food additives. Drugs used in food-producing animals have to meet not only drug standards but also food additive standards.
1960: Color Additive Amendment	
1962: Kefauver-Hams Drug Amendment	Extended authority of the Food and Drug Administration (FDA) to require manufacturers to demonstrate efficacy as well as safety as a condition of drug approval.
1970: Controlled Substance Act	Regulated manufacture, distribution, and dispensing of controlled substances.
1988: Generic Animal Drug Patent Term Restoration Act	Enabled approval of abbreviated new animal drug application (ANADA) for generic products of approved off-patent animal drugs. Also defined prescription animal drugs.
1994: Animal Medicinal Drug Use Clarification Act	Enabled licensed veterinarians to use and prescribe animal and human drugs for extra-label drug use under defined conditions.
1996: Animal Drug Availability Act	Reformed FDA evaluation and approval process for animal drugs to facilitate approval of new animal drugs and feed additives. In addition, this act defined a new class of approved animal drugs (veterinary feed directive [VFD] drugs). VFD drugs are approved for use in or on animal feed under the supervision of a licensed veterinarian.
2003: Animal Drug User Fee Act	Authorized FDA to collect fees from pharmaceutical firms to support the review of new animal drugs, accelerating and improving the review process.
2004: Minor Use/Minor Species Animal Health Act	Provided greater flexibility for making drugs available for minor species (i.e., agriculture, zoo, or wildlife species) or for use in uncommon disease conditions in a major species. Alternative categories for approval are provided, including conditional approval, drug indexing, and drug designation.

a valid **veterinarian-client-patient relationship** (VCPR). A valid VCPR is defined as outlined in Box 27-1.

The Durham-Humphrey Amendment of 1951 gave the FDA power to designate approved human drugs as OTC or prescription. Before the Durham-Humphrey Amendment was enacted, drug manufacturers decided whether a drug would be made available OTC or by prescription. It was not until 1988 under the Generic Animal Drug Patent Term Restoration Act that a similar legal designation was made for regulating the distribution of animal drugs.

Prescription animal drugs are defined as approved drugs that may be dispensed only by or under the direction of a licensed veterinarian because of their potential for toxicity or abuse. Use of a prescription drug requires an intervention by a veterinarian to establish a diagnosis (preliminary or specific) and to monitor the patient's response to therapy, including potential adverse reactions. Veterinary prescription drugs can be dispensed only in association with a valid VCPR. All veterinary prescription drug labels contain the following warning statement: "Caution: Federal law restricts this drug to use by or on the order of a licensed veterinarian." An equivalent warning label, "Caution: Federal law prohibits dispensing without a prescription," or "Rx only," is on all approved human prescription drugs.

BOX 27-1	Components of a Valid Veterinarian-Client-Patient Relationship as Defined by FDA Code of Federal Regulations*

1. A veterinarian has assumed the responsibility for making medical judgments regarding the health of (an) animal(s) and the need for medical treatment, and the client (the owner of the animal or animals or other caretaker) has agreed to follow the instructions of the veterinarian;
2. There is sufficient knowledge of the animal(s) by the veterinarian to initiate at least a general or preliminary diagnosis of the medical condition of the animal(s); and
3. The practicing veterinarian is readily available for follow-up in case of adverse reactions or failure of the regimen of therapy.

Such a relationship can exist only when the veterinarian has recently seen and is personally acquainted with the keeping and care of the animal(s) by virtue of examination of the animal(s), and/or by medically appropriate and timely visits to the premises where the animal(s) are kept.

*Title 21 CFR 530.3(i).

TABLE 27-19	Controlled Substances Categorized by Schedule Under the Controlled Substances Act (CSA)		
SCHEDULE	ABUSE POTENTIAL	SUBSTANCES	COMMENTS
I	High	Heroin, LSD, marijuana, mescaline, methaqualone, peyote	• Use not accepted in a practice setting in the United States • Research use only
II	High	Opium, morphine, hydromorphone, cocaine, methadone, meperidine, fentanyl Barbiturates: pentobarbital, amobarbital, secobarbital Amphetamines	• Risk for severe psychic or physical dependence in humans • Amphetamines no longer available under Schedule II for veterinary use • Require a written prescription, no refills permitted
III	Moderate	Anabolic steroids—boldenone, mibolerone, stanozolol, tenbolone, testosterone Opioids—nalorphine, opium combination products (acetaminophen and codeine, hydrocodone) Barbiturates—thiamylal, thiopental Non-narcotic drugs—tiletamine, zolazepam, phencyclidine, ketamine, benzphetamine	• Risk for moderate to low physical dependence but high psychological dependence in humans • Anabolic steroids added in 1991 under Anabolic Steroids Control Act (ASCA); progesterones and estrogens are not subject to ASCA or CSA • Oral or written prescription permitted with a maximum of 5 refills in 6 months
IV	Low	Barbital, phenobarbital, methylphenobarbital, chloral hydrate Butorphanol, meprobamate, chlordiazepoxide, diazepam, midazolam	• Risk for limited physical or psychological dependence in humans • Oral or written prescription permitted with a maximum of 5 refills in 6 months
V	Low	Codeine, dihydrocodeine, diphenoxylate	• No DEA limit on prescriptions

DEA, Drug Enforcement Administration; *LSD*, lysergic acid diethylamide.

Animal drugs approved as OTC products are recognized as safe and effective for the labeled indication only. Use of OTC drugs by a layperson is considered safe provided directions on the label are followed; therefore, the use of OTC drugs does not require a veterinarian's intervention.

Veterinary feed directive (VFD) drugs were defined in 1996 under the Animal Drug Availability Act (ADAA). VFD drugs are used under the order of a veterinarian in animal feed. This class of approved drugs was developed to enable the distribution of animal feeds containing a VFD drug because VFD drugs are not subject to regulation by state pharmacy laws. No **extra-label drug use** is permitted for VFD drugs, and their use requires a valid VCPR.

> **TECHNICIAN NOTE** Use of prescription and veterinary feed directive (VFD) drugs by a veterinarian requires a valid veterinarian-client-patient relationship (VCPR).

CONTROLLED SUBSTANCES

The **Controlled Substance Act** (CSA) was introduced in 1970 to regulate the manufacture, distribution, and dispensing of controlled substances. A detailed publication on proper handling of controlled substances, entitled "Practitioner's Manual," is provided online by the Drug Enforcement Agency (DEA) (see "Recommended Readings"). The CSA broadened the definition of a controlled substance to include opiates, barbiturates, hallucinogens, methadone,

stimulants (amphetamines), and other addictive or habit-forming drugs. Under the CSA, identified drugs are controlled by restricting their use to a defined group of individuals registered with the Drug Enforcement Agency (DEA), which includes manufacturers, distributors, pharmacists, and licensed practitioners. Controlled substances are categorized into five schedules (I, II, III, IV, and V) by the DEA based on their potential for abuse. Table 27-19 summarizes the five schedules assigned to controlled substances and the drugs that fall into each category.

Manufacturers and distributors of controlled substances are required to label the original containers of controlled substances with the schedule drug classification assigned to its contents (a capital "C" followed by a Roman numeral from I through V). Both veterinarians and pharmacists are responsible for proper use and handling of controlled substances in their possession. For example, a licensed veterinarian must be registered with the DEA as an individual or through their hospital to legally use or prescribe controlled substances. At the time of registration with the DEA, the practitioner must request certification for those schedules of drugs that he or she expects to purchase, store, prescribe, dispense, or use (Schedules II through V). Once registered, a DEA certificate and registration number will be provided. In addition, an official DEA form is required to order and purchase controlled substances.

All controlled substances must be stored in a locked cabinet, box, or safe; if possible, the locked container should be secured to a concrete floor. Use of controlled substances by a registered individual requires accurate record keeping of orders, receipts, and usage. Inventory must be reconcilable with records, and all records must be available for inspection at any time by the DEA.

> **TECHNICIAN NOTE** All controlled substances must be stored in a locked cabinet, box, or safe; if possible, the locked container should be secured to a concrete floor.

EXTRA-LABEL DRUG USE

In 1994, the FFD&C Act was amended to include extra-label drug use by veterinarians as provided under the **Animal Medicinal Drug Use Clarification Act (AMDUCA)**. Under the AMDUCA, veterinarians can legally use or prescribe certain approved animal and human drugs for the treatment of veterinary species in an extra-label fashion, provided specific conditions are met. Before the AMDUCA was signed, this practice was illegal.

Extra-label drug use is defined as follows: "actual use or intended use of a drug in an animal in a manner that is not in accordance with the approved labeling. This includes but is not limited to use in a species not listed in the labeling, use for indications (disease and other conditions) not listed on the labeling, use at dosage levels, frequencies, or routes of administration other than those stated in the labeling, and deviation from labeled withdrawal time based on these different uses." Withdrawal time is the time interval between the last administered drug dose to a food-producing animal and the time that animal can be slaughtered, or animal products such as eggs or milk can be used. When a drug is used in an extra-label fashion in food-producing animals, the veterinarian is responsible for making every effort to determine an extended withdrawal time. Resources such as the Food Animal Residue Avoidance Database (FARAD) are available for consultation in determining withdrawal times (see "Recommended Readings").

Extra-label drug use enables the veterinarian to use his or her professional judgment in the treatment of veterinary species under certain conditions but requires the veterinarian to make every effort to initially use an approved drug at an approved dosage. Specific conditions that must be met when an approved drug is used include a valid veterinarian-client-patient relationship, appropriate animal identification, and documentation such as drug labeling and record keeping. Box 27-2 provides additional information on specific criteria that must be met for extra-label drug use in veterinary species, as well as additional criteria needed for extra-label use in food-producing animals. In addition, extra-label use is limited to ill patients whose life or health is threatened, or that are suffering if treatment is withheld. Extra-label drug use is prohibited for enhancement of animal production or reproduction, growth promotion, routine disease prevention, alteration of cost of therapy, or as a feed additive. In addition, as stated under AMDUCA, the FDA CVM may prohibit the extra-label drug use of approved new

---

> **BOX 27-2** | Criteria Used to Determine Extra-Label Drug Use in Veterinary Species and Additional Criteria Required for Food-Producing Animals Under AMDUCA

Criteria Used to Determine Extra-Label Drug Use in Veterinary Species

1. There is no approved new animal drug that is labeled for such use and that contains the same active ingredient in the required dosage form and concentration, except where a veterinarian finds, within the context of a valid veterinary-client-patient relationship, that the approved new animal drug is clinically ineffective for its intended use.
2. Before prescribing or dispensing an approved new animal or human drug for an extra-label use in food animals, the veterinarian must:
   a. Make a careful diagnosis and evaluation of the conditions for which the drug is to be used.
   b. Establish a substantially extended withdrawal period prior to marketing of milk, meat, eggs, or other edible products supported by appropriate scientific information, if applicable.
   c. Institute procedures to assure that the identity of the treated animal or animals is carefully maintained; and
   d. Take appropriate measures to assure that assigned time frames for withdrawal are met and no illegal drug residues occur in any food-producing animal subjected to extra-label treatment.

Additional Criteria Used to Determine Extra-Label Drug Use in Food-Producing Animals

1. Such use must be accomplished in accordance with an appropriate medical rationale; and
2. If scientific information on the human food safety aspect of the use of the drug in food-producing animals is not available, the veterinarian must take appropriate measures to assure that the animal and its food products will not enter the human food supply.
3. Extra-label use of an approved human drug in a food-producing animal is not permitted if an animal drug approved for use in food-producing animals can be used in an extra-label manner for the particular use.

---

animal or human drugs under other circumstances. For example, specific drugs or drug classes are prohibited for use in food-producing animals (Table 27-20) because of their potential to adversely affect human health. Extra-label use of a prohibited drug in food-producing animals is considered one of the FDA's highest regulatory violations.

> **TECHNICIAN NOTE** Specific drugs or drug classes are prohibited for use in food-producing animals because of their potential to adversely affect human health. Extra-label use of a prohibited drug in food-producing animals is considered one of the FDA's highest regulatory violations.

TABLE 27-20	Drugs Prohibited for Use in Food-Producing Animals Under AMDUCA
ALL FOOD-PRODUCING ANIMALS	**COMMENTS**
• Diethylstilbestrol (DES)	• Banned in 1979 because of an identified link between in utero exposure to DES and rare vaginal cancer. DES is no longer marketed.
• Chloramphenicol	• Banned in 1984 because of observed reversible, dose-related bone marrow suppression in many species. Humans may develop an idiosyncratic bone marrow toxicosis that can be fatal.
• Nitroimidazoles	• Include metronidazole, dimetridazole, ipronidazole. Risk for mutagenicity and carcinogenicity.
• Clenbuterol	• Toxicity and death associated with human consumption of edible tissues (liver).
• Nitrofurans	• Include furazolidone and nitrofurazone. Banned in 1991 because of concerns about carcinogenicity and mutagenicity.
• Fluoroquinolones	• Banned in 1997 because of concerns for microbial drug resistance in humans (e.g., *Salmonella* spp.). Fluoroquinolones are the mainstay therapy for the treatment of antibiotic-resistant *Salmonella* infection in humans.
• Glycopeptides	• Vancomycin. Banned in 1997 because of concerns about microbial drug resistance in humans. Considered treatment of last resort for methicillin-resistant *Staphylococcus aureus* (MRSA) infection in humans.
• Cephalosporins (not including cephapirin)	• Prohibited in 2012 in cattle, swine, chickens, and turkeys (major species of food-producing animals) because of concern for microbial drug resistance in humans. Prohibited uses include (1) for disease prevention purposes, (2) at unapproved doses, durations, or routes of administration, and (3) if the drug is not approved for that species and production class.
DAIRY CATTLE	**COMMENTS**
• Sulfonamides	• Prohibited in lactating dairy cows. Concerns of carcinogenicity. Exception: sulfonamides with an approved labeled indication for use in lactating dairy cows (sulfadimethoxine, sulfabromomethazine, sulfaethoxypyridazine).
• Phenylbutazone	• Use prohibited in female dairy cattle, 20 months of age or older.
CHICKENS, TURKEYS, AND DUCKS	**COMMENTS**
• Adamantanes • Neuraminidase inhibitors	• Drugs used for treating or preventing influenza A

AMDUCA, Animal Medicinal Drug Use Clarification Act.

DRUG RESIDUES IN FOOD-PRODUCING ANIMALS

Chemical adulteration of, or the presence of residues in, edible products derived from food-producing animals (meat, poultry, egg, and milk) is regulated by the FDA and the EPA to protect the public food supply. Enforcement of these regulations minimizes the effects that food residues have on public health, as well as their economic impact. Drugs of concern that are commonly used in veterinary food-producing animals include antimicrobials, pesticides, and herbicides. Environmental contaminants of concern include heavy metals, dioxins, and mycotoxins.

A *chemical residue* is defined as the presence of a drug or its metabolite in cells, tissues, organs, or any edible products of an animal. The FDA and the EPA have established tolerances for drugs, pesticides, and other chemicals in tissues of food-producing animals that are used to determine safe drug withdrawal times. Use of drugs in food-producing animals requires establishment of drug withdrawal times (based on pharmacokinetics data) as a condition for approval. In addition, as has been mentioned, some approved drugs (animal and human) used in veterinary species are prohibited for use (including extra-label use) in food-producing animals because of the significant threat that they pose to human

health. Drugs with no approved labeled veterinary indication are considered illegal for use in food-producing animals. Drugs prohibited for use in food-producing animals are listed in Table 27-20.

ADVERSE DRUG EVENT REPORTING

Veterinary drug approval requires review and assessment of animal studies evaluating the safety and efficacy of a drug in the target species. In addition, for drugs used in food-producing animals, food safety studies are required. When a drug is approved, a new animal drug application (NADA) number is generated, and any post-approval information about the drug is recorded under the NADA number. Despite studies conducted before the time of drug approval, post-approval surveillance is important to further assess the safety and efficacy of an approved drug. The system put in place by the FDA CVM is termed **adverse drug event** (ADE) reporting.

An ADE is any adverse event associated with a drug that may or may not be drug related and that occurred regardless of whether the drug was used according to "FDA-approved" labeling. Adverse events associated with extra-label drug use should not be a deterrent for reporting an ADE. Goals of ADE are to capture any clinical manifestations of a drug that were too infrequent to be detected by small pre-approval studies, to identify alternative conditions for use that were not predicted during pre-approval, and to identify any other confounding factors. ADE reporting enables identification of the frequency, similarity, and severity of clinical signs associated with a post-approval ADE to determine whether the ADE is drug related. The FDA uses a standard algorithm (list of instructions used to solve a problem) to facilitate an objective review process.

In the United States, ADE reporting is a voluntary process. ADEs most commonly are reported by an owner or a veterinarian to the manufacturer, who then subsequently reports the ADE to the FDA via the CVM. Direct reporting to the FDA CVM is also possible but generally accounts for only a small percentage of ADE reporting. Outcomes associated with significant ADEs for a drug may result in a change in the drug label, or in recall or withdrawal of the drug. Veterinary ADE reporting is considered a valuable tool for communicating drug risks to both veterinarians and consumers.

> **TECHNICIAN NOTE** Adverse drug event reporting through the Food and Drug Administration (FDA) Center for Veterinary Medicine (CVM) in the United States is voluntary but is encouraged to identify significant post-approval drug risks, which then can be communicated across the profession and to the consumer.

DRUG COMPOUNDING

Drug compounding is defined as any manipulation of a drug other than that described on the approved drug label. This practice is sometimes necessary to ensure that a particular patient receives an appropriate amount of a drug. Circumstances under which a drug may be compounded include those in which a drug cannot be accurately dosed (e.g., because available tablets cannot be cut into small enough pieces to ensure that the correct amount is given) or will not be accepted (e.g., because the available form has an offensive taste). Drug compounding raises concerns, however. For example, of primary concern is the development of adverse reactions or treatment failures associated with loss of the drug's stability, purity, and potency after alteration of the original dosage form.

The FDA CVM has recognized the need for drug compounding in veterinary medicine to more effectively meet the medical needs of our diverse patient populations, and considers compounding of a drug under the classification of extra-label drug use. Consequently, under AMDUCA rules, a veterinarian can legally compound an approved animal or human drug for use in a veterinary species.

In addition, the FDA CVM has developed Compliance Policy Guidelines (CPG) on compounding drugs for animals (see "Recommended Readings"). CPG indicate that drug compounding cannot be done from bulk chemicals (raw chemical ingredients used to produce the manufactured dosage form). It is also stated under AMDUCA that extra-label drug use is not allowed for bulk drugs. Compounding cannot be used to produce a new animal drug. Compounding of bulk drugs and mass marketing of compounded drugs to avoid the FDA drug approval process are illegal practices.

Drug compounding in veterinary medicine is limited to FDA-approved drugs and to custom compounding for a particular patient. It requires a prescription issued by a licensed veterinarian and is limited to the needs of the particular patient designated on the prescription. A common example of the use of a compounded product in veterinary medicine is the preparation of an oral flavored suspension of an FDA-approved drug to facilitate accurate oral dosing in small patients or in noncompliant patients (e.g., cats). Drugs used in veterinary medicine that commonly require compounding and that are recognized by the FDA as essential in the treatment of companion animals include potassium bromide, cisapride, phenylpropanolamine (PPA), and diethylstilbestrol (DES).

Although compounded products are not regulated by the FDA, compounding must be performed in compliance with regulations stated for extra-label drug use. For example, compounded drugs used in food animals cannot violate tissue or milk residues. Thus, if a product is compounded, the compounder is required to establish an expiration date and an appropriate withdrawal time for food-producing animals.

> **TECHNICIAN NOTE** The Food and Drug Administration (FDA) Center for Veterinary Medicine has recognized the need for drug compounding in veterinary medicine to more effectively meet the medical needs of our diverse patient populations. Drugs commonly used in veterinary medicine that require compounding and that are recognized by the FDA as essential in the treatment of companion animals include potassium bromide, cisapride, phenylpropanolamine (PPA), and diethylstilbestrol (DES).

The act of compounding is regulated at the state level by the board of pharmacy; as has been mentioned, state rules and regulations may vary among states. State regulations are intended to ensure that compounded protocols are followed, and to document the ingredients in a compounded product; however, in most cases, they do not require quality assurance of drug content.

Veterinarians may prescribe compounded drugs through compounding pharmacies, which are businesses that prepare and sell compounded drugs for veterinary patients. Accreditation of a compounding pharmacy by a compounding accreditation board is obtained at the discretion of the pharmacy. Compounding pharmacies that have undergone accreditation show their willingness to follow compounding recommendations, assuring as much as possible that their compounding methods are ethical and that they follow established regulations and are based on available science.

DIETARY SUPPLEMENTS/NUTRACEUTICALS

Dietary supplements fall somewhere between the category of food and the category of drugs; in some cases, only a fine line divides a dietary supplement from a drug. **Nutraceuticals**, along with vitamins, minerals, and herbs, fall under the category of *dietary supplements*. Nutraceutical products commonly used in veterinary patients include S-adenosylmethionine (SAMe), milk thistle, and glucosamine and chondroitin.

A *nutraceutical*, as defined by the North American Veterinary Nutraceutical Council, is a "nondrug substance that is produced in a purified or extracted form and administered orally to provide agents required for normal body structure and function with the intent of improving the health and well-being of animals." Legally, nutraceuticals are not considered prescription or OTC medications, and they are dispensed and administered without medical supervision. Although they are readily available to consumers, no efficacy or safety evaluations from the FDA are required before marketing and sale of nutraceuticals. In addition, raw materials, the manufacturing process, and product stability are not evaluated or standardized; therefore, products may vary, and bioequivalence between products cannot be ensured.

The FDA Center for Food Safety and Applied Nutrition regulates human dietary supplements and is responsible for the accuracy of label claims, monitoring of safety through postmarketing surveillance, and confirmation that manufacturing facilities meet standards of suitability. Of particular concern are nutraceuticals marketed as pet products because they do not require the same scientific and clinical evaluations required of human nutraceutical products. Nutraceuticals and/or nutritional supplements are used at the risk and discretion of the user; therefore, before a particular product is used or recommended, consideration should be given to the need for supplementation in a specific patient and the source of the product.

> **TECHNICIAN NOTE** Although nutraceuticals are readily available to consumers, no efficacy or safety evaluations from the FDA are required before marketing and sale of these products. In addition, raw materials, the manufacturing process, and product stability are not evaluated or standardized; therefore, products may vary, and bioequivalence between products cannot be ensured.

THE VETERINARY PHARMACY

DRUG PROCUREMENT

Veterinary and human approved drugs can be obtained directly from the drug manufacturer or through drug distributors, which provide access to a variety of products through a single source. The Compendium of Veterinary Products provides a comprehensive list of veterinary pharmaceutical companies and their available product lines (see "Recommended Readings").

Human approved products—both prescription and OTC—are available to veterinarians and owners through local retail pharmacies. However, routinely available products are limited to oral, ophthalmic, and topical preparations. Oftentimes, owners may prefer the convenience of their local retail pharmacy (based on location) rather than the veterinary clinic. In addition, human hospital pharmacies may serve as a valuable resource for veterinarians. Most human pharmacists acquire some training in the area of veterinary pharmacology and welcome the opportunity to dispense products for veterinary patients.

Other sources of veterinary pharmaceutical products available to owners are local feed stores, mail order suppliers, and Internet pharmacies. Of particular note are the increasing numbers of Internet pharmacies that provide convenience, enable easy cost comparisons, and, in some cases, offer cost savings. Online sites can also serve as a source of health care information. Despite the perceived convenience of information and products available over the Internet, the information provided may not always be accurate and products can be of questionable quality. Thus the consumer of information and goods must maintain healthy objectivity and a cautious perspective when exploring Internet sources.

Regulation of online pharmacies is primarily in the hands of the state board of pharmacy, although some federal oversight is required. The National Association of Boards of Pharmacy (NABP) does not have a role in regulating online pharmacies. Hallmarks of a reputable Internet pharmacy are that it (1) requires a valid hard copy or verbal prescription provided directly from the prescriber with a valid VCPR; (2) provides a toll-free telephone number and street address on its website; (3) allows direct contact with its pharmacists for consultation; and (4) is certified as a Verified Internet Pharmacy Practice Site (VIPPS).

VIPPS is a voluntary accreditation program of the NABP that provides a VIPPS seal of verification to Internet pharmacies that are appropriately licensed and legitimately operated. To attain the VIPPS seal, the online pharmacy is required to undergo and successfully complete a thorough review to ensure compliance with the same state and federal laws and regulations that a traditional local retail pharmacy must observe. A VIPPS also provides a mechanism for reporting any errors or inconsistencies made by a VIPPS-certified pharmacy.

> **TECHNICIAN NOTE** Hallmarks of a reputable Internet pharmacy are that it (1) requires a valid hard copy or verbal prescription provided directly from the prescriber with a valid veterinarian-client-patient relationship (VCPR); (2) provides a toll-free telephone number and street address on its website; (3) allows direct contact with its pharmacists for consultation; and (4) is certified as a Verified Internet Pharmacy Practice Site (VIPPS).

DRUG DOSAGE FORMS

Different drug dosage forms are available for delivery of drugs by a variety of routes. Oral dosage forms are most commonly used and include tablets (flavored and unflavored), capsules, and oral suspensions. Depending on the drug's stability at low gastric pH and the preferred site of intestinal absorption, some oral dosage forms are enteric coated to prevent drug exposure to the low pH of the stomach and to delay absorption until the drug reaches the higher pH of the small intestine. Oral tablets that are enteric coated should not be split or crushed for oral administration.

Injectable products are available for administration via subcutaneous (SQ), intramuscular (IM), or intravenous (IV) injection. Injectable preparations may be provided as sterile solutions or as fine (or **lyophilized**) powders that require dissolution in a sterile diluent before administration. A few injectable drugs are well absorbed when administered transmucosally because of the ability of the drug to cross the oral mucous membranes in some species. An example of a commonly used drug with good transmucosal absorption is buprenorphine in cats. Other commonly used dosage forms include topical preparations such as ophthalmic ointments or solutions and topical creams, lotions, or sprays.

A few drugs such as fentanyl and methimazole will be absorbed systemically when delivered by the transdermal route. Transdermal drug delivery in veterinary species is limited by the ability of the drug to absorb across the skin's surface. Therefore, although many drugs can be formulated for transdermal delivery, therapeutic systemic drug levels are rarely achieved.

Antibiotic formulations are available for intrauterine or intramammary infusion in large animal medicine. Remember that withdrawal times remain important in food-producing animals, even when local antibiotic therapy such as this is used.

DRUG STORAGE AND DISPOSAL

The storage recommendation for a drug is established by the drug manufacturer on the basis of results of stability studies conducted on the manufactured finished product. To ensure the safety and potency of a drug for the lifetime of the product, storage recommendations must be followed to prevent premature degradation. Storage recommendations for a particular drug product are available in the package insert accompanying the product.

Product expiration dates are provided by the manufacturer to ensure the purity and potency of the final dosage form based on controlled stability studies. The expiration date ensures product purity and potency only if the product is stored in accordance with the manufacturer's recommendations. The FDA requires standard expiration dates (month, day, and year) on all approved drug products. Exceptions to this rule are drugs regulated by the EPA (pesticides, rodenticides, and insecticides), for which no expiration date is included on the manufactured product, but the required shelf life is a minimum of 5 years.

Drug disposal is governed by the Department of Environmental Quality (DEQ), the EPA, the FDA, and local boards of pharmacy. Disposal of controlled substances is regulated by the DEA. Expired drugs and unused drugs should not be dumped down the drain, flushed down the toilet, placed in the trash, or discarded in the ground.

Expired drug should be returned to the manufacturer or the distribution company for credit, or should be sent to a reverse distribution company (RDC). An RDC functions as the intermediary between the drug purchaser and the drug vendor. The RDC provides credit to the drug purchaser for a returned drug; when credit is not acceptable, the RDC discards or destroys a returned drug on a per pound cost basis. Approved disposal of a controlled substance is provided only through an RDC.

> **TECHNICIAN NOTE** Expired drugs and unused drugs should not be dumped down the drain, flushed down the toilet, placed in the trash, or discarded in the ground. Expired drug should be returned to the manufacturer or the distribution company for credit, or should be sent to a reverse distribution company (RDC).

PRESCRIPTION DRUGS

PRESCRIPTION WRITING AND DISPENSING

Correct prescription writing and reading are essential for accurate dosing and dispensing of drugs. A veterinary prescription is valid only if written or authorized by a licensed veterinarian. Essential elements required by law on a prescription written for a noncontrolled substance include (1) the printed or stamped name, address, and telephone number of the licensed veterinarian; (2) the DEA registration number of the licensed veterinarian (required on all prescriptions for controlled substances); (3) the legal signature of the licensed veterinarian; (4) the drug name, concentration, and quantity (#); (5) directions for use; (6) the full name and address of the client; (7) identification of the animal (name and species); (8) any cautionary statements (e.g., withdrawal times for food animals); and (9) the number of refills (if applicable). Prescriptions for dispensing controlled substances require all the same elements required for noncontrolled substances, with the following additional requirements for items 3 and 9. Not only is the legal signature of the licensed veterinarian required for item 3, the licensed veterinarian's name must also be printed. Regarding item 9, the number of refills allowed is dictated by the controlled substance being dispensed. No refills are allowed for Schedule II drugs, and refills are limited to 5 times or 6 months (whichever comes first) for Schedule III and Schedule IV drugs. Figure 27-2 shows the essential parts of a prescription form.

Legal prescription writing allows the use of standardized abbreviations. Table 27-21 provides a list of recognized and accepted abbreviations commonly used in prescription writing. It is best to spell out any term that does not have an accepted abbreviation, or to ask the prescribing veterinarian for clarification of unrecognized or unreadable abbreviations or terms. An example of a properly written prescription that uses common abbreviations to describe directions for use and correct interpretation of that prescription for accurate filling are shown in Figure 27-3.

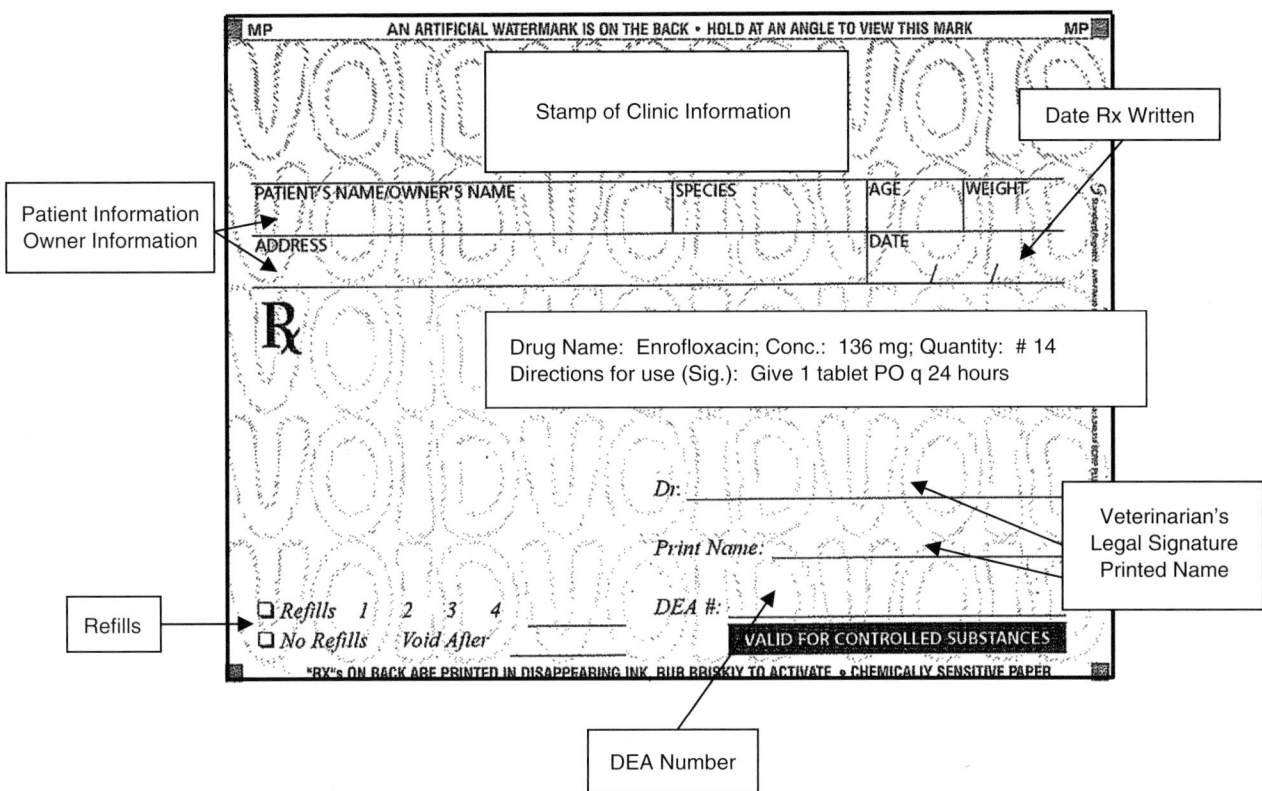

FIGURE 27-2 The parts of a prescription form. Note, when a tamper resistant prescription pad is used any reproductions of the prescription paper (ex. photocopying) activated the hidden watermark "VOID."

TABLE 27-21	Latin Abbreviations Commonly Used and Accepted in Prescription Writing.		
LATIN ABBREVIATION	**INTERPRETATION**	**LATIN ABBREVIATION**	**INTERPRETATION**
a.c.	before meals	o.d.	right eye
a.d.	right ear	o.s.	left eye
a.s.	left ear	o.u.	both eyes
a.u.	both ears	p.c.	after meals
amp.	ampule	p.o.	by mouth
b.i.d.	twice a day	p.r.n.	as needed
c.	with	q. (q. × hour)	every (every × hour)
cap	capsule	q.i.d	4 times a day
cc	cubic centimeter	q.o.d.	every other day
disp.	dispense	q.s.	a sufficient quantity
g or gm	gram	Rx	recipe
ggt(s)	drop(s)	Sig.	directions to patient
h.	hour	stat	immediately
h.s.	at bedtime	SubQ, SQ	subcutaneous
IM	intramuscular	SC, Subcut.	subcutaneous
IO	intraosseous	susp.	suspension
IP	intraperitoneal	t.i.d.	3 times a day
lb.	pound	tab	tablet
m²	meter squared	Tbsp., T	tablespoon (15 ml)
mg	milligrams	tsp., t	teaspoon (5 ml)
ml or mL	milliliter	UT dict	as directed

When medications are dispensed that are intended to go home with the patient to be administered by the owner, a label must be affixed to the bottle or vial with the following information: (1) the name, address, and phone number of the dispensing veterinary clinic or pharmacy; (2) the name of the client; (3) identification of the animal (name and species); (4) the date dispensed; (5) directions for use; (6) the name, concentration, and quantity of the drug dispensed; (7) the name of the prescribing veterinarian; and (8) if the dispensed drug is a controlled substance, the label must contain the following statement: "Caution: Federal law prohibits transfer of this drug to any person other than the patient for whom it was prescribed." In addition, any medication that is dispensed for home use must be provided in a child-resistant container, as required by the Poison Prevention Packaging Act. Other label requirements include precautions, requirements for refrigeration, and for liquid suspensions and other liquids that require them, directions to shake well before use. Figure 27-4 shows a sample prescription label for a noncontrolled drug dispensed for an outpatient.

> **TECHNICIAN NOTE** The abbreviation "s.i.d." is not a universally accepted abbreviation for "once a day" outside of veterinary medicine; therefore, it should not be used in prescription writing. Alternatively, the language "every 24 hours" should be used.

DRUG CALCULATIONS

An important aspect of dispensing and administering drugs is calculating accurate doses, infusion volumes, and

> **Rx:** Enrofloxacin, 136 mg, # 14; **Sig:** give 1 tab PO q 24 hours
>
> **Interpretation:** Dispense 14, 136 mg tablets of enrofloxacin with the following directions for use: Give 1 tablet orally every 24 hours.

FIGURE 27-3 Example of a properly written prescription using common abbreviations to describe directions for use and the correct interpretation of that prescription for accurate filling.

conversions between units of measure. Correctly calculating doses is just as essential to a patient's outcome as is determining an accurate diagnosis and treatment plan. Outlined below are some of the most common calculations made by a veterinary technician, including (1) converting between units of measure; (2) converting the recommended dosage for a patient into the correct drug dose; (3) performing calculations using percent solutions; and (4) performing calculations needed to successfully delivery a drug by constant rate infusion (CRI).

Converting Between Units of Measure

Conversions are most commonly performed between units of measure within the metric system because most drug dosages are expressed as the number of milligrams (mg) of drug per unit body weight in kilograms (kg). By using known conversion factors and keeping track of the units carefully, one can readily calculate conversions between units of measure. Box 27-3 contains some common units of conversion. Conversions between metric and English systems of measures are sometime necessary, especially in association with body weight (pounds to kilograms and kilograms to pounds), or for dispensing medications that use grains as a unit of measure (e.g., aspirin). Sample calculations for converting between units of measure are provided in Box 27-4 and Table 27-22.

Calculating the Correct Drug Dose

Most often, the veterinarian will prescribe the dose of a drug in milligrams (mg) or will indicate the dosage to be

Patient's Name: _____ ; Species: _____

Rx # _____ ; MR # _____ ; Date: _____

_____ ; Drug Name: _____ ; Concentration: _____

Sig: _____

Prescribed By: _____

Special Instructions: _____

Refill # _____ ; Refill Exp. Date: _____ ; Drug Exp. Date: _____

Rx Dispensed By: _____ ; Drug Mfg.: _____

Stamp of Clinic's Name; Address; Phone Number

FIGURE 27-4 Sample prescription label for a drug (noncontrolled substance) dispensed for an outpatient. *Definitions:* Rx #: prescription number; MR #: medical record number; #: quantity of tablets dispensed; Sig: directions for use; Prescribed by: name of prescribing doctor; Dispensed by: name of person who dispensed the medication; Drug Mfg: Drug manufacturer. Note that the "patient's name" should include the client's last name.

BOX 27-3	Common Units of Conversion

Metric System Conversions
1 kilogram (kg) = 1000 grams (g)
1 g = 1000 milligrams (mg)
1 mg = 1000 micrograms (μg or mcg)
1 μg = 1000 nanograms (ng)
1 liter (L) = 1000 milliliters (ml)
100 ml = 1 deciliter (dl)
1 ml = 1000 microliters (μl or mcl)
1 cc = 1 ml

Metric-to-English System Conversions
1 kg = 2.2 lb
1 grain (gr) = 64.8 mg

BOX 27-4	Sample Calculations for Conversion Between Units of Measure

I. A dog's body weight was recorded in the medical record in pounds (lb). Convert this dog's weight (95 lb) to kilograms (kg).

$$95 \text{ lb } (1 \text{ kg}/2.2 \text{ lb})$$

Cancelling units = 95 l̶b̶ (1 kg/2.2 l̶b̶) = 43.2 kg

II. A cat is prescribed buprenorphine at a dosage of 30 mcg/kg for transmucosal administration. The concentration of buprenorphine in the vial is 0.3 mg/ml. Convert the dosage of buprenorphine from mcg/kg to mg/kg.

$$30 \text{ mcg/kg } (1 \text{ mg}/1000 \text{ mcg})$$

Cancelling units = 30 m̶c̶g̶/kg (1 mg/1000 m̶c̶g̶)
= 0.03 mg/kg of buprenorphine

III. A dog is prescribed cephalexin at a dosage of 1000 mg orally twice a day. The pharmacy has 1-gram capsules of cephalexin. Convert the dosage of cephalexin from milligrams (mg) to grams (g), so that you can determine the number of capsules to dispense for a 3-week course of therapy.

$$1000 \text{ mg } (1 \text{ g}/1000 \text{ mg})$$

Cancelling units = 1000 m̶g̶ (1 g/1000 m̶g̶)
= 1 gram of cephalexin per dose

IV. Most drug dosages are expressed as the number of milligrams of drug per kilogram of body weight (mg/kg), but many chemotherapeutic agent dosages are expressed as the number of milligrams/body surface area. Using Table 27-22, calculate the body surface in m^2 for a dog weighing 25 kg.

$$25 \text{ kg } (0.85 \text{ m}^2/25 \text{ kg})$$

Cancelling units = 25 k̶g̶ (0.85 m^2/25 k̶g̶)
= 0.85 m^2 of body surface area

TABLE 27-22	Converting Body Weight (kg) to Body Surface Area (m²)				

WEIGHT, KG	SURFACE AREA, M²	WEIGHT, KG	SURFACE AREA, M²
DOGS		CATS	
0.5	0.06	2	0.159
1	0.1	2.5	0.184
2	0.15	3	0.208
3	0.2	3.5	0.231
4	0.25	4	0.252
5	0.29	4.5	0.273
6	0.33	5	0.292
7	0.36	5.5	0.311
8	0.4	6	0.33
9	0.43	6.5	0.348
10	0.46	7	0.366
11	0.49	7.5	0.383
12	0.52	8	0.4
13	0.55	8.5	0.416
14	0.58	9	0.432
15	0.6	9.5	0.449
16	0.63	10	0.464
17	0.66		
18	0.69		
19	0.71		
20	0.74		
21	0.76		
22	0.78		
23	0.81		
24	0.83		
25	0.85		
26	0.88		
27	0.9		
28	0.92		
29	0.94		
30	0.96		
32	1.01		
34	1.05		
36	1.09		
38	1.13		
40	1.17		
42	1.21		
44	1.25		
46	1.28		
50	1.36		
54	1.44		
58	1.51		
62	1.58		
66	1.65		
70	1.72		
74	1.78		
80	1.88		

administered in milligrams per kilogram of body weight (mg/kg). In either case, depending on the formulation of the drug, the veterinary technician administering the drug will need to calculate the amount of drug to be administered to the patient in milligrams (mg) or milliliters (ml). Calculating the dose of an oral drug in milligrams (mg) or the dose of an injectable solution in milliliters (ml) requires careful unit conversions, knowledge of the patient's weight, and knowledge of the concentration of the drug in a solid dosage form (tablet or capsule), or in the case of an injectable drug, the concentration of the drug dissolved in solution (Box 27-5).

> **TECHNICIAN NOTE** Most often, the veterinarian will prescribe the dose of a drug in milligrams (mg) or will indicate the dosage to be administered in milligrams per kilogram of body weight (mg/kg). In either case, depending on the formulation of the drug, the veterinary technician administering the drug will need to calculate the amount of drug to be administered to the patient in milligrams (mg) or milliliters (ml).

BOX 27-5	Sample Calculations for Calculating Correct Drug Dosage

I. Dr. Smith just diagnosed pneumonia in a 30-kg dog and would like to prescribe doxycycline at a dosage of 5 mg/kg orally every 12 hours. Calculate the dose of doxycycline (in mg) that needs to be administered twice a day.

$$5 \text{ mg/kg (30 kg)}$$

Cancelling units = 5 mg/~~kg~~ (30 ~~kg~~) = 150 mg of doxycycline

II. You need to administer 30 mcg/kg of buprenorphine via the transmucosal route to a cat that weighs 5 kg. Buprenorphine is available as a 0.3-mg/ml solution. Calculate the volume (in ml) of buprenorphine that needs to be administered to this cat.

$$30 \text{ mcg/kg (5 kg)}$$

Cancelling units = 30 mcg/~~kg~~ (5 ~~kg~~)
= 150 ~~mcg~~ (1 ~~mg~~/1000 ~~mcg~~)/0.3 ~~mg~~/ml)
= 0.5 ml of buprenorphine

III. As mentioned previously, most drug dosages are expressed as the number of milligrams of drug per kilogram of body weight (mg/kg), but many chemotherapeutic agent dosages are expressed as the number of milligrams/body surface area. Using Table 27-22, calculate the dose of vincristine (recommended dosage of 0.5 mg/m²) to be administered to a 50-kg dog.

$$50 \text{ kg (1.36 m}^2/50 \text{ kg)}$$

Cancelling units − 50 ~~kg~~ (1.36 m²/50 ~~kg~~)
= 1.36 ~~m²~~ (0.5 mg/~~m²~~)
= 0.68 mg of vincristine

Using Percent Solutions

Use of injectable drugs with concentration expressed as percent of the drug in solution can create much confusion for many technicians and veterinarians alike. The fundamental concept to keep in mind when working with percent solutions is that this way of expressing concentration is equivalent to a ratio of parts of the drug per 100 parts of solution.

Percent solutions can be expressed as vol/vol, meaning the number of milliliters of a drug in 100 ml of solution. For example, a 10% solution (vol/vol) contains 10 ml of drug in 100 ml of solution. Percent solutions can also be expressed as weight/vol, meaning the number of grams of drug in 100 ml of solution. For example, a 10% (weight/vol) solution contains 10 g of drug in a total of 100 ml of solution. Percent solutions can be expressed as weight/weight, meaning the number of grams of drug in 100 g of a mixture. For example, a 10% weight/weight solution contains 10 g of drug in a total of 100 g of a mixture (Box 27-6).

BOX 27-6	Sample Calculation Using Percent Solutions

I. You need to administer a 140-mg/kg loading dose of N-acetylcysteine (NAC) to a 20-kg dog by IV infusion over 1 hour. The NAC must be diluted in 5% dextrose solution to a concentration of 5%. NAC is commercially available as a 20% solution.
  a. Calculate the loading dose of NAC to be administered to this patient.

$$140 \text{ mg/kg (20 kg)}$$

Cancelling units = 140 mg/~~kg~~ (20 ~~kg~~) = 2800 mg NAC

  b. Determine the volume of 20% NAC solution that needs to be drawn up for dilution to 5%.

$$2800 \text{ mg NAC (1 g/1000 mg)/(20 g/100 ml)}$$

Cancelling units = 2800 ~~mg~~ NAC (1 ~~g~~/1000 ~~mg~~)/
(20 ~~g~~/100 ml)
= 14 ml of 20% NAC

  c. Determine the total infusion volume of 5% NAC to be administered, and determine the infusion rate to complete the 5% NAC infusion over 1 hour.

$$14 \text{ ml (20 g/100 ml)/(5 g/100 ml)}$$

Cancelling units = 14 ~~ml~~ (20 ~~g~~/100 ~~ml~~)/(5 ~~g~~/100 ml)
= 56 ml of infusion volume
Infusion rate of 56 ml/hour

  d. Determine the volume of 5% dextrose that needs to be added to the calculated volume of 20% NAC solution to provide the appropriate dose of NAC to this dog as a 5% solution.

$$56 \text{ ml total volume} − 14 \text{ ml 20\% NAC}$$
= 42 ml of 5% dextrose to be added

BOX 27-7	Sample Calculation of Constant Rate Infusions

I. A 30-kg dog was just diagnosed with ventricular tachycardia and requires an immediate IV infusion of lidocaine. An initial loading dosage of 1.5 mg/kg is recommended, followed by a constant rate infusion (CRI) of 50 mcg/kg/minute.
   a. Calculate the loading dose of lidocaine for this dog.

$$30 \text{ kg } (1.5 \text{ mg/kg})$$

$$\text{Cancelling units} = 30 \cancel{\text{ kg}} (1.5 \text{ mg/}\cancel{\text{kg}}) = 45 \text{ mg of lidocaine}$$

   b. Calculate the amount of lidocaine (in mg) that needs to be added to a 1000-ml bag of Normosol R, which is currently running at an infusion rate of 65 ml/hour.

$$M = (D \times W \times V)/(R) = (50 \text{ mcg/kg/minute}) (30 \text{ kg}) (1000 \text{ ml})/(65 \text{ ml/hour}) (1 \text{ hour/}60 \text{ minutes})$$

$$\text{Cancelling units} = (50 \text{ mcg/}\cancel{\text{kg}}/\cancel{\text{minute}}) (30 \cancel{\text{ kg}}) (1000 \cancel{\text{ ml}})/(65 \cancel{\text{ ml}}/\cancel{\text{hour}}) (1 \cancel{\text{ hour}}/60 \cancel{\text{ minutes}})$$

$$= 1,384,615 \cancel{\text{ mcg}} (1 \text{ mg/}1000 \cancel{\text{ mcg}})$$

$$= 1384 \text{ mg of lidocaine needs to be added to } 1000 \text{ ml of Normosol R}$$

   c. Calculate the volume (in ml) of a 2% lidocaine solution that would need to be added to the 1000-ml bag of Normosol R to provide 1384 mg of lidocaine.

$$= 1384 \text{ mg of lidocaine/}(2 \text{ g/}100 \text{ ml lidocaine solution}) (1000 \text{ mg/}1 \text{ g})$$

$$\text{Cancelling units} = 1384 \cancel{\text{ mg}}/(2 \cancel{\text{ g}}/100 \text{ ml lidocaine solution}) (1000 \cancel{\text{ mg}}/1 \cancel{\text{ g}}) = 65.9 \text{ ml of lidocaine}$$

II. In some cases, an IV infusion pump may not be available. Therefore, it may be necessary to convert an infusion rate from milliliters/hour to drops/minute. Convert an infusion rate of 10 ml/hour to drops/minute with a drip set capable of delivering 15 drops/ml.

$$10 \text{ ml/hour} (15 \text{ drops/ml}) (1 \text{ hour/}60 \text{ minutes})$$

$$\text{Cancelling units} = 10 \cancel{\text{ ml}}/\cancel{\text{hour}} (15 \text{ drops/}\cancel{\text{ml}}) (1 \cancel{\text{ hour}}/60 \text{ minutes})$$

$$= 2.5 \text{ drops/minute}$$

Constant Rate Infusion (CRI)

Some drugs are delivered intravenously using a constant rate infusion (CRI) of drug (usually expressed in micrograms or milligrams per unit time). Drugs are delivered as CRI for a variety of reasons. Some drugs such as fentanyl and dobutamine are given by CRI because their half-life is so short that intermittent bolus dosing is not effective. Other drugs such as metoclopramide are more efficacious when given by CRI. CRIs are also used when dehydration is severe enough to impair absorption of a drug given subcutaneously or intramuscularly (as may happen when regular insulin is used to treat a diabetic ketoacidotic patient that is dehydrated). When CRI is given, an appropriate volume of the drug must be added to an appropriate volume of base solution (often a bag of IV fluids). The following equation can be used to calculate the amount of drug (in micrograms or milligrams) that should be added to the base solution when a CRI is prepared (Box 27-7).

$M = (D \times W \times V)/(R)$

M = Amount of drug (mcg or mg) to be added to the base solution

D = Dosage (mcg/kg/minute or mg/kg/minute)

W = Body weight (kg)

V = Volume of base solution (ml)

R = Infusion rate (ml/minute)

> **TECHNICIAN NOTE** When a CRI is calculated, the formula $M = (D \times W \times V)/(R)$ can be used to calculate the amount of drug (in micrograms or milligrams) to be added to the base solution (often a bag of fluids); where:
> M = Amount of drug (**mcg** or **mg**) to be added to the base solution
> D = Dosage (**mcg/kg/minute** or **mg/kg/minute**)
> W = Body weight in **kg**
> V = Volume of base solution (**ml**)
> R = Infusion rate (**ml/minute**)

> **TECHNICIAN NOTE** The single most important rule in successfully performing drug calculations is to keep track of the units; this oftentimes requires writing out the equations and cancelling the units.

RECOMMENDED READINGS

American Veterinary Medical Association: Best management practices for pharmaceutical disposal, 2009. Available at: https://www.avma.org/KB/Policies/Pages/Best-Management-Practices-for-Pharmaceutical-Disposal.aspx (accessed on September 28, 2012).

Dowling P: Geriatric pharmacology, Vet Clin Small Anim 35:557, 2005.

Food and Drug Administration: Animal Medicinal Drug Use Clarification Act (AMDUCA), 1994. Available at: http://www.fda.gov/RegulatoryInformation/Legislation/FederalFoodDrugandCosmeticActFDCAct/SignificantAmendmentstotheFDCAct/AnimalMedicinalDrugUseClarificationActAMDUCAof1994/default.htm (accessed on September 16, 2012).

Food and Drug Administration, Center for Veterinary Medicine: Compliance policy guides (CPG), 2012. Available at: http://www.fda.gov/ICECI/ComplianceManuals/CompliancePolicyGuidanceManual/ucm117042.htm (accessed on September 28, 2012).

National Association of Boards of Pharmacy: Verified Internet Pharmacy Practice Sites (VIPPS), 2011. Available at: http://www.nabp.net/programs/accreditation/vipps/ (accessed on September 16, 2012).

Nicholson BT, Center SA, Randolph JF, et al: Effects of oral ursodeoxycholic acid in healthy cats on clinicopathological parameters, serum bile acids and light microscopic and ultrastructural features of the liver, Res Vet Sci 61:258, 1996.

North American Compendiums: Compendium of veterinary products, Port Huron, MI, 2010, North American Compendiums.

Occupational and Safety Health Administration: OSHA technical manual: controlling occupational exposure to hazardous drugs, Washington, DC, 2005, U.S. Department of Labor, OSHA.

Papich M: Drug compounding for veterinary patients, The AAPS Journal 7:E281, 2005.

Papich M: Saunders handbook of veterinary drugs, St Louis, 2006, Saunders.

Plumb D: Veterinary drug handbook, ed 7, White Bear Lake, MN, 2011, Wiley-Blackwell.

Rannazzisi JC, Caverly MW: Practitioner's Manual- an informational outline of the controlled substance act of 1970, Springfield, VA, 2006. U.S. Department of Justice, Drug Enforcement Administration. Available at http://www.deadiversion.usdoj.gov/pubs/manuals/pract/index.html (accessed on Septermber 28, 2012).

Slater MG, Rogers K: Long-term health and predictors of survival for hyperthyroid cats treated with iodine 131, J Vet Intern Med 15:47, 2001.

Thomson A: Back to basics: pharmacokinetics, Pharm J 272:769, 2004.

Thomson A: Why do therapeutic drug monitoring? Pharm J 273:153, 2004.

U.S. Department of Agriculture: Food Animal Residue Avoidance Database (FARAD), 2011. Available at: http://www.farad.org/ (accessed on September 16, 2012).

28 Pain Management

Nancy Shaffran and Tamara Grubb

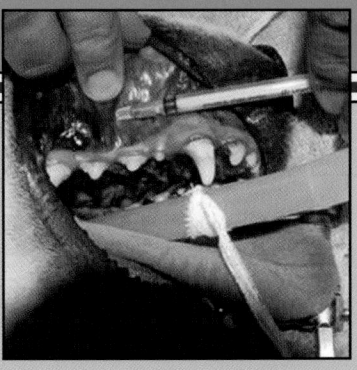

OUTLINE

The Role of the Veterinary Technician as a Patient Advocate, 1047
Communication, 1047
Patient Assessment, 1047
Signs of Pain, 1048
The Science of Pain Management, 1049
Pain Is Bad, 1049
Physiology of Pain, 1051
Treatment of Pain in Small Animals, 1053
Environmental and Emotional Care, 1053
Principles of Administering Analgesia, 1053

Administration of Analgesics and Analgesic Techniques, 1054
Treatment of Pain in Large Animals, 1062
Identifying and Anticipating Pain, 1062
Treating Pain in Large Animals, 1064
Species-Specific Information, 1071
Horses, 1071
Cattle, Sheep, and Goats, 1071
Camelids, 1073
Pigs, 1073
Summary, 1073

KEY TERMS

Agonist
Allodynia
Antagonist
Dysphoria
Hyperalgesia
Modulation
Multimodal analgesia
Neurotransmitter
Nociception
Preemptive Analgesia
Transduction
Transmission
Wind-up phenomenon

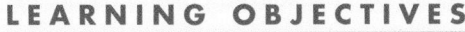

LEARNING OBJECTIVES

When you have completed this chapter, you will be able to:

1. Pronounce, define, and spell all Key Terms in the chapter.
2. Explain how the technician can use effective communication, observation, and interpretation skills to advocate for the patient and to help provide effective and appropriate analgesia.
3. List common causes and physiologic and behavioral signs of pain in small animals, including the negative effects of untreated pain.
4. Describe the physiologic aspects of pain, including the phases of nociception in mammals; and, compare and contrast acute, chronic, inflammatory, neuropathic, somatic, and visceral pain, and explain the significance of the "wind-up phenomenon."
5. Do the following regarding treatment of pain in small animals:
   • Describe the basic principles of effective analgesia protocol design and pain management, including the concepts of preemptive and multimodal analgesia.
   • Compare and contrast agents used to treat pain in small animals, including nonsteroidal anti-inflammatory drugs (NSAIDs), local anesthetics, opioids, and alpha$_2$ agonists.
   • List the analgesics commonly given by constant rate infusion (CRI), and perform the calculations required to administer a drug by CRI.
   • List the "adjunctive analgesics" and nonpharmacologic treatment options for pain control; describe the uses and benefits of each.
6. Do the following regarding the treatment of pain in large animals:
   • List causes and signs of pain in large animals, and explain why large animals often are undertreated for pain.
   • Compare and contrast agents used to treat pain in large animals, including NSAIDs, opioids, alpha$_2$ agonists, and local anesthetics.
   • Discuss the role of joint supplements, chondroprotective agents, miscellaneous agents, alternative and complementary therapy, and good husbandry in the treatment of pain in large animals.
7. Describe analgesic agents and techniques commonly used in horses, cattle, sheep, goats, camelids, and pigs; and, explain how economics and drug residues influence the decision to treat pain in food animals.

INTRODUCTION

In recent years, the practice of pain management has become mainstream in veterinary medicine. Optimal use of analgesic drugs, combinations, methods of administration, and alternative therapies are still being developed as more is learned about the way animals feel and express pain. The search also continues for the most objective, scientific methods of measuring and assessing pain in nonverbal patients. Technicians continue to play a vital part in the field of pain management. Many veterinarians rely heavily on the ability of the veterinary technician to recognize and report animal pain and use this input to guide decision making. This is not surprising given the huge role that nurses have played in pain management for nonverbal human patients. Human neonatal and pediatric nurses and veterinary technicians share the position of patient advocate, giving patients a voice and attending to their needs. However, unlike in human medicine, veterinary technicians typically do this without the help of parents, who play a large role in advocating for their hospitalized children.

The role of advocate for a nonverbal patient can be daunting. Veterinary technicians are responsible for the quality of patient care and the overall condition of patients but do not have the freedom to prescribe or initiate therapy. This sometimes can result in frustration while the technician pursues a positive response from veterinarians toward giving analgesia. Knowledge of the physiology of pain and the pharmacology of analgesics is essential for good communication between veterinarians and veterinary technicians. Optimally, the veterinarian regards the technician as an integral member of the pain management team. The skilled technician is a source of vital information required to choose and administer appropriate analgesics. He or she is a trusted caretaker for recovering patients. The success of this relationship is terribly important for all hospitalized patients regardless of whether the case is elective, routine, or extraordinary.

THE ROLE OF THE VETERINARY TECHNICIAN AS A PATIENT ADVOCATE

COMMUNICATION

Technicians use critical thinking, observation, and interpretation skills to make important pain management recommendations. Discussion about each case directly with the clinician might include the technician's particular concerns about a patient or a general approach to managing different types of pain. Based on his or her interaction with patients, the technician may offer suggestions for adjustments in analgesic regimens, changes or additions to drug protocols, or the possible addition of sedatives, if needed.

Veterinary technicians often complain that their requests for patient analgesia go unheeded. The actual method of communication used plays a large part in achieving a positive outcome. For example, "Can I give Charlie something for pain?" is inadequate to convey the situation and often results in the response, "No." To be effective, technicians must present two sets of information: what the patient is doing that indicates painfulness, and what has already been done that is considered inadequate. For example, "Dr. X, yesterday's cruciate repair, the black Lab, Charlie, is not doing as well as I would like. Despite the fact that his bladder is empty and I have offered him food and water, he seems restless and has difficulty getting comfortable. He is panting excessively, although his temperature is normal. I checked the bandage, and it does not seem too tight. The record says he received morphine last night at midnight, which allowed him to sleep for 4 hours, but he has not had any since. May I give him a repeat dose to see if it makes him more comfortable?" This approach delivers the necessary information to gain the veterinarian's confidence in the technician's assessment skills and knowledge of the case. He or she is much more likely to agree to administer pain medication under these circumstances.

Technicians can also play a vital role in the administration of preemptive medication, which is often overlooked in a busy hospital setting. For example, "I have noticed a difference in the recovery of animals that are given a dose of NSAID [nonsteroidal anti-inflammatory drug] before surgery. Would you like me to give an NSAID to this patient now?" This approach also applies to the placement of transdermal analgesic patches, the administration of constant rate infusions (CRIs), and the performance of local or regional nerve blocks. Technicians should provide as much feedback as possible as to which analgesic protocols are working well, and which need to be improved to increase patient comfort.

PATIENT ASSESSMENT

Historically, animal pain has been recognized and treated only in those patients that display overt behavioral signs, such as vocalization. When clinicians wait for signs, patients are forced to prove that they are in pain before they are given analgesics. In reality, dogs and cats instinctively hide pain just as they would in the wild to avoid becoming prey. Once animals display obvious signs of pain, the pain intensity that they are experiencing is likely to be severe. Old or severely debilitated patients may be too ill or weak to display changes in behavior. Patients should never be required to prove that they are in pain. A sound approach to pain management favors anticipation of the severity and duration of pain that is likely to occur with any procedure, condition, or surgery. In many cases, animals do "appear" to tolerate pain better than humans. Several explanations may be put forth for this. In contrast to the pain detection threshold (the point at which pain nerve fibers are stimulated to send signals), pain tolerance (the greatest intensity of pain that is voluntarily tolerated) varies widely between species and between individuals within a species. Like humans, animals tolerate pain to a certain point before they show changes in their behavior. Awareness that patients may exhibit a wide range of pain tolerance and a broad spectrum of behaviors can improve pain recognition and treatment. Recently, research in pain management has shifted toward identifying and even predicting known painful events. For example, severe pain is expected with cervical disc herniation, extensive inflammation, medical or surgical fracture repair, limb amputation, declawing, ear canal ablation, and so forth. Moderate to mild pain is expected with cruciate repair, laparotomy, mass removal, castration, dental procedures, and so forth. This approach encourages us to treat patients that undergo painful procedures or disease processes without requiring proof. It does not, however, consider the vast variation in pain tolerance among individuals. It seems reasonable to incorporate both concepts to develop a truly effective analgesic plan (i.e., to have direction given by what are known to be painful events and to be prepared to provide adequate analgesia for the expected level of pain, but also to look at the individual and to tailor analgesic protocols accordingly). A more complete list of anticipated levels of pain associated with surgical procedures, illnesses, or injuries is available in *Veterinary Clinics of North America*, July 2000.

Technicians observe patients closely for extended periods and usually are the first to notice changes in status. Familiarity with individual patients' personalities and usual reactions to stimuli gives insight into the meaning of behaviors. Experience establishes expectations of how particular patients may react to painful stimuli. This includes differences in expression between dogs and cats and young and old, and variations among certain breeds. For example, Siberian Huskies and Dobermans, which vocalize regularly, are thought to be more "sensitive" to pain or to possess a lower pain threshold than other breeds, whereas Pit Bulls and Labrador Retrievers appear to remain stoic in the face of pain. The skilled technician factors this into his or her pain assessments.

> **TECHNICIAN NOTE**　Companion animals retain survival instincts despite being bred into captivity. These instincts include a drive to hide pain from potential predators so that they do not appear to be weak compared with the rest of the pack. Much to their detriment in a setting without predators, dogs and cats attempt to hide pain from us. Because of this, many animals probably reach a high threshold of pain before showing changes in behavior. Conversely, some animals express more pain than expected. This may indicate an unusually low pain threshold, and the situation should be managed appropriately.

SIGNS OF PAIN

Pain is seldom diagnosed in veterinary medicine on the basis of a single observation or physiologic value. Because pain is an individual, subjective experience, assessment depends on the combination of good examination skills; familiarity with species, breed, and individual behavior; knowledge of the degree of pain associated with particular surgical procedures or illnesses; and recognition of the signs of stress and pain.

Signs of pain in animals can be categorized as physiologic or behavioral (Table 28-1). Physiologic pain signs may be obvious and include increased heart rate and blood pressure, increased respiratory rate, and vocalization. More subtle behavioral changes, such as general restlessness, decreased appetite, not sleeping, resenting handling, and not assuming a normal position, may be even more significant. Clinical signs of pain in dogs and cats most often reported include tachycardia, increased respiratory rate, restlessness, increased temperature, increased blood pressure, abnormal posturing, inappetence, aggression, frequent movement, facial expression, trembling, depression, and insomnia. Less frequently reported are anxiety; nausea; pupillary enlargement; licking, chewing, and staring at the surgical site or wound; poor mucous membrane (MM) color; salivation; decreased carbon dioxide (CO_2); and head pressing.

Clinical manifestations may be different between species and even among different members of the same species. For dogs, standing or sitting for long periods and sleeping in an atypical position are considered pain signs. For cats, abnormal posture, hiding, and aggression are ranked as common pain signs. Because the signs of pain are so varied and diverse, any abnormal sign in a veterinary patient that cannot be attributed to another cause is suspected of indicating pain.

> **TECHNICIAN NOTE**　Signs of pain vary among animals. Patients should assume normal positions (what you would expect to see at home) while caged in the hospital. Standing for long periods or sleeping in an abnormal position indicates discomfort. Normal posture and behavior is a good indication that the patient is comfortable.

All patients should be evaluated for pain upon admission and at regular intervals throughout the hospitalization period. The observer's subjective opinion and physiologic signs can be described using a pain scale, such as a visual analogue scale (VAS). A good pain scale for dogs and cats developed at Colorado State University (CSU) uses numeric, pictorial, and descriptive assessments (Figure 28-1).

Veterinary technicians are trained to recognize animal pain. By nature, technicians are skillful observers of behavioral changes in patients, noticing the subtlest expressions of potential pain. Most experienced technicians have an innate sense of how painful most procedures, conditions, and surgeries are likely to be based on repeated prolonged exposure to animals in the recovery phase. However, it is often difficult for even the most experienced technician to distinguish between pain and other stress. For example, postoperative patients frequently display aberrant behavior for several minutes up to hours after surgery. These behaviors may

TABLE 28-1	Behavioral Signs of Pain in Dogs and Cats			
POSTURE	**TEMPERAMENT**	**VOCALIZATION**	**LOCOMOTION**	**OTHER**
Dogs				
Tail between legs	Aggressive	Barking	Reluctance to move	Unable to perform normal
Arched or hunched back	Clawing	Howling	Carrying one leg	tasks
Twisted body to protect pain site	Attacking, biting	Moaning	Lameness	Attacks other animals or
Drooped head	Escaping	Whimpering	Unusual gait	people if pain site is
Prolonged sitting position			Unable to walk	touched (self-trauma)
Tucked abdomen			Chewing painful areas	No interest in food or play
Lying in flat, extended position				
Cats				
Tucked limbs	Aggressive	Crying	Reluctance to move	Attacks if pain site is
Arched or hunched head and	Biting	Hissing	Carrying one leg	touched
neck or back	Scratching	Spitting	Lameness	Failure to groom
Tucked abdomen	Chewing	Moaning	Unusual gait	Dilated pupils
Lying flat	Attacking	Screaming	Unable to walk	No interest in food or play
Slumped body	Escaping	Purring	Inactive	
Drooped head	Hiding			

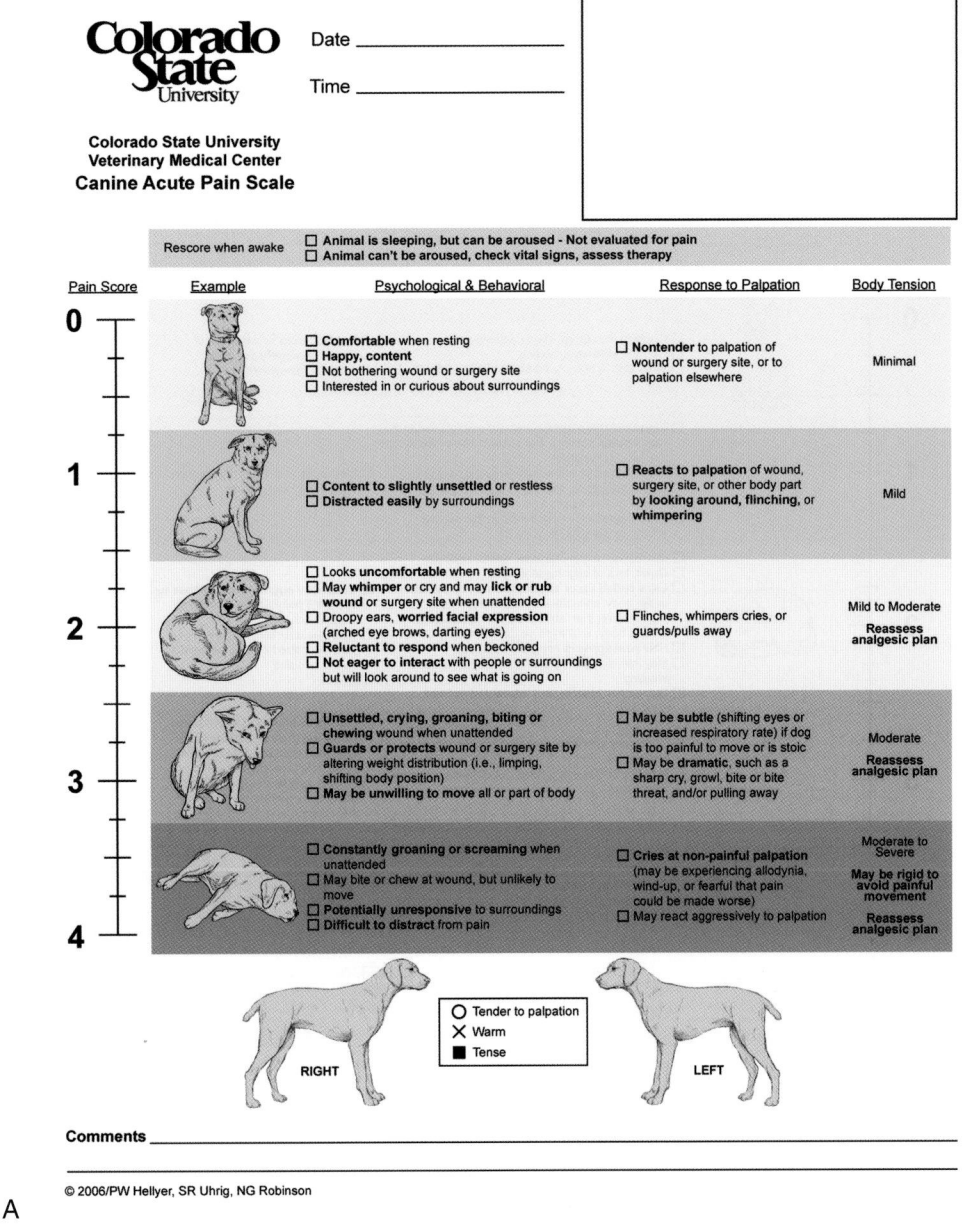

Colorado State University

Date _____

Time _____

Colorado State University
Veterinary Medical Center
Canine Acute Pain Scale

Rescore when awake

☐ Animal is sleeping, but can be aroused - Not evaluated for pain
☐ Animal can't be aroused, check vital signs, assess therapy

Pain Score	Example	Psychological & Behavioral	Response to Palpation	Body Tension
0		☐ **Comfortable** when resting ☐ **Happy, content** ☐ Not bothering wound or surgery site ☐ Interested in or curious about surroundings	☐ **Nontender** to palpation of wound or surgery site, or to palpation elsewhere	Minimal
1		☐ **Content to slightly unsettled** or restless ☐ **Distracted easily** by surroundings	☐ **Reacts to palpation** of wound, surgery site, or other body part by **looking around, flinching,** or **whimpering**	Mild
2		☐ Looks **uncomfortable** when resting ☐ May **whimper** or cry and may **lick or rub** wound or surgery site when unattended ☐ Droopy ears, **worried facial expression** (arched eye brows, darting eyes) ☐ **Reluctant to respond** when beckoned ☐ **Not eager to interact** with people or surroundings but will look around to see what is going on	☐ Flinches, whimpers cries, or guards/pulls away	Mild to Moderate **Reassess analgesic plan**
3		☐ **Unsettled, crying, groaning, biting or chewing** wound when unattended ☐ **Guards or protects** wound or surgery site by altering weight distribution (i.e., limping, shifting body position) ☐ **May be unwilling to move** all or part of body	☐ May be **subtle** (shifting eyes or increased respiratory rate) if dog is too painful to move or is stoic ☐ May be **dramatic**, such as a sharp cry, growl, bite or bite threat, and/or pulling away	Moderate **Reassess analgesic plan**
4		☐ **Constantly groaning or screaming** when unattended ☐ May bite or chew at wound, but unlikely to move ☐ **Potentially unresponsive** to surroundings ☐ **Difficult to distract** from pain	☐ **Cries at non-painful palpation** (may be experiencing allodynia, wind-up, or fearful that pain could be made worse) ☐ May react aggressively to palpation	Moderate to Severe **May be rigid to avoid painful movement** **Reassess analgesic plan**

RIGHT   LEFT

○ Tender to palpation
✕ Warm
■ Tense

Comments _____

© 2006/PW Hellyer, SR Uhrig, NG Robinson

A

FIGURE 28-1 Colorado State University (CSU) pain scale for dogs **(A)** and cats **(B)**. (Acute animal pain scales developed by P. Hellyer, et al, at CSU for assessment of pain in dogs and cats. Available at: www.IVAPM.org [accessed on September 16, 2012].)

include vocalization, thrashing, rolling, self-mutilation, and tachypnea. When these behaviors are thought to be related to stress other than pain, they are often referred to as **dysphoria** (an emotional state characterized by anxiety, depression, or unease). *Dysphoria* is a general term that does not specify a cause. Abnormal postoperative behaviors sometimes are referred to as *emergence delirium* attributed to residual gas anesthetics. Some animals do in fact display this response upon awakening, but anesthetic-related behaviors should resolve within several minutes. Behaviors that persist beyond a few minutes require further investigation and attention. In any case, it can be difficult to discern between pain, dysphoria, and reaction to narcotics or general anesthetics. Rapid control of the patient using sedation and analgesia is essential, regardless of the cause of pain.

THE SCIENCE OF PAIN MANAGEMENT

PAIN IS BAD

Today in human medicine, preventing and treating pain are recognized as essential parts of overall patient management. Pain is considered to play such an important role in overall health and well-being that pain is now regarded as a fifth vital sign, ranking it of equal importance with temperature, pulse, respiration, and blood pressure. Not only do human

FIGURE 28-1, cont'd

health care providers view pain as a symptom of an underlying disease or condition, they view pain as an important syndrome in its own right because of the vast array of negative physiologic events attributable to pain, regardless of the patient's underlying disease or condition.

Pain triggers a series of physiologic changes that increase stress. Although the nervous system is the main target of pain transmission and provides the means for the body to react to that information, the body's response to pain signals is not limited to the nervous system. Most, if not all, of the body's major systems are affected by inadequately controlled pain (Box 28-1). For example, increased cortisol levels that accompany pain may interfere with wound healing and may reduce the immune system's ability to work effectively. In addition to suppressing the immune system, increased sympathetic nervous system activity associated with unrelieved pain may result in increased catabolism and metabolic rate, anorexia, ileus, and atelectasis. The cardiovascular system can also be adversely affected, resulting in increased heart rate and blood pressure, irregular heart rhythms, and coagulopathies. Reducing or suppressing the stress response by managing pain can minimize adverse effects on the entire body. Given the potential consequences listed previously, it becomes obvious that, as with humans, animals in pain require more intensive medical care than those in which pain is adequately managed. The standards of the American Animal Hospital Association (AAHA) require pain assessment in every patient, regardless of the presenting

Cardiovascular System
Arrhythmias

Gastrointestinal System
Nausea, vomiting

Pulmonary System
Tachypnea
Hypoxemia
Pulmonary edema
Pulmonary hypertension
Respiratory acid-base imbalance

Renal System
Renal hypertension

Metabolic System
Cachexia
Increased oxygen demand
Negative nitrogen balance

Immune Function
Hemorrhage

Sleep Pattern
Behavior changes

| BOX 28-2 | Summary of AAHA Pain Management Standards |

- Pain assessment for every patient, regardless of presenting complaint
- Assessment recorded in the medical record
- Use of preemptive pain management
- Appropriate pain management for anticipated level and duration
- Pain management with ALL surgical procedures
- Reassessment for pain throughout procedures
- Medical and chronic pain also treated
- Written protocols
- Teaching clients to recognize pain in their pets

AAHA, American Animal Hospital Association.

complaint. Other requirements include making repeat regular assessments throughout hospitalization and recording those assessments in the medical record. A full listing of AAHA pain management standards can be found on its website at www.aahanet.org/ (Box 28-2).

PHYSIOLOGY OF PAIN
Nociception and the Pain Pathway

From a physiologic standpoint, pain is processed identically in all mammals. **Nociception**, derived from the Latin word *nocere* ("to injure"), includes three distinct phases: **transduction**, **transmission**, and **modulation**. The pain pathway begins at the site of tissue damage (evidenced by localized redness, heat, and swelling—classic signs of inflammation).

Regardless of the cause of inflammation (e.g., injury, tumor, surgical incision), nociceptors (pain receptors) are stimulated. These specialized nerve endings convert mechanical, chemical, and thermal energy into electrical impulses (transduction) once their threshold is exceeded. If the noxious stimulus is large enough to exceed the nociceptor's threshold, a nerve impulse is generated and transmitted along peripheral nerves to the spinal cord (transmission). These nerve fibers are highly specialized to carry pain information and are distinct from other nerve fibers that typically carry pleasant or neutral sensations. Once at the spinal cord, a nerve impulse may be projected upward to the thalamus and then to other parts of the brain, or it may be transmitted to a nerve cell located entirely within the central nervous system (CNS) that activates sympathetic reflexes (Figure 28-2). In this way, the sensation of pain is dampened (modulation).

The fourth phase of the pain pathway is perception. Perception occurs in the conscious brain and is the awareness that "I hurt." Although the terms *pain* and *nociception* are often used interchangeably, they are not synonymous. What differentiates nociception from pain is consciousness. This means that patients under a general anesthetic (unconscious) do not perceive that they are in pain. However, nociception occurs even when an animal is in a state of unconsciousness.

> **TECHNICIAN NOTE**   Without the benefits of analgesia, the nervous system is still activated to process pain signals, triggering negative physiologic effects, even though no pain-related behaviors are seen.

As anesthesia wears off and consciousness returns, postoperative pain perception occurs. This explains why many patients display pain signs immediately upon waking. Good pain management is designed to interrupt nociception, even if the patient is under a general anesthetic, and should be initiated whenever pain is anticipated. When analgesia is provided to surgical patients, recovery typically is much more comfortable.

Neuropathic Pain and Wind-Up Phenomenon

Pain traditionally has been subdivided into acute and chronic types; acute pain is described as a sharp stabbing sensation, and chronic as dull, persistent throbbing. Most pain is related to inflammation, but unpleasant sensations may arise directly from nerves involved in pain transmission. When attributed to nerves, these sensations are generally described as "neuropathic." Therefore, it may be more appropriate to classify pain as inflammatory (with subsets of acute and chronic) or neuropathic (present in the nerves, irrespective of ongoing inflammation). Neuropathic pain is described as a persistent stabbing, aching, burning, itching, or tingling sensation with or without an observable cause; it can occur along with inflammatory pain, or as a separate syndrome. Treating neuropathic pain may allow patients to return to a state of normal or near normal. A commonly used neuropathic pain

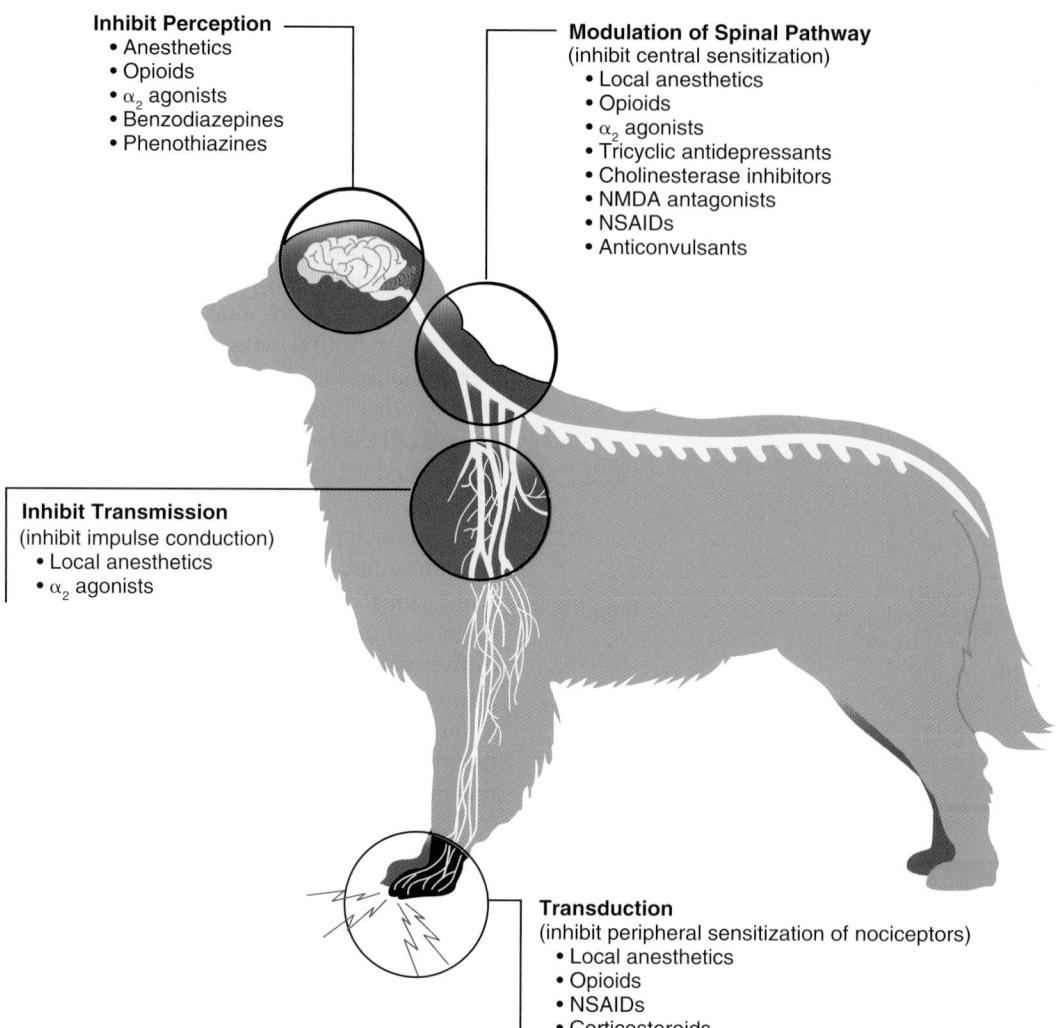

Inhibit Perception
- Anesthetics
- Opioids
- α_2 agonists
- Benzodiazepines
- Phenothiazines

Modulation of Spinal Pathway
(inhibit central sensitization)
- Local anesthetics
- Opioids
- α_2 agonists
- Tricyclic antidepressants
- Cholinesterase inhibitors
- NMDA antagonists
- NSAIDs
- Anticonvulsants

Inhibit Transmission
(inhibit impulse conduction)
- Local anesthetics
- α_2 agonists

Transduction
(inhibit peripheral sensitization of nociceptors)
- Local anesthetics
- Opioids
- NSAIDs
- Corticosteroids

FIGURE 28-2 Nociception. Sites of analgesic action along the pain pathway. (From Tranquilli WJ, Grimm KA, Lamont LA: Pain management for the small animal practitioner, Jackson, WY, 2004, Teton NewMedia.)

reliever in human and veterinary medicine is gabapentin (Neurontin), which is discussed in the analgesia section of this chapter.

An extreme form of neuropathic pain occurs when the CNS is bombarded by persistent pain impulses. This can have a profound effect on the architecture of the nervous system, altering pain processing. When spinal neurons are subjected to repeat or high-intensity nociceptive impulses, these neurons become progressively and increasingly excitable, even after the stimulus is removed. This condition is known as *central sensitization* or **wind-up phenomenon** and leads to nonresponsive or chronic intractable pain. Wind-up is the culmination of two distinct phases of change in the nervous system. First, the pain-transmitting nerve fiber threshold is reset to a lower level. This resetting results in **hyperalgesia**, where less and less stimulation is required to initiate pain. In the second phase, nerve fibers that normally carry pleasant or neutral information are recruited and become part of the pain transmission process. This phase is termed **allodynia** and results in interpretation of

normally harmless sensations as pain. The presence of hyperalgesia and allodynia collectively is considered wind-up phenomenon. This is apparent, for example, in the Dachshund with vertebral disc disease that cries out in pain when any part of its body is touched, or in the Cocker Spaniel with a chronic ear infection that can no longer tolerate normal petting. People suffering from a migraine headache can attest to both the increase in pain sensitivity and the feeling that normally innocuous feelings (light touch, clothing, wind, etc.) have become unpleasant. Wind-up phenomenon highlights the need for effective analgesia to treat pain before it begins and at regular intervals once it occurs. Wind-up phenomenon is an important concept in pain management. The vast majority of patients experiencing acute pain can be managed using common analgesics, such as NSAIDs. Patients experiencing wind-up require additional therapy, just as the migraine sufferer would not likely be helped by taking two ibuprofen tablets, even though this approach would be adequate to treat a common headache. A variety of approaches can be used to "unwind" the patient, aimed at resetting neurologic processing so that conventional medications will work again. These are discussed in the analgesia section of this chapter.

TREATMENT OF PAIN IN SMALL ANIMALS

ENVIRONMENTAL AND EMOTIONAL CARE

Pain has both physical and psychological components. Fear and anxiety can exacerbate pain and vice versa. Attending to an animal's physical and perceived emotional needs can reduce stress and consequently minimize pain levels. Environmental factors seem to affect the perception of pain in pets. The hospitalized patient in unfamiliar surroundings may be comforted by a favorite blanket or toy. Veterinary technicians must be adept at "reading" patients because the emotional needs of individual dogs and cats vary greatly. Environmental care, such as providing a clean cage of appropriate size, extra padding, and careful positioning to reduce pressure on painful areas, is important. Designate the patient's cage as a safe zone so that animals do not associate contact with an unpleasant experience. Any procedure that might be considered noxious should be performed by taking the patient outside the cage, if possible. This allows the animal to feel comfortable and safe when in the cage. Nonpharmacologic actions can reduce pain by removing other stressors. However, tending to a patient's comfort needs should not be seen as a substitute for analgesia.

PRINCIPLES OF ADMINISTERING ANALGESIA

Improved understanding of the impact of pain on the body is shaping new philosophies in managing patients' pain. Several basic principles are used in the approach to designing analgesic protocols and are particularly important in managing pain effectively.

1. *The best way to treat pain is to prevent it.* This is the concept of **preemptive analgesia.** All research in human and veterinary medicine shows that preventing pain is unquestionably the best approach to treatment. It is an easy concept to grasp, but not so easy to remember to implement. That is because we have become used to treating animal pain on "request" (i.e., when we see overt signs of pain), even though we rationally know that once we see the signs, it is already too late. We have already missed the opportunity to most effectively manage pain in that patient. Administering preemptive analgesics whenever possible appears to be much more effective than using the same agent to treat pain once it occurs. Analgesia given before a noxious stimulus reduces postprocedure analgesia requirements, minimizes detrimental effects of pain, improves handling of patients, and potentially lowers sedation or anesthetic requirements. Reducing pain signaling helps to prevent hypersensitization at the spinal cord and neuropathic pain syndromes.

> **TECHNICIAN NOTE** Imagine that tomorrow at 5 PM, you were going to have an excruciating headache, guaranteed. What would you do at 4:30? Probably, you thought, "I would take something," such as ibuprofen or another NSAID. You would make that choice because the looming headache is an example of a planned painful event. Knowing that the pain is coming allows you the opportunity to stop that pain before it starts. Elective surgery is also a planned painful event. It makes sense to preempt the pain that is associated with *all* surgical procedures.

2. *Drug combinations often produce better pain relief than single agents.* The physiology of nociception gives rise to the concept of **multimodal analgesia.** Multimodal analgesia takes advantage of the synergistic effects obtained by combining two or more classes of analgesic drugs to alter more than one phase (transduction, transmission, modulation, and perception). Attacking pain from many angles is more effective than from only one. Because the pain pathway has distinct phases, pain can be interrupted at various points. For example, in addition to preemptive NSAIDs (transduction), we may want to do a local block (transmission) and administer opioids (modulation and perception). Using drugs from three different classes provides better pain control and confers the added benefit of allowing the use of lower doses of individual agents, thereby reducing side effects. Effective analgesia can also reduce the amount of gaseous anesthetic required for a procedure.

3. *Matching analgesics* (based on dosage and duration of action) to the degree of expected surgical pain rather than to the patient's ability to express pain in a recognizable way is a more effective way to ensure pain relief.

4. *Maintaining an analgesic plane once pain control is established.* This may include the use of epidurals, CRIs, or continued bolus dosing. Pain management is weaned off as patients are transitioned out of the intensive care unit (ICU). Regimented treatment (i.e., dosing at regular intervals) is helpful in maintaining an analgesic plane. Otherwise, a roller coaster effect occurs, leaving the patient in varying degrees of pain between treatments. Keeping a patient out of pain is always more efficacious than continually taking the patient out of pain.

5. *"Don't quit till the pain quits."* Send pain relief home with the patient. Many professionals agree that most soft tissue procedures, such as spaying or neutering, require 3 to 4 days of postoperative analgesia, whereas orthopedic procedures probably require a 1-week supply. Of course, individual patients may vary, and owners should be advised to request additional analgesia if they perceive their pet to be in pain beyond the anticipated period.

Dispelling the pain myth that *pain is beneficial in limiting a recovering animal's activity* is critical in patient care. Although this is one of the mostly widely held myths about pain, studies demonstrate that animals in pain tend to be restless, change positions frequently, and bite and/or chew and/or lick at painful sites, whereas pain-managed animals tend to rest quietly. Aside from being morally questionable, allowing animals to remain in pain for the purpose of restraint is not medically sound. The type of pain produced by tissue injury, inflammation, or direct damage to the nervous system is never beneficial. The previously described negative effects of pain far outnumber any possible benefit, real or imagined. Providing effective analgesia reduces the pain-induced stress response, thereby enhancing patient comfort and recovery.

ADMINISTRATION OF ANALGESICS AND ANALGESIC TECHNIQUES

The basic principles of current pain management have just been described to include preemptive (preventive) analgesia, multimodal analgesia (using different classes of drugs simultaneously to interrupt the pain pathway at various points), and appropriate follow-up analgesia (postoperative and take-home). Using this strategy, an analgesic plan is designed for each patient that maximizes pain control, maintains patients on an analgesic plane, and reduces unwanted side effects (Table 28-2).

Choosing the correct analgesic therapy requires an understanding of both the pharmacokinetics of a wide range of drugs and the levels or types of pain associated with various conditions. The four categories of drugs—NSAIDs, local anesthetics, opioids, and α_2 **agonists**—are used in various combinations to inhibit the nociceptive process at more than one site. For this reason, combinations are more effective than single agents. Ultimately, pain relief, as assessed by the criteria previously described, is the only true measure of successful treatment. More recently, several classes of drugs have been added to the pain management regimen as adjunctive therapy in nonresponsive cases, including N-methyl-D-aspartate (NMDA)-receptor **antagonists** (which have efficacy against wind-up) and anticonvulsants (which have efficacy against neuropathic pain).

Anticipating pain level and duration provides a starting point for analgesic protocols. The initial approach is based on knowledge of the mechanisms of pain, drug dosages and expected duration, pain assessment, and knowledge of expected levels of pain for injuries, surgery, and diseases. Patients should be continually evaluated for breakthrough pain (exceeding usual protocol) or pain that persists beyond the expected period. Categorization of the expected severity (mild, moderate, severe) of pain is used to establish the initial type of analgesia and the duration of treatment. Later dosages can be adjusted according to individual patient response. For example, mild pain may be manageable with NSAIDs alone or in combination with a weak opioid, whereas moderate pain may require the addition of a stronger opioid. Severe pain might be best approached with an NSAID and a full opioid agonist, or may require CRI or additional therapies. Local and regional blocks can and should be added to the pain management plan, whenever feasible. When specific nerves cannot be identified for block, lidocaine can be administered by CRI for excellent systemic analgesia (Box 28-3).

TABLE 28-2	Monitoring Patients Taking Analgesics	
ADVERSE EFFECT	**MONITORING**
Opioids	
Sedation, low blood pressure, respiratory depression	Mentation, blood pressure, respiratory rate and nature
Local Anesthetics	
None unless given by CRI. Then nausea, vomiting, neurologic signs, and seizures	Observe regularly for muscle tremors and GI upset
NSAIDs	
GI disturbances, GI bleeding, renal disturbances	General observation, hydration status, stool quality, and urine production
α_2 Agonists	
Bradycardia, cardiac arrhythmias, hypertension, peripheral vasoconstriction	Palpate femoral pulse rate and quality, auscultate heart, blood pressure

CRI, Constant rate infusion; *GI,* gastrointestinal; *NSAIDs,* nonsteroidal anti-inflammatory drugs.

A variety of techniques may be used to administer analgesics. Experienced veterinary technicians are able to deliver drugs by oral, transmucosal, subcutaneous (SQ), intramuscular (IM), intravenous (IV), transcutaneous, and epidural routes, and by constant rate infusion (CRI).

BOX 28-3	Sound Approach to Developing an Individual Pain Management Protocol

The initial approach should be based on the following questions:

- How painful is the condition, procedure, or surgery expected to be?
- Are there any underlying factors, such as stress, anxiety, fear, or preexisting chronic pain conditions, that could be causing an increased pain response?
- What is the normal behavior and disposition of the particular breed and for this animal in particular?
- Are there any contraindications to particular drugs or drug classes for this patient's condition?
- Does this animal have a history of drug sensitivities?

NSAIDs

Nonsteroidal anti-inflammatory drugs provide analgesia by modifying the inflammatory response. Pharmacologic actions of NSAIDs include analgesia, antipyresis (fever reduction), and control of inflammation. Because they treat the underlying problem (inflammation) and pain is diminished as a result, NSAIDs are considered to be a therapeutic class of analgesics. Since NSAIDs approved for use in dogs were introduced into the market, they have been universally accepted as the treatment of choice for osteoarthritis. NSAIDs remain the most widely used analgesics in the treatment of chronic pain. However, they are also extremely effective in reducing acute pain in the perioperative period (around surgery). Recent changes in our understanding of animal pain and the best ways to manage it and new Food and Drug Administration (FDA) drug approvals have led to NSAIDs becoming one of the most widely used classes of veterinary analgesics in a variety of situations.

Research shows that pretreatment with NSAIDs greatly reduces intraoperative and postoperative pain from soft tissue or orthopedic procedures. Therefore, patients undergoing everything from spaying to neutering to cruciate ligament repair potentially benefit from NSAID administration, especially when given preemptively, and NSAIDs have been shown to have a synergistic effect when combined with other classes of drugs, such as opioids. Often, patients with severe acute pain can be weaned to NSAIDs alone as their pain diminishes. NSAIDs have an onset of action of 45 to 60 minutes. The duration of action is typically 24 hours in the dog and varies from 8 to 96 hours in the cat. NSAIDs are best suited for mild to moderate pain, whether acute or chronic in nature. In addition to controlling postsurgical pain, NSAIDs are extremely effective in controlling inflammatory pain associated with traumatic soft tissue injury, ophthalmic conditions, otitis, and gingivitis, as well as some cancer pain.

Current commonly used veterinary NSAIDs include Rimadyl (carprofen), Metacam (meloxicam), Deramaxx (deracoxib), and Previcox (firocoxib). Regardless of the NSAID, patients should be normotensive (normal blood pressure), with normal renal and liver function, without bleeding abnormalities, and without evidence of or concern for gastric ulceration. Patients that receive NSAIDs preoperatively MUST have blood pressure monitored intraoperatively, and IV access must be maintained for administration of IV fluids if necessary. Patients that are receiving corticosteroids or aspirin should not be given NSAIDs. Two different NSAIDs should not be administered concurrently.

The most commonly reported adverse events in the dog are related to the gastrointestinal (GI) tract and include vomiting, diarrhea, GI bleeding, and GI perforation, whereas in the cat, signs are more commonly related to the renal system and include renal failure.

> **TECHNICIAN NOTE** Cats can safely receive approved nonsteroidal anti-inflammatory drugs (NSAIDs) on a one-time basis because of their varying metabolic rate of excretion for this drug class (7 to 96 hours). Repeat dosing is not recommended in cats at this time because this may result in renal failure. Cats should *never* receive Tylenol (acetaminophen). Cats lack an enzyme required to metabolize acetaminophen, resulting in liver toxicity and an inability of the red blood cells to carry oxygen. One regular-strength tablet (325 mg) may be toxic to cats, and a second could be lethal. The most common signs of acetaminophen toxicity observed upon physical examination of cats are increased respiratory rate; pale, muddy mucous membranes; hypothermia; and tachycardia. Other signs include central nervous system (CNS) depression, anorexia, vomiting, swollen face and paws, salivation, diarrhea, coma, and death.

Take-Home Analgesia

The availability of NSAIDs has greatly improved outpatient pain management. These drugs are convenient to administer (once a day, chewable), are relatively inexpensive, and provide long-lasting pain relief compared with other analgesics. The current anecdotal recommendation for dogs from pain management experts is that elective soft tissue procedures, such as spaying or castration, require 3 to 4 days of postoperative treatment with NSAIDs. Orthopedic procedures may require treatment for 1 week or longer. Of course, each individual animal must be evaluated for the presence of pain that persists beyond the expected time, or that is of significant intensity and requires additional analgesics.

Local and Regional Anesthetics

Local anesthetics work by totally disrupting neural transmission of information. Blocking transmission of painful signals is one of the most effective ways of managing pain. Nerve blocks routinely performed by veterinary technicians include canine and feline dental blocks and feline declaw blocks. The use of lidocaine as a systemic blocking agent given by CRI is increasingly popular. A great deal of recent work has revived the use of local or regional analgesia. Applying analgesia directly to affected nerve endings can provide excellent pain control while reducing the need for systemic drugs.

Lidocaine, the most widely used local anesthetic, takes effect in 3 to 5 minutes and is effective for 60 to 90 minutes. The duration of lidocaine can be extended by combination with a 1:200,000 dilution of epinephrine. Epinephrine should *never* be used in circumferential limb blocks, such as feline declaw blocks. Marcaine (bupivacaine) takes longer to take effect (15 to 20 minutes), but its anesthetic and analgesic effects last 6 to 8 hours. Bupivacaine is not effective as a topical analgesic but is an excellent choice for local infiltration.

Drugs such as lidocaine and bupivacaine are relatively safe if correctly administered. Most cases of toxicity in small animals occur as a result of accidental overdose or inadvertent IV administration. Signs of toxicity include seizures, coma, neurotoxicity, and cardiovascular collapse.

> **TECHNICIAN NOTE**   If it ends in "-caine," it blocks a nerve. All local anesthetics end in the suffix "-caine" and block nerve transmission via sodium channels. Differences between individual agents are noted in time to onset and duration of action. Most procedures in small animals are best performed using the longest-acting agent possible (bupivacaine), although mixing local anesthetics to get faster onset is not uncommon.

Routes of Administration

Topical. Application of topical analgesia to the surface skin or mucosa can reduce pain associated with minor procedures, such as wound suturing, venipuncture, arterial puncture, nasal cannulation, and urinary catheterization. Solutions of lidocaine, bupivacaine, tetracaine, and epinephrine can be used alone or in various combinations to provide desensitization at the application site. Gauze pads soaked with solutions can be applied directly to the site. Alternatively, several commercially prepared topical anesthetic creams and jellies can be applied as a thick paste. Regardless of the application method selected, 20 to 30 minutes of direct contact time is required to ensure effective analgesia.

Local infiltration. Injection of lidocaine or bupivacaine into local tissue can reduce pain associated with various painful procedures. This technique is useful for small mass removal, digit amputation, arterial catheter placement, thoracocentesis, abdominocentesis, bone marrow sampling, and so forth. The entry area is infiltrated with small amounts of anesthetic before tissue penetration. An appropriate waiting time must be observed to ensure adequate desensitization of the area, as described earlier.

Circumferential ring block. This block is especially effective for use in feline declawing and involves subcutaneous (SQ) injection of bupivacaine or a bupivacaine and lidocaine combination just above the carpal bend on the top of the paw, and just above the accessory carpal pad on the underside (Figure 28-3). The dosage is 1 ml of 0.5% bupivacaine/10 lb of body weight divided among injection sites. Sterile saline can be added to achieve sufficient coverage for smaller cats. Injections are made just above the carpal bend on the top side of the paw and just above the accessory carpal pad on the underside. The skin is tented horizontally, and the needle is fed under the skin. As the needle is withdrawn, the drug is injected slowly to leave behind a "line." When this is done on both surfaces, the lines will connect, creating a bracelet or ring block around the limb. This four-injection technique provides regional nerve block sufficient to eliminate pain for up to 8 hours after surgery.

Dental nerve block. The entire muzzle can be anesthetized by blocking the infraorbital and mandibular foramen. This

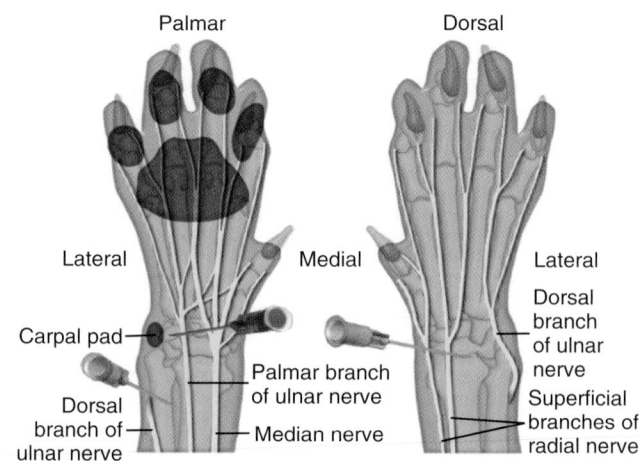

FIGURE 28-3 Circumferential block for feline declawing. Landmarks are shown indicating proper site for SQ injection of local anesthetic to provide block of the three major nerves in the feline forelimb.

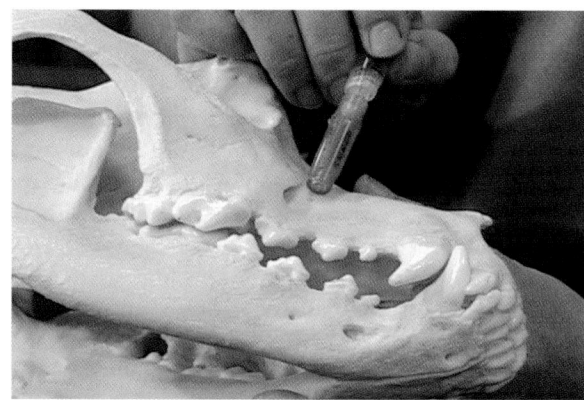

FIGURE 28-4 Location for blocking the infraorbital foramen in the dog. Infraorbital foramina are the sites for injection to provide nerve block to the entire maxilla. The left and right foramen can be located easily just above the third premolar and about midway up the gum line.

relatively simple technique is effective for dental extractions, oral mass removal, fracture repair, mandibulectomy, maxillectomy, and nasal biopsy (Figures 28-4 and 28-5). Lidocaine or bupivacaine can be used. Epinephrine can be added to reduce bleeding by coating the syringe with epinephrine before local anesthetic is drawn up. Volume of administration is limited by the size of the foramen. Typically, about 0.5 ml per site is appropriate for a 50-lb dog, whereas about 0.1 ml per site is adequate in the cat.

Intra-articular (joint space). Effective analgesia in preoperative and postoperative orthopedic cases has been achieved by injection of local anesthetics directly into the joint space, as in cruciate ligament repair. Intra-articular morphine has also been shown to effectively reduce joint pain. The effectiveness of this technique when used preoperatively is evident in the smooth plane of anesthesia maintained when the joint capsule is incised. This is in sharp contrast to the spike in heart rate and "lightness" that is observed when the joint capsule is entered without using local anesthetics

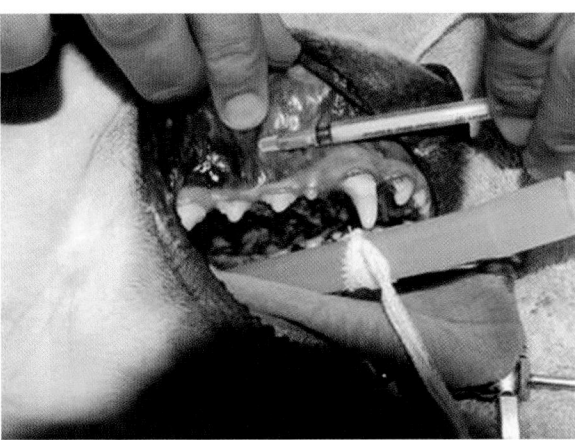

FIGURE 28-5 Blocking the foramen in the dog. Photo shows needle inserted into the foramen to block the right maxilla. Care must be taken in shorter muzzled dogs to avoid overinserting the needle and entering the ocular orbit.

and/or morphine, indicating that these responses are likely due to pain.

Pleural space. Interpleural bupivacaine infusion following thoracotomy surgery may have some analgesic benefit. Bupivacaine (1.5 to 2 mg/kg) is injected via an indwelling chest tube into the pleural space. Analgesia is thought to occur by direct blocking of the intercostal nerves. For maximum coverage, patients are held in sternal recumbency for 5 to 10 minutes after injection and are gently rolled from side to side. Drug absorption through the pleural tissue should be considered.

Epidural nerve block. Injection of opioids (morphine, fentanyl) and/or local anesthetics (lidocaine, bupivacaine) directly into the epidural space has been used to provide analgesia to the caudal half of the body while minimizing sedative effects. This is a fairly simple and safe technique. Injection is generally performed at the lumbosacral space. Epidural catheters can be inserted to allow long-term analgesic administration.

Intravenous. Intravenous (IV) administration of lidocaine by CRI is an effective technique for managing a variety of pain states. At the cardiac dose of 30 to 80 µg/kg/minute, lidocaine provides excellent analgesia for visceral pain (e.g., pancreatitis, parvovirus) and in procedures with extensive nerve damage, such as limb amputation. Lidocaine given by CRI can be administered as a sole agent or in conjunction with other analgesics.

> **TECHNICIAN NOTE**   The addition of 0.1 ml of sodium bicarbonate per 10 ml of local blocking agents may reduce the stinging sensation and is advised when blocking agents are administered to awake patients.

Opioids

Opioids are the most commonly used analgesics in hospitalized patients because of their efficacy, rapid onset of action, and safety.

The efficacy of various opioids is determined by the specific receptors in the brain and spinal cord that they affect. Receptors are classified as mu, kappa, or sigma. Mu receptors are chiefly responsible for providing analgesia. Kappa receptors are chiefly responsible for providing sedation. Sigma receptors are less clinically relevant and are thought to be responsible for the adverse effects of opioid administration, such as dysphoria, excitement, restlessness, and anxiety. Opioid drugs are classified as agonists (meaning that they stimulate the opioid receptors) or antagonists (meaning that they block particular opioid receptors). Also, mixed agonist-antagonist opioids stimulate some receptors while blocking others and partial agonists with overall decreased effects at all receptor sites. In general, pure agonists (working at all receptors) are the most potent of the opioids, but they also cause the most severe adverse effects. Mixed agonist-antagonist and partial agonist opioids can provide reasonably good analgesia without many of the deleterious side effects of pure agonists. Side effects may include vomiting, constipation, excitement, respiratory depression, bradycardia, and panting. The type of opioid is chosen on the basis of the degree of analgesia required and the specific needs or limitations of the individual patient. The most commonly used pure agonists in the United States are morphine, hydromorphone, oxymorphone, and fentanyl.

> **TECHNICIAN NOTE**   Emesis (vomiting) is a common side effect of some opioids, particularly morphine and hydromorphone. It occurs most frequently when an opioid is used as a premedication rather than when an opioid is administered as an analgesic to an animal already in pain.

Pure antagonists have the effect of reversing the narcotic properties of agonists. The availability of opioid antagonists makes opioid use extremely safe because drug effects can be rapidly removed. Opioids are metabolized by the liver and excreted via the kidneys and should be used with caution in patients with renal or hepatic disease. Opioids are most effective when administered before the onset of pain. As a class, these drugs produce minimal side effects in animals. Virtually any animal patient experiencing pain is a candidate for opioid analgesia.

Opioids can be administered through numerous routes, including intravenous (IV), intramuscular (IM), transcutaneous, epidural, and oral routes, and by CRI. Opioids can be administered concurrently with all other analgesics.

Severe Pain

Morphine sulfate (pure opioid agonist). Morphine is the gold standard for pure opioid agonists. All other drugs in this class are compared with morphine in terms of efficacy, duration of action, and cost. Morphine is commonly used to provide maximal analgesia and sedation. Its relatively low cost and excellent efficacy cause it to be preferred over other opioids in some cases. However, morphine has additional side effects, particularly systemic hypotension and vomiting, which make it less desirable in many instances. Cats are particularly sensitive to morphine; therefore, lower doses are used in the cat. It is common for cats to become hyperthermic from morphine. The typical dosage for dogs is 1.0 to 1.5 mg/kg IV every 4 to 6 hours. The dosage in cats is 0.25 to 1.0 mg/kg SQ or IM every 4 to 6 hours.

Hydromorphone (pure opioid agonist). Hydromorphone has similar properties to morphine in terms of providing analgesia, but it is thought to have fewer side effects. Specifically, hydromorphone is less likely than morphine to induce vomiting or hypotension. Elevated body temperature has been noted, especially in cats. The typical dosage in dogs is 0.1 to 0.2 mg/kg SQ or IM and 0.03 to 0.1 mg/kg IV. Cat dosage is 0.05 to 0.1 mg/kg SQ or IM and 0.01 to 0.025 mg/kg IV. The duration of action is 3 to 4 hours.

Fentanyl citrate (pure opioid agonist). Fentanyl is an extremely potent synthetic opioid with rapid onset but short duration of action when administered IV or IM. It is most efficaciously used as a transdermal patch for long-term (3 days) analgesia. Fentanyl is contained in adhesive patches of varying concentrations to deliver 25, 75, or 100 µg/hour. Once applied to shaved, cleaned skin, the drug is continually absorbed. Onset of action is from 12 to 24 hours; therefore, supplemental analgesia is recommended during the initial treatment period. Use of mixed agonist-antagonist opioids reverses the effects of the fentanyl patch and should be avoided. Fentanyl can also be delivered as a CRI; its use in this manner will be described later in the chapter.

Moderate to Severe Pain

Buprenorphine (buprenex) (partial mu agonist). Buprenorphine is a partial mu agonist that is of longer duration than morphine as a result of its slow dissociation from receptors, providing analgesia for approximately 6 to 8 hours. Partial agonists avidly bind and partially activate mu receptors. Buprenorphine is recommended for moderate pain in the dog and for moderate to severe pain in the cat. Buprenorphine is readily absorbed across mucous membranes in the feline as a result of the unique oral pH in this species. This allows for transmucosal administration in the cat, providing analgesia for up to 8 hours from a single appropriate dose. Transmucosal buprenorphine is the primary analgesic for take-home use in cats. It is extremely easy for owners to administer and provides long-lasting analgesia (Figure 28-6). The dose for buprenorphine in dogs and cats is 0.02 to 0.06 mg/kg administered IM, IV, or transmucosally (cat only). Duration of action is directly related to dose.

Mild Pain

Butorphanol tartrate (torbugesic) (mixed agonist/antagonist). Butorphanol is a kappa agonist and a mu

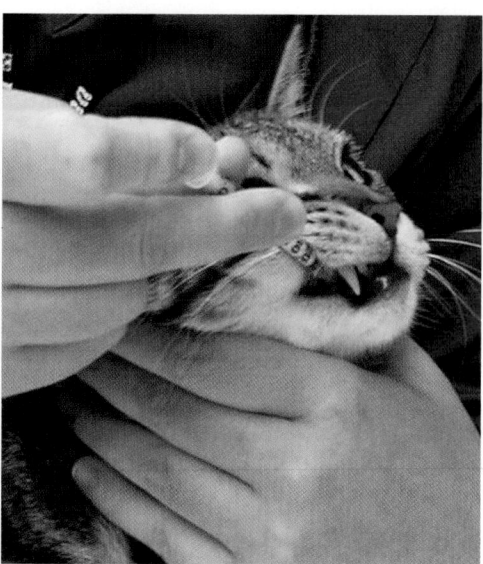

FIGURE 28-6 Administering transmucosal buprenorphine to a cat. Transmucosal delivery of buprenorphine is extremely efficacious in the cat and provides up to 8 hours of pain relief in the hospital or at home.

antagonist. As a kappa agonist, it is a mild analgesic with marked sedative properties. Whereas the sedative effects of butorphanol may last for 2 or more hours, the effect of analgesia is only about 45 minutes—an important consideration for managing pain of any greater duration. As a mu antagonist, butorphanol can be used to reverse adverse events thought to be associated with mu opioid agonists, such as morphine. The dosage is 0.2 to 0.8 mg/kg given SQ, IM, or IV.

> **TECHNICIAN NOTE** Butorphanol should not be used as the sole analgesic unless mild pain of short duration (less than 1 hour) is expected.

Opioid Reversal

Naloxone hydrochloride (pure opioid antagonist). One of the reasons why opioid use is safe is the clinician's ability to rapidly reverse sedation and adverse side effects. Antagonists work by blocking opioid action at the receptors. Onset of reversal occurs within 1 to 2 minutes of IV administration and can last for 1 to 4 hours. Treatment may be repeated when narcotics with a longer duration are reversed. The typical dosage is 2 µg/kg IV.

Butorphanol tartrate (torbugesic) (mu antagonist). See preceding comments under "Mild Pain."

Synthetic Opioid

Tramadol. Tramadol is a synthetic drug with analgesic effects. Tramadol has opioid-like activity at the mu receptor in cats but not in dogs. It has serotonin and norepinephrine reuptake inhibition in both species. Tramadol can be effective in controlling moderate pain, especially when used in conjunction with an NSAID. It is available in oral form, making it suitable for long-term at-home management of postoperative, cancer, orthopedic, and other chronic pain. A wide variety of dosages have been tried and reported in both the dog and the cat. The current dosing recommendation calls for 4 mg/kg PO given 3 to 4 times daily in the dog and the cat.

α_2 Agonists

Xylazine, medetomidine (Domitor), and dexmedetomidine (Dexdomitor) are α_2 agonists that have been widely used in veterinary medicine. Dexdomitor is the first premedication labeled for use as a sedative/analgesic in dogs and cats, and the most potent and selective α_2 agonist available in the United States. α_2 agonists, which are non-narcotic and non-scheduled agents, can be useful as adjuncts in a balanced analgesic protocol. The main effect is to produce significant sedation accompanied by visceral and somatic analgesia. A variety of new ways are available to use this drug class as a premedication and for rough recovery rescue and ongoing management of in-hospital pain and anxiety. α_2 agonist combinations are also extremely effective in cats for a variety of surgical and nonsurgical procedures.

α_2 agonists inhibit release of the excitatory **neurotransmitter** norepinephrine to produce analgesia and sedation. α_2 agonists are short-duration analgesics and can be rapidly reversed with α_2 antagonists. This characteristic makes these drugs suitable for procedures requiring short-term restraint and analgesia. α_2 agonists may bind to the same receptors as opioids and act synergistically with them. Dosages of other analgesic and anesthetic agents can be significantly reduced if given concurrently with α_2 agonists. α_2 agonists can have profound effects on the cardiovascular and nervous systems, but these adverse events can be minimized by using low dosages. Bradycardia and vomiting are the side effects most commonly seen with α_2 agonists.

> **TECHNICIAN NOTE** α_2 agonists cause vasoconstriction; as when a water hose is kinked, the narrowed vessels result in increased blood pressure or hypertension. Because heart rate normally goes up when blood pressure is low and down when pressure is high, slowed heart rate is expected. Bradycardia is considered a normal finding when α_2 agonists are used.

Advantages of α_2 Agonists Over Other Sedatives

Other commonly used sedatives (e.g., acepromazine, diazepam) do not provide pain relief. Analgesia achieved with α_2 agonists is of moderate intensity and moderate duration. Even more important, α_2 agonists work synergistically with opioids (such as butorphanol or morphine) and improve both the intensity and the duration of pain relief. Other advantages are that the degree of sedation can be "tailored" or "titrated" by using different dosages and/or different drug combinations to provide mild to profound sedation, and

that α_2 agonists are reversible. Antisedan (atipamezole) is most commonly used to reverse Dexdomitor. Antisedan is the safest of all the reversal agents because it works almost exclusively by simply displacing Dexdomitor from the α_2 receptors, so that nerve function can return to normal. After administration of Antisedan, patients usually awaken in about 5 to 10 minutes and are able to stand or walk within 10 minutes.

α_2 agonists are used in a variety of ways to provide patient comfort, including as a premedicant before surgery combined with an opioid, as a stand-alone sedative or analgesic for short procedures such as x-rays, and as a rescue drug for patients experiencing rough recovery from anesthesia. α_2 agonists are most commonly used in cats in a combination called "kitty magic," which consists of an α_2 agonist, an opioid (most commonly buprenorphine), and ketamine. The addition of ketamine makes the combination a general anesthetic protocol rather than just a sedative protocol. Minor surgical procedures can be performed under kitty magic, or kitty magic can be used before a gas anesthetic for more advanced procedures. α_2 agonists can also be administered as a CRI for patients with continual anxiety or pain.

> **TECHNICIAN NOTE** Like any sedative, α_2 agonists work best when they are administered to an animal that is not overly agitated. Agitated patients should be placed in a quiet place for 15 minutes after administration to allow the drug to take effect. Handling, loud noises, or any other sudden stimuli may cause a startle reaction, even if the animal is sedated. Caution should be used, especially around the animal's head and neck.

Dexdomitor has been extensively used and valued as a "rescue" drug for patients that are experiencing rough recovery after anesthesia. Excitement in recovery (sometimes called "emergence delirium") is not appropriate whether it is caused by pain or by residual effects of anesthesia because both cause tremendous physiologic stress and side effects that include tachycardia (high heart rate), hypertension (high blood pressure), cardiac arrhythmias (abnormal electrical activity of the heart), ventilation abnormalities (e.g., increased respiratory rate [i.e., tachypnea] with decreased volume of breaths [i.e., tidal volume]), cortisol release (which impairs proper healing), and a predisposition for GI ileus and ulceration. Dexdomitor is an excellent choice (in heart-healthy patients) for treatment because it provides both sedation and analgesia. Patients who require repeated rescue doses of Dexdomitor can be placed on low-dose CRI for continued sedation and analgesia.

Constant Rate Infusion

Constant rate infusion allows continuous low-dose administration of various analgesics. Optimally, CRIs are established before tissue damage occurs (i.e., preoperatively) and are run for 6 to 12 hours postoperatively. CRI analgesia is also effective in the management of hospitalized patients

BOX 28-4	Calculating Constant Rate Infusions

Step 1. Set up equation based on dosage: μg/kg/minute = μg to add to bag
Step 2. Replace hash marks with time signs: μg × kg × minutes = μg to add to bag
Step 3. Enter known information: dose and weight
Step 4. Solve for hours: Fluid bag size ÷ Hourly rate = # hours bag will last
Step 5. Solve for minutes: # hours above × 60 min/hour
Step 6. Solve equation: μg × kg × minutes = μg to add to bag
Step 7. Convert μg to mg; divide answer by 1000.
Step 8. Calculate drug volume and add to bag desired: mg ÷ Concentration in mg/ml = ml

A controlled rate infusion pump is required because the rate of drug delivery must be precisely controlled. This can be a syringe pump, a cassette pump, or a rotary pump.

with preexisting or persistent medical pain. Many agents can be delivered, but this method most commonly uses local anesthetics (lidocaine), opioids (morphine or fentanyl), NMDA antagonists (ketamine), and α_2 agonists (Dexdomitor). These drugs can be used as single agents or in combination with one another. Technicians should be adept at calculating CRIs (Box 28-4).

Morphine
The main advantage of giving morphine as a CRI is that it prevents the peaks and valleys typically seen with opioid bolus dosing. A lower dose of morphine can be used in a CRI; this can reduce unwanted side effects, such as dysphoria or panting. Morphine by CRI is useful for managing any severe pain and can be safely combined with ketamine and/or lidocaine. The CRI dose for morphine in dogs is 0.2 to 0.5 mg/kg SLOW IV loading bolus, followed by 0.1 to 0.3 mg/kg/hour CRI. For cats, the dose is 0.05 to 0.1 mg/kg IV loading bolus, followed by 0.025 to 0.2 mg/kg/hour CRI. *Fentanyl* is a full opioid agonist with similar properties to morphine. The main advantage of fentanyl over morphine is its rapid onset of action and short half-life, which allows for rapid cessation of unwanted side effects. The CRI dose for fentanyl in dogs is 2 to 5 μg/kg IV loading dose, followed by 5 to 20 μg/kg/hour CRI intraoperatively; for cats, the dose is 1 to 2 μg/kg IV loading dose, followed by 5 to 20 μg/kg/hour CRI.

Lidocaine is a local anesthetic that provides excellent systemic analgesia when delivered IV. Because it is safe for use in patients with GI disturbances, lidocaine is a good choice for analgesia in patients with gastric dilatation-volvulus (GDV), pancreatitis, or similar disorders. Lidocaine seems to also provide benefit for patients undergoing procedures with excessive nerve trauma, such as complicated back surgeries or limb amputations. IV lidocaine is extremely short acting and can be discontinued without residual effect almost immediately. Lidocaine CRI should be discontinued if the

TABLE 28-3	Recipe for MLK	
AMOUNT OF EACH DRUG ADDED TO A 500-ML BAG OF LACTATED RINGER'S SOLUTION (LRS)	**RATE AT WHICH EACH DRUG IS INFUSED, PROVIDED FLUIDS ARE ADMINISTERED AT A RATE OF 10 ML/KG/HOUR**
10 mg morphine (.66 ml)	Morphine 0.2 mg/kg/hour
120 mg lidocaine (6 ml 2%)	Lidocaine 2.5 mg/kg/hour
100 mg ketamine (1 ml)	Ketamine 2 mg/kg/hour

patient shows signs of toxicity, including muscle tremors, seizures, nausea, or vomiting. The CRI dose for lidocaine in the dog is 1 to 2 mg/kg IV, followed by 30 to 50 μg/kg/minute. Lidocaine CRI dosages have been reported for cats, but typically, lidocaine is not recommended for use in cats because of the potential for severe cardiotoxic effects.

Ketamine at CRI dosing is an NMDA receptor antagonist and as such is used to reverse or prevent wind-up phenomenon, which causes stimulation of NMDA receptors in the spinal cord. "Wind-up" will be most evident in the postoperative period once the patient has regained consciousness. However, as an NMDA receptor antagonist, ketamine, given as an intraoperative CRI, binds at these CNS receptors and prevents "wind-up." Ketamine should always be given in combination with other analgesics and can be delivered in the same infusion. The CRI dosage for ketamine in the dog and the cat is 0.5 mg/kg IV loading bolus, followed by 10 μg/kg/minute CRI during surgery and 2 μg/kg/minute for 24 hours after surgery.

Morphine-Lidocaine-Ketamine (MLK)
The MLK infusion combines an opioid (morphine), a local anesthetic (lidocaine), and ketamine to provide optimal analgesia and to treat wind-up. The recipe for MLK is shown in Table 28-3.

Dexmedetomidine
CRIs of dexmedetomidine are commonly used in human patients, including children who are agitated in the hospital, resistant to ventilators, or in narcotic withdrawal. Similar success has been reported in veterinary patients, particularly in anxious breeds. The CRI dose for continued dysphoria/anxiety/pain in dogs and cats is 1 to 3 μg/kg/hour. Dexdomitor can be added to other CRIs, including MLK.

Adjunctive Agents
The vast majority of patients experiencing acute pain can be managed with conventional analgesics, such as NSAIDs, opioids, and local anesthetics. Patients in which pain is unmanaged or that are in preexisting pain states may require additional therapy. In addition to the classic analgesic agents, medications with other indications can be used to help manage pain. These drugs are referred to as *adjunctive analgesics* and come from many separate classes of pharmacologic compounds. Adjuvant analgesics are agents that can enhance analgesic drugs when co-administered but have few or no analgesic properties

when given alone. Examples of adjunctive and adjuvant analgesics are as follows:

- *Tranquilizers* (phenothiazines, benzodiazepines), which alter an animal's response to pain and can relax muscles, are used in combination with true analgesics. These drugs also reduce anxiety and fear, which can exacerbate pain.
- *NMDA receptor antagonists*, such as CRI of ketamine or oral administration of amantadine, can enhance analgesia by blocking sensitization of neurons in the spinal cord and are especially useful for managing patients that have experienced wind-up phenomenon.
- *Corticosteroids* (prednisolone) have powerful anti-inflammatory and immunosuppressive effects, "dampening the fires" of acute inflammation.
- *Tricyclic antidepressants* (amitriptyline, imipramine) are effective analgesics for chronic pain, especially neuropathic or cancer-related pain.

Neuropathic Pain Reliever

Gabapentin (an anticonvulsant) plays an important role in reducing neuropathic pain and central sensitization. Gabapentin is becoming increasingly popular in both human and veterinary medicine as the first choice in patients whose pain does not respond to conventional therapies, especially when nerve involvement or neuropathic pain is suspected. Indications for initiating gabapentin therapy include the following:

- Chronic degenerative conditions such as osteoarthritis and cancer
- Dermatologic conditions such as lick granuloma and chronic skin or ear infection
- Persistent biting, licking, chewing, and scratching at body areas
- Resistance to being touched at unaffected body sites
- Limping or obvious signs of pain not associated with current inflammation

A typical starting dose is 5 to 10 mg/kg PO 2 to 3 times per day in dogs and 2.5 to 5 mg/kg 2 to 3 times per day in cats. Patients should be reevaluated for response frequently, with dose adjustments made every 5 to 7 days until full efficacy is reached. Sleepiness is the side effect most commonly reported at higher doses. Gabapentin should not be stopped abruptly; patients should be weaned off. *Caution*: Neurontin elixir contains xylitol and can be used in cats but is not recommended for use in dogs.

Nonpharmacologic Treatment Options[1]

When possible, multimodal therapy that includes both pharmacologic and nonpharmacologic modalities should be used to treat pain, whether acute or chronic. Nonpharmacologic options include thermotherapy, massage, therapeutic exercise, aquatic therapy, acupuncture, electrical stimulation, therapeutic ultrasound, extracorporeal shock-wave therapy, and low-level laser, among others. Many of these modalities (e.g., acupuncture) provide direct pain relief; others (e.g., many therapeutic exercises) are associated with pain relief secondary to improved function and strength.

- *Thermotherapy* includes the use of both heat and cold for treatment of pain, injury, surgical incisions, and so forth.
- *Massage* decreases pain and accelerates recovery by relieving muscle tension, increasing blood flow to painful muscles, and mobilizing adhesions.
- *Therapeutic exercises* are a part of physical therapy that is designed to improve active pain-free range of motion and flexibility; use of limbs while reducing lameness; muscle mass and muscle strength; and daily function, while helping to prevent further injury. Forms of therapeutic exercise include passive exercises, proprioceptive training exercises, active exercises to improve limb use, and speed and strengthening exercises.
- *Aquatic therapy*, such as underwater treadmill exercises and swimming, may be used for rehabilitation after orthopedic surgery and after neurologic injury for muscle strengthening, and to attain improved joint function. Water is an excellent medium for therapy because the body bears less weight in water, which reduces the load on painful joints and allows the patient to exercise more comfortably and to do exercises that were not possible for the patient on land.
- *Electrical stimulation* indications include pain management (especially in arthritis, spondylosis, spondyloarthrosis, recovery from orthopedic surgery, and nerve regeneration), facilitation of fracture healing, relief of muscle tension, prevention of muscle atrophy from disuse, and muscle strengthening. Treatment modalities include neuromuscular electrical stimulation (NMES), transcutaneous electrical stimulation (TENS), and electrical muscle stimulation (EMS).
- *Acupuncture* has been used for thousands of years to treat pain, yet the mechanism of action is still not completely understood. The efficacy of acupuncture in relieving pain, especially chronic pain, is documented in the veterinary literature, and many veterinarians support its use.
- *Therapeutic ultrasound* has numerous applications but seems to be especially effective in treating diseased and dysfunctional joints and joint components and certain muscle diseases. Goals of treatment are to reduce pain, increase the elasticity of fibrous structures, promote blood flow, and improve tissue nutrition.
- Indications for *extracorporeal shock-wave therapy* (ESWT) include joint disease (e.g., arthritis of the hip, knee, or elbow) and tendinopathy.
- *Low-level laser therapy* is increasing in popularity and has many possible applications. Anecdotally, laser therapy has been shown to reduce pain and inflammation, promote healing, and stimulate nerve regeneration, muscle relaxation, and immune system response.

See Case Presentations 28-1, 28-2, and 28-3 for examples of analgesic protocols designed to manage pain associated with a feline onychectomy, a canine ovariohysterectomy with tooth extraction, and surgical repair of a herniated disc in a dog, respectively.

CASE PRESENTATION 28-1 FELINE ONYCHECTOMY (DECLAW)*

An 8-lb, 3-year-old spayed female Siamese is seen for destructive behavior at home, and the owners have elected declawing as an alternative to euthanasia. Pain is expected to be severe immediately after surgery and for 3 to 5 days postoperatively. How would you design an analgesic protocol that provides maximum preemptive, multimodal, and take-home analgesia for this cat?

Preemptive Pain Management
- Give one dose of NSAIDs SQ 1 to 2 hours before surgery.
- Administer 0.02 to 0.03 mg/kg buprenorphine IM with sedation 30 to 45 minutes before anesthesia.
- Perform circumferential ring block using 0.8 ml of 0.5% bupivacaine and allow 15 minutes to onset of action.

Postoperative Pain Management
- Administer subsequent doses of buprenorphine SQ or transmucosally every 6 to 8 hours until discharge.

Take-Home Pain Management
- Dispense buprenorphine to be given every 8 hours transmucosally by owners for 3 days.
- Reevaluate at day 4 and continue buprenorphine as needed. May repeat NSAID at this time if deemed necessary.*

*Declawing is one of the most painful procedures performed electively in veterinary medicine. Maximum analgesia should be administered to every cat undergoing this procedure to minimize associated pain.

CASE PRESENTATION 28-2 CANINE OVARIOHYSTERECTOMY (SPAY) AND TOOTH EXTRACTION

A 2-year-old Golden Retriever is being spayed, but physical examination reveals a fractured premolar tooth that needs to be removed while she is under a general anesthetic. What analgesia do you think would be appropriate for these two procedures?

Preemptive Pain Management
- Give NSAIDs SQ 1 to 2 hours before surgery.
- Administer a premedication combination of a strong opioid, such as morphine, combined with an α_2 agonist for sedation and analgesia about 15 minutes before induction.
- Perform an infraorbital nerve block on the affected maxillary side using approximately 0.5 ml of 0.5% bupivacaine. (Rinse syringe with epinephrine before drawing up bupivacaine to reduce bleeding from extraction.)

Postoperative Pain Management
- Administer additional doses of morphine every 4 to 6 hours for 12 to 24 hours.
- Can change to buprenorphine for its longer-lasting effects (6 to 8 hours) in the evening if personnel are unavailable to assess during the night.

Take-Home Pain Management
- Continue once-daily NSAIDs for 3 to 4 days postoperatively (longer, if indicated).

TREATMENT OF PAIN IN LARGE ANIMALS

As poor as pain management can be in some small animal practices, the situation in large animal medicine generally is even worse. Although we do not know exactly how many large animal patients receive analgesia in the United States, a survey of Canadian veterinarians sheds some insight on just how few horses, steers, and piglets actually receive analgesic drugs. For routine procedures, such as castrations in patients younger than 6 months, only 0.001% of piglets, 6.9% of beef calves, and 18.7% of dairy calves received pain medication.[2] Analgesia improved slightly in older patients, among which 19.9% of beef calves and 33.2% of dairy calves older than 6 months received some analgesic drugs. In horses, 95.8% of patients received analgesics for castration, and more than 90% of veterinarians used analgesic drugs for other equine surgeries, for cesarean sections in sows and cows, and for bovine claw amputations and omentopexies. However, even when analgesia was provided, it was often inadequate. In most cases, a single agent was used to treat levels of pain that would have required multimodal analgesia for adequate pain control, and often that agent was a drug with a short duration of action.

IDENTIFYING AND ANTICIPATING PAIN

Why is large animal pain so grossly undertreated? Fortunately, some of the reasons are exactly the same in large animals as they are in small animals, so we can use our existing small animal knowledge to educate our large animal colleagues. However, species-specific treatment differences have been noted, along with differences in the economic perceptions of veterinarians and producers. Here are the main reasons why large animal pain is not addressed:

1. "Animals don't feel pain." As with pain in small animals, this is absolutely false. All mammals have the same pain pathway, so if a procedure or injury would be painful to you, it will be painful to other mammals, including large animals.
2. "Animals don't show pain." As occurs in small animals, this one is often true, but it is absolutely no excuse for not treating pain. Unless an animal is in so much pain that it can no longer hide the pain, it is instinctual for them not to show pain. Remember, most farm animals are "prey," and in their world, the weakest member of the herd might be lunch for a "predator." It is in their best interest to be stoic. Thus each patient should be treated on the expected pain intensity and should not be forced to prove that it is in pain.

CASE PRESENTATION 28-3
HERNIATED DISC, SURGICAL REPAIR

A 9-year-old male castrated Dachshund has acute lameness progressing within several hours to inability to walk. Owners report that the dog has been walking "funny" for several weeks. After an MRI confirms a herniated disc, surgery is scheduled ASAP. How do you think this dog's pain should be managed before, during, and after surgery?

Presurgery
- The dog is started on steroids immediately and therefore should *not* receive additional NSAIDs.
- Morphine, lidocaine, and ketamine CRI is started to treat existing pain and prevent wind-up phenomenon.
- Epidural block is performed using 0.5% bupivacaine and morphine.

During Surgery
- Continue MLK infusion throughout surgery.

Postoperative Pain Management
- MLK infusion is continued for 12 to 24 hours postoperatively.
- Steroids are continued.

Take-Home Pain Management
- Send home on once-daily NSAIDs for several weeks.
- Give tramadol as needed for multimodal pain control.
- After 2 weeks, the dog is able to walk and does not appear to be in pain, but is chewing persistently at his left hind toes. What could be added to treat this assumed nerve pain?
- Gabapentin is added, and signs resolve in 2 days.

3. "A limited number of analgesic drugs are available for farm animals." This one is also often true but is absolutely no excuse for not treating pain. The analgesic drug classes that are available in small animal medicine (NSAIDs, opioids, local anesthetic agents, α_2 agonists, etc.) are available in large animal medicine. However, it is true that some species differences have been reported in how patients respond to a drug (e.g., horses can get excited after opioid administration) and in how drugs are "handled" in the body (e.g., orally administered drugs may be inactivated in the rumen). However, effective drugs are available for each species; they are listed in specific species discussions provided later in the chapter.

4. "Owners or producers won't pay for analgesia." This one may be true if we let it be true. It is definitely not true for most horses, and this is reflected by the large percentage of veterinarians in the Canadian study who provided at least some analgesia for their equine patients.[2] However, most farm animals have an absolute economic value (which is generally low), and the value to the producer is in the herd rather than in each individual animal; thus individual animal medicine is not a priority, and pain

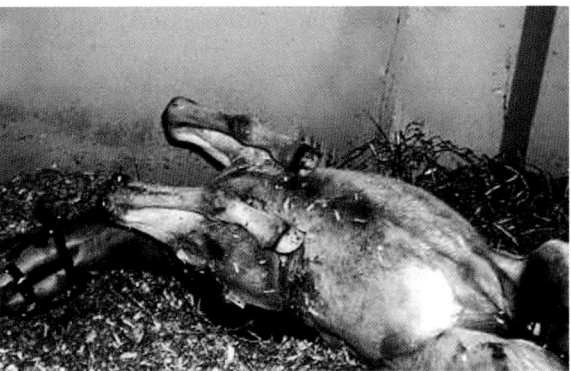

FIGURE 28-7 Painful horse rolling in the stall. Horses occasionally will roll in the pasture, presumably as a way to scratch an itchy back. However, horses that are rolling and thrashing violently and repeatedly are generally in pain, and the source of the pain is almost always the gastrointestinal tract. This degree of pain requires immediate attention.

relief falls in the category of individual animal medicine. However, to counter that argument, many analgesic drugs (e.g., lidocaine) are inexpensive and can be used without significant added costs. Furthermore, the stress of pain causes decreased food intake, weight loss, decreased milk production, and other side effects, which can be expensive for the producer. Additional information on this topic is provided under the "Cattle, Sheep, and Goats" section of this chapter.

As troubling as the situation seems, in a few instances, the practice of large animal pain medicine might be slightly ahead of that in small animals. For instance, equine practitioners are extremely comfortable with the use of NSAIDs for acute and chronic musculoskeletal pain and with the use of α_2 agonists for control of acute abdominal pain (or colic). Of course, this perceived comfort level with analgesics sometimes stems from issues other than concern over the welfare of the patient. As an example, NSAIDs are administered because lame horses are not highly functional and certainly will not perform well if they are in competition. Colic pain is treated because severe GI pain can make horses become extremely violent and dangerous to humans. But for whatever reason analgesic agents are administered, the benefit to the patient is the same. Veterinarians and veterinary technicians should continue to stress the message that large animals do indeed feel pain, and that pain should be treated in all animals (Figure 28-7).

> **TECHNICIAN NOTE** All mammals, including large animals, have the same pain pathway and do experience pain, although they may not show signs of pain. Pain causes deleterious effects (e.g., hypertension, arrhythmias, GI ulceration, ileus, delayed healing) and should be treated on the basis of what we expect the pain level to be after a given painful stimulus—not on the basis of what the patient actually exhibits.

Identifying pain in large animals can be extremely difficult because these animals evolved in a prey-predator society, and all are in the "prey" group. This means that they instinctively hide weakness (and pain is a weakness) to survive. However, because the pain pathway is the same in all mammals, the phrase, "If it hurts you, it hurts them," is appropriate in determining whether a patient might be in pain, regardless of whether the patient shows pain. Unfortunately, as with small animals, the negative effects of pain (see Box 28-1) occur any time pain occurs (whether or not the patient shows pain) and cause detrimental effects to the patient, including delayed healing. Treatment of pain is not just an ethical issue—it is also a medical issue. Species-specific signs of pain are listed in Box 28-5.

Furthermore, because these animals often do not show pain until the pain is too severe to be hidden, the sequelae of pain may well be advanced by the time a human realizes that the patient is in pain. The degree of pain that we expect the patient to be in should be anticipated and analgesia administered on the basis of that expectation, rather than on the basis of exhibited pain. Species-specific, commonly encountered painful conditions and surgical procedures and the degree of pain expected with each condition are listed in Tables 28-4 and 28-5.

TREATING PAIN IN LARGE ANIMALS

All of the analgesic drug classes used to treat small animals can be used to treat large animals, but fewer FDA-approved drugs are available, and, in general, less is known about the use of these drugs in large animal species (Box 28-6). However, affordable and effective analgesic drugs are available for all species, and "lack of drugs" is not a viable excuse for withholding analgesia.

As with small animals, the principles of pain management include use of the following:
1. Preemptive analgesia (for surgical pain).
2. Multimodal analgesia (any time pain is moderate to severe).

3. Analgesia of a duration that covers the entire painful period (this applies to both acute and chronic pain).

Regardless of which analgesic drugs are chosen for the patient, these principles should be addressed every time an analgesic protocol is formulated. Drug classes that can be

---

BOX 28-5	Signs of Pain in Horses and Farm Animals

General Signs of Pain
Decreased interest in food or anorexia
Lethargy
Excitement, restlessness
Pawing
Vocalizing (especially cattle)
Bruxism
Reluctance to move
Lying down more frequently or for longer periods than usual
Any abnormal behavior

Additional Signs of Gastrointestinal (GI) Pain
Kicking at or looking at abdomen
Violently trying to roll
Stretching out in abnormal posture (especially horses)
Standing with abdomen "tucked" (especially cattle)
Dog sitting (especially foals with GI pain)

Additional Signs of Musculoskeletal Pain
Lameness
Abnormal gait
Positive response to hoof testers or flexion tests

Other Signs of Pain (Horses Only)
Reluctance to be bridled (may be head or tooth pain)
Reluctance to be saddled (may be back pain)
Reluctance to be ridden (may be back pain, lameness, or general pain)

TABLE 28-4	Most Commonly Occurring Painful Conditions in Horses, Cattle, Sheep, Goats, and Camelids	
SOURCE OF PAIN	**SIGNS/SEVERITY**	**TREATMENT**
Horses		
Musculoskeletal Pain: Conditions of the Foot		
Acute: sole abscess	Severe lameness of sudden onset.	Treat source—remove abscess; treat with NSAIDs for 2 to 3 days to control inflammation.
Chronic: laminitis or navicular disease	Mild, moderate to severe lameness of long duration; may have bouts of severe lameness that must be treated more aggressively; these are extremely difficult conditions to treat.	Use NSAIDs to control inflammation; shoeing and hoof care are extremely important; local anesthetic blockade; opioids; other therapies (e.g., vasodilators); alternative care (e.g., acupuncture)—all may be necessary.
Musculoskeletal/Joint Pain		
Acute: OCD	Moderate to severe lameness that occurs with exercise; joint effusion.	Surgery is required for resolution of lesion; NSAIDs may be necessary long term; joint supplements and chondroprotective agents may help.
Chronic: osteoarthritis	Mild to severe lameness that may decrease during exercise.	NSAIDs long term; joint supplements and chondroprotective agents may help.

TABLE 28-4	Most Commonly Occurring Painful Conditions in Horses, Cattle, Sheep, Goats, and Camelids—cont'd	
SOURCE OF PAIN	**SIGNS/SEVERITY**	**TREATMENT**
Soft Tissue Pain GI pain: colic	Moderate to severe pain; may have recurring episodes with chronic cases; restlessness, pawing, looking and/or kicking at abdomen; frequently lying down and rising; trying to roll; violent movements; bruxism; tachycardia; etc.	Requires treatment, may require surgery. For acute pain: NSAIDs, opioids, α_2 agonists, antispasmodic agents, CRIs, alternative therapy, etc.—all may be included in the protocol. For chronic pain: depends on cause of colic.
Cattle *Musculoskeletal Pain* Foot (claw) and joint problems	Moderate to severe lameness; lying down more frequently than usual; anorexia; decreased milk production (dairy cattle).	NSAIDs; general foot care; may require antibiotics; local anesthetics for diagnostics; may need surgery.
Soft Tissue Pain GI pain: colic	Mild to severe pain; general restlessness; standing with abdomen "tucked"; bruxism.	Requires treatment, may require surgery. For acute pain: NSAIDs, opioids, α_2 agonists, antispasmodic agents, CRIs, alternative therapy, etc.—all may be included in the protocol. For chronic pain: depends on cause of colic.
Mastitis	Mild to severe depending on degree of inflammation; stilted gait; unwillingness to move; kicking at udder; redness and swelling of udder.	NSAIDs, antibiotics; stripping of affected quarter.
Sheep and Goats Urolithiasis	Mild, progressing to severe if urinary tract is blocked; spraying urine or inability to urinate; abdominal pain; restlessness moving to recumbency; anorexia.	Requires treatment, may require surgery; NSAIDs, opioids, epidural analgesia.
Foot (claw) and joint pain	Moderate to severe lameness; lying down more frequently than usual; anorexia; decreased milk production (dairy goats).	NSAIDs; general foot care; may require antibiotics, local anesthetics for diagnostics; may need surgery.
GI pain: colic	Moderate to severe lameness; lying down more frequently than usual; anorexia	Requires treatment, may require surgery. For acute pain: NSAIDs, opioids, α_2 agonists, antispasmodic agents, CRIs, alternative therapy, etc.—all may be included in the protocol. For chronic pain: depends on cause of colic.
Camelids Dental pain	Mild to severe, depending on severity of disease; anorexia; lethargy; swelling of jaw; nasal discharge.	Generally requires surgery, NSAIDs, antibiotics, opioids, and oral blockade with local anesthetics.
Dystocia	Can be severe during the actual dystocia; moderate to severe (depending on tissue trauma) following dystocia; signs of GI pain, lethargy, anorexia.	Dystocia requires treatment and fetal manipulation; may require surgery; NSAIDs and epidural analgesia.
Foot and joint pain	Moderate to severe lameness; lying down more frequently than usual; anorexia	NSAIDs, general foot care, may require antibiotics, local anesthetics for diagnostics; may need surgery.
GI pain: colic	Mild to severe pain; general restlessness; standing with abdomen "tucked"; bruxism.	Requires treatment, may require surgery. For acute pain: NSAIDs, opioids, α_2 agonists, antispasmodic agents, CRIs; alternative therapy, etc.—all may be included in the protocol. For chronic pain: depends on cause of colic.

CRI, Constant rate infusion; *GI,* gastrointestinal; *NSAIDs,* nonsteroidal anti-inflammatory drugs; *OCD,* osteochonditis dissecans.

TABLE 28-5 | Most Commonly Occurring Painful Surgeries in Horses, Cattle, Sheep, Goats, and Camelids

SURGERY	PAIN SEVERITY	TREATMENT EXAMPLES
Horses		
Colic surgery	Severe	Opioids, α_2 agonists, NSAIDs, CRIs
Joint surgery	Moderate to severe	Opioids, α_2 agonists, NSAIDs, intra-articular analgesia, epidural analgesia for rear limb pain
Sinus surgery	Moderate to severe	Opioids, α_2 agonists, NSAIDs
Castration	Mild to moderate	Butorphanol + α_2 agonist premedication, NSAIDs, testicular block
Cattle		
GI or colic surgery	Severe	Opioids, α_2 agonists, NSAIDs, CRIs
Abomasopexy	Moderate	Local anesthetics, NSAIDs
Claw removal	Moderate to severe	Local anesthetics, NSAIDs, opioids + α_2 agonists during surgery
Dehorning	Moderate to severe	Local anesthetics, NSAIDs
Teat surgery	Moderate to severe	Local anesthetics, NSAIDs, opioids + α_2 agonists during surgery
Castration	Moderate	Local anesthetic block, NSAIDs
C-section	Moderate to severe	Local anesthetics, epidural, NSAIDs, opioids + α_2 agonists during surgery
Sheep, Goats		
C-section	Moderate to severe	Local anesthetics, epidural, NSAIDs, opioids + α_2 agonists during surgery
Perineal urethrostomy	Moderate to severe	Epidural analgesia, NSAIDs, opioids + α_2 agonists during surgery
Castration	Moderate	Local anesthetic blockade, NSAIDs, opioids + α_2 agonists during surgery
Dehorning (goats)	Moderate to severe	Local anesthetic blockade, NSAIDs, opioids + α_2 agonists during surgery
Claw removal	Severe	See comments under "Cattle"
Camelids		
Dental surgery	Moderate to severe	NSAIDs, local anesthetic blockade, α_2 agonists, and opioids during surgery
C-section	Moderate to severe	Epidural analgesia, NSAIDs, opioids, and α_2 agonists during surgery

CRI, Constant rate infusion; *NSAIDs,* nonsteroidal anti-inflammatory drugs.

BOX 28-6 | What FDA Approval Means

Food and Drug Administration (FDA) approval of a drug for use in a particular species is gained only after a rigorous amount of research has proved that the drug is both safe and effective in that species. Thus FDA approval guarantees that the drug has been studied in the target species. However, many "off-label" or nonapproved FDA drugs are used when no approved drug is available for treatment, or when nonapproved drugs may be more effective or safer than approved drugs. Approved drugs may also be used in a nonapproved way (e.g., medetomidine is approved for use in dogs, but not as a premedicant to anesthesia, yet it is commonly used this way) or at a nonapproved dose (e.g., the dose of butorphanol used clinically in horses is generally lower than the FDA-approved dose). Not all of the products mentioned in this chapter are FDA approved, but all are commonly used in veterinary practice, and all can be referenced in the veterinary literature.

used in large animal analgesic protocols are listed in Tables 28-6 and 28-7 and include the following.

NSAIDs

NSAIDs are an ideal choice for most painful conditions because they are anti-inflammatory and analgesic. Thus, any time pain is caused by inflammation, NSAIDs are treating the source of pain, as well as the pain itself (Figure 28-8). NSAIDs are relatively safe, easy to administer, inexpensive, and long lasting (12 to 24 hours). Because of their long duration, NSAIDs are ideal to pair with more potent but short-acting drugs, such as opioids and α_2 agonists. Depending on which drug is chosen, NSAIDs can be used IV, IM, SQ, PO, or transdermally. The most commonly used NSAIDs in large animals are phenylbutazone ("bute") and flunixin meglumine ("Banamine"), but other NSAIDs are also available (see Tables 28-6 and 28-7). The primary side effect of NSAIDs in large animals is GI ulceration.

TECHNICIAN NOTE The most common side effect associated with NSAIDs in all species is GI upset or ulceration; large animals are more likely to experience ulceration. Patients with GI ulceration tend to stop eating and appear lethargic. Pain may cause animals to stand with backs "hunched" (especially ruminants) or to stretch out in abnormal postures (especially horses). Adult horses often grind their teeth when they are in pain, and foals may "dog sit" when they have stomach pain. Anorexia, lethargy, and/or abnormal behavior in any patient that is on therapy should prompt immediate evaluation of the patient and assessment for possible drug side effects.

TABLE 28-6	Analgesic Drug Dosages for Horses			
DRUG CLASS/DRUG	**DOSE (MG/KG UNLESS STATED)**	**ROUTE**	**DOSING INTERVAL**	**COMMENTS**
NSAIDs				
Phenylbutazone	2-4	PO, IV	q12hours	FDA approved for use in horses; reduce dose to 2 mg/kg on second day; used most commonly for musculoskeletal pain.
Flunixin meglumine	1	PO, IV, IM	q12hours or q24hours	FDA approved for use in horses. Used most commonly for GI pain and treatment of endotoxemia.
Ketoprofen	2-3	IV	q24hours	FDA approved for use in horses.
Firocoxib	0.1	PO	q24hours	FDA approved for use for up to 14 days for control of pain and inflammation associated with equine osteoarthritis.
Diclofenac sodium	5-inch ribbon of cream	Topical, over painful joint	q12hours	FDA approved for treatment of joint pain and inflammation for up to 10 days.
Carprofen	0.7	IV	q24hours	Approved for horses in countries other than the United States.
Meloxicam	0.6	IV	q12hours	Approved for horses in countries other than the United States.
Opioids				
Morphine	0.1-0.3		q3-4hours	Inject slowly if administered IV; horses may have excitatory response.
	0.1-0.2	Epidural	q24hours	qs to 10-30 ml with sterile saline.
	0.1	Intra-articular	Once, intraoperative	
Butorphanol	0.02-0.1	IM, IV	q2-3hours	FDA approved for relief of pain associated with colic at 0.1 mg/kg; ataxia associated with label dose; lower dosages are generally used clinically.
	23.7 µg/kg/minute (0.013 mg/kg/hour)	IV	CRI	Loading dose 0.02 mg/kg.
Fentanyl	2 of the 100-µg patches/450 kg	Transdermal	Change patches at 48 hours	Can be used without sedation—no excitement noted.
Buprenorphine	0.004-0.006	IV, IM, SQ		
Tramadol	2	IV		Analgesic effects unknown.
α_2 Agonists				
Detomidine	0.01-0.02	IV	q2-4hours	FDA approved as a sedative-analgesic.
	0.02-0.04	IM		
	0.06	PO		
	0.15-0.3 µg/kg/minute		CRI	Loading dose 6-10 µg/kg; adjust CRI to achieve desired sedation.
Romifidine	0.04-0.120	IM, IV	q2-4hours	FDA approved as sedative-analgesic and as a preanesthetic.
Xylazine	0.5-1.0	IV	q2-4hours	FDA approved as a sedative-analgesic.
	1.0-2.2	IM		
	0.17	Epidural		Generally added to lidocaine.
Medetomidine	0.005-0.007	IV	q2-4hours	Loading dose 5 µg/kg.
	3-5 µg/kg/hour	IV	CRI	

Continued

TABLE 28-6	Analgesic Drug Dosages for Horses—cont'd			
DRUG CLASS/DRUG	**DOSE (MG/KG UNLESS STATED)**	**ROUTE**	**DOSING INTERVAL**	**COMMENTS**
Local Anesthetic Drugs				
Lidocaine	As needed for tissue infiltration; total dose <5 mg/kg	Tissue		
	50 µg/kg/hour	IV	CRI	Intraoperative or postoperative or for medical pain.
	0.35	Epidural		May be combined with morphine or
	0.35	Intra-articular		xylazine.
Bupivacaine	As needed for tissue infiltration; total dose 2 mg/kg			Longer duration of action than lidocaine; can also be used for epidural and intra-articular administration.
Mepivacaine	2-15 ml	Tissue		FDA approved for use in horses;
	5-20 ml	Epidural		dosages are from label.
	10-15 ml	Intra-articular		
Joint Supplements and Chondroprotective Agents*				
Sodium hyaluronate	10-40 mg/joint	Intra-articular	Every 7 days	
Polysulfated GAGs	250 mg/joint	Intra-articular	Every 7 days	
	500 mg	IM	Every 5 days	
Other Agents				
Ketamine	40 µg/kg/minute	IV	CRI	FDA approved for one-time injection
Antispasmodic agents (Buscopan)	0.3	IV	One dose	for spasmodic, flatulent, or impaction colic in horses. Administer slowly.

CRI, Constant rate infusion; *FDA,* Food and Drug Administration; *GAGs,* glycosaminoglycans; *NSAIDs,* nonsteroidal anti-inflammatory drugs.
*Numerous products are included in this category, and two examples are listed here. Use of these products should be governed by proven efficacy.

TABLE 28-7	Analgesic Drug Dosages for Farm Animals (Cattle, Sheep, Goats, and Pigs) and Camelids				
DRUG CLASS/DRUG	**SPECIES**	**DOSE (MG/KG UNLESS STATED)**	**ROUTE**	**DOSING INTERVAL**	**COMMENTS**
NSAIDs					
Phenylbutazone	All	4-6	PO	q24-48hours	Prohibited in dairy cattle older than 20 months of age.
		2-4	IV		
Flunixin meglumine	All	1	PO, IV, IM	q12-24hours	FDA approved in some species; withdrawal times are published.
Ketoprofen	All	2-3	PO, IV, IM, SQ	q24hours	Widely used because of low cost, but absorption may be erratic.
Aspirin	Cattle, sheep, goat	100	PO	q12hours	
Carprofen	All	0.7	IV	q24-48hours	
Meloxicam	Cattle	0.5 mg/kg	SQ, IV	q24hours	
	Pig	0.4 mg/kg	IM	q24hours	
Opioids					
Morphine	All	0.05-0.1	IV	q3-4hours	Inject slowly if administered IV. May cause excitement, especially in pigs.
		0.1-0.4	IM		
		0.1	Epidural		Commonly combined with local anesthetic agent.
	All	0.1-0.2	Epidural	q6-12hours	Dilute with 0.05 ml/kg sterile saline or combine with bupivacaine at 1.5 mg/kg.
	All	0.1	Intra-articular	Once, intraoperative	

TABLE 28-7	Analgesic Drug Dosages for Farm Animals (Cattle, Sheep, Goats, and Pigs) and Camelids—cont'd				
DRUG CLASS/DRUG	**SPECIES**	**DOSE (MG/KG UNLESS STATED)**	**ROUTE**	**DOSING INTERVAL**	**COMMENTS**
Butorphanol	All	0.01-0.2	IM, IV	q2-3hours	Camelids are extremely sensitive to sedative properties.
	Pig	0.2 mg/kg	IM, IV	q2-3hours	
Fentanyl	Sheep, goat	50 µg/hour	Transdermal	48-72 hours	Dosage is for adult animals of the respective species.
	Pig	50 µg/hour			
	Camelid	150-225 µg/hour			
Buprenorphine	Sheep, goat	0.015	IV, IM		Rarely causes sedation or excitement.
	Pig	0.01	IV, IM		
	Camelid	0.01	IV, IM		
α₂ Agonists*					
Detomidine	Cattle, sheep, goat	0.003-0.01	IM, IV	q2-4hours	
	Pig	0.1	IM, IV	q2-4hours	
Romifidine	Cattle, sheep, goat	0.003-0.005	IM, IV	q2-4hours	
	Pig	0.1	IM, IV	q2-4hours	
Xylazine	Cattle, sheep, goat	0.1-0.3	IM	q2-4hours for all	Alpacas are more resistant than llamas and require a dose of 0.3-0.6 mg/kg IV or IM.
	Camelid	0.05-0.1	IV		
	Pig	0.2-0.4	IV, IM		
		2.2-4.4	IM Epidural		
Medetomidine	Camelid	0.01-0.03	IV, IM	q2-4hours	
	Pig	0.08	IV, IM	q2-4hours	
	Sheep, goat	0.004-0.01	IV, IM	q2-4hours	
Dexmedetomidine	Camelid	0.005-0.015	IV, IM	q2-4hours	
	Sheep, goat	0.002-0.005	IV, IM	q2-4hours	
	Pig	0.04	IV, IM	q2-4hours	
Local Anesthetic Agents					
Lidocaine	All	As needed for tissue infiltration; total dose, ≤5 mg/kg	Tissue	q1-3hours	Goats sensitive to side effects—dose carefully.
	All	0.2-0.4	Epidural	q1-3hours	
	All	0.1	Intra-articular	q1-3hours	
Bupivacaine	All	As needed for tissue infiltration; total dose, ≤2 mg/kg	Tissue	q4-6hours	Goats sensitive to side effects—dose carefully; do not give IV.

*α₂ agonists cause profound sedation in ruminants and camelids, but pigs are fairly insensitive to α₂ agonist–induced sedation.

Opioids

Opioids are the most potent class of analgesic drugs and should be used to treat all moderate to severe cases of pain, especially acute pain. The opioid most commonly used in large animals is butorphanol, but morphine, buprenorphine, and fentanyl are also used. Although the side effect is rare in painful patients, opioids may cause excitement in large animal species, especially horses and pigs, and are often used with a sedative (e.g., xylazine, romifidine, detomidine) in these species. Cattle, sheep, and goats generally become lightly sedated with opioids but may exhibit behavioral changes, such as restlessness and vocalization. Camelids are sensitive to the sedating properties of opioids. Opioids can be administered IV, IM, SQ, transdermally, epidurally, intra-articularly, and by CRI. Opioids are used primarily for acute medical or surgical pain. Other than butorphanol, opioid use in large animals has been fairly uncommon but is increasing.

α₂ Agonists

α₂ agonists, such as detomidine, xylazine, and romifidine, are used more commonly in large animals than in small animals; although they are generally considered sedatives, they actually provide moderate pain relief. α₂ agonists are often combined with opioids (primarily butorphanol) for improved sedation and enhanced analgesia in patients that are experiencing acute pain (e.g., patients with colic) and patients that will undergo minor procedures (e.g., wound repair). The dosage of α₂ agonists is highly variable between species because the response to α₂ agonists is highly variable. Ataxia secondary to profound sedation is the most common side effect of this class of drugs in large animals. The decrease in heart rate that often follows administration of α₂ agonists is rarely a matter of concern because it is a normal physiologic response to increased blood pressure caused by α₂ agonist–mediated vasoconstriction.

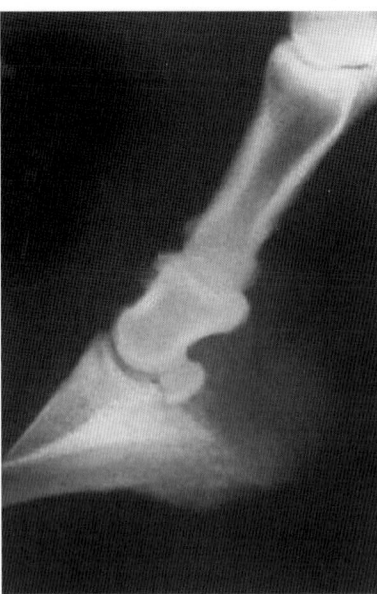

FIGURE 28-8 Radiograph of the pastern joint of a horse with "high ringbone." This is a slowly progressive disease that causes mild to severe lameness (depending on the degree of the pathologic condition) that will limit the usefulness of the horse. Mild pain generally can be controlled with nonsteroidal anti-inflammatory drugs (NSAIDs) and light use, but more severe pain requires multimodal therapy.

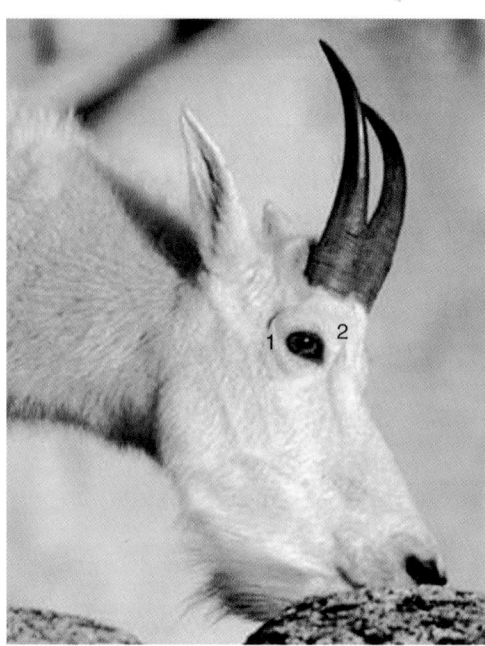

FIGURE 28-9 Locations for blocking the nerves supplying the horns in a goat. The number *1* indicates the location to block the cornual branch of the zygomaticotemporal nerve, and the number *2* indicates the location to block the cornual branch of the infratrochlear nerve. It is important to note that both nerves must be blocked in goats, as opposed to cattle, in which only the cornual branch of the zygomaticotemporal nerve supplies the horns.

> **TECHNICIAN NOTE**   Wide variation in species' response to the sedative effects of α_2 agonists has been reported. Pigs are most resistant and require high dosages for sedation. Horses are next in sensitivity and require moderately high dosages. Cattle, sheep, and goats are the most sensitive, and all of these species require approximately one-tenth of the horse dose. Dose sensitivity of camelids falls right in between that of horses and ruminants.

Local Anesthetic Drugs

Local anesthetic drugs are some of the most effective and least expensive (yet underused) analgesic drugs available. Local anesthetic drugs are ideal for pain control in all species because they block the transmission of painful impulses without causing systemic effects. Lidocaine, bupivacaine, and mepivacaine are used locally in large animals, and lidocaine can be used IV as a CRI. Mepivacaine is often chosen for diagnostic nerve blocks because it has an intermediate duration of action between lidocaine and bupivacaine (Figure 28-9). For true analgesia (i.e., blocking nerves to control the pain of laminitis), longer-lasting drugs, such as bupivacaine, should be used. Lidocaine CRI is fairly commonly used to control intraoperative and postoperative pain, especially GI pain in horses.

Joint Supplements and Chondroprotective Agents

Joint supplements and chondroprotective agents, such as nutraceuticals, chondroitin sulfate, hyaluronic acid, and glycosaminoglycans (GAGs), are used more commonly in horses than in any other species, although they can be used in all of the species mentioned in this chapter. These products generally are not truly analgesic agents, but they may help to improve joint health, thereby decreasing pain. However, some may have an anti-inflammatory or other medical effect. These products are appropriate to add to a multimodal protocol (e.g., with NSAIDs) and sometimes are used alone for mild to moderate pain, especially in performance horses that cannot receive other pharmaceuticals because of drug administration rules. A large number of products are included in this category. The choice of which one(s) to use should be based on proven efficacy of the product.

> **TECHNICIAN NOTE**   Most nutraceuticals and other feed additives are not FDA regulated; thus research proving their efficacy and safety is not required by law. Reports of efficacy generally are anecdotal and are not backed by research. Furthermore, the true content of the product is not regulated, and some products have been shown to have a lower percentage of active ingredients than the percentage listed on the label. This does not mean that these products do not work. However, it means that only products that are shown to be safe and effective and products that come from reputable companies should be used.

Miscellaneous Agents
Ketamine
Ketamine is an NMDA receptor antagonist that is used as a CRI to treat the pain of "wind-up" (see p. 1060 in this chapter). Ketamine CRIs can be added to multimodal analgesic protocols in patients that are experiencing pain that is difficult to control. Ketamine CRIs have been shown to be useful in a variety of large animal species, including horses and llamas.

Antispasmodic Agents
Antispasmodic agents (e.g., Buscopan) are frequently administered as part of a multimodal plan in the initial treatment phases of colic in horses.

Alternative and Complementary Therapy
Alternative and complementary therapy encompasses many modalities, including acupuncture, chiropractics, massage, low-level laser therapy, extracorporeal shock-wave therapy, magnetic therapy, and many others (see "Nonpharmacologic Treatment Options" in the small animal section of this chapter). However, not all of the alternative modalities have scientific credibility, and all treatment modalities should be carefully researched before they are endorsed. These treatments may be used for acute pain, but more commonly, they are added to a multimodal protocol for chronic pain or are used when pharmaceuticals are not allowed (e.g., in performance horses that will be drug tested).

Good Husbandry
Good husbandry and nursing care are always a major part of an effective pain management program. This includes not only attention to comfort, as in small animals, but also attention to species-specific details, such as proper shoeing in horses with foot and limb pain and proper udder care in lactating dairy cattle.

More species-specific information on each drug class is available later in the species section and in Tables 28-6 and 28-7.

SPECIES-SPECIFIC INFORMATION

HORSES
Horses generally receive better analgesic treatment than is received by other large animals for several reasons:
1. They are more likely to be treated as "companion animals," such as dogs and cats.
2. Horses generally are performance animals, and pain can affect their performance.
3. Horses may become violent and dangerous when in acute pain—especially with GI pain.
4. Unlike cattle and pigs, most horses do not have an absolute economic value; thus, the owners are more likely to spend money on care.

A greater number of analgesic agents have been researched in the horse; thus we have more information about how to use these drugs in this species. NSAIDs are the mainstay for both acute and chronic pain, and equine practitioners are often better than small animal practitioners in prescribing NSAIDs. Opioids are used with increasing frequency in horses. Morphine is a potent analgesic drug that is used intraoperatively as an IV injection or in the epidural or intra-articular space. Morphine is often used IM in patients with postoperative pain or in patients with chronic pain. When morphine is used parenterally in the horse, it is often combined with an α_2 agonist or acepromazine to reduce the chance of an excitatory response. Butorphanol is the most commonly used opioid in the horse; it is routinely combined with an α_2 agonist for the treatment of acute pain. Buprenorphine, albeit somewhat expensive in adult horses, has been shown to provide analgesia and has a longer duration of analgesia than butorphanol. Fentanyl patches have been used in adult horses and in foals for acute pain; tramadol has been used in a few horses (with mixed success) for control of chronic pain. Other agents that are routinely used in horses include chondroprotective agents for joint pain and antispasmodic agents for GI pain. Ketamine and lidocaine CRIs are used more and more commonly for intraoperative and postoperative pain and for medical pain (e.g., nonsurgical colic). Local and regional types of blockade (e.g., epidurals, intra-articular blocks) are fairly standard treatments for pain in horses.

See Case Presentation 28-4 for an example of an analgesic protocol designed to manage pain associated with severe colic in a horse, and Case Presentation 28-5 for an example of an analgesic protocol designed to manage pain associated with osteoarthritis in a horse.

> **TECHNICIAN NOTE** Do not be afraid to use potent opioids (e.g., morphine) in horses, especially for intraoperative and postoperative pain. These drugs are highly effective and extremely inexpensive. However, like cats, horses may exhibit excitement after receiving a potent opioid, so generally, a sedative (e.g., xylazine, romifidine, detomidine) should be administered at the same time. Excitement is rare in painful horses but is fairly common in nonpainful horses.

CATTLE, SHEEP, AND GOATS
With the exception of animals kept as individual pets, valuable beef herd sires, and high-producing dairy cows, food-producing herd animals, such as cattle, sheep, and goats, are the least likely large animal patients to receive analgesia, because these animals often have an absolute economic value with a narrow profit margin, and pharmaceutical residue is not generally accepted in the food chain. The latter issue means that some drugs are totally prohibited in this group of patients, whereas other drugs have a withdrawal time that must be observed between administration of the drug and the time that meat and/or milk can be used.

CASE PRESENTATION 28-4 SEVERE COLIC

Lightning, a 4-year-old quarter horse gelding, was found 1 hour ago kicking at his abdomen and trying to lie down and roll. His respiratory rate is 30 breaths/minute, his heart rate is 80 beats/minute, and his capillary refill time is 3 seconds. All other physiologic parameters are normal, but the horse is now pawing and is aggressively trying to throw himself down to roll. On rectal palpation, the veterinarian discovers a great deal of large intestine distention, and she decides to send the horse to a surgical referral center. How will you make the horse comfortable for the ride to the referral center?

ANSWER: Multimodal therapy is required for this degree of pain. Potent analgesic drugs that act quickly are the best choice. A combination of an α_2 agonist (xylazine, detomidine, and romifidine are all appropriate) and an opioid (most likely butorphanol) should be administered IV. NSAIDs do not work fast enough and are not potent enough to treat this horse's pain when used alone. However, they are long lasting and will become effective as the other drugs wear off, so an NSAID (most likely flunixin) should also be considered. An antispasmodic agent would be a good addition.

CASE CONTINUED: The horse arrives at the referral center, and the surgeon determines that he needs to go to surgery immediately. What analgesic protocol will you recommend preoperatively and intraoperatively?

ANSWER: Preemptive, multimodal analgesia is required. Some analgesia is most likely still present from the α_2 agonist–opioid combination and the NSAID administered by the referring veterinarian. However, more α_2 agonist will be needed for induction of anesthesia, and the opioid will

have to be repeated at induction or just before the surgeon makes an incision. IV morphine just before the incision would be an excellent choice because it is a potent, long-lasting opioid. Although the previously administered butorphanol is an agonist-antagonist opioid and could potentially decrease the effectiveness of the pure opioid agonist morphine, butorphanol has a fairly short duration, and any clinical effects are likely minimal within 1 to 2 hours. An NSAID should be administered if one was not administered before arrival at the referral center. CRI of lidocaine with or without ketamine could be administered intraoperatively.

CASE CONTINUED: The horse had an obstructed bowel, which was corrected during surgery. He recovered well, but now, 6 hours after surgery, he seems a bit uncomfortable. What can be done postoperatively to control his pain?

ANSWER: Unless the horse is only mildly uncomfortable and would need only one dose of analgesic drugs, CRI is the best choice. Lidocaine, ketamine, or butorphanol (or a combination of two or three of these drugs) can be used. The best choice is probably lidocaine because it is inexpensive, is not controlled, and causes neither sedation nor excitement (unless overdosed). Ideally, in our attempt to anticipate pain rather than force the patient to show pain, CRI should have been started *before* the horse became uncomfortable. Multimodal analgesia will be required, so the horse should be continued on an NSAID (long duration and anti-inflammatory properties). Flunixin is the most commonly used NSAID for colic pain.

CASE PRESENTATION 28-5 OSTEOARTHRITIS

Rajah, an 11-year-old Arabian mare, has been diagnosed with osteoarthritis of the pastern joint ("high ringbone"). She has been a competitive endurance horse, but her owner is willing to retire her. However, she still wants a "performance" horse, in that she would like to do some light trail riding with Rajah. What will you recommend to control chronic pain in this horse?

ANSWER: NSAIDs will be the mainstay of treatment because they will help to control both the pain and the inflammation associated with this disease. Phenylbutazone is the most likely choice. Nutraceuticals added to the feed, GAGs administered IM, and hyaluronic acid with or without steroids injected directly into the joint are all excellent additions to the NSAIDs. Proper shoeing will also greatly benefit Rajah. An increased dose of NSAIDs may be needed immediately before and the day after long rides to keep Rajah comfortable and able to enjoy the trail.

Economics

Although it is true that many farm animals have an absolute economic value with a low profit margin, it is also true that several of the analgesic drugs are inexpensive (e.g., local anesthetic drugs), and the side effects of pain (e.g., anorexia, weight loss) can be as or more costly than the analgesia. In many other countries of the world (e.g., the United Kingdom, many European countries), analgesia is required by law for surgical procedures done on farm animals. Most commonly, the use of local anesthetic drugs is required. Local anesthetics provide good analgesia for the duration of the block (albeit this may be fairly short), have been shown to decrease the side effects associated with pain, and have minimal tissue uptake, so that drug residues are of decreased concern. Analgesia may be difficult to regulate in the United States because many routine procedures (e.g., castration in calves, pigs, and lambs) are done by producers, not by veterinarians. However, as a profession, we should strive to ensure that all procedures done by a veterinarian are accompanied by analgesia. Unfortunately, even this seemingly simple step may be difficult, as evidenced by a few of the swine practitioners who participated in the Canadian study, who were concerned about loss of professional time and income while waiting for local anesthetics to take effect—a delay that is only 2 to 5 minutes in duration.

Drug Residues in Meat and Milk

Because drug residues in the human food chain could be harmful to human beings, strict regulations regarding the use of many pharmaceuticals in food-producing (meat and milk) animals have been put forth. For instance, the use of phenylbutazone is completely prohibited in dairy cattle 20 months of age or older. On the other hand, some forms of flunixin (but not all brands) are approved for use in cattle and pigs, with withdrawal times of 72 hours for milk and 10 days for meat in cattle, and 12 days for meat in pigs. Because regulations change, people dealing with food-producing animals should routinely update withdrawal information on the drugs they are using. The best source for information is the Food Animal Residue Avoidance Databank (FARAD) at www.farad.org.

Finally, many food-producing animals are ruminants, and delivery of oral drugs into the rumen can inactivate them, slow their absorption, or otherwise alter the drug or patient response to the drug. Fortunately, most oral drugs that are available to treat pain can be used in ruminants; of course, IV, IM, SQ, transdermal, epidural, intra-articular, and local tissue infusion routes of administration can all be used as well.

> **TECHNICIAN NOTE** The latest guidelines for withdrawal times of drugs in food-producing animals can be obtained from the Food Animal Residue Avoidance Databank (FARAD) at www.farad.com.

All of the drug classes used in horses can be used in ruminants. The most commonly used NSAIDs are phenylbutazone, flunixin, and aspirin. α_2 agonists are commonly used for acute pain, but this group of animals is extremely sensitive to the sedating effect of α_2 agonists, so low dosages should be used. Butorphanol is also commonly used for acute pain, and morphine is used occasionally. Fentanyl patches, buprenorphine, and both ketamine and lidocaine CRIs have been used to control pain in small ruminants (sheep and goats), but use of these drugs and techniques is not as common in adult cattle simply because treatment of pain in this group is not as common. By far, the most commonly used analgesic drugs in ruminants are local analgesic agents (primarily lidocaine and bupivacaine); techniques include local field blocks (tissue block at the site of surgery or injury), IV regional blocks, epidurals, paravertebral blocks, and cornual blocks, among others. For a description of these blocks and how to perform them, see the chapter by Dr. Skarda and Dr. Tranquilli (full citation under "Recommended Readings" in this chapter). Alternative and complementary techniques, such as acupuncture, are also appropriate for analgesia in ruminants.

See Case Presentation 28-6 for an example of an analgesic protocol designed to manage pain associated with dehorning a goat.

CASE PRESENTATION 28-6 DEHORNING

Bucky, a 6-month-old Spanish goat, comes to your practice for dehorning. How will you manage surgical pain?

ANSWER: For multimodal, preemptive analgesia, sedate Bucky with an α_2 agonist (xylazine, medetomidine, dexmedetomidine, or romifidine would be a good choice) combined with butorphanol. Use bupivacaine to block the nerves to the horn, and give one dose of flunixin or ketoprofen IV.

> **TECHNICIAN NOTE** Local anesthetic agents are an excellent choice for analgesia in all ruminants. However, keep in mind that sheep and goats are easily overdosed, so drug dosages in these species must be calculated carefully.

CAMELIDS

Camelids (e.g., llamas, alpacas) are more likely than cattle, sheep, and goats (but not as likely as horses) to receive analgesic treatment because they generally are constrained neither by an absolute economic value nor by entry into the human food chain. These animals have a GI tract similar to that found in ruminants with a "third compartment" that functions like a rumen. Thus drug administration issues are the same in camelids as they are in ruminants, in which orally administered drugs may be inactivated. All drugs used in other ruminant types of species can be used in camelids. NSAIDs are generally the first treatment for both acute and chronic pain. α_2 agonists and butorphanol are used to treat acute pain, but these drugs cause fairly profound sedation in camelids, so they are used only when sedation is appropriate. Other treatment modalities include fentanyl patches, lidocaine CRIs, ketamine CRIs, local or regional blockade, and alternative and complementary therapies, such as acupuncture.

See Case Presentation 28-7 for an example of an analgesic protocol designed to manage pain associated with surgery to repair a bone fracture in a llama.

PIGS

Lack of good pain management in swine practice rivals its lack in cattle practice, but high-producing boars and sows, along with pot-bellied pigs kept as pets, may receive better treatment. Like ruminants, pigs generally have an absolute economic value and are affected by their likely entry into the human food chain. All of the drugs discussed previously for use in other species can be used in pigs.

SUMMARY

Providing effective pain management is not an individual endeavor. It requires a team approach involving everyone who participates in patient care. As true patient advocates, veterinary technicians constitute a vital force in this effort.

CASE PRESENTATION 28-7 BONE FRACTURE

Willow, an 8-year-old adult female llama, has a fractured tibia that will be surgically repaired today. How will you handle the pain associated with this surgery?

ANSWER: For preemptive, multimodal analgesia, administer butorphanol and xylazine (or medetomidine, dexmedetomidine, or romifidine) as a premedicant to anesthesia, and give a dose of an NSAID IV. Once the patient has been anesthetized, administer an epidural block of morphine and bupivacaine. For pain after the epidural wears off, there are three options: (1) place an epidural catheter (*easy* to do in large animals and my personal favorite for this case) and administer morphine twice daily for 2 to 3 days; (2) place a fentanyl patch for 72 hours of analgesia; or (3) keep Willow on a lidocaine-ketamine CRI (this is probably the least practical because this patient will not likely be on fluids postoperatively). Whichever method is chosen, it should be combined with IV NSAIDs. Subsequently, the patient should be discharged from the hospital with instructions to be given oral NSAIDs for 10 to 14 days.

A successful technician understands the goals of pain control and the analgesic options. Combining keen observation with good technical skills, the technician appropriately assesses pain and then requests and administers analgesics to his or her patients. Paying attention to environmental and emotional needs and differentiating other stress from pain is part of a technician's daily routine (Box 28-7). Veterinary technicians have played a vital role in bringing animal pain management to the forefront of veterinary practice. Through continued teaching and vigilant practice, technicians no doubt will be credited in large part with continuing improvements in the practice of veterinary pain management. Much work is still to be done, particularly in the arena of large animal practice. Although it is true that large animals hide pain (often even better than small animals), and some economic constraints and species-specific limitations have been applied in drug use or administration, it is not true that large animals do not feel pain. Pain management is often initiated by the technician because he or she is often the person who spends the most time with the patient and is most likely to recognize pain in the patient.

BOX 28-7	Summary of Technician's Responsibilities

Technicians typically are responsible for the following:
- Assessing patients
- Identifying (or predicting) pain
- Providing nonpharmacologic comfort and care
- Differentiating pain from other stress
- Requesting appropriate analgesia and/or sedation
- Helping to develop appropriate protocols for pain management
- Administering medications, performing analgesic techniques
- Monitoring and treating drug effects
- Assessing patients postoperatively
- Communicating with clients
- Logging controlled substances

REFERENCES

1. Bockstahler B, Levine D, Millis D: Essential facts of physiotherapy in dogs and cats: rehabilitation and pain management, Höst, Germany, 2004, BE VetVerlag.
2. Hewson CJ, Dohoo IR, Lemke KA, et al: Canadian veterinarians' use of analgesics in cattle, pigs, and horses in 2004 and 2005, Can Vet J 48:155, 2007.

RECOMMENDED READINGS

Bath GF: Management of pain in production animals, Appl Anim Behav Sci 59:147, 1998.
Benson GJ, Rollin BE, editors: The well-being of farm animals: challenges and solutions, Ames, IA, 2004, Blackwell Publishing.
Mama K, Hendrickson D: Pain management and anesthesia, Vet Clin North Am Eq Pract 27:ix, 2002.
Skarda RT, Tranquilli WJ: Local and regional anesthetic and analgesic techniques: ruminants and swine. In Tranquilli WJ, Thurmon JC, Grimm, KA, editors: Lumb & Jones' veterinary anesthesia and analgesia, ed 4, Ames, IA, 2007, Blackwell Publishing.
U.S. Department of Agriculture: Animal Welfare Act and Regulations. Available at http://awic.nal.usda.gov/government-and-professional-resources/federal-laws/animal-welfare-act (accessed on September 30, 2012).
Valverde A, Gunkel CI: Pain management in horses and farm animals, J Vet Emerg Crit Care 15:295, 2005.
Wildlife Information Network: Pain management in ruminants. Available at: www.wildlifeinformation.org (accessed on September 16, 2012).

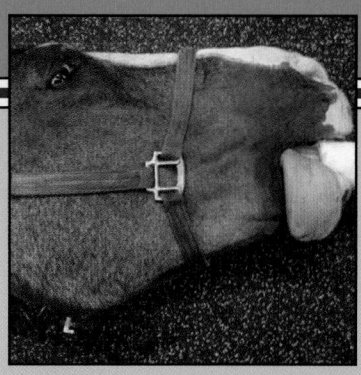

29 Veterinary Anesthesia

John A. Thomas and Phillip Lerche

OUTLINE

What Is Anesthesia? *1078*
Patient Preparation, *1078*
Fasting Recommendations, *1078*
Gathering Historical Information, *1079*
Physical Assessment, *1079*
Diagnostic Testing, *1079*
Patient Stabilization, *1079*
Physical Status Classification, *1079*
Anesthetic Agents, *1080*
Agonists, Partial Agonists, Mixed Agonist-
Antagonists, and Antagonists, *1080*
Anticholinergics, *1080*
Tranquilizers and Sedatives, *1081*
Phenothiazine Tranquilizers, *1081*
Benzodiazepine Tranquilizers, *1081*
Alpha$_2$-Adrenergic Drugs, *1082*
Opioids, *1083*
Propofol, *1084*
Dissociatives, *1084*
Barbiturates, *1085*
Etomidate, *1085*
Guaifenesin, *1086*
Inhalant Anesthetics, *1086*
Halogenated Anesthetics, *1086*
Nitrous Oxide, *1087*
Anesthetic Equipment, *1087*
Endotracheal Tubes, *1087*
Laryngoscopes, *1087*
Masks, *1087*
Anesthetic Chambers, *1088*
The Anesthetic Machine, *1089*
Preparing the Machine, *1090*
The Carrier Gas Supply, *1091*
Anesthetic Vaporizers, *1093*
Breathing Circuits, *1094*
Rebreathing Circuit Parts, *1096*
Scavenging System, *1097*
Anesthetic Machine Maintenance, *1097*
**Principles of Endotracheal
Intubation,** *1098*
Selecting a Tube, *1098*
Preparing the Tube, *1098*
Intubation Procedures, *1098*
Checking for Proper Placement, *1100*
Cuff Inflation, *1101*
Laryngospasm, *1101*
Complications of Intubation, *1101*

Anesthetic Monitoring, *1102*
Stages and Planes of Anesthesia, *1102*
Principles of Monitoring, *1102*
Vital Signs, *1104*
Indicators of Circulation, *1104*
Indicators of Oxygenation, *1105*
Indicators of Ventilation, *1105*
Reflexes and Other Indicators of Anesthetic
Depth, *1106*
Monitoring Equipment, *1107*
Mechanical Indicators of Circulation, *1107*
Mechanical Indicators of
Oxygenation, *1110*
Mechanical Indicators of Ventilation, *1111*
Small Animal Anesthesia, *1112*
Selecting a Protocol, *1112*
Equipment Preparation, *1113*
The Preanesthetic Period, *1115*
Anesthetic Induction, *1115*
Maintenance of Anesthesia, *116*
Patient Positioning, Comfort, and
Safety, *1117*
Anesthetic Recovery, *1117*
Equine Anesthesia, *1118*
Selecting a Protocol, *1118*
Equipment Preparation, *1119*
The Preanesthetic Period, *1119*
Anesthetic Induction, *1119*
Maintenance of Anesthesia, *1120*
Anesthetic Recovery, *1121*
Ruminant Anesthesia, *1122*
Selecting a Protocol, *1122*
Preanesthetic Fasting, *1122*
Equipment Preparation, *1122*
The Preanesthetic Period, *1122*
Anesthetic Induction, *1122*
Maintenance of Anesthesia, *1125*
Anesthetic Recovery, *1125*
Manual and Mechanical Ventilation, *1125*
Manual Ventilation, *1125*
Mechanical Ventilation, *1125*
Periodic Ventilation, *1126*
Intermittent Mandatory Ventilation, *1126*
Complications of Ventilation, *1126*
**Anesthetic Problems and
Emergencies,** *1126*
A Patient That Will Not Stay Asleep, *1127*

KEY TERMS

Analgesia
Apnea
Atelectasis
Ayre's T-piece
Bain coaxial circuit
Cyanosis
Hypercarbia
Hypnotic
Hypothermia
Hypoventilation
Hypoxia
Miosis
Mydriasis
Non-rebreathing system
Oxygen saturation
Pneumothorax
Rebreathing system
Respiratory minute
volume (RMV)
Tachycardia
Tachypnea
Tidal volume
Vasodilatation

LEARNING OBJECTIVES

When you have completed this chapter, you will be able to:

1. Pronounce, define, and spell all Key Terms in the chapter.
2. Differentiate general anesthesia, sedation, tranquilization, neuroleptanalgesia, local anesthesia; differentiate the periods of a general anesthetic event (premedication, induction, maintenance); and list the objectives of anesthesia and techniques used to achieve these objectives, including the concept of balanced anesthesia.
3. Discuss each aspect of patient preparation for an anesthetic procedure, including fasting, gathering historical information, physical assessment, stabilization, and physical status classification.
4. Do the following regarding injectable anesthetic agents:
   - Describe the ways anesthetic agents are classified, and differentiate agonists, partial agonists, agonist-antagonists, and antagonists.
   - Describe the effects, adverse effects, properties, and uses of anticholinergics, phenothiazine and benzodiazepine tranquilizers, alpha2-adrenergic agents, opioids, propofol, dissociatives, barbiturates, etomidate, and guaifenesin.
5. Explain how vapor pressure, blood-gas partition coefficient, and minimum alveolar concentration (MAC) influence the way inhalant anesthetics are used; and, describe the effects, adverse effects, properties, and uses of halogenated inhalant anesthetics and nitrous oxide.
6. Do the following regarding the use of anesthetic equipment:
   - Discuss the characteristics, uses, and maintenance of endotracheal tubes, laryngoscopes, anesthetic masks, and anesthetic chambers.
   - Describe the characteristics of an anesthetic machine, including the four general machine systems.
   - Explain how to assemble an anesthetic machine, check for leaks, and set the pop-off valve before use.
   - Describe the structure, function, and use of each component of the carrier gas supply, including compressed gas cylinder, pressure gauge, pressure-reducing valve, flowmeter, and oxygen flush valve.
   - List and calculate the oxygen flow rates used for various species, systems, and periods of an anesthetic procedure.
   - Describe the structure, function, and uses of precision and nonprecision vaporizers.
   - Discuss rebreathing and non-rebreathing systems, and explain the criteria used to choose an appropriate breathing system for any given patient.
   - Describe the structure, function, and use of each component of the breathing system, including unidirectional flow valves, reservoir bag, pop-off valve, carbon dioxide absorber canister, pressure manometer, negative pressure relief valve, and breathing tubes.
   - Discuss the function and uses of passive and active scavenging systems.
   - Describe the procedures used to maintain anesthetic machines.
7. Do the following regarding endotracheal intubation:
   - Discuss the principles of endotracheal intubation, including the equipment needed to place an endotracheal tube and the criteria used to select and prepare an appropriate endotracheal tube for any given patient.
   - Describe placement of an endotracheal tube in a small animal, horse, adult ruminant, and small ruminant; how to check an endotracheal tube for proper placement; and how to inflate the cuff.
   - Discuss laryngospasm and other complications of intubation, including causes and methods of prevention.
8. Do the following regarding anesthetic monitoring:
   - Explain the principles of anesthetic monitoring and how monitoring parameters can be used to identify the classic stages and planes of anesthesia.
   - Identify physical monitoring indicators of circulation, oxygenation, and ventilation.
   - Discuss the methods used to assess vital signs, including normal values, and common causes of abnormal values.
   - Describe methods used to assess reflexes and other monitoring indicators, and explain how they are used to determine anesthetic depth.

- Discuss the function and setup of monitoring equipment used to assess circulation, oxygenation, and ventilation, and interpretation of data generated by these instruments.
9. Do the following regarding small animal anesthesia:
   - Describe the sequence of events required to take a small animal patient from consciousness to surgical anesthesia and back to consciousness.
   - Describe agents and methods commonly used to induce a small animal patient by IM or IV injection, mask, or chamber.
   - Describe agents and methods used to maintain anesthesia in a small animal patient and considerations for patient positioning, comfort, safety, and recovery.
10. Explain the sequence of events for an anesthetic event in a horse, including ways in which an equine anesthetic procedure differs from that of a small animal patient.
11. Explain the sequence of events for an anesthetic event in a ruminant, including ways in which a ruminant anesthetic procedure differs from that for a small animal patient.
12. Differentiate manual, mechanical, periodic, and intermittent mandatory ventilation, and explain the indications for and principles of manual and mechanical ventilation.
13. List common anesthetic problems and emergencies, associated causes, and interventions.

INTRODUCTION

Anesthesia is a unique discipline for several reasons. First, anesthetic procedures are performed not for their own sake, but to allow veterinary professionals to do things that otherwise would not be possible. For instance, anesthesia enables surgery, dentistry, endoscopy, and other procedures that require patient immobility and unconsciousness, and pain control. It enables treatment, handling, and transport of exotic and feral animals. In some patients, it is necessary to perform procedures such as nail trims, grooming, and radiographic studies, which—although not painful—evoke fear, cause discomfort, and are unwelcome. This wide range of indications makes anesthesia a constant presence in the professional life of the veterinary technician.

Second, the practice of anesthesia involves much more than choosing machine settings, checking reflexes, or watching monitoring devices. It is an extremely complex discipline that involves use of complicated equipment, administration of potentially dangerous drugs, and awareness of an intricate set of monitoring parameters that enable the anesthetist to assess the well-being of the patient.

Also, general anesthesia is by nature a high-risk procedure. Anesthetic drugs cause adverse physiologic changes in cardiac output, blood pressure, respiratory drive, and central nervous system (CNS) function that can be dangerous and even life threatening if not monitored and managed. Although a competent anesthetist is never controlled by fear, a healthy respect for the risks of anesthesia must be maintained at all times to keep the "edge" required for best performance.

Finally, changes in the status of anesthetized patients occur quickly and unexpectedly—often within minutes or even seconds. This urgency demands a high level of awareness and an ability to make critical decisions rapidly and effectively to ensure patient safety.

This unique combination of frequent use, complexity, high risk, and fast pace of veterinary anesthesia tests the knowledge and abilities of even the most experienced veterinary technician. Therefore, the successful practice of anesthesia demands that the technician be prepared, skillful, alert, and attentive. The purpose of this chapter is to provide the reader with the information needed to reach this end.

WHAT IS ANESTHESIA?

Anesthesia is defined as an absence of sensation that affects the whole body or an isolated part or region of the body. Tranquilization and sedation are by convention included in the study of anesthesia because these techniques are frequently used in conjunction with anesthesia. Effects appropriate for each patient vary depending on the procedure and may include light to heavy sedation, local anesthesia, general anesthesia, muscle relaxation, **analgesia**, or a combination thereof.

General anesthesia is characterized by unconsciousness and insensibility to feeling and pain induced by administration of anesthetic agents given alone or in combination. General anesthesia provides an environment in which general surgery or other painful procedures can be performed without the danger of patient movement or injury to personnel. Anesthetic induction is the process used to take the patient from a state of consciousness to general anesthesia. Anesthetic maintenance is the process used to keep the patient under general anesthesia until recovery.

In contrast, local anesthesia is the loss of sensation in a localized body part or region induced by administration of a drug or other agent without loss of consciousness. Local anesthesia is used for procedures that do not require the patient to be unconscious, and for adjunct pain control. Administration of local anesthetic to remove a skin tumor, a nerve block performed on a horse to localize lameness, and an epidural used to provide analgesia for a patient undergoing an orthopedic procedure are all examples of local anesthesia.

Premedication refers to the administration of an agent or agents before induction of general anesthesia to calm and relax the patient, ease induction and recovery, minimize adverse effects, reduce the amount of general anesthetic needed, provide muscle relaxation, or provide pain control. A variety of tranquilizers, sedatives, anesthetics, and anticholinergics are used alone or in combination for this purpose. Premedication is also referred to as preanesthesia.

Sedation is a state of calm or drowsiness; tranquilization is a state of relaxation and reduced anxiety. Many tranquilizers also produce some degree of sedation. Consequently, these terms are often used interchangeably, even though they have somewhat different meanings.

Neuroleptanalgesia is a state of profound sedation and analgesia produced by simultaneous administration of an opioid and a tranquilizer. Neuroleptanalgesia is commonly used to perform minor procedures, such as wound treatment or radiography, and to induce general anesthesia in compromised patients.

The objectives of anesthesia are to produce loss of sensation in the whole body or a body part or region, and to provide muscle relaxation, analgesia, and alteration of consciousness appropriate to the procedure. In addition, patient safety must be preserved and adverse effects minimized, with special attention to respiratory and cardiovascular function. This can seldom be achieved with the use of only one drug.

This is why concurrent administration of two or more anesthetic drugs is commonplace. The use of drugs with complementary effects, referred to as balanced anesthesia, enables the anesthetist to fulfill these diverse objectives. Although many protocols are commonly used, premedication with acepromazine, anesthetic induction with a ketamine-diazepam mixture, anesthetic maintenance with sevoflurane gas, and administration of a morphine infusion for pain control constitute one example of balanced anesthesia.

PATIENT PREPARATION

The technician must accurately identify factors that can compromise a patient and must effectively communicate this information to the veterinarian before beginning any anesthetic procedure. Specifically, careful patient preparation is important for the following reasons:

- To minimize the likelihood of preventable complications, such as aspiration
- To allow treatment of any problems that may endanger the patient, such as dehydration, bleeding, organ dysfunction, or organ failure
- To allow the veterinarian to make anesthetic drug choices based on facts about the patient's condition
- To make the anesthetist aware of potential problems that the patient may experience during the procedure

FASTING RECOMMENDATIONS

Swallowing reflexes become sluggish, lower esophageal sphincter tone decreases, and patients may experience nausea or vomiting during anesthetic procedures. This combination of factors may allow stomach contents to reflux into the esophagus and the pharynx, resulting in a range of mild to devastating complications, including aspiration of stomach contents into the lungs, postanesthesia esophagitis, and esophageal stricture. Therefore, it is vital to observe fasting recommendations before any anesthetic procedure is performed in common domestic species. Fasting recommendations vary widely from practice to practice; however, guidelines may be found in Table 29-1.

TABLE 29-1	Fasting Recommendations	
SPECIES	**FOOD WITHHOLDING TIME, hours**	**WATER WITHHOLDING TIME, hours**
Dogs and cats	8-12*	2-4
Horses	8-12	0-2
Cattle	24-48	8-12
Small ruminants	12-18	8-12
Neonates and pediatric patients (<8 weeks old)	None	None

*Note that patients weighing less than 2 kg should be fasted for shorter lengths of time.

> 📎 *TECHNICIAN NOTE* Make certain that fasting instructions have been observed before admitting *any* patient for anesthesia.

GATHERING HISTORICAL INFORMATION

In addition to the usual historical information needed for any patient, such as vaccine status and medical and surgical history, several other pieces of information must be obtained before an anesthetic is administered. Following is a list of questions that should be asked of a client at the time of patient drop-off:

- Has the patient been fasting for the recommended time?
- How is the patient feeling today?
- Have any changes in the patient's condition been noted since the procedure was scheduled?
- Is the patient up to date on routine preventive care?
- What is the patient in for today (including left or right side if the procedure involves a limb, eye, or ear; and including the location of tumors or other localized lesions)?
- Is the patient taking any medications?

Unless asked, a client may not reveal this information at the time of drop-off for a variety of reasons. For example, an owner who failed to observe fasting recommendations may be unwilling to admit the lack of willpower to withhold food, may not realize the importance of fasting, or may simply have forgotten to tell you. An owner may not think to inform you that the patient worsened or developed vomiting, coughing, or some other sign of significant illness. If the procedure is not verbally confirmed, the surgeon could mistakenly perform a procedure on the incorrect limb, or the wrong surgery altogether. Thus any missing piece of information can make the difference between a successful and a potentially serious outcome.

PHYSICAL ASSESSMENT

A physical assessment should be performed immediately before any anesthetic is administered to uncover any problems that may increase patient risk or may necessitate a change in patient management (see Box 29-1 for physical

---

BOX 29-1	Physical Findings That Should Be Reported to the Veterinarian

- Dehydration, obesity, or cachexia
- Change in consciousness or any other sign of neurologic disease (e.g., seizures, ataxia, abnormal pupil size)
- Pale mucous membranes or prolonged capillary refill time (CRT)
- Cyanosis or icterus
- Abnormal heart rate (HR) or rhythm, or heart murmur
- Weak or irregular pulse
- Increased respiratory effort or rate
- Abnormal lung sounds, such as wheezing or crackles
- Marked hypothermia or hyperthermia

---

findings that should be reported to the veterinarian). This assessment should focus on the nervous, cardiovascular, and pulmonary systems because the health status of these systems is closely associated with the outcome of any anesthetic procedure. Below is a list of important components of a preanesthetic physical assessment:

- Observe the patient's level of consciousness (e.g., bright, alert, and responsive; quiet, alert and responsive; lethargic; obtunded; stuporous; comatose).
- Observe the general body condition, including body weight and hydration.
- Note weakness, abnormal gait, or recumbency.
- Look for parasites, wounds, tumors, or other external lesions.
- Examine body orifices for external signs of disease, such as diarrhea, nasal discharge, hematuria, or vaginal discharge.
- Determine vital signs (temperature, pulse, respiratory rate [RR]).
- Assess mucous membrane color and capillary refill time (CRT).
- Watch the patient breathe, noting respiratory effort.
- Auscultate the lungs for abnormal respiratory sounds.
- Concurrently palpate the pulse and auscultate the heart.

DIAGNOSTIC TESTING

When a patient is prepared for surgery, diagnostic tests are often needed to supplement the history and physical assessment. The purpose of these tests is to uncover abnormalities that may impair the patient's ability to compensate, that may lead to unanticipated complications, or that may impair the patient's ability to eliminate the anesthetics. Testing recommendations vary widely from practice to practice. Most diagnostic testing recommendations are based on the signalment and physical status class and may include blood work, urinalysis, thoracic radiographs, serology, electrocardiography, and other tests as indicated. In general, young, healthy patients receive relatively fewer tests, and patients that are older or sick, or that have other risk factors, receive more tests.

PATIENT STABILIZATION

Abnormalities identified during patient evaluation must be treated before the anesthetic is administered. This patient stabilization includes treatment or correction of dehydration, anemia, cardiac arrhythmias, respiratory compromise, major organ failure, or electrolyte or acid-base imbalance, and may involve administration of antibiotics, analgesics, fluids, blood, oxygen, or a wide variety of other agents. The veterinary technician will be intimately involved in this stabilization process and must be prepared to accurately calculate doses, place intravenous (IV) catheters, set fluid administration rates, and administer drugs, blood, and oxygen as ordered by the veterinarian.

PHYSICAL STATUS CLASSIFICATION

Information gleaned from the patient evaluation is used to determine a physical status classification. This system,

TABLE 29-2	ASA Physical Status Classifications		
CLASSIFICATION	**RISK**	**CRITERIA**	**REPRESENTATIVE CONDITIONS**
P1	Minimal	Normal, healthy patient	Patients undergoing elective procedures (OHE, castration, or declaw)
P2	Low	Patient with mild systemic disease	Neonatal, geriatric, or obese patients Mild dehydration Skin tumor removal
P3	Moderate	Patient with severe systemic disease	Anemia Moderate dehydration Compensated major organ disease
P4	High	Patient with severe systemic disease that is a constant threat to life	Ruptured bladder Internal hemorrhage Pneumothorax Pyometra
P5	Extreme	Moribund patient that is not expected to survive without the operation	Severe head trauma Pulmonary embolus Gastric dilatation-volvulus End-stage major organ failure

ASA, American Society of Anesthesiologists; *OHE*, ovariohysterectomy.

developed by the American Society of Anesthesiologists (ASA), is a subjective rating of the patient's condition based on historical, physical, and laboratory findings that places the patient into one of five classes (Table 29-2). This system is a tool that can be used to guide the anesthetist in appropriate patient management because anesthetic protocols are often based on physical status classification. This classification is somewhat subjective, so the technician must use her or his best judgment based on the criteria listed. Any surgery that is an emergency, regardless of ASA class, is additionally assigned the letter "E."

ANESTHETIC AGENTS

Anesthetic agents used in veterinary patients may be classified in one of several ways. They may be grouped according to the route of delivery (topical, oral, injectable, or inhalant) or by primary use (preanesthetic, sedative, induction agent, or maintenance agent). Anesthetics may also be grouped into drug classes based on chemistry. Agents in any given class tend to have similar actions, properties, uses, and effects, so this system will be used to classify the anesthetic agents described.

AGONISTS, PARTIAL AGONISTS, MIXED AGONIST-ANTAGONISTS, AND ANTAGONISTS

Anesthetic drugs work by binding to specific receptors on or inside the cells of target tissues. In the case of many anesthetics, these target tissues are located in the central or peripheral nervous system. Most anesthetic agents are agonists (drugs that bind to receptors and exert one or more effects). Some drug classes, such as opioids and alpha$_2$-adrenergics, include drugs called antagonists that block or reverse the action of the corresponding agonist. These antagonists are referred to

as *reversal agents*. In the opioid class are agents that are classified as partial agonists and those that are classified as mixed agonist-antagonists. Partial agonists bind to receptors and exert a partial or milder effect, whereas mixed agonist-antagonists partially reverse the effects of pure agonists.

ANTICHOLINERGICS

Although not true anesthetic agents, anticholinergics are used to counteract effects of parasympathetic nervous system stimulation, such as bradycardia and excess salivation. Although many anesthetics cause these effects to some degree, barbiturates and dissociatives have a notable tendency to cause excess salivation, and opioids and alpha$_2$-adrenergic agonists are especially likely to cause bradycardia. Atropine and glycopyrrolate are the most commonly used anticholinergics in veterinary patients.

Anticholinergics have many effects expected to result from a parasympathetic nervous system blockade, including increased heart rate (HR), reduced tear secretions and salivation, reduced gastrointestinal (GI) activity, and dilatation of the pupils, especially in cats. Protective ophthalmic ointment should be applied to patients receiving these agents to prevent drying of the corneas.

Many potential adverse effects, including **tachycardia**, cardiac arrhythmias, bronchodilation, **mydriasis**, and ileus, are known. Bronchodilation caused by these drugs can increase anatomic dead space, which increases the risk for hypoxemia. Mydriasis may render the pupillary light reflex unreliable. Anticholinergics may cause thickening of mucus in the airways, especially in cats, and this can result in blockage. Some anesthetists use anticholinergics routinely in small animal (SA) patients, whereas others do not.

In ruminants, copious salivary secretions become more viscid, pool in the pharynx, and may be aspirated, thus predisposing the patient to airway blockage. Horses may develop colic from GI stasis. For these reasons, anticholinergics are avoided in these species unless they are necessary to treat bradycardia.

Atropine is a rapid-acting agent that is available in SA and large animal (LA) strengths (0.54 mg/ml and 15 mg/ml, respectively). Glycopyrrolate is similar to atropine with the following differences: glycopyrrolate has a slower onset and a longer duration. It is less likely to cause tachycardia, cardiac arrhythmias, and ileus, and it suppresses salivation more effectively. Unlike atropine, it does not cross the placental barrier and will not adversely affect fetuses if used for cesarean section (C-section). It also does not cross the blood-brain barrier and thus has less impact on vision than atropine.

> **TECHNICIAN NOTE** Anticholinergics are used to counteract bradycardia and hypersalivation. LA and SA concentrations of injectable atropine differ in strength by a factor of almost 30. Do *not* mix them up.

TRANQUILIZERS AND SEDATIVES

Tranquilizers and sedatives are commonly used to provide patient restraint for minor procedures such as grooming, diagnostic imaging, blood draws, nail trims, and wound treatment. They are used as premedications and to produce specific effects, such as analgesia and muscle relaxation. Each of these drugs has unique properties and must be chosen on the basis of the particular effects desired. For instance, dexmedetomidine (an alpha$_2$-adrenergic agonist) produces analgesia and muscle relaxation, whereas acepromazine minimizes vomiting and development of cardiac arrhythmias. Often tranquilizers and sedatives are used in combination or with other anesthetic agents to produce a combination of effects that cannot be achieved by using one drug alone.

PHENOTHIAZINE TRANQUILIZERS

Phenothiazine tranquilizers (also classified as major tranquilizers) are used to calm and sedate patients before general anesthesia. This helps to improve the quality of anesthetic induction and recovery by reducing anxiety. The phenothiazine tranquilizer used most commonly for this purpose is acepromazine. In addition to its use alone, it is often used in combination with other agents. Combinations include "RAT" (Rompun [generic name, xylazine], acepromazine, and Torbugesic [generic name, butorphanol]) and "BAG" (butorphanol, acepromazine, and glycopyrrolate).

Acepromazine induces mild to moderate sedation and is antiemetic and antiarrhythmic. Unlike many other agents, it causes little respiratory or cardiac depression. It has a relatively long duration.

Acepromazine blocks alpha$_1$-adrenergic receptors in the sympathetic nervous system, resulting in dose-dependent peripheral **vasodilatation**. Consequently, the main adverse effect of acepromazine is hypotension, which can lead to cardiovascular collapse. Acepromazine also can cause

hypothermia or hyperthermia, changes in HR, prolapse of the third eyelid, and paradoxical excitement or aggression. Adverse effects specific to horses include excitement, sweating, **tachypnea**, and protrusion of the penis, which can lead to permanent injury. Therefore, some clinicians will not use this drug in breeding stallions.

Give acepromazine IM at least 15 minutes before induction and allow the patient to remain in a quiet area, because the tranquilizing effect may be overridden, especially in excited patients. Note that the commonly used dose of the injectable form of acepromazine is significantly less than the dose on the label. Use of higher doses will not increase the level of sedation, but will cause increased hypotension.

When administering acepromazine IV, give it slowly and avoid intra-arterial injection. Boxers, Greyhounds, giant breed dogs, and debilitated, young, or geriatric patients may be sensitive to this drug, whereas terriers and cats are relatively resistant. Acepromazine should not be given to patients with seizure disorders because it may lower the seizure threshold. Instruct owners to use caution when handling patients that have received this drug because personality changes may occur, resulting in aggression.

> **TECHNICIAN NOTE** The commonly used dose of acepromazine (about 0.05 to 0.1 mg/kg in small animals, with a maximum dose of 3 mg in dogs and 1 mg in cats; 0.03 to 0.05 mg/kg in horses) is significantly lower than the labeled dose. Higher doses will increase hypotension, but not sedation.

BENZODIAZEPINE TRANQUILIZERS

Benzodiazepines (also classified as minor tranquilizers) most often are used in combination with other agents, such as opioids and dissociatives, to produce a range of effects from sedation to general anesthesia. Benzodiazepines are controlled substances. Diazepam, midazolam, and zolazepam are benzodiazepines commonly used in veterinary patients. Zolazepam is one of the two components in the product Telazol. The other component of this product is tiletamine (see "Dissociatives" for a discussion of this drug). Although benzodiazepine antagonists (flumazenil and sarmazenil) are available, they are seldom used because of the expense.

Effects of benzodiazepines include anxiety reduction and mild to moderate sedation, although young healthy dogs are resistant to these drugs, and sedation in cats is often unpredictable. Other effects include appetite stimulation in cats, skeletal muscle relaxation, and anticonvulsant activity. Effects generally last no longer than a few hours.

Benzodiazepines are relatively safe and minimally affect the cardiopulmonary system, but they can produce adverse effects that vary among species. Dogs tend to experience CNS excitement, anxiety, and fear, especially if young and healthy, and may become more difficult to control. Aggressive animals may lose inhibition, prohibiting use in these patients. Horses may experience muscle fasciculations, weakness, and mild ataxia.

After intramuscular (IM) injection, diazepam is erratically absorbed and causes pain. It can also cause bradycardia, **apnea**, hypotension, and pain if given rapidly intravenously as a result of the propylene glycol vehicle.

Do not store diazepam in syringes or IV bags because it is soluble in plastic and will lose potency. Diazepam commonly is mixed with ketamine (a dissociative anesthetic) in equal volumes and given intravenously to induce general anesthesia in small animals (see Boxes 29-7 and 29-8).

Midazolam is more potent than diazepam but can be used with ketamine in place of diazepam for anesthetic induction. Midazolam is water soluble and is compatible with a variety of agents, unlike diazepam, which is not water soluble and therefore cannot be mixed with other agents except ketamine.

> **TECHNICIAN NOTE** As a result of incompatibility with most other agents, injectable diazepam can be mixed only with ketamine. When administering diazepam by IV injection, give it slowly.

ALPHA₂-ADRENERGIC DRUGS

Alpha₂-adrenergic agonists are sedatives that are used alone or in combination with opioids, dissociatives, and other agents to produce a wide spectrum of effects from mild sedation to general anesthesia, including analgesia and muscle relaxation. Xylazine and dexmedetomidine are alpha₂-agonists most commonly used in SA patients. Xylazine, detomidine, and romifidine are used most commonly in LA patients.

The main therapeutic effects of alpha₂-agonists are sedation (CNS depression), analgesia, and muscle relaxation. These agents may cause vomiting in dogs and cats. Effects on the cardiovascular system include initial hypertension followed by prolonged hypotension. Bradycardia is common, and cardiac output is decreased. At high doses, these drugs cause a decrease in both respiratory rate and depth. In horses, xylazine causes lowering of the head and relaxation of the facial muscles, leading to drooping of the ears and lower lip. Relaxation of limb muscles leads to ataxia and a wide-based stance.

Alpha₂-agonists can cause significant bradycardia, reduced cardiac output, hypotension, and cardiac arrhythmias, including heart block. They can cause respiratory depression, especially when administered with other agents, and respiratory distress in brachycephalic dogs. Other adverse effects include pain upon IM injection, muscle tremors, and changes in body temperature. Dogs may bloat secondary to aerophagia, and horses may sweat. Ruminants may experience profound respiratory depression, hypersalivation, bloat, diarrhea, premature delivery, or abortion. Because sedated patients are sensitive to auditory stimuli, horses may kick, small animals may move, and aggressive patients may bite in response to loud noises.

Sedation produced by these drugs can be profound and prolonged, as can cardiovascular depression. Therefore, give standard doses only to young, healthy patients, and use cautiously in geriatric, diabetic, pregnant, pediatric, or sick patients. Most clinicians do not recommend routine use of anticholinergics with alpha₂-agonists because they can predispose the patient to development of arrhythmias and hypertension.

Xylazine is used in many domestic and exotic species as one component of anesthetic mixtures and is also used to induce vomiting in cats after ingestion of toxins. Xylazine is available in SA (2% or 20 mg/ml) and LA (10% or 100 mg/ml) concentrations. Ruminants are extremely sensitive to this drug, requiring about one-tenth of the dose used for horses. Swine require a high dose, so xylazine usually is given in combination with other drugs in this species.

Dexmedetomidine is used primarily in small and exotic animal species. When compared with xylazine, it is more potent and is less likely to produce side effects. It can be used in equal volumes with the reversal agent atipamezole to sequentially sedate and awaken patients undergoing minor procedures. Sudden arousal has been reported in patients heavily sedated with dexmedetomidine, resulting in bites.

Detomidine (Dormosedan) and romifidine (Sedivet) are alpha₂-agonists used in horses to produce sedation for procedures, such as dental work, and as a part of anesthetic combinations. Detomidine has a longer duration of action and provides more profound sedative and analgesic activity than xylazine. Romifidine generally causes less muscle relaxation than is produced by xylazine or detomidine.

> **TECHNICIAN NOTE** When giving alpha₂-agonists, monitor closely for hypotension, cardiac arrhythmias, bradycardia, and abnormal temperatures. Use special caution in geriatric, pediatric, and sick patients. Both LA and SA concentrations of xylazine are available—do *not* mix these up.

Alpha₂-adrenergic antagonists increase HR, increase blood pressure, and stimulate the CNS. They are used to "wake" patients after sedation or anesthesia, and to reverse adverse effects of alpha₂-agonists. Unfortunately, these agents also reverse desirable effects, such as analgesia. Therefore, an alternative analgesic must be administered if pain control is warranted. Adverse effects include apprehension caused by rapid arousal, excitement, muscle tremors, and salivation.

Yohimbine is an alpha₂-antagonist used to reverse the effects of xylazine. Although it is labeled for use in dogs, it is also used in other species. It should be used cautiously in patients with seizure disorders. Atipamezole (Antisedan) is used to reverse the effects of dexmedetomidine (Dexdomitor). The dose and the concentration of this drug are 10 times those of dexmedetomidine, so these two drugs are administered in equal volumes. Cats are more sensitive to this drug and are given a reduced dose. In addition to the general adverse effects of alpha₂-antagonists listed earlier, this drug can cause vomiting or diarrhea. Atipamezole may also be used to reverse detomidine. Tolazoline is used to reverse the effects of alpha$_2$-agonists in a variety of species.

Alpha$_2$-antagonists may be given IM in all species. When given IV, alpha$_2$-antagonists should be given slowly to effect (see page 1115) to avoid the excitation and aggression that are sometimes seen with rapid reversal. IV use in cats may cause unwanted severe salivation and excitement and thus is contraindicated.

OPIOIDS

Opioids (also known as narcotics) are drugs related to morphine. Opioids may be classified as agonists, partial agonists, mixed agonist-antagonists, and antagonists. Morphine, fentanyl, oxymorphone, and hydromorphone are examples of pure agonists. Buprenorphine is a partial agonist, butorphanol is a mixed agonist-antagonist, and naloxone is an antagonist. Opioids provide analgesia and sedation and are combined with tranquilizers to produce neuroleptanalgesia. With the exception of naloxone, most opioids commonly used in veterinary patients are controlled substances.

Opioids work by stimulating specific opioid receptors in the brain and spinal cord, each of which produces distinct effects. For instance, stimulation of μ-opioid receptors produces analgesia, euphoria, dependence, **miosis**, hypothermia, and respiratory depression. κ-Receptor stimulation produces analgesia, miosis, and sedation. σ-Receptor stimulation produces dysphoria, hallucinations, respiratory and cardiac stimulation, and mydriasis. Thus, the effects of each opioid depend on its affinity for each of the various receptors.

Opioid agonists primarily stimulate μ-receptors. They are used as sedatives, analgesics, and—when combined with tranquilizers—neuroleptanalgesics. Effects of opioid agonists vary according to species. Cats and large animals tend to experience anxiety, excitement, hyperthermia, and mydriasis, whereas dogs and primates experience sedation, hypothermia, and miosis. High doses of opioid agonists can induce narcosis in dogs—a state in which the patient appears profoundly sedated but can be aroused by loud noises or other stimulation. CNS effects may include euphoria and dysphoria. Euphoria is an exaggerated sense of well-being, whereas dysphoria is restlessness or discomfort. Opioid agonists are among the best analgesics available and are often used to control moderate to severe pain. Opioid agonists cause a variety of other effects, including cough suppression, respiratory depression, bradycardia, hypotension, and changes in urination and GI tract activity, which vary from agent to agent.

Opioid agonists have many adverse effects, including significant CNS and respiratory depression, which are of concern, especially when morphine is used. Peristalsis initially increases then decreases in dogs, causing defecation followed by constipation. Dogs may pant or—if not in pain—may whine or bark. Other adverse effects of opioids include vomiting, excessive salivation, and, in horses, sweating and increased locomotor activity. Special caution must be used in neonatal, geriatric, and debilitated patients;

patients with head trauma or respiratory disease; and patients with various other major organ diseases. Rapid IV administration of morphine may cause histamine release and bronchoconstriction.

Morphine, hydromorphone, fentanyl, and many other pure agonists are class II controlled substances and consequently are subject to special record keeping requirements. As a result of respiratory depression, monitor patients closely and be prepared to provide ventilatory support. Opioid agonists must be used with caution and in lower doses in cats and horses. GI activity should be monitored closely in horses receiving μ-agonist opioids because decreased motility may lead to colic.

Most opioid agonists have a duration of only a few hours, necessitating administration by constant rate infusion for sustained effect. When used for analgesia, morphine may be administered by epidural injection, and fentanyl may be administered via transdermal patch (Duragesic). Oxymorphone and hydromorphone are used in a similar fashion to morphine.

Opioid partial agonists exert partial activity at the μ-receptors but cannot stimulate receptors to the same degree as a full or pure agonist, and thus cannot provide the same degree of analgesia. The partial agonist buprenorphine is available only as a solution for injection, but it can be given orally for pain control in cats. Buprenorphine has a long duration of action and so is given only every 8 to 12 hours. At high doses, this drug can cause respiratory depression that is difficult to reverse with naloxone because buprenorphine binds tightly to the μ-receptors.

Opioid mixed agonist-antagonists exert agonist activity at the κ-receptors and antagonist activity at the μ-receptors. This results in many of the same effects as are caused by opioid agonists (sedation, analgesia, and cough suppression) but to a lesser degree. If given after a pure opioid agonist, they partially reverse the effects of these agents, including the analgesic effects. In other words, if given after a pure agonist, they decrease—not increase—their beneficial effects.

Butorphanol, the representative drug in this class, is used as a premedicant, an analgesic for mild to moderate pain, an antitussive, and, when given with tranquilizers, neuroleptanalgesia. In small animals, adverse effects of this agent are rare but may include transient sedation and ataxia. Horses may experience excitement at high doses. Because the analgesic effects of butorphanol last only about 1 to 2 hours, frequent administration is necessary for adequate pain control.

Butorphanol is available in oral and injectable forms. The injectable form is available in multiple strengths: 0.5 mg/ml, 2 mg/ml, and 10 mg/ml. It is important to be sure that you select the correct strength.

> **TECHNICIAN NOTE** Concurrent administration of opioid partial agonists or mixed agonist-antagonists (e.g., buprenorphine or butorphanol, respectively) and opioid agonists (e.g., morphine, hydromorphone, fentanyl) may decrease analgesia and other beneficial effects.

Opioid antagonists are used to "wake" patients after sedation with opioid agonists, partial agonists, or mixed agonist-antagonists, and to reverse undesirable effects of these agents. Naloxone is the opioid antagonist most commonly used in veterinary patients. Adverse effects of this drug are uncommon. Naloxone may be administered by giving the calculated dose slowly intravenously to effect, and the remainder by the subcutaneous route. The duration of effect is about 1 to 2 hours, so if the opioid you are reversing is of a longer duration than this, repeat doses may be needed. One to two drops under the tongue can be used to revive neonates delivered by C-section if the dam received opioids.

PROPOFOL

Propofol is an ultra-short-acting IV anesthetic used to induce general anesthesia in a variety of species. It may also be used to maintain general anesthesia by administering repeat boluses to effect or a constant rate infusion. Propofol is a phenolic compound that is chemically unlike any other anesthetic. It is not a controlled substance.

After slow IV injection, it induces a state of general anesthesia in 30 to 60 seconds with duration of approximately 2 to 5 minutes. The patient rapidly recovers when drug administration is stopped, will sit up within about 10 minutes, and will stand within about 15 to 30 minutes. Propofol decreases intracranial and intraocular pressure, provides muscle relaxation, and exhibits antiemetic and anticonvulsant properties. It does not provide significant analgesia. Although propofol is safe when used as directed, it has a relatively narrow therapeutic index and so must be given with caution.

Respiratory depression including apnea may occur and can be severe after rapid injection or with high doses. Therefore, it is important to monitor RR and depth carefully, especially during the first 1 to 2 minutes after initial injection. Cardiac effects include bradycardia and decreased strength of contraction. It causes hypotension, which can be significant after rapid injection. Propofol should be given with caution to patients with preexisting hypotension.

Propofol can cause seizure-like symptoms after induction and allergic reactions in some patients. Transient excitement and muscle tremors may occur during induction if the drug is given slowly, or if the patient is not premedicated. Cats can develop Heinz body anemia (a specific type of anemia induced by exposure to certain drugs or toxins), anorexia, lethargy, and diarrhea after repeat doses or use on a daily basis.

Unlike barbiturates, propofol is not cumulative and may be used in Greyhounds and other sight hounds. It is available only as an IV injectable in the form of a milky emulsion containing soybean oil and egg lecithin and is an exception to the rule that cloudy liquids should never be administered IV.

Propofol will support bacterial growth. Therefore, it is important to handle containers not containing a preservative with strict aseptic technique. The manufacturer recommends discarding unused portions more than 6 hours old, although some clinicians believe that propofol can be kept in the refrigerator for up to 24 hours if sterile technique is observed. PropoFlo™ 28 (Abbott Laboratories, Abbott Park, Illinois) is a propofol product that contains benzyl alcohol as a preservative. Once opened, the container can be stored at room temperature for 28 days. It is only licensed for use in dogs due to toxicity of benzyl alcohol in cats.

Propofol must be well mixed before use. If the patient experiences apnea or is given an overdose, treat with supportive care (intubation, oxygen administration, manual or mechanical ventilation, fluid therapy, and diuresis) until vital signs normalize.

> **TECHNICIAN NOTE** For induction of general anesthesia, give about one-fourth of the calculated dose of propofol every 30 seconds to effect. For maintenance, give boluses about every 3 to 5 minutes to effect or a constant rate infusion of about one-tenth of the induction dose per minute. Monitor for respiratory depression or apnea.

DISSOCIATIVES

Dissociatives (also known as *cyclohexamines*) are a unique group of injectable anesthetic agents used alone to immobilize patients for minor or brief procedures. They are also used in combination with opioids and tranquilizers to induce and maintain anesthesia and to provide analgesia or other specific effects. Ketamine and tiletamine (one of two agents contained in Telazol) are the dissociatives most often used in veterinary patients. Both are controlled.

When used alone, dissociatives produce immobilization, but not surgical anesthesia. Ketamine and other dissociatives induce a state known as *catalepsy* or *dissociative anesthesia*, in which the patient appears awake but is immobilized and does not respond to its surroundings. Catalepsy is also characterized by open, central, and dilated eyes; nystagmus; normal or increased muscle tone; increased sensitivity to light and sound; and intact palpebral, pedal, and laryngeal reflexes.

Dissociatives increase HR and blood pressure without the decrease in cardiac output characteristically seen with most other agents. Other effects include increased cerebrospinal fluid (CSF) pressure and intraocular pressure and superficial analgesia. They may also induce apneustic breathing—a pattern in which a prolonged pause follows inspiration and a short pause follows expiration.

Dissociatives can induce respiratory depression, cardiac arrhythmias, hypersalivation, vomiting, vocalization, prolonged recoveries, jerking movements, tremors, and pain upon IM injection. Increased salivation can be prevented by premedicating with a low dose of an anticholinergic. Dissociatives may induce seizure-like activity during recovery and should not be used in patients with seizure disorders. Ketamine may also cause behavioral changes that can, in some cases, last for days or weeks.

Tranquilizers or sedatives should be used with or before administration of dissociatives in dogs and horses to decrease adverse effects. Because the eyes remain open, a corneal lubricant should be used during dissociative anesthesia.

Ketamine can be given at a rate of 100 mg/5 kg orally for restraint of fractious cats.

The product Telazol contains tiletamine in combination with zolazepam (a benzodiazepine) and, when reconstituted, contains 50 mg of each drug/ml. Once reconstituted, Telazol is stable for 14 days if refrigerated. Telazol is used as an induction agent in healthy dogs and cats, especially if aggressive. Because it causes hypothermia, body temperature must be closely monitored.

A mixture of ketamine and diazepam (or midazolam) is commonly used to induce general anesthesia in dogs, cats, and horses. This combination has an onset of about 30 to 90 seconds, and 5 to 10 minutes of working time. In small animals, the two drugs are mixed in a 1:1 volume ratio and are given at a dosage of about 1 ml of the mixture/20 lb of body weight, IV slowly to effect (over 30 to 90 seconds). Diazepam or midazolam (0.03 to 0.05 mg/kg) can be added to ketamine (2.2 mg/kg) for induction of anesthesia in horses.

Ketamine–alpha$_2$-adrenergic agonist mixtures are used to provide anesthesia in dogs, cats, horses, and exotics. These mixtures cause significant cardiovascular and respiratory depression and must be used cautiously. Other dissociative mixtures include TKX (Telazol-ketamine-xylazine) and TKD (Telazol-ketamine-Dexdomitor).

> **TECHNICIAN NOTE** Unlike most other anesthetics, dissociative agents cause normal or increased muscle tone, sensitivity to light and sound, intact reflexes, increased HR, and increased blood pressure.

BARBITURATES

Barbiturates, a class of drugs developed in the early 1900s, are used for a variety of purposes, including induction of general anesthesia, treatment of seizures, and euthanasia. All barbiturates are controlled. These agents are classified as ultra-short-, short-, intermediate-, and long-acting according to their duration of action.

The ultra-short-acting barbiturates, thiopental sodium and methohexital, are used for induction of general anesthesia. Thiopental sodium* is rapidly absorbed into the brain, is redistributed into muscle and fat, and later is metabolized and excreted. The patient recovers as the drug is redistributed to muscle and fat, thus decreasing the amount in the brain tissue. This results in rapid onset (30 to 60 seconds) and short duration (5 to 20 minutes) after a single dose.

Effects of thiopental are cumulative if multiple doses are given, however, because fat and muscle become saturated with the drug until it is metabolized and excreted. The result of this saturation is prolonged recovery time. Sight hounds have low body fat levels and decreased hepatic metabolism of thiobarbiturates; thus saturation occurs more quickly and

results in even longer recovery times than are seen in other breeds.

Thiopental sodium causes a dose-dependent decrease in cardiac output, blood pressure, RR, and **tidal volume** (V$_T$). It does not produce significant analgesia, however, and is a poor muscle relaxant. Adverse effects include hypotension, bradycardia, salivation, coughing, laryngospasm, and arrhythmias, particularly ventricular premature contractions (VPCs) and bigeminy (alternating normal complexes and VPCs). It can also cause severe respiratory depression, including a period of apnea after induction, which may require ventilatory support. Thiopental sodium is cumulative if multiple doses are given, should not be used in sight hounds, and must *not* be injected out of the vein. Several other important cautions must be observed, so the reader should consult an anesthesia text before using this drug.

Methohexital is an ultra-short-acting barbiturate used for induction and maintenance of anesthesia in SA patients; it has an onset of about 15 to 60 seconds and duration of about 5 to 10 minutes. This drug is reconstituted to a 1% solution and has a shelf life of 6 weeks at room temperature. It is considered safe in sight hounds because it is rapidly metabolized; therefore, repeat doses are not cumulative. Because it can cause excitement and seizures during induction or recovery, patients should be premedicated before administration.

Pentobarbital sodium is an intermediate-acting barbiturate that, although it is no longer used for routine anesthesia in clinical settings, is given intraperitoneally to induce general anesthesia in laboratory animals. It is also given intravenously to treat status epilepticus in small animals and is used in a concentrated form as a euthanasia agent.

> **TECHNICIAN NOTE** The ultra-short-acting barbiturate thiopental sodium is cumulative if multiple doses are given, should not be used in sight hounds, and must *not* be injected out of the vein. Several important cautions must be observed, so the reader should consult an anesthesia text before using this drug.

ETOMIDATE

Etomidate is a short-acting, injectable, imidazole-derivative sedative-**hypnotic** used for induction of anesthesia in dogs and cats. It is not a controlled substance. Etomidate causes minimal changes in cardiovascular and respiratory function and decreases both intracranial and intraocular pressure. It has a significantly wider therapeutic index than propofol and thiopental sodium. It is therefore the agent of choice for patients with severe heart disease or shock. Etomidate produces good muscle relaxation, but no analgesia.

Although etomidate has a wide margin of safety, adverse effects include vomiting, muscle movements, sneezing, and excitement during induction and recovery. It also suppresses adrenocortical function. Premedication is recommended to reduce these adverse effects. IV injections may be painful and may cause phlebitis; rapid injection or repeat doses can cause

---

*Thiopental sodium has become increasingly difficult to obtain in recent years, and so has been gradually replaced by other IV induction agents and combinations listed in Box 29-7 and Box 29-10.

hemolysis. Administration through a running IV fluid line will decrease pain and hemolysis. Etomidate is not in common use because of its relatively higher cost and adverse effects.

GUAIFENESIN

Guaifenesin, also known as "GG," or glyceryl guaiacolate, is an injectable muscle relaxant and sedative used in combination with other agents for short procedures or to improve the quality of induction and recovery in large animals. It is also used as an expectorant to treat respiratory conditions.

Adverse effects on the cardiovascular, respiratory, and GI systems are mild and of little consequence. If injected out of the vein, guaifenesin is irritating to the tissues. Solutions of greater than 7% strength cause hemolysis in ruminants, whereas solutions with greater than 15% strength cause hemolysis in horses.

Guaifenesin is often administered as a 5% to 10% solution in dextrose by rapid IV infusion before ketamine or barbiturate induction to produce muscle relaxation in LA species. Several combinations are also commonly used. "Double drip" (ketamine and GG) is used for induction and/or maintenance of anesthesia in ruminants. "Triple drip" (xylazine, ketamine, and GG) is used for IV maintenance of anesthesia in horses.

INHALANT ANESTHETICS

Inhalant anesthetics are liquid agents that are vaporized in oxygen and administered via an anesthetic breathing system by endotracheal tube, mask, or chamber. Vapor pressure, blood-gas partition coefficient, and minimum alveolar concentration (MAC) measure properties of these agents that influence the way they are used. Therefore a basic knowledge of these concepts is necessary to use inhalant anesthetics effectively and safely.

Vapor pressure is a measurement of the tendency of a liquid to evaporate. Agents with high vapor pressure evaporate readily, reaching dangerously high concentrations if not regulated, and therefore must be administered using an agent-specific precision vaporizer. Conversely, low vapor pressure agents may be administered with a nonprecision vaporizer.

The blood-gas partition coefficient is a measurement of the tendency of an agent to dissolve in blood. It is associated with the speed of induction, recovery, and change in anesthetic depth, each of which is faster when agents with a low partition coefficient are used, and slower when agents with a high partition coefficient are used.

The MAC is the percent concentration of an agent required to prevent a response to surgical stimulation in 50% of patients, and therefore is a measurement of the potency of an agent. An agent with high MAC is less potent (more of the agent is required to attain surgical anesthesia) than an agent with low MAC. Typically, a dial setting of approximately 1.5 times the MAC is required to reach surgical anesthesia in most patients.

HALOGENATED ANESTHETICS

These inhalant agents are used in a wide variety of species to induce and maintain general anesthesia. Isoflurane and sevoflurane are the halogenated anesthetics most commonly used in veterinary patients.

Halogenated anesthetics cause CNS depression, hypothermia, respiratory depression, hypotension, and muscle relaxation. Although they cause myocardial depression, cardiac function is maintained close to preanesthetic levels. These agents have little or no analgesic effect postoperatively.

Both isoflurane and sevoflurane have high vapor pressures (240 mm Hg and 160 mm Hg, respectively) and must be administered via a precision vaporizer. Both agents also have low blood-gas partition coefficients (1.46 and 0.68, respectively) resulting in relatively rapid inductions, recoveries, and changes in anesthetic depth.

Halogenated anesthetics induce dose-dependent hypotension, which is more prominent with sevoflurane than isoflurane. They can also cause vomiting, nausea, and ileus, in addition to dose-dependent respiratory depression that can progress to apnea. Although the primary route of excretion for these agents is through the lungs, the amount that is metabolized by the liver and excreted by the kidneys varies from agent to agent. About 2% to 5% of sevoflurane is metabolized, whereas only about 0.2% of isoflurane is metabolized, making it an excellent anesthetic choice for patients with kidney or liver disease.

Reports have described fire or extreme heat production when sevoflurane is used with desiccated carbon dioxide (CO_2) absorbent. This problem is more common when low oxygen flow rates are used over a long time. To prevent this complication, turn off the machine when not in use, replace absorbent granules regularly, avoid the use of low oxygen flow for protracted periods, and monitor the temperature of the absorbent canister. Sevoflurane also reacts with chemicals in CO_2 absorbent to produce compound A, a chemical that causes renal damage in rats. This effect has not been found to be clinically significant in other species.

Although isoflurane and sevoflurane are similar, subtle differences have been noted in the way they are used. Because isoflurane is irritating to mucous membranes, patients may struggle and hold their breath during mask or chamber induction. In contrast, sevoflurane is not irritating, making it ideal for anesthetic induction. Some of the chief advantages of sevoflurane are the rapid inductions, recoveries, and changes in anesthetic depth associated with this agent. Therefore, safe use of this agent requires subtle dial changes and vigilant monitoring on the part of the veterinary anesthetist.

> **TECHNICIAN NOTE**   Although the perception frequently is that sevoflurane is safer than isoflurane, it causes more hypotension and must be monitored even more closely than isoflurane as a result of the more rapid response time.

Halothane was used extensively in veterinary anesthesia for many years, but it is no longer available in the United States. Halothane has a similar vapor pressure to isoflurane, necessitating use of a precision vaporizer. It can be used for mask or chamber induction but has a higher blood-gas partition coefficient (2.54) than isoflurane. Consequently, inductions, recoveries, and changes in anesthetic depth take somewhat longer. Halothane has similar effects to isoflurane but causes less respiratory depression, has a greater tendency to induce cardiac arrhythmias, and is a more potent cardiac depressant.

Methoxyflurane currently is off the market but was used for many years to maintain anesthesia. Because of its low vapor pressure (23 mm Hg), methoxyflurane can be administered from a nonprecision vaporizer in-circle (VIC). It cannot be used for mask or chamber inductions, however, because of a high blood-gas partition coefficient (15). Methoxyflurane is 50% to 75% metabolized and has been linked to organ damage.

Desflurane is similar to isoflurane but has an extremely high vapor pressure and a low blood-gas partition coefficient. Because the boiling point of this agent is near room temperature, desflurane requires a special, expensive electronic vaporizer. Inductions and recoveries are even more rapid than with sevoflurane, producing what is sometimes referred to as "one-breath anesthesia." Desflurane is not arrhythmogenic but causes a dose-related respiratory depression.

Enflurane has not found wide acceptance in veterinary medicine because of adverse effects.

NITROUS OXIDE

Nitrous oxide (N_2O), sometimes referred to as "laughing gas," is a gas at room temperature and is stored in compressed gas cylinders identified by a deep blue color. N_2O is administered along with oxygen through a gas-specific blue flowmeter.

N_2O is one of the oldest inhalant anesthetics, its use dating back to the mid-1800s. N_2O will not produce general anesthesia alone, but it speeds the uptake of other agents into the bloodstream and allows lower doses to be used because it has analgesic properties. In the past, it was administered in conjunction with older halogenated agents such as methoxyflurane. When used with newer agents, these benefits are of less clinical importance. In addition, its use can potentially result in hypoxemia unless the user is appropriately trained. It is seldom used in practice for these reasons. The interested reader should consult a veterinary anesthesia textbook for a detailed discussion of N_2O.

ANESTHETIC EQUIPMENT

ENDOTRACHEAL TUBES

An endotracheal tube is a device that is placed inside the trachea of an unconscious patient, attached to a breathing circuit, and is used to administer oxygen and inhalant anesthetics. Endotracheal tubes increase patient safety because they maintain an open airway; minimize the likelihood of pulmonary aspiration of blood, stomach contents, and other substances; facilitate administration of supplemental oxygen; and allow the anesthetist to ventilate the patient when necessary. Because of these benefits, many veterinarians prefer to place an endotracheal tube in all patients undergoing general anesthesia, even those not receiving inhalant anesthetics.

Endotracheal tubes are available in a variety of sizes, lengths, and types to accommodate the wide size variation of veterinary patients; they may be made of red rubber (Figure 29-1, *D*), silicon rubber (Figure 29-1, *A*), or polyvinyl chloride (PVC) (Figure 29-1, *C* and *E*). Murphy tubes have a side hole called the Murphy eye (Figure 29-2, *J*) at the beveled end that permits airflow in the event of blockage of the tip. The patient end of a Cole tube is tapered and has no cuff (Figure 29-1, *B*). This type is used for small patients and for birds, which do not have an expandable trachea.

An endotracheal tube consists of the following parts: the connector (Figure 29-2, *D*) is attached to the breathing circuit of the anesthetic machine or to an Ambu bag. The cuff (Figure 29-2, *H*) is a balloon-like part at the beveled patient end (Figure 29-2, *I*), which, when inflated, creates a seal between the tube and the tracheal mucosa. This prevents mixing of room air and anesthetic gases and aspiration of liquid or solid materials around the tube. The cuff is connected by a small tube to the pilot balloon (Figure 29-2, *B*) and a valve (Figure 29-2, *A*), which is used to inflate the cuff. The pilot balloon allows the anesthetist to monitor cuff inflation.

Although several different scales may be used to measure the diameter of an endotracheal tube, internal diameter (ID) is most common (Figure 29-2, *G*). Tubes for dogs and cats range in size from 3.0 to 14 mm ID. Small ruminants, swine, and foals require tubes between 6 and 18 mm ID. Small exotic animals may require tubes as small as 1.0 mm ID. Horses and mature cattle require sizes ranging from 16 to 30 mm ID.

LARYNGOSCOPES

Laryngoscopes are used to visualize the larynx while placing endotracheal tubes. A laryngoscope consists of a handle and a blade that is used to depress the tongue; it also includes a light-source for illuminating the throat (Figure 29-3). Common blade sizes range from 0 (small) to 5 (large), although longer blades are available for use in swine and some exotics. Miller blades are straight (Figure 29-3, *A* and *C*) and McIntosh blades are curved (Figure 29-3, *B* and *D*). Laryngoscopes are often used in small ruminants, camelids, and swine, may be helpful in dogs and cats, but are not used in adult cattle, which are intubated by digital palpation, and horses, which are intubated blindly.

MASKS

Masks are cone-shaped devices used to administer oxygen and anesthetic gases to patients that are not intubated

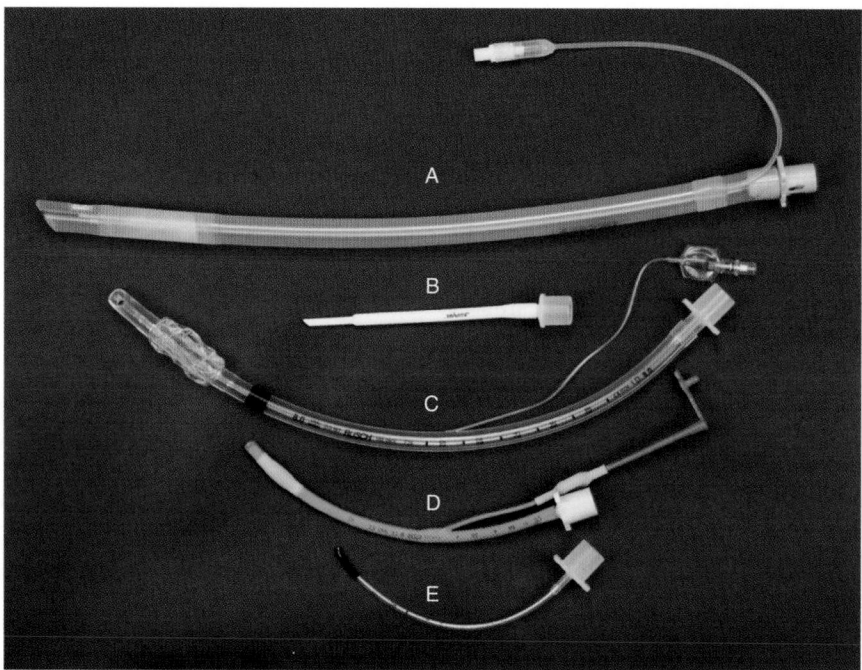

FIGURE 29-1 Endotracheal tube type, material, and size comparison. *A,* Cuffed 11-mm silicone rubber tube. *B,* 2.5-mm Cole tube. *C,* Cuffed 8-mm polyvinylchloride (PVC) tube. *D,* Cuffed 4-mm red rubber tube. *E,* Uncuffed 2-mm PVC tube.

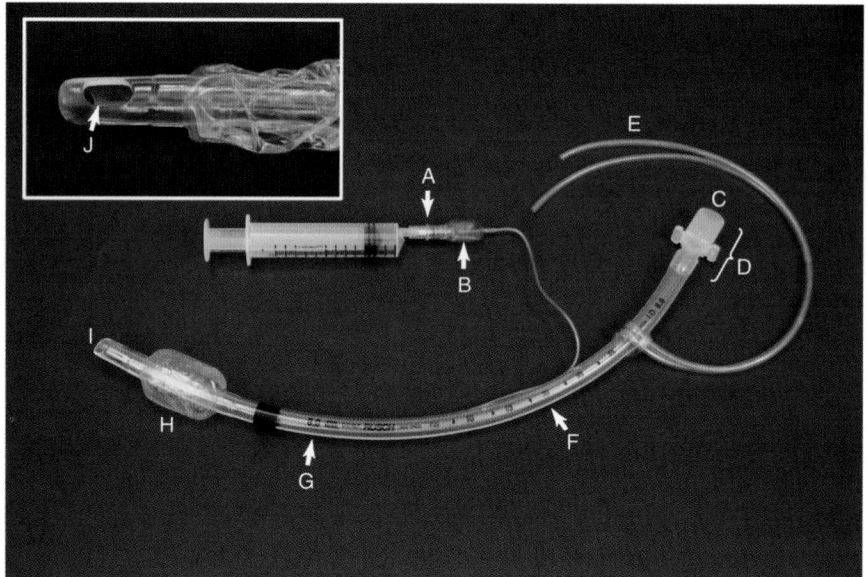

FIGURE 29-2 Endotracheal tube parts. *A,* Valve with syringe attached. *B,* Pilot balloon. *C,* Patient end. *D,* Connector. *E,* Tie. *F,* Measurement of length from the patient end (cm). *G,* Measurement of internal diameter (ID) (mm). *H,* Inflated cuff. *I,* Patient end. *J,* Murphy eye.

(Figure 29-4). They are usually made of plastic or rubber, come in a variety of sizes, and have a rubber gasket designed to create a seal around the patient's muzzle. The smallest mask that comfortably fits the patient should be selected. Masks may be used to induce or maintain anesthesia. They are frequently used to administer anesthetic gases to small patients in which intubation is difficult. Masks may also be used to administer oxygen during the preanesthetic and postanesthetic periods. Masks do not maintain an open airway, do not protect against aspiration, and do not afford the ability to ventilate the patient, as does an endotracheal tube.

ANESTHETIC CHAMBERS

Anesthetic chambers are solid boxes used to induce general anesthesia in small patients that are feral, vicious, or intractable, or cannot be handled without undue stress (Figure 29-5). Chambers are usually clear to allow the anesthetist to observe the patient. They have two ports: one is attached to a fresh gas source, and the other allows the exit of waste gas. A common way to set up a chamber is to attach the inhalation tube and the exhalation tube of a semi-closed **rebreathing system** to each port in place of the Y-piece. Chambers prevent close monitoring of the patient during induction,

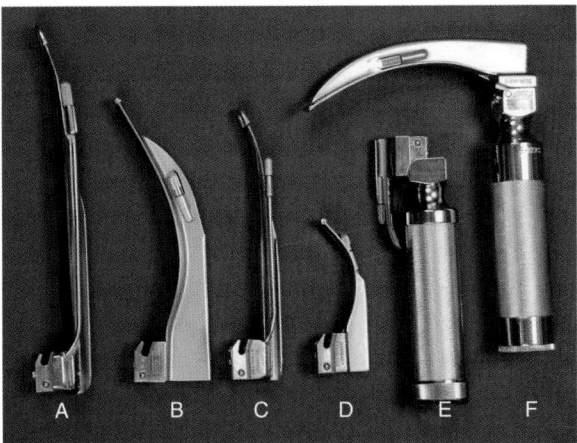

FIGURE 29-3 Laryngoscope handles and blades. *A,* Size 4 Miller blade. *B,* Size 4 McIntosh blade. *C,* Size 2 Miller blade. *D,* Size 1 McIntosh blade. *E,* Laryngoscope handle with size 00 Miller blade in unlocked position. *F,* Laryngoscope handle with size 3 McIntosh blade in locked position (note that the light turns on when the blade is locked).

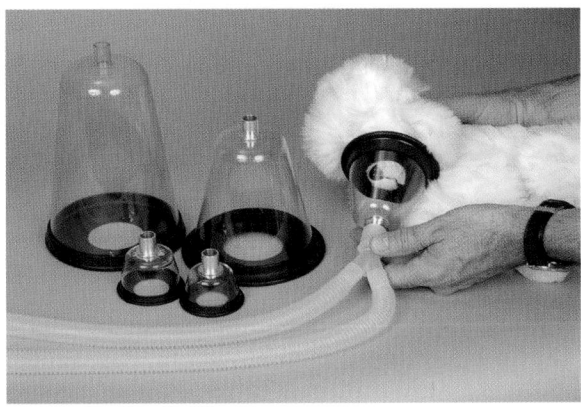

FIGURE 29-4 Anesthetic masks. Note the good fit around the patient's muzzle to minimize leakage.

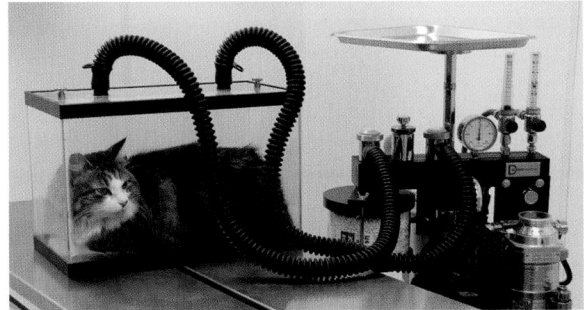

FIGURE 29-5 Anesthetic chamber attached to the corrugated breathing tubes of a semi-closed rebreathing circuit in place of the Y-piece.

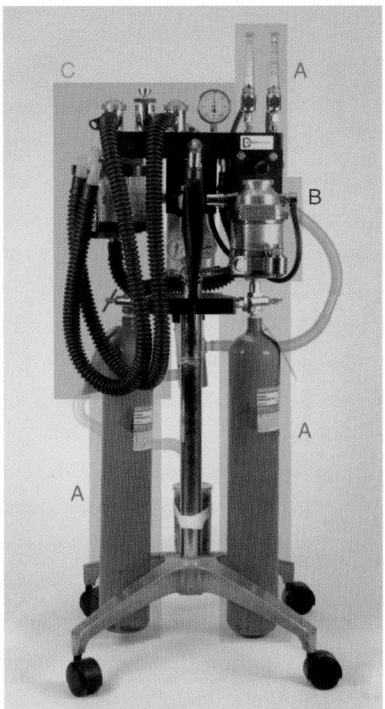

FIGURE 29-6 Anesthetic machine systems. *A,* Carrier gas supply: Note the two size E compressed gas oxygen cylinders beside the "As" at the bottom of this image. *B,* Anesthetic vaporizer. *C,* Breathing circuit. Note that the scavenging system (see Figure 29-8) is not visible in this view.

thus necessitating extreme care when patients are anesthetized by this method.

THE ANESTHETIC MACHINE

Anesthetic machines are used to deliver inhalant anesthetics and oxygen to patients during general anesthesia. These machines are complex and have many specialized and distinct parts that must be properly used and maintained to ensure patient safety. Many different makes and models are in common use, ranging from state-of-the-art machines to those that have been in service for many years, so the veterinary technician may encounter machines of highly varied appearance, size, and age. The basic function and uses are similar, however, and have not changed significantly over the past several decades. For this reason, complete knowledge of anesthetic machine systems and associated equipment, along with a review of the owner's manual, will prepare the technician for operation of any machine that he or she may encounter.

An anesthetic machine consists of the following general systems:
1. The carrier gas supply (Figure 29-6, *A*) delivers oxygen and other carrier gases to the patient at a controlled flow rate. Compressed gas cylinders, the pressure-reducing valve, the tank and line pressure gauges, the flowmeters, and the oxygen flush valve are part of this system.
2. The anesthetic vaporizer (Figure 29-6, *B*) vaporizes a precise concentration of liquid inhalant anesthetic and mixes it with carrier gases.
3. The breathing circuit (Figure 29-6, *C*) delivers the anesthetic and oxygen mixture to the patient via endotracheal tube, mask, or chamber and conveys expired gases away from the patient. Breathing circuits may be classified as rebreathing circuits (see Figure 29-6) or as non-rebreathing circuits (Figure 29-7).

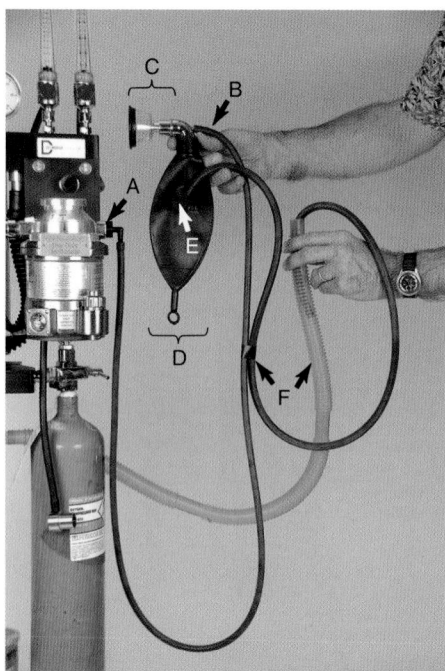

FIGURE 29-7 Parts of a non-rebreathing circuit. *A,* Outlet port of the vaporizer with keyed fitting. *B,* Fresh gas inlet. *C,* Connector with mask attached. *D,* Reservoir bag. *E,* Pressure relief valve. *F,* Scavenging hose.

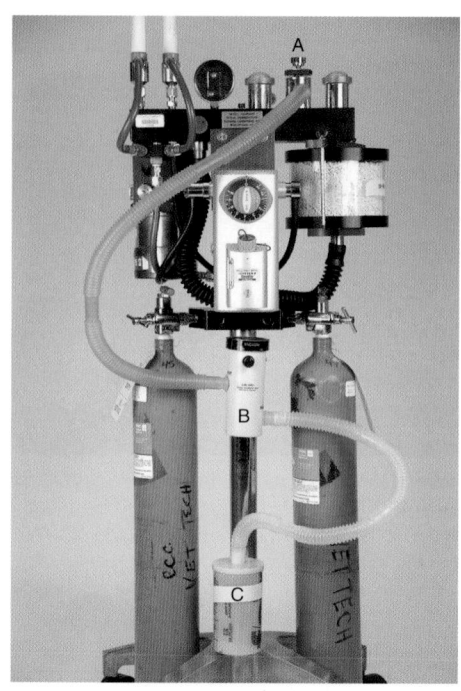

FIGURE 29-8 Scavenging system. Waste gas exits from the pop-off valve *(A)* of this rebreathing system (or the discharge hose of a non-rebreathing system), flows through the vacuum regulator *(B)*, and finally into a charcoal canister *(C)* or, alternatively, into an outlet pipe in the ceiling or wall.

4. The scavenging system disposes of waste and excess anesthetic gases (Figure 29-8).

PREPARING THE MACHINE

Box 29-2 highlights the steps required to prepare an anesthetic machine for use.

Machine Assembly

Before using any anesthetic machine, attach all necessary parts, including the vaporizer inlet and outlet port hoses, the reservoir bag, the corrugated breathing tubes, the scavenging system hoses, and any other parts required for the machine that you are using.

Checking for Leaks

To check the low-pressure system of a **non-rebreathing system** for leaks, occlude the patient connector and the scavenging hose or pressure relief valve. Turn the oxygen on to fill the bag. When the bag is full, turn the flowmeter off. The system has no leaks if the bag remains inflated for at least 10 seconds.

To check the low-pressure system of a rebreathing system for leaks, assemble the machine and secure all connections. Close the pop-off valve completely. Place your thumb over the Y-piece, and use the oxygen flush valve and the oxygen flowmeter to fill the reservoir bag until the pressure manometer indicates a pressure of 30 cm of water. Turn off the flowmeter. No leaks are present if the pressure decreases by no more than 5 cm of water (to the 25 cm of water mark) in 10 seconds. As an alternative, when pressure in the system reaches 30 cm of water, you may turn the flowmeter back on

BOX 29-2	Preparing an Anesthetic Machine for Use

1. Check the quantity of carrier gases in the compressed gas cylinders, and replace them if needed.
2. Check the level of inhalant anesthetic in the anesthetic vaporizer, and refill it if necessary.
3. Select a rebreathing system or a non-rebreathing system based on patient size and requirements.
4. If using a rebreathing system, select an appropriately sized reservoir bag and breathing tubes.
5. Assemble the machine and check the low-pressure system for leaks.
6. Set the pop-off valve.
7. Assemble, turn on, and adjust the scavenging system.

just enough to maintain pressure. A leak is present if more than 200 ml/minute is necessary to do so.

Setting the Pop-off Valve

When using a semi-closed rebreathing system, adjust the pop-off valve immediately after checking the low-pressure system for leaks. With the Y-piece occluded, turn the oxygen flow back on to the anticipated maximum for that procedure. A general rule of thumb is about 1 to 3 L/minute for patients weighing less than 30 kg, about 3 to 5 L/minute for patients weighing 30 kg or more, and 10 L/minute for large animal patients. Then open the pop-off valve gradually until the pressure manometer indicates pressure of 1 to 2 cm of water.

THE CARRIER GAS SUPPLY

The gases into which the liquid inhalant anesthetic evaporates and that carry the vaporized anesthetic to the patient are referred to as *carrier gases*. Oxygen is the carrier gas used during all anesthetic procedures. Oxygen administration is necessary throughout anesthesia not only to carry the anesthetic, but also to compensate for the diminished RR, V_T, and available oxygen that most patients experience during anesthesia. In some circumstances, N_2O may be used with oxygen, although in recent years, use of N_2O in veterinary patients has declined.

Compressed gas cylinders store carrier gases at high pressure (see Figure 29-6, *A*). They may be attached to the yoke (Figure 29-9, *A*) of the anesthetic machine or may be stored in a remote location and connected to the machine via gas lines. An outlet valve is located on the top of all compressed gas cylinders (Figure 29-9, *C*). This valve must be opened when the cylinder is in use by turning the valve stem counterclockwise until it is fully open. When opened, gas will flow through the yoke and into the anesthetic machine. The valve is closed by turning it clockwise (see Figure 29-9, *right side*).

> **TECHNICIAN NOTE** The mnemonic "left-loose, right-tight" (loose meaning open and tight meaning closed) may be used to remember the proper direction to turn the compressed gas cylinder outlet valve, flowmeter dials, and the pop-off valve.

Compressed gas cylinders are usually owned by a supplier that will pick up and refill them as needed. Always be sure that you have at least one spare full tank before commencing any anesthetic procedure. If the primary tank runs out, you will always have a second tank available.

Three holes are visible on the face of the outlet valve. The large hole is the valve port where the gas exits the cylinder (Figure 29-9, *D*). This port fits onto the nipple of the yoke (Figure 29-9, *F*) with a nylon washer in between (Figure 29-9, *H*). The two smaller holes (Figure 29-9, *E*) fit onto index pins (Figure 29-9, *G*), which hold the cylinder in place. These holes and pins are a specific distance apart for each gas—a feature that prevents a cylinder containing the wrong gas from being attached to the yoke.

When removing a cylinder from the machine, make sure the outlet valve is closed and the oxygen is evacuated ("bled off") from the system (see later section on tank pressure gauges for a review of this procedure). Support the cylinder, loosen the wing nut (Figure 29-9, *B*), and back the valve port off of the yoke. Carefully lower the tank until the valve clears the yoke. When attaching a full cylinder, first inspect the valve port for cleanliness, then place a clean, undamaged nylon washer between the valve port and the nipple. Gently raise the tank into place, lining up the valve port and the pin holes with corresponding structures on the yoke. Tighten the wing nut as securely as you can by hand. Open the valve slowly and listen for leaks. If a leak is present, recheck the holes for proper alignment, tighten the wing nut further, or use a new washer.

Compressed gas cylinders may contain different gases. To prevent confusion, cylinders are color coded as follows: green (United States) or white (international) is oxygen; blue is N_2O. These cylinders are available in two sizes, called E tanks (see Figure 29-6, *A*, at the bottom) and H tanks. E tanks are stored on the yoke of the anesthetic machine or in a rack. H tanks are much larger and are stored on a movable cart or chained to the wall and are often used to feed centralized oxygen sources. A centralized oxygen source is one in which

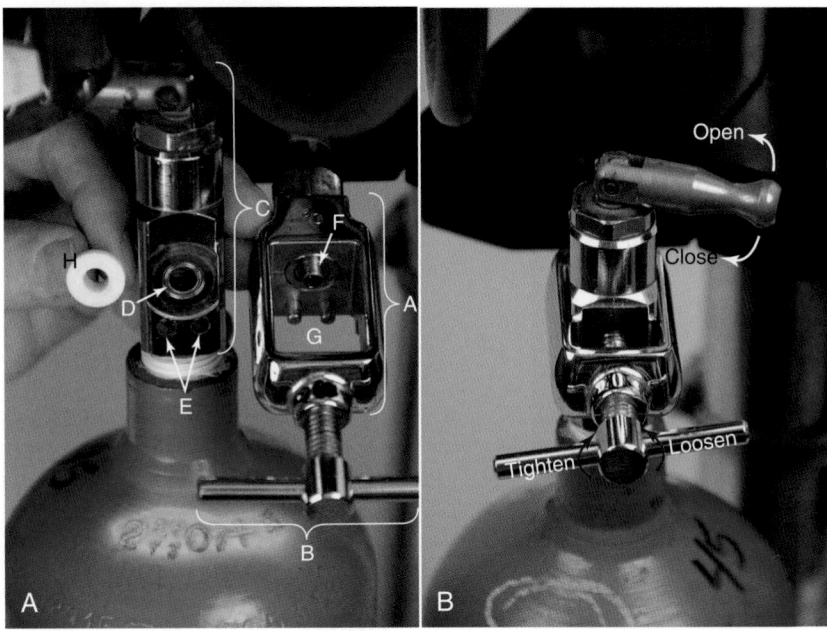

FIGURE 29-9 A *(right image)*, Parts of compressed gas cylinder and yoke. *A*, Yoke. *B*, Wing nut. *C*, Outlet valve. *D*, Valve port. *E*, Pin holes. *F*, Nipple of yoke. *G*, Index pins. *H*, Nylon washer. **B**, Opening-closing the outlet valve; loosening-tightening the wing nut.

the oxygen from an H tank is piped to outlets at various points around the hospital. These outlets are then connected to anesthetic machines via quick-release connectors.

> **TECHNICIAN NOTE** The following rules must be observed when compressed gas cylinders are used, to prevent injury. Never leave an unattended compressed gas cylinder unsupported or lying on its side. Never attempt to remove the valve or index pins. When turning a tank on, keep skin and eyes clear of the valve port. Do not use oxygen near any source of ignition.

Some larger practices use an oxygen concentrator or a bulk oxygen tank as a primary oxygen source. An oxygen concentrator is a machine that extracts oxygen from room air, and a bulk oxygen tank contains a large quantity of oxygen in liquid form.

The tank pressure gauge (Figure 29-10, B) indicates the pressure in a compressed gas cylinder. When full, a cylinder contains oxygen at a pressure of approximately 2200 pounds per square inch (psi). As oxygen is used, cylinder pressure gradually decreases. Oxygen cylinders should be changed when pressure reaches 500 psi, or a level at which the tank does not contain enough gas to last the anticipated length of the procedure. It is important to check the pressure before and throughout the anesthetic period to make sure that there is enough oxygen to complete the procedure.

The volume of oxygen contained in an E tank (expressed in liters) can be estimated by multiplying the pressure in psi by a factor of 0.3. Therefore, a full tank contains about 660 L of oxygen (2200 psi × 0.3 = 660). At a flow rate of 1 L/minute, this will last about 660 minutes, or 11 hours. The volume of oxygen in an H tank in liters is about 3 times the pressure in psi. Therefore, an H tank with a pressure of 2200 psi contains about 6600 L of oxygen (2200 psi × 3 = 6600). When a compressed gas cylinder is turned off, the tank pressure gauge will continue to register pressure until the system is evacuated or "bled off." This is accomplished by depressing the oxygen flush valve until the gauge reads 0 psi.

The pressure-reducing valve (Figure 29-10, C) reduces the pressure of gas exiting the compressed gas cylinder to 40 to 50 psi. This pressure is maintained regardless of the pressure in the cylinder. The line pressure gauge (Figure 29-10, A) indicates pressure in the line connecting the pressure-reducing valve and the flowmeter(s). When the oxygen is turned on, this gauge should read 40 to 50 psi. Both of these parts function passively and require no action on the part of the machine operator.

The flowmeter (Figure 29-11) controls the rate at which carrier gas is delivered to the patient, and reduces the pressure from 40 to 50 psi to 15 psi. Carrier gas flow rates are expressed in liters per minute (L/minute). Flowmeters are gas specific and are color coded to match the compressed gas cylinders (green for oxygen and blue for N_2O). Therefore, if N_2O is used, in addition to oxygen, flowmeters can be used to adjust the flow separately for each carrier gas. Some machines, such as the one pictured, have two oxygen flowmeters. The meter on the right is used for flow rates greater than 1 L/minute, and the meter on the left is used for flow rates less than 1 L/minute.

Turn on a flowmeter by turning the dial counterclockwise. All flowmeters have a ball or rotor indicator that rises to a height proportional to the flow of gas. Read the *center*

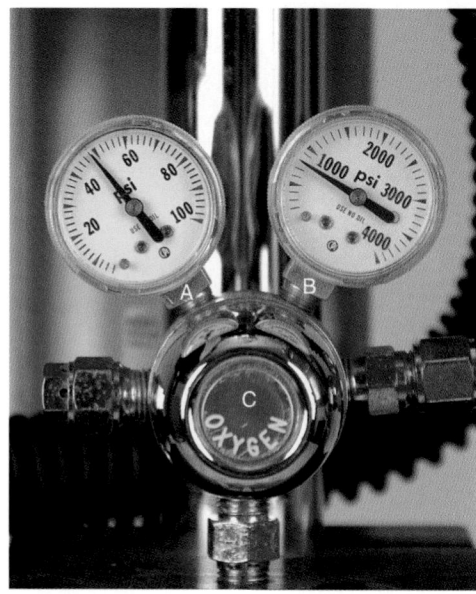

FIGURE 29-10 *A,* Line pressure gauge (registering 48 psi). *B,* Tank pressure gauge (registering 800 psi). *C,* Pressure-reducing valve.

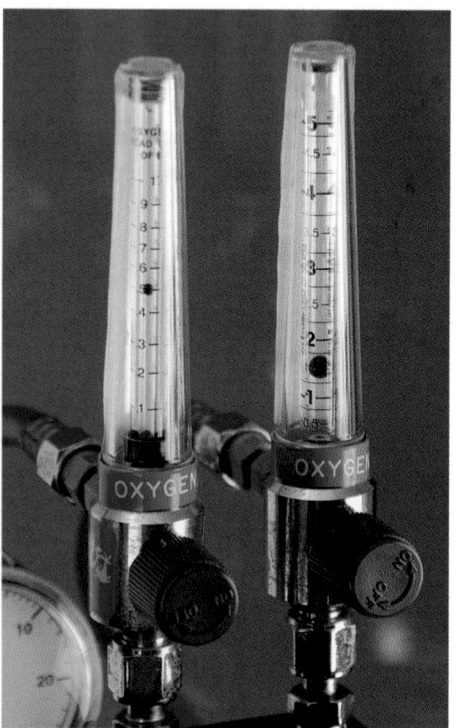

FIGURE 29-11 Oxygen flowmeters with ball indicators. The flowmeter on the left is adjusted to 0.5 L/minute, and flowmeter on the right is adjusted to 1.5 L/minute, for a total oxygen flow of 2 L/minute.

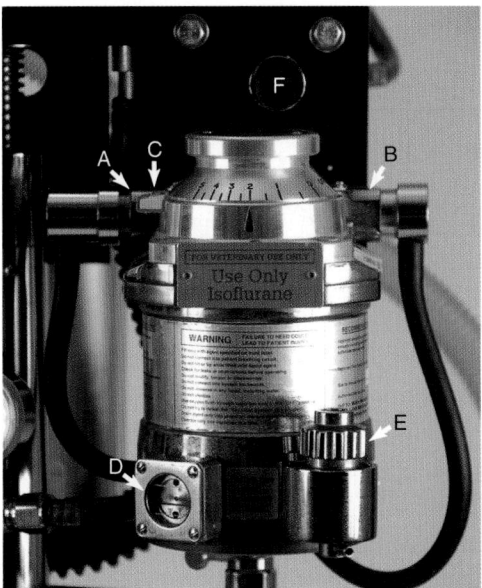

FIGURE 29-12 Precision anesthetic vaporizer for isoflurane set on 2%. *A,* Inlet port with keyed fitting leading from the flowmeters. *B,* Outlet port with keyed fitting leading to the fresh gas inlet. *C,* Safety lock. *D,* Indicator window. *E,* Fill port. *F,* Oxygen flush valve (part of the compressed gas supply).

of a ball indicator or the *top* of a rotor indicator. When turning off these meters, turn clockwise just until the ball or rotor drops to zero. Even though the knob can still be turned, do *not* turn it any further, to prevent damage to the valve.

Oxygen flow rates must be carefully chosen to ensure patient safety, produce desired changes in anesthetic depth, and conserve carrier and anesthetic gases. Although in some practices it is common to use a standard rate of 1 to 2 L/minute for most SA patients, using specific rates will improve patient response, cost savings, and safety. Oxygen flow rates depend on the type of equipment and system used. When a rebreathing system is used, higher rates should be used during induction and recovery, and when changing anesthetic depth. Lower rates may be used during maintenance (Box 29-3 lists recommended oxygen flow rates).

The oxygen flush valve (Figure 29-12, *F*) delivers pure oxygen at 35 to 75 L/minute directly to the breathing circuit, bypassing the flowmeter and the vaporizer. The oxygen flush valve is used to quickly fill an empty reservoir bag with fresh oxygen but will dilute the concentration of inhalant anesthetic in the breathing circuit. It is also used to deliver fresh oxygen to a critically ill patient or to flush inhalant anesthetic out of the circuit during anesthetic recovery or during a crisis. To flush the circuit, turn off the vaporizer, force the gases out of the reservoir bag using gentle hand pressure, and press the valve to refill the bag with fresh oxygen. When using this valve, use only short bursts to avoid overfilling the bag and damaging the patient's lungs as a result of a buildup of pressure.

ANESTHETIC VAPORIZERS

The anesthetic vaporizer holds liquid inhalant anesthetic and adds controlled amounts of vaporized anesthetic to the

---

BOX 29-3 | Oxygen Flow Rates

Oxygen Flow Rates for Small Animals, Foals, Calves, and Small Ruminants
Chamber and Mask Inductions
Chamber induction: 5 L/minute
Mask induction: (300 ml/kg/minute or 30 times V_T)
- 1 to 3 L/minute for patients ≤10 kg
- 3 to 5 L/minute for patients >10 kg

Rebreathing Systems
Semi-closed system after induction, during a change in anesthetic depth, or during recovery: (50 to 100 ml/kg/minute up to a maximum of 5 L/minute. This is approximately equal to ¼ to ½ of the RMV.)
- ≈0.5 to 1 L/10 kg body weight/minute up to a maximum of 5 L/minute
Semi-closed system during maintenance: (20 to 40 ml/kg/minute)
- ≈0.2 to 0.4 L/10 kg body weight/minute with a minimum of 250 ml/minute regardless of patient size
  Note: The use of a maintenance rate of 0.2 L/10 kg/minute is sometimes referred to as "low flow."
Semi-closed system during maintenance with minimal rebreathing: (200 to 300 ml/kg/minute)
- ≈2 to 3 L/10 kg body weight/minute up to a maximum of 5 L/minute
  Note: At this flow, the machine functions in a manner similar to a non-rebreathing system.

Non-Rebreathing Systems (used only for patients weighing 7 kg or less)
Mapleson A (Magill), modified Mapleson A (Lack), and modified Mapleson D (Bain) systems: (150 to 200 ml/kg/minute. This is equal to approximately 0.75 to 1.0 times the RMV.)
- ≈0.5 to 1.5 L/minute
Modified Mapleson D systems (Bain) with no rebreathing, Mapleson E systems (Ayre's T-piece), and Mapleson F systems (Jackson-Rees and Norman mask elbow): (400 to 600 ml/kg/minute. This is equal to approximately 2 to 3 times the RMV.)
- ≈1 to 3 L/minute)

Oxygen Flow Rates for Large Animals
Rebreathing Systems:
Note: Only rebreathing systems are used in LA patients.
Semi-closed system after induction, during a change in anesthetic depth, or during recovery:
- ≈8 to 10 L/minute
Semi-closed system during maintenance:
- ≈3 to 5 L/minute

LA, Large animal; *RMV,* respiratory minute volume; *V_T,* tidal volume.

---

carrier gas. Vaporizers may be classified as precision or as nonprecision.

Precision Vaporizers

The inhalant anesthetics isoflurane and sevoflurane require the use of a precision vaporizer designed and color coded

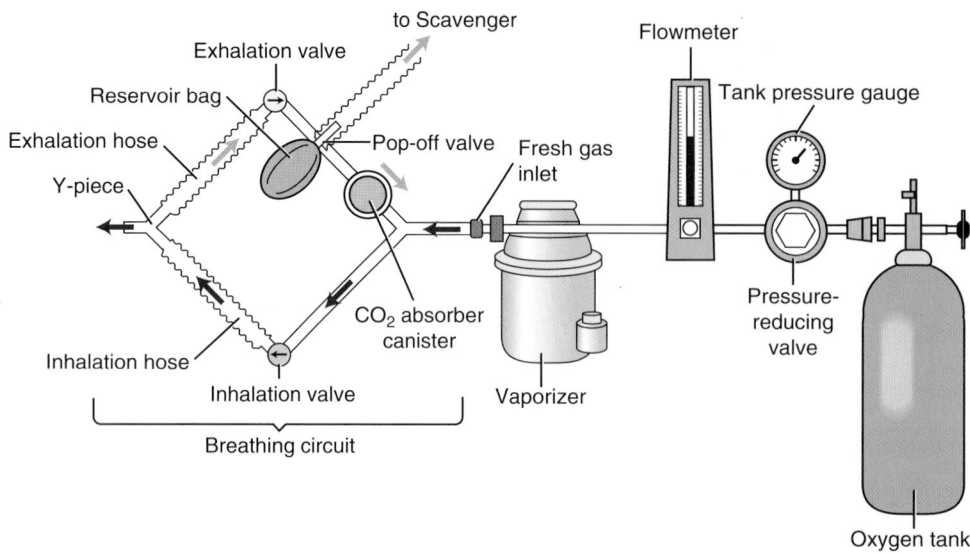

FIGURE 29-13 Diagram of an anesthetic machine with a rebreathing circuit and vaporizer out-of-circle (VOC). Note that the vaporizer is located outside the breathing circuit.

specifically for the agent used (purple is isoflurane; yellow is sevoflurane) (see Figure 29-12). Turn on the vaporizer by disengaging the safety lock (Figure 29-12, *C*) and turning the dial to the desired percent concentration.

> **TECHNICIAN NOTE**　The level of liquid anesthetic in the vaporizer should be noted before each procedure. To function properly, it must be between the upper and lower lines of the window (see Figure 29-12, *D*). Refill as needed, but keep the vaporizer at least one-half full at all times. Overfilling a vaporizer will result in anesthetic overdose; underfilling will lead to an inability to keep the patient anesthetized.

With the exception of some older models, the amount of inhalant anesthetic gas vaporized by a precision vaporizer is independent of variables such as ambient temperature, oxygen flow rate, RR, depth, and back pressure. This allows precise delivery of high vapor pressure inhalant agents, such as isoflurane and sevoflurane. Precision vaporizers are located out of the breathing circuit because of their high resistance to gas flow and are therefore known as vaporizer out-of-circle, or VOC (Figure 29-13).

All precision vaporizers will be somewhat affected by very high or very low carrier gas flow rates. Specifically, oxygen flows in excess of 10 L/minute or lower than 250 mL/minute may affect output. When flows are significantly less than the patient's **respiratory minute volume** (RMV) (200 mL/kg/minute), output will decrease slightly as a result of a dilution effect by expired gases. Therefore, higher dial settings may be needed under these circumstances.

Nonprecision Vaporizers

Nonprecision vaporizers are intended to be used only with low vapor pressure anesthetics, such as the discontinued agent methoxyflurane and, in contrast with precision

vaporizers, are located in the breathing circuit (VIC) because they do not impede the flow of gases around the circuit as the patient breathes. These vaporizers do not measure a precise concentration and are affected by ambient temperature, oxygen flow rate, back pressure, and patient RR and respiratory depth. Although infrequently encountered, these vaporizers may be used with high vapor pressure anesthetics, such as isoflurane, if specifically adapted for this purpose.

Vaporizer Inlet Port and Outlet Port, and the Fresh Gas Inlet

The vaporizer inlet port (see Figure 29-12, *A*) is the point where oxygen and other carrier gases enter the vaporizer from the flowmeters. The vaporizer outlet port (see Figure 29-12, *B*) is the point where oxygen, inhalant anesthetic, and other carrier gases exit the vaporizer. The point at which these gases enter the breathing circuit is referred to as the *fresh gas inlet*. Vaporizer outlet and inlet ports are connected to hoses with keyed fittings that prevent the operator from inadvertently attaching the wrong hose to the wrong vaporizer port.

BREATHING CIRCUITS

Breathing circuits circulate fresh gases to the patient and convey waste gases to the scavenging system. During inhalation and exhalation, the patient's lungs act like a bellows to move air through the breathing circuit. Non-rebreathing systems do not resist air movement and are generally used for smaller patients because they minimize the work required to breathe. In contrast, rebreathing systems resist air movement, thus impairing the ability of small patients to move gases through the circuit.

Use of a non-rebreathing system (Figure 29-14) is recommended for patients weighing less than 7 kg. A non-rebreathing circuit is attached to the outlet port of the anesthetic vaporizer in place of the keyed fitting of a

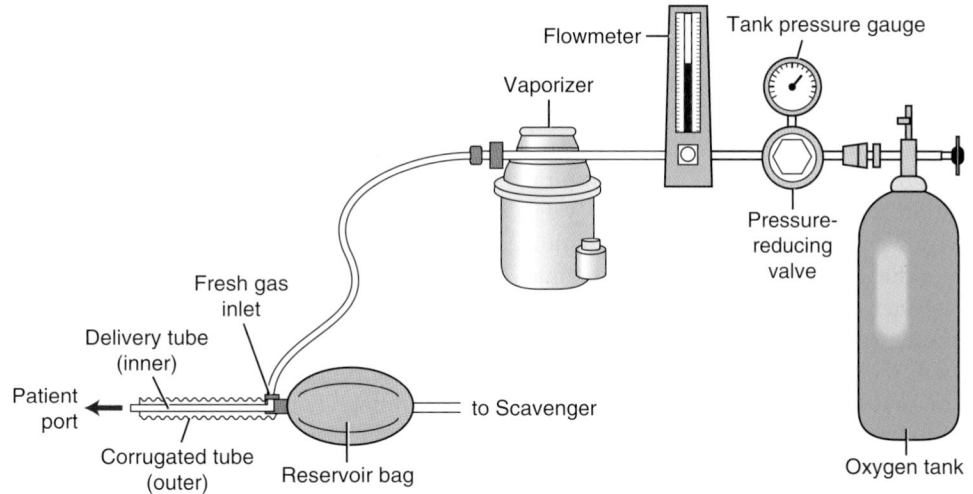

FIGURE 29-14 Diagram of an anesthetic machine with a non-rebreathing system attached to the vaporizer outlet port.

rebreathing circuit (see Figure 29-7, *A*). Fresh oxygen and inhalant anesthetic are delivered to the patient through a fresh gas inlet (see Figure 29-7, *B*), while exhaled gases pass into the scavenging system (see Figure 29-7, *F*), often after passing through a reservoir bag (see Figure 29-7, *D*). These systems flush out expired gases with the use of a relatively high oxygen flow rate (150 to 600 ml/kg/minute) and consequently do not require a CO_2 absorbent canister or unidirectional valves. Non-rebreathing circuits are available in a variety of configurations in which the position of some parts, including the fresh gas inlet, the reservoir bag, and the scavenger outlet, varies. These circuits are grouped using the Mapleson classification system into classes A through F based on the position of the parts. The Magill circuit (Mapleson A), Lack circuit (modified Mapleson A), **Bain coaxial circuit** (modified Mapleson D), **Ayre's T-piece** (Mapleson E), Jackson-Rees circuit (Mapleson F), and Norman Mask elbow (Mapleson F) are non-rebreathing circuits in common use.

Non-rebreathing systems have disadvantages. They do not conserve gases, moisture, or body heat, thus increasing the vigilance required to maintain patient body temperature. Manual ventilation and waste gas scavenging are more difficult.

> **TECHNICIAN NOTE** After a non-rebreathing circuit is removed, the keyed fitting leading to the fresh gas inlet of a rebreathing circuit may be inadvertently left unattached to the vaporizer outlet port. If this happens, anesthetic gas will discharge into the room instead of into the circuit, resulting in an inability to keep the patient anesthetized and exposure of personnel to anesthetic gas. Checking the machine for leaks before each procedure will prevent this error.

Rebreathing systems deliver anesthetic gases to the patient, remove CO_2, and recirculate carbon dioxide–free exhaled gases to the patient. These systems are also called "circle

systems" because the gases move in a modified circular pattern (see Figure 29-13). Fresh oxygen and inhalant enter the breathing circuit through the fresh gas inlet, and excess and waste gases exit the circuit through the pop-off valve. A rebreathing system may be used for patients weighing 2.5 kg or more, provided it is fitted with pediatric breathing tubes when used to anesthetize patients between 2.5 kg and 7 kg.

Rebreathing systems offer several advantages. They may be operated with lower gas flow rates and therefore are more economical than non-rebreathing systems. They allow waste anesthetic gas to be efficiently and easily scavenged. These systems also minimize body heat and moisture loss, and allow observation and control of patient ventilation. These systems also bring disadvantages. Infectious agents may be transferred from patient to patient via microbe-laden moisture that condenses inside the machine parts and is inhaled by subsequent patients. Because the parts of these systems restrict air movement, they are not intended for use in small patients.

A semi-closed rebreathing system (partial rebreathing system) is a safe, practical, and economical system used in general practice in all patients with body weight of 2.5 kg or more. When a semi-closed rebreathing system is used, the pop-off valve is partially open, the oxygen flow rate is higher than the metabolic needs of the patient (greater than 10 ml/kg/minute), and waste gases exit through the pop-off valve.

A closed rebreathing system (total rebreathing system) is identical to the semi-closed system with two exceptions. The pop-off valve is nearly or entirely closed, and the oxygen flow rate is just enough to meet the metabolic needs of the patient (5 to 10 ml/kg/minute). In other words, in this system, approximately the same amount of fresh gas is added to the circuit as the patient consumes. With the exception of equine and bovine anesthesia, closed systems are infrequently used in practice because of the constant monitoring required, although most veterinary anesthesia texts include a detailed protocol for using these systems.

REBREATHING CIRCUIT PARTS

Unidirectional flow valves keep the flow of gases in a rebreathing circuit going one way as the patient breathes. The inhalation (inspiratory) valve (Figure 29-15, *C*) opens to allow gas to flow through the corresponding corrugated breathing tube and into the patient's lungs during inspiration. During expiration, the exhalation (expiratory) valve (Figure 29-15, *A*) opens to allow expired gases to flow through the corresponding corrugated breathing tube into the CO_2 absorbent canister. Thus inhalation of expired gases containing CO_2 is prevented.

The reservoir bag or rebreathing bag (Figure 29-15, *E*) is a storage reservoir for anesthetic gases. It holds gases that fill the patient's lungs during inspiration, and receives gases breathed out by the patient during expiration. It therefore should deflate during inspiration and inflate during expiration. The reservoir bag allows the anesthetist to visually observe patient respirations and to manually ventilate for the patient, when necessary. Reservoir bags are available in a variety of sizes.

The bag should contain enough gas to fill the patient's lungs during inhalation, but it should not be so large as to prevent visualization of respiratory movements. The following rules of thumb can be used when selecting a bag: 500 ml for up to 3 kg; 1 L for 4 to 7 kg; 2 L for 8 to 15 kg; 3 L for 16 to 50 kg; 5 L for 51 to 150 kg. Patients weighing more than 150 kg or that are intubated with at least an 18-mm endotracheal tube require an LA anesthesia machine that uses 30-L bags.

> **TECHNICIAN NOTE** The V_T is the amount of air that passes into or out of the lungs during a normal breath. Normal V_T is about 10 to 15 mL/kg body weight. The size of the reservoir bag ideally should be at least 6 times the patient's V_T, although this is not always practical or necessary.

When in use, the reservoir bag should be approximately three-fourths full at peak expiration. The amount of gas in the bag is influenced by a variety of factors, including oxygen flow, pop-off valve adjustment, and scavenging system adjustment. Low oxygen flows, a fully-open pop-off valve, or a maladjusted scavenging system can cause the bag to empty. This will prevent the patient from filling its lungs with anesthetic gases during inspiration and will impair manual ventilation of the patient. In contrast, high oxygen flows, a closed pop-off valve, or a malfunctioning scavenging system may result in an overfilled bag. This may impair the patient's ability to exhale or may cause a buildup of pressure within the lungs and will impair monitoring of respirations by sight.

The pop-off valve or the pressure relief valve (Figure 29-15, *B*) allows excess gases to exit the breathing circuit, transfers these waste gases to the scavenging system, and prevents buildup of excess pressure within the circuit. The pop-off valve allows a range of settings from fully closed to fully open to maintain optimum volume in the reservoir bag. When fully open, it releases when gas pressure in the circuit exceeds 0.5 to 1 cm of water. As the valve is tightened, more pressure is required for release. When a semi-closed rebreathing system is used, the valve is kept partially open when the patient is spontaneously breathing. It is closed *only* when manual ventilation is provided so that gases may be forced into the patient's lungs with the use of hand pressure. After each breath provided by manual ventilation, it must be opened again to allow the escape of gases and to prevent excess pressure in the chest, which can lead to decreased cardiac output and death.

The CO_2 absorbent canister (Figure 29-15, *F*) is connected to the exhalation valve and receives expired gases. The canister holds absorbent granules, such as calcium hydroxide, which passively remove CO_2 from expired air. Be sure to purchase an absorbent intended specifically for the inhalant agent that you are using.

Absorbent granules in the canister must be fresh to prevent the patient from rebreathing toxic levels of CO_2. When saturated, the granules will no longer absorb waste CO_2 and therefore should be changed after 6 to 8 hours of use, or when one-third to one-half of the granules become saturated. Fresh absorbent granules can be crushed and are white but when saturated, they become hard and turn an off-white color that is visibly distinguishable from the original. Most absorbents also contain a pH indicator that will cause a color change to blue or violet when saturated. The color reaction does not always occur, however, and will dissipate after a few hours if not noted.

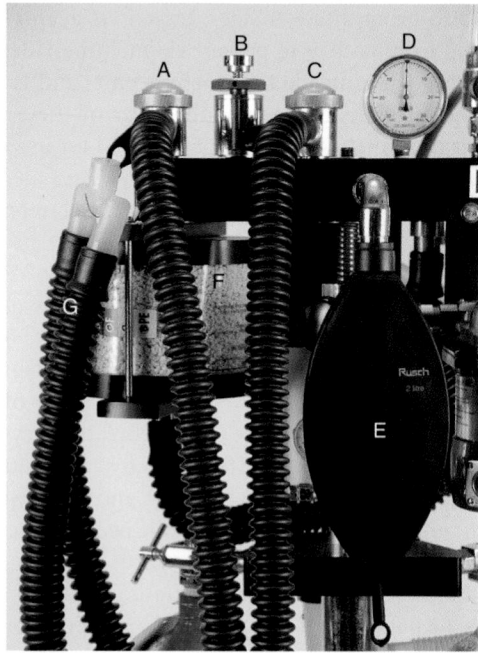

FIGURE 29-15 Parts of a rebreathing circuit. *A*, Exhalation unidirectional flow valve. *B*, Pop-off valve. *C*, Inhalation unidirectional flow valve. *D*, Pressure manometer. *E*, 2-L reservoir bag. *F*, CO_2 absorbent canister. *G*, Small animal (SA) corrugated breathing tubes.

The pressure manometer (Figure 29-15, *D*) indicates pressure (expressed in centimeters of water) in the breathing circuit and in the patient's lungs. This pressure is influenced primarily by oxygen flow and pop-off valve adjustment. The pressure manometer should read 0 to 2 cm of water when the patient is breathing spontaneously. It should read no more than 20 cm of water in small animals, or 40 cm of water in large animals, when manual or mechanical ventilation is provided, unless the chest cavity is open, in which case the pressure can be somewhat higher. Excessive pressure in the circuit can result in dyspnea, lung damage, **pneumothorax**, and decreased cardiac output. Therefore, frequent monitoring of the pressure is critical during any anesthetic procedure.

The negative pressure relief valve admits room air into the breathing circuit if a vacuum is detected, thus preventing patient asphyxiation. A vacuum may occur if the scavenging system exerts excessive suction, if the oxygen flow is too low, or if the oxygen cylinder is empty.

The corrugated breathing tubes (Figure 29-15, *G*) complete the breathing circuit by carrying anesthetic gases to and from the patient. The Y-piece connects the inhalation and exhalation corrugated breathing tubes. Opposite ends of the breathing tubes attach to the unidirectional valves. The remaining port of the Y-piece is then connected to a mask or to an endotracheal tube. LA tubes are 50 mm in diameter. SA tubes (Figure 29-16, *A*) are 22 mm in diameter. Pediatric tubes (Figure 29-16, *B*), which are shorter and smaller than conventional SA tubes, decrease mechanical dead space and are intended for patients weighing between 2.5 and 7 kg. The universal F-circuit (Figure 29-16, *C*) is a type of SA breathing tube in which the inhalation tube is located within the exhalation tube. This arrangement is designed to conserve body heat. As cold inspired gases travel through the inner turquoise tube, warm expired gases travel through the outer, transparent tube, warming inspired gases.

SCAVENGING SYSTEM

The scavenging system is connected to the pop-off valve (see Figure 29-8, *A*) or another breathing circuit outlet and transfers waste gas outside the building through a system of hoses and pipes. Active scavenging systems use a fan to remove waste gas, whereas passive scavenging systems work by gravitational flow. Some active scavenging systems have a vacuum regulator (see Figure 29-8, *B*) that can be adjusted to prevent inadequate or excessive vacuum.

All scavenging systems must be checked periodically to ensure that the tubes are not blocked, and that the vacuum is properly adjusted. Excess vacuum from an active scavenging system will draw all gas out of the breathing circuit. This may lead to asphyxiation and can be recognized by a collapsed reservoir bag. Obstruction of the scavenging system will have the same effect as a closed pop-off valve and is indicated by a full reservoir bag or pressure buildup in the circuit.

An activated charcoal cartridge (see Figure 29-8, *C*) is attached to the discharge hose of the scavenging system and may be used as an alternative when a conventional scavenging system is not available. Activated charcoal will absorb most commonly used inhalant anesthetics (except N_2O) as waste gas is filtered through the cartridge. Activated charcoal cartridges should be weighed before use and must be replaced after a weight gain of 50 g.

ANESTHETIC MACHINE MAINTENANCE

All anesthetic machines require regular maintenance to keep them functioning properly. Whereas much of the maintenance of individual parts can be performed by the anesthetist, the machine should be inspected and maintained by a repair professional at least once a year to ensure proper operation.

The tank pressure gauge, line pressure gauge, pressure-reducing valve, flowmeters, oxygen flush valve, pop-off valve, negative pressure relief valve, and pressure manometer do not require regular maintenance, but should be checked by a repair professional for proper function annually, or when a problem is suspected. Corrugated breathing tubes, reservoir bags, and other detachable rubber parts should be cleaned periodically with a mild disinfectant, such as chlorhexidine, rinsed, dried, inspected for holes or defects, and replaced as necessary.

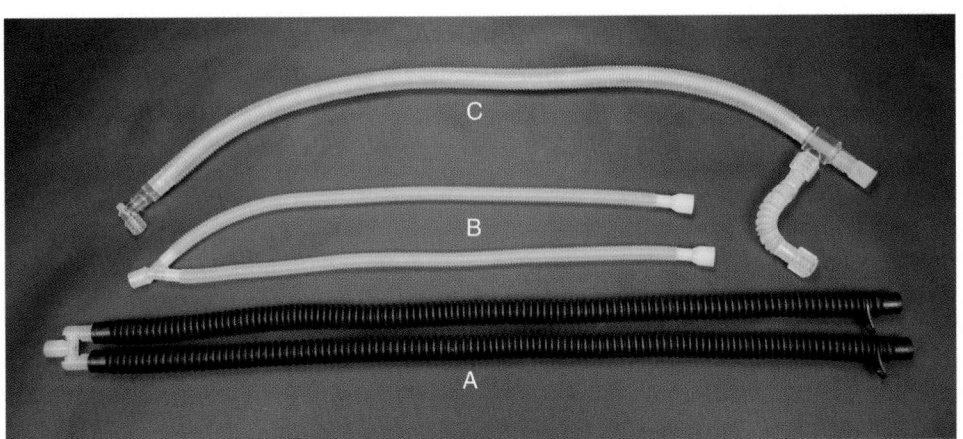

FIGURE 29-16 Corrugated breathing tubes. *A,* Standard 22-mm small animal (SA) breathing tubes. *B,* 15-mm pediatric tubes. *C,* Universal F-circuit.

Unidirectional flow valves should be disassembled, cleaned with 70% isopropyl alcohol or mild disinfectant, dried, and inspected before reassembly to ensure that neither the valve nor the valve seat is damaged or warped. An incompetent valve will allow rebreathing of expired CO_2—a serious and potentially fatal complication.

To change the CO_2 absorbent, disassemble the canister, dispose of the exhausted granules, check the gaskets for damage, and clean each part with mild soap and water. Rinse, dry, and reassemble the parts. Fill the canister loosely with fresh absorbent granules, leaving at least one-half inch of air space at the top. After reassembly, the canister must be air-tight.

PRINCIPLES OF ENDOTRACHEAL INTUBATION

Placement of an endotracheal tube offers several important advantages. It helps to maintain an open airway and allows inhalant anesthetics and oxygen to be administered precisely. It prevents pulmonary aspiration of stomach contents, blood, fluid, or other debris. It permits careful observation of RR and respiratory depth and gives the anesthetist the ability to ventilate the patient when needed. The following equipment is required to perform endotracheal intubation:

- Appropriately sized endotracheal tubes
- Hard roll of gauze or IV tubing to secure the tube
- A gauze sponge to grasp the tongue
- A syringe to inflate the cuff (12 ml for small animals and 20 ml for large animals)
- A good examination light
- Some species require a laryngoscope with an appropriately sized blade.
- Prepare a stylet if intubating small ruminants or swine, if using a tube of narrow diameter, or if using any other tube that requires additional support.
- Lidocaine to control laryngospasm (cats, small ruminants, and swine)

SELECTING A TUBE

Select a tube of appropriate diameter and length. Always prepare at least three tubes of different sizes so that you are prepared if your first choice does not fit the patient's trachea. The following rules of thumb may be used to select the diameter. Most cats require a 3- to 4.5-mm tube. The appropriate size for a dog is based on the patient's body weight. Prepare a 9.5- to 10-mm tube for a patient weighing 20 kg. Increase or decrease the size by approximately 1 mm for each 5 kg body weight less than or more than 20 kg. In other words, prepare a 7.5- to 8-mm tube for a 10-kg patient or a 10.5- to 11-mm tube for a 25-kg patient. Be aware that usefulness of this rule of thumb depends on a variety of factors, including body condition and conformation, and the rule may not apply to all patients, particularly brachycephalic breeds and small or obese animals.

Prepare a 7- to 12-mm tube for sheep and goats; a 6- to 14-mm tube for swine; a 9- to 16-mm tube for foals; a 9- to 18-mm tube for calves; and a 22- to 30-mm tube for adult horses and cattle.

Next, determine whether the tube is of appropriate length. The endotracheal tube should ideally extend from the tip of the nose to the thoracic inlet. If the tube is too long, one of two problems may occur. If inserted too far, the beveled end may inadvertently be advanced into only one mainstem bronchus, thus supplying only one lung with oxygen and anesthetic. If inserted cranial to the thoracic inlet, the portion of the tube extending from the mouth will increase mechanical dead space. Either situation will predispose the patient to **hypoventilation** and **hypoxia**. If the tube is too short, it may not be long enough to reach the trachea.

Dead space is defined as breathing passages and tubes that convey fresh oxygen to the alveoli but in which no gas exchange can occur. Increased dead space decreases the amount of fresh air that reaches the alveoli and is therefore available to the patient. Mechanical dead space is produced by the Y-piece, the portion of the endotracheal tube extending beyond the mouth, and anything placed between these structures, such as an apnea or capnograph monitor sensor, whereas anatomic dead space includes the mouth, nasal passages, pharynx, trachea, and bronchi. It is to the patient's advantage to decrease dead space as much as possible.

PREPARING THE TUBE

Check each tube for blockages, holes, or other damage. Check to make sure that the connector is securely attached, and check the cuff by inflating it. If intact, the cuff should remain inflated after the syringe is detached from the valve. If the tube is soft or narrow, use a stylet that does *not* extend beyond the end of the tube, to stiffen it during placement. The tube can be lubricated with a small amount of sterile water-soluble lubricant or with the patient's saliva immediately before placement.

> **TECHNICIAN NOTE** Before placing an endotracheal tube, check the length, diameter, and cuff. Make sure that the connector is not loose and that the tube is not damaged or blocked with dried mucus.

Successful endotracheal tube placement requires knowledge of the anatomy of the pharynx and larynx, including glottis, epiglottis, vocal folds, and soft palate (Figure 29-17, *B* and *C*). Proper restraint, positioning, and visualization are also critical for success. The induction agent must be administered until the patient is in a state of readiness for intubation. Readiness for intubation is characterized by unconsciousness, lack of voluntary movement, sufficient muscle relaxation to allow the mouth to be held open, and absent pedal and swallowing reflexes.

INTUBATION PROCEDURES
Intubation Procedure for Small Animals
(See Figure 29-17)
- Place the patient in sternal recumbency.
- Have an assistant grasp the maxilla behind the canine teeth, extend the neck, and raise the head.

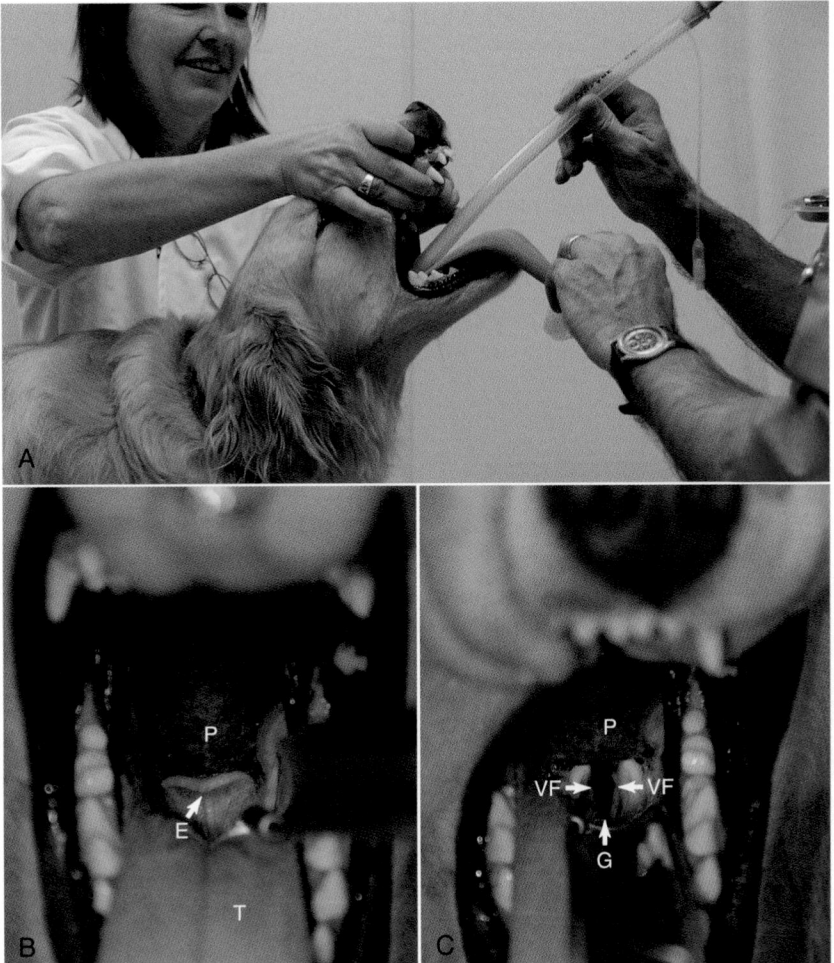

FIGURE 29-17 *A,* Proper position for endotracheal intubation in a small animal. **B,** The anatomy of the pharynx and larynx: *P,* palate; *T,* tongue; *E,* epiglottis, which in this view is covering the glottis. **C,** In this view, the epiglottis has been displaced ventrally with a laryngoscope. The glottis (G) is visible as the dark, oval opening between the vocal folds (VF), which move apart when the patient inspires and relax as the patient expires.

- Grasp the tongue with a gauze sponge and open the mouth fully by firmly pulling the tongue out and down.
- Adjust the light so that you have good illumination of the larynx.
- If necessary, use the tube or laryngoscope to gently displace the epiglottis ventrally or the soft palate dorsally until the glottis can be visualized (see Figure 29-17, *C*).
- Gently insert the tube past the vocal folds using a rotating motion. If the tube is too large to pass easily, exchange the tube for one of smaller diameter, but *never force the tube.*
- After the tube is placed, gently transfer the patient into lateral recumbency.
- Check the tube to ensure that it is in the appropriate distance and is oriented to match the natural curve of the trachea.
- Secure the tube with roll gauze or used IV tubing (over the nose for dolichocephalic dogs and behind the head for cats and brachycephalic dogs). Make sure that the tie is secure enough not to slip but does not compress the tube.
- Connect the tube connector to the breathing circuit.
- Inflate the cuff and check for leaks.

- Ensure a patent airway by checking the position of the patient and tube. The neck and tube should assume a gentle natural curve.

Intubation Procedure for Horses (Figure 29-18)
Endotracheal intubation is performed blindly in this species because the larynx is impossible to see.
- Extend the head to line up the mouth, oropharynx, and larynx.
- Place a speculum or mouth gag.
- Advance the tube over the tongue taking care to stay in the center of the oropharynx so that the molar teeth do not damage the cuff.
- During inspiration, advance the tube *gently.*
- If resistance is encountered, stop and pull the tube back 10 to 15 cm.
- Repeat if unsuccessful, each time rotating the tube 90 degrees.
- Once the tube passes easily into the larynx and trachea, check for correct replacement by feeling air passing out of the tube on expiration. If the horse is apneic, pressure on the thorax will produce the same effect.

It may be helpful to apply gentle pressure externally on the larynx (cricoid pressure) or to flex, then reextend the head if intubation is difficult.

Intubation Procedure for Adult Cattle
(Figure 29-19)

Endotracheal intubation is also performed blindly in this species.

- Place a speculum or mouth gag.
- Extend the head and neck.
- Insert your arm into the mouth.
- Palpate, then reflect the epiglottis forward.

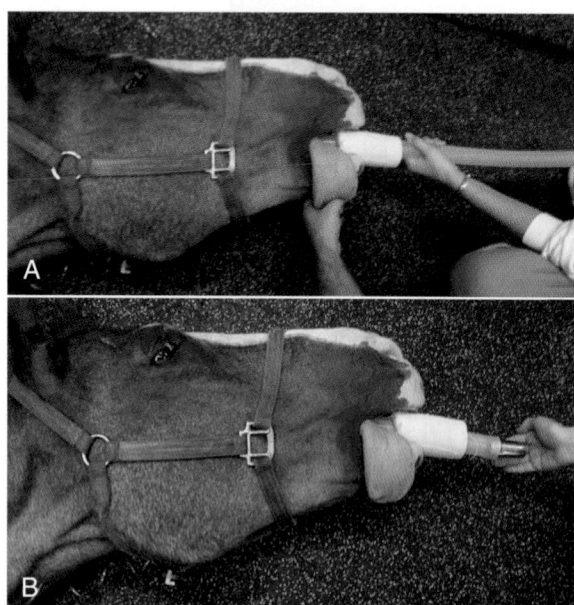

FIGURE 29-18 Equine intubation. **A,** The anesthetist advances the endotracheal tube blindly through a speculum in the mouth and into the larynx with the head extended. **B,** The anesthetist feels for movement of air when the horse breathes out, to confirm correct placement of the tube in the trachea.

- Remove your arm and grasp the endotracheal tube with the beveled end protected in your palm.
- Guide the tube into the larynx using the hand that is in the mouth, while using your other hand to advance the tube into the trachea.

Intubation Procedure for Small Ruminants and Small or Young Cattle

These patients are intubated using a technique similar to that used for SA patients. The oral cavity is long and narrow in these animals, so visualization of the larynx requires use of a laryngoscope with a long blade, and intubation is facilitated using a stylet.

- Extend the head and neck.
- Hold the mouth open.
- Gently pull the tongue down and out by grasping it with a gauze sponge.
- Insert a stylet that protrudes from the patent end of the endotracheal tube to facilitate intubation.
- Once the larynx is visualized, insert the stylet no more than 2 to 5 cm into the trachea.
- While holding the stylet firmly in position, pass the tube over the stylet into the larynx.

Because of limited space in the mouth, it may be necessary to remove the laryngoscope while passing the endotracheal tube. Goats may develop laryngospasm, so topical lidocaine may be used to desensitize the larynx before intubation. It is imperative to inflate the cuff as soon as the patient is intubated to prevent aspiration of regurgitated material or saliva.

CHECKING FOR PROPER PLACEMENT

An endotracheal tube can be easily misplaced in the esophagus and therefore may appear to be correctly placed when it is not. This will result in an inability to keep the patient anesthetized. Therefore, confirmation of proper placement is essential. The following techniques may be used to confirm proper placement:

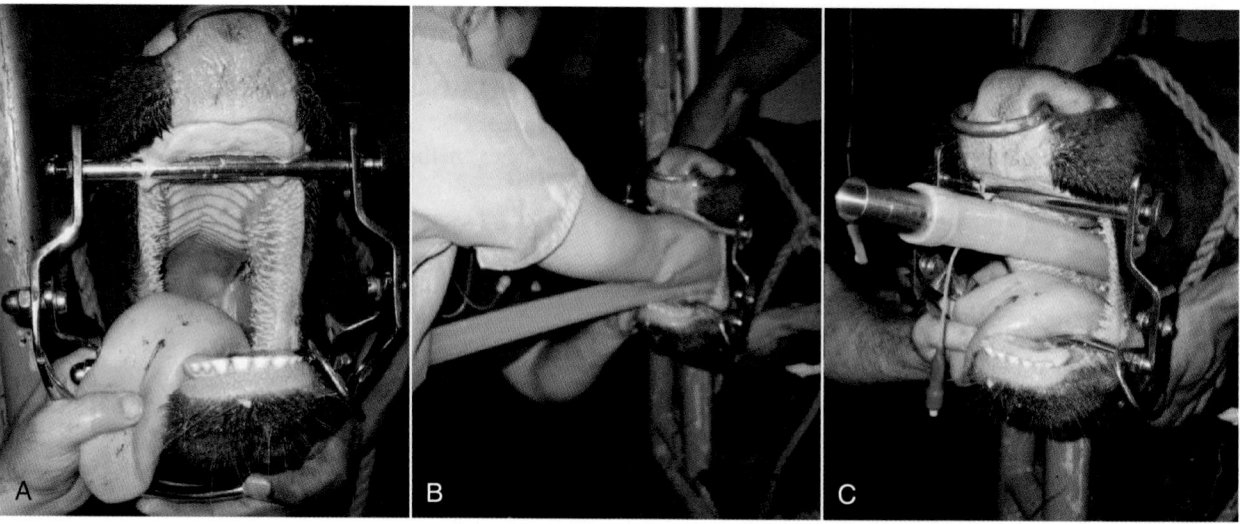

FIGURE 29-19 Bovine intubation. **A,** A mouth gag is placed and the head extended by an assistant. **B,** The anesthetist palpates the larynx with her fingers and directs the endotracheal tube into the trachea. **C,** With the tube in place, the cuff can be inflated and the mouth gag removed.

- Revisualize the larynx to confirm successful intubation (dogs, cats, and small ruminants).
- Watch for expansion and contraction of the reservoir bag as the animal breathes.
- Feel for air movement from the tube connector as the patient exhales.
- Check that the motion of the unidirectional valves coincides with breathing.
- Palpate the neck. The only naturally firm structure in the neck is the trachea. If the tube is properly placed, only one firm structure should be palpable. Palpation of two firm structures (the tube and the trachea) indicates placement of the tube inside the esophagus.
- If the patient can vocalize (whine or cry), the tube is not in the correct location (this most commonly applies to dogs).
- Although a cough reflex during intubation is indicative of proper placement, not all patients exhibit this sign.
- When using an end-tidal CO_2 monitor, the presence of a normal waveform indicates proper placement.

CUFF INFLATION

The cuff of the endotracheal tube must be gently inflated until a seal is formed between the trachea and the cuff. This will prevent leakage of anesthetic gases and mixing with room air, which will result in a variety of complications, including contamination of the surgery suite with waste gases and difficulty keeping the patient asleep. To inflate the cuff, extend the patient's head to straighten the airway. Attach an air-filled syringe to the valve port. Have an assistant close the pop-off valve and gently compress the reservoir bag. Listen for gas leakage around the tube, which may sound like a soft hiss or gurgling. Slowly inflate the cuff until the leaking just ceases at a pressure of 20 cm of water. Avoid overinflation of the cuff, which can result in a variety of mild to serious complications.

LARYNGOSPASM

Laryngospasm is a complication in which the glottis forcibly closes during intubation. This complication is most commonly encountered in cats, swine, and small ruminants. It is extremely difficult to place a tube in a patient experiencing laryngospasm because the glottis closes as soon as it is touched and cannot be safely forced open. Laryngospasm can lead to hypoxia and **cyanosis** in severe cases, but it is prevented using one or more of the following strategies:

- Apply 2% injectable lidocaine via a syringe directly to the glottis before placement. Wait 30 to 60 seconds for the lidocaine to take effect before attempting intubation; 0.1 ml is appropriate for cats, whereas 1 to 2 ml can be used in sheep, goats, and pigs.
- Make sure that the patient is adequately anesthetized before attempting intubation because laryngospasm decreases with increasing depth of anesthesia.
- Prepare carefully, wait for the glottis to open before attempting placement, and try to get the tube in the first time. Repeat attempts worsen laryngospasm.

- *Do not force the tube.* This can lead to severe and potentially life-threatening complications, including tracheal rupture, pneumothorax, and pneumomediastinum.

COMPLICATIONS OF INTUBATION (Box 29-4)

Numerous hazards are associated with endotracheal intubation. Most are associated with tracheal irritation, trauma, or

BOX 29-4	Complications of Endotracheal Intubation

Cuff Not Inflated/Underinflated
- Inability to create a seal between cuff and trachea
- Difficulty with or inability in keeping the patient anesthetized
- Aspiration of stomach contents
- Aspiration of foreign material and fluid during dental cleaning
- Pollution of the work space with anesthetic gas

Tube Diameter Too Small
- Inability to create a seal between cuff and trachea, leading to the same complications listed earlier
- Small tubes are more likely to block with mucus.
- Increased resistance to breathing with increased respiratory effort

Cuff Overinflated/Tube Diameter Too Large
- Necrosis of the tracheal mucosa
- Possibility of tracheal rupture in extreme situations

Tube Too Long
- If placed past the thoracic inlet, intubation of only one mainstem bronchus, leading to hypoxia and difficulty in keeping the patient anesthetized
- If extending beyond the mouth, increased mechanical dead space, leading to hypoventilation and hypoxia

Tube Too Short
- Inability to intubate the patient successfully
- Changes in patient position may dislodge the tube from the glottis.

Overzealous Intubation
- Tracheal irritation, leading to tracheitis and postoperative cough
- Trauma or tracheal rupture, resulting in pneumomediastinum and/or pneumothorax

Tube Kinked or Obstructed
- Dyspnea and hypoxia
- Asphyxia and cardiac arrest if not corrected

Tube Not Removed Before Return to Consciousness
- Damage to the tube from chewing
- Blockage of the airway
- In extreme situations, a severed portion of the tube can be aspirated or swallowed

Tube Not Cleaned and Disinfected
- Transmission of infectious agents, leading to tracheitis, bronchitis, or pneumonia
- Blockage of the tube with dried mucus or other foreign material

failure to protect the airway. Although the larynx and the trachea of mammals are relatively resilient structures, excessive force will result in damage, perforation, rupture, or irritation of the delicate mucosa. An endotracheal tube therefore must be chosen, maintained, placed, and monitored with care.

ANESTHETIC MONITORING

The common perception is that modern anesthetic agents are safe. Although this belief can lead to the erroneous assumption that careful monitoring is not important, anesthetic monitoring is and always has been one of the cornerstones of the successful practice of anesthesia, because conditions that may lead to serious complications are often subtle but must be recognized and corrected without delay. Serious anesthetic complications often develop rapidly and, if not prevented, are devastating for the patient, the owner, and the anesthetist. Consequently, the anesthetist must develop the ability to endure long periods of relative boredom in a state of readiness to manage periods of urgency and crisis. This requires that the anesthetist be knowledgeable, alert, and watchful for subtle changes in the condition of the patient.

During any general anesthetic procedure, the anesthetist must strike a delicate balance of sufficient depth of anesthesia to produce unconsciousness and insensitivity to pain without endangering the life of the patient by compromising cardiovascular and respiratory system function. Monitoring allows the anesthetist to achieve this balance through careful observation and precise regulation of the amount of anesthetic administered.

The American College of Veterinary Anesthesiologists (ACVA) has published a set of anesthetic monitoring guidelines entitled "Recommendations for Monitoring Anesthetized Veterinary Patients" (available at http://www.acva.org/). These guidelines are designed to improve the level of patient care and to decrease the incidence of anesthetic complications by providing specific recommendations for monitoring, including methods, frequency, and record keeping. Familiarity with this reference will help the veterinary anesthetist provide state of the art care for all anesthetized and sedated patients.

> **TECHNICIAN NOTE** Principles of patient monitoring:
> - Monitor patients frequently using your hands, eyes, and ears.
> - Always check multiple parameters.
> - Never depend on instrumentation alone.
> - Do not attempt to judge anesthetic depth by drug doses or dial settings.

STAGES AND PLANES OF ANESTHESIA

In the early 1900s, a system of stages and planes of general anesthesia was developed to describe patient responses to diethyl ether, an early inhalant anesthetic that is no longer used in clinical practice. Changes in patient behavior, body movements, ocular signs, reflexes, and vital signs in response to the progression from consciousness to deep surgical anesthesia were observed and documented. Under this system, general anesthesia was divided into four stages (I to IV), and stage III was subdivided into four planes (1 to 4).

Stage I—Period of Voluntary Movement
During this stage, the patient gradually loses consciousness. This stage is usually characterized by fear, excitement, and struggling. HR and RR increase, and the patient may pant, urinate, or defecate. Near the end of stage I, the patient loses its ability to stand and becomes recumbent.

Stage II—Period of Involuntary Movement
During this stage, also known as the excitement stage, the patient loses voluntary control and assumes an irregular breathing pattern. It is usually characterized by involuntary reactions in the form of vocalizing, reflex struggling, or paddling. HR is often elevated, pupils are dilated, muscle tone is marked, and reflexes are present.

Stage III—Period of Surgical Anesthesia
During this stage, the patient is unconscious and progresses gradually from light to deep surgical anesthesia. This stage is characterized by progressive muscle relaxation, decreasing HR and RR, and loss of reflexes. The pupils gradually dilate, tear production decreases, and the pupillary light reflex is lost. The increase in HR and RR seen in response to surgical stimulation during light anesthesia is gradually lost. Many authors now divide this stage into three planes corresponding to light (stage III, plane 1), medium (stage III, plane 2 and early in plane 3), and deep (stage III, late in plane 3 and plane 4) surgical anesthesia.

Stage IV—Period of Anesthetic Overdose
During this stage, the nervous, cardiovascular, and respiratory systems are extremely depressed. Breathing stops, muscle tone is flaccid, pupils are widely dilated, and all reflexes are absent. The heart stops, and death follows quickly unless rapid action is taken.

PRINCIPLES OF MONITORING

Healthy patients (physical status class P1) should be monitored at least every 5 minutes during any general anesthetic procedure. Higher-risk patients (physical status classes P2 to P5) must be monitored more frequently and in some cases continuously. Ultimately, the anesthetist must judge the frequency of monitoring that is appropriate for each patient. An anesthetic record should be used to document monitoring parameters, drug administration, and other information pertinent to the procedure (Figure 29-20).

At any given time during anesthesia, the patient should be somewhere between consciousness and deep surgical anesthesia (stage III, plane 3). Careful observation of the patient based on expected responses enables the anesthetist

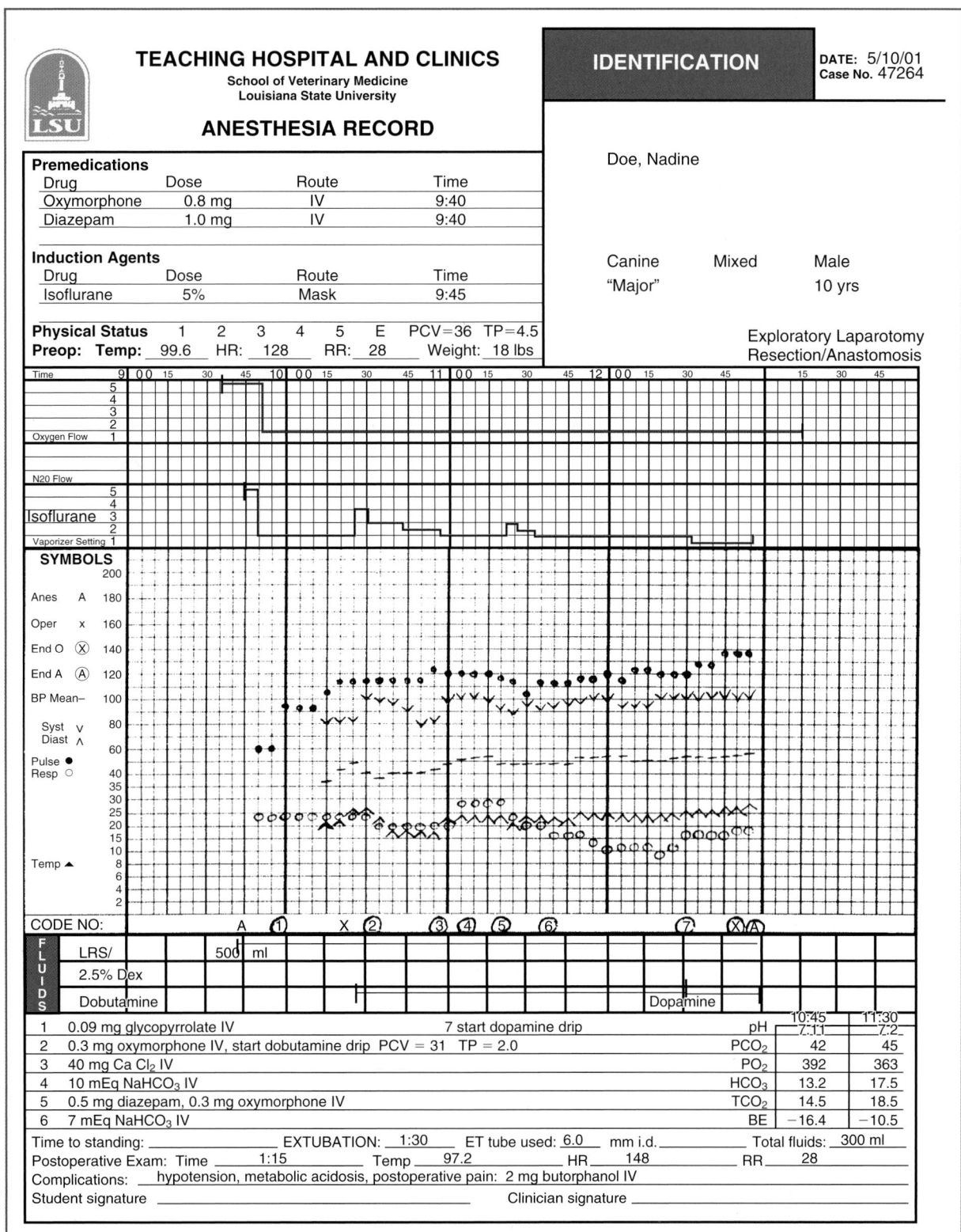

FIGURE 29-20 Anesthesia record: The form is used to document the anesthetic protocol, monitoring parameters, treatments, and other information pertinent to the procedure.

to determine the stage that the patient is in. For instance, unconsciousness, intact reflexes, eyes in a central position, marked jaw tone, and movement in response to stimulation are all expected responses from a patient in light surgical anesthesia (stage III, plane 1)—a point inappropriate to perform surgery. In contrast, absent palpebral, pedal, and swallowing reflexes; moderate jaw tone; eyes in a ventromedial position; and an intact corneal reflex are all expected responses from a patient in medium surgical anesthesia (stage III, plane 2)—an appropriate stage to begin the procedure.

Many factors can influence progression through the stages of anesthesia and interpretation of physical signs. For instance, patients induced using IV agents often pass through stages I and II so quickly that they are minimally noticeable. In contrast, patients induced with an inhalant agent take longer to reach surgical anesthesia and may be difficult to control while passing though these stages. Administration of premedications generally decreases the excitement seen during stages I and II and therefore eases passage into surgical anesthesia.

In addition, the anesthetic protocol will influence interpretation of physical signs. For example, a patient induced with an alpha$_2$-adrenergic agonist will often have a much lower HR than one induced with an inhalant agent. A patient may have dilated pupils if given a dissociative agent, but conversely may have constricted pupils if given an opioid. Consequently, physical signs must be interpreted in light of the agents administered.

After considering each of these factors, the anesthetist must ultimately answer two questions:
1. Is the patient safe or in danger?
2. Is the anesthetic depth inadequate, excessive, or appropriate for the procedure performed?

Monitoring parameters are the physical signs used to answer these questions. They are subdivided into vital signs, reflexes, and other indicators of anesthetic depth. Although all monitoring parameters are evaluated together, some are more useful for answering the first question, whereas others are more useful for answering the second.

VITAL SIGNS

Vital signs are used primarily to evaluate the cardiovascular and pulmonary systems. Vital signs include HR and heart rhythm, RR and respiratory depth, mucous membrane color, CRT, blood pressure, and temperature. These parameters are used principally to answer the question, "Is the patient safe or in danger?" They are only loosely correlated with the depth of anesthesia. Specifically, patients in lighter planes of anesthesia tend to have higher HR, RR, and blood pressure; pinker mucous membranes; and more rapid CRT, whereas patients in deeper planes experience opposite effects (Table 29-3). However, other factors may change this association. For example, a patient in light surgical anesthesia given an opioid agonist may have a decreased HR. Conversely, a patient in deep surgical anesthesia may have an elevated HR if in shock. Although vital signs are helpful in determining

TABLE 29-3	Relationship Between Vital Signs and Anesthetic Depth		
VITAL SIGN	**DEPTH: TOO LIGHT**	**DEPTH: SURGICAL ANESTHESIA**	**DEPTH: TOO DEEP**
Heart rate	Usually elevated	Variable	Usually decreased
Respiration rate	Usually elevated	Variable	Usually decreased
Pulses	Strong	Palpable but often less strong	Weak/nonpalpable
Mucous membrane color/capillary refill time	Normal/normal	Normal but may be somewhat paler/normal	Pale/prolonged

TABLE 29-4	Normal and Abnormal Heart Rate (HR) and Rhythm		
SPECIES	**NORMAL HR, bpm (awake/at rest)**	**NORMAL HR, bpm (anesthetized)**	**REPORT TO THE VETERINARIAN IF***
Dog†	60-180	60-150	<60 (large); <70 (small) or >140 (large); >160 (small)
Cat	120-240	120-180	<100 or >200
Horse	30-45	28-40	<25 or >60
Cattle	60-80	50-80	<40 or >100

*In addition to the rates listed, any arrhythmia should be reported to the veterinarian.
†Because of the extreme variability of size, large dogs tend to have lower rates, whereas small dogs and puppies have higher rates.

anesthetic depth, other parameters are better suited to this purpose.

The ACVA Recommendations for Monitoring Anesthetized Veterinary Patients group vital signs into three classifications: (1) indicators of circulation, (2) indicators of oxygenation, and (3) indicators of ventilation.

INDICATORS OF CIRCULATION

Indicators of circulation include heart rate and rhythm, mucous membrane color and CRT, pulse strength, and blood pressure. Heart rate measured in beats/minute (bpm), and heart rhythm (Table 29-4) may be monitored by palpation of the chest wall, palpation of the pulse, auscultation, or use of monitoring equipment. HR generally decreases gradually in response to increasing anesthetic depth because most anesthetic agents are cardiovascular depressants. This effect is extremely variable, however, and is influenced by the specific agents used, blood pressure, preexisting illness, and other factors. Although bradycardia is caused to some degree by most anesthetic agents, opioids and alpha$_2$-adrenergic agonists are particularly likely to have this effect. Conversely, dissociatives and anticholinergics may cause tachycardia.

TABLE 29-5	Normal and Abnormal Mucous Membrane Color, CRT, and Pulse Strength		
VITAL SIGN (all species)	**NORMAL (awake/at rest)**	**NORMAL (anesthetized)**	**REPORT TO THE VETERINARIAN IF**
Mucous membrane color	Pink (often described as "bubblegum pink")	Pink (may be somewhat paler than when awake)	Pale or blue
CRT	<2 seconds	<2 seconds	>2 seconds
Pulse strength	Palpable with one pulse closely following each heartbeat	Often somewhat decreased in strength but still palpable	Nonpalpable Irregular Excessively weak

CRT, Capillary refill time.

TABLE 29-6	Normal and Abnormal Respiratory Rate, Effort, and Tidal Volume (V_T)		
SPECIES	**NORMAL (awake/ at rest)**	**NORMAL (anesthetized)**	**REPORT TO THE VETERINARIAN IF**
Dogs	10-30 (panting is normal)	8-20	<6 or >20
Cats	15-30	8-20	<6 or >20
Horses	8-20	6-12	<6 or >20
Cattle	8-20	6-12, although rapid, shallow breathing is common	<6 or >20
All species	Normal effort and V_T	Normal effort ≈25% decrease in V_T	Increased effort >25% decrease in V_T

During anesthesia, the normal heart rhythm is normal sinus rhythm (NSR) or sinus arrhythmia in dogs and NSR in cats. Large animals typically exhibit NSR, but sinus arrhythmia may also be observed. Athletic horses may exhibit first- or second-degree atrioventricular (AV) block. Cardiac arrhythmias can be induced by anesthetic agents, particularly alpha$_2$-adrenergic agonists, barbiturates, anticholinergics, and dissociatives, but can also be caused by other conditions such as hypoxia, gastric dilatation-volvulus, **hypercarbia**, preexisting heart disease, and trauma.

Mucous membrane color (Table 29-5) is monitored by observing the color of the oral mucous membranes. Capillary refill time (see Table 29-5) is the time it takes (in seconds) for normal color to return after digital pressure is applied to the gums near the base of a tooth. If oral tissues are pigmented, the tongue, conjunctiva, or mucous membranes of the prepuce or vulva can be used as alternatives.

Pale mucous membranes indicate poor capillary perfusion or anemia resulting from any cause. Prolonged CRT indicates poor capillary perfusion.

Blood pressure can be monitored by indirect measurement (obtained with a Doppler or oscillometric monitor) or by direct measurement (obtained with an arterial catheter) (see "Monitoring Equipment"). Pulse strength (see Table 29-5) as determined by palpation of a peripheral artery (such as the lingual, femoral, carotid, or dorsal pedal artery in small animals, or the facial, auricular, digital, or dorsal pedal artery in large animals) gives the anesthetist a crude indication of blood pressure. A strong pulse is suggestive of normal blood pressure, and a weak pulse is suggestive of hypotension. Pulse strength varies widely among individuals, so the anesthetist should assess the pulse as a point of reference before administering an anesthetic.

INDICATORS OF OXYGENATION

Pulse oximetry and measurement of dissolved blood oxygen through blood gas analysis are the best indicators of oxygenation. Pulse oximetry is discussed in the section, "Monitoring Equipment" (see p. 1110). Mucous membrane color, the only physical indicator of oxygenation, will change from pink to cyanotic in severely deoxygenated nonanemic patients, but this does not warn of deoxygenation in sufficient time to permit timely intervention and is not accurate in the presence of anemia. It is therefore, at best, a very crude indicator of tissue oxygenation.

INDICATORS OF VENTILATION

Indicators of ventilation include RR, respiratory effort, V_T, capnography, and blood gas analysis. Respiratory rate measured in bpm, respiratory effort, and V_T (Table 29-6) are monitored by observing movement of the chest wall, expansion and contraction of the reservoir bag, or movement of unidirectional flow valves, or by using monitoring equipment. Auscultation—an important tool for evaluating lung sounds—does not work well for monitoring RR and respiratory depth. It is advisable to observe the patient's respiratory depth and quality while awake as a point of reference.

Because many anesthetic agents are respiratory system depressants, anesthetized patients often experience a decrease in RR and about a 25% decrease in V_T directly related to anesthetic depth. This hypoventilation can lead to **atelectasis**. Atelectasis results in decreased gas exchange, which may lead to hypoxemia. This effect is common during anesthesia, particularly in the dependent lung (the one nearest the table). Many clinicians recommend gentle inflation of the lungs by periodic manual ventilation about every 2 to 5 minutes during anesthesia to prevent this complication. This technique is referred to as "bagging" or "sighing" the patient.

In addition to the effects of anesthetic agents, many other potential causes of hypoventilation are known, including postinduction apnea. As the name implies, postinduction apnea is a phenomenon that commonly occurs after anesthetic induction for the following reason. During induction, all patients pass through lighter stages of anesthesia, during

TABLE 29-7	Normal and Abnormal Body Temperatures		
SPECIES	**NORMAL (awake/at rest)**	**NORMAL (anesthetized)**	**REPORT TO THE VETERINARIAN IF**
Dog and cat	37.8° C-39.2° C (100° F-102.5° F)	Variably decreased	>39.7° C (103.5° F) or <36.1° C (97° F)
Horse	37.2° C-38° C (99° F-100.5° F)	Variably decreased	>38.6° C (101.5° F) or <36.1° C (97° F)
Cattle	37.8° C-39.2° C (100° F-102.5° F)	Variably decreased	>39.7° C (103.5° F) or <36.1° C (97° F)

which hyperventilation occurs for a period ranging from several seconds to a few minutes. Hyperventilation of sufficient length will cause the patient to expire excessive quantities of CO_2, resulting in a decreased concentration of CO_2 in the blood. In response to this decreased concentration, the patient hypoventilates or stops breathing until a normal CO_2 level is reestablished.

Postinduction apnea can be frightening and dangerous if not understood and must be managed promptly with supportive care. Supportive care involves careful monitoring of other parameters, including **oxygen saturation**, and periodic manual ventilation about 2 to 4 times/minute to maintain adequate oxygen levels until the patient begins to breathe spontaneously. When managing postinduction apnea, avoid ventilating too frequently, so that the normal CO_2 level can be reestablished. Use of a capnograph allows precise measurement of CO_2 levels and is a useful tool for managing this problem.

During anesthesia, the patient should exhibit normal respiratory effort. Dyspnea indicates a serious patient problem or machine malfunction that must be addressed promptly. Abdominal breathing is a unique breathing pattern associated with dangerously excessive anesthetic depth. It is characterized by a rocking motion of the abdomen and chest as a result of paralysis of the respiratory muscles and must be acted upon immediately.

Body temperature (Table 29-7) should be monitored about every 15 to 30 minutes with a rectal thermometer or probe. Although body temperature can be estimated by touching the skin of the paw or ear, it cannot be accurately determined this way. Hypothermia is experienced by most patients during anesthesia but can lead to prolonged recovery and predisposition to anesthetic overdose if severe. Hypothermia usually occurs rapidly after induction and is often of a relatively large magnitude. Therefore, the following steps should be taken to reduce heat loss during all anesthetic procedures:

- Do not allow the patient's body to contact stainless steel.
- Place a heat-retaining surface under the patient, such as a warm-water circulating blanket, a blanket, a towel, or lamb's wool.
- Warm IV fluids before administration.
- During preparation of the surgery site, avoid the use of alcohol as a rinsing agent and avoid wetting the hair excessively.
- Avoid excessively low ambient temperatures in the surgical suite.

Malignant hyperthermia (MH) is a complication of general anesthesia in which the body temperature progressively rises to dangerous levels. MH is due to a genetic defect in muscle metabolism that occurs in the presence of some anesthetic drugs such as halothane and neuromuscular blockers. It is most common in pigs but has been reported in other species. MH is a medical emergency that must be promptly recognized, reported, and treated. Early signs include muscle rigidity, skin that is red and hot to the touch, and excessive production of CO_2, which leads to exhaustion of the CO_2 absorbent.

REFLEXES AND OTHER INDICATORS OF ANESTHETIC DEPTH (Table 29-8)

Reflexes are involuntary protective responses to stimuli (such as the "kick" response when your physician taps your knee with a neurologic hammer). Reflexes and other indicators of anesthetic depth are used to answer the question, "Is the anesthetic depth inadequate, excessive, or appropriate for the procedure being performed?"

The palpebral reflex is induced by gently tapping the skin at the medial or lateral canthus of the eye with your finger. This reflex is present when the patient is too light, progressively diminishes with increasing depth, and is generally absent in surgical anesthesia in small animals, but it may still be present in horses and ruminants until they are in a moderately deep plane of anesthesia.

The swallowing reflex is a normal reflex that occurs in response to the presence of saliva or food in the pharynx. It is detected by watching the throat for swallowing motions. The swallowing reflex is present when anesthetic depth is inadequate, but is absent in surgical and deeper stages of anesthesia and therefore is used to determine whether the patient is too light.

The pedal reflex is the withdrawal of a limb in response to a painful stimulus. To induce this reflex, place a limb in a relaxed position and vigorously pinch a toe. Withdrawal of the limb indicates inadequate depth of anesthesia.

The corneal reflex is induced by placing a drop of sterile artificial tears on the cornea. When the reflex is present, the eyeball will retract slightly within the orbit. When in lighter planes of anesthesia, a blink response may also occur. This response is difficult to interpret when the eyes are in a ventromedial position and is not reliable in small animals, but it should be present during all planes of surgical anesthesia in large animals, and therefore helps to determine whether a large animal patient is too deep.

Muscle tone is most frequently determined in small animals by assessing jaw tone. Open the jaw with the fingers, and feel for resistance. Muscle tone is high when the patient is too light, gradually diminishes with increasing anesthetic

TABLE 29-8	Interpretation of Reflexes and Other Indicators of Anesthetic Depth		
INDICATOR	**INADEQUATE DEPTH**	**SURGICAL ANESTHESIA**	**EXCESSIVE DEPTH**
Palpebral reflex	Present	Decreased or absent*	Absent
Swallowing reflex	May be present	Absent	Absent
Pedal reflex	Present	Absent	Absent
Corneal reflex[†]	Present	Present	Absent
Muscle tone	Marked	Moderate	Flaccid
Eyeball position	Usually central	Usually ventromedial	Central
Pupil size	Constricted	Gradually larger	Widely dilated
PLR	Present	Gradually nonresponsive	Absent
Lacrimal secretions	Present	Gradually decreased	Absent
Nystagmus[‡] (horses)	Fast	Slow or absent	Absent
Response to surgical stimulation	Marked increase in HR, RR, or V_T	Mild or no increase in HR No increase in RR or V_T	No increase in HR, RR, or V_T

HR, Heart rate; *PLR*, pupillary light reflex; *RR*, respiratory rate; V_T, tidal volume.

*Absent when halogenated inhalant agents are used (small animals); may be sluggish when other agents are used to maintain anesthesia or in large animals.

[†]The corneal reflex is not reliable in small animals.

[‡]Nystagmus may also be caused by severe hypoxia or hypercarbia in horses.

depth, and is described using the terms *marked, moderate, loose,* and *flaccid.* Muscle tone alternatively may be assessed by observing the size of the anal opening, which will be closed at lighter planes and progressively more open at deeper planes.

Eye position and pupil size are also useful in determining anesthetic depth. Eye position is central (straight forward) in light anesthesia, gradually shifts to a ventromedial position (toward the chin), and finally shifts back to a central position in deep anesthesia. In most patients, ventromedial deviation is common during surgical anesthesia. In some horses, eye position may change from ventromedial to central, and back again. This is usually indicative of surgical anesthesia. The presence of nystagmus usually indicates a light plane of anesthesia in any patient.

Response to Surgical Stimulation

When stimulated by cutting or manipulation of viscera, HR, RR, V_T, or blood pressure may increase. A sudden marked increase in any of these parameters indicates inadequate depth of anesthesia. Mild changes in HR may occur, however, even in surgical anesthesia. Realize that the appropriate depth for each patient may vary somewhat according to the degree of surgical stimulation and pain associated with the procedure.

MONITORING EQUIPMENT

Monitoring equipment is a useful addition to physical assessment but should never be used alone. The main advantages of this equipment are that it gives early warning of impending problems before serious consequences develop, and it allows measurement of certain physical parameters, such as blood pressure, oxygen saturation, or expired CO_2, which is not possible with physical assessment. Monitoring equipment allows the anesthetist to assess the patient more

precisely than would be otherwise possible. For instance, a pulse oximeter can detect hypoxemia long before cyanosis is visible. A capnograph can accurately and rapidly warn of inadequate or excessive ventilation, and an oscillometric monitor can detect subtle changes in blood pressure before a change in pulse strength is evident. In this section, use of this equipment is reviewed.

MECHANICAL INDICATORS OF CIRCULATION

An esophageal stethoscope (Figure 29-21) is a device designed to amplify the sound of the heartbeat, so the anesthetist can monitor the heart from a distance. Although this device is not capable of determining heart rhythm, the anesthetist can be alerted to a possible arrhythmia by noting changes in rate, irregularity, or interruption in heart sounds. Esophageal stethoscopes are inexpensive and are easy to operate and maintain.

Parts include esophageal catheters of various sizes, a sensor, and a base unit, which amplifies and converts heart sounds into an audible electronic signal. To use an esophageal stethoscope, lubricate the closed end of an appropriately sized catheter and insert it into the esophagus to the level of the heart (about the 5th rib). Attach the free end to the electronic base via the sensor. Adjust the position of the catheter and the volume until the signal is audible.

The base should be cleaned as needed, and batteries must be changed periodically. Catheters should be washed with a disinfectant and dried after use. Avoid immersing the catheter or introducing water inside the catheter.

An electrocardiographic (ECG) monitor is used to monitor HR and heart rhythm. Electrodes are attached to specific locations on the patient's skin, and electrical activity of the heart and HR are displayed on a screen in real time.

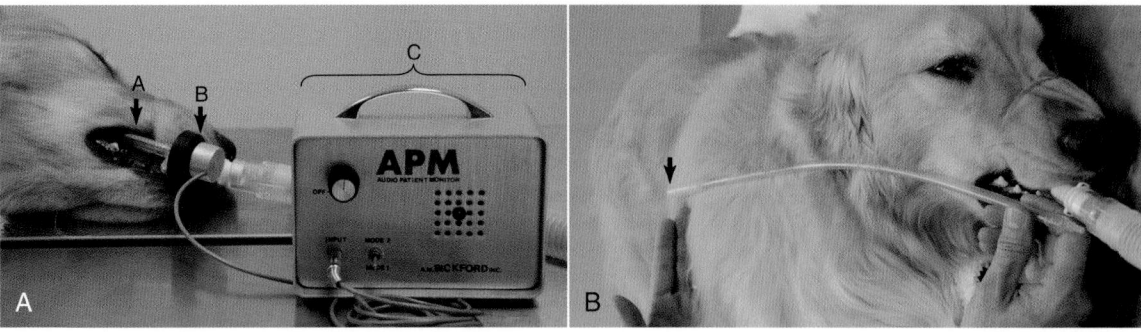

FIGURE 29-21 **A,** Esophageal stethoscope. *A,* Catheter. *B,* Sensor. *C,* Base unit. **B,** Measurement of the catheter to the level of the 5th rib or the caudal border of the scapula *(arrow).*

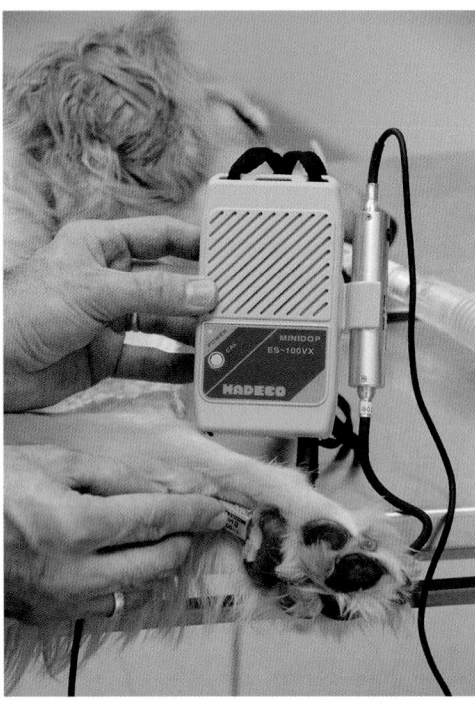

FIGURE 29-22 Doppler monitor: Base unit with the probe positioned over the ventral surface of the metacarpus proximal to the metacarpal pad.

These monitors generally require little care. When using an ECG monitor, realize that it is possible for the heart to stop beating and for electrical activity to continue for a time after the heart has stopped. Therefore, never depend on this monitor alone as a guarantee of patient safety.

An ultrasonic Doppler monitor (Figure 29-22) is a device that detects the flow of blood through small arteries and converts this motion into an audible signal. Blood flow is converted to a continuous sound similar to that of a heart murmur. Parts include an electronic base unit that processes the signal and a probe that emits and receives an ultrasonic wave. The hair overlying a small artery must be clipped and the skin cleaned and covered with a generous amount of ultrasonic gel. The probe is positioned over the artery, is adjusted until an audible signal is detected, and then is taped in place.

Placement of an ultrasonic Doppler probe requires patience and finesse. It must be oriented parallel to and precisely over the artery and must make firm but not excessive contact. Sometimes, subtle differences in position of only a millimeter or two can make the difference between success and failure in acquiring a signal.

Ultrasonic Doppler probes are delicate and expensive and must be handled carefully. They should be cleaned by wiping gently with a gauze sponge. Gentle cleaning with tap water is acceptable, but the probe must not be immersed, scrubbed, or autoclaved.

In SA patients, ultrasonic Doppler probes may be placed on the ventral surface of a paw proximal to the metacarpal or metatarsal pad, on the ventral surface of the tail base, on the dorsomedial surface of the hock, or on the medial surface of the thigh in patients weighing less than 10 lb. In LA patients, the ventral tail is the most frequently used site (Figure 29-23 shows common locations for placement of the probe).

When used with a sphygmomanometer, the Doppler monitor can also be used to determine blood pressure (see Figure 29-23, *top left*). Place a properly fitted cuff on the foreleg, metatarsus, or tail base with the cuff balloon centered over the artery. The width of the cuff should be 30% to 50% of the circumference of the extremity (Figure 29-24, *inset*). After establishing a good Doppler signal, inflate the cuff until the artery is occluded (the signal can no longer be heard). Gradually decrease the pressure until the audible signal can be heard again. This represents the systolic pressure. These instruments tend to consistently underestimate systolic blood pressure in cats but are fairly accurate in dogs. All indirect blood pressure measurements are subject to many inaccuracies, however, and must be interpreted in light of other signs (Table 29-9 provides normal blood pressure values during anesthesia).

An oscillometric blood pressure monitor (see Figure 29-24) is a device that is used to measure blood pressure and HR. Parts include a blood pressure cuff and a computerized base unit that inflates and deflates the cuff and analyzes signals received by the cuff.

A cuff is placed around a leg or a tail with the balloon centered over an artery, and the unit is turned on. The cuff

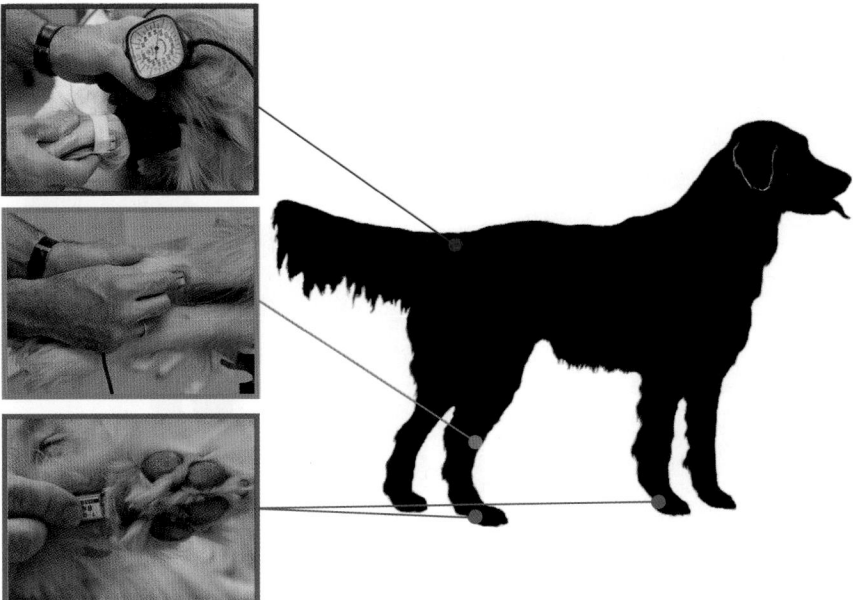

FIGURE 29-23 Locations for Doppler probe placement. *Red,* Determination of systolic blood pressure with the use of a sphygmomanometer with the cuff placed around the tail base and the probe placed on the ventral surface of the tail distal to the cuff. *Green,* Probe over the dorsomedial surface of the hock. *Blue,* Probe proximal to the metatarsal pad or the metacarpal pad.

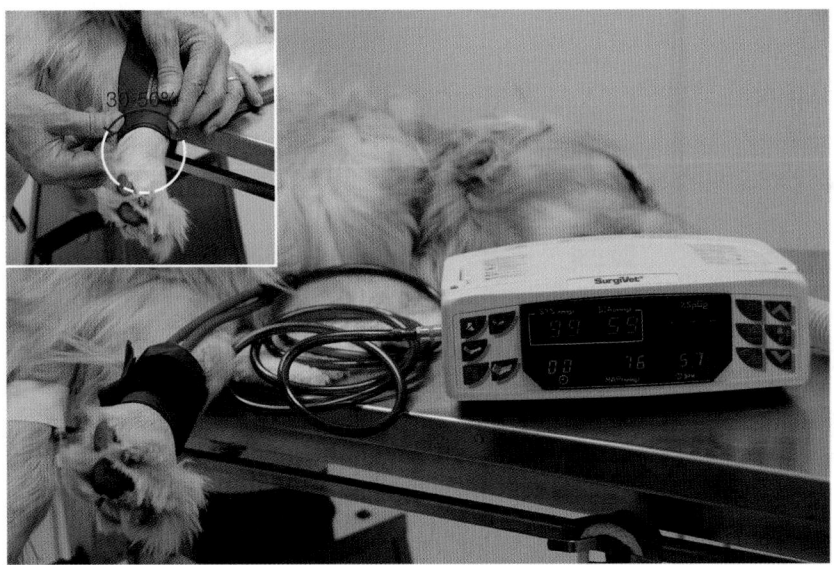

FIGURE 29-24 Oscillometric blood pressure (BP) monitor with a cuff placed on the metacarpus. The following measurements are indicated: systolic BP: 99 mm Hg; diastolic BP: 59 mm Hg; mean arterial pressure (MAP): 76 mm Hg; heart rate (HR): 57 bpm. *Inset,* Select an appropriately sized blood pressure cuff, the width of which should be 30% to 50% of the circumference of the extremity.

is inflated and deflated automatically by the machine. The unit detects oscillations within the cuff bladder caused by pulsations of the arteries. Based on changes in intracuff pressure, systolic, mean, and diastolic pressures are calculated. The cuff can be placed around the foreleg, metatarsus, metacarpus, or tail of small and large animal patients (Figure 29-25 shows examples of locations for placement of the cuff). For proper operation, the cuff should be at the same horizontal plane as the heart. This device is more accurate in patients weighing more than 7 kg.

TABLE 29-9	Normal Blood Pressure Values During Anesthesia	
BLOOD PRESSURE VALUE, mm Hg	**SMALL ANIMAL**	**EQUINE**
Systolic	100-160	100-120
Mean	80-120	80-100
Diastolic	60-100	60-80
Minimum acceptable mean during anesthesia	60	70
Hypertension	Systolic >160	Systolic >140

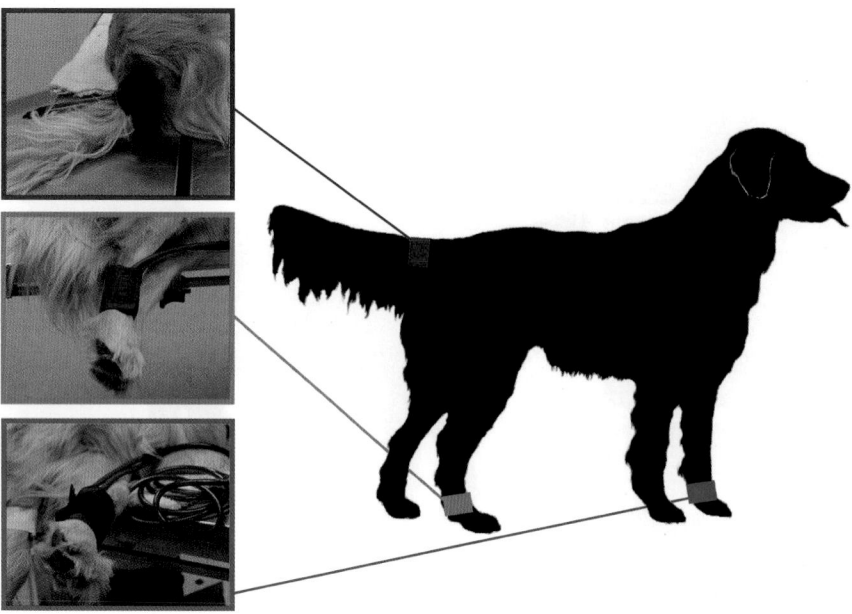

FIGURE 29-25 Locations for placement of a blood pressure cuff. *Red,* Base of the tail. *Green,* Metatarsus. *Blue,* Metacarpus.

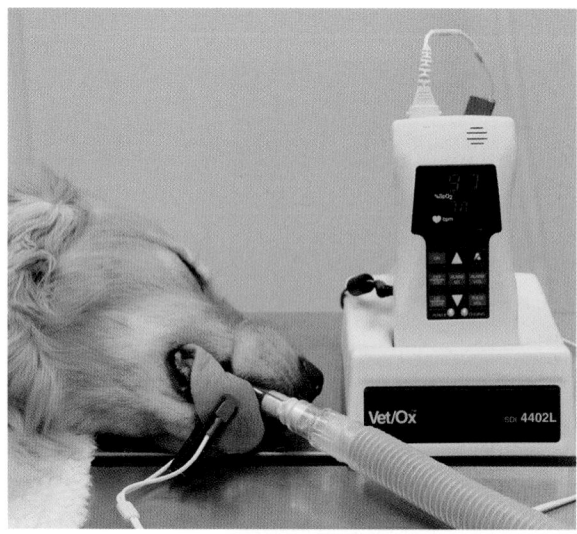

FIGURE 29-26 Pulse oximeter with transmission lingual probe. The upper number (97) represents the percent oxygen saturation (%SpO$_2$). The lower number (70) represents the heart rate (HR) in beats per minute.

MECHANICAL INDICATORS OF OXYGENATION

A pulse oximeter (Figure 29-26) is a device that is designed to detect changes in the oxygen saturation of hemoglobin. Red and infrared wavelength light is passed through or reflected off of a tissue bed, detected by a sensor, and analyzed. The sensor is sensitive to blood pulsation in the arteries, so it also determines HR. The machine determines the percent oxygen saturation (%SpO$_2$) by calculating the difference between levels of oxygenated and deoxygenated hemoglobin. Both HR and oxygen saturation are digitally displayed.

Normally, when one is breathing pure oxygen, hemoglobin in the lungs is at least 97% saturated with oxygen.

Therefore, during oxygen administration, oxygen saturation should be greater than 95%. Saturation between 90% and 95% indicates desaturation and signals the need to determine a cause. Saturation less than 90% indicates hypoxemia that requires treatment. Saturation less than 85% for longer than 30 seconds is a medical emergency.

Parts include a computerized base unit and a variety of probes. Pulse oximeter probes are classified as transmission or reflective. Transmission probes are constructed in a clamp-like configuration. One of the jaws houses a light source, and the other houses a sensor that detects the transmitted light. Transmission probes must be applied over a nonpigmented tissue bed that is thin enough to allow light transmission, such as the tongue, lip, ear, flank fold, prepuce, vulva, digital web, nasal septum, or foot of smaller patients. Although these probes can function through a thin hair coat, excessive hair will prevent operation. The lingual probe and the "C" probe are examples of transmission probes (Figure 29-27 shows examples of probe types and placement).

Reflective probes are often long and narrow. The light source and the sensor are located next to each other on one side of the probe. These probes are placed inside a hollow organ, such as the esophagus or rectum, with the side housing the light source and sensor in contact with a tissue bed. When a reflective probe is placed in the rectum, care must be taken to digitally displace the feces from the wall of the rectum and place the correct side of the probe against the tissue. A reflective probe may also be taped against the ventral surface of the tail (see Figure 29-27).

Pulse oximeter probes can be frustrating to work with because of the high incidence of signal loss. When this happens, values will no longer appear on the display, the numbers will be incorrect, or an alarm may sound, and the probe must be readjusted or moved to a different location. Probe function is adversely affected by many factors,

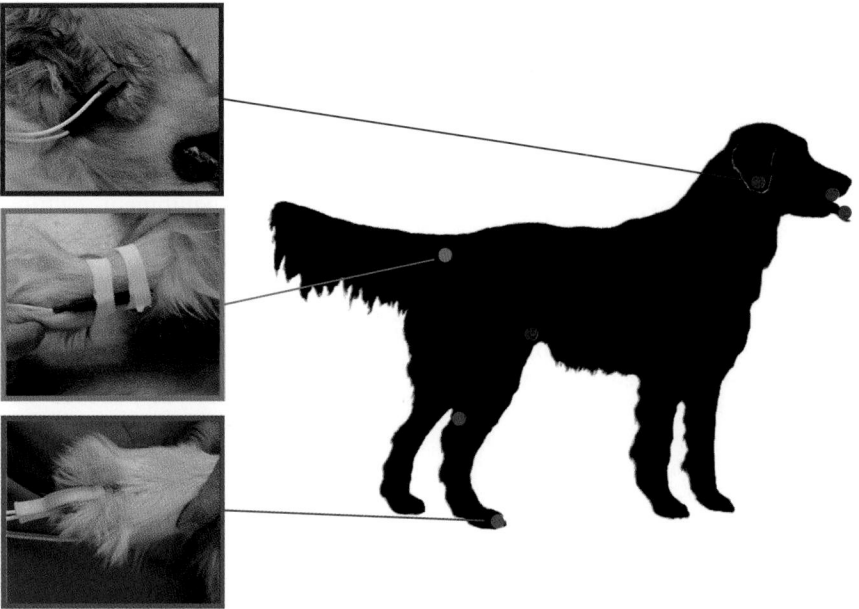

FIGURE 29-27 Examples of pulse oximeter probes and locations for placement. *Red,* Transmission probe on the ear flap. Additional red dots show alternate placement locations for this probe (tongue, lip, and flank fold). *Green,* Reflective probe taped to the ventral surface of the tail base. *Blue,* "C-probe" (a transmission probe) on the toe web. The other blue dot shows an alternate placement location for this probe (the skin fold between the Achilles tendon and the tibia).

BOX 29-5	Suggestions for Troubleshooting Pulse Oximeter Signal Loss

Transmission Probes
- Make sure the patient is safe by assessing vital signs.
- Remove and replace the probe.
- If the tongue is dry, rewet it.
- Be sure that no excessive or inadequate pressure is placed on the tissue.
- When possible, the jaw with the sensor should be oriented toward the ceiling to avoid interference from ambient light.
- Choose a different area that is not pigmented, covered with excessive hair, icteric, or edematous.
- If the area is heavily haired, clip and gently cleanse the area.

Reflective Probes
- Make sure the patient is safe by assessing vital signs.
- Make sure the side with the light source and sensor is oriented toward the tissue.
- Check for adequate tissue contact.
- When placed in the rectum, make sure that feces are not between the probe and the tissue.

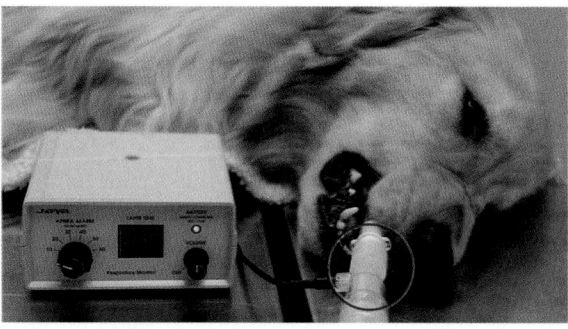

FIGURE 29-28 Apnea monitor. The probe *(circled)* is located between the breathing circuit and the endotracheal tube connector. Lapse time indicates the time in seconds since the previous breath. This alarm is set to sound if the interval between breaths exceeds 10 seconds.

MECHANICAL INDICATORS OF VENTILATION

As its name implies, an apnea monitor (Figure 29-28) is used to warn the anesthetist of apnea. Parts include a base unit and a sensor. The sensor, which is placed between the endotracheal tube connector and the breathing circuit, detects temperature changes between warm expired and cold inspired air. It emits an audible beep when the patient breathes and will sound an alarm when no breath is detected for a preset time.

The sensor increases mechanical dead space, which can be significant, especially in small patients. For this reason, special endotracheal tube connectors are available that accommodate the sensor and minimize dead space. Although apnea monitors do not warn of inadequate respiratory depth, they may have difficulty detecting respirations if the patient's V_T is significantly decreased or if the patient

including tissue pigmentation, motion, excessive pressure, orientation in relation to ambient light, and patient conditions, such as anemia, icterus, vasoconstriction, or edema. Box 29-5 contains suggestions for troubleshooting signal loss.

Pulse oximeters require little maintenance but must be handled with care. Probes should be cleaned with alcohol or another mild disinfectant, but must not be immersed, scrubbed, or autoclaved. (Case Presentation 29-1 shows an example of a pulse oximeter used to monitor oxygenation.)

CASE PRESENTATION 29-1
ANESTHESIA OF A CANINE

Cocoa, a 2-year-old, female, 15.2-kg Spaniel mix, was anesthetized in preparation for a routine OHE. Based on preanesthetic assessment, she was classified as a physical status class P1 patient. Cocoa was premedicated with 0.1 mg/kg acepromazine IM 15 minutes before anesthetic induction and was induced with a mixture of 5 mg/kg ketamine and 0.25 mg/kg diazepam IV. After reaching surgical anesthesia, she was maintained with isoflurane at 2.5% and oxygen at a rate of 0.5 L/minute. Pulse oximetry was used to monitor Cocoa via a transmission probe placed on the tongue. After surgical preparation, she was transferred to the operating room. For the first 10 minutes of surgery, Cocoa's oxygen saturation (SpO_2) was in the range of 96% to 99%. Then over a 3-minute period, SpO_2 gradually fell to 92%, although HR (85 bpm), RR (8 bpm), mucous membrane color, and refill remained normal.

Normal SpO_2 for patients breathing oxygen is 95% or greater. Low SpO_2 can be caused by many factors, including preexisting disease, pulmonary edema, loss of signal, airway blockage, lack of adequate oxygen flow, and respiratory depression. When in this situation, the veterinary technician must rapidly determine whether the decrease is real or an artifact, and then if real, must explore possible causes and correct the problem without delay.

The technician determined that the patient was in no immediate danger, based on assessment of the other vital signs. Preexisting disease was deemed unlikely based on this patient's medical history. She rapidly checked the airway, checked the oxygen supply, turned the oxygen up to 3 L/minute, and ruled out pulmonary edema based on normal lung sounds. Because pulse oximeter probe signals are frequently lost as a result of excess probe pressure, drying of the tissue, patient movement, interference from ambient light, and other factors, the technician removed the probe, rewetted the tongue, and replaced the probe with careful attention to location, orientation, and pressure.

Despite these measures, SpO_2 remained between 90% and 93%. Although RR was normal, careful observation revealed a V_T estimated to be less than 50% of normal. Manual ventilation was initiated with a maximum inspiratory pressure of 20 cm of water. After the first breath, SpO_2 rapidly returned to 96%. Intermittent positive-pressure breaths were given about every 30 seconds for the first 2 minutes, and then about every 5 minutes for the duration of the procedure. Oxygen saturation remained in the normal range. This case illustrates the importance of careful observation of respiratory depth during anesthesia, which in this patient was insufficient to maintain an adequate oxygen level.

The capnograph enables the anesthetist to estimate the partial pressure of CO_2 in the patient's bloodstream and is one of the best indicators of adequate respiration. Because CO_2 is produced at the tissue level, is carried by the vascular system, and is eliminated by the lungs, abnormal readings may be caused by disease of the lungs, cardiovascular system, or tissues and by equipment malfunction.

In normal animals during inspiration, the level should be 0 mm Hg, and at the end of expiration, the level should rise to 35 to 45 mm Hg when awake, and to 40 to 55 mm Hg when anesthetized. This increase during anesthesia occurs as the result of the respiratory depression that accompanies general anesthesia. Any change in the configuration of the curve can indicate a problem and should be explored. Interpretation of capnograph tracings is complex and is beyond the scope of this chapter. The student is encouraged to explore the recommended readings for additional information.

SMALL ANIMAL ANESTHESIA

A successful anesthetic procedure requires not only careful preparation, but also a good understanding of the sequence of events involved in taking a patient from consciousness to surgical anesthesia and back to consciousness. Procedure 29-1 summarizes these events when an SA patient is induced with injectable agents and maintained with an inhalant agent.

SELECTING A PROTOCOL

An anesthetic protocol is a list of premedications and anesthetics for a particular patient, including dosages, routes, and order of administration. Anesthetic protocols are commonly selected by the veterinarian in charge based on training and clinical experience. A suitable protocol takes into account the patient signalment, preexisting problems, the physical status class, and the procedure to be performed (see Procedure 29-2 for sample protocols used in physical status class P1 and P2 dogs, and Box 29-6 for sample protocols used in physical status class P1 and P2 cats).

After the protocol is known, calculate all drug dosages, oxygen flow rates, and fluid administration rates, and check them *carefully*, because most anesthetic agents have narrow therapeutic indices and can easily be overdosed.

TECHNICIAN NOTE The volume (in milliliters) of each injectable anesthetic drug to be given must be calculated with extreme care. The general formula for most injectable anesthetics is as follows:

Volume (ml) = Drug dosage (mg or μg/kg or lb body wt) × Patient body weight (kg or lb) ÷ Drug concentration (mg or μg/ml)

---

becomes hypothermic, and will sound the apnea alarm. Consequently, as with any monitor, alarm signals must be confirmed by physical examination of the patient.

A capnograph, also known as an end-tidal CO_2 monitor (Figure 29-29), is a device that measures the level of CO_2 present in inspired and expired air. Parts include a computerized base unit and a fitting that is placed between the endotracheal tube connector and the breathing circuit.

Note: When this calculation is performed, drug dosage and body weight units must be the same (kg or lb), as must drug dosage and drug concentration units (mg or μg).

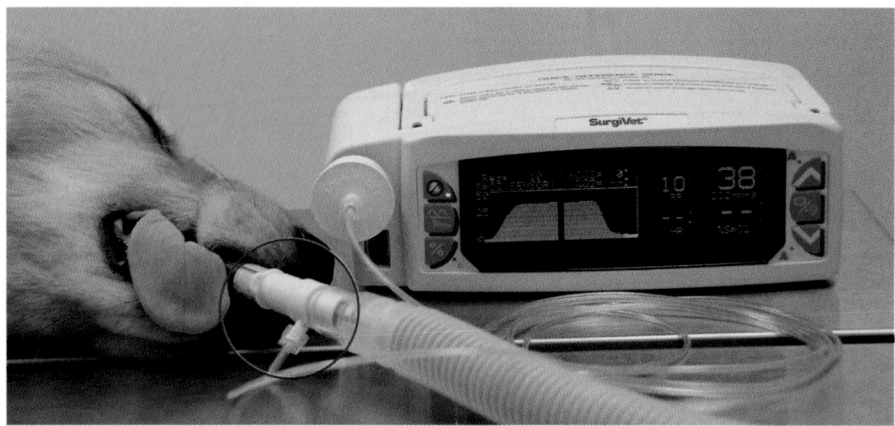

FIGURE 29-29 Capnograph registering an end-tidal CO_2 level of 38 mm Hg and a respiratory rate (RR) of 10 bpm *(upper right)*. The sensor *(circled)* is located between the breathing circuit and the endotracheal tube connector. The graph indicates CO_2 levels throughout the respiratory cycle, which in normal awake patients is 35 to 45 mm Hg during expiration and 0 mm Hg during inspiration.

PROCEDURE 29-1	Sequence of Events for a Small Animal Anesthetic Procedure*

1. Assess, prepare, and weigh the patient (see Patient Preparation, p. 1078, for a discussion of patient assessment, preparation, and stabilization).
2. Determine the protocol (anesthetic agents, including dosages, routes, and sequence of administration).
3. Calculate the volume of each agent to be given, including fluid administration rates (preanesthetic, induction, maintenance, and analgesic agents).
4. Calculate the oxygen flow rates (see Box 29-3).
5. Prepare equipment required to administer drugs (scales, syringes, needles, agents, reversal agents, emergency cart, controlled substance log).
6. Prepare fluid administration equipment (clippers, antiseptic scrub, intravenous [IV] catheters, tape, heparinized saline, catheter cap, administration extension set, fluids).
7. Prepare equipment for endotracheal intubation (see Principles of Endotracheal Intubation, p. 1098, for an equipment list).
8. Prepare monitoring equipment, including anesthesia record, stethoscope, monitors, and probes (see Anesthetic Monitoring, p. 1107, for a discussion of monitoring equipment).
9. Assemble and test the anesthetic machine (see Anesthetic Equipment, p. 1090, for a discussion of these procedures).
10. Administer premedications approximately 15 to 20 minutes intramuscularly (IM) or 5 to 10 minutes IV before anesthetic induction.
11. Place an IV catheter, attach the fluid administration set, and begin fluid administration.
12. Administer the induction agent.
13. Check the patient's readiness for intubation.
14. Place and secure the endotracheal tube (see Principles of Endotracheal Intubation, p. 1098, for a discussion of this procedure).
15. Turn on the oxygen and connect the endotracheal tube to the breathing circuit.
16. Check the patient's vital signs.
17. Turn on the inhalant anesthetic to the appropriate level.
18. Determine the patient's anesthetic depth and commence regular monitoring.
19. Position and secure the patient for the procedure with attention to padding, maintenance of an open airway, unrestricted blood flow, and unrestricted chest excursions.
20. Attach monitoring devices.
21. Continue to monitor and adjust anesthetic and oxygen levels as needed until completion of the procedure.
22. Prepare the patient for recovery.
23. Discontinue the anesthetic and extubate the patient at the appropriate time.
24. Remove monitoring equipment, IV catheters, and any other equipment no longer needed.
25. Prepare the patient for continued hospitalization or discharge by applying bandages, administering medications, and performing any other procedures ordered by the veterinarian.

*Induction with an IV agent and maintenance with an inhalant agent.

Physical status class P3 to P5 patients require use of modified protocols based on the patient's primary condition (Table 29-10). Management of these cases can be challenging and requires customization of the anesthetic protocol by the veterinarian in charge.

EQUIPMENT PREPARATION

During a typical anesthetic induction, anesthetic agents are administered; the patient becomes unconscious and recumbent; the endotracheal tube is placed, secured, cuffed, and attached to the machine; the anesthetic gas level is adjusted; the patient is positioned and monitored; and adjustments are made as needed—all within the first few minutes of the procedure. Because these events follow one another so rapidly, the technician has little to no time to leave the patient to locate necessary equipment. Consequently, all equipment must be carefully gathered, checked, and organized before the procedure is begun.

| **PROCEDURE 29-2** | Protocols for Premedication, Sedation, and General Anesthesia in Physical Status Class P1 and P2 Dogs |

Protocols for Mild to Moderate Sedation or for Premedication

1. Acepromazine: 0.05 to 0.1 mg/kg IM with a maximum dose of 3 mg (not for use in old or debilitated patients or in sensitive breeds).
2. Dexmedetomidine: 0.0015 to 0.003 mg/kg IM (equivalent to 1.5 to 3 µg/kg).
3. Midazolam 0.2 mg/kg IM and butorphanol 0.2 mg/kg IM.
   Can add glycopyrrolate 0.01 mg/kg or atropine 0.04 mg/kg to this mixture. Halve the doses for IV administration.

Protocols for Moderate to Heavy Sedation (for Minor Procedures such as Radiography or Grooming) or for Premedication

1. "BAG" (butorphanol 0.2 mg/kg, acepromazine 0.05 mg/kg, and glycopyrrolate 0.005 mg/kg mixed in one syringe and given IM or IV).
   As an alternative, mix 1 ml acepromazine, 4 ml butorphanol (10 mg/ml), and 5 ml glycopyrrolate, and give this mixture in a volume of 0.5 ml/10-20 lb of body weight.
2. Dexmedetomidine: 0.005 to 0.01 mg/kg IM and butorphanol: 0.2 to 0.4 mg/kg IM.
   Note: Can use hydromorphone 0.1 mg/kg in place of butorphanol.
3. Dexmedetomidine: 0.015 mg/kg IM and ketamine: 3 mg/kg IM.

Halve the doses for IV administration. Do not reverse the dexmedetomidine until at least 40 minutes later.
4. Telazol: 4 mg/kg IM or IV to effect (for aggressive patients).

Protocols for Anesthetic Induction

1. Ketamine: 5.5 mg/kg IV and diazepam*: 0.28 mg/kg IV mixed in the same syringe. (This is equivalent to 1 ml of the mixture/20 lb of body weight.)
   Butorphanol at a dose of 0.1 to 0.2 mg/kg can be given IV before induction, in a separate syringe, for additional analgesia.
   *Note: An equivalent volume of midazolam can be used in place of diazepam.
2. Propofol: 6 to 8 mg/kg IV to effect if not premedicated or 2 to 4 mg/kg IV after premedication.
3. Thiopental sodium: 4 to 8 mg/kg IV to effect after premedication or 10 to 15 mg/kg if not premedicated.
   Note that administration without premedication is not recommended.
4. Isoflurane 3% to 5% or sevoflurane 4% to 6% by mask or chamber.
5. Etomidate: 1 to 3 mg/kg to effect.

Protocols for Anesthetic Maintenance

1. Isoflurane 1.5% to 2.5% or sevoflurane 2.5% to 4%.
2. Propofol: 0.2 to 0.4 mg/kg/minute by constant rate infusion or by repeat bolus to effect every 3 to 5 minutes.

IM, Intramuscular; *IV,* intravenous.

| **BOX 29-6** | Protocols for Premedication, Sedation, and General Anesthesia in Physical Status Class P1 and P2 Cats |

Protocols for Mild to Moderate Sedation or Premedication

1. Acepromazine: 0.05 to 0.1 mg/kg IM up to a maximum dose of 1 mg.
2. "BAG" (same dose as for the dog).
3. Dexmedetomidine: 0.005 to 0.02 mg/kg IM.

Protocols for Moderate to Heavy Sedation (for Minor Procedures such as Radiography or Grooming) or for Premedication

1. Dexmedetomidine: 0.005 to 0.025 mg/kg IM and ketamine: 5 mg/kg IM.
2. Dexmedetomidine: 0.005 to 0.01 mg/kg IM and butorphanol: 0.2 mg/kg IM.
3. Ketamine: 10 to 20 mg/kg IM (causes immobilization with muscle rigidity).
4. Telazol: 4 mg/kg IM or IV to effect (for aggressive patients).

Protocols for Anesthetic Induction
Use the same protocols as for the dog.

Protocols for Anesthetic Maintenance
Use the same protocols as for the dog.

Protocols for Injectable Anesthesia

1. Dexmedetomidine: 0.03 mg/kg with ketamine: 5 mg/kg and butorphanol: 0.2 mg/kg IM for elective surgeries.
2. "TKX": Add 4 ml of ketamine and 1 ml 10% (LA) xylazine to 1 vial of Telazol powder. Give at a dose of 0.015 ml/kg IM (must dose accurately).
3. Add 2.5 ml butorphanol (10 mg/ml) and 2.5 ml dexmedetomidine to 1 vial of Telazol powder. Give at a rate of 0.015 ml/kg IM for castration and 0.02 ml/kg IM for OHE.

BAG, Butorphanol, acepromazine, and glycopyrrolate; *IM,* intramuscular; *IV,* intravenous; *LA,* large animal; *OHE,* ovariohysterectomy; *TKX,* Telazol-ketamine-xylazine.

TABLE 29-10	Recommendations for Physical Status Class P3 to P5 Small Animal Patients	
PRIMARY CONDITION	**EXAMPLE PROTOCOLS AND OTHER CONSIDERATIONS**	**AVOID THESE AGENTS/CIRCUMSTANCES**
Cardiac disease	Premedicate with opioids and benzodiazepines Etomidate or propofol induction Ketamine/diazepam induction acceptable except in feline patients with hypertrophic cardiomyopathy Maintain with isoflurane or sevoflurane Maintain blood pressure in normal range	Acepromazine in patients with congestive heart failure Alpha$_2$-agonists Mask/chamber induction (as a result of stress) Ketamine/Telazol Thiopental sodium without premedication
Liver disease	No premedication or use opioids if needed Preoxygenation before induction Propofol or etomidate induction if mild to moderate Mask induction if severe Maintain with isoflurane or sevoflurane Maintain blood pressure and fluid balance	Acepromazine Barbiturates
C-section	Propofol or mask induction Maintain with isoflurane or sevoflurane Epidural analgesia is helpful to reduce the need for other analgesics Minimize anesthetic time If opioids used before delivery, administer 1 to 2 drops of naloxone sublingually to neonates If needed to stimulate breathing, administer 1 drop doxapram sublingually to neonates	Thiopental sodium and other barbiturates Alpha$_2$-agonists Opioids before delivery
Respiratory disease	Preoxygenate and minimize stress Premedicate with opioids and benzodiazepines Any induction agent that allows rapid control of the airway and ventilation Place endotracheal tube rapidly and be prepared to ventilate if needed Maintain with isoflurane or sevoflurane	Alpha$_2$-agonists N$_2$O
Kidney disease	Premedicate with opioids + or − benzodiazepines Mask or propofol induction Maintain with isoflurane or sevoflurane Maintain blood pressure and fluid balance	Alpha$_2$-agonists Ketamine in blocked cats

THE PREANESTHETIC PERIOD

The preanesthetic period is the time before induction of general anesthesia. During this period, a physical assessment is performed, patient history and results of laboratory tests are reviewed, the patient is stabilized, an IV catheter is placed, and fluid administration is started. Premedications, including tranquilizers, alpha$_2$-agonists, opioids, dissociatives, anticholinergics, or a combination thereof, are administered to calm and prepare the patient for anesthetic induction. Premedications are chosen to produce a specific set of desired effects, such as sedation, analgesia, and muscle relaxation. Most are given IM, although some may be administered IV. After IM injection, place the patient in a quiet but observable location for about 15 to 20 minutes for the agents to take effect before proceeding; otherwise, the patient may partially override the beneficial effects.

ANESTHETIC INDUCTION

During anesthetic induction, the patient is taken from consciousness to unconsciousness. Agents commonly used for anesthetic induction in small animals include a ketamine and diazepam mixture, propofol, neuroleptanalgesics, and inhalant anesthetics. Except for inhalant anesthetics, these agents are most often given IV.

IV Induction

To induce general anesthesia by the IV route, draw up the calculated volume and administer it *to effect* until you are able to intubate the patient, or until the patient is at an adequate plane of anesthesia for completion of the planned procedure. The term "to effect" means that the drug is administered gradually in increments until the desired stage of anesthesia is reached. The entire calculated dose may or may not be given.

Immediately after giving the patient an initial dose, check HR and RR to ensure that the patient is stable and breathing. Remove muzzles and other restraint devices. Make sure that the patient has passed through stage II and is deep enough to intubate. While the drug is given, there must be interplay between administration of the drug and monitoring of the patient. Give the initial dose; then rapidly check the vital signs, pedal reflex, palpebral reflex, and jaw tone; give more if needed; check again, etc. If the patient is light and needs more drug or starts to wake up while being intubated, give a much smaller amount to effect (about one-fifth to one-tenth of the original volume) until the patient is in an adequate plane of anesthesia. Although all are given to effect, different induction agents are given at slightly different rates.

Propofol

Give one-fourth of the calculated dose every 30 seconds to effect until the patient is at an adequate depth for endotracheal intubation. Be sure to give it rapidly enough to take the patient through stage II and into stage III.

Ketamine-Diazepam or Ketamine-Midazolam

Give slowly to effect over 60 to 120 seconds.

Thiopental Sodium

In healthy patients, give one-half of the calculated dose over 10 to 15 seconds, then to effect. Old, ill, and debilitated patients may need much less and may require that the drug be given much more cautiously and slowly.

IM Induction

To induce anesthesia by the IM route, draw up and administer the entire calculated volume. In general, the dosage for IM injection is about 2 to 3 times the corresponding IV dosage. When given IM, anesthetic agents have a slower onset and a longer duration than when given IV. A typical induction will take 5 to 20 minutes. After peak effect, if the patient is still too light, administer additional drug or an inhalant agent with a mask until you are able to intubate the patient. Remember that some drugs, such as propofol, thiopental sodium, and etomidate, *must not* be given IM.

Mask Induction

Mask induction requires the use of a rapid-acting inhalant anesthetic, such as isoflurane, sevoflurane, or desflurane. Once induced, an endotracheal tube can be placed to maintain the patient for the duration of the procedure. Mask induction is a special challenge for several reasons. Many patients struggle, necessitating skillful restraint (enough to prevent operator and patient injury, but not so much as to restrict chest excursions or the airway). It is more challenging to monitor mucous membrane color and refill and ocular indicators of anesthetic depth because the mask partially obscures the eyes and the muzzle. Therefore, monitor carefully and do not be lulled into the belief that monitoring requirements are less with this method of induction than with others.

To induce a patient by mask, first attach a well-fitted mask to the breathing circuit. Hold the mask over the patient's muzzle. Administer pure oxygen for 2 to 3 minutes at the recommended rate, and then turn on the vaporizer to 0.5% to 1% for about 30 seconds to allow the patient to become accustomed to the smell of the gas. Increase the setting to 3% to 5% if using isoflurane and 4% to 6% with sevoflurane. Some clinicians recommend a gradual increase over several minutes; this allows the patient time to become accustomed to the gas. Other anesthetists increase the vaporizer setting

immediately, especially if the patient is difficult to handle, when using the gradual method. If the patient struggles, monitor carefully for cyanosis or other problems, and be ready to act quickly if the patient becomes compromised. As soon as the patient is laterally recumbent, assess readiness for intubation and adjust the anesthetic level as appropriate. From this point on, the patient is managed much the same as for IV induction. Mask induction generally is *not* appropriate for brachycephalic breeds.

Chamber Induction

Chamber induction may be used only for patients small enough to fit comfortably into the chamber. This technique is commonly used in place of a mask for small patients that are aggressive or difficult to handle. Once induced, an endotracheal tube can be placed to maintain the patient for the duration of the procedure.

To induce a patient using this method, place the patient in the chamber, close the lid, and attach to the ports the breathing tubes of a semi-closed rebreathing system. Deliver oxygen at 5 L/minute and isoflurane at 3% to 5% or sevoflurane at 4% to 6%. As soon as the patient can no longer stand, shake the chamber gently to assess the patient's mobility. When the patient is immobile enough to allow it to be safely handled, remove the patient from the chamber, place a mask, and proceed as with mask induction.

Patients can easily get into trouble while inside a chamber from stress, trauma, vomiting, airway blockage, or other issues. Because it is impossible to accurately assess most monitoring parameters while inside a chamber, the anesthetist must be vigilant and prepared to act quickly if the patient shows signs of compromise.

> **TECHNICIAN NOTE** Patients must be restrained and watched *carefully* during both mask and chamber inductions because they can get into trouble suddenly and unexpectedly and cannot be monitored closely under these circumstances.

MAINTENANCE OF ANESTHESIA

After anesthetic induction and endotracheal intubation, the patient must be maintained with injectable anesthetics, inhalant anesthetics, or a combination thereof. The goal during maintenance is to administer enough anesthetic to keep the patient in the desired plane of surgical anesthesia. This requires that the anesthetist frequently evaluate the patient by watching for subtle changes, then adjust the amount of anesthetic administered based on this observation.

Most patients are light immediately after intubation and must be brought to surgical anesthesia. Because inhalant anesthetics are most commonly used to maintain anesthesia, this discussion will focus on maintenance with the use of these agents. During maintenance with inhalant agents, a delayed effect is noted between the time the vaporizer dial setting is changed and the time the anesthetic depth is changed, because it takes time for the new concentration to fill the breathing circuit, reach the patient's lungs, and equilibrate with blood and tissues. The time required is influenced by several factors, including the patient's respiratory drive, the agent used, the carrier gas flow rate, and the volume and type of breathing circuit used. For this reason, vaporizer setting adjustments must be anticipated as much as possible through close monitoring. In general, if a patient is significantly light or deep, larger dial changes are indicated, whereas if the patient is slightly too light or deep, more subtle changes are needed. Familiarity with appropriate dial changes is acquired through experience.

IV maintenance agents such as propofol may be used to maintain general anesthesia by repeat boluses administered every few minutes to effect or by constant infusion via a syringe pump. A syringe pump is a device that automatically delivers the drug through an IV line at a calculated infusion rate.

PATIENT POSITIONING, COMFORT, AND SAFETY

Below are some considerations that must be observed throughout the anesthetic induction and maintenance periods.

- Prevent patient trauma by supporting the patient's body as consciousness is lost.
- When using an IV agent for induction: as soon as the patient is intubated, remove the needle and syringe to prevent accidental overdose.
- Following intubation, lay the patient in lateral recumbency, and secure and cuff the tube.
- Before surgery begins, check the tube for proper placement and cuff inflation.
- Check the endotracheal tube for kinks or bends. An open airway must be maintained at all times.
- Temporarily disconnect the endotracheal tube from the breathing circuit while turning the patient to prevent trauma to the trachea caused by torsion of the tube.
- Support the corrugated breathing tubes so that they do not exert traction on the endotracheal tube.
- Place the patient in a position that is as normal as possible during the procedure without hyperflexion or hyperextension of the neck or limbs.
- Do not compress the chest with restraint devices or instruments.
- Place the patient on a heat-retaining surface, such as a warm-water circulating blanket. Do *not* use an electric heating pad, which can burn the patient.
- Do not restrict blood flow by overtightening leg restraint ropes.
- Place sterile lubricant in the eyes every 90 minutes.
- If one lung is diseased, place the normal side up to maximize oxygen exchange.
- Avoid elevation greater than 15 degrees in the caudal aspect of the body to prevent pressure on the diaphragm.

ANESTHETIC RECOVERY

The recovery period is the time between discontinuation of the anesthetic and the time when the patient is able to walk without assistance. Many factors affect recovery, including length of the procedure, anesthetic protocol, patient condition, body temperature, and patient signalment.

Preparation for Recovery

Upon completion of the procedure, transfer the patient to a recovery area, where it can be extubated and monitored. Turn off the inhalant anesthetic, but continue oxygen administration at a rate of 50 to 100 ml/kg/minute (0.5 to 1 L/10 kg body weight up to a maximum of 5 L/minute) for 5 minutes after discontinuation of the anesthetic, or until the animal swallows. If the patient is light and must be extubated, administer oxygen by mask, or place an oxygen source close to the nose for 5 minutes. Remove all ties, catheters, monitoring devices, and other unnecessary equipment. Keep the patient warm. Turn the patient at least every 10 to 15 minutes.

Monitoring During Recovery

During recovery, the patient must be watched on a continual basis at close range. Put the patient in the cage in a position that allows observation of the mucous membranes and respirations, but never leave the patient in an open cage or on a table unattended because a recovering patient may fall and be injured. Monitor at least every 5 minutes, paying particular attention to vital signs. Watch for and report unusual signs, such as vomiting or hemorrhage.

> **TECHNICIAN NOTE** Many anesthetic accidents occur during recovery. Monitor at close range, and do not let down your guard. Never leave a patient unattended on a table or in an open cage because patients may awake rapidly, chew the tube, fall, or be injured.

Signs of Recovery

During recovery, gently comfort and reassure the patient. Recovery may be hastened through gentle stimulation by talking softly to the patient, by rubbing or patting the chest, and by turning the patient. Gentle movement of the endotracheal tube will stimulate breathing.

As the patient recovers, it will progress back through the stages and planes of anesthesia. Passage through stage II during recovery may result in a variety of alarming signs, including excitement, vocalization, hyperventilation, and head thrashing. Be prepared to prevent self-trauma if the recovery is unusually violent or stormy.

Extubation

To prepare the patient for extubation, deflate the cuff by drawing out all the air until the pilot balloon is empty. Untie the tube to prepare for rapid removal. Both before and after removal, keep the neck in a natural but extended position to protect the airway. Remove the endotracheal tube gently when the swallowing reflex returns, using a slow, steady motion. You may also remove it when signs of imminent

---

PROCEDURE 29-3 | Sequence of Events for an Equine Anesthetic Procedure*

1. Assess, prepare, and weigh the patient (see Patient Preparation, p. 1078, for a discussion of patient assessment, preparation, and stabilization).
2. Prepare equipment and place intravenous (IV) catheter, which may require IV or intramuscular (IM) sedation in some horses (clippers, local anesthetic, antiseptic scrub, IV catheters, tape, heparinized saline, suture material, catheter cap, and/or extension line with three-way stopcock).
3. Rinse the horse's mouth, clean the hooves, and remove or wrap shoes when appropriate.
4. Determine the protocol (anesthetic agents, including dosages, routes, and sequence of administration).
5. Calculate the volume of each agent to be given, including fluid administration rates (preanesthetic, induction, maintenance, and analgesic agents).
6. Review oxygen flow rates (see Box 29-3).
7. Prepare equipment required to administer drugs (scales, syringes, needles, agents, reversal agents, emergency cart, controlled substance log).
8. Prepare fluid administration equipment (fluids, administration extension set, syringe pump, tape, heparinized saline).
9. Prepare equipment for endotracheal intubation (see Principles of Endotracheal Intubation, p. 1098, for an equipment list).
10. Prepare monitoring equipment, including arterial catheterization materials, anesthesia record, monitors, and probes (see Anesthetic Monitoring, p. 1107, for a discussion of monitoring equipment).
11. Assemble and test the anesthetic machine and ventilator (see Anesthetic Equipment, p. 1090, and Manual and Mechanical Ventilation, p. 1125, for a discussion of these procedures).
12. Administer premedications approximately 20 to 30 minutes IM or 5 to 10 minutes IV before anesthetic induction.
13. If the horse is adequately sedate, administer the induction agent; otherwise, give additional IV sedation before inducing.
14. Check the patient's readiness for intubation.
15. Place and secure the endotracheal tube (see Principles of Endotracheal Intubation, p. 1098, for a discussion of this procedure).
16. Check the patient's vital signs.
17. Hoist, position, and secure the patient for the procedure with attention to padding of the face and limbs if the horse is in lateral recumbency, maintenance of an open airway, unrestricted blood flow, and unrestricted chest excursions.
18. Remove the halter.
19. Turn on the oxygen and connect the endotracheal tube to the breathing circuit.
20. Turn on the inhalant anesthetic to the appropriate level.
21. Determine the patient's anesthetic depth and commence regular monitoring.
22. Attach monitoring devices, including placement of an arterial catheter.
23. Continue to monitor and adjust the anesthetic and oxygen levels as needed until completion of the procedure.
24. Prepare the patient for recovery, including placement of a nasopharyngeal tube and removal of monitoring equipment, and ensure that the recovery area has been prepared.
25. Discontinue the anesthetic and transfer the horse to the recovery area, paying attention to positioning.
26. Extubate the patient at the appropriate time and ensure that the horse can breathe through its nostrils without obstruction.
27. Assist the horse until it stands as directed by the veterinarian.
28. Prepare the patient for continued hospitalization or discharge by applying bandages, administering medications, and performing any other procedures ordered by the veterinarian.

*Induction with an IV agent and maintenance with an inhalant agent.

---

arousal are present, such as voluntary movement of the limbs or head, movement of the tongue, or chewing. Delay extubation in brachycephalic dogs until the patient is able to lift its head unassisted.

The Postanesthetic Period

After recovery, most SA patients should be given nothing by mouth for the first hour or two and no food for at least several hours. Upon discharge, instruct the client to reintroduce water gradually after arriving home and to feed a small meal after several hours. Exceptions to these rules include small and neonatal patients, which require shorter withholding times. Monitor the patient for signs of pain, and administer analgesics as prescribed.

EQUINE ANESTHESIA

All of the basic principles discussed under SA anesthesia apply to anesthesia of the horse. Additional challenges for the equine anesthetist include temperament and physical size of the patient, effects of inhalant anesthetics on cardiorespiratory physiology, and management of recovery. As with SA anesthesia, a successful anesthetic procedure requires careful preparation and a good understanding of the sequence of events involved in taking a horse from consciousness to surgical anesthesia and back to consciousness. Procedure 29-3 summarizes these events when a horse is induced with injectable agents and is maintained with an inhalant agent.

SELECTING A PROTOCOL

As for SA anesthesia, protocols are commonly selected by the veterinarian in charge. A suitable protocol takes into account patient signalment, preexisting problems, physical status class, and the procedure to be performed (Box 29-7 offers sample protocols used in physical status class P1 and P2 horses). After the protocol is known, calculate all drug dosages, oxygen flow rates, and fluid administration rates, and check them *carefully*.

BOX 29-7	Protocols for Premedication, Sedation, and General Anesthesia in Physical Status Class P1 and P2 Horses

Protocols for Mild to Moderate Sedation
1. Acepromazine: 0.03 to 0.05 mg/kg IV or IM (not for use in debilitated patients, or in breeding stallions).
2. Xylazine: 0.1 to 0.3 mg/kg IV.
3. Detomidine: 0.005 to 0.01 mg/kg IV.
4. Butorphanol: 0.02 to 0.05 mg/kg can be combined in the same syringe with any of the sedatives listed above and given IV for additional sedation.

Protocols for Moderate to Heavy Sedation (for Minor Procedures such as Wound Débridement or Radiography) or for Premedication
1. Xylazine: 1.1 mg/kg IV.
2. Detomidine: 0.01 to 0.02 mg/kg IV.
3. Romifidine: 0.05 to 0.1 mg/kg IV.
4. Butorphanol: 0.05 to 0.2 mg/kg IV or morphine: 0.05 to 0.1 mg/kg IV can be added to any of the alpha$_2$-agonists listed previously, to provide neuroleptanalgesia.

Protocols for Anesthetic Induction
1. Ketamine: 2.2 mg/kg IV.
2. Guaifenesin: IV to effect followed by ketamine: 2.2 mg/kg IV.
3. Diazepam: 0.03 to 0.05 mg/kg IV with ketamine: 2.2 mg/kg IV (midazolam can be used in place of diazepam).

Protocols for Anesthetic Maintenance
1. Isoflurane 1.5% to 2.5% or sevoflurane 2.5% to 4%.
2. "Triple drip" IV to effect: 500 mg ketamine and 250 mg xylazine are added to 500 ml of 5% guaifenesin. The mixture is then administered at 1 to 2 ml/kg/hour.

IM, Intramuscular; *IV,* intravenous.

Physical status class P3 to P5 patients require use of modified protocols based on the primary condition (Table 29-11).

EQUIPMENT PREPARATION

It is critical in equine anesthesia to be prepared and to check equipment before use, including any hoists and hydraulic tables that are to be used for lifting and positioning horses. Recovery pads, ropes, and other equipment, if used, should be organized before induction, if possible.

THE PREANESTHETIC PERIOD

The preanesthetic procedure in horses differs slightly from that in small animals. After appropriate patient assessment, the first step is placement of an IV catheter, almost always in one of the jugular veins. Some horses object to venipuncture and must be sedated first. Xylazine IV or IM is commonly used for this purpose. Once the horse is cooperative, a small bleb of local anesthetic is administered over the proposed site of catheterization to desensitize the skin.

After catheterization, the horse's mouth should be rinsed out with a dose syringe placed between the cheek and the

TABLE 29-11	Recommendations for Physical Status Class P3 to P5 Equine Patients	
PRIMARY CONDITION	**EXAMPLE PROTOCOLS AND OTHER CONSIDERATIONS**	**AVOID THESE AGENTS/ CIRCUMSTANCES**
Colic	Premedicate with xylazine to effect Induce with a ketamine-based protocol Maintain blood pressure in normal range	Acepromazine Thiopental
C-section	Premedicate with xylazine to effect Induce with ketamine Maintain with isoflurane or sevoflurane Epidural analgesia is helpful to reduce the need for other analgesics Minimize anesthetic time Monitor oxygenation	Thiopental sodium Opioids before delivery

teeth on each side of the mouth to flush out any feed material. This prevents aspiration of the material during intubation or in recovery. Feet should be cleaned before sedation, and then shoes should be removed or wrapped. Just before or immediately after premedication, the horse is positioned in an induction area or is placed adjacent to a tilt table. Some horses startle easily in a strange environment, and some breeds (such as Arabians and thoroughbreds) have a higher drug tolerance. An excited horse should never be induced to anesthesia because this will increase the anesthetic maintenance requirement. This may result in difficulty keeping the patient anesthetized as a result of high levels of circulating catecholamines, requiring dangerously deep levels of anesthesia. Sedation is considered to be adequate when the horse's head (and lower lip) droops, the horse no longer pays attention to its surroundings, and the horse demonstrates a wide-based stance or reluctance to move (Figure 29-30).

> **TECHNICIAN NOTE**   *Never* induce anesthesia in a horse that is not adequately sedated.

ANESTHETIC INDUCTION

Horses are generally induced to anesthesia by intravenous administration of drugs.

IV Induction

Induction typically occurs in a special induction stall that has padded walls and often a padded floor. Induction may be done "free fall" or behind a gate that restrains the horse. Sometimes the induction stall is also used for recovery. In comparison with small animals, in which IV induction is given to effect, the goal of induction in horses is to rapidly

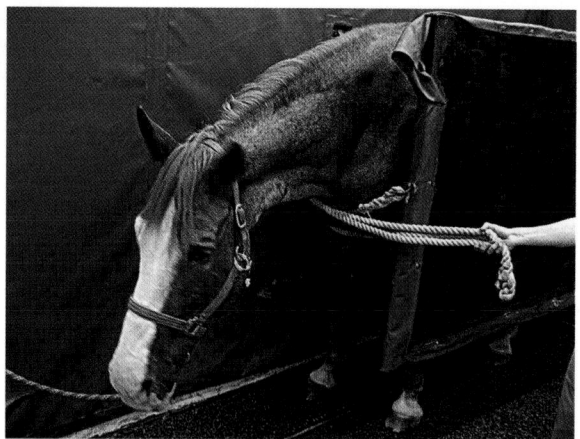

FIGURE 29-30 The horse is positioned behind a gate, which is secured to the fixed wall of the induction stall with a rope. Note the relatively wide-based stance and the lowered head position. The horse is not particularly interested in its surroundings. This indicates that the horse is adequately sedate before induction.

take the horse from standing (sedated) to lateral recumbency (unconscious) so as to minimize excitement, which can cause the horse to injure itself or personnel. All drugs are thus given as a bolus, with the exception of the muscle relaxant guaifenesin, which is administered rapidly intravenously to effect by placing it in a pressure bag. Once the horse shows signs of ataxia—typically knuckling of the forelimbs at the fetlocks—the induction agent is given as a bolus.

Once the horse has been induced, vital signs should be briefly checked. The horse is then intubated (see Figure 29-18, *A* and *B*).

In some practices, the floor of the induction stall forms part of the surgery table, but in many, the horse must be hoisted onto a table (Figure 29-31, *A*). It is important to understand how the hoist functions, so the horse can be transported safely and any problems can be resolved rapidly.

It is essential to ensure that muscles and prominent nerves are protected when a horse is placed on a surgical table or surface (Figure 29-31, *B*). Many table designs are available, and the anesthetist should make sure that muscle groups are well supported to prevent myopathy ("tying up"), and that facial and radial nerves are supported. Horses in lateral recumbency should have the forelimb closest to the table pulled forward, if possible, to decrease pressure placed on it by the chest and the opposite limb.

MAINTENANCE OF ANESTHESIA

Of all domestic species, horses present the biggest challenge to the anesthetist. Sudden unexpected movement can occur with no change in signs of depth. As a result of large breathing circuit volume and patient size, response to changes in inhalant anesthetic and oxygen flow rates occur too slowly to return the patient to surgical anesthesia simply by altering machine settings. A syringe of ketamine or thiopental is typically drawn up before anesthesia and may be attached to a three-way stopcock in the fluid administration line or kept close to the IV port for this purpose. Approximately one-fifth

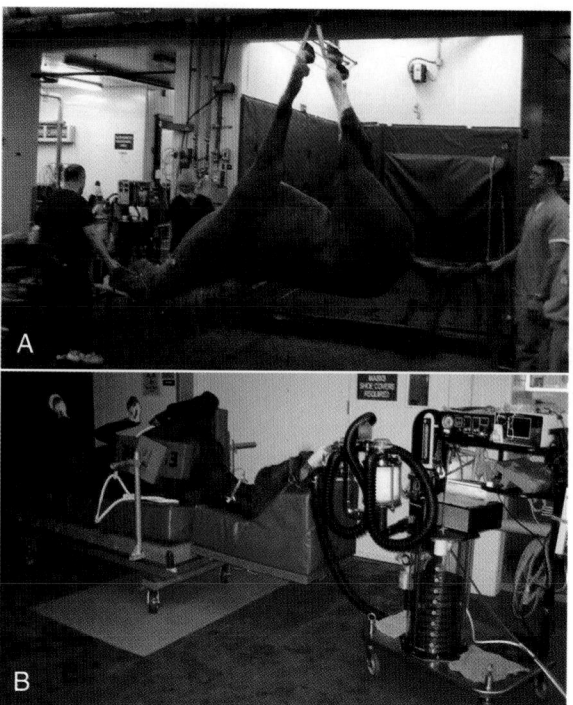

FIGURE 29-31 A, Once the horse is intubated and the anesthetist confirms that it is stable after induction, it is hoisted for placement on the surgery table. The anesthetist controls and supports the head while the patient is on the hoist. **B,** The horse is positioned on a thick foam pad to prevent muscle damage. Side paddles are used to keep the horse in dorsal recumbency on the table, and smaller foam pads support the large muscles of the upper forelimbs. Once the horse is positioned, it is connected to a large animal (LA) anesthesia machine.

of the IV induction dose is administered to the horse to return it to surgical anesthesia.

Compared with other species, horses are more likely to develop hypoxemia, hypoventilation, and hypotension during maintenance of anesthesia, particularly when inhalant agents are used. To monitor blood pressure more accurately and to obtain arterial blood gas values, it is recommended that horses anesthetized with inhalants for procedures lasting longer than 1 hour have an arterial catheter placed in a peripheral artery (facial, transverse facial, or dorsal pedal) (Figure 29-32). Blood gas samples should be taken every 30 to 60 minutes, or more frequently if the situation warrants.

Hypoventilation is so common in anesthetized horses, particularly those placed in dorsal recumbency, that a ventilator is often used to maintain normal ventilation. Hypotension (mean arterial blood pressure less than 70 mm Hg) has been shown to contribute to myopathy, so treatment with drugs is frequently indicated if increased IV fluid rate, decreased anesthetic depth, and surgical stimulation do not increase blood pressure. The drug most often used to support blood pressure is the positive inotrope dobutamine (typically administered via a syringe pump). Dobutamine and many other positive inotropes may cause arrhythmias, so it is important to monitor the electrocardiogram (ECG) closely when starting an infusion.

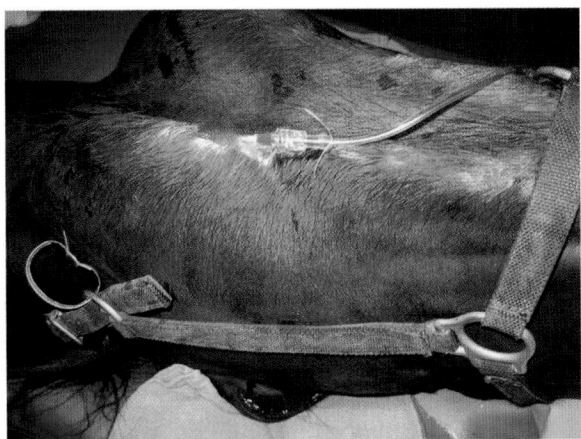

FIGURE 29-32 Placement of a catheter in the facial artery for monitoring blood pressure and taking blood samples for arterial blood gas analysis.

Hypoxemia can occur in any horse, regardless of the physical status class, but is more common in horses that are obese or pregnant, or have torsed intestines, and in those that are placed in dorsal recumbency. Hypoxemia has several possible causes, including hypoventilation, lung disease, and low cardiac output. Wherever possible, the cause should be investigated and corrected.

IV maintenance of anesthesia in horses is generally reserved for shorter procedures (less than 1 hour) in healthy patients and for procedures done away from a veterinary practice ("field anesthesia"). "Triple drip" is the mainstay of IV anesthesia in horses; it is generally characterized by higher blood pressure, better breathing, and more active palpebral reflexes than are seen with inhalant anesthesia. Use of "triple drip" for short procedures is also associated with recoveries of good quality.

ANESTHETIC RECOVERY

Horses have an instinctive need to stand shortly after awakening from anesthesia, and it is this that makes recovery particularly dangerous. Some steps can be taken to minimize injury to the horse and the anesthetist, but a high incidence of complications results from anesthetic recovery in horses, and clients should be informed of the risks.

Preparation for Recovery

Replace the halter. Place a nasopharyngeal tube before movement if nasal edema is present (Figure 29-33, *A*). Upon completion of the procedure, turn off the inhalant anesthetic and transfer the horse to a padded recovery stall, where it can be extubated and monitored. If possible, and particularly if the horse was hypoxemic during anesthesia, provide oxygen support using a demand valve or insufflation (5 to 10 L/minute delivered nasally or through the endotracheal tube via tubing that is connected to an oxygen flowmeter) until the horse is extubated or is too light to tolerate an insufflation hose. If recovery is assisted by ropes, a head rope should be attached to the halter and another rope tied to the tail (Figure 29-33, *B* and *C*).

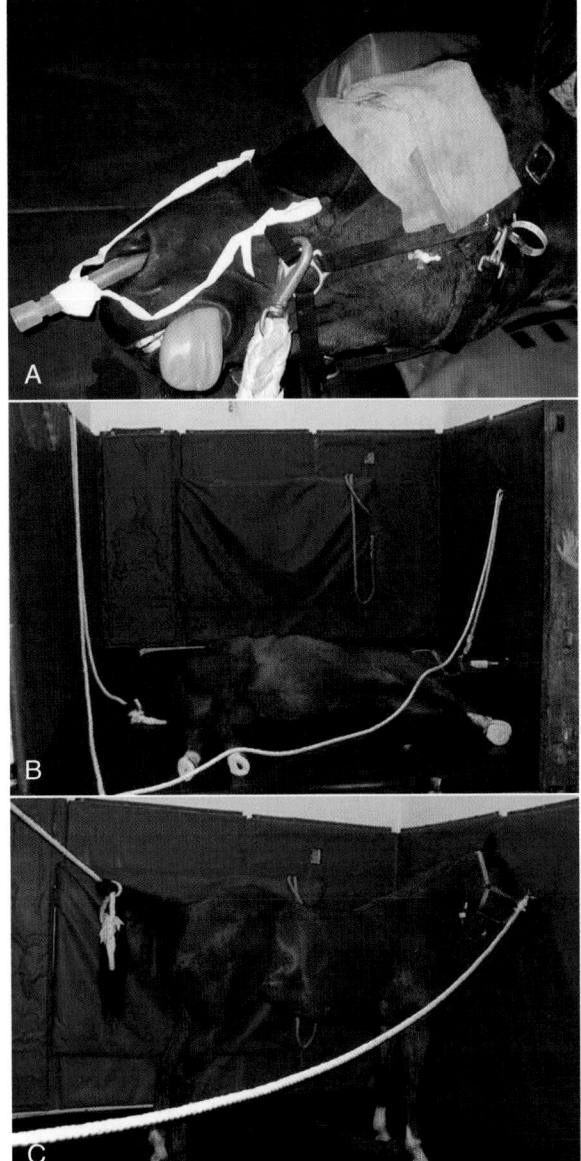

FIGURE 29-33 Recovery. **A**, A nasopharyngeal tube is placed and secured to the halter to ensure a patent airway. Note that the eye is covered to decrease stimulation during recovery. **B**, Placement of head and tail ropes for recovery. **C**, Recovered horse standing quietly. The nasopharyngeal tube stays in place until the horse is fully recovered.

Monitoring During Recovery

During recovery, it is ideal to watch the horse continuously so that it can be assisted or sedated, if necessary. While the horse is lying quietly, the anesthetist should watch respirations to make sure that the horse is breathing normally; the anesthetist should also take the pulse (facial artery) and assess the eye for depth of anesthesia.

Signs of Recovery

As the horse recovers, it will progress back through the stages and planes of anesthesia. Many horses develop nystagmus during recovery, and rapid nystagmus accompanied by "paddling" of the limbs generally means that a horse will try to get up too soon and will have a "rough" recovery. In this event, it may be prudent to sedate the horse with 50 to 100 mg xylazine IV. Generally, maintaining control of the head by sitting on the neck or holding the head up off the floor will provide some control over the horse. However, once the horse is strong enough to lift an anesthetist off its neck, the anesthetist should retreat to a safe distance from which to observe the remainder of recovery.

Extubation

To prepare the patient for extubation, deflate the cuff by drawing out all of the air until the pilot balloon is empty. Both before and after removal, keep the neck in a natural but extended position to protect the airway. Remove the endotracheal tube gently when the swallowing reflex returns, using a slow, steady motion. You may also remove it when signs of imminent arousal are present, such as voluntary movement of the limbs or head, movement of the tongue, or chewing. Check to make sure that the horse can breathe without obstruction. Horses can breathe only through their noses and will become distressed and compromised if they are unable to do so. If a nasopharyngeal tube has not been placed and the nasal passages are or become obstructed, one must be placed immediately. In the event that a nasopharyngeal tube does not alleviate the obstruction, a tracheostomy must be performed by the veterinarian, so materials for performing this procedure must be close to the recovery stall at all times.

The Postanesthetic Period

Once the horse is standing and is able to walk steadily, it can be returned to its stall. This can be assessed by walking the horse in a circle inside the recovery stall. Once back in its own stall, the horse should be muzzled for 1 to 3 hours but should have free access to water.

RUMINANT ANESTHESIA

Ruminants do not pose the same challenge to the anesthetist as is posed by horses; however, an understanding of their unique digestive physiology is important because it affects the well-being of the patient under general anesthesia. Additionally, ruminants present for general anesthesia less frequently than small animals or horses do, so it takes longer to gain anesthetic experience. Several reasons for this are known. Because of their relatively calm nature, ruminants require general anesthesia for relatively few procedures. Many surgeries can be conducted using local or regional anesthetic techniques. A discussion of local and regional anesthesia is beyond the scope of this chapter; this subject is covered in most veterinary anesthesia textbooks. Finally, administration of general anesthesia to production animals is often uneconomical.

The general principles discussed for other species also apply to ruminants, and careful preparation and planning are important for a successful anesthetic outcome. Procedure 29-4 summarizes the sequence of events involved when a ruminant is induced with injectable agents and is maintained with an inhalant agent.

SELECTING A PROTOCOL

As with other species, protocols are commonly selected by the veterinarian in charge. A suitable protocol takes into account patient signalment, preexisting problems, physical status class, and the procedure to be performed (see Box 29-8 for sample protocols used in physical status class P1 and P2 ruminants, and Table 29-12 for physical status P3 to P5). After the protocol is known, calculate all drug dosages, oxygen flow rates, and fluid administration rates, and check them *carefully*.

PREANESTHETIC FASTING

It is essential to ensure that ruminants have been adequately fasted before anesthesia. Fasting reduces the size of the rumen and decreases microbial activity. This in turn decreases gas production during anesthesia. Normally, ruminants eructate to expel gas from the rumen; however, under anesthesia, this does not happen, and bloating may occur. A bloated rumen can put pressure on the diaphragm and large blood vessels (aorta, caudal vena cava) in the abdomen, resulting in respiratory and circulatory compromise. Once an anesthetized ruminant develops severe bloat, it can be difficult to treat and may lead to death if it goes unnoticed or untreated.

EQUIPMENT PREPARATION

Any specialized equipment required for restraining or positioning anesthetized ruminants, such as head gates, transporters, and tilt tables, should be checked. In addition to the standard equipment, it is extremely helpful to have suction available for small ruminants to allow feed material, regurgitus, or saliva to be removed from the pharynx during intubation.

THE PREANESTHETIC PERIOD

Many ruminants are calm and tractable enough to allow IV catheterization and induction of anesthesia with minimal or no premedication and with mild restraint. Adult cattle are typically restrained using the head gate of a transporter or chute. Premedication is often reserved for patients that are aggressive, excited, or stressed. Although many ruminants do not require sedation before anesthesia, premedication will provide benefits, such as decreased dose of induction and maintenance drugs and improved muscle relaxation (Figure 29-34).

> **TECHNICIAN NOTE** Ruminants are sensitive to xylazine, requiring at most one-tenth of the dose that horses do.

ANESTHETIC INDUCTION
IV Induction

Induction of large cattle may occur in a special induction stall that has padded walls, in a transporter, or on a tilt table.

PROCEDURE 29-4	Sequence of Events for a Ruminant Anesthetic Procedure*

1. Assess, prepare, and weigh the patient (see Patient Preparation, p. 1078, for a discussion of patient assessment, preparation, and stabilization).
2. Prepare equipment and place intravenous (IV) catheter, which may require restraint in a chute with a head gate for larger or aggressive cattle (clippers, local anesthetic, antiseptic scrub, IV catheters, tape, heparinized saline, suture material, catheter cap, and/or extension line with three-way stopcock).
3. Determine the protocol (anesthetic agents, including dosages, routes, and sequence of administration).
4. Calculate the volume of each agent to be given, including fluid administration rates (preanesthetic, induction, maintenance, and analgesic agents).
5. Review the oxygen flow rates (see Box 29-3).
6. Prepare equipment required to administer drugs (scales, syringes, needles, agents, reversal agents, emergency cart, controlled substance log).
7. Prepare fluid administration equipment (fluids, administration extension set, syringe pump, tape, heparinized saline).
8. Prepare equipment for endotracheal intubation. Have suction equipment assembled and turned on for small ruminants. Remove jewelry and watch, and ensure that fingernails are trimmed short for digital intubation of adult cattle (see Principles of Endotracheal Intubation, p. 1098, for an equipment list).
9. Prepare monitoring equipment, including arterial catheterization materials, anesthesia record, monitors, and probes (see Anesthetic Monitoring, p. 1107, for a discussion of monitoring equipment).
10. Assemble and test the anesthetic machine and ventilator (see Anesthetic Equipment, p. 1090, and Manual and Mechanical Ventilation, p. 1125, for a discussion of these procedures).

11. Administer premedications approximately 20 to 30 minutes IM or 5 to 10 minutes IV before anesthetic induction, if this is considered necessary.
12. Administer the induction agent.
13. Check the patient's readiness for intubation.
14. Place and secure the endotracheal tube (see Principles of Endotracheal Intubation, p. 1098, for a discussion of this procedure).
15. Check the patient's vital signs.
16. Hoist or lift (as appropriate), position, and secure the patient for the procedure. It is imperative that the pharynx be positioned higher than the head, whenever possible.
17. Turn on the oxygen and connect the endotracheal tube to the breathing circuit.
18. Turn on the inhalant anesthetic to the appropriate level.
19. Determine the patient's anesthetic depth, and commence regular monitoring.
20. Attach monitoring devices and place an arterial catheter.
21. Continue to monitor and adjust anesthetic and oxygen levels as needed until completion of the procedure.
22. Prepare the patient for recovery, including removal of monitoring equipment, and ensure that the recovery area has been prepared.
23. Discontinue the anesthetic, and transfer the patient to the recovery area.
24. Place and support the patient in sternal recumbency so that it can eructate. Extubate the patient at the appropriate time with the cuff partially inflated.
25. Prepare the patient for continued hospitalization or discharge by applying bandages, administering medications, and performing any other procedures ordered by the veterinarian.

*Induction with an IV agent and maintenance with an inhalant agent.

BOX 29-8	Protocols for Premedication, Sedation, and General Anesthesia in Physical Status Class P1 and P2 Ruminants

Protocols for Mild to Moderate Sedation*
1. Acepromazine: 0.02 to 0.03 mg/kg IV (may increase regurgitation).
2. Xylazine: 0.01 to 0.05 mg/kg IV or IM (unlikely to cause recumbency).
3. Detomidine: 0.005 to 0.02 mg/kg IV.

Protocols for Moderate to Heavy Sedation (for Minor Procedures such as Radiography or Wound Assessment) or for Premedication†
1. Acepromazine: 0.03-0.05 mg/kg IV.
2. Xylazine: 0.05-0.1 mg/kg IV or 0.05-0.2 mg/kg IM (likely to cause recumbency and potentially light anesthesia).
3. Detomidine: 0.01-0.03 mg/kg IV.
4. Midazolam: 0.1 mg/kg plus butorphanol: 0.1-0.2 mg/kg IV (may produce ataxia, so recommended for small ruminants or restrained cattle).

Protocols for Anesthetic Induction
1. Ketamine: 2.5 mg/kg IV and diazepam: 0.12 mg/kg IV mixed in the same syringe. (This is equivalent to 1 ml of the mixture/20 kg of body weight and is given most commonly to small ruminants. Note the difference from SA dosage.)
Note: An equivalent volume of midazolam can be used in place of diazepam.
2. "Double drip" administered IV to effect (approximately 1 to 2 ml/kg). "Double drip" can be made by adding 500 mg ketamine to a 500-ml bag of 5% guaifenesin.
3. Telazol: 1 to 4 mg/kg IV or IM (lower dose after xylazine premedication).

Protocols for Anesthetic Maintenance
1. Isoflurane 1.5% to 2.5% or sevoflurane 2.5% to 4%.
2. "Double drip" can be used to maintain anesthesia at 1 to 2 ml/kg/hour.

IM, Intramuscular; *IV,* intravenous.
*Note that many ruminants require no sedation for standing procedures performed with local anesthetic.
†Note that many ruminants do not require premedication before anesthesia.

TABLE 29-12	Recommendations for Physical Status Class P3 to P5 Ruminant Patients	
PRIMARY CONDITION	EXAMPLE PROTOCOLS AND OTHER CONSIDERATIONS	AVOID THESE AGENTS/CIRCUMSTANCES
C-section requiring general anesthesia (live calf)	No premedication Induce with ketamine-based protocol Maintain with isoflurane or sevoflurane Epidural analgesia is helpful to reduce the need for other analgesics Minimize anesthetic time	Thiopental sodium and other barbiturates Alpha$_2$-agonists Acepromazine Opioids before delivery
C-section requiring general anesthesia (dead calf, septicemic cow)	No premedication or benzodiazepines Induce with ketamine-based protocol Maintain with isoflurane or sevoflurane Support blood pressure	Thiopental sodium and other barbiturates Alpha$_2$-agonists Acepromazine
Urethral obstruction	No premedication or premedicate with benzodiazepines (e.g., diazepam) Induce with "double drip" or diazepam-ketamine Maintain with isoflurane or sevoflurane Monitor electrolytes preoperatively and intraoperatively Maintain blood pressure and fluid balance	Acepromazine Alpha$_2$-agonists

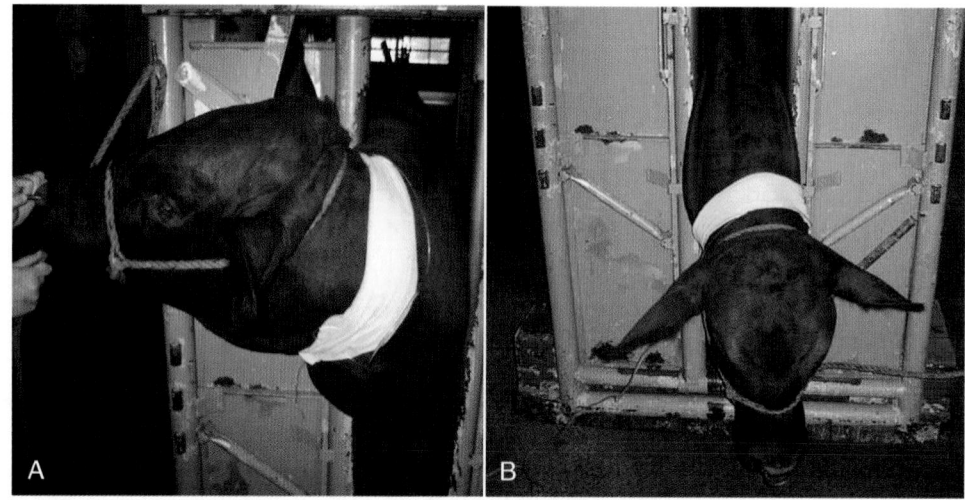

FIGURE 29-34 A, A 500-kg bull is restrained for jugular catheterization in a transporter with a head gate. B, The same bull after sedation with 25-mg xylazine IV.

Smaller ruminants can generally be induced next to the surgery table or, if small or severely compromised, while lying on it. Although ruminants do not typically become excited during induction of anesthesia, the goal with larger patients is similar to that in horses: to rapidly produce unconsciousness and while minimizing injury to the patient and to personnel. Drugs are thus given as an IV bolus, with the exception of "double drip," which is administered rapidly IV to effect. Smaller ruminants, particularly those that are compromised, can be given induction drugs IV to effect, as for SA patients.

Once the patient is unconscious, it should be kept in sternal recumbency for intubation whenever possible. It is important to be vigilant for regurgitation, which can occur at any point in the anesthetic procedure but occurs most frequently when anesthesia is light or too deep. If regurgitation occurs, the head should immediately be positioned so that it is lower than the body, to prevent aspiration.

Once the patient has been induced, vital signs should be briefly checked before intubation (see Figure 29-19).

All ruminants should be positioned for surgery with the mouth lower than the pharynx to allow drainage of saliva and any regurgitated material from the mouth, preventing buildup in the pharynx, which could lead to aspiration during recovery. Ruminants produce copious amounts of saliva each day, which is normally swallowed. Under anesthesia, this cannot occur, so it must be allowed to drain. Ruminants, even large cattle, are not predisposed to developing myopathy or neuropathy, as horses are; however, appropriate physical support and padding during anesthesia are prudent.

MAINTENANCE OF ANESTHESIA

Healthy ruminants typically have relatively few problems during the maintenance phase of anesthesia. Blood pressure is usually well maintained and often is much higher than that seen in SA and equine patients. However, ruminants do tend to hypoventilate and are often observed to breathe rapidly and shallowly, somewhat like a panting dog. This type of breathing pattern tends to lead to hypoxemia and difficulty keeping the patient anesthetized because of inadequate delivery of inhalant anesthetic to the lungs. Patients that demonstrate this breathing pattern should be placed on a ventilator.

Most ruminants have accessible arteries in their ears; these are often catheterized so that blood pressure can be monitored directly and blood samples can be taken for blood gas analysis.

IV maintenance of anesthesia in ruminants is generally reserved for shorter procedures (less than 20 minutes) in healthy patients, although if the patient is intubated, the duration of anesthesia can be extended. "Double drip" is commonly used for this purpose.

ANESTHETIC RECOVERY

Unlike horses, ruminants are generally content to lie in sternal recumbency after they wake up from anesthesia. Complications from anesthetic recovery are generally limited to the residual effects of bloat. Ruminants rarely develop nasal edema during anesthesia and usually do not require nasal intubation.

Preparation for Recovery

Upon completion of the procedure, turn off the inhalant anesthetic and transfer the patient to a padded recovery stall, where it can be extubated and monitored (large cattle), or to a quiet, clean area on the floor (small ruminant). If possible, support or prop the patient in sternal recumbency.

Monitoring During Recovery

The patient should be monitored for signs of excessive bloating (visually large abdomen that feels tight to the touch).

Signs of Recovery

As the patient recovers, it will progress back through the stages and planes of anesthesia. Generally, this is not as dramatic an event in ruminants as it is in horses, even if the patient did not receive premedication. Eructation of rumen gas commonly occurs during the recovery period.

Extubation

In contrast to other species, the endotracheal tube cuff should be kept inflated or only partially deflated to prevent aspiration of any material that may have become lodged in the pharynx during anesthesia. The anesthetist should wait for strong swallowing movements or coughing before extubation. Both before and after removal, keep the neck in a natural but extended position to protect the airway. Remove the endotracheal tube gently, using a slow, steady motion. If removing the tube is difficult, remove some more air from the cuff, and try again.

The Postanesthetic Period

Once a ruminant is lying in sternal recumbency without support and is no longer in danger of bloating, it can be left unattended. Many ruminants will lie quietly after anesthesia, standing only after some time has passed, unless they are stimulated to rise. It is not necessary to withhold food or water from ruminants postoperatively unless specifically instructed to do so.

MANUAL AND MECHANICAL VENTILATION

Ventilation is a process in which air or anesthetic gases are artificially forced into a patient's lungs. Although ventilatory support is necessary in patients with preexisting problems, such as lung disease, obesity, abdominal distention, or brain trauma, some ventilatory support is needed even in healthy patients to compensate for the respiratory depression that accompanies general anesthesia. This is especially true in healthy LA patients; therefore, many practices will ventilate all horses and ruminants under general anesthesia.

Under certain circumstances, such as loss of a normal vacuum in the chest cavity (e.g., thoracotomy for repair of diaphragmatic hernia, thoracic injury, or pneumothorax) or paralysis of the respiratory muscles when neuromuscular blockers are used as part of the anesthetic protocol, a patient may be unable to breathe. At these times, ventilation is mandatory throughout the procedure to keep the patient alive.

This support can be provided by the anesthetist by applying pressure to the reservoir bag with the pop-off valve fully or partially closed (manual ventilation), or by using a ventilator (mechanical ventilation).

MANUAL VENTILATION

Manual ventilation is used when a mechanical ventilator is not available, to provide ventilatory support to patients with temporary apnea or inadequate respiratory depth, or to prevent atelectasis in any patient. Depending on the need, manual ventilation may be periodic or mandatory.

MECHANICAL VENTILATION

Mechanical ventilation is routinely used for large animals and at other times when mandatory ventilation is required. Different types of ventilators function in different ways. Pressure cycle ventilators force air into the lungs until a set pressure is reached. Volume cycle ventilators deliver a preset volume (usually 10 to 15 ml/kg). Time cycle ventilators force air into the lungs according to a set inspiratory time, regardless of the volume delivered or the pressure generated. Because of the wide variety of ventilators available, safe use requires careful review of the operating instructions in the owner's manual. To prepare for mechanical ventilation, follow the procedure below:

- Connect the ventilator to an electrical supply, an oxygen source, and the scavenging system.

- Insert the pressure feedback sensor between the expiratory valve and the corrugated breathing tube.
- Remove the reservoir bag from the anesthetic machine, and attach in its place the tube that connects to the bellows of the ventilator.
- Close the pop-off valve.
- Check that the endotracheal tube cuff is inflated and that the entire breathing circuit is air-tight.
- Set RR, maximum inspiratory pressure, V_T, and/or inspiratory time as indicated in the owner's manual.
- Turn on the ventilator and adjust the settings to achieve target volume, pressure, and/or time.

PERIODIC VENTILATION

Periodic ventilation is used to support normal healthy patients and patients that are experiencing apnea or hypoventilation. As mentioned earlier, healthy SA patients should receive a breath once every 2 to 5 minutes to prevent atelectasis. In contrast, hypoventilating or apneic patients may require breaths at 15-second to 5-minute intervals depending on the specific need, as determined by observation of monitoring parameters and monitoring equipment. To provide periodic manual ventilation, first close the pop-off valve and gently squeeze the bag until the patient's chest rises as in a normal breath. Then immediately after each breath, reopen the pop-off valve.

INTERMITTENT MANDATORY VENTILATION

Intermittent mandatory ventilation is used for most LA patients, which are extremely prone to hypoventilation under inhalant anesthesia. It is also needed during procedures in which the thoracic cavity is exposed to the atmosphere and during those in which neuromuscular blockers are used. To provide intermittent mandatory ventilation, do the following:

- Ventilate at a rate of 8 to 20 until spontaneous breathing ceases.
- Lower the rate to 6 to 12 bpm.
- For the duration of the procedure, adjust the rate based on data from blood gas analysis, capnography, pulse oximetry, and other monitoring parameters.
- When you are ready for the patient to resume spontaneous breathing, gradually reduce the rate to about 4 bpm (SA) or 2 bpm (LA).
- When the patient begins to spontaneously breathe, support the patient with periodic ventilation as needed.
- Discontinue ventilation when rate and V_T are normal.

COMPLICATIONS OF VENTILATION

Use of manual and mechanical ventilation is not without risk. Positive pressure is generated in the chest during the inspiratory phase of normal ventilator cycling. This leads to a reduction in venous return to the heart and a temporary drop in blood pressure. Therefore, ventilation should be used cautiously in the hypotensive patient.

If excessive pressure is applied to the airways, alveoli can rupture, resulting in pneumothorax or pneumomediastinum.

Additionally, high positive pressure in the thorax will decrease the return of blood to the heart. This may lead to a life-threatening reduction in cardiac output. For these reasons, never allow pressure in the breathing circuit to exceed 15 to 20 cm of water in small animals or 30 to 40 cm of water in large animals, unless the chest is open, in which case, higher pressures may be required.

If respiratory minute volume (RMV) is excessive, respiratory alkalosis can occur as a result of loss of CO_2. In contrast, if RMV is inadequate, the patient can develop hypercarbia and respiratory acidosis. For this reason, use of an appropriate RR and V_T is critical for maintaining patient safety during ventilation. Capnography is the best noninvasive tool for judging the appropriateness of the rate and volume, with the gold standard of measurement of arterial CO_2 through blood gas analysis.

If a nonprecision VIC is used, anesthetic overdose is possible if the patient receives an excessive minute volume. Therefore, careful monitoring of anesthetic depth is important in these patients.

Finally, artificial ventilation is generally more efficient at delivering anesthetic gas, even from a precision VOC. A ventilator will thus deliver more inhalant anesthetic to the patient, which may lead to exacerbation of side effects, such as hypotension. Conversely, ventilators are often used in LA patients as anesthetic delivery devices to maintain a smoother plane of anesthesia than sometimes occurs with spontaneous breathing, particularly if the patient is hypoventilating.

ANESTHETIC PROBLEMS AND EMERGENCIES

Most general anesthetic procedures are uneventful, but from time to time, problems develop that have the potential to cause transient or permanent harm to the patient. Most studies show that although as many as 1 out of 10 patients have complications of one sort or another, on average only 1 or 2 out of 1000 healthy patients die as a result of anesthesia. Therefore, it is likely that a technician will have experience with many successful anesthetic procedures before a serious complication ever occurs. This can easily lead to a false sense of security, which, unless tempered with increased watchfulness, may impair readiness to handle a crisis.

Although patients with preexisting conditions, such as major organ disease, are more likely to develop complications, healthy patients may be at greater risk by reason of species, age, breed, reproductive status, body conformation, or a variety of other factors. For instance, brachycephalic dogs and geriatric, young (less than 8 weeks old), obese, and pregnant patients are at greater risk. Ruminants may bloat, leading to cardiorespiratory compromise, and equine anesthetic recovery poses many risks, including myopathy and neuropathy. Therefore, the anesthetist must approach any anesthetic procedure prepared for problems that are likely to arise.

Adverse drug reactions, equipment malfunctions, anesthetic overdose, complications of surgery, and human error are other possible causes of anesthetic problems and emergencies. Most can be managed successfully, however, if recognized early and acted upon before they reach a crisis level. Many indicators of developing problems may be detected by careful and frequent observation throughout the procedure. These indicators usually come from the machine (e.g., an overfilled reservoir bag, exhausted CO_2 granules), the patient (e.g., a patient that will not stay anesthetized or that is experiencing a rough recovery), or monitoring devices (e.g., an SpO_2 below 95%, a cardiac arrhythmia).

The anesthetist may be able to manage some problems independently and quickly, whereas others require rapid and effective communication with the veterinarian in charge, in addition to further exploration. For instance, mildly excessive or inadequate anesthetic depth in most cases can be managed by the anesthetist by simply adjusting the vaporizer setting and oxygen flow or by altering the administration of injectable agents. On the other hand, problems such as hypotension or cardiac arrhythmias may require more complex action, such as changing the anesthetic protocol, treating blood loss, or interpreting data from a monitoring device. The remainder of this section highlights causes, solutions, and prevention of common anesthetic problems and emergencies.

A flowmeter or oxygen tank pressure gauge that registers zero indicates that the flowmeter is turned off, or that the oxygen tank is empty or turned off. If the primary tank is empty, open the reserve tank. If it is impossible to solve the problem right away (there is no reserve tank on the machine and only one machine at your disposal), you should disconnect the endotracheal tube from the breathing system until the problem is rectified, although there is a risk that the patient may wake up or become hypoxemic in the interim.

Lack of movement of the reservoir bag or of the unidirectional valves when the patient breathes usually indicates that the endotracheal tube is not in the trachea, is disconnected, or is blocked. A disconnected or misplaced tube will result in difficulty keeping the patient anesthetized. A blocked tube will usually cause dyspnea and cyanosis. To manage this problem, first check that the tube is connected to the breathing circuit and is correctly placed. Next, disconnect the tube and listen or feel for airflow when the patient breathes, to rule out a blockage. If the tube is blocked or is incorrectly placed, immediately remove the tube and reintubate the patient. If reintubation is not possible (e.g., no one to help you), administer oxygen and anesthetic via mask until the tube can be replaced.

An overinflated reservoir bag or a pressure manometer reading greater than 2 cm of water while the patient is breathing spontaneously occurs most commonly because the pop-off valve has inadvertently been left too far closed. Occlusions of the scavenging system, high oxygen flow, and overzealous use of the oxygen flush valve are other possible causes. If the pop-off valve is closed, open it immediately. If the pressure is dangerously high (more than 20 cm of water), immediately disconnect the endotracheal tube from the breathing circuit, and then correct the primary problem. If

pressure builds again when the tube is reconnected, check the scavenging system for a blockage. If high oxygen flow is causing the bag to overfill, the pressure in the circuit should not increase but will remain less than 2 cm of water, even though the bag appears to be overinflated. In this case, gently press the bag to empty it as needed and—if safe to do so—reduce the oxygen flow.

An underinflated reservoir bag indicates inadequate oxygen flow, a leak in the system, a maladjusted scavenging system, or a pop-off valve that is too far open. If it is completely deflated, immediately increase the oxygen flow or use the oxygen flush valve to fill the bag one-half to three-fourths full. Then check pop-off valve, machine assembly, and scavenging system adjustments. If the problem cannot be corrected quickly, change to another machine.

Violet or off-white, brittle absorbent granules indicate saturation of the CO_2 absorbent. The resulting increase in CO_2 in the breathing circuit will cause increased inspired and expired CO_2 levels on a capnograph and may also cause tachypnea or tachycardia. The solution to this problem is to change the granules as soon as the machine is no longer in use. For the duration of the procedure, change the patient to another machine. If you have only one machine, use high oxygen flow (1 L/5 kg body weight/minute), continue close monitoring, and wake the patient as soon as possible, or, if the patient weighs less than 7 kg, change to a non-rebreathing system.

A PATIENT THAT WILL NOT STAY ASLEEP

Difficulty keeping a patient adequately anesthetized is most often related to problems with the machine and associated equipment. Check that the oxygen is on and flow is adequate, the vaporizer is not empty and is turned on, the machine is correctly assembled, no system leaks are present, and the endotracheal tube is properly placed and cuffed. Also check the RR and respiratory depth, which, if decreased, may be insufficient to draw enough anesthetic into the lungs. If this is the case, manually ventilate the patient every 5 to 10 seconds until in surgical anesthesia. If light, it may be necessary to prevent the patient from chewing the tube by applying gentle but firm pressure to the muzzle, and to give additional injectable anesthetic until the source of the problem is identified and corrected.

Excessive anesthetic depth is usually due to excessively high vaporizer settings, equipment problems, or preexisting medical problems. Immediately inform the veterinarian, stop administration of all anesthetics, increase the flow of oxygen, and proceed as ordered by the veterinarian. Excessively deep patients may require bagging, IV fluid support, measures to increase body temperature, reversal agents or other drug therapy, and even resuscitation in extreme situations. If a vaporizer problem (overfilled, tipped over, out of calibration) is suspected, change to another machine until the problem is corrected.

Cardiopulmonary arrest (CPA) most often follows uncorrected excessive anesthetic depth but can happen at any time during anesthesia. Patients in physical status classes P3 to P5 are at especially high risk for CPA. A patient that has arrested has no heartbeat, pulse, or respirations and requires prompt initiation of cardiopulmonary-cerebral resuscitation (CPCR). The reader is directed to Chapter 25 for a complete discussion of CPCR.

Apnea or hypoventilation commonly occurs after any episode of hyperventilation as a result of a decrease in blood CO_2 levels. Apnea or hypoventilation is also common after induction with drugs that depress the respiratory system but can indicate excessive anesthetic depth and in some cases even respiratory arrest. To manage apnea, rapidly inform the veterinarian, check other vital signs, and then determine the anesthetic depth by assessing other monitoring parameters. If the patient is stable and at an appropriate depth, it may be necessary to "bag" the patient 2 to 10 times/minute until normal respirations resume. Use the low end of this range if apnea is secondary to hyperventilation to allow normalization of CO_2 levels.

Hypotension is a common anesthetic complication caused by preexisting conditions, blood loss, shock, cardiac arrhythmias, excessive anesthetic depth, and adverse effects of drugs. Hypotension is confirmed with Doppler, oscillometric, or direct blood pressure monitoring but may be suspected on the basis of pale mucous membranes, increased CRT, and weak pulses. After informing the veterinarian, treat hypotension as ordered. Treatment often includes IV fluid therapy, decreased delivery of anesthetic, administration of additional oxygen, warming of the patient, and drug therapy.

Cyanosis or low oxygen saturation indicates hypoxemia and can be caused by cardiopulmonary disease, ineffective respirations, airway blockage, or machine problems. Cyanosis is a medical emergency that requires immediate action. Dyspnea often accompanies or precedes cyanosis and must also be treated aggressively. Low oxygen saturation is defined as SpO_2 less than 95% on a pulse oximeter. If you believe that the value is correct and is not due to a machine or probe problem, first inform the veterinarian and then check the oxygen flow, machine assembly, and endotracheal tube for blockage. Also check that RR and V_T are adequate.

Vomiting or regurgitation may occur at any time during an anesthetic procedure and can result in serious complications from pulmonary aspiration if the airway is not protected with a cuffed endotracheal tube. Vomiting is more common during induction and recovery, whereas regurgitation is more common during surgical anesthesia because of relaxation of the lower esophageal sphincter. Keep the tube cuffed at all times, and position the head level with or slightly higher than the rest of the body during surgical anesthesia to decrease the likelihood of regurgitation. If the patient begins to retch or vomit at any time during general anesthesia, quickly position the patient's head lower than the body, so that the vomitus flows out of the oral cavity and away from the pharynx. When the vomiting stops, carefully clean the oral cavity and the pharynx with swabs, gauze, or suction.

Prolonged recovery may be seen in patients with preexisting disease or hypothermia and in those that have received barbiturates or dissociatives, or after prolonged procedures. Patients must be supported with IV fluids, good nursing care, measures to treat hypothermia, administration of reversal agents if indicated, and careful monitoring.

A rough or stormy recovery is one in which a patient thrashes, vocalizes, paddles, tries to bite, falls over, or exhibits any other uncontrolled behavior that can result in injury of the patient or of personnel during the recovery period. Rough recoveries are more common in non-premedicated patients and may result from pain, fear, or disorientation. To manage a rough recovery, approach the patient with caution, administer sedatives or analgesics as ordered by the veterinarian, calm the patient, and use padding, restraint, and bandaging techniques to prevent self-trauma.

ACKNOWLEDGMENTS

The authors would like to acknowledge Steven Ahern, AA, AAB, and William Fogarty, MEd, at Cuyahoga Community College, for photography and art direction for many of the figures in this chapter (Figures 29-1 through 29-29, with the exception of 29-13, 29-14, 29-18, 29-19, and 29-20).

RECOMMENDED READINGS

American College of Veterinary Anesthesiologists (ACVA): Small animal monitoring guidelines, 2009. Available at: www.acva.org (accessed on May 15, 2011).

Blaze CA, Glowaski MM: Veterinary anesthesia drug quick reference, St Louis, 2004, Saunders.

Greene SA: Veterinary anesthesia and pain management secrets, St Louis, 2002, Hanley and Belfus.

Love L, Harvey R: Arterial blood pressure measurement: physiology, tools, and techniques, Compend Cont Educ Pract Vet 28:450, 2006.

Marshall M: Capnography in dogs, Compend Cont Educ Pract Vet 26:761, 2004.

Muir WW, Hubbell JAE: Equine anesthesia, ed 4, St Louis, 2009, Saunders.

Muir WW, III, Hubbell JAE, et al: Handbook of veterinary anesthesia, ed 4, St Louis, 2007, Mosby.

Thomas JA, Lerche P: Veterinary anesthesia and analgesia for veterinary technicians, ed 4, St Louis, 2011, Mosby.

Thurmon JC, Tranquilli WJ, Benson GJ: Essentials of small animal anesthesia and analgesia, Baltimore, 1999, Lippincott Williams & Wilkins.

Tranquilli WJ, Thurmon JC, Grimm KG: Lumb & Jones' veterinary anesthesia and analgesia, ed 4, Ames, IA, 2007, Blackwell.

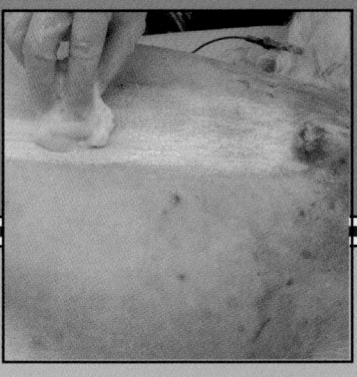

PART SEVEN
Surgical Nursing

30 Surgical Instruments and Aseptic Technique

James A. Perry, William T.N. Culp, and Daniel J. Burba

OUTLINE

INSTRUMENTATION, *1131*
General Surgery Instruments, *1131*
Scalpel, *1131*
Electrosurgery, *1131*
Biomedical Lasers and Laser Safety, *1131*
Scissors, *1136*
Needle Holders, *1137*
Thumb Forceps, *1138*
Tissue Forceps, *1139*
Hemostatic Forceps, *1139*
Retractors, *1140*
Suction Tips, *1140*
Stapling Equipment, *1141*
Vascular Sealing Devices, *1142*
Ophthalmic Instruments, *1142*
Orthopedic Instruments, *1143*
Periosteal Elevators, *1143*
Rongeurs, *1143*
Curettes, *1143*
Bone-Holding Forceps, *1144*
Osteotomes and Chisels, *1144*
Gigli Wire, *1144*
Trephines and Jamshidi Needles, *1145*
Power Equipment, *1145*
Orthopedic Implants, *1145*
Bone Pins, *1145*
Interlocking Nails, *1146*
Orthopedic Wire, *1146*
External Fixators, *1146*
Bone Screws, *1146*
Bone Plates, *1148*
Total Hip Prosthesis, *1149*
Arthroscopic Instruments and Equipment, *1149*
Arthroscope, *1149*
Ancillary Arthroscopic Equipment, *1150*
Fluid Delivery Systems, *1151*

Hand Instruments for Arthroscopic Surgery, *1153*
Laparoscopic Instruments and Equipment, *1154*
Laparoscope, *1154*
Laparoscopic Trocars and Cannulas, *1154*
Instrument Packs, *1155*
Instrument Care, *1157*
Drapes and Gowns, *1158*

ASEPTIC TECHNIQUE, *1158*
Physical Methods of Sterilization, *1161*
Filtration, *1161*
Radiation, *1161*
Heat, *1162*
Chemical Methods of Sterilization, *1164*
Ethylene Oxide, *1165*
Hydrogen Peroxide Gas Plasma, *1166*
Chemical Disinfection, *1166*
Antiseptic and Disinfectant Compounds, *1166*
Sterilization of Arthroscopic/Laparoscopic Equipment, *1168*
Operating Room Preparation, *1169*
Small Animal Patient Preparation, *1169*
Skin Preparation—Surgical Clip, *1169*
Skin Preparation—Surgical Scrub, *1170*
Small Animal Positioning, *1171*
Equine Patient Preparation, *1171*
Patient Positioning, *1171*
Skin Preparation, *1172*
Surgical Team Preparation, *1174*
Attire, *1174*
Hand Scrub, *1175*
Gowning and Gloving, *1176*
Maintaining Sterility, *1176*
The Patient, *1183*
Opening Sterile Items, *1184*

The authors and publisher wish to acknowledge the contribution of Jacqueline R. Davidson to previous editions of this chapter.

KEY TERMS

Asepsis
Aseptic technique
Assisted gloving
Box lock
Chemical sterilization
Closed gloving
Flash sterilization
Gas sterilization
Incise drape
Ingress port
Insufflate
Joule
Obturator
One-step prep
Open gloving
Osteochondral fragments
Paralumbar fossa
Peritoneal lining
Physical sterilization
Plume
Prosthesis
Ratchet
Recumbency
Residual activity
Scrub in
Scrub suit
Sterile field
Sterile technique
Strike-through
Subchondral bone
Triangulation

LEARNING OBJECTIVES

When you have completed this chapter, you will be able to:

1. Pronounce, define, and spell all Key Terms in this chapter.
2. Do the following regarding general surgery instruments and stapling equipment:
   - Name and describe commonly used surgical instruments
   - Know the basic operation and properties of CO_2 and diode lasers and develop a basic knowledge of laser safety protocol.
   - State advantages of surgical stapling and list common surgical stapling devices.
3. List commonly used instruments and equipment for ophthalmic, orthopedic, arthroscopic, and laparoscopic procedures.
4. Do the following regarding surgical instrument packs, instrument care, and the use of surgical drapes and gowns:
   - List surgical instruments and supplies routinely included in general and emergency surgical packs for small and large animals.
   - Describe procedures for cleaning, packing, and sterilizing instruments.
   - Describe procedures for folding and packing cloth surgical drapes and gowns.
5. Do the following regarding the processes of sterilization and disinfection as part of aseptic technique:
   - Differentiate between sterilization and disinfection.
   - List and describe physical and chemical methods of sterilization and methods of quality control of sterilization methods.
   - Know the appropriate sterilization processes for sensitive equipment.
   - State safe storage times and conditions for sterile packs.
   - List and describe common antiseptic and disinfectant agents.
   - Describe requirements for preparation of the operating room and maintenance of operating room sterility.
6. Describe preparation requirements for patients, including skin preparation, patient positioning, and draping.
7. Describe preparation requirements for the surgical team and explain the procedures that may be used for hand scrubbing before surgery, the procedure for donning surgical attire, and the procedures for opening sterile items.

INTRODUCTION

To be thoroughly prepared for surgery, it is critical that the veterinary technician be comfortable with all types of equipment and the steps involved in ensuring that **aseptic technique** is maintained. Instrumentation is constantly being changed and improved, and it is often the responsibility of the veterinary technician to prepare, handle, and maintain instruments before, during, and after surgery. Additionally, patients need to be appropriately prepared for surgery, and meticulous dedication to the proper techniques of surgical preparation is essential to decrease the incidence of surgical site infection; the veterinary technician plays a crucial role in all of these steps, and this chapter focuses on these principles.

Instrumentation

A complete description of all possible surgical instruments is well beyond the scope of this chapter. The goal of this section is to familiarize the technician with the most commonly used instruments in general small and large animal practices; additionally, some of the more advanced items of equipment will be briefly discussed to familiarize the surgical technician with these new devices. Because each instrument has a unique purpose and requirements for care, the veterinary technician should become acquainted with different types of instrumentation so that he or she can be prepared for the myriad of situations that may be encountered.

> **TECHNICIAN NOTE** Each instrument is designed for a specific purpose, such as cutting, holding, clamping, or retracting.

GENERAL SURGERY INSTRUMENTS

SCALPEL

Scalpels (or blades) are the instruments used to make most incisions. Scalpels are available in a variety of different sizes and shapes, and disposable versions are placed onto scalpel handles. Although the choice of scalpel blade is clinician dependent, certain blades are used for particular tasks. The most commonly used scalpel handles include the Bard-Parker No. 3 (for scalpel blades #10, #11, #12, and #15) and No. 4 (for scalpel blades #20, #21, and #22). Small animal surgeries are generally performed with a No. 3 handle, whereas large animal surgeons usually use a No. 4 handle (Figure 30-1).

ELECTROSURGERY

Electrocautery has become common in both general and specialty veterinary practice. The main advantage of this

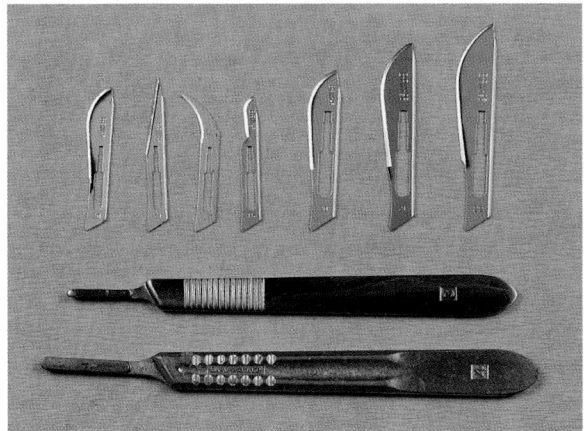

FIGURE 30-1 Scalpel handles and attachable surgical blades. Surgical blades #10, #11, #12, and #15 fit the Bard-Parker No. 3 scalpel handle, and surgical blades #20 to #22 fit the Bard-Parker No. 4 handle. The No. 3 handle and the #10 blade are commonly used in small animal surgery. The No. 4 handle and the #20 blade are commonly used in large animal surgery.

technology is that it allows the clinician to cut while simultaneously limiting bleeding through electrocoagulation. This is made possible through the passing of a high-frequency alternating electrical current through the tissue from the handpiece to the electrical ground plate located under the patient. Cutting and/or coagulation can be performed through the same handpiece, and the surgeon can activate it by using a switch on the sterile handpiece or a foot pedal. A nonsterile technician is required to adjust the power level for most units (Figure 30-2, *A* and *B*); however, newer electrosurgery systems also allow this task to be performed by the surgeon on the handpiece (Figure 30-2, *C*). It is of utmost importance that adequate contact is made between the patient's skin and the ground plate because the patient can be burned at the site of the ground plate. Good contact can be made by placing a damp surgical towel between the patient and the ground plate, or by using electrocautery gel (Figure 30-2, *D*). It is not necessary to clip the hair between the patient and the ground plate. In *bipolar electrosurgery*, the current passes between two tips on the handpiece (Figure 30-2, *E*), which grasp the tissue. The most common application of bipolar cautery is for delicate sealing of small vessels in areas where cauterization of surrounding tissues must be minimized (e.g., neurosurgery, cardiosurgery). No ground plate is needed for bipolar electrosurgery.

BIOMEDICAL LASERS AND LASER SAFETY
Laser Properties

Laser is an acronym for *light amplification by stimulated emission of radiation*. Several different types of lasers are used in veterinary medicine. Energized light coming from a laser unit is generated from gas, liquid, or crystal. The beam of light coming from a laser is highly focused and intense, with very little divergence of a laser beam. Unlike light from a flashlight, the light from a laser is uniform in wavelength and frequency. This is referred to as *coherent light*. Thus it does not scatter in different directions as it is emitted from a laser unit.

The effect of a laser on tissue depends on its wavelength within the light spectrum. Its interactions with tissues may result in beam scatter, transmission, reflection, or absorption. The resulting interaction depends on the density and makeup of the tissue. For example, bone is more likely than muscle to cause scatter. However, most lasers have a thermal effect, resulting in cutting, vaporizing, coagulating, or welding. The amount of laser energy applied to tissue is measured in **joules, or watts (W) per unit time (seconds)**. As an example, if a laser is set at 20 watts of power and is applied to tissue for 4 seconds, 80 joules of energy has been applied to the tissue.

An important property of laser surgery is latent and collateral thermal damage. Some lasers cause delayed cellular death, which is referred to as *latent thermal damage*. Lasers can also cause cellular damage or death wider than the actual path of the laser beam; this is referred to as *collateral thermal damage*. The desired effects determine whether a laser can be used for a surgical procedure.

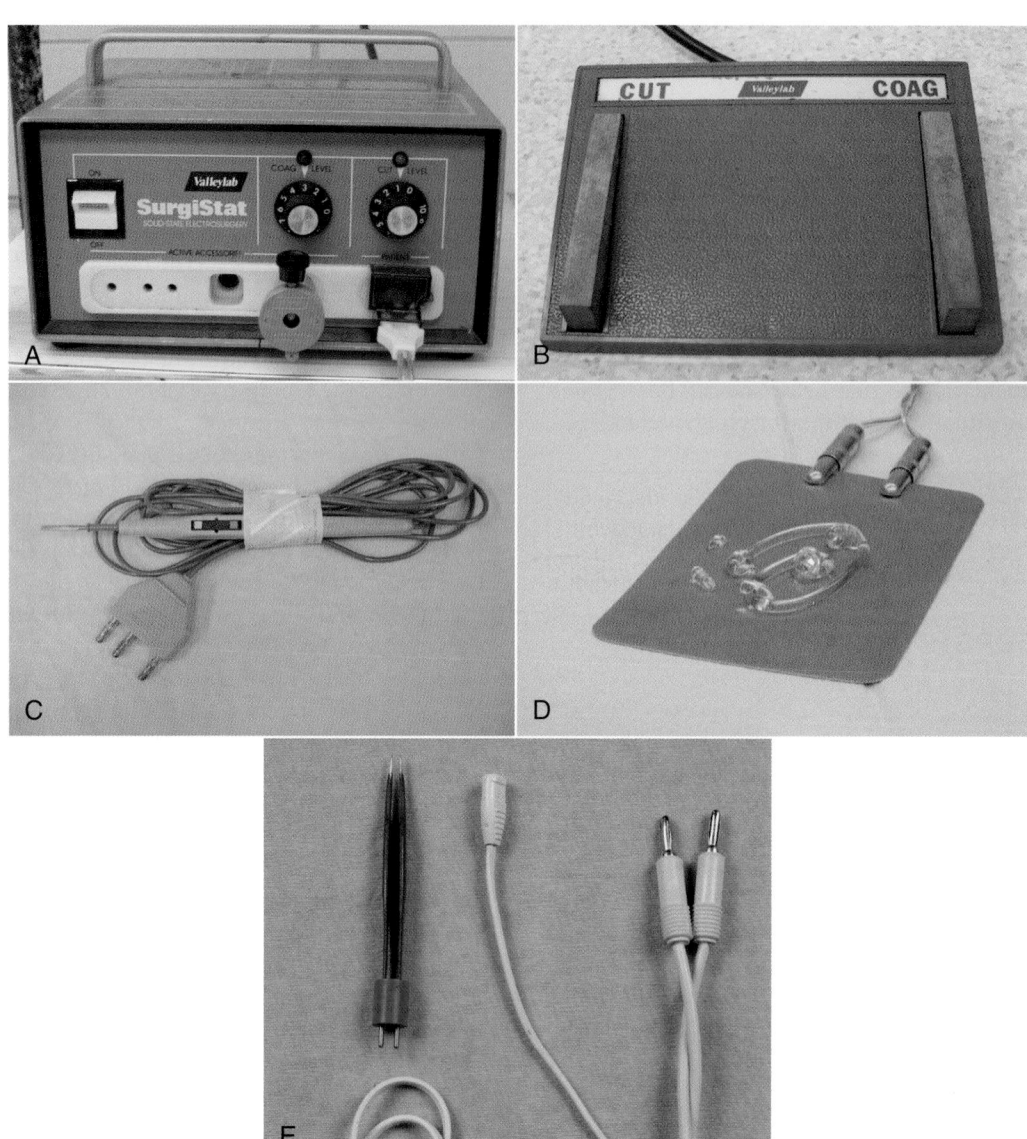

FIGURE 30-2 Electrosurgical equipment. **A,** Settings on electrosurgical unit are adjusted by nonsterile technician. **B,** Electrosurgical foot switch is placed near the surgeon's foot. **C,** Monopolar electrosurgery handpiece. If the handpiece has a cutting coagulation button, a foot switch is not needed. The handpiece is sterilized and is given to the surgeon. The surgeon passes the end of the cord to a nonsterile assistant, who plugs it into the electrosurgical unit. **D,** Ground plate on surgery table with gel to improve skin contact when the animal lies on it. Good contact is important for proper function. **E,** Bipolar handpiece is sterilized for use. A nonsterile foot switch is needed for activation.

Types of Lasers

The most commonly used lasers in the veterinary field include CO₂, neodymium: yttrium-aluminum-garnet (Nd:YAG), and diode lasers. The CO_2 laser is a free beam laser directed by a handpiece, which is held slightly above the tissue surface. Because it does not touch the tissue directly, it is categorized as a noncontact laser (Figure 30-3). YAG and diode lasers, on the other hand, are directed by a hand-held quartz fiber whose tip can be directly applied to tissue (Figure 30-4). Lasers are activated with a foot or hand switch. Most laser beams are invisible, so laser units are built with a helium-neon (He-Ne) visible guide light (Figure 30- 5).

CO₂ Laser

The laser beam is produced from a gas medium (CO_2). The beam is then transmitted down an arm with reflective mirrors or it can pass through a tube called a *reflective waveguide* (Figure 30-6). The CO_2 laser is emitted as a free beam, which means that the beam travels freely a short distance through air before it contacts the surgical tissue. It is ideal for both cutting and vaporizing. CO_2 lasers create minimal latent and collateral thermal damage, thus it can be used for precise cutting. It does not penetrate deep into tissues. CO_2 lasers range in power from 20 W to more than 100 W. Generally, the smaller units are used in small animal surgery and the larger units for horses.

Nd:YAG and Diode Lasers

YAG and diode lasers are very similar in their properties because their wavelengths are very similar (1064 μm vs. 980 μm). The laser beam of the Nd:YAG is produced from a crystal of yttrium, aluminum, and garnet "doped" with

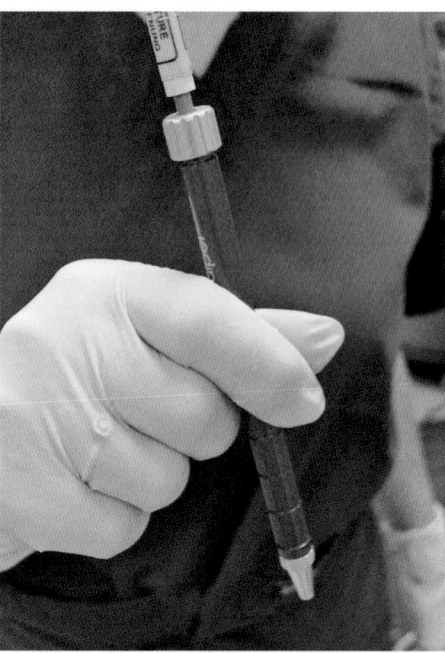

FIGURE 30-3 A handpiece directs an operating CO_2 laser (noncontacting laser), which is held slightly above the surface of the surgical tissue.

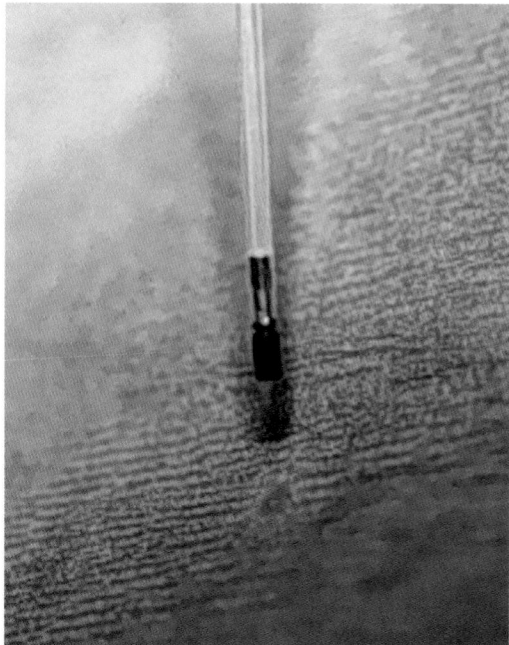

FIGURE 30-5 The beam from lasers is invisible, but the use of a helium-neon (He-Ne) guide light generates a visible red color that allows the surgeon to see the direction of the laser beam during operations.

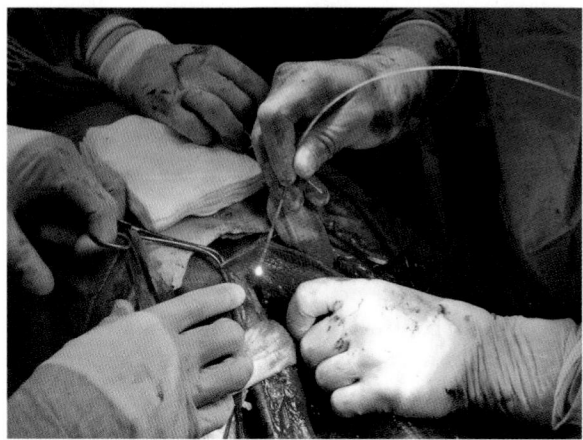

FIGURE 30-4 The beam of a diode laser is directed by a quartz fiber. The tip of the fiber is applied directly to the surgical tissue.

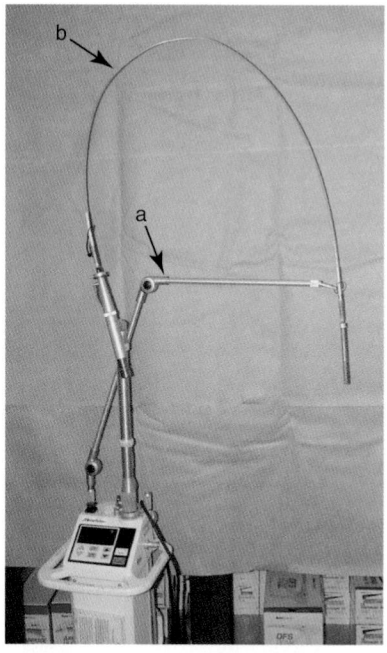

FIGURE 30-6 CO_2 laser can pass through an arm with reflective mirrors (a) or through a flexible tube called a *reflective wave guide* (b).

neodymium. The diodes are gallium (indium) aluminum arsenide lasers (Figure 30-7). Both transmit the laser beam through a quartz fiber (Figure 30-8). The quartz fiber can be specially designed with tips made of sapphire to emit the laser as a free beam, or the bare quartz fiber can be used in a direct contact mode. The beam can be used for transendoscopic surgery because it is fiber transmitted (Figure 30-9). The quartz fiber is coated with polyethylene that must be stripped away near the tip of the fiber as it is being used, or it will ignite (Figure 30-10). Nd:YAG and diode lasers create greater latent and collateral thermal damage than is produced by the CO_2 laser, and they are very effective in tissue vaporization. These lasers range in power from 20 to 50 W up to 100 W (Nd:YAG).

Laser Safety

The importance of safety when one is working with lasers cannot be stressed enough. Serious injury can occur as a result of contact with a surgical laser beam. All veterinary technicians working with lasers must be trained to take important safety measures each and every time a laser is used in the operating room. In addition, veterinary technicians should know whom to contact immediately in the event that a laser-related issue develops during surgery. The veterinary

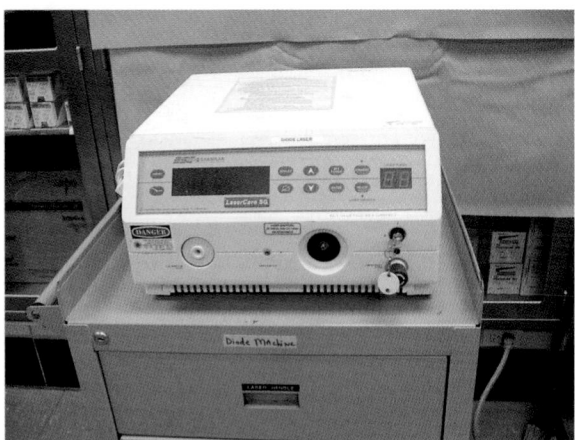

FIGURE 30-7 Diode laser unit.

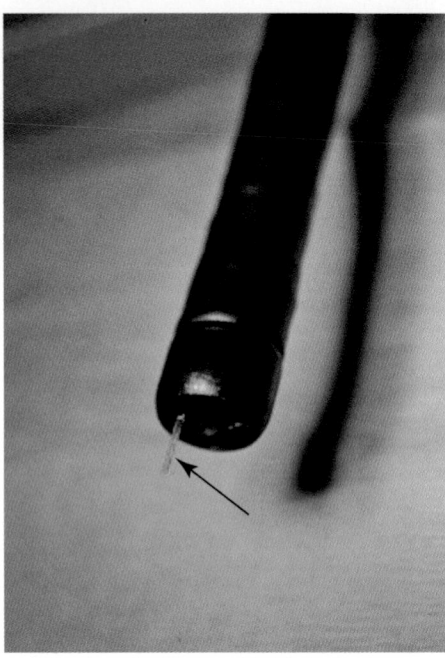

FIGURE 30-8 A diode laser fiber is passed through the biopsy channel of an endoscope in preparation for transendoscopic laser surgery in a pony.

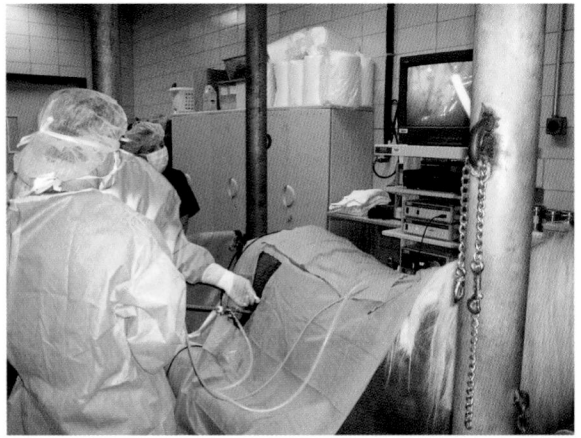

FIGURE 30-9 Transendoscopic laser surgery. A fiberoptic endoscope fitted with a laser has been introduced into the abdominal cavity of a pony. Notice that the tip of the laser is visible on the monitor screen in the background.

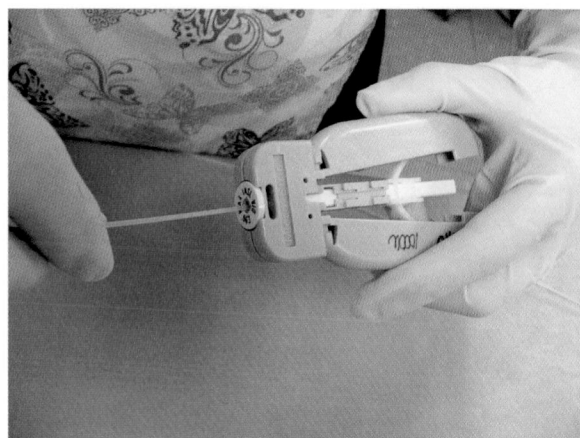

FIGURE 30-10 Flammable polyethylene coating is stripped off a laser fiber before it is used.

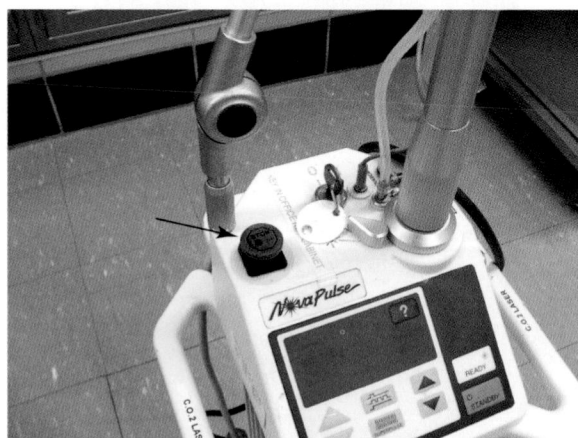

FIGURE 30-11 Emergency shutdown button on a laser unit.

technician who controls the laser unit during surgery must be skilled in its operation and emergency shutdown. Most lasers are equipped with an emergency shutdown button, as illustrated in Figure 30-11. It is a good idea for a technician to be assigned the role of "laser safety officer." As a technician, it will be your responsibility to know the safety protocols and to make sure they are followed while the laser is in use.

> **TECHNICIAN NOTE**   All veterinary technicians working with lasers must be trained to take important safety measures each and every time a laser is used in the operating room. In addition, they must make use of the emergency shutoff button, if an emergency develops during an operation.

Laser Hazard Classification

Lasers are divided into four classes according to their ability to inflict damage to skin or eyes (Table 30-1). Most medical lasers, which are class IV lasers, can cause skin and eye damage.

TABLE 30-1	Laser Hazard Classification
CLASS	**DESCRIPTION**
I	Not harmful for direct viewing or skin contact
II	Not harmful for vision if momentary
III	Harmful for direct viewing
IV*	Will cause skin or eye damage
	Any laser with power greater than 0.5 W for longer than 0.25 seconds
	May pose fire hazard

*Includes most surgical lasers.

BOX 30-1	Laser Safety Protocol for Personnel

- Laser surgical procedures are to be performed exclusively in an operating room or in another room specifically designed for the purpose.
- Person at the laser control must be familiar with the operation and shut down, including emergency shutdown of the laser.
- Laser warning signs are to be posted on the operating room door.
- All personnel must wear wavelength-specific eye protection.
- All windows in the operating room are to be covered with a nonreflective material during laser use.
- Laser is placed on "stand-by" by control operator when not being actively used by the surgeon.
- Plume evacuator must be in use during lasing.
- Laser-specific face masks should be worn during laser procedures.

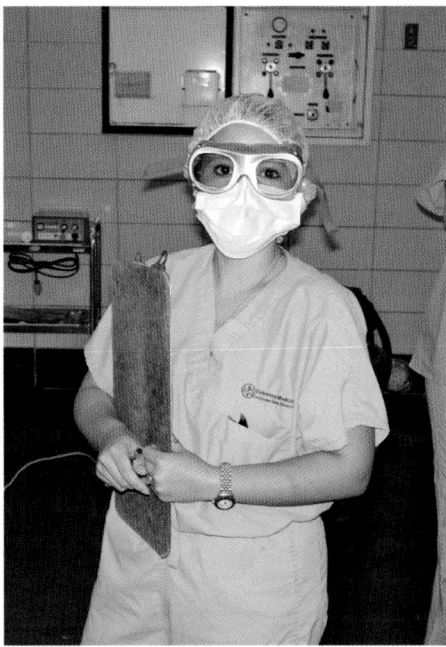

FIGURE 30-12 Laser eye protection must be worn by all surgical staff whenever a laser is in use. The type of eye protection to be worn varies with the type of laser being used. It is therefore important to be sure to wear the **correct eye protection.**

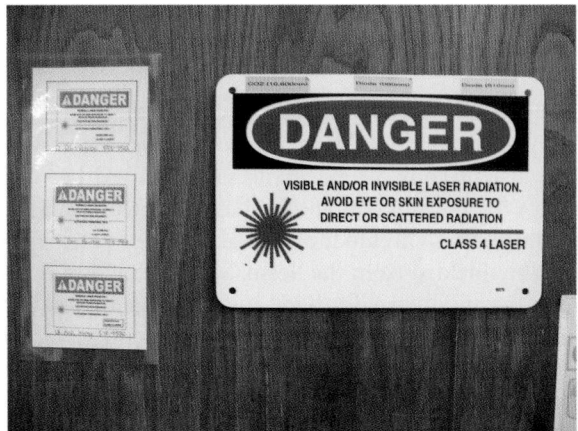

FIGURE 30-13 A warning sign alerts staff when a laser is in use.

Laser Safety Protocol for Personnel

Protocols for the safety of personnel should be developed in each hospital regarding laser use (Box 30-1). These should be tailored to the specifications of each practice, but regardless of the type of practice, all practices must provide a safe working environment by utilizing appropriate safety equipment and gear. It is often the veterinary technician who is responsible for enforcing the safety protocol. Safe use of lasers has been outlined by the American National Standards Institutes (ANSI). The ANSI defines the area of risk during laser operation as the nominal hazard zone (NHZ). The NHZ is the space within the level of direct, reflected, or scattered radiation during normal operation that exceeds the applicable maximum permissible exposure level (MPE). The MPE is the maximum laser radiation exposure that can occur without adverse biologic effects to the eyes or skin. The eyes are most vulnerable to laser injury. It is important to note that *wavelength-specific eye protection* is available for each laser and must be consistently employed during surgeries that involve lasers (Figure 30-12). Using one type of eye protection does not protect staff from all types of lasers. Thus it is important that the staff is aware of which type of laser is in use and which eye protection should be worn. *Laser warning signs* should be posted at the door of the

operating room, stating that a laser is in use and that proper eye protection is required (Figure 30-13). To prevent accidental transmission of a laser through a surgery window, nonreflective material (i.e., cloth) should be placed over them (Figure 30-14). Some lasers, such as the diode laser, can penetrate clear glass.

Laser Plume Control

Another hazard associated with lasers is the generation of **plume**, or smoke. Plume generated from lasering tissue may contain toxic substances that can have deleterious effects on personnel and on the patient. Plume can be controlled with the use of a plume evacuator (Figure 30-15, *A*). A plume evacuator creates suction to pull the plume into a hand-held

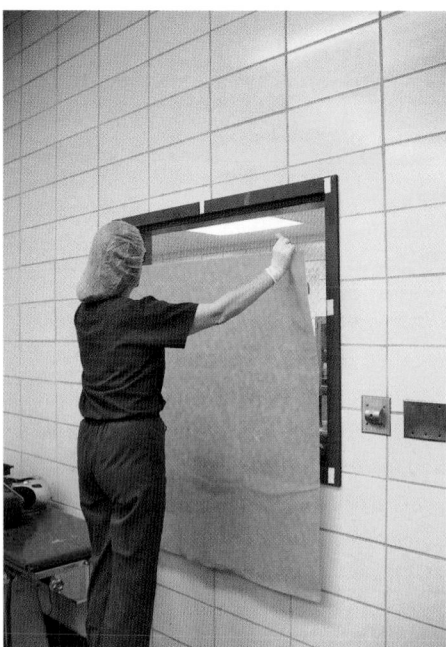

FIGURE 30-14 All windows in the surgery suite must be covered with nonreflective material to prevent inadvertent laser beam transmission through the glass.

sterile tube and into a filtered container (Figure 30-15, *B*). Filtering face masks specifically made for lasering should be worn in lieu of conventional surgical masks.

Laser Safety Protocol for the Patient

A safety protocol should be established for the patient, which is also at risk (Box 30-2). Sterile saline should be readily available for the surgeon at all times to protect against the possibility of flash fires in the surgical field. The patient's eyes should be shielded from the beam. Special shields are available for the anesthetized patient, and moistened sponges can be used to cover the eyes of an awake patient. Flammable anesthetic agents such as pressurized oxygen should never come in contact with the laser beam because this creates an explosive fire hazard. Shielded endotracheal tubes must be used if laser penetration of the trachea or upper respiratory tract is possible.

SCISSORS

Surgical scissors are among the most commonly used surgical instruments in small animal and large animal surgery alike. Each type of scissors has a function and should be used only to perform that function (Figure 30-16). Operating scissors are classified by multiple features, including blade type (straight or curved), the character of their points (blunt-blunt, blunt-sharp, or sharp-sharp), and the design of the cutting edge of the blades (plain or serrated). *Mayo dissecting scissors* are heavy-duty operative scissors used primarily for cutting fascia and other, more dense tissues. The blades may be straight or curved, blunt or sharp, and plain or serrated. Their size and length may also vary according to surgeon preference. *Metzenbaum dissecting scissors* are fine,

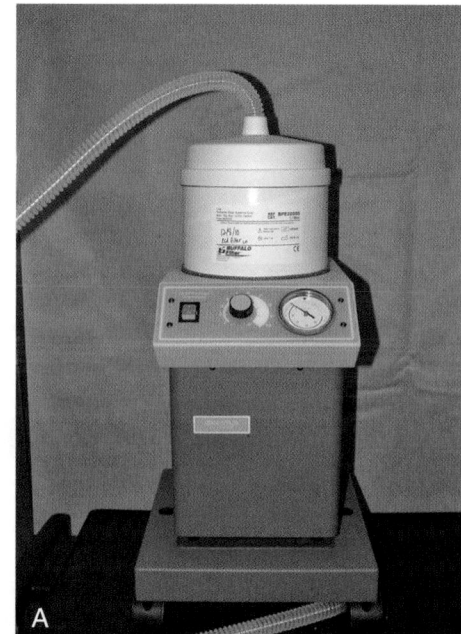

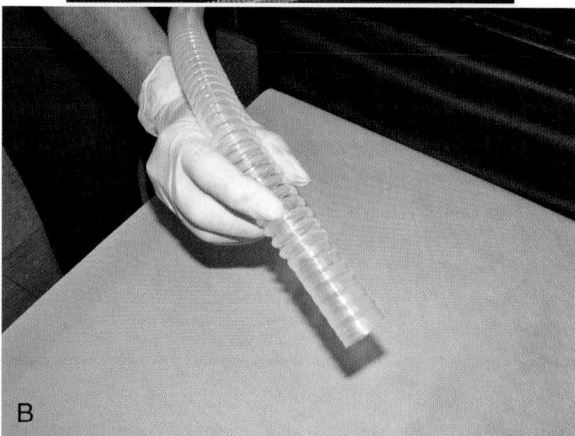

FIGURE 30-15 A, Plume evacuator. **B,** The plume evacuator hose is sterilized so that it can be used as the surgical site and directed by sterile personnel. The circulating nurse attaches the hose to the evacuator and controls the unit.

| **BOX 30-2** | Laser Safety Protocol for Patients |

- Sterile saline must be available for the surgeon at all times.
- The patient's eyes are to be shielded during laser use.
- Tissues surrounding the laser surgical field are to be covered with moistened sponges.
- A backstop such as moistened gauze sponges is to be used to prevent laser penetration beyond the desired depth. This is especially important when working over hollow organs.
- Flammable anesthetic agents including pressurized oxygen are not to come in contact with the laser beam.
- Shielded endotracheal tubes must be used if laser penetration of the trachea or the upper respiratory tract is possible.

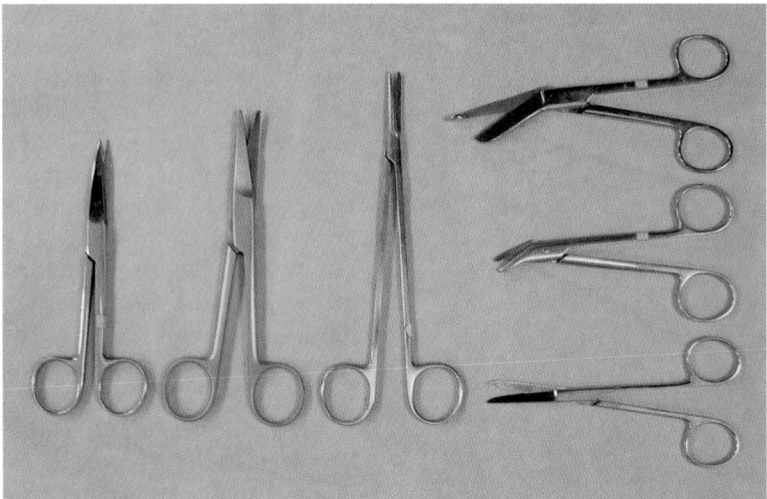

FIGURE 30-16 *Scissors. Left to right:* Sharp-sharp operating scissors. Mayo dissecting scissors and Metzenbaum dissecting scissors. *At right, from top to bottom:* Lister bandage scissors, wire-cutting scissors, Littauer suture removal scissors.

straight or curved scissors used for cutting delicate tissue, such as fat or thin muscle. Metzenbaum scissors are preferred for most soft tissue dissection and come in a wide variety of sizes. Most have rounded points and plain blades. They should never be used for cutting suture because this dulls the edges and causes the blades to separate and lose effectiveness. *Stitch scissors* or *Littauer suture removal scissors* are used to cut all sutures except wire sutures. *Wire suture–cutting scissors* can cut wire suture. *Lister bandage scissors* are available to cut bandage material. One blade of the Lister scissors is blunted to facilitate sliding under a bandage without poking the skin. To prolong the life of any scissors, it should be used only for its intended purpose.

> **TECHNICIAN NOTE** Scissors are specifically designed for many purposes, including dissecting tissue and cutting suture or bandage materials. Each pair of scissors should be used only for its intended purpose.

NEEDLE HOLDERS

Needle holders, also commonly called *needle drivers*, are used to grasp and pass suture needles with suture through tissue; needle holders can also be used to perform tying of suture knots. The two most commonly used needle holders in veterinary medicine are *Mayo-Hegar and Olsen-Hegar* (Figure 30-17). Various other designs have been manufactured for specific uses such as microsurgery and ophthalmic surgery. The primary difference between Mayo-Hegar and Olsen-Hegar needle holders is the presence of built-in scissors. The Olsen-Hegar needle holder contains built-in scissors, and close attention needs to be paid when they are used because suture can be inadvertently cut. Advantages of the Olsen-Hegar needle holder include a potential increase in surgical speed and the fact that the surgeon can work alone without the assistance of another individual to cut suture.

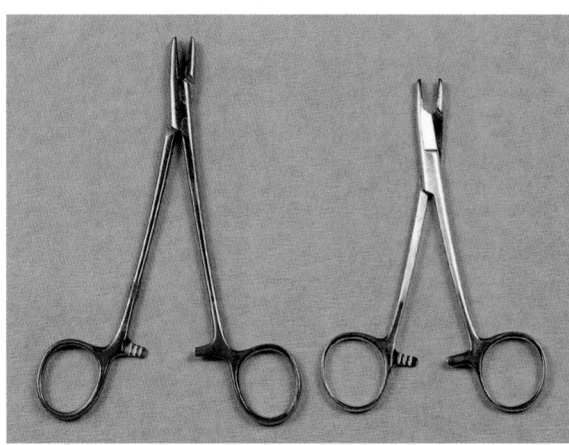

FIGURE 30-17 Needle holders. Mayo-Hegar needle holder *(left)*, Olsen-Hegar needle holder *(right)*.

Similar to other instruments described below, needle holders have a set of jaws and a **box lock**; further, a ratcheted locking device allows suture needles to be held within the jaws of the needle holder without falling out or twisting (Figure 30-18). Improper use of needle holders (such as using a needle holder that is too small for the size of the needle or using a needle holder to bend or twist wire) not only may damage the jaws but also may spring the box lock and **ratchet**, thereby ruining the instrument. High-quality needle holders often contain within their jaws tungsten carbide inserts that are replaceable. These inserts allow for excellent grip and are resistant to wear. When jaws or inserts become worn down, the jaws of a needle holder may close incorrectly, preventing appropriate grasping of the needles or accidental cutting of suture; it is important to replace worn down inserts to prevent these potential complications.

> **TECHNICIAN NOTE** Needle holders are designed for handling the suture needle and performing instrument suture ties.

THUMB FORCEPS

Thumb forceps have a spring action, and the jaws are opposed by manually compressing the two metal handles together. These forceps are important in the manipulation of tissues and are designed in several different sizes and grasping surfaces to be selected according to the intended use (Figure 30-19, *A* through *C*). *Brown-Adson thumb forceps* are used very commonly in veterinary medicine. They have multiple intermeshing teeth with a broad tip to provide good tissue and suture needle handling for most routine suturing and wound/incisional closures. *Rat-tooth thumb forceps* have large interdigitating teeth and are used primarily for skin or fascia. *Adson thumb forceps* have delicate intermeshing teeth that provide a good, atraumatic grasp of delicate tissues. They are commonly used during dissection of muscle and more delicate connective tissues. *Cooley* and *DeBakey thumb forceps* have long, narrow jaws with multiple delicate sets of teeth, are relatively atraumatic, and are especially good for vascular surgery. *Russian thumb forceps* have a broad curved surface that is good for needle handling, but they are traumatic when used to hold tissues. Additionally, many thumb forceps intended for skin manipulation (e.g., Brown-Adson thumb forceps) contain replaceable tungsten carbide inserts that facilitate secure needle handling during suture application, similar to those present on quality needle holders.

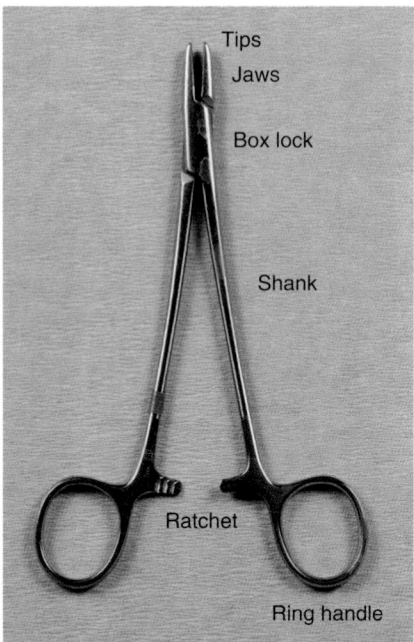

FIGURE 30-18 Basic components of a surgical instrument.

> ⓘ **TECHNICIAN NOTE** Thumb forceps are commonly used in the surgeon's nondominant hand to hold tissues while dissecting or suturing.

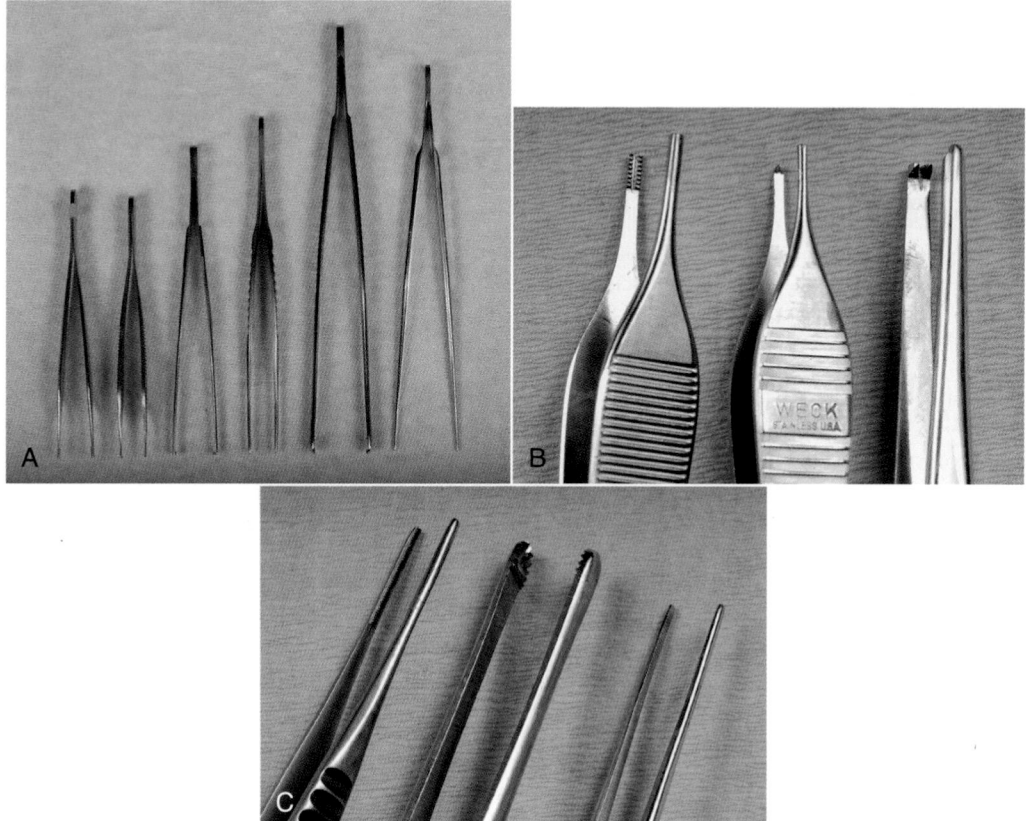

FIGURE 30-19 Thumb forceps. **A,** *Left to right:* Brown-Adson thumb forceps, Adson thumb forceps, rat-tooth thumb forceps, DeBakey vascular thumb forceps, Russian thumb forceps, dressing thumb forceps. **B,** Close-up of tips *(left to right):* Brown-Adson thumb forceps, Adson thumb forceps, rat-tooth thumb forceps. **C,** Close-up of tips *(left to right):* DeBakey vascular thumb forceps, Russian thumb forceps, dressing thumb forceps.

TISSUE FORCEPS

Tissue forceps are locking instruments that clamp tissues (Figure 30-20). Similar to needle holders, they contain a set of jaws, a box lock, and handles with a ratcheted locking device. Various tooth patterns allow different types of tissue forceps to grip tissue with variable strength and secondary tissue trauma. *Allis tissue forceps* securely grasp tissue but cause significant tissue crushing. Allis tissue forceps are therefore considered to be "traumatic forceps" and should be used only on tissues that are being removed from the patient (e.g., tumors, damaged bowel, etc.). These tissue forceps are also commonly used to secure patient drapes and instrument cords (e.g., cautery and suction). *Babcock forceps* are similar in shape to Allis tissue forceps but are considerably less traumatic for tissues at the expense of reduced tissue security. Babcock forceps are less traumatic as a result of their smoother grasping surface and less stiff design. *Doyen intestinal tissue forceps* are designed with flexible, atraumatic jaws

that allow them to safely clamp off viable portions of bowel and other delicate tissues. As has been discussed, generally speaking, the less traumatic the forceps, the less tissue holding security they afford.

> **TECHNICIAN NOTE** Tissue forceps use a self-locking mechanism to clamp and hold tissues.

HEMOSTATIC FORCEPS

Hemostatic forceps, also known simply as *hemostats*, are tissue forceps named for their function—to stop bleeding by crushing tissues and associated blood vessels (Figures 30-21 and 30-22). Types of hemostatic forceps are classified according to their size, the pattern of the grooves on the inside surface of the jaws, and whether they are straight or curved. Most hemostats have transverse grooves on the inside surface of the jaws to better grasp the tissue. *Halsted mosquito*

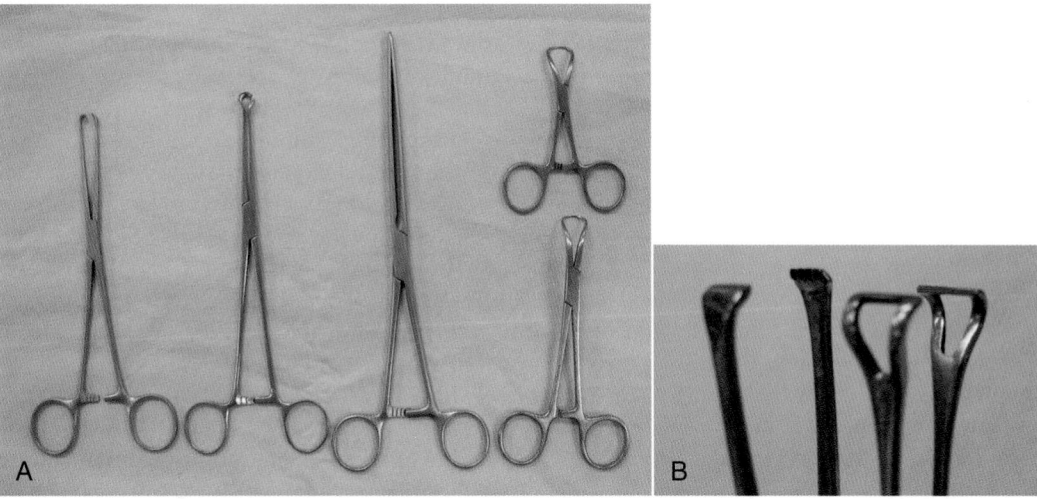

FIGURE 30-20 Tissue forceps. **A,** *Left to right:* Allis tissue forceps, Babcock tissue forceps, Doyen intestinal tissue forceps, Backhaus towel clamps (two sizes). **B,** *Close-up of tips:* Allis tissue forceps *(left)*, Babcock tissue forceps *(right)*.

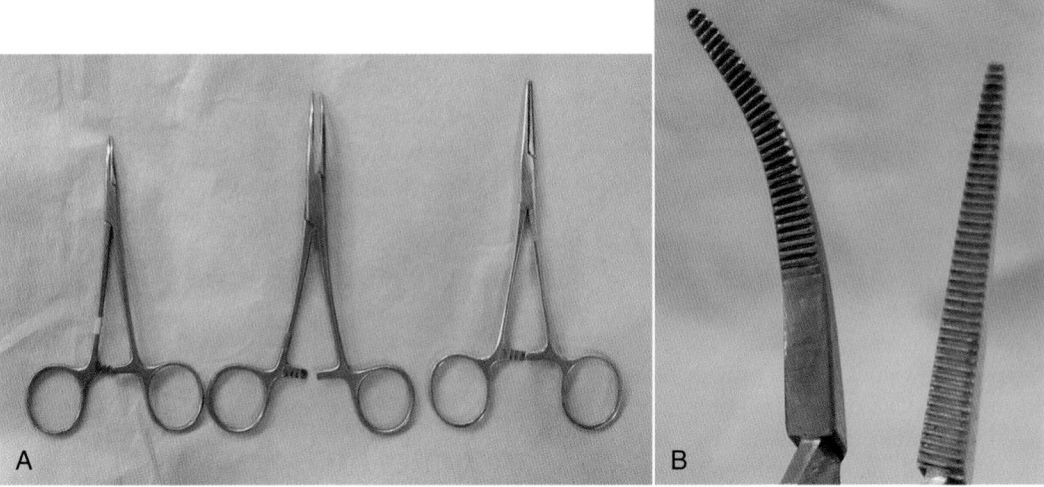

FIGURE 30-21 Hemostatic forceps. **A,** *Left to right:* Halsted mosquito hemostatic forceps, Kelly forceps, Crile forceps. **B,** *Close-up of jaws:* curved Kelly *(left)*, straight Crile *(right)*.

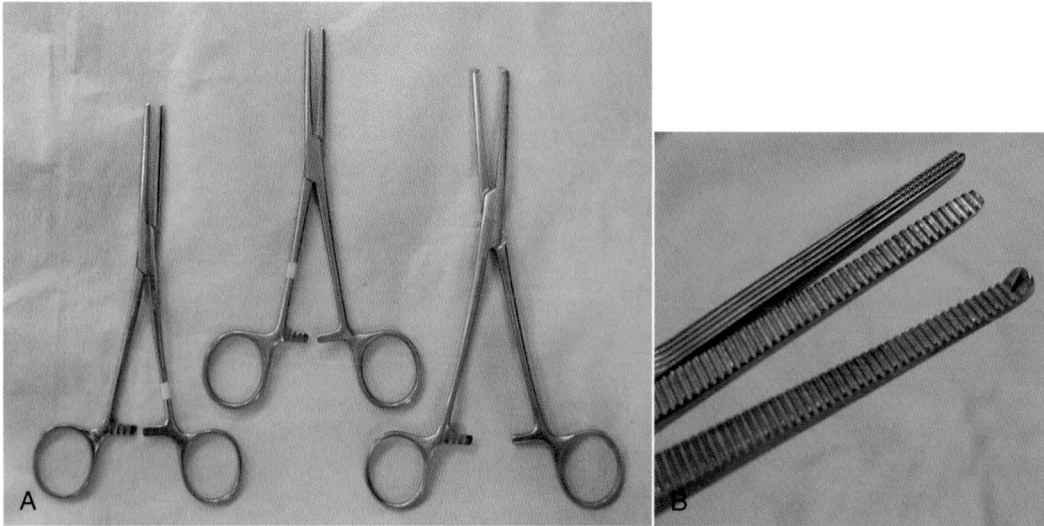

FIGURE 30-22 Hemostatic forceps. **A,** *Left to right:* Rochester-Carmalt forceps, Rochester-Péan forceps, Rochester-Ochsner forceps. **B,** Close-up of jaws *(left to right):* Rochester-Carmalt forceps, Rochester-Péan forceps, Rochester-Ochsner forceps.

hemostats are small and are designed to occlude small vessels. *Crile forceps* and *Kelly forceps* are similar in design to mosquito hemostats but are larger for use in crushing larger tissues and vessels. Crile and Kelly forceps differ in their jaw tooth pattern. Crile forceps contain transverse grooves that extend the entire length of the jaws. Kelly forceps contain grooves associated with only the distal-most aspect of the jaws. *Rochester-Péan forceps* are large, transversely grooved forceps that are used to clamp tissue bundles and large vessels. *Rochester-Ochsner forceps* are similar to Rochester-Péan forceps, but they have interdigitating teeth at the tips that aid in grasping the tissue. Rochester-Ochsner forceps are used most commonly in orthopedic or large animal surgery. *Rochester-Carmalt forceps* are large, crushing forceps with longitudinal grooves and cross-grooves at the tip to provide greater traction. These forceps are used for clamping across tissue that contains vessels. The most common use of Rochester-Carmalt forceps is to crush and hold the tissues and vessels of the ovary during routine spay in small animals.

> **TECHNICIAN NOTE** Hemostatic forceps are used to clamp, crush, and hold blood vessels with a self-locking mechanism.

RETRACTORS

Surgical retractors are used to atraumatically improve the field of visualization and are commonly used both in soft tissue and during orthopedic surgical procedures. Properly placed hand-held or self-retaining retractors should not interfere with surgery but rather should provide more room for the surgeon to work. The most commonly used hand-held retractors are shown in Figure 30-23. The *Army-Navy retractor* and the *Senn retractor* are double-ended hand-held retractors commonly used to retract skin, fat, or muscle. The Army-Navy retractor has smooth blades, whereas the Senn

has one smooth blade and one blade with three sharp or blunt prongs. The *malleable retractor* is made of thin metal that is easily bent to the desired shape and is especially useful for retracting abdominal and thoracic organs. The *Snook ovariohysterectomy hook*, or spay hook, is a specialized type of hand-held retractor used to grasp the horn of the uterus during an ovariohysterectomy. The *Hohmann retractor* consists of a single blade and a handle that are used to lever tissues out of the way for better visibility. It is used almost exclusively in orthopedic surgery and can provide good visibility in certain joint surgeries.

In contrast to hand-held tissue retractors, self-retaining retractors (Figures 30-24 and 30-25) can be locked in place and maintained in an optimal position without the need for a surgical assistant for tissue retraction. The *Balfour retractor* provides increased exposure of the abdominal cavity. The two wire-like blades are used to distract the abdominal incision, and the solid spoon-like blade is hooked onto the sternum to distract it cranially. It is important to ensure that no abdominal contents (e.g., bowel, spleen) are entrapped between the body wall and the retractor during placement. The *Finochietto rib spreader* retracts the ribs to expose the surgical field within the thoracic cavity. The ratcheted part of the retractors is positioned at the dorsal or cranial aspect of the thoracic incision so that it does not interfere with the surgeon. *Gelpi retractors* and *Weitlaner retractors* are self-retaining retractors commonly used for muscle retraction, especially in orthopedic and neurologic surgery.

> **TECHNICIAN NOTE** Retractors rather than hands are used to retract tissues and provide good visibility of the surgical site.

SUCTION TIPS

Various suction tip designs are commonly used in both small and large animal surgery (Figure 30-26). The suction tip is

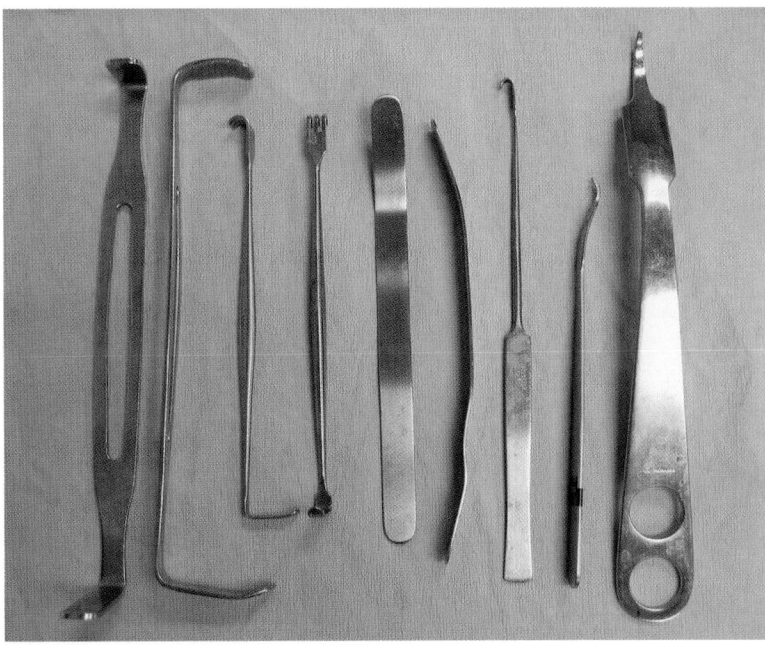

FIGURE 30-23 Hand-held retractors. *Left to right:* Two Army-Navy retractors, two Senn retractors, two small malleable retractors, Snook ovariohysterectomy hook (spay hook), two Hohmann retractors (different sizes).

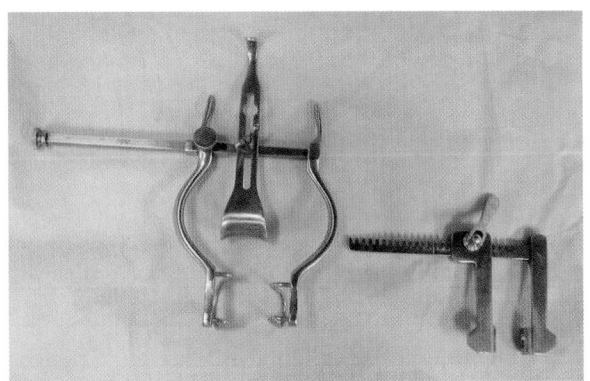

FIGURE 30-24 Self-retaining retractors. Balfour abdominal retractor *(left)*, Finochietto rib retractor *(right)*.

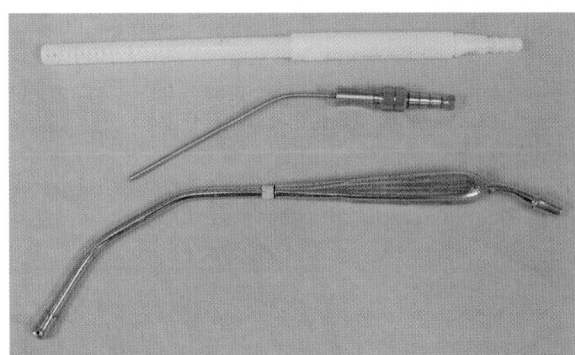

FIGURE 30-26 Suction tips. *Top to bottom:* Poole, Frazier, Yankauer. The suction tip is attached to a sterile hose. The surgeon hands the other end of the hose to a nonsterile assistant to plug it into the suction unit.

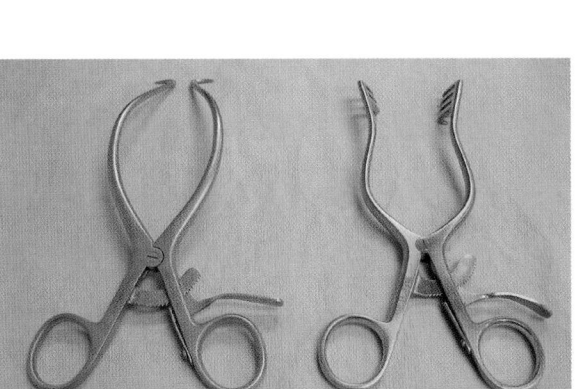

FIGURE 30-25 Self-retaining retractors. Gelpi retractor *(left)*, Weitlaner retractor *(right)*.

attached to a long, sterile suction tube that is connected to a vacuum source, often by the nonsterile surgical nurse or anesthesia technician. The *Poole suction tip* is used primarily in the abdominal or thoracic cavity because it has an outer sleeve with small holes to prevent tissue, such as fat, from becoming entrapped in the tip. The *Frazier tip* is used most commonly in orthopedic and neurologic surgery. The *Yankauer tip* is a general purpose suction tip.

STAPLING EQUIPMENT

Several different surgical stapling devices are available for an array of purposes (Figures 30-27 and 30-28) and offer the advantage of fast and easy application relative to hand suturing. The most commonly used stapling devices include the ligate-divide-separate (LDS), thoracoabdominal (TA) and

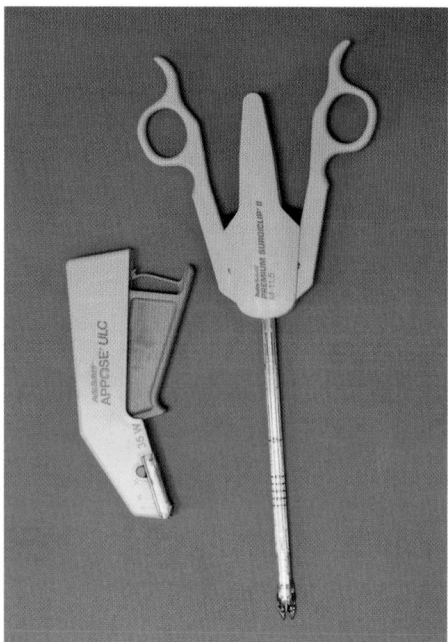

FIGURE 30-27 Skin *(top)* and vascular "hemo" clips *(bottom)*.

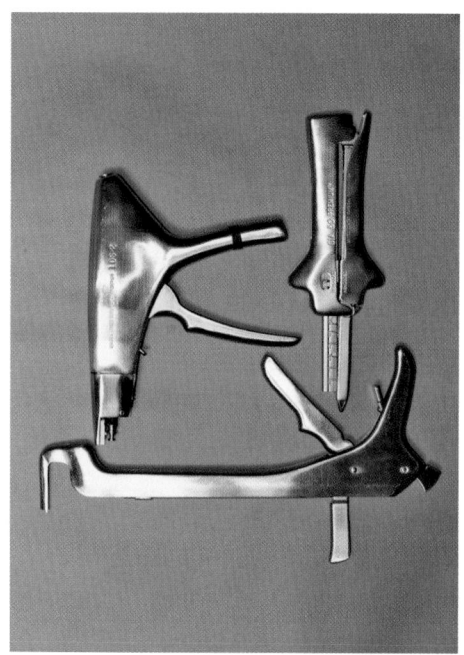

FIGURE 30-28 Surgical stapling equipment. *Left,* Ligate-divide-separate (LDS) stapling device applies two staples to tissue and cuts between staples. *Right,* Gastrointestinal anastomosis (GIA) gastrointestinal stapler. Cartridge of staples for one-time use is purchased in a presterilized package. *Bottom,* Thoracoabdominal stapler (TA). Staple cartridges are purchased as for GIA. Shown here without staple cartridges in place.

gastrointestinal anastomosis (GIA), as well as surgical clips (Ligaclip, Ethicon, Somerville, NJ) and skin staples. Some stapling devices (LDS and GIA) also cut tissue after stapling. The staplers are named by an abbreviation of their designed function (Table 30-2). A number may be used after the name "thoracoabdominal stapler (TA)" or "gastrointestinal stapler (GIA)" to indicate the length of the row of staples (e.g., a TA 30 places rows of staples in a line 30 mm long).

VASCULAR SEALING DEVICES

Various vascular sealing devices allow for ligation of vessels much larger than that afforded by traditional bipolar and monopolar electrocautery units. Such devices use a combination of pressure and energy output to achieve adequate vessel fusion (e.g., sealing of vessels upward of 7 mm in diameter compared with 1 to 2 mm, which is achievable with traditional monopolar and bipolar cautery) (Figure 30-29, *A* and *B*). Many of these devices have been designed for both open surgical techniques (e.g., laparotomy, thoracotomy) and minimally invasive surgical techniques (e.g., laparoscopy, thoracoscopy).

OPHTHALMIC INSTRUMENTS

Ophthalmic surgery, like many other surgical subspecialties, requires highly specialized and often delicate instruments. Gentle and safe handling of such instruments is necessary to keep them functioning properly for extended periods. Basic ophthalmic operative packs include specialized scalpels (e.g., No. 7 scalpel handle), fine scissors (e.g., iris and strabismus scissors), thumb forceps, needle holders (e.g., Castroviejo ophthalmic needle holders), retractors

TABLE 30-2	Stapling Equipment		
DERIVATION OF NAME	**COMMON USE**	**COMMENTS**	
TA			
Thoracoabdominal	Lung and liver lobe resection	Places double or triple row of staples	
GIA			
Gastrointestinal anastomosis	Gastrointestinal resection and anastomosis	Places four rows of staples and cuts between the middle two rows	
EEA			
End-to-end anastomosis	Gastrointestinal anastomosis	Staples two intestinal segments together in a circular manner with a functional lumen	
Ligaclip stapler	Vessel ligation	Places a single staple	
Skin stapler	Skin and fascia closures	Places a single staple	
LDS			
Ligate-and-divide stapler	Blood vessel ligation	Places two staples on a vessel and cuts between them	

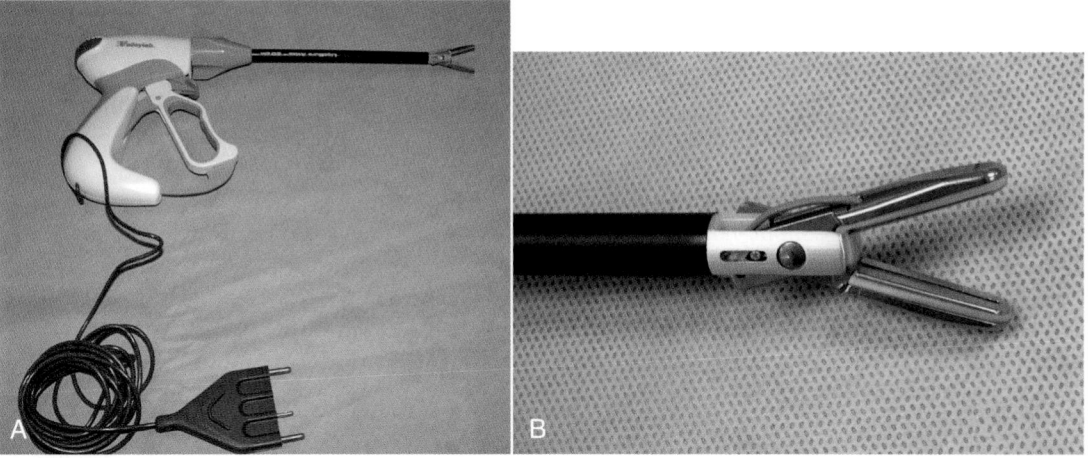

FIGURE 30-29 Vascular sealing device (Ligasure Atlas, Covidien, Irvine, California). Hand-held unit **(A)**, close-up of sealing tip **(B)**.

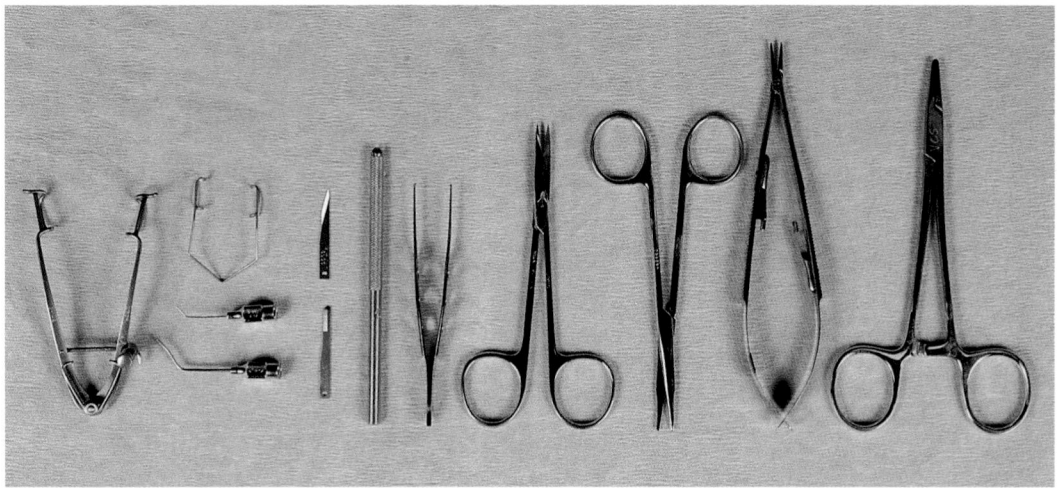

FIGURE 30-30 Common ophthalmic instruments. *Left to right:* Lid speculum, small lid speculum *(above)* and lacrimal cannulas *(below)*, beaver blade handle with #64 and #65 surgical blades, Bishop-Harmon thumb forceps, iris scissors, tenotomy scissors, Castroviejo needle holder, and Derf needle holder.

(e.g., Chalazion and Graeffe eyelid retractors), and lacrimal duct cannulas (Figure 30-30).

ORTHOPEDIC INSTRUMENTS

PERIOSTEAL ELEVATORS

Periosteal elevators are instruments that are used to pry periosteum or muscle from the bone surface. They have a blade-like structure at one or both ends of a handle. The blades have sharp or blunt edges and are available in various sizes (Figure 30-31). The Freer elevator is the most commonly used periosteal elevator in small animal orthopedics.

RONGEURS

Rongeurs are hand-held instruments with sharp, cupped tips that are used to cut small pieces of dense tissue, such as bone, cartilage, or fibrous tissue (Figure 30-32, *A* and *B*). *Bone-cutting forceps* are similar to rongeurs but have paired chisel-like tips. They are used for cutting bone and should not be

mistaken for wire cutters (Figure 30-33). Rongeurs have a double-action or single-action mechanism. *Double-action rongeurs* have a smooth cutting action and are mechanically stronger than single-action rongeurs, and they are also larger. Double-action rongeurs are preferred for removing large amounts of dense tissue. *Single-action rongeurs* are more commonly used in confined areas such as joints and the spinal canal. *Kerrison rongeurs*, which have a gun-shaped appearance, are used specifically in spinal surgery.

CURETTES

Curettes are used to scrape hard tissue, such as bone or cartilage. These instruments are often included in both orthopedic and arthroscopic surgical packs. Curettes are designed with a small, cup-like structure at one or both ends of a handle (similar to an ice cream scoop). The cup has a sharp cutting edge and is available in various sizes (Figure 30-34). Bone curettes are commonly used to retrieve cancellous bone from the medullary cavity (tibia, humerus, ilium) for use as a bone graft. Cancellous bone grafts are often used during fracture repair. Curettes are also commonly used during arthroscopic surgery to débride joint surfaces and to dislodge loose, bony fragments within joints.

BONE-HOLDING FORCEPS

Bone-holding forceps are designed to hold bone and bone fragments in alignment while orthopedic implants (screws, pins, wires, or plates) are applied. Most bone-holding forceps are self-retaining. Bone-holding forceps are available in a variety of designs and sizes. The most commonly used types are displayed in Figure 30-35. *Kern bone-holding forceps* have a ratcheted handle that allows them to be clamped securely onto the bone. Clam shell and point-to-point bone-holding

forceps have a locking mechanism similar to that of needle holders and hemostatic forceps. *Self-retaining bone-holding forceps*, also known as *speed locks*, have a nut that tightens against one handle to squeeze the handles together.

OSTEOTOMES AND CHISELS

Osteotomes and chisels are used to cut bone. Osteotomes and chisels are used by pounding on the flat or flared end of the instrument with a mallet (Figure 30-36). The cutting edge of the osteotome is tapered on both sides, whereas the chisel is tapered only on one side. Osteotomes and chisels are made from relatively soft metal and should not be used for purposes other than their intended use.

GIGLI WIRE

Gigli wire is used to cut bone by placing the wire around the bone and drawing it back and forth in a sawing fashion.

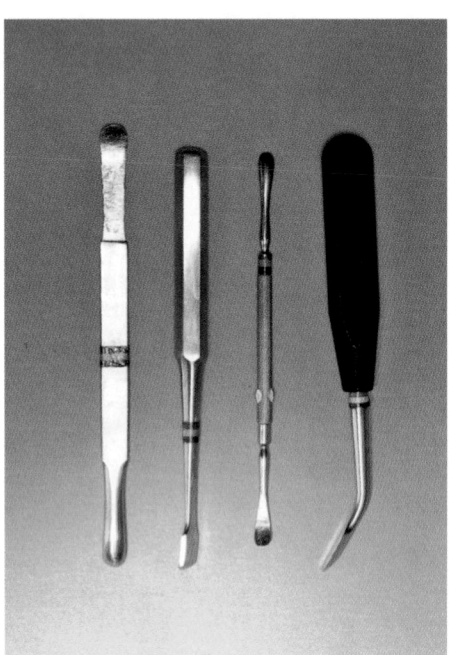

FIGURE 30-31 Periosteal elevators. *Top to bottom:* Seldin retractor, Key elevator, Freer elevator, and AO-round edge periosteal elevator.

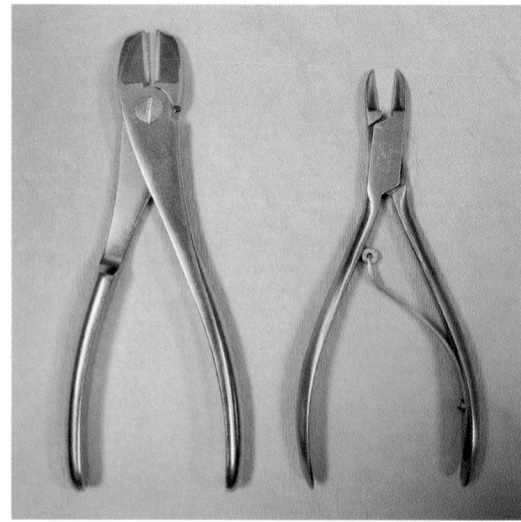

FIGURE 30-33 Wire cutters *(left)* and bone cutters *(right)*. They look similar but should not be confused. Bone cutters have finer jaws.

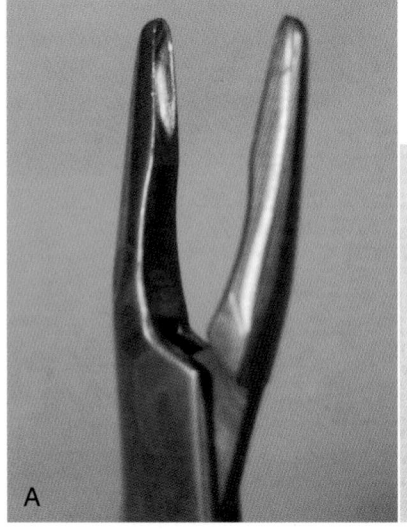
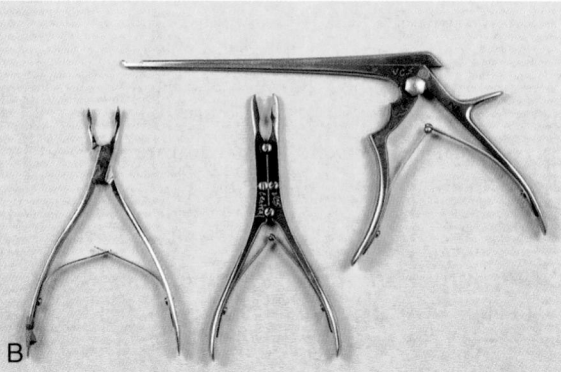

FIGURE 30-32 Rongeurs. **A,** Close-up of tips. **B,** *Left to right:* Single-action rongeur, double-action rongeur, Kerrison rongeur.

T-shaped handles hook onto the wire to allow the surgeon to firmly grasp the wire.

TREPHINES AND JAMSHIDI NEEDLES

Trephines and Jamshidi needles are specially designed to remove a core of bone for biopsy. Trephines are T-shaped, reusable, stainless steel tubular instruments with a cylindrical cutting blade similar to a traditional punch biopsy (Figure 30-37). The Jamshidi is a similar instrument but is often single use and disposable.

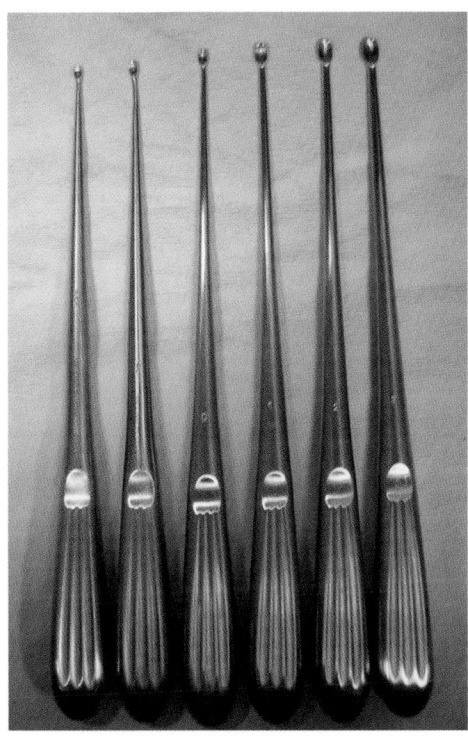

FIGURE 30-34 Bone curettes of various sizes.

POWER EQUIPMENT

Power equipment is commonly used in orthopedic and neurologic surgery. Although some drills are electric or battery powered (Figure 30-38, *A* and *B*), many orthopedic drills and saws are powered by nitrogen gas that is supplied via a sterile hose (Figure 30-38, *C*). The Hall air drill is a specialized high-speed bur that grinds bone (Figure 30-38, *D*). It is used most commonly for spinal surgery. Many of these instruments cannot tolerate autoclave steam sterilization; therefore, **gas sterilization** or covering with sterile coverings is required for their use in sterile procedures. This is discussed in detail in the next section.

ORTHOPEDIC IMPLANTS

Orthopedic surgery sometimes involves the use of various products that are placed into or around the bone and are left in place permanently or for an extended time. Metal implants usually are made of stainless steel alloy, cobalt-chromium alloy, or titanium. Of these three types, titanium is the most resistant to corrosion and has the best fatigue life. It is also the most expensive. Although it is beyond the scope of this chapter to go into great detail regarding various orthopedic implants, it is important to be conceptually familiar with general implant types and uses.

BONE PINS

Bone pins vary in diameter, length, and types of points. *Steinmann pins* are smooth, stainless steel pins ranging in diameter from $\frac{1}{16}$ to $\frac{1}{4}$ inch. Three different types of pin points are available, including chisel, trocar, or threaded trocar. Steinmann pins may also be called *intramedullary (IM) pins* because they are often placed in the medullary cavity of long bones for fracture fixation. *Kirschner wires (K-wires)* are similar to Steinmann pins, but they are smaller and can be used to pin small bone fragments. Available sizes

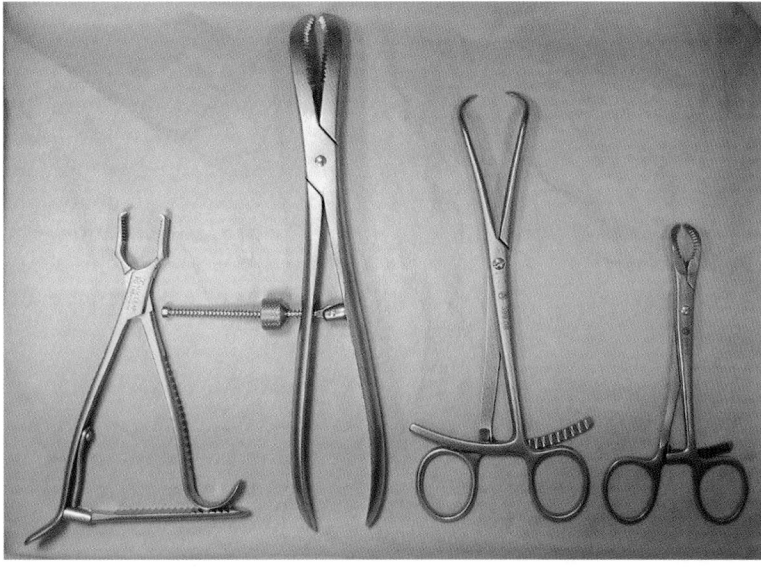

FIGURE 30-35 Bone-holding forceps. *Left to right:* Small Kern forceps, large speed-lock forceps, large point-to-point forceps, small clamshell forceps.

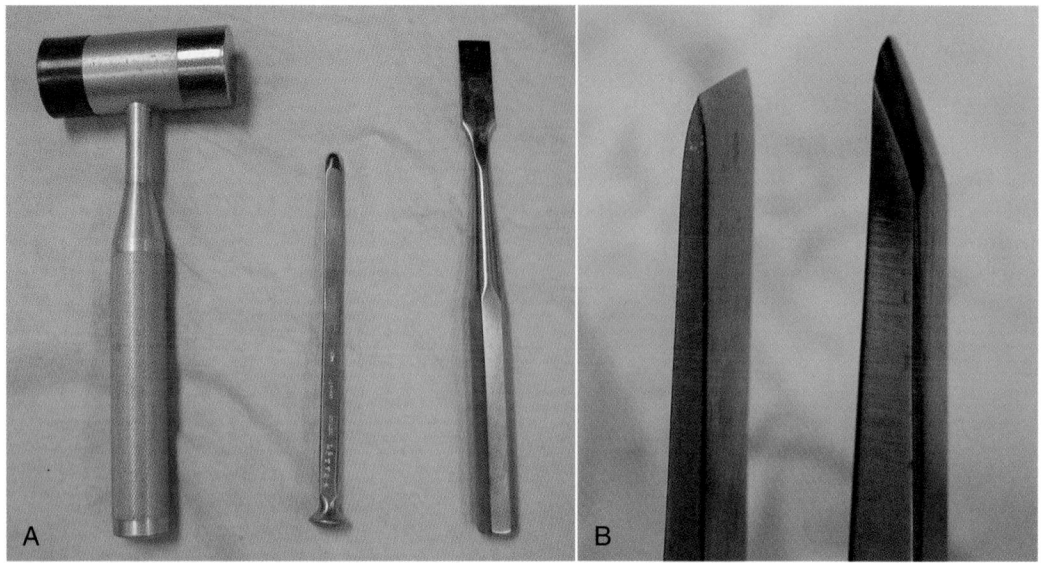

FIGURE 30-36 A, Mallet, chisel, and osteotome. B, Osteotome *(left)* and chisel *(right).*

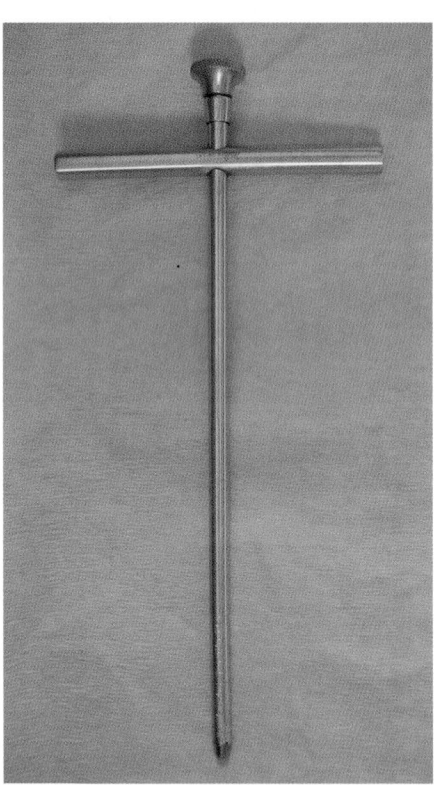

FIGURE 30-37 Michel trephine.

TABLE 30-3	Commonly Used Orthopedic Wire Sizes	
GAUGE	**INCHES**	**MILLIMETERS**
22	0.025	0.64
20	0.032	0.81
18	0.040	1.02

INTERLOCKING NAILS

Interlocking nails are similar to IM pins but have preplaced holes through the pin that allow screw placement. Interlocking nails provide more rigid fixation than is provided by IM pins alone, and they provide resistance to compression and rotational forces. Equipment is similar to that required for pins, but specialized equipment is needed to guide screw placement.

ORTHOPEDIC WIRE

Stainless steel orthopedic wire or cerclage wire is supplied on spools (Figure 30-41); sizes most commonly used in small animal surgery are 22 gauge, 20 gauge, and 18 gauge (Table 30-3). It is most commonly applied in a cerclage fashion by encircling the bone or bone fragments and twisting the ends in a twist-tie. Special wire twisters, similar in appearance to standard needle holders, are used to fasten cerclage wire in their twist-tie fashion.

EXTERNAL FIXATORS

External fixators have gained popularity in recent years because of their ease of placement and their use as a means of providing fixation without disrupting the fracture site (e.g., closed fracture reduction techniques). External fixation is a means of stabilizing fractures using pins or wire placed through skin and bone. The pins or k-wires are held rigid by

are 0.035 inch, 0.045 inch, and 0.062 inch diameter. Some pins have threads, similar to a screw, which are used most commonly for extraskeletal fixator placement (Figure 30-39). The threads can be located at the end of a pin or in the middle, and they can have a positive or negative profile. A power drill or a Jacobs hand chuck is required to insert the pin into bone, and a pin cutter is necessary to cut it to the proper length (Figure 30-40).

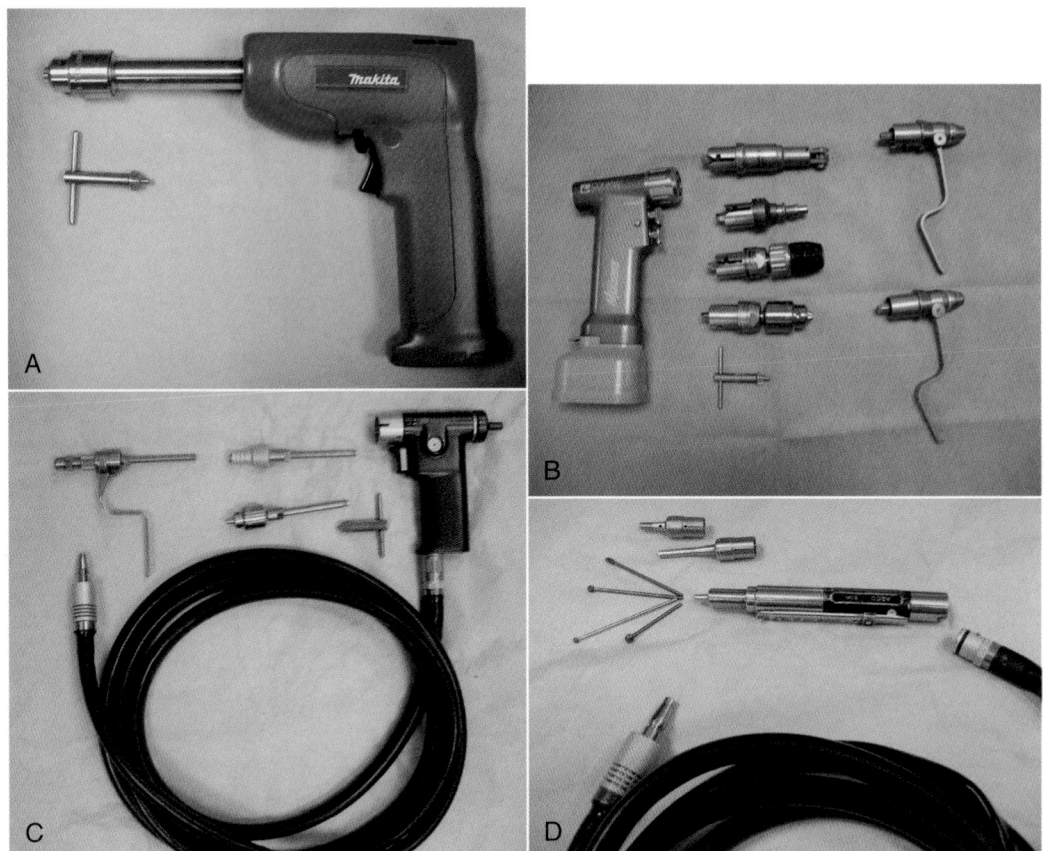

FIGURE 30-38 Power equipment. **A,** The Makita drill is an example of a battery-powered drill. **B,** ConMed Linvatec battery-powered handpiece *(left).* Attachments shown include *(center, top to bottom)* saw blade attachment, quick release for drill bit, keyless chuck, and Jacobs chuck with key, and *(right)* pin and wire drivers. **C,** The 3M mini-driver is powered by a tank of pressurized nitrogen gas. It has an attachment for K-wires and quick-release or chuck attachments for drill bits. **D,** The Hall air drill has various sizes and shapes of burs, and two bur guards of different lengths.

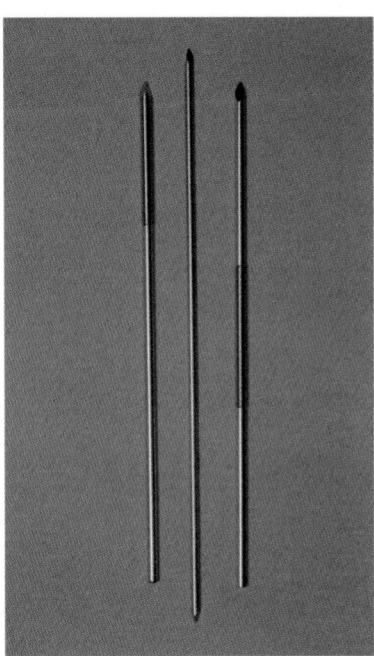

FIGURE 30-39 Various pin types. *Top to bottom:* Positive end-threaded pin, smooth pin, and positive central-threaded pin.

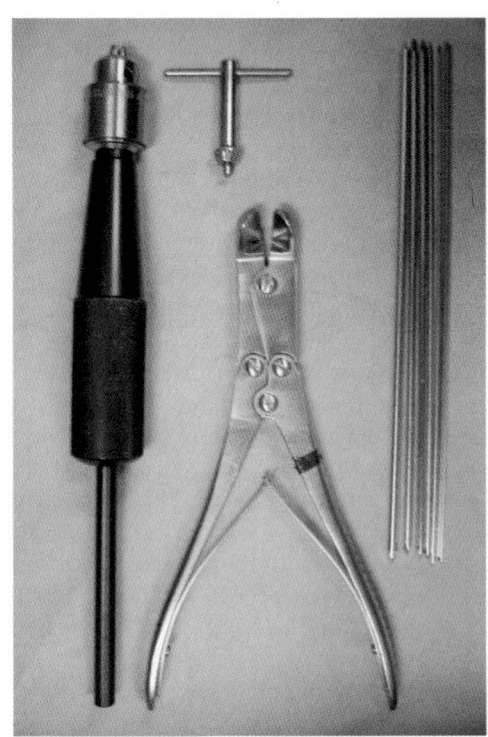

FIGURE 30-40 Jacobs hand chuck, key, pin cutter, and various sizes of Steinmann pins and K-wires.

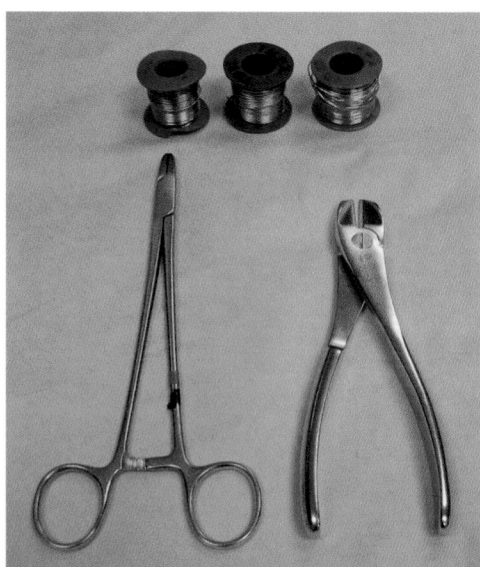

FIGURE 30-41 Orthopedic wire, wire twisters, wire cutters. Wire twisters look similar to needle holders but are more rugged and are designed to withstand higher forces.

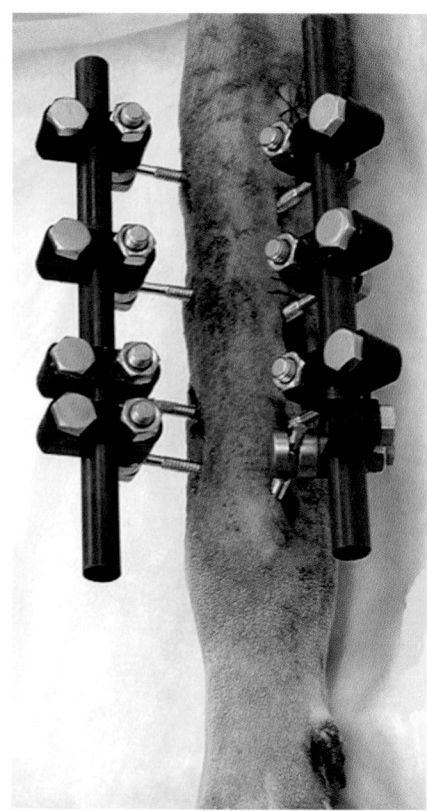

FIGURE 30-42 An external fixator on the radius of a dog. Pins that penetrate the skin and bone are fixed to bars with the use of special clamps. (Courtesy Dr. James Toombs.)

metal bars, rings, or by acrylic connecting bars attached to the pins at least 1 cm from the skin (Figure 30-42). If metal apparatus is used, special clamps are placed to attach a metal connecting bar to each pin.

BONE SCREWS

Orthopedic screws are available in many different lengths, diameters, and head patterns. Additionally, two basic screw designs are available: cortical and cancellous. Cortical screws are fully threaded screws that are designed for dense (cortical) bone. Cancellous screws may be fully threaded or partially threaded (e.g., lag style) and are made with wider threads to allow a better grip in softer cancellous bone (Figure 30-43).

The general steps of screw placement include drilling a hole in the bone, measuring the hole with a depth gauge to determine proper screw length, using a bone tap (a screwlike instrument with sharp threads) to cut a screw path in the bone, and inserting the screw with a specialized screwdriver. Newer screw designs include a self-tapping screw (negating the need for a bone tap), as well as locking screws, in which separate threads engage the bone and the plate. These two newer designs allow more rapid placement and a more stable fixation construct, respectively. Bone screws may be used alone or in conjunction with a bone plate or an interlocking nail.

Bone screws are named by both screw length and thread diameter (in millimeters). Screws commonly used in small animal surgery are 1.5-, 2.0-, 2.7- and 3.5-mm-diameter cortical screws and 4.0-mm-diameter cancellous screws. Larger (2.7- and 3.5-mm) screws often have hexagonal heads and are driven by the same hexagonal screwdriver; smaller screws (1.5- and 2.0-mm-diameter) have cruciate heads and require a small, cruciate screwdriver. Larger screws (4.5-, 5.5-, and

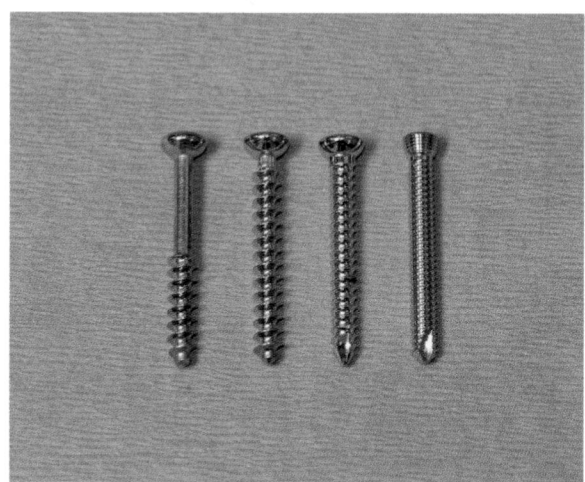

FIGURE 30-43 Bone screws. *Left to right:* Partially threaded 4.0-mm cancellous screw, fully threaded 4.0-mm cancellous screw, fully threaded 3.5-mm nonlocking cortical screw, and fully threaded 3.5-mm locking cortical screw.

6.5-mm-diameter) are used in large animal surgery. These screws use a large hexagonal screwdriver.

BONE PLATES

Bone plates come in many shapes, sizes, and types (Figure 30-44). First, bone plates are named by the number of screw holes and by the screw diameter size that best fits the plate.

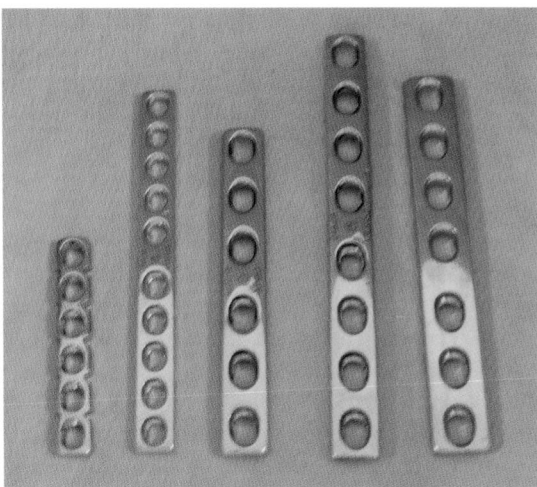

FIGURE 30-44 Bone plates of various sizes.

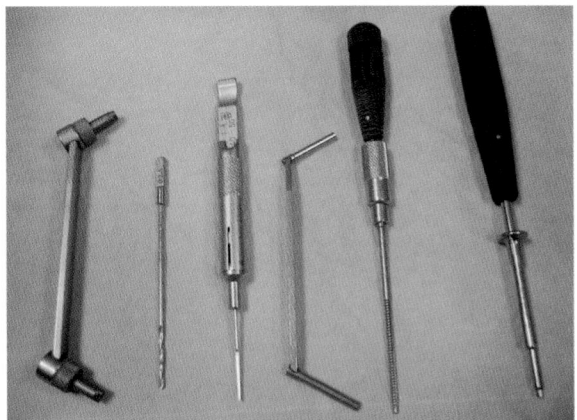

FIGURE 30-45 Bone plating equipment. *Left to right:* Drill guide, drill bit, depth gauge, tap sleeve (to prevent soft tissues from being caught on the bone tap), bone tap, and screwdriver.

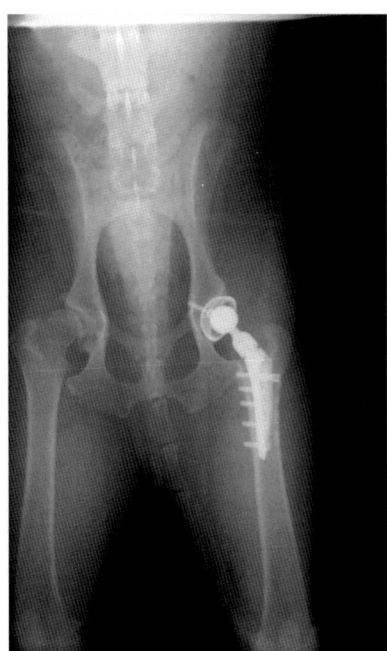

FIGURE 30-46 Radiograph of a dog with a total hip prosthesis.

For example, a seven-hole, 3.5-mm plate would have holes for seven 3.5-mm-diameter screws. Additionally, bone plates are classified according to whether they provide compression or not, and whether they house locking or nonlocking screws. Bone plates must be bent to match the curve of the bone and fastened to it with bone screws. Locking plates have specialized inserts that are placed into the threaded screw holes during bending to maintain the correct thread pattern.

Instrumentation required to apply a bone plate is highly specialized and includes drills, drill bits, drill guides, depth gauges, bone taps, tap sleeves, screws, screwdrivers, and plate benders (Figure 30-45), all of which are included in most general orthopedic plating packs. Although bone plating is more complex than other types of orthopedic fixation, and requires an extensive "inventory" of implants, the final result is often a more stable construct for healing.

TOTAL HIP PROSTHESIS

The hip joint may be replaced with a **prosthesis** in some dogs with severe arthritis (Figure 30-46). This procedure is done by highly trained veterinary surgeons and requires the use of specialized orthopedic equipment, in addition to the prosthesis itself. The femoral prosthesis consists of a long stem placed inside the proximal femur using bone cement or screws (cementless) and a ball that replaces the femoral head. A special cup replaces the acetabulum.

ARTHROSCOPIC INSTRUMENTS AND EQUIPMENT

The arthroscope is used as a diagnostic and surgical tool in veterinary surgery. It is used to examine various joints of the horse, including the scapulohumeral, humeroradial, carpal, fetlock, distal interphalangeal, coxofemoral (foals only), stifle, and tarsocrural joints. It is also used to examine various joints in the dog. Arthroscopy has many uses in both small and large animal surgery but classically is performed to remove **osteochondral fragments** and osteochondritic lesions on the articular surface in joints of young horses and dogs. Advances in technology and in surgeon proficiency have allowed arthroscopy to be performed in any joint for both diagnostic and treatment purposes. The arthroscope has been used to visualize intra-articular fractures during lag screw fixation, such as third carpal bone slab fractures in the carpus (knee) of horses, and to identify meniscal and cruciate injuries in dogs. Most of the equipment used in veterinary arthroscopy has been adapted from human arthroscopy. New technology is constantly being developed that will no doubt influence the veterinary field. This section is intended to allow the veterinary technician to become more familiar with the instruments and techniques of arthroscopy.

ARTHROSCOPE

The arthroscope is a rigid telescope that carries light into a joint cavity and produces a magnified image of the internal structures that is displayed on a viewing monitor. Different types of arthroscopes with various diameters and viewing angles have been developed, including a 5-mm-outer-diameter (OD) arthroscope with a 10-degree, 25-degree, or 70-degree lens viewing angle; a 4-mm OD with a 10-degree, 30-degree, 70-degree, or 110-degree lens angle; a 2.7-mm OD with a 5-degree, 30-degree, or 70-degree lens angle; and a 1.9-mm OD with a 5-degree or 30-degree lens angle. A 4-mm OD, 25-degree or 30-degree angled lens scope is generally used by most equine surgeons (Figure 30-47), whereas a 2.7-mm OD, 30-degree angled lens scope is commonly used for canine arthroscopy. Most arthroscopes have a small video camera that can be coupled to them, which allows the surgeon to view the joint on a video monitor (Figure 30-48). A video monitor offers the advantage of a larger, more crisp image. This greatly improves visualization of the intra-articular space compared with direct viewing through the eyepiece of the arthroscope. This method also allows better aseptic technique because the surgeon's face is not near the surgical field, and an assistant can operate the camera-scope unit, allowing the surgeon more freedom. A monitor also allows several persons to observe the procedure simultaneously, and a digital record can be made for future replay.

ANCILLARY ARTHROSCOPIC EQUIPMENT

Along with the arthroscope come various instruments used to introduce the scope into the joint and to work inside the joint. Stab incisions are made in the skin over the joint space through which the arthroscope and hand instruments will be inserted once the site has been surgically prepared and the animal has been positioned and draped for surgery.

Sharp Trocar and Sleeve

The *sharp trocar* is a pointed instrument that is inserted into a hollow, cannula-type instrument called the *arthroscope sleeve* (Figure 30-49). The trocar and the sleeve unit are used to penetrate the fibrous portion of the joint capsule through a stab incision.

Blunt Obturator

Once the sharp trocar has penetrated the fibrous joint capsule, the sharp trocar is replaced with a *conical* (blunt-tipped) **obturator** (Figure 30-50), which is used to penetrate

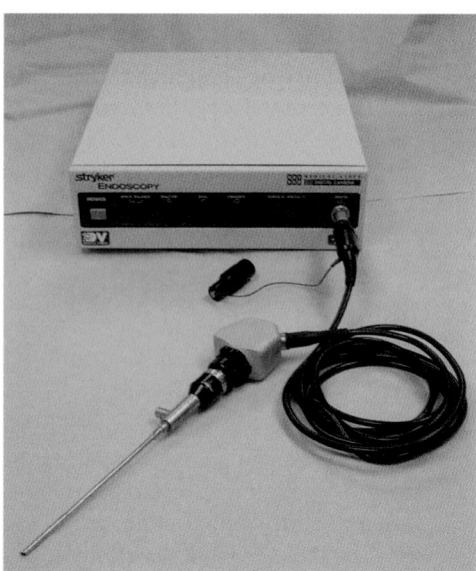

FIGURE 30-47 Video camera attached to a 4 mm-OD arthroscope.

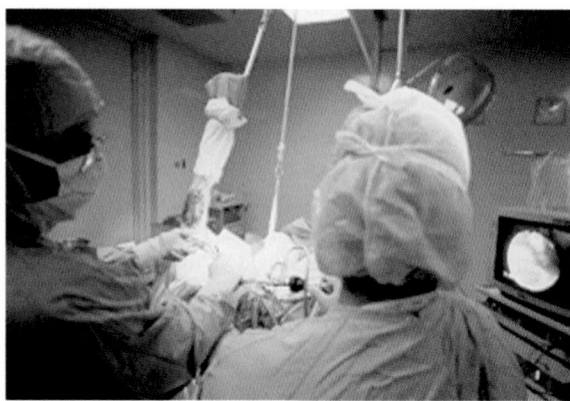

FIGURE 30-48 Most arthroscopic procedures are viewed on a monitor.

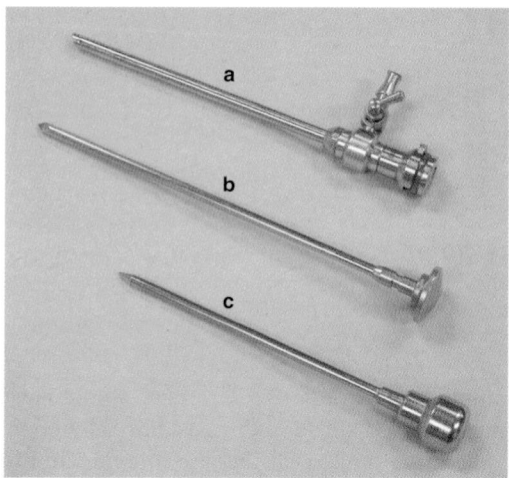

FIGURE 30-49 The sharp trocar (b) fits inside the arthroscope sleeve (a). The unit is used to penetrate the fibrous joint capsule through a stab incision in the skin. The conical obturator (c) replaces the sharp trocar in the sleeve once the fibrous joint capsule has been penetrated.

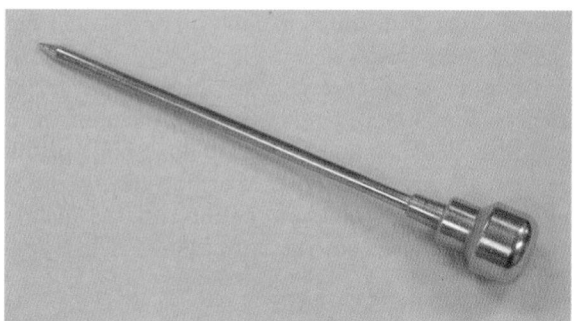

FIGURE 30-50 The conical obturator replaces the sharp trocar in the sleeve and is used to penetrate the synovial membrane portion of the joint capsule and to advance the sleeve farther into the joint.

the synovial membrane of the joint capsule and advance the arthroscope sleeve into the joint space with less risk of damaging the articular cartilage. At this point, the obturator is withdrawn from the sleeve. The joint space is distended with a sterile, balanced electrolyte solution (fluids) before placement of the sleeve in the joint, so a rush of fluid through the barrel of the sleeve will occur as the obturator is removed. The obturator is replaced with the *arthroscope* (Figure 30-51), which is designed to lock onto the sleeve once it is slid into position inside the sleeve.

Light Cable, Light Projector, and Video Camera

Modern arthroscopy is performed with the use of a light source, a video camera and viewing monitor, and ancillary power equipment. These are collectively stacked on a specially designed cart called the *tower* (Figure 30-52). A fiberoptic *light cable* (Figure 30-53) is attached directly to the optical light port on the arthroscope (Figure 30-54). A high-intensity light generated from a specially designed *light*

projector is fed through the fiberoptic cable and arthroscope to illuminate the joint space (Figure 30-55). It is important to note that fiberoptic cables are easily damaged if excessive bending or kinking occurs.

FLUID DELIVERY SYSTEMS

Sterile fluid—usually a balanced electrolyte solution—is infused into the joint under pressure to maintain distention

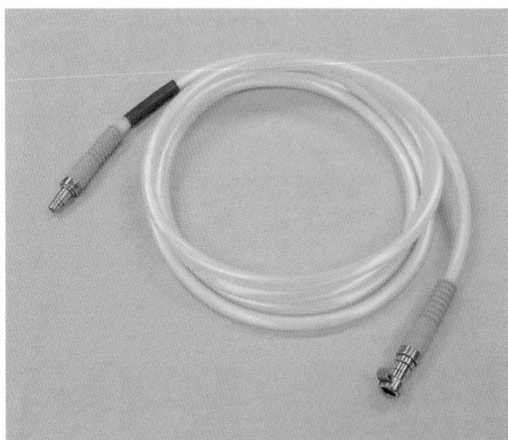

FIGURE 30-53 Fiberoptic light cable.

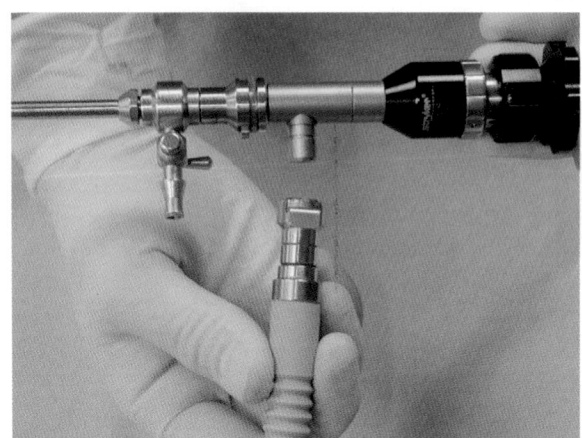

FIGURE 30-54 The fiberoptic light cable attaches to the light port of the arthroscope.

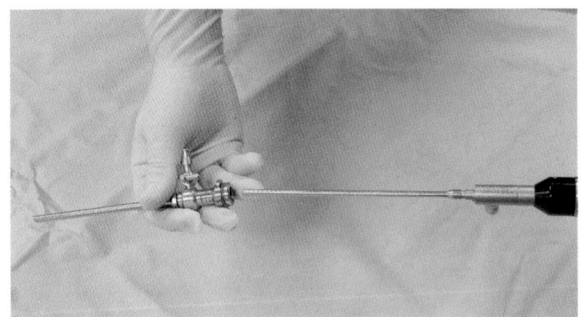

FIGURE 30-51 Once the sleeve is in position in the joint, the obturator is removed, and the arthroscope is placed into the sleeve.

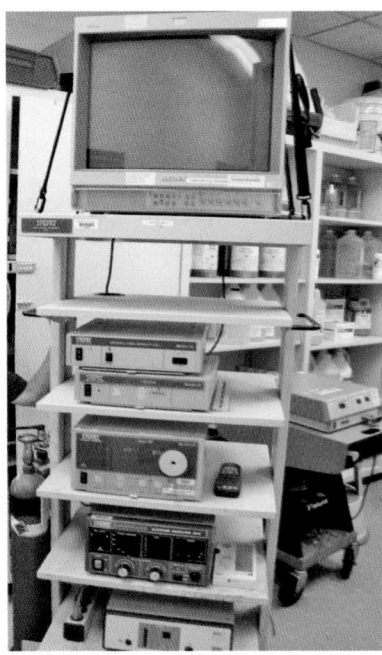

FIGURE 30-52 The arthroscopy tower containing the stacked power units.

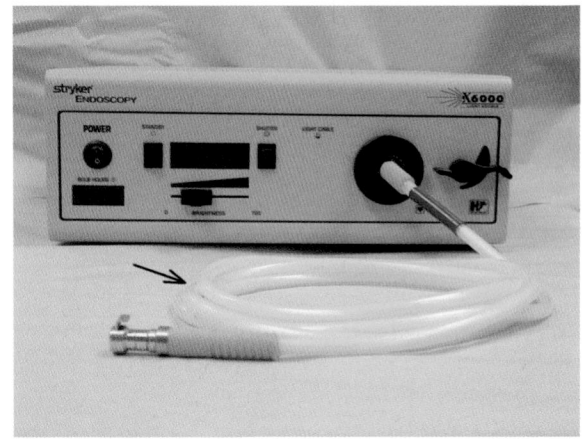

FIGURE 30-55 Light projector that projects light through a fiberoptic light cable *(arrow)* of the arthroscope.

of the joint capsule, which is essential for visualization of the intra-articular space. The fluid is infused into the joint space through the sleeve, around the arthroscope. The sleeve has at least one stopcock that is used as an **ingress port** to connect a sterile fluid line (Figure 30-56). Gas insufflation, performed using CO_2 or nitrous oxide, has also been used as a method of distending the joint. However, a special system with a pressure-regulating device is required. One disadvantage of gas is that it does not allow for lavage of the joint space if osteochondral fragments become detached within the joint.

Pressurized Bag System

Various systems are available to deliver fluid to the joint. One system is a pressurized bag design. A pneumatic pressure cuff

is slipped around a bag containing sterile fluid. The cuff is inflated with air, which squeezes the fluid bag, thus pressurizing the fluid (Figure 30-57). The amount of pressure is regulated by the amount of cuff inflation.

Automated Pump System

Another type of system uses a motorized pump to regulate the fluid rate through fluid lines connected to the arthroscope. One example of this type of system is the Hydroflex (Davol, Inc., Warwick, Rhode Island) (Figure 30-58). Pressure volume and fluid volume going into the joint are automatically regulated within the fluid pump via a pressure feedback control. This allows the pump to maintain a preset pressure within the joint without the need for the surgeon to adjust fluid pressure.

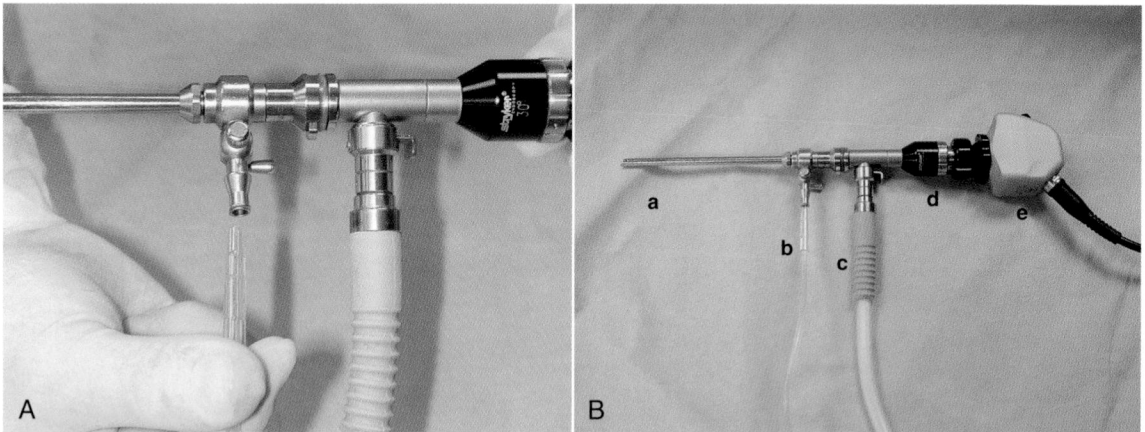

FIGURE 30-56 A, The fluid line is connected to the stopcock of the arthroscope. **B,** Arthroscopic sleeve (a), fluid line (b), light cable (c), arthroscope (d), and camera (e).

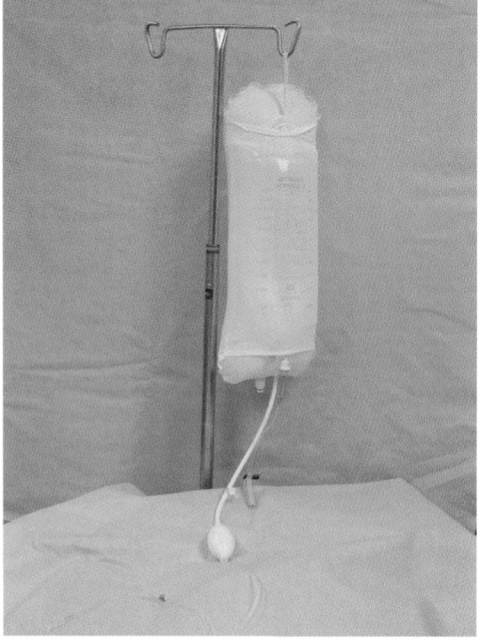

FIGURE 30-57 Pressurized bag of fluid can be used to distend a joint during arthroscopy.

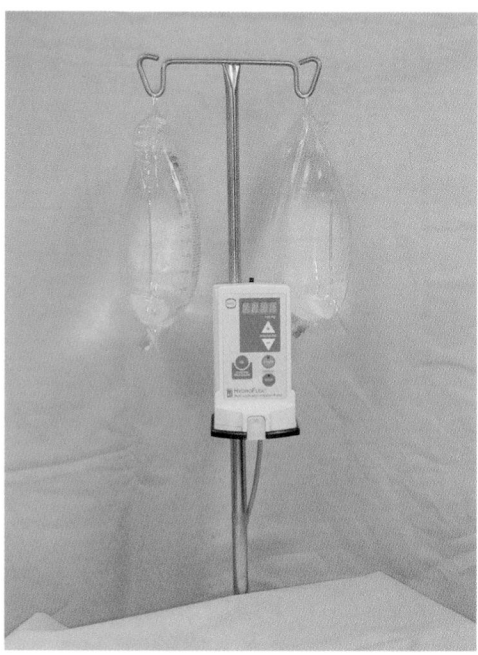

FIGURE 30-58 Automated fluid pressure pump can be used to infuse sterile fluid into a joint during arthroscopy. Pressure within the joint is automatically regulated by the pump.

HAND INSTRUMENTS FOR ARTHROSCOPIC SURGERY

Numerous hand instruments of various types are available or have been adapted for arthroscopy. They are used to remove or retrieve osteochondral fragments, to débride articular cartilage or **subchondral bone**, or to probe cartilage or cartilage lesions. These instruments are inserted into the joint through a separate stab incision, and the arthroscopic operation is performed via a technique called **triangulation**. The hand instruments are often placed in a separate pack from the arthroscope and accessories. The surgeon or surgical assistant will place these instruments onto the instrument table for easy access during surgery. The most commonly used instruments are described here.

Blunt Probe

The *blunt probe* is used to probe cartilage and subchondral bone in the joint to determine such aspects as cartilage integrity or the extent of a cartilage lesion (Figure 30-59).

Rongeurs and Grasping Forceps

Various types and sizes of *rongeurs* have been adapted for use in arthroscopy. These instruments have a beveled edge along cupped jaws to cut the attachments of an osteochondral fragment as it is removed (Figure 30-60). Forceps are used to retrieve loosely attached fragments (see Figure 30-22).

Elevators and Osteotomes

These instruments have small beveled heads that are designed to cut or break down the attachments of an osteochondral fragment and elevate it from the parent subchondral bone bed (Figure 30-61).

Curettes

Curettes are inserted into the joint to débride a defect left in the articular cartilage or subchondral bone after removal of an osteochondral fragment or osteochondritic lesion (Figure 30-62).

Motorized Burs

Motorized burs are often referred to as a *motorized arthroplasty system*. The system consists of a small, rounded bur attached to a power-driven shaft. The bur and shaft are enclosed in a sleeve, with a portion of the bur protected to prevent inadvertent damage to surrounding articular cartilage (Figure 30-63). The bur is also used to débride a defect left in the articular cartilage or subchondral bone after removal of an osteochondral fragment or osteochondritic

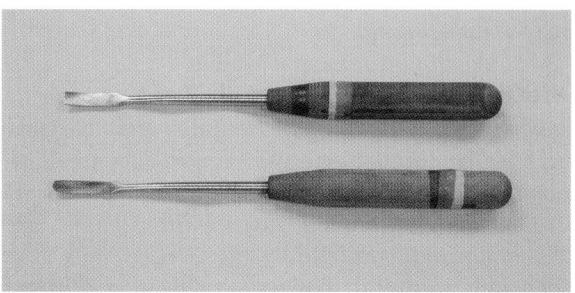

FIGURE 30-61 Elevator and osteotome used in arthroscopy.

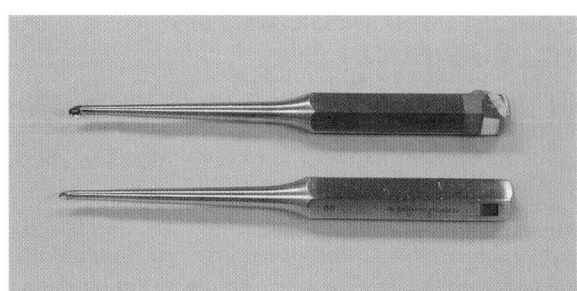

FIGURE 30-62 Small cupped bone curettes used in arthroscopy.

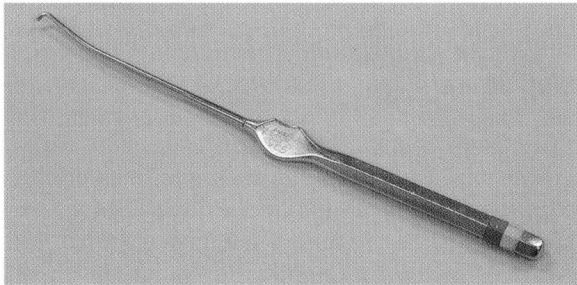

FIGURE 30-59 Blunt arthroscopy probe.

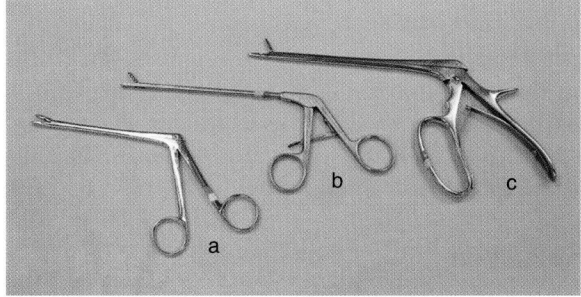

FIGURE 30-60 Rongeurs used in arthroscopy: Love-Gruenwald (a), grasping forceps (b), and Ferris-Smith (c).

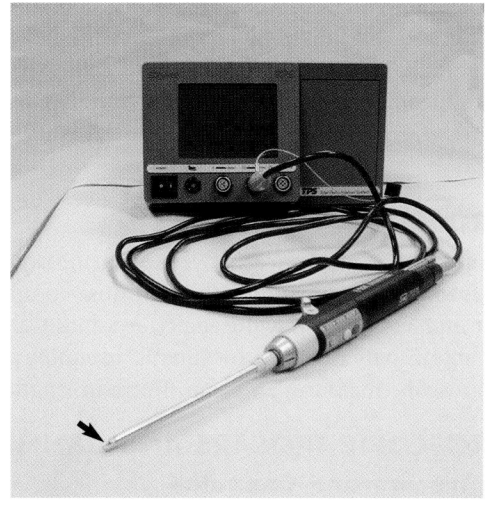

FIGURE 30-63 Motorized arthroplasty system with bur attachment (arrow).

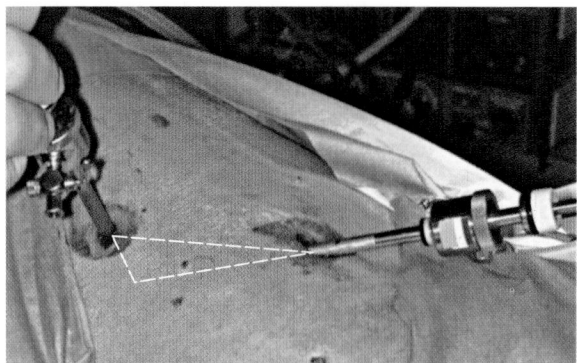

FIGURE 30-64 Laparoscopic surgery being performed on a pony showing abdominal portals.

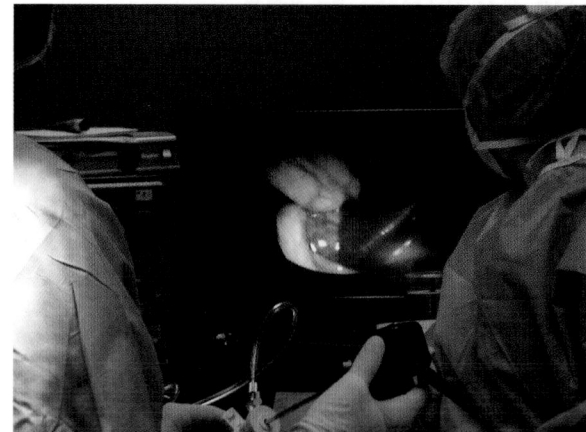

FIGURE 30-65 Laparoscopic imaging.

lesion. The speed of rotation of the bur can be adjusted; it is usually operated at several thousand revolutions per minute. Most systems operate with an on-off foot pedal or hand switch for the surgeon.

Radiofrequency Arthroscopic Probes

Intra-articular electrosurgical cutting and coagulation devices are used under arthroscopic guidance to allow for hemostasis of blood vessels, as well as débridement or resection of damaged soft tissue structures within a joint. Similar to the motorized burs already mentioned, most systems operate with an on-off foot pedal or hand switch for the surgeon.

LAPAROSCOPIC INSTRUMENTS AND EQUIPMENT

Similar to the arthroscope, the laparoscope is used as a diagnostic and surgical tool in veterinary surgery. It is used to examine the abdominal and thoracic cavities. The abdominal cavity is accessed via the **paralumbar fossa** (equine) or the ventral abdomen (canine and equine). Laparoscopy is performed primarily to remove ovaries and retained testicles, to examine/biopsy diseased organs, to repair damaged organs (urinary bladder), and to look for tumors or adhesions. Laparoscopy is performed most often with the patient under general anesthesia; however, it is sometimes performed in sedated horses with local anesthesia (Figure 30-64). The laparoscope is coupled with a small video camera that sends the image to a monitor for viewing (Figure 30-65). Laparoscopy uses gas (CO_2) to distend (**insufflate**) the abdomen.

LAPAROSCOPE

The laparoscope is in essence an oversized arthroscope. Different viewing angles may be selected. Most common are 0-degree and 30-degree viewing angles. A 5-mm OD is used in small animal patients and a 10-mm OD in equine patients. The laparoscope measures 33 cm or 57 cm in length.

LAPAROSCOPIC TROCARS AND CANNULAS
Sharp Trocars and Cannulas

Various trocars (Figure 30-66) and cannulas (Figure 30-67) are used as portals for the laparoscope and for hand

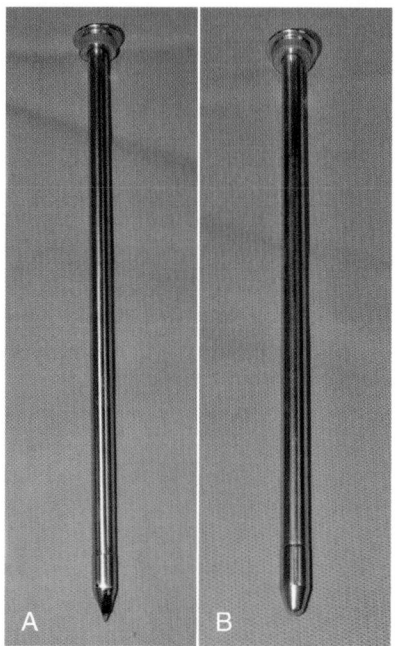

FIGURE 30-66 A, Sharp laparoscopic trocar. B, Blunt laparoscopic trocar.

instruments. *Sharp trocars* and *cannulas* are used to penetrate subcutaneous tissue and the **peritoneal lining** through a skin incision. Sharp trocars are manufactured with a conical or pyramidal tip. Cannulas are equipped with a valve that prevents escape of gas when a scope or an instrument is not occupying its barrel. Disposable trocars are available but are usually reserved for the human field.

Blunt Trocar

Once the perineum has been entered, the sharp trocar is exchanged for a *blunt trocar* so as to avoid inadvertent puncture of a visceral organ (see Figure 30-66, *B*). This allows the cannula to be advanced safely.

Light Cable, Light Projector, and Video Camera

As with arthroscopy, it is necessary to have a light source, a video monitor, ancillary power equipment, and a gas insufflator. These electrical units are collectively stacked on a cart, and this is also called the *tower*. Once the laparoscope has been introduced into the abdomen, a *small video camera* is attached to the eyepiece of the scope. This small camera feeds an image to a *monitor* through a cable for viewing. To illuminate the abdominal cavity, a *light cable* is attached to the light port on the laparoscope and is run to a *light generator*.

Insufflator

Distention of the abdominal cavity is necessary to obtain a safer distance for manipulation of the laparoscope and instruments and to allow better visualization of the viscera. This is accomplished with an *insufflator* (Figure 30-68). The insufflator creates and automatically maintains the desired degree of abdominal distention during a laparoscopic procedure. CO_2 is the most widely used gas because it is not combustible. CO_2 is fed into the abdomen through a sterile line (hose) connected to the insufflator and to a port on the cannula. Intra-abdominal pressure generally is maintained at between 10 and 15 mm Hg; higher abdominal pressures decrease ventilation and should be avoided. A flow rate of 9 L/minute is used to insufflate.

Hand Instruments for Laparoscopic Surgery

Numerous hand instruments are available for laparoscopic surgery. They are used to grasp organs or structures, and to cut, cauterize, staple, or biopsy (Figure 30-69). Shafts of most laparoscopic instruments are designed to rotate to attain the most effective angle for use in the abdomen. Because of their length, these instruments are stored in specialized containers (Figure 30-70).

INSTRUMENT PACKS

Most veterinary hospitals organize surgical instruments into several different instrument packs. Surgical pack

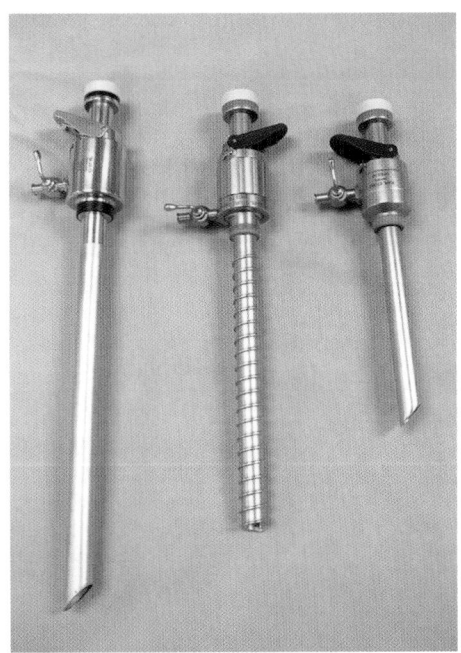

FIGURE 30-67 Laparoscopic cannulas.

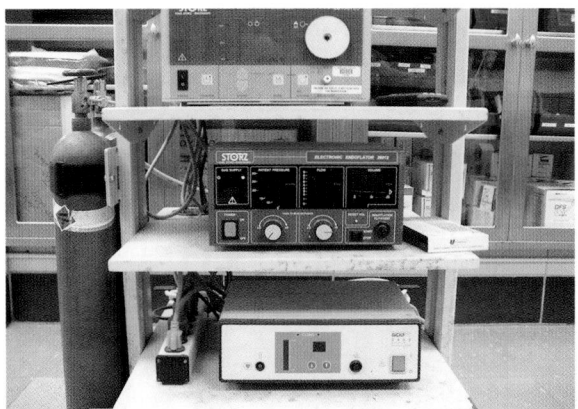

FIGURE 30-68 Laparoscopic insufflator and air line.

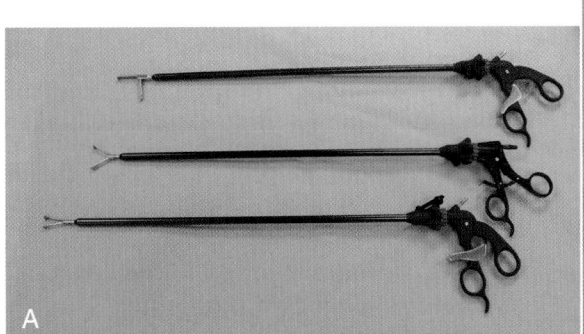
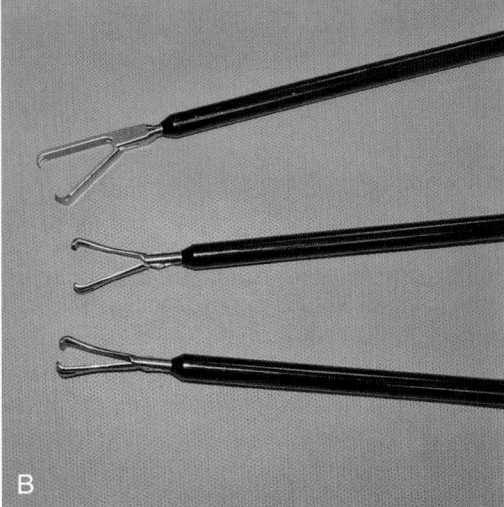

FIGURE 30-69 A, Hand-held laparoscopic grasping forceps. B, Close-up of laparoscopic grasping forceps.

TABLE 30-4	Small Animal Instrument Packs		
SPAY/NEUTER PACK	**SOFT TISSUE/GENERAL PACK**	**EMERGENCY PACK**	**ORTHOPEDIC**
No. 3 scalpel handle	No. 3 scalpel handle	No. 3 scalpel handle	Army-Navy retractors
Brown-Adson thumb forceps	Brown-Adson thumb forceps	Brown-Adson thumb forceps	Senn retractors
Needle holder, Mayo-Hegar	Adson thumb forceps	Needle holder, Olsen-Hegar	Rongeurs
Metzenbaum scissors	Needle holder, Mayo-Hegar	Mayo scissors, curved	Large Kern bone-holding forceps
Sponges (standard count)	Mayo scissors	Mosquito hemostats (3 curved, 3 straight)	Small Kern bone-holding forceps
Sterilization indicator	Metzenbaum scissors	Crile or Kelly forceps (1 curved, 1 straight)	Bone curette
Mosquito hemostats (2 curved, 2 straight)	Wire-suture scissors	Allis forceps	Periosteal elevator
Carmalt forceps (2 curved)	Mosquito hemostats (4 curved, 4 straight)	Towel clamps (4)	Steinmann pins ($\frac{5}{64}$, $\frac{3}{32}$, $\frac{7}{64}$, $\frac{1}{8}$, $\frac{9}{64}$, $\frac{5}{32}$, $\frac{3}{16}$, $\frac{1}{4}$)
	Carmalt forceps (2 curved)	Crile forceps (1 curved, 1 straight)	Wire (0.035, 0.045, 0.062)
	Allis forceps (2)	Sponges (standard count)	Jacobs chuck and key
	Towel clamps (8)	Sterilization indicator	Roll 18-gauge stainless
	Towels (6)		Roll 20-gauge stainless
	Stainless steel bowl		Roll 22-gauge stainless
	Sponges (standard count)		Metal ruler
	Lap sponges (2)		Michel clips and applicator
	Sterilization indicator		Sterilization indicator

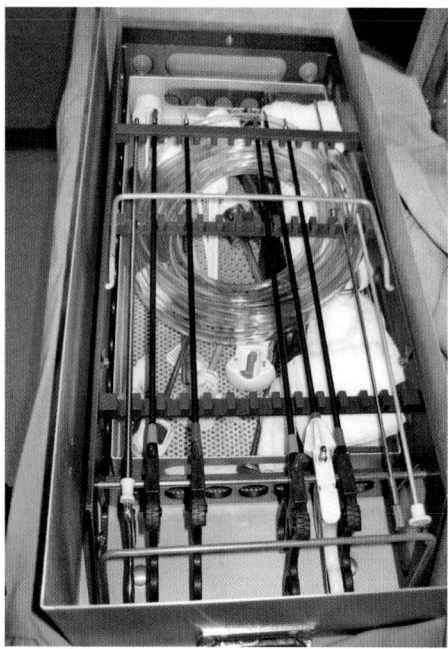

FIGURE 30-70 Laparoscopic instrument tray.

TABLE 30-5	Large Animal Standard and Emergency Packs
STANDARD PACK	**EMERGENCY PACK**
No. 3 scalpel handle	No. 3 scalpel handle
No. 4 scalpel handle	No. 4 scalpel handle
Rat-tooth thumb forceps (3)	Rat-tooth thumb forceps
Adson thumb forceps (3)	Brown-Adson thumb forceps
Needle holders (2)	Needle holder
Mayo scissors (1 curved, 1 straight)	Mayo scissors (1 curved, 1 straight)
Operating scissors (2 curved, 2 straight)	Mosquito hemostats (sharp-sharp)
Metzenbaum scissors (1 curved, 1 straight)	Allis tissue forceps (2)
Bandage scissors	Towel clamps (4)
Mosquito hemostats (4 straight, 4 curved)	Towel
Kelly or Crile forceps (2 straight, 2 curved)	Sponges (standard count)
Ochsner forceps, 15 cm (1 curved, 1 straight)	Sterilization indicator
Allis tissue forceps (2)	
Towel clamps (16)	
Towels (4)	
Saline bowl	
Sponges (standard count)	
Sterilization indicator	

organization is dependent on the type of practice and the types of surgeries performed. Examples include the following: minor packs (e.g., spay/neuter packs, laceration packs), general packs for more involved soft tissue surgeries, and bone packs for orthopedic procedures. Depending on the practice, other, more specialized packs such as neurologic packs for spinal and brain surgeries and vascular packs may be required (Tables 30-4 and 30-5). A pack system helps staff members to organize the instruments so that the most commonly used instruments are readily available, and infrequently used instruments are not contaminated and resterilized unnecessarily. For example, all commonly used instruments for spinal surgery are in one pack, so it is

opened, used, cleaned, sterilized, and repacked only when necessary. Infrequently used instruments are typically wrapped individually for use as needed. Large and bulky instruments are also packed separately. In addition, some commonly used instruments (e.g., scalpel handle, hemostats, thumb forceps, scissors, needle holders, sponges)

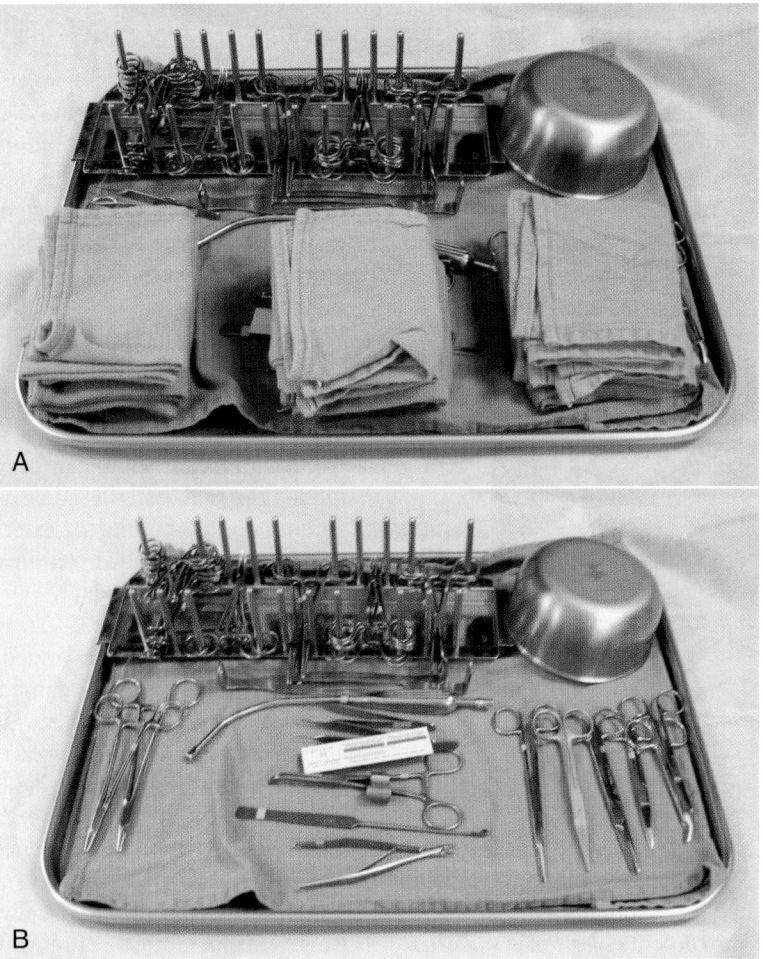

FIGURE 30-71 A, Properly organized surgery tray. B, Same tray, but towels have been removed.

may be wrapped individually to provide access to an additional instrument without the need to open an entire instrument pack.

Each type of pack should be organized in such a way that items are always placed in the same location on the tray (Figure 30-71). This makes it easier to inventory the instruments and facilitates finding the instruments quickly during surgery. Sponges may be counted at the beginning and at the end of each surgery to ensure that none has been left in the patient. It is often recommended to have a list of instruments and ancillary items (towels, sponges, etc.) and a picture of each pack available for review in the preparation area to ensure that each pack is correctly and consistently organized after each procedure, before resterilization.

INSTRUMENT CARE

Quality surgical instruments are expensive and require specific care and maintenance to keep them functioning properly for their expected lifetime. All instruments should be handled gently, and particularly delicate instruments should be separated from general instruments before cleaning. Additionally, multiple-component instruments should be disassembled before cleaning. Power equipment should be cleaned separately to ensure that water does not get inside the components. Most surgical instruments are made of satin finished stainless steel. Stainless steel is relatively rust resistant and retains sharp edges when properly sharpened. The satin or dull finish is often favored over polished to reduce glare. However, satin finished instruments are less resistant to spotting and discoloration, and therefore require more vigilant cleaning and care.

After each surgical procedure, all instruments that were used or soiled should be rinsed free of blood and organic debris with the use of cold, distilled, or deionized water. Use of tap water can increase staining and rust formation because of the high iron content. Instruments should be soaked in a commercial instrument detergent if there is a delay between completion of a surgical procedure and thorough cleaning of the instruments. After it has been rinsed in cold water or soaked in detergent, each instrument should be inspected and scrubbed with a soft brush in warm water using a neutral pH instrument detergent. Abrasive cleaning agents should never be used on surgical instruments. After manual cleaning is done to remove blood and debris, an ultrasonic (high-frequency sound) cleaner (Figure 30-72) is used to further

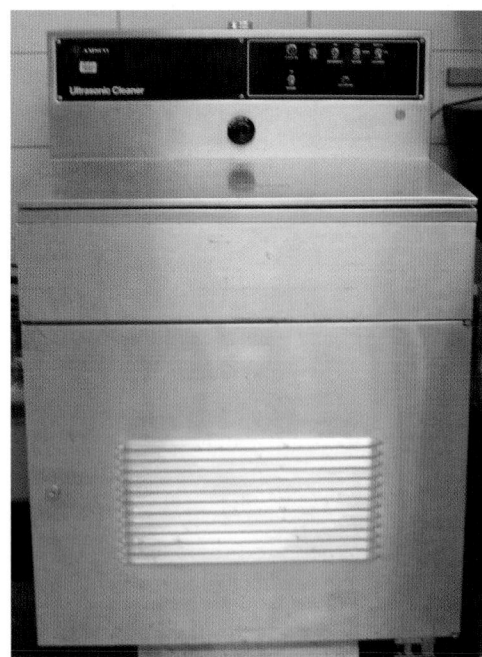

FIGURE 30-72 Ultrasonic cleaners are available in different sizes and models. Follow manufacturer's recommendations regarding use.

remove tightly bound debris and to clean areas that the brush cannot effectively reach. When instruments are placed into the ultrasonic cleaner, box locks should be in the open position. Additionally, only instruments of similar material should be put together in the ultrasound unit (e.g., stainless steel with stainless steel, chrome with chrome) because intermixing of instruments with different material composition may result in scratching and pitting of the instruments composed of softer material. If an ultrasonic cleaner is not available, all instruments should be cleaned as thoroughly as possible by hand, but this may shorten the overall functional life of the instrument.

Once properly cleaned, instruments should be thoroughly rinsed with deionized water and allowed to air dry before autoclaving to prevent rust formation. Wiping instruments dry rather than air drying is not performed because this can leave lint residue. Instruments with a working action, such as a hinge or a box lock, should be treated with a water-soluble instrument lubricant such as a sterile spray lubricant. Milk baths are known to harbor bacteria and must be changed frequently, if used at all. Instrument lubricants limit rust formation and keep moving parts fluid. Spray lubricants are not oily or sticky, and they do not interfere with steam sterilization. Working components of power equipment should be lubricated to maximize efficiency and to prolong the working lifetime of the equipment. Before instruments are repacked for sterilization, they should be thoroughly inspected for cleanliness, stiff or "frozen" hinges, improper jaw alignment, rust spots, and worn or broken parts. Defective instruments should be repaired or replaced.

DRAPES AND GOWNS

Surgical drapes and gowns may be made of paper or cloth. Paper drapes and gowns are designed to be disposable and are purchased prepackaged and sterilized for one-time use. Cloth drapes and gowns are designed for repeated use, but they require washing after each use. Immediately soaking the cloth in cold water will prevent blood and other fluid from setting. All cloth drapes and gowns should be washed in a mild detergent and thoroughly dried before sterilization, ideally in a clean, dedicated washer and dryer. They should be inspected for holes or other signs of wear and repaired or replaced as needed.

Cloth gowns must always be folded and packed in a correct and consistent manner (Figure 30-73). This technique allows the sterile gown to be unfolded and put on without contaminating the exterior surface. A cloth or paper towel is often included within the gown pack to facilitate hand drying immediately after scrubbing and before "gowning-up."

Cloth drapes must be folded and packed in such a way that sterility can be maintained as they are unfolded and applied to the patient or surgical table. *Accordion folding* allows easy unfolding and placement of the drape (Figure 30-74). Many specifically designed drapes are available, including adhesive drapes (e.g., povidone-iodine impregnated), transparent drapes, fenestrated drapes, stockinettes, and compressive wraps. After drapes and gowns have been properly folded, they are usually double-wrapped in tightly woven muslin fabric or a nonwoven disposable barrier before sterilization (Figure 30-75).

> **TECHNICIAN NOTE** Accordion folding of drapes allows easy unfolding and placement on the patient.

Aseptic Technique

Postsurgical infection can have disastrous consequences for an otherwise perfectly performed surgery. **Asepsis** is a condition of sterility whereby no living organisms are present. Aseptic technique includes all steps taken to prevent contamination of the surgical site by infectious agents. A thorough understanding of aseptic technique is required throughout the entire surgical process, from proper sterilization of surgical equipment and cleaning of the operating room to scrubbing and draping of the patient.

The technician may need to act as a circulating nurse by getting the patient into the operating room and opening sterile equipment for the surgeon. Additionally, the technician may be called upon to **scrub in** as a scrub nurse or surgical assistant to organize and pass instruments to the surgeon, or to assist with the surgical procedure. A working knowledge of aseptic technique is necessary to perform these tasks correctly and to monitor for inadvertent "breaks" in **sterile technique**.

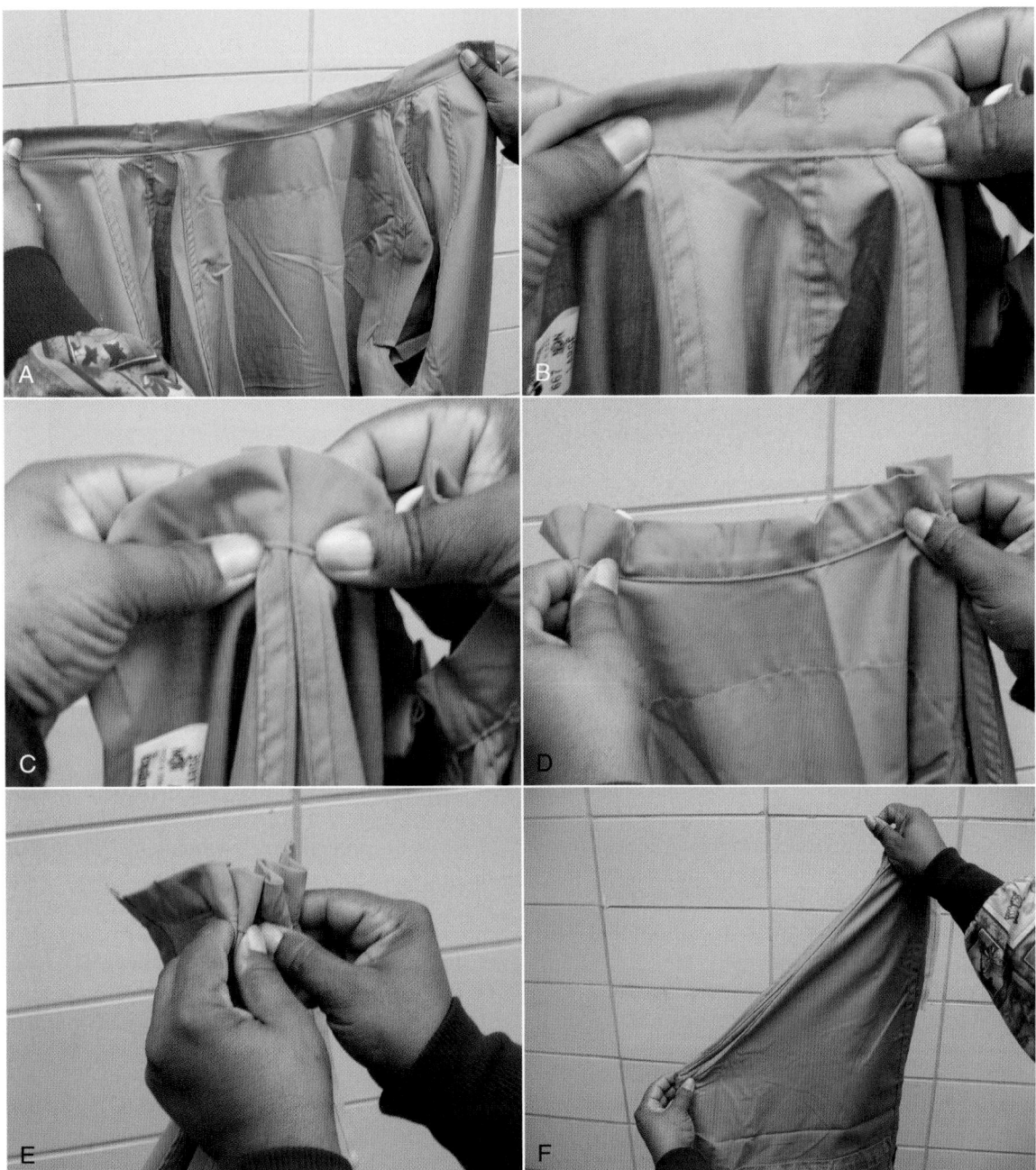

FIGURE 30-73 Method of folding a cloth surgical gown. **A,** The gown is held by the neck so the shoulder seams on the inside of the gown can be seen. **B,** Close-up of the three seams of one shoulder. **C,** The gown is folded so the outer two seams of one shoulder are touching. **D,** The same fold is done with the other shoulder. **E,** The gown is folded so the seams of both shoulders are touching. **F,** The shoulders are held in one hand while the other hand aligns the armpit seams.

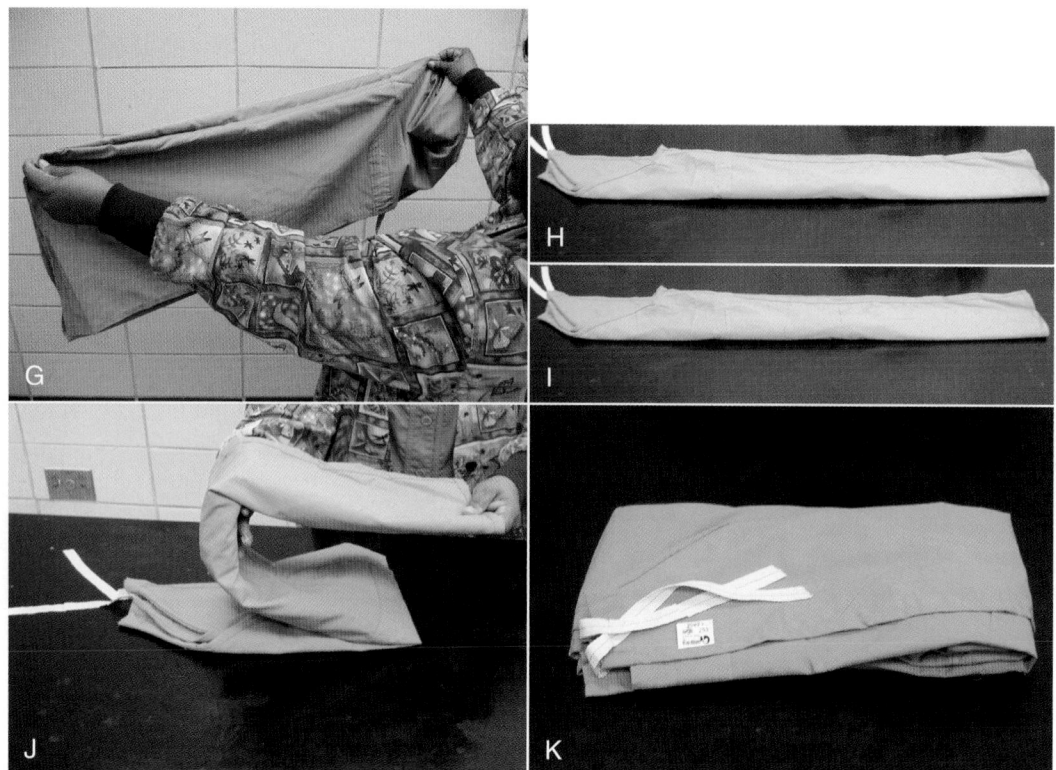

FIGURE 30-73, cont'd **G,** The shoulders and armpits are held in one hand while the other hand aligns the gown hem. **H,** The gown is laid flat on the table. (A tabletop method of folding is to first lay the gown open flat on the countertop with the outside of the gown facing up, sleeves on top. The side edges of the gown are each folded to meet near the middle, and then the gown is folded in half.) Only the inside surfaces of the gown are now exposed. **I,** The gown is folded in half lengthwise. **J,** The gown is folded in accordion fashion. **K,** The gown is laid on the table so the neck ties are uppermost. Proceed to Figure 30-75 to wrap the gown.

Microorganisms must be introduced into the surgical site for infection to develop. Sources of microorganisms include *exogenous* and *endogenous* routes. Exogenous sources of contamination include air, surgical instruments and supplies, the patient's skin, and the surgical team. Endogenous contamination arises from within the patient and reaches the wound as a result of bacteremia (through the bloodstream). Examples of endogenous sources are bacteria from the oral cavity (gingivitis) or the skin (dermatitis).

During every surgery, it is likely that some bacterial contamination will occur at the surgical site regardless of vigilance toward asepsis. The factor most consistently observed to influence the incidence of wound contamination and subsequent infection is the length of time the patient is under general anesthesia. Risk for infection roughly doubles every hour that the patient is under general anesthesia. This fact affirms the importance of an efficient and effective surgical team. Whether contamination progresses to infection depends on many factors, including the general health of the patient, the degree of tissue damage present in the wound, the virulence of the infectious agent, the number of infectious agents, and the use of perioperative antimicrobial agents. The factor over which the surgical team has greatest control is the number of infectious agents that are introduced into the wound by an exogenous route. Strict adherence to the principles of aseptic technique will minimize exogenous wound contamination and will prevent infection.

All procedures do not require the same degree of vigilance regarding aseptic technique. Whether surgery is considered *clean*, *clean-contaminated*, *contaminated*, or *dirty* determines the appropriate degree of asepsis and the need for perioperative antimicrobials. For example, débridement of a cutaneous abscess is considered to be a dirty surgery, so aseptic technique would not be strictly followed. The wound would be scrubbed, but surgical instruments may be disinfected (cold sterilization) rather than sterilized (steam autoclave or gas sterilization), and the surgeon may wear sterile gloves but may forgo complete sterile surgical attire. It may be preferable for such a patient to remain outside the operating room to prevent contamination of an otherwise clean surgical suite. In stark contrast, for clean surgeries, especially procedures involving placement of permanent implants (e.g., total hip replacement surgery), the surgical team must adhere strictly to aseptic protocol. Contamination and subsequent infection during these types of procedures can lead to devastating consequences. In each case, the surgeon will determine the degree to which principles of asepsis are to be followed.

Sterilization is defined as the *elimination or destruction* of all living organisms (including viruses) from a material being sterilized; this contrasts with *disinfection*, which is the

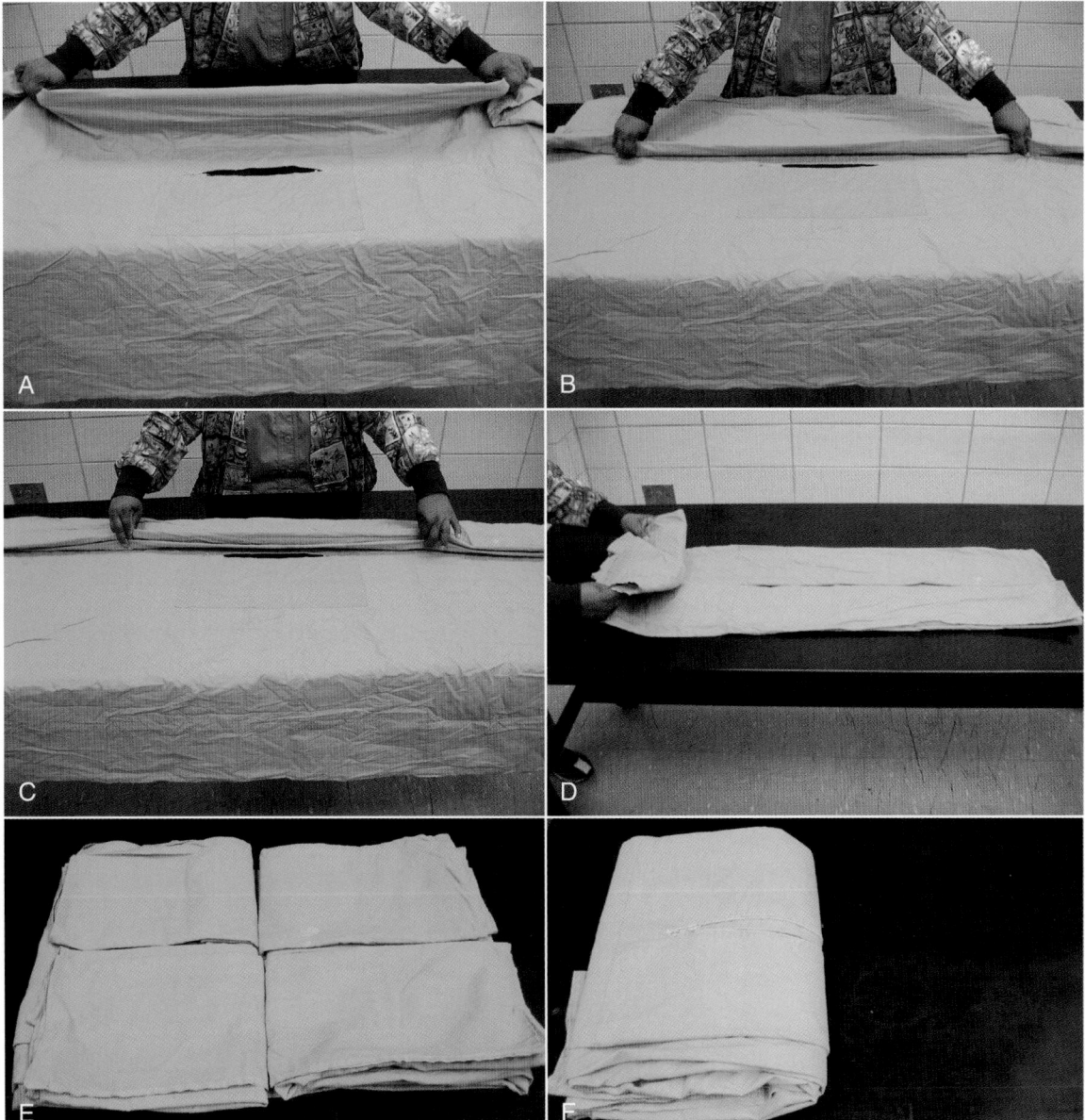

FIGURE 30-74 Cloth drapes are folded in accordion fashion so that they are easily unfolded onto the patient. **A** and **B,** A lengthwise fold is created in the drape (approximately 30 cm from the middle), and the folded edge is brought to the fenestration at the middle of the drape. **C,** This is repeated with a second fold, creating an accordion folding. Each section of folded drape is approximately 15 cm wide. **D,** The opposite side is folded in a similar manner. Then one end of the drape is folded to the center in accordion fashion. **E,** The opposite end is folded in the same manner. **F,** The drape is folded in half (half of the fenestration is visible), and it is ready to be wrapped as in Figure 30-75.

destruction of vegetative forms of bacteria but not the spores. Both sterilization and disinfection are used to prepare medical and surgical materials. The process selected depends on the nature of the material and its intended use. Methods of sterilization and disinfection can be classified as *physical* or *chemical.*

PHYSICAL METHODS OF STERILIZATION

The three general methods of **physical sterilization** include filtration, radiation, and heat. Filtration and radiation are used primarily during the production and packaging of certain surgical products.

FILTRATION

The term *filtration* refers to the use of a filter to separate particulate material from liquids or gases. Pharmaceuticals are commonly sterilized by filtration.

RADIATION

Some materials that would be damaged by other methods of sterilization can be safely sterilized by radiation. Radiation destroys microorganisms without causing significant temperature elevation. Gloves and some suture materials are sterilized by radiation during the manufacturing process.

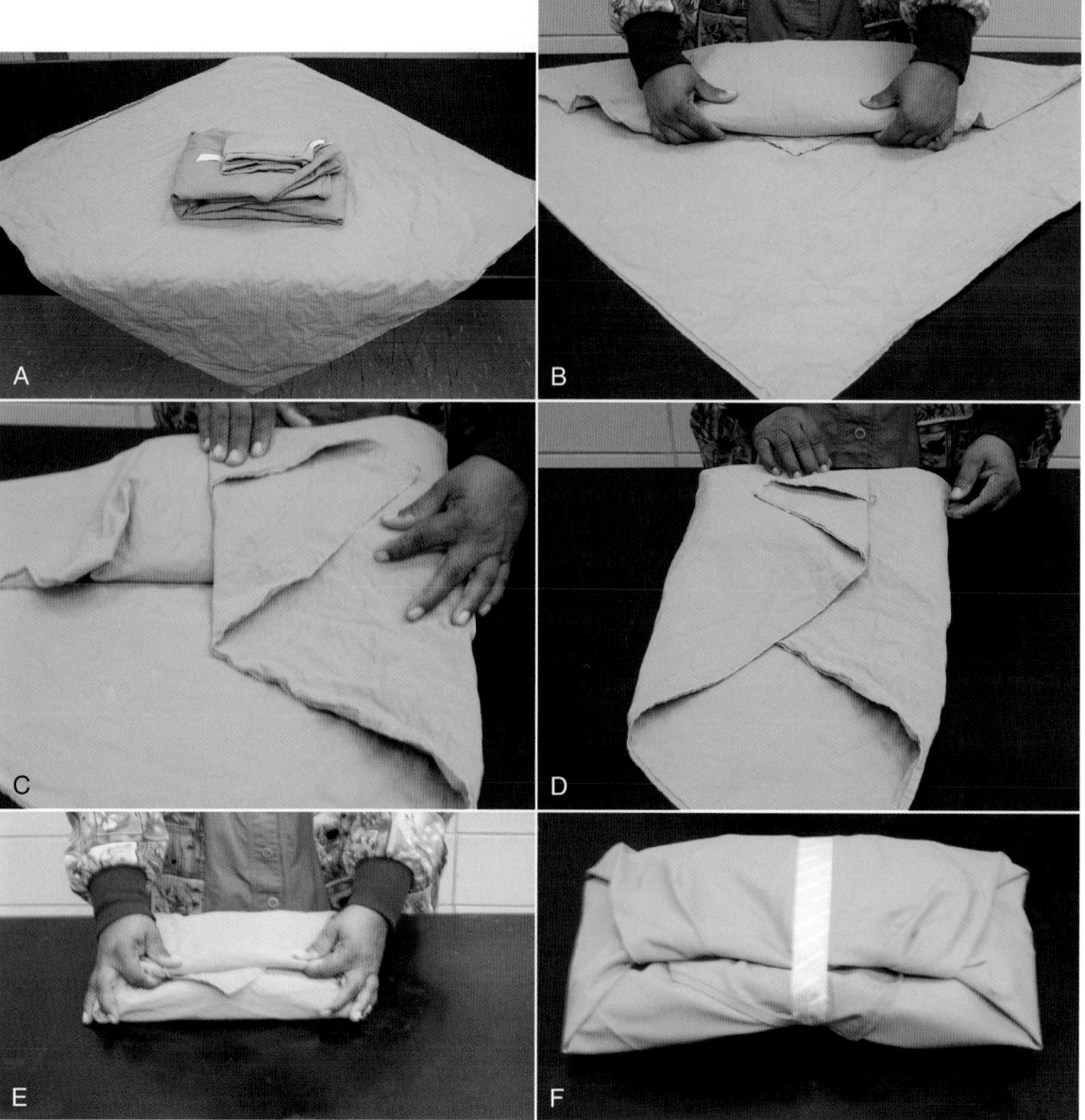

FIGURE 30-75 Wrapping a cloth drape or gown or an instrument pack. **A,** The gown along with an accordion-folded hand towel and a sterilization indicator is placed diagonally onto the drapes. **B,** One corner is folded over the entire pack and tucked under it, leaving the tip visible. **C,** An adjacent corner is folded over the end of the pack and the tip folded back so the drape is flat on top of the pack. **D,** The opposite corner is folded the same way. **E,** The pack is turned around, and the final corner is folded over the top of the pack and tucked under the folded drape edges, leaving the tip visible. **F,** The pack is then wrapped in a second layer in the same manner. The pack is secured with autoclave tape and is then labeled with contents, date, and the initials of the individual preparing the pack.

HEAT

The method used most commonly for sterilization is heat. There is no one temperature at which all microorganisms are killed instantaneously because death of bacteria and spores is a function of temperature and duration of heat exposure.

The two basic types of heat sterilization are wet heat and dry heat. Dry heat is used to sterilize materials that cannot tolerate moist heat but can withstand high temperatures. Oils, powders, and petroleum products are most effectively sterilized by dry heat, whereas rubber, fabrics, and some metals may be damaged by high temperatures.

An advantage of dry heat is that it will not rust or corrode needles or sharp instruments. Dry heat is more difficult to control than moist heat, and the sterilization time is longer.

Moist heat sterilization can be accomplished by boiling water or by steam under pressure. Using boiling water at ambient pressures is not a reliable means of sterilization because of its relatively low temperature (100° C); it likely results in disinfection rather than sterilization. The bactericidal effect of boiling water can be enhanced by alkalinization with sodium hydroxide (0.1 g/dl) or sodium carbonate (2 g/dl). The addition of these agents reduces instrument corrosion, but they cannot be used with glassware or rubber goods.

The most common method of moist sterilization involves use of saturated steam under pressure. Most commonly used autoclaves sterilize by using this mechanism. Increased pressure causes steam to achieve a higher temperature. Materials to be sterilized in this manner must be penetrable by steam and must not be damaged by heat or moisture.

Dry heat and moist heat destroy bacteria through protein denaturation; more specifically, dry heat kills by protein oxidation, whereas moist heat kills by coagulation of critical cellular proteins. Moisture facilitates the coagulation of protein; thus moist heat kills bacteria and spores at lower temperatures and at shorter exposures than dry heat.

Autoclave Sterilization

Autoclave sterilization is technique sensitive, so operating instructions accompanying the autoclave should be followed. An autoclave load is not sterile unless steam has penetrated the packs completely, so that all materials have been exposed to steam at the proper temperature and for the proper duration. Adequate steam penetration requires that packs be properly prepared and loaded into the autoclave. Most autoclaves used in veterinary practice are *gravity displacement* or downward displacement sterilizers, which means that steam is introduced into the top of the chamber and forces air to the bottom. With *prevacuum sterilizers*, a vacuum pump evacuates the air before steam is introduced. This provides more rapid and even penetration of steam than occurs with gravity displacement, permitting higher temperatures and shorter duration.

Proper pack preparation begins with checking that all materials are thoroughly cleaned and free of grease, oil, or protein residues, and are functioning properly. Complex instruments should be disassembled, and any box locks should be open. Packs must be properly wrapped with steam-permeable wrappers, such as double-thickness muslin (thread count of 140 threads per 6.45 cm^2), or a nonwoven barrier (crepe paper or polypropylene fabric). Muslin wrappers can be washed and reused, but nonwoven barriers are designed for single use. Packs are usually wrapped in two layers of muslin or nonwoven wrappers. External wraps are folded around a large pack in the same manner as described for drape and gown packs (see Figure 30-75). Heat-sealable paper or plastic or plastic peel pouches may be used for individual instruments (Figure 30-76). Each pack must be labeled to identify pack contents, the person who prepared it, and the date it was sterilized. Paper wraps provide longer storage times relative to fabric wraps regardless of the number of layers. See Table 30-6 for safe storage times for sterile packs.

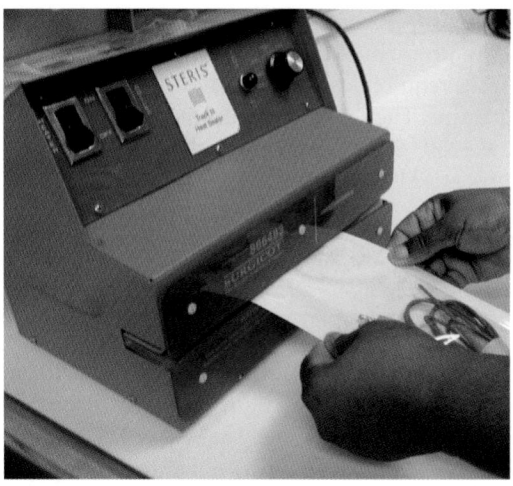

FIGURE 30-76 Individual instruments may be heat sealed in plastic or paper pouches in preparation for steam or gas sterilization. The instrument should be positioned in the pouch so that the handle will be presented to the surgeon when the pouch is opened.

TABLE 30-6	Safe Storage Times for Sterile Packs	
WRAPPER	**CLOSED CABINET**	**OPEN CABINET**
Single-wrapped muslin	1 week	2 days
Double-wrapped muslin	7 weeks	3 weeks
Single-wrapped crepe paper	At least 8 weeks	3 weeks
Single-wrapped muslin sealed in 3-ml polyethylene		At least 9 months
Heat-sealed paper and transparent plastic pouches		At least 1 year

Materials need to be packed as loosely as is practical to ensure good steam penetration. There should be 2.5 to 7.5 cm of space around each pack, and packs should be arranged to allow steam to flow readily from top to bottom. For example, a large pack should not be placed on top of several small ones because it will block the flow of steam down to the smaller packs. Steam flow may be facilitated by positioning packs vertically (on edge). It is recommended that packs be no larger than 30 cm × 30 cm × 50 cm, and that they weigh no more than 5.4 kg, depending on the type of material being autoclaved. In many practices, pack size is limited by the size of the autoclave.

Various minimum time-temperature standards have been established for routine sterilization of surgical packs. Exposure to saturated steam at 121° C (250° F) for 13 minutes is considered to be a safe minimum standard. Five to 10 minutes at 121° C will destroy most resistant microbes, and an additional 3 to 8 minutes provides a margin of safety. When the temperature in the exhaust line reaches the desired level, the entire content of the sterilizing chamber has been exposed to steam, so this is the beginning of exposure time. The time required to reach the sterilizing temperature is

---

TECHNICIAN NOTE Instruments with hinges or box locks should remain in the unlocked position during autoclaving.

referred to as *heat-up time* and is extremely short (about 1 minute) in prevacuum and pulsing types of sterilizers. Large linen packs require both a longer heat-up time and a longer exposure time. They should be saturated for 30 to 45 minutes at 121° C (250° F) in gravity displacement sterilizers and for 4 minutes at 131° C (270° F) in prevacuum sterilizers.

> **TECHNICIAN NOTE** The safe minimum standard for autoclave sterilization is 121° C (250° F) for 13 minutes.

Emergency sterilization, also called **flash sterilization**, is usually performed in prevacuum sterilizers. Recommended exposure time is 3 minutes at 131° C (270° F). Unwrapped instruments are placed in a perforated metal tray for sterilization and then are carried to the operating room with the use of detachable handles.

After sterilization, it is necessary to allow the packs to slowly cool, thereby reducing condensation formation that can occur as a result of too rapid exposure to cool air. This is done by slightly cracking open the autoclave door for a minimum of 20 minutes after the sterilization cycle. If the autoclave door is opened wide, cool outside air will condense steam in the materials, making them soggy and promoting corrosion of metal instruments. Paper-wrapped products should not be left in the autoclave longer than 15 to 20 minutes after the door is cracked. If they are left too long, heat will dry the paper, making it brittle and likely to crack and split when handled.

> **TECHNICIAN NOTE** Packs should be allowed to cool slowly to reduce condensation formation.

Sterilization Quality Control

Certainty that sterilization has been achieved is attained through use of proper technique and dependable sterilization indicators. Indicators should always be checked before materials are used.

Four types of sterilization indicators are used in autoclaves: (1) autoclave tape, (2) fusible melting pellet glass, (3) culture tests, and (4) **chemical sterilization** indicators. These indicators are meant to be used in combination because no one test alone can provide quality assurance of sterility.

> **TECHNICIAN NOTE** The four types of sterilization indicators are (1) autoclave tape, (2) melting pellet glass, (3) culture tests, and (4) chemical sterilization indicators.

Autoclave tape is useful for identifying packs and articles that have been exposed to steam, but it does not indicate whether proper requirements related to time, temperature, and steam have been met (Figure 30-77). The fusible melting pellet glass type of indicator indicates that a temperature of approximately 118° C (244° F) was reached but does not show whether proper time or steam saturation was achieved.

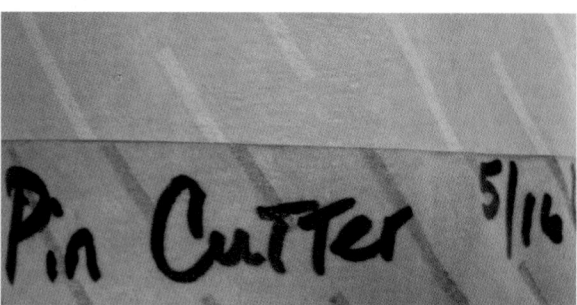

FIGURE 30-77 Autoclave tape before *(above)* and after *(below)* sterilization. Note the appearance of the black stripes, indicating exposure to steam.

Culture test indicators are strips that contain a controlled-count spore population of some particular strain of bacterium (e.g., *Bacilis subtilis* var.). This biological challenge test is useful because it is the only test that proves microorganisms were killed. Disadvantages of this test are that results are not immediately available (results require 1 to 7 days), and it does not assess steam penetration. Chemical sterilization indicators are available in many types, and they undergo color changes when subjected to saturated steam for adequate periods of time (Figure 30-78). Most practices use a combination of autoclave tape on the outside of the pack and a chemical sterilization indicator in the center of the pack to assess sterility.

With prevacuum sterilizers, an air removal test can be run daily to ensure that air is sufficiently removed from the autoclave. With gravity displacement sterilizers, temperature graphs can be kept as a record of autoclave performance. Therefore, quality assurance occurs at two levels: one to ensure that the pack runs through a sterilization cycle, and another to ensure that the autoclave system is working properly. Quality control is essential for any surgical practice because failure to ensure proper sterilization can have far-reaching consequences.

Care and Handling of Sterile Packs

Sterile packs should be stored in a dust-free, dry, well-ventilated area away from contaminated equipment. Closed cabinets provide cleaner storage area than is provided by open shelving. Safe pack storage times are listed in Table 30-6. If a pack is dropped, the tape sealing the pack is broken, or the pack wrap becomes wet, punctured, or torn, the pack should be considered contaminated. If there is any doubt as to the sterility of an item, consider it to be nonsterile.

CHEMICAL METHODS OF STERILIZATION

Chemical sterilization is performed with certain liquids or gases. Liquid chemicals can be used for instrument sterilization. The agent most commonly used for liquid sterilization is glutaraldehyde. Gas sterilization is used for items that cannot tolerate the high temperatures or steam associated with autoclaving (some power equipment or plastic

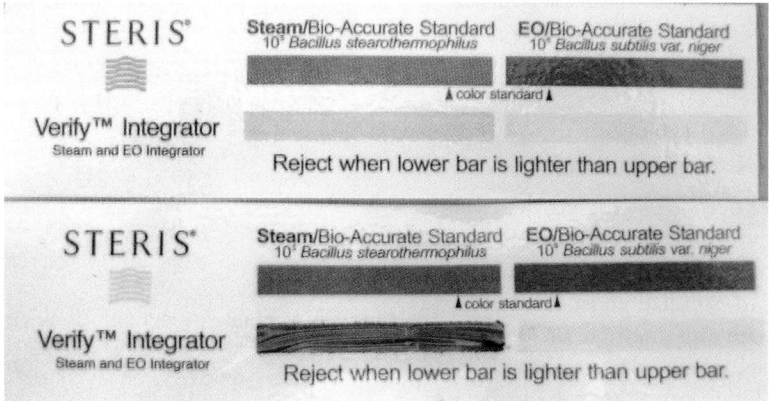

FIGURE 30-78 Chemical indicator strip to be placed inside pack. This strip can monitor steam *(left)* or gas *(right)* sterilization. Lower strip has been exposed to adequate steam, as indicated by the darkened bar.

products). The agents most commonly used for gas sterilization are ethylene oxide and hydrogen peroxide gas plasma.

ETHYLENE OXIDE

Ethylene oxide is a colorless gas at room temperature. It is flammable, explosive, and toxic. It can cause skin burns, respiratory irritation, vomiting, headaches, and birth defects. Refer to Chapter 4 regarding the occupational hazards associated with ethylene oxide. The manufacturer's guidelines should be followed carefully to prevent injury to hospital personnel and to patients. Ethylene oxide penetrates paper and plastic film packaging. The item to be gas sterilized is wrapped in plastic packaging (polyethylene, polycoated paper, and Mylar) and is sealed with adhesive or heat sealed before sterilization.

Ethylene oxide destroys metabolic pathways within cells by alkylation, and it is capable of killing all microorganisms. Effective sterilization with ethylene oxide is proportionate with the concentration of gas, exposure time, temperature, and relative humidity. Ethylene oxide activity is enhanced by increasing the temperature or the gas concentration. Ethylene oxide sterilizers usually operate at temperatures between 21° C and 60° C (70° F and 140° F). The activity of ethylene oxide approximately doubles with each 10° C increase in temperature. Doubling the ethylene oxide concentration decreases sterilization time by approximately one-half. Moisture is necessary for the lethal action of ethylene oxide; optimum relative humidity for sterilization with ethylene oxide is 40%, and a minimum of 35% humidity is required for effective sterilization. Exposure time varies from 48 minutes to several hours, but 12 hours of exposure is commonly used for sterilization at room temperature. Specific positioning of packs within the sterilization unit is not as important for ethylene oxide sterilization as it is for steam sterilization. In most ethylene oxide sterilizers, packs are placed inside an air-tight plastic bag, which is then sealed with the vacuum/gas unit in place (Figure 30-79).

After ethylene oxide sterilization, materials should be quarantined in a well-ventilated area for a minimum of 7 days, or in an aerator for 12 to 18 hours. Recommended aeration time varies with the type of material and other

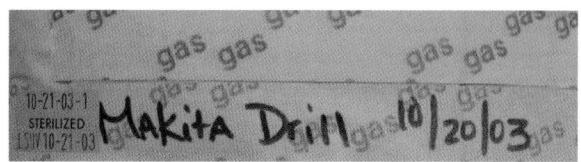

FIGURE 30-79 Gas tape before *(above)* and after *(below)* sterilization. Note the change in color of the word *gas*, indicating exposure.

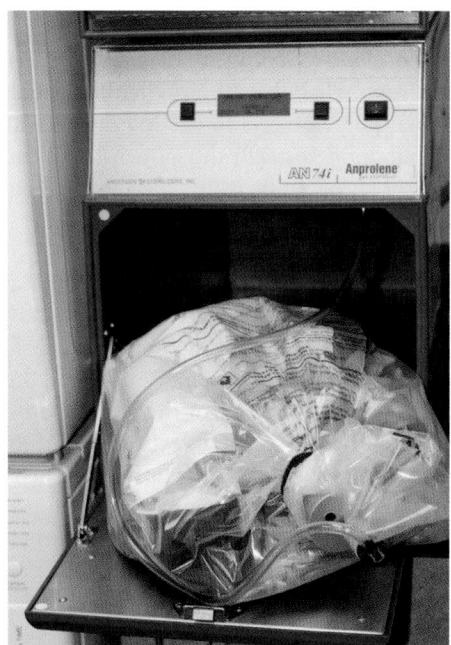

FIGURE 30-80 Ethylene oxide gas sterilizer.

factors. Color-coded chemical sterilization indicators are commonly placed within the packs when ethylene oxide sterilization is used. Biological indicators are available for ethylene oxide sterilization and are the only truly reliable test for sterility. Because results are unavailable for several days, as has been discussed, biological indicators are most commonly used to evaluate the sterilization system, not individual packs. External tape can be used to indicate exposure to gas sterilization (Figure 30-80).

> **TECHNICIAN NOTE** Because of the high toxicity of ethylene oxide, it is being replaced by hydrogen peroxide gas plasma sterilization.

HYDROGEN PEROXIDE GAS PLASMA

Gas plasma sterilization has been replacing ethylene oxide because it is safer for the environment and for personnel. It can inactivate mycobacteria, bacterial spores, fungi, and viruses and can be used to sterilize most items. Items that cannot be sterilized with this method include linen, wood or paper, endoscopes, some plastics, liquids, and tubes or catheters that are long (longer than 12 inches) or of small diameter (less than 3 mm). Items to be sterilized are wrapped in nonwoven polypropylene fabric or plastic (Tyvek-Mylar) pouches and are placed in the sterilization chamber. A vacuum is drawn, and hydrogen peroxide is injected and vaporized. After 50 minutes, pressure is lowered and radio waves are applied to the chamber, creating gas plasma. This creates free radicals, which kill the microorganisms. The process takes about an hour and requires no aeration. A biological indicator is used to test for sterility, and a chemical indicator is used to show that hydrogen peroxide was present.

CHEMICAL DISINFECTION

Again, a *disinfectant* is an agent that destroys bacteria or inactivates viruses. Disinfectants are chemical agents that are applied to inanimate objects to destroy the vegetative form of bacteria, but not necessarily the spore forms. Disinfectants that are capable of destroying vegetative bacteria plus spores, tubercle bacilli, and viruses may be used as chemical sterilizers.

Disinfection time is the time required for a particular agent to produce its maximal effect. It is influenced by many factors, including the nature of the material disinfected, the degree of soil and microbial contamination, and the concentration and germicidal potency of the disinfectant.

Antisepsis is prevention of infection by inhibiting the growth of infectious agents. Antiseptic agents, such as iodine or chlorhexidine, are substances used to effect antisepsis in living tissue. A glossary of key terms used in describing aseptic technique may be found in Box 30-3.

ANTISEPTIC AND DISINFECTANT COMPOUNDS

Iodine

Iodine compounds are effective antimicrobial agents but have limited activity against bacterial spores. Iodine solutions are used for surgical preparation, topical wound therapy, and joint and body cavity lavage. Iodine compounds are available as aqueous solutions, tinctures, and iodophors. *Aqueous solutions* contain higher levels of free iodine than iodophors and therefore have greater bactericidal activity. However, aqueous solutions are also cytotoxic and cannot be used in living tissue unless they are greatly diluted. Aqueous iodine stains materials and is corrosive to instruments.

BOX 30-3	Glossary of Key Terms Associated With Aseptic Technique

Antiseptic—Agent capable of preventing infection by inhibiting the growth of infectious agents. This term is generally applied to living tissues.
Autoclave—Sterilizer that uses saturated steam under pressure to achieve high temperatures for sterilization. Minimum exposure to saturated steam is 13 minutes at 121° C (250° F).
Disinfectant—Agent that destroys or inhibits microorganisms. Typically refers to inanimate objects.
Ethylene oxide—Gas chemical sterilization agent used to sterilize objects that cannot withstand heat. A good exhaust system must be used.
Flash sterilization—Emergency sterilization in which an object (instrument) is placed unwrapped in an autoclave and is taken directly to surgery after sterilization. Recommended exposure is 3 minutes at 131° C (270° F).
Sterilization—Destruction of all microorganisms. This term is generally applied to inanimate objects.

Tincture of iodine is a solution of 2% iodine in 50% ethyl alcohol and is intended for use on intact skin. It is not commonly used in veterinary practices.

Iodophors contain iodine complexed with surfactants or polymers so free iodine is slowly released. Adverse properties of staining and irritation are reduced, and delivery of iodine to tissues is enhanced. *Povidone-iodine*, the most commonly used iodophor, is available in the form of scrubs or solutions. Dilution of stock solutions (common dilutions include 1:10, 1:50, and 1:100) increases bactericidal activity and decreases cytotoxicity. Residual bactericidal activity (i.e., continued action when left on the skin) of povidone-iodine is 4 to 6 hours, but this is greatly diminished in the presence of organic matter.

Povidone-iodine is one of the most common surgical scrubs used in veterinary hospitals (Table 30-7). Although it is a relatively safe skin preparation, several matters regarding its use must be considered. Alcohol, lavage solutions, or organic debris, such as blood, will destroy residual bactericidal activity. Povidone-iodine can cause skin irritation or acute contact dermatitis in up to 50% of canine patients, and it may be a problem for some hospital staff. Rarely, individuals who have repeated contact with iodine scrub solutions may develop systemic iodine toxicity, resulting in metabolic acidosis and thyroid dysfunction.

> **TECHNICIAN NOTE** The two most commonly used antiseptic agents are povidone-iodine and chlorhexidine.

Chlorhexidine

Chlorhexidine is an antiseptic agent that is available in aqueous, tincture, and detergent formulations. It is an effective antimicrobial agent with activity against bacteria, molds, yeasts, and viruses. Chlorhexidine has a rapid onset and long

TABLE 30-7	Common Antiseptic and Disinfectant Agents		
EXAMPLES	**COMMON USES**	**SPECTRUM OF ACTIVITY**	**RESIDUAL ACTIVITY**
Povidone-Iodine Detergent Betadine scrub (Purdue Frederick, Stamford, Connecticut) (brown sudsy solution)	Preoperative scrubs	Bacteria, viruses, fungi, protozoa, yeasts	4-6 hours, but inactivated by organic debris and alcohol
Povidone-Iodine Solution Betadine solution (Purdue Frederick) (brown solution)	Preoperative skin preparation; wound lavage when diluted 1 : 100	Bacteria, viruses, fungi, protozoa, yeasts	4-6 hours, but inactivated by organic debris and alcohol
Chlorhexidine Detergent Nolvasan scrub (Fort Dodge Laboratories, Madison, New Jersey) (blue solution), Hibiclens scrub (Stuart Pharmaceuticals, Pasadena, California) (pink solution)	Preoperative scrubs	Bacteria, viruses, fungi, yeasts	2 days; not inhibited by organic matter or alcohol; less skin irritation
Isopropyl Alcohol-Iodine Povacrylex DuraPrep (3M, Maplewood, Minnesota)	Preoperative skin preparation—one step Do not use in open wounds	Bacteria	Rapid onset; at least 1 day residual
Isopropyl Alcohol–Povidone-Iodine Prevail-Fx (Cardinal Health, Dublin, Ohio)	Preoperative skin preparation—one step Do not use in open wounds	Bacteria	Rapid onset; at least 1 day residual
Isopropyl Alcohol–Chlorhexidine Gluconate ChloraPrep (Cardinal Health)	Preoperative skin preparation—one step Do not use in open wounds	Bacteria	Rapid onset; 2-day residual; not inhibited by organic matter
Chlorhexidine Nolvasan solution (Fort Dodge Laboratories) (nonsudsy blue solution)	Preoperative skin preparation; wound lavage when diluted 1 : 40	Bacteria, viruses, fungi, yeasts	2 days; bactericidal, but solution not cytotoxic in open wounds at diluted concentrations
Alcohol, Isopropyl and Ethanol Many manufacturers	Surgical preparations; disinfection antisepsis; do not use in open wounds	Bacteria, some fungi	Rapid onset, but no residual activity
Ethyl Alcohol–Chlorhexidine Gluconate Avagard (3M)	Preoperative hand scrub—waterless	Bacteria	Rapid onset, with some residual activity
Phenol, Hexachlorophene pHisoHex scrub (Sanofi, Paris, France; Winthrop, Surrey, UK) (white)	Preoperative hand scrub	Bacteria (more effective against Gram-positive than Gram-negative species)	Up to 2 days
Phenol, Glutaraldehyde	Cold sterilization; not intended for living tissues	Bacteria, viruses, fungi, yeasts, spores	None; causes skin irritation

residual activity that is not affected by alcohol, lavage solutions, or organic debris. It has become a popular surgical scrub because of its effectiveness, and because it is nonirritating to the skin. In several human studies, chlorhexidine has been found to be superior to povidone-iodine as a surgical hand scrub. The effectiveness of chlorhexidine is similar to that of povidone-iodine when they are used as surgical scrubs for canine surgery.

> ⌇ *TECHNICIAN NOTE* Chlorhexidine is an effective antimicrobial agent with rapid onset and long residual activity.

As a lavage solution for open wounds, chlorhexidine must be diluted 1:40 with sterile water or saline to produce a 0.05% solution. At this concentration, chlorhexidine has significant antibacterial activity with no cytotoxicity and is superior to povidone-iodine, saline, and other antiseptics. Higher concentrations can cause inflammation and cytotoxicity and are not recommended in open wounds. When chlorhexidine is mixed with electrolyte solutions (such as lactated Ringer's solution), it will precipitate, but this does not affect antimicrobial activity, and the solution can still be used for wound lavage.

Alcohols

Alcohols are used as disinfectant and antiseptic agents. They are organic solvents that evaporate rapidly and leave no residue. Alcohols are bactericidal but are ineffective against spores and fungi. They have no residual effects and are inhibited by organic debris. Ethyl and isopropyl alcohols are more effective than methyl alcohol as disinfecting agents. Alcohols should never be used in open wounds because they are both painful and cytotoxic.

Phenols

Phenols (carbolic acid) have been used historically as both antiseptics and disinfectants but have been routinely replaced by newer, safer, and more effective agents. Hexachlorophene, a skin preparation, was one of the most popular phenols, but it has been replaced by povidone-iodine and chlorhexidine.

Quaternary Ammonium

Quaternary ammonium compounds are synthetic cationic detergents that act on cell membranes and are effective against bacteria, but not against spores and some viruses. Bland and nontoxic, these agents are popular. Benzalkonium chloride, the most commonly used quaternary ammonium compound, is used as a disinfectant.

Chloride

Chloride compounds, some of the first agents to be used as medical disinfectants, found popularity for wound treatment during World War I as Dakin's solution. Antimicrobial chlorine compounds, specifically the hypochlorites, have broad bactericidal and virucidal activity, but they can be

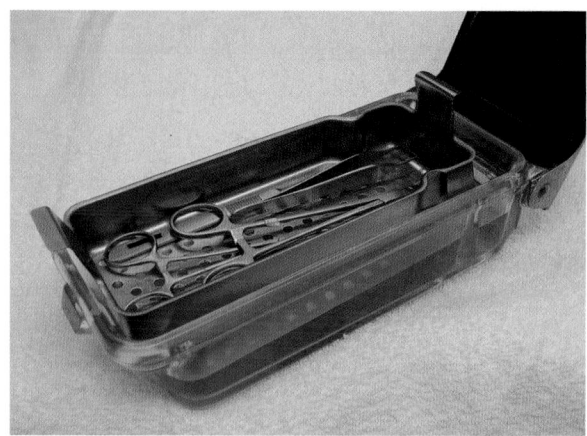

FIGURE 30-81 Cold sterilization tray. Instruments are kept submerged in disinfectant and are retrieved by lifting the rack.

cytotoxic when improperly used on living tissues. Presently, sodium hypochlorite (bleach) is commonly used as a disinfectant in many hospitals.

Aldehyde

Formaldehyde and glutaraldehyde are the most commonly used aldehydes in veterinary medicine. They are both toxic and irritating, which restricts them from use on living tissues. They are effective antimicrobial agents but may require several hours of exposure time. Formaldehyde is commonly used in the preservation of tissue specimens. Glutaraldehyde is commonly used for chemical sterilization in cold trays and for endoscopic equipment.

Cold Sterilization

Cold sterilization refers to soaking instruments in disinfecting solutions such as chlorhexidine and glutaraldehyde. Metal trays used to soak instruments in disinfectant are called *cold trays* (Figure 30-81). Because sterility cannot be guaranteed, cold-sterilized instruments should be used only for minor procedures (superficial lacerations, dental procedures) or for equipment that cannot tolerate other forms of sterilization, such as endoscopic equipment. Exposure times should exceed 3 hours, and the equipment must be rinsed thoroughly before use.

STERILIZATION OF ARTHROSCOPIC/ LAPAROSCOPIC EQUIPMENT

All endoscopic cannulas and hand instruments (particularly laparoscopic instruments) should be completely disassembled, if applicable, before cleaning and disinfecting. Particular attention should be paid to the jaws because this is where blood and tissue will accumulate. Most hand instruments and ancillary equipment items can be steam sterilized. They can also be gas sterilized with ethylene oxide or cold sterilized with a glutaraldehyde-based solution (CidexPlus, Johnson & Johnson Medical Inc., Arlington, Texas). Gas sterilization is the preferred method for arthroscopic and laparoscopic equipment, but in some situations cold sterilization is an alternative. Cold sterilization, unlike steam and gas sterilization in most situations, affords the ability to use equipment more than once in a single day. The arthroscope or laparoscope, light cable, and the camera can be gas sterilized or cold sterilized, but not steam sterilized.

> **TECHNICIAN NOTE** The arthroscope or laparoscope, fiberoptic light cable, and the camera should never be steam sterilized.

With cold sterilization, instruments are soaked a minimum of 20 minutes in the CidexPlus just before surgery. The electrical plug of the camera cable is not submerged in the cold sterilization solution (this would damage it). The end is draped out over the top of the container with the CidexPlus. It is important to use deep, wide containers so no solution splashes out of the container during transfer of the instruments and equipment. The surgeon or assistant double gloves and removes the instruments from the solution. The instruments are then placed in a sterile autoclave tray containing sterile water. Once the instruments have been submerged in the sterile water, each piece is gently agitated, individually removed from the tray, rinsed with sterile water by a scrub nurse or other assistant, and transferred to the instrument table. The surgeon or assistant removes his or her outer gloves and dries the instruments. It is important that the CidexPlus is thoroughly rinsed from the instruments. Glutaraldehyde, which is included in CidexPlus, can cause a chemical synovitis and is injurious to chondrocytes. A double rinse further reduces the amount of glutaraldehyde residue remaining on the instruments.

> **TECHNICIAN NOTE** Glutaraldehyde is carcinogenic, causes a chemical synovitis, and is injurious to chondrocytes.

OPERATING ROOM PREPARATION

Operating room design is important for ease of cleaning. The operating room should be simple and uncluttered. Commonly used equipment and materials should be readily available, but excess stock should not be stored in the operating room. When additional equipment is needed, it is brought to the operating room by the circulating nurse.

Operating room cleanliness is essential for proper aseptic technique. A routine daily and weekly cleaning schedule should be established to keep the operating room clean and dust free. The surgery table should be cleaned and disinfected, and soiled areas of the floor should be cleaned and disinfected by damp mopping immediately after each surgery. It is preferable to perform a thorough daily cleaning at the end of each day because cleaning creates airborne dust that takes several hours to settle. Buckets should be emptied and cleaned. The operating table and all equipment should

be cleaned and wiped with a disinfectant solution. (The operating room is never dry mopped or dusted because this produces excessive airborne dust.) The casters on equipment should be cleaned, and the entire floor should be mopped.

Once a week, the operating room should undergo a thorough cleaning in which movable equipment is removed and cleaned with a disinfectant solution. Permanent structures, such as walls, air vents, window sills, light fixtures, and the surgical table, should be wiped clean. Cabinets should be emptied, washed, and restocked. The operating room floor should be scrubbed and disinfected. Disinfectant can be applied with a mop, although this may actually spread dirt and microorganisms throughout the room. To prevent this, the mop head should be laundered daily and not stored in used disinfectant solution. The wet vacuum method in which the clean floor is flooded with disinfectant solution and then vacuumed is superior to mopping. Cleaning equipment used in the operating room should be kept separate from all other cleaning equipment.

Daily cleaning of the surgical preparation room is important because this room is subject to continual contamination. Sinks and plumbing fixtures should be scrubbed. Buckets and vacuum canisters should be emptied. Furniture and cabinets should be wiped clean and the floor scrubbed. If holding cages are kept in the preparation room, they should be cleaned and disinfected. All surgical preparation solutions and supplies should be replenished.

> **TECHNICIAN NOTE** Daily and weekly cleaning schedules should be established for the operating room.

SMALL ANIMAL PATIENT PREPARATION

SKIN PREPARATION—SURGICAL CLIP

Preparation of small animals for surgery usually ensues after the patient has been induced with general anesthesia—before transport into the operating suite. With a #40 clipper blade, the hair is first clipped in the same direction as hair growth; this is followed by clipping against the direction of hair growth to achieve the closest shave possible. The surgical clip should be thorough but gentle. Unnecessary roughness will result in inflamed or traumatized skin, which can cause greater postoperative complications. Razors are not recommended because they have been shown to increase surgical site infections up to 10-fold through the creation of microlacerations in the skin, which are easily colonized by bacteria. The size of the clip is determined on the basis of an estimation of the proposed surgical incision. Long hair growing near the periphery of the clipped area should be cut short enough that it cannot hang over the clipped area. As a general rule, a perimeter of at least 5 to 15 cm is clipped around the proposed incision site. Even larger preparations may be indicated when large masses are being removed, or when skin flaps or grafts are being performed. For abdominal procedures, the clip should extend several centimeters cranial to the xiphoid, caudal to the pubis, and lateral to the nipples. For orthopedic procedures, the entire circumference of the limb is clipped from the foot up onto the body. In cases where the proposed surgical field includes an open wound and needs to be prepared, sterile, water-soluble lube should be used to cover the wound before clipping, thereby providing a barrier between exposed tissues and hair clippings. Once the clip has been performed, the water-soluble lube is rinsed away and the site is prepared routinely, as discussed later. Areas that appear to be particularly contaminated or grossly infected should be clipped last. This prevents iatrogenic spread of potentially infectious material across the prepared surgical site. After clipping, a vacuum cleaner may be used to eliminate loose hairs on the skin.

SKIN PREPARATION—SURGICAL SCRUB

Initial skin preparation is done in the preparation room to remove gross contamination. Before the abdomen of a male dog is scrubbed, the prepuce should be flushed with an antiseptic solution, if it is to be in the surgical field. This is done by using a syringe of preferably 0.05% chlorhexidine gluconate solution to fill the prepuce while sealing the end of the prepuce, allowing the solution to contact the entire area for several seconds. This takes place several times before the patient is transferred to the operating room. Chlorhexidine gluconate has been shown to be superior to povidone-iodine for this purpose. Examination gloves are worn to decrease contamination from the hands during preparation. The presurgical scrub can be performed in the patient preparation area or inside the operating room, and is performed by alternating an antiseptic scrub (such as povidone-iodine or chlorhexidine scrub) with alcohol or sterile saline. (Remember not to use alcohols or detergents in open wounds, eyes, or mucous membranes.) Scrubbing should begin over the proposed incision site (Figure 30-82) and should extend outward in a spiraling pattern, never going back toward the center with the same gauze sponge. The gauze sponge is then replaced with a clean one, and the process is repeated until

no dirt is visible on the discarded sponges—often for three to five cycles.

The final sterile surgical scrub is performed only after the animal has been properly positioned on the operating table. Sterile gloves should be worn, and sterile gauze sponges are used. If the sterile surgical scrub is performed by alternating povidone-iodine with alcohol, the total contact time of the povidone-iodine should be at least 5 minutes. After the final povidone-iodine scrub, a 10% povidone-iodine solution should be sprayed or painted onto the skin. Alternatively, the sterile surgical scrub may be performed by alternating chlorhexidine gluconate with alcohol or sterile saline. Chlorhexidine or sterile saline may be left on the skin at the end of preparation. Povidone-iodine and chlorhexidine are effective scrub solutions, but the contact time for chlorhexidine is less critical than for povidone-iodine.

> **TECHNICIAN NOTE** It is generally recommended that the surgical site be scrubbed and rinsed at least 3 times. The sterile scrub should provide at least 5 minutes of contact time for povidone-iodine. An antiseptic solution is often applied to the skin after the scrubs.

Several skin preparations are now available that enable a **one-step prep**. The solution is packaged in a small plastic bottle that is directly attached to an applicator sponge. After the bottle is squeezed to activate solution flow, the sponge is used to "paint" a single uniform coat of solution on the skin, starting at the incision site and working outward in a circular motion (Figure 30-83). The solution requires a 30-second application time and dries within 2 to 3 minutes, so the preparation time is much faster than for the traditional

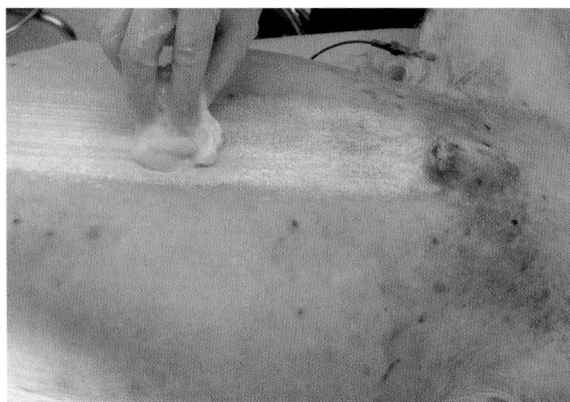

FIGURE 30-82 Surgical preparation should begin at the proposed incision site and should progress outward, never returning to the proposed incision line with the same gauze sponge. Gloves are worn during the preparation to decrease contamination from the hands.

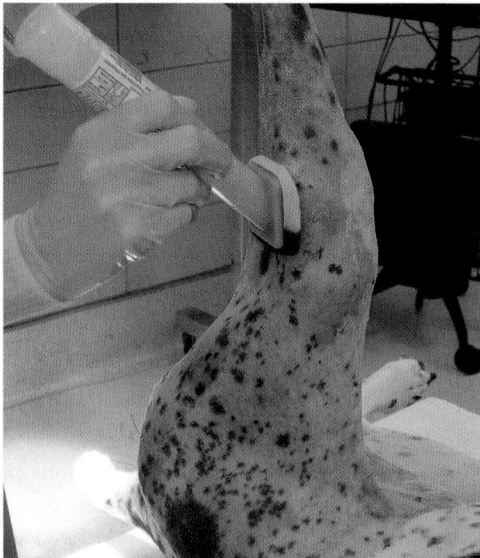

FIGURE 30-83 Skin preparation using a one-step prep method. In this case, the planned incision will be made along the lateral aspect of the femur. The applicator sponge is used to paint a single uniform coat of antiseptic solution on the skin, starting at the planned incision site and working outward in a circular pattern. (Photo courtesy Dr. Susanne Lauer.)

alternating scrub described earlier. These one-step solutions contain isopropyl alcohol, which is a broad-spectrum antimicrobial with rapid onset of activity. The other substances in these preparations result in further antimicrobial action and the formation of a film that adheres strongly to the skin and provides long residual activity. These solutions should be applied to clean, dry skin, and the skin should *not* be scrubbed beforehand with povidone-iodine or chlorhexidine gluconate scrub because residues of these may prevent the one-step preparation from adhering and disinfecting appropriately. These one-step preparations should be applied to intact skin and are not appropriate for use in open wounds or near sensitive eye tissues and other mucous membranes because of the high alcohol content (70% to 74%). These preparations enhance the skin adherence of **incise drapes**. The region will be flammable until it dries, so caution should be taken when electrocautery is used until the scrubbed area is completely dry. Alcohol-free solutions are being developed to reduce this flammable risk.

> **TECHNICIAN NOTE** *One-step preps are easy to apply, much faster than traditional scrubbing techniques, and effective for antimicrobial kill. They have a rapid onset and a long residual effect.*

The surgical preparation technique has many modifications. For example, in preparation for feline orchiectomy (castration), the scrotal hair is plucked rather than clipped. Feline onychectomy (declawing), tail docking, and dewclaw removal of neonatal puppies are commonly performed without clipping the hair. In these cases, the unclipped surgical site is soaked or gently scrubbed with antiseptic solution and is swabbed with alcohol only before the procedure. When surgery is to be performed on digits, or when the entire foot is required to be uncovered in the surgical field, the clipped foot should be soaked in dilute 0.05% chlorhexidine gluconate or 1% povidone-iodine. This can be facilitated by filling an examination glove with the antiseptic of choice and sealing the foot within the glove using surgical tape before the traditional presurgical and sterile scrubs. Bovine and porcine castrations are performed without clipping the hair, and an alcohol or antiseptic wash is usually used. Equine castrations may be prepared with three thorough washes using dilute chlorhexidine or povidone-iodine solution.

SMALL ANIMAL POSITIONING

Patient positioning for small animal surgical procedures is highly dependent on the procedure being performed and surgeon preference. Generally speaking, the position of the animal is described by the region of the body that contacts the table. For example, right lateral **recumbency** means the animal is lying on its right side, dorsal recumbency means the animal is on its back, and sternal recumbency means the animal is on its belly. Maintaining patient positioning is facilitated by the use of adjustable surgical tables, portable tabletop V troughs, sand bags, or vacuum-activated "beanbags." It is important to anticipate how the patient should be positioned before patient preparation is begun so that catheters, monitoring equipment, and the like are readily accessible throughout the surgical procedure.

> **TECHNICIAN NOTE** The dorsal recumbent position is commonly used for abdominal surgical procedures.

In orthopedic surgery, the affected leg is often suspended from an overhead support or intravenous (IV) stand during skin preparation and initial surgical draping. The advantage of hanging the leg is that it allows aseptic preparation of the entire circumference of the limb, so the surgeon can manipulate the entire leg during surgery. To hang the leg, the distal unclipped portion of the limb is first covered with an examination glove, followed by white tape and vetwrap. Additional strips of tape (stirrups) are extended from the end of the foot. The limb is then suspended by these stirrups, allowing for circumferential scrubbing of the limb (Figure 30-84) from the foot to the level of the inguinal or axillary region. If the distal aspect of the foot needs to be exposed, the preclipped and soaked foot is hung using one or two towel clamps affixed to the skin or the cornified portion of the toenail.

EQUINE PATIENT PREPARATION

PATIENT POSITIONING

Positioning of the equine patient for surgery can be a highly involved process. It requires more personnel than are needed for small animal patients. In most situations, the minimum number of persons required to position a horse on a surgery table is three. A horse can be moved or transported to the surgical suite and ultimately onto the surgical table in various ways. The method used is determined by the physical setup of the surgical facility. An overhead hoist system greatly facilitates lifting and positioning of the horse onto the surgery table. As an example, the horse is walked into a padded induction room and is anesthetized while several persons push the horse against one of the walls (Figure 30-85, *A*). As the animal becomes anesthetized, supporting personnel allow it to collapse to the floor and then roll into lateral recumbency. At some surgical facilities, the horse is positioned in the center of the movable induction room floor that rolls into the surgical suite. Nylon leg bands are strapped to the front and rear feet, and an overhead chain hoist is hooked to the bands (Figure 30-85, *B*). The horse is raised off the floor and is moved onto the surgical table by way of a rail system on which the chain hoist moves. In other facilities, the horse is lifted off the induction floor with a hoist and is transported into the surgery room. Once the animal is over the surgical table, it is gently lowered onto the table in the desired recumbency. If the horse is to be in dorsal recumbency, it is maintained in this position with the use of side poles, with pads wedged between the poles and the horse

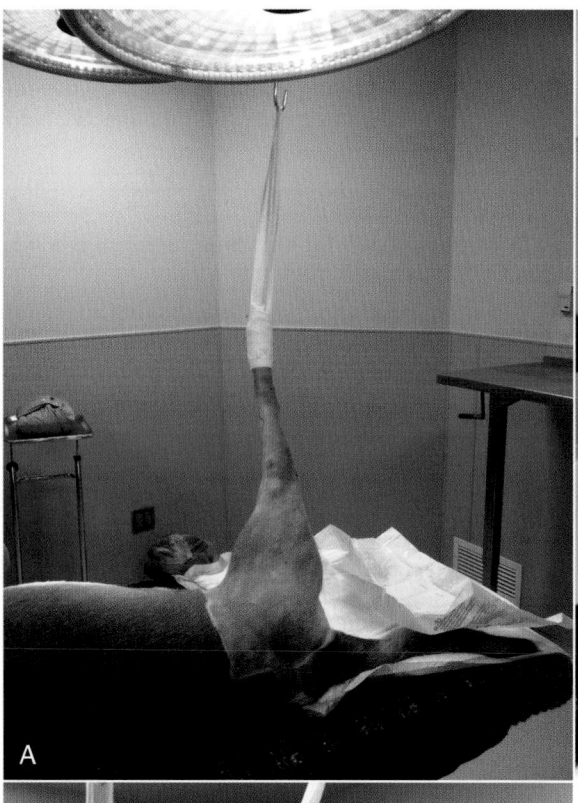

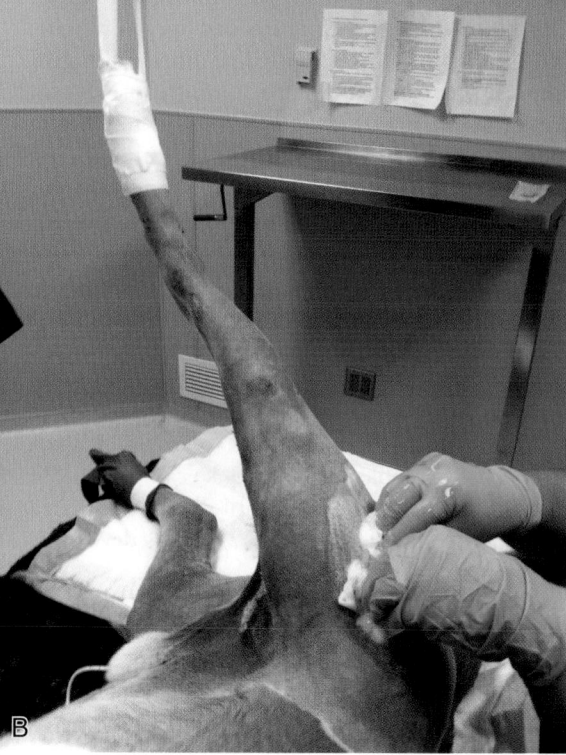

FIGURE 30-84 Hanging leg surgical preparation. This is commonly used for orthopedic surgeries of legs, including procedures involving the shoulder and hip. **A,** Taped stirrups are applied to the distal aspect of a clipped limb. The limb is suspended from the ceiling (pictured) or from a fluid stand or pole attached to the surgical table. **B,** A surgical scrub is applied to the leg working from the distal aspect of the limb downward in a circular pattern. **C,** Using sterile vet wrap, the surgeon covers the distal aspect of the limb prior to cutting of the taped stirrups. The leg will then be draped and positioned on the surgery table. (Courtesy Veterinary Specialty and Emergency Center, Langhorne, PA.)

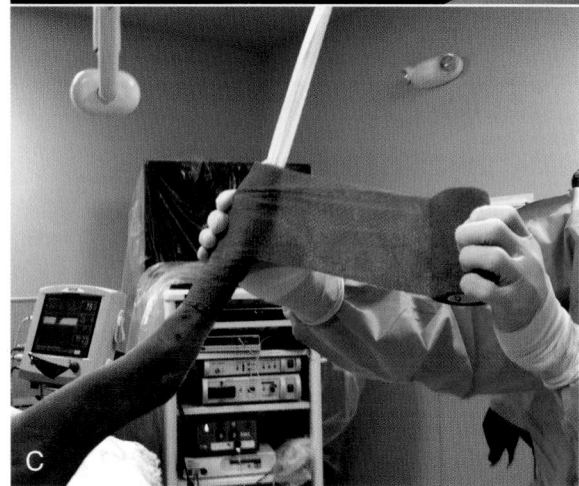

(Figure 30-85, *C*). Once the horse is positioned on the table, the leg bands are removed, and the legs may be secured to the positioning poles or table to reduce shifting of the horse during surgery. The chain hoist is rolled away, the rolling floor is pushed back into the padded induction room, and the surgical doors are closed. Large examination gloves or obstetrical (OB) sleeves are used to cover the feet of the horse to reduce contamination of the surgical suite. As with proper surgery room technique, personnel remaining in the surgical suite must wear proper surgical attire, including caps and masks. The surgical nurse should take charge to make sure that all personnel in the surgery suite are following protocol. During this preparation time, an anesthesiologist or anesthesiology technician is often placing arterial catheters in the hindlimb or facial artery, attaching the electrocardiographic (ECG) monitor, and attaching fluid lines to the IV catheters, which the scrub nurse must work around.

> **TECHNICIAN NOTE** The surgical nurse should take charge to make sure that all personnel in the surgery suite are following protocol.

SKIN PREPARATION

For some equine surgical procedures, particularly *abdominal surgeries*, it is difficult to clip the hair and perform an initial skin preparation before the horse is anesthetized; thus this must be done in the surgical suite. A wide area of hair at the intended surgical site is removed with electric clippers (Figure 30-85, *D*). The hair is collected with a portable vacuum. The initial skin preparation is performed by using chlorhexidine or povidone-iodine scrub with a rinse and wipe-down of alcohol. Next, a sterile skin preparation is performed with sterile gloves and sterile sponges. Three to five surgical scrubs alternating with chlorhexidine and

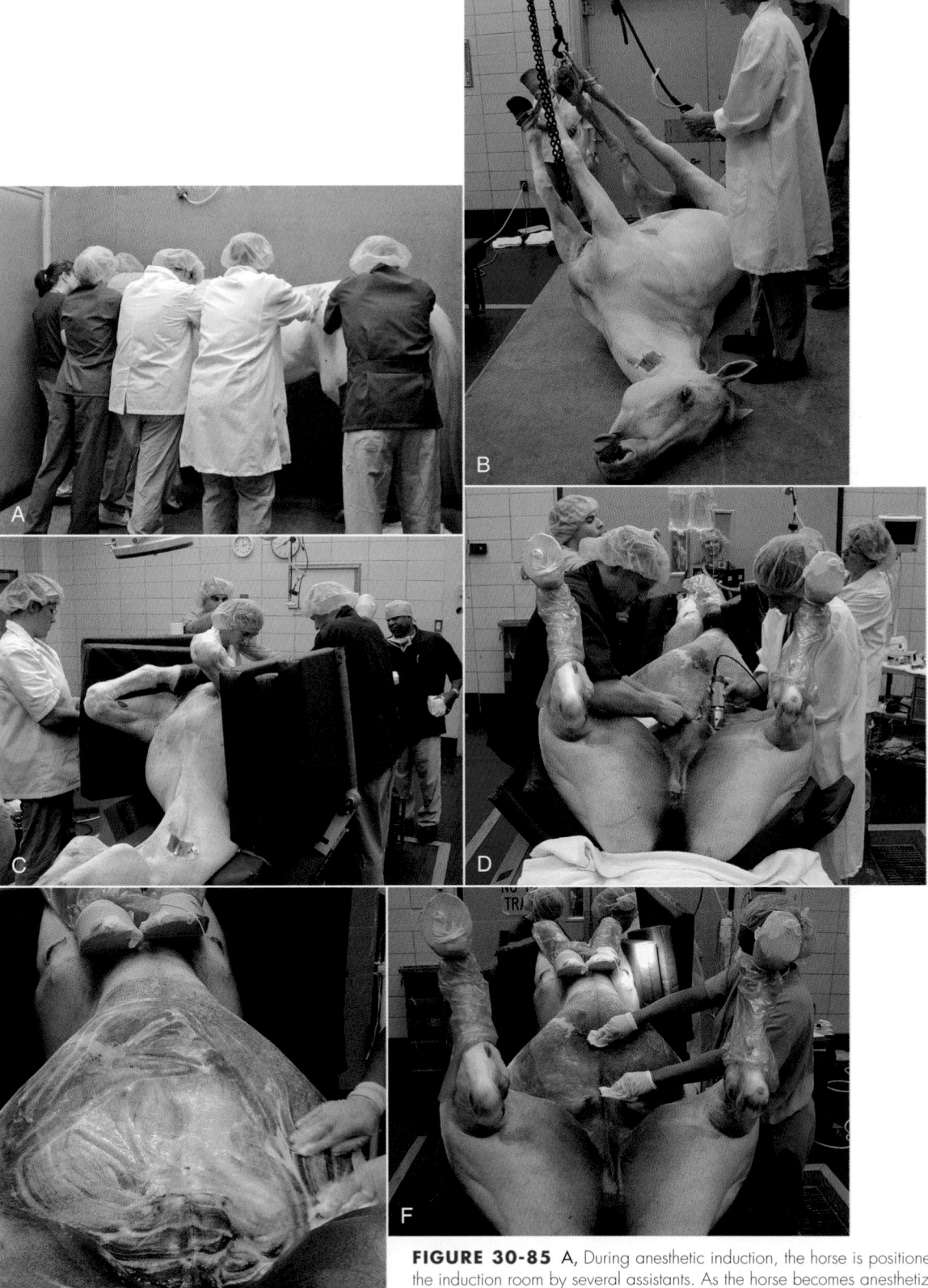

FIGURE 30-85 A, During anesthetic induction, the horse is positioned against the wall of the induction room by several assistants. As the horse becomes anesthetized, the assistants will keep the horse pressed to the wall as it slides to the floor. **B,** Nylon webbing leg bands are strapped to the horse's limbs at the pastern using double half-hitch loops. The leg bands are then attached to a chain hoist to transport the horse to the surgery table. **C,** The horse is maintained in dorsal recumbency for surgery using side poles with pads wedged between the poles and the horse. **D,** Large examination gloves or obstetrical (OB) sleeves are used to cover the feet of the horse to reduce contamination of the surgical suite. A wide area of hair is removed with electric clippers, and a surgical scrub of the area is subsequently performed. **E,** Three to five surgical scrubs are performed using chlorhexidine. **F,** The surgical area is rinsed with alcohol between scrubs.

alcohol are performed, starting at the center of the surgical site and moving outward in a circular fashion (Figure 30-85, *E*). Preparation is complete when the sponges no longer visibly collect dirt (Figure 30-85, *F*). A sterile bowl and gauze sponges are used to complete the final preparation of the surgical site on a horse. The inner sterile wrapping is opened with sterile gloves (Figure 30-86). After the final preparation

has been completed, the surgical area is sprayed with a chlorhexidine solution, which is left on the skin.

Before surgeries are performed on stallions and geldings, the opening of the prepuce sheath is packed with gauze sponges and is sutured closed. This prevents urine and smegma from contaminating the surgical field (Figure 30-87). With female horses, it is imperative that the mammary area is cleaned thoroughly.

SURGICAL TEAM PREPARATION

ATTIRE

Correct surgical attire and proper scrubbing, gowning, and gloving procedures are important aspects of aseptic technique. Street clothing, especially shoes, are a major source of contamination and should not be worn into the operating room. Ideally, each person should have a pair of shoes designated for use only in the operating room. Disposable shoe covers may be worn in the operating room and discarded upon leaving the room. Lint-free **scrub suits** should be worn in the operating room. The shirt should be tucked into the pants to reduce the amount of skin debris dispersed into the room. Outside the operating room, scrub suits should be protected by a laboratory coat to reduce contamination.

During surgery, surgical caps, masks, and booties are worn by all persons in the room. The surgical cap covers the hair to reduce airborne contamination. Different types of surgical head covers are available to cover short hair, long hair, or beards (Figure 30-88). The mask protects the wound from saliva droplets, primarily by redirecting airflow out the sides of the mask. It is important that one should not face

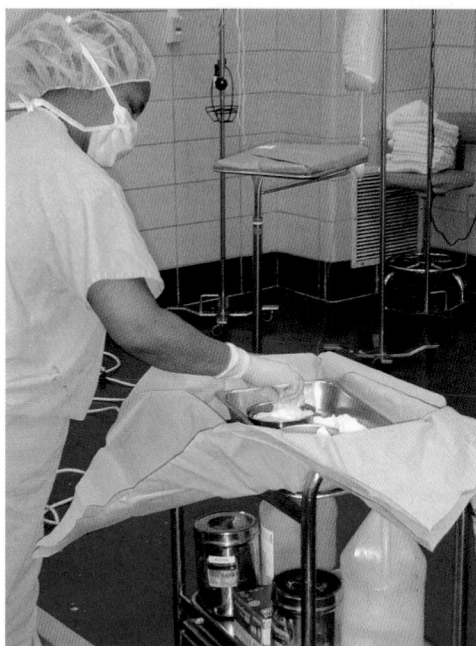

FIGURE 30-86 A sterile bowl and gauze sponges are used to do the final preparation of the surgical site on a horse. The inner sterile wrapping is opened with sterile gloves. Note that all personnel in the operating room wear caps and masks.

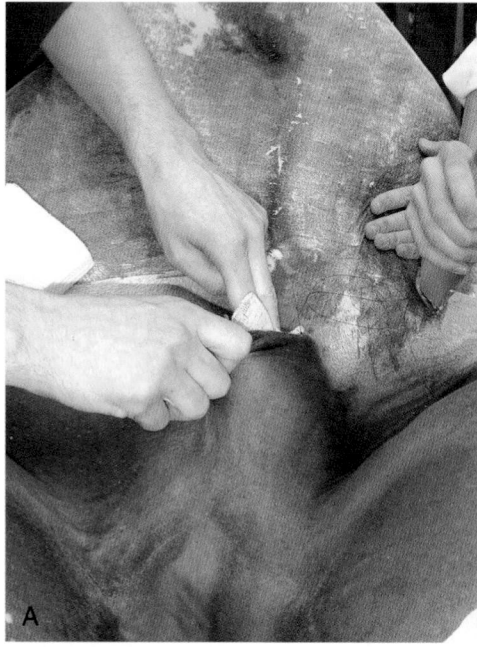

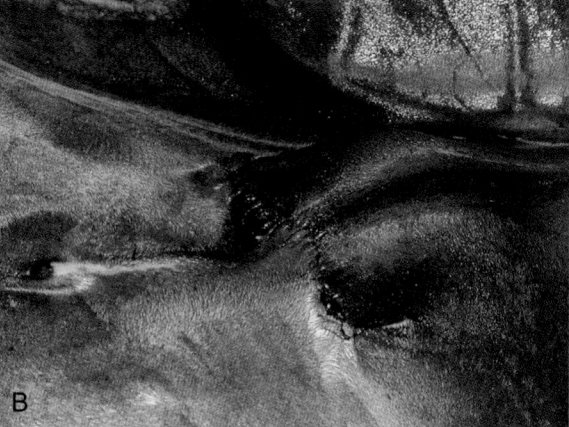

FIGURE 30-87 Surgical preparation of the ventral abdomen of a horse. **A,** During initial preparation of the ventral abdomen of a horse for surgery, the opening of the male's sheath (gelding or stallion) is packed with gauze sponges. **B,** It is sutured closed to prevent urine and smegma from contaminating the surgical field.

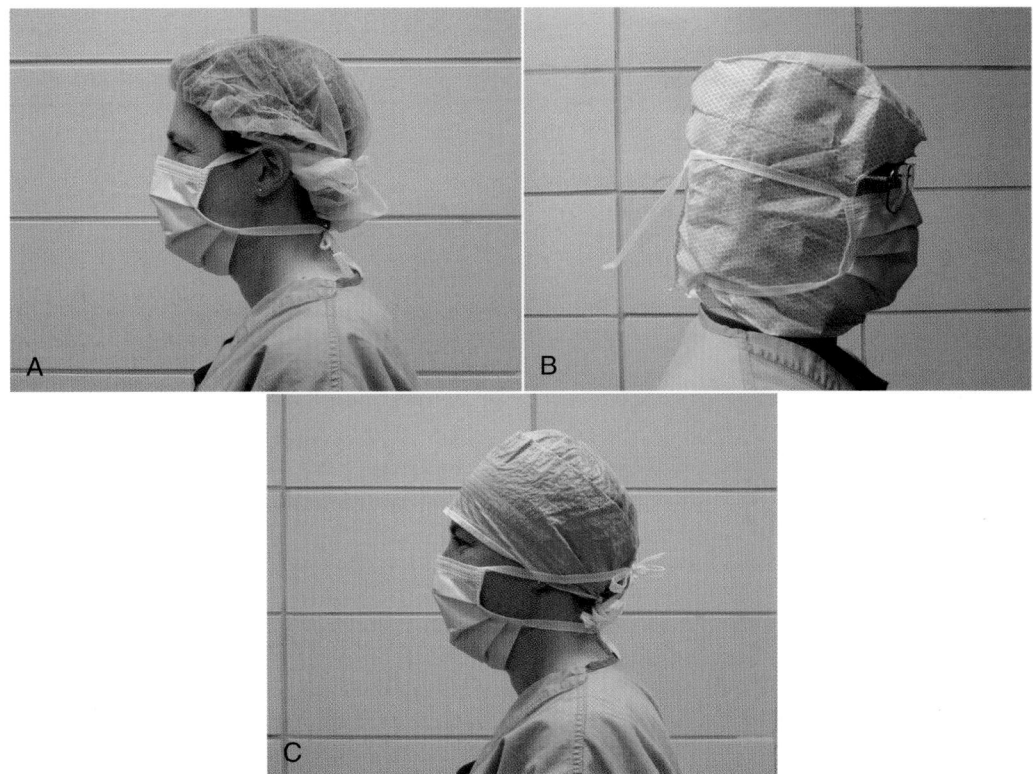

FIGURE 30-88 Surgical caps and masks. **A,** Bouffant head cover is used to cover long or short hair. **B,** Hoods are available for individuals with sideburns or a beard. **C,** A cap may be suitable for covering short hair.

away from the patient when talking, coughing, or sneezing because this allows debris to flow from the side of the mask potentially into the surgical field. Masks are effective for relatively short periods and should be changed between procedures.

> **TECHNICIAN NOTE** Anyone entering the operating room should wear a cap, mask, booties, and scrub suit.

HAND SCRUB

The purpose of the surgical hand scrub is to clean and remove debris and excessive oils from all skin surfaces distal to the surgeon's or surgical assistant's elbows. A properly performed surgical hand scrub also provides a prolonged antimicrobial effect on the previously scrubbed surface. Scrubbing should be performed before each procedure and should be followed by gowning and gloving. The surgical scrub provides protection from spreading microorganisms should a breach in sterile technique occur (e.g., torn glove, poor gowning and gloving technique), and even if an overt breach has not occurred. This scrub is done because gloves can contain microscopic perforations within the latex and should not be relied upon as the sole mechanism of preventing iatrogenic surgical site contamination from a surgeon's or assistant's hands.

Before the surgical scrub is begun, a surgical cap and mask should be donned, all jewelry removed, and each fingernail cleaned using a nail pick. Nail picks are typically included with individually wrapped scrub sponges. Additionally, the gown pack and gloves should be opened before scrubbing to facilitate gowning and gloving once the surgical scrub has been performed (Figure 30-89, A and B). During and after the surgical scrub, the hands should always be held above the level of the elbows so that any water or soap runs down the arm from "sterile to not sterile."

Surgical scrub brushes are commonly purchased as individual, prepackaged, antiseptic-soaked brushes. However, many practices still purchase reusable brushes, which require the application of antiseptic before the scrub is performed. If reusable scrub brushes are used, they should be thoroughly washed and resterilized between uses.

The surgical scrub begins distally at the fingers. All four sides of each finger should be scrubbed in a thorough and consistent manner (Figure 30-90, A). The back, both sides, and the palm of the hand are then scrubbed. Next, the wrist and forearm are scrubbed, working toward the elbow to complete the scrub (Figure 30-90, B). After completion of the scrub, the hands are rinsed in water so that the water flows from the fingers to the elbow (e.g., from clean to dirty) (Figure 30-90, C and D).

The two basic methods of surgical scrubs are *counted brush strokes* and *timed*. The counted brush strokes method is performed by counting the number of brush strokes used on each skin surface. Ten to 25 brush strokes are made on each surface of the fingers, hands, and arms before rinsing. This is done 4 times. The timed method is used more commonly and is done by repeatedly scrubbing and rinsing for

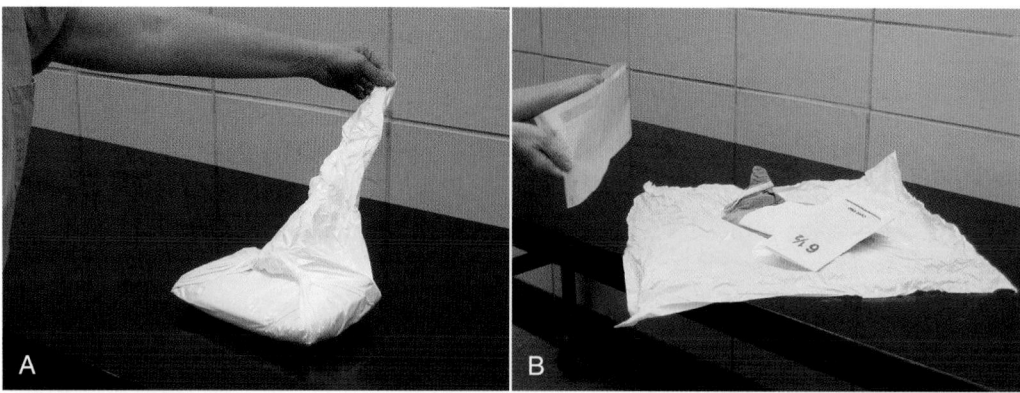

FIGURE 30-89 Open gown pack. **A,** The gown pack may be opened before scrubbing so that the hand towel is available. When opening a pack, always open the flap away from you first. Keep the arm off to the side, not directly over the pack. Then open the other three sides, touching only the corners of the wrap on the outside surface. **B,** The sterile gloves are opened onto the gown. With the package positioned at the edge of the sterile filed, it is opened symmetrically. This gives the contents enough forward momentum to fall onto the sterile field without the need for the clinician to reach over it.

a set period of time. The initial scrub of the day should last about 5 minutes. For subsequent scrubs during the day, 2 to 3 minutes is adequate.

> **TECHNICIAN NOTE** The surgical hand scrub requires that all surfaces of the fingers, hand, and forearm be scrubbed. Skin-soap contact time should last 5 minutes.

Waterless hand antiseptics can be considered an alternative or supplement to traditional scrubbing. These newer, alcohol- and chlorhexidine-based antiseptics have been shown to be at least as effective, if not more effective, in reducing skin bacterial numbers. The alcohol solution provides rapid bactericidal and other antimicrobial functions. Similar to traditional surgical scrubbing, hands must be clean and free of debris. In general, it is recommended that a traditional scrub be performed before the first procedure of the day to remove any debris; waterless hand antiseptics can be used for subsequent procedures throughout the day as hands remain clean. The solution is rubbed briskly and evenly over one hand and forearm; a second scrub is applied to the other hand and forearm. A final application is applied to both hands and is allowed to air dry. Waterless antiseptics are fast, effective, easy to apply, and nonirritating.

> **TECHNICIAN NOTE** Waterless hand antiseptics are easy to apply, faster than traditional hand-scrubbing techniques, effective against microorganisms, and nonirritating to the skin.

GOWNING AND GLOVING

The hands and arms are thoroughly dried with a sterile towel (Figure 30-91, *A* through *D*) before gowning and gloving. Gowning is performed as shown in Figure 30-92, *A* through *G*. First, the folded gown is grasped at the upside surface, and sleeve openings are identified. While the gown is held in this

region, it is allowed to unfold without touching any nonsterile surfaces. Arms are then inserted into each sleeve, and gowning is completed with the help of a nonsterile assistant by tying or fastening the gown around the surgeon's or surgical assistant's neck and waist.

The two methods used for gloving yourself are **closed gloving** and **open gloving**. The risk for contamination is minimized with closed gloving (Figure 30-93) because the outside of the gloves never contacts the skin. The risk for contamination is much higher during open gloving (Figure 30-94), and it is generally reserved for minor procedures for which a gown is not worn (e.g., sterile patient scrub, urinary catheterization). If it is necessary to replace gloves during surgery, it is preferable to have a nonsterile assistant remove the old gloves and simultaneously pull the gown sleeve so that the hands remain inside the sleeves (Figure 30-95). If the old gloves are removed in this manner, new gloves can be put on by the closed gloving method or by **assisted gloving** (Figure 30-96).

> **TECHNICIAN NOTE** The two methods of gloving yourself are *closed gloving* and *open gloving*. *Assisted gloving* requires the help of a sterile assistant.

MAINTAINING STERILITY

It is important for all members of the surgical team to be conscientious about sterility, even if they are not "scrubbed in" (i.e., gowned and gloved). Nonsterile personnel should touch only nonsterile items or areas and should not lean over or reach across **sterile fields**. Those who are scrubbed in should touch only sterile items or areas and should always face the sterile field. Only sterile items can be placed on a sterile field. If anyone on the surgical team notices a potential source of contamination or "break" in sterile technique, this should be mentioned immediately, so that steps can be taken to reduce the risk for further

Text continued on p. 1182

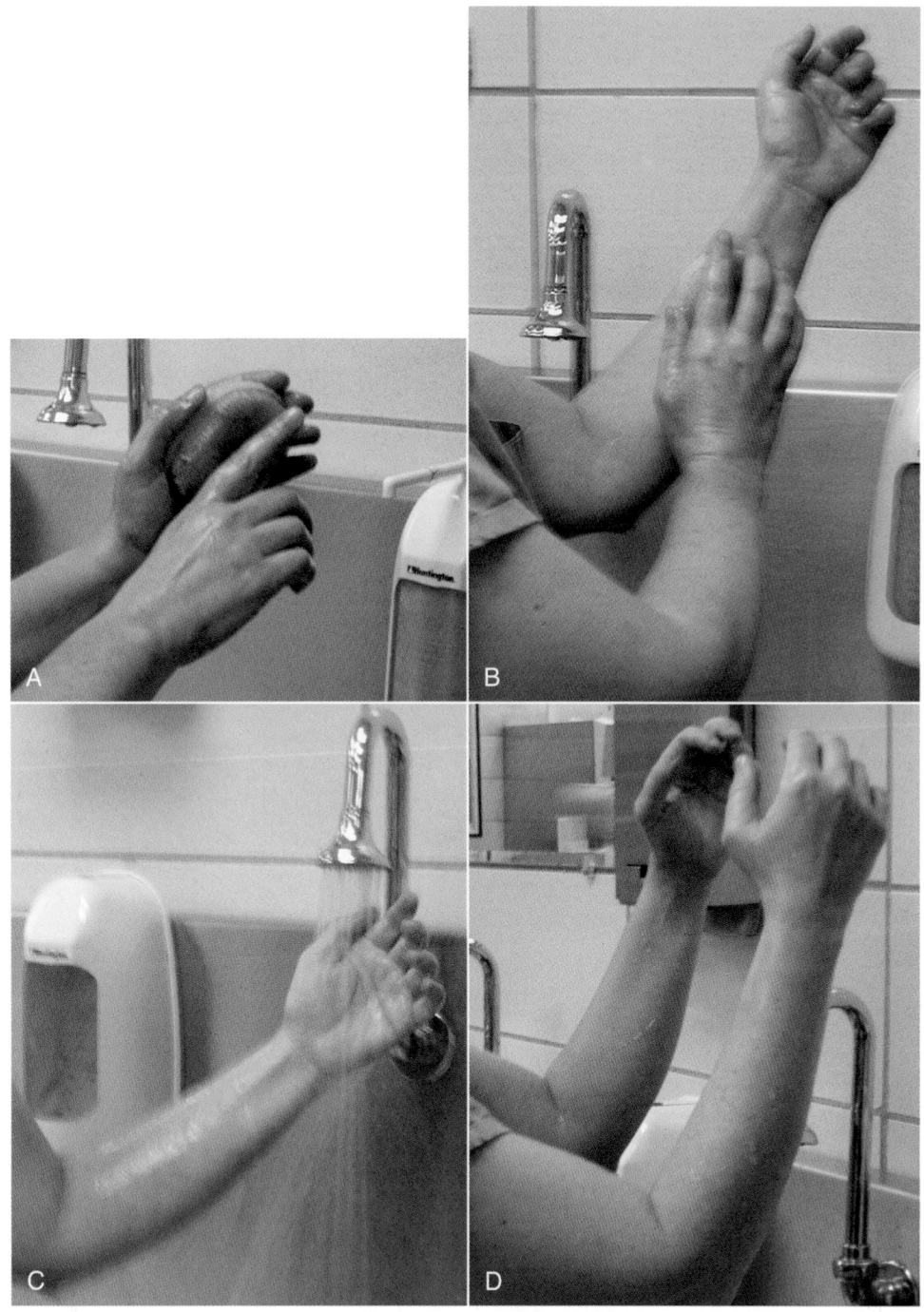

FIGURE 30-90 Surgical hand scrub. **A,** Imagine each finger as having a tip and four sides. Scrub each surface of each finger. Also scrub the palm, back, and sides of the hand. **B,** Imagine the forearm as having four sides, and scrub each side. **C,** After scrubbing both hands and arms, rinse the brush, hands, and forearms. The hands are always kept above the elbows. **D,** After the last scrub, drop the brush, rinse, and let the excess water drip off the elbows.

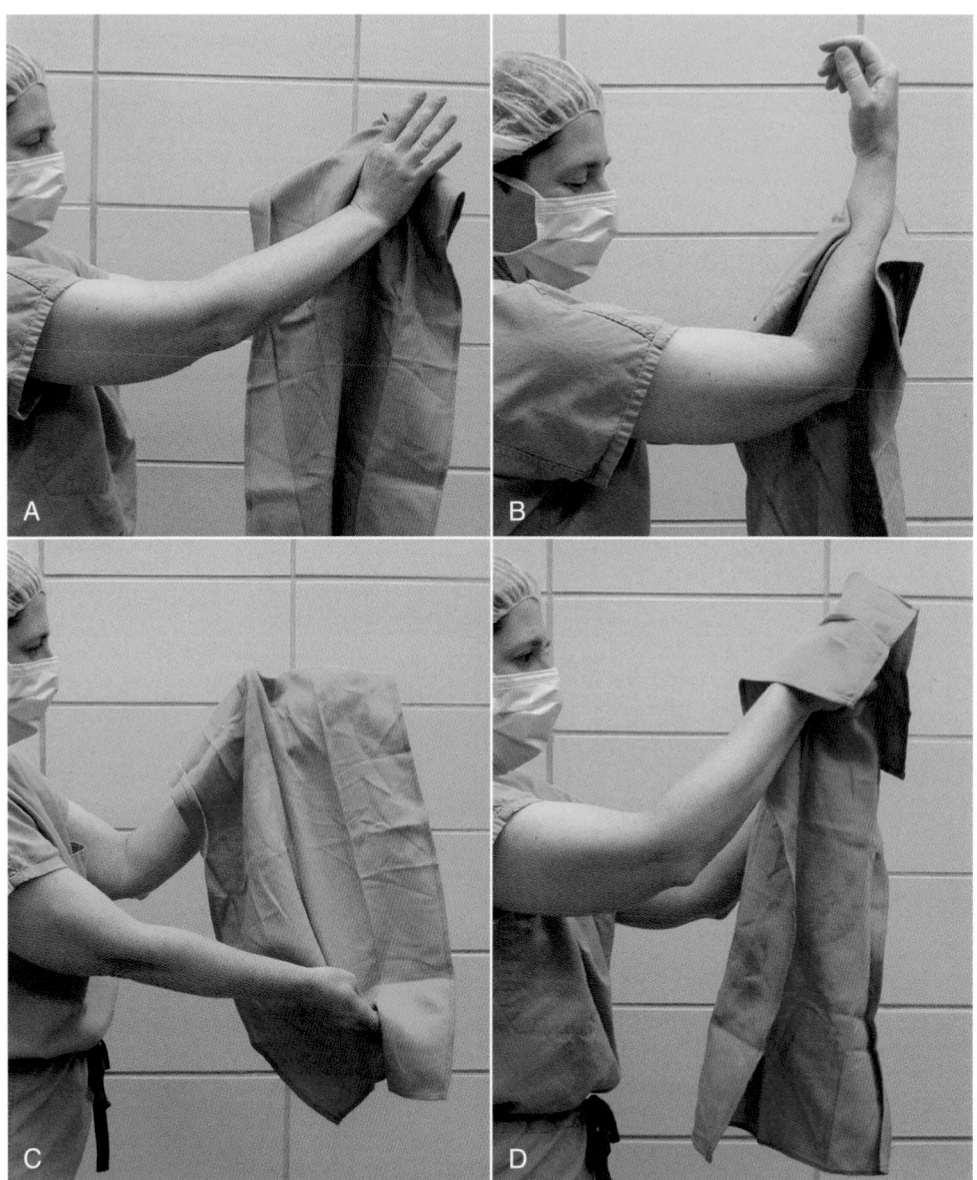

FIGURE 30-91 Towel dry. **A,** One hand is dried first, with the towel held away from the body. **B,** Move the towel down to dry the arm, using only the top end of the towel. **C,** The dry hand now grasps the dry end of the towel. **D,** The other hand and arm are dried. Note that the hands do not switch sides of the towel during the process.

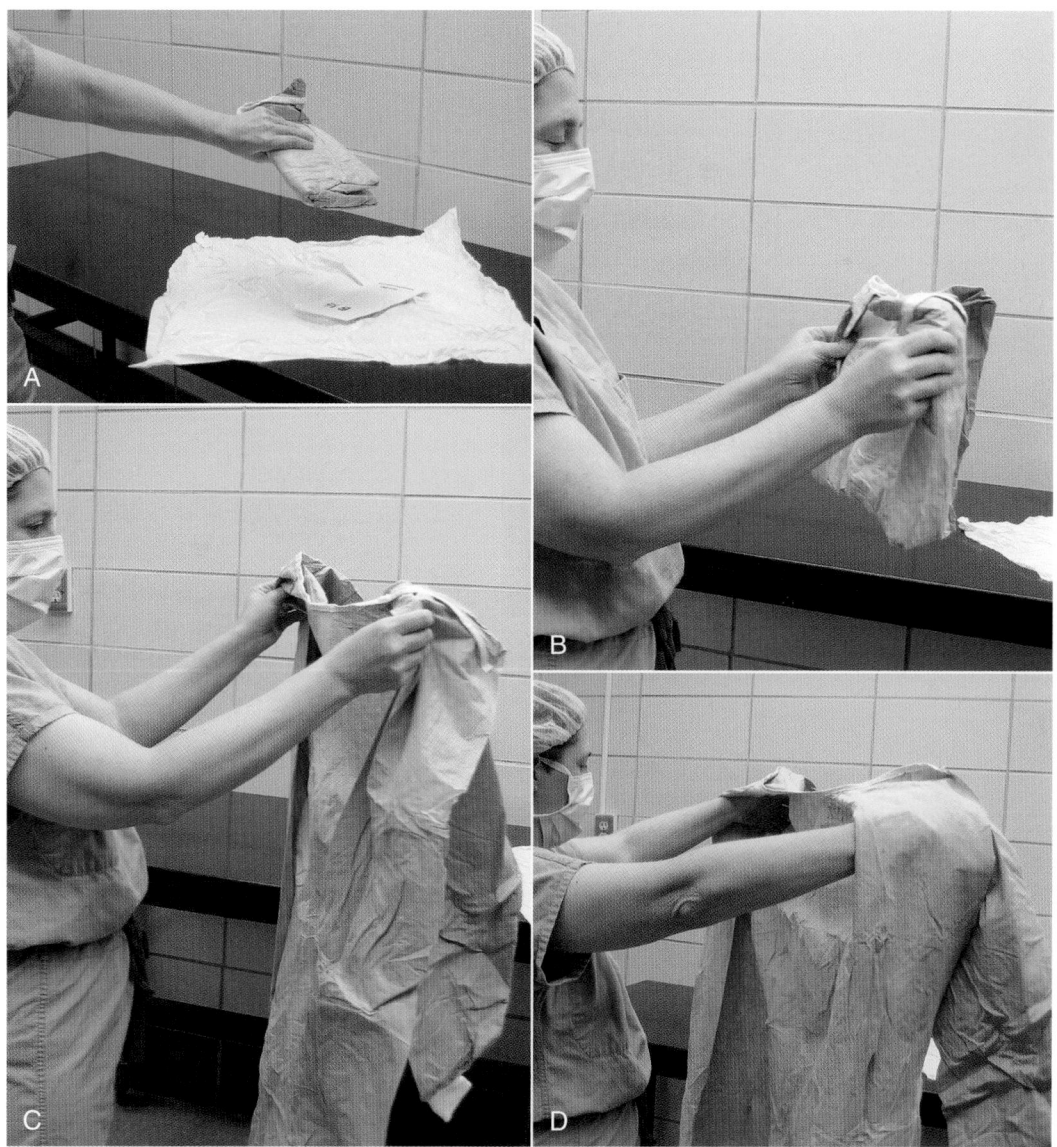

FIGURE 30-92 Gowning. **A,** The gown is picked up in its folded state. This same technique is used when picking up sterile folded towels or drapes. This reduces the risk for accidental contamination. **B,** Move to a spacious area to reduce the risk for contamination. **C,** The gown is held away from the body by the inside shoulder seams and is allowed to unfold. **D,** The arms are slid into the sleeves, but the hands should not extend through the cuff openings.

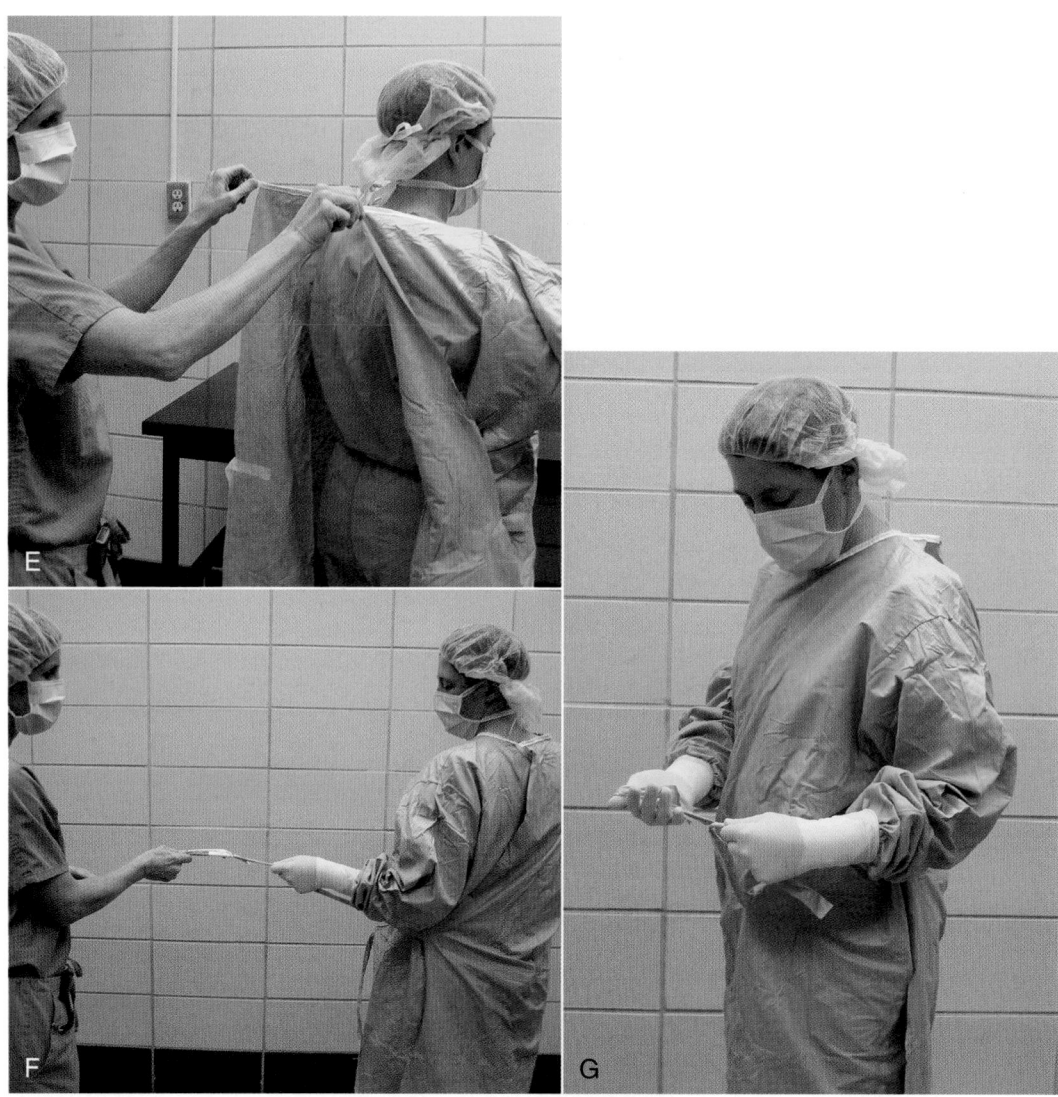

FIGURE 30-92, cont'd E, A nonsterile assistant pulls the gown over the shoulders and ties the back of the gown at the neck and waist. F, If the gown has a wraparound back, the last tie is performed after the surgeon has gloved. The surgeon hands the sterile tag to a nonsterile assistant. The assistant holds the end of the tag while the surgeon turns around, causing the gown to cover the surgeon's back. The surgeon takes the gown tie and pulls, releasing it from the tag that is still in the assistant's hand. G, The final tie is done in front by the surgeon.

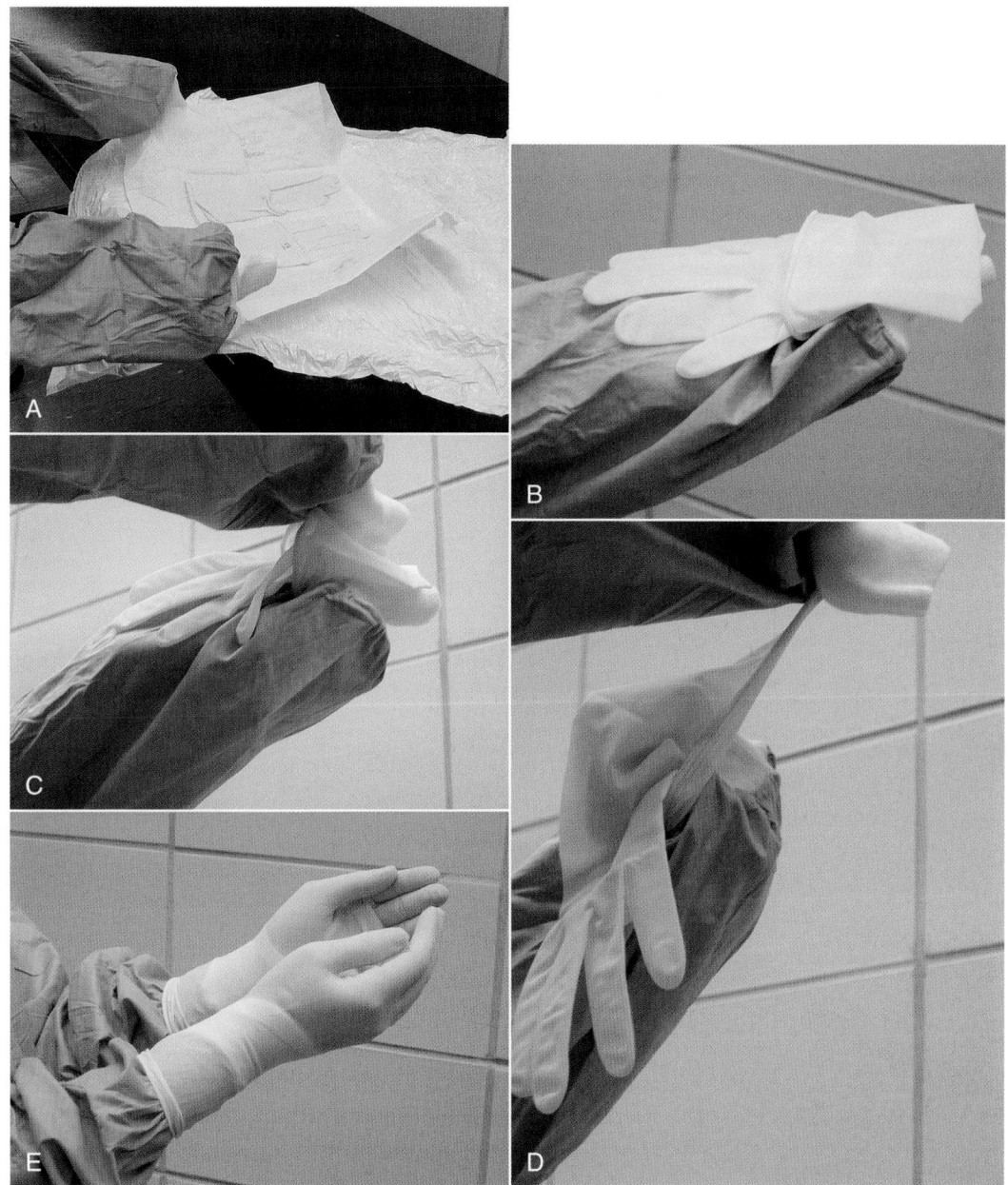

FIGURE 30-93 Closed gloving. **A,** The sterile pack is close to the table edge so that the surgeon can maintain some distance from the table to prevent contaminating the sterile gown. The sterile paper wrap containing the gloves is unfolded, and one glove is picked up. It is easiest for most people to glove their nondominant hand first. The fingers must be kept inside the sleeves at all times during closed gloving. **B,** The glove is laid on the hand to be gloved, with the glove fingers pointing toward the elbow and the glove thumb lying against the sleeve. The edge of the glove cuff is grasped through the gown sleeve. **C,** The opposite side of the cuff is grasped in the other hand. **D** and **E,** The glove is pulled over the hand. Now the gown and the glove cuff may be grasped together to pull the glove completely onto the hand.

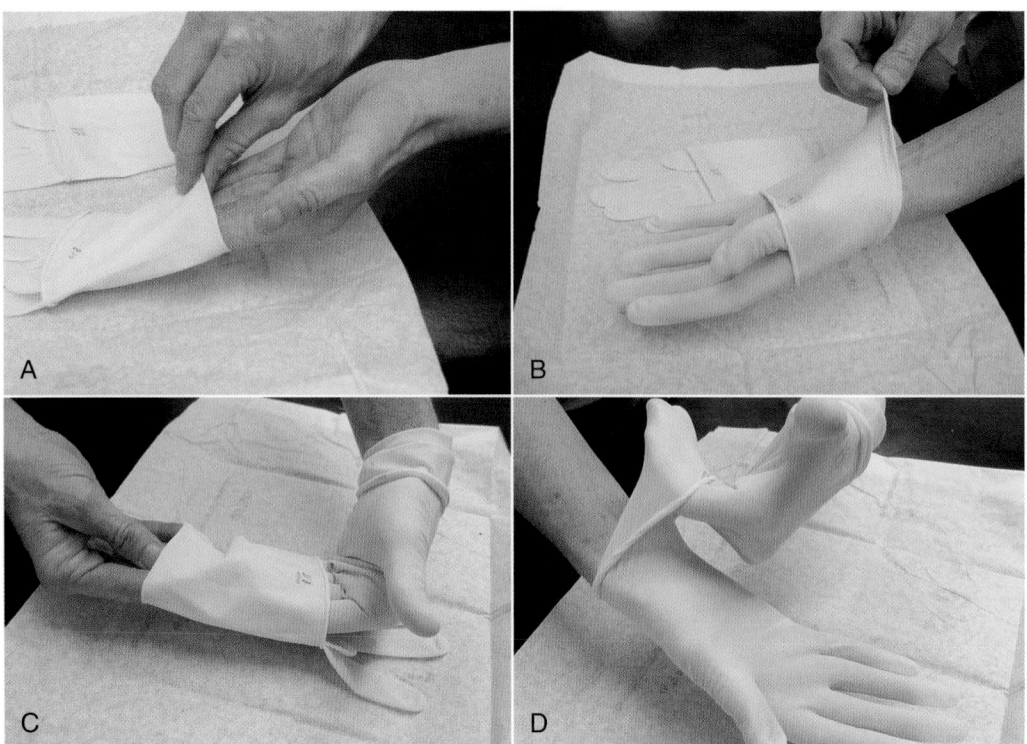

FIGURE 30-94 Open gloving. **A,** The glove pack is opened near the edge of a table. The hand is inserted into the glove opening, taking care not to touch the outside of the glove. The inside of the glove will not be sterile, so the cuff may be touched. **B,** The glove is pulled on by grasping the cuff fold with the other hand. The cuff will still be folded, but the glove is on well enough to allow use of the hand. **C,** The gloved hand is placed between the cuff and the palm of the glove to assist gloving of the other hand. This protects the gloved hand from accidental contamination on the arm. **D,** The cuff can be unfolded. Now adjustments can be made to both gloves, taking care to touch only the sterile areas of the gloves.

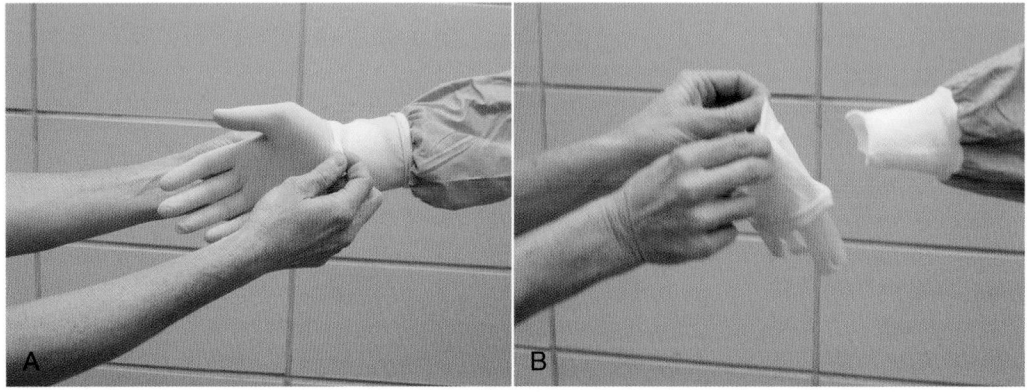

FIGURE 30-95 Removing gloves aseptically. **A,** A nonsterile assistant grasps the glove and gown cuff together without touching the gown sleeve. **B,** As the glove is removed, the gown is pulled over the fingers. The gown cuff is considered contaminated. The surgeon can reglove, taking care not to contaminate anything with the gown cuff. It may be preferable to perform an assisted gloving as shown in Figure 30-96.

contamination. To reduce contamination, only essential personnel should be present in the operating room, and excessive movement should be avoided. Conversation should be kept to a minimum.

> **TECHNICIAN NOTE** Nonsterile personnel should not lean over or reach across sterile fields.

Scrubbed-In Personnel

The sterile area on a person is considered to be the front of the gown, from just below the shoulders (the neckline is not sterile) to the waist or the level of the table. The gown sleeves are also considered to be sterile. Note that the back of a gowned person is considered to be nonsterile, so it should not be turned to face any sterile field. Gloved hands may be rested on a sterile drape or clasped in front of the body in the zone between the shoulders and the waist. The arms

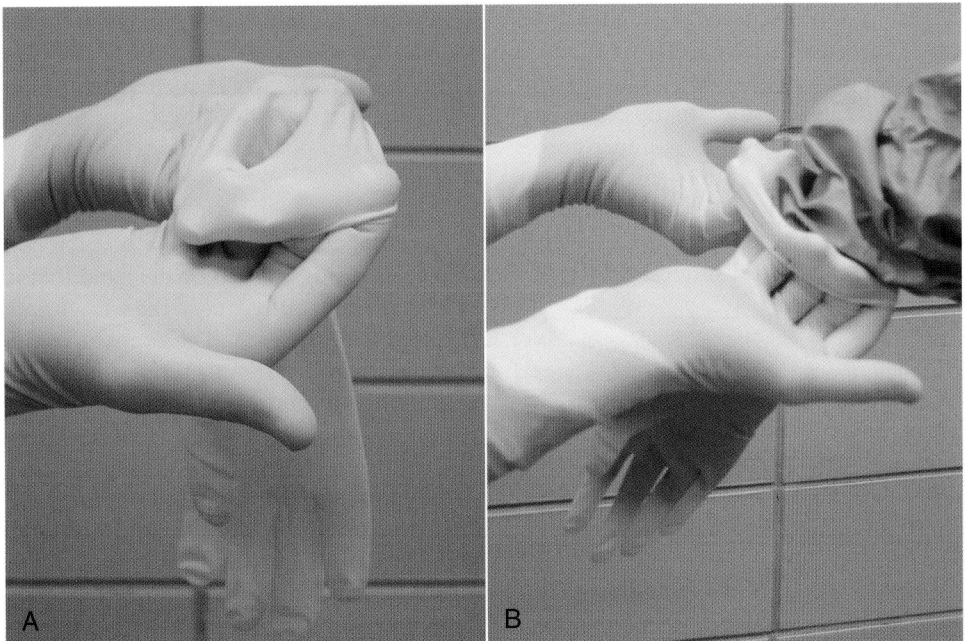

FIGURE 30-96 Assisted gloving. **A,** A sterile assistant picks up the appropriate sterile glove, holding it so the location of the glove thumb is apparent. The assistant hooks his or her fingers under the glove cuff and pulls to make the glove opening as large as possible. **B,** The surgeon slides his or her hand into the glove while the assistant pulls the glove cuff up to be sure it covers the gown cuff before releasing.

should not be folded across the chest because the armpit region is considered to be nonsterile, and the hands should not drop below waist level.

> **TECHNICIAN NOTE** After gowning and gloving, the sterile region is the front of the gown between the waist and just below the shoulders. Gown sleeves are also sterile, but not the back.

THE PATIENT

Sterile surgical drapes are used to maintain a sterile field around the surgical site. Draping is performed by personnel who have scrubbed in. First, four small towels (cloth or paper) are placed to surround the area where the surgical incision will be made. These are called *quarter drapes*, and they are secured to the skin using towel clamps. *Towel clamps* are forceps used to attach towels and drapes to the patient. These forceps have pointed tips that curve and join like ice tongs. They are available in different sizes. *Backhaus towel clamps* and *Roeder towel clamps* are two common designs. The Roeder towel clamp has a metal bead or ball stop attached to the jaws that prevents deep tissue penetration and prevents the towel from slipping toward the box lock of the forceps.

During this procedure, one must be careful to avoid brushing the front of the surgical gown against the surgical table. A large drape is placed over the animal, the surgical table, and the instrument stand to provide one continuous sterile field. Cloth drapes have an opening or *fenestration*, which is positioned over the surgical site. If a disposable paper drape is used, an appropriately sized hole may be cut

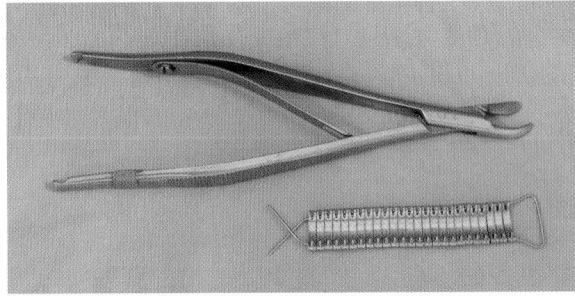

FIGURE 30-97 Michel skin clips and Michel clip forceps.

after the drape has been placed. Because skin preparations do not sterilize but only disinfect the skin, additional incisional drapes or plastic incise drapes may be used to provide a sterile surface at the start of surgery. Incisional drapes are attached at the incision edges using *Michel clips* (Figure 30-97), scalp clamps, or towel clamps. Such incisional drapes have largely been replaced by translucent, self-adhesive coverings. These newer skin coverings are used to completely cover any visible skin after the barrier drapes have been applied before the skin incision is made. Additionally, incise drapes are often impregnated with an antiseptic (e.g., Ioban, 3M Products, St Paul, Minnesota). The surgeon can cut through the incise drape while making the skin incision. Refer to Chapter 31 for additional details on draping procedures.

If a limb has been suspended in preparation for an orthopedic procedure (as described under "Patient Positioning"), quarter drapes are placed on the body at the base of the limb. The nonscrubbed, distal portion of the limb is then covered first with an impermeable sterile material (e.g., aluminum foil), followed by covering with a sterile towel or adhesive material (e.g., gas sterilized Vetrap [3M]). During this process, a nonsterile assistant cuts the stirrups, allowing complete covering of the distal limb with the impermeable sterile material and wrap. A sterile cotton stockinette or adhesive incise drape may be used to cover the entire limb. Finally, the limb is passed through a hole in the large sterile drape that covers the entire animal and surgical field.

> **TECHNICIAN NOTE** The *optimal* approach to draping includes isolating the surgical site with two layers of drapes: (1) four quarter drapes, and (2) a large drape that covers the entire animal and the instrument table. Additional incisional drapes or antiseptic-impregnated adhesive drapes can be added to further improve aseptic technique.

After draping is completed, sterile instrument packs, light handles, and other sterile equipment may be opened. Draped tables and instrument trays are considered to be sterile only on the top of the draped surface, so if part of a sterile item slips below the level of the tabletop, it is considered to be contaminated and should no longer be touched by the surgeons.

OPENING STERILE ITEMS

Nonsterile assistants must open all sterile items for the surgeon. Nonsterile assistants can touch only the outside of sterile packs and should never reach over a sterile field. Large or heavy packs, such as an instrument pack, may be set on a table to be opened. The four folded edges of the outer wrap are opened one at a time, and the hand and arm are never extended over the top of the pack in a fashion similar to opening a sterile gown. If the pack can be placed on a *Mayo*

instrument stand, this can be accomplished by moving around the stand and pulling each fold away from the center. The inner wrap may be opened by the surgeon or by a nonsterile assistant. Once the instrument tray is exposed, the surgeon can pick it up and set it on the draped instrument stand.

A smaller wrapped pack may be opened while it is held in one hand (Figure 30-98). As each corner of the pack is unfolded, it is grasped by the hand that is holding the pack. This prevents the edges of the wrap from contaminating the contents of the pack. The exposed item may be grasped by the surgeon or carefully set on the sterile field.

To open a plastic or paper pouch, scalpel blade, or suture package, the edges of the wrapper should be peeled back slowly and symmetrically, keeping the package opening directed away from the body. Some items may be dropped onto the sterile field; be careful not to lean or reach across the sterile field. If the item is small or awkward to handle, the surgeon can grasp it with a gloved hand or a sterile instrument. The item should not be allowed to touch the peeled edges of the pouch because the edges are considered contaminated.

> **TECHNICIAN NOTE** While opening a pack, make sure that the opening faces away from you.

Sterile saline may be poured into the sterile saline bowl. To avoid reaching over the sterile field with the saline container or spilling onto the draped surface, the surgeon may hold the bowl away from the instrument tray or position it on the tray at the edge of the sterile field. The lip of the saline container should be a few inches above the rim of the bowl to reduce the risk of touching it, but not so high that the saline splashes as it is poured. If drapes or gowns (especially

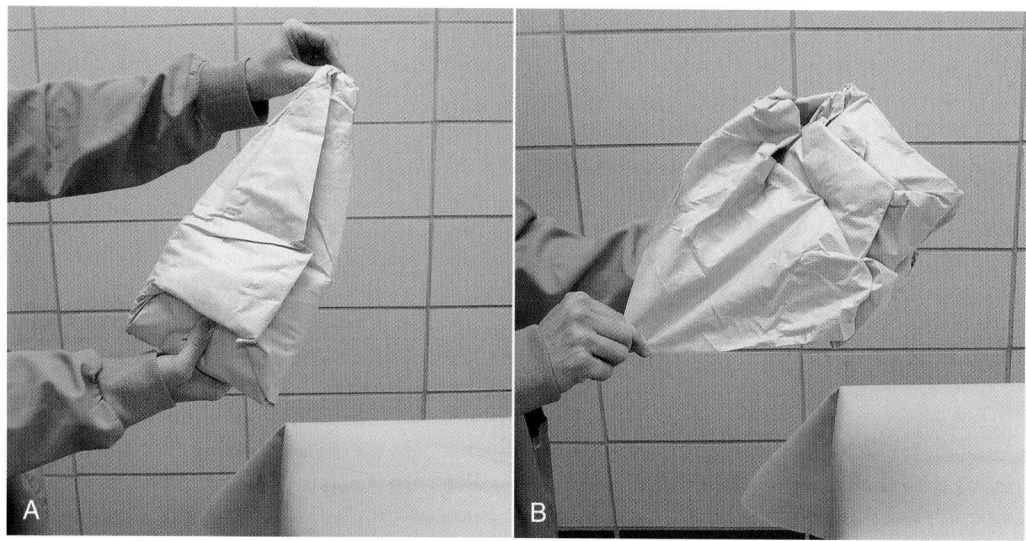

FIGURE 30-98 Opening a sterile pack that can be held in one hand. **A,** Open the first flap away from you. **B,** As each flap is opened, it is held together with the hand holding the pack. After the fourth flap is pulled back and secured, the inner package may be grasped by the surgeon. Move the wrap down and toward you as the surgeon lifts the contents up and toward him or her. Alternatively, the package may be set on a sterile field near its edge to avoid reaching over the field.

those made of cloth) become wet with saline or blood, they may no longer be impermeable to bacteria and are said to have **strike-through**. If this occurs, the instruments in contact with the region of strike-through should no longer be considered sterile and should be removed from the surgical field.

> **TECHNICIAN NOTE** If drapes or gowns (especially those made of cloth) become wet with saline or blood, they may no longer be impermeable to bacteria and are said to have *strike-through*.

RECOMMENDED READINGS

Bartels KE: Lasers in veterinary medicine—where have we gone, and where are we going? In Bartels KE, editor: The Veterinary Clinic of North America, Small Animal Practice, Philadelphia, 2002, Saunders.

Beale BS, Hulse DA, Schulz KS, et al: Small animal arthroscopy, St Louis, 2003, Saunders.

Chamness CJ: Nondisposable instrumentation for equine laparoscopy. In Fischer AT, Jr, editor: Equine diagnostic surgical laparoscopy, Philadelphia, 2002, Saunders.

Cockshutt J: Principles of surgical asepsis. In Slatter D, editor: Textbook of small animal surgery, ed 3, St Louis, 2003, Saunders.

Fry TR: Laser safety. In Bartels KE, editor: The Veterinary Clinic of North America, Small Animal Practice, Philadelphia, 2002, Saunders.

Hobson HP: Surgical facilities and equipment. In Slatter D, editor: Textbook of small animal surgery, ed 3, St Louis, 1993, Saunders.

Kronberger C: The veterinary technician's role in laser surgery. In Bartels KE, editor: The Veterinary Clinic of North America, Small Animal Practice, Philadelphia, 2002, Saunders.

Lemarie RJ, Hosgood G: Antiseptics and disinfectants in small animal practice, Compend Cont Educ Pract Vet 17:1339, 1996.

McIlwraith CW, Nixon AJ, Wright IM, et al: Diagnostic and surgical arthroscopy in the horse, ed 3, Philadelphia, 2005, Mosby.

Mitchell SL, Berg J: Sterilization. In Slatter D, editor: Textbook of small animal surgery, ed 3, Philadelphia, 2003, Saunders.

Nieves MA, Wagner SD: Surgical instruments. In Slatter D, editor: Textbook of small animal surgery, ed 3, Philadelphia, 2003, Saunders.

Pavletic MM: Surgical stapling, Vet Clin North Am 24:225, 1994.

Shmon C: Assessment and preparation of the surgical patient and the operating team. In Slatter D, editor: Textbook of small animal surgery, ed 3, Philadelphia, 2003, WB Saunders.

Sonsthagen TF: Veterinary instruments and equipment: a pocket guide, ed 2, St Louis, 2011, Mosby.

Tear M: Small animal surgical nursing, ed 2, St Louis, 2012, Mosby.

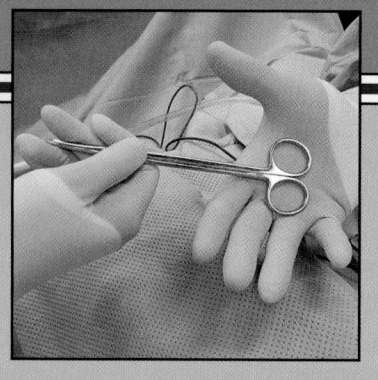

William T.N. Culp and Daniel J. Burba

KEY TERMS

Fenestrated
Impervious
Ingesta
Laparotomy
Orthopedic
Swaged

OUTLINE

General Concepts in Veterinary Surgical Assisting, *1188*
Role of the Surgical Assistant, *1188*
Preoperative Preparation, *1188*
Preparation of the Surgical Patient, *1188*
Operating Room Sterility, *1193*
Surgical Instruments and Instrument Table Organization, *1193*
Intraoperative Techniques, *1194*
Surgical Lighting, *1194*
Instrumentation Cords and Tubing, *1194*
Scalpel Use, *1195*
Instrument Passing, *1195*
Retraction, *1196*
Hemostasis, *1196*
Suture Cutting, *1197*
Lavage and Suction, *1197*
Camera Manipulation, *1197*

Tissue Manipulation, Retraction, and Organ Positioning, *1197*
Surgical Implants, *1199*
Postoperative Management, *1200*
Suture Material, *1201*
Considerations When Choosing Suture, *1201*
Suture Classification and Examples, *1202*
Suture Needles, *1203*
Suture Placement and Removal, *1204*
Surgical Assisting for Equine Patients, *1204*
Draping for Abdominal Surgery, *1204*
Draping for Orthopedic Surgery, *1205*
Instrument Setup and Handling, *1207*
Tissue Handling Techniques, *1208*
Suture Materials Used in Horses, *1210*

LEARNING OBJECTIVES

When you have completed this chapter, you will be able to:

1. Pronounce, define, and spell all Key Terms in this chapter.
2. Describe the role of the veterinary technician in surgical assistance for large and small animal patients.
3. Explain preoperative preparation, including preoperative preparation of the surgical patient, clipping, and surgical scrub techniques. Discuss considerations for operating room sterility and instrument table organization.
4. Discuss the following intraoperative techniques of the surgical assistant: surgical lighting, instruments, hemostasis, suture cutting, lavage and suction, camera manipulation, tissue manipulation, retraction, and organ positioning.
5. Describe the most common permanent and temporary forms of surgical implants and their uses.
6. Describe the role of the surgical assistant in the postoperative management of patients.
7. Discuss the considerations involved in choosing a type of suture material, and list and describe commonly used suture materials and needles and their application.
8. Discuss the differences associated with surgical assisting in equine patients, including draping techniques, instrument setup, tissue handling, and suture materials used in horses.

The authors and publisher wish to acknowledge the contribution of Susanne K. Lauer to previous editions of this chapter.

INTRODUCTION

Small and large animal patients are anesthetized, positioned on the operating table, and prepared for surgery by veterinary technicians who serve as anesthetist, operating room technician, and surgical assistant. Their role in the operating room (OR) is indispensable. In some practices, a single veterinary technician may juggle all three of these roles; at other practices, specialized veterinary technicians carry out the roles individually.

Excellent veterinary operating room technicians and surgical assistants improve surgical outcomes by ensuring that effective sterile techniques and proper operating room conduct are carried out before, during, and after each and every surgical procedure. This chapter focuses on the role of the surgical assistant and presents surgery-specific techniques, types and characteristics of suture material, and correct instrument handling.

Refer to Chapter 30 for information about surgical instrumentation and aseptic preparation of the patient. The duties of the anesthetist are covered in Chapter 29.

GENERAL CONCEPTS IN VETERINARY SURGICAL ASSISTING

ROLE OF THE SURGICAL ASSISTANT

While the veterinary operating room technician prepares surgical instrument tables on which all of the required instruments, tools, and materials are placed, the surgical assistant collaborates with the surgeon to ensure that patients are properly clipped, scrubbed, and positioned. The surgical assistant is also responsible for confirming that all of the equipment needed to perform a particular surgical procedure is nearby to allow quick and easy access throughout the surgical procedure. Veterinary technicians who serve as surgical assistants possess a thorough understanding of preoperative patient preparation, positioning, intraoperative techniques, instrumentation, instrument handling, and postoperative wound and patient care. Veterinary technicians who are skilled in carrying out duties required during preoperative, intraoperative, and postoperative surgical phases increase the likelihood of a positive surgical outcome.

PREOPERATIVE PREPARATION

PREPARATION OF THE SURGICAL PATIENT
Assessment of Clipping and Surgical Scrub

Instructions for clipping hair from the incision site, performing an initial scrub, and transporting the patient to the operating room from the prep area are presented in Chapter 30. When the patient has been moved to the operating room, it is important for the surgical assistant to take responsibility for assessing the clipped area for proper dimensions and thoroughness of hair removal. The surgical assistant will be able to determine whether sufficient hair has been removed, thus preventing contamination of the surgical site. For procedures involving the hanging-limb technique, the surgical assistant should particularly focus on aseptic preparation of the distal limb because this portion of the limb will be located within the sterile field.

Positioning and Draping

Before surgery, the operating room technician positions the surgical patient on the basis of several factors:
1. The surgical approach
2. The particular surgery to be performed
3. The draping technique for that procedure
4. The number of surgeries to be performed on the patient

During positioning of the patient, the veterinary technician may place a warming blanket and an electrocautery plate, if required for the procedure. The warming blanket must be located away from the surgical site and should not be turned on until the patient has been properly draped to prevent contamination of the surgical field. Electrocautery plates should be in direct contact with the patient at all times (Figure 31-1). Poor contact with the patient may affect the

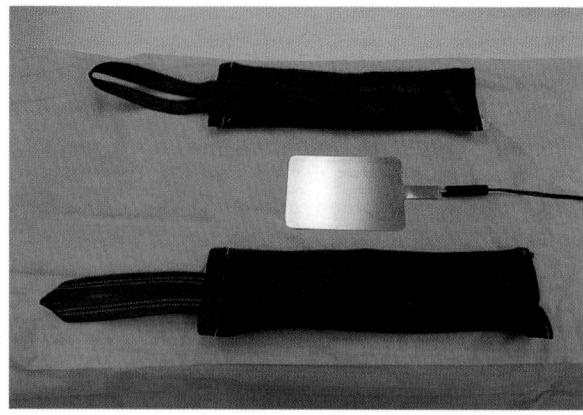

FIGURE 31-1 The surgery table has been prepared with the cautery plate in the center of the table. Additionally, sandbags are used to stabilize the patient in the proper position.

function of the electrocautery unit. This is a particular concern in patients with long, thick hair coats.

> **TECHNICIAN NOTE**   Assess the location of the warming blanket and the electrocautery plate before draping.

Patients can be maintained in the desired position by a variety of means. Tape can be passed over the patient and secured to the table to prevent the patient from moving. Alternatively, sandbags can be used to prevent movement of a patient (see Figure 31-1). Vacuum bags are a useful alternative to tape and sandbags (Figure 31-2). These bags are generally placed under the patient, and the patient is held in position by OR nurses while air is evacuated from the bag. When air has been sufficiently removed from the bag, the bag will maintain rigid positioning of the patient.

Placement of sterile surgical drapes increases asepsis during surgery and diminishes postoperative complications from infection. Drapes are typically wrapped and sterilized in a package that can be opened before surgery and placed on an instrument table (Figure 31-3). When preparation of the surgical site is finished, and after the surgeon and the surgical assistant are fully gowned and gloved, the patient can be draped by the surgeon and the surgical assistant. Care should be taken to establish a sterile surgical field. Because skin cannot be sterilized, it is considered nonsterile. Sterile drapes are therefore placed around the surgical site to cover the nonsterile skin and to establish an **impervious** barrier. In this way, surgical drapes effectively decrease the contact of sterile instruments and gloved hands with nonsterile skin and hair.

Specific drapes are designed for particular procedures. Surgical assistants and circulating OR technicians should be familiar with the different types of drapes and should understand how they are to be used. Quarter drapes, towel clamps, and a single large surgical drape that is capable of covering the patient and the entire surgery table should be available to the surgical team (Figure 31-4).

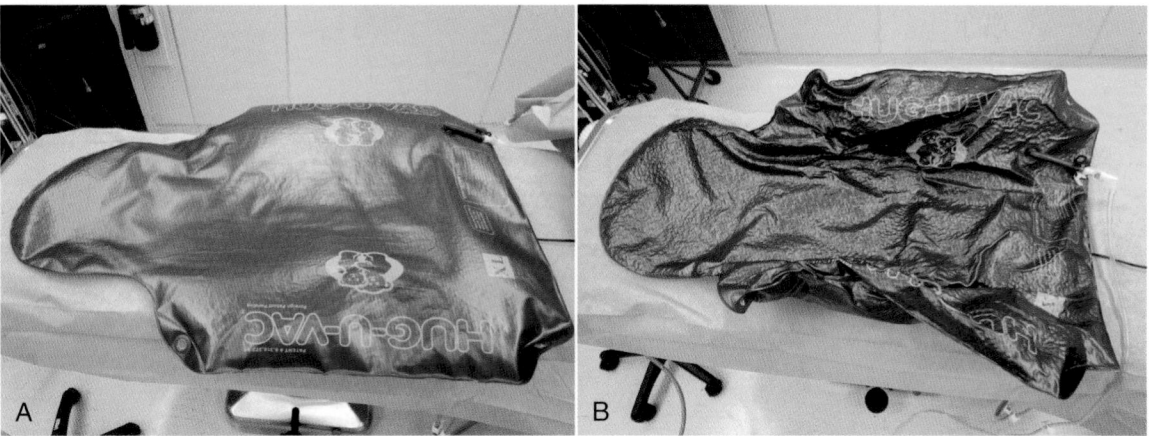

FIGURE 31-2 **A,** A vacuum bag is present on the table. The patient will be placed on the bag and held in position by operating room (OR) technicians; air will be evacuated from the bag by attaching suction tubing to the bag. **B,** This bag was held in position, and the air was evacuated. The bag is maintained in position after removal of the air.

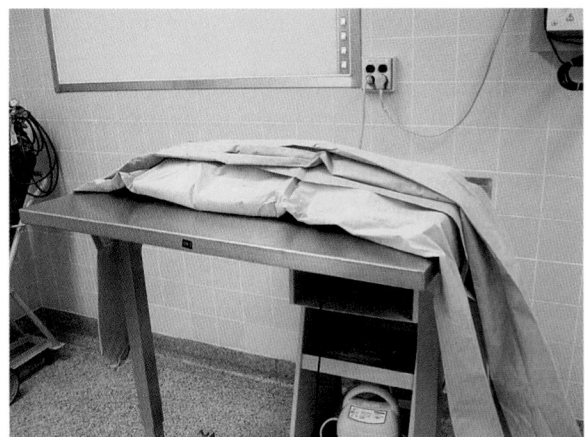

FIGURE 31-3 The pack has been placed on the instrument table and contains the drapes and instrumentation needed by the surgeon and the surgical assistant to drape at the surgical site.

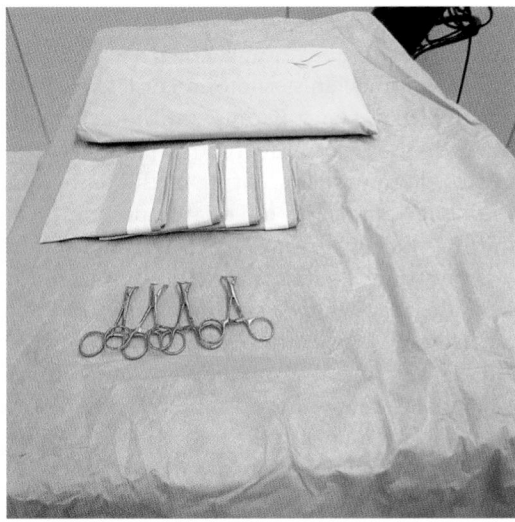

FIGURE 31-4 Necessary equipment for draping (quarter drapes, towel clamps, and a large surgical drape) is located on the instrument table.

Use of quarter drapes is the most common way of generating a sterile surgical field. Each drape is laid down and secured with Backhaus towel clamps. Appropriate technique for placement of a quarter drape is critical for preventing contamination. To do this, the surgical assistant grasps the quarter drape, steps away from the instrument table, and gently opens it to its fullest length and width. The top edge of the drape is folded under, away from the surgical assistant. The corners of the drape are grasped by extended fingers and rolled outward so that the drape wraps around the palms and fingers to protect them from contamination (Figure 31-5). The drape is then floated above the patient before it is placed so that it is not dragged along the contaminated body of the patient. During this process, it is important that the assistant maintain a safe distance away from the patient to prevent contamination of the assistant's gown.

The quarter drape is positioned a few centimeters from the proposed incision site and once placed should never be advanced toward the proposed incision because this action would drag contaminants toward the incision site. The double layer of inwardly folded drape provides extra protection in the surgical region, where the drape is most likely to absorb fluids from blood and sterile saline lavages. Once positioned, the four quarter drapes are secured to the patient and to each other with Backhaus towel clamps (Figure 31-6). These towel clamps should not be moved once placed because the tips are considered nonsterile once they perforate skin. If they must be removed, they should be handed off the table to a nonsterile circulating OR technician, and a new clamp should be used.

After quarter drapes have been secured, a large final drape is placed over the patient, the surgical table, and the instrument table. To ensure sterility, draping the patient and the tables generally requires two people (Figure 31-7). After the instrument table is covered, sterile instrument packs are opened and instruments are organized on the table. Some large surgical drapes are available with fenestrations (see Figure 31-7), but others are not. After a nonfenestrated drape

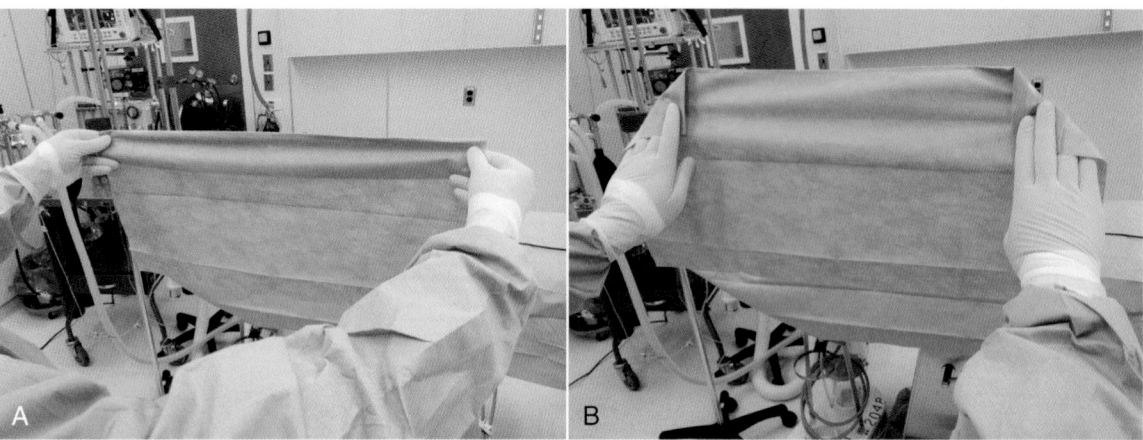

FIGURE 31-5 Proper technique for grasping and placing the quarter drapes. **A,** The quarter drape has been opened to maximum width, and a fold has been maintained in the region closest to the incision. **B,** The assistant's fingers are wrapped around the end of the drape that is going to be placed down. The palms are now facing the patient, but the hands are protected by the drape from touching the contaminated skin of the patient.

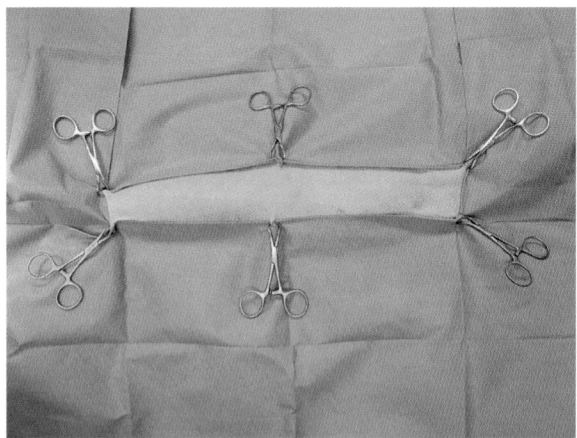

FIGURE 31-6 All four quarter drapes have been placed and secured by Backhaus towel clamps to isolate the region where the incision will be made.

has been placed, scissors can be used to make a fenestration over the surgical site.

Additional drapes or sterile covers can be placed. Some surgeons elect to attach drapes or sterile towels to an incision using Michel clips. This technique prevents any skin from being exposed and provides an additional layer of protection against surgical site infection. Drapes that have a sticky surface, such as Ioban (3M, St Paul, Minnesota), can also be used after placement of surgical drapes. These sticky drapes allow the entire skin surface to be covered, and an incision can be made directly through Ioban because it is translucent. For extremity surgeries, stockinettes may be used. These allow the surgeon and the surgical assistant to maneuver the leg without touching the skin (Figure 31-8).

If penetration of a previously sterile field is noted, action should be taken to secure the field. Sterile drapes can be added to the region that has been contaminated and secured with nonpenetrating clamps. If a surgeon's or surgical assistant's gown or glove has come into contact with a contaminated region, that item should be removed and a sterile replacement obtained. Depending on the location and the

degree of contamination, postoperative antibiotics should be considered but are not mandatory in all cases of contamination.

Specific examples of patient positioning and draping of each body part are discussed in the following sections.

Abdomen

For most abdominal approaches in which a ventral midline incision is being performed, such as ovariohysterectomy, gastrotomy, and abdominal exploration, patients are placed in dorsal recumbency with the ventrum oriented to the ceiling. This position allows access to all organs of the peritoneal cavity and retroperitoneal space. Four quarter drapes should be placed as previously described, and this should be followed by placement of a large drape over the surgical site (see Figure 31-7). If a positioning device has been used to maintain patient positioning, inflation should not be taken to a point that allows the device to interfere with access to the abdomen.

Thorax

Most approaches to the thorax are performed with the patient in dorsal (median sternotomy) or lateral (intercostal thoracotomy) recumbency. Because the thorax tends to have greater length in a dorsal-to-ventral plane, especially in deep-chested dogs, proper securing of the thorax during a ventral midline approach is essential to prevent the patient from shifting during surgery. When an intercostal thoracotomy is performed, patients are placed in lateral recumbency with the surgical approach facing up. During a right lateral intercostal thoracotomy, for example, the patient is placed in left lateral recumbency. For both thoracic approaches, the patient is draped as described for an abdominal approach with four quarter drapes and a large drape to cover the entire patient and the instrument table.

Extremity

For some extremity surgeries, it is desirable for the surgeon to maintain mobility of the limb. In these instances, the leg

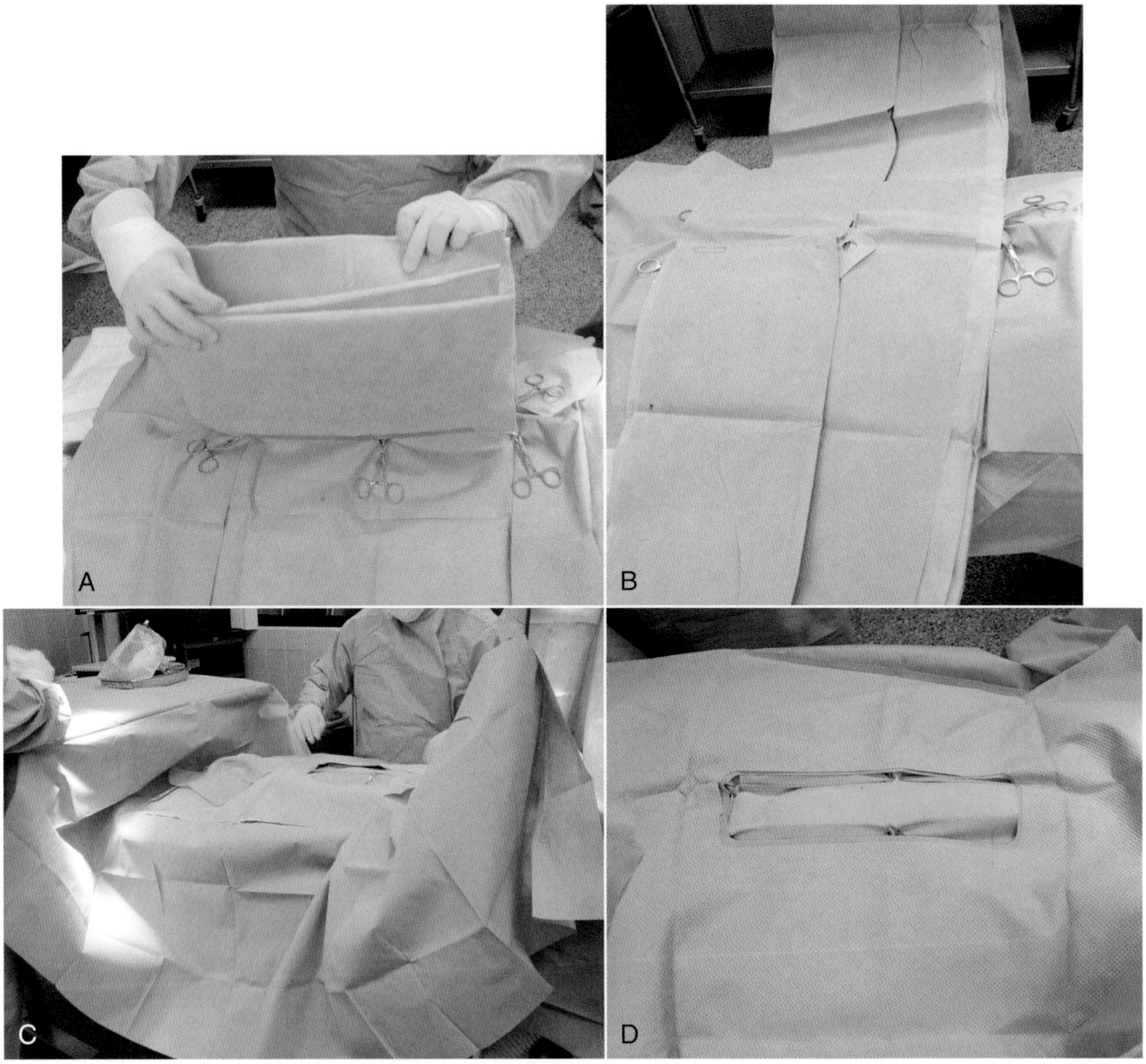

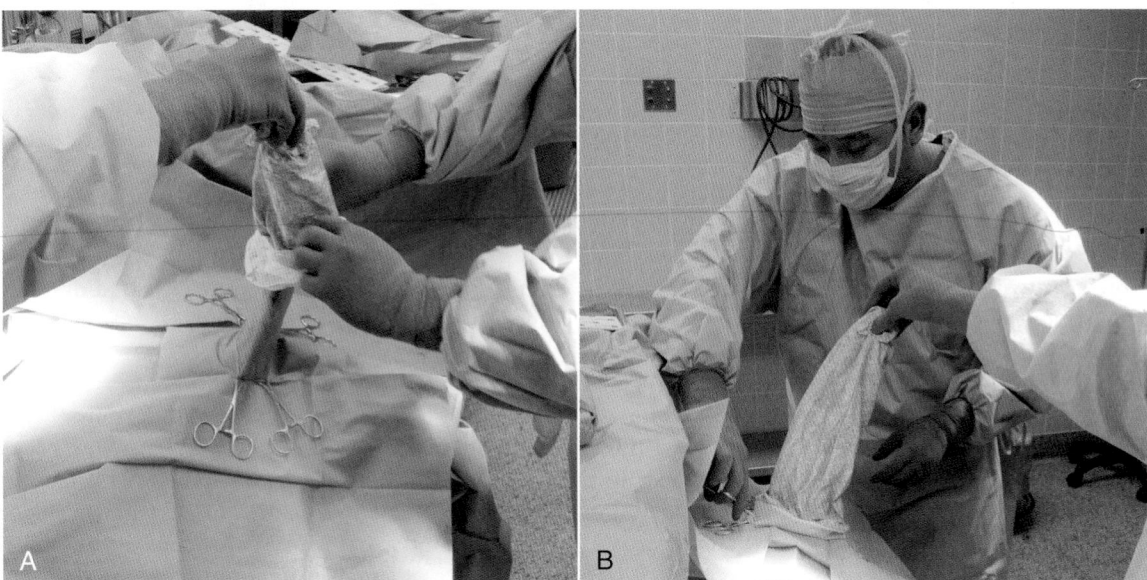

FIGURE 31-7 A, The quarter drapes have been placed. A single, large drape is positioned so that its fenestration covers the proposed incision site. B, The surgeon and the surgical assistant have extended the drape out from the patient. C, The drape has been placed over the patient and instrument table and has been secured to prevent it from moving. The front part of the drape has been elevated to allow the anesthesia team to have access to the patient. D, The large drape is covering the quarter drapes and the towel clamps while allowing access to the proposed incision site.

FIGURE 31-8 A, A stockinette has been added to cover the leg and to decrease the chance that a surgical site infection may develop. B, The stockinette is being clamped to the other drapes to prevent it from slipping during the procedure.

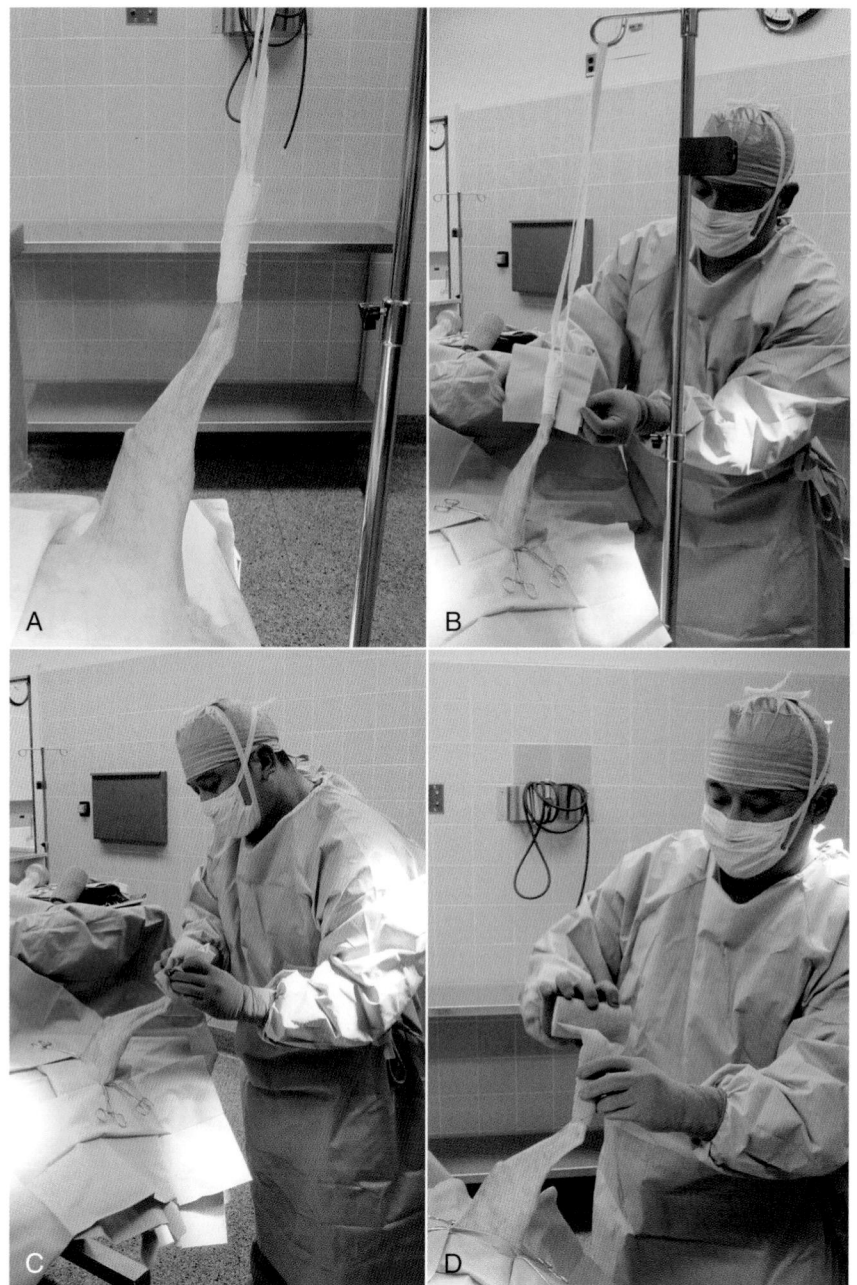

FIGURE 31-9 "Hanging-limb" draping technique. **A,** The lower limb has been taped and attached to an intravenous pole to allow for preparation with aseptic technique and draping. **B** and **C,** After draping-in the limb with quarter drapes, a sterile drape is being placed around the distal limb to allow grasping of the limb and subsequent draping. **D,** A sterile outer layer of a self-adherent wrap is then placed over the sterile distal limb drape to maintain the quarter drape in position.

should be prepared with a hanging-limb technique (Figure 31-9). This technique allows the limb to be held away from the body (generally attached to an intravenous pole or ceiling hook) so that the leg can be prepared with aseptic technique and draped into the sterile field. As the surgeon or the surgical assistant is draping the extremity, it is essential that the leg not be touched until it has been properly draped. If surgery is not being performed on the distal limb, the foot should be encompassed with an impervious drape that is secured with sterile bandaging material such as Vetrap (3M; see Figure 31-9). After the foot has been draped, the entire limb can be passed through a **fenestrated** drape to include the limb within the surgical field.

Spine

The spine can be approached both dorsally (hemilaminectomy and dorsal laminectomy) and ventrally (cervical ventral slot). For both approaches, four quarter and large patient drapes are used. Many surgeons elect to use an added layer of drapes (attached with Michel clips or Ioban) to decrease the chance of surgical site infection because the spinal cord is often exposed after neurologic surgery.

Perineum

For certain surgical procedures (anal sacculectomy, episioplasty, rectal pull-through), patients may be placed in ventral recumbency on a perineal stand. The perineal stand allows the patient to be in a raised position and prevents the hindlimbs from interfering with the surgery. Patients positioned in a perineal stand are draped with the previously described technique; however, the instrument table cannot be draped with the usual large patient drape unless it is placed over the patient. Often, a second instrument table drape is used because the table is off to the side of the surgeon and surgical assistant.

When a patient is positioned in a perineal stand, it is essential that the ventral abdomen be cushioned. Because the hindlimbs are often hanging free, pressure on the pelvis and the abdomen can increase during surgery. Placing padding or several soft towels under the abdomen often provides sufficient cushioning of these patients.

Oral Surgery

Positioning for oral surgery depends on the procedure that is to be performed because patients may be in dorsal, ventral, or lateral recumbency. Draping can be difficult because the anatomy of the nose, mouth, and orbit prevents easy drape positioning. Most oral surgeries are not considered sterile procedures, but surgeons and surgical assistants should attempt to perform these surgeries with as clean a technique as possible.

OPERATING ROOM STERILITY

The surgeon, surgical assistant, and operating room technician are responsible for maintaining operating room sterility. For the surgeon and the surgical assistant, the focus should be on maintaining the sterility of gowns, gloves, drapes, and instruments. Circulating OR technicians should police the surgeon and the surgical assistant, as well as the anesthesia team and any other observers in the room. The most likely time for breaks in sterility to occur is when the patient is being draped and surgical and instrument tables are being set up.

The hands of those scrubbed into surgery should always be maintained above the waist and below the shoulders (Figure 31-10). The only part of the surgery gown considered sterile is the front region from shoulders to waist; the back of the surgery gown is not sterile.

> **TECHNICIAN NOTE** The surgery gown is considered sterile only in the front from shoulders to waist.

SURGICAL INSTRUMENTS AND INSTRUMENT TABLE ORGANIZATION

The surgical assistant should be responsible for the instruments that are chosen for a particular procedure. To aid this process, a "pick sheet" for each surgical procedure can be established that contains the instruments used or needed during a particular surgery. For example, when a

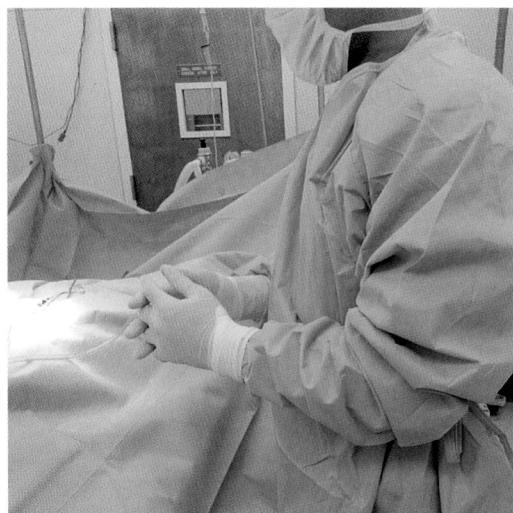

FIGURE 31-10 The surgical assistant is maintaining proper hand position while facing the operating table. Anything below the waist is considered nonsterile, so it is important for all sterile personnel to keep their hands above the waist.

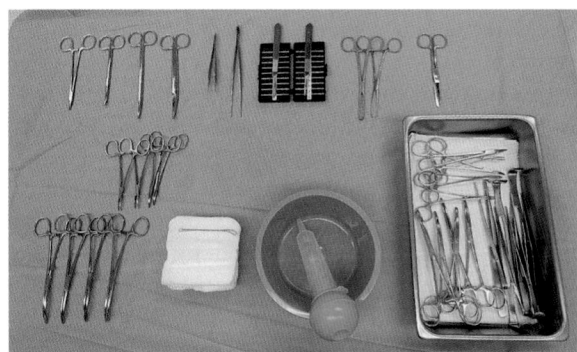

FIGURE 31-11 An organized instrument table.

hemilaminectomy is performed to treat intervertebral disc disease, Gelpi retractors, rongeurs, and a surgical drill are often needed; if they are included on a pick sheet, the surgical assistant can make sure that these instruments are available to the surgeon when he or she needs them by having them close by in the room or already opened on the instrument table. For a review of the most commonly used surgical instruments, refer to Chapter 30.

Many veterinary hospitals maintain surgical packs that contain surgical instruments commonly used in most surgeries. When these packs have been opened onto the sterile instrument table, the surgical assistant can take responsibility for organizing the instrument table.

Although all surgeons and surgical assistants may have different techniques of organization, a few general principles should be considered. The most commonly used instruments should be placed in a location that is easily accessible by both the surgeon and the surgical assistant. This equipment often includes thumb forceps, scissors, and needle holders that are used on a regular basis (Figure 31-11). As instruments are placed on the instrument table after use,

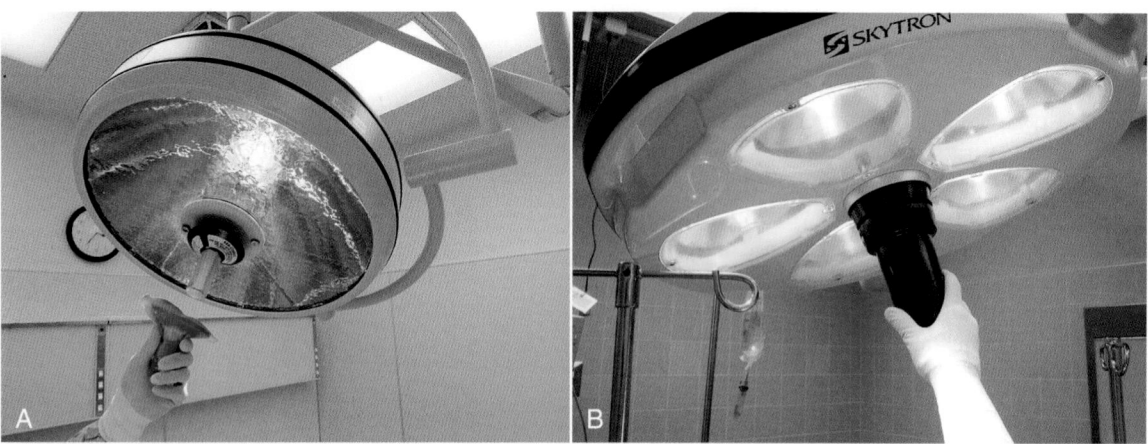

FIGURE 31-12 Light handle sterile technique. **A,** This light maintains a permanent handle, and a temporary collapsible sterile light handle cover is placed during every surgery. **B,** A sterile light handle sleeve is placed to control this light. This particular light has a camera incorporated into the design that allows video capturing of a procedure.

they should be organized. Replacing an instrument to the predetermined location prevents delays in accessing that instrument at a future time, or in a situation where the instrument is needed quickly. Sharp instrumentation (such as blades and needles) should be located in a region where the surgeon and the surgical assistant cannot inadvertently poke themselves or the patient. A magnetic box used to hold sharp instruments is preferable because this will decrease the likelihood of an accident (see Figure 31-11).

When an instrument is contaminated by a dirty wound or tumor cells, it should be removed from the instrument table (passed off to an operating room technician) or placed on an isolated region of the instrument table that will not be accessed again. The surgical assistant is responsible for ensuring that contaminated instruments are not used again in a surgical wound because this can increase the chance of a surgical site infection or seeding of tumor cells. Additionally, if surgical gloves have been in contact with a contaminated instrument or wound, they should be changed.

> **TECHNICIAN NOTE** Instruments that are contaminated should be passed off the instrument table to an operating room technician or placed in an isolated region of the instrument table.

Surgical sponges and gauze should be counted before surgery is begun. Additionally, gauze that is placed into a cavity should be accounted for and tracked closely. Before closure of that cavity, the surgical assistant should ensure that the gauze has been removed and that all gauze is accounted for. Gauze may contain radiopaque strips (see Figure 31-11) that are capable of being visualized on radiographs should they be left inside a patient accidentally.

INTRAOPERATIVE TECHNIQUES

A proficient and conscientious surgical assistant can be the key to a successful surgery. Immediately after draping, the surgical assistant should work with the surgeon to perform certain tasks, including setup of suction and electrocautery, placement of light handles, orientation of lighting, and appropriate placement of scalpel blades on scalpel handles. Attention to detail during hemostasis and suturing can lead to improved surgical outcomes.

SURGICAL LIGHTING

Light handles or sterile light covers should be placed after the patient has been draped (Figure 31-12). Waiting until drapes are placed over the patient prevents accidental contamination of surgical gowns and gloves when reaching up to adjust the lights. After light handles or sterile light covers have been placed, the surgical lights can be focused and aimed at appropriate sites.

> **TECHNICIAN NOTE** Light handles or sterile light covers should be placed after the patient has been draped.

In certain procedures, it may be necessary for the surgeon or the surgical assistant to wear a head lamp to improve lighting. These lamps can dramatically improve visualization in surgeries that take place in a deeply positioned surgical field, such as neurologic and aural surgeries.

INSTRUMENTATION CORDS AND TUBING

Suction may not be necessary during all surgical procedures, but when it is needed, it is important to secure the suction tubing to the surgical drapes to prevent contamination (Figure 31-13). Tubing can be prevented from falling off the table with a nonpenetrating instrument such as an Allis tissue forceps to attach the tubing to a secure section of drape.

When an electrocautery handpiece is used, it is generally necessary to pass the plug for the device off the surgical table. The electrocautery cord should be secured to the drape or the table to prevent contamination (see Figure 31-13). To lower the risk of pulling on the cord by the surgeon or the

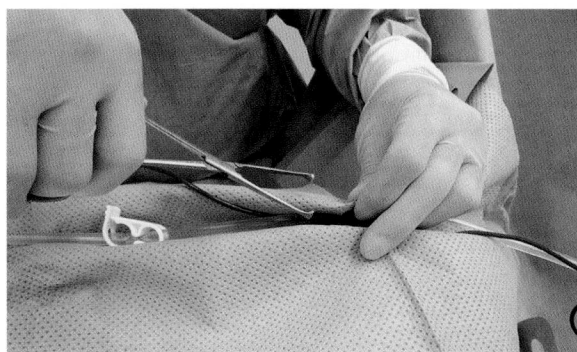

FIGURE 31-13 Suction tubing and the electrocautery cord are secured to the drape by means of a sterile instrument such as an Allis tissue forceps.

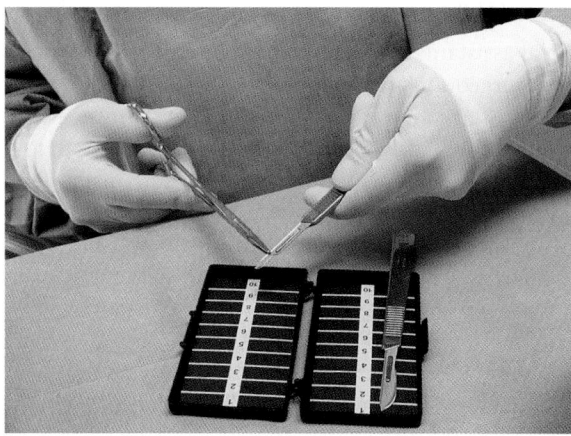

FIGURE 31-14 Proper placement of a scalpel blade onto a scalpel handle.

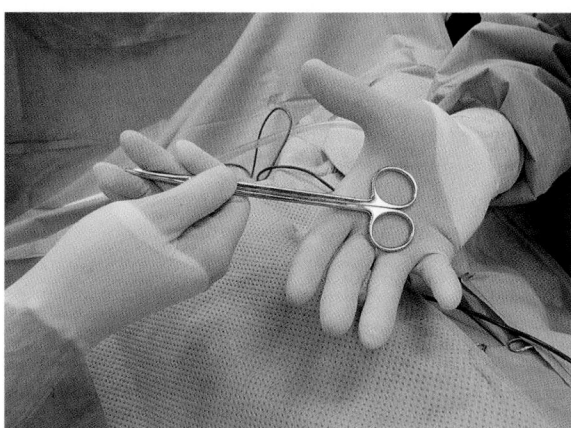

FIGURE 31-15 The instrument is being passed to the surgeon in the proper orientation. Note that the instrument is being placed into his open hand to allow more immediate usage.

surgical assistant, the unit containing the outlet should be strategically placed; often the best location is behind the instrument table, not on the patient's sides.

Similarly, drills and saws may contain tubing that needs to be attached to a tank that is off the instrument table. This tubing should be safely secured to the drapes and/or to the instrument table. Further, this tubing should not be attached in a position where it can be inadvertently pulled, resulting in loss of the instrument off the table or, worse, trauma to the patient.

Minimally invasive procedures such as arthroscopy, laparoscopy, and thoracoscopy are being performed regularly and require specialized equipment that includes additional tubing and cords. When a pneumoperitoneum is required for visualization during laparoscopy, carbon dioxide is delivered to the port via tubing; similarly, fluid delivered to a joint for arthroscopy is transported via tubing attached to the port. In addition, these procedures require use of a camera and a light source, both of which have cable attachments that must be passed off the table to a nearby tower.

SCALPEL USE

Numerous scalpel blades are available. The blade chosen depends on the indication for use. Scalpel blades are placed onto scalpel handles using needle holders. To prevent accidental injury while attaching scalpel blades to the handle, always be sure to use an instrument, not hands alone, to place the blade (Figure 31-14).

Three primary grips may be used to hold the scalpel blade: pencil grip, fingertip grip, and palm grip. The pencil grip is employed when the surgeon is attempting to make a very precise cut, or when a "stab" incision is necessary, for instance, during a cystotomy or gastrotomy approach. The fingertip grip is recommended for longer incisions such as the skin approach to a ventral celiotomy. The palm grip is rarely used but allows the surgeon to generate greater force because the palm is positioned directly over and onto the scalpel handle.

Great care should be taken when passing a scalpel blade to a surgeon. Excessive speed should be avoided, and the blade should be passed when the surgeon is aware and ready

to receive the blade. The scalpel blade should be passed with the blade away from the surgeon's hand to prevent accidental injury.

INSTRUMENT PASSING

The surgical assistant is often requested to hand instruments to the surgeon; this responsibility requires anticipation and proper placement of the instrument in the surgeon's hand. As a surgical assistant gains more experience with a particular procedure, he or she will begin to anticipate subsequent steps, and the instrument required next will be readily available. Efficient surgical assisting decreases surgical time, and this benefits the patient.

Instruments should be placed in the open palm of the surgeon in a position that allows easy manipulation and usage of the instrument. The instrument should be passed with sufficient forcefulness to allow the surgeon to be able to grasp the instrument and prevent it from falling (Figure 31-15). When sharp instruments (needles) or scalpel blades are passed, the sharp component should be passed away from the surgeon's hand to prevent accidental injury.

RETRACTION

Surgical assistants are often called upon to retract organs to allow a surgeon to access certain regions or to ligate a bleeding vessel. Retraction is a learned skill that requires attention to detail and a focused mind to prevent damage to surrounding tissues while allowing sufficient exposure of the surgical site. Proper use of retractors such as Army-Navy retractors, Senn retractors, and malleable retractors takes practice but can be a crucial component of successful surgery (Figure 31-16).

HEMOSTASIS

Hemostasis can be achieved through a variety of techniques. Applying pressure via gauze sponges may be sufficient for certain bleeding vessels. When gauze is used, it is critical to blot the area of interest as opposed to wiping, because wiping removes blood clots that have been established. When a blood vessel is not going to be spared, hemostats can be placed directly on the vessel to cause hemostasis. Further hemostasis may not be necessary for small blood vessels. Hemostats contain a ratchet that allows them to be placed onto a vessel and maintained in position. The tips of hemostats should be used to clamp the vessel to prevent inadvertent clamping of nontarget tissue.

With vessels that are slightly larger, the use of suture ligation, vascular clips, or electrocautery may be warranted. When ligating a blood vessel, the surgical assistant is often called upon to hold the vessel away from the body (using hemostats or forceps) to allow the surgeon to access the vessel with suture. Gentle manipulation of the vessel is necessary to prevent tearing of the vessel or release of the vessel back into the surgical wound. Vascular clips can be placed with the use of a clip applier, and, similar to ligation, the clip should be placed only on the bleeding vessel, not indiscriminately on surrounding normal tissue.

Cauterization of blood vessels via electrocautery is an excellent technique for controlling blood loss and decreasing surgical time. Electrocautery is a process by which heat is conducted through a metal probe by an electrical current with the goal of destroying bleeding tissue.

Electrocauterization can be performed with monopolar or bipolar coagulation devices (Figure 31-17). Monopolar electrocautery involves the use of a handpiece that passes a current through the target tissue (bleeding vessel) and disperses the current through the patient to a ground pad underneath the patient's body. When monopolar electrocautery is used, the patient is acting as part of the electrical circuit. Monopolar electrocautery handpieces are often equipped with both cutting and coagulation modes.

For best functioning of monopolar electrocautery, a dry surgical site is necessary. The surgical assistant may need to use a gauze blotting technique or gentle suction at first to decrease blood in the region. Removing blood first allows monopolar electrocautery to work with greater efficiency. Additionally, the monopolar electrocautery probe can be applied to an instrument that is clamped to a blood vessel. For precise cauterization of a blood vessel, the vessel can be grasped with a thumb (DeBakey) or hemostatic forceps, and the tip of the monopolar electrocautery handpiece can be touched to the instrument to induce cauterization.

A bipolar electrocautery unit passes a current between two tips of a forceps. The current is often controlled by a foot switch. Bipolar electrocautery is generally employed in situations where precisely targeted cauterization is necessary, as during ophthalmic and neurologic procedures.

Several hemostatic agents have been designed to assist with control of intraoperative bleeding. Bone wax is a mixture of beeswax, paraffin, isopropyl palmitate, and a wax-softening agent that can be applied to actively bleeding bone. Bone wax functions by occluding the bleeding channel and effectively controls bleeding that is occurring from medullary bone (e.g., during hemilaminectomy) or from within a

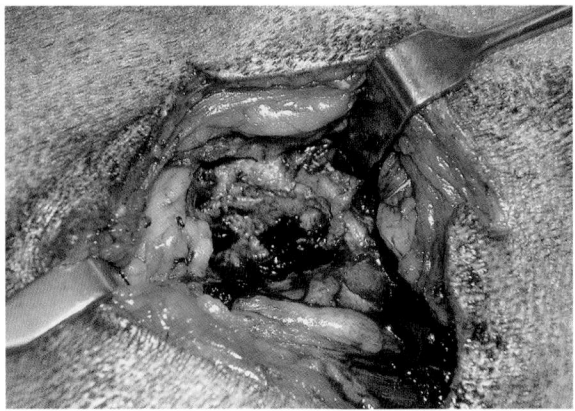

FIGURE 31-16 Use of hand-held retractors (Senn retractors) to expose a surgical site while a biopsy is being obtained.

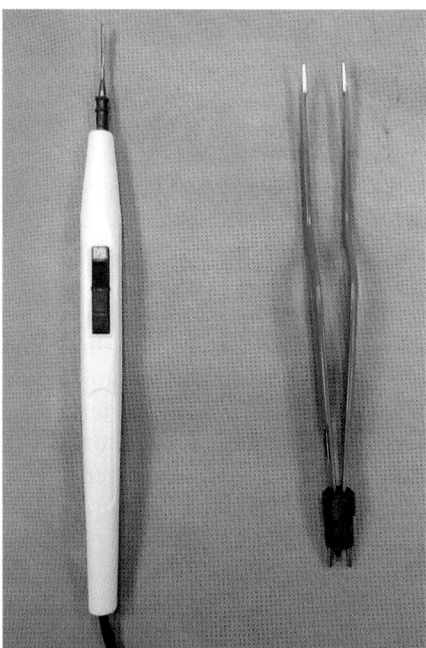

FIGURE 31-17 Examples of handpieces used for performing cauterization: monopolar *(left)* and bipolar *(right)*.

cut bone (e.g., mandibulectomy). Gelatin foams (Gelfoam) can be placed onto regions of bleeding and provide a framework for the initiation of clotting. Gelatin foams can be cut or torn into shapes that can be placed more effectively into a bleeding site. These materials are absorbed over time. Oxidized cellulose (Surgicel) is made into a sheet that can be laid on organ surfaces and cut to specific sizes. It most likely works by generating artificial clots.

SUTURE CUTTING

In general, when a surgeon is suturing, suture scissors should be picked up by the assistant when possible. Suture cutting should be performed with scissors that are designed for that specific purpose, not with scissors that are designed for dissecting or cutting of tissue. The tips of the scissors should be used to cut suture to prevent accidental trauma to adjacent normal tissue.

> **TECHNICIAN NOTE** Surgical assistants should focus on using the tips of scissors to cut suture.

LAVAGE AND SUCTION

Use of fluid to lavage a wound is routine. Lavage fluids should be sterile and iso-osmotic. Examples include lactated Ringer's and normal strength saline. These fluids are kept on the instrument table in a sterile bowl and can be transferred to the surgical site via a bulb syringe or by direct pouring of the lavage fluid into a body cavity.

Suction is essential for removing lavage fluid or body fluids that have accumulated in a body cavity or wound site. Suction tubing can be attached to suction tips that have different configurations and functions (see Chapter 30). Large suction tips with multiple holes, such as the Poole tip, are effective for suctioning large amounts of fluid that may accumulate in the abdominal or thoracic cavity. Smaller suction tips with a single end-on hole, such as the Frazier tip, may be used for more focal suctioning, such as that required during many neurosurgeries.

In situations where bleeding becomes excessive, surgical assistants often play a key role in controlling visualization by suctioning blood while the source of bleeding is being identified. Two hands are often necessary to find the offending vessel: one hand to retract surrounding tissue and one hand to grasp the vessel. Targeted suctioning by a well-trained assistant can be the key to isolating and controlling bleeding vessels.

CAMERA MANIPULATION

With increased use of minimally invasive procedures such as arthroscopy, laparoscopy, and thoracoscopy, the surgical assistant is asked to take on a more active role in visualization (see Chapter 30). During these procedures, a camera is placed into the body cavity or joint that is being evaluated, and an image is generated and viewed on a monitor positioned near the surgery table. The assistant is often responsible for pointing the camera in the appropriate direction

because the surgeon typically uses both hands to perform the procedure.

TISSUE MANIPULATION, RETRACTION, AND ORGAN POSITIONING
Skin

Although it is necessary to incise the skin during initiation of surgery, surgeons and assistants should avoid regular contact with the skin during surgery. The skin is prepared with aseptic technique before surgery, but the skin should never be considered sterile. Minimizing skin contact will improve the chance of not developing a postoperative surgical site infection. Once incised, the skin edges should be handled gently and as atraumatically as possible. Each manipulation of the skin results in trauma, and excessive force should be avoided.

Abdomen

Surgical assistance during many abdominal procedures is essential. Most abdominal surgeries are started with an abdominal exploration, and although each surgeon has his or her preferred approach to exploration, certain principles of organ positioning should be known.

The liver is a fairly mobile organ consisting of six major lobes. The left side of the liver can be gently retracted to the right for viewing of the abdominal esophagus and the stomach (Figure 31-18). When the liver is examined, the gallbladder is also evaluated and can be expressed for assessment of the patency of cystic and common bile ducts.

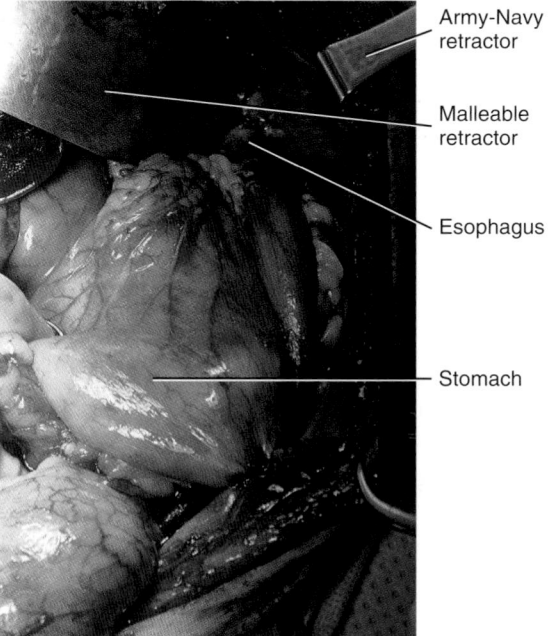

Army-Navy retractor

Malleable retractor

Esophagus

Stomach

FIGURE 31-18 During this celiotomy to correct a hiatal hernia, an esophagopexy and a gastropexy have been performed. The malleable retractor is being used to retract the left side of the liver to the right to allow visualization of the abdominal esophagus. The Army-Navy retractor is retracting the left body wall to further increase visualization.

The pancreas consists of right and left limbs and a central body. The right limb is easily visible because of its close association with the duodenum. The left limb is located caudal to the stomach and can be viewed by entering the omental bursa. Because over-manipulation of the pancreas can result in pancreatitis, palpation of the pancreas should be kept to a minimum.

The spleen can vary in size even within the same animal because it has the capacity to contract and expand. The spleen is a highly mobile organ and can often be lifted out of the abdomen. During splenectomies, the assistant is often responsible for handling the spleen and allowing the surgeon to view the splenic vascular supply.

The gastrointestinal tract should be fully evaluated for any abnormalities. Surgical gloves should be wet when abdominal organs are touched, particularly the gastrointestinal tract, because dry gloves can cause drying of the organs or tearing of the serosal layer. The gastrointestinal tract can be palpated along its entire length. However, surgeons and assistants should focus on gentle palpation of each organ and should avoid overstretching of the intestines. The surgical assistant is often asked to hold intestinal loops for the surgeon during enterotomies and intestinal resections and anastomoses. It is important that microbe-rich intestinal contents **not** be released into the abdominal cavity during these procedures. It is the surgical assistant's responsibility to ensure that this does not happen.

To allow viewing of the retroperitoneal structures (kidneys, ureters, adrenal glands, aorta, caudal vena cava), the more ventrally located organs need to be moved aside. Right-sided retroperitoneal structures can be viewed most easily by retracting the duodenum ventrally and to the left. Left-sided retroperitoneal structures are best viewed by retracting the descending colon and spleen to the right. These structures can prevent other abdominal organs from sitting on top of the retroperitoneal organs; their retraction allows better visualization of them.

The urinary bladder is located in the caudal abdomen, and in certain situations (some cystotomies), this organ is approached via a minimal caudal celiotomy incision. The urinary bladder is often manipulated with the use of stay sutures; these allow both ventral and dorsal aspects of the bladder to be seen. The ureters enter the urinary bladder on the dorsal surface, so careful attention is necessary when surgery of the dorsal bladder is performed.

Stay sutures are commonly placed during abdominal surgery. Stay sutures are sutures that are placed into the lumen of a hollow organ, such as the stomach or the bladder, to allow that organ to be manually manipulated (Figure 31-19). When stay sutures are used, the assistant is responsible for clamping the free ends of the suture together with a hemostat and cutting the suture ends for removal. Once stay sutures have been placed, the surgical assistant is often asked to hold the organ in a particular position to allow completion of the next stage of surgery.

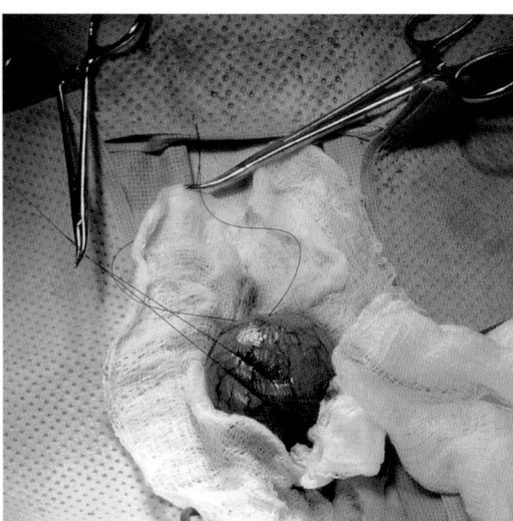

FIGURE 31-19 Stay sutures attached to hemostats have been placed in the bladder. Stay sutures are commonly used to facilitate manipulation of hollow organs.

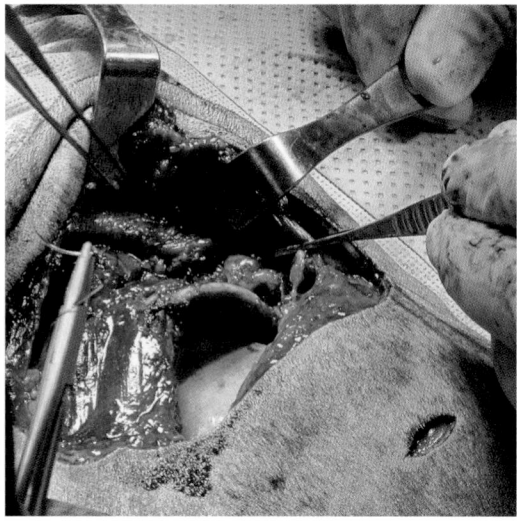

FIGURE 31-20 Two Army-Navy retractors are being used to improve visualization during repair of a region of thoracic trauma secondary to bite wounds.

Thorax

Although gentle retraction is always important, this principle becomes amplified within the thorax because over-manipulation of the heart or lungs can result in life-threatening consequences. Most retraction in the thorax is related to the movement of lung lobes to improve access to the heart, cranial mediastinal structures, or other lung lobes. Large retractors (such as flat malleable retractors) are often used in the thorax, particularly when a median sternotomy has been performed. It is often advisable to surround the malleable retractor with a moistened **laparotomy** pad to decrease the chance of iatrogenic trauma to intrathoracic organs. Retraction may also be necessary when surgery is performed to stabilize fractured ribs (Figure 31-20).

Musculoskeletal

Muscle can undergo repair and regeneration, and gentle manipulation will decrease trauma and lower the chance of iatrogenic bleeding. Additionally, when excessive force or traction is applied to muscle, tearing can occur, further exacerbating trauma. When surgical approaches to bones and joints are taken, muscles are often retracted by the surgical assistant (see Figure 31-16). It is important to keep muscle tissue moist because drying can result in further damage.

Although they are generally more resistant to iatrogenic injury than muscle, bones should be treated with care. In general, soft tissue attachments to bones should be preserved as much as possible. Bones may be grasped with forceps specifically designed for that purpose (refer to Chapter 30), and it may be necessary for the surgical assistant to hold fractured bones in reduction during repair. Additionally, it may be necessary to distract bones during certain joint surgeries to improve visualization.

Vascular and Nervous System

During vascular and neurologic surgeries, the surgeon is responsible for manipulation of involved structures and placement of retraction devices in the correct location. It is crucial for the surgical assistant to maintain the position of retraction devices. Enhanced focus is often required to decrease the chance of iatrogenic injury to the vasculature or nervous system.

SURGICAL IMPLANTS

Many surgeries require the use of permanent or temporary surgical implants. Implants are devices that are left in the surgical wound to perform a function. Use of these devices is widespread, and the demand for improved implants is increasing.

Permanent

Permanent implants are placed with the intention of being left in place for the patient's life; however, when failure or infection occurs, these implants may have to be removed. Many **orthopedic** procedures involve the placement of permanent implants such as plates, pins, wires, and screws. Surgical assistants should familiarize themselves with these different implants and their basic uses. Although each fracture repair or joint stabilization surgery may be unique, having a basic knowledge of the steps involved in the repair process and of the instruments and implants that are used will enhance the efficiency of the procedure.

Temporary

Drains are likely the most common temporary implant used in veterinary medicine. Drains are devices inserted into post-surgical wounds or body cavities to allow for drainage of fluid accumulations and to help eliminate dead space. Drains are generally classified as passive or active. Neither passive nor active drains are benign, and both must be removed. Drains are generally removed when fluid production has

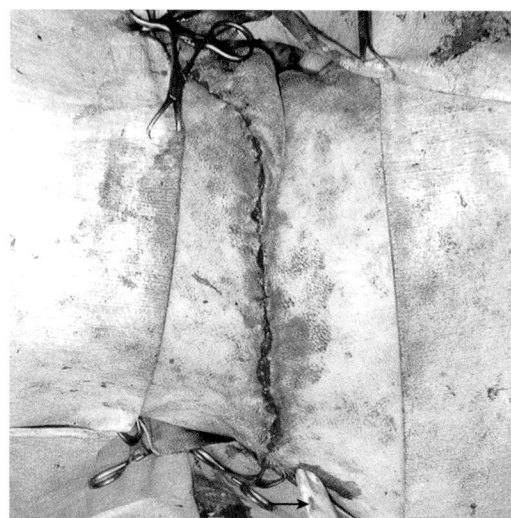

FIGURE 31-21 A passive drain (Penrose) has been placed to allow drainage of a wound that has been débrided and closed after a traumatic bite wound.

slowed or ceased, and it should be remembered that drains present within tissue stimulate fluid production.

> **TECHNICIAN NOTE** Drains are not benign, and, when present in tissue, they may stimulate fluid production.

Passive Drains

Passive drains are used most often to drain subcutaneous wounds (Figure 31-21). Because these drains tend to be less rigid then active drains, they need to be secured in place. It is important to remember that the drain ultimately will be removed, and that the location for securing the drain should be readily accessible. Passive drains are gravity dependent; this requires that they be placed in a dependent location. Passive drains should never be used to drain the abdomen.

Penrose drains are the most common type of passive drain (see Figure 31-21). Penrose drains are made of soft latex and can be stocked in a variety of sizes. Penrose drains should generally be exited out of a single hole in a dependent location (occasionally a two-hole technique can be used). These drains can be secured by placing a suture percutaneously through the nonvisible or upper aspect of the drain. An additional suture can be placed in the visible or lower aspect of the drain; however, this suture should not cause closure of the drain's exit site in the skin.

Active Drains

Active drains use negative pressure to suction fluid and air from a wound. Active drains can be used in medium to large subcutaneous wounds and are the drain-of-choice for abdominal drainage. For smaller wounds, an active drain can be created by placing the tubing from a butterfly catheter into the wound, and attaching the needle to a blood collection tube that has maintained negative suction; alternatively,

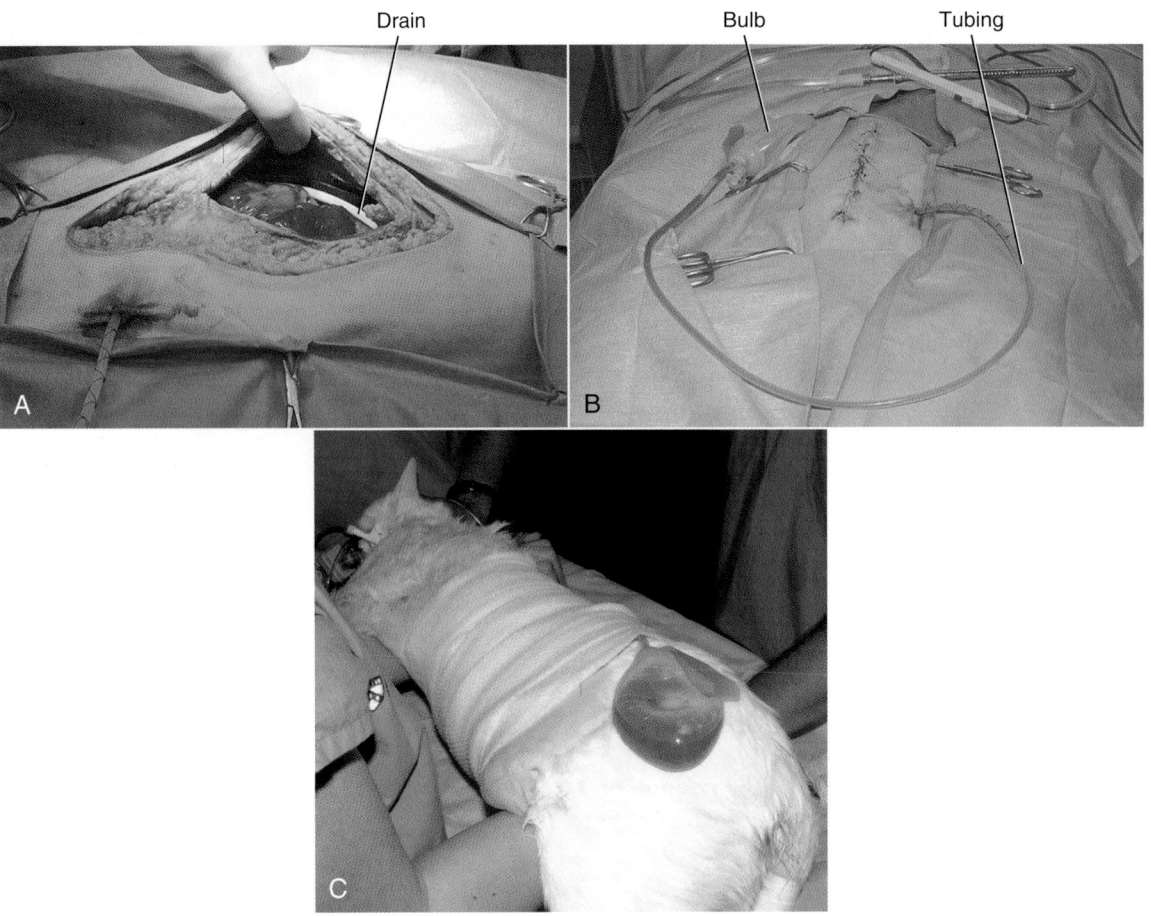

FIGURE 31-22 A Jackson-Pratt drain has been placed intra-abdominally in this feline patient to allow active drainage postoperatively. **A,** The drain component can be seen intra-abdominally before closure of the abdomen. **B,** The tubing is exiting through a hole lateral to midline. The tubing is sutured to the skin to prevent inadvertent removal. The suction canister (bulb) is gently squeezed and capped to generate suction. **C,** Postoperatively, the patient is bandaged to decrease the likelihood of inadvertent removal, to decrease the chance of infection, and to diminish pain associated with the drain.

the hub from the butterfly catheter tubing can be attached to a syringe that is pulled back to negative pressure and secured in place with a needle.

Larger, commercially available drains are also available. These drains consist of a multifenestrated component that is placed within the wound and attached to tubing. The external aspect of the tubing is attached to a suction canister (bulb) that continually generates a negative pressure, causing air and fluid that within the wound to be evacuated. Like passive drains, active drains need to be secured to the skin to prevent inadvertent removal (Figure 31-22).

> **TECHNICIAN NOTE**   Both passive and active drains need to be secured to the skin to prevent premature removal.

POSTOPERATIVE MANAGEMENT

Because the surgical assistant is familiar with the surgical procedure performed, it is often helpful for him or her to be actively involved in immediate postoperative management

of the patient. The wound and surrounding skin should be cleaned immediately after closure because this region is likely to be too painful for cleaning when the patient is fully awake. Sterile, clean lavage fluid is generally sufficient to remove any remaining blood or debris that is present on the wound.

A sterile wound cover can be placed on the incision after cleaning to prevent the wound from coming into direct contact with the environment postoperatively. When surgery has been performed on a mid to distal limb, these limbs are often bandaged postoperatively to decrease swelling and to protect the wound. The surgical assistant can place the bandage or discuss the surgical procedure that was performed with another technician, who may be responsible for placing the bandage.

If a biopsy sample has been obtained during surgery, the surgical assistant can ensure that the sample has been appropriately identified and submitted. If surgical margins are to be evaluated, the assistant can mark the margins with ink and properly orient the sample for histopathologic evaluation.

The surgical assistant may be asked to participate in writing the surgical report, which is an account of all procedures performed during surgery and includes any implants or sutures that were used. The surgical report is an important component of any patient's medical record in that it may be necessary to refer back to the report in the future should a problem arise. Additionally, if the patient is evaluated at another clinic, the clinic can receive a written account of the surgical procedure that was performed.

> **TECHNICIAN NOTE** The surgical assistant can assist in the postoperative care of a surgical patient by cleaning the wound, placing a bandage, submitting a biopsy sample, or writing the surgical report.

SUTURE MATERIAL

Suturing is the act of joining two surfaces together with a stitch or a series of stitches. The goal of a suture is to hold the wound edges in apposition to one another until the tissue has sufficient time to heal. Suturing is a learned skill, and a myriad of options are available when suture type, suture size, and suture pattern are considered. Sutures are not simply used to close skin or body cavities, they may also be used to reappose the edges of organs that have been incised, to reattach transected or avulsed ligaments and tendons, to perform "pexy" techniques, to eliminate dead space, and to support hernia repairs. Although it is likely that personal preference plays a role in the type of suture selected, many factors should be considered to ensure that the most effective suture is chosen.

CONSIDERATIONS WHEN CHOOSING SUTURE

Wound Type

Sutures have the ability to enhance the development of wound infections. When placing sutures into an infected wound, it is best to use sutures that have a greater ability to withstand infection; multifilament sutures are less advisable in a contaminated wound because they are more susceptible to contamination because of increased capillary action. In wounds that may have delayed wound healing, as in patients undergoing long-term steroid use or in patients that have diabetes, sutures that last a long time should be considered.

The type of organ being sutured is an important factor when choosing a suture material. Sutures placed into hollow organs are often exposed to intraluminal materials that may degrade the suture. Sutures that can withstand degradation by intraluminal substances should therefore be chosen. Foreign material placed into contaminated tissue may cause inflammation and may exacerbate the problem, leading to infection. Additionally, certain sutures have been shown to break down easily in infected environments. Tissues that heal quickly, such as those of the stomach, intestine, and bladder, are often closed with absorbable sutures, whereas nonabsorbable sutures may be prudent in tissues that heal more slowly, such as fasciae and tendons.

Construction

Sutures can be monofilament (composed of a single strand) or multifilament (several filaments twisted or braided together). Monofilament sutures are generally considered easier to pass through tissue because they cause less resistance, but greater attention is needed during knot tying of monofilament sutures because they tend to be slippery and have a propensity to untie. Multifilament sutures have greater capillary action, making them more susceptible to bacterial colonization than monofilament sutures. Use of multifilament sutures in infected wounds should therefore be avoided.

> **TECHNICIAN NOTE** Sutures are constructed in monofilament or multifilament forms. Multifilament sutures are less resistant to contamination in infected wounds.

Size and Strength

The nomenclature of suture sizes has been derived by the United States Pharmacopeia (USP). Most sutures are referred to in terms of their USP size, which correlates with a millimeter diameter size; for instance, a size 1 suture has a diameter of 0.4 mm, and a size 7-0 suture has a diameter of 0.05 mm. Originally, sutures were made only in large sizes (size 1 to 6); however, as smaller suture sizes were developed, a "0" was added to sizes to define those smaller than 1. This means that a size 3 suture is larger than a size 2; however, a size 2-0 suture is larger than a size 3-0 suture. The greater the number of zeroes, the thinner is the suture. Sutures are available in sizes from 11-0 (thinnest) to the largest of 7 (thickest).

The strength of a suture is measured by the force required to break a knotted suture strand. Factors that can weaken a suture include knotting, wetting, absorption, placement in an environment that can break the suture down, such as inflamed and infected tissue, and inappropriate manipulation of the suture with instruments.

The suture selected should be at least as strong as the normal tissue through which it has been placed. However, the smallest diameter suture that will adequately hold healing tissues together should be used. Larger sutures and needles increase trauma induced during placement, resulting in a greater quantity of foreign material left inside the patient.

> **TECHNICIAN NOTE** The suture that is selected to close a wound should be at least as strong as the tissue that it is holding together.

Handling

Suture handling is related to memory (the capacity of returning to a previously determined shape after undergoing deformation) of the suture. Having a "lower" memory (or no memory) is considered a beneficial trait because these sutures are much easier to handle, and the quality of the knots is improved. To decrease memory and improve handling, sutures are sometimes gently pulled to remove some of the curl.

Knot Security

Knots are formed when "throws" or wrappings of strands of suture are formed around each other and pulled together. The knot is the weakest point in a tied suture. The security of a knot is affected by the quality of the knot, knot tying technique, the coefficient of friction, and the size of the suture material. Additionally, some sutures have poor knot security when placed in tissue fluids.

SUTURE CLASSIFICATION AND EXAMPLES

Sutures can be classified by numerous different methods, including type of material (natural or synthetic), biological behavior (absorbable or nonabsorbable), and method of construction (monofilament or multifilament). For purposes of this text, sutures will be classified into broad categories of absorbable and nonabsorbable, and specific examples of each will be discussed.

Absorbable

Absorbable sutures are those that lose most of their breaking strength within 60 days of placement. Both synthetic and natural versions of absorbable sutures, as well as monofilament and multifilament forms, are available. These sutures are absorbed by enzymatic degradation (natural) or by hydrolysis (synthetic).

Natural

Natural absorbable sutures consist of catgut or collagen. Catgut is a multifilament suture constructed from the intestines of sheep, goats, or cattle and consists mostly of collagen. Catgut sutures are packaged in solutions of alcohol. The strength of catgut is maintained for only a short time (plain gut: 7 to 10 days; chromic gut: 10 to 14 days) and is essentially gone after 2 weeks; the rate of absorption is variable and unpredictable. Rapid loss of strength calls into question the use of catgut for securing support layers, and use of catgut to close layers such as the linea alba is not recommended. Catgut can stimulate a severe inflammatory reaction.

Reconstituted collagen is an alternative natural absorbable suture to catgut. This suture is made from bovine flexor tendon and has a similar rate of absorption to catgut. This type of suture is generally only used in microsurgeries (e.g., ophthalmic surgery).

Synthetic

Synthetic absorbable sutures offer an advantage over natural absorbable sutures in terms of predictable degradability in a biological environment; wounds that are infected or inflamed do not significantly affect the degradation of these sutures. The most commonly used synthetic absorbable sutures in veterinary medicine include polyglactin 910, polyglycolic acid, poliglecaprone 25, polydioxanone, and polyglyconate.

Polyglactin 910 (Vicryl) is a braided multifilament suture. Polyglactin 910 has several advantageous characteristics, including good handling characteristics and stimulation of minimal tissue inflammation. Although it is stable in contaminated wounds, the multifilament construction of polyglactin 910 causes it to be less resistant to contamination than monofilament sutures. Absorption of polyglactin 910 is generally complete at 60 to 70 days. An antibacterial version of polyglactin 910 (Vicryl Plus) has been developed that is coated with triclosan.

Polyglycolic acid (Dexon) is also a braided multifilament suture. Polyglycolic acid rapidly loses strength and is less strong than other synthetic absorbable sutures. Polyglycolic acid may cut through friable tissue, and knot security is considered relatively poor. Polyglycolic acid loses approximately 35% of its tensile strength by 14 days and is usually completely absorbed between 60 and 120 days. This suture is not recommended for use in the oral cavity or in infected urine because the rate of breakdown may be increased by the alkaline pH of the urine.

Poliglecaprone 25 (Monocryl) is a monofilament suture that is one of the strongest absorbable sutures made. However, tensile strength is lost rapidly; by 14 days, approximately 80% is lost. Poliglecaprone 25 has good knot security and handling characteristics. Poliglecaprone 25 is absorbed by 90 to 120 days after placement in tissues.

Polydioxanone (PDS) is a monofilament suture that has greater initial tensile strength than polyglactin 910 and polyglycolic acid. Although polydioxanone has poor knot security, this suture has excellent maintenance of strength after placement; approximate strength loss at 14 days is only 14%. This suture is generally completely absorbed at 180 days. Polydioxanone is often used to close the bladder even in the presence of infected urine.

Polyglyconate (Maxon) is a monofilament suture that is very similar to polydioxanone. Polyglyconate has excellent strength when placed, and absorption occurs by 180 days post placement. Polyglyconate maintains approximately 70% strength 14 days after placement.

Nonabsorbable
Natural

Silk is a multifilament suture that consists of braided or twisted strands. Silk has no memory, which makes it the near-perfect suture to handle. Silk offers several disadvantages, including poor strength, high capillarity, and the ability to stimulate an intense inflammatory reaction. The tissue reaction that it causes results in loss of tensile strength by 180 days and increases the risk for contamination.

Metallic sutures (stainless steel) are available in monofilament and multifilament forms. Stainless steel has the greatest tensile strength and knot security of all suture materials. Stainless steel sutures result in virtually no inflammatory reaction and can be used in contaminated or infected wounds. Disadvantages of stainless steel sutures include the poor handling quality and the tendency of the suture to kink or break when bent repeatedly. Additionally, tissue necrosis can occur from tissue movement over knot ends.

Synthetic

Polyamide (Nylon) is available in both monofilament and multifilament forms. Polyamide sutures cause minimal tissue reaction, and the monofilament form has no capillarity. Although polyamide is considered a nonabsorbable suture, 30% of its tensile strength is lost by 2 years after placement. Polyamide has poor handling characteristics and knot security.

Polypropylene (Prolene) is a monofilament suture that has the greatest strength of the synthetic nonabsorbable sutures. Other advantages of polypropylene include minimal tissue reactivity, ability to resist weakening by tissue enzymes, and low thrombogenic potential. Polypropylene has high memory and slippery handling characteristics. Polyamide and polypropylene are suitable sutures for use in the skin.

Polybutester (Novafil) is a monofilament suture that has excellent stretching ability; this characteristic makes it an excellent choice for suturing tendons and ligaments. Polybutester stimulates minimal tissue reaction and has good tensile strength, knot security, and handling characteristics.

Polyester (Mersilene) is a braided multifilament suture. This suture retains excellent strength and is suitable for use in slowly healing tissues. Polyester provides the disadvantages of stimulating a tissue reaction that is greater than that of other synthetic suture materials, and poor handling and knot security. Additionally, polyester sutures should not be used in infected wounds because bacteria can be trapped between the fibers, essentially keeping them protected from phagocytic cells.

SUTURE NEEDLES

Suture needles can be preloaded with suture (i.e., **swaged**) or can require loading onto an eyed needle (Figure 31-23). Most needles are swaged; they are considered less traumatic than eyed needles because the tissue damage produced is minimal. Eyed needles can be closed or French (contain a slit to ease threading). In certain surgeries (e.g., cardiovascular), a double-armed suture, which contains a needle on both ends of the suture, may be used.

> **TECHNICIAN NOTE** Eyed needles cause greater tissue trauma than swaged needles.

Suture needles are classified according to their size and shape and type of needle point. Length and diameter of the needle should be considered when needle size is discussed. The smallest needle that can effectively reach both sides of the incision should be used to decrease needle-induced tissue trauma. Tissue thickness and depth of the incision also need to be considered when needle size is determined.

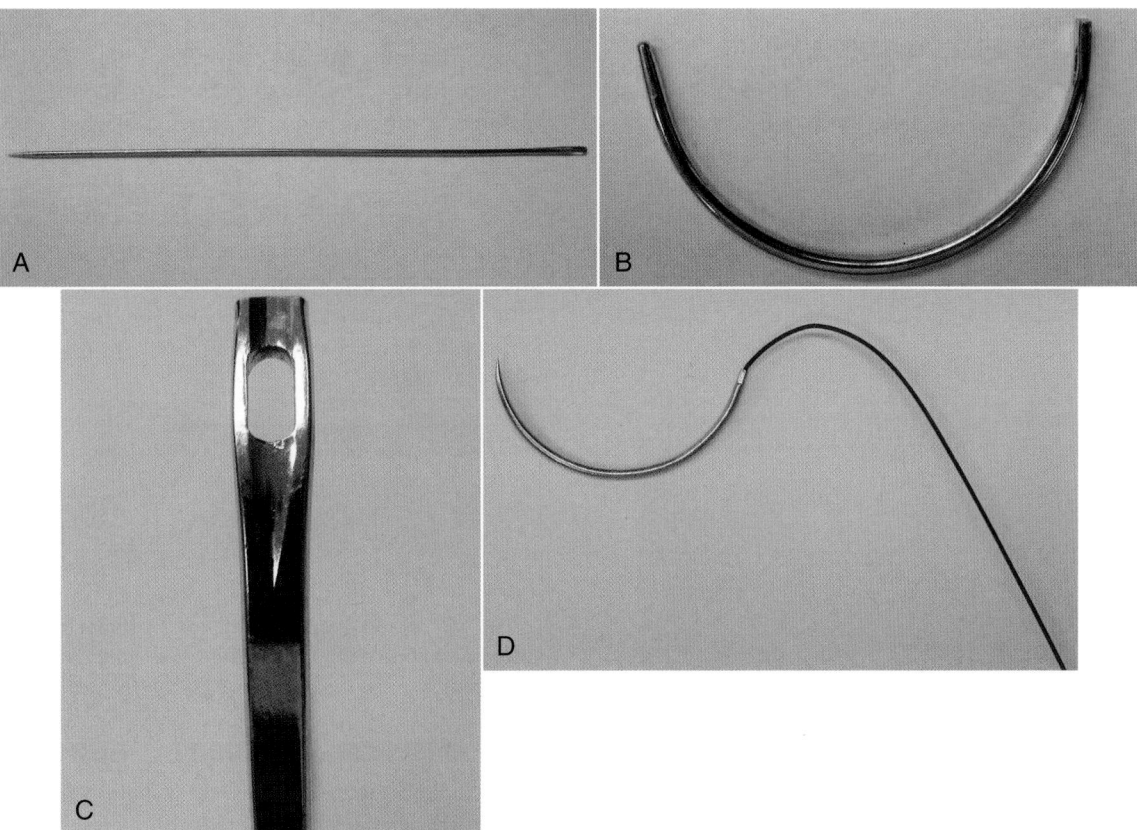

FIGURE 31-23 Surgical needles. **A,** Straight surgical needle. **B** and **C,** A ½-circle eyed needle. Note the hole or eye in part **C** to allow suture passage. **D,** A swaged ½-circle needle.

Several needle shapes are available; common shapes include straight, half-curved, and parts of a circle ($\frac{1}{4}$-circle, $\frac{3}{8}$-circle, $\frac{1}{2}$-circle, and $\frac{5}{8}$-circle). Straight needles are generally used only in locations where the fingers can be used (surface of the body) to pass the sutures, whereas curved needles are manipulated with needle holders. Three-eighths and $\frac{1}{2}$ needles are most commonly used (see Figure 31-23).

Needle points are categorized as cutting, tapered, or blunt. Cutting needles are recommended for tough tissue (e.g., skin) and are available in conventional and reverse-cutting forms. Conventional cutting needles have three cutting edges, with the third edge on the inside concave curvature. Reverse-cutting needles have three cutting edges as well; however, the third edge is on the outer convex curvature of the needle. Reverse-cutting needles are designed to resist cutout as compared with conventional cutting needles. Taper needles contain a sharp tip that is capable of piercing and spreading tissue, but surrounding tissues are not cut. Locations where taper needles are commonly used include the intestines, subcutaneous tissue, and fascia. Blunt-point needles have a tapered body with a rounded, blunt point. These needles dissect through friable tissue without cutting the tissue and are generally recommended for suturing the liver and kidney.

> **TECHNICIAN NOTE** Reverse-cutting needles resist cutting out of tissues more effectively when compared with conventional cutting needles.

SUTURE PLACEMENT AND REMOVAL

Suture packages are generally opened by operating room staff in a sterile manner and can be passed directly to a surgeon or surgical assistant or can be dropped onto the instrument table (Figure 31-24). Suture packages are designed to have their outer packaging peeled back to expose the inner packaging, which houses the suture. The surgical assistant can grasp the inner packaging and position the needle (visible within the package) to be grasped by needle holders. The suture needle is generally grasped perpendicular to the long axis of the needle holder. The position in which the needle is placed within the tips varies on the task; the needle should be positioned near the tip when the needle is passed through dense tissue, near the middle for most general purpose suturing, and near the eye for fine suturing of delicate tissues.

Once a suture has been chosen, the surgeon and the surgical assistant should consider the pattern and the technique that will be used to close the wound. As a rule-of-thumb, tissue should be handled as infrequently as possible, and forceps should contain teeth for improved grasping ability. Needles should be inserted perpendicular to the skin, and grasping of the needle with the gloved hand should be avoided.

Basic suture patterns include interrupted and continuous forms; both patterns have advantages. Interrupted suture patterns allow increased control of suture tension and apposition of wounds as compared with continuous suture patterns. Additionally, use of interrupted suture patterns avoids the potentially catastrophic complications that can occur when a single continuous strand breaks. In this instance, wound dehiscence would occur with subsequent tissue herniation and/or infection. Continuous suture patterns decrease operative time and form an air-tight and water-tight seal.

SURGICAL ASSISTING FOR EQUINE PATIENTS

It is important, particularly with large animal surgeries, that the veterinary technician, whether an operating room technician or a surgical assistant, anticipates what is needed with regard to preparation of the equine patient, and what will be needed during surgery (i.e., instrumentation) to reduce anesthesia time. This will lessen the potential for postanesthetic recovery complications that can occur with large animals under general anesthesia for prolonged periods of time. Surgeons rely instinctively on veterinary technicians in surgery to be prepared and to keep things moving in an efficient manner.

> **TECHNICIAN NOTE** It is important, particularly with large animal surgeries, that veterinary technicians, whether serving as operating room technicians or surgical assistants, anticipate what is needed with regard to preparation of the equine patient, and what will be needed during surgery (i.e., instrumentation) to reduce anesthesia time. This will lessen the potential for postanesthetic recovery complications that can occur with large animals under general anesthesia for prolonged periods of time.

DRAPING FOR ABDOMINAL SURGERY

As in small animal surgeries, the function of draping is to separate the sterile surgical site from the rest of the contaminated area around the patient. Draping should be performed only by members of the surgical team who are aseptically

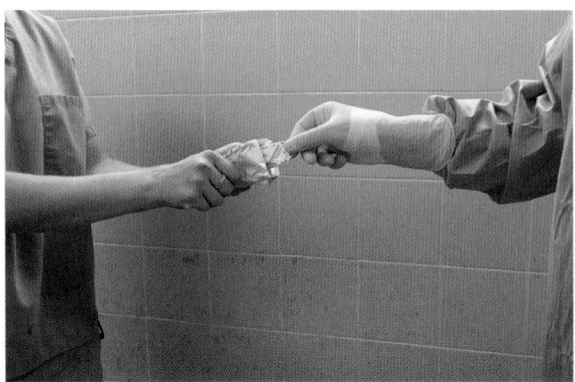

FIGURE 31-24 The outer layer of a pack of suture material is being opened by the operating room technician and is offered to the surgeon or the surgical assistant using proper sterile technique. The inner lining of the suture pack is sterile and can be grasped by sterile personnel.

gowned and gloved. In most cases, it takes at least two persons to correctly perform draping of a horse because of the size of the drapes. Abdominal surgery is one of the most common surgical procedures performed on a horse.

Once the animal has been prepared with aseptic technique, sterile stockinettes or leg drapes are placed individually over each hindlimb (Figure 31-25). Next, the horse is draped in a similar manner as a small animal would be, with hand towels placed in a four-quarter fashion around the incision site (Figure 31-26). These are secured with several Backhaus towel clamps. Then a large laparotomy drape is placed, with individuals positioned on opposite sides of the patient carefully unfolding the large drape over the horse. The most effective way of doing this is to place the drape over the center of the surgical site, on top of the already secured hand towels, and to carefully unfold the large drape with a backward step away from the horse. Then, in a coordinated fashion, the drape is unfolded longitudinally to cover the entire animal (Figure 31-27). Equine laparotomy drapes are already fenestrated, so no cuts are needed to create the fenestration. Towel clamps are used to secure the

laparotomy drape by clamping to the towel clamps underneath the drape (Figure 31-28, *A*). Each exposed towel clamp is covered with a single 4 × 4 gauze sponge (Figure 31-28, *B*), and an adhesive, impervious drape is placed directly over the incision site (Figure 31-28, *C*). An adhesive spray is needed for good contact. The gauze sponge prevents the adhesive drape from sticking to the clamp. However, it is important that none of these gauze sponges fall into the abdominal cavity unnoticed. Serious life-threatening consequences could occur.

> **TECHNICIAN NOTE** It is important that no gauze sponges fall into the abdominal cavity without being retrieved.

DRAPING FOR ORTHOPEDIC SURGERY

The way in which a horse is positioned on the surgery table for an orthopedic procedure depends on which part of the affected limb is to be addressed. Nevertheless, arthroscopic procedures are commonly performed in dorsal recumbency (Figure 31-29). When the patient is positioned on the surgery table, an electocautery plate with contact gel is placed underneath the patient by a circulating OR technician, and associated cords are connected to the nearby unit. Impervious plastic drapes are used to reduce strike-through contamination and tearing. An adhesive, impervious type of drape is used directly over the surgical site (Figure 31-30). If the horse is positioned in lateral recumbency, the affected limb is prepped for surgery by suspending it from an IV fluid pole using tape placed around the hoof (Figure 31-31). Once the limb has been aseptically prepared, the area proximal to the surgery site is draped off with sterile hand towels (Figure 31-32). The circulating OR technician removes the limb from the IV pole by removing the foot from the hanger and grasping a nonprepped area of the limb. The surgeon or the surgical assistant grasps the limb with a sterile hand towel or drape (Figure 31-33). A sterile surgical glove is placed over the hoof by the surgeon or the surgical assistant; a sterile

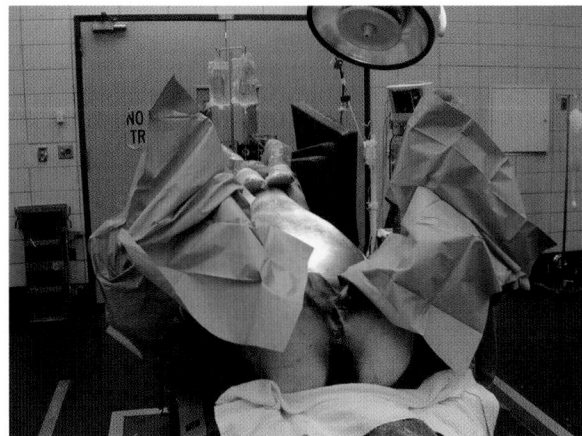

FIGURE 31-25 Draping of an equine surgery patient. Leg drapes are used to cover the rear limbs of the patient.

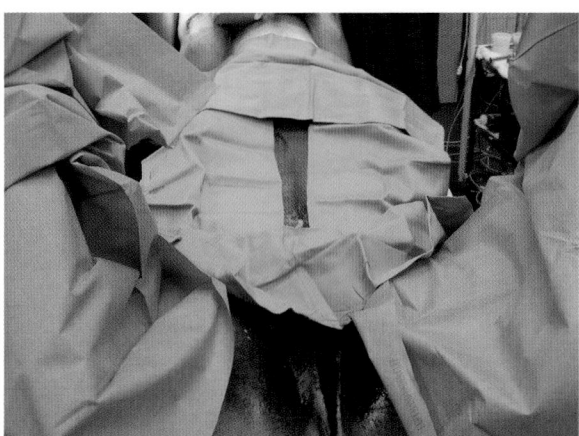

FIGURE 31-26 Draping the ventral abdomen of an equine surgery patient. Hand towels are placed in a four-quarter fashion around the incision site.

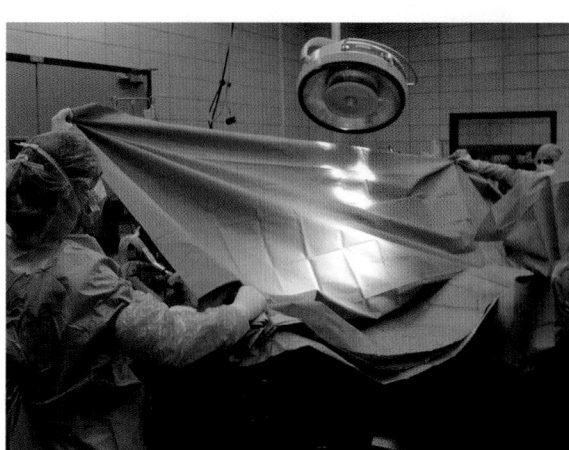

FIGURE 31-27 Draping of an equine surgery patient. Two persons are required to drape the patient.

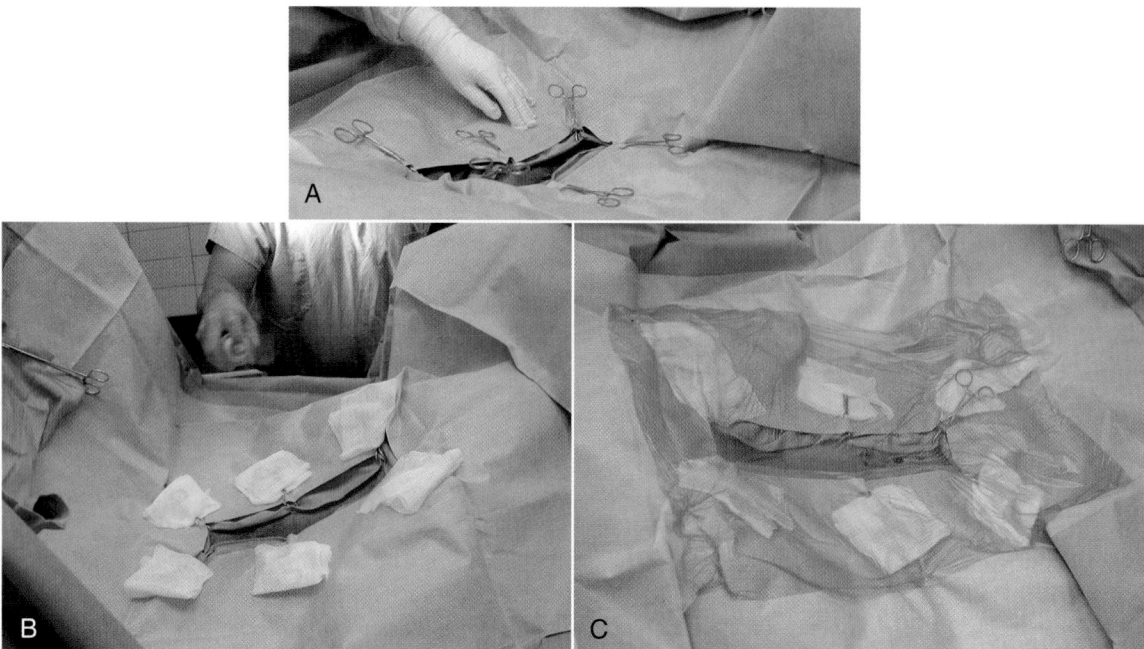

FIGURE 31-28 Draping the ventral abdomen of an equine surgery patient. **A,** Towel clamps are used to secure the laparotomy drape by clamping to the towel clamps underneath the drape. **B,** Exposed towel clamps are covered with a single 4 × 4 gauze, and an adhesive spray is used to improve the adhesiveness of the adhesive drape. **C,** An adhesive, impervious drape is placed directly over the incision site. Gauze prevents the adhesive drape from sticking to the clamp.

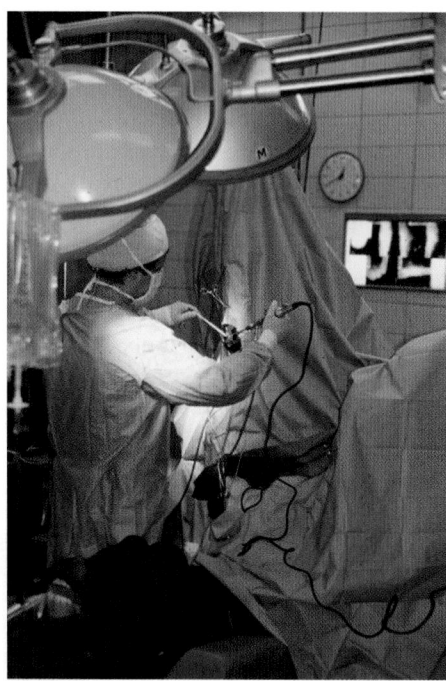

FIGURE 31-29 Arthroscopic surgery performed on the carpus of a horse.

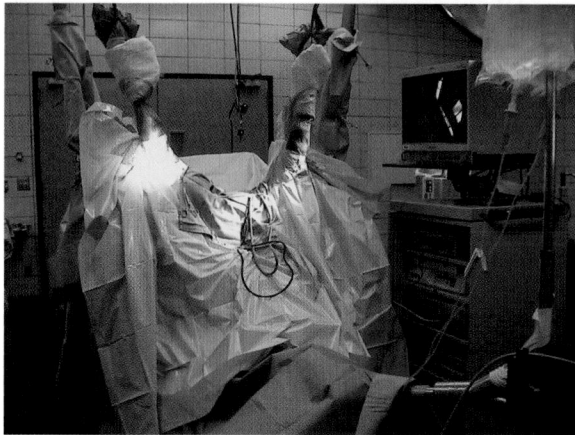

FIGURE 31-30 The horse is draped for arthroscopic surgery of the carpi. Adhesive, impervious drapes are placed around the carpi to reduce surgical wound contamination.

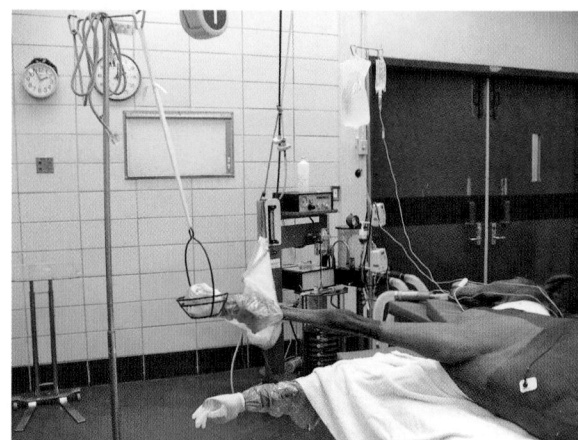

FIGURE 31-31 Intravenous (IV) fluid pole used to suspend the horse's limb for surgical preparation.

hand towel is then wrapped around the hoof, or an impervious orthopedic stockinette is placed over the limb. A large drape is fenestrated by cutting a "cross" in the center of the drape to accommodate the limb (Figure 31-34). The limb is then fed through the fenestration up to the sterile hand towels, and the entire animal is draped off (Figure 31-35). The drape is secured at the top of the surgical field with towel clamps. An adhesive, impervious plastic, iodine-impregnated drape is then wrapped over the incision site.

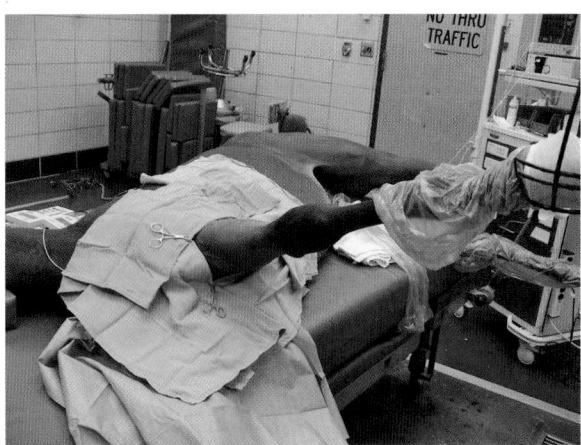

FIGURE 31-32 The area proximal to the surgery site is draped off with sterile hands towels.

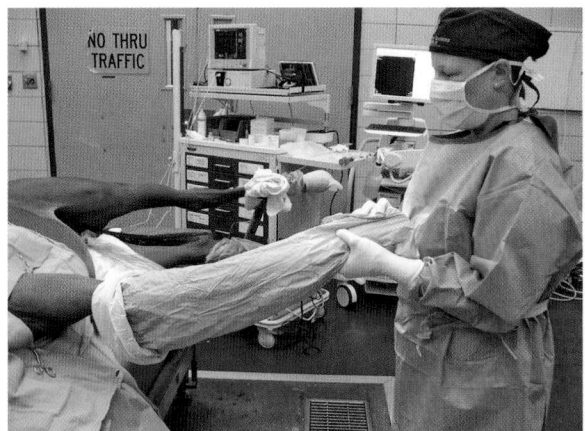

FIGURE 31-33 During draping of the horse's limb for surgery, the surgeon or assistant grasps the limb with a sterile, impervious orthopedic stockinette.

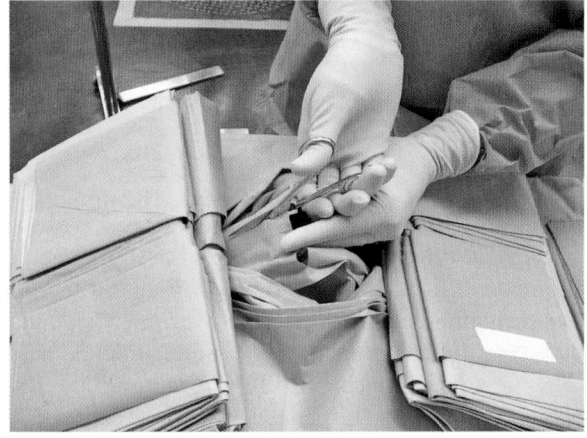

FIGURE 31-34 A large drape is fenestrated by cutting a "cross" in the center of the drape to accommodate the limb.

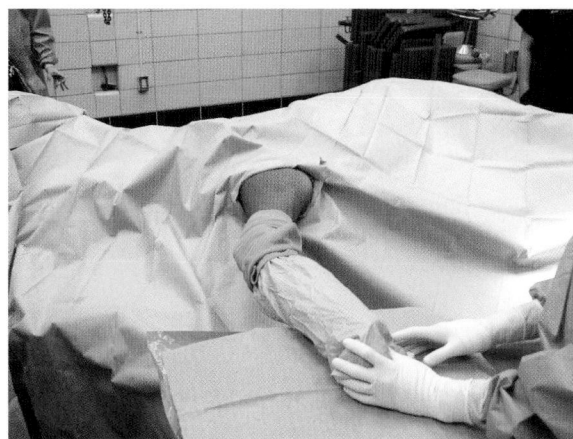

FIGURE 31-35 To drape a limb for orthopedic surgery, the limb is placed through a fenestrated drape.

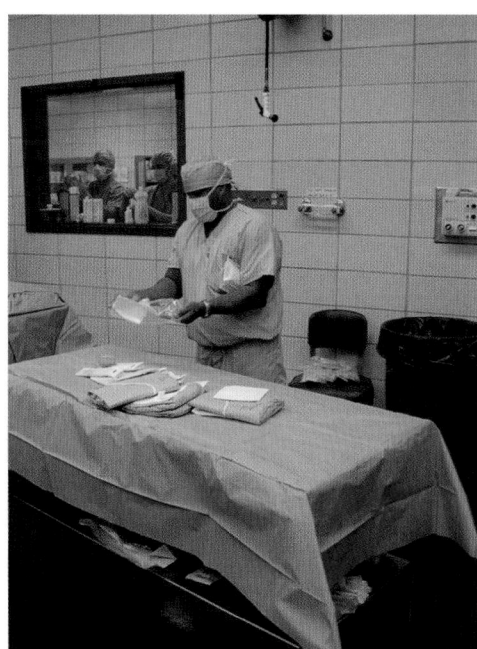

FIGURE 31-36 Instrument table is being set up for equine surgery by an operating room technician.

INSTRUMENT SETUP AND HANDLING

If adequate numbers of surgical technicians are present, the surgical instrument packs are opened during the time that the surgeon and the surgical assistant are draping the horse. This reduces anesthesia time. Occasionally, as during some orthopedic surgeries, two tables may be draped, depending on the number of instruments needed for the procedure. The instrument table is draped by a nongloved or gowned operating room technician (Figure 31-36). The surgical instrument packs needed for the surgery are placed on a Mayo instrument stand or a similar type of table, and with careful sterile technique, the outer wrap <u>only</u> is opened by the operating room technician (Figure 31-37). Subsequently, the gloved surgical assistant opens the sterile inner wrap and removes the sterile instrument tray, which is placed onto the draped instrument table. Sterile light handles, suction hose, electrocautery, fluid bowl, gauze sponges, scalpel blade, and suture are arranged on the instrument table. If the horse is draped for abdominal surgery, the surgeon and the surgical assistant create a pouch between the back legs of the horse by clamping a hand towel folded to the drape using a

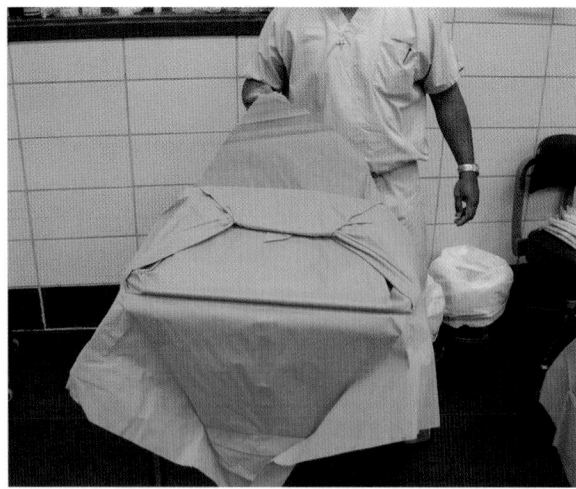

FIGURE 31-37 Preparing for equine surgery. The operating room technician opens the outer wrap of the instrument pack. One member of the surgical team will aseptically open the inner wrap and move the pack onto the instrument table.

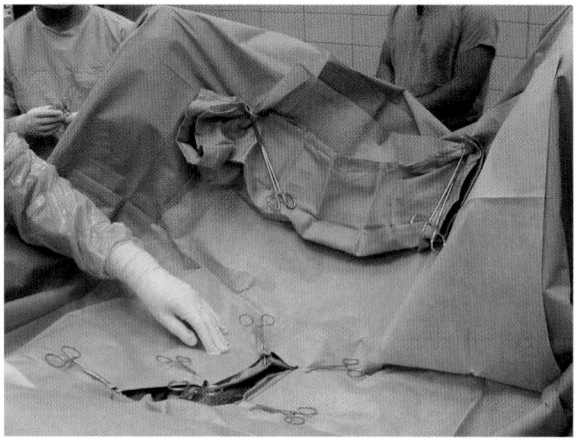

FIGURE 31-38 A pouch is made from a sterile folded hand towel and is clamped to the surgery drape by nonpenetrating clamps between the horse's rear limbs to hold the suction hose and cautery line.

nonpenetrating instrument, such as an Allis tissue forceps (Figure 31-38). The suction hose and the electrocautery line are held in this pouch. The ends of these are then run over the drapes between the legs of the horse and are connected by the operating room technician. A sterile IV fluid line, used to lavage the abdominal organs, may also be set up at this time. The surgical assistant organizes the surgical instruments on the instrument table. During this time, the instrument tray is placed on the back of the surgical table, a hand towel is placed in front of the tray, and frequently used instruments are placed on the towel to allow immediate access (Figure 31-39). Disposable scalpel blades are attached to the scalpel handles. The bowl is positioned on the back edge of the table so that sterile saline can be poured into the bowl by a circulating operating room technician. It is important during the surgical procedure, particularly in horses, that the instruments be kept clean. This is done by taking a wet 4 × 4 sponge and gently wiping the blood from the used

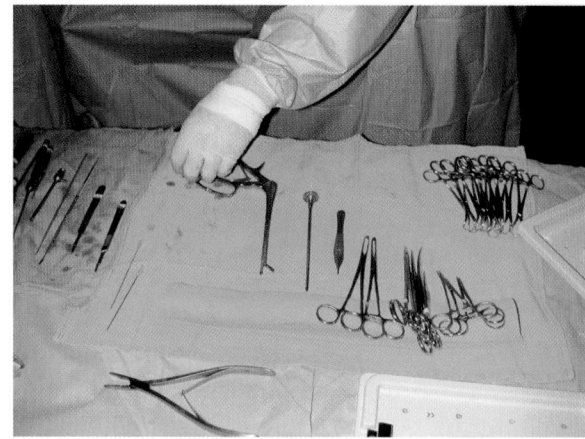

FIGURE 31-39 For efficiency in retrieving, the most frequently used instruments are placed in front of the instrument pack on a hand towel.

surgical instrument and placing it back onto the instrument table. However, if an instrument becomes contaminated during the surgical procedure, the instrument is discarded from the surgical table. At any time in which a break in asepsis occurs, whether a glove or a gown becomes contaminated, these need to be immediately discarded and replaced. It is important during the surgical procedure that the surgical assistant work efficiently and develop a thoughtful process of anticipating the next move of the surgeon. This will create a more efficient surgical environment and will reduce the length of time that the animal is anesthetized.

> **TECHNICIAN NOTE**   Any instrument that becomes contaminated during surgery is immediately discarded from the surgical table.

TISSUE HANDLING TECHNIQUES

Surgical manipulation of tissue in the horse is similar to that in the small animal. However, there are differences, which are discussed in the next section.

Hollow Organ Surgery

Surgical procedures involving hollow organs, especially intestinal structures, are complicated in the horse because of the sheer size, weight, and length of the intestinal tract. The small intestine, for example, is more than 80 feet in length. Additionally, the large intestine contains many pounds of **ingesta**, creating a problem during manipulation. Because of the weight of the large colon in the horse, for example, the risk that it may tear and ultimately contaminate the abdominal cavity is high. Thus, surgical assistants must be both strong and careful when handling the large colon (Figure 31-40). If the contents from the large intestine are to be evacuated, a colon tray is positioned alongside the horse and is draped with sterile impervious drapes that allow the large colon to be placed onto the tray away from the abdominal opening. This allows the colon to be evacuated without risk for contamination of the abdominal cavity (Figure 31-41).

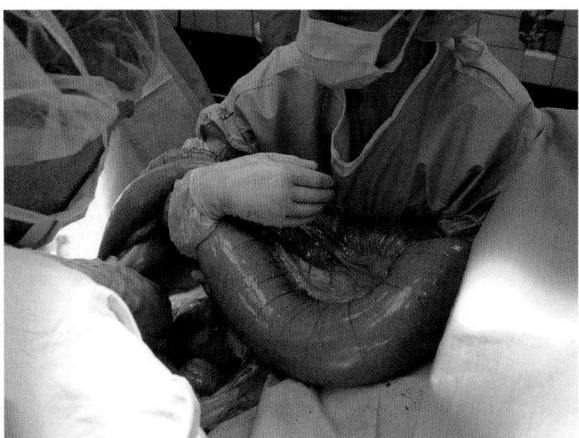

FIGURE 31-40 During abdominal surgery, the large intestines must be carefully handled during exploration of the abdominal cavity. In this photo, the large colon is being cradled by the surgical assistant.

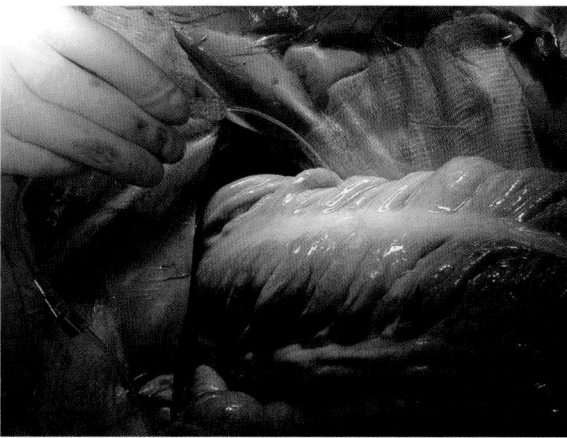

FIGURE 31-42 Photo of a segment of the large colon of a horse. It is imperative that the surface of the intestines be kept moist to prevent drying and subsequent tissue damage.

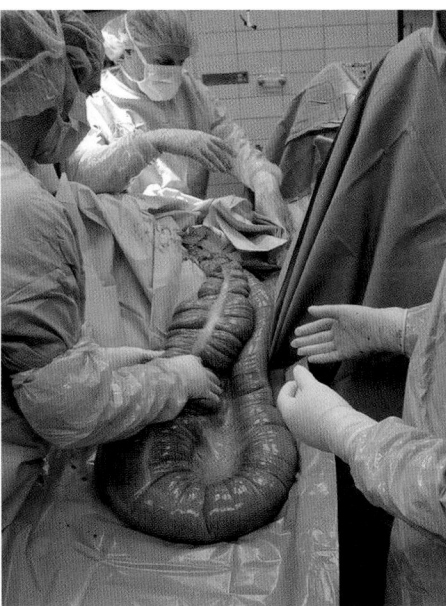

FIGURE 31-41 The large colon is placed on the colon tray in preparation for an enterotomy and content evacuation. Note that the opening of the abdominal cavity is being draped off.

It is the responsibility of the surgical assistant to maintain the large colon on the tray during the evacuation process so that it is not unintentionally pulled back into the abdominal cavity. If a small intestinal resection is performed in a horse, this segment of small intestine is isolated from the rest of the abdominal cavity as much as possible with laparotomy sponges and impervious drapes. It becomes a coordinated effort between the surgeon and the surgical assistant to ensure that the portion of the small intestine that is undergoing surgery be kept on the table, and that most of the intestine in the abdominal cavity be kept there as well. In addition, it is important for the surgical assistant to maintain proper orientation of the segments during intestinal resection and anastomosis and to maintain their proper positioning for the surgeon during closure and suturing of the enterotomy site.

Any instruments that come in contact with the ingesta should be discarded from the surgical table. Also, immediately after closure of the intestine, the surgeon and the surgical assistant must change gloves and gowns for clean, sterile ones before the abdomen is closed.

The intestinal organs can easily become dehydrated if they are left outside the abdominal cavity for an extended time. In addition, damage to the organ and possible risk of creating areas for adhesion formation may develop without proper care of the organs. It is important therefore that the surgical assistant be aware of tissue dehydration during the entire surgical procedure, and that the exposed intestinal segments be kept moist. This can be accomplished by applying sterile saline via a pressurized fluid bag or bulb syringe (Figure 31-42).

> **TECHNICIAN NOTE** It is imperative that a torn glove be replaced immediately during surgery.

Bone and Joints

Because of the severe consequences of infection in bone and joints, aseptic technique is an absolute must during orthopedic surgeries. Instrument handling or sharp ends of fracture bones can result in glove tearing. It is imperative that torn gloves be replaced immediately. Frequent irrigation of the tissue is absolutely vital. Irrigation is mandatory during bone drilling (Figure 31-43) because heat generated from drilling can cause thermal damage to bone, resulting in tissue necrosis. Being proactive in keeping blood removed from the surgical field, via suction or blotting, allows the surgeon to visualize affected structures and will lead to more efficient surgery. In addition, the surgical assistant is responsible for keeping the surgical table in order and the instruments clean and free of blood each time they are used. Proper tissue retraction and fragment reduction during fracture repair are also important roles of the surgical assistant during equine orthopedic surgery.

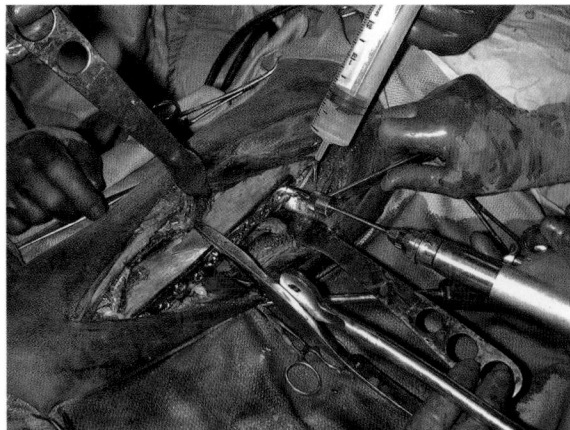

FIGURE 31-43 Repair of a radial fracture in a foal. Note that the drill bit is bathed with sterile saline to reduce thermal damage to the bone. Surgeons are using sterile, transparent gloves (note the powder on the hand to the right).

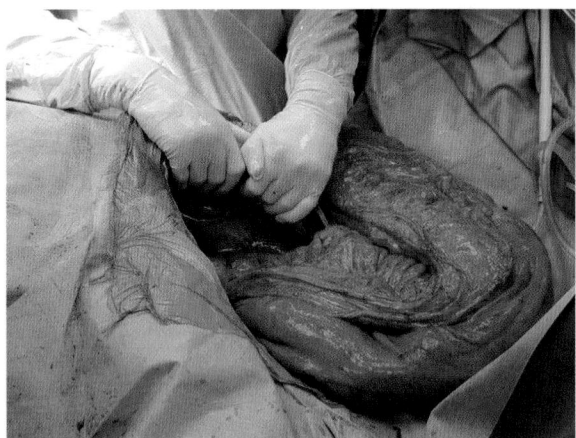

FIGURE 31-44 Abdominal exploration on a horse. Retraction of the ventral abdominal wall is performed by an assistant, who grasps it with the hands.

> **TECHNICIAN NOTE** Constant irrigation of the drill bit is necessary while bone drilling is performed during fracture repair.

Retraction Techniques

Retraction techniques in equine surgery are, for the most part, similar to those in small animal surgery, except during abdominal surgery. Because of the sheer size of the incision sites, it is difficult to maintain self-retaining retractors of any type. The surgical assistant therefore may be called upon to retract the abdominal wall with the hands (Figure 31-44). As with small animal orthopedics, retraction of muscle and tendon is necessary for visualization of fractures in horses. Hohmann retractors are effective hand-held retractors for deep tissues surrounding bone.

Hemostasis

Because of the size of the horse, loss of blood in most surgical procedures is not a major concern. However, it can become a concern, particularly during certain procedures such as open sinusotomies, nasal septum resections, ovariectomies,

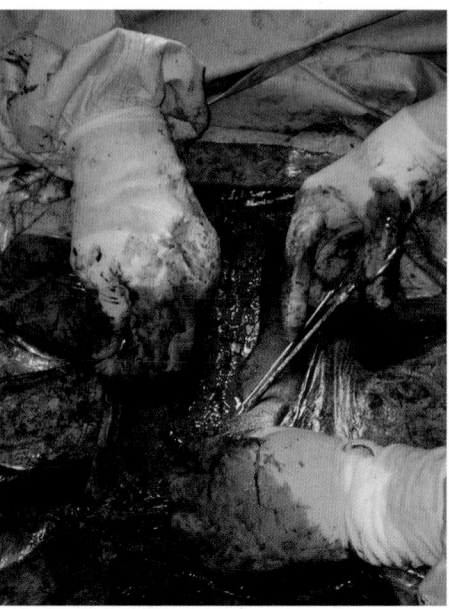

FIGURE 31-45 Closure of a ventral abdominal incision. Large suture material is needed to maintain closure.

castration, uterine trauma repair, and cesarean sections (C-sections). Sponge hemostasis is avoided in abdominal surgery because of the potential for loss of a sponge within the abdominal cavity, which can be devastating and life threatening to the horse. Lost sponges cause severe inflammatory reactions, resulting in peritonitis and intra-abdominal adhesions that could impair the normal function of the equine gastrointestinal tract. Therefore, during abdominal surgery, suction is used to evacuate fluids from the area. When hemorrhage from large vessels occurs, the vein or the artery is clamped and ligated with suture material, as is done in small animals. With small vessel bleeding, however, it is common to apply hemostats in combination with electrocautery to fuse the vessel walls together. Refer to the "Small Animal" section of this chapter for more information regarding hemostasis.

SUTURE MATERIALS USED IN HORSES

Because of the large size of horses, strong, thick suture material is required during equine surgeries. For closure of abdominal organs, a 2-0 absorbable material is commonly used. Closure of the ventral abdominal wall of a horse requires at least a No. 2 or a No. 3 absorbable suture material (Figure 31-45). PDS and Vicryl are commonly used suture materials. For closure of the subcutaneous space, often a 0 absorbable suture material is used. Zero or 2-0 nonabsorbable material (nylon or Prolene) is used for apposition of the skin; however, skin staples are commonly used. In most cases, suture material with swaged needles is used. This saves time and improves efficiency. It is important for surgical assistants to have the proper suture material readily available for the surgeon as it is needed. Often, the required sutures are discussed before surgery. It is a common practice for the surgical assistant to open the suture material and have it ready by arming a needle holder with needle and suture before it is requested by the surgeon.

ACKNOWLEDGMENT

The authors wish to acknowledge the veterinary technicians who assisted in the preparation of this chapter.

RECOMMENDED READINGS

Evans HE, Christenson GC: Miller's anatomy of the dog, ed 3, Philadelphia, 1993, Saunders.
Fossum TW: Small animal surgery, ed 3, St Louis, 2007, Mosby.
Auer JA, Stick JA: Equine surgery, ed 3, Philadelphia, 2006, Saunders.

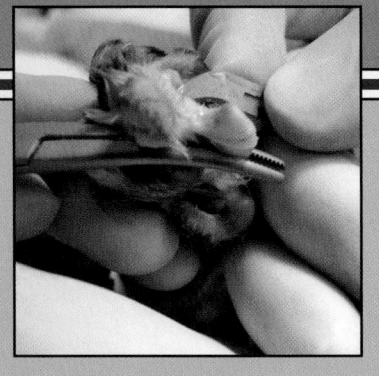

32 Small Animal Surgical Nursing

Loretta J. Bubenik-Angapen

OUTLINE

Preoperative Patient Assessment, *1215*
**Surgical Preparation and Animal
   Positioning,** *1215*
Perioperative Antibiotics, *1215*
Monitoring, *1216*
Blood Loss, *1217*
Hypothermia, *1217*
Pain, *1218*
Incision Evaluation, *1219*
Suture Removal, *1221*
Bandage Care, *1221*
Drain Care, *1222*
Restraint, *1223*
Common Surgical Procedures, *1223*
Elective Versus Nonelective Surgery, *1223*
**Tail Docking and Dewclaw Removal
   in Puppies,** *1224*
Definition, *1224*
Indications, *1224*
Preoperative Considerations, *1224*
Teaching and Intraoperative
   Considerations, *1224*
Postoperative Considerations, *1224*
**Tail Docking and Dewclaw Removal in
   the Adult,** *1224*
Indications, *1224*
Preoperative Considerations, *1224*
Technique and Intraoperative
   Considerations for Dewclaw Removal in
   the Adult, *1225*
Technique and Intraoperative
   Considerations for Tail Amputation in
   the Adult, *1225*
Postoperative Considerations, *1225*
Feline Onychectomy, *1225*
Definition, *1225*
Indications, *1225*
Preoperative Considerations, *1225*
Technique and Intraoperative
   Considerations, *1225*
Postoperative Considerations, *1227*
Celiotomy, *1228*
Definition, *1228*
Indications, *1228*
Preoperative Considerations, *1228*

Technique and Intraoperative
   Considerations, *1228*
Postoperative Considerations, *1229*
Gastrointestinal Surgery, *1229*
Definition, *1229*
Indications, *1230*
Preoperative Considerations, *1230*
Technique and Intraoperative
   Considerations, *1230*
Postoperative Considerations, *1231*
Gastric Dilatation-Volvulus, *1231*
Definition, *1231*
Preoperative Considerations, *1232*
Technique and Intraoperative
   Considerations, *1232*
Postoperative Considerations, *1233*
**Ovariohysterectomy in the Dog
   and Cat,** *1233*
Definition, *1233*
Indications, *1233*
Preoperative Considerations, *1234*
Technique and Intraoperative
   Considerations, *1234*
Postoperative Considerations, *1235*
Pyometra, *1235*
Definition, *1235*
Indications, *1235*
Preoperative Considerations, *1235*
Technique and Intraoperative
   Considerations, *1236*
Postoperative Considerations, *1236*
Canine Castration, *1236*
Definition, *1236*
Indications, *1236*
Preoperative Considerations, *1236*
Technique and Intraoperative
   Considerations, *1239*
Postoperative Considerations, *1240*
Feline Castration, *1240*
Definition, *1240*
Indications, *1240*
Preoperative Considerations, *1240*
Technique and Intraoperative
   Considerations, *1241*
Postoperative Considerations, *1241*

Cesarean Delivery, *1241*
Definition, *1241*
Preoperative Considerations, *1241*
Technique and Intraoperative
  Considerations, *1242*
Postoperative Considerations for
  the Neonate, *1243*
Postoperative Considerations for
  the Dam, *1243*
Cystotomy, *1243*
Definition, *1243*
Indications, *1243*
Preoperative Considerations, *1243*
Technique and Intraoperative
  Considerations, *1244*
Postoperative Considerations, *1244*
Urethrostomy, *1245*
Definition, *1245*
Indications, *1245*
Preoperative Considerations, *1245*
Technique and Intraoperative
  Considerations, *1245*
Postoperative Considerations, *1246*
Hernias, *1247*
Umbilical Hernia, *1247*
Inguinal Hernia, *1247*
Diaphragmatic Hernia, *1248*
Lumpectomy, *1249*

Definition, *1249*
Indications, *1249*
Preoperative Considerations, *1249*
Technique and Intraoperative
  Considerations, *1250*
Postoperative Considerations, *1250*
Removal of Mammary Neoplasia, *1250*
Definition, *1250*
General Information and Indications, *1250*
Technique and Intraoperative
  Considerations, *1250*
Postoperative Considerations, *1251*
Amputation, *1251*
Definition, *1251*
Indications, *1251*
Preoperative Considerations, *1251*
Technique and Perioperative
  Considerations, *1252*
Postoperative Considerations, *1252*
Neurologic Patient Care, *1253*
Surgical Technique and Perioperative
  Considerations, *1253*
Postoperative Considerations, *1254*
Orthopedic Surgery, *1255*
Long-Bone Fractures, *1255*
Joints, *1257*
Client Education, *1257*
Guidelines for Discharge Instructions, *1258*

LEARNING OBJECTIVES

When you have completed this chapter, you will be able to:

1. Pronounce, spell, and define all Key Terms in the chapter.
2. Do the following regarding surgical preparation and animal positioning:
   - Describe the preoperative, intraoperative, and postoperative responsibilities of the veterinary technician in surgical assistance.
   - Describe indications and use of prophylactic antibiotics for surgical patients.
   - Describe signs of blood loss in the postoperative patient.
   - Discuss concerns related to hypothermia in anesthetized patients and describe methods for increasing patient body temperature intraoperatively and postoperatively.
   - Describe postoperative abnormalities that can occur in surgical incisions, the procedure for removal of skin sutures, and general considerations for care of bandages and drains.
   - Discuss the proper use of animal restraint with regard to surgical technique, and patient safety and comfort.
3. Differentiate between elective and non-elective surgery.
4. List and describe indications and preoperative, intraoperative, and postoperative considerations for the following procedures in dogs and cats: tail docking and dewclaw removal in puppies and adults, feline onychectomy, and celiotomy.
5. List and describe indications and preoperative, intraoperative, and postoperative considerations for the following procedures in dogs and cats: gastrointestinal surgery, gastric dilatation-volvulus, ovariohysterectomy, and pyometra.
6. List and describe indications and preoperative, intraoperative, and postoperative considerations for the following procedures in dogs and cats: canine and feline castration, cesarean delivery, cystomy, and urethrostomy.

7. List and describe indications and preoperative, intraoperative, and postoperative considerations for the following procedures in dogs and cats: hernia repair, lumpectomy, removal of mammary neoplasia, amputation, neurologic patient care, and orthopedic surgery.
8. List considerations related to client education for discharged surgical patients.

INTRODUCTION

The veterinary technician's role in surgical nursing is an important part of hospital and patient management. Preoperative, intraoperative, and postoperative responsibilities should be considered for a successful outcome. The surgical candidate must undergo preoperative assessment, including examination and laboratory evaluation and appropriate positioning and preparation for surgery. The technician's responsibilities during surgery include patient monitoring and surgeon assistance. In the postoperative period, patient monitoring and supportive care are important for postsurgical recovery and healing. Duties of the veterinary technician include appropriate animal restraint; appropriate sample collection and diagnostic evaluation; administration of sedation, anesthesia, and pain medication; instrument preparation; operating room preparation; appropriate patient preparation and positioning for surgery; aseptic patient and instrument handling; patient monitoring; direct surgical assistance; patient recovery; and securing of the operating room. Many of these topics are covered in Chapters 6, 18, 26, 28, 29, 30, and 31. This chapter focuses on familiarizing the veterinary technician with specific surgical procedures and relevant anatomy and highlighting technician responsibilities in the preoperative, intraoperative, and postoperative periods. A working knowledge of common surgical procedures will ensure proficiency in surgical assistance, decrease surgery time, enhance the flow of surgery, and improve the quality of patient care.

PREOPERATIVE PATIENT ASSESSMENT

The veterinary surgical candidate should undergo a complete preoperative assessment. It is important to know what the primary problem is so that the specific needs of the patient and the surgeon can be anticipated and met. Elective surgical procedures do not have the same demands as emergency or urgent surgical procedures. Nevertheless, a good patient history is important in all cases. Eating, drinking, urination, and defecation habits of the animal should be ascertained. An animal that has not been eating or drinking will likely require rehydration before anesthesia and surgery. Rehydration may necessitate a blood or plasma transfusion because dilution of the blood cell volume occurs with rehydration. Fluids should not be withheld, to prevent anemia. If the animal has eaten on the day of scheduled surgery, the procedure will have to be delayed to decrease the risk for aspiration of stomach contents into the trachea and lungs. The animal should not have food for at least 12 hours before anesthesia. However, water does not need to be withheld. Emergency surgeries will have to be performed whether the animal has eaten or not, but owners should be warned of the increased risk for aspiration. In addition, it is important to know what medications the animal is currently taking or has taken because this may affect what medications are administered before and after surgery. A history of previous medical problems and surgical procedures should be noted and brought to the attention of the surgeon. Vaccine status should be ascertained. A young puppy or kitten is best vaccinated at least 2 weeks before surgery rather than on the day of surgery because the immune system can be suppressed by anesthesia and surgery, making the patient less responsive to immunization. Temperature, pulse rate and quality, respiration rate and character, **capillary refill time**, mucous membrane color, body weight, and demeanor should be assessed before surgery. Abnormalities should be brought to the attention of the surgeon.

Preanesthetic screening will depend on the animal's condition and the reason for surgery. Specifics of this are covered in Chapter 29. From a nursing standpoint, it is important to discuss with the surgeon what diagnostics are appropriate before surgery and to ensure that they are performed in a timely manner. Diagnostics might include blood work, such as packed cell volume (PCV), total plasma protein (TP) concentration, blood urea nitrogen (BUN) concentration, blood glucose concentration, complete blood count (CBC), complete biochemical analysis, and the heartworm test; blood gas analysis; electrocardiogram (ECG); radiographs; ultrasound and fine-needle mass aspiration; fecal analysis; and/or urinalysis. Abnormalities detected on the preanesthetic screen should be brought to the attention of the surgeon.

SURGICAL PREPARATION AND ANIMAL POSITIONING

It is the veterinary technician's responsibility to inquire about the surgical procedure to be performed and what

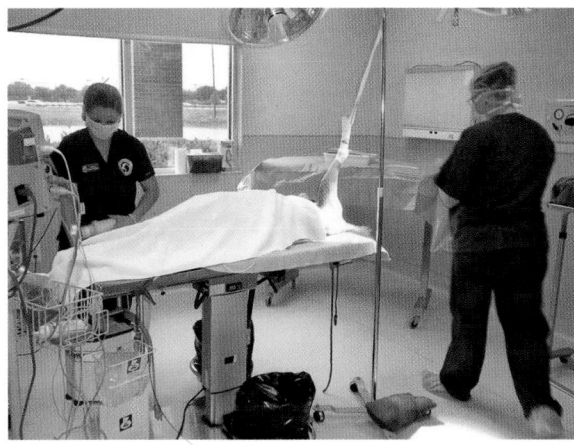

FIGURE 32-1 This dog has been appropriately covered with a warming-air blanket and a towel over the blanket to provide additional warmth during surgery. All areas of the body not involved in the surgical field can be covered. This dog is also lying on a heated surgery table.

instrumentation will be required. The technician should have all the necessary equipment readily accessible for use. The operating room should be clean and anesthesia equipment checked for functionality and ready for use. A heated circulating water blanket should be placed on the operating table, turned on, and covered with a towel so that it is warm by the time the animal is positioned on the table. Appropriate blankets should be set up and placed over the patient before draping (Figure 32-1). Clean surgical hair clippers and skin cleansing solutions should be made available for use. Dirty clipper blades should not be used to prepare a surgical incision.

The postoperative cage should be set up with appropriate warming equipment turned on (Figure 32-2, *A*). Warm-air blankets should be nearby when accessible to cover the patient if needed when they return to the cage (Figure 32-2, *B*).

Inadequate animal preparation or inappropriate positioning can hinder surgical technique, increase the risk for surgical infection, and result in wasted time spent correcting deficiencies. Aseptic protocol should always be followed with animal preparation and draping and surgical instrument handling. The hair should be liberally clipped around the surgical site and the skin cleansed appropriately (refer to Chapters 30 and 31). The veterinary technician should be familiar with the type of surgery to be performed so that animal preparation is consistent and adequate.

> **TECHNICIAN NOTE** Inadequate surgical preparation can hinder surgical technique, increase risk for infection, and result in prolonged anesthesia.

PERIOPERATIVE ANTIBIOTICS

Prophylactic antibiotics are used to decrease the risk for infection in clean or clean-contaminated surgeries, but their use will not entirely eliminate infections associated with a surgical procedure. Using antibiotics to treat active infection

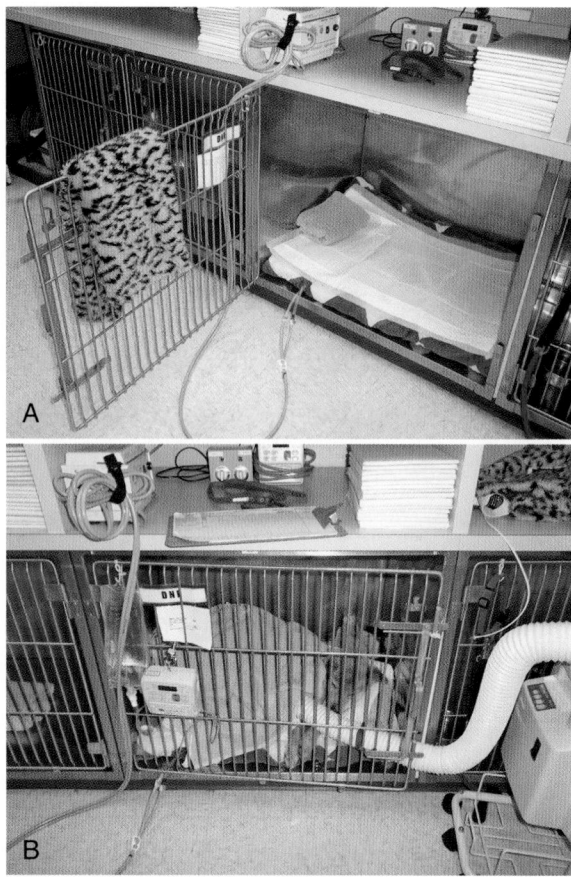

FIGURE 32-2 A, This cage has been set up for a postoperative patient. The cage heat is turned on, and adequate bedding is provided. Note the blanket hanging over the door, ready to be placed over the patient at recovery. **B,** When this animal was placed in the cage for recovery, a warming-air blanket was close by and was immediately placed over the animal for additional heat support.

is a completely different process and will not be discussed here. Antibiotics should never be given indiscriminately to animals undergoing surgery. All antibiotics have potential side effects, and their use increases the cost of surgery. More important, indiscriminant use of antibiotics contributes to the development of resistant strains of bacteria (hospital "superbugs") that are difficult to treat.

> **TECHNICIAN NOTE** Antibiotics should never be given indiscriminately to animals undergoing surgery because this contributes to the development of resistant strains of bacteria (hospital "superbugs") that are difficult to treat.

Indications for Prophylactic Antibiotics

- Operative time is longer than 90 minutes. Open surgical wounds are constantly exposed to bacteria from the animal's skin, the operative team, and the air. The longer the wound is open, the higher is the chance of infection. Prolonged anesthesia also increases the risk for infection.

- The patient may be immunosuppressed. Factors that suppress the immune system include use of immunosuppressive drugs (steroids), Cushing's disease (hyperadrenocorticism), some cancers, chemotherapy or radiation therapy, feline leukemia virus (FeLV), and feline immunodeficiency virus (FIV).
- A hollow viscus (e.g., gastrointestinal [GI] tract, urinary bladder) is to be entered.
- The incision is to involve an area that is difficult to aseptically prepare (such as a toe or an ear).
- Orthopedic implants are placed.
- Joint procedures that are long and aggressive and certain joint procedures require multiple entrances into the joint (arthroscopy).
- If the consequences of infection could be devastating to the surgical outcome, examples include total hip replacement and spinal surgery of any kind.
- Prophylactic antibiotics are not recommended for short, clean surgical procedures, such as simple mass removal, osteochondritis, cartilage flap removal, **ovariohysterectomy**, castration, and simple biopsies.

Therapeutic drug levels must be present in the wound fluid (serum and interstitial tissues) at the time of surgical incision, or the antibiotics will not be effective. They should be given at least 20 minutes before the surgical incision is made. Antibiotics given 3 or more hours before the procedure select for resistant bacteria. Prophylactic antibiotics given more than 3 to 5 hours after the surgical incision has been made will likely not be effective in preventing infection. No advantage is associated with continuing antibiotics beyond 6 to 24 hours after surgery unless it is necessary to treat an active infection, or a break in sterile technique occurred during surgery. The appropriate antibiotic should be effective against the potential contaminant (usually broad spectrum), achieve good tissue concentrations, and cause minimal side effects. The veterinarian in charge should be questioned as to what antibiotic is appropriate for what surgical procedure, and when antibiotic prophylaxis is needed. If a break in sterile technique has occurred or an active infection has developed, antibiotics are continued in the postoperative period according to the manufacturer's dosing recommendations and under the supervision of the veterinarian in charge. Continuing antibiotics for other reasons (e.g., you want to be on the safe side) is a misuse of prophylactic antibiotics.

MONITORING

Intraoperative and postoperative monitoring is critical for proper surgical nursing care. Chapter 29 covers anesthetic monitoring in detail, and the reader should refer to that chapter for further information. Some important components of patient monitoring as they pertain to surgery and recovery after surgery will be discussed here.

During surgery, a surgical plane of anesthesia is crucial for appropriate surgical technique and animal well-being. Careful monitoring during this time and afterward can alert the observer to potential fatal complications. Anesthesia and surgery can result in several potential problems, including blood loss, hypothermia, pain, and cardiac and respiratory problems. The veterinary surgical technician must be prepared to deal with changes in animal status during and after surgery and to address issues as the need arises. Monitoring should involve a series of evaluations and tests. Suspected complications during anesthesia and recovery are based on a group of signs consistent with a problem and abnormal trends in values—not just one abnormality. The postoperative phase is a critical transition period from general anesthesia to consciousness, and continual monitoring should be provided until the animal is safely extubated, normothermic, and in sternal recumbency.

Patient monitoring does not stop once the animal has recovered from anesthesia. As long as the animal is hospitalized, vital signs, behavior, appetite, and the surgical incision should be evaluated. Depending on animal status, daily or more frequent observation of these parameters is performed. Diagnostic tests may be warranted. Abnormalities should be reported to the veterinarian in charge.

> **TECHNICIAN NOTE** A single abnormal vital sign does not necessarily identify a significant clinical problem. All indicators (temperature, pulse, respiration, mucous membranes) should be evaluated serially to detect a trend in the animal's condition. It is this trend that will determine the severity of the postoperative problem and will dictate appropriate treatment.

BLOOD LOSS

Many procedures can result in substantial blood loss as a complication, or blood loss may be due to the inherent nature of the procedure or disease. PCV and TP should always be assessed before surgery to obtain a baseline value. Preoperative anemia should be brought to the attention of the veterinarian in charge, and, if present, a CBC should be performed. If substantial blood loss occurred during surgery, PCV and TP should also be assessed serially in the postoperative period. It can be difficult to determine whether an animal is hemorrhaging or has lost a substantial amount of blood immediately postoperatively because a painful, recovering animal can have similar clinical signs. Furthermore, it is not unusual for PCV and TP to drop up to 10% as a result of anesthesia and surgery, even when no major blood loss has occurred. Temperature, heart rate, pulse quality, respiration, and character of mucous membranes should be examined periodically during and after surgery. Animals with substantial blood loss may experience continued hypothermia or a drop in body temperature, rapid heart rate with weak peripheral pulses, rapid respiratory rate, and pale or white mucous membranes. Abnormalities should be promptly reported to the veterinarian in charge. Other signs include abdominal enlargement if intra-abdominal hemorrhage occurs, incisional swelling or oozing of blood, and dyspnea and decreased ventral lung sounds if intrathoracic hemorrhage occurs. Another important thing to remember

is that changes in PCV and TP may not occur immediately with blood loss, and these tests may have to be repeated a few hours after the incident of blood loss to document abnormalities or to assess continued blood loss.

Besides PCV and TP determination, **abdominocentesis** (aspiration of fluid from the abdomen), thoracocentesis (aspiration of fluid from the thoracic cavity), or fine-needle aspiration beneath the incision can be performed when the patient is suspected of having substantial bleeding. If the sampled fluid has a PCV nearly equal to the systemic PCV and clinical signs are consistent with hemorrhage, the index of suspicion should be high. Treatment strategies include crystalloid fluid bolus, colloidal fluid administration, blood transfusion, oxygen carrier fluid administration (oxyglobin, which may no longer be available), pressure bandages, and/or reoperation—in some cases, to stop the source of hemorrhage. The treatment of choice depends on the animal's status and ability to maintain a stable condition. The reader should review the clinical signs and treatment strategies for various types of fluid therapy and shock as discussed in Chapters 24 and 25.

HYPOTHERMIA

Hypothermia is defined as a subnormal body temperature. Once an animal is anesthetized, its body temperature begins to drop. It is important to monitor body temperature throughout general anesthesia and during recovery. All anesthetized animals, especially small dogs and all cats, should be actively warmed during anesthesia and surgery to help maintain body temperature. Small animals become hypothermic quickly when placed under general anesthesia, especially if a body cavity is opened. It is important to remember that the more surface area is exposed (e.g., large incision exposing the abdominal organs), the faster and lower the body temperature is expected to drop. If the exposed area is moist, evaporative cooling occurs. Mechanisms to maintain body temperature include placing animals on heated circulating water blankets; wrapping paws and the body in plastic wrap to prevent heat loss (Figure 32-3); wrapping warm water bottles (or gloves filled with warm water) with a towel and placing them next to the animal; covering areas not involved in the surgical procedure with an insulated blanket;

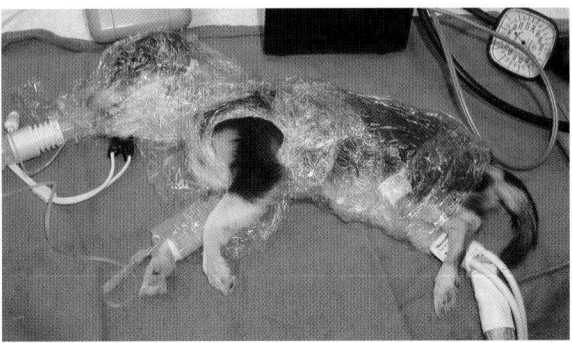

FIGURE 32-3 One method of heat retention during surgery is wrapping the animal in plastic. This works well for small dogs and cats.

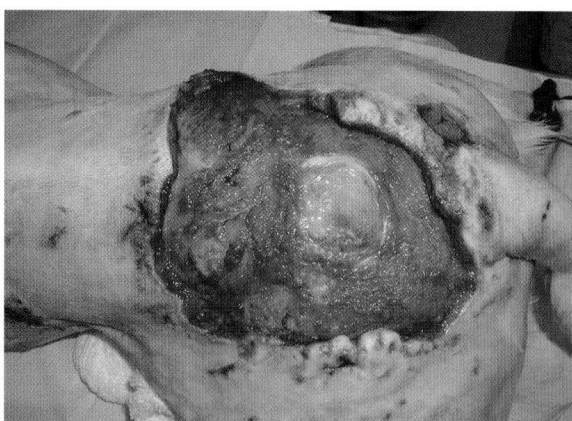

FIGURE 32-4 The area of denuded skin over the rump of this dog is a result of a thermal burn sustained from an electric heating pad used to maintain body temperature during ovariohysterectomy.

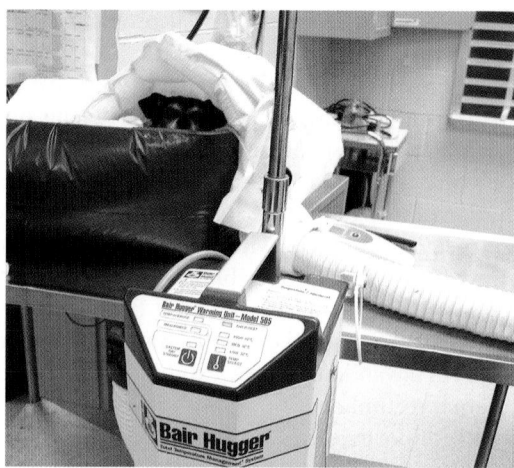

FIGURE 32-5 Blankets that blow warm air and warm-water baths can be used to bring the body temperature up quickly. Note that the dog is placed under the blue hot-air blanket in a well-constructed water bath. This is a close-up of a water bath. A large container is filled with warm water and is covered with thick plastic and a towel. The dog or cat is placed on the towel in the container and is allowed to sink down into the warm water, with the plastic preventing soaking. The animal must be monitored carefully to prevent accidental puncture of the plastic and drowning.

using actively warmed cages and surgery tables; and using a warm-air blanket (Bair Hugger, Arizant Healthcare, Inc., Eden Prairie, Minnesota) on areas not involved in the surgical procedure. Heat lamps are not recommended because they can cause thermal burns, especially in an anesthetized animal that cannot respond to painful, concentrated heat. It must be remembered that electric heating pads should never be used to warm anesthetized animals. Electric heating pads concentrate heat and may cause thermal burns (Figure 32-4). The veterinarian is liable for burns caused by electric heat units because they are a known cause of thermal skin injury during anesthesia. Unless a warm-air blanket is used, all heat sources should be applied with a towel between the heat source and the animal. Although rare, if the body temperature rises above normal during the procedure, the heat source can be turned off.

After surgery, the animal is placed in a warm area to recover, and any necessary heat sources are used. If the patient is severely hypothermic, a warm-air blanket and/or a warm-water bath can be used to raise the temperature quickly (Figure 32-5). A warm-water bath is made by filling a large, deep pan—big enough to place the entire animal in—three-fourths full with warm water, placing a thick garbage bag over the pan and water, and placing a towel over the garbage bag where the animal is to be placed (similar to a heated water bed). The animal is placed in the water bath, allowing the warm water to "wrap" around the animal; the plastic prevents soaking. The animal must be monitored closely to prevent accidental puncture of the plastic and drowning. Only small dogs and cats can be warmed in this way.

Body temperature should show a steady rise as the animal recovers. When the animal's temperature approaches 100° F, heating sources should be discontinued, but the animal should be kept covered, and body temperature should be reevaluated periodically to ensure that it returns to and remains normal. If the temperature remains low or continues to fall, this may be an indication of a potential problem, and the veterinarian in charge should be alerted. Heat should

be reapplied if the animal's body temperature begins to drop after heat sources are removed.

PAIN

Intraoperative and postoperative pain assessment is important for animal well-being and health. During surgery, increases in heart rate, respiratory rate, and blood pressure and lightening of the anesthetic plane can indicate that the animal is in pain. However, it is important to remember that trends and a combination of factors should be used to determine what problem is actually present. Increased heart rate alone, for example, does not indicate pain. Increased heart rate also occurs with hypotension, so all parameters should be assessed before a decision is made regarding treatment. A drop in blood pressure may indicate a need to turn the patient's anesthetic down, whereas an increased heart rate with other parameters of pain or awakening may indicate the need to increase anesthesia. During recovery, animals that are in pain, among other things, may vocalize, have elevated heart and respiratory rates, thrash, bite or chew at the surgery site, and/or become aggressive. Other signs of pain include disinterest in the environment, crying upon manipulation of the painful area, insomnia, and lack of appetite (Figure 32-6). It should be remembered that changes in vital signs can mean numerous things, and the animal should be carefully evaluated by the technician and the surgeon before drug administration. It is best not to allow the animal to experience pain before pain medication is given. If an incision was made, pain is going to be experienced by the animal. It is up to the veterinary technician and the surgeon to decide how much pain a particular procedure might cause. Painful procedures include fracture repair, amputation, declaw, joint surgery, and any major abdominal procedure. Moderately

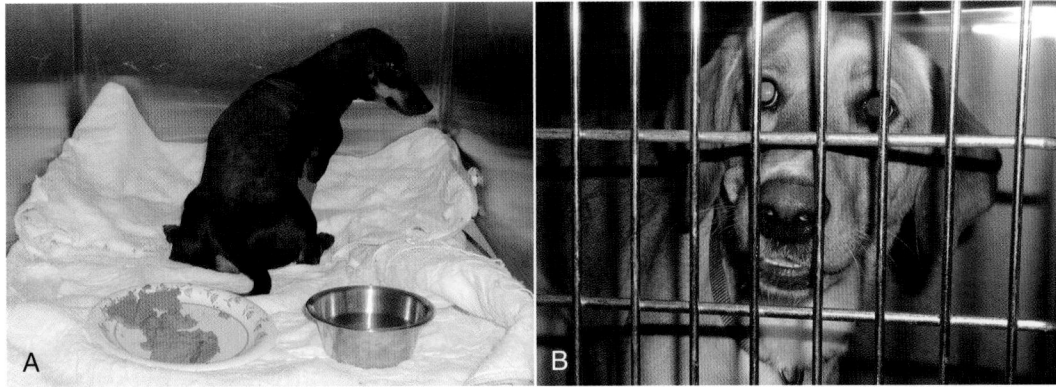

FIGURE 32-6 Note how the dog in **(A)** does not turn to face the door, even when it is opened. Also note the full food dish in the front of the cage. This dog is suffering from severe spinal pain and is not interested in her environment. Comfortable animals are often interested in their surroundings and will come to the cage door to greet you. In spite of her fracture of the tibia, the dog in **(B)** is more than willing to interact with those around her.

painful procedures include minor abdominal procedures (spay, **cystotomy**) and simple body wall hernia repair. Mildly painful procedures might include simple mass removal or biopsy. It can be difficult to determine how much pain an animal is in because animals respond so differently to pain. Animals may vocalize or pant during recovery as a side effect of drugs given for anesthesia and pain control. Use of a pain scale that assesses a combination for parameters such as vital signs, behavior, mobility, and sensitivity to touching the incision or painful site can help the veterinary team make decisions on the need for relief of pain. See Chapter 28 for more information on treatment of pain.

Pain treatment is accomplished in several ways; the animal, the availability of pain medications, and the type of procedure that was performed determine what sort of regimen is chosen. Most soft tissue surgical pain will last 4 to 5 days after surgery. For bone and joint procedures, an additional 4 to 5 days might be expected. It is best to preemptively manage pain rather than wait for the animal to show pain before administering pain medication. If the animal is allowed to experience pain before administration of pain medication, the pain is harder to treat and may not be relieved by the medication administered (see Chapter 28). Pain medication should be administered before surgery in premedicants, and they should be continued throughout the surgical procedure and into the postoperative period according to the dosing regimen for the particular drug used. A wait-and-see attitude should never be adopted because this allows the animal to experience pain before treatment is given.

Another misconception is that animals will stay quiet and calm if they are in pain, so avoidance of pain medication is a form of treatment. You would never be treated that way in a hospital, and animals should not be treated that way. This is an ethical dilemma that many veterinarians and technicians must face. An appropriately managed surgical patient will likely sleep for several hours after surgery, should be comfortable when manipulated, should be alert and interested in its environment when aroused, and will often be

willing to eat and drink, although this depends on the nature of the problem being treated.

> **TECHNICIAN NOTE** The animal should not be allowed to experience pain before medication is given. Pain medication should be administered at dosing intervals appropriate for the medication—not as needed.

INCISION EVALUATION

The surgical wound should be visually and palpably inspected daily (see Chapter 26 for detailed information on wounds and healing). The surgical incision is usually left uncovered after surgery. The incision can be covered with an adhesive or a wrap bandage for the first few days after surgery to keep the incision clean, prevent contact with the hospital environment, and absorb seepage. Ointments and creams (even antibiotic topicals) should not be placed on the incision because this can cause irritation, and components of the ointment can delay wound healing.

Abnormalities that can occur in the early postoperative period (1 to 3 days) include redness, swelling, drainage, and **dehiscence** (wound breakdown). An incision should be evaluated with respect to the type of surgical procedure performed. Elective operations, such as ovariohysterectomy and castration, can be expected to produce mild redness and swelling with no drainage from the incision site (Figure 32-7). However, if the wound was contaminated (e.g., laceration, perianal wound), or if surgical exposure was extensive, the incision is expected to be somewhat swollen, reddened, and warm to the touch and may have mild to moderate drainage in the first 24 to 48 hours postoperatively. Swelling secondary to surgical trauma will usually resolve within 3 to 7 days after surgery. However, **seromas** (serum accumulation under the incision) and hematomas (blood accumulation under the incision) may persist for weeks.

It is surprising to note that most animals will not lick or chew at the surgical incision. Animals usually lick or chew at the incision only if the character of the incision is irritating.

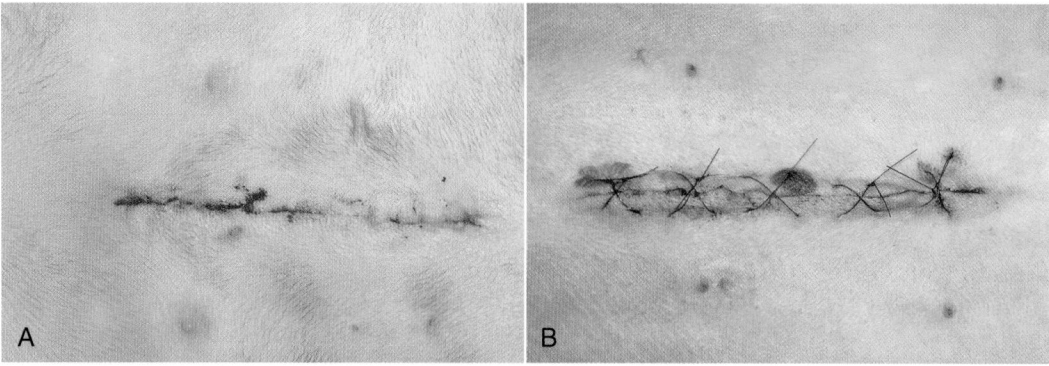

FIGURE 32-7 These photographs were taken 4 hours after surgery. **(A)** shows a celiotomy incision after routine ovariohysterectomy, whereas **(B)** shows a celiotomy incision after severe traction on the skin during surgery for exposure. Note the minimal redness, swelling, and drainage from incision **(A)** compared with incision **(B)**.

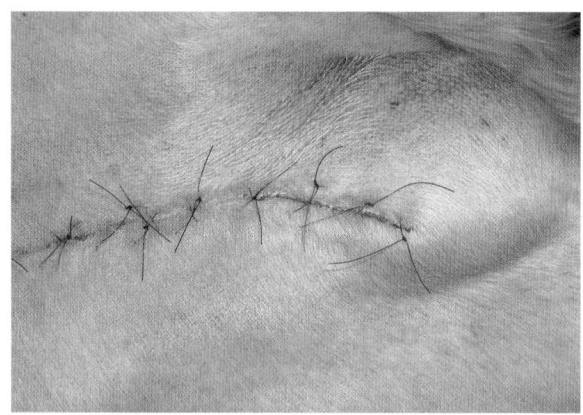

FIGURE 32-8 Note the swelling on right beneath the incision. The swelling was nonpainful, and the dog's vital signs were normal. The swelling was diagnosed as a seroma.

Contributors to incision irritation include sutures placed too tight, traumatic tissue handling, suture reaction, tension on the suture line, clipper burn, prepping irritation (clipper burn and solution reaction), incision infection, and seroma formation. Only rarely will an animal chew the sutures just because it can. Using appropriate suture technique minimizes incision self-trauma. However, if an animal begins to traumatize the incision via licking or scratching, an Elizabethan collar, bandage, neck brace, T-shirt, and/or chemical restraint should be used to protect the incision.

Seromas can form if extensive surgical dissection occurred beneath the incision, tissue planes could not be or were not adequately closed, or excessive motion occurs at the incision site. Seromas are recognized as localized areas of fluctuant swellings that are not usually painful or warm to the touch (Figure 32-8). Seromas usually resolve without treatment in a few weeks. Warm compresses, hydrotherapy, and bandaging may aid in resolution. Seromas are not typically drained because of the increased chance for infection and self-resolution. If the seroma is very large and/or is causing impairment, drainage is warranted. Drainage should be performed aseptically, and an active, closed drain should be

placed. It is important to keep animals calm during the postoperative period to decrease the chance of seroma formation. Hematomas are treated the same way.

> **TECHNICIAN NOTE** Repeated aspiration of seromas can result in infection and should be avoided. If an area must be aspirated, it should be aseptically prepared before aspiration. Suspected abscesses should be aseptically aspirated for cytology and culture, but there is no reason to aspirate a suspected seroma except for the purpose of treatment, which is rare.

If incision swelling occurs 4 to 6 days postoperatively, is warm to the touch, is associated with an elevated body temperature, or is reddened and/or draining, the possibility of infection or **cellulitis** (infection along tissue planes) must be considered (Figure 32-9). Abscess/infection must be treated by drainage, warm compresses, and systemic antibiotics. Cellulitis typically is not drained but otherwise is treated similarly. Aseptic aspiration of fluid or tissues beneath the incision should be performed for cytology and culture before empirical antibiotic therapy is started where possible. Some infected incisions can be flushed and managed with an active, closed suction drain, but others will require open wound management (see Chapter 26 for details on infected and open wound management).

Wound dehiscence is the separation of the layers of an incision or wound. Early recognition is imperative in any wound, but especially in abdominal and thoracic incisions. Dehiscence is most often due to technical error in suture technique, but incision complications can play a role. Things that contribute to wound dehiscence include use of inappropriate suture to close a wound, inappropriate suturing technique, tension on the incision line, incision infection, seroma formation, and disease and/or drug therapy leading to delayed wound healing. Rarely an animal self-mutilates an incision, causing dehiscence (see previous discussion). It is important to promptly apply an Elizabethan collar or another protective device if licking or chewing at the incision is noted.

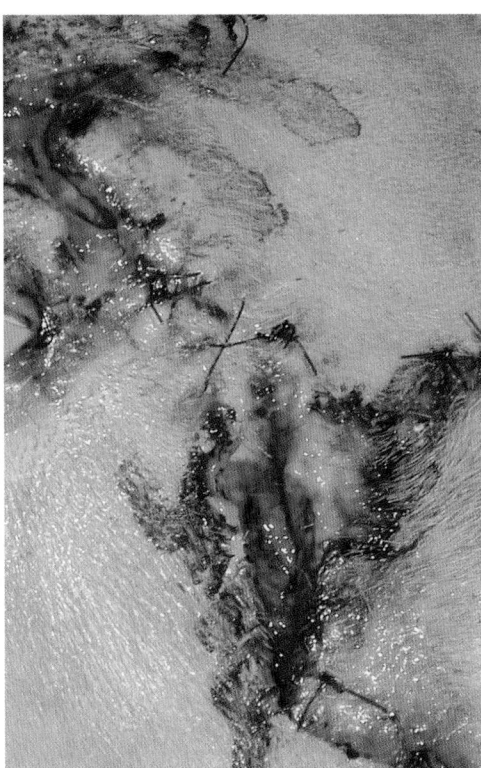

FIGURE 32-9 Incisional infection is recognized by drainage, redness, swelling, fever, dehiscence, and/or abscess formation. Note the purulent discharge and partial dehiscence of the incision.

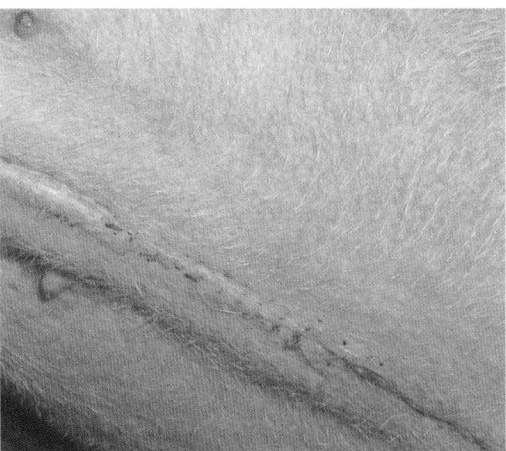

FIGURE 32-10 Healed incision. Note that the incision is not red, swollen, or draining. The skin edges are apposed, and the scar is slightly raised. This photo was taken 12 days after surgery.

Early detection of surgical incision problems is of paramount importance to help prevent more serious complications. If dehiscence is suspected, the reason for dehiscence should be ascertained. If the external suture layer (skin) is dehiscing and it is only partial, conservative management may be possible. The open portion of the wound will heal by second intention. However, the open wound will likely need to be bandaged and the animal placed in an Elizabethan collar to prevent licking of the open wound and further dehiscence. In some cases, cleansing and closure of the incision may be necessary depending on the degree of dehiscence and contamination of the wound. Dehiscence of deeper layers can be more serious and should be brought to the attention of the veterinarian in charge as soon as possible, especially if the incision involves the abdominal or thoracic cavity. Complete dehiscence of an abdominal wound can result in **evisceration** (exposure) of the abdominal organs, with subsequent contamination and infection. Complete dehiscence of a thoracic wound will result in a pneumothorax (air within the chest causing collapse of the lungs), a problem that may result in sudden death.

TECHNICIAN NOTE Dehiscence of an abdominal wound or thoracic wall can result in life-threatening complications. The veterinarian should be alerted immediately of impending complications.

SUTURE REMOVAL

Suture removal is commonly performed by the veterinary technician. The procedure is usually performed 10 to 14 days after surgery because this is the approximate time that the wound is beginning to strengthen (see Chapter 26). If internal sutures were placed in the dermis in addition to external sutures, suture removal can be performed in 5 to 7 days because the internal suture layer will hold the incision closed while healing continues. The incision should be inspected carefully for adequate healing before removal. A healed incision is usually confluent, slightly raised, and whitish in color and has no gaps between skin edges (Figure 32-10). An appropriately healed incision should not be draining, severely reddened, or severely swollen. However, if complications are encountered, some reddening, swelling, and excessive scarring are expected. Incisions that are swollen, draining, or reddened, or that have obvious separation should be inspected by the veterinarian in charge before suture removal.

Skin sutures are usually easy to remove in the calm animal. Suture scissors are simple to use and allow removal with minimal discomfort. The suture should be grasped with thumb forceps or your finger. Gentle traction is placed on the suture, and the suture is cut near the skin surface (Figure 32-11). The suture is manually pulled out of the skin after cutting. If metal staples were placed, a staple remover should be used to allow removal with minimal discomfort. The staple remover is placed under the staple according to manufacturer instructions (Figure 32-12, *A*) and is squeezed to bend the staple ends up and out of the skin (Figure 32-12, *B*).

BANDAGE CARE

If a bandage was placed on a limb, that limb should be monitored carefully. The bandage should be kept clean and dry. A plastic bag or other water-resistant covering should be placed over the bandage when the animal is walked outside and removed once back inside. The plastic will prevent the bandage from getting wet, but it should not be left in place because moisture will accumulate under the plastic if left on for an extended time. The animal's toes should be checked at least twice daily for swelling or coldness. This is especially important immediately after placement. Swollen toes might be an indication that the bandage is too tight. If the bandage gets wet or dirty, or has an odor, or if the toes become swollen or cold, the bandage should be changed. A soiled, wet bandage can lead to formation of sores and incision infection. Bandages placed too tight can result in vascular compromise to the skin with death and sloughing. Bandages are changed at intervals designated by the veterinarian in charge and depending on the reason for placement. Bandages covering open wounds often have to be changed more frequently than other types of bandages. Wounds can drain excessively, causing serum to seep through the bandage and extend to the external environment. This is called *strike-through* (Figure 32-13). Strike-through must be prevented to help prevent wound infection because bacteria have better access to a wound or incision when they can migrate through the moisture of a wet bandage. See Chapter 26 for more information on bandaging.

DRAIN CARE

Drains are placed to collect fluid under a wound or surgical incision. They are often placed when large amounts of tissue are resected (mammary chains, some amputations, large skin masses) or when a large amount of drainage is expected (a contaminated or infected wound). If a drain is placed, the drain exit site should be kept covered with a bandage. Additionally, the animal should be placed in an Elizabethan collar to prevent premature removal or drain trauma by the animal. Active drains (drains that are sealed to the environment and actively collect fluid from the wound into a reservoir) should be emptied as needed (Figure 32-14, *A*). Passive drains (drains that provide an exit port for fluid to the external environment) should be avoided because of the risk for ascending bacterial infection and their difficult maintenance as a result of constant drainage of fluid through the drain exit site, although they are placed under some circumstances (Figure 32-14, *B*). If passive drains are used, the bandage should be changed frequently to prevent strike-through. Drains are removed when the amount of drainage has substantially decreased. Some drainage is expected as long as a drain is in place as a result of tissue irritation by the drain, but it should be minimal.

> **TECHNICIAN NOTE**   Some drainage is expected as long as a drain is in place as a result of tissue irritation by the drain, but it should be minimal.

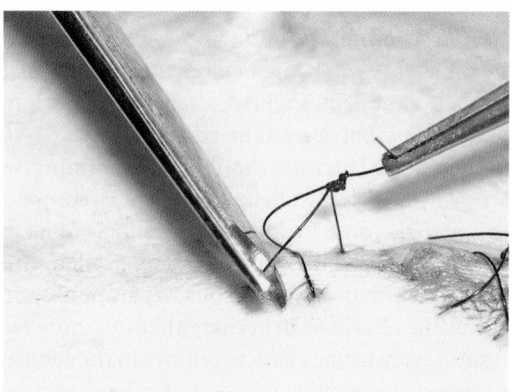

FIGURE 32-11 Suture removal. The suture is grasped with forceps or fingers and is gently tensioned. It is cut with suture scissors near the skin and then is pulled with slow, steady traction until completely removed.

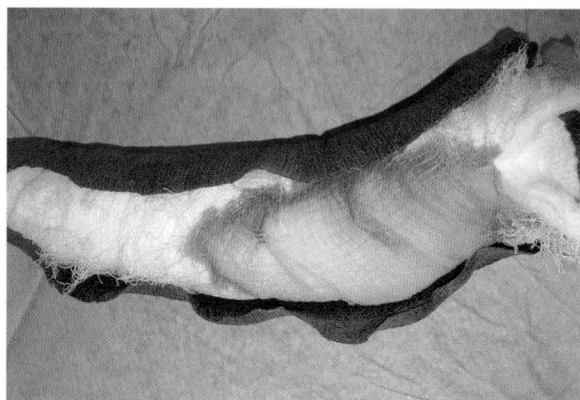

FIGURE 32-13 Strike-through. Note the red-tinged fluid seeping through the bandage from the wound bed.

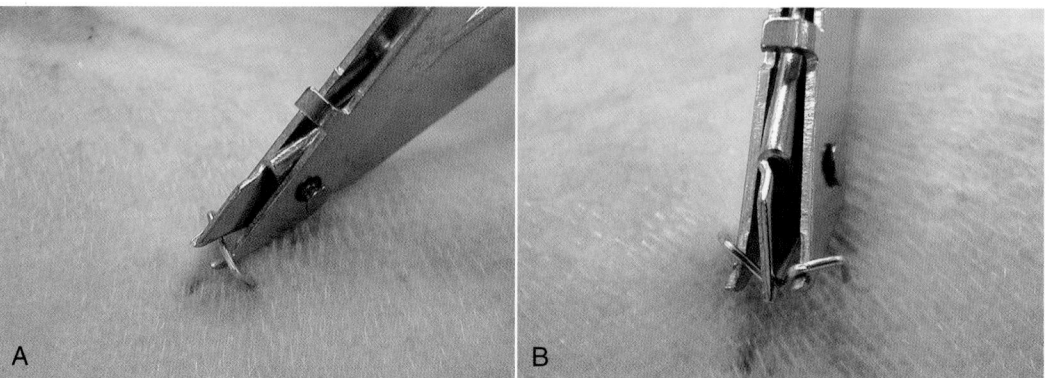

FIGURE 32-12 Staple removal. Staple remover is used. **A,** Staple remover is slipped under the staple. **B,** Staple remover is closed, causing the staple to be folded at its midsection and the teeth on either end of the staple to be dislodged from the skin.

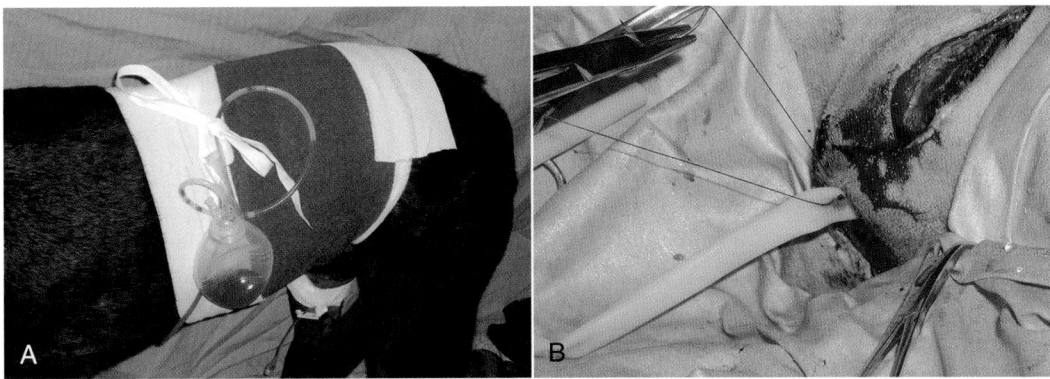

FIGURE 32-14 Drains. **A,** Active drains actively suck fluid from the wound bed into a sealed reservoir and are preferred over passive drains. **B,** Passive drains are placed under incisions and just provide surface area for fluid to drain from the wound with gravitational forces. They are more prone to ascending infection and are more difficult to manage. In photo **(B),** the wound is being closed over a rubber drain *(yellow)*. The incision and the drain will be bandaged afterward.

RESTRAINT

Animal restraint is important for appropriate surgical technique, patient safety, and patient comfort. All animals should be well controlled after surgery to minimize complications. The length and degree of confinement depend on the type of procedure performed. Animals undergoing routine sterilization or simple mass removal usually require 10 to 14 days of restricted activity, whereas animals undergoing orthopedic surgery will likely require 6 to 8 weeks of confinement. No animal should be allowed to roam free immediately after surgery to help prevent trauma to healing tissues.

Besides crate, leash, and room confinement, chemical agents and mechanical devices can be used for restraint. Tranquilizers and noxious-tasting substances are commonly used chemical restraints. Refer to Chapter 29 for more information on drugs used for sedation. Appropriate crate or room confinement usually will suffice without the addition of tranquilization.

Noxious-tasting agents are used to prevent animals from licking or chewing, and they must be used with discretion. Commonly used substances include Bandguard Cream (Schering-Plough), Bitter Apple (Grannick's), Tabasco, and various thumb-sucking preparations. The agent can be impregnated into bandage material, and some can be placed directly on the skin around the incision. These agents should never be placed directly on the incision because they can burn or irritate the incision, and they have the potential to delay wound healing. Caution should be used when any chemical is directly placed on the skin because a reaction can occur even if it is labeled for such.

Mechanical restraint devices include the Elizabethan collar, the body brace, the side bar, the neck brace, hobbles, and various bandages. These devices are used to limit motion, prevent licking and chewing, and prevent weight bearing. The assembly, materials necessary, specific indications, contraindications, and complications have been adequately described elsewhere (see Chapter 26 and "Recommended Readings"), and further discussion is beyond the scope of this chapter. A properly selected, constructed, and applied device will be well tolerated by the animal and effective for its desired purpose.

COMMON SURGICAL PROCEDURES

The veterinary technician must have a working knowledge of common surgical procedures to properly prepare an animal preoperatively, act as an efficient surgical assistant, manage immediate and long-term postoperative care, and be able to clearly converse with pet owners about a performed procedure. The remainder of this chapter reviews common small animal surgical procedures performed in veterinary practice. A brief description of the procedure, with emphasis on the role of the veterinary technician, will be given. Details on aseptic technique, surgical site preparation, gowning, and gloving are discussed in other sections of this book and will not be covered here (see Chapters 30 and 31).

> **TECHNICIAN NOTE** The veterinary technician must have a working knowledge of common surgical procedures to properly prepare the animal for surgery, act as an efficient surgical assistant, converse with the owner, and manage immediate and long-term postoperative care.

ELECTIVE VERSUS NONELECTIVE SURGERY

Surgical procedures are divided into elective and nonelective types. Elective procedures are performed at the veterinarian's and the owner's convenience, usually in healthy animals. Spay, castration, and declaw are examples of such procedures. Some procedures must be done to improve the animal's quality of life but are not necessarily urgent; these include stifle stabilization for cranial cruciate ligament rupture, correction of patellar luxation, and cancer resection. For these procedures, if animals are not ideal candidates for surgery at the time of presentation, surgery can be delayed. However, ideally, surgery would be performed at some point to improve the animal's quality of life. Nonelective surgical procedures must be done urgently. These are usually emergency procedures performed on compromised animals.

TAIL DOCKING AND DEWCLAW REMOVAL IN PUPPIES

DEFINITION

Tail docking refers to partial amputation (removal) of the tail. Dewclaw removal is amputation of the vestigial first digit located on the medial aspect of the front and hind legs.

INDICATIONS

Tail docking and dewclaw removal in young puppies are performed primarily for aesthetic reasons. Dog breeders have traditionally developed breed standards through alteration of the breed character with surgery. Tails are docked and dewclaws removed according to breed standards set forth by the American Kennel Club. It should be remembered that in certain breeds, such as Great Pyrenees and Newfoundland, the presence of dewclaws is necessary for proper show quality.

> **TECHNICIAN NOTE**   Hunting dogs may have dewclaws removed for practical reasons because rapid movement through dense brush may snag and tear dewclaws away from the foot. Preemptive removal of dewclaws in hunting dogs is thought to spare them this painful possibility.

PREOPERATIVE CONSIDERATIONS

The dam can get upset as puppies are removed from her presence for these procedures. Some dams will even become aggressive. Care must be taken with removal and replacement of puppies from the nest. If the dam becomes too upset, it may be necessary to place her in another room while procedures are performed on the puppies. Alternatively, some dams are more comfortable in the same room with the puppies.

Tail docking and dewclaw removal should be performed during the first week of life (3 to 5 days of age). At this age, the procedures can be performed without general anesthesia and are minimally traumatic to the dam and puppies. It must be remembered that puppies of this age are immunogenetically naïve. It is important to perform the procedures in an area where the puppies will not be exposed to high concentrations of infectious agents.

TECHNIQUE AND INTRAOPERATIVE CONSIDERATIONS

The puppy should be cradled in the palm of both hands and the surgical site prepared using aseptic technique. The limb or tail is extended toward the surgeon for improved accessibility.

Tail Docking

The desired length of remaining tail is marked, and the skin of the tail is retracted craniad (toward the base of the tail). The tail is amputated with a pair of scissors, bleeding is controlled with electrocautery or pressure, and the skin is released, allowing it to retract over the exposed bone. One simple interrupted absorbable suture is placed to appose the skin edges, or the edges are glued with a tissue adhesive.

Dewclaw Removal

The puppy is cradled in the palm of one hand, and the extremity is extended with the other hand. Scissors are used to amputate the claw. Hemorrhage is controlled with electrocautery or pressure. The skin edges may be left to heal by second intention or apposed with one absorbable suture.

If a surgical laser is used to remove the tail and dewclaws, the technician should ensure that appropriate equipment and eye protection are available for the surgical team, and that the surgery site is not prepared with alcohol. Plenty of saline-soaked sponges should be available to cover exposed areas close to the laser beam, instruments, and the surgeon's fingers if need be, to absorb extraneous laser energy and prevent iatrogenic laser burns. It is best to use instruments approved for laser surgery to prevent reflected laser beams from inappropriately penetrating objects and tissues if an instrument must be close to the laser's path. Furthermore, the technician must be available to vacuum the emitted plume (smoke) from the laser because it is harmful to people and animals.

POSTOPERATIVE CONSIDERATIONS

Puppies should be returned to the mother as soon as hemorrhage is controlled. Surgical sites should be monitored for the first few hours for excessive bleeding. During the week after surgery, the tail and the feet should be monitored daily for drainage, redness, and swelling. The suture remains until it is absorbed or licked out by the mother. Complications are not expected after tail docking or dewclaw removal, but might include hemorrhage and infection. In some animals, too much skin is removed during amputation of the tail. These animals may have chronic wound healing problems and bone exposure at the amputation site. Revision of the surgery site may be necessary to correct the problem.

TAIL DOCKING AND DEWCLAW REMOVAL IN THE ADULT

Tail docking and dewclaw removal should ideally be done within the first week of life if performed for aesthetic purposes. In some instances, adult dogs are seen for one or both procedures.

INDICATIONS

Indications for tail docking or dewclaw removal in the adult dog include aesthetics, trauma, infection, and neoplasia.

PREOPERATIVE CONSIDERATIONS

One must consider the reason for tail or claw amputation before animal prepping and initiation of the procedure. If it is done to treat cancer, acceptable tumor-free margins should be taken with the diseased tissue, and the appropriate amount of skin must be prepared before surgery. Removed tissues will have to be placed in formalin at a 1:10 ratio for eventual histopathologic evaluation. If trauma is the reason for the procedure, the animal may have to be stabilized before anesthesia can safely be performed. If amputation is performed as treatment for infection, the veterinary technician should have culture swabs available so that the veterinarian can obtain appropriate cultures at the time of surgery.

TECHNIQUE AND INTRAOPERATIVE CONSIDERATIONS FOR DEWCLAW REMOVAL IN THE ADULT

The animal must be placed under general anesthesia. The surgical site is clipped and prepared using aseptic technique. The surgeon will make an elliptical incision at the base of the dewclaw. The dewclaw is dissected free and is transected at the carpometacarpal joint in the front paw or at the tarsometatarsal joint in the hind paw. Hemorrhage is controlled with suture, electrocautery, laser, and/or direct pressure. If a surgical laser is used, the same precautions already noted under puppy tail and dewclaw removal should be taken. The skin edges are apposed with suture. The paw is usually bandaged to control swelling.

TECHNIQUE AND INTRAOPERATIVE CONSIDERATIONS FOR TAIL AMPUTATION IN THE ADULT

The tail should be clipped and hung from an intravenous stand or other secure object. The skin should be prepared using aseptic technique. If the tail is to be amputated near the base, the rump adjacent to the tail base must also be clipped and aseptically prepared. A tourniquet may be placed at the base of the tail to help control hemorrhage and is placed before the animal is draped for surgery if the base of the tail is not to be included in the surgical field. The surgeon can use a sterile tourniquet otherwise. A tourniquet should not stay in place longer than 90 minutes in people, but no particular safety time has been reported in animals. Alert the surgeon after 30 to 60 minutes so the tourniquet can be released for a time and then repositioned to improve the tissue environment.

The tail is amputated at the desired location by skin incision and disarticulation of the caudal vertebra at the appropriate site. The skin incision is made 1 or 2 cm distal to the expected amputation site to ensure adequate skin coverage of the stump. Blood vessels are identified and ligated. Skin edges are sutured over the remaining vertebrae, and the tourniquet is removed.

POSTOPERATIVE CONSIDERATIONS

Surgical sites should be monitored for hemorrhage, swelling, drainage, redness, evidence of self-trauma, and dehiscence. Elizabethan collars should be placed on those animals attempting to traumatize the surgical site. Bandages placed on the foot should be maintained as previously discussed and as directed in Chapter 26. If placed, skin sutures are removed in 7 to 14 days, depending on how the incision was

closed. Pain medication is generally needed for 4 to 5 days after the procedure. Complications are rare for these procedures, even in adult animals.

FELINE ONYCHECTOMY

DEFINITION

Onychectomy (declawing) is removal of the claw and its associated distal phalanx on each digit.

INDICATIONS

Onychectomy is an elective procedure done to prevent scratching of owners and household items. Most veterinarians recommend declawing the front feet only. This does not significantly impair the cat's ability to climb trees or defend itself from intruders. Onychectomy is often performed at the same time as castration or ovariohysterectomy.

PREOPERATIVE CONSIDERATIONS

Onychectomy is a painful procedure. Preoperative analgesics should be administered.

TECHNIQUE AND INTRAOPERATIVE CONSIDERATIONS

The cat is placed under general anesthesia. The feet are surgically scrubbed but need not be clipped unless the cat is a long-haired breed. If a laser is to be used during the procedure, alcohol should not be used to prepare the toes because it is flammable and is likely to ignite when the laser beam strikes the soaked area. The nails are left long to facilitate nail manipulation during the procedure. A tourniquet is usually placed to control hemorrhage during the procedure. It should be placed over the foot before aseptic preparation, but tightened when the surgeon is ready to perform the procedure. The surgeon will squeeze the distal limb to help decrease pooling blood (Figure 32-15). The tourniquet should always be placed distal to the elbow to prevent nerve

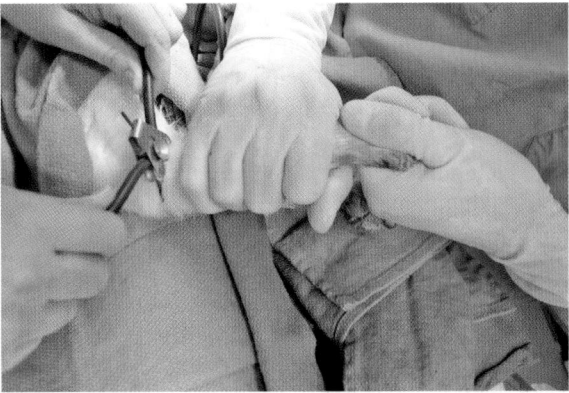

FIGURE 32-15 Declaw. The surgeon or another assistant is squeezing the distal limb before the tourniquet is tightened to help move blood out of the distal limb. The tourniquet should always be placed distal to the elbow (*as shown*) rather than proximal to the elbow to help prevent permanent radial nerve damage.

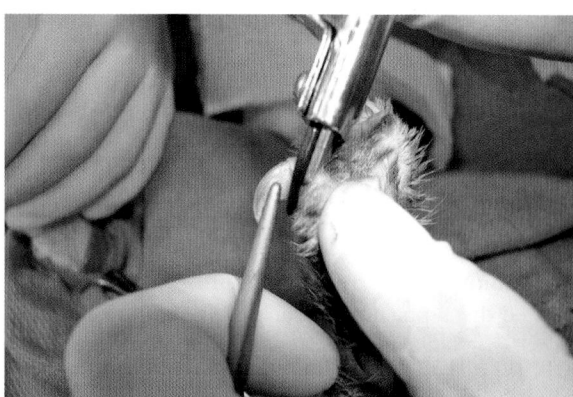

FIGURE 32-16 Declaw. The nail trimmer has been placed over the claw in such a way that the blade is between the second and third phalanges, and the bottom support is in front of the digital pad. The nail will be pulled forward as the nail trimmer is squeezed to remove the claw.

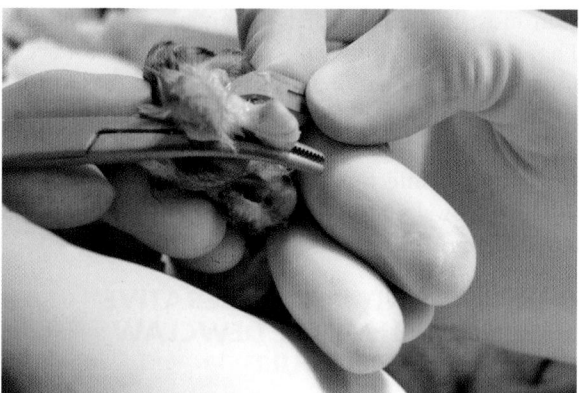

FIGURE 32-17 Declaw. The scalpel blade was positioned dorsally between the second and third phalanges and the dorsal joint capsule severed along with the collateral ligaments. The blade is subsequently manipulated dorsally to avoid cutting the digital pad located ventral to the blade.

damage. The radial nerve is more superficial just proximal to the elbow and can be permanently damaged if the tourniquet is tightened over that area. The tourniquet should be managed as discussed for tail amputation.

Three techniques can be used to remove the claws. The Rescoe (nail trimmer technique), the scalpel blade, and CO_2 laser techniques are all effective means of performing the procedure. For the nail trimmer technique (Rescoe), a guillotine-type nail trimmer is positioned snugly onto the dorsal surface of the toe between the second phalanx and the third phalanx (Figure 32-16). During positioning of the nail trimmer, the claw should be pulled cranially. As little skin as possible should be excised. The cutting edge of the nail trimmer is positioned at the cranial edge of the footpad. As the cutting edge is advanced, the pad is moved caudally while the nail is rotated dorsally and caudally. The third phalanx is then excised by the nail trimmer. Care is taken to prevent cutting the footpad. Each nail is amputated in a similar fashion. A portion of the third phalanx is usually left behind with this technique, but the entire germinal layer is removed to prevent regrowth of the nail.

The blade technique amputates the entire third phalanx using a #12 scalpel blade. The phalanx is disarticulated dorsolaterally, first by cutting through the joint capsule between phalanges 2 and 3, and then by cutting the collateral ligaments (Figure 32-17); afterward, the nail is cut away from the underlying tissue and digital pad. The pad is moved out of the way by positioning the blade more dorsal to prevent inadvertent laceration of the pad.

The laser technique is similar to the blade technique except that it uses laser energy instead of a sharp edge to dissect the third phalanx free from the second phalanx. The surgical site usually does not bleed with the laser technique, so a tourniquet is not necessary (Figure 32-18). If laser is used, precautions as previously discussed for tail removal in puppies should be taken into account. The technician should be familiar with laser safety before use.

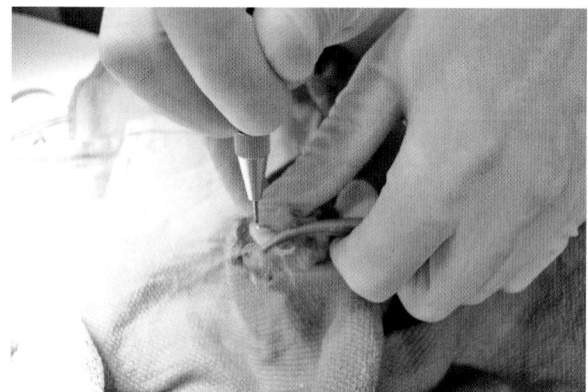

FIGURE 32-18 Declaw. The laser pictured here is used to remove the third phalanx during declaw. Note the lack of blood. A tourniquet is not required.

One to two sutures are often placed to appose the skin edges after nail removal. Surgical glue (cyanoacrylic tissue adhesive) is used instead of sutures in some instances. If surgical glue is used, it should never be placed on the exposed bone of the second phalanx or dropped inside the void (wound) created by removal of the third phalanx. Instead, the wound should be manually closed and a drop of glue placed only on the skin edges of the closed wound (Figure 32-19). Dropping glue into the wound can cause chronic lameness and foreign body reaction. Some veterinarians do not appose the skin edges with anything other than a bandage. The tourniquet is removed as soon as the sutures are placed and bandaging is initiated.

TECHNICIAN NOTE Do not place tissue glue into the open wound formed after a claw is removed. The wound should be manually apposed and the glue placed only on the skin edges. Placing surgical glue internally can result in chronic lameness and foreign body reaction.

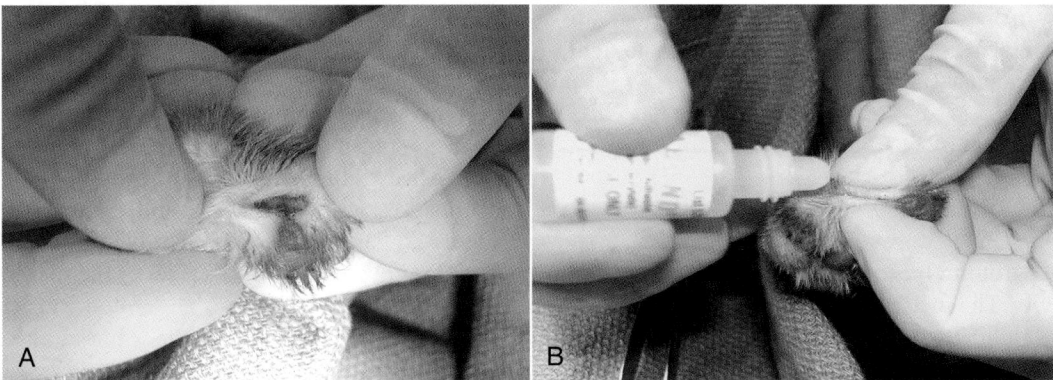

FIGURE 32-19 Declaw. **A,** When tissue adhesive is applied to a wound, the glue should never be placed inside the wound created by removing the claw. **B,** The wound should be manually apposed and the glue placed along the skin edges.

After surgery, the paws are bandaged snugly with a gauze sponge and strips of tape. The sponge is placed over the ends of the digits. Strips of tape are placed longitudinally along the leg and distally around the paw. Tape is then placed circumferentially around the paw up to the elbow. Care is taken to lay tape on the leg and not to pull too tightly. Bandages placed too tightly can result in vascular compromise to the foot with skin sloughing. The tourniquet is removed as soon as bandaging is complete.

POSTOPERATIVE CONSIDERATIONS

Onychectomy is painful. Pain medication should be administered to all cats in the postoperative period. It is appropriate to administer a pure opioid agonist for the first 24 hours after surgery (see Chapter 28 for details on administration, advantages, and disadvantages of specific pain medications). A fentanyl patch can be placed the day before surgery to allow the fentanyl to take effect and can last up to 3 days postoperatively, but pain control can be variable with the patch, and the cat should be monitored closely for continued pain in spite of having a patch in place. Alternatively, injectable or oral pain medication can be given. Some nonsteroidal anti-inflammatory drugs can also be used in cats; however, care must be taken to avoid overdosage because cats are very sensitive to these drugs. Most nonsteroidal anti-inflammatories given to cats are given for off-label use. A wait-and-see attitude regarding pain medication for this procedure is not acceptable. Instead, medication should be given at appropriate dosing intervals for at least 4 to 5 days postoperatively. Because this procedure is not sterile, some surgeons will also send the cat home on a short course of antibiotics.

Bandages are kept in place for 24 hours and then are removed. The cat should be hospitalized while the bandages are in place. After surgery, litter should consist of shredded paper or pellets to prevent accumulation of clay or sand in the surgical wounds with resultant irritation and infection. Normal litter should not be reintroduced until 10 days after surgery. The paws should be monitored for hemorrhage, swelling, drainage, and redness. Cats will be fairly sensitive on the front legs after surgery, but this should start improving within 2 weeks of surgery. An Elizabethan collar may be necessary for the first 5 to 10 days for those cats causing self-trauma. If sutures were placed, suture removal generally is not necessary because cats will remove them on their own. Sutures can be removed by the veterinary team if they are still in place after 20 days.

> **TECHNICIAN NOTE** Bandages from onychectomy should be removed within 24 hours. The cat should remain in the hospital until the bandages have been removed.

Most cats allow removal of the bandages performed by carefully cutting the bandage apart longitudinally and gently peeling it off the leg. If the cat is intractable, the bandage may be cut and the cat returned to its cage. The cat will then remove the bandage on its own. If this technique is used, however, the cat will have to be monitored to ensure that bandage ingestion does not occur. In severely intractable patients, a light dose of a tranquilizer may be necessary to remove the bandages safely. Cats are monitored carefully for 8 to 12 hours after bandage removal for hemorrhage. Rebandage with prolonged hospitalization will be necessary if hemorrhage occurs.

Onychectomy complications can be divided into those that occur in the early postoperative period and those that occur in the late postoperative period. Early complications include loose bandages, self-bandage removal, and postoperative bleeding. Cats should be checked frequently for these problems. In the event of hemorrhage, the paws should be rebandaged snugly. Infection can occur and generally becomes evident within the first 3 weeks of surgery. Infection requires antibiotic therapy and/or wound débridement. A swab for bacterial culture and sensitivity should be taken from any draining toes. Late complications include regrowth of the claws, chronic lameness, or both. Claw regrowth requires reoperation and removal of remaining germinal epithelium. Chronic lameness without evidence of regrowth may be seen with incomplete removal of the phalanx or cut footpads. The nail trimmer technique is more likely to result in lameness associated with residual tissue. Other complications include radial nerve damage secondary to tourniquet placement and skin sloughing secondary to tight, prolonged bandage placement.

CELIOTOMY

DEFINITION

Celiotomy (laparotomy) is a surgical incision into the abdominal cavity. The incision can be made at several locations: ventral midline, paramedian, paracostal, parapreputial, and flank (Figure 32-20). The most commonly used incision site is ventral midline.

INDICATIONS

A celiotomy is performed for both elective and nonelective procedures. Some of the common elective procedures include ovariohysterectomy, organ biopsy, cystotomy, planned cesarean delivery, gastropexy, and removal of retained abdominal testicles. Common nonelective procedures include emergency cesarean delivery, gastric dilatation-volvulus (GDV) (bloated, twisted stomach), **intussusception**, gastrointestinal foreign bodies, ruptured spleen, penetrating foreign bodies (e.g., knife wound, arrow wound, bullet wound), severe abdominal bleeding, and diaphragmatic hernia. In some instances, the animal is seen for an unknown abdominal problem. Patients may need elective or nonelective celiotomy, referred to as an *exploratory celiotomy*. Exploratory celiotomy is often performed to treat abdominal masses of unknown origin and to obtain biopsies for disease diagnosis.

PREOPERATIVE CONSIDERATIONS

Animals should always be clipped widely for abdominal incisions. At times, the incision must be extended, and an inappropriate prep will hinder surgical exposure. Animals undergoing abdominal incision because of illness or trauma may have to be stabilized before anesthesia is administered. If biopsies or cultures are to be taken, the veterinary technician should make sure that culture supplies and tissue sample cups with formalin are available.

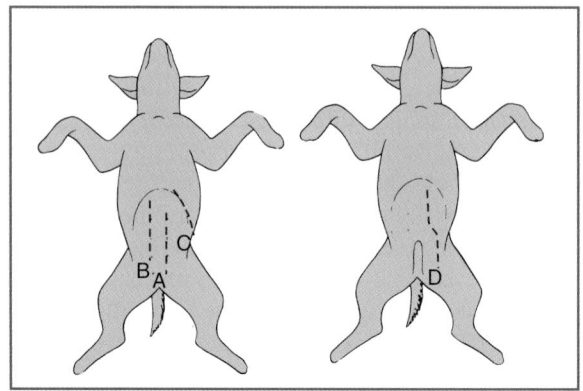

FIGURE 32-20 Locations for celiotomy incisions. **A,** Ventral midline. **B,** Paramedian. **C,** Paracostal. **D,** Parapreputial.

TECHNIQUE AND INTRAOPERATIVE CONSIDERATIONS

For ventral midline celiotomy, the patient is placed in dorsal recumbency. Some animals can be difficult to stabilize in this position, but many techniques can be used to facilitate this process, including use of V-troughs, foot ties, bean bags, sandbags (Figure 32-21, *A*), and tables with raised sides. Figure 32-21, *B*, shows a patient held in dorsal recumbency with foot ties and the raised sides of the surgery table, which forms a stabilizing V shape. The abdomen is clipped lengthwise from 2 cm cranial to the xiphoid cartilage to 2 cm caudal to the pubis. The side clip should extend at least 2 to 4 cm lateral to the nipples. The skin is aseptically prepared for surgery.

Various incisions (paramedian, paracostal, etc.) are variations of the ventral midline incision and are less commonly used (see Figure 32-23). The surgeon should be asked about the approach if it is not clear, so that adequate surgical preparation can be performed. Emphasis will be given to the ventral midline incision in this chapter.

The line of the incision extends from the xiphoid process to the pubis. The length used varies with the type of

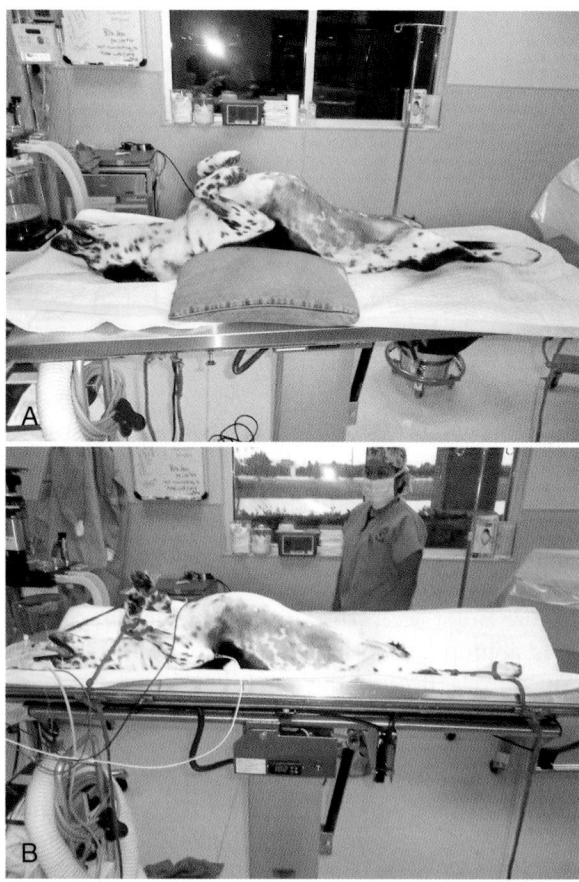

FIGURE 32-21 For abdominal and other procedures that require an animal to stay in dorsal recumbency, numerous options are available to help maintain the position of that animal during surgery, including **(A)** positioned with sandbags (homemade from old jeans here) and **(B)** positioned with the aid of a surgical table and foot ties, with the sides raised forming a V shape.

procedure (see specific procedures). A surgical sponge count should be performed before entry into the abdominal cavity, but this is surgeon dependent. The incision is made with a scalpel blade, electrocautery in the cutting mode, or laser. The incision is carried through the subcutaneous tissue to the level of the linea alba, which is elevated with forceps (tented) to pull it away from the underlying abdominal viscera while abdominal entry is accomplished. This will prevent the inadvertent puncture of abdominal organs when the peritoneal cavity is entered. A scalpel blade is then used to penetrate the linea alba and enter the peritoneal cavity (Figure 32-22). The incision is extended the desired length with scissors or scalpel blade and forceps. Moistened laparotomy pads (sponges) are placed along the incision edges for protection during major abdominal procedures. This usually is not necessary during ovariohysterectomy because the incision is small and manipulation is minimal. A Balfour self-retaining abdominal retractor can be introduced into the incision to facilitate visualization of abdominal structures. Surgical lights and air exposure of abdominal organs will quickly dry out abdominal structures. It is important for the surgical assistant to keep exposed tissues moist to prevent damage and decrease adhesion formation. The technician should pay special attention to viscera moved external to the abdominal cavity. Viscera temporarily moved to outside the abdominal cavity should be covered with warm, moist laparotomy pads. They should also be monitored for cyanosis because of kinking of the blood supply. Abdominal viscera should be handled carefully and as little as possible. Whenever retraction or manipulation of structures is necessary, atraumatic technique is mandatory. Retract viscera with moistened laparotomy pads, manipulate viscera with moistened gloves, blot any excess hemorrhage with moistened sponges (do not wipe surfaces with sponges because this causes tissue trauma and dislodges blood clots), and, when using suction, be careful to avoid sucking the walls of visceral structures against the suction orifice. A thorough inspection of the abdomen is performed. If a preoperative sponge count was performed, it should be repeated before abdominal closure to ensure that all sponges are accounted for.

> **TECHNICIAN NOTE** Tissues exposed to the air during surgery should be kept moist to help prevent tissue desiccation with subsequent death or irritation.

The abdomen is sutured closed in at least three layers most of the time. The linea alba is the layer of strength and must be securely closed. The subcutaneous tissues are then sutured to decrease the amount of dead space. This helps reduce the frequency of postoperative hematoma or seroma formation. The skin is sutured to complete the celiotomy closure.

> **TECHNICIAN NOTE** A thorough inspection of the abdomen should be made before closure to prevent leaving instruments or sponges in the abdominal cavity. Preoperative and postoperative sponge counts are recommended.

POSTOPERATIVE CONSIDERATIONS

During the first 24 hours, the skin incision should be examined carefully for swelling, drainage, excessive redness, dehiscence, and evidence of self-trauma. An Elizabethan collar should be considered if the animal appears to lick or chew the incision. Incision problems should be brought to the attention of the veterinarian. Incision monitoring should be continued for 2 weeks after surgery or until suture removal. Animals should be exercise restricted until the abdominal wound is healed. If evidence of dehiscence is noted, the veterinary technician should notify the veterinarian immediately. Emergency closure may be necessary.

Some animals may be inappetent or may vomit after celiotomy. Intestinal and pancreatic manipulation can lead to intestinal **ileus** (temporary loss of intestinal motility), nausea, and/or pancreatitis. One or two episodes of vomiting or lack of appetite for the first 24 to 48 hours after celiotomy is usually not a matter of concern in and of itself. However, if the animal appears ill or is vomiting, and if inappetence continues, further evaluation should be performed. Animals that are not eating or drinking after surgery should be supported with intravenous fluid therapy until oral alimentation is resumed.

GASTROINTESTINAL SURGERY

DEFINITION

Gastrotomy is incision (opening) into the stomach. **Enterotomy** is incision into the intestine. These are often done to obtain biopsies or to retrieve foreign material. **Anastomosis** is suturing portions of the gastrointestinal tract together to allow confluent ingesta flow. Anastomosis is performed after damaged tissue or tumor requires a segment of the gastrointestinal tract to be removed.

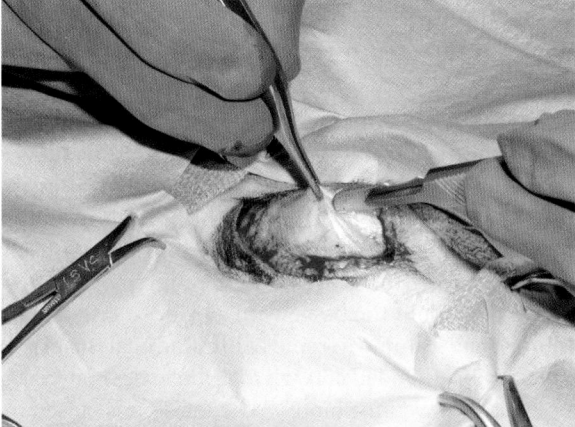

FIGURE 32-22 This image shows the linea alba tented (raised) with forceps and a scalpel blade in position to penetrate the linea to enter the abdominal cavity.

INDICATIONS

Gastrointestinal surgery has many indications. Gastrointestinal foreign body lodgment, neoplasia, biopsy for vomiting or diarrhea of unknown origin, GDV, gastrointestinal trauma, and gastrointestinal obstruction of unknown cause can all be reasons for abdominal exploration and gastrointestinal surgery.

PREOPERATIVE CONSIDERATIONS

Many animals undergoing gastrointestinal surgery have been recently vomiting or not eating for several days. The veterinary technician should stabilize the animal with appropriate fluid management to correct dehydration before surgery. The animal should be intubated as soon as possible with a cuffed endotracheal tube to help ward off aspiration of stomach contents should the animal vomit during induction. The veterinary technician should make sure that extra instruments are available in case the primary pack is contaminated with intestinal contents during the procedure. Prophylactic antibiotics are used if the gastrointestinal tract is to be entered.

> **TECHNICIAN NOTE**   It is important to remember that gastrointestinal contents are not sterile. Materials that touch intestinal contents are considered contaminated and are removed from or kept in a separate place on the surgical field.

TECHNIQUE AND INTRAOPERATIVE CONSIDERATIONS

The animal is prepared for a full midline celiotomy. The procedure is initiated with an incision made in the linea alba (see Figure 32-22) with care taken to avoid damaging underlying structures. An abdominal exploration is performed. The normal gastrointestinal tract is pink, has visible vasculature on the surface, and has active motility (Figure 32-23, A). Abnormalities are noted. Foreign bodies leading to gastrointestinal obstruction are removed via gastrotomy or enterotomy. In some instances, devitalized tissue must be removed via resection and anastomosis. Devitalized intestine is discolored and lacks blood supply. Purple and red discoloration does not necessarily imply devitalization; blood supply must be evaluated by direct visualization of cut sections, Doppler, or injection of vital stains. If the tissue is questionable, it should be resected (Figure 32-23, B).

Characteristics of intestinal devitalization include the following:
- Lack of motility
- Gray, green, or black discoloration
- Severe thinning of the visceral wall
- Lack of bleeding on cut section
- Lack of fluorescein dye uptake
- Lack of Doppler blood flow

For biopsy or foreign body removal, the affected portion of the gastrointestinal tract is isolated with laparotomy pads (Figure 32-24). Laparotomy pads are placed to prevent

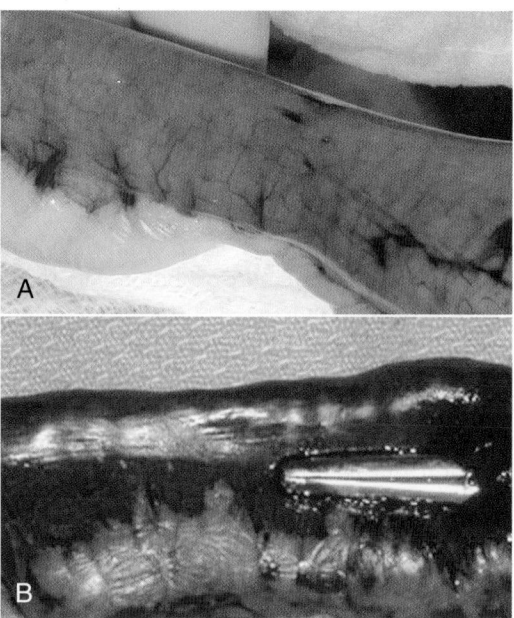

FIGURE 32-23 The normal intestine is pink with visible vessels and motility. Note the difference in color between **(A)** the normal intestine and **(B)** the devitalized segment of bowel.

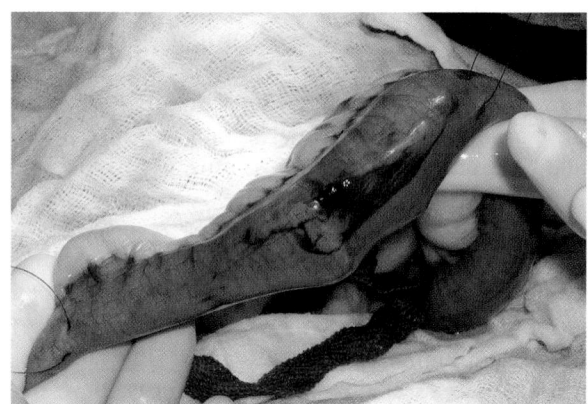

FIGURE 32-24 If a biopsy is to be performed on the gastrointestinal tract, the segment is packed off with laparotomy pads to prevent leaking ingesta from contaminating the abdominal cavity. Note the white pads surrounding the intestine. Ingesta is prevented from leaking from the cut surface of the intestine by placement of intestinal clamps, or by having an assistant gently pinch off the intestinal lumen on either side of the incision with fingers.

intestinal contents from leaking into the abdomen if accidental spillage occurs. Stay sutures are placed to steady the tissue on either side of the incision. The surgical assistant holds the stay sutures steady during the procedure. Biopsy is performed by making a stab incision into the stomach or intestine between the stay sutures and removing a full-thickness portion of the tissue with a blade or scissors. If the incision is made simply to remove intraluminal material, the stab incision is extended enough to remove the material, and no tissue is removed for biopsy. The incision is closed in an interrupted pattern with absorbable, monofilament suture.

If resection and anastomosis is to be performed, the vasculature to the portion of the intestine to be removed is

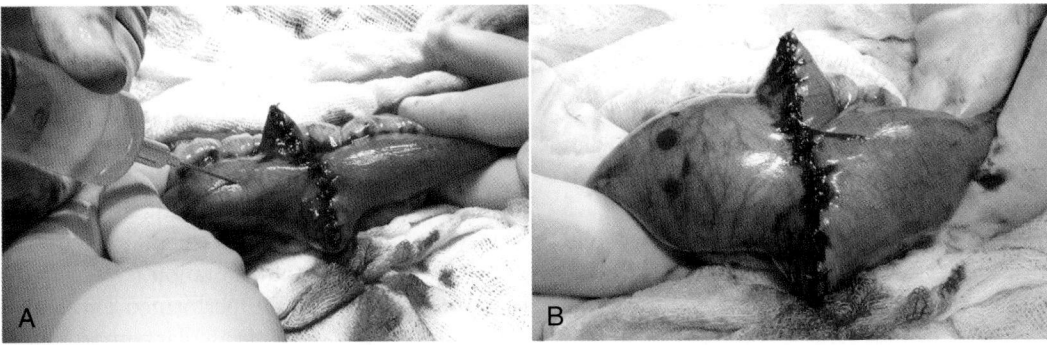

FIGURE 32-25 **A,** To check for leaks after intestinal anastomosis, the intestine is occluded on either side of the incision, and the occluded segment of intestine is filled with sterile saline. **B,** The incision is checked for leakage while the segment is filled with saline.

ligated; the intestines are clamped with Doyen forceps, or the surgical assistant supports the intestines with fingers to prevent ingesta from leaking onto the surgical field; the portion of the intestines to be removed is excised; and the viable intestinal ends are sutured together in an interrupted pattern similar to a biopsy site. After completion of the anastomosis, the intestine is evaluated for leakage. This is accomplished by occluding the intestine on either side of the anastomosis site and filling the enclosed space with sterile saline using a syringe and a small-gauge needle (Figure 32-25). The surgeon and the surgical assistant check for leaks along the incision. Leaks are sealed with additional suture. The intestine is flushed, and the laparotomy pads are removed from the abdomen and surgical field, with care taken to avoid contaminating the rest of the abdomen or the surgical field with ingesta that might have leaked onto the pads. The technician should ensure that warm isotonic saline is available for flushing the abdominal cavity. The abdomen is flushed and omentum is placed over intestinal incisions. The celiotomy is closed routinely. Many surgeons will ask for a clean surgical pack, gloves, and drape to perform the celiotomy closure to prevent contamination of the celiotomy wound with ingesta from instruments used during the intestinal procedure.

POSTOPERATIVE CONSIDERATIONS

Careful patient monitoring is important after intestinal surgery. The main consideration is evaluation for intestinal leakage. If intestinal dehiscence or leakage occurs, septic peritonitis will develop. Animals should be monitored for inappetence, vomiting, fever, painful abdomen, abdominal enlargement, incision drainage, and shock, all of which are potential indicators of peritonitis. Most animals are willing to eat within 24 hours of intestinal surgery. Minor vomiting (1 to 2 times) might be expected. However, protracted vomiting and inappetence should alert the technician to a potential impending problem with the intestinal surgery site. If intestinal leakage is suspected, abdominal ultrasound or abdominocentesis is performed. Material collected is evaluated for cell population and bacteria. If material obtained for evaluation from simple abdominocentesis is not sufficient, but leakage is still suspected, a diagnostic peritoneal lavage should be performed. A septic abdominal tap warrants emergency abdominal exploration and correction of the problem.

Feeding animals after intestinal surgery is another consideration. The gastrointestinal tract requires food for cellular health and proper function. Intestinal surgery can result in ileus and may cause inappetence, nausea, and vomiting. However, animals without complications are most often willing to eat within 24 hours. Unless the animal is vomiting, oral alimentation should be initiated as soon as the animal has an appetite. Animals should be introduced to water first. If no vomiting occurs after water intake, then food is introduced. A small amount of highly digestible, bland food should be fed initially. Many diets are available, and preference is up to the surgeon. If no vomiting occurs over 2 to 4 hours, another small amount can be fed. If vomiting does not occur, the amount fed can be gradually increased and frequency decreased. Animals are reintroduced to their normal or another maintenance diet gradually after recovery.

Monitoring as discussed for routine celiotomy should also be done.

GASTRIC DILATATION-VOLVULUS

DEFINITION

Gastric dilatation-volvulus is dilatation of the stomach with ingesta and gas, with rotation of the stomach into an abnormal position. This life-threatening condition typically occurs in deep-chested, large, and giant breed dogs. The cause is not specifically known, but genetics and chest/abdomen configuration may play a role. Some animals have eaten a large meal, drunk a large portion of water, and/or engaged in heavy exercise following either; however, others have not. Some animals develop the condition during times of stress, such as hospitalization or boarding. Vomiting, retching, and bloating (severe distention of the stomach) are classic clinical signs. Gastropexy is attachment of the stomach to the body wall with the goal of creating a permanent adhesion. It is performed to substantially decrease the chance of stomach rotation, but it does not prevent bloating. Partial gastrectomy is removal of part of the stomach. Splenectomy is removal of the spleen.

PREOPERATIVE CONSIDERATIONS

Animals suffering from GDV usually are in shock. If left untreated, these animals will die from cardiovascular collapse. The enlarged stomach compresses the caudal vena cava and affects venous return to the heart, leading to hypovolemic shock. Large-bore catheters should be placed immediately. It is important to place the catheters in the front legs or jugular vein because venous return from the caudal half of the body is impaired by the dilated stomach. These dogs are often large and require a substantial amount of fluid. It is best to place at least two catheters. Baseline blood work, coagulation assessment, ECG, and blood gas are typically obtained shortly after presentation. The veterinary technician should review treatment of hypovolemic shock (see Chapters 24 and 25).

> **TECHNICIAN NOTE** Intravenous catheters should be placed in the front half of an animal suffering from gastric dilatation-volvulus (GDV). Venous return is compromised from the back half of the dog as a result of compression of the vena cava from the dilated stomach.

After fluids are started, the stomach must be decompressed to help stabilize the animal and decrease the chance of gastric wall necrosis secondary to vascular compromise from severe distention. An orogastric tube is placed. Refer to Chapter 18, "Diagnostic Sampling and Treatment Techniques," for detailed instructions on placing orogastric tubes.

If the tube cannot be passed after sedation, the stomach should be decompressed by trocarization. The disadvantage of trocarization is potential leakage of gastric contents into the abdominal cavity at the stomach puncture site or stomach rupture. For trocarization, the right side of the stomach is aseptically prepared behind the last rib. Decompression is performed by passage of a large-bore needle or a large-bore intravenous (IV) catheter attached to a 60-ml syringe with a three-way stopcock gently passed into the dilated stomach percutaneously. Air is aspirated until the stomach is decompressed enough to stabilize the dog.

After stabilization is under way and vital signs are improving, right lateral abdominal radiographs are obtained. This view is best for evaluating whether rotation of the stomach or simple bloat without rotation is present. Thoracic radiographs should also be performed because aspiration is a possibility. As a result of vascular compromise to the stomach wall, the animal should also be started on broad-spectrum antibiotics to help prevent septicemia should intestinal compromise lead to bacterial translocation from the gastrointestinal tract to the bloodstream. The animal is further stabilized and prepared for emergency surgery.

Anesthesia can be challenging in these cases. Respiratory compromise often occurs as a result of compression of the diaphragm by the gas-distended stomach. Blood pressure is often low and difficult to maintain. If possible, an arterial access port should be established for continuous pressure and blood gas monitoring. Additionally, cardiac arrhythmias can occur and may need to be treated. The veterinary technician should review Chapter 29 for details of specific anesthetic techniques and monitoring.

TECHNIQUE AND INTRAOPERATIVE CONSIDERATIONS

The dog is prepared for a full ventral midline celiotomy. The abdomen is opened carefully to prevent puncture of the stomach because gas distention pushes the stomach against the ventral aspect of the abdomen (Figure 32-26). The veterinary technician should make sure that a stomach tube, bucket, and pump are available in the operating room because if the stomach is substantially distended at the time of surgery, further decompression will be needed to make manipulation easier. The tube should be gently passed down

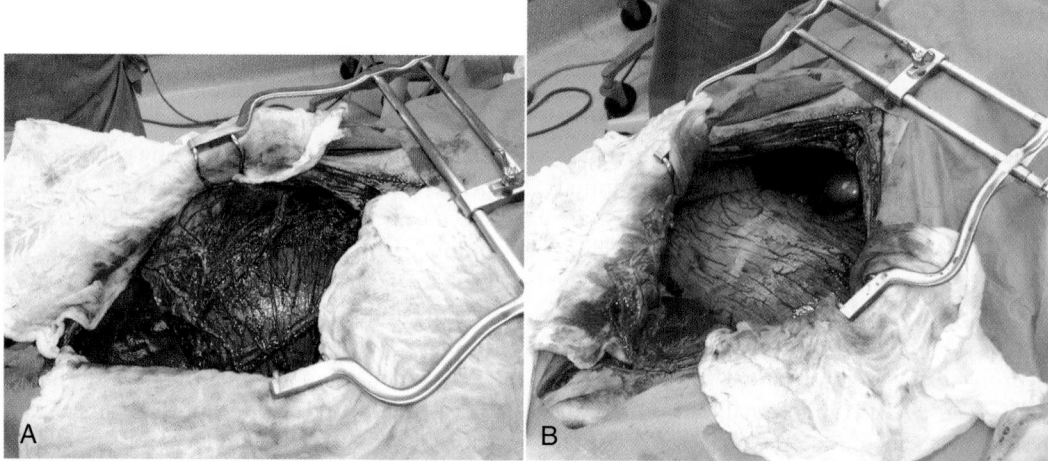

FIGURE 32-26 **A,** Note how the dilated, rotated stomach is pressed against the ventral abdominal wall and protrudes out of the abdomen. Inadvertent stomach puncture can occur if the abdomen is not entered carefully. **B,** The normally positioned stomach is still dilated but recesses back away from the ventral incision and lies completely within the abdomen.

the esophagus after lubrication while the veterinarian manipulates the tube into position within the stomach. The veterinarian can often gently express gas and fluid from the stomach through the tube. If decompression cannot be achieved in this manner, it can be performed with a syringe, three-way stopcock, and needle under direct visualization by the surgeon. The stomach must be handled with care. The stomach wall is often friable as a result of vascular compromise of the tissues. Additionally, ingesta and fluid that accumulate in the stomach after GDV are heavy and can contribute to tissue tearing during manipulation of the stomach back into the normal position. Extreme care must be taken to prevent inadvertent damage. Once the stomach is in its normal position, it is evaluated for viability. The stomach is often discolored at the start of the procedure, but this usually improves as blood supply and venous drainage return. A complete abdominal exploratory is performed while circulation is allowed to return to the stomach. The spleen is carefully evaluated. Vascular compromise to the spleen can occur with dilatation and rotation of the stomach, or the spleen may rotate. If the spleen is discolored, the vascular pedicle is relieved of compromise, and the spleen is gently placed out of the abdomen and covered with moistened laparotomy pads while a gastropexy is performed. In most instances, the spleen will return to its normal character once the blood supply has been reestablished. After abdominal exploration, the stomach is reevaluated for viability. Partial resection is performed, if needed.

A gastropexy is then performed on the right ventrolateral aspect of the body wall near the last rib. Many different techniques may be used to perform gastropexy, and a discussion of each technique is beyond the scope of this chapter. The technique used depends on the comfort level and skill of the surgeon performing the procedure. Fixation of the stomach into the celiotomy incision at the time of closure is not recommended because future abdominal surgery can result in accidental perforation of the stomach when the abdominal cavity is entered. The surgical assistant is responsible for retraction of tissues and suture manipulation to keep the procedure running smoothly. It will often help the veterinary surgeon if the assistant stands on the right side of the dog and holds the body wall up with towel clamps during the gastropexy. This will often expose the entire surgical field for the surgeon. After gastropexy, the spleen is reevaluated. If all or a portion of the spleen does not appear viable, all or part of the spleen is removed, respectively. The abdomen is flushed, and the celiotomy incision is closed routinely.

POSTOPERATIVE CONSIDERATIONS

Dogs suffering from GDV can have many postoperative complications. Arrhythmias can continue for 2 to 3 days postoperatively. Treatment of arrhythmias should be initiated if vascular compromise is present or is expected on the basis of the type of arrhythmia present and cardiovascular stability. The veterinarian should be alerted as to the type of arrhythmia present. Hypotension and hypovolemia can continue postoperatively and should be treated as needed.

Urination should be monitored because prolonged hypotension under anesthesia can affect renal function. A urinary catheter should be placed if urine production is questionable. Some dogs will require a blood transfusion because of hemorrhage associated with tearing of blood vessels during bloating and rotation of the stomach and/or spleen. If a partial gastrectomy was performed, the dog should be monitored for evidence of gastric wall dehiscence. Some dogs continue to develop gastric wall compromise after decompression and surgery. Fever, persistent inappetence, and vomiting may indicate that this is occurring. Signs are similar to intestinal incision dehiscence, as previously discussed. Antibiotics should be continued for at least 7 days postoperatively. Immediately after surgery, antibiotics should be given intravenously to avoid oral administration. Gastrointestinal protectants, such as H_2 blockers, should be administered for 2 to 4 days postoperatively. Some surgeons prefer to place these animals on a gastric motility modifier to help treat ileus. Finally, gastric dilatation can again occur in the postoperative period, necessitating decompression. However, gastropexy should prevent rotation of the stomach.

Oral alimentation should be initiated slowly. Water is given in small amounts at first. If no vomiting occurs, food is gradually introduced. Feeding can start as soon as the animal is willing to eat—often within 24 hours of surgery. Some animals may require antiemetics in the perioperative period to help control nausea and vomiting. Long-term dietary management should be considered. When home, dogs should be on a 3- to 4-times-a-day feeding schedule. If possible, a 2- to 3-times-a-day feeding schedule should be continued for the rest of the dog's life. Once-a-day feedings should be avoided. Water should always be available, but gulping of water should be avoided. Heavy activity should be avoided after feeding. Owners should be warned that bloating can still occur, even though gastropexy was performed, but surgery is likely to prevent gastric rotation, which is life threatening. Stomach decompression may be needed if bloat is severe.

OVARIOHYSTERECTOMY IN THE DOG AND CAT

DEFINITION

Ovariohysterectomy (spay) is surgical removal of the uterus and ovaries.

INDICATIONS

The primary indication for ovariohysterectomy is prevention of pregnancy and subsequent production of unwanted puppies and kittens. Other indications for ovariohysterectomy include endocrine imbalance, infection, injury, cyst, tumor, prevention of unwanted behavior, and congenital abnormalities. Endocrine disturbances are associated with varied clinical manifestations, such as sterility, skin lesions, mammary tumors, **pseudocyesis** (false pregnancy), and nymphomania. Ovariohysterectomy before the first estrus will greatly decrease the chance of mammary neoplasia in dogs. Uterine diseases that may require ovariohysterectomy include metritis, **pyometra**, uterine prolapse, endometrial hyperplasia, neoplasia, injury, neglected dystocia, and congenital abnormalities.

PREOPERATIVE CONSIDERATIONS

Ovariohysterectomy is usually performed between 5 and 6 months of age, but it can be performed at almost any age and during any phase of the reproductive cycle. Performing ovariohysterectomy around 6 months of age decreases anesthetic risk in younger animals and usually allows the procedure to be performed before the first estrus. If performed during estrus or pregnancy, increased vasculature may be encountered with the potential for increased hemorrhage. This is more important for dogs than for cats. The most favorable time to spay a mature dog is 3 to 4 months after estrus. After whelping, the operation should be done as soon as the puppies or kittens have been weaned and lactation has ceased—about 6 to 8 weeks after parturition.

TECHNIQUE AND INTRAOPERATIVE CONSIDERATIONS

The animal is clipped and aseptically prepared for a ventral midline celiotomy. The skin incision extends caudally 3 to 6 cm from the umbilicus in the dog and from 2 cm caudad to the umbilicus caudally 3 to 4 cm in the cat. When the abdominal cavity is entered, the uterine horns are located and exteriorized from the abdomen using a spay hook or digital manipulation (Figure 32-27, A). The suspensory ligament holds each ovary tight in the abdominal cavity and must be severed or torn to exteriorize the ovaries, especially on the right, for proper ligation. This is often the most painful part of the procedure and the animal may begin to wake up. The anesthetist should be prepared for this. The ovarian arteries and veins (pedicles) are ligated with absorbable suture material of appropriate size (Figure 32-27, B) and are severed. Usually, two circumferential ligatures are placed. The broad ligament is broken down, and the uterine body is exteriorized and ligated with transfixation and or circumferential sutures (Figure 32-27, C and D). The uterus is removed with the ovaries, and the assistant or surgeon checks to

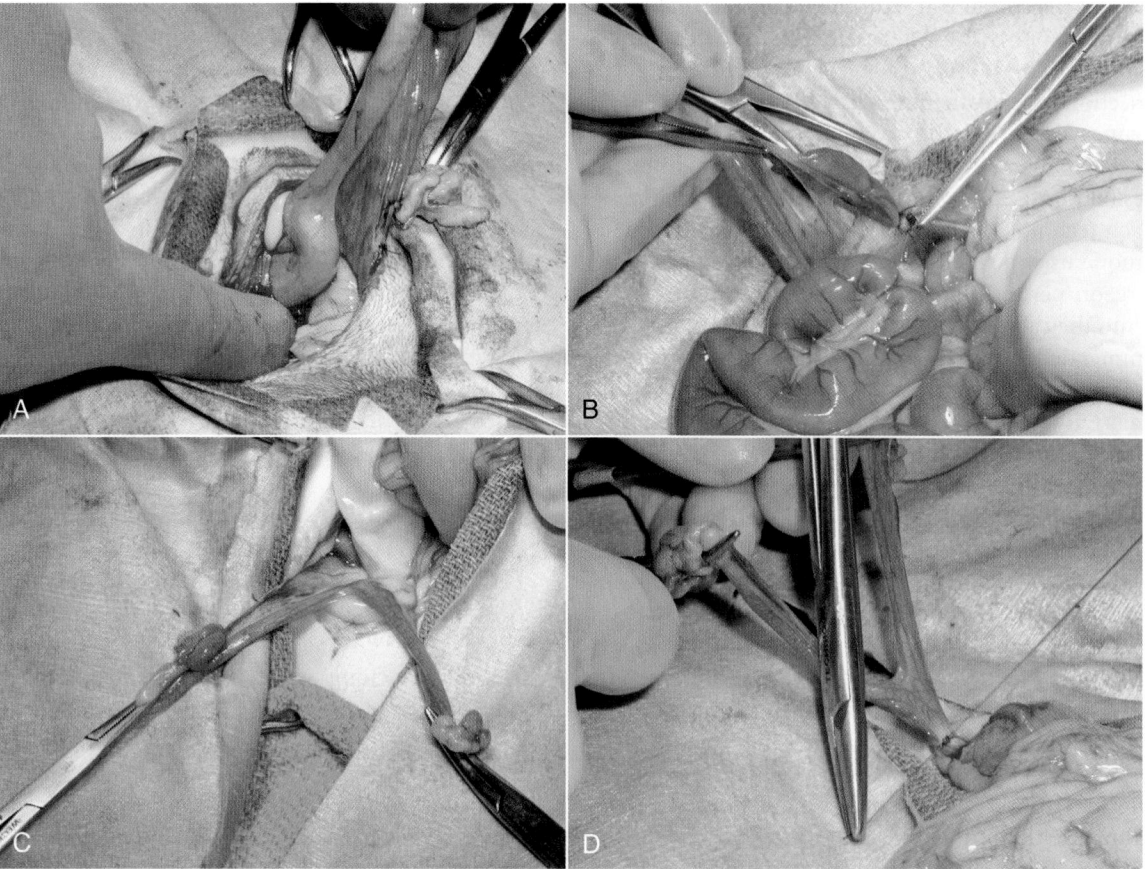

FIGURE 32-27 Ovariohysterectomy. **A,** The uterine body is exposed and the suspensory ligament broken down so the ovarian pedicles can be ligated. Both uterine horns are shown in this figure as digital manipulation is used to bring the uterus out of the abdomen. **B,** Once the ovarian pedicle is freed, two circumferential sutures are secured on the portion that will remain in the animal. The ovarian pedicle would be severed proximal to the ovary but distal to the placed ligatures. **C,** The uterine body is fully exposed with gentle traction once the ovarian pedicles are ligated and severed and after the broad ligament is broken down. **D,** The uterine vessels are ligated with tranfixation sutures that individually ligate the vessels on either side of the uterine body and/or as shown with circumferential ligatures that encircle the entire uterine body and the uterine vessels.

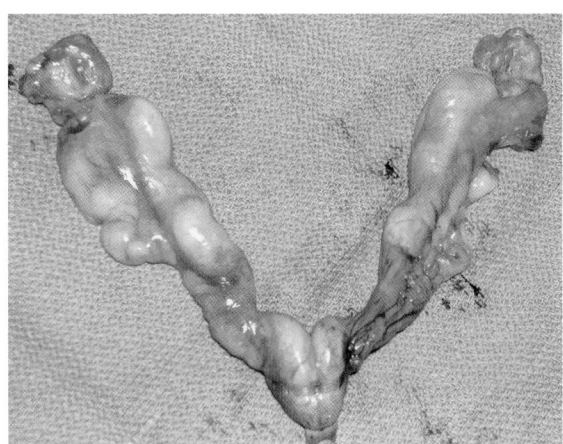

FIGURE 32-28 Ovariohysterectomy. The uterus is positioned with the ovaries to the top of the picture. Note that the ovaries are not well visualized and look like a continuation of the uterine horns. The ovaries should be exposed from their bursae to ensure that ovarian tissue was not left behind.

ensure that both ovaries were completely removed (Figure 32-28). Leaving ovarian tissue behind can lead to recurrent heat cycles and stump pyometra due to the presence of hormones that can influence any remaining uterine tissue. The abdominal cavity is carefully examined for hemorrhage. The celiotomy incision is closed routinely.

Intraoperative complications include hemorrhage and anesthetic problems. If excessive intra-abdominal blood is seen during surgery, both ovarian pedicles and the uterine stump should be evaluated before celiotomy closure. The abdominal incision will likely have to be extended cranially. This is why adequate preparation before surgery is important. The left ovarian pedicle is evaluated by retraction of the descending colon to the right and viewing of the pedicle just caudal to the left kidney. The right pedicle is evaluated by retraction of the descending duodenum to the left and viewing of the pedicle just caudal to the right kidney. The uterine stump is visualized between the urinary bladder ventrally and the colon dorsally. Bleeding stumps are re-ligated before abdominal closure.

POSTOPERATIVE CONSIDERATIONS

Postoperative, intra-abdominal hemorrhage can occur and can be fatal if not treated appropriately (see the section on monitoring blood loss). After ovariohysterectomy, the technician should monitor the animal carefully for the first 24 hours. Abnormalities should be promptly reported to the veterinarian in charge.

Incision complications can also occur after ovariohysterectomy. These include irritation, premature suture removal by the animal, seroma formation, infection, suture reaction, and dehiscence. Only rarely are these complications serious. The veterinarian should be alerted to impending incision complications.

Some animals experience renal dysfunction secondary to accidental ureteral ligation during surgery. Ligation typically occurs when overzealous attempts are made to alleviate

hemorrhage from a bleeding stump with mass ligation of tissues and poor visualization. It is important to ensure that the ureters are visualized and are not in the mass of tissue to be ligated when hemorrhage from bleeding ovarian or uterine stumps is controlled. Animals are unlikely to show signs of renal failure if only one ureter is ligated, but they may be seen at a later date for abdominal enlargement, abdominal pain, or signs consistent with renal infection. If both ureters are inadvertently ligated, the animal will begin to show signs within 24 hours and will die if steps are not taken to alleviate the obstruction of urine flow.

Body weight gain may occur as a late sequela to ovariohysterectomy. Reasons for this excessive weight gain are poorly understood, but it may be caused in part by ovarian endocrine deficiency. In actuality, obesity can be controlled by proper diet and exercise. Other late complications include loss of stamina in working dogs (eunuchoid syndrome) and urinary incontinence. Although incompletely understood, urinary incontinence may be related to endocrine alteration after ovariohysterectomy or scar tissue formation around the urinary bladder and proximal urethra. These appear to be rare complications.

PYOMETRA

DEFINITION

Pyometra is a condition of the uterus in which endometrial hyperplasia has resulted in increased uterine secretions and accumulation of fluid in the uterus with secondary infection. Progesterone production from the ovaries during diestrus contributes to uterine gland hyperplasia and the disease process. The process typically occurs in middle-aged to older dogs 4 to 8 weeks after estrus. **Mucometra** or **hydrometra** is enlargement of the uterus with a sterile mucoid or serous fluid, respectively.

INDICATIONS

Ovariohysterectomy is the recommended treatment for pyometra. This is especially true for closed (nondraining) pyometra. Some owners will elect conservative management for open (draining) pyometras in valuable breeding dogs, but this should be discouraged because septicemia and endotoxemia are possible, and the incidence of recurrence is high. Conservative management of closed pyometras is not recommended because of the risk for uterine rupture, septicemia and endotoxemia, and possible death.

PREOPERATIVE CONSIDERATIONS

An intact female dog with fever, lethargy, polyuria, polydipsia, vaginal discharge, abdominal pain, abdominal enlargement, inappetence, vomiting, and/or diarrhea should be evaluated carefully for pyometra. Animals with closed pyometra are more likely to have severe clinical signs. Baseline biochemical values and blood cell counts should be obtained. Many of these animals are dehydrated or inappetent, and have metabolic and/or electrolyte abnormalities at the time

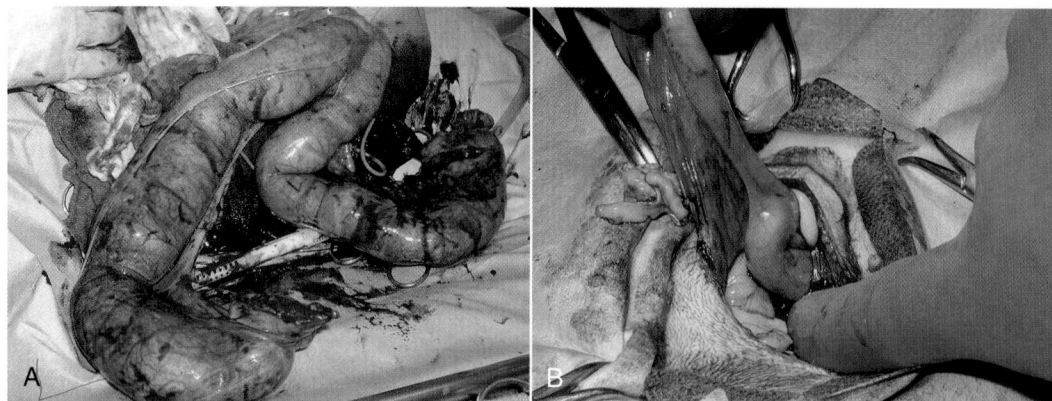

FIGURE 32-29 Pyometra. The uterus must be carefully handled in cases of pyometra because it is often large, friable, and heavy. Compare (A) the pyometra uterus with (B) the normal uterus.

of presentation (renal or hepatic dysfunction, glucose imbalance, etc.). They should be started on intravenous fluids and their metabolic/electrolyte abnormalities corrected, if possible, before surgery. If left untreated, pyometra can result in septicemia and/or endotoxemia and possible death. Additionally, uterine rupture and peritonitis are possible. Palpation of the abdomen should be done with extreme care, and cystocentesis to collect urine should be avoided in animals suspected of having pyometra. Broad-spectrum intravenous antibiotic therapy is initiated before surgery.

TECHNIQUE AND INTRAOPERATIVE CONSIDERATIONS

The animal is prepped for a ventral midline celiotomy. A routine ovariohysterectomy is performed with some exceptions. The uterus is usually large, heavy, and friable (Figure 32-29). It should be manipulated with extreme care during the procedure to prevent rupture and contamination of the abdomen. This means that the celiotomy incision should extend from the xiphoid to the pubis so that excessive tension is not placed on the uterus during manipulation. Vessels are usually prominent and may be increased in number, so care must be taken to ligate and separate vessels appropriately to prevent hemorrhage. Uterine contents should be cultured for aerobic and anaerobic bacteria and a bacterial sensitivity test performed after the uterus is removed from the surgical field. This is done via aseptic aspiration of the fluid with a needle and syringe before the uterus is contaminated, but after removal from the surgical field to prevent contamination of the abdomen with purulent material. The uterus can be placed sterilely on a surgical drape on a table away from the sterile operating field, and an assistant can take the samples needed using aseptic technique. The abdomen should be flushed before closure. Abdominal closure is routine.

POSTOPERATIVE CONSIDERATIONS

Animals should be monitored as for ovariohysterectomy. Special considerations include continued antibiotic therapy in the postoperative period. Septicemia can lead to severe

complications such as shock, disseminated intravascular coagulation, and death. Antibiotics are given intravenously until the animal is stable and eating. Antibiotic therapy is continued for 7 to 10 days after surgery according to culture and sensitivity results. Electrolyte and metabolic abnormalities can continue postoperatively, and monitoring for this is important. Abnormalities should be corrected. Intravenous fluids should be given until the animal is stable, eating, and drinking.

CANINE CASTRATION

DEFINITION

Orchidectomy (castration or neuter) is the removal of both testicles. Scrotal ablation is removal of the scrotum with the testicles at the time of castration.

INDICATIONS

Numerous indications for canine castration are known; the most common is an elective procedure in the young male dog to help prevent roaming, aggressiveness, unwanted breeding, or a combination of these. Several medical problems may also be treated by castration, including prostate disorders, anal and perianal tumors, perineal hernias, and testicular tumors. Older dogs with a well-developed scrotum and animals with scrotal abnormalities should undergo scrotal ablation to prevent severe scrotal swelling, improve postoperative aesthetics, and/or treat disease.

PREOPERATIVE CONSIDERATIONS

An optimal age for canine castration is not known, but the procedure is often performed at around 6 months of age. Performing castration before the development of unwanted male behavior—before sexual maturity—may help prevent this behavior from occurring. Castration after development of this behavior will often improve behavior but may not eliminate it in all male dogs. Before surgery, a careful examination should be performed to ensure that both testicles lie within the scrotum.

CASE PRESENTATION 32-1

Signalment: Lady, 6-year-old female Labrador Retriever (Figure 1)

History: Two-week history of increased drinking and urination. Lady showed progressive lethargy and decreased appetite over the 3 days before presentation. For 24 hours before presentation, Lady was inappetent, depressed, and extremely lethargic. The owner noticed some blood-tinged fluid coming from the vulva 4 days ago, and that Lady has been licking her vulva regularly. The owner has noticed some blood in the urine when Lady has accidents in the house, which started happening about 1.5 weeks before presentation.

Technical considerations: The dog is an intact female, she has not been eating or drinking for 24 hours, she has blood in her urine, she has a bloody discharge from her vulva, and she had been drinking and urinating more frequently than she normally does.

Other questions asked:

1. Is Lady current on vaccinations? *Yes, rabies, distemper, and Bordetella*
2. Has Lady ever had puppies? *Yes, two litters, all healthy*
3. When was her last heat cycle? *About 8 weeks ago*
4. When was the last time Lady was bred? *3 years ago*
5. Are there toxins around your home, and can Lady free roam? *No toxins that owners are aware of, and Lady stays indoors or in a fenced yard*
6. Has she had any other illnesses? *No*
7. Did Lady have any dietary items out of the ordinary before this started? *No, she eats adult maintenance dry (1 cup twice a day) and milk bones only. The owner did try to feed her steak last night because she was not eating, but Lady turned that down.*
8. Any coughing, sneezing, runny eyes, vomiting, or diarrhea? *No*

Examination: Physical examination revealed Lady to be depressed and her abdomen to be tense and painful; Lady had a mucopurulent discharge coming from her vulva. Other findings include fleas, waxy debris in both ears, and moderate dental tarter.

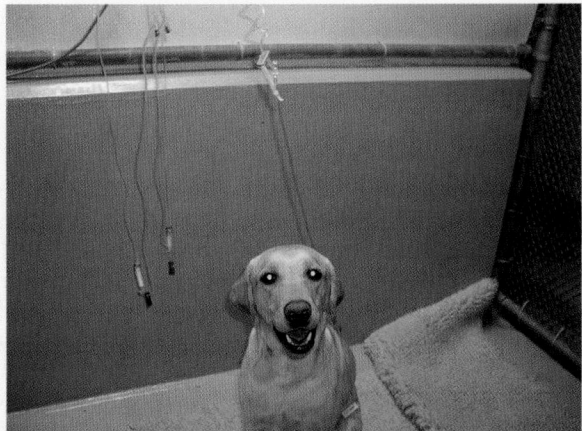

FIGURE 1 Lady: 6-year-old female Labrador Retriever that came for treatment of inappetence and lethargy.

Temperature: 104.5° F
Pulse: 110 bpm, pulses weak and thready
Respiratory rate: 50 bpm
Mucous membranes: pale and tacky
Capillary refill time: 3 seconds

Technical assessment: Lady is febrile, tachycardic, and tachypneic; has weak and thready pulses; and is painful in the abdomen. Lady appears to be dehydrated and in early shock.

Diagnostic Tests and Findings

- *CBC:* Mild nonregenerative anemia; mildly low TP; leukocytosis (increased white blood cell count) consisting of a neutrophilia (a high neutrophil count) with a left shift (too many immature neutrophils) and toxic changes to the neutrophils; and a mild thrombocytopenia (low platelets)
- *Biochemistry panel abnormalities:* Elevated Na and Cl, mildly low potassium, elevated BUN (meaning high-protein diet, renal insufficiency, gastrointestinal bleeding, and or dehydration), elevated creatinine (kidney value—high means renal insufficiency or the animal is dehydrated), mildly low albumin, mildly low TP, and elevated alkaline phosphatase (liver enzyme)
- *Abdominal radiographs:* tissue-dense mass in the caudal abdomen displacing the intestines cranial and dorsal and the intestinal ileus. The mass is consistent with an enlarged uterus (Figure 2).
- *Abdominal ultrasound:* enlarged, fluid-filled uterus
- *Urinalysis collected at the time of ultrasound by cystocentesis:* numerous bacteria, increased white blood cells, hematuria (blood in the urine), urine specific gravity of 1.012 (urine is not concentrated—in a dehydrated dog, this number should be higher. This means that the kidneys may not be functioning normally, or the toxins from the disease are causing diuresis—increased filtration of fluid through the kidneys).

Veterinarian's diagnosis: pyometra, anemia, possible renal insufficiency, possible sepsis.

Technical considerations: Lady has been diagnosed with a pyometra. She will require emergency surgery to remove the source of infection (her uterus). However, she is azotemic (has an elevated BUN and creatinine), dehydrated, potentially septic, anemic, thrombocytopenic, and in the early stages of shock. This makes her a poor anesthetic candidate because she is systemically unstable.

Veterinarian's Treatment Orders

1. Place an intravenous catheter.
2. Give shock dose of intravenous crystalloid therapy (may consider adding in a colloid because the protein is low).
3. Begin a cooling process with fans and fluid therapy.
4. Obtain an ECG and blood pressure.
5. Obtain a coagulation profile to check for evidence of early disseminated intravascular coagulation (a disease that involves severe metabolic disruptions that leads to generalized blood clotting throughout the body followed by hemorrhage).
6. Start on intravenous, broad-spectrum antibiotics.

Continued

CASE PRESENTATION 32-1—cont'd

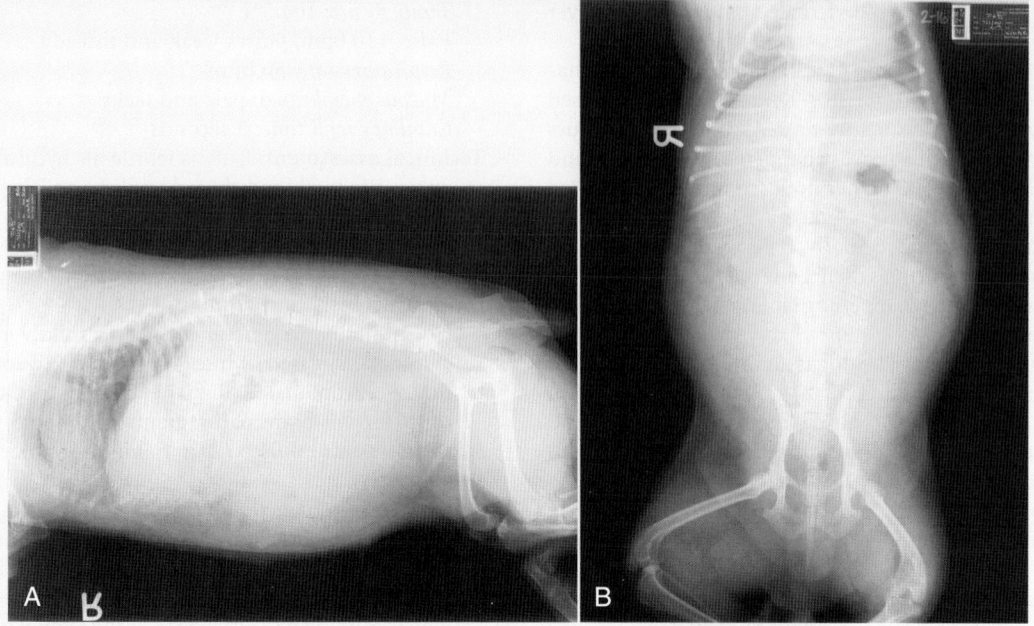

FIGURE 2 Abdominal radiographs of Lady showing a large tissue-dense mass in the caudal abdomen (large dense [more white] structure that is irregular and is pushing the intestines cranial and dorsal). **(A)** is a lateral radiograph, and **(B)** is a ventrodorsal view.

7. Continue crystalloid and/or colloid therapy until improvements in body temperature, pulses, and respiration are noted.
8. Initiate pain control.
9. Start gastrointestinal protectants because of GI stasis and inappetence caused by the stress of being in the hospital.
10. Repeat CBC and chemistry panel after Lady's condition begins to stabilize.

What to consider at this point: Lady's systemic condition should begin to stabilize within a few hours of admission to the hospital. She has a life-threatening infection of her uterus and must go to surgery sooner rather than later. As soon as she appears to be out of shock and rehydrated (it is hoped that BUN and creatinine would come down), she should be prepared for surgery. Lady has bacteria in the urine, and a urine sample should be turned in for culture and sensitivity.

Anesthetic considerations: Lady is not a stable patient. *Adequate monitoring:* blood pressure, temperature, pulse, oxygen saturation, and vitals should be monitored. Only light anesthetics would likely be required and are desired. Instead of using rapid inducing agents that lead to apnea and decreased blood pressure, a muscle relaxant (like midazolam) and a dissociative anesthetic (like ketamine) have the potential to better maintain blood pressure. Because inhalant anesthetics are notorious for dose-dependent effects on the cardiovascular system, a constant rate infusion of pain medication and high epidural should also be considered to keep gas anesthetic administration to a minimum.

Surgical considerations: Lady should be prepped quickly and moved into the OR for surgery. The technician should ensure that the OR is set up with all necessary equipment

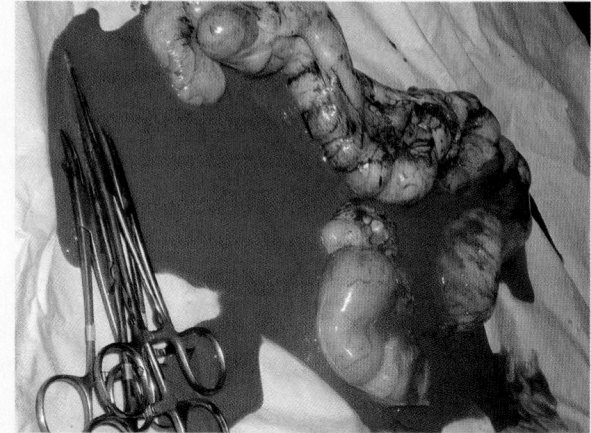

FIGURE 3 This uterus has been cut open with sterile instruments. Note the brown fluid that exudes from the cut uterus. The fluid should be cultured using sterile technique by sticking a culture swab into the uterine lumen through an aseptically made incision.

and suture so that the surgery proceeds quickly. A general abdominal pack would be required. Culture swabs and a bucket for the uterus should be available. The surgeon would likely hand the infected uterus to the technician, and the technician would have to cut into the uterus with sterile technique and obtain a culture—this should be done outside of the OR (Figure 3). The surgical technique would be ovariohysterectomy. However, a wide abdominal preparation will be required because a large incision will be needed for gentle uterine handling and abdominal exploration (Figure 4). A sponge count should be performed before abdominal incision and before incision closure to ensure that none were left in the abdomen. The surgical

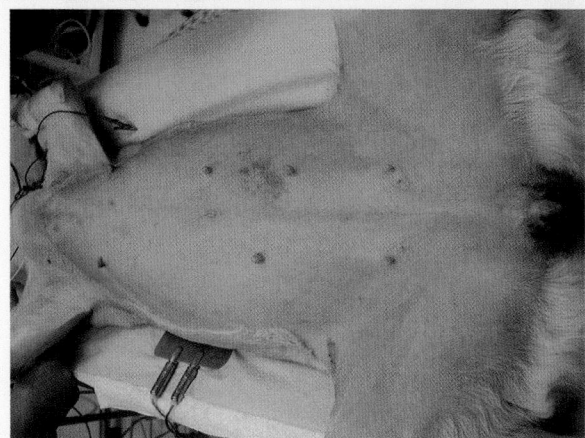

FIGURE 4 This dog's abdomen has been aseptically prepared for pyometra surgery. Note the wide abdominal clip, so a full surgical approach to the abdomen can be made.

assistant should remember to keep the tissues moist and to avoid pulling on the uterus because it will be friable and will tear easily (this would cause septic fluid to leak onto the surgical field and into the sterile abdominal cavity). Tissue and culture samples should be promptly submitted.

Considerations for recovery: Lady will likely be hypothermic, even though she had a fever before surgery. She should be warmed appropriately. Although the infected uterus was removed, she could still experience complications of septicemia and her illness, such as fever, low blood pressure, anemia, shock, organ failure, and death. All vitals, PCV, TP, ECG, blood pressure, and mucous membranes should continue to be monitored until Lady is stable.

Other postoperative care: Pain should be controlled with injections rather than orally, and injections should be administered on a routine schedule (do not wait for Lady to be painful). Intravenous fluids should be continued until Lady is eating and drinking. Food and water should be offered 12 hours after surgery. PCV and TP should normalize within a few days, but if they drop too low, colloidal fluid support and/or blood transfusion may be necessary. Coagulation times, CBC, and biochemistry panel should be reevaluated 24 hours after surgery to ensure that improvements are noted. The incision should be monitored for oozing of fluid (which might occur in a dog with low protein and platelets—this should improve in 24 to 48 hours). A bandage should be placed around the belly if incisional oozing occurs. Gastrointestinal protectants are continued until Lady's appetite returns to normal. As she improves over 24 to 48 hours and begins to eat and drink, fluid therapy is decreased and then stopped, and oral antibiotic therapy is continued on the basis of culture and sensitivity results.

Postoperative events and client education: Surgery was a success, and Lady recovered without complications. Her blood work abnormalities began to normalize, and her appetite returned within 36 hours. She was discharged from the hospital 3 days after surgery taking enrofloxacin and tramadol. Initial culture results from urine and uterus revealed *Escherichia coli* sensitive to enrofloxacin. The owners were instructed to monitor the incision daily and to return for suture removal and blood work in 7 days. Lady was back to normal at that time.

Note: Pyometra generally has a good prognosis if caught early and treated appropriately. Recovery is often quick so long as the animal does not have complications with septicemia.

TECHNIQUE AND INTRAOPERATIVE CONSIDERATIONS

The abdomen is clipped from the tip of the prepuce to the margin of abdominal skin and scrotal skin. The clipped area should extend widely into the inguinal region. The scrotum typically is not draped into the surgical field and is not normally clipped during surgical preparation. The scrotum has delicate, thin skin that is easily subject to clipper burn and laceration. If, however, long scrotal hairs are protruding into the surgical field, they should be trimmed without touching the clippers to the scrotal skin. If scrotal ablation is to be performed, the scrotum is clipped and prepared aseptically, along with the rest of the surgical field (Figure 32-30).

For simple castration, the dog is secured in dorsal recumbency, and standard surgical preparation of the prescrotal skin (craniad to the scrotum) is performed. A testicle is pushed cranial beneath the prescrotal skin. A midline incision is made in the prescrotal skin centrally and over the cranially displaced testicle. With gentle pressure, the testicle

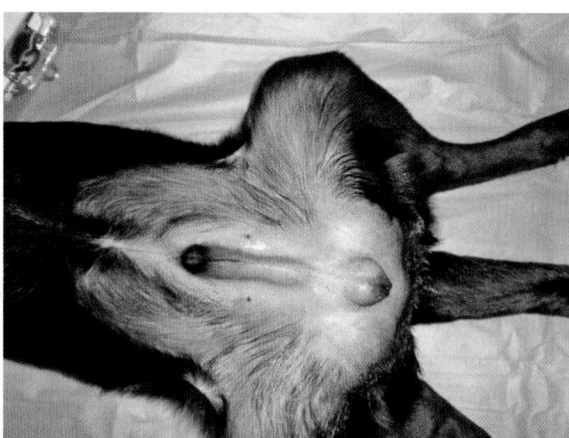

FIGURE 32-30 Canine castration. Proper positioning and preparation for canine castration via scrotal ablation. Note that the scrotum is clipped. The same positioning is used for routine castrations, but the scrotum does not require clipping.

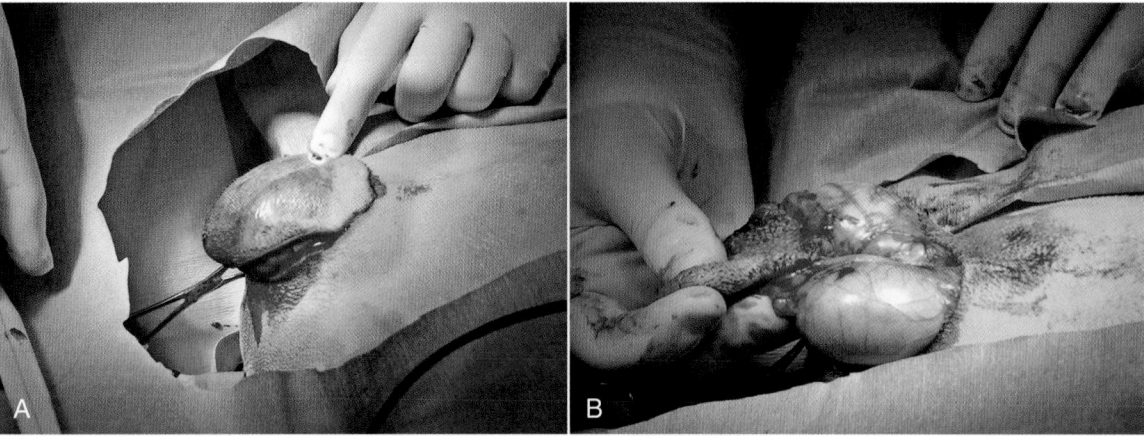

FIGURE 32-31 Canine scrotal ablation. **A,** An incision has been made around the scrotum, ensuring that enough skin would be available for closure post castration. **B,** The testicles are exposed through blunt and sharp dissection after the skin incision is made.

is exteriorized through the incision by carefully incising over the common tunic (tissue that encases the testicle). The testicle is pulled away from the body for ligation as the remaining scrotal ligament is gently dissected from the testicle. Ligation can proceed with an open technique or a closed technique. For the closed technique, two ligatures are placed external to the tunics of the pedicle such that all the vessels and the vas deferens are ligated as a unit. This technique is fast, but if it is not carefully done, the vascular pedicle can slip inside the tunics and into the abdominal cavity, causing uncontrolled hemorrhage. The closed technique is best used on very small patients. The open technique allows individual ligation of the vas deferens and its blood supply and the pampiniform plexus. The testicle is then removed with sharp severance distal to the ligatures. The opposite testicle is handled in a similar fashion and is exteriorized through the same incision as the first. The incision is closed with a continuous subcuticular suture pattern. It is best to bury suture here because potential irritation might lead to a greater desire to lick.

For scrotal ablation, the incision is made circumferentially around the base of the scrotum (Figure 32-31, *A*). Care must be taken to avoid removal of too much skin around the scrotum to prevent excessive tension on the closure. The subcutaneous tissue is bluntly dissected to expose the testicles and associated structures. Castration is carried out via ligation of these structures, as for simple castration (Figure 32-31, *B*). The testicles and scrotum are removed and the incision closed in two to three layers.

POSTOPERATIVE CONSIDERATIONS

Several postoperative complications can occur. If the presurgical preparation is not done carefully so as to preclude scrotal dermatitis (clipper burn, excessive scrubbing), the dog will lick aggressively at the scrotum and the incision. This often results in severe inflammation and swelling of scrotal and prescrotal skin. If this problem is not detected early, results can include premature suture removal and wound dehiscence. The best treatment is prevention. If

scrotal dermatitis does occur, the dog should be placed in an Elizabethan collar.

Another less common complication is hemorrhage. When the testicles are removed from the scrotal sac, free space remains in the scrotum. If any hemorrhage occurs from the subcutaneous tissue or the common tunic, the space will fill with a considerable amount of blood before enough pressure is present to create hemostasis, resulting in a large hematoma within the scrotum. If a hematoma is detected early, before the scrotum is full, cold compresses can be applied with slight pressure to the scrotal area to encourage hemostasis. If the scrotum becomes excessively large, not only is it unsightly, but trauma and skin sloughing may occur. At this point, removal of the scrotum may be necessary.

A scrotal seroma is more likely to occur than hemorrhage and can result in scrotal swelling. In older dogs with well-developed scrotal tissue, fluid accumulation after castration can be excessive. Some advocate performing scrotal ablation at the time of castration to help prevent this complication in older animals. Treatment is the same as for hematoma. It is important to restrict activity in these dogs to decrease the amount of fluid accumulation.

FELINE CASTRATION

DEFINITION

Feline orchidectomy (neuter) is the removal of both testicles.

INDICATIONS

Major indications for feline castration are to prevent fighting, roaming, and urine spraying and to decrease urine odor. Castration in the cat may lead to a rapid response (2 to 4 weeks) to these objectionable characteristics, although complete resolution may not occur.

PREOPERATIVE CONSIDERATIONS

The cat is usually castrated at around 6 months of age. Preanesthetic evaluation should include palpation of both

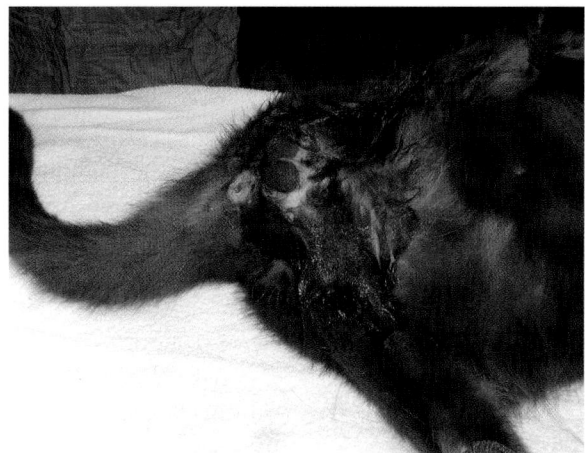

FIGURE 32-32 Proper positioning for feline castration. The legs are pulled forward, and the cat is in dorsal recumbency.

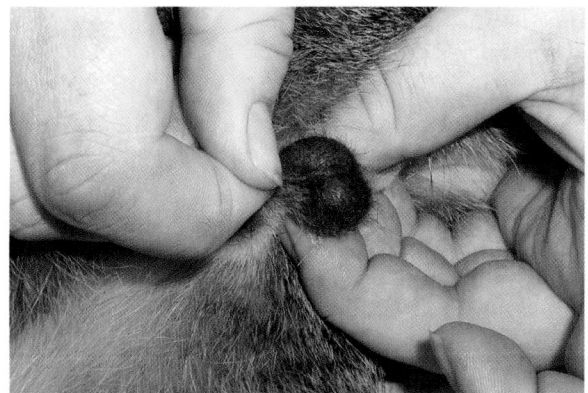

FIGURE 32-33 Technique for scrotal plucking to remove hair in preparation for surgery.

testicles to confirm the gender of the cat and to detect retained testicles before surgery.

TECHNIQUE AND INTRAOPERATIVE CONSIDERATIONS

Several acceptable techniques may be used for feline castration. The patient is generally placed in dorsal recumbency with the legs tied craniad (Figure 32-32). Unlike in the dog, the scrotum is the site of the primary incision and should be aseptically prepared for surgery. Scrotal dermatitis is not a major concern in the cat, although you should avoid putting alcohol on the scrotum during surgical preparation. Warmed sterile saline is a good substitute for alcohol. Scrotal hairs are gently plucked from the scrotum with the thumb and finger (Figure 32-33). This is easily accomplished by grasping the base of the scrotum with the thumb and index finger of one hand and gently pushing the testicles into the scrotum. With the other hand, the thumb and finger are used to gently strip hair from the scrotal skin. The scrotum is then scrubbed and draped in an aseptic manner.

An incision is made directly through the scrotum, and then the testicle is pushed through the incision by gentle pressure with the thumb and index finger (Figure 32-34, *A*

and *B*). The testicle and its spermatic cord (vessels) are exteriorized with gentle traction and striping (Figure 32-34, *C*). The spermatic cord may be ligated with suture, ligated with metal clips, or tied in a knot on itself, or the vessels can be separated from the vas deferens and tied in a square knot. The testicle is then removed by severing the spermatic cord with a blade distal to the ligation site. The scrotum is left unsutured (Figure 32-34, *D*).

POSTOPERATIVE CONSIDERATIONS

Scrotal swelling and bleeding are the two most common complications of feline castration. Scrotal swelling is due primarily to traumatic surgical preparation and hair plucking. An Elizabethan collar may be necessary to control licking. If scrotal hemorrhage is noted after surgery, cold compresses on the scrotum for 5 to 7 minutes will help to encourage hemostasis (but practically, this is difficult to accomplish). Severe hemorrhage can also occur and may actually occur intra-abdominally. The veterinary technician should monitor these animals carefully (see discussion on blood loss) and should bring clinical abnormalities to the attention of the veterinarian. Scrotal infection occurs rarely and should be treated with drainage (if not already draining), scrotal flushing, Elizabethan collar, and appropriate antibiotics.

When the cat is sent home, the owner should be informed to change the litter from a gravel type of litter to a shredded or pelleted type of litter for the first 5 to 7 days. This will prevent pieces of litter from contaminating the surgical site.

CESAREAN DELIVERY

DEFINITION

Cesarean delivery derived its name from Caesar, who allegedly was the first to be born by such a technique. The procedure involves making an incision into the abdominal cavity and then into the uterus to deliver a neonate. It is usually performed on animals experiencing dystocia. Dystocia (Greek: *dys*, "difficult" + *tokos*, "birth") literally translated means "difficult birth."

INDICATIONS

Cesarean delivery is indicated when a bitch or queen cannot deliver puppies or kitttens through the birth canal by normal uterine contractions because of maternal or fetal abnormalities. Some breeders schedule planned cesarean deliveries in dog breeds that might typically have birthing problems, such as Bulldogs. Common causes of dystocia are presented in Table 32-1. Normal stages of parturition are discussed in Chapter 11.

PREOPERATIVE CONSIDERATIONS

The aim of treatment should be the successful delivery of live and undamaged puppies or kittens without harm to the dam. Medical therapy to increase uterine contractures or to treat metabolic abnormalities in the dam should be

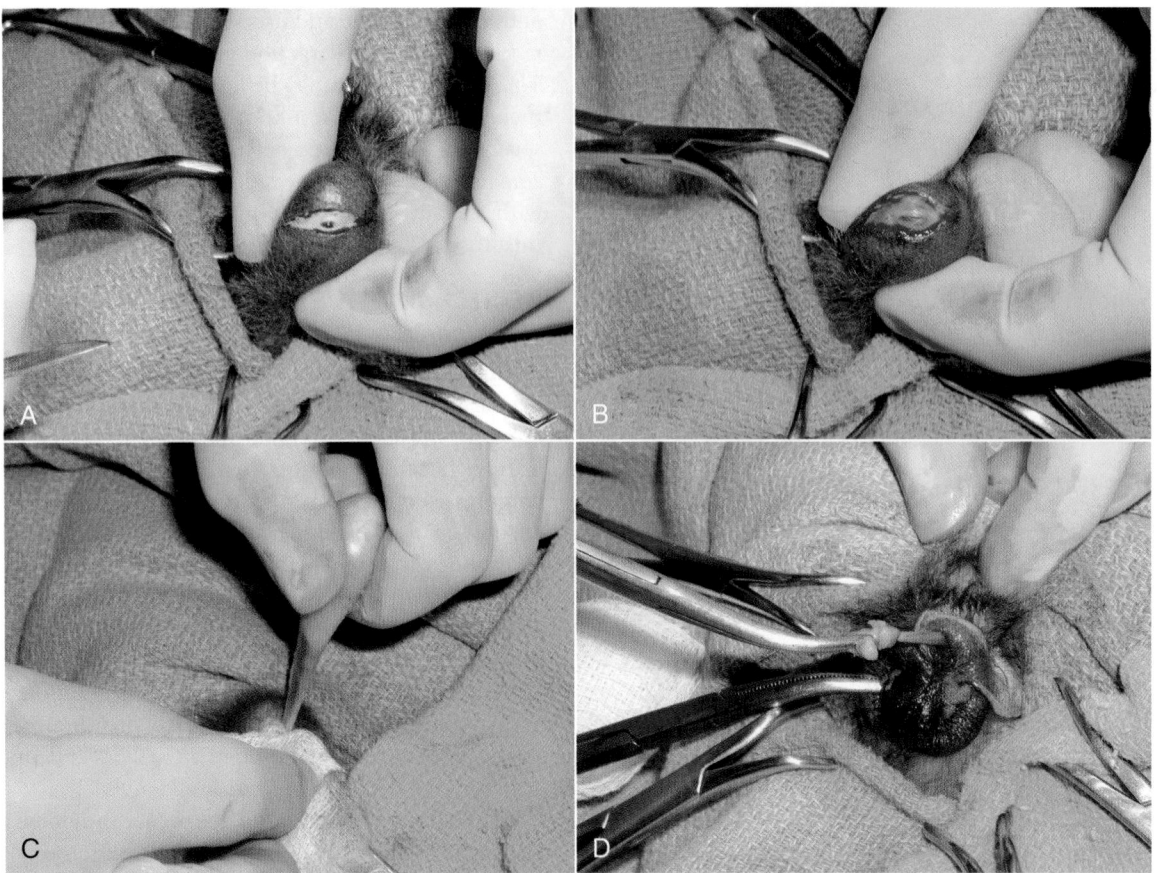

FIGURE 32-34 Feline castration. **A,** A skin incision is made directly over the scrotum as pictured. **B,** Manual pressure is applied to the testicle to exteriorize it through the incision. **C,** Traction is then applied to the testicle to pull it out of the scrotal sac for ligation. **D,** In this image, the spermatic cord has been knotted on itself and then will be released to go back into the scrotal sac. The scrotal sac will be left unsutured.

TABLE 32-1	Common Causes of Dystocia		
MATERNAL FACTORS		**FETAL FACTORS**	
CONTRACTION FORCES	**BIRTH CANAL**	**OVERSIZE FETUS**	

Uterine inertia (lack of contractions)
• First degree (primary)
Uterine muscle defect
Oxytocin deficiency
Premature birth
• Second degree
	Inadequate pelvis
	• Immature
	• Fracture
	• Breed
	• Disease
		Faulty pelvic presentation
		• Caudal simultaneous
		  • Head flexion
		  • Limb flexion	

Abdominal • Age • Pain • Hernia of uterus • Uterine rupture	Insufficient dilatation • Uterus • Cervix • Vagina • Vulva		

considered before surgery; however, a diagnosis of the cause of dystocia must be made first. Medical therapy may do more harm than good when used in the wrong type of dystocia (e.g., giving a drug [oxytocin] that would increase uterine muscular contractions to a dam that has a uterine obstruction from a malpositioned or too large fetus, or that has uterine torsion). When proper diagnosis of the type of dystocia is made and medical therapy is contraindicated or is not effective, the dam should be prepared for surgery. Dehydration and other metabolic alterations should be addressed before anesthesia, if possible. If not, treatment during and after surgery may be necessary.

The anesthetic regimen is of prime importance when cesarean delivery is considered. The dam that is dehydrated and exhausted with potential metabolic abnormalities from a prolonged attempted delivery is a poor anesthetic candidate. Anesthetic complications may be encountered. Selected anesthetic agents should have minimal effects on the newborn and should be safe for the dam.

TECHNIQUE AND INTRAOPERATIVE CONSIDERATIONS

The animal is clipped before anesthesia. Care should be taken to avoid damaging enlarged mammary glands and nipples. After anesthetic induction and maintenance, the dam is placed in dorsal recumbency. It is important to remember that increased weight of the gravid uterus on the diaphragm may compromise the normal breathing capacity of the dam, and intermittent manual respiration or a ventilator should be considered.

A ventral midline celiotomy is performed. The uterus is exteriorized and isolated with moistened surgical towels. Uterine isolation helps prevent uterine contents from entering the abdominal cavity. An incision is made into the ventral aspect of the uterine body. Care is taken to avoid cutting a fetus. A neonate and its associated fetal membranes are advanced through the uterine incision by applying gentle manual traction and pressure to the uterine wall. On fetal presentation, the fetal membranes are removed, the umbilicus is clamped or ligated, and the neonate is handed to an assistant. Fetal membranes can be firmly attached to the uterus if the fetus was not full term. Severe hemorrhage can result if membranes are pulled from the uterus under these circumstances. Each successive neonate is handled in a similar fashion until all are delivered. The birth canal (uterine body and vagina) is checked carefully before closure to ensure that a fetus is not wedged there. The uterine incision is closed in two layers. The abdominal cavity is flushed to remove any debris that might have leaked into it from the gravid uterus. The celiotomy incision is closed in a routine fashion. The skin should be closed internally with an absorbable suture to prevent premature removal by puppies or kittens during nursing. Puncture of swollen mammary tissue with the needle during closure should be avoided because puncture can lead to milk leakage and subsequent irritation of tissues.

Some owners prefer that the dam be spayed at the time of cesarean delivery. This can be accomplished in two ways: en bloc removal of the gravid uterus with secondary extraction of the neonates, or cesarean section followed by uterine body closure and ovariohysterectomy. En bloc resection entails clamping both ovarian pedicles and the uterine body, cutting the gravid uterus out of the dam, then going back and ligating all vasculature in the dam. The gravid uterus is given to an assistant, and the assistant cuts each neonate carefully from the uterus using sterile instruments and ligates or clamps the umbilicus. The technique chosen by the surgeon depends on preference and assistance available to care for the neonates. No proven benefit or downfall is associated with either technique if it is performed appropriately. Removal of the uterus and ovaries at the time of neonate delivery does not affect milk production or motherly instincts. Alternatively, the dam can be returned for ovariohysterectomy after the neonates have been weaned.

POSTOPERATIVE CONSIDERATIONS FOR THE NEONATE

The assistant should be ready to grasp the neonate from the surgeon and immediately place it in a dry towel. The assistant can then massage the animal gently to stimulate respiration, dry any secretions around the mouth and nose, and dry the remainder of the body to decrease the chance of hypothermia. The mouth should be inspected for evidence of mucus that may be plugging the airway. Gentle suction of the nostrils or mouth may be necessary to remove debris. Weak neonates and those with faint respirations may be stimulated by placing doxapram (a respiratory stimulant)

under the tongue. A thorough examination for congenital defects is performed, and the neonate is placed in an incubator or a warm, padded area. Neonates stressed from the prolonged attempted delivery may not survive or may already be dead by the time cesarean delivery is attempted.

Neonates should be returned to the dam as soon as she has recovered from anesthesia. Care should be taken to avoid returning them so early that the dam may unknowingly harm them by stepping or lying on them. The dam should be returned to her home environment as soon as possible so that she can begin caring for the neonates, and to prevent transmission of hospital organisms to immune-challenged neonates.

POSTOPERATIVE CONSIDERATIONS FOR THE DAM

The dam should be awakened from anesthesia as soon as possible so that the neonates can begin to nurse. The mother and neonates should be monitored carefully as they are introduced. Most dams accept the young readily, but some may be aggressive. Pain medication should be administered, but judiciously, because most medications are secreted in the milk and can affect the neonates. Epidural drug administration before surgery can provide pain relief for 4 to 8 hours and will minimize the need for pain medication and transmission of these drugs to the neonate (see section, "Anesthetic Management of Cesarean Delivery," Chapter 29). Other considerations include the development of metritis secondary to retained fetal membranes or infection, excessive uterine hemorrhage from overzealous fetal membrane removal, and all potential complications discussed for routine celiotomy or ovariohysterectomy, if that was performed at the same time. Some dogs may experience infertility after cesarean delivery as a result of scar tissue formation.

CYSTOTOMY

DEFINITION

Cystotomy means incision into the urinary bladder to expose the lumen or interior of the urinary bladder.

INDICATIONS

The most common indication for cystotomy in small animals is for removal of cystic calculi (bladder stones). A cystotomy is also indicated to remove tumors, to correct congenital defects, or to repair traumatic rupture of the urinary bladder. A final indication for cystotomy is placement of a cystostomy tube (a tube exiting the urinary bladder and abdominal wall) to provide an alternate outlet of urine in the case of tumor, calculi, or scar tissue causing obstruction of urine flow through the urethra.

PREOPERATIVE CONSIDERATIONS

Animals undergo cystotomy for various reasons. If urinary flow was obstructed, the animal should be stabilized before anesthesia, and surgery should be performed. Severe metabolic and/or electrolyte abnormalities might be present. Imaging studies may be necessary to identify the extent of disease and its exact location.

TECHNIQUE AND INTRAOPERATIVE CONSIDERATIONS

The abdomen is widely clipped from the xiphoid to the pubis. In male dogs, care is taken to clip the hair from the prepuce. The preputial orifice and the penis are then gently flushed with a 1% povidone-iodine (Betadine) solution.

The animal is placed in dorsal recumbency and is prepared for surgery with a standard skin preparation. For males, the abdominal skin incision will curve laterally to avoid the prepuce (refer to Figure 32-21, *D*). Care should be taken to thoroughly prepare this area aseptically. The prepuce is draped into the surgical field in the case of urinary calculi removal. This allows placement of a urinary catheter through the urethra for flushing of the urethra to aid in calculi removal. Although it is more common for urinary stones to lodge in the urethra of the male, a urethral catheter should be passed in the female because urethral calculi have been reported to lodge there occasionally. The urinary catheter in the female dog is usually placed aseptically before surgery. Care should be taken if bladder expression is attempted before celiotomy because an outflow obstruction from tumor, calculi, or scar tissue may result in inadvertent bladder rupture. Bladder expression should be avoided in those cases or when urinary bladder wall fragility is expected (e.g., urinary flow obstruction or tumor).

In the female, a standard caudal midline celiotomy is performed (see Figure 32-21, *A*). In the male, a caudal midline skin incision is made from the umbilicus to the sheath of the penis and is then extended lateral to the sheath. The caudal superficial epigastric artery and vein lateral to the prepuce are encountered. These are ligated and transected. The sheath is retracted laterally, and a ventral midline celiotomy is performed. The bladder is exteriorized and is packed off with laparotomy pads to preclude urine spillage into the abdominal cavity. If urinalysis and urine culture were not obtained before surgery, a syringe and needle are used to obtain a urine sample before cystotomy. An avascular area on the ventral aspect of the bladder is visualized and two stay sutures placed along the intended incision line (Figure 32-35, *A*). An incision is made along the proposed incision line between preplaced stay sutures (Figure 32-35, *B*). If cystic calculi are present, they are removed and submitted for stone analysis. If biopsies are taken for a suspected tumor, samples are placed in formalin and submitted for histologic analysis. Sample collection containers should be readily available; urinary calculi are not typically placed in formalin, and it is best to ask for appropriate sampling technique from the laboratory to which they will be submitted. Crushed stone, bladder wall, and urine samples are cultured.

Because calculi can lodge in the urethra, after removal, the entire lower urinary tract (bladder to urethra) is flushed

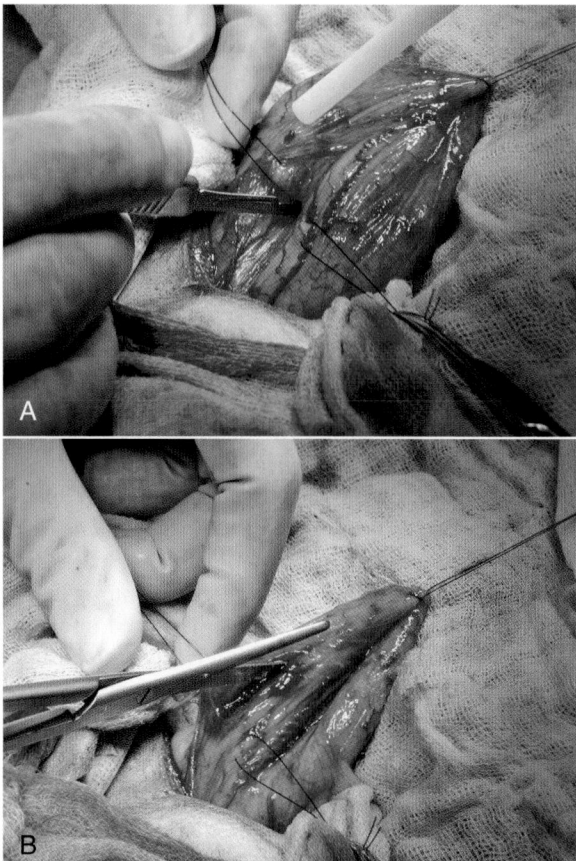

FIGURE 32-35 Cystotomy. **A,** Note the stay sutures in the urinary bladder. Stay sutures are held by the surgical assistant to help stabilize the tissue for the surgeon. This technique can be used for any hollow organ, including the stomach, small intestine, colon, and gallbladder. **B,** An incision has been made into the urinary bladder between the two stay sutures and is being extended with scissors.

with sterile physiologic saline solution until all calculi have been removed. The bladder wall is inspected for abnormalities and is then closed with a simple interrupted or inverted suture pattern. Laparotomy pads are removed, the abdomen is lavaged with sterile physiologic saline solution, and the abdominal incision is closed in a routine fashion. A postoperative imaging study may be necessary to determine whether all calculi were removed.

POSTOPERATIVE CONSIDERATIONS

The animal should be placed on intravenous fluids after cystotomy to help dilute blood clots and flush the urinary bladder. Urine production should be carefully monitored. If the incision was close to or involved the proximal urethra, postoperative swelling can obstruct urine flow. Also, blood clots can accumulate in the bladder and migrate into the urethra, obstructing urine flow. The veterinarian in charge should be alerted if the animal is straining to urinate and does not produce a urine stream or has not produced urine in 12 hours. Some straining to urinate can be expected after cystotomy as a result of swelling and bladder irritation, but a urine stream should accompany the straining, and the bladder should be nearly empty afterward. During the first week postoperatively, mild hematuria (bloody urine) with or without blood clots and frequent urination can be expected. If this continues or worsens instead of improving, the animal should be reevaluated.

> **TECHNICIAN NOTE** For the first week after cystotomy, mild hematuria with or without blood clots and frequent urination can be expected.

Treatment ultimately depends on urinalysis, urine culture, and identification of the type of disease present (type of calculi, type of tumor, type of congenital defect). If cystic calculi were removed, stone analysis must be performed before an appropriate treatment regimen can be initiated. Therapy will likely involve dietary alterations and/or antibiotics. Owners should be informed that recurrence of calculi is a possibility, and that dietary recommendations should be followed strictly to help decrease that chance.

Postoperative complications are rare after cystotomy. They include urinary outflow obstruction as a result of swelling or lodging of blood clots in the urethra, celiotomy incision complications, uroabdomen secondary to urine leakage through the cystotomy incision, and recurrence of the primary problem. If the animal is unable to urinate after cystotomy, a temporary urinary catheter may have to be placed to keep the bladder decompressed until surgical swelling decreases. This is not done routinely because catheter placement can cause further irritation to the healing cystotomy incision, and because it increases the chance of infection. An animal that could not urinate before surgery and had blood work abnormalities should have blood work (renal values, electrolytes, and PCV/TP) reassessed serially postoperatively to ensure that values are returning to normal. If the animal is not producing urine or is producing minimal urine and abdominal distention is detected, a complete biochemistry panel, CBC, and paracentesis should be performed. Fluid taken from the abdomen should be spun for PCV determination and should undergo creatinine and BUN determination. Values higher than serum values indicate a problem and should be reported to the veterinarian in charge. Urine leakage through a cystotomy incision is treated with an indwelling urinary catheter or reoperation and appropriate urinary bladder incision closure.

URETHROSTOMY

DEFINITION

Perineal **urethrostomy** is the process of making an external opening in the urethra in the area of the perineum that is large enough for passage of urine, mucus, crystals, and small calculi without obstruction. It bypasses the narrow penile urethra, where obstruction often occurs. The procedure is performed in male cats with recurrent urethral obstruction secondary to feline urologic syndrome. Urethrostomy is also performed in other locations and procedures are named by their location (scrotal urethrostomy, prescrotal urethrostomy, antepubic urethrostomy, etc.). Scrotal urethrostomy rather than perineal urethrostomy is performed in male dogs prone to calculi obstruction or with penile scar tissue preventing normal urination, because this location provides the best functional outcome. The general technique is the same.

INDICATIONS

The primary indication for a perineal urethrostomy is multiple episodes of obstruction in association with feline urologic syndrome. Other less common indications include rupture of the penile urethra secondary to traumatic catheterization or blunt trauma (e.g., hit by a car, abdominal kick), stricture of the penile urethra, and obstruction secondary to cancer.

PREOPERATIVE CONSIDERATIONS

A cat with feline urologic syndrome can come in for examination with an array of clinical findings, as can dogs with urethral obstruction. The presentation often depends on the duration and completeness of the urinary obstruction. A common factor is straining to urinate. If the animal is brought for examination early, there is little chance that other organ systems are affected. If the animal is brought in 12 to 24 hours after a complete obstruction, severe electrolyte abnormalities, cardiac arrhythmias, kidney dysfunction, and shock can be present. These animals must have the obstruction removed and must be stabilized with establishment of improved or normal renal function before surgery when possible. Catheterization with or without light sedation may be necessary. Intravenous fluid therapy to help remove toxins is also needed. Some animals will require lifesaving measures to protect the heart from severe electrolyte abnormalities (high potassium). ECG monitoring and blood work are key diagnostics preoperatively to determine the state of the patient. Obstruction of urine flow is an emergency situation in both cats and dogs.

Depending on the suspected cause and location of the obstruction, preoperative imaging studies will be necessary to determine the exact location and extent of the problem.

TECHNIQUE AND INTRAOPERATIVE CONSIDERATIONS

The hair on the perineum and external genitalia is clipped. For perineal urethrostomy, the cat is placed in ventral recumbency with the perineum elevated approximately 30 degrees (Figure 32-36). The tail is extended directly over the dorsal midline and is immobilized with tape. A purse-string suture is placed in the anus to eliminate fecal contamination of the surgical field. Standard skin preparation is performed. For scrotal urethrostomy in male dogs, the animal is placed in dorsal recumbency, and the area is prepped as for castration and scrotal ablation.

For perineal urethrostomy, an elliptical skin incision is made around the scrotum and prepuce. The testicles are removed if the cat is intact. The penis is dissected free from

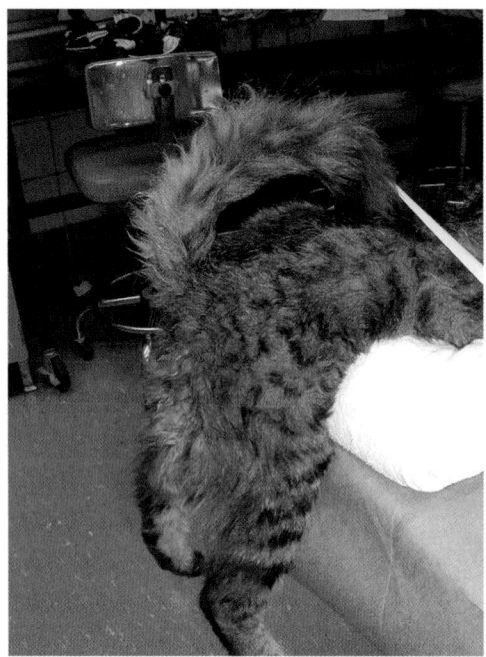

FIGURE 32-36 The perineal position can be used in the dog or cat.

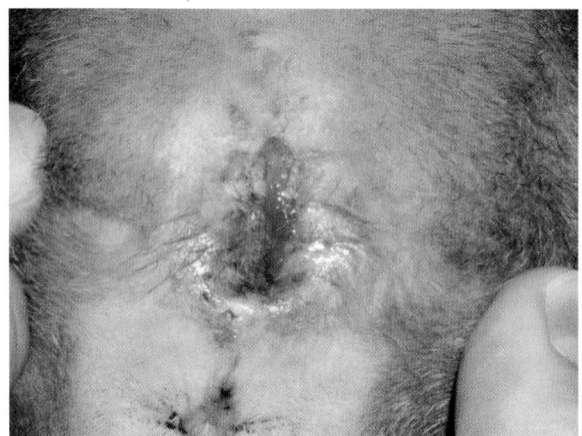

FIGURE 32-37 This is the appearance of the urethrostomy opening 14 days after surgery.

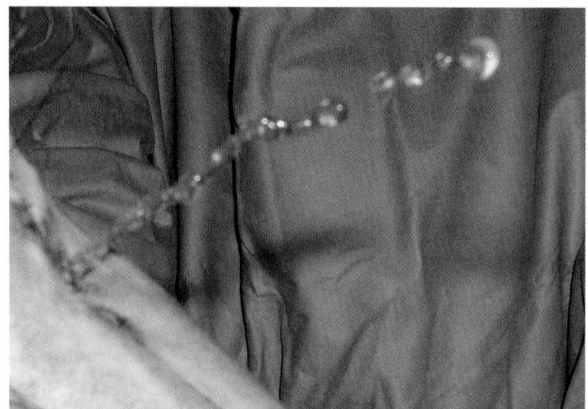

FIGURE 32-38 After urethrostomy in cats, the bladder should be gently expressed to ensure easy urine passage.

its pelvic attachments. A catheter is placed in the urethra, and a longitudinal incision is made through the penile urethra extending craniad to the level of the pelvic urethra. The diameter of the pelvic urethra is approximately 2 times that of the penile urethra. This allows normal urination in the face of crystalluria (sand-like material in the urine) and mucous plugs. The urethral mucosa is sutured to the skin. The remaining portion of the penis is amputated during urethral suturing, and the urinary catheter is removed. This results in a new, permanent opening that will accommodate the excess mucus and crystals (Figure 32-37). The bladder should be expressed at completion of the procedure to ensure that a good urine stream is obtained (Figure 32-38). Scrotal urethrostomy in male dogs is performed the same way, except that the penis is not amputated. A skin incision is made in the area of the scrotum (castration with scrotal

ablation is performed in intact dogs); this is followed by a urethral incision over a presurgically placed urethral catheter, then suturing of the urethral mucosa to the skin as for perineal urethrostomy.

POSTOPERATIVE CONSIDERATIONS

The purse-string suture is removed. Immediate postoperative care includes placement of an Elizabethan collar and examination of the surgical site for evidence of hemorrhage. The Elizabethan collar is essential to keep the animal from licking the sutures. Mild hemorrhage during urination is expected for the first 1 to 2 weeks after surgery. Blood dripping is possible, mostly after urination. This usually is of no consequence and will resolve on its own. Rarely is the bleeding severe enough to require additional surgery or transfusion. Animals should be placed on intravenous fluids for at least 24 hours after surgery, especially if urinary outflow obstruction was encountered, to maintain normal renal function and flush the urinary bladder and urethra.

The animal should be monitored carefully for normal urination in the early postoperative period. If no urine is produced for 12 hours after surgery, the bladder should be manually expressed until normal urination is seen. Postoperative catheters are discouraged because of the increased incidence of strictures at the surgery site. Some animals will have a distended and flaccid urinary bladder that will not contract normally after surgery because of overstretching of the bladder and loss of neuromuscular connections, damaged muscle tissue, and formation of scar tissue. The bladder may not function normally for several days in these animals, and manual expression and possible catheterization may be needed. Animals are prone to urinary tract infection and potential overflow incontinence. The urethrostomy site should be manipulated as little as possible. Ointments and warm cleansings are discouraged. These may delay healing or aggravate hemorrhage. For cats, the use of shredded paper or pellets in the litter box is recommended for the first 7 to 10 days. Dietary alterations will likely be necessary, depending on the composition of the mucous plug, grit, or calculi causing the obstruction, and the presence or absence of a urinary tract infection. Owners will have to be counseled on the importance of dietary modification.

The most common late postoperative complication is stricture, a narrowing of the urethral opening caused by excessive scar tissue formation. Self-mutilation of the surgery site by licking can increase the chance of stricture formation and must be prevented. Strictures typically manifest as chronic stranguria (straining to urinate). Complete obstruction of urine flow may also be noted. Stricture requires reoperation.

HERNIAS

The strict definition of *hernia* is protrusion of tissue from its normal cavity (generally the abdominal cavity) through a congenital or acquired defect in the wall of that cavity. Common hernias in the dog and cat include umbilical hernias, inguinal hernias, and diaphragmatic hernias.

UMBILICAL HERNIA
Definition
An umbilical hernia is one in which bowel or, more commonly, omentum and intra-abdominal fat protrude through a defect in the abdominal wall under the skin at the umbilicus. This hernia is most commonly congenital, and it is recognized on physical examination by the presence of swelling at the umbilicus (Figure 32-39).

Preoperative Considerations
Most umbilical hernias are not life threatening and are surgically repaired at the time of ovariohysterectomy or castration. Small hernias in young dogs (2 to 4 months of age) may be self-limiting. Larger hernias or those in older dogs (6 to 9 months of age) generally require surgical repair. Large umbilical hernias can result in intestinal entrapment (incarceration) within the confines of the hernia with resultant **strangulation** (loss of intestinal blood supply with devitalization and possible intestinal perforation). If intestinal strangulation occurs, surgical repair becomes an emergency.

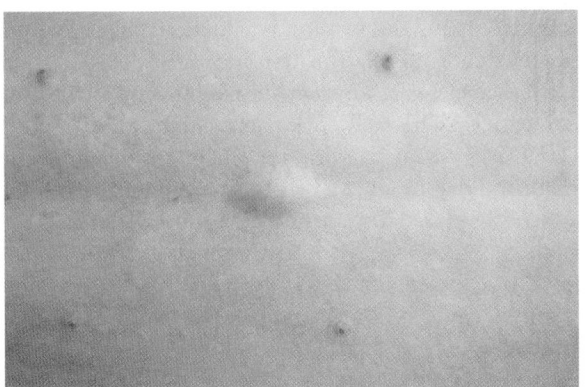

FIGURE 32-39 Note the raised lesion in the region of the umbilicus (umbilical hernia) on the ventral abdomen.

Technique and Intraoperative Considerations
The abdomen is widely clipped from xiphoid to pubis. The patient is placed in dorsal recumbency, and standard skin preparation is performed. A ventral midline incision is made directly over the hernia, with care taken to avoid perforating hernia contents. The skin is dissected away from the hernial sac; the contents are then exposed and may be replaced into the abdominal cavity (intestine) or excised (falciform or omental fat). The edges of the hernial ring are trimmed to ensure healing of the defect. The abdomen is closed in a routine fashion, as for the celiotomy incision.

Postoperative Considerations
Postoperative care is similar to that provided for any celiotomy incision. Recurrence is a rare complication of repair, and reoperation is necessary for correction.

INGUINAL HERNIA
Definition
An inguinal hernia is one in which intestine, uterus, broad ligament, intra-abdominal fat, and/or another abdominal organ protrudes through the inguinal canal as a result of a defect in the constraints of the canal. This is more common in the bitch than in the male dog. An inguinal hernia is diagnosed on physical examination by the presence of a soft, doughy, nonpainful mass in the inguinal region. Inguinal hernias can develop early or late in life. They do not spontaneously regress, and surgical correction is necessary.

Preoperative Considerations
The opposite inguinal ring should be carefully palpated for weakness. Owners should be told that hernias can develop bilaterally, even if a hernia is not present on the opposite side at the time of presentation. Owners should also be told that recurrence is rare but possible.

Technique and Intraoperative Considerations
The abdomen is widely clipped from the umbilicus to and including the inguinal area. The animal is placed in dorsal recumbency, and standard skin preparation is performed. A midline skin incision is made in the caudal abdomen between the inguinal folds. The abdominal cavity is not entered. Lateral dissection is performed carefully to expose the affected inguinal ring with its hernial sac and external pudendal vessels. The hernial sac is emptied of its contents with gentle manipulation and pressure toward the abdominal cavity. The empty sac is then excised and sutured along with the margin of the inguinal ring. Care is taken during closure to avoid the external pudendal vessels that exit from the caudal medial aspect of the ring. The skin incision is closed as for celiotomy.

Postoperative Considerations
The incision is monitored similarly to any abdominal incision. The owner should monitor for recurrence or occurrence on the opposite side.

DIAPHRAGMATIC HERNIA

Definition

A diaphragmatic hernia exists when abdominal contents protrude through an opening in the diaphragm into the thoracic cavity. Diaphragmatic hernias may be congenital or traumatic.

Preoperative Considerations

Any animal with a history of trauma or suspected trauma should be examined for the presence of a diaphragmatic hernia. Diaphragmatic hernias can be life threatening or insidious and difficult to identify. Signs can be masked by other problems. Presumptive diagnosis is based on a thorough physical examination. Classic signs of diaphragmatic hernia include a "tucked-up" abdomen (thin, empty abdomen), intestinal sounds in the chest, muffled heart and lung sounds, and dyspnea. However, some animals have only decreased lung sounds over the area of the hernia and mild exercise intolerance, if that. The diagnosis is confirmed by thoracic radiographs.

> **TECHNICIAN NOTE** Animals with a diaphragmatic hernia should have oxygen and cage confinement to allow maximal oxygenation, minimal stress, and constant monitoring for respiratory insufficiency before surgery.

An animal with a massive hernia will have a diminished intrathoracic space as a result of the presence of abdominal contents within the thoracic cavity. The resultant space-occupying mass does not allow the lungs to expand normally and compromises delivery of oxygen to the blood. These animals can have life-threatening respiratory compromise and should be treated appropriately. Any animal with respiratory compromise should be stabilized. This consists of minimal stress, oxygen cage or nasal oxygen insufflation, confinement, sternal recumbency, and constant monitoring for respiratory insufficiency or arrest. Sometimes holding the animal gently and with the head up and the rear legs hanging down will allow some abdominal contents to shift back into the abdomen. Along the same lines, the animal can be propped up in such a way that the front half of the chest and shoulders is higher than the hindquarters. Intravenous access should be established in case of an emergency, so long as the stress of catheter placement does not cause further respiratory embarrassment. Thoracic radiographs will be necessary for diagnosis and to assess for other pathologic conditions, but the animal should be stabilized to the greatest extent possible—before anesthesia. Rarely is diaphragmatic hernia repair an emergency. Mortality is actually higher in those animals operated on acutely for the problem. Only in cases of massive hernia with severe respiratory distress or severe gas distention of a herniated viscus (stomach) is immediate operation necessary. On the other hand, animals with chronic hernias have a greater chance of severe complications that could result in death. In general, operation for a diaphragmatic hernia should occur 1 to 3 days after presentation if the animal is stable. Blood work should be obtained in all traumatized animals to assess overall heath and organ function.

> **TECHNICIAN NOTE** Positioning an animal with a diaphragmatic hernia in sternal recumbency with the shoulders higher than the pelvis or gently raising the animal up from the front end may help reduce abdominal structures back into the abdomen from the thoracic cavity and improve respiration.

Technique and Intraoperative Considerations

One of the most critical times for an animal with a diaphragmatic hernia is anesthetic induction. It is important to be thoroughly familiar with induction procedures and resuscitative techniques in the event of respiratory or cardiac arrest. The animal is placed in dorsal recumbency on an incline, with the head slightly higher than the hindquarters. It is important to remember that severe respiratory compromise may result when the animal is placed in dorsal recumbency, and the technician should be prepared to breathe for the animal. Mechanical ventilation or intermittent manual respiration will be necessary throughout the procedure.

The skin is widely clipped from about 3 inches cranial to the xiphoid to the pubis. The lateral thoracic wall on at least one side, preferably the side of the hernia, should be clipped and aseptically prepared for potential chest tube placement. A ventral midline celiotomy from xiphoid to umbilicus is performed. The edges of the incision are protected with laparotomy pads, and a Balfour self-retaining abdominal retractor is placed to enhance visualization. The diaphragmatic defect is inspected, and any herniated contents are gently reduced into the abdominal cavity. If the herniated contents do not reduce easily, the diaphragmatic defect is enlarged slightly to allow easy reduction. A thorough inspection of abdominal and thoracic viscera is made to rule out organ rupture or vascular compromise.

Diaphragmatic hernia repair can require working in a deep cavity if the tear is found along the dorsal or lateral components of the diaphragm. Ventral hernias are more easily exposed for repair. Gentle retraction of viscera to expose the defect during repair is necessary to preclude damage to abdominal organs and to allow adequate visualization by the surgeon (Figure 32-40). The diaphragmatic defect is sutured with a nonabsorbable suture material in a simple continuous suture pattern. This will create an air-tight and water-tight seal. Air is evacuated from the chest by thoracocentesis through the diaphragm or with chest tube placement. The celiotomy is closed in a routine fashion. After celiotomy closure, the chest cavity is once again aspirated from the lateral thoracic wall. If a chest tube was placed, evacuation of the thoracic cavity is done through the chest tube.

Postoperative Considerations

The animal should be monitored carefully for signs of respiratory distress. It is best to waken the animal with oxygen

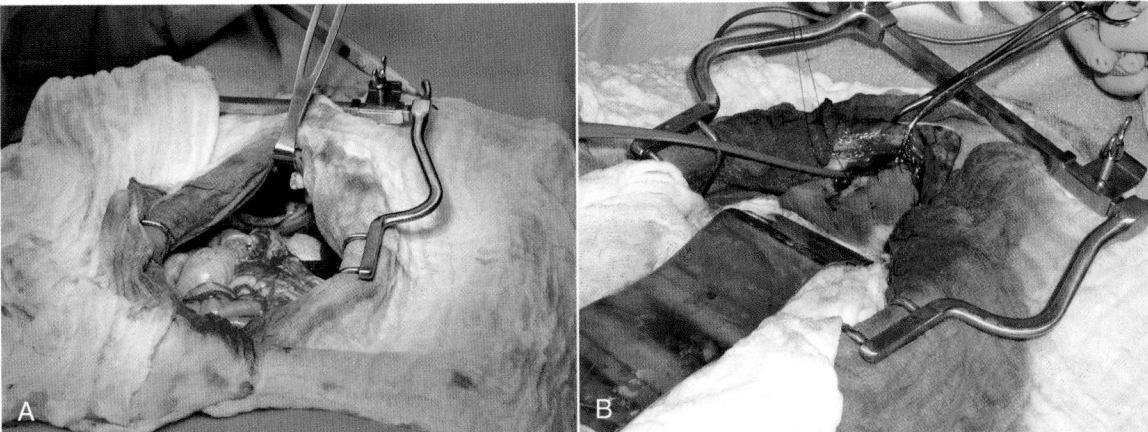

FIGURE 32-40 Diaphragmatic hernia. **A,** An Army-Navy retractor is positioned to show a large hole in the diaphragm at the cranial edge of the incision *(top of picture)*. The abdominal contents have been removed from the chest cavity and have been returned to the abdominal cavity. **B,** The defect in the diaphragm has been closed and a red-rubber catheter has been inserted into the right side of the defect near the sternum *(the left side of the picture)* for restoration of normal intrathoracic pressure before the abdominal cavity is closed.

supplementation provided through placement in an oxygen cage or through nasal insufflation. If a pulse oximeter is available, oxygen saturation should be checked frequently, especially as an attempt is made to wean the animal off oxygen. If dyspnea occurs or if the animal cannot maintain normal oxygen saturation, the chest should be evacuated with a hypodermic needle, a three-way stopcock, and a large syringe, or evacuation can be done through the chest tube. A rapid return to normal negative thoracic pressure and normal lung capacity should be seen with evacuation of air and fluid. In some cases, pulmonary trauma may also be present. This could lead to continued respiratory compromise and or pneumothorax in the early postoperative period. Most traumatic lung lesions will reseal within a week of the trauma.

If an indwelling chest tube was placed, periodic aspiration using positional changes (right lateral recumbency, left lateral recumbency, standing on hind legs, standing on front legs) will afford maximal removal of air and fluid. It is of utmost importance to keep the animal from chewing a hole in the drain or removing it from the chest cavity, and those involved in tube management should be informed on how the tube should be handled. An Elizabethan collar may be necessary, and the chest tube should be covered with a bandage. It is imperative to keep all connections on the chest drain air-tight. A security clamp should be placed on the tube to keep air from leaking into the chest if the free end of the tube is inadvertently opened. Premature removal, puncture, or inappropriate management (leaving the three-way stopcock open to the atmosphere) can result in acute animal death secondary to pneumothorax and resultant pulmonary dysfunction. Proper management of a chest tube requires full-time patient monitoring. A chart quantitating the amount of air and fluid removed during a given period (12 to 24 hours) will help to determine when the tube should be removed. Most chest tubes are removed immediately after surgery once negative intrathoracic pressure is obtained or within 12 hours of hernia repair. Otherwise, the tube can

be removed safely as the amount of air and fluid decreases toward zero.

> **TECHNICIAN NOTE** The animal with a chest tube should be handled carefully to prevent inadvertent introduction of air around the lungs and potential death of the animal. Make sure the tube is air-tight, that all connections to the environment are closed, and that it is equipped with a protective clamp.

LUMPECTOMY

DEFINITION

Lumpectomy refers to local surgical resection of a mass. The term often refers to cutaneous or subcutaneous masses.

INDICATIONS

Indications for lumpectomy include masses of cancerous origin, masses that appear to be changing over time, rapidly growing masses, ulcerative masses, or masses that are impairing function.

PREOPERATIVE CONSIDERATIONS

Some masses are related to biochemical or blood cell alterations. Blood work should be performed to evaluate for these abnormalities. Where possible, abnormalities should be corrected before anesthesia. Additionally, many animals undergoing surgery for mass resection are older and may have organ system failure, which should be evaluated before anesthesia. After a mass has been diagnosed, fine-needle aspiration of the mass may be performed. If the mass is considered benign (e.g., lipoma), resection can proceed or the owner can monitor the mass. If the mass has suspicious characteristics and may be cancerous, or if it is in a location at which future resection may not be possible if growth occurs, resection should be considered. If the mass is suspected of being cancerous, further workup for detection of metastasis should be considered. This would involve blood work, urinalysis, three-view thoracic radiographs, abdominal radiographs, and possibly abdominal ultrasound. Advance imaging or sampling of other areas may also be needed, depending on the location and character of the mass. All surgically resected masses should be submitted for histologic evaluation. Removed masses are placed in formalin at a 1:10 ratio of mass to fluid.

TECHNIQUE AND INTRAOPERATIVE CONSIDERATIONS

The skin around the area to be resected is prepared for surgery. It should be remembered that a generous clip needs to be performed because normal margins will have to be removed with the mass. Additionally, large mass resections will require that normal skin around the mass be pulled into the surgical field during closure. If the skin was not prepared aseptically before surgery, this will contaminate the surgical field. Masses should be manipulated as little as possible before surgery. A sterile marker may be used to draw an elliptical pattern around the mass to be removed after the animal is draped for surgery (Figure 32-41). One to 3 cm of normal tissue is included in the resection plane; large margins are reserved for cancerous lesions. The mass is removed and the wound closed in three or more layers, depending on the depth of dissection and resected tissue. Where large amounts of tissue were resected, active drains may have to be placed beneath the wound to prevent fluid accumulation (see Figure 32-15), or advanced surgical techniques may be needed to close the area. Rarely, some excised areas may have to be managed as an open wound. The mass is marked with ink or suture to note cranial and lateral margins for the pathologist evaluating the mass. This will facilitate future surgical planning if the mass was found to be incompletely resected.

POSTOPERATIVE CONSIDERATIONS

The surgical wound should be monitored as during any other surgical procedure. Large resections will result in

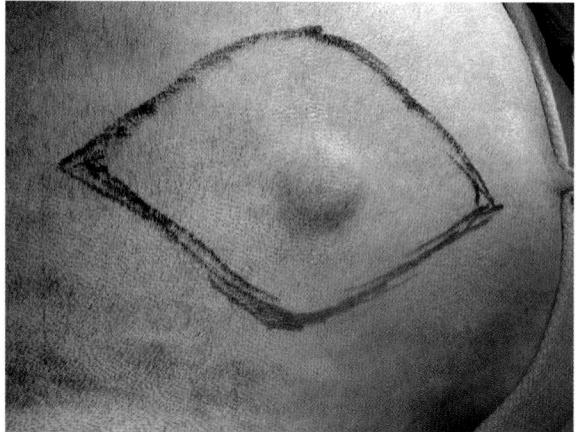

FIGURE 32-41 Surgical margins have been outlined around this skin mass for removal of the mass and a margin of normal tissue.

tension on the incision line, making dehiscence more likely. Animals should be exercise restricted until the wound is healed and sutures have been removed. Owners should be told that additional steps for treatment may be needed once a diagnosis has been obtained (future surgery if complete resection was not obtained, chemotherapy, radiation therapy, etc.).

REMOVAL OF MAMMARY NEOPLASIA

DEFINITION

Mammary neoplasia is cancer of the mammary gland. It is the most frequently occurring neoplasm in the female dog and the third most frequently found tumor in the female cat. Mastectomy is removal of a mammary gland. Radical mastectomy is removal of a chain of mammary glands on one or both sides of the animal. Lumpectomy is removal of a mammary tumor with approximately 1 cm of normal marginal tissue—not the entire mammary gland.

GENERAL INFORMATION AND INDICATIONS

In dogs, a significantly higher incidence of mammary gland tumor has been noted in nonspayed females and in females that are spayed after their first estrus. Spaying before the first estrous cycle provides a definite protective factor against mammary tumor development.

In initial stages, the tumor usually appears as a small, pea-shaped, firm mass in one or more of the glands of the mammary chain. Long-standing or fast-growing tumors may present a sizable mass with ulceration and drainage. Early diagnosis and therapy are best with mammary neoplasia.

Before surgery is considered, an examination is done to detect possible metastasis of the tumor. Malignant tumors generally metastasize to the lymph nodes and lungs. Chest radiographs may detect pulmonary metastases, and abdominal radiographs may show iliac lymph node enlargement suggestive of metastasis, but abdominal ultrasound may more clearly identify subtle abdominal abnormalities. About 50% of mammary tumors in dogs are malignant, and about 80% to 90% of mammary tumors in cats are malignant. Surgical resection of tumors that have already metastasized does not improve prognosis. At the time of surgery, biopsy of regional lymph nodes should always be performed.

Surgery is currently considered the most effective therapy. The primary objectives of surgical treatment are to remove completely the tumor tissue for potential cure, and to obtain a histologic diagnosis of tumor type and behavior.

TECHNIQUE AND INTRAOPERATIVE CONSIDERATIONS

Two techniques are available for tumor resection. In dogs, there appears to be no advantage of radical gland resection versus lumpectomy unless the tumor is incompletely excised.

Lumpectomy affords the same long-term outcome associated with varying forms of mastectomy as long as the tumor is freely movable, small, and on the periphery of the gland. If the tumor is centralized within a gland, if multiple tumors are present within a gland or a chain of glands, or if the tumor is large and/or fixed, a more radical excision is warranted. In cats, unlike in dogs, recurrence is decreased if a unilateral mastectomy is performed rather than local excision of the mass. If bilateral radical mastectomy is necessary, the procedure must be staged (removal of one side at a time) to allow less tension on the skin closure. The skin is clipped widely to include all affected mammary glands. The animal is placed in dorsal recumbency, and a standard skin preparation is performed. An elliptical incision is made, attempting to include a 1-cm margin around the tumor. The skin and tumor, with or without the mammary gland, are gently undermined and removed. The skin incision is often gaping after tumor excision if an entire gland is removed, requiring meticulous subcutaneous closure. Subcutaneous tissues are closed with a simple interrupted pattern using absorbable suture material. An active drain may be placed if a large amount of tissue is removed to help prevent fluid accumulation under the skin. The skin is closed in a routine fashion. The excised mammary masses are placed in formalin and sent to a laboratory for histopathologic evaluation.

POSTOPERATIVE CONSIDERATIONS

Major complications that can occur postoperatively are generally related to tension placed on the skin to adequately close the wound when large amounts of tissue are removed. Seroma formation is common, especially if a drain was not placed at the time of surgery and the resection was large. It is best to bandage these animals for 48 to 72 hours postoperatively to help prevent large amounts of fluid from accumulating under the incision, and to make the animal more comfortable if radical excision was performed. Warm compresses may be needed after seroma development. Dehiscence is not common, but the incision should be examined daily for evidence of separation, especially if a large amount of tissue is removed. Bruising along the incision edges is common and should be expected. Immediate postoperative hemorrhage can occur. In the event of oozing blood, an abdominal bandage should be applied with gentle pressure. If a drain was placed, a bandage should be placed over the drain. The drain is emptied several times a day and is removed when minimal drainage is noted. If the animal irritates the incision by licking, an Elizabethan collar should be applied until suture removal. An Elizabethan collar should be applied as long as a drain is in place to prevent self-inflicted pulling or breaking of the drain. The animal should be exercise restricted, especially if a large incision under tension is present, to help prevent dehiscence and seroma formation. Radical mastectomy is a painful procedure, and pain management should be continued for at least 5 days postoperatively.

AMPUTATION

DEFINITION

Amputation refers to partial or complete removal of a body part, such as a limb or a toe. This section covers limb amputation.

INDICATIONS

Indications for amputation include appendicular cancer not amenable to local excision or another treatment modality (amputation may be curative or may be done as palliative therapy in some instances); severe neurologic dysfunction resulting in repeated trauma to a limb; nonunion fractures that will not result in limb function with orthopedic repair; irresolvable osteomyelitis; vascular disease of the limb, such as thrombosis or arteriovenous fistula; and congenital deformity resulting in a nonfunctional limb that is not amenable to orthopedic repair. Simple limb fracture is not an indication for amputation, although some veterinarians may perform the procedure for that problem.

PREOPERATIVE CONSIDERATIONS

Amputation can involve considerable blood loss. It is important to perform presurgical blood work, including assessment of ability to coagulate, to determine the animal's overall heath and to identify any concerns for anesthesia. Abnormalities should be corrected where possible before anesthesia. Furthermore, transfusion should be given or anticipated depending on the animal's preoperative values. Additionally, coagulation times should be assessed. A thorough orthopedic examination should be done to evaluate concurrent orthopedic problems. The owner needs to be aware of other orthopedic conditions that are diagnosed and how they may affect function after amputation. Orthopedic problems in other limbs can make ambulation after amputation difficult, depending on the severity and the type of problem. The owner should be made aware of neurologic problems affecting other limbs. This too can lead to difficult ambulation after amputation. When amputation is done because of neoplasia, the animal should be screened appropriately for metastasis before undergoing surgery. The amputation must be planned so that adequate margins of normal tissue are obtained if cancer is involved. Amputation is a painful procedure, and analgesics are best initiated before surgery and continued without interruption in the postoperative period.

For rear limb amputations with disarticulation of the coxofemoral joint in intact male dogs, scrotal swelling is a major concern. Seroma formation after amputation is common, and fluid tends to accumulate in the scrotum. Scrotal swelling can become so severe that ablation is necessary. Additionally, the scrotum is more visible after amputation and may not be aesthetically pleasing to some owners. It is best to perform a scrotal ablation and castration at the time of amputation in these dogs.

TECHNIQUE AND PERIOPERATIVE CONSIDERATIONS

The limb is suspended from an intravenous fluid stand as for an orthopedic procedure. The limb is clipped and aseptically prepared for surgery. The clip should be generous and should include the skin around the base of the limb to prevent contamination during closure. In general, a skin incision is made around the limb in the area to be amputated. A surgical assistant is needed to help hold the limb in various positions during surgery while dissection occurs. Vessels are ligated and transected, and nerves are blocked with local anesthetic and then transected. Subcutaneous and muscle tissues are dissected and transected for removal of the limb. Depending on the site of amputation, the limb may have to be disarticulated or the bone severed to remove the limb. Remaining muscle and subcutaneous tissue are closed over the bone and/or the wound bed. The skin is closed in three layers. If a large amount of dead space is present at the time of closure, a closed, active drain may have to be placed.

Thoracic limb amputation can be done by removal of the scapula and the entire forelimb (forequarter amputation), by disarticulation of the scapulohumeral joint, or by **ostectomy** (excision and removal of all or part of the bone) at the level of the proximal humerus. Forequarter amputation offers the advantages that major vessels and nerves are well visualized, sectioning of the bone is not required, and the prominent scapular spine will not be present as the scapular muscle mass atrophies. It is also indicated in neoplastic diseases of the humerus (especially proximal) or of the scapula. Disarticulation leaves a more full appearance to the thorax and requires less extensive dissection, but muscle atrophy over the scapula can be unsightly in some cases. If disarticulation is performed, the acromion process should be excised to improve appearance. Proximal humeral amputation may be faster for some.

Pelvic limb amputation can be accomplished by disarticulation of the coxofemoral joint or by proximal femoral osteotomy. Proximal femoral osteotomy yields a more cosmetic result, particularly in an intact male dog. It is faster and easier than disarticulation. However, the remaining stump will move as the animal ambulates, and owners must be made aware of this. Neoplastic diseases of the femur will require disarticulation to obtain a normal margin of tissue.

POSTOPERATIVE CONSIDERATIONS

Postoperative complications are not a major concern but should not be ignored. Animals undergoing amputation are painful, and analgesics must be given. It is best to give analgesics as scheduled doses rather than on an "as needed" basis. Analgesics will likely be required after surgery.

Seroma formation is common. The area can be cold compressed for the first 24 hours after surgery, and if a seroma forms, warm compresses can be initiated. The limb should be bandaged for the first 24 to 48 hours, if possible (Figure 32-42). This will provide some comfort for the animal and will help minimize seroma formation. The animal should be exercise restricted because motion will increase the size of the seroma. Hematoma is also a possibility.

Seroma or formation of hematoma after surgery can increase the chance of infection. If infection occurs, the incision site may have to be opened and drained, and a culture and sensitivity obtained. Anemia can occur in the postoperative period as a result of blood loss at the time of surgery. Transfusion may be necessary. Intravenous fluids should be administered postoperatively until eating and drinking are

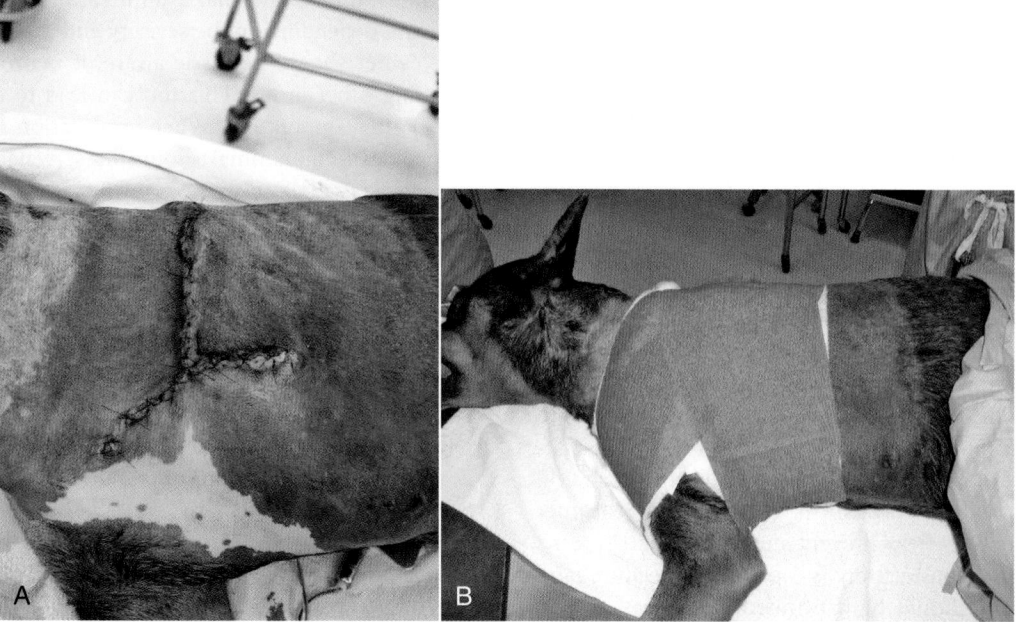

FIGURE 32-42 A, Amputation incision immediately postoperatively. B, A bandage has been applied to the surgical area to provide compression and incisional protection.

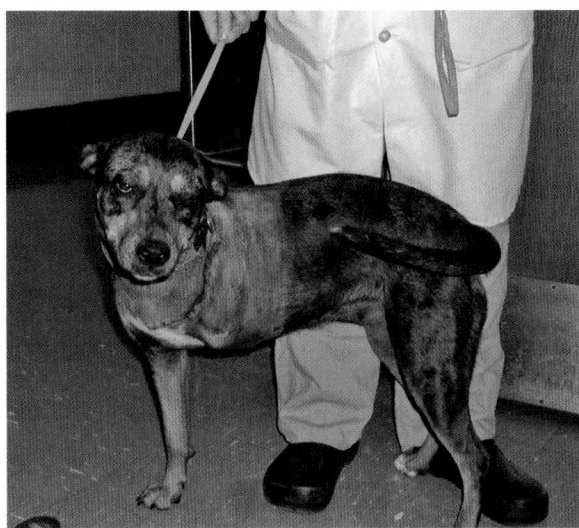

FIGURE 32-43 This dog's front leg was amputated the day before this picture was taken. Note how willing the dog is to be up and moving around, and that support is not needed even 1 day postoperatively.

resumed. Additionally, the animal should be kept in a well-padded area and supported with a sling when taken out for a walk (until the animal learns to ambulate on three legs). Tension on the incision line, seroma formation, or infection may lead to dehiscence. Depending on the cause and degree of dehiscence, this is managed conservatively or with surgical closure. Animals with neoplasia may develop metastatic disease or may have tumor recurrence at the surgery site.

Amputation is generally more traumatic for the owner than for the pet. Three-legged dogs and cats are excellent pets, and it is important to help the owner understand this. Most animals are ambulating within 24 hours of surgery (Figure 32-43), but some may take a little longer. Almost all are ambulatory within 2 days of surgery. Animals should be kept in the hospital until they are ambulating and their pain seems well controlled. Amputees have an excellent prognosis unless the limb was amputated for neoplastic disease. For neoplasia, the prognosis depends on the type of tumor. Most owners are satisfied regardless of the reason for amputation; the age, breed, or weight of the animal; or the animal's survival time after surgery.

NEUROLOGIC PATIENT CARE

The most common neurologic disorder in the dog is spontaneous intervertebral disc rupture. Discs are normally found between vertebral bodies in the spine and act as shock absorbers during spinal movement. Over time, discs can undergo degeneration and calcification. When this occurs, the normal shock absorber–like effect is impaired, and extrusion (rupture) of disc material into the spinal canal can occur. This puts pressure on the spinal cord and can cause an array of neurologic deficits or pain. Other neurologic disorders that may be encountered include atlantoaxial subluxation in toy breeds (abnormal articulation between the first and second cervical vertebrae); acute spinal trauma

(fracture or luxation); lumbosacral stenosis/malarticulation or cauda equina (compression of the lumbosacral nerve roots); cervical vertebral malarticulation/malformation; spinal cyst; cancers of the spinal column, brain, nerves, or spinal cord; malformation of the caudal brain fossa; and hypdrocephalus. Many animals with neurologic problems are referred to specialty hospitals for surgery. However, the veterinary technician should be familiar with some of the procedures that might be performed and should understand how to manage neurologic patients in general, so that when they return to the veterinary hospital for care after surgery, the technician knows what to do.

One neurosurgical procedure that is occasionally performed in small animal practice is intervertebral disc fenestration. During this procedure, each disc that is calcified or that may become calcified is removed (scraped) from the intervertebral space. This procedure is performed under some circumstances to help deter rupture of the disc material into the spinal canal, although its benefit is unproven. Dogs may develop spontaneous intervertebral disc extrusions in the cervical spine (neck) or the thoracolumbar spine (lower back). If the disc has already ruptured and the animal's ability to ambulate is affected, a decompressive procedure must be performed to alleviate compression on the spinal cord. The most common decompressive procedures are ventral slot (for cervical disc rupture) and hemilaminectomy (for thoracolumbar disc rupture). For acute disc herniation, the most commonly affected breed is the Dachshund, but the Beagle, Pekingese, Poodle, Spaniel, and Terrier breeds also frequently experience disc herniation.

SURGICAL TECHNIQUE AND PERIOPERATIVE CONSIDERATIONS

When an animal with spinal column instability is anesthetized, the normal protective abilities of muscle support and conscious perception of pain are removed. Conditions that can result in instability include spinal fracture or luxation and atlantoaxial instability. Animals with simple disc herniation or spinal malformation can be worsened by excessive manipulation while under anesthesia. It is the responsibility of the veterinary technician, the anesthesiologist, and the surgeon to protect the animal from further neurologic damage by handling the spine with care while under anesthesia. It is important to keep the neck and the back as straight as possible when moving the animal from one location to another. To accomplish this, the animal can be taped to a rigid, flat surface; can be carefully cradled in the arm; or can be placed in a stiff blanket sling supported on all sides. No matter how the animal is carried, one should be careful to avoid manipulation of the affected area. The means of transportation is often dictated by the size of the animal, but a rigid, flat surface is the preferred method for transporting animals with severe instability of the thoracolumbar spine. For cervical instability, a neck brace can be placed. Sometimes however, it is easiest to place the unrestrained animal on blankets or on a firm surface in a basket or a topless carrier, so the blanket or hard surface can just be lifted out

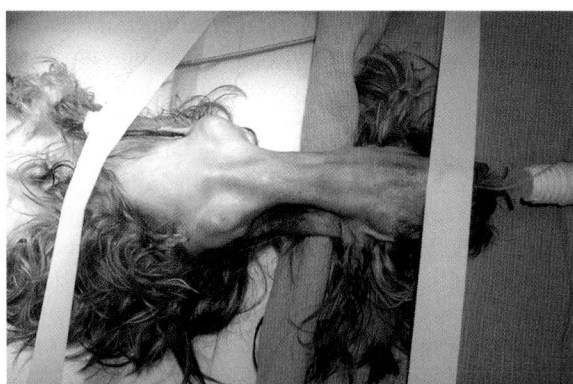

FIGURE 32-44 Proper positioning for cervical disc surgery.

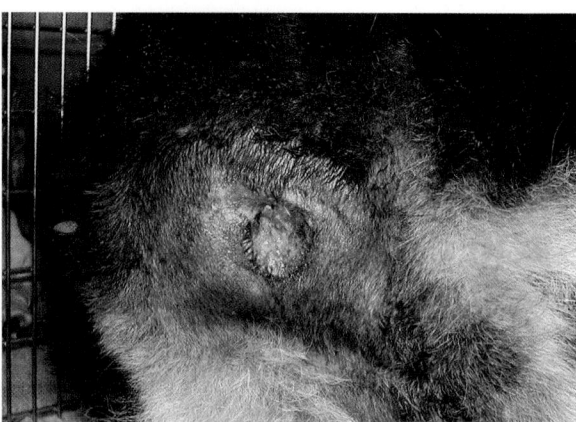

FIGURE 32-45 Decubital ulcer (pressure sore). The ulcer developed over the greater trochanter of this dog as a result of improper care during recovery from spinal surgery.

with the animal supported on top. The awake animal will often protect a painful spinal fracture to prevent excess motion and will lie mostly still without the need to be taped down. Greater concern is evoked by the animal that is thrashing, severely sedate, or anesthetized.

Animals undergoing cervical disc surgery are placed in dorsal recumbency with the head and neck in slight extension (Figure 32-44). The ventral aspect of the neck is widely clipped from the manubrium sterni to the cranial aspect of the larynx. Standard skin preparation is performed. A ventral midline incision is made through the skin and muscles to expose the intervertebral spaces. For fenestration, a dental tartar scraper, a curved needle, a fenestration hook, or a curette can be used to remove disc material from the interspace. Fenestration is carried out from the C2-3 to C6-7 disc space. If decompression is needed, an oblong slot is made through vertebral bodies into the spinal canal using a pneumatic or electrically powered bur. The disc material is then carefully removed from the spinal canal. A fat graft is placed over the spinal cord in the defect to prevent restrictive scar formation. The surgical wound is closed in layers with a continuous suture pattern using an absorbable suture. The skin is closed in a routine fashion.

Animals undergoing thoracolumbar disc surgery are placed in ventral recumbency. For fenestration, the dorsum over the back is widely clipped from the midthoracic region to the pelvis. Standard skin preparation is performed. A skin incision is made from T11 to L6. Careful dissection between epaxial muscles (muscles of the back) allows palpation and limited visualization of the disc spaces. For fenestration, each space between T10 and L5 is curetted with a technique similar to that described for cervical disc fenestration. If decompression is needed, a portion of the bony lamina covering the spinal cord is removed with a pneumatic or electrically powered bur or bone rongeurs. The ruptured disc material is then carefully removed from the spinal canal. A fat graft is placed in the defect over the spinal cord. Muscles, subcutaneous tissue, and skin are closed in a routine fashion.

POSTOPERATIVE CONSIDERATIONS

Preoperative and postoperative care of neurologic patients depends on their neurologic status and the type of

neurologic disease that they have. Management for the non-ambulatory animal is demanding. Animals are subject to decubital ulcers or pressure sores (Figure 32-45), urinary bladder infections, joint stiffness, muscle atrophy (muscle wasting), pneumonia, and gastrointestinal ulceration. Preventing these conditions from occurring is the main objective of proper postoperative management, and steps should include the following:

- Passive range-of-motion exercises, muscle massages, underwater treadmill activity, sling walking, and whirlpool baths encourage joint motion and muscular activity and help decrease the occurrence of pressure sores. Passive range of motion should be performed at least 3 times a day on all affected limbs until the animal is able to ambulate normally.
- Urinary bladder expression should be performed 4 or 5 times per day to keep the urinary bladder empty. This will help keep the animal clean, will prevent detrusor muscle atony secondary to bladder overdistention (which can lead to permanent bladder dysfunction), and might lower the incidence of infection resulting from urine retention.

> **TECHNICIAN NOTE**   For animals that cannot consciously urinate, it is important to keep the urinary bladder empty by urinary catheterization or manual expression. This will prevent overdistention with permanent urinary bladder dysfunction, will keep the animal clean, and will help decrease the infection rate.

- Flip the animal frequently (every 4 hours) to reduce the incidence of pneumonia and to help prevent pressure sore formation. Slings and wheelchairs can be used to get the animal up and off pressure points for a time if the spinal injury is stable.
- Monitor the animal daily for fever, cough, or respiratory distress. The down animal is at risk for pneumonia. Daily coupage and getting the animal up will help prevent this. Fever may be an indication of severe gastrointestinal ulcer formation.

- Keep the animal in a well-padded area to prevent the formation of sores. A water bed mattress works well for large dogs.
- Keep the animal clean and dry. Soiling will increase the chance of pressure sore formation. This can be challenging when incontinence and immobility play a role.
- Observe the stool daily for evidence of fresh blood (bright red on feces or thermometer) or digested blood (dark, tarry feces), which may be an indicator of colonic or gastric ulceration, respectively, which can occur after spinal cord injury, hospital stress, and/or steroid therapy.
- Observe vomiting. If the vomitus contains coffee ground–like material, it is indicative of gastric bleeding secondary to ulcer formation.
- Observe the animal daily for evidence of pressure sores. Sores tend to form over bony prominences, especially in large dogs. Formation of pressure sores can lead to sepsis and death if severe, and their presence should not be taken lightly. Prompt treatment should be initiated to prevent severe complications. Treatment consists of frequent flipping, whirlpool baths, massages, antibiotics, clipping and cleaning of the area, surgical débridement, and/or bandages placed to alleviate pressure over a prominence, depending on the severity of the lesion. Prevention is the best form of therapy.

TECHNICIAN NOTE It is better to prevent pressure sore formation than to have to treat a pressure sore once it occurs.

- Animals that have lost pain sensation in one or more limbs should be monitored carefully. These animals may begin to lick or chew the asensory (lack of feeling) portions of their limbs, especially if the area becomes traumatized. Some will even chew off toes or whole limbs. If an animal without sensation to a limb begins to lick the limb, an Elizabethan collar should be placed immediately.
- Animals that cannot feel their legs may develop ascending or descending myelomalacia. This rare problem is associated with severe spinal cord damage with loss of deep pain sensation, in which progressive loss of spinal cord function occurs as the result of progressive hemorrhage and destruction of normal tissue by inflammatory mediators. Animals that develop this unfortunate complication may be very painful, may show progression from rear limb paralysis to forelimb involvement, may exhibit a change from upper motor neuron myotactic reflexes to lower motor neuron, and may exhibit gradual loss of panniculus (fly twitch) response along the back. It is important to alert the surgeon if this is suspected because the problem is progressive, and animals eventually suffocate because of loss of diaphragm function. Euthanasia before this occurs is recommended.
- Animals that cannot walk should never be allowed to roam free. They will traumatize their skin as they drag themselves around and can develop serious abrasions and ulcers.
- Animals with some motor function in the limbs and a stable spinal injury should be gotten up at least 3 times a day and encouraged to use their limbs. Ambulatory but ataxic animals should be supported when ambulating to help prevent falls that might lead to further spinal damage. Rehabilitation through specialized centers offering underwater treadmill work and other rehabilitation techniques should be considered.

TECHNICIAN NOTE Animals with injuries to the cervical spine should always be placed in a harness rather than in a collar to prevent further cervical damage.

All animals with neurologic injuries require cage rest and controlled activity to allow the spinal column to heal. All should be leashed when outdoors (animals with cervical problems should always be placed in a harness rather than in a neck collar to prevent further cervical damage), crated when indoors, and restricted according to the surgeon's protocol. Owners should be carefully counseled on the importance of confinement for prevention of further spinal injury.

TECHNICIAN NOTE All animals with a spinal injury will require cage rest, whether or not surgery is done. It is important to emphasize to owners that cage rest is important for proper healing, even if the pet is walking and feeling normal.

As can be seen from the preceding list, the veterinary technician and the veterinarian must work diligently and continually to properly manage animals with neurologic dysfunction.

ORTHOPEDIC SURGERY

LONG-BONE FRACTURES

Preoperative Considerations

When an animal is brought to the veterinary hospital with a fracture, several steps must be taken to ready the animal for a permanent repair. First, the animal must be stabilized with respect to all other body systems (treated for shock, chest injuries, and abdominal injuries). Second, any open wounds associated with the fracture should be managed. Third, the fracture must be immobilized by means of a bandage, cast, or sling if the fracture is in a location amenable to bandaging (review Chapter 26). Once these three steps have been achieved, fracture repair can be safely considered. Most long-bone fractures are not life threatening and do not require emergency surgery. Stability of the animal determines when the fracture is repaired.

> **TECHNICIAN NOTE** Most long-bone fractures are not life threatening and do not require emergency surgery.

Intraoperative Considerations

The limb is usually suspended from the foot. An extensive hair clip is required on all limb preparations. The limb will usually undergo extensive manipulation during reduction and repair. For this reason, the limb is clipped from the level of the metacarpus or metatarsus to the scapula or pelvis, respectively, including medial and lateral aspects of the extremity. This may vary slightly, depending on the particular bone that is fractured, but the general rule should be to perform a wide and thorough clip. Remaining hair at the tip of the paw is covered with a rubber glove or plastic wrap that is taped to the clipped skin. Refer to Chapter 31, "Surgical Assistance and Suture Material," for detailed instructions on preparing limbs for orthopedic surgery.

Positioning

Animal positioning depends on the specific bone that is fractured. Generally, the following positions are recommended for different types of fractures:

- Femur: lateral recumbency, affected side up
- Tibia-fibula: lateral recumbency, affected leg down (it may be easiest to start with the patient in dorsal recumbency and to roll the animal over after draping)
- Humerus: lateral recumbency, affected leg up
- Radius-ulna: dorsal recumbency, affected leg craniad; or lateral recumbency, affected leg up
- Pelvis: lateral recumbency, affected leg up

With so much skin exposed, skin preparation is time-consuming, but it must be meticulous. The surgeon eventually covers the extremity with a sterile stockinette, but this should not preclude adequate skin preparation.

Surgical Assistance

Orthopedic procedures are often difficult and time-consuming and may demand the help of an assistant. Often, the veterinary technician is called on to participate as a surgical assistant and therefore should have a general understanding of orthopedic tissue handling and instrumentation (specifics of intraoperative assistance are covered in Chapters 30 and 31).

Several basic maneuvers commonly required by the surgeon are often performed by the veterinary technician. They include retraction, muscle fatigue, alignment and reduction, and suction of the field. Proper techniques for each are discussed separately.

Retraction

Care should be taken to preserve soft tissues in the operative field. It will be necessary to have functional muscle groups remaining when the bone is repaired. Retraction should be firm but not so traumatic as to bruise or tear the muscle. The tissues should be kept moist. Tissue desiccation can cause tissue death and loss of function.

Muscle Fatigue

Fractures in large breed dogs or fractures that are 3 to 5 days old may be difficult to reduce because of heavy muscle mass or severe muscle contraction, respectively. In such cases, constant, steady traction on the muscle groups will cause them to fatigue and relax, thus facilitating reduction. Epidural anesthetics and/or paralytics can be used to aid in muscle reduction (review Chapter 29).

Alignment and Reduction

For repair of fractured bones, the ends must be reduced and aligned. It is often necessary for an assistant to hold reduction during fixation of the fracture. Pins, wires, screws, and plates of stainless steel may be used to achieve the necessary fixation.

Suction

Whenever a fracture occurs, bleeding into the fracture site can be massive. Some continuous oozing occurs during fixation. A clean surgical field is of the utmost importance in facilitating early and accurate reduction and fixation. Pay particular attention to ensuring that fracture lines remain visible because the surgeon needs to see them for reduction and alignment.

Postoperative Considerations

Some postoperative orthopedic patients may require external coaptation. Applied bandages should be managed as previously discussed (refer to Chapter 26). Animals undergoing orthopedic surgery will likely require limited passive activity. Animals should be encouraged to use the operated limb to increase blood supply to the fracture site, to maintain joint and muscle health, and to speed fracture healing. However, limb use should be slow, deliberate, and well controlled. No off-leash activity, running, jumping, or playing with other animals should be allowed. A crate is the best place for animals that are recovering from an orthopedic procedure when the veterinarian, the veterinary technician, or the owner is not strictly controlling them. The only orthopedic procedure in which activity is strongly encouraged is femoral head and neck excision, for which rehabilitation, building of muscle mass, and encouragement of weight bearing are extremely important for optimal limb function. It is also important to realize the relatively unsure gait of a three-legged dog or cat, and, when exercising the animal, one must be certain to avoid slippery surfaces (vinyl or wet floors). Cement, grass, dirt, carpet, or rubber matting provides a much more sure-footed environment.

Rehabilitation is an important part of recovery. Slowly flexing and extending of affected joints along with muscle massage will improve limb blood flow, maintain joint health, improve joint range of motion, improve muscle tone, and reduce muscle contraction. Range-of-motion exercises should be repeated 2 to 3 times per day with 10 to 15 repetitions of the exercise. A demonstration by the technician of proper technique will aid the client in understanding the therapy. Slow leash walking is performed to encourage limb use. The faster the animal is walked, the more likely it will carry the affected limb.

JOINTS

Preoperative Considerations

Most orthopedic procedures involving a joint are elective and patients rarely need emergency care. Traumatic fractures and luxations, however, do require urgent treatment. Preoperative management should include limiting the animal's activity and controlling pain. External coaptation is rarely necessary for nonurgent cases but will make the traumatically injured animal (animals with luxations or fractures) more comfortable if the particular area involved is amenable to bandaging. For some injuries, such as cranial cruciate ligament tear, joint range of motion can be done before surgery to improve joint health. Indications for joint surgery include dislocations, ligament ruptures, infections, fractures, synovial biopsy, **arthrodesis** (surgical fusion of a joint), and treatment of **osteochondrosis** (abnormally thickened portion of the articular cartilage).

Intraoperative Considerations

An extensive clip, as for fractures, should be done for joint surgery. Positions will vary depending on the joint involved. Generally, the following positions are recommended:

Hip: lateral recumbency, affected leg up

Stifle: lateral recumbency, affected leg up; or dorsal recumbency, leg hanging off the end of the table

Shoulder: lateral recumbency, affected leg up

Tarsus: lateral recumbency, affected leg up

Elbow: lateral recumbency, affected leg up (or down for medial approaches)

Carpus: lateral recumbency, affected leg up; or dorsal recumbency

Intraoperative assistance in joint surgery is similar to that necessary in fracture repair. Some special precautions should be taken while joints are exposed.

Retraction

Care should be taken to avoid placing retractors in direct contact with the articular cartilage. This would damage the cartilage, and cartilage has a relatively poor response to trauma. When exposure of the joint is necessary, sharp retraction of the joint capsule will decrease trauma while increasing exposure.

> **TECHNICIAN NOTE** Care should be taken to avoid placing retractors in direct contact with the articular cartilage, and the cartilage should be kept moist to prevent permanent cartilage damage.

Flush

The cartilage should be frequently flushed with saline to keep it from drying out during the procedure. This is true of all tissues, especially the articular cartilage because of its poor regenerative ability.

Postoperative Considerations

Postoperative care of animals undergoing joint surgery is variable, depending on the surgical procedure, the joint involved, and the surgeon's preference. Early passive range-of-motion activity with light joint usage is recommended for most animals undergoing joint surgery. Heavy joint use is discouraged in the early postoperative period. Animals should be encouraged to use the affected joint during slow, leash-controlled walks but are discouraged from running or jumping on the limb. Joint use is increased gradually over the course of recovery, which is variable depending on the procedures performed. Joint immobilization is necessary in some cases, such as luxation, but is discouraged in most instances and can result in severe limitations in joint range of motion after recovery if care is not taken to rehabilitate the joint carefully.

> **TECHNICIAN NOTE** It is important to encourage limb use for optimal recovery after long-bone or joint surgery. This is best done by slow, controlled leash walking at limited times throughout the day. Running, jumping, and off-leash activity are not allowed.

CLIENT EDUCATION

The care an animal receives at home can be just as important as the care it received at the veterinary clinic. In a matter of seconds, a surgery can be "undone" with inappropriate care. Failure to communicate concerns associated with the patient's primary problem and postoperative care can make the clinic liable for some complications.

The surgical patient has special needs. Some of these needs are general for all surgical patients, and others are specific to the surgical procedure performed. The following questions help guide client education and communication with the pet owner at the time of discharge.

1. What is the intensity of patient care required after discharge?

Veterinary technicians communicate to clients the level of patient care required at home. Simple procedures require minor confinement, few medications, and incision monitoring; other patients may require more intensive home care. If the intensity of care needed is beyond the level that a layperson can be expected to provide, discharge should be reconsidered and postponed until the level of care needed is reduced to a manageable level. Transfer to a specialty clinic for 24-hour care may be another option, although the cost of prolonged care or specialized care may be challenging or prohibitive for the client.

2. Can the owner provide the needed home care?

Different pet owners are more or less capable of providing home care, depending on the individual's physical abilities, as well as time constraints and circumstances. Veterinary technicians should confirm that if the owner is not able to care for the pet, alternate sources of care are provided.

3. What form of communication is best for helping the client understand the animal's needs at the time of dismissal?

Several methods of client education are available; what works best will depend on the nature of the surgical procedure performed and the personality of the client. Forms of communication include written instructions, handouts, verbal instructions, personal demonstrations, computer-based resources, and videos. In some cases, more than one form of communication may be needed.

4. What major concerns should be relayed to the owner for monitoring purposes?

Not only should general care be relayed to the client, but pet owners should also be made aware of potential complications, symptoms of concern, and particular concerns that the surgeon may have relative to the surgical procedure. The owner should be instructed on how to best monitor the patient for these potential complications.

5. If complications or emergencies arise, what should the client do?

The veterinary clinician should make sure that owners receive clear contact instructions in case of an emergency or complication, depending on the time of day that the emergency occurs. Also, the clinician should educate clients about on-call emergency schedules and let them know that the pet's surgeon may not be available during an emergency. Clients should be given numbers to call for general concerns and questions.

6. When should the animal return to the clinic for repeat evaluation?

If bandage changes or rechecks will be needed, those visits ideally should be set up on the day of discharge. Veterinary technicians should keep a list of animals that were discharged, so that a call-back system can be established to check on the client and the pet 1 to 2 days after discharge.

GUIDELINES FOR DISCHARGE INSTRUCTIONS

Discharge instructions should be tailored to the procedure performed. A single form should not be used for every procedure because specialized care may be required for some patients. However, general instructions that can be followed for every procedure should be provided, along with modifications based on need. Basic instructions would include medication administration, incision monitoring, activity restriction, and contact information in the event of a problem. Refer to Chapter 3 and to the Evolve Site for specific examples of discharge instructions. If some form of rehabilitation is required, instructions and methods should be both written and demonstrated for the client. The same holds true for any specialized treatment technique such as feeding tube management, wound care, drain care, and feeding instructions.

The veterinary technician should include in the medical record all communications and a copy of the discharge instructions. Maintaining appropriate medical record details is important for future reference and is a legal responsibility. Discharge instructions are generally posted as the last entry in the medical record before the patient's return for the follow-up visit. Ensure that the record is complete with a surgery report from the surgeon, a list of treatments performed, and signed consent forms. Remember to place the client on a future communication reminder for a follow-up phone call 1 to 2 days after discharge.

RECOMMENDED READINGS

Dunning D: Surgical wound infection and the use of antimicrobials. In Slatter D, editor: Textbook of small animal surgery, ed 3, vol 1, St Louis, 2002, Saunders.

Licroy MD, Bartels KE: Surgical lasers. In Slatter D, editor: Textbook of small animal surgery, ed 3, vol 1, St Louis, 2002, Saunders.

Quandt JE: Postoperative patient care. In Slatter D, editor: Textbook of small animal surgery, ed 3, vol 1, St Louis, 2002, Saunders.

Seim HB III, Creed JF: Restraint techniques for prevention of self-trauma. In Bojrab MJ, editor: Current techniques in small animal surgery, ed 4, St Louis, 1998, Lea & Febiger.

Shmon C: Assessment and preparation of the surgical patient and the operating team. In Slatter D, editor: Textbook of small animal surgery, ed 3, vol 1, St Louis, 2002, Saunders.

Tear M: Small animal surgical nursing: skills and concepts, ed 2, St Louis, 2011, Mosby.

33 Large Animal Surgical Nursing*

Colin F. Mitchell

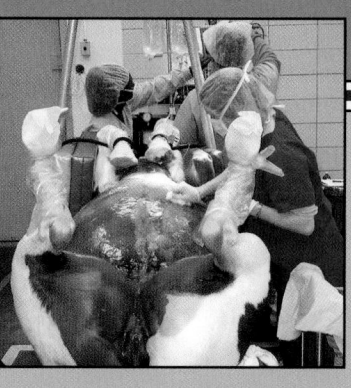

OUTLINE

SURGICAL NURSING OF HORSES, *1261*
Overview, *1261*
Preoperative Preparation, *1261*
Intraoperative Nursing, *1261*
Postoperative Nursing, *1262*
Surgical Considerations, *1263*
Gastrointestinal Tract Surgery, *1263*
Urogenital Tract Surgery, *1266*
Orthopedic Surgery, *1269*
Upper Respiratory Tract Surgery, *1276*

**SURGICAL NURSING OF FOOD
ANIMALS,** *1278*
Preoperative Preparation, *1278*
**Conditions of the Gastrointestinal
Tract,** *1279*
Oral Lacerations, *1279*
Mandibular Fractures, *1279*
Laparotomies, *1280*
Regional Analgesic Techniques for
Abdominal Surgery, *1280*
Surgical Approaches to the Abdomen, *1280*
Rumenotomy for Grain Overload, *1281*
Traumatic Reticuloperitonitis, *1281*
Abomasal Displacements and Volvulus, *1281*
Aftercare Following a Laparotomy, *1282*
Other Gastrointestinal Conditions, *1282*
**Conditions of the Musculoskeletal
System,** *1283*
Lameness, *1283*
Regional Analgesia and Antibiotic
Perfusion Techniques and PMMA
Implants, *1283*

Surgical Diseases of the Hoof and
Phalanges, *1283*
**Conditions of the Respiratory
System,** *1286*
Conditions of the Urogenital System, *1286*
Anesthesia of the Urogenital and
Reproductive Systems, *1286*
Urolithiasis, *1287*
Ruptured Bladder, *1288*
Urovagina, *1288*
**Conditions of the Reproductive
System,** *1288*
Supernumerary Teat Removal, *1288*
Ovarian Disease, *1288*
Dystocia, *1289*
Uterine Torsion, *1289*
Vaginal and Uterine Prolapse, *1289*
Fibropapillomas of the Penis, *1290*
Preputial Prolapse, *1291*
**Conditions of the Ophthalmic
System,** *1291*
Ocular Squamous Cell Carcinoma
(Cancer Eye), *1291*
Surgical Procedures of Young Stock, *1292*
Dehorning, *1292*
Castration, *1292*
Umbilical Hernias and Infections, *1293*
**Selected Conditions of Small
Ruminants,** *1293*
Urinary System, *1293*
Ophthalmic System, *1295*
**Surgical Procedures Commonly
Performed on Small Ruminants,** *1295*

LEARNING OBJECTIVES

When you have completed this chapter, you will be able to:
1. Pronounce, spell, and define all Key Terms in this chapter.
2. Describe the preoperative preparation needed for equine patients, as well as the
   responsibilities of the veterinary technician before, during, and after equine surgery,
   including postoperative monitoring, medication administration, bandage care, and
   grooming.

*The authors and publisher wish to acknowledge Rustin M. Moore for his contributions to previous
editions of this chapter.*

KEY TERMS

Abomasopexy
Colpotomy
Laparotomy
Omentopexy
Pyloropexy
Rumenostomy
Rumenotomy

3. List surgical procedures commonly performed in equine patients, and describe indications and preoperative, intraoperative, and postoperative considerations for common surgical procedures in equine patients.
4. List surgical procedures commonly performed in bovine patients, and describe indications and preoperative, intraoperative, and postoperative considerations for common surgical procedures in bovine patients.
5. List surgical procedures commonly performed in small ruminants, and describe indications and preoperative, intraoperative, and postoperative considerations for common surgical procedures in small ruminants.

INTRODUCTION

As with all aspects of veterinary technology, large animal surgical nursing relies heavily upon the observational skills, clinical knowledge, and technical ability of the veterinary technician to ensure that all large animal patients receive optimal medical care. Technicians are expected to provide patient monitoring, treatment, surgical assistance, nursing care, and client education. Providing veterinary care for large animals is particularly cumbersome because they are massive, fractious, and at the same time, fragile animals. Skilled technical support with expertise in patient handling, restraint, and the use of specialized instrumentation is crucial for the practitioner to provide quality preoperative, intraoperative, and postoperative intensive care. Familiarity with large animal behavior will allow the veterinary technician to quickly recognize abnormal behavior, such as early signs of pain, and neurologic and respiratory disorders. The technician is often the first to identify a change in patient status and may save valuable time at a crucial turning point for therapeutic intervention. In addition, recognition of the unique layperson's language will help the veterinary technician communicate with the client and recognize the significance of patient historical data. In these ways, large animal nursing imparts an essential contribution to the quality and efficiency of patient care in a hospital setting.

This chapter addresses the most commonly seen surgical conditions among large animal species and includes the steps taken by veterinary technicians in the support and care of surgical patients. In this chapter, these steps begin after completion of a thorough physical examination and the acquisition of results from hematology, clinical chemistry, and imaging tests.

Surgical Nursing of Horses

OVERVIEW

PREOPERATIVE PREPARATION

Numerous procedures are required in preparation of the equine patient for anesthesia and surgery. Many if not all of these procedures involve the veterinary technician. It is probably wise that a checklist be developed that the veterinary technician can use to make sure that all procedures are performed. This is particularly helpful in a hospital where more than one technician is working on the same case. Because of the dense hair coat of horses, thorough grooming is necessary. This may include simply brushing or currying the horse's coat, or it may require that the horse be bathed. The aim of grooming is to remove as much loose hair, dander, and dirt from the horse's body as possible, thereby keeping such material out of the operating room (OR). If the horse is shod, the shoes are generally removed before surgery to prevent injury to the horse during recovery from anesthesia and damage to the recovery stall flooring. Some therapeutic shoes may not be removed to prevent damage to the hooves. If the shoes must be left on, wrapping them with gauze and elastic tape will provide some protection from injury from the shoes during recovery. The horse's feet need to be picked out and cleaned. One of the main responsibilities of the technician is to clip a wide area of hair in the vicinity of the surgery site before anesthetic induction. If surgery will be performed on a limb, the hair can be clipped the day before surgery, and the limb can be cleaned and a bandage placed to keep the site clean. The final aseptic preparation is performed once the horse is under anesthesia. Clipping the hair and cleaning the surgery site before anesthetic induction will reduce anesthesia time.

It is important that the technician consult the clinician regarding the specific site that should be clipped. Areas of the mane and tail should be clipped only under special circumstances. Most owners are adamant that these areas should not be clipped for cosmetic purposes. The hair of the mane and tail takes months to years to grow out, and unnecessarily clipping these areas may cause needless delay in a show horse's convalescence. The location of the skin incision and the appropriate part of the horse to clip before surgery can usually be found in equine surgical textbooks. However,

because of variation among surgeons, the technician should always consult the surgeon before clipping the patient.

Unlike ruminants and small animals, horses do not regurgitate or vomit. For elective surgical procedures, adult horses are generally held off feed for approximately 4 to 6 hours to allow time for emptying of the stomach, which may enable the horse to ventilate more easily. Horses are generally provided water during this time. Young foals that are still nursing are generally not held off feed before anesthesia, but if they are, it is usually only for 1 to 2 hours. For emergency surgical procedures, this period of feed restriction is not usually possible. A complete physical examination should be performed, including auscultation of the heart and lungs. In adult horses, a rebreathing bag may have to be used to increase the respiratory effort sufficiently to hear air moving through the lung fields. An electrocardiogram should be performed if any evidence of an abnormal heart rhythm is detected during auscultation. Preoperative blood work usually includes a complete blood count (CBC) and fibrinogen determination. Some clinicians also perform a chemistry profile depending on the age and health of the horse. A tetanus vaccination should have been given within the previous 3 months. If the date is not known, a booster should be given intramuscularly.

Before general anesthesia is given, an intravenous (IV) catheter is placed in one of the jugular veins. The location of the catheter is important to provide access without compromising the surgical site. Anesthetic agents for induction are administered through the catheter. Some anesthetic agents (thiobarbiturates) and perioperative medications (phenylbutazone) are irritating if injected perivascularly. Therefore, it is imperative that the veterinary technician place the catheter into the vein and secure it appropriately. Perioperative medications such as antibiotics and nonsteroidal anti-inflammatory drugs (NSAIDs) are usually administered before anesthetic induction. However, if an infectious process is suspected, the surgeon may opt to start antibiotics after a sample has been obtained at surgery for culture and susceptibility testing. In this case, the medication can be administered during anesthesia or after recovery; this will depend on the medication and the condition of the patient while under anesthesia. Because horses are generally intubated with an endotracheal tube through the oral cavity, it is important that the mouth be thoroughly washed out before anesthetic induction; this will reduce the chance that feed material will be carried into the airway during intubation. Once the horse is intubated, the cuff should be inflated to prevent saliva and other materials from draining into the lower airway and leading to aspiration pneumonia.

INTRAOPERATIVE NURSING

The OR technician should consult the surgeon regarding which instruments will be required. In a hospital where many OR technicians and surgeons are present, an organized system should be used to delineate various instrument preferences and glove sizes of surgeons. This will allow the technician to know the different requirements of individual surgeons. One common difference among surgeons is the type of suture material chosen to close wounds. The technician must learn to adapt to these individual preferences. It is recommended that the technician have all available instruments close to the location of surgery. Even if the instrument is used infrequently, it is better to have it nearby rather than waste time looking for it when it is needed. Time-wasting activities lead to prolonged anesthetic time, which could lead to increased morbidity or mortality. Correctly labeled radiographs are essential for most limb surgery procedures. Radiographs should be placed on a radiographic view box, or, if digital radiography systems are used, opened on a computer in the OR. The technician should have available gloves, gowns, and drapes and all other supplies anticipated to be used. In some lower limb surgeries, an Esmarch bandage (Latex Rubber Bandage/Tourner Wrap, Smiths & Nephew Richards, Memphis, Tenn) and a tourniquet are used to assist with hemostasis during surgery. An Esmarch bandage is a flat, gum-rubber elastic bandage that is wrapped around the limb in a spiral fashion from distal to proximal to a point above the surgical site. At this point, an apneumatic tourniquet is applied and secured. The aim of the Esmarch bandage is to force blood out of the limb, and the tourniquet prevents blood from entering into the site. The Esmarch bandage is removed after the tourniquet is fully inflated. Use of an Esmarch bandage and tourniquet enables the surgeon to operate in a bloodless field, resulting in a shorter surgery time. An Esmarch bandage can be used instead of a pneumatic tourniquet and can be secured in place with adhesive tape once it has been applied. It is important to use a relatively wide Esmarch for this because narrow tourniquets cannot adequately restrict blood flow.

After surgery, a pressure bandage is applied, and the tourniquet is released. It is strongly recommended that the tourniquet be used for a maximum period of 2 hours to prevent potentially serious side effects.

> **TECHNICIAN NOTE**   In a hospital where many operating room (OR) technicians and surgeons are present, an organized system should be used to delineate the various instrument preferences and glove sizes of surgeons.

Because of their immense body weight, horses are prone to myositis (muscle damage) during recumbency, and this can be life threatening. Therefore, the OR technician must ensure that the patient is well padded on the surgery table. For a horse in lateral recumbency, it is important that the dependent forelimb is pulled as far forward as possible to minimize pressure over the triceps and the radial nerve. Rear limbs should be supported so that both are extended perpendicular to the body and parallel to the ground. When in dorsal recumbency, adequate padding is necessary underneath the horse's back, and the horse must be supported so that it cannot rotate to one side or the other because this can unevenly load the muscles of the croup or shoulder regions. The limbs in this situation are allowed to flex to a relaxed position. Extending the rear limbs out behind the horse

(e.g., for a femoropatellar arthroscopy) should be done only for aseptic preparation or for surgery; maintaining the limb in this position for prolonged periods often leads to severe myopathy or neuropathy of the rear limbs. The pressure of the horse's body and the hypotension that can occur during anesthesia can result in hypoperfusion of the muscles. If this condition is prolonged, the muscles can undergo metabolic change, resulting in extreme soreness and pain. In severe cases, muscle pigment (myoglobin) is released into the bloodstream and is excreted in the urine (coffee-colored urine); the pigment can lead to kidney damage. The first sign that muscle damage has occurred during anesthesia is manifested during recovery. Usually the front or rear limb, or both, on the side on which the horse is lying on will be affected. However, the uppermost limb or any limb in a horse in dorsal recumbency can be involved. The horse may be unable to bear weight on the limb. If a forelimb is involved, the horse will drag the limb in a flexed position and will be unable to bear weight; this is an indication of triceps damage. If the hindlimb is involved, the horse may knuckle in the lower joints and walk on the dorsal aspect of the fetlock, and the limb will collapse as the horse tries to bear weight. Both myopathy and neuropathy will affect the horse's ability to bear weight on the affected limb, but myopathies tend to cause increased pain and distress, whereas neuropathies seem to be less painful. Most horses show some improvement over the first few days, but some horses are unable to rise. Management of a postoperative recumbent patient presents a number of problems for clinicians and technicians. Appropriate padding materials include an inflatable water bed, semi-inflated inner tubes under the shoulder and hip, dunnage bags, and foam rubber pads.

The patient and the surgery site must be positioned so that it is comfortable for the surgeon and safe for the patient. This will help ensure that the surgeon does not become fatigued or frustrated, and that a subsequent compromise in technique does not occur. It is not wise to overextend, overflex, abduct, or adduct the limbs because of potential complications of myopathy and neuropathy.

Aseptic preparation of the surgery site, surgical instruments, and the surgeon is imperative for a successful and uncomplicated surgery. It is the responsibility of all personnel involved to maintain asepsis, but OR technicians should assume primary responsibility for ensuring that the surgical site is properly prepared and that instruments are properly sterilized and packaged. The OR technician must be cognizant of all activities in preparation for surgery and during the surgical procedure. If the technician observes a break in aseptic technique, it should be brought to the attention of the surgeon, so the problem can be remedied. Techniques involved in sterilization of surgical instruments and supplies and in aseptic preparation of the surgery site are covered in Chapter 30.

POSTOPERATIVE NURSING

Technicians play a vital role in the postoperative care of the equine patient. Although veterinarians are responsible for patient care, technicians are often primarily involved with postoperative monitoring, administering medications, changing bandages, grooming, and other tasks required in caring for postoperative patients. Monitoring the postoperative patient is similar to previously discussed patient monitoring. Although all body systems should be evaluated, important things to consider in the postoperative patient are the presence and magnitude of postoperative pain, whether the patient is febrile, and whether any signs of infection (swelling, erythema, heat, pain) are evident at the incision site. The postoperative patient should be examined for any complications, such as pneumonia, diarrhea, jugular vein thrombophlebitis, or laminitis.

> **TECHNICIAN NOTE** Although veterinarians are responsible for patient care, technicians are often primarily involved with postoperative monitoring, administering medications, changing bandages, grooming, and other tasks required in caring for postoperative patients.

Technicians are generally responsible for administering medications postoperatively. This may involve giving antibiotics or NSAIDs orally, intravenously, or intramuscularly, or IV catheter maintenance (flushing should be performed at least every 6 hours). Many horses that undergo surgery have an IV catheter that is used in the postoperative period to administer perioperative antibiotics. The duration of antibiotic therapy depends on clinician preference and the type and severity of the underlying disease process. Many horses are administered NSAIDs in the postoperative period for their anti-inflammatory and analgesic properties.

Horses undergoing limb surgery generally have a bandage placed on the limb at the conclusion of surgery before recovery from anesthesia. The limbs are often kept bandaged until skin sutures are removed 10 to 14 days postoperatively. The bandages should probably be changed every 2 to 3 days initially, or more frequently if they become wet or soiled from the outside, or if wound drainage soaks through from the inside. Several types of materials may be used for limb bandages in horses as well as several methods of application (see Chapter 26). In general, a sterile nonadherent material is usually placed directly against the incision and is held in place with sterile, soft roll gauze (Kling, Johnson & Johnson, New Brunswick, New Jersey). The next layer of the bandage is usually a sterile, soft combine that covers the circumference of the limb for the entire distance of the bandage, which is held in place with soft roll gauze. This layer can be skipped if the outer bandage that is placed is a thick, sterile combine material. Next, a thick layer of rolled cotton, sheet cottons, or combine material is placed on the limb and secured with soft roll gauze. An Ace bandage, Elasticon (Johnson & Johnson), or Vetwrap (Animal Care Products/3M, St Paul, Minnesota) can be used as the final layer of the bandage. Elasticon is useful for securing the top of the bandage to the skin above it and the bottom of the bandage to the foot below. This helps seal the bandage and prevents debris from getting between the skin and the bandage. All layers of the bandage should be applied in the same direction (dorsal to palmar or plantar) and with even tension; this should help prevent constriction of the tendons in the metacarpal or metatarsal area and subsequent tendonitis (bandage bow). When bandages are changed postoperatively, the incision should be examined for swelling, heat, exudate, and pain on palpation. The limb should be monitored for excessive swelling above and below the bandage. Exudate should be removed, the wound gently cleaned, and the bandage reapplied. If an appreciable change in the horse's gait is noted, or if the incision appears different than it did at the last bandage change, this should be brought to the immediate attention of the veterinarian.

SURGICAL CONSIDERATIONS

GASTROINTESTINAL TRACT SURGERY

Abdominal surgery is a major undertaking, and a full team is required to perform it in an effective and efficient manner. Adult horses and foals frequently undergo abdominal surgery for gastrointestinal and urogenital tract disease. Although a flank incision in a standing, sedated horse is sometimes used for horses with colic or other abdominal disease, the most common approach to the abdominal cavity is through a ventral midline incision with the horse under general anesthesia and positioned in dorsal recumbency (Figure 33-1). Because most horses with colic requiring surgery will be operated on with the patient under general anesthesia, the veterinary technician will be involved in preparation of the

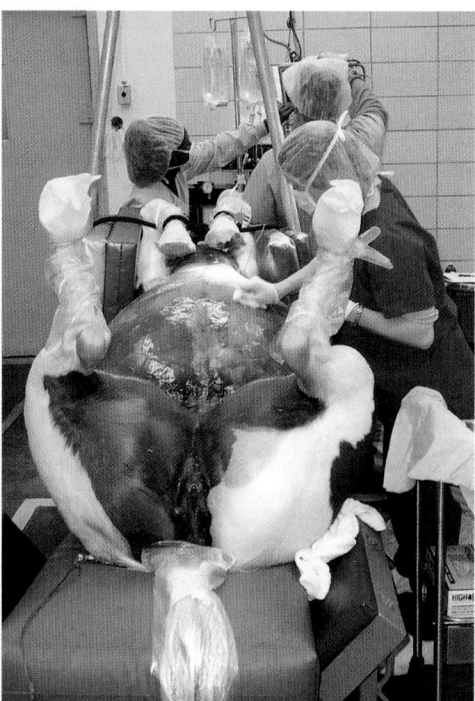

FIGURE 33-1 Preparation of the ventral abdominal area for abdominal surgery in a horse with colic that is under general anesthesia and is positioned in dorsal recumbency.

horse for surgery. This will include placing a catheter, administering perioperative medications, passing a nasogastric tube, washing out the mouth, clipping the hair, preparing the anesthetics, aseptically preparing the incision site, and opening surgical packs at the time of surgery. Most colic patients can be clipped before anesthesia, but if the horse is in severe pain, this may be done after anesthetic induction for the safety of the horse and personnel. The hair should be clipped from rostral to the xiphoid area to the udder or preputial area and to the flank folds on either side; clipped hair and other debris can be removed with a vacuum before aseptic preparation. The incision is draped with four small drapes or towels, and a large, water-impermeable drape is placed that covers the entire horse. The incision is usually made from the umbilicus rostrally toward the xiphoid until the necessary exposure is achieved, but the incision can be extended caudal to the umbilicus. This is particularly necessary for urogenital tract surgery, such as a cystotomy for removal of cystic calculi. Once the incision has been made, a thorough exploration is usually performed, depending on the reason for surgery. Once the abnormality has been identified, it is corrected. Suction is often necessary to decompress gas from the gastrointestinal tract or aspirate fluid such as urine from the bladder during a cystotomy.

> **TECHNICIAN NOTE**   The most common approach to the abdominal cavity is through a ventral midline incision with the horse under general anesthesia and positioned in dorsal recumbency.

The surgeon may perform numerous surgical techniques and manipulations with which the OR veterinary technician becomes familiar through experience. Many specialized instruments are required for abdominal surgery (see Chapter 30). One group of instruments that has become increasingly popular with veterinary surgeons for use in equine abdominal surgery is gastrointestinal stapling equipment. The technician must become familiar with the different instruments and cartridges. Intestinal resection and anastomosis often require specialized instruments and supplies.

Once the cause of colic or another abdominal problem has been corrected and the horse has recovered from anesthesia, the veterinary technician becomes even more closely involved with patient management. Horses usually require administration of IV fluids, antibiotics, anti-inflammatory drugs, and other medications in the postoperative period. The veterinary technician usually administers or oversees administration of these medications. The technician may also perform nasogastric intubation, blood collection, IV catheterization, and bandage changes.

Fortunately, most horses with colic respond to conservative medical treatment, and only a small percentage require surgical intervention. Surgical treatment of colic is necessary for intestinal volvulus and incarceration, enterolithiasis, fibrous foreign body obstruction, and some intestinal displacements (Case Presentation 33-1).

Hernia Repair

Herniation of omentum or abdominal viscera through the abdominal wall can occur with an umbilical hernia, an

CASE PRESENTATION 33-1

A 4-year-old thoroughbred filly was seen for evaluation of colic-like symptoms of 8 hours' duration. The horse had been eating and behaving normally the night before, but was found to be uncomfortable (restless, rolling, and looking at his flank) the next morning. Medical therapy with flunixin did not resolve the horse's clinical signs, so the owners brought her to the clinic for further evaluation.

Upon presentation, the filly's parameters were as follows:
Heart rate: 58 beats per minute
Respiratory rate: 24 breaths per minute
Mucous membranes: pale and tacky to the touch
CRT: prolonged (greater than 3 seconds)
Gut sounds were identified only on the left side and were decreased.
Dehydration: Skin tent was prolonged, and the horse is estimated to be between 5% and 10% dehydrated.
Weight: 465 kg
Blood was collected from the left jugular vein and was submitted for CBC and serum biochemistry. While results were pending, a nasogastric tube was placed using a twitch for restraint, and after the tube was primed, 16 L of net reflux was obtained. Before the rectal examination, the filly was sedated with 200 mg of xylazine administered IV and placed in a set of stocks. The veterinarian performed the rectal examination using a well-lubricated sleeve and identified a thick loop of small diameter in the right side of the abdomen, running

vertically. This loop appeared to be fixed in place at this location. An IV jugular catheter was placed by the technician, and the horse was bolused with 10 L of lactated Ringer's solution. Abdominal ultrasound identified distended, amotile loops of small intestine throughout the ventral abdomen and a loop of thickened small intestine within the lumen of larger viscera (creating a "target lesion") (Figure 1). The combination of

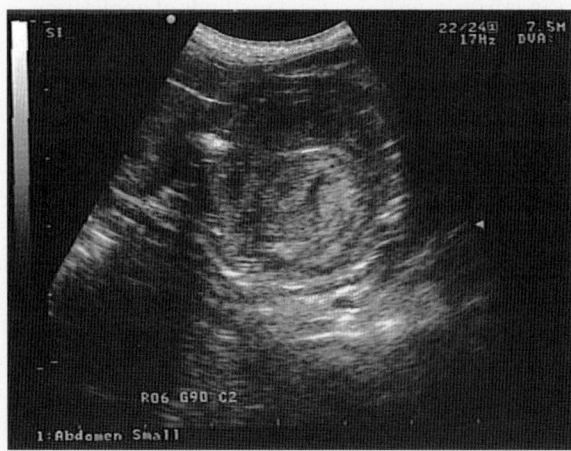

FIGURE 1 The smaller hyperechoic (white) circular structure is a loop of jejunum within a larger hyperechoic circle, which is otherwise known as a "target" lesion. This is a cross-sectional view of an intussusception.

ultrasonographic results, rectal examination findings, and the presence of a small intestinal obstruction (demonstrated by the volume of reflux) justified the need for an exploratory celiotomy to treat a suspected ileocecal intussusception. Blood work revealed signs of dehydration and a prerenal azotemia.

The need for surgical therapy and the risks associated with surgery and anesthesia were explained to the client, and permission was granted to proceed. The filly's belly was clipped while preoperative antibiotics (penicillin and gentamicin IV) and fluids were administered. A rough prep using iodine scrub was then applied to the abdomen and left in place. The filly was moved to the induction box, and general anesthesia was induced. The horse was moved onto the surgery table using a hydraulic hoist and was secured in dorsal recumbency. A sterile prep using chlorhexidine scrub was applied and was finally rinsed off with sterile saline while surgical team members scrubbed their hands and arms.

Once the horse was draped, a ventral midline incision was made, and the abdomen was explored. A jejunocecal intussusception was identified, but it could not be manually reduced. This was blindly resected off within the cecum, and a jejunocecostomy was performed (Figure 2). The linea was sutured closed, the skin was stapled (Figure 3), and the horse was moved back into the recovery stall, where she recovered uneventfully after 90 minutes.

Postoperatively, the filly was maintained on IV fluids at 1½ times daily maintenance, antibiotics were continued for 72 hours, and she received another dose of flunixin. Fluids were supplemented with potassium chloride and calcium gluconate. Physical examinations, including PCV and TP, were performed every 6 hours. The filly remained comfortable and quiet for the first 36 hours postoperatively, but then an increased respiratory rate (30 breaths per minute) and signs of discomfort (pawing, circling in the stall) were noted. A nasogastric tube was passed, and 14 L of net reflux was obtained, indicating that the horse had an obstruction of her small intestine. At this time after surgery, this was most likely secondary to ileus, which is related to inflammation within the intestinal wall interfering with its function. The nasogastric tube was secured to the horse's halter and was left in place to allow frequent gastric decompression (every 3 hours). The filly was no longer given access to any feed, and the fluid rate was increased to counter the increased fluid loss that was occurring. A constant rate infusion of lidocaine was given to try to reduce inflammation and stimulate normal gastrointestinal motility when discontinued. The filly's fecal output decreased over the next 48 hours because she was no longer eating anything.

The filly remained comfortable, although she would grind her teeth and would salivate excessively because of the indwelling nasogastric tube. After refluxing for 36 hours, the volume obtained began to decrease each time, and by 48 hours after it began, the net reflux obtained at each interval was less than 3 L, which was within normal limits. The nasogastric tube was removed, and water was offered in small amounts to the horse. At this time, the lidocaine infusion was discontinued, and the dose of flunixin she received was halved. She drank this water willingly, but to reduce the risk for recurrence of the ileus, only small volumes were offered for the first afternoon. Because her gut managed to tolerate this, the volume of water offered was increased, and she was taken outside to graze for a few minutes. This improved her demeanor considerably, and over the next couple of days, she was gradually returned to a full level of feeding with no additional complications. As her water intake increased, she was weaned off IV fluids, and the jugular catheter was subsequently removed.

When she was back to eating a normal ration and had not been on any medication for at least 24 hours, the filly was discharged to her owners. They were given a printed and signed discharge letter that included specific instructions for her aftercare and things about which to be vigilant. The filly left the clinic and has not had additional episodes of colic.

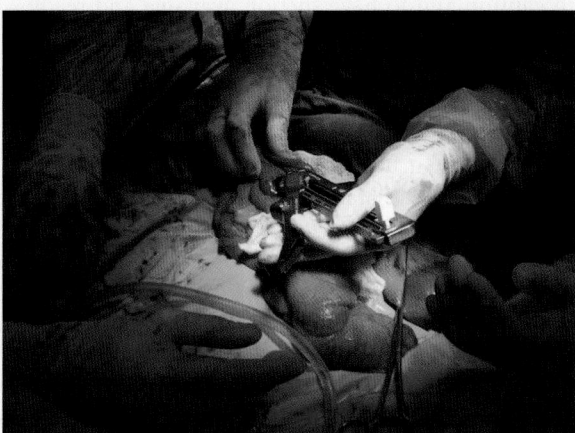

FIGURE 2 An intestinal stapling device (GIA 90) is used to anastomose the jejunum to the cecum.

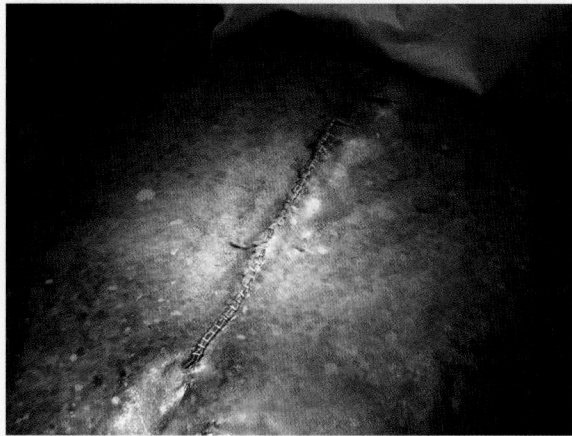

FIGURE 3 The skin incision has been stapled. This can be performed faster than skin suturing.

inguinal (scrotal) hernia, or an incisional hernia. Umbilical hernias are usually congenital and are relatively common in foals. Small hernias may close spontaneously as the foal grows, whereas others require surgical intervention. Umbilical hernias can be repaired through several different methods. Generally, the body wall is closed with interrupted or continuous absorbable suture. Some surgeons open the peritoneum (open herniorrhaphy), and others leave the peritoneum intact (closed herniorrhaphy). If an umbilical hernia is large, or if it has not closed by several months of age, it should probably be surgically repaired. The owner should be instructed to manually reduce hernial contents at least daily; if at any time the hernia cannot be reduced, the horse should be examined immediately by a veterinarian. If intestine becomes incarcerated in the hernia, vascular compromise can occur, leading to ischemic injury.

Inguinal or scrotal hernias can occur in horses of any age, but newborn foals and adult breeding stallions are probably most commonly affected. Frequently, herniated contents do not become incarcerated and can be easily reduced. The hernia should be reduced at least daily in foals because intestine could become incarcerated, and this would necessitate emergency surgery. Sometimes these hernias will spontaneously resolve in foals, but many foals require surgical repair. Because the tissues are friable in foals, successful surgical repair can be difficult. Scrotal hernias in adult horses most commonly occur in stallions shortly after breeding. In most instances, the herniated structure or structures become incarcerated (not reducible), which necessitates immediate surgery. Incarceration of intestine within the scrotum will result in a large, firm, and cold scrotum on the affected side secondary to compromised testicular blood flow. The blood supply to the intestine also becomes compromised, resulting in ischemic injury. Generally, the testicle on the affected side is removed, and the affected segment of intestine often requires resection. This requires preparation of the horse for inguinal and ventral midline surgery.

Acquired body wall herniation occurs in horses subsequent to trauma and after surgery. Blunt trauma, such as a kick, can lead to disruption of the body wall musculature. Body wall hernias can appear secondary to abdominal incisions; these occur more frequently in horses that develop incisional infection or other complicating factors. Small body wall hernias can be repaired primarily by suturing the defect. Larger body wall defects require the use of mesh implants. It is critical that no residual incisional infection is present at the time of mesh herniorrhaphy, and that aseptic technique is followed during placement of the mesh.

UROGENITAL TRACT SURGERY
Urinary Calculi
Urinary calculi are found infrequently in horses. Urinary calculi in horses are usually composed of calcium carbonate and have a spicular appearance. These calculi may develop in the kidney or the urinary bladder. Small-diameter calculi can be passed during normal urination and may go unnoticed. Clinical signs of urinary calculi include stranguria

(slow and difficult urination or straining to urinate), pollakiuria (frequent urination), and hematuria (bloody urine). Horses that develop renal calculi will develop signs of abdominal discomfort when stones become lodged in the ureter. In addition, cystic (urinary bladder) calculi that become lodged in the urethra in male horses cause an inability to urinate and subsequent abdominal pain. Urinary calculi can be diagnosed on the basis of clinical signs, urinalysis, palpation of the urinary bladder per rectum, and endoscopic evaluation of the urethra and urinary bladder. Occasionally, a calculus can be palpated in the proximal urethra of male horses at the level of the ischial arch. Several techniques and specific instruments are available for removing urinary tract calculi.

> **TECHNICIAN NOTE**   Urinary calculi occur infrequently in horses. Urinary calculi in horses are usually composed of calcium carbonate and have a spicular appearance. These calculi may develop in the kidney or the urinary bladder.

Umbilical Repair
Foals commonly develop diseases of the umbilical remnants, including infection (navel ill) in the umbilical arteries, veins, and urachus. These foals often become depressed, inappetent, and febrile. Many foals also develop secondary septicemia and septic arthritis. Umbilical remnant infection may be diagnosed on the basis of clinical signs of swelling, heat, or drainage in the umbilical area. However, foals can have infection within these structures and may be normal on palpation. Transabdominal ultrasonography is helpful in diagnosing diseases of the umbilical structures. Foals with umbilical remnant infection require treatment with broad-spectrum antibiotics; many require surgical removal of affected structures. Surgery for umbilical remnant disease involves an approach and instrumentation similar to those used to repair an umbilical hernia. It is necessary to proceed with caution and to have suction available and ready when umbilical structures are dissected, to prevent contamination of the abdominal cavity.

Patent urachus is a condition wherein foals dribble urine from the umbilicus because a patent canal between the urachus and the urinary bladder is present at birth or develops during the postnatal period. Because those that develop in the postnatal period often occur secondary to an infectious process, it is imperative to rule out umbilical remnant infection and systemic infectious disease. Foals with a patent urachus may be treated nonsurgically by applying an irritant, such as iodine solution, or by using silver nitrate sticks on the external surface of the urachus to promote scarification and closure. This is probably most effective in foals that have a patent urachus at birth. Caution should be used with these agents, and application should be limited to once daily. If a rapid response is not observed, or if an infectious process is occurring in the umbilical remnants of the foal, surgical resection should be performed.

Castration

Castration is one of the most commonly performed surgeries in horses. It is usually performed in the field and does not require extensive surgical facilities or instrumentation. Although under most circumstances castration is performed with short-acting IV general anesthesia, it can be performed in the standing horse with heavy sedation and infiltration of a local anesthetic into the scrotum and spermatic cord. Drugs most commonly used for castration with the horse under IV anesthesia include xylazine-ketamine and xylazine-thiobarbiturate; both combinations can be used with or without guaifenesin. It is important to document that both testicles have descended into the scrotum before commencing with castration in the field. One needs to be prepared for a more extensive surgery requiring entrance into the abdominal cavity (as in a retained testicle); this needs to be planned for because it often takes more time than is needed for a routine castration. If both testicles cannot be palpated in the scrotum, the testicle may be located intra-abdominally, in the inguinal canal, or immediately outside the external inguinal ring. A horse with a testicle located outside the abdominal cavity but not within the scrotum is referred to as a *high flanker*. If the testicle cannot be palpated in the scrotum, sedation may relax the horse and the cremaster muscle and allow the examiner to palpate the testicle or a portion of it. If the testicle still cannot be palpated after sedation, a rectal examination with or without ultrasonography may help confirm the location of the testicle. Involvement of the veterinary technician during castration includes general restraint, handling, administering and monitoring of anesthesia, preparation of the surgical site, and preparation of instruments.

Castration is usually performed with the horse in lateral recumbency with the upper rear limb pulled forward and tied around the horse's neck. Castration involves making an incision over each testicle parallel to the median raphe through the skin and subcutaneous tissue. The testicles are removed by crushing then cutting the spermatic cord proximal to the testicle and the epididymis using emasculators (Figure 33-2, *A*). The emasculators should be placed on the spermatic cord so that the cord is crushed on the side toward the body wall and is cut on the side toward the scrotum (Figure 33-2, *B*). Numerous types of emasculators are available, and each surgeon may have an individual preference. The entire spermatic cord may be crushed and cut simultaneously within the tunic (closed castration), or the tunica albuginea may be opened, and the emasculators can be applied to the vascular structures separately (open castration); this is often done in aged stallions that have an excessively large-diameter spermatic cord. The spermatic cord should be examined after the emasculator is removed to ensure that no bleeding is occurring. The skin incisions are stretched manually to promote drainage.

Postoperative care usually includes strict stall confinement for 24 hours followed by controlled exercise (hand walking) once or twice daily for 1 to 2 weeks to promote drainage, prevent excessive swelling, and prevent or reduce

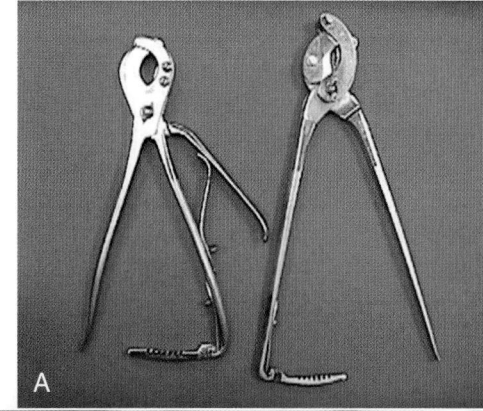

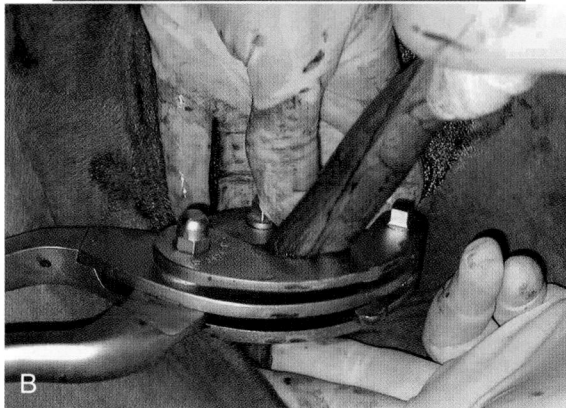

FIGURE 33-2 A, Emasculators used to crush and cut the spermatic cord of horses during castration. B, Use of emasculators during castration of a horse: emasculators are placed around the spermatic cord so that the nut on the emasculators is located toward the testicle, ensuring that the spermatic cord is crushed toward the body side, and that the cord is cut toward the testicle side.

stiffness and soreness. The horse should be monitored closely during the first day after surgery for signs of excessive hemorrhage, evisceration of intestine or omentum (herniation), or excessive swelling.

> **TECHNICIAN NOTE** Post-castration hemorrhage is a potentially life-threatening complication. Hemorrhage should stop rapidly after surgery, and anything more frequent than an occasional drip should be monitored closely.

If the testicle has not descended (cryptorchidism), surgery is more involved and requires anesthesia of longer duration. Cryptorchidectomy (removal of a cryptorchid testicle) also requires the surgeon to use a different surgical technique than is used for routine castration. The testicle can be approached through various incisions, but an approach through the inguinal ring is used most often. A sponge forceps is used to grasp the structures that lead to the scrotum (gubernaculum), and the testicle is extracted from the inguinal canal. In some horses, the testicle cannot be retrieved in this manner, and the surgeon must manually explore the inguinal canal or the caudal abdominal cavity. Once the testicle has been retrieved, it is removed using a similar technique as described for routine castration. After removal of the retained testicle, the other one is removed in a routine manner. Occasionally, horses have both testicles retained. More recently, laparoscopic cryptorchidectomy techniques have been described that can be performed in the standing, sedated horse. The testicle is removed via a flank incision, with care taken to avoid enlargement or damage to the inguinal canal. Laparoscopy can also be used in an anesthetized patient, particularly in cases where locating an abdominal testicle is difficult.

It is believed that cryptorchid horses are at greater risk for evisceration after surgery. To prevent this, some surgeons may elect to temporarily pack a length of gauze soaked in sterile saline or an antiseptic into the subcutaneous areas of the inguinal canal. The gauze packing is held in place with large sutures in the skin and is usually removed in 24 to 72 hours. Other surgeons place interrupted absorbable sutures in the external inguinal ring.

Ovariectomy

Ovariectomy is performed in mares with diseased ovaries, in mares with normal reproductive tracts for use as teaser mares, and in some mares used as performance horses that have unacceptable behavior associated with estrus. An ovariectomy can be performed unilaterally or bilaterally, depending on the reason for the procedure. Laparoscopic techniques have been described that allow an ovariectomy to be performed in the standing horse. This provides excellent visualization of the ovary, good access to the associated artery and vein to ensure that adequate hemostasis is achieved, and a shorter convalescence. Diseased ovaries usually are enlarged and require removal through an incision in the ventral body wall (caudal midline or diagonal paramedian) or the flank. The most common cause of ovarian disease necessitating removal is neoplasia; the most common types of ovarian neoplasia include granulosa theca cell tumors and teratomas. Mares with granulosa theca cell tumors often display abnormal behavior, such as anestrus, persistent estrus or nymphomania, or stallion-like behavior. Ovarian tumors and other ovarian diseases are diagnosed on the basis of clinical signs, rectal examination, and transrectal ultrasonography. Nondiseased ovaries of normal size usually can be removed through a flank incision or via an incision in the vaginal wall (**colpotomy**) in standing, sedated mares with local anesthetic infiltration in the body wall or a caudal epidural anesthetic. Hemostasis of the ovarian pedicle may be provided by transfixing with multiple sutures, by applying an automatic stapling device, or by crushing with a chain écraseur. Complications include hemorrhage, abdominal pain, myositis, and other problems related to anesthesia and abdominal surgery.

> **TECHNICIAN NOTE**   Mares are often uncomfortable after ovariectomy, but laparoscopic techniques are followed by much shorter and better quality postoperative recoveries, requiring fewer analgesics and characterized by a more rapid return to function.

Perineal Surgery

Perineal surgery is relatively common in equine practice. Primiparous mares develop rectovaginal and cervical lacerations during foaling. Abnormal perineal conformation can lead to reproductive unsoundness. Mares with abnormal conformation can develop pneumovagina or pneumouterus secondary to aspirating air into the reproductive tract. They also can develop vesicovaginal reflux, in which urine pools in the cranial vaginal cavity; this can drain into the uterus during estrus when the cervix is opened, leading to endometrial inflammation. Most surgical procedures to correct these caudal reproductive tract abnormalities are performed in standing mares that have been sedated, and a caudal epidural anesthesia is used.

A caudal epidural anesthesia is provided after the hair over the tail head is clipped and the skin is aseptically prepared. An 18-gauge, 1.5-inch needle is inserted through the skin between the last sacral and first coccygeal vertebrae, or between the first and second coccygeal vertebrae, and is advanced (Figure 33-3). Longer spinal needles (18 gauge, 3 inch) may be necessary in large or obese horses. The correct location can be confirmed by checking to see whether local anesthetic placed in the hub of the needle is drawn into the epidural space. Once the correct location has been identified, the local anesthetic is injected. Agents most commonly used for horses include lidocaine, mepivacaine, and xylazine. A caudal epidural anesthetic will desensitize the perineal region. Because horses also develop incoordination in their rear limbs after the procedure, care should be taken when moving them until the effects of the anesthetic have dissipated.

Several surgical procedures may be used to correct caudal reproductive tract abnormalities. The most important factor in the eventual success of repairing a rectovaginal tear is that the mare's feces must be made soft (cow patty consistency) and kept soft for at least 30 days after surgery. This decreases straining and tension placed on the repaired rectal shelf. The most effective method for getting the feces soft involves removing hay and other coarse roughage from the diet and feeding the mare on lush pasture or a complete pelleted feed.

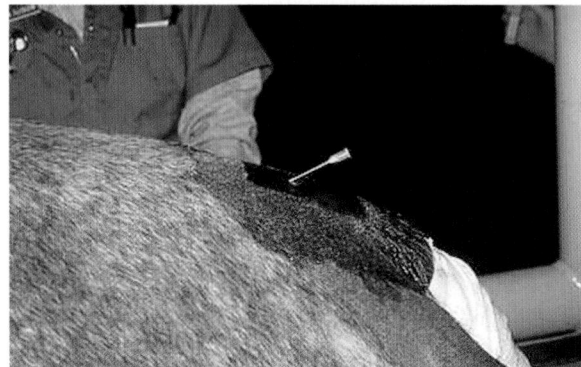

FIGURE 33-3 Technique for injecting a caudal epidural anesthetic between the first and second coccygeal vertebrae in a horse using an 18-gauge, 1½-inch needle.

Administration of mineral oil or magnesium sulfate to the diet also helps soften the feces.

Caslick's Procedure

The most commonly performed perineal surgery is Caslick's operation. This is performed in many fillies on the racetrack and in mares with poor vulvar conformation to prevent pneumovagina and fecal contamination of the vagina, respectively. This procedure is usually performed with sedation and local anesthetic infiltration of the edge of the vulva. The edges of the dorsal vulvar labia are incised and then are sutured with a continuous suture pattern. Closure is extended down to the level of the pelvic floor. Suture should not be placed any lower than this because it may interfere with urination and contribute to urine pooling.

Dystocia: Fetotomy and C-Section

Dystocia means "difficult birth" and is relatively uncommon in horses compared with cattle. However, when dystocia occurs in mares, it is usually a serious problem. Because parturition is rapid in horses and the expulsive efforts of the mare are violent, veterinary obstetric manipulations are difficult and exhausting. Care must be taken at all times to prevent injuring the reproductive tract of the mare. Dystocia in the mare may result from many causes; the most frequent of these include premature placental separation and abnormal presentation of the fetus, especially when either head or limbs or both are deviated. Because the neck of the foal is relatively long, it can easily become twisted. Sometimes the foal may come hind feet first (rare), or if the hind feet are retained, the tail may come first. This latter situation is true breech position. Transverse presentation is also rare in mares. Other occasional causes of dystocia include an excessively large fetus or fetal monsters (e.g., hydrocephalus). An anatomic or physiologic abnormality in the mare herself may cause dystocia. For example, a mare that has sustained a pelvic fracture can develop calluses; these impair the shape and size of the birth canal. Another cause of dystocia is torsion of the uterus. This may occur during gestation, particularly in the last trimester.

Dystocia in mares may be corrected by a variety of methods, depending on the cause of the dystocia, the status of the foal, and the condition of the mare. Sometimes dystocia can be corrected by manipulating fetal position or presentation with the mare standing, with or without the use of sedation or an epidural anesthetic. Placement of a nasotracheal tube will prevent the mare from exerting an abdominal press and will relieve straining. Sometimes a short-acting anesthetic protocol combined with rolling the mare on her back or hoisting her hindlimbs is enough to relieve the dystocia and provide the veterinarian with sufficient relaxation in the mare to deliver the fetus. Fetotomy is sometimes performed to relieve dystocia, particularly if the fetus is dead. Fetotomy is the process in which a dead foal is cut into pieces while within the uterus and is removed. Caution must be taken when a fetotomy is performed, to prevent serious injury to the reproductive tract of the mare.

> **TECHNICIAN NOTE** Most cesarean (C-section) deliveries are performed in the mare with the use of general anesthesia. Generally, time is critical for saving the foal and for ensuring the overall health and well-being of the mare. The technician must be prepared for the surgery and must have the necessary equipment, personnel, and drugs ready for reviving the foal if necessary.

Most C-section deliveries are performed in the mare with the use of general anesthesia. Generally, a C-section delivery is performed through a caudal ventral midline or flank incision in mares. Time is usually critical for saving the foal and for ensuring the overall health and well-being of the mare. The technician must be prepared for the surgery and must have the necessary equipment, personnel, and drugs ready for reviving the foal if necessary. The same instruments that are used for colic surgery are often used for C-section delivery, but additional instruments may be necessary. If the foal is alive, the technician or other personnel must be prepared and equipped to revive it. The foal will usually be depressed from the effects of general anesthesia and may need vigorous rubbing and drying. Oxygen should be available as well as heat lamps and a nasotracheal tube and Ambu bag to ventilate the foal. Forceps to clamp the umbilicus should be readily available if excessive bleeding occurs. A suction device to remove mucus and stomach contents from the airway should be attended to by a technician while the other technicians continue to be cognizant of and attentive to the needs of the surgeons.

ORTHOPEDIC SURGERY

Horses frequently sustain severe musculoskeletal injuries, such as long-bone fractures or disruption of tendons or ligaments. These injuries often require stabilization with the use of bandages, splints, or casts before transport to a referral hospital. Successful stabilization of these injuries and safety of transport are important considerations in the outcome of these cases. Most severe injuries should be bandaged and splinted or casted to a level at least one joint above the injury. A heavy Robert Jones bandage should be applied and rigid splints placed on the lateral and dorsal or palmar aspects of the limb to provide appropriate support. Splints can be made out of rigid materials, such as wood, steel, or aluminum. They should not be excessively heavy or bulky but must provide appropriate support. Horses with phalangeal fractures can be casted with their distal limb in flexion or can be placed in a commercially available device, such as a Kimsey splint (Figure 33-4). Horses with limb injuries should be hauled in a trailer with partitions to provide some support for them to balance themselves. The head should be tied loosely enough to enable the horse to use the head and neck for balance. Horses with front limb injuries should be transported with their head toward the rear of the trailer, and those with rear limb injuries should be transported with their head toward the front of the trailer. This positioning

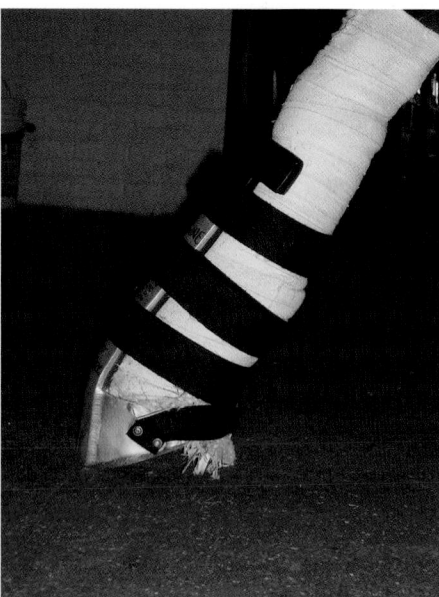

FIGURE 33-4 Use of Kimsey splint to stabilize fractures or joint subluxations in the lower limb of horses.

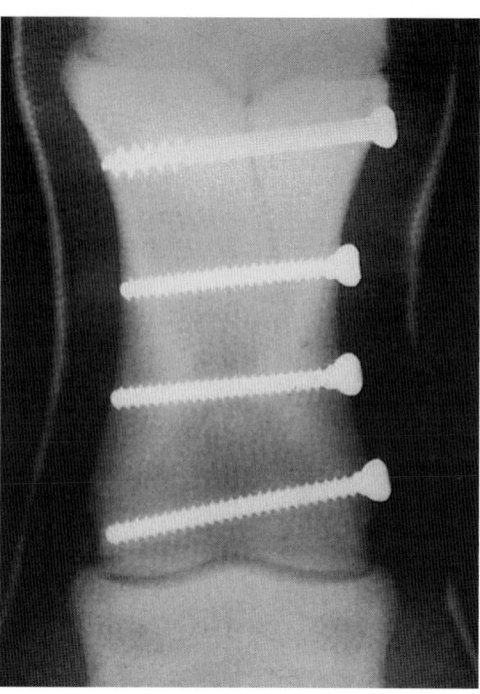

FIGURE 33-5 A proximal phalanx fracture in a horse repaired with cortical bone screws placed in lag fashion to compress the fracture line.

allows the horse to use its healthy limbs to balance itself if the trailer has to brake or stop suddenly.

Orthopedic surgery has become more commonplace among horses. Athletic horses develop numerous orthopedic conditions that are amenable to surgical correction. Historically, fractures of long bones in adult horses were considered irreparable. However, with advanced techniques and more rigid surgical implants, many of these injuries are potentially correctable.

Major fractures of long bones in horses are best repaired with screws and bone plates to prevent movement at the fracture site while the bone heals under rigid fixation (Figure 33-5). Although aseptic technique is imperative for all surgical procedures, it is especially crucial for the overall success of orthopedic surgery in horses. If bony infection develops, it can lead to instability of the implants and fixation failure, which often necessitates euthanasia. It is the responsibility of all personnel to follow aseptic protocol. The technician should strive to maintain asepsis by monitoring the activities of all personnel involved in surgery. Orthopedic surgery requires the use of several specialized instruments and implants; because many of these surgeries are performed on an emergency basis, it is imperative that the technician make sure that instruments are available and ready for use. Many orthopedic injuries that are surgically repaired require the use of external coaptation (cast) for anesthetic recovery or for longer periods postoperatively (see Chapter 26). The technician should anticipate this need and should have appropriate materials available at the conclusion of surgery. The technician may also be needed to assist with anesthetic recovery of the orthopedic equine patient.

Postoperative monitoring of the orthopedic patient is vital for early detection of potential problems. It is particularly important to observe how the horse is using the affected limb in the stall; any dramatic change in use of the limb may signal an impending problem (infection or cast sores). The cast should be monitored for heat, odor, or exudate, which would indicate the development of cast sores. The most common locations for sores to develop in association with a half-limb cast are at the proximal, dorsal aspect of the metacarpus or metatarsus, at the palmar or plantar aspect of the fetlock over the sesamoid bones, and over the heel bulbs. As healing progresses, swelling of the limb will decrease, and this can make the case slightly looser than it was when applied. This can also increase motion of the limb within, which can accelerate the formation of cast sores at the previously mentioned locations. For this reason, casts are often changed routinely before any cast-related complications are observed. Bandages need to be changed frequently, and incision sites should be monitored for swelling, erythema, and discharge. Drains are commonly used in orthopedic surgery after repair of a long bone. Drains can be useful in preventing seroma formation, and they can serve as potential routes for inoculation of the surgery site. Therefore, it is important to ensure that drains are sterile by keeping a clean, sterile bandage on the leg. This may require changing the bandage more frequently than once daily.

> **TECHNICIAN NOTE** Postoperative monitoring of the orthopedic patient is vital for early detection of potential problems. It is particularly important to observe how the horse is using the affected limb in the stall; any dramatic change in use of the limb may signal an impending problem (infection or cast sores).

Arthroscopic Surgery

Arthroscopy is commonly performed for the diagnosis and treatment of joint disease, including removing osteochondral chip fractures, treating cartilaginous and bony abnormalities associated with osteochondrosis, treating septic arthritis, and evaluating causes of joint lameness that have no definitive radiographic abnormalities. Depending on the joint evaluated and the type and location of the lesion, the horse may be positioned in dorsal or lateral recumbency. It is necessary to have the radiographs on a view box or on a computer monitor in the OR, so the surgeon can evaluate them intraoperatively. During arthroscopy, the technique of triangulation is used, whereby the lesion forms one corner of the triangle, and the arthroscope and surgical instruments serve as the other two corners of the triangle. Generally, the arthroscope is placed in the joint on the side opposite the lesion, and the surgical instrument is placed in the joint on the same side as the lesion. The portal for placement of the arthroscope is usually formed by making a small (1-cm) incision in the skin and subcutaneous tissue, and then using a sharp trocar to advance the arthroscopic cannula through the fibrous joint capsule and synovial lining. Once the cannula has penetrated the joint cavity, the sharp trocar is replaced with a blunt obturator to pass the cannula across the joint; this prevents iatrogenic damage to the cartilage. Skin incisions are usually made before joint distention in the carpus, but after joint distention in other joints. The joint is distended with sterile polyionic fluid to facilitate placement of the arthroscope. Once the arthroscope is in place, the joint is evaluated; once the lesion is identified, the most appropriate location for the instrument portal is determined by using a needle to triangulate the lesion with the arthroscope. Once the appropriate location for the instrument portal has been identified, the instrument portal is made with a scalpel blade (#11 or #15). The appropriate instrument is placed into the joint. Instruments commonly used in arthroscopy include a blunt probe for palpating intra-articular structures, rongeurs for removing osteochondral fragments, and curettes for débriding diseased cartilage and bone. A fenestrated cannula is often used at the end of surgery to facilitate removal of cartilage and bone debris via lavage. Motorized equipment is available and is sometimes necessary for débridement of large areas of diseased bone.

The surgeon uses specific instruments for arthroscopy; these may vary depending on the joint involved and the individual surgeon's preference. Generally, a standardized set of arthroscopy instruments are packaged together. Instruments are steam-sterilized, but if they are to be used for more than one case per day, they are sterilized with a cold sterilization solution before each use. After sterilization, the instruments are packed in a sterile stainless steel pan that is later used to rinse disinfecting solution off the arthroscopy instruments. One of the most important and most expensive instruments is the arthroscope; it should be handled carefully to prevent damage. Additional necessary items include a sterile needle (usually 18 gauge) and syringe, which are used for distending the joint. During arthroscopic surgery,

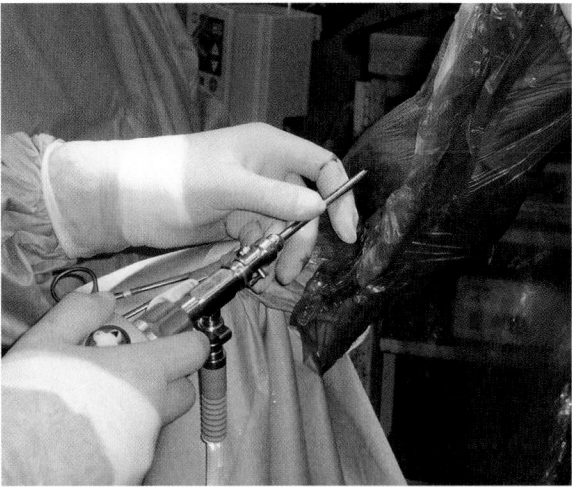

FIGURE 33-6 Use of arthroscopy for evaluating joint disease in horses. The arthroscope is inserted into the joint and is attached to a camera that projects the image on a television screen for easy viewing by the surgeon and other personnel.

the joint is kept distended with sterile physiologic solution, which is usually delivered with a pump through a sterile IV set.

Many hospitals perform arthroscopy using a video camera, so the entire procedure can be viewed on a television screen or a computer monitor (Figure 33-6). This places less strain on the surgeon's eye, makes the procedure more educational for surgery assistants and technical staff, provides an opportunity to videotape or digitally record images from the procedure, and probably allows the procedure to be performed with fewer breaks in aseptic technique. To provide the intense light required to illuminate the inside of the joint, a fiberoptic light source and a light cable are required. It is essential that the technician be familiar with assembly and function of the arthroscopic equipment, as well as proper care, cleaning, and disinfecting of the instruments. Arthroscopy instruments are disinfected using a cold sterilization solution, such as activated dialdehyde (Cidex, Surgikos, Arlington, Texas); instruments, arthroscope, and light cables are soaked for a minimum of 10 minutes. One should read manufacturer recommendations regarding the time required for disinfecting. To prevent delays, the instruments can be placed in sterilizing solution at the start of anesthesia. This will ensure adequate sterilization time. Before the instruments are used, they are transferred sterilely into an empty sterile tray. They are then rinsed with sterile saline to remove the sterilization solution.

After the surgical site has been aseptically prepared and draped and instruments removed from the sterilizing solution, the technician will be responsible for attaching the fiberoptic cable to its light source. The system that delivers fluid to distend the joint must also be connected to the appropriate fluid source. Once the system has been connected to the fluid source, the surgeon must run fluid through the system to flush all air bubbles out of the tubing, so they do not enter the joint. Electric fluid pumps are

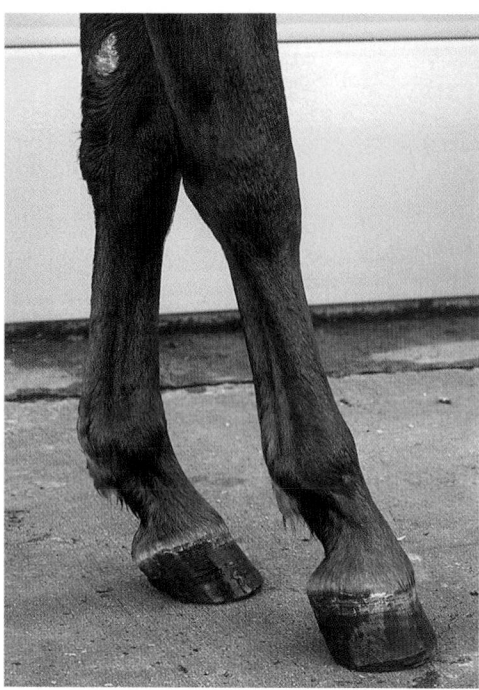

FIGURE 33-7 Flexural deformity of the distal interphalangeal (coffin) joint of the right front limb in a horse.

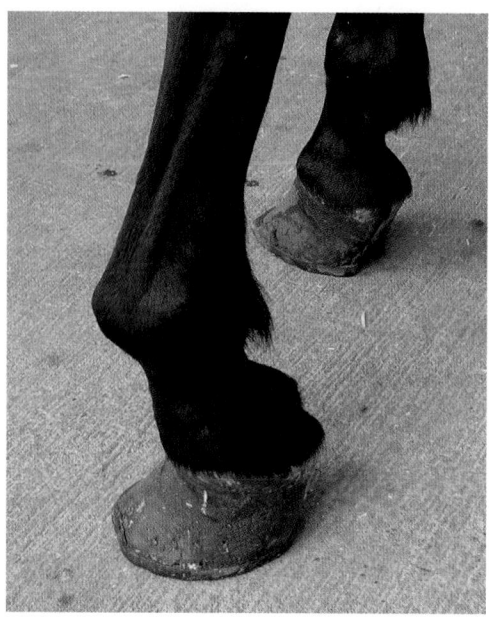

FIGURE 33-8 A flexural deformity of the metacarpophalangeal (fetlock) joint.

generally used to maintain joint distention; they may be manually or pressure controlled.

After surgery, all specialized arthroscopy equipment and instruments must be cleaned. The arthroscope lens should be examined for scratches, and the video camera should be dried carefully. If several arthroscopy surgeries are scheduled the same day, instruments are placed in cold sterilization solution in preparation for the next surgery.

Flexural Deformities

Flexural and angular limb deformities (crooked legs) are abnormalities of the limbs that arise from abnormal development of bones and musculotendinous structures in the limbs. Flexural limb deformities result in overflexion of certain joints. Three main manifestations of flexural limb deformities may be noted in horses. They can be present at birth or may develop during the first few months or years of life. Carpal flexural deformities result in front limbs that are flexed or buckled forward at the carpus. This may range from mild deformity to a severe deformity that prevents the foal from standing. Mild to moderate cases are often amenable to treatment with controlled exercise combined with application of bandages and splints that extend from the ground to the elbow, or tube casts that extend from just above the fetlock to the middle portion of the antebrachium. IV administration of oxytetracycline may be beneficial to help relax the musculotendinous structures.

The second type involves flexural deformity of the distal interphalangeal (coffin) joint, which results in a characteristic clubfoot-shaped hoof (Figure 33-7). This often is first noticed when the foal is a few months of age and can progress to the point that the foal walks on the toe or on the dorsum of the hoof wall. Mild to moderate cases (those in which the foot has not passed the vertical plane) often respond to corrective trimming (lower heel) and application of an extended toe shoe, which helps to stretch out the deep digital flexor tendon. More advanced cases usually require surgical transection of the inferior check ligament, which lengthens the deep digital flexor musculotendinous unit.

The third type of flexural deformity involves the metacarpophalangeal joint and is characterized by increased steepness to the pastern and fetlock (Figure 33-8). This usually begins to develop around 1 year of age but may occur as late as 2 years. It can progress until the horse knuckles over at the fetlock. This condition commonly occurs in rapidly growing, heavily muscled horses such as 1- to 2-year-old quarter horses. Conservative treatment involves controlled exercise, dietary management (balanced minerals, low energy and protein), management of pain (arising from osteochondrosis or physitis) with NSAIDs, and application of bandages and splints that extend from the ground to the elbow. More severely affected horses and those that do not respond to conservative treatment may be successfully treated surgically by performing a superior check or inferior check ligament desmotomy or both, depending on whether superficial digital flexor or deep digital flexor tendons or both are involved.

> **TECHNICIAN NOTE** When evaluating a foal with a flexural or angular limb deformity, it is often easiest to perform this with the foal standing on a firm surface with no bedding. This allows accurate evaluation of foot and limb placement and conformation.

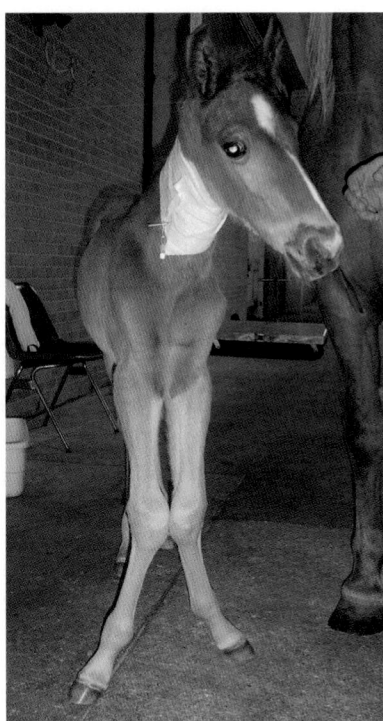

FIGURE 33-9 Bilateral carpal valgus deformity in a foal.

Angular Limb Deformities

Angular limb deformities are deformities that develop in the appendicular skeleton in a medial-to-lateral direction. These deviations can be present at birth or may develop during the first few months of life. Mild deformities may self-correct, others may persist but not worsen, and still others may become more severe with time. These deformities are named in reference to the joint involved and the direction of the deviation. The most common deviation is carpal valgus, where the limb distal to the carpus deviates laterally (Figure 33-9). Other common deviations include fetlock varus, where the limb distal to the fetlock deviates medially (Figure 33-10), and tarsal valgus. These deviations can occur because of disproportionate growth of bone on either side of the growth plate, incompletely ossified cuboidal bones in the carpus and tarsus, or ligamentous laxity. Deviations in foals with incompletely ossified cuboidal bones or ligamentous laxity can usually be manually straightened, whereas those with disproportionate growth at the physis cannot.

Treatment for mild to moderate angular deviations may include stall rest with controlled exercise, depending on the age of the foal. Successful surgical procedures have been developed to treat moderate to severe deformities. Transection and elevation of the periosteum near the affected growth plate on the concave (short) side of the limb will stimulate more rapid bone growth, which usually leads to correction of disproportionate growth. Periosteal transection and elevation can be repeated in 4 to 6 weeks if the deformity has not been completely corrected. Deformities do not overcorrect with this procedure. With more severe deformities or in older foals with less growth potential, growth on the convex

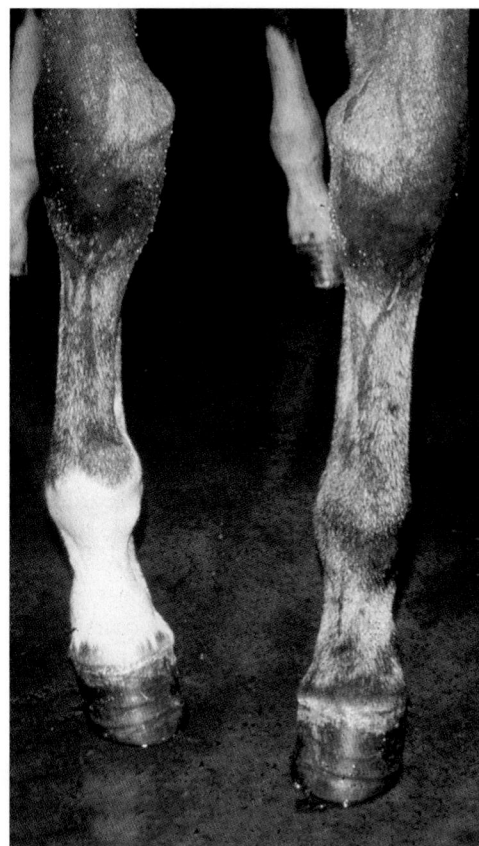

FIGURE 33-10 Varus deformity of the right fetlock in a foal.

(or long) side of the bone can be slowed by performing transphyseal bridging. This is usually done by placing a screw on either side of the growth plate and then tightening a figure-eight wire around the screw heads to provide compression to the growth plate. Use of transphyseal bridging can lead to correction of more severe deformities, but it is imperative that these implants be removed at the correct time to prevent overcorrection leading to the opposite type of deformity. Foals with deviations of the carpus or tarsus subsequent to ligamentous laxity or incompletely ossified cuboidal bones are best treated with stall rest with controlled exercise combined with application of full-limb bandages and splints or tube casts extending from the distal cannon bone to the proximal radius or tibia.

Laminitis

Laminitis (founder) is a serious, often life-threatening disease of horses involving inflammation of the sensitive laminae of the feet. It often involves both front feet or all four feet. However, it can occur in only one forefoot or rear foot if severe lameness is present in the opposite limb. The exact cause of laminitis is unknown, but horses with serious infectious or inflammatory disease resulting in endotoxemia, such as ischemic or inflammatory bowel disease, pleuropneumonia, septic metritis, and grain overload, are predisposed. Laminitis occurs almost exclusively in adult horses; it rarely occurs in horses younger than 1 year of age. In geriatric horses, laminitis may occur secondarily to Cushing's disease or equine metabolic syndrome. Horses often present only with signs of laminitis, but good outcomes can be difficult to achieve unless the underlying condition is accurately identified and treated (see Chapter 35).

TECHNICIAN NOTE Laminitis (founder) is a serious, often life-threatening disease of horses involving inflammation of the sensitive laminae of the feet. It often involves both front feet or all four feet.

Acute laminitis occurs at initial stages of the disease, resulting in extreme pain and reluctance to move. Horses often have increased heat in the hooves and have a pronounced or bounding digital pulse. They are reluctant to walk, turn, or allow their feet to be picked up. They stand with a characteristic stance with their rear legs camped underneath their torso and their front feet camped out in front (Figure 33-11). Chronic laminitis occurs when, because of degeneration of the sensitive laminae on the coffin bone (distal phalanx), dorsal laminar attachments to the

insensitive laminae of the hoof detach and the coffin bone rotates. In severe chronic laminitis, the rotated coffin bone may protrude through the sole of the foot. A lateral radiograph of the foot is usually required to determine whether coffin bone rotation has occurred (Figure 33-12, A and B). In more severe cases, all laminar attachments may become detached, and the coffin bone is displaced distally within the hoof wall. Horses that have distal displacement of the coffin bone develop a characteristic depression at the coronary band and are termed *sinkers*. Horses with chronic laminitis develop characteristic concentric rings on the hooves and an abnormal shape of the hooves (Figure 33-13).

The main focus of treatment of horses with laminitis involves reducing inflammation and providing analgesia with anti-inflammatory drugs (NSAIDs such as phenylbutazone), promoting digital blood flow with vasodilator drugs (acepromazine, isoxsuprine, topical glyceryl trinitrate), reducing inflammatory enzyme activity (pentoxifylline) and mechanically supporting the distal phalanx by providing frog support (frog pads or insulation foam pads). Nursing care is also an important component of the therapeutic regimen, particularly in chronic laminitis. Because laminitis

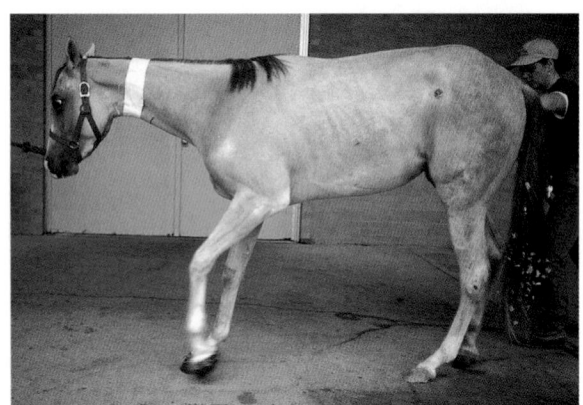

FIGURE 33-11 Typical posture of a horse with laminitis walking or turning on a hard surface.

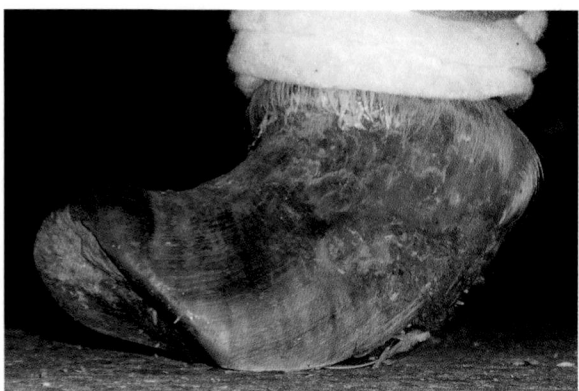

FIGURE 33-13 Abnormal hoof growth in a horse with chronic laminitis in both front feet.

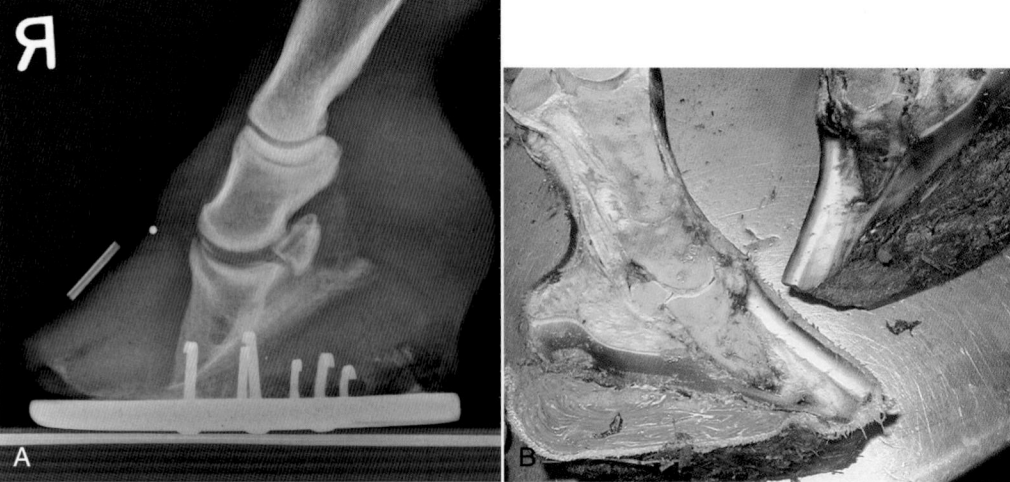

FIGURE 33-12 A, Lateral radiograph of the front foot of a horse with laminitis that has evidence of coffin bone rotation. **B,** Gross pathologic photograph of the sagittal section of both front feet of a horse with bilateral laminitis that has undergone coffin bone rotation.

is extremely painful, horses often spend long periods of time lying down. This necessitates care of decubital ulcers. Deep bedding is necessary, and using straw on top of shavings, padded mats, or a water bed can help prevent the development of these ulcers. In addition, horses often develop subsolar abscesses that require daily soaking and bandaging. The prognosis for return of the horse to athletic competition depends on the occurrence and severity of rotation or sinkage of the coffin bone. Most horses that have appreciable rotation do not return to athletic function. The prognosis for horses that develop distal displacement of the coffin bone is poor. Corrective shoes (heart bars) or clogs are usually placed once the acute, painful stage of laminitis has passed.

Arthritis

Degenerative joint disease (arthritis) is a common performance-limiting condition of horses that can affect numerous joints. The disease is characterized by damage to the articular cartilage and subchondral bone. This is usually secondary to accumulated wear and tear on the joint, although it can occur after a single serious injury, such as an articular fracture. *Bone spavin* refers to arthritis in the distal intertarsal and tarsometatarsal joints of the hock. *High ring-bone* and *low ring-bone* refer to arthritis in the proximal interphalangeal (pastern) and distal interphalangeal (coffin) joints, respectively. *Osselet* is the term used to describe arthritis in the metacarpophalangeal or metatarsophalangeal (fetlock) joint. Diagnosis is often based on historical information and physical examination, but radiographs are necessary to confirm the presence of arthritic changes. The degree of lameness seen with this can vary, but horses often improve slightly as they warm up. Treatment options vary depending on the affected joint, the severity of the condition, use of the horse, and owner expectations. Conservative therapy includes exercise modifications (stall rest tends to exacerbate clinical signs), NSAIDs, disease-modifying treatments (polysulfated glycosaminoglycans, hyaluronic acid), and intra-articular medication (corticosteroids or hyaluronic acid). When cases are severe, arthrodesis can be performed on select joints (pastern, fetlock, carpus), although these procedures often result in a horse that at best will be pasture sound. Intra-articular therapy with interleukin-1 receptor antagonist protein (IRAP) specifically inhibits one of the main inflammatory cytokines responsible for pain and inflammation in the process of arthritis. IRAP therapy is provided by collecting blood from the patient in a special syringe containing glass beads that activate certain cells. This blood is incubated and processed before plasma is drawn off and frozen. This plasma can be thawed and injected into the patient's affected joints, once weekly for 3 weeks. IRAP therapy has been very useful in alleviating clinical signs in horses that were no longer responsive to intra-articular steroids or other therapies, and yields greater benefit if used earlier in the disease process.

Tendonitis

Tendonitis (bowed tendons) is an injury involving primarily the superficial digital flexor tendon and occasionally the deep digital flexor tendon of the front limbs. This injury is usually sustained secondary to racing or other strenuous activity. Degrees of tendonitis range from mild edema and inflammation to tendon fiber separation to tendon fiber tearing or disruption. When tendon fibers tear, hemorrhage and inflammatory debris accumulate in a cavity within the tendon; this is known as a *core lesion*. Treatment for tendonitis includes hydrotherapy, NSAIDs, support bandages, topical anti-inflammatory agents (sweats, poultices), and exercise restriction or controlled exercise. Regenerative therapies, such as stem cell and platelet-rich plasma injections, are gaining acceptance; these are helping to improve the prognosis for treated horses. Several surgical procedures have been used to treat tendonitis or prevent its recurrence. The most commonly performed surgery is tendon splitting, which evacuates the core lesion and allows rapid vascularization and healing of the area. The prognosis for return to athletic function depends on the severity of the injury; some horses with severe core lesions can return to athletic function if given appropriate treatment and time for convalescence.

Osteochondrosis

Osteochondrosis is a form of developmental orthopedic disease in which the articular cartilage and underlying subchondral bone do not develop appropriately. This can result in the formation of osteochondritis dissecans (cartilage flaps), osteochondral fragments, cartilage erosion, and subchondral bone cysts. These abnormalities often manifest as joint effusion and lameness when young horses are first put into strenuous exercise. Many of these lesions are amenable to treatment via arthroscopy, resulting in return of the horse to athletic function. *Bog spavin* is the term used to describe the accumulation of synovial fluid (effusion) in the tarsocrural joint of the hock (Figure 33-14); this is the most common clinical sign observed in horses with osteochondrosis.

Subsolar Abscess

Subsolar abscess is a common cause of severe lameness. Horses usually will not bear weight on the limb. Heat is palpable in the hoof, and the bounding digital pulse is similar to that noted in a horse with laminitis. However, the difference is that subsolar abscesses usually occur in only one foot. Pain can be localized by applying focal pressure to the sole of the foot with hoof testers. Occasionally, purulent debris will accumulate and migrate, and an area will break open at the coronary band and drain (gravel). Treatment involves establishing drainage by paring out the sole or opening the dorsal hoof wall, until the abscess cavity has been located and has drained. The foot should be kept bandaged to keep it dry and clean. The affected foot can be soaked daily in a solution of povidone-iodine (Betadine) and magnesium sulfate (Epsom salts) and then rebandaged. The horse should be given analgesics (phenylbutazone) for a few days. Appropriate tetanus prophylaxis should be administered. The foot needs to be protected from dirt and debris until the area fills

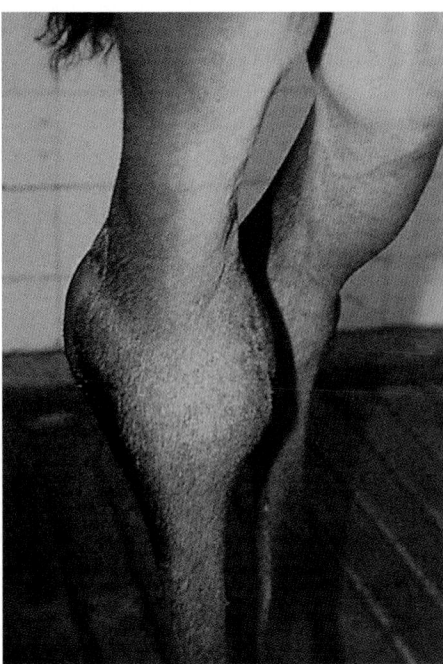

FIGURE 33-14 A young horse with a marked tibiotarsal joint effusion, otherwise known as *bog spavin*.

in with granulation tissue and is covered with cornified tissue.

> **TECHNICIAN NOTE**   The horse with non–weight-bearing lameness is always an emergency because the differential diagnosis list includes severe laminitis, hoof abscess, septic arthritis, and fracture.

Septic Arthritis

Septic arthritis is a common occurrence in adult horses secondary to iatrogenic inoculation of joints during arthrocentesis or joint surgery, or subsequent to traumatic joint injury. It occurs commonly in foals subsequent to hematogenous spread from a focus of infection, such as the umbilicus (navel ill), the lungs (pneumonia), or the intestinal tract (enteritis). The cornerstone of treatment for septic arthritis includes broad-spectrum antibiotics administered systemically, intra-articular antibiotics, NSAIDs, IV regional perfusion with antibiotics, and joint drainage and lavage.

UPPER RESPIRATORY TRACT SURGERY

Abnormalities of the upper respiratory tract can be performance limiting for athletic horses and, if severe, can be life threatening. Many obstructive diseases of the upper respiratory tract are amenable to surgical correction. The most common of these are left laryngeal hemiplegia, epiglottic entrapment, dorsal displacement of the soft palate (DDSP), and arytenoid chondritis. Others include subepiglottic cysts, guttural pouch empyema, guttural pouch tympany, and guttural pouch mycosis.

> **TECHNICIAN NOTE**   Many upper airway diseases can be diagnosed using upper airway endoscopy. Because many of these conditions manifest as functional problems, sedation cannot be used to facilitate the examination because this can abnormally affect the function of the larynx. Other forms of restraint must be used until conditions such as laryngeal hemiplegia, dorsal displacement of the soft palate, and epiglottic entrapment have been eliminated from the differential diagnosis list.

Left laryngeal hemiplegia ("roarer") is a condition that results in paralysis of the left arytenoid cartilage, which prevents it from being abducted during inspiration. This causes the arytenoid to collapse and be pulled into the airway secondary to the negative pressure generated during inspiration. The cause of this condition is unknown, but it results in a recurrent laryngeal neuropathy. Because this nerve normally provides innervation to the major abductor muscle of the arytenoid cartilage, the cricoarytenoideus dorsalis, a neuropathy results in muscle atrophy and an inability to abduct the arytenoid. As the name implies, this condition occurs almost exclusively on the left side (95%); it is believed that this is related to the longer length of the nerve on the left when compared with the nerve on the right side. This condition is diagnosed using endoscopy at rest or during exercise on a high-speed treadmill; the left arytenoid cartilage is not fully abducted during inspiration and in severe cases actually collapses into the airway. Horses with this condition make a characteristic inspiratory noise (roaring) and develop exercise intolerance. In performance horses, appropriate surgical treatment consists of a prosthetic laryngoplasty, which involves placing a suture between the cricoid cartilage and the muscular process of the arytenoid cartilage to mimic the action of the cricoarytenoideus dorsalis and to abduct the arytenoid cartilage (tie-back). Intraoperative visualization with the endoscope, placed up the dependent nostril, is helpful because this can be used to ensure that the suture does not penetrate the tracheal mucosa, and that adequate abduction of the arytenoid is achieved. This is done to try to minimize resistance to airflow, which occurs during inhalation, but it does not always prevent horses from making respiratory noise during fast work.

The laryngeal ventricles (saccules) can be everted and resected (ventriculectomy or sacculectomy), sometimes in combination with the left vocal cord (vocal cordectomy), through a ventral laryngotomy or with the use of an endoscopically guided laser. If laser resection is performed, pretreating the horse with steroids can be helpful in reducing the risk for postoperative airway obstruction. The combination of a sacculectomy and a vocal cordectomy can be helpful in reducing respiratory noise produced when the horse works but does not improve airflow in the way that a prosthetic laryngoplasty does. Approximately 70% of horses treated with a prosthetic laryngoplasty and sacculectomy return to athletic function. The laryngotomy incision is usually left open to heal by second intention. This requires daily cleaning with gauze sponges with saline or water, followed by application of petrolatum to the skin around the incision and on the mandible and neck to prevent skin scald from the drainage. It usually takes approximately 3 weeks for the incision to heal. Some clinicians partially close the incision; this reportedly shortens the time required to heal.

> **TECHNICIAN NOTE** Left laryngeal hemiplegia ("roarer") is a condition resulting in paralysis of the left arytenoid cartilage, which prevents it from being abducted during inspiration.

Epiglottic entrapment is a condition wherein the aryepiglottic membrane that extends from the arytenoid cartilage to the ventral surface of the epiglottis hypertrophies and rolls upward to envelop the rostral and abaxial portions of the epiglottis. Normally, the epiglottis should have a serrated edge and a distinct vascular pattern on the dorsal surface. When the epiglottis becomes entrapped, the serrated edge and the vascular pattern can no longer be seen. The shape or outline of the epiglottis can still be observed (unlike that seen with a DDSP), but the tip appears more rounded, and the abaxial surface is smooth rather than serrated. In chronic cases, the tip of the epiglottis may become ulcerated. The cause of epiglottic entrapment is unknown, but it is believed that these horses have instability between the caudal edge of the soft palate and the epiglottis, and that the aryepiglottic membrane hypertrophies and makes the epiglottis more rigid. Epiglottic entrapment can be intermittent or permanent. Some horses continue to perform athletically with an entrapped epiglottis, but it does appear to affect performance in most horses.

Treatment for epiglottic entrapment includes transecting the aryepiglottic membrane to release the epiglottis. This can be done by using several techniques. First, it can be performed with a hooked bistoury placed through the nasal passages in a standing, sedated horse with or without endoscopic guidance; care must be taken to prevent trauma to other structures and to prevent laceration of the soft palate. Second, it can be performed in an anesthetized horse with a mouth speculum by manually guiding a hooked bistoury and transecting the membrane on midline. Third, it can be performed by using an endoscopically guided laser in a standing, sedated horse. Finally, in more severe or chronic recurring cases, the aryepiglottic membrane can be resected through a ventral laryngotomy. The prognosis for return to athletic performance is good, but entrapment can recur. Some horses may develop DDSP after the entrapment is released. Horses that have the entrapment released by the hooked bistoury or laser can generally resume training in a few days, whereas those treated via resection through a laryngotomy require approximately 3 weeks before training can be resumed.

DDSP is generally a dynamic obstructive disease of the upper respiratory tract that occurs during exercise. Normally, the soft palate remains ventral to the epiglottis.

However, if the epiglottis is small or flaccid, or if the caudal edge of the soft palate is flaccid, the soft palate can become displaced dorsal to the epiglottis during strenuous exercise. The cause of this condition is unknown, but it is believed that the factors listed previously predispose the palate to become displaced during inspiration when negative pressure is generated in the upper airway. This condition usually is intermittent, occurring during strenuous exercise and dissipating once exercise has stopped and the horse swallows. Because horses are obligate nasal breathers, DDSP interferes with their breathing. Horses with DDSP usually make a characteristic gurgling or snoring type of noise, which dissipates as soon as they swallow and replace the palate into its normal position.

Treatment options for a horse with DDSP include placing a cloth or leather tie on the horse's tongue and pulling the tongue rostrad, then tying the tongue to the mandible in the interdental space. The epiglottis, tongue, and sternothyrohyoideus muscles are attached to the hyoid apparatus. Because the tongue is attached at the rostral aspect of the hyoid apparatus, and the sternothyrohyoideus muscles are attached at its caudal aspect, a tongue tie prevents caudal retraction of the hyoid apparatus, including the epiglottis. This seems to help approximately 50% of horses with DDSP because it prevents caudal retraction of the epiglottis and maintains normal epiglottic-palate alignment. Because of its noninvasive nature, the tongue tie is generally the first treatment attempted in horses with DDSP. If this does not work, a section of the sternothyrohyoideus muscles can be resected in the midcervical region; this also prevents caudal retraction of the hyoid apparatus. This myectomy procedure helps in approximately 50% of horses with DDSP that fail to respond to a tongue tie. If this procedure does not work, the caudal margin of the soft palate can be resected (staphylectomy). Two theories have been put forth as to why this may help prevent DDSP. First, it is believed that the caudal edge of the palate becomes more fibrous as it heals with scar tissue; this makes the caudal edge more rigid and therefore more resistant to displacement. The other theory is that if the palate does displace, the palate can be replaced more easily. Regardless of the mechanism, it seems that it helps to prevent DDSP in approximately half of horses that do not respond to the tongue tie or myectomy. A laryngeal tie forward procedure reportedly has achieved a higher success rate in horses with DDSP and should now be considered the surgery of choice if no other source of inflammation is present in the upper respiratory tract. However, general anesthesia is required, so some of the alternative procedures may be performed initially in the standing patient.

Arytenoid chondritis is an inflammatory, degenerative condition of arytenoid cartilages that results in a proliferative mass on one or both arytenoids. It usually leads to obstructive disease of the upper airway with signs similar to the conditions described earlier. These cartilages usually are enlarged and more fibrous than normal, and this prevents them from being effectively treated with a tie-back. The treatment of choice is to remove the affected arytenoid cartilage through a ventral laryngotomy. Performing this surgery with the endoscope passed up one nostril can be helpful because the light from the endoscope will significantly improve visualization of the surgery site. Because of the time required for dissection in the laryngeal region during an arytenoidectomy, a tracheotomy is usually performed in the middle or proximal trachea to provide a mechanism for ventilation during anesthesia. The tracheotomy can be performed before anesthetic induction or once the horse has been anesthetized. These horses are prone to upper airway obstruction postoperatively and need to be closely monitored. The tracheotomy tube is usually left in place, at least for a couple of days, until it is believed that the horse has an airway of adequate diameter for breathing. It is imperative that these horses be monitored closely while the tracheotomy tube is in place to ensure that it does not become dislodged or obstructed with mucus or another discharge. Laryngotomy and tracheotomy sites require daily cleaning and application of petrolatum on the skin around the incisions. Both of these incisions heal by second intention in approximately 3 weeks.

Bacterial infection of the guttural pouch (empyema) usually is a sequela to strangles or retropharyngeal lymph node abscess. Clinical signs include swelling in the throatlatch region and a bilateral mucopurulent nasal discharge. Horses with guttural pouch empyema can be treated conservatively with antibiotics and guttural pouch lavage; this may be effective in many horses that are treated early in the course of the disease. However, in chronic cases, the mucopurulent material becomes inspissated and forms gelatinous concretions (chondroids) that lie in the floor of the guttural pouches. Resolution of empyema requires removal of the chondroids, and long-term effective drainage usually can be achieved only with surgical drainage. Several approaches have been reported for surgical drainage of the guttural pouches, but the most common surgical approach for guttural pouch empyema is the modified Whitehouse technique; an incision is made in the skin on the ventrum of the throat region just axial to the linguofacial vein, and this is followed by blunt dissection into the pouch. The guttural pouch is lavaged intraoperatively. Indwelling catheters can be placed into the guttural pouches in standing, sedated horses under endoscopic guidance; these catheters enable frequent lavage of the pouches. The guttural pouches should not be lavaged with irritating solutions because of the proximity of blood vessels and nerves coursing through the area. The incision is managed similarly to a laryngotomy or tracheotomy incision.

Guttural pouch tympany is an accumulation of air in the guttural pouches; this occurs in foals and weanlings and is usually associated with an abnormality of the opening to the pouches. It can occur on one or both sides and is characterized by a fluctuant, nonpainful swelling in the throat-latch region. If unilateral guttural pouch tympany is present, it is usually treated by surgically creating an opening in the septum between the left and right pouches; this is usually approached through an incision in Viborg's triangle on the affected side. If bilateral tympany is present, creating an opening in the septum will not effectively drain the two sides. Therefore, the opening to one or both of the guttural pouches is surgically revised through a Viborg's triangle approach or by using an endoscopically guided laser. Surgical revision of the guttural pouch opening may be performed on only one side with creation of an opening in the septum to enable both pouches to evacuate the air through one opening.

Guttural pouch mycosis can be life threatening. Fungal plaques form in the lining of the guttural pouches; if the plaques involve vascular structures, such as the internal carotid artery, severe fatal hemorrhage can occur. Fatal hemorrhage is often preceded by several episodes of substantial epistaxis. However, once the diagnosis has been made, surgery should not be delayed. The most accepted method of surgical treatment is vascular occlusion of the internal carotid artery, the external carotid artery, or both, depending on which vessels are affected. This can be done by placement of an intra-arterial balloon-tipped catheter, or by placement of newer springs or coils that stimulate local occlusion. Both internal and external carotid arteries can be ligated unilaterally with no untoward effects. The major potential complication of external carotid artery occlusion is blindness. Once the affected vessels have been ligated, the fungal infection is treated by lavage of the guttural pouches and instillation of antifungal medication into the pouch via indwelling catheters or via the endoscope, although these infections often regress without further specific antifungal therapy.

Surgical Nursing of Food Animals

As in equine practice, veterinary technicians are vital team members in food animal practices. Their roles and responsibilities are identical to those in other fields of veterinary nursing; the principal goal is to safely provide optimal nursing care to patients. Familiarity with food animal species (the emphasis of this section of the chapter will be bovine) is important because they act and behave differently from each other, particularly from horses. To ensure personnel safety, the practice must be equipped with appropriate chutes and stocks so that animals can be examined and restrained. Additional equipment, such as tilt tables, will allow additional surgical or diagnostic procedures to be performed with the use of sedation or general anesthesia. This equipment is invaluable in allowing veterinarians and technicians to examine and work on even the largest bulls in relative safety. Smaller stocks and restraint devices are available for small ruminants but should be used only for these species.

PREOPERATIVE PREPARATION

In nonemergency situations, the following tasks should be routinely performed before any surgical intervention is provided. A physical examination must be performed, and packed cell volume (PCV) and total protein are recommended if risk for significant blood loss is present, or if general anesthesia will be used. Further blood work, such as CBC and a full biochemistry panel, is indicated for most complicated gastrointestinal disturbances because electrolyte abnormalities or infectious processes can influence the surgical outcome and postoperative convalescence. The position of the patient during surgery needs to be considered, so that feed can be withheld for an appropriate time to reduce the risks for regurgitation and aspiration pneumonia. If the adult patient will be in dorsal or lateral recumbency or under general anesthesia, 36 to 48 hours of fasting is indicated. Because of the capacity of the rumen, water should be removed 12 hours preoperatively. For standing procedures, no fasting is required. IV catheterization should be performed shortly before surgery if a catheter is necessary. Either jugular vein can be used, but because of the thickness of cow skin, a stab incision is often made with a scalpel blade to prevent burring of the edges of the catheter. IV catheters can be displaced or pulled out, even when sutured or superglued to the skin. In most cases where IV fluid therapy is indicated, the cow will remain quiet and usually will not move around excessively or rub at the catheter site.

If antibiotics, analgesics, or anesthetics are to be used, care should be taken to ensure that all drugs administered are licensed for use in this species (refer to Chapters 20, 27, 28, and 29). The technician and the veterinarian must be conscious of withdrawal times for all drugs that are used because these may influence postoperative management. Penicillin and ceftiofur tend to be the most widely used antibiotics, and high doses of ceftiofur will provide reasonable Gram-negative coverage. Other alternatives include oxytetracycline, but it has only bacteriostatic properties. Flunixin is the only licensed NSAID; the use of phenylbutazone should be avoided. Anesthetic drugs are used off-label in cattle (see Chapter 29).

Given the environment in which cattle live, they are often dirtier or dustier than animals that are maintained on pasture. If possible, clipping the hair before entering the OR is preferable, to minimize the risk for contamination of the surgery suite. Skin preparation is performed initially to remove any gross skin contaminants and dander, and immediately before surgery, a sterile prep of povidone-iodine or chlorhexidine scrub solution should be applied by standard technique, once the cow has been restrained for surgery (e.g., stocks, tilt table). Iodine scrub should be rinsed with alcohol, and chlorhexidine should be rinsed off with saline.

Preparation of the surgical room or area is important. Having all of the necessary supplies nearby will improve efficiency and prevent surgery from beginning with some important instrument or piece of equipment unavailable. If the animal is to be recumbent for the procedure, the patient must be placed on adequate padding to prevent anesthetic-related complications such as myopathy or myositis and neuropathies (particularly radial nerve paresis or paralysis) from developing. If in lateral recumbency, the distal forelimb should be pulled cranially, and the uppermost hindlimb should be elevated off the most dependent hindlimb with pads or a bale of straw. Even with appropriate padding and support, complications can develop and need to be addressed.

Surgical preparation for the veterinarian must include an appropriate surgical scrub of the hands and forearms. Sterile gloves should be worn, and, where possible, the patient should be draped, and the surgeon should be wearing a sterile gown, cap, and mask.

CONDITIONS OF THE GASTROINTESTINAL TRACT

Abnormalities in the gastrointestinal tract make up the majority of surgeries performed in cattle. For a discussion of actinomycosis and pharyngeal injuries, refer to Chapter 20.

ORAL LACERATIONS

Cattle, especially calves, are not discriminate eaters and often consume debris, such as hardware, found in the pasture. Lacerations or injuries can occur on the tongue, cheeks, or palate when pieces of wire or other sharp objects are chewed and potentially swallowed. Excess salivation or bloody oral discharge may be seen, along with varying degrees of dysphagia and malodorous breath if feed is accumulating within the wound. Diagnosis is usually easy once an oral examination has been performed. With appropriate wound care, many of these lacerations will heal without much treatment because of the excellent blood supply to the oral cavity. Flushing with copious amounts of water (usually via a hose) will prevent accumulation of feedstuff within the wound. Changing the diet to softer feed rather than course roughage will limit feed buildup within the wound. Severe lacerations or punctures may require surgical débridement and repair, and if the tongue is involved, application of a tourniquet may help limit blood loss during the repair.

MANDIBULAR FRACTURES

Fractures may be traumatic or may occur secondary to other pathologic processes, such as lumpy jaw. Fracture location and type and the ability of the animal to eat and drink usually dictate whether surgical repair is necessary. Clinical signs observed include dysphagia, salivation, and often crepitus or palpable instability. Oral examination is important for identifying any communication with the oral cavity because this is a route for secondary bacterial infection, which can complicate the healing process. Radiographs will help confirm the diagnosis and will aid in identification of optimal therapy. If displacement or instability of the mandible is noted, and if the animal is having difficulty eating and drinking, some form of stabilization is indicated.

Surgical options include figure-eight wiring with orthopedic cerclage wire, screw fixation, and application of an external fixation device. The choice is made depending on the location of the fracture, the degree of comminution, the level of involvement of tooth roots, whether the fracture is open or closed, and the cost of the procedure. External fixators are inexpensive, effective, and relatively easily applied.

Most fractures will heal with some form of stabilization, and many cows will resume eating immediately after fixation. If the cow remains anorexic, offering different types of feed is recommended because some cows will eat only their usual ration. If necessary, the oral cavity can be bypassed completely by performing a **rumenostomy**. Potential complications of mandibular fractures include osteomyelitis, sequestrum formation, and abscessation of involved tooth roots. Failure or loosening of the implants often is not a problem because these injuries heal rapidly. The implants can be removed with sedation once healing has occurred.

LAPAROTOMIES

Numerous surgical approaches to the bovine abdomen have been described, and all provide various advantages and disadvantages. Most procedures can be performed via a flank **laparotomy** in the standing patient, but ventral midline or paramedian approaches are necessary in specific situations. Clipping a much larger area than is necessary will prevent any problems if the incision has to be extended and will limit contamination of tissue if any of the drapes used should slip. Local anesthetic techniques can be used to facilitate surgery in the standing patient. IV sedation is sometimes required so the patient tolerates this, but once the area is successfully anesthetized, most patients will settle down, often to the point that some will begin to ruminate.

REGIONAL ANALGESIC TECHNIQUES FOR ABDOMINAL SURGERY

For a flank incision, lidocaine can be injected directly over the line of the incision. Local anesthetic must be placed under the skin, into the muscle, and to the level of the peritoneum if complete analgesia is to be achieved. This is effective and simple but may lead to increased risk for incisional complications, such as infection or dehiscence. An alternative that does not involve injection directly into the surgical site is an inverted-L block. Local anesthetic is injected into all layers of tissue in an inverted-L pattern, vertically behind the last rib, and then horizontally below the transverse processes of the lumbar vertebrae. This blocks nerve fibers at a site distant from the location of the incision, and for this reason, the block must be continued at least a few centimeters distal and caudal to the edge of the incision. If these blocks do not provide adequate analgesia, more local anesthetic can be placed easily and quickly, but because a large volume of local anesthetic can be used, care must be taken to avoid exceeding the toxic dose of lidocaine (6 to 8 mg/kg).

Paravertebral analgesia can be performed; this requires the use of less local anesthetic and can provide a larger area of surgical analgesia than is provided by other techniques. Two techniques are described, and the simplest to perform in dairy cattle (tend to be thinner and the landmarks are easily palpable) is the distal paravertebral technique. Here the transverse processes of lumbar vertebrae 1, 2, and 4 are palpated through the skin. An 18-gauge, 1½-inch needle is then inserted completely, so that it lies parallel to and just below the palpable tip of the transverse process of L1. About

20 ml of 2% lidocaine is injected in a fan pattern; the needle is then withdrawn so that it can be relocated in the same fashion above the transverse process. Ten to 15 ml of lidocaine can be injected into the area in the same fan-like pattern. This process is repeated over the transverse processes of L2 and L4. The technique anesthetizes nerves T13, L1, and L2 at a site distal to where they exit the vertebral column.

The proximal paravertebral technique requires a longer needle; an 18-gauge, 5-inch spinal needle passed through a 14-gauge, 1-inch guide needle is used for this technique. The 14-gauge needle is placed 2 cm lateral to midline at the cranial edge of the transverse process of L1. The spinal needle is then inserted through the 14-gauge needle down onto the transverse process. The spinal needle is walked cranially, off the edge of the process. A "pop" will be felt as the needle penetrates the thick fascial layer, and 15 ml of lidocaine should be injected in this location. Withdrawing the needle roughly 1 to 2 cm will place it above the fascia, and another 15 ml of lidocaine should be injected at this site. The technique should be repeated over the transverse processes of L2 and L3.

Successful placement of either paravertebral block will result in analgesia of the flank, but this can take between 15 and 30 minutes and can be confirmed by observation of scoliosis (the side that is blocked will relax, making the spine bend laterally the other way); vasodilatation, which will make the side palpably warmer (particularly in cool weather); and lack of response to noxious stimuli. Incomplete analgesia may resolve if more time is allowed for diffusion of the anesthetic to occur.

SURGICAL APPROACHES TO THE ABDOMEN

Most abdominal exploratory laparotomies are performed through the right flank (Figure 33-15). This approach provides access to most of the abdominal viscera, although only certain structures can actually be exteriorized. The proximal extent of the incision is approximately one handbreadth below the transverse processes and one handbreadth behind

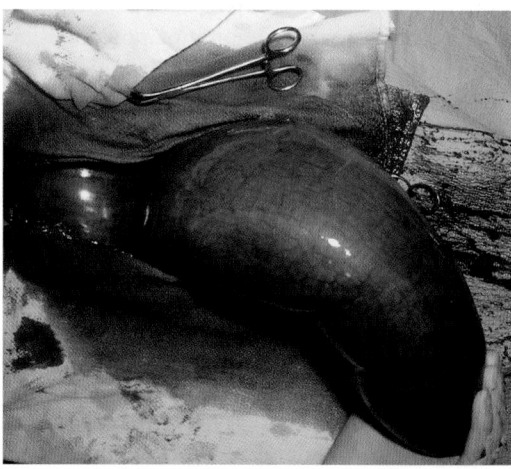

FIGURE 33-15 A right flank laparotomy approach for correction of an intestinal obstruction (cecal volvulus) in a cow.

the caudal edge of the ribs. A 15-cm vertical incision will allow passage of an arm into the abdominal cavity. Keeping the incision located higher in the flank is desirable to limit the ability of the intestine to prolapse out of the incision. Procedures commonly performed from the right flank include abdominal exploratories and correction of abomasal displacements and torsions. An approach through the left flank is used for C-sections, rumenotomies, or rumenostomies.

Some procedures may require a ventral midline or paramedian celiotomy. Sedation is essential for these, as is some form of restraining device to maintain the cow's position. Tilt tables can be used, or the cow can be propped up in dorsal recumbency with bales of straw or ropes. Abomasopexies, C-sections, and umbilical procedures sometimes require this approach. Instead of paravertebral analgesia, local infiltration is often used, or lidocaine is infiltrated on either side of the incision with a portion that converges together at the most cranial aspect of the incision.

RUMENOTOMY FOR GRAIN OVERLOAD

A **rumenotomy** is performed via a left flank laparotomy with the cow standing. A broad area should be clipped and prepped for surgery. The skin incision is oriented vertically and often needs to be bigger than usual flank laparotomy incisions (may need to be 20 cm) so that the rumen can be exteriorized and then secured. The rumenotomy site is the dorsal sac of the rumen. This is secured using one of two recommended rumenotomy procedures: use of a rumen board (Weingarth apparatus) or suturing of the rumen wall to the skin. This is important to prevent contamination of the peritoneal cavity or the skin and muscle layers with rumen contents. Ensuring that enough rumen is exposed beyond the site of fixation will help make closure easier. The contents of the rumen have to be evacuated manually, which is time-consuming. Placing rumen contents into specially designed feed bins can be helpful. A normal trash can with multiple holes drilled through its bottom and a chicken-wire mesh insert to hold fiber in the can may be used to allow fluid to drain out and to hold in most of the fibrous portion of the rumen contents. This will make movement and subsequent disposal of rumen contents easier. Siphoning off the fluid can be performed with a larger-bore tube, such as a Kingman tube, placed into the rumen via the rumenotomy. Once the rumen has been emptied, transfaunation of ruminal fluid from a normal cow can be beneficial. This can be given orally or via the rumenotomy before closure. Removing any gross contamination from the edges of the rumenotomy is important before it is sutured closed in two layers. The body wall and the skin can then be closed in a routine fashion.

A rumenostomy, or permanent rumen fistula, can be created using a similar technique. Commercial rubber rumen fistulas and plugs are available, and if one of these is to be used, close attention to the size of the surgical incision is necessary. The skin incision needs to be longer and should measure about 15 cm. This will allow the fistula to form a tight seal and will prevent leakage of rumen contents. The skin incision is continued through the external abdominal oblique muscle; then the deeper muscles are separated in the direction of their fibers. After opening of the peritoneum, a three-layer closure technique can be used. The peritoneum is sutured to the abdominal muscles using an absorbable suture. After exteriorization of part of the rumen, the rumen is sutured to the subcutaneous tissue, then the rumen is incised and the mucosa is sutured to the skin. Ensuring that the second layer is tight before incising the rumen will help minimize the risk of contaminating the abdomen with rumen contents. Placement of the rubber fistula and plug will now allow the rumen to be sealed, but accessible when necessary. This is usually done for research purposes but can be helpful when one is treating sick cattle because it makes collection of ruminal contents for rumen transfaunation considerably easier.

TRAUMATIC RETICULOPERITONITIS

For information on diagnosis and medical treatment of this condition, please see Chapter 20. Surgical intervention may be necessary if traumatic reticuloperitonitis (TRP) fails to respond to conservative treatment, if a foreign body is observed outside the reticulum on radiography, or if an intra-abdominal or thoracic abscess is suspected. The approach of choice is a left flank exploratory laparotomy and rumenotomy using transruminal exploration. The technique required for rumenotomy is the same as that described for treating grain overload, with the exception that the incision is located a little more cranially to ensure that the reticulum can be reached by the surgeon. Most abscesses that form secondary to TRP are located on the medial wall of the reticulum and are tightly adhered. These abscesses are the most common causes of vagal indigestion associated with TRP. These tightly adhered abscesses can be lanced and drained into the reticulum or omasum and then explored for the presence of a foreign body. Lancing these abscesses can be difficult and requires a blind technique. Providing a scalpel blade on a loop of suture will allow the loop to be placed over the surgeon's wrist to reduce the risk of dropping it into the rumen.

> **TECHNICIAN NOTE** TRP (hardware disease) may lead to peritonitis, liver or reticular abscesses, pericarditis, vagal indigestion, or other secondary problems.

ABOMASAL DISPLACEMENTS AND VOLVULUS

Abomasal displacement is a common problem of high-producing dairy cows fed high-concentrate, low-roughage diets. Displacements are most likely to occur in the first 6 weeks after calving. Predisposing factors include high-grain diets with increased quantities of volatile fatty acids in the abomasum; hypocalcemia; concurrent diseases, such as mastitis, metritis, and ketosis; and lack of exercise. Increased volatile fatty acids, histamine release with concurrent diseases, and hypocalcemia may lead to abomasal dilatation and atony and subsequent displacement of the abomasum from its normal right paramedian position to the left or right paralumbar area. Left displaced abomasum (LDA) is much more common than right displaced abomasum (RDA). Abomasal volvulus (AV) may occur after displacement to the right and carries a poorer prognosis than LDA or RDA because of compromise of the innervation and blood supply that occurs when the abomasum twists. AV can quickly lead to development of shock and toxemia if not diagnosed and treated early.

LDA, RDA, or AV can be diagnosed by auscultation of a distinct "ping" in the left or right paralumbar fossa area because gas trapped in the abomasum produces a characteristic "metallic pinging" sound when the area over the gas cap is percussed while simultaneous auscultation is performed with a stethoscope.

The Liptak test can be used as an aid in diagnosing LDA. After percussion of the abomasum on the left side under the last few ribs, an area just below the gas ping, which corresponds to the fluid level in the abomasum, is clipped and surgically prepared. Centesis is performed using an 18-gauge, 10- to 12-cm needle. Fluid with a pH less than 4.5 confirms the presence of an LDA. Aspiration of gas with a characteristic "burnt almond" odor is indicative of an LDA.

Surgery is usually necessary to correct abomasal displacements, and AV requires immediate surgical intervention. Choices of surgical approach and technique depend on the direction of the displacement, the presence of volvulus, the condition of the animal, and the surgeon's preference. Traditionally, a right flank laparotomy is performed to correct the displacement. The most helpful piece of equipment is a piece of surgical tubing (must be long enough to reach to the far side of the cow and then extend well clear of the surgical incision) attached to a large needle. This is taken into the abdomen, guarded by the surgeon's hand, and carried around the caudal edge of the rumen and omentum. It is then tunneled through the abomasal wall to decompress it. Once decompressed, the abomasum can be swept or pulled back to the left side, where an **omentopexy** or a **pyloropexy** can be performed to the abdominal wall. A right-sided displacement or volvulus needs to be decompressed and repositioned before pexying to the body wall. Surgical approaches using a left and right flank laparotomy or laparoscopic approaches have been described and are beyond the scope of this text. If a cow has had a recurrence of an abomasal displacement after a left-sided approach, a paramedian **abomasopexy** may be indicated. In this situation, the cow is sedated and is rolled into dorsal recumbency on a tilt table or by casting with ropes. The ventral abdomen is clipped and prepped for a paramedian incision roughly 10 cm behind the xiphoid process and 10 cm to the right of midline. The surgical site is anesthetized using local infiltration of local anesthetic, and the site is sterilely prepped. An incision is made into the body wall, and the abomasum is exposed through this incision. An abomasopexy is performed by suturing the abomasum and the body wall closed simultaneously, resulting in a strong adhesion that will prevent future displacements. After surgery, the diet should be restricted to roughage only, and grain should be introduced gradually into the diet once recovery is complete.

AFTERCARE FOLLOWING A LAPAROTOMY

Feed can be reintroduced once the cow has recovered from any sedation or general anesthesia. It is usually ideal to withhold feed and water until the cow no longer shows any signs of sedation, which can be prolonged with xylazine. The goal is to return the cow to full feed, but this should be done gradually over a few days. Cows that are relatively healthy will often eat well after surgery and will require little further management. If they have been anorexic for a prolonged period, offering different feed is important to try to tempt the cow to eat something. If necessary, force feeding can be performed via a large-bore stomach tube. Slurries made from alfalfa meal or a pelleted feed can be used but can be difficult to pump through the tube. Constant stirring or increasing the fluid content of the feed can be helpful to ease its passage through the tube. Rumen fluid transfaunation can also be helpful for these cows, if possible. Keeping the cow in a well-bedded, dry, draft-free environment will ensure that it is comfortable and should help it to recover. The incision usually will need little if any care. Infection of the surgical site can be identified by swelling, discomfort upon palpation of the area, and usually some discharge. Flank incisions can be treated by creating ventral drainage and allowing any purulent material to drain out. This is often all that is needed, and the incision will heal by second intention with routine wound management.

OTHER GASTROINTESTINAL CONDITIONS

The remainder of the gastrointestinal tract can also require surgical therapy. In the small intestine, intussusceptions, volvulus, or hemorrhagic bowel syndrome can occur. Cecal tympany or displacement can sometimes be mistaken for an RDA (ping in this case will be farther caudal and dorsal on the flank than for an abomasal problem), or this can even become intussuscepted into itself. Obstructions or intussusceptions of the spiral colon can also occur. These often are evaluated surgically, and an approach through the right flank is most commonly used. Exposure of the entire gastrointestinal tract is not always possible, so if the incision needs to be elongated ventrally, general anesthesia may be indicated to prevent sudden movement or to keep the cow from becoming sternal, which could allow (uncontrolled evisceration) parts of the intestines to fall onto nonsterile surfaces.

Adhesion formation can be a sequela of abdominal surgery or can follow a separate disease process. This will often lead to signs of an abomasal outflow obstruction, general colic, or weight loss. An exploratory laparotomy can be performed to evaluate this, but treatment options are limited. Adhesions can be broken down, but the risk for recurrence is high.

CONDITIONS OF THE MUSCULOSKELETAL SYSTEM

LAMENESS

Lameness is commonly encountered in cattle and most often (88%) is caused by lesions or problems in the foot. Most of these conditions have been discussed in Chapter 20. Upper leg problems, such as anterior cruciate ligament rupture, coxofemoral (hip) luxation, fracture, and arthritis, account for the remaining 12% of cases of lameness seen. When foot problems occur, they are most often seen in the claws that bear the most weight—front medial and hind lateral claws. It is important to examine all foot problems early because many conditions can progress to osteomyelitis and/or septic arthritis if not properly treated. Regardless of the cause of lameness, it can lead to loss of production as a result of decreased milk production, weight loss, delayed breeding or anestrus, and culling. Intensive housing and feeding of large groups of animals have led to an increased incidence of lameness.

> **TECHNICIAN NOTE** Lameness is commonly encountered in cattle and most often is caused by lesions or problems in the foot.

REGIONAL ANALGESIA AND ANTIBIOTIC PERFUSION TECHNIQUES AND PMMA IMPLANTS

Regional analgesia (IV retrograde analgesia) of the foot and/or distal limb is commonly performed before claw amputation or corn removal, although regional block can be used for other surgeries or painful techniques of the foot or distal limb, or as a diagnostic aid in lameness examinations. A tourniquet is applied distal to the hock or carpus in the midmetatarsal or midmetacarpal area. A superficial vein is located—the common dorsal metacarpal (metatarsal) vein or the palmar or plantar metacarpal (metatarsal) vein—and is surgically prepared. An IV injection of 15 to 30 ml of 2% lidocaine will provide analgesia in 5 minutes, and this will persist until the tourniquet is released (the tourniquet should not be left in place for longer than an hour) (Figure 33-16). It is ideal to have the cow's leg secured to prevent extravascular placement of the local anesthetic. Even with restraint, movement is often still possible, so use of a butterfly catheter with a short extension can be helpful.

An alternative to this technique involves placing the tourniquet above the tarsus or carpus to achieve analgesia more proximally. Accordingly, more lidocaine should be used to block this larger area (may need 30 to 60 ml of perfusate). This same technique can be used to provide regional perfusion of antibiotics to the distal limb for the purpose of treating localized infection, such as foot rot with cellulitis. An antibiotic with an IV formulation should be used and can

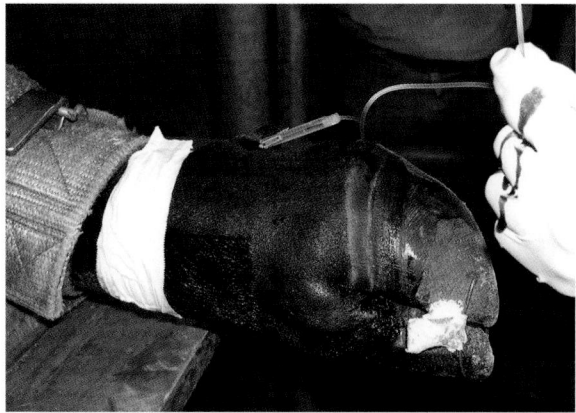

FIGURE 33-16 Injection of lidocaine for IV retrograde analgesia of the bovine foot after placement of a tourniquet above the fetlock.

be diluted with sterile saline to produce a perfusate volume of at least 20 to 30 ml. Cephalosporins can be injected through the catheter and allowed to perfuse the limb distal to the tourniquet for approximately 45 minutes. Both of these techniques are used primarily in cattle, but they can be applied to all food animal species. Implantation of antibiotic-impregnated polymethylmethacrylate (PMMA) beads subcutaneously near infected joints has shown promise for treatment of septic arthritis in calves. The beads slowly release antibiotics into the joint and appear to be more effective than systemic antibiotic treatment or joint flushing alone. Techniques such as joint flushing, PMMA bead implants, regional perfusion, and systemic antibiotics used in combination work well to resolve septic arthritis. After the sepsis has resolved, the beads can be removed, but they should cause no problem if left in place.

SURGICAL DISEASES OF THE HOOF AND PHALANGES

Interdigital Hyperplasia

Interdigital hyperplasia (interdigital fibroma, corn) is a thickening of the interdigital skin that causes a mass to protrude between the claws (Figure 33-17). One or more feet may be involved, but the hind feet are more commonly affected. Beef breeds, especially bulls, have a higher incidence of corns. Fibromas develop in response to chronic irritation between the claws. Hereditary predisposition is suspected. Spreading of the toes and other conformational problems probably contribute to irritation of the interdigital skin.

The size of the mass varies from a noticeable thickening of the skin to a size of 3 cm or larger. A large mass can cause pain, and the fibroma may become eroded, ulcerated, and even infected, leading to increased swelling and pain. Lameness varies, depending on the size of the mass, from absent to severe. The size of the corn and the degree of lameness are guides in determining whether removal is necessary. Surgical excision is accomplished using IV retrograde analgesia, and care should be taken to ensure that all hyperplastic tissue is excised. Excision of part of the fat pad in the interdigital

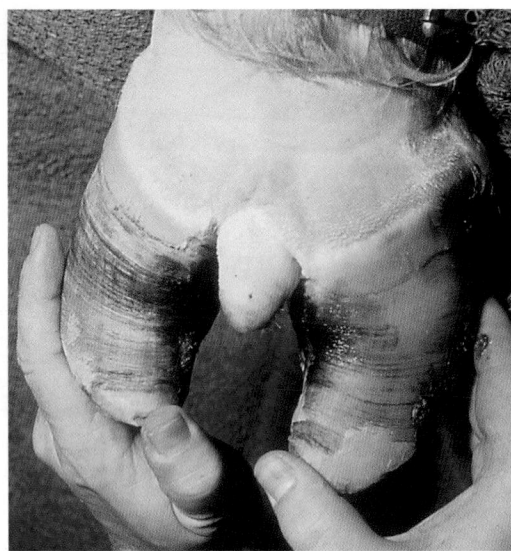

FIGURE 33-17 Interdigital hyperplasia (fibroma or corn) between the toes of a bull's foot.

space will help to improve wound healing by preventing fat from protruding between healing skin edges. To reduce the discomfort associated with outward displacement of the toes, the toes can be wired together by drilling holes at the toe region and securing them using cerclage wire. Placement of wires on the abaxial side of the claws will reduce the risk that the wire may pull through the hoof capsule prematurely.

Claw Amputation

Diseases of the foot may become so severe that they cannot be treated, thus necessitating amputation of the affected digit. Any of the previously discussed conditions of the foot (see Chapter 20) and other diseases may lead to infection of deeper tissues with resulting osteomyelitis of the first phalanx (P1), second phalanx (P2), or third phalanx (P3) and/or septic arthritis of the proximal or distal interphalangeal joints (pastern or coffin joint). In cases of advanced infection, removal of the infected claw may be the only treatment option. This procedure is performed with IV retrograde analgesia (as described earlier). A full-thickness skin incision is made on the axial aspect of the claw, perpendicular to the bone's long axis, down to the bone of the distal first phalanx. The affected claw is then removed at a level necessary to remove all infected tissue using obstetrical (OB) wire (it should be noted that amputation can be performed only distal to the fetlock joint). The claw should be removed at a cosmetic angle and through bone rather than through a joint. The foot is then bandaged snugly after topical antibiotic application. Bandage changes should be done every 3 days until any exposed bone is covered with granulation tissue. The entire healing process takes about 6 weeks. Cattle can support weight on one claw but eventually will experience breakdown of supporting structures of the remaining claw. The time it takes for breakdown depends on the claw removed, the weight and use of the animal, and the surface

on which the animal must stand. It is undesirable to remove any claw in a bull, except for salvage purposes, and it is not generally a good choice to remove a weight-bearing claw (front medial or hind lateral) in cows, although sometimes there is no choice.

> **TECHNICIAN NOTE** Diseases of the foot may become so severe that they cannot be treated, thus necessitating amputation of the affected digit.

Foot Block Application and Casting

Wooden or acrylic blocks or commercial rubber shoes may be glued to the bottom of healthy claws to reduce or eliminate weight bearing on a diseased or painful claw. These devices are adhered to the claw using an acrylic material (Technovit, Jorgensen Laboratories, Inc., Loveland, Colorado) or products such as Equithane adhesives. Wooden blocks may last as long as 6 weeks and may be allowed to wear off naturally unless they are wearing abnormally, in which case they may be manually removed earlier. Blocks or shoes help promote healing of affected claws and make the animal more comfortable when standing or moving.

An additional method of immobilizing the claws is application of a hoof cast. A wound dressing should be applied to the surgery site, if one is present, and a layer of cast padding material should be placed between the claws. The claws can be wired together, stockinette can be applied up to the distal metacarpal or metatarsal bone, and then cast padding material can be applied to the proximal extent of the area to be cast (usually level of mid-P1). This material should overlap approximately 50% with the previous layer. Fiberglass cast material can then be applied to immobilize the distal limb. Applying the material while it is still wet will prevent it from curing too rapidly because this can keep it from adhering to itself, which can result in a weaker cast. The cast can remain in place for 10 to 14 days, after which time it should be removed. Cast removal can be performed with a cast saw or Gigli wires, if they were placed between the cast padding and the cast tape at the time of application.

Obturator and Sciatic Nerve Paresis and Paralysis

The obturator and/or sciatic nerves may sustain damage during dystocia or forced fetal extraction, resulting in "calving paralysis." Treatment consists of NSAIDs given early, good nursing care, housing the animal on a soft surface with good footing, using flotation devices, lifting the cow or heifer for short periods of time at least a couple of times a day, rolling the cow from side to side several times daily to prevent severe muscle compression, and hobbling cows or heifers that can stand but cannot adduct their hind legs.

> **TECHNICIAN NOTE** During dystocia or forced fetal extraction, the obturator and/or sciatic nerves may sustain damage, resulting in "calving paralysis."

Radial Nerve Paralysis

Radial nerve paralysis is most commonly seen after a period of lateral recumbency, with the most dependent forelimb being exposed to excessive or prolonged pressure (the weight of the animal itself can be enough) over the upper forelimb. The most obvious clinical sign is an inability to bear any weight on the affected limb if an attempt to stand is made. The elbow will appear to be dropped, and the cow will be unable to maintain its carpus or elbow in extension, thereby preventing weight bearing. This often does not appear to be painful, but it can be stressful if multiple attempts to stand or move are made. Treatment is supportive. Systemic NSAIDs should be administered, and a Robert Jones bandage and splint should be applied to the limb. The bandage should extend from the proximal radius to the hoof, and the splint can be placed on the dorsal or palmar surface. The goal is to lock the carpus in extension with the splint; this will allow weight bearing to resume while limiting mobility. This is often all that is necessary, and the condition usually will show signs of improvement within 24 hours of onset. The duration of neurologic deficits will depend on the severity of the injury, but a full recovery is usually possible. The most important other cause of radial nerve deficits is an upper limb fracture (humerus, proximal radius or ulna), but these cases can often be distinguished by marked local swelling, pain upon palpation, or manipulation and often crepitus.

Fractures

Trauma from a kick or a fall can result in long-bone, spinal, or pelvic fracture. An acute-onset, severe lameness is observed, with the animal often non–weight bearing in the affected limb or recumbent. Soft tissue swelling tends to be marked, and as a result of limited soft tissue coverage, many fractures will be open. Before any fracture repair is attempted, the weight, size, age, disposition, and financial value of the animal need to be taken into consideration. Radiographs should be taken to allow accurate classification of the fracture (displaced or nondisplaced, open or closed, simple or comminuted). Injury to associated soft tissues can delay healing if the vasculature has been compromised; if excessive tissue is injured, it can predispose to infection. Some form of support should be applied to the limb until fixation is attempted; this can range from a Robert Jones bandage with or without splints, cast material, or, for some fractures (femur, humerus, and pelvis), simple stall confinement.

Feed should be withheld if anesthesia is going to be necessary for fracture stabilization, systemic antibiotics should be initiated, and analgesia should be provided. If the cow is dehydrated or is showing signs of shock, IV fluids may be administered via a jugular catheter.

Fracture stabilization can be achieved using internal fixation devices (screws and bone plates) or external fixation (casts, Thomas splints, or transfixation casts). If stabilization is adequate and no infection is present, the bones will often be able to heal with time.

Osteomyelitis should be considered if after fracture stabilization, a sudden increase in the degree of lameness is noted.

Signs of inflammation and swelling are often present at the surgical site (assuming this is visible and not underneath a cast), but radiographs are often necessary to confirm the presence of infection. Radiographic evidence of osteomyelitis usually is observed only once the infection is well established—roughly 10 to 14 days after its onset. Systemic or local antibiotics should be administered, drainage should be established to prevent accumulation of purulent material, and, in severe cases, internal implants may have to be removed or replaced. Before radiographic changes become evident, the patient may be febrile or may have an altered leukogram. Aggressive therapy is necessary if there is to be any chance of success, but the prognosis is often poor.

Strict stall rest is needed until radiographic evidence of fracture healing is found, and the patient may still be reluctant or unable to move easily. Ensuring that the cow has easy access to feed and water is essential to prevent it from struggling or moving excessively and risking damage to healing bone. Keeping these cows on deep bedding is important to reduce the risk for decubital ulcers, so rolling the cow may be required to prevent or reduce their occurrence. Excessively deep bedding can actually make it more difficult for the cow to stand or move, especially if it is wearing a cast. When possible, slings or flotation devices may be helpful in preventing prolonged periods of recumbency.

Septic Arthritis

Septic arthritis is a common cause of severe, acute-onset lameness in cattle. In calves, it is usually secondary to infection elsewhere in the body and spreads hematogenously. In adults, it is often secondary to a puncture wound or trauma. Diagnosis is based on severe lameness, local swelling, and often an obvious wound. Confirmation of synovial involvement can be obtained by performing a sterile arthrocentesis at a site distant from any puncture or wound. If possible, a sample of the synovial fluid should be obtained for cytology, white blood cell count, total protein, and culture and sensitivity. In a septic joint, white blood cells will be preponderantly neutrophils (greater than 75%), the white blood cell count is greater than $3000/\mu l$, total protein is greater than 40 g/L, and bacteria may or may not be cultured. Attempts to distend the joint with saline will not succeed if the joint is open and if it communicates with a wound. In this case, when saline is injected, it will be seen exiting the joint via the wound, confirming involvement of the joint. If the joint is intact, sterile saline can be injected into the joint to distend it, and the increase in pressure should allow the syringe to fill back up if it remains attached and pressure is removed from the plunger. Care should be taken when identifying a site for arthrocentesis so as to prevent iatrogenic infection of the joint; the needle should not be passed through any infected tissue. Identification of infected tissue can be difficult, so if there is any doubt, arthrocentesis may be contraindicated.

Treatment revolves around removing bacteria and inflammatory mediators from within the joint. The joint can be flushed under sedation using sterile fluids and through-and-through lavage with multiple needles placed within the joint. Large needles (14 to 16 gauge) often are needed because smaller needles often become blocked by fibrin or other debris from the joint. If this occurs, or if the infection is chronic, arthrotomies may be necessary to establish adequate drainage. These may have to be protected by bandages or stent dressings between joint flushes. If arthroscopic lavage is performed, general anesthesia may be indicated to prevent damage to the equipment. After lavage, antibiotics can be placed directly into the joint to achieve high concentrations that will persist. Ceftiofur or penicillin can be used for this purpose. Joint lavage is usually performed once daily and should be repeated until no lameness is evident. Other cost-effective methods of antibiotic delivery include regional IV antibiotic perfusion and insertion of PMMA antibiotic-impregnated beads. These techniques are beneficial, but if they cannot be used, systemic antibiotics should be administered in conjunction with lavage. In joints that do not respond to therapy, or that develop secondary osteoarthritis after resolution of the infection, arthrodesis and claw amputation are treatment options to try to improve the level of comfort. Coffin joint arthrodesis has been performed after resolution of septic coffin joints, using Acutrak Plus screws. This procedure is more expensive than claw amputation, but it results in much longer survival times and increased productivity.

> **TECHNICIAN NOTE** Septic arthritis can occur secondary to a penetrating wound or hematogenously in young stock. This must be a differential diagnosis in acute-onset, severe lameness.

CONDITIONS OF THE RESPIRATORY SYSTEM

Surgical conditions of the respiratory tract are rare in cattle. Tracheostomies may be the most useful techniques for this body system, but they will be performed infrequently. Any obstruction of the upper respiratory tract may necessitate this, and surgical preparation, such as clipping, often cannot be performed. In true emergencies, reestablishing a patent airway is more important than having a neatly clipped or scrubbed surgical site. The most appropriate location at which to perform a tracheostomy is on the ventral midline—roughly halfway between the larynx and the thoracic inlet. Palpation of tracheal rings in this region that have the least soft tissue overlying them will help locate the ideal surgical site. Placing a line block with local anesthesia under the skin will facilitate the procedure. If possible, the trachea should be grasped with one hand through the skin and stabilized before the skin is incised over it (about 8 to 10 cm). Ensuring that the incision is on midline will expose a muscle layer that should be split, either sharply or bluntly, until the trachea is exposed. The trachea should be opened by making a stab incision (just big enough to insert a tracheostomy tube) into it through the membrane between the cartilaginous tracheal rings. A temporary tracheotomy tube, a piece of stomach

tube, or another semi-rigid, hollow piece of tubing can then be used to establish a patent airway. If the skin or deeper incision is off the ventral midline, exposing the trachea can be difficult, and other vital structures (jugular veins, carotid artery, etc.) can be damaged. In most situations, a temporary tracheotomy should be performed; a permanent tracheostomy, if indicated, can be performed in a more controlled manner at a later time.

The tracheostomy site will have to be cleaned frequently because most normal respiratory secretions will exit through this site. Application of petroleum jelly to the skin around the site will prevent scalding. After resolution of the inciting cause, the tube can be removed, and the tracheostomy site will heal by second intention. A permanent tracheostomy can be performed in a similar location, but instead of incising between the tracheal rings, the opening into the tracheal lumen removes a portion of three to four tracheal rings to allow the tracheal mucosa to be sutured to the skin edges. Aftercare of this stoma is the same as for a temporary tracheostomy.

CONDITIONS OF THE UROGENITAL SYSTEM

ANESTHESIA OF THE UROGENITAL AND REPRODUCTIVE SYSTEMS

A caudal or low epidural provides loss of sensation to the anus, vulva, and perineum, and to caudal aspects of the thighs. It is used for relief of tenesmus and obstetric straining; vaginal, rectal, and uterine prolapse repair; and surgical procedures of the perineal area. Injection is made between the first and second coccygeal (Cy1 to Cy2) vertebrae or in the sacrococcygeal space. The space is located by moving the tail up and down while palpating for the first obvious articulation caudal to the sacrum. With aseptic technique, an 18-gauge, $1\frac{1}{2}$-inch needle is inserted through the space at the midline at a 10-degree angle (tip of the needle directed cranially) until a drop of lidocaine placed in the hub of the needle is sucked into the space. An alternative approach involves inserting the needle until it hits the floor of the spinal canal, at which time the needle is backed out slightly to enter the epidural space. There should be no resistance to injection. The dose of lidocaine used is 0.5 to 1 ml of 2% lidocaine per 45 kg body weight, with which the animal should have adequate analgesia but remain standing. If sedation is helpful, or if a longer duration of action is indicated, xylazine can be given alone (0.05 mg/kg diluted to 5 ml in sterile saline) or in combination (use a lower dose, 0.03 mg/kg) with the lidocaine.

A bilateral, internal pudendal nerve block can be performed to facilitate examination or surgery of a bull's penis. This nerve can be palpated via a rectal examination, on either side of the pelvic canal, dorsal to the pudendal artery where it is associated with the lesser sciatic foramen. Care must be taken to inject only the area around the nerve; about 15 ml is injected in the region of the nerve and slightly caudally.

UROLITHIASIS

Urolithiasis is the result of formation of calculi (uroliths) within the urinary tract. Uroliths may result in conditions ranging from minor urinary tract irritation to complete obstruction of urine flow. The nonclinical manifestation of this condition is referred to as *urolithiasis*, whereas the clinical form is termed *obstructive urolithiasis*. When complete obstruction occurs, marked distention of the urinary bladder is noted, with eventual rupture of the bladder, the urethra, or both. Depending on the site of rupture, urine accumulates in the ventral subcutaneous tissues (urethra) or in the abdomen (bladder), resulting in swelling that is commonly referred to as *water belly*.

Although no sex predilection for the development of calculi has been noted, males are much more likely to become obstructed as a result of the length, shape, and size of their urethra. The most common site of obstruction in cattle is the distal sigmoid flexure of the penis (Figure 33-18). Feedlot animals receiving grain rations with high phosphorus levels are predisposed to development of phosphate calculi.

Clinical signs of acute urethral obstruction are attributable to trauma to the urinary tract epithelium and to bladder distention. Early in the course, the animal repeatedly assumes a posture for urination, but little or no urination results from these attempts to void. As bladder distention progresses, the animal may tread, stretch, tail swish, and kick at its abdomen. Blood and/or crystals may be present on the preputial hairs. Nonspecific signs such as anorexia, mild bloat, and lethargy are also common. Owners often misinterpret these signs as evidence of acute gastrointestinal disorders, especially because affected animals may show signs similar to colic. After the bladder or urethra ruptures, straining ceases, and the animal may go through a brief phase of euphoria; however, azotemia (increased blood urea nitrogen [BUN] and creatinine) and dehydration quickly develop. If urethral obstruction is diagnosed early, before azotemia develops, or before the bladder or urethra ruptures, the animal may be immediately slaughtered. If not, medical and/or surgical treatment should be initiated quickly.

Medical management involves the use of muscle relaxants to facilitate passage of the calculi, antimicrobial therapy for urinary tract infection, and the use of a urinary acidifier, such as ammonium chloride. Medical therapy alone is rarely successful, so it may be necessary to consider surgery in some cases. Perineal urethrostomy may be chosen as a salvage procedure, particularly for feedlot steers and bulls of low economic value (Figure 33-19). This surgical approach allows for relief of obstruction and resolution of the uremia before slaughter. Long-term urethral stricture has been a problem with this technique. The procedure is performed with the animal standing and analgesia provided by a caudal or low epidural block.

The low approach is often preferred for perineal urethrostomy. This allows the penis to be diverted caudally at such an angle as to prevent urine scald to the hind legs. It also makes it possible to perform repeated procedures higher, if necessary. The skin incision is made beginning at the dorsal aspect of the scrotum or scrotal remnant, and extending dorsally on the midline for 10 to 15 cm. The incision is continued until the penis is encountered. The retractor penis muscles may be the first structures seen and are frequently mistaken for the penis. These muscles are superficial to the penis, pink, soft, and easily separated into two structures. The penis is a relatively firm, single structure covered by the white tunica albuginea. Once the penis has been located, it is bluntly dissected from the surrounding tough fascia and is pulled caudally out of the incision. The penis is transected at a length adequate to allow the transected end to exit the perineal incision without tension, leaving a 2- to 3-cm stump exposed. The stump is sutured to the skin of the lower part of the incision using a mattress suture that surrounds the corpus cavernosum penis (CCP) and passes under the

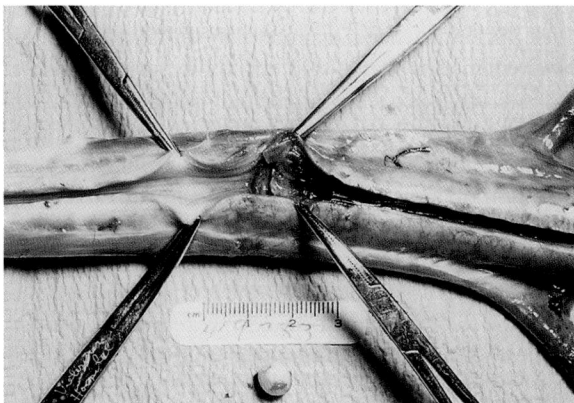

FIGURE 33-18 Identification of a calculus causing obstructive urolithiasis at the distal sigmoid flexure in a bull. Note urethral necrosis at the site where the calculus was lodged.

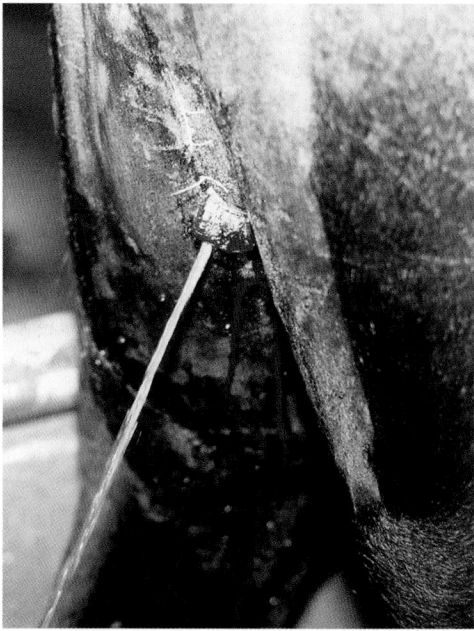

FIGURE 33-19 Perineal urethrostomy performed as a salvage procedure for treatment of obstructive urolithiasis in a steer.

urethra. This suture limits hemorrhage from the CCP. In addition, the urethra can be split for several centimeters and spatulated by suturing the urethral mucosa and the tunica albuginea to the skin using 2-0 or 3-0 absorbable suture material. This optional technique is intended to limit stricture of the urethral opening. The remaining skin incision is closed with simple interrupted sutures of nonabsorbable suture material. Urethral obstruction may recur as a result of additional calculi, or because of stricture of the urethrostomy site.

An alternative surgical procedure that can be used for valuable breeding bulls or "pets" is the ischial urethrostomy, a temporary urethrostomy with catheter placement. This technique allows for urine egress through a Foley catheter placed in the urethra at the level of the ischium, just below the anus, and antegrade or retrograde flushing of the distal urethra to remove calculi. When the tube is pulled, the urethrostomy usually heals by second intention without stricture formation. This procedure can be useful for preservation of fertility in valuable breeding bulls.

Dietary management is the key to control and prevention of obstructive urolithiasis. The calcium-to-phosphorus ratio of the overall diet should be in the range of 2:1 to 2.5:1. A continuous supply of fresh, clean water should be available at all times, and salt may be added to the ration up to 4% to promote water intake and diuresis. In addition, vitamin A may be added to the ration to help prevent desquamation of epithelial cells in the bladder. Prophylactic use of urinary acidifiers is advocated; administration of ammonium chloride at 1% to 1.5% of the ration is recommended.

> **TECHNICIAN NOTE** Perineal urethrostomy may be chosen as a salvage procedure for feedlot steers with obstructive urolithiasis.

RUPTURED BLADDER

This is seen as a secondary complication of obstructive urolithiasis that is not treated promptly enough. In adults, this complication is diagnosed by clinical signs of progressive abdominal distention, dehydration, anorexia, and depression. Confirmation often requires abdominocentesis, which produces a clear, yellow fluid with a peritoneal-to-serum creatinine ratio of 2:1 or greater. Urinary catheterization is reported to be an effective treatment to allow the bladder time to heal if a dorsal tear is present. Ventral tears usually require surgical repair, but gaining access to this region of the bladder can sometimes be challenging via a flank laparotomy, necessitating a ventral approach.

UROVAGINA

Older cows with poor perineal conformation and those in poor condition may be more susceptible to urovagina. Urine accumulates in the vagina, resulting in marked inflammation, which can lead to infertility. A vaginal examination will reveal the presence of urine in the vagina, which is considered to be diagnostic. If the cow is to be treated, surgical correction is necessary, to elongate the urethra or to elevate the transverse fold to redirect the urine externally. Anesthesia can be provided by performing a caudal or low epidural, or by locally infiltrating lidocaine along the site of the incisions. Restraining the cow in stocks is preferable to limit their movement. Before surgery is begun, the rectum should be emptied, and the tail should be restrained so that it is clear from the surgery site. Self-retaining retractors can be helpful for this procedure, or, alternatively, stay sutures can be placed to hold the vulva open against the perineum. Adequate lighting is best provided by the surgeon wearing a head lamp. Other forms of lighting are difficult to aim properly, and the surgeon's head usually obstructs the beam. Urethral extensions can be created by splitting the transverse fold, which is located above the urethral orifice in the vagina, and then creating a new shelf by continuing this incision laterally along the vaginal wall on both sides. Dissection of these shelves distally is performed bluntly to allow them to meet at the midline with no tension, and then the mucosal sheets are sutured in a Y pattern. Leaving a urinary catheter in place for a period postoperatively is helpful to ensure that urination can occur, because some postoperative swelling may occur.

CONDITIONS OF THE REPRODUCTIVE SYSTEM

SUPERNUMERARY TEAT REMOVAL

Removal of extra teats is of greatest value in young dairy heifers, but it is also performed in beef heifers intended for show. Often this procedure is performed at the time of brucellosis vaccination. The extra teats are removed flush with the skin and parallel to the normal folds of the udder using curved scissors. In young calves, suturing the skin is not usually necessary. Care must be taken to avoid removing any of the four normal teats.

OVARIAN DISEASE

Ovarian cysts, abscesses, or neoplasms occur in cattle. Other indications for ovariectomy include preventing pregnancy and trying to improve fattening of feedlot cows. To minimize the risk for hemorrhage, ovariectomy should ideally be performed when the ovary is in the follicular or early luteal phase. A flank approach is often used if a unilateral ovariectomy is performed or in situations where the ovary is enlarged. A colpotomy can be used for a bilateral ovariectomy if both ovaries are of normal size, but this will require a caudal epidural. Achieving good hemostasis is essential, especially in pathologic ovaries. To minimize discomfort during this process, applying a gauze or lap sponge soaked in lidocaine to the ovarian pedicle may reduce movement by the patient. This gauze or sponge should be attached to the surgeon to prevent it from being lost inside the abdomen. Holding this sponge over the pedicle for at least a minute may be beneficial. Transfixation sutures and application of a chain écraseur or emasculators can be used if a flank approach is selected. Specific instruments, such as a Kimberly-Rupp or a Willis rod, should be reserved for normal ovaries.

Postoperatively, these patients should be monitored for signs of hemorrhage because inadequate hemostasis can be life threatening.

DYSTOCIA

C-section is indicated when there is a chance of delivering a live calf during a dystocia, malposition, or presentation, or when the calf is excessively large. Several approaches are available for C-section, including flank approaches (right or left), paramedian approaches (right or left), and the ventral midline approach. The technique used is determined by the size, temperament, and physical condition of the cow and the veterinary surgeon's preference. Most commonly, an approach is made in the standing patient via an incision through the left paralumbar fossa, using the landmarks described earlier in this chapter for a right-sided flank laparotomy. One of the benefits of using a left flank approach is that the rumen will obstruct other viscera, such as small intestine, from eviscerating through the incision. This is of particular concern if the incision has to be extended distally as a result of the size of the fetus (this incision will be considerably larger than that necessary for an abdominal exploratory). The limbs of the fetus are used to maneuver the uterus to the body wall. The limb is then pulled through the incision and is used to lock the uterus and calf in place. The uterus is incised over the metacarpus or metatarsus, and the calf can be exteriorized with minimal abdominal contamination. Closure of the uterus is performed in two layers, with at least one layer in an inverting pattern. The uterus is then lavaged and replaced into the abdomen before routine closure of the laparotomy site. If available, oxytocin can be administered at this stage to aid uterine involution and to minimize hemorrhage. This will also encourage passage of the placenta, as long as it has not been sutured during the uterine closure. If the calf is not viable or is emphysematous, alternative surgical approaches may be indicated, but selection is often limited by available facilities, equipment, or personnel.

> **TECHNICIAN NOTE** During forced fetal extraction, obstetric chains should be looped above the calf's fetlocks and half-hitched below the fetlocks to more evenly distribute pulling forces on the legs to prevent physeal fracture.

UTERINE TORSION

This is an infrequent cause of dystocia that, if present, will prevent parturition from proceeding. It is most commonly seen during early labor and is identified when an animal that is having a prolonged labor is evaluated rectally or rarely during a vaginal examination. Torsion is identified by the location of the broad ligaments because one of these is pulled tight as the uterus rotates away from its origin, whereas the other broad ligament is less taut. This also provides information on the direction of the torsion—clockwise or counterclockwise (when viewed from behind the cow). If the calf's limbs can be palpated through the cervix, attempts can be made to swing the calf and uterus to reduce torsion. This can be difficult when the calf is large or the cow is small. Rolling the cow while placing pressure on the flank (usually with an assistant standing on a plank of wood placed over the flank and paralumbar fossa) to unwind the torsion can be attempted, but only if the direction of the torsion has been correctly identified. For example, to reduce a clockwise torsion, the cow should be placed in right lateral recumbency and then rolled onto her left side while pressure is applied to try to stabilize the calf. The rectal examination should then be repeated to see whether torsion has been reduced. If this is not successful, it can be repeated, but a flank celiotomy and C-section may be necessary.

VAGINAL AND UTERINE PROLAPSE

Vaginal prolapse is a fairly common occurrence in cattle (Figure 33-20). It usually occurs in pluripara cows during the last 2 months of gestation and tends to recur during subsequent pregnancies. Hereford, Santa Gertrudis, and Holstein breeds seem to be more commonly affected. Factors that influence the development of vaginal prolapse include increased estrogen levels in late pregnancy, increased fetal size with increased intra-abdominal pressure in late pregnancy, bulky diets causing increased intra-abdominal pressure, recumbency that forces the urinary bladder and other organs into the pelvic cavity and places pressure on the constrictor vestibuli muscle, and obesity with proliferation of pelvic fat (vaginal prolapse can occur in overconditioned, nonpregnant heifers). A new population of vaginal prolapse cows is emerging in embryo donor cows that are superovulated. Hormonal extremes are a suggested cause of vaginal prolapse in these cows.

Initially, the vaginal prolapse may be intermittent, protruding only when the animal is lying down, but eventually

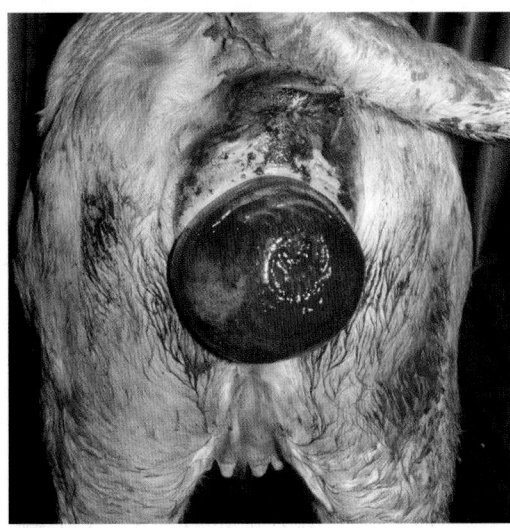

FIGURE 33-20 Vaginal prolapse in a prepartum cow. Recurrence during subsequent pregnancies is common.

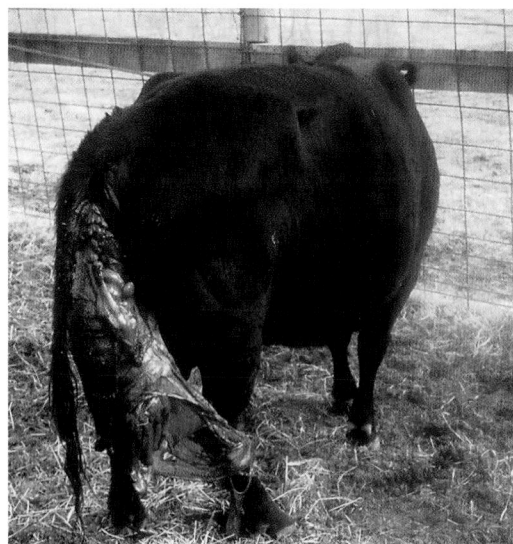

FIGURE 33-21 Uterine eversion with exposure of the caruncles in a postpartum cow.

it progresses to the point that the vagina remains prolapsed at all times. Although vaginal prolapse is not an emergency, it should be repaired soon after it is noticed by the owner. The most common method of repair is the Buhner technique (see later). Because this condition usually occurs before calving, the cow will have to be observed closely for signs of impending parturition. Owners should be advised to cull these cows because this is likely to recur with subsequent pregnancies.

Uterine prolapse is common in the cow as a result of anatomic suspension of the uterus (Figure 33-21). It occurs at parturition or shortly thereafter while the cervix is fully dilated. The uterus invaginates, and the uterine mucosa protrudes through the vulvar lips. Uterine prolapse is more likely to occur in first-calf heifers and is not likely to recur at subsequent calvings. Factors playing a role in the development of uterine prolapse include concurrent hypocalcemia, recumbency, such as that resulting from obturator nerve paralysis, dystocias with excessive straining, excessive force used during fetal extraction, and unnecessary traction on retained placentas.

Uterine prolapse is considered an emergency because of the possibility of shock from exposure of uterine mucosa, fatal hemorrhage from rupture of the middle uterine arteries, and concurrent hypocalcemia. In addition, the urinary bladder and/or intestines may be involved within the prolapse.

To prevent uterine prolapse, it is wise to force the animal to stand as soon as possible after calving and to administer oxytocin to begin uterine involution.

Treatment consists of replacement of the prolapsed portion and application of a retention suture (Buhner) to prevent recurrence. This is best accomplished with the animal in a standing position with the aid of a caudal epidural. If the cow is already down and cannot get up, attempt to elevate the hind quarters or pull the cow's hind legs

straight out behind her as she lies in sternal recumbency; an epidural helps maintain this position. Before replacement of the uterus, the placenta is removed atraumatically, if possible; the uterus is cleansed with warm water and a mild disinfectant; and the uterus is lubricated to facilitate replacement. Elevation of the uterus makes it easier to replace. The uterus is inserted a little at a time, making certain that the apical end of each horn has been completely returned to its normal position. Oxytocin (40 IU), calcium, if necessary, intrauterine antibiotics, and systemic antibiotics should be administered. The vulva is then sutured using the Buhner suture technique.

The Buhner suture technique is useful for retention of both vaginal and uterine prolapse. It is a buried purse-string suture that simulates the action of the constrictor vestibuli muscle. To begin the suture pattern, a 1-cm horizontal skin incision is made midway between the dorsal commissure of the vulva and the anus. Another horizontal incision is made at the ventral commissure of the vulva. The Buhner needle is inserted into the ventral incision, driven deeply (5 to 8 cm), and directed out of the dorsal skin incision. The eye of the needle is threaded with Buhner suture tape, and the needle is pulled out through the ventral incision. The procedure is repeated on the opposite side, resulting in two free ends of tape from the ventral incision. The suture is tightened so that only two to three fingers can be inserted into the vagina. This allows normal urination but prevents reprolapse of the vagina or uterus. This suture may be completely buried and left in place indefinitely. Buhner suture tape is particularly strong, will not disintegrate, and is well tolerated by the tissues. The tape may be tied in such a way that it can be untied as the cow begins to calve, as in the case of prepartum vaginal prolapse.

> **TECHNICIAN NOTE**   Uterine prolapse is considered an emergency because of the possibility of shock from exposure of uterine mucosa, fatal hemorrhage from rupture of the middle uterine arteries, and concurrent hypocalcemia.

FIBROPAPILLOMAS OF THE PENIS

Fibropapillomas of the penis in bulls are caused by the bovine papillomavirus (Figure 33-22). They tend to occur in young bulls housed together and are contracted from warts on other parts of the body when the bulls display homosexual behavior by "riding" each other. The warts may result in hesitancy or refusal to breed and may become large enough that they prevent extension (phimosis) or retraction (paraphimosis) of the penis. Surgical removal of the wart(s) is one treatment option and may be performed in conjunction with vaccination with a commercial or autogenous wart vaccine. Warts can be removed in the standing animal using local anesthetic (bilateral internal pudendal nerve block or anesthesia of the dorsal penile nerve) and restraint. The fibropapilloma can be excised, and the penile mucosa should

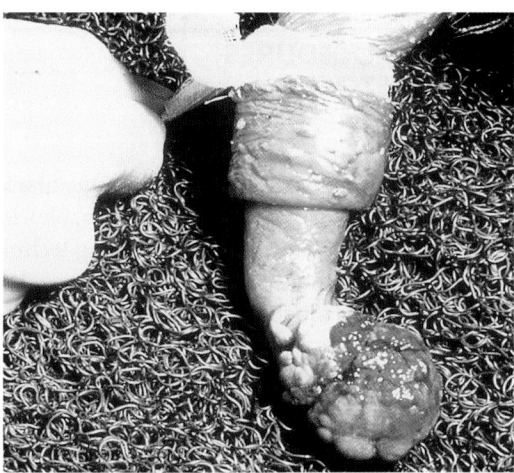

FIGURE 33-22 Fibropapillomas (warts) of the glans penis in a bull.

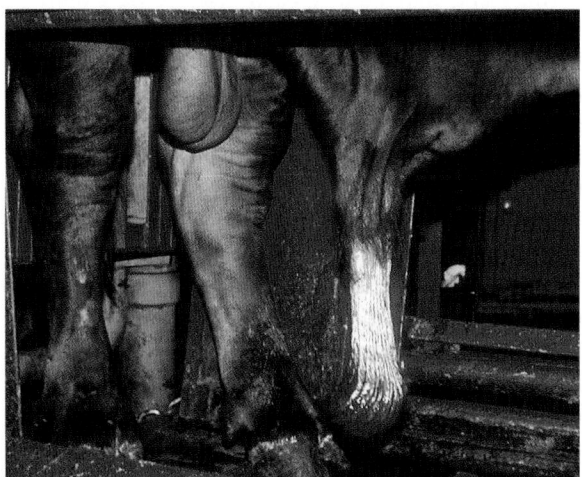

FIGURE 33-23 Prolapse of the prepuce of a *Bos indicus* bull with a pendulous sheath.

be sutured using an absorbable suture. Recurrence is not uncommon.

PREPUTIAL PROLAPSE

Preputial prolapse tends to occur in bulls of *Bos indicus* influence (i.e., Brahman, zebu) as a result of several predisposing breed-related factors, including a pendulous sheath, a long prepuce, a large preputial orifice, and the absence of retractor prepuce muscles. The prepuce may become traumatized as a result of environmental exposure because of the inability of the bull to keep the prepuce within the preputial cavity, or trauma may occur as an accident during breeding. Once traumatized, the prepuce begins to swell and prolapses further, making it susceptible to further injury (Figure 33-23). The affected prepuce is treated initially by soaking in warm water with Betadine and Epsom salts to reduce swelling and to control infection. The prepuce is returned to the preputial cavity and is wrapped with a tube in place to prevent further trauma. Once inflammation and infection are under control, surgery (reefing) to remove scar tissue and

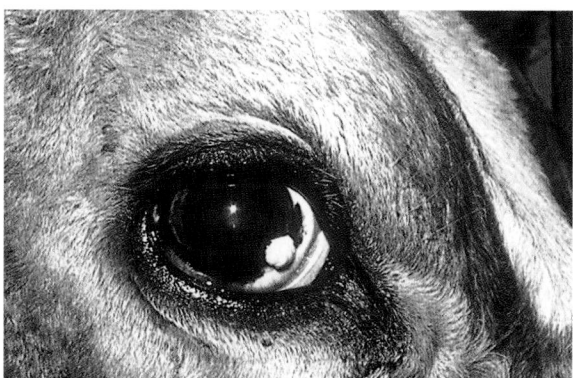

FIGURE 33-24 Ocular squamous cell carcinoma (OSCC) of the medial canthus of the eye of a cow.

to shorten the prepuce may be considered if the bull is valuable. Without surgery, the recurrence rate for preputial trauma and reprolapse is high.

> **TECHNICIAN NOTE** Preputial prolapse occurs most commonly in bulls of *Bos indicus* influence as a result of several breed-related factors, including a pendulous sheath, a long prepuce, a large preputial orifice, and the absence of retractor prepuce muscles.

CONDITIONS OF THE OPHTHALMIC SYSTEM

OCULAR SQUAMOUS CELL CARCINOMA (CANCER EYE)

Ocular squamous cell carcinoma (OSCC), the most common tumor of cattle, is estimated to cause annual losses of $20 million in beef cattle in the United States. Losses result from condemnation of affected carcasses and loss of prime breeding stock.

The cause is multifactorial; there appears to be a genetic predisposition for the development of ocular squamous cell tumors, and exposure to ultraviolet radiation (amount and intensity) and lack of protective pigmentation around the eye play an important role. Tumors occur predominantly in Herefords, but also in other breeds with similar patterns of periocular pigmentation, such as Simmentals and Holsteins. They are seldom seen in animals younger than 4 years of age, and the peak age of occurrence is 8 years. Tumors begin as benign plaques or papillomas that often progress quickly to squamous cell carcinoma. Common sites for development of malignancy in decreasing order of prevalence are the lateral and medial limbus (Figure 33-24), the eyelids (especially lower), the third eyelid, and the medial canthus.

Treatment modalities include cryotherapy, radiofrequency hyperthermia, immunotherapy, chemotherapy, radiation therapy, and surgery (keratectomy, lid resection, or extirpation). Although commonly referred to as enucleation, the term *extirpation* is more accurate. Extirpation is removal of all contents of the bony orbit. Because this procedure is commonly performed for advanced cases of OSCC where removal of all ocular tissue is crucial, and because cosmetic appearance is not as important in cattle, we are more likely to perform extirpation rather than evisceration or enucleation of the eye.

Extirpation is performed with the aid of a retrobulbar or Peterson eye block. To perform the Peterson block, an 18-gauge, 12-cm needle bent to a slight curve is used to block cranial nerves II, IV, V, and VI as they emerge from the round foramen. The needle enters the skin at the angle produced by the supraorbital process and the zygomatic arch and is directed medially. The concavity of the needle is directed caudally so that the point of the needle will pass around the cranial border of the coronoid process of the mandible and to the pterygopalatine fossa of the skull. A reliable indication of proper position is severe twitching of the eyelids. Once the proper position is located, 5 ml of local anesthetic is injected. The needle is repositioned slightly 2 more times with injection of 5 ml of local anesthetic each time. Aspiration is essential before injection to prevent depositing of lidocaine in the cerebrospinal fluid (CSF), possibly resulting in sudden death. Before the needle is withdrawn completely, it is redirected caudally just beneath the skin along the zygomatic arch to block the auriculopalpebral nerve. The four-point retrobulbar block is performed by injecting through the eyelids, both dorsally and ventrally, and at the medial and lateral canthi, using a slightly curved, 18-gauge, 12-cm needle that is directed to the apex of the orbit. Five to 10 ml of local anesthetic is injected at each site. Exophthalmos, corneal anesthesia, and mydriasis indicate a satisfactory retrobulbar block.

The eye is surgically prepared, and the lids are sutured or clamped together. A transpalpebral incision is made approximately 1 cm from the lid margins (unless the disease extends beyond this margin). The skin incision is full thickness but does not penetrate the palpebral conjunctiva; the conjunctival sac helps contain contaminated ocular structures during surgery. Sharp dissection is continued 360 degrees around the bony orbit. The orbital ligament is incised at the medial canthus, and muscles, adipose, lacrimal glands, and fasciae are removed. The optic artery can be ligated, significantly reducing hemorrhage, or the lids can be tightly closed and a gauze stent placed over the incision to provide pressure and hemostasis. The lids are closed with appositional or everting interrupted sutures using nonabsorbable No. 3 suture material. If excessive skin must be removed such that the incision cannot be closed, the orbit can be packed with gauze that is removed in 48 to 72 hours. The incision is left to heal by second intention. NSAIDs and antibiotics may be administered before surgery.

> **TECHNICIAN NOTE**   OSCC, the most common tumor of cattle, results in large economic losses for cattle producers.

SURGICAL PROCEDURES OF YOUNG STOCK

DEHORNING

If possible, calves should be dehorned within the first month of life (or when the horn buds are first palpable) using a dehorning iron. The electrothermal dehorning technique is easy to perform when the calf is young; produces desirable cosmetic results; and is much less stressful for the young calf. Dehorning of beef calves is commonly performed at the time of weaning in conjunction with castration, vaccination, and other management procedures. This age group is usually dehorned using a Barnes dehorner or scoop to remove the horn (Figure 33-25). Hemostasis, which is crucial, is provided by pulling or twisting the cornual artery. Calves older than 6 months may have exposed frontal sinuses after dehorning and may be at greater risk for development of sinusitis. Dehorning of mature cattle often requires analgesia given via a cornual nerve block. The block is performed by injecting 10 ml of 2% lidocaine under the frontal crest halfway between the lateral canthus of the eye and the base of the horn. Large horns are removed with a dehorning saw or Gigli wire. Another method of dehorning cattle is surgical or cosmetic dehorning, which is usually performed on show cattle. This method requires local or regional analgesia. An elliptical incision is made around the base of the horn, the horn is removed, and the skin incision is closed. This surgical technique allows for a more cosmetic appearance of the poll and reduces the chance of postoperative hemorrhage or infection.

CASTRATION

Several techniques are available for castration of calves. As with dehorning, castration is best performed when the calf is young, because it is easier and less stressful for the calf at that time. Castration of young calves is often done without

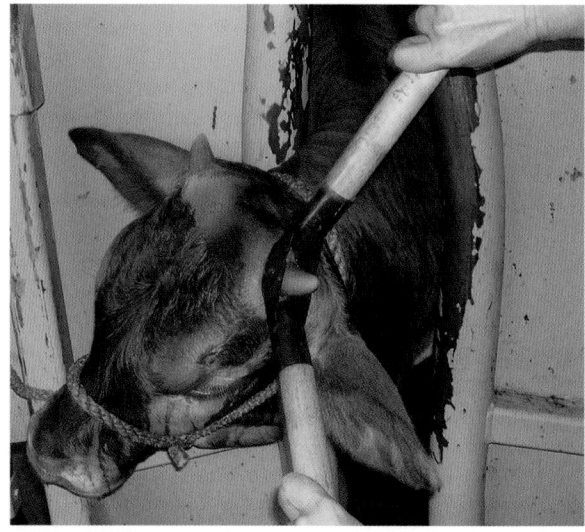

FIGURE 33-25 Use of a Barnes dehorner or scoop for removal of the horns in a young calf.

analgesia. Small calves can be adequately restrained on the ground, whereas larger calves are restrained in a chute with the tail pushed tightly up over the back. A technique commonly employed is the "open" method, in which the bottom one-third to one-half of the scrotum is excised, exposing the testicles. In young calves, the testicles are pulled until the cords break. In older calves, the cord can be sharply transected, or an emasculator that crushes and cuts can be used to separate the cord (Figure 33-26). Another less commonly used technique is a "closed" castration using an emasculotome, which crushes the cord within the scrotum without cutting the scrotal skin. This technique is also referred to as *bloodless castration* or *pinching*. Castration in young calves has also been performed by the application of an elastrator band. It is important to make certain that both testicles are below the band when the procedure is completed. It takes 2 to 3 weeks for the scrotum and testicles to slough. This technique has been associated with the development of tetanus; therefore, vaccination for tetanus may be advisable.

UMBILICAL HERNIAS AND INFECTIONS

As in other species, the umbilicus consists of paired umbilical arteries, a urachus, and an umbilical vein. The foramen where these exit the body wall is a common site of herniation, and this is considered to be a hereditary defect in some breeds, such as Holsteins. Any increase in size of the umbilical stalk, discharge from it, or swelling associated with adjacent tissue warrants closer investigation. Simple umbilical hernias do occur and if small can be managed with application of belly wraps, hernia clamps, or elastrator bands. Close examination and palpation of the hernia and its ring is vital to ensure that it is completely reducible, that no intestines appear to be in the hernia sac, that no evidence of infection is evident, and that the hernia is small (less than 5 cm in length). Ultrasonographic examination can be useful to identify structures within the hernia sac. Hernias that are longer than 5 cm often benefit from an umbilical herniorrhaphy.

Most hernias or umbilical swellings are associated with infection in one or more of the umbilical remnants. Palpation of the mass is often of limited use diagnostically because it is firm, hot, and swollen, and the patient usually resents palpation. Ultrasonographic examination allows the umbilical structures to be visualized and any enlargement or involvement of bladder or liver to be identified before treatment is initiated. Medical treatment can be started in an attempt to treat the infection, but surgical resection may be necessary for severely affected patients.

Omphalectomy or umbilical herniorrhaphy can be performed with the calf in dorsal recumbency using sedation and a local block or general anesthesia. Feed does not have to be withheld for as long as for adult patients, but this should be removed approximately 6 to 8 hours before surgery. A large area should be clipped and prepped for surgery as if the umbilical vein or urachus is infected; the surgical incision may have to extend as far cranially as the xiphoid process or caudally to the pelvis. If the vein is infected up to the liver, a marsupialization may need to be performed that will require a second incision lateral to the main site. Attempts should be made to remove the infected tissue intact; this may necessitate resection of the apex of the bladder. After removal of infected tissue, the body wall will be repaired. Some defects may be large enough to require a mesh herniorrhaphy, but most can be sutured closed.

After surgery, the calf must be maintained in a stall for a month. Allowing excessive exercise will often lead to incisional complications, such as edema, seroma formation, or dehiscence. If umbilical vein marsupialization was performed, the stoma must be cleaned daily, and low-pressure lavage with sterile fluid can be performed to try to treat the infected structures that could not be removed. This stoma will often need to be repaired in the future because it may form a small hernia when the infection has resolved.

SELECTED CONDITIONS OF SMALL RUMINANTS

URINARY SYSTEM

Male small ruminants are at high risk for developing urolithiasis as a result of feeding of excessive grain in the diet. The cause and clinical presentation are similar to those described in cattle. Goats that are obstructed tend to vocalize because of pain. Small ruminants are small enough that it is possible to palpate and/or ultrasound their urinary bladders, which further aids diagnosis of the condition. Management of this condition is somewhat different in small ruminants. Small ruminants possess a urethral process or vermiform appendage, which usually is the first place at which obstruction occurs. The second most common site of obstruction is the distal sigmoid flexure. Oftentimes calculi resemble sand and may block most of the distal portion of the urethra.

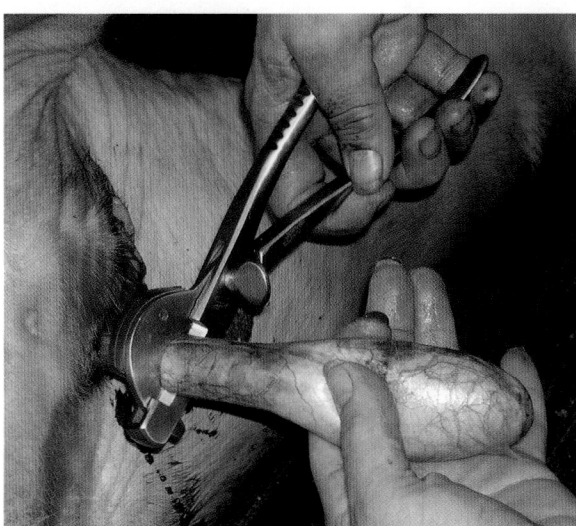

FIGURE 33-26 Castration of a calf by emasculation after removal of the bottom half of the scrotum.

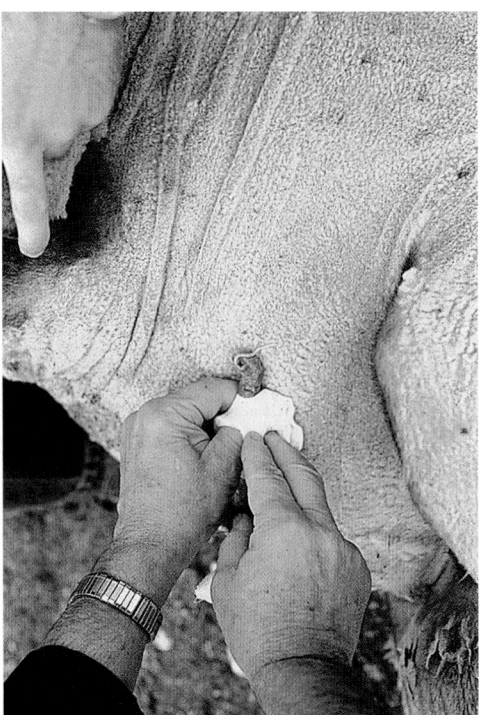

FIGURE 33-27 Examination of the urethral process in a wether for the presence of calculi (urolithiasis).

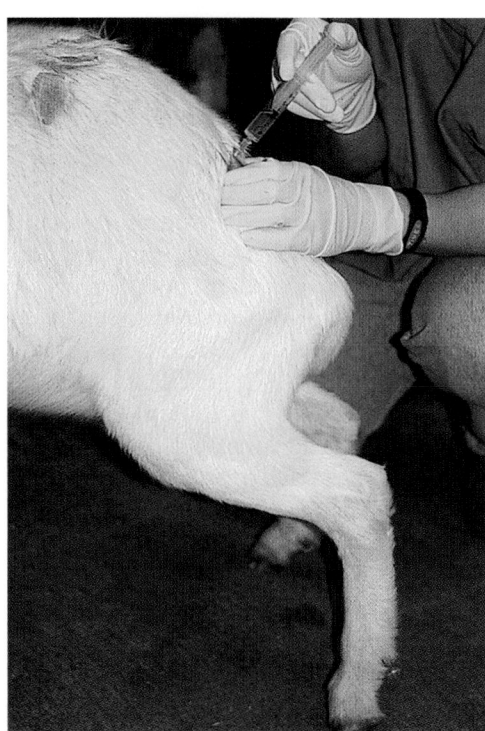

FIGURE 33-28 Administration of a lumbosacral epidural in a goat results in loss of motor control in the hind legs.

The urethral process should be examined in all cases of suspected urolithiasis in small ruminants because this is the most common location for calculi to lodge. The penis and the urethral process can be exteriorized by placing the animal in a sitting position on its rump (Figure 33-27). If necessary, a lumbosacral epidural can be performed. Epidural anesthesia provides analgesia and prevents resistance to exteriorization of the penis caused by the retractor penis muscles. Lidocaine (2%, 1 ml/20 lb, not to exceed a total dose of 15 ml in any small ruminant) is injected into the epidural space at the lumbosacral junction (Figure 33-28). Loss of motor control to the hind legs lasts from 1 to 3 hours, so the patient should be recovered on a well-bedded surface to prevent trauma to the rear legs. Once the penis has been exteriorized, it can be grasped with dry gauze. If the urethral process is obstructed, it can be amputated close to its attachment to the glans. If the urethral process is not present, this may mean that it had already been amputated, or that it may have necrosed and sloughed by itself during a previous episode of obstruction. Immediate urethral patency may occur after urethral process amputation; however, reobstruction is common. Consequently, it appears that urethral process amputation alone rarely results in a long-term cure.

Urethral catheterization with saline flushing may be attempted to relieve obstruction; however, the bladder is difficult to catheterize because of the presence of the suburethral diverticulum in ruminants, and complications associated with catheterization include urethritis, urethral rupture, and urethral damage leading to stricture.

Perineal urethrostomy may be suitable in cattle as a salvage procedure (Figure 33-29). Urethrostomy frequently

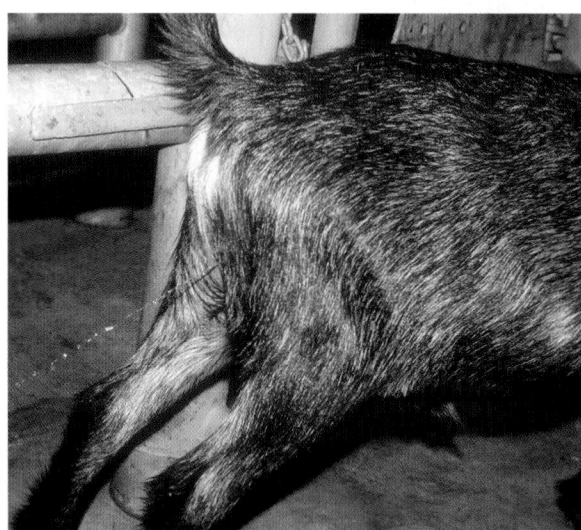

FIGURE 33-29 Perineal urethrostomy, a surgical treatment for obstructive urolithiasis, is prone to stricture formation in small ruminants.

results in stricture formation in the urethra and probably is not a good choice for pets because of a shortened life span.

Cystotomy and tube cystostomy have become the procedures of choice for treatment of obstructive urolithiasis and often result in prolonged life and preservation of breeding capability in breeding males. With this procedure, calculi can be removed from the bladder, and normograde and retrograde urethral flushing can be attempted. In addition, a Foley catheter placed in the bladder allows urine egress while the urethra and the bladder heal (Figure 33-30). The catheter

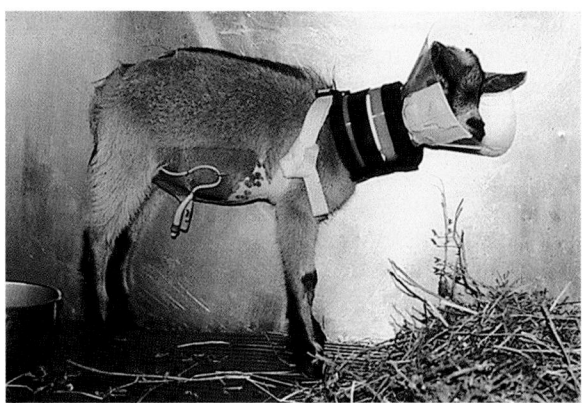

FIGURE 33-30 Temporary tube cystostomy allows urine egress while the urethra and the bladder heal post obstruction.

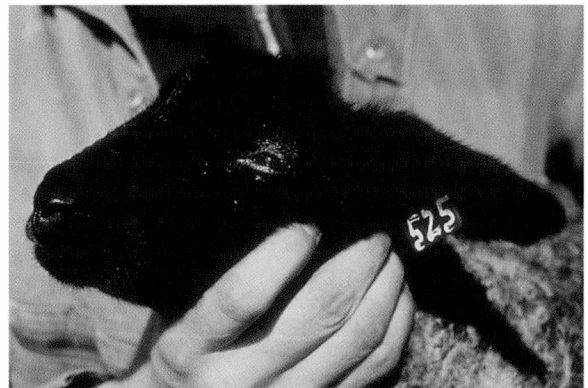

FIGURE 33-31 A lamb with corneal irritation from congenital entropion or inward rolling of the lower eyelid.

is removed when it is determined that the animal can urinate a normal stream consistently from the urethra.

> **TECHNICIAN NOTE** Male small ruminants are at high risk for development of obstructive urolithiasis as a result of feeding of excessive grain in the diet.

OPHTHALMIC SYSTEM
Entropion

Entropion, or inward rolling of the eyelid, has been reported to be the most common ocular disease of neonatal lambs (Figure 33-31). The congenital or primary form involves only the lower lid, but it is usually bilateral. Clinical signs of blepharospasm, photophobia, eye rubbing, and keratoconjunctivitis are ordinarily observed in lambs during the first few days to weeks of life. Initial treatment is conservative and involves administering ophthalmic antibiotics and manually rolling the lower lid outward. If this is unsuccessful, other treatment options include injection of penicillin or tetracycline in a linear fashion parallel to the lower lid or clamping of the skin of the lower lid below and parallel to the lid margin with mosquito forceps for 30 seconds. Both techniques should create sufficient inflammation and fibrosis

to keep the lower lid rolled out. Another technique involves placement of two or three vertical mattress sutures in the lower lid to roll out the lid margin. Congenital entropion is considered to be a heritable trait, so affected animals should not be kept for breeding.

SURGICAL PROCEDURES COMMONLY PERFORMED ON SMALL RUMINANTS

Lumbosacral epidurals are useful for alleviating pain during procedures performed caudal to the umbilicus. The animal will lose motor control to the hind legs and should be confined to a small, well-bedded area to prevent injury. A lumbosacral epidural is performed at the lumbosacral junction, which can easily be palpated in small ruminants. A 20-gauge, 3.8-cm needle is used for this technique. The needle is inserted perpendicular to the dorsal midline until a slight popping sensation is encountered. If the epidural space has been entered, injection should be easy. An alternative is to advance the needle until bone is felt, then back the needle out slightly and attempt injection. If CSF is encountered, the subarachnoid space rather than the epidural space has been entered. It is acceptable to inject lidocaine into this area if aseptic technique has been used during the procedure, but the lidocaine dose should be reduced to half of that used for epidural injection. Analgesia will take several minutes if in the epidural space and will be almost immediate if injected into the subarachnoid space. The dose of lidocaine used for this procedure is 5 to 8 ml/45 kg body weight.

The optimal time for disbudding or dehorning kids is 3 to 5 days in buck kids and 5 to 7 days in doe kids. At this age, the procedure is less invasive because the horn buds have not yet attached to the underlying bone, and there is less chance of regrowth if the kid is dehorned properly at this age. Many owners perform this procedure with restraint only; however, the kid may be sedated with xylazine and butorphanol. In addition, a ring block of 1% lidocaine around the base of the horn will provide local analgesia. The horn bud is removed by first burning with the dehorning iron and allowing the bud to slough, or by excising the bud after burning around its base. Care should be taken to avoid leaving the iron on too long (5 to 10 seconds per side), to prevent thermal meningitis. The burning procedure may be repeated, allowing the area to cool between burns, until a uniform ring of copper-colored skin is apparent around the entire horn bud base (Figure 33-32).

C-section is indicated in cases of dystocia. A left flank laparotomy can be used to approach the uterus and, with sedation and an inverted-L block, can be rapidly performed. After incision of the skin, the flank muscles can be bluntly separated along the direction of their fibers, and the uterus can be brought into the surgical field. It is important that the uterus is carefully palpated before closure to prevent leaving a fetus in the contralateral horn. Alternatively, a ventral midline or ventral paramedian approach can be used.

Factors causing rectal prolapse in sheep include short tail docking, overconditioning of lambs (increased pelvic fat),

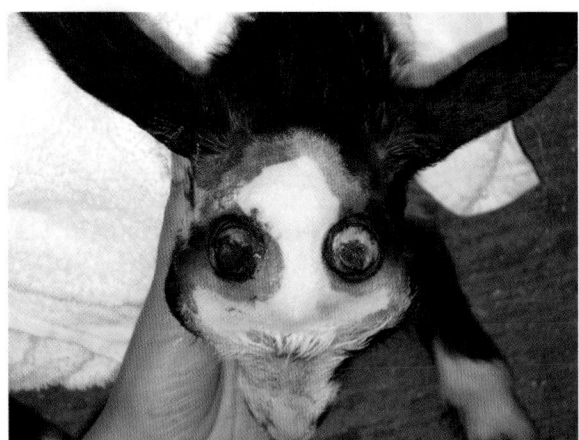

FIGURE 33-32 Disbudding of kids is performed by burning the horn buds with an electric dehorning iron before 2 weeks of age. The goat is looking toward the ground, and its ears are pointing toward the top corners of the image.

straining as a result of urolithiasis, diarrhea, dystocia, and conditions that increase abdominal pressure, such as coughing.

Short tail docks are performed strictly for cosmetic reasons in show lambs and may result in loss of innervation to the rectum and anal sphincter, which comes from S3 to Cy5. A resolution of the American Veterinary Medical Association (AVMA) suggests that lamb tails not be docked shorter than the distal end of the caudal tail fold. Methods for rectal prolapse repair include purse-string suture after replacement (strictly a salvage procedure), injection of irritating solutions (tetracycline, strong iodine in oil) at three to four points perirectally, and rectal amputation.

> **TECHNICIAN NOTE** The optimal time for disbudding or dehorning kids is 3 to 5 days in buck kids and 5 to 7 days in doe kids.

RECOMMENDED READINGS

Auer JA, Stick JA, editors: Equine surgery, ed 3, Philadelphia, 2006, Saunders.

Divers TJ, Peek SF: Rebhun's diseases of dairy cattle, ed 2, St Louis, 2008, Saunders.

Fubini SL, Ducharme NC: Farm animal surgery, St Louis, 2004, Saunders.

Hanie EA: Large animal clinical procedures for veterinary technicians, St Louis, 2006, Mosby.

Koterba AM, Drummond WH, Kosch PC, editors: Equine clinical neonatology, Philadelphia, 1990, Lea & Febiger.

Orsini JA, Divers TJ: Manual of equine emergencies, ed 3, St Louis, 2008, Saunders.

Pugh DG: Sheep and goat medicine, ed 2, St Louis, 2012, Saunders.

Reed S, Bailey W, Sellon D, editors: Equine internal medicine, ed 3, St Louis, 2009, Saunders.

Smith BP: Large animal internal medicine, ed 4, St Louis, 2009, Mosby.

34 Veterinary Dentistry

John R. Lewis and Bonnie R. Miller

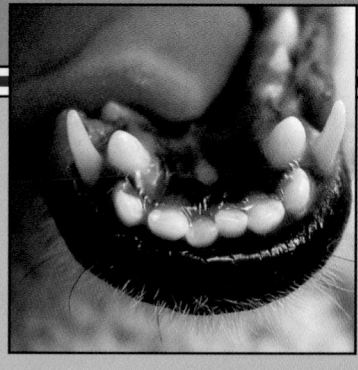

OUTLINE

Ethical and Legal Aspects, *1299*
Veterinary Dental Organizations, *1299*
Dental Morphology, *1299*
Occlusion, *1302*
Oral Examination and History, *1303*
Extraoral Examination, *1304*
Intraoral Examination, *1309*
Dental Radiography, *1315*
Equipment, *1316*
Film, *1317*
Film Processing, *1317*
Digital Radiography, *1318*
Techniques, *1319*
Exposure and Processing Errors, *1319*
Radiographic Interpretation, *1320*
Periodontal Disease, *1321*
Periodontal Débridement, *1322*
Power Scaling, *1323*
Sonic Scaler, *1323*
Ultrasonic Scaler, *1323*
Safety Precautions, *1324*
Tip Designs, *1324*
Energy Dispersion, *1324*
Types of Ultrasonic Scalers, *1325*
Knob Settings, *1326*
Hand Scaling, *1326*
Supragingival Instruments, *1327*
Subgingival Curettes, *1328*
Principles of Scaling, *1329*

Sharpening, *1330*
Polishing, *1330*
Regional Nerve Blocks for Oral Surgery in Dogs and Cats, *1331*
Infraorbital Nerve Block, *1332*
Middle Mental Nerve Block, *1332*
Inferior Alveolar Nerve Block, *1332*
Maxillary Nerve Block, *1332*
Periodontal Surgery, *1333*
Home Care, *1335*
Restorative Dentistry, *1336*
Endodontics, *1336*
Exodontics, *1340*
Closed Extractions, *1341*
Surgical Extractions, *1342*
Common Dental Problems in Dogs and Cats, *1343*
Tooth Resorption, *1343*
Orthodontic Problems, *1344*
Dental Trauma, *1347*
Oral Neoplasia, *1348*
Stomatitis, *1349*
Masticatory Myositis, *1350*
Jaw Fractures, *1350*
Equine Dentistry, *1351*
Dental Anatomy and Physiology, *1351*
Dental Examination and Imaging, *1352*
Common Dental Problems of Horses, *1352*

KEY TERMS

Anisognathism
Apex
Brachycephalic
Brachygnathism
Calculus
Caries
Cementum
Diastema
Dolichocephalic
Enamel
Endodontics
Exodontics
Furcation
Hypsodont
Malocclusion
Mesaticephalic (mesocephalic)
Periodontium
Plaque
Pulp
Triadan system

LEARNING OBJECTIVES

When you have completed this chapter, you will be able to:
1. Pronounce, spell, and define all Key Terms in this chapter.
2. Describe ethical and legal issues related to dental procedures performed by veterinary technicians, and list professional organizations related to veterinary dentistry.
3. Be familiar with terminology used in veterinary dentistry to designate location and direction; describe the modified Triadan system for numbering teeth; and, describe normal occlusion in dogs and cats, common malocclusions, and orthodontic treatment in small animals.
4. Discuss aspects of the complete medical history as they relate to veterinary dentistry. and describe aspects of extraoral and intraoral examinations in dogs and cats.
5. Describe equipment and supplies used for dental radiography (both film and digital radiography); and, compare and contrast paralleling, bisecting angle, and occlusal techniques in dental radiography.

6. Differentiate between the types of periodontal disease seen in dogs and cats, including stomatitis, gingivitis, and periodontitis; and, state the goal of periodontal débridement.
7. Describe equipment and procedures for professional dental cleaning using power and hand scalers, and explain methods for sharpening dental instruments.
8. Discuss the rationale and procedures for polishing teeth.
9. Compare and contrast regional nerve blocks for oral surgery for dogs and cats.
10. Explain the grading system for periodontal disease and the importance of home care in veterinary dentistry.
11. Discuss indications for restorative dentistry, endodontics, and exodontics.
12. Describe common dental problems seen in small animals.
13. List and describe equine dental clinical practices, as well as common problems and treatments.

INTRODUCTION

Veterinary dentistry has been in existence as a specialty for more than 20 years. However, few veterinarians and technicians have received formal training in dentistry and oral surgery because of the relative paucity of educational opportunities. Dentistry has become a significant part of nearly every small animal practice, and more attention is paid to dental disease of other species, such as horses and exotic animals. Veterinary technicians play a vital role in veterinary dentistry. Common tasks include (1) performing professional dental cleanings, including periodontal débridement and polishing; (2) obtaining diagnostic information through dental charting and dental radiography; (3) providing intraoperative assistance with dental and oral surgeries; (4) in some states, where allowed by law, extracting **(exodontics)** diseased teeth; and (5) providing client education, including proper use of appropriate dental home care products and preventive techniques. Most veterinary practices provide professional dental cleanings for their patients. Some practices also provide advanced dental care, such as **endodontics,** exodontics, and advanced periodontal therapy. In the process of providing routine dental care, technicians have an opportunity to identify disease in its early stages. Therefore, a strong foundation in oral anatomy and oral pathologic conditions is important. Because technicians are often on the front line of identifying oral disease, this chapter provides a strong foundation in disease recognition and treatment principles.

This chapter also provides a detailed discussion of periodontal disease, including pathophysiology, treatment, follow-up, and prevention. Because scaling and polishing procedures are the most common dental procedures performed in practice, special attention is paid in this chapter to instrumentation and techniques of proper periodontal therapy. These procedures are often mistakenly referred to as *prophylaxis*, or "prophy." Because of the variation in severity of disease at the time of treatment, the term "dental prophylaxis" is largely being replaced with the term "professional dental cleaning." The technician who is involved in performing a professional dental cleaning should be capable of performing assessment, periodontal débridement (supragingival and subgingival scaling), polishing, home care education, and counseling about proper diet, treats, and toys as they relate to dentistry. Dental radiology is extremely important in veterinary dentistry because disease is often missed or underestimated when teeth are not examined beneath the gingival margin. Techniques for taking diagnostic dental radiographs are covered, and interpretation of normal and abnormal dental radiographic anatomy is discussed. This chapter also addresses other subspecialties of dentistry, including endodontics, exodontics, orthodontics, and restorative dentistry. Equine dental anatomy and pathologic conditions are discussed, along with preventive and therapeutic treatments for common equine dental problems.

ETHICAL AND LEGAL ASPECTS

The level of dental care a veterinary technician may provide varies from state to state, and the laws and regulations for the state of practice must be understood before dental care is provided. The American Veterinary Dental College (AVDC) published a position statement in 1998 regarding veterinary dental health care providers. This statement provides recommendations for the qualifications of persons who perform veterinary dental procedures. The AVDC considers it appropriate for the veterinarian to delegate certain dental tasks to veterinary technicians. Tasks appropriately performed by veterinary technicians include professional dental cleanings and certain procedures that do not result in alterations in the shape, structure, or positional location of teeth in the dental arch. The American Veterinary Medical Association has created a resource which describes the scope of what veterinary technicians and non-veterinarians can do in each state: see https://www.avma.org/Advocacy/StateAndLocal/Pages/sr-dental-procedures.aspx.

> **TECHNICIAN NOTE** The level of dental care the technician can legally provide varies from state to state. Become familiar with laws regulating veterinary dentistry in your state: see https://www.avma.org/Advocacy/StateAndLocal/Pages/sr-dental-procedures.aspx.

In addition, the AVDC supports advanced training of veterinary technicians to perform additional dental services, such as taking impressions, making models, charting veterinary dental lesions, taking and developing dental radiographs, and performing nonsurgical subgingival root planing.

VETERINARY DENTAL ORGANIZATIONS

Opportunities exist for veterinary technicians to achieve advanced training and recognition in dentistry. The National Association of Veterinary Technicians in America (NAVTA) governs technicians who have completed credential requirements and passed specialty examinations to be considered veterinary technician specialists (VTS). Technicians interested in pursuing the dental specialty must secure a mentor, maintain case logs, write case reports, and attend continuing education courses as part of the credentials process of the Academy of Veterinary Dental Technicians (AVDT). Before beginning the credentialing process, the technician must have completed 3000 hours of dental experience. For further information about becoming a member of the AVDT, visit the website at www.avdt.us.

> **TECHNICIAN NOTE** The Academy of Veterinary Dental Technicians (AVDT) consists of technicians who have completed a credentials process and passed a specialty examination.

The American Veterinary Dental Society (AVDS) is an organization that was created to advance awareness and knowledge of veterinary dentistry among members of the profession and the public. Membership in the AVDS is open to all veterinarians, veterinary technicians, and dental hygienists. Membership includes a subscription to the *Journal of Veterinary Dentistry*, the official journal of many national and international dental societies and colleges. More information can be found at the AVDS website at www.avds-online.org.

The first organization established to provide dental knowledge to veterinary technicians and assistants was the American Society for Veterinary Dental Technicians (ASVDT). Membership includes a self-taught home study course that serves as a good introduction to basic dentistry. The ASVDT provides a baseline level of dental knowledge and is open to staff members who may or may not have formal veterinary education, whereas members of the AVDT have an advanced level of dental knowledge and are required to hold a certification or a state license for membership.

DENTAL MORPHOLOGY

Morphology refers to the form and structure of an organism or its parts. Teeth can be classified as brachyodont or **hypsodont** on the basis of their crown and root structure (Figure 34-1). All teeth of humans, carnivores, and pigs are brachyodont teeth. Brachyodont teeth have a relatively small, distinct crown compared with the size of their well-developed roots. The apices (singular, **apex**) of the roots are open for a limited time during eruption and development of the teeth; therefore, the teeth do not continually grow or erupt. This contrasts with hypsodont teeth (seen in horses, rodents, and lagomorphs), which have a comparatively large reserve crown beneath the gingival margin and root structure that allows for continued growth and/or continued eruption during all or most of an animal's lifetime. Hypsodont teeth can be divided further into two categories: radicular and aradicular hypsodont teeth. The cheek teeth of horses are an example of radicular hypsodont teeth. The apices of these teeth remain open for a significant portion of adult life, but they eventually close, after which continued growth of the tooth ceases, and occlusal wear is offset only by continued eruption. Cheek teeth and incisors of rabbits and some rodents are aradicular hypsodont (also called *elodont*) teeth, indicating lack of true root structure along with lifelong tooth growth, which compensates for occlusal wear.

Dogs and cats have four types of teeth: incisors, canines, premolars, and molars. Incisor teeth are the most rostral teeth and are used for gnawing and grooming. Canine teeth are distal to the incisors. They are long and are used for prehending and holding. Premolars and molars (often referred to as "cheek teeth") are used for shearing and grinding.

Most mammals are diphyodont, meaning that they have two sets of teeth. The first set of teeth is referred to as *deciduous* (also referred to as *primary* or *baby teeth*); these are

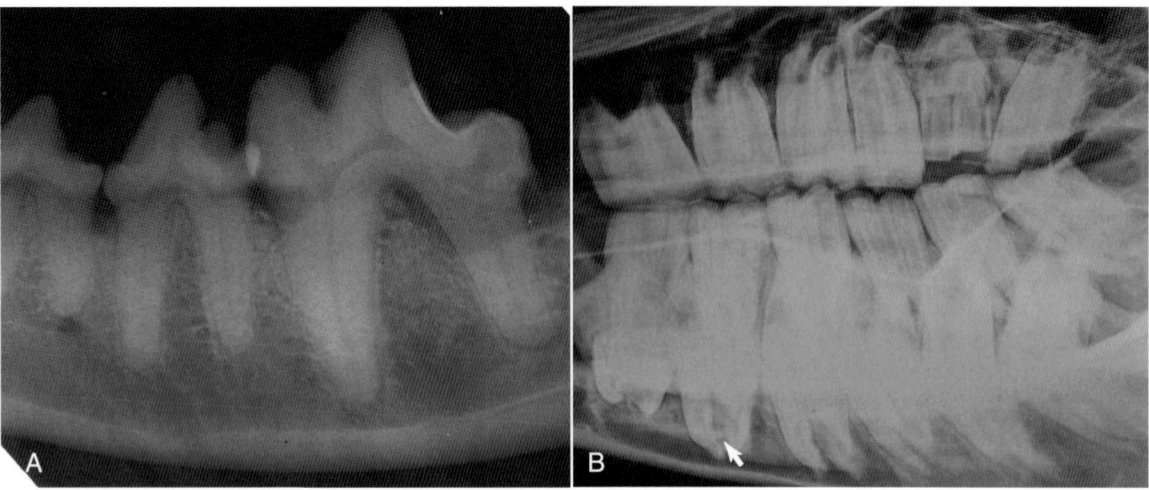

FIGURE 34-1 Radiograph of brachyodont teeth of the dog **(A)** and hypsodont teeth of the horse **(B)**.

BOX 34-1	Dental Formulas

Dog: *Deciduous teeth* 2 × (I 3/3, C 1/1, P 3/3) = 28 teeth
    Permanent teeth 2 × (I 3/3, C/1/1, P 4/4, M 2/3) = 42 teeth
Cat: *Deciduous teeth* 2 × (I 3/3, C 1/1, P 3/2) = 26 teeth
    Permanent teeth 2 × (I 3/3, C 1/1, P 3/2, M 1/1) = 30 teeth
Horse: *Deciduous teeth* 2 × (I 3/3, C 0/0, P 3/3) = 24 teeth
    Permanent teeth 2 × (I 3/3, C 1/1 or 0/0, P 3 or 4/3 or 4, M 3/3) = 36 to 44 teeth (depending on the presence of canine and wolf teeth)

C, Canines; I, incisors; M, molars; P, premolars.

TABLE 34-1	Approximate Eruption Schedule for Teeth of Dogs and Cats (in weeks)

	DECIDUOUS TEETH		PERMANENT TEETH	
	PUPPY	**KITTEN**	**DOG**	**CAT**
Incisors	4-6	3-4	12-16	11-16
Canines	3-5	3-4	12-16	12-20
Premolars	5-6	5-6	16-20	16-20
Molars	—	—	16-20	20-24

replaced with permanent teeth (also referred to as *secondary* or *adult teeth*). Mammals show great variety in numbers and types of teeth, depending on the species. Dental formulas used to classify numbers and types of teeth are seen in Box 34-1. Normal eruption times of deciduous and permanent teeth in dogs and cats are provided in Table 34-1, although it should be mentioned that some normal variation exists.

It is important to be aware of the number of roots of each tooth. Table 34-2 lists the number of roots of each tooth of cats and dogs. Anatomic variation does occur, so preoperative dental radiographs are important to confirm numbers

---

TABLE 34-2	Permanent Dentition of the Dog and Cat

Dog Permanent Dentition

MANDIBLE	TOOTH	ROOTS
Incisors	1st, 2nd, 3rd	1
Canines	1	1
Premolars	1st	1
Premolars	2nd, 3rd, 4th	2
Molars	1st, 2nd	2
Molars	3rd*	1 (or 2)
MAXILLA	**TOOTH**	**ROOT**
Incisors	1st, 2nd, 3rd	1
Canines	1	1
Premolars	1st	1
Premolars	2nd, 3rd*	2
Premolars	(3rd*), 4th	3
Molars	1st, 2nd	3

Cat Permanent Dentition

MANDIBLE	TOOTH	ROOTS
Incisors	1st, 2nd, 3rd	1
Canines	1	1
Premolars	1st, 2nd	Not present
Premolars	3rd, 4th	2
Molars	1st	2
MAXILLA	**TOOTH**	**ROOTS**
Incisors	1st, 2nd, 3rd	1
Canines	1	1
Premolars	1st	Not present
Premolars	2nd*	1 (or 2)
Premolars	3rd*	2 (or 3)
Premolars	4th	3
Molars	1st*	1 (or 2)

*Anatomic variation in root numbers is common. An extra root may be present, or it may be partially fused to the normal root(s).

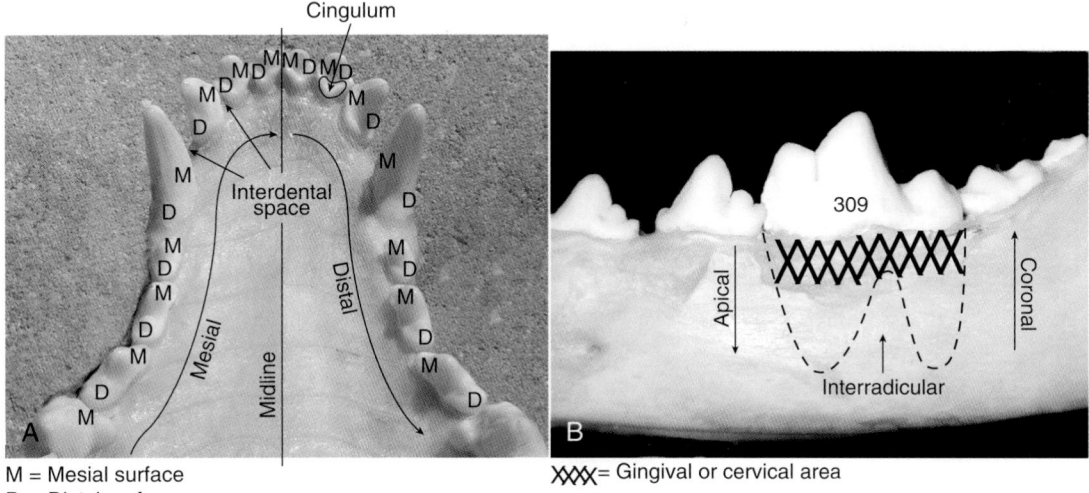

FIGURE 34-2 Positional terminology commonly used in dentistry. **A,** Palatal view of the canine maxilla. *D,* Distal; *M,* mesial. **B,** Mandibular left first molar.

and shapes of tooth roots before extraction or other procedures involving subgingival pathologic conditions. For example, the maxillary third premolar is usually a two-rooted tooth in dogs and cats, but it is not uncommon to see a third root in some dogs and cats.

The veterinary dental technician must have an understanding of dental anatomic terminology to accurately describe the location of a structure or lesion. "Rostral" is a term that when used to describe cranial anatomy refers to a structure that is closer to the front of the head in comparison with another structure. "Caudal" is a term that is used to describe a structure that is toward the back of the head when compared with another structure. "Vestibular" is a term that describes the tooth surface facing the lips or vestibule (acceptable alternatives are "buccal" and "labial"). "Facial" is a term that describes the vestibular surface of teeth visible from the front (incisors). "Lingual" refers to the surface of the mandibular teeth adjacent to the tongue. "Palatal" refers to the surface of maxillary teeth adjacent to the palate. "Mesial" refers to the portion of the tooth in line with the dental arcade that is closest to the most rostral portion of the midline of the dental arch. "Distal" refers to the portion of the tooth that is closest to the most caudal portion of the dental arch. The concepts of mesial and distal surfaces are difficult to describe without referring to a diagram. Figure 34-2 shows a diagram on which these terms appear. It may help to remember that the terms "mesial" and "distal" are used to describe surfaces of the teeth where adjacent teeth touch or nearly touch. "Apical" refers to a portion of the tooth that is closer to the apex (tip of the root). "Coronal" refers to a structure with a location that is closer to the crown of the tooth in relation to another structure.

Referring to the teeth by using a numeric system rather than descriptive terminology saves time when detailed charting is performed. The most commonly used numbering system is the modified **Triadan system**. Teeth in the maxillary right quadrant are considered the 100 series, and the left maxillary quadrant is called the 200 series. The left mandibular quadrant is the 300 series, and the right mandibular quadrant is the 400 series. Each tooth within the quadrant has a two-digit number, starting at the anterior midline and moving along the dental arch in a caudal direction. The right maxillary first incisor is 101, right maxillary second incisor 102, right maxillary third incisor 103, right maxillary canine 104, and so on. The left maxillary canine is 204, left mandibular canine 304, and right mandibular canine 404 (Figure 34-3). Deciduous teeth are assigned the 500 series for the right maxillary quadrant, 600 series for the left maxillary quadrant, 700 series for the left mandibular quadrant, and 800 series for the right mandibular quadrant.

> **TECHNICIAN NOTE** Knowledge of the Triadan tooth numbering system saves time during charting of oral pathologic conditions.

Cats have fewer teeth than dogs, but even when teeth are missing, those that are present will have a predictable number with the Triadan system. For example, tooth 108 always refers to the right maxillary fourth premolar whether one is discussing a dog, a hyena, a cat, or a lion. Because the cat does not have a maxillary first premolar, the premolar closest to the canine tooth is tooth 106 (Figure 34-4). Cats are missing their mandibular first and second premolars, so the premolars closest to the mandibular canine teeth are numbered 307 and 407, respectively, for the left and right mandible. Keeping these numbers consistent among species allows veterinary professionals to quickly equate a tooth number with an anatomic location. When someone says that tooth 208 is fractured, one should think of the left maxillary fourth premolar, regardless of species.

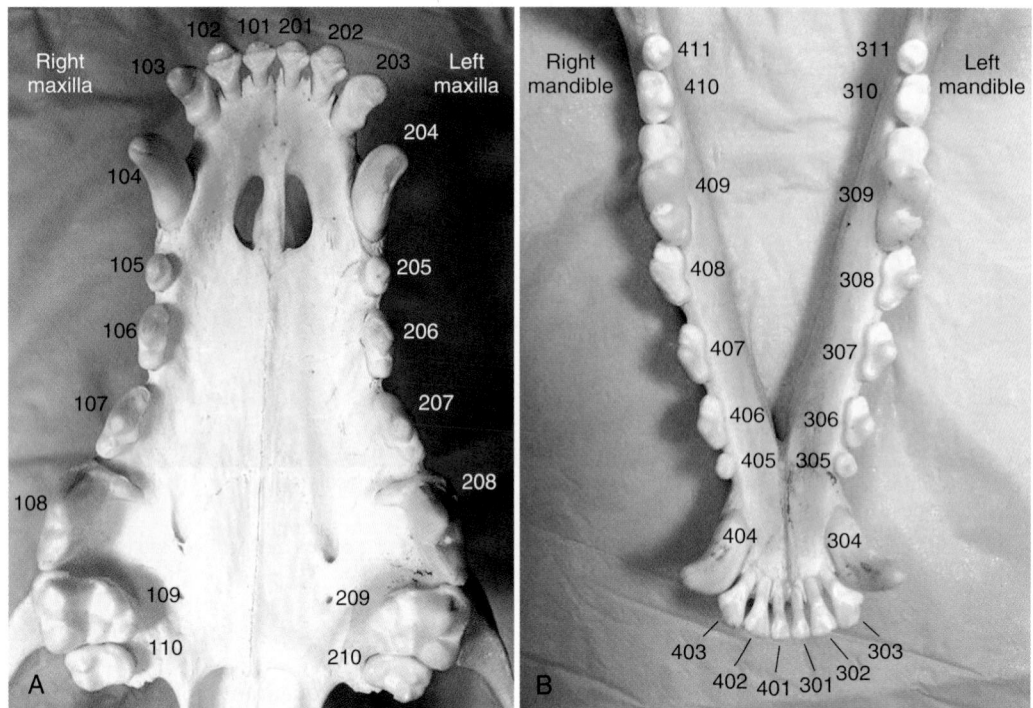

FIGURE 34-3 Triadan tooth numbering system in the dog. **A**, Maxilla. **B**, Mandible.

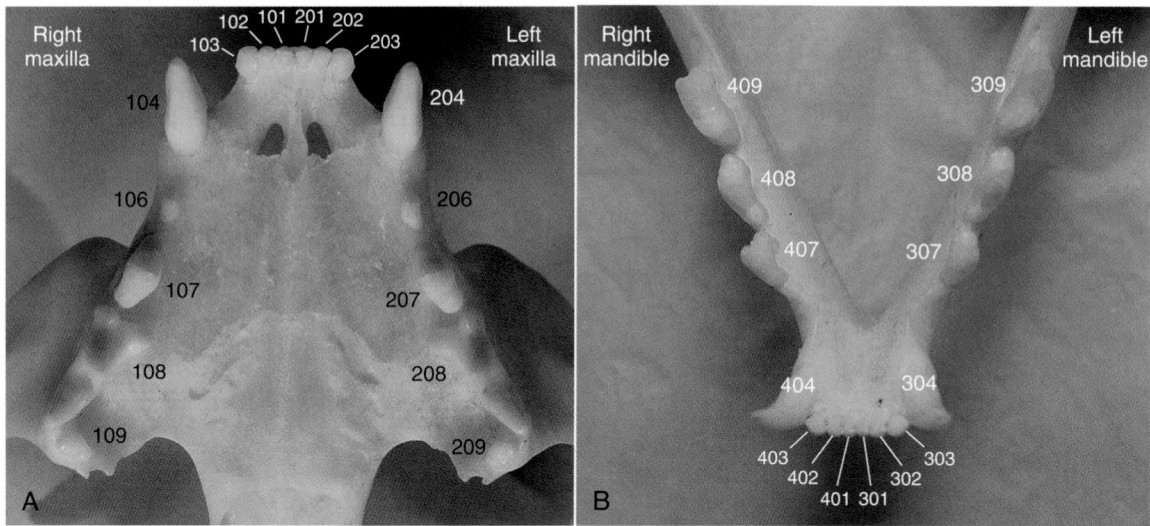

FIGURE 34-4 Triadan tooth numbering system in the cat. **A**, Maxilla. **B**, Mandible. Note that the canine tooth always ends with the numbers "04," and the first molar always ends with the numbers "09," regardless of species.

OCCLUSION

Occlusion refers to the spatial relationship of teeth within the mouth. **Malocclusion** refers to the situation when teeth or jaws are not correctly aligned. Although cosmetic issues of misaligned teeth are not typically a concern in dogs and cats, malocclusions can result in discomfort from impingement of teeth on soft tissue structures of the opposing dental arcade. Dogs and cats with a normal occlusion have a scissors bite, in which the incisors come together to closely overlap like blades of a scissors (Figure 34-5, *A* and *B*). When teeth are properly aligned in scissors occlusion, there is maximal function of all teeth with no occlusal trauma. Variations of dental occlusion in dogs and cats occur, depending on the breed and the skull type. The relationships of brachyodont teeth in normal occlusion are discussed below.

Incisors

The mandibular incisors should be palatal to (behind) the maxillary incisors, and the coronal third of the mandibular incisors should rest on the cingulum of the maxillary incisors. The cingulum is a smooth convex bulge located on the palatal side of the gingival third of the incisor teeth.

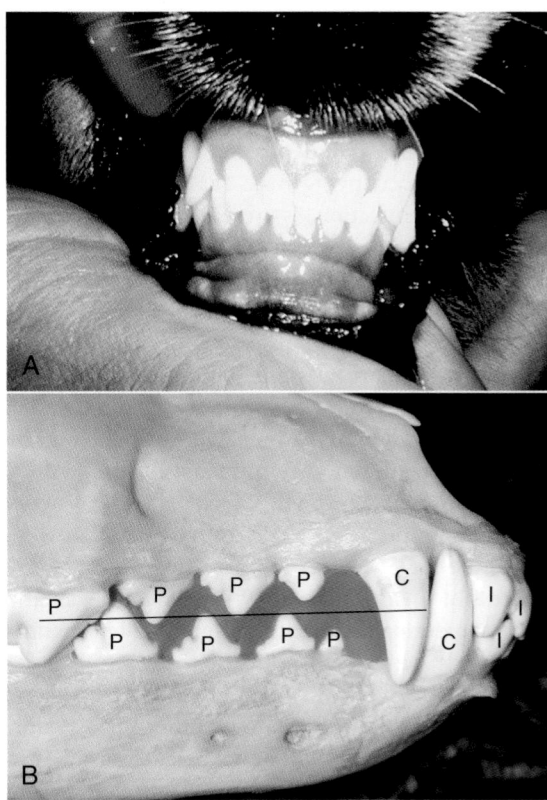

FIGURE 34-5 Normal scissors occlusion in a dog. **A,** Rostral view of incisor and canine teeth in a dog. **B,** Lateral view of a dog skull. Premolar cusps interdigitate toward the opposing interdental space. *C,* Canine; *I,* incisor; *M,* molar; *P,* premolar.

Canines

When the mouth is closed, the mandibular canine tooth is distal to the maxillary third incisor and mesial to the maxillary canine, and it should be centered between these two teeth without touching either of them.

Premolars

The premolar cusps point to the interdental space of the opposing premolar teeth. The mandibular fourth premolar cusp points in the interdental space between the maxillary third and fourth premolars. When the mouth is closed, the mandibular first premolar is mesial to the maxillary first premolar. The premolars are not in occlusion with the opposing premolar teeth, but when the mouth is closed, the cusp tips should intersect a plane drawn midway between mandibular and maxillary occlusal planes (see Figure 34-5, B).

Carnassial Teeth

The term *carnassial,* interpreted literally, means "tearing of flesh." This adjective is used to describe the largest shearing tooth of the upper and lower jaw in dogs, cats, and other carnivores. These teeth work together during mastication and contribute most significantly to the masticatory effort. The carnassial teeth of dogs and cats are the maxillary fourth premolar and the mandibular first molar teeth. In most

species, the upper jaw is wider than the lower jaw; this is referred to as **anisognathism**. Therefore, the maxillary fourth premolar tooth normally occludes lateral (buccal) to the mandibular first molar tooth.

Molars

Humans have many flat occlusal surfaces of the maxillary and mandibular molars that come together during chewing to crush food particles. In contrast, carnivores have sharp, shearing cusps and less-flat occlusal surfaces. Two maxillary and three mandibular molars of dogs have flat occlusal surfaces that are capable of grinding and crushing hard food particles. Cats, having the dentition of a true carnivore, have molars with few flat occlusal surfaces. Flat occlusal surfaces are often susceptible to the development of **caries** lesions (also referred to by the term *cavities*) in pits and fissures that occur as a result of incomplete development of **enamel** on the occlusal surface. The relative lack of occlusal surfaces in dogs and cats partly explains their decreased susceptibility to caries lesions compared with humans.

ORAL EXAMINATION AND HISTORY

The patient's medical history should be assessed before dental procedures are performed because dental procedures require elective anesthesia. The technician can obtain a complete medical history and a history specifically pertinent to dentistry. Clinical symptoms to inquire about include pawing at the mouth, dropping food, walking away from the food bowl after showing initial interest in food, rubbing the face along furniture, and showing uncharacteristic aggression when approached or touched around the facial region (Box 34-2). These signs can indicate oral disease and may manifest earlier in the disease process than would anorexia or oral bleeding. A history of sneezing after drinking water is suggestive of the presence of an oronasal fistula—a common problem in small breed dogs with severe periodontal disease.

History regarding oral home care can also be obtained by the technician. Inquire about whether a home care regimen is currently performed. If not, delve further to determine whether the client is willing or able to provide oral care at home. If the client has attempted home care and was not successful, find out what was tried, so that alternative methods may be suggested. If the client is currently providing home care, ask how frequently and what techniques and products are being used. History pertaining to diet, treats, and toys is also important. Ask if the pet is fed dry, canned, or semi-moist food. Inquire about the kinds of treats the pet is eating to determine what role treats are playing in the development or prevention of dental disease. Ask what kinds of toys the pet plays with and if it has any inappropriate habits that may increase the risk for dental fracture. Once the dental history has been established, the veterinary technician is in a perfect position to provide counseling on proper home care techniques, diets, and toy products.

The dental or oral surgical procedure, whether routine or emergency, should begin with a comprehensive extraoral and intraoral examination. The mouth can be an indicator of general health, and a thorough oral examination is an integral part of any diagnostic sequence. The technician plays a crucial role in providing dental care and services, so it is imperative that the technician becomes familiar with the normal anatomy of the oral cavity and surrounding structures. By performing examination techniques on a regular basis and by establishing a routine sequence of examination, the clinician can efficiently and accurately recognize abnormalities. All information gathered during the examination should be recorded on a dental record—the legal document of clinical data and dental services that becomes part of the patient's medical record (Figures 34-6, *A* and *B*, and 34-7, *A* and *B*). Any abnormalities should be brought to the attention of the veterinarian, so that a diagnosis and a proper treatment plan can be established for the patient.

> **TECHNICIAN NOTE** Every dental procedure should begin with a comprehensive oral examination to evaluate extraoral structures of the face, head, and neck, and intraoral structures, including soft tissues of the oral cavity, the teeth, and their supporting structures.

EXTRAORAL EXAMINATION

The examination begins with extraoral observation of the head, face, eyes, ears, and neck using direct visual observation, palpation, and smell. Using both hands, palpate each side of the face, head, and neck for symmetric comparison. Feel the temporal and masseter muscles for the presence of atrophy, enlargement, or pain. Palpate the ventral, lateral, and medial surfaces of the left and right mandibles for the presence of swelling, which could suggest neoplasia or fracture. Small breed dogs with advanced periodontal disease are commonly affected by bone loss and pathologic fracture of the mandible, which may be found as an incidental finding in the examination room.

Visually inspect the ears, and note evidence of discharge, odor, or pain on palpation because middle ear disease may

be a cause for the presenting complaint of pain on opening the mouth. Visually inspect the eyes, and palpate using your thumbs on the closed eyelids to gently push (retropulse) both eyes at the same time. Bilateral retropulsion allows for symmetric comparison of depth and firmness (Figure 34-8). Often if a space-occupying mass (as a result of neoplasia, inflammation, or infection) is present behind or beneath the eye, retropulsion may reveal decreased ability of the globe to move caudally in the orbit on one side when compared with the opposite side. Ability to retropulse varies depending on facial conformation. Retropulsion of the eyes of **brachycephalic** dogs and cats results in less movement of the globe, so comparison of both eyes is important for determining relative differences. Observe for evidence of ocular discharge, which may be due to blockage of the nasolacrimal duct by a pathologic process, such as a tooth root abscess or neoplasia. Palpate the soft tissue in the area ventral to the medial canthus of the eye. Swelling in this area may be due to a tooth root abscess of the maxillary fourth premolar. Evaluation of the neck includes palpation of the right and left mandibular salivary glands beneath the skin of the ventral neck. The mandibular salivary gland is the only easily palpable major salivary gland in dogs and cats. The other three major salivary glands may be too diffuse to palpate easily (parotid, sublingual glands) or not superficial enough to palpate (zygomatic gland). The mandibular gland is easily distinguished from the mandibular lymph nodes because it is softer, larger than, and caudomedial to the mandibular lymph nodes. Once the salivary glands are located, the mandibular lymph nodes can be identified by moving the fingertips cranially. Palpate the lymph nodes bilaterally for symmetry and firmness. In the cat, mandibular lymph nodes are difficult to palpate unless they are enlarged. In the dog, mandibular lymph nodes are almost always palpable, ranging in size from 0.5 to 1.5 cm in diameter, depending on the size of the patient. Although we often refer to the mandibular lymph "node," in reality, the area contains anywhere from one to five nodes. Other nodes that drain the head (retropharyngeal, parotid) are not normally palpable. Nine percent of dogs have another lymph node that is palpable in the subcutaneous tissue dorsal to the maxillary third premolar tooth. This node is referred to as the *facial* or *buccal lymph node* and is often bilateral, when present.

> **TECHNICIAN NOTE** The major salivary glands of the dog and cat are the paired mandibular, sublingual, zygomatic, and parotid glands.

The occlusion should be evaluated before intubation by noting any teeth that are positioned incorrectly. The technician should pay particular attention to discrepancies of jaw length, the spatial relationships of the teeth as they erupt, and the relationships of erupting teeth with the soft tissues of the opposing jaw. Note any deciduous teeth that have not exfoliated by the time their permanent counterpart

Text continued on page 1309

VHUP DENTAL RECORD

R L

Date:

Staff:
(circle primary staff)

Chief Complaint:

(Addressograph)

Awake   Sedated   Anesthetized

MAL/1   MAL/2   MAL/3   MAL/WRY
MAL/BN Malocclusion/base narrow mand. canines
MAL/ABX, PBX Mal/anterior, posterior crossbite
OC   Orthodontic/genetic consultation
OR   Orthodontic recheck
SN   Supernumerary tooth
DT   Deciduous tooth
RD   Retained deciduous tooth
PD0   No perio dx (maybe calculus)
PD1   Gingivitis (no bone loss)
PD2   Mild periodontitis (<25% attach loss)
PD3   Mod periodontitis (<50% attach loss)
PD4   Severe periodontitis (>50% attach loss)
GH   Gingival hyperplasia
GR   Gingival recession
ST   Stomatitis
ST/CU   Stomatitis – contact ulcer
ST/FFS   Stomatitis – Feline faucitis-stomatitis
OM   Oral mass:
    OM/EPA OM/EPF OM/EPO
    OM/MM OM/FS OM/SCC OM/OS
    OM/AD OM/LS OM/PAP
DTC   Dentigerous cyst
O   *Missing Teeth*

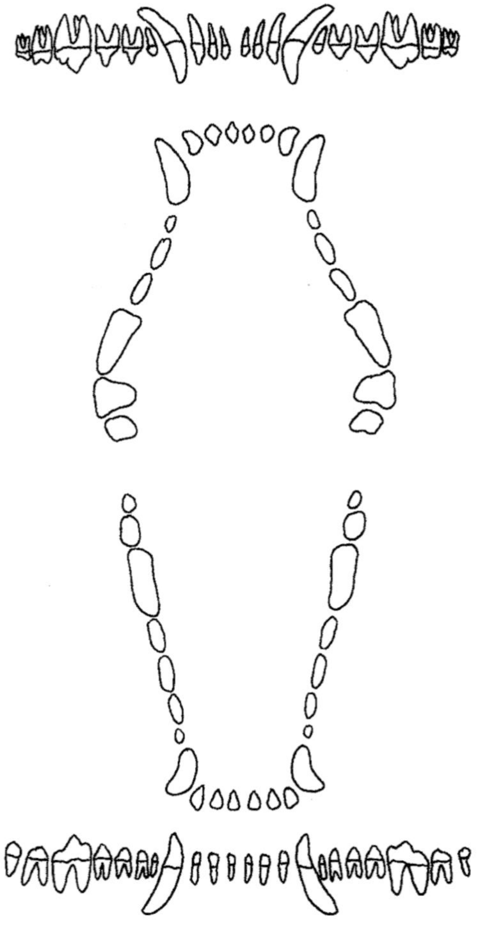

AT / AB   Attrition/abrasion
E/D, H   Enamel/defect, hypoplasia
CA   Caries
RL 1, 2, 3, 4, 5   Resorptive lesion (grade)
RR   Internal root resorption
RTR   Retained tooth root
RRT   Retained root tip
T/A, I, LUX   Tooth/ avulsed, impacted, luxated
T/FX, PE, NE   Tooth/frac., pulp exposure, near PE
T/NV, V   Tooth/non-vital, vital
G/B, L   Granuloma/buccal, sublingual
G/E/L, P, T   Eosinophilic gran./lip, palate, tongue
FB   Foreign body
OST   Osteomyelitis
LAC/B, L, T   Laceration/buccal, lip, tongue
MN/FX   MX/FX   Jaw fractures
SYM/S   Symphyseal separation
CFP CFL   Cleft palate, Cleft lip
ONF   Oronasal fistula
CMO   Cranio-Mandibular Osteopathy
TMJ/D, FX, LUX   TMJ/dysplasia, fracture, luxation
OTH:

N   A - Extraoral/facial

N   A – Lymph nodes

N   A – Buccal mucosa

N   A – Tongue

N   A – Palate

N   A – Tonsils

N   A – Pharynx

Tooth	M2	M1	P4	P3	P2	P1	C	I3	I2	I1	I1	I2	I3	C	P1	P2	P3	P4	M1	M2	M3
Triadan	110	109	108	107	106	105	104	103	102	101	201	202	203	204	205	206	207	208	209	210	211
Mobility																					
Recession																					
Pocket																					
Furcation																					
Hyperplasia																					
Calculus																					
Plaque																					
Gingivitis																					

Right   Left

Tooth	M3	M2	M1	P4	P3	P2	P1	C	I3	I2	I1	I1	I2	I3	C	P1	P2	P3	P4	M1	M2	M3
Triadan	411	410	409	408	407	406	405	404	403	402	401	301	302	303	304	305	306	307	308	309	310	311
Mobility																						
Recession																						
Pocket																						
Furcation																						
Hyperplasia																						
Calculus																						
Plaque																						
Gingivitis																						

R   L

FIGURE 34-6 Canine dental chart. This form is also available on the Evolve site. A, Front used to document diagnosis.

A

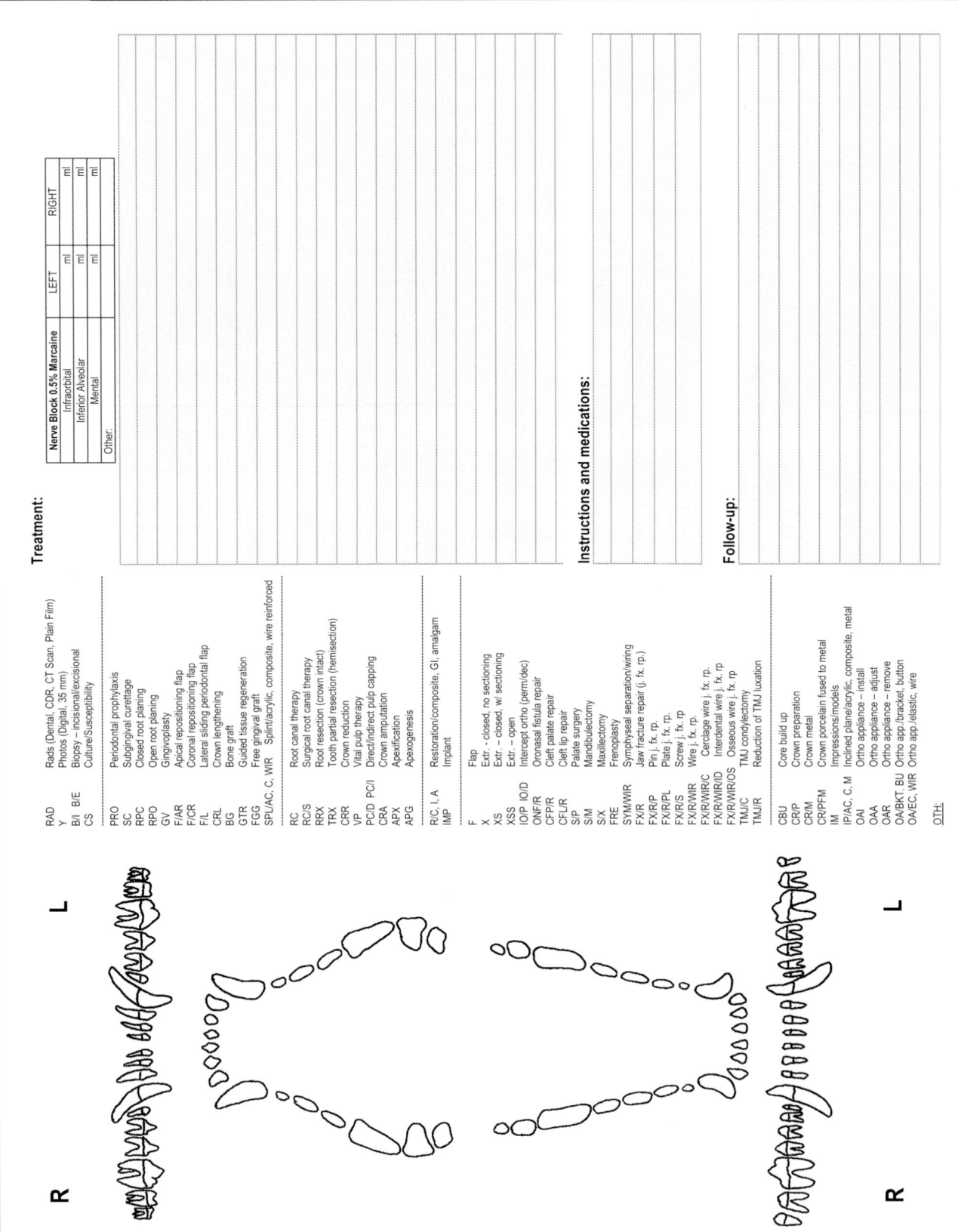

Treatment:

Nerve Block 0.5% Marcaine	LEFT		RIGHT	
Infraorbital		ml		ml
Inferior Alveolar		ml		ml
Mental		ml		ml
Other:				

R **L**

RAD Rads (Dental, CDR, CT Scan, Plain Film)
Y Photos (Digital, 35 mm)
B/I B/E Biopsy – incisional/excisional
CS Culture/Susceptibility

PRO Periodontal prophylaxis
SC Subgingival curettage
RPC Closed root planing
RPO Open root planing
GV Gingivoplasty
F/AR Apical repositioning flap
F/CR Coronal repositioning flap
F/L Lateral sliding periodontal flap
CRL Crown lengthening
BG Bone graft
GTR Guided tissue regeneration
FGG Free gingival graft
SPL/AC, C, WIR Splint/acrylic, composite, wire reinforced

RC Root canal therapy
RC/S Surgical root canal therapy
RRX Root resection (crown intact)
TRX Tooth partial resection (hemisection)
CRR Crown reduction
VP Vital pulp therapy
PC/D PC/I Direct/indirect pulp capping
CRA Crown amputation
APX Apexification
APG Apexogenesis

R/C, I, A Restoration/composite, GI, amalgam
IMP Implant

F Flap
X Extr. - closed, no sectioning
XS Extr. - closed, w/ sectioning
XSS Extr. – open
IO/P IO/D Intercept ortho (perm/dec)
ONF/R Oronasal fistula repair
CFP/R Cleft palate repair
CFL/R Cleft lip repair
S/P Palate surgery
S/M Mandibulectomy
S/X Maxillectomy
FRE Frenoplasty
SYM/WIR Symphyseal separation/wiring
FX/R Jaw fracture repair (j. fx. rp.)
FX/R/P Pin j. fx. rp.
FX/R/PL Plate j. fx. rp.
FX/R/S Screw j. fx. rp
FX/R/WIR Wire j. fx. rp
FX/R/WIR/C Cerclage wire j. fx. rp.
FX/R/WIR/ID Interdental wire j. fx. rp
FX/R/WIR/OS Osseous wire j. fx. rp
TMJ/C TMJ condylectomy
TMJ/R Reduction of TMJ luxation

CBU Core build up
CR/P Crown preparation
CR/M Crown metal
CR/PFM Crown porcelain fused to metal
IM Impressions/models
IP/AC, C, M Inclined plane/acrylic, composite, metal
OAI Ortho appliance – install
OAA Ortho appliance – adjust
OAR Ortho appliance – remove
OA/BKT, BU Ortho app./bracket, button
OA/EC, WIR Ortho app./elastic, wire

OTH:

Instructions and medications:

Follow-up:

R **L**

FIGURE 34-6, cont'd B, Back used to document treatment.

B

VHUP DENTAL RECORD

R   L

Date:

Staff: (circle primary staff)

Chief Complaint:

| | Awake | Sedated | Anesthetized |

(Addressograph)

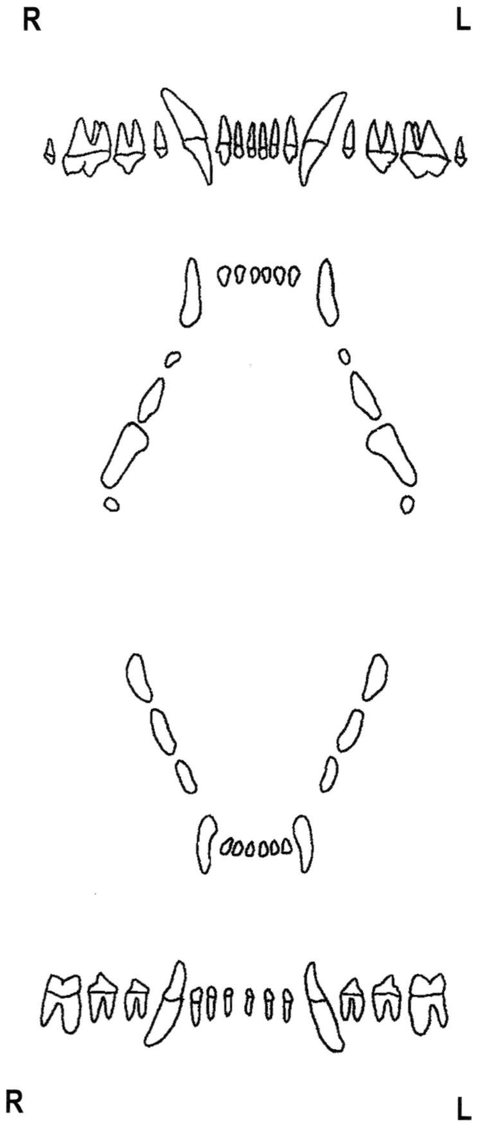

MAL/1   MAL/2   MAL/3   MAL/WRY
MAL/BN   Malocclusion/base narrow mand. canines
MAL/ABX, PBX   Mal/anterior, posterior crossbite
OC   Orthodontic/genetic consultation
OR   Orthodontic recheck
SN   Supernumerary tooth
DT   Deciduous tooth
RD   Retained deciduous tooth
PD0   No perio dx (maybe calculus)
PD1   Gingivitis (no bone loss)
PD2   Mild periodontitis (<25% attach loss)
PD3   Mod periodontitis (<50% attach loss)
PD4   Severe periodontitis (>50% attach loss)
GH   Gingival hyperplasia
GR   Gingival recession
ST   Stomatitis
ST/CU   Stomatitis – contact ulcer
ST/FFS   Stomatitis – Feline faucitis-stomatitis
OM   Oral mass:
    OM/EPA   OM/EPF   OM/EPO
    OM/MM   OMFS   OM/SCC   OM/OS
    OM/AD   OM/LS   OM/PAP
DTC   Dentigerous cyst
O   *Missing Teeth*

AT / AB   Attrition/abrasion
E/D, H   Enamel/defect, hypoplasia
CA   Caries
RL1, 2, 3, 4, 5   Resorptive lesion (grade)
RR   Internal root resorption
RTR   Retained tooth root
RRT   Retained root tip
T/A, I, LUX   Tooth/ avulsed, impacted, luxated
T/FX, PE, NE   Tooth/frac., pulp exposure, near PE
T/NV, V   Tooth/non-vital, vital
G/B, L   Granuloma/buccal, sublingual
G/E/L, P, T   Eosinophilic gran./lip, palate, tongue
FB   Foreign body
OST   Osteomyelitis
LAC/B, L, T   Laceration/buccal, lip, tongue
MN/FX MX/FX   Jaw fractures
SYM/S   Symphyseal separation
CFP CFL   Cleft palate, Cleft lip
ONF   Oronasal fistula
CMO   Cranio-Mandibular Osteopathy
TMJ/D, FX, LUX   TMJ/dysplasia, fracture, luxation
OTH:

N   A - Extraoral/facial
N   A – Lymph nodes
N   A – Buccal mucosa
N   A – Tongue
N   A – Palate
N   A – Tonsils
N   A – Pharynx

Upper right quadrant

Tooth	M1	P4	P3	P2	C	I3	I2	I1
Triadan	109	108	107	106	104	103	102	101
Mobility								
Recession								
Pocket								
Furcation								
Hyperplasia								
Calculus								
Plaque								
Gingivitis								

Upper left quadrant

Tooth	I1	I2	I3	C	P2	P3	P4	M1
Triadan	201	202	203	204	206	207	208	209
Mobility								
Recession								
Pocket								
Furcation								
Hyperplasia								
Calculus								
Plaque								
Gingivitis								

Lower right quadrant

Tooth	M1	P4	P3	C	I3	I2	I1
Triadan	409	408	407	404	403	402	401
Mobility							
Recession							
Pocket							
Furcation							
Hyperplasia							
Calculus							
Plaque							
Gingivitis							

Lower left quadrant

Tooth	I1	I2	I3	C	P3	P4	M1
Triadan	301	302	303	304	307	308	309
Mobility							
Recession							
Pocket							
Furcation							
Hyperplasia							
Calculus							
Plaque							
Gingivitis							

Right   Left

R   L

A

FIGURE 34-7 Feline dental chart. This form is also available on the Evolve site. **A,** Front used to document diagnosis.

Treatment:

Nerve Block 0.5% Marcaine	LEFT		RIGHT	
Infraorbital		ml		ml
Inferior Alveolar		ml		ml
Mental		ml		ml
Other:				

Instructions and medications:

Follow-up:

RAD	Rads (Dental, CDR, CT Scan, Plain Film)
Y	Photos (Digital, 35 mm)
B/I B/E	Biopsy – incisional/excisional
CS	Culture/Susceptibility

PRO	Periodontal prophylaxis
SC	Subgingival curettage
RPC	Closed root planing
RPO	Open root planing
GV	Gingivoplasty
F/AR	Apical repositioning flap
F/CR	Coronal repositioning flap
CRL	Lateral sliding periodontal flap
F/L	Crown lengthening
BG	Bone graft
GTR	Guided tissue regeneration
FGG	Free gingival graft
SPL/AC, C, WIR	Splint/acrylic, composite, wire reinforced

RC	Root canal therapy
RC/S	Surgical root canal therapy
RRX	Root resection (crown intact)
TRX	Tooth partial resection (hemisection)
CRR	Crown reduction
VP	Vital pulp therapy
PC/D PC/I	Direct/indirect pulp capping
CRA	Crown amputation
APX	Apexification
APG	Apexogenesis

R/C, I, A	Restoration/composite, GI, amalgam
IMP	Implant

F	Flap
X	Extr. - closed, no sectioning
XSS	Extr. - closed, w/ sectioning
IO/P IO/D	Extr. – open
ONF/R	Intercept ortho (perm/dec)
CFP/R	Oronasal fistula repair
CFL/R	Cleft palate repair
S/P	Cleft lip repair
S/M	Palate surgery
S/X	Mandibulectomy
FRE	Maxillectomy
SYM/WIR	Frenoplasty
FX/R	Symphyseal separation/wiring
FX/R/PL	Jaw fracture repair (j. fx. rp.)
FX/R/S	Pin j. fx. rp.
FX/R/WIR	Plate j. fx. rp.
FX/R/WIR/C	Screw j. fx. rp
FX/R/WIR/ID	Wire j. fx. rp.
FX/R/WIR/OS	Cerclage wire j. fx. rp.
TMJ/C	Interdental wire j. fx. rp
TMJ/R	Osseous wire j. fx. rp
	TMJ condylectomy
	Reduction of TMJ luxation

CBU	Core build up
CR/P	Crown preparation
CR/M	Crown metal
CR/PFM	Crown porcelain fused to metal
IM	Impressions/models
IP/AC, C, M	Inclined plane/acrylic, composite, metal
OAI	Ortho appliance – install
OAA	Ortho appliance – adjust
OAR	Ortho appliance – remove
OA/BKT, BU	Ortho app./bracket, button
OA/EC, WIR	Ortho app./elastic, wire

OTH:

FIGURE 34-7, cont'd B, Back used to document treatment.

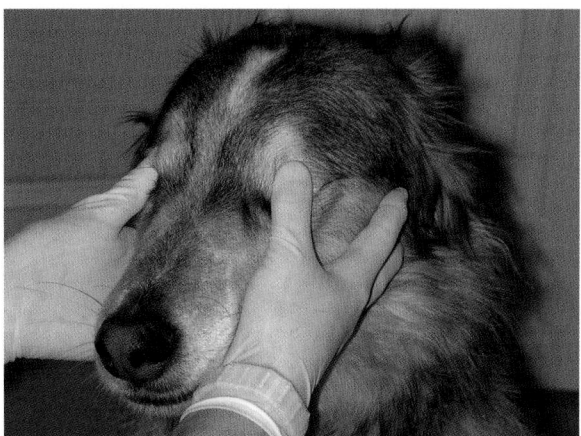

FIGURE 34-8 Retropulsion of both eyes is an important component of the extraoral examination.

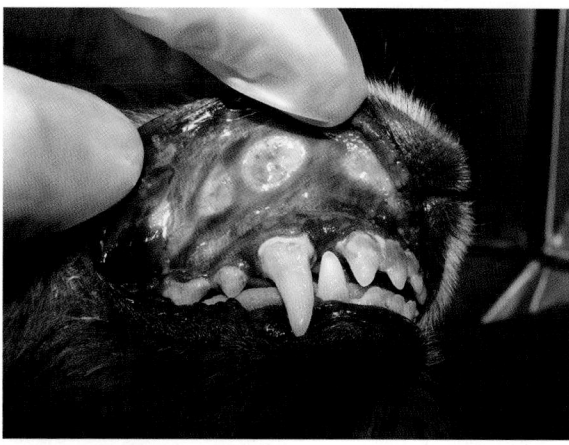

FIGURE 34-9 Chronic ulcerative paradental stomatitis in a dog (CUPS).

has erupted because persistent deciduous teeth may create situations of periodontal disease and redirection of permanent tooth eruption. Once the deciduous and permanent canines begin to erupt, routinely monitor the relationship of the mandibular canines and the space between the maxillary third incisor and the canine teeth. Deviations from normal canine positioning can cause trauma to the palate and require treatment.

INTRAORAL EXAMINATION

The intraoral examination consists of evaluations of the soft tissues of the oral cavity, the dental structures, and the **periodontium**, a term that describes the supporting structures of the teeth. A standard approach to the oral examination allows for efficiency and thoroughness. Begin by observing the skin and mucosa of the upper and lower lips. Some breeds are prone to lip fold dermatitis of the lip area caudal to the mandibular canine tooth that can cause oral malodor unrelated to periodontal disease. *Buccal mucosa* refers to the mucosa that begins at the mucocutaneous junction and lines the cheeks and lips. *Alveolar mucosa* refers to the mucosa that lies against the bone of the upper or lower jaw and meets the gingiva at the mucogingival junction. The normal appearance of the mucosa may be pink or pigmented, and the mucosa should exhibit no lesions, ulcerations, or swellings. Pay particular attention to areas of mucosa that lay adjacent to periodontally diseased teeth, because the bacteria in the **plaque** may contribute to painful mucosal ulcerations, often referred to as *chronic ulcerative paradental stomatitis* (CUPS) (Figure 34-9). Observe the caudal cheek lining in the region of the carnassial and molar teeth. This mucosa frequently becomes pressed between the teeth during chewing, creating a condition known as "cheek chewing lesions" (Figure 34-10). Similarly, mucosa beneath the tongue may show signs of chewing lesions referred to as "tongue chewing lesions," which are usually bilateral (Figure 34-11). These lesions usually do not require treatment unless they are not bilaterally similar or are ulcerated. In these cases, the affected mucosa may be removed and submitted for histopathologic evaluation.

Two raised bumps are found on the alveolar mucosa dorsal to the maxillary fourth premolar and first molar teeth. Salivary secretions from the parotid and zygomatic salivary glands travel through ducts leading to these duct openings (Figure 34-12).

The roof of the mouth is composed of the hard and soft palate. The hard palate forms the rostral two-thirds and is covered by palatal mucosa arranged in prominent ridges, called *rugae* (Figure 34-13). These rugae range from eight to ten in number. In brachycephalic dogs, the rugae are closely positioned, and hair and debris can accumulate in these rugal folds. At the midline of the hard palate, just caudal to the incisor teeth, the incisive papilla is a round, slightly raised structure (Figure 34-14). Lateral to the incisive papilla, a small bilateral communication with the incisive duct and the vomeronasal organ can be found. The vomeronasal organ is a sensory organ involved in detection of pheromones and other chemical compounds. Palpation of the area lateral to the incisive papilla may normally feel as if air is trapped beneath the mucosa as a result of the communication between the mouth and these nasal structures. The soft palate consists of mucosa and muscle that separate the oropharynx from the nasopharynx. Two prominent bony structures can be palpated just lateral to the midline of the soft palate; these are the hamular processes of the bilateral pterygoid bones. One or both hamular processes may be difficult to palpate because of the presence of a nasopharyngeal mass.

> **TECHNICIAN NOTE** The incisive papilla is a raised structure located at the midline behind the maxillary incisors in dogs and cats.

The pharynx should be evaluated for evidence of inflammation or neoplasia. When the patient's mouth is open, bilateral folds of pharyngeal mucosa will be evident lateral to the tongue. These are referred to as the *palatoglossal folds*, and this area and the mucosa lateral to these folds may be inflamed in cats with lymphocytic-plasmacytic stomatitis (LPS) (Figure 34-15).

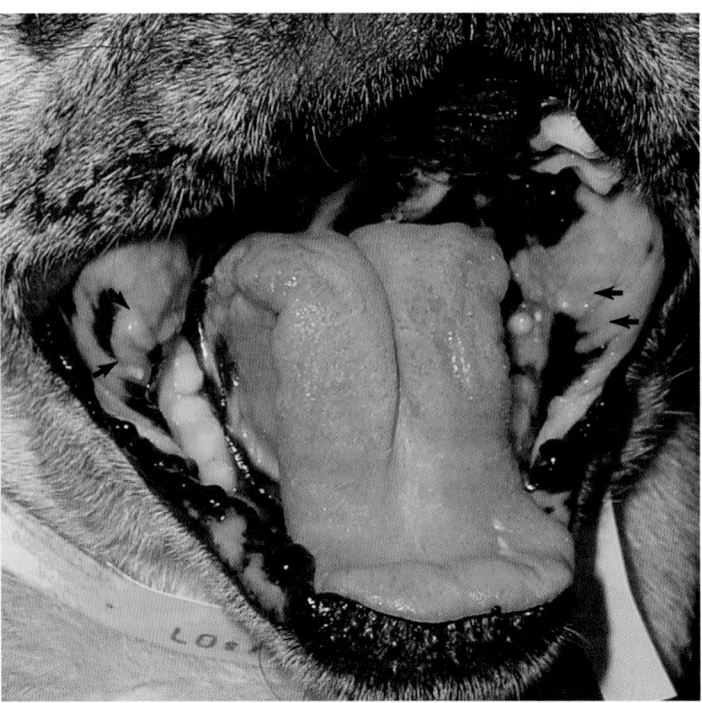

FIGURE 34-10 Bilateral cheek chewing lesions in a dog (arrows). These lesions can be proliferative and sometimes ulcerated.

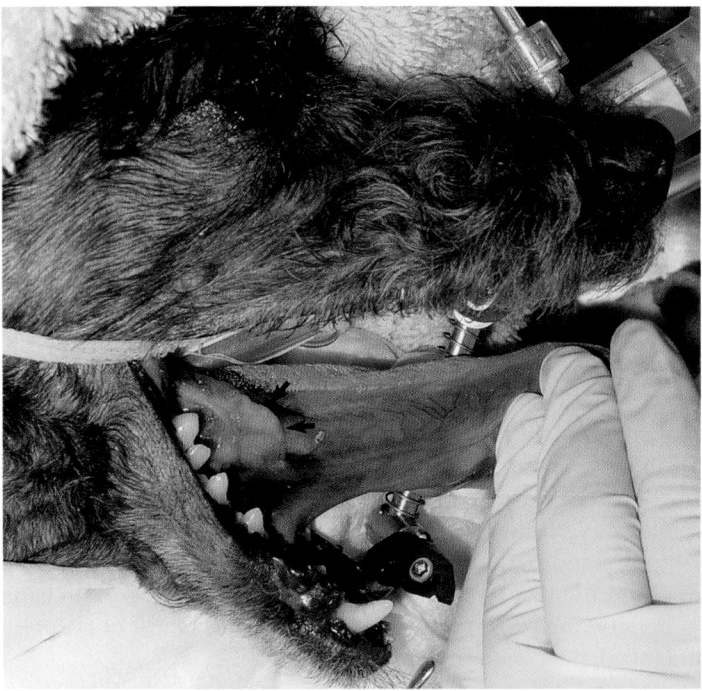

FIGURE 34-11 Tongue chewing lesion in a dog (arrows).

Gently hold the tip of the tongue to enable visual examination of the dorsal, ventral, and lateral surfaces. Lift the tongue to observe the mucosa of the floor of the mouth and the base of the tongue. In the conscious patient, the examiner's thumb may be used extraorally to push the tongue dorsally for better visualization of the ventral surface of the tongue. The dorsal surface of the tongue is covered by thousands of papillae, some of which contain taste buds. The large, distinctive papillae located at the caudal third of the tongue are the vallate papillae, which are spaced in a curved line separating the body from the root of the tongue. Depress the tongue to visualize the tonsils, noting any enlargement or change in color or texture. The color of a normal tonsil typically is more hyperemic than the color of adjacent mucosa. Normal tonsils may be fully contained within the tonsillar crypt and may be difficult to visualize.

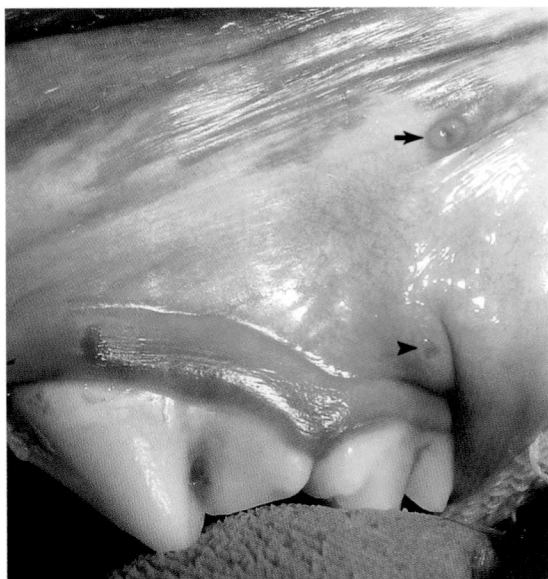

FIGURE 34-12 Parotid *(arrow)* and zygomatic duct *(arrowhead)* openings in a dog. When the mucosa is not retracted caudally, the parotid opening is rostral and dorsal to the zygomatic duct opening.

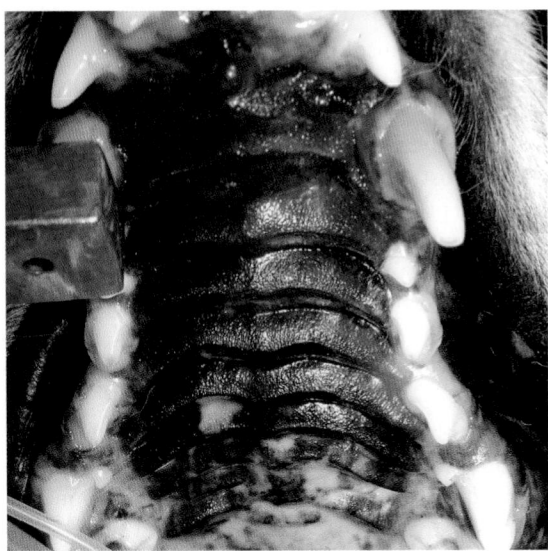

FIGURE 34-13 Palatal rugae in a dog. The rugae may be widely spaced in dolichocephalic dogs or close together in brachycephalic dogs.

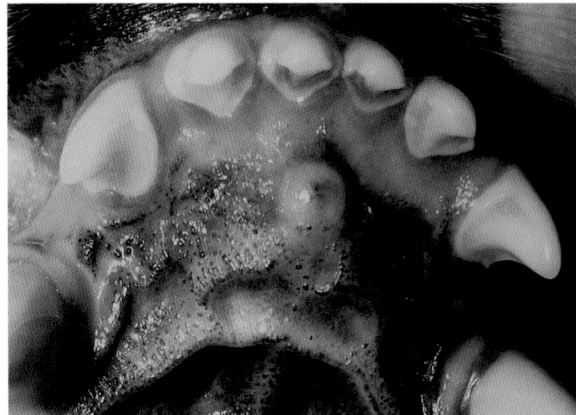

FIGURE 34-14 Incisive papilla in a dog. The left and right incisive ducts open on the lateral aspects of the papilla.

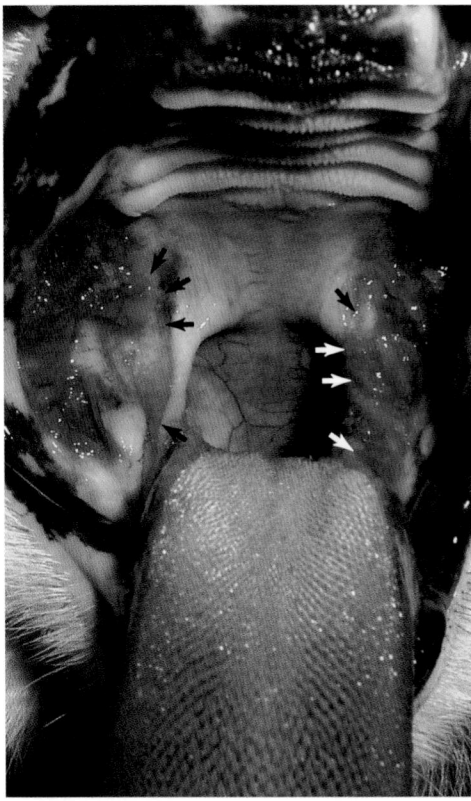

FIGURE 34-15 Caudal stomatitis in the area lateral to the palatoglossal folds *(arrows)* in a cat.

During the soft tissue examination, any tissue variations from normal should be described by recording size, shape, color, surface texture, and consistency (e.g., soft, firm, hard, fluctuant). A dedicated area on the dental record may be created to allow for documentation of any abnormalities of oral soft tissue structures (see Figures 34-6, *A*, and 34-7, *A*).

The next step in the intraoral examination is evaluation of the teeth and their supporting structures. First, determine the presence or absence of teeth in each quadrant. Missing teeth can be documented on the dental chart by darkening or circling them. Further radiographic evaluation of areas of missing teeth is imperative because dentigerous cysts can develop as a result of an unerupted tooth. To evaluate the condition of the teeth and the periodontium, the technician must use a periodontal probe and a dental explorer. These dental instruments are important clinical tools for obtaining data about the health status of each tooth. Consider the canine mouth as containing 42 patients, and the feline mouth as containing 30 patients, with each patient requiring a thorough evaluation. The periodontal probe has a round or flat working end that is marked in millimeter increments, ending in a blunt tip. The probe is used as a miniature intraoral ruler to measure attachment levels, sulcus and pocket depths, loss of bone in **furcation** areas, and size of oral

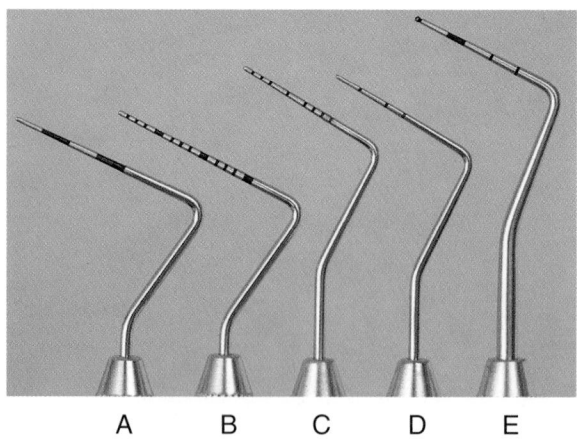

FIGURE 34-16 Periodontal probes with different calibrations. *A,* Tufts 17; *B,* Shepherd's hook 23; *C,* ODU 11/12; *D,* 3A; *E,* 2A Pigtail. The blunt-tipped working end is used to measure sulcus or pocket depth, tooth mobility, furcation involvement, gingival recession, and gingival hyperplasia. (From Darby ML, Walsh MM: Dental hygiene theory and practice, ed 3, St Louis, 2010, Saunders.)

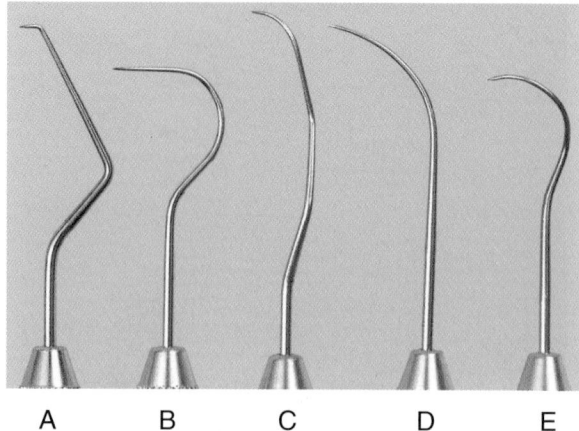

FIGURE 34-17 Dental explorers with sharp, wire-like tips are used to explore the topography of tooth surfaces. (From Darby ML, Walsh MM: Dental hygiene theory and practice, ed 3, St Louis, 2010, Saunders.)

lesions. It is also used to assess the mobility of teeth and the presence of gingival bleeding. Periodontal probes are available in an assortment of design styles, with variations in the thickness of the diameter of the working end and variations in increments of millimeter markings (Figure 34-16). Probes with Williams' markings have millimeter increments at 1, 2, 3, 5, 7, 8, 9, and 10 mm. The UNC 15 probe has millimeter markings at 1, 2, 3, 4, 5, 6, 7, 8, 9, 10, 11, 12, 13, 14, and 15 mm; it is useful for large dogs and patients with deep periodontal pockets. Some probes have a small, 0.5-mm ball on the end to minimize tissue trauma; however, these probes typically have markings at 3.5, 5.5, 8.5, and 11.5 mm, resulting in inexact determination of pocket depth. Although many probes are available, a probe with markings beginning at 1 mm is necessary for assessing subtle pocket depths in cats. The Michigan "O" probe with Williams' markings is best suited for use in cats because the diameter of the working end of the probe is narrowest. Some styles contain color-coded bands for easier viewing of calibrations. Naber's probe is a curved furcation probe that is used to assess the extent of bone loss in the furcation area where multiple roots converge.

> **TECHNICIAN NOTE** Normal sulcus depth is 0 to 3 mm in dogs and 0 to 1 mm in cats. Probing depths greater than normal are documented on the chart as pockets.

The dental explorer has a slender, wire-like working end that tapers to a sharp point and is used to explore the topography of the tooth surface. When the explorer is held with a light modified pen grasp, the technician will acquire a tactile sense to locate tooth surface irregularities, such as caries, feline resorption, **calculus** deposits, and **pulp** exposure. Tactile sensitivity is achieved when the flexible working end of the explorer vibrates as it detects surface irregularities.

Vibrations are transmitted from the tip to the handle as felt by the technician. The explorer is also used to determine the completeness of treatment after calculus débridement and to ensure smooth transitions of dental restoratives (fillings). Several designs of explorers are available (Figure 34-17). Varying degrees of flexibility contribute to the degrees of tactile sensitivity. The shepherd's hook is the most common explorer in most veterinary practices and is often paired with a periodontal probe as a double-ended instrument. Although it is convenient to have a shepherd's hook on the opposite end of a probe, it is bulky, inflexible, and less adaptable for subgingival use when compared with other explorers. The Orban explorer has a 2-mm tip that is bent at a 90-degree angle from the shank, allowing it to be used subgingivally with little tissue distention (stretching of the gingiva away from the tooth) or trauma to the epithelial lining of the sulcus. The 2-mm tip may be a limitation when the Orban is used to determine the depth of a dental lesion, such as caries or feline resorption. The curved 11/12 ODU explorer is an ideal choice for veterinary use. The curvature of the long shank and the working ends make it adaptable for use on rostral and caudal teeth, supragingivally and subgingivally, and its smaller working end allows detection of subtle hard tissue defects.

Periodontal instruments, including the probe and the explorer, are held with a modified pen grasp (Figure 34-18), which is a variation of the grasp used for writing. This recommended grasp facilitates good fingertip tactile sensitivity and precise control of the instrument's working end, decreasing risk of trauma to the tissues. The modified pen grasp uses three fingertips placed in a triangular (tripod) position, plus a rest finger. The pads of the index finger and the thumb rest on the instrument where the handle and shank meet to hold the instrument. The pad near the fingernail of the middle finger rests on the shank. The shank is the portion of the instrument that connects the handle with the working end (Figure 34-19). Proper placement of the middle fingertip pad

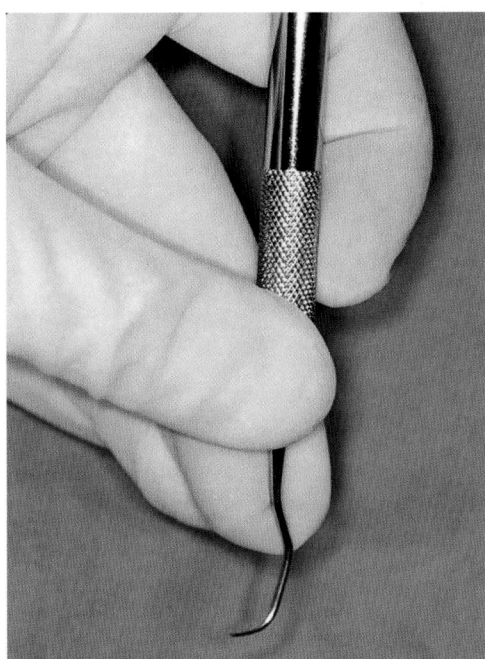

FIGURE 34-18 Modified pen grasp hand position for periodontal instrumentation: the thumb and index finger hold the instrument handle; the corner of the middle finger rests on the shank. The ring finger is used as a fulcrum and for control.

against the shank is important for enhancing tactile sensitivity and helping to guide and control the working end. The ring finger should rest on an oral structure, such as a tooth located close to the working area, to provide stability to the hand for added control. Keeping the ring finger in contact with the middle finger will ensure proper wrist motion by limiting the amount of finger motion and will prevent finger fatigue. The little finger should be relaxed and has no specific function in this grasp.

Assessment of the periodontium and teeth should begin at the midline of the mouth; each tooth should be systematically evaluated, one at a time, through visual observation and tactile use of the probe and explorer. Begin to detect excessive tooth mobility by placing the tip of the probe against the tip of the tooth and gently attempting to move the tooth in a buccolingual direction. Movement is estimated on a scale of 1, 2, or 3, on the basis of the number of millimeters beyond normal physiologic mobility that the tooth moves in a single direction (Box 34-3). A slight amount of movement is normal because of the periodontal ligament that connects the tooth to alveolar bone. The most severe mobility, with a classification of 3, includes any tooth with vertical movement. As you evaluate each tooth for mobility, visually notice the characteristics of the gingiva for color, shape, texture, and consistency. Healthy gingival tissues are pink (except where normally pigmented), stippled (orange peel appearance), firm, tapered to a thin margin, and scalloped to follow the contour of the cementoenamel junction (CEJ) and underlying alveolar bone. Any area of the gingiva that deviates from these normal characteristics should be examined more closely with the probe.

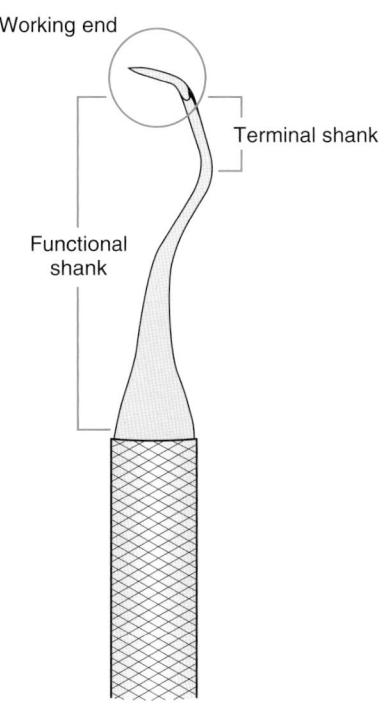

FIGURE 34-19 Parts of the instrument include the handle, shank, and working end. The functional shank extends from the handle to the working end, and the terminal shank is the part of the shank closest to the working end. (From Daniel SJ, Harfst SA, Wilder R: Mosby's dental hygiene: concepts, cases, and competencies, ed 2, St Louis, 2008, Mosby.)

BOX 34-3	Mobility Scoring Index

- Stage 0 (M0): physiologic mobility up to 0.2 mm
- Stage 1 (M1): mobility is increased in any direction other than axial* over a distance of more than 0.2 mm and up to 0.5 mm
- Stage 2 (M2): mobility is increased in any direction other than axial over a distance of more than 0.5 mm and up to 1.0 mm
- Stage 3 (M3): mobility is increased in any direction other than axial over a distance exceeding 1.0 mm or any axial movement

With permission of AVDC (www.AVDC.org/Nomenclature.pdf).
*Axial movement refers to movement in the long axis of the tooth.

TECHNICIAN NOTE The *periodontium*, the term that describes the attachment structures of the teeth, includes gingival connective tissue, alveolar bone, periodontal ligament, and cementum.

The probe is gently inserted into the sulcus or pocket, with the probe kept as close to parallel to the long axis of the root as possible, and with the side of the probe tip in contact with the tooth. When physical resistance is felt at the base of the sulcus or pocket, note the marking level on the probe that is adjacent to the gingival margin. The probe is then "walked" around the tooth with up and down bobbing

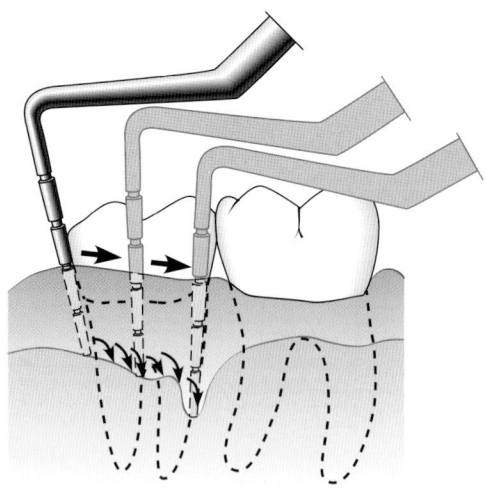

FIGURE 34-20 While keeping the side of the tip of the probe in contact with the tooth and using a light touch, the probe is "walked" around the circumference of the tooth with short up-and-down strokes every few millimeters. (From Newman MG, Takei H, Klokkevold PR, et al: Carranza's clinical periodontology, ed 10, St Louis, 2006, Saunders.)

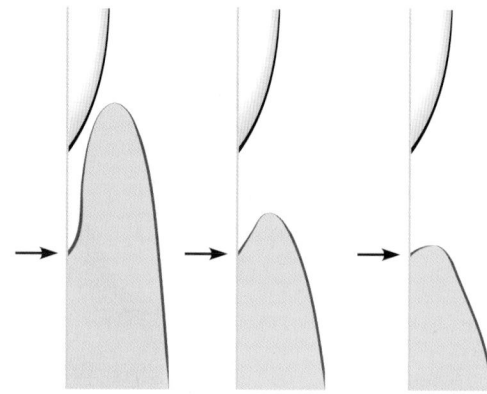

FIGURE 34-21 Attachment level is measured from the bottom of the pocket *(arrows)* to a fixed point on the tooth, such as the cementoenamel junction (CEJ). Attachment level is a better indicator of periodontal status than is pocket depth because gingival recession or hyperplasia can greatly affect pocket depth measurement. Note that the three examples have the same level of attachment loss yet different pocket depths, as a result of gingival recession. (From Newman MG, Takei H, Klokkevold PR, et al: Carranza's clinical periodontology, ed 11, St Louis, 2012, Saunders.)

strokes approximately 1 to 2 mm in height ($\updownarrow$) and in 1- to 2-mm horizontal steps ($\leftrightarrow$) to assess the entire circumference of the tooth (Figure 34-20). Abnormal measurements (those greater than 3 mm in dogs, greater than 1 mm in cats) should be noted on the dental chart, along with the specific location of the pocket measurement (e.g., MB for mesiobuccal). Probe measurements between millimeter markings are rounded up to the larger measurement. For accurate readings, it is essential for the technician to develop skill in consistently probing forces (between 10 and 20 *g* of pressure). This amount of pressure can be attained by pressing the probe tip into the pad of a thumb until the skin is depressed approximately 2 mm.

In areas where the height of the free gingival margin has migrated apically toward or beyond the CEJ, the probe is used to measure gingival recession. Recession is measured in millimeters from the CEJ to the level of the gingival margin. *Attachment loss* is a term that truly describes the periodontal state of a tooth because it accounts for both pocket depth and gingival recession (Figure 34-21). Gingival hyperplasia occurs when the free gingival margin migrates coronally, toward the crown of the tooth. Hyperplasia is measured in millimeters from the CEJ to the gingival margin, which is covering a portion of the tooth crown. Increased pocket depth may be due to hyperplasia or attachment loss, so clinical examination findings are necessary to determine whether the increased probing depth is due to a true pocket or to a pseudopocket.

When multi-rooted teeth are approached, the probe is used to assess loss of bone in the areas between and around the roots. A bifurcation, which is the furcation between two-rooted teeth, should be assessed from the buccal and lingual-palatal surfaces. Trifurcations of three-rooted teeth should be assessed between each of the three roots. The extent of

BOX 34-4	Furcation Involvement/Exposure Index

- Stage 1 (F1, furcation involvement) exists when a periodontal probe extends less than halfway under the crown in any direction of a multi-rooted tooth with attachment loss.
- Stage 2 (F2, furcation involvement) exists when a periodontal probe extends more than halfway under the crown of a multi-rooted tooth with attachment loss, but not through and through.
- Stage 3 (F3, furcation exposure) exists when a periodontal probe extends under the crown of a multi-rooted tooth, through and through from one side of the furcation out the other.

With permission of AVDC (www.AVDC.org/Nomenclature.pdf).

bone loss determines the furcation classification (Box 34-4). Naber's furcation probe is curved to fit over the dental bulge of the crown, so that the side of the tip can be held as parallel as possible to the long axis of the tooth. The tip is dragged horizontally across a root, dipping into the furcation area and continuing to the adjacent root. The depth of penetration into the furcation area determines the classification. If a straight probe is used, care must be taken to minimize tissue distention.

During the periodontal evaluation of each tooth, also observe the hard structures of the tooth, and use the dental explorer when noticing any chips, fractures, pulp exposure, or abnormal wear patterns of abrasion or attrition. *Abrasion* refers to tooth wear associated with aggressive chewing on external objects, such as toys, rocks, and ice cubes. *Attrition* refers to two possible scenarios. *Physiologic attrition* refers to the normal wear associated with tooth-to-tooth contact of a patient over time with normal mastication. *Pathologic*

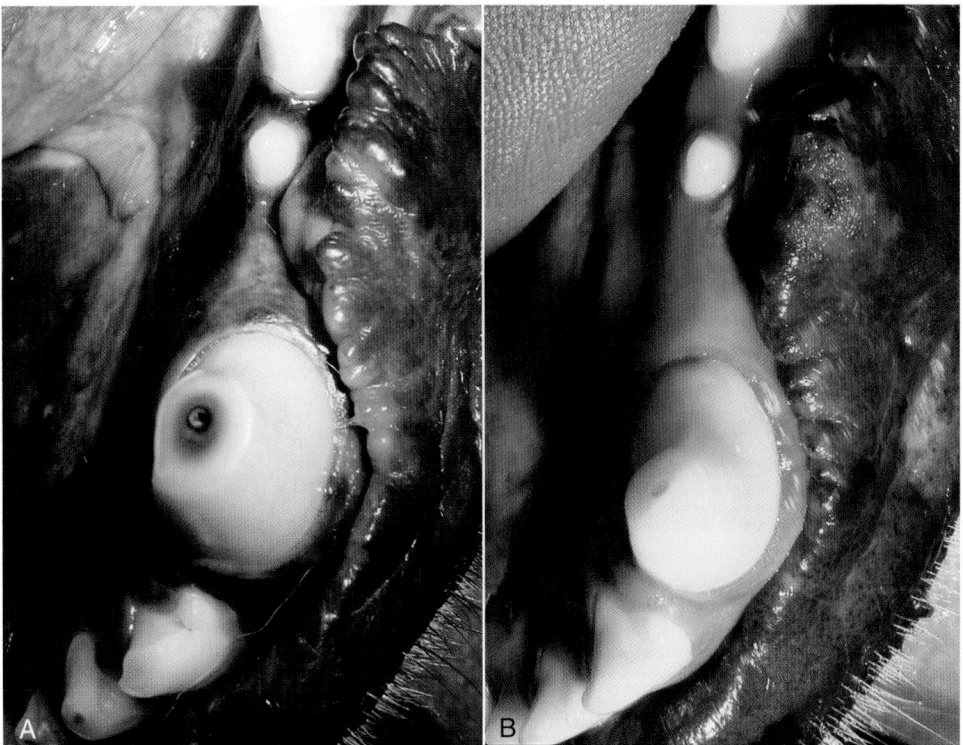

FIGURE 34-22 Abrasion of two canine teeth from different patients. **A,** Abrasion has occurred rapidly enough to result in pulp exposure; this is determined by running an explorer over the flat surface and "falling into" the pulp chamber. **B,** Abrasion has occurred slowly enough to allow the tooth to respond by producing tertiary (reparative) dentin, which feels smooth as glass when explored. Both teeth should be radiographed to assess for endodontic pathologic conditions, but the pulp-exposed tooth definitely requires extraction or root canal therapy.

attrition is caused by a malocclusion that results in abnormal wear of teeth as a result of contact with teeth of the opposing jaw.

Dental caries (commonly referred to by the lay term of "cavities") result from demineralization of the enamel and dentin from acids produced by certain oral bacteria. These lesions occur most commonly on occlusal (flat) surfaces of the molar teeth. Gently explore for pits and fissures of the occlusal surfaces of the maxillary first and second molars and the distal half of the mandibular first molar, feeling for areas of demineralization. Use the explorer to check for clinical signs of feline resorptive lesions by dragging the sharp point horizontally across the cervical portion of each tooth. Sometimes it is challenging to determine whether a concavity in the area of a furcation is a resorptive lesion or merely mild furcation exposure. If a resorptive lesion is present, the explorer tip will "catch" on the edge of the concavity, whereas the explorer will freely move out of the concave area as easily as it fell into it when mild furcation exposure is encountered. When tooth fractures are present, gently drag the sharp point of the explorer across the tooth surface, feeling for any openings into the pulp. Teeth with significant abrasion may have a brown or black dot in the center of the worn tooth. This can be a sign of chronic pulp exposure, or it may be a reparative material produced by the tooth in response to chronic wear (tertiary dentin). Pulp exposure can be distinguished from tertiary dentin with the use of an explorer. If a tooth

has pulp exposure, the tip of the explorer will "fall into a hole," whereas a discolored area caused by tertiary dentin will feel smooth as glass when the explorer is run over this area. This is an important clinical distinction because treatment of pulp-exposed teeth is necessary, but worn teeth with tertiary dentin usually do not require treatment (Figure 34-22, *A* and *B*).

DENTAL RADIOGRAPHY

Intraoral radiographs are essential for planning and assessing outcomes of dental treatment for dogs, cats, and exotic species. Intraoral radiography is also used in horses but is limited to the most rostral teeth because of difficulties in accessing the caudal teeth and small film size. Radiographs provide the clinician with an important diagnostic tool to detect pathologic conditions that are not clinically visible in the mouth. The following are types of pathologic findings for which dental radiographs are useful: root resorption, caries, periapical radiolucency (often seen with tooth root abscesses), periodontal bone loss, retained root tips, unerupted teeth, osteomyelitis, neoplasia, tooth and jaw fractures, foreign bodies, and disease of the temporomandibular joint (TMJ). The veterinary patient must be sedated or anesthetized for quality dental radiographs to be obtained. Intraoral dental radiography is becoming more routine in general veterinary practice.

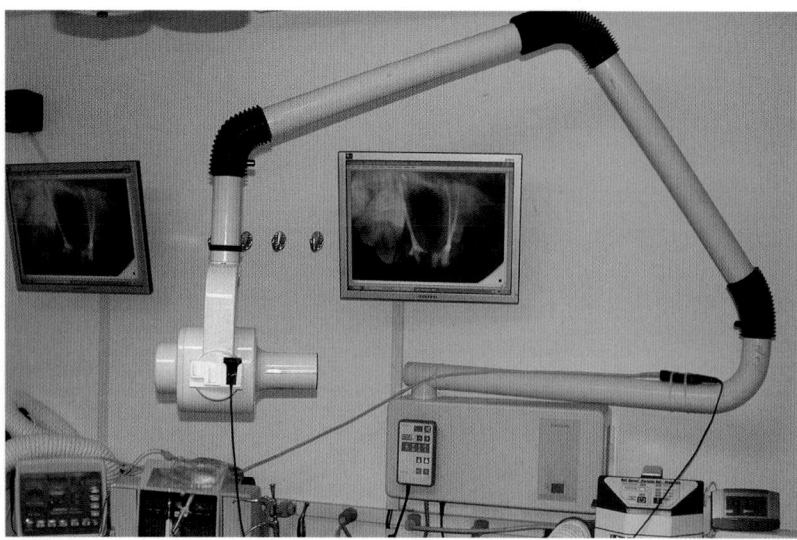

FIGURE 34-23 Intraoral radiograph machine control panel, arm, and tube head. (From DuPont GA, DeBowes LJ: Atlas of dental radiography in dogs and cats, St Louis, 2009, Saunders.)

EQUIPMENT

The dental x-ray machine may be wall mounted, or it may stand on the floor with wheels that permit storage when not in use. The unit is composed of three primary parts: the control panel, a long (72- to 86-inch) arm that extends from the control panel, and a tube head that is attached to the end of the arm (Figure 34-23). The control panel, which typically is mounted to a wall near the dental workstation, contains the power switch, selector buttons for kilovoltage and milliamperes, a dial or buttons for changing exposure time, and a button that is located at the end of a 6-foot coiled cord. Many dental x-ray units have an internally set level of kilovoltage and milliamperes, and only exposure time may be changed for a darker or lighter technique. The timing selection may be located at the end of the cord of some newer models. An indicator light and an audible sound are emitted from the control panel when exposure is attained.

> **TECHNICIAN NOTE**   The dental radiograph machine should be inspected regularly for leakage. Many states require such inspections.

The milliamperage (mA) setting regulates the intensity of the electrical current that heats the filament (cathode), thus controlling the quantity of electrons produced and available to bombard the target (anode). Milliampere seconds (mAs) describes the quantity of radiation, which is determined by multiplying the milliamperes by the exposure time. For example, a film exposed for $\frac{1}{2}$ second at 10 mA would have an exposure of 5 mAs.

The peak kilovoltage (kVp) is a measure of electrical force that regulates the speed at which electrons travel between the negatively charged cathode (filament) and the positively charged anode (target), thus controlling the quality of the x-ray beam. When electrons hit the anode at a higher force, x-rays produced have greater penetrating power at the surface of the skin. Most dental machines operate at 60 or 70 kVp. Low kilovoltage settings result in images with high black-white contrast; this is useful in detecting caries or resorption. High kilovoltage settings result in low contrast with a wider gray scale between black-white densities; this is useful in monitoring periodontal disease.

The cathode and the anode are housed in the Coolidge tube, which is located in the tube head at the end of the articulating arm. Within the tube head, the Coolidge tube is immersed in oil to help absorb the heat produced at the target. The position-indicating device (PID) contains a collimator that controls the beam size. Ranging from 8 to 16 inches in length, the PID extends from the tube head to the patient's mouth and aids in minimizing scattered radiation.

The timer switch starts production of the x-rays. Timers may be calibrated in fractions of seconds or numbers of impulses. Once the timer is activated, a short delay occurs while the filament is preheating. With experience in using the radiograph machine, the technician will be able to determine proper exposure times based on the size of the patient and the density of the tissues through which the x-ray beam must penetrate. It is helpful to create an exposure time chart to post near the control panel for quick reference. New machine models marketed for veterinary use provide timers with preset exposure times associated with pictures of the dental arcade. The technician needs only to select dog or cat, patient size, and the specific tooth.

All veterinary staff members must become familiar with radiation safety guidelines. The timer switch can be remotely wired and mounted outside of the dental treatment room, or at least 6 to 8 feet away from the tube head. Standing at a distance behind a barrier or at a 90-degree to 130-degree angle that is perpendicular to the beam will place the technician in a safe position, away from the direction of the beam.

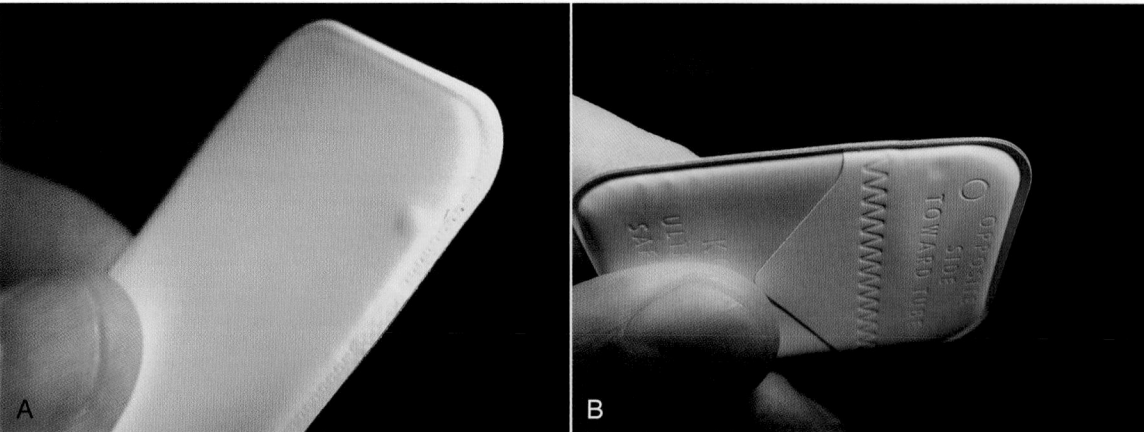

FIGURE 34-24 Two sides of a dental x-ray film packet. **A,** Convex (raised) dot is placed toward the beam. **B,** Concave (indented) dot is placed away from the beam.

The film should never be held in the patient's mouth by the technician while the radiograph is taken; therefore, anesthesia is necessary not only to ensure diagnostic quality films, but also for safety reasons. The machine should be inspected regularly for leaks by a competent radiation expert, as may be required by state regulations. Development of skills will minimize unnecessary radiation from retakes resulting from poor technique or positioning.

FILM

Intraoral film consists of a plastic base covered on both sides with emulsion of silver halide crystals. The film is wrapped in black paper with a lead foil backing placed on the side that will be farthest from the beam. The lead foil prevents scatter radiation from affecting the back side of the film. Film, paper, and foil are wrapped in a plastic or paper packet. This type of film is considered direct exposure or nonscreen film. The white surface of the film wrapper should always be placed in the mouth so that it faces the beam, and the colored surface of the film wrapper is placed away from the beam. A raised (convex) dot is present on the white surface of the film wrapper, and a recessed (concave) dot is present on the colored surface (Figure 34-24, *A* and *B*). The raised dot will always be placed so that it faces the beam, and the concave dot will be farthest from the beam.

> **TECHNICIAN NOTE** When intraoral film is placed into the mouth, the white surface of the x-ray film (the surface with the raised dot) always faces toward the beam.

Dental film is available in several sizes, ranging from 0 to 4; to accommodate variation in the size of veterinary patients, it is important to keep all sizes of film in stock. Intraoral film also comes in several speeds. The *speed* refers to sensitivity to radiation exposure, or the amount of radiation required to produce the image. Less radiation is required to produce an image using fast film; however, faster film, such as E-speed, contains larger silver halide crystals; thus the appearance of

the image is grainier than that of D-speed. Very slow speed films (speeds A, B, and C) are associated with higher radiation exposure and are no longer used. Current choices include D-, E-, and F-speed film. Recent advances in F-speed film have allowed for reduction in radiation requirements up to 60% compared with D-speed film while maintaining good image quality. Film is sensitive to heat and moisture and should be stored in a dry, clean, cool place. Observe time limits printed on the boxes, and discard the film when expired. The contents of a dental film packet are shown in Figure 34-25.

FILM PROCESSING

To convert the latent image into a visual image, the film is processed using chemicals that convert silver halide crystals to metallic silver and preserve the image. Processing of intraoral film can be accomplished in a dark room, with a manual chairside developer (Figure 34-25, *A*), or with an automatic processor.

Use of the chairside developer allows rapid evaluation of radiographs after approximately 1 minute of processing time. Premixed chemicals (developer and fixer) are available from veterinary distributors. An orange filtering lid is used with D-speed film, whereas a red lid is used with E- and F-speed film. The films are opened inside the chairside developer and are attached to a film clip. Inside are four cups into which the film will be dipped. Working from left to right, the first cup is filled with developer solution. The second cup contains water for rinsing. The third cup contains fixer solution that will halt the development process, wash off silver halide crystals that were not exposed to radiation, and preserve the image on the film. The fourth cup contains water for rinsing (Figure 34-25, *B*). Films must be developed from left to right without backtracking to prevent contamination of the solutions. One exception is that films in the fourth cup may be placed back into the third cup (fixer) without a problem. The timing of each step is critical, and manufacturers' directions should be followed. Keep in mind the possible need for adjustments in time when the temperature of the

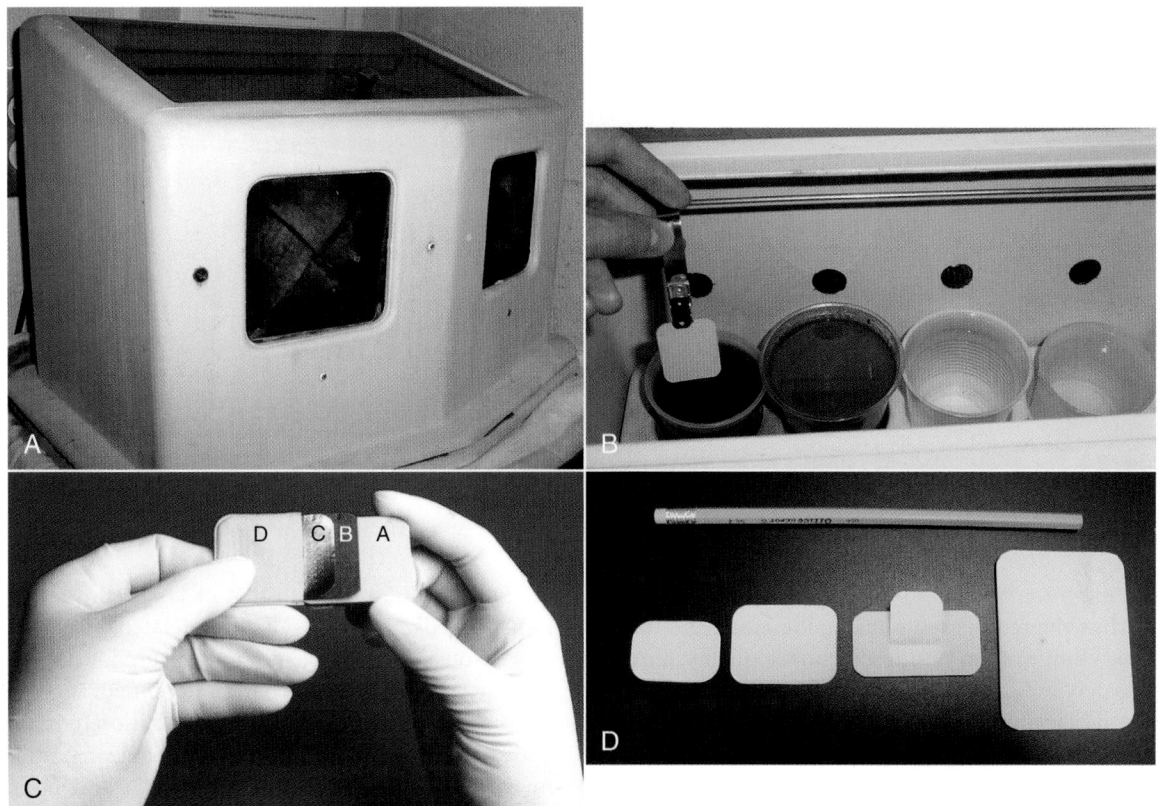

FIGURE 34-25 **A,** The chairside developer is convenient and more rapid than an automatic processor. **B,** Inside, the four containers are filled with developer, water rinse, fixer, and water rinse. The film is processed from left to right, with no movement of films in the opposite direction to prevent mixing of solutions. **C,** The dental film packet contains the following: *A,* Film; *B,* protective black paper; *C,* lead foil; and *D,* outer paper or plastic wrapping. **D,** Size 0, 2, 3, 4 film placed near a pencil for size comparison. (C from Robinson DS, Bird DL: Essentials of dental assisting, ed 4, St Louis, 2007, Saunders.)

chemicals is not the optimal 68° F. After fixation, the films should be rinsed in slowly running water for 20 minutes before they are hung on a film rack to dry. Once completely dry, films can be placed into film mounts or small coin envelopes to be filed with the patient's dental record.

> *TECHNICIAN NOTE*   After initial viewing of the newly developed radiograph, the radiograph should be placed in fixer for 10 minutes so that archive-quality films can be obtained.

Automatic processors used for standard x-ray films may be used to develop dental films by taping the dental film to the back end of a standard film and having it tag along with the larger film. This process is sometimes unreliable because it may cause the dental film to get lost in the rollers of the processor.

DIGITAL RADIOGRAPHY

Use of computed digital radiography (CDR) in the veterinary practice is increasing in favor as practitioners become more aware of the benefits when compared with conventional radiographic techniques. The quality of the digital images is improving since its first introduction into dentistry; today the resolution is good but does not always approximate that of nonscreen film. Direct method CDR technology, which is most commonly used today, requires an electronic intraoral sensor, a computer, and the x-ray machine. The sensor, called a charged coupled device (CCD), may be cordless or may be attached to a cord that connects to the computer. After the sensor is covered with a plastic infection barrier, the sensor is placed into the mouth to capture the image and convert it to the digital format of "pixels"—picture elements in various shades of gray. A remote module transmits the data to the computer so the image can be immediately viewed, manipulated, and stored. The images can be magnified, and enhancements in contrast or darkness can be made. The sensors are available in sizes comparable with those used with traditional dental film sizes 0, 1, and 2, limiting application in large breed dogs, which typically require size 4 films for viewing of the entire tooth image. Because use of a size 2 sensor for larger mouths requires additional exposures to accomplish the task, it is practical to use standard radiography for some patients and CCD digital radiography for other patients. A digital option that allows for digital size 4 films is an indirect digital system that uses phosphor plate technology and a scanner to produce digital images within seconds of processing a reusable plate through a specially devised digital scanner. When digital technology is used, caution must be taken to ensure that

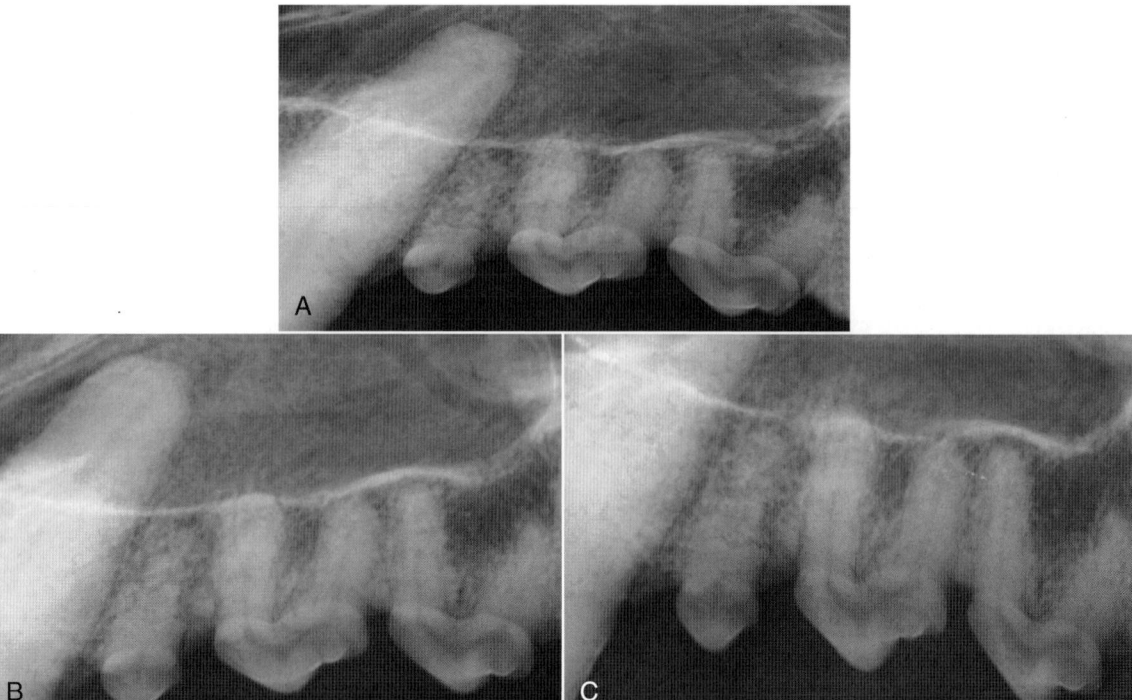

FIGURE 34-26 Three radiographs taken using the bisecting angle technique on the maxilla of a dog with three different position-indicating device (PID) angles. **A,** Foreshortened image from PID positioned too dorsally. **B,** Correctly determining the bisecting angle results in an image that most closely represents the size and shape of subgingival structures. **C,** Elongated image from PID positioned too ventrally.

patients have adequate anesthesia depths, because replacement of a damaged sensor is costly.

Digital technology reduces radiation exposure by 50% to 90% when compared with use of D- and E-speed film. Most modern dental x-ray machines are compatible with digital radiology if they have timers that allow the exposure setting in a $\frac{1}{100}$ of a second time frame. A disadvantage of digital radiography is the high initial cost of the sensor and software. However, the expense is offset by the cost of film and processing chemicals.

Exposure and Processing Errors

Errors in film exposure and processing account for unnecessary radiation exposure and additional anesthetic time for the patient. Cone cutting occurs when the beam misses portions of the film, resulting in clear areas of film. Elongation and foreshortening (stretched and shortened images, respectively) are caused by inaccurate vertical angulation during PID alignment (Figure 34-26, *A* through *C*). Images that are too dark or too light can result from errors in kVp and mA settings, or in exposure and processing times. If the film is placed in the mouth with the wrong surface facing the beam, dotted streaks from the lead foil will appear across the film surface. Care must be taken when multiple films are placed into the fixer cup, to prevent scratches that appear as white lines when emulsion is removed from the film surface.

> **TECHNICIAN NOTE** A film that appears too dark is often the result of greater than necessary exposure time, excessive time in the developing solution, or leakage of light during developing.

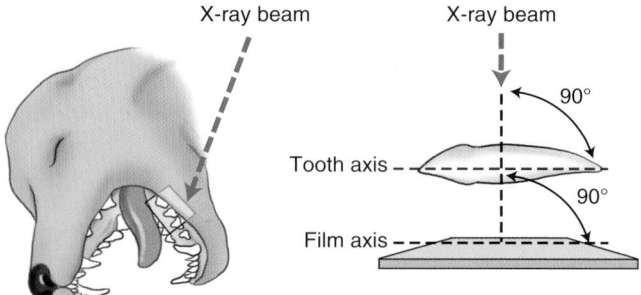

FIGURE 34-27 Paralleling technique is useful for caudal mandibular teeth for which the film is placed parallel to the teeth; the beam is directed at a 90-degree angle to the film and teeth.

TECHNIQUES

Three techniques are commonly used to obtain dental radiographs. Each technique varies in the relationship of the beam to the film and the teeth to be imaged. Film of proper size is placed into the mouth and is held in position with gauze. The paralleling technique requires the film to be placed parallel to the long axis of the tooth. The beam is then directed at a right angle to the film and teeth and is positioned to aim for the center of the film (Figure 34-27). Parallelism can be used only on the mandibular teeth, caudal to the second premolars, where the film can easily slide toward the floor of the mouth.

The symphysis at the rostral portion of the mandible and the flat palate of the maxilla prevent use of the paralleling technique. To minimize inherent distortion of dental structures when the paralleling technique is not an option, the

bisecting angle technique is used. The x-ray beam is projected at a right angle to an imaginary line that cuts in half (bisects) the angle formed by the plane of the film and the long axis of the tooth (Figure 34-28).

The occlusal technique places the film on the occlusal plane and directs the beam at a right angle to the film (Figure 34-29). Typically, this view is of value in showing larger areas on one film, with applications available to view nasal disease and to identify root remnants.

RADIOGRAPHIC INTERPRETATION

To assess the presence of intraoral pathologic conditions on radiographs, it is essential to have knowledge of the appearance of normal radiographic anatomic structures (Figure 34-30). The radiodensity of the components of the teeth and supporting structures varies widely; therefore, the terms

radiopaque and *radiolucent* are used to describe the relative radiographic appearance of oral and dental structures. Radiopaque structures, such as **cementum**, dentin, and bone, block or absorb the radiation, causing that portion of the processed radiograph to appear light or white. The thin layer of enamel covering the crown is the most radiodense structure of the tooth. The lamina dura, which is a cribriform plate of bone lining the tooth socket, appears as a white line adjacent to the periodontal space surrounding a healthy tooth. Beyond the lamina dura, the trabecular pattern of bone may vary in radiodensity. The cortex of the mandible is radiodense.

In contrast, radiolucent structures, such as soft tissue and periodontal ligament space, appear dark or black because

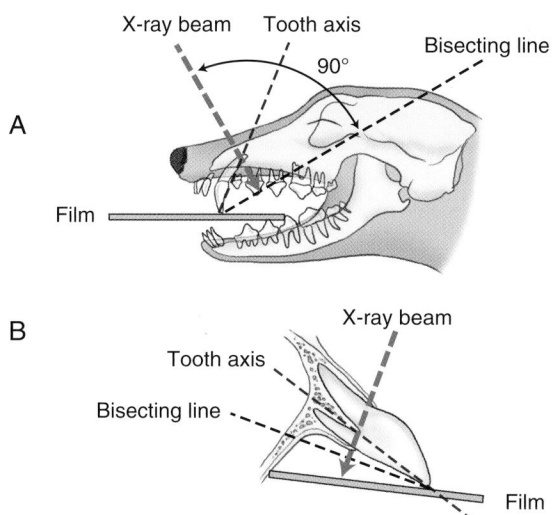

FIGURE 34-28 Bisecting angle technique is used for the maxilla and the rostral mandible, for which the film cannot be placed parallel to the roots. First, determine the angle created by the plane of the tooth and the plane of the film. Bisect that angle and direct the beam at a right angle to the bisecting line.

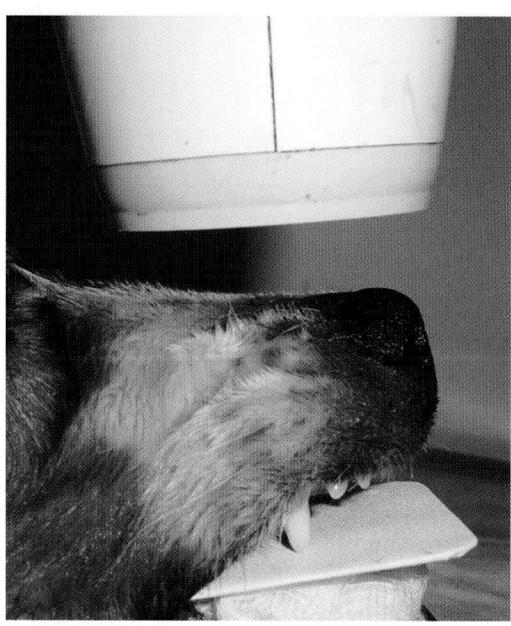

FIGURE 34-29 Occlusal technique is often used on the maxilla to provide an additional view of a tooth of interest, or for imaging of the nasal cavity. The film is placed in the mouth parallel to the palate. The beam is directed down at a right angle to the film.

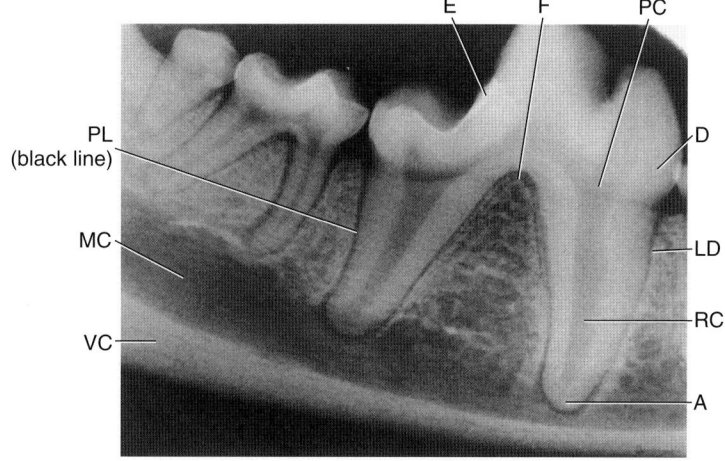

FIGURE 34-30 Normal radiopaque and radiolucent structures: *A,* Root apex; *D,* dentin; *E,* enamel; *F,* furcation area; *LD,* lamina dura; *MC,* mandibular canal; *PC,* pulp chamber; *PL,* periodontal ligament; *RC,* root canal; *VC,* ventral cortex.

x-ray photons can easily pass through to the film. The periodontal ligament fibers are not visible on the film; however, the space they occupy can be traced as a black line surrounding the roots. Because pulp is soft tissue, it appears as a dark area (less radiodense) in the center of the tooth.

The radiolucent mandibular canal lies apical to most of the mandibular tooth roots. In small breed dogs, the apices of the mandibular first molar roots may be seen at a level at or even below the mandibular canal, extending into the ventral cortex. Normal anatomic structures must be distinguished from pathologic structures. For example, the middle mental foramen is located apical to the mandibular second premolar in dogs and can be misinterpreted as a periapical pathologic condition if superimposed over a tooth root (Figure 34-31). It is helpful to refer to a textbook with normal and pathologic radiographic appearances (see "Recommended Readings").

PERIODONTAL DISEASE

The periodontium is composed of four supporting structures of the tooth: (1) periodontal ligament; (2) gingival connective tissue; (3) alveolar bone forming the tooth socket;

and (4) cementum covering the surface of the root. Healthy gingiva has a sharp, tapered edge (margin) that lies closely against the crown of the tooth. The free gingiva forms a moat around the tooth, called the *gingival sulcus*. The epithelial attachment to the tooth crown forms the bottom of the gingival sulcus. The depth of this sulcus varies (up to 3 mm in the healthy mouth of a dog, and up to 1 mm in the cat).

Gingivitis refers to inflammation of the gingiva. *Periodontitis* describes inflammation not only of the gingiva, but also of other structures of the periodontium. Gingivitis represents the earliest stages of periodontitis and is easily reversible with proper treatment and home care. Once advanced periodontitis occurs, these changes are more difficult to reverse. Periodontitis is the most common disease of animals.

Periodontitis is caused by accumulation of subgingival plaque and the body's response to it. Plaque is a white-tan film that collects around and within the gingival sulcus of the tooth. It is composed of bacteria, food debris, exfoliated cells, and salivary glycoproteins. Within as quickly as 24 hours if left undisturbed, plaque will mineralize on the teeth to form dental calculus (sometimes referred to by the term "tartar")—a light brown or yellow, raised, irregular deposit adherent to the tooth and root surfaces (Figure 34-32). This

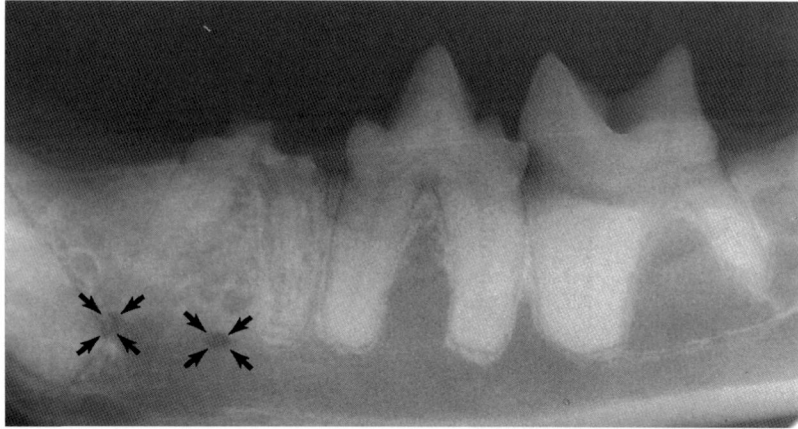

FIGURE 34-31 Normal anatomic structures may appear as periapical pathologic conditions if superimposed over a root. The middle mental foramen and the caudal mental foramen are labeled with arrows. The middle mental foramen is superimposed over the apex of the canine tooth root.

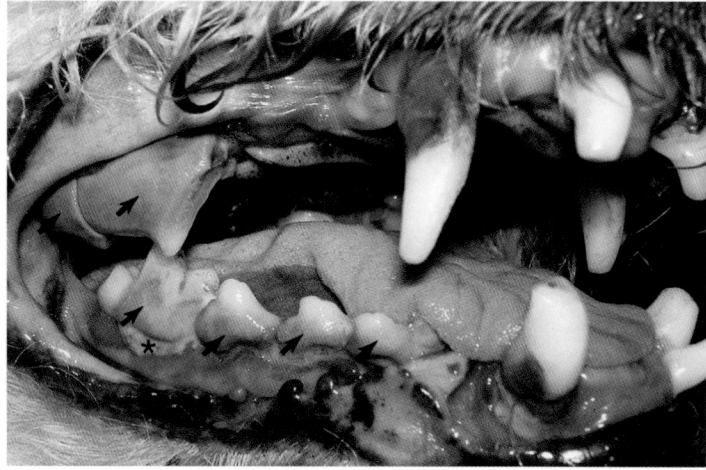

FIGURE 34-32 Plaque and calculus in a dog. Plaque is white-tan *(asterisk)* and accumulates on the rough surface of calculus. Plaque that is not removed within approximately 24 hours will become mineralized, adherent calculus *(arrows)*.

irregular, plaque-retentive surface of calculus allows for further plaque accumulation. As plaque accumulates within the gingival sulcus, it damages the gingival tissues by releasing bacterial by-products that can damage the periodontium. The patient's immune response may also cause tissue damage through the release of inflammatory cytokines from white blood cells as they attempt to destroy the bacteria. In the early stages, the gingiva becomes inflamed and bleeds easily (Figure 34-33). Progression of periodontitis results in loss of attachment. Attachment loss is clinically detectable in its earliest stages by measuring pocket depths with a periodontal probe in the anesthetized patient (Figure 34-34, A and B).

> **TECHNICIAN NOTE** Plaque begins to mineralize as early as 24 hours after it adheres to the tooth surface. Therefore, daily brushing is necessary to minimize calculus formation.

Periodontal disease is difficult to control once it has developed. For this reason, great emphasis must be placed on its prevention. Other diseases can contribute to the

severity of periodontal disease, but bacteria in plaque are the primary cause. Early in the formation of plaque, the bacterial population consists mainly of Gram-positive aerobic bacteria. Once these bacteria accumulate in substantial numbers, the oxygen gradient of the subgingival environment changes to support a shift to predominantly Gram-negative anaerobic rods and spirochetes. Gram-negative bacteria are capable of producing endotoxin, which has direct adverse effects on cells of the periodontium, resulting in a more severe immune response. Endotoxins are believed to be attached to the tooth surface, loosely embedded in cementum, and unattached in the sulcular space. When periodontitis is already present, destruction of the junctional epithelium at the base of the gingival sulcus has begun and will continue if not treated. Once the junctional epithelium and the periodontal ligament become destroyed, it is difficult to stimulate regeneration. As the tooth begins to lose its periodontal attachment, it becomes more susceptible to plaque accumulation in the deep periodontal pockets that form around the tooth roots. When the tooth loses a significant portion of its periodontium, it becomes mobile. The infection and inflammation associated with periodontitis are present for months to years before the tooth is eventually lost. Throughout the duration of the periodontitis, bacteremia occurs with the potential for colonization of bacteria at distant sites, including liver, kidneys, heart, and lungs.

For patients with periodontal disease, the treatment goal is removal of plaque and calculus from the teeth both supragingivally and subgingivally. General anesthesia is necessary to provide access to subgingival areas, where bacteria can contribute to local and sometimes systemic inflammation. A second and equally important goal is minimization of plaque reattachment through proper home care and appropriate follow-up treatment.

PERIODONTAL DÉBRIDEMENT

Removal of bacterial plaque, endotoxins, and hard calculus deposits is essential to halting the disease process. Home care can be effective in removing supragingival debris when the

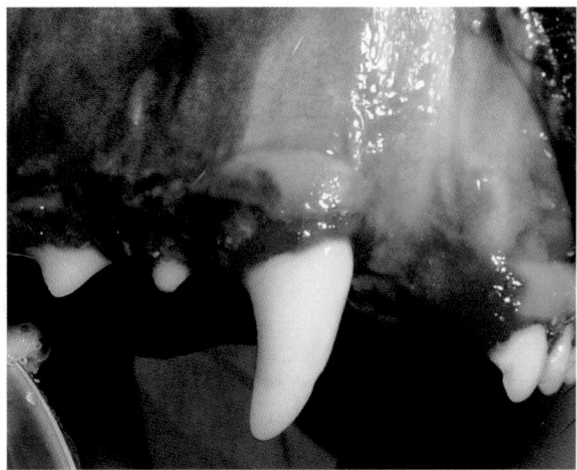

FIGURE 34-33 Gingivitis in a dog. Inflammation is limited to the gingival tissue and does not cross the mucogingival junction.

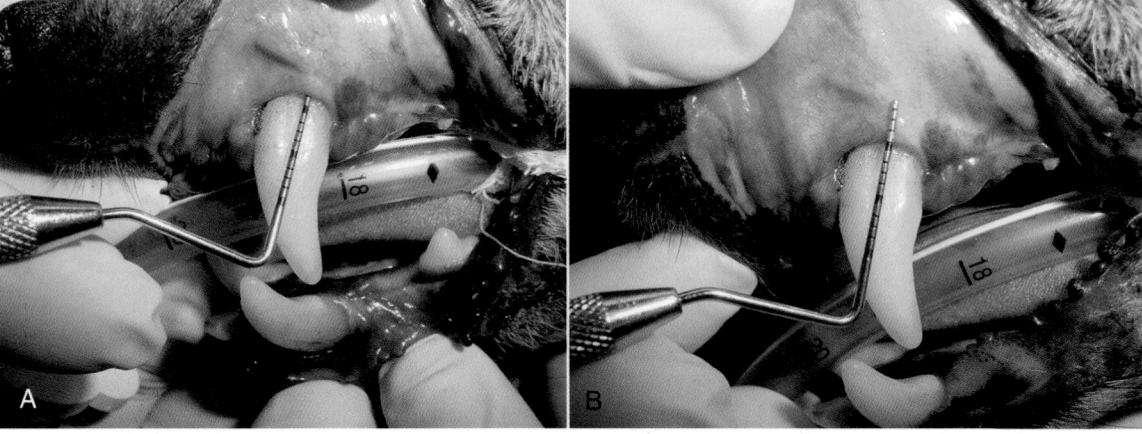

FIGURE 34-34 A, Probe is inserted to determine pocket depth. **B,** Probe is removed to show degree of attachment loss, which is pocket depth plus gingival recession.

client is educated to perform the procedures on a daily basis. If oral hygiene is not performed thoroughly, subgingival biofilm will mature and within 48 hours will contain enough periodontal pathogens to cause gingivitis. Professional clinical care is required to remove pathogens and calculus that harbor bacteria.

Periodontal débridement is the term used to refer to nonsurgical instrumentation that focuses on removal of hard and soft deposits from supragingival and subgingival surfaces of teeth, along with disruption of nonadherent bacteria within the sulcus. The goal of periodontal débridement is to prevent or arrest the infection and restore oral soft tissues to health. Hand and power instruments are used to remove plaque, scale, root plane, and polish. The traditional approach of scaling and root planing was based on the belief that bacterial endotoxins were firmly attached to the pitted, irregular surfaces of cementum. Instrumentation with a curette included root planing to remove all damaged layers of cementum, resulting in a glossy, smooth surface that would be less plaque retentive. Current research has shown that endotoxins are only lightly adherent, and that removal of superficial layers of cementum is adequate to achieve the goals of periodontal débridement.

POWER SCALING

Ultrasonic devices, mechanized instruments currently used for periodontal débridement, were first introduced in the early 1950s to remove tooth material during treatment for caries in human patients. When high-speed air-driven handpieces were introduced shortly thereafter, the ultrasonic application was deemed to be too slow for removal of tooth structure. In 1955, ultrasonic scalers were introduced. As a result of their bulky tip design, the capabilities of original scalers were limited to removing supragingival deposits. More definitive scaling was routinely accomplished with hand scalers and curettes. During the 1980s, thinner, probe-like tips were developed, and today, continued advances in technology have expanded their application to subgingival use. Knowledge of the instrument and of tooth morphology is critical for safe use. No longer considered to be an adjunct to hand instrumentation, ultrasonic scalers are now considered to be the primary instrument in veterinary practice for use in routine débridement and advanced periodontal therapy.

> **TECHNICIAN NOTE** When performing periodontal débridement, you should use a cuffed endotracheal tube and gravity (tipping the nose lower than the rest of the head) to prevent aspiration of fluids and debris.

Power scaling instruments use a water-cooled vibrating tip to remove hard and soft deposits from teeth and periodontal pockets. Vibrations are measured by frequency, or the number of times that the tip moves back and forth in 1 second (cycles per second [cps], also called *Hertz* [Hz]).

Most units used in veterinary medicine are automatically tuned and have frequencies that are controlled by the unit. Manually controlled units are available and are used mostly in the human field in advanced periodontal therapy. Research indicates that when skillfully used, ultrasonic instrumentation is as effective as hand instrumentation. Box 34-5 lists the benefits of power scaling.

Two types of power scalers—sonic and ultrasonic—are categorized by frequency of tip vibrations and the type of power used to create movement at the working end.

SONIC SCALER

The sonic scaler is powered by an air compressor on a dental unit and is attached to the high-speed air-line. It operates with a frequency between 2000 and 9000 cps. The tip vibrates in an elliptical pattern, with all surfaces around the diameter of the tip active. The vibrations are audible to the human ear, creating a sound that may be uncomfortable to some operators. As a result of the low frequency, the sonic scaler has less ability to remove heavy, tenacious calculus and is slow to accomplish its task. It is best suited for use in cats and dogs with light accumulations.

ULTRASONIC SCALER

Ultrasonic devices use electrical energy that converts the working tip to mechanical energy in the form of rapid vibrations to effectively remove biofilm and calculus deposits. Ranging in frequency from 18,000 to 50,000 cps—above the audible human range—they are more popular and practical for veterinary use when compared with the sonic scaler. The ultrasonic scaling unit contains the electronic generator inside plastic housing. A hose connects the unit to the water supply, which may consist of a portable pressure tank or a quick disconnect at the sink pipes. A cable attaches the unit to a foot pedal, and the handpiece is attached by tubing that transports the water for coolant. A power cord is also attached. Unlike hand scalers that only remove debris with direct contact, ultrasonic scalers provide the additional benefit of a stream of water coming from the tip that acts as a coolant and lavage, flushing debris from the sulcus. The flushing action is destructive to the biofilm by causing acoustic turbulence and cavitation. Acoustic turbulence, also known as *acoustic microstreaming*, is disruption of bacteria in plaque caused by streaming of fluid over the tooth surface, or churning of fluid within the confined pocket space.

BOX 34-5	Benefits of Power Scaling

- Ergonomically superior in reducing hand fatigue and the need for repetitive, intricate hand movements
- Reduces total time patient must remain anesthetized
- Causes less tissue distention than curettes (when slim tips are used subgingivally)
- Causes less root surface damage when used correctly
- Lavage is destructive to bacteria (cavitation, acoustic turbulence, and streaming).

Cavitation is the energy that is created from the mist of water. As the water coolant exits the handpiece and strikes the vibrating working end, it creates thousands of water bubbles. These water bubbles implode with enough energy to disrupt bacterial cell walls.

> ▌*TECHNICIAN NOTE*   The transducer in a magnetostrictive ultrasonic scaler may be a metal stack or a ferrite rod. The transducer in a piezoelectric ultrasonic scaler may be a quartz crystal or a ceramic disc.

SAFETY PRECAUTIONS

Because water is a necessary part of the dental cleaning, appropriate safety precautions must be taken for the technician and the patient. To reduce the quantity of aerosolized bacteria, the mouth can be rinsed with chlorhexidine (0.1% to 0.2%) before scaling. This preemptive rinse may reduce the severity of bacteremia in the patient (this invariably occurs during a dental cleaning). The technician and all coworkers in the vicinity of the workstation should wear gloves, masks capable of high bacterial filtration, and eye protection, such as plastic goggles or disposable face shields. The patient's eyes should be lubricated and covered to protect against entry of debris and contaminated fluid. The single most important safety precaution involves intubating the patient and checking to ensure that the endotracheal cuff is fully inflated. The air-tight seal of the cuff should be checked occasionally to prevent the patient from developing aspiration pneumonia. However, care should be taken to avoid excessive inflation of the cuff, which may result in excess pressure on the tracheal lining, or a tracheal tear. Placement of a radiopaque laparotomy sponge in the back of the throat before scaling will filter loosened debris; however, remembering to remove the sponge after scaling is critical.

TIP DESIGNS

Standard-size "universal" and broad tips are designed for removing medium and heavy deposits, whereas slim tip designs allow better access to subgingival pockets and furcation areas. Approximately 30% to 40% more narrow than standard tips, slim tips are approximately 0.5 mm in diameter at the blunt end and are designed to mimic periodontal probes. The slim profile enables easier access to the base of deeper pockets and improves tactility for better detection of calculus. Tips are available in straight and curved designs. Precision tips are available in diameters as narrow as 0.2 mm at the tip for use in advanced periodontal procedures. They are extremely fragile and must be used with a light touch. Another tip option is the diamond-coated tip. If used incorrectly during a nonsurgical procedure, the diamond coating can cause soft tissue damage and excessive loss of tooth substance; therefore, this design should be reserved for use during open-flap procedures and should be used only by highly skilled clinicians. Some tips have a built-in light-emitting diode (LED) light (Figure 34-35). LED technology tends to offer only minimal additional light when used with a good surgical overhead light. A new tip designed for use in furcations has a 0.8-mm ball on the end that may be too large to allow access to the furcations of the teeth in some animals.

Tips should be replaced at least annually, or when they are bent or worn down (Figure 34-36). As the tip wears, it becomes shorter, and the effectiveness of scaling diminishes. One ultrasonic manufacturer offers a wear indicator that helps to measure the amount of wearing of the tip. For each millimeter of wear, a 25% decrease in efficiency has been noted.

ENERGY DISPERSION

For hand scalers to be effective, the sharp cutting edge of the working end must contact the calculus. In contrast, ultrasonic scalers disperse energy over a 360-degree circle around

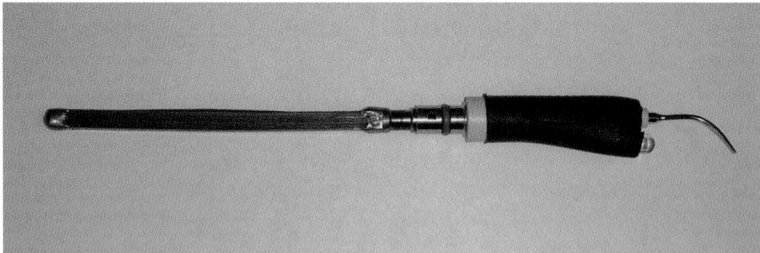

FIGURE 34-35 Magnetostrictive ultrasonic insert: metal stack transducer and light-emitting diode (LED) light at working end.

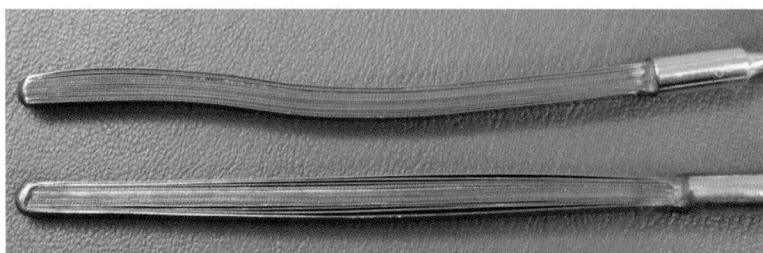

FIGURE 34-36 Damaged ultrasonic inserts; magnetostrictive inserts should be discarded when metal stack becomes bent or splayed.

the tip of power instruments. Vibrating activity occurs on the back, face (concave surface), and two side (lateral) surfaces, and on the point; however, each surface has varying degrees of vibration, depending on the type of scaler used. Typically, the strongest vibrations are concentrated 2 to 4 mm from the tip. Technicians must know the specific type of unit with which they are working and must understand the differences in energy dispersal among different tip surfaces to correctly adapt the tip to the tooth for efficient scaling.

TYPES OF ULTRASONIC SCALERS

Ultrasonic scalers are available in two types: magnetostrictive and piezoelectric; each type is distinct in its mechanism of action, type of transducer, and direction of tip movement. The transducer is the portion of the handpiece that converts electrical energy into mechanical energy.

The magnetostrictive scaler is the most common type of power scaler used in human and veterinary dentistry. The typical magnetostrictive unit has an insert that slides into the handpiece. The insert has two connected parts: the transducer and the working end. The magnetostrictive transducer is a stack of thin nickel alloy metal strips. When a magnetic field is created from the copper coil inside the handpiece, the dimension of the strips is altered by lengthening and shortening, sending vibrations to the tip. Movement of the tip occurs in an elliptical pattern with energy dispersion around the entire diameter of the tip, providing vibrations on all 5 surfaces. The point of the tip, having the highest power dispersion, can cause damage when directed at a 90-degree angle to the tooth, acting like a jackhammer on hard dental tissue (Figure 34-37). The face (concave surface) has the next highest powerful vibrations, followed by the back. The two

side surfaces have the least powerful vibrations. The back and side surfaces are used most often for scaling, as it is good practice to adapt the surface with the least amount of vibrations that will accomplish the task of debris removal. Magnetostrictive units range in frequency from 18,000 to 42,000 cps (18 to 42 kHz). Another type of magnetostrictive scaler uses a transducer that is a ferrite rod that produces rotational tip movement. Differences in operation between magnetostrictive units require close attention to manufacturers' recommendations. See Procedure 34-1 for preparation guidelines for a magnetostrictive unit with a metal stack transducer.

> **TECHNICIAN NOTE** The ultrasonic scaler tip should never be directed at a 90-degree angle toward the tooth surface because the tip will cause damage to the enamel.

The piezoelectric scaler uses a ceramic disc or crystal as the transducer to produce the straight, linear movement of the tip. Electrical energy causes the discs to alter dimension by expanding and contracting, sending vibrations to the tip at a frequency ranging from 25 to 50 kHz. Because of the back-and-forth motion, the tip is active only on the two lateral surfaces, forcing the operator to pivot the wrist as the tip is moved around the tooth. If the other surfaces are accidentally adapted to the tooth, the operator will be warned by a different sound and by incomplete removal of debris. Limitations of effective vibrating surfaces cause the piezoelectric scaler to be more technique sensitive than other power scalers. The ceramic disc of the transducer is fragile and is easily breakable if the handpiece is accidentally dropped.

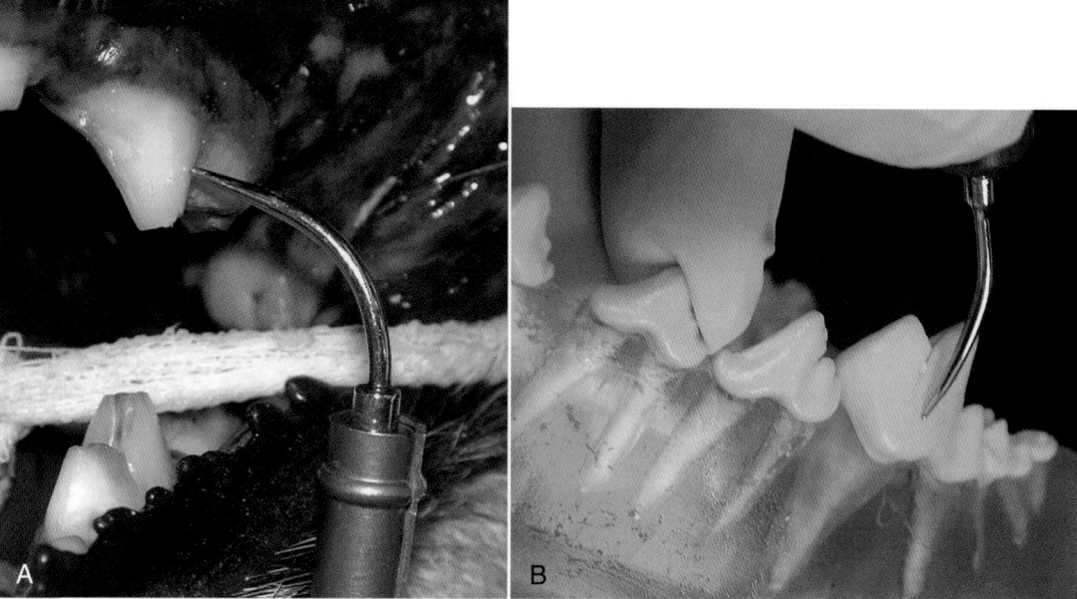

FIGURE 34-37 **A,** The tip of the ultrasonic insert will cause damage when directed at a 90-degree angle to the tooth surface. **B,** Correct angulation of the tip: the insert tip should be held at an angle of 0 to 15 degrees from the long axis of the tooth.

PROCEDURE 34-1	Techniques for Preparation and Instrumentation When Magnetostrictive Ultrasonic Scaling Unit Is Used With Metal Stack Transducer*

- Plug the electrical cord into the outlet.
- Run water through the handpiece for a minimum of 2 minutes (each morning) to flush the biofilm, draining into the sink.
- Disinfect the handpiece.
- Hold the handpiece upright, perpendicular to the floor, while stepping on the pedal, to completely fill the handpiece with water.
- Choose the tip design.
- Remove foot from the pedal, and slide the insert into the handpiece until resistance is met at the rubber "O" ring. Gently twist as the insert is completely seated (if using a metal stack transducer).
- If using a unit with screw-in tip, insert the tip and tighten with the supplied wrench.
- Hold the handpiece parallel to the floor to adjust the power to low-medium and water to a spray. Use the lowest power setting that will accomplish the task.
- Wear gloves, mask, and face shield or goggles.
- Place gauze or a lap sponge in the back of the patient's throat.
- Protect the patient's eyes (lubricate and cover).
- Check the endotracheal cuff for leakage, and make adjustments if necessary.
- Flush the patient's mouth with chlorhexidine (0.12%).
- To reduce the pulling weight of the cord, wrap the cord around the forearm or pinky finger, or drape over the neck.
- Hold the handpiece lightly with a pen or modified pen grasp.
- Establish a comfortable finger rest.
- Retract the patient's cheeks, tongue, and lips to prevent contact with any portion of the metal tip. A dental mirror is useful for retraction.
- Activate the tip before touching the tooth or calculus.

- Adapt the side of the tip to the tooth in a similar fashion to using a periodontal probe, at an angle of 0 to 15 degrees to the tooth.
- With light pressure, move the tip in a sweeping motion as if using a pencil eraser, keeping the end 2 mm of the tip in constant contact with the tooth surface. Use of hard pressure is counterproductive because this will diminish the vibrations. Vertical, horizontal, or oblique strokes may be used.
- REMEMBER: Never hold the point at a 90-degree angle to the tooth because scratching and gouging of the enamel or cementum may occur.
- Move the tip in a direction beginning on the crown and advancing toward the apex of the tooth to the bottom of the sulcus or pocket. This is opposite to the approach used with hand instrumentation, in which the curette is adapted at the base of the pocket and is moved coronally.
- Assess the surface of the tooth for smoothness by using the tip without activating the vibrations—similar to using an explorer.
- When encountering stubborn tenacious pieces of calculus, use light tapping motions against the surface of the calculus, or increase the power setting.
- Check for remaining residual calculus by using compressed air from the air or water syringe on the dental unit. Missed calculus will appear chalky white.
- Rinse the mouth with chlorhexidine, flushing any loose debris from tongue, cheek, and lip vestibules.
- Remove gauze from the throat, checking for debris before extubation.
- Wipe the unit, handpiece, and cords with federally approved nonimmersion type of disinfectant. Observe the manufacturer's instructions for sterilizing the handpiece and tips.

*Slight variations may be seen with other types of units; please follow the manufacturer's instructions.

KNOB SETTINGS

The power knob adjusts the amplitude—the distance the tip is moving back and forth in one cycle. Greater distance is higher power. Higher power is necessary to remove heavy deposits, whereas low power is satisfactory for removing plaque. It is good principal to use the lowest power setting that will accomplish the task. Low power should always be used with thin tips to prevent the tips from breaking.

The water knob adjusts the flow of water through the handpiece. Because ultrasonic scalers produce heat, fluid must be adequate to prevent pulp damage caused by heat during scaling. Pressure of the water supply line to the unit must measure a minimum of 25 psi. A warm or hot handpiece is an indication that water pressure is inadequate, and the clinician must immediately stop and make adjustments by increasing the amount of water and checking the water pressure (if a portable water tank is used). With magnetostrictive units, the water knob should be turned until water exits the tip as a mist, rather than just as a straight stream. Water on the piezoelectric unit should be adjusted to a steady drip.

HAND SCALING

Periodontal débridement may be accomplished with the use of hand instrumentation. Successful use of hand instruments is dependent on the technician's understanding of instrument design and knowledge of the basic principles of instrumentation.

In general, dental instruments consist of three parts: the handle, the shank, and the working end (see Figure 34-19). The handle contains the instrument's identification, a description of the instrument with abbreviations that include the name of the designer or the school where it was designed, the manufacturer, the classification type, and the design number. Classifications are determined by the design of the working ends and the intended purpose of the instrument. Examination instruments include probes and explorers.

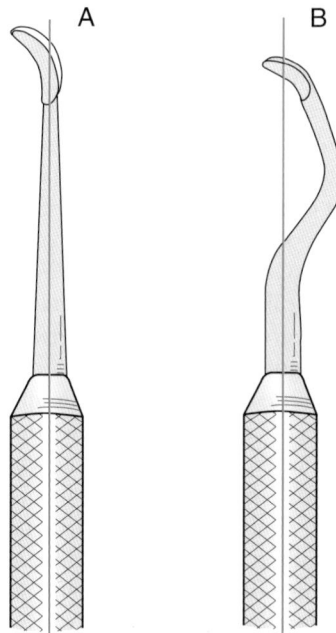

FIGURE 34-38 A straight shank (**A**) is best used for scaling teeth in the rostral portion of the mouth. A bent shank (**B**) is designed for working on premolars and molars. (From Daniel SJ, Harfst SA, Wilder R: Mosby's dental hygiene: concepts, cases, and competencies, ed 2, St Louis, 2008, Mosby.)

Scaling instruments include curettes, sickles, files, and hoes. Current trends in handles include hollow, lightweight designs that are more efficient in transmitting vibrations detected through tactile sensitivity. Use of wider handle sizes minimizes finger pinching and hand fatigue. Various patterns of surface texture are knurled into the handle to prevent fingers from slipping.

The shank connects the handle to the working end. The curvature of the shank determines the best location within the mouth for use of the instrument. In relation to the long axis of the handle, a straight shank is used for rostral teeth; an angled shank is used for caudal teeth (Figure 34-38). When the shank is bent to form an angle, the terminal shank is the portion below the bend and closest to the working end. Length and diameter of shanks vary; therefore, the instrument of choice may depend on the situation for which the instrument is needed. Elongated shanks are useful for accessing deeper pockets and reaching farther caudal in the mouth. A thick, rigid shank is useful for removing heavy tenacious calculus because the shank will not flex when pressed against the tooth. Thin, flexible shanks are better suited for removing light calculus deposits or plaque.

The working end of an instrument may be blunt, as in a probe, or pointed, as in an explorer, or it may have sharp cutting edges like those of scaling instruments. An instrument handle may have a single working end (SE), or it may be double-ended (DE) with two working ends. The working end of a hand scaling instrument is called the *blade*, and it has several parts: the two lateral sides, the face, the back, the heel, and the toe or point (Figure 34-39). The face and lateral

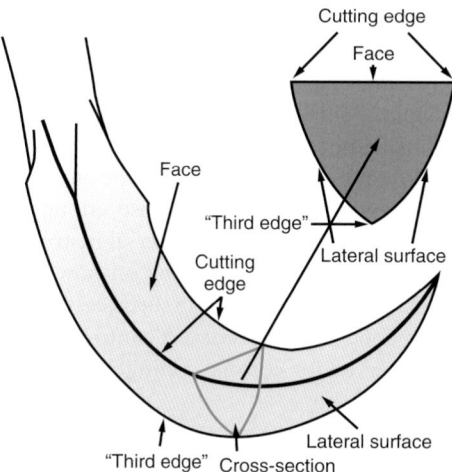

FIGURE 34-39 The parts of the working end of a hand instrument include the face, cutting edges, lateral sides, back, and toe (tip). (From Darby ML, Walsh MM: Dental hygiene theory and practice, ed 3, St Louis, 2010, Saunders.)

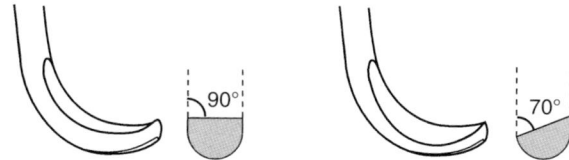

FIGURE 34-40 Universal versus area-specific (Gracey) curettes: the angle between the face and the terminal shank is 90 degrees on the universal and 70 degrees offset on the area specific. Note that one cutting edge is lower when the face is offset. The lower cutting edge is the correct one when an area-specific curette is used. (From Nelson DM: Saunders review of dental hygiene, Philadelphia, 2000, WB Saunders.)

surfaces meet to form a cutting edge. The back is formed by the convergence of the two lateral surfaces. Instruments used for supragingival scaling have a pointed tip, whereas subgingival scalers, known as *curettes*, have a rounded tip. The tip of a curette (known as the *toe*) is designed to minimize trauma to the soft tissue lining the sulcus or pocket.

The angulation of the face of the blade in relation to the terminal shank will classify the instrument as universal or area specific. To determine this classification, position the instrument handle so the terminal shank is perpendicular to the floor, then identify the face. If the angle between the face and the terminal shank is 90 degrees, the instrument is universal, meaning that when in use, the handle is placed parallel to the long axis of the tooth, and then is slightly tipped left or right to permit either cutting edge to be adapted to the tooth. If the face is offset at an angle of 60 to 70 degrees, as in Gracey curettes, the instrument is considered to be area specific, and only one of the cutting edges may be adapted to the tooth (Figure 34-40).

SUPRAGINGIVAL INSTRUMENTS

Sickle scalers are used to scale the crowns of the teeth. The flat face may be straight or curved lengthwise; the straight lateral surfaces are flat and converge to form a pointed back and tip. When the cross section of a sickle is envisioned, the instrument is characteristically triangular in shape with 70- to 80-degree internal angles between the face and lateral surfaces (Figure 34-41, *A*). The sharp tip will cause lacerations if the instrument is used subgingivally; however, it may be used with caution slightly below the gingival margin, where the gingiva is spongy and loose enough to permit insertion. Because the sickle is a universal instrument, either cutting edge may be used, depending on how the handle is tipped. Because of the straight side surfaces, the sickle is not conducive to following the curved contours of roots and therefore is reserved for coronal scaling.

> ⚕ *TECHNICIAN NOTE*   Scalers are designed to be used on the tooth crown, and curettes are designed to be used subgingivally.

When the handle, shank, and blade are on the same plane, the instrument is designed for use toward the front of the mouth. For caudal teeth, the shank will be angled and the instrument will be double-ended to provide mirror images. This style is useful for veterinary patients during scaling of the buccal groove of maxillary carnassial teeth. One working end is contoured for scaling the mesial edge of the groove, and the contralateral end contours with the distal edge of the groove.

When the blade is placed against the tooth, the face should be at an angle between 45 degrees and 90 degrees with the tooth surface. The cutting edge is directed to the apical edge of the calculus, lateral pressure is placed against the tooth, and the instrument is used with a short pull stroke to disengage the debris.

SUBGINGIVAL CURETTES

Curettes may be used for supragingival scaling, although they are designed for subgingival scaling and root planing. The flat face is curved lengthwise from the heel to the toe, meeting the lateral surfaces to create a cutting edge that extends around the toe. Unlike the flat lateral sides of the sickle scaler that converged to form a pointed back, the sides of the curette are rounded, creating a round back that is easier to insert into a sulcus or pocket. The cross section of the curette is classically shaped like a semi-circle with internal angles of 70 degrees to 80 degrees between the face and lateral surfaces (Figure 34-41, *B*).

A universal curette can be adapted for all surfaces of the teeth, whereas use of an area-specific curette would require several different instruments to scale each tooth in the mouth. Use of area-specific instruments is an advanced concept, and they should be used only by technicians who have an understanding of the inherent design features and a thorough knowledge of root anatomy and shape. Incorrect use of an area-specific instrument can cause trauma to the hard and soft tissues.

The terms *site-specific* and *area-specific* are often interchanged with Gracey instruments, although other area-specific instruments are available. Gracey curettes are designed to be used as a set, with each instrument having a complex curvature of the shank for better access to specific teeth. Unlike the universal curette, which is curved only on the plane of the face, the Gracey is also curved on the plane of the lateral surface. To help identify the two curved planes, hold the instrument with the terminal shank perpendicular to the floor, and view the face at eye level. The face will slope downward, rather than be parallel with the floor and perpendicular to the terminal shank, and the lateral surfaces will

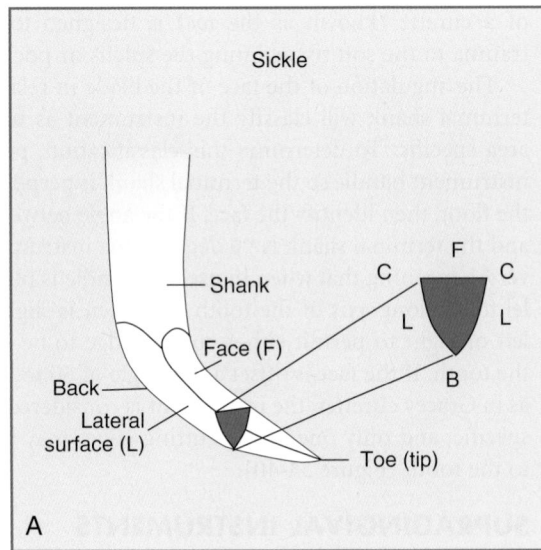
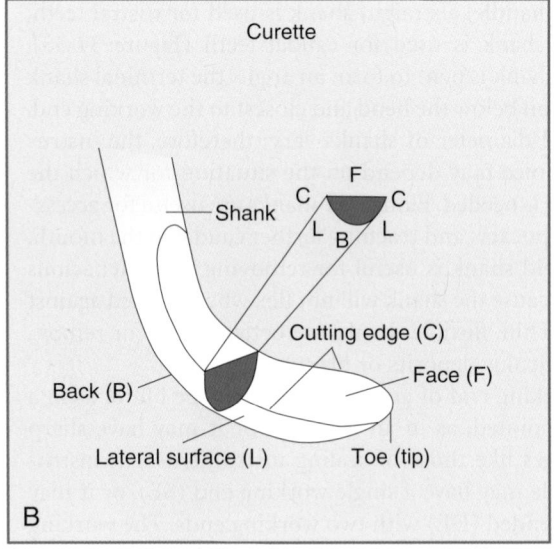

FIGURE 34-41 *A,* The cross section of a sickle scaler is triangular in shape. The sickle is used for supragingival scaling and has a pointed tip. *B,* The cross section of a curette is half-moon shaped. The curette is used for subgingival scaling and has a rounded toe. (From Novack DE: *Contemporary dental assisting,* St Louis, 2001, Mosby.)

be curved to the left or right. This curvature enables adaptation around the contours of roots. As with universal curettes, site-specific curettes have two cutting edges; however, the site-specific curette is unique in that only one edge is designed for use. Before adapting the blade to the tooth, the technician must confirm that the appropriate edge is chosen. To determine the correct cutting edge, hold the terminal shank perpendicular to the floor to view the honed face from above, enabling the lateral curves to be seen. One cutting edge forms an inner curve; another edge forms an outer curve that appears larger and closer to the floor. The proper cutting edge is always the curve that appears lower and farther from the terminal shank. Unlike universal instruments, which require parallelism of the handle with the tooth, area-specific instruments require parallelism of the terminal shank with the tooth. When in this position against a tooth surface, if the correct edge has been chosen, only the back should be visible. If the face is visible (reflecting light), flip the instrument to use the contralateral working end.

> **TECHNICIAN NOTE** When an area-specific curette is used, the proper cutting edge is the lower edge, as determined by holding the terminal shank perpendicular to the floor. The terminal shank of an area-specific curette is kept parallel to the long axis of the tooth during a vertical scaling stroke. The handle of the universal scaler is kept parallel to the long axis of the tooth during a vertical scaling stroke.

Langer curettes have a combination of universal curette qualities (face 90 degrees to shank) with the Gracey curvature of shanks. Langers and Graceys are available with blades that are shorter (mini), which makes them particularly suitable for use on small dogs and cats.

PRINCIPLES OF SCALING

Adaptation of hand scaling instruments involves the application of the cutting edge against the tooth. Approximately one-third of the cutting edge of the tip should remain in contact with the tooth; constant attention to this detail will prevent damage to the soft tissues as a result of trauma from the tip or toe (Figure 34-42). As the curvature of the tooth changes, adjustments must be made to that portion of the cutting edge that is adaptable to the tooth. Use of the thumb

against the handle will enable the instrument to be rolled to maintain the contact of the cutting edge around curves.

Angulation refers to the relationship of the face of the instrument to the tooth. When a curette is inserted into a pocket, the angulation of the face should be as close to zero as possible (Figure 34-43). In this position, the face would be parallel with the root surface, and the back of the blade would be against the soft tissue lining of the pocket. When the blade is positioned at the bottom of the pocket or apical to the intended piece of calculus, the angle should be opened by tilting the handle to the scaling and root planing angle of 45 to 90 degrees—more often between 60 and 80 degrees. Using an angle that is too closed will cause burnishing (smoothing) of the calculus, rather than biting into it for removal. An angle that is too open will place the noncutting edge sharply against the lining of the pocket when a curette is used. This technique is useful if the operator deliberately desires to perform a gingival curettage.

Strokes used when dental procedures are performed will vary according to the task. With hand scaling, the initial stroke assesses tooth surface topography by lightly feeling for irregularities. This exploratory stroke is also performed with an explorer or with the tip of a power scaler when the power

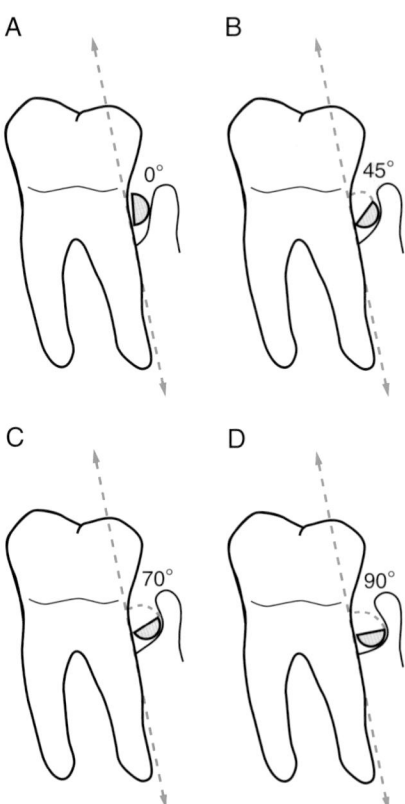

FIGURE 34-43 A, The angle formed by the tooth surface and the face of the instrument should begin at insertion into the sulcus or pocket at 0 degrees. B, The minimum angle when the curette is used is 45 degrees. The maximum angle when the curette is used is 70 degrees. C, An angle greater than 90 degrees will cause (D) damage to adjacent soft tissue. (Adapted from Daniel SJ, Harfst SA, Wilder R: Mosby's dental hygiene: concepts, cases, and competencies, ed 2, St Louis, 2008, Mosby.)

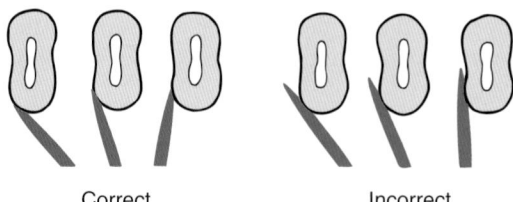

Correct   Incorrect

FIGURE 34-42 Correct adaptation: the lower third of the working end of the instrument must remain in contact with the tooth surface to prevent trauma to soft tissues. (From Novak DE: Contemporary dental assisting, St Louis, 2001, Mosby).

is not activated. When scalers and curettes are used, once an irregularity is detected, the working stroke is performed by applying lateral pressure against the tooth and pulling the blade vertically, horizontally, or obliquely in a short, controlled stroke. A root planing stroke is longer, and light lateral pressure is used. Apply the minimum number of strokes necessary to accomplish the task.

SHARPENING

Thorough periodontal débridement with use of scalers and curettes can be accomplished only with the use of sharp instruments. Each stroke of a sharp instrument against the tooth will wear away the metal of the cutting edge, causing it to transform from a precise sharp line at the junction of the face and lateral surfaces into a dull, rounded surface. Using a dull surface requires heavier lateral pressure against the tooth, reducing tactile sensitivity and creating hand fatigue. The dull surface will burnish the calculus, rather than causing it to be shaved off. Once burnished, this calculus is difficult to detect and remove.

Instrument sharpening can be accomplished manually using sharpening stones or with the help of mechanical sharpening devices. Either way, it is critical to have a thorough understanding of the instrument design, including the cross-sectional shape and the line angles between surfaces, to enable a sharp cutting edge to be reestablished without creating changes in the instrument's original design.

Sharpening stones typically used for dental instruments include Arkansas, India, ceramic, and a synthetic composition, each differing in coarseness. A few drops of lubricant are required on most stones to keep metal particles from embedding into the stone and to reduce heat friction. Lubricate with sharpening oil on Arkansas and India stones; the ceramic stone can be lubricated with water or used dry, and the composition stone requires water.

Several methods of manual sharpening can be used; however, the technique that requires the instrument to be held stationary while the stone is moved provides a good view of the blade so that the angle can be precisely controlled. Hold the instrument in a palm grasp with the blade facing you and the face parallel to the floor. Elbows should be braced against the side of the body for stability, and the procedure should be performed under good lighting that is reflecting off the face. Hold the stone perpendicular to the face (Figure 34-44), beginning at a right angle (90 degrees), then tilt the stone against the lateral surface so the angle opens to 100 to 110 degrees. An angle guide can be purchased or made by using a protractor to aid in visualizing correct angles.

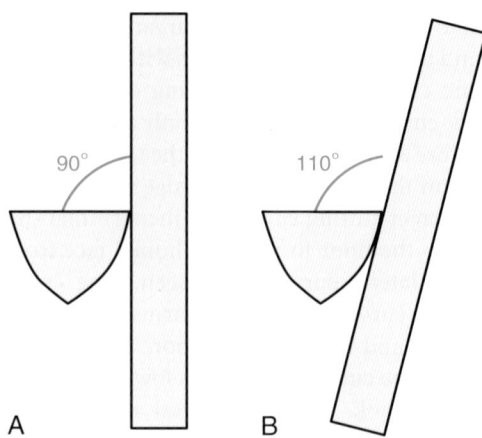

FIGURE 34-44 **A,** Initial setup of sharpening stone is 90 degrees to the face of the instrument. **B,** Open the angle to 110 degrees for sharpening. (From Daniel SJ, Harfst SA, Wilder R: Mosby's dental hygiene: concepts, cases, and competencies, ed 2, St Louis, 2008, Mosby.)

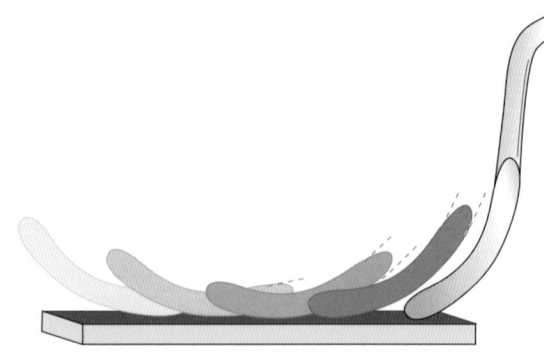

FIGURE 34-45 To maintain the original design of the instrument, when sharpening curved curettes, begin at the heel, sharpening small sections while working toward the toe. (From Nelson DM: Saunders review of dental hygiene, Philadelphia, 2000, WB Saunders.)

Using light pressure, move the stone in short up-and-down strokes against the lateral surface of the instrument, beginning at the heel of the instrument and working toward the toe, continuing around the toe when sharpening curettes (Figure 34-45). At the point where sharpening allows the lateral surface to meet sharply with the face, a black "sludge" will appear on the face. Finish with a few more light strokes, ending with a down stroke of the stone to remove wire particles that have been lifted from the metal.

Sharpening methods that include sharpening of the face should be avoided because the blade will be weakened and may break during débridement. Instruments that have been oversharpened and are excessively thin should be discarded.

POLISHING

Polishing is the final but critical step performed on an anesthetized dental patient as part of routine cleaning or advanced periodontal therapy. During non-routine dental procedures, such as endodontic therapy or jaw fracture repair, polishing

---

> **TECHNICIAN NOTE**   When hand instruments are sharpened, the angle between the stone and the face should be approximately 110 degrees. When sharpening curettes, remember to continue sharpening around the toe while maintaining this angle.

may be the initial procedure performed to remove plaque from the treatment area. In human dentistry, the need for routine polishing has become controversial, and selective polishing is becoming standard procedure to minimize the amount of enamel lost by frequent polishing.

The rationale for polishing veterinary mouths is to smooth surfaces that have been microscopically scratched during scaling procedures and to remove any extrinsic stains that were not removed with hand or power scalers. Extrinsic stains are discolorations that accumulate on the surfaces from pigments in food, blood, and some antiplaque products, such as chlorhexidine rinses. Intrinsic stains, often seen on the occlusal surface of maxillary molars in dogs, are within the tooth substance and are not removable by polishing procedures. Causes of intrinsic staining include exposure to certain drugs during tooth development (e.g., tetracyclines), trauma, and developmental defects.

Two methods of polishing are currently used in veterinary practices. The most common method is driven by an electrical motor or an air compressor from a dental unit. A low-speed handpiece is used with a rubber cup. A prophylaxis angle, also called a *prophy angle*, is the attachment that is connected to the handpiece and holds the rubber cup. The cup is available in soft, flexible rubber or firm rubber. Prophy angles may consist of single-use plastic disposable or autoclavable metal. The rubber cup can be filled with a polishing paste that contains an abrasive agent available in fine, medium, and coarse grits. Because the act of polishing removes tooth substance, the prophy paste chosen should contain the least abrasive agent that will accomplish the task.

Friction from the rotating rubber cup creates heat that has the potential to injure the pulp. New prophy angles have been developed with cups that oscillate back and forth rather than rotating. Use the handpiece on a low rpm (revolutions per minute) level to minimize adverse effects. Also use adequate paste, refilling the cup for each tooth, especially when polishing large dog teeth. When using a low-speed handpiece without a gauge, activate the handpiece to full speed before touching the rubber to the tooth by depressing the foot pedal. Listen for the pitch clues of the highest rpm level of the low-speed unit, and then ease off the pedal to less than one-quarter of the maximum rpm. Use light pressure against the tooth—just enough to cause the rim of the cup to flare slightly, and polish each tooth surface for only 1 to 3 seconds. Complete the procedure with a gentle rinse of water or chlorhexidine to flush residual prophy paste from the mouth. Eye protection should be worn by the operator, and the patient's eyes should be protected during the polishing procedure.

The second polishing method involves the use of an air polisher. An abrasive agent, sodium bicarbonate, is mixed with water to form a slurry that is propelled by air against the tooth. The tip of the nozzle is kept approximately 4 mm from the tooth surface. To prevent sloughing of soft tissues, the nozzle must never be directed toward the gingiva or into the sulcus or pocket. Air polishing may be quicker and has

been determined to be as effective as rubber cup polishing. However, the procedure is messy, and problems of clogging the equipment have plagued practitioners.

REGIONAL NERVE BLOCKS FOR ORAL SURGERY IN DOGS AND CATS

Regional nerve blocks are an essential tool for controlling intraoperative and postoperative pain in dogs and cats during oral surgery. Benefits include preemptive analgesia and prevention of "wind-up pain," postoperative analgesia when long-acting anesthetics are used, and decreased concentration of inhalant anesthetic gas needed during the procedure (therefore potentially safer and cost effective).

Local anesthetics have three basic uses. A "splash block" refers to wound irrigation directly into an open incision, providing topical anesthesia. "Local anesthesia" refers to infiltration of local anesthetic along planned incision lines or into the periodontal ligament of a tooth of interest. "Regional anesthesia" (the most commonly performed technique in our veterinary practice) refers to the delivery of local anesthetic to specific nerves to block an entire region of the body. Box 34-6 lists materials needed to perform regional nerve blocks for oral surgery. Bupivacaine 0.5% is the most commonly used local anesthetic because of its long duration of action, providing intraoperative and postoperative pain relief. Bupivacaine takes effect in 4 to 20 minutes and lasts from 4 to 10 hours. Lidocaine 2% takes effect in 3 to 5 minutes and lasts from 1.5 to 2 hours. The maximum safe dose of bupivacaine is considered to be 2 mg/kg in dogs and 1.5 mg/kg in cats. If blocks are required in all four oral quadrants, it is important to keep in mind that the total possible volume should be divided by 4 to ensure that each quadrant can be effectively blocked. In general, the authors use 0.1 to 0.2 ml of 0.5% bupivacaine for any of the regional blocks described later in cats, and 0.2 to 0.8 ml for a regional oral block in the dog, depending on the size of the patient. Box 34-7 provides an example calculation of four-quadrant nerve blocks in a cat.

BOX 34-6	Materials Needed for Regional Nerve Blocks Used for Oral Surgery

- Dental aspirating syringe (optional): allows aspiration and injection with one hand
- 27-Gauge, ½-inch hypodermic needles attached to a 1-ml syringe
- 27-Gauge, 1¼-inch hypodermic needles attached to a 3-ml syringe
- Bupivacaine 0.5%: takes effect in 4 to 20 minutes; duration of effect, 4 to 10 hours
- Lidocaine 2%: takes effect in 3 to 5 minutes; duration of effect, 1.5 to 2 hours
- Dog and cat skulls: valuable in learning the location of anatomic landmarks

---

| **BOX 34-7** | Calculating Amounts of Regional Anesthesia per Oral Surgery Quadrant |

Example: A 3-kg cat suffering from severe stomatitis presents for full-mouth extraction. How much 0.5% bupivacaine can you use in each quadrant?
- Maximum safe dose = 1.5 mg/kg × 3 kg = 4.5 mg
- 0.5% solution = 5 mg/ml
- Therefore, a total of 0.9 ml can be used in the cat.
- Divided by four quadrants = 0.225 ml/quadrant (maximum)

INFRAORBITAL NERVE BLOCK

The infraorbital nerve block prevents sensation from the tip of the needle rostrally on the ipsilateral maxilla. The infraorbital foramen is located dorsal to the roots of the maxillary third premolar tooth. Palpate the foramen through the oral mucosa. Insert the needle through the mucosa into the foramen at the level of the mesial root of the third premolar. Gently redirect the needle if its tip does not advance easily. The needle tip is advanced caudal to the level where the caudal-most extent of oral surgery will be performed, so a $1\frac{1}{4}$-inch needle is usually necessary in dogs. In cats, the infraorbital canal is shorter and wider; therefore, care should be taken to avoid angulation of the needle tip toward the ocular structures. Aspirate before injecting to ensure that the needle is not in a blood vessel. If blood is aspirated, reposition and try again, or obtain a new needle and syringe. Use digital pressure over the site after the needle is removed to encourage caudal diffusion and decrease hematoma formation. The foramen is large enough that a 27-gauge needle can be inserted with minimal risk of causing damage to the nerve. The extent of the region blocked depends on how far the needle is inserted into the foramen.

MIDDLE MENTAL NERVE BLOCK

The middle mental nerve block prevents sensation of the ipsilateral rostral lower lip from the labial frenulum rostrally; this block may also provide decreased sensation of the ipsilateral incisors and canine teeth, although not predictably. The foramen is palpable below the mesial root of the mandibular second premolar in medium-size and large dogs within the labial frenulum. The foramen is not easily palpable in cats and small dogs. Significant resistance may be felt when the needle is inserted because of the narrowness of the foramen. It is advisable to avoid forceful insertion of the needle. Instead, placement of a bleb of anesthetic at the opening of the foramen with a 27-gauge needle is followed by massage of the anesthetic into the foramen. Insert the needle into the region of the foramen, and infuse with anesthetic. Aspirate before injecting to prevent intravascular infusion.

INFERIOR ALVEOLAR NERVE BLOCK

The inferior alveolar nerve block prevents sensation of the soft tissue and bone of the entire ipsilateral mandible. This nerve block has the potential to result in self-trauma to the tongue upon recovery, of which patients are not aware, because patients cannot feel self-inflicted trauma when the tongue is numb. This potential complication is rare, but any person who performs nerve blocks should be aware of it. This complication may be avoided by staying close to the medial surface of the mandible and using a small volume of anesthetic to prevent medial diffusion, which results in loss of sensation not only of the inferior alveolar nerve, but also of the lingual nerve. Lidocaine, rather than bupivacaine, may be a good option for this block when the procedure is of short duration, and whether the block will be placed in the correct position is a matter of concern. To perform this block, palpate the foramen intraorally on the medial surface of the caudal mandible. The foramen is caudal and ventral to the mandibular third molar in the dog, and caudal and ventral to the mandibular first molar in the cat. In a mid-size dog, the foramen is approximately 1 cm dorsal to the ventral cortex of the caudal mandible, where the ventral cortex of the mandible curves slightly dorsally. No attempt is made to enter the foramen with the needle; instead, a bleb of anesthetic is placed at the foramen, close to the medial surface of the mandible. Two approaches may be used for placement of this bleb. The intraoral approach involves insertion of a 27-gauge needle along the medial surface of the bone into the region of the foramen. The needle is inserted at a 20-degree angle from the long axis of the mandible approximately 1 cm caudal to the M3 (dog), or $\frac{1}{2}$ cm caudal to the M1 (cat). The extraoral approach involves a two-handed technique. Palpate the midpoint of the zygomatic arch, between rostral and caudal aspects, and move ventrally to the mandible. This should approximate the location of the facial vascular notch on the ventral cortex of the mandible—a dorsal deviation of the ventral cortex of the mandible. Insert a 27- or 25-gauge needle through the skin at this region (25-gauge may be necessary to penetrate tough skin), staying as close as possible to the medial surface of the mandible. Use the gloved index finger of your opposite hand to feel for the foramen and to assess whether the tip of the needle is in the correct position. The extraoral technique is a good option for beginners because it allows the operator to feel where the bleb is being deposited.

MAXILLARY NERVE BLOCK

The maxillary nerve block prevents sensation of the entire maxillary quadrant on buccal and palatal sides of the teeth. The same area may be blocked by performing an infraorbital block with a long needle. The approach to the maxillary block is an intraoral approach using a 27-gauge, $1\frac{1}{4}$-inch needle on a 3-ml syringe (dog), or a 27-gauge, $\frac{1}{2}$-inch needle on a 1-ml syringe (cat). The needle is bent approximately 1 cm from the tip. The most caudal aspect of the hard palate is identified just caudal to the maxillary second molar (dog) or the maxillary first molar (cat). Insert the needle perpendicular to the soft palate just caudal to the molar approximately $\frac{1}{2}$ cm deep in cats and 1 cm deep in dogs. Be careful to avoid inserting the needle too far because you are

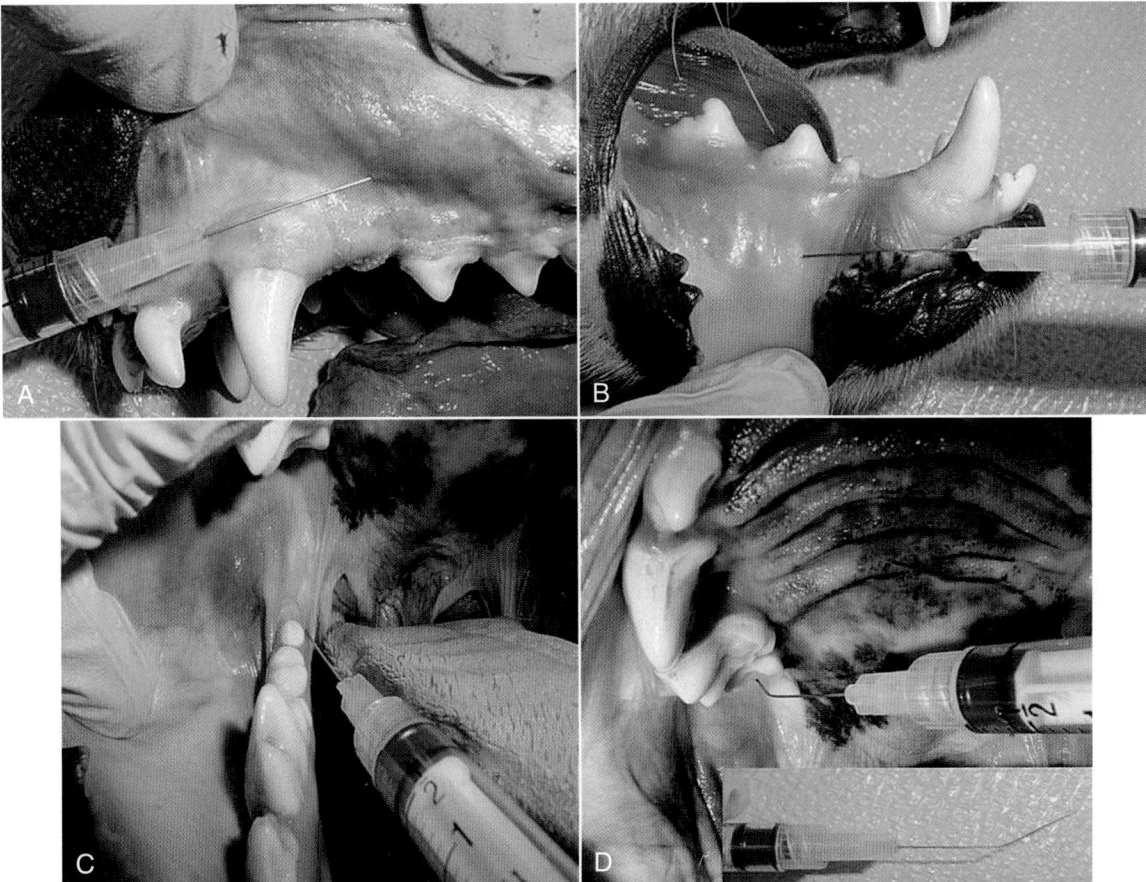

FIGURE 34-46 Common regional nerve blocks used in dentistry and oral surgery. **A,** Infraorbital nerve block. **B,** Middle mental nerve block. **C,** Inferior alveolar nerve block. **D,** Maxillary nerve block (note that the needle is bent 1 cm from the tip).

directly ventral to the eye. Bending the needle 1 cm from the tip provides a reference point as to how far the needle has been inserted. Be careful when bending the needle to avoid creating a rough edge at the tip of the needle, which might result in undue trauma when inserted. As with all blocks described here, aspirate on the plunger of the syringe before placement of the bleb to ensure that the needle tip is not in a vessel. Figure 34-46 shows intraoral approaches to the most common regional nerve blocks used in oral surgery.

PERIODONTAL SURGERY

A grading system that has been created to categorize periodontal disease helps to provide generalizations for appropriate treatment (Box 34-8). Grade I periodontal disease refers to inflammatory changes confined to the gingiva (gingivitis); this is an easily reversible sign that suggests the need for a routine dental cleaning and increased home care regimens. Grade II periodontal disease is an early form of periodontitis wherein evidence of loss of attachment is noted, and root débridement or subgingival curettage may be required. Grade III periodontal disease is considered moderate periodontitis in which 25% to 50% of the attachment structures of the tooth have been lost; root débridement, gingival curettage, and periodontal surgery are often

BOX 34-8	Periodontal Disease Classification

- PD 0: clinically normal
- PD 1: gingivitis with no attachment loss
- PD 2: <25% attachment loss—mild periodontitis
- PD 3: 25% to 50% attachment loss—moderate periodontitis
- PD 4: >50% attachment loss—advanced periodontitis

required. Grade III teeth have a fair to guarded prognosis. Grade IV periodontal disease is considered severe periodontitis. With attachment loss of 50% or greater, these teeth often require extraction.

Deep periodontal pockets may warrant involved periodontal surgery. One technique for dealing with unexpected periodontal pocketing in the context of a busy private practice is staging of the procedure over two visits. Visit 1 involves baseline charting, radiographs, cleaning, and polishing, along with closed root planing, gingival curettage, and placement of a doxycycline gel, with a return visit for more involved periodontal surgery to be scheduled 1 to 2 months later. Doxycycline gel may be placed into a freshly débrided periodontal pocket, provided that the pocket is 4 mm or deeper to allow for retention of the product. The product labeled for use in dogs carries the trade name Doxirobe; it is a doxycycline gel mixed with a slowly absorbable polymer. The polymer allows delivery of the product in gel form, and, once placed in the sulcus, spraying the product with water causes the polymer to harden, allowing for compaction of the product into the pocket. This provides several beneficial effects. Doxycycline is an antimicrobial with good spectrum against various periodontal pathogens. Doxycycline has anti-inflammatory effects that are beneficial in decreasing damage to periodontal tissues that may be mediated by the response of the immune system to periodontal pathogens. Finally, the space-occupying effect of the polymer prevents the treated pocket from filling with food and debris immediately after the procedure, allowing the site to heal from the most apical aspect coronally. A similar product containing clindamycin is available with the trade name of Clindoral.

Upon return in 1 to 2 months, pocket depth should be gently probed once the patient is under general anesthesia. If the pocket depth is normal, no further treatment is necessary, and home care can be continued with routine checkups and periodontal débridement as necessary. If the abnormal pocket depth is still 5 mm or greater in dogs, or 3 mm or greater in cats, periodontal surgery is indicated if the client would like to save the affected tooth. A variety of periodontal surgical procedures have been documented, and each technique is appropriate in different situations. Creation of a flap and open root planing usually are necessary with pocket depths of 5 mm or greater. In the past, periodontal disease was considered to be irreversible. Now, with advances in surgical technique and materials, periodontal disease may be considered to be reversible if it is dealt with before severe damage to the periodontium occurs; without proper postoperative home care, the condition will invariably recur. Pets with advanced periodontal disease may require periodontal débridement every 3 to 4 months until evidence suggests that the disease is controlled. A periodontitis treatment decision tree is provided in Figure 34-47.

Vertical bone loss and horizontal bone loss represent two very different challenges in periodontal surgery. Vertical bone loss occurs along the long axis of the tooth root and is easier to deal with than widespread horizontal bone loss, wherein multiple furcations are exposed. After débridement of the vertical infrabony defect, an osteoconductive or osteoinductive material may be placed in the defect. Osteoconductive materials will not induce new bone, but will act as scaffolding for new bone cells to traverse the defect. In contrast, osteoinductive materials stimulate progenitor cells of osteoblasts to differentiate and form new bone in an area. Multiple products are available on the human dental market. In veterinary dentistry, an example of an osteoconductive product is Consil (Nutramax Laboratories, Edgewood, Maryland). An example of an osteoinductive material is Osteoallograft (Veterinary Transplant Services, Kent, Washington). These products generally require a means of retention, which may be an absorbable or nonabsorbable membrane or flap that is repositioned in a coronal location

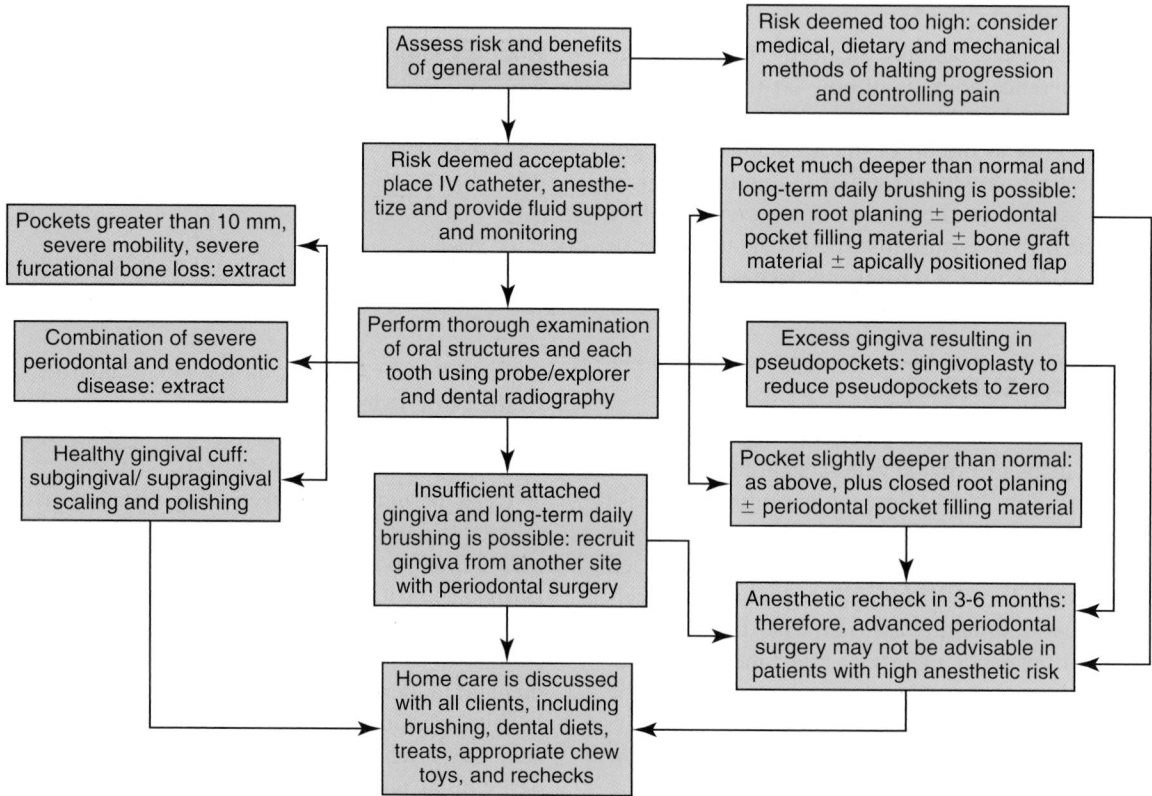

FIGURE 34-47 Decision tree for patients with periodontal disease.

to contain the material once placed. Any foreign material may act as a nidus for continued infection, so the placement site must be able to be adequately débrided before placement of these products is considered. The surgery site may be lavaged with 0.12% chlorhexidine, followed by lactated Ringer's solution to minimize the cytotoxic effects of chlorhexidine. The flap is closed with 4-0 or 5-0 absorbable monofilament suture material placed interdentally in a simple interrupted pattern, and digital pressure is applied to the gingiva for 60 seconds. Occasionally, a sling suture may be used to provide a purse-string effect to encourage the gingival portion of the flap to reattach. The patient should be placed on a soft-food diet with no hard toys or treats for 2 weeks, and antibacterial mouth rinses (0.12% chlorhexidine) may be prescribed. The owner should start to brush the teeth 1 week postoperatively using the modified Stillman technique at the surgery site (Figure 34-48, A).

> **TECHNICIAN NOTE** Attempts should not be made to save teeth with advanced periodontal surgery unless the client is able to perform daily brushing.

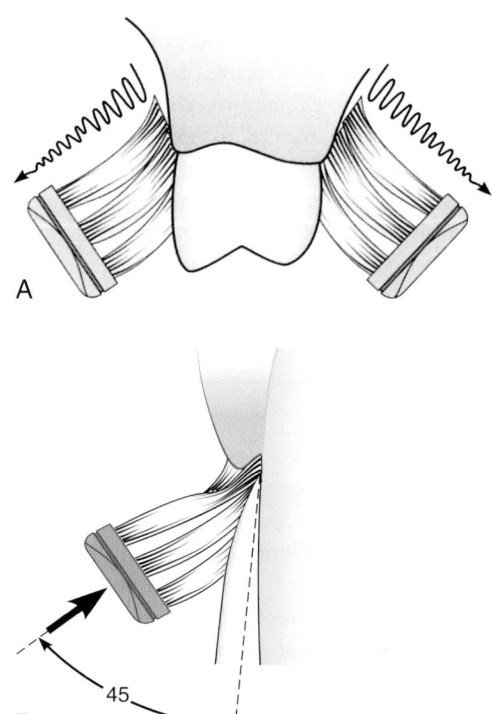

FIGURE 34-48 A, The modified Stillman brushing technique of placing the sides of the bristles along the tooth and gums and moving in a coronal direction provides gingival stimulation without traumatizing a periodontal surgery site. **B,** The 45-degree angle of the toothbrush in the Bass technique aims the soft bristles toward the gingival margin and into the sulcus. Use short back-and-forth motions without dislodging the bristles from the sulcus. Gentle pressure should elicit blanching of the gingival tissues. In the modified Bass technique, the Bass method is followed by gentle rolling of the bristles over the coronal portion of the teeth. (From Newman MG, Takei H, Klokkevold PR et al: Carranza's clinical periodontology, ed 11, St Louis, 2012, Saunders.)

HOME CARE

Client communication regarding dental home care is an important technician intervention. The technician will spend time with the client to demonstrate brushing techniques and to provide recommendations for various diets and products that can be used at the patient's home to reduce accumulations of plaque and calculus. Reduction of bacteria in the mouth can be accomplished through brushing, diets, and use of toys.

The mechanical cleansing provided by daily tooth brushing provides the most thorough method of plaque control for pets. Several methods may be used; the most widely accepted is the Bass technique, which concentrates the bristles along the gingival margin and in the sulcus (Figure 34-48, B). With a soft toothbrush, the bristles are directed at a 45-degree angle toward the gingival margin, so that some of the bristles enter the sulcus while other bristles are resting on the tooth adjacent to the margin. While pressing lightly, use short back-and-forth strokes and maintain the 45-degree angle for 5 to 10 seconds before repositioning the brush along the next group of teeth. Veterinary patients are reluctant to keep their mouth open, so it is best to brush while the mouth is closed with access to the teeth gained by gentle lifting of the lips. Perform this brushing technique with the bristles rinsed in water rather than covered with a veterinary dentifrice (toothpaste); patients try to eat the brush if its bristles are covered with dentifrice. When brushing is completed, the dentifrice can be applied into the mouth as a treat and to confer enzymatic or antiseptic benefits. Human toothpastes may cause stomach upset if swallowed and should not be used. Instruct the client to prioritize brushing in areas that collect the heaviest debris (usually the buccal surfaces of the caudal teeth) in case the patient becomes uncooperative before the task is completed, then to move to lingual and palatal surfaces as the patient allows. Brushing should be initiated at a young age to allow the patient to become accustomed to oral care. Before a toothbrush is introduced, the puppy or kitten should be given gum massages so they have the experience of the mouth being manipulated. The modified Stillman technique is sometimes used in areas of periodontal surgery to minimize plaque accumulation while preventing trauma to the reattaching gingival tissue (see Figure 34-50, A). This technique involves placement of the bristles apical to the gingival margin with a gentle sweeping motion in the coronal direction against the gingiva and crown of the tooth without placement of bristles into the healing sulcus.

> **TECHNICIAN NOTE** The Bass technique of tooth brushing places the bristles of the brush at a 45-degree angle against the tooth along the gingival margin to enable some bristles to slide into the sulcus. The Stillman technique is used in areas of periodontal surgery where bristles apical to the gingival margin are moved with a gentle sweeping motion in the coronal direction against the gingiva without placement of bristles into the healing sulcus.

Feeding a diet of soft food that adheres to tooth surfaces may contribute to periodontal disease. Plaque control can be augmented by feeding a hard dental diet that has been manufactured and tested to reduce accumulations. The Veterinary Oral Health Council (VOHC) was established in 1997 by veterinary dentists and researchers to recognize products that have been shown to meet predetermined standards for plaque and calculus retardation. The VOHC seal of acceptance is issued to products that have proved to reduce plaque and/or calculus on the basis of generally accepted protocols. For a complete list of VOHC-approved products, visit its website at www.VOHC.org.

Diets reduce accumulation through mechanical or chemical action. The first dental diet was created to take advantage of mechanical cleansing. Long fibers within large pieces of kibble oriented in one direction help to keep the biscuit from crumbling readily when a dog or cat bites into it. This design allows the biscuit to mechanically scrape the sides of the teeth clean as the teeth penetrate the biscuit. An example of a chemical used to provide anticalculus effects is hexametaphosphate (HMP), which works by sequestering the calcium in plaque fluids to reduce formation of calculus by preventing mineralization of plaque. Use of dental diets alone is generally not as effective as tooth brushing. A regimen that combines special diets with tooth brushing is recommended for optimal plaque control.

Many home care products, including treats, rinses, and water additives, are available. Technicians should assess each product before offering recommendations to their clients. During home care instructions, the technician should also offer counseling regarding which types of toys may be harmful to the pet's teeth. Rawhide has an excellent cleansing action. However, the size and shape of the product must be correctly matched with the chewing habits of the dog. Rawhide should be taken away after 20 to 30 minutes of gnawing to decrease the likelihood of gastrointestinal problems caused by ingestion of a large piece. Allowing the rawhide to dry overnight and repeating the process will minimize the chance that the pet may encounter gastrointestinal or choking problems associated with ingestion of a large piece of rawhide.

Many toys found in pet stores, including cow hooves, hard nylon bones, and natural sterilized bones, are harmful to the teeth; each is capable of causing dental fractures. Aggressive chewing of tennis balls causes abrasion of teeth, especially when dirt and sand become incorporated within the felt of the ball. Instruct clients to always monitor their pets when providing chew toys.

RESTORATIVE DENTISTRY

Restorative dentistry is the subspecialty of dentistry that restores or maintains the structure and function of a tooth. No restorative material is as strong as the original tooth structure, so an attempt is always made to preserve as much of the original tooth as possible. Indications for restorative dentistry include teeth with

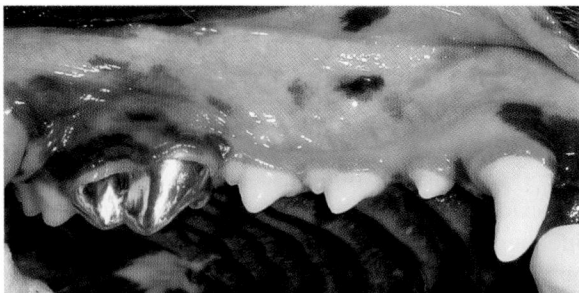

FIGURE 34-49 A full metal jacket crown has been placed over an endodontically treated maxillary fourth premolar tooth. Metal crowns rather than tooth-colored crowns are chosen because of their strength and the need for less tooth removal.

dental caries (cavities), fractured teeth, and endodontically treated teeth.

Fractured teeth may be restored to function while periodontal health is maintained. The cheek teeth (premolars and molars) have a natural design called the *dental bulge* that deflects food away from the gingival sulcus. When teeth lose this natural contour, they can become predisposed to periodontal disease. Fractured teeth can be restored with restorative materials alone or in combination with retention pins, posts, or both. Pins and posts do not add strength to the restoration, but they aid in retention of the restoration.

Metal or zirconium crowns are placed on fractured teeth to protect the tooth, especially in working dogs or in cases where repeated tooth trauma is expected. Metal crowns made of a mixture of metals are more common than porcelain or zirconium crowns because of their greater strength and requirements for less tooth removal than with crowns that have a porcelain exterior fused to metal. Crowns are most commonly placed in dogs on the canine and maxillary fourth premolar teeth (Figure 34-49).

ENDODONTICS

Endodontics deals with the study and treatment of the inside of the tooth (pulp) and periapical tissues. Periapical tissue is located around the tip (apex) of the tooth root. The tooth pulp consists of nerves, blood vessels, lymphatics, and connective tissue. Pulp tissue is found in the pulp chamber (crown) and root canal (root) of the tooth and enters the tooth through numerous small openings in the apex of the tooth root called the *apical delta*.

The dental pulp is important for the development of the tooth in a young animal. It supplies nutrients needed by the odontoblasts to deposit secondary dentin. This makes the walls of the root and crown thicker, so the tooth is stronger. Once the dog or cat is 10 to 18 months of age, the root apex should be closed. As the animal continues to age, the pulp chamber and canal will become smaller because odontoblasts will continue to produce secondary dentin, which makes the tooth stronger (Figure 34-50, *A* and *B*).

Treatment options for teeth with endodontic disease depend on the age of the animal, the duration of endodontic

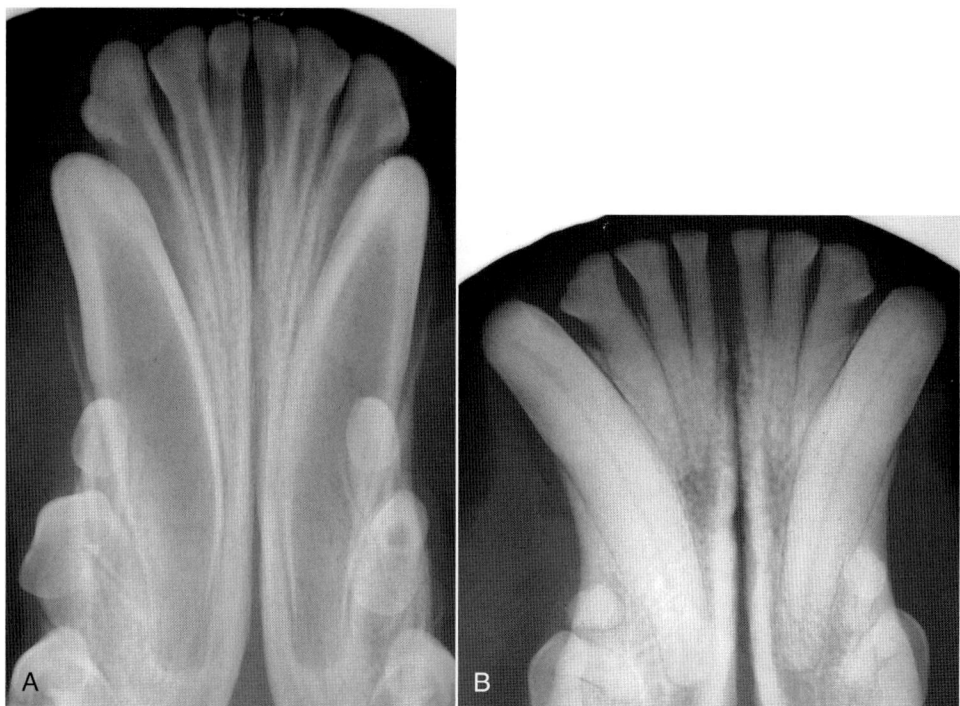

FIGURE 34-50 A, Radiographs of immature permanent teeth of a 6-month-old dog and of (B) permanent teeth of a 6-year-old dog. Note that the secondary dentin produced in the older dog has strengthened the tooth and narrowed the pulp chamber and root canal.

BOX 34-9	Endodontic Instrument and Materials Setup

- Dental radiography
- High-speed handpiece and burs
- Barbed broaches
- Endodontic files and file organizer
- Rubber stops
- Endodontic ruler
- Canal lubricant, irrigant, and irrigation needles
- Paper points
- College pliers
- Zinc oxide, eugenol
- Glass slab, mixing spatula
- Gutta percha points
- Lentulo, paste fillers
- 10 : 1 reduction gear contra angle
- Pluggers and spreaders
- Heating instrument
- Restorative materials and instruments

disease, and the anatomy of the tooth. Conventional root canal therapy is usually performed on dogs and cats 12 months of age and older with endodontic disease. Treatment involves removing dead or dying pulp tissue from the tooth, disinfecting and shaping the root canal, and filling the canal (obturation) with an appropriate material to seal the apex from periapical tissues. Radiographs are necessary to ensure that a proper apical seal has been achieved.

Box 34-9 lists equipment and supplies needed for conventional root canal therapy. These items should be ready for use before root canal treatment is started. A preoperative radiograph is taken to evaluate the tooth root and periapical region. The veterinarian will gain appropriate access to the root canal through the crown of the tooth with a dental bur. The canal may have partially necrotic pulp that will require removal with a barbed broach (Figure 34-51). The broach is placed in the canal and is rotated to ensnare the pulp. The broach and pulp tissue are removed from the canal. This step is repeated until all pulp has been removed. Many teeth will not have any visible pulp tissue remaining (necrotic pulp), and barbed broaches will not be needed. When a barbed broach is used, it is important to avoid binding the broach in the walls of the canal because the broach may break off in the canal. The canal is cleaned with files and irrigant to sterilize the canal, and the files are used to shape the canal to allow for proper obturation. Several types and sizes of files are available. Hedström (H) and Kerr (K) files are the most commonly used hand files (Figure 34-52). H-files have a sharper edge and can remove dentin faster than K-files. They are used in a push-pull motion. H-files are more susceptible to file breakage than K-files. K-files are inserted to the apical extent of the canal, turned one-quarter turn, and removed, allowing for shaping of the apical portion of the canal. The edges of K-files are less sharp, so dentin removal is less efficient than with H-files. K-files are structurally more sound and are less likely to fracture in the canal. These files are available in different lengths and diameters. The smallest-diameter file is a number 6 ($\%_{100}$ of a millimeter at the tip). Files increase in diameter by even number increments from 6 to 10, and then they increase by increments of 5. For instance, the following diameters are available: 6, 8, 10, 15,

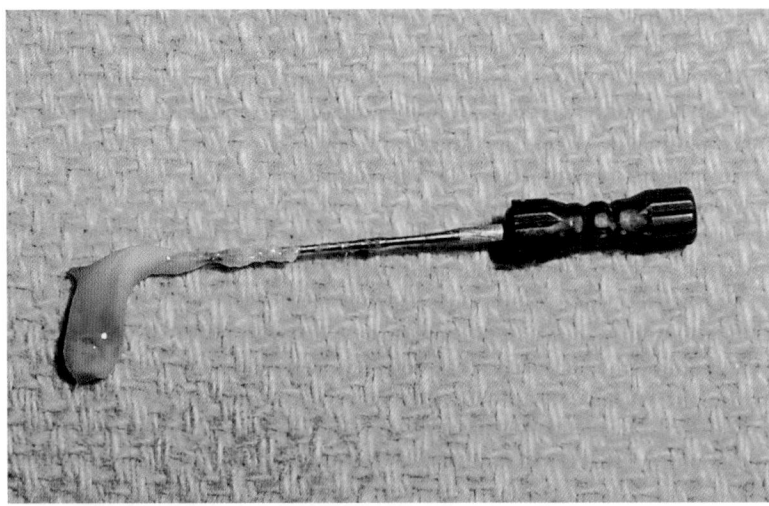

FIGURE 34-51 Partially necrotic pulp retrieved with a barbed broach.

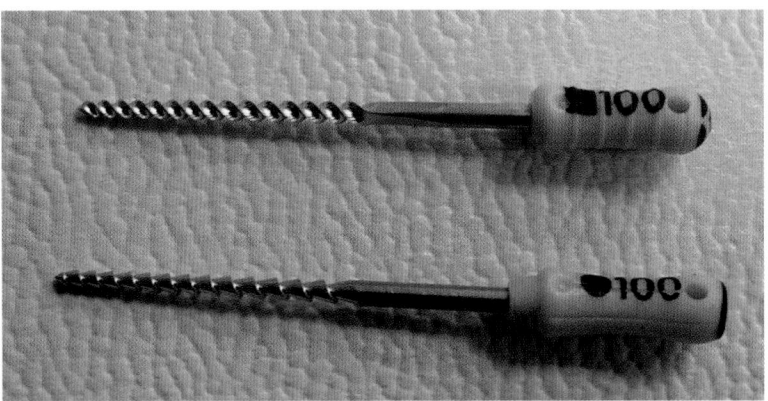

FIGURE 34-52 H- and K-endodontic files: H-files *(lower file)* are designed to be used in a push-pull manner, whereas K-files *(upper file)* are used to shape the apical canal with quarter-turn advances.

20, 25, 30, 35, 40, and so on until file 60, at which point the diameter increases by 10. The largest-diameter file is a 140. Files made for human root canals are available in lengths of 21 mm, 25 mm, and 31 mm. Special veterinary files are available for teeth in which human files would not reach the apex (Figure 34-53). This variation in length is necessary so that the apex of the tooth root can be reached in long teeth (canines). The variation in diameter is necessary so that the narrow canals of old and/or small animals and the large canals of young or large animals can be properly filed.

> **TECHNICIAN NOTE** H-files are used in a push-pull motion and are more susceptible to file breakage than K-files. K-files are inserted to the apical extent of the canal, turned one-quarter turn, and removed, allowing for shaping of the apical portion of the canal.

Files should be removed from the package and placed in an organized manner. Files of similar length may be placed in a piece of autoclavable foam in order of increasing diameter. The files can be autoclaved, and when the veterinarian

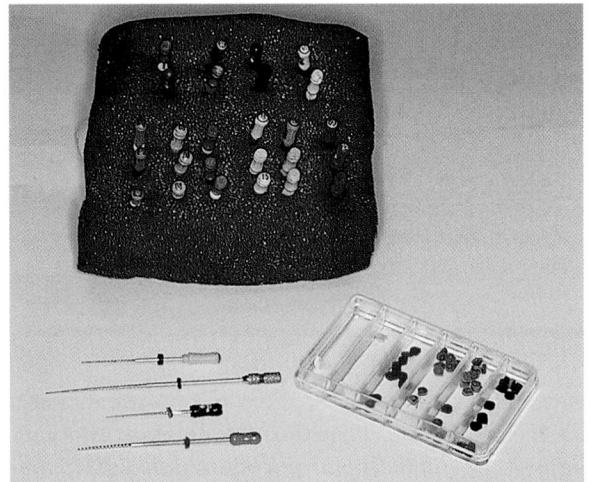

FIGURE 34-53 Endodontic files are made in human and veterinary lengths. Files should be arranged by size for easy identification. Endodontic stops *(right)* are placed on each file to determine and maintain working length.

is ready to perform the root canal, the files will be sterile and prepared in an organized manner. Preoperative planning and technician assistance during the procedure are helpful in minimizing anesthesia time.

Endodontic stops are small pieces of rubber that go around the file to mark a specific length (see Figure 34-51). The file is placed in the root canal, and a radiograph is taken to make sure that the file goes all the way to the apical extent of the root canal system (Figure 34-54). The distance from the endodontic stop to the file tip is called the *working length*. The rest of the files are set to this length to ensure that the root canal is filed to the proper depth. Measuring gauges are available that allow quick adjustment of the endodontic stop to the proper working length (Figure 34-55).

Canal lubricants are used to soften the dentinal walls to ease filing and help prevent file breakage. An irrigant is used between file sizes to rinse the canal of dentinal shavings and other debris. The most common irrigant is sodium hypochlorite because of its excellent disinfecting properties and ability to break down organic debris (pulp). Endodontic irrigation needles are placed on the syringe that contains the irrigant. These needles have a blunt end with a side opening to prevent forcing noxious irrigant periapically (Figure 34-56).

> **TECHNICIAN NOTE** Sodium hypochlorite is irritating to soft tissue. Contact with oral soft tissues should be avoided, as should forceful irrigation of the canal to prevent periapical migration of the irrigant.

After the canal has been properly cleaned and shaped by the files, it is ready for obturation. *Obturation* refers to filling the canal with a material that will seal it from the periapical area. The canal should have a final rinse of sterile water, and then it is dried with sterile paper points. Successive paper points are inserted and removed until the points come out of the canal dry. An endodontic sealer is applied to the canal walls. Sealer application can be done with a sterile paper point, a K-file, or a spiral paste filler on a slow-speed handpiece (Figure 34-57). Gutta percha should make up the bulk of the filling agent. It is a radiopaque rubber-like material that can be vertically and laterally condensed to adapt to the shape of the root canal. The material can be heated to allow it to flow into the canal and adapt more easily to the shape of the canal. Vertical and lateral condensation is performed with pluggers and spreaders, and additional gutta percha is added as needed to fill the entire canal. Pluggers have a blunt end that pushes the gutta percha vertically in an apical

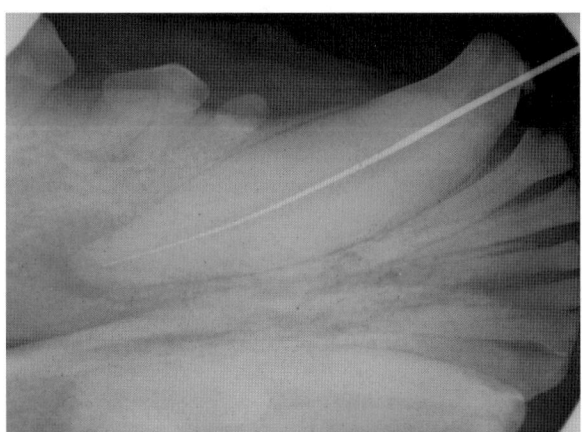

FIGURE 34-54 An endodontic file is placed to the apex, and a radiograph is taken to determine the working length.

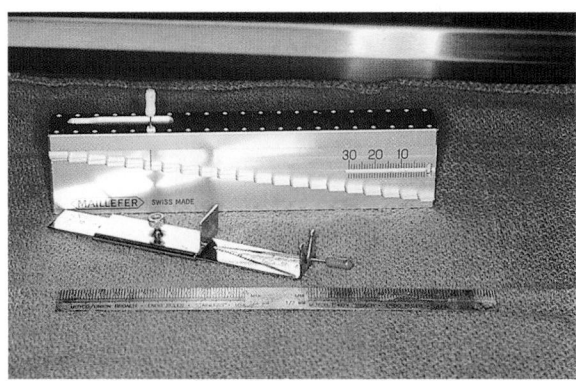

FIGURE 34-55 Measuring gauges and rulers are used to measure the working length of the root from the access site to the apex.

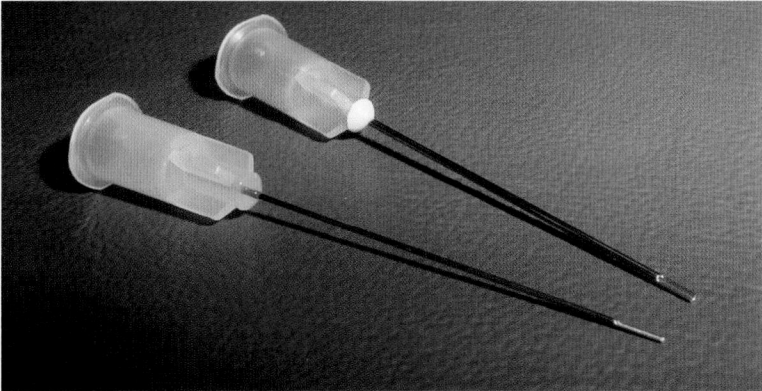

FIGURE 34-56 Endodontic needles are open on the side of the tip to prevent inadvertent forcing of sodium hypochlorite through the apical delta.

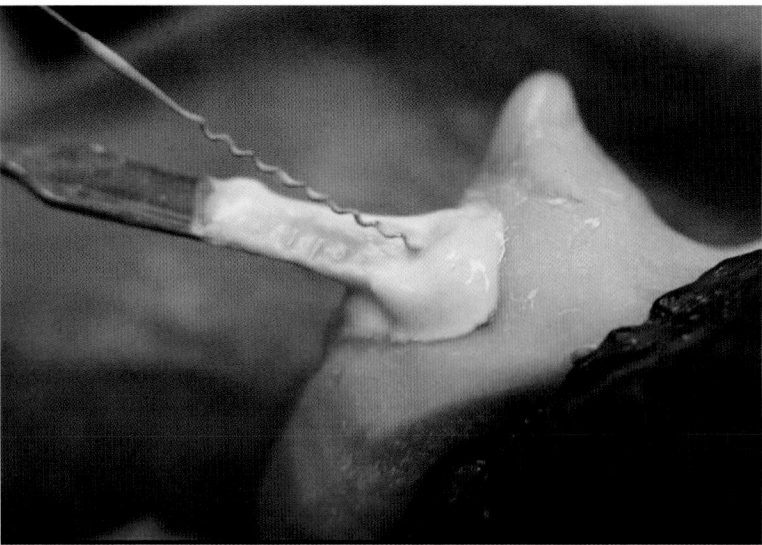

FIGURE 34-57 Lentulo spiral paste filler for delivery of cement. A spatula loaded with cement is placed near the spiral filler, which pushes the cement apically. Care should be taken to use a contra angle with reduction gear to decrease chances of the filler breaking in the canal. A composite splint is seen at the gingival margin, resulting from a healing jaw fracture in the area of the canine tooth.

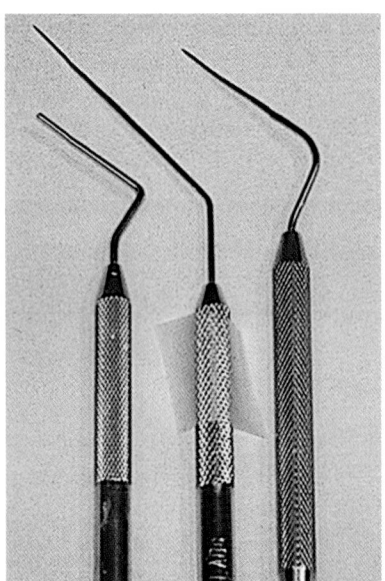

FIGURE 34-58 An endodontic plugger and endodontic spreaders. Spreaders have a pointed tip and are used for lateral compaction. Pluggers have a flat tip and are used for vertical compaction.

direction. Spreaders have a pointed tip and push the gutta percha laterally to create room for more gutta percha for a solid fill. Spreaders and pluggers come in a variety of lengths and diameters (Figure 34-58). Extra-long veterinary length spreaders and pluggers are available.

Once obturation of the canal has been accomplished, the restorative filling material is placed. This can be done with a single filling material or in two layers with intermediate and final filling material used. Composite fillings cannot be placed next to eugenol because eugenol interferes with hardening of the composite. Glass ionomers are a commonly used intermediate filling material. A light-cured composite

filling material is often used as the final restorative at the surface of the access site and fracture site.

Teeth that have undergone pulp death become more brittle over time because they lack the hydration that was originally provided by the pulp tissue. A good history should always be taken to try to determine how the pet fractured the tooth. If inappropriate chew toys are in the environment, these toys should be removed. A metal crown may be indicated to minimize the likelihood of repeat fracture of the tooth. Endodontically treated teeth should be assessed radiographically at least yearly.

EXODONTICS

Although attempts should be made to save teeth whenever possible, extraction (exodontics) is necessary when the prognosis for saving the tooth is grave, and when financial constraints or medical conditions prevent multiple anesthetic episodes that may be necessary to salvage the teeth. Extraction of a tooth with severe periodontal disease may be straightforward if many of the attachment structures of the tooth have been lost, but as a result of their large root surface area, extraction of canine or feline teeth can be challenging. The extraction process begins with placement of a regional nerve block to decrease inhalant anesthesia requirements.

Serious complications can arise from extraction. Possible complications should be discussed with the owner before the procedure is begun. Complications include those associated with anesthesia, hemorrhage, ocular trauma, jaw fracture, and displacement of a root into an inaccessible area such as the nasal passage. Iatrogenic jaw fracture can occur easily when diseased mandibular first molars or mandibular canine teeth are extracted in cats and small breed dogs, especially when significant periodontal disease already exists.

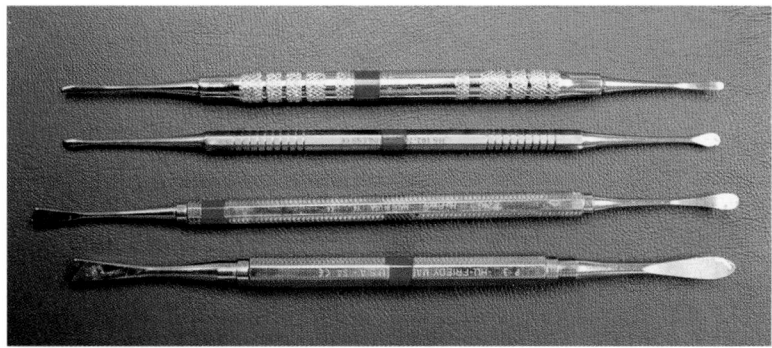

FIGURE 34-59 Various periosteal elevators used in oral surgery.

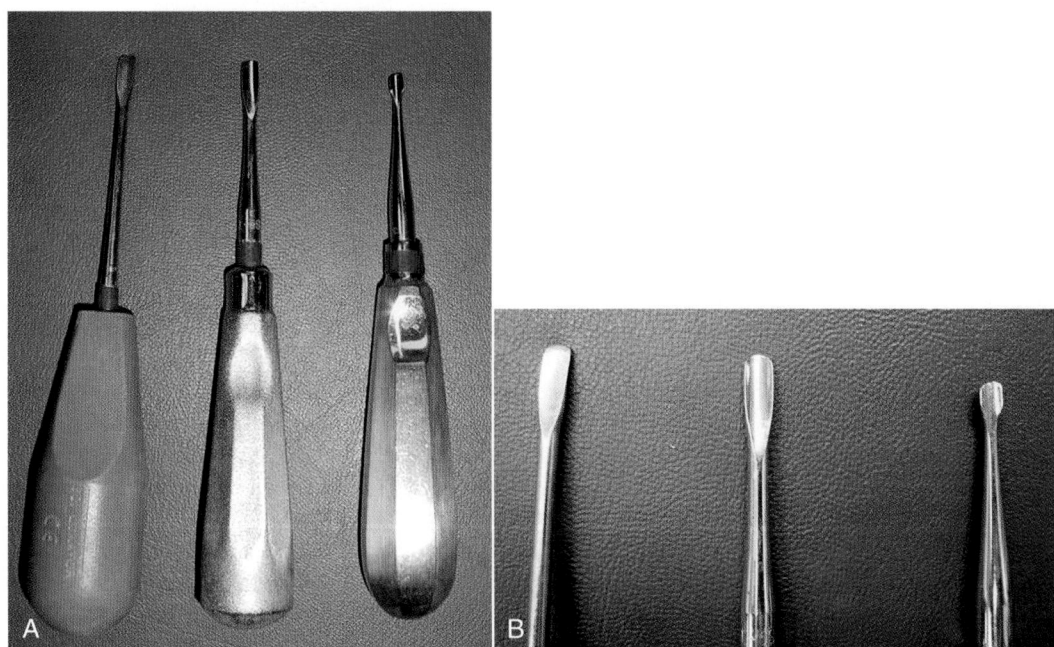

FIGURE 34-60 **A,** Dental luxator, straight elevator, and winged elevator. **B,** Working end of each.

> **TECHNICIAN NOTE** Never extract a tooth without the direct permission of the client. Always obtain a contact phone number to discuss any unexpected findings.

> **TECHNICIAN NOTE** Regional nerve blocks not only lower inhalant requirements, they also provide postoperative pain relief.

CLOSED EXTRACTIONS

While the regional block is taking effect, a pre-extraction radiograph should be taken of the tooth to assess for evidence of root pathologic conditions that may affect the surgical approach. A closed technique is best reserved for single-rooted teeth and for teeth that have severe periodontal disease. Once the regional nerve block has been placed, the gingival attachments around the tooth are separated with a periosteal elevator (Figure 34-59), a dental luxator, or a scalpel blade. After the soft tissue attachments have been severed, a dental elevator of appropriate size and shape (Figure 34-60, *A* and *B*) is placed in the periodontal space on the mesial or distal surface of the crown. Once placed in the space, gentle pressure is placed to seat the elevator within the tooth and alveolar bone, and the handle of the elevator is rotated slightly to stretch the periodontal ligament fibers. If elevation is done correctly, the tooth will be observed to move slightly when the elevator is rotated. Pressure is held for 10 seconds, and then the elevator is advanced apically and is rotated against the root in the opposite direction to create pressure, and pressure is held again. The goal is to fatigue the periodontal ligament and prevent tooth root fracture. Larger elevators are used as the periodontal ligament breaks down, which allows more room for placement of a larger instrument. The temptation to wiggle the elevator in an attempt to obtain a deeper position in the periodontal space should be avoided because this will often cause breakdown of the alveolar bone and loss of leverage. The elevator may also be placed on the palatal or lingual surface and the vestibular surface within the periodontal space to stretch

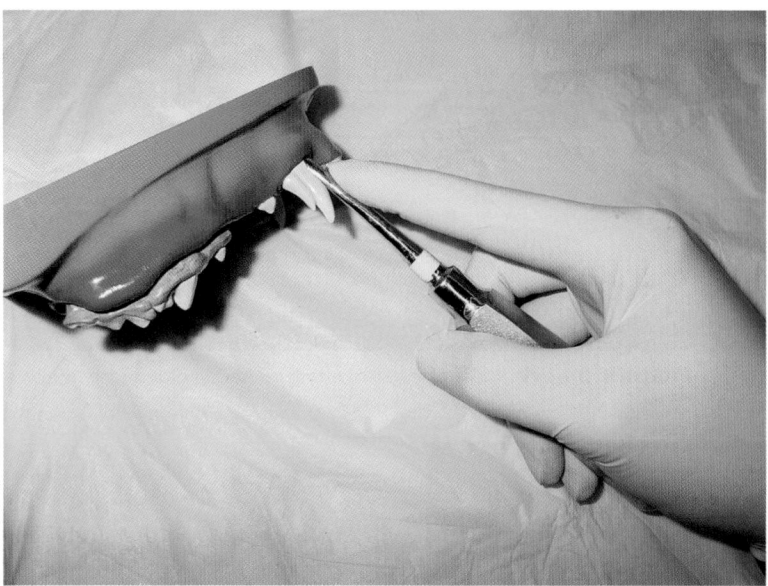

FIGURE 34-61 Proper grasp of a dental elevator. The index finger is extended to minimize soft tissue trauma if the elevator should slip.

BOX 34-10 | Extraction Instrument Setup

- High-speed handpiece
- Burs: fissure and round in assorted sizes, carbide and diamond coated
- Periosteal elevators
- Dental luxators
- Dental elevators
- Extraction forceps
- Root tip elevators, root tip forceps
- Absorbable monofilament suture
- Metzenbaum scissors
- Needle holders
- Tissue forceps
- Suture scissors
- Blade handle and blade

---

periodontal ligament fibers around the entire circumference of the tooth. Elevators come in a variety of shapes and sizes, and it is important to have access to different sizes for different situations. When a dental elevator is grasped, the handle should rest securely in the palm of the hand. The index finger should be extended so that if the elevator slips, the index finger will help to stop the advancing of the elevator into deeper structures (Figure 34-61). Ocular trauma and brain trauma have been documented in cases where dental elevators have slipped during extraction procedures. To prevent this, forces used must be well controlled and should be generated in the lateral, medial or coronal direction rather than in the apical direction. The gingival tissue is apposed to close the extraction site with 4-0 or 5-0 monofilament absorbable suture in a simple interrupted pattern. Sterile extraction packs that contain the necessary instruments may be wrapped and prepared for use (Box 34-10).

SURGICAL EXTRACTIONS

As a result of the large surface area and multi-rooted nature of carnivore teeth, surgical extraction is often a less traumatic option than attempts to remove a firmly rooted tooth by closed extraction. As with closed extraction, gingival attachments are separated from the tooth crown with a periosteal elevator, a dental luxator, or a scalpel blade. A flap is created, depending on the location and the underlying root structure. A flap with no releasing incisions is called an *envelope flap*. A flap with one releasing incision is a *triangle flap*, and a flap with two releasing incisions is called a *pedicle flap*. Each situation should be assessed individually to decide which type of flap is necessary to provide optimal access and tension-free tissue closure while inflicting the minimum amount of soft tissue trauma. Pedicle flaps are created with a broad base to ensure good blood supply and adequate tissue for closure. Once the flap is raised, a round carbide bur is used in a water-cooled, high-speed handpiece to create a window in the buccal bone of roots to be extracted. Multi-rooted teeth are separated with a tapered fissure bur. Once the window is created and roots are sectioned, minimal force is necessary to gently pry the roots and attached crown segments from their sockets. Once the roots have been removed in their entirety, rough bone edges are smoothed with a large round diamond bur. The alveolus of each root is curetted and lavaged with sterile isotonic solution or 0.12% chlorhexidine. The periosteum is separated from the mucosa to provide adequate tension-free tissue to close the defect. The flap is closed with 4-0 or 5-0 absorbable monofilament suture in a simple interrupted pattern. Occasionally, osteoconductive or osteoinductive products may be placed in the alveolus before closure if it is suspected that the product will not act as a nidus; they will help to prevent significant bone loss in the area of the extraction. A postextraction radiograph should be taken to

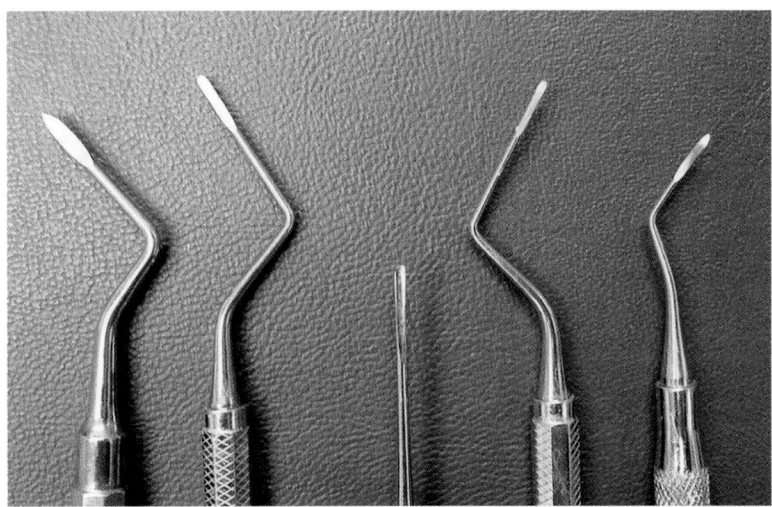

FIGURE 34-62 Root tip elevators in various shapes and sizes. These instruments are fragile and are meant to be used with minimal force.

document complete removal of the roots in cases where the roots were not retrieved easily.

When a root fractures, additional instruments will be needed to retrieve the retained tooth root. Root tip elevators and root tip forceps are valuable tools in root tip retrieval (Figure 34-62). Care should be taken to prevent dislodging the root tip into the nasal passage or the mandibular canal. Cotton-tipped applicators are helpful for controlling hemorrhage in the alveolar socket to allow visualization of the root tip. Avoid blowing air from an air or water syringe into the socket. Although this may facilitate visualization of the root, a fatal air embolism may occur. The pet should be given no hard food or treats for 14 days postoperatively. Postoperative antibiotics generally are not necessary after extraction procedures. The AVDC has put forth a position statement regarding the use of antibiotics in dental patients (Box 34-11).

COMMON DENTAL PROBLEMS IN DOGS AND CATS

TOOTH RESORPTION

Tooth resorption is common in cats and rare in dogs. Prevalence studies have found that 20% to 70% of cats are affected by this problem, depending on the population of cats and the investigative methods employed. The lesions are usually appreciated clinically at the cervical portion of the tooth (the junction of where the crown meets the root, sometimes referred to as the "neck" of the tooth), which is often hidden by the gingiva. However, recent histologic studies have found that these lesions begin on the root surface, and radiographic changes can often be seen before a clinical lesion is obvious. When a lesion develops at the gingival margin, the adjacent gingiva often covers these lesions with a combination of hyperplastic gingiva and granulation tissue (Figure 34-63, *A*).

BOX 34-11	American Veterinary Dental College (AVDC) Position Statement Regarding Use of Antibiotics in Veterinary Dentistry

The AVDC endorses the use of systemic antibiotics in veterinary dentistry for treatment of some infectious conditions of the oral cavity. Although culture and susceptibility testing is rarely performed on individual patients that have an infection extending from or to the oral cavity, selection of an appropriate antibiotic should be based on published data regarding susceptibility testing of the spectra of known oral pathogens.

Patients that are scheduled for an oral procedure may benefit from pretreatment with an appropriate antibiotic to improve the health of infected oral tissues. Bacteremia is a recognized sequela to dental scaling and other oral procedures. Healthy animals are able to overcome this bacteremia without the use of systemic antibiotics. However, use of a systemically administered antibiotic is recommended to reduce bacteremia for animals that are immune compromised or have underlying systemic disease (such as clinically evident cardiac, hepatic, and renal diseases), and/or when severe oral infection is present.

Antibiotics should never be considered a monotherapy for treatment of oral infection and should not be used as preventive management of oral conditions.

With permission of AVDC (www.AVDC.org/position-statements.html).

> **TECHNICIAN NOTE** The cause of feline tooth resorption is still unknown, but recent research suggests that vitamin D levels in commercial cat food may play a role (see "Recommended Readings").

A fine explorer should be used to check for irregularities, as described earlier in this chapter. In the past, restorations have been placed in lesions, but follow-up studies have shown poor long-term results with restoration. Therefore, extraction is the treatment of choice. Dental radiographs of

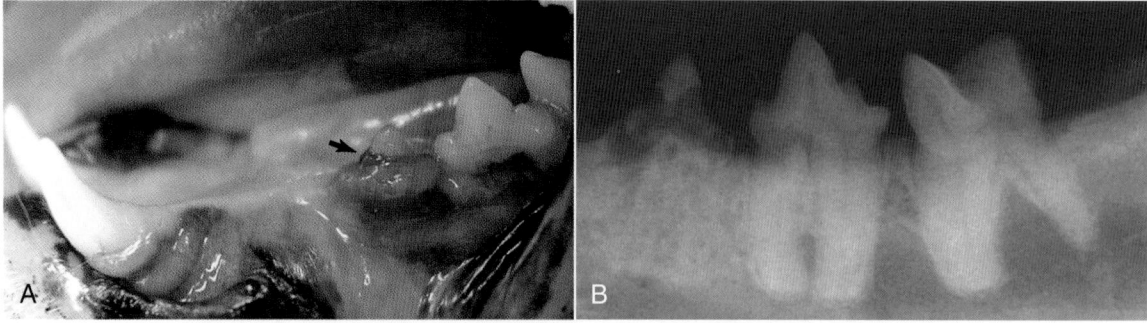

FIGURE 34-63 **A,** Photograph of a mandibular third premolar affected by idiopathic feline tooth resorption (*arrow*). **B,** Radiograph of the left mandible using the paralleling technique. The mandibular left third premolar has undergone significant root replacement resorption, as seen by decreased root density and loss of the normal periodontal space.

these teeth are necessary to evaluate the severity of resorption and to guide treatment.

Sometimes it is not possible to perform a complete tooth extraction because of severe root resorption, wherein a portion of the root has been replaced by a reparative bone-cementum material. When this occurs, the tooth root becomes incorporated into the adjacent alveolar bone. Radiographic evidence of this is seen by loss of periodontal ligament space and decreased root density, approximating that of surrounding bone density (Figure 34-63, *B*). When this radiographic appearance is seen, in the absence of periodontal or endodontic disease, it is possible to perform a crown amputation, during which hard tissue with characteristics of tooth root is removed, and resorbed root that has been replaced by bone is not removed. The tooth crown and the coronal root segment are removed with a dental bur and a high-speed handpiece. The crestal alveolar bone is smoothed with a dental bur, and the gingiva is closed with absorbable suture over the crown amputation site.

ORTHODONTIC PROBLEMS

Malocclusions

Four classes of malocclusions are used. Class I malocclusion occurs when the maxillary and mandibular jaw lengths are normal but one or more teeth are in an abnormal position. Class I malocclusions (also referred to as *neutroclusion*) are the most common type of malocclusion receiving orthodontic correction in pets. Common examples of Class I malocclusions are lingually displaced (base-narrow and/or in-standing) mandibular canines, anterior cross-bite, and lance canine teeth. When the mandibular canines are displaced lingually, they often cause occlusal trauma to palatal mucosa and/or gingiva because of their long crown height. Severe cases can result in complete penetration of the palatine process of the maxillary bone and/or the incisive bone, resulting in an oronasal fistula.

A rostral cross-bite (referred to as *anterior cross-bite* in humans) occurs when closed-mouth examination reveals that one or more maxillary incisors are positioned lingual to the mandibular incisors. A caudal cross-bite (called *posterior cross-bite* in humans) occurs when one or more maxillary

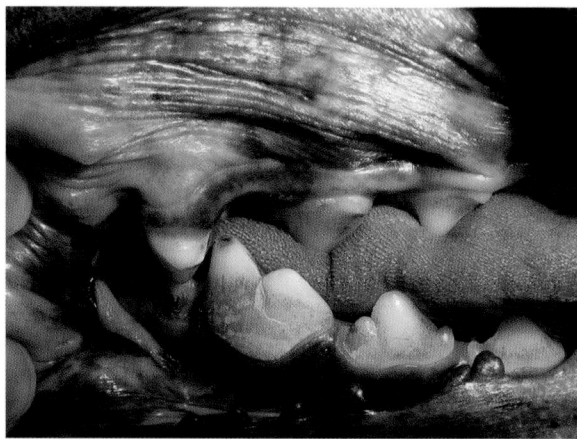

FIGURE 34-64 Caudal cross-bite: the mandibular first molar is buccal, or vestibular, to the maxillary fourth premolar. This may result in abnormal accumulation of plaque and calculus on the buccal surface of the mandibular molars, increasing the need for brushing in this area.

premolar or molar teeth are positioned lingual to the opposing mandibular premolar or molar (Figure 34-64).

It is important to evaluate the entire dentition and jaw length relationships if proper classification is to be made because clinical presentations similar to those described earlier can occur as a result of abnormalities in jaw length rather than abnormalities in tooth position. The remaining classes refer to skeletal malocclusions associated with jaw length discrepancies. A Class II malocclusion is also referred to as *distoclusion, overjet,* or *overshot,* and sometimes is incorrectly referred to as an *overbite* (Figure 34-65). In a Class II malocclusion, the mandible is relatively shorter than the maxilla; this can be the result of an abnormally long maxilla (maxillary prognathism) or an abnormally short mandible (mandibular **brachygnathism**). The AVDC accepted term for this occlusion is mandibular distoclusion.

A Class III malocclusion is also referred to as *mesioclusion, underjet,* or *undershot,* and sometimes is incorrectly referred to as an *underbite* (Figure 34-66). In a Class III malocclusion, the maxilla is relatively shorter than the mandible; this can be the result of an abnormally long mandible (mandibular prognathism) or an abnormally short maxilla (maxillary

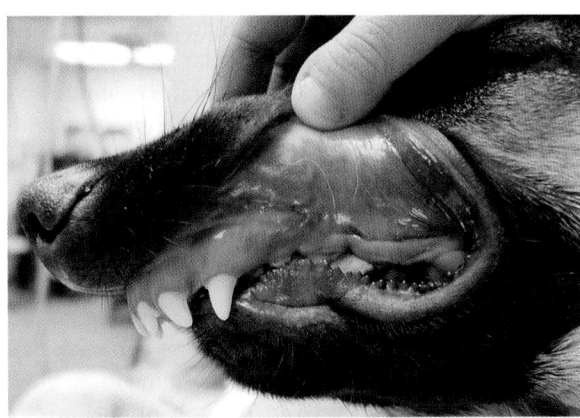

FIGURE 34-65 Class II malocclusion (mandibular distoclusion). The mandible is relatively shorter than the maxilla; this results in palatal trauma from the mandibular canine and sometimes mandibular incisor teeth.

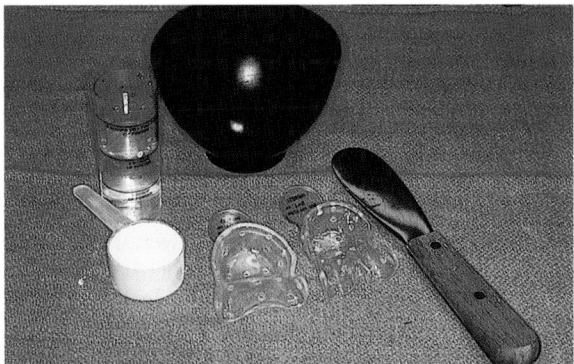

FIGURE 34-67 Materials and equipment used to take an alginate impression: rubber mixing bowl, spatula, impression trays, alginate scoop, and water-measuring cylinder.

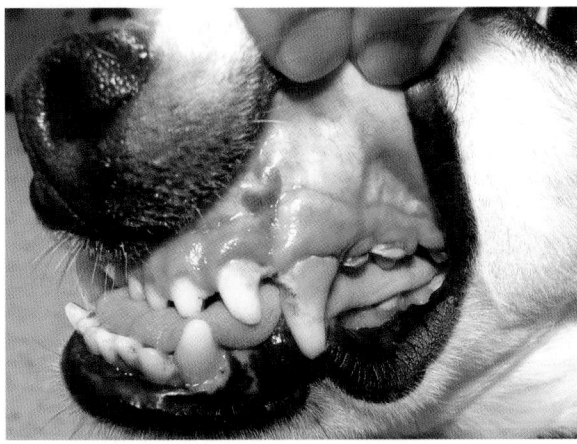

FIGURE 34-66 Class III malocclusion (mandibular mesioclusion). The maxilla is relatively shorter than the mandible; this may result in attrition of the teeth or trauma to the mandibular mucosa beneath the tongue.

brachygnathism). The AVDC accepted term for this occlusion is *mandibular mesioclusion.*

Mandibular mesioclusion is an accepted breed standard of some breeds, including Boxers, Boston Terriers, Bulldogs, and Pugs. Therefore, brachycephalic breeds are referred to as a normal Class III occlusion.

A general understanding of these terms allows veterinary professionals and personnel to communicate with breeders and pet owners who may use lay or scientific terms to describe a malocclusion. A detailed study of occlusion is necessary before orthodontic treatment for pets or counseling breeders on the role of genetics in malocclusion is considered. Although the genetics of malocclusion in dogs and cats has not been fully elucidated, skeletal malocclusions (Class II to IV) are considered to be of genetic origin, and some Class I malocclusions (such as lance canines in Shetland Sheepdogs) are considered to have a genetic component.

The shape of a dog's or a cat's skull must be evaluated when a dental occlusion evaluation is performed. We recognize three types of skulls: brachycephalic, **mesaticephalic** (or **mesocephalic**), and **dolichocephalic.** Brachycephalic breeds

have a wide skull with a short maxilla. Examples of these breeds are Boxers, Bulldogs, and Persian cats. Mesaticephalic breeds have well-proportioned skull width and maxillary length. Examples include Beagles, Labrador Retrievers, and German Shepherd dogs. Dolichocephalic breeds have a narrow skull and a long maxilla; examples include Sight Hounds (Greyhound, Whippet) and Siamese cats.

Wry bite is a non-specific term for a form of unilateral maxillary-mandibular asymmetry wherein one segment of the jaw is disproportionate to the other segment (e.g., the left mandible is longer than the right mandible). The disproportionate jaw length can occur in the maxilla or the mandible, resulting in what appears to be a curvature of the jaw toward the shorter side.

Impressions and Models

Impressions and models are important in treatment planning of orthodontic disease and in creation of orthodontic devices and restorations. Veterinary technicians and dental assistants can play an important role in obtaining impressions and pouring stone models. Stone dental models also serve as a part of the medical record for documentation of the starting point and of treatment progress.

Alginate is the material that records the imprint of the teeth when full-mouth impressions are taken. The teeth should be cleaned before the impressions are taken. A dental impression tray of appropriate size is selected for the patient. The area of interest must fit into the tray without touching the sides of the tray, and the tray must completely cover the teeth. Impression trays for dogs and cats can be purchased or fabricated.

The jar of alginate should be agitated (fluffed) with the top on before use and should be allowed to sit for at least 5 minutes after agitation, so the dust will settle. Alternatively, a dustless alginate product is available. Level scoops contained within the jar of alginate are placed in a rubber mixing bowl. A proper scoop of alginate will be level on the surface and will not contain filling voids. Gently tap the scoop of alginate to eliminate any voids, and then level the surface with the blade of the alginate spatula (Figure 34-67).

Alginate spatulas have a wide blade that is used to blend alginate powder with water. A cylinder comes with the alginate to measure out the proper amount of water. The amount of alginate used is based on the size of the impression tray, and 8 to 12 scoops are usually necessary for a full-mouth impression of the maxilla or mandible. Water is added to the alginate all at once, and the spatula is used in a stirring action to wet the powder. Once the powder is wet, the wide blade is used to start spatulating. The bowl is held in the palm of the hand while the dominant hand works the spatula, smearing the alginate from one side of the bowl to the other in a back-and-forth motion. Once the alginate is mixed to the consistency of cake frosting, it is loaded into the impression tray with the spatula. The lips of the animal are held away from the teeth, and the tray is placed over the teeth. The tray should be held steady while the material sets. This takes about 5 minutes from the start of the mix. Cold water will increase the set time, and warm water will shorten the set time. The extra alginate around the rim of the impression tray can be touched periodically to determine when it is set. Once the material sets, it is similar to rubber and will not stick to the finger when touched. The impression tray and the alginate are then removed from the teeth in one quick pulling motion in the direction of the long axis of the teeth.

Once removed from the teeth, the impression should be inspected to ensure that the area of interest was adequately recorded (Figure 34-68). The material should then be rinsed off and wrapped in a moist paper towel until the stone can be poured into it. The sooner the stone is poured, the more accurate the impression will be, because alginate is susceptible to desiccation and overhydration. Most technicians pour the stone as soon as the animal is recovered from anesthesia or sooner.

Dental stone is used to make the positive image of the mouth. The stone comes in a powder form and is mixed with water. The powder can be weighed out and mixed with a specified volume of water. Experienced technicians can determine approximate amounts of water and stone powder by the thickness of the mix. A good mix will slowly run off the mixing blade when held above the bowl.

Once the stone is mixed, the bowl containing the stone is placed on the vibrator until all visible air bubbles have been released from the mixture. The alginate impression should be cleared of excess water by gently tapping or shaking it. The impression is then held on a laboratory vibrator while small amounts of stone are placed on the impression and are allowed to run into the teeth. This step is critical because if an air bubble gets trapped in the teeth, the stone model will be missing part of the tooth. The vibrator serves two purposes. First, it helps to remove bubbles from the stone, and second, it causes the stone to flow into the teeth. Once the teeth have been filled with stone, the rest of the stone can be added at a faster rate because this step is less critical. The stone mix can then be made thicker by adding more powder. This portion can be placed on the top of the model to give it a strong base. Optimal working time for the stone is about 10 minutes. Complete set of the stone takes about 1 to 2 hours.

The model should be removed from the alginate impression after the stone has had 45 to 60 minutes to set. An exothermic reaction will occur, causing the model to feel warm. The model can be separated once the stone has cooled. Do not wait several hours because the alginate will dry and will stick to the stone model. The model should be carefully pulled from the alginate and inspected to ensure that all teeth are adequately recorded. If a portion of a tooth is missing, this could be the result of an air bubble, or the tooth could have broken off and still remains in the impression. The canine teeth are particularly susceptible to fracture because of their long curved anatomy. If a tooth from the stone model breaks, it can be glued back onto the model. The model should then be labeled with the pet's name and the date.

Interceptive Orthodontics

Interceptive orthodontics involves the extraction of persistent deciduous or adult teeth that are causing or will cause problems associated with malocclusion (Figure 34-69). Interceptive orthodontics can be extremely beneficial, and abnormally erupting permanent teeth sometimes will correct

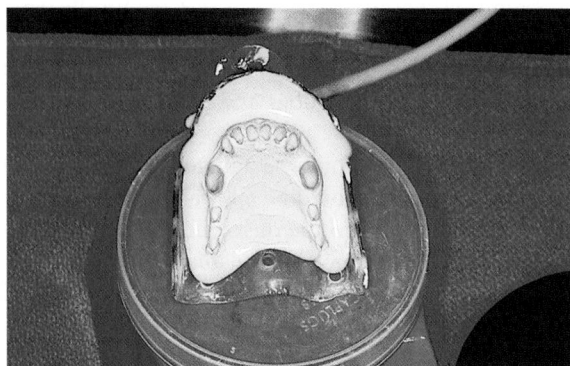

FIGURE 34-68 Alginate impression of the rostral maxilla is inspected and prepared for pouring of dental stone.

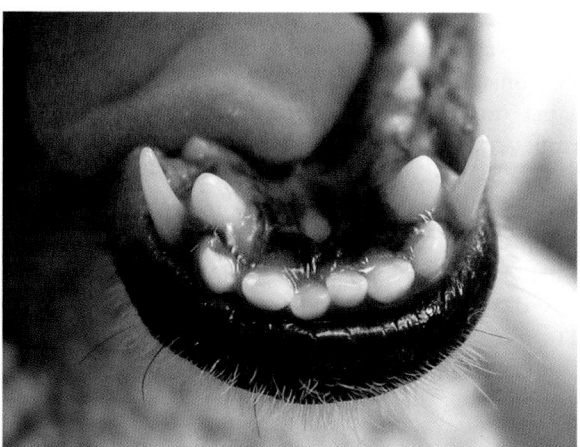

FIGURE 34-69 Persistent deciduous teeth may contribute to orthodontic (linguoverted or base-narrow permanent canine teeth) and periodontal problems.

after extraction of retained deciduous teeth. The most important factor determining success with this treatment is early detection of the problem. Many puppies and kittens have completed their vaccination series by the time they reach this mixed dentition stage and will not be seen again before spay or neuter unless a dental examination can be scheduled to ensure that early orthodontic problems do not go undetected.

Persistent deciduous teeth can occur in any breed of dog or cat, but they are seen most commonly in small breed dogs, such as Yorkshire Terriers, Poodles, and Dachshunds. Deciduous teeth should be shed before eruption of their permanent counterpart. When persistent (previously and mistakenly referred to as "retained") deciduous teeth are identified, they should be extracted before they cause misalignment of their permanent counterparts. Most permanent teeth will erupt lingual or palatal to the retained deciduous teeth, with one exception. Maxillary canine teeth erupt mesial to the persistent deciduous teeth. This is noteworthy because misalignment will decrease the space between the maxillary canine and the third incisor tooth, where the mandibular canine occludes. When this space is too narrow, one or both maxillary teeth will interfere with the mandibular canine tooth, and tooth wear (attrition) can occur.

Extraction of persistent deciduous teeth is a challenge because of their long, thin roots, which can fracture easily. The goal is to remove the entire tooth root to provide space into which the permanent tooth can move. The immature jaw contains numerous developing permanent tooth buds that can be damaged by dental elevators. Clients need to be cautioned about the possibility of permanent tooth damage or discoloration during extraction of deciduous teeth. A skilled veterinary dental surgeon can significantly minimize these complications.

Base-Narrow or In-Standing Mandibular Canine Teeth

Lingually displaced mandibular canine teeth may result from deciduous teeth that do not exfoliate properly, but other factors may play a role, including the genetics responsible for the development of normal mandibular width. These malocclusions can be corrected by orthodontics in most cases, but clients must be willing to invest the time and expense necessary to clean the oral appliance and return for rechecks as needed. Orthodontic treatment generally is more expensive than tooth extraction and involves additional anesthetic procedures. Orthodontics can be an important treatment option when alternatives to extraction of large teeth, such as canine teeth, are considered.

Crown height reduction, along with partial pulpectomy, and direct pulp capping under sterile conditions may be an option for animals with malocclusions. This combination of procedures entails shortening the tooth to remove the interference it is causing with another tooth or surrounding soft tissue. This method is less invasive than extraction, removes the animal's source of discomfort, and achieves results more rapidly than orthodontic movement. However, it does permanently alter the appearance and, to some degree, the function of the tooth. The pulp chamber is exposed when the crown is reduced, and a small percentage of these teeth may become nonvital after this procedure.

DENTAL TRAUMA

Dogs and cats can generate large quantities of biting, pulling, and grinding forces, and their teeth are often the recipients of dental trauma. This trauma can be exhibited as wear (attrition or abrasion), uncomplicated tooth fracture (no pulp exposure), or complicated fracture (pulp exposure).

Many dogs will cause severe abrasion of their teeth by chewing on inappropriate objects, such as rocks or fences. The teeth most commonly fractured are canines and maxillary fourth premolar teeth (see Figure 34-22, A). Attrition and abrasion usually occur on incisors and canines but can be seen on premolars and molars. If dental wear occurs slowly, odontoblasts will deposit tertiary (reparative) dentin within exposed dentinal tubules to prevent pulp exposure as enamel and dentin are lost. Tertiary dentin may be seen on the surface of worn teeth as a brown or black dot (see Figure 34-22, B). A dental explorer is dragged over the tooth surface to ensure that the pulp tissue is not exposed. When the pulp tissue is exposed, the tip of the dental explorer will fall into the pulp chamber as it crosses the surface of the tooth, whereas tertiary dentin feels smooth as glass with the explorer.

In acute fractures with pulp exposure, the tooth may bleed from the exposed pulp surface. If the tooth is treated within the first 48 hours, vital pulp therapy may be successful. This procedure involves removing the coronal pulp tissue (the pulp tissue in the tooth root remains), covering the pulp tissue with a medicament, and sealing the coronal exposure site with appropriate dental restorative materials.

All teeth with exposed pulp tissue should be treated with endodontic treatment (conventional root canal, vital pulp therapy) or by extraction. If left untreated, infection from the exposure site will spread to the periapical tissues, and a periapical abscess will develop over time. The client may notice ipsilateral facial swelling or a draining tract just below the medial canthus of the pet's eye (Figure 34-70, A and B). Most periapical abscesses will not form a fistula through the skin; this means that unless the teeth of these pets are examined for endodontic disease, many abscesses will go untreated. These abscesses can be painful and serve as a source of infection, which can spread to other areas of the body.

> **TECHNICIAN NOTE** A tooth with pulp exposure requires endodontic treatment or extraction. A "wait and see" approach is not appropriate because dogs and cats disguise their level of discomfort.

Discoloration is another sign of endodontic disease; it is commonly seen as a result of prior trauma to the pulp, resulting in pulpitis (Figure 34-71). Ninety-two percent of discolored teeth show evidence of partial or complete pulp

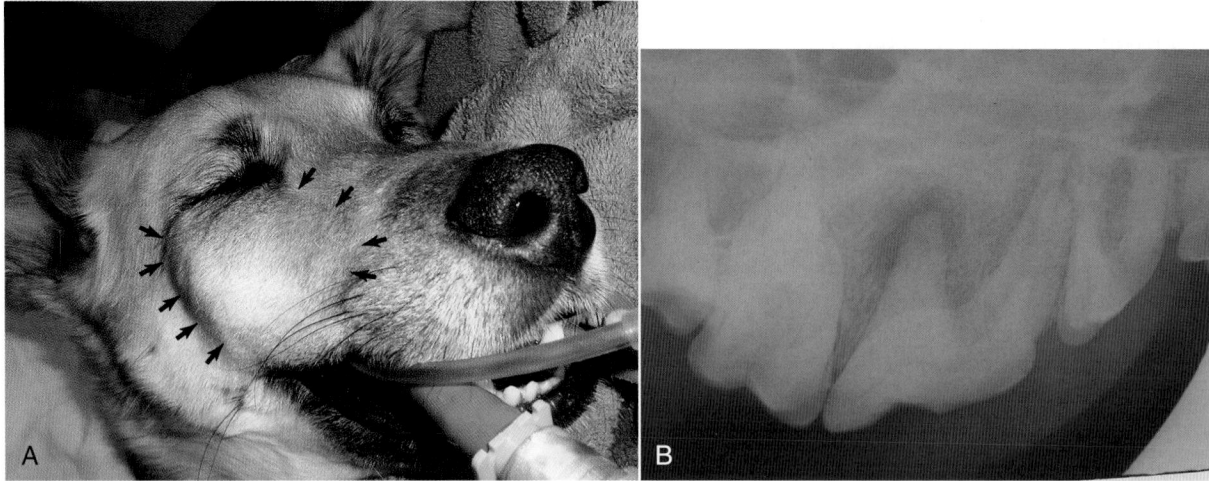

FIGURE 34-70 A, Facial swelling associated with a periapical abscess of the right maxillary fourth premolar tooth *(arrows)*. **B,** Radiograph shows severe periapical lucencies (bone loss at root tips as a result of infection).

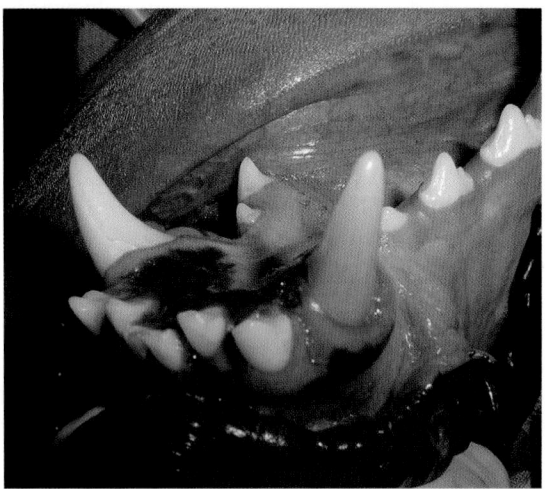

FIGURE 34-71 Discoloration of the left mandibular canine tooth from pulpitis (inflammation of the tooth often as a result of blunt trauma).

necrosis on exploratory pulpotomy. Because dogs and cats do not articulate their discomfort, evidence of pulpitis warrants endodontic or exodontic therapy to relieve possible pain in a tooth affected by pulpitis.

ORAL NEOPLASIA

Oral tumors account for only 6% of all cases of neoplasia in dogs and 3% to 12% in cats; these tumors are often aggressive, and prognosis depends on early detection. The most common oral tumor in cats is squamous cell carcinoma (SCC), which accounts for approximately 70% of all oral tumors in cats (Figure 34-72). If a cure for SCC is to be provided, early detection is particularly important in smaller patients (cats and small dogs) because of the need to obtain clean surgical margins while maintaining adequate function.

> **TECHNICIAN NOTE** Squamous cell carcinoma (SCC) accounts for approximately 70% of oral tumors in cats.

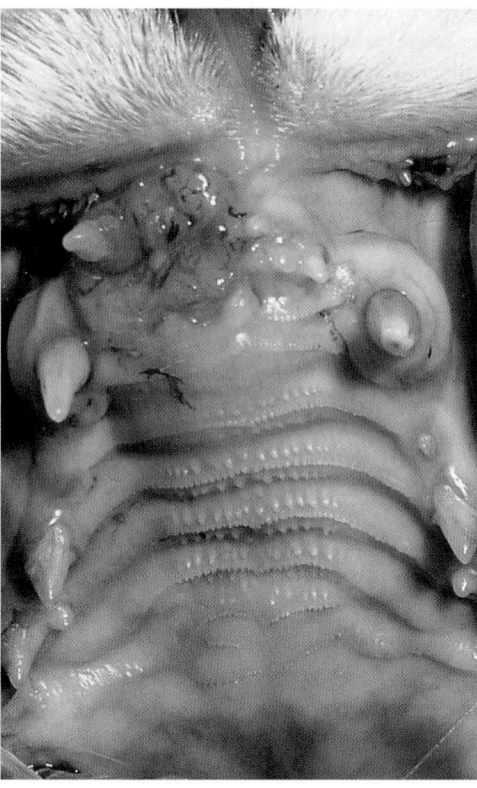

FIGURE 34-72 Squamous cell carcinoma (SCC) of the maxilla in a cat. SCC accounts for approximately 70% of oral tumors in cats.

In dogs, tumors may be benign or malignant. The most common benign tumor in dogs is a gingival tumor that in the past has been referred to as an *epulis* (plural: *epulides*). The epulides were categorized as fibromatous, ossifying, and acanthomatous; the latter is the most locally invasive. Fibromatous and ossifying epulides are also sometimes referred to as "peripheral odontogenic fibromas." Acanthomatous epulis is now referred to as canine acanthomatous ameloblastoma. Peripheral odontogenic fibromas do not typically invade bone and usually do not recur if the tooth of origin

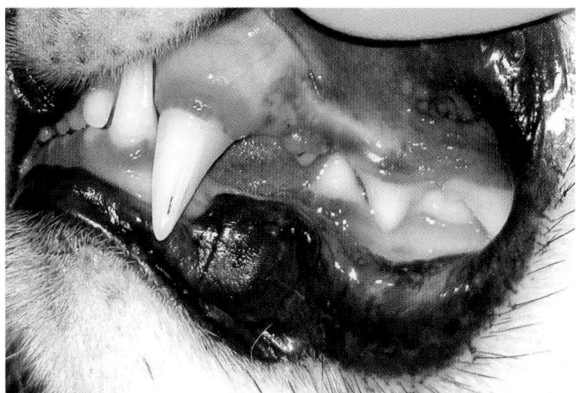

FIGURE 34-74 Stomatitis in a cat. Inflammation extends beyond the gingiva into the alveolar mucosa; often the buccal mucosa lateral to the palatoglossal folds is also inflamed.

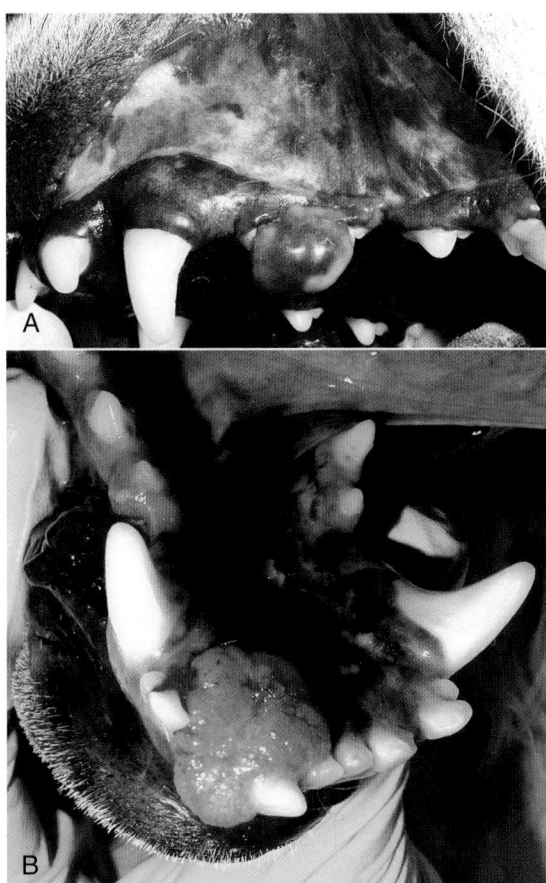

FIGURE 34-73 A, Peripheral odontogenic fibroma (also referred to as an *ossifying epulis*) in a dog. B, Acanthomatous ameloblastoma in a dog (previously referred to as *acanthomatous epulis*). Acanthomatous ameloblastoma is locally invasive but does not metastasize, making these patients good candidates for surgery if margins are attainable.

and its periodontal ligament are removed (Figure 34-73, *A*). Canine acanthomatous ameloblastoma requires removal of the tumor with a minimum of 1 cm of normal tissue in all directions to prevent recurrence (Figure 34-75, *B*). Most oral tumors are not entirely responsive to chemotherapy or radiation, but canine acanthomatous ameloblastoma often responds to radiation. Surgery (mandibulectomy or maxillectomy) is often the treatment of choice, however, because development of malignant tumors at the site of radiation has been reported with this tumor type.

The most common malignant oral tumors in dogs are malignant melanoma, SCC, fibrosarcoma, and osteosarcoma. These tumors are locally invasive and have the potential to metastasize to regional lymph nodes or to the lungs. After the patient is staged to determine the extent of disease, surgery or radiation is usually recommended to deal with the primary tumor, and metastases are dealt with by chemotherapy, radiation of metastatic nodes, or immunotherapy. Malignant melanoma may be pigmented or amelanotic. A vaccine that has been developed for treatment of dogs with malignant melanoma has shown increased survival times.

Dogs and cats that undergo radical maxillectomy and mandibulectomy for removal of an oral tumor generally function well postoperatively, and most clients are pleased with long-term quality of life and appearance. Cats recover more slowly from maxillectomy and mandibulectomy and often require placement of a feeding tube (usually an esophagostomy tube) during the recovery period, whereas dogs usually eat and drink within 24 hours after surgery.

STOMATITIS

Diffuse inflammation of the entire oral cavity is seen commonly in cats and occasionally in dogs. Inflammation confined to the gingiva is referred to as *gingivitis*. Inflammation that extends beyond the mucogingival junction is called *stomatitis* (Figure 34-74). Stomatitis may be due to a variety of causes, including ingestion of a caustic substance, uremia, viral exposure, plant foreign bodies, allergic response to drugs, and, most commonly, immune-mediated causes. Cats are often affected by a type of stomatitis referred to as *lymphocytic-plasmacytic stomatitis*, which can involve gingiva, alveolar mucosa, buccal mucosa, sublingual mucosa, and even the mucosa of the caudal oral cavity lateral to the palatoglossal folds. Cats often have decreased appetite or anorexia, halitosis, dehydration, and blood-tinged saliva.

The cause of LPS is not clear, but it appears that cats develop inappropriate inflammation in the presence of even small amounts of plaque accumulation. Many cats with LPS concurrently shed both herpesvirus and calicivirus. These viruses may have an effect on the immune system, resulting in an overzealous or deficient immune response to bacterial plaque. Therefore, plaque control in the form of frequent dental cleanings and home care is important. Unfortunately, many LPS cats are so painful that home care is not feasible. Immunosuppressive agents, such as corticosteroids and cyclosporine, help in many cases, but when medical therapy fails or causes unacceptable side effects, full-mouth extractions or nearly full-mouth extractions have been shown to provide resolution of oral discomfort in approximately 80% of cases. When seen in dogs, stomatitis may be due to autoimmune diseases, such as pemphigus vulgaris or bullous pemphigoid.

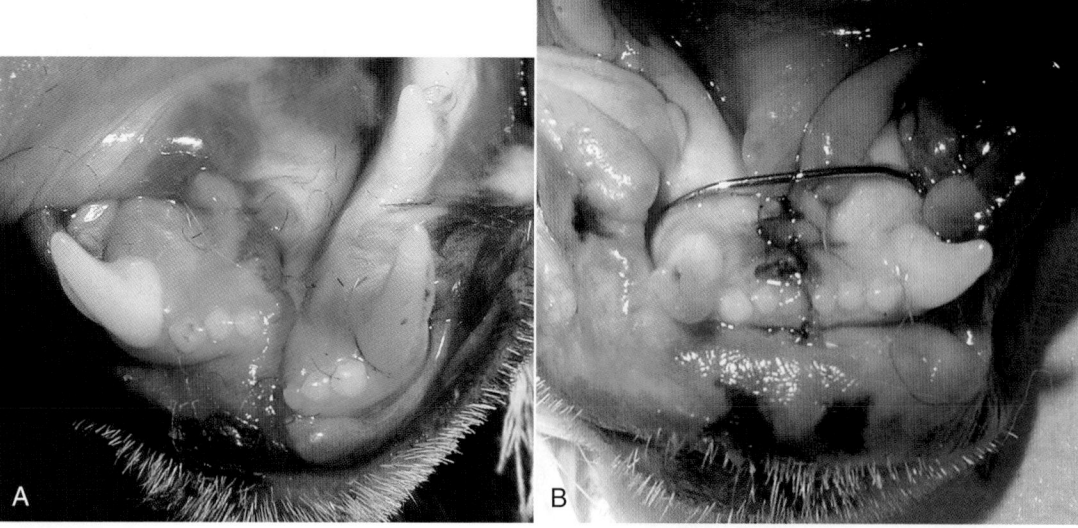

FIGURE 34-75 A, Photograph of a symphyseal separation in a cat. B, Photograph after repair with cerclage wire.

> 📎 *TECHNICIAN NOTE* Full-mouth extractions and nearly full-mouth extractions for treatment of feline stomatitis have been shown to provide resolution of oral discomfort in approximately 80% of cases.

MASTICATORY MYOSITIS

Masticatory myositis is an immune-mediated disease whereby the immune system forms antibodies toward a specific component of myosin found only in muscles of mastication. Patients affected by this disease may be seen in the acute phase of the disease, which is painful, or in the chronic phase of the disease, where much scarring has already taken place. Patients in the acute phase often d exhibit pain upon opening the mouth, decreased appetite, or dropping of food. They often have swelling of the temporal, masseter, and/or pterygoid muscles, which occasionally may also cause exophthalmos. Patients in the chronic phase often have severe temporal and masseter muscle atrophy and inability to open the mouth as a result of severe scar tissue formation. The goal is to diagnose the disease before these chronic changes occur because this condition is difficult to deal with in the chronic phase. A diagnosis is made by sending serum and muscle samples to the Comparative Neuromuscular Laboratory at the University of California, San Diego. Treatment at the acute phase involves a long, slow taper of oral corticosteroids, beginning at an immunosuppressive dose of 1 mg/kg twice daily. To prevent recurrence, some patients need to be taking some level of steroids for life.

JAW FRACTURES

Jaw fractures are common in dogs and cats with motor vehicle trauma, high-rise syndrome, or severe periodontal disease resulting in a pathologic fracture. Most jaw fractures benefit from some type of rigid fixation. One of the most common types of jaw trauma is a symphyseal separation, wherein the right and left mandibles separate at their rostral

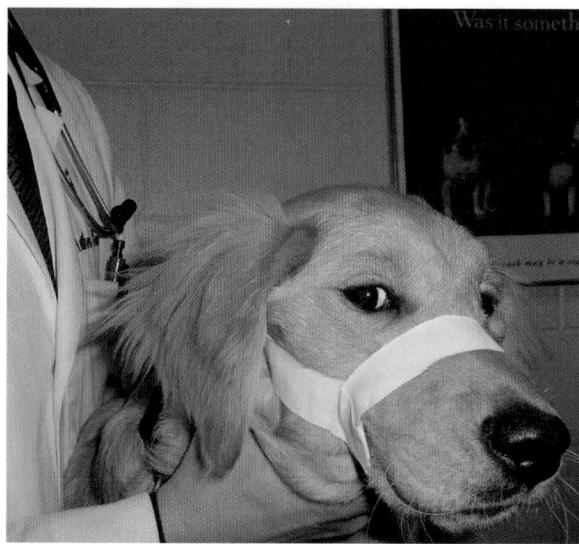

FIGURE 34-76 Tape muzzle for stabilization of a mandibular fracture in a young dog.

fibrous union, called the *symphysis*. A cerclage wire placed behind the canine teeth for no longer than 4 weeks provides stability while the symphysis heals (Figure 34-75, *A* and *B*).

More involved jaw fractures may be repaired with the use of interdental wire and acrylic composite, transosseous wiring, miniplates, external fixation, or maxillomandibular fixation. Sometimes teeth along the fracture line can be used as anchor points, but teeth affected by severe periodontal disease should be removed because the fracture likely will not heal when the diseased tooth acts as a nidus for infection.

Patients who present acutely with a mandibular fracture may benefit from placement of a tape muzzle (Figure 34-76) to stabilize the fracture until surgical treatment is performed. The tape muzzle is created using one piece of tape (adhesive side outward) around the muzzle itself, which is attached to a second piece that wraps around the head below the ears. The muzzle should be tight enough to minimize motion but loose enough to prevent irritation of the soft tissue, and to allow the tongue to move between the incisor teeth to allow for drinking and eating food of a slurry consistency. Tape muzzles are sometimes considered the definitive treatment of choice in young patients for whom rigid fixation may adversely affect growth of the healing mandible.

> **TECHNICIAN NOTE** Tape muzzles are often used as the definitive treatment of mandibular fractures in puppies because rigid fixation may arrest growth of the mandible.

EQUINE DENTISTRY

DENTAL ANATOMY AND PHYSIOLOGY

Horses have 24 deciduous teeth and 36 to 44 permanent teeth, depending on the presence or absence of canine and first premolar teeth. At eruption, the occlusal surfaces of equine teeth are fully covered by cementum, compared with dogs and cats, in which cementum covers only the root. Beneath the crown cementum, a thin layer of crown enamel is present. Both of these layers get worn away, exposing an intricate, wavy combination of cementum, dentin, and enamel on the occlusal surface. Equine mandibular incisor teeth develop features of their occlusal surface that have been traditionally used to estimate age. However, because much variation is seen in the rate of tooth wear based on breed, type of food, and environment, the age of the horse determined via this technique is an estimate at best. Eruption times provide the most accurate method of determining age but can be used only in horses that have not erupted their complete permanent dentition. Of all changes on the occlusal surface of the incisors, the appearance of the dental star is one of the more reliable features. The dental star is composed of dentin, and the position of the star moves from the lingual edge of the occlusal surface to the center as the horse ages. Galvayne's groove, a groove that appears on the labial surface of the third incisor in some horses older than age 10, was once considered to be an excellent method of aging horses between 10 and 30 years of age. It has since been determined that its presence is inconsistent and is of little value in determining the age of a horse.

The canine teeth are usually absent or rudimentary in female horses, but males typically have four permanent canine teeth that erupt at 4 to 6 years of age in the **diastema** between the incisors and the cheek teeth. The permanent first premolars, which are referred to as "wolf teeth," are much smaller and located rostral to the other premolars. The first premolar has no deciduous precursor. Wolf teeth are present in 24.4% of female and 14.9% of male horses. Wolf teeth occur more commonly on the maxilla. These teeth are often extracted because of concern for causing oral discomfort, especially when the bit contacts the tooth. The premolars and molars are collectively referred to as the

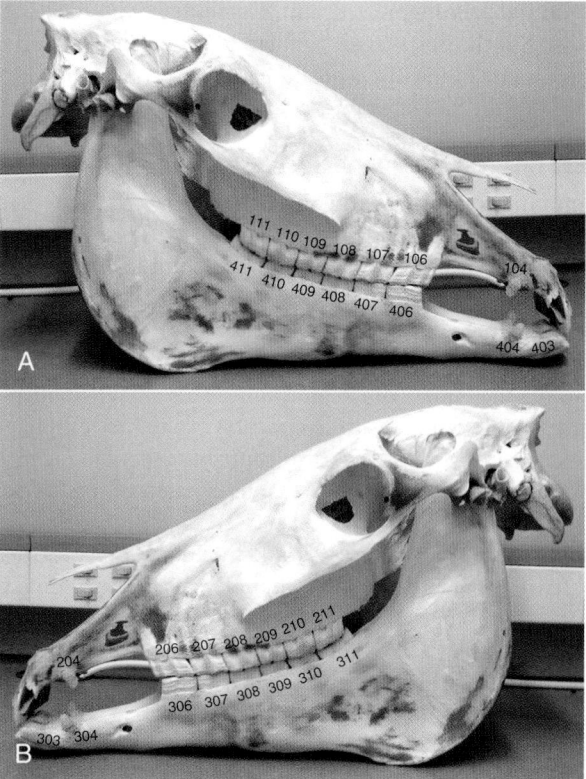

FIGURE 34-77 Skull of a horse showing the Triadan tooth numbering system. **A**, Right side. **B**, Left side. Wolf teeth, when present, end in the numbers "05."

"cheek teeth." Not including the wolf teeth, each quadrant should contain six cheek teeth (second, third, and fourth premolars, and first, second, and third molars). A numbering system has been developed for equine teeth that is based on the Triadan system (Figure 34-77, *A* and *B*). The cheek teeth are closely arranged with no spaces in between them, so the six teeth in one quadrant function as a single unit. The occlusal surfaces of the cheek teeth have many grooves and ridges composed of enamel, cementum, and dentin, which provide varied surfaces for grinding of food material. The upper jaw is wider than the lower jaw—a condition referred to as *anisognathism*. The occlusal surface is normally angled at 10 to 15 degrees in a downward slope toward the buccal aspect of the teeth. In horses with painful dental disease or in those fed an inappropriate diet (too little forage), this angle may be increased, resulting in more vertical angulation of the occlusal surface. This condition is termed *shear mouth*.

In horses, the left and right mandibles are not separated by a symphysis as in dogs and cats. The mandibles fuse at the midline at approximately 3 months of age in the horse. In contrast to carnivores, the TMJ is designed for horizontal movement, and the muscles necessary to provide this movement are more developed. Dogs and cats have large temporal muscles on the top of their head that provide strength in vertical movement of the mandible, whereas horses have well-developed masseter and pterygoid muscles that allow horizontal grinding movement. Horses have well-developed muscles of the lips that allow them to prehend food, and the commissure of the lips is positioned rostrally, making examination of the caudal cheek teeth challenging.

DENTAL EXAMINATION AND IMAGING

Common presenting problems of horses with severe dental disease include weight loss, dropping of food (quidding), head shaking, and tilting of the head during mastication. Routine oral examinations are helpful in detecting dental abnormalities at early stages. Dental disease interferes with normal mastication, resulting in larger feed particle size at the time of deglutition. This may predispose horses and donkeys to impaction colic or esophageal choke. Dental disease may also contribute to systemic infection as a result of hematogenous spread of periodontal pathogens.

Extraoral examination should include observation for evidence of facial swelling, atrophy of masticatory muscles, and the presence of ocular, nasal, or oral discharge. The patient's stable floor should be evaluated for evidence of quidding, such as dropped grain and partially chewed boluses. Feces should be evaluated for particle size because large stems of hay and whole grain indicate incomplete mastication. Young horses between 2.5 and 4 years of age will have symmetric, nonpainful bony enlargement of the mandible and/or maxilla associated with eruption of the permanent cheek teeth. Sharp points of the buccal surface of the maxillary teeth may be palpable extraorally. Palpation may cause the horse to resist if points are present. They should be removed before placement of a full-mouth speculum because the cheeks will be pushed tightly against the points once the mouth is opened. Observe the lips for evidence of ulcers, tumors, or bit injuries, especially in the area of the commissure.

Thorough examination of the oral cavity of the horse requires sedation. A self-supporting mouth speculum, a strong light source, a dental mirror, and long-handled dental picks are helpful in assessing hard and soft tissue structures and in removing food material from areas of interest. Intraoral cameras are available to provide visualization and magnification of difficult areas. Skull radiographs are helpful in diagnosing subgingival abnormalities (Figure 34-78). Various views, including lateral, lateral oblique, dorsoventral, open- and closed-mouth views, may be necessary. A radiopaque object (such as a needle or a gutta percha point) placed in the center of a facial swelling or draining tract before a radiograph is taken may help to reveal the tooth of origin.

As a result of the large patient size, small film size, and limited intraoral access, intraoral dental radiography is limited to use in imaging of the incisor teeth. If skull radiographs do not show obvious pathologic conditions in a case in which dental disease is suspected, other imaging techniques, including nuclear scintigraphy, computed tomography (CT), and magnetic resonance imaging (MRI), may be options.

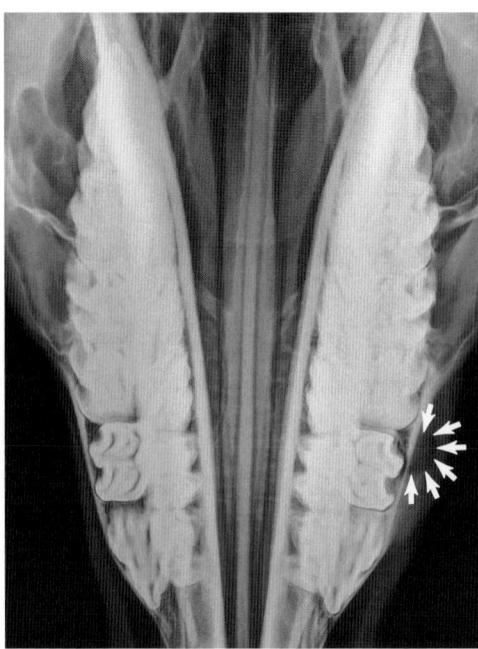

FIGURE 34-78 Radiograph of a horse with facial swelling caused by a periapical abscess. Arrows point to bone loss associated with an infected maxillary third premolar.

COMMON DENTAL PROBLEMS OF HORSES

Endodontic abnormalities occur as a result of disease of the inner chamber of the tooth, which is most commonly seen in the form of a tooth root abscess. Tooth root abscesses occur as a result of exposure of the pulp to the oral environment or death of a tooth with hematogenous spread of bacteria to the compromised site. Pulp exposure may occur as a result of tooth fracture, excessive wear, or decay. Tooth root abscesses may cause a large swelling of the surrounding bone and soft tissue.

The caudal maxillary tooth roots (fourth premolar and first, second, and third molar) are located just ventral to the maxillary sinus, so infection of any of these teeth may lead to sinusitis and chronic unilateral nasal discharge. Infection caused by a tooth root abscess will not permanently resolve with administration of antibiotics, although antibiotics may provide temporary improvement. Extraction or endodontic therapy is necessary for long-term success. Extraction is often difficult because of limited access and the large amount of subgingival tooth structure. Cheek teeth often are approached through an extraoral technique. Although incisors, wolf teeth, and canines can usually be extracted via an intraoral technique, cheek teeth most often need to be approached by buccotomy or repulsion.

Orthodontic abnormalities refers to those abnormalities of occlusion (the normal spatial relationship of teeth and jaws) caused by abnormal development, eruption, or wear. Mandibular brachygnathism (or mandibular distoclusion) is a developmental disorder in which the lower jaw is relatively shorter than the upper jaw. A common term for this condition is "parrot mouth." One goal of treatment is to prevent or minimize the degree of abnormal tooth wear that can

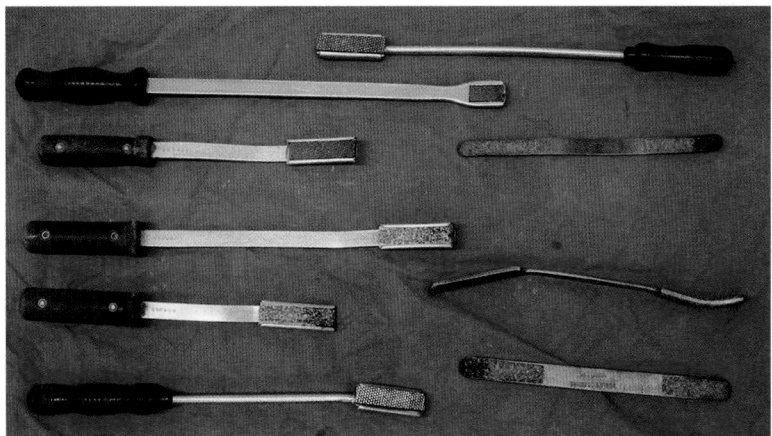

FIGURE 34-79 Various dental floats used for occlusal equilibration in horses.

occur from malocclusion. Orthodontic procedures can be performed to prevent or correct ventral deviation of the incisive bone and upper incisors, and to attempt to overcome the jaw length discrepancy early in life while growth is still occurring. The opposite of parrot mouth is referred to as "monkey mouth"; this occurs when the maxilla is relatively shorter than the mandible (resulting from maxillary brachygnathism or mandibular mesioclusion). This condition is seen most commonly in miniature horses.

Horses with jaw length discrepancies require more frequent occlusal adjustments, but any horse should be evaluated at least yearly for abnormal wear patterns. *Floating* is the term used to describe the process of mechanically adjusting the occlusal surfaces of the teeth. Flat files (floats), which are available in hand and electrically driven versions, are used to remove raised areas, such as hooks, ramps, or points (Figure 34-79). Removal or loss of a tooth can result in drift of adjacent teeth into the vacancy, leading to abnormal occlusion patterns. Similarly, the tooth from the opposing arcade may overgrow into this void as a result of lack of normal wear. Patients with these problems will require more frequent examinations and occlusal equilibrations as necessary (Box 34-12).

Another orthodontic problem seen in foals is wry nose. Wry nose is a deviation of the incisive bone, maxilla, and nasal septum laterally from the midline. Affected foals may have difficulty suckling or prehending forage, and dyspnea resulting from deviation of the nasal septum can be so severe that a tracheostomy may be necessary. This is believed to be a hereditary condition most commonly seen in Arabians and miniature horses. Orthognathic surgical correction often requires two separate surgeries and usually is attempted between 5 and 7 months of age.

Periodontal abnormalities refers to loss of or damage to the attachment structures of the teeth, which consist of the periodontal ligament, cementum, alveolar bone, and gingival connective tissue. Gingivitis is one of the earliest signs of periodontal disease; the gingiva may appear hyperemic, edematous, and bleeding more readily than normal. Gingival recession may be seen, or, alternatively, loss of periodontal

---

BOX 34-12 | Suggested Schedule for Routine Dental Examination of Horses

- *Birth:* Examine for malocclusions and congenital defects affecting the tongue, lips, and palate.
- *6 to 8 months:* Examine for eruption of incisors, check occlusion, remove sharp points or hooks if present (float teeth).
- *16 to 24 months:* Examine for presence of wolf teeth, ulcers, points, or hooks; float if necessary.
- *2 to 3 years:* Examine for presence of wolf teeth, bit injuries, deciduous eruption, points, or hooks. Remove wolf teeth; float if necessary.
- *3 to 4 years:* Examine size and shape of jaws; check for retained third premolars, blind wolf teeth, bit injuries, points, or hooks. Remove wolf teeth, caps; float if necessary.
- *4 to 5 years:* Examine all teeth for proper eruption, occlusion, and presence of cysts; remove deciduous teeth and hooks; float if necessary. Remove tissue of cyst structure if present.
- *5 years +:* Evaluate jaw excursion; examine mouth for hooks, abnormal wear patterns, periodontal disease, dental decay. Correct uneven wear patterns, float teeth; shorten incisors if necessary.

Adapted from Easley KJ: Equine dental development and anatomy, Proc Am Assoc Equine Pract 42:1, 1996.

---

ligament attachment may result in development of a periodontal pocket. Although the cause of periodontal disease in horses is similar to that described for dogs and cats earlier in this chapter, treatment is challenging because of limited accessibility of the cheek teeth of horses. The tooth-cleansing process associated with mastication of abrasive substances is an important part of keeping teeth periodontally sound. Therefore, any dental pathologic condition, such as abnormal wear and oral ulceration, should be corrected to prevent preferential use of certain teeth and disuse of others. Depending on their accessibility, deep periodontal pockets may be débrided and lavaged. Off-label use of a canine doxycycline gel (Doxirobe) has been described to deal with periodontally affected teeth that have not lost enough attachment to require extraction. Teeth with severe attachment loss and mobility require extraction.

Cemental hypoplasia is a developmental abnormality that can occur in all equine teeth and may predispose maxillary cheek teeth to endodontic disease, tooth fracture, abnormal occlusal patterns, and caries. Caries are a result of tooth decay caused by bacterial fermentation of food. When a carious lesion occurs within the infundibulum (the infoldings of the occlusal surface of incisors and cheek teeth) of a tooth, this is referred to as *infundibular decay*. Restoration of these lesions with composite filling material has been advocated by some equine dentists, but treatment is controversial.

> **TECHNICIAN NOTE** Infundibular decay in horses is most likely to affect the maxillary first molar tooth.

RECOMMENDED READINGS

Baker GJ, Easley J: Equine dentistry, ed 2, Philadelphia, 2005, Elsevier.

Beckman B, Legendre L: Regional nerve blocks for oral surgery in companion animals, Compend Cont Educ Pract Vet 24:439, 2002.

Bellows J: Small animal dental equipment, materials and techniques: a primer, Ames, IA, 2004, Blackwell.

DuPont GA, DeBowes LJ: Atlas of dental radiography in dogs and cats, St Louis, 2009, Saunders.

Harvey CE, Emily PP: Small animal dentistry, Philadelphia, 1993, Mosby.

Holmstrom SE: Veterinary dentistry for the technician & office staff, Philadelphia, 2000, Saunders.

Holmstrom SE: Veterinary dentistry: a team approach, St Louis, 2013, Elsevier Saunders.

Mulligan TW, Aller MS, Williams CA: Atlas of canine & feline dental radiography, Yardley, PA, 1998, Veterinary Learning Systems.

Nield-Gehrig JS: Fundamentals of periodontal instrumentation, ed 6, Baltimore, 2008, Lippincott Williams & Wilkins.

Niemiec BA: A color handbook of small animal dental, oral and maxillofacial disease, London, UK, 2010, Manson.

Reiter AR, Lewis JR, Okuda A: Update on the etiology of tooth resorption in the domestic cat, Vet Clin North Am Small Anim Pract 35:913, 2005.

Torres HO, Ehrlich A, Bird D: Essentials of dental assisting, ed 2, Philadelphia, 1996, Saunders.

Verstraete FJM: Self-assessment colour review of veterinary dentistry, London, UK, 1999, Manson Publishing.

Wiggs RB, Lobprise HB: Veterinary dentistry: principles and practice, Philadelphia, 1997, Lippincott-Raven.

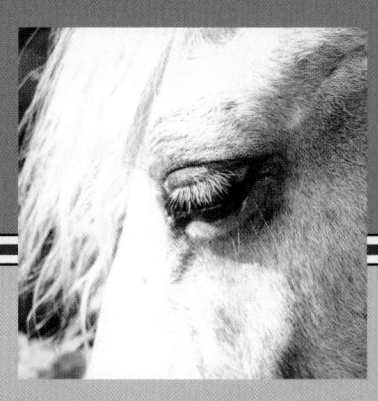

35 Geriatric and Hospice Care: Supporting the Aged and Dying Patient

Karen Todd-Jenkins and Amy I. Bentz

KEY TERMS

Geriatric
Hirsutism
Hospice
Incontinence

OUTLINE

GERIATRIC CATS AND DOGS, *1357*
Life Stages Guidelines, *1357*
Integrating Geriatric Care, *1357*
Common Problems in Aging Pets, *1358*
Oral Problems, *1360*
Cardiac Disease, *1360*
Respiratory Disease, *1360*
Neoplasia, *1360*
Kidney Disease, *1360*
Urinary and Fecal Incontinence, *1360*
Neurologic Abnormalities, *1360*
Orthopedic Disease, *1361*
Endocrine Conditions, *1361*
**Changing Nutritional Needs of Aging
 Pets,** *1361*
**Hospice Care for the Aged and Dying Cat
 and Dog,** *1363*
Pain Medications, *1363*
Nursing Care for the Hospice Patient, *1363*
Decubital Ulcers, *1364*
Subcutaneous Fluids, *1364*
Expressing Bladders, *1364*
Urine Scalding, *1365*
Appetite Stimulants, *1365*
Feeding Tubes, *1365*
Carts and Slings, *1366*
**When Is the Right Time for
 Euthanasia?** *1366*

GERIATRIC HORSES, *1368*
Physical Examination, *1368*
Common Problems in Aging Horses, *1368*
Oral and Nasal Health, *1368*
Vision, *1369*
Cardiac Disease, *1370*
Respiratory Disease, *1370*
Gastrointestinal Disease, *1370*
Kidney Disease, *1370*
Skin Disorders, *1370*
Neurologic Abnormalities, *1370*
Orthopedic Disease, *1370*
**Chronic Diseases of the Geriatric
 Horse,** *1371*
Equine Cushing's Disease (Pituitary Pars
 Intermedia Dysfunction), *1371*
Heaves (Recurrent Airway
 Obstruction), *1372*
Laminitis (Founder), *1373*
Dental Problems and Sinusitis, *1374*
Equine Recurrent Uveitis (ERU, or Moon
 Blindness), *1374*
Neurologic Deficits, *1374*
Musculoskeletal System, *1374*
**Management, Nutrition, and Nursing Care
 of the Geriatric Horse,** *1375*
End of Life Issues, *1375*

LEARNING OBJECTIVES

When you have completed this chapter, you will be able to:
1. Pronounce, define, and spell all Key Terms in the chapter.
2. List the life stages of dogs and cats, and describe the effects of aging on body systems.
3. Identify and explain the oral, cardiac, respiratory, orthopedic, renal, neoplastic, neurologic, and endocrine disorders commonly seen in geriatric dogs and cats.

*The authors and publisher wish to acknowledge the contributions of Tara K. Trotman, whose work
served as a foundation for this chapter.*

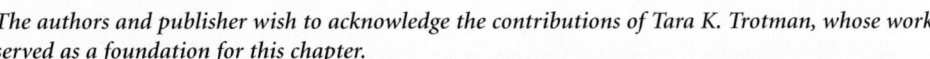

4. Explain the changing nutritional needs of aging pets.
5. Discuss components of hospice nursing care for geriatric dogs and cats, including how to identify the appropriate time to discuss euthanasia with a pet's owner.
6. Discuss components of the physical examination of a geriatric horse.
7. List and describe disorders commonly seen in geriatric horses, including oral/nasal, vision, cardiac, respiratory, gastrointestinal, kidney, skin, neurologic, and orthopedic problems.
8. Identify and explain the chronic conditions that most commonly affect geriatric horses such as equine Cushing's disease, heaves, laminitis, dental problems and sinusitis, equine recurrent uveitis (ERU), and neurologic and musculoskeletal defects.
9. Discuss the management, nutrition, and nursing care of geriatric horses, including end of life issues.

INTRODUCTION

The term **geriatric** is used to describe "a branch of medicine that deals with the problems and diseases of old age." With the advances we have seen in veterinary medicine, the number of geriatric pets is growing. Not only is pet ownership at an all-time high, but dogs, cats, and horses are living longer as a result of our ability to understand and treat diseases.

Hospice, or hospice care, is defined as "a facility or program designed to provide a caring environment for meeting the physical and emotional needs of the terminally ill." Because of the rise in the number of geriatric pets combined with the increased commitment that owners feel toward their pets, the need for "hospice care" is increasing. As members of the veterinary community, it is our job to provide relief to animals that suffer and to ensure a good quality of life for geriatric pets. One must be aware, however, that it is also our duty to provide support when it is time to end the suffering of dying patients via euthanasia. Pet owners often rely on veterinary personnel to help them make the difficult decision to euthanize their pet.

Routine preventive health programs should be followed for all patients (see Chapter 8), but this is especially important for geriatric pets. The effects of aging in animals are similar to those in people and include overall deterioration in physical and mental condition, organ function, and immunity. Although it is important to treat conditions once they become apparent, it is equally important to teach owners about how to recognize early signs of disease. Early identification and treatment of disease can dramatically improve quality of life and can increase longevity for geriatric patients.

The purpose of this chapter is to present common health problems of geriatric cats, dogs, and horses, and to give some specific nursing techniques that support the chronically ill or recumbent patient. In addition, this chapter describes techniques for supporting owners who are facing the end of their pet's life.

TECHNICIAN NOTE Companion animals are considered by many pet owners to be part of the family. Pets are living longer due to advances in veterinary medicine, and special needs must be taken into account for the geriatric patient.

Geriatric Cats and Dogs

LIFE STAGES GUIDELINES

A lifetime incorporates the sum of the various life stages of dogs and cats. Age by itself is not a disease, but understanding the changing physiologic functioning of aging pets requires an appreciation of the effect that aging has on body systems. Aging is a continuum, so although organized veterinary medicine has attempted to categorize life stages, these categories should be considered estimations. General health, size, breed variations, and other factors affect life expectancy and how quickly animals age. Refer to Box 35-1 for a list of the recognized life stages in dogs and cats.

INTEGRATING GERIATRIC CARE

Care for aging dogs and cats consists of a proactive comprehensive health care program that addresses the older animal's special needs. This specialized medical service is based on two premises: first, fundamental differences in specific diseases, behavior traits, and nutritional needs are seen in the older animal; second, prevention, early detection, and timely intervention for medical problems can have a significant impact on the life span and quality of life of an older dog or cat.

Care for older dogs and cats should incorporate owner education, disease prevention strategies, and detection of medical and behavioral problems at the earliest possible stage, when the prognosis may be more favorable and treatment options are likely to be more numerous. The term "senior" or "geriatric" describes the life stage of progressive decline in physical condition, organ function, sensory function, mental function, and immunity. Although it is generally accepted that the senior life stage begins around 7 years of age for the average dog or cat, several interrelated factors, including size and individual genetics, may affect the onset and rate of this progressive decline. Refer to Box 35-2 for a list of age-related changes in the body.

Starting at 7 years, many veterinarians recommend routine physical examination of healthy animals on a twice-a-year basis and advocate routine diagnostic screening for developing diseases. For patients with chronic illnesses, more frequent examinations and diagnostic assessment may be warranted.

BOX 35-1 | Life Stages for Dogs and Cats

- Cats
  - Pediatric: Birth-6 months
  - Young adult: 7 months-6 years
  - Mature adult: 7-10 years
  - Senior: 11-14 years
  - Geriatric: 15 years and older
- Dogs (general)
  - Pediatric: Birth-6 months
  - Young adult: 7 months-5 years
  - Mature adult: 6-9 years
  - Senior: 9-12 years
  - Geriatric: 12 years and older
- Dogs (large and giant breed)
  - Pediatric: Birth-6 months
  - Young adult: 7 months-2 years
  - Mature adult: 3-5 years
  - Senior: 6-9 years
  - Geriatric: 9 years and older

BOX 35-2 | Common Effects of Aging

Metabolic Effects
- Decreased metabolic rate plus lack of activity decreases caloric needs by 30% to 40%.
- Immune competence decreases, despite normal numbers of lymphocytes.
- Phagocytosis and chemotaxis decrease, and older animals are less able to ward off infection.
- Autoantibodies and immune-mediated diseases develop.

Physical Effects
- Percentage of body weight that is represented by fat increases.
- Skin becomes thickened, hyperpigmented, and inelastic.
- Foot pads become hyperkeratinized, and claws become brittle.
- Muscle, bone, and cartilage mass are lost, with subsequent development of osteoarthritis.
- Dental calculus results in tooth loss and gingival hyperplasia (see Figure 32-34).
- Periodontitis results in gingival retraction and atrophy.
- Gastric mucosa becomes atrophic and fibrotic.
- Hepatocyte numbers are decreased, and hepatic fibrosis occurs.
- Pancreatic enzyme secretion is diminished.
- Lungs lose elasticity, fibrosis occurs, and pulmonary secretions become more viscous. Vital capacity is decreased.
- Cough reflex and expiratory capacity are decreased.
- Kidney weight is decreased, glomerular filtration rate is decreased, and tubules atrophy.
- Urinary incontinence frequently develops.
- Prostate gland is enlarged, testes atrophy, and the prepuce becomes pendulous.
- Ovaries are enlarged, and mammary glands become fibrocystic or neoplastic.
- Cardiac output is decreased, and valvular fibrosis and intramural coronary arteriosclerosis develop.
- Bone marrow becomes fatty and hypoplastic, and nonregenerative anemia develops.
- The number of cells in the nervous system is decreased. Senility causes loss of house training.

COMMON PROBLEMS IN AGING PETS

Conditions that occur commonly in our aging pet population include oral health abnormalities, vision loss, hearing loss, cardiac disease, respiratory disease, neoplasia, kidney disease, urinary and fecal incontinence, dermatologic disease, orthopedic disease, and metabolic conditions. It is important for owners to be aware of these issues and to seek veterinary attention if any of them should arise. It is equally important for members of the veterinary community to question owners closely regarding their pet's health status, so that early detection of disease is possible.

Frequently, ill geriatric animals have vague symptoms, including inappetence, lethargy, and weight loss. Therefore, it is important to acquire a thorough history from owners and to perform a complete physical examination with routine screening tests. Refer to Tables 35-1 and 35-2 for a list of key points to address when carrying out nursing

TABLE 35-1	Nursing Assessment of the Geriatric Cat and Dog: Medical History

Providing adequate nursing care for geriatric or hospice cats and dogs requires periodic assessments. The frequency of assessments should be determined in part by the pet's current condition, an understanding of potential complications associated with the patient's illnesses, and an appreciation for medication side effects or monitoring considerations. Assessments can be performed daily, weekly, monthly, or on a flexible schedule. Whether the veterinary technician is assessing a hospitalized patient, evaluating a pet during an outpatient appointment, or conducting a home visit for a hospice patient, the key points to address during an assessment are similar.

MEDICAL HISTORY	WHAT TO ASK THE OWNER	OBJECTIVES AND CONSIDERATIONS
Appetite and bowel movements	• "What are you feeding your pet?" • "How much are you feeding?" • "How often is the pet eating?" • "Is the pet eating normal amounts?" • "Has he/she eaten today? If so, when? If not, when was the last meal?" • "Has there been any vomiting or diarrhea?" • "When was the most recent bowel movement?" • "Have the stools been normal in appearance and frequency?" • "Have you noticed any straining or other changes in defecation?"	Simply asking "Is the pet eating" will likely yield inadequate information. Asking more specific questions can facilitate a more productive discussion.
Drinking and urination	• "Is the pet drinking any more or less than usual?" • "Is fresh water available at all times?" • "How often do you change or freshen the pet's water?" • "Have there been any changes in urination (amount, effort, or frequency)?"	Considerations are the same as with eating. If any changes in appetite or drinking are noted, try to determine when the change occurred and whether something could have precipitated the change (e.g., a new medication, a diet change).
Activity level	• "Have there been any changes in the pet's attitude or activity level?" • "Are you happy with the pet's current activity level?"	Lethargy may go unnoticed by some pet owners. Others may note decreased activity but dismiss it as simply "slowing down" or "getting old." Although pets do become less active with age, sudden changes in activity level should be investigated.
Interactions with the family	• "Does the pet seem to be interacting in his/her customary way?" • "If not, what is the pet doing that is different?"	Some pets hide or become detached when they are not feeling well, whereas other pets may become "clingy" and may demand more attention from the owner. Sudden changes in interactions with other pets or family members could indicate a problem.
Medication administration	• "Are you having any problems with your pet's medication?" • "How does he/she seem to be tolerating the medication?" • "Do you remember what side effects to watch for?"	Review the list of medications the pet is supposed to be receiving, and make sure the dosages are correct. Ask the owner about side effects. Many pet owners may not be fully aware of medication side effects or other things to watch for after a pet begins a new medication. For pets that are receiving injections (such as insulin or subcutaneous fluids), observe the owner administering the injection. This can be a good way to make sure the procedure is being done properly.

TABLE 35-1	Nursing Assessment of the Geriatric Cat and Dog: Medical History—cont'd	
MEDICAL HISTORY	**WHAT TO ASK THE OWNER**	**OBJECTIVES AND CONSIDERATIONS**
General owner feedback	• "Is there anything new that you would like to bring to the doctor's attention?" • "Do you have any additional questions or concerns that we haven't addressed?"	Even the most thorough medical history is improved when pet owners get a chance to address their personal concerns. When possible, owners should be provided an opportunity to ask general questions and to provide their own feedback on the pet's condition and behavior at home.

TABLE 35-2	Nursing Assessment of the Geriatric Cat and Dog: Physical Assessment	
PHYSICAL ASSESSMENT	**WHAT TO CHECK**	**OBJECTIVES AND CONSIDERATIONS**
Vital signs	Temperature, pulse, respiration, blood pressure (if recommended)	Vital signs (especially blood pressure) should be checked when the patient is minimally stressed. Depending on the pet, this may be at the beginning of the appointment or at the end (after the pet has gotten used to new people and started to settle down).
Hydration status	Mucous membrane color and capillary refill time, skin turgor	Pet owners may assume that if a pet seems to be drinking (especially drinking more, as with diabetes, kidney disease, or feline hyperthyroidism) that dehydration should not be possible. Owners may need help understanding that their pet's illnesses may be affecting his/her ability to maintain adequate hydration. If dehydration becomes a concern, subcutaneous fluid injections can be helpful.
Pain	Increased pulse rate; increased respiratory rate; changes in mobility, body posture, or attitude; vocalization; changes in grooming habits; and changes in appetite or drinking are just a few indicators of pain.	Pain assessment (especially chronic pain) can be subjective and difficult to quantify. When in doubt about whether to provide pain medication, it is recommended to err on the side of caution and presume that a pet may be painful even if this cannot be confirmed.
Cardiorespiratory system	Thoracic auscultation to assess heart rate and rhythm, to detect heart murmurs, or to assess pulmonary sounds	Respiratory distress can be subtle, and pet owners can easily overlook minor changes in breathing effort.
Abdomen	Abdominal palpation to assess for pain, distention	Abdominal palpation may be limited in pets that are obese, but gentle palpation to assess for pain or distention is recommended.
Body condition	If possible, patients should be weighed at each assessment. Standardized body condition scoring charts can be incorporated into this evaluation. A chart is available at http://vet.osu.edu/vmc/body-condition-scoring-chart.	Weight loss or gain can be easy to overlook. If practical, owners should weigh their pets in between assessments, so that weight changes can be monitored.
Mental status	Observe the pet for signs of disorientation or other altered behavior.	Pet owners may report that their pet "doesn't seem to be himself." Although a full neurologic assessment may not be practical, obvious signs of disorientation or altered mental state should be evaluated more thoroughly by a veterinarian.

Plan: What's Next?

• Address immediate concerns.
• Determine whether more in-depth evaluation and/or diagnostic testing may be warranted.
• Recommend adjustments to current treatment regimen.
• Develop a contingency plan if the pet's condition should deteriorate.
• Manage the owners' expectations so they know what is coming next.
• Schedule follow-up assessment.

assessments of geriatric cats and dogs. Ideally, a complete blood count (CBC), chemistry screen, urinalysis, and blood pressure measurement should be performed annually for older dogs and cats (those older than 7 years of age). Blood and urine tests screen for dysfunction in the major organ systems, including kidneys and liver. Some specialists also recommend thyroid screening, especially for cats, and some practices include ocular pressure screening, chest and abdominal radiographs, and an electrocardiogram among their recommendations. If a pet owner is unable to pursue all of the recommended screening tests, an abbreviated "senior screen" (perhaps a chemistry profile and a CBC) may be fiscally feasible for the owner. It is important to involve owners in the decisions regarding their pets and to teach them about the importance of screening tests. Partial information is preferable to no information, so skill in the art of negotiation with pet owners is often helpful in obtaining the necessary monitoring tests associated with an annual geriatric patient assessment.

> **TECHNICIAN NOTE** As in humans, multi-systemic abnormalities increase in frequency with advancement of age, making screening tests an essential part of the annual geriatric patient evaluation.

ORAL HEALTH

Good oral health is essential in ensuring that veterinary patients will continue to eat and drink well. Owner complaints of halitosis, difficulty chewing, dropping food from the mouth, or excessive salivation should prompt a thorough oral examination. Signs of periodontal inflammation, tartar and calculus accumulation, and/or fractured teeth may require intervention. Although geriatric patients may present more of an anesthetic risk, these patients are more likely to require routine dental procedures to ensure oral comfort. Owners should be made aware of at-home prophylaxis that they can perform, such as daily tooth brushing and oral rinses, to limit the progression of dental disease. In addition, owners should be instructed to periodically check their pet's gums and tongue for growths or lesions, and to contact the veterinarian if they should note signs of oral discomfort.

CARDIAC DISEASE

The heart is an organ that is commonly affected by age. Chronic valvular disease (CVD) resulting from thickening of the heart valves affects many older dogs, especially smaller breeds, but occurs less commonly in cats. Larger-breed dogs, although also affected by CVD, may develop different cardiac disease, such as dilated cardiomyopathy. Cats are more likely to develop hypertrophic cardiomyopathy (HCM)—a condition in which the heart muscle becomes thickened. Hypertrophic cardiomyopathy can affect younger cats, but many are middle-aged at the time of initial presentation. Cardiac disease in pets can lead to arrhythmias, congestive heart failure, and other complications, such as renal damage

secondary to reduced renal perfusion. It is important that a thorough auscultation is performed in every geriatric patient, and testing should be discussed if a murmur or arrhythmia is heard. Additionally, any reports of fatigue, exercise intolerance, collapse, or cough should be investigated further, because all of these may be secondary to cardiac disturbances. These clinical signs, with or without evidence of an arrhythmia or murmur, warrant diagnostic investigation.

RESPIRATORY DISEASE

Similar to heart disease, respiratory disease is commonly reported in older patients and may be due to chronic lower airway disease, such as bronchitis, or upper airway disease, such as a collapsing trachea or laryngeal paralysis. Any abnormal lung sounds or owner complaints of coughing, exercise intolerance, or change in breathing rate or effort should be evaluated immediately.

NEOPLASIA

Neoplasia is one of the most common diseases of geriatric patients. Cancer may affect a single organ or multiple organs, depending on the type and stage of disease. Early detection is crucial in providing appropriate therapeutic measures to increase life span and improve quality of life.

> **TECHNICIAN NOTE** In addition to organ failure, cancer is increasingly common with age, and owners should seek veterinary care if they notice any abnormal behavior in their pet.

KIDNEY DISEASE

Chronic renal disease is one of the diseases seen most commonly in geriatric patients, especially cats. In addition to causing increased urination (polyuria) and water intake (polydipsia), kidney disease can cause complications, such as anemia, gastric upset, anorexia, weight loss, and muscle weakness. Routine screening for proteinuria, azotemia, and other abnormalities associated with kidney disease should be part of any diagnostic evaluation in a senior pet. With early detection, diet changes, fluid support, and specific medications may be used to slow progression.

URINARY AND FECAL INCONTINENCE

As veterinary patients age, degenerative neurologic diseases and spinal cord problems may lead to difficulties with urination and defecation. This is discussed in greater depth later.

NEUROLOGIC ABNORMALITIES

In addition to spinal cord abnormalities leading to incontinence, paresis, or paralysis, diseases of the brain occur with increasing frequency in the geriatric patient. Development of inflammatory or neoplastic lesions in the brain may lead to altered mentation or behavior changes. Any onset of behavior or mentation change should prompt a veterinary evaluation in an effort to find a medical cause. Veterinary patients, like humans, can display signs of cognitive dysfunction with age. Clinical signs such as altered sleep-wake cycles, house soiling, confusion, and irritability can strain the critical human-animal bond. Pet owners should be counseled about how to manage cognitive changes in their aging pets, and veterinary professionals should strive to manage owner expectations regarding this condition.

ORTHOPEDIC DISEASE

As our pet population ages, one of the problems most commonly seen is osteoarthritis. Osteoarthritis is also known as degenerative joint disease (DJD), and it can affect cats and dogs of any breed. Animals that are overweight tend to be more severely affected because excess weight leads to increased stress on joints. Use of nutraceuticals, anti-inflammatory medications, and other medications to control discomfort has dramatically improved the quality of life of many geriatric veterinary patients with DJD. Additionally, with the introduction of physical therapy and rehabilitation centers in veterinary medicine, strides have been made in the management of orthopedic problems. Household modifications can help pets with joint pain and limited mobility; these include ramps, skid-proof mats placed on the floor, and elevated food and water bowls (for pets with neck pain).

TECHNICIAN NOTE Orthopedic disease is one of the most common debilitating diseases in older animals; it may be managed with appropriate medical and nursing care. It is important for clinicians to make patient comfort a priority.

ENDOCRINE CONDITIONS

Endocrine diseases in general can be managed once diagnosed, but they can be life threatening if proper attention is not given. Because these diseases occur with increasing frequency in middle-aged to older veterinary patients, owners should be made aware of their clinical signs and should visit a veterinarian for evaluation if one of these diseases is suspected. The following sections discuss some common endocrine disorders seen in geriatric veterinary patients.

Hyperthyroidism

A common disease in middle-aged and older cats, the clinical syndrome of hyperthyroidism is caused by excessive production of thyroid hormone. This leads to an increase in metabolic rate and clinical signs including increased appetite with concurrent weight loss, polyuria and polydipsia, lack of grooming, and vomiting. Life-threatening cardiac complications can also occur. Early detection of hyperthyroidism is important because excellent therapeutic options are available. Therapy, such as administration of radioactive iodine, can be curative, and if done early enough, some of the cardiac changes induced by the disease may be reversible.

Hypothyroidism

Hypothyroidism is relatively common among middle-aged and older dogs, although younger dogs can also be affected. The condition is caused by inadequate production of thyroid hormone. Clinical signs include weight gain, lethargy, and muscle weakness—changes that pet owners may mistake for simple signs of aging, or "slowing down." Screening of patients that exhibit clinical signs is an important step toward confirming a diagnosis, initiating therapy, and improving quality of life for dogs with this disease. Hypothyroidism is well managed with oral thyroid hormone supplementation.

Diabetes Mellitus

Diabetes mellitus, caused by insufficient production of insulin or by an inability of insulin to work at its receptors, affects middle-aged to older dogs and cats. Insulin is required for glucose to enter cells, and glucose is the nutrient needed by body cells to perform their normal functions. Diabetes mellitus leads to polyuria, polydipsia, and increased appetite (polyphagia), along with weight loss. It predisposes animals to infection, especially in the urinary tract, because glucose overloads the kidneys and is spilled into urine. Glucose is an excellent source of nutrients for bacteria, so animals with diabetes mellitus are at risk for urinary tract infection. Diabetic animals typically require daily injections of insulin by their owners to properly manage the disease. Dietary modification can also be beneficial in many cases.

Hyperadrenocorticism

Hyperadrenocorticism, also known as *Cushing's disease*, is caused by excessive production of glucocorticoids, such as cortisol, released from the adrenal cortex. Elevations in blood glucocorticoid levels cause a variety of clinical signs, such as polyuria, polydipsia, muscle wasting, and increased appetite. In addition, elevated glucocorticoid levels inhibit the function of neutrophils and diminish their ability to adequately protect against infection. With appropriate treatment, hyperadrenocorticism can be managed, and infection and other complications limited. Refer to Chapter 19 for additional information about Cushing's disease.

TECHNICIAN NOTE Veterinary technicians are responsible for teaching owners about early signs of age-related disorders. Changes in eating, drinking, and urination habits, for example, may be associated with conditions that can be managed well, if identified and treated early.

CHANGING NUTRITIONAL NEEDS OF AGING PETS

Inappropriate nutrition can adversely affect the health and longevity of all pets, particularly elderly ones. Nutritional assessment therefore is an important part of veterinary geriatrics. Each assessment begins with a medical history, a physical examination, and laboratory screening tests. Because numerous dietary formulations are available for senior cats and dogs, the ideal nutritional regimen should meet the nutritional and caloric needs of each individual patient, taking into account the animal's specific health challenges, such as obesity, diabetes or heart disease. The 2008 Senior Care Guidelines of the American Association of Feline Practitioners (AAFP) recommend that each geriatric patient be placed on a dietary regimen that supports an ideal body condition score, and that addresses underlying health risks and illnesses. Although these guidelines are intended for elderly cats specifically, their underlying principles are appropriate for elderly dogs as well. Meeting the nutritional needs of this diverse population of elderly patients can be challenging. Refer to Chapter 9, "Companion Animal Nutrition," and to Box 35-3 for detailed information about feeding geriatric cats and dogs.

BOX 35-3 | Meeting the Nutritional Needs of the Geriatric Patient

Many pet food manufacturers promote the concept of "life stages nutrition," which includes developing diets specifically formulated for aging dogs and cats. However, little consensus has been reached among veterinary nutritionists and food manufacturers about the best way to feed healthy senior pets. Recommendations become even more complicated when nutritional management of diseases (or multiple diseases in the same pet) becomes a factor. No single "senior diet" formulation can be ideal for all geriatric pets. However, here are several factors to consider when determining how to best feed a particular animal:

- *Energy needs:* Maintenance energy requirement (MER) is the amount of energy needed for a normal animal to survive with minimal activity. MER has been shown to decrease as dogs age; this can contribute to obesity if caloric/food intake remains the same. However, studies in cats have suggested that MER decreases in older cats until approximately 11 or 12 years of age, after which it may increase. This means that older cats may be at risk for obesity, but after the age of 11 or 12, they are more likely to lose weight as they continue to age. In an effort to help control obesity in aging pets, most senior pet foods provide reduced fat and calories. However, this is not optimal for pets that are underweight or at ideal weight.
- *Ability to digest nutrients:* Senior cats have a reduced ability to digest fat (and possibly protein). Senior cat foods that are too low in fat may increase the risk for excessive weight loss, so some nutritionists recommend a higher fat intake for geriatric cats. Despite age-related reductions in MER, geriatric dogs can also be underweight, possibly owing to factors such as reduced food intake. In general, a senior pet diet should be highly digestible to help compensate for illness and other variables that affect ability to digest food.
- *Protein:* Because of the prevalence of kidney disease in older pets, some senior pet foods are formulated to contain reduced levels of protein. Reduced protein diets can help slow the progression of kidney disease. However, protein restriction in a pet that does not already have kidney disease has not been shown to reduce the risk of developing the condition. Additionally, senior pets tend to lose muscle mass, so reducing protein is not necessarily beneficial. In fact, some nutritionists suggest that older dogs may need more protein than their younger counterparts. Inadequate protein intake can contribute to further reductions in muscle mass (as the body uses skeletal muscle to supply protein and amino acids) and can exacerbate muscle weakness and mobility issues. The ideal protein content of senior dog and cat foods remains an active area of research.

- *Fiber:* Some senior pet foods contain additional fiber, which can help manage obesity, promote water absorption in the colon (helping to reduce constipation), and promote colon motility. However, fiber can also reduce food digestibility, so senior pets that are underweight or at ideal weight may not require as much fiber.
- *Other nutrients:* Senior diets may be supplemented with antioxidants, certain fatty acids, and joint-protective compounds (such as glucosamine and chondroitin). Some senior diet manufacturers modify amounts of sodium, calcium, phosphorus, and other nutrients in an effort to optimize benefits to senior pets.
- *Home-cooked diets:* Home-cooked diets can be risky; if the diet is not formulated precisely, or if the pet does not consume enough of each component, malnutrition can result. If a pet owner prefers to feed the senior pet home-cooked food, a nutritionist should ideally be involved in formulation of the diet. Another option may be referring pet owners to www.balanceit.com, a Web-based nutritional consultation service that can help pet owners (and veterinarians) formulate home-cooked diets for pets.
- *Illness and hospice conditions:* For pets in hospice care, appetite inconsistency, underlying illnesses, and the effect of illness on the body's metabolism are just a few factors to consider when determining how best to feed them. A feeding regimen should be individualized to meet the individual pet's needs. For pets that stop eating, a feeding tube or other nutritional support may be warranted.
- *Other considerations:* Even if the "perfect" diet is available for a particular pet, the patient may be unwilling to eat the food consistently, so adjustments may be necessary. This can include offering a different formulation of the same diet (canned vs. dry), pureeing food for pets with dental disease, heating canned food to increase aroma, or selecting a different diet that the pet is more willing to eat. Nutritional needs can change as a pet ages or develops new illnesses, so what is ideal for a pet today may not be ideal months or years into the future. Also, nutraceuticals and supplements have a role in promoting health in aging pets and in managing illnesses (such as osteoarthritis and kidney disease), so these products are worth investigating.

Providing adequate nutrition requires a sound understanding of the needs of geriatric pets, cooperation from pet owners, and the ability to remain flexible as conditions change. The ideal nutritional plan should be individualized to meet the specific needs of the patient.

HOSPICE CARE FOR THE AGED AND DYING CAT AND DOG

Despite the best efforts of veterinary professionals, at some point many companion animals develop terminal diseases. Technicians play a large role in ensuring that aged and dying patients are kept as comfortable as possible at home.

PAIN MEDICATIONS

A primary goal of the veterinarian and the veterinary technician is to provide medical care and comfort to the sick patient. In some cases, particularly in the terminally ill patient, controlling pain is all that can be done. However, one of the most difficult challenges is to accurately assess the level of pain experienced by a particular patient. Unlike humans, dogs and cats have subtle ways of expressing their discomfort, and owners may not be aware that their pet is in pain. However, owners may report general malaise, inappetence, or decreased activity in their pet, or they may notice an unwillingness to climb stairs or jump onto or off of the couch. When assessing patients, veterinary technicians should be able to recognize signs of discomfort that may include tachycardia, tachypnea, elevated temperature, unwillingness to use a limb or to posture for normal eliminations (especially in pets with severe hip osteoarthritis or lumbar pain), and yelping when a limb is manipulated (see Table 35-1).

The decision to start a geriatric patient on medications to control pain should not be taken lightly. Many geriatric patients have underlying organ insufficiency, and nearly all pain medications used in veterinary medicine have some potential for organ toxicity or other adverse effects. Careful patient monitoring is essential for detecting complications early and reducing the likelihood of permanent damage. Complete blood work should be performed before any type of pain medication is used in a geriatric patient and should be performed serially while the animal is receiving these medications.

The most common drug classes that veterinarians prescribe to manage pain in geriatric patients are (1) nonsteroidal anti-inflammatory drugs (NSAIDs), (2) steroids, and (3) opiates. Each has its own potential benefits and risks. NSAIDs are typically administered orally or parenterally and are potent analgesic, anti-inflammatory agents. Some have antipyretic activity as well. They are the medications used most commonly for managing the pain of DJD, chronic intervertebral disc disease, and other forms of osteoarthritis. Side effects are rare and may include gastrointestinal (GI) ulceration and renal and hepatic toxicity. In the past, these drugs have rarely been used to manage pain in older cats. However, the development of newer formulations of NSAIDs has made their use a practical option in some cats.

Steroids, more specifically, glucocorticoids, also have potent anti-inflammatory effects. Unfortunately, long-term use of steroids (in some cases, even short-term use) may lead to significant side effects that can detrimentally affect quality of life in these patients. Glucocorticoid side effects may include excessive thirst and urination, increased susceptibility to systemic infection, increased panting, muscle weakness, GI ulceration, and thromboembolic complications. For these reasons, glucocorticoids are usually given for pain control only as a last resort.

Opiates are narcotic drugs that produce some degree of analgesia. In humans, these drugs are known to have the potential to become habit forming and to cause sedation and respiratory depression. Several types of opiate receptors are present in the brain, and different opiates have been developed to work in the area of interest in specific patients.

Refer to Chapter 28 for additional information regarding recognition and assessment of pain, and on specific analgesic drugs.

Finally, nutraceutical products are becoming more popular as adjunct therapies for managing DJD in dogs and cats. Although nutraceuticals are not "medicines," they can improve quality of life for senior patients by supporting improved joint functioning and having a positive effect on joint cartilage.

> **TECHNICIAN NOTE** Providing pain relief is one of the most important responsibilities of veterinary professionals. When uncertain about whether a pet is in pain, err on the side of caution; assume that the pet is painful, and provide appropriate analgesia.

NURSING CARE FOR THE HOSPICE PATIENT

Many animals that are at the point of needing hospice care have their normal mental faculties but have physical disabilities that prevent them from performing typical daily activities. This is seen commonly in animals with severe orthopedic or spinal cord disease, in cases where the patient is mentally appropriate and has a good appetite but cannot ambulate on its own. Teaching pet owners to care for their recumbent pets at home is therefore critical if the animal is to survive and live comfortably. Veterinary technicians play a key role in providing this valuable instruction. Pet owners need to know how to keep their animals clean and comfortable and how to determine when they should give pain medications. In addition, owners should be taught to turn recumbent animals on a regular basis—at least every 4 to 6 hours—to limit formation of decubital ulcers, or bed sores (see later discussion). Animals that spend more time on one side than on the other can also develop atelectasis in the lung lobes on the "down" side, which can lead to respiratory compromise and pneumonia. Therefore, recumbent patients should be encouraged to ambulate regularly, if at all possible. Animals should always be in sternal recumbency when fed, to help prevent accidental aspiration of food material or vomitus. Appetite should be monitored closely because a decline in appetite may indicate that the pet's condition is deteriorating.

DECUBITAL ULCERS

As has been mentioned, one of the more common reasons why animals need at-home hospice care is that they have lost their ability to ambulate well and thus spend a significant amount of time in recumbency. This can be especially worrisome in large dogs, which are more prone to developing sores and ulcers at pressure points along their bodies. These "decubital ulcers" develop most commonly around the elbows, shoulders, tarsi, and hips. Decubital ulcers result from pressure and/or rubbing against a surface, so they can be found anywhere on the body that spends a large amount of time adjacent to the floor.

The best way to prevent such ulcers is to encourage the pet to stand and walk on a regular basis—at least every 4 to 6 hours—and to ensure that the animal does not spend excessive time lying on one side of the body. Extra pads and cushioning, such as an air mattress or a thick comforter, should be provided. Keeping the pet clean and dry of urine and feces is essential to help prevent development of sores and skin infections. Shaving the hair near the perineum, groin, and rear legs can facilitate bathing and drying, and corn starch can be applied to help reduce moisture.

If ulceration does occur, a topical antibiotic ointment and a protective bandage may be applied to reduce further trauma to the area. The difficulty with bandaging the area is that often the bandage itself causes skin trauma because the sore remains in close contact with the bandaging material, and healing is delayed. If the sore is noted over a joint, such as the elbow or tarsus, a doughnut type of bandage can be fashioned, so that the sore itself remains exposed but cannot rub against surfaces, thus limiting continued trauma.

SUBCUTANEOUS FLUIDS

A vast majority of dogs and cats receiving at-home care are eating and drinking on their own, but some pets require additional fluid support to maintain adequate hydration. Many of the geriatric diseases commonly seen in veterinary medicine (such as chronic kidney disease) can predispose to dehydration. If a patient is at risk for inadequate fluid intake or dehydration, owners may be taught to administer subcutaneous fluids. One or more in-office training sessions may be needed before owners are comfortable administering injections to their pet. However, the steps involved are relatively simple, and most owners can master this skill. Refer to Chapter 24, "Fluid Therapy and Transfusion Medicine," for detailed instructions on giving subcutaneous fluids.

Owners should be advised that warming fluids before administration can make the procedure more pleasant for the pet. Also, owners should be warned that the fluid will often become dependent. In other words, although fluid injections are usually given between the shoulder blades or along the back, before they are absorbed into the body, gravity often causes fluids to travel down the side of the animal and settle ventrally. If fluids are administered too far forward in the scruff area, the front limbs may swell as the fluid settles ventrally into the legs. This is not a matter of pathologic significance, but it is something owners often recognize. Owners should also be aware that administering excessive quantities of fluid, especially in cats, can be detrimental and may lead to fluid overload if cardiac function is compromised. Owners of any animal receiving subcutaneous fluid should report any change in respiratory pattern to the veterinarian because this could indicate fluid overload or heart disease.

EXPRESSING BLADDERS

Pets with orthopedic diseases, such as hip osteoarthritis, may have a difficult time posturing to urinate and/or defecate. Additionally, animals that are recumbent or have spinal cord injuries or other forms of spinal cord disease may be unable (or unwilling) to urinate on their own. Owners can be taught to express their pet's bladder to allow complete voiding. Bladder expression is a painless procedure if done correctly. Different methods may be used to perform this procedure, with the main focus on applying gentle pressure to the urinary bladder by squeezing both sides of the bladder in a front-to-back motion. Bladder expression can be performed with the pet standing, or in recumbent patients lying in lateral recumbency. Place one hand on each side of the patient's abdomen and move the hands caudally toward the pelvis until a soft, round structure that feels similar to a water balloon is palpable. This is the urinary bladder, and once it is found, gentle pressure (directed toward the rear of the patient) should be applied to it. The amount of pressure that should be applied varies with the individual, but with the right amount of pressure, urine will be expressed through the urethra, and a nice stream should be maintained until the "balloon" feels empty. Excessive pressure should never be applied because it is possible to rupture the urinary bladder.

It is always important to express as much urine as possible from the bladder. When urine sits in the bladder, especially in a patient that is unable to void on its own, cystitis becomes more likely. Therefore, any animal that requires regular bladder expression should be evaluated by the veterinarian on a routine basis, and urine cultures should be performed periodically. Additionally, it is important that owners routinely clean the patient's fur and skin of urine after expressing the bladder to prevent urine scalding (see later discussion).

> **TECHNICIAN NOTE** Veterinary technicians who teach owners about how to care for their pet at home help to extend the life of the pet and avoid costly hospitalizations or premature euthanasia. Administering subcutaneous fluids and medications, expressing bladders, tending to bed sores, and rotating recumbent animals are particularly helpful skills for clients to learn.

URINE SCALDING

Patients that have limited mobility or are recumbent may have urinary incontinence or may consciously urinate in a recumbent position. Urinary incontinence is common among patients that have spinal cord disease. Innervation to the external urethral sphincter arises from spinal cord segments at S1 to S3; therefore, spinal cord disease in this area often leads to "lower motor neuron" bladder dysfunction, whereby the sphincter does not close tightly, and urine leaks. Additional causes of urinary incontinence include decreased mobility, such that the bladder becomes too full and begins to leak. Without proper attention, such as regular expression of the bladder or frequent walks to allow elimination, the animal may dribble urine uncontrollably.

If urine leakage occurs, it may stain and soak the fur and scald the skin. If left untreated, this can eventually lead to sores and skin infections. This condition is painful and contributes to a poor quality of life. This situation becomes quickly intolerable for many pet owners and serves as a reason for choosing euthanasia over continued attempts to care for a sick pet. It is important to keep these patients clean and dry at all times. Shaving the perineum, groin, and rear legs and applying corn starch as described earlier can facilitate keeping the patient clean and dry. Some pet owners prefer to use diapers to help keep the area around the pet clean, but these must be checked and changed frequently. Bladder expression may lead to urine on the fur and skin; it is important for the clinician to be aware of this when expressing the bladder, and to always clean and dry the patient afterward.

APPETITE STIMULANTS

Decreased appetite with associated weight loss is a serious problem in some geriatric cats and dogs. The first thing to bear in mind when an animal's appetite begins to wane is that there is usually an underlying cause, such as a systemic illness, orthopedic pain, or a central neurologic depression. Every effort should be made to identify and treat an underlying condition. If no underlying cause is found, or if the appetite remains poor even with treatment of the underlying illness, medications such as antiemetics and appetite stimulants may be administered.

FEEDING TUBES

The use of feeding tubes for the geriatric patient is a controversial issue. Although providing basic nutrition is regarded by some as a medical obligation, except in extreme circumstances, others may consider nutritional support in the hospice care setting to be inhumane if the patient is otherwise debilitated. Veterinary patients cannot talk, and one of the most important indicators of how an animal feels is the presence or absence of an appetite. However, some pets are more "finicky" than others, so an apparent loss of appetite should be considered in the context of what is normal for the pet. Also, appetite loss can result from various factors, including diet change and certain medications, so it is not always an indication of a pet's sense of well-being. In a recumbent, debilitated patient, anorexia may mark the time to consider euthanasia of the pet. However, this approach cannot be applied in every case. If pet owners are not ready to consider euthanasia, efforts must be directed toward maintaining the patient's ability to obtain nutrition.

Feeding tubes are necessary sometimes, as in cases in which the animal's alimentary tract is abnormal (megaesophagus) but the patient is otherwise enjoying a good quality of life. As we discussed earlier, animals often need subcutaneous fluids at home to maintain proper hydration. Feeding tubes may be used for providing fluid and nutritional support to select animals. Feeding tubes can also facilitate administration of oral medications, which can be particularly problematic in cats.

Many types of feeding tubes are available in veterinary medicine. Some are used for short-term management, others for long-term support. The most common short-term feeding tube is a nasoesophageal tube. Animals may be sent home with this type of feeding tube, but it is typically used on a temporary basis when the animal is expected to begin eating on its own relatively soon. This flexible, soft, thin-diameter tube is introduced into the nasal cavity and then is advanced past the nasopharynx and into the esophagus. The external end of the tube is generally held in place by a suture (or surgical glue) to the side of the pet's face. Because of their location, animals can easily paw at nasoesophageal tubes, causing early removal; therefore, an Elizabethan collar must be worn at all times. Additionally, types of food given through the tube are limited and must be of liquid consistency.

A more permanent type of tube is an esophagostomy tube, which is placed while the patient is under general anesthetic through an incision directly into the esophagus from the neck. A slightly larger tube may be used for this type of feeding supplementation, and thus the choice of a liquid or slurry diet is more varied. The external end of the tube is generally sutured to the skin under the neck, and a bandage is placed around the neck to reduce the risk of accidental dislodging. Animals tend to tolerate these tubes well because they do not interfere with the pet's nostrils/face and they cause minimal discomfort. Esophagostomy tubes can be left in place for several months, and pet owners can use these tubes at home to facilitate administration of oral medication, as well as fluids and food.

Finally, the most permanent type of feeding tube is one that goes directly into the stomach. A gastrostomy tube may be placed surgically or with endoscopic assistance and typically is an even larger-diameter tube. It is away from the face and neck and rarely interferes with normal daily activities of the patient. It is ideal for patients with esophageal disorders because the esophagus is avoided entirely. Its drawback is that its placement is much more invasive, and complications, although uncommon, can be devastating and life threatening (e.g., bacterial infection in the abdomen if the tube leaks).

Feeding tubes are reserved for specific occasions and generally are not recommended as a "life support" type of measure. The animal should have a reasonable quality of life other than its inability to adequately obtain nutrition.

CARTS AND SLINGS

As animals age, orthopedic and neurologic disease can lead to severe impairment in ambulatory abilities. Small dogs and cats can be carried to some extent, but this may be difficult or impossible with large dogs. Products have been developed that make this type of problem manageable for many owners, while still providing a good quality of life for the pet.

Slings can be used to support the hind end of an animal that has normal use of the front end of its body and still maintains some control of the hind end. Typically, slings fit around the caudal portion of the body, just cranial to the hindlimbs, allowing the caretaker to simply support the hindlimbs while the animal ambulates. A sling works best if the animal can still use the hindlimbs to some extent, and often the sling is used merely as a support and fail-safe device if the pet is prone to falling. If the animal is only mildly affected, a Bottom's Up leash (Watson's Pet Co., Santa Monica, CA) and a soft blanket or towel can be used as a sling (Figure 35-1).

For animals that maintain little to no function of their hindlimbs, as often occurs with spinal cord injuries, carts are available for purchase. The hindlimbs fit into the apparatus, allowing the animal to use its front limbs to move around (Figure 35-2). Animals typically adapt to these devices quite

well. Additional styles of carts are available for pets that have difficulties with all four limbs.

> **TECHNICIAN NOTE** In addition to caring for the needs of geriatric patients, veterinary personnel should address the needs, fears, and concerns of pet owners who provide home care for their elderly or hospice animals.

WHEN IS THE RIGHT TIME FOR EUTHANASIA?

Pets are often thought of as members of a family and therefore are provided excellent veterinary medical care throughout their lifetime. Some owners go to extreme lengths to save the life of a seriously ill pet; other owners do not want their pet to suffer or cannot afford expensive medical care. Regardless of the situation, veterinary personnel are often asked when the time is right for a pet to be euthanized. Refer to Chapter 36 for a detailed discussion about client communication regarding euthanasia.

> **TECHNICIAN NOTE** The decision to euthanize a beloved family pet is a difficult one, and owners often seek guidance from veterinarians and veterinary technicians whom they know and have grown to trust.

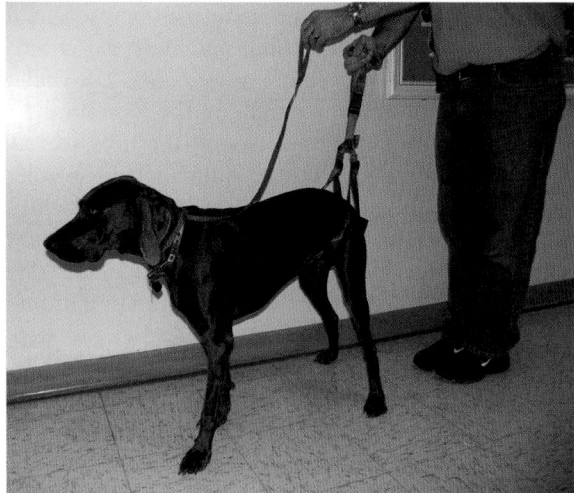

FIGURE 35-1 Bottom's Up leash (Watson's Pet Co., Santa Monica, CA) is being used in this patient for support of the hindlimbs. Alternatively, depending on the severity of hindlimb weakness, a towel or a soft blanket may be used as a temporary sling. The sling should be used for support only and not as a replacement for walking unless the animal is unable to use its limbs entirely.

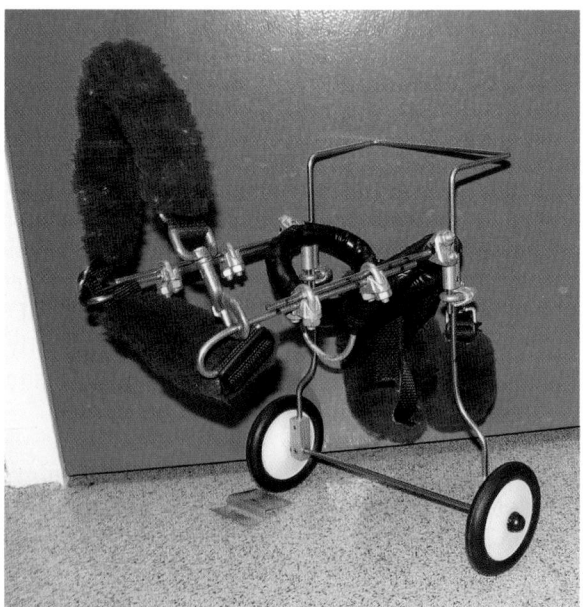

FIGURE 35-2 This cart is used for an animal with hindlimb paresis. For the cart to work properly, the animal must have normal mobility of the front limbs. The patient's head and front limbs fit through the soft red padding to the left of the picture, and the hindlimbs fit through the black doughnut-shaped holes to the right. Normal mobility in the front limbs allows the animal to ambulate fairly well and to control direction changes. These carts can be sized for the particular patient, such that the fitting can actually encourage use of the hindlimbs.

CASE PRESENTATION 35-1 "MISSY"

Signalment: 21-year-old, spayed female, 8-pound (3.6-kg), domestic short-haired cat

History: Missy was diagnosed with chronic renal failure approximately 3 years before presentation. She had been well managed on a prescription renal diet, subcutaneous fluid injections (100 ml lactated Ringer's solution every other day), an aluminum hydroxide antacid for phosphorus binding (1.0 ml PO SID), and an omega-3 fatty acid supplement. At approximately the same time that renal disease was diagnosed, Missy was diagnosed with borderline hyperthyroidism (T_4 2.5 µg/dl [range, 0.5 to 5.8 µg/dl], free T_4-ed 4.5 ng/dl, and 57.0 pmol/L [range, 1.2 to 4.3 ng/dl and 15.4 to 55.3 pmol/L]). However, because hyperthyroidism-associated modification of renal blood flow was expected to help support her renal functioning, and because Missy's values indicated only borderline thyroid disease, medication for hyperthyroidism was not initiated. Missy was also receiving a glucosamine/chondroitin/ASU supplement and aspirin ($\frac{1}{2}$ of an 81-mg tablet every 3 days) for osteoarthritis affecting her hips and knees, lactulose (3 ml PO SID) for periodic episodes of constipation, and famotidine (2.5 mg PO SID) as needed for occasional vomiting.

Overall, her owners were very happy with her condition, appetite, energy level, and quality of life at home. Regular monitoring consisted of physical examinations every 3 months and checking a chemistry profile, CBC, urinalysis, T_4, free T_4, and blood pressure every 3 months. Urine cultures were checked every 6 months.

Approximately 6 months before presentation, a grade II/V left-sided systolic heart murmur was detected. Because Missy was not exhibiting any clinical signs consistent with heart disease and her other monitoring parameters were unchanged, the owners decided not to pursue a cardiac evaluation right away. However, follow-up blood pressure readings increased, so Missy's owners decided to pursue thoracic radiographs and echocardiography.

Presentation: On physical examination, Missy was well hydrated and in reasonable body condition given her illnesses (BCS, 2.5/5). The cardiac murmur was consistent with previous assessments, and her resting heart rate was approximately 200 beats per minute. Her blood pressure was also elevated (systolic pressure, 190 mm Hg).

Diagnostic evaluation: Thoracic radiographs revealed mild pulmonary edema and mild cardiac enlargement. Additional radiographic findings included degenerative joint disease involving several thoracic and lumbar vertebrae. Echocardiography revealed moderate left ventricular and mild left atrial enlargement with mild mitral valve insufficiency. A mild pericardial effusion was also identified. A presumptive diagnosis of hypertrophic cardiomyopathy with congestive heart failure was made.

Treatment: In addition to continuing previous medications and supplements, amlodipine (0.625 mg PO SID) and furosemide (3.1 mg PO SID) were given.

Outcome: Initially, Missy responded well to management of her heart condition, hypertension, and renal disease. A recheck examination 2 weeks after the echocardiogram indicated that pulmonary edema and pericardial effusion had resolved, and her blood pressure was normalizing in response to medication. However, follow-up blood work 3 months later showed an increase in renal values (BUN 88 mg/dl [range, 15 to 34 mg/dl], creatinine 4.8 mg/dl [range, 0.8 to 2.3 mg/dl]), and Missy's owners reported that her appetite had tapered off. She had also developed anemia secondary to renal compromise (HCT 21% [Range 29%-45%]). The owners were aware of her worsening condition but were not yet ready to consider euthanasia. Appetite stimulants were prescribed but were variably effective, so during the following several weeks, the owners attempted to offer her different things to eat and syringe-fed her for a time. However, this was becoming difficult for them, and Missy was starting to resent being syringe-fed. Follow-up examination showed that Missy had lost weight (6.3 lb; weighing 1.7 lb less than previously). Her blood work showed renal values that continued to be high, and her hematocrit had fallen further (17.6%), so erythropoietin injections were initiated (215 U SC 3 times/week) and Missy was started on an oral iron supplement. The owners were advised that end of life choices should be discussed at home because Missy's condition was not expected to improve significantly for the duration of her life.

Within a few weeks, Missy had stopped eating completely, and appetite stimulants were ineffective. She was becoming progressively lethargic. Her owners were not yet ready to euthanize, so an esophagostomy feeding tube was placed. For approximately 9 weeks, the owners used the feeding tube to administer oral medications and regular feedings. They reported that the feeding tube made caring for Missy much easier and much less stressful. Missy gained some weight (7.8 lb—an increase of 1.5 lb) and was also regaining some of her strength. The owners reported that she was jumping onto furniture for the first time in months, and she seemed to enjoy being with them. She enjoyed being brushed daily and spending quiet time on the sun porch with her owners. Because of her weakened condition, the owners had moved her food, water, beds, and litter box into the common area of the home, so Missy could spend more time with the family and could be observed more closely. Despite initially responding well to treatment, Missy exhibited periodic episodes of weakness and difficulty breathing. Approximately 9 weeks after the esophagostomy tube was placed, Missy developed respiratory distress and died at home from cardiac complications.

Discussion: Missy's case illustrates the importance of addressing not just the primary problem (renal disease), but also underlying medical issues and hospice care that affect the patient's quality of life and well-being, while continuing to manage owner expectations. As with many geriatric patients, chronic illnesses progressed in this case and new illnesses developed; all of these changes must be managed with the patient *and owners* in mind. This case also shows how a feeding tube can facilitate owners' continuing to care for a sick pet and is an easy-to-use method of providing fluids and medication. Hospice care in this situation

Continued

Geriatric Horses

As a result of advances in equine management and nutrition over the past few decades, many horses are living beyond 30 years of age. Some of these horses are pasture pets and are well loved by their owners but are not referred to a veterinary hospital when problems arise. Factors such as advanced age, inability to ride in a trailer, and economics play a part in the owner's decision to not refer the patient. Therefore, many equine veterinarians in private practice manage geriatric horses on the farm.

Aged horses are often defined as greater than 20 years old. Many of these horses are older than 30 years of age; they often live into their late 30s or even early 40s. Aged horses suffer from a myriad of problems, including poor body condition, lack of teeth, Cushing's disease (pituitary pars intermedia dysfunction), musculoskeletal disease such as degenerative joint disease (DJD or osteoarthritis), and chronic laminitis. Cushing's disease, a common disease of older horses, is discussed in detail in this chapter.

PHYSICAL EXAMINATION

An annual physical examination is crucial in maintaining good health of the aged horse. Often problems are found on a thorough examination. Refer to Chapter 7 for a detailed description of physical examination of the equine patient. An annual body condition score is helpful in determining whether the aged horse is maintaining an adequate body condition. Acute or chronic weight loss indicates an underlying problem, such as lack of teeth, inability of the GI tract to absorb nutrients, or neoplasia. The horse's hair coat should be short and smooth. If it is long and wavy and is not shedding out completely in the spring, the horse has Cushing's disease, which is discussed later in the chapter. Common problems in older horses include heaves, laminitis, dental problems, sinusitis, equine recurrent uveitis (ERU), neurologic deficits, and DJD.

COMMON PROBLEMS IN AGING HORSES

The general physical examination of a geriatric horse follows the same guidelines as an examination performed on a younger horse. However, aged horses are more prone to

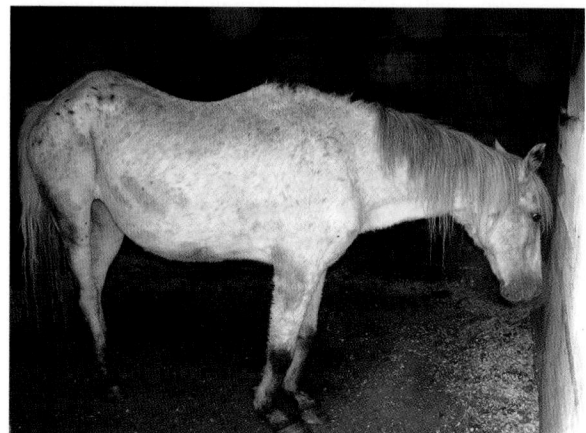

FIGURE 35-3 Geriatric horse with poor body condition and depressed attitude. (Courtesy Katie Costanzo, CVT.)

certain problems, which are highlighted in the following discussion. Also, refer to Tables 35-3 and 35-4 for a list of questions that aid in performing nursing evaluations of geriatric horses.

The horse should have a body score performed on physical examination. This system offers an objective way to determine the horse's condition and to assess whether weight loss occurs over time. Refer to Chapter 10, Table 10-3, for the Equine Body Condition Score scale. A score of 1 indicates that the horse is emaciated, and 9 indicates obesity. The horse's attitude is assessed as bright and alert or depressed (Figure 35-3). Many older horses appear quiet and depressed, but this attitude is often due to Cushing's disease and can improve with treatment. The hair coat should be short and shiny. If it is dull, is excessively long and wavy, and is not shedding completely in the spring (**hirsutism**), the horse has Cushing's disease.

ORAL AND NASAL HEALTH

Performing an oral examination is important because older horses often are in poor body condition, are unable to chew properly, and drop food when chewing. Many older horses are missing teeth or have sharp points (hooks) on their teeth, preventing normal chewing (Figure 35-4). The most severe change is called a *wave mouth*. This condition occurs when the horse's teeth are of different lengths, preventing normal chewing action. Geriatric horses are prone to chronic sinus

TABLE 35-3	Nursing Assessment of a Geriatric Horse: Medical History

Providing adequate nursing care for a geriatric horse requires periodic assessments of key points, whether the clinician is assessing a patient that is hospitalized or during a farm call.

MEDICAL HISTORY	WHAT TO ASK THE OWNER	NURSING ASSESSMENT QUESTIONS
Attitude, appetite, and manure production	• "Have there been any changes in the horse's attitude or activity level?" • "What are you feeding right now?" • "How much and how often are you feeding?" • "Is the horse eating readily?" • "Has he/she eaten today?"	• "Is the horse bright and alert or dull and depressed?" • "Does the horse appear comfortable and eating readily or is he reluctant to move or eat?" • "Is the manure normal in appearance and frequency?"
Drinking and urination	• "Is the horse drinking any more or less than usual?" • "Is fresh water available at all times (especially in cold weather)?" • "How often do you change the water bucket?" • "Have any changes in urination (amount, effort, or frequency) been noted?"	• "How is the water provided—by a bucket or by an automatic waterer?" • "Is fresh water available?" • "Is the stall excessively wet or dry?"
Medication administration	• "Is the horse receiving any medication or supplements?" • "Do you remember what side effects to watch for?"	• Is the medication stored and administered correctly?

TABLE 35-4	Nursing Assessment of a Geriatric Horse: Physical Assessment

PHYSICAL ASSESSMENT	WHAT TO CHECK	NURSING ASSESSMENT QUESTIONS
Mentation and walking	Observe the horse for signs of dullness, depression, and reluctance to move; palpate distal limbs for bounding digital pulses.	• "Is the horse quiet and depressed or reluctant to move?" (Horses with laminitis or degenerative joint disease will be reluctant to move or walk.)
Body condition and hair coat	A body condition score should be determined on a scale of 1 (emaciated) to 9 (obese); the horse's weight should be assessed using a weight tape.	• "Does the horse have poor body condition or muscle atrophy?" • "Does the horse have a long, wavy hair coat?"
Vital signs	Temperature, pulse, and respiration	• "Does the horse have a fever (>101.5° F)?" • "Is the horse's heart rate increased (>44 beats/minute) or respiratory rate increased (>20 breaths/minute)?"
Hydration status and cardiorespiratory system	Mucous membrane color and quality; capillary refill time (CRT) and jugular vein refill time; pulse quality; thoracic auscultation to assess heart rate and rhythm, to detect heart murmurs, or to assess pulmonary sounds	• "Are the horse's mucous membranes pink and moist with a CRT <2 seconds?" • "Are the horse's heart rate and rhythm within normal limits?" • "Are nasal discharge, coughing, and abnormalities evident on thoracic auscultation of the respiratory system?"
Abdomen	Signs of abdominal pain such as pawing or rolling; auscultate both sides of the abdomen to determine whether borborygmi are present, and note distention	• "Is the horse comfortable or painful?" • "Are borborygmi present, or is abdominal distention noted?"

infection, so the presence of nasal discharge and a dull sound when the sinuses are percussed indicate that the sinus cavity contains fluid.

VISION

An ophthalmic examination is performed to check the horse's eyes for diseases such as ERU and cataracts. It is not uncommon for an older horse to have significant visual impairment that is discovered only during an ophthalmic examination. Many older horses are housed on the same farm for years and are able to compensate for loss of vision. If they are moved to a new location, the owner will discover that the horse has difficulty maneuvering in the new environment as a result of decreased vision.

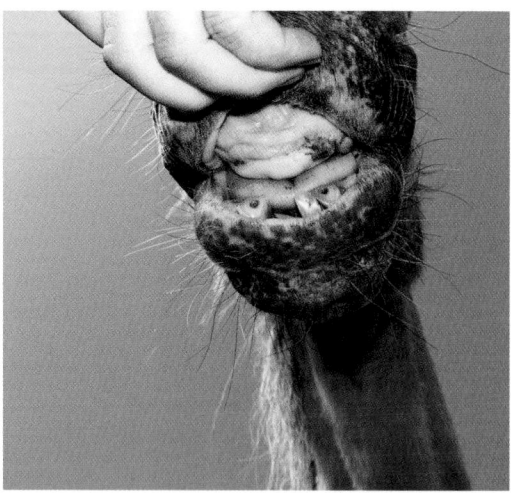

FIGURE 35-4 Note the lack of multiple incisors. (Courtesy Katie Costanzo, CVT.)

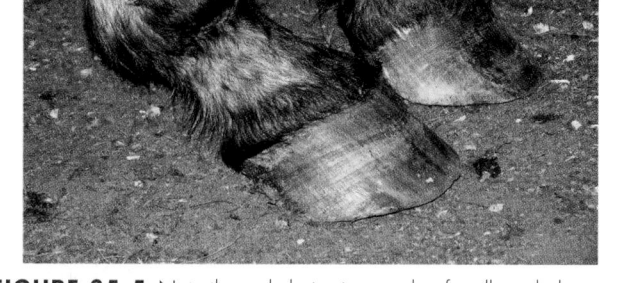

FIGURE 35-5 Note the curly hair, rings on hoof wall, and abnormal angle of the distal limb as a result of suspensory tendon deterioration. (Courtesy Katie Costanzo, CVT.)

CARDIAC DISEASE

Cardiac auscultation is important for assessing a resting heart rate and the presence of murmurs or arrhythmias. It is helpful to feel the pulse at the same time that the heart rate is auscultated to ensure that they are synchronous with one another. Feeling the pulse also ensures that the pulse is strong and has a normal rhythm. Mitral regurgitation is the most common valvular lesion in horses older than 15 years of age. This condition gives rise to a systolic murmur on the left side of the thorax. Aortic regurgitation also occurs in older horses and is clinically associated with a diastolic murmur on the left side. The most common arrhythmia in older horses is atrial fibrillation. It is often an incidental finding on physical examination. The rhythm is irregularly irregular, and the horse has an elevated resting heart rate (>44 beats/minute). Many horses can tolerate this arrhythmia for years and appear healthy but may exhibit exercise intolerance at high levels of exercise.

RESPIRATORY DISEASE

A respiratory examination evaluates respiratory rate, respiratory effort, and the presence of nasal discharge or coughing. Older horses often have heaves (recurrent airway obstruction) and will have an increased respiratory rate and effort. Chronic cases develop a heave line (hypertrophy of abdominal muscles) resulting from increased effort to exhale.

GASTROINTESTINAL DISEASE

The GI tract is assessed initially by evaluating the consistency and amount of manure. Manure should have a normal consistency and should not contain large pieces of hay or grain. If large pieces are present, the horse has poor chewing ability to grind food well and needs an oral examination. The presence of diarrhea may indicate chronic colitis or malabsorptive disease.

KIDNEY DISEASE

The horse's renal system can be assessed by evaluating the amount of water consumed daily and the frequency of urination. Annual urinalysis is important to assess the concentrating ability of the kidneys and to ensure that urine does not contain substances such as protein or glucose.

SKIN DISORDERS

The horse's integument is examined for dermatitis and abrasions, especially around bony areas, such as the pelvis. Reproductive organs are visually examined. Elderly male horses may develop tumors on their sheath (prepuce) or penis. These tumors are often squamous cell carcinoma and require treatment. The rectal area is evaluated for the presence of melanomas and normal anal tone.

NEUROLOGIC ABNORMALITIES

On general neurologic examination, older horses may drag their hind feet and may have blunted toes. This change may be due to neurologic deficits or musculoskeletal pain (e.g., DJD in the hocks). The horse's neck should be examined for evidence of pain. Offer the horse a carrot or a handful of grain to encourage the horse to touch nose to shoulder. If the horse is reluctant or is unable to perform this action, this may indicate the presence of neck pain. Sometimes this is due to fracture of the cervical vertebrae that can be diagnosed on cervical radiographs.

ORTHOPEDIC DISEASE

The musculoskeletal examination is an important part of a general physical examination. Older horses are prone to laminitis and may have changes, such as rings on the hoof wall, indicating chronic laminitis (Figure 35-5). They also often have DJD in multiple joints (e.g., carpus, hock) and become stiff without regular pasture turnout (Figure 35-6). Muscle atrophy is common, especially on the dorsum and around the gluteal area (Figure 35-7).

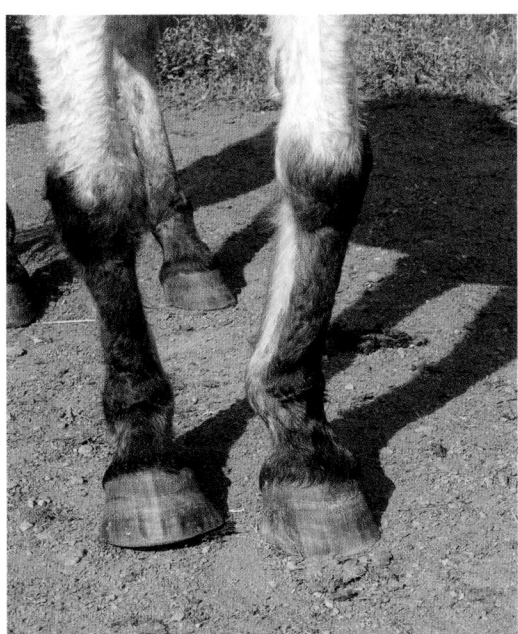

FIGURE 35-6 Severe carpal bone degeneration causing a bow-legged appearance. (Courtesy Katie Costanzo, CVT.)

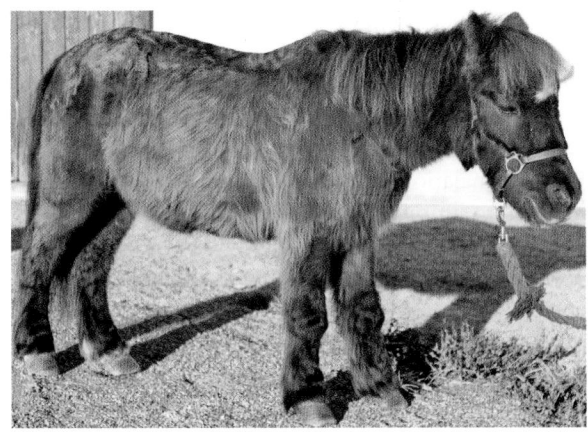

FIGURE 35-7 Note this geriatric pony's long, wavy hair coat, typical of horses with Cushing's disease (pituitary pars intermedia dysfunction). (Courtesy Katie Costanzo, CVT.)

TECHNICIAN NOTE Geriatric horses are likely to have general health problems. An annual physical examination is important to identify and treat problems early.

CHRONIC DISEASES OF THE GERIATRIC HORSE

Geriatric horses often have multiple problems that require close attention to minimize complications. Cushing's disease is common in older horses and can cause immunosuppression. It also leads to or exacerbates other diseases, such as heaves (recurrent airway obstruction), ERU, laminitis, and sinusitis. For successful management of these other

conditions, Cushing's disease requires treatment with pergolide to minimize immunosuppression.

EQUINE CUSHING'S DISEASE (PITUITARY PARS INTERMEDIA DYSFUNCTION)

Equine Cushing's disease, also known as pituitary pars intermedia dysfunction (PPID), is a common disease in horses, especially among those older than 15 years of age. Certain breeds, such as Quarter Horses, are more predisposed to the disease than other breeds such as Thoroughbreds. It is caused by excessive hormonal secretions (pro-opiomelanocortin [POMC]-derived peptides) from the pituitary pars intermedia (PI), which stimulate excessive cortisol release from the adrenal glands.

In the brain, the hypothalamus is the master endocrine gland; it controls many activities of other endocrine glands. The hypothalamus resides above the pituitary gland and has neurons with long axons that synapse on melanotrophs in the pituitary PI. Dopamine secreted by these hypothalamic neurons inhibits the production of POMC by the pituitary PI. However, loss of dopamine in Cushing's disease leads to excessive production of POMC by the pituitary gland. POMC is converted into different hormones, including adrenocorticotropic hormone (ACTH), which stimulates the adrenal glands to produce excessive cortisol.

Clinical signs of Cushing's disease vary among patients. The affected horse may exhibit one or more clinical signs, including hirsutism (over-long hair coat), patchy sweating, lethargy, polyuria/polydipsia (PU/PD), laminitis, "potbelly" appearance, and muscle wasting on the dorsum. Other possible clinical signs include spontaneous lactation in mares without foals, tachypnea (increased respiratory rate), and immunosuppression resulting in parasitism. Horses with Cushing's disease are more prone to concurrent diseases, such as recurrent uveitis, heaves (recurrent airway obstruction), and sinusitis. Abnormalities noted on blood work (CBC and chemistry profile) include hyperglycemia (blood glucose level >180 mg/dl), increased liver enzymes, neutrophilia, lymphopenia, and anemia.

In the past, many older horses with Cushing's disease were misdiagnosed as having hypothyroidism (low thyroid hormone levels). One of the common clinical signs thought to indicate hypothyroidism in horses was the presence of a thickened crest neck. It is now recognized, however, that hypothyroidism is not common in horses, and the thick neck is due to abnormal fat deposition. Measuring baseline thyroid hormone levels (e.g., thyroxine [T_4], triiodothyronine [T_3]) is not reliable in horses. These levels can be decreased for many reasons and should not be used as a screening test. Thyroid supplementation should be used only when indicated in equine patients.

Diagnosis of Cushing's disease is made on the basis of the horse's history, signalment, physical examination, and ancillary diagnostic blood tests. Three tests are typically used: dexamethasone suppression test (DST) to assess cortisol response; serial measurements of ACTH, insulin, and dextrose; and thyrotropin-releasing hormone (TRH) stimulation. The DST is not always reliable and can yield inconsistent results. This test requires steroid administration, and steroids are associated with laminitis in horses. Horses with Cushing's disease are prone to laminitis and/or may have a current episode of laminitis, so steroid administration is often contraindicated. Serial measurements of ACTH, insulin, and dextrose can be more accurate than DST findings. Steroids are not used in this test, so it is a good option for many horses with Cushing's disease. However, one sample may not be diagnostic, so taking three blood samples in one day (AM, noon, PM) is optimal. ACTH levels increase in the fall as compared with January or May, so results should be interpreted on the basis of time of year. Despite various available diagnostic tests, owners of geriatric horses sometimes refuse diagnostic tests. Empirical treatment should be considered if the owner refuses diagnostic tests, and the horse's history, signalment, and physical examination findings are consistent with Cushing's disease.

The primary treatment for Cushing's disease is a dopamine agonist, pergolide. The authors recommend use of Prascend® (pergolide mesylate) since it is the only FDA approved treatment for Cushing's disease, rather than continued use of compounded pergolide. Many 450-kg horses respond well to 1 mg or 1.5 pergolide orally once a day, but the dose needs to be altered on the basis of response to treatment. Many clinical signs will improve with treatment, but hirsutism usually remains. Numerous horses with Cushing's disease appear quiet and depressed, but once treatment is initiated, they become much more alert and act younger. Rechecking blood tests after starting medication will aid in determining the optimum pergolide dose. Another medication, cyproheptadine, was used in the past to treat Cushing's disease. It is not as effective as pergolide and is more expensive.

General management is important for horses with Cushing's disease. The horse should have his teeth floated every 6 months or yearly to maintain oral health. Regular foot care every 4 to 5 weeks will keep him more comfortable and will prevent an over-long toe, which can aggravate lameness or laminitis. Regular deworming and manure management, such as weekly removal from the pasture, will aid in parasite control. Horses with Cushing's disease have poor thermoregulation and patchy sweating associated with hirsutism. These patients are more comfortable with regular body clipping to minimize hirsutism and using blankets in the winter. Clipping also permits better assessment of the horse's body condition.

Nutrition is important with aged equine patients and those with Cushing's disease. Feeding small amounts of a senior diet often, adding corn oil ($\frac{1}{4}$ cup daily) and grass pasture, and avoiding lush pastures are beneficial. Alfalfa hay or soaked alfalfa cubes or pellets can help maintain an older horse's body condition. Alternate sources include processed hay, such as Dengie hay.

> **TECHNICIAN NOTE** Cushing's disease is common in older horses. Clinical signs vary, but horses often have hirsutism (excessive long hair growth) and depression. Cushing's disease can cause immunosuppression and can exacerbate other diseases, so diagnosis and treatment are imperative to maintain the health of the geriatric horse.

HEAVES (RECURRENT AIRWAY OBSTRUCTION)

This disease can be acute or chronic in nature. Some horses are affected only a few weeks each year, other horses are affected year-round. Usually, if a horse acutely develops signs of heaves, it eventually becomes a chronic condition and requires careful management to minimize clinical signs. Horses with heaves are often allergic to dust or mold in the environment. Horses living in a dusty stable with minimal pasture turnout, exposed to cobwebs, straw, and hay, are prone to developing heaves. This allergic reaction leads to inflamed airways and constriction of smooth muscle in the airways, causing narrowed airways and difficulty breathing, especially during exhalation. Clinical signs on physical examination include increased respiratory rate (tachypnea) and increased effort (dyspnea), nostril flare, and dry cough. The horse will not have a fever and may have a clear nasal discharge. Horses with chronic heaves are often in poor body condition with a heave line (extreme development of the external abdominal oblique muscles as a result of increased effort on exhalation). The horse may extend his head on exhalation to improve airflow. On thoracic auscultation, wheezes will be heard on both sides of the chest, especially on expiration. A rebreathing bag (large trash bag) may be used to encourage the horse to inhale deeply, permitting better thoracic auscultation. After the bag is removed, a horse with heaves will cough and will take a long time to return to normal breathing. Additional diagnostic tests include blood tests (CBC, chemistry profile), transtracheal wash, bronchoalveolar lavage (BAL), and thoracic radiographs. Abnormalities on blood tests include increased total protein and increased fibrinogen concentration. Samples of airway secretions can be obtained on transtracheal wash or BAL and submitted for cytology and culture to differentiate heaves from infection (e.g., pneumonia). Changing the horse's environment to minimize allergens is the most important part of therapy. Increasing pasture turnout, soaking hay for 4 hours before feeding, and eliminating dusty bedding are vital for minimizing clinical signs. Medication to control inflammation and bronchoconstriction is administered systemically (e.g., IV, IM, PO) or locally (e.g., using an inhaler). Steroids (e.g., dexamethasone, fluticasone) are used to decrease inflammation, and bronchodilators (e.g., clenbuterol, albuterol) dilate narrowed airways. Local treatment using an Equinehaler (Equine Health, Hørsholm, Denmark) or an AeroMask Equine Medical System (Trudell Medical International, London, Ontario, Canada) provides effective treatment while minimizing possible side effects. However, this method is expensive because inhalers for human patients are used. It also requires a dedicated caregiver initially giving medications a few times daily. Systemic steroids are effective but have been associated with laminitis in horses. Horses with heaves require management changes, close monitoring, and early treatment at onset of clinical signs, but can live comfortably for a long time if treated properly.

LAMINITIS (FOUNDER)

Laminitis is a devastating, sometimes fatal disease in young and older horses. Although extensive research has been conducted, the pathophysiology of laminitis is not clear. It may be acute or chronic in nature, and all four feet may be affected or just one or two feet. Ultimately, the soft tissue in the foot (laminae) holding the bone (distal phalanx, or P3) and hoof wall together becomes inflamed and necrotic. The horse initially may develop separation of the hoof wall from the bone. In severe cases, the bone will rotate, sink, and penetrate the bottom of the foot (sole), necessitating euthanasia. Laminitis may be a complication of a primary problem (e.g., postcolic surgery) or may develop acutely with no apparent cause. However, laminitis most commonly occurs

in the geriatric horse as a result of Cushing's disease. Some breeds (e.g., Quarter Horse, ponies) are more prone to developing laminitis. Laminitis is a painful condition because the horse is standing on the affected foot and often cannot find relief from pain. Clinical signs of laminitis include reluctance to walk and turn, bounding digital arterial pulses (palpated over the fetlock near the sesamoid bones), rings on the hoof wall, depression, and inappetence resulting from discomfort. Diagnostic tests include radiographs of the feet and additional tests to diagnose the inciting cause. If the inciting cause is identified, treatment is directed at the disease. For example, if Cushing's disease is diagnosed, treatment with pergolide is paramount to control laminitis. Treatment for laminitis is often symptomatic and includes shoeing changes (e.g., blunting the toe), footpads, deep bedding in the stall (e.g., sand), and use of NSAIDs (e.g., phenylbutazone). It is ideal if the horse will lie down to relieve pressure from affected feet. Laminitis may be acute or chronic; geriatric horses often develop chronic laminitis and require regular foot care every 4 weeks to minimize clinical signs. Recovery can be complete, or permanent damage to the laminae may occur, so long-term care is directed at the individual patient.

CASE PRESENTATION 35-2 CUSHING'S DISEASE IN A QUARTER HORSE MARE

A 32-year-old Quarter Horse mare appeared depressed and inappetent, so the owner called her equine veterinarian and veterinary technician (Figure 1). On physical examination, the mare had poor body condition (body score, 4/9), hirsutism, a wave mouth, and rings on the dorsal hoof wall of her front feet. Initial blood work was performed, and no abnormalities were noted. Samples were submitted for ACTH, insulin, and dextrose. Samples were drawn 3 times in a single day (AM, noon, PM), and dextrose was performed stall-side using a dextrometer. Insulin levels were within normal limits, but dextrose was greater than 200 mg/dl for each sample; ACTH levels were greater than 300 for each sample. The mare was diagnosed with Cushing's disease, and treatment was started (1 mg PO SID pergolide). She was sedated with 2 mg detomidine and 1 mg butorphanol IV for a thorough

dental float to correct the wave mouth. Radiographs of her front feet showed chronic laminitic changes but minimal rotation of P3 (coffin bone). Her feet were in poor condition, so the farrier trimmed her feet and agreed to return every 4 weeks. Her diet was evaluated, and her ration of Equine Senior was increased, with ¼ cup corn oil added daily. The owner also clipped the mare and agreed to place a blanket on her in the winter. Within a week after starting pergolide treatment, the mare became much more active and bright. She nickered to everyone who came to her stall and ate readily, no longer dropping grain from her mouth. She began to play with the other horses again. After 3 months on her new diet, she was in better condition (grade 6/9), and the grateful owner was happy to have her beloved horse back (Figure 2).

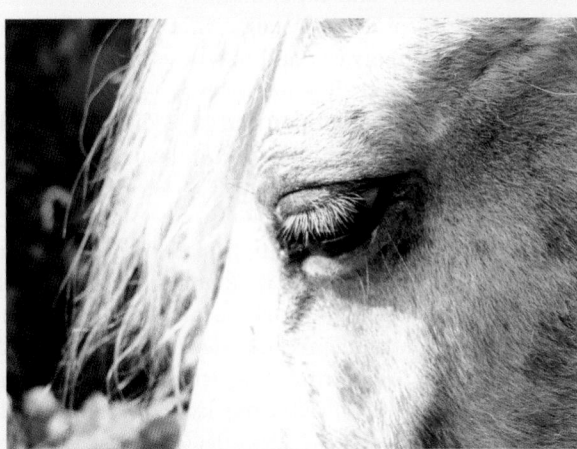

FIGURE 1 Depressed geriatric mare with hirsutism.

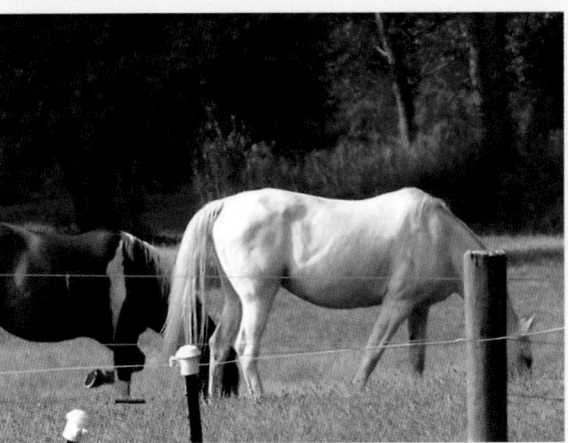

FIGURE 2 A picture of good health. (Courtesy Katie Costanzo, CVT.)

DENTAL PROBLEMS AND SINUSITIS

Geriatric horses often develop dental disease as they age. As their teeth wear down or fall out, the opposing tooth will become too long or will develop points (sharp areas on the tooth). This causes abnormal occlusion, and the horse will not be able to chew properly. The most severe abnormality is called *wave mouth*. The horse will have abnormal occlusion of all teeth and extreme difficulty chewing food. Wave mouth is a common problem in geriatric horses. Clinical signs of oral abnormalities include poor body condition, slow chewing, dropping a lot of grain or hay from the mouth, discomfort when chewing, and whole grain in manure. A thorough dental examination should be performed at least annually on horses 20 years of age or older to prevent oral abnormalities. When proper dental care is provided, many older horses are able to chew their food well and maintain their body condition.

Chronic sinusitis is common in older horses and is often caused by tooth root abscessation or immunosuppression due to Cushing's disease. One or more sinuses may be affected. Clinical signs include purulent, unilateral nasal discharge, and a reddish color may be present. Percussing the sinuses in the middle of the horse's head will elicit a dull sound, indicating fluid accumulation. Diagnostic tests include an oral examination to look for tooth root abscessation, upper airway endoscopy, skull radiographs, and evaluation for Cushing's disease. Treatment includes administration of long-term antimicrobials, flushing the sinuses under general anesthetic, removal of an infected tooth root, and pergolide if Cushing's disease is present.

EQUINE RECURRENT UVEITIS (ERU, OR MOON BLINDNESS)

Geriatric horses often develop eye problems, and the leading cause of blindness in horses is equine recurrent uveitis. ERU is a progressive disease that causes frequent episodes of inflammation and degeneration in one or both eyes. Some breeds, such as Appaloosas, are more commonly affected. Clinical signs include a swollen and painful eye, photophobia, corneal edema (blue tint to cornea), a corneal abrasion or ulceration, miosis (constricted pupils), neovascularization (blood vessel growth on cornea), anterior uveitis (inflammation in the front chamber of the eye), hypopyon (cellular debris in the eye), and hyphema (hemorrhage in the eye). A horse with a swollen, painful eye is treated as an emergency because the cornea is thin (1.5 mm thick) and has no blood supply, and the eye can rupture if not treated quickly. Horses live in a contaminated environment and may develop bacterial and fungal ulcers that can be resistant to therapy. Diagnostic evaluation includes sedating the horse to perform a thorough ophthalmologic examination, applying fluorescein stain to evaluate the cornea for ulceration, and taking samples for cytology and culture. When a corneal ulcer is present, the damaged corneal epithelium will stain bright green, showing the extent of the ulcer. Both eyes should be evaluated because many geriatric horses will have cataracts and degenerative retinal changes. If the horse lacks vision in the clinically unaffected eye and the other eye is swollen and painful, the horse may become scared and may react differently than it normally would. Treatment depends on whether primarily inflammatory changes or a corneal ulcer is present. If no ulcer is present, topical steroids (e.g., dexamethasone, prednisolone) and other medications (atropine, serum, and systemic NSAIDs, such as flunixin meglumine) are used to eliminate inflammation and dilate the pupil. If an ulcer is present, topical antimicrobials and other medications (atropine, serum, and systemic NSAIDs, such as flunixin meglumine) are given until the ulcer resolves, and then steroids can be used if needed. Mild cases can be treated with topical ointments or solutions. Severe cases require frequent treatment; it is often difficult to treat a horse with a painful eye, so a subpalpebral catheter can be placed for ease of treatment. Sometimes surgery is also required to aid healing. Once the episode has resolved, preventive treatment, such as using a fly mask and anti-inflammatory medications, is often needed to minimize additional inflammatory flares. Enucleation (removal of the affected eye) is the last resort in older horses because both eyes are often affected. Without treatment, the horse will be in pain, and the affected eye will become smaller over time.

> **TECHNICIAN NOTE**   A horse with a swollen, painful eye is considered an emergency because the eye can rupture if it is not treated quickly.

NEUROLOGIC DEFICITS

Older horses can develop mild or progressive neurologic deficits as a result of trauma or chronic changes, such as cervical fractures compressing the spinal cord. Clinical signs in an affected horse include depression, decreased proprioception, dragging toes, ataxia, and reluctance to turn the neck. Diagnostic tests include a thorough physical and neurologic examination, blood tests such as liver function tests, cervical radiographs, and cerebrospinal fluid aspiration. Treatment includes anti-inflammatory medications and small paddock turnout and stall confinement, if needed. These horses are often weak and may lose their position in the hierarchy. Therefore, it is important to place them with other horses in similar condition and to feed them individually to ensure that they are receiving adequate nutrition.

MUSCULOSKELETAL SYSTEM

Geriatric horses often have multiple sites of DJD (osteoarthritis) and can be lame at the walk and trot. Lower limbs, hocks, carpi, and cervical vertebrae are most commonly affected. Soft tissue problems include degeneration of the suspensory tendon. Diagnostic tests include lameness examination, local anesthetic for nerve blocks, sonographic evaluation, and radiographs to identify affected areas. Treatment includes local joint injection of steroids to relieve clinical signs, but this cannot be repeated too many times. Many of these horses require long-term NSAIDs (e.g., phenylbuta-zone, firocoxib) to have a good quality of life. Monitoring the horse using diagnostic tests, such as chemistry profile, packed cell volume (PCV), total protein, and urinalysis, is an important part of using these medications. Although side effects, such as renal insufficiency or right dorsal colitis, may be noted with long-term NSAID use, it is paramount to keep these geriatric horses comfortable at the end of their lives. Firocoxib is a cyclooxygenase (COX)-2 inhibitor that should spare gastric mucosal protection and renal blood flow. Pasture turnout as much as possible is important because older horses become stiff when standing in the stall for too long. Regular foot trimming every 4 weeks and use of shoes are often vital in maintaining the horse's comfort.

> **TECHNICIAN NOTE** Geriatric horses often have multiple problems that require careful monitoring and treatment to ensure optimal health and longevity.

MANAGEMENT, NUTRITION, AND NURSING CARE OF THE GERIATRIC HORSE

Management of the aged horse is paramount in maintaining optimal health and keeping the horse comfortable. Frequent hoof trimming every 4 weeks is important to maintain the horse's comfort, especially when he has DJD and lameness. If the horse's foot grows too long, this changes the angle of the leg and makes walking more difficult. Routine dental floating every 6 months will keep the horse comfortable and eating well, and will prevent problems such as wave mouth.

It is notoriously difficult to maintain weight and body condition in older horses. It is especially difficult to improve a horse's condition if he has lost weight or is already thin.

Additional considerations must be noted in treating geriatric horses. These horses seem more sensitive to certain medications, such as sedation and NSAIDs. This sensitivity may be seen as a combination of decreased muscle mass and renal and/or liver insufficiency, but many geriatric horses tolerate only one-half of a typical dose of sedative given intravenously. For example, the clinician should give only 75 mg xylazine and 1 mg butorphanol *or* 2 mg detomidine and 1 mg butorphanol to an average 450-kg (1000-lb) horse. Many of these horses receive daily NSAID treatment for chronic DJD (osteoarthritis). They may be given 1 g of phen-ylbutazone orally daily for a few years, because without medication they are in significant pain. When administering NSAID medication, the owner should be aware of potential side effects, such as renal failure or right dorsal colitis. It is important to monitor the horse's attitude, appetite, manure production, renal values (creatinine, blood urea nitrogen [BUN]), urinalysis, and PCV and total protein. If any changes in these values are reported, the patient and the treatment protocol should be reassessed.

General management recommendations include regular deworming, frequent manure removal, and low stocking density (e.g., a few horses in a large pasture) to minimize parasite burden in a pasture. Performing periodic fecal egg counts is helpful in assessing whether the deworming schedule is adequate. It is not uncommon to have a false-negative test result from fecal examination, but the horse has a parasite burden, so regular deworming is important, even if the fecal examination test result is negative, and fecal egg counts offer a quantitative method that can be used to assess deworming protocols.

Regular vaccination is recommended, using the recom-mended vaccine protocol for the area. If the horse has a history of vaccine reactions, pretreatment with an NSAID, such as phenylbutazone or flunixin meglumine, is recom-mended. Many horses develop more severe reactions over time, so geriatric horses with a history of vaccine reaction are at higher risk. If the horse still shows a reaction despite pretreatment, only necessary vaccines should be adminis-tered to minimize complications. Annual physical examina-tions are important in maintaining the health of a geriatric horse and in detecting problems. Many geriatric horses seem to develop renal and liver insufficiency over time, so annual blood tests (e.g., CBC, chemistry profile) are important for monitoring their health.

Management is paramount to maintaining a healthy geri-atric horse. Geriatric horses can have a good quality of life with proper care, but they require close monitoring. Many are turned out in pasture and are not monitored well. They may have poor body condition hidden by a thick hair coat, so it is best to train the owner to assess the horse's body condition. Clipping older horses and placing a blanket in the winter keep these older horses comfortable. Geriatric horses with an over-long hair coat are not able to thermoregulate well, may have patchy sweating, and are prone to develop dermatitis. It is also advisable to clip over the jugular vein before administering intravenous medications to easily visu-alize the vein and avoid the carotid artery. Frequent pasture turnout is ideal for maintaining body condition and GI tract health, and for minimizing stiffness. It is important to turn the geriatric horse out with other horses in equal condition. Otherwise, the older horse will be at the bottom of the hier-archy and may not have adequate access to food. If the older horse is in poor body condition, feeding him individually is important to ensure that the horse is receiving enough food and to assess appetite. Feeding free-choice high-quality hay with supplementation of alfalfa (hay or soaked alfalfa cubes or pellets) will aid in maintaining weight. Feeding an equine senior feed is also important for maintaining weight or pro-viding calories when the horse has lost teeth. Corn oil ($\frac{1}{4}$ to $\frac{1}{2}$ cup per day) added to the feed provides additional calories.

END OF LIFE ISSUES

When a geriatric horse is no longer enjoying a good quality of life, euthanasia may be considered by the owner and/or recommended by the veterinarian. Considerations for eutha-nasia include poor body condition or rapidly losing weight, refractory pain (e.g., acute, severe laminitis), and severe DJD, leading to chronic, severe lameness. Additional considerations include episodes of the horse falling frequently and impending cold weather. Cold weather, snow, and icy conditions are difficult for older horses to manage. If the horse slips on the ice, it may be impossible to lift the horse up again, necessitating euthanasia. These geriatric horses have often been a part of the family for years, and the entire family would like to be present for the horse's final moments. A scheduled euthanasia can allow the family to say goodbye and can offer a peaceful end to a beloved horse.

SUMMARY

The veterinary community can contribute to the health and well-being of geriatric veterinary patients in many ways. Because pets have become an integral part of modern family life, the need for home and barn support for these animals is increased today. Veterinary technicians can help to provide at-home hospice care for these patients, in addition to the routine geriatric care provided at veterinary hospitals. It is important to remember that hospice care should be provided only while the animal maintains a good quality of life. Once the quality of life declines to an unacceptable level, euthanasia should be considered.

Geriatric horses are living longer today; many are living well into their 20s and 30s when properly cared for and closely monitored. They often make excellent companions for younger horses and provide much enjoyment for their owners. Medical problems must be detected early and treatment initiated promptly to provide optimal quality of life for the geriatric equine patient. As in small animals, once the horse's quality of life declines to an unacceptable level, euthanasia should be considered. The veterinary technician can provide thorough patient assessment and nursing care, and can teach clients how to provide care at home.

RECOMMENDED READINGS

Geriatric Cats and Dogs

Debraekeleer J, Gross KL, Zicker SC: Feeding mature adult dogs: middle aged and older. In Hand MS, Thatcher CD, Remillard RL, et al, editors: Small animal clinical nutrition, ed 5, Topeka, KS, 2010, Mark Morris Institute, p 273.

Fahey GC, Barry KA, Swanson KS: Age-related changes in nutrient utilization by companion animals, Annu Rev Nutr 28:425, 2008.

Gross KL, Becvarova I, Debraekeleer J: Feeding mature adult cats: middle aged and older. In Hand MS, Thatcher CD, Remillard RL, et al, editors: Small animal clinical nutrition, ed 5, Topeka, KS, 2010, Mark Morris Institute, p 390.

Hancock CG, McMillan FD, Ellenbogen TR: Owner services and hospice care. In Hoskins JD, editor: Geriatrics & gerontology of the dog and cat, ed 2, St Louis, 2004, Saunders, p 5.

McMillan FD: The concept of quality of life in animals. In McMillan FD, editor: Mental health and well-being in animals, Ames, IA, 2005, Blackwell Publishing, p 183.

Yazbek KVB, Fantoni DT: Validity of a health-related quality-of-life scale for dogs with signs of pain secondary to cancer, J Am Vet Med Assoc 226:1354, 2005.

Pittari J, Rodan I, Beekman G, et al: 2008 AAFP senior care guidelines. Available at: catvets.com/professionals/guidelines/publications/?Id= 398 (accessed on April 18, 2011).

Geriatric Horses

Beech J, Boston RC, McFarlane D, et al: Evaluation of plasma ACTH, α-melanocyte–stimulating hormone, and insulin concentrations during various photoperiods in clinically normal horses and ponies and those with pituitary pars intermedia dysfunction, JAVMA 235:715, 2009.

Bentz AI: Fare thee well: how to help owners (and yourself) deal with the death of a horse, Compend Cont Educ Vet 31:514, 2009.

Bertone J, editor: Equine geriatric medicine and surgery, Philadelphia, 2006, Elsevier.

Donaldson MT: Equine Cushing's disease: diagnosis, treatment, pathogenesis and clinical signs, Proc North Am Vet Conference 2004.

Donaldson MT, Jorgensen AJ, Beech J: Evaluation of suspected pituitary pars intermedia dysfunction in horses with laminitis, J Am Vet Med Assoc 224:1123, 2004.

McCarthy C: Geriatric horses: maintaining a good quality of life, Vet Tech 30:36, 2009.

McFarlane D: Endocrine and metabolic diseases. In Smith BP, editor: Large animal internal medicine, ed 4, St Louis, 2009, Mosby.

36 The Human-Animal Bond, Bereavement, and Euthanasia

Joseph Taboada and Stephanie W. Johnson

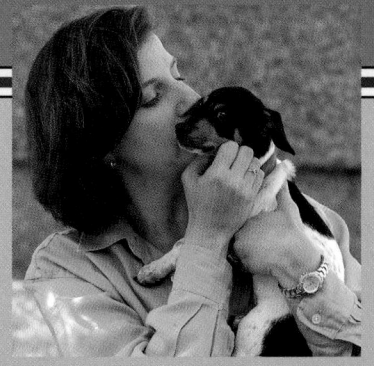

OUTLINE

The Human-Animal Bond, *1378*
The Attachment Between Animals and
  Humans, *1378*
Benefits of Attachment, *1379*
Pet Loss and Veterinary Medicine, *1379*
When the Bond Is Broken, *1379*
Pet Loss and the Grief Process, *1380*
The Normal Grief Process, *1381*
**Grief and the Veterinary
  Professional,** *1385*
Euthanasia, *1387*

The Decision, *1387*
As the End Draws Near: The Beginning
  of the End, *1388*
At the End, *1390*
The End as a Beginning … After the
  End, *1391*
The Stress of Euthanasia, *1392*
Euthanasia in the Shelter and
  Research Facility, *1393*
Euthanasia of Large Animals, *1396*

KEY TERMS

Anger
Barbiturate
Bargaining
Bereavement
Catharsis
Compassion
Denial
Depression
Drug Enforcement
  Agency (DEA)
Euthanasia
Grief process
Resolution
Validation

LEARNING OBJECTIVES

When you have completed this chapter, you will be able to:
1. Pronounce, define, and spell each of the Key Terms in this chapter.
2. Discuss aspects of strong attachments to animals.
3. List and describe the stages of grief and the role of veterinary professionals in grief counseling.
4. Do the following regarding euthanasia:
   • Discuss the impact of euthanasia and client grief on members of the veterinary health care team.
   • Discuss the legal and ethical issues related to euthanasia.
   • Discuss the role of the veterinary health care team in counseling owners considering euthanasia of their pet, and factors that owners need to consider when making decisions regarding euthanasia.
   • Describe considerations in scheduling euthanasia appointments and in preparing for unexpected events during euthanasia.
   • List signs and symptoms of staff burnout.
   • List and describe acceptable methods of euthanasia in animals.
   • Discuss special considerations related to euthanasia of large animals.

INTRODUCTION

Today, with more than 72.9 million households owning one or more companion animals, pets are considered part of the extended family network.[1] Surveys and clinical experience indicate that many people consider their pets to be like children, partners, or best friends. Because of changing family structure and increasing numbers of persons who live alone, companion animals have taken on larger roles in people's support systems. With these changes have come added expectations of veterinary health care professionals. Members of the veterinary medical profession must realize that they are treating not just dogs, cats, birds, rabbits, or horses, but important members of their clients' family and an important part of their clients' support system (Figure 36-1).

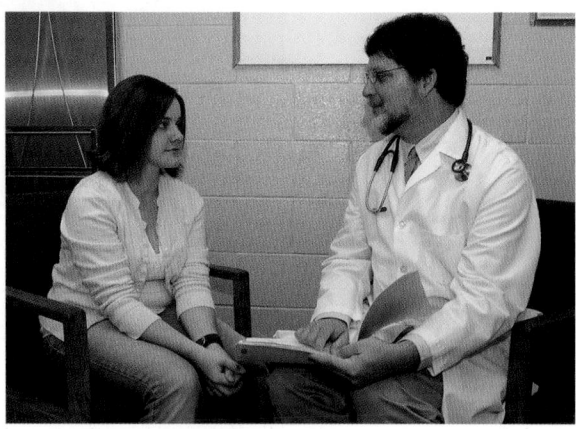

FIGURE 36-1 The diagnosis of a disease can be a difficult time for both clients and veterinary professionals. It is important to respond to both the pet's and the owner's needs.

THE HUMAN-ANIMAL BOND

Today, modern society is largely urban rather than rural. Through world urbanization, people tend to live in neighborhoods rather than on farms. Animals live with their owners in apartments or houses, thus increasing familiarity, dependency, and bonding. Eighty percent of our animal companions live inside.

Companion animals provide both parents and children with stability, constancy, and security. It is not unusual for families to change locales and residences several times within a 10-year period. As a result, most people no longer live within a short distance of their extended families. The nuclear family is smaller, consisting of an average of fewer than two children. The single-parent family is becoming common. Because an increasing number of U.S. women work outside the home, many school-age children return home to be greeted not by their mother but by the family pet. An increasing number of adults live alone, and couples opt to remain childless. More and more, people are filling these voids with pets, which provide a unique outlet for their owners' needs to nurture and be loved. As health and medical care improves, the number of persons in the age group older than 60 years has increased to more than 16% of the population. Pets fulfill many needs for elderly people, including needs for interaction, exercise, companionship, protection, and motivation to remain active and independent.

It is becoming increasingly recognized that physically and mentally disabled individuals benefit from contact with animals. As society has realized the special talents of pets, new utilitarian functions have been found for them. Dogs are used with success to assist blind, hearing impaired, and physically disabled persons. These specially trained animals provide their owners with independence, companionship, social lubrication, protection, and love. Horses, cats, and dogs have been used successfully in animal-assisted therapy programs for people with all types of physical and mental disabilities. Animals facilitate interaction with people who may be reluctant to interact, and their presence reduces anxiety, lowers blood pressure, and decreases heart rate. Results of some studies indicate that animals may alleviate or prevent **depression**. Survival rates for cardiac patients who are pet owners are higher than for those who do not own pets. Pet ownership is considered an important predictor of survival for patients with coronary artery disease.

In short, the relationships between people and animals have become physically closer, and the role of animals in the daily lives of their owners has become more emotional as society has changed. Of the more than 72.9 million families owning at least one pet, one-third of companion animal pet owners describe their pets as family members and cite companionship, love, affection, and fun as the most important derivatives of the relationship. Further, it has been shown that 83% of pet owners refer to themselves as mom or dad; 93% buy their pets gifts; 84% treat them as children; and 63% say, "I love you," at least once daily to their pets.

> **TECHNICIAN NOTE**   Many people consider their pets to be like children.

THE ATTACHMENT BETWEEN ANIMALS AND HUMANS

Strong attachments can form between owners and any type of animal, but they are probably recognized most commonly in veterinary practices with dogs, cats, and horses. The degree of attachment varies greatly from the utilitarian attachment between a rancher and his or her cattle to the parent-child type of bonding that occurs between some people and their dog or cat. In 2010, 72% of the 117.5 million households in the United States had owned at least one pet.[1] It is estimated that about 50% of these pet owners classify their attachment to their pet as strong. Of these "strong attachment" owners, about half see their pets as reflections of themselves or of their tastes with the pet depending on the owner for love, affection, and care. The other half of the strong attachment owners report a reliance on their pets as an emotional crutch, supplying unconditional love and affection, and sometimes acting as a substitute for family, friends, or children.

As pets are used to meet many of the changing psychosocial needs of modern society, the intensity of attachment has increased. When pet loss occurs, the intensity and duration of attachment determine the significance of the loss and the intensity of the grief that follows. Attachment is more intense when the animal has functioned in many roles for the owner. The owner of an assistance dog therefore may suffer more intense **bereavement** than the owner of a dog used only for herding or hunting. Owners who have experienced previous significant losses, adjustments, or traumas and have been comforted by their pet's presence may also exhibit strong attachment and thus intense bereavement.

> **TECHNICIAN NOTE**   If a pet is associated with an important person or a significant life stage or event, it can take on added significance.

BENEFITS OF ATTACHMENT

As reminders of both pleasant and traumatic events in people's lives, pets can take on symbolic meaning. Several keys are helpful in assessing the level of attachment between an owner and his or her animal or animals (Box 36-1). Even when the pet is simply another family member, grief can be intense. Grief is also individual, and each family member may grieve in a unique way. (Case Presentation 36-1 can be studied to further understand the attachment between owners and animals.)

BOX 36-1 | Keys to Attachment

The levels of attachment are different for each pet and owner. Human-animal relationships may be perceived as stronger and more important when the following aspects are present:

- Owners believe that they rescued their companion animals from death or near death.
- Owners believe that their companion animals got them through a difficult period in life.
- Owners spent their childhood with their companion animals.
- Owners have relied on their companion animals as their most significant source of support.
- Owners anthropomorphize their companion animals.
- Owners have invested extensive time, effort, or financial resources into their companion animals' long-term medical care.
- Owners view their companion animal as a symbolic link to significant people who are no longer part of their lives or to significant times in their lives.

CASE PRESENTATION 36-1

Sneaky, a 12-year-old female domestic shorthair cat, is brought into the practice for lethargy and anorexia. After a workup, she is diagnosed as having cardiomyopathy. Even with appropriate treatment, the prognosis for a long lifetime is poor.

Sneaky is owned by a 73-year-old widow named Ruth. The cat was a gift from her husband, Ralph, who died of cancer 2 years earlier. During her husband's fight against the disease, Sneaky was his constant companion. Ruth can still vividly remember how Sneaky, as a kitten, used to make her husband laugh by hiding in his boots and jumping out at him when he leaned down to pick them up.

Sneaky was brought to the veterinarian for what was perceived to be a minor problem, but a severe, life-threatening disease was diagnosed. Ruth is likely to feel numb initially. The diagnosis is likely to be hard to accept. An important part of Ruth's attachment to Sneaky comes from her relationship with her late husband. Sneaky represents a tangible link between Ruth's life now and the many memories of her life with her husband. Not only is Sneaky's death going to be hard because of the loss of a faithful companion and family member, but it is also going to bring back many of the emotions that were associated with the death of her husband.

PET LOSS AND VETERINARY MEDICINE

Veterinarians and veterinary technicians are confronted daily with complex issues of attachment, loss, and grief in the course of their patients' illness and death. The diagnosis of life-threatening or terminal disease can be a difficult time for both the client and the veterinary professional (see Figure 36-1).

> **TECHNICIAN NOTE** Veterinary technicians are confronted daily with complex issues of attachment, loss, and grief.

Given all the emotional and utilitarian aspects of the human-animal relationship in modern society, it is not surprising that breaking of the bond caused by the death of the pet is a significant event in the lives of many pet owners. Loss of the pet for many owners is made even more intense and personal in that the pet is often grieved by no one other than themselves. Daily routines are filled with reminders of activities once performed for or with the pet. The loss of a pet often means that a unique, irreplaceable member of the family is gone.

A person's support system is made up of people (and pets) that interact with one another on a daily basis, providing support, comfort, and social interaction. Support systems are especially important during times of loss. Unfortunately, many people who make up these support systems do not understand the full extent of attachment between a pet owner and a pet. This lack of understanding can present serious problems for the owner who is facing the odyssey of grief after the death of a pet. As a result, pet owners often turn to veterinary professionals as sources of support, comfort, and understanding at and around the time of their pet's death.

> **TECHNICIAN NOTE** People tend to turn to the veterinary staff during grief over a pet because they believe that the veterinary technician understands their attachment and loss.

Pet owners tend to turn to veterinary staff members when they are grieving the death of their pet. This can place veterinary professionals in an awkward position because the situation demands knowledge that is typically outside the boundaries of veterinary medicine and requires confidence in talking about death and the **grief process**. This is why the areas of attachment, animal behavior, human bereavement, and grief counseling are becoming increasingly relevant to veterinary medicine.

WHEN THE BOND IS BROKEN

In general, people in U.S. society are uncomfortable talking about death. We know little about the experience of death, and we fear the unknown, yet veterinarians and their staff must frequently discuss death, participate in causing it, witness it, and deal with the emotions triggered by these experiences.

Although people in the midst of grief have a need and a right to understand what is happening to them, there are few places that they can go to get helpful, supportive information about grief. This is particularly true when the loss that they are grieving is that of a beloved pet. Like most of society, veterinarians and veterinary technicians rarely have formal training in this area. Despite this fact, veterinary professionals are often the people clients instinctively turn to for support.

Making the job more difficult is the fact that grief and bereavement are emotional and often irrational areas of human interaction. Bereaved individuals at times may seem out of control or out of touch with reality. When this happens, those around the griever, including the veterinary professional, may feel uncomfortable; few veterinary professionals are taught how to support or deal with people who are irrational or emotional. **Compassion** is an important sensitivity to draw on when interacting with clients experiencing grief.

> **TECHNICIAN NOTE** Compassion is an important sensitivity to draw on when interacting with clients experiencing grief.

Grief is the companion to death. It is the mental anguish experienced by any human who is confronted with the loss of an object of attachment. Grief may ensue as an effect of any loss, including loss through death, divorce, loss of a job, or even moving or having friends move away. It can be intensely emotional and can affect mind, body, and spirit. When confronted with grief, the bereaved individual goes through a grief process. The term *grief process* implies that there is an intended end or result to be produced through grieving. Thus the grief process is the means of letting go of the object of attachment to feel better, reinvest, emotionally grow, and attach again.

The veterinary staff is in a unique position to assist clients as they go through the process of grief as it relates to the loss of a pet. By way of their unique role in the life of both the owner and the pet, veterinary professionals are in a unique position to understand the bond that had developed. In addition, the veterinarian and the owner may have interacted uniquely in choosing the time of the pet's death (as occurs when **euthanasia** is performed). To assist clients during the difficult bereavement period, it is helpful to understand the normal grief process and its manifestations as applied to pet loss.

PET LOSS AND THE GRIEF PROCESS

The death of a pet is all too often regarded as a trivial loss by society, perhaps in part because of the mistaken belief that pets can be easily replaced. There are no socially sanctioned rituals, such as funerals or memorial services, to help grieving pet owners gain support once the bonds between them and their animal have been broken. Further, people are rarely granted time off from their jobs to care for sick animals or to make arrangements for them after their death. Society also does not allow adequate time for mourning the death of a pet. Most people feel pressured to be "back to normal" within a few days of their pet's death to avoid being labeled as neurotic, hysterical, or overly attached. However, crying, taking time away from work, and wanting to memorialize a pet are healthy responses to the death of a pet. People should not be discouraged, nor should they be judged.

One of the most effective ways for veterinary professionals to assist grieving clients is to educate and reassure them that their feelings and behaviors are normal parts of the grief process. Other ways that veterinary professionals can help are listed in Box 36-2.

> **TECHNICIAN NOTE** Veterinary professionals can assist clients by normalizing their feelings.

| **BOX 36-2** | Stages of Grief: How Veterinary Professionals Can Help |

Denial

What the client needs most is time, support, understanding, and permission to grieve.

Before Death

- Arrange to communicate with the client in person, if possible, where both of you can sit down to talk without interruption or distraction. Recognize denial as a normal part of grief.
- Communicate clearly and reiterate patiently. Phrase statements in words that are concrete and simple for the layperson. Avoid using medical jargon and lapsing into complicated medical explanations.
- Listen actively: maintain eye contact, use attentive body language, and paraphrase or clarify the client's statements as you respond. Give him or her permission to express feelings.

- Give the client time to think about and to grasp the reality of information that has been given. Some clients need only a slight pause in the conversation or a few minutes alone. Other clients may need more time to themselves before they comprehend the news of severe illness or actual death.
- Refrain from judging the client as "stupid" or "out of it."
- Remain nonjudgmental and unhurried toward the client, and state that you are available to talk about specifics or about his or her feelings whenever the time is right.
- Never attempt to force clients to "come to their senses" or to move out of denial. Clients will comprehend at their own pace.

After Death

- Encourage the client to view the body and say goodbye.
- Give permission to grieve.

BOX 36-2 | Stages of Grief: How Veterinary Professionals Can Help—cont'd

Bargaining

- Understand that bargaining is an attempt to control or reverse a dire situation. The client feels irrationally compelled to bargain during the grief process and does not mean to doubt the professionals involved.
- When the patient is terminally ill, do not become defensive or threatened when clients ask for other opinions or consider alternative treatments. Giving information, materials to read, and referral for second opinion will ameliorate bargaining attempts and facilitate commitment to treatment.
- After the death, be empathetic and educate about the stage of bargaining when clients confide their feelings and bargaining behaviors, such as prayers and dreams (or daydreams) of the pet still alive. Reassure them that the emotional basis for their behaviors and feelings is normal even though it may seem irrational.
- When clients inquire as to when to "replace" their pet, educating them about the role bargaining plays in shopping for a new pet can alleviate future disappointment. State that their dead pet was unique and cannot be replaced, but encourage them to obtain a new pet whenever all members of the family feel ready. Help them to find the type of animal that they are looking for while gently steering toward one that is slightly dissimilar to the dead pet. Encourage them to choose a different breed, color, or gender, and a new name should be chosen.

Anger

- Listen actively, and let the client know that you understand.
- Arrange for communication in a private room with no distractions. Sit at eye level, and use attentive body language. Take notes if the client is complaining or criticizing.
- Give the client permission to vent feelings. Listen actively while using attentive body language, eye contact, nodding, and responses that paraphrase, clarify, and indicate your understanding of the client's feelings (e.g., "I can see that you're angry...," or "You feel that diagnosis could have been made sooner...").
- If the client is directly angry at the veterinarian, the technician, or the clinic staff, take a mental step backward and pause with a deep breath or by counting to 10.
- Do not become defensive or respond in like manner to the client.
- Relieve guilt by assuring the client that he or she did the right thing, and that what he or she is feeling is a normal part of the grief process.

Depression

- Encourage depressed clients to talk about their feelings with regard to their pet. Follow up with clients whose pets have died with a telephone call in a few days, and then 2 weeks afterward.
- Listen actively.
- Attend to the client by positioning yourself at eye level, offering tissues or a drink of water, and leaning slightly toward the client. A nonthreatening yet compassionate touch on the forearm or on the shoulder communicates empathy and understanding.
- Offer a place to sit, a place to be out of the "public eye."
- Tell the client that it is all right and even good to cry. Listen supportively and actively, and touch the client gently on the shoulder or forearm. Some clients are known well enough to embrace, and this can be helpful.
- Validate feelings of sadness by letting the client know that this is normal.
- Offer to call a family member or friend.
- Encourage and suggest means by which clients can memorialize their pet. Making scrapbooks, planting a tree, writing a letter to the pet, and writing the pet's life story all are cathartic activities that alleviate depression caused by grief.
- If a client expresses continued depression several weeks after the death of a pet, if his or her support system is poor, or if a client expresses a personal wish to die, referral to a compassionate professional counselor is necessary. Although referral may feel awkward, many clients appreciate the technician who states, "Grief as a result of pet loss is normal, but sometimes there can be no one to talk to, or the grief can be overwhelming. I know of a person who understands what you're going through. Would you like her (his) telephone number, or may I have her (him) call you?" Today, several schools of veterinary medicine employ counselors experienced in pet loss. Many communities have established support groups, and private counselors increasingly view pet loss as significant bereavement.

Resolution

- Acceptance is achieved once the previous four stages have fallen into the background of the client's life. At this point, the bereaved person can channel emotional energy into a new relationship. The veterinary professional can help clients reach the resolution stage by offering insight into the grief process through his or her actions and by offering suggestions of reading material or seminars on the grief process.

THE NORMAL GRIEF PROCESS

As stated earlier, the word *process* implies movement toward some end or result. With regard to grief, this movement is accomplished by passing through what have been termed *stages, phases,* or *tasks.* Although there are a few differences, the basic emotional process experienced in pet loss is the same as in human loss.

Several models of the grief process can be modified to describe the emotional process that occurs during pet loss. The following discussion uses the classic model supplied by Elisabeth Kübler-Ross (see "Recommended Readings").

Dr. Kübler-Ross was one of the first to work extensively with dying persons and their families during the late 1960s. She described the grief process as consisting of five stages:

denial, **bargaining**, **anger**, depression, and **resolution**. She used these stages to describe the passage through grief, but it is helpful to remember that the stages are not a linear odyssey. Although people may travel through the grief process in a straight line, they more often fluctuate between stages, bounce back and forth, and feel the entire gamut of grief within minutes, days, or months.

> **TECHNICIAN NOTE** The grief process consists of five stages: denial, bargaining, anger, depression, and resolution.

Denial and Bargaining

Case Presentation 36-2 can be studied to further understand the types of reactions that a client might exhibit during denial and/or bargaining.

Denial is a normal defense mechanism that buffers humans from some unbearable news or reality. It is important to recognize the word *normal* here because many individuals experiencing denial at the time a poor prognosis is given or during bereavement will seem to all observers to be out of touch with reality. The veterinary staff may wonder

---

CASE PRESENTATION 36-2

Captain, a 9-year-old Boxer, is brought into the practice for a checkup and vaccinations. His owner, Don, tells you that 1 year ago, Captain was treated for lymphosarcoma. The cancer went into remission, and Captain has been doing fine ever since. However, it is obvious to you that Captain is not feeling well.

Examination reveals that the cancer has returned. It takes Don some time to accept that fact. It is agreed that treatment should start again immediately. After a lack of response to a rescue phase of chemotherapy, it is clear that Captain's death is imminent. When the news is given to Don, he insists over and over again that the treatment should be continued. "If it worked before, it will work again—just keep on trying." If the treatment really is not working, Don believes that changing Captain's diet to one he read about on the Internet will have better results.

Don brought Captain in for a routine examination. It was immediately obvious to you that Captain was not feeling well. However, Don either could not recognize any of the symptoms or was denying that Captain was sick again. Despite the fact that Don went into the initial treatment protocol knowing that relapse was eventually inevitable, he still exhibits signs of denial. It is obvious that he is not ready to accept Captain's impending death. It is important for the clinician to realize that Don's response is a normal part of the grief process. He will not be able to understand the seriousness of the situation until he is ready. Don also shows signs of bargaining when he wants other treatment options to be explored even though it is clear that nothing can be done at this point to save Captain.

---

whether the client has even heard the veterinarian stating the seriousness of an animal's illness. A client in denial may listen attentively to a diagnosis of cancer with a poor prognosis, but may ask only if the toenails can be clipped, or if the flea shampoo currently being used is correct. A client informed of the death of his or her pet while it was hospitalized may chatter on about activities for the weekend. A simple form of denial is exemplified by the client who states repeatedly, "It can't be. I don't believe it."

It is tempting when presented with a client who is experiencing denial to insist that he or she recognize the seriousness of the situation. Many veterinarians and veterinary technicians worry that the client does not comprehend or has not heard correctly. There is no harm in repeating oneself to a client in denial. Restating diagnoses, prognoses, treatment plans, and particulars is advisable. However, clients in denial will accept the unbearable reality of the situation only when they are ready internally; attempts to push them may backfire, resulting in frustration. Usually a client will begin to ask appropriate questions about the time he or she arrives home and may telephone the veterinary office. Some may even seem to return to reality before your eyes while those toenails are attended to. The veterinary professional must be assured that the client has been told the basic information that needs to be given. Remember, however, that it may not have been fully understood; therefore, always leave the door open for further communication.

Denial is reflected by the client's eyes and demeanor and by incongruous questions. The veterinary staff should not believe that they are responsible to "break through" a client's denial. The client will move out of denial, accepting the reality of the situation, when he or she is ready. The veterinary staff's recognition of the client's denial can prevent impatience and frustration during the veterinary contact.

> **TECHNICIAN NOTE** Even when dealing with attentive clients, veterinary professionals may be required to repeat themselves several times while clients decide on a course of treatment for their pet. Clients overwhelmed with emotion may have difficulty comprehending information. Members of the team must be patient.

Once the reality of death or impending death is realized, the client may show various impotent attempts to control or reverse the reality. The client is grappling with the stage of the grief process that Dr. Kübler-Ross called *bargaining*. During this stage, the client maneuvers personally and privately, possibly praying and negotiating with God for miracles. The client might add various herbs and old family remedies to food. Children behave like little angels, hoping to be rewarded with a reversal of bad news. The veterinary staff may be subject to various inquiries by the client at this stage, relative to the latest "miracle cure" that the client has discovered on the Internet. It is while bargaining that a pet owner may request permission to obtain a second (and sometimes third, fourth, or fifth) opinion. During this time, be compassionate, and when possible, answer clients' questions. Help clients to understand that this stage of grief is normal.

Seeking to replace the lost animal without grieving at all is a form of bargaining. Many pet owners seek a new pet too soon; they purchase the same species and the same color, and they name the pet the same or a similar name.

It is important to recognize denial and bargaining as part of the normal grief process. Veterinary professionals who understand these stages will avoid frustration in their attempts to provide quality patient care and client service.

Anger

Case Presentation 36-3 can be studied to further understand the types of reactions that a client might exhibit during the anger stage.

During the grief process, clients may move into and out of the stage called *anger*. Clients coping with this stage may exhibit anger in a wide variety of direct or indirect ways. The anger may be specific or nonspecific in the way that it is directed. Anger may also be exhibited in the form of guilt, which can be defined as anger turned inward.

Anger is a particularly difficult emotion to deal with when a client directs it toward the veterinary professional. Regardless of whether the client is justified in his or her stated cause

---

CASE PRESENTATION 36-3

John brings Sparky, a 3-year-old Dalmatian, into the practice. Sparky got out of the yard this afternoon because the gate was left open. He ran across the street and was hit by a car. His spine is fractured, and his spinal cord is severely injured. A substantial amount of internal bleeding has been noted.

John is informed that Sparky has only a slim chance of surviving surgery. He elects for any measure to be taken regardless of cost. Unfortunately, Sparky dies during the procedure. When you tell John, he immediately begins yelling at you, "How dare you let Sparky die? There must have been something else that could have been done!" He then refuses to pay the bill and storms out of the practice.

The next day, John calls and apologizes for his rude outburst. He lets you know that he realizes that every measure was taken to save Sparky. He also admits to feeling guilty for having left the gate open. Then he requests that the bill be mailed to him.

John is expressing his anger over Sparky's death, which should be recognized as a stage of grief. Although John initially expressed his anger at you, it should not be taken personally. It is not necessarily directed at you. You should not react defensively, but instead listen politely, and let John know that you empathize and understand. Realize that part of his anger may come from guilt that he left the gate open.

His call on the following day emphasizes that anger can be an uncomfortable but transient part of the grief process. He admits that his anger was not really caused by you. He attributes it to his feelings of guilt.

---

for anger, staff members must use tolerance and patience to avoid responding defensively. Bereaved clients may complain that the illness that resulted in death should have been discovered sooner, should have been treated differently, or should not have been allowed to happen. They may complain that their pet died while hospitalized because of neglect or inappropriate treatment rather than because of the tumor revealed by necropsy.

> **TECHNICIAN NOTE** Regardless of whether the client is justified in his or her stated cause for anger, staff members must use tolerance and patience to avoid responding defensively.

Anger may be apparent in the form of guilt. Clients who are feeling guilt use language with an abundance of "I should've" statements. They often seek the listening ear of the veterinary professional, looking for absolution from guilt. They may ask whether the food that they fed their pet could have contributed to the illness or death. They often ask whether it was the pesticide in their home or in the shampoo that caused a tumor or cardiac arrest. Clients may believe that they allowed their pet to be too active or too fat; others may believe that they caused kidney failure in their cat by feeding an insufficient diet. These clients can direct anger at themselves, but frequently they cannot find a specific crime that they committed. When possible, the veterinary professional can assist clients by assuaging their guilt. Reassuring clients that, in your opinion, they did everything possible for their pet, that they did only what they thought would benefit their pet, and that they made the right decisions for their pet will relieve much of clients' guilt or anger and will assist them in moving through the grief process.

> **TECHNICIAN NOTE** Veterinary professionals can help by reassuring clients that they did everything possible and made the right decisions.

The client in this stage may be gruff or rude and generally difficult to get along with. Stating that he or she is angry, the client may be at a loss to express the object of the anger. These clients may yell at the cashiers, the hospital manager, the receptionist, the technicians, and the veterinarian. Giving the angry client an opportunity to express feelings (venting) is an effective way for the veterinary professional to help. At times, all that is needed is for the sensitive veterinary professional to explain that given the client's loss, anger is a normal feeling.

Anger is often exhibited by reluctance to pay the bill. On receiving an inquiry by telephone, the client implies that nonpayment is due to anger at treatment provided by the veterinarian or technician, or because the pet was neglected, the illness was mistreated, or the client was treated insensitively. Bereavement support can alleviate this client's anger. Listen attentively, state your apologies, if any, and follow up with this client. No admission of mistakes need be made, but the client needs to feel significant and understood.

Anger is difficult to work through, but it is guilt that may be hardest for the client to relinquish. In continuing to feel guilt and anger, the client avoids letting go of the beloved pet, and the grief process is stymied. Once the client is able to relinquish the guilt or anger, the grief process can continue.

The veterinary professional can assist the client with all types of exhibited anger by taking a mental step back and a deep breath, committing to a nondefensive attitude, and simply listening. Take notes, if possible, and reassure the client of follow-up if anger is directed at veterinary staff. Assuage any guilt if the opportunity arises, and allow the client to vent. A few minutes on the telephone or in person may salvage a client relationship and may go a long way in assisting the client through the grief process.

Depression

Case Presentation 36-4 can be studied to further understand the types of reactions that a client might exhibit during the depression stage.

The stage of the grief process that is termed *depression* has also been called *grief*. Clients who are experiencing depression describe their mood as complete, overwhelming sadness. Intense grief can result in depression, which prohibits a client from functioning normally. Appetite is changed, energy level is lowered, the client withdraws from others; sometimes the client is unable to go to work. More subtle symptoms of depression include irritability, sleep irregularity, restlessness, and inability to concentrate.

CASE PRESENTATION 36-4

Two weeks ago, Micah brought her 10-year-old barrel racing horse, Lightning, to the practice. Lightning had colic. Every possible remedy was explored; however, Lightning had to be euthanized. Micah was extremely distraught over the loss of Lightning, whom she described as "the other half of my soul."

You have a couple of free minutes, so you decide to call to see how Micah is doing. Micah is still upset about the loss of Lightning. She says that she has no desire to ever barrel race again and cannot even stand to go to the barn to visit the other horses. She also tells you that she has not been eating or sleeping well. Her parents and friends all think that she is overreacting. At that, Micah begins to cry and immediately apologizes. You respond, "It's OK. I know Lightning was special to you. It is normal to still be grieving. I know of someone who specializes in pet loss counseling. Would you like her phone number?"

If you had not taken the time to call, Micah's depression might have gone unnoticed. Many times, clients suffer through depression feeling alone. Depression may occur on and off during the entire grief process. Micah also explained to you that support was not available from her friends and family. It is important to follow up on clients who have poor support systems or who are attached to their animals like Micah. Referral to a professional counselor can be of great assistance in helping clients such as Micah in resolving the grief process.

TECHNICIAN NOTE   Depression has been described as complete, overwhelming sadness.

The veterinary professional has occasion to recognize depression as a result of pet loss when follow-up contacts are made with the client. Depression, when severe, usually sets in some time after the loss. Clients with poor social support systems, elderly clients, and clients with intense or symbolic attachment to the pet may experience clinical depression.

TECHNICIAN NOTE   Follow-up is important for clients with poor support systems or unusual attachments.

When contacts are made several days or weeks after bereavement, and it is suspected that a client is depressed, referral can be made to a counselor or a hot line specializing in pet loss (Box 36-3). Although referral sometimes is awkward, it might be gently phrased as, "I know a person experienced in counseling people who have lost their pets." Reassurance that grief is normal is beneficial.

TECHNICIAN NOTE   If severe depression is suspected, referral can be made to a counselor or hot line.

Most clients feel overwhelmed by their emotions because of grief. They describe feeling as if their emotions are out of control. They may state surprise and worry that they are

---

BOX 36-3   Places to Contact for Help and Referral Sources for Clients Needing Help With Grief-Related Information*

The Delta Society
ATTN: Librarian
289 Perimeter Road East
Renton, WA 98055-1329
Telephone: (206) 226-7357
www.deltasociety.org

Veterinary Grief Counseling Hot Lines
ASPCA National Pet Loss Hotline
424 East 92nd Street
New York, NY 10128
Telephone: (877) 474-3310

Websites
American Veterinary Medical Association: www.avma.org
   (Look under "Care for pets.")
Argus Institute for Families and Veterinary Medicine:
   www.argusinstitute.colostate.edu
Grief Healing: www.griefhealing.com
Pet Bereavement Counseling: www.petloss.org
Pet Grief Support and Candle Ceremony: www.petloss.com
Pet Loss Help: www.petlosshelp.org

---

*For more grief-related resources, see the Evolve site.

reacting with such intensity to the death of an animal. They may be embarrassed. It comforts clients when veterinary professionals confide that most pet owners feel and act similarly after the loss of a pet. Assuring them of your knowledge of their pet's importance and your respect for their grief is valuable to them. This assurance validates their emotions and responses.

Grief must be worked through, not avoided; thus it is a process requiring some emotional **catharsis**. Many clients cry, and some are uninhibited about expressing anger and sadness. Becoming comfortable with one's own emotions facilitates comfort with others' emotions. It is human and necessary to feel empathy for grieving clients, but it can also be uncomfortable and painful. Separating your own feelings from theirs will allow you to transform empathy into sympathetic gestures that help the client.

Resolution or Acceptance

Case Presentation 36-5 can be studied to further understand the types of reactions that a client might exhibit during the stage of resolution or acceptance.

The stage of resolution or acceptance is marked by the belief that everything is OK, normal functioning is restored, and emotional energy is reinvested. This does not mean that the pet is forgotten, but that it has been assigned to a special place in the bereaved individual's heart. New attachments can be made without regret and hesitation. Resolution may come easily for some and may be difficult for others. In general, children reach the stage of acceptance and resolution more quickly and more easily than do adults. (For more information on how to help children when a pet dies, see Box 36-4.) As has been stated, the grief process is not linear, and bits of this stage occur with greater and greater

---

CASE PRESENTATION 36-5

Two months later, Micah (the client in the previous case study) calls back to let you know how she is doing. She expresses gratitude for your concern and compassion while she was grieving over losing Lightning. In his memory, she has decided to donate Lightning's winnings from last year to the Colic Research Foundation. She has also made a memorial plaque with Lightning's shoe on it to hang on his stall door. She would like for you and the veterinarian to come out to the farm to examine the soundness of a horse, Blaze, that she thinks has barrel potential. She is beginning to realize that Lightning would like for her to ride again.

Micah is doing well. She has gone through the process of grieving over Lightning. By memorializing Lightning with the plaque, she has a special way to remember him. Through the donation, she is able to believe that both she and Lightning have made an important contribution to equine medicine. Micah experienced a degree of personal growth through the process of grieving. Resolution and acceptance for Micah are symbolized by focusing her emotional energy into potentially developing a relationship with Blaze. It is important that Lightning is not forgotten.

---

frequency and with longer durations throughout the grief process. Eventually the client who successfully resolves the grief process experiences few, if any, of the first four stages.

Many factors may complicate the grief process (Box 36-5). These complicating factors may lengthen the time it takes to reach resolution or, in severe cases, may arrest progress through the grief process without allowing the individual to reach a resolution. Situations in which the grief process is complicated may not affect some individuals' ability to progress but may drastically affect the ability of others. Few veterinary professionals are equipped to give the special kind of help that these complicated situations may require, but most have empathy and the ability to listen for signs that indicate someone may need help. Early recognition of factors that may complicate the grief process can be helpful when a person appears not to be progressing well through the process. Early recognition may also be important for timely referral in situations in which further assistance is required. Keeping on hand a list of professional alternatives for referral to someone who can give the help that is needed is advised (see Box 36-3 and the Evolve site for a short list of potential sources of help).

> **TECHNICIAN NOTE**   Keeping on hand a list of professional alternatives for referral to someone who can give the help that is needed is advised.

The question is often raised whether clients should get a new pet before they reach resolution of the grief process (Figure 36-2). The process itself is highly variable in length. It can be as short as a few weeks to as long as many years. Most pet owners are able to reinvest and reattach to a new pet at any time, but only after they become aware that replacement of their unique loved one is impossible. If companionship, tactile closeness, and friendship are desired while grieving, these qualities can be obtained through a new pet. Cautioning and encouraging clients to choose animals somewhat dissimilar to their dead pet can be helpful. Having a new pet forced on the grieving individual who is not ready to reinvest in a new relationship will only end up furthering heartache in the bereaved and causing unhappiness in the new pet.

GRIEF AND THE VETERINARY PROFESSIONAL

Individuals in the veterinary profession deal with client grief on an almost daily basis. Rarely do they think about their own. The veterinary professional must realize that the grief process the client is struggling with is not taking place in an emotional vacuum. It is real and touches not only the bereaved person, but also those around him or her, including the veterinary professional. It is common for veterinarians and veterinary technicians to cry with clients, to feel a lump in the throat, and to feel guilty or depressed or experience a sense of failure. The fact that veterinary professionals may go through a grief process each time a patient is lost must

---

BOX 36-4 | How to Help Children When a Pet Dies

When a child's companion animal dies, many parents follow their instincts to protect the child from pain and grief. Some parents make decisions regarding the pet without discussing them with their children. Some may even lie to their children about the actual circumstances of the pet's "disappearance," preferring to tell them that a beloved pet ran away or was stolen rather than died. These tactics are not used maliciously by parents. They develop from a desire to spare children feelings of pain, and from a belief that the parents, as parents, are inadequately prepared to discuss loss, death, and grief with their children.

Children, however, are tuned into their parents' emotions and, almost without exception, know that something is going on in the family. They do not know what that something is, but they do know that it upsets Mom and Dad. Consequently, children may feel anxious, confused, left out, and even guilty because without honest explanations of a family crisis, children often believe that they are somehow responsible for the tension level in the home. At later ages, children may also believe that they were betrayed by the parents whom they trusted when they discover the truth about their childhood pet's disappearance.

The knowledge, skills, and tools for dealing with loss and grief that are developed in childhood are the same ones used in adolescence and adulthood. It is of utmost importance that children be given honest support and information about loss and death, so that their grief-coping strategies will be healthy, rather than unhealthy, ones.

How Technicians Can Help

Parents will often turn to veterinary professionals for assistance in telling their children about the death of a pet. Having books available for them to read and having information that you can share can help ease an otherwise traumatic situation. Here are some suggestions:

- Always encourage parents to be honest with their children throughout a companion animal's illness, treatment, and death. Never agree to participate in a lie that the parents may want to tell their children to protect them. In the long run, lies create more problems for everyone involved and

can be more damaging to children than the pet's death itself.

- Children younger than 8 years of age do not really understand that death is final. They may believe that a dead pet can return, or that they will need food in their grave with them. Young children are egocentric and believe quite strictly in the law of cause and effect. Thus they may develop the idea that they did something to cause the pet's death. Therefore, they must be reassured repeatedly that the pet died because it had a disease or an accident or was old.
- Straightforward explanations and concrete words, such as "dead" and "died," should be used when talking to children about death. Young children do not understand euphemisms and can become upset when they hear terms such as "put to sleep." Because they go to sleep every night and do not want to die like their pet did, attempts at softening the blow can actually make the situation more difficult and frightening for children.
- Children need to be held, reassured, and allowed to ask questions. Open communication about death is important for keeping death anxiety manageable. Pets' names should be used in conversation whenever possible, and memories of them should be shared by the whole family. Older children should be included in the euthanasia process, the memorial ceremonies, and the goodbye rituals to whatever extent they wish to be, and should be encouraged to demonstrate their sensitivity and compassion.
- It is always helpful to contact children's teachers, care providers, relatives, and other significant adults so that they can help acknowledge the loss and grief process. Adults may observe children playing funeral or may overhear them talking to friends about a pet's death. Although these activities may seem alarming and even morbid to adults, they are normal, healthy responses for children. Children deal with issues through play and experimentation. Unless they are in physical danger, their activities do not in most cases require interference. Refer to the "Recommended Readings" section at the end of this chapter for a list of books and publications about helping children cope with loss.

BOX 36-5 | Factors That May Complicate the Grief Process

- Multiple losses occurring within a related time frame
- Loss of a pet that was associated with a special person or event
- Loss of a pet on a day that is important, such as a birthday or a holiday
- Loss of a pet because of factors that may have been preventable
- Feelings of guilt about the death of a pet
- An inability to afford expensive care that was offered
- Loss of a pet because of an illness or a situation that previously caused the loss of another pet
- Sudden illness or trauma resulting in loss
- Witnessing the violent or unnecessary death of a pet

- Disappearance of a pet
- Lack of explanation as to why a pet died
- Situations in which the person experiencing loss has little or no support
- Insensitive comments from others who may not understand the bond between owner and pet
- Getting incorrect or bad information about the loss of a pet and/or the grieving process
- No previous experience with grief
- Not present at the time the pet dies or not having the opportunity to view the body
- Not able to say goodbye

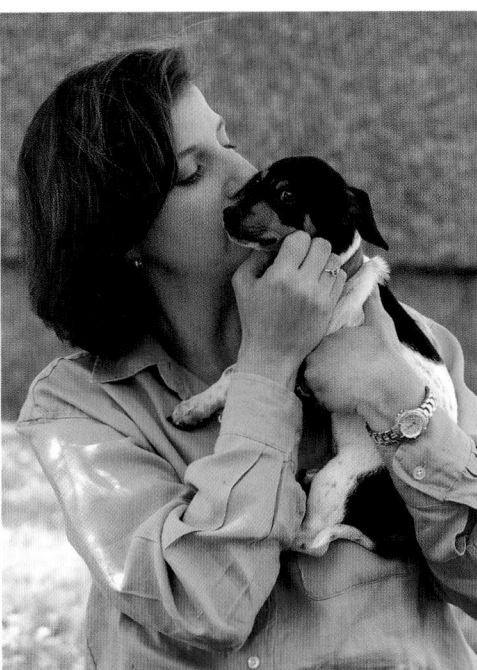

FIGURE 36-2 The decision to bond with a new animal should be left to the client who is experiencing the loss. Bonding with a new pet should be viewed as a tribute to the love and companionship shared with the previous animal.

BOX 36-6	Taking Care of You and Your Team

- Recognize that you will grieve too.
- Give yourself permission to grieve.
- Acknowledge your feelings.
- Write a condolence card to the owner(s).
- Memorialize pets in some way. You may even want to develop some way to memorialize that affords that opportunity to the entire clinic (e.g., bulletin board, scrapbook, monthly ceremony).
- Be patient with yourself.
- Take time to de-stress from work through journaling, drawing, painting, exercise, vacation time, laughing, recreation, or contact with nature.
- Validate each other's feelings.

---

be recognized and accepted. Time should be spent thinking about these feelings and responses. **Validation** of the process within the profession, by way of staff meetings, discussions, and support sessions, can be important in recognizing and dealing with the stresses of "professional grief." Left unacknowledged, the grief process encountered by veterinary professionals can become destructive and may lead to burnout (Box 36-6).

TECHNICIAN NOTE Left unacknowledged, the grief process encountered by veterinary professionals can become destructive.

EUTHANASIA

Perhaps no single issue in veterinary medicine conjures up the range of emotion, ethical deliberation, and stress occasioned by euthanasia. Euthanasia was defined by the 2001 American Veterinary Medical Association (AVMA) panel on euthanasia as "the act of inducing painless death," but the act is only one small aspect of the larger issue facing the profession.

The word "euthanasia" is derived from the Greek root "eu," meaning "good," and "thanatos," which refers to "death." Few in the veterinary profession would argue that when used in the context of relieving suffering, the word runs counter to its Greek roots; however, as the word is currently defined, it also pertains to the killing of unwanted, abandoned, stray, or phenotypically undesired animals by veterinary professionals. It is not always in the common interest of the patient, client, and veterinarian that euthanasia is performed, and in this way, problems can arise in balancing conflicting interests. Euthanasia is an emotionally charged issue, with members of the profession varying significantly in their acceptance of the practice and in their views as to its usefulness. On the one hand, it might be viewed simply as "convenience killing," whereas on the other, it might be viewed as a means of furthering respect and love through the compassionate termination of hopeless suffering. No matter how one looks at it, the animal health professional may be caught in the middle, experiencing doubts, confusion, and moral questions over participation in the ending of an animal's life. It is an ethical dilemma that does not have an easy or even an absolutely right or wrong answer. It is an issue that all veterinary professionals must wrestle with, individually and collectively.

TECHNICIAN NOTE Euthanasia is an issue that all veterinary professionals must wrestle with, individually and collectively.

THE DECISION

The decision to perform euthanasia is one of the most difficult decisions that the owner of a companion animal will ever face. Some owners may make the decision quickly because of financial constraints or fear of what the illness may eventually cause, whereas others may never be able to make the decision, preferring to let their pet die naturally. The decision is often made more difficult because few pet owners have an adequate support group available that understands the bond that develops between an animal and the recipient of its unconditional love.

Most owners who elect to have euthanasia performed make the decision because they perceive that their pet's illness involves some degree of suffering. Suffering is difficult to define, and perceptions of animal suffering differ greatly between individuals and from case to case. The place the pet holds in the owner's family circle, how long the pet has been owned, the relationship between the pet and other loved ones, the financial resources available to the owner, and the disease process afflicting the pet are other factors that most owners take into consideration when trying to make the decision.

The veterinary team (veterinarian, veterinary technician, animal health care providers) can play an important role in the decision-making process. The veterinary staff often serves as a sounding board for the client who is trying to make the decision. Staff members can help with the decision by approaching the subject professionally with compassion and respect. The most important help that the team can give is to provide information. What the owner can expect from the disease process, what treatments are available, the prognosis with and without treatment, and what costs are involved are all questions that should be answered by the veterinarian. The veterinary technician can play a vital role as a client resource by answering questions about euthanasia. How euthanasia is performed, whether the animal will feel pain, how long the procedure will take, and what happens to the body afterward are all areas that a technician may be asked to address.

> **TECHNICIAN NOTE** Veterinary technicians, as professionals, can help clients with euthanasia decisions by approaching the subject professionally with compassion and respect.

When interacting with an owner who is considering euthanasia, the veterinary professional should go to great lengths to lay out all available options while being careful not to make the decision for the client. Too many veterinary professionals make judgments as to the value of an animal (both monetary and personal) that only the owner can make. Questions such as "What would you do if he were your animal?" are difficult to address and perhaps are best answered by urging the client to verbalize what he or she sees as the pros and cons of each choice. In doing this, it may become obvious that the client has already made the decision and is looking for support or validation. The client may feel guilt, anger, sadness, depression, pain, and helplessness during the decision-making process and after euthanasia has been performed. The veterinary professional can help by assuring owners that these feelings are normal and indeed are expected and by letting them know that they are not alone in the pain that they are feeling.

Once an informed decision has been made, it should be supported, even if it may not have been the decision that the veterinarian or veterinary staff would have made. Pet owners are sensitive to the actions of hospital personnel, and for this reason, it is extremely important that persons interacting with the client or handling the animal in the presence of the owner be supportive, gentle, and empathetic.

At times, decisions concerning euthanasia may be made on the basis of convenience factors. Convenience euthanasia

for reasons such as a client moving and not being able to take the animal, new furniture in the house, or an inability to effectively house train an animal is something that most veterinary professionals will have to face. It is up to each practice to decide how they are going to deal with these issues. Some practices will decide that they are going to follow the owner's wishes no matter what, and others will decide that they are not going to euthanize animals in these settings. Often situations are looked at on a case-by-case basis, and although this may result in an inconsistent approach, it may be best, especially if all members of the practice understand how decisions are made. Questioning a client concerning his or her reasons for choosing euthanasia in these situations will sometimes bring out that they are making the decision because they really do not know that there are other options. Education about what other options are available will sometimes result in a happier outcome.

AS THE END DRAWS NEAR: THE BEGINNING OF THE END

The death of a pet can be a devastating experience that can drastically affect the relationship between client and veterinarian. As many as 40% of clients change veterinarians after a pet has died. This number probably approaches 100% if euthanasia is handled in a manner that causes the client to perceive lack of care, concern, or respect on the part of the veterinarian or other staff members. On the other hand, much can be done to foster a long-lasting relationship through the professional and compassionate handling of euthanasia. It is often true that the client who loudly sings the praises of a veterinarian and staff is not the owner of an animal saved through long hours of hard work and outstanding medical care, but rather the owner who was treated with compassion, care, and concern at and around the time of the loss of a pet (Box 36-7).

> **TECHNICIAN NOTE** Many clients change veterinarians after the death of a pet, especially if euthanasia is handled without the utmost care and respect.

Preparations for pet loss should begin as soon as it becomes apparent that death is a possibility. The veterinarian should discuss euthanasia with a client early so that the client understands that it is an available option. However, it is important to discuss all other medical or surgical options first. Euthanasia should not be presented in such a manner that it is completely discounted or is viewed as the only reasonable course. Remember that the initial reaction of a client receiving bad news is often denial or feelings of numbness or shock. It is important to allow time for this initial reaction to fade and for the entire family to discuss the various options before the client makes such a difficult and important decision.

While discussing options with the client, the veterinarian should not use alternative jargon for euthanasia, such as "put

BOX 36-7 | Are You Facilitating Compassionate Euthanasia?

Before

- Has euthanasia previously been mentioned with the client in a chronic disease situation?
- Does the client understand what euthanasia entails/what to expect?
- Did you offer the option for the client to be present for the euthanasia?
- Did you take care of the bill?
- Did you offer options for body disposition?
- Does your practice offer a cremation option?
- Did you offer options for the location of the euthanasia?
- Is there anyone else the client would like present for the euthanasia?
- Would they like to talk, or would they like you to talk, to family members and friends before they make the final decision?

During

- Is there comfortable seating for the client(s) and others who might be present?
- Are you in a quiet place without potential for interruptions?
- Is the staff well trained and do they know their roles?
- Have you planned for the unexpected?
- Have you allowed time for visitation before the procedure?
- Do you have tissues in the room?
- Are you talking the client through the process?
- Have you checked to make sure that the patient has died, and have you shared this with the client?
- Have you validated the client's grief response?

After

- Have you asked the client if he or she wants a moment alone with the body?
- Have you done the appropriate paperwork for body disposition?
- Have you asked the client if he or she has any questions?
- Have you made a paw print?
- Have you sent a condolence card?
- Does your practice participate in a memorial program?
- Have you informed the rest of the staff that the patient has been euthanized?
- Is it obvious when someone pulls up the medical record that the animal is deceased?
- Have you made sure to take care of each other?

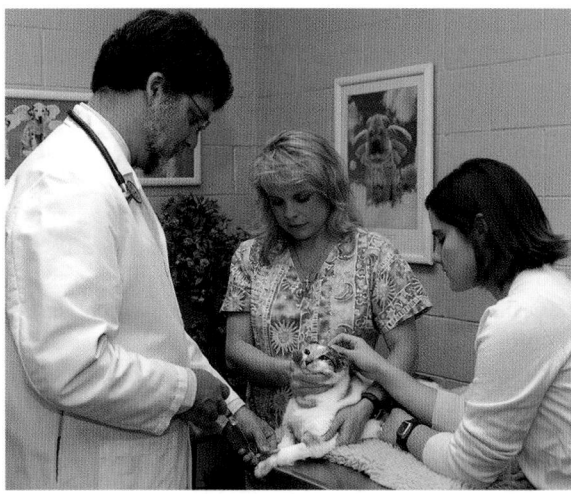

FIGURE 36-3 Clients' presence during the euthanasia of their companion animal helps them to say goodbye. Allow the client to make as many decisions, with guidance, about the site, time, and tempo of the euthanasia process; this makes the event more personal and meaningful.

TECHNICIAN NOTE Communication is critical to a smooth euthanasia when owners are present.

Once the decision has been made to have an animal undergo euthanasia, a client must make many decisions. When and where should the euthanasia take place? Should the client or other family members be present during the euthanasia? What is to happen to the body after euthanasia? Should a necropsy examination be allowed? What special method, if any, will the client use to memorialize the pet? It is best to discuss these concerns thoroughly in advance so that everyone understands precisely the wishes of the client.

The client together with the veterinarian should decide who will be present during the euthanasia. This is sometimes a difficult decision for both the client and the veterinarian. Some veterinarians do not offer this option to the client in the mistaken view that it will be too difficult for the client to watch. Contrary to this view, many clients will grieve more easily and accept more quickly the loss of their pet if they have had the opportunity to say goodbye in this most personal way (Figure 36-3). The chance to hold their pet and let it know that it is loved dearly while sharing its last moments is sometimes an important first step in the grief process. However, with the benefits to the client can come problems for the veterinarian and staff. Veterinary team members must realize that having the client present can increase their own stress level associated with euthanasia, and every attempt should be made to understand and minimize its effects.

TECHNICIAN NOTE Many clients will go through the grief process more easily if they are present at the euthanasia.

When the client or family members are to be present, euthanasia should be scheduled for a time of day when interruptions are unlikely, the waiting room is empty, and the

to sleep," "put down," "put away," "humanely destroy," "rock," and "shoot," unless its meaning is understood by all individuals involved. Confusion will result from the use of a term such as "put to sleep" when talking to a companion animal owner who perceives the phrase to refer to anesthesia instead of euthanasia. Children are especially confused by the term "put to sleep" and may associate death with sleeping, causing them to be afraid that they might die when going to sleep at night. Whatever term is used to describe the act of euthanasia, it is important that it be fully understood by all parties involved.

potential for embarrassment by public exposure is minimized. Early mornings, evenings, or during the lunch hour may be suitable. It is best to schedule at least 30 minutes. The most important aspect of the euthanasia to consider is communication. The unexpected should be avoided at all costs, and before the procedure, the client should be given a detailed explanation of exactly what is about to happen to the pet, and what he or she is about to see. Then the client should be talked through each step of the procedure. The euthanasia should proceed at a pace with which the client feels comfortable. Occasionally, pets will urinate, defecate, vocalize, twitch, or gasp after they have become unconscious. Although these reflex acts can be minimized, they will occasionally occur and will have a far less negative effect if they are expected, and if the client is told ahead of time that they are not a reflection of pain or suffering.

It is important for the veterinary team to effectively recognize signs of pain, fear, and distress, so that they might be minimized in relation to the disease process or during euthanasia. Distress vocalization, struggling, attempts to escape, aggression, panting, salivation, urination, expression of anal sacs, tremoring, tachycardia, and dilation of the pupils may all indicate distress, pain, or fear. Awareness of these signs can help to minimize stress during the euthanasia process.

Deciding where the euthanasia is to take place can be important. Using a hospital space that is less stark than the typical stainless steel hospital examination room is preferred. If the examination room is to be used, at least a blanket should be placed over the table, and a chair should be provided for the client to sit down. Some clients will request that the euthanasia be performed at home or at some special place. Many veterinarians will honor these requests or will use the services of a house call practice for this need. Sometimes just to be outside the "normal" environment of the veterinary facility is a fair and acceptable compromise. A blanket on the floor, the lawn beside the practice, and even the back seat of the family car might serve this purpose. One important consideration for the veterinarian in choosing the place is that many clients will feel uncomfortable coming back into the room where a pet previously underwent euthanasia. Indeed, many clients switch veterinarians because of lack of sensitivity to this fact by the veterinary staff. To minimize this potential conflict in the future, it is best to choose a space that will not be used routinely for other client-related activities.

Clients who choose not to be present during euthanasia may still wish to see the body of the animal after it is dead. Seeing the animal dead conveys finality and allows the client the opportunity to say goodbye. Many clients have a difficult time proceeding through the grief process if they have not been given this chance.

> **TECHNICIAN NOTE** Clients who choose not to be present for euthanasia often still wish to see the body afterward.

Make arrangements in advance concerning how payment for services is to be made. Discuss with the client whether payment is going to be made in advance, at the time of services, or by a later bill. This can be an uncomfortable subject to broach after euthanasia has occurred.

AT THE END

Once all preparations have been made, the euthanasia should be performed with skill and concern. Each member of the veterinary team should be well trained, know his or her responsibilities, and be available. The key, as already mentioned, is to expect and plan for the unexpected. Although many methods of euthanasia are deemed acceptable by the AVMA panel on euthanasia, only those that are aesthetically acceptable should be used when the client is going to be present.

> **TECHNICIAN NOTE** Expect and plan for the unexpected.

If the examination room is to be used, the table should be covered with a cloth or a blanket. Some owners will want to bring a favorite blanket for the pet to spend its last few moments on. It is important that they understand that it is possible, indeed likely, that the blanket will be soiled by feces or urine when euthanasia occurs. If the pet is likely to be aggressive or extremely apprehensive, sedating it ahead of time should be considered. If the client is to be present, the animal should be taken away briefly, so that a peripheral vein can be catheterized for smooth delivery of the euthanasia solution. It is advisable to put the catheter into a vein in a back leg; this will allow the client to hold the animal and pet its head without getting in the way of the veterinarian while the injections are given. Once the catheter has been placed, the client should be given the opportunity to be alone with the pet for a few moments.

Before the euthanasia solution is administered, a saline solution should be injected into the catheter to ensure its patency. Next, the patient should be anesthetized with propofol or an ultra-short-acting **barbiturate**. This will decrease the incidence of excitement after the euthanasia solution is injected. Once the animal is anesthetized, the euthanasia solution can be injected. Sodium pentobarbital is the most commonly used euthanasia solution. It is a member of the barbiturate family of drugs that depress the entire central nervous system.* When large doses of this drug are

---

*Note that all barbiturates are strictly controlled by federal regulations, and accurate accounting for the use of these agents is required. The **Drug Enforcement Agency (DEA)** of the U.S. Department of Justice is responsible for enforcement of laws governing the user of barbiturates. Sodium pentobarbital is a Schedule II controlled substance and can be obtained only by a licensed medical practitioner, such as a physician, dentist, veterinarian, or approved institution. In addition to the DEA paperwork involved in procuring barbiturates such as sodium pentobarbital, careful handling of the drug is necessary after the drug is on the hospital premises. Thorough record keeping is required by law.

administered, as for euthanasia, unconsciousness occurs first, and then breathing stops because of depression of the respiratory center. This is followed by cardiac arrest. The pentobarbital dose, concentration, and rate of administration determine the speed of action. When the drug is administered intravenously, animals die swiftly and quietly. Although intravenous administration is preferred, the drug is also effective when injected by an intrahepatic or intracardiac route, and, to a lesser extent, into the peritoneal cavity. Intracardiac and intrahepatic injections, although effective, are not considered appropriate for euthanasia of awake animals because it can be difficult to accurately inject euthanasia solutions into these organs consistently. Intraperitoneal injection of nonirritating solutions is considered appropriate in situations where intravenous injection is not possible. Death after intraperitoneal injection may take as long as 15 minutes, however, because of relatively slow absorption. Pentobarbital for euthanasia is available alone or in combination with other drugs. The concentration of pentobarbital in most euthanasia solutions is approximately 20% by weight. The recommended dose is 2 ml for the first 4.5 kg of body weight and 1 ml for each additional 4.5 kg of body weight. Sodium pentobarbital should be administered as rapidly as possible to provide the quietest and swiftest form of euthanasia. The veterinary team should be completely familiar with the use of the euthanasia solution chosen and the possible reactions.

Because the cerebral cortex is affected by general anesthetic, predominant emotions may take over and the animal may show fear behavior, which is usually characterized by struggling and vocalization. Experimental studies indicate that the animal is not conscious of these feelings at the time. People who have undergone the "excitement" phase during general anesthesia do not remember that it took place. Although trained individuals may understand this excitement phase from the clinical standpoint, it is difficult for the owner to understand that the struggling and vocalization seen are not due to pain, fear, or discomfort. Thus the owner's perception is that the animal is not experiencing a peaceful death. Clients who choose to be present should be warned that this phase may occur. Use of an ultra-short-acting barbiturate first will minimize the excitement phase.

THE END AS A BEGINNING ... AFTER THE END

Many veterinary professionals are good at the technical aspects of euthanasia but fall short in supplying what the client needs after euthanasia has been performed. The animal's death is often only the beginning of a long and difficult odyssey that the client is about to face. Some clients will feel a great sense of relief immediately after the pet's death, but most will soon feel empty, numb, or alone. They may question whether they did the right thing. Veterinary professionals can help them by again stressing that the pet's death was painless, assuring them that they did the right thing, and focusing on the positive things that the pet brought to their life. At the time of euthanasia, it is important that an

environment be fostered that says, "It's all right to cry, it's all right to be emotional, it's all right to begin to grieve." This process is known as *validation*. Few of us have the gift of the ability to say the right thing at the right time, so sometimes consolation can best be offered in a touch or an embrace. A touch on the arm or a simple embrace will often express best what the client needs to hear, "We care, and you are not alone."

> **TECHNICIAN NOTE** The pet's death is often only the beginning of a long and difficult odyssey.

Many clients, whether present for the euthanasia or not, need assurance that the animal is dead. Clients will feel more assured by the veterinarian who takes the time to listen to the animal's thorax with a stethoscope and shine a penlight into the animal's eyes before pronouncing the patient dead. For those who choose not to be present, allowing them to view the animal's body can alleviate some of this fear. Before the body is brought to the client, it should be made as presentable as possible. It must always be treated with dignity and respect. Clean any blood from the fur, remove any catheters or bandages, place the tongue in the mouth, and close the eyes. Placing a drop of cyanoacrylate glue (Krazy Glue, Super Glue) in each eye will keep the eyelids closed. If time permits, bathe and brush the animal before laying it on a clean paper, blanket, or towel in a sturdy box. This will help to make the viewing as pleasant an experience as possible. This last, and often lasting, impression that the client takes away from the practice may go a long way toward determining whether he or she returns with another pet. If the animal's body is sealed in a box (commercially made boxes for home burial are available), let the client know how the body is wrapped, and whether any signs of trauma or surgery are present. Even clients who assure the veterinarian that they will not open the box before burial or cremation often change their mind after leaving the office.

> **TECHNICIAN NOTE** Always treat the pet's body with dignity and respect.

Having the client bring someone who will be able to drive him or her home will help ease the feeling of being alone and will ensure a safe trip. It is nice to call clients after they have arrived home to check on them. Attempts should be made to call all clients who have lost a pet to answer any questions and to show concern. The veterinarian or a staff member may call. The show of concern is always appreciated; it helps clients who are having difficulty dealing with grief and assures clients that a relationship with the practice fostered in life has not been ended by the death of their pet. Most clients will eventually choose to get another pet. A sympathy card or a handwritten note is usually appreciated. Many beautiful sympathy cards designed for veterinary use are available (Figure 36-4).

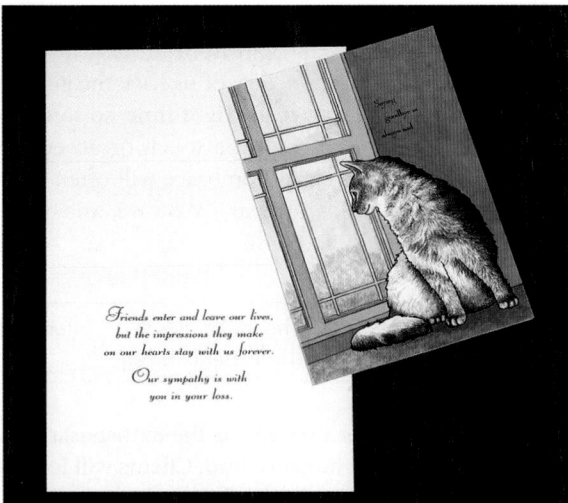

FIGURE 36-4 Follow-up communication is important for the client and the veterinary team. A condolence card lets the client know that you care, and this gesture often brings clients back to your practice when they eventually invest in a new relationship with another pet. In addition, sending a card allows practice team members to empathize, express their own grief, and experience some degree of closure.

| BOX 36-8 | Memorialize With Clay Paw Imprints |

World by the Tail, Inc., offers ClayPaws®, a paw print kit that allows owners or veterinary personnel to make an impression in clay of the pet's paw. These products, and others like them, help owners process their loss.

ClayPaws Kits are available by phone at (888) 271-8444, or online at VeterinaryWisdom.com for veterinary professionals, and at VeterinaryWisdomforPetParents.com for pet owners.

One of the biggest concerns of clients who have just lost a pet is disposition of the body. When possible, all arrangements should be made in advance. The veterinary staff should be prepared with information to assist the client in making these arrangements. Know the laws concerning burial in the practice area. Make available names and telephone numbers of places that offer cremation and pet cemetery burial. If the client chooses to have the veterinarian handle the remains, it is best not to lie to the client concerning the disposal of the animal's body.

Memorializing the pet is a step that many clients find comforting. It can be an important part of grieving for many clients. Offering the client a lock of hair or a clay paw print, and returning collars or leashes may facilitate these wishes. Refer to the end of the chapter and to the Evolve site for sources of additional information related to grief management and support (Box 36-8). Having a memorial service, planting a special plant in memory of the pet, framing a photograph, keeping a lock of hair, writing a poem or special letter, offering a memorial scholarship at a veterinary school, and making a donation to

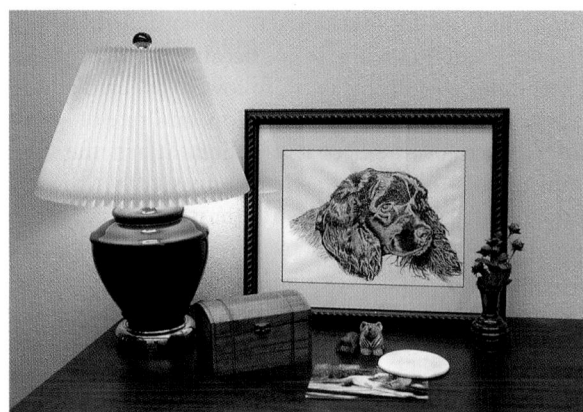

FIGURE 36-5 Memorializing a pet that has died is important in the grief response. Cremains, a paw print, and a framed picture are comforting ways to memorialize.

| BOX 36-9 | Signs and Symptoms of Burnout |

Physical Symptoms
- Headaches
- Gastrointestinal disturbance
- Muscle tightness
- High blood pressure
- Nausea
- Skin disorders
- Ulcers
- Heartburn

Emotional Symptoms
- Reduced sleep (inability to sleep/stay asleep)
- Irritability
- Crying spells
- Physical fatigue
- Withdrawal from family and friends
- Increased alcohol intake
- Eating disturbance (overeating/inability to eat)
- Loss of interest in things usually enjoyed
- Persistent thoughts and images related to the problems of others
- Distraction
- Aggressive behavior

organizations, such as the American College of Veterinary Internal Medicine Foundation, a veterinary school foundation, or a local animal shelter/humane society, are actions that clients may use to memorialize their pet (Figure 36-5).

> **TECHNICIAN NOTE**   Memorializing the pet can be an important part of grieving for many clients.

THE STRESS OF EUTHANASIA

Euthanasia is stressful not only for the client, but also for the veterinarian and veterinary staff. Frequent performance of euthanasia is a primary cause of burnout within animal control facilities, shelters, and small animal practices (Box 36-9). It is at times even more stressful for the technical staff than it is for the veterinarian because staff members usually have little control over the situation. Euthanasias that go smoothly and difficult euthanasias will create stress. Difficult or inherently stressful euthanasias include euthanasia in which technical problems arise, instances in which the animal reacts badly to the injections in the presence of the client, and the euthanasia of one's own pet, healthy animals, young animals, and animals for whom one has put a great deal of time and medical effort into fighting their disease. Euthanasia with the client present usually creates more stress on the veterinary staff than when the procedure is performed in the absence of the owner.

Each individual will have to decide what type of euthanasia he or she is able to participate in, and his or her personal tolerance for euthanasia. A technician may not be able to work effectively in a practice in which the veterinarian's views on euthanasia are vastly different from his or her own. Stress can become intense if these differences are not discussed and reconciled. Veterinarians differ greatly in their views on euthanasia. A survey of British veterinarians revealed that 74% would perform euthanasia on a healthy animal if the owner requested it. A similar survey in Japan revealed that 63% would not. There is room within the veterinary profession for this divergence of views; indeed, the diversity of opinions is one of the strengths of the profession.

One of the most important mechanisms of coping with the stress brought on by euthanasia is discussion with colleagues. Sessions for the hospital staff in which people can openly express their feelings provide a good outlet for emotions that if unexpressed can cause further stress and may lead to burnout. This type of communication allows members of the veterinary team to understand their colleagues' feelings and tolerances for different situations. Members of the team may need to temporarily pass responsibility for euthanasia to their colleagues when they have reached the limit of their tolerance. Other mechanisms of managing stress include taking time off, making time for self, adopting recreational habits, helping clients deal with their grief, and finding strength in relationships formed with colleagues who experience the same stresses.

EUTHANASIA IN THE SHELTER AND RESEARCH FACILITY

Technicians in veterinary practice participate in an average of three to six euthanasias per week; however, shelter technicians and potentially research technicians experience much more death than this. Millions of animals must be euthanized each year because there are no homes for them, because of overpopulation, or because of the needs of certain research protocols. These deaths can be difficult to rationalize, making euthanasia a stressful event for these technicians. The fact that different euthanasia methods are employed depending on the species or facility is a complicating stressor (Table 36-1). This factor brings up a wide range of both psychosocial and safety issues that need to be addressed.

The stress associated with euthanasia is exemplified in that staff turnover is higher in shelters where euthanasia

TABLE 36-1	Summary of Agents and Methods of Euthanasia: Characteristics and Modes of Action				
ACCEPTABILITY	**MODE OF ACTION**	**EASE OF PERFORMANCE**	**SAFETY FOR PERSONNEL**	**SPECIES SUITABILITY**	**EFFICACY AND COMMENTS**
Barbiturates Acceptable	Direct depression of cerebral cortex, subcortical structures, and vital centers; direct depression of heart muscle	Animal must be restrained; personnel must be skilled to perform intravenous injection	Safe except human abuse potential; DEA-controlled substance	Most species	Highly effective when appropriately administered; acceptable by intravenous and in small animals
Benzocaine Acceptable	Depression of CNS	Easily used	Safe	Fish and amphibians	Effective but expensive
Carbon Dioxide Acceptable	Direct depression of cerebral cortex, subcortical structures, and vital centers; direct depression of heart muscle	Used in closed container	Minimal hazard	Small laboratory animals, birds, cats, small dogs, mink (high concentrations), zoo animals, amphibians, fish, some reptiles, swine; conditionally acceptable for nonhuman primates and free-ranging wildlife	Effective, but time required may be prolonged in immature and neonatal animals

Continued

TABLE 36-1	Summary of Agents and Methods of Euthanasia: Characteristics and Modes of Action—cont'd				
ACCEPTABILITY	**MODE OF ACTION**	**EASE OF PERFORMANCE**	**SAFETY FOR PERSONNEL**	**SPECIES SUITABILITY**	**EFFICACY AND COMMENTS**
Carbon Monoxide (Bottled Gas Only)					
Acceptable	Combines with hemoglobin, preventing its combination with oxygen	Requires appropriately maintained equipment	Extremely hazardous, toxic, and difficult to detect	Most small species, including dogs, cats, rodents, mink, chinchillas, birds, reptiles, amphibians, zoo animals, rabbits; conditionally acceptable for nonhuman primates and free-ranging wildlife	Effective; acceptable only when equipment is properly designed and operated
Cervical Dislocation					
Conditionally acceptable	Direct depression of brain	Requires training and skill	Safe	Poultry, birds, laboratory mice and rats less than 200 g, or rabbits less than 1 kg	Irreversibile, violent muscle contractions can occur after cervical dislocation
Chloral Hydrate					
Conditionally acceptable	Direct depression of brain	Requires skill in IV injection techniques	Safe	Horses, ruminants, and swine	Animals should be sedated before administration
Decapitation					
Conditionally acceptable	Direct depression of brain	Requires training and skill	Guillotine poses potential employee injury hazard	Laboratory rodents, small rabbits, birds, fish, amphibians, reptiles	Irreversibile, violent muscle contractions can occur after decapitation
Electrocution					
Conditionally acceptable	Direct depression of brain and cardiac fibrillation	Not easily performed in all instances	Hazardous to personnel	Used primarily in foxes, sheep, swine, mink (with cervical dislocation), ruminants	Violent muscle contractions can occur at same time as loss of consciousness
Gunshot					
Conditionally acceptable	Direct concussion of brain tissue	Requires skill and appropriate firearm	May be dangerous	Large domestic and zoo animals, reptiles, wildlife	Instant unconsciousness, but motor activity may continue
Inhalant Anesthetics					
Acceptable	Direct depression of cerebral cortex, subcortical structures, and vital centers	Easily performed with closed container; can be administered to large animals by mask	Must be properly scavenged or vented to minimize exposure to personnel	Some amphibians, birds, cats, dogs, fur-bearing animals, rabbits, some reptiles, rodents and other small animals, zoo animals, fish, free-ranging wildlife	Highly effective provided subject is sufficiently exposed
Microwave Irradiation					
Acceptable	Direct inactivation of brain enzymes by rapid heating of brain	Requires training and highly specialized equipment	Safe	Mice and rats	Highly effective for special needs

TABLE 36-1	Summary of Agents and Methods of Euthanasia: Characteristics and Modes of Action—cont'd				
ACCEPTABILITY	**MODE OF ACTION**	**EASE OF PERFORMANCE**	**SAFETY FOR PERSONNEL**	**SPECIES SUITABILITY**	**EFFICACY AND COMMENTS**
Nitrogen, Argon					
Conditionally acceptable	Reduced partial pressure of oxygen available to blood	Use closed chamber with rapid filling	Safe if used with ventilation	Cats, small dogs, birds, rodents, rabbits, other small species, mink, zoo animals, nonhuman primates, free-ranging wildlife	Effective except in young and neonates; an effective agent, but other methods preferable; not acceptable in most animals younger than 4 months of age
Penetrating Captive Bolt					
Acceptable	Direct concussion of brain tissue	Requires skill, adequate restraint, and proper placement of captive bolt	Safe	Ruminants, horses, swine	Instant unconsciousness, but motor activity may continue
2-Phenoxyethanol					
Acceptable	Depression of CNS	Easily used	Safe	Fish	Effective but expensive
Pithing					
Conditionally acceptable	Trauma of brain and spinal cord tissue	Easily performed, but requires skill	Safe	Some ectotherms	Effective, but death not immediate unless brain and spinal cord are pithed
Potassium Chloride					
Acceptable	Direct depression of cerebral cortex, subcortical structures, and vital centers secondary to cardiac arrest	Requires training and specialized equipment for remote injection anesthesia and ability to give IV injection of potassium chloride	Anesthetics may be hazardous with accidental human exposure	Most species	Highly effective, some clonic muscle spasms may be observed
Thoracic Compression					
Conditionally acceptable	Physical interference with cardiac and respiratory function	Requires training	Safe	Small to medium-size free-ranging birds	Apparently effective
Tricane Methane Sulfonate					
Acceptable	Depression of CNS	Easily used	Safe	Fish and amphibians	Effective but expensive

Modified from 2007 AVMA Guidelines on Euthanasia.
CNS, Central nervous system; *DEA,* Drug Enforcement Administration.

rates are high compared with those with lower euthanasia rates. Practices that have been associated with decreased turnover rates include provision of a designated euthanasia room, exclusion of other live animals from the vicinity during euthanasia, and removal of euthanized animals from a room before entry of another animal to be euthanized. Staff members involved in the types of euthanasia occurring in shelters or research settings often cope by shifting moral responsibility for killing animals away from themselves. Shelter technicians view their acts as a crusade for animals and against the ignorant public, whereas research technicians may view the euthanasia as necessary for the "greater good." To prevent burnout, they must see themselves as generators of medical knowledge beneficial to humans and animals, combatants of pet overpopulation, or providers of humane death. These technicians must remember their objectives in their work. Their objective, like every other technician's, is to prevent and release animals from suffering.

The mechanisms for coping with the stress of euthanasia mentioned previously are important for both shelter and research technicians. Perhaps one of the most important coping strategies is for the team to rotate euthanasia responsibilities. This rotation releases technicians from the moral stress of euthanasia and reschedules them to a more hopeful task, such as education or adoption responsibilities or other important research missions; it is hoped that giving them a break will prevent burnout. Dark humor is also used to relieve stress. Such humor reduces tension by acknowledging death as part of the setting while minimizing, for the moment, its tragedy and finality. Although this humor may appear callous and may be misunderstood by those outside the shelter or research culture, it has been shown to be an effective coping strategy. It is important to recognize this humor for what it is—a coping mechanism. These technicians care tremendously but find themselves in an environment without much societal support.

> **TECHNICIAN NOTE**   Open discussion of issues surrounding euthanasia can help hospital staff deal with the stress.

EUTHANASIA OF LARGE ANIMALS

Euthanasia of large domestic animals presents specific hazards and problems not encountered in companion small animals. Safety must be a major consideration. The jugular vein should be used for injection whenever possible because this will place the person injecting the euthanasia solution in the safest position. On rare occasions, thrombosis of the jugular veins may have occurred from disease, and the cephalic vein must be used. However, this puts the individual under the animal's forequarters and in a dangerous position.

Euthanasia-strength pentobarbital can be administered with a large-gauge needle (14 to 16 gauge). The volume of solution is large, and even with a large-gauge needle, the time it takes to inject the solution is relatively long. The animal may go through the same excitement phase as that experienced by small animals, and it may come crashing to the ground on becoming unconscious. Generally, large animal euthanasia should be performed in an area with vehicle access to allow removal of the body. In some instances, the client may wish to bury a large animal. It should be remembered that all the same emotional concerns encountered in small animal euthanasia pertain to large animals when a bond has formed between the owner and the animal.

SUMMARY

The loss of a pet and the grieving associated with it constitute a difficult process, both for the pet owner and for veterinary personnel. Despite this difficulty, veterinary professionals deal with the illness, loss, and euthanasia of their patients on a daily basis, yet they are rarely trained in how best to address the grief of their clients. Nevertheless, it is important for veterinarians and veterinary technicians to provide a positive, supportive environment for pet euthanasia and to help clients with their subsequent loss. If euthanasia is performed poorly, it can be a disastrous experience for both the client and the veterinary practice. If performed with practiced care and gentle concern, it can be remembered positively for a long time. The ability to empathize, maintain a balanced perspective, and be compassionate is essential. The veterinary technician can be available and can listen; assure/validate clients that their feelings, emotions, and struggles are normal; and offer referral when clients think that they need more help than their available support group is able to provide. This form of client assistance strengthens the bond that develops between the client and the veterinary staff and results in positive growth and added fulfillment for both the client and the veterinary professional.

REFERENCE

1. American Pet Product Manufacturers Survey, March 2011.

RECOMMENDED READINGS

Anderson M: Coping with sorrow on the loss of your pet, Los Angeles, 1994, Peregrine Press.

Arluke A: Coping with euthanasia: a case study of shelter culture, J Am Vet Med Assoc 198:1176, 1991.

AVMA: AVMA guidelines on euthanasia. 2007. Available at: www.avma.org/issues/animal_welfare/euthanasia.pdf (accessed on October 10, 2012).

Brackenridge SS, Elkins AD: Euthanasia and patient death: stressors in veterinary practice, Vet Pract Staff 4:1, 1992.

Church JA: Joy in a wooly coat, Tiburon, CA, 1987, HJ Kramer.

Cohen SP, Fudin CE, editors: Animal illness and human emotions, Prob Vet Med 3:1, 1991.

Cusack O: Pets and mental health, New York, 1988, Haworth Press.

Fogle B, Abrahamson D: Pet loss: a survey of the attitudes and feelings of practicing veterinarians, Anthrozoos 3:143, 1990.

Fogle B, Abrahamson D: Pet loss: attitudes and feelings of practicing veterinarians, Anthrozoos 3:143, 1990.

Grier RL, Schaffer CB: Evaluation of intraperitoneal and intrahepatic administration of a euthanasia agent in animal shelter cats, J Am Vet Med Assoc 197:1611, 1990.

Harris JM: Nonconventional human/companion animal bonds. In Kay WJ, Nieburg HA, Kukscher AH, editors: Pet loss and human bereavement, Ames, IA, 1984, Iowa State University Press.

Hart LA, Hart BL, Mader B: Humane euthanasia and companion animal death: caring for the animal, the client, and the veterinarian, J Am Vet Med Assoc 197:1292, 1990.

Katcher A: Interactions between people and their pets: form and function. In Fogle B, editor: Interrelations between people and pets, Springfield, IL, 1981, Charles C Thomas.

Kay WJ: Euthanasia, Trends 1:52, 1985.

Kay WJ, Cohen SP, Nieburg HA, editors: Euthanasia of the companion animal: the impact on pet owners, veterinarians, and society, Baltimore, 1988, The Charles Press.

Kogure N, Yamazaki K: Attitudes to animal euthanasia in Japan: a brief review of cultural influences. Anthrozoos 3:151, 1990.

Kübler-Ross E: On death and dying, New York, 1969, Macmillan.

Lagoni L, Butler C, Hetts S: The human animal bond and grief, Philadelphia, 1994, WB Saunders.

Lawrence EA: Love for animals and the veterinary profession, J Am Vet Med Assoc 205:970, 1994.

Milani M: A loss for words: remembering animals loved and lost, Westmoreland, NH, 2011, Fainshaw Press.

Milani M: A veterinarian's guide to pet loss, Westmoreland, NH, 2011, Fainshaw Press.

Nieburg HA, Fischer A: Pet loss: a thoughtful guide for adults and children, New York, 1982, Harper & Row.

Peters TG: Commander, JAMA 260:1460, 1988.

Quackenbush JE, Glickman L: Helping people adjust to the death of a pet, Health Soc Work 9:42, 1984.

Quackenbush JE, Graveline D: When your pet dies: how to cope with your feelings, New York, 1985, Simon & Schuster.

Ramsey EC, Wetzel RW: Comparison of five regimens for oral administration of medication to induce sedation in dogs prior to euthanasia, J Am Vet Med Assoc 213:1170, 1998.

Randolph JW: Learning from your own pet's euthanasia, J Am Vet Med Assoc 205:544, 1994.

Rogelberg SG, Reeve CL, Spitzmüller C, et al: Impact of euthanasia rates, euthanasia practices, and human resource practices on employee turnover in animal shelters, J Am Vet Med Assoc 230:713, 2007.

Rosenberg MA: Clinical aspects of grief associated with loss of a pet: a veterinarian's view. In Kay WJ, Neiburg HA, Kukscher AH, editors: Pet loss and human bereavement, Ames, IA, 1984, Iowa State University Press.

Stewart MF: Companion animal death, Woburn, MA, 1999, Butterworth-Heinemann.

Tannenbaum J: Veterinary ethics, Baltimore, MD, 1989, Williams & Wilkins.

Veevers JE: The social meanings of pets: alternative roles for companion animals. In Sussman MB, editor: Pets and the family, Marriage Family Rev 8:11, 1985.

Voith VL: Attachment of people to companion animals, Vet Clin North Am Small Anim Pract 15:289, 1985.

Walshaw SO: Role of the animal health technician in consoling bereaved clients. In Kay WJ, Nieburg HA, Kukscher AH, editors: Pet loss and human bereavement, Ames, IA, 1984, Iowa State University Press.

For adult information about helping children deal with pet loss, consult the following books:

Barton C: Pet loss and children: establishing a health foundation, New York, 2005, Routledge.

Jewett CL: Helping children cope with separation and loss, Boston, 1982, Harvard Common Press.

Nieburg HA, Fischer A: Pet loss: a thoughtful guide for adults and children, New York, 1982, Harper & Row.

Quackenbush J, Graveline D: When your pet dies: how to cope with your feelings, New York, 1985, Simon & Schuster.

Shirl-Potter JW, Koss GJ: Death of a pet: answers to questions for children and animal lovers of all ages, Stamford, CT, 1991, Guideline Publications.

Tousley M: Children and pet loss, Scottsdale, AZ, 1996, Companion Animal Association of Arizona.

Tuzeo-Jarolmen J: When a family pet dies: a guide to dealing with children's loss, Philadelphia, 2007, Jessica Kingsley Publishers.

The following children's books may be helpful in explaining the loss of a pet to children:

Brackenridge SS: Because of flowers and dancers, Santa Barbara, CA, 1994, Veterinary Practice Publishing.

Dalpra-Berman G: Remembering pets, Brandon, OR, 2010, Robert Reed Publishers.

Davis C: For every dog an angel, Portland, OR, 2004, Light Hearted Press.

Disalvo-Ryan D: A dog like Jack, New York, 1999, Holiday House.

Morehead D: A special place for Charlie, Broomfield, CO, 1996, Partners in Publishing.

Rylant C: Cat heaven, New York, 1997, Scholastic.

Rylant C: Dog heaven, New York, 1995, The Blue Sky Press.

Viorst J: The tenth good thing about Barney, New York, 1971, Aladdin Books.

Abaxial Facing away from the axis of an organ.

Abdominal pinging Technique of identifying abdominal gas accumulations by simultaneous percussion and auscultation of the abdominal wall.

Abdominocentesis Sampling of free fluid within the peritoneal space.

Aberrant/erratic parasite Parasite that has wandered into an organ or location in which it is not normally found.

Abomasopexy Surgical fixation of the abomasum to the body wall.

Abomasum The "true stomach" of the ruminant; secretes acids, mixes and contracts ingesta, and moves liquid chyme into the small intestine.

Abrasion An area of skin that has been superficially scraped, creating a wound. Also, tooth wear associated with chewing on objects, such as rocks, ice cubes, toys, and bones.

Abscess Localized collection of pus (composed of dead neutrophils) in any part of the body, usually associated with bacterial infection, inflammation, and swelling around the site.

Absorption Uptake of substances into or across tissue.

Acanthocephalan A "thorny-headed" worm. *Macracanthorhynchus hirudinaceus* is a "thorny-headed" worm parasite found in the small intestine of pigs.

Acanthocytes Red blood cells (RBCs) with multiple, irregularly spaced, club-shaped projections from the cell surface.

Acariasis Any infestation/infection with acarines—mites or ticks. For example, infestation with *Demodex canis*, the follicular mite of dogs, is referred to as demodectic acariasis.

Accessory motion Refers to the spin, roll, and gliding motions of one joint surface on another.

Accounts receivable Money that is due to the practice from the sale of goods or services.

Acid-base Metabolic status associated with pH of blood or tissue.

Acidemic Serum pH above the reference interval.

Acid-fast stain Stain that distinguishes bacteria that have mycolic acid incorporated into their cell walls.

Acidosis Elevated levels of metabolic acids within the blood or tissue.

Acids Compounds whose water-based solutions have a sour taste, turn blue litmus paper red, and can combine with metals to form salts and yield hydrogen ions or protons when dissolved in water.

Aciduria Condition in which the urine is acidic (pH below 7).

Acoustic impedance Attenuation of the energy of the ultrasound beam as it passes through different tissues. It is specific for each tissue type (fluid, air, bone, fat, etc.).

Acoustic shadow Ultrasound beam interaction with a highly reflective surface, such as bone, foreign material, or gas, causing a high degree of attenuation of the beam and blocking of the pathway of the beam to deeper tissue.

Activated clotting time (activated coagulation time, ACT) Inexpensive but relatively insensitive test to evaluate the intrinsic and common pathways of coagulation. The test uses a special ACT Vacutainer tube containing a diatomaceous earth activator that must be prewarmed before use. The test should not be performed in animals that are severely thrombocytopenic.

Activated partial thromboplastin time (APTT) Test used to evaluate the intrinsic and common pathways of coagulation. The test requires citrated plasma and careful adherence to collection and processing requirements.

Active assisted range of motion (AAROM) Patient is assisted manually or mechanically to achieve a normal range of motion when the prime muscle mover is weak or injured.

Active immunity Production of substances in the body such as antibodies and interferon that render the animal immune from disease. Active immunity can occur via immunization, as an immune response caused by natural exposure to the antigen, or as a sequela of the disease.

Active listening skills Combination of acutely paying attention to what another is saying plus demonstrating this focused attention through body language and verbal feedback while maintaining a nonjudgmental attitude.

Active range of motion (AROM) Ability of a patient to voluntarily move a limb through a range of motion.

Acupuncture Use of needles (or injection of fluid, laser, ultrasound, surgically implanted material, or electrical stimulation) to stimulate specific predetermined "acupuncture" points in the body to produce chemical or physiologic changes in the body. It is combined with herbs and massage to make up traditional Chinese medicine (TCM).

Acute radiation toxicity Side effects caused by radiotherapy that occur between day 1 (the start of radiotherapy) and day 90. They are characterized by toxicity to rapidly proliferating normal tissues, such as skin, mucous membranes, intestinal tract, and bone marrow, and often resolve within days to weeks.

Adaptation Adjustment to a dental instrument that accounts for curvature of the tooth.

Adjunctive agent Medication other than those commonly used that may assist primary treatment.

Adjuvant Substance, such as aluminum phosphate, that increases the efficacy of a vaccine without having any immunologic property of its own.

Adjuvant therapy   Cancer treatment that is given in addition to the primary or initial treatment. The most common examples are radiotherapy that is given to treat residual cancer remaining after an incomplete surgical resection and postoperative chemotherapy that is administered to prevent or treat systemic metastasis. The overall purpose of adjuvant therapy is to decrease the likelihood of cancer recurrence.

Adrenocortical   Pertaining to the cortex or the outermost layer of the adrenal gland.

Adsorbent   Solid substance that attracts and holds a substance to its surface.

Adulticide   The suffix "-cide" means "kill." Therefore, an *adulticide* will kill adult forms of a parasite, a larvicide will kill larval forms of a parasite, and a microfilaricide will kill microfilarial forms of a parasite.

Adverse drug event (ADE)   Any adverse event associated with a drug that may or may not be drug related and that occurred regardless of whether the drug was used according to Food and Drug Administration (FDA)-approved labeling.

AE title   Name assigned to each modality so that it can communicate electronically with the picture archiving and communication system (PACS) in digital imaging.

Aerobe   Bacterial organism that can grow in the presence of oxygen.

Aerophagia   Swallowing an excessive volume of air.

Affiliative behaviors   Behaviors performed by two individuals such as grooming or nuzzling that serve to maintain social bonds.

Agammaglobulinemic   Description of a pathologic condition in which the body forms few or no γ-globulins or antibodies.

Agglutination   Visible or microscopic clumping of red blood cells.

Aggression   Behavior that is angry, destructive, and intended to be injurious. Behaviors that result in harm to the opponent. Threats and aggression exist along a continuum. An inhibited bite that leaves a red mark or indentation in the skin or that only pulls hair from another animal usually reflects an intent to warn (threat) rather than to harm (aggression).

Agonist   Substance such as a drug that produces a physiologic or pharmacologic effect characteristic of the receptor to which it binds.

Agonistic behaviors   Behaviors related to social conflict, which typically include avoidance, appeasement, threats, and aggression.

Air gap technique   By increasing the distance between the patient and the cassette, scatter produced by the patient does not reach the cassette as easily, thereby improving image quality.

Alkalemic   Serum pH above the reference interval.

Alkali   Alkaline substances produce hydroxide ions on contact with water.

Alkalosis   Elevated pH (decreased acid) within blood or tissue.

Alkaluria   Condition in which the urine is alkaline (pH above 7).

Allantois   Innermost portion of the fused chorioallantoic membrane, which assists in the transfer of nutrients, oxygen, and waste products to and from the fetus.

Allodynia   Recruitment of nonpainful nerve fibers that transmit information as pain, resulting in previously pleasant or neutral sensations experienced as unpleasant.

Allogrooming   Grooming performed by one animal on another animal of the same species.

Alopecia   The partial or complete absence of hair from regions of the body where it normally grows.

Altrenogest   Synthetic progestin administered orally and indicated mainly to suppress estrus in mares. It is also used commonly to help prevent loss of pregnancy in the mare.

Alveolar   Pertaining to the air sacs that are anatomically located in clusters at the end of the smallest airways within the lungs.

Ambu bag   Equipment used to provide manual ventilations; usually attached to the patient via an endotracheal tube or face mask and connected to an oxygen source. Brand name of a self-inflating reservoir bag used to provide manual ventilation when an anesthetic machine is not available.

American Animal Hospital Association (AAHA)   Small animal veterinary association that provides veterinary professionals with resources, including member services, continuing education, and hospital accreditation standards.

Amino acids   Nitrogen-containing compounds that constitute the "building blocks" or units from which more complex protein is formed. They contain both an amino (NH_2) group and a carboxyl (COOH) group. Approximately 11 essential amino acids must be provided in the diet, along with approximately 10 nonessential amino acids, which can be synthesized in the body.

Aminoglycoside antibiotics   Group of broad-spectrum antibiotics. Common examples are streptomycin, gentamicin, amikacin, kanamycin, tobramycin, and neomycin.

Ammonium sulfate precipitation test   Used to differentiate hemoglobinuria from myoglobinuria; hemoglobin is expected to clear in contrast to myoglobin.

Amnion   Membrane that separates the amniotic lubricating fluid surrounding the fetus from the urine-like fluid within the allantoic membrane.

A-mode   Amplitude-mode image display in ultrasound imaging. The energy of the returning echo is shown as an amplitude spike at each tissue interface.

Amplitude   The distance the tip of a power scaler is moving back and forth in one cycle as adjusted by the power knob.

Ampulla   Portion of the uterine tube (oviduct) that connects to the uterus.

Amputation   Removal of a body part (limb, toe, ear, tail, etc.).

Anaerobe   Bacterial organism that is unable to grow in the presence of oxygen.

Analgesia   Pain relief.

Analgesic   Drug that alleviates pain.

Anaphylactic   Exaggerated allergic reaction to a foreign protein or substance in the body.

Anaphylaxis   Hypersensitivity (to foreign proteins or drugs) resulting from sensitization after prior contact with the causative agent. Severe anaphylaxis can be fatal if untreated because of hypoxia.

Anastomosis   Reconnecting (suturing) of bowel after resection of a portion of bowel.

Anechoic   Structure in an ultrasound image that does not produce echoes and appears black.

Anemia   Condition in which the blood is deficient in red blood cells or hemoglobin.

Anestrus   Period of no or least reproductive activity.

Anger   Stage of grief during which anger is the primary emotion expressed directly, indirectly, and specifically or generally.

Angulation   Relationship of the face of the instrument to the tooth surface.

Animal Medicinal Drug Use Clarification Act (AMDUCA)   Amendment to the Federal Food, Drug, and Cosmetic (FFD&C) Act that regulates extra-label drug use for the treatment of veterinary species, provided specific conditions are met.

Anisocytosis   Variation in red blood cell (RBC) size that can be detected by examining a blood smear or by measuring an increase in the RBC distribution width (RDW). Anisocytosis often is increased in animals with regenerative anemia but may occur in other conditions such as iron deficiency.

Anisognathism   Condition in which the maxilla and the mandible are not equally wide.

Anisokaryosis   Variation in nuclear size.

Anode   Positively charged side of the x-ray tube that receives oncoming electrons from the cathode. Both heat and x-rays are produced as a result of interactions between electrons and the metal anode.

Anoplurans   Sucking lice that are members of the insect order Anoplura.

Anorexia   Loss of appetite or absence of food, especially when prolonged.

Antagonist   Drug that blocks activation of a receptor by its agonists (including the receptor's endogenous substrate).

Anterior pituitary gland   Adenohypophysis; the rostral portion of the pituitary gland that produces seven hormones, many of which influence other endocrine glands.

Anterior uveitis   Inflammation of the uvea.

Anthelminthic/anthelmintic   Compound or drug that can be used to kill helminths, such as nematodes, trematodes, cestodes, acanthocephalans, pentastomes, and hirudineans.

Anthropomorphism   The attribution of human characteristics to animals.

Antibiogram   Pattern of in vitro susceptibilities resulting from laboratory testing of an isolated bacterial strain for susceptibility to different antimicrobial drugs.

Antibiotic   Substance produced by a microorganism that inhibits or kills other microorganisms.

Antibody   Immunoglobulin formed in blood or tissue that interacts only with antigens that induced its synthesis.

Anticholinergic agent   Drug that inhibits the action of acetylcholine by competing at the receptor sites, producing increased heart rate, dry mouth, blurred vision, urinary retention, and constipation.

Anticoagulants   Additives used in blood collection bags for blood banking to keep blood from clotting.

Antiemetic   Drug used to treat or prevent vomiting.

Antigen   Molecule or substance that is recognized by the immune system as foreign (nonself) and that elicits an immune response or a specific antibody response.

Anti-inflammatory agents   Drugs that reduce or remedy pain by reducing inflammation.

Antimicrobial   Drug that destroys or inhibits the growth of microorganisms.

Antimicrobial susceptibility test   Test performed to determine whether an antimicrobial agent will kill or inhibit the growth of a bacterial organism.

Antipyretics   Drugs that lower body temperature from a raised state.

Antiseptic   Antimicrobial agent that kills or inhibits the growth of microorganisms on external surfaces of the body. Antiseptics generally should be distinguished from drugs such as antibiotics, which destroy microorganisms internally, and from disinfectants, which destroy microorganisms found on nonliving objects.

Antitoxin   Antibody produced in response to a toxin, such as tetanus, and capable of neutralizing the toxin.

Anxiety   Anticipation of future or potential danger that may be unknown, imagined, or real. Leads to a physiologic response similar to that of fear.

Aortic stenosis   Congenital cardiac anomaly resulting in resistance to flow of blood from the left ventricle into the aorta.

Apex   Tip of the root of a tooth.

Apical   Positional term referring to an area of the tooth or root that is closer to the apex.

Apnea   Temporary absence of spontaneous breathing.

Appendicular skeleton   Bones of the limbs (appendages).

Application software   Programs that help a user perform certain tasks. Common examples of application software include word processing software, bookkeeping software, and practice management information systems.

Applied kinesiology   Form of medicine that includes joint mobilizations or manipulations, myofascial therapy, cranial techniques, meridian therapy, clinical nutrition, dietary management, and reflex procedures.

Appointment system   System by which clients call ahead and are given a specific time and date to come into the practice.

Aquatic physical therapy   Specific treatment interventions in which a water-filled pool is used.

Argasid ticks   Soft ticks or members of the tick family Argasidae. Only a few of the ticks that parasitize domesticated animals are soft ticks. Soft ticks are periodic parasites that attach to their hosts only to take a blood meal. An example of a soft tick is *Otobius megnini*, the spinous ear tick.

Aroma therapy   Use of essential oils to bring about a physiologic or psychological response in the body.

Arrhythmia   Abnormal heartbeat rhythm detected during palpation of the chest or pulse during auscultation or recorded on an electrocardiogram (ECG).

Arterial blood gases   Measurement of partial pressure of oxygen and carbon dioxide, total bicarbonate, and blood pH in an arterial blood sample that helps determine the metabolic acid-base status of a patient; usually used to monitor patients with severe respiratory disease.

Arthrocentesis   Aspiration of fluid from a joint.

Arthrodesis   Surgical fusing of a joint together such that all motion at the joint is lost.

Arthropod   Any member of the phylum Arthropoda. Most of the members of this phylum have jointed appendages in the adult stage. Relative to veterinary parasitology, arthropods include a wide variety of creatures with "jointed feet," such as centipedes, millipedes, crustaceans, insects, and mites and ticks.

Artificial insemination   Placement of semen within the uterus or oviduct by other than natural means, so fertilization of oocytes can occur.

Ascarid   Specific type of nematode often referred to as a *roundworm*. *Ascaris suum*, the porcine ascarid, is a roundworm parasite found in the small intestine of pigs.

Ascites   Abnormal buildup of fluid in the abdominal cavity.

Asensory   Lacking sensation.

Asepsis   Condition of sterility wherein no living organisms are present.

Aseptic technique   Methods used to prevent contamination of a surgical site or wound by disease-producing organisms.

Asphyxiation   The act of cutting off the supply of oxygen; suffocation.

Aspiration   1. Removal of tissue or fluid from a tissue.
2. Accidental inhalation of material (liquid, food, gastrointestinal contents) down the trachea.

Assisted feeding   Providing energy and nutrients when animals are not eating adequate amounts. Enteral feeding uses the gastrointestinal tract, and parenteral feeding uses the venous (blood circulatory) system.

Assisted gloving   Method of putting on sterile gloves in which a sterile, gloved assistant holds the glove open to allow the surgeon to advance his or her hand into the glove without touching the outside.

Association of American Feed Control Officials (AAFCO)   Association that establishes standards for label information and the description of ingredients on pet food sold in the United States.

Asystole   Type of arrhythmia characterized by a "flat line," or the absence of heartbeats.

Ataxia   Uncoordinated gait usually associated with neurologic dysfunction.

Atelectasis   Collapse of a portion of or all of one or both lungs.

Atlas   First cervical vertebra. It forms the atlantooccipital joint with the occipital bone of the skull, and the atlantoaxial joint with the axis (2nd cervical vertebra).

Atrial fibrillation   Very rapid, uncoordinated contractions of the atria of the heart, resulting in lack of synchronism between heartbeat and pulse beat.

Atrial premature complexes   Premature contractions of the atria initiated by one of the atria from a location other than the normal sinus heartbeat, which originates in the sinoatrial node.

Atrioventricular (AV) valve   Heart valve located between an atrium and a ventricle. The right AV valve is the tricuspid valve, and the left AV valve is the mitral valve.

Atrophy   Wasting away of a cell, tissue, organ, or part.

Attachment loss   In dental terms, a true indicator of the periodontal status of the tooth. Attachment loss is calculated by adding together recession and pocket depth.

Attenuation   Decrease in the energy of x-ray photons as they pass through matter.

Attrition   Tooth wear associated with tooth-to-tooth contact.

Atwater factors   Average energy content of macronutrients. For human foods, the Atwater factors are as follows: 4.0 kcal for 1 g protein or 1 g carbohydrate, and 9.0 kcal for 1 g fat. For commercial pet foods, modified Atwater factors are used, including 3.5 kcal for 1 g protein or 1 g carbohydrate, and 8.5 kcal for 1 g fat.

Aural   In or of the ear.

Auscult   To listen to sounds made by internal organs, especially the heart and lungs.

Auscultation   Listening with a stethoscope (usually to heart and lung sounds).

Autoclave   Machine that uses pressurized steam to sterilize objects.

Autogenous   Originating or derived from sources within the same individual (e.g., an *autogenous* graft, *autogenous* vaccine),

Autolysis   Self-digestion of tissues or cells by enzymes that are released by their own lysosomes.

Autonomic nervous system   Serves to monitor and control internal body functions such as digestive processes, blood volume, cardiac output, and kidney function.

Autotomize   The act of reflex separation of a part from the body. In the case of lizard or snake tails, to disengage part of the distal part of the tail when stressed or held.

Axial   Along the same line as a center line.

Axillary   Under the armpit.

Axis   Second cervical vertebra. It forms the atlantoaxial joint with the 1st cervical vertebra (the atlas).

Ayre's T-piece   Non-rebreathing circuit with corrugated tubing, but no reservoir bag or pressure relief valve, in which the fresh gas inlet is located near the patient, and the waste gas exits away from the patient; Mapleson E circuit.

Ayurvedic medicine   The ancient Hindu art of practicing medicine and prolonging life. Diagnosis is done by palpation of the pulses in different positions.

Azotemia   Condition in which blood has increased concentrations of nitrogenous wastes such as urea nitrogen (BUN). Azotemia may be further characterized as prerenal azotemia caused by dehydration, as renal azotemia caused by impaired kidney function, or as postrenal azotemia caused by obstruction of the urinary tract.

Bacterial translocation   Movement of bacteria from a normal location to an undesirable location (translocation of bacteria from a compromised gastrointestinal tract into the bloodstream).

Bacteriostatic   Inhibition of bacterial multiplication.

Baermann technique   Collection technique that uses the force of gravity to concentrate nematode larvae (most often lungworm larvae) from within a liquid medium. The larvae of *Aelurostrongylus abstrusus* are often concentrated and collected using Baermann apparatus.

Bain coaxial circuit   Non-rebreathing circuit with a reservoir bag and corrugated tubing in which the fresh gas inlet is located near the patient and the pressure relief valve is located away from the patient; Mapleson D circuit.

Band/stab   Developmental stage before the segmenter with an incompletely segmented band-shaped nucleus.

Band neutrophil   Immature neutrophil characterized by a U- or S-shaped nucleus with generally parallel sides. The number of band neutrophils increases in some animals with inflammation.

Barbering   Behavioral problem in which the animal obsessively grooms to the point of damaging the hair and skin.

Barbiturates   Nervous system depressants used to induce sleep, and in high doses as anesthetics and euthanasia agents.

Bargaining Stage of grief experienced as conscious or unconscious attempts to control the situation or refute the loss.

Barr body Small drumstick-appearing nuclear appendage representative of an inactivated X chromosome that may be present in neutrophils from females.

Barrier nursing Collection of techniques employed during nursing of a contagious patient to limit transmission of an infectious pathogen to other patients. Involves erecting a barrier between patients and includes use of isolation wards and separate equipment and wearing of protective (barrier) gear, including shoe covers, gowns, and gloves.

Basilic vein Large vein on the ventral surface of a bird's wing that courses over the humeral-ulnar joint (elbow).

Basophil Type of granulocyte with a segmented nucleus and granules that stain blue to purple with Wright's stain or quick stains. Marked species variation in the appearance of the granules has been noted. Basophils from dogs have a few darkly purple–staining granules, basophils from cats have numerous gray to lavender granules, and basophils from horses and cows have numerous darkly purple–staining granules.

Basophilic stippling Multiple tiny, lightly basophilic red blood cell (RBC) inclusions resulting from staining of small amounts of cytoplasmic ribonucleic acid (RNA) in RBCs in the RBC cytoplasm. May be seen in cases of markedly regenerative anemia and occasionally in cases of lead poisoning.

Behavior wellness Condition or state of normal and acceptable pet conduct that enhances the human-animal bond and the pet's quality of life.

Behavior wellness care Planned attention to a pet's conduct and active integration of behavior wellness programs into the delivery of pet-related services, including routine veterinary medical supervision.

Behavior wellness programs Protocols, procedures, services, and systems that teach pet owners and professionals about what constitutes the behaviorally healthy or well pet. Promote behavioral wellness through positive proaction, behavior assessments, early intervention, and timely referrals, and decrease unrealistic human expectations and interpretations of pet behavior.

Behavioral needs In this context, opportunities and experiences that support the development of healthy behaviors.

Benign A benign cancer is one that may grow but does not invade surrounding normal tissues and does not spread (metastasize) to other parts of the body.

Bereavement State of sadness, grief, and mourning after the loss of a loved one.

Binocular vision Vision in which both eyes are used synchronously to produce a single image.

Bioavailability (F) Fraction of a drug dose that reaches the bloodstream.

Biological value Percentage of protein of a feed that is usable as a protein by the animal. A protein that has a high biological value is said to be of good quality.

Biosecurity Series of steps implemented to prevent or reduce the spread of infectious disease. Veterinary personnel who travel between production farms are required to implement biosecurity practices such as changing or sanitizing boots, changing coveralls, and, on some farms, driving through an antiseptic tire bath when entering a farm.

Biotoxin or toxin Noxious or poisonous substance that is formed or elaborated during the metabolism and growth of certain microorganisms and some higher plant and animal species.

Biotransformation Chemical modification of a drug to an active, inactive, or toxic metabolite.

Blepharospasm Spasmodic blinking from involuntary contraction of the orbicularis oculi muscle of the eyelids.

Blind spot Area directly in front of or behind the horse, where the field of vision is extremely limited and the horse is unable to see a person.

Bloat Accumulation of gas within certain portions of the gastrointestinal tract that produces visible enlargement of the abdomen.

Blood smears Thin films of anticoagulated blood prepared on glass slides that are air dried, stained, and evaluated for cell morphology and differential leukocyte counts.

Blood type Reflects the presence of specific erythrocyte antigens that have the potential to cause immune stimulation.

Blood urea nitrogen (BUN) Product of protein metabolism that is normally filtered by the kidneys for excretion. This blood value is elevated when the animal is on a high-protein diet, is dehydrated, or has renal insufficiency.

B-mode Brightness-mode ultrasound image display. It forms the basis of two-dimensional ultrasound images so that anatomic structures can be assessed in real time on a monitor.

Board Administrative agency that governs the practice of veterinary medicine and technology in each state. The formal name of this administrative agency may vary from state to state; names such as "Board of Veterinary Medical Examiners," "State Board of Veterinary Medicine," and "Licensing Board of Veterinary Medicine" are common.

Body condition score Estimate of body fat composition, with higher scores indicating overweight or obese animals, and lower scores indicating thin or emaciated animals.

Body condition scoring system System that can subjectively assess a pet's fat stores and muscle mass.

Borborygmi Rumbling noises caused by propulsion of gas and ingesta through the intestines (sing. borborygmus).

Box lock Hinged part of a needle holder, tissue forceps, or hemostatic forceps.

Brachycephalic Head shape that is shortened in the rostrocaudal dimension, as seen with breeds such as Pugs, Boston Terriers, and Boxers.

Brachygnathism Occurs when one of the jaws is caudal to its normal relationship with the other jaw; mandibular brachygnathism (retrognathism, Class II occlusion) exists when the mandible is shorter than the maxilla.

Brachyodont Tooth type with a small, distinct crown compared with large, well-developed roots.

Bradyzoite Literally, "a slow growing, tiny organism." This is a term for a tissue stage, for example, a slow growing developmental stage that occurs in cysts in the life cycle of *Toxoplasma gondii*.

Bronchopneumonia Pneumonia involving many relatively small areas of lung tissue.

Broodmare Adult female horse used for breeding.

Buccal Pertaining to the inside of the cheek or mouth.

Buccotomy Surgical incision through the cheek.

Bulbus glandis Expanded "bulb" of the proximal canine penis.

Bursae Fluid-filled sacs that decrease friction between structures.

Bursitis Inflammation of bursae.

CAAHTT Canadian Association of Animal Health Technologists and Technicians.

Cabergoline Synthetic dopamine agonist that is therefore a prolactin inhibitor.

Cachexia Weight loss, loss of muscle mass, and general debilitation that may accompany chronic disease.

Calculus Plaque that has become calcified and is firmly adhered to the teeth.

Calibrator Standardized material with known quantitative or qualitative characteristics (such as concentration, activity, reactivity, intensity, size, etc.) that is used to adjust (or calibrate) an instrument or a measurement procedure. The instrument or procedure is adjusted to yield results that match the calibrator.

Calorie Amount of heat energy needed to increase the temperature of 1 g of water from 14.5° C to 15.5° C. In nutrition, the kilocalorie (1000 calories) is used as the basic unit of energy.

Camelid "Camel-like" animals that include llamas and alpacas.

Cancer One of many diseases characterized by uncontrolled growth and spread of abnormal cells within the body. If local growth, invasion, and spread of cancer are not controlled, death may result.

Canthus Either of the angles formed by the meeting of the upper and lower eyelids. Each eye has a medial and a lateral canthus.

Capillaria Roundworm parasite located in the intestinal tract of infected birds. The double-operculated eggs can be identified in a fecal flotation examination.

Capillary refill time Time required for blood to refill the small capillary beds of the mucous membranes after digital blanching.

Capnograph Instrument that noninvasively measures carbon dioxide in exhaled air. This value is an indirect assessment of ventilation status.

Carbohydrate One of the essential nutrients necessary for all life functions. They are a quick source of energy and may be stored in the body as glycogen or sugars.

Carcinogen Substance or agent that causes cancer in animals or people.

Carcinogenesis Complex process by which normal cells are transformed into cancer cells.

Cardiopulmonary arrest Cessation of breathing and absent heartbeat.

Cardiopulmonary cerebrovascular resuscitation Emergency procedure performed in an effort to manually preserve intact brain function until further measures are taken to restore spontaneous blood circulation and breathing.

Caries Tooth decay caused by bacterial acid production and demineralization of tooth substance.

Carpal flexion sling Forelimb sling used in small animals that flexes the wrist joint and is used to protect flexor tendon repair and prevent weight bearing while allowing movement of the elbow and the shoulder.

Carpal tunnel syndrome (CTS) Medical condition in which the median nerve of the hand is compressed at the wrist, leading to pain, paresthesias, and muscle weakness in the forearm and hand. CTS is the best known of the ergonomic injuries classified as repetitive motion disorders (RMDs).

Carpus The knee on the forelimb of a horse.

Cash flow Measurement of a practice's inflow and outflow of cash over a period of time.

Catalase Enzyme required to convert hydrogen peroxide to hydrogen gas and water.

Catarrhal Inflammation of mucous membranes with discharge, especially inflammation of the air passages of the nose and trachea.

Catharsis The release of pent-up emotions with resulting alleviation of symptoms.

Cathartics Medications that through their chemical effects serve to promote the clearing of intestinal contents.

Cathode Negatively charged side of the x-ray tube that produces electrons from a metal filament when it is heated.

Cationic detergents Nonsoap surfactants that are in a positive state.

Caudal Positional term referring to a structure toward the back of the head or the hind end.

Cavitation Rapid collapse of a bubble in a liquid that produces a shock wave. Ultrasonic dental scalers cause cavitation.

Celiotomy Surgical opening of a coelomic cavity (e.g., the abdominal cavity).

Cellular casts Casts that contain recognizable cells embedded in the protein matrix.

Cellulitis Sterile or nonsterile inflammation of the interstitial tissues.

Cementoenamel junction Portion of brachyodont teeth at which the enamel of the crown meets the cementum of the root.

Cementum Hard tissue that covers the root of brachyodont teeth and portions of the crown of some hypsodont teeth.

Center for Veterinary Medicine (CVM) Governing body that regulates the manufacture and distribution of drugs, food additives, and medical devices used in veterinary species under the Federal Food, Drug, and Cosmetic (FFD&C) Act.

Centers for Disease Control and Prevention (CDC) Agency of the U.S. Department of Health and Human Services that works to protect public health and the safety of people by conducting research and providing information on health issues of concern.

Centesis Surgical puncture (as of a tumor or membrane); usually used in compounds (e.g., para*centesis*, thoraco*centesis*).

Central nervous system Includes the brain and spinal cord and serves to monitor, convey, and process signals from receptors throughout the body.

Central venous pressure (CVP) Blood pressure measurement taken from intrathoracic portions of the cranial vena cava; normal range is 0 to 10 cm H_2O.

Cerumen Waxy secretion found in the external ear canal.

Ceruminolytics Agents that dissolve cerumen in the external ear canal.

Cervical In reference to teeth, the portion of the tooth where the crown meets the root of a brachyodont tooth.

Cestode   Adult stage of a tapeworm. Usually found in the intestinal tract of the definitive host. Tapeworms are long and flattened parasites. The three basic parts of a tapeworm are the scolex, the neck, and the strobila. The strobila is composed of proglottids. Three types of proglottids are known: immature, mature, and gravid.

Chelate   To bind to a metal.

Chelonian   Turtle.

Chemical sterilization   Use of liquid or gas to sterilize surgical materials. Glutaraldehyde is a liquid that is commonly used to sterilize surgical instruments. Ethylene oxide and hydrogen peroxide are vaporized to sterilize delicate equipment, instruments, and plastic items that cannot tolerate the high temperatures, pressures, and steam associated with autoclaving.

Chemosis   Edema of the conjunctiva (swollen tissue around the eye).

Chemotherapy   Use of chemical substances to treat disease, primarily with cytotoxic drugs used to treat cancer. Chemotherapy is usually systemic therapy and is given intravenously or by mouth.

Chest tube   Flexible tube inserted through the intercostal muscles into the pleural space.

Chiropractic therapy   Form of medicine that manually restores reduced motion in the spine and limbs, thereby improving patient mobility, comfort, and, in many cases, nervous system function.

Chlamydophila psittaci   Intracellular bacterium that is a zoonotic disease (psittacosis) and commonly infects avian species (avian chlamydiosis).

Choke   Obstruction of the esophagus by a foreign body.

Cholinomimetic agents   Drugs that mimic the stimulatory effects of acetylcholine (ACh), such as salivation, lacrimation, urination, and defecation.

Chondroprotective   Term that refers to drugs and other agents (e.g., nutraceuticals) that promote joint health by "protecting" the joint by slowing or stopping degradation of articular cartilage.

Chorioallantoic   Extraembryonic membrane formed by the fusion of the allantois with the serosa or false chorion. In mammals, it forms the fetal portion of the placenta.

Chorioallantois   Membrane formed by the fusion of the chorionic and allantoic membranes.

Chorion   Membrane that attaches to the endometrium and aids in the transfer of nutrients, oxygen, and waste products from fetus to dam.

Chromosome   Nuclear portion of the cell that contains the genes.

Cingulum   Smooth convex bulge on the palatal side of the incisor teeth.

Classical conditioning   Also known as *respondent conditioning*. The animal learns the association between events—one event (the conditioned stimulus) predicts another (the unconditioned stimulus). Emotional behaviors are easily classically conditioned.

Clinic   A veterinary or animal clinic is a facility in which the practice conducted may include inpatient and outpatient diagnosis and treatment.

Cloaca   In birds and reptiles, a single terminus of the urinary, intestinal, and reproductive tracts.

Cloprostenol   Potent synthetic prostaglandin.

Closed gloving   Method of putting on sterile gloves in which the hands are kept hidden within the sleeves of a sterile gown during gloving.

Closed kinetic chain exercise   Exercise in which the distal limb segment is fixed.

Coagulase   Enzyme required to convert fibrinogen to fibrin.

Coagulation   Blood clotting.

Coagulation cascade   Term used to describe the interaction of multiple activated proenzymes (clotting factors) involved in secondary hemostasis, resulting in cross-linked fibrin strands that stabilize the primary platelet plug.

Coagulopathy   Disease or condition that affects the ability of the blood to coagulate.

Coccidia   Microscopic, single-celled parasites that spread from one animal to another (including humans) by contact with infected feces.

Coenurus   Type of metacestode stage found in the intermediate host in the life cycle of a tapeworm. The coenurus is usually found within a vertebrate intermediate host. A coenurus is a large, fluid-filled vesicle, cavity, or bladder with multiple invaginated scolices budding out from its wall. In its life cycle, *Multiceps multiceps* uses the coenurus, which may be found within the brain or nervous tissue of its intermediate host—a sheep. This coenurus has a scientific name, *Coenurus cerebralis*. See **Metacestode stage.**

Colic   Severe abdominal pain of sudden onset caused by a variety of conditions, including obstruction, twisting, and spasm of the intestine.

Colitis   Inflammation of the colon.

Collagen   Proteins that make up most of the skin, bone, cartilage, tendons, and other connective tissue.

Collimator   Device that filters or "focuses" a stream of x-rays, so that only those inside the open part of the device are allowed through.

Colloid   Substance that consists of particles that are dispersed throughout a solution and are too small for resolution with an ordinary light microscope but are incapable of passing through a semi-permeable membrane.

Colloid fluids   Category or type of IV fluid solution that contains large particles that help retain fluid within vessels.

Colonic wash   Fluid lavage of the reptile's distal intestinal tract in an attempt to collect a sample for parasite examination.

Colostrum   The first milk, which contains the antibodies.

Colpotomy   Incision through the wall of the vagina.

Colt   Male horse younger than 4 years of age, usually noncastrated.

Comatose   In a coma, a state of unconsciousness from which the patient cannot be aroused.

Combination therapy   Administration of two or more drugs concurrently to treat a particular condition.

Commensal   Relation between two types of organisms in which one obtains food or other benefits from the other without damaging or benefiting it.

Commissure   Area where the upper and lower lips meet.

Compassion   The quality of understanding the suffering of others and wanting to do something about it.

Complete and balanced   Refers to a pet food that supplies at least 100% of all daily nutrients without excesses or deficiencies.

Complete blood count (CBC)   Test used to evaluate peripheral blood that typically includes packed cell volume (or hematocrit), a red blood cell (RBC) count, hemoglobin concentration, RBC indices, a platelet count, a white blood cell (WBC) count, and a WBC differential.

Complex metamorphosis   Type of developmental change used by many insects. Four developmental stages are seen in complex metamorphosis: egg, larva, pupa, and adult. Each of these stages is drastically different from each of the other stages. The orders of parasitic insects that undergo complex metamorphosis include Dipterans (two-winged flies) and Siphonapterans (fleas).

Computed radiography   Similar to digital radiography except that an x-ray receiver similar to a film cassette is used and must be processed in a special machine. The special cassette contains a photostimulable phosphor that changes x-ray photons into a latent electronic image when read by a laser.

Concentrates   Broad classification of feedstuff that is high in energy and low in fiber.

Conflict   Occurs when an individual is motivated to perform two opposing behaviors.

Conflict-related aggression   Aggression toward people, often over resources and in similar contexts as dominance aggression, but with the dog showing ambivalent visual cues. These dogs are often submissive or fearful in other contexts and are likely to act submissive or fearful immediately after an attack. Many clients will say that the dog acted like it "was sorry for what it did."

Congenital   Born with a specific condition. Can be genetic or environmentally induced.

Conjunctivitis   Inflammation of the tissue under the lid margins and surrounding the visible globe.

Conserved gene   Gene that is evolutionarily very similar among bacterial species but usually is different enough to identify a specific species.

Conspecies   Animals belonging to the same species. Species belonging to the same genus.

Constant rate infusion (CRI)   Administration of low doses of drugs in intravenous (IV) fluids at a fixed rate over time.

Consultation   Specific period of time that the veterinarian meets with the client and the patient for the purpose of diagnosis/treatment.

Contamination   The presence of disease-producing bacteria or other microorganisms on the surface of a wound or surgical field.

Contralateral   The opposite side.

Contrast   Density or opacity differences between neighboring areas on the radiographic image. Large differences result in high-contrast images, whereas small differences result in low-contrast images.

Control   Standardized material that is used to monitor an assay to ensure that it is working correctly, consistently, and within desired limits. Controls are used to determine whether the instrument or the measurement procedure is yielding expected results for a sample with known characteristics. Controls are usually within the range of what you might expect to see in your patients. At least two control levels (normal and abnormal) are run. Low, normal, and high controls may be run if both high and low values of the analyte are clinically important. Control materials should be different from calibrator materials to ensure independent assessment of performance of the procedure.

Control solutions   Quality control products that may report a given expected concentration of the analyte of interest; alternatively, a laboratory may use a sample, possibly pooled, from representative animal(s) that has had its concentration repeatedly determined by the analyzer itself.

Controlled Substance Act (CSA)   Federal law regulating the manufacture, distribution, and dispensing of controlled substances.

Conviction   Process of convicting an individual of a crime in a court of law.

Coombs' test   Species-specific test performed to detect red blood cell (RBC) surface-bound antibodies and/or complement; it is most frequently used to support the diagnosis of immune-mediated hemolytic anemia.

Corium   Sensitive lamina.

Cornify   Cellular change indicative of cell proliferation and death. The vaginal epithelium of the bitch cornifies during estrus.

Coronal   Positional term referring to an area of the tooth or root closer to the crown.

Corpora lutea   Plural of corpus luteum.

Corpus hemorrhagicum   Structure formed within the ruptured follicle immediately after ovulation.

Corpus luteum   Structure that replaces the corpus hemorrhagicum and is capable of the production of progesterone.

Corrosive   Highly reactive substance that causes obvious damage to living tissue.

Corticotropin-releasing hormone   Secreted by the hypothalamus, it causes the fetal adrenal gland to produce high concentrations of cortisol.

Cortisol   Natural glucocorticoid produced by the adrenal cortex of the adrenal gland; major functioning hormone that participates in many life-sustaining processes in the body, such as maintaining blood glucose levels.

Coupage   The act of striking the chest wall rhythmically with cupped hands. Cupping the hands creates an air cushion on impact so that tenacious mucus is dislodged.

Cow kick   A kick from a rear leg directly to the side and the back.

Cradle   A barred restraint device. The bars are tied together like a nonridged fence. It is tied around the neck of a horse like a loose splint and prevents the horse from biting or licking itself.

Creatinine   Natural waste product of muscle tissue.

Crimes of depravity This group includes murder, rape, and distribution of drugs, as well as misdemeanor offenses, such as stalking, harassment, and assault.

Crimes of moral turpitude Crimes that involve dishonesty or deception. All theft offenses, such as shoplifting, theft by unlawful taking, theft by deception, forgery, writing bad checks, and embezzlement, as well as false swearing, are considered crimes of moral turpitude because they involve dishonesty.

Crop Dilatation of the esophagus of birds at the base of the neck, where food is stored, is softened with fluids, and is passed to the stomach in small amounts.

Cross-match Testing of compatibility of the blood of a transfusion donor and the blood of a recipient by mixing the serum of each with the red cells of the other, and examining the samples for the presence or absence of agglutination reactions.

Cross-ties Common method of restraining a horse for simple procedures such as grooming. The horse is tied to a pillar on either side by the square metal pieces on either side of the halter.

Crown Portion of the tooth above the gingival margin. Hypsodont teeth as a result of their continual growth and/or eruption have reserve crown beneath the gingival margin.

Cryoprecipitate Frozen plasma product containing concentrated factor VIII, factor XIII, fibrinogen, and von Willebrand factor.

Cryotherapy Therapeutic techniques used to decrease tissue temperature; cold therapy.

Cryptorchid A male with one or both testes not in the scrotum.

Crystalloid fluid Solution composed of electrolytes and water.

Crystalluria The presence of crystals in the urine.

Curative therapy Cancer treatment whose purpose is to permanently control the tumor. Because the goal is long-term survival, aggressive therapies are often recommended, and more than one modality (e.g., surgery, radiotherapy, chemotherapy) may be employed.

Curette Hand instrument designed with a rounded toe for subgingival scaling.

Cushing's disease (hyperadrenocorticism) Disease of the adrenal or pituitary gland that causes production of too much of the endogenous steroids.

Cutaneous larva migrans Zoonotic skin condition caused when an infective third-stage larva of a hookworm (usually *Ancylostoma braziliense*) penetrates the skin of a human being and travels within the superficial layers of the epidermis, producing highly pruritic, serpentine (twisting) tracts in the skin. Common names for this skin condition include sandworms, creeping eruption, and plumber's itch.

Cyanosis Bluish discoloration of the mucous membranes or skin caused by severe reduction of hemoglobin in the blood.

Cylindruria The presence of casts in the urine.

Cysticercoid Type of metacestode stage found in the intermediate host in the life cycle of a tapeworm. The cysticercoid is usually found within an invertebrate intermediate host, such as a flea or a grain mite. A cysticercoid is a single, non-invaginated scolex within a small, fluid-filled vesicle, cavity, or bladder. In its life cycle, *Dipylidium caninum* uses the cysticercoid stage, which may be found within the intermediate host, an adult flea. See **Metacestode stage**.

Cysticercus A type of metacestode stage found in the intermediate host in the life cycle of a tapeworm. The cysticercus is usually found within a vertebrate intermediate host. A cysticercus is a single, invaginated scolex within a large, fluid-filled vesicle, cavity, or bladder. In its life cycle, *Taenia pisiformis* uses the cysticercus stage, which may be found within the omentum of its intermediate host—a rabbit. This cysticercus has a scientific name, *Cysticercus pisiformis*. See **Metacestode stage**.

Cystocentesis Method of obtaining a urine sample by inserting a needle through the abdominal wall and into the urinary bladder and withdrawing urine from the bladder into a syringe. The bladder may be located by palpation or by ultrasound guidance.

Cystotomy Incision into the urinary bladder.

Cytology Microscopic evaluation of cell morphology in samples collected by fine-needle aspiration or impression smears of tissue or fluid accumulations. Cytology often is used as a screening test to determine whether inflammation or neoplasia is present, although definitive diagnosis of specific causative agents or neoplasms sometimes can be made.

Cytopathic Of, relating to, characterized by, or producing pathologic changes in cells.

Cytoplasmic basophilia Neutrophils with increased amounts of cytoplasmic ribonucleic acid (RNA).

Cytoplasmic vacuolation/foaminess Neutrophils with secondary organelle abnormalities.

Cytotoxic Agent or process that kills cells. Chemotherapy and radiotherapy are forms of cytotoxic therapy.

Cytotoxic drugs (CDs) Class of drugs that is toxic to cells. In modern medicine, CDs are used primarily to treat cancer.

D-Dimers Specific proteolytic fragments that result from plasmin digestion of cross-linked fibrin and contain two D domains and one E domain of the original fibrinogen molecule. D-Dimers are sometimes measured in animals with suspected disseminated intravascular coagulation (DIC) or other diseases associated with increased fibrinolysis.

Dead space Space between tissues created by a wound, allowing accumulation of fluid.

Debilitated Lacking strength; weak.

Débride To cleanse by removal (usually surgical) of lacerated, devitalized, or contaminated tissue.

Débridement Removal of foreign matter and dead tissue from a wound.

Decibel (dB) A measure of noise volume.

Deciduous Refers to primary or "baby" teeth, which exfoliate before eruption of permanent (adult) teeth.

Decontamination Removal or neutralization of injurious agents.

Decubitus ulcers Pressure sores (bed sores) that develop when an animal lies on a bony prominence for too long.

Defensive aggression Behaviors that result in harm to another individual as a result of defending oneself. Defensively aggressive animals are both fearful and aggressive.

Defibrillation Process of converting a fibrillation arrhythmia to a normal heartbeat (usually via electrical shock with a defibrillator).

Definitive diagnosis With respect to oncology, a completely accurate and reliable diagnosis of cancer that is established after thorough evaluation of the patient's history, physical examination findings, and laboratory diagnostics. A tissue biopsy with histopathologic examination is usually required for a definitive diagnosis.

Definitive host Within the *life cycle of a p*arasite, the host that harbors the adult, sexual, or mature stage of a parasite is the definitive host. For example, the definitive host for *Dirofilaria immitis*, the canine heartworm, is the dog. Adult male and female heartworms are found within the right ventricle and pulmonary arteries of the canine definitive host.

Definitive therapy Treatment intended to cure or permanently control a cancer. One or a combination of anticancer therapies may be used, including surgery, radiotherapy, and chemotherapy.

Degenerate left shift Left shift in the absence of increased segmenters (i.e., mature neutrophils).

Degenerate neutrophil Dying neutrophils displaying nuclear dissolution.

Degloving injury Injury—typically to the distal limb—in which a large section of skin is torn off the underlying tissue in a glove-like fashion.

Deglutition Medical term that refers to the act of swallowing.

Dehiscence Loss of integrity of the sutured layers of an incision.

Dehydration Abnormal depletion of body fluids.

Denial Normal defense that serves to buffer an individual from some unbearable news or shock.

Density Degree of blackness of a radiographic image. Denser areas are blacker and are noted in areas of the image where little x-ray absorption occurred. Whiter areas are less dense and are noted in areas of greater x-ray absorption.

Dentifrice Paste, liquid, or powder used to help maintain good oral hygiene.

Dentigerous cyst Cyst that forms around an unerupted tooth, which rarely may transform into a malignant tumor.

Dentin Hard tissue that makes up the bulk of a mature tooth.

Depression Actual grief; sorrow.

Dermatophyte Fungus that infects the skin and nails.

Designated assembly area The place where occupants of a building will gather for accountability if a general evacuation of the facility was ordered.

Detail Degree of sharpness that defines the edge of an anatomic structure in the radiographic image.

Diagnostic peritoneal lavage Insertion of fluid into the peritoneal cavity; fluid is allowed to dwell for a short time and then is drained. Gross, microscopic, and chemical analyses are performed on the returned fluid.

Diaphragm Thin, dome-shaped sheet of muscle that forms the boundary between thoracic and abdominal cavities; it helps to produce inspiration when it contracts. The diaphragm is dome shaped at rest, with its convex surface directed cranially. When it contracts, the dome of the diaphragm flattens out; this increases the volume of the thoracic cavity and causes air to be drawn into the lungs.

Diastema Gap between teeth, as seen between incisors and the cheek teeth of a rabbit.

Diastolic blood pressure Measurement of blood pressure when the heart is in diastole or dilatation.

DICOM (Digital Imaging and Communications in Medicine) A standard for handling, storing, and transmitting medical images.

Differential medium Medium that detects differences between two organisms on the basis of a biochemical test, for example, MacConkey's agar differentiates between lactose-fermenting bacteria and lactose nonfermenters on the basis of color (positive organisms are pink on this medium, and negative organisms are white).

Digenetic fluke Digenetic trematode that has two intermediate hosts—a first intermediate host and a second intermediate host—in addition to the definitive host.

Digestible energy Energy that remains after the energy lost in feces is subtracted from gross energy.

Digestion Process of protein, carbohydrate, and fat breakdown into absorbable nutrients.

Digital Image Communications in Medicine (DICOM) DICOM 3.0 is the current standard format for digital images in veterinary and medical fields.

Digital radiography A digital imaging technique in which the x-ray tube is coupled to a specialized receiver that changes x-rays into electrical signals. The analogue image is digitalized and is displayed on the integrated computer screen.

Dipterans Two-winged flies. *Anopheles quadrimaculatus*, the malaria mosquito, is a Dipteran fly.

Direct life cycle Life cycle that does not use an intermediate host, for example, *Ancylostoma caninum*, the canine hookworm, uses a direct life cycle.

Disc diffusion test Antimicrobial susceptibility test that uses paper discs impregnated with a specific concentration of an antimicrobial agent.

Disinfectant Antimicrobial agent that is applied to nonliving objects to destroy disease-causing microorganisms and their spores by physical or chemical means.

Disinfection Destruction of vegetative forms of bacteria, but not of the spores.

Displacement behaviors Behaviors observed in dogs and cats that serve as a coping mechanism intended to help the pet reduce its anxiety level. Displacement behaviors include grooming (in cats), yawning, scratching, and licking lips (in dogs).

Disseminated intravascular coagulation (DIC) Pattern of generalized concurrent intravascular thrombosis and bleeding. This is among the most serious complications of shock.

Disseminated intravascular coagulopathy (DIC) Disorder in which excessive coagulation of blood is followed by hemorrhage and lack of coagulation of blood because the clotting factors have been used up. DIC usually occurs secondary to excessive turbulent blood flow or to a severe infectious, immune-mediated, or neoplastic process.

Distal In dentistry, a positional term that refers to the surface of the tooth farthest from the rostral midline of the dental arch.

Distemper virus inclusions Distinct, spherical, eosinophilic to lightly basophilic inclusions that may be seen in red blood cells (RBCs) or in white blood cells (WBCs); may be more readily appreciated with some of the rapid Wright stains.

Distribution Dispersion of a drug that is systemically available from the intravascular space and of extravascular fluids and tissues to target receptor sites.

Diuresis Increased excretion of urine.

Diuretic Drug that increases the rate of urine output.

Diversionary restraint Type of restraint in which varying techniques or devices are used to distract the horse.

Döhle bodies Neutrophils with pale, bluish-gray, irregular cytoplasmic inclusions of ribonucleic acid (RNA) containing rough endoplasmic reticulum.

Dolichocephalic Head shape that is longer than average in the rostrocaudal dimension, as is seen in Greyhounds and Collies.

Dominance aggression Aggression against other members of an animal's social group to prevent subordinate individuals from performing actions or engaging in activities for which the higher-ranking individual claims priority.

Dominant role A superior position in a rank order or social hierarchy. Note that dominance describes a social position (role in a relationship), not a personality trait.

Dopamine A prolactin inhibitor.

Dose-dependent drug reaction Predictable reaction to a drug, the likelihood of which increases as the drug dose increases; may or may not be associated with the action of the drug.

Dosimetry badge Device worn by personnel when potentially exposed to radiation; measures the dose of radiation received.

Double barrel kick Kicking out with both hind legs simultaneously.

Down animals Animals that cannot stand.

Drug Any chemical agent that affects living processes.

Drug clearance (Cl) The rate at which a drug is removed from an organ or from the body, expressed as the volume of plasma cleared of drug per unit time (ml/minute). This value is used to measure the efficiency of drug elimination.

Drug compounding Any manipulation of a drug (combining, mixing, or altering) other than that provided for on the approved drug label.

Drug distribution Movement of an absorbed drug from the blood to various tissues of the body.

Drug Enforcement Agency (DEA) Agency in the U.S. Department of Justice that is responsible for enforcement of laws governing the user of barbiturates.

Duodenum The first segment of the small intestine after the stomach. Chyme enters the duodenum from the stomach.

Dynamic range The number of shades of gray in an image. The larger the number, the greater is the dynamic range.

Dysbiosis Imbalance in intestinal bacteria that precipitates changes in the normal activities of the gastrointestinal tract.

Dysphagia Difficulty in swallowing.

Dysphoria Uneasy emotional state characterized by anxiety and abnormal behavior.

Dyspnea Difficult or labored breathing.

Dystocia Difficult birth. This term can be applied to difficult birth in any species, which can be due to a number of causes such as large fetus, small dam, or malpositioning.

Ecchymotic hemorrhage Visible hemorrhage lesions 1 mm to 1 cm in diameter.

Ecdysis Shedding of the outer integument (layer of skin).

Echinocytes Crenated red blood cells (RBCs) that have multiple spicule-appearing projections.

Echocardiography Real-time imaging of the heart with ultrasound waves that reflect the heart tissue and blood, providing a picture of heart function.

Eclampsia Postpartum complication caused by a deficiency of blood calcium (hypocalcemia). Also called "milk fever." Low blood calcium levels give rise to tonoclonic muscle contractions that inhibit mobility. Often caused by an underactive parathyroid gland in the dog.

Ectoparasite Parasite that is found on the exterior of the definitive host. Ectoparasites *infest* the host; they produce an *infestation* or *ectoparasitism*. For example, *Ctenocephalides felis*, the cat flea, is an ectoparasite found within the pelage (hair coat) of the cat.

Edema Accumulation of fluid in a space that is not normally fluid-filled, resulting from venous or lymphatic obstruction or increased vascular permeability (e.g., pulmonary edema is fluid in the lungs, whereas cerebral edema is fluid accumulation within brain tissue).

Efficacy A drug's capacity, once bound to its receptor, to produce an effect.

Effleurage Form of massage that consists of gliding strokes that follow the contour of the body.

Effusion Escape of a fluid from anatomic vessels by rupture or exudation.

Egg/Larva/Nymph/Adult The four developmental stages in the life cycle of a mite or tick.

Egg/Larva/Pupa/Adult The four developmental stages in the life cycle of some insects. Collectively, these stages are known as *complex metamorphosis*. During their life cycle, fleas undergo complex metamorphosis.

Egg/Nymph/Adult The three developmental stages in the life cycle of some insects. Collectively, these stages are known as *simple metamorphosis*. During their life cycle, lice undergo simple metamorphosis.

Egg packet The typical reproductive "offspring" produced by adult *D. caninum*. Egg packets are discharged through either of the lateral genital pores of this tapeworm.

Ehmer sling Pelvic limb sling used in small animals that prevents weight bearing and helps force the femoral head into the acetabulum by abduction and internal rotation of the femur.

Ejection murmur Normal heart sound in large animals produced by large volumes of blood moving at high speeds through the heart valves. Because of the large heart size, these sounds are amplified and are readily heard with a stethoscope.

Electrical mechanical dissociation (EMD) Arrhythmia characterized by electrical waveforms on the electrocardiogram (ECG) without a corresponding mechanical heartbeat or pulse. Also called "pulseless electrical activity (PEA)."

Electrical stimulation Use of electricity to stimulate soft tissues to facilitate healing and reduce pain.

Electrocardiogram Tracing made by an electrocardiograph that reflects electrical activity in the heart.

Electrocardiography (ECG) Measurement of the electrical conductance of the heart; ECG rhythm strips.

ELISA E̲nzyme-L̲inked I̲mmunos̲orbent A̲ssay is a method used to measure a substance (antigen or antibody) by linking formation of an antigen-antibody complex to a detection method, typically a color change mediated by an enzymatic reaction (see Figure 13-3).

Embryo Structure formed by fertilization of the oocyte by sperm.

Emergence delirium Delirious behavior resulting from incomplete recovery from gas anesthesia. Usually lasts 1 to 2 minutes after removal from anesthesia.

Emergency facility A veterinary emergency facility is one with the primary function of receiving, treating, and monitoring emergency patients during its specified hours of operation. A veterinarian is in attendance at all hours of operation, and sufficient staff is always available to provide timely and appropriate care. Veterinarians, support staff, instrumentation, medications, and supplies must be sufficient to provide an appropriate level of emergency care. A veterinary emergency service may be an independent, after-hours service; an independent 24-hour service; or part of a full-service hospital or a large teaching institution.

Emesis Vomiting.

Emetics Agents used to induce vomiting.

Emphysematous Condition characterized by air-filled expansions in interstitial or subcutaneous tissues.

Enamel Hard tissue of high mineral content that covers the crown of a tooth.

Endemic Restricted or peculiar to a specific locality or region.

Endodontics Branch of dentistry dealing with disease of the pulp.

Endogenous Arising from within the body.

Endogenous substrate Natural substance in the body that triggers a cascade of cellular events by binding to a cell receptor.

Endometrial Belonging to the mucous membrane lining the uterus.

Endoparasite Parasite that is found on the interior of the definitive host. Endoparasites *infect* the host; they produce an *infection* or *endoparasitism*. For example, *Dirofilaria immitis*, the canine heartworm, is an endoparasite found within the right ventricle and pulmonary arteries of the dog.

Endotoxemia The presence of poisonous substances in bacteria; separable from the cell body only upon its disintegration.

Endotracheal tube Tube inserted into the trachea to ensure an open airway and to assist with anesthesia or breathing support.

Energy All body processes—building up of cells, motion of the muscles, maintenance of body temperature—require energy, and the body derives this energy from the food it consumes.

Energy density The number of calories provided in foods. For pet diets, energy density is expressed as kcal/kg.

Enrichment medium Culture medium used to enhance the growth of specific bacteria.

Enteral feeding Use of the upper alimentary tract (mouth, esophagus, stomach, and small intestine) for assisted feeding.

Enterohepatic recirculation Occurs with some compounds that are metabolized in the liver. The metabolites are emptied in the bile and are reabsorbed in the small intestines.

Enteropathy Disease of the intestinal tract.

Enterotomy Incision into a small intestinal lumen.

Enterotoxemia Disease (e.g., pulpy kidney disease of lambs) attributed to absorption of a toxin from the intestine—also called *overeating disease*.

Environmental Protection Agency (EPA) Government agency charged with protecting human health and the environment. The Pesticide Regulation Division, under the Federal Insecticide, Fungicide, and Rodenticide Act, oversees pesticides.

Enzootic Animal diseases peculiar to or constantly present in a locality.

Eosinophil Type of granulocyte with a segmented nucleus and granules that stain pink to red with Wright's stain or quick stains. Marked species variation in the appearance of the granules has been noted. Eosinophils from dogs have numerous round reddish granules; eosinophils from cats have numerous rod-shaped reddish granules; eosinophils from horses have numerous large, round reddish granules; and eosinophils from cows have numerous small, round reddish granules.

Epidermal membrane Thin, semi-transparent membrane that covers the camelid fetus and is attached at mucocutaneous junctions, at the coronet of the nails, and at the umbilicus.

Epidural anesthesia Local anesthesia that is injected into the epidural space to achieve desensitization of the perineal region. Epidural anesthesia is commonly used in cases of dystocia to decrease pain associated with delivery and to decrease straining.

Epiphora Tearing of the eyes as a result of excessive secretion of tears or obstruction of the lacrimal passages.

Epistaxis An attack of bleeding from the nose.

Epithelialization Process of wound coverage by epithelial cells during the final stage of the proliferative phase of wound healing.

Epizootic An outbreak of disease that affects many animals of one kind at the same time.

Equine chorionic gonadotropin (ECG) Glycoprotein hormone secreted by specialized cells of the equine chorion that have embedded into the endometrium. They exhibit luteinizing hormone activity in the horse, but follicle-stimulating hormone activity when administered to other species.

Ergonomic injury Injury involving the musculoskeletal system of the body, including muscle injuries, such as back strains, and repetitive motion injuries, such as carpal tunnel syndrome.

Ergonomics The study of how the human body moves. This term is commonly used to describe how the human body interacts with inanimate objects during work or play.

Erratic (or aberrant) parasite Parasite that has wandered into an organ or tissue in which it does not ordinarily live, for example, *Cuterebra* species, which is usually found in the skin of dogs and cats, wandering aberrantly into the brain of a dog.

Eructate To eject gas from the stomach; to burp.

Eructation Act or instance of belching.

Esophagostomy feeding tube Tube placed into an artificial opening in the esophagus when oral feeding is impossible because of injury or surgery.

Estrogen Hormone found in both males and females that primarily encourages female characteristics and aids in the signs of estrus.

Estrone sulfate Hormone secreted by the equine fetal-placental unit. It is a good indicator of fetal viability.

Estrus Period of sexual activity in nonhuman, female mammals that includes proliferation of uterine mucosa, swelling of the vulva, ovulation, and acceptance of coitus.

Ethylene oxide (EO)   Gaseous substance used as a sterilant for instruments and articles that would be damaged by steam sterilization. EO is suspected to cause cancer in some animals in cases involving very large or long exposures.

Etiology   Study of the cause of disease.

Euthanasia   Greek for "good sleep." Method of intentionally ending a life to relieve suffering.

Evisceration   Uncontrolled exposure of organs through an incision as a result of dehiscence or trauma.

Excoriation   Skin lesions caused by the self-trauma of scratching.

Excretion   Process by which drugs are eliminated from the body.

Exodontics   Extraction of teeth via closed or surgical techniques.

Exogenous   Arising from outside the body.

Exophthalmos   Outward protrusion of the eye.

Expectorant   Drug that liquefies respiratory secretions, promoting elimination.

Explorer   Sharp, fine-tipped instrument used to examine irregularities in dental hard tissue.

External coaptation   Use of a rigid external device such as a bandage, splint, or cast to align fractures.

Extracellular matrix   Meshwork-like substance attached to the outer cell surface that provides support and anchorage.

Extra-label drug use   Actual use or intended use of a drug in an animal in a manner that is not in accordance with approved labeling.

Extravasation   Leakage of something out of its container or normal location, such as a drug out of a vein.

Exuberant granulation tissue   Excessive formation of vascularized fibrous tissue (granulation tissue) in an open wound. Granulation tissue is considered exuberant when it grows above the level of the skin. Also referred to as *proud flesh*.

Exudate   Material composed of serum, fibrin, and white blood cells (WBCs) that escapes from blood vessels into a superficial lesion or area of inflammation.

Face   The flat surface of a hand scaler that lies between the two cutting edges.

Facial   Positional term in dentistry that describes the vestibular surface of the incisor teeth.

Facultative parasite   Organism that is capable of living free or as a parasite, for example, *Pelodera strongyloides*, a free-living soil nematode that may cause rhabditic dermatitis in downer cows.

Failure of passive transfer   Deficient levels of antibodies absorbed by the gut in animals dependent upon colostrum for immunologic protection. Failure can occur because colostrum contains inadequate levels of antibodies, or because the animal is not able to absorb adequate quantities of antibodies.

Fasciculation   Involuntary muscle twitching.

Fastidious   Describes bacteria that have specific growth requirements.

Fats   Energy-producing component of the diet; can be broken down into triglycerides.

Fatty acid   Building block of animal or vegetable fats and oils with varying carbon chain length. Several essential fatty acids must be provided in the diet.

Fatty casts   Casts that contain fat globules from degenerating tubular epithelial cells.

Fear   Feeling of apprehension experienced when an animal perceives that some nearby place, thing, or event may be dangerous. This emotion usually leads to avoidance of fear-inducing stimuli. Physiologic changes (increased heart rate, respiratory rate, and blood pressure, and dilated pupils) involve autonomic arousal, stimulation of the hypothalamic-pituitary-adrenal axis (HPA), and release of stress hormones.

Fear biting   The tendency of a fearful animal to bite. Anxious and fearful animals are more likely to defend themselves when they feel threatened. Perceived threats may include: a reaching hand or being cornered or restrained.

Fear-related (defensive) aggression   Aggression displayed when the dog perceives a threat. Most dogs demonstrate fearful body postures and possibly physiologic signs. Over time, as the dog learns that these behaviors are effective, it can begin to demonstrate more offensive body postures.

Federal Food, Drug, and Cosmetic (FFD&C) Act   Federal law regulating drug approval, use, safety, and efficacy.

Feeder calf   Steer or heifer, 6 to 9 months of age, 600 to 800 lb, that goes directly to a feedlot to promote fattening.

Felony   Grave crime declared to be a felony by common law or statute.

Fenestrated   Having a window or one created in a surgical drape.

Fetal membranes   Membranes that support fetal development by providing nutrition and enabling respiration and excretion. Fetal membranes include yolk sac, allantois, amnion, and chorion.

Fetatome   Device used to cut a fetus into smaller parts that can be more easily extracted vaginally when a fetotomy is performed.

Fetotomy   Procedure in which a dead fetus is cut into smaller pieces so that it can be extracted vaginally.

Fetus   Stage of development in which the species is recognizable.

Fever   Elevation of body temperature caused by a temporary increase in the body's thermoregulatory set point, usually caused by infection, inflammation, or neoplasia.

Fibrillation   Disorganized, rapid, random, and ineffective contraction of cardiac muscle cells.

Fibrin(ogen) degradation products (FDPs)   Small-molecular-weight polymers that result from plasmin cleavage of fibrinogen and fibrin. FDPs sometimes are measured in animals suspected of having disseminated intravascular coagulation (DIC) or other disorders of fibrinolysis.

Fibrinolysis   Enzymatic breakdown of fibrin, usually by plasmin. Fibrinolysis is the part of normal coagulation that results in dissolution of clots as part of the healing process. Some diseases are associated with increased fibrinolysis.

Fibroblasts   Cells that are recruited into a wound during the proliferative phase of wound healing that help form granulation tissue.

FIFO   First in, first out for inventory stock rotation.

Fight-or-flight response   Reaction in animals presented with a perceived threat. In livestock species, this response is used in low-stress handling to direct animals in a calm and efficient manner.

Filly   Female horse younger than 4 years of age.

Flaccid   Lacking any muscle tone.

Flail chest   Freely movable segment of the chest wall caused by segmental fracture of two or more ribs.

Flash sterilization   Emergency sterilization in which the instrument is placed unwrapped in an autoclave and is taken directly to surgery after sterilization. It is not recommended as a routine sterilization procedure.

Flexibility   Ability of a limb to move through a specific range of motion.

Flight zone   Area surrounding a livestock animal that, when entered by a predator, will cause the animal to move.

Fluctuant   Term used to describe a mass that is movable and compressible, such as an abscess.

Fluid resuscitation   Use of fluid therapy to treat low blood pressure or severe dehydration.

Fluoroscopy   Presentation of a continuous x-ray image, which involves directing the x-ray beam through the patient and onto an image intensifier.

Foal   Juvenile horse nursing from its mother.

Focal film distance   Distance between the target in the x-ray tube and the surface of the x-ray cassette.

Focal spot   Region on the anode that is bombarded by electrons. A large and a small focal spot correspond to the sizes of the filaments of the cathode.

Focusing cup   Hollowed-out metal surrounding the cathode filament that holds the electron cloud before its rapid acceleration toward the anode.

Fogged film   Partially exposed film that causes poor contrast in the resulting radiographic image.

Foley catheter   Catheter threaded through the urethra to the bladder, where it is held in place with a tiny, inflated balloon.

Follicle   Structure on the ovary within which the oocyte develops.

Follicle-stimulating hormone   Hormone produced in the anterior pituitary that when released encourages follicular development and spermatogenesis.

Fomite   An object that in itself is harmless, such as clothing or instruments, but is able to harbor pathogenic or infectious agents and serve as an agent of transmission of infection.

Food and Drug Administration (FDA)   Government agency charged with ensuring the safety and efficacy of human and animal drugs, and the safety of cosmetics, foods, and other consumer items.

Food-related aggression   Aggression demonstrated only in the presence of food, bones, rawhides, human food, or other high-value food items to prevent real or perceived attempts by others to access the food.

Forage   Vegetative portion of plants in a fresh, dried, or ensiled state; it is fed to livestock (as pasture, hay, or silage).

Foramen magnum   Large hole in the occipital bone through which the spinal cord exits the skull.

Forestomach   Prestomach chambers in a ruminant animal. Includes reticulum, rumen, and omasum.

Formalin   Aqueous solution of formaldehyde used as a disinfectant and tissue fixative in medicine. Formaldehyde is also used in the manufacture of building materials and adhesives. Formaldehyde is suspected to cause cancer in some animals in cases involving very large or long exposures.

Free catch   Urine obtained when the animal voids spontaneously or is assisted by gentle manual expression.

Friction massage   Form of massage in which the tissue is manipulated to increase circulation. This method is commonly used over tendons when tendonitis is present, over knots and trigger points, and over joint capsules with excessive fibrous tissue. It is also used to break up skin adhesions and scar tissue.

Frustration   Experienced when an animal is in a situation in which it is prevented from performing a behavior that it is highly motivated to perform.

Furcation   Region of a multi-rooted tooth where the roots diverge from the crown.

Galactostasis   Cessation of milk production (lactation) in the dam.

Gametogony   Type of sexual reproduction used by coccidian parasites, such as *Isospora* and *Eimeria* species.

Gangrenous mastitis   Necrosis of a large area of a mammary gland or glands secondary to infection. One or more anaerobic bacteria are often attributed to the infection. It is known as "blue bag" because of the dark blue color of the necrotic mammary tissue.

Gas sterilization   Use of chemical vapors to sterilize surgical materials and instruments that cannot withstand the high temperatures associated with stream sterilization in autoclaves. The most commonly used chemical gas is ethylene oxide.

Gastric dilatation-volvulus   A dangerous gastrointestinal condition that occurs primarily in deep-chested large breed dogs, in which the stomach swells with air and twists on its long axis, leading to shock, loss of blood supply, and other serious consequences.

Gastric gavage   Feeding by passing a feeding tube into the stomach.

Gastroenteritis   Inflammation of the lining membrane of the stomach and the intestines.

Gastrostomy   Method of enteral feeding in which a tube is surgically introduced through the abdominal wall.

Gastrostomy feeding tube   Gastric feeding tube inserted directly into the stomach.

Gastrotomy   Incision into the stomach.

Gelding   Castrated male horse; reproductive organs, the testes, have been removed.

Genetic   Inherited. In general, one parent or both parents transmit disease-causing genes to the offspring, unless it is a new mutation in the patient. The disease may not show up until much later in life.

Genital tubercle   Embryonic precursor of the penis and scrotum in the male, and of the caudal vagina, vestibule, and vulva in the female.

Geriatric   Branch of medicine that deals with the problems and diseases of old age and aging people.

Giardia Flagellated protozoal parasite of the small intestine. Animals with giardiasis may have watery diarrhea. *Giardia* can be spread to humans via contaminated water.

Gilt Female pig that has not yet produced a litter.

Glandular therapy Type of supplement that consists of animal products to supply nutrients (steroids, enzymes, and raw materials of some organs, such as liver) to the patient to help restore health.

Glottis Opening of the trachea within the oral cavity of birds. Usually located at the base of the tongue.

Glucocorticoids Group of steroid hormones (like cortisone) that bind to the glucocorticoid receptor. Glucocorticoids are used for physiologic replacement, and for their anti-inflammatory or immunosuppressive effects.

Gluconeogenesis Formation of glucose within the animal body from precursors other than carbohydrates, especially by the liver and kidney, using amino acids from protein, glycerol from fats, or lactate produced by muscle during anaerobic glycolysis—called also *glyconeogenesis*.

Glucosuria The presence of glucose in the urine.

Glutaraldehyde Chemical disinfection solution used to sterilize hard surface instruments by immersion. Glutaraldehydes are suspected to cause cancer in some animals in cases involving very large or long exposures.

Gonadotropin-releasing hormone Hormone produced in the hypothalamus that when released can initiate the release of follicle-stimulating hormone or luteinizing hormone in the male or female.

Goniometer Tool used to measure joint range of motion.

Goniometry Technique used to measure range of motion at a joint.

Gram stain Stain used to differentiate bacteria on the basis of the composition of their cell walls. Gram-positive organisms have peptidoglycan in their cell wall and lack an outer cell membrane. Gram-negative bacteria have an outer cell wall that comprises a lipid bilayer with lipopolysaccharide. Gram-positive bacteria retain crystal violet in the Gram stain reaction and stain blue, whereas Gram-negative bacteria do not and stain red.

Granular casts Degenerating cellular casts characterized by a nonspecific granular matrix and designated as coarsely or finely granular.

Granulation tissue Vascularized fibrous tissue that covers a full-thickness skin wound if the wound is left to heal by second intention.

Granulomatous Of, relating to, or characterized by a mass or nodule of chronically inflamed tissue with granulations that is usually associated with an infective process.

Granulosa cell layer Luminal cell layer in the follicle that converts testosterone to estradiol, a specific steroid hormone that is produced by the mature follicle (and the placenta in some species near parturition).

Gravel Foot infection that gains access to the foot through the white line traveling up the sensitive lamina underneath the hoof wall, forming an abscess that drains at the coronet.

Grid A thin sheet of lead strips with radiolucent spacers encased in an aluminum cover, giving the appearance of a thin, flat rectangular tray. A grid is placed between the patient and the film cassette to absorb scatter radiation so it does not reach the cassette and affect image quality.

Grid ratio Height of the lead strip compared with the width of the spacers between strips. A 12:1 ratio means that the lead strip is 12 times higher than the width of the spacers. The higher the ratio, the more efficient is the grid in removing scatter radiation.

Grief process The emotional process that one experiences when anticipating or following the loss of an object of attachment.

Gross energy Total potential energy of a foodstuff determined by measuring the total heat produced when the food is burned in a bomb calorimeter.

Gross income Total income before expenses.

Gross pathology Refers to pathologic changes in tissue that are visible with the unaided eye.

Gross revenue total Money generated by a business through the sale of goods or services before any expenses are deducted.

Ground fault circuit interruption (GFCI) Type of outlet or circuit designed to prevent electrocution by detecting the leakage current, such as what happens when an electrical current comes in contact with water. GFCI-protected outlets are common near sinks and tubs, and in wet areas of buildings.

Half-life (t₁/₂) Time required for the amount of a drug in the body to decrease by one-half, or 50%. Used to estimate the dosing interval.

Halitosis A foul odor to the breath.

Halogenated anesthetic agents Class of chemicals used to induce and maintain anesthesia in animals and humans. Halogenated anesthetic agents differ from earlier forms of anesthesia, such as diethyl ethers, in that they contain at least one halogen atom in each molecule that makes them generally nonflammable. Examples of halogenated ethers include the general anesthetics halothane, isoflurane, desflurane, and sevoflurane.

Hanging surgical preparation Process of preparing a limb for surgery by first suspending it from a point above the surgery table. Once hung, the limb is subjected to a sterile scrub, in which the veterinary technician makes a circuitous pattern around the limb, starting at the top and moving down to the proximal portion of the limb. The veterinary technician must take into account the force of gravity on scrub liquids because "dirty fluids" will flow proximally.

Hardware Parts of the system that you can touch: the monitor, the hard drive, the mouse, the printers, the modem, the discs, and the scanner.

Haul-in facility Large animal facility to which animals are brought to the practice for examination or treatment.

Hazardous chemical Any chemical or chemical product that may present a physical or health hazard, including but not limited to carcinogens, irritants, sensitizers, toxins, flammable materials, and products that may be reactive with other common chemicals.

Hazardous materials plan Written plan required by the Right to Know law. The hazardous materials plan is prepared by the employer to inform employees of the warning, training, and safe use procedures for hazardous chemicals in the workplace.

Hazmat—short for "hazardous materials" Also commonly used as an acronym for hazardous chemicals.

Heel effect The x-ray beam produced through interactions with the anode has a spectrum of x-ray energies. The x-ray beam is more intense at the side of the cathode than in the center of the beam or on the anode side.

Heifer Bovine female that has not yet had a calf.

Heinz bodies   Denatured hemoglobin that has fused to the red blood cell (RBC) membrane; appear as lightly eosinophilic spherical inclusions on standard Wright's stain, and as distinct, darkly staining inclusions on new methylene blue (NMB) stain.

Helminth   A worm. There are many types of worms, including nematodes (roundworms), trematodes (flukes), cestodes (tapeworms), acanthocephalans (thorny-headed worms), pentastomes (tongue worms), and hirudineans (leeches).

Hemacytometer   Counting chamber used for microscopic determination of cell concentration in fluids.

Hematemesis   Vomiting blood.

Hematochezia   Frank, red blood in feces.

Hematocrit (HCT)   The percentage of a specific volume of blood that consists of packed red blood cells (RBCs). Although hematocrit often is used synonymously with packed cell volume, it is used most correctly to refer to a value measured by an automated hematology analyzer and calculated from the mean cell volume multiplied by the RBC count.

Hematoma   Blood clot.

Hematuria   Blood in the urine.

Hemoabdomen   Abnormal accumulation of blood in the abdomen.

Hemocytometer   Specialized counting chamber with a surface that contains a pair of etched counting grids and a special weighted coverglass used for manual determination of cell counts. Detailed manufacturer instructions must be followed carefully for accurate results.

Hemodynamics   The interplay of factors that affect blood flow and fluid balance in the body.

Hemoglobin   Specialized, iron-containing protein in red blood cells (RBCs) that binds oxygen in the lungs for transport to tissues. Hemoglobin concentration is measured by most automated hematology analyzers as an index of RBC mass.

Hemoglobin saturation   Measured with a pulse oximeter to evaluate the amount of hemoglobin in blood in the peripheral tissues; measurement of perfusion of blood in the peripheral tissues.

Hemoglobinemia   The presence of free hemoglobin in blood plasma resulting from the solution of hemoglobin out of the red blood cells (RBCs), or from their disintegration.

Hemoglobinuria   Hemoglobin in the urine.

Hemolysis   Destruction of red blood cells with liberation of hemoglobin. In microbiology, clearing of media around a bacterial colony.

Hemoptysis   Coughing up blood, or blood in sputum.

Hemostasis   Process of vasoconstriction, platelet plug formation, and blood coagulation resulting in clot formation in response to vascular injury.

Hepatic encephalopathy   Altered cognitive and neurologic function due to buildup of toxins in the bloodstream that are normally removed by the liver.

Hepatotoxic   Compound that is toxic to liver cells.

Hermaphrodite   Intersex condition in which testicular and ovarian tissues exist in the same animal.

Hermaphroditic   Refers to the condition in which a single adult organism has the reproductive organs of both the male and the female of the species. Cross-fertilization and self-fertilization are possible with hermaphrodites. Most digenetic flukes of domesticated animals are hermaphroditic.

Hernia   Abnormal protrusion of an organ or other body structure through a defect or natural opening in a covering, muscle, or bone.

Hertz (Hz) cycles per second   Unit of measurement used to quantify the frequency of ultrasound waves.

Heterogonic life cycle   One of two pathways in the life cycle of *Strongyloide sstercoralis*. The heterogonic cycle takes place when environmental temperatures are fair (not extremely cold or hot).

Heterophil   Type of granulocyte in birds, guinea pigs, and rabbits. Heterophils have bilobed or segmented nuclei and numerous red-staining seed-shaped or rod-shaped granules. Heterophils function similarly to neutrophils, but there are differences in the granule content.

Hirsutism   Abnormally excessive hair growth associated with Cushing's disease in horses and ponies.

Hirudiniasis   Infestation with blood-sucking leeches.

Histopathology   Refers to pathologic changes in tissue that are microscopic and can be seen only with the use of a microscope.

Hobbles   Leather straps fastened around the pasterns of horses; can be placed on all four limbs and tied together with a rope, or just on front limbs or hindlimbs to keep a horse from kicking.

Holistic   Form of medicine that concentrates on the "whole" animal and animal wellness, rather than concentrating on clinical signs of disease.

Homeopathy   System of medicine that is based on the principle that "like cures like."

Homogonic life cycle   One of two pathways in the life cycle of *Strongyloide sstercoralis*. The homogonic cycle takes place when environmental temperatures are adverse (harsh weather).

Homotoxicology   Form of homeopathy that uses multiple remedies at the same time to promote healing in the body.

Hooks   Raised area of the tooth resulting from incomplete occlusal wear; most commonly seen in the rostral maxillary cheek tooth of horses.

Horizontal bone loss   Dental radiography term that refers to alveolar bone loss along the long axis of the jaw, affecting multiple teeth.

Hospice   Facility or program designed to provide a caring environment to meet the physical and emotional needs of the terminally ill.

Hospital   A veterinary or animal hospital is a facility in which the practice conducted typically includes inpatient and outpatient diagnostics and treatment.

Hospital safety manual   A collection of written safety "do's and don'ts" unique to a specific workplace.

Host   See **Parasitism.**

Howell-Jolly bodies   Small, often singular, deeply basophilic nuclear remnants that are occasionally seen in red blood cells (RBCs) on normal blood films; increased numbers may be seen with regenerative anemias and in splenectomized animals.

Human chorionic gonadotropin (hCG)   Glycoprotein hormone secreted from the human chorion. It has luteinizing hormone activity when injected into most animals.

Humane twitch   Restraint device with a hinged metal device that is placed over the upper lip of the horse and clipped to the halter.

Hyaline casts   Colorless, homogeneous, and semi-transparent casts.

Hydatid cyst/Multilocular hydatid cyst   Type of metacestode/larval tapeworm that is closely associated with *Echinococcus multilocularis*.

Hydatid cyst/Unilocular hydatid cyst   Type of metacestode/larval tapeworm that is closely associated with *Echinococcus granulosus*.

Hydrocarbons   Any of a large class of organic compounds that contain only carbon and hydrogen. Examples include natural gas, propane, butane, kerosene, gasoline, and motor oil.

Hydrometra   A condition in which the uterus fills with sterile fluid that causes mild to moderate distention.

Hydronephrosis   Dilatation and distention of the renal pelvis and calices usually caused by obstruction of the flow of urine from the kidney.

Hydrophilic   Having an affinity for water; soluble in water. Hydrophilic drugs often are poorly absorbed and distributed, and therefore require administration by injection (parenteral administration) to achieve effective therapeutic levels.

Hydrophobia   A morbid dread of water.

Hydrotherapy   Use of water for therapeutic effects.

Hyoid bone   Bone in the neck region that supports the base of the tongue, the pharynx, and the larynx and aids the process of swallowing. The hyoid is usually referred to as a single bone, but it is composed of several portions. The hyoid bone is attached to the temporal bone by two small rods of cartilage.

Hyperalgesia   Lowering of the pain threshold resulting in less stimulation required to produce pain.

Hypercarbia   Elevated carbon dioxide levels in the blood.

Hyperchromasia   Increased mean corpuscular hemoglobin concentration (MCHC); artifact secondary to hemolysis, lipemia, icterus, and Heinz body formation.

Hyperechoic   Structure in the ultrasound image that appears bright or white compared with adjacent structures.

Hypermobile joint   Excessive motion at a joint.

Hyperplasia   Too much growth of something.

Hyperpnea   Abnormal increase in the depth and rate of respiratory movements.

Hyperproteinemia   Excessive protein concentrations in the blood.

Hypersegmentation   Nuclei with five or more lobes.

Hypersensitivity   Exaggerated immune response to some source of stimulation.

Hypertension   Elevated blood pressure.

Hyperthermia   Elevation of body temperature caused by inadequate heat-dissipating mechanisms to overcome excessive ambient heat, without a change in the body's thermoregulatory set point.

Hypertonic   Having an osmolality higher than that of blood.

Hyperventilation   Increased ventilation; a respiratory pattern that results in lower carbon dioxide blood levels.

Hypnotic   Drug that induces sleep.

Hypobiosis   A life cycle term that means "being in suspended animation" or "undergoing arrested development."

Hypocerebellum   Decreased size of the cerebellum; the cerebellum is stunted in growth in the fetus.

Hypochromia   Decreased mean corpuscular hemoglobin concentration (MCHC); red blood cells (RBCs) may have an increased area of central pallor.

Hypoechoic   Structure in the ultrasound image that appears darker than adjacent structures.

Hypoglycemia   Lower than normal levels of blood glucose resulting in lack of fuel to the brain and other organ systems.

Hypomobile joint   Less than functional range of motion at a joint.

Hypophyseal portal vessels   Circulatory network that moves small quantities of releasing hormones from the hypothalamus to the anterior pituitary.

Hypoproteinemia   Condition with low blood protein.

Hypopyon   An accumulation of white blood cells (WBCs) in the anterior chamber of the eye.

Hyposthenuric urine   Specific gravity (SG) of less than 1.008.

Hypotension   Low blood pressure; the opposite of hypertension.

Hypothalamus   Specialized portion of the ventral brain that secretes releasing hormones to the anterior pituitary via the hypophyseal-portal vessels.

Hypothermia   Abnormally low body temperature. The measured body temperature must be compared with what is normal for the age group because neonates have lower body temperatures than adults.

Hypotonic   Having an osmolality lower than that of blood.

Hypoventilation   Decreased ventilation; a respiratory problem that results in higher blood levels of carbon dioxide.

Hypovolemia   Decreased circulating blood volume.

Hypoxemia   Low blood oxygen levels.

Hypoxia   Low tissue oxygen levels.

Hypoxic   Deficient in the amount of oxygen reaching body tissues.

Hypsodont   Tooth type with a long reserve crown and roots that allow for continued growth and/or continued eruption.

Icterus   Yellow discoloration of tissues, serum, or plasma due to the presence of bilirubin (see Figure 13-1). Icterus, also referred to as *jaundice*, may develop as a result of hemolytic disease (prehepatic), liver disease (hepatic), or cholestasis (posthepatic or obstruction of bile flow).

Idiopathic aggression   Unpredictable and severe aggression that occurs in the absence of stimuli that would allow the aggression to be categorized otherwise. The type of aggression commonly referred to as "Springer rage" is likely a form of aggression that could be called *idiopathic*.

Idiosyncratic drug reaction   An unpredictable reaction to a drug that does not occur immediately, but after several days of treatment, and that is often associated with an immune system response.

Ileus   Functional loss of intestinal motility.

Immunoglobulins   Group of large glycoproteins that are secreted into blood and tissue fluids by plasma cells, and that function as antibodies in the immune response by binding with specific antigens.

Immunohistochemical stain   Method of analyzing and identifying microbial or cellular components based on the binding of antibodies to a specific antigenic marker.

Impervious   Waterproof. Does not allow water to penetrate.

In situ In its normal place; confined to the site of origin.

Incidental parasite Parasite in a host in which it does not usually live, for example, the canine heartworm, *Dirofilaria immitis*, localizing in the lungs of humans.

Incise drape A sterile, adherent, plastic surgical drape. It is often impregnated with an antiseptic. The drape is incised along with the skin.

Incontinence Involuntary urination or defecation.

Indigenous flora Bacteria that normally inhabit an anatomic site. Also called *normal flora* or *microflora*.

Indirect life cycle Life cycle that uses an intermediate host, for example, *Dirofilaria immitis*, the canine heartworm, uses an indirect life cycle.

Infection Growth of disease-producing bacteria or other microorganisms in the tissues. Parasitism by an internal parasite, for example, canine heartworms infect dogs. Endoparasites, such as the canine heartworm, *Dirofilaria immitis*, infect their hosts.

Infestation Parasitism by an external parasite, for example, fleas infest dogs. Ectoparasites, such as the cat flea, *Ctenocephalides felis*, infest their hosts.

Inflammation Response of body tissues to injury or irritation; characterized by pain, swelling, redness, and heat.

Inflammatory phase The first phase of wound healing. Characterized by formation of a blood clot within the wound, release of growth factors, and recruitment of macrophages and neutrophils to clean up the wound and to modulate healing.

Infundibulum Finger-like portion of the uterine tube (oviduct) that captures the ova upon ovulation.

Ingesta Food material in the intestinal tract.

Ingress port Port on a tubular instrument used to infuse a solution into a cavity, such as a joint.

Inguinal Pertaining to the groin area.

Inhibin Glycoprotein hormone that inhibits release of follicle-stimulating hormone.

Initiation Process by which normal cells are changed so that they have the potential to form cancers. Not all initiated cells go on to become cancer.

Inpatient Patient that comes into the practice and is hospitalized for further treatment or workup.

Insufflate To pump a gas or medicinal substance into a body cavity.

Insurance examination Required by an insurance company before an animal can receive insurance coverage. Most commonly performed in the equine industry.

Inter-dog (male/male) aggression As the term implies, may occur because of fear of strange dogs, or may be related to hormonal influences when it occurs between two intact male dogs. Inter-dog aggression within a household may develop because of a changing hierarchy between the dogs.

Interference with justice Includes eluding a police officer or interfering with the conduct of a criminal investigation.

Interferon Protein manufactured by cells exposed to viruses. Uninfected cells are protected from viral infection by interferon.

Intermediate host Within the life cycle of a parasite, the host that harbors the immature, asexual, or larval stage of a parasite.

Intermediate to large lymphocytes Intermediate to large mononuclear cells that have clear cytoplasm, moderate nuclear-to-cytoplasmic (N/C) ratios, and centralized oval nuclei with a brushed chromatin pattern, and may display a focal accumulation of low numbers of small reddish granules.

Interradicular Referring to the space between the roots of teeth.

Intra-articular Within the joint space.

Intracranial pressure Pressure within the bony vault of the skull that contains the brain and other soft tissues. Increases in intracranial pressure can damage the brain.

Intralingual Within the tongue.

Intramedullary catheter Catheter placed into the medullary canal of a bone (i.e., bone marrow catheter).

Intraosseous Administration of a drug or fluid into the bone.

Intraperitoneal Situated within or administered by entering the peritoneum.

Intravenous pyelogram (IVP) Iodinated contrast medium is injected intravenously to assess the kidneys. Also called an excretory urogram, or EU.

Intubation Placement of an endotracheal tube into the trachea.

Intussusception Telescoping of a portion of the bowel into another.

Ionizing radiation Any radiation that is capable of displacing electrons from atoms or molecules, thereby producing ions. Examples include alpha particles, beta particles, gamma rays or x-rays, and cosmic rays. In medicine, ionizing radiation arises from radiotherapy, x-ray machines, and radioactive substances. Ionizing radiation also enters the atmosphere of the earth from outer space. At high doses, ionizing radiation increases specific types of chemical activity inside cells. This effect can be used to treat cancer, but it also leads to health risks such as the induction of cancer.

IP address The "Internet protocol" address. The series of numbers specific to each computer of each modality for electronic communication with the picture archiving and communication system (PACS) in digital imaging.

Irritable aggression Can be similar to pain-related aggression, but may occur simply because a dog is tired or just is not desiring interaction. May be more common in older dogs and/or in dogs living with small children. May be difficult to differentiate from pain- or fear-related aggression.

Irritant Agent that causes pain or inflammation at the site of injection.

Ischemia Deficient supply of blood to a body part, such as the heart or brain, caused by obstruction of the inflow of arterial blood.

Ischemic compression Use of manual pressure on trigger points to bring about muscle relaxation and to relieve pain.

Isoechoic Structure in the ultrasound image that is of equal echogenicity to another structure.

Isosthenuria Refers to urine with a specific gravity (SG) of 1.008 to 1.012. Indicates that relative amounts of solute and water in the urine are similar to those in plasma.

Isosthenuric urine Specific gravity (SG) of 1.008 to 1.012.

Isotonic Having the same osmolality as that of blood.

Isthmus Portion of the uterine tube (oviduct) that connects the infundibulum to the ampulla.

IVNTA International Veterinary Nurses and Technicians Association.

Ixodid ticks Hard ticks or members of the tick family Ixodidae. Most of the ticks that parasitize domesticated animals are hard ticks. Hard ticks usually attach to their hosts to take a blood meal.

Jackson-Rees circuit Nonrebreathing circuit with a reservoir bag and corrugated tubing but no pressure relief valve, in which the fresh gas inlet is located near the patient, and waste gas exits near the bag; Mapleson F circuit.

Jejunostomy feeding tube Tube that is surgically positioned in the jejunum and is used for enteral feeding when it is necessary to bypass the upper gastrointestinal tract.

Joint mobilization Very specific passive movements applied to the joint.

Joule Unit of energy or work. The amount of work required or energy needed to produce 1 watt of power for 1 second.

Jugular vein Consists of paired veins running in the neck that drain the brain, face, and neck.

Junctional epithelium Thin layer of epithelium that attaches to the tooth just coronal to the cementoenamel junction.

Keratoconjunctivitis Combined inflammation of the cornea and the conjunctiva.

Ketonemia Condition marked by an abnormal increase in ketone bodies within the circulating blood. Ketones are acids that build up in the blood when glucose is not used by cells; can be a result of lack of insulin needed to shuttle glucose into most cells of the body; complication in a patient with diabetes mellitus.

Ketonuria The presence of excess ketone bodies in the urine in conditions such as diabetes mellitus and starvation, which involve reduced or disturbed carbohydrate metabolism.

Ketosis, or acetonemia Nutritional disease of cattle and sometimes sheep, goats, or swine that is marked by reduction of blood glucose and the presence of ketone bodies in the blood, tissues, milk, and urine; it is associated with digestive and nervous disturbances.

Kilocalorie Amount of heat (energy) needed to raise the temperature of 1 kg of water by 1° C.

Kilojoule Amount of mechanical energy needed for a force of 1 newton to move a weight of 1 kg a distance of 1 m. Used as a measure of food energy in Europe, with conversions of 1 kcal = 4.184 kJ and 1 kJ = 0.239 kcal.

Kilovoltage Quality factor that regulates the energy of the x-ray beam. The higher the kVp (kilovoltage), the higher the energy of the x-ray photons. Regulates contrast in the radiographic image. The higher the kVp, the lower the contrast.

Kyphosis Exaggerated upward curvature of the thoracic region of the spinal column, resulting in a rounded upper back.

Laceration Sharp cut or tear through the skin and possibly deeper tissues.

Lacrimation The secretion of tears, *specifically,* abnormal or excessive secretion of tears resulting from local or systemic disease.

Lamina dura Cortical plate of alveolar bone surrounding the tooth.

Laminae Interdigitations between the corium and the hoof that serve as attachment sites between the hoof and the coffin bone. Also bony plates that form the roof of the arch of each spinal vertebra.

Laminar flow Nonturbulent flow of a viscous fluid in layers near a boundary.

Laminitis Inflammation of a lamina, especially in the hoof of a horse, cow, or goat, typically caused by excessive ingestion of a dietary substance (e.g., carbohydrate); called also *founder.*

Laparotomy Surgical incision into the abdominal wall.

Larvicide Preventive compound that will kill the migrating, larval stages of a parasite.

Larviparous nematodes Nematodes that bear live larvae. *Filaroides osleri* is a larviparous nematode that produces L_1 larvae that are infective to the canine host.

Laryngoscope Instrument used to visualize the larynx during endotracheal intubation.

Laser (light amplification by stimulated emission of radiation) Use of a coherent, monochromic, polarized light to bring about a physiologic change in the body.

Late-phase radiation toxicity Side effects caused by radiotherapy that occur more than 90 days after the start of treatment. They are generally characterized by permanent changes such as tissue fibrosis, atrophy, necrosis, and ischemia. They often develop months to years after completion of therapy.

Left shift An increased number of immature granulocytes, typically used to refer to an increased number of band neutrophils. The presence of a left shift often indicates inflammation.

Legend drug A prescription drug. A drug that must be prescribed by a veterinarian, as opposed to an over-the-counter (OTC) drug.

Leptocytes Red blood cells (RBCs) with an increased surface area; target cells (codocytes) and cells with a transverse fold are two common types of leptocytes.

Lesions Alterations or abnormalities in a tissue (pathologic changes); for example, wounds, sores, ulcers, tumors, cataracts, and any other tissue damage.

Leukocytosis Condition characterized by an abnormally high total number of circulating leukocytes. Neutrophilia indicates increased numbers of circulating neutrophils.

Leukoencephalomyelitis Concurrent inflammation of the white matter of the brain and spinal cord.

Levy-Jennings chart Graph on which quality control data are sequentially plotted for rapid visual inspection (see Figure 13-2). The *x*-axis may show the date or control run number, whereas the *y*-axis depicts the concentration of the control. The mean and ±1, 2, or 3 standard deviations from the expected mean of the control material are indicated on the graph.

Life cycle The development of a parasite through its various life stages (e.g., the life cycle of the canine heartworm). In the life cycle of *Dirofilaria immitis,* the dog is the definitive host, and the mosquito is the intermediate host.

Ligament Structure that connects bone to bone.

Limbus Corneal-scleral junction of the eye.

Lingual Positional term in dentistry that refers to the surface of mandibular teeth adjacent to the tongue.

Lipemia Turbidity of serum or plasma due to the presence of lipids that contain a high concentration of triglycerides (see Figure 13-1). Lipemia may occur after a meal or in association with various metabolic diseases.

Lipid   Any fat or oil or related compound that is insoluble in water but soluble in nonpolar solvents.

Lipophilic   Soluble in lipids. Drug absorption across cell membranes is most effective for drugs that are lipophilic.

Local area network (LAN)   The LAN is the connection of the workstation to the picture archiving and communication system (PACS) server for image transfer.

Locomotor   Movement from place to place.

Lordosis   Condition in which the back is arched in such a way that the head and the tail are elevated, and the back is dropped. It is a characteristic sign of estrus in the queen.

Lumen   The cavity of a tubular organ (e.g., the *lumen* of a blood vessel).

Lumpectomy   Removal of a small mass of tissue that is freely movable, such as a small skin tumor or a small mammary mass.

Luteinizing hormone   Hormone produced in the anterior pituitary that when released can initiate follicular maturation, ovulation, and spermatogenesis.

Lyme disease   Also called *borreliosis*; an infectious disease caused by bacteria from the genus *Borrelia*. The bacteria typically are spread through the bite of an infected deer tick.

Lymphoblasts   Intermediate to large lymphoid cells with moderate nuclear-to-cytoplasmic (N/C) ratios, moderately to darkly basophilic cytoplasm, frequent Golgi zones, close nuclear to plasma membrane apposition along most of the perimeter of the round to oval nucleus, and finely stippled chromatin patterns; defined by the presence of one or more variably sized usually round to oval basophilic nucleoli within their nuclei.

Lymphocyte   Variably sized, round leukocyte with a round nucleus, condensed chromatin, and minimal pale cytoplasm, resulting in a relatively high nuclear-to-cytoplasmic ratio. Most lymphocytes normally present in the circulation are small. B and T lymphocytes mediate humoral and cell-mediated immunity, respectively.

Lymphosarcoma   Also known as *lymphoma*; cancer of lymphocytes and lymphoid tissues and the third most commonly diagnosed cancer in dogs.

Lyophilized   Freeze-dried.

Macrocytic   Larger than normal cells.

Macrominerals   Minerals such as calcium, phosphorus, magnesium, sodium, potassium, chlorine, and sulfur that are required in larger quantities than other minerals.

Magill circuit   A non-rebreathing circuit with a reservoir bag and corrugated tubing in which the fresh gas inlet is located near the bag, and the pressure relief valve is located near the patient; Mapleson A circuit.

Magnetostrictive ultrasonic   Type of power scaler that uses a metal stack or a ferrite rod as a transducer to create vibrations of the tip for periodontal débridement.

Maintenance fluid requirement   The amount of fluid typically required to support a healthy animal.

Maintenance nutrient requirements (MNRs)   Levels of nutrients needed to sustain body weight without gain or loss.

Maintenance rate   The amount of fluid needed to fulfill the physiologic requirement for water.

Malignant   A malignant cancer is one that can invade and destroy surrounding normal tissues. Some malignant cancers also have the ability to spread (metastasize) to other parts of the body.

Mallophagans   Chewing lice that are members of the insect order Mallophaga.

Malnutrition   Condition caused by a diet that contains all of the essential nutrients but in suboptimal amounts.

Malocclusion   Incorrect alignment of jaws or specific teeth within the jaws.

Malpractice   Practicing beyond the scope of the license granted by the state, or negligence in carrying out the duties of the license.

Manometer   Instrument used to measure the pressure of liquids such as blood.

Manual muscle testing   Technique used in applied kinesiology to test muscle weakness or paresis that may be affected by functional imbalances in the structural, chemical, mental, and energetic systems of the patient.

Manual therapy   Type of treatment performed with the hands, such as massage and chiropractic.

Many-host tick   An individual tick that is capable of feeding on many different hosts. Many-host ticks make frequent visits to different hosts.

Mapleson circuit   Any one of a number of non-rebreathing circuits in which the position of the fresh gas inlet, the reservoir bag, and the scavenger outlet varies as classified by W.W. Mapleson.

Mare   Adult female horse.

Marketing   All forms of client communication (i.e., signs, business cards, treatment plans, website, etc.).

Massage   Varying types of manual strokes applied to the body to promote relaxation, to decrease pain, or to promote circulation to surrounding tissues.

Masseter muscle   Large bilateral muscle of mastication positioned ventral to the zygomatic arch, which functions to close the mouth.

Mastectomy   Removal of a mammary gland.

Master problem list   Complete list of diagnoses given to a patient during its lifetime.

Mastication   Term used to describe chewing and breakdown of food material by the teeth.

Mastitis   Inflammation of the mammary gland. Typically occurs during lactation. If endotoxins are absorbed from septic secretions within the udder, endotoxemia can result, and the condition is termed *toxic mastitis*.

Material safety data sheet (MSDS)   Form prepared by the manufacturer of a product that contains data regarding the properties of the product; it is intended to provide workers and emergency personnel with procedures for handling or working with that substance in a safe manner.

Maternal aggression   Aggression typical of a female that is attempting to prevent access to her offspring (usually neonates). May also occur during pseudopregnancy (pseudocyesis), when females nest and guard items as if they are neonates, in the absence of actual pregnancy.

Maturation phase   The third and final phase of wound healing. During this phase, collagen fibers remodel and align, and there is a final gain in wound strength.

Maxillomandibular fixation Type of jaw fracture fixation that immobilizes the jaws with the mouth slightly open, allowing the patient to eat and drink through a narrow space between the incisors.

Mean corpuscular hemoglobin concentration (MCHC) The average concentration of hemoglobin in a volume of blood. MCHC is calculated from the hemoglobin concentration divided by the packed cell volume (hematocrit) and is used to characterize red blood cells (RBCs) in anemic patients.

Mean corpuscular volume (MCV) Average volume of red blood cells (RBCs). MCV is measured by most automated hematology analyzers and is used to characterize the RBCs in anemic patients. It also may be calculated by dividing the packed cell volume by RBC count obtained through manual methods.

Medial metatarsal vein The vein in birds that is found on the medial aspect of the tarsometatarsal bone.

Mediastinum Space in the thorax between the lungs that contains the trachea, esophagus, heart, nerves, lymphatic vessels, and major blood vessels.

Medical administration and order records (MAOR) Records used by the entire veterinary health care team to help organize the management and care of hospitalized patients.

Megestrol acetate Synthetic progestagen used to suppress estrus in the bitch.

Melatonin Hormone produced in the pineal gland during hours of darkness. It is involved with the seasonality of estrus in many species.

Melena Passage of dark tarry stools that contain decomposing blood; usually an indication of bleeding in the upper part of the alimentary tract, especially the esophagus, stomach, and duodenum.

Meninges Connective tissue layers that cover the brain and spinal cord.

Mentation Mental activity or acuity of a patient.

Meridian Line drawn to connect a group of acupuncture points named for the organ on which they have the greatest effect.

Mesial Positional term in dentistry that refers to the surface of the tooth along the dental arch that is closest to the rostral midline of the dental arch.

Mesocephalic Also called *mesaticephalic*; refers to a head shape of moderate length in the rostrocaudal dimension, as is seen in Beagles.

Metabolic acidosis Acidosis resulting from excess acid in the blood caused by abnormal metabolism, excessive acid intake, renal retention, or excessive loss of bicarbonate (as in diarrhea).

Metabolism (biotransformation) The ability of a living organism to modify the chemical structure of drugs, so that they are no longer active.

Metabolizable energy Energy available to the animal after energy from feces, urine, and combustible gases has been subtracted from gross energy. Used to express the energy content of foods and commercial diets.

Metabolizable (maintenance) energy requirement Average amount of energy used by an animal with normal activity, exercise, and growth, or other energy demands beyond resting.

Metacestode A larval tapeworm. Stage of the tapeworm found within the vertebrate or invertebrate intermediate host. Examples of metacestode stages include cysticercoid, cysticercus, coenurus, and the hydatid cyst (both unilocular and multilocular).

Metamyelocyte Developmental stage before the band with a bean-shaped or butterfly-shaped nucleus.

Metaphylaxis Use of antimicrobial treatment for subclinical manifestation of bovine respiratory disease (BRD) complex in cattle.

Metastasis Process by which a malignant cancer spreads from the primary or original site to a distant location in the body.

Metritis Inflammation of the uterus. This condition can be associated with buildup of septic fluid within the uterus. If endotoxins are absorbed from the septic uterine fluid, endotoxemia can result, and the condition is termed *toxic metritis*.

MHz Abbreviation for megahertz—the unit of frequency for diagnostic ultrasound waves.

Mibolerone Synthetic androgen used to suppress estrus in the bitch.

Microbiology The study of microorganisms (bacteria, fungi, and viruses) and their interactions within ecosystems.

Microcytic Smaller than normal cells.

Microfilaria (pl. microfilariae) This "prelarval" developmental stage is often associated with *Dirofilaria immitis*, the canine heartworm.

Microfilaricide Therapeutic compound that will kill the microfilarial stages of a parasite.

Microflora Microorganisms (mostly bacteria) with intimate and permanent associations with epithelial surfaces. Also called *normal flora*, *indigenous flora*, or *autochthonous flora*.

Microminerals Group of minerals called "trace elements," such as copper, iron, boron, molybdenum, and cobalt, all of which are required in minute amounts.

Microorganisms Organisms that are too small to be seen with the naked eye. Group includes bacteria, viruses, fungi, and protozoa.

Microsporum sp. Genus of fungi that can cause ringworm. Most common in cats and horses, but dogs and other species of animals (including humans) are susceptible.

Milliamperage The milliamperage setting controls the quantity of electrons boiled off the filament in the x-ray tube.

Mineralocorticoids Group of hormones (like aldosterone) that regulate body water and electrolytes.

Minerals Nonorganic solid substances that occur naturally in food and form the mineral composition of the animal body; at least 13 are essential to health.

Minimum inhibitory concentration (MIC) Lowest concentration of an antimicrobial agent that will inhibit the visible growth of a microorganism after overnight incubation.

Miosis Constriction of the pupil of the eye.

Miracidium A ciliated, motile stage that emerges from the operculated egg of a digenetic fluke. The miracidium is covered with tiny moving hairs that allow it to swim in the water and to come in contact with the first intermediate host of the fluke, which is usually a snail.

Mitchell markers   Special radiographic markers used primarily in standing radiography of the equine head to assist in identifying fluid levels in paranasal sinuses.

M-mode   Time-motion ultrasound imaging mode wherein motion of the body, usually the heart, is observed by scanning a thin slice of it over time.

Mobile facility   A mobile practice is a veterinary practice conducted from a vehicle with special medical or surgical facilities, or from a vehicle suitable for making house or farm calls. Regardless of mode of transportation, such practices shall have a permanent base of operations with a published address, and telecommunication capabilities for making appointments or responding to emergency situations.

Modality   Method of application of or use of any therapeutic agent, usually physical agents.

Modified Robert Jones bandage (soft-padded bandage)   Bandage that is similar to a Robert Jones bandage but with a much thinner secondary layer.

Modified Thomas splint   Traction splint constructed of rods; used to stabilize long-bone fractures in large animals.

Modulation   Process of amplifying or dampening incoming pain signals after arrival to the spinal cord.

Moist wound healing   Maintaining a moist wound environment by using an occlusive or semi-occlusive primary bandage layer.

Monoclonal antibodies   Antibodies that recognize a single antigen.

Monocyte   Largest circulating leukocyte in health; monocytes are characterized by abundant basophilic cytoplasm that often contains clear vacuoles and/or small pink granules. Nuclei are oval, indented, or amoeboid in shape and have chromatin that is less condensed than in lymphocytes.

Monotherapy   Administration of a single drug to treat a particular condition.

Morbidity   Incidence of disease; rate of sickness (as in a specified community or group).

Moribund   Near death.

Mortality   Number of deaths in a given time or place.

MPD   Maximum permissible dose (MPD). This is the maximum allowed radiation exposure a person can receive during occupational exposure over a specified time.

Mucin clot test   Used to evaluate joint fluid viscosity; formation and integrity of a mucin clot upon addition of joint fluid to an acidic reagent are evaluated.

Mucogingival junction   The line created at the place where the alveolar mucosa meets the gingiva.

Mucometra   Sterile mucus within the uterus causing mild to moderate distention.

Mucositis   Inflammation of mucous membranes lining the digestive tract from the mouth to the anus. Mucositis is a possible side effect of chemotherapy or radiotherapy that involves any part of the digestive tract.

Mucous membrane   Moist body surface associated with an orifice (e.g., oral cavity, genitourinary cavity).

Müllerian duct   Embryologic precursor of the female tubular reproductive tract (uterine tubes, uterus, cranial vagina).

Multilocular hydatid cyst   A type of metacestode/larval tapeworm that is closely associated with *Echinococcus multilocularis*. The multilocular hydatid cyst consists of many, tiny, spherical, fluid-filled vesicles or cysts; however, these cysts are NOT enclosed by a thick, fibrous cyst wall of host origin, as in the case of *Echinococcus granulosus*.

Multimodal analgesia   Use of two or more drugs to affect different phases of nociception simultaneously.

Multi-modality therapy   Cancer treatment that combines more than one form of therapy (e.g., surgery, radiotherapy, and chemotherapy).

Multiparous   An animal that has given birth multiple times.

Multiple organ dysfunction syndrome (MODS)   A complication of shock in which generalized microvascular clotting causes sufficient organ damage to result in failure of multiple organs.

Mutagen   Chemical or physical agent that causes permanent deoxyribonucleic acid (DNA) injury and alteration within a cell. These changes are separate and distinct from those that normally occur during genetic recombination.

Mycosis   Fungal infection in or on a part of the body.

Mydriasis   Dilatation of the pupil of the eye.

Myelocyte   Developmental stage before metamyelocyte with oval-shaped nuclei.

Myelosuppression   Condition in which normal bone marrow activity is decreased, resulting in fewer white blood cells (WBCs; especially neutrophils), platelets, and red blood cells (RBCs) in the circulation. Myelosuppression is a potential side effect of some cancer therapies (e.g., radiotherapy, chemotherapy).

Myiasis   Infection or infestation of Dipteran larvae (maggots) into the organs or tissues of humans, domesticated animals, or wild animals.

Myocardium   Middle layer of the heart and the main muscle layer responsible for contraction during systole.

Myofibroblast   Type of fibroblast with contractile properties similar to those of smooth muscle cells, which are responsible for wound contraction.

Myoglobinuria   Myoglobin in the urine.

Myositis   Inflammation of muscle.

Myotherapy (aka *trigger point therapy*)   Form of massage that uses ischemic compression to relieve pain and muscle spasms.

Nadir of leukopenia   Lowest circulating neutrophil count after administration of a chemotherapy drug. The nadir occurs at a predictable time point after therapy that varies depending on exactly what drug has been given.

Nares   Nostrils.

Nasal cannula   Catheter or tube inserted into the nasal passages to supply oxygen.

Nasogastric feeding tube   Flexible tube with a rounded end that is passed through the nasal cavity to the stomach.

Nasolacrimal duct   Duct that travels from the medial canthus of the eye to the rostral nasal passage; responsible for drainage of tears.

National Commission on Veterinary Economic Issues (NCVEI) A nonprofit organization formed jointly in 2000 by the American Veterinary Medical Association (AVMA), the American Animal Hospital Association (AAHA) and the Association of American Veterinary Medical Colleges (AAVMC) to study and support economic growth and the delivery of excellent patient care in veterinary medicine.

National Fire Protection Association (NFPA) Organization with the mission of reducing incidence of and damage from fire by providing and advocating scientifically based codes and standards, research, training, and education.

National Institute for Occupational Safety and Health (NIOSH) As part of the Centers for Disease Control and Prevention (CDC), NIOSH is responsible for conducting research and making recommendations for the prevention of work-related illnesses and injuries.

Navicular bursa Closed fibrous sac lined with a smooth membrane, producing a viscous lubricant known as *synovial fluid*, and located between the deep digital flexor tendon and the navicular bone.

NAVTA National Association of Veterinary Technicians in America.

Necropsy Examination of an animal after it has died to determine abnormal and disease-related changes that occurred during its life. The term *necropsy* originates from the Greek language and means "viewing the dead." Necropsy is also known as *autopsy*, which is Greek for "seeing with one's own eyes."

Necrosis Tissue or cellular death.

Necrotizing Causing, associated with, or undergoing necrosis (death of living tissue).

Needle teeth Deciduous third incisors and canines of piglets. These "baby teeth" are very sharp and should be nipped to protect the sow during suckling.

Negative punishment Decreases the frequency of a behavior because something *pleasant* is *taken away (subtracted)* after that behavior.

Negative reinforcement Increases the frequency of a behavior because something *unpleasant* is *taken away or avoided (subtracted)* after that behavior.

Nematode A roundworm.

Neonatal Pertaining to the time immediately after birth.

Neonatal isoerythrolysis (NI) Uncommon, complex disorder of newborns that results from blood group incompatibility between the dam and the offspring; NI occurs after the neonate suckles and absorbs antibodies from the dam's colostrum, which then attack the red blood cells (RBCs) of the neonate, resulting in destruction of RBCs of the baby and subsequent anemia (decrease in RBCs).

Neonatal period In puppies and kittens, the first 2 to 4 weeks of life are characterized by complete dependence on the mother because of incomplete neurologic functions, such as audio and visual abilities and proper spinal reflexes.

Neoplasm Abnormal growth of tissue that may be benign or malignant.

Nephrectomy Surgical removal of a kidney.

Nephrotoxic Toxic or destructive to kidney cells.

Net energy Energy available to the animal after energy from feces, urine, combustible gases, and loss of body heat has been subtracted from gross energy.

Net income Total income less all expenses and taxes.

Network Where veterinary software is stored and the associated patient-client database.

Neurologic larva migrans Term that describes a zoonotic condition caused by ingestion of an egg that contains an infective second-stage larva of the roundworm *Baylisascaris procyonis*, which is commonly referred to as the *raccoon ascarid*.

Neuromuscular blocker Drug that relaxes and paralyzes muscles and causes cessation of breathing as a result of paralysis of the muscles of respiration.

Neuromuscular electrical stimulation (NMES) A modality of physical therapy in which small electrical impulses are sent through the skin to underlying nerves and muscles, creating an involuntary muscle contraction. NMES is helpful in maintaining muscle tone in patients with muscle atrophy caused by disuse and incapacitation.

Neurons Nerve cells that relay information from the central nervous system to the rest of the body.

Neurotransmitter Chemical substance released from the axon terminal of a presynaptic neuron; diffuses across the synaptic cleft to excite or inhibit the target cell.

Neutroclusion Malocclusion in which no jaw length discrepancy is evident, but one or more teeth are in an abnormal position.

Neutropenia Abnormal decrease in the number of neutrophils (the most common type of white blood cells [WBCs]) in the blood.

Neutrophil Type of granulocyte characterized by a segmented nucleus with condensed chromatin and cytoplasm that contains numerous granules. In most species, the granules are neutral staining and are not readily visible with routine stains. Neutrophils are the most abundant cell type in circulation in healthy dogs, cats, and horses.

Nidus Place where bacteria and other organisms can lodge and replicate.

Nit The egg of an Anopluran (sucking) or Mallophagan (chewing) louse. The adult female louse cements the nit to a hair shaft or to a feather of the infested host.

N-methyl-D-aspartate (NMDA) receptor One of several receptors in the central nervous system that secrete excitatory neurotransmitters. NMDA receptors play a large role in the processing of pain signals.

Nociception Term used to describe three neuralgic phases of the pain pathway: transduction, transmission, and modulation.

Nonadherent dressing Primary layer that does not adhere firmly to the wound surface.

Nonionic Without a charge. Used in reference to drugs that are uncharged.

Non-rebreathing system Breathing circuit in which exhaled gases are carried away from the patient into a scavenging system.

Nonscreen film Radiographic film that requires direct exposure to x-rays to create an image. They are insensitive to visible light from screens. Used mainly for the oral cavity.

Nonshopped fees Fees for which clients do not call the practice to find out the cost. They make up the largest percentage of the fee schedule.

Nonsteroidal anti-inflammatory drugs (NSAIDs) Large group of anti-inflammatory agents that work by inhibiting the production of prostaglandins. Examples include ibuprofen, ketoprofen, naproxen, and aspirin. These compounds also possess analgesic, antipyretic, and anti-inflammatory effects; they reduce pain, fever, and inflammation.

Nonthreatening greeting behaviors When greeting dogs and cats, technicians should look off to the side or down (avoid eye contact), stand up straight or bend at the knees (avoid bending at the waist and leaning over the pet), stroke the pet under the chin at first (do not reach over the animal's head to pet it), and turn the side of their bodies to face the pet (avoid approaching front to front).

Normothermic Normal body temperature

Nosocomial infection Infection acquired during hospitalization.

Nucleated RBCs (NRBCs) Immature red blood cells (RBCs) before developmental stage to the reticulocyte; usually metarubricytes if associated with regenerative anemia or bone marrow toxicity.

Nutraceutical Nondrug substance administered orally to provide substances required for normal body structure and function with the intent of improving the health of animals.

Nutrients Substances that provide nourishment for growth and maintenance of life.

Nutritional myodegeneration Degeneration of muscle tissue usually associated with vitamin E and selenium deficiency.

Nymphomania Behavior state in which a female is in continuous estrus or estrus for prolonged periods.

Nystagmus Rhythmic, involuntary oscillation of both eyes.

Obesity Body composition with a ratio of too much fat to lean tissue, or body weight 15% to 20% greater than optimal.

Obligatory parasite Organism that must live a parasitic existence (e.g., the canine heartworm, *Dirofilaria immitis*, in dogs).

Obstructive urolithiasis Condition characterized by the formation or presence of calculi in the urinary tract that cause complete obstruction of urinary flow.

Obtunded Mentally dull.

Obturator Stylus or removable plug used during insertion of a tubular instrument.

Occlusal Positional term that refers to the part of a tooth that meets with, or occludes with, the teeth of the opposite dental arcade.

Occlusive Impermeable to moisture. Used in reference to bandage materials. An occlusive primary layer is used for moist wound healing.

Occupational Safety and Health Act Law in the United States that established the Occupational Safety and Health Administration. It gives every American worker protections and responsibilities in the area of safety. The Act applies to all workplaces in the United States and its territories that have at least one employee.

Occupational Safety and Health Administration (OSHA) Agency of the U.S. government that is charged with enforcing the Occupational Safety and Health Act. Twenty-one states and territories have OSHA programs administered by the state; the remainder fall under federal OSHA jurisdiction.

Ocular larva migrans, Visceral larva migrans Zoonotic condition caused by the migration of nematode larvae (usually *Toxocara canis*) through the eyes of children. Children become infected with these larvae by ingestion of eggs containing the infective second-stage larvae of *T. canis*.

Odontoblasts Cells that line the pulp cavity and root canal and are responsible for the production of dentin.

Odontoclasts Cells of the macrophage lineage (similar to osteoclasts) that cause resorption of the tooth.

Offensive aggression Behaviors that result in harm done to another individual when the aggressor initiates the conflict. Offensive animals are not fearful and will move toward rather than away from an opponent.

Office A veterinary office is a veterinary practice in which a limited or consultative practice is conducted and that typically provides no facilities for housing or for inpatient diagnostics or treatment.

Omentopexy Surgical fixation of the omentum to the body wall.

Omentum Supportive mesenteries, which arise from the greater and lesser curvatures of the stomach.

Omphalophlebitis Condition (e.g., navel ill) characterized by or resulting from inflammation and infection of the umbilical vein.

On-call emergency service Veterinary medical service in which veterinarians and staff members are not necessarily on the premises during all hours of operation, or one where, after initial triage and treatment are provided, veterinarians leave orders for continued patient care by staff and remain available on-call.

Oncosphere The "growth ball." Many tapeworm eggs are referred to as *oncospheres*.

Oncotic pressure The portion of total osmotic pressure contributed by colloids.

One-handed method Technique of replacing the cap on a used hypodermic needle using only one hand. This technique is used to prevent accidental insertion of the needle into the opposite hand while one is holding a cap.

One-host tick An individual tick that will feed on a single animal or on a single species of animal.

One-step prep Alcohol-based solutions containing other antiseptics that form a film when painted on the skin. Provide rapid onset of antiseptic effect and a long residual effect.

Onychectomy Removal of a claw.

Oocyst The "egg-like offspring" produced by coccidial parasites such as *Cystoisospora (Isospora)*.

Oocyte Female component of the embryo that originates from the follicle of the ovary.

Open gloving Method of putting on sterile gloves when the person is not wearing a sterile gown or when the hands are protruding through the ends of the gown sleeves.

Open kinetic chain exercise Exercise in which the distal limb segment is free.

Operant conditioning Also known as *instrumental conditioning*; based on the principle that the consequences of a behavior will influence its frequency; known as the Thorndike law of effect. Behaviors that result in pleasant outcomes will increase in frequency, whereas those that result in unpleasant outcomes will decrease.

Operating software Tells the different parts of the hardware how to communicate with one other. For instance, the operating system translates strikes on the keyboard to letters seen on the screen. It monitors and organizes files and directories, and it controls peripheral devices, such as printers, scanners, and disc drives.

Operculated egg An egg that possesses a "tiny, cap-like door" at one pole. Operculated eggs are produced by digenetic trematodes and pseudotapeworms.

Operculum The "door" on one end of a trematode egg or the egg of a pseudotapeworm. The miracidium of the juvenile fluke will exit via the operculum of the fluke egg; the coracidium of the juvenile pseudotapeworm will exit via the operculum of the pseudotapeworm egg.

Opioids Analgesics that remedy pain by affecting pain receptors in the brain.

Opisthotonos Condition of spasm of the muscles of the back, causing the head and limbs to bend backward and the trunk to arch forward.

Opportunistic infection Infection caused by an organism that is usually harmless, but that causes disease under certain circumstances, such as failure of host defenses.

Orchidectomy Removal of the testicles.

Oronasal fistula Abnormal communication between the mouth and the nasal passage, usually caused by severe periodontal disease or palatal trauma.

Orthopedic Related to surgery on the skeleton.

Orthopnea Shortness of breath when lying down. Animals in congestive heart failure will stand and will resist lying down, to facilitate respiration.

Osmolality Concentration of osmotically active particles in solution expressed in osmoles or milliosmoles per kilogram.

Osmotic Having the ability to retain or pull water.

Ostectomy Removal of a portion of bone.

Osteochondral fragments Fracture involving the articular cartilage and underlying bone.

Osteochondrosis Defect in cartilage maturation that causes lack of ossification of maturing cartilage.

Osteoconductive Term that refers to a material that does not stimulate bone formation but facilitates movement of bone cells to traverse a defect.

Osteoinductive Term that refers to a material that stimulates bone formation in areas where no bone is present.

Osteomyelitis Infection of the bone.

Otoacariasis Infestation of the external ear canal with mites or ticks. *Otobius megnini*, the spinose ear tick, and *Otodectes cynotis*, the ear mite of dogs and cats, produce otoacariasis.

Outpatient Patient that comes into the practice and is treated and leaves without staying.

Ovariohysterectomy Spay; removal of the uterus.

Over-the-counter (OTC) drug A nonprescription drug, as opposed to a legend drug.

Overhydration The opposite of dehydration. Condition characterized by fluid retention or overload.

Oxidase An enzyme such as cytochrome oxidase that catalyzes an oxidation-reduction reaction using oxygen as the electron acceptor.

Oxygen free radicals Highly reactive compounds or molecules that cause tissue damage.

Oxygen saturation The amount of hemoglobin bound to oxygen at any given moment. This value is measured in percent, and it reflects the degree of blood oxygenation.

Oxytocin Hormone produced in the hypothalamus and stored in the posterior pituitary, which, when released, enhances milk "letdown" into the teat canal and uterine contractility.

Packed cell volume (PCV) The percentage (%) of red blood cells (RBCs) in a specific volume of blood; determined by centrifugation of a microhematocrit tube filled with anticoagulated blood. PCV is used commonly in veterinary medicine as an index of RBC mass.

PACS (picture archiving and communication system, picture archival computing systems) A computer system used to store, transmit, and access digital medical images.

Pain detection threshold The point at which pain nerve fibers are stimulated enough to send pain signals to the central nervous system.

Pain tolerance The greatest intensity of pain that can be tolerated by an individual.

Pain-related aggression Aggression similar to fear-related aggression in that the dog may be aggressing because of discomfort, pain, or fear of pain (e.g., a dog with a history of painful ears may display aggression when the owner approaches with ear medication).

Palatability Description of the taste, texture, aroma, and other characteristics of pet food. Highly palatable foods tend to be rich in fat and have added flavor enhancers.

Palatal Positional term in dentistry that describes the surface of maxillary teeth adjacent to the palate.

Palatoglossal folds Bilateral bands of soft tissue that run from the roof of the mouth to beneath the tongue. The area lateral to the palatoglossal folds is often affected in cats with stomatitis.

Palliative therapy Cancer treatment administered to relieve symptoms and reduce suffering caused by cancer. The primary goal of palliative therapy is to improve quality of life; it is not intended to cure cancer or even to extend survival time.

Palpation The sense of touch used to assess what structures lay below the skin and the potential for injury to those structures.

Palpebral edema Swelling of the eyelids.

Pancytopenia A decrease to below normal in the concentration of the three major blood cell types: red cells, white cells, and platelets.

Panleukopenia Viral infection of cats that is not considered zoonotic but is highly contagious from cat to cat.

Paracentesis Surgical puncture of a body cavity (e.g., the abdomen) with a trocar, an aspirator, or another instrument usually to draw off an abnormal effusion for diagnostic or therapeutic purposes.

Paralumbar fossa Depression in the dorsocaudal abdominal body wall of quadrupeds bordered by the costal processes of the lumbar vertebrae, the last thoracic rib, and the tuber coxae.

Paralysis Nervous or musculoskeletal problem that prevents any movement of the affected body part.

Paramedian Situated adjacent to the midline.

Paraneoplastic syndrome   Symptoms that result from effects on organs or tissues distant from the site of a primary tumor or its metastases. The underlying cause is usually a substance that is produced by the tumor and then is released into the systemic circulation. Almost any organ or tissue can be affected.

Paraphimosis   Condition in which the penis is extended and cannot be retracted to its normal position within the prepuce.

Parasite   See **Parasitism**.

Parasitism   Association between two organisms of different species in which one member (the parasite) lives on or in the other member (the host) and may cause harm. Parasitism implies a metabolic dependency.

Parasitology   The study of parasitic relationships.

Paratenic host/Transport host   A host in which a parasite does not undergo further development, but in which it remains encysted or in "suspended animation," serving as a source of the definitive host when the definitive host ingests the paratenic host.

Parenteral administration   Administration by injection.

Parenteral feeding   The delivery of nutrients intravenously.

Paresis   Incomplete paralysis (i.e., some function is still possible).

Parthenogenesis   Modified form of sexual reproduction characterized by the formation of an ovum without the fertilization of a male's spermatozoan.

Parturition   Process by which delivery of mammalian offspring occurs.

Parvoviral enteritis   Viral infection of dogs that is not considered zoonotic but is highly contagious from dog to dog.

Passerine   Of or related to the largest order (Passeriformes) of birds, which includes more than half of all living birds and consists chiefly of altricial songbirds.

Passive immunity   Type of immunity incurred via one of the following ways:

1. In utero when antibodies pass through the placenta from the dam to the fetus.

2. In newborns from the consumption of antibody-rich colostrum (first milk).

3. By intravenous infusion of antibody-rich plasma (usually given to neonates that failed to gain adequate levels of antibodies in steps 1 and 2 here).

Passive range of motion (PROM)   Joint movement caused by a therapist who moves a limb with no assistance from the patient.

Passive transfer   Absorption of protective antibodies from the colostrum by the newborn.

Patent ductus arteriosus   Congenital cardiac anomaly that results in persistent vascular communication between the aorta and the pulmonary artery.

Pathogenesis   Sequence of events that leads to or underlies a disease.

Pathogenic organism   Biological agent (fungus, bacterium, virus, etc.) that causes disease or illness.

Pathognomonic   Feature or abnormality that specifically denotes a single disease or condition.

Pathology   The science and study of disease, especially the causes and development of abnormal conditions.

PCV (packed cell volume)   Percent of blood volume composed of red blood cells.

Peak serum concentration   Point of maximum concentration of drug on the time-versus-serum concentration curve.

Pediatric period   Pediatrics covers the period from birth to puberty and is concerned with development and disease during this period. Puppies and kittens are considered pediatric patients during the first 7 to 12 months of life (puberty sets in later in giant breed dogs; thus they may be considered pediatric patients until 1.5 to 2 years of age).

Pediculosis   Infestation with Anopluran (sucking) or Mallophagan (chewing) lice.

Pemphigus vulgaris   Vesicular autoimmune disease of the skin and oral mucosa that also causes pyrexia, depression, and anorexia.

Pentastomes (tongue worms)   A unique group of parasites (distantly related to the arthropods) that infect the lungs of snakes and other reptiles.

Pepsinogen   A granular zymogen of the gastric glands that is readily converted into pepsin in a slightly acid medium.

Percutaneous   Term that refers to something passing through the skin.

Periapical lucency   Term in dental radiography that refers to decreased radiodensity at the tip of a tooth root, which is suggestive of its pathologic condition.

Pericardiocentesis   Surgical puncture of the pericardium, especially to aspirate pericardial fluid.

Pericardiotomy   Surgical incision of the pericardium.

Pericarditis   Inflammation of the pericardium.

Pericardium   The sac of serous membrane that encloses the heart and the roots of the great blood vessels of vertebrates and consists of an outer fibrous coat, which loosely invests the heart, and a double inner serous coat, of which one layer is closely adherent to the heart; the other lines the inner surface of the outer coat with the intervening space filled with pericardial fluid.

Perineal   The area between the anus and the dorsal part of the external genitalia, especially in the female.

Perineal hernia   Herniation of abdominal contents through the pelvic diaphragm, resulting in swelling on either side of the anus.

Perineum   An area of tissue that marks externally the approximate boundary of the outlet of the pelvis and gives passage to the urogenital ducts and rectum.

Periodic parasite   Parasite that makes short visits to its host to obtain nourishment or some other benefit (e.g., female mosquitoes alighting on the vertebrate host to obtain a blood meal).

Periodontal débridement   Nonsurgical instrumentation for removal of hard and soft deposits from teeth and surrounding spaces.

Periodontium   Supporting structures of the tooth, including the periodontal ligament, gingival connective tissue, alveolar bone, and cementum.

Periparturient   Period of time that surrounds parturition or birth.

Peritoneal cavity   The abdominal cavity (lined by a membrane known as the *peritoneum*).

Peritoneal lining A thin transparent membrane (serosa) that lines the peritoneal cavity. It is also called the *parietal peritoneum*.

Peritonitis Inflammation of the serosa (peritoneum) that lines the walls of the abdominal cavity and covers the abdominal organs and mesenteries.

Perjury Making a false statement under oath.

Persistent deciduous tooth Primary or "baby" tooth that has not been lost by the time the adult tooth is erupting. Previously and incorrectly referred to as *retained*.

Persistent infection (PI) Chronic infection that does not resolve despite use of antimicrobials.

Personal protective equipment (PPE) Any piece of clothing or article worn by the user that is designed to prevent injury. Typically, PPE would not remove the hazard at hand, but merely places a physical barrier between the wearer and the hazard. Examples include gloves, glasses or goggles, aprons, boots, smocks, masks, etc.

Petechiation, or petechial hemorrhage Small, visible, pinpoint hemorrhage lesions less than 1 mm in diameter.

Pétrissage Type of massage that consists of kneading, rhythmic lifting, squeezing, and releasing of tissue. It assists in removing metabolic waste and increasing circulation.

Petty cash Small discretionary funds in the form of cash that are used to buy items at times when it is not practical to write a check or use a credit card.

Peyer patches Aggregations of lymphoid tissue that are usually found in the lowest portion of the small intestine (ileum).

pH Measurement of the concentration of hydrogen ions in a solution. The pH indicates whether a solution is acidic (pH < 7.0), neutral (pH = 7.0), or basic (pH > 7.0).

Pharmacodynamics (PD) Study of the biochemical and physiologic effects of drugs.

Pharmacognosy Aspect of pharmacology that includes the history and sources of drugs.

Pharmacokinetics (PK) Study of the movement of drugs in the body (i.e., absorption, distribution, metabolism, and excretion).

Pharmacology The study of drugs.

Pharmacotherapeutics Therapeutic uses of drugs.

Pharynx The part of the digestive and respiratory tracts that extends from the back of the nasal cavity and mouth to the esophagus, more specifically delineated as the nasopharynx and the oropharynx.

Pheromone Substance that is secreted by an animal and is detected by the olfactory system of another animal. Usually provides sexual signals.

Phimosis Condition in which an animal is unable to extend the penis, perhaps as a result of the presence of masses on the penis or secondary to balanoposthitis.

Phlebitis Inflammation of a vein.

Phobia Fear of a specific stimulus that is excessive and persistent. The response usually seems out of proportion to the threat.

Photophobia Intolerance to light; painful sensitivity to strong light.

Physical sterilization Use of filtration, radiation, and heat applied to medical products. Filtration is often used to sterilize pharmaceuticals, radiation is used to sterilize packaged products such as sterile bandaging material, and heat is used to sterilize surgical instruments and materials that cannot withstand the high temperatures, pressure, and heat of autoclaving.

Physiologic age An individual's age as estimated in terms of organ and body function and translated into probable life expectancy. The physiologic age may be shorter or longer than the actual chronological age, as measured in months and years.

Picture archival computing systems (PACS) Required to store, send, receive, print, and view images from all imaging modalities.

Piezoelectric ultrasonic Type of power scaler that uses a ceramic disc or a quartz crystal as a transducer to create vibrations of the tip for periodontal débridement.

Pineal gland The endocrine structure within the brain that acts to correlate the length of daylight to reproduction.

Pinocytosis Uptake of fluid and dissolved substances by a cell through invagination and pinching off of the cell membrane.

Pituitary gland The "master endocrine gland." A pea-sized endocrine gland located at the base of the brain, made up of the anterior pituitary gland, which produces seven known hormones, and the posterior pituitary gland, which stores and releases two hormones from the hypothalamus; also called the *hypophysis*.

Placenta Structure that consists of the yolk sac, the amnion, the allantois, and the chorion; responsible for the passage of oxygen, nutrients, and waste products between fetus and dam.

Placentomes Placental structures in ruminants formed by the fusion of caruncles and cotyledons.

Plaque An accumulation of food particles, saliva, minerals, and bacteria that appears as a white-tan, easily removable film on the teeth.

Plasmin Proteolytic enzyme formed from plasminogen in blood. Plasmin cleaves fibrin to dissolve clots and reestablish blood flow in areas of vascular injury.

Platelet concentrate Prepared by centrifugation of platelet-rich plasma or by plateletpheresis.

Platelet-rich plasma Concentrated source of platelets prepared by centrifugation or filtration of fresh whole blood.

Platelets Non-nucleated fragments of megakaryocyte cytoplasm that circulate in blood and are involved in primary hemostasis. Platelets usually are smaller than red blood cells (RBCs), and the cytoplasm contains numerous small blue to purple granules, the contents of which are important in hemostasis.

Play-related aggression Behavior typical of play, usually nonaffective, and often simply referred to as inappropriate play behavior when directed toward humans.

Pleural effusion Fluid buildup in the space surrounding the lungs within the thorax.

Pleural space The small potential space between the rib cage and the lung that is lined by a membrane called the *pleura*.

Plerocercoid (Sparganum) The infective developmental stage that parasitizes the second intermediate host in the life cycle of a pseudotapeworm.

Plume Smoke created from laser application on tissue.

Pneumomediastinum The presence of air in the space between the lungs that contains the heart and great vessels.

Pneumothorax Abnormal accumulation of air in the space between the rib cage and the lung. This abnormal air pocket compresses the lung, resulting in respiratory distress. The lung may collapse. This condition may be caused by injury to lung tissue, rupture of air-filled pulmonary cysts, or puncture of the chest wall.

Pocket Pathologic condition wherein the normal sulcus depth increases as a result of loss of attachment of junctional epithelium to periodontal ligament (compare: pseudopocket).

Poikilocytosis Abnormal cell shape of a red blood cell (RBC).

Point of balance The point on a livestock animal that if you took a step in either direction, the animal would move in the opposite direction.

Points Raised areas of teeth associated with incomplete wear of the occlusal surface of horses and exotic species, usually on the vestibular surface of maxillary cheek teeth and the lingual surface of mandibular cheek teeth.

Polioencephalomalacia (PEM) Also known as *cerebrocortical necrosis*, and characterized by altered function of the central nervous system. Brain swelling and inflammation lead to necrosis of brain tissue and death. Diagnosis is confirmed postmortem. Causes may include ingestion of grain diets and plants high in thiaminases, which inactivate vitamin B$_1$.

Pollakiuria Abnormally frequent urination.

Poloxalene Nonionic surfactant that lowers the surface tension of a frothy mass (such as frothy bloat) so that the bubble film is weakened and can no longer contain the gas.

Polyarthritis Arthritis (inflammation of the joints) involving two or more joints.

Polychromatophils Large basophilic and eosinophilic immature anucleate red blood cells (RBCs) seen on standard Wright-stained blood smears; corresponds to the reticulocyte.

Polycythemia Condition in which an abnormally large number of red blood cells (RBCs) are present within the circulatory system.

Polydipsia A condition evidenced by increased levels of thirst and excessive drinking (adj. polydipsic).

Polyestrus Having multiple estrous cycles throughout the year.

Polymerase chain reaction (PCR) An in vitro technique that is used to rapidly synthesize large quantities of a given deoxyribonucleic acid (DNA) segment. This involves separating the DNA into its two complementary strands, binding a primer to each single strand at the end of the given DNA segment where synthesis will start, using DNA polymerase to synthesize two-stranded DNA from each single strand, and repeating the process.

Polyuria Excessive production of urine.

Polyvalent Effective against, sensitive toward, or counteracting more than one exciting agent (as a toxin or antigen) (e.g., a *polyvalent* vaccine).

Position-indicating device (PID) Term that describes the cone at the end of a dental x-ray machine, which exhibits the area of exposure.

Positive inotrope Drug that increases the force of contraction of the heart muscle.

Positive punishment Decreases the frequency of behavior because something *unpleasant* is *added* after a behavior.

Positive reinforcement Increases the frequency of behavior because something *pleasant* is *added* after a behavior.

Possessive aggression Aggression demonstrated in the presence of any highly valued resource used to prevent real or perceived attempts by others to access the resource.

Potency Strength of a homeopathic preparation.

Potter-Bucky diaphragm Movable grid that is timed with the exposure, so that it moves across the cassette and the lead lines of the grid are not visible in the resulting image because of blurring.

Practice acts Primary laws or statutes written and passed by the legislature to govern the practice of a profession. Typically, each state has its own practice act for each licensed profession.

Predatory aggression Aggression-consistent hunting; usually quiet, staring, and stalking with tail twitching and body lowered. When directed at small children or infant humans, this should be considered an emergency situation in need of immediate assessment and management.

Preemptive analgesia Pain management administered before any trauma occurs to prevent expected pain.

Pregnancy toxemia Sudden demand for energy by fast-growing fetuses that can occur in the last few weeks of pregnancy. Occurs more commonly in ewes with twins than with a single fetus. Rapid breakdown of body stores releases ketones, leading to ketoacidosis.

Pregnant mare serum gonadotropin (PMSG) Hormone that originates from the uterus of pregnant mares and that circulates in the bloodstream from day 40 to day 140 of pregnancy. PMSG is used pharmaceutically to stimulate follicle growth in inactive ovaries and to superovulate cows.

Prehend To take hold of or grab, as when cattle eat grass or hay.

Prep Abbreviation for aseptic skin preparation in anticipation of surgery or another sterile procedure.

Prepatent period Period between the time the infective stage of a parasite is ingested by a host and the time that the infective stage develops to the adult stage of the parasite, becomes sexually mature, breeds, and begins to produce offspring (eggs or larvae).

Prepurchase examination Examination conducted before the sale of an animal is completed; a common procedure in equine practice.

Prescription drug (Rx drug) See **Legend drug**.

Previous history The medical history of a patient that precedes the events surrounding the current problem.

Primary closure Surgical closure of a fresh, clean wound, leading to primary intention healing.

Primary dentin The first dentin produced during development of the tooth.

Primary intention wound healing Healing of a wound across a surgically closed incision.

Primiparous Describes an animal that has given birth once.

Probe A blunt, narrow instrument with markings used to assess the periodontal status of a tooth and its surrounding soft tissue.

Problem-oriented veterinary medical record (POVMR) A record keeping system in which clinical data are organized by medical problem. This approach is more labor-intensive and generates more voluminous records than the source-oriented veterinary medical record (SOVMR), but it offers a comprehensive written evaluation of the patient.

Procercoid The developmental stage that parasitizes the first intermediate host in the life cycle of a pseudotapeworm. This host is usually an aquatic crustacean.

Profits The amount left over after all normal and necessary operating expenses of a business are subtracted from the gross revenue.

Progesterone Hormone present primarily in the female that is related to the presence of a corpus luteum and to pregnancy.

Proglottid One of the individual units of the tapeworm that make up the strobila. Proglottids are arrayed in a chainlike manner (much like boxcars in a freight train).

Prognathism Condition marked by abnormal protrusion of one or both jaws, particularly the mandible, relative to the facial skeleton and soft tissues.

Progress notes Chronologically ordered notations made in the medical record that describe the events of each patient's examination, diagnosis, and treatment.

Prolactin Hormone secreted by the pituitary that, in concert with progesterone and estrogen and other hormones, stimulates milk formation.

Proliferative phase The second phase of wound healing; characterized by invasion of fibroblasts, formation of granulation tissue, deposition of collagen, epithelialization across healthy granulation tissue, and wound contraction by myofibroblasts.

Promotion Process by which initiated cells that have damaged deoxyribonucleic acid (DNA) are stimulated to grow into cancer. Tumor promoters cannot cause the development of cancer by themselves.

Proprioception Awareness of body position and movement in space.

Proprioceptive Activated by, or related to, stimuli that arise within an animal.

Prosector The person performing the necropsy.

Prosecution Process of pursuing formal charges against an offender to final judgment.

Prostaglandin Twenty-carbon fatty acid produced in the uterus and involved in luteolysis.

Prosthesis Synthetic material used to replace some tissue or part of the body.

Protein Long chains of amino acids held together by peptide bonds.

Protein efficiency ratio The number of grams of body weight gain per unit of protein consumed.

Prothrombin time (PT) Test used to evaluate extrinsic and common pathways of coagulation. This test requires citrated plasma and careful adherence to collection and processing requirements.

Protozoan A unicellular (one-cell) organism.

Pruritic Itchy.

Pruritus Localized or generalized itching resulting from irritation of sensory nerve endings.

Pseudocyesis False pregnancy.

Pseudoparasite Object that is mistaken for a parasite.

Pseudopocket Pathologic condition whereby sulcus depth increases as a result of gingival enlargement in the coronal direction (compare: pocket).

Pseudopregnancy Anestrous state resembling pregnancy that occurs in various mammals, usually after an infertile copulation; pseudocyesis, false pregnancy.

Pseudotapeworm A member of the order Cotyloda. Pseudotapeworms are unusual in that the scolex possesses two slitlike, hold-fast organelles called bothria. They are also unusual in that they produce an operculated ovum, very similar to that of the digenetic trematodes. An excellent example of a pseudotapeworm is *Spirometra mansonoides*.

Psittacine Of or related to parrots.

Pulmonary artery Artery arising from the right ventricle that delivers blood into the pulmonary circulation.

Pulmonary edema Fluid buildup within the alveoli or interstitial spaces of the lung.

Pulmonary thromboembolism Formation of a blood clot in the lumen of a blood vessel in the lung tissue, causing decreased function of that portion of the lung.

Pulp Soft tissue within the center of a tooth, consisting of cells, vessels, and nerves.

Pulse deficit As detected by simultaneous cardiac auscultation and pulse palpation, a condition wherein each audible heartbeat is not accompanied by a palpable pulse wave.

Pulse oximeter Instrument used to noninvasively measure the oxygen saturation of hemoglobin. This value serves as an indirect assessment of the animal's oxygenation status.

Pulse pressure The difference between systolic and diastolic pressures. This determines the intensity of the sensation when peripheral pulses are palpated.

Pulsed electromagnetic field therapy (PEMF) Complementary therapy that directs electromagnetic pulses through injured tissue, stimulating cellular repair. PEMF is used in healing soft tissue wounds, suppressing inflammatory responses, alleviating pain, and increasing range of motion.

Purulent Containing, consisting of, or being pus (e.g., a *purulent* discharge).

Pyloropexy Surgical fixation of the pylorus to the body wall.

Pyometra Bacterial infection of the uterus with purulent fluid accumulation.

Pyrethrin A natural insecticide derived from plants, used to control various ectoparasites.

Pyriform apparatus Pear-shaped, innermost covering of certain tapeworm ova. The pyriform apparatus is found in such genera as *Anoplocephala* species of horses and *Moniezia* species of cattle and sheep.

Pyuria Refers to the presence of inflammatory cells (neutrophils) in the urine.

Quality control (QC) Method or program that uses specific decision criteria or rules to determine whether an analytical test is producing accurate, consistent, and reliable results. QC uses control materials to determine whether a procedure is in control (performing acceptably) or out of control (failing to perform within acceptable control limits). A QC system is designed to detect problems before test results are transmitted to the clinician, thus avoiding implementation of treatment based on erroneous test results.

Quidding   Dropping of food during mastication.

Rabies   Viral disease spread by the saliva of infected animals, primarily through bite wounds. Human and animal vaccines are available and effective, but once symptoms of the disease appear in a patient, mortality is nearly 100%.

Rad   Unit of absorbed dose of ionizing radiation.

Radiation sensitizer   Compound or agent that acts by any of a number of mechanisms to make cancer cells more susceptible to death by ionizing radiation.

Ramp   Pathologic exaggeration of the upward slope of the distal mandibular cheek teeth of the horse.

Range of motion (ROM)   Movement at a joint.

Raptorial species   Of, related to, or being a bird of prey.

Rare earth screens   Screens that contain a phosphor that is highly efficient in transforming energy into light compared with calcium tungstate screens. Rare earth screens emit green light and require less radiation exposure to produce a radiographic image.

Ratchet   Part of an instrument—usually located near the rings or handles—that allows the instrument to be maintained in one position after it has grasped or retracted the tissue.

Reactive lymphocytes   Lymphocytes with a slight increase in cytoplasm, which is frequently basophilic and may display a small, pale perinuclear zone (Golgi zone).

Rebreathing system   Breathing circuit in which exhaled gases are recirculated to the patient after carbon dioxide is removed.

Recent history   Events surrounding the current medical problem.

Recession   Pathologic condition in which the height of the gingiva is decreased as a result of periodontal disease or focal trauma to the gingiva.

Reconstitute   To mix a dry lyophilized powder form of a drug with a diluent for administration orally, parenterally, or topically.

Recumbency   Lying down. This adjective indicates which part of the body is on the ground or table. For example, *lateral recumbency* means that the animal is lying on its side, and *dorsal recumbency* means that the animal is lying on its back.

Red blood cell (RBC) indices   Measurements or calculations that are part of the complete blood count (CBC). Mean corpuscular volume (MCV; see earlier) and mean corpuscular hemoglobin concentration (MCHC; see earlier) are used to describe the average RBC volume and hemoglobin concentration, respectively. Red blood cell indices may be useful in the classification of anemia.

Red blood cells (RBCs; also called *erythrocytes*)   Circulating cells that contain hemoglobin to carry oxygen from lungs to tissues. In most mammals, RBCs are round and anucleate, although in camelids, RBCs are oval. In nonmammalian species, RBCs are oval and have nuclei.

Red cell distribution width (RDW)   Coefficient of variation of the mean corpuscular volume (MCV); a measure of anisocytosis.

Redirected aggression   Aggression toward a nearby individual that occurs when an animal is highly emotionally aroused, usually because of some other stimulus (e.g., the dog that bites its owner when he or she tries to intervene in a dog fight).

Redirected behaviors   Occur when an animal is highly motivated to perform a particular behavior but for some reason is prevented from doing so. The animal subsequently redirects the behavior to another target.

Reepithelialization   Regrowth of epithelial cells over a wound. Cells advance in a single layer across the wound until they meet in the middle when migration stops as the result of contact inhibition.

Referral facilities   Provide services by veterinarians with a special interest in certain species or a particular area of veterinary medicine.

Reflux   Backward or return flow, as from the small intestine into the stomach.

Refractometer   Instrument that measures the bending of light (angle of refraction) as it passes between liquid and air. Because the angle of refraction and the concentration of solutes are relatively linear, refractometry can be used to approximate total protein concentration in serum or plasma.

Regional nerve block   Procedure whereby a relatively small amount of local anesthetic is injected near a nerve, causing desensitization to a larger area on the body. Proximal and distal paravertebral nerve blocks are examples of regional nerve blocks used to anesthetize the flank area.

Regurgitation   Flow of stomach contents into the esophagus and mouth unaccompanied by retching, as distinguished from vomiting, which occurs as forceful expulsion of stomach contents into the esophagus and mouth preceded by retching.

Rehabilitation   Restoration of health.

Relaxin   Hormone secreted by the corpus luteum in the ovaries of pregnant animals. It relaxes the pubic symphysis, softens the cervix, and inhibits uterine contractions.

Rem   Abbreviation for roentgen equivalent man; it is the product of the dose in rads and the relative biological effectiveness of the radiation used.

Remedy   Term for the homeopathic product used to treat the patient's symptoms.

Renal   Related to the kidneys.

Renomegaly   Enlargement of one or both kidneys.

Reperfusion injury   Tissue injury resulting from the reestablishment of blood flow after a period of oxygen deprivation.

Replacement   Volume and rate of fluids needed to replenish fluid deficit and replace ongoing losses.

Repulsion   In dental terms, extraction of a tooth by pushing it from the bottom of its socket. Repulsion is necessary for removal of some equine teeth.

Reservoir host   Vertebrate host in which a parasite (or disease) occurs naturally and that is a source of infection for humans and their domestic animals, as the case may be, for example, birds are reservoir hosts for West Nile virus. Mosquitoes pick up the virus from birds and transmit it to horses and sometimes to humans.

Residual activity   Continued bactericidal activity that persists after antiseptic or disinfectant has been applied.

Resolution   Stage during which there is no longer anger or depression, but acceptance.

Resorption   In dental terms, destruction of the roots and sometimes the crown of a tooth by odontoclasts. Resorption may be external (on the root surface) or internal (within the pulp).

Respiratory minute volume (RMV)   The amount of air that moves into and out of the lungs in a minute; tidal volume multiplied by respiratory rate.

Resting energy requirement (RER) Average amount of energy used by an animal while resting in a thermoneutral environment. The formula used to estimate RER for dogs and cats is $RER = 70 \times BW_{kg}^{0.75}$ kcal/day.

Resuscitation (fluid) The volume of fluids needed to replace vascular volume and restore cardiovascular stability.

Reticulocyte Red blood cells (RBCs) stained with new methylene blue or other vital stains that form visible aggregates of ribosomal ribonucleic acid (RNA; reticulum). RBCs that contain reticulum are immature and are counted as an index of a bone marrow regenerative response to anemia.

Rhabdomyolysis Breakdown of striated muscle that leads to excretion of myoglobin in the urine.

Right to Know law Common name for the hazard communication standard of the Occupational Safety and Health Administration (OSHA). This standard requires an employer to inform employees when they may be exposed to hazardous chemicals while performing their duties.

Ringwomb Condition in which the cervix does not dilate at parturition. It is most common in sheep.

Ringworm Contagious fungal infection of the skin. Fungal spores of the genera *Trichophyton* and *Microsporum* are the most common causative agents.

RIS Radiology information system. The RIS is a computer-based patient record system that allows integration of patient details (examination findings, tests performed, results) that incorporate the imaging information. Once a user enters patient information into the system, it is coordinated with the programs with other users in the hospital.

Robert Jones bandage Distal limb bandage for which a large amount of rolled cotton is used; aids in immobilization of fractures. Rigid material can be incorporated into this bandage.

Roentgen Measure of radiation exposure or x-ray machine output.

Root planing Technique of hand scaling to remove superficial layers of cementum for root debridement.

Rostral Positional term that refers to a structure toward the front of the head: analogous to the positional term *cranial*, used in areas of the body other than the head.

Rotating anode Anode plate in an x-ray tube that rotates around a stem made of molybdenum to aid in heat dissipation.

Rouleaux Rouleaux formation refers to red blood cells (RBCs) in chains that resemble a stack of coins. In horses and cats, rouleaux formation is common, whereas in dogs, rouleaux formation may be an indication of inflammation or an artifact of smear preparation.

Rugae Prominent ridges of palatal mucosa covering the hard palate.

Rules and regulations Secondary mandates written by the state board.

Rumen The first chamber of the ruminant digestive tract; used for storage of ingested food and initial digestion of protein and simple carbohydrates.

Rumen trocarization Placement of a trocar, needle, or cannula in the rumen for the purpose of relieving free gas bloat.

Rumen tympany Rumen distention with air; commonly referred to as *bloat*.

Rumenostomy Surgical procedure whereby a permanent hole is created from the skin into the rumen.

Rumenotomy Surgical incision into the rumen.

Safelight Light bulb in the darkroom that is shielded by a plastic filter that stops light that the film is sensitive to from penetrating and exposing the film.

Sanctions Disciplinary actions carried out by the board.

Sanitizer An antimicrobial product, often a detergent, that reduces the number of bacteria on a treated surface to a safe level but does not completely eliminate them.

Sarcoptic mange Also called *scabies*, sarcoptic mange is a parasitic infestation of the skin of animals with the mite *Sarcoptes scabiei canis*. Common symptoms include hair loss, itching, and inflammation.

Sarcoptiform mites Parasitic mites belonging to assorted genera, including *Sarcoptes*, *Notoedres*, *Cnemidocoptes*, *Psoroptes*, *Chorioptes*, and *Otodectes* species. These microscopic mites are round to oval in silhouette, have unique suckers on pedicels (stalks) at the tips of certain legs, and may produce dermatitis in domesticated animals.

Scattered radiations Lower-energy x-ray photons that have undergone a change in direction after interacting with structures in the patient's body.

Scavenger or scavenging system Device or system used to capture, transport, or remove waste anesthetic gases from an anesthesia machine.

Schistocytes Red blood cell (RBC) fragments.

Schistosome A "blood fluke" that inhabits the blood vasculature of its definitive host.

Schistosome cercarial dermatitis Zoonotic condition resulting from repeated penetration of the cercarial stage of blood flukes of birds, usually migratory aquatic birds. This condition manifests as papular or pustular areas in the skin of humans who have come in contact with infested waters containing these cercarial stages of avian schistosomes.

Schizogony Type of asexual reproduction used by coccidian parasites, such as *Isospora* or *Eimeria* species.

Sciatic nerve Nerve that runs along the caudal aspect of the femur beneath the biceps. It is important to avoid this nerve when giving intramuscular injections.

Scientific name Several million species of animals and plants exist here on the planet earth. They may have different common names in different regions of the world. Sometimes a common name may refer to different organisms in different places. The solution to this problem is to give each organism a scientific name that does not vary. A scientific name consists of two Latin words and is usually written in *italics* or *underlined*. The first word is capitalized and the genus name. The genus indicates the group to which a particular type of animal belongs. The second word is not capitalized. It is the specific epithet and indicates the type of animal itself. Examples: the dog, *Canis familiaris*; the cat, *Felis catus*; the housefly, *Musca domestica*; and a bacterium normally found in the gut, *Escherichia coli*. All species of animals that look and behave similarly are placed in the same genus. Likewise, all genera that look and behave similarly are placed in the same family. All families that look and behave similarly are placed in the same order. All orders that look and behave similarly are placed in the same class. All classes that look and behave similarly are placed in the same phylum. All phyla that look and behave similarly are placed in the same kingdom. There are five kingdoms: Plants, Animals, Fungi, Protists, and Monerans.

Scolex   The holdfast organelle of an adult true tapeworm. The scolex of a true tapeworm has four suckers (acetabula), and many have an armed rostellum (possess additional hooks for attachment to the gut of the definitive host). If the hooks are lacking, the rostellum is said to be unarmed.

Scoliosis   Lateral deviation of the spinal column.

Screen film   Radiographic film that is sensitive to wavelengths of light emitted from the intensifying screen.

Screen speed   The ability of the intensifying screen in a film cassette to convert absorbed x-ray energy into visible light. Fast screens require less radiation to expose the film because of better conversion to light than slow screens. However, fast screens produce poorer radiographic detail than slow screens.

Scrub   Applying an antiseptic to disinfect the animal's skin in preparation for a sterile procedure. Also refers to disinfecting the hands of the personnel who will be involved in a sterile procedure.

Scrub-in   The process of disinfecting the hands and donning sterile gown and gloves to participate in a sterile procedure.

Scrub suit   Shirt and pants worn into the operating room. Usually made of a lint-free cotton or polyester material.

Seasonally polyestrus   Repeated estrous cycles that occur during the breeding season of a species.

Second intention healing   Healing of a wound by granulation tissue formation, epithelialization, and contraction.

Secondary closure   Wound that has formed healthy granulation tissue and is then closed by apposing the skin over the granulation tissue.

Secondary dentin   Dentin that is produced after eruption and throughout the working life of the tooth.

Seed ticks   The six-legged larval stages of ticks.

Segmenter (seg)   Mature neutrophil.

Segregated early weaning   The practice of weaning piglets from the sow at an early age and moving them to a distant nursery that is isolated from the breeding and/or grow-out herd to limit vertical transmission of disease from older pigs to young pigs.

Selective medium   Culture medium that reduces the growth of unwanted bacteria to allow the growth of other bacteria. MacConkey's agar is selective because it inhibits the growth of Gram-positive organisms.

Semi-occlusive   Allowing air and moisture to move through. Used in reference to bandage materials. A semi-occlusive primary layer is used for moist wound healing.

Sepsis   A state of systemic inflammation characterized by deteriorating vital signs and the presence of infection.

Septicemia   Invasion of the bloodstream by microorganisms (usually bacteria) from a focus of infection. It is accompanied by fever, chills prostration, pain, nausea, and diarrhea.

Sequestrum   A piece of dead bone that has become separated from the surrounding bone during the process of necrosis.

Serology   When used to denote laboratory diagnostic tests, it is concerned with the quantitative and qualitative detection of antibody in serum that reacts with a known antigen, usually as an indication of infection.

Seroma   Sterile fluid accumulation beneath an incision after surgery.

Serosanguineous   Containing or consisting of both blood and serous fluid (e.g., a *serosanguineous* discharge).

Serous   Of, related to, producing, or resembling serum.

Shank   Portion of the dental instrument that connects the handle with the working end.

Shock   A condition of decreased perfusion and decreased oxygen delivery to vital organs.

Shopped fees   Fees for which clients call the practice to find out the charge before the visit (e.g., physical examination, elective surgery, vaccinations).

Sickle scaler   Hand instrument with a pointed tip used for supragingival scaling.

Signalment   The patient species, breed, age, sex, and reproductive status.

Simian   Relating to an ape or monkey.

Simple metamorphosis   Type of developmental change used by many insects. Simple metamorphosis consists of three developmental stages: egg, nymph, and adult. The nymphal and adult stages are similar to each other in form and structure; however, the nymphal stages tend to be smaller than the adult stages. The adult stages are sexually mature, whereas the nymphal stages are not. The orders of parasitic insects that undergo simple metamorphosis include Hemipterans (true bugs), Mallophagans (chewing lice), and Anoplurans (sucking lice).

Siphonaptera   The order that contains fleas. Fleas are Siphonapterans.

Siphonapterosis   Infestation with fleas within the hair coat or feathers of a host.

Skin preparation   The process of mechanical and chemical cleansing of the skin.

Small lymphocyte   Small mononuclear cells with a thin rim of light blue cytoplasm and high nuclear-to-cytoplasmic (N/C) ratios, with close nuclear-to-plasma membrane apposition along most of the perimeter of the round nucleus.

Smegma   Thick, cheesy secretion found under the prepuce of males and around the labia of females.

SOAP   Acronym for subjective, objective, assessment, and plan. The SOAP format is used to evaluate hospitalized or sick patients.

Social hierarchies   Social structures that allow for division of resources, rights, and privileges. Animals in higher social positions tend to have priority access to resources. However, social hierarchies are flexible, not absolute. Hierarchies can change over time and can be different in different contexts; they vary according to the specific individuals that make up the hierarchy.

Social status/Dominance aggression   Aggression toward people in an attempt to acquire or maintain resources. Dogs that display this form of aggression should be demonstrating offensive rather than defensive or fear-related visual cues.

Socialization   Process by which an animal develops appropriate social behaviors toward members of its own and other species. The process of socialization requires providing to the young animal pleasant experiences with people, situations, inanimate elements of the environment, and other animals.

Soda lime   White, granular agent used in anesthetic machines to absorb carbon dioxide expelled from the patient in a rebreathing circuit.

Software   Relates to the computer instructions contained within or added to the hardware.

Somatotropin   Growth hormone.

Source-oriented veterinary medical record (SOVMR) Record keeping system that enters medical information from multiple sources in chronological order.

Sparganosis A zoonotic condition resulting from a second intermediate host (sometimes a human) becoming infected with the plerocercoid or sparganum in the life cycle of a pseudotapeworm. Sparganosis is a condition that is commonly associated with the pseudotapeworm, *Spirometra mansonoides.*

Sparganum See **plerocercoid.**

Specialty facilities A veterinary/animal facility in which services are provided by board-certified veterinarians/specialists.

Species-typical behaviors Behaviors that are characteristic of a particular species. Some definitions limit species-typical behaviors to behaviors that are *exclusive* to a species, whereas other definitions use the term *species-specific behaviors* for the latter.

Specific gravity (SG) The ratio of the density of a fluid to the density of pure water. SG depends on both the number and the molecular weight of solutes found in the solution. SG is used as an indicator of solute concentration in the urine and, by extension, the concentrating ability of the kidney.

Spectrophotometry Measurement of the amount of light that a substance absorbs. Spectrophotometers are instruments that pass a beam of light of a specific wavelength through a substance such as serum or plasma. The amount of light that passes through the sample is then measured by a photodetector. Typically, an analyte will absorb some of the photons from the light beam, thus reducing the light that reaches the detector in proportion to the quantity of analyte present in the sample.

Spherocytes Red blood cells (RBCs) that lack a central zone of pallor and appear slightly smaller and denser than normal RBCs. Spherocytes result from binding of antibody to the RBC surface and removal of a portion of cell membrane by macrophages in the spleen. This occurs most commonly in immune-mediated hemolytic anemia.

Sphygmomanometer A gauge and cuff used to measure blood pressure.

Spica splint Full-limb bandage, including a lateral splint that reaches over the shoulder or hip that is used to aid in immobilization.

Splenectomy Removal of the spleen.

Sprain Excessive stretching of a ligament.

Stallion Noncastrated male horse used for breeding.

Standard solutions Quality control products that contain the analyte of interest at a validated "true" concentration, as determined by the manufacturer using "gold standard" methods.

Stationary anode Anode block in an x-ray tube that does not move and is embedded in copper to aid in heat dissipation. Found exclusively in portable equipment used in fieldwork.

Status epilepticus Continuous seizure activity.

Statute Law.

Steady state After repeated drug dosing, a drug's plasma concentration reaches steady state (or stable concentration in the blood) when the amount of drug administered equals the amount of drug eliminated.

Steady-state serum concentration Values that recur with each dose and represent a state of equilibrium between the amount of drug administered and the amount eliminated over a given time interval.

Sterile Free from any living microorganisms.

Sterile field An area that has been prepared for the use of sterile equipment. This includes the area around the wound, incision site, or body orifice into which an instrument or catheter will be passed. It also includes the area covered by sterile drapes and the sterile region of properly attired personnel.

Sterile technique Creating a sterile field and working within it by not contaminating it with nonsterile objects.

Sterilization The destruction of all disease-producing organisms and spores on an object.

Sternum The breastbone. The series of rod-like bones called *sternebrae* that form the floor of the thorax.

Steroid hormone A group of hormones that have a common four-ring structure and a similar synthetic pathway. They are normally produced in the gonads and adrenal glands.

Stertor Inspiratory noise similar to snoring usually caused by obstruction to airflow at the pharynx or larynx.

Stocker calf A steer or heifer, 6 to 9 months of age, weighing 400 to 700 lb, and bought to be fed on pasture or forage to promote growth rather than fattening at a rate of 1 to 1.5 lb/day.

Stocks Vertical metal or wooden pillars, arranged in a rectangular shape and connected by horizontal bars, designed to restrain horses or cattle standing within.

Stoma A surgically created opening from an area inside the body to the outside.

Stomatitis Inflammation of the oral soft tissue, which is not confined to the gingiva.

Stopcock Small, valve-like apparatus used to control flow through a syringe or tube.

Strabismus Abnormal position of the eyes (medial strabismus is also called *cross-eye*).

Strain Excessive stretch of a muscle that may cause tearing of muscle fibers.

Strangulation Encircling of a tissue with suture or internal structures (such as slipping of bowel into a hernia, or through scar tissue) such that blood supply to the tissue is lost and death of the tissues ensues, unless the tissue is released and blood flow can resume.

Stranguria The act of straining to urinate.

Strategic planning An organization's process for defining or updating its vision, mission, and strategy and allocating resources toward achievement of these goals.

Stress Any pressure or strain placed on a system. If pressure is great enough or persistent enough, for example, an animal that is unable to escape from a fear-inducing stimulus, constant stimulation of the hypothalamic–pituitary–adrenal axis (HPA) can lead to immune suppression and increased susceptibility to disease. Animals that experience frequent frustration or conflict are likely to be stressed.

Stridor A harsh, high-pitched respiratory sound usually caused by obstruction of airflow at the pharynx or larynx.

Strike Any cutaneous myiasis in sheep. This myiasis is usually due to infestation of a wound by fly larvae (maggots) of species of the genera *Lucilia, Phormia, Sarcoptes, Calliphora,* and *Phaenicia.*

Strike-through When fluid penetrates a surgical drape or gown, it creates a pathway by which organisms can invade the sterile field.

String test   Used to evaluate joint fluid viscosity; a stick is placed into joint fluid and then is withdrawn, with a string longer than 2 to 3 cm considered adequate.

Strobila   The entire body of the tapeworm is called the *strobila*. The scolex is at the anterior (front) end of the tapeworm. Behind the scolex is the chain of proglottids, the total of which is called the strobila. The youngest proglottids are at the anterior end of the tapeworm; the oldest proglottids are at the posterior end of the tapeworm.

***Strongylus*-type ovum**   Ovum produced by nematodes that are members of the family Strongylidae—members of the genus *Strongylus* and a variety of small strongyli. Adult nematodes parasitize the alimentary tracts of horses. The ova of these nematodes are similar in morphology, so it is not feasible to categorize them within a specific genus. The ova are simply reported as "*Strongylus*-type ova."

Stuporous   Characterized by decreased responsiveness to stimulation.

Subchondral bone   The bone that lies just beneath joint cartilage.

Subcutaneous emphysema   Abnormal accumulation of air underneath the skin, usually resulting from traumatic airway rupture.

Subgingival   Positional term that refers to below the gumline (i.e., toward the root).

Subinvolution of placental sites (SIPS)   Failure of involution of the sites of placental attachment in a postpartum bitch causes persistent intrauterine bleeding for longer than 12 weeks.

Submissive behaviors   Also known as *appeasement behaviors*, they function as signals to "turn off" threatening and aggressive behaviors from other individuals.

Subordinate role   A lower position in a rank order or social hierarchy. Note that "subordinate" describes a social position (role in a relationship), not a personality trait.

Sulcus   The normal trough that exists around a tooth between the crown and the free gingiva. Normal sulcus depth is less than 3 mm in dogs and less than 1 mm in cats.

Superfecundation   Successive fertilization of ova involving multiple episodes of coitus during the same heat. Fertilization is provided by different males.

Superfetation   Fertilization of two or more ova in the same female during different heats. In this way, a pregnant dam may ovulate and become pregnant a second time.

Supragingival   Positional term that refers to "above the gum line" (i.e., toward the crown).

Surge suppressor   Device designed to protect sensitive electronic devices, such as computers, from voltage spikes. A surge suppressor is not intended to be a substitute for a permanent outlet because it cannot carry the same amperage as solid wiring inside the walls of a building.

Surgical drape   Cloth or paper fabric used to create a barrier that inhibits migration of microorganisms into the sterile field.

Swaged   Squeezed-on, as with a suture needle onto suture.

Symphysis   Fibrous joint between the right and left mandible seen in dogs, cats, and some other species.

Syncope   Fainting.

Syndesmochorial   Having fetal epithelium in contact with maternal submucosa (as is seen in ruminants).

Systemic inflammatory response syndrome (SIRS)   Widespread inflammation caused by an underlying disease process. Often causes generalized tissue damage and can be a complication of shock.

Systolic blood pressure   Measurement of blood pressure when the heart is in systole or contraction.

Tachycardia   Rapid heart rate; the opposite of bradycardia.

Tachypnea   Fast, shallow breathing.

Tachyzoite   Literally "a fast growing, tiny organism." This is a term for a tissue stage, for example, a fast growing developmental stage that occurs in cysts in the life cycle of *Toxoplasma gondii*.

Tail tie   Restraint of an equine or bovine tail by tying a quick release knot in the switch and the free end to the animal, often the neck.

Tapotement   Form of massage that uses tapping motions of the hands or fingers. When done for a short time, it stimulates nerve endings; when done longer, it has a more sedative effect.

Targeted therapy   Use of a drug designed to act on a specific cellular molecule.

Tarsorrhaphy   Operation that consists of suturing the eyelids together entirely or in part.

Technician assessment   Clinical judgment that the veterinary technician makes regarding the physiologic and psychological problems and needs of a patient. The technician assessment comprises the "A" portion of the veterinary technician SOAP—the list of technician evaluations arranged in order of priority with reference to the psychological and physiologic needs of the patient.

Technician evaluation   The second phase of the veterinary technician practice model. Conclusions drawn from patient assessment and analysis of the database related to the animal's (or the owner's) physical and psychological response to a veterinary medical condition. Refer to Table 1-2 for a list of approved technician evaluations.

Technician intervention   The third phase of the veterinary technician practice model. An action planned and implemented by the veterinary technician using independent critical thinking to address a patient's reaction to illness and risk for future problems, as well as owner knowledge deficits. Typically, a technician intervention is carried out to address each of the technician evaluations.

Teleradiology   Transmission of digital images from one hospital to the next via computer cable connections. Teleradiology allows rapid turnaround in assessment of images and improves access to expert opinions on patient findings.

Temporal muscle   Large bilateral muscle of mastication on the top of the head that functions to close the mouth.

Temporomandibular joint (TMJ)   Articulation between the upper jaw and the lower jaw.

Tendon   Structure that connects muscle to bone.

Tendonitis   Inflammation of a tendon.

Tenesmus   Distressing but ineffectual urge to evacuate the rectum or urinary bladder.

Teratogen Agent or substance that may cause physical defects in a developing embryo when a pregnant female is exposed to that substance.

Terminal shank Portion of a hand instrument closest to the working end.

Territorial aggression Aggression demonstrated only in a particular, circumscribed area when approached by a perceived threat.

Tertiary dentin Reparative dentin produced in response to tooth trauma. Tertiary dentin may be darker in color than primary or secondary dentin because of its more rapid, less organized development, and because of its potential to become stained a brown or black color.

Thecal cell layer Inner cell layer of a follicle that converts cholesterol to testosterone.

Therapeutic blood level Range of concentrations of a drug in the bloodstream at which it is expected to have the desired effect.

Therapeutic drug monitoring Periodic measurement of the amount of a drug in the blood.

Therapeutic index Ratio between toxic and therapeutic doses of a drug used to measure relative safety; thus a drug with a wide therapeutic index (much more of the drug is required to intoxicate a patient than is required to treat it) is relatively safer than a drug with a narrow therapeutic index (one for which toxic and therapeutic doses are similar).

Therapeutic range Range of concentrations at which a drug is effective with minimal toxicity to the patient.

Therapeutic window Range of a drug serum concentration associated with a high degree of efficacy and low risk for undesired dose-related adverse reactions.

Thermal agents Tools used to modify tissue temperature and change blood flow to surrounding tissues.

Thermogenesis The ability to generate heat through physiologic processes, such as shivering or intake of food.

Third intention wound healing Healing of a wound that has already formed granulation tissue and undergone secondary closure.

Thoracocentesis A procedure in which air or fluid is removed from the chest (pleural space) using a syringe and needle aseptically.

Threatening behavior Behavior that signals an intent or willingness to attack or become aggressive. Like aggression, threats can be defensive or offensive in nature.

Three-host tick An individual tick that will feed on three individual animals or three different species of animal.

Thrombocytopenia Occurs as a decrease in the number of platelets in the blood.

Thromboembolism Formation of a blood clot that lodges in or obstructs a blood vessel.

Thrombophlebitis Inflammation of the vein associated with a thrombus.

Thrombosis Clotting of blood within a vessel that results in obstruction of blood flow.

Thrombus A clot consisting of fibrin, platelets, red blood cells (RBCs), and white blood cells (WBCs) that forms within a blood vessel or a chamber of the heart and can obstruct blood flow. **Thrombogenicity** refers to the tendency of a material in contact with the blood to produce a thrombus or clot.

Tick paralysis An ascending, flaccid, motor paralysis in humans, domesticated animals, and wild animals caused by the attachment of a tick, usually a female tick. The agent that produces this paralysis may be an ovarian toxin or a salivary toxin. Upon detachment of the tick, the paralysis usually dissipates.

Tidal volume The volume of a normal breath ($\approx$10 to 15 ml/kg body weight).

Time-out from reinforcement For a designated time, the animal is prevented from receiving any reinforcement for any behavior. This can be accomplished by removing the animal from a reinforcing situation (e.g., confinement in a small bathroom) or by removing the reinforcing environment from the animal (e.g., all members of the animal's social group leave).

Titer The dilution of serum containing a specific antibody at which the solution retains a specific activity (such as neutralizing or precipitating an antigen) that it loses at a greater dilution (a test for toxoplasmosis antibodies yielded a *titer* of 1:1024).

Tort A wrong or injury for which a court will provide a remedy.

Tortoise A land turtle.

Total digestible nutrients (TDN) Term that indicates the energy value of a feedstuff. TDN is calculated by using the following formula: % TDN = % DCP + % DCF + % DNFE + (%DEE × 2.25), where DCP = digestible crude protein, DCF = digestible crude fiber, DNFE = digestible nitrogen-free extract, and DEE = digestible ether extract.

Total plasma protein (TP) The total protein content of blood.

Toxic change Occurs when several morphologic abnormalities indicate intense stimulation of neutrophil production and shortened maturation time. Toxic changes include Döhle bodies, cytoplasmic basophilia and vacuolation, toxic granules and nuclear vacuolation, hyposegmentation, ring formation, and fragmentation. Rarely, formation of giant neutrophils occurs.

Toxic dose Dose greater than the upper limit of the therapeutic range that causes poisonous symptoms.

Toxic granulation Neutrophils with retention of fine reddish primary granules.

Toxic line A continuous line of purple gum color that appears along the margins of the teeth and gums; unique characteristic finding of endotoxic shock in equines.

Toxicant Any substance that when introduced into or applied to the body can interfere with the life processes of cells of the organism. Toxicants may be of biological origin, or they may be manufactured chemicals or naturally occurring chemicals.

Toxicology Study of the symptoms, mechanisms, treatments, and detection of biological poisoning.

Toxicosis (pl. toxicoses) Any disease of toxic origin.

Toxin A poisonous substance.

Toxoid A toxin that has been altered so that it does not cause disease but is able to induce the production of protective antibodies. The immunogenicity, however, remains intact and makes toxoids suitable for use as vaccines. Immunizations against tetanus and botulism are examples of toxoids.

Toxoplasmosis Infestation with a single-celled parasite called *Toxoplasma gondii*. Toxoplasmosis is a disease of concern primarily for pregnant women and for people with compromised immune systems.

Tracheostomy   Surgical creation of a hole from the skin to the trachea.

Tracheostomy tube   Large-bore tube inserted into the cervical trachea to bypass the upper airways. A treatment for upper airway obstruction.

Tracheotomy   Surgical act of making an incision on the ventral aspect of the neck and opening a direct airway through an incision in the trachea.

Traditional Chinese medicine (TCM)   Form of medicine that combines acupuncture, herbology, and massage therapy.

Traffic flow   Pattern of movement of patients through the practice (e.g., reception to examination room, ward to reception).

Transdermal   Delivered via absorption through the skin, such as in a patch.

Transducer   In power scalers, the portion that converts electrical energy to mechanical energy.

Transduction   Conversion of unpleasant stimuli into nerve signals at the point of injury.

Transfaunation   Transfer of beneficial microorganisms from the rumen of one individual to that of another.

Transformation   Change that occurs in a normal cell as it becomes malignant.

Transfusion reaction   Adverse events that occur as a result of receiving a transfusion.

Transmammary infection   Infection by a nematode using the milk of a lactating female dog given to her nursing puppies. *Ancylostoma caninum canis* uses transmammary infection.

Transmission   The sending of pain signals via nerve fibers to the spinal cord.

Transmucosal   Delivered via absorption through mucous membranes, such as the gums.

Transplacental infection   Infection by a nematode using the migration of larvae across the placenta of a female dog into her developing puppies. *Toxocara canis* uses transplacental infection.

Transport host   See **Paratenic host.**

Transport medium   Medium that maintains bacteria in original concentrations without encouraging growth or causing death of the bacteria.

Transtracheal aspirate   Passing through or administered by way of the trachea.

Transtracheal cannulas   Catheters or other narrow-diameter breathing tubes used to supply oxygen to a patient.

Transudate   Fluid that passes through a membrane and filters out many of the proteins and cellular elements to yield a watery solution. A transudate results from increased pressure in the veins and capillaries forcing fluid through the vessel walls, or from low levels of protein in the blood serum. It is a filtrate of blood.

Travel sheet   A sheet of specific charges for a patient that follows the patient (travels with the patient) in the practice facility to capture all charges.

Trematode   Digenetic fluke. See **Digenetic fluke.**

Triadan system   Tooth numbering system applicable to multiple veterinary species.

Triage   The act of sorting patients quickly into groups on the basis of a rapid initial assessment of disease or injury severity.

Triangulation   Technique used in laparoscopic and arthroscopic surgery that establishes two reference points—one using the scope and the other the surgical hand instrument—to target a third point, the surgical site. This enables the surgeon to visualize the site of interest while at the same time manipulating surgical instruments inside a body cavity to make surgical corrections.

***Trichostrongylus*-type ovum**   An ovum produced by nematodes that are members of the family Trichostrongylidae. Adult nematodes parasitize the alimentary tracts of cattle, sheep, horses, and other vertebrates. The ova of these nematodes are similar in morphology, so it is not feasible to identify them in relation to a specific genus. The ova are simply reported as "*Trichostrongylus*-type ova." The most common genera of importance are *Trichostrongylus*, *Haemonchus*, *Ostertagia*, and *Cooperia* species. The eggs of *Nematodirus* and *Marshallagia* species are similar in appearance to those of the other trichostrongyli; however, the eggs of *Nematodirus* and *Marshallagia* species are much larger than those of their familial counterparts.

***Trombicula* species**   Chiggers. The six-legged larval chigger is the only stage of this mite that is parasitic. Chiggers are periodic parasites that attach to the skin of their hosts. Their salivary secretions liquefy the host tissue, which is sucked up by the feeding larval mite.

Trophozoite   Literally, "a tiny, moving organism." This is term for a tissue stage, for example, a fast growing developmental stage that occurs in cysts in the life cycle of Toxoplasma gondii and other similar apicomplexan parasites.

Tube cystostomy   Surgical procedure in which a Foley catheter is placed through the abdominal wall and into the bladder. The catheter allows urine to passively drain from the bladder while urolithiasis is managed.

Tumor grade   Microscopic assessment of the degree to which particular cancer cells are similar in appearance and function to normal cells of the same tissue type. In general, cancer cells that differ markedly from normal cells or are poorly differentiated (high grade) have a more malignant clinical behavior.

Tumor stage   Clinical assessment of how much cancer a patient has (volume of disease) and how much it has spread. Tumor stage is determined by the results of diagnostic tests, such as blood work, radiographs, and tissue biopsy. Stage takes into account the size and degree of invasion of the primary tumor, whether it has metastasized to any lymph nodes, and whether it has spread to distant organs. In general, the higher or more advanced the tumor stage, the worse is the patient's prognosis.

Turbinate   Of, related to, or being a nasal concha.

Turtles   Any of an order (Testudinata) of land, freshwater, and marine reptiles that have a toothless horny beak and a shell of bony dermal plates usually covered with horny shields enclosing the trunk, and into which the head, limbs, and tail usually may be withdrawn.

Twitch   Device used in restraining horses; consists of a wooden handle and a chain loop or rope loop that gets twisted around a horse's nose; it is believed that the nose is a pressure point, and once it is squeezed by the twitch, endorphins are released, relaxing the horse.

Two-host tick   An individual tick that will feed on two individual animals or two different species of animal during its life cycle.

Tympanic membrane   Tissue that separates the internal and middle ear canal from the external ear canal; also referred to as the *eardrum.*

Tympany Hollow sound produced when a body cavity containing air is sharply tapped.

Ultrasound (therapeutic) Penetrating tissue through high-frequency sound waves to decrease pain and improve healing of tissues.

Unilocular hydatid cyst A type of metacestode/larval tapeworm that is closely associated with *Echinococcus granulosus*.

Urethral process Small appendage extending from the tip of the penis in sheep and goats; represents the distal end of the urethra in these species. This is the primary location for urinary calculi to lodge in these animals.

Urethrostomy Surgical formation of a new opening into the urethra to allow urine diversion.

Urine protein-to-urine creatinine ratio (UPC) Used to quantitate protein loss in the urine.

Urolithiasis Condition that is characterized by the formation or presence of calculi in the urinary tract.

U.S. Department of Agriculture (USDA) Government agency that regulates veterinary biologics (vaccines, antitoxins, and diagnostics that are used to prevent, treat, or diagnose animal diseases).

U.S. Pharmacopoeia (USP) National Formulary (NF) The official legal drug compendium for the United States. A compilation of all drug substances and products focused on providing active ingredients.

Uterine prolapse Condition that occurs when the uterus folds inside-out through an open cervix and protrudes through the vulvar lips.

Uterine torsion Condition in which the uterus twists, preventing delivery of the fetus. Uterine torsion occurs in cattle and in camelids and can be a cause of dystocia.

Vagus indigestion Characterized by gradual development of ruminoreticular and abdominal distention thought to be the result of lesions affecting the vagus nerve.

Validation Process of understanding and expressing acceptance of another person's emotional state.

Vasoconstriction Constriction of blood vessels.

Vasodilatation Dilatation of the blood vessels; the opposite of vasoconstriction.

Vasopressor Category of drugs used to increase blood pressure and cardiac output.

Vector Arthropod that mechanically transmits bacteria, viruses, *Chlamydia*, and spirochetes from one host to another. *Musca autumnalis*, the face fly, transmits the bacterium *Moraxella bovis*, the causative agent of pinkeye, from one cow to another. The face fly has sticky feet to which bacteria adhere, thus allowing mechanical transmission of this pathogen.

Velpeau sling Non–weight-bearing forelimb sling that flexes the entire limb; primarily used for medial shoulder luxation.

Ventilation This term generally refers to breathing. It can describe spontaneous breathing or breathing that is assisted by a caregiver with equipment. In some instances, *ventilation* refers specifically to the carbon dioxide status of an animal as determined by an arterial blood gas analysis.

Ventricular premature complexes Premature contraction of the ventricles, initiated by one of the ventricles from a location other than the normal cardiac conduction system.

Ventricular tachycardia An abnormally high heart rate initiated and sustained by one of the ventricles outside the normal cardiac conduction system.

Vertebral subluxation complex (VSC) An abnormal relationship between two adjacent vertebrae consisting of muscles, ligaments, connective tissue, a spinal nerve, blood vessels, lymphatics, and cerebrospinal fluid.

Vertical bone loss Dental radiography term that refers to bone loss along the long axis of a tooth root.

Vesicant Agent that causes tissue destruction or necrosis on extravasation.

Vestibular Positional term in dentistry that refers to the surface of the teeth facing the buccal mucosa. *Buccal* and *labial* are alternate terms.

Veterinarian A graduate of an accredited school of veterinary medicine. Veterinarians typically complete 4 years of undergraduate study and acquire a bachelor's degree before completing an additional 4 years of postgraduate study in veterinary medicine.

Veterinarian-client-patient relationship (VCPR) Set of requirements that must be met for a veterinarian to use a prescription or a veterinary feed directive drug.

Veterinary assistant The adjectives "animal," "veterinary," "ward," and "hospital" combined with the nouns "attendant," "caretaker," and "assistant" are titles sometimes used for individuals for whom training, knowledge, and skills are less than those required for identification as a veterinary technician or a veterinary technologist.

Veterinary feed directive (VFD) drug Drug used under the order of a veterinarian in animal feed.

Veterinary Medical Database (VMDB) National data bank located at Purdue University that includes medical data supplied by veterinary medical schools in the United States and Canada.

Veterinary teaching hospital A facility at which consultative, clinical, and hospital services are rendered, and in which a large staff of basic and applied veterinary scientists perform significant research and teaching of professional veterinary students (DVM or equivalent degree) and house officers.

Veterinary team Made up of veterinarians, practice managers, veterinary technicians, veterinary assistants, ward attendants, and receptionists.

Veterinary technician Carries out the Veterinary Technician Practice Model and completes all patient care duties except those exclusive to the practice of veterinary medicine. Veterinary technicians are graduates of American Veterinary Medical Association (AVMA)-accredited programs of veterinary technology and have successfully completed the Veterinary Technician National Examination.

Veterinary Technician Practice Model Serves as the foundation for the practice of veterinary technology and includes a series of prescribed steps taken by veterinary technicians engaged in patient care. These include the following:

1. Helps to generate a database (history, physical examination findings, and test results) for each animal patient.

2. Assesses subjective and objective information to generate a list of technician evaluations related to a patient's reaction to illness, risk for future problems, and the owner's knowledge and/or limitations in coping at home with pet care.

3. Uses critical thinking to formulate and enact a technician plan of action that includes a series of technician interventions designed to improve patient health and comfort.

4. Reevaluates the patient and adjusts the plan of action to address changes in patient status.

Veterinary technician specialist   Credentialed veterinary technician who has completed the requirements established by an academy of veterinary technician specialists, the Canadian Association of Animal Health Technologists and Technicians (CAAHTT). Requirements typically include completion of several years of postgraduate clinical work at the level of a specialist, documentation of 50 or more advanced cases, and successful completion of an examination offered by the related academy.

Veterinary technologist   A graduate of a 4-year baccalaureate American Veterinary Medical Association (AVMA)-accredited program in veterinary technology.

Veterinary technology   The science and art of providing professional support to veterinarians. The American Veterinary Medical Association (AVMA) accredits programs in veterinary technology that graduate veterinary technicians and/or veterinary technologists.

Visceral   Of, related to, or located on or among the viscera (e.g., *visceral* organs).

Visceral larva migrans, Ocular larva migrans   Both of these terms describe zoonotic conditions caused by ingestion of an egg that contains an infective second stage larva of a roundworm (usually *Toxocara canis*).

Viscid   Thick and sticky.

Viscus   Any large internal organ (i.e., the intestines) in any of the body cavities.

Visual analogue scale (VAS)   Scoring system used to give objective value to a subjective concept, such as pain. Usually a scale of 1 to 10, but may be pictorial.

Vitamins   Organic compounds necessary for normal physiologic function.

Volatile fatty acids   Fatty acids with a carbon chain of six carbons or fewer that are created through fermentation in the rumen; examples include acetate, propionate, and butyrate.

Volume of distribution (Vd)   Estimate of the distribution of a drug in the body (relationship between the amount of drug in the body and the drug plasma concentration).

von Willebrand's disease   Inherited disorder of platelet function that may result in clinically abnormal bleeding.

VTNE   Veterinary Technician National Examination. This national examination for veterinary technicians is offered in the United States and Canada on the third Friday in June and January each year.

Walk-in system   Clients come into the practice at will with no appointment needed.

Walter E. Collins, DVM   Considered the father of veterinary technology in the United States.

Waste anesthetic gas (WAG)   Gas used in inhalation anesthetic machines that is not metabolized by the patient and is given off in respiration.

Waterless hand prep   Alcohol-based antiseptic solution that provides a very rapid onset of activity. It is rubbed on the hands and forearms and is allowed to dry. No water rinsing is needed.

Waxy casts   Wide and homogeneous casts, usually with distinct blunt or squared ends.

Weanling   Young horse (usually 6 to 12 months old) that is not nursing from its mother.

White blood cells (also called *leukocytes*)   Nucleated cells, including neutrophils, eosinophils, basophils, lymphocytes, and monocytes. These cells are produced in the bone marrow and are involved in the immune response, as well as in inflammation, allergic responses, coagulation, and tissue repair.

Wind-up phenomenon   Alterations in the nervous system (hyperalgesia and allodynia) that occur as a result of untreated or inadequately treated pain, leading to untreatable pain states.

Wolffian duct   Embryologic precursor of the male tubular reproductive tract (epididymis, ductus deferens).

Working problem list   List of problems in a patient that is pertinent to the current hospital stay.

Wry malocclusion   Jaw length discrepancy in which one mandible or maxilla is shorter than the other, often resulting in a bending of the jaw to one side.

X-rays   Form of electromagnetic radiation that can be used in diagnostic imaging to produce radiographs or computed tomographic images.

Xiphoid   Small cartilaginous extension of the caudal part of the sternum.

Yearling   A 1-year-old horse.

Yeast   Unicellular fungal organisms that reproduce by budding.

Zoonosis   Any disease that is transmissible from lower animals to humans (e.g., rabies, plague, trichinosis). *Visceral larva migrans* caused by *Toxocara canis* is a zoonotic condition that may be transmitted from dogs to humans.

Zoonotic disease   Disease that is common to both animals and humans. Commonly used to describe a disease that is easily transmissible between animals and humans.

A

A-a gradient, 920-921
AAFCO. *See* Association of American Feed Control Animals
AAVSB. *See* American Association of Veterinary State Boards
Abbreviations, for prescriptions, 1039t, 1040b
Abdomen
  auscultation of
    in horses, 251-252, 252b, 252f
    in ruminants, 256, 256f
  bovine, 958
  draping of, 1190, 1204-1205
  necropsy examination of, 572, 572f, 578-579, 578f
  organs in, 237-238, 237f
  palpation of
    description of, 237-238, 238f
    per rectum, 947
Abdominal aorta, 578
Abdominal breathing, 1106
Abdominal cavity dissection, in necropsy, 576
Abdominal effusion, 419-420
Abdominal pinging, 256, 256f
Abdominal surgery
  adhesion formation after, 1282
  approaches for, 1280-1281
  in cattle, 1280-1281
  in horses, 1263-1264
Abdominal tap. *See* Abdominocentesis
Abdominocentesis, 664-669
  in alpacas, 668f
  in bovine, 668
  in camelids, 668, 668f
  in cattle, 668
  complications of, 669
  definition of, 610
  female canine urinary catheter method, 665-666
  in foals, 667-668
  in goats, 668-669
  in horses, 665-668, 947
    18- to 22-gauge × 1.5-inch needle method, 666-667
    18-gauge × 3.5-inch spinal needle method, 667
    indications for, 746
    supplies for, 945b, 948f
    teat cannula method, 665-666
  indications for, 665
  peritoneal fluid obtained with, 664
  in sheep, 668-669
  in small animals, 610-611, 916, 916f
  supplies for, 665f
  technique for, 916
Abducens nerve, 243t
Aberrant parasite, 461b
Abomasopexy, 1282

Abomasum
  displaced, 339t-340t, 1281-1282
  necropsy examination of, 578-579
  volvulus of, 1281-1282
Abrasions, 978, 1314-1315, 1315f, 1347
Abscess
  bacterial species associated with, 486t-487t
  periapical, 1347
  subsolar, 1275-1276
Absorption of drugs, 1011
Academy of Veterinary Behavior Technicians, 135, 136b
Academy of Veterinary Dental Technicians, 1299b
Acanthocheilonema reconditum, 462
Acanthocytes, 409-410, 409f-410f
Acanthomatous epulis, 1348-1349
Acariasis, 463, 466
Accelerate idioventricular rhythm, 941
Accessory sex glands, 371-372
Accordion folding, of cloth drapes, 1158, 1161f
Accounting, 68
Accounts receivable, 41
  aging of, 70
  description of, 41
  practice information management systems monitoring of, 78
Accreditation, 6
Acepromazine, 145t-146t, 968, 1081, 1081b, 1114b
Acetaminophen, 1016t
Acetic acid, 420
Acetylcholine receptors, 701
Acid-fast bacteria, 503
Acid-fast stain, 478, 490, 492, 492b
Aciduric, 431-432
Acoustic enhancement, 555, 555f
Acoustic microstreaming, 1323-1324
Acoustic nerve, 243t
Acoustic shadowing, 555
Acquired body wall herniation, 1266
ACT. *See* Activated clotting time
ACTH stimulation test, 699
Actinobacillosis, 751t-752t
Actinobacillus spp.
  A. lignieresii, 751t-752t
  A. pleuropneumoniae, 775t-776t
  description of, 504
Actinomyces spp.
  A. bovis, 751t-752t
  description of, 503
Actinomycosis, 751t-752t
Actions, responsibility for, 32
Activated clotting time, 417
Activated partial thromboplastin time, 417-418

Active drains, 1199-1200, 1222
Active immunity, 262
Active listening, 56-57
Acupressure, 860
Acupuncture, 858-860, 1061
  autonomic nervous system theory of, 859
  bioelectrical theory of, 859
  cardiopulmonary cerebrovascular resuscitation and, 924
  definition of, 858
  dry needling, 859-860, 859f
  endogenous opioid theory of, 859
  gate theory of, 859
  herbal medicine versus, 852
  history of, 858
  humoral theory of, 859
  laser, 860, 860f
  meridians, 858-859
  needle placement, 860
  record keeping, 858-859
  techniques used in, 859-860
  terminology associated with, 858-859
  theories of, 859
Acute abdomen, 932, 932b
Acute enteritis, 692t
Acute gastritis, 692t
Acute hemolytic transfusion reactions, 903-904
Acute kidney injury, 926
Acute lymphoid leukemia, 416
Acute pain, 1051-1052
Acute renal failure, 735
Acute respiratory distress syndrome, 461
Addison's disease, 699
Additives, food
  description of, 1070b
  for parasites, 284
  in pet food, 314
Adhesive drapes, 989
Adjunctive agents, 1060-1061
Adjuvants, 263
Administration, fluid/medication
  aural, 588
  epidural, 639-641
    in bovine, 640, 640f
    in camelids, 640-641, 640f
    description of, 639-640
    in goats, 641
    in horses, 640, 640f
    locations for, 639-640
    in pigs, 641
    in sheep, 641
  guidelines for, 586
  intradermal
    in large animals, 635-636, 636f
    in small animals, 589
  intramammary, 638

Administration, fluid/medication *(Continued)*
  intramuscular. *See* Intramuscular administration
  intranasal
    in large animals, 638
    in small animals, 589
  intraosseous
    in birds, 818, 818f
    description of, 890-891
    sites for, 599
    in small animals, 599
  intraperitoneal
    in bovine, 637
    in goats, 637
    in horses, 636, 637f
    in large animals, 636-638
    in pigs, 638
    in sheep, 637
    in small animals, 599
  intrarectal
    in large animals, 641-642
    medications, 641-642
    in small animals, 588-589
  intrasynovial, 641
  intratracheal, 598-599
  intravenous. *See* Intravenous administration
  nasogastric intubation. *See* Nasogastric intubation
  oral
    balling guns for, 621, 621f
    in cats, 586-587, 587f
    in cattle, 203, 203f
    in dogs, 586-587, 587f
    drench for, 621, 621f
    in large animals, 620-621, 620f
    pill gun for, 203
    in small animals, 586-587
    syringes for, 620-621, 620f
  orogastric intubation for. *See* Orogastric intubation
  in small animals
    aural, 588
    intradermal, 589
    intramuscular, 590
    intranasal, 589
    intraosseous, 599
    intrarectal, 588-589
    oral, 586-587
    orogastric intubation, 587-588
    subcutaneous, 589
    transdermal, 588
  subcutaneous
    in bovine, 634
    in camelids, 634, 635f
    in goats, 634, 635f
    in horses, 634, 635f
    in large animals, 634-635, 635f
    in pigs, 635
    in sheep, 635, 636f

Note: Page numbers followed by "f" refer to illustrations; page numbers followed by "t" refer to tables; page numbers followed by "b" refer to boxes.

Administration, fluid/medication (*Continued*)
sites for, 589
in small animals, 589
topical ophthalmic
in large animals, 638-639, 639f
in small animals, 590-598, 591f
transdermal, 588, 641
of vaccines, 264-265
Adrenal gland diseases, 1021-1022
Adson thumb forceps, 1138, 1138f
Advanced life support, 924-926, 924f, 925t
Adverse drug reactions
description of, 1015-1016, 1016t
reporting of, 1035-1036
Adverse vaccine events, 273-274
Advertising, 66-67
newspaper, 67
radio, 67
television, 67
Aerobic swabs, 488
Aeromonas spp., 504
Affiliative behaviors, 156
Agammaglobulinemic, 748
Agglutination, 400-401, 405-406, 406f, 896-897
Aggravation, 856
Aggression
in bulls, 202
in cats, 156, 159-161, 159f
in cattle, 173
definition of, 153
in dogs, 153-154, 153b-154b
fear-related, 149, 149f
in horses, 172, 190-191
human-directed, 172, 174-175
play-related, 151, 153b, 160
in swine, 777-778
Aging, 1015, 1357b
Agonists, 1013-1014, 1080
α_2-Agonists, 1054, 1054t, 1059, 1067t-1068t, 1069
Air Muzzle, 184, 185f
Air-handling system, 49
Airway obstruction, recurrent, 723t-724t, 726, 742-744, 1372-1373
Alanine aminotransferase, 425, 802
ALARA principle, 544-545
Albendazole, 1029t
Albumin
description of, 425
transfusion of, 896
Alcohol dehydrogenase, 1012t
Alcohols, 1168
Aldehyde, 1168
Aldehyde dehydrogenase, 1012t
Alginate impression, 1345, 1345f-1346f
Alkaluric, 431-432
Allantois, 389
Allergic skin disease, 702t-703t
Allergy history, 225-226
Allis tissue forceps, 1139, 1139f
Allodynia, 1052-1053
Allogrooming, 173
Allometric scale, 886
All-purpose pet food, 305, 336
Alopecia, 240, 240f
Alpacas. *See also* Camelids; Crias
abdominocentesis in, 668f
cerebrospinal fluid collection in, 671
gestation in, 781, 781b
heat stress in, 781f, 782-784, 784f

Alpacas (*Continued*)
restraint of, 209-210, 210f
ribs of, 661f
urine catheterization in, 655-656
Alpha₂-adrenergic drugs, 1082-1083
Alpha-hemolysis, 497f
Alpha-linoleic acid, 294b, 299, 319, 326, 342
Alprazolam, 145t-146t
ALT. *See* Alanine aminotransferase
Alveolar mucosa, 1309
Amblyomma americanum, 467t
Ambu bag, 923, 923f
Ambulatory practices, 111-112, 111f
American Animal Hospital Association
description of, 44
pain management standards of, 1050-1051, 1051b
American Association for Laboratory Animal Science, 17
American Association of Equine Professionals, 35
American Association of Feline Practitioners, 1361-1362
American Association of Veterinary State Boards, 9, 26b
American College of Veterinary Anesthesiologists, 1102
American College of Veterinary Behaviorists, 135, 136b
American College of Veterinary Surgeons, 15
American National Standards Institutes, 1135
American Society of Anesthesiologists physical status classification, 1079-1080, 1080t, 1119t
American Veterinary Dental College, 1299
American Veterinary Dental Society, 1299
American Veterinary Medical Association
description of, 39
ethics, 83b
House of Delegates, 3
scope of practice, 9
veterinary practices, 39, 39b
American Veterinary Society of Animal Behavior, 136b
Amino acids, 293, 297-298, 297t, 1023
Aminoglycosides, 735, 1016t-1019t
Amiodarone, 925t
Amitraz, 1030t
Amitriptyline, 145t-146t
Amlodipine, 1026
Ammonium biurate crystals, 433-435, 436f
Ammonium sulfate test, 431b
Amnion, 389
A-mode, 553
Amphenicols, 1018t-1019t
Amphotericin B, 1020t
Ampicillin, 507t
Amputation
claw, 1284
pelvic limb, 1252
in small animals, 1251-1253, 1253f
Anaerobic pathogens, 504-505
Anaerobic swabs, 488

Anal sacs
in dogs, 238-239, 239f
in ferrets, 834f
Analgesia
multimodal, 1053
paravertebral, 1280
preemptive, 1053
Analgesics. *See also specific analgesic*
administration of, 1054-1061, 1054b
in cattle, 1068t-1069t
circumferential ring block, 1056, 1056f
dental nerve block, 1056, 1056f-1057f
epidural nerve block, 1057
in goats, 1068t-1069t
in horses, 1067t-1068t
for hospitalized horses, 744
intra-articular administration of, 1056-1057
intravenous administration of, 1057
local anesthetics for, 1055-1057, 1070
local infiltration of, 1056
monitoring of, 1054t
nonsteroidal anti-inflammatory drugs. *See* Nonsteroidal anti-inflammatory drugs
in pigs, 1068t-1069t
pleural space administration of, 1057
regional anesthetics for, 1055-1057
in sheep, 1068t-1069t
in swine, 1068t-1069t
topical application of, 1056
transdermal administration of, 588
Analyzers
automated hematology, 400-401
clinical chemistry, 426-427
Anaphylactoid reactions, 276
Anaphylaxis, 903
definition of, 273-274
vaccine-related, 273-274
Anaplasma spp.
A. marginale, 412
A. phagocytophilum, 728
Anaplasmosis, 728, 763
Anaplastic mast cell tumor, 421f
Anastomosis, 1229
Ancylostoma spp.
A. braziliense, 455-457
A. caninum, 455-457, 455f
A. tubaeforme, 455-457
Anechoic, 554
Anemia
equine infectious, 428, 727-728
immune-mediated hemolytic, 405-406, 407b, 700, 898
Anesthesia. *See also* Regional nerve blocks
agents used in. *See* Anesthetic agents
in birds, 817-818
blood pressure in, 1109t
cardiopulmonary arrest during, 1127-1128
in cats, 1114b
caudal epidural, 1268, 1268f
chamber induction of, 1116
of chelonians, 826, 826t
cyanosis during, 1128
definition of, 1078

Anesthesia (*Continued*)
depth of
excessive, 1127
eye position as indicator of, 1107
reflexes as indicator of, 1106-1107, 1107t
vital signs and, 1104t
description of, 1077
diagnostic testing, 1079
difficulty in maintaining, 1127-1128
dissociative, 1084
in dogs, 1112b, 1114b
emergencies, 1126-1128
fasting recommendations for, 1078, 1078t, 1122
in ferrets, 833
general, 1077-1078
history-taking, 1079
in horses, 1118-1122
general anesthesia, 1261
induction of, 1119-1120, 1119b, 1261
maintenance of, 1119b, 1120-1121
physical status considerations, 1119t
preanesthetic period, 1119
protocol for, 1118-1119, 1119b
recovery of, 1121-1122, 1121f
sequence of events for, 1118b
hypotension secondary to, 1128
indications for, 1077
induction of
in horses, 1119-1120, 1119b
in ruminants, 1122-1124, 1123b
in small animals, 1115-1116
intramuscular induction of, 1116
intravenous induction of
in horses, 1119-1120
in ruminants, 1122-1124
in small animals, 1115-1116
in lizards, 826, 827t
local, 1331
definition of, 1078
in horses, 993
for magnetic resonance imaging, 559-560
maintenance of
in horses, 1119b, 1120-1121
in ruminants, 1123b, 1125
in small animals, 1116-1117
mask induction of, 1116
monitoring of, 129f
blood pressure, 1105
circulation, 1104-1105, 1107-1109
equipment for, 1107
mucous membranes, 1105, 1105t
overview of, 1102-1112
oxygenation, 1105, 1110-1111
principles of, 1102-1104, 1102b
ventilation, 1105-1106, 1111-1112, 1111f
vital signs, 1104, 1104t
objectives of, 1078
patient positioning during, 1117
patient preparation for, 1078-1080
patient stabilization, 1079
physical assessment before, 1079, 1079b
physical status classification, 1079-1080, 1080t, 1119t

Anesthesia (Continued)
planes of, 1102
postanesthetic period
in horses, 1122
in ruminants, 1125
in small animals, 1118
preanesthetic period
in horses, 1119
in ruminants, 1122
in small animals, 1115
premedication, 1078, 1114b, 1123b
problems during, 1126-1128
progression of, 1104
protocols for, 127-129
of rabbits, 836
recovery from
in horses, 1121-1122, 1121f
monitoring during, 1117, 1121, 1125
prolonged, 1128
rough/stormy, 1128
in ruminants, 1125
signs of, 1117, 1121-1122, 1125
in small animals, 1117-1118
regurgitation during, 1128
in reptiles, 826-827, 826t
respiratory effort during, 1105-1106
in rodents, 838
in ruminants
induction of, 1122-1124, 1123b
maintenance of, 1123b, 1125
overview of, 1122
physical status classification, 1124t
protocol for, 1122
recovery of, 1125
sequence of events for, 1122, 1123b
safety during, 127-129, 1117
in small animals
equipment preparation, 1113
induction of, 1115-1116
intramuscular induction of, 1116
intravenous induction of, 1115-1116
maintenance of, 1116-1117
patient positioning, 1117
preanesthetic period, 1115
premedication, 1114b
protocol for, 1112-1113
recommendations, 1115t
recovery, 1117-1118
sequence of events, 1113b
of snakes, 826-827
stages of, 1102
urogenital system, 1286
veterinary technician's responsibilities, 13f
vomiting during, 1128
waste anesthetic gases, 127
Anesthesia log, 109
Anesthesia machine, 127, 128b
Anesthesia record, 1103f
Anesthetic agents
agonists, 1080
alpha$_2$-adrenergic drugs, 1082-1083
anticholinergics, 1080-1081, 1081b
barbiturates, 1085
classification of, 1080
dissociatives, 1084-1085
etomidate, 1085-1086
guaifenesin, 1086
halogenated, 1086-1087

Anesthetic agents (Continued)
inhalant, 1086-1087
mixed agonist-antagonists, 1080
nitrous oxide, 1087
opioids, 1083-1084
partial agonists, 1080
propofol, 826t, 1084, 1116
respiratory system affected by, 1105
safety of, 1102
sedatives, 1081
tranquilizers, 1081-1082
Anesthetic equipment
anesthetic chambers, 1088-1089, 1089f
endotracheal tubes, 1087.
See also Endotracheal tubes
laryngoscopes, 1087, 1089f
masks, 1087-1088, 1089f
preparation of
for ruminants, 1122
for small animals, 1113
Anesthetic machine
assembly of, 1090
breathing circuits, 1094-1097, 1094f, 1096f
carrier gas supply for, 1091-1093, 1091f, 1093f
components of, 1089-1090, 1089f
description of, 1089-1090
leaks in, 1090
maintenance of, 1097-1098
nonrebreathing circuits, 1090, 1090f, 1094-1095, 1095f
oxygen flow rates, 1093, 1093b
pop-off valve, 1090, 1096
preparation of, 1090, 1090b
rebreathing systems, 1095, 1096f
scavenging system, 127, 1090f, 1097
systems, 1089-1090
Anesthetic protocol
in horses, 1118-1119, 1119b
in ruminants, 1122
in small animals, 1112
Anesthetic vaporizers, 1089, 1089f, 1093-1094
Anesthetist, 13
Anestrus, 169
in bitch, 372, 378
definition of, 372
Anger stage, of grief, 1380b-1381b, 1383-1384
Angiotensin-converting enzyme inhibitors, 1026
Angulation, 1329, 1329f
Animal abuse, 30
Animal Behavior Society, 136b
Animal care talks, 66
Animal cruelty, 35-36
Animal Health Technology/
Veterinary Technician
Program Accreditation
Committee, 6
Animal Medicinal Drug Use
Clarification Act, 1034
Animal welfare, 36
Animal Welfare Act, 35
Animal-related hazards, 123-126
minimization of, 123
noise, 123
Anipryl. See Selegiline
Anisocoria, 232
Anisognathism, 1303, 1351
Annealing temperature, 512-513
Anode, 520
Anogenital reflex, 791b

Anorexia, 675t-679t
in cats, 682-684
in horses, 738t-739t
Antacids, 691t
Antagonist, 1013-1014
Anterior cross-bite, 1344
Anterior uveitis, 702t-703t
Anthelmintics, 284, 453, 755
Anthrax
description of, 763
vaccine for, 277t-283t, 284
Anthropomorphizing, 135-136
Antiarrhythmics, 1026-1027, 1026t
Antibacterial agents, 1018
Antibiotic perfusion techniques, 1283
Antibiotic-associated colitis, 729t-730t
Antibiotics
dentistry use of, 1343b
prophylactic use of, 1215-1216
Antibody screen, 898
Anticholinergics, 1080-1081, 1081b
Anticonvulsants, 1027
Anti-DEA 1.1 antibody, 896-897
Antidiarrheal drugs, 691t
Antiemetics, 1024t
Antifibrotic therapy, 1024
Antifungals, 1018, 1020t
Antigen tests, 478
Antihypertensives, 1026
Antimicrobial susceptibility
testing, 505-507
breakpoints, 507
broth dilution method, 505, 508f
definition of, 505
disc diffusion method, 506, 506b-507b
in hospitalized horses, 746
illustration of, 508f
indications for, 505
interpretive criteria for, 507t
methods of, 505-507
microbroth dilution, 505
quality assurance, 505
zones of inhibition, 506, 507b, 508f
Antimicrobials, 1017
Antioxidants, 295
Antiparasitics, 1029t
Antipsychotics, 145t-146t
Antisepsis, 1166
Antiseptics
definition of, 1166b
types of, 1166-1168
waterless hand, 1176, 1176b
Antispasmodic agents, 1067t-1068t, 1071
Antitoxin, 276
Anxiety
behavior and, 138-139
in dogs, 151-152
minimizing of, 180
separation, 152
Apathetic hyperthyroidism, 698
Apical delta, 1336
Apnea, 1128
Apnea monitor, 1111, 1111f
Apomorphine, 933
Appearance, professional, 18-20
Appendicular skeleton, 580
Appetite stimulants, 1365
Applied kinesiology, 846, 862-865
definition of, 862-864
manual muscle testing, 864-865
Appointment scheduling, 71-72, 76, 77f
Apron, lead, 545, 545f

APTT. See Activated partial thromboplastin time
Aquapuncture, 860
Aquatic therapy, 1061
Arachidonic acid, 299, 326
Arcanobacterium pyogenes, 760
Army-Navy retractors, 1140, 1141f, 1198f
Arnica montana, 856-857
Aromatherapy, 853, 854t-855t
Arrhythmias. See Cardiac arrhythmias
Arterial blood pressure
monitoring, 928-930, 929f-930f
Arterial blood samples
in bovine, 654
in camelids, 654
catheter placement for, 604
from dorsal metatarsal artery, 603-604, 604f
from femoral artery, 604
in foals, 652-653, 653f-654f
in goats, 654
in horses, 652-654, 653f
indications for, 651
in large animals, 651-654
needles used for, 651
sample collection for, 603-604
in sheep, 654
site preparation, 651-652
in small animals, 603-604
syringes for, 651, 652f
Arterial pulse, 230, 248-249, 249f
Arthritis
in horses, 1275
osteoarthritis, 701, 1064t-1065t, 1072b, 1361
septic, 803b, 1276, 1285-1286
Arthrocentesis
carpus joint, 614
in cats, 614-616, 615f
definition of, 614
in dogs, 614-616, 615f
in horses, 956
in small animals, 614-616
stifle joint, 614-616
tarsus joint, 614
Arthropods, 462-467
chiggers, 465, 465f, 466b
definition of, 462b
mites. See Mites
Sarcoptes scabiei, 462-467, 463f, 464b
ticks, 466-467, 467t
Arthroscope, 1149-1150, 1150f
Arthroscopic surgery
in horses, 1271-1276, 1271f
instruments and equipment for, 1149-1155, 1271
arthroscope, 1149-1150, 1150f
blunt obturator, 1150-1151
conical obturator, 1150-1151, 1150f
elevators, 1153, 1153f
fluid delivery systems, 1151-1152
grasping forceps, 1153, 1153f
hand instruments, 1153-1154
light cable, 1151, 1151f
light projector, 1151, 1151f
motorized burs, 1153-1154, 1153f
radiofrequency probes, 1154
sharp trocar, 1150, 1150f
sterilization of, 1168-1169
technique for, 1271, 1271f

Artifacts
  radiographic, 527-529, 528b, 541
  reverberation, 554-555, 555f
  ultrasound, 554-555
Artificial insemination
  of bitch, 378
  in cattle, 388
  of mare, 386
Artificial vagina, 393f
Arytenoid chondritis, 1277-1278
Ascarids, 452-454, 452f
Ascending myelomalacia, 1255
Ascending placentitis, 797-798
Ascites, 1025
Ascorbic acid, 302, 839
Asepsis, 1158
Aseptic technique, 1158-1185
  procedures and, 1160
  sterilization
    autoclave, 1163-1164, 1163f
    chemical, 1164-1168
    cold, 1168, 1168f
    definition of, 1160-1161, 1166b
    ethylene oxide, 1165, 1165f
    filtration, 1161
    flash, 1164, 1166b
    heat for, 1162-1164
    hydrogen peroxide gas plasma, 1166
    indicators of, 1164, 1165f
    physical methods of, 1161-1164
    quality control, 1164
    radiation, 1161
"Ash", 295, 295b
Aspartate aminotransferase, 425
Aspiration, risk for, 680t
Aspiration pneumonia, 592b-594b
Assets, 68
Assisted feeding, 329-335
  enteral, 330-334
    enterostomy tubes for, 333b
    esophagostomy tubes for, 331, 331f, 333
    gastrostomy tubes for, 331, 332f, 333
    indications for, 332
    jejunostomy tubes for, 332-334
    liquid diets, 332-333, 332t, 333b
    nasoesophageal tubes for, 330-332
    nasogastric tubes, 330-332
  parenteral, 334-335, 334f
Assisted gloving, 1176, 1183f
Association of American Feed
  Control Animals, 309-310, 312, 322
Association of Pet Dog Trainers, 136b
Associative learning, 137
AST. See Aspartate aminotransferase
Asystole, 924-925, 924f
Ataxia
  definition of, 228, 242
  spinal, 734
Atelectasis, 1105
Atenolol, 1026t
Atipamezole, 827t, 1082-1083
Atlantooccipital joint, 574f
Atlantooccipital tap, 669
Atrial fibrillation, 727, 939-940, 940f
Atrial flutter, 939
Atrial premature complexes, 939, 939b, 939f

Atrial standstill, 942-943, 942f
Atrial tachycardia, 939, 940f
Atrioventricular valve, 575
Atrophic rhinitis, 775t-776t
Atropine, 925t, 1081
Attendants, 43-44
Attorney, right to, 33
Attrition, 5-6, 1314-1315
Atwater factors, 296, 296b
Aujeszky's disease, 772
Aural administration, 588
Aural hematoma, 702t-703t
Aural temperature, 228-229
Auricular vein, intravenous
  administration using, 628
Auscultation
  of cardiovascular system, 235, 248, 248f, 1370
  of respiratory system, 234-235, 674t, 1105
Authorization forms, 83-85
Autoclave, 1166b
Autoclave sterilization, 1163-1164, 1163f
Autoclave tape, 1164, 1164f
Autolysis, 563-564
Automated hematology analyzers, 400-401
Automated platelet count, 407-408
Automated pump systems, for
  fluid delivery, 1152, 1152f
Automatic film processor, 538, 538f, 542b
Autonomic nervous system theory,
  of acupuncture, 859
AV block
  first-degree, 943
  second-degree
    in cats, 943, 943f
    in dogs, 943, 943f
    in horses, 250, 727
  third-degree, 943, 943f
Avermectins, 1029t-1030t
Avian beak speculum, 814
Avian schistosomes, 443-445, 444f
Avidin, 302
AVMA. See American Veterinary
  Medical Association
Axillary lymph nodes, 240-241
Axillary temperature, 228-229
Ayre's T-piece, 1094-1095
Ayurvedic herbs, 852-853, 853t
Azapirones, 145t-146t
Azathioprine, 1016t-1017t, 1017
Azotemia, 424, 695, 912

B
Babcock forceps, 1139, 1139f
Bach, Edward, 857
Bacillus spp.
  B. anthracis, 503, 763
  description of, 503
Back injuries, 117-118, 118f
Background checks, 28
Backhaus towel clamps, 1183, 1189
Bacteria. See also specific bacteria
  acid-fast, 503
  anaerobes, 504-505
  curved, 505
  Gram-negative, 503-504
  Gram-positive, 499, 499t-501t, 502-503
  nosocomial infections and, 515
  obligate intracellular, 505
  in periodontal disease, 1322
  spirochetes, 505

Bacterial culture and
    identification, 492-505
  blood culture, 501-502
  collection methods, 488f
  disposal, 492, 492b
  equipment for, 493
  evaluation of, 497-498, 497f
  fecal culture, 501
  flow chart for, 498f
  in hospitalized horses, 746
  identification procedures, 498-501
    catalase test, 498, 498f
    commercial kits, 500-501
    definitive, 500
    Gram reaction, 498
    oxidase test, 498-499, 499f
    presumptive, 499-500, 499t-500t
  media for
    description of, 493-497
    differential, 495
    enrichment, 495
    incubation conditions, 496
    inoculation of, 495-496, 495f-496f, 502f
    primary isolation, 497
    selective, 495
    types of, 493t-494t
  preliminary evaluation of, 497-498, 497f
  results of, 498
  urine culture, 502, 502f
Bacterial cystitis, 697
Bacterial enteritis, 710t, 749f
Bacterial infections, 124, 1018
Bacterial pneumonia, 723t-724t, 726-727, 740b-741b
Bacterial pyoderma, 702t-703t
Baermann technique, 459, 479, 479f
Bain coaxial circuit, 1094-1095
Balance sheet, 68
Balfour retractor, 1140, 1141f
Balling guns, 621, 621f
Band neutrophils, 413
Bandages/bandaging
  adherent primary layer of, 980-981
  aftercare for, 990-993
  in cattle, 1002-1007
  chest, 990, 992f
  distal limb, 981-986, 984f, 986b, 991-993
  functions of, 980b
  head, 989-990, 992f
  indications for, 979
  layers of, 980, 980t
  lower limb wound, 995
  nonadherent primary layer of, 981
  onychectomy, 1227
  padded layer of, 997f
  postoperative care of, 1221-1222
  primary layer of, 980-981, 980t
  principles of, 979-981
  Robert Jones, 981, 985f, 1269-1270
  secondary layer of, 980t
  semi-occlusive, 979-980
  tail, 990, 993f
  tertiary layer of, 980t
  three-layer soft-padded, 989-990
  tie-over, 988-989
  wet-to-dry, 980-981
Bands, 168
Bangs vaccination, 286-287
Barbed broach, 1337-1338, 1338f

Barbering, 240, 841f
Barbiturates, 1085, 1390-1391, 1393t-1395t
Bargaining stage, of grief, 1380b-1381b, 1382-1383
Barium enema, 548-549
Barium sulfate, 547-548
Barking, 123, 151
Barn attendants, 43-44
Barnes dehorner, 1292, 1292f
Barrier nursing, 704-705, 705b
Bartonella spp., 710t
Basal metabolic rate, 820
Base-narrow mandibular canine
  teeth, 1347
Basil, 854t-855t
Basilic vein, 816, 816f
Basket muzzle, 184
Basophilic stippling, 411-412
Basophils, 414f-415f, 416
Bass technique, 1335, 1335b
Bastard strangles, 722
Bathing, 124
Baylisascaris procyonis, 454-455, 455b
Beef cattle. See also Bovine(s);
    Cattle; Ruminants
  calves, 352, 352b
  cow-calf production in, 349-351
  energy requirements for, 351
  handling of, 201-202
  nutrition for, 349-353
    energy, 351
    grain, 351, 351b
    guidelines, 353t
    minerals, 351, 352f
    protein, 351
    vitamins, 351
  undernutrition in, 351b
Behavior(s)
  anxiety and, 138-139
  displacement, 178-179
  eliciting of, 140
  fear-related, 178t
  inappropriate
    minimizing of, 140-141
    "take-away" method for
      discouraging, 142
  reinforcing of, 140
  resources about, 136b
  veterinary technician's role in, 135
Behavior counseling, 135
Behavior modification, 136-139
Behavior problems
  in cats
    aggression, 156, 159-161, 159f
    chewing, 158
    clawing, 158
    cognitive dysfunction, 164
    destructive behavior, 158-159
    house soiling, 161-164, 162t
    scratching, 158, 159f
    unruly behavior, 158
  in cattle, 174-175
  in dogs
    aggression, 153-154, 153b-154b
    anxiety, 151-152
    barking, 151
    in clinic, 149-150
    cognitive dysfunction, 154-155, 155b
    destructive behavior, 152-153
    fear, 151-152
    house soiling, 154
    phobia, 151-152
    unruly behaviors, 150-151
  in horses, 171-172
    aggression, 172, 191

Behavior problems (Continued)
  cribbing, 171-172
  human-directed aggression, 172
  inter-horse aggression, 172
  kicking, 172, 190
  repetitive behaviors, 171-172
  stable vices, 171-172
  medications for, 144
  prevention of, 139-144
  proaction plan for handling, 140-143, 140b
  socialization to prevent, 143
Behavior technician, 135
Behavioral history, 135-136, 136b
Behavioral information, 224-225
Behavioral needs, 141-142
Benazepril, 1026
Bence Jones proteins, 432
Benefits, employment-related, 60
Bennett's reflexes, 864
Benzocaine, 1393t-1395t
Benzodiazepines
  description of, 145t-146t
  as tranquilizers, 1081-1082
Bereavement, 1378
Beta blockers, 1026, 1027b
Beta-lactams, 1018t-1019t
Bicarbonate, 892-893, 893b
Bigeminy, 940-941
Bilirubin, serum, 432
Bilirubinuria, 432-435
Bill, 24
Billing, 78
Binocular vision, 190
Bioavailability, 1011, 1011b
Bioelectrical stimulation, 872
Bioelectrical theory, of acupuncture, 859
Biological challenge test, 1164
Biological safety cabinet, 131f
Biological value, 299t, 341
Biological waste, 492, 492b
Biopsy
  endometrial, 394-395, 395f
  uterine, 394-395, 394f
Biosecurity, 286
Biotin, 294t, 302, 347t
Biotransformation, 1011-1012
Bipolar coagulation devices, 1196, 1196f
Bipolar electrocautery, 1196
Birch, 854t-855t
Birds, 812-823
  ambient temperature for, 822-823
  anesthesia of, 817-818
  basal metabolic rate in, 820
  basilic vein in, 816, 816f
  capture of, 813
  in carrier, 812f, 813
  chemical restraint of, 213
  diagnostic procedures in, 814-817
  dietary management in, 819-822, 821f
  examination of
    behavior considerations during, 813
    crop wash, 814-816, 815f
    hematology, 816-817, 816f
    oral, 814-816, 814f
  flight feathers, 818
  glottis of, 815-816
  history-taking, 812-813
  hospital treatment, 818-820
  hospitalization of, 822-823
  husbandry for, 818-820
  intraosseous catheter placement in, 818, 818f

Birds (Continued)
  intubation in, 817-818
  jugular vein in, 816, 816f
  mineral grit for, 822, 822f
  nail trimming of, 818-819, 819f
  necropsy examination of, 581
  nucleated red blood cells in, 404
  nutrition for, 819-822
  protein requirements for, 821
  psittacines. See Psittacines
  radiography of, 817, 817f-818f
  red blood cells in, 408f
  restraint of, 211-214, 813
  sample collections in, 814-817
    blood, 817, 817f
    choanal culture, 814
    cloacal swab, 814
    fecal flotation, 814
  schistosomes in, 443-445, 444f
  seed diet in, 821, 821f
  toenail-clipping blood sample in, 816-817
  types of, 812b
  venipuncture in, 816
  water for, 822
  wing clipping in, 818, 819f
  zoonotic diseases, 823
Birds of prey, 213-214
Bisecting angle technique, 1319f
Bitch. See also Dog(s)
  artificial insemination of, 378
  breeding of, 378
  cesarean delivery in, 1241-1243
  definition of, 372
  dystocia in, 379
  estrous cycle in, 372-378, 374f
  feeding of, 323
  mastitis in, 699-700
  ovariectomized, 372
  parturition in, 377-378
  puberty of, 372
Bite wounds, 979
Black tongue disease, 302
Blackleg, 769-770
Bladder
  anatomy of, 1198
  catheterization of, 430
  contrast agents used in radiography of, 549
  expressing of, 1364
  necropsy examination of, 577, 577f
  palpation of, 238
  rupture of, 803b, 1288
Bladder marsupialization, 969
Bladder spoon, 969f
Bladder stones
  cystotomy for, 1243-1245
  description of, 238, 735-736
Blastomyces dermatitidis
  microscopic appearance of, 510, 511f
Blind spots, 190
Blind staggers, 363
Blister beetle toxicity, 729t-730t
Bloat
  in cattle, 256, 256f, 958-959
  free gas, 754
  in ruminants, 339t-340t, 751t-752t, 754
Blood agar plate, 493t-494t
Blood collection tubes, 399t
Blood culture
  description of, 501-502
  specimen collection, 489
Blood gas analysis, 745, 913, 919-920, 920f
Blood glucose, 927

Blood pressure
  in anesthesia, 1109t
  monitoring of, 928-930, 929f-930f, 1105
Blood pressure cuff, 1110f
Blood products
  administration of, 901-904
  description of, 900-901
Blood samples
  arterial
    in bovine, 654
    in camelids, 654
    catheter placement for, 604
    from dorsal metatarsal artery, 603-604, 604f
    from femoral artery, 604
    in foals, 652-653, 653f-654f
    in goats, 654
    in horses, 652-654, 653f
    indications for, 651
    in large animals, 651-654
    needles used for, 651
    sample collection for, 603-604
    in sheep, 654
    site preparation, 651-652
    in small animals, 603-604
    syringes for, 651, 652f
  collection of
    in birds, 817, 817f
    in bovine, 645-647, 646f
    in camelids, 647-648, 647f-648f
    in ferrets, 833, 833f
    in goats, 648
    in horses, 644-645
    in large animals, 642-671
    in pigs, 648-651
    in rabbits, 836-837, 837f
    in reptiles, 825-826, 825f
    in sheep, 648, 648f-649f
    site preparation for, 643
    in small animals, 599-604
    technique for, 600b
    Vacutainer system for, 600f
    vein selection for, 643-644
    venipuncture for. See Venipuncture
  concentration techniques for, 480-481, 480f-481f, 481t
  description of, 642-643
  filter techniques for, 481
  heartworm detection using, 479-480
Blood smear, 399
  counting area of, 406
  direct, 479-480
  drying of, 405
  evaluation of, 405-417, 405f
  feathered edge of, 406, 406f
  heartworm disease diagnosis using, 479-480
  platelets, 407-408
  preparation of, 404-405, 404f
  red blood cells, 408-412, 408f-411f
  regions of, 405, 405f
  Romanowsky-type stains, 405
  thick, 480
  thin, 480
Blood transfusion, 895-904
  administration of, 901-904, 902b, 902f
  antibody screen, 898
  blood collection for, 898-899
  blood typing, 896-898, 896b, 897f
  cross-matching, 898
  donors, 896, 896t
  goal of, 895

Blood transfusion (Continued)
  in horses, 903b
  indications for, 895-896
  monitoring of, 903-904
  plasma
    administration of, 902
    indications for, 895-896, 895b
    rate determinations, 902-903
    reactions to, 903-904, 903f
    testing before, 896-898
    volume determinations, 902-903, 902b
  blood typing, 896-898, 896b, 897f
Bloodless castration, 1292-1293
Blunt probe, 1153, 1153f
Blunt trocar, 1154, 1154f
B-mode, 553
Boarding kennels, 50
Boars, 778, 840
Body cavities, necropsy examination of, 570-573, 572f
Body condition score, 228, 320, 321f
  for camelids, 786
  for cats, 321f, 335
  for dogs, 320, 321f, 322, 335
  for horses, 359-361, 360t-361t
  for sheep, 762b
Body fluid compartments, 883, 883f
Body language
  of cats, 156-157, 157f, 182
  of dogs, 148-149, 149f
  of lizards, 217
Body surface area, 1041t
Body temperature. See also Hyperthermia; Hypothermia
  abnormalities in, 229-230
  aural, 228-229
  axillary, 228-229
  in cats, 229-230, 230t, 1106t
  in cattle, 248t, 1106t
  in dogs, 229-230, 230t, 1106t
  in goats, 248t
  in horses, 247-248, 247f-248f, 248t, 722b
  in kittens, 789-790
  measurement of, 228, 230f
  physical examination of, 228-230
  postoperative recovery of, 1218
  in puppies, 789-790
  rectal measurement of, 228-229, 230f
  in sheep, 208b, 248t
  variations in, 229-230
Body weight, 1041t
Bone cutters, 1144f
Bone marrow aspiration
  complications of, 617
  contraindications, 617
  femoral, 618f, 619
  fine-needle, 619-620
  humeral, 618f, 619
  iliac, 617-619, 618f
  indications for, 616-617
  needles for, 617, 617b, 617f
  in reptiles, 825
  sample, 618f-619f
  sites for, 617, 618f
  in small animals, 616-620
Bone pins, 1145-1146, 1147f
Bone plates, 1148-1149, 1149f
Bone screws, 1148, 1148f
Bone spavin, 1275
Bone spurs, 701
Bone wax, 1196-1197
Bone-cutting forceps, 1143
Bone-holding forceps, 1144, 1145f

Bookkeeping, 68
Boosters, 286
Borborygmi, 252, 946
Bordetella spp.
  B. bronchiseptica, 706t, 775t-776t
  canine, 268t-269t, 273
  description of, 504
  feline, 266t-267t, 271
Borrelia burgdorferi
  description of, 709t
  Lyme disease caused by. *See* Lyme disease
  vaccine for, 268t-269t, 273
Botulism
  in horses, 735
  vaccine for, 277t-283t, 283-284
Bouin's fixative, 566
Bovine. *See also* Beef cattle; Cattle
  abdomen of, 958
  abdominocentesis in, 668
  blood sample collection in
    arterial, 654
    venous, 645-647, 646f
  cesarean section in, 966, 966b
  epidural administration in, 640, 640f
  infectious bovine keratoconjunctivitis, 767-768, 768f
  intramuscular administration in, 632-633
  intraperitoneal administration in, 637
  intravenous administration in
    auricular vein, 628
    catheterization, 628, 628b, 628f
    cephalic vein, 628
    coccygeal vein, 627-628, 628f
    jugular vein, 627
    subcutaneous abdominal vein, 628
  reproduction in
    artificial insemination in, 388
    estrous cycle, 387-388
    gestation, 389
    overview of, 387-389
    parturition, 389
    terminology associated with, 373t
    udder enlargement, 389
  rumen fluid collection in, 659-660
  subcutaneous administration in, 634
  thoracocentesis in, 660-661
  urine collection in, 656-657
  venipuncture in
    coccygeal vein, 645-646, 646f
    jugular vein, 645, 646f
    subcutaneous abdominal, 646-647
Bovine diarrhea virus, 286-287
Bovine herpesvirus-1, 757t
Bovine keratoconjunctivitis, 287-288
Bovine leukosis virus, 762
Bovine respiratory disease syndrome, 756-758, 758f
Bovine spongiform encephalopathy, 580b
Bovine viral diarrhea, 751t-752t, 755-756, 757t
Box lock, 1137
Box stalls, 201, 201f
Braces, 877
Brachycephalic airway syndrome, 686t-687t

Brachycephalic dogs, 1304
Brachygnathism, 1344
Brachyodont teeth, 1299, 1300f
Brachyspira hyodysenteriae, 505, 775t
Bradycardia, 910, 1104
Bradypnea, 908-909
Bradyzoites, 471, 471b
Brain
  disorders of, 732-734
    head trauma, 733
    leukoencephalomalacia, 733
    rabies, 732-733
    temporohyoid osteoarthropathy, 733-734
    viral equine encephalitis, 733
  necropsy examination of, 573-574, 574f
Brainstem disorders, 732-734
Brainstem lesions, 732
Breathing circuits, 1089, 1090f
Breathing tubes, 1097, 1097f
Breech, 965
Breeding soundness examination
  in females, 394-395, 394f
  in males, 392-394
Bronchoalveolar lavage, 489, 663-664, 664f
Bronchodilation, 1080
Broth dilution, 505, 508f
Brown-Adson thumb forceps, 1138, 1138f
Brucella abortus, 286-287
Brucella blood agar plate, 493t-494t
Brucella spp., 504
Brucellosis, 286-287
Buccal lymph nodes, 1304
Buccal mucosa, 1309
Buck, 245t, 391
Budgeting, 70
Buffered formalin, 566, 566b
Buffy coat method, 480, 480f
Buhner suture technique, 1290
Bulbourethral glands, 371-372
Bull. *See also* Cattle
  aggression by, 202
  breeding soundness examination in, 392-393
  definition of, 245t, 387
  handling of, 202
  ischial urethrostomy in, 1288
  nutrition for, 350t, 353t
  penile fibropapillomas in, 1290-1291, 1291f
  preputial prolapse in, 1291, 1291f
  teaser, 388
  urolithiasis in, 1287, 1287f
  vaccinations for, 288
Buller steer syndrome, 174
BUN, 402, 424
Bundle branch block, 943, 944f
Bupivacaine, 1055-1056, 1067t-1069t, 1331
Buprenorphine, 1058, 1067t-1069t, 1083
Buretrol, 889-890, 889f
Burley method, 205
Burnout, 1392b
Burns, 979
Business plan, 58
Business planning, 58-59
Buspirone, 145t-146t
Butorphanol tartrate, 827t, 1058, 1058b, 1067t-1069t, 1073, 1083, 1114b, 1375
By-products, 314

C

Cachexia, 329, 713
Cage
  description of, 49
  removing a pet from, 182
  reptile, 824, 824f
Cage cards, 98
Calcitriol, 301
Calcium
  in alfalfa, 363
  description of, 302-303
  for foals, 363
  for kittens, 326-327
  for livestock, 344t
  puppy requirements for, 319
  recommended allowance of, 303t
Calcium channel blockers, 1026
Calcium gluconate, 925t, 932
Calcium oxalate, 433-435, 436f
Calcium tungstate screen, 534, 534t
Calculi
  cystic, 696-697
  definition of, 696-697
  urinary
    cystostomy for, 1243-1245
    in horses, 735-736, 1266
    in ruminants, 339t-340t
Calibration of instruments, 427
Calibrator, 427
California mastitis test, 658-659, 658f, 759, 759f
Calorie, 295
Calves. *See also* Cattle
  beef, 352, 352b
  care of, 747-749
  castration of, 1292-1293, 1293f
  colostrum for, 286, 348, 748, 748b
  definition of, 245t, 387
  dehorning of, 287, 1292, 1292f
  diseases and conditions that affect, 747-749
    bacterial enteritis, 749f
    enterotoxemia, 750, 751t-752t
    failure of passive transfer, 748
    scours, 748-749, 749f
    white muscle disease, 749
  feeding of, 348, 352b
  halter for, 201
  milk replacers for, 348
  in sternal recumbency position, 747-748
  vaccines for, 286-287
  weaning of, 286-287
Camelids. *See also* Alpacas; Llamas
  abdominocentesis in, 668, 668f
  analgesics for, 1068t-1069t
  approaching, 208
  blood sample collection from
    arterial, 654
    venous, 647-648, 647f-648f
  body condition scoring of, 786
  body language of, 208
  body temperature of, 781b
  capture of, 208
  catheterization in, 629
  cerebrospinal fluid collection in, 671
  classification of, 779, 779b
  diseases and conditions that affect, 779-786
    dental, 785-786
    digestive system, 782
    heat stress, 781f, 782-784, 784f
    hepatic lipidosis, 782

Camelids *(Continued)*
    meningeal worm, 784-785, 785f
    metabolic, 782-784
    nervous system, 784-785, 785f
    rabies, 785
  epidural administration in, 640-641, 640f
  feces of, 779, 779f
  foot trimming in, 786
  health maintenance in, 785-786
  intramuscular administration in, 634, 634f
  intravenous administration in, 628-629
  pain management in, 1064t-1065t, 1073
  parasites in, 785
  pulse rate in, 780b
  red blood cells in, 408-409, 408f
  respiratory rate in, 781b
  restraint of, 209-210, 210f
  shearing of, 784b
  South American, 779, 779b
  subcutaneous administration in, 634, 635f
  surgery-related pain in, 1066t
  thoracocentesis in, 661-662
  uterine torsion in, 966
  venipuncture in, 647-648, 647f-648f
Campylobacter jejuni, 501, 710t
Canadian Association of Animal Health Technologists and Technicians, 23
Canadian Association of Laboratory Animal Science, 17
Canadian Food Inspection Agency, 36
Canadian Meat Inspection Act, 36
Canadian Veterinary Medical Association, 3
Canal lubricants, 1339
Cancer, 705-717. *See also* Tumor(s)
  cachexia caused by, 713
  canine, 711t
  chemotherapy for. *See* Chemotherapy
  clinical manifestations of, 713
  definition of, 705
  diagnosis of, 713-715, 713b
  feline, 711t
  in geriatric cats and dogs, 1360
  pain caused by, 713
  radiotherapy for, 714
  surgery for, 714
  treatment of, 713-717
Candida albicans, 510, 511f
Canine. *See* Dog(s)
Canine adenovirus
  type 1, 707t
  type 2, 706t
  vaccine for, 268t-269t, 272
Canine antibiotic-responsive encephalopathy, 692t
Canine chronic hepatitis, 693-694, 694t
Canine coronavirus vaccine, 266t-267t, 273
Canine demodicosis, 464
Canine distemper
  description of, 707t-708t
  vaccine for, 268t-269t, 271-272, 835
Canine ehrlichiosis, 709t
Canine *Giardia* vaccine, 264t, 266t-267t

Canine infectious hepatitis, 707t
Canine infectious tracheobronchitis, 706t
Canine influenza vaccine, 268t-269t, 273
Canine intervertebral disc disease, 876b-877b
Canine monocytic ehrlichiosis, 468t-469t
Canine parainfluenza vaccine, 268t-269t, 272
Canine parvoviral enteritis, 707t
Canine parvovirus
    description of, 707t
    vaccine, 268t-269t, 272
Canine prostatic disease, 700
Canine reproduction. See Reproduction, canine
Canines (teeth), 1303, 1303f
Cannulas, 1154, 1155f
Cantharidin, 729t-730t
Capacitation, 371-372
Capillary refill time, 893, 910
    in cats, 674t
    in dogs, 674t
    gingival mucous membranes as indicator of, 235, 236f
    in horses, 253
Capnograph/capnography, 919, 1112, 1113f
Caprine. See Goats
Caprine arthritis encephalitis, 765t-766t, 767
Capture, 180-182
    of birds, 813
    of camelids, 208
    of cats, 181-182
    of dogs, 181
    of foals, 193
    of goats, 208
    of horses, 192-194, 192f-193f
    of piglets, 207
    of sheep, 208
    of swine, 205-207
Capture antibody, 510-512
Capture-resistant equipment, 123
Carbamates, 1030t
Carbohydrates, 300
    complex, 294, 300
    as concentrates, 342
    for dairy cattle, 346
    description of, 294
    dietary requirements, 300
    engorgement of. See Grain overload
    feedstuff energy, 342-343
    fermentable, 342
    hydrolyzable, 342
    for large animals, 342-343
    simple, 294
Carbon dioxide, 910b, 1393t-1395t
Carbon dioxide absorbent canister, 1096, 1096f
Carbon monoxide, 1393t-1395t
Carbonized billing sheets, 112f
Carboplatin, 1028t-1029t
Carcinogenesis, 705-706
Carcinogens, 705-706
Cardiac arrhythmias
    atrial fibrillation, 939-940, 940f
    atrial flutter, 939
    atrial premature complexes, 939, 939b, 939f
    atrial tachycardia, 939, 940f
    bundle branch block, 943, 944f
    classification of, 938b
    definition of, 938
    escape rhythms, 944
    first-degree AV block, 943
    junctional escape beats, 944

Cardiac arrhythmias (Continued)
    junctional escape rhythms, 944
    junctional tachycardia, 940, 940f
    second-degree AV block, 943, 943f
    sick sinus syndrome, 944
    supraventricular tachycardia, 940f
    third-degree AV block, 943, 943f
    ventricular asystole, 942
    ventricular fibrillation, 941-942, 942f
    ventricular premature complexes, 940-941, 941f
    ventricular tachycardia, 941
Cardiac conduction, 935-936, 936f
Cardiac insufficiency, 675t-679t
Cardiogenic shock, 915
Cardiomyopathy, 688
    definition of, 688
    dilated, 235-236, 683t, 688
    hypertrophic, 683t, 688, 1360
Cardiopulmonary arrest, 921
    during anesthesia, 1127-1128
    central nervous system affected by, 926-927
    description of, 921
    organs affected by, 927
    respiratory system after, 926
Cardiopulmonary cerebrovascular resuscitation
    abdominal compressions, 922-923
    acupuncture and, 924
    acute kidney injury after, 926
    advanced life support, 924-926, 924f, 925t
    Ambu bag, 923, 923f
    basic life support, 922-924
    care after, 926-927
    chest compressions, 922, 922f
    closed-chest compressions, 923
    definition of, 921
    description of, 914, 921-922
    drugs used in, 925, 925t
    electrical defibrillator, 924-925
    fluid resuscitation during, 926
    gastrointestinal tract injury after, 926
    hand placement for, 922f
    ventilatory support during, 923
Cardiovascular disease. See also Cardiac arrhythmias; cardiomyopathy. See Cardiomyopathy
    congestive heart failure, 685-688
    degenerative atrioventricular valve disease, 683t, 688
    in geriatric patients
        cats and dogs, 1360
        horses, 1370
    heart disease, 685-688
    heart failure, 685-688
    heartworm disease. See Heartworm disease
    in horses, 727, 1370
    mitral valve insufficiency, 688
    pharmacokinetics affected by, 1014-1015
    in ruminants, 763-764
    in small animals, 685-689
    systemic hypertension, 689
Cardiovascular drugs, 1024-1027
    antiarrhythmics, 1026-1027, 1026t
    antihypertensives, 1026
    diuretics, 1025, 1025b, 1025t
    inotropic agents, 1025

Cardiovascular system
    heart murmur, 236-237, 237t
    physical examination of, 235-237, 236f
Carnassial teeth, 1303
Carotenoids, 295, 300-301
Carotid artery, 249
Carpal flexion slings, 988, 991f
Carpal tunnel syndrome, 118
Carprofen, 1016t, 1067t-1069t
Carpus joint, 614
Carrier
    acclimating cat to, 179b
    bird, 812f, 813
    description of, 157
    removing cat from, 181-182
Carrier gases, 1091
Carts, 1366, 1366f
Caruncle, 389
Caseous lymphadenitis, 762-763, 763b
Cash flows, statement of, 68-69
Caslick's procedure/surgery, 385, 1269
Cast(s), 433, 435f, 986-987
    aftercare for, 990-993
    for cattle, 1002-1007
    forelimb, 986-987, 986f-987f
    hoof, 1284
    for horses, 994-1002
        application of, 997-1002, 998f-1001f
        bottom of, 1002, 1002f
        fiberglass, 997-998, 1001
        foot preparation, 998
        orthopedic felt application, 1000, 1000f
        removal of, 1002, 1003f
        stockinette placement, 998-999, 999f-1000f
        support foam, 1000, 1000f
        immobilization using, 997-998
Cast padding, 985-986, 985f
Casting of cattle, 204-205
Castration
    aggression and, 154b
    of calves, 1292-1293, 1293f
    of cats, 1240-1241, 1241f-1242f
    of dogs, 1236-1240, 1239f-1240f
    hemorrhage after, 1267b
    of stallions, 170, 1267-1268, 1267f
Cat(s). See also Feline; Kittens; Queen
    abdominal palpation in, 237-238, 238f
    affiliative behaviors in, 156
    aggression in, 156, 159-161, 159f
    aging effects, 1357b
    anesthesia in, 1114b
    anorexia in, 682-684
    arthrocentesis in, 614-616, 615f
    behavior problems in
        aggression, 156, 159-161, 159f
        chewing, 158
        clawing, 158
        cognitive dysfunction, 164
        destructive behavior, 158-159
        house soiling, 161-164, 162t
        scratching, 158, 159f
        unruly behavior, 158
    blood collection in, 900b
    blood groups in, 897-898
    blood typing of, 897f
    body condition score for, 321f, 335
    body language of, 156-157, 157f, 182

Cat(s) (Continued)
    body temperature in, 229-230, 230t, 1106t
    cancers in, 711t
    capture of, 181-182
    cardiac arrhythmias in
        atrial fibrillation, 939-940, 940f
        atrial flutter, 939
        atrial premature complexes, 939, 939b, 939f
        atrial tachycardia, 939, 940f
        bundle branch block, 943, 944f
        classification of, 938b
        definition of, 938
        escape rhythms, 944
        first-degree AV block, 943
        junctional escape beats, 944
        junctional escape rhythms, 944
        junctional tachycardia, 940, 940f
        second-degree AV block, 943, 943f
        sick sinus syndrome, 944
        supraventricular tachycardia, 940f
        third-degree AV block, 943, 943f
        ventricular asystole, 942
        ventricular fibrillation, 941-942, 942f
        ventricular premature complexes, 940-941, 941f
        ventricular tachycardia, 941
    as carnivores, 305b
    carrier for, 157, 179b, 181-182
    castration of, 1240-1241, 1241f-1242f
    in clinic, 157
    cough in, 684t
    declawing of. See Onychectomy
    dental chart for, 1307f-1308f
    dental problems in
        malocclusion, 1344-1345, 1344f-1345f
        masticatory myositis, 1350
        oral neoplasia, 1348-1349, 1348f
        stomatitis, 1349, 1349f
        tooth resorption, 1343-1344, 1344f
        trauma, 1347-1348
    development of, 155-156
    diabetes mellitus in, 683t, 698-699, 1022-1023, 1361
    digestive diseases in, 689-695, 707t, 849b-850b
    Dipylidium caninum in. See Dipylidium caninum
    domestication of, 156
    electrocardiography in
        acquisition of, 935, 935f
        analysis, 936-938, 936f
        cardiac conduction, 935-936, 936f
        indications for, 933-935
        lead, 935
        principles of, 935
        rhythm evaluation, 936-938, 937f
        waveforms, 935
    elimination by, 162, 164
    endotracheal intubation in, 1098
    energy requirements, 327
    escape by, 182
    fasting in, 1078t

Cat(s) (Continued)
  fat requirements for, 299-300,
      300t, 327
  fear in, 156, 178t
  feeding of
      adult maintenance, 327-328
      description of, 304
      free-choice, 327
      growth, 327
      neonatal period, 325
      during reproduction, 328-329
      seniors, 329
  fiber requirements, 327-328
  full-service care for, 64
  gastrointestinal disease in,
      849b-850b
  geriatric. See Geriatric care, cats
      and dogs
  heart rate in, 230t, 674t, 1104t
  heartworm disease in, 688-689
  hepatobiliary diseases in,
      689-695, 707t
  human-directed aggression by,
      160-161, 160f
  hyperthyroidism in, 1021t
  hypertrophic cardiomyopathy
      in, 1360
  joint fluid in
      analysis of, 616
      collection of, 614-616, 614f
  jugular venipuncture in, 601,
      602f
  life stages of, 260, 1357b
  litter boxes for, 163, 163b
  lower urinary tract disease in,
      697-698
  lung flukes in, 441-443, 443f
  mammary glands in, 239
  marking by, 162, 164
  minerals for, 328
  nail trimming in, 188-189, 188f,
      190f
  neutrophils from, 414f-415f
  new, 156-158
  nonsteroidal anti-inflammatory
      drugs in, 1055b
  onychectomy in. See
      Onychectomy
  oral administration in, 586-587,
      587f
  ovariohysterectomy in,
      1233-1235, 1234f-1235f
  pain in, 1048t, 1049f-1050f
  panleukopenia in, 125-126
  pleural effusion in, 684
  predatory aggression in, 157
  preventive health programs for
      grooming, 262
      immunity, 262-274
      wellness visits, 260-261
  protein requirements of, 298t,
      327
  pulse rate in, 230t
  redirected aggression by, 161
  reproduction in. See
      Reproduction, feline
  respiratory diseases in, 706t,
      1360
  respiratory rate in, 230t, 674t
  resting energy requirements for,
      297, 328
  restraint of. See Restraint, of
      cats
  senior. See also Geriatric care,
      cats and dogs
      definition of, 261-262
      feeding of, 329
  social behavior in, 156
  submissive, 159-160
  symphyseal separation in, 1350f

Cat(s) (Continued)
  teeth in
      description of, 1299, 1300b
      eruption schedule for, 1300t
      numbering of, 1301
      permanent, 1300t
  territoriality of, 156
  unruly behavior in, 158
  urinary catheterization in
      females, 609
      males, 608-609, 609f
  urinary tract disorders in, 162
  urine marking by, 162, 164
  urolithiasis in, 696-697
  venipuncture in, 600-601
      positioning for, 188
      restraint for, 188
  vitamins for, 328
  vomiting in, 684t
  water in, 293, 328
Cat bags, 187-188, 187f
Cat food
  history of, 304
  types of, 305
Catabolism, 293
Catalase test, 498, 498f
Catalepsy, 1084
Cataracts, 702t-703t
Catgut sutures, 1202
Catharsis, 1385
Catheter(s)
  arterial, 604
  intravenous
      aseptic technique with,
          887-888
      central line catheters, 887
      central venous, 889
      chemotherapy agents, 597
      flushing of, 596
      in jugular vein, 594-596, 595f
      maintenance of, 596
      monitoring of, 889
      multi-lumen, 591, 591f, 887,
          887f
      observation of, 596
      over-the-needle, 591, 591f,
          610f
      in peripheral vein, 591-594
      placement of, 591-596
      through-the-needle, 591, 591f
      types of, 591f
      winged needle, 591, 591f
  urethral, 607t
  urinary, 606-607
Catheterization
  intravenous
      in bovine, 628, 628b, 628f
      in camelids, 629
      complications of, 629
      in goats, 629
      in horses, 625-627, 626f, 744
      in pigs, 629, 630f
      in sheep, 629
  urinary. See Urinary
      catheterization
Cathode, 520
Cathode assembly, 520f
Cat-scratch fever, 710t
Cattle. See also Bovine(s); Bull;
      Calves; Dairy cattle; Heifers
  abdominal surgery in, 959b,
      1280-1281
  abdominocentesis in, 668
  aggressive behaviors in, 173-175
  allogrooming in, 173
  analgesics for, 1068t-1069t
  approaching, 199
  artificial insemination in, 388
  bandages in, 1002-1007
  behavior problems in, 174-175

Cattle (Continued)
  blood sample collection in
      arterial, 654
      venous, 645-647, 646f
  body temperature in, 248t,
      1106t
  bovine respiratory disease
      syndrome in, 756-758, 758f
  bovine viral diarrhea in,
      751t-752t, 755-756, 755f,
      757t
  capture of, 199-205
  casting of, 204-205
  casts in, 1002-1007
  cesarean delivery in, 1289
  claw block in, 1002-1003,
      1003f-1004f
  coccygeal vein in
      blood sample collection from,
          645-646, 646f
      intravenous administration
          using, 627-628, 628f
  dehorning of, 287
  diarrhea in, 959
  dominant behaviors by, 173
  dorsal recumbency position,
      204-205
  down animals, 963, 963f
  dystocia in, 964-967, 1289
  endotracheal intubation in,
      1100, 1100f
  estrous cycle in, 387-388
  fasting in, 1078t
  fear response in, 199
  finishing, 352-353
      definition of, 352
      energy for, 352
      minerals for, 352-353
      protein for, 352
      vitamins for, 352-353
  flight zone of, 199, 199f
  foot control and restraint in,
      204
  gestation in, 389
  handling of, 199-200
  head restraint in, 203
  heart rate in, 248t, 1104t
  heat in, 388
  hoof diseases in, 1283-1284,
      1284f
  interdigital necrobacillosis in,
      768, 768f
  intestinal obstruction in, 1280f
  intramuscular administration
      in, 632-633
  intravenous administration in
      auricular vein, 628
      catheterization, 628, 628b,
          628f
      cephalic vein, 628
      coccygeal vein, 627-628, 628f
      jugular vein, 627
      subcutaneous abdominal
          vein, 628
  lameness in, 204, 1283
  lateral recumbency position,
      204-205
  low-stress handling of, 199-200
  mastitis in, 758-760, 967
  maternal behavior in, 174
  modified Thomas splint in,
      1003-1007, 1004f-1008f
  moving of, 200, 200f
  musculoskeletal injuries in,
      962-964
  musculoskeletal pain in,
      1064t-1065t
  nasogastric intubation in, 622f
  ophthalmic conditions in,
      1291-1292

Cattle (Continued)
  oral administration in, 203,
      203f
  pain in, 1064t-1065t, 1071-1073
  physical examination of,
      254-257, 256f
  reproduction in
      artificial insemination, 388
      estrous cycle, 387-388
      gestation, 389
      overview of, 387-389
      parturition, 389
      terminology associated with,
          373t
      udder enlargement, 389
  reproductive system disorders
      in, 1288-1291, 1289f-1291f
  respiratory rate in, 248t
  respiratory system conditions
      in, 1286
  sexual behavior in, 174
  social hierarchies in, 173
  species-typical behaviors in,
      172-174
  subcutaneous abdominal vein
      blood sample collection from,
          646-647
      intravenous drug
          administration in, 628
  subcutaneous administration in,
      634
  submissive behaviors by,
      173-174
  supernumerary teat removal in,
      1288
  surgery-related pain in, 1066t
  surgical nursing of
      abdomen, 1280-1281
      abomasal displacements,
          1281-1282
      abomasal volvulus,
          1281-1282
      bladder rupture, 1288
      cesarean delivery, 1289
      claw amputation, 1284
      dystocia, 1289
      foot blocks, 1284
      fractures, 1285
      gastrointestinal tract,
          1279-1282
      hoof casts, 1284
      lameness, 1283
      laparotomies, 1280
      mandibular fractures,
          1279-1280
      musculoskeletal conditions,
          1283-1286
      obturator nerve paresis and
          paralysis, 1284
      oral lacerations, 1279
      ovarian disease, 1288-1289
      penile fibropapillomas,
          1290-1291, 1291f
      preoperative preparation,
          1278-1279
      preputial prolapse, 1291,
          1291f
      radial nerve paralysis, 1285
      reproductive system
          conditions, 1288-1291,
          1289f-1291f
      respiratory system conditions,
          1286
      rumenotomy for grain
          overload, 1281
      sciatic nerve paresis and
          paralysis, 1284
      septic arthritis, 1285-1286
      supernumerary teat removal,
          1288

Cattle *(Continued)*
traumatic reticuloperitonitis, 1281
urogenital system conditions, 1286-1288
urolithiasis, 1287-1288, 1287f
urovagina, 1288
uterine prolapse, 1289-1290, 1290f
uterine torsion, 1289
vaginal prolapse, 1289-1290, 1289f
terminology associated with, 245t
thoracocentesis in, 660-661
tracheostomy in, 962
urine catheterization of, 657
vaccines for, 286-287, 287t
water intake by, 346b
Cattle chute, 52f, 200f, 201-202, 862
Caudal, 1301
Caudal epidural anesthesia, 1268, 1268f
Caudal tail vein, 825
Cecal volvulus, 958
Cefazolin, 507t
Cefovecin, 507t
Celiotomy, 1197f
definition of, 1228
exploratory, 1228
indications for, 1228
intraoperative considerations, 1228-1229
paramedian, 1281
postoperative considerations, 1229
preoperative considerations, 1228
technique for, 1228-1229, 1228f
Cell receptors, 1013-1014
Cell therapy, 848-850
Cellulitis, 1220, 1221f
Cemental hypoplasia, 1354
Cementoenamel junction, 1313-1314
Center, 40b
Center for Veterinary Medicine, 309, 1031, 1036, 1036b
Central line catheters, 887
Central sensitization, 1052-1053
Central venous catheters, 889
Central venous pressure
definition of, 927-928, 928b
description of, 894, 921
measurement of, 928
monitoring of, 927-928
Centrifugal fecal flotation, 478
Centrifugation, 901
Cephalic venipuncture
in bovine, 628
in camelids, 647
in dogs, 188
in horses, 627, 627f, 644-645, 646f
in small animals, 601
Cephalosporins, 1035t
Cephalothin, 507t
Cercarial stages, 443, 443b
Cerebrospinal fluid
collection of
in alpacas, 671
atlantooccipital, 669
in camelids, 671
in horses, 669-671
indications for, 669
in llamas, 671
lumbosacral, 669-671, 670f
neurologic diseases diagnosed using analysis of, 746

Cerebrovascular resuscitation. *See* Cardiopulmonary cerebrovascular resuscitation
Certificates, 26-28
Certification, 42
Certification Council for Professional Dog Trainers, 136b
Certified Applied Animal Behaviorists, 136b
Certified veterinary practice managers, 42
Cervical dilatation, 389
Cervical disc surgery, 1254, 1254f
Cervical dislocation, 1393t-1395t
Cervical vertebral malformation, 734
Cervids
handling of, 210-211
restraint of, 210-211
Cesarean delivery
in bovine, 966, 966b, 1289
in cattle, 1289
in horses, 1269, 1269b
in small animals, 1241-1243
in small ruminants, 1295
Cestodes, 445-451
definition of, 445, 445b
diagnosis of, 445
Dipylidium caninum. See Dipylidium caninum
Echinococcus granulosus, 448-450, 448f-449f, 450b
Echinococcus multilocularis, 448-450, 448f-449f, 450b
proglottids, 445-446, 446b, 446f
pseudotapeworms, 450-451, 451f
Spirometra mansonoides, 450-451, 450b, 451f
Chain shanks, 194, 194f
Chamomile, 854t-855t
Champing, 164
Chapman's reflexes, 864
Charged coupled device, 1318-1319
Chelating agents, 1024
Chelonians
anesthetic agents for, 826, 826t
diets for, 828-829, 828b
Chemical(s), 122-123
definition of, 1031
ethylene oxide, 122
formalin, 122
glutaraldehyde, 122-123
hazardous, 121-122
in pet food, 313
radiographic processing, 127
spill of, 122, 122b
Chemical disinfection, 1166
Chemical residue, 1035
Chemical restraint
of birds, 213
of cats, 187-188
of cervids, 210-211
of dogs, 185
of ferrets, 216
of horses, 191, 195
of rabbits, 215
for radiography, 550-551
Chemistry. *See* Clinical chemistry
Chemotherapy, 714-715
administration of, 596-598, 597f-598f, 715, 715b
agents used in
definition of, 1027
handling of, 715, 715b
nursing considerations for, 716b

Chemotherapy *(Continued)*
parenterally administered, 1027
reactions associated with, 716-717
toxicities associated with, 716-717, 716t
types of, 1027, 1028t-1029t
complications of
alopecia, 717
hypersensitivity reactions, 715-716
local tissue necrosis, 715
definition of, 714-715
indications for, 714-715
intravenous administration of, 596-598, 597f-598f
safety considerations, 130
Chest bandage, 990, 992f
Chest compressions, 922, 922f
Chewing
by cats, 158
by dogs, 142
by ferrets, 835
by horses, 171
Cheyletiella parasitivorax, 464, 465f
Cheyne-Stokes breathing, 909
Chief complaint, 226, 245
Chiggers, 465, 465f, 466b
Chinchillas, 215
Chinese Crested Water Dragons, 217, 217f
Chinese herbal medicine, 851-852, 852t
Chiropractic
definition of, 860
history of, 860-861
in large animals, 862
philosophy of, 861
theory of, 861
treatment applications of, 861-862
veterinary technician's role in, 862
Chiropractic subluxation, 861b
Chisels, 1144, 1146f
Chlamydiosis, avian, 823
Chlamydophila
C. felis, 266t-267t, 271
C. psittaci, 823
Chloral hydrate, 1393t-1395t
Chlorambucil, 1017, 1017t, 1028t-1029t
Chloramphenicol, 1016t, 1035t
Chlorhexidine, 1166-1168, 1167t
Chloride, 303, 303t, 1168
Chlorine, 344t
Chlorpromazine, 1024t
Choanal atresia, 781, 962
Choke, 731-732, 732b, 959-960
Cholangiohepatitis, 690-691, 694-695
Cholangitis, feline, 694-695
Choleretic drugs, 1024
Choline, 294t, 295, 302, 302t
Chondroids, 724
Chondroprotective agents, 1067t-1068t, 1070
Chorioallantois, 378, 389
Chorion, 380
Christensen's urea agar slant, 493t-494t
"Christmas tree" adaptor, 891, 891f
Chromium, 345t-346t
Chronic hepatitis, 683t, 693-694, 694t
Chronic kidney disease, 695-696, 695b, 695t-696t

Chronic pain, 1051-1052
Chronic renal failure, 683t
Chronic ulcerative paradental stomatitis, 1309, 1309f
Chronic valvular disease, 1360
Chronic wasting disease, 580b
Chute
cattle, 52f, 200f, 201-202, 202f
for deer, 210-211, 210f
squeeze, 202, 202f
Chylothorax, 686t-687t
Cingulum, 1302
Circulation, 1104-1105
Circumferential ring block, 1056, 1056f
Cisapride, 1024t
Cisplatin, 1028t-1029t
Citrate test media, 493t-494t
Citrate-phosphate-dextrose, 899
Citrate-phosphate-dextrose-adenine, 899
Civil penalty, 34
Class I malocclusion, 1344
Class II malocclusion, 1344, 1345f
Class III malocclusion, 1344-1345, 1345f
Classical conditioning, 137, 137b
Classical homeopathy, 857
Claw amputation, 1284
Claw block, 1002-1003, 1003f-1004f
Clean wound, 976b
Clean-contaminated wound, 976b
Cleanliness, 118
Clearance, 1013
Clenbuterol, 1035t
Client(s), 54-57
communication, 55-57, 78
difficult, 57
education of, 65, 705
financial information from, 68
hand-out materials given to, 64-65, 64f-65f
information gathering, 86-88, 89f
rapport with, 223
relationships with, 63
sympathy communications to, 65
thank you notes sent to, 65
Client payments, 72-73
Client reminders, 64, 77
Clindamycin, 507t
Clinic, 40b
Clinical chemistry, 424-428
alanine aminotransferase, 425
analytical factors, 426
analyzers for, 426-427
aspartate aminotransferase, 425
case presentation of, 424b
definition of, 424
electrolytes, 425
gamma glutamyltransferase, 425
preanalytical factors that affect, 425-426
quality control, 427-428
serum proteins, 425
total proteins, 425
Clinical mastitis, 759
Clinical nutrition. *See also* Nutrition
assisted feeding. *See* Assisted feeding
description of, 329-336
Cloacal probes, 823f
Cloacal swab, 814
Clomipramine (Clomicalm), 144, 145t-146t
Closed extractions, 1341-1342
Closed gloving, 1176

Closed rebreathing system, 1095
Closed-suction drains, 978
Clostridial diseases
    in goats, 288
    in sheep, 288
Clostridiosis, 729t-730t
Clostridium spp.
    C. botulinum, 283-284, 305
    C. chauvoei, 769-770
    C. difficile, 504-505, 729t-730t
    C. perfringens, 356, 504-505,
        729t-730t, 749-750,
        751t-752t, 773t-774t, 783t,
        785
    C. septicum, 769-770
    C. tetani, 276, 749, 765t-766t,
        766
Cloth drapes, 1158, 1161f-1162f
Clotrimazole, 1020t
CO₂ laser, 1132, 1133f
Coagulase, 499-500
Coagulation cascade, 417-418
Coagulation factors, 417
Coagulation testing, 417-418
Coagulopathy, 884-885
Coat, 240, 240f
Cobalamin, 302, 302t, 347t
Cobalt, 347t
Coccidia, 125, 289
Coccidian parasites, 478
Coccidioides immitis, 510, 511f
Coccidiosis, 773t-774t, 783t
Coccygeal vein
    blood sample collection from,
        645-646, 646f
    intravenous drug
        administration in, 627-628,
        628f
Coconut oil, 298-299
Cod liver oil, 301
Code of ethics, 18b
Codocytes, 409
Coggin's test, 727-728
Cognitive decline, 154-155
Cognitive dysfunction
    in cats, 164
    in dogs, 154-155, 155b
Colchicine, 1024
Cold sterilization, 1168, 1168f
Colibacillosis, 773t-774t, 783t
Colic
    in horses, 944-945, 1072b,
        1263-1264
    lactate levels in, 745
Colic pain, 1063, 1064t-1065t
Colic surgery, 1066t
Colitis, 692t
    causes of, 729t-730t
    in foals, 803b
    in horses, 728-730, 729t-731t,
        730f
    right dorsal, 728, 729t-730t
    treatment of, 731t
Collagenase, 976
Collateral thermal damage, 1131
Collimator, 545, 545f
Collins, Walter E., 3, 4b
Colloids, 884-885, 885t, 894
Colonic ulcers, 728
Colonic wash, 825
Colony-forming units, 502
Colostrum, 262
    for calves, 286, 348, 748, 748b
    for kittens, 325
    nutritional composition of, 317
    for piglets, 771
    for puppies, 317
    sample collection, 659
Colpotomy, 1268, 1288-1289
Colts, 244t, 380-381

Committee on Veterinary
    Technician Education and
    Activities, 6
Committee on Veterinary
    Technician Specialties, 3-4
Communication
    aspects of, 55-57
    clarity of, 56
    client, 55-57, 78
    courtesy in, 56
    e-mail, 21
    empathy in, 57
    medical records, 20-21, 82
    myths regarding, 55
    nonverbal, 56, 142
    open-ended inquiry, 56
    professionalism in, 20-21
    text messaging, 21
    verbal, 20
    written, 20-21
Community activities, 67
Community-acquired infections, 514
Companion Animal Parasite
    Council, 453
Compassion, 1380
Compensation, 60
Complete blood count, 398-399,
    399t, 802
Complex carbohydrates, 294, 300
Compounding, drug, 1036
Compressed gas
    in cylinders, 1091-1092, 1091f
    description of, 129, 129f
Computed digital radiography,
    1318-1319
Computed radiography, 526-527
    cassettes for, 527f
    description of, 517, 526
    equipment for, 526-527, 527f
Computed tomography
    helical scanners, 557-558
    patient positioning for, 557-558,
        558f
    principles of, 557-558
    radiography versus, 557
    veterinary technician's
        responsibilities, 11
Computer, 75-78
    billing uses of, 78
    practice information
        management systems.
        See Practice information
        management systems
    reminders, 77
Computer workstations, 75
Conditioned response, 137
Conditioned stimulus, 137
Conditioning
    classical, 137, 137b
    operant, 137-138
Conduct, professional, 20, 20b
Conflict aggression, 153b
Congestive heart failure
    coughing as sign of, 687b
    signs and symptoms of, 687
    in small animals, 685-688
Conical obturator, 1150-1151,
    1150f
Conjunctiva, 232, 253f
Conjunctival hyperemia, 232
Conjunctivitis, 486t-487t,
    702t-703t
Connective tissue tumors, 712t
Consent forms, 83-84
Conspecies, 165
Conspecifics, 172
Constant rate infusions
    description of, 887, 1043, 1043b,
        1047, 1054, 1059-1060
    morphine sulfate, 1060

Constipation
    characteristics of, 690
    in small animals, 690
    technician evaluation of,
        675t-679t
Consultants, 92
Consultation, 47
Contagious ecthyma, 770, 770b,
    770f
Contagious mastitis, 759
Contingency, 137
Continuing education, 5, 7, 29
Continuous reinforcement, 138
Contrast agents, 547-550, 547f
    barium sulfate, 547-548
    for esophagus, 548
    for large bowel, 548-549
    nonionic organic iodides, 548
    organic iodides, 548
    radiolucent gases, 547
    for small bowel, 548
    soluble radiopaque ionic, 548
    for spinal cord, 549-550
    for stomach, 548
    types of, 547
    for urinary bladder, 549
    for urinary tract, 549
Controlled internal drug release
    preparations, 388
Controlled substance log, 109
Controlled substances, 34-35, 109,
    1033-1034, 1033t
Controlled Substances Act, 34-35,
    1033
Cooley thumb forceps, 1138,
    1138f
Copper, 303t, 304
    for livestock, 345t-346t
    for mares, 362
    toxicity, 763, 763f
Core lesion, 1275
Core vaccines, 265
Corneal reflex, 242, 791b, 1106,
    1107t
Corneal ulcers, 486t-487t,
    702t-703t, 737, 737f
Coronavirus
    in camelids, 783t
    canine, 266t-267t, 273
    feline
        description of, 707t-708t
        vaccine for, 271
    in ruminants, 757t
    in swine, 773-777
Corpus hemorrhagicum, 368,
    369f, 384
Corpus luteum, 368-369,
    368f-369f
Corticosteroids, 744
Cortisol, 1050-1051
Corynebacterium
    pseudotuberculosis, 762
Corynebacterium spp.
    C. renale, 503, 770
    description of, 503
Cosmetic necropsy, 582
Costoabdominal breathing, 250
Cough, 684, 684t
Coulomb, 542, 544b
Counted brush strokes method, of
    hand scrub, 1175-1176
Counter-commanding, 139
Counter-conditioning, 139
Coupage, 612, 869, 870f
Courtesy, 56
Cow, 245t. *See also* Cattle; Dairy
    cattle
Cow kick, 190
Cow-calf production, 349-351
Coxiella burnetii, 468t-469t

Coxofemoral joint, 188-189
Cradle, 198, 198f
Cranial nerves, 242, 243t
Crash cart, 914, 914f
Crate training, 140-141, 141b
Creams, 588
Creatine phosphokinase, 745
Creep feeding, of foals, 362-363,
    363b
Crias. *See also* Camelids
    body temperature of, 780b
    care of, 780-781
    choanal atresia in, 962
    congenital abnormalities in, 781
    description of, 391, 623f,
        647-648, 780f
    diarrhea in, 782
    diseases in, 780-781
    failure of passive transfer in,
        780
    orphaned, 780
    prematurity in, 781, 781f
    pulse rate in, 780b
    respiratory rate in, 780b
Cribbing, 171-172
Crile forceps, 1139-1140
Crimes of depravity, 28
Crimes of moral turpitude, 28, 30
Critical care diet, 333, 333t
Crop wash, 814-816, 815f
Cross-bite, 1344
Cross-matching, 898
Cross-tie, 196-197, 197f
Crown height reduction, 1347
Crowns, 1336, 1336f
Crust, 240
Cryoprecipitate, 895, 901
Cryosurgery, 714
Cryotherapy, 874-875
Cryptococcus neoformans, 510, 511f
Cryptorchid, 370, 380-381
Cryptorchidectomy, 1267-1268
Cryptosporidiosis, 472-473, 473f,
    783t
Cryptosporidium parvum, 472-473,
    473f, 478
Crystalloids, 883-885, 884t, 890f
Crystalluria, 433-435
Ctenocephalides felis, 447, 447f
Cucumber seed tapeworm.
    See Dipylidium caninum
Culicoides hypersensitivity, 736
Culture
    bacterial. *See* Bacterial culture
        and identification
    dermatophyte, 509, 509b
    fecal, 501
    general information about,
        485-488
    media for
        description of, 493-497
        differential, 495
        enrichment, 495
        incubation conditions, 496
        inoculation of, 495-496,
            495f-496f, 502f
        primary isolation, 497
        selective, 495
        types of, 493t-494t
    milk, 502
    routine systems, 496-497
    swabs for, 488, 489f
    urine, 488, 502, 502f
Culturette, 815f
Curettes
    dental, 1327-1329, 1328f
    Gracey, 1327-1329
    subgingival, 1328-1329, 1328f
    surgical, 1143-1144, 1145f,
        1153, 1153f

Curved bacteria, 505
Cushing's disease, 1368, 1371-1372, 1372b-1373b
Cushing's syndrome, 699
Cutaneous hypersensitivity reaction, 909f
Cutaneous larva migrans, 125, 455-456, 457f
Cutaneous papillomas, 770
Cutaneous trunci reflex, 242-243
Cyanosis, 1128
Cyclohexamines. See Dissociatives
Cyclophosphamide, 1028t-1029t
Cyclosporine A, 1017, 1017t
Cylindruria, 433
Cypress, 854t-855t
Cystic calculus, 696-697
Cysticercoid, 447, 447b, 447f
Cystine crystals, 436f
Cystine urolithiasis, 683t
Cystitis, feline idiopathic, 698b
Cystocentesis, 430, 435, 488, 604-605, 606f
    in turtles, 825
    ventral, 606b, 606f
    ventrolateral, 606b, 606f
Cystostomy, 1243-1245, 1294-1295
Cytauxzoon felis, 468t-469t
Cytauxzoonosis, 468t-469t
Cytochrome P450 enzymes, 1012-1013, 1012t
Cytologic examination
    endometrial, 394-395
    samples for, at necropsy, 568-569
    vaginal, 374b-377b
Cytology, 418-422
    abdominal effusion, 419-420
    definition of, 418
    description of, 398
    enlarged organs, 418-419
    otic, 421-422
    sample submission to reference laboratory, 420-421
    smears, 419f
    solid tissue masses, 418-419
    stains, 420
    synovial fluid, 420
    thoracic effusion, 419-420
Cytoplasmic basophilia, 413
Cytotoxic drugs
    administration of, 130
    safety considerations, 130

D

Dairy cattle
    calves, 352b. See also Calves
    capture of, 200-202
    drugs prohibited for use in, 1035t
    flight zone of, 199
    handling of, 175
    head-lock system for, 202, 202f
    hoof trimming, 288
    ketosis in, 761
    lactating, 350t, 353t
    mastitis vaccinations, 288
    milk samples from
        California mastitis test, 658-659, 658f, 759, 759f
        collection of, 658-659
        colostrum, 659
        nonsterile, 658-659
        sterile, 658
    nutrition for, 343-348
        dry-matter intake, 346b
        energy, 346-348
        forage, 346-348
        guidelines, 350t

Dairy cattle (Continued)
        minerals, 348, 349t-350t
        protein, 348, 349t-350t
        vitamins, 348, 350t
        water, 346b
        water-soluble vitamins, 347t
    reproduction in. See Reproduction, bovine
    tail vein injections in, 628
    vaccinations in, 286-287, 287t
Darkroom, 537-539
    automatic film processor, 538, 538f, 542b
    equipment used in, 537
    film storage in, 538, 538f
    importance of, 537
    safelight used in, 537, 537f
    worktable in, 537
Database, 86-92
D-dimers, 418
Dead space, 978, 1098
DeBakey thumb forceps, 1138, 1138f
Débridement
    periodontal, 1322-1323, 1326, 1330
    wound, 976, 976b, 976f
Decanting method, 478-479
Decapitation, 1393t-1395t
Deceit, 29
Decerebellate posturing, 911
Decerebrate posture, 911
Deciduous teeth, 1299-1300, 1347
Declawing. See Onychectomy
Decontamination, 933
Decubitus ulcers, 979, 1254f, 1364
Deer
    handling of, 210-211
    restraint of, 210-211
Degenerative atrioventricular valve disease, 683t, 688
Degenerative joint disease. See Osteoarthritis
Degenerative left shift, 413
Degloving injuries, 977f, 978, 982b-984b
Dehiscence of wound, 1219-1220, 1221b
Dehorning
    of calves, 287, 1292, 1292f
    of goats, 1073b
    of kids, 1295
Dehydration
    assessment of, 912b
    causes of, 911
    definition of, 293, 911
    estimation of, 911-912
    in horses, 253, 738t-739t
    hypovolemia versus, 912
    in kittens, 793-794, 794b
    laboratory abnormalities in, 912
    mild, 911
    in puppies, 793-794, 794b
    signs of, 911-912
    technician evaluation of, 675t-679t
    treatment of, 912
Delayed hemolytic transfusion reactions, 904
Delegation, 40, 42
Delta Society, 136b
Demodex canis, 464, 464f
Denaturing, 512-513
Denial stage, of grief, 1380b-1381b, 1382-1383
Density, radiographic, 540
Dental bulge, 1336
Dental calculus, 1321-1322, 1321f
Dental care, 284-285
Dental caries, 1303, 1315

Dental chart
    for cats, 1307f-1308f
    for dogs, 1305f-1306f
Dental explorer, 1312, 1312f
Dental extractions
    closed, 1341-1342
    complications of, 1340
    indications for, 1340
    surgical, 1342-1343
    for tooth resorption, 1344
Dental floats, 1353f
Dental formulas, 1300b
Dental instruments
    curettes, 1327-1329, 1328f
    description of, 1326-1327, 1327f
    elevators, 1341f-1343f
    sharpening of, 1330, 1330f
Dental luxator, 1341-1342, 1341f
Dental morphology, 1299-1303
Dental nerve block, 1056, 1056f-1057f
Dental occlusion, 1302-1303, 1303f
Dental organizations, 1299
Dental pad, 203
Dental pain, 1064t-1065t
Dental procedures
    description of, 126
    eye protection during, 126f
    veterinary technician's responsibilities, 12-13, 12f
Dental pulp, 1336
Dental radiography, 1315-1321
    bisecting angle technique, 1319f-1320f
    digital, 1318-1319
    equipment used in, 1316-1317, 1316f
    film
        chairside developer for, 1317, 1318f
        description of, 1317, 1317f
        errors involving, 1319
        processing of, 1317-1319, 1318f
    interpretation of, 1320-1321, 1320f-1321f
    occlusal technique, 1320, 1320f
    paralleling technique, 1319f
    pathologic findings identified using, 1315
    radiolucent structures on, 1320-1321, 1320f
    radiopaque structures on, 1320, 1320f
    techniques of, 1319-1320, 1319f-1320f
Dental stone, 1346
Dentin, tertiary, 1315
Dentistry. See also Teeth
    antibiotics use in, 1343b
    endodontics. See Endodontics
    ethical considerations, 1299
    exodontics, 1340-1343
    home care, 1335-1336
    in horses
        anatomy of, 1351-1352, 1351f
        common problems, 1352-1354
        examination, 1352, 1353b
        imaging, 1352
        jaw length discrepancies, 1353
        oral cavity, 1352
        orthodontic abnormalities, 1352-1353
        periodontic abnormalities, 1353-1354
        physiology of, 1351-1352

Dentistry (Continued)
    impressions used in, 1345-1346, 1345f-1346f
    interceptive orthodontics, 1346-1347, 1346f
    legal considerations, 1299
    models used in, 1345-1346
    positional terminology used in, 1301f
    restorative, 1336, 1336f
Department of Environmental Quality, 1038
Depression stage, of grief, 1380b-1381b, 1384-1385
Dermacentor spp.
    D. andersoni, 467t
    D. variabilis, 466, 466b, 467t
Dermatitis
    flea allergy, 274
    foot pad, 840, 840f
    miliary, 464
    papillomatous digital, 769, 769f
    schistosome cercarial, 443-445, 445f
Dermatologic diseases
    in horses, 736-737
    in small animals, 240b
Dermatophilus congolensis, 736
Dermatophyte culture, 509, 509b
Dermatophytosis, 770, 770f
Descending myelomalacia, 1255
Desflurane, 1087
Desoxycorticosterone, 1021-1022
Destructive behavior
    in cats, 158-159
    in dogs, 152-153
Detomidine, 1067t-1069t, 1082
Developmental needs, 141-142
Dewclaw removal, 1224-1225
Dexamethasone suppression test, 1371-1372
Dexmedetomidine, 1059-1060, 1081-1083, 1114b
Dextrose, 892
Dextrose 5% in water, 883-884
Diabetes mellitus
    in cats, 683t, 698-699, 1022-1023, 1361
    definition of, 1022
    in dogs, 683t, 698-699, 1022-1023, 1361
    signs of, 698b
Diabetic ketoacidosis, 592b-594b, 699, 892
Diagnostic nuclear medicine, 556
Diagnostic peritoneal lavage
    procedure for, 611
    in small animals, 611
Diaphragm, necropsy examination of, 572-573, 572f
Diaphragmatic hernia, 686t-687t, 1248-1249, 1249f
Diarrhea
    bovine viral, 751t-752t, 755-756, 755f, 757t
    in calves, 748-749
    in camelids, 782
    in cattle, 959
    characteristics of, 690
    large bowel, 690t
    in small animals, 690
    small bowel, 690t
    technician evaluation of, 675t-679t
Diastema, 1351
Diastolic murmurs, 236-237

Diazepam, 145t-146t, 1016t, 1082, 1114
  intranasal administration of, 589
  intrarectal administration of, 588-589
Diclofenac sodium, 1067t-1068t
DICOM, 518, 528-529
Diestrus
  in bitch, 372, 377-378
  in cattle, 388
  in goats, 391
  in mare, 383-385, 384f
  in sheep, 390
Diet, holistic, 847. See also Feeding; Nutrition
Diet history, 335
Dietary supplements, 1037
Diethylstilbestrol, 1035t
Differential medium, 495
Diff-Quik stain, 490-491, 491b
Diflubenzuron, 1030t
Digenetic flukes, 441b
Digestible energy, 342
Digestion, 341
Digestive diseases
  in camelids, 782
  in ruminants, 750-756
  in small animals, 689-695, 707t
Digital imaging and communications in medicine. See DICOM
Digital photographs, 110, 110f
Digital radiography, 526
  artifacts with, 527-529, 528b
  clinical uses of, 526
  control system for, 526f
  dental applications of, 1318-1319
  description of, 517, 526
  disadvantages of, 526
  in electronic medical records, 110f
  image quality in, 527
  "look-up table", 527-528
Digoxin, 1017t, 1025
Dihydrofolate reductase inhibitors, 1018t-1019t
1,25-Dihydroxycholecalciferol, 301
Dilated cardiomyopathy, 235-236, 683t, 688
Diltiazem, 1026t, 1027
Diode lasers, 1132-1133, 1134f
Dipetalonema reconditum, 480-481, 480f
Dipping, 124
Dipylidium caninum, 445-448
  abbreviated life cycle of, 446-447, 446f-447f
  Ctenocephalides felis, 447, 447f
  diagnosis of, 448b
  illustration of, 445f-446f
  laboratory tests for, 447-448
  prevention of, 448
  proglottids, 445-446, 446b, 446f, 448
  segments of, 446f, 475f
  signs of, 445-446
  species affected by, 445
  treatment of, 448
  zoonotic potential of, 448
Direct smear, 476-477, 479-480
Dirty shadowing, 554-555
Disbudding, 1295, 1296f
Discharge instructions, 94, 98-105, 104f, 1258

Disciplinary action
  grounds for, 29-32
    animal abuse, 30
    committing or aiding illegal professional acts, 30
    crimes of moral turpitude, 28, 30
    deceit, 29
    fraud, 29
    incompetence, 32
    malpractice, 31-32
    misrepresentation, 30
    negligence, 31-32
    practicing beyond the scope of practice, 31
    responsibility for actions, 32
    substantive violations, 29-32
    technical violations, 29
    unprofessional conduct, 31
    working impaired, 30
  hearing on, 32-33
  notice of, 32
  process of, 32-34
  right to hearing on, 32-33
Disciplinary sanctions, 33-34
Disease, 681. See also specific disease
Disinfectant, 1166b
Disinfection
  chemical, 1166
  definition of, 1160-1161
Displacement behaviors, 178-179
Dissection, in necropsy, 570
Disseminated intravascular coagulation, 915-916
Dissociative anesthesia, 1084
Dissociatives, 1084-1085
Distal, 1301
Distal forelimb fracture, 954, 954f
Distal hindlimb fracture, 955
Distal limb bandages, 981-986, 984f, 986b, 991-993
Distal urethra, 239
Distance education, 7
Distemper, canine
  description of, 707t-708t
  vaccine for, 268t-269t, 271-272, 835
Distribution, 1012
Diuretics, 1025, 1025b, 1025t
Diversionary restraint, 191
DMSO, 744
DNA sequencing, 513-514
DNA template, 512-513
Docking of tail
  in dogs, 1224-1225
  in piglets, 772f
  in puppies, 1224
  in sheep, 288-289, 1296
Docosahexaenoic acid, 299, 319, 326
Documentation
  complaints and, 84
  litigation protection uses of, 84
Doe, 245t, 391
Dog(s). See also Bitch; Canine; Puppies; specific canine entries
  abdominal palpation in, 237-238, 238f
  aggression, 153-154, 153b-154b
  aging effects, 1357b
  anal sacs in, 238-239, 239f
  Ancylostoma caninum in, 455-457, 455f
  anesthesia in, 1112b, 1114b
  arthrocentesis in, 614-616, 615f
  barking by, 123, 151

Dog(s) (Continued)
  behavior problems in
    aggression, 153-154, 153b-154b
    anxiety, 151-152
    barking, 151
    in clinic, 149-150
    cognitive dysfunction, 154-155, 155b
    destructive behavior, 152-153
    fear, 151-152
    house soiling, 154
    phobia, 151-152
    unruly behaviors, 150-151
  blood collection in, 899b
  blood typing of, 896-897, 897f
  body condition score for, 320, 321f, 322, 335
  body language of, 148-149, 149f
  body temperature in, 229-230, 230t, 1106t
  brachycephalic, 234
  breeding of, 378
  breeding soundness examination in, 392-393
  cancers in, 711t
  capillary refill time assessments in, 236f
  capture of, 181
  cardiac arrhythmias in
    atrial fibrillation, 939-940, 940f
    atrial flutter, 939
    atrial premature complexes, 939, 939b, 939f
    atrial tachycardia, 939, 940f
    bundle branch block, 943, 944f
    classification of, 938b
    definition of, 938
    escape rhythms, 944
    first-degree AV block, 943
    junctional escape beats, 944
    junctional escape rhythms, 944
    junctional tachycardia, 940, 940f
    second-degree AV block, 943, 943f
    sick sinus syndrome, 944
    supraventricular tachycardia, 940f
    third-degree AV block, 943, 943f
    ventricular asystole, 942
    ventricular fibrillation, 941-942, 942f
    ventricular premature complexes, 940-941, 941f
    ventricular tachycardia, 941
  castration of, 1236-1240, 1240f
  chronic hepatitis in, 693-694, 694t
  chronic ulcerative paradental stomatitis in, 1309, 1309f
  crate training of, 141
  dental chart for, 1305f-1306f
  dental problems in
    base-narrow canine teeth, 1347
    jaw fractures, 1350-1351, 1350f
    malocclusion, 1344-1345, 1344f-1345f
    masticatory myositis, 1350
    oral neoplasia, 1348-1349, 1349f
    stomatitis, 1349, 1349f

Dog(s) (Continued)
    tooth resorption, 1343-1344, 1344f
    trauma, 1347-1348, 1348f
  destructive behavior in, 152-153
  development of, 146-147
  dewclaw removal in, 1224-1225
  diabetes mellitus in, 683t, 698-699, 1022-1023, 1361
  digestive diseases in, 689-695, 707t
  Dipylidium caninum in. See Dipylidium caninum
  domestication of, 147-148
  electrocardiography in
    acquisition of, 935, 935f
    analysis, 936-938, 936f
    cardiac conduction, 935-936, 936f
    indications for, 933-935
    lead, 935
    principles of, 935
    rhythm evaluation, 936-938, 937t
    waveforms, 935
  energy requirements of, 321
  esophageal obstruction in, 227b, 227f
  estrous cycle in, 372-378, 374f
  fasting in, 1078t
  fat requirements for, 299-300, 300t, 322
  fear biting by, 181
  fearful, 148-152, 149b, 149f, 178f
  feeding of, 317-325
    adult maintenance, 320-323
    description of, 304
    energy, 321
    fat, 322-323
    fiber, 322
    free-choice, 323-324
    gestation, 323
    growth, 318-320
    hand-feeding, 318
    lactation, 323-324
    minerals, 322
    neonatal period, 317-318
    overfeeding, 322
    parturition, 323
    protein, 321-323
    raw foods, 307-308, 308b
    vitamins, 322
  gastric dilatation-volvulus in, 1233
  geriatric. See Geriatric care, cats and dogs
  greeting of, 150
  growth of, 318-319
  heart rate in, 230t, 1104t
  heart valves in, 235, 236f
  hepatobiliary diseases in, 689-695, 707t
  housetraining of, 155b
  hypothyroidism in, 1021t
  intervertebral disc disease in, 876b-877b
  intervertebral disc rupture, 1253
  intravenous administration in, 590
  joint fluid in
    analysis of, 616
    collection of, 614-616, 614f
  jugular venipuncture in, 601, 601f
  lateral recumbency position, 189f
  leash walking of, 151
  life stages of, 1357b
  lifting of, 183

Dog(s) *(Continued)*
lung flukes in, 441-443, 443f
lymph nodes in, 240-241, 241f
mammary glands in, 239
mammary neoplasia in, 1250
mandibular lymph nodes in, 240-241, 241f
nail trimming in, 188-189, 189f, 878, 878f
neurologic disorders in, 1253
neutrophils from, 414f-415f
new, 150
occlusion in, 1303f
oral administration in, 586-587, 587f
orogastric intubation in, 587-588, 587f-588f
ovariohysterectomy in, 1062b, 1233-1235, 1234f-1235f
overfeeding of, 322
oxygen therapy in, 918f
packed red blood cells in, 901
pain in, 1048t, 1049f-1050f
parvoviral enteritis in, 125-126
performance, 324
preventive health programs for
grooming, 262
immunity, 262-274
wellness visits, 260-262
problem behaviors in, 149-150
prostatic disease in, 700
protein requirements of, 298t, 321-322
pulse rate in, 230t
rectal examination in, 238-239, 239f
red blood cells in, 408-409, 408f
respiratory diseases in, 706t, 1360
respiratory rate in, 230t
resting energy requirements for, 297
restraint of. *See* Restraint, of dogs
selection considerations, 143
senior. *See also* Geriatric care, cats and dogs
definition of, 261-262
feeding of, 324-325
separation anxiety in, 152
sinus rhythm in, 938, 938f
sniffing by, 148
social behavior of, 147-148, 148f
socialization of, 147
submissiveness by, 148, 148f
tail docking in, 1224-1225
tapeworms in. *See* Tapeworms
teeth in
description of, 1299, 1300b
eruption schedule for, 1300t
numbering of, 1301
permanent, 1300t, 1337f
unruly behaviors in, 150-151
urinary catheterization in
females, 608, 608f
males, 607-608, 607f
urine marking by, 154
urolithiasis in, 696-697
venipuncture in, 600-601
cephalic, 188
positioning for, 188
restraint for, 188, 188f
vocalizations by, 1047
water for, 293
white blood cells in, 414f-415f
working, 324
Dog attacks, 963-964
Dog erythrocyte antigens, 896-897, 897b

Dog food
history of, 304
types of, 305
Döhle bodies, 413
Dolasetron, 1024t
Dolichocephalic, 1345
Doll's eye reflex, 242
Dominance aggression, 153b
Dominant role, 147-148
Dopamine, 927
Doppler blood pressure monitoring, 929, 929f
Doppler monitor, ultrasonic, 1108, 1108f
Dorsal displacement of the soft palate, 1276-1277
Dorsal metatarsal artery
blood sample collection from, 603-604, 604f, 652-653, 653f-654f
description of, 249
Dose creep, 546
Dose-dependent drug reactions, 1016, 1016t
Dosimetry badge, 127
Double barrel kick, 190
Double exposures, 528
Double-action rongeurs, 1143, 1144f
Double-contrast cystography, 549
Doughnuts, 985-986
Down animals, 963
Doxapram hydrochloride, 747-748
Doxorubicin, 1028t-1029t
Doxycycline, 1333-1334
Doyen intestinal tissue forceps, 1139, 1139f
D-penicillamine, 1024
Drains, 1199-1200, 1199f-1200f, 1222, 1223f, 1270
Drapes, 1158, 1161f-1162f, 1183
Draping
of abdomen, 1190
description of, 1184b, 1188-1193, 1189f, 1191f-1192f
in equine surgery, 1204-1206, 1205f-1207f
of extremity, 1190-1192
for oral surgery, 1193
for orthopedic surgery, 1205-1206, 1205f-1207f
of perineum, 1193
of spine, 1192
of thorax, 1190
Drench, 621, 621f
"Drop-offs", 72
Drug(s)
absorption of, 1011
adrenal gland diseases treated with, 1021-1022
adverse reactions, 1015-1016, 1016t, 1035-1036
cardiovascular disease treated with, 1024-1027
categories of, 1031-1033
chemical residue of, 1035
commonly used types of, 1014t
controlled substances, 1033-1034, 1033t
disposal of, 1038
dosage adjustments, 1015t
dosage forms, 1037-1038
elimination of, 1013
endoparasites treated with, 1027-1030
expired, 1038
extra-label use of, 1034, 1034b
in food-producing animals, 1035, 1035t

Drug(s) *(Continued)*
gastrointestinal disease treated with, 1023
immune-mediated diseases treated with, 1016-1017
immunosuppressive, 1016-1017, 1017t
infectious diseases treated with, 1017-1018
liver disease treated with, 1023-1024
mechanism of action of, 1013-1014
metabolism of, 1012-1013, 1012t
neoplastic disease treated with, 1027, 1028t-1029t
neurologic disease treated with, 1027
new animal, 1031-1032
parasitic disease treated with, 1027-1031
prescription animal, 1032
procurement of, 1037
storage of, 1038
Drug administration
aural, 588
epidural, 639-641
in bovine, 640, 640f
in camelids, 640-641, 640f
description of, 639-640
in goats, 641
in horses, 640, 640f
locations for, 639-640
in pigs, 641
in sheep, 641
guidelines for, 586
intradermal
in large animals, 635-636, 636f
in small animals, 589
intramammary, 638
intramuscular. *See* Intramuscular administration
intranasal
in large animals, 638
in small animals, 589
intraosseous
in birds, 818, 818f
of fluids, 890-891
sites for, 599
in small animals, 599
intraperitoneal
in bovine, 637
in goats, 637
in horses, 636, 637f
in large animals, 636-638
in pigs, 638
in sheep, 637
in small animals, 599
intrarectal
in large animals, 641-642
medications, 641-642
in small animals, 588-589
intrasynovial, 641
intratracheal, 598-599
intravenous. *See* Intravenous administration
nasogastric intubation. *See* Nasogastric intubation
oral
balling guns for, 621, 621f
in cats, 586-587, 587f
in cattle, 203, 203f
in dogs, 586-587, 587f
drench for, 621, 621f
in large animals, 620-621, 620f
pill gun for, 203

Drug administration *(Continued)*
in small animals, 586-587
syringes for, 620-621, 620f
orogastric intubation for. *See* Orogastric intubation
in small animals
aural, 588
intradermal, 589
intramuscular, 590
intranasal, 589
intraosseous, 599
intrarectal, 588-589
oral, 586-587
orogastric intubation, 587-588
subcutaneous, 589
transdermal, 588
subcutaneous
in bovine, 634
in camelids, 634, 635f
in goats, 634, 635f
in horses, 634, 635f
in large animals, 634-635, 635f
in pigs, 635
in sheep, 635, 636f
sites for, 589
in small animals, 589
topical ophthalmic
in large animals, 638-639, 639f
in small animals, 590-598, 591f
transdermal, 588, 641
of vaccines, 264-265
Drug clearance, 1013
Drug compounding, 1036
Drug Enforcement Agency, 34-35, 1390-1391
Drug laws, 1031, 1031b
Drug regulations, 1031
Drug residue, 1035, 1073
Dry heat, 1162-1163
Dry matter, 297-298
Dry reagent systems, 427
Dry-matter intake, 346b
Duodenum, 576
Durham-Humphrey Amendment, 1032
Dysbiosis, 836
Dysphoria, 1048-1049
Dyspnea, 684, 1106
Dystocia, 760, 760f
in bitch, 379
in cattle, 964-967
causes of, 1242t
examination for, 965
fetotomy for, 1269
in food animals, 964-967
in horses, 1269
pain associated with, 1064t-1065t
in queen, 380
in small ruminants, 966, 1295
Dystocia box, 964-965, 964b, 964f
Dystrophic calcification, 836

E

Ear(s)
in cats, 232
disorders of, in small animals, 701, 702t-703t
in dogs, 232
physical examination of, 232-233, 233f
Ear mites, 275t, 421-422, 422f, 463, 463f, 464b, 837, 837f

Eastern equine encephalitis/
    encephalomyelitis
    description of, 733
    vaccines for, 276-279, 277t-283t
Eccentrocytes, 409f-410f, 410-411
Ecchymotic hemorrhage, 252-253
Echinococcus spp.
    E. granulosus, 448-450,
        448f-449f, 450b
    E. multilocularis, 448-450,
        448f-449f, 450b
Echinocytes, 409-410
Echogenicity, 554-555, 556b
Eclampsia, 700
Ectoparasites
    classification of, 1030
    definition of, 439
    drugs for, 1030t
    veterinary technician's role in
        educating clients about,
        441
Ectoparasiticides, 1030, 1030t
Edge artifact, 555
EDTA. *See*
    Ethylenediaminetetraacetic
    acid
Education, 6-7
    continuing, 7, 29
    coursework, 6b
    degrees, 14t
    distance, 7
    four-year program, 6
    standard criteria for, 7
    two-year program, 6
    veterinary technology programs,
        6-7
Effleurage, 869
Egg packet, 447b
Ehmer sling, 987-988
Ehrlichia canis, 468t-469t, 709t
Ehrlichiosis
    canine, 468t-469t, 709t
    equine granulocytic, 728
Eicosapentaenoic acid, 299, 319,
    326
Eimeria spp., 783t
Ejaculation of sperm, 371-372
Ejection murmurs, 251
Elbow fracture, 955
Electrical defibrillator, 924-925
Electrical hazards, 119
Electrical stimulation, 1061
Electrical therapies, 871-873
Electroacupuncture, 860
Electrocardiography
    acquisition of, 935, 935f
    analysis, 936-938, 936f
    cardiac conduction, 935-936,
        936f
    heart rate monitoring using,
        1107-1108
    indications for, 933-935
    lead, 935
    principles of, 935
    rhythm evaluation, 936-938,
        937f
    waveforms, 935
Electrocautery, 1131, 1194-1196
Electrocautery cord, 1194-1195
Electrocution, 1393t-1395t
Electro-ejaculation, 392-393, 393f
Electrolytes, 425
    imbalance of, 675t-679t
    for working horses, 365
Electromagnetic stimulation,
    872-873
Electronic medical records, 76f
    advantages of, 111
    backup, 111, 111f
    digital photographs, 110, 110f

Electronic medical records
    (Continued)
    digital radiographs, 110f
    illustration of, 76f, 110f
    management of, 109-111
    overview of, 109-110
    risk of loss, 111
    validating of, 110-111
    voice recognition software used
        with, 109
Electrosurgery instruments, 1131,
    1132f
Elevators
    arthroscopic, 1144f, 1153, 1153f
    dental, 1341f-1342f
    periosteal, 1143, 1144f, 1341f
    root tip, 1343f
Elimination
    by cats, 162, 164
    description of, 1013
ELISA. *See* Enzyme-linked
    immunosorbent assay
Elizabethan collar, 1220, 1251
E-mail, 21
Emasculators, 1267f
Emergence delirium, 1048-1049
Emergency care station, 914
Emergency exits, 120, 120b
Emergency facilities
    definition of, 40b
    description of, 39
Emergency practices, 51-52
Emergency warning system, 120
Emesis, 933
Empathy, 57
Employee(s), 39-44
    compensation for, 60
    delegation to, 40, 42
    employment positions for,
        39-44
    feedback given to, 61
    hiring of, 59-60
    interviewing of, 60
    management of, 60-61
    management personnel, 40-42
    ongoing training of, 60
    orientation of, 60
    performance appraisals of, 61
    personal appearance of, 64
    retention of, 60-61
    safety training to, 117
    self-appraisal by, 61
    stress on, 61-62
    substance abuse by, 62
    training of, 60
Empyema, guttural pouch,
    722-724, 1278
En bloc excision, 976b, 976f
Enalapril, 1026
Enamel, 1303
Encephalitozoon cuniculi, 837
Endangered Species Act, 35
Endocrine diseases, 1020-1023
    adrenal gland diseases,
        1021-1022
    diabetes mellitus. *See* Diabetes
        mellitus
    in geriatric cats and dogs, 1361
    hyperadrenocorticism, 699,
        1361
    hyperthyroidism, 698, 1020,
        1021t, 1361
    hypoadrenocorticism, 699
    hypothyroidism, 698, 1020,
        1021t, 1361
    in small animals, 698-699
    thyroid disease, 1020-1021
Endocrinopathies, 974
Endodontic plugger, 1340f
Endodontic sealer, 1339-1340

Endodontic spreaders, 1339-1340,
    1340f
Endodontic stops, 1339
Endodontics, 1298, 1336-1340
    definition of, 1336
    files, 1337-1338, 1338b,
        1338f-1339f
    instruments for, 1337-1338,
        1337b, 1338f
    needles, 1339f
    options for, 1336-1337
Endogenous opioid theory, of
    acupuncture, 859
Endogenous substrate, 1013-1014
Endometrial biopsy, 394-395, 395f
Endometrial cytologic
    examination, 394-395
Endometrial folds, 381f
Endometritis, 760
Endoparasites
    cestodes. *See* Cestodes
    classification of, 1027-1029
    definition of, 439
    diagnosis of, 474-481
        antigen tests, 478
        Baermann technique, 479,
            479f
        blood sample examination,
            479-480
        fecal samples for. *See* Fecal
            samples
        necropsy sample collection,
            478-479
        staining procedures, 478
    drugs for, 1027-1030
    nematodes. *See* Nematodes
    pentastomes, 473-474,
        473f-474f, 474b
    protozoa. *See* Protozoa
    in ruminants, 751t-752t, 755
    shipping samples of, 479
    trematodes. *See* Trematodes
    veterinary technician's role in
        educating clients about,
        441
Endoscopy
    lower airway, 950
    upper airway, 950
    veterinary technician's
        responsibilities, 12f
Endotoxemia, 738t-739t, 742, 743f
Endotracheal intubation,
    1098-1102
    advantages of, 1098
    in cattle, 1100, 1100f
    complications of, 1101-1102,
        1101b
    equipment needed for, 1098
    in horses, 1099-1100, 1100f
    laryngospasm as complication
        of, 1101
    in small animals, 1098-1099,
        1099f
    in small ruminants, 1100
Endotracheal tubes
    cuff inflation, 1101
    definition of, 1087
    diameter of, 1087
    parts of, 1087, 1088f
    placement of, 1100-1101
    preparation of, 1098, 1099f
    selection of, 1098
    sizes of, 1087, 1088f
End-tidal carbon dioxide, 919
Enema
    barium, 548-549
    description of, 589
    in foals, 799-800
    indications for, 691t
    in neonates, 642, 799-800

Enema *(Continued)*
    rectal administration of, 642
    retention, 642, 643f
    warm-water, 589
Energy
    food intake and regulation for,
        295
    gross, 295-296
    metabolizable, 295-296
    partitioning of, 295-296
    in pet food, 296t
    puppy requirements, 318-319
Energy density, 296, 336
Energy expenditure, 296-297
Energy requirements
    beef cattle, 351
    cats, 327
    dairy cattle, 346-348
    dogs, 321
    factors that affect, 343b
    finishing cattle, 352
    foals, 808
    horses, 359-362
    sheep, 354b
    swine, 357-358
    working horses, 363, 364t
Energy units, 295
Enflurane, 1087
Enrofloxacin, 507t
Enteral feeding, 330-334
    enterostomy tubes for, 333b
    esophagostomy tubes for, 331,
        331f, 333
    foals, 808
    gastrostomy tubes for, 331, 332f,
        333
    indications for, 332
    jejunostomy tubes for, 332-334
    liquid diets, 332-333, 332t, 333b
    nasoesophageal tubes for,
        330-332
    nasogastric tubes, 330-332
Enteritis, 692t
Enterobius vermicularis, 460-461,
    461f
Enterococcus spp., 503
Enterotomy, 1229
Enterotoxemia
    in calves, 750, 751t-752t
    in camelids, 783t
    characteristics of, 751t-752t
    in ruminants, 339t-340t
    in swine, 773t-774t
Enterotoxigenic *E. coli*, 773,
    773t-774t
Entropion, 803b, 1295, 1295f
Envelope flap, 1342-1343
Environmental enrichment, 142
Environmental modifications, 155
Environmental Protection Agency,
    34
Enzymatic agents, 976
Enzyme-linked immunosorbent
    assay
    description of, 429, 429f
    viral detection using, 510-512
Eosinophilia, 416
Eosinophils, 414f-415f, 416
Ephedra, 852
Epididymis, 370
    canine, 371f
Epidural administration, 639-641
    in bovine, 640, 640f
    in camelids, 640-641, 640f
    description of, 639-640
    in goats, 641
    in horses, 640, 640f
    locations for, 639-640
    in pigs, 641
    in sheep, 641

Epidural analgesia, 965
Epidural nerve block, 1057
Epiglottic entrapment, 1277
Epinephrine, 925t
Epithelial tissue tumors, 712t
Epithelialization, 974
Epulis, 1348-1349
Equine chorionic gonadotropin, 386
Equine degenerative myelopathy, 735
Equine encephalitis vaccines, 276-279, 277t-279t, 733
Equine granulocytic ehrlichiosis, 728
Equine herpesvirus
    description of, 723t-724t, 725-726, 734-735
    respiratory disease caused by, 725-726
    vaccine for, 277t-283t, 279, 725-726
Equine herpesvirus-4, 723t-724t
Equine hyperimmune plasma, 900-901
Equine infectious anemia, 428, 727-728
Equine influenza
    description of, 723t-724t
    vaccine for, 277t-283t, 279
Equine protozoal myelitis, 734, 861
Equine recurrent uveitis, 737, 1374
Equine sarcoid, 736
Equine viral arteritis
    description of, 723t-724t, 727
    vaccine for, 277t-283t, 283
Equipment
    anesthesia. See Anesthetic equipment
    arthroscopic. See Arthroscopic surgery, instruments and equipment for
    cleaning of, 44
    computed radiography, 526-527, 527f
    darkroom, 537
    dental radiography, 1316-1317, 1316f
    endotracheal intubation, 1098
    maintenance of, 44
    personal protective, 116
    power, 1145, 1147f
    safety considerations for, 119
    stapling, 1141-1142, 1142f, 1142t
    x-ray. See X-ray(s), equipment for
Ergonomic injuries, 118
Ergosterol, 1018
Erratic parasite, 461b
Eructation, 959
Erysipelas, 286, 772
Erysipelothrix rhusiopathiae, 503
Escape rhythms, 944
Escherichia coli, 770
Esmarch bandage, 1261-1262
Esophageal catheters, 1107
Esophageal obstruction
    choke, 731-732, 732b
    in dogs, 227b, 227f
    in horses, 731-732, 732b
Esophageal stethoscope, 1107, 1108f
Esophagitis, 692t
Esophagostomy tubes, 331, 331f, 333, 1365

Esophagus
    contrast agents used in radiography of, 548
    necropsy examination of, 573, 573f
Estimates for services, 72-73
Estrogen
    description of, 369
    toxicity, in ferrets, 833-834
Estrous cycle
    in bitch, 372-378, 374f
    in cattle, 387-388
    in cows, 387-388
    in dogs, 372, 374f
    in goats, 391
    in mare, 381-385
    in sheep, 390
Estrus
    in bitch, 369, 377
    in mare, 383-385
    in queen, 379
Ethics
    code of, 18b
    professional, 23-24
Ethyl alcohol–chlorhexidine gluconate, 1167t, 1168
Ethylene oxide
    description of, 122
    sterilization using, 1165, 1165f
Ethylenediaminetetraacetic acid, 399, 419
Etiology, 681
Etomidate, 1085-1086
Euthanasia, 1387-1396
    agents used in, 1393t-1395t
    clients' presence during, 1389f, 1391
    compassionate, 1389b
    decision to perform, 1387-1388
    definition of, 1387
    follow-up after, 1391, 1392f
    of large animals, 1396
    memorializing of pet after, 1392, 1392b, 1392f
    methods of, 1393t-1395t
    pentobarbital for, 1390-1391, 1396
    preparations for, 1388
    procedure for, 1390-1391
    in research facility, 1393-1396
    in shelter, 1393-1396
    site for, 1390
    stress of, 1392-1393, 1396
    timing of, 1366
Evacuation, 119-120
Evisceration, 1221
Ewe. See also Sheep
    breeding season for, 390-391
    definition of, 245t, 389
    energy requirements of, 354
    ewe-lamb bond, 749, 750b
    lactating, 355t
    nutrition for, 353-354, 355t
    reproduction in. See Reproduction, sheep
    scrapie in, 764f
    for sheep, 762b
Examination. See Physical examination
Examination areas
    in large animal practices, 53, 53f
    in small animal practices, 46, 47f
Examination rooms, 9-11
Excitement-induced hyperglycemia, 425
Excoriation, 232
Exercise-induced pulmonary hemorrhage, 723t-724t, 726, 1025

Exercises, therapeutic, 866-867, 867f, 867t
Exocrine pancreas disorders, 690-695
Exocrine pancreatic insufficiency, 683t, 691
Exodontics, 1298, 1340-1343
Exploratory celiotomy, 1228
Exposure artifacts, 528
Extensor reflex, 791b
Extensor tone, 791b
External coaptation, 972
External fixators, 1146-1148, 1148f
External marketing, 66-68
External parasites, 125
Extinction, 138
Extinction burst, 138, 138b
Extirpation, 1291-1292
Extracellular fluid, 883
Extracellular matrix, 974
Extracorporeal shock-wave therapy, 1061
Extractions, dental
    closed, 1341-1342
    complications of, 1340
    indications for, 1340
    surgical, 1342-1343
    for tooth resorption, 1344
Extrahepatic shunts, 694
Extra-label drug use, 1034, 1034b
Extraoral examination, 1304-1309, 1352
Extravasations, 597
Extremity draping, 1190-1192
Extrinsic pathway, 417
Extubation
    in horses, 1122
    in ruminants, 1125
    in small animals, 1117-1118
Exuberant granulation tissue in open wounds, 994, 994f
Eye(s)
    anatomy of, 232
    physical examination of, 231-232, 232f
    squamous cell carcinoma of, 1291-1292, 1291f
Eye disorders
    in ruminants, 767-768, 768f
    in small animals, 701, 702t-703t
Eyewash station, 124

F

Facial lymph nodes, 1304
Facial nerve, 243t
Facilitative incision, 594
Fading puppy syndrome, 795
Failure of passive transfer
    in calves, 748
    in crias, 780
    in foals, 801
Famotidine, 1024t
Farriers, 172
Farrowing crate, 206f
Fasting, 1078, 1078t
Fasting hyperbilirubinemia, 747b
Fats, 293-294, 298-300
    for cats, 299-300, 300t, 327
    dietary requirements, 299-300, 300t
    for dogs, 299-300, 300t, 322-324
    for kittens, 326
    for large animals, 342
    for puppies, 319
    for senior dogs, 324
    structure of, 298-299
Fat-soluble vitamins, 294t
Fatty acids, 294, 298-299

Fear, 137
    aggression secondary to, 149, 149f, 153b
    in cats, 156
    in dogs, 148-152, 149b, 149f
Fear biting, 181
Febantel, 1029t
Fecal culture, 501
Fecal flotation
    in birds, 814
    centrifugal, 478
    diagnostic uses of, 472-473, 473f
    standard, 477-478, 477f
Fecal incontinence, 1360
Fecal samples
    collection of, 474, 489, 657-658
    concentration methods for, 477-478, 477f
    direct smear of, 476-477
    examination of, 474-475
    ferrets, 835
    handling of, 474-475
    small animal, 474, 609
Fecal sedimentation, 478
Feces
    in cattle, 257
    direct smear of, 476-477
    in goats, 257
    gross examination of, 475, 475f
    microscopic examination of, 475-476
    protozoa examination, 478
    in reptiles, 832
    in sheep, 257
Federal Food, Drug, and Cosmetic Act, 1031, 1031b, 1032t
Federal Trade Commission, 310
Fee estimates for services, 72-73, 84
Feed, 341. See also Feeding; Nutrition
Feeding. See also Nutrition
    assisted. See Assisted feeding
    of calves, 348
    of cats
        adult maintenance, 327-328
        description of, 304
        free-choice, 327
        growth, 327
        neonatal period, 325
        during reproduction, 328-329
        seniors, 329
    of dairy cattle, 343-348
        dry-matter intake, 346b
        energy, 346-348
        forage, 346-348
        minerals, 348, 349t-350t
        protein, 348, 349t-350t
        vitamins, 348, 350t
        water, 346b
        water-soluble vitamins, 347t
    of dogs, 317-325
        adult maintenance, 320-323
        description of, 304
        energy, 321
        fat, 322-323
        fiber, 322
        free-choice, 323-324
        gestation, 323
        growth, 318-320
        hand-feeding, 318
        lactation, 323-324
        minerals, 322
        neonatal period, 317-318
        overfeeding, 322
        parturition, 323
        protein, 321-323
        raw foods, 307-308, 308b
        vitamins, 322

Feeding (Continued)
  enteral. See Enteral feeding
  of horses, 284, 742-744
  of kittens, 325-327
  of lambs, 356, 749-750
  pasture, 354b
  of puppies, 317-318
Feeding standards, 341
Feeding tubes. See also
    Tube-feeding
  complications of, 333-334
  enterostomy, 333b
  esophagostomy, 331, 331f, 333
  flushing of, 332
  gastrostomy, 331, 332f, 333
  in geriatric cats and dogs,
    1365-1366
  jejunostomy, 332-334
  nasoesophageal, 330-332
  nasogastric, 330-332
  securing of, 333
Feedstuff energy, 342-343
Feline bronchitis, 686t-687t
Feline calicivirus
  description of, 706t
  vaccine for, 266t-267t, 270
Feline cholangitis, 694-695
Feline coronavirus
  description of, 707t-708t
  vaccine for, 271
Feline development, 155-156
Feline hepatic lipidosis, 693, 694t
Feline herpesvirus-1, 706t
Feline idiopathic cystitis, 698b
Feline idiopathic megacolon, 692t
Feline immunodeficiency virus
  description of, 707t-708t
  vaccine for, 264t, 266t-267t
Feline infectious peritonitis,
    707t-708t
Feline leukemia virus
  administration of, 264t
  characteristics of, 707t-708t
  description of, 260
  vaccine for, 266t-267t, 270
Feline lower urinary tract disease,
    697-698
Feline orchiectomy, 1171
Feline panleukopenia, 266t-267t,
    270, 707t
Feline parvovirus, 707t
Feline reproduction. See
    Reproduction, feline
Feline upper respiratory tract
    disease, 706t
Feline urologic syndrome, 1245
Feline viral rhinotracheitis
    vaccine, 264t, 270
Female(s). See also Bitch; Mare;
    Queen; Sows
  breeding soundness
    examination in, 394-395,
    394f
  reproduction in
    anatomy of, 368
    estrous cycle, 369
    ovulation, 368-369
    physiology of, 368-370, 368f
  reproductive tract in, 577
Femoral artery, blood sample
    collection from, 604
Fenbendazole, 284, 1029t
  Toxocara spp. treated with,
    453
  Trichuris vulpis treated with,
    458
Fenced enclosures, 50
Fentanyl citrate, 1038, 1058,
    1067t-1069t, 1071
Fermentable carbohydrates, 342

Ferrets
  acute respiratory distress
    syndrome in, 461
  anal sac removal from, 834f
  anesthesia of, 833
  blood collection in, 833, 833f
  canine distemper vaccinations
    in, 835
  chewing by, 835
  estrogen toxicity in, 833-834
  estrus prolongation in, 834
  fecal samples from, 835
  fluid administration in, 835
  human influenza susceptibility
    in, 834-835
  nail trimming in, 833
  nutrition for, 833
  parasites in, 835
  restraint of, 215-216
  scruffing of, 215-216, 215f
  venipuncture in, 833f
Fescue toxicosis, 339t-340t
Fetal membranes
  description of, 389
  retained, 760, 760f
Fetal necropsy, 581
Fetatome, 965
Fetotomy, 965, 1269
Fever, Potomac horse, 277t-283t,
    283, 729t-730t, 730
Fiber
  for cats, 327-328
  dietary requirements, 300
  for dogs, 322, 324-325
  insoluble, 294, 300
  for senior dogs, 324-325
  soluble, 294, 300
Fiberglass cast, 997-998, 1001
Fibrinogen
  description of, 418
  in foals, 802
  heat precipitation
    determination of, 403b
  plasma concentration of, 402
Fibrinogen degradation products,
    418
Fibrinolysis, 417
Fibroblastic sarcoid, 736
Fibroblasts, 974
Fibropapillomas, of penis,
    1290-1291, 1291f
"Fight or flight" response, 180
File, 1337-1338, 1338b, 1338f-
    1339f, 1353, 1353f
Filly, 244t, 380-383
Film
  artifacts, 541
  automatic processor of,
    534-535, 535f, 542b
  contrast, 540
  density, 540
  dental radiography
    chairside developer for, 1317,
    1318f
    description of, 1317, 1317f
    errors involving, 1319
    processing of, 1317-1319,
    1318f
  detail, 539-540
  handling of, 538-539
  identification of, 518, 519f
  intraoral, 1317, 1317f
  labeling of, 518, 518f-519f
  magnification, 540-541
  nonscreen, 532f, 534-535, 535f
  preparation of, 534
  screen, 534-535, 535f
  storage of, 538
  technical errors associated with,
    541, 541b-542b

Film badge, 544, 544f
Filtration, 1161
Financial management
  accounting, 68
  balance sheet, 68
  bookkeeping, 68
  budgeting, 70
  income statement, 68-69
  key performance indicators,
    69-70, 70b
  overview of, 68-71
  price setting, 70-71
  profitability calculations, 69
  statement of cash flows, 68-69
Fine screens, 534
Fine-needle aspiration, 619-620
Finishing cattle, 352-353
  definition of, 352
  energy for, 352
  minerals for, 352-353
  protein for, 352
  vitamins for, 352-353
Finochietto rib spreader, 1140,
    1141f
Fipronil, 1030t
Fire, 119-120
Fire extinguisher, 120, 120b
Fireworks phobia, 144
Firocoxib, 1067t-1068t
First aid, 913
First heart sound, 235-236
First-degree burns, 979
Fish oil, 301
Flail chest, 923
Flammable liquids, 119-120
Flash sterilization, 1164, 1166b
Flat files, 1353
Flavonoids, 295
Flea allergy dermatitis, 274
Flehmen response, 167, 169,
    383f
Flexor tone, 791b
Flexural limb deformities, in
    horses, 1272, 1272f
Flight feathers, 818
Flight zone
  of cattle, 199, 199f
  of horses, 192
Floating, 1353
Flooding, 139
Florfenicol, 507t
Flower essences, 853-858, 858t
Flowmeter, 1092-1093, 1092f, 1127
Fluconazole, 1020t
Fludrocortisone acetate,
    1021-1022, 1022t
Fluid balance, 931
Fluid delivery systems, 1151-1152
Fluid pump, 890f
Fluid therapy, 883-895, 883b
  additives, 891-893
    dextrose, 892
    potassium chloride, 891-892,
    892t
    sodium bicarbonate, 892-893,
    893b
  body fluid compartments, 883,
    883f
  case studies of, 888b
  colloids, 884-885, 885t, 894
  complications of, 894-895
  crystalloids, 883-885, 884t, 890f
  drip set calculations, 889b
  enteral administration of, 891,
    891f
  importance of, 882
  intramedullary administration
    of, 890-891
  intraosseous administration of,
    890-891

Fluid therapy (Continued)
  intravenous administration of,
    883-885, 887-890
  maintenance phase of, 886-887,
    886b, 887t
  monitoring of, 893-894
  phases of, 885-887
  replacement phase of, 886, 894
  resuscitation phase of, 885,
    893-894
  subcutaneous administration of,
    890, 890b
Flukes, lung, 441-443, 443f
Flunixin meglumine, 744, 1066,
    1067t-1069t
Fluorine, 345t-346t
Fluoroquinolones, 1018t-1019t,
    1035t
Fluoroscopy, 525-526, 525f
Fluoxetine, 144, 145t-146t
Foal(s). See also Horse(s)
  abdominocentesis in, 667-668
  angular limb deformities in,
    1272b, 1273, 1273f
  arterial blood sample collection
    from, 652-653, 653f-654f
  behaviors by, 193, 193f
  body temperature in, 248,
    800-801
  capture of, 193
  creep feeding of, 362-363, 363b
  critically ill, 803-805
  definition of, 244t
  diseases that affect, 803b
  dysmaturity of, 803b
  enema in, 799-800
  failure of passive transfer in,
    801
  flexural limb deformities in,
    1272b
  hospitalization of, 805
  hyperimmune plasma
    administration in, 902
  infections in, 802
  intravenous administration in,
    805-806, 805f
  neonatal care of, 797-809
    antibody levels, 801
    assessments, 807t
    behavior, 800-801
    diseases, 803b
    dysmaturity, 803b
    energy requirements for, 808
    enteral nutrition for, 808
    failure of passive transfer, 801
    history-taking, 806t
    immunoglobulin levels, 801
    laboratory evaluation,
    801-802
    mare's milk for, 808-809,
    809b
    normal behaviors, 799-802
    nutrition, 808-809
    prematurity, 800b, 803b
    routine care, 801
    sickness, 802-808
    weight gain, 808
  neurologic system of, 801
  normal, 799-802
  nursing care for, 805-808
  nutrition for, 362-363, 364t
  oral administration in, 620f
  patent urachus in, 1266
  postnatal changes in, 799-800
  premature, 800b, 803b
  pulse rate in, 249, 800-801
  rejection of, 171
  respiratory rate in, 250, 800-801
  restraint of, 193, 193f, 196, 197f,
    805f, 806-808

Foal(s) (Continued)
sick, 802-808
sternal recumbency of, 806f
umbilical repair in, 1266
vaccinations for, 277t-279t
water for, 363
weaning of, 170, 364t
Foal heat, 387
Foaling, 380-381, 798-799, 799b
Focal distance, 536
Focal point, 536
Focal spot, 520-521, 522f, 539
Focal-film distance, 530-531, 539
Focused assessment with
sonography in trauma, 913,
913b
Focusing cup, 520, 520f
Foley catheter, 607, 969b
Folic acid, 294t, 302, 302t, 347t
Follicle-stimulating hormone, 370,
372-373
Fomites, 283, 514, 704
Food. See Pet food
Food allergy, 315
Food and Drug Administration
approval from, 1066b
Center for Veterinary Medicine,
309
pet food regulation by, 309
psychotropic drugs approved
by, 144, 145t-146t
Food Animal Residue Avoidance
Databank, 1073
Food animals. See also Cattle;
Goats; Pig(s); Sheep; Swine
considerations for, 957
dog attacks on, 963-964
drugs prohibited for use in,
1035, 1035t
dystocia in, 964-967
fractures in, 962-963, 1285
gastrointestinal injuries in
ancillary diagnostics for, 958
choke, 960, 960f
diarrhea, 959
emergency intervention for,
958-959
parasitism, 959
physical examination of, 958
rumenostomy, 959-960, 960f
ruminal tympany, 959
joint luxations in, 962-963
medicine for, 747-786
musculoskeletal injuries in,
962-964
obstetrical emergencies in
cesarean section, 966, 966b
epidural analgesia, 965
examination for, 965
uterine prolapse, 966-967
uterine torsion, 966
respiratory injuries in, 961-962
restraint of, 957
rumen fluid analysis in,
960-961, 961f
surgical nursing of, 1278-1296
vaginal delivery in, 965
wild animal attacks on, 963-964
Food intake, 295
Food intolerance, 315
Food labels
description of, 296
feeding directions on, 312-313
guaranteed analysis on,
311-312, 311t
illustration of, 311f
information panel of, 310
ingredient statement, 312
net weight, 311
principal display panel of, 310

Food labels (Continued)
product identity on, 310-311
statement of nutritional
adequacy, 312
Food rewards, 140, 140b, 157
Food-related aggression, 153b, 154
Foot blocks, 1284
Foot pad dermatitis, 840, 840f
Foot rot, 768-769, 768f
Foot trimming
in camelids, 786
in cattle, 288
Foot-stomping, 164
Forage
for dairy cattle, 346-348, 351t
description of, 342
for horses, 359
quality of, 351t
vitamins in, 353
Foramen magnum, 573-574
Forceps
bone-holding, 1144, 1145f
grasping, 1153, 1153f
hemostatic, 1139-1140,
1139f-1140f
Michel clip, 1183f
thumb, 1138, 1138f
tissue, 1139, 1139f
Forelimb cast, 986-987, 986f-987f
Forelimb reflexes, 242-243
Forelimb splint, 988f
Formaldehyde, 566
Formalin, 122, 566, 566b
Founder. See Laminitis
Fractional inspiration of oxygen,
920-921
Fracture(s)
in cattle, 1285
in food animals, 962-963,
1285
in horses, 954-955
jaw, 1340, 1350-1351, 1350f
long-bone
in horses, 1270
in small animals, 1255-1257
mandibular, 1279-1280,
1350-1351, 1350f
phalangeal, 1269-1270, 1270f
root, 1343
in ruminants, 962-963
stabilization of, 954b
tooth, 1336, 1347
Francisella tularensis, 468t-469t
Fraud, 29
Frazier tip, 1140-1141, 1141f
Free gas bloat, 754
Free-choice feeding
of cats, 327
of dogs, 323-324
Freer elevator, 1144f
Fresh frozen plasma, 895b, 900,
902
Frick speculum, 203, 659b
Friction, 869
Front desk management, 71-73
Frothy bloat, 959
Full-service care, 63-64
Full-time-equivalent, 69
Fungal cultures, 509-510
dermatophytes, 509, 509b
safety considerations for,
509
Fungal infections, 125, 1018
Fur slip, 216
Furcation involvement,
1314b
Furosemide, 927, 1025, 1025t
Fusarium moniliforme, 733
Fusobacterium necrophorum,
768

G
Gag reflex, 242
Gait assessment, 242
Galactostasis, 700
Gallbladder diseases, 691-693
Gallop rhythm, 235-236
Galvayne's groove, 1351
Gamma glutamyltransferase, 425
Gangrenous mastitis, 759, 760b
Gas sterilization, 1164-1165
Gastric dilatation-volvulus, 915,
932, 1231-1233, 1232f
Gastric lavage, 933
Gastric reflux, 946
Gastric ulcers, 728
Gastritis, 692t
Gastroenteritis, 486t-487t
Gastrointestinal anastomosis
stapler, 1141-1142, 1142f
Gastrointestinal diseases and
disorders, 692t
in cats, 849b-850b
constipation, 690
diarrhea, 690
drugs for, 1023
in horses, 728-732, 944-949,
1370
management of, 691t
in ruminants, 750-756
in small animals, 689-690, 692t
in swine, 773
treatment of, 690, 691t
Gastrointestinal injuries
in food animals
ancillary diagnostics for, 958
choke, 960, 960f
diarrhea, 959
emergency intervention for,
958-959
parasitism, 959
physical examination of, 958
rumenostomy, 959-960, 960f
ruminal tympany, 959
in horses, 944-949
abdominal exploration,
948-949
abdominal palpation per
rectum, 947
abdominal radiography, 948
abdominal ultrasound, 947
colic, 944-945, 945b
conditions, 948
lesions, 948b
nasogastric intubation,
946-947, 946t
Gastrointestinal motility, 251-252,
946
Gastrointestinal neoplasia, 732
Gastrointestinal obstruction, 692t
Gastrointestinal surgery
in horses, 1263-1266
in small animals, 1229-1231
Gastrointestinal system, 792b
Gastrointestinal tract
evaluation of, 1198
physical examination of, 238
Gastrointestinal ulcers, 692t
Gastropexy, 1233
Gastrostomy tubes
feeding using, 331, 332f, 333
in geriatric cats and dogs,
1365-1366
placement of, 331
Gastrotomy, 1229
Gate theory, of acupuncture, 859
Gauntlets, 182f, 187
Gauze, 1194
Gauze muzzle, 184, 185f
Gelatin foams, 1196-1197

Gelding, 244t, 380-381
Gelpi retractor, 1140, 1141f
General anesthesia, 993
General history, 245
Genital tract infections, 486t-487t
Gentamicin, 507t
Gerbils, 216, 841, 841f
Geriatric care
cats and dogs, 1357-1366
appetite stimulants, 1365
assessments, 1358-1361,
1358t-1359t
bladder expression, 1364
cardiac disease, 1360
carts, 1366, 1366f
common problems,
1358-1361
decubital ulcers, 1364
endocrine conditions, 1361
euthanasia, 1366
fecal incontinence, 1360
feeding tubes, 1365-1366
history-taking, 1358t-1359t
hospice care, 1363-1366
hypertrophic
cardiomyopathy, 1360
integration of, 1357
kidney disease, 1360
life stages guidelines, 1357,
1357b
neoplasia, 1360
neurologic abnormalities,
1360-1361
nursing care, 1363
nutritional needs, 1361-1362,
1362b
oral health, 1360
orthopedic disease, 1361,
1361b
pain medications, 1363
respiratory disease, 1360
slings, 1366, 1366f
subcutaneous fluids, 1364
urinary incontinence, 1360,
1365
urine scalding, 1365
definition of, 1356
horses, 1368-1376
assessments, 1369t
cardiac disease, 1370
chronic diseases, 1371-1375
common problems, 1368-1370
Cushing's disease, 1371-1372,
1372b-1373b
dental problems, 1374
end of life issues, 1375-1376
equine recurrent uveitis, 1374
gastrointestinal disease, 1370
heaves, 723t-724t, 726,
742-744, 1372-1373
history-taking, 1369t
kidney disease, 1370
management of, 1375
musculoskeletal system, 1374
nasal health, 1368-1369
neurologic abnormalities,
1370
neurologic deficits, 1374
nutrition for, 1375
oral health, 1368-1369, 1370f
orthopedic disease, 1370,
1370f-1371f
osteoarthritis, 1374-1375
physical examination of, 1368
respiratory disease, 1370
sinusitis, 1374
skin disorders, 1370
vision, 1369
wave mouth, 1368-1369, 1374
integration of, 1357

Gestation. *See also* Reproduction
  in alpacas, 781, 781b
  in camelids, 391, 781
  in cats, 380
  in cattle, 389
  in dogs, 323, 378
  in llamas, 781, 781b
  in mare, 797
  in mares, 386, 386f
  in sheep, 391
  in swine, 773
Giardia spp., 125, 467-471, 470f,
    478
  vaccine for, 264t, 266t-267t, 271
Giardiasis, 783t
Gigli wire, 1144-1145
Gilt, 778
Gingiva
  hyperplasia of, 1314
  mucous membranes of, 235,
    236f
  recession of, 1353-1354
Gingival sulcus, 1321
Gingivitis, 1321, 1322f, 1349,
    1353-1354
Glandular-like products, 848-850
Glandulars, 848-850
Glass ionomers, 1340
Glaucoma, 702t-703t
Glossopharyngeal nerve, 242, 243t
Glottis
  of birds, 815-816
  of snakes, 827
Gloves, lead, 545, 545f
Gloving, 1176, 1181f-1182f
Glucocorticoids, 1017, 1363
Glucose, in urine, 432
Glucosuria, 432
Glucuronide conjugation, 1012t,
    1013
Glutaraldehyde, 122-123,
    1164-1165
Glutathione conjugation, 1012t,
    1013
Gluteal muscles, intramuscular
    administration in, 632, 633f
Glycopeptides, 1035t
Glycoproteins, 293
Glycopyrrolate, 1081
Glycosaminoglycans, 1067t-1068t,
    1070
Goats. *See also* Kid(s)
  abdominocentesis in, 668-669
  aggression in, 173
  analgesics for, 1068t-1069t
  approaching, 208
  arterial blood sample collection
    in, 654
  blood sample collection in, 654
  body temperature in, 248t
  capture of, 208
  catheterization in, 629
  dehorning of, 1073b
  endotracheal intubation in,
    1098
  epidural administration in, 641
  feces in, 257
  heart rate in, 248t
  horns in, 289
  intramuscular administration
    in, 633, 633f
  intraperitoneal administration
    in, 637
  intravenous administration in,
    629
  mastitis in, 760
  parasitism in, 289
  perineal urethrostomy in, 1294f
  pulse in, 255
  reproduction in, 373t, 391

Goats *(Continued)*
  respiratory rate in, 248t
  restraint of, 209, 209f
  subcutaneous administration in,
    634, 635f
  submissive behaviors by, 173
  surgery-related pain in, 1066t
  terminology associated with, 245t
  urinary catheterization in, 657
  urine collection in, 657
  urolithiasis in, 967-969,
    1064t-1065t, 1293
  vaccines used in, 289t
  venipuncture in, 648
Gonadotropin-releasing hormone,
    370, 381
Goniometry, 865
Goodheart, George, 864
Gown pack, 1176f
Gowning, 1176, 1179f-1180f
Gowns, 1158, 1159f-1160f
Gracey curettes, 1327-1329
Grain, 351, 351b
Grain overload
  description of, 750, 751t-752t,
    753-754
  rumenotomy for, 1281
Grain-free diet, 848
Gram reaction, 498
Gram stain, 490-491, 491b, 491f,
    814
Gram-negative bacteria, 503-504
Gram-negative rods, 501t, 504
Gram-positive cocci, 499,
    499t-501t, 502-503
Gram-positive rods, 503
Granular casts, 433, 435f
Granulation tissue, 974
Granulocytes, 413
Grasping forceps, 1153, 1153f
Grass tetany, 339t-340t
Gray, 542, 544b
Green Iguana, 216-217, 217f
Grids, 523, 535-537, 536f
Grief
  in children, 1386b
  complicating factors, 1385,
    1386b
  description of, 1380
  normal process of, 1381-1385
  referral sources for dealing with,
    1384b
  stages of, 1380b-1381b,
    1382-1385
  in veterinary professional,
    1385-1387, 1387b
Grooming, 50, 262
Gross energy, 295-296
Gross pathology, 562
Gross revenue total, 68-69
Ground-fault circuit interruption,
    119
Growing-finishing swine, 358-359
  energy requirements, 358
  minerals, 359
  protein for, 358
  vitamins, 359
Guaifenesin, 1086
Guaranteed analysis, on pet food
    label, 311-312, 311t
Guilt, 1383
Guinea pigs
  description of, 839
  foot pad dermatitis in, 840, 840f
  nutrition for, 839-840
  restraint of, 215, 215f
  sexing of, 840
  vitamin C supplementation for,
    839
  water for, 839-840

Gutta percha, 1339-1340
Guttural pouch diseases, 722-725
Guttural pouch empyema,
    722-724, 1278
Guttural pouch mycosis, 722-725,
    1278
Guttural pouch tympany, 725,
    1278

H

Habituation
  definition of, 143
  to handling, 143
Haemonchus contortus, 755, 959
Haemophilus spp., 504
Hahnemann, Samuel, 853, 855
Hair, 19-20, 240, 240f
Half-life, 1013
Halitosis, 231
Hall air drill, 1145, 1147f
Halogenated anesthetics,
    1086-1087
Halothane, 1087
Halsted mosquito hemostatic
    forceps, 1139-1140, 1139f
Halters
  bovine, 200-201, 201f
  calves, 201
  equine, 194, 194f
Hamsters, 216, 840-841, 840f
Hand(s)
  scrub of, 1175-1176, 1177f,
    1188
  of veterinary professional, 19
Hand scaling, 1326-1333
Handling
  of beef cattle, 201-202
  of bull, 202
  of cattle, 199-200
  of cervids, 210-211
  of dairy cattle, 175
  of deer, 210-211
  habituation to, 143
  of reptiles, 216-219
  of snakes, 218, 219f
Hand-out materials, 64-65,
    64f-65f
Hands (measurement), 253
Hanging leg surgical preparation,
    1171, 1172f, 1192f
Hard palate, 1309, 1311f
Hardware disease, 751t-752t,
    754-755, 754f
Harnesses, 875
Hazard warning labels, 121f
Hazardous chemicals, 121-122
Hazardous drugs, 130
Hazardous materials plan, 121
Head bandages, 989-990, 992f
Head halters, 151, 151b
Head trauma, 733
Head-lock system, 202, 202f
Healing, wound. *See* Wound
    healing
Hearing
  procedures for, 33
  right to, 32-33
Hearing protectors, 123f
Heart
  apex of, 250, 250f
  atrioventricular valve of, 575
  auscultation of
    in horses, 248f, 250-251,
      250f-251f
    in ruminants, 255
  development of, 792b
  necropsy examination of,
    575f-576f

Heart disease
  description of, 1024-1025
  progression of, to heart failure,
    687b
  signs of, 682
  in small animals, 685-688
Heart failure
  heart disease progression to,
    687b
  in small animals, 685-688
Heart murmurs, 236-237, 237t,
    251
Heart rate
  calculation of, 936
  in cats, 230t, 1104t
  in cattle, 248t, 1104t
  definition of, 248
  in dogs, 230t, 1104t
  in goats, 248t
  in horses, 248t, 250-251, 1104t
  in sheep, 248t
Heart sounds, 235-236, 250-251
Heart valves
  chronic disease of, 1360
  in dogs, 235, 236f
  endocarditis of, 763-764
Heartworm disease, 688-689
  blood sample examination for
    detection of, 479-480
  in cats, 688-689
  definition of, 688
  Dirofilaria immitis, 461-462, 479
  pathogenesis of, 682
  prevention of, 275t, 462
  serologic tests for, 429-430
  signs of, 688
  treatment of, 462, 688-689
Heat lamps, 1217-1218
Heat sterilization, 1162-1164
Heat stress, 781f, 782-784, 784f
Heaves, 723t-724t, 726, 742-744,
    1372-1373
Hedgehogs, 216, 842-843, 843f
Hedström file, 1337-1338
Heel effect, 522, 522f, 528
Heifers
  definition of, 245t, 387
  nutrient guidelines for, 353t
  puberty in, 387
Height measurements, in horses,
    253-254
Heimlich valve, 661f
Heinz bodies, 410-411, 411f
Hektoen enteric agar, 493t-494t
Hemangiosarcoma, 711t
Hematemesis, 689
Hematochezia, 690
Hematology, 399-417
  automated analyzers, 400-401
  in birds, 816-817, 816f
  blood collection tubes, 399t
  complete blood count, 399, 399t
  hemoglobin concentration, 401
  in horses, 744-745
  packed cell volume, 399-401,
    401f
  plasma protein concentration,
    402, 403f
  platelet count, 404
  red blood cell count, 401
  red blood cell indices, 399,
    401-402, 402b
  red cell distribution width, 402
  white blood cell count, 403-404,
    404f
Hematuria, 430
Heme, 432-433
Hemocytometer, 403
Hemoglobin concentration, 401
Hemoglobinuria, 430, 431b, 735

Hemolymphatic diseases
   in ruminants, 762-763
   in small animals, 727-728
Hemolysis, 896-897
   alpha-, 497f
   characteristics of, 426
   in venipuncture, 600
   virulence and, 497
Hemolytic anemia, immune-
      mediated, 700
Hemoptysis, 684
Hemostasis, 417, 1196-1197, 1196f
Hemostatic forceps, 1139-1140,
      1139f-1140f
Heparinized samples, 426
Hepatic encephalopathy, 691-693,
      1024
Hepatic lipidosis
   in camelids, 782
   feline, 693, 694t
Hepatitis, chronic, 683t, 693-694,
      694t
Hepatobiliary system
   diseases of, 689-695, 707t
   functions of, 693t
Hepatoprotectants, 1023-1024
Herbal medicine, 850-853
   acupuncture versus, 852
   administration of, 851
   ayurvedic herbs, 852-853, 853t
   Chinese, 851-852, 852t
   definition of, 850
   ingredients, 852, 852t
   regulation of, 851
   Western herbs, 851, 851f, 852t
Herd health history, 245-246
Hermaphroditic flukes, 441
Hernia
   acquired body wall, 1266
   definition of, 1247
   diaphragmatic, 686t-687t,
      1248-1249, 1249f
   in horses, 1264-1266
   inguinal, 1247, 1264-1266
   scrotal, 1266
   umbilical, 1247, 1247f, 1293
Hertz, 551, 1323
Heterogonic life cycle, 459, 459b
Heterophils, 413, 414f-415f
Hexachlorophene, 1167
Hexametaphosphate, 1336
H-file, 1337-1338, 1338b, 1338f
High ring-bone, 1275
Hindlimb fracture, 955
Hip lifters, 963, 963f
Hiring, of employees, 59-60
Hirsutism, 1368
Histopathology, 562
Histophilus somnus, 757t,
      765t-766t
Histoplasma capsulatum, 510, 511f
History
   agent information, 244
   allergy, 225-226
   background information,
      224-243
   behavioral information
      included in, 224-225
   birds, 812-813
   chief complaint, 226, 245
   of current problem, 245
   documenting of information in,
      224
   general, 245
   geriatric cats and dogs,
      1358t-1359t
   herd health, 245-246
   household information
      included in, 225
   of large animals, 243-257, 246b

History (Continued)
   medications, 226, 245
   open-ended questions used in,
      223-224
   owner information, 244
   past pertinent, 226
   presenting complaint, 226
   preventive medicine, 224
   questions asked during, 223-224
   reproductive, 226
   reptiles, 824
   sample, 225f
   signalment
      in large animals, 244
      in small animals, 224
   of small animals, 223-226, 227b
   systems review, 226
   treatment, 245
   urolithiasis, 967
   veterinary technician's role in,
      223-224
Hobbles, 197-198, 988, 991f
Hog snare, 207, 207f
Hohmann retractor, 1140
Holistic, 846
Holistic pet foods, 307
Hollow organ surgery, 1208-1209,
      1209f
Homeopathy, 846, 853-858
   applications of, 856-857, 857t
   classical, 857
   definition of, 853
   history of, 853-855
   modern, 857
   potencies, 856
   practice of, 855-857
   preparations, 856, 856f, 856t
   principles of, 853-855
   remedies, 856, 856t
   scientific research on, 857
Home-prepared pet food, 313-317,
      847
Homogonic life cycle, 459
Homotoxicology, 853-858, 857t
Hoof
   care of, 285
   cleaning of, 285
   diseases of, 1283-1286, 1284f
   interdigital hyperplasia of,
      1283-1284, 1284f
   regional analgesia of, 1283
   trimming of, 288, 878. See also
      Foot trimming
Hoof cast, 1284
Hookworms
   Ancylostoma caninum, 455-457,
      455f
   prevention of, 275t
   in puppies, 442b
Hopping reflex, 791b
Horizontal bone loss, 1334-1335
Hormones, 145t-146t, 368
Horse(s). See also Mare; Stallion;
      specific equine entries
   abdomen in
      exploration of, 948-949
      palpation of, per rectum, 947
      radiography of, 948
      ultrasound of, 947
   abdominocentesis in, 665-668,
      947
      18- to 22-gauge × 1.5-inch
         needle method, 666-667
      18-gauge × 3.5-inch spinal
         needle method, 667
      indications for, 746
      supplies for, 945b, 948f
      teat cannula method, 665-666
   aged, 1368
   aggression by, 172, 190-191

Horse(s) (Continued)
   analgesics in, 1067t-1068t
   anesthesia in, 1118-1122
      caudal epidural, 1268, 1268f
      general anesthesia, 1261
      induction of, 1119-1120,
         1119b, 1261
      maintenance of, 1119b,
         1120-1121
      physical status considerations,
         1119t
      preanesthetic period, 1119
      protocol for, 1118-1119,
         1119b
      recovery of, 1121-1122, 1121f
      sequence of events for, 1118b
   approaching, 190, 191f
   arterial blood sample collection
      in, 652-654, 653f
   arthritis in, 1275
   arthrocentesis in, 956
   arytenoid chondritis, 1277-1278
   atrioventricular block in, 250
   auscultations in
      abdomen, 251-252, 252b,
         252f
      heart, 248f, 250-251,
         250f-251f
      lung, 251, 251f
   bandages for, 994-1002, 995f
   behavior modification
      techniques in, 172b
   binocular vision of, 190
   blind spots for, 190
   blood collection in, 901b
   blood sample collection in
      arterial, 652-654, 653f
      venous, 644-645, 644f
   blood transfusion in, 903-904,
      903b
   body condition score of,
      359-361, 360t-361t, 1368
   body temperature of, 247-248,
      247f-248f, 248t, 722b
   brachial artery in, 653-654
   breeding season for, 384
   bronchoalveolar lavage in, 664f
   capillary refill time in, 253
   capture of, 192-194, 192f-193f
   carotid artery in, 652
   castration of, 170, 1267-1268,
      1267f
   casts for, 994-1002
      application of, 997-1002,
         998f-1001f
      bottom of, 1002, 1002f
      fiberglass, 997-998, 1001
      foot preparation, 998
      orthopedic felt application,
         1000, 1000f
      removal of, 1002, 1003f
      stockinette placement,
         998-999, 999f-1000f
      support foam, 1000, 1000f
   catheterization of
      arterial blood sample
         collection, 654
      in facial artery, 1121f
      intravenous drug
         administration, 625-627,
         626f
      urinary, 654-655, 656f
   cerebrospinal fluid collection in,
      669-671
   colic in, 944-945, 945b, 946f,
      1072b, 1263-1264
   communication by, 164-168,
      165f-166f
   conjunctiva examination in,
      253f

Horse(s) (Continued)
   dehydration in, 253
   dental care in, 284-285
   deworming of, 284
   diseases and conditions that
      affect, 722-737
      anaplasmosis, 728
      atrial fibrillation, 727
      bacterial pneumonia,
         723t-724t, 726-727,
         740b-741b
      botulism, 735
      brain disorders. See Brain,
         disorders of
      cardiovascular, 727, 1370
      choke, 731-732
      chronic, 1371-1375
      colic. See Colic
      colitis, 728-730, 729t-731t,
         730f
      colonic ulcers, 728
      corneal ulcers, 737, 737f
      culicoides hypersensitivity,
         736
      Cushing's disease, 1371-1372,
         1372b-1373b
      dermatologic, 736-737
      equine degenerative
         myelopathy, 735
      equine infectious anemia,
         727-728
      equine protozoal myelitis,
         734
      equine recurrent uveitis, 737
      gastric ulcers, 728
      gastrointestinal, 728-732
      gastrointestinal neoplasia,
         732
      guttural pouch empyema,
         722-724, 1278
      guttural pouch mycosis,
         722-725, 1278
      guttural pouch tympany, 725,
         1278
      heaves, 723t-724t, 726,
         742-744, 1372-1373
      hemolymphatic, 727-728
      herpesvirus, 723t-724t,
         725-726, 734-735
      inflammatory airway disease,
         723t-724t, 726
      laminitis, 769, 769b, 769f,
         1064t-1065t, 1273-1275,
         1274f, 1370, 1370f, 1373
      liver disease, 732
      lower airway disease, 725f
      Lyme disease, 728
      lymphosarcoma, 732
      melanoma, 736-737
      neurologic, 732-735
      ophthalmologic, 737
      pleuropneumonia, 726-727
      Potomac horse fever,
         277t-283t, 283,
         729t-730t, 730
      rain rot, 736
      respiratory, 722-727,
         723t-724t, 1370
      ringworm, 736
      sarcoid, 736
      second-degree
         atrioventricular block,
         727
      skull fractures, 733
      spinal cord disorders,
         734-735
      strangles. See Strangles
      temporohyoid
         osteoarthropathy,
         733-734

Horse(s) (Continued)
  tetanus, 735
    urinary tract, 735-736
    vertebral fracture, 735
    viral arteritis, 723t-724t, 727
    wobbler syndrome, 734
  distal forelimb fracture in, 954, 954f
  distal hindlimb fracture in, 955
  distal to mid forelimb fracture in, 954-955
  distal to mid hindlimb fracture in, 955
  dominance hierarchy of, 168
  dorsal displacement of the soft palate in, 1276-1277
  dorsal metatarsal artery in, 652-653, 653f
  dystocia in, 1269
  ears of, 164, 165f-166f
  elbow fracture in, 955
  emergencies and emergency nursing in, 944-957
    gastrointestinal, 944-949
      abdominal exploration, 948-949
      abdominal palpation per rectum, 947
      abdominal radiography, 948
      abdominal ultrasound, 947
      colic, 944-945, 945b
      conditions, 948
      lesions, 948b
      nasogastric intubation, 946-947, 946t
    musculoskeletal
      arthrocentesis, 956
      description of, 953-957, 1269-1270
      fractures, 954-955
      soft tissue injuries, 955-957
    physical examination, 945-946, 945b
    respiratory
      description of, 949
      lower airway endoscopy, 950
      oxygen administration, 951-952
      physical examination of, 949-950
      radiography of, 950
      thoracic ultrasound, 950
      thoracocentesis, 950-951
      tracheotomy, 952-953
      transtracheal wash, 951
      upper airway endoscopy, 950
    types of, 944
  endotracheal intubation in, 1099-1100, 1100f
  epidural administration in, 640, 640f
  extubation in, 1122
  facial artery in, 249f, 652, 653f
  fasting in, 1078t
  flehmen response in, 167, 169, 383f
  flexural limb deformities in, 1272, 1272f
  flight zone of, 192
  foot-stomping by, 164
  fractures in, 954-955
  gestation in, nutrition during, 361-362
  grooming by, 167-168, 168f
  guttural pouch tympany, 725, 1278

Horse(s) (Continued)
  heart auscultation in, 248f, 250-251, 250f-251f
  heart rate in, 248t, 250-251, 1104t
  height measurements in, 253-254
  herd behavior of, 164, 190f
  hernia repair in, 1264-1266
  hierarchy of, 168, 190
  hospitalized, 737-747
    analgesics for, 744
    anorexia in, 742-744
    antimicrobials for, 744
    bacterial culture and susceptibility testing in, 746
    blood gas analysis in, 745
    body fluid evaluations, 746
    corticosteroids for, 744
    endotoxemia, 742, 743f
    feeding of, 742-744
    hematology studies, 744-745
    isolation procedures for, 739, 742b
    laboratory studies, 744-747
    lactate studies, 745
    monitoring of, 737-744
    polymerase chain reaction testing in, 746-747
    pressure sores in, 739-742
    recumbency, 738t-739t, 739-742
    serum chemistry panel for, 745
    technician evaluations and interventions for, 738t-739t
    therapeutics for, 744
    urinalysis in, 746
  hyperthyroidism in, 1021t
  infundibular decay in, 1354, 1354b
  intradermal administration in, 636
  intramuscular administration in
    gluteal muscles, 632, 633f
    lateral cervical muscles, 631, 631f
    pectoral muscles, 632, 632f
    semimembranosus/ semitendinosus muscles, 631, 632f
  intraperitoneal administration in, 636, 637f
  intravenous administration in, 624-627
    catheterization, 625-627, 626f, 744
    cephalic vein, 627, 627f
    jugular vein, 625
    lateral thoracic vein, 627
    restraint for, 624
  juvenile, 193. See also Foal(s)
  kicking by, 172, 190
  lactation in, nutrition during, 361-362
  lameness in, 863b-864b
  laminitis in, 1273-1275, 1274f, 1370, 1370f, 1373
  limb deformities in
    angular, 1272b, 1273, 1273f
    flexural, 1272, 1272f
  lower limb support bandage for, 996
  lower limb wound bandage for, 995
  lung auscultation in, 251, 251f
  maintenance, 359-361
  mandible in, 1351-1352

Horse(s) (Continued)
  maneuvering around, 190, 191f
  maternal behavior by, 170-171
  mid forelimb fracture in, 955, 955f
  mid hindlimb fracture in, 955
  mucous membranes of, 252-253, 253f
  nasogastric intubation in, 622-624, 622f, 946-947, 946t
  necropsy examination of, 580
  nicker by, 165-166
  nonsteroidal anti-inflammatory drugs in, 1067t-1068t
  nutrition for, 359-365
    age-specific, 364t
    energy, 359-362
    forage, 359
    during gestation and lactation, 361-362
    maintenance horses, 359-361
    minerals, 361
    protein, 361-362
    during sickness, 365
    vitamins, 361
    water, 359
    working horses, 363-365
  odor recognition by, 167
  olfaction sense of, 167
  opioids in, 1067t-1068t
  oral administration in, 620-621, 620f
  osteochondrosis in, 1275, 1276f
  ovary in, 381f
  pain management in, 1064t-1065t, 1067t-1068t, 1071
  palmar artery in, 653
  pawing by, 164, 171
  periodontal disease in, 1353-1354
  personal safety during, 192
  phalangeal fractures in, 1269-1270, 1270f
  physical examination of, 246-248, 275, 945-946, 945b
    abdominal auscultation, 251-252, 252b, 252f
    body temperature, 247-248, 247f-248f
    geriatric patients, 1368
    heart auscultation, 248f, 250-251, 250f-251f
    heart rate in, 248-250, 248t
    height measurements, 253-254
    hydration status, 253
    mucous membranes, 252-253, 253f
    preventive health purposes of, 275
    pulse rate, 248-250, 248f-249f, 248t
    rectal thermometers for, 247-248, 247f-248f
    respiratory rate, 250
    weight measurements, 253-254
  pneumothorax in, 949
  preventive health programs for, 275-285
    dental care, 284-285
    hoof care, 285
    nutrition, 285
    outline of, 276b
    parasites, 284
    physical examination, 275
  prey behavior, 168-169
  problem behaviors in, 171-172

Horse(s) (Continued)
  aggression, 172, 190-191
  cribbing, 171-172
    human-directed aggression, 172
    inter-horse aggression, 172
    kicking, 172, 190
    repetitive behaviors, 171-172
    stable vices, 171-172
  proximal forelimb fracture in, 955
  proximal hindlimb fracture in, 955
  pulse rate in, 248-250, 248f-249f, 248t, 722b
  rectal thermometer insertion in, 247-248, 247f-248f
  recumbency, 738t-739t, 739-742, 742f-743f
  reproduction in. See Reproduction, equine
  reproductive tract examination in, 385-386
  respiratory rate in, 248t, 250, 722b
  restraint of. See Restraint, of horses
  senses of, 164-168
  serum in, 747b
  sick, feeding of, 365
  skin of, 167-168
  skull fractures in, 733
  snapping by, 164
  social behavior in, 168
  splints for, 994-1002, 998f
  squeal by, 166
  striking by, 190
  subcutaneous administration in, 634, 635f
  subsolar abscess in, 1275-1276
  surgery and surgical nursing in
    abdominal, 1263-1264
    angular limb deformities, 1272b, 1273, 1273f
    arthritis, 1275
    arthroscopic, 1271-1276, 1271f
    case study of, 1264b-1265b
    castration, 1267-1268, 1267f
    cesarean delivery, 1269, 1269b
    for dystocia, 1269
    fasting before, 1261
    gastrointestinal tract, 1263-1266, 1263f
    hernia repair, 1264-1266
    intraoperative nursing, 1261-1262
    laminitis, 1273-1275, 1274f
    limb surgery, 1263
    orthopedic, 1269-1276
    osteochondrosis, 1275, 1276f
    ovariectomy, 1268
    pain caused by, 1066t
    patent urachus, 1266
    perineal surgery, 1268-1269, 1268f
    postoperative nursing, 1262-1263
    preoperative preparation, 1261
    septic arthritis, 1276
    subsolar abscess, 1275-1276
    tendonitis, 1275
    umbilical repair, 1266
    upper respiratory tract, 1276-1278
    urinary calculi, 1266
    urogenital tract, 1266-1269
  tail positions associated with, 167f

Horse(s) (Continued)
  tapeworms in, 475f
  teeth in, 284-285, 1351, 1351f
  tendonitis in, 1275
  terminology associated with, 244t
  thoracocentesis in, 660-661, 950-951
  transtracheal wash in, 662-663, 663f, 951
  transverse facial artery in, 249, 652, 653f
  transverse facial vein in, 644, 645f
  urinary calculi in, 735-736, 1266
  urinary catheterization in, 654-655, 656f
  venipuncture in
    cephalic vein, 644-645, 646f
    jugular vein, 644, 644f
    saphenous vein, 645
    transverse facial vein, 644, 645f
  vision of, 164, 190, 1369
  vocalizations by, 165-166
  water for, 359
  weight measurements in, 253-254, 255f, 359-361
  wood chewing by, 171
  working, 363-365
  wound care in, 993-994, 994f
Horse Protection Act, 35
Hospice/hospice care
  of cats and dogs, 1363-1366
  definition of, 1356
  nursing care, 1363
Hospital
  cleanliness of, 44
  definition of, 40b
  design of, 45
  examination rooms, 46, 47f
  grooming services, 50
  inpatient areas in, 47-50, 48f
  isolation ward in, 49
  laboratories in, 47, 47f
  management of, 14
  outpatient areas in, 45-47, 45f
  pharmacy areas in, 47, 48f
  radiology suite in, 47-49, 48f
  reception area in, 46, 46f
  storage area of, 51
  support area of, 51
  surgical area of, 50-51, 51f
  treatment area in, 47, 48f
  waiting area in, 46, 46f
Hospital administrators, 41
Hospital information system, 529
Hospital Safety Manual, 117
Hospitalization
  of birds, 822-823
  of foals, 805
  of horses. See Horse(s), hospitalized
  of reptiles, 827-828
Hospitalized patient records
  cage cards, 98
  discharge instructions, 94, 98-105, 104f
  medication administration/ order record, 98, 99f-100f
  notations, 96-97
  overview of, 94-105
  SOAP notes, 94-96, 95f
  summary forms, 98-105
Hostile work environment, 34
House call services, 51
House soiling
  in cats, 161-164, 162t
  in dogs, 154

House training, 155b
Howell-Jolly bodies, 411-412
Human resources, 59-62
  compensation determinations by, 60
  definition of, 59-62
  hiring, 59-60
  management of employees by, 60-61
  retention of employees by, 60-61
  stress management role of, 61-62
  training and orientation of employees by, 60
Human resources manager, 41
Human-animal bond, 1378-1385
Human-directed aggression, 172, 174-175
Humane Methods of Slaughter Act, 35-36
Humane twitch, 194-195, 196f
Humoral theory, of acupuncture, 859
Husbandry, 1071
Hutch, 201, 201f
Hyaline casts, 433, 435f
Hybridomas, 512
Hydralazine, 1026
Hydration status, 253
Hydrochlorothiazide, 1025, 1025t
Hydrogen peroxide
  description of, 498b
  gas plasma sterilization, 1166
Hydrolyzable carbohydrates, 342
Hydrometra, 1235
Hydromorphone, 1058
Hydronephrosis, 582
Hydrophilic drugs, 1011
Hydrotherapy, 867-868, 868f
Hyoid bones, 573
Hyperadrenocorticism, 683t, 699, 1021, 1361
Hyperalgesia, 1052-1053
Hyperbilirubinemia, 747b
Hyperechoic, 554
Hyperemia, 232, 235
Hyperglycemia, stress-induced, 698
Hyperkalemia, 892, 932, 967-968
Hypernatremia, 883-884
Hyperproteinemia, 425
Hypersensitivity reactions, 715-716
Hypertension, systemic, 689
Hyperthermia
  description of, 229-230
  technician evaluation of, 675t-679t
Hyperthyroidism, 683t, 698, 1020, 1021t, 1361
Hypertonic crystalloids, 884, 885t
Hypertrophic cardiomyopathy, 683t, 688, 1360
Hypervitaminosis A, 300-301
Hypoadrenocorticism, 683t, 699, 1021
Hypoalbuminemia, 425
Hypobiosis, 453, 453b
Hypocalcemia, periparturient, 761
Hypochromic, 402
Hypoglossal nerve, 243t
Hypoglycemia
  in kittens, 794
  in lambs, 749-750
  in puppies, 794
  treatment of, 794
Hypokalemia, 892
Hypomagnesemia, 339t-340t
Hypotension, 1120, 1128

Hypothalamic-pituitary-adrenal axis, 151
Hypothermia
  anesthesia-related, 1106
  definition of, 1217-1218
  description of, 229-230
  in kittens, 793
  in lambs, 749-750
  in puppies, 793
  in surgery, 1217-1218, 1217f-1218f
  technician evaluation of, 675t-679t
  treatment of, 793
Hypothyroidism, 683t, 698, 1020, 1021t, 1361
Hypotonic fluids, 883-884
Hypoventilation, 1098, 1105-1106, 1120, 1128
Hypovolemia, 230
  dehydration versus, 912
  technician evaluation of, 675t-679t, 738t-739t
  treatment of, 912
Hypovolemic shock, 915
Hypoxemia, 685, 908-909, 913
Hypoxia
  description of, 685, 915-916, 1098
  technician evaluation of, 675t-679t, 738t-739t

I

Icterus, 232, 232f, 252-253
Idiopathic, 681
Idiopathic aggression, 153b
Idiopathic megacolon, 683t
Idiosyncratic drug reactions, 1016, 1016t
Iguanas, 216-217, 217f, 829
Ileitis, 775t
Ileus, 946, 1229
Iliac bone marrow aspiration, 617-619, 618f
Illegal professional acts, 30
Imidacloprid, 1030t
Immune system, 792b
Immune-mediated diseases
  definition of, 700
  drugs for, 1016-1017
  myasthenia gravis, 701
  in small animals, 700-701
Immune-mediated hemolytic anemia, 405-406, 407b, 700, 898
Immunoradiometric assay, 429
Immunosuppressive drugs, 1016-1017, 1017t, 1349
Implants
  orthopedic. See Orthopedic implants
  surgical, 1199-1200, 1199f-1200f
Import Drug Act, 1031
Impression smears, 419, 419f
Impressions, 1345-1346, 1345f-1346f
Imprint training, 170-171
Incision
  celiotomy, 1220f
  complications of, 1220-1221
  dehiscence of, 1219
  healed, 1221f
  postoperative evaluation of, 1219-1221, 1220f-1221f
  swelling of, 1220f-1221f
Incisive papilla, 1309, 1309b
Incisors, 1302
Income statement, 68-69

Incompetence, 32
Incontinence, 1360, 1365
Indigenous flora, 484, 485t
Indole test media, 493t-494t
Infections
  community-acquired, 514
  nosocomial, 514-515
    agents of, 515
    bacteria associated with, 515
    control of, 515
    definition of, 44b, 514
    description of, 484
    pathogen transmission methods, 515
    prevention of, 44b
    recognition of, 515
    sources of, 44b
    viruses as cause of, 515
  risk for, 680t
  steps of, 701-704, 704f
  wound, 978, 978b
Infectious bovine keratoconjunctivitis, 287-288, 767-768, 768f
Infectious bovine rhinotracheitis, 286-287, 757t
Infectious diseases, 701-705
  bacterial, 1018
  client education about, 705
  control of, 704
  definition of, 701-704
  drugs for, 1017-1018
  host susceptibility to, 704
  isolation facilities and procedures for, 704-705, 742b
  nursing care for, 705
  risk for, 680t
  in small animals, 705, 706t-710t
  transmissible, 704
  vector-borne, 704, 709t
Inferior alveolar nerve block, 1332, 1333f
Inflammatory airway disease, 723t-724t, 726
Inflammatory bowel disease, 683t, 692t
Informed consent, 83-84
Infraorbital nerve block, 1332, 1333f
Infundibular decay, 1354, 1354b
Ingredient statement, 312
Inguinal hernia, 1247, 1264-1266
Inguinal lymph nodes, 240-241
Inhalant anesthetics, 827, 1086-1087, 1393t-1395t
Inhibin, 388
In-hospital triage, 908-911
Injection site sarcoma, 711t
Inoculation, of culture media, 495-496, 495f-496f, 502f
Inotropic agents, 1025
Inpatient areas, 47-50, 48f
Insect growth regulators, 1030t
Insecticides, 124
Insoluble fiber, 294, 300
In-standing mandibular canine teeth, 1347
Institutional Animal Care and Use Committees, 35
Instrument(s)
  dental, 1326-1327, 1327f
  endodontics, 1337-1338, 1337b
  surgical. See Surgical instruments
Instrument packs, 1155-1157, 1156t, 1163t
Instrumental conditioning, 137-138
Insufflator, 1155, 1155f

Insulin, 1022-1023, 1023t
Insurance, 72-73
　　large animal, 244
　　loss of use, 244
　　mortality, 244
　　surgical, 244
Insurance examination, 246
Integumentary system, 240, 240f
Intensifying screens, 533-534, 533f
Interceptive orthodontics, 1346-1347, 1346f
Interdigital hyperplasia, 1283-1284, 1284f
Interdigital necrobacillosis, 768-769, 768f
Inter-dog aggression, 153b
Interleukin-1 receptor antagonist protein, 1275
Interlocking nails, 1146
Intermittent mandatory ventilation, 1126
Intermittent reinforcement, 138
Internal marketing, 63-66
Internal parasites, 125
International Renal Interest Society, 695-696
International Veterinary Acupuncture Society, 858
Intervertebral disc fenestration, 1253
Intervertebral disc rupture, 1253
Intestinal tract dissection, 577
Intracellular fluid, 883
Intradermal administration
　　in large animals, 635-636, 636f
　　in small animals, 589
Intramammary administration, 638
Intramedullary pins, 1145-1146
Intramuscular administration
　　advantages of, 630
　　anesthetic induction, 1116
　　in bovine, 632-633
　　in camelids, 634, 634f
　　in cattle, 632-633
　　in goats, 633, 633f
　　in horses
　　　　gluteal muscles, 632, 633f
　　　　lateral cervical muscles, 631, 631f
　　　　pectoral muscles, 632, 632f
　　　　semimembranosus/ semitendinosus muscles, 631, 632f
　　in large animals, 630-634
　　in pigs, 633-634
　　procedure for, 630
　　in sheep, 633, 633f
　　in small animals, 590
　　in swine, 633-634
Intraoral examination, 1309-1315, 1309f-1311f
Intraoral film, 1317, 1317f
Intraosseous administration
　　in birds, 818, 818f
　　of fluids, 890-891
　　sites for, 599
　　in small animals, 599
Intraperitoneal administration
　　in bovine, 637
　　in goats, 637
　　in horses, 636, 637f
　　in large animals, 636-638
　　in pigs, 638
　　in sheep, 637
　　in small animals, 599
Intrarectal administration
　　enema, 642
　　in large animals, 641-642
　　in small animals, 588-589

Intrasynovial administration, 641
Intratracheal administration, 598-599
Intravenous administration
　　access devices for, 591, 591f
　　analgesics, 1057
　　anesthetic induction, 1115-1116, 1119-1120
　　in bovine
　　　　auricular vein, 628
　　　　catheterization, 628, 628b, 628f
　　　　cephalic vein, 628
　　　　coccygeal vein, 627-628, 628f
　　　　jugular vein, 627
　　　　subcutaneous abdominal vein, 628
　　in camelids, 628-629
　　catheterization
　　　　in bovine, 628, 628b, 628f
　　　　in camelids, 629
　　　　complications of, 629
　　　　in goats, 629
　　　　in horses, 625-627, 626f, 744
　　　　in pigs, 629, 630f
　　　　in sheep, 629
　　catheters
　　　　aseptic technique with, 887-888
　　　　central line, 887
　　　　central venous, 889
　　　　chemotherapy agents, 597
　　　　flushing of, 596
　　　　in horses, 625-627, 626f
　　　　in jugular vein, 594-596, 595f
　　　　maintenance of, 596
　　　　monitoring of, 889
　　　　multi-lumen, 591, 591f, 887, 887f
　　　　observation of, 596
　　　　over-the-needle, 591, 591f, 610f
　　　　in peripheral vein, 591-594
　　　　placement of, 591-596
　　　　through-the-needle, 591, 591f
　　　　types of, 591
　　　　winged needle, 591, 591f
　　chemotherapy agents, 596-598, 597f-598f
　　in coccygeal vein, 627-628, 628f
　　in dogs, 590
　　of fluids, 887-890
　　in foals, 805-806, 805f
　　in goats, 629
　　in horses, 624-627
　　　　catheterization, 625-627, 626f
　　　　cephalic vein, 627, 627f
　　　　jugular vein, 625
　　　　lateral thoracic vein, 627
　　　　restraint for, 624
　　jugular vein
　　　　in bovine, 627
　　　　catheter placement in, 594-596, 595f
　　　　in horses, 625
　　peripheral vein, 591-594
　　in pigs, 629, 630f
　　in sheep, 629
　　sites for, 590
　　in small animals, 590
　　in swine, 629, 630f
　　technique for, 590b
Intravenous pyelogram, 549
Intrinsic pathway, 417
Intubation
　　in birds, 817-818
　　nasogastric. See Nasogastric intubation
　　orogastric. See Orogastric intubation

Inventory
　　computer management of, 78
　　management of, 73-75, 78
　　theft of, 74
Iodine, 303t, 304, 345t-346t, 1166
Iodophors, 1166
Ionizing radiation, 714
IRMA. See Immunoradiometric assay
Iron, 303-304, 303t, 345t-346t
Iron deficiency anemia, 357b
Iron dextran, 771-772, 771f
Irritable aggression, 153b, 160
Isoechoic, 554
Isoerythrolysis, neonatal, 794, 803b
Isoflurane, 826, 826t, 1086, 1093-1094
Isolation
　　of hospitalized horses, 739, 742b
　　for infectious diseases, 704-705
　　ward for, 49
Isopropyl alcohol, 1167t
Isospora spp., 478, 773t-774t
Isothenuria, 912
Isothenuric urine, 431
Isotonic crystalloids, 884-885, 885t, 975
Itraconazole, 1016t, 1020t
Ivermectin, 284
Ixodes scapularis, 467t

J

Jackson-Pratt drain, 1200f
Jacobs hand chuck, 1145-1146, 1147f
Jacobson's organ, 167
Jamshidi needles, 1145
Jaw fractures, 1340, 1350-1351, 1350f
Jejunostomy tubes, 332-334
Jewelry, 19-20
Job description, 40, 59
Job opportunities, 5-6, 5t
Johne's disease
　　case study of, 756b
　　in cattle, 288, 756, 756b, 756f
　　description of, 751t-752t
Joint diseases
　　osteoarthritis, 701
　　in small animals, 701
Joint fluid
　　analysis of
　　　　in cats, 616
　　　　in dogs, 616
　　collection of
　　　　in cats, 614-616, 614f
　　　　description of, 489
　　　　in dogs, 614-616, 614f
　　　　gross appearance of, 616
Joint luxations, 962-963
Joint supplements, 1067t-1068t, 1070
Joint surgery, in small animals, 1257
Joules, 1131
Jugular veins
　　in birds, 816, 816f
　　distended, 237
　　physical examination of, 237
Jugular venipuncture
　　in bovine, 645, 646f
　　in camelids, 647, 647f
　　in cats, 601, 602f
　　in dogs, 601, 601f
　　in horses, 644, 644f
　　in pigs, 650
　　in small animals, 601, 601f-602f
　　in turtles, 826f

Junctional escape beats, 944
Junctional escape rhythms, 944
Junctional tachycardia, 940, 940f

K

Kelly forceps, 1139-1140
Kennel attendants, 43-44
Kennel cough. See Canine infectious tracheobronchitis
Kennels, 50
Keratoconjunctivitis, 767-768, 768f
Keratocytes, 409-410, 409f-410f
Kern bone-holding forceps, 1144, 1145f
Kerr file, 1337-1338
Kerrison rongeurs, 1143, 1144f
Ketamine, 826t-827t, 833, 1059-1060, 1067t-1068t, 1071, 1084, 1114b, 1116
Ketoconazole, 1013, 1016t, 1020t
Ketones, 432, 761
Ketonuria, 432, 699
Ketoprofen, 1067t-1069t
Ketosis, 339t-340t, 761, 761f
Key elevator, 1144f
Key performance indicators, 69-70, 70b
K-file, 1337-1338, 1338f
Kicking
　　by cows, 190
　　by horses, 172, 190
Kid(s). See also Goats
　　definition of, 391
　　dehorning of, 1295
　　disbudding of, 1295, 1296f
　　diseases and conditions that affect, 749-750
　　as hiders, 174
　　subcutaneous administration in, 635f
Kidney(s)
　　acute renal failure, 735
　　aging changes in, 1015
　　development of, 792b
　　necropsy examination of, 577, 577f
　　palpation of, 238
Kidney disease
　　chronic, 695-696, 695b, 695t-696t
　　in geriatric patients
　　　　cats and dogs, 1360
　　　　horses, 1359
　　pharmacokinetics affected by, 1015
Kilocalorie, 295, 295b
Kilojoule, 295
Kilovoltage, 520, 530, 540
Kimsey splint, 1269-1270, 1270f
Kingman tube, 959-960, 960f
Kinyoun's modified Ziehl-Nielsen acid-fast stain, 492, 492b
Kirby-Bauer method, 506, 506b
Kirschner wires, 1145-1146
Kitchen, 50, 50f
Kittens. See also Cat(s)
　　Ancylostoma caninum in, 457b
　　ascarids in, 454b
　　body temperature in, 789-790
　　colostrum for, 325
　　death of, 795
　　dehydration in, 793-794, 794b
　　development of, 155-156, 790-791, 792b
　　energy of, 325
　　fading kitten syndrome, 795
　　fat requirements of, 326

Kittens (Continued)
  feeding of, 325-327, 794-795, 795t
  hypothermia in, 793
  milk replacers for, 325, 327f, 797t
  neonatal care of. See Neonatal care, of kittens
  neonatal isoerythrolysis in, 794
  neurologic examination in, 791b
  nutritional requirements, 795t, 796b
  overfeeding of, 796-797
  play by, 156
  protein requirements of, 325
  sex determination in, 790
  socialization of, 156
  weaning of, 325
  wellness visits for, 260-262
Kleiber-Brody equation, 296-297
Köhler illumination, 490
Krey-hook, 965
Kübler-Ross, Elisabeth, 1381-1382
Kussmaul's breathing, 909

L

Labor laws, 34
Laboratories
  quality assurance in, 509
  quality control testing, 509
  in small animal practices, 47, 47f
  uniforms worn in, 19
  veterinary technician's responsibilities, 11, 11f
Laboratory animal technicians, 17
Laboratory diagnostic flow sheet, 91
Labored breathing, 908-909
Lacerations, 955, 978, 1279
Lactate, 745, 893-894
Lactation
  in dogs, 323-324
  feeding during, 323-324
Lactic acidosis, 753-754
Lactobacillus spp., 753
Lactulose, 1024
Lamb(s). See also Sheep
  definition of, 245t
  diseases and conditions that affect, 749-750
  entropion in, 1295f
  ewe-lamb bond, 749, 750b
  feeding of, 356, 749-750
  as followers, 174
  milk replacers for, 749-750
  nutrition for, 356
  weaning of, 356
Lambing
  definition of, 389
  paralysis during, 354
Lameness
  in cattle, 204, 1283
  in horses, 863b-864b
  in ruminants, 767
Lamina dura, 1320
Laminitis, 769, 769b, 769f, 1064t-1065t, 1273-1275, 1274f, 1370, 1370f, 1373
Land treadmill, 868
Langer curettes, 1329
Laparoscope, 1154
Laparoscopic instruments, 1154-1155, 1156f, 1168-1169

Laparotomy
  aftercare following, 1282
  description of, 1198, 1230, 1280f
  exploratory, 1282
Laptop computers, 111-112
Large animal(s). See also Beef cattle; Bovine; Camelids; Cattle; Dairy cattle; Horse(s)
  carbohydrates for, 342-343
  euthanasia of, 1396
  facilities for
    examination areas, 53, 53f
    haul-in, 52-54, 53f
    inpatient treatment areas, 53
    mobile units, 52
    necropsy area, 54
    surgical room, 54, 54f
    traffic flow patterns, 54
    treatment areas, 53
  fats for, 342
  fecal sample collection in, 657-658
  hazards associated with, 123
  history of, 243-257, 246b
  insurance status of, 244
  intradermal administration in, 635-636, 636f
  intranasal administration in, 638
  minerals for, 343
  nutrients for, 340-343
  orogastric intubation in, 624, 624f
  physical examination of, 246-257, 254b
  protein for, 341-342
  subcutaneous administration in, 634-635, 635f
  terminology associated with, 244t-245t
  thoracocentesis/thoracentesis in, 660-662
  topical ophthalmic administration in, 638-639, 639f
  transtracheal wash in, 662-663
  vitamins for, 343
Large animal practices
  client service attributes of, 55
  medical records used in, 112, 112f
Large granular lymphocytes, 416
Large intestine
  contrast agents used in radiography of, 548-549
  diarrhea of, 690t
  palpation of, 238
Larval cyathostomiasis, 729t-730t
Larval migrans, 125
Laryngeal hemiplegia, 1276
Laryngeal paralysis, 234-235, 686t-687t
Laryngeal ventricles, 1276-1277
Laryngoscopes, 1087, 1089f
Laryngospasm, 1101
Larynx, 573, 573f
Laser(s)
  CO$_2$, 1132, 1133f
  definition of, 1131
  diode, 1132-1133, 1134f
  eye protection for, 1135
  hazard classification for, 1134, 1135t
  low-level therapy, 874, 874f
  Nd:YAG, 1132-1133
  onychectomy performed using, 1226, 1226f
  plume control, 1135-1136, 1136f

Laser(s) (Continued)
  properties of, 1131
  safety of, 1133-1136, 1135f-1136f, 1136b
  thermal damage caused by, 1131
  tissue effects of, 1131
  types of, 1132-1133, 1133f
Laser acupuncture, 860, 860f
L-Asparaginase, 1028t-1029t
Latent thermal damage, 1131
Lateral cervical muscles, 631, 631f
Latitude, 540
Lavender, 854t-855t
Laws
  animal-related, 35-36
  Canada, 36
  Endangered Species Act, 35
  Horse Protection Act, 35
Lawsonia intracellulans, 775t
L-carnitine, 295, 336
Lead apron, 545, 545f
Lead gloves, 545, 545f
Lead (rope), 192, 192f, 194
Leadership, 116-117
Learned helplessness, 139
Learning
  associative, 137
  methods of, 136-139
  operant, 138-139, 138t
Leash walking, 151
Left displaced abomasum, 1281-1282
Left laryngeal hemiplegia, 1276, 1277b
Legal document, medical record as, 82
Legend drug, 1031-1032
Lemon, 854t-855t
Leptocytes, 409
Leptospira interrogans, 268t-269t
Leptospirosis, 272-273, 707t-708t, 710t, 777
Lesions
  brainstem, 732
  definition of, 562
Leukocyte casts, 433, 435f
Leukocytes, 433
Leukoencephalomalacia, 733
Levothyroxine, 1017t
Levy-Jennings chart, 428, 428f
Liabilities, 68
Licensee, probation of, 33-34
License/licensure
  refusal of, 28
  renewal of, 29
  revocation of, 33
  suspension of, 33
  of veterinarian, 26-28
Licorice, 853
Lidocaine, 925t, 927, 1026, 1026t, 1055, 1060, 1067t-1069t, 1283f, 1331
Lift table, 181f
Light cable, 1149f, 1151, 1151f, 1154-1155
Light handles
  placement of, 1194
  sterile technique for, 1194f
Light projector, 1151, 1151f, 1154-1155
Limbs
  forelimb. See Forelimb
  hindlimb fracture, 955
  neurologic examination of, 242-243
Limited-grain diet, 848
Lincosamides, 1018t-1019t
Linear array transducers, 553
Linguatula serrata, 473-474, 474f
Linoleic acid, 294b, 299, 326, 342

Lipemia, 425-426
Lip/gum chain, 194, 194b, 195f
Lipids, 293-294
Lipophilic drugs, 1011
Lipoproteins, 293
Liptak test, 1282
Listening
  active, 56-57
  importance of, 56
  reflective, 56-57
Listeria monocytogenes, 503, 765t-766t, 767
Listeriosis, 765t-766t, 767, 767f
Lithotripsy, 696-697
Littauer suture removal scissors, 1136-1137, 1137f
Litter boxes, 163, 163b
Liver
  development of, 792b
  diseases of, 691-693, 732
  palpation of, 238
Liver disease
  drugs for, 1023-1024
  pharmacokinetics affected by, 1015
Livestock. See also Beef cattle; Cattle; Dairy cattle
  macrominerals for, 344t
  microminerals for, 345t-346t
Lizards
  anesthesia of, 826, 827t
  body language of, 217
  herbivorous, 829
  nutrition for, 829-832
  restraint of, 216-218, 217f
  venipuncture in, 217-218, 217f-218f
  water for, 829-832
Llamas. See also Camelids
  cerebrospinal fluid collection in, 671
  description of, 779
  gestation of, 781, 781b
  heat stress in, 781f, 782-784, 784f
  restraint of, 209-210, 210f
  subcutaneous administration in, 634f
  urine catheterization in, 655-656
Local anesthesia, 1331
  definition of, 1078
  in horses, 993
Local anesthetics
  analgesic use of, 1055-1057, 1067t-1068t, 1070
  monitoring of, 1054t
Logs, 107-109
  anesthesia, 109
  controlled substance, 109
  necropsy, 109
  purposes of, 107
  radiology, 107, 108f
  surgery, 107
Lomustine, 1028t-1029t
Long yearling, 244t
Long-bone fractures
  in horses, 1270
  in small animals, 1255-1257
"Look-up table", 527-528
Loop diuretics, 1025
Loop of Henle, 1025
Loss of pets, 1379-1385. See also Euthanasia; Grief
Loss of use insurance, 244
Lost records, 107
Low ring-bone, 1275
Lower airway disease, 725f
Lower airway endoscopy, 950
Lower limb support bandage, 996

Lower limb wound bandage, 995
Lower urinary tract disease, feline, 697-698
Low-level laser therapy, 874, 874f, 1061
Lufenuron, 1030t
Lugol's iodine, 478
Lumbar reflex, 791b
Lumbosacral epidural, 1295
Lumbosacral epidurals, 1295
Lumbosacral tap, 669-671, 670f
Lumpectomy, 1249-1250
Lung(s)
  anatomy of, 235f
  auscultation of, in horses, 251, 251f
Lung flukes, 441-443, 443f
Lung sounds, 234-235
Luteinizing hormone, 370, 377, 379
Lyme disease, 124, 709t, 728
Lymph nodes
  in dogs, 240-241, 241f
  physical examination of, 240-241
Lymphocytes, 414f-415f, 416
Lymphocytic-plasmacytic stomatitis, 1309, 1311f, 1349
Lymphocytosis, 416
Lymphoma, 711t
Lymphosarcoma, 732, 762, 762f
Lysine iron agar slant, 493t-494t

M

Ma huang, 852
Macaws. See Psittacines
MacConkey's agar plate, 493t-494t, 495, 495f, 502
Machinery safety, 119
Macrocyclic lactones, 1029-1030
Macrocytic red blood cells, 401-402
Macrolides, 1018t-1019t
Macrominerals, 302, 344t
Macronutrients, 293
Macroplatelets, 407
Magnesium, 303, 303t, 344t
Magnesium sulfate, 925t
Magnet-based therapy, 872-873
Magnetic resonance imaging, 558-560
  anesthesia for, 559-560
  description of, 558-559
  disadvantages of, 558-559
  high field strength, 559, 559f
  low field strength, 559, 559f
  magnetic field, 559-560, 560f
  safety considerations, 559-560, 560f
  veterinary technician's responsibilities, 11, 12f
Magnetostrictive scalers, 1325, 1326b
Magnification, 540-541
Magnus reflex, 791b
Maintenance nutrient requirements, 340-341
Malassezia pachydermatis, 421-422, 510, 510b, 511f
Male(s). See also Bull; Stallion
  breeding soundness examination in, 392-394
  reproduction in
    anatomy of, 370
    physiology of, 370-372, 371f
    spermatogenesis, 370, 372
    semen analysis in, 393-394
Malignant edema, 769-770

Malignant hyperthermia, 777, 1106
Malnutrition
  in kittens, 794-795
  in puppies, 794-795
  in sugar gliders, 844
Malocclusion, 1302, 1344-1345, 1344f-1345f
Malpractice, 31-32
Mammary glands
  adenocarcinoma of, 711t
  in cats, 239
  in dogs, 239
Mammary neoplasia removal, 1250-1251
Management personnel, 40-42
Mandible
  fracture of, 1279-1280, 1350-1351, 1350f
  in horses, 1351-1352
Mandibular brachygnathism, 1352-1353
Mandibular lymph nodes, 240-241, 241f
Mandibular mesioclusion, 1344-1345
Mandibular molars, 1303
Mandibulectomy, 1349
Manganese, 303t, 304, 345t-346t
Mange, sarcoptic, 125, 215b
Mannheimia haemolytica, 757t
Mannitol, 927, 1013
Manual muscle testing, 864-865
Marcaine. See Bupivacaine
Mare. See also Horse(s)
  artificial insemination of, 386
  ascending placentitis in, 797-798
  colostrum sample collection from, 659
  definition of, 244t, 380-381
  dystocia in, 1269
  estrous cycle in, 381-385
  estrus inducement in, 385
  foal rejection by, 171
  foaling by, 798-799, 799b
  gestation in, 797
  heat in, 381-383
  high-risk, 797-799, 799b
  maternal behavior of, 170-171
  milk dripping in, 797-798, 798b
  minerals for, 362
  nutrition for, 361-362
  ovariectomy in, 380-381, 1268
  ovulation by, 383-384
  parturition in, 387, 387f
  perinatal period, 797-799
  placenta in, 386
  pregnancy diagnosis in, 386
  protein for, 362
  as seasonal polyestrous, 384
  sexual behavior of, 169
  urinary catheterization in, 655, 656f
  vaginal examination in, 385-386, 386f, 798
  vitamins for, 362
  vulva conformation in, 385, 385f
Marketing, 62-68
  advertising, 66-67
  animal care talks, 66
  client education view of, 62-63
  community activities, 67
  components of, 62-63
  external, 66-68
  hand-out materials, 64-65, 64f-65f
  internal, 63-66
  newsletters, 65

Marketing (Continued)
  newspapers, 67
  pet portals, 68
  point-of-sale displays, 66, 66f
  radio advertising, 67
  targeted mail, 65-66
  television advertising, 67
  web-based, 67-68
Maropitant, 1024t
Masks
  anesthesia induction using, 1116
  oxygen therapy using, 1087-1088, 1089f
Maslow, Abraham, 96
Massage, 868-870, 869f-870f
Mast cell tumor, 711t
Mast cells, 417
Master problem list, 92-93, 93f
Masticatory myositis, 1350
Mastitis, 288
  bacterial species associated with, 486t-487t, 502b
  in bitch, 699-700
  in cattle, 758-760
  classification of, 759
  clinical, 759
  contagious, 759
  culture for, 502
  definition of, 758-759
  gangrenous, 759, 760b
  in goats, 760
  intramammary drug administration for, 638
  laboratory tests for, 758, 758f
  pain associated with, 1064t-1065t
  prevention of, 759-760
  in sheep, 760
  signs of, 699-700
  in small ruminants, 760
  subclinical, 759, 759f
  toxic, 967
  treatment of, 759
Masturbation, 170
Material safety data sheets
  definition of, 121
  illustration of, 121f
  in pharmacy area, 47
Materials storage, 118, 118f
Maternal aggression, 153b
Maternal behavior
  in cattle, 174
  in horses, 170-171
  in ruminants, 174
Maxillary molars, 1303
Maxillary nerve block, 1332-1333, 1333f
Maxillectomy, 1349
Maximum permissible dose, 543
Mayo dissecting scissors, 1136-1137, 1137f
Mayo instrument stand, 1184
Mayo-Hegar needle holder, 1137, 1137f
Mean corpuscular hemoglobin concentration, 402, 402b
Mean corpuscular volume, 402b
Mean electrical axis, 937-938
Measles virus, 268t-269t
Measurements, 1040
Meat Inspection Act, 36
Mechanical dead space, 1098
Mechanical débridement, 976b
Mechanical ventilation, 1125-1126
Mechanism of action, 1013-1014
Meconium, 799-800
Meconium retention, 803b
Medetomidine, 826t-827t, 1067t-1069t

Medial metatarsal vein, 816
Mediastinum, 574-575
Medical devices, 131t
Medical hazards, 123-126
Medical record, 20-21
  alphabetic filing of, 106
  ambulatory practices, 111-112, 111f
  business activities supported with, 82
  color-coding systems for, 106f
  communications documented using, 82
  copying of, 85
  definition of, 81
  description of, 681
  electronic. See Electronic medical records
  errors in, 84, 85b
  ethics, 83b
  filing of, 105-107
  format of, 86
  functions of, 82, 83b
  hospitalized patients. See Hospitalized patient records
  large animal practices, 112, 112f
  as legal document, 82, 84
  letter-size folders, 105, 106f
  lost, 107
  management of, 105-109
  medical care uses of, 82
  newborn, 789f
  numeric filing of, 106-107, 106f
  organization of, 105-107
  ownership of, 85
  problem-oriented. See Problem-oriented veterinary medical record
  purging of, 107
  purposes of, 82, 83b
  release of medical information from, 85
  research uses of, 82
  source-oriented, 86
Medical waste, 129-130, 131t
Medical waste management laws, 34
Medical Waste Tracking Act, 34
Medicated pet food, 309
Medication administration/order record, 98, 99f-100f
Medications
  administration of. See Drug administration
  behavior problems treated with, 144
  history-taking about, 226, 245
Medium-chain triglycerides, 298-299
Megacalories, 343
Megaesophagus, 701
Melamine, 314-315
Melanoma, 736-737
Melarsomine, 462
Melatonin, 385
Melena, 690
Meloxicam, 1067t-1069t
Menace reflex, 232, 791b
Meningeal worm, 765t-766t, 784-785, 785f
Meninges, 573-574, 574f
Meningiomas, 558f, 706
Mentation, 228, 242, 910
Mepivacaine, 1067t-1068t, 1070
Meridians, 858-859
Mesaticephalic, 1345
Mesial, 1301
Mesioclusion, 1344-1345

Metabolic bone disease, 828, 828f, 830-831
Metabolic diseases
    in camelids, 782-784
    in ruminants, 761-762
Metabolism, 1012-1013, 1012t
Metabolizable energy, 295-297, 327, 342
Metacarpophalangeal joint deformity, in horses, 1272, 1272f
Metacercariae, 443
Metacestodes
    definition of, 445, 445b
    diagnosis of, 445
Metal chelation therapy, 1024
Metallic sutures, 1202-1203
Metamyelocytes, 413
Metaphylaxis, 758
Metarubricytes, 411
Metastasis, 706
Metestrus, 388
Methimazole, 1016t, 1020, 1038
Methohexital, 1085
Methoprene, 1030t
Methoxyflurane, 1087
Methylation, 1012t
Methylene blue stain, 478
Metoclopramide, 1024t
Metric system, 1041b
Metritis, 700, 760, 967
Metzenbaum dissecting scissors, 1136-1137, 1137f
Mice, 216, 841-842, 841f
Michel clip forceps, 1183f
Michel skin clips, 1183, 1183f
Microbroth dilution, 505
Microfilariae, 461-462, 461f, 480, 481t
Microhematocrit tube, 401f
Micronutrients, 293
Microscope
    calibration of, 476, 476f
    description of, 405
    fecal examination, 475-476
    specimen examination, 490
    urinalysis use of. See Urinalysis
Microsomal cytochrome P450 enzymes, 1012t
Microsporum spp.
    characteristics of, 709t
    M. canis, 509f
Microwave irradiation, 1393t-1395t
Mid forelimb fracture, 955, 955f
Midazolam, 1082
Middening, 162
Middle mental nerve block, 1332, 1333f
Milbemycins, 1029t
Miliary dermatitis, 464
Milk culture, 502
Milk dripping in mares, 797-798, 798b
Milk fever, 339t-340t, 761
Milk replacers
    for kittens, 325, 327f, 797t
    for lamb, 749-750
    for piglets, 778, 778b
    for puppies, 318, 797t
Milk samples
    California mastitis test, 658-659, 658f, 759, 759f
    collection of, 489, 658-659, 759f
    colostrum, 659
    nonsterile, 658-659
    sterile, 658
Milk thistle, 851
Milliamperage, 520, 523, 530, 1316
Milligrams, 1040-1042, 1042b

Mineral(s), 295, 302-304
    for beef cattle, 351, 352f
    calcium, 302-303
    for cats, 328
    for dairy cattle, 348, 349t-350t
    dietary requirements, 302-304
    for dogs, 322
    for finishing cattle, 352-353
    for foals, 363
    for horses, 361
    for large animals, 343
    macrominerals, 302, 344t
    for mares, 362
    microminerals, 345t-346t
    for senior dogs, 325
    for sheep, 356
    for swine
        breeding herd, 357-358
        growing-finishing, 359
    trace, 302
    for working horses, 365
Mineral block, 822, 822f
Mineral grit, 822, 822f
Minimum alveolar concentration, 1086
Minimum inhibitory concentration, 505
Miracidium, 443, 443b
Mirror-image artifact, 555
Misconduct, 30b
Misrepresentation, 30
Mites, 462-467
    Cheyletiella parasitivorax, 464, 465f
    Demodex canis, 464, 464f
    ear, 421-422, 422f, 463, 463f, 464b
    Otodectus cynotis, 421-422, 422f, 463, 463f, 464b
    Sarcoptes scabiei, 462-467, 463f, 464b
    Trombicula spp., 465, 465f
Mitotane, 1021
Mitoxantrone, 1028t-1029t
Mitral regurgitation, 1370
Mitral valve insufficiency, 688
Mixed agonist-antagonists, 1080, 1083
Mixed animal practices, 39
    definition of, 39
    traffic flow patterns, 54
Mixed practice, 3
M-mode, 553
Mobile facility
    definition of, 40b
    description of, 51
Mobile x-ray unit, 524-525
Mobility scoring index, 1313b
Models, dental, 1345-1346
Modern homeopathy, 857
Modified Knott's technique, 480-481, 481t
Modified Robert Jones bandage, 981, 985f, 986-987
Modified Stillman tooth brushing technique, 1335, 1335f
Modified Thomas splint, 1003-1007, 1004f-1008f
Moist heat sterilization, 1162-1163
Molars, 1303
Molybdenum, 347t
Monitor lizards, 217, 217f
Monoamine oxidase inhibitors, 145t-146t
Monoamine oxidases, 1012t
Monoclonal antibodies, 512
Monocytes, 414f-415f, 416
Monofilament sutures, 1201
Monopolar electrocautery, 1196
Moral character, 28

Moral turpitude, crimes of, 28, 30
Morantel, 1029t
Moraxella bovis, 767
Morphine sulfate, 1057-1058, 1060, 1067t-1069t, 1071
Morphine-lidocaine-ketamine, 1060
Mortality insurance, 244
Motorized burs, 1153-1154, 1153f
Moxibustion, 860
Moxidectin, 284
99mTc. See Technetium 99m
Mucin, 420
Mucometra, 1235
Mucosal protectants, 691t
Mucositis, 714
Mucous membranes
    color of, 252-253, 674t, 1105t
    in foals, 800-801
    gingival, 235, 236f
    in horses, 252-253, 253f
    icteric, 909-910
    in kittens, 789-790, 790f
    pale, 1104
    in puppies, 789-790, 790f
    in ruminants, 255-256, 255f
Multicentric lymphoma, 711t
Multifilament sutures, 1201
Multi-lumen catheters, 591, 591f
Multimodal analgesia, 1053
Multiparous, 174
Multiple organ dysfunction syndrome, 915-916
Mu-receptors, 1083
Murmur, heart, 236-237, 237t
Muscle tone, 242, 1106-1107, 1107t
Musculoskeletal diseases and disorders
    in cattle, 1283-1286
    in ruminants, 768-770
    in swine, 777
Musculoskeletal infections, 486t-487t
Musculoskeletal injuries
    in food animals, 962-964
    in horses
        arthrocentesis, 956
        description of, 953-957
        fractures, 954-955
        soft tissue injuries, 955-957
Musculoskeletal system
    physical examination of, 241-242
    surgical retraction, 1197-1199
Muzzle restraint
    of cats, 185f, 186, 187f
    of dogs, 184, 185b, 185f, 1350-1351
Myasthenia gravis, 701
Mycobacterium spp.
    description of, 503
    M. paratuberculosis, 751t-752t, 756
Mycoplasma spp.
    description of, 505
    M. bovis, 757t
    M. conjunctivae, 767
    M. haemocanis, 412f
    M. hyopneumoniae, 775t-776t
Mydriasis, 1080
Myelocytes, 413
Myelography, 549-550
Myelomalacia, 1255
Myofibroblasts, 974
Myoglobinuria, 430, 431b
Myositis, 1262
    masticatory, 1350
Myotherapy, 869

N
N-acetylation, 1012t
Nails
    description of, 19
    physical examination of, 240
    trimming of. See also Foot trimming
        in birds, 818-819, 819f
        in cats, 188-189, 188f
        in dogs, 188-189, 189f, 878, 878f
        in ferrets, 833
        habituation to, 143
        in rabbits, 835
        restraint for, 188-189, 188f-189f
Naloxone hydrochloride, 1058, 1084
Naltrexone, 145t-146t
Nares, 234
Nasal cannula, 952
Nasal discharge, 682-684
Nasoesophageal tubes
    feeding uses of, 330-332, 331f
    in geriatric cats and dogs, 1365
    in puppies, 326f
Nasogastric intubation, 621-624
    in cattle, 622f
    gastric lavage using, 624
    in horses, 622-624, 622f-623f, 946-947, 946t
    tubes
        feeding uses of, 330-332
        in puppies, 326f
Nasolacrimal duct lavage, 639
Nasopharyngeal polyp, 702t-703t
National Association of Boards of Pharmacy, 1037
National Association of Veterinary Technicians in America, 3-4, 21, 1299
    Committee on Veterinary Technician Specialties, 3-4
    description of, 43
    model rules and regulations, 27b, 31
    terminology approved by, 43
National Commission on Veterinary Economic Issues, 5-6, 69
National Farm Animal Care Council, 36
National Formulary, 1031
National Research Council, 310
National Veterinary Associates, 39
Natural pet foods, 307
Navicular disease, 1064t-1065t
NCVEI. See National Commission on Veterinary Economic Issues
Nd:YAG laser, 1132-1133
Neck, necropsy examination of, 574-576
Necropsy
    ancillary procedures, 567-569
    in birds, 581
    cosmetic, 582
    definition of, 562
    diagnostic samples, shipping of, 569
    dissection, 570
    external examination during, 570
    facilities for, 566-567, 566f
    in fetus, 581
    fixatives used in, 566
    in horses, 580
    instruments used in, 566-567, 567b, 567f

Necropsy (Continued)
knowledge required for, 563
in laboratory animals, 581-582
outline of, 569b
personal protective clothing worn during, 566, 566f
in pig, 580-581
preparations for, 561f, 563, 564f
prosector performing, 566
in rabies, 568, 568b
refrigeration of body before, 563-564, 564b
in ruminants, 578-580
sample collection at, 478-479
in small animals
abdomen, 572, 572f
abdominal aorta, 578
abdominal cavity, 576
body cavities, 570-573, 572f
brain, 573-574, 574f
diaphragm, 572-573, 572f
dissection, 570
external examination, 570
female reproductive tract, 577
heart, 575f-576f
incisions, 570, 571f
intestinal tract, 577
joint examination, 570-572
kidneys, 577, 577f
limb reflection, 570-573, 571f-572f
male reproductive organs, 577
meninges, 573-574, 574f
neck, 574-576
outline of, 569b
patient positioning, 570, 571f
pituitary gland, 574
preliminary observations, 570
skin reflection, 570-573, 571f-572f
skull, 573-574, 574f
spinal cord, 573, 574f, 578, 582
superficial organs, 570-573
thoracic viscera, 574-576
tissue collection, 569-570
ureters, 577
urinary bladder, 577, 577f
urinary tract, 577
vertebral column, 578
specimen collection during, 568
tissue collection during, 569-570
Necropsy area, 54
Necropsy log, 109
Necropsy report, 564-565, 565f
Needle(s)
disposal of, 129-130
endodontic, 1339f
recapping of, 130b
Needle holders, 1137, 1137f
Needle teeth, 285, 772f
Negative punishment, 137b, 142
Negative reinforcement, 137-138, 137b
Negligence, 31-32
Nematodes, 451-462
Ancylostoma spp.. See Ancylostoma spp.
Baylisascaris procyonis, 454-455, 455b
characteristics of, 451
definition of, 451
Dirofilaria immitis, 461-462, 479
Enterobius vermicularis, 460-461, 461f
Toxocara spp.. See Toxocara spp.
Trichuris vulpis, 457-458, 457f-458f

Neomycin, 1024
Neonatal care
after cesarean delivery, 1243
definition of, 789
enema administration, 642
of foals, 797-809
antibody levels, 801
assessments, 807t
behavior, 800-801
diseases, 803b
dysmaturity, 803b
energy requirements for, 808
enteral nutrition for, 808
failure of passive transfer, 801
history-taking, 806t
immunoglobulin levels, 801
laboratory evaluation, 801-802
mare's milk for, 808-809, 809b
normal behaviors, 799-802
nutrition, 808-809
prematurity, 800b, 803b
routine care, 801
sickness, 802-808
weight gain, 808
of kittens, 789-797, 793b
body temperature, 789-790
dehydration, 793-794
diagnostics, 791
fading kitten syndrome, 795
fluid requirements, 794
history-taking, 789
hypoglycemia, 794
hypothermia, 793
maintenance, 791-793
malnutrition, 794-795
mucous membranes, 789-790, 790f
orphan care, 795-797
physical examination, 789-790, 790f
tube feeding, 795, 795b, 796f
of puppies, 789-797, 793b
body temperature, 789-790
dehydration, 793-794
diagnostics, 791
fluid requirements, 794
history-taking, 789
hypoglycemia, 794
hypothermia, 793
maintenance, 791-793
malnutrition, 794-795
mucous membranes, 789-790, 790f
orphan care, 795-797
physical examination, 789-790, 790f
tube feeding, 795, 795b, 796f
Neonatal encephalopathy, 803b
Neonatal gastroenteropathy, 803b
Neonatal isoerythrolysis, 794, 803b
Neonatal nephropathy, 803b
Neoplasia
chemotherapeutic drugs for, 1027, 1028t-1029t
definition of, 705
gastrointestinal, 732
in geriatric cats and dogs, 1360
mammary, 1250-1251
in mice, 841-842
oral, 1348-1349, 1348f
Neoplastic lymphocytes, 414f-415f
Neorickettsia risticii, 728-730
Nerve blocks, 966, 1331-1333
inferior alveolar, 1332, 1333f
infraorbital, 1332, 1333f
materials needed for, 1331b
maxillary, 1332-1333, 1333f
middle mental, 1332, 1333f

Nervous ketosis, 761, 765t-766t
Nervous system
diseases that affect. See Neurologic diseases
physical examination of, 242-243, 243t
Net energy, 342
Net income, 69
Net protein utilization, 299t
Netobimin, 1029t
Neuroleptanalgesia, 1078
Neurologic diseases, 1027
in camelids, 784-785, 785f
cerebrospinal fluid analysis for diagnosis of, 746
in geriatric cats and dogs, 1360-1361
in horses, 732-735, 746, 1374
in ruminants, 764-767
in swine, 777
temporohyoid osteoarthropathy, 733-734
viral equine encephalitis, 733
Neurologic larva migrans, 454-455, 455b
Neurolymphatic reflexes, 864
Neuromuscular stimulation, 871-872, 871b, 872f
Neuropathic pain, 1052-1053
Neurovascular reflexes, 864
Neuter. See Castration
Neutrophilia, 413
Neutrophils, 413, 414f-415f
New animal drug, 1031-1032
New animal drug application, 1035
Newsletters, 65
Newspaper advertising, 67
Niacin, 302, 302t, 347t
Nicker, 165-166
Nictitating membrane, 232
Nitenpyram, 1030t
Nitrofurans, 1035t
Nitrogen, 297, 1393t-1395t
Nitroimidazoles, 1018t-1019t, 1035t
Nitrous oxide, 1087
N-methyl-D-aspartate receptor antagonists, 1054, 1061
Nocardia spp., 503
Nociception, 1051, 1052f
Noise, 123
Nonadherent dressing, 995, 995f
Nongovernmental animal welfare organizations, 36
Nonhemolytic transfusion reactions, 904
Nonprecision vaporizers, 1094
Nonprotein nitrogen, 355b
Non-rebreathing circuit, 1090f
Nonscreen film, 534-535, 535f
Nonshivering thermogenesis, 793
Nonsterile milk sample, 658-659
Nonsteroidal anti-inflammatory drugs
adverse effects of, 1055, 1066b
in cats, 1055b
in geriatric cats and dogs, 1363
glucocorticoids and, 1017b
in horses, 1067t-1068t
kidney disease and, 1015
monitoring of, 1054t
pain management using, 1055, 1066
in ruminants, 1073
side effects of, 1066b
take-home analgesia using, 1055
types of, 1055
Nonverbal communication, 56, 142

Nonzoonotic diseases, 125-126
Normochromic, 402
Normocytic red blood cells, 401-402
Nose tongs, 203
Nose twitch, of horse, 195f
Nosocomial infections, 514-515
agents of, 515
bacteria associated with, 515
control of, 515
definition of, 44b, 514
description of, 484
pathogen transmission methods, 514
prevention of, 44b
recognition of, 515
sources of, 44b
viruses as cause of, 515
Notice of disciplinary action, 32
Nuclear medicine, 556-557
diagnostic, 556
therapeutic, 556
Nuclear sclerosis, 232
Nursing care plan, 675-679, 682b
Nutraceuticals, 848, 848t, 1037, 1070b, 1363
Nutrients
amino acids, 293
carbohydrate, 294
classification of, 293b, 293f
definition of, 293
fat, 293-294
fiber, 294
for large animals, 340-343
lipids, 293-294
lipoproteins, 293
macronutrients, 293
maintenance nutrient requirements, 340-341
measurement of, 297
micronutrients, 293
minerals, 295
in pet food, 307
protein. See Protein
supplements, 295
vitamins, 294-295, 294t
water, 293
Nutrition. See also Feeding
alternative types of, 847-850
for beef cattle, 349-353
energy, 351
grain, 351, 351b
guidelines, 353t
minerals, 351, 352f
protein, 351
vitamins, 351
for birds, 819-822
for dairy cattle, 343-348
dry-matter intake, 346b
energy, 346-348
forage, 346-348
guidelines, 350t
minerals, 348, 349t-350t
protein, 348, 349t-350t
vitamins, 348, 350t
water, 346b
water-soluble vitamins, 347t
for ferrets, 833
for foals, 362-363, 808-809
for geriatric patients
cats and dogs, 1361-1362, 1362b
horses, 1375
for guinea pigs, 839-840
for horses, 285, 1375
for kittens, 795t, 796b
for lizards, 829-832
obesity managed with, 335-336, 335f
for potbellied pigs, 778-779

Nutrition (Continued)
  for puppies, 795t, 796b
  for rabbits, 835-836
  in recumbent patients, 931
  for reptiles, 828-832
  for snakes, 829
  for swine
    description of, 356
    energy, 357
    feed rations, 357t
    growing-finishing pigs,
      358-359
    minerals, 357-358
    protein, 357
    vitamins, 357-358
  for tortoises, 828
Nutritional assessment, 329
Nutritional secondary
  hyperparathyroidism, 361
Nystagmus, 242
Nystatin, 1020t

O
Obesity
  diet history in, 335
  maintenance diets for, 335-336
  nutritional strategies for,
    335-336, 335f
Object film distance, 539
Obligate intracellular bacteria, 505
Observation, 179
Obstetrical chains, 965
Obstetrical emergencies
  cesarean section, 966, 966b
  epidural analgesia, 965
  examination for, 965
  uterine prolapse, 966-967
  uterine torsion, 966
Obstructive shock, 915
Obstructive urolithiasis,
  1287-1288
Obturation, 1339-1340
Obturator nerve paresis and
  paralysis, 1284
Occlusal technique, 1320, 1320f
Occlusion, 1302-1309, 1303f
Occlusive bandages, 979-980
Occupational Safety and Health
  Act, 116
Occupational Safety and Health
  Administration, 34
  functions of, 116
  "right to know" laws, 121
Ocular larva migrans, 452-453,
  454b
Ocular squamous cell carcinoma,
  1291-1292, 1291f
Oculomotor nerve, 243t
Offensive aggression, 153
Office, 40b
Office manager, 41
Oils, 294
Olfactory nerve, 242, 243t
Olsen-Hegar needle holder, 1137,
  1137f
Omega-3 fatty acids, 299
Omentopexy, 1282
Omentum, 578-579, 579f
Omeprazole, 728, 1024t
Omphalectomy, 1293
On-call emergency service, 40b
Oncology, 705
Ondansetron, 1024t
One-host ticks, 466, 466b
Ongoing training, 60
Onychectomy
  circumferential ring block for,
    1056f
  complications of, 1227-1228

Onychectomy (Continued)
  definition of, 1225
  description of, 1062b
  indications for, 1225
  intraoperative considerations,
    1225-1227
  laser technique for, 1226, 1226f
  postoperative considerations,
    1227-1228
  preoperative considerations,
    1225
  technique for, 1225-1227,
    1225f-1227f
Oocysts, 471
Oocyte, 369-370
Open gloving, 1176
Open gown pack, 1176f
Open wounds, exuberant
  granulation tissue in, 994,
  994f
Open-ended inquiry, 56
Open-ended questions, 223-224
Operant conditioning, 137-138
Operant learning, 138-139, 138t
Operating profit, 69
Operating room
  air-handling system in, 51
  description of, 50-51
  preparation of, 1169
  sterility of, 1193, 1193f
  veterinary technician's
    responsibilities, 13
Operculated eggs, 441
Ophthalmic disorders, 1291-1292
Ophthalmic instruments,
  1142-1143, 1143f
Ophthalmic medications, 590-598,
  591f
Opiates, 1363
Opioid(s)
  adverse effects of, 1083
  anesthetic uses of, 1083-1084
  antagonists, 145t-146t, 1057
  buprenorphine, 1058,
    1067t-1069t, 1083
  butorphanol tartrate, 1058,
    1058b, 1067t-1069t, 1073,
    1083
  classification of, 1057, 1083
  efficacy of, 1057
  fentanyl citrate, 1038, 1058,
    1067t-1069t
  in horses, 1067t-1068t
  hydromorphone, 1058
  in large animals, 1069
  mechanism of action, 1083
  mixed agonist-antagonists, 1083
  monitoring of, 1054t
  morphine sulfate, 1057-1058
  mu-receptors stimulated by,
    1083
  partial agonists, 1080, 1083
  reversal of, 1058
  side effects of, 1057, 1083
  synthetic, 1058-1059
Opisthotonus, 911
Opportunistic infections
  description of, 485
  nosocomial transmission of, 514
Optic nerve, 243t
Oral administration
  balling guns for, 621, 621f
  in cats, 586-587, 587f
  in cattle, 203, 203f
  in dogs, 586-587, 587f
  drench for, 621, 621f
  in large animals, 620-621, 620f
  pill gun for, 203
  in small animals, 586-587
  syringes for, 620-621, 620f

Oral disease
  in geriatric cats and dogs, 1360
  signs of, 1303, 1303b
Oral examination, 1303-1315
  extraoral, 1304-1309
  intraoral, 1309-1315,
    1309f-1311f
Oral lacerations, 1279
Oral neoplasia, 1348-1349, 1348f
Oral surgery, 1193
Orchidectomy. See Castration
Orf, 289, 770, 770b, 770f
Organic pet foods, 307
Organizational chart, 59
Organophosphates, 1030t
Orogastric intubation
  in dogs, 587-588, 587f-588f
  in large animals, 624, 624f
  in sheep, 660f
  in small animals, 587-588
  tubes for
    rumen fluid collection from,
      659
    in small animals, 587-588,
      588f
Oropharyngeal system, 231
Orthodontics, interceptive,
  1346-1347, 1346f
Orthopedic disease
  in geriatric cats and dogs, 1361,
    1361b
  in geriatric horses, 1370,
    1370f-1371f
Orthopedic implants, 1145-1149
  bone pins, 1145-1146, 1147f
  bone plates, 1148-1149, 1149f
  bone screws, 1148, 1148f
  external fixators, 1146-1148,
    1148f
  interlocking nails, 1146
  titanium, 1145
  total hip prosthesis, 1149, 1149f
Orthopedic surgery
  draping for, 1205-1206,
    1205f-1207f
  in horses
    conditions, 1269-1276
    description of, 1209, 1210f
    draping for, 1205-1206,
      1205f-1207f
  instruments used in, 1143-1145,
    1144f-1147f
  in small animals, 1255-1257
Orthopedic wire, 1146, 1146t,
  1148f
Orthopnea, 684, 908-909
Orthotics, 877
Oscillometric blood pressure
  monitor, 1108, 1109f
Osmolality, 594
Osselet, 1275
Ostectomy, 1252
Osteoarthritis, 701, 1064t-1065t,
  1072b, 1361, 1374-1375
Osteochondral fragments, 1149
Osteochondrosis, 362-363, 1275,
  1276f
Osteoconductive materials,
  1334-1335
Osteomyelitis, 1285
Osteosarcoma, 711t, 712
Osteotomes, 1144, 1146f, 1153
Otic cytology, 421-422
Otitis externa, 702t-703t
Otitis interna, 702t-703t
Otitis media, 702t-703t
Otoacariasis, 466
Otodectus cynotis, 421-422, 422f,
  463, 463f, 464b
Otoscopes, 233, 233f-234f

Outpatient areas, in small animal
  practices, 45-47, 45f
Outpatient clinic, 40b
Outpatient technicians, 39-40
Outpatients, 9-11
Ovarian cysts, 1288-1289
Ovariectomized bitch, 372
Ovariectomy, 1268, 1288-1289
Ovariohysterectomy, 1062b,
  1233-1235, 1234f-1235f
Overbite, 1344, 1345f
Overeating disease, 339t-340t
Over-the-counter drug, 1031-1032
Over-the-needle catheters, 591,
  591f, 610f
Overweight, 675t-679t
Oviduct, 369f
Ovine. See Sheep
Ovine progressive pneumonia,
  758, 760
Ovulation
  definition of, 368-369
  in mare, 383-384
Ovulation depression, 388
Oxacillin, 507t
Oxidase test, 498-499, 499f
Oxygen cage, 919f
Oxygen flow rates, 1093, 1093b
Oxygen flush valve, 1093, 1093f
Oxygen therapy
  delivery methods for, 918-919
  in horses, 951-952, 952f
  intranasal administration, 638
  nasal cannula delivery of, 952
  in small animals, 917-921, 918f
Oxygen transport, 303-304
Oxygenation, 1105, 1110-1111
Oxytocin, 379-380

P
P wave, 937-938
Packed cell volume, 399-401, 401f,
  480, 894-895, 912-913, 1217
Packed red blood cells, 899, 901
Pain
  acute, 1051-1052
  anticipating of, 1062-1064
  assessment of, 1047
  behavioral, 1048
  cancer-related, 713
  chronic, 1051-1052
  clinical manifestations of, 1048
  colic, 1063, 1064t-1065t
  in horses, 738t-739t
  identification of, 1062-1064
  in large animals, 1062-1064
  negative effects of, 1049-1051,
    1051b
  neuropathic, 1052-1053
  phases of, 1051
  physiologic, 1048
  physiology of, 1050-1053
  risk for, 680t
  signs of, 1048-1049, 1048t,
    1218-1219
  technician evaluation of,
    675t-679t
  tolerance to, 1047
Pain management
  adjunctive agents, 1060-1061
  American Animal Hospital
    Association standards,
    1050-1051, 1051b
  in camelids, 1064t-1065t, 1073
  in cats, 1363
  in cattle, 1064t-1065t,
    1071-1073
  in dogs, 1363
  in geriatric cats and dogs, 1363

Pain management (Continued)
in goats, 1064t-1065t,
1071-1073
in horses, 1064t-1065t,
1067t-1068t, 1071
in large animals, 1062-1071
chondroprotective agents,
1070
identification and
anticipation of pain,
1062-1064
joint supplements, 1067t-
1068t, 1070
local anesthetics, 1070
opioids, 1069
principles of, 1064-1071
nonpharmacologic options,
1061
opioids for. See Opioid(s)
overview of, 1046
in pigs, 1073
postoperative, 1062b, 1218-
1219, 1219f-1220f
preemptive, 1062b
protocol for, 1054b
science of, 1049-1053
in sheep, 1064t-1065t,
1071-1073
in small animals, 1053-1061
analgesia administration,
1053
analgesics for. See Analgesics
environmental and emotional
care, 1053
in swine, 1073
veterinary technician's role and
responsibilities, 1047-1049,
1074b
Pain pathway, 1051
Pain receptors, 1051
Pain scale, 1048, 1049f-1050f
Pain-related aggression, 153b
Palatal, 1301
Palatal rugae, 1309, 1311f
Palatoglossal folds, 1309
Palpation
abdomen, 237-238, 238f
bladder, 238
kidneys, 238
large intestine, 238
liver, 238
lymph nodes, 241
prostate gland, 238
small intestines, 238
spleen, 238
stomach, 238
Palpebral reflex, 242, 791b, 1106,
1107t
Pancreas, 1198
Pancreatitis, 690-691
Panleukopenia, 125-126
Pansteatitis, 299-300
Pantothenic acid, 294t, 302, 302t,
347t
Papillomatous digital dermatitis,
769, 769f
Papule, 240
Paragonimus kellicotti, 441-443,
443f
Parainfluenza virus, 757t
Parakeets. See Psittacines
Parallel grid, 536
Paralumbar fossa, 1154
Paraneoplastic syndromes, 713,
713b
Paraphimosis, 1290-1291
Parasites, 284. See also
Ectoparasites; Endoparasites
anthelmintics, 284
in camelids, 785

Parasites (Continued)
in cattle, 959
deworming programs for, 284
external, 125
feed additives for, 284
in ferrets, 835
internal, 125
prevention of, 274-275, 275t, 284
veterinary technician's role in
educating clients about,
441
Paravertebral analgesia, 1280
Parelaphohstrongylus tenuis,
765t-766t, 784-785
Parenteral assisted feeding,
334-335, 334f
Paroxetine, 145t-146t
Parrot mouth, 1352-1353
Parrots, 212. See also Psittacines
Partial agonists, 1080, 1083
Partial parenteral nutrition,
334-335
Partial pressure of carbon dioxide,
920
Parturition
in camelids, 391-392
in cattle, 389
in dogs, 323, 378-379, 379f
feeding during, 323
in mares, 387, 387f
in queen, 380
Parvoviral enteritis, 125-126
Parvovirus
canine, 268t-269t, 272, 707t
feline, 707t
porcine, 773-777
Passerines, 213
Passive drains, 978, 1199, 1199f,
1222
Passive immunity, 262
Passive range of motion, 870-871,
871f
Past pertinent history, 226
Pasteurella spp.
description of, 504, 504b
P. multocida, 126, 757t,
775t-776t, 837
Pasture feeding, 354b
Patent ductus arteriosus, 230
Patent urachus, 803b, 1266
Pathogenesis, 562, 681
Pathologic attrition, 1314-1315
Pathology, 562
Patient
identification of, 87-88, 98
information gathering, 86-88,
89f-90f
Patient evaluations, 96, 96b
Pawing, 164, 171
Payment options, 72
PCR. See Polymerase chain
reaction
PCV. See Packed cell volume
Peak kilovoltage, 1316
Pectoral muscles, 632, 632f
Pectus excavatum, 789-790
Pedal reflex, 1106, 1107t
Pedicle flap, 1342-1343
Pelger-Huet anomaly, 413
Pellagra, 302
Pelvic limb amputation, 1252
Penalty, civil, 34
Penetrating captive bolt,
1393t-1395t
Penicillin
antimicrobial susceptibility
testing for, 507t
Gram-positive pathogens
treated with, 744
procaine, 744

Penis, 371
fibropapillomas of, 1290-1291,
1291f
physical examination of, 239
Penrose drains, 1199
Pentastomes, 473-474, 473f-474f,
474b
Pentobarbital, 1085, 1390-1391,
1396
Peppermint, 854t-855t
Percent solutions, 1042, 1042b
Performance appraisals, 61
Performance dogs, 324
Pergolide, 1372
Perianal adenoma, 711t
Periapical abscesses, 1347
Periapical tissue, 1336
Pericarditis, 764, 764f
Perineal draping, 1193
Perineal surgery, in horses,
1268-1269, 1268f
Perineal urethrostomy, 968-969,
1245-1247, 1246f, 1287-1288,
1287f, 1294, 1294f
Periodic ventilation, 1126
Periodontal débridement,
1322-1323, 1326, 1330
Periodontal disease
algorithm for, 1334f
classification of, 1333b
description of, 1321-1322,
1321f
in horses, 1353-1354
Periodontal instruments,
1312-1313, 1313f
Periodontal ligament, 1313
Periodontal pocket, 1322f,
1333-1334, 1353-1354
Periodontal probe, 1311-1314,
1312f, 1322f
Periodontal space, 1320
Periodontal surgery, 1334-1335
Periodontitis, 1321-1322
Periodontium
assessment of, 1313
definition of, 1309, 1313b
Periosteal elevators, 1143, 1144f,
1341f
Periparturient hypocalcemia, 761
Peripheral arterial pulse, 230
Peripheral odontogenic fibromas,
1348-1349, 1349f
Peripheral vein
blood collection from, 600-601
intravenous administration
using, 591-594
Peritoneal fluid
analysis of, for traumatic
reticuloperitonitis, 754-755
description of, 664
values for, 948t
Permanent teeth, 1299-1300, 1337f
Personal appearance, 64
Personal protective equipment,
116
Personnel. See Employee(s)
Pertechnetate, 556-557
Pet(s). See also specific type of pet
approaching toward, 179-180
attachment with, 1378-1379,
1379b
human-animal bond,
1378-1385
loss of, 1379-1385
selection of, 143-144
Pet food
additives in, 314
advertising of, 305
all-purpose, 305
"ash" in, 295, 295b

Pet food (Continued)
Association of American Feed
Control Animals regulation
of, 309-310
by-products in, 314
carbohydrate levels in, 296t
chemicals in, 313
companies that produce, 305
contaminants in, 314-315
cost of, 315
energy content of, 296t
energy from, 295
fat levels in, 296t
fiber types in, 300
flavors of, 306
Food and Drug Administration
regulation of, 309
history of, 304
holistic, 307
home recipe formulations,
317
home-prepared, 313-317,
847
ingredients in, 307
marketing of, 305-308
medicated, 309
National Research Council and,
310
natural, 307
nutrients in, 305, 307, 323
organic, 307
palatability of, 306, 315
people food design of, 306
premium, 306, 306f
preservatives in, 313
protein in, 296t, 307
for puppies, 318
quality issues, 314
raw, 307-308, 308b
recipes for, 315-317
regulation of, 309-310
semi-moist, 305
specific-purpose, 306
therapeutic diets, 308-309
toxins in, 314-315
types of, 305
U.S. Department of Agriculture
regulation of, 309
value-priced, 306
varieties of, 306
veterinary therapeutic diets,
308-309
water content in, 293
Pet food labels
description of, 296
feeding directions on, 312-313
guaranteed analysis on,
311-312, 311t
illustration of, 311f
information panel of, 310
ingredient statement, 312
net weight, 311
principal display panel of,
310
product identity on, 310-311
statement of nutritional
adequacy, 310
Pet health insurance, 72-73
Pet portals, 68
Petechial hemorrhages,
252-253
Petechiation, 232, 233f
Pétrissage, 869
Petting-related aggression, 160
Petty cash, 68
pH
rumen fluid, 750-753
urine, 431-432
Phalangeal fractures, 1269-1270,
1270f

Pharmacodynamics, 1010
    definition of, 1013
    mechanism of action,
        1013-1014
    side effects, 1014
Pharmacokinetics, 1010
    absorption, 1011
    aging effects on, 1015
    cardiovascular disease effects
        on, 1014-1015
    definition of, 1011
    disease effects on, 1014-1015
    distribution, 1012
    elimination, 1013
    kidney disease effects on, 1015
    liver disease effects on, 1015
    metabolism, 1012-1013, 1012t
    schematic diagram of, 1011f
Pharmacology, 1010
Pharmacy
    in small animal practices, 47,
        48f
    veterinary technician's
        responsibilities, 11
Pharyngeal abscessation,
    751t-752t, 753
Pharyngeal masses, 231
Pharynx, 1309
Phenobarbital, 1016t-1017t, 1027
Phenols, 1167t, 1168
Phenothiazine tranquilizers, 1081
2-Phenoxyethanol, 1393t-1395t
Phenylbutazone, 1016t, 1035t,
    1066, 1067t-1069t
Phenylbutazone toxicosis, 728
Phimosis, 1290-1291
Phlebitis, 594, 596, 892
Phobias, 151-152
Phosphorus, 303, 303t, 319,
    326-327
    for foals, 363
    for livestock, 344t
Physical dysfunction, 866b
Physical examination
    body temperature, 228-230
    cardiovascular system, 235-237,
        236f
    of cattle, 254-257, 256f
    cranial nerves, 242, 243t
    documentation of information
        from, 228, 229f
    ears, 232-233, 233f
    eyes, 231-232, 232f
    form for, 92f
    gastrointestinal system, 237-238,
        237f-238f
    of horses, 246-254
        abdominal auscultation,
            251-252, 252b, 252f
        body temperature, 247-248,
            247f-248f
        geriatric patients, 1368
        heart auscultation, 248f,
            250-251, 250f-251f
        heart rate in, 248-250, 248t
        height measurements,
            253-254
        hydration status, 253
        mucous membranes,
            252-253, 253f
        preventive health purposes
            of, 275
        pulse rate, 248-250,
            248f-249f, 248t
        rectal thermometers for,
            247-248, 247f-248f
        respiratory rate, 250
        weight measurements,
            253-254
    importance of, 226-228

Physical examination (Continued)
    integumentary system, 240, 240f
    jugular veins, 237
    of kittens, 789-790, 790f
    of large animals, 246-257,
        254b
    lymph nodes, 240-241
    musculoskeletal system, 241-242
    nervous system, 242-243, 243t
    oropharyngeal system, 231
    pulse, 230
    of puppies, 789-790, 790f
    rectal examination, 238-239,
        239f
    respiratory rate, 230
    respiratory system, 234-235,
        234f
    of ruminants, 254-257, 256f
    sample form for, 229f
    scrotum, 239
    skin, 240
    of small animals, 226-243
    surroundings noted in, 228
    systems review, 230-243
    testes, 239
    urogenital, 239
    urolithiasis, 967
    vagina, 239
    veterinary technician's
        responsibility for, 46-47
Physical therapy and
    rehabilitation, 865-878
    after orthopedic surgery,
        1256-1257
    assistive devices, 875-878
        braces, 877
        harnesses, 875
        orthotics, 877
        protective devices, 875-877
        slings, 875
        TTouch wrap, 877-878, 878f
        wheelchairs, 875, 875f
    bioelectrical stimulation, 872
    definition of, 865
    electrical therapies, 871-873
    electromagnetic stimulation,
        872-873
    exercise-based therapy, 866
    history of, 865
    hydrotherapy, 867-868, 868f
    indications for, 865, 866b
    land treadmill, 868
    low-level laser therapy, 874,
        874f, 1061
    magnet-based therapy,
        872-873
    massage, 868-870, 869f-870f
    neuromuscular stimulation,
        871-872, 871b, 872f
    passive range of motion,
        870-871, 871f
    superficial thermal therapy,
        874-875
    therapeutic exercises, 866-867
    therapeutic ultrasound, 873,
        873b, 873f
    veterinary technician's role in,
        865, 866b
Physiologic attrition, 1314-1315
Picture archival computing
    system, 526, 528-529
Piezoelectric effect, 551
Piezoelectric scaler, 1325
Pig(s). See also Piglets; Sows;
    Swine
    analgesics for, 1068t-1069t
    behaviors in, 777-778
    blood sample collection in,
        648-651
    catheterization in, 629, 630f

Pig(s) (Continued)
    diseases and conditions that
        affect
        Aujeszky's disease, 772
        diarrhea, 773, 773t-775t
        erysipelas, 286, 772
        gastrointestinal, 773
        iron deficiency anemia, 357b
        leptospirosis, 777
        musculoskeletal, 777
        nervous system, 777
        neurologic, 777
        pleuropneumonia, 775t
        porcine parvovirus, 773-777
        porcine reproductive and
            respiratory syndrome,
            286, 772
        porcine stress syndrome, 777
        pseudorabies virus, 772, 772b
        reproductive, 773-777,
            775t-776t
        respiratory, 773, 775t-776t
        salt poisoning, 777
    epidural administration in, 641
    finisher, 773, 775t
    flight zone of, 206
    growing-finishing, 358-359, 773,
        775t
        energy requirements, 358
        minerals, 359
        protein for, 358
        vitamins, 359
    intramuscular administration
        in, 633-634
    intraperitoneal administration
        in, 638
    intravenous administration in,
        629, 630f
    moving of, 206
    necropsy examination of,
        580-581
    in open pens, 206, 206f
    orbital sinus of, venipuncture
        in, 651, 651f
    pain management in, 1073
    potbellied, 778-786, 779f
    reproduction in. See
        Reproduction, swine
    restraint of, 207
    subcutaneous administration in,
        635
    urine collection in, 657
    vaccinations for, 286
    venipuncture in, 648-651
        auricular vein, 650
        coccygeal vein, 651
        cranial vena cava, 649-650,
            649f-650f
        jugular vein, 650
        orbital sinus, 651, 651f
        peripheral leg veins, 650-651,
            651f
Pig board, 206, 206f
Piglets
    approaching, 205f
    capture of, 207
    care of, 771-772, 771f-772f
    colostrum for, 771
    diarrhea in, 773, 773t-774t
    iron dextran injections for,
        771-772, 771f
    milk replacer for, 778, 778b
    restraint of, 207, 208f
    tail docking in, 772f
    weaning of, 358
Pill gun, 203
Pimobendan, 1025
PIMS. See Practice information
    management systems
Pineal gland, 368

Pinkeye, 287-288, 767
Pinworms, 460-461, 461f
Pithing, 1393t-1395t
Pituitary gland, necropsy
    examination of, 574
Pituitary pars intermedia
    dysfunction. See Cushing's
    disease
Placenta, retained, 760, 760f
Placentome, 389
Plague, 710t
Plan of care, 9
Planking, 528
Planning, 58-59
Plaque, 1321-1322, 1321f, 1322b,
    1336
Plasma protein concentration, 402,
    403f
Plasma transfusions
    administration of, 902
    indications for, 895-896, 895b
Plasmin, 417
Platelet(s)
    automated counts, 407-408
    blood smear evaluation of,
        407-408, 408f
    description of, 407
    in hemostasis, 417
    transfusion of, 895
Platelet concentrate, 901
Platelet count, 404
Platelet-rich plasma, 901
Play, 156
Play-related aggression, 151, 153b,
    160
Plerocercoid, 450
Pleural effusion, 234-235, 684
    thoracentesis for, 609-610, 609b,
        610f
Pleural space, 1057
Pleuritis, 486t-487t
Pleuropneumonia
    in horses, 726-727
    in swine, 775t
Plume, laser, 1135-1136, 1136f
PMMA implants, 1283
PMSG. See Pregnant mare serum
    gonadotropin
Pneumonia
    bacterial, 486t-487t, 723t-724t,
        726-727, 740b-741b
    characteristics of, 949
    ovine progressive, 758, 760
    Pasteurella, 775t-776t
    pleuropneumonia, 726-727, 775t
    in small animals, 686t-687t
Pneumothorax, 234-235
    in horses, 949
    in small animals, 686t-687t
    thoracentesis for, 609-610, 609b,
        610f
Podiatry, 878, 878f
Poikilocytosis, 409
Point of maximal intensity, 236-237
Point-of-care instruments, 428
Point-of-sale displays, 66, 66f
Poliglecaprone, 1202
Polioencephalomalacia, 753,
    765t-766t, 767
Polishing, 1330-1331
Poloxalene, 959
Polyamide sutures, 1203
Polybutester sutures, 1203
Polychromasia, 412
Polyclonal antibodies, 512
Polydioxanone, 1202
Polydipsia, 736, 1360
Polyester sutures, 1203
Polyglactin 910, 1202
Polyglycolic acid, 1202

Polyglyconate, 1202
Polymerase chain reaction,
    512-513, 513f, 657, 746-747
Polymorphic ventricular
    tachycardia, 942f
Polymorphonuclear neutrophils,
    616
Polyphenols, 295
Polypropylene sutures, 1203
Polysulfated glycosaminoglycans,
    1067t-1068t
Polyunsaturated fatty acids, 299
Polyuria, 736, 1360
Poole suction tip, 1140-1141,
    1141f
Popliteal lymph nodes, 240-241,
    241f
Porcine. *See* Pig(s); Swine
Porcine parvovirus, 773-777
Porcine reproductive and
    respiratory syndrome, 286,
    772
Porcine stress syndrome, 206-207,
    777
Portable x-ray unit, 523-524, 525f
Portosystemic shunts
    congenital, 683t
    description of, 433-435, 694
    diagnosis of, 694
Position-indicating device, 1316
Positive punishment
    after unwanted behavior, 142
    avoidance of, 143b
    correct use of, 142-143
    definition of, 137b
Positive reinforcement, 137b
Positive-pressure ventilation, 826
Possessive aggression, 153b
Posterior cross-bite, 1344
Postinduction apnea, 1106
Postoperative pain management,
    1062b
Postpartum disorders, 699-700
Potassium, 303, 303t, 344t
Potassium bromide, 1017t, 1027
Potassium chloride, 891-892, 892t,
    1393t-1395t
Potbellied pigs, 778-786, 779f
Potencies, 856
Potomac horse fever, 277t-283t,
    283, 729t-730t, 730
Potter-Bucky diaphragm, 536-537
Povidone-iodine, 1166, 1167t
Power equipment, 1145, 1147f
Power scaling, 1323-1326
    benefits of, 1323b
    history of, 1323
    safety precautions for, 1324
    sonic scaler, 1323
    ultrasonic scalers. *See* Ultrasonic
       scalers
PR interval, 937
Practice acts
    description of, 8, 24
    model, 24, 25b-26b
    purpose of, 24
Practice information management
    systems
    accounts receivable monitoring
       using, 78
    appointment scheduling using,
       76, 77f
    billing use of, 78
    definition of, 75
    doctor production tracked
       using, 78
    inventory management using, 78
    patient locations in hospital
       managed with, 76, 77f
    reminders, 77

Practice management, 57-78
    finances
       accounting, 68
       balance sheet, 68
       bookkeeping, 68
       budgeting, 70
       income statement, 68-69
       key performance indicators,
          69-70, 70b
       overview of, 68-71
       price setting, 70-71
       profitability calculations, 69
       statement of cash flows,
          68-69
    human resources, 59-62
       compensation determinations
          by, 60
       definition of, 59-62
       hiring, 59-60
       management of employees
          by, 60-61
       retention of employees by,
          60-61
       stress management role of,
          61-62
       training and orientation of
          employees by, 60
    marketing. *See* Marketing
    operations
       appointment scheduling,
          71-72
       client payments, 72-73
       description of, 71-75
       estimates for services, 72-73
       front desk management,
          71-73
       inventory management,
          73-75
       payment options, 72
    planning, 58-59
Practice manager, 41
    certification of, 42
    duties of, 41
    veterinary technician as, 41
Prairie dogs, 842
Praziquantel, 284, 451, 1029t
Preanesthetic period, 1115
Precision vaporizers, 1093-1094
Predatory aggression
    in cats, 157
    in dogs, 153b, 154
Prednisone, 1022t, 1028t-1029t
Preemptive analgesia, 1053
Preemptive pain management,
    1062b
Pregnancy. *See also* Reproduction
    in bitch, 323
    in mare, 386
Pregnancy toxemia, 761-762
Pregnant mare serum
    gonadotropin, 386
Premium pet foods, 306, 306f
Premolars, 285, 1303, 1303f
Preputial prolapse, 1291, 1291f
Prescapular lymph nodes, 240-241
Prescription animal drugs, 1032
Prescription drugs
    calculations, 1040-1043,
       1041b-1042b, 1041t
    dispensing of, 1038-1040, 1039f,
       1039t
    label of, 1040f
Prescription writing, 1038-1040
Presenting complaint, 226
Preservatives, 313
Pressing reflex, 791b
Pressure manometer, 1097
Pressure sores, 979, 1255
    in dogs, 1254f
    in hospitalized horses, 739-742

Pressured bag system, 1152, 1152f
Pressure-reducing valve, 1092,
    1092f
Prevacuum sterilizers, 1163-1164
Preventive care, 42
Preventive health programs
    for cats
       grooming, 262
       parasite prevention, 274-275,
          275t
       vaccines, 263-267
    for cattle, 286-288
    for dogs
       grooming, 262
       parasite prevention, 274-275,
          275t
       vaccines, 263-267
       wellness visits, 260-262
    for horses
       dental care, 284-285
       hoof care, 285
       nutrition, 285
       outline of, 276b
       parasites, 284
    for sheep, 288-289
    for swine, 285-286
Price setting, 70-71
Primary antibody, 510-512
Primary spermatocytes, 372
Primiparous, 174
Prions, 580b
Probiotics, 691t
Problem list, 92-93, 93f-94f
Problem-oriented veterinary
    medical record
    client information, 86-88, 89f
    communication use of, 86
    components of, 86-105, 87b
    consultants, 92
    database, 86-92
    description of, 86
    laboratory diagnostic flow
       sheet, 91
    master problem list, 92-93, 93f
    patient information, 86-88,
       89f-90f
    working problem list, 92-93, 94f
Procaine penicillin, 744
Procercoid, 450
Prochlorperazine, 1024t
Proestrus, 372, 375f
Professional ethics, 23-24
Professional organizations, 21-23,
    22t
Professionalism, 17-21
    in appearance, 18-20
    in communication, 20-21
    in conduct, 20, 20b
Profitability, 69
Profits, 38
Progesterone, 368, 379-380
Progestins, 145t-146t
Progestogens, 385
Proglottids, 445-446, 446b, 446f
Progress notes, 95f
    case study of, 102f-103f
    notations in, 96-97
    SOAP, 94-96, 95f
Prolactin, 379-380
Proliferative enteropathy, 775t
Promotion, 705-706
Prophy angle, 1331
Propofol, 826t, 1084, 1116
Propranolol, 1026t
Proprioceptive exercises, 867
Prosector, 566
Prostaglandin F2α, 380, 390-391
Prostate gland, 238
Prostatic abscesses, 700
Prostatic disease, 700

Protein, 293
    amino acids, 293, 297, 297t
    in animal feed, 341
    for beef cattle, 351, 351b
    for birds, 821
    for cats, 298t, 327
    for dairy cattle, 348, 349t-350t
    definition of, 293, 341
    dietary, 293, 297-298
    digestibility of, 298
    for dogs, 298t, 319, 321-322,
       324
    excessive, 298
    for finishing cattle, 352
    food sources of, 293
    for horses, 361-364
    for kittens, 325
    for large animals, 341-342
    in pet food, 307
    for puppies, 319
    quality of, 298, 299t
    for ruminants, 341-342
    for senior dogs, 324
    serum, 425
    for sheep, 354, 355b
    for swine
       breeding herd, 357
       growing-finishing, 358
    for working horses, 363-364
Protein-efficiency ratio, 299t
Proteus spp., 504
Prothrombin time, 417-418
Protozoa, 125, 467-473
    Cryptosporidium parvum,
       472-473, 473f, 478
    definition of, 467b
    fecal examination to detect, 478
    Giardia spp., 467-471, 470f, 478
    Toxoplasma gondii, 471-472
Proving, 855
Provitamin A, 300-301
Proximal forelimb fracture, 955
Proximal hindlimb fracture, 955
Pseudocyesis, 1233-1234
Pseudomonas spp.
    description of, 504
    P. aeruginosa, 497-498
Pseudoparasite, 460b
Pseudopregnancy, 760-761
Pseudorabies virus, 772, 772b
Pseudotapeworms, 450-451, 451f
Psittacines
    approaching, 211
    body temperature of, 815
    diet for, 813t
    observation of, 211
    restraint of, 211-213, 212f-213f
    stool of, 814f
    tube feeding of, 815, 815f,
       819-820
Psoroptes cuniculi, 837f-838f
Psychotropic drugs
    behavior problems treated with,
       144
    FDA-approved, 144, 145t-146t
    types of, 144, 145t-146t
Puberty
    in camelids, 391
    definition of, 369
    in dogs, 372
    in heifers, 387
    in queen, 379
    in sheep, 389
Public Broadcasting System, 67
Pudendal nerve block, 1286
Pulmonary artery, 575
Pulmonary edema, 234-235
Pulmonary thromboembolism,
    688-689
Pulpitis, 1347-1348, 1348f

Pulse
    arterial, 230, 248-249
    in cattle, 255, 255f
    in dogs, 230t
    in goats, 255
    in horses, 248-250, 248f-249f,
        248t, 722b
    measurement of, 230
    peripheral arterial, 230
    quality of, 250
    in ruminants, 255, 255f
    in sheep, 255
Pulse deficit, 230, 248
Pulse oximeter, 913, 919,
    1110-1111, 1110f-1111f,
    1111b
Pulse pressure, 230
Pulse strength, 1105
Pulsed electromagnetic field
    therapy, 872-873
Pulsed signal therapy, 873f
Pulseless electrical activity, 924f
Puncture wounds, 964
Punishment
    definition of, 137-138, 137b
    reinforcement versus, 138
    remote, 143
Pupillary light reflex, 242
Pupillary light response, 926-927
Pupils, 911
Puppies
    Ancylostoma caninum in, 457b
    ascarids in, 454b
    body temperature in, 789-790
    calcium requirements of, 319
    chewing by, 142
    death of, 795
    dehydration in, 793-794, 794b
    development of, 146, 790-791,
        792b
    dewclaw removal in, 1224
    energy requirements of,
        318-319
    fat requirements of, 319
    feeding of, 317-320, 794-795
    hand-feeding of, 318
    hookworms in, 442b
    hypothermia in, 793
    mental stimulation for, 142
    milk replacers for, 318, 797t
    neonatal care of. See Neonatal
        care, of puppies
    neurologic examination in,
        791b
    nutritional requirements, 795t,
        796b
    overfeeding of, 796-797
    physical stimulation for, 142
    protein requirements of, 319
    roundworms in, 442b
    selection considerations, 143
    socialization of, 147
    solid food for, 318
    tail docking in, 1224
    weaning of, 318
    wellness visits for, 260-261
Purkinje fibers, 935-936
Purpura hemorrhagica, 283
Pustule, 240
Pyelonephritis, 770
Pyloropexy, 1282
Pyometra, 226, 239, 915f,
    1235-1236, 1236f
Pyothorax, 686t-687t
Pyrantel, 453, 1029t
Pyrethrins, 464-465, 1030t
Pyrethroids, 1030t
Pyridoxine, 302, 302t, 347t
Pyriproxifen, 1030t
Pyuria, 433

Q
Q fever, 468t-469t
Q wave, 935-936
QRS complex, 937-938
Quality control, 427-428
Quarter drapes, 1183-1184,
    1189-1190, 1190f-1191f
Quaternary ammonium, 1168
Queen. See also Cat(s)
    cesarean delivery in, 1241-1243
    definition of, 379
    dystocia in, 380
    estrous cycle in, 379-380
    fertilization in, 380
    parturition in, 380
    puberty of, 379
    as seasonal polyestrous, 379
Queening, 379
Quinidine, 727, 1026t
Quinine, 853

R
R wave, 935-936
Rabbits, 836
    anesthesia for, 836
    blood collection in, 836-837,
        837f
    dental procedures in, 837-838,
        838f
    description of, 835
    diet for, 836
    diseases that affect, 837-838
    general procedures for, 836-837,
        837f
    intravenous injections in,
        836-837
    malocclusion in, 837-838
    nail trimming of, 835
    nutrition for, 835-836
    perineal examination in, 215
    Psoroptes cuniculi in, 837f-838f
    restraint of, 214-215, 214f
    snuffles in, 837
    stress levels in, 214
    thumping by, 214
    towel restraint of, 214, 214f
Rabies, 124
    in camelids, 785
    carriers of, 732-733
    characteristics of, 267, 709t
    diagnosis of, 733, 764
    in horses, 732-733
    necropsy considerations in, 568,
        568b
    postexposure prophylaxis, 733
    in ruminants, 764, 764f,
        765t-766t
    signs of, 267
    vaccine for
        in dogs and cats, 266t-269t,
            267, 271
        in horses, 277t-283t, 284, 733
        postexposure, 733
    as zoonotic disease, 710t
Raccoons, 454, 455b
Rad, 542, 544b
Radial nerve paralysis, 1285
Radiation
    adverse effects of, 714
    ALARA principle for, 544-545
    film badge, 544, 544f
    filtration of, 542
    maximum permissible dose of,
        543
    measurement of, 542-544, 544b
    secondary, 546-547
    tissue necrosis caused by, 975
    tissue sensitivity to, 541-542
Radiation exposure records, 116

Radiation safety, 541-547,
    1316-1317
    ALARA principle for, 544-545
    apron, 545, 545f
    film badge, 544, 544f
    gloves, 545, 545f
    measurements, 542-544, 544b
    nuclear medicine, 557
    positioning devices, 546f-547f
    practices for, 545-547, 545f
    protection officer in charge of,
        544-545
Radio advertising, 67
Radiofrequency identification,
    563-564
Radiofrequency probes, 1154
Radiographic contrast, 540
Radiographic density, 540
Radiographic detail, 539-540
Radiographic developing
    solutions, 127
Radiography/radiographs. See also
    X-ray(s)
    of birds, 817, 817f-818f
    case study of, 543b
    computed tomography versus,
        557
    contrast agents used in,
        547-550, 547f
        barium sulfate, 547-548
        for esophagus, 548
        for large bowel, 548-549
        nonionic organic iodides, 548
        organic iodides, 548
        radiolucent gases, 547
        for small bowel, 548
        soluble radiopaque ionic, 548
        for spinal cord, 549-550
        for stomach, 548
        types of, 547
        for urinary bladder, 549
        for urinary tract, 549
    digital. See Digital radiography
    filing of radiograph, 519
    film
        artifacts, 541
        automatic processor of,
            534-535, 535f, 542b
        contrast, 540
        density, 540
        detail, 539-540
        handling of, 538-539
        identification of, 518, 519f
        labeling of, 518, 518f-519f
        magnification, 540-541
        nonscreen, 532f, 534-535,
            535f
        preparation of, 534
        screen, 534-535, 535f
        silver recovery, 539
        storage of, 538
        technical errors associated
            with, 541, 541b-542b
    film quality in, 539-541
    as legal records, 518
    positioning for, 550
    of reptiles, 826
    restraint for, 550-551
    of wounds, 957
Radioimmunoassay, 429
Radiology, 126-127. See also
    X-ray(s)
    darkroom. See Darkroom
    portable machines for, 127
    safety considerations, 126-127
    veterinary technician's
        responsibilities, 11, 11f
Radiology information system,
    529
Radiology log, 107, 108f

Radiology suite, 47-49, 48f
Radiolucent, 1320
Radionuclides, 557, 557b
Radiopaque, 1320
Radiotherapy, 714
Rain rot, 736
Ram, 245t, 389
Ranitidine, 1024t
Ranula, 231
Rare earth screens, 534-535, 534b
Rats, 842, 842f
Raw bones, 847, 847b
Raw pet foods, 307-308, 308b
Rawhide, 1336
RDW. See Red cell distribution
    width
Reactive lymphocytes, 416
Rebreathing bag, 1096, 1096f
Rebreathing systems, 1088-1089,
    1095
Recapping of needles, 130b
Reception area, 9, 46, 46f
Receptionists, 43, 46, 72
Reconcile. See Fluoxetine
Reconstituted collagen, 1202
Record. See Medical record
Recovery diet, 333, 333t
Rectal examination, 238-239, 239f
Rectal prolapse, 1295-1296
Rectal tears, 947
Rectal thermometer
    for large animals, 247-248,
        247f-248f
    for small animals, 228-229, 230f
Recumbency, 738t-739t
Recumbent horses, 738t-739t,
    739-742, 742f-743f
Recumbent small animals,
    930-931
Recurrent airway obstruction,
    723t-724t, 726, 742-744
Red blood cell(s)
    agglutination of, 400-401
    blood smear of, 408-412,
        408f-411f
    in camelids, 408-409, 408f
    crenated, 409-410, 409f-410f
    in dogs, 408f
    microcytic, 408-409
    morphologic abnormalities in,
        409, 409f-410f
    parasites, 412
    in urine, 434f
Red blood cell count, 401
Red blood cell indices, 399,
    401-402, 402b
Red cell distribution width, 402
Redirected aggression, 153b, 161
Redirected behaviors, 171
Reepithelialization, 974, 979
Referral facility, 40b
    caseloads in, 43
    definition of, 40b
    description of, 39
Referral pain, 859
Referral practices, 39
Reflective listening, 56-57
Reflective waveguide, 1132
Reflex responses, 243t
Reflexes. See also specific reflex
    anesthetic depth and,
        1106-1107, 1107t
    definition of, 1106
    description of, 242-243, 243t
Refraction, 555
Refractometer, 402, 430, 431t
Regional anesthesia, 1331, 1332b
Regional anesthetics
    abdominal surgery using, 1280
    analgesic use of, 1055-1057

Regional nerve blocks, 966, 1331-1333
  inferior alveolar nerve block, 1332, 1333f
  infraorbital nerve block, 1332, 1333f
  materials needed for, 1331b
  maxillary nerve block, 1332-1333, 1333f
  middle mental nerve block, 1332, 1333f
Registrations, 26-28
Registry of Continuing Education, 29
Regurgitation, 689
Rehabilitation. See Physical therapy and rehabilitation
Reinforcement
  continuous, 138
  definition of, 137b
  intermittent, 138
  punishment versus, 138
Relaxin, 378
Release of medical information, 85
Rem, 542, 544b
Remote punishment, 143
Renal diseases. See Kidney disease
Renomegaly, 238
Reperfusion injury, 916
Repertorizing, 856
Reportable diseases, 85
Reprimand, 34
Reproduction. See also Gestation
  bovine
    artificial insemination in, 388
    estrous cycle, 387-388
    gestation, 389
    overview of, 387-389
    parturition, 389
    terminology associated with, 373t
    udder enlargement, 389
  camelids
    breeding of, 391
    gestation in, 391
    overview of, 391-392
    parturition in, 391-392
    terminology associated with, 373t
  canine, 372-379
    artificial insemination, 378
    breeding, 378
    estrous cycle, 372-378, 374f
    gestation, 378
    overview of, 372-373
    parturition, 378-379, 379f
    terminology associated with, 373t
    vaginal cytologic examination, 374b-377b
    whelping, 372
  caprine, 373t
  cattle
    artificial insemination in, 388
    estrous cycle, 387-388
    gestation, 389
    overview of, 387-389
    parturition, 389
    terminology associated with, 373t
    udder enlargement, 389
  corpus luteum, 368-369, 368f-369f
  embryo, 369-370
  equine
    artificial insemination, 386
    breeding season, 384
    estrous cycle, 381-385
    gestation, 386, 386f
    overview of, 380-387

Reproduction (Continued)
  parturition, 387, 387f
  physiology of, 382f
  reproductive tract examination, 385-386
  terminology associated with, 373t
  estrous cycle
    in bitch, 372-378, 374f
    description of, 369
    hormones involved in, 369
    in queen, 379-380
  feline
    dystocia, 380
    estrous cycle, 379-380
    feeding during, 328-329
    gestation, 380
    overview of, 379-380
    terminology associated with, 373t
  female
    anatomy of, 368
    estrous cycle, 369
    ovulation, 368-369
    physiology of, 368-370, 368f
  goats, 373t, 391
  male
    anatomy of, 370
    physiology of, 370-372, 371f
    spermatogenesis, 370, 372
  ovine
    breeding season, 390-391
    estrous cycle, 390
    gestation, 391
    overview of, 389-391
    terminology associated with, 373t
  sheep
    breeding season, 390-391
    estrous cycle, 390
    gestation, 391
    overview of, 389-391
    terminology associated with, 373t
  swine, 373t
  terminology associated with, 373t
Reproductive diseases
  in ruminants, 758-761
  in small animals, 699-700
  in swine, 773-777, 775t-776t
Reproductive history, 226
Reptiles. See also Chelonians; Lizards; Snakes; Tortoises; Turtles
  anesthetic agents for, 826-827, 826t
  blood samples from, 825-826, 825f
  bone marrow specimens from, 825
  cage for, 824, 824f
  colonic wash in, 825
  diagnostic procedures in, 824-826
  equipment for, 823
  feces of, 832
  handling of, 216-219
  history-taking, 824
  hospital cage for, 824, 824f
  hospital husbandry for, 827-828
  injections in, 827-828, 828f
  metabolic bone disease in, 828, 828f
  nucleated red blood cells in, 404
  nutrition for, 828-832
  ownership statistics for, 823
  radiography of, 826
  red blood cells in, 408-409, 408f
  restraint of, 216-219

Reptiles (Continued)
  sample collection in, 824-826
  sexing of, 823f
  skin for, 832
  sputum sample in, 832
  stomach lavage in, 825
  tube-feeding of, 827
  types of, 823b
  urine samples from, 825
  venipuncture in, 825-826
  zoonotic diseases in, 832
Rescue Remedy, 857
Research, 82
Reservoir bag, 1127
Resolution stage, of grief, 1380b-1381b, 1385
Respiratory diseases and disorders
  in cats, 706t, 1360
  in cattle, 1286
  in dogs, 706t, 1360
  in food animals, 961-962, 1286
  in horses, 722-727, 723t-724t, 1370
  in ruminants, 756-758, 757t
  in small animals, 682-685, 685t-687t
  in swine, 773, 775t-776t
  therapeutic approach to, 685t
Respiratory distress, 931-932, 961
Respiratory minute volume, 1094, 1126
Respiratory rate
  in cats, 230t
  in dogs, 230t
  in horses, 250, 722b
  measurement of, 230
Respiratory sinus arrhythmia, 235
Respiratory syncytial virus, 757t
Respiratory system
  auscultation of, 234-235, 674t
  physical examination of, 234-235, 234f
Response blocking, 139
Responsibility for actions, 32
Resting energy requirements, 296-297, 297t, 320, 328
Restorative dentistry, 1336, 1336f
Restraint
  approach to, 178-180
  of birds, 211-214
  of camelids, 209-210, 210f
  of cats, 186-188
    "burrito style" wrap, 186, 187f
    cat bags, 187, 187f
    chemical restraint, 187-188
    muzzle, 186, 187f
    scruffing, 186, 186f-187f
    towel, 186, 186f
    uncooperative pet, 186-188
    for venipuncture, 188
    well-behaved pet, 186
  of cattle
    box stalls, 201, 201f
    casting, 204-205
    chute, 200f, 201-202, 202f
    foot control and restraint, 204
    halter, 200-201, 201f
    head, 203
    head-lock system, 202, 202f
    hutch, 201, 201f
    tail restraint, 203-204, 204f.
      See also Tail jack
    techniques for, 202-205, 202f
    for venipuncture, 204, 204f
  of cervids, 210-211
  chemical
    of birds, 213
    of cats, 187-188

Restraint (Continued)
  of dogs, 185
  of ferrets, 216
  of horses, 191, 195, 247
  of rabbits, 215
  for radiography, 550-551
  of chinchillas, 215
  of Cockatoos, 212f-213f, 213
  definition of, 191
  diversionary, 191, 194-195
  of dogs, 183-185
    chemical restraint, 185
    muzzle, 184, 185b, 185f
    for nail trimming, 188-189, 189f
    tips for, 184b
    towel, 184-185
    uncooperative pet, 184-185
    for venipuncture, 188, 188f
    well-behaved dog, 183, 183f
  of ferrets, 215-216
  of foals, 193, 193f, 196, 197f, 805f, 806-808
  of gerbils, 216
  of goats, 209, 209f
  of guinea pigs, 215, 215f
  of hamsters, 216
  of hedgehogs, 216
  of horses, 190-199
    approach for, 191-192
    brown gauze tail tie, 198, 198f
    chain shanks, 194, 194f
    chemical restraint, 191, 195, 247
    cradle, 198, 198f
    diversionary techniques, 191, 194-195
    foreleg lift, 197-198, 198f
    halter, 194, 194f
    hind leg lift, 197-198
    hobbles, 197-198
    humane twitch, 194-195, 196f
    juvenile horses, 193, 195-196
    lead rope for, 192, 192f, 194
    lip/gum chain, 194, 194b, 195f
    manual twitches, 194-195, 195f
    personal safety during, 192
    physical restraint, 191, 194
    stocks, 198, 198f
    tail tie, 198, 198f
    techniques for, 194-195, 194f-196f
    ties, 196-197, 197f
    twitches, 194-195, 195f-196f
  indications for, 178-182
  of lizards, 216-218, 217f
  mechanical devices for, 1223
  of mice, 216
  of piglets, 207, 208f
  of pigs, 205-207, 207f
  of psittacines, 211-213, 212f-213f
  of rabbits, 214-215, 214f
  for radiography, 550-551
  of reptiles, 216-219
  of sheep, 209, 209f
  of small ruminants, 208-211
  of snakes, 218, 219f
  of sugar gliders, 216
  for surgery, 1223
  of swine, 205-207, 207f
  tail, 203-204, 204f
  tips for, 184b
  of tortoises, 218-219
  of turtles, 218-219, 219f
Restrictive breathing, 908-909

Resuscitation. *See*
　　Cardiopulmonary
　　cerebrovascular resuscitation
Retained placenta, 760, 760f
Retention enema, 642, 643f
Retention of employees, 60-61
Reticulocyte count, 412b
Reticulocytes, 411f, 412
Reticuloperitonitis, traumatic,
　　1281
Retort, 305
Retractors, 1140, 1141f, 1196,
　　1196f
Retrobulbar block, 1292
Retroperitoneal structures, 1198
Reverberation artifact, 554-555,
　　555f
Reversal agents, 1080
Reverse distribution company,
　　1038
Reverse zoonoses, 704
Reverse-cutting needles, 1204
Rhinitis, 686t-687t
Rhipicephalus sanguineus, 467t
Rhodococcus equi, 503
RIA. *See* Radioimmunoassay
Riboflavin, 302, 302t, 347t
Ribosomal DNA, 513-514
Rickets, 301, 339t-340t
Rickettsia rickettsii, 468t-469t, 709t
Right displaced abomasum,
　　1281-1282
Right dorsal colitis, 728, 729t-730t
"Right to know" laws, 121
Ringworm, 125, 709t-710t, 736,
　　770, 770f
Robert Jones bandage, 954-955,
　　981, 984f, 1269-1270
　　modified, 981, 985f, 986-987
Rochester-Carmalt forceps,
　　1139-1140
Rochester-Ochsner forceps,
　　1139-1140
Rochester-Péan forceps,
　　1139-1140
Rocky Mountain spotted fever,
　　468t-469t, 709t
Rodents
　　anesthesia for, 838
　　antibiotics for, 838
　　antiparasitic agents for, 838
　　types of, 838
Roeder towel clamps, 1183
Roentgen, 542, 544b
Rolled conforming gauze, 995
Romanowsky-type stains, 405
Romifidine, 1067t-1069t, 1082
Rongeurs, 1143, 1144f, 1153, 1153f
R-on-T phenomenon, 941b
Root abscesses, 1352
Root fractures, 1343
Root tip elevators, 1343f
Rosemary, 854t-855t
Rostral, 1301
Rotating anode x-ray tube,
　　520f-521f, 521-522
Rotavirus
　　diarrhea in swine caused by,
　　　773t-774t
　　vaccine for, 277t-283t
Rouleaux formation, 405-406,
　　406f
Roundworms
　　Baylisascaris procyonis, 454-455,
　　　455b
　　characteristics of, 451, 451b
　　prevention of, 275t
　　in puppies, 442b
　　Toxocara spp.. *See Toxocara* spp.
Rugae, 1309, 1311f

Rules and regulations
　　description of, 8, 25-26
　　model, 27b
　　National Association of
　　　Veterinary Technicians in
　　　America, 27b, 31
Rumen, 622
Rumen contractions, 256
Rumen fluid
　　analysis of, 750, 960-961
　　collection of, 659-660
　　　in bovine, 659-660, 660f
　　　indications for, 659
　　　orogastric tube method, 659
　　　in sheep, 660
　　　in small ruminants, 660
　　pH, 750-753
Rumen indigestion, 751t-752t, 753
Rumen trocarization, 754
Rumen trocars, 959, 960f
Rumen tympany, 751t-752t, 754,
　　958-959
Rumenocentesis, 660
Rumenostomy, 959-960, 960f,
　　1280
Ruminants. *See also* Beef cattle;
　　Cattle; Dairy cattle; Ewe;
　　Goats; Horse(s); Large
　　animal(s); Sheep; Small
　　ruminants
　　abdominal examination in, 256,
　　　256f
　　contact calls by, 172-173
　　diseases and conditions that
　　　affect, 747-771
　　anaplasmosis, 763
　　anthrax, 763
　　blackleg, 769-770
　　bloat, 751t-752t, 754
　　bovine respiratory disease
　　　syndrome, 756-758, 758f
　　bovine viral diarrhea,
　　　751t-752t, 755-756, 755f,
　　　757t
　　caprine arthritis encephalitis,
　　　765t-766t, 767
　　cardiovascular, 763-764
　　caseous lymphadenitis,
　　　762-763, 763b
　　contagious ecthyma, 770,
　　　770b, 770f
　　copper toxicity, 763, 763f
　　cutaneous papillomas, 770
　　dermatophytosis, 770, 770f
　　digestive system, 750-756
　　endoparasitism, 751t-752t,
　　　755
　　foot rot, 768-769, 768f
　　grain overload, 750,
　　　751t-752t, 753-754, 1281
　　hemolymphatic system,
　　　762-763
　　infectious bovine
　　　keratoconjunctivitis,
　　　767-768, 768f
　　interdigital necrobacillosis,
　　　768-769, 768f
　　Johne's disease, 288, 756,
　　　756b, 756f
　　keratoconjunctivitis, 767
　　ketosis, 339t-340t, 761, 761f
　　lameness, 768, 1283
　　laminitis, 769, 769b, 769f
　　listeriosis, 767, 767f
　　lymphosarcoma, 762, 762f
　　malignant edema, 769-770
　　mammary gland, 758-761
　　mastitis. *See* Mastitis
　　metabolic, 761-762
　　metritis, 760

Ruminants *(Continued)*
　　milk fever, 339t-340t, 761
　　musculoskeletal, 768-770
　　nervous system, 764-767
　　neurologic, 764-767
　　ophthalmologic, 767-768,
　　　768f
　　ovine progressive pneumonia,
　　　758, 760
　　papillomatous digital
　　　dermatitis, 769, 769f
　　pericarditis, 764, 764f
　　periparturient hypocalcemia,
　　　761
　　pharyngeal abscessation,
　　　751t-752t, 753
　　pharyngeal trauma,
　　　751t-752t, 753
　　pinkeye, 767
　　polioencephalomalacia,
　　　765t-766t, 767
　　pregnancy toxemia, 761-762
　　pseudopregnancy, 760-761
　　pyelonephritis, 770
　　rabies, 764, 764f, 765t-766t
　　reproductive system, 758-761
　　respiratory, 756-758, 757t
　　retained placenta, 760, 760f
　　rumen indigestion, 751t-752t,
　　　753
　　rumen tympany, 751t-752t,
　　　754
　　salmonellosis, 729t-730t,
　　　751t-752t, 755
　　scrapie, 764-766, 764f
　　skin, 770, 770f
　　tetanus, 765t-766t, 766, 766f
　　traumatic reticuloperitonitis,
　　　751t-752t, 754-755, 754f,
　　　755b
　　urinary, 770-771, 1293-1295
　　urolithiasis, 771, 771f
　　vegetative endocarditis,
　　　763-764
　　endotracheal intubation in,
　　　1100
　　fasting in, 1078t
　　feeding problems in,
　　　339t-340t
　　fractures in, 962-963
　　heart auscultation in, 255
　　joint luxations in, 962-963
　　maternal behavior in, 174
　　mucous membranes in,
　　　255-256, 255f
　　musculoskeletal injuries in,
　　　962-964
　　necropsy examination of,
　　　578-580
　　nonsteroidal anti-inflammatory
　　　drugs in, 1073
　　olfaction capabilities of, 172
　　physical examination of,
　　　254-257, 256f
　　protein for, 341-342
　　pulse in, 255, 255f
　　respiratory injuries in,
　　　961-962
　　rumen contractions in, 256
　　social facilitation of, 173
　　social hierarchies in, 173
　　surgical procedures in,
　　　1295-1296
　　terminology associated with,
　　　245t
　　vocalizations by, 172-173
Run
　　description of, 49
　　removing a pet from, 182
"Running W" method, 205

S
S-Adenosylmethionine, 851,
　　1023-1024
Safelights, 537, 537f
Safety
　　anesthesia, 127-129
　　compressed gases, 129, 129f
　　laser, 1135-1136, 1135f-1136f
　　leadership's rights and
　　　responsibilities, 116-117
　　medical waste, 129-130, 131t
　　radiology, 126-127
　　rights to, 116-117
　　sharps, 129-130
　　workplace, 34
Safety program
　　objectives of, 116
　　veterinary technician's
　　　responsibilities, 116
Safety training, 117
Salary, 5-6, 5t
Salmonella spp., 504, 710t,
　　729t-730t
Salmonellosis, 729t-730t,
　　751t-752t, 755, 775t
Salt mannitol agar, 493t-494t
Salt poisoning, 777
Sample
　　anticoagulants added to, 485
　　blood. *See* Blood sample
　　bone marrow aspirate,
　　　618f-619f
　　bronchoalveolar lavage, 489
　　collection of
　　　blood, 489
　　　dermatophytes, 509
　　　feces, 489
　　　general information about,
　　　　485-488
　　　joint fluid, 489
　　　milk, 489
　　　at necropsy, 568
　　　swabs used in, 488, 489f
　　　tissue, 488
　　direct microscopic examination
　　　of, 490
　　fecal. *See* Fecal samples
　　Gram stain, 490-491, 491b, 491f
　　milk. *See* Milk sample
　　processing of, 490-492
　　tissue, 488
　　transportation, 489-490, 489f
　　transtracheal wash, 489
　　urine. *See* Urine sample
Sanctions, disciplinary, 33-34
Sarcocystis neurona, 734
Sarcoid, 736
Sarcoma
　　hemangiosarcoma, 711t
　　injection site, 711t
　　lymphosarcoma, 732, 762, 762f
　　osteosarcoma, 711t, 712
Sarcopenia, 324
Sarcoptes scabiei, 462-467, 463f,
　　464b
Sarcoptic mange, 125, 215b
Saturated sodium chloride
　　solution, 477
Scale of contrast, 530
Scale (skin), 240
Scalers, 1327-1328, 1328b, 1328f
Scaling
　　hand, 1326-1333
　　power. *See* Power scaling
　　principles of, 1329-1330,
　　　1329f
　　subgingival, 1328-1329, 1328f
　　supragingival, 1327-1328
Scalpel, 1131, 1131f, 1195, 1195f

Scatter radiation, 522-523, 523f, 532, 537

Scavenging system, 127, 1090f, 1097

Scheduling of appointments, 71-72, 76, 77f

Schiff-Sherrington posture, 911

Schistosome cercarial dermatitis, 443-445, 445f

Schistosomes, 443-445, 444f

Schroeder-Thomas splint, 987

Sciatic nerve paresis and paralysis, 1284

Scissors, 1136-1137, 1137f

Scope of practice
  description of, 9
  practicing beyond, 31

Scours, calf, 748-749, 749f

Scrapie, 580b, 764-766, 764f

Scratching, 158, 159f

Scratching posts, 159f

Screen craze, 534

Screen film, 534-535, 535f

Screens, intensifying, 533-534, 533f

Screws, bone, 1148, 1148f

Scrotal hernia, 1266

Scrotal urethrostomy, 1245

Scrotum
  ablation of, 1240, 1240f
  physical examination of, 239

Scrub in, 1158

Scrub suits, 1174

Scruffing
  of cats, 186, 186f-187f
  of ferrets, 215-216, 215f
  of hamsters, 216

Second heart sound, 235-236

Second intention wound healing, 973, 977-978, 977b

Secondary radiation, 546-547

Secondary spermatocytes, 372

Second-degree AV block
  in cats, 943, 943f
  in dogs, 943, 943f
  in horses, 250, 727

Second-degree burns, 979

Sedation, 1078

Sedatives, 1081

Seed ticks, 466

Segmented neutrophils, 413

Selamectin, 463

Seldin retractor, 1144f

Seldinger technique, 595, 595f

Selective serotonin reuptake inhibitors, 145t-146t

Selegiline, 144, 145t-146t

Selenite, 493t-494t

Selenium, 303t, 304
  acute toxicity from, 363
  for livestock, 345t-346t

Self-appraisal, 61

Self-mutilation, in stallions, 170

Self-retaining retractors, 1140, 1141f

Self-trauma, risk for, 680t

Semen analysis, 393-394

Semi-closed rebreathing system, 1095

Semimembranosus muscle, 631, 632f

Semi-moist pet food, 305

Semi-occlusive bandages, 979-980

Semitendinosus muscle, 631, 632f

Senior cats. *See also* Geriatric care, cats and dogs
  feeding of, 329
  wellness of, 261-262

Senior dogs. *See also* Geriatric care, cats and dogs
  energy of, 324
  fat requirements, 324
  feeding of, 324-325
  fiber for, 324-325
  minerals for, 325
  protein requirements, 324
  vitamins for, 325
  wellness of, 261-262

Senn retractor, 1140, 1141f

Separation anxiety, 152

Sepsis, 803b, 915-916

Septic arthritis, 803b, 1276, 1285-1286

Septic metritis, 760

Septic physitis, 803b

Septic shock, 803b, 915

Septicemia, 745

Serologic tests, 428-430, 429f

Serology, 428-430

Seromas, 1219-1220, 1220b, 1252-1253

Sertoli cells, 370

Serum chemistry panel, 745

Settlement agreements, 33

Sevoflurane, 826, 1086, 1093-1094

Sexual behavior
  in cattle, 174
  of mare, 169
  of stallion, 169-170

Shadowing, 555

Shared-vector zoonoses, 704

Sharp trocar
  for arthroscopy, 1150, 1150f
  for laparoscopy, 1154, 1154f

Sharpening of dental instruments, 1330, 1330f

Sharps, 129-130, 131t

Sharps container, 129-130

Sheep. *See also* Ewe; Lamb(s)
  abdominocentesis in, 668-669
  analgesics for, 1068t-1069t
  approaching, 208
  blood sample collection in
    arterial, 654
    venous, 648, 648f-649f
  body condition score for, 762b
  body temperature of, 208b, 248t
  breeding flock, 353-356, 355t
    energy for, 354, 354b
    minerals for, 356
    protein for, 354, 355b
    vitamins for, 356
  breeding season for, 390-391
  breeds of, 354b
  capture of, 208
  catheterization in, 629
  dominant behaviors in, 173-174
  endotracheal intubation in, 1098
  energy requirements for, 354b
  epidural administration in, 641
  estrous cycle in, 390
  feces in, 257
  gestation in, 391
  heart rate in, 248t
  intramuscular administration in, 633, 633f
  intraperitoneal administration in, 637
  intravenous administration in, 629
  mastitis in, 760
  nonprotein nitrogen use in, 355b
  nutritional considerations in, 355t
  orogastric intubation in, 660f

Sheep *(Continued)*
  ovine progressive pneumonia, 758, 760
  pain management in, 1064t-1065t, 1071-1073
  parasitism in, 289
  pasture feeding of, 354b
  preventive health programs for, 288-289
  puberty in, 389
  pulse in, 255
  rectal prolapse in, 1295-1296
  reproduction in. *See* Reproduction, goats
  respiratory rate in, 248t
  restraint of, 209, 209f
  rumen fluid collection in, 660
  scrapie in, 764f
  subcutaneous administration in, 635, 636f
  surgery-related pain in, 1066t
  tail docking in, 288-289, 1296
  terminology associated with, 245t
  urinary catheterization in, 657
  urine collection in, 657
  urolithiasis in, 967-969, 1064t-1065t, 1294f
  vaccines used in, 289t
  venipuncture in, 648, 648f-649f

Shepherd's hook, 1312

Shiatsu, 869

Shock, 230
  cardiogenic, 915
  definition of, 914-915
  distributive, 915
  hypovolemic, 915
  inflammatory response during, 915-916
  obstructive, 915
  septic, 915
  in small animals, 914-916
  stages of, 914-915

Short-chain fatty acids, 298-299

SI units, 542, 544b

Sick sinus syndrome, 944

Sickle scalers, 1327-1328, 1328f

Side effects, 1014

Sieverts, 542, 544b

Sieving method, 478-479

Signage, 66-67, 67f

Signalment, 87-88
  of large animals, 244
  of small animals, 224

Sildenafil, 1026

Silent heat, 169

Silicon, 345t-346t

Silk sutures, 1202

Silymarin, 1023-1024

Simple carbohydrates, 294

Sinoatrial node, 935-936

Sinus arrhythmia, 938-939, 938f

Sinus bradycardia, 939

Sinus rhythm, 938, 938f

Sinus tachycardia, 939

Sinusitis, 686t-687t, 1374

Skin
  of horses, 167-168
  physical examination of, 240
  reflection of, during necropsy, 570-573, 571f-572f
  of reptiles, 832

Skin diseases
  in horses, 1370
  in ruminants, 770, 770f
  in small animals, 701, 702t-703t, 709t

Skin masses, 240

Skin papules, 240

Skin pinch test, 253

Skin snap test, 253

Skin turgor, 253, 894

Skin twitch, of horse, 195f

Skin wounds, 486t-487t

Skinks, 218f

Skinnerian conditioning, 137-138

Skull
  axis of, 573-574
  fracture of, in horses, 733
  necropsy examination of, 573-574, 574f

Slice-thickness artifact, 555

Slings, 875, 987-988
  aftercare for, 990-993
  carpal flexion, 988, 991f
  in geriatric cats and dogs, 1366, 1366f
  90/90 flexion, 988
  Velpeau, 988, 990f

Slipper, 786

Small animal(s). *See also* Cat(s); Dog(s); *specific small animal*
  abdominocentesis in, 610-611, 916, 916f
  anesthesia in
    equipment preparation, 1113
    induction of, 1115-1116
    intramuscular induction of, 1116
    intravenous induction of, 1115-1116
    maintenance of, 1116-1117
    patient positioning, 1117
    preanesthetic period, 1115
    premedication, 1114b
    protocol for, 1112-1113
    recommendations, 1115t
    recovery, 1117-1118
    sequence of events, 1113b
  arthrocentesis in, 614-616
  bone marrow aspiration in, 616-620
  diagnostic peritoneal lavage in, 611
  diseases in, 681-717. *See also specific disease*
    cardiovascular, 685-689
    digestive, 689-695, 707t
    ears, 701, 702t-703t
    endocrine, 698-699
    etiology, 681
    eyes, 701, 702t-703t
    hepatobiliary, 689-695
    immune-mediated, 700-701
    joint-related, 701
    reproductive, 699-700
    respiratory, 682-685, 685t-687t
    skin, 701, 702t-703t, 709t
    urinary, 695-698
  drug administration in
    aural, 588
    intradermal, 589
    intramuscular, 590
    intranasal, 589
    intraosseous, 599
    intraperitoneal, 599
    intrarectal, 588-589
    oral, 586-587
    orogastric intubation, 587-588
    subcutaneous, 589
    transdermal, 588
  emergency and critical care nursing, 908-933
    abdominocentesis, 916, 916f
    acute abdomen, 932, 932b
    advanced life support, 924-926, 924f, 925t

Small animal(s) (Continued)
arterial blood gas analysis, 913, 919-920, 920f
arterial blood pressure monitoring, 928-930, 929f-930f
cardiopulmonary arrest, 921
cardiopulmonary cerebrovascular resuscitation. See Cardiopulmonary cerebrovascular resuscitation
cardiovascular system triage, 910
central venous pressure monitoring, 927-928
crash cart, 914, 914f
dehydration, 912b
electrocardiography, 913
emergencies, 931-933
emergency care station, 914
first aid, 913
gastric dilatation-volvulus, 932
hydration assessments, 911-912
hypovolemia assessments, 911-912
initial diagnostics, 912-913
neurologic system, 910-911
oxygen therapy, 917-921
patient monitoring, 927-930
pulmonary function, 920
reperfusion injury, 916
respiratory distress, 931-932
respiratory system
support of, 917-921
thoracic auscultation, 910
triage of, 908-910
shock. See Shock
standard of care, 931-933
systemic inflammatory response syndrome, 914-916, 915b-916b
thoracic drain placement, 917, 917f
thoracocentesis, 916-917
toxin exposure, 932-933, 933b, 934t
tracheostomy tubes, 917, 918f
triage, 908-911
definition of, 908
in-hospital, 908-911
telephone, 908
urethral obstruction, 932
endotracheal intubation in, 1098-1099, 1099f
fecal sample collection in, 474, 609
infectious diseases in, 705, 706t-710t
long-bone fractures in, 1255-1257
necropsy of. See Necropsy, in small animals
recumbent, 930-931
surgery/surgical nursing in
amputation, 1251-1253, 1253f
antibiotic prophylaxis, 1215-1216
bandage care, 1221-1222, 1222f
blood loss concerns, 1217
castration
in cats, 1240-1241, 1241f-1242f
in dogs, 1236-1240, 1239f-1240f

Small animal(s) (Continued)
celiotomy. See Celiotomy
cervical disc surgery, 1254, 1254f
cesarean delivery, 1241-1243
client education about, 1257-1258
cystostomy, 1243-1245
dewclaw removal, 1224-1225
discharge instructions, 1258
dorsal recumbency for, 1171, 1171b
drain care, 1222, 1223f
elective, 1223
gastrointestinal surgery, 1229-1231
hanging leg surgical preparation, 1171, 1172f, 1192f
heat retention methods, 1217-1218, 1217f
hernia. See Hernia
hypothermia, 1217-1218, 1217f-1218f
incision evaluation, 1219-1221, 1220f-1221f
instrument packs for, 1156t
joints, 1257
lumpectomy, 1249-1250
mammary neoplasia removal, 1250-1251
monitoring, 1216-1217
neurologic care, 1253-1255
nonelective, 1223
onychectomy. See Onychectomy
orthopedic, 1255-1257
ovariohysterectomy, 1233-1235, 1234f-1235f
pain management, 1218-1219, 1220f
patient preparation for, 1169-1171
perioperative antibiotics, 1215-1216
positioning, 1215-1223
positioning for, 1171
preoperative assessments, 1215
pyometra, 1235-1236
restraint for, 1223
skin preparation, 1169-1171, 1170f
staple removal, 1221, 1222f
surgical clip, 1169-1170
surgical preparation, 1215-1223
surgical scrub for, 1170-1171, 1170f
suture removal, 1221, 1222f
tail docking, 1224
thoracolumbar disc surgery, 1254
urethrostomy, 1245-1247, 1246f
warming equipment, 1215, 1216f
thoracocentesis in, 609-610, 609b, 610f, 916-917
transtracheal wash in, 611-614
indications for, 611
percutaneous technique, 612-613, 612f
sample
cytologic interpretation of, 613-614
handling of, 613
through-the-needle catheter system for, 613
two-catheter system for, 612, 612f

Small animal practices
description of, 44-45
examination rooms, 46, 47f
exercise area in, 50
exterior of, 45, 45f
fenced enclosures in, 50
grooming services, 50
house call services, 51
inpatient areas in, 47-50, 48f
isolation ward in, 49
kitchen in, 50, 50f
laboratories in, 47, 47f
maintenance of, 45
outpatient areas in, 45-47, 45f
pharmacy areas in, 47, 48f
reception area in, 46, 46f
treatment area in, 47, 48f
waiting area in, 46, 46f
Small intestine
contrast agents used in radiography of, 548
diarrhea of, 690t
palpation of, 238
Small ruminants. See also Small animal(s); specific small ruminant
approaching, 208
capture of, 208-211
flight zones of, 208
observation of, 208
restraint of, 208-211
Smears
blood. See Blood smear
cytology, 419f
impression, 419, 419f
otic cytology, 421-422
Smudge cells, 417
Snakes
anesthesia of, 826-827
handling of, 218, 219f
nutrition for, 829
restraint of, 218, 219f
venipuncture in, 825
SNAP4Dx test, 429-430
Sneeze, 684
Snook ovariohysterectomy hook, 1140, 1141f
Snuffles, 837
SOAP notes
definition of, 81
description of, 49
elements of, 94-96, 95f
Social behavior
in cats, 156
in dogs, 147-148, 148f
in horses, 168
Social play, 142
Social status aggression, 153b
Socialization
behavior problems prevented through, 143
of kittens, 156
of puppies, 147
Society of Veterinary Behavior Technicians, 136b
Sodium, 303, 303t, 344t
Sodium bicarbonate, 892-893, 893b, 1331
Sodium hyaluronate, 1067t-1068t
Sodium hypochlorite, 1339b
Sodium ion toxicosis, 777
Sodium nitrate solution, 477
Soft palate
anatomy of, 1309
dorsal displacement of, 1276-1277
Soft tissue injuries, 955-957
Solid phase immunoassays, 510-512
Solid tissue masses, 418-419

Soluble fiber, 294, 300
Somatic migration, 456
Sonic scaler, 1323
Sore mouth, 289
Sotalol, 1026, 1026t
Sound waves, 551, 551f
Source-oriented medical record, 86
South American camelids, 779, 779b
Sows
milk from, 357-358
vaccines for, 286
Sparganosis, 450
Sparganum, 450
Spay hook, 1140, 1141f
Specialties, 3
Specialty facility, 39, 40b, 51-52
caseloads in, 43
definition of, 40b
description of, 39
Specific gravity, 424, 431, 477
Specific-purpose pet food, 306
Specimen. See also Sample
diagnostic, shipping of, 569
direct microscopic examination of, 490
fecal. See Fecal samples
tissue, 488
Spectrophotometry, 427
Speed locks, 1144
Sperm
analysis of, 393-394
concentration tests, 394
ejaculation of, 371-372
emission of, 371-372
maturation of, 372
motility assessments, 393-394
production of, 370
Spermatocytes, 372
Spermatogenesis, 370, 372
Spermatogonia, 372
Spermatozoan, 372
Spherocytes, 409f-411f, 410
Sphygmomanometer, 1108, 1109f
Spica splint, 987
Spinal accessory nerve, 242, 243t
Spinal ataxia, 734
Spinal column instability, 1253-1254
Spinal cord
contrast agents used in radiography of, 549-550
necropsy examination of, 573, 574f, 578, 582
Spinal cord disorders
cervical vertebral malformation, 734
in horses, 734-735
Wobbler syndrome, 734
Spinal neurons, 1052-1053
Spine, draping of, 1192
Spirochetes, 505
Spirometra mansonoides, 450-451, 450b, 451f
Spironolactone, 1025, 1025t
Spleen, 1198
necropsy examination of, 576
palpation of, 238
Splints
aftercare for, 990-993
for cattle, 1002-1007
description of, 986-987
forelimb, 988f
for horses, 994-1002, 998f
Kimsey, 1269-1270, 1270f
modified Thomas, 1003-1007, 1004f-1008f
non–weight-bearing, 988b
prefabricated, 987

Splints *(Continued)*
  Schroeder-Thomas, 987
  spica, 987
Sporothrix schenckii, 510, 511f
Sporozoites, 472
Sports massage, 869
Spraying, 124
Sputum sample, 832
Squamous cell carcinoma, 711t, 732
  ocular, 1291-1292, 1291f
  oral, 1348, 1348f
Squeeze chute, 202, 202f
ST segment, 937
Stable vices, 171-172
Stage micrometer, 476
Staged surgical débridement, 976b
Stains, 420
  acid-fast, 478, 490, 492, 492b
  for coccidian parasites, 478
  Gram, 490-491, 491b, 491f
  Romanowsky-type, 405
  Wright, 405
  Wright-Giemsa, 405, 420
Stallion. *See also* Horse(s)
  breeding of, 169-170
  breeding soundness
    examination in, 392-393
  castration of, 170, 1267-1268, 1267f
  definition of, 244t, 380-381
  libido of, 169-170
  masturbation by, 170
  self-mutilation in, 170
  sexual behavior of, 169-170
  teasing of mare by, 383, 383f
  urinary catheterization in, 655
Standard fecal flotation, 477-478, 477f
Standard operating procedure, 427
Staphylococcus spp.
  S. aureus, 502-503, 759
  S. pseudintermedius, 502-503
Staple removal, 1221, 1222f
Stapling equipment, 1141-1142, 1142f, 1142t
Statement of cash flows, 68-69
Statement of nutritional adequacy, 312
Stationary anode x-ray tube, 520f, 521
Stay sutures, 1198, 1198f
Steady state, 1013
Steam sterilization, 1163-1164
Steer, 245t, 387
Sterile fields
  description of, 1176-1182
  maintenance of, 1183
Sterile items, 1184-1185, 1184f
Sterile milk sample, 658
Sterile packs, 1163t, 1164
Sterilization
  arthroscopic equipment, 1168-1169
  autoclave, 1163-1164, 1163f
  chemical, 1164-1168
  cold, 1168, 1168f
  definition of, 1160-1161, 1166b
  ethylene oxide, 1165, 1165f
  filtration, 1161
  flash, 1164, 1166b
  heat for, 1162-1164
  hydrogen peroxide gas plasma, 1166
  indicators of, 1164, 1165f
  laparoscopic equipment, 1168-1169
  physical methods of, 1161-1164
  quality control, 1164
  radiation, 1161

Stertor, 234, 684
Stethoscope, 234, 234f, 251, 251f, 789-790
Stifle joint
  arthrocentesis of, 614-616
  description of, 523f
Stimulus-response relationships, 137
Stitch scissors, 1136-1137, 1137f
Stockinette, 998-999, 999f-1000f, 1191f
Stocks, 198, 198f
Stomach
  contrast agents used in radiography of, 548
  gastric dilatation-volvulus of, 915, 932, 1231-1233, 1232f
  lavage of, in reptiles, 825
  palpation of, 238
  squamous cell carcinoma of, in horses, 732
Stomatitis
  in cats, 1349, 1349f
  in dogs, 1349, 1349f
  lymphocytic-plasmacytic, 1309, 1311f, 1349
Stomatocytes, 409
Storage area, 51
Straight shank, 1327, 1327f
Strangles
  bastard, 722
  description of, 722, 723t-724t
  vaccine for, 277t-283t, 283
Stranguria, 770
Strategic planning, 41
Streptococcus spp.
  description of, 503
  S. agalactiae, 499, 759
  S. bovis, 753
  S. equi, 722, 723t-724t
Stress
  addressing of, 61-62
  reduction of, 62, 62b
  stressors, 61-62
Stress-induced hyperglycemia, 698
Stridor, 234, 684, 917-918
Strike-through, 1184-1185, 1221-1222, 1222f
Striking, 190
Strongyloides spp., 729t-730t
  S. cati, 458-460, 460f
  S. ransomi, 773t-774t
  S. stercoralis, 458-460, 460f
Strongyloidosis, 458-460, 460f
Struvite, 433-435, 436f
Struvite urolithiasis, 683t
Subchondral bone, 1153
Subclinical mastitis, 759, 759f
Subcutaneous abdominal vein
  blood sample collection from, 646-647
  intravenous drug administration using, 628
Subcutaneous administration
  of fluids, 890, 890b
  sites for, 589
  in small animals, 589
Subgingival curettes, 1328-1329, 1328f
Submissive behaviors
  in cats, 159-160
  in cattle, 173-174
  description of, 142
  in dogs, 148, 148f
Subordinate role, 147-148
Subsolar abscess, 1275-1276
Substance abuse, 62
Substantive violations, 29-32
Suckling reflex, 791b, 799-800
Sucralfate, 1024t

Suction tips, 1140-1141, 1141f
Sugar gliders, 216, 843-844, 843f, 844b
Sulcus depth, 1312b
Sulfonamides, 1018t-1019t, 1035t
Sulfonation, 1012t
Sulfur, 344t
Summary forms, 98-105
Superfecundation, 368b, 369
Superfetation, 369
Superficial thermal therapy, 874-875
Supernumerary teat, 1288
Supplements, 295
Support area, 51
Suppositories, 588
Supragingival instruments, 1327-1328
Supragingival scaling, 1327
Supraventricular tachycardia, 940, 940f
Surge suppressors, 119, 119f
Surgery
  abdominal, 1197-1198
    adhesion formation after, 1282
    approaches for, 1280-1281
    in cattle, 1280-1281
    in horses, 1263-1264
  antibiotic prophylaxis, 1215-1216
  arthroscopic. *See* Arthroscopic surgery
  blood loss during, 1217
  cancer treated with, 714
  cryosurgery, 714
  gastrointestinal
    in horses, 1263-1266
    in small animals, 1229-1231
  hemostasis during, 1196-1197, 1196f, 1210
  in horses
    draping of, 1204-1206, 1205f-1207f
    hemostasis, 1210
    hollow organ surgery, 1208-1209, 1209f
    instrument setup and handling, 1207-1208, 1207f-1208f
    orthopedic surgery, 1209, 1210f
    overhead hoist system for, 1171-1172, 1174f
    patient positioning, 1171-1172, 1173f
    retraction techniques, 1210, 1210f
    skin preparation, 1172-1174, 1173f
    surgical assisting, 1204-1211
    suture materials, 1210-1211, 1210f
  intraoperative techniques, 1194-1200
    camera manipulation, 1197
    hemostasis, 1196-1197, 1196f, 1210
    instrumentation cords and tubing, 1194-1195, 1195f
    lavage, 1197
    lighting, 1194, 1194f
    passing of instruments, 1195, 1195f
    retraction, 1196, 1196f
    scalpel, 1195, 1195f
    suctioning, 1197
    suture cutting, 1197
    tissue manipulation, 1197-1199

Surgery *(Continued)*
  in large animals, 1156t. *See also specific animal*
  operating room for. *See* Operating room
  positioning for
    description of, 1188-1193
    horses, 1171-1172, 1173f
    small animals, 1171
  postoperative management, 1200-1201
  preoperative preparation
    clipping, 1188
    draping, 1188-1193, 1189f, 1191f-1192f
    positioning, 1188-1193
    quarter drapes, 1183-1184, 1189-1190, 1190f-1191f
    surgical scrub, 1188
  in ruminants, 1124. *See also specific ruminant*
  in small animals
    dorsal recumbency for, 1171, 1171b
    hanging leg surgical preparation, 1171, 1172f, 1192f
    instrument packs for, 1156t
    patient preparation for, 1169-1171
    positioning for, 1171
    skin preparation, 1169-1171, 1170f
    surgical clip, 1169-1170
    surgical scrub for, 1170-1171, 1170f
  suction during, 1194
Surgery log, 107
Surgery table, 1188f, 1193-1194, 1193f
Surgery tray, 1157, 1157f
Surgical areas
  in large animal practices, 54, 54f
  in small animal practices, 50-51, 51f
Surgical assistant, 1188
Surgical assisting
  in equine surgery, 1204-1211
  surgical assistant's role, 1188
Surgical cap, 1174-1175, 1175f
Surgical implants, 1199-1200, 1199f-1200f
Surgical instruments
  arthroscopic. *See* Arthroscopic surgery, instruments and equipment for
  cannulas, 1154, 1155f
  care of, 1157-1158, 1158f
  chisels, 1144, 1146f
  components of, 1138f
  curettes, 1143-1144, 1145f, 1153, 1153f
  electrosurgery, 1131, 1132f
  in equine surgery, 1207-1208, 1207f-1208f
  Gigli wire, 1144-1145
  hemostatic forceps, 1139-1140, 1139f-1140f
  Jamshidi needles, 1145, 1146f
  laparoscopic, 1154-1155, 1156f
  lasers. *See* Laser(s)
  needle holders, 1137, 1137f
  ophthalmic instruments, 1142-1143, 1143f
  organization of, 1193-1194, 1193f
  orthopedic, 1143-1145, 1144f-1147f
  osteotomes, 1144, 1146f, 1153
  packs, 1155-1157, 1156t, 1163t

Surgical instruments (Continued)
  passing of, 1195, 1195f
  periosteal elevators, 1143, 1144f
  power equipment, 1145, 1147f
  retractors, 1140, 1141f, 1196, 1196f
  rongeurs, 1143, 1144f, 1153, 1153f
  scalpel, 1131, 1131f
  scissors, 1136-1137, 1137f
  stapling equipment, 1141-1142, 1142f, 1142t
  suction tips, 1140-1141, 1141f
  on surgery tray, 1157, 1157f
  thumb forceps, 1138, 1138f
  tissue forceps, 1139, 1139f
  trephines, 1145, 1146f
  ultrasonic cleaners for, 1157-1158, 1158f
  vascular sealing devices, 1142, 1143f
Surgical insurance, 244
Surgical lighting, 1194, 1194f
Surgical masks, 1175f
Surgical nursing
  of cattle. See Cattle, surgical nursing of
  of horses. See Horse(s), surgery and surgical nursing in
  of small animals. See Small animal(s), surgery/surgical nursing in
Surgical scrub, 1177f-1178f, 1188
Surgical site infection, 1160
Surgical sponges, 1194
Surgical team, 1174-1185
  attire of, 1174-1175, 1175f
  gloving, 1176, 1181f-1182f
  gowning, 1176, 1179f-1180f
  hand scrub, 1175-1176, 1177f
  scrubbed-in personnel, 1182-1183
  sterility maintenance in, 1176-1183
Suture(s)
  absorbable, 1202
  catgut, 1202
  classification of, 1202-1203
  cutting of, 1197
  handling of, 1201-1202
  in horses, 1210-1211, 1210f
  knots, 1202
  metallic, 1202-1203
  monofilament, 1201
  multifilament, 1201
  natural, 1202-1203
  nonabsorbable, 1202-1203
  placement of, 1204
  polyamide, 1203
  polybutester, 1203
  polyester, 1203
  polypropylene, 1203
  purpose of, 1201
  removal of, 1204, 1221, 1222f
  selection considerations for, 1201-1202
  silk, 1202
  size and strength of, 1201
  stay, 1198, 1198f
  synthetic, 1203
  wound type and, 1201
Suture needles, 1203-1204, 1203f
Suture packages, 1204, 1204f
Suturing, 1201
Swabs, 488, 489f
Swallowing reflex, 1078, 1106, 1107t
Swedish massage, 869-870

Swine. See also Pig(s); Piglets; Sows
  aggressive behavior by, 777-778
  analgesics for, 1068t-1069t
  approaching, 205-206
  behaviors in, 777-778
  blood sample collection in, 648-651
  breeding herd
    description of, 356-357
    energy, 357
    feed rations, 357t
    minerals, 357-358
    protein, 357
    vitamins, 357-358
  capture of, 205-207
  diseases and conditions that affect
    Aujeszky's disease, 772
    diarrhea, 773, 773t-775t
    erysipelas, 286, 772
    gastrointestinal, 773
    leptospirosis, 777
    musculoskeletal, 777
    nervous system, 777
    neurologic, 777
    pleuropneumonia, 775t
    porcine parvovirus, 773-777
    porcine reproductive and respiratory syndrome, 286, 772
    porcine stress syndrome, 777
    pseudorabies virus, 772, 772b
    reproductive, 773-777, 775t-776t
    respiratory, 773, 775t-776t
    salt poisoning, 777
  epidural administration in, 641
  flight zone of, 206
  gestation in, 773
  growing-finishing, 358-359
    energy requirements, 358
    minerals, 359
    protein for, 358
    vitamins, 359
  intramuscular administration in, 633-634
  intraperitoneal administration in, 638
  intravenous administration in, 629, 630f
  lactation, 357
  moving of, 206
  necropsy examination of, 580-581
  nutrition for
    description of, 356
    energy, 357
    feed rations, 357t
    growing-finishing pigs, 358-359
    minerals, 357-358
    protein, 357
    vitamins, 357-358
  observation of, 205
  pain management in, 1073
  pet, 207
  preventive health program for, 285-286
  reproduction in. See Reproduction, swine
  restraint of, 205-207, 207f
  senses in, 777
  starter, 358
  subcutaneous administration in, 635
  urine collection in, 657
  venipuncture in, 648-651
    auricular vein, 650
    coccygeal vein, 651

Swine (Continued)
  cranial vena cava, 649-650, 649f-650f
  jugular vein, 650
  orbital sinus, 651, 651f
  peripheral leg veins, 650-651, 651f
Swine dysentery, 775t
Swine influenza, 775t-776t
Sympathy card, 65
Symphyseal separation, 1350, 1350f
Syncope, 933
Synovial fluid
  analysis of
    in cats, 616
    in dogs, 616
  description of, 420
  normal values for, 616b, 956t
Syringes
  for arterial blood sample collection, 651, 652f
  for oral administration, 620-621, 620f
Systematic desensitization, 138-139
Systemic hypertension, 689
Systemic inflammatory response syndrome
  causes of, 915b
  definition of, 916b
  inflammatory mediators in, 915-916
  in small animals, 914-916, 915b-916b
Systems review, 226
Systolic murmurs, 236-237

T

T coat, 534
Tablets, 586, 587f
Tachyarrhythmias, 938
Tachycardia, 910
  atrial, 939, 940f
  junctional, 940, 940f
  sinus, 939
  supraventricular, 940, 940f
  ventricular, 924-925, 941
Tachypnea, 908-909
Tachyzoites, 471
Taenia pisiformis, 447, 448f, 475f
Taenia taeniaeformis, 447, 475f
Tail bandage, 990, 993f
Tail docking
  in dogs, 1224-1225
  in piglets, 772f
  in puppies, 1224
  in sheep, 288-289, 1296
Tail jack, 204, 204f, 628, 645-646
Tail restraint, 203-204, 204f
Tail tie, 198, 198f
"Take-away" method, 142
Tank pressure gauge, 1092, 1092f
Tapeworms
  calcareous bodies associated with, 475, 475f
  Dipylidium caninum. See Dipylidium caninum
  Echinococcus granulosus, 448-450, 448f-449f, 450b
  Echinococcus multilocularis, 448-450, 448f-449f, 450b
  fecal examination for, 475
  in horses, 475f
  pseudotapeworms, 450-451, 451f
  segments of, 475f
  Spirometra mansonoides, 450-451, 450b, 451f

Tapeworm (Continued)
  Taenia pisiformis, 447, 448f, 475f
  Taenia taeniaeformis, 447, 475f
Tapotement, 869, 870f
Targeted mail, 65-66
Tarsus joint, 614
Taurine, 297
Tea pills, 852
Teat, supernumerary, 1288
Teat cannula method, of abdominocentesis, 665-666
Technetium 99m, 556-557
Technical violations, 29
Technician evaluations
  description of, 96, 97t
  horses, 738t-739t
Teeth. See also Dentistry
  attachment level of, 1314f
  brachyodont, 1299, 1300f
  in camelids, 785-786
  canines, 1303, 1303f
  carnassial, 1303
  deciduous, 1299-1300, 1347
  eruption of, 1300t
  examination of, 1311-1312
  fractured, 1336, 1347
  in horses, 284-285, 1351, 1351f
  hypsodont, 1299
  incisors, 1302
  molars, 1303
  morphology of, 1299-1303
  multi-rooted, 1314
  needle, 285
  numeric system for, 1301, 1302f
  permanent, 1299-1300, 1337f
  premolars, 285, 1303, 1303f
  root abscesses, 1352
  Triadan system for, 1301, 1302f
Telephone triage, 908
Teleradiology, 528-529
Temporohyoid osteoarthropathy, 733-734
Tendonitis, 1275
Tenesmus, 690
TENS. See Transcutaneous electrical nerve stimulation
Territorial aggression, 153b
Territoriality, 156
Tertiary dentin, 1347
Testes
  anatomy of, 370
  canine, 371f
  enlargement of, 392f
  physical examination of, 239
Testicular biopsy, 394
Testosterone, 370
Tetanus
  characteristics of, 276, 735
  in horses, 735
  in ruminants, 765t-766t, 766, 766f
  "sawhorse" stance associated with, 766, 766f
  treatment of, 766
  vaccine for, 276, 277t-283t, 766
Tetanus antitoxin, 735
Tetanus toxoid, 735
Tetracyclines
  antimicrobial susceptibility testing for, 507t
  description of, 1018t-1019t
Tetrathionate broth, 493t-494t
Text messaging, 21
Thank you notes, 65
Theft of inventory, 74
Theophylline, 1017t
Therapeutic diets, 308-309
Therapeutic drug monitoring, 1016, 1017t

Therapeutic exercises, 866-867, 867f, 867t, 1061
Therapeutic ultrasound, 873, 873b, 873f, 1061
Thermocycler, 512-513
Thermogenesis, 793
Thermometer, rectal
    for large animals, 247-248, 247f-248f
    for small animals, 228-229, 230f
Thermotherapy, 1061
Thiamine, 294t, 301-302, 347t
Thiamine-deficiency polio, 339t-340t
Thiopental sodium, 1085, 1085b, 1116
Third heart sound, 235-236
Third intention wound healing, 977
Third-degree burns, 979
Thirty-party medical payment plans, 72
Thoracic auscultation, 910
Thoracic compression, 1393t-1395t
Thoracic drain placement, 917, 917f
Thoracic effusion, 419-420
Thoracic ultrasound, 950
Thoracocentesis/thoracentesis, 684
    in camelids, 661-662
    definition of, 950-951
    in horses, 660-661, 950-951
    indications for, 609
    in large animals, 660-662
    nursing care after, 610
    procedure for, 610
    in small animals, 609-610, 609b, 610f, 916-919
    technique for, 918-919
Thoracolumbar disc surgery, 1254
Thorax
    draping of, 1190
    surgical retraction of, 1198
Threadworms, 773t-774t
Three-host ticks, 466, 466b
Thrombin, 417
Thrombocytes, 407, 408f
Thrombocytopenia, 407-408
Thrombocytosis, 407-408
Thrombophlebitis, 586, 596
Thrombo-Wellcotest, 418
Through-the-needle catheters
    intravenous administration using, 591, 591f
    transtracheal wash through, 613
Through-transmission, 555
Thumb forceps, 1138, 1138f
Thumping, 214
Thunderstorms phobia, 144
Thyme, 854t-855t
Thyroid disease, 1020-1021
Thyroid gland, 792b
Thyroid hormones, 1020
Thyroxine, 698, 1020
Tibial plateau leveling osteotomy, 865
Tick paralysis, 468t-469t
Ticks, 466-467, 467t
    prevention of, 275t
Tie-over bandage, 988-989
Tiletamine, 826t-827t, 1085
Tilmicosin, 507t
Time cycle ventilators, 1125-1126
Timed method, of hand scrub, 1175-1176
Time-gain compensation control, 554
Tincture of iodine, 1166

Tissue
    chemotherapy-induced necrosis of, 715
    collection of, at necropsy, 569-570
    radiation sensitivity of, 541-542
    sample of, 488
    ultrasound interaction with, 551-553
Tissue forceps, 1139, 1139f
Tissue necrosis, 975
Tissue perfusion, 893
TNM staging, 712-713
α-Tocopherol, 301
Tolazoline, 1082-1083
Tom, 379
Tongue
    examination of, 1310
    necropsy examination of, 573, 573f
Tongue depressors, 219b
Tonic neck reflexes,. 791b
Tonification, 851
Tonsils, 573, 573f
Tooth brushing, 1335, 1335f
Tooth resorption, 1343-1344, 1344f
Topical medications
    nonsteroidal anti-inflammatory drugs, 1056
    transdermal administration of, 588
Topical ophthalmic administration
    in large animals, 638-639, 639f
    in small animals, 590-598, 591f
Tortoises. See also Turtles
    nutrition for, 828
    restraint of, 218-219
Total body water, 883
Total digestible nutrients, 342-343
Total hip prosthesis, 1149, 1149f
Total mixed ration, 343
Total parenteral nutrition, 334
Total proteins, 425, 912-913, 1217
Towel clamps, 1183, 1189
Towel restraint
    of cats, 186, 186f
    of dogs, 184-185
    of lizards, 217, 217f
    of psittacines, 212-213, 212f-213f
    of rabbits, 214, 214f
Toxemia, pregnancy, 761-762
Toxic line, 252-253
Toxic mastitis, 967
Toxic metritis, 967
Toxin exposure, 932-933, 933b, 934t
Toxocara spp.
    T. canis, 452-454, 452f-453f
    T. cati, 452-454, 452f
Toxoplasma gondii, 125, 471-472, 710t
Toxoplasmosis, 125, 710t
Trace minerals, 302
Trach wash. See Transtracheal wash
Tracheal migration, 452-453
Tracheal rings, 1286
Tracheal wash. See Transtracheal wash
Tracheostomy
    description of, 1286
    tubes for, 917, 918f, 962
Tracheotomy, 952-953
Traditional Chinese medicine, 851-852, 858-859
Training of employees, 60
Tramadol, 1058-1059, 1067t-1068t
Tranquilizers, 1061, 1081-1082

Transcutaneous electrical nerve stimulation, 872
Transdermal administration, 588, 641
Transendoscopic laser surgery, 1134f
Transfaunation, 960-961
Transfusion(s)
    albumin, 896
    blood, 895-904
        administration of, 901-904, 902b, 902f
        antibody screen, 898
        blood collection for, 898-899
        blood typing, 896-898, 896b, 897f
        cross-matching, 898
        donors, 896, 896t
        goal of, 895
        in horses, 903b
        indications for, 895-896
        monitoring of, 903-904
        plasma
            administration of, 902
            indications for, 895-896, 895b
        rate determinations, 902-903
        reactions to, 903-904, 903f
        testing before, 896-898
        volume determinations, 902-903, 902b
Transfusion-associated circulatory overload, 904
Transfusion-related acute lung injury, 904
Transitional epithelial cells, 433, 434f
Transmissible gastroenteritis, 773t-774t
Transmissible spongiform encephalopathy, 580b
Transportation, 36
Transtracheal wash
    endoscopic method of, 662-663
    in horses, 662-663, 663f, 951
    in large animals, 662-663
    percutaneous technique
        in large animals, 662
        in small animals, 612-613, 612f
    sample, 489
        cytologic interpretation of, 613-614
        handling of, 613
    in small animals, 611-614
        indications for, 611
        percutaneous technique, 612-613, 612f
        sample
            cytologic interpretation of, 613-614
            handling of, 613
        through-the-needle catheter system for, 613
        two-catheter system for, 612, 612f
Transverse facial artery, 249
Transverse facial vein, 644, 645f
Trauma
    dental, 1347-1348, 1348f
    head, 733
Traumatic brain injury, 910
Traumatic reticuloperitonitis, 751t-752t, 754-755, 755b, 1281
Treadmill, 868
Treatment areas
    in large animal practices, 53
    in small animal practices, 47, 48f

Treatment history, 245
Treatment plan estimate, 72
Treatment room, 11-13
Trematodes, 441-445
    definition of, 441
    Paragonimus kellicotti, 441-443, 443f
    schistosomes, 443-445, 444f
Trephines, 1145, 1146f
Triadan system, 1301, 1302f
Triage, 908-911
    definition of, 908
    in-hospital, 908-911
    telephone, 908
Triangle flap, 1342-1343
Triangulation, 1153
Tricane methane sulfonate, 1393t-1395t
Trichophyton spp., 709t, 770
Trichuriasis, 457-458, 457f-458f
Trichuris spp.
    T. campanula, 458b
    T. suis, 775t
    T. vulpis, 457-458, 457f-458f
Tricuspid valve insufficiency, 688
Tricyclic antidepressants, 145t-146t
Trigeminal nerve, 243t
Trigger-point massage, 869
Triiodothyronine, 698
Trilostane, 1021
Trimethoprim-sulfamethoxazole, 507t
Trimming. See Foot trimming; Nails, trimming of
Triple sugar iron agar slant, 493t-494t
Triplet, 940-941
Trochlear nerve, 243t
Trombicula spp., 465, 465f, 466b
Trophozoites, 470, 470b, 478
Trueperella pyogenes, 503
Trypsin, 976
TTEAM, 869, 877-878
TTouch wrap, 877-878, 878f
Tube cystotomy, 969, 1294-1295, 1295f
Tube-feeding. See also Feeding tubes
    of geriatric cats and dogs, 1365-1366
    of kittens, 795, 795b, 796f
    of psittacines, 815, 815f, 819-820
    of puppies, 795, 795b, 796f
    of reptiles, 827
Tubular epithelial cells, 433, 435f
Tularemia, 468t-469t
Tulathromycin, 507t
Tumor(s). See also Cancer
    biology of, 705-706
    categorization of, 712, 712t
    classification of, 712-713, 712t
    connective tissue, 712t
    epithelial tissue, 712t
    malignant, 706
    metastasis of, 706
    TNM staging of, 712-713
Tunica albuginea, 370, 380-381
Turtles. See also Tortoises
    cystocentesis in, 825
    restraint of, 218-219, 219f
    shell repair in, 823-824, 824f
Twitches, 194-195, 195f-196f
Two-host ticks, 466, 466b
Tympany, 911
    guttural pouch, 725, 1278
    rumen, 751t-752t, 754, 958-959
Tyzzer's disease, 837, 841

U

Uberschwinger artifact, 528
Ulcers
    colonic, 728
    corneal, 486t-487t, 702t-703t
    decubitus, 979, 1254f, 1364
    gastric, 728
Ultrasonic cleaners, 1157-1158,
    1158f
Ultrasonic scalers
    description of, 1323-1324
    energy dispersion, 1324-1325
    knob settings of, 1326
    magnetostrictive, 1325, 1326b
    piezoelectric, 1325
    tip designs for, 1324, 1324f
    types of, 1325
Ultrasound, 551-556
    abdominal, 947
    A-mode, 553
    artifacts on, 554-555
    basics of, 551, 551f
    B-mode, 553
    clinical uses of, 556, 556b
    display modes for, 553-554
    dynamic focusing technology,
        553
    echogenicity, 554-555, 556b
    examination, 555-556
    image, 552, 554
    M-mode, 553
    patient positioning for, 553f
    patient preparation for,
        552-553, 552f
    piezoelectric effect, 551
    portable machine, 554f
    real-time, 551
    terminology associated with,
        554
    therapeutic, 873, 873b, 873f,
        1061
    time-gain compensation
        control, 554
    tissue interaction with, 551-553
    transducers for, 553, 554b
Umbilical hernia, 1247, 1247f,
    1293
Umbilical herniorrhaphy, 1293
Umbilical repair, 1266
Uncinaria stenocephala, 455-457
Unconditioned response, 137
Unconditioned stimulus, 137
Underbite, 1344-1345, 1345f
Undernutrition, 351b
Underweight, 675t-679t
Uniform, 18-19, 19f
Universal curettes, 1328-1329
Unprofessional conduct, 31
Unruly behaviors
    in cats, 158
    in dogs, 150-151
Upper airway endoscopy, 950
Upper respiratory tract
    emergencies of, 949
    infections of, 486t-487t
    surgery of, in horses,
        1276-1278
Upregulation, 1026
Urate urolithiasis, 683t
Urethra
    obstruction of, 675t-679t, 697,
        932, 967, 1287
    physical examination of, 239
Urethral catheter, 607t
Urethral process, 968, 1294
Urethrography, 549
Urethrostomy, 968-969, 969b,
    1245-1247, 1246f, 1287-1288,
    1294

Urinalysis, 430-435
    chemical evaluations, 431-433
        bilirubin, 432
        blood, 432-433, 434f
        glucose, 432
        heme, 432-433
        ketones, 432
        pH, 431-432
        protein, 432
    description of, 430
    equipment for, 430
    in horses, 746
    microscopic examination,
        433-435
        casts, 433, 435f
        cells, 433, 434f
        crystals, 433-435, 436f
        microorganisms, 435
    urine
        collection of, 430
        color of, 430
        pH, 431-432
        specific gravity of, 431
        turbidity of, 430
Urinary bladder. See Bladder
Urinary calculi
    cystostomy for, 1243-1245
    in horses, 735-736, 1266
    in ruminants, 339t-340t
Urinary catheter(s)
    illustration of, 655f
    indwelling, 606-607
    in recumbent patients, 931
Urinary catheterization, 606-609
    in camelids, 655-656
    in cats
        female, 609
        male, 608-609, 609f
    complications of, 606, 654
    in cows, 657
    in dogs
        female, 608, 608f
        male, 607-608, 607f
    in goats, 657
    in horses, 654-655, 656f
    indications for, 606
    in llamas, 655-656
    in sheep, 657
Urinary diseases
    bacterial cystitis, 697
    chronic kidney disease, 695-696,
        695b, 695t-696t
    feline lower urinary tract
        disease, 697-698
    in ruminants, 770-771,
        1293-1295
    in small animals, 695-698
    urolithiasis, 696-697
Urinary incontinence, 1360,
    1365
Urinary tract diseases
    acute renal failure, 735
    in cats, 162
    in horses, 735-736
    polydipsia, 736
    polyuria, 736
    urinary calculus, 735-736
Urinary tract infection
    case study of, 506b
    description of, 486t-487t
Urinary tract radiography, using
    contrast agents, 549
Urine
    in cattle, 257
    crystals in, 433-435, 436f
    glucose in, 432
    ketones in, 432
    pH, 431-432
    protein in, 432
    red blood cells in, 434f

Urine collection
    in bovine, 656-657
    in camelids, 655-656
    catheterization for. See Urinary
        catheterization
    cystocentesis for, 430, 435, 488,
        604-605, 606f
    free-catch method
        in bovine, 656-657
        in camelids, 655
        description of, 488
        in goats, 657
        in horses, 654
        in sheep, 657
    in large animals, 654-657
    manual expression, 605
    midstream method of, 488, 654
    in pigs, 657
    from reptiles, 825
    in small animals, 604-609
    in swine, 657
    voided, 604-605
Urine culture, 488, 502, 502f
Urine marking
    in cats, 162, 164
    in dogs, 154
Urine sample, 654
Urine scalding, 1365
Urine specimen, 430
Urogenital system
    anesthesia of, 1286
    physical examination of, 239
Urogenital tract conditions
    in cattle, 1286-1288
    in horses, 1266-1269
Urogenital tract surgery, in horses,
    1266-1269
Urohydropulsion, 696-697
Urolithiasis, 683t, 696-697
    in cattle, 1287-1288, 1287f
    in food animals, 1287-1288,
        1287f
    in goats, 967-969, 1064t-1065t
    prevention of, 969
    in ruminants, 339t-340t, 771,
        771f, 1293
    in sheep, 967-969, 1064t-1065t
Urovagina, 1288
Ursodiol, 1024
U.S. Pharmacopoeia, 1031
Uterine biopsy, 394-395, 394f
Uterine prolapse, 966-967,
    1289-1290, 1290f
Uterine torsion, 965-966, 1289
Uveitis, 1374

V

Vaccines
    administration of, 264-265,
        264f, 589
    adverse events, 273-274
    anthrax, 277t-283t, 284
    bangs, 286-287
    Bordetella
        canine, 268t-269t, 273
        feline, 266t-267t, 271
    botulism, 277t-283t, 283-284
    canine adenovirus, 268t-269t,
        272
    canine coronavirus, 266t-267t,
        273
    canine distemper, 268t-269t,
        271-272
    canine influenza, 268t-269t, 273
    canine parainfluenza, 268t-269t,
        272
    canine parvovirus, 268t-269t
    for cattle, 286-287, 287t
    core, 265

Vaccines (Continued)
    dosing of, 263-264
    duration of immunity with,
        265-267
    equine encephalitis, 276-279,
        277t-279t, 733
    equine herpesvirus, 277t-283t,
        279
    equine influenza, 277t-283t, 279
    equine viral arteritis, 277t-283t,
        283
    feline calicivirus, 266t-267t, 270
    feline immunodeficiency virus,
        264t, 266t-267t
    feline leukemia virus, 264t,
        266t-267t, 270
    feline panleukopenia, 266t-267t,
        270
    feline viral rhinotracheitis, 264t,
        270
    Giardia
        canine, 264t, 266t-267t
        feline, 271
    intranasal administration of,
        589
    leptospirosis, 272-273
    lyophilized, 263f
    noncore, 265
    onset of immunity with,
        265-267
    panleukopenia, 266t-267t, 270
    rabies
        in dogs and cats, 266t-269t,
            267, 271
        in horses, 277t-283t, 284
    reconstitution of, 263-264
    rotavirus, 277t-283t
    storage of, 263-264
    strangles Streptococcus equi,
        280t-283t, 283
    tetanus, 276, 277t-283t
    types of, 263
    West Nile virus, 277t-283t, 284
Vacutainer blood collection
    system, 600f
Vacuum bags, 1188, 1189f
Vaginal examination
    cytologic, 374b-377b
    description of, 239
    in mares, 385-386, 386f, 798
Vaginal prolapse, 1289-1290,
    1289f
Vagus nerve, 243t
Valerian, 854t-855t
Value-priced pet food, 306
Valvular endocarditis, 763-764
Vapor pressure, 1086
Vascular sealing devices, 1142,
    1143f
Vasodilatation, 600
Vasopressin, 925t, 927
VCPR. See Veterinary-client-
    patient relationship
Vector-borne infectious diseases,
    704, 709t
Vegetables, 847
Vegetative endocarditis, 763-764
Velpeau sling, 988, 990f
Venezuelan equine encephalitis/
    encephalomyelitis, 276-279,
        277t-279t, 733
Venipuncture
    auricular
        in camelids, 647
        in pigs, 650
    in birds, 816
    in bovine. See Bovine,
        venipuncture in
    in camelids, 647-648, 647f-648f
    in cats, 600-601

Venipuncture (Continued)
cephalic
in bovine, 628
in camelids, 647
in dogs, 188
in horses, 627, 627f, 644-645, 646f
in small animals, 601
coccygeal
in camelids, 647
in pigs, 651
in dogs, 600-601
femoral, 602
in ferrets, 833f
in goats, 648
jugular
in bovine, 645, 646f
in camelids, 647, 647f
in cats, 601, 602f
in dogs, 601, 601f
in horses, 644, 644f
in pigs, 650
in small animals, 601, 601f-602f
in turtles, 826f
lateral saphenous, 601-602, 602f
in lizards, 217-218, 217f-218f
marginal vein, 602-603, 603f
medial saphenous, 602, 603f
middle coccygeal vein, in camelids, 647
orbital sinus, in pigs, 651, 651f
in pigs. See Pig(s), venipuncture in
in reptiles, 825-826
saphenous vein
in camelids, 647
in horses, 645
in small animals, 601-602, 602f
in sheep, 648, 648f-649f
in snakes, 825
Ventilation, 1125-1126
anesthesia monitoring, 1105-1106, 1111-1112, 1111f
complications of, 1126
definition of, 1125
intermittent mandatory, 1126
manual, 1125
mechanical, 1125-1126
periodic, 1126
Ventral cystocentesis, 606b, 606f
Ventricular asystole, 942
Ventricular escape beats, 944
Ventricular escape rhythms, 944
Ventricular fibrillation, 941-942, 942f
Ventricular fibrillator, 924-925, 924f
Ventricular premature complexes, 940-941, 941f, 1085
Ventricular tachycardia, 924-925, 941
Ventrolateral cystocentesis, 606b, 606f
Verbal communication, 20
Verified Internet Pharmacy Practice Site, 1037
Verrucous sarcoids, 736
Vertebral column dissection, 578
Vertebral fracture, 735
Vertebral subluxation complex, 861
Vertical bone loss, 1334-1335
Vestibular, 1301
Veterinarian, 14-15, 42
delegation of responsibilities by, 42
education of, 14-15
as general practitioner, 39

Veterinarian (Continued)
licensure of, 14-15
personal appearance of, 64
responsibilities of, 42
substance abuse by, 62
wellness care by, 42
Veterinarian-client-patient relationship, 1031-1032, 1032b
Veterinary assistant
description of, 16-17, 43
role and responsibilities of, 43
Veterinary feed directive, 1031-1032
Veterinary Hospital Managers Association, 42
Veterinary Medical Database, 112
Veterinary Oral Health Council, 1336
Veterinary practice
appearance of, 63
cleanup in, 43-44
client service attributes of, 55
employee positions in. See Employee(s)
facilities, 44-54
full-service care from, 63-64
hours of operation, 39
large animals. See Large animal practices
management of. See Practice management
marketing of. See Marketing
medium-sized, 41
mixed animal, 39
referral practices, 39
signage of, 66-67, 67f
size of, 41
small animals. See Small animal practices
types of, 39, 39b
Veterinary spinal manipulative therapy. See Chiropractic
Veterinary teaching hospital, 40b
Veterinary technician, 15-16, 42-43
anesthetist duties of, 13f
attrition rate, 5
client education by, 65
definition of, 42
employment benefits for, 5
history-taking by, 223-224
job opportunities for, 5, 5t
management role of, 58
oath of, 3
occupational settings for, 5
physical examination by, 46-47
present-day status of, 3-6
role and responsibilities of, 9-14, 42-43, 46-47, 1074b
safety responsibilities, 116
salary for, 5t
scope of practice, 9
in specialty practices, 3
Veterinary technician national examination, 7-8
Veterinary technician practice model, 8-9, 10t, 674-681
data gathering, 674
interventions, 681b
nursing care plan, 675-679, 682b
reevaluation of patient, 679-681
technician evaluations, 674-675, 675t-679t
Veterinary technician specialist, 15
definition of, 3-4
description of, 39
initials used to designate, 15
requirements for becoming, 15, 16b

Veterinary technologist, 15, 42-43
definition of, 15
role and responsibilities of, 42-43
Veterinary technology
features of, 8
history of, 3
as profession, 8-14
Veterinary therapeutic diets, 308-309
Veterinary-client-patient relationship, 82-83
Vetstarch, 884-885
Vibration, 869-870
Video camera, 1154-1155
Vinblastine, 1028t-1029t
Vincristine, 1028t-1029t
Violations
substantive, 29-32
technical, 29
Violence, 120-121, 120f
Viral antigen, 510-512
Viral equine encephalitis, 733
Viral infections, 124
Virology, 510-512
Virus. See also specific virus
detection of, 510-512
immunohistochemical staining of, 512
isolation of, 512
nosocomial infections caused by, 515
Visceral larva migrans, 125, 452-453, 454b
Viscosity, 420
Vision, in horses, 164, 190, 1369
Visual analogue scale, 1048
Vital signs, 1104, 1104t
Vitamin(s)
for beef cattle, 351
for cats, 328
characteristics of, 294
for dairy cattle, 348, 350t
description of, 294-295
dietary requirements, 300-302
for dogs, 322
fat-soluble, 294t
for finishing cattle, 352-353
for foals, 363
for horses, 361
for large animals, 343
for mares, 362
for senior dogs, 325
for sheep, 356
for swine
breeding herd, 357
growing-finishing, 358
water-soluble, 294t
Vitamin A
for beef cattle, 351
chemical names of, 294t
deficiency of, 828-829, 836
dietary requirements, 300-301
for foals, 363
recommended allowance for, 301t
Vitamin B, 294t
Vitamin B₁, 294t, 301-302, 347t
Vitamin B₂, 294t, 302, 302t, 347t
Vitamin B₃, 294t, 302, 302t
Vitamin B₆, 294t, 302, 302t, 347t
Vitamin B₁₂, 347t
Vitamin C, 294t, 347t, 839
Vitamin D, 294t, 301, 301t
Vitamin E, 294t, 301, 301t
Vitamin K, 294t, 301
Vocalizations
by dogs, 1047
by horses, 165-166
by ruminants, 172-173

Voice recognition software, 109
Voided urine sample, 604-605
Volume cycle ventilators, 1125-1126
Volume of distribution, 1012
Vomeronasal organ, 167, 1309
Vomiting
during anesthesia, 1128
antibacterial-associated, 1018
in cats, 684t
definition of, 689
opioid-related, 1057b
in small animals, 689
technician evaluation of, 675t-679t

W

Waiting area, 46, 46f
Walking dandruff. See Cheyletiella parasitivorax
Walk-ins, 71
Ward, 13
Ward attendants, 43-44
Ward treatment sheet, 98
Warm-water enema, 589
Warts, 770
Waste anesthetic gases, 127
Water, 293, 328
for birds, 822
for cattle, 346b
for foals, 363
for guinea pigs, 839-840
for horses, 359
for lizards, 829-832
for working horses, 363
Water belly, 339t-340t, 1287
Water deprivation, 777
Water manometer, 928f
Waterless hand antiseptics, 1176, 1176b
Water-soluble drugs, 1011
Water-soluble vitamins
description of, 294t
for livestock, 347t
Wave mouth, 1368-1369, 1374
Waxy casts, 433, 435f
Weaning
of foals, 170
of kittens, 325
of lambs, 356
of piglets, 358
of puppies, 318
Weanlings
capture of, 193
definition of, 244t, 380-381
restraint of, 195-196
Web-based marketing, 67-68
Weight measurements, in horses, 253-254, 255f, 359-361
Weight-loss diets, 336
Weitlaner retractor, 1140, 1141f
Wellness care, 42
West Nile virus
encephalitis caused by, 733
vaccine for, 277t-283t, 284
Western equine encephalitis/encephalomyelitis
description of, 733
vaccines for, 276-279, 277t-283t, 733
Western herbs, 851, 851f, 852t
Wether, 245t, 389, 391
Wet-to-dry bandage, 980-981
Wheelchairs, 875, 875f
Whelping, 372
Whipworms, 457-458, 457f-458f, 775t
prevention of, 275t

White blood cell count, 403-404, 404f, 413
White blood cells, 413-417
  basophils, 414f-415f, 416
  in dogs, 414f-415f
  eosinophils, 414f-415f, 416
  lymphocytes, 414f-415f, 416
  monocytes, 414f-415f, 416
  morphologic features of, 413
  neutrophils, 413, 414f-415f
White muscle disease, 339t-340t, 749
Wild animal attacks, 963-964
Wind-up phenomenon, 1051-1053
Wing clipping, 818, 819f
Winged needle catheter, 591, 591f
Winter dysentery, 751t-752t
Wire cutters, 1144f
Wobbler syndrome, 734
Wolf packs, 147-148
Wolf teeth, 285, 1351
Working dogs, 324
Working horses
  minerals for, 365
  nutrition for, 363-365
  protein for, 363-364
  work classification for, 363, 364t
Working length, 1339, 1339f
Working problem list, 92-93, 94f
Workplace
  professional conduct in, 20, 20b
  safety in, 34
Workplace hazards, 117-123
  back injuries, 117-118, 118f
  chemicals, 121-122
  cleaning up, 118
  dressing to prevent, 117
  electrical, 119
  equipment, 119
  evacuation considerations, 119-120
  fire, 119-120
  machinery, 119
  materials storage and, 118, 118f
  violence, 120-121, 120f
Workstations, 75
Wound(s)
  abrasions, 978
  bite, 979
  burns, 979
  classification of, 976b
  clean, 976b
  clean-contaminated, 976b
  closure of, 957, 976-978, 977b, 993
  contaminated, 974-975, 976b-977b, 1160, 1219

Wound(s) (Continued)
  débridement of, 976, 976b, 976f
  decubitus ulcers, 979
  degloving injuries, 977f, 978, 982b-984b
  dehiscence of, 1219-1220, 1221b
  description of, 955
  dirty, 976b
  drainage of, 978
  en bloc excision of, 976b, 976f
  in horses, 955-956
  immediate care of, 975
  infected, 976b
  infiltration of, 994f
  lacerations, 978
  lavage system for, 975, 975f
  open, exuberant granulation tissue in, 994, 994f
  preparation of, 993-994
  pressure sores, 979
  radiography of, 957
  secondary closure of, 977
  sterile cover on, 1200
  surgical, 1200
  sutures matched to type of, 1201
  types of, 978-979
  ultrasonography of, 957
Wound bandages. See Bandages
Wound healing, 973-975
  factors that affect, 974-975
  inflammatory phase of, 973-974, 973b, 973f
  maturation phase of, 973b, 973f, 974
  moist environment for, 974
  phases of, 973-974, 973b, 973f
  primary, 974, 976
  proliferative phase of, 973b, 973f, 974
  second intention, 973, 977-978, 977b
  third intention, 977
Wound infection, 978, 978b
Wound management
  in horses, 993-994, 994f
  in small animals, 956, 975-979, 975b
Wright stain, 405
Wright-Giemsa stain, 405, 420
Wry bite, 1345

X

X-ray(s). See also Radiography/radiographs

X-ray(s) (Continued)
  definition of, 519-520
  equipment for producing, 523-527
    features of, 523, 524f
    fluoroscopy, 525-526, 525f
    mobile unit, 524-525
    portable unit, 523-524, 525f
    stationary unit, 525, 525f
  exposure factors, 529-532
    exposure time, 530
    focal-film distance, 530-531, 539
    kilovoltage, 520, 530, 540
    milliamperage, 530
  grids, 535-537, 536f
  intensifying screens for, 533-534, 533f
  as legal records, 518
  physics of, 522
  principles of, 519-520
  production of, 519-523
  scatter radiation, 522-523, 523f, 532, 537
  technique charts, 531-532, 532b, 535t
  veterinary technician's responsibilities, 11, 11f
X-ray cassette
  description of, 532-533, 532f-533f
  loading and unloading of, 538, 539f
X-ray film
  automatic processor of, 534-535, 535f, 542b
  handling of, 538-539
  identification of, 518, 519f
  labeling of, 518, 518f-519f
  nonscreen, 532f, 534-535, 535f
  preparation of, 534
  screen, 534-535, 535f
  silver recovery, 539
  storage of, 538, 538f
X-ray tube, 520-522
  cathode assembly, 520f
  filament, 520
  focal spot, 520-521, 522f, 539
  focusing cup, 520, 520f
  heel effect, 522, 522f, 528
  rating chart for, 522
  rotating anode, 520f-521f, 521-522
  stationary anode, 520f, 521
Xylazine, 1059, 1067t-1069t, 1082

Y

Yankauer tip, 1140-1141, 1141f
Yearlings
  capture of, 193
  definition of, 244t, 380-381
  nutrients for, 364t
  restraint of, 195-196
Yeasts
  description of, 509
  microscopic appearance of, 510
Yersinia pestis, 710t
Yohimbine, 1082-1083

Z

Zebu, 387
Ziehl-Neelsen procedure, 490, 492b
Zinc, 303t, 304, 345t-346t
Zinc sulfate, 477, 769
Zipper tapeworm. See Spirometra mansonoides
Zirconium crowns, 1336
Zona pellucida, 369-370
Zonary placentation, 378, 379f
Zone of inhibition, 506, 507b, 508f
Zoonotic diseases, 124-125, 710t
  bacterial infections, 124
  birds, 823
  cutaneous larva migrans, 125
  definition of, 124, 704
  external parasites, 125
  fungal infections, 125
  internal parasites, 125
  Lyme disease, 124
  neurologic larva migrans, 454-455, 455b
  ocular larva migrans, 452-453, 454b
  protozoal infections, 125
  rabies, 124
  reptiles, 832
  ringworm, 125
  sarcoptic mange, 125
  schistosome cercarial dermatitis, 445, 445f
  Spirometra mansonoides, 451
  strongyloidosis, 458-460, 460f
  toxoplasmosis, 125
  viral infections, 124
  visceral larva migrans, 125, 452-453, 454b

1989

The Canadian Association of Animal Health Technologists and Technicians (CAAHTT) is formed.

The AVMA House of Delegates approves use of the term veterinary technician, which replaces the term animal health technician.

Consequently: CATAT name is changed to CVTEA, ATTC is changed to VTTC, and ATNE is changed to VTNE

1990

NAVTA adopts its official mission statement and begins a strategic planning process.

NAVTA produces "The World of the Veterinary Technician" videotape and other promotional materials.

The Ontario Association of Animal Health Technicians (OAAHT) establishes a registry.

First annual liaison meeting of NAVTA and AVMA representatives is held at AVMA headquarters in Schaumberg, IL.

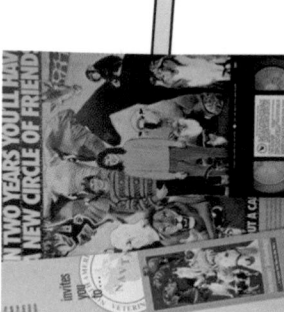

1991

The OAAHT changes its title to the Ontario Association of Veterinary Technicians (OAVT).

The Norwegian Veterinary Nurse and Technician Association is formed.

Patrick Navarre, BS, RVT, becomes NAVTA's first Executive Director.

1992

The New Zealand Veterinary Nursing Association is formed.

1993

In England, Parliament approves change of the nomenclature from Royal Animal Nursing Auxiliaries to Registered Veterinary Nurse.

Veterinary nurses and technicians from around the world meet in England and establish the International Veterinary Nurses and Technicians Association (IVNTA).

The Ontario Association of Veterinary Technicians Act is passed, recognizing the title "Registered Veterinary Technician (RVT)."

NAVTA declares the third week in October to be National Veterinary Technician Week.

1994

NAVTA creates the Committee on Veterinary Technician Specialties (CVTS) to oversee the development of veterinary technician academics and guidelines for specialty certification.

The first "National Veterinary Technician Week" is celebrated (October 16-22).

The American Society of Veterinary Dental Technicians is formed.

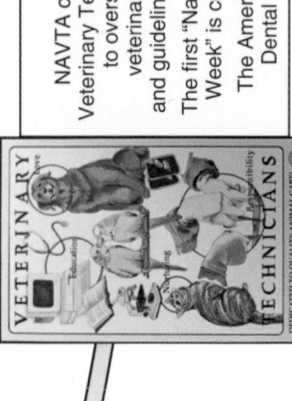

1995

The American Association of Veterinary State Boards (AAVSB) replaces the AVMA in its oversight of the VTNE.

Canadian provincial associations grant reciprocity of credentials for their respective members.

The Veterinary European Transnational Network for Nursing Education and Training (VETNNET) is established.

The AVMA accredits the first distance learning program in veterinary technology at St. Petersburg Junior College.

The Japanese Veterinary Nurses and Technician Association is established.

The first meeting of the Pennsylvania Association of Veterinary Technician Educators (PAVTE) is held.

1996

The first specialty in veterinary technology is established; the Academy of Veterinary Emergency and Critical Care Technicians is granted provisional recognition by NAVTA.

NAVTA is named cosponsor of National Pet Week.

1998

NAVTA's Committee on Veterinary Technician Specialties recognizes the Academy of Veterinary Technician Anesthetists.

NAVTA holds its first state representative workshop that included representatives from 27 states and Canada.

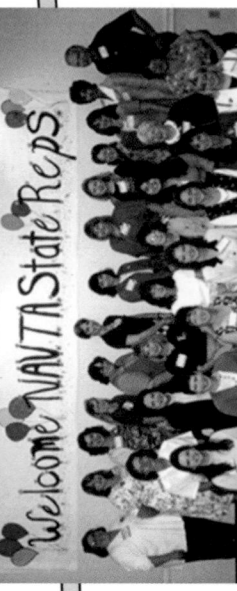
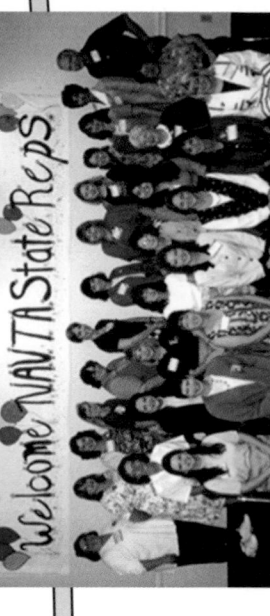

1999

Eighty programs of veterinary technology are accredited by the AVMA.

The AVMA incorporates language recommended by NAVTA in the AVMA's model practice act, which delineates the roles of the veterinary technician and the veterinary assistant.

The Academy of Veterinary Technician Anesthetists (AVTA) is recognized by NAVTA.

The American Association for Laboratory Animal Science creates National Laboratory Animal Technician Week.